EMERGING SCIENCE BOX

McCance & Huether's

PATHOPHYSIOLOGY

The Biologic Basis for Disease in Adults and Children

9th EDITION

McCance & Huether's
PATHOPHYSIOLOGY
The Biologic Basis for Disease in Adults and Children

Julia L. Rogers, DNP, APRN, CNS, FNP-BC, FAANP
Assistant Professor, College of Nursing
Purdue University Northwest
Hammond, Indiana;
Certified Nurse Practitioner
Northwest Medical Group Pulmonary and Critical Care Medicine
Valparaiso, Indiana

SECTION EDITOR
Valentina L. Brashers, MD, FACP, FNAP
Professor Emerita, School of Nursing
Attending Physician in Internal Medicine
University of Virginia Health System
Charlottesville, Virginia

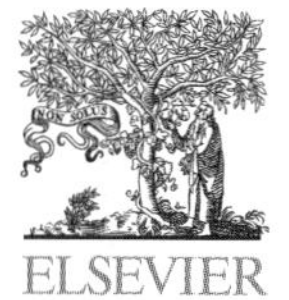

ELSEVIER

Elsevier
3251 Riverport Lane
St. Louis, Missouri 63043

MCCANCE & HUETHER'S PATHOPHYSIOLOGY: THE BIOLOGIC BASIS FOR DISEASE IN ADULTS AND CHILDREN, NINTH EDITION ISBN: 978-0-323-78987-5

Previous editions copyrighted 2019, 2014, 2010, 2006, 2002, 1998, 1994, and 1990.

Executive Content Strategist: Sonya Seigafuse
Senior Content Development Specialist: Laura Goodrich
Publishing Services Manager: Julie Eddy
Senior Project Manager: Rachel E. McMullen
Design Direction: Maggie Reid

Printed in Canada
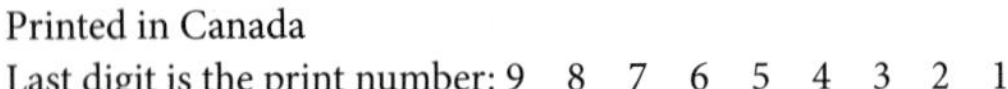
Last digit is the print number: 9 8 7 6 5 4 3 2 1

This book is dedicated to all those who think they can't: guess what—YOU CAN!

To my family, Dwayne, Zachery, and Shane. Your willingness to support this endeavor means more than I can express. I appreciate all the time and space you provided me to work on and complete this project. Your love surrounds me in every aspect of my life and inspires me to be a better human.

Dwayne, thanks for always letting me know that everything will be alright. I guess you were right. You have always been my rock, and I couldn't have made it the last 22 years without you believing in me.

Shane, thanks for never giving up and being the strongest woman I have ever known. Your beautiful smile brightens even the worst of days. You are loved more than you know. P.S. Please call your parents more often.

Last, but not least, my dearest Zachery, the calm in my storm, you have always amazed me with your uncanny ability to see the best in everyone. Never lose your gentle spirit and do not let anyone steal your joy. Believe in yourself and finish writing your own story. You are an inspiration.

P.S. Thanks for introducing me to dunking Oreos; life has not been the same since, Oh, and I almost forgot: you have lost the game.

J.L.R.

CONTRIBUTORS

Jodi A. Allen, DNP, RN, FNP-C
Assistant Professor and FNP Program Coordinator
College of Nursing
Purdue University Northwest
Hammond, Indiana

Rose Ann U. Baker, PhD, PMHCNS-BC
Assistant Lecturer, School of Nursing
College of Health Professions
University of Akron
Akron, Ohio

Casey Bor, MS, CPNP-AC, BSN, RN
Pediatric Cardiothoracic Surgery Nurse Practitioner
Pediatric Cardiothoracic Surgery and Pediatric Critical Care
University of Maryland Medical Center
Baltimore, Maryland

Valentina L. Brashers, MD, FACP, FNAP
Professor Emerita, School of Nursing
Attending Physician in Internal Medicine
University of Virginia Health System
Charlottesville, Virginia

Dennis J. Cheek, PhD, RN, FAHA
Professor
Harris College of Nursing and Health Sciences
Texas Christian University
Fort Worth, Texas

Devra Davis, PhD, MPH, FACE
Visiting Professor
Ondokuz Mayis Medical University
Samsun, Turkey;
President, Environmental Health Trust
Teton Village, Wyoming

Corinne M. Djuric, MSN, FNP-C
Assistant Clinical Professor
College of Nursing
Purdue University Northwest
Hammond, Indiana

Linda Felver, PhD, RN
Associate Professor
School of Nursing
Oregon Health & Science University
Portland, Oregon

Diane P. Genereux, PhD
Scientist
Vetebrate Genome Biology
Broad Institute of MIT and Harvard
Cambridge, Massachusetts

Victoria Gray, MS
Biologist
Science Department
Michigan City High School
Michigan City, Indiana

Anne Harvey, DNP
Nurse Practitioner
Hematology
Primary Children's Hospital;
APP Director—Pediatric Hem/Onc/BMT
Intermountain Healthcare
Salt Lake City, Utah

Mary Fran Hazinski, RN, MSN, FAAN, FAHA, FERC
Professor
Vanderbilt University School of Nursing
Assistant
Departments of Surgery and Pediatrics
Vanderbilt University School of Medicine;
Clinical Nurse Specialist
Monroe Carell, Jr. Children's Hospital at Vanderbilt
Nashville, Tennessee

Kathleen E. Hubner, DNP, APRN, ACNS-BC, ANVP, CNRN
Clinical Assistant Professor
Science of Nursing Care
Indiana University School of Nursing
Indianapolis, Indiana

Sue E. Huether, MS, PhD
Professor Emeritus
College of Nursing
University of Utah
Salt Lake City, Utah

Lynn B. Jorde, PhD
Mark and Kathie Miller Presidential Professor and Chair
Department of Human Genetics
University of Utah School of Medicine
Salt Lake City, Utah

Lauri A. Linder, PhD, APRN, CPON
Associate Professor
College of Nursing
University of Utah;
Clinical Nurse Specialist
Center for Cancer and Blood Disorders
Primary Children's Hospital
Salt Lake City, Utah

Kathryn L. McCance, RN, MS, PhD
Professor Emeritus
Nursing
University of Utah
Salt Lake City
Utah

Sean McConnell, PhD
President
Genomics
McConnell Consulting
Valparaiso, Indiana

Mary A. Mondozzi, MSN, BSN, WCC
Burn Center Education/Outreach Coordinator
The Paul and Carol David Foundation Burn Institute
Akron Children's Hospital
Akron, Ohio

Noreen Heer Nicol, PhD, RN, FNP, NEA-BC
Associate Professor
College of Nursing
University of Colorado
Aurora, Colorado

Judith O'Haver, PhD, RN, CPNP-PC, FAANP, FAAN
Pediatric Nurse Practitioner
Pediatric Dermatology
Phoenix Children's Hospital,
Assistant Professor of Pediatrics
Mayo Clinic College of Medicine,
Clinical Assistant Professor
Department of Child Health
University of Arizona College of Medicine
Phoenix, Arizona;
Nurse Scientist
Rady Children's Hospital
San Diego, California

Jan Powers, PhD, RN, CCNS, CCRN, NE-BC, FCCM
Director Nursing Research and Professional Practice
Nursing, Patient Care System
Parkview Health
Fort Wayne, Indiana

Geri Cage Reeves, PhD, APRN, FNP-BC
Associate Professor
School of Nursing
Vanderbilt University
Nashville, Tennessee

George W. Rodway, PhD
Adjunct Professor of Family Medicine—Sports Medicine
School of Medicine
University of Nevada—Reno
Reno, Nevada

Julia L. Rogers, DNP, APRN, CNS, FNP-BC, FAANP
Assistant Professor, College of Nursing
Purdue University Northwest
Hammond, Indiana;
Certified Nurse Practitioner
Northwest Medical Group Pulmonary and Critical Care Medicine
Valparaiso, Indiana

Kaveri Roy, DNP, RN
Assistant Professor
School of Nursing
MGH Institute of Health Professions
Boston, Massachusetts

John Ruge, MD, FAANS
Chairman
Neurosurgery
Advocate Lutheran General;
Chief
Pediatric Neurosurgery
Advocate Children's Hospital
Park Ridge, Illinois

Suzanne M. Ruiz, MBA, MSN, NP-C
Adjunct Faculty, Nursing
Purdue University Northwest
Hammond, Indiana

Melanie L. Scala, MS, CRNP-AC
Senior Nurse Practitioner II
Pediatric Cardiac Surgery Nurse Practitioner
University of Maryland Medical Center
Baltimore, Maryland

Mary C. Selzer, DNP, APRN, ACNP-BC
Assistant Professor Professional Practice
Nursing
Texas Christian University;
Manager
Trauma & Acute Care Surgery Advanced Practice Surgery
John Peter Smith Hospital
Fort Worth, Texas

Benjamin Allan Smallheer, PhD, RN, ACNP-BC, FNP-BC, CCRN, CNE
Associate Professor
School of Nursing
Duke University,
Acute Care Nurse Practitioner
Critical Care Medicine
Duke Regional Hospital
Durham, North Carolina;
Acute Care Nurse Practitioner
Critical Care Medicine
Duke Raleigh Hospital
Raleigh, North Carolina

William E. Somerall, Jr., MD, MAEd
Associate Professor of Nursing
Acute, Chronic, and Continuing Care
University of Alabama at Birmingham
Birmingham, Alabama

Scarlet R. Spain, DNP, RN, CNS, FNP-BC
Assistant Professor
CONHP
Valparaiso University
Valparaiso, Indiana;
Occupational Health Nurse Practitioner
Community Healthcare Systems
Hobart, Indiana;
Occupational Health Consultant
Medix
Chicago, Illinois

Lorey K. Takahashi, PhD
Professor of Psychology
Department of Psychology
University of Hawaii at Manoa
Honolulu, Hawaii

Karen C. Turner, BS
Freelance Editor
TurnKey Content, LLC
Melbourne, Florida

Mary Beth Winton, PhD, RN, ACANP-BC
Associate Professor
School of Nursing
Tarleton State University
Stephenville, Texas

PREFACE

The intent of the ninth edition of *Pathophysiology* is to continue the extraordinary work of Kathy McCance and Sue Huether, which started 30 years ago, by illustrating the principles of pathophysiology with clarity and accuracy.

Pathophysiology incorporates basic, translational, and clinical research to advance the understanding of disease and dysfunction. The study of pathophysiology involves many biomedical sciences and a wide range of research activities. Multiple aspects of cellular physiology are progressing rapidly, generating vast amounts of data to understand. This was made ever more present during the writing of this edition, when the world began to see the effects of cellular changes and adaptations from the coronavirus (COVID-19; severe acute respiratory syndrome coronavirus 2 [SARS-CoV-2]) pandemic. The information gained provided a greater understanding of the behavior of individual cells, their neighboring microenvironment, and the molecules that not only make up those cells but also communicate with their surroundings. Importantly, the forward movement of biomedical sciences occurs within the context of social, economic, and political processes that determine how disease is defined, experienced, and treated.

Interdisciplinary research has led to significant advancements in genetics, epigenetics, cell signaling and communication, control of cell behavior, metabolism, and cell fate. Knowledge about normal cell structures, function, and signaling pathways is at the forefront of translational science and foundational to the understanding of pathophysiology. Advancements in technology that allow close observation of cells are providing new understanding of cellular processes, including how cells function and prioritize their activities, monitor their environment, move, differentiate, and regenerate. Advances in the molecular mechanisms of disease, particularly cell signaling, genetic directives, and immune and metabolic modulators, are providing an understanding of individual differences in disease risk, biologic markers, diagnostic strategies, and individualized treatment.

Although these advancements have created an ever-increasing state of excitement, they have also created the problem of how students, professors, and clinicians can cope with the expanding new information. Translating and compressing these data into simplified discussions for students and clinicians is challenging. The approach for this edition of the book was to streamline the content and present the information in an organized, logical sequence of content based on current literature and research reports with understandable explanations and accompanied by illustrations and summary tables. The primary focus is on pathophysiology, and there is less emphasis on the evaluation and treatment that is found in clinical management textbooks.

This edition has been extensively revised with the following specific goals:

- Organize the content in a logical and uniformed format to facilitate learning and teaching.
- Place emphasis on the readability of the material for improved comprehension.
- Focus on updating outdated terminology and use inclusive language.
- Present emerging new data on disease including controversial topics.
- Provide the most current and relevant information on the etiology, epidemiology, pathophysiology, clinical manifestations, and treatment for disease processes.
- Integrate health promotion and disease prevention by updating risk factors, explaining relationships between nutrition and disease, and referencing screening recommendations.

ORGANIZATION AND CONTENT: WHAT'S NEW IN THE NINTH EDITION

The book is organized into two parts. Part One presents the cellular and tissue responses common to disease. Normal organ system structure and function and the pathophysiology of disease, organized by body systems, are presented in Part Two. All content has been reviewed and updated with extensive new references and revised figures. The previous Chapter 18 in the eighth edition titled *Disorders of the Central and Peripheral Nervous Systems and the Neuromuscular Junction* has been renamed in the ninth edition as *Alterations of the Brain, Spinal Cord, and Peripheral Nerves.* Alterations of the hematologic system, which were previously discussed over two chapters, have been combined into one chapter.

PART ONE: CENTRAL CONCEPTS OF PATHOPHYSIOLOGY: CELLS AND TISSUES

Part One begins with an in-depth study of the cell and progresses to cover the underlying processes of disease. Concepts covered include cell signaling and cell communication processes; genes and common genetic diseases; epigenetics and disease; fluid, electrolyte, and acid-base balance; inflammation, cytokines and their biologic functions, and normal and altered immunity; infection, stress, coping, and immunity; and tumor biology, epidemiology of cancer, and cancer in children. Revisions and updated additions to Part One include the following:

- Updated content on cellular organelles, the plasma membrane, cell signaling, and communication (Chapter 1)
- Reorganized with extensive updates throughout the chapter with close attention to air pollution and climate change (Chapter 2)
- Updated content on fluids, electrolytes and acids and bases (Chapter 3)
- Updated content on genes and diseases related to genetics, the environment and lifestyle patterns (Chapter 4 and 5)
- Updated content on epigenetics and disease (Chapter 6)

- Updated to content on normal innate and adaptive immunity (Chapters 7 and 8)
- Extensively updated to content on alterations of immunity and inflammation including up-to-date information on coronavirus (COVID-19) and severe acute respiratory syndrome coronavirus 2 (SARS-CoV-2) (Chapter 9)
- Extensively revised with up-to-date information on COVID-19 and SARS-CoV-2 (Chapter 10)
- Updated content on stress and disease (Chapter 11)
- Updated content on tumor biology and invasion and metastases (Chapter 12)
- Updated content on the epidemiology of cancer (Chapter 13)

PART TWO: PATHOPHYSIOLOGIC ALTERATIONS: ORGANS AND SYSTEMS

Part Two is a systematic survey of diseases within body systems. Each unit focuses on a specific body system and begins with an anatomy and physiology chapter to provide a basis of comparison for understanding the alterations created by disease. A brief summary of geriatric considerations is included at the end of the section on anatomy and physiology. The discussion of each disease in the alterations chapters is developed in a logical manner that begins with an introductory paragraph on etiology and epidemiology, followed by pathophysiology, clinical manifestations, and evaluation and treatment. Separate chapters are dedicated to pediatric pathophysiology, with a particularly sensitive approach to sex at birth and age. Significant revisions and updated additions to Part Two include the following:

- Updated content on pediatric cancers (Chapter 14)
- Updated content on the anatomy and physiology of the neurologic system (Chapter 15)
- Updated content on pain syndromes and sleep disorders (Chapter 16)
- Rewritten and extensively revised content on Parkinson disease, Huntington disease, amyotrophic lateral sclerosis, multiple sclerosis, and myasthenia gravis with updates to content on consciousness, memory, dementia, and delirium syndromes (Chapter 17)
- Chapter renamed as Alterations of the Brain, Spinal Cord, and Peripheral Nerves. Rewritten and extensively revised content on the manifestations for specific central and peripheral nervous system disorders including brain and spinal cord injury, stroke, seizure, and headache syndromes (Chapter 18)
- Updated content and terminology on schizophrenia, mood disorders, and anxiety (Chapter 19)
- Updated content on cerebral palsy, seizure disorders, and pediatric brain tumors (Chapter 20)
- Updated content on the mechanisms of hormonal regulation (Chapter 21)
- Extensive updates on diabetes mellitus, insulin resistance, and thyroid and adrenal gland disorders (Chapter 22)
- Updated content on obesity and disorders of nutrition (Chapter 23)
- Updated content on anatomy and physiology of the reproductive system (Chapter 24)
- Updated content on female reproductive disorders including cancers, benign breast diseases, and breast cancer (Chapter 25)
- Updated content on male reproductive disorders and cancer with extensive updating and reorganization (Chapter 26)
- Extensive updating of sexually transmitted infections (Chapter 27)
- Updated content on the anatomy and physiology of the hematologic system (Chapter 28)
- Extensively rewritten chapter on the alterations of hematologic function, combining two previous chapters into one with updated content on anemia (Chapter 29)
- Updated content on alterations of hematologic function in children (Chapter 30)
- Updated chapter on the anatomy and physiology of the cardiovascular and lymphatic systems (Chapter 31)
- Updated content on atherosclerosis, endothelial injury and dysfunction, coronary artery disease, myocardial infarction, and heart failure (Chapter 32)
- Updated content on the alterations of cardiovascular function in children (Chapter 33)
- Updated content on the anatomy and physiology of the pulmonary system (Chapter 34)
- New content on COVID-19 and SARS-CoV-2, and updated content on pulmonary embolism asthma, chronic lung disease, respiratory tract infection, pulmonary hypertension, and lung cancers (Chapters 35)
- New content on COVID-19 and SARS-CoV-2 with updated content on childhood asthma, respiratory distress syndrome, cystic fibrosis, lung infections, and sudden infant death syndrome (Chapter 36)
- Updated content on the anatomy and physiology of the renal and urologic system (Chapter 37)
- Updated content on kidney stones, urinary tract infection, glomerulopathies, acute and chronic renal failure, and bladder and kidney tumors (Chapter 38)
- Updated content on urinary tract infection and renal failure in children (Chapter 39)
- Updated content on the anatomy and physiology of the digestive system (Chapter 40)
- Updated content on gastroesophageal reflux disease, peptic ulcer disease, irritable bowel syndrome, inflammatory bowel disease, colon cancer, and hepatitis (Chapter 41)
- Updated content on gluten-sensitive enteropathy, necrotizing enterocolitis, infections of the intestine, and liver disease in children (Chapter 42)
- Updated content on the anatomy and physiology of the musculoskeletal system (Chapter 43)
- Updated content on alterations of the musculoskeletal system (Chapter 44)
- Updated content on alterations of the musculoskeletal system in children (Chapter 45)
- Updated content on integumentary system disorders including pressure ulcers, dermatitis, psoriasis, scleroderma, and melanoma (Chapter 46)

- Updated content on childhood atopic dermatitis, skin infections, and immune drug reactions (Chapter 47)
- Extensively updated content on septic shock, multiple organ dysfunction syndrome, included recent guideline updates, and burns for adults (Chapters 48)
- Extensively updated content on septic shock, multiple organ dysfunction syndrome, included recent guideline updates, and burns for children (Chapters 49)

FEATURES TO PROMOTE LEARNING

Ease of learning has been enhanced by designing a number of features that guide and support understanding, including:

- *Chapter Outlines* for each chapter
- *Consistent Headings* to underscore the consistent treatment of each disease—Pathophysiology, Clinical Manifestations, and Evaluation and Treatment
- More than 70 *Emerging Science* boxes that review the most current research and clinical developments of disease.
- End-of-chapter *Summary Review* sections that summarize the content in each chapter and serve as built-in content review guides
- Boldface *Key Terms* found within all the chapters
- A comprehensive *Glossary* with approximately 1000 terms to help students with the often-difficult terminology related to pathophysiology

ART PROGRAM

The art program is extensive and has received as much attention and revision as the narrative. Nearly 100 new or revised full-color illustrations were created and strategically placed throughout the textbook. Also included are many new high-quality, full-color photographs of clinical manifestations, pathologic specimens, and clinical imaging techniques. The combination of illustrations, algorithms, and photographs and the use of color for tables and boxes allow clarification for complex concepts and the emergence of easily recognized essential information.

ANCILLARIES

For Students

On **Evolve**, at http://evolve.elsevier.com/Rogers/pathophysiology/, students can access Evolve-only figures, tables, and boxes, 570 review questions, 100 animations to help them master the text content, 26 case studies with questions and answers, and downloadable chapter summaries documents for each chapter.

The **Study Guide** includes a variety of question styles, aiming to help the diverse way students learn. Question types include the following:

- Respond to Clinical Scenarios
- Categorize Clinical Examples
- Match the Definitions
- Order the Steps
- Choose the Correct Words
- Complete These Sentences
- Explain the Pictures
- Teach People About Pathophysiology
- Plus many more…

Answers are found in the back of the Study Guide for easy reference for students.

For Instructors

The **Evolve Instructor Resources** for this textbook provide the following teaching aids:

- Image Collection with all of the approximately 1200 figures from the text
- PowerPoint lecture slides for each chapter (approximately 3300 slides total), including integrated Audience Response Questions in each chapter (218 total), and integrated case studies at the end of each unit (15 total)
- Teach for Nurses Instructor's Manual, broken down by chapter, detailing the resources available to instructors for their lesson planning, and including unique case studies and class activities they can share with students
- Test Bank in ExamView with 1560 questions (in multiple-choice and multiple-response formats) with answers, rationales, and textbook page references

Evolve is an Internet-based learning environment that works in coordination with the text. This resource enables you to publish your class syllabus, outline, and lecture notes; set up "virtual office hours" and e-mail communication; share important dates and information through the online class calendar; and encourage student participation through chat rooms and discussion boards. Free with qualified adoption. Contact your sales representative or visit http://evolve.elsevier.com for more information about integrating **Evolve** into your curriculum.

ACKNOWLEDGMENTS

It is with gratitude that I dedicate this book to the creative pioneers who started it all, Kathy McCance and Sue Huether. Over the last 30 years, you have worked tirelessly to update the textbook to remain relevant using the most current research advancements, and I applaud your dedication. Thanks for having the confidence to pass the torch to me.

To Tamara, thank you for taking a chance on me. You are a sparkle in this world that can light up an entire room. I am forever grateful for your kindness.

To Tina Brashers, a mentor throughout this journey that had several sharp turns. Thank you for your devotion to the book and passion to create. You are brilliant, and I could not have done it without you. I appreciate you more than you will ever know and will forever be slightly envious.

To Melanie, the eagle eyes of the project. Thank you for all the time and commitment you put into this textbook. Words cannot express the gratitude I have for all your hard work.

To the Development and Production teams—Laura, Laurie, Rachel, artists, and editors, thanks for your mastery and caring about this project as much as I do.

To all the contributors—thanks for hanging in there over the last few years. It was a time of change and constraints with COVID, but all of you produced phenomenal work. Thank you!

To my amazing father, who provided me with strength and courage throughout the entire project.

To the WOW women, thanks for helping me pick up the broken pieces and make time for what is most important in life.

To Patti Ludwig-Beymer thank you for taking the time to guide me. You have been a true mentor and reminded me to breathe, believe, and be the very best version of me.

To Dr. Douglas Mazurek, you have been an inspiration to me. You believed in me since the beginning of my nursing career and opened the door to see the possibilities as a nurse practitioner. Thanks for igniting my passion and love for pathophysiology.

To Emily, thanks for making sure everything was in order. You are a gem in the world.

Seek joy. Live your life as your message. Be the change in the world that you wish to see. Most of all......be kind.

Julia L. Rogers

CONTENTS

UNIT II Genes and Gene-Environment Interaction

UNIT III Mechanisms of Self-Defense

UNIT IV Cellular Proliferation: Cancer

PART TWO: Structure, Function, and Pathophysiologic Alterations: Organs and Systems

UNIT V The Neurologic System

UNIT VI The Endocrine System

UNIT VII The Reproductive Systems

UNIT VIII The Hematologic System

1

Cellular Biology

Victoria Gray and Kathryn L. McCance

http://evolve.elsevier.com/Rogers/pathophysiology/

CHAPTER OUTLINE

All body functions are dependent on the integrity of cells. These trillions of complex cells are the basic building blocks of the human body. Therefore an understanding of cellular biology is fundamental to understanding health, wellness, and disease processes. Cells behave as a multicellular "social" organism in that they message between, among, and within one another through cellular communication (cellular "crosstalk"). Cells have the ability to originate, transmit, receive, interpret, and use information to maintain cellular function and specialization. Cells must demonstrate a "chemical fondness" for other cells to maintain the integrity of the entire organism. When they no longer tolerate this fondness, the conversation breaks down, and cells either adapt (e.g., altering function) or become vulnerable to isolation, injury, or disease.

PROKARYOTES AND EUKARYOTES

Living cells generally are divided into eukaryotes and prokaryotes. The cells of animals and plants are eukaryotes, as are the single-celled organisms, fungi, protozoa, and most algae. Prokaryotes include bacteria and archaea. Prokaryotes traditionally were studied as core subjects of molecular biology, which generated an abundance of data related to prokaryotic genomes (a set of genes carried on molecules of deoxyribonucleic acid [DNA]). Currently, emphasis is on the eukaryotic cell, which contains genomes that are more complex.[1]

Eukaryotes (*eu* = true; *karyon* = nucleus; also spelled "eucaryotes") are larger and have more extensive intracellular anatomy and organization than prokaryotes. Eukaryotic cells have a characteristic set of membrane-bound intracellular compartments, called *organelles*, that includes a well-defined nucleus. The prokaryotes contain no organelles, and their nuclear material is not encased by a nuclear membrane.

Besides having structural differences, prokaryotic and eukaryotic cells differ in chemical composition and biochemical activity. The *nuclei* of prokaryotic cells carry genetic information in a single circular chromosome, and they lack a class of proteins called *histones*, which in eukaryotic cells bind with DNA and are involved in the supercoiling of DNA. Eukaryotic cells have several chromosomes, the number of which is dependent on species. Protein production, or synthesis, in the two classes of cells also differs because of major structural differences in ribonucleic acid (RNA) protein complexes. Other distinctions include differences in mechanisms of transport across the outer cellular membrane and in enzyme content.

CELLULAR FUNCTIONS

Cells become specialized through the process of differentiation, or maturation, so that some cells eventually perform one function and other cells perform other functions. Cells with a highly developed function, such as movement, often lack some other property, such as hormone production, which is more highly developed in other cells.

The eight chief cellular functions are as follows:

- *Movement.* Muscle cells can generate forces that produce motion. Muscles that attach to bones produce limb movements, whereas muscles that enclose hollow tubes or cavities move or empty contents when they contract (e.g., the colon).
- *Conductivity.* Conduction as a response to a stimulus is manifested by a wave of excitation, an electrical potential that passes along the surface of the cell to reach its other parts. Conductivity is the chief function of nerve cells. (e.g., the brain or heart).
- *Metabolic absorption.* All cells can take in and use nutrients and other substances from their surroundings. (e.g., cells of the intestines or kidneys).
- *Secretion.* Certain cells, such as mucous gland cells, can synthesize new substances from substances they absorb and then secrete the new substances to serve elsewhere as needed.
- *Excretion.* All cells can rid themselves of waste products resulting from the metabolic breakdown of nutrients. Membrane-bound sacs (lysosomes) within cells contain enzymes that break down, or digest, large molecules, turning them into waste products that are released from the cell (e.g., urine).
- *Respiration.* Cells absorb oxygen, which is used to transform nutrients into energy in the form of adenosine triphosphate (ATP). Carbohydrates, fats, and proteins can be used as fuels. Cellular respiration, or oxidation, occurs in organelles called *mitochondria* (e.g., glucose).
- *Reproduction.* Tissue growth occurs as cells enlarge and reproduce themselves. Even without growth, tissue maintenance requires that new cells be produced to replace cells that are lost normally through cellular death. Not all cells are capable of continuous division (see Chapter 2) (e.g., mitosis and meiosis).
- *Communication.* Communication is vital for cells to survive as a society of cells. Appropriate communication allows the maintenance of a dynamic steady state. Table 1.1

STRUCTURE AND FUNCTION OF CELLULAR COMPONENTS

Fig. 1.1A shows a "typical" eukaryotic cell, which consists of three components: an outer membrane called the plasma membrane; a fluid "filling" called cytoplasm (see Fig. 1.1B); and the "organs" of the cell—the membrane-bound intracellular organelles, among them the nucleus.

Nucleus

The nucleus, which is surrounded by the cytoplasm and generally is located in the center of the cell, is the largest membrane-bound organelle. Two pliable membranes compose the nuclear envelope (Fig. 1.2A). The nuclear envelope is pockmarked with pits, called nuclear pores, which allow chemical messages to exit and enter the nucleus (see Fig. 1.2A, B, and D). The outer membrane is continuous with membranes of the endoplasmic reticulum (see Fig. 1.1). The nucleus contains the nucleolus (a small dense structure composed of DNA, RNA, and ribosomal proteins), most of the cellular DNA, and the DNA-binding proteins (i.e., the histones) that regulate its activity. The DNA chain in eukaryotic cells is so long that it is easily broken. Therefore the histones that bind to DNA cause DNA to fold into chromosomes (see Fig. 1.2C). The wrapping of DNA into tight packages of chromosomes is essential for cell division in eukaryotes. The primary functions of the nucleus are cell division and control of genetic information. These functions include the replication and repair of DNA and the transcription of the information stored in DNA into RNA.

Cytoplasmic Organelles

Cytoplasm is an aqueous solution (cytosol) that fills the cytoplasmic matrix—the space between the nuclear envelope and the plasma membrane. The cytosol represents approximately half the volume of a eukaryotic cell. It contains thousands of enzymes involved in intermediate metabolism and is *crowded* with ribosomes making proteins (see Fig. 1.1B). Newly synthesized proteins remain in the cytosol if they lack a signal for transport to a cell organelle.[2]

The organelles suspended in the cytoplasm are enclosed in biologic membranes, so they can simultaneously carry out functions requiring different biochemical environments. Many of these functions are directed by coded messages carried from the nucleus by RNA. Functions of organelles can be divided into four major categories: (1) genetic control; (2) manufacturing, distributing, and breaking down molecules; (3) energy processing; and (4) structural support, movement, and communication between cells. The cytosol is a storage unit for fat, carbohydrates, and secretory vesicles. Table 1.1 lists the principal cytoplasmic organelles.

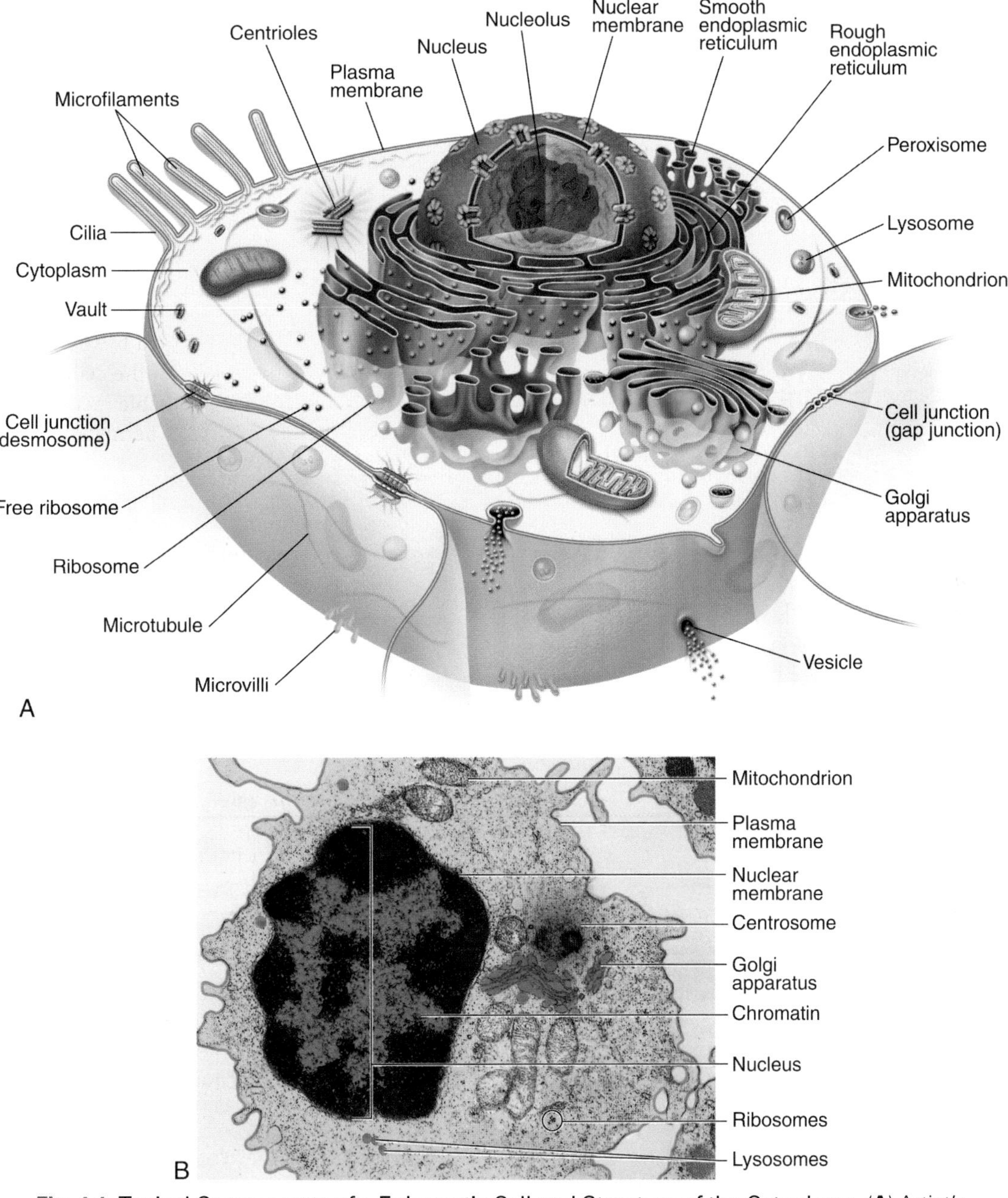

Fig. 1.1 Typical Components of a Eukaryotic Cell and Structure of the Cytoplasm. (**A**) Artist's interpretation of cell structure. (B). Color-enhanced electron micrograph of a cell. Both show the many mitochondria known as the "power plants" of the cell. Note, too, the innumerable dots bordering the endoplasmic reticulum. These are ribosomes, the cell's "protein factories." (**B**, From Patton KT, Thibodeau GA. *Anatomy & physiology*, 9th edition. St. Louis: Mosby; 2016.

Plasma Membranes

Membranes define the cell's boundaries. Membranes surround the cell or enclose an intracellular organelle and are exceedingly important to normal physiologic function because they control the composition of the space, or compartment, they enclose. Membranes can allow or exclude various molecules, and because of selective transport systems, they can move molecules in or out of the space (Fig. 1.3). By controlling the movement of substances from one compartment to another, membranes exert a powerful influence on metabolic pathways. Directional transport is facilitated by polarized domains, distinct apical and basolateral domains. The plasma membrane also has an important role in cell-to-cell recognition, cellular mobility, and the maintenance of cellular shape (Table 1.2).

Membrane Composition

The main components of cell membranes are lipids and proteins. The cell membrane is a lipid bilayer, composed of two opposing leaflets and proteins that span the bilayer or interact with the lipids on either side of the two leaflets (Fig. 1.4). Historically, the plasma membrane was described as a fluid lipid bilayer *(fluid mosaic model)* composed of a uniform lipid distribution with

TABLE 1.1 Principal Cytoplasmic Organelles

Genetic Control

Organelle	Characteristics and Description
Nucleus 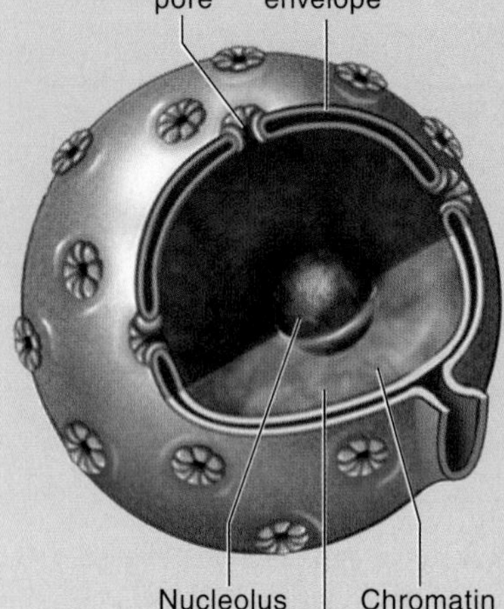 (From Patton KT: *Anatomy & Physiology, 10 ed.,* Mosby, 2019, Elsevier.)	*(See text for further description of function and structure)*
Nucleolus	*(See text for further description of function and structure)*

Manufacturing, Distributing and Breaking Down Molecules

Organelle	Characteristics and Description
Ribosomes	Ribonucleic acid (RNA)-protein complexes (nucleoproteins) synthesized in nucleolus and secreted into cytoplasm. Provide sites for cellular protein synthesis. Uses the information from deoxyribonucleic acid (DNA), written in messenger RNA (mRNA), to build proteins.
Endoplasmic reticulum (rough and smooth) 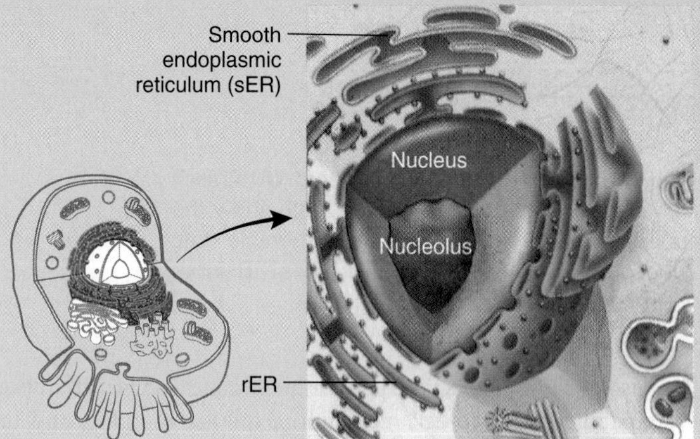 (From McCance KL, Huether S: *Pathophysiology: the biologic basis for disease in adults and children,* St. Louis, 2019, Elsevier.)	Network of tubular channels (cisternae) that extend throughout the outer nuclear membrane. **Rough Endoplasmic Reticulum (RER)**—bumpy exterior due to ribosomes and ribonucleoprotein particles attached to it; is responsible for much of a cell's protein synthesis and folding. **Smooth Endoplasmic Reticulum (SER)**—does not contain ribosomes or ribonucleoprotein particles. Rather, membranous surfaces of the SER contain enzymes involved in the synthesis of steroid hormones and are responsible for a variety of reactions required to remove toxic substances from the cell. The SER communicates with the Golgi complex and interacts with other organelles, particularly lysosomes and peroxisomes.

Continued

TABLE 1.1 Principal Cytoplasmic Organelles—cont'd

Manufacturing, Distributing and Breaking Down Molecules	
Organelle	**Characteristics and Description**
Golgi complex 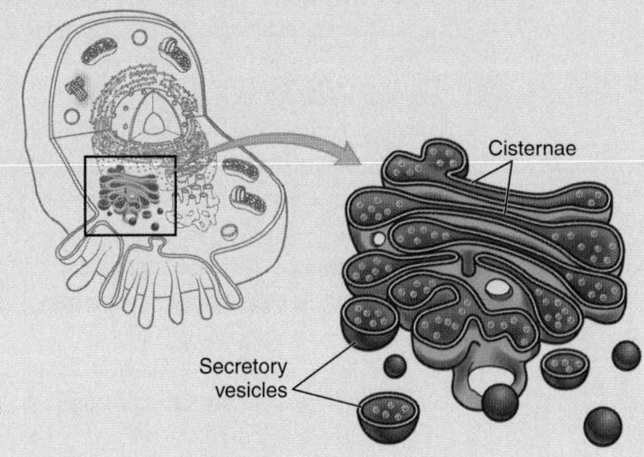 (From McCance KL, Huether S: *Pathophysiology: the biologic basis for disease in adults and children*, St. Louis, 2019, Elsevier.)	Network of flattened, smooth membranes and vesicles located neared the nucleus and the RER. Proteins from the endoplasmic reticulum are processed and packaged into small membrane-bound sacs or vesicles called **secretory vesicles**, which collect at the end of the membranous folds of the Golgi bodies—called **cisternae** (like a stack of pita breads). The secretory vesicles then break off from the Golgi complex and migrate to a variety of intracellular and extracellular destinations, including the plasma membrane. The vesicles fuse with the plasma membrane, and their contents are released from the cell. The best-known vesicles are those that have coats made largely of the protein **clathrin** and are called *clathrin-coated vesicles*. The Golgi complex is a refining plant and directs cellular traffic (e.g., protein, polynucleotide, polysaccharide molecules) in the cell.
Lysosomes 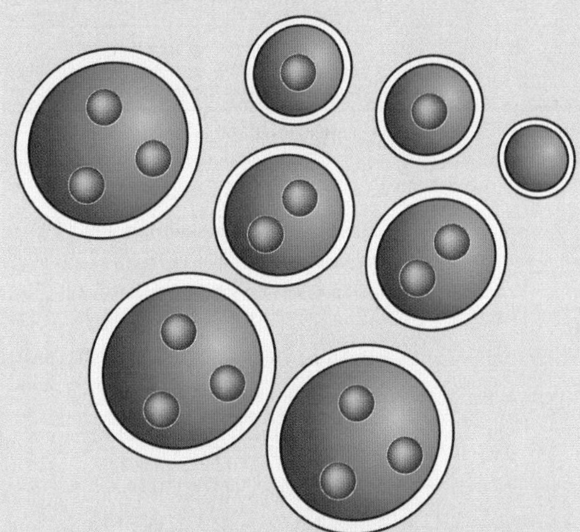 (From McCance KL, Huether S: *Pathophysiology: the biologic basis for disease in adults and children*, St. Louis, 2019, Elsevier.)	Sac-like, membrane-bound structures containing enzymes for digesting most cellular substances to their basic forms, such as amino acids, fatty acids, and carbohydrates (sugars). The lysosomal membrane acts as a protective shield between the powerful digestive enzymes within the lysosome and the cytoplasm, preventing their leakage into the cytoplasmic matrix. Lysosomes maintain cellular health because of efficient removal of toxic cellular components, removal of useless organelles, termination of signal transduction, and maintenance of metabolic homeostasis. Aging can lead to progressive loss of lysosomal efficiency and decline of the regenerative capacity of organs and tissues. Cellular injury leads to release of lysosomal enzymes that cause cellular self-digestion.
Peroxisomes	Similar to lysosomes in appearance but contain several oxidative enzymes (e.g., catalase, urate oxidase) that can detoxify compounds and fatty acids. Peroxisomes are so named because they usually contain enzymes that use oxygen to remove hydrogen atoms from specific substrates in an oxidative reaction that produces hydrogen peroxide (H_2O_2). Hydrogen peroxide is a powerful oxidant, potentially destructive if it accumulates or escapes from peroxisomes. Peroxisomes also have an important role in the synthesis of specialized phospholipids necessary for nerve cell myelination. Such reactions are important in detoxifying various wastes within the cell or foreign components that enter the cell, such as ethanol. Impairment of peroxisomes can lead to disease (see Fig. 1.1A).

TABLE 1.1 Principal Cytoplasmic Organelles—cont'd

Organelle	Characteristics and Description
Energy Processing	
Mitochondria 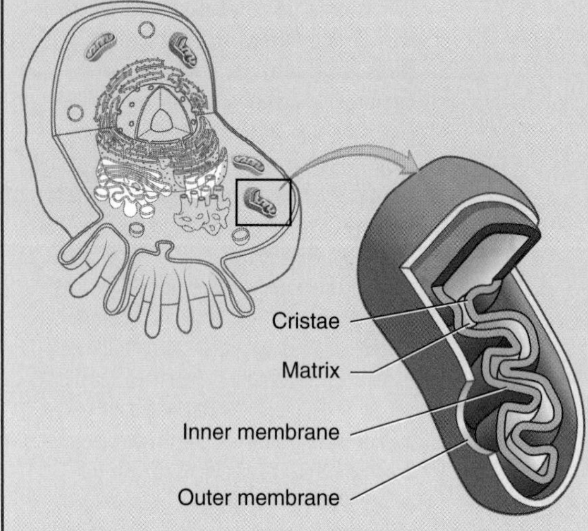 (From McCance KL, Huether S: *Pathophysiology: the biologic basis for disease in adults and children*, St. Louis, 2019, Elsevier.)	Organelles, found in large numbers in most cells, are responsible for cellular respiration and energy production. These cytoplasmic organelles appear as spheres, rods, or filamentous bodies that are bound by a double membrane. The **outer membrane** is smooth and surrounds the mitochondrion itself; the inner membrane is convoluted in the mitochondrial matrix to form partitions called **cristae**. The **inner membrane** contains the enzymes of the **respiratory chain**—the name given to the electron transport chain. These enzymes are essential to the process of oxidative phosphorylation that generates most of the cell's adenosine triphosphate. Metabolic pathways involved in the metabolism of carbohydrates, lipids, and amino acids and special pathways involving urea and heme synthesis are located in the mitochondrial matrix. Mitochondria contain their own DNA that codes for enzymes needed for oxidative phosphorylation.
Structural Support, Movement, and Communication Between Cells	
Structures	**Characteristics and Description**
Cytoskeleton (From McCance KL, Huether S: *Pathophysiology: the biologic basis for disease in adults and children*, St. Louis, 2019, Elsevier.)	All eukaryotic cells contain elaborate and specialized internal structures in the cytosol that provide the "bones and muscles" of the cell—the **cytoskeleton**. The cytoskeleton maintains the cell's shape and internal organization, and it permits movement of substances within the cell and movement of external projections (cilia or microvilli; flagella in sperm) outside the plasma membrane. The internal skeleton is composed of a network of protein filaments; the three main types of filaments include actin filaments, microtubules, and intermediate filaments. These filaments collectively promote cell strength, shape, and movement. Intermediate filaments bridge the cytoplasm from one cell junction to another, strengthening and supporting the sheet of epithelium.

inserted moving proteins. Although the notion is controversial, it now appears that the lipid bilayer is a much more complex structure where lipids and proteins are not uniformly distributed, but may separate into discrete units called *microdomains*, differing in their protein and lipid compositions. Different membranes have varying percentages of lipids and proteins. Intracellular membranes may have a higher percentage of proteins than do plasma membranes, presumably because most enzymatic activity occurs within organelles. The membrane organization is achieved through noncovalent bonds that allow different physical states called phases (solid gel, fluid liquid–crystalline, and liquid ordered). These phases can change under physiologic factors, such as temperature and pressure fluctuations. Carbohydrates are mainly associated with plasma membranes, in which they are chemically combined with lipids, forming glycolipids, and with proteins, forming glycoproteins (Fig. 1.5).

The outer surface of the plasma membrane in many types of cells, especially endothelial cells and adipocytes, is not smooth

TABLE 1.2 Plasma Membrane Functions

Cellular Mechanism	Membrane Functions
Structure	Usually thicker than membranes of intracellular organelles
	Containment of cellular organelles
	Maintenance of relationship with cytoskeleton, endoplasmic reticulum, and other organelles
	Maintenance of fluid and electrolyte balance (ion channels)
	Outer surfaces of plasma membranes in many cells are not smooth but are dimpled with cave-like indentations called *caveolae;* they are also studded with cilia or even smaller cylindrical projections called *microvilli;* both are capable of movement
Protection	Barrier to toxic molecules and macromolecules (proteins, nucleic acids, polysaccharides)
	Barrier to foreign organisms and cells
Activation of cell	Hormones (regulation of cellular activity)
	Mitogens (cellular division; see Chapter 2)
	Antigens (antibody synthesis; see Chapter 7)
	Growth factors (proliferation and differentiation; see Chapter 11)
Storage	Storage site for many receptors
	Transport (e.g., sodium [Na^+] pump)
	Diffusion and exchange diffusion
	Endocytosis (pinocytosis, phagocytosis)
	Exocytosis (secretion)
	Active transport
Cell-to-cell interaction	Communication, anchors (integrins), and attachment at junctional complexes
	Symbiotic nutritive relationships
	Release of enzymes and antibodies to extracellular environment
	Relationships with extracellular matrix

Modified from King DW, Fenoglio CM, Lefkowitch JH. *General pathology: Principles and dynamics.* Philadelphia: Lea & Febiger; 1983.

but dimpled with flask-shaped invaginations known as *caveolae* ("tiny caves"). Caveolae, considered to serve as a storage site for many receptors, provide a route for transport into the cell and may act as the initiator for relaying signals from several extracellular chemical messengers into the cell's interior.

Lipids. Each lipid molecule is polar, or amphipathic, which means that one part is hydrophobic (uncharged, or "repelled by water") and another part is hydrophilic (charged, or "attracted to water") (see Fig. 1.4B). The membrane spontaneously organizes itself into two layers because of these two incompatible solubilities. The hydrophobic region (hydrophobic tail) of each lipid molecule is protected from water, whereas the hydrophilic region (hydrophilic head) is immersed in it. The bilayer serves as a barrier to the diffusion of water and hydrophilic substances, while allowing lipid-soluble molecules, such as oxygen (O_2) and carbon dioxide (CO_2), to diffuse through the membrane readily.

Cell membranes may contain many different lipid classes, but in animals, the main ones are phospholipids, cholesterol, and glycolipids. Phospholipids, the most abundant lipids, have a phosphate-containing hydrophilic head connected to a hydrophobic tail. Phospholipids and glycolipids form self-sealing lipid bilayers. Lipids along with protein assemblies act as "molecular glue" for the structural integrity of the membrane. Phospholipids are key for repairing the membrane—they tend to spontaneously rearrange themselves to avoid a tear by folding on themselves and forming a sealed compartment.[2]

Proteins. Proteins perform most of the plasma membrane's tasks and are the major workhorses of the cell. A protein is made from a chain of amino acids, known as polypeptides. There are 20 types of amino acids in proteins and each type of protein has a unique sequence of amino acids. After translation (the synthesis of protein from RNA, see Chapter 4) of a protein, posttranslational modifications (PTMs) are the methods used to diversify the limited numbers of proteins generated. These modifications alter the activity and functions of proteins. PTMs have become very important in understanding disease processes. An emerging field of study in science is proteomics, the study of the proteome. This molecular approach is used to study an entire set of proteins expressed by a genome from synthesis, translocation, and modification (e.g., folding). Biologists are analyzing and uncovering information related to the roles of proteomes in a staggering number of diseases.

Membrane proteins associate with the lipid bilayer in different ways (Fig. 1.6), including:

1. Transmembrane proteins that extend across the bilayer and are exposed to an aqueous environment on both sides of the membrane (see Fig. 1.6A)
2. Proteins located almost entirely in the cytosol and associated with the cytosolic half of the lipid bilayer by an α helix exposed on the surface of the protein (see Fig. 1.6B)
3. Proteins that exist outside the bilayer, on one side or the other, and attached to the membrane by one or more covalently attached lipid groups (see Fig. 1.6C)
4. Proteins bound indirectly to one or the other bilayer membrane face and held in place by their interactions with other proteins (see Fig. 1.6D).[3]

Proteins directly attached to the membrane bilayer can be removed by dissolving the bilayer with detergents called

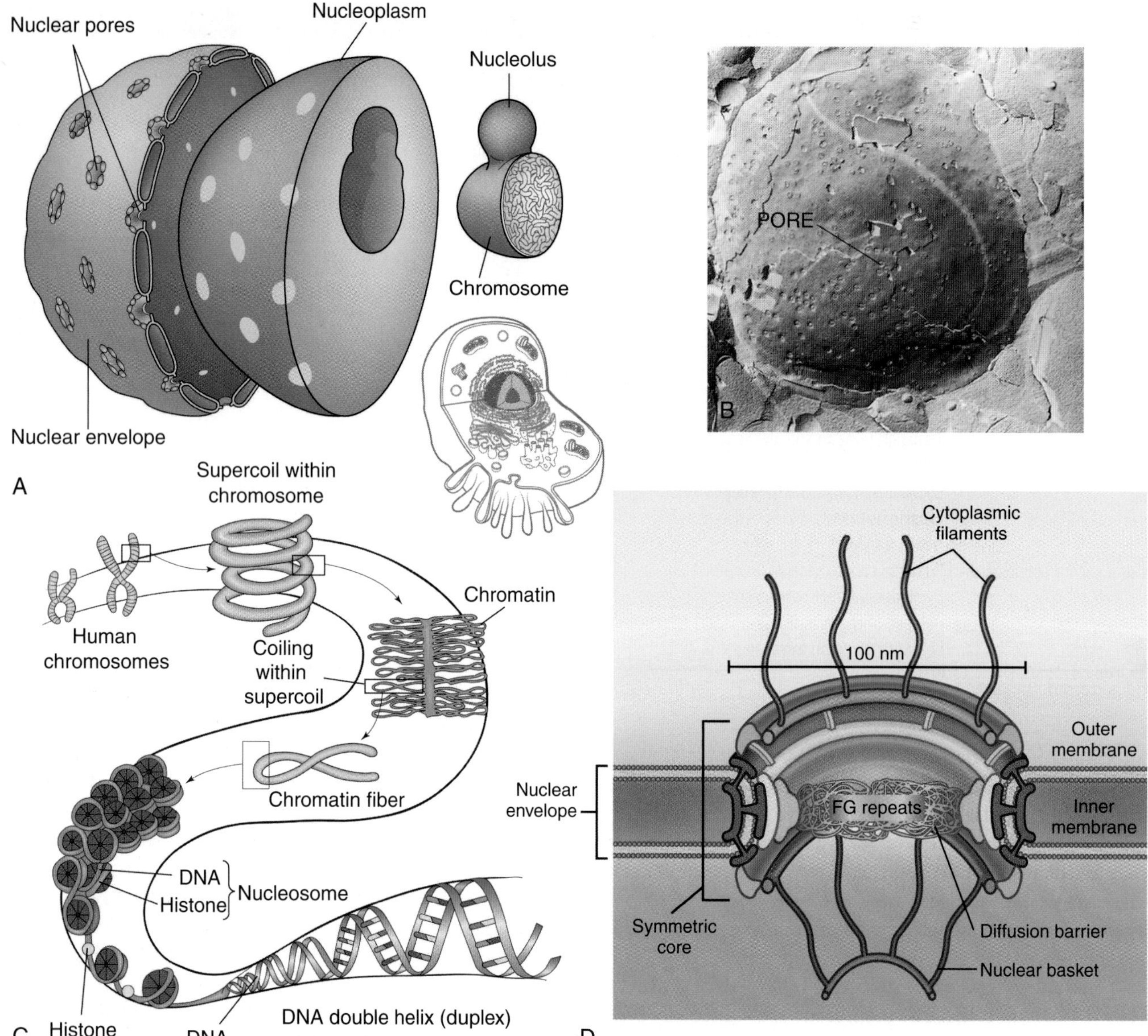

Fig. 1.2 The Nucleus. The nucleus is composed of a double membrane, called a nuclear envelope, which encloses the fluid-filled interior, called *nucleoplasm*. The chromosomes are suspended in the nucleoplasm (illustrated here much larger than actual size to show the tightly packed deoxyribonucleic acid [DNA] strands). Swelling at one or more points of the chromosome, shown in **(A)** occurs at a nucleolus where genes are being copied into ribonucleic acid. The nuclear envelope is studded with pores. **(B)** The pores are visible as dimples in this freeze-etch of a nuclear envelope. **(C)** Histone-folding DNA in chromosomes. **(D)** Nuclear pore complex. (A, C, From McCance KL, Huether S *Pathophysiology: The biologic basis for disease in adults and children*. St. Louis: Elsevier; 2019 B, From Raven PH, Johnson GB. *Biology*. St. Louis: Mosby; 1992. D, Adapted from The-scientist infographic: the nuclear pore complex. Available at https://www.The-scientist.com/infographics/infographic-the-nuclear-pore-complex-32456)

integral membrane proteins. The remaining proteins that can be removed by gentler procedures, that interfere with protein-protein interactions, but do not dissolve the bilayer, are known as peripheral membrane proteins.

Proteins exist in densely folded molecular configurations rather than straight chains; thus most hydrophilic units are at the surface of the molecule, and most hydrophobic units are inside. Membrane proteins, like other proteins, are synthesized by the ribosome and translocate, called *trafficking*, to different membrane locations of a cell. Trafficking puts unique demands on membrane proteins for folding, translocation, and stability.

Although membrane structure is determined by the lipid bilayer, membrane functions are determined largely by proteins (see Fig. 1.3). Proteins act as:

1. Recognition and binding units (receptors) for substances moving into and out of the cell

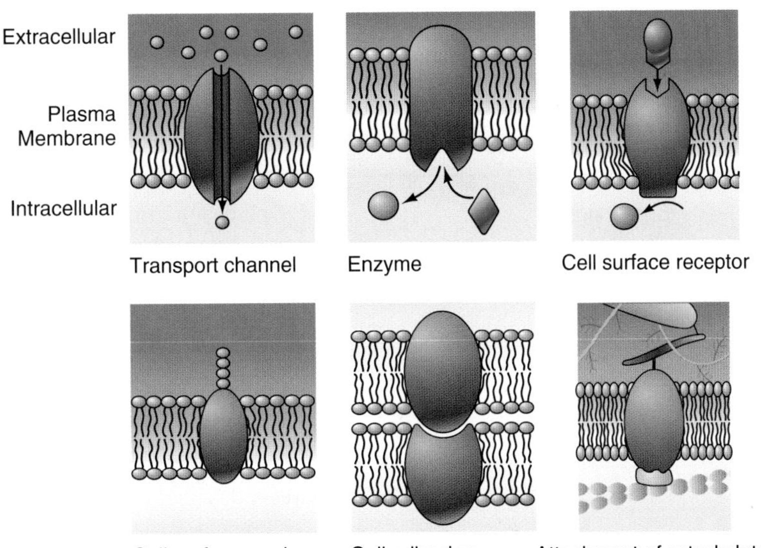

Fig. 1.3 Functions of Plasma Membrane Proteins. The plasma membrane proteins illustrated here show a variety of functions performed by the different types of plasma membranes. (From Raven PH, Johnson GB. *Understanding biology,* 3rd edition. Dubuque, IA: Brown; 1995.

2. Pores or transport channels for various electrically charged particles, called ions or *electrolytes*, and specific carriers for amino acids and monosaccharides
3. Specific enzymes that drive active pumps to promote concentration of certain ions, particularly potassium (K^+), within the cell while keeping concentrations of other ions (e.g., sodium [Na^+]), less than concentrations found in the extracellular environment
4. Cell surface markers, such as glycoproteins (proteins attached to carbohydrates), which identify a cell to its neighbor
5. Cell adhesion molecules (CAMs), or proteins that allow cells to hook together and form attachments of the cytoskeleton for maintaining cellular shape
6. Catalysts of chemical reactions (e.g., conversion of lactose to glucose)

Membrane proteins are key components of energy transduction, converting chemical energy into electrical energy, or electrical energy into either mechanical energy or synthesis of ATP. Investigators are studying ATP enzymes and the changes in shape of biologic membranes, particularly mitochondrial membranes, and their relationship to aging and disease.[4]

In animal cells, the plasma membrane is stabilized by a meshwork of proteins attached to the underside of the membrane called the cell cortex. Human red blood cells have a cell cortex that maintains their flattened biconcave shape.[3]

The cellular protein pool is in constant change or flux. Proteostasis is the process that regulates protein synthesis, folding, and degradation within and around a cell. This adaptable system depends on how quickly proteins are made, how long they survive, or when they are broken down. The proteostasis network comprises ribosomes (makers); chaperones (helpers); and two protein breakdown systems or proteolytic systems—lysosomes and the ubiquitin-proteasome system (UPS). These systems regulate protein homeostasis under a large variety of conditions, including variations in nutrient supply, the existence of oxidative stress or cellular differentiation, changes in temperature, and the presence of heavy metal ions and other sources of stress. Proteostasis is vital to health, and failure to maintain protein homeostasis is associated with aging and numerous degenerative diseases (Fig. 1.7).

Carbohydrates. The short chains of sugars or carbohydrates *(oligosaccharides)* contained within the plasma membrane are mostly bound to membrane proteins (glycoproteins) and lipids (glycolipids). Long polysaccharide chains attached to membrane proteins are called *proteoglycans*. All of the carbohydrate on the glycoproteins, proteoglycans, and glycolipids is located on the outside of the plasma membrane and the carbohydrate coating is called the glycocalyx. The glycocalyx helps to protect the cell from mechanical damage.[5] In addition, the layer of carbohydrate gives the cell a slimy surface that assists the mobility of other cells, such as leukocytes, to squeeze through the narrow spaces.[3] Other functions of carbohydrates include specific cell-to-cell recognition and adhesion. Intercellular recognition is an important function of membrane oligosaccharides; for example, the transmembrane proteins called *lectins*, which bind to a particular oligosaccharide, recognize neutrophils at the site of bacterial infection. This recognition allows the neutrophil to adhere to the blood vessel wall and migrate from blood into the infected tissue to help eliminate the invading bacteria.[3]

Cellular Receptors

Cellular receptors are protein molecules on the plasma membrane, in the cytoplasm, or in the nucleus that can recognize and bind with specific smaller molecules called ligands (from the Latin *ligare*, "to bind") (Fig. 1.8). The region of a protein that associates with a ligand is called its binding site. For example, hormones are ligands. Numerous receptors are found in

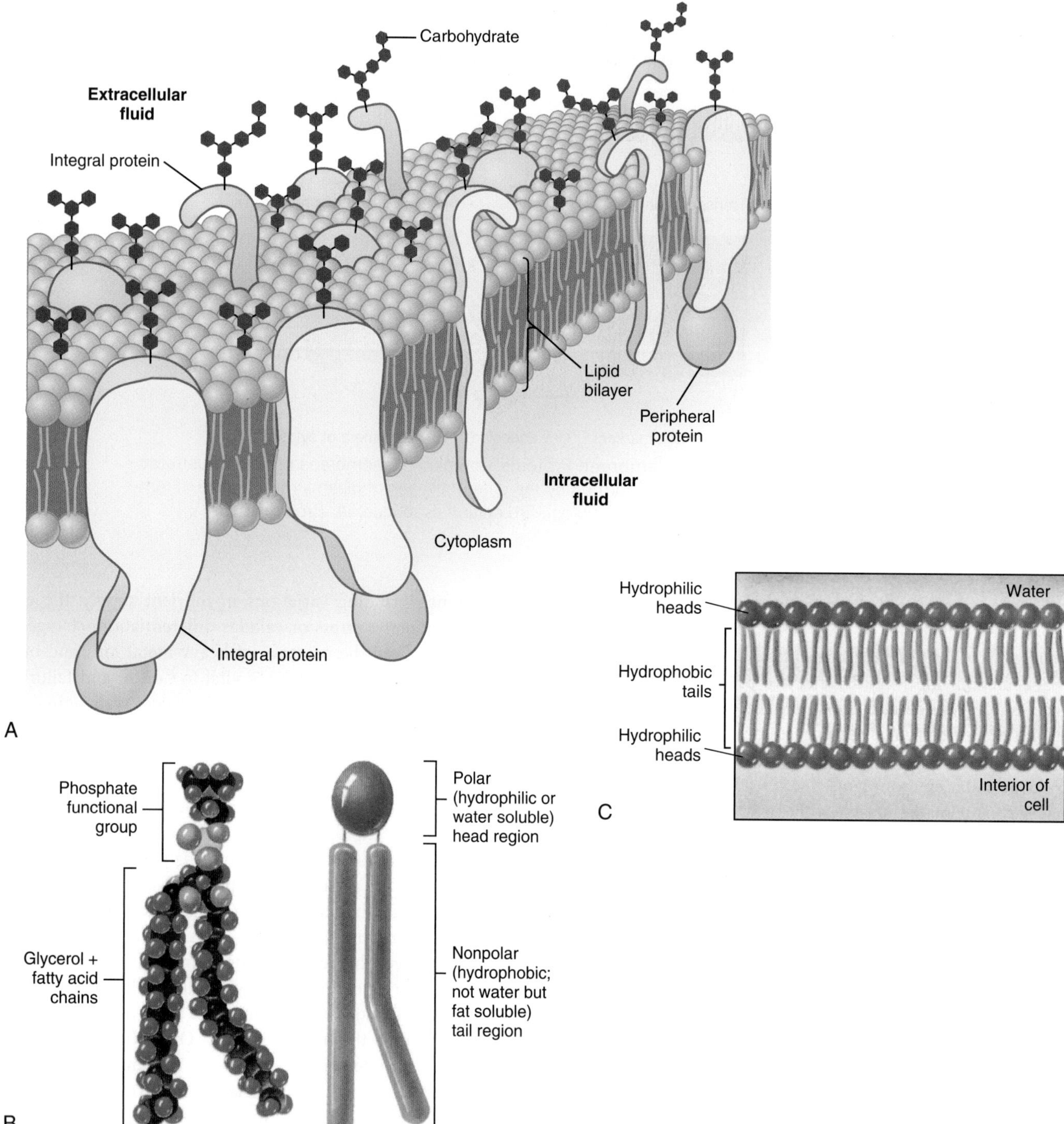

Fig. 1.4 Lipid Bilayer Membranes. (A) The structure of a cell membrane showing the lipid bilayer, embedded proteins, and attached extracellular carbohydrates. **(B)** Each phospholipid molecule consists of a phosphate functional group and two fatty acid chains attached to a glycerol molecule. **(C)** The fatty acid chains and glycerol form nonpolar, hydrophobic "tails," and the phosphate functional group forms the polar, hydrophilic "head" of the phospholipid molecule. When placed in water, the hydrophobic tails of the molecule face inward, away from the water, and the hydrophilic head faces outward, toward the water. (A, From Guyton AC, Hall JE. *Textbook of medical physiology,* 11th edition. Amsterdam: Elsevier Saunders; 2006. B and C, From Raven PH, Johnson GB. *Understanding biology,* 3rd edition. Dubuque, IA: Brown; 1995.

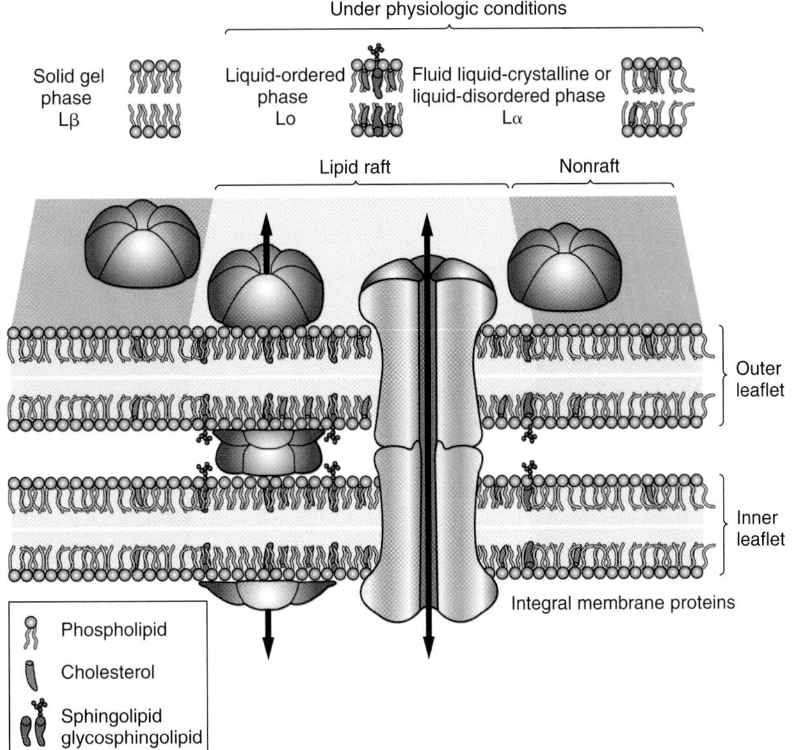

Fig. 1.5 Lipid Bilayer Membranes. Concepts of biologic membranes have markedly changed in the last two decades, from the classic fluid mosaic model to the current model that lipids and proteins are not evenly distributed but can isolate into microdomains, differing in their protein and lipid composition. The three major phases of lipid bilayer organization include a solid gel phase (e.g., with low temperatures), a liquid-ordered phase (high temperatures), and a fluid liquid-crystalline (or liquid-disordered) phase.

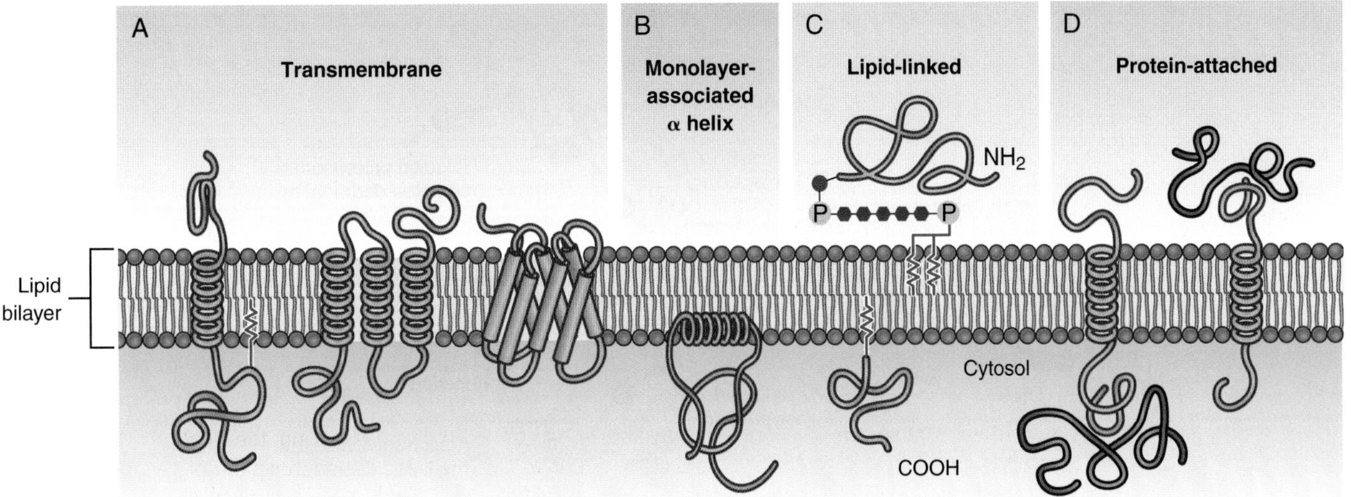

Fig. 1.6 Proteins Attach to the Plasma Membrane in Different Ways. (A) Transmembrane proteins extend through the membrane as a single α helix, as multiple α helices, or as a rolled-up barrel-like sheet called a β barrel. **(B)** Some membrane proteins are anchored to the cytosolic side of the lipid bilayer by an amphipathic α helix. **(C)** Some proteins are linked on either side of the membrane by a covalently attached lipid molecule. **(D)** Proteins are attached by weak noncovalent interactions with other membrane proteins. (D, Adapted from Alberts B, Bray D, Hopkin K, et al. *Essential cell biology,* 4th edition. New York: Garland; 2014.

most cells. Ligand binding to receptors activates or inhibits the receptor's associated signaling or biochemical pathway (see the Cellular Communication and Signal Transduction section). Recognition and binding depend on the chemical configuration of the receptor and its smaller ligand, which must fit together somewhat like the pieces of a jigsaw puzzle. Binding selectively to a protein receptor with high affinity to a ligand depends on formation of weak, noncovalent interactions—hydrogen bonds, electrostatic attractions, and van der Waals attractions—and favorable hydrophobic forces.[3]

Plasma membrane receptors protrude from or are exposed at the external surface of the membrane and are important for cellular uptake of ligands (see Fig. 1.8). The ligands that bind with membrane receptors include hormones, neurotransmitters, antigens, complement components, lipoproteins, infectious agents, drugs, and metabolites. Specific interactions of cellular receptors with their respective ligands have provided a basis for understanding disease.

Although the chemical nature of ligands and their receptors differs, receptors are classified based on their location and function. Cellular type determines overall cellular function, but plasma membrane receptors determine which ligands a cell will bind with and how the cell will respond to the binding. Specific processes also control intracellular mechanisms.

Receptors for different drugs are found on the plasma membrane, in the cytoplasm, and in the nucleus. Membrane receptors have been found for certain anesthetics, opiates, endorphins, enkephalins, antibiotics, cancer chemotherapeutic agents, digitalis, and other drugs. Membrane receptors for endorphins, which are opiate-like peptides isolated from the pituitary gland, are found in large quantities in pain pathways of the nervous system (see Chapters 15 and 16). With binding to the receptor, the endorphins (or drugs, e.g., morphine) change the cell's permeability to ions, increase the concentration of molecules that regulate intracellular protein synthesis, and initiate molecular events that modulate pain perception.

Receptors for infectious microorganisms, or antigen receptors, bind bacteria, viruses, and parasites to the cell membrane. Antigen receptors on white blood cells (lymphocytes, monocytes, macrophages, granulocytes) recognize and bind with antigenic microorganisms and activate the immune and inflammatory responses (see Chapter 7).

CELL-TO-CELL ADHESIONS

Cells are small and squishy, *not* like bricks. They are enclosed only by a flimsy membrane, yet the cell depends on the integrity of this membrane for its survival. How can cells be connected strongly, with their membranes intact, to form a muscle that can lift this textbook? Plasma membranes not only serve as the outer boundaries of all cells but also allow groups of cells to be held together robustly, in cell-to-cell adhesions, to form tissues and organs (Box 1.1). Once arranged, cells are linked by three different means: (1) the extracellular matrix (ECM), (2) CAMs in the cell's plasma membrane, and (3) specialized cell junctions.

Extracellular Matrix and Basement Membrane

Cells can be united by attachment to one another or through the ECM (including the basement membrane), which the cells secrete around themselves. The extracellular matrix (ECM) is an intricate meshwork of fibrous proteins embedded in a watery, gel-like substance composed of complex carbohydrates (Fig. 1.9).

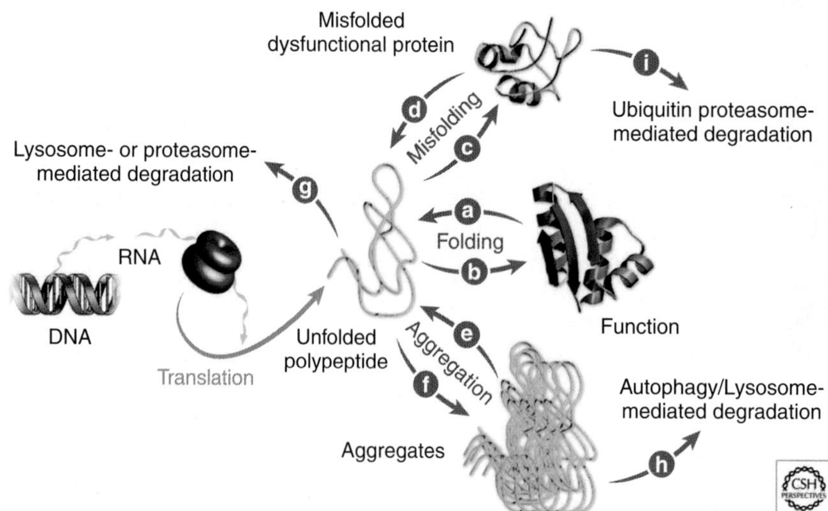

Fig. 1.7 Protein Homeostasis System and Outcomes. A main role of the protein homeostasis network *(proteostasis)* is to minimize protein misfolding and protein aggregation. The network includes ribosome-mediated protein synthesis, chaperone (folding helpers in the ER) and enzyme mediated folding, breakdown systems of lysosome and proteasome-mediated protein degradation, and vesicular trafficking. The network integrates biologic pathways that balance folding, trafficking, and protein degradation depicted by *arrows a, b, c, d, e, f, g, h,* and *i. ER,* Endoplasmic reticulum. (Adapted from Balch WE, Morimoto RI, Dillin A, et al. Adapting proteostasis for disease intervention. *Science* 2008;319:916 -919.)

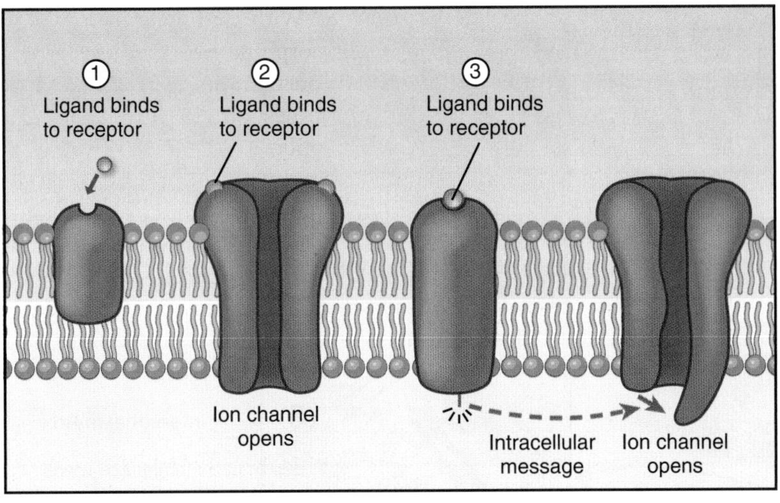

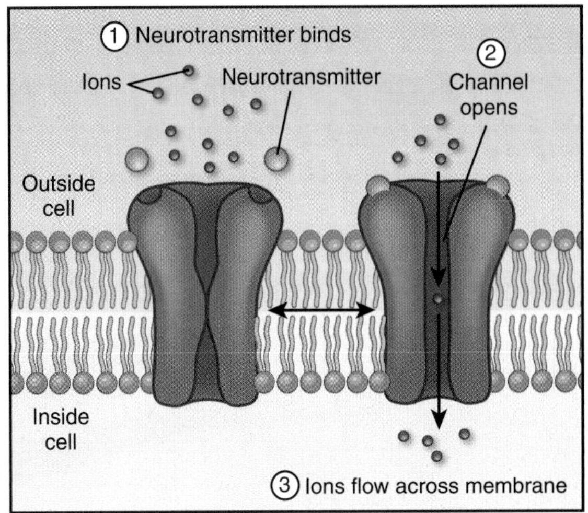

Fig. 1.8 Cellular Receptors. (A) ***1,*** Plasma membrane receptor for a ligand (here, a hormone molecule) on the surface of an integral protein. A neurotransmitter can exert its effect on a postsynaptic cell by means of two fundamentally different types of receptor proteins. ***2,*** Channel-linked receptors. ***3,*** Non–channel-linked receptors. Channel-linked receptors are also known as *ligand-gated channels.* **(B)** Example of ligand-gated ion channels. The channel structure is changed when, for example, a neurotransmitter binds and ions can now enter.

BOX 1.1 Cell Adhesion Molecules

Cell adhesion molecules (CAMs) are cell surface proteins that bind the cell to an adjacent cell and to components of the extracellular matrix (ECM). CAMs include four protein families: (1) the integrins, (2) the cadherins, (3) the selectins, and (4) the immunoglobulin superfamily CAMs (IgSF CAMs). Integrins are receptors within the ECM and regulate cell-ECM interactions with collagen. Cadherins are calcium (Ca^{2+})-dependent glycoproteins throughout tissue (e.g., epithelial [E-cadherin]). Selectins are proteins that bind some carbohydrates (e.g., mucins). The IgSF CAMs bind integrins and other IgSF CAMs.

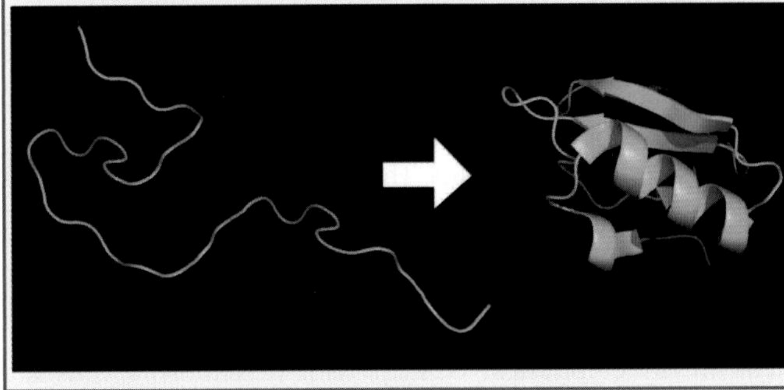

The basement membrane (BM) (also known as basal lamina) is a specialized type of ECM. This sheet of matrix is very thin, tough, and flexible; lies beneath epithelial cells; occurs between two cell sheets (kidney glomerulus); and surrounds individual muscle cells, fat cells, and Schwann cells (which wrap around peripheral nerve cell axons) (Fig. 1.10). The ECM is similar to glue; however, it provides a pathway for diffusion of nutrients, wastes, and other water-soluble substances between the blood and tissue cells. Interwoven within the matrix are three groups of large molecules or macromolecules: (1) fibrous structural proteins, including collagen and elastin; (2) adhesive glycoproteins, such as fibronectin; and (3) proteoglycans and hyaluronic acid.

1. Collagen forms cable-like fibers or sheets that provide tensile strength or resistance to longitudinal stress. Collagen breakdown, such as occurs in osteoarthritis, destroys the fibrils that give cartilage its tensile strength.
2. Elastin is a rubber-like protein fiber most abundant in tissues that must be capable of stretching and recoiling, such as found in the lungs.
3. Fibronectin, a large glycoprotein, promotes cell adhesion and cell anchorage. Reduced amounts have been found in certain types of cancerous cells; this allows cancer cells to travel, or metastasize, to other parts of the body. All of these macromolecules occur in intercellular junctions and cell surfaces and may assemble into two different components: interstitial matrix and BM (see Fig. 1.9).

The ECM is secreted by fibroblasts ("fiber formers") (Fig. 1.11), local cells that are present in the matrix. The matrix and the cells within it are known collectively as *connective tissue* because they interconnect cells to form tissues and organs. Human connective tissues are enormously varied. They can be hard and dense (e.g., bone), flexible (e.g., tendons or the dermis of the skin), resilient and shock absorbing (e.g., cartilage), or soft and transparent, similar to the jelly-like substance that fills the eye. In all these examples, the majority of the tissue is composed of ECM, and the cells that produce the matrix are scattered within it like raisins in a pudding (see Fig. 1.11).

The matrix is not just passive scaffolding for cellular attachment but also helps to regulate the function of the cells with which it interacts. The matrix helps to regulate important functions, such as cell growth and differentiation.

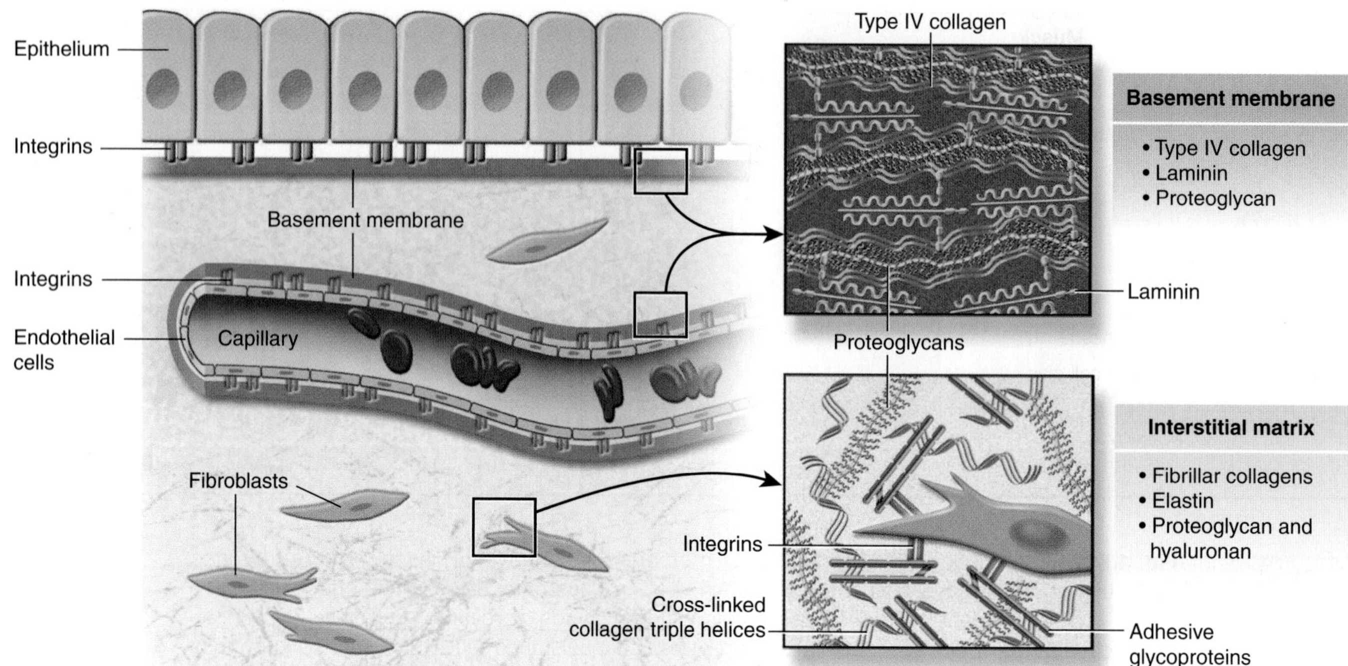

Fig. 1.9 Extracellular Matrix. Tissues are not just cells but also extracellular space. The extracellular space is an intricate network of macromolecules called the *extracellular matrix (ECM)*. The macromolecules that constitute the ECM are secreted locally (by mostly fibroblasts) and assembled into a meshwork in close association with the surface of the cell that produced them. Two main classes of macromolecules include proteoglycans, which are bound to polysaccharide chains called *glycosaminoglycans;* and fibrous proteins (e.g., collagen, elastin, fibronectin, and laminin), which have structural and adhesive properties. Together the proteoglycan molecules form a gel-like ground substance in which the fibrous proteins are embedded. The gel permits rapid diffusion of nutrients, metabolites, and hormones between blood and the tissue cells. Matrix proteins modulate cell-matrix interactions, including normal tissue remodeling (which can become abnormal, for example, with chronic inflammation). Disruptions of this balance result in serious diseases such as arthritis, tumor growth, and other pathologic conditions. (Adapted from Kumar A, Abbas K, Jon C. *Robbins and Cotran pathologic basis of disease*, 9th edition. Philadelphia: Saunders; 2015.

Cell Adhesion Molecules

Cell adhesion molecules (CAMs) are cell surface proteins that bind the cell to adjacent cells and to components of the ECM. CAMs are divided into four protein families: integrins, cadherins, selectins, and the immunoglobulin superfamily (IgSF).[6] Integrins are a major class of molecules that typically bind to the ECM, whereas selectins, cadherins, and IgSF are associated with cell-to-cell adhesion. Integrins regulate cell interactions with collagen, fibronectin, vitronectin, and fibrinogen in the ECM. Cadherins, an abbreviation of "calcium-dependent adherent proteins," are associated with cell-cell adhesive bonds in solid tissues. They are calcium-dependent glycoproteins that have specific functions and distributions within tissues. For example, epithelial cells express E-cadherin, which cause tight adhesions between cells that interface between the body and the environment to create a protective barrier. Neural and endothelial cells express N-cadherin which helps to maintain the structural integrity of nerve cells and blood vessels.[7] Selectins are a family of proteins that bind certain carbohydrates. Selectins are divided into subgroups based on which cell types they are found in: P—platelets, E—endothelial, and L—leukocytes. Their primary function is to allow blood cells to bind to the endothelial surfaces of blood vessels during the inflammatory response (see Chapter 7). The immunoglobulin superfamily CAMs (IgSF CAMs) is one of the largest and most diverse protein families. These CAMs include vascular (VCAM), intercellular (ICAM), neural (NCAM), and nectins. Their functions include adhesion between immune and endothelial cells, neural development, and cellular migration and growth.

Specialized Cell Junctions

Cells in direct physical contact with neighboring cells are often interconnected at specialized plasma membrane regions called cell junctions. Cell junctions are classified by their function:

1. Tight Junction: To hold cells together and form a tight seal and to maintain apicobasal polarity of individual epithelial cells (Fig. 1.12)
2. Adherens junctions, desmosomes, hemidesmosomes: To provide strong mechanical attachments
3. Gap junctions: To provide a special type of chemical communication (e.g., inorganic ions and small water-soluble molecules to move from the cytosol of one cell to the cytosol of another cell), such as those causing an electrical wave

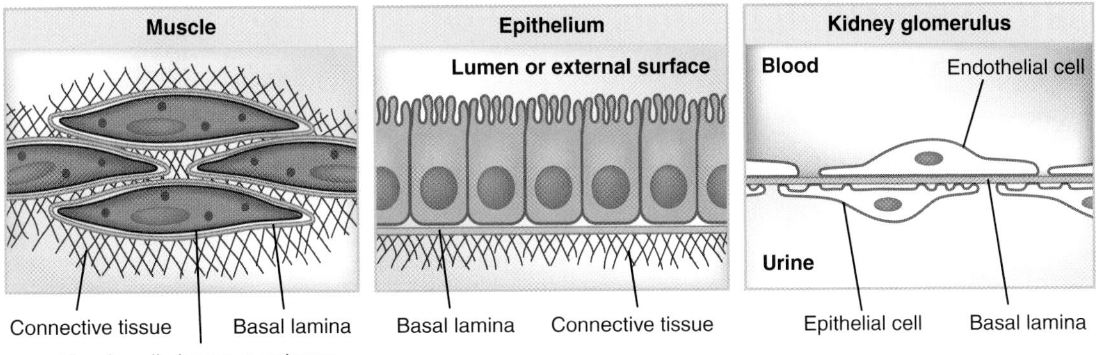

Fig. 1.10 Three Ways Basement Membranes (Basal Laminae) Are Organized. Basal laminae *(yellow)* surround certain cells like skeletal cells, underlie epithelia, and occur between two cell sheets (kidney glomerulus). (Adapted from Alberts B, Bray D, Hopkin K, et al. *Essential cell biology*, 4th edition. New York: Garland; 2014.

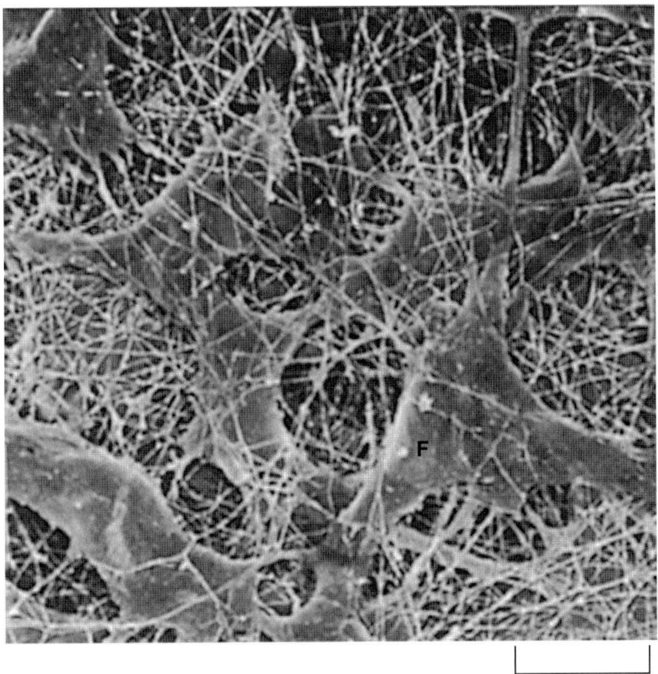

Fig. 1.11 Fibroblasts in Connective Tissue. This micrograph shows tissue from the cornea of a rat. The extracellular matrix surrounds the fibroblasts *(F)*. (Adapted from Nishia T, et al. The extracellular matrix of animal connective tissues. *Invest Ophthalmology Visual Science*, 1998; 29:1887-1880.)

In summary, cell junctions make the epithelium leak-proof and mediate mechanical attachment of one cell to another, allowing communicating tunnels and maintaining cell polarity.[8]

Cell junctions can be classified as symmetric and asymmetric. Symmetric junctions include tight junctions (zonula occludens), the belt desmosome (zonula adherens), desmosomes (macula adherens), and gap junctions (also called *intercellular channel* or *communicating junctions*). An asymmetric junction is the hemidesmosome (see Fig. 1.12A). Together they form the junctional complex. Tight junctions are barriers to diffusion, prevent the movement of substances through transport proteins in the plasma membrane, and prevent the leakage of small molecules between the plasma membranes of adjacent cells.[9] Desmosomes unite cells either by forming continuous bands or belts of epithelial sheets or by developing button-like points of contact. Desmosomes also act as a system of braces to maintain structural stability (see Fig. 1.12B). Gap junctions are composed of integral membrane proteins called connexins. Connexins are hemichannels that extend outward from each of the adjacent plasma membranes (see Fig. 1.12C). Gap junctions facilitate intercellular communication by allowing small ions and signaling molecules to pass directly from the inside of one cell to the inside of another. This process of cell communication is a critical feature for the development, function, and homeostasis of tissues and organs.[10] Multiple factors regulate gap junction intercellular communication, including voltage across the junction, intracellular pH, intracellular calcium (Ca^{2+}) concentration, and protein phosphorylation. Cell polarity, the direction of cellular transport, maintains normal cell and tissue structure for numerous functions (e.g., movement of nutrients in and out of the cell) and becomes altered with diseases (see Fig. 1.12D).

The junctional complex is a highly permeable part of the plasma membrane where permeability is controlled by a process called gating. Increased levels of cytoplasmic calcium cause decreased permeability at the junctional complex. Gating enables uninjured cells to protect themselves from injured neighbors.

CELLULAR COMMUNICATION AND SIGNAL TRANSDUCTION

Cells need to communicate with each other to maintain a stable internal environment, or homeostasis; to regulate their growth and division; to oversee their development and organization into tissues; and to coordinate their functions. Cells communicate by using hundreds of signal molecules (e.g., insulin-like growth factor 1). Cells communicate in three main ways:

1. They display plasma membrane–bound signaling molecules (receptors) that affect the cell itself and other cells in direct physical contact (Fig. 1.13A).

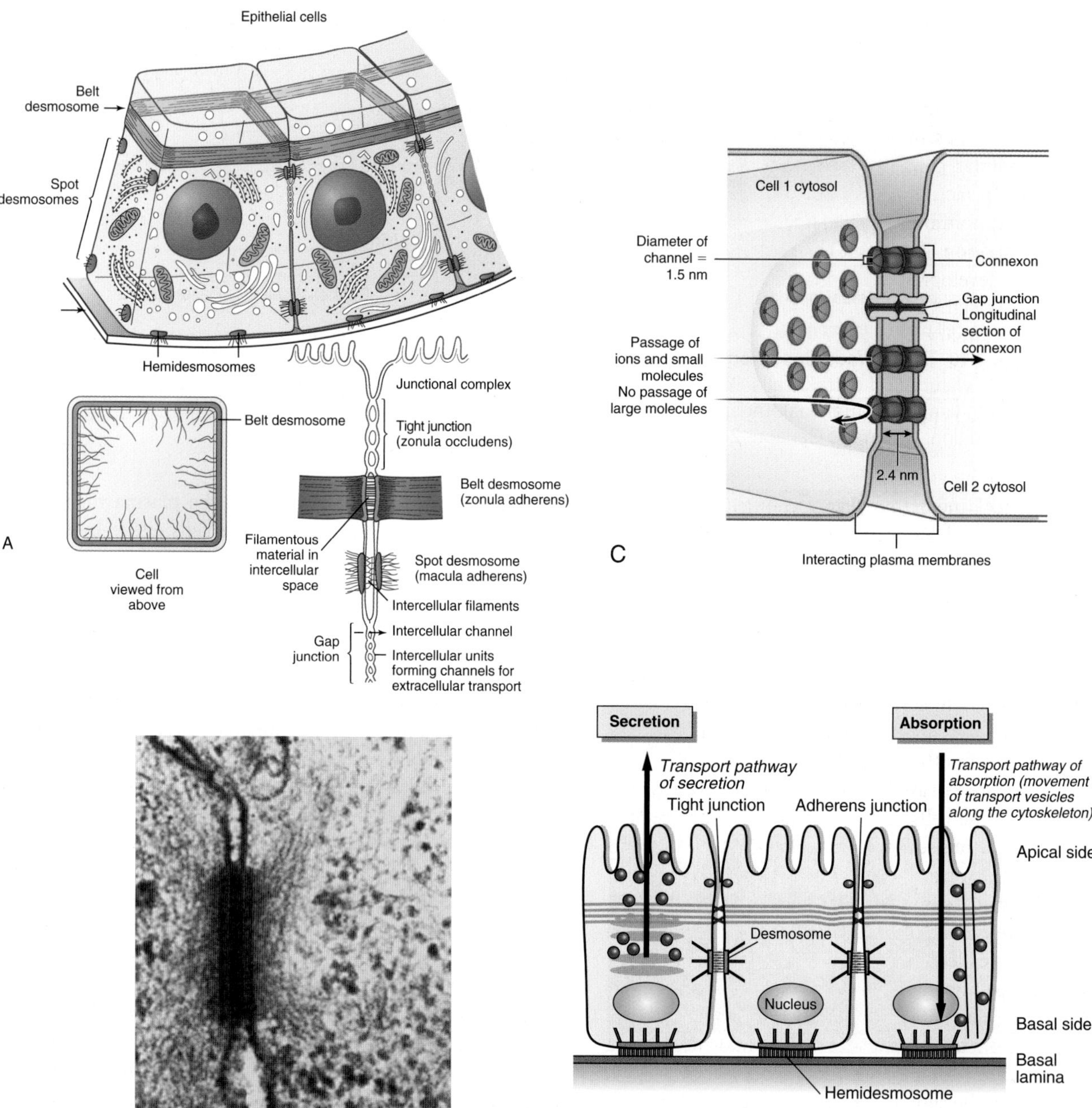

FIG. 1.12 Junctional Complex. (A), Schematic drawing of a belt desmosome between epithelial cells. This junction, also called *zonula adherens*, encircles each interacting cell. The spot desmosomes and hemidesmosomes, like the belt desmosomes, are adhering junctions. The tight junction is an impermeable junction that holds cells together but seals them in such a way that molecules cannot leak between them. The gap junction, as a communicating junction, mediates the passage of small molecules from one interacting cell to the other. **(B)** Electron micrograph of desmosomes. **(C)** Connexons. The connexin gap junction proteins have four transmembrane domains, and they play a vital role in maintaining cell and tissue function and homeostasis. Cells connected by gap junctions are considered ionically (electrically) and metabolically coupled. Gap junctions coordinate the activities of adjacent cells; for example, they are important for synchronizing contractions of heart muscle cells through ionic coupling and for permitting action potentials to spread rapidly from cell to cell in neural tissues. The reason gap junctions occur in tissues that are not electrically active is unknown. Although most gap junctions are associated with junctional complexes, they sometimes exist as independent structures. **(D)** Cell Polarity of Epithelial Cells. Schematic of cell polarity (cell direction) of epithelial cells. Shown are the directions of the basal side and the apical side. Organelles and cytoskeleton are also arranged directionally to enable, for example, intestinal cell secretion and absorption. (A and B, From Raven PH, Johnson GB. *Biology*. St. Louis: Mosby; 1992.; C, Adapted from Gartner LP, Hiatt JL. *Color textbook of histology*, 3rd edition. St. Louis: Saunders Elsevier; 2006; Sherwood L. *Learning*, 8th edition. Belmont, CA: Brooks/Cole CENGAGE; 2013; D, Adapted from *Life science web textbook*, The University of Tokyo.)

2. They affect receptor proteins *inside* the target cell and the signal molecule has to enter the cell to bind to them (see Fig. 1.13B).
3. They form protein channels (gap junctions) that directly coordinate the activities of adjacent cells (see Fig. 1.13C). Alterations in cellular communication affect disease onset and progression. In fact, if a cell cannot perform gap junctional intercellular communication, normal growth control and cell differentiation is compromised, thereby favoring cancerous tumor development (see Chapter 12).

Secreted chemical signals involve communication locally and at a distance. Primary modes of intercellular signaling are contact dependent, paracrine, hormonal, neurohormonal, and neurotransmitter. Autocrine stimulation occurs when the secreting cell targets itself (Fig. 1.14).

Contact-dependent signaling requires cells to be in close membrane-to-membrane contact. In paracrine signaling, cells secrete local chemical mediators that are quickly taken up, destroyed, or immobilized. Paracrine signaling usually involves different cell types; however, cells also can produce signals to which they alone respond, and this is called autocrine signaling (see Fig. 1.14). Cancer cells use this form of signaling to stimulate their survival and proliferation. The mediators act only on nearby cells. Hormonal signaling involves specialized endocrine cells that secrete chemicals called *hormones;* hormones are released by one set of cells and travel through the bloodstream to produce a response in other sets of cells. In neurohormonal signaling hormones are released into blood by neurosecretory neurons. Like endocrine cells, neurosecretory neurons release blood-borne chemical messengers, whereas ordinary neurons secrete short-range neurotransmitters into a small discrete space (i.e., synapse). Neurons communicate directly with the cells they innervate by releasing chemicals or neurotransmitters at specialized junctions called chemical synapses; the neurotransmitter diffuses across the synaptic cleft and acts on the postsynaptic target cell (see Fig. 1.14). Many of these same signaling molecules are receptors used in hormonal, neurohormonal, and paracrine signaling. Important differences lie in the speed and selectivity with which the signals are delivered to their targets.[2]

Plasma membrane receptors belong to one of three classes that are defined by the signaling (transduction) mechanism used. Table 1.3 summarizes these classes of receptors. Cells respond to external stimuli by activating a variety of signal transduction pathways, which are communication pathways, or signaling cascades (Fig. 1.15). Signals are passed between cells when a particular type of molecule is produced by one cell—the signaling cell—and received by another—the target cell—by means of a receptor protein that recognizes and responds specifically to the signal molecule (see Fig. 1.15A and B). In turn, the signaling molecules activate a pathway of intracellular protein kinases that results in various responses, such as growing and reproducing, dying, surviving, or differentiating (see Fig. 1.15). If deprived of appropriate signals, most cells undergo a form of cell suicide known as *programmed cell death*, or *apoptosis* (see Chapter 2).

Binding of the extracellular signaling messenger (i.e., ligand), or first messenger, to the membrane receptors causes (1) opening or closing of specific channels in the membrane to regulate the movement of ions into or out of the cell; and (2) transfer of the signal to an intracellular messenger or second messenger, which triggers a cascade of biochemical events within the cell (Fig. 1.16).

CELLULAR METABOLISM

All of the chemical tasks of maintaining essential cellular functions are referred to as cellular metabolism. The energy-using process of metabolism is called anabolism (*ana* = upward), and the energy-releasing process is known as catabolism (*kata* = downward). Metabolism provides the cell with the energy it needs to produce cellular structures.

Dietary proteins, fats, and starches (i.e., carbohydrates) are hydrolyzed in the intestinal tract into amino acids, fatty acids, and glucose, respectively. These constituents are then absorbed, circulated, and incorporated into the cell, where they may be used for various vital cellular processes, including the production of ATP. The process by which ATP is produced is one example of a series of reactions called a metabolic pathway. A metabolic pathway involves several steps whose end products are not always detectable. A key feature of cellular metabolism is the directing of biochemical reactions by protein catalysts or enzymes. Each enzyme has a high affinity for a substrate, a specific substance converted to a product of the reaction.

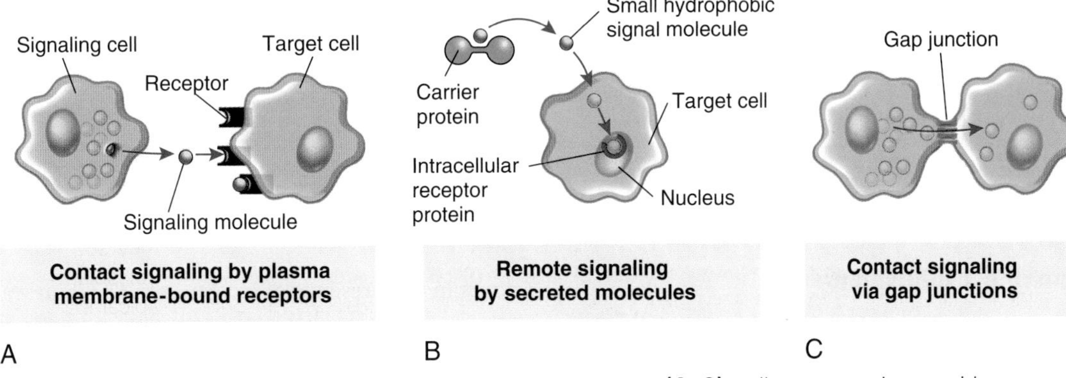

Fig. 1.13 Cellular Communication. Three primary ways **(A–C)** cells communicate with one another. (B, Adapted from Alberts B, Johnson A, Lewis J, et al. *Molecular biology of the cell*, 5th edition. New York: Garland; 2008.

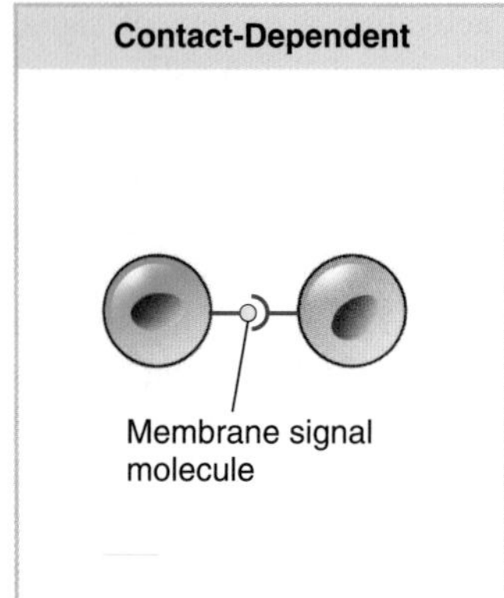

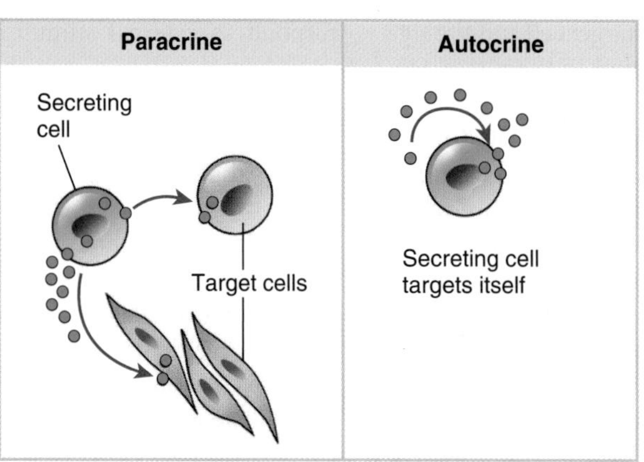

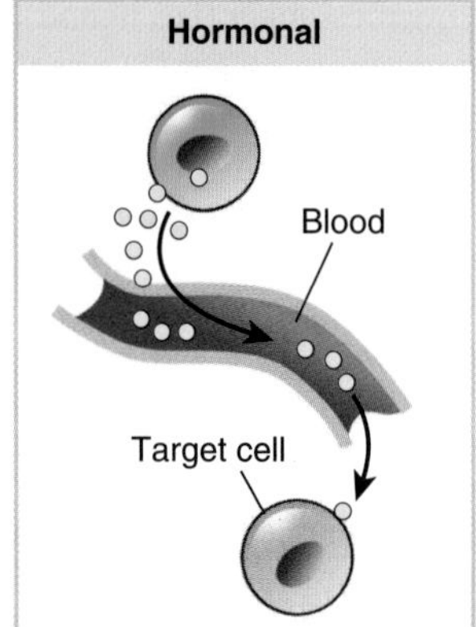

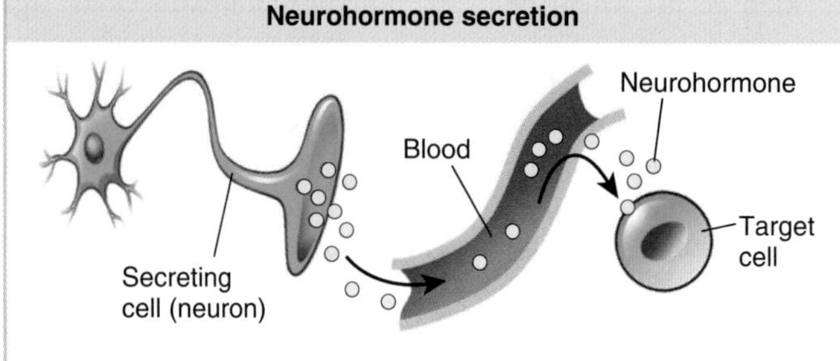

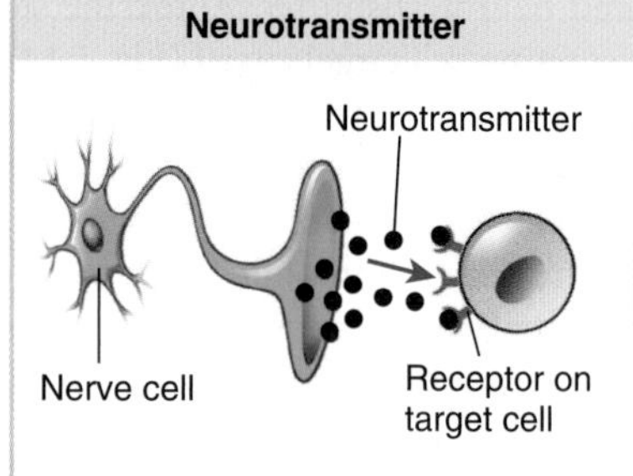

Fig. 1.14 Primary Modes of Chemical Signaling. Five forms of signaling mediated by secreted molecules. Hormones, paracrines, neurotransmitters, and neurohormones are all intercellular messengers that accomplish communication between cells. Autocrines bind to receptors on the same cell. Not all neurotransmitters act in the strictly synaptic mode shown; some act in a contact-dependent mode as local chemical mediators that influence multiple target cells in the area.

TABLE 1.3 Classes of Plasma Membrane Receptors

Type of Receptor	Description
Channel linked	Also called *ligand-gated channels;* involve rapid synaptic signaling between electrically excitable cells. Channels open and close briefly in response to neurotransmitters, changing ion permeability of plasma membrane of postsynaptic cell.
Catalytic	Once activated by ligands, function directly as enzymes. Composed of transmembrane proteins that function intracellularly as tyrosine-specific protein kinases.
G-protein linked	Indirectly activate or inactivate plasma membrane enzyme or ion channel; interaction mediated by guanosine triphosphate (GTP)-binding regulatory protein (G protein). When activated, a chain of reactions occurs that alters concentration of intracellular messengers, such as cyclic adenosine monophosphate (cAMP) and calcium, or signaling molecules. Behaviors of other target proteins are also altered. May also interact with inositol phospholipids, which are significant in cell signaling, and molecules involved in the inositol-phospholipid transduction pathway.
	A G-protein–linked receptor activates the enzyme phosphoinositide-specific phospholipase, which, in turn, generates two intracellular messengers: (1) inositol triphosphate (IP_3) releases calcium (Ca^{2+}), and (2) diacylglycerol remains in the plasma membrane and activates protein kinase C. Protein kinase C further activates various cell proteins. Several different plasma membrane receptors are known to use the inositol-phospholipid transduction pathway.

Data from Alberts B, Bray D, Hopkin K, et al. *Molecular biology of the cell*, 5th edition. New York: Garland; 2008.

Role of Adenosine Triphosphate

What is best known about ATP is its role as a universal "fuel" *inside* living cells. This fuel, or energy, drives biologic reactions necessary for cells to function. For a cell to function, it must be able to extract and use the chemical energy in organic molecules. When 1 mole (mol) of glucose metabolically breaks down in the presence of oxygen into CO_2 and water, 686 kilocalories (kcal) of chemical energy are released. The chemical energy lost by one molecule is transferred to the chemical structure of another molecule by an energy-carrying or energy-transferring molecule, such as ATP. The energy stored in ATP can be used in various energy-requiring reactions and in the

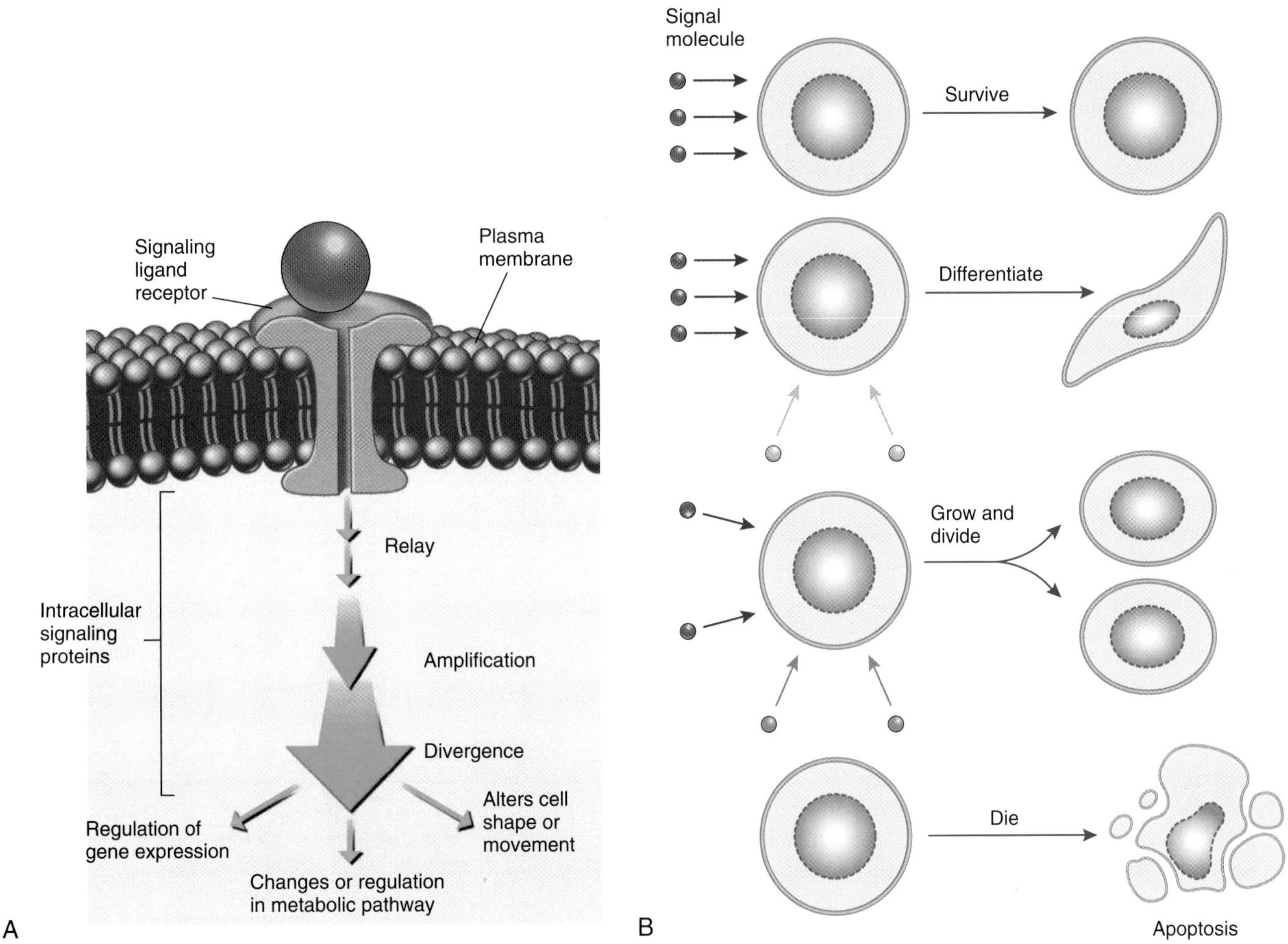

Signaling ligand receptor
Plasma membrane
Intracellular signaling proteins
Relay
Amplification
Divergence
Regulation of gene expression
Changes or regulation in metabolic pathway
Alters cell shape or movement
A

Signal molecule
Survive
Differentiate
Grow and divide
Die
Apoptosis
B

Fig. 1.15 Schematic of a Signal Transduction Pathway. Like a telephone receiver that converts an electrical signal into a sound signal, a cell converts an extracellular signal. **(A)** An extracellular signal molecule (ligand) binds to a receptor protein located on the plasma membrane, where it is transduced into an intracellular signal. This process initiates a signaling cascade that relays the signal into the cell interior, amplifying and distributing it during transit. Amplification is often achieved by stimulating enzymes. Steps in the cascade can be modulated by other events in the cell. **(B)** Different cell behaviors rely on multiple extracellular signals.

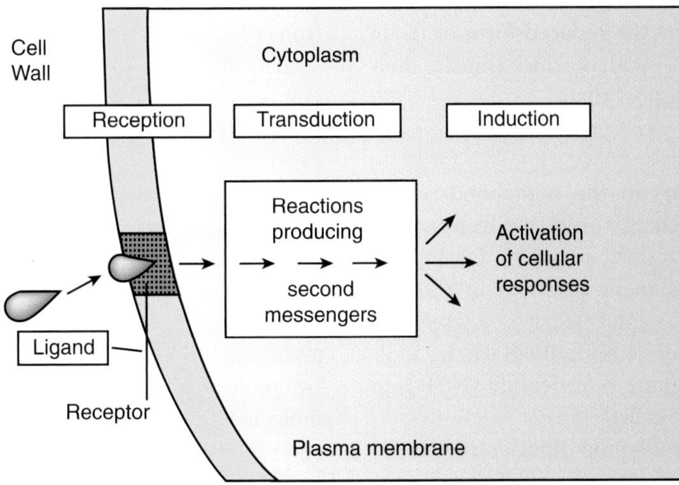

Fig. 1.16 First and Second Messengers. The first messenger or ligand attaches to the membrane receptor relaying the message across the membrane and intracellular messengers or second messengers trigger the cascade of intracellular events. The two major second-messenger pathways are cyclic adenosine monophosphate and calcium. A large number of human disorders involve problematic signaling.

process is generally converted to adenosine diphosphate (ADP) and inorganic phosphate (Pi). The energy available as a result of this reaction is approximately 7 kcal/mol of ATP. The cell uses ATP for muscle contraction and active transport of molecules across cellular membranes. ATP not only stores energy but also *transfers* it from one molecule to another. Energy stored by carbohydrate, lipid, and protein is catabolized and transferred to ATP.

ATP can also be found outside of cells. *Extracellular ATP* is released from cells in a variety of conditions and is considered important in inflammation and immunity. High levels of extracellular ATP may contribute to chronic inflammatory responses and to metastasis of cancer cells.[11]

Food and Production of Cellular Energy

Catabolism of the proteins, lipids, and polysaccharides found in food must be broken down into smaller molecules before cells can use them as a fuel source for energy or as building blocks for other molecules. The process can be divided into the following three phases (Fig. 1.17):

Phase 1: Digestion. Large molecules are broken down into smaller subunits: proteins into amino acids, polysaccharides into simple sugars (i.e., monosaccharides), and fats into fatty acids and glycerol. These processes occur outside the cell within the intestines or within the specialized lysosome organelle within the cell and are activated by secreted enzymes.

Phase 2: Glycolysis and oxidation. The most important part of phase 2 is glycolysis, the splitting of one glucose molecule into two molecules of pyruvate. During pyruvate formation, ATP and reduced nicotinamide adenine dinucleotide (NADH) are produced through oxidation, or the removal and transfer of a pair of electrons. The total process is called *oxidative cellular metabolism* and involves 10 biochemical reactions (see Fig. 1.17).

Phase 3: Citric acid cycle (Krebs cycle, tricarboxylic acid cycle). Most of the ATP is generated during this final phase, which begins with the citric acid cycle and ends with oxidative phosphorylation. Approximately two-thirds of the total oxidation of carbon compounds in most cells is accomplished during this phase. The major end products are CO_2 and two dinucleotides—NADH and the reduced form of flavin adenine dinucleotide ($FADH_2$)—both of which transfer their electrons into the electron transport chain.

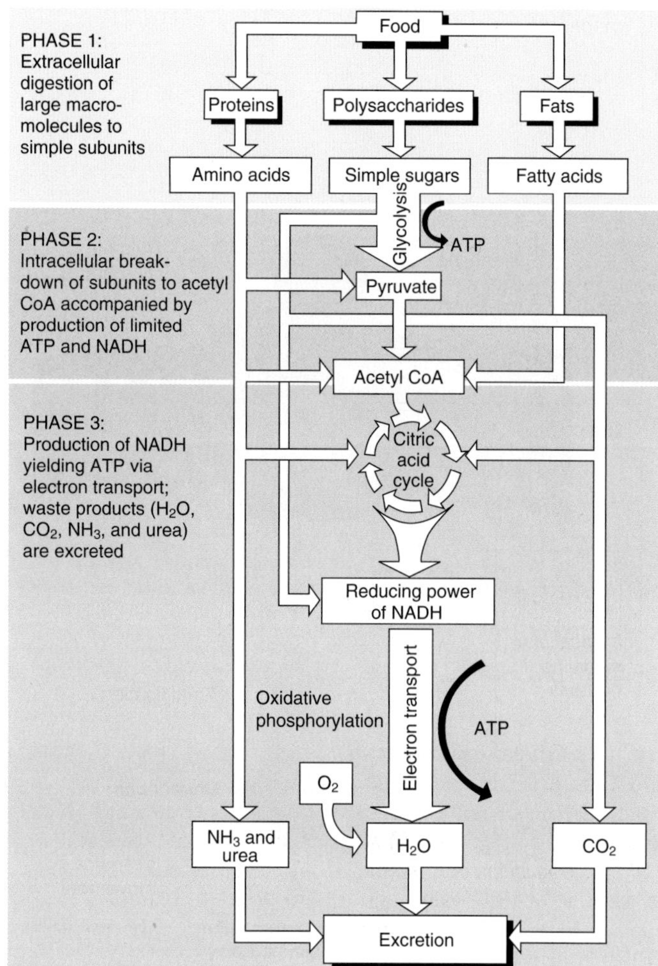

Fig. 1.17 Three Phases of Catabolism, Which Lead From Food to Waste Products. These reactions produce adenosine triphosphate *(ATP)*, which is used to power other processes in the cell. *NADH*, Nicotinamide adenine dinucleotide.

Oxidative Phosphorylation

Oxidative phosphorylation occurs in the mitochondria and is the mechanism by which the energy produced from carbohydrates, fats, and proteins is transferred to ATP. During the breakdown (catabolism) of foods, many reactions involve the removal of electrons from various intermediates. These reactions generally require a coenzyme (a nonprotein carrier molecule), such as nicotinamide adenine dinucleotide (NAD), to transfer the electrons and thus are called transfer reactions.

Molecules of NAD and flavin adenine dinucleotide (FAD) transfer electrons they have gained from the oxidation of substrates to molecular O_2. The electrons from reduced NAD and FAD, NADH and $FADH_2$, respectively, are transferred to the electron transport chain on the inner surfaces of the mitochondria with the release of hydrogen ions. Some carrier molecules are brightly colored, iron-containing proteins known as cytochromes, which accept a pair of electrons. These electrons eventually combine with molecular oxygen.

If O_2 is not available to the electron transport chain, ATP will not be formed by the mitochondria. Instead, an anaerobic (without O_2) metabolic pathway synthesizes ATP. This process, called substrate-level phosphorylation or anaerobic glycolysis, is linked to the breakdown (glycolysis) of carbohydrate (Fig. 1.18). Because glycolysis occurs in the cytoplasm of the cell, it provides energy for cells that lack mitochondria. The reactions in anaerobic glycolysis involve the conversion of glucose to pyruvic acid (pyruvate) with the simultaneous production of ATP. With the glycolysis of one molecule of glucose, two ATP molecules and two molecules of pyruvate are liberated. If O_2 is present, the two molecules of pyruvate move into the mitochondria, where they enter the citric acid cycle (Fig. 1.19).

If O_2 is absent, pyruvate is converted to lactic acid, which is released into the extracellular fluid (ECF). The conversion of pyruvic acid to lactic acid is reversible; therefore, once O_2 is restored, lactic ACID is quickly converted back to either pyruvic

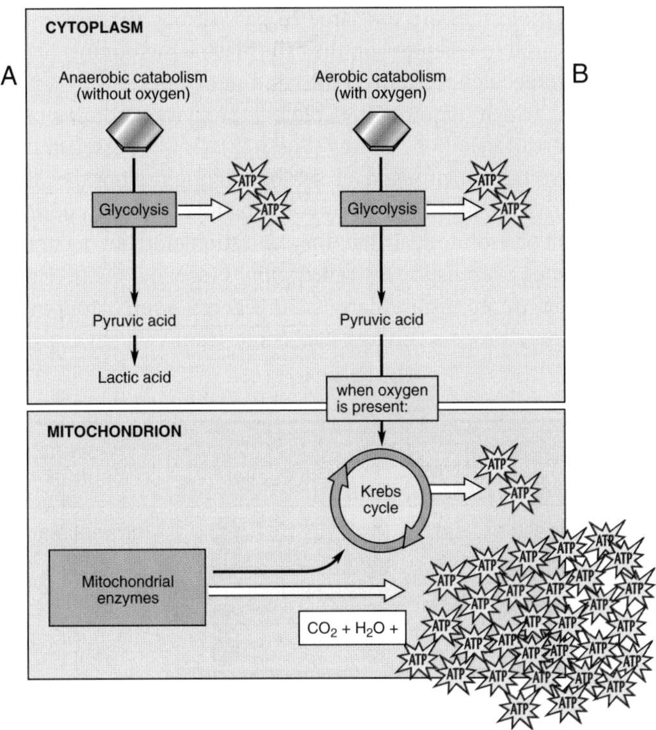

Fig. 1.18 Glycolysis. Sugars are important for fuel or energy, and they are oxidized in small steps to carbon dioxide and water. Glycolysis is the process for oxidizing sugars or glucose. Breakdown of glucose. **(A)** Anaerobic catabolism, to lactic acid and little adenosine triphosphate (ATP). **(B)** Aerobic catabolism, to carbon dioxide, water, and lots of ATP. (From Herlihy B. *The human body in health and illness*, 5th edition. St. Louis: Saunders; 2015.

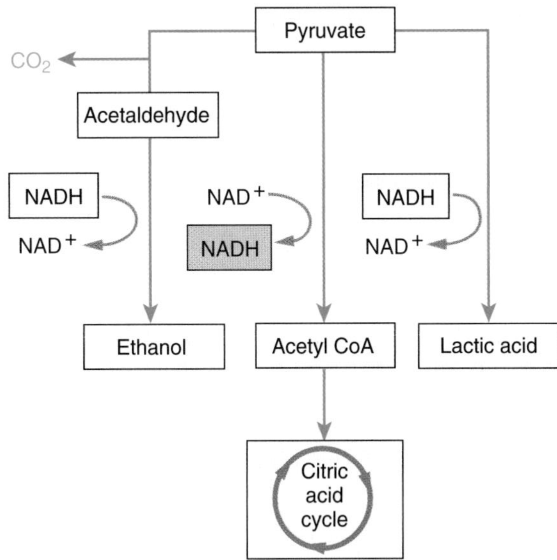

Fig. 1.19 What Happens to Pyruvate, the Product of Glycolysis? In the presence of oxygen, pyruvate is oxidized to acetyl coenzyme A *(Acetyl CoA)* and enters the citric acid cycle. In the absence of oxygen, pyruvate instead is reduced, accepting the electrons extracted during glycolysis and carried by reduced nicotinamide adenine dinucleotide *(NADH)*. When pyruvate is reduced directly, as it is in muscles, the product is lactic acid. When carbon dioxide *(CO_2)* is first removed from pyruvate and the remainder is reduced, as it is in yeasts, the resulting product is ethanol.

acid or glucose. The anaerobic generation of ATP from glucose through glycolysis is not as efficient as the aerobic generation process. Adding an oxygen-requiring stage to the catabolic process (phase 3; N see Fig. 1.18) provides cells with a much more powerful method for extracting energy from food molecules. A field of cancer research examines how tumor cells are able to alter their metabolic pathways (metabolic reprogramming) to promote cancer progression (see the Emerging Science Box: Metabolic Reprogramming and Cancer Cells box).[12]

MEMBRANE TRANSPORT: CELLULAR INTAKE AND OUTPUT

Cell survival and growth depend on the constant exchange of molecules with their environment. Cells continually import nutrients, fluids, and chemical messengers from the extracellular environment and expel metabolites, or the products of metabolism, and end products of lysosomal digestion. Cells also

EMERGING SCIENCE BOX

Metabolic Reprogramming and Cancer Cells

Proliferating cancer cells require a great deal of cellular energy to support their rapid growth and spread through the body. Cancer cells create more energy by altering their metabolic pathways for all types of fuel sources, including carbohydrates, proteins, and lipids. These alterations are known as metabolic reprogramming. An example of metabolic reprogramming is the ability of tumor cells to greatly increase their uptake of glucose and to use it in multiple alternative pathways for generating energy and the molecules required for rapid growth. Not only do cancer cells use glucose to generate ATP in mitochondria, they also can convert glucose-derived pyruvate into lactate even in the presence of oxygen (Warburg effect) and can use nonmitochondrial pathways that do not require high levels of oxygen in order to generate energy and important metabolites. These nonmitochondrial pathways are stimulated by mutated genes (oncogenes such as c-MYC) and by growth factors that promote cancer cell proliferation. Glutamate, serine, and amino acid metabolic pathways may also be altered in cancer cells. An increasing understanding of metabolic reprogramming is leading to innovative experimental approaches toward slowing cancer growth.

Data from DeBerardinis RJ, et al. We need to talk about the Warburg effect. *Nature Metabolism*, 2020; 2:127–129; Dong Y, et al. Regulation of cancer cell metabolism: oncogenic MYC in the driver's seat. Signal Transduction and Targeted Therapy, 2020;5:124; Lin X, Xiao Z, Chen T, et el. Glucose metabolism on tumor plasticity, diagnosis, and treatment. Frontiers in Oncology, 2020; 10:317; Orang AV, et al. Micromanaging aerobic respiration and glycolysis in cancer cells. Molecular Metabolism, 2019; 23:98–125; Samec M, et al. Flavonoids against the Warburg phenotype—concepts of predictive, preventive and personalised medicine to cut the Gordian knot of cancer cell metabolism. EPMA Journal, 2020; 11:377–398

must regulate ions in their cytosol and organelles. Simple diffusion across the lipid bilayer of the plasma membrane occurs for such important molecules as O_2 and CO_2. However, the majority of molecular transfer depends on specialized membrane transport proteins that span the lipid bilayer and provide private conduits for select molecules.[3]

Membrane transport proteins occur in many forms and are present in all cell membranes. Transport by membrane transport proteins is sometimes called mediated transport. Most of these transport proteins allow selective passage (e.g., Na^+ but not K^+, or K^+ but not Na^+). Each type of cell membrane has its own transport proteins that determine which solute can pass into and out of the cell or organelle.[3] The two main classes of membrane transport proteins are *transporters* and *channels.* These transport proteins differ in the type of solute—small particles of dissolved substances—they transport. A transporter is specific, allowing only those ions that fit the unique binding sites on the protein (Fig. 1.20A). A transporter undergoes conformational changes to enable membrane transport. A channel, when open, forms a pore across the lipid bilayer that allows ions and selective polar organic molecules to diffuse across the membrane (see Fig. 1.20B). Transport by a channel depends on the size and electrical charge of the molecule. Some channels are controlled by a gate mechanism that determines which solute can move into it. Ion channels are responsible for the electrical excitability of nerve and muscle cells and play a critical role in the membrane potential.

The mechanisms of membrane transport depend on the characteristics of the substance to be transported. In passive transport, water and small electrically uncharged molecules move easily through pores in the plasma membrane's lipid bilayer (Fig. 1.21). This process occurs naturally through any semipermeable barrier. Molecules will easily flow "downhill" from a region of high concentration to a region of low concentration; this movement is called *passive* because it does not require expenditure of energy or a driving force. It is driven by osmosis, hydrostatic pressure, and diffusion, all of which depend on the laws of physics and do not require life (see the Passive Transport: Diffusion, Filtration, and Osmosis section).

Other molecules are too large to pass through pores or are ligands bound to receptors on the cell's plasma membrane. Some of these molecules are moved into and out of the cell by active transport, which requires life, biologic activity, and the cell's expenditure of metabolic energy (Fig. 1.22). Unlike passive transport, active transport occurs across only living membranes that have to drive the flow "uphill" by coupling it to an energy source. Movement of a solute against its concentration gradient occurs by special types of transporters called *pumps* (see Fig. 1.22). These transporter pumps must harness an energy source to power the transport process. Energy can come from ATP hydrolysis,

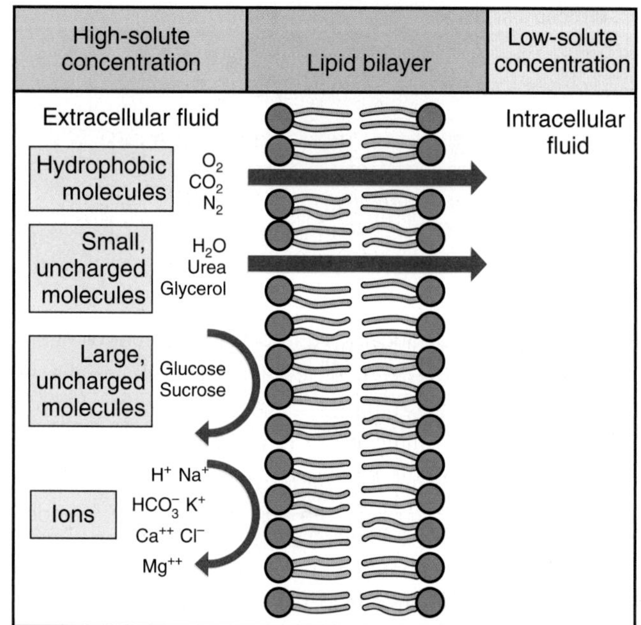

Fig. 1.21 Passive Diffusion of Solute Molecules Across the Plasma Membrane. Oxygen, nitrogen, water, urea, glycerol, and carbon dioxide can diffuse readily down the concentration gradient. Macromolecules are too large to diffuse through the pores in the plasma membrane. Ions may be repelled if the pores contain substances with identical charges. If the pores are lined with cations, for example, other cations will have difficulty diffusing because the positive charges will repel one another; diffusion can still occur, but it occurs more slowly.

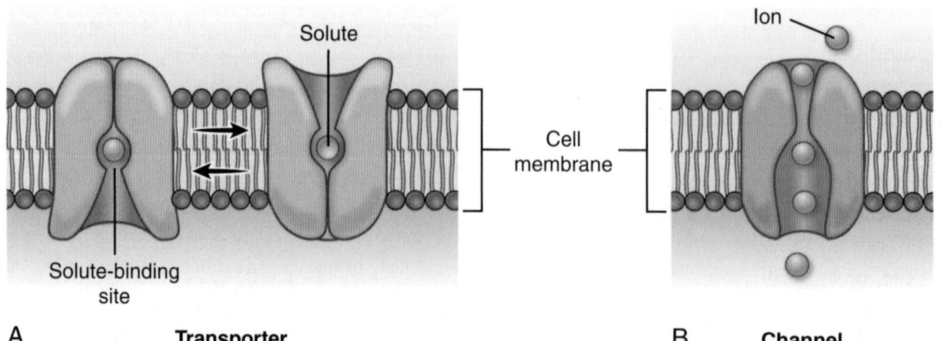

Fig. 1.20 Inorganic Ions and Small, Polar Organic Molecules Can Cross a Cell Membrane Through Either a Transporter or a Channel. (Adapted from Alberts B, Bray D, Hopkin K, et al. *Essential cell biology*, 4th edition. New York: Garland; 2014.

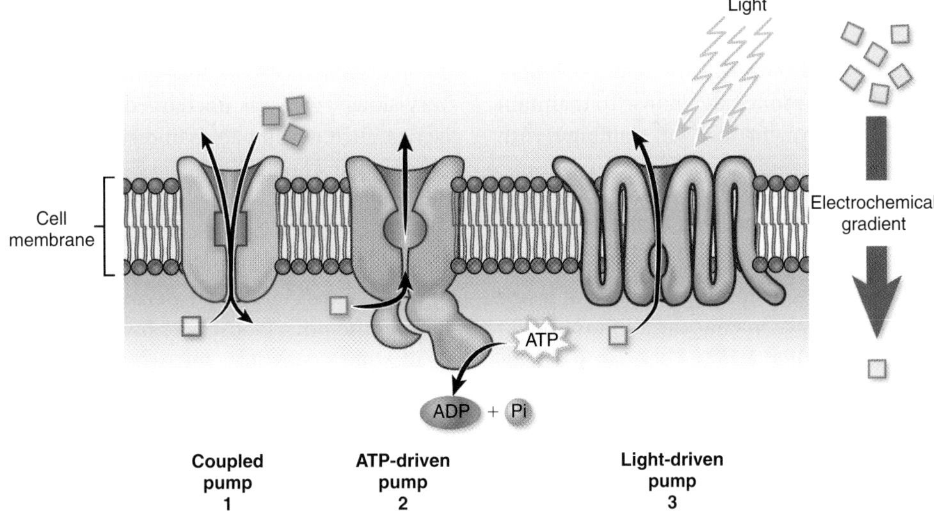

Fig. 1.22 Pumps Carry Out Active Transport in Three Ways. *1, Coupled pumps* link the uphill transport of one solute to the downhill transport of another solute. *2, Adenosine triphosphate (ATP)-driven pumps* drive uphill transport from hydrolysis of ATP. *3, Light-driven pumps* are mostly found in bacteria and use energy from sunlight to drive uphill transport. (Adapted from Alberts B, Bray D, Hopkin K, et al. *Essential cell biology*, 4th edition. New York: Garland; 2014.

a transmembrane ion gradient, or sunlight (see Fig. 1.22). The best-known energy source is the Na^+-K^+–dependent adenosine triphosphatase (ATPase) pump. It continuously regulates the cell's volume by controlling leaks through pores or protein channels and maintaining the ionic concentration gradients needed for cellular excitation and membrane conductivity (see the Active Transport of Na^+ and K^+ section). The maintenance of intracellular K^+ concentrations is required also for enzyme activity, including enzymes involved in protein synthesis. Large molecules (macromolecules), along with fluids, are transported by endocytosis (taking in) and exocytosis (expelling) (see the Transport by Vesicle Formation section). Receptor-macromolecule complexes enter the cell by means of receptor-mediated endocytosis.

Mediated transport systems can move solute molecules singly or two at a time. Two molecules can be moved simultaneously in one direction (a process called symport; e.g., sodium-glucose in the digestive tract) or in opposite directions (called antiport; e.g., the sodium-potassium pump in all cells), or a single molecule can be moved in one direction (called uniport; e.g., glucose) (Fig. 1.23).

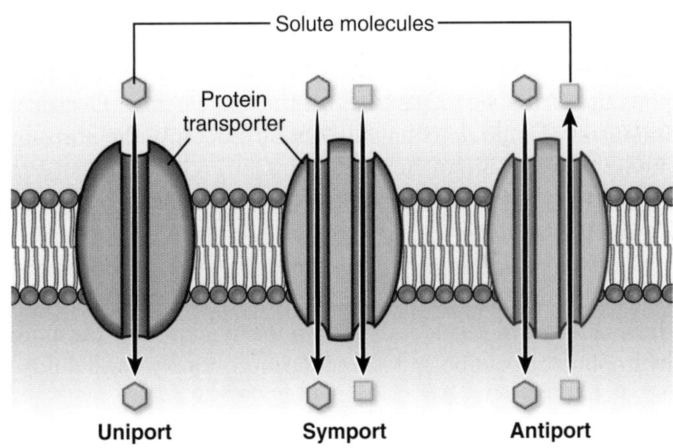

Fig. 1.23 Mediated Transport. Illustration shows simultaneous movement of a single solute molecule in one direction *(uniport)*, of two different solute molecules in one direction *(symport)*, and of two different solute molecules in opposite directions *(antiport)*.

Electrolytes as Solutes

Body fluids are composed of electrolytes, which are electrically charged and dissociate into constituent ions when placed in solution. Nonelectrolytes, such as glucose, urea, and creatinine, do not dissociate. Electrolytes account for approximately 95% of the solute molecules in body water. Electrolytes exhibit polarity by orienting themselves toward the positive or negative pole. Ions with a positive charge are known as cations and migrate toward the negative pole, or cathode, if an electrical current is passed through the electrolyte solution. Anions carry a negative charge and migrate toward the positive pole, or anode, in the presence of electrical current. Anions and cations are located in both the intracellular fluid (ICF) and the ECF compartments, although their concentration depends on their location. (Fluid and electrolyte balance between body compartments is discussed in Chapter 3). For example, Na^+ is the predominant extracellular cation, and K^+ is the principal intracellular cation. The difference in ICF and ECF concentrations of these ions is important to the transmission of electrical impulses across the plasma membranes of nerve and muscle cells.

Electrolytes are measured in milliequivalents per liter (mEq/L) or milligrams per deciliter (mg/dL). The term *milliequivalent* indicates the chemical-combining activity of an ion, which depends on the electrical charge, or valence, of its ions. In abbreviations, valence is indicated by the number of plus or minus signs. Monovalent ions, or ions with one charge, include sodium (Na^+), chloride (Cl^-), and potassium (K^+). Divalent ions, which have two charges, include calcium (Ca^{2+}) and magnesium (Mg^{++}). One milliequivalent (mEq) of any cation can combine chemically with 1 mEq of any anion: one monovalent anion will combine with one monovalent cation. Divalent ions combine more strongly than monovalent ions. To maintain electrochemical balance, one divalent ion will combine with two monovalent ions (e.g., $Ca^{2+} + 2\ Cl^- = CaCl_2$).

Passive Transport: Diffusion, Filtration, and Osmosis

Diffusion. Diffusion is the movement of a solute molecule from an area of greater solute concentration to an area of lesser solute concentration. This difference in concentration is known as a concentration gradient (see Fig. 1.21). Although particles in a solution move randomly in any direction, if the concentration of particles in one part of the solution is greater than that in another part, the particles distribute themselves evenly throughout the solution. According to the same principle, if the concentration of particles is greater on one side of a *permeable membrane* than on the other side, the particles diffuse spontaneously from the area of greater concentration to the area of less concentration until equilibrium is reached. Molecules still move back and forth to maintain this equilibrium; however, there is no net change in concentration of the molecules on either side of the permeable membrane. The higher the concentration on one side, the greater is the diffusion rate.

The diffusion rate is influenced by differences of electrical potential across the membrane (see the Movement of Electrical Impulses: Membrane Potentials section). Because the pores in the lipid bilayer are often lined with Ca^{2+}, other cations (e.g., Na^+ and K^+) diffuse slowly because they are repelled by positive charges in the pores.

The rate of diffusion of a substance depends also on its size (diffusion coefficient) and its lipid solubility (Fig. 1.24). Usually, the smaller the molecule and the more soluble it is in oil, the more hydrophobic or nonpolar it is, and the more rapidly it will diffuse across the bilayer. Oxygen, CO_2, and the steroid hormones (e.g., androgens and estrogens) are all nonpolar molecules. Water-soluble substances, such as glucose and inorganic ions, diffuse very slowly, whereas uncharged lipophilic ("lipid-loving") molecules, such as fatty acids and steroids, diffuse rapidly. Ions and other polar molecules generally diffuse across cellular membranes more slowly compared with lipid-soluble substances.

Water readily diffuses through biologic membranes because water molecules are small and uncharged. The dipolar structure of water allows it to rapidly cross the regions of the bilayer containing the polar phosphate head groups. The polar phosphate head groups constitute the two outer regions of the lipid bilayer.

Filtration: hydrostatic pressure. Filtration is the movement of water and solutes through a membrane because of a greater pushing pressure (force) on one side of the membrane than on the other side. Hydrostatic pressure is the mechanical force of water pushing against cellular membranes (Fig. 1.25A). In the vascular system, hydrostatic pressure is the *blood pressure* generated in vessels when the heart contracts. Blood reaching the capillary bed has a hydrostatic pressure of 25 to 30 millimeters of mercury (mm Hg), which is sufficient force to push water across the thin capillary membranes into the interstitial space. Hydrostatic pressure is partially balanced by osmotic pressure, whereby water moving *out* of the capillaries is partially balanced by osmotic forces that tend to *pull* water *into* the capillaries (Fig. 1.25B). Water that is not osmotically attracted back into the capillaries moves into the lymph system (see the discussion of Starling forces in Chapter 3).

Osmosis. Osmosis is the movement of water "down" a concentration gradient—that is, across a semipermeable membrane from a region of higher water concentration to one of lower concentration. For osmosis to occur, (1) the membrane must be more permeable to water than to solutes, and (2) the concentration of solutes on one side of the membrane must be greater than that on the other side so that water moves more

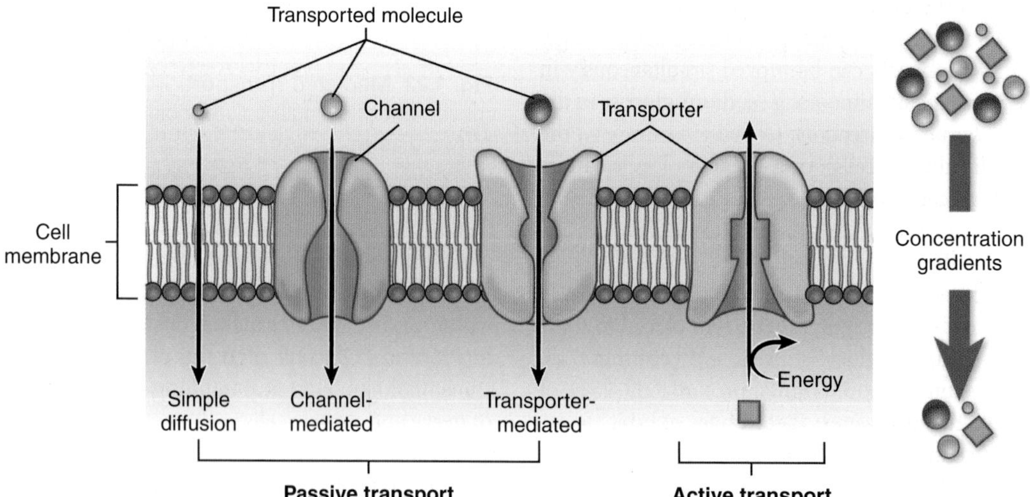

Fig. 1.24 Passive Diffusion of Solute Molecules Across the Plasma Membrane. Oxygen, nitrogen, water, urea, glycerol, and carbon dioxide can diffuse readily down the concentration gradient. Macromolecules are too large to diffuse through pores in the plasma membrane. Ions may be repelled if the pores contain substances with identical charges. If the pores are lined with cations, for example, other cations will have difficulty diffusing because the positive charges will repel one another. Diffusion can still occur, but it occurs more slowly.

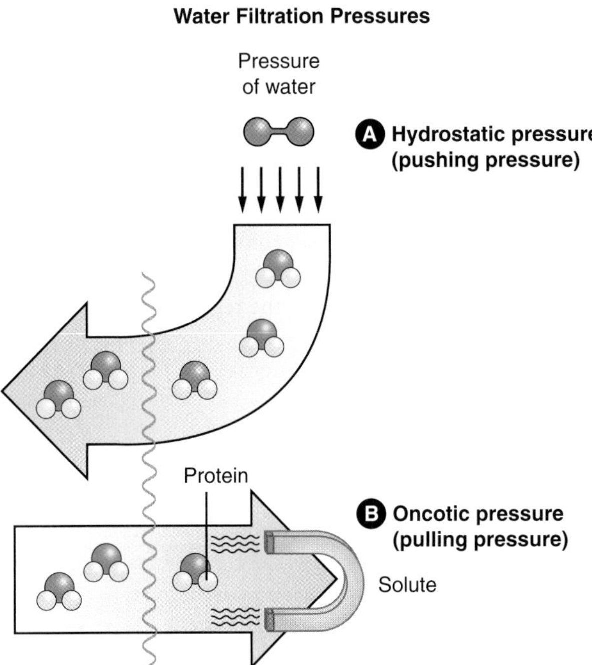

Fig. 1.25 Hydrostatic Pressure and Oncotic Pressure in Plasma. (A) Hydrostatic pressure in plasma is a pushing pressure in relation to water. **(B)** Oncotic pressure exerted by proteins in the plasma usually tends to *pull* water into the circulatory system. Individuals with low protein levels (e.g., starvation) are unable to maintain a normal oncotic pressure; therefore water is not reabsorbed into the circulation and, instead, causes body edema.

easily. Osmosis is directly related to both hydrostatic pressure and solute concentration but *not* to particle size or weight. For example, particles of the plasma protein albumin are small but are more concentrated in body fluids compared with the larger and heavier particles of globulin. Therefore albumin exerts a greater osmotic force compared with globulin.

Osmolality controls the distribution and movement of water between body compartments. The terms *osmolality* and *osmolarity* often are used interchangeably in reference to osmotic activity, but they define different measurements. Osmolality measures the number of milliosmoles per kilogram (mOsm/kg) of water, or the concentration of molecules per *weight* of water. Osmolarity measures the number of milliosmoles per liter (mOsm/L) of solution, or the concentration of molecules per *volume* of solution.

In solutions that contain only dissociable substances, such as Na^+ and Cl^-, the difference between the two measurements is negligible. When considering all the different solutes in plasma (e.g., proteins, glucose, lipids), the difference between osmolality and osmolarity becomes more significant. Less of plasma's weight is water, and the overall concentration of particles is therefore greater. The osmolality will be greater than the osmolarity because of the smaller proportion of water. Osmolality is thus preferred in human clinical assessment.

The normal osmolality of body fluids ranges from 280 to 294 mOsm/kg. The osmolalities of ICF and ECF tend to equalize, providing a measure of body fluid concentration and thus the body's hydration status. Hydration is affected also by hydrostatic pressure because the movement of water by osmosis can be opposed by an equal amount of hydrostatic pressure. The amount of hydrostatic pressure required to oppose the osmotic movement of water is called the osmotic pressure of the solution. Factors that determine osmotic pressure are the type and thickness of the plasma membrane, the size of the molecules, the concentration of molecules or the concentration gradient, and the solubility of molecules within the membrane.

Effective osmolality is sustained osmotic activity and depends on the concentration of solutes remaining on one side of a permeable membrane. If the solutes penetrate the membrane and equilibrate with the solution on the other side of the membrane, the osmotic effect will be diminished or lost. For example, urea is a small solute that readily diffuses across cellular membranes. Solutions containing urea quickly lose their effective osmolality because they rapidly equilibrate. Solutes too large to pass through the membrane sustain an effective osmolality, meaning that they enhance osmotic activity. Plasma proteins are examples of molecules that provide effective osmolality because they normally do not cross cellular membranes.

Plasma proteins influence osmolality because they have a negative charge (Fig. 1.25B). The principle involved is known as *Gibbs-Donnan equilibrium;* it occurs when the fluid in one compartment contains small, diffusible ions, such as Na^+ and Cl^-, together with large, nondiffusible, charged particles, such as plasma proteins. Because the body tends to maintain an electrical equilibrium, the nondiffusible protein molecules cause asymmetry in the distribution of small ions. Anions such as Cl^- are thus driven out of the cell or plasma, and cations, such as Na^+, are attracted to the cell. The protein-containing compartment maintains a state of electroneutrality, but the osmolality is higher. The overall osmotic effect of colloids, such as plasma proteins, is called the oncotic pressure, or colloid osmotic pressure.

Tonicity describes the effective osmolality of a solution. (The terms *osmolality* and *tonicity* may be used interchangeably.) Solutions have relative degrees of tonicity. An isotonic solution (or isosmotic solution) has the same osmolality or concentration of particles (285 mOsm) as ICF or ECF (Fig. 1.26A). Examples of isotonic solutions include 5% dextrose in water and normal (0.9%) saline solution. A hypotonic solution has a lower concentration and is thus more dilute than body fluids (Fig. 1.26B). Water is a hypotonic solution. Consequently, water is osmotically pulled into the cells, causing cells to swell or burst. A hypertonic solution has a concentration of more than 285 to 294 mOsm/kg (Fig. 1.26C). An example of a hypertonic solution is 3% saline solution. Cells shrink in a hypertonic solution because water is being pulled out of the cells. The concept of tonicity is important when correcting water and solute imbalances by administering different types of replacement solutions (see Chapter 3).

Active Transport of Na^+ and K^+

The active transport system for Na^+ and K^+ is found in virtually all mammalian cells. The Na^+-K^+–antiport system (i.e., Na^+ moving out of the cell and K^+ moving into the cell) uses the direct energy of ATP to transport these cations. The transporter protein is ATPase, which requires Na^+, K^+, and magnesium (Mg^{++}) ions. The concentration of ATPase in plasma membranes is directly related to Na^+-K^+–transport activity. Approximately

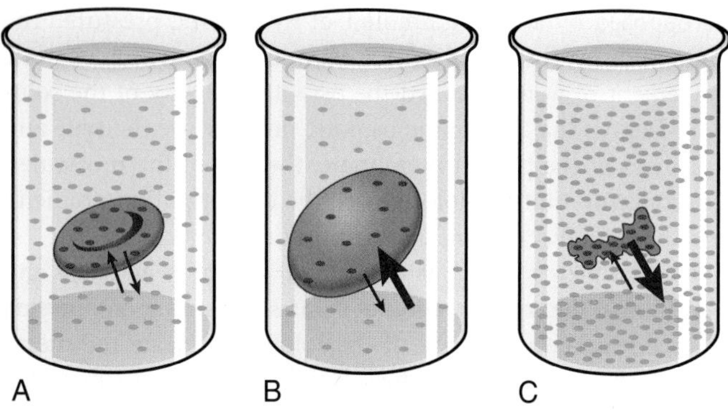

Fig. 1.26 Tonicity. Tonicity is important, especially for red blood cell function. **(A)** Isotonic solution. **(B)** Hypotonic solution. **(C)** Hypertonic solution. (From Waugh A, Grant A. *Ross and Wilson anatomy and physiology in health and illness*, 12th edition. London: Churchill Livingstone; 2012.

60% to 70% of the ATP synthesized by cells, especially muscle and nerve cells, is used to maintain the Na^+-K^+–transport system. Excitable tissues have a high concentration of Na^+-K^+ ATPase, as do other tissues that transport significant amounts of Na^+ (e.g., kidneys and salivary glands). For every ATP molecule hydrolyzed, three molecules of Na^+ are transported out of the cell, whereas only two molecules of K^+ move into the cell. The process leads to an electrical potential and is called *electrogenic*, with the inside of the cell more negative than the outside. Although the exact mechanism for this transport is uncertain, it is possible that ATPase induces the transporter protein to undergo several conformational changes, causing Na^+ and K^+ to move short distances (Fig. 1.27). The conformational change lowers the affinity for Na^+ and K^+ to the ATPase transporter, resulting in the release of the cations after transport.

Table 1.4 summarizes the major mechanisms of transport through pores and protein transporters in the plasma membranes. Many disease states are caused or manifested by loss of these membrane transport systems.

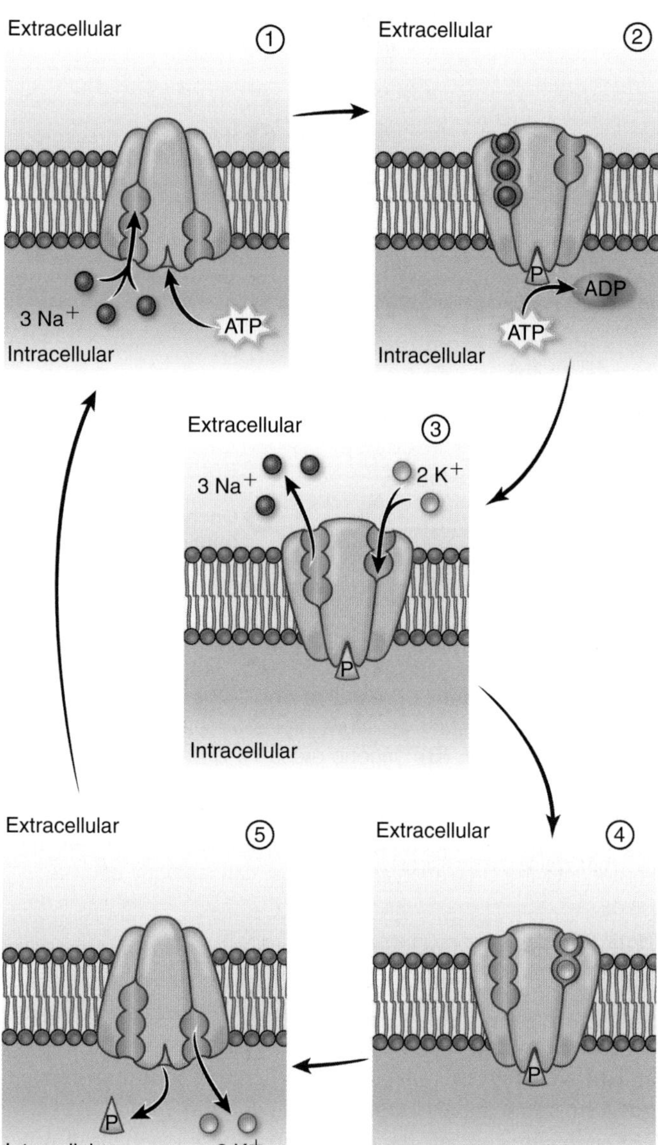

Fig. 1.27 Active Transport and the Sodium–Potassium (Na+–K+) Pump. ***1,*** Three sodium (Na^+) ions bind to Na-binding sites on the carrier's inner face. ***2,*** At the same time, an energy-containing adenosine triphosphate *(ATP)* molecule produced by the cell's mitochondria binds to the carrier. ATP dissociates, transferring its stored energy to the carrier, and changes shape. ***3*** and ***4,*** The ATP releases the three Na^+ ions to the outside of the cell, and attracts two potassium *(K^+)* ions to its potassium-binding sites. *5,* The carrier then returns to its original shape, releasing the two K^+ ions and the remnant of the ATP molecule to the inside of the cell. The carrier is now ready for another pumping cycle.

Transport by Vesicle Formation

Endocytosis and Exocytosis

The active transport mechanisms by which the cells move large proteins, polynucleotides, or polysaccharides (macromolecules) across the plasma membrane are very different from those that mediate small solute and ion transport. Transport of macromolecules involves the sequential formation and fusion of membrane-bound vesicles.

In endocytosis, a section of the plasma membrane enfolds substances from outside the cell, invaginates (folds inward), and separates from the plasma membrane, forming an endocytic vesicle that moves into the cell (Fig. 1.28).

Two types of endocytosis are designated based on the size of the vesicle formed. Pinocytosis (cell drinking) involves the ingestion of fluids, bits of the plasma membrane, and solute molecules through formation of small vesicles; phagocytosis (cell eating) involves the ingestion of large particles, such as bacteria, through formation of large vesicles (vacuoles).

Because most cells continually ingest fluid and solutes by pinocytosis, the terms *pinocytosis* and *endocytosis* often are used interchangeably. In pinocytosis, the vesicle containing fluids, solutes, or both fuses with a lysosome, and lysosomal enzymes digest the vesicle's contents for use by the cell. Vesicles that bud from membranes have a particular protein coat on their cytosolic surface and are called coated vesicles. The best studied are those that have an outer coat of bristle-like structures—the protein clathrin. Pinocytosis occurs mainly by the clathrin-coated pits and vesicles (Fig. 1.29). After the coated pits pinch off from the plasma membrane, they quickly shed their coats and fuse

TABLE 1.4 Major Transport Systems in Mammalian Cells

Substance Transported	Mechanism of Transport[a]	Tissues
Carbohydrates		
Glucose	Passive: protein channel Active: symport with Na^+	Most tissues
Fructose	Active: symport with Na^+ Passive	Small intestines and renal tubular cells Intestines and liver
Amino Acids		
Amino acid specific transporters	Coupled channels	Intestines, kidney, and liver
All amino acids except proline	Active: symport with Na^+	Liver
Specific amino acids	Active: group translocation Passive	Small intestine
Other Organic Molecules		
Cholic acid, deoxycholic acid, and taurocholic acid	Active: symport with Na^+	Intestines
Organic anions (e.g., malate, α-ketoglutarate, glutamate)	Antiport with counter-organic anion	Mitochondria of liver cells
ATP-ADP	Antiport transport of nucleotides; can be active	Mitochondria of liver cells
Inorganic Ions		
Na^+	Passive	Distal renal tubular cells
Na^+/H^+	Active antiport, proton pump	Proximal renal tubular cells and small intestines
Na^+/K^+	Active: ATP driven, protein channel	Plasma membrane of most cells
Ca^{2+}	Active: ATP driven, antiport with Na^+	All cells, antiporter in red cells
H^+/K^+	Active	Parietal cells of gastric cells secreting H^+
Cl^-/HCO_3 (perhaps other anions)	Mediated: antiport (anion transporter–band 3 protein)	Erythrocytes and many other cells
Water	Osmosis passive	All tissues

[a]NOTE: The known transport systems are listed here; others have been proposed. Most transport systems have been studied in only a few tissues and their sites of activity may be more limited than indicated.

ADP, Adenosine diphosphate; *ATP*, adenosine triphosphate; *Ca^{2+}*, calcium; *Cl^-/HCO_3*, chloride/bicarbonate; *H^+*, hydrogen; *K^+*, potassium; *Na^+*, sodium.
Data from: Alberts B, Bray D, Hopkin K, et al. *Molecular biology of the cell*, 4th edition. New York: Wiley; 2001; Alberts B, Bray D, Hopkin K, et al. *Essential cell biology*, 4th edition. New York: Garland; 2014; Devlin TM. *Textbook of biochemistry: With clinical correlations*, 3rd edition. New York: Wiley; 1992; Raven, PH, Johnson GB. *Understanding biology*, 3rd edition. Dubuque, IA: Brown; 1995.

with an endosome. An endosome is a vesicle pinched off from the plasma membrane from which its contents can be recycled to the plasma membrane or sent to lysosomes for digestion. In phagocytosis, the large molecular substances are engulfed by the plasma membrane and enter the cell so that they can be isolated and destroyed by lysosomal enzymes (see Chapter 7). Substances that are not degraded by lysosomes are isolated in residual bodies and released by exocytosis. Both pinocytosis and phagocytosis require metabolic energy and often involve binding of the substance with plasma membrane receptors before membrane invagination and fusion with lysosomes in the cell. New data are revealing that endocytosis has an even larger and more important role than previously known (Box 1.2). Exosomes are small membrane vesicles of endocytic origin containing protein, lipid, and RNA species in a single unit. Exosomes are secreted by many cell types and confer messages between cells as mediators of cell-to-cell communication. Researchers are revealing this communication through exosomes, including those released from cancer cells, taken up by neighboring cells, and capable of inducing pathways involved in cancer initiation and progression (Fig. 1.30).[13] Many new exosome-based therapies are being developed (Emerging Science Box: Exosome-Based Therapies).

In eukaryotic cells, secretion of macromolecules almost always occurs by exocytosis (see Fig. 1.28). Exocytosis has two main functions: (1) replacement of portions of the plasma membrane that have been removed by endocytosis and (2) release of molecules synthesized by the cells into the ECM.

Receptor-Mediated Endocytosis

The internalization process, called receptor-mediated endocytosis (ligand internalization), is rapid and enables the cell to ingest large amounts of receptor-macromolecule complexes in clathrin-coated vesicles without ingesting large volumes of ECF (see Fig. 1.29). For example, the cellular uptake of cholesterol depends on receptor-mediated endocytosis. In addition, many essential metabolites (e.g., vitamin B_{12} and iron) depend on receptor-mediated endocytosis and, unfortunately, the influenza virus.

Movement of Electrical Impulses: Membrane Potentials

The movement of ions through various channels and transporters results in electrostatic charges across the cell membrane. The electrical potential difference across the plasma

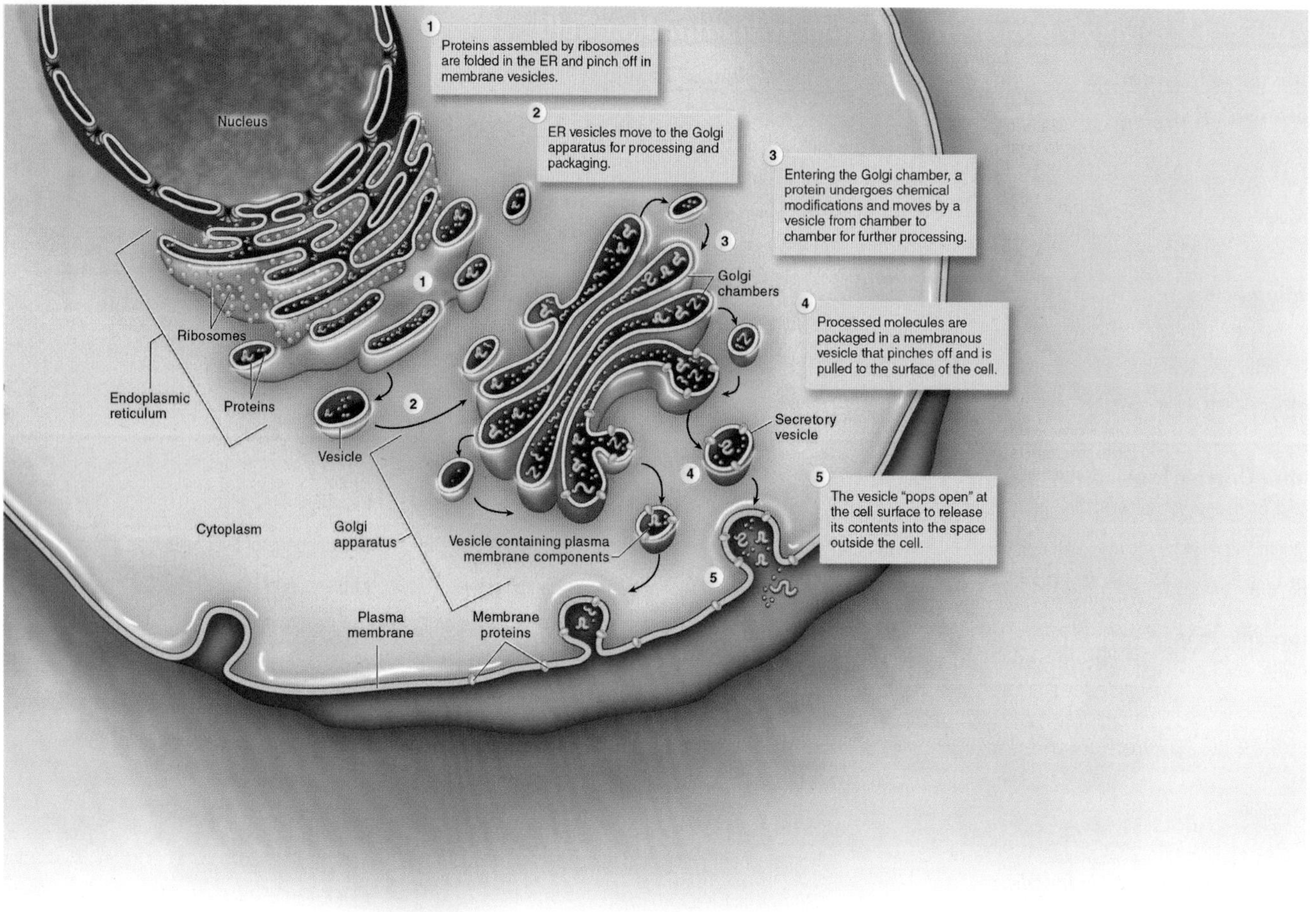

1 Proteins assembled by ribosomes are folded in the ER and pinch off in membrane vesicles.
2 ER vesicles move to the Golgi apparatus for processing and packaging.
3 Entering the Golgi chamber, a protein undergoes chemical modifications and moves by a vesicle from chamber to chamber for further processing.
4 Processed molecules are packaged in a membranous vesicle that pinches off and is pulled to the surface of the cell.
5 The vesicle "pops open" at the cell surface to release its contents into the space outside the cell.
Nucleus
Golgi chambers
Ribosomes
Endoplasmic reticulum
Proteins
Vesicle
Secretory vesicle
Cytoplasm
Golgi apparatus
Vesicle containing plasma membrane components
Plasma membrane
Membrane proteins

A

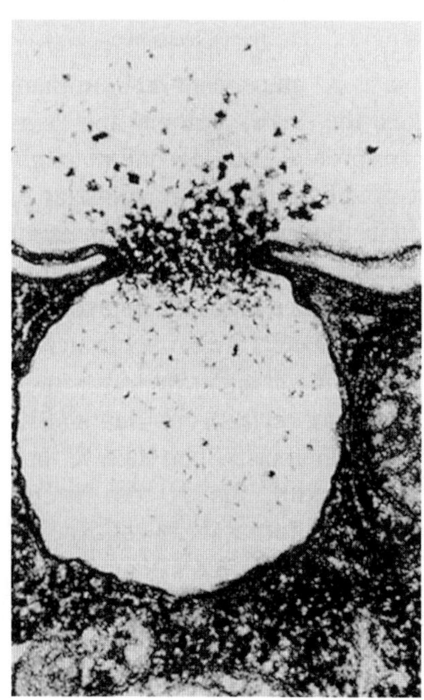

B

Fig. 1.28 Endocytosis and Exocytosis. (A) Endocytosis and fusion with lysosome and exocytosis. **(B)** Electron micrograph of exocytosis. (A, From Patton KT, Thibodeau GA. *The human body in health & disease*, 7th edition. St Louis: Mosby; 2018. B, From Raven PH, Johnson GB. *Biology*, 5th edition. New York: McGraw-Hill; 1999.)

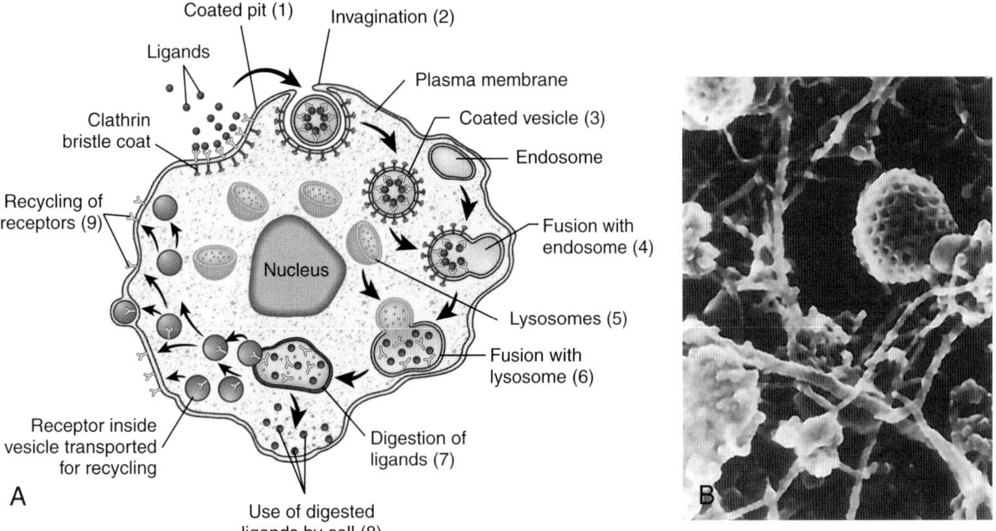

Fig. 1.29 Ligand Internalization by Means of Receptor-Mediated Endocytosis. (A) The ligand attaches to its surface receptor (through the bristle coat or clathrin coat **(1)** and receptor-mediated endocytosis), invagination **(2)** and coated pit **(3)**, and enters the cell. The ingested material fuses **(4)** with an endosome and lysosomes **(6)** and is processed by hydrolytic lysosomal enzymes **(7)**. Processed molecules can then be transferred to other cellular components **(8 and 9)**. **(B)** Electron micrograph of a coated pit showing different sizes of filaments of the cytoskeleton (×82,000). (B, From Erlandsen SL, Magney JE. Color of histology. St. Louis: Mosby; 1992.)

EMERGING SCIENCE BOX

Exosome-Based Therapies

An increased understanding of the role of exosomes in intercellular communication has led to new therapeutic approaches for a number of diseases including cancer. Exosomes are capable of carrying nuclear material (DNA, RNA), lipids, metabolites, proteins, and medications. They can be engineered to deliver therapeutic "payloads" that can promote or constrain a variety of pathophysiologic processes. These payloads may include nucleotides, chemotherapeutic drugs, and immune modulators. They can be administered orally, intranasally, intravenously, or intramuscularly depending on their specific characteristics. The goal is to target and maximize the therapeutic response while reducing adverse reactions. Research areas of particular promise for exosome-based therapies include neurogenerative diseases, cancer, and infection. In addition, exosomes produced by diseased cells can be detected in biologic fluids and be used for early detection. Most recently, a vaccine for coronavirus disease 2019 (COVID-19) that uses exosomes to deliver severe acute respiratory syndrome coronavirus 2 (SARS-CoV-2) spike protein messenger RNA is being evaluated in research trials. Many other new therapeutic uses for exosomes are being explored.

Data from Dai J, et al. Exosomes: Key players in cancer and potential therapeutic strategy. *Signal Transduction and Targeted Therapy*, 2020; 5:145; Kalluri R, et al. The biology, function, and biomedical applications of exosomes. *Science*, 2020; 367:6478–6977; Patil SM, et al. Exosomes as drug delivery systems: a brief overview and progress update. *European Journal of Pharmaceutics and Biopharmaceutics*, 2020; 154:259-269; Tsai SJ, et al. Exosome-Mediated mRNA Delivery For SARS-CoV-2 Vaccination. *bioRxiv*, 2020; 11.06.371419.

BOX 1.2 The New Endocytic Matrix

An explosion of new data is disclosing a much more involved role for endocytosis than just a simple way to internalize nutrients and membrane-associated molecules. These new data show that endocytosis not only is a master organizer of signaling pathways but also has a major role in managing signals in time and space. Endocytosis appears to control signaling; therefore it determines the net output of biochemical pathways. This occurs because endocytosis modulates the presence of receptors and their ligands as well as effectors at the plasma membrane or at intermediate stations of the endocytic route. The overall processes and anatomy of these new functions are sometimes called the "endocytic matrix." All of these functions ultimately have a large impact on almost every cellular process, including the nucleus.

membrane when the cell is in a nonexcited state is the resting membrane potential and is approximately −70 to −85 millivolts (mV).[14] The difference in voltage across the plasma membrane results from the differences in ionic composition of ICF and ECF. The positively charged sodium ions are more concentrated in ECF, and positively charged potassium ions are in greater concentration in ICF. Negatively charged intracellular proteins and organic phosphates that cannot cross the cell membrane are also contributory. The concentration difference is maintained by the active transport of Na^+ and K^+ (the sodium-potassium [Na^+-K^+] pump), which transports Na^+ outward and K^+ inward (Fig. 1.31A *and* B). Because the resting plasma membrane is more permeable to K^+ than to Na^+, K^+ diffuses easily from ICF to ECF. The movement of only the cation from the inside of the cell to the outside of the cell leaves behind a negative anion, leaving the inside of the cell more negative and the outside of the cell more positive. The change generates an electrostatic gradient that builds up over time. Because both Na^+ and K^+ are cations, the net result is an excess of anions inside the cell, resulting in the resting membrane potential.

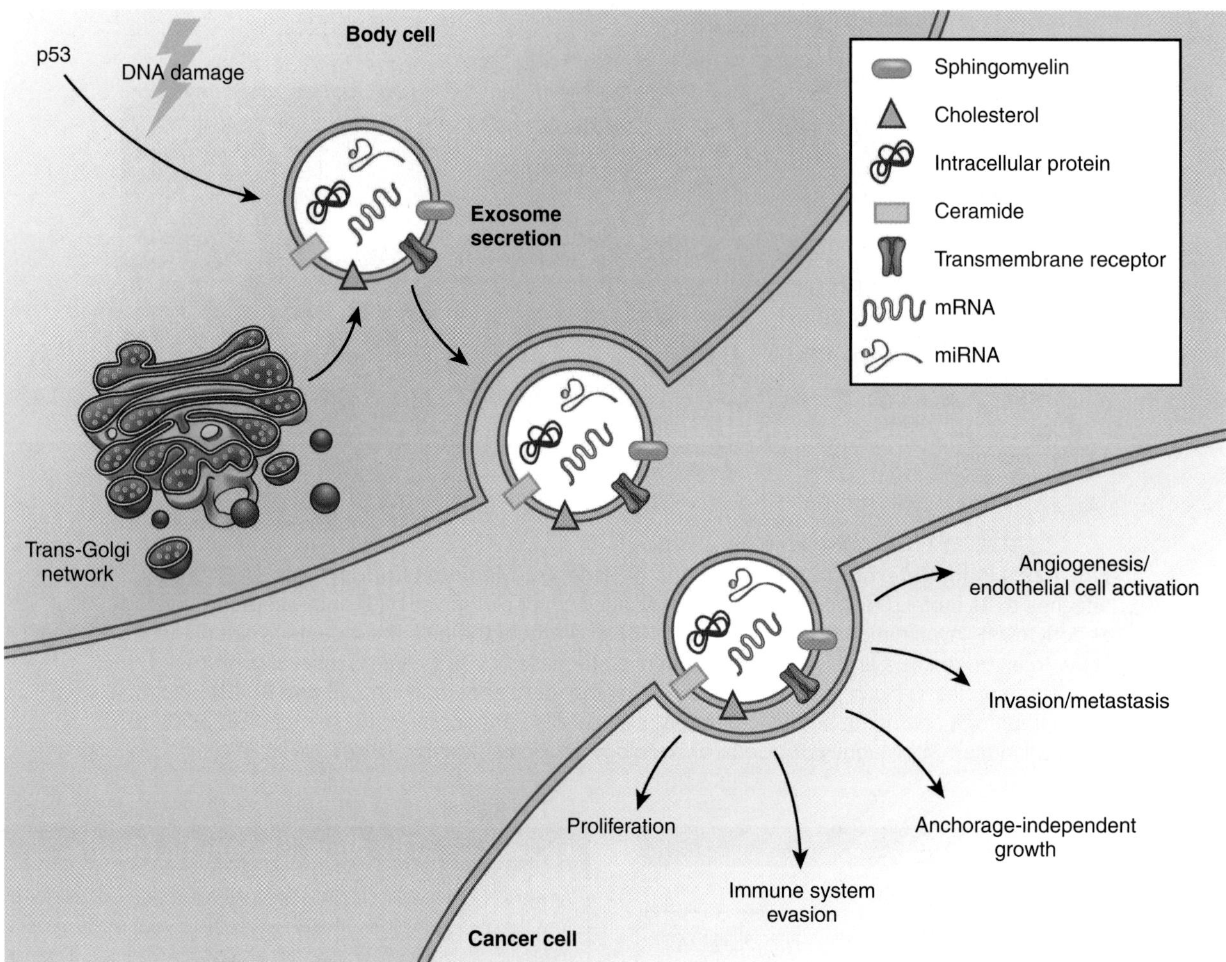

Fig. 1.30 Exosomes and Cell Signaling. Cancer. From a model of cancer cell signaling, exosomes are secreted with characteristic protein and ribonucleic acid (RNA) components. Exosomes that are released from body cells and taken up by neighboring cancer cells and are capable of inducing pathways in cancer initiation and progression. A growing interest in defining the clinical relevance of exosomes in cancers is based partially on their ability to alter tumor microenvironment by regulating immunity, angiogenesis, and metastasis. (From Henderson M, Azorsa D. The genomic and proteomic content of cancer cell-derived exosomes. *Frontiers in Oncology*, 2012; 2:38.)

All cells within the body are electrically polarized and have a characteristic resting membrane potential dependent on cell type. The resting membrane potentials of neurons and the three types of muscle cells—smooth, skeletal, and cardiac—are crucial to the proper functioning of the nervous and muscular systems.[14] Nerve and muscle cells are excitable and can change their resting membrane potential in response to electrochemical stimuli. Changes in resting membrane potential convey messages. For neurons, the firing of an action potential allows cell-to-cell communication by the release of various neurotransmitters. In muscle cells, the generation of an action potential causes the muscle to contract. When a nerve or muscle cell receives a stimulus that exceeds the membrane threshold value, a rapid change occurs in the resting membrane potential, known as the action potential. Nerve impulses are described in Chapter 15.

An action potential has three main stages: depolarization, repolarization, and hyperpolarization. Increased levels of K^+ result in depolarization of the membrane of cells. This depolarization inactivates sodium channels, which increases the refractory period.[15] When a resting cell is stimulated through voltage-regulated channels, the cell membranes become more permeable to Na^+, so a net movement of Na^+ into the cell occurs causing the interior of the cell to become more positively charged. The membrane becomes less polarized (less negative) than at resting potential. The membrane potential has *decreased*, moving closer to 0 mV (the potential is less than −70 mV, such as −60 mV). The membrane polarity is neutralized. This decrease is known as depolarization (Fig. 1.31C). Initially, depolarization proceeds slowly until it reaches a critical level known as threshold potential (usually between −50 and −55 mV). In general, this occurs when the cell has depolarized by 15 to 20 mV. At threshold potential, an explosive depolarization takes place. The sharp upward deflection then reverses itself and the inside of the cell becomes more positive. Just as rapidly, the potential drops back to resting potential as the membrane repolarizes. Repolarization is when the membrane returns to resting potential after depolarization. The forces that drive the membrane back to resting potential push it too far, causing a transient hyperpolarization.

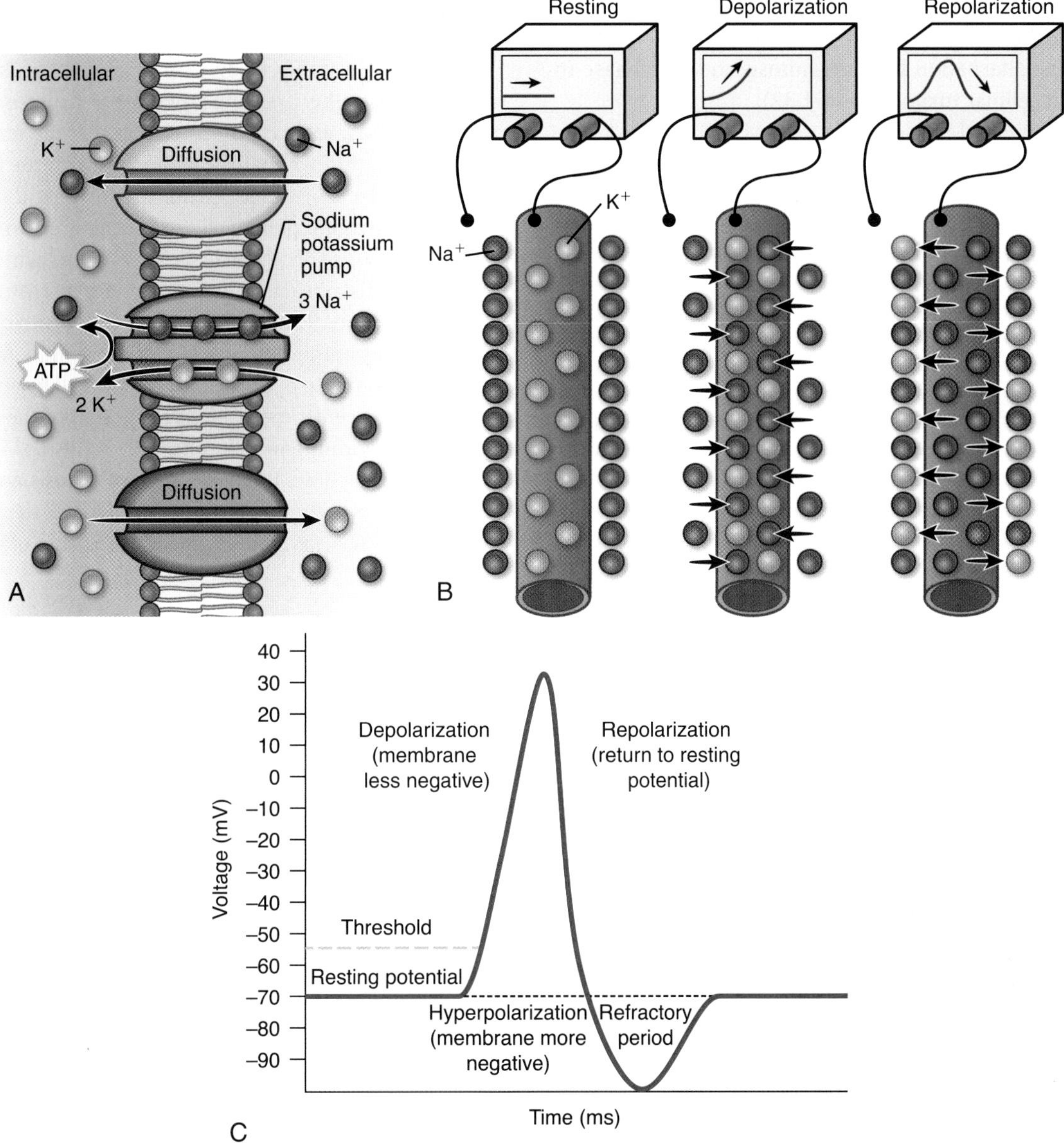

Fig. 1.31 Sodium-Potassium (Na+-K+) Pump and Propagation of an Action Potential. **(A)** Concentration difference of sodium *(Na^+)* and potassium *(K^+)* intracellularly and extracellularly. The direction of active transport by the Na^+-K^+ pump is also shown. **(B)** The left diagram represents the polarized state of a neuronal membrane when at rest. The middle and right diagrams represent changes in sodium and potassium membrane permeabilities with depolarization and repolarization. **(C)** The process for generating an action potential includes depolarization, repolarization, and hyperpolarization. From a recording device, a decrease in potential (i.e., the inside of the cell being less negative than at resting) is represented as an upward deflection, whereas an increase in potential (i.e., the inside being more negative than at resting) is represented by a downward deflection.

At this stage, the inside of the membrane becomes even more negative (more polarized) than normal. The rapid change in potential from threshold to peak reversal and then back to resting is called the action potential (see Fig. 1.31C).

During most of the action potential, the plasma membrane cannot respond to an additional stimulus. This time is known as the absolute refractory period (see Fig. 1.31C) and is related to changes in permeability to Na^+. During the latter phase of the action potential, when permeability to K^+ increases, a stronger-than-normal stimulus can evoke an action potential; this time is known as the relative refractory period.

CELLULAR REPRODUCTION: THE CELL CYCLE

Humans must make millions of cells every second to just survive.[2] Continuity of life depends on constant rounds of cell growth and division. In most tissues, new cells are created as fast as old cells die. The cycle of repeated rounds of duplication and division is called the cell cycle. Reproduction of gametes (sperm and egg cells) occurs through a process called *meiosis*, which is described in Chapter 4. The reproduction, or division, of other body cells (somatic cells) involves two sequential phases—mitosis, or nuclear division, and cytokinesis, or cytoplasmic division. However, before a cell can divide, it must double its mass and duplicate all its contents. Most of the work preparing for division occurs during the growth phase, called interphase. The cell cycle drives the alternation between mitosis and interphase in all tissues with cellular turnover (Fig. 1.32).

The four designated phases of the cell cycle (Fig. 1.33A) are (1) the G1 phase (G = gap), which is the period between the M phase and the start of DNA synthesis; (2) the S phase (S = synthesis), in which DNA is synthesized in the cell nucleus; (3) the G2 phase, in which RNA and protein synthesis occurs, the period between the completion of DNA synthesis and the next phase (M); and (4) the M phase (M = mitosis), which includes both nuclear and cytoplasmic division.

Phases of Mitosis and Cytokinesis

Interphase (the G_1, S, and G_2 phases) is the longest phase of the cell cycle. During interphase, the chromatin consists of very long, slender rods jumbled together in the nucleus. Late in interphase, strands of chromatin (the substance that gives the nucleus its granular appearance) begin to coil, causing them to shorten and thicken.

The M phase of the cell cycle, mitosis and cytokinesis, begins with prophase, the first appearance of chromosomes. As the phase proceeds, each chromosome is seen as identical halves called chromatids, which lie together and are attached by a spindle site called a centromere. (The two chromatids of each chromosome, which are genetically identical, are sometimes called *sister chromatids.*) The nuclear membrane, which surrounds the nucleus, disappears. Spindle fibers are microtubules formed in the cytoplasm. They radiate from two centrioles located at opposite poles of the cell. The role of the spindle fibers is to pull the chromosomes to opposite sides of the cell by attaching to the chromosome's centromere. The production of the spindle fibers signals the beginning of metaphase.

During metaphase, the next phase of mitosis and cytokinesis, the centromeres become aligned in the middle of the spindle, which is called the equatorial plate (or metaphase plate) of the cell. In this

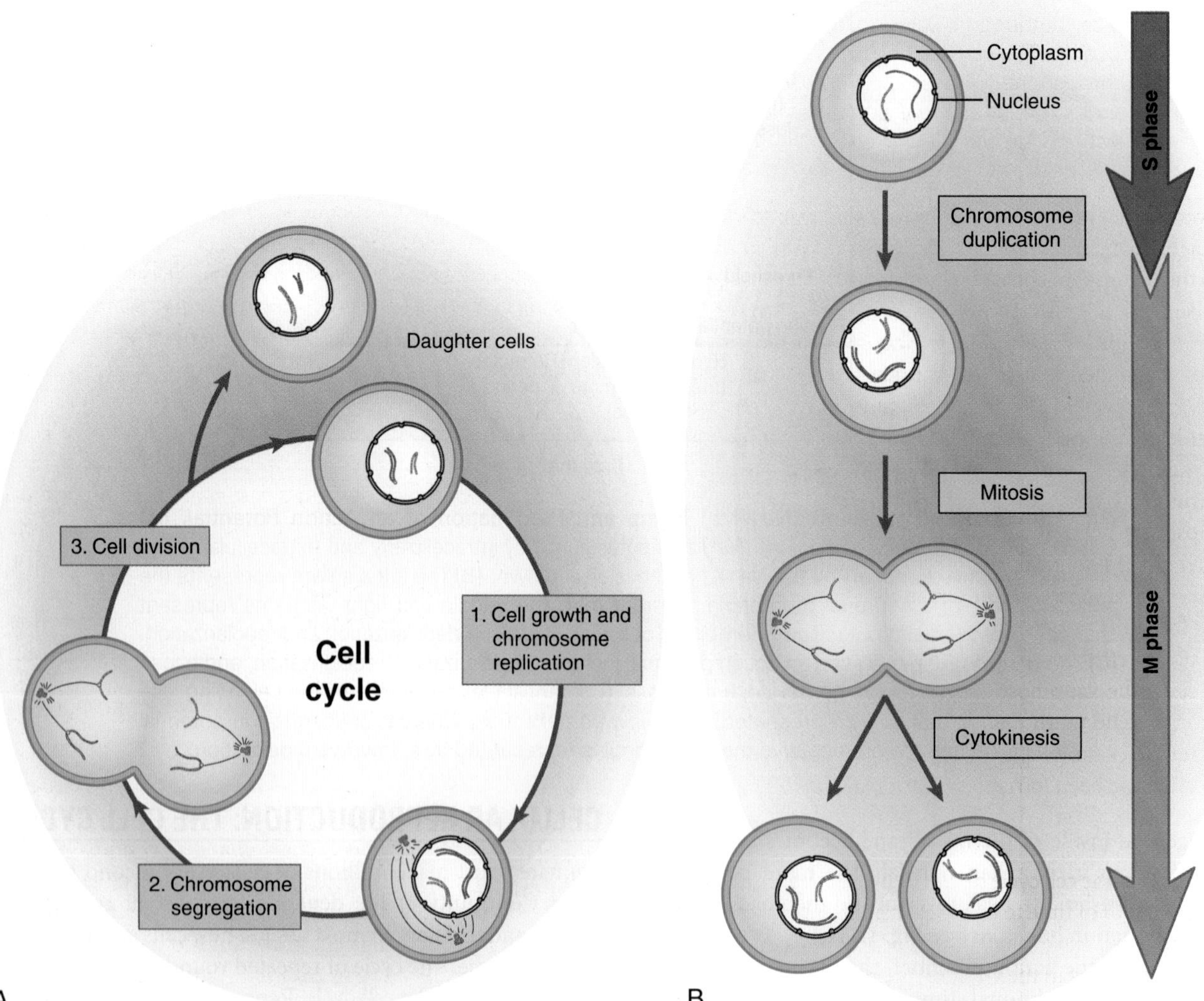

Fig. 1.32 The Cell Cycle. (A) Simplified figure of schematic cell with one green chromosome and one yellow chromosome to show how two genetically identical daughter cells are produced in each cycle. **(B)** Cell cycle events: mitosis and cytokinesis. (Adapted from Alberts B, Bray D, Hopkin K, et al. *Molecular biology of the cell*, 6th edition. New York: Garland Science; 2015.)

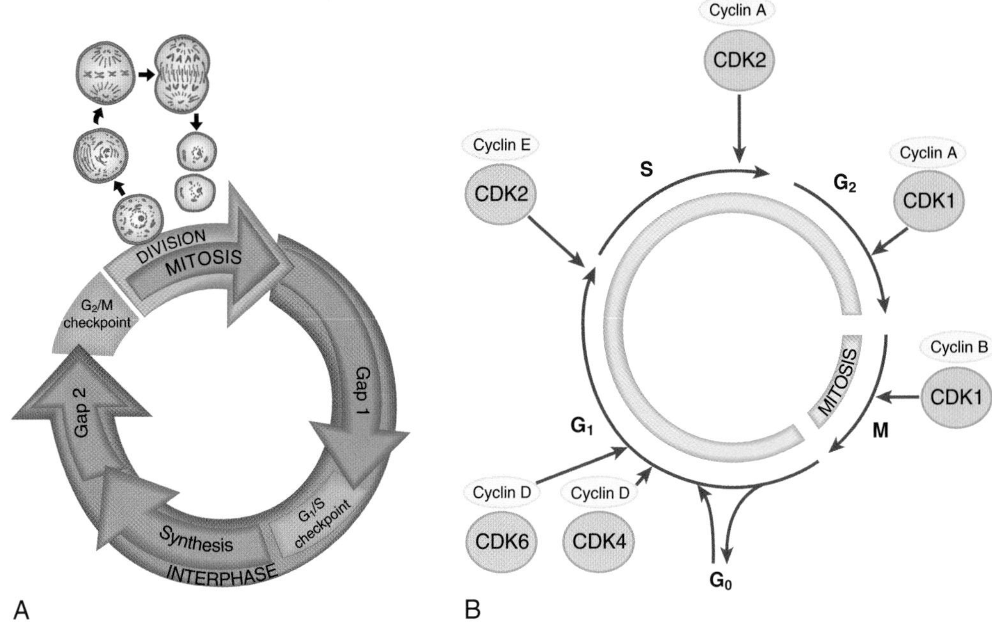

Fig. 1.33 Interphase and the Phases of Mitosis. (A) The G_1/S checkpoint is to "check" for cell size, nutrients, growth factors, and deoxyribonucleic acid (DNA) damage. See text for resting phases. The G_2/M checkpoint checks for cell size and DNA replication. **(B)** The orderly progression through the phases of the cell cycle is regulated by *cyclins* (so called because levels rise and fall) and *cyclin-dependent protein kinases* (CDKs) and their inhibitors. When cyclins are complexed with CDKs, cell cycle events are triggered.

stage, chromosomes are easiest to observe microscopically because they are highly condensed and arranged in a relatively organized fashion in the two-dimensional equatorial plate. The attached spindle fibers begin to pull the centromeres of the chromosomes.

Anaphase begins when the centromeres split and the sister chromatids are pulled apart. The spindle fibers shorten, causing the sister chromatids to be pulled, centromere first, toward opposite sides of the cell. With sister chromatid separation, each is considered to be a chromosome. Thus the cell has 92 chromosomes during this stage. By the end of the anaphase, there are 46 chromosomes lying at each side of the cell. Barring mitotic errors, each of the two groups of 46 chromosomes is identical to the original 46 chromosomes present at the start of the cell cycle.

During the telophase, the final stage, a new nuclear membrane is formed around each group of 46 chromosomes, the spindle fibers disappear, and the chromosomes begin to uncoil. Cytokinesis causes the cytoplasm to divide into almost equal parts during this phase. At the end of the telophase, two identical diploid cells, called daughter cells, have been formed from the original cell.

The Cell Cycle Control System

Various features of the cell cycle differ from one cell type to another including the length of time to complete certain functions. Most of the variability in cell cycle length in the adult body occurs during the time the cell spends in the G_1 or G_0 phase of the cell cycle. This length of time is different from the brief time a cell takes to progress from the beginning of the S phase through mitosis—typically 12 to 24 hours. Cells are capable of disassembly of their cell cycle control system and can withdraw from the cycle to a nondividing state called G0. The reversibility of the G_0 state varies in different types of cells. For example, most of the neurons and skeletal muscle cells are in a *terminally differentiated* G_0 state; with their cell cycle control system disassembled, the molecular regulatory switches (cyclin-dependent kinases [CDKs] and cyclins, see following text) become permanently turned off and cell division rarely occurs.[2]

The cell cycle control system triggers the essential events of the cell cycle. The system operates like a timer that triggers the constant sequence of events. Although early embryonic divisions are independent of feedback controls, in most cells the control system responds to feedback (information) from the processes it controls. For example, if some malfunction occurs with DNA synthesis, signals are sent to the control system to delay progression to the M phase.[2] Such delays allow repair and prevent progression of cellular disasters.

The cell cycle control system works because of a connected series of biochemical switches that either activate or inhibit cell events. Two classes of *switches* or regulatory molecules that determine a cell's progress through the cell cycle are CDKs and cyclins (Fig. 1.33B).

Cyclin-dependent kinases (CDKs) are protein kinases, and their functions rise and fall as the cell moves through the cycle. The rise and fall leads to cyclical changes in phosphorylation of intracellular proteins that start or regulate the events of the cell cycle. Many enzymes and other proteins regulate the different CDKs, and the most important are proteins called cyclins.[2] CDK activity is dependent on binding of cyclins *(cyclin-CDK complexes)*. For example, activation of S-phase cyclin-CDK complexes (s-CDKs) initiates the S phase. Without cyclin, CDK is inactive. Binding of *CDK inhibitor proteins (CKIs)* inactivates cyclin-CDK complexes. Two other essential enzyme complexes that regulate the cell cycle control system are the APC/C and SCF ubiquitin ligases, which promote ubiquitylation (process of marking for destruction) and subsequent destruction of various proteins that modulate the cell cycle (Fig. 1.33B).

Control of Cell Division and Cell Growth: Mitogens, Growth Factors, and Survival Factors

Organ size and body size are determined by three main processes: (1) cell growth, (2) cell division, and (3) cell survival.[2] These processes are tightly regulated by intracellular programs and extracellular signal molecules, usually soluble proteins, proteins bound to cells, or molecules of the ECM. The molecules comprise three main classes: (1) mitogens, (2) growth factors, and (3) survival factors. A mitogen is a chemical agent that induces or stimulates mitosis (cell division). Mitogens act as an extracellular signal and they usually come from another neighboring cell. Mitogens can stimulate cell growth, differentiation, migration, and survival.[2]

Growth factors (also called *cytokines*) stimulate an increase in cell mass or cell growth by fostering the synthesis of proteins and other macromolecules and inhibiting their breakdown (Table 1.5), including examples of mitogens and growth factors. Cells starved of growth factors come to a halt after mitosis and enter the arrested, or G_0, state of the cell cycle. Survival factors promote cell survival by inhibiting programmed cell death, or *apoptosis* (see Chapter 2).

DNA Damage Response: Blocks Cell Division

The DNA damage response occurs when DNA is damaged, with recruitment of protein kinases to the site of damage and signaling that promotes a stop to the progression of the cell cycle, called cell cycle arrest (Fig. 1.34).

TABLE 1.5 Examples of Mitogens and Growth Factors and Their Actions

Growth Factor	Physiologic Actions
Platelet-derived growth factor (PDGF)	Stimulates proliferation of connective tissue cells and neuroglial cells
Epidermal growth factor (EGF)	Stimulates proliferation of epidermal cells and other cell types
Insulin-like growth factor 1 (IGF-1)	Collaborates with PDGF and EGF; stimulates proliferation of fat cells and connective tissue cells
Insulin-like growth factor 2 (IGF-2)	Collaborates with PDGF and EGF; stimulates proliferation of fat cells and connective tissue cells
Transforming growth factor-beta (TGF-β)	Stimulates or inhibits response of most cells to other growth factors; regulates differentiation of some cell types (e.g., cartilage)
Fibroblast growth factor (FGF)	Stimulates proliferation of fibroblasts, endothelial cells, myoblasts, and other cell types
Interleukin-2 (IL-2)	Stimulates proliferation of T lymphocytes
Nerve growth factor (NGF)	Promotes axon growth and survival of sympathetic and some sensory and CNS neurons
Hematopoietic cell growth factors (IL-3, GM-CSF, M-CSF, G-CSF, erythropoietin)	Promotes growth of white and red blood cells

CNS, Central nervous system; *CSF*, colony-stimulating factor; *G*, granulocyte; *GM*, granulocyte-macrophage; *M*, macrophage.

TISSUES

Cells of common structure and function are organized into tissues, of which there are four primary types: *muscle, neural, epithelial*, and *connective*. Epithelial, connective, and muscle tissues are summarized in Tables 1.6, 1.7, and 1.8, respectively. Different types of neurons have special characteristics that depend on their distribution and function within the nervous system (see Chapter 15). Different types of tissues compose organs. Finally, organs are integrated to perform complex functions as tracts or systems.

All cells are in contact with a network of extracellular macromolecules known as the ECM (see the Extracellular Matrix and Basement Membrane section). This matrix results in mechanical strength by holding cells and tissues together.[16] It also provides an organized latticework in which cells can migrate and interact with one another.

Tissue Formation and Differentiation

To form tissues, cells must exhibit intercellular recognition and communication, adhesion, and memory. Specialized cells sense their environment through signals, such as growth factors, from other cells. This type of communication ensures that new cells are produced only when and where they are required. Different cell types have different adhesion molecules in their plasma membranes, sticking selectively to other cells of the same type. They can also adhere to the ECM components. Because cells are tiny and squishy and enclosed by a flimsy membrane, it is remarkable that they form a strong human being. Strength can

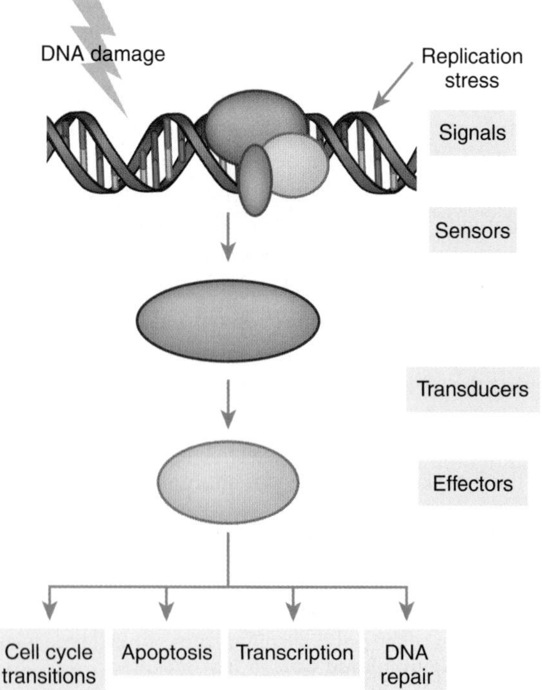

Fig. 1.34 Deoxyribonucleic Acid Damage Response. Several injurious agents can damage deoxyribonucleic acid (DNA). These include exogenous agents such as ultraviolet light; ionizing radiation; chemicals and endogenous agents; oxidative damage; and replicative stress. Protein kinases are activated and serve as sensors and transducers causing many effector responses. The cell cycle arrest prevents entry into mitosis and several cell fates occur including DNA repair and apoptosis or cell death.

TABLE 1.6 Characteristics of Epithelial Tissues

Simple Squamous Epithelium

Structure

Single layer of cells

Location and Function

Lining of blood vessels leads to diffusion and filtration

Lining of pulmonary alveoli (air sacs) leads to separation of blood from fluids in tissues

Bowman capsule (kidney), where it filters substances from blood, forming urine

Stratified Squamous Epithelium

Structure

Two or more layers, depending on location, with cells closest to basement membrane tending to be cuboidal

Location and Function

Epidermis of skin and linings of mouth, pharynx, esophagus, and anus provide protection and secretion

Transitional Epithelium

Structure

Vary in shape from cuboidal to squamous depending on whether basal cells of bladder are columnar or are composed of many layers; when bladder is full and stretched, the cells flatten and stretch like squamous cells

Location and Function

Linings of urinary bladder and other hollow structures stretch, allowing expansion of the hollow organs

Simple Cuboidal Epithelium

Structure

Simple cuboidal cells; rarely stratified (layered)

Location and Function

Glands (e.g., thyroid, sweat, salivary) and parts of the kidney tubules and outer covering of ovary secrete fluids

Simple Columnar Epithelium

Structure

Large amounts of cytoplasm and cellular organelles

Location and Function

Ducts of many glands and lining of digestive tract allow secretion and absorption from stomach to anus

Ciliated Simple Columnar Epithelium

Structure

Same as simple columnar epithelium but ciliated

Location and Function

Linings of bronchi of lungs, nasal cavity, and oviducts allow secretion, absorption, and propulsion of fluids and particles

Stratified Columnar Epithelium

Structure

Small and rounded basement membrane (columnar cells do not touch basement membrane)

Location and Function

Linings of epiglottis, part of pharynx, anus, and male urethra provide protection

Pseudostratified Ciliated Columnar Epithelium

Structure

All cells in contact with basement membrane

Nuclei found at different levels within cell, giving stratified appearance

Free surface often ciliated

Location and Function

Linings of large ducts of some glands (parotid, salivary), male urethra, respiratory passages, and eustachian tubes of ears transport substances

TABLE 1.7 Connective Tissues

Loose or Areolar Tissue

Structure

Unorganized; spaces between fibers

Most fibers collagenous, some elastic and reticular

Includes many types of cells (fibroblasts and macrophages most common) and large amount of intercellular fluid

Location and Function

Attaches skin to underlying tissue; holds organs in place by filling spaces between them; supports blood vessels

Intercellular fluid transports nutrients and waste products. Fluid accumulation causes swelling (edema)

Dense Irregular Tissue

Structure

Dense, compact, and areolar tissue, with fewer cells and greater number of closely woven collagenous fibers than in loose tissue

Location and Function

Dermis layer of skin; acts as protective barrier

Dense, Regular (White Fibrous) Tissue

Structure

Collagenous fibers and some elastic fibers, tightly packed into parallel bundles, with only fibroblast cells

Location and Function

Forms strong tendons of muscle, ligaments of joints, some fibrous membranes, and fascia that surrounds organs and muscles

Elastic Tissue

Structure

Elastic fibers, some collagenous fibers, fibroblasts

Location and Function

Lends strength and elasticity to walls of arteries, trachea, vocal cords, and other structures

Adipose Tissue

Structure

Fat cells dispersed in loose tissues; each cell containing a large droplet of fat flattens nucleus and forces cytoplasm into a ring around cell's periphery

Location and Function

Stores fat, which provides padding and protection

Cartilage (Hyaline, Elastic, Fibrous)

Structure

Collagenous fibers embedded in a firm matrix (chondrin); no blood supply

Location and Function

Gives form, support, and flexibility to joints, trachea, nose, ear, vertebral disks, embryonic skeleton, and many internal structures

Bone

Structure

Rigid connective tissue consisting of cells, fibers, ground substances, and minerals

Location and Function

Lends skeleton rigidity and strength

Special Connective Tissues

Plasma

Structure

Fluid

Location and Function

Serves as matrix for blood cells

Macrophages in Tissue, Reticuloendothelial, or Macrophage System

Structure

Scattered macrophages (phagocytes) called *Kupffer cells* (in liver), alveolar macrophages (in lungs), microglia (in central nervous system)

Location and Function

Facilitate inflammatory response and carry out phagocytosis in loose connective, lymphatic, digestive, medullary (bone marrow), splenic, adrenal, and pituitary tissues

TABLE 1.8 Muscle Tissues

Skeletal (Striated) Muscle

Structure Characteristics of Cells

Long, cylindrical cells that extend throughout length of muscles
Striated myofibrils (proteins)
Many nuclei on periphery

Location and Function

Attached to bones directly or by tendons and provide voluntary movement of skeleton and maintenance of posture

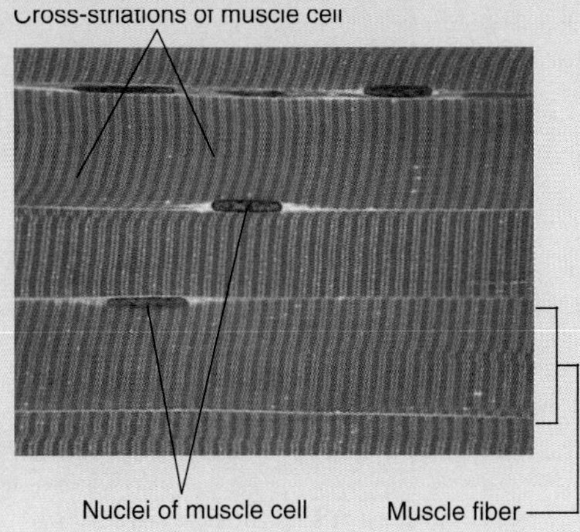

Skeletal (Striated) Muscle. From Thibodeau GA, Patton KT. *Anatomy & physiology*, 6th edition. St. Louis: Mosby; 2007.

Cardiac Muscle

Structure Characteristics of Cells

Branching networks throughout muscle tissue
Striated myofibrils

Location and Function

Cells attached end-to-end at intercalated disks with tissue forming walls of heart (myocardium) to provide involuntary pumping action of heart

Smooth (Visceral) Muscle

Structure Characteristics of Cells

Long spindles that taper to a point
Absence of striated myofibrils

Location and Function

Walls of hollow internal structures, such as digestive tract and blood vessels (viscera), provide voluntary and involuntary contractions that move substances through hollow structures

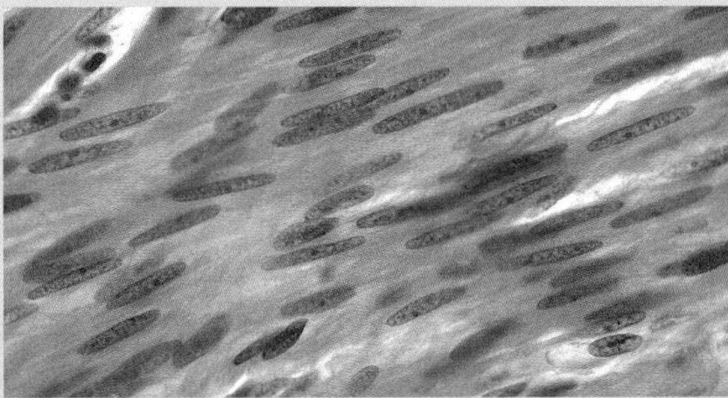

Smooth (Visceral) Muscle. From Young B, Woodford P. *Wheater's functional histology*, 6th edition. Philadelphia: Churchill Livingstone; 2014.

occur because of the ECM and the strength of the cytoskeleton with cell-to-cell adhesions to neighboring cells. Cells have memory because of specialized patterns of gene expression evoked by signals that acted during embryonic development. Memory allows cells to autonomously preserve their distinctive character and pass it on to their offspring.[2]

Fully specialized, or terminally differentiated cells that are lost, are regenerated from proliferating *precursor cells.* These precursor cells have been derived from a smaller number of stem cells.[2] Stem cells are unspecialized cells of the human body and have the ability to differentiate into any type of cell.[17] Stem cells exist in both embryos and adult tissues. In many tissues, stem cells serve as an internal repair and maintenance system, dividing indefinitely. However, in some organs (e.g., pancreas), stem cell division occurs only under special physiologic conditions. These cells can maintain themselves by dividing and perpetuating the stem cell pool over very long periods (throughout life), an ability that is referred to as self-renewal. This requires cell control by dividing and developing into multiple specialized cell types in specific tissues or organs, known as multipotency, or dividing and developing into the three primary germ cell layers of the early embryo and therefore into all cells of the adult body, which is known as pluripotency.[18] This stem cell–driven tissue renewal is very evident in the epithelial lining of the intestine, stomach, blood cells, and skin, which is continuously exposed to environmental factors. When a stem cell divides, each daughter cell has a choice: It can remain as a stem cell, or it can follow a pathway that results in terminal differentiation (Fig. 1.35).

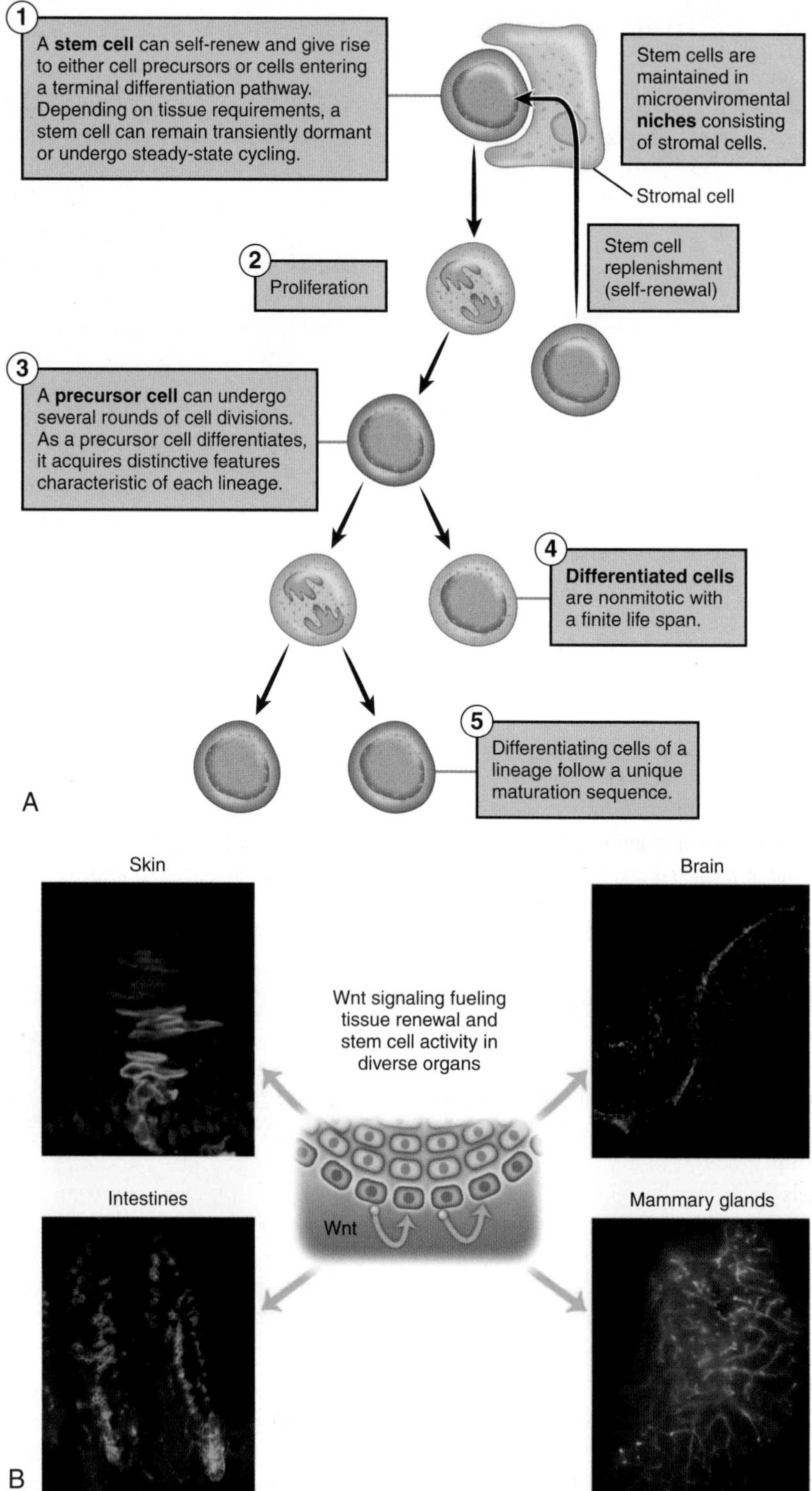

FIG. 1.35 Properties of Stem Cell Systems. (A) Stem cells have three characteristics: *self-renewal, proliferation*, and *differentiation* into mature cells. Stem cells are housed in *niches* consisting of *stromal cells* that provide factors for their maintenance. Stem cells of the embryo can give rise to cell precursors that generate all the tissues of the body. This property defines stem cells as *multipotent*. Stem cells are difficult to identify anatomically. Their identification is based on specific *cell surface markers* (cell surface antigens recognized by specific monoclonal antibodies) and on the lineage they generate following *transplantation*. **(B)** Wnt signaling fuels tissue renewal. (A, From Kierszenbaum A. *Histology and cell biology: An introduction to pathology*, 3rd edition. St. Louis: Elsevier; 2012. B, From Clevers H, Loh KM, Nusse R. Stem cell signaling. An integral program for tissue renewal and regeneration: Wnt signaling and stem cell control. Science, 2014; 346:6205, 1248012.)

SUMMARY REVIEW

Prokaryotes and Eukaryotes

1. Eukaryotes are the cells of higher animals and plants, fungi, protozoa, and most algae. These cells are larger and have membrane-bound intracellular compartments (organelles) and a well-defined nucleus. Genetic information is contained in several or many chromosomes.
2. Prokaryotes include bacteria and archaea. They contain no organelles, and their nucleus is not well defined. Genetic information is contained in a single circular chromosome.

Cellular Functions

1. Cells become specialized through the process of differentiation, or maturation, so that they perform one kind of function.
2. The eight specialized cellular functions are movement, conductivity, metabolic absorption, secretion, excretion, respiration, reproduction, and communication.

Structure and Function of Cellular Components

1. The eukaryotic cell consists of three general components: the plasma membrane, cytoplasm, and intracellular organelles.
2. The nucleus is the largest membrane-bound organelle and is found usually in the cell's center. The chief functions of the nucleus are cell division and control of genetic information.
3. Cytoplasm, or the cytoplasmic matrix, is an aqueous solution (cytosol) that fills the space between the nucleus and the plasma membrane. It represents about half of the volume of the cell.
4. The organelles are suspended in the cytoplasm and are enclosed in biologic membranes.
5. Ribosomes are RNA-protein complexes that use the information from DNA, written in messenger RNA (mRNA), to build proteins and provide sites for cellular protein synthesis.
6. The endoplasmic reticulum (rough and smooth) is a network of tubular channels (cisternae) that extend throughout the outer nuclear membrane. The rough endoplasmic reticulum (RER) specializes in the synthesis, folding, and transport of protein components. The smooth endoplasmic reticulum (SER) is involved in the synthesis of steroid hormones and is responsible for a variety of reactions required to remove toxic substances from the cell.
7. The Golgi complex is a network of flattened, smooth membranes and vesicles located near the nucleus. The Golgi complex is responsible for processing and packaging proteins into secretory vesicles that break away from the Golgi complex and migrate to a variety of intracellular and extracellular destinations, including the plasma membrane.
8. Lysosomes are sac-like structures that contain digestive enzymes. These enzymes are responsible for digesting most cellular substances to their basic form, such as amino acids, fatty acids, and carbohydrates (sugars). Cellular injury leads to a release of the lysosomal enzymes, causing cellular self-digestion. They also serve as signaling hubs in a network for cellular adaptation.
9. Peroxisomes appear similar to lysosomes but contain several enzymes that either produce or use hydrogen peroxide and their reactions detoxify waste products.
10. Mitochondria contain the metabolic machinery necessary for cellular energy metabolism. The enzymes of the respiratory chain (electron transport chain), found in the inner membrane of the mitochondria, generate most of the cell's adenosine triphosphate (ATP).
11. The cytoskeleton is the "bone and muscle" of the cell. The internal skeleton is composed of a network of protein filaments, including microtubules and actin filaments (microfilaments). They also form cell extensions (microvilli, cilia, flagella).
12. The plasma membrane encloses the cell and, by controlling the movement of substances across it, exerts a powerful influence on metabolic pathways. Other important functions include cell-to-cell recognition, cellular mobility, and maintenance of cellular shape.
13. The basic structure of plasma membrane is the lipid bilayer, which is studded with various proteins. Carbohydrates contained within the plasma membrane are generally bound to membrane proteins (glycoproteins) and lipids (glycolipids).
14. The lipid bilayer determines the structure of the membrane. Each lipid molecule is polar, or amphipathic: the head is hydrophilic ("water loving") and the tail is hydrophobic ("water hating"). The membrane is organized in two layers, with the tails inward and the heads outward. This provides a barrier to the diffusion of hydrophilic substances, while allowing lipid-soluble molecules to diffuse through readily.
15. Membrane proteins can extend across the bilayer, be in the bilayer but primarily on one side or the other, or can exist outside of the bilayer. Membrane proteins, like other proteins, are synthesized by the ribosome and then translocate, called trafficking, to different locations in the cell. Trafficking places unique demands on membrane proteins for folding, translocation, and stability. Misfolded proteins are emerging as an important cause of disease.
16. Proteins determine the functions of the membrane. Proteins perform most of the plasma membrane's tasks. Proteins act as recognition and binding units for substances moving in and out of the cell, pores and transport channels, enzymes that drive pumps or maintain ion concentrations, cell surface markers, cell adhesion molecules, and catalysts of chemical reactions. Proteins form cellular receptors that recognize and bind with smaller molecules called ligands.
17. Proteostasis is the state of cell balance of the processes of protein synthesis, folding, and dehydration (protein homeostasis). The proteostasis network is composed of ribosomes (makers), chaperones (helpers), and protein breakdown or proteolytic systems. Malfunction of these systems is associated with disease.
18. The carbohydrates on the outside of the plasma membrane form a coating (glycocalyx) that protects the cell from mechanical damage and creates a slimy surface that assists in mobility. Carbohydrates also function in cell-cell recognition and adhesion.

Cell-to-Cell Adhesions

1. Cell-to-cell adhesions are formed on plasma membranes, thereby allowing the formation of tissues and organs. Cells are held together by three different means: (1) the extracellular membrane, (2) cell adhesion molecules in the cell's plasma membrane, and (3) specialized cell junctions.
2. The extracellular matrix (ECM) is secreted by cells and is a meshwork of fibrous proteins in a gel-like substance. It provides a pathway for diffusion of nutrients, wastes, and other water-soluble substances. The ECM includes three groups of macromolecules: (1) fibrous structural proteins (collagen and elastin), (2) adhesive glycoproteins, and (3) proteoglycans and hyaluronic acid. The matrix helps regulate cell growth, movement, and differentiation.
3. Basement membrane is a specialized type of ECM that is very thin, tough, and flexible. It lies under the epithelium of many organs and is also called the basal lamina.
4. Cell adhesion molecules (CAMs) are cell surface proteins that bind the cell to an adjacent cell and to components of the ECM. CAMs include four protein families: the integrins, cadherins, selectins, and IgSF.
5. Cell junctions are the contacts between neighboring cells. They can hold cells together with a tight seal, provide strong mechanical attachments, provide a chemical communication, and maintain polarity of cells. Cell junctions can be classified as symmetric and asymmetric. Symmetric junctions include tight junctions, the belt desmosome, desmosomes, and gap junctions. An asymmetric junction is the hemidesmosome.

Cellular Communication and Signal Transduction

1. Cells communicate in three main ways: (1) they form protein channels (gap junctions); (2) they display receptors that affect intracellular processes or other cells in direct physical contact; and (3) they use receptor proteins inside the target cell.
2. Primary modes of intercellular signaling include contact-dependent, paracrine, hormonal, neurohormonal, and neurotransmitter.
3. Signal transduction involves signals or instructions from extracellular chemical messengers that are conveyed to the cell's interior for execution. If deprived of appropriate signals, cells undergo a form of cell suicide known as programmed cell death or apoptosis.
4. Binding of the extracellular signaling messenger (first messenger) to the membrane receptors causes (1) the opening or closing of channels that regulate ion movement and (2) the transfer of the signal to an intracellular messenger (second messenger) that triggers a cascade of events in the cell.

Cellular Metabolism

1. The chemical tasks of maintaining essential cellular functions are referred to as cellular metabolism. Anabolism is the energy-using process of metabolism, whereas catabolism is the energy-releasing process.
2. ATP functions as an energy-transferring molecule. It is fuel for cell survival. Energy is stored by molecules of carbohydrate, lipid, and protein, which, when catabolized, transfers energy to ATP. The phases of catabolism are digestion, glycolysis and oxidation, and the citric acid cycle.
3. Oxidative phosphorylation occurs in the mitochondria and is the mechanism by which the energy produced from carbohydrates, fats, and proteins is transferred to ATP.

Membrane Transport: Cellular Intake and Output

1. Cell survival and growth depend on the constant exchange of molecules with their environment. The majority of molecular transfer depends on specialized membrane transport proteins. The two main classes of membrane transport proteins are transporters and channels.
2. Passive transport does not require the expenditure of energy; rather, it is driven by physical effects. Passive transport mechanisms include diffusion, filtration, and osmosis. Water and small, electrically uncharged molecules move through pores in the plasma membrane's lipid bilayer via passive transport.
3. Diffusion is the passive movement of a solute from an area of greater solute concentration to an area of lesser solute concentration, a difference known as the concentration gradient.
4. Filtration is the movement of water and solutes through a membrane because of a greater pushing pressure on one side. Hydrostatic pressure is the force of water pushing against a cellular membrane.
5. Osmosis is the movement of water across a semipermeable membrane from a region of lower solute concentration to a region of higher solute concentration. The amount of hydrostatic pressure required to oppose the osmotic movement of water is called the osmotic pressure of solution. The overall osmotic effect of colloids, such as plasma proteins, is called the oncotic pressure or colloid osmotic pressure.
6. Active transport requires expenditure of metabolic energy by the cell by means of ATP. Larger molecules and molecular complexes are moved into the cell by active transport.
7. The active transport of Na^+ and K^+ is found in virtually all cells. Approximately 60% to 70% of ATP synthesized by cells is used to maintain the transport of Na^+ and K^+.
8. The largest molecules (macromolecules) and fluids are transported by membrane-bound vesicles through the processes of endocytosis (ingestion) and exocytosis (expulsion).
9. Endocytosis, or vesicle formation, occurs when the substance to be transported is engulfed by a segment of the plasma membrane, forming a vesicle that moves into the cell. Pinocytosis is a type of endocytosis in which fluids and solute molecules are ingested through formation of small vesicles. Phagocytosis is a type of endocytosis in which large particles, such as bacteria, are ingested through formation of large vesicles, called vacuoles.
10. In receptor-mediated endocytosis, the plasma membrane receptors are clustered, along with bristle-like structures, in specialized areas called coated pits. Endocytosis occurs when the coated pits invaginate, internalizing ligand-receptor complexes in coated vesicles.

11. Inside the cell, lysosomal enzymes process and digest material ingested by endocytosis.
12. In exocytosis, a membrane-bound vesicle carries macromolecules to the outer cell membrane. It has two main functions: it releases molecules synthesized by the cells into the ECM and replaces portions of the plasma membrane that have been removed by endocytosis.
13. Two types of solutes exist in body fluids: electrolytes and nonelectrolytes. Electrolytes are electrically charged and dissociate into constituent ions when placed in solution. Nonelectrolytes do not dissociate when placed in solution.
14. All body cells are electrically polarized, with the inside of the cell more negatively charged than the outside. The difference in voltage across the plasma membrane is the resting membrane potential.
15. When an excitable (nerve or muscle) cell receives an electrochemical stimulus, cations enter the cell and cause a rapid change in the resting membrane potential known as the action potential. The action potential "moves" along the cell's plasma membrane and is transmitted to an adjacent cell. This is how electrochemical signals convey information from cell to cell.

Cellular Reproduction: The Cell Cycle

1. Cellular reproduction in body tissues involves mitosis (nuclear division) and cytokinesis (cytoplasmic division).
2. Only mature cells are capable of division. Maturation occurs during a stage of cellular life called interphase (growth phase).
3. The cell cycle is the reproductive process that begins after interphase in all tissues with cellular turnover. There are four phases of the cell cycle: (1) the G_1 phase (G = gap), the period between the M phase and the start of DNA synthesis; (2) the S phase (S = synthesis), during which DNA synthesis takes place in the cell nucleus; (3) the G_2 phase, the period between the completion of DNA synthesis and the next phase in which RNA and protein synthesis occurs; and (4) the M phase (M = mitosis), which involves both nuclear and cytoplasmic division.
4. The M phase (mitosis) involves four stages: prophase, metaphase, anaphase, and telophase.
5. Cellular division and growth are regulated by intracellular programs and several extracellular signal molecules (cell cycle control system). The cell cycle control system works because of a connected series of biochemical switches that either activate or inhibit cell events. Two classes of *switches*, or regulatory molecules that determine a cell's progress through the cell cycle, are CDKs and cyclins.
6. Organ size and body size are determined by three main processes: (1) cell growth, (2) cell division, and (3) cell survival. Mitogens induce or simulate mitosis. Growth factors stimulate an increase in cell mass or cell growth. Survival factors inhibit the programmed cell death called apoptosis.

Tissues

1. Cells of one or more types are organized into tissues, and different types of tissues compose organs. Organs are organized to function as tracts or systems.
2. Three key factors that maintain the cellular organization of tissues are (1) recognition and cell communication, (2) selective cell-to-cell adhesion, and (3) memory.
3. Fully specialized or terminally differentiated cells that are lost are generated from proliferating precursor cells and they, in turn, have been derived from a smaller number of stem cells. Stem cells are cells with the potential to develop into many different cell types during early development and growth. In many tissues, stem cells serve as an internal repair and maintenance system dividing indefinitely. These cells can maintain themselves over very long periods of time, called self-renewal, and can generate all the differentiated cell types of the tissue or multipotency.
4. The four basic types of tissues are epithelial, muscle, nerve, and connective tissues.
5. Neural tissue is composed of highly specialized cells called neurons that receive and transmit electrical impulses rapidly across junctions called synapses.
6. Epithelial tissue covers most internal and external surfaces of the body. The functions of epithelial tissue include protection, absorption, secretion, and excretion.
7. Connective tissue binds various tissues and organs together, supporting them in their locations and serving as storage sites for excess nutrients.
8. Muscle tissue is composed of long, thin, highly contractile cells or fibers. Muscle tissue that is attached to bones enables voluntary movement. Muscle tissue in internal organs enables involuntary movement, such as the heartbeat.

REFERENCES

1. Setubal JC, Almeida NF, Wattam AR. Comparative genomics for prokaryotes. *Methods Mol Biol.* 2018;1704:55–78.
2. Alberts B, et al. *Molecular biology of the cell.* ed 6 New York: Garland Science; 2015.
3. Alberts B, et al. *Essential cell biology.* ed 5, New York: W.W. Norton & Company; 2019.
4. Vyssokikh MY, et al. Mild depolarization of the inner mitochondrial membrane is a crucial component of an anti-aging program. *Proc Natl Acad Sci U S A.* 2020;117:6491–6501.
5. Cao RN, et al. Endothelial glycocalyx as a potential therapeutic target in organ injuries. *Chin Med J (Engl).* 2019;132:963–975.
6. Harjunpää H, et al. Cell adhesion molecules and their roles and regulation in the immune and tumor microenvironment. *Front Immunol.* 2019;10:1078.
7. Loh CY, et al. The E-cadherin and N-cadherin switch in epithelial-to-mesenchymal transition: signaling, therapeutic implications, and challenges. *Cells.* 2019;8(10):1118.
8. Angulo-Urarte A, van der Wal T, Huveneers S. Cell-cell junctions as sensors and transducers of mechanical forces. *Biochim Biophys Acta Biomembr.* 2020;1862(9):183316.
9. Díaz-Coránguez M, Liu X, Antonetti DA. Tight junctions in cell proliferation. *Int J Mol Sci.* 2019;20(23):5972.
10. Tschernig T. Connexins and gap junctions in cancer of the urinary tract. *Cancers (Basel).* 2019;11(5):704.
11. Manica A, et al. High levels of extracellular ATP lead to chronic inflammatory response in melanoma patients. *J Cell Biochem.* 2018;119(5):3980–3988.

12. Dong Y, et al. Regulation of cancer cell metabolism: oncogenic MYC in the driver's seat. *Signal Transduct Target Ther*. 2020;5:124.
13. Tang Z, et al. The cancer exosomes: clinical implications, applications, and challenges. *Int J Cancer*. 2020;146:2946–2959.
14. Chrysafides SM, et al. *Physiology, resting potential. StatPearls*. Treasure Island (FL): StatPearls Publishing; June 28, 2020. Available at: https://www.ncbi.nlm.nih.gov/books/NBK538338/.
15. Simon LV, Hashimi MF, Farrell MW. *Hyperkalemia. StatPearls*. Treasure Island (FL): StatPearls Publishing; February 11, 2021. Available at. https://www.ncbi.nlm.nih.gov/books/NBK470284/.
16. Nourian Dehkordi A, et al. Skin tissue engineering: wound healing based on stem-cell-based therapeutic strategies. *Stem Cell Res Ther*. 2019;10:111.
17. Zakrzewski W, et al. Stem cells: past, present, and future. *Stem Cell Res Ther*. 2019;10:68.
18. Das D, Fletcher RB, Ngai J. Cellular mechanisms of epithelial stem cell self-renewal and differentiation during homeostasis and repair. *WIREs Dev Biol*. 2020;9:e361.

2

Altered Cellular and Tissue Biology: Environmental Agents

Victoria Gray, Kathryn L. McCance, and Julia L. Rogers

http://evolve.elsevier.com/Rogers/pathophysiology/

CHAPTER OUTLINE

Most diseases are caused by multiple factors acting together *(multifactorial)* or a single factor interacting with a genetically susceptible person. Injury to cells or their surrounding environment, the *extracellular matrix (ECM)*, leads to tissue and organ damage. Although the normal cell is characterized by a narrow range of structural and functional constraints, cells can *adapt* to increased demands and stress to maintain a steady state, called *homeostasis*. Adaptation is a reversible response involving structural or functional modifications to accommodate both physiologic (normal) demands and pathologic (adverse) conditions. For example, the uterus adapts to pregnancy—a normal physiologic state—by enlarging. Pregnancy triggers an increase in the size and number of cells to accommodate a growing fetus. Adaptation to a pathologic condition occurs with high blood pressure or hypertension. Myocardial cells become enlarged, resulting in a larger, thicker left ventricle to accommodate the increased workload of the heart. Cellular adaptations to pathologic conditions are usually only temporarily successful. If the stressor is eliminated, cells can return to normal state without lasting injury; however, severe or long-term stressors can overwhelm the adaptive processes, resulting in cellular injury or death. Common sources of cell stress include structural damage, neoplasia, fluid/solute accumulations, genetic influences, and aging.

Cellular injury can result from any factor that disrupts cellular structures or deprives the cell of oxygen and essential nutrients. Resultant injury may be *sublethal* (reversible) or *lethal* (irreversible). Common sources of cell injury are classified broadly as ischemic–hypoxic (lack of sufficient oxygen), ischemia–reperfusion, free radical, immunologic, infectious, intentional or unintentional, and inflammatory. Clinical manifestations and alteration to normal physiology will vary with the type of injury. Stress from metabolic derangements is linked to intracellular excessive *accumulations* of carbohydrate, protein, and lipids. Cell death can result in calcium accumulation within surrounding damaged tissue, a condition referred to as *pathologic calcification*. The two main types of cell death are necrosis and apoptosis. A third process, autophagy, occurs during times of cellular stress and is typically triggered by deficiency of nutrients or growth factors. The various forms of cell death are discussed in greater detail later in this chapter.

Cellular aging causes structural and functional changes that may result in decreased capacity to recover from injury and, ultimately, cell death. The exact mechanisms governing cellular aging is unclear; distinguishing pathologic changes from age-associated physiologic changes can be challenging. Aging clearly results in alterations to cellular structure and function, yet senescence (growing old) is both inevitable and normal.

CELLULAR ADAPTATION

Cells have the remarkable capacity to adapt to their environment to avoid injury. An adapted cell is neither normal nor injured; its status falls somewhere between these two states. Adaptations are reversible changes affecting the size, number, phenotype, metabolic activity, or function of cells.[1]

Adaptive responses have limits; additional stress can compromise essential cell functions leading to cell injury or death. Cell adaptation may be the central component in many disease states. In the early stages of successful adaptation, cells may have enhanced function, making it difficult to distinguish a pathologic response from vigorous adaptation. Over time, the adaptive response may fail, and pathology will ensue. The most significant adaptive changes in cells include the following:

- Atrophy—decrease in cell size
- Hypertrophy—increase in cell size
- Hyperplasia—increase in cell number
- Metaplasia—reversible replacement of one differentiated cell type by another cell type
- Dysplasia—or deranged cellular growth, is not considered a true cellular adaptation but rather atypical hyperplasia

These changes are shown in Fig. 2.1.

Atrophy

Atrophy refers to *decrease* in cell *size*. If atrophy affects enough cells, the affected organ decreases in size and is said to be atrophic. Atrophy can affect any organ, but it occurs most commonly in skeletal muscle, heart muscle, secondary sex organs, and the brain. Atrophy is classified as either *physiologic* or *pathologic*, depending on the underlying cause, and regardless of whether atrophy results from normal physiologic or pathologic conditions, identical changes to cellular structure will occur. Physiologic atrophy occurs with normal development. In early development, embryonic structures (i.e., notochord) undergo atrophy, whereas during early childhood the thymus gland involutes, and in adolescence, the tonsils shrink. In women, the uterus decreases in size shortly after childbirth.

Pathologic atrophy occurs in organs as a result of decreases in workload, pressure, use, blood supply, nutrition, hormonal stimulation, or neural stimulation. *Disuse atrophy* (decreased workload) occurs when a limb is placed in a cast for an extended period with prolonged bed rest or immobilization. Pressure can cause tissue to atrophy and is often seen in pressure ulcers. Chronic ischemia can result in senile atrophy from a decrease in blood supply to the brain (Fig. 2.2). The lack of hormonal stimulation results in atrophic changes that occur more readily with age. In postmenopausal women, the ovaries atrophy secondary to a lack of estrogenic stimulation. In men, the gonads shrink secondary to decreases in hormonal stimulation. Aging also results in atrophic changes to brain cells. *Denervation atrophy* is seen with peripheral neuropathies. Atrophic muscle cells contain less endoplasmic reticulum (ER), fewer mitochondria, and fewer *myofilaments* (the contractile components of the muscle fiber) compared with normal cells. Muscle atrophy, caused by decreased neural stimulation, results in reduced oxygen consumption and decreased amino acid uptake. The mechanisms of atrophy for such changes include a decrease in protein synthesis, an increase in protein degradation, or both. The degradation of proteins occurs mainly by the ubiquitin–proteosome pathway (see Chapter 1).

Atrophy, secondary to chronic malnutrition, is associated with a process called *autophagy* ("self-eating"), where self-destructive autophagic vacuoles are created within the cell. These membrane-bound vesicles contain cellular debris and hydrolytic enzymes that degrade substances into simple units of fat, carbohydrate, or protein. Isolation of these enzymes within autophagic vacuoles prevents uncontrolled cell destruction in neighboring cells and tissue. Some substances contained within autophagic vacuole may resist destruction, persisting as membrane-bound residual bodies within tissues. Lipofuscin refers to yellow-brown pigmented granules; lipid-containing residue that persists after lysosomal destruction. These granules tend to accumulate in liver, myocardial, renal, retinal, adrenal, and neural tissues as individuals age. When they accumulate in

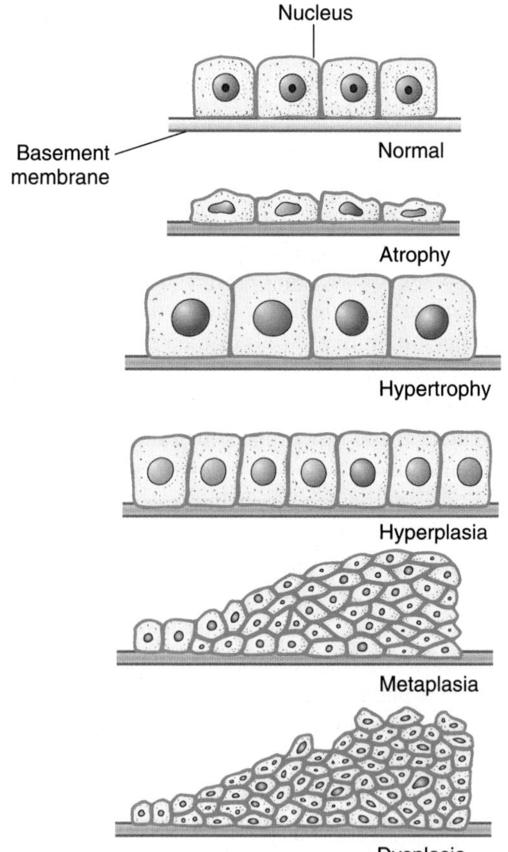

Fig. 2.1 Adaptive and Dysplastic Alterations in Simple Cuboidal Epithelial Cells.

the skin, they are the basis of the so-called age spots appearing in older individuals.

Hypertrophy

Hypertrophy is a compensatory *increase* in the *size* of cells, occurring in response to mechanical load or stress, and results in increased size of the affected organ. Common triggers include repetitive stretching, chronic pressure, and volume overload. The cells of the heart and kidneys are particularly prone to enlargement. Hypertrophy, as an adaptive response, occurs in the striated muscle cells of both the heart and skeletal muscles. It presents clinically as muscle enlargement. In the case of cardiac muscle hypertrophy, typically left ventricular hypertrophy (LVH), an increased synthesis of cardiac muscle proteins follows, allowing muscle fibers to do more work (Fig. 2.3). Hypertrophy may be *physiologic* or *pathologic.* Physiologic hypertrophy results from increased demand, stimulation by hormones, and growth factors. An example of physiologic hypertrophy is enlargement secondary to aerobic exercise or a "runner's heart." In this case, no pathology is present, and normal structure and function are preserved. Pathologic hypertrophy results from chronic hemodynamic overload, such as from hypertension or heart valve dysfunction. When LVH occurs secondary to hypertension, it represents *pathologic hypertrophy.* The initial adaptation, in the form of cardiac enlargement with dilated ventricles, is short lived. Prolonged cardiac hypertrophy progresses to contractile dysfunction and finally heart failure. In contrast to physiologic hypertrophy, where the myocardial matrix is preserved, pathologic hypertrophy is associated with increased interstitial fibrosis, cell death, and abnormal cardiac function (see Fig. 2.3). After a *unilateral nephrectomy* (removal of one kidney), compensatory hypertrophy occurs in the remaining kidney, which preserves renal structure and function.

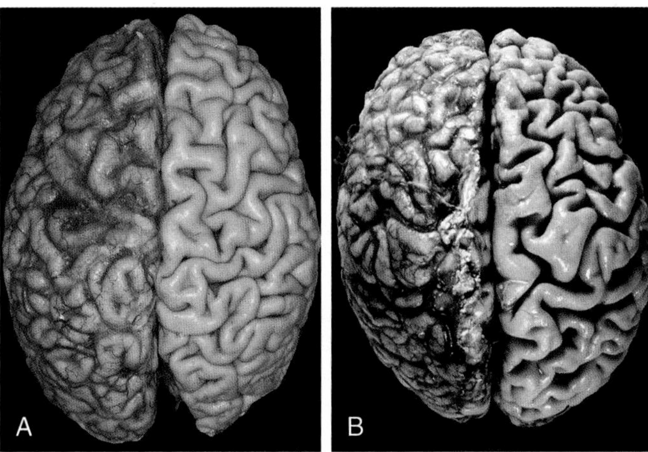

Fig. 2.2 Atrophy. (A) Normal brain of a young adult. **(B)** Atrophy of the brain in an 82-year-old male with atherosclerotic cerebrovascular disease, resulting in reduced blood supply. Note that loss of brain substance narrows the gyri and widens the sulci. The meninges have been stripped from the right half of each specimen to reveal the surface of the brain. (From Kumar V, Abbas AK, Aster JC. *Robbins & Cotran pathophysiologic basis of disease*, 10th edition. Philadelphia: Elsevier; 2020:60.)

Hyperplasia

Hyperplasia is an *increase* in the *number* of cells, resulting from an increased rate of cellular division. As a response to a stimulus (e.g., injury), hyperplasia occurs when the damage is severe or prolonged or when it results in cell death. Hyperplasia requires that cells undergo mitosis, a process wherein a single cell divides into two identical cells. The main mechanism for hyperplasia is the production of hormones or growth factors, which stimulate the remaining cells after injury or cell loss to synthesize new cell components and, ultimately, to divide. Another mechanism is increased output of new cells from tissue stem cells. For example, if liver cells are injured, new cells can regenerate from intrahepatic stem cells.[1] Mature cells have differing capacity for hyperplastic (mitotic) growth. Although hyperplasia and hypertrophy have distinct processes, they can occur together within the same tissue.

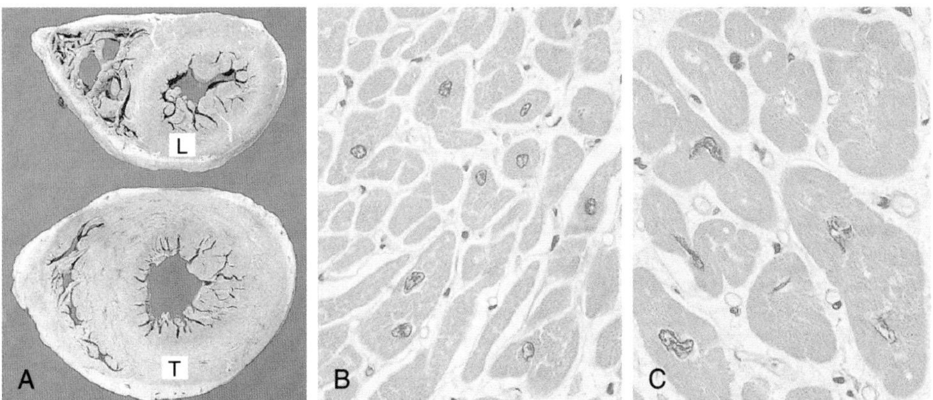

Fig. 2.3 Hypertrophy of Cardiac Muscle in Response to Valve Disease. (A) Transverse slices of a normal heart and a heart with hypertrophy of the left ventricle (*L*, normal thickness of left ventricular wall; *T*, thickened wall from heart in which severe narrowing of aortic valve caused resistance to systolic ventricular emptying). **(B)** Histology of cardiac muscle from the normal heart. **(C)** Histology of cardiac muscle from a hypertrophied heart. (From Stevens A, Lowe J. *Pathology: Illustrated review in color*, 2nd edition. Edinburgh: Mosby; 2000.)

Two types of physiologic (normal) hyperplasia occur: compensatory hyperplasia and hormonal hyperplasia. Compensatory hyperplasia is an adaptive mechanism that enables organs to regenerate. Removal of part of the liver leads to rapid hyperplasia of the remaining hepatocytes (liver cells). Even with removal of 70% of liver mass, regeneration is complete in about 2 weeks. Significant compensatory hyperplasia readily occurs in epidermal and intestinal epithelia, hepatocytes, bone marrow cells, and fibroblasts. Loss of cells within an organ triggers deoxyribonucleic acid (DNA) synthesis, mitotic division, and hyperplasia. To a lesser extent, hyperplasia occurs in bone, cartilage, and smooth muscle cells. A callus, or thickening of the skin, is an example of compensatory hyperplasia. It occurs in response to injury from a mechanical stimulus. Another example is the response to wound healing secondary to the inflammation process (see Chapters 7 and 9).

Hormonal hyperplasia occurs chiefly in estrogen-dependent organs, such as the uterus and breast. For example, during pregnancy and puberty in the female, proliferation of the glandular epithelium occurs, causing hypertrophy (enlargement) of the female breasts. Similarly, after ovulation, estrogen stimulates the endometrium to grow and thicken for reception of the fertilized ovum. If pregnancy occurs, hormonal hyperplasia, as well as hypertrophy, enables the uterus to enlarge. (Hormone function is discussed further in Chapters 21, 22, 24–26.)

Pathologic hormonal hyperplasia is the abnormal proliferation of normal cells, usually in response to excessive hormonal stimulation or to the action of growth factors on target cells. Hyperplastic cells are identified by pronounced enlargement of the nucleus, clumping of chromatin, and the presence of one or more enlarged nucleoli. The most common example is pathologic hyperplasia of the endometrium, which is caused by an imbalance between estrogen and progesterone levels with relative increases of estrogen (see Chapter 25). Pathologic endometrial hyperplasia, which causes excessive menstrual bleeding, is under the influence of regular growth-inhibition controls. The resulting endometrial hyperplasia commonly presents as erratic or excessive uterine bleeding, known as *dysfunctional uterine bleeding*. Left unchecked, the regular growth-inhibiting control mechanisms can fail over time, producing malignant transformation or endometrial cancer.[1]

Benign prostatic hyperplasia (BPH) is another example of pathologic hyperplasia and results from changes in hormone balance (Fig. 2.4). The incidence of BPH increases with age, secondary to age-related hormonal imbalances that result in epithelial and stromal proliferation or impaired apoptosis. Similarly, thyroid enlargement, including thyroid goiters, can result from excessive levels of pituitary thyroid-stimulating hormone (TSH). In the absence of malignant transformation, when the predisposing factors are corrected, pathologic hyperplasia will typically regress.

Dysplasia: Not a True Adaptive Change

Dysplasia refers to abnormal changes in the *size, shape, and organization* of mature cells (Fig. 2.5). Dysplasia is not considered a true adaptive process but is related to hyperplasia and is often referred to as atypical hyperplasia. Although dysplastic tissue appears disorderly, the term *dysplasia* does not refer to cancer. Dysplastic changes are common in the epithelial tissue of the uterine cervix, the endometrium, and the gastrointestinal (GI) and respiratory tract mucosa. Dysplasia that does not involve the entire thickness of epithelium may be completely reversible.[1] When dysplastic changes penetrate the basement membrane, it is considered an invasive neoplasm. Dysplasia is described as "low grade" or "high grade," depending on the degree of variation from normal. If the triggering stimulus is removed—for example, certain hormonal stimuli—dysplastic transformation may be reversible. (Dysplasia is discussed further in Chapter 12.)

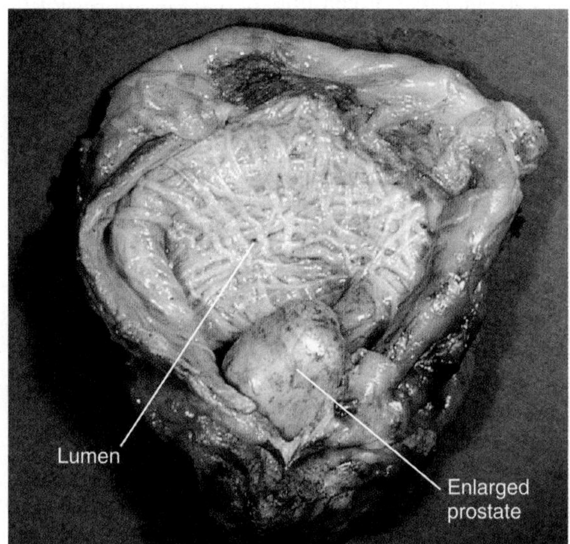

Fig. 2.4 Hyperplasia of the Prostate with Secondary Thickening of the Obstructed Urinary Bladder (Bladder Cross-Section). The enlarged prostate is seen protruding into the lumen of the bladder, which appears trabeculated. These "trabeculae" result from hypertrophy and hyperplasia of smooth muscle cells that occur in response to increased intravesical pressure caused by urinary obstruction. (From Damjanov I. *Pathology for the health professions*, 4th edition. St Louis: Saunders; 2012.)

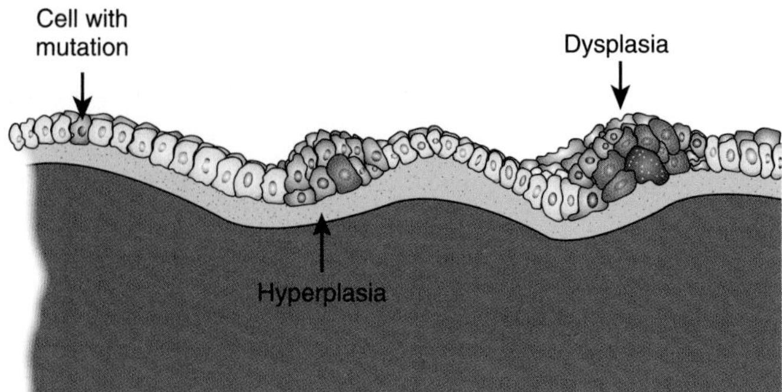

Fig. 2.5 Dysplasia. Abnormal changes in the size, shape, and organization of cells. Dysplasia is related to hyperplasia and called atypical hyperplasia. (Adapted from http://www.ndhealthfacts.org/wiki/Oncology_%28Cancer%29.)

Metaplasia

Metaplasia is the *reversible* replacement of one mature cell type (epithelial or mesenchymal) by another cell type that can survive in an adverse environment. It is found in association with tissue damage, repair, and regeneration.[1] Usually, however, the change is not beneficial. For example, in the long-term cigarette smoker, the chronic irritation from smoke causes the normal ciliated columnar epithelial cells of the trachea and bronchi to become replaced by stratified squamous epithelial cells (Fig. 2.6). The newly formed squamous epithelial cells do not secrete mucus or have cilia, causing a loss of a critical protective mechanism. Bronchial metaplasia can be reversed if the inducing stimulus, usually cigarette smoking, is removed. If the inducing stimulus is persistent, it can initiate malignant transformation in the metaplastic epithelium. At certain times, the adaptive replacement cell type may be more suitable to the changed conditions in the surrounding environment. For example, gastroesophageal reflux damages squamous epithelium of the esophagus, and the adapted change or replacement by glandular epithelium may better tolerate the acidic environment.

Metaplasia results from a reprogramming of *stem cells* present in most epithelia or colonization by differentiated cell populations from adjacent sites.[1] These precursor cells mature along a different pathway with metaplastic change. Differentiation of stem cells from a particular cell lineage responds to signals generated by growth factors, cytokines, and ECM components in the cell's environment.

CELLULAR INJURY

Injury to cells and to the ECM leads to injury of tissues and organs and ultimately determines the structural patterns of disease. Cellular injury occurs when the cell is unable to maintain *homeostasis* (a normal or adaptive steady state). The injury may be reversible injury (the cell can recover) or irreversible injury (cellular death). Loss of function is the result of cell and ECM injury and cell death. Cellular injury may occur secondary to a variety of factors: chemical agents, hypoxia, free radicals, infectious agents, physical and mechanical factors, immunologic reactions, genetic factors, and nutritional imbalances. Types of cell injuries and their responses are summarized in Table 2.1 and Fig. 2.7.

The extent of cellular injury is a function of cell type, level of differentiation, and adaptive mechanisms of the cell. Also important are the nature, severity, and duration of the injury. Fully differentiated, mature cells are more susceptible to injury

TABLE 2.1 Types of Progressive Cell Injury and Responses

Type	Responses
Adaptation	Atrophy, hypertrophy, hyperplasia, metaplasia
Active cell injury	Immediate response of "entire" cell
Reversible	Loss of ATP, cellular swelling, detachment of ribosomes, autophagy of lysosomes
Irreversible	"Point of no return" structurally when severe vacuolization of mitochondria occurs and Ca^{++} moves into cell
Necrosis	Common type of cell death with severe cell swelling and breakdown of organelles
Apoptosis, or programmed cell death	Cellular self-destruction for elimination of unwanted cell populations
Autophagy	Eating of self, cytoplasmic vesicles engulf cytoplasm and organelles, recycling factory
Chronic cell injury (subcellular alterations)	Persistent stimuli response may involve only specific organelles or cytoskeleton (e.g., phagocytosis of bacteria)
Accumulations, or infiltrations	Water, pigments, lipids, glycogen, proteins
Pathologic calcification	Dystrophic and metastatic calcification

ATP, Adenosine triphosphate; *Ca^{++}*, calcium.

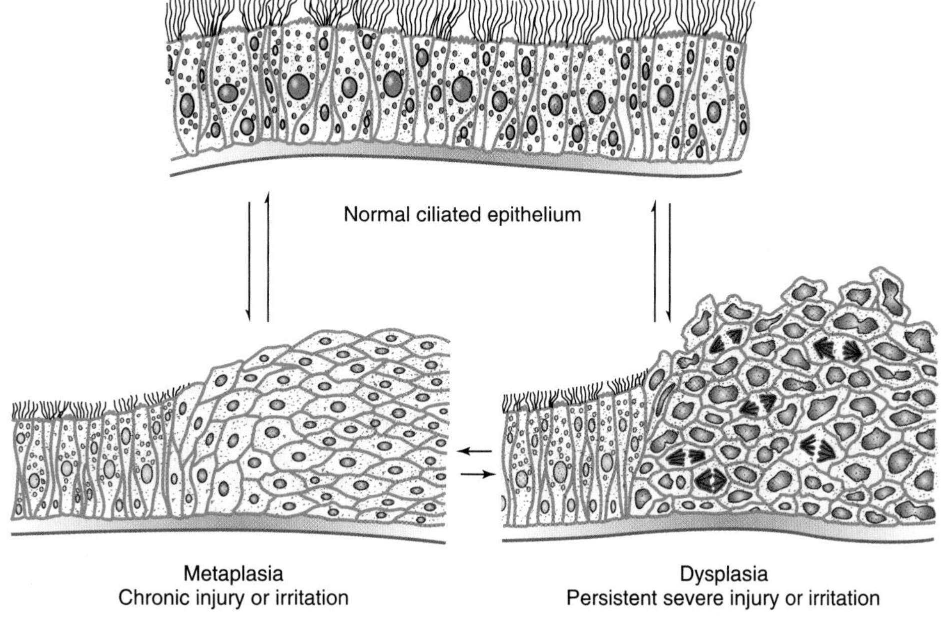

Fig. 2.6 Reversible Changes in Cells Lining the Bronchi.

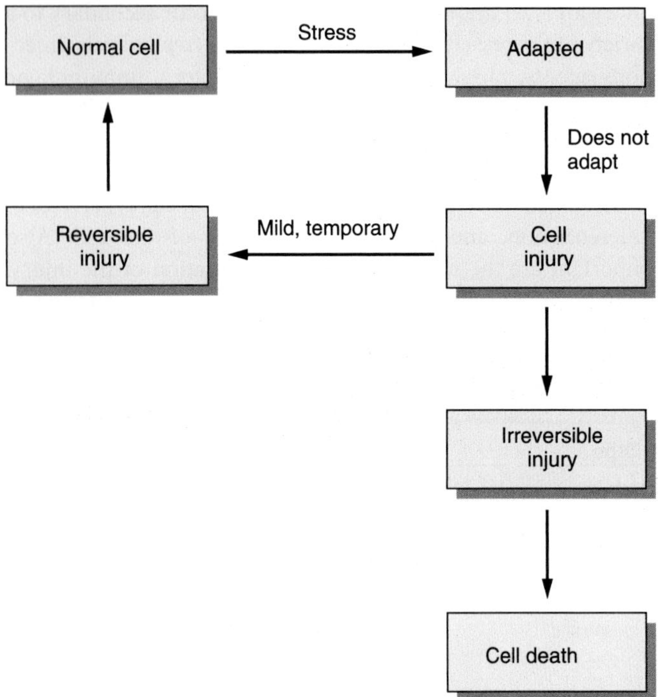

Fig. 2.7 Stages of Cellular Adaptation, Injury, and Death. The normal cell responds to physiologic and pathologic stresses by adapting (atrophy, hypertrophy, hyperplasia, metaplasia). Cell injury occurs if the adaptive responses are exceeded or compromised by injurious agents, stress, and mutations. The injury is reversible if it is mild or transient, but if the stimulus persists, the cell suffers irreversible injury and eventually death.

TABLE 2.2 Common Themes in Cell Injury and Cell Death

Theme	Comments
ATP depletion	Loss of mitochondrial ATP and decreased ATP synthesis; results include cellular swelling, decreased protein synthesis, decreased membrane transport, and lipogenesis, all changes that contribute to loss of integrity of plasma membrane
Reactive oxygen species (↑ROS)	Lack of oxygen is key in progression of cell injury in ischemia (reduced blood supply); activated oxygen species (ROS, O_2, H_2O_2, OH^-) cause destruction of cell membranes and cell structure
Ca^{++} entry	Normally intracellular cytosolic calcium concentrations are very low; ischemia and certain chemicals cause an increase in cytosolic Ca^{++} concentrations; sustained levels of Ca^{++} continue to increase with damage to plasma membrane; Ca^{++} causes intracellular damage by activating a number of enzymes
Mitochondrial damage	Can be damaged by increases in cytosolic Ca^{++}, ROS; two outcomes of mitochondrial damage are loss of membrane potential, which causes depletion of ATP and eventual death or necrosis of cell, and activation of another type of cell death (apoptosis) (see p. 7 and p. 46)
Membrane damage	Early loss of selective membrane permeability found in all forms of cell injury, lysosomal membrane damage with release of enzymes causing cellular digestion
Protein misfolding, DNA damage	Proteins may misfold, triggering *unfolded protein response* that activates corrective responses; if overwhelmed, response activates cell suicide program or apoptosis; DNA damage (genotoxic stress) also can activate apoptosis (see p. 46)

ATP, Adenosine triphosphate; *Ca^{++}*, calcium; *DNA*, deoxyribonucleic acid; *H_2O_2*, hydrogen peroxide; O_2, superoxide radical; *OH^-*, hydroxyl radical; *ROS*, reactive oxygen species.

than are cell precursors. Two individuals exposed to an identical stimulus may incur varying degrees of cellular injury. Individual differences, including genetics, nutritional status, and immunologic competency, can profoundly influence the extent of cell injury. The precise "point of no return" with respect to cell death remains unclear. Once changes to the nucleus have occurred or cell membranes are disrupted, or both, irreversible injury and cell death are inevitable.

General Mechanisms of Cell Injury

Regardless of the cause of injury, a host of biochemical events results in cell injury and death. Such events include adenosine triphosphate (ATP) depletion, damage from oxygen-derived free radicals, and alterations in calcium level. Injury to cell components includes membrane damage, protein folding defects, mitochondrial compromise, and DNA damage (see Table 2.2). The most common forms of cell injury include (1) ischemic and hypoxic injury, (2) ischemia–reperfusion injury, (3) oxidative stress or accumulation of oxygen-derived free radicals-induced injury, and (4) chemical injury.

Ischemic and Hypoxic Injury

Hypoxia, or the lack of sufficient oxygen within cells, is the single most common cause of cellular injury and is a prominent feature of pathological states encountered in bacterial infection, inflammation, wounds, cardiovascular defects, and cancer (Fig. 2.8).[2] Hypoxia can result from several circumstances, such as reduced oxygen content in the ambient air, loss of hemoglobin, decreased red blood cell (RBC) production, respiratory and cardiovascular diseases, and poisoning of the cellular oxidative enzymes (cytochromes). The most common cause of hypoxia is ischemia, or a reduced supply of blood and therefore oxygen. Hypoxia negatively impacts normal physiologic processes: differentiation, angiogenesis, proliferation, erythropoiesis, and overall cell viability. Mitochondria are the primary consumers of oxygen. Hypoxia triggers the mitochondrial complex to produce reactive oxygen species (ROS). From a physiologic perspective, ROS can be both beneficial and harmful, for example, by promoting *oxidative stress*, which can damage cells (oxidative stress is discussed in the next section). The relationship between hypoxia and inflammation has been linked to inflammatory bowel disease, certain cancers, and infection. Ongoing research seeks to clarify how tumors adapt to low oxygen levels, including angiogenesis, increasing glucose consumption, and promoting the metabolic state of glycolysis.

Arteriosclerosis (narrowing of blood vessels) and thrombus (blood clots within vessels) can result in localized tissue ischemia. Progressive hypoxia, caused by gradual arterial narrowing, is better tolerated than the acute anoxia (total lack of oxygen) caused

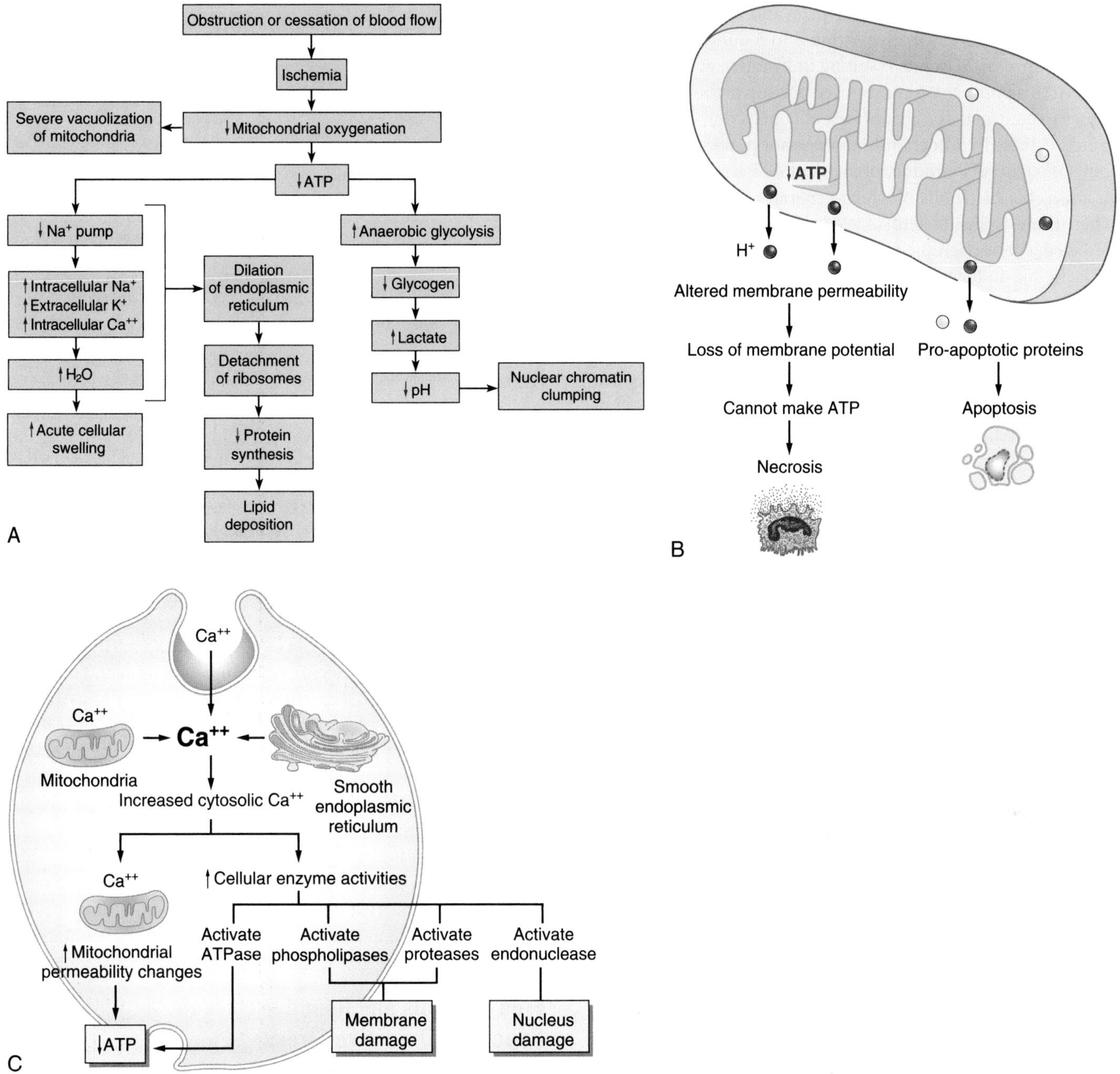

Fig. 2.8 Hypoxic Injury Induced by Ischemia. **(A)** Consequences of decreased oxygen delivery or ischemia with decreased adenosine triphosphate *(ATP)*. The structural and physiologic changes are reversible if oxygen is delivered quickly. Significant decreases in ATP result in cell death, mostly by necrosis. **(B)** Mitochondrial damage can result in changes in membrane permeability, loss of membrane potential, and decrease in ATP concentration. Between the outer and inner membranes of the mitochondria are proteins that can activate the cell's suicide pathways, called *apoptosis*. **(C)** Calcium ions are critical mediators of cell injury. Calcium ions (Ca^{++}) are usually maintained at low concentrations in the cell's cytoplasm; thus ischemia and certain toxins can initially cause an increase in the release of Ca^{++} from intracellular stores and later an increased movement (influx) across the plasma membrane. (Adapted from Kumar V, Abbas AK, Aster JC. *Robbins & Cotran pathophysiologic basis of disease*, 9th edition. St. Louis: Saunders; 2014.)

by an acute obstruction, or a thrombus. An acute obstruction in a coronary artery can result in a rapidly evolving *myocardial infarction* ("heart attack") if the blood supply is not restored. Irreversible myocardial cell death, with loss of heart function, will follow. Gradual onset of ischemia, however, usually results in myocardial adaptation. Myocardial infarction and stroke are frequent causes of mortality in the United States and generally result from atherosclerosis and consequent ischemic injury.[3]

Cellular responses to hypoxic injury occur rapidly. Within 1 minute after the blood supply to the myocardium is interrupted, the heart becomes pale and dysfunctional and unable to contract normally. Within 3 to 5 minutes, mitochondrial compromise occurs, resulting in insufficient ATP production. At this point, the compromised portion of the myocardium ceases to contract. The abrupt lack of contraction is caused by a rapid decrease in mitochondrial phosphorylation, which results in insufficient ATP production. Lack of ATP leads to an increase in anaerobic metabolism, which generates ATP from glycogen when there is insufficient oxygen. When glycogen stores are depleted, even anaerobic metabolism ceases.

Ischemia-induced reduction in ATP levels causes a failure of the plasma membrane's sodium–potassium (Na^+-K^+) pump and sodium–calcium (Na^+-Ca^{++}) exchange mechanisms. Sodium and calcium influx into and accumulate in the cell. Potassium (K^+) diffuses out of the cell. Without the pump mechanism, sodium and water can freely enter the cell resulting in cellular swelling and dilation of the ER. With dilation, ribosomes detach from the rough ER, reducing protein synthesis. If hypoxia persists, the entire cell becomes markedly swollen. These disruptions are reversible if oxygen (O_2) is restored. If oxygen is not restored, vacuolation (formation of vacuoles or cytoplasmic small cavities) occurs within the cytoplasm. The damaged outer membrane causes lysosomes to swell; marked swelling occurs to the mitochondria. With continued hypoxia, cell death rapidly follows as calcium accumulates within the cell, essential metabolic processes cease, and cell membranes become dysfunctional (see Fig. 2.8C). Influx of calcium into the cell activates enzymes that trigger apoptosis. Restoration of blood flow and oxygen can actually result in additional injury known as *ischemia–reperfusion injury.*

Ischemia–Reperfusion Injury

Restoration of blood flow and oxygen to ischemic tissues can increase recovery of cells reversibly injured, but paradoxically result in additional injury known as ischemia–reperfusion injury (reperfusion [reoxygenation] injury) and cause cell death (Fig. 2.9). Reperfusion is a serious complication and an important mechanism of injury in instances of tissue transplantation and other ischemic syndromes (e.g., hepatic, intestinal, renal). Several mechanisms are proposed for reperfusion injury, including the following:

- *Oxidative stress:* Reoxygenation induces *oxidative stress* by generating ROS and nitrogen species. Reactive oxygen intermediates include hydroxyl radical (OH^-), superoxide radical anion (O_2^-), nitric oxide-derived peroxynitrite ($ONOO^-$), and hydrogen peroxide (H_2O_2), and all have been shown to increase within minutes of reperfusion. They cause damage to the myocytes by altering membrane proteins and phospholipids.[1]
- Nitrogen-based free radicals present mostly in the form of nitric oxide (NO) and are generated by endothelial cells, macrophages, neurons, and other cells. The radicals further damage the already compromised membrane and facilitate calcium overload within the mitochondria. Additionally, reperfusion injury promotes proinflammatory neutrophil adhesion to the endothelium where they release toxic oxidants and harmful proteases. Antioxidant agents, such as vitamin C and vitamin E, reverse neutrophil adhesion. They also reverse neutrophil-mediated reperfusion injury in cardiac muscle.[4,5]

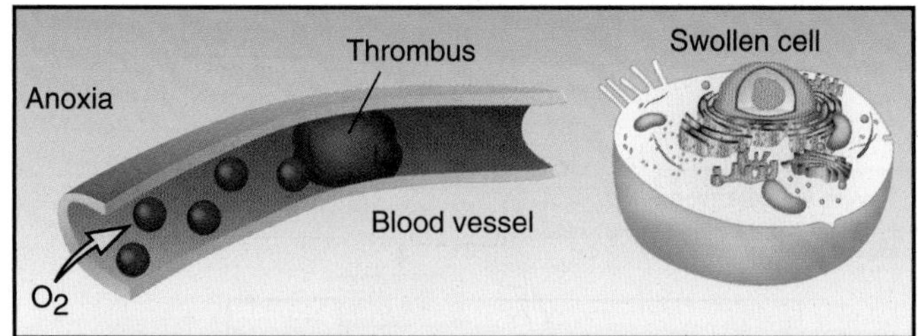

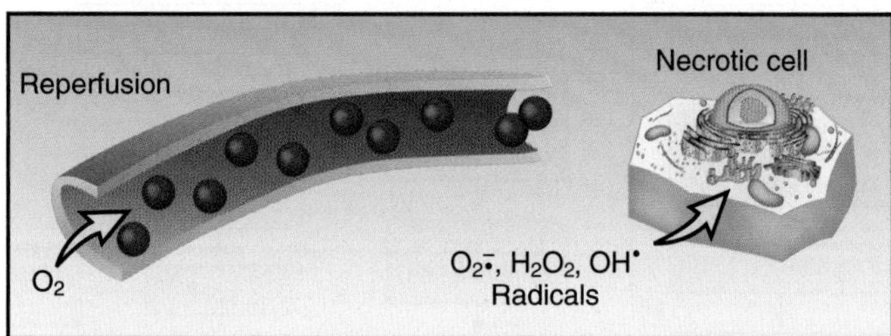

Fig. 2.9 Reperfusion Injury. Without oxygen, or in anoxia, the cells display hypoxic injury and become swollen. With reoxygenation, risk of reperfusion injury increases because of the formation of reactive oxygen radicals that can cause cell necrosis. (Redrawn from Damjanov I. *Pathology for the health professions*, 3rd edition. St Louis: Saunders; 2006.)

- *Increased intracellular calcium concentration*: Intracellular and mitochondrial calcium accumulate within the cell during acute ischemia. Reperfusion results in even more calcium influx because of damaged cell membranes and ROS-mediated injury to the sarcoplasmic reticulum. The increased calcium enhances mitochondrial permeability; damaged mitochondria have decreased or ceased production of ATP.
- *Inflammation*: Ischemic injury promotes inflammation. Dead cells stimulate immune cells to release cytokine-mediated danger signals, thus initiating an inflammatory response.
- *Complement activation*: Complement activation may exacerbate microvascular damage that has occurred secondary to reperfusion injury.[1]

Free Radicals and Reactive Oxygen Species—Oxidative Stress

Free radicals are an important mechanism of cellular injury, especially injury caused by ROS. This form of injury is called oxidative stress. Reactive oxygen species (ROS) are reactive molecules from molecular oxygen formed as a natural oxidant species in cells during mitochondrial respiration and energy generation. The intracellular sources of oxidants are numerous and include (1) cellular organelles with mitochondria (thought to be the largest contributor), ER (particularly during endoplasmic stress), and peroxisomes; (2) nicotinamide adenine dinucleotide phosphate (NADPH) oxidases (NOX enzymes); and (3) other enzymes (Fig. 2.10). From oxidative phosphorylation, mitochondria utilize oxygen to generate ATP from organic fuel molecules and, in the process, produce ROS. Oxidative stress is caused by an increase in different reactive species, depletion of antioxidant defense, or both. Oxidative stress results in detrimental oxidation of different molecules, including proteins, lipids, nucleic acids, and others. Oxidative stress can activate several intracellular signaling pathways because ROS can regulate enzymes and transcription factors. This process is an important mechanism of

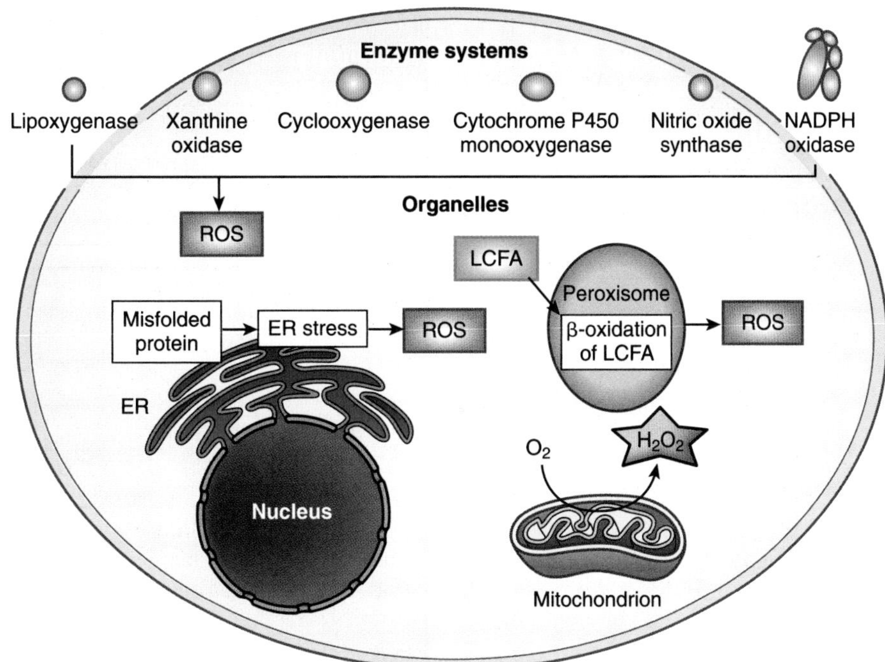

Fig. 2.10 Intracellular Sources of Reactive Oxygen Species and Sites of Generation of Reactive Oxygen Species from Mitochondria. The intracellular sources of reactive oxygen species *(ROS)* include some organelles: mitochondria, endoplasmic reticulum *(ER)* (particularly ER stress), and peroxisomes (metabolizing long-chain fatty acids *[LCFAs]*). As part of the enzymatic reaction cycles, various enzymes generate ROS, including oxidases and oxygenases. H_2O_2, Hydrogen peroxide; *NADPH*, nicotinamide adenine dinucleotide phosphate. (Adapted from Homstrom KM, Finkel T. Cellular mechanisms and physiological consequences of redoxdependent signalling. *Nature Reviews*, 2014;15(6):411–421.)

cell damage in many conditions, including cell injury, cancer, certain degenerative diseases (e.g., Alzheimer disease), and aging.

A free radical is an electrically uncharged atom, or group of atoms, which has an unpaired electron. Having one unpaired electron makes the molecule unstable; the molecule becomes stabilized either by donating or by accepting an electron from another molecule. The free radical has the potential to form a damaging chemical bond with proteins, lipids, and carbohydrates found within the cell membrane. Free radicals are highly reactive. They have low chemical specificity—that is, they can react with most molecules in their proximity. Reactions involving free radicals are difficult to control, and they initiate chain reactions. Free radicals are generated in a variety of conditions, including chemical and radiation injury, ischemia–reperfusion injury, cellular aging, and microbial destruction by phagocytes.

Free radicals are generated within cells by a number of mechanisms. These mechanisms are as follows:

1. *Reduction–oxidative reactions* (redox reactions): An oxidative-reduction reaction is a type of biochemical reaction involving the transfer of elections between two species (molecule, atom, or ion). A species may either gain or lose an electron. All biologic membranes contain redox systems, which serve to support cellular activity (Fig. 2.11).
2. *Absorption of extreme energy sources* (ultraviolet light, radiation) produces free radicals.
3. *Enzymatic metabolism of exogenous chemicals or drugs:* Many exogenous (outside the body) substances within the environment readily generate free radicals. As an example, CCL_3, a byproduct of carbon tetrachloride [CCl_4]) (Fig. 2.12), forms free radicals known to damage the liver, predisposing this organ to cancer. Accordingly, CCL_4 is classified by the

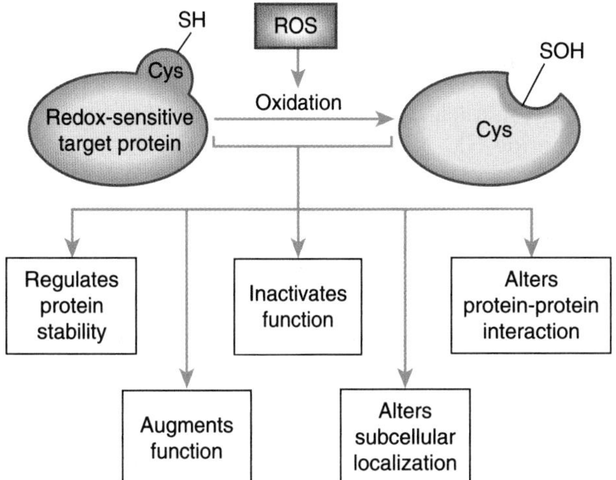

Fig. 2.11 Redox-Dependent Signaling: Biologic Mechanisms and Consequences. The oxidation and reduction (redox) of sensitive targets or proteins with cysteine *(Cys)* residues provide a mechanism to rapidly and reversibly alter protein function. Cys residues can function as redox-dependent "switches." Oxidation of Cys residues (SH [thiol]) to *SOH* (sulfenic acid) leads to alterations in the redox-sensitive target that result in many effects on protein stability, activity, and protein-protein interaction. (Adapted from Homstrom KM, Finkel T. Cellular mechanisms and physiological consequences of redoxdependent signalling. *Nature Reviews*, 2014;15(6):411–421.)

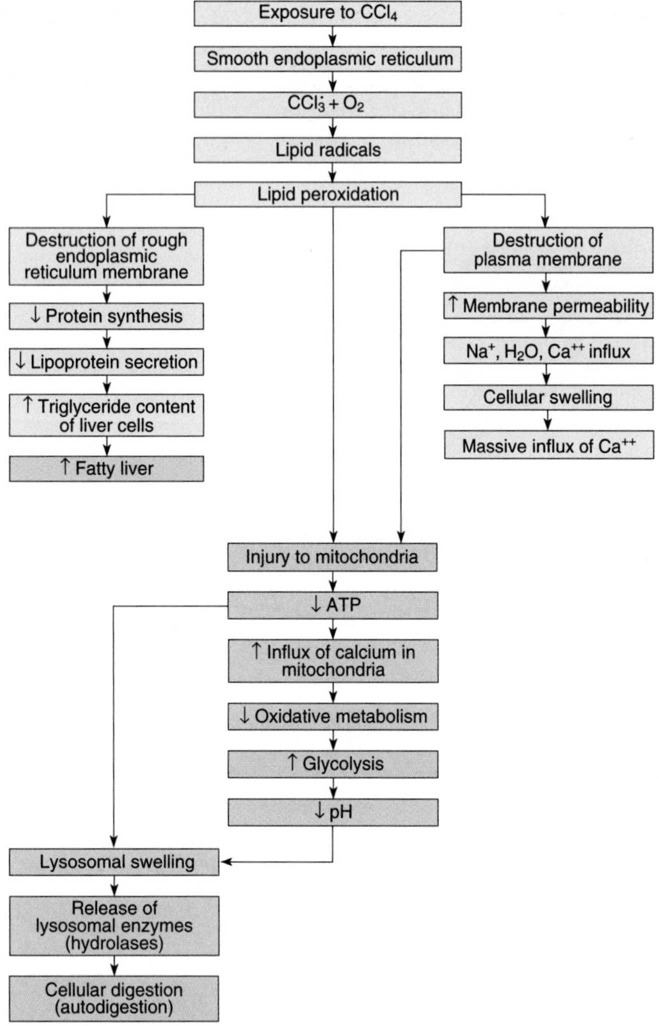

Fig. 2.12 Chemical Injury of Liver Cells Induced by Carbon Tetrachloride (CCl_4) Poisoning. Light blue boxes are mechanisms unique to chemical injury, purple boxes involve hypoxic injury, and green boxes are clinical manifestations. *ATP,* Adenosine triphosphate.

TABLE 2.3 Biologically Relevant Free Radicals

Reactive oxygen species (ROS) Superoxide radical $O_2^{\bar{\cdot}}\ O_2 \xrightarrow{\text{Oxidase}} O_2^{\bar{\cdot}}$	Generated either (1) directly during autoxidation in mitochondria or (2) enzymatically by enzymes in cytoplasm, such as xanthine oxidase or cytochrome p450; once produced, it can be inactivated spontaneously or more rapidly by enzyme superoxide dismutase (SOD): $O_2^{\bar{\cdot}} + O_2^{\bar{\cdot}} + -H_2^{\bar{\cdot}} \xrightarrow{\text{SOD}} H_2O_2 + O_2$
Hydrogen peroxide (H_2O_2) $O_2^{\bar{\cdot}} + O_2^{\bar{\cdot}} + -H \xrightarrow{\text{SOD}} H_2O_2 + O_2$ *Or* Oxidases present in peroxisomes O_2 peroxisome $O_2^{\bar{\cdot}} \xrightarrow{\text{SOD}} H_2O_2$	Generated by SOD or directly by oxidases in intracellular peroxisomes (NOTE: SOD is considered an antioxidant because it converts superoxide to H_2O_2); catalase [another antioxidant] can then decompose H_2O_2 to $O_2 + H_2O$.)
Hydroxyl radicals (OH^-) $H_2O \rightarrow H\cdot + OH\cdot$ *Or* $Fe^{++} + H_2O_2 \rightarrow Fe^{++} + OH\cdot + OH^-$ *Or* $H_2O_2 + O_2^{\bar{\cdot}} \rightarrow OH\cdot + OH^- + O_2$	Generated by hydrolysis of water caused by ionizing radiation or by interaction with metals—especially iron (Fe) and copper (Cu); iron is important in toxic oxygen injury because it is required for maximal oxidative cell damage
Nitric oxide (NO) $NO\cdot + O_2^{\bar{\cdot}} \rightarrow ONOO^- + H^+$	NO by itself is an important mediator that can act as a free radical; it can be converted to another radical—peroxynitrite anion ($ONOO^-$), as well as nitrogen dioxide (NO_2) and carbonate radical (CO_3^-)

Data from Cotran RS, et al. *Robbins pathologic basis of disease,* 6th edition. Philadelphia: Saunders; 1999.

International Agency for Research on Cancer (IARC; Group 2B) as a possible carcinogenic and by the Environmental Protection Agency (EPA) as a probable human carcinogen. Many reported cases of CCL_4 toxicity are associated with drinking alcohol.

4. *Transition metals* (iron and copper) donate or accept free electrons during intracellular reactions, generating free radicals in the process. As an example, the Fenton reaction, involving iron and H_2O_2, produces the potentially damaging hydroxyl radical and higher oxidation states of the iron. It has been implicated in iron accumulation disease.
5. *NO,* a colorless gas, acts as an intermediate in reactions involving endothelial cells, neurons, macrophages, and other cell types. NO can act as a free radical and convert to highly reactive compounds, including peroxynitrite anion ($ONOO^-$), nitrogen dioxide (NO_2), and nitrate (NO_3). Table 2.3 describes the most significant free radicals.

Free radicals also cause several damaging effects, such as the following:

1. Lipid peroxidation—the destruction of polyunsaturated lipids, which leads to membrane damage and increased permeability. This same process causes fats to become rancid.
2. Protein alteration—a process whereby polypeptide chains become fragmented, leading to protein loss, protein misfolding, and alters protein–protein interaction.
3. DNA damage—results in mutations (Fig. 2.13 and Chapter 4).
4. Mitochondrial effects—mitochondria are organelles that generate ATP. They can become damaged by ROS compromising available energy for the cell. Increases in intracellular calcium also damage mitochondria (see Fig. 2.8A and B). Box 2.1 summarizes the major types of mitochondrial damage. Cell damage from ROS can extend to neighboring cells.

The toxicity of certain drugs and chemicals can be attributed to free radicals. The drug/chemical may be converted to a free radical, or it may generate oxygen-derived metabolites. Free radicals have been either directly or indirectly linked with a growing number of diseases and disorders (see Box 2.2). The body has various mechanisms to eliminate free radicals. As an example, the oxygen free radical *superoxide* may spontaneously decay into oxygen and hydrogen peroxide. Table 2.4 summarizes other methods that contribute to inactivation or termination of free radicals.

Chemical or Toxic Injury

Humans are exposed to thousands of chemicals that have insufficient toxicologic data.[6] Time, cost, and an interest in reducing animal testing dictate the need to develop new methods for toxicity testing. To meet public health concerns, many agencies have collaborated to investigate how chemicals interact with biologic systems. Advances in molecular and systems biology, computational toxicology, and bioinformatics have aided investigators' efforts. Mechanisms of cell stress from chemical agents include oxidative stress, ER stress, heat shock response, DNA damage response, mental stress, inflammation, and osmotic stress (sudden change in solute concentration). Chemicals are being classified under these types of cell stress mechanisms.

Xenobiotics (from Greek *xenos*, "foreign"; *bios*, "life") are compounds and chemicals that have toxic, mutagenic, or carcinogenic

BOX 2.1 Three Major Types and Consequences of Mitochondrial Damage

1. Damage to the mitochondria results in the formation of the *mitochondrial permeability transition pore,* a high-conductance channel or pore. The opening of this channel results in the loss of mitochondrial membrane potential, causing failure of oxidative phosphorylation, depletion of adenosine triphosphate (ATP), and damage to mitochondrial DNA (mtDNA), leading to necrosis of the cell.
2. Altered oxidative phosphorylation leads to the formation of reactive oxygen species (ROS) that can damage cellular components.
3. Because mitochondria store several proteins between their membranes, increased permeability of the outer membrane may result in leakage of pro-apoptotic proteins and cause cell death by apoptosis.

Data from Kumar V, et al, eds. *Robbins and Cotran pathologic basis of disease*, 9th edition. Philadelphia: Elsevier; 2015.

BOX 2.2 Diseases and Disorders Linked to Oxygen-Derived Free Radicals

- Deterioration in aging
  - Atherosclerosis
  - Ischemic brain injury
  - Alzheimer disease
- Neurotoxins
- Cancer
- Cardiac myopathy
- Chronic granulomatous disease
- Diabetes mellitus
- Eye disorders
  - Macular degeneration
  - Cataracts
- Inflammatory disorders
- Iron overload
- Lung disorders
  - Asbestosis
  - Oxygen toxicity
  - Emphysema
- Nutritional deficiencies
- Radiation injury
- Reperfusion injury
- Rheumatoid arthritis
- Skin disorders
- Toxic states
  - Xenobiotics (tetrachloride [CCl_4], paraquat, cigarette smoke, etc.)
  - Metal irons (nickel [Ni], copper [Cu], iron [Fe], etc.)

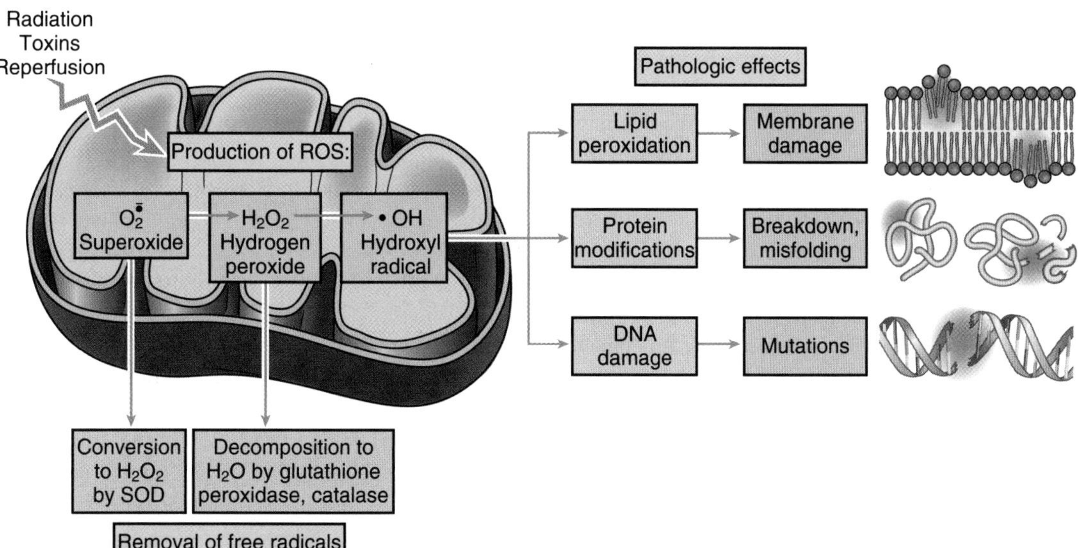

Fig. 2.13 The Role of Reactive Oxygen Species in Cell Injury. The production of reactive oxygen species *(ROS)* can be initiated by many cell stressors, such as radiation, toxins, and reperfusion of oxygen. Free radicals are removed by normal decay and enzymatic systems. ROS accumulates in cells because of insufficient removal or excess production leading to cell injury, including lipid peroxidation, protein modifications, and DNA damage or mutations. (Adapted from Kumar V, et al., eds. *Robbins and Cotran pathologic basis of disease*, 10th edition. Philadelphia: Elsevier; 2020.)

TABLE 2.4 Methods Contributing to Inactivation or Termination of Free Radicals

Method	Process
Antioxidants	Endogenous or exogenous; either blocks synthesis or inactivates (e.g., scavenges) free radicals; includes vitamin E, vitamin C, cysteine, glutathione, albumin, ceruloplasmin, transferrin, γ-lipoacid, others
Enzymes	Superoxide dismutase,[a] which converts superoxide to hydrogen peroxide (H_2O_2); catalase[a] (in peroxisomes) decomposes H_2O_2; glutathione peroxidase[a] decomposes hydroxyl radical (OH^-) and H_2O_2

[a]These enzymes are important in modulating the cellular destructive effects of free radicals; also released in inflammation.

properties (Fig. 2.14). A few of these compounds include pesticides, antibiotics, steroids, and biomedical waste compounds.[7] Some of these chemicals are found in the human diet, for example, the fungal mycotoxin, aflatoxin B_1. Many xenobiotics are hepatotoxic (toxic to the liver). The liver is the initial site of contact for many ingested compounds—xenobiotics, drugs, and alcohol—predisposing this organ to chemically induced injury. Once absorbed by the GI tract, the liver is the initial site of contact. This dynamic is called *first-pass effect*. A frequent cause for withdrawing medications from the market is hepatotoxicity. Herbal products are less subject to regulation by the U.S. Food and Drug Administration (FDA). There are several classes of dietary, weight reduction, and body building supplements that have compounds that are listed as potentially hepatotoxic. Several marketed herbal medicines, such as ma huang (ephedra), kava Huang, Lipokinetix, and Hydroxycut, have been identified as harmful by the FDA and other health authorities, and subsequently, the FDA has requested these products be removed.[8]

Many chemical compounds used in household cleaning, insect control, outdoor maintenance, or chemical manufacturing are potential carcinogens. Many such agents are absorbed in the body through the skin or by inhalation; ubiquitous in the environment, some agents have been linked with liver and other organ damage. The extent of chemically induced liver injury varies from minor liver injury to acute liver failure, cirrhosis, and liver cancer.[9,10]

Hepatic detoxification occurs through enzyme-mediated biotransformation and antioxidant systems. Biotransformation is a process whereby enzymatic reactions convert one chemical into a less toxic or nontoxic compound. The liver has the highest supply of biotransformation enzymes of all organs and plays a key role in protecting the host from chemical toxicity. Fig. 2.15 provides a summary of chemically induced liver injury.

Antioxidants are molecules that inhibit the oxidation of other molecules, thereby preventing the formation of free radicals. Antioxidants often terminate a chain reaction, which would otherwise result in free radical formation. *Endogenous antioxidants* are antioxidants produced by the body. The five most powerful endogenous antioxidants are *superoxide dismutase (SOD), alpha lipoic acid (ALA), catalase, coenzyme Q 10 (CoQ10),* and *glutathione peroxidase (GPX)*. Exogenous antioxidants are antioxidants that originate from outside the body, typically from dietary sources, such as vitamin C. Foods rich in antioxidants are appropriately encouraged as part of a healthy diet.

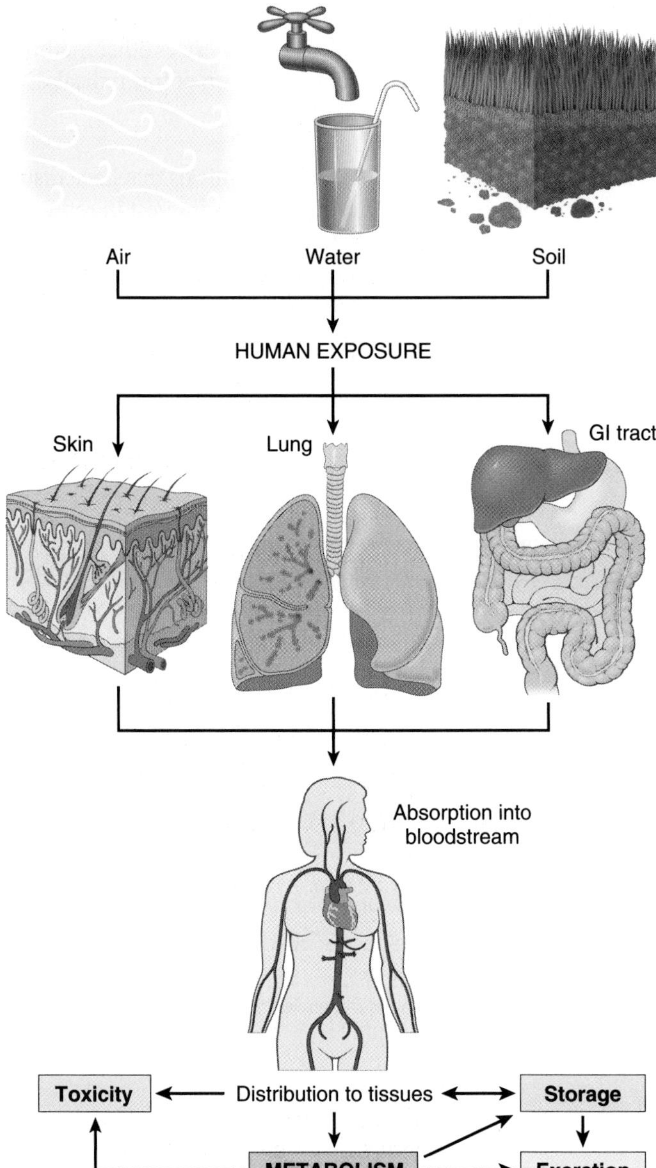

Fig. 2.14 Metabolism of Xenobiotics. Pollutants contained in air, water, and soil are absorbed through the lungs, gastrointestinal tract, and skin. In the body, the pollutants may act at the site of absorption but are generally transported through the bloodstream to various organs where they can be stored or metabolized. Metabolism of xenobiotics may result in the formation of water-soluble compounds that are excreted, or a toxic metabolite may be created by activation of the agent. (From Kumar V, et al., eds. *Robbins and Cotran pathologic basis of disease*, 10th edition. Philadelphia: Elsevier; 2020:407.)

Chemical Agents Including Drugs

Numerous chemical agents cause cellular injury. Minute amounts of some, such as arsenic and cyanide, can rapidly destroy cells and cause death of the individual. Chronic exposure to air pollutants, insecticides, and herbicides can cause cell injury (see Fig. 2.14). Carbon tetrachloride, alcohol, and social drugs can significantly alter cellular function and injure cellular structures. Over-the-counter (OTC) and prescribed drugs are an important cause of cellular injury. The abuse and addiction to opioids, such as heroin, morphine, and fentanyl, and other

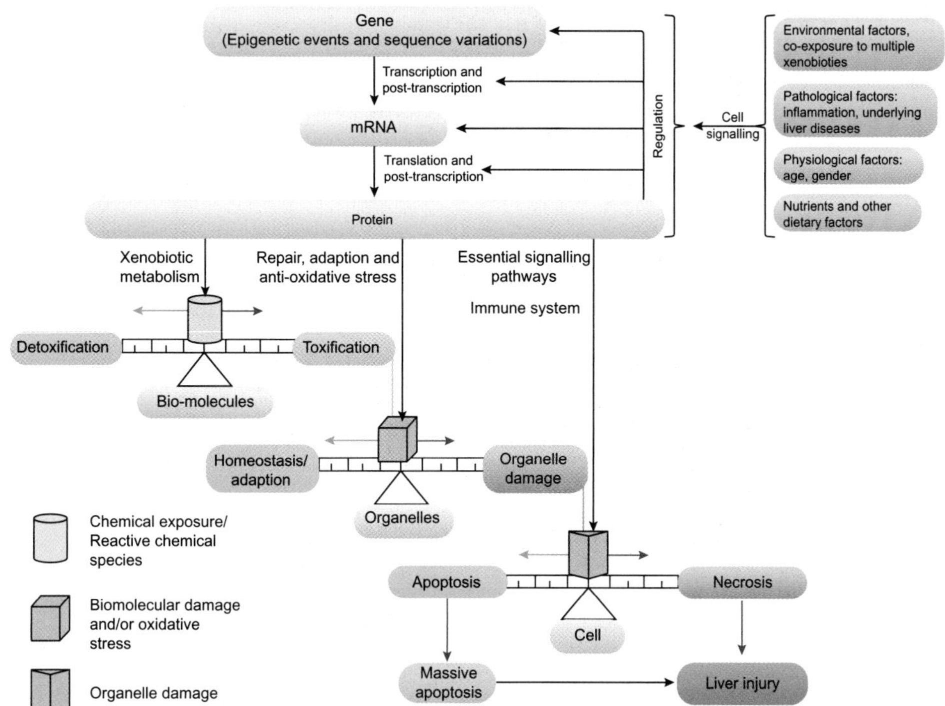

Fig. 2.15 Chemical Liver Injury. Liver injury is a result of genetic, environmental, biologic, and dietary factors. Certain chemicals can form toxic or chemically reactive metabolites. The risk of liver injury also can increase with increasing doses of a toxicant. Xenobiotic enzyme induction can lead to altered metabolism of chemicals, and drugs can either inhibit or induce drug-metabolizing enzymes. These changes can lead to greater toxicity. The dose at the site of action is controlled by phase I to III xenobiotic metabolites, and metabolizing enzymes are encoded by numerous different genes. Additionally, all aspects of xenobiotic metabolism are regulated by certain transcription factors (cellular mediators of gene regulation). Overall, the extent of cell damage depends on the balance between reactive chemical species and protective responses aimed at decreasing oxidative stress, repairing macromolecular damage, or preserving cell health by inducing apoptosis or cell death. Significant clinical outcomes of chemical-induced liver injury occur with necrosis and the immune response. Covalent binding of reactive metabolites to cellular proteins can produce new antigens (haptens) that initiate autoantibody production and cytotoxic T-cell responses. Necrosis, a form of cell death (see the Cellular Death section), can result from extensive damage to the plasma membrane with altered ion transport, changes of membrane potential, cell swelling, and eventual dissolution. Green arrows are pathways leading to cell recovery; red arrows indicate pathways to cell damage or death; black arrows are pathways leading to chemically induced liver injury. (Adapted from Gu X, Manautou JE. Molecular mechanisms underlying chemical liver injury. *Expert Reviews in Molecular Medicine*, 2013;14:e4.)

prescription pain relievers, are a serious global problem that affects all societies. Millions of people abuse opioids worldwide. The issue has become a public health crisis. In the United States, drug overdoses dramatically increased over the last 2 years, with the COVID-19 pandemic as a contributing factor.[11] Over the last two decades, deaths related to opioids more than tripled.[12]

The leading cause of poisoning in children is cosmetics and personal care products in children under 6 years of age, followed by cleaning substances and analgesic medications, including inappropriate administration of OTC preparations containing acetaminophen.[13] Social or street drugs are listed in Table 2.5. The use of e-cigarettes or vaping has become one of the leading causes of lung injury. In 2019, there were 6401 e-cigarette exposures, with nearly 45% involving children less than 5 years of age and another 23% in children 6 to 19 years of age. The exposure rate is up from 2018, when the number of e-cigarette exposures was 3142, causing acute lung injuries disproportionally affecting adolescents, children, and young adults. Hence, the Centers for Disease Control and Prevention (CDC) has classified this injury as e-Cigarette or Vaping Product Use-Associated Lung Injury (EVALI).[14]

Snakebite: Envenoming

Snakebite envenoming, poisoning by venom from either the bite of a venomous snake or by spraying venom into the victim's eyes, can have potentially deadly effects.[15] Snakes have hollow fangs in their anterior mouth that they use to inject venom into the subcutaneous tissue of their prey. Snake venom is composed primarily of proteins (e.g., metalloproteinases) and other complex substances with enzymatic activity. Available global data show that 4.5 to 5.4 million people per year are bitten by snakes. The majority (>99%) of snakebites in the United States are from pit vipers, with the majority (56.3%) occurring from rattlesnakes.[16] The chemistry and resulting

TABLE 2.5 Social or Street Drugs and Their Effects

Type of Drug	Description and Effects
Marijuana (pot)	*Active substance:* Δ9-Tetrahydrocannabinol (THC), found in resin of *Cannabis sativa* plant. With smoking (e.g., "joints"), about 5%–10% is absorbed through lungs; with heavy use, the following adverse effects have been reported: alterations of sensory perception; impairment of cognitive and psychomotor judgments (e.g., inability to judge time, speed, distance); increases in heart rate and blood pressure; increased susceptibility to laryngitis, pharyngitis, bronchitis; cough and hoarseness; possibility of lung cancer (dosages levels not determined); contains large number of carcinogens; data from animal studies only indicate reproductive changes include reduced fertility, decreased sperm motility, and decreased levels of circulatory testosterone; fetal abnormalities include low birth weight; increased frequency of infectious illness is thought to be result of depressed cell-mediated and humoral immunity; beneficial effects include decreased nausea secondary to cancer chemotherapy and decreased pain in certain chronic conditions.
Methamphetamine ("meth")	An amine derivation of amphetamine ($C_{10}H_{15}N$) used as crystalline hydrochloride CNS stimulant: in large doses causes irritability, aggressive (violent) behavior, anxiety, excitement, auditory hallucinations, and paranoia (delusions and psychosis); mood changes are common, and abuser can swiftly change from being friendly to being hostile; paranoiac swings can result in suspiciousness, hyperactive behavior, and dramatic mood swings. Appeals to abusers because body's metabolism is increased and produces euphoria, alertness, and perception of increased energy Stages: *Low intensity:* User is not psychologically addicted and uses methamphetamine by swallowing or snorting. *Binge and high intensity:* User has psychological addiction and smokes or injects to achieve a faster, stronger high. *Tweaking:* Most dangerous stage; user is continually under the influence, not sleeping for 3–15 days, extremely irritated, and paranoid.
Cocaine and crack	Extracted from leaves of cocoa plant and sold as a water-soluble powder (cocaine hydrochloride) liberally diluted with talcum powder or other white powders; extraction of pure alkaloid from cocaine hydrochloride is "free-base" called *crack* because it "cracks" when heated. Crack is more potent than cocaine; cocaine is widely used as an anesthetic, usually in procedures involving oral cavity; it is a potent CNS stimulant, blocking reuptake of neurotransmitters norepinephrine, dopamine, and serotonin; also increases synthesis of norepinephrine and dopamine; dopamine induces sense of euphoria, and norepinephrine causes adrenergic potentiation, including hypertension, tachycardia, and vasoconstriction; cocaine can therefore cause severe coronary artery narrowing and ischemia; reason cocaine increases thrombus formation is unclear; other cardiovascular effects include dysrhythmias, sudden death, dilated cardiomyopathy, rupture of descending aorta (i.e., secondary to hypertension); effects on fetus include premature labor, retarded fetal development, stillbirth, hyperirritability.
Heroin	Opiate closely related to morphine, methadone, and codeine Highly addictive, and withdrawal causes intense fear ("I'll die without it"); sold "cut" with similar-looking white powder; dissolved in water, it is often highly contaminated; feeling of tranquility and sedation lasts only a few hours and thus encourages repeated intravenous or subcutaneous injections; acts on the receptors enkephalins, endorphins, and dynorphins, which are widely distributed throughout body with high affinity to CNS; effects can include infectious complications, especially *Staphylococcus aureus* infections, granulomas of lung, septic embolism, and pulmonary edema—in addition, viral infections from casual exchange of needles and HIV; sudden death is related to overdosing secondary to respiratory depression, decreased cardiac output, and severe pulmonary edema.
Fentanyl	Synthetic opioid analgesic similar to morphine but is 50–100 times more potent. The synthetic opioid fentanyl and its analogs have risen across the United States in a variety of forms. Currently, it is documented in connection with a growing number of overdoses and overdose deaths.

CNS, Central nervous system; *HIV*, human immunodeficiency virus.
Data from Kumar V, Abbas A, Aster J. *Robbins and Cotran pathologic basis of disease*, 9th edition. Philadelphia: Saunders; 2015; Nahas G, Sutin K, Bennett WM. Review of marihuana and medicine. *New England Journal of Medicine*, 2000;343(7):514..

cellular levels effects of snake venom can vary between species of snakes, but most pit viper envenomation has little neurotoxic effects. Box 2.3 shows the pathophysiology, clinical manifestations, evaluation, and treatment for snakebite envenoming. Fig. 2.16 presents a step-by-step management approach to snake (crotalid) envenomation.

Common Environmental Toxins

Air Pollution

Ambient fine particle air pollution. The world's largest single environmental health risk is air pollution. Air pollution is contamination of the indoor or outdoor environment by any chemical, physical, or biologic agent that modifies natural characteristics of the atmosphere. Air pollution was the fourth leading risk factor for premature death globally, with nearly 12% of all deaths, and more than 6.67 million in 2019 alone (Fig. 2.17). Early deaths from air pollution were surpassed only by high blood pressure, tobacco use, and poor diet.[17] The percentage of Global Deaths attributed to air pollution in 2019 was:

- 40% of chronic obstructive pulmonary disease (COPD) deaths
- 20% of diabetes deaths
- 20% of ischemic heart disease deaths
- 19% of lung cancer deaths
- 26% of stroke death
- 30% of lower-respiratory deaths
- 20% of neonatal deaths

The EPA has identified the following six pollutants as "criteria" air pollutants: carbon monoxide, lead, nitrogen oxides, photochemical oxidants, ground-level ozone particle pollution known as particulate matter, and sulfur oxides (Figs. 2.18 through 2.20).[18]

BOX 2.3 Snakebite Envenoming

Pathophysiology

Examples of pathophysiological effects from snake envenomation:

- Necrosis of cells due to toxic tissue enzymes
- Increased permeability of cell membranes leading to increased localize spread of venom
- Pit viper venom has both fibrinolytic and protein C activation effects, causing **coagulopathy** (impaired ability to clot blood)
- Mohave rattlesnake envenomation can produce cranial nerve dysfunction, weakness, and paralysis
- Timber rattlesnakes can induce *myokymia*, an involuntary quivering of muscles or localized muscle fibers

Clinical Manifestations

- Fang marks are usually identifiable
- Local symptoms include pain, swelling, and bleeding from the bite site
- With severe presentations, there may be local tissue necrosis and ecchymosis
- Systemic manifestations include angioedema, bleeding from other orifices (hematemesis, hematochezia), nausea, vomiting, diarrhea, dyspnea, and anaphylaxis

Evaluation and Treatment

- Individuals need immediate and rapid transport for evaluation by a qualified medical provider
- Wounds should be cleaned, and severity of envenomation should be assessed
- Persons should be given intravenous fluid and blood drawn for complete laboratory evaluations of snakebite
- Persons who are asymptomatic should be observed for at least 12 hours before safe discharge
- The leading edge of the swelling should be marked, time of observation recorded, and circumference of extremity measured every 30 minutes
- Persons with bites from snakes with neurotoxic venom should be observed for at least 24 hours
- Antivenin should be administered for venomous snakebites within 4 hours of snakebite, but it is still effective for at least the first 24 hours; identification of the snake is helpful in knowing which antivenin to administer

Data from Corbett B, Clark RF. North American snake envenomation. *Emergergency Medicine Clinics of North America*, 2017;35(2):54. https://doi.org/10.1016/j.emc.2016.12.003; Juckett G, Hancox J. Venomous snakebites in the United States: Management review and update. *American Family Physician*, 2002;65(7):1367–1375. PMID: 11996419; Lavonas EJ, Ruha AM, Banner W, et al. Rocky mountain poison and drug center, Denver health and hospital authority: Unified treatment algorithm for the management of crotaline snakebite in the United States: Results of an evidence-informed consensus workshop. *BMC Emergency Medicine*, 2011;11:2; Patel V, Kong EL, Hamilton RJ. Rattle snake toxicity. StatPearls [Internet]. Treasure Island, FL: StatPearls; 2021; Vohra R, Cantrell FL, Williams SR. Fasciculations after rattlesnake envenomation: A retrospective statewide poison control system study. *Clinical Toxicology*, 2008;46(2):117–121. https://doi.org/10.1080/15563650701638925. World Health Organization (WHO). Snakebite. Geneva, Switzerland: World Health Organization; 2021. https://www.who.int/healthtopics/snakebite#tab=tab_1. Accessed October 1, 2021.

Table 2.6 defines each of the criteria pollutants with sources and known human health impacts.

Household air pollution. From the most recent report, 3.8 billion people cook using solid fuels (e.g., coal, charcoal, wood, dung, kerosene, agricultural residue) (Fig. 2.21). Nearly 50% of the world's population is exposed to household air pollution from the burning of solid fuels, which contributes to 3.8 million premature deaths per year (2018) from illnesses caused by these practices.[19] These inefficient practices produce high levels of household air pollution with a range of health-damaging pollutants, including carbon monoxide and small soot particles that penetrate deep into the lungs. Indoor smoke can be 100 times higher than acceptable levels for fine particles.[17] These exposures are particularly high for women and young children. Most individuals exposed to indoor pollutants live in developing countries. Individuals exposed to indoor pollution along with outdoor pollution face a double health burden.[20] Household air pollution is a significant contributor to ambient $PM_{2.5}$.[21]

Reducing outdoor emissions from household coal and biomass energy systems, agricultural waste incineration, forest fires, and certain agroforestry activities (e.g., charcoal production) would reduce key rural and peri-urban air pollution sources in developing regions.[17] Reducing outdoor air pollution decreases emissions of CO_2 and short-lived climate pollutants; for example, black carbon particles and methane. These actions would contribute to mitigating climate change. Since 2010, the use of solid fuels has fallen slowly and steadily in most regions, especially in South Asia, Southeast Asia, East Asia, and Oceania Super Regions (see Fig. 2.21B).

COVID-19 infection has raised awareness to an invisible threat to our respiratory and cardiovascular health and has brought renewed attention to air pollution. Although COVID-19's effects may appear in a few weeks, the health consequences of air pollution may take years to manifest in the form of chronic diseases (see Emerging Science Box: Long-Term Exposure to Air Pollution and Increased Risk of Severe COVID-19 Outcomes). Respiratory and cardiovascular health have made individuals more vulnerable to the effects of COVID-19.[21]

Heavy Metals as Environmental Pollutants

The most common heavy metals associated with harmful effects in humans include lead, mercury, arsenic, and cadmium. Damage from metals includes involvement of DNA repair mechanisms, tumor suppressor functions, and interference with signal transduction pathways.

Lead. Lead (Pb) is a heavy toxic metal present in paint of older homes (built before 1978), the environment, and the workplace. Lead may be found in hazardous concentrations in food, water, and air, and it is one of the most common overexposures found in industry.[22] Despite efforts to reduce exposure through government regulation, lead exposure persists in homes, the environment, and the workplace for many people, and lead toxicity is still a primary hazard to children. Older buildings, where lead-based paint is peeling from the walls, are a particular hazard to children (see Emerging Science Box: Lead Poisoning). Lead-based paint has a sweet taste, and toddlers are apt to find paint chips on the floor and put them into their mouths. Although Pb was removed from paint in the United States in 1978, many homes in the United States still contain leaded paint, and chipped and peeling leaded paint constitutes a significant source of current childhood exposure.[23,24]

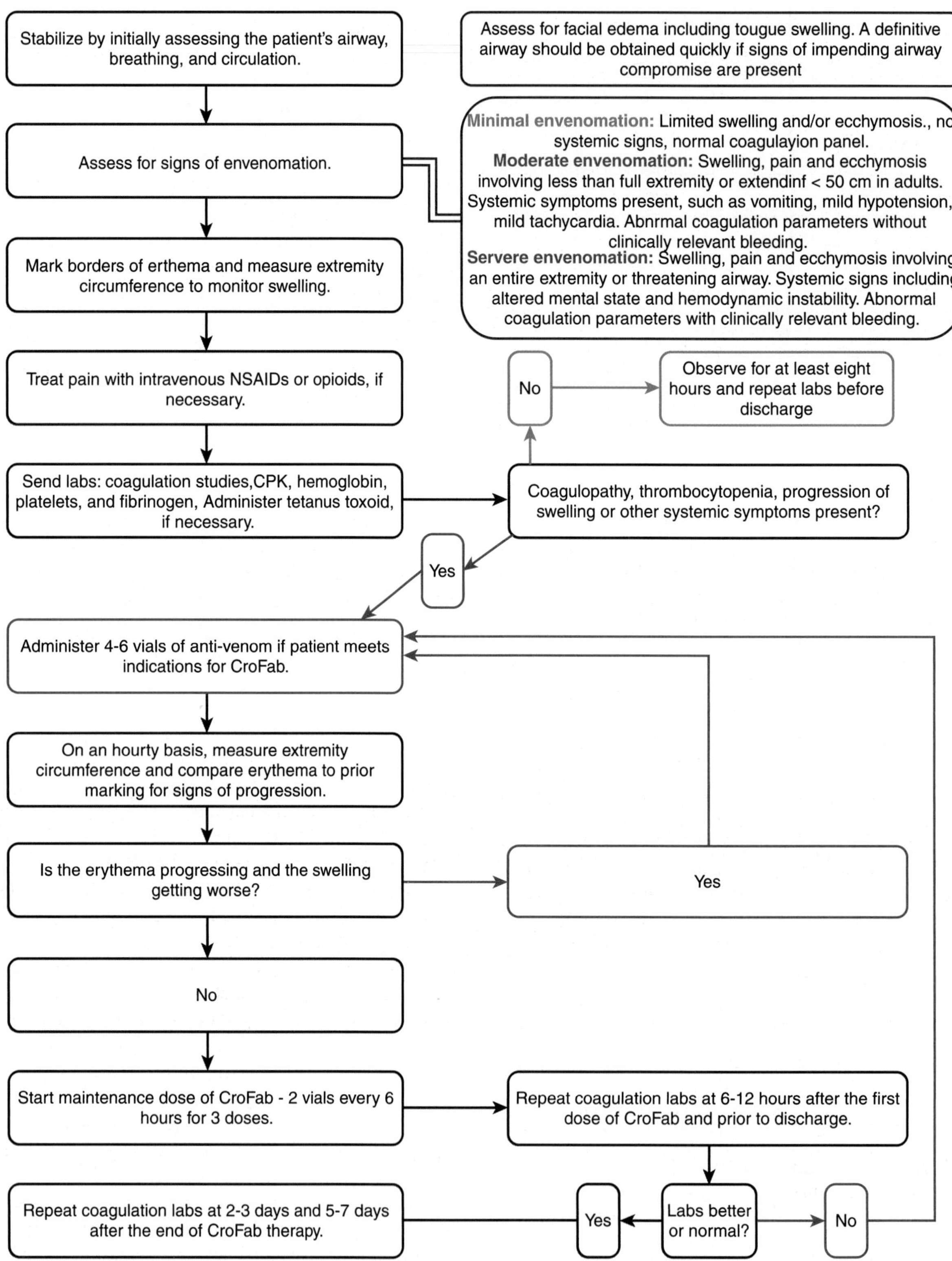

Fig. 2.16 Algorithm Snake (Crotalid) Envenomation Management. Crotalid venom causes various local, hematologic, neurologic, and system effects requiring a step-by-step approach to treatment. (From Patel V, Kong EL, Hamilton RJ. *Rattle snake toxicity. StatPearls [Internet].* Treasure Island, FL: StatPearls; 2021.)

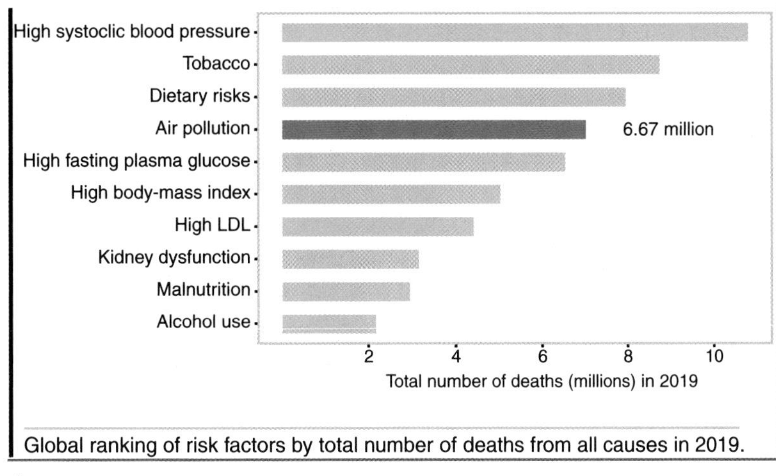

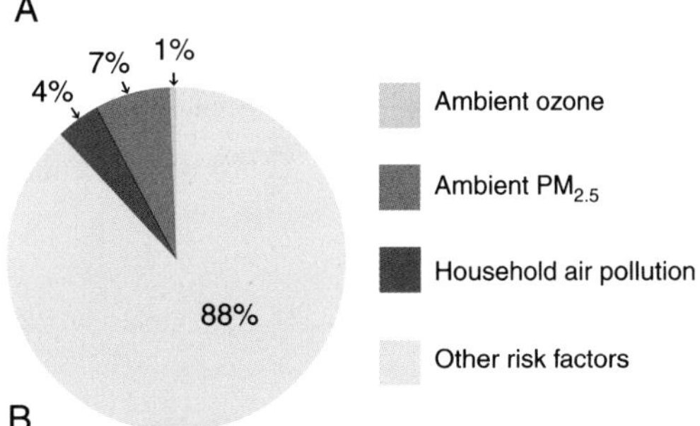

Fig. 2.17 Global Ranking of Risk Factors and Deaths from Air Pollution. **(A)** Bar graph showing rankings by total numbers of deaths in 2019. **(B)** Percentage of global deaths from individual pollutants. (Data from Health Effects Institute. State of Global Air 2020 Report. Data source: Global Burden of Disease Study. IHME; 2020. https://www.stateofglobalair.org/resources.)

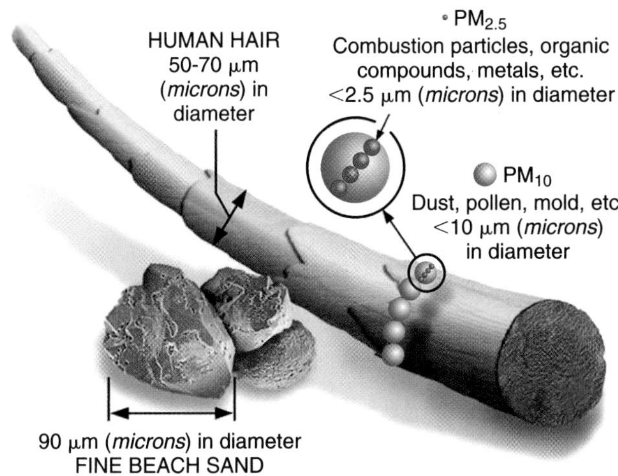

Fig. 2.18 Particle Sizes and Pollution. (From Environmental Protection Agency. Particulate matter updated March 18, 2013. Washington, DC; 2013.)

The chipped paint can disintegrate at friction surfaces to form lead dust. Another source of contamination is lead dust dispersed along roadways from previous leaded gasoline emissions. When lead was removed from gasoline, blood lead levels (BLLs) dropped significantly.[25]

Previous emissions of leaded fuel created large dispersions of lead dust in the environment. Particulate lead (2 to 10 μm) does not degrade and persists in the environment, making it a notable source of human exposure.[26] Other airborne sources include smelters and piston-engine airplanes.[27] Drinking water exposed to lead occurs from outdated fixtures, plumbing without corrosion control, and solders. Because well water is not subject to EPA regulation, it may not be tested for lead. Although the average blood levels of lead in children in the United States have dropped since the 1970s, there are at-risk populations with higher-than-average BLLs. Children living at or below the poverty line who live in older housing are at greatest risk. Importantly, the CDC reports "no safe blood lead level in children has been identified."[28] Millions of children are being exposed to lead in their homes, increasing their risks for damage to the brain and nervous system, slowed growth and development, learning and behavior problems (e.g., reduced IQ, attention-deficit/hyperactivity disorder [ADHD], juvenile delinquency, and criminal behavior), and hearing and speech problems.

The neurologic effect of lead in exposed children is the driving force for reducing lead levels in the environment. Children are more susceptible than adults to the effects of lead for several reasons:

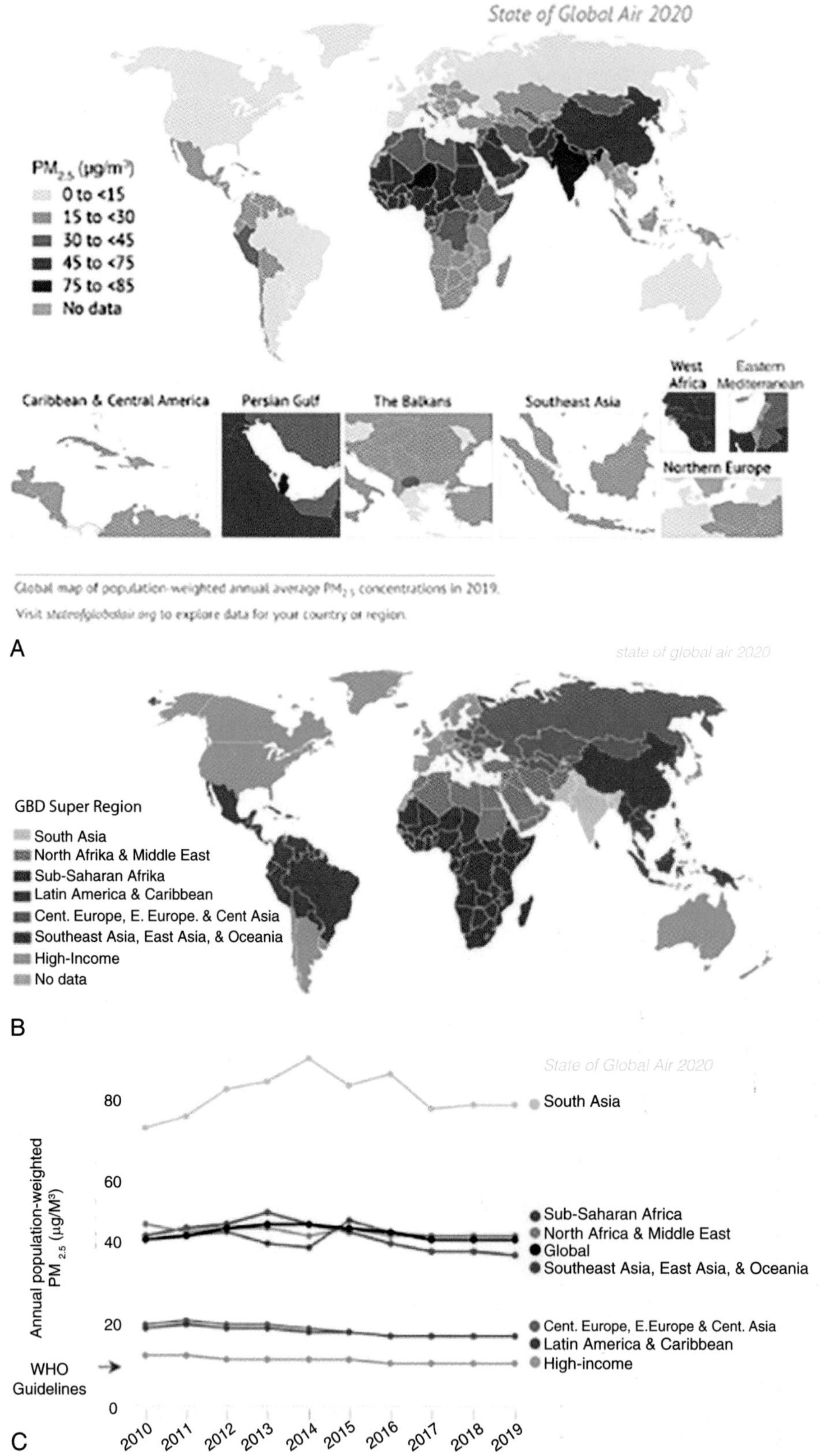

Fig. 2.19 Air Pollution Globally. (A) Global map of population-weighted annual average $PM_{2.5}$ concentrations in 2019. **(B)** Countries included in the seven Global Burden of Disease (GBD) Super Regions. That is, countries grouped by similar cause-of-death patterns. **(C)** Trends in population-weighted annual average PM 2.5 concentrations globally and in the GBD Super Regions, 2010–2019. (Data from Health Effects Institute. *State of Global Air 2020 Report.* Data source: Global Burden of Disease Study. IHME; 2020. https://www.stateofglobalair.org/resources, to explore data for a certain country or region.)

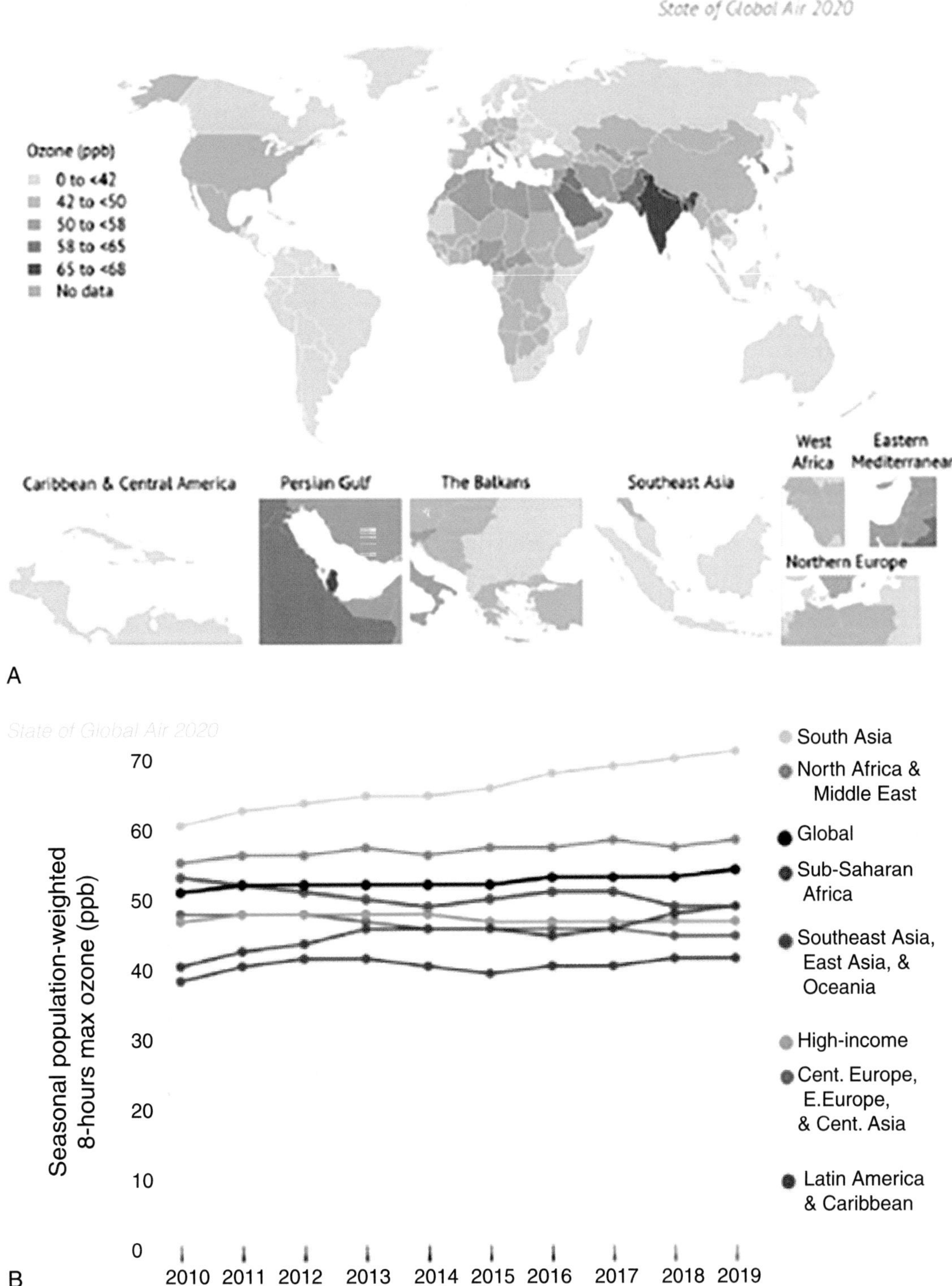

Fig. 2.20 Ozone Globally. **(A)** Global map of population-weighted average seasonal 8-hour maximum ozone concentrations in 2019. **(B)** Trends in population-weighted average seasonal 8-hour maximum ozone concentration globally and in the Global Burden of Disease (GBD) Super Regions, 2010–2019. (Data from Health Effects Institute. *State of Global Air 2020 Report*. Data source: Global Burden of Disease Study. IHME; 2020. https://www.stateofglobalair.org/resources.)

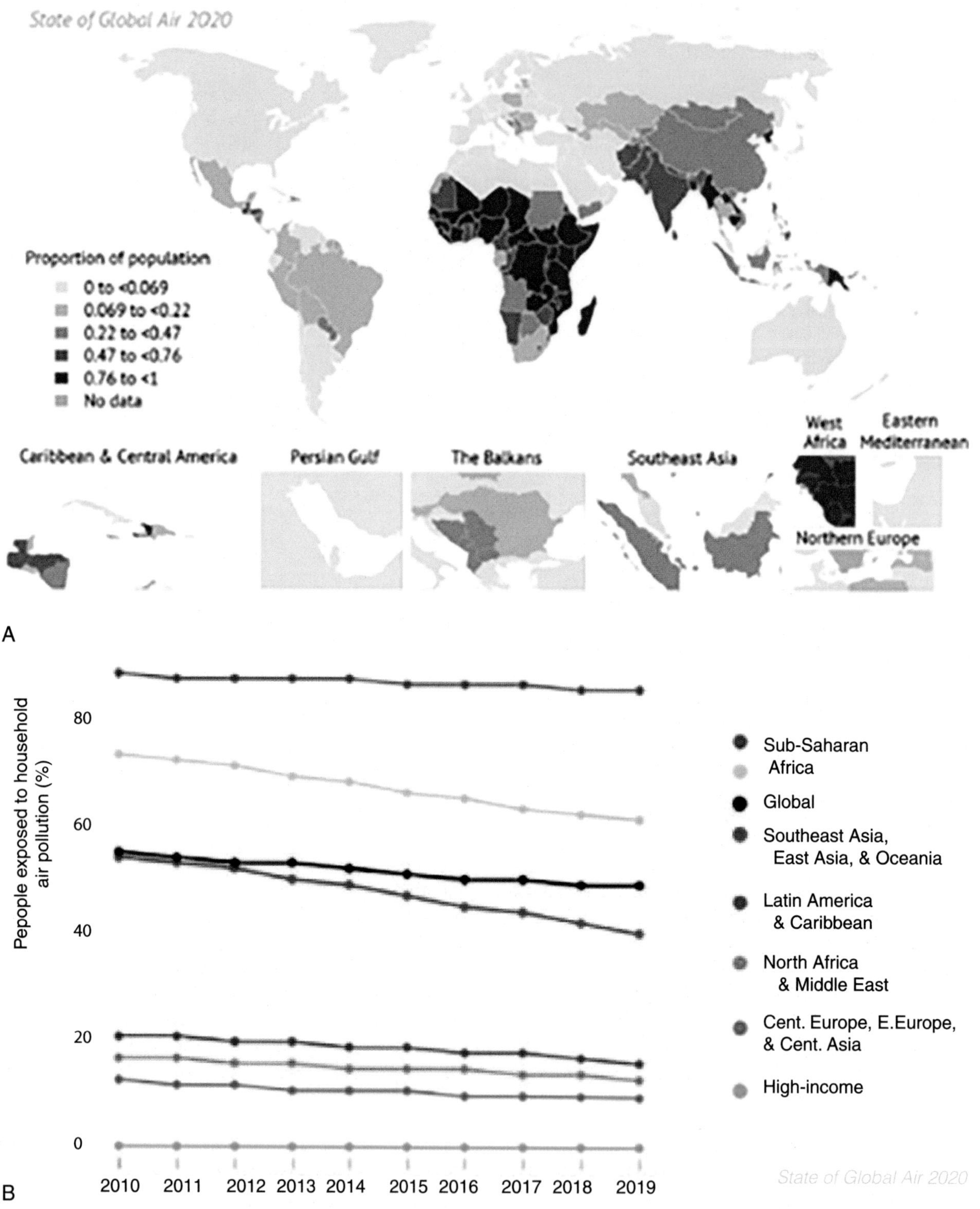

Fig. 2.21 Household Air Pollution. (A) Global map of the proportion of each country's population cooking with solid fuels in 2019. **(B)** Trends in the proportion of population cooking with solid fuels globally and in the GBD Super Regions, 2010–2019. (Data from Health Effects Institute. *State of Global Air 2020 Report*. Data source: Global Burden of Disease Study. IHME; 2020. https://www.stateofglobalair.org/resources.)

EMERGING SCIENCE BOX

Long-Term Exposure to Air Pollution and Increased Risk of Severe COVID-19 Outcomes

Past findings have indicated that long-term air pollution exposure (especially fine particulate matter, $PM_{2.5}$) increases the risk of severe outcomes during outbreaks of infectious diseases, such as with the 2003 outbreak of severe acute respiratory syndrome (SARS) caused by a type of coronavirus called SARS-CoV. Locations in China with "moderate or high long-term air pollution index (API) had SARS case fatality rates 126% and 71% higher, respectively than locations with low AP" (Cui et al., 2003). Late December 2019, an outbreak of a novel coronavirus, COVID-19 (close relative to SARS-CoV), originated in Wuhan, China, and then rapidly spread to many other countries. By late 2020, 215 countries and territories reported having cases of COVID-19. This disease mainly affects the respiratory system and lung function (same as SARS-CoV), but many cases have shown this virus to attack other parts of the body, such as the brain causing anosmia (loss of smell and taste); has formed blood clots causing stroke and heart attacks; and even damaged kidneys requiring persons to be on dialysis. A study *(pre-print)* conducted by researchers from the Harvard T.H. Chan School of Public Health (2020) has findings consistent with the study conducted in China by Cui et al. (2003). They found statistically significant evidence that an increase of 1 $\mu g/m^3$ in long-term $PM_{2.5}$ exposure was associated with an 8% increase in the COVID-19 mortality rate. Long-term exposure to $PM_{2.5}$ is associated with cardiovascular and respiratory comorbidities that have been found to dramatically increase the risk of death in COVID-19 affected individuals. All of these results highlight the importance of continuing to enforce existing air pollution regulations and to work on improving air quality in areas with the highest rates of air pollution-related deaths, such as in China or India.

Data from Cui Y, et al. Air pollution and case fatality of SARS in the People's Republic of China: An ecologic study. *Environmental Health,* 2003;2(1):15. doi:10.1186/1476-069X-2-15; Wu X, et al. Exposure to air pollution and COVID-19 mortality in the United States: A nationwide cross-sectional study. Preprint. medRxiv, 2020;2020.04.05.20054502. doi:10.1101/2020.04.05.20054502.

EMERGING SCIENCE BOX

Lead Poisoning

In 2012, the Centers for Disease Control and Prevention (CDC) updated recommendations on children's blood lead levels. The shift is to focus on primary prevention of lead exposure to reduce or eliminate dangerous and toxic sources in children's environments. At least 4 million households have children living in houses where they are being exposed to high levels of lead. Experts now use a reference level of 5 micrograms per deciliter (mcg/dL) to identify children with blood lead levels that are much higher than most children's levels. (This new level is based on the US population of children ages 1–5 years who are in the highest percentile [2.5% of children] when tested for lead.) The CDC will update the reference value every 4 years using the most recent National Health and Nutrition Examination Survey (NHANES) based on the 97.5th percentile of blood lead distribution in children.

The recommendation for when medical treatment is advised for children with high blood lead levels has not changed. Chelation therapy is recommended in a child with blood lead test result showing ≥45 mcg/dL.

Data from National Center for Environmental Health, Division of Environmental Health Science and Practice. *Childhood Lead Poisoning Program.* https://www.cdc.gov/nceh/lead/default.htm; Centers for Disease Control and Prevention (CDC). *Lead: What Do Parent's Need to Know to Protect Their Children?* Atlanta, GA; May 14, 2021. https://www.cdc.gov/nceh/lead/docs/lead-levels-in-children-fact-sheet-508.pdf.

1. Children have increased hand-to-mouth behavior and thus are prone to putting objects found in their environment into their mouths.
2. The blood–brain barrier in children is immature during fetal development, contributing to greater accumulation in the developing brain.
3. Infant absorption of lead is greater than that in adults. In adults, the body burden of lead is found in bone. In children, growth results in a rapid turnover in skeletal bone, causing a continuous leaching of lead into blood.[29,30]
4. In cases of compromised nutrition, where dietary intake of iron and calcium is insufficient, children are more likely to have elevated BLLs.[29]

Elevated BLLs in children are linked to cognitive deficits and behavioral changes, including antisocial behavior, acting out in school, and attention deficits.[29] These deficits can persist even after the individuals are no longer exposed to lead within their environment. Lead interferes with the normal remodeling of cartilage and bone in children (remodeling increases lead reintroduction). Radiologic studies often reveal *lead lines* in children. Lead accumulates in gums, causing hyperpigmentation. Particularly worrisome is lead exposure during pregnancy because the developing fetal nervous system is especially vulnerable to lead toxicity. Lead can cross the placental barrier, exposing the fetus *in utero*, which may result in significant cognitive impairment and subsequent learning disabilities.

From the most recent National Health and Nutrition Examination Survey (NHANES) data set, approximately 535,000 children between 1 and 5 years of age have an elevated blood lead concentration.[24,31] Blood levels of lead were defined by the Advisory Committee on Childhood Lead Poisoning Prevention of the CDC as greater than or equal to 5 mcg/dL based on the 97.5 percentile of blood lead concentrations.[32] The rates in adults of elevated BLLs in 2013 was 20.4 per 100,000 employed adults (16 years and older). These levels showed a blood lead concentration over 10 mcg/dL.[33] Higher risk occupations include metal welding, battery manufacturing and recycling, shipbuilding and shipbreaking, firing range instruction and bullet salvaging, lead smelting and refining, painting and construction work, pipefitting, and plumbing.[24,34] Less common exposures occur from contaminated pewter and ceramic dining ware, imported spices and cosmetics, folk remedies, ingestion of lead foreign bodies, and retained leaded bullets.[24,35] As demonstrated by the Flint, Michigan water crisis, soluble lead concentrations in drinking water can be at critical levels. Lead poisoning from degrading lead pipes is a

TABLE 2.6 Environmental Protection Agency Criteria of Ambient Air Pollutants

Air Pollutant	Criteria and Sources	Human Health Impacts
Carbon Monoxide (CO)	• Colorless, odorless gas • Sources: emitted during combustion processes, defective furnaces, occupation exposure (coal mining, firefighting, welding, engine repair), or exposure to tobacco smoke (first or secondhand)	• Unborn babies, infants, people with chronic heart disease or lung disease, and anemia are at the highest risk of CO poisoning • Causes reduction of oxygen delivery to organs, such as the heart and brain, by binding to hemoglobin (**carboxyhemoglobin**) reducing the blood's oxygen-carrying capacity • Disruption of cellular oxidative processes • Binding to myoglobin and hepatic cytochromes • Lipid peroxidation of brain lipids • At very high levels can cause death
Nitrogen Oxides (NO_X)	• Emitted from cars, trucks, buses, power plants, and off-road equipment • Industrial sources include power plants, industrial boilers, cement kilns, and turbines • Natural sources include biological decay processes and lightning strikes	• People with asthma, children, and the elderly are generally at greater risk for the health effects of NO_2 • Exposures over short periods can aggravate respiratory diseases, particularly asthma, leading to respiratory symptoms (such as coughing, wheezing or difficulty breathing) • Longer exposures to elevated concentrations of NO_2 may contribute to the development of asthma and potentially increase susceptibility to respiratory infections
Ground-level/Tropospheric Ozone (O_3)	• Ground-level ozone is created by chemical reactions between oxides of nitrogen (NOX) and volatile organic compounds (VOCs) in the presence of sunlight. • The main sources of NOX and VOCs are emissions from industrial facilities and electrical utilities, motor vehicle exhaust, gasoline vapors, and chemical solvents.	• People with asthma, children, older adults, and people active outdoors are highest health risk from inhalation of ozone • Can cause coughing and sore or scratchy throat • Inflame and damage the airways making it difficult to breathe deeply • Aggravate existing lung diseases • Increases frequency of asthma attacks
Particulate Matter (PM); PM_{10} and $PM_{2.5}$	• PM is a complex mixture of extremely small particles and liquid droplets that get into the air. • $PM_{2.5}$ poses the greatest risk to health and are the main cause of haze or reduced visibility. • Most particles form in the atmosphere as a result of combustion reactions from power plants, industries, and automobiles. • Over 90% of the world's population live in areas where ambient particulate matter ($PM_{2.5}$) levels are above the WHO guideline for healthy air	• Irritation of eyes, nose, and throat • Respiratory effects (asthma, bronchitis) • Cardiac arrhythmias and heart attacks • Can get deep into the lungs and even get into the bloodstream
Sulfur Dioxide (SO_2)	• Largest source of SO_2 in the atmosphere is the burning of fossil fuels by power plants and other industrial facilities • Smaller sources of SO_2 emissions include industrial processes such as extracting metal from ore • A natural source of SO_2 is from volcanic eruptions	• Children, the elderly, and those who have asthma are most sensitive to SO_2 health impacts • Short-term exposure can cause respiratory dysfunction and difficulty breathing • SO_2 can react with other compounds in the atmosphere to form fine particles that may get deep into the lungs causing additional health concerns
Lead	See text under Lead	See text under Lead

pervasive problem that needs immediate scientifically based, data-driven risk assessments that inform decisions involving drinking water systems.[36]

Pathophysiology. The pathogenic effects of lead are multifactorial and complex. Lead is an easily absorbed metal that binds to sulfhydryl groups in proteins and interferes with calcium (Ca^{++}) metabolism. A key event underlying the effects of lead exposure in humans is the alteration of cellular ion status (disruption of divalent cations, altered ion transport mechanisms, and disruption of protein function from displacement of metal enzyme cofactors). Because calcium (Ca++) is a crucial cell signal carrier and regulates critical cellular functions, its interference leads to hematologic, skeletal, neurologic, GI, and renal toxicities.[37] The change in intracellular Ca^{++} concentrations is most likely due to alterations in ion transport mechanisms and, importantly, the inhibition of transport proteins such as Na^+, K^+ - ATPase, and Ca^{++} channels. Specifically, Pb interferes with these proteins by displacing or competing with normal metal cofactors (e.g., lead binds to calcium-activated proteins with higher affinity than Ca^{++}) or through proteins important in Ca^{++}-dependent cell signaling (protein kinase C or calmodulin).[37] Lead disrupts other divalent metals, including zinc and magnesium, leading to alterations in neurotransmitter function, inhibiting heme synthesis, and, from impaired mitochondrial function, decreasing cellular energy. Lead is toxic to multiple enzyme systems. Lead causes abnormal conformational changes in the protein structure, resulting in altered protein functions.

Antagonism of normal metal ion functions by lead leads to oxidative stress.[37,38] Lead-induced oxidative stress is possibly the result of a multi-pathway process and results from binding to and subsequent inhibition of the function of *delta aminolevulinic acid dehydratase (ALAD)* because of competition of lead ions with normal zinc ions leading to the accumulation of *delta-aminolevulinic acid (δ-ALA)* in blood and urine. With accumulation of δ-ALA, it undergoes conformational protein change and autooxidation resulting in the generation of ROS.[38] Other sources of lead-induced oxidative stress are membrane lipid oxidation, NADPH oxidation, and antioxidant depletion.[37]

ROS causes the following changes:

- DNA damage, impaired DNA repair, cell apoptosis, or carcinogenesis
- Peroxidation of cell membrane lipids and cell damage
- Inactivation of enzyme proteins
- Prevention of protein folding
- Protein aggregation
- Conformational changes affecting cell structure and function and cause cell damage[38]

These *key* events from lead exposure affect the nervous, immune, endocrine, cardiovascular, musculoskeletal, renal, and reproductive systems and have negative developmental effects, such as delayed puberty onset, as well as cancer. A causal relationship is determined for lead and cardiovascular effects.[37]

Clinical Manifestations. Lead affects the nervous, cardiovascular, reproductive, endocrine, musculoskeletal (including teeth), renal, and immune systems. The clinical manifestations vary depending on the dose and chronicity of exposure. Most children are asymptomatic; however, the primary concern, even at low BLLs, is the intelligence quotient (IQ) scores and markers of academic achievement.[32,39,40]

Evaluation, Prevention, and Treatment. Diagnosis involves the medical history, clinical signs, and determination of routes of exposure. The main method of evaluation is laboratory analysis of the BLL. According to the CDC, experts now use a reference level of 5 mcg/dL to identify children with BLLs that are much higher than normal.[28]

The most important strategy for lowering exposures to lead is prevention. Prevention methods include individual and family prevention, preventive medicine, and public health. There is an urgent need to focus on preventive strategies, especially for fetal development and the developing child. The key for adults is prevention of exposures at the workplace and home. The main methods of treatment are removal of the source of exposure and, for those with high blood levels, chelation therapy. Additionally, treatment may include correcting deficiencies of iron, calcium, and zinc; irrigating the bowel; removing strategic bullets or shrapnel; and administering medications for control of seizures.

Cadmium and arsenic. See Table 2.7 for a summary of the toxic effects of cadmium and arsenic.

Mercury. Mercury (quicksilver) is a neurotoxic elemental metal liquid at room temperature and is widely present in the environment. Mercury is a global threat to human and environmental health. It can be released into the air, water, and soil through industrial processes, including mining, metal and cement production, fuel extraction, and combustions of fossil fuels (especially coal). Sources of exposure include natural geologic sources, vehicle emissions, consumer products, industrial waste, and landfills and disposal sites. Climate change and thawing of enormous areas of frozen lands may release long-stored mercury into lakes, rivers, and oceans.

Mercury also is found in dental amalgam; some vaccine preservatives; food products (e.g., rice); and terrestrial and marine animals, some of which are consumed by humans. The previously common practice of allowing school children to handle mercury in chemistry classes is no longer permitted. Similarly, the once ubiquitous mercury-filled household thermometer is being phased out of production. There are safe and cost-effective replacements for mercury for many healthcare applications and for pharmaceuticals; goals have been set to phase out some mercury-containing devices altogether. Since 2001, thimerosal (a preservative in multidose vials of vaccines containing ethyl mercury) was removed from childhood vaccines in the United States.[41]

There are three forms of mercury: metallic mercury (elemental mercury), inorganic mercury compounds (mostly mercuric chloride), and organic mercury. A prominent source of mercury is contaminated fish (mostly methylmercury, [MeHg]). Inorganic mercury is converted to organic mercury, such as methylmercury, by bacteria. Methylmercury enters the food chain and, in carnivorous fish (especially swordfish and shark), it may be concentrated to high levels greater than the surrounding water.[1]

Acute exposures from release of methylmercury from industrial sources caused the disaster at Minamata Bay and the Agano River in Japan and led to widespread mortality and morbidity. Known as *Minamata disease*, the disorders included deafness, blindness, intellectual disability, cerebral palsy, and central nervous system (CNS) defects in children exposed in utero. The developing brain is extremely sensitive to methylmercury.[1] Mercury is found in many species of fish, including grouper, tuna, seabass, marlin, halibut, tilefish, swordfish, shark, and king mackerel.[42] The FDA has recommended that women planning to become pregnant, pregnant women, nursing mothers, and young children avoid eating fish with a high mercury content (>1 part per million [ppm]), such as shark, swordfish, tile fish, and king mackerel. Fish that are lower in methylmercury include shrimp, canned light tuna, salmon, pollock, and

TABLE 2.7 Summary of Toxic Effects of Cadmium and Arsenic

Metals	Key Concepts
Arsenic	Arsenic salts were the poison of choice during the Renaissance in Italy. Deliberate poisoning by arsenic is rare today; however, its exposure is an important health concern in many areas worldwide. Arsenic is found naturally in soils and water and used in products (wood preservers, herbicides, agricultural products). It can be released from mines and smelting industries and may be present in some Chinese and Indian herbal medicines. Inorganic arsenic may be present in ground water with large concentrations found in Bangladesh, Chile, and China. Most toxic forms are the trivalent compounds arsenic trioxide, sodium arsenate, and arsenic trichloride. Arsenic trioxide is used as a therapy for acute promyelocytic leukemia; ingestion of large quantities of arsenic causes acute gastrointestinal, cardiovascular, and CNS toxicities that often are fatal. These effects are partially attributed to replacement of phosphates in ATP and interference of mitochondrial oxidative phosphorylation and the function of some proteins. Chronic exposure causes skin lesions (hyperpigmentation, hyperkeratosis) and the development of cancers (lung, bladder, skin). The mechanism for arsenic carcinogenesis has not been fully defined. Arsenic present in drinking water has been correlated with nonmalignant respiratory disease.
Cadmium	Compared with the other metals discussed, cadmium poisoning is a more modern problem. Pollution in the environment and occupationally is from mining, electroplating, and production of nickel-cadmium batteries, which are often disposed of in household waste. Food is an important source of cadmium because cadmium can contaminate soil and plants directly or from fertilizers and irrigation water. The most probable mechanism of toxicity is the generation of ROS. The main toxic effects of excess cadmium are obstructive lung disease and renal tubular damage. It also can cause skeletal abnormalities associated with calcium loss. In Japan, cadmium-containing water used to irrigate rice fields caused a disease in postmenopausal women known as "Itai-Itai" (ouch-ouch), a combination of osteoporosis and osteomalacia associated with renal disease. Cadmium is associated with higher risk of lung cancer in populations living near zinc smelters.

ATP, adenosine triphosphate; *CNS*, central nervous system; *ROS*, reactive oxygen species.
Data from Kumar V, Abbas A, Aster J, eds. *Robbins & Cotran pathologic basis of disease*, 9th edition. Philadelphia: Saunders; 2015.

catfish.[43] Like Pb, mercury binds with high affinity to sulfhydryl groups in some proteins, leading to tissue damage in the CNS and kidney.[1]

Lipid solubility of methylmercury and metallic mercury increases their accumulation in the brain, altering neuromotor, cognitive, and behavioral functions. An antioxidant, intracellular glutathione acting as a sulfhydryl donor, is the main protective mechanism from mercury-induced CNS and kidney damage.

Ethanol. Alcohol (ethanol) is the primary choice of mood-altering drugs available in the United States. According to the 2019 National Survey on Drug Use and Health (NSDUH), 85.6% of people aged 18 or older reported that they drank alcohol at some point in their lifetime; 69.5% reported that they drank in the past year; and 54.9% reported that they drank in the past month.[44] An estimated 95,000 people (approximately 68,000 men and 27,000 women) die from alcohol-related causes annually, making alcohol the third leading preventable cause of death in the United States. The first is tobacco, and the second is poor diet and physical inactivity.[45] A blood alcohol concentration of 80 mg/dL is the legal definition for driving while intoxicated in the United States. The amount of alcohol intake required to achieve this blood level will vary, depending on age, sex, percent body fat, metabolic rate, and genetically controlled factors influencing alcohol metabolism.[46]

Nutritional deficiencies remain one of the most frequent complications of alcohol-related disease. Although inadequate dietary intake is a significant cause of the vitamin deficiency, other possible mechanisms may also be involved. Alcohol is absorbed by diffusion in the stomach, duodenum, and jejunum. Chronic alcohol consumption breaks down the gut barrier function (causing leaky gut), which leads to impaired gut motility, delaying gastric emptying time; induces chemical gastritis; and increases the orocaecal transit time leading to impaired absorption of nutrients (e.g., folic acid, thiamine, vitamin B_6, magnesium, and phosphorus).[47,48] Folic acid deficiency, in particular, is problematic in persons consuming large quantities of alcohol. Ethanol alters folic acid (folate) homeostasis by decreasing intestinal absorption of folate, increasing liver retention of folate, and increasing the loss of folate through urinary and fecal excretion. Folic acid deficiency becomes especially serious when alcohol is consumed during pregnancy and may contribute to fetal alcohol syndrome.[49] Thiamine (vitamin B1) deficiencies result in significant neurologic sequela, common in persons with alcohol abuse. Wernicke encephalopathy is an acute neurological crisis that results from depleted thiamine stores and is characterized by the clinical triad of encephalopathy, oculomotor dysfunction, and gait ataxia.[47] Magnesium is the second most abundant micronutrient in the human body, and deficiency is almost universal in individuals with high levels of alcohol consumption and/or liver disease. Urinary excretion of magnesium is increased secondary to alcohol consumption, and total body stores of magnesium become depleted. Most of the alcohol ingested is metabolized to *acetaldehyde* in the liver. Acetaldehyde is a highly toxic substance and known carcinogen, with particular implications for head and neck cancer. It is responsible for both the acute effects of alcohol ingestion and for numerous disease processes associated with chronic alcohol consumption. The major pathway involves alcohol dehydrogenase (ADH), an enzyme located in the cytosol of hepatocytes. The microsomal ethanol-oxidizing system (MEOS) depends on cytochrome P-450 (CYP2E1), an enzyme needed for cellular oxidation. Activation of CYP2E1 requires a high ethanol concentration and thus is thought to be important in the accelerated ethanol metabolism (i.e., tolerance) noted in persons with chronic alcoholism (Fig. 2.22).

The major effects of acute alcoholism involve the CNS. The result of ethanol breakdown is thought to be the result of hepatic aldehyde dehydrogenase 2 (ALDH2) and contributes to alcohol's behavioral effects and alcoholism.[50] ALDH2 mediates low-dose ethanol induced increases in GABA levels, affecting tonic inhibition and alteration of balance and coordination skills.

After alcohol is ingested, it is absorbed, unaltered, from the stomach and small intestine. Fatty foods and milk slow absorption. After absorption, alcohol is distributed to all body tissues and fluids in direct proportion to blood concentration levels. Individuals differ widely in their capability to metabolize alcohol. Genetic differences in the hepatic metabolism of alcohol are related to levels of hepatic aldehyde dehydrogenases. There is considerable variability in alcohol tolerance among different ethnic groups. Persons with chronic alcoholism tend to develop an increased tolerance because of the enhanced production of metabolic enzymes.

Alcohol may exert both positive and negative effects on cardiovascular system. While numerous studies have validated the so-called *J-curve* or *U-shaped* inverse association between alcohol and overall or cardiovascular mortality, there are several factors that may modulate this effect. Among light to moderate drinkers, in the absence of binge drinking, mortality rates tend to be lower than in nondrinkers; mortality rates are higher among heavy drinkers. These findings, however, may be confounded by medical care and social relationships. The proposed mechanisms for observed cardiovascular benefit includes one or more of the following effects: increased levels of high-density lipoprotein–cholesterol (HDL-C), decrease in levels of low-density lipoprotein (LDL), prevention of clot formation, reduction in platelet aggregation, decrease in blood pressure, increase in coronary vessel vasodilation, increase in coronary blood flow, decrease in coronary inflammation, decrease in atherosclerosis, limited ischemia–reperfusion injury, and decreased diabetic vessel pathology. According to the Dietary Guidelines for Americans, recent evidence reveals that even drinking within the recommended limits may increase risks, including cancer, cardiovascular disease, and death.[51] The current recommendation is no more than two drinks per day for men and no more than one drink per day for women. One drink is defined as 12 oz 5% ABV beer, 5 oz 12% ABV wine, 1.5 oz of 40% ABV (80-proof) spirits, or 8 oz 7% ABV malt liquor.[52] Consuming

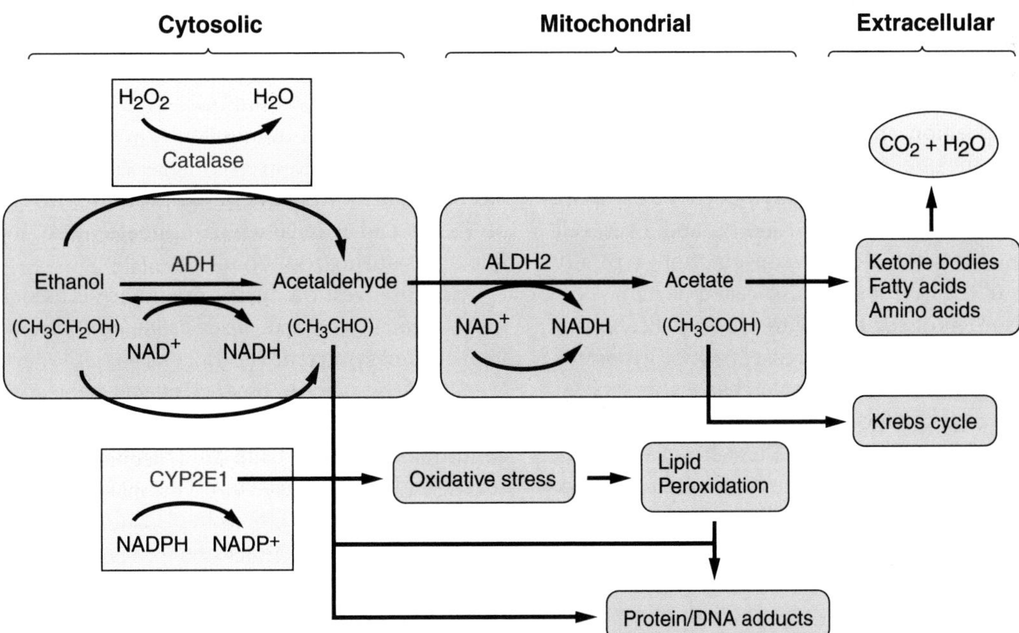

Fig. 2.22 Ethanol Metabolism Pathway. Ethanol is metabolized into acetaldehyde through the cytosolic enzyme alcohol dehydrogenase *(ADH)*, the microsomal enzyme cytochrome P-450 2E1 (CYP2E1), and the peroxisomal enzyme catalase. The ADH enzyme reaction is the main ethanol metabolic pathway involving an intermediate carrier of electrons, namely, nicotinamide adenine dinucleotide (NAD +), which is reduced by two electrons to form NADH. Acetaldehyde is metabolized mainly by aldehyde dehydrogenase 2 (ALDH2) in the mitochondria to acetate and NADH before being cleared into the systemic circulation. (Adapted from Zhang Y, Ren J. ALDH2 in alcoholic heart diseases: Molecular mechanism and clinical implications. *Pharmacology and Therapeutics*, 2011;132[1]:86–92.)

alcohol in greater than recommended amounts is associated with numerous health hazards, including increased risk for alcoholism, high blood pressure, obesity, stroke, breast cancer, suicide, and accidents.

Acute alcohol intoxication (drunkenness) primarily affects the CNS, causing dose-related CNS depression. Alcohol consumption induces varying levels of sedation, drowsiness, loss of motor coordination, delirium, altered behavior, and loss of consciousness. Alcohol blood levels of approximately 200 g/dL causes drowsiness, and toxic blood levels (300 to 400 mg/dL) result in a lethal coma or respiratory arrest caused by medullary center depression. Additionally, acute alcoholism may induce reversible hepatic and gastric changes.[1]

Binge drinking, defined as four standard alcoholic drinks on one occasion for women and five drinks for men, has significant health hazards. Chronic drinking and binge drinking cause alcoholic liver disease (ALD) with the spectrum ranging from *hepatic steatosis* (fatty change) and *steatohepatitis* (fatty and inflammatory changes) to cirrhosis of the liver. These alterations can lead to hepatocellular carcinoma. Alcohol can induce damage to mitochondrial DNA, lipid accumulation, and oxidative stress. Additionally, there is evidence that alcohol drinking in adolescents, especially binge drinking, can result in neurocognitive changes affecting both gray and white brain matter and may result in risk-taking behaviors.

Chronic alcoholism causes structural alterations in practically all organs and tissues in the body because most tissues contain enzymes capable of ethanol oxidation or nonoxidative metabolism. The most significant changes, however, occur in the liver. Excessive consumption of alcohol is the leading cause of alcohol-related liver disease, morbidity, and mortality.[53] Hepatic changes, initiated by acetaldehyde, are far reaching and include inflammation, fat deposition, and liver enlargement. On the cellular level, changes include protein transport malfunctions, increased intracellular water, decreased mitochondrial fatty acid oxidation, excessive membrane rigidity, and liver cell necrosis. Chronic, excessive alcohol consumption typically results in cirrhosis of the liver and the associated portal hypertension. Other disorders associated with chronic alcoholism include alcoholic cardiomyopathy; increased risk of hypertension, gastritis, and pancreatitis; regressive changes in skeletal muscle; and an increased risk for oral, esophagus, pharynx, larynx, liver, and breast cancer (Fig. 2.23).[54] The risk is even greater with concurrent smoking or use of smokeless tobacco. Chronic alcoholism can lead to massive bleeding from gastritis, gastric ulcer, and esophageal varices (associated with cirrhosis).

Over long periods, excessive alcohol intake weakens the immune system, putting persons at increased risk of a variety of immune defects, including cytokine production, inflammation, increased susceptibility to infection, increased incidence and severity of pneumonia, and enhanced progression of human immunodeficiency disease.[55–57] The immune system is weakened because chronic ethanol abuse causes a decrease in the number of circulating T cells (responsible for cell mediated immunity) and B cells (responsible for antibody-mediated immunity). Despite reduced B-cell numbers, serum concentrations of immunoglobulins (IgA, IgG, and IgE) are increased. In

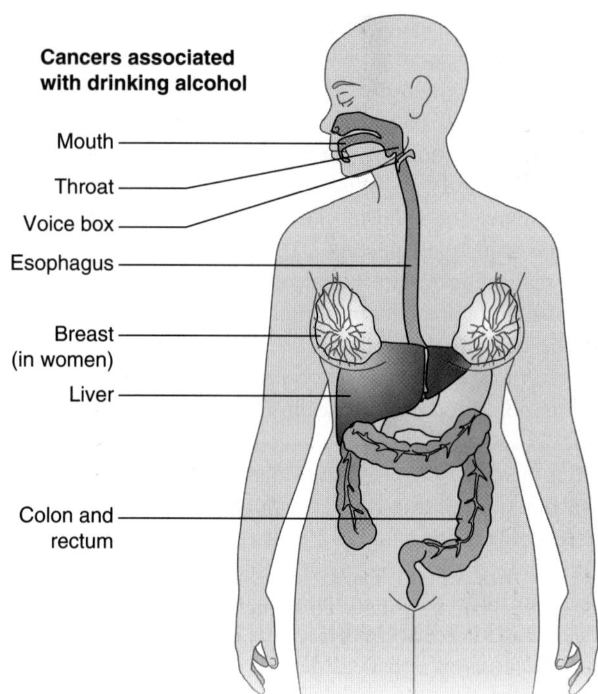

Fig. 2.23 Cancers Associated with Drinking Alcohol. (Data from National Cancer Institute Alcohol and Cancer Risk National Cancer Institute, National Institutes of Health. U.S. Department of Health and Human Services; 2018. https://www.cancer.gov/about-cancer/causes-prevention/risk/alcohol/alcohol-fact-sheet. Accessed October 1, 2021.)

particular, the levels of antibodies against liver-specific autoantigens are increased in individuals with ALD, which may promote alcohol-related liver damage. Alcohol exposure in utero has been shown to interfere significantly with the development of T cells and B cells, which ultimately may increase risk for infections during adulthood.[55]

Alcohol ingestion during pregnancy is associated with *cognitive deficiencies* and *neurobehavioral disorders*, including fetal alcohol syndrome (FAS). Fetal alcohol spectrum disorders (FASDs) are a range of physical effects, behavioral disorders, or cognitive deficits caused by prenatal alcohol exposure. These conditions can range from mild to severe with FAS at the more severe end of the spectrum. Conservative estimates indicate that up to 1 in 20 U.S. schoolchildren may be affected by FASDs, making these disorders more common than autism spectrum disorder, currently estimated to affect 1 in 54 children.[58,59]

FAS syndrome is characterized by growth retardation, facial anomalies, cognitive impairment, and ocular malformations. A diagnosis of FAS is made based on identifying one or more structural, neurologic, or functional CNS abnormalities (e.g., small head size, problems with attention and hyperactivity, poor coordination); prenatal or postnatal growth deficit in height, weight, or both; and abnormal facial features (e.g., smooth philtrum (ridge between nose and upper lip, thin vermillion border, and small palpebral fissures) (Fig. 2.24) with confirmed prenatal

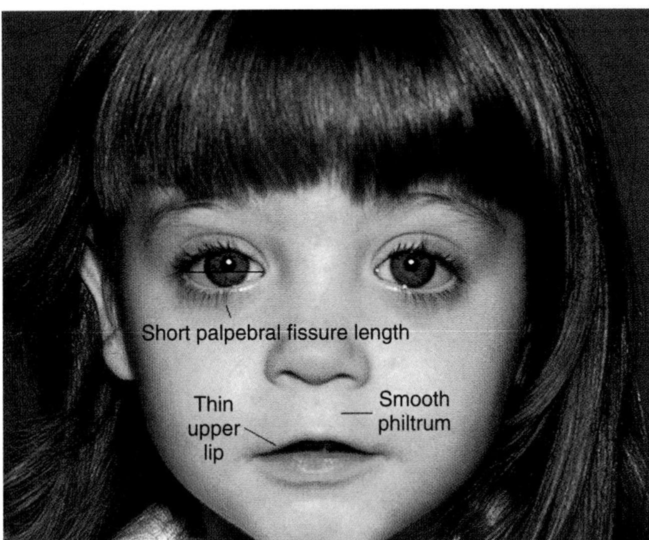

Fig. 2.24 Diagnostic Facial Features of Fetal Alcohol Syndrome. Three diagnostic facial features of fetal alcohol syndrome: (1) short palpebral fissure lengths, (2) smooth philtrum, and (3) thin upper lip. (© 2022 Susan (Astley) Hemingway PhD, University of Washington.)

alcohol exposure; although confirmation is not required to make a diagnosis.[60] Alcohol readily crosses the placenta, reaching the fetus in 1 to 2 hours, and produces fetal blood levels that are equivalent to maternal alcohol levels. Amniotic fluid acts as a reservoir for alcohol, prolonging fetal exposure.[61] Overall, maternal ingestion of alcohol can be catastrophic for the developing fetus. Autopsies of children with FAS have revealed widespread, severe damage, including failure of certain brain regions to develop, malformations of brain tissue, and failure of certain cells to migrate to their necessary location during development.[62] Imaging studies reveal that in addition to an overall reduction in brain size, the corpus callosum is reduced in size or missing, the cerebellum is significantly reduced in size, and the basal ganglia and caudate nucleus are significantly reduced.

Social or Street Drugs

The social or recreational use of psychoactive and narcotic drugs is a major problem in many parts of the world. Popular drugs are methamphetamine ("meth"), marijuana, cocaine, heroin, and, increasingly, fentanyl. Many of these drugs have a high risk for addiction and dependence, and some can cause respiratory distress and death. The 10 drugs most frequently involved in overdose deaths include heroin, oxycodone, methadone, morphine, hydrocodone, and fentanyl; the benzodiazepines alprazolam and diazepam; and the stimulants cocaine and methamphetamine.[63] Although opiates, both prescription and illicit, are causes of drug overdose deaths, recent increases in drug overdose deaths are driven by continuing increases in synthetic opioids other than methadone, such as illicitly manufactured fentanyl (IMF) (Fig. 2.25).[64] Overall, drug overdose deaths rose from 2018 to 2019, with 70,630 deaths reported in 2019.

Opioid-involved overdose deaths rose from 21,088 in 2010 to 47,600 in 2017 and remained steady in 2018 with 46,802 deaths. A significant increase occurred in 2019 to 49,860 overdose deaths.[65]

Although this increase affected all ethnic groups, non-Hispanic whites experienced the most devastating increase, with adults ages 45 to 54 suffering the highest rates of mortality, according to the National Center for Health Services.[63] Increases in drug overdose deaths are seen more in males, with female rates remaining steady. Drug overdoses from heroin and natural and semisynthetic opioids (e.g., oxycodone and hydrocodone) have started to decline over the last several years.[66]

Unintentional and Intentional Injuries

Unintentional and intentional injuries are an important health problem in the United States. In 2019, there were 220,551 deaths from injury. This breaks down to 173,040 deaths from unintentional injury (3rd leading cause of death in the United States) and another 47,511 deaths from intentional injury (10th leading cause of death in the United States).[67] In 2019. the number of deaths because of unintentional poisoning was 65,773, at a rate of 20.0 deaths per 100,000. Motor vehicle accident-related deaths accounted for 37,595, with a rate of 11.5 deaths per 100,000. Fatalities caused by firearms in 2018 were 39,740, with many more individuals reporting nonfatal firearm-related injuries.[67] The rate of deaths attributable to drug overdose in 2019 was reported to be 70,630, with a rate of 21.6 per 100,000.[66]

Death rates because of unintentional falls were reported, in 2019, to be 39,433, or a rate of 12.0 per 100,000, which has continued to increase over the last 5 years. Fall death rates increased 30% from 2007 to 2016 for older adults. Each year 7 million individuals are treated in emergency departments for fall injuries, with 3.1 million being greater than age 65.[68] More than 95% of hip fractures are caused by falls, and falls are the leading cause of traumatic brain injuries (TBI).

Sexual violence affects millions of people each year in the United States. Specifically, more than 1 in 3 women and nearly 1 in 4 men have experienced sexual violence involving physical contact. Furthermore, 1 out of every 5 women and 1 in 38 men have experienced an attempted or completed rape.[69] In 2019, rape or sexual assault victimizations declined to 1.7 per 1000 from 2.7 per 1000 persons aged 12 or older in 2018.[70] Child sexual abuse is when a child younger than 18 years of age experiences sexual violence without consent. Sexual violence includes sex trafficking, which is the use of force, fraud, or coercion to make an individual engage in commercial sex.[69] Sports- and recreation-related injuries accounted for 2.7 million visits to the emergency department between 2010 and 2016 for individuals 5 to 24 years of age. The top five most frequent activities that caused ED visits for sports injuries were football (14.1%), basketball (12.5%), pedal cycling (9.9%), soccer (7.1%), and ice or roller skating or skateboarding (6.9%).[71]

The 10 leading causes of death (heart disease, cancer, unintentional injuries, chronic lower respiratory diseases, stroke, Alzheimer disease, diabetes, influenza and pneumonia, kidney disease, and suicide) have remained constant over the last few years. These 10 leading causes accounted for 73.8% of all deaths in the United States in 2018.[72]

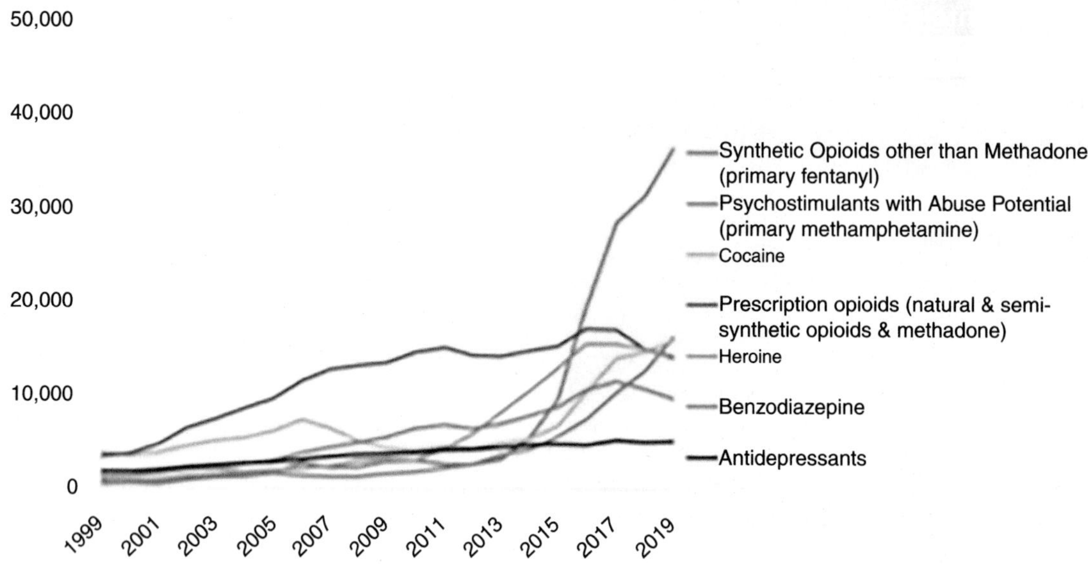

Fig. 2.25 Drug-Involved Overdose Deaths by Specific Category All Ages, 1999–2019. (From Centers for Disease Control and Prevention, National Center for Health Statistics. Multiple Cause of Death 1999–2019 on CDC WONDER Online Database, released December 2020. https://wonder.cdc.gov/controller/datarequest/D77.)

In 2020, COVID-19 was the third leading cause of death, following heart disease and cancer, respectively. The COVID-19 pandemic caused approximately 375,000 deaths in the United States during 2020. The overall age-adjusted death rate in 2020 increased by 15.9%. Overall death rates were highest among non-Hispanic Black persons and non-Hispanic American Indian or Alaska Native persons.[73]

Unintentional injury is the fourth leading cause of death and highest among those between ages 1 and 34 years; intentional injury (suicide, homicide) ranks between the second and fourth leading causes of death in these age groups. Unintentional hospital-acquired conditions do occur and can have severe consequences, including death and long-term injury, as well as contribute to adverse mental and emotional effects on the individual and the healthcare providers.[74] Examples of hospital-acquired conditions include adverse drug events, catheter-associated urinary tract infections, central-line-associated bloodstream infections, pressure injuries, and surgical site infections, among others. The magnitude of healthcare-associated morbidity and mortality can be linked to healthcare-associated infections (HAI). While progress has been made to decrease HAI, every year, 1 in 25 hospitalized persons will acquire at least one infection related to hospital care; additional infections occur in other healthcare settings.[75] Many HAIs are caused by antibiotic-resistant microbials, which lead to complications such as sepsis and eventually death.

The Agency for Health Care Research and Quality (AHRQ) report found that overall hospital-acquired infections and adverse drug events dropped from 99 per 1000 acute care discharges to 86 per 1000 discharges between 2014 and 2017, representing a decrease in 910,000 healthcare-associated conditions. Opportunities to improve patient safety by reducing infections, pressure injuries, and other healthcare-related conditions exist.[76]

Medical errors are a serious public health problem and a leading cause of death in the United States.[77] It is challenging to know a consistent cause of errors and minimize the effects on patient safety. According to the WHO, globally, as many as 4 in 10 persons are harmed in primary and outpatient health care.[78] In high-income countries, it is estimated that 1 in 10 persons is harmed while receiving hospital care,[79] and nearly 50% of harms are preventable.[80] The most detrimental errors are related to diagnosis, prescription, and the use of medicines.[79] Recognizing, improving, and ensuring patient safety is a growing challenge to health service delivery. The 72nd World Health Assembly in 2019 adapted resolution WHA72.6 on global action on patient safety, the Global Patient Safety Action Plan 2021 to 2030. It has urged member states, and where applicable, regional economic integration organizations to recognize patient safety as a health priority.[81] Maintaining a culture that works toward recognizing safety challenges and implementing solutions, rather than harboring a culture of blame, shame, and punishment, is important. Healthcare organizations and hospitals need a culture that focuses on patient safety and system improvement by viewing medical errors as challenges that must be overcome.[77]

The more common terms used to describe and classify unintentional and intentional injuries, and brief descriptions of important features of these injuries are presented in Table 2.8.

Asphyxiation

Asphyxial injuries are caused by the failure of cells to receive or use oxygen. Deprivation of oxygen may be partial *(hypoxia)* or total *(anoxia)*. Asphyxiation can be grouped into four general categories: *suffocation, strangulation, chemical asphyxiants*, and *drowning*.

Suffocation. Suffocation, or the process of dying as a result of lack of oxygen, can result from either a *lack of oxygen in the*

TABLE 2.8 Unintentional and Intentional Injuries

Type of Injury	Description
Blunt-Force Injuries 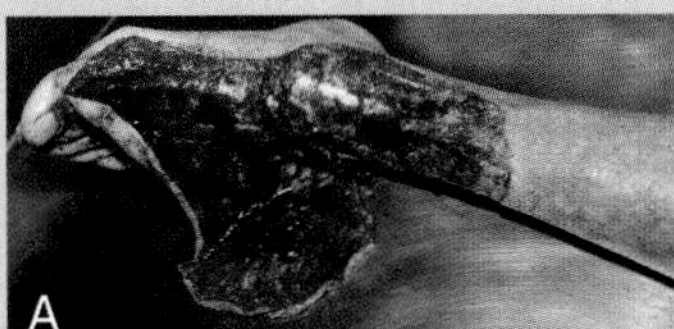	Mechanical injury to body resulting in tearing, shearing, or crushing; most common type of injury seen in healthcare settings; caused by blows or impacts; motor vehicle accidents and falls most common cause (see Photo A) *Contusion (bruise):* Bleeding into skin or underlying tissues; initial color will be red-purple, then blue-black, then yellow-brown or green; duration of bruise depends on extent, location, and degree of vascularization; bruising of soft tissue may be confined to deeper structures; *hematoma* is collection of blood in soft tissue; *subdural hematoma* is blood between inner surface of dura mater and surface of brain; can result from blows, falls, or sudden acceleration/deceleration of head as occurs in *shaken baby syndrome; epidural hematoma* is collection of blood between inner surface of skull and dura; is most often associated with a skull fracture *Laceration:* Tear or rip resulting when tensile strength of skin or tissue is exceeded; is ragged and irregular with abraded edges; an extreme example is *avulsion*, where a wide area of tissue is pulled away; lacerations of internal organs are common in blunt-force injuries; lacerations of liver, spleen, kidneys, and bowel occur from blows to abdomen; thoracic aorta may be lacerated in sudden deceleration accidents; severe blows or impacts to chest may rupture heart with lacerations of atria or ventricles *Fracture:* Blunt-force blows or impacts can cause bone to break or shatter (see Chapter 44)
Sharp-Force Injuries 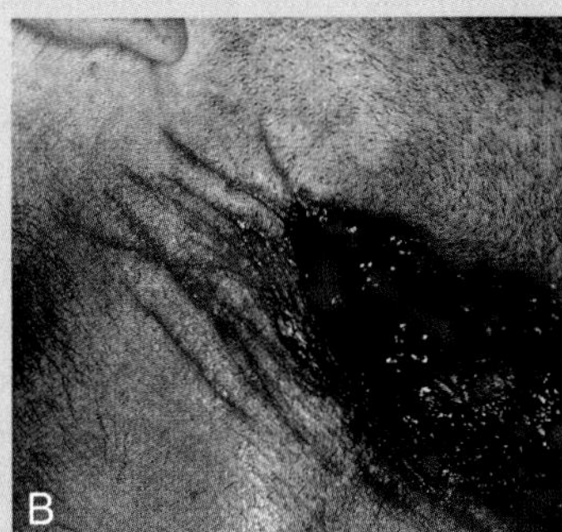	Cutting and piercing injuries accounted for 2734 deaths in 2007; men have a higher rate (1.37/100,000) compared with women (0.44/100,000); differences by race are as follows: whites 0.71/100,000; blacks 2.12/100,000; and other groups 0.80/100,000 *Incised wound:* A wound that is *longer* than it is *deep;* wound can be straight or jagged with sharp, distinct edges without abrasion; usually produces significant external bleeding with little internal hemorrhage; these wounds are noted in sharp-force injury suicides; in addition to a deep, lethal cut, there will be superficial incisions in same area called *hesitation marks* (see Photo B) *Stab wound:* A penetrating sharp-force injury that is *deeper* than it is *long;* if a sharp instrument is used, depths of wound are clean and distinct but can be abraded if object is inserted deeply and wider portion (e.g., hilt of a knife) impacts skin; depending on size and location of wound, external bleeding may be surprisingly small; after an initial spurt of blood, even if a major vessel or heart is struck, wound may be almost completely closed by tissue pressure, thus allowing only a trickle of visible blood despite copious internal bleeding *Puncture wound:* Instruments or objects with sharp points but without sharp edges produce puncture wounds; classic example is wound of foot after stepping on a nail; wounds are prone to infection, have abrasion of edges, and can be very deep *Chopping wound:* Heavy, edged instruments (axes, hatchets, propeller blades) produce wounds with a combination of sharp- and blunt-force characteristics
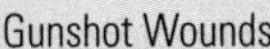 Gunshot Wounds 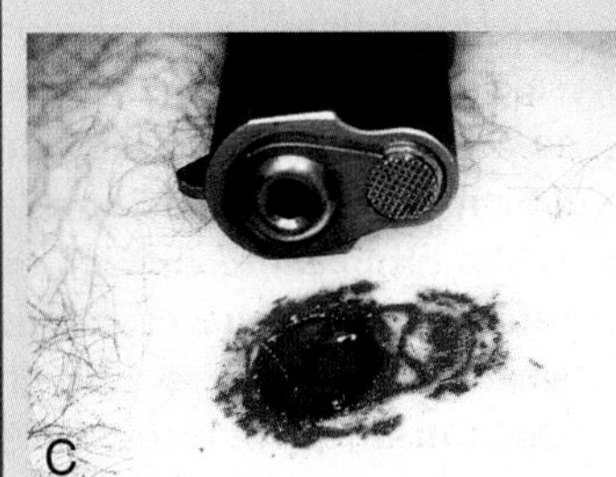 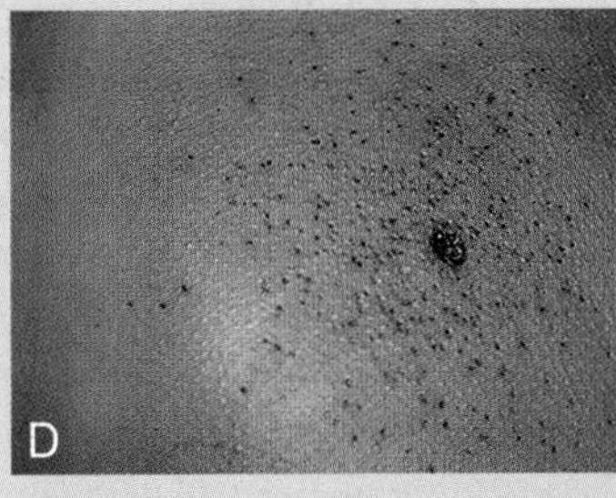	Accounted for >33,636 deaths in the United States in 2015; men more likely to die compared with women (18.16 vs. 2.73/100,000); black men ages 15–24 years have greatest death rate (86.95/100,000); gunshot wounds are either penetrating (bullet remains in body) or perforating (bullet exits body); bullet also can fragment; most important factors or appearances are whether it is an entrance or exit wound and range of fire *Entrance wound:* All wounds share some common features; overall appearance is most affected by range of fire *Contact range entrance wound:* Distinctive type of wound when gun is held so muzzle rests on or presses into skin surface; there is searing of edges of wound from flame and soot or smoke on edges of wound in addition to hole; hard contact wounds of head cause severe tearing and disruption of tissue (because of thin layer of skin and muscle overlying bone); wound is gaping and jagged, known as *blow back;* can produce a patterned abrasion that mirrors weapon used (see Photo C) *Intermediate (distance) range entrance wound:* Surrounded by gunpowder tattooing or stippling; *tattooing* results from fragments of burning or unburned pieces of gunpowder exiting barrel and forcefully striking skin; *stippling* results when gunpowder abrades but does not penetrate skin (see Photo D) *Indeterminate range entrance wound:* Occurs when flame, soot, or gunpowder does not reach skin surface, but bullet does; *indeterminate* is used rather than *distant* because appearance may be same regardless of distance; for example, if an individual is shot at close range through multiple layers of clothing, the wound may look the same as if the shooting occurred at a distance *Exit wound:* Has the same appearance regardless of range of fire; most important factors are speed of projectile and degree of deformation; size cannot be used to determine whether hole is an exit or entrance wound; usually has clean edges that can often be reapproximated to cover defect; skin is one of toughest structures for a bullet to penetrate; thus it is not uncommon for a bullet to pass entirely through body but stopp just beneath skin on "exit" side *Wounding potential of bullets:* Most damage done by a bullet is a result of amount of energy transferred to tissue impacted; speed of bullet has much greater effect than increased size; some bullets are designed to expand or fragment when striking an object, for example, *hollow-point* ammunition; lethality of a wound depends on what structures are damaged; wounds of brain may not be lethal; however, they are usually immediately incapacitating and lead to significant long-term disability; a person with a "lethal" injury (wound of heart or aorta) also may not be immediately incapacitated

environment or from a *blockage of the respiratory airways* (see Choking Asphyxiation section below). Persons can become entrapped in an enclosed space that is lacking in adequate oxygen. This scenario will occur if a child becomes trapped in an abandoned refrigerator or if a toddler's head becomes entangled in a plastic bag. Both scenarios have been linked to fatalities. Unintentional suffocation is the leading cause of injury death among infants <1 year old in the United States, and about 82% are attributable to accidental suffocation and strangulation in bed. Investigators analyzed data from 2011 to 2014 and found cases were most frequently attributed to soft bedding (69%), followed by overlay (19%) and wedging. Soft bedding deaths occurred most often in an adult bed (49%), in a prone position (82%), with a blanket/s obstructing the airway (34%). Overlay deaths occurred most often in an adult bed (71%), overlaid by the mother (47%). Wedging deaths occurred most often when the infant became entrapped between the mattress and a wall (48%).[82] Suffocation also can occur when another gas displaces oxygen in the environment. Methane, the largest component of sewer gas, has caused fatal asphyxiation when it has displaced atmospheric oxygen. Children have died from methane asphyxiation shortly after falling into a pit containing sewage; rescue workers have a very narrow time frame in which to save the child. Volcanos have been known to belch carbon dioxide (CO_2) gas in amounts sufficient to displace the normal oxygen level in the atmosphere for several miles, resulting in widespread death of humans and animals within the area. Normal ambient oxygen level in the atmosphere is 21%. A reduction to a level of 16% poses immediate danger. If the level drops below 5%, death can ensue within minutes. History and forensic examination are important in diagnosing suspected asphyxiation because even autopsy may not demonstrate specific physical findings in such cases.

Choking asphyxiation occurs when there is an obstruction of the pulmonary airways. An object may become lodged in a large airway, directly obstructing breathing. Injury or disease also may result from soft tissue swelling surrounding the airway, leading to a partial or complete obstruction and subsequent asphyxiation. Treatment requires locating and removing the obstructing object immediately or, in the case of airway swelling, reversing the swelling before asphyxiation occurs. *Compressional asphyxiation* occurs when mechanical compression of the chest or abdomen prevents normal respiratory movements. Usual signs and symptoms include florid facial congestion and *petechiae* (pinpoint skin hemorrhages) of the eyes and face. An individual entrapped beneath a heavy object, which impairs chest expansion, may become asphyxiated.

Strangulation. Strangulation is caused by compression of the blood vessels and air passages resulting from external pressure on the neck. The compression causes hypoxia from impaired blood flow to the brain. The amount of force needed to compress the jugular veins (2 kg) or carotid arteries (5 kg) is significantly less than the force required to crush the trachea (15 kg). Injury or death, which occurs secondary to strangulation, results from the impaired cerebral blood flow, not from lack of airflow. With a complete blockage of the carotid arteries, unconsciousness will typically occur within 10 to 15 seconds.

Hanging strangulation occurs when a noose or similar object is placed around the neck, after which the support under the victim's feet is suddenly removed so that the body falls freely. Death or severe injury results as the noose tightens, cutting off airflow through the trachea. Hanging strangulation is usually an intentional event, such as suicide, homicide, or a judicial hanging. However, it can also be accidental. This form of strangulation typically produces severe soft tissue injury and cervical spinal trauma. The body does not need to be completely suspended for death to occur. Hanging may cause petechiae in the eyes or face; however, this finding is uncommon. More typically, an inverted V-shaped ligature mark about the neck is seen at autopsy.

Ligature strangulation does not require suspension. Instead, some form of cord encircles and tightens about the neck. This event may be intentional, as in the case of homicide with use of a garrote from behind the victim. It also may be accidental, as when a child becomes accidentally entangled in cords of window blinds. Autopsy will reveal a horizontal mark about the neck, without an inverted V pattern. Petechiae are more common in this scenario because intermittent opening and closure of the blood vessels may occur as a result of the victim's struggle. Internal injuries of the neck are rare.

Manual strangulation occurs when an assailant's hands compress the neck of the victim to the point where death by asphyxiation occurs. There is evidence of variable amounts of external trauma to the neck. Contusions and abrasions are either caused directly by the assailant or by the victim clawing at their own neck in an attempt to remove the assailant's hands. Internal damage can be quite severe; bruising of deep structures, including fractures of the hyoid bone, the tracheal cartilage, and the cricoid cartilages occur. Petechiae are common. Non-fatal strangulation (NFS) can be a cause of serious injury.[83]

Chemical asphyxiants. A number of substances can act as chemical asphyxiants. They either prevent the delivery of oxygen to the tissues or block oxygen utilization. Carbon monoxide is the most common chemical asphyxiant. Carbon monoxide (CO) is an odorless, colorless, nonirritating, and undetectable gas; it is often mixed with a visible or odorous compound. CO is produced by incomplete combustion of fuels, such as gasoline. CO produces hypoxic injury, specifically, oxygen deprivation. As a systemic asphyxiant, CO causes death by inducing CNS depression. Normally, oxygen molecules are carried to tissues bound to the hemoglobin in RBCs. Because the affinity of CO for hemoglobin is 300 times greater than that of oxygen, CO quickly binds with hemoglobin, preventing oxygen molecules from binding to hemoglobin, and they are thus transported to tissues. Minute amounts of CO can produce a significant percentage of *carboxyhemoglobin* (carbon monoxide bound with hemoglobin). With increasing levels of carboxyhemoglobin, hypoxia occurs insidiously, evoking widespread ischemic changes in the CNS. Individuals are often unaware of exposure. Death may occur in an individual who believes they are simply feeling sleepy; thus no evasive action is taken. The use of CO monitors in homes is therefore strongly recommended. Diagnosis can be made from the measurement of carboxyhemoglobin levels in blood. Victims of CO poisoning may have a cherry red coloration to the skin and mucous membranes.

Symptoms related to CO poisoning include headache, giddiness, tinnitus (ringing in the ears), chest pain, confusion, nausea, weakness, and vomiting. CO is an environmental air pollutant found in combustion fumes produced by cars and trucks, small gasoline engines, stoves, gas ranges, gas refrigerators, heating systems, lanterns, burning charcoal or wood, and cigarette smoke. Chronic exposure can occur in people working in confined spaces, such as underground garages and tunnels. Fumes can accumulate in enclosed or semi-enclosed spaces. Individuals most susceptible to CO poisoning are fetuses, infants, and people with chronic heart disease, respiratory problems, and anemia.

Cyanide is an extremely toxic salt. Cyanide acts as an asphyxiant by combining with the ferric (iron) ion in hemoglobin, facilitating its transport to tissues. When present in tissues, cyanide inhibits the formation of cytochrome oxidase by interrupting the electron transport chain within the mitochondria. As a result, the mitochondria can no longer aerobically generate ATP, and oxygen can no longer bind to the final molecule in the electron transport chain. The host dies from oxygen deprivation, even though abundant oxygen may be present. As with CO poisoning, victims of cyanide poisoning may have a cherry red coloration to the skin and mucus membranes. With the presence of cyanide, an odor of bitter almonds may be detected; however, the ability to smell cyanide is a genetic trait that is present in only 20% to 40% of the general population.

Hydrogen sulfide, one of several sewer gases, is a chemical asphyxiant and neurotoxin; it interferes with the body's ability to carry oxygen. It has a characteristic "rotten egg" odor that is detectable even at very low levels. Victims of hydrogen sulfide poisoning may have brown-tinged blood in addition to the nonspecific signs of asphyxiation. Methane, another sewer gas, is nontoxic but readily causes asphyxiation by displacing oxygen. Because of the presence of asphyxiant gases, caution is indicated when working in areas containing septic tanks, cesspools, and manure pits. Numerous fatalities have occurred in persons working in these environments.

Drowning. Drowning is death from inhalation of and suffocation by a liquid, usually water. Drowning ranks fifth among the unintentional injury death in the United States[84] and is the third leading cause of unintentional injury death worldwide, accounting for 7% of all injury-related deaths.[85,86] An estimated 236,000 annual drowning deaths occur worldwide. In the United States, drowning is the second leading cause of unintentional injury death in children aged 1 to 14 years. Males have the highest risk of drowning, with twice the mortality rate of females.[85] The major mechanism of injury is hypoxemia (low blood oxygen levels). Contrary to previous prevailing views, there is no evidence that drowning deaths result from fluid and electrolyte disturbances or from blood hemolysis. In freshwater drownings, large amounts of water can pass through the alveolar–capillary interface. Even in this setting, there is no evidence that an increase in blood volume results in either hemolysis or electrolyte derangements. With drowning, airway obstruction is the more important consideration because, in as many as 15% of drownings, little or no water enters the lungs. Vagal-mediated laryngospasms may close off the airway producing a phenomenon known as dry-lung drowning.

Regardless of the mechanism, cerebral hypoxia leads to unconsciousness in a matter of minutes. Whether this status progresses to death depends on several factors, including the age and the health of the individual. One of the most important determinants is water temperature. Irreversible injury develops much more rapidly in warm water than in cold water. Survival after up to 1 hour has been reported in children who were submerged in very cold water. Complete submersion is not enough to cause drowning. An incapacitated or helpless individual (e.g., persons with epilepsy or alcoholism, infants) may drown in water only a few inches deep.

No specific or diagnostic findings *prove* that a person recovered from the water is actually a drowning victim. In cases where water has entered the lung, there may be large amounts of foam exiting the nose and mouth. This same phenomenon, however, could occur with other causes of death, including drug overdoses. A body recovered from water could have been that of a victim of some other type of fatal injury. Drowning may represent an effort to obscure the actual cause of death. When treating a living victim recovered from water, it is essential to keep an index of suspicion for any underlying condition that may have predisposed the person to become incapacitated, causing him or her to fall into the water.

Infectious Injury

The pathogenicity (virulence) of microorganisms lies in their ability to survive and proliferate within the host. The disease-producing potential of a microorganism is a function of its ability to (1) invade and destroy cells, (2) produce toxins, and (3) produce damaging hypersensitivity reactions (see Chapter 9).

Immunologic and Inflammatory Injury

Cellular membranes are injured as a result of direct contact with immune or inflammatory-mediated responses, such as phagocytes (lymphocytes and monocytes) and biochemical substances generated during an inflammatory response. Potentially injurious biochemical agents include histamine, antibodies, lymphokines, complement system products, and proteases (see Chapter 7). A variety of mechanisms for potential cellular injury exist. The complement system is responsible for several membrane alterations associated with immunologic injury. Membrane alterations can facilitate a rapid leakage of potassium out of the cell, along with an influx of water. Antibodies can bind and occupy receptor molecules located on the plasma membrane, interfering with its function. Antibodies also can block or destroy cellular junctions, obstructing intercellular communication. Other mechanisms include genetic and epigenetic factors, nutritional imbalances, and physical agents, which are summarized in Table 2.9.

Impacts of Climate Change on Human Health

Climate conditions are changing globally due to increasing levels of greenhouse gases (carbon dioxide, methane, nitrous oxide, and fluorinated gases) in the atmosphere, trapping more and more heat. Anthropogenic activities producing these greenhouse gases have increased (e.g., combustion of fossil fuels, raising of livestock, especially cattle, agricultural practices), and studies indicate a strong correlation between increasing

TABLE 2.9 Examples of Mechanisms of Cellular Injury

Mechanism	Characteristics	Examples
Genetic factors	Alter cell's nucleus and plasma membrane's structure, shape, receptors, or transport mechanisms	Sickle cell anemia, Huntington disease, muscular dystrophy, abetalipoproteinemia, familial hypercholesterolemia See Chapters 4 and 5
Epigenetic factors	Induction of mitotically heritable alterations in gene expression without changing DNA	Gene silencing in cancer See Chapter 6
Nutritional imbalances	Pathophysiologic cellular effects develop when nutrients are not consumed in diet and transported to body's cells *or* when excessive amounts of nutrients are consumed and transported	Protein deficiency, protein-calorie malnutrition, glucose deficiency, lipid deficiency (hypolipidemia), hyperlipidemia (increased lipoproteins in blood causing deposits of fat in heart, liver, and muscle), vitamin deficiencies
Physical Agents		
Temperature extremes	*Hypothermic injury* results from chilling or freezing of cells, creating high intracellular sodium concentrations; abrupt drops in temperature lead to vasoconstriction and increased viscosity of blood, causing ischemic injury, infarction, and necrosis; reactive oxygen species (ROS) are important in this process	Frostbite (see Chapter 46)
	Hyperthermic injury is caused by excessive heat and varies in severity according to nature, intensity, and extent of heat	Burns, burn blisters, heat cramps usually from vigorous exercise with water and salt loss; heat exhaustion with salt and water loss causes heme contraction; heat stroke is life-threatening with a clinical rectal temperature of 106°F
	Tissue injury caused by compressive waves of air or fluid impinging on body, followed by sudden wave of decreased pressure; changes may collapse thorax, rupture internal solid organs, and cause widespread hemorrhage: carbon dioxide and nitrogen that are normally dissolved in blood precipitate from solution and form small bubbles (gas emboli), causing hypoxic injury and pain	*Blast injury* (air or immersion), decompression sickness (caisson disease or "the bends"); recently reported in a few individuals with subdural hematomas after riding high-speed roller coasters
Illumination	Fluorescent lighting and halogen lamps create harmful oxidative stresses; ultraviolet light has been linked to skin cancer. Blue light induces ROS and S-opsin (light sensitive protein) aggregation.	Eyestrain, obscured vision, cataracts, headaches, melanoma
Mechanical stresses	Injury is caused by physical impact or irritation; they may be overt or cumulative. *Compression* is a perpendicular force, *tension* is a stretching force, *torsion* is a twisting force. Fluid *shear forces* or layers rubbing against each other.	Faulty occupational biomechanics, leading to overexertion disorders A pile of material squished or compressed together Pulling on a rope is a tension force Torsion when wringing something dry like a wet towel Shear forces in the vascular channels from endothelial cells
Noise	Can be caused by acute loud noise or cumulative effects of various intensities, frequencies, and duration of noise; considered a public health threat	Hearing impairment or loss; tinnitus, temporary threshold shift (TTS), or loss can occur as a complication of critical illness, from mechanical trauma, ototoxic medications, infections, vascular disorders, and noise

greenhouse gas concentrations in the atmosphere (especially carbon dioxide) and increasing global temperatures. Climate change affects social and environmental determinants of human health, including clean air, safe drinking water, sufficient food, and secure shelter. Climate change will have both direct and indirect effects on human health, and a summary of the main expected health impacts from climate change and climate variability is outlined in the table below (Table 2. 10).

Wildfires are becoming more common and are projected to worsen with climate change. Wildfire smoke can increase ambient air pollution (see section on air pollution). Fires will increase excess mortality and morbidity from burns, smoke, and mental health effects[88–90]; however, data are needed on long-term health effects of wildfire smoke on individuals, including vulnerable populations.[87,91]

Ionizing Radiation

Ionizing radiation (IR) is any form of radiation capable of removing orbital electrons from atoms, resulting in the production of negatively charged free electrons and positively charged ionized atoms. Ionizing radiation is emitted by x-rays, γ-rays, and alpha and beta particles (which are emitted from atomic nuclei in the process of radioactive decay). Ionizing radiation of three types (x-radiation, gamma radiation, and neutrons) was classified as a carcinogen in 2004.

The environment is a source of exposure to IR through emissions from radioactive material, primarily uranium, thorium, and potassium. Other sources of IR are from medical procedures (e.g., x-rays, computed tomography [CT] scans) used to aid in the diagnosis and treatment of disease. Medical radiation now comprises about 48% to 50% of the per capita radiation doses

TABLE 2.10 Summary of Expected Health Impacts of Climate Variability and Climate Change

	Climate Change Effects	Health Risks	Health Impacts
Direct Effects	Increased number of warm days and nights; increased frequency and intensity of heat waves; increased fire risk in low rainfall conditions	Excess heat-related mortality; increased incidence of heat exhaustion and heat stroke; exacerbated circulatory, cardiovascular, respiratory, and kidney diseases; increased premature mortality related to ozone and air pollution produced by fires, particular during heat waves	Increased risk of injury, disease, and death due to more intense heat waves and fires
	Decreased number of cold days and nights	Lower cold-related mortality and reduced cardiovascular and respiratory diseases particularly for the elderly in cold and temperate climates	Modest improvements in cold-related mortality and morbidity
Effects mediated through natural systems	Higher temperatures and humidity; changing and increasingly variable precipitation; higher sea surface and freshwater temperatures	Accelerated microbial growth, survival, persistence, transmission, virulence of pathogens; shifting of geographic and seasonal distributions of diseases (e.g., cholera, schistosomiasis) and ecological changes (e.g., harmful algal blooms); lack of water leading to poor hygiene; flood damage to water and sanitation infrastructures contamination of water sources through overflow	Increased risks of food- and water-borne diseases
	Higher temperatures and humidity; changing and increasingly variable precipitation	Accelerated parasite replication and increased biting risks; prolonged transmission seasons; re-emergence of formerly prevalent diseases; changing distribution and abundance of disease vectors; reduced effectiveness of vector control interventions	Increases risks of vector-borne diseases
Effects heavily mediated by human systems	Higher temperatures and changes in precipitation	Lower food production in the tropics; lower access to food due to reduced supply and higher prices; combined effects of undernutrition and infectious diseases; chronic effects of stunting and wasting in children	Increased risk of undernutrition resulting from diminished food production in poor regions
	Higher temperatures and humidity	Outdoor and unprotected workers obliged to work either in physiologically unsafe conditions or to lose income and livelihood opportunities	Consequences on workers' health include lost work capacity and reduced labor productivity in vulnerable populations

Note. Table adapted from World Health Organization. 2.1 Public health rational. *Operational framework for building climate resilient health systems*; 2015. https://www.who.int/publications-detail-redirect/operational-framework-for-building-climate-resilient-health-systems. Accessed October 1, 2021.

compared with 15% in the 1980s; since 1980, medical radiation exposure has increased 600% in the U.S. population.[92]

The main determinants of the biologic effects of ionizing radiation depend on several factors and include the following:

1. *Rate of delivery*. Because the effect of radiant energy is cumulative, divided doses may allow cells to repair between exposures, called *fractionated doses. Field size*. Doses of radiation delivered to shielded smaller fields are safer than smaller doses delivered to larger fields, which may be lethal.[1]
2. *Cell proliferation*. Rapidly dividing cells are more vulnerable to injury because ionizing radiation damages DNA. Vulnerable tissues have a high rate of cell division and include *gonads, bone marrow, lymphoid tissue*, and the *mucosa of the gastrointestinal tract*. Injury is manifested early after exposure.
3. *Oxygen effects and hypoxia*. A main mechanism of damage to DNA by ionizing radiation is from generation of ROS from reactions with free radicals by radiolysis of water. Tissue with low oxygenation (hypoxia) is less sensitive to radiation, for example, the center of rapidly growing tumors.
4. *Vascular damage*. Endothelial cell damage is an important effect of radiotherapy and can result in narrowing or occlusion of blood vessels, leading to impaired healing, fibrosis, and chronic ischemic atrophy. These changes can appear months or years after exposure. Radiation both initiates and accelerates atherosclerosis, leading to stroke, coronary artery disease, and peripheral artery disease (Fig. 2.26).[93–95]

Late effects in tissues with a low rate of cell proliferation (brain, kidney, liver, muscle, subcutaneous tissue) may include cell death, atrophy, and fibrosis. These effects are associated with vascular damage from the release of proinflammatory mediators in irradiated tissue.[1]

Cellular damage from IR in the absence of effective repair involves two types of damage: (1) early or late tissue reactions (previously called *deterministic*) and (2) stochastic (those that occur by chance) or random effects. High doses of radiation cause substantial cell death and result in detectable tissue reactions within days (early) or sometimes months to years (late) after exposure (Fig. 2.27).

IR can cause a large spectrum of genetic changes because all phases of the cell cycle can be affected. Irradiation during mitosis induces chromosomal aberrations. DNA may be damaged *directly* or *indirectly* by interaction with reactive products (e.g., free electrons, hydroxyl radicals, hydrogen free radicals) (Fig. 2.28).

Stochastic effects are produced at random, without a threshold level of dose, and the main effects include carcinogenesis and genetic mutation. The severity of the outcome is *not* related to

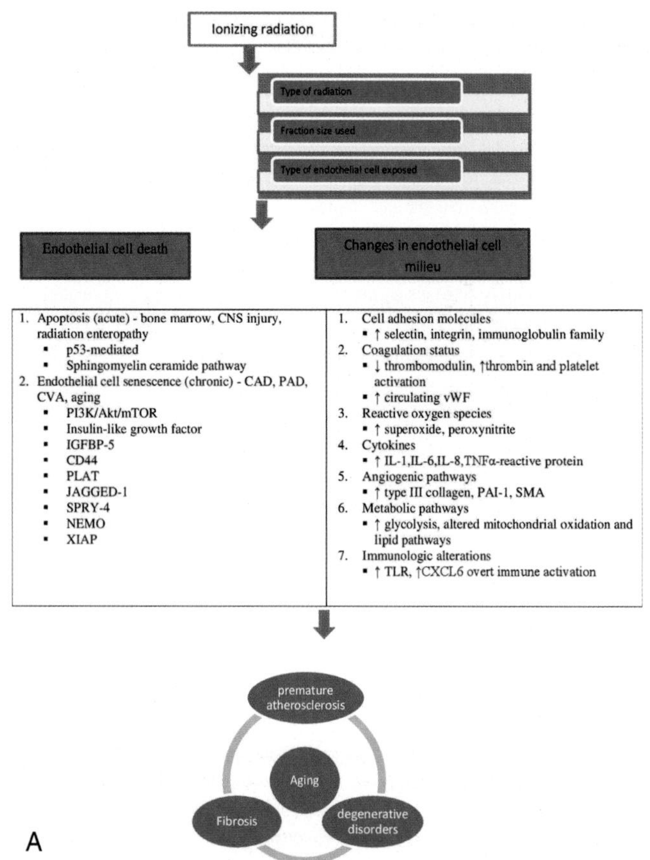

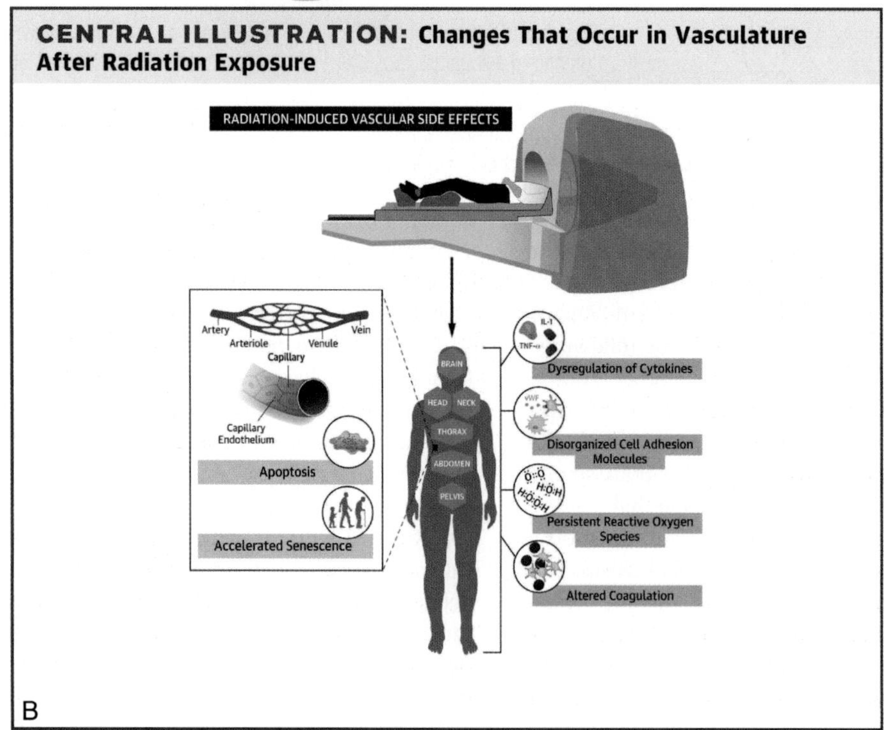

Fig. 2.26 Radiation and Vascular Damage: A Working Model. **(A)** Proposed Changes in Endothelial Cells. **(B)** Changes that occur in vasculature after radiation. *IGFBP5*, Insulin-like growth factor binding protein 5; *PLAT*, tissue plasminogen activator; *JAGGED-1*, a cell surface protein; *SPRY4*, gene; *NEMO*, NF-kappa-B essential modulator; *XIAP*, X-linked inhibitor of apoptosis; *vWF*, Von Willebrand factor; *IL*, interleukin; *TNFα*, tumor necrosis factor alpha; *TLR*, toll-like receptors. (B, From Venkatesulu BP, Mahadevan LS, Aliru ML, et al. Radiation-induced endothelial vascular injury. *JACC: Basic to Translational Science*, 2018;3[4]:563–572.)

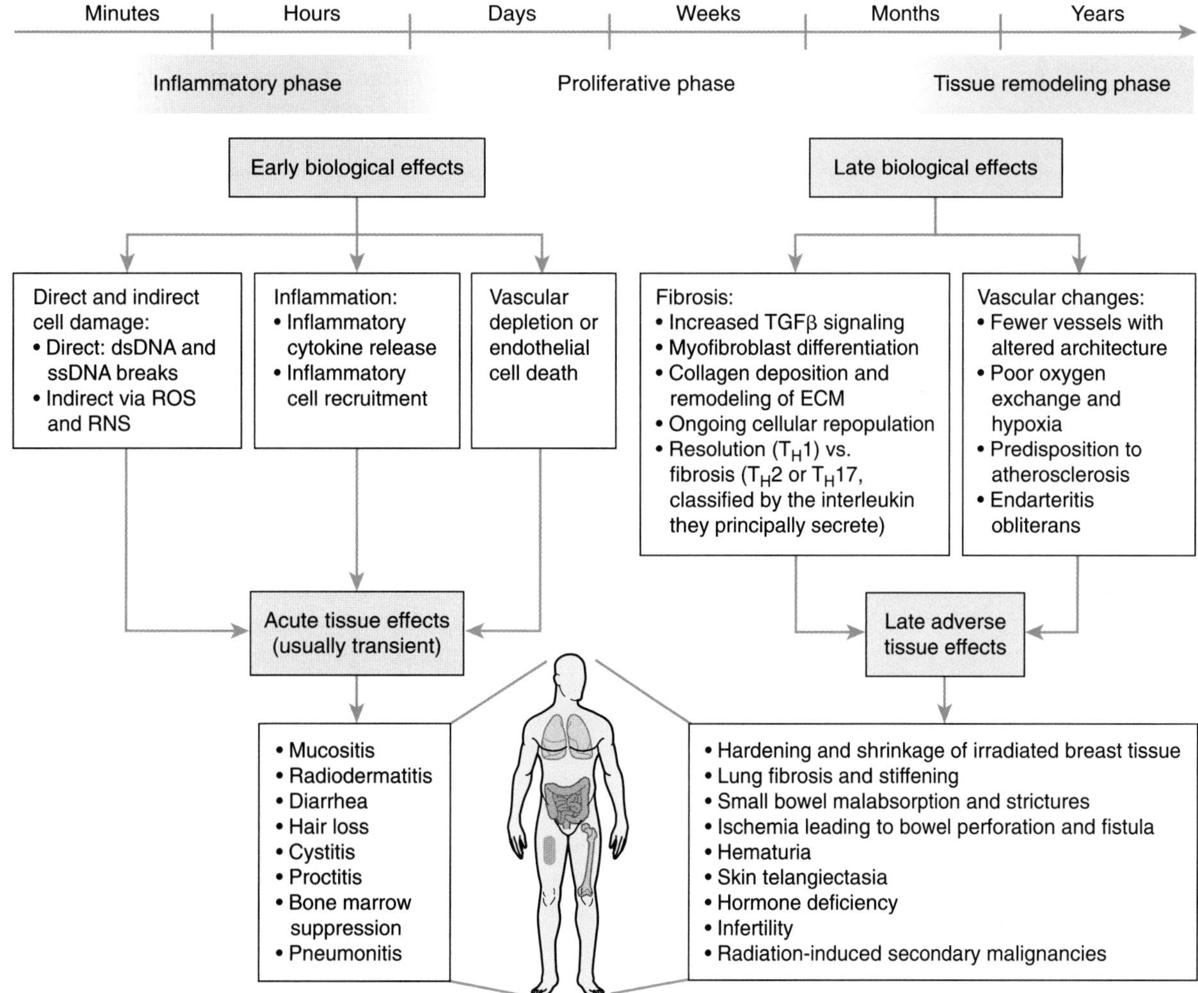

Fig. 2.27 Early and Late Tissue Effects of Radiation. Early biologic events cause acute effects that are normally transient and resolve within 3 months of completing therapy. These events can lead to biologic effects over time, for example, fibrosis, vascular changes, and secondary malignancies. Severity is increased for these biologic effects with higher radiation dose per fraction. *dsDNA*, Double-stranded DNA; *ECM*, extracellular matrix; *ROS*, reactive oxygen species; *RNS*, reactive nitrogen species; *ssDNA*, single-stranded DNA; *TGFβ*, transforming growth factor-beta; *TH*, T helper cell. (From International Commission on Radiological Protection. Ann ICRP. 2012;41[1/2]).

dose but rather to the entire tissue and stress response.[96,97] More simply, IR causes damage that initiates DNA repair mechanisms, alterations in gene expression, and various stress responses.

The nontargeted effects of IR include bystander effects and genomic instability. Bystander effects, or effects on cells not directly in the radiated field, are affected by the radiation and show high levels of mutations, chromosomal aberrations, and membrane signaling changes leading to what some call "horizontal transmission." Stress response signals can generate between cells damaged by targeted effects of IR.[98] Current study includes the bystander effects and the role of exosomes mediating microRNA transfer and communication between the directly irradiated cells and the nonirradiated cells (also see Chapters 12 and 13).[99]

Radiation-induced genomic instability (RIGI) is where generations of cells derived from an irradiated progenitor cell appear normal, but time-lethal (i.e., irreversible) and nonlethal mutations appear in distant offspring, sometimes called "vertical transmission."[100,101] Genomic instability is associated with a diverse set of biological endpoints (see Chapter 4) and is present in the majority of cancers, which drive tumor development and evolution.[101] Importantly, a new paradigm shift of the effects of IR or radiobiology is occurring (also see Chapter 13). These effects represent a tissue response or cell stress response from IR. Not all cells and tissues have the same sensitivity to radiation, although all cells can be affected. Radiosensitivity depends partly on the rate of mitosis and cellular maturity. Because fetal cells are both immature and undergoing rapid cycling, the fetus is at great risk for injury caused by IR. Particularly vulnerable are embryonic germ cells, which are precursors of ova and sperm. Throughout life, cells of the bone marrow, intestinal mucosa, testicular seminiferous epithelium, and ovarian follicles are susceptible to injury because they are always undergoing mitosis, which ensures the presence of vulnerable, immature daughter cells. In utero radiation exposure in the Japanese A-bomb survivors was associated with an increased adult-onset risk of solid tumors.[102] The studies of diagnostic x-rays in utero revealed a risk of pediatric leukemia and other cancers.[97]

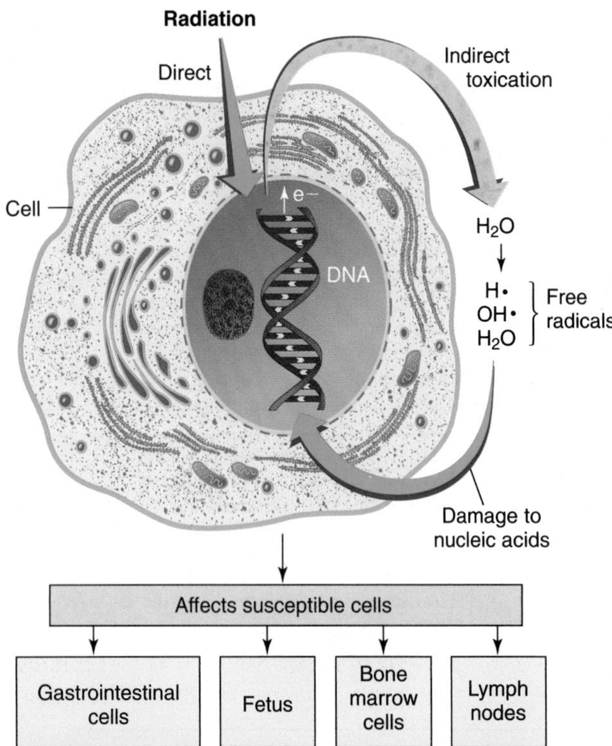

Fig. 2.28 Cellular Damage Caused by Ionizing Radiation. Radiation can damage macromolecules in two ways: (1) directly, in which the micromolecules are ionized and (2) indirectly, in which water is ionized and produces free radicals that in turn damage macromolecules. Cells that are particularly susceptible to damage are those of the gastrointestinal tract, bone marrow, lymph nodes, fetus, and ovarian follicles.

Therefore, other imaging modalities, including magnetic resonance imaging (MRI), plain radiograph, ultrasound, and nuclear medicine studies, should be considered first before performing CT.[103] For example, presentations such as appendicitis first require evaluation with MRI instead of CT.[104] For evaluating intra-abdominal trauma, it is crucial to optimize CT setting to minimize the dose. CT protocols should be optimized to minimize unnecessary radiation exposure, and unnecessary multiphasic protocols should get simplified into a single-phase protocol. Plain films are obtained more frequently than CTs, but multiple plain films can easily accumulate. Technologists should optimally position individuals to avoid repeat examinations. Radiographs are only obtained when it is critical for clinical management.[103]

The International Commission on Radiological Protection (ICRP) emphasizes that protection should be optimized for whole-body exposures and for specific tissues, particularly the lens of the eye, the heart, and the cerebrovascular system.[105]

Radiation-induced cancers are also found in the "cancer-prone" ages (usually 50 to 80 years of age), independent of age at exposure; therefore, the latency period between radiation exposure and the potential appearance of a cancer decreases significantly with increasing age at exposure.[106]

Changes in Atmospheric Pressure

Sudden increases or decreases in atmospheric pressure cause blast injury, which can be transmitted by either air (air blast) or water (immersion blast). With sudden increases in pressure, tissue injury is caused by compressive waves of air impinging on the body, followed by a sudden wave of decreased pressure. The pressure changes may collapse the thorax, rupture internal solid organs, and cause widespread hemorrhage. In increased pressure caused by immersion blast, water pressure is applied suddenly to all sides of the body, forcing the body up out of the water. The positive pressure compresses the abdomen and ruptures hollow internal organs, such as the spleen, kidneys, and liver.

Decompression Sickness

Decompression sickness (DCS) (diver disease, the bends, or caisson disease) is a condition arising with sudden decreases in pressure; carbon dioxide and nitrogen that are normally dissolved in the blood come out of solution and form tiny bubbles called *gas emboli*. Deep-sea divers, scuba divers, and underwater construction workers who return to the surface too quickly develop DCS. The incidence of DCS is rare with a greater (2.5 times) risk for males than females.[107] Individuals presenting with clinical manifestations involving only the skin, musculoskeletal system, or lymphatic systems are considered to have Type I DCS; individuals with type II DCS have symptoms associated with the CNS (headache and visual disturbances).[107] Oxygen is quickly redissolved, but nitrogen bubbles may persist and obstruct blood vessels. Ischemia resulting from gas emboli causes cellular hypoxia, particularly in the muscles, joints, and tendons. Emboli and interstitial gas accumulate around the joints and skeletal muscles, causing the individual to bend in pain. Tissues of the heart and brain also may be affected by emboli, causing necrosis. Dehydration increases the risk of decompression sickness because immersion of the body in water increases venous return to the heart. As a counter-regulatory measure, the cardiac atria secrete atrial natriuretic peptide (ANP), causing diuresis (the Gauer-Henry reflex). At the same time, with a decreased secretion of ADH from the hypothalamus, the kidneys excrete water. The result is a reduction of blood volume. During ascent, fluid is lost in expired air. The total volume deficiency changes the rheological (flow of matter) dynamics in blood and promotes the onset of decompression sickness.[108,109] The gases can be promptly redissolved in blood by raising the atmospheric pressure, which is accomplished by placing the individual in a decompression chamber and increasing the pressure until it approximates pressure at the depth to which the diver had descended. This redissolves the gas bubbles in the blood. Pressure is then decreased gradually until it equals the pressure at the surface of the water. This slows the release of gas bubbles out of solution.

Nitrogen concentrations can have a crippling anesthetic effect on the brain. This narcosis has been referred to as "rapture of the deep," where both physical and cognitive abilities may be seriously impaired.[110] Thus, when a person dives to great depths, both the volume of nitrogen and the volume of oxygen must be decreased. This is accomplished by the addition of an "inert" gas (one that has no metabolic activity within the body). It has been suggested that problems associated with deep, long-duration dives could be avoided by replacing the nitrogen in a diver's gas supply with helium, an inert gas and nature's second lightest gas.[111] Helium has not been shown to have an anesthetic or narcotic effect on divers at depth breathing compressed gases, but it does inflict a greater decompression burden upon divers as compared to nitrogen.[112] Decompression sickness also can happen with very rapid ascent to high altitude in an aircraft that is not properly pressurized.[113] Although decompression sickness is not a concern when people ascend slowly (e.g., on foot) to a low atmospheric pressure environment, such as altitudes higher than 10,000 feet, there is a significant decrease in available oxygen because of decreased partial pressure of the inspired gases. The hypoxemia that occurs may result in pathologic conditions unique to the hypoxic environment at high altitude.

High-Altitude Illness: HAPE, HACE, AMS

High-altitude illness, in the form of high-altitude pulmonary edema (HAPE) or high-altitude cerebral edema (HACE), is potentially fatal.[114] A less serious and more common form of HAI is acute mountain sickness (AMS). HAI is due to hypobaric (having a specific gravity lower than that of cerebrospinal fluid) hypoxia, is not associated with age or physical conditioning, and is easily treated when mild.[115] Several factors are proposed to influence AMS, including rate of ascent to altitude, final altitude reached, altitude at which a person sleeps, and individual physiologic differences.[116] Other risk factors that magnify the effects of hypoxia include certain preexisting cardiopulmonary conditions, residence at low altitude, prior history of high-altitude illness, and level of exertion at altitude.[114,117]

AMS is defined as the presence of a combination of nonspecific symptoms that appear within a few hours after ascent to altitude and may include headache, loss of appetite, nausea, vomiting, weakness, lassitude, dizziness, and difficulty sleeping.[117,118] Fig. 2.29 summarizes current hypotheses of the pathophysiology of AMS and HACE. Symptoms are usually most noticeable during the first few days at altitude and may reappear on further ascent to a higher altitude. AMS is usually a relatively benign, self-limited condition and does not include abnormal neurologic symptoms or signs. An increase in severity of symptoms or signs of neurologic dysfunction, such as ataxia or altered consciousness, indicates transition to HACE.[119]

HACE is a clinical diagnosis defined as the onset of ataxia, altered consciousness (including confusion, impaired mentation, stupor, and coma), and severe lassitude. Frequently present are severe headache, nausea, and vomiting. In both AMS and HACE, headache is most likely initially produced by hypoxemia-induced cerebral vasodilation and a significant increase in blood flow. In

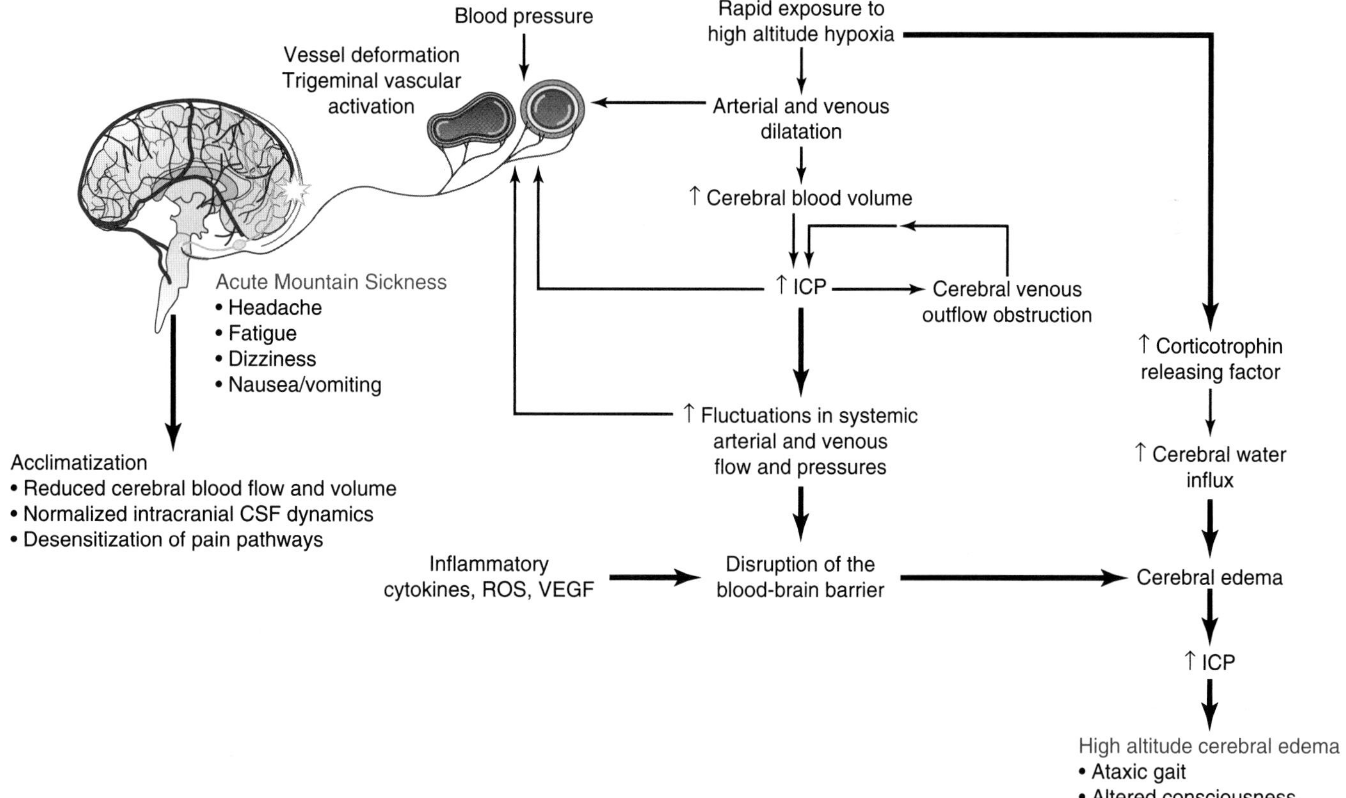

Fig. 2.29 Working Model of Pathophysiology of Acute mountain Sickness and High-Altitude Cerebral Edema. Rapid exposure to high-altitude hypoxia results in changes in cerebral blood flow and volume that can cause acute mountain sickness. With acclimatization, most individuals will recover. Some individuals progress to sustained increases in ICP with decreased cerebral venous outflow, alterations in vascular pressures and flow, inflammation, loss of the integrity of the blood brain barrier, and changes in hypothalamic hormone release. The result is high-altitude cerebral edema, which can be fatal. *ICP*, Intracranial pressure; *ROS*, reactive oxygen species; *VEGF*, vascular endothelial growth factor. (Modified from Davis, C, Hackett, P. Advances in the prevention and treatment of high-altitude illness. *Emergency Medicine Clinics of North America*, 2017;35[2]:241–260.)

addition, recent MRI studies suggest that in persons ascending to high altitudes and suffering moderate to severe AMS, some degree of cerebral edema occurs. However, in milder forms of AMS (a subjective distinction), brain edema is present in some MRI studies, but not in all.[117] The cerebral edema may be either cytotoxic or vasogenic in nature (see Chapter 17).

As potentially lethal as HACE can be, HAPE is thought to account for most deaths from high-altitude illness.[118] HAPE is a noncardiogenic pulmonary edema associated with pulmonary hypertension and elevated capillary pressure. The proposed mechanism for HAPE is uneven hypoxia-induced vasoconstriction, which increases capillary bed pressures and promotes a shift in fluid and vascular leakage (Fig. 2.30).[120] The disruption to the endothelial barrier causes an influx of fluid, proteins, and hemorrhage into alveolar spaces.[121] At a molecular level, the proposed mechanisms for the development of pulmonary edema at altitude include the nitric oxide pathway, the renin-angiotensin system, heat shock protein, pulmonary surfactant proteins, and hypoxia inducible factor.[115] The incidence of HAPE also is related to the rate of ascent, the ultimate altitude reached, and the individual's susceptibility to HAPE (e.g., congenital or acquired pulmonary circulation abnormalities increases susceptibility).

MANIFESTATIONS OF CELLULAR INJURY

Cellular Manifestations: Accumulations

Metabolic disturbances can result from cell injury, particularly where there is excessive intracellular accumulation of biochemical substances. Cellular accumulations, also known as infiltrations, can occur with both sustained cell injury and with normal but inefficient cell function. Two categories of substances can produce infiltrations:

1. *Normal cellular substances*—excess water, proteins, lipids, and carbohydrates
2. A*bnormal substances*—including *endogenous* substances (products of abnormal metabolism and synthesis) and *exogenous* substances (infectious agents or minerals)

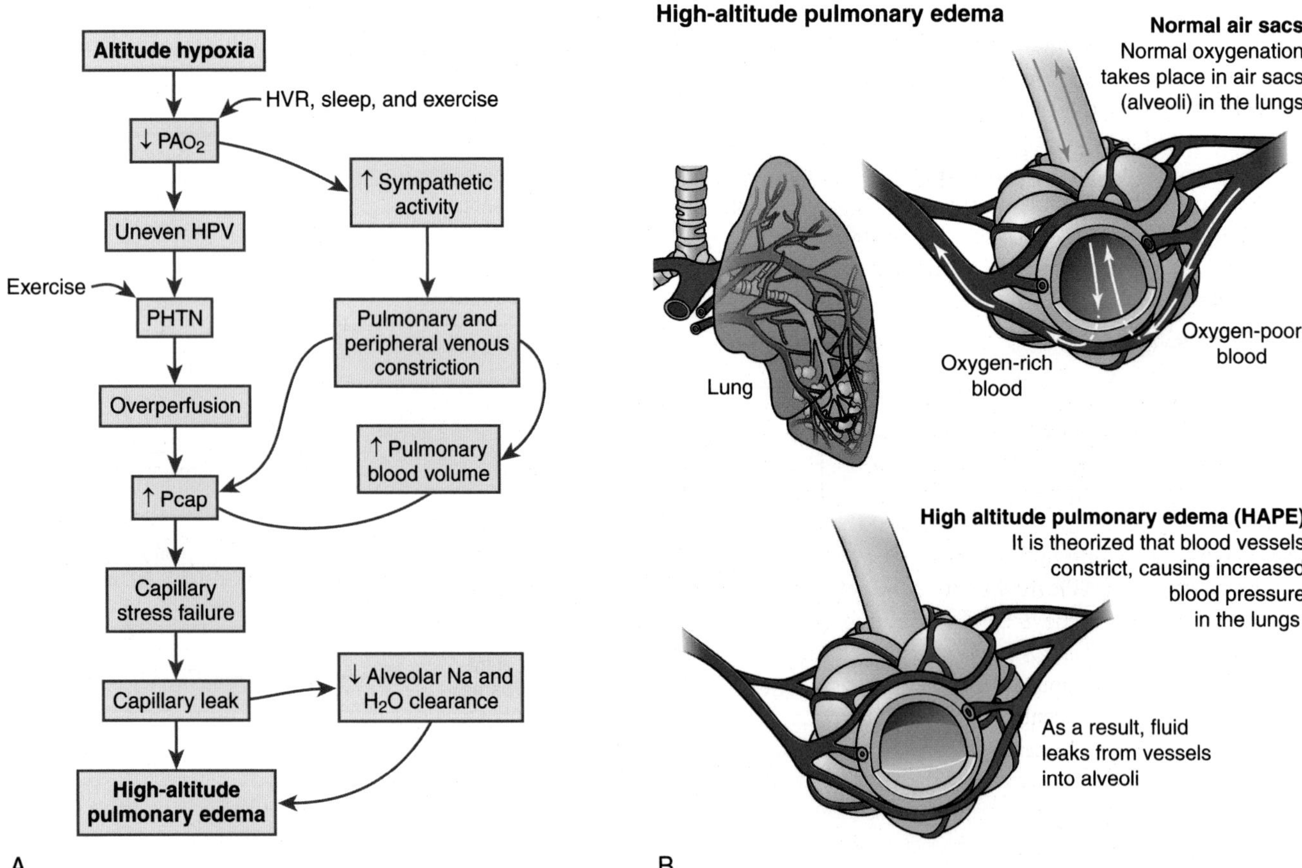

Fig. 2.30 High-Altitude Pulmonary Edema. (A) In high-altitude pulmonary edema (HAPE), the proposed mechanism is uneven pulmonary vasoconstriction, such that high microvascular pressure occurs in the pulmonary capillary beds that are not protected by arteriolar vasoconstriction. Capillary hypertension results in fluid shifts via Starling principles and stretching or disruption of cellular junctions and pores. Other factors involved include inadequate ventilatory response, increased sympathetic nervous system tone, inadequate production of endothelial nitric oxide and impaired or delayed clearance of alveolar fluid. **(B)** Schematic of high-altitude pulmonary edema. *HPV,* Hypoxic pulmonary vasoconstriction; *HVR,* hypoxic ventilatory response; *PHTN,* pulmonary hypertension. (A, From Davis, C, Hackett, P. Advances in the prevention and treatment of high-altitude illness. *Emergency Medicine Clinics of North America*, 2017;35[2]:241–260.)

Products can accumulate transiently or permanently and can be toxic or harmless. Infiltrations may occur in the cytoplasm, typically within the lysosomes, or in the nucleus. Most accumulations result from four main types of mechanisms, all of which lead to abnormal intracellular accumulations (Fig. 2.31). The four mechanisms are

1. Insufficient removal of the normal substance because of altered configuration or transport. Example: steatosis, fatty changes in the liver.
2. Accumulation of abnormal substance because of defects in protein folding, packaging, transport, secretion, or abnormal degradation. Such occurrences are usually secondary to gene mutation. Example: *α_1- antitrypsin.*
3. Inadequate degradation of metabolites because of a lack of enzymes, usually a lysosomal enzyme. Example: *storage diseases.*
4. Accumulation of harmful exogenous materials. Example: heavy metals and mineral dust inhalation and ingestion or the presence of pathogenic microorganisms.

In all storage diseases, the cells attempt to digest, or catabolize, the "stored" substances resulting in excessive amounts of metabolites accumulating within the cells. These metabolites are expelled into the ECM, where they are attacked by phagocytic cells, usually macrophages (see Chapter 7). Some of these scavenger cells circulate throughout the body; others remain fixed in tissues, particularly in liver or spleen tissue. As more and more macrophages and other phagocytes migrate to tissues that are producing excessive metabolites, the affected tissues begin to swell. The engorgement results in organ enlargement. This mechanism causes hepatomegaly (enlarged liver) or splenomegaly (enlarged spleen). Enlargement of one or both organs is a clinical manifestation of many storage diseases.

Water

Cellular swelling is the most common degenerative change; it results from a shift of extracellular water into the cells. In hypoxic injury, the movement of fluid and ions into the cell is associated with acute metabolic failure and the loss of ATP production. The energy-dependent sodium pump, which transports sodium ions out of the cell, requires ATP. Adenosine triphosphatase (ATPase) is the active transport enzyme; it is reduced with hypoxia. Inadequate levels of ATP and ATPase permit sodium to accumulate within the cell while potassium diffuses outward. Increased intracellular sodium concentration raises osmotic pressure, drawing more water into the cell. The cisternae of the ER become distended and are predisposed to rupture. Once ruptured, the cisternae reunite, forming large vacuoles that isolate water, a process called *vacuolation*. Progressive vacuolation results in cytoplasmic swelling, termed oncosis *(hydropic degeneration)* or vacuolar degeneration (Fig. 2.32). If cellular swelling affects the majority of cells within an organ, the organ increases in weight, becomes distended, and takes on a pale appearance.

Cellular swelling is reversible or sublethal. It is an early manifestation of almost all types of cellular injury, including injuries that are severe or lethal. Cellular swelling is associated with high fever, hypokalemia (decreased blood potassium), and certain infections.

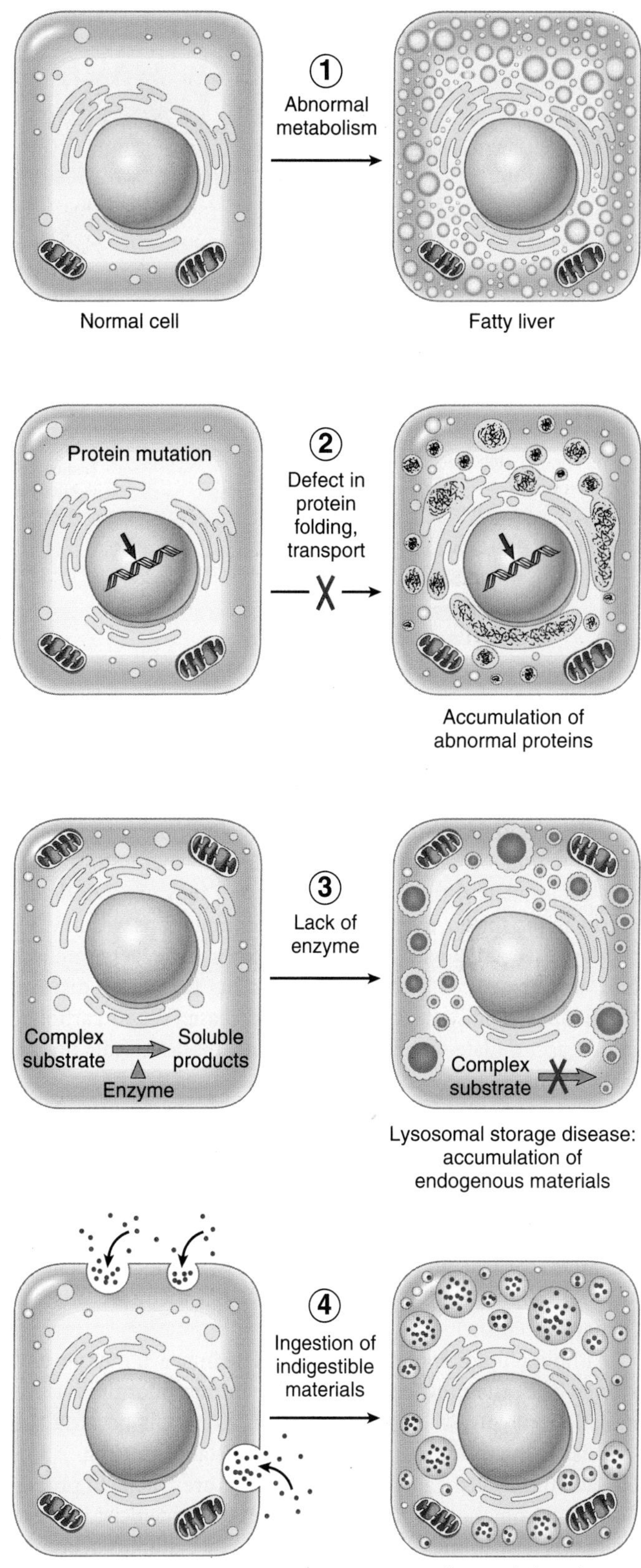

Fig. 2.31 Mechanisms of Intracellular Accumulations. (From Kumar V, Abbas AK, Aster JC. Robbins & *Cotran pathophysiologic basis of disease*, 10th edition. Philadelphia: Elsevier; 2020.)

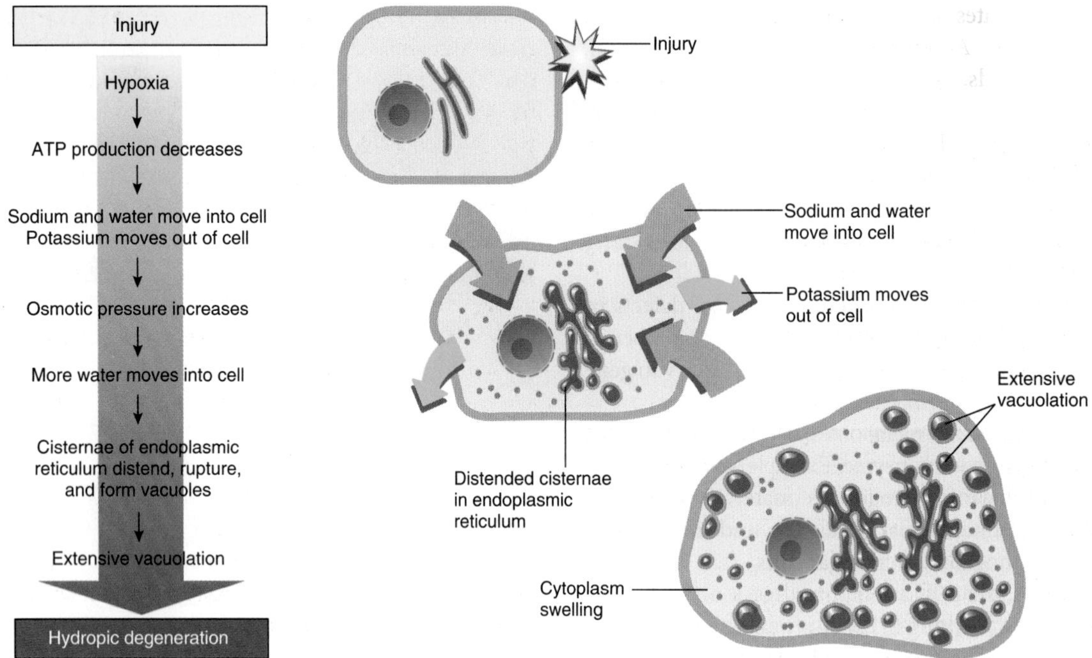

Fig. 2.32 The Process of Oncosis or Vacuolar Degeneration. *ATP,* Adenosine triphosphate.

Lipids and Carbohydrates

Certain metabolic disorders result in an abnormal intracellular accumulation of carbohydrates and lipids. These substances may accumulate throughout the body, but they are found primarily in the spleen, liver, and CNS. Accumulations within CNS cells are associated with neurologic deficits and severe intellectual impairment. Lipids accumulate in Tay-Sachs disease, Niemann-Pick disease, and Gaucher disease. When carbohydrates accumulate, mucopolysaccharide diseases (mucopolysaccharidoses) result. Mucopolysaccharidoses are progressive disorders, typically affecting multiple organs and, particularly, the liver, spleen, heart, and blood vessels. Mucopolysaccharides accumulate at various sites throughout the body: reticuloendothelial cells, endothelial cells, intimal smooth muscle cells, and fibroblasts. Carbohydrate accumulations are associated with cataracts (corneal clouding), joint stiffness, intellectual deficits, and the characteristic eye changes seen in Graves' disease (hyperthyroidism).

Although lipids sometimes accumulate in heart, muscle, and kidney cells, the most common site of intracellular lipid accumulation, or fatty change (steatosis), is liver cells because the liver is the main organ involved in fat metabolism (Fig. 2.33). Hepatic metabolism and secretion of lipids are crucial to proper body function; therefore, any imbalances or deficiencies in these processes lead to major pathologic changes. As lipids accumulate in the cells, increased vacuolation pushes the nucleus and other organelles aside. The outward appearance of the liver becomes yellow and greasy. In developed countries, the most common causes of fatty changes to the liver are alcohol abuse and nonalcoholic fatty liver disease, often associated with obesity and diabetes (see Chapters 22, 23, and 41). Other causes include protein malnutrition, toxins, and anoxia. Mechanisms for lipid accumulation in the liver include the following:

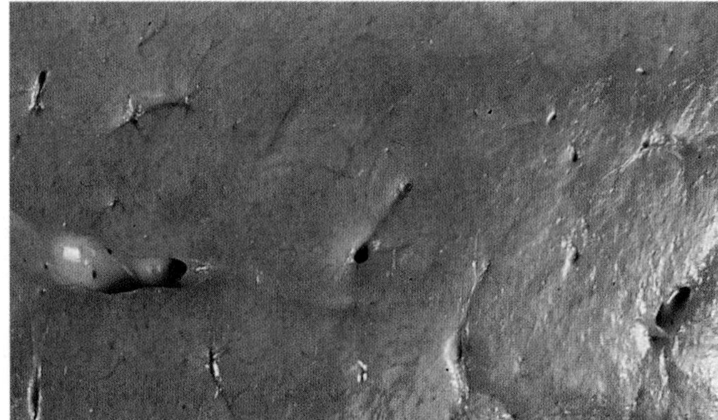

Fig. 2.33 Fatty Liver. The liver appears yellow. (From Damjanov I, Linder J. *Pathology: A color atlas.* St. Louis: Mosby; 2000.)

1. Increased movement of free fatty acids into the liver (for example, starvation increases triglyceride metabolism in adipose tissue, and fatty acids are released and enter liver cells)
2. Failure to convert fatty acids to phospholipids results in (preferential) conversion into triglycerides
3. Increased synthesis of triglycerides from fatty acids
4. Decreased synthesis of apoproteins (lipid-acceptor proteins)
5. Failure of lipids to bind with apoproteins to form lipoproteins
6. Failure of mechanisms that transport lipoproteins out of the cell
7. Direct damage to the ER by free radicals released by alcohol's toxic effects

Many pathologic states show accumulation of cholesterol and cholesterol esters. Atherosclerosis is characterized by plaques containing lipids, cholesterol, calcium, macrophages, and other substances. The coronary and carotid arteries are particularly prone to plaques. Their presence in these vessels can result in myocardial infarction and stroke. Cholesterol-rich deposits in the gallbladder commonly lead to obstruction from cholelithiasis (gall stones). Niemann-Pick disease is characterized by lipid accumulation in the spleen, liver, lungs, bone marrow, and brain, secondary to a genetic lack of sphingomyelinase, an enzyme that affects cholesterol transport.

Glycogen

Glycogen is the storage form of glucose, with 90% found in the liver. Glycogen serves as a readily available source of energy needed for normal cell function. Intracellular accumulations of glycogen are seen in a large group of genetic disorders called *glycogen storage diseases.* Accumulations also are noted disorders affecting glucose and glycogen metabolism. Glycogen storage diseases have profound detrimental effects on growth and development and negatively impact various organ and body system functions. As with water and lipid accumulation, glycogen accumulation results in excessive vacuolation in the cytoplasm. Excess glycogen accumulation is evident in 80% of persons with diabetes. The high levels of blood glucose and excess glycogen cause a multiplicity of problems in the individual with diabetes (see Chapter 22).

Proteins

Proteins provide cellular structure and account for most of the cell's dry weight. Proteins are synthesized on ribosomes from the essential amino acids. Intracellular accumulation of excess protein damages cells in two ways. First, protein metabolism results in the release of lysosomal enzymes, which can damage cellular organelles. Second, excessive amounts of protein in the cytoplasm crowd cell organelles, disrupting their function and intracellular communication.

Protein excess accumulates primarily in two locations: in the epithelial cells of the renal convoluted tubules and in the antibody-forming plasma cells (B lymphocytes) of the immune system. A variety of renal disorders result in excessive excretion of protein molecules into urine (proteinuria) (see Chapter 38). Normally, protein is conserved with little or no protein escaping into urine. Proteinuria suggests cellular injury or altered cellular function, or both. Excess protein aggregates can accumulate in and distend the ER, producing *Russell bodies,* large homogenous eosinophilic inclusions. Russell bodies have been identified in multiple myeloma, which is a cancer of the plasma cells.

A number of disease states result from mutations, which impair protein folding. Partially folded intermediates accumulate within the cell. Emphysema without a history of smoking can result from α_1-antitrypsin deficiency, a genetic mutation that impairs protein folding. Cell injury is associated with the accumulation of cytoskeleton proteins. The *neurofibrillary tangle* found in the brain in Alzheimer disease contains these types of proteins.

Pigments

Pigment accumulations may be normal or abnormal, endogenous (produced within the body), or exogenous (produced outside the body). Endogenous pigments, derived from amino acids (tyrosine, tryptophan), include melanin and blood proteins (porphyrins, hemoglobin, and hemosiderin). Lipofuscin, a lipid-rich pigment known as the "aging pigment," imparts a yellow-brown color to cells, which are undergoing slow, regressive, or atrophic changes. The most common exogenous pigment is carbon black (coal dust), a pervasive air pollutant in urban areas. Inhaled carbon black interacts with lung macrophages. Lymphatics transport it to regional pulmonary lymph nodes where it accumulates. This accumulation blackens lung tissues and pulmonary nodes, causing a variety of respiratory disorders. Other exogenous pigments include mineral dusts: silica, iron particles, lead, silver salts, and dyes used for tattoos.

Melanin

Melanin is a brown-black pigment derived from the amino acid *tyrosine.* Melanin is synthesized by epidermal cells called *melanocytes* and is stored in membrane-bound cytoplasmic vesicles called *melanosomes.* It accumulates in epithelial cells (keratinocytes) of the skin and retina where it serves to protect the tissue from the harmful effects of prolonged exposure to sunlight. Melanin is essential in the prevention of skin cancer. Persons with absent or low levels of melanin (lighter-skinned persons) are more susceptible to skin cancer (see Chapters 13 and 46). Particularly hazardous are episodes of sunburn during the early years of life because these events increase the life-long risk for developing skin cancer. Ultraviolet radiation from nonnatural sources (tanning salon lamps) also is associated with an increased risk for skin cancer. Individuals who have more darkly pigmented skin because of the presence of higher levels of melanin are proportionately less susceptible to skin cancers.

Ultraviolet light from sunlight and other sources stimulates the synthesis of melanin. Melanin absorbs ultraviolet rays during subsequent exposures. Melanin also may serve to trap harmful free radicals derived by the action of ultraviolet light on skin. Melanin accounts for the brown to black coloration seen in *pigmented nevi,* benign skin moles. Melanin also is found in cancerous skin lesions, particularly *malignant melanoma,* a highly aggressive and lethal form of skin cancer. It is characterized by irregular black skin lesions, which rapidly metastasize to other organs.

Albinism is a congenital inherited disorder characterized by the complete or partial absence of melanin. Individuals with albinism are extremely predisposed to developing skin cancer because they experience sunburn upon even minimal exposure to sunlight. In humans, the disorder is inherited as either an autosomal recessive or a sex-linked recessive genetic disorder, depending on the type of albinism involved. The mechanism for albinism is a defect in tyrosinase, a copper-containing enzyme, which catalyzes the production of melanin from the amino acid tyrosine.

Hemoproteins

Hemoproteins are essential endogenous pigments. They include hemoglobin and oxidative enzymes, the cytochromes. Numerous disorders result from abnormalities involving these pigments, particularly iron uptake, metabolism, excretion, and storage (see Chapter 28). Excessive intracellular iron storage results from accumulations of hemoprotein, originating when this substance is transferred from the bloodstream into cells. Iron enters blood from three primary sources: (1) tissue stores, (2) the intestinal mucosa, and (3) macrophages. Macrophages remove and destroy dead or defective RBCs. The amount of iron in blood plasma also depends on the metabolism of the major iron-transport protein, *transferrin*.

Iron is stored in tissue cells in two forms: ferritin, the major vehicle for iron storage, and with greater levels of iron present, as hemosiderin, an intracellular, yellow-brown pigment. Excess accumulation of hemosiderin usually occurs in the mononuclear phagocyte systems (MPSs) and, to a lesser extent, in the liver, kidneys, lungs, spleen, lymph nodes, and bone marrow. Iron overload, also known as hemochromatosis, refers to an accumulation of iron within the body and results from a variety of mechanisms (see Chapter 29).

In contrast to hemochromatosis, a chronic and systemic disorder, hemosiderosis is a transient, localized deposition of iron. It usually does not result in tissue damage. Transient hemosiderin accumulation within tissues can be seen in bruising where ruptured blood vessels result in RBCs exiting the circulatory system. The RBCs diffuse into tissues surrounding the site of injury. A local hemorrhage (bruise) forms after a contusion. The skin surrounding the site of impact injury first appears red or dark blue, or both, or, in lay terminology, "black and blue" as blood accumulates under the skin. Depending on the nature of the trauma, the color change can be quite profound (deep, blackish blue) and extend over a large area (Fig. 2.34). Over the course of a few days to several weeks, the blue coloration is gradually replaced by characteristic color changes—green, yellow, and brown-pigmentation to the skin. The colors reflect the sequential degradation of hemoglobin (red–blue) to biliverdin (green) to bilirubin (yellow) and, finally, to hemosiderin (golden brown). Eventually, the abnormal pigmentation resolves, and the normal skin color returns.

Bilirubin is a normal, yellow-to-green pigment of bile derived from the porphyrin structure of hemoglobin. Excess bilirubin within cells and tissues causes jaundice (icterus), a yellowing of the skin, and sclera of the eye. Jaundice occurs when the bilirubin level exceeds 2 mg/dL of plasma, compared with the normal values of 0.4 to 1 mg/dL. Hyperbilirubinemia develops because of one of several mechanisms: (1) destruction of erythrocytes (RBCs) causing *hemolytic jaundice;* (2) diseases affecting the metabolism and excretion of bilirubin in the liver (e.g., cirrhosis); and (3) diseases causing obstruction of the common bile duct (e.g., gallstones or pancreatic tumors). Various drugs can cause the obstruction of normal bile flow through the liver, increasing blood levels of bilirubin.

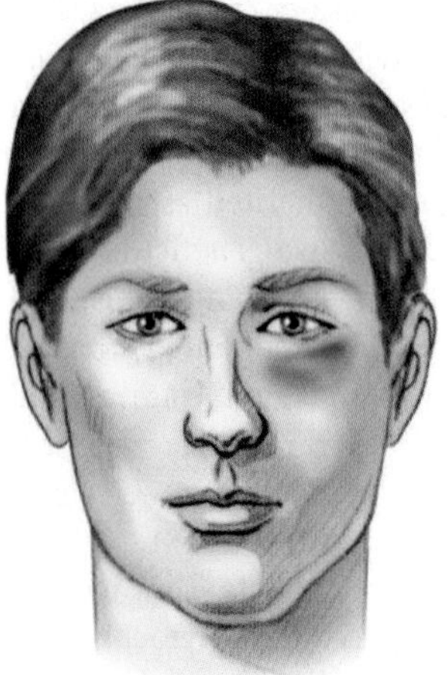

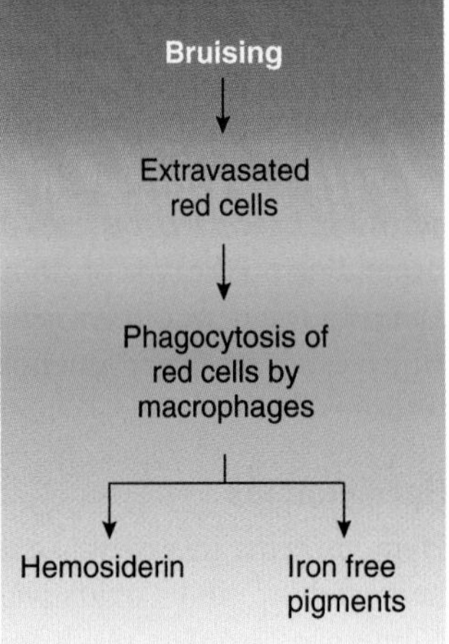

Fig. 2.34 Hemosiderin Accumulation as Noted as the Color Changes in a "Black Eye."

Calcium

Calcium salts accumulate in both injured and dead tissues (Fig. 2.35), a process that results in *cellular calcification.* An important mechanism for cellular calcification is the influx of extracellular calcium in injured mitochondria. Another mechanism that causes calcium accumulation in alveoli, gastric epithelium, and renal tubules is the excretion of acid at these sites, leading to the local production of hydroxyl ions. Hydroxyl ions result in precipitation of calcium hydroxide ($Ca[OH]_2$) and hydroxyapatite ($Ca_5[PO_4]_3[OH]$), a mixed salt. Damage occurs when calcium salts clump and harden, interfering with normal cellular structure and function. Pathologic calcification can be dystrophic or metastatic. Dystrophic calcification refers to calcification occurring in dying or necrotic tissues. It is present in chronic tuberculosis of the lungs, lymph nodes, arteries with advanced atherosclerosis (narrowing as a result of plaque accumulation), and in injured heart valves (Fig. 2.36). Calcification impedes the smooth opening or closing of heart valves and presents clinically as a heart murmur (see Chapter 32). Calcification of the coronary arteries predisposes them to severe narrowing and thrombosis, which can lead to myocardial infarction. Dystrophic calcification is frequently found in the center of tumors. Over time, necrosis and subsequent calcification occur in the inner regions of growing tumors as they are progressively deprived of oxygen. Calcium salts appear as gritty, clumped granules that can become stone-like. Psammoma bodies (named for the Greek word denoting "sand") are laminated, calcified structures, which resemble grains of sand. They are concentric and commonly found within tumors; however, the exact mechanism responsible for their formation remains unclear.

Metastatic calcification consists of mineral deposits that occur in undamaged, normal tissues secondary to hypercalcemia (excess calcium in the blood). Frequent causes of hypercalcemia include hyperparathyroidism, toxic levels of vitamin D, hyperthyroidism, Addison disease (adrenocortical insufficiency), and excess calcium supplementation. Hypercalcemia can develop secondary to the increased bone demineralization, resulting from bone tumors, leukemia, and disseminated cancers. It also may occur in advanced renal failure with phosphate retention. As phosphate levels increase, the activity of the parathyroid gland increases resulting in higher levels of circulating calcium.

Urate

In humans, uric acid (urate) is the major end product of purine catabolism. Humans lack the enzyme urate oxidase present in most other mammals. This enzyme is needed to convert uric

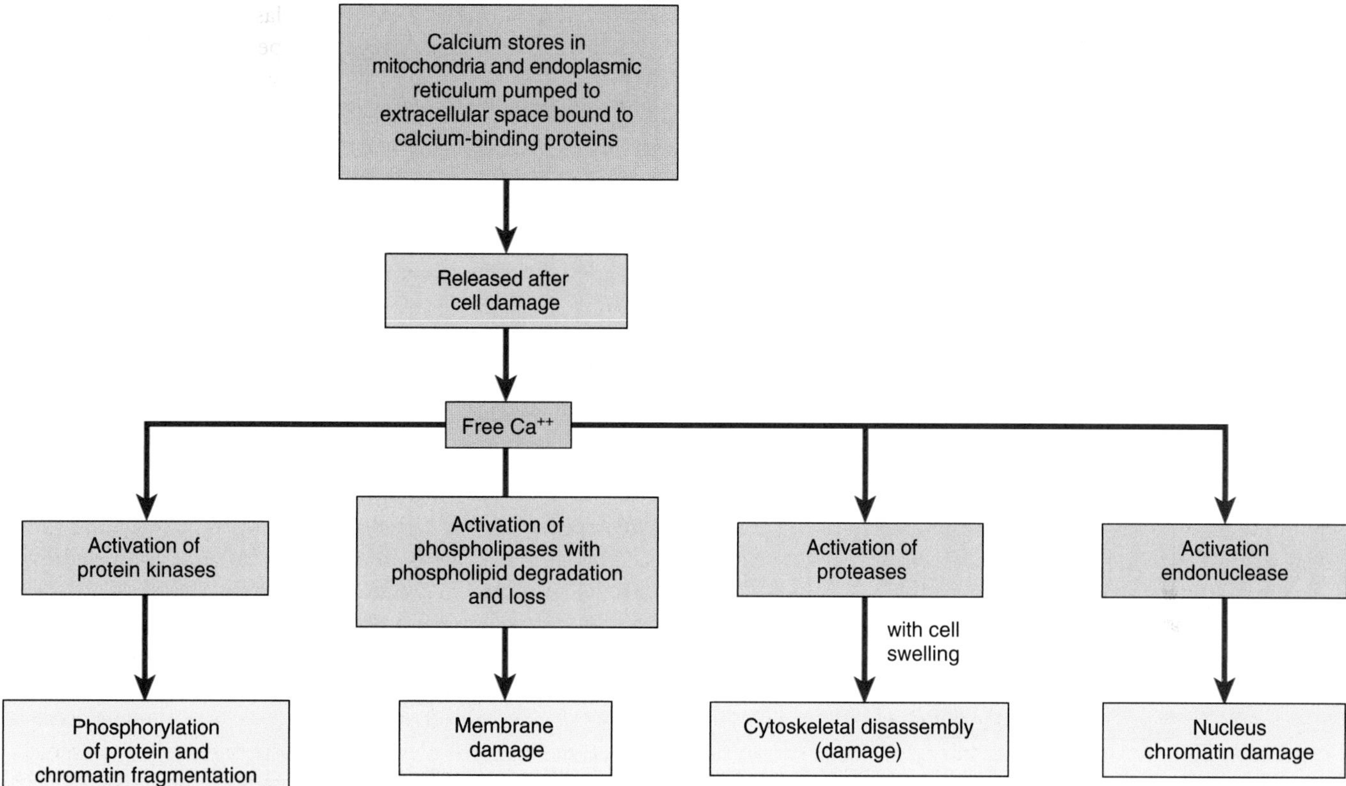

Fig. 2.35 Free Cytosolic Calcium: A Destructive Agent. Normally, calcium is removed from the cytosol by adenosine triphosphate (ATP)–dependent calcium pumps. In normal cells, calcium is bound to buffering proteins, such as calbindin or parvalbumin and is contained in the endoplasmic reticulum and the mitochondria. If there is abnormal permeability of calcium ion channels, direct damage to membranes, or depletion of ATP (i.e., hypoxic injury), calcium increases in the cytosol. If the free calcium cannot be buffered or pumped out of cells, uncontrolled enzyme activation takes place, causing further damage. Uncontrolled entry of calcium into the cytosol is an important final common pathway in many causes of cell death.

acid to allantoin. Because urate crystals are not degraded by lysosomal enzymes, they persist in dead cells. Normally, serum urate concentration is stable, measuring approximately 5 mg/dL in postpubertal males and 4.1 mg/dL in postpubertal females. With elevated serum urate levels, sodium urate crystals accumulate in tissues, leading to a group of painful disorders collectively called gout. These disorders include acute arthritis, chronic gouty arthritis, tophi (firm, nodular, subcutaneous deposits of urate crystals surrounded by fibrosis), and nephritis (inflammation of the nephron). In all these disorders, cell injury and inflammation are characteristic findings (see Chapters 38 and 44).

Systemic Manifestations of Cellular Injury

Dead and injured cells initiate local inflammation and, with more severe injury, cause systemic inflammation. Inflammation promotes systemic manifestations of cellular injury, including fatigue, malaise, altered appetite, and fever. Fever may occur because of endogenous pyrogens (fever-inducing substances) released during the inflammatory response. Table 2.11 summarizes the most significant systemic manifestations of cellular injury.

CELLULAR DEATH

With sufficient structural or physiologic damage, cell injury becomes irreversible, and cells die. Cells die from accidental cell death (ACD) or regulated cell death (RCD).[122] There are two main types of cell death, necrosis or apoptosis (Fig. 2.37 and Table 2.12). Historically, necrosis has been referred to as "accidental" cell death, whereas apoptosis is known as "regulated" cell death. Although necrosis was considered passive or accidental, occurring after severe and sudden injury, some forms of necrosis are genetically controlled through a defined molecular pathway called necroptosis. Also, the distinction between apoptosis and necrosis may not always be clear; cells may progress from one to the other. Usually, however, they are considered non-overlapping pathways of cell death because their morphological features and functional consequences are mostly different.[1] An increased understanding of RCD is emerging with associative distinct morphological changes and immunologic consequences.[122]

Necrosis

Necrosis is the cellular consequence of severe injury. Causes of necrosis include ischemia, exposure to microbial toxins,

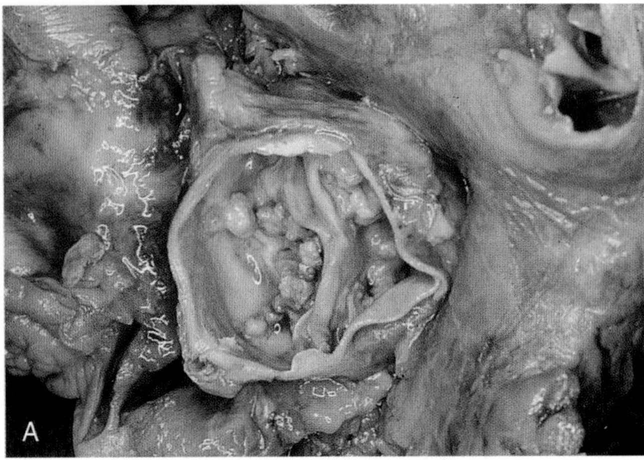

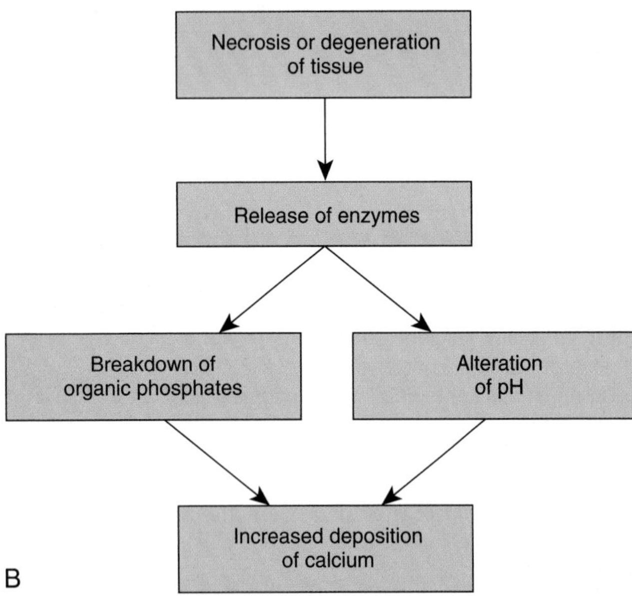

Fig. 2.36 **Aortic Valve Calcification.** **(A)** Calcified aortic valve is an example of dystrophic calcification. **(B)** Algorithm showing the dystrophic mechanism of calcification. (A, From Damjanov I. *Pathology for the health professions*, 4th edition. St Louis: Saunders; 2012.)

TABLE 2.11 Systemic Manifestations of Cellular Injury

Manifestation	Cause
Fever	Release of endogenous pyrogens (interleukin-1, tumor necrosis factor-α, prostaglandins) from bacteria or macrophages; acute inflammatory response
Increased heart rate	Increase in oxidative metabolic processes resulting from fever
Increase in leukocytes (leukocytosis)	Increase in total number of white blood cells because of infection; normal is 5000–9000/mm^3 (increase is directly related to severity of infection)
Pain	Various mechanisms, such as release of bradykinins, obstruction, pressure
Presence of cellular enzymes	Release of enzymes from cells of tissue[a] in extracellular fluid
Lactate dehydrogenase (LDH) (LDH isoenzymes)	Release from red blood cells, liver, kidney, skeletal muscle
Creatine kinase (CK) (CK isoenzymes)	Release from skeletal muscle, brain, heart
Aspartate aminotransferase (AST/serum glutamic-oxaloacetic transaminase [SGOT])	Release from heart, liver, skeletal muscle, kidney, pancreas
Alanine aminotransferase (ALT/serum glutamic pyruvic transaminase [SGPT])	Release from liver, kidney, heart
Alkaline phosphatase (ALP)	Release from liver, bone
Amylase	Release from pancreas
Aldolase	Release from skeletal muscle, heart

[a]The rapidity of enzyme transfer is a function of the weight of the enzyme and the concentration gradient across the cellular membrane. The specific metabolic and excretory rates of the enzymes determine how long levels of enzymes remain elevated.

chemical and physical agents (e.g., burns), and rare occurrences such as when active proteases leak out from cells and damage the surrounding tissues (for example, pancreatitis).[1] Necrosis is a form of cell destruction characterized by ruptured plasma and lysosomal membrane structures, denaturation of cellular proteins, leakage of cellular contents, rapid loss of ATP, swelling of organelles, severe mitochondrial damage, and local inflammation. Certain substances released from injured cells are called damage-associated molecular patterns (DAMPs) (see Chapter 7). DAMPs include ATP released from damaged mitochondria, uric acid from the breakdown of DNA, and many other molecules usually shielded within healthy cells that, when released, become an indicator of severe cell injury.[1] DAMPs are recognized by macrophage receptors and other cells and trigger phagocytosis of the debris and production of cytokines that prompt inflammation (see Chapter 7). The processes of inflammatory cells and release of proteolytic enzymes, phagocytosis, and enzymatic digestion lead to clearance of the necrotic tissue.[1]

Necrosis is the sum of cellular changes occurring after local cell injury (see Fig. 2.37). In the later stages of necrosis, when most organelles are disrupted, karyolysis (enzymatic hydrolysis of nuclear chromatin) is well underway. In some cells, pyknosis, a process where the nucleus shrinks into a small, dense mass of genetic material, occurs. Eventually, lysosomal enzymes break up the pyknotic nucleus. Karyorrhexis is fragmentation of the nucleus into small particles or "nuclear dust."

Different patterns of necrosis tend to occur in different organs or tissues, sometimes indicating the mechanism or cause of cellular injury. The main forms of necrosis are *coagulative, liquefactive, caseous, fat*, and *fibrinoid* (Fig. 2.38A–E). These forms of necrosis occur mostly in the kidneys, heart, and adrenal glands. Another form, gangrenous necrosis, is not a distinctive type of cell death but, instead, refers to large areas of tissue death.

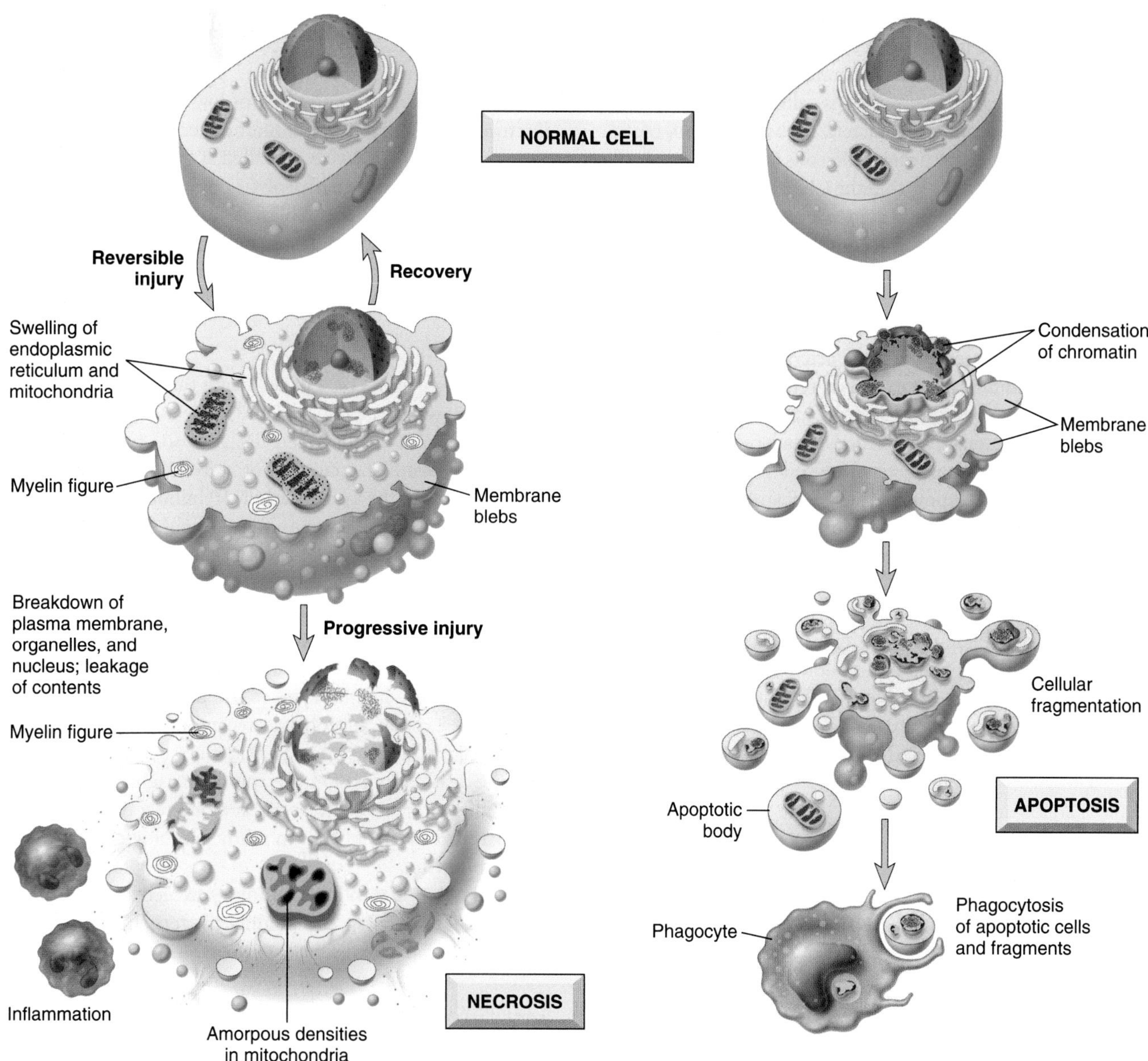

Fig. 2.37 Schematic Illustration of the Morphologic Changes in Cell Injury Culminating in Necrosis or Apoptosis. Myelin figures come from degenerating cellular membranes and are noted within the cytoplasm or extracellularly. (From Kumar V, Abbas AK, Aster JC. *Robbins & Cotran pathophysiologic basis of disease*, 10th edition. Philadelphia: Elsevier; 2020:38.)

TABLE 2.12 Features of Necrosis and Apoptosis

Feature	Necrosis	Apoptosis
Cell size	Enlarged (swelling)	Reduced (shrinkage)
Nucleus	Pyknosis, karyorrhexis, karyolysis	Fragmentation into nucleosome-size fragments
Plasma membrane	Disrupted	Intact; altered structure, especially orientation of lipids
Cellular contents	Enzymatic digestion; may leak out of cell	Intact; may be released in apoptotic bodies
Adjacent inflammation	Frequent	No
Physiologic or pathologic role	Usually pathologic (culmination of irreversible cell injury)	Often physiologic, means of eliminating unwanted cells; may be pathologic after some forms of cell injury, especially deoxyribonucleic acid (DNA) damage

From Kumar V, et al. Cellular responses to stress and toxic insults: Adaptation, injury, and death. In: Kumar V, Abbas AK, Aster JC, eds. *Robbins & Cotran pathophysiologic basis of disease*, 10th edition. Philadelphia: Elsevier; 2020.

Coagulative necrosis occurs as a result of protein denaturation, where albumin is transformed from a gelatinous, transparent state into a firm, opaque substance (see Fig. 2.38A). The localized area of coagulative necrosis is called an infarct.

Liquefactive necrosis is characterized by digestion of the dead cells transforming tissue into a viscous liquid. It commonly results from hypoxic injury within the CNS (see Fig. 2.38B). It is also seen in focal bacterial and sometimes in fungal infections because microbes stimulate the accumulation of leukocytes and their release of enzymes. The necrotic material is called pus, which is creamy and yellow.

Caseous necrosis commonly results from pulmonary tuberculosis or infection caused by *Mycobacterium tuberculosis* (see Fig. 2.38C). Caseous, Latin for cheese, refers to the curdled or cheese-like gross appearance. It combines elements of both coagulative and liquefactive necrosis. Dead cells disintegrate, but the debris is not completely hydrolyzed. Instead, a granulomatous inflammatory response ensues. Soft and granular tissues form the end-product, resembling clumped cheese. An inflammatory wall encloses the areas of caseous necrosis, forming the characteristic granulomas of pulmonary tuberculosis (see Chapter 35).

Fatty necrosis is cellular dissolution caused by lipases, potent enzymes found in the breast and abdominal structures, especially within the pancreas (see Fig. 2.38D). Lipases break down triglycerides, releasing free fatty acids. The fatty acids combine with calcium, magnesium, and sodium ions, creating soaps, a process known as *saponification*. The necrotic tissue formed appears opaque and chalky white.

Fibrinoid necrosis is a unique form of vascular damage typically seen in immune reactions involving blood vessels (see Fig. 2.38E). It occurs from injury, and complexes of antigens and antibodies are deposited in the walls of arteries. The type of injury is often called immunologically-mediated vasculitis syndromes.

Gangrenous necrosis refers to tissue death but does not denote a specific pattern of cell death. It results from severe hypoxic injury, commonly secondary to the blockage of major arterial vessels supplying a region of the body. Gangrenous necrosis is particularly common with severely compromised circulation of the lower leg, either from acute or chronic disorders. With hypoxia, bacterial invasion, which enters a wound, can readily result in gangrenous necrosis. *Dry gangrene* typically results from coagulative necrosis. The skin becomes very dry and shriveled, and skin coloration in such cases is brown or black. *Wet gangrene*, the more lethal form, develops secondary to necrotizing bacterial infections, particularly infection with gram-positive cocci, gram-negative rods, or anaerobic microorganisms, especially *Clostridium* spp. These microorganisms invade the site, causing a liquefactive necrosis. Wet gangrene causes the affected tissues to become cold, swollen, and black, and a foul odor is present. Wet gangrene also can affect internal organs, usually secondary to hypoxia. The presentation is similar regardless of the site involved. Wet gangrene is an aggressive disorder, which spreads rapidly to surrounding tissue. Left untreated, it can rapidly progress to death.

Gas gangrene refers to a type of wet gangrene caused by tissue infection with *Clostridium* spp., most commonly *Clostridium perfringens*. These microorganisms are widely present in soil and proliferate under conditions of low oxygen tension. Deep puncture wounds from soil-contaminated objects are common sources of infection. Once established at the site of infection, the microorganisms produce hydrolytic enzymes and toxins, which destroy tissue and cause bubbles of gas to form in the affected region. The infection progresses rapidly, spreading to adjacent tissue. Untreated, death typically occurs within 12 hours secondary to overwhelming sepsis, shock, and renal shutdown

Apoptosis

Apoptosis is a distinct type of cell death that differs from necrosis in several ways (see Fig. 2.37 and Table 2.12). Apoptosis is an active process of cellular self-destruction, resulting in *programmed cell death*. It occurs in both physiologic and pathologic tissue changes. In the average adult, 10 billion new cells are created every day, and the same number of cells are destroyed daily. If cells did not undergo apoptosis, endless cell proliferation would result. Normal physiologic death by apoptosis occurs during embryogenesis; involution of hormone-dependent tissue after hormone withdrawal, such as involution of the lactating breast after weaning; cell loss in proliferating cell populations, such as immature lymphocytes in the bone marrow or thymus that do not express appropriate receptors; and elimination of possibly harmful lymphocytes that may be self-reactive and cause the death of cells after they perform useful functions (e.g., neutrophils after an acute inflammatory reaction).[1] Death by apoptosis causes loss of cells in many pathologic states, including the following:

- *Severe cell injury:* When cell injury exceeds the capacity for repair mechanisms, cell signaling triggers apoptosis.
- *Accumulation of misfolded proteins:* This condition results from either genetic mutations or free radicals. Excessive accumulation of misfolded proteins in the ER leads to a condition known as endoplasmic reticulum stress (ER stress) (see Chapter 1). ER stress culminates in cell death secondary to apoptosis. It has been linked to several degenerative diseases of the CNS and other organs (Fig. 2.39).
- *Infections (particularly viral):* Apoptosis may be the result of the host's immune response to the presence of a virus infecting the cell. Cytotoxic T lymphocytes respond to viral infections by inducing apoptosis, thus eliminating infectious cells. This process, however, can result in tissue damage. The same mechanism can result in cell death in tumor-related disease and organ transplant rejection.
- *Obstruction in tissue ducts:* Obstruction of blood flow to an organ results in pathologic atrophy, a process commonly noted in the pancreas, kidney, or parotid gland.

Excessive or insufficient apoptosis is known as *dysregulated apoptosis*. A low rate of apoptosis can encourage survival of abnormal cells, particularly mutated cells, which predispose the individual to develop cancer. Similarly, defective apoptosis may fail to eliminate lymphocytes implicated in attacking host tissue (self-antigens), thus leading to autoimmune disorders. Excessive

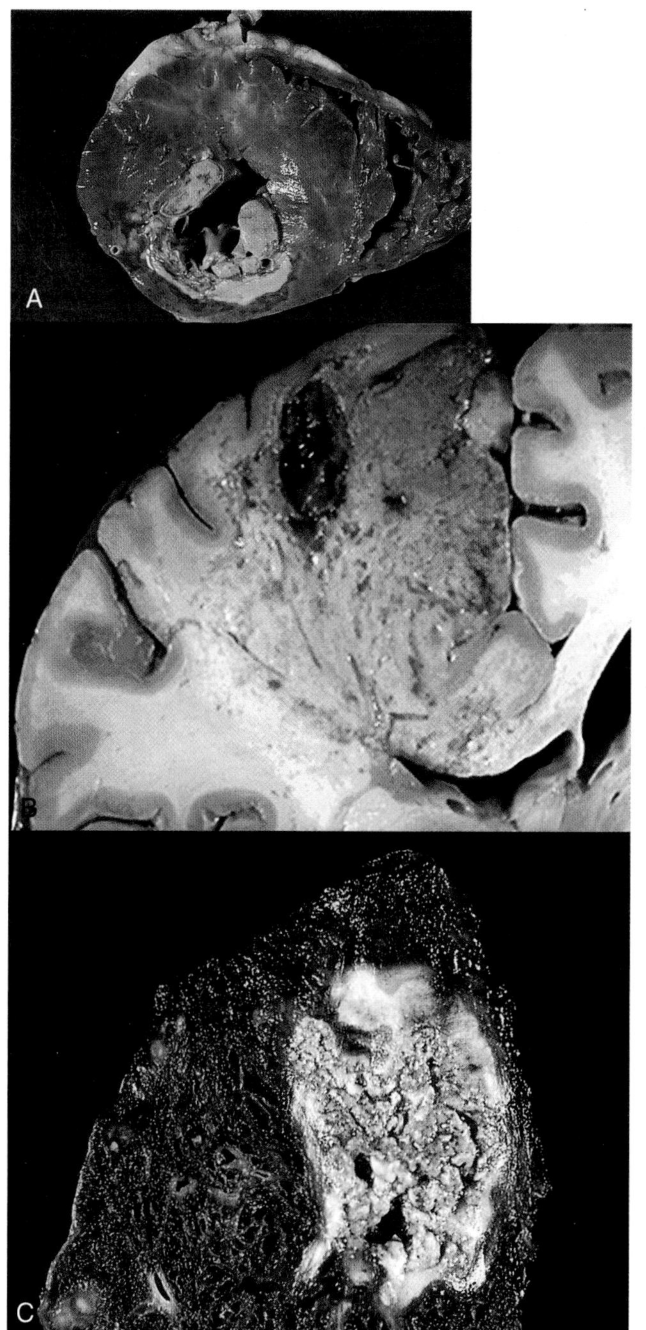

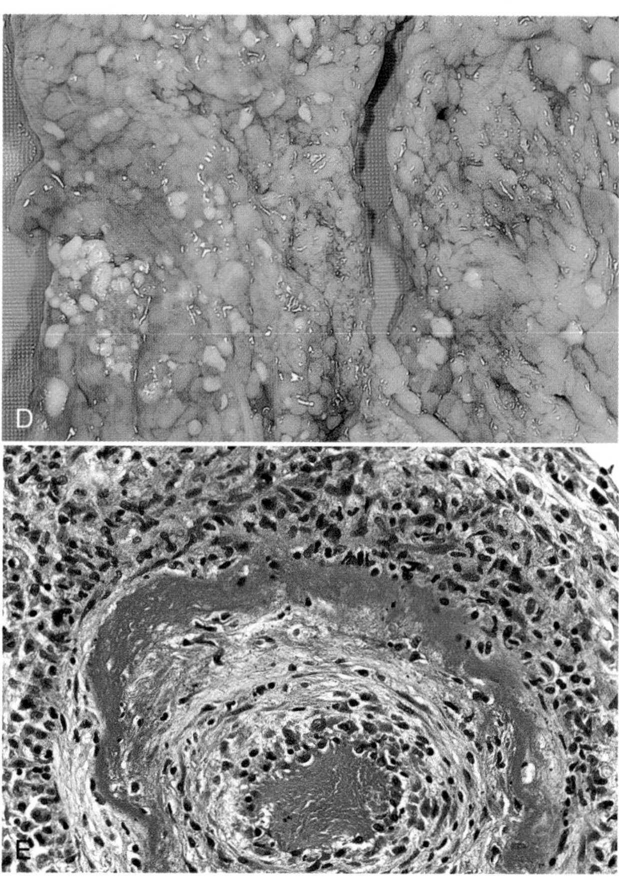

Fig. 2.38 Types of Necrosis. (A) Coagulative necrosis of myocardium of posterior wall of left ventricle of heart. A large anemic *(white)* infarct is readily apparent; note also the necrosis of papillary muscle. (From **(B)** Liquefactive necrosis of the brain. The area of infarction is softened as a result of dissolution of tissue. (From **(C)** Caseous necrosis. Tuberculosis of the lung, with a large area of caseous necrosis containing yellow-white and cheesy debris (From **(D)** Fat necrosis. Areas of white chalky deposits represent foci or fat necrosis with calcium soap formation (saponification) at sites of lipid breakdown in the mesentery. (From **(E)** Fibrinoid Necrosis in an Artery. Wall of the artery shows a circumferential bright pink area of necrosis with inflammation (neutrophils with dark nuclei). It occurs when complexes of antigens and antibodies are deposited in the walls of arteries. The type of injury is often called immunologically mediated vasculitis syndromes. (From (A, From Damjanov I, Linder J, eds. Anderson's pathology, 10th edition. St Louis: Mosby; 1996; B to E from Kumar V, Abbas AK, Aster JC. *Robbins & Cotran pathophysiologic basis of disease,* 10th edition. Philadelphia: Elsevier; 2020:41.)

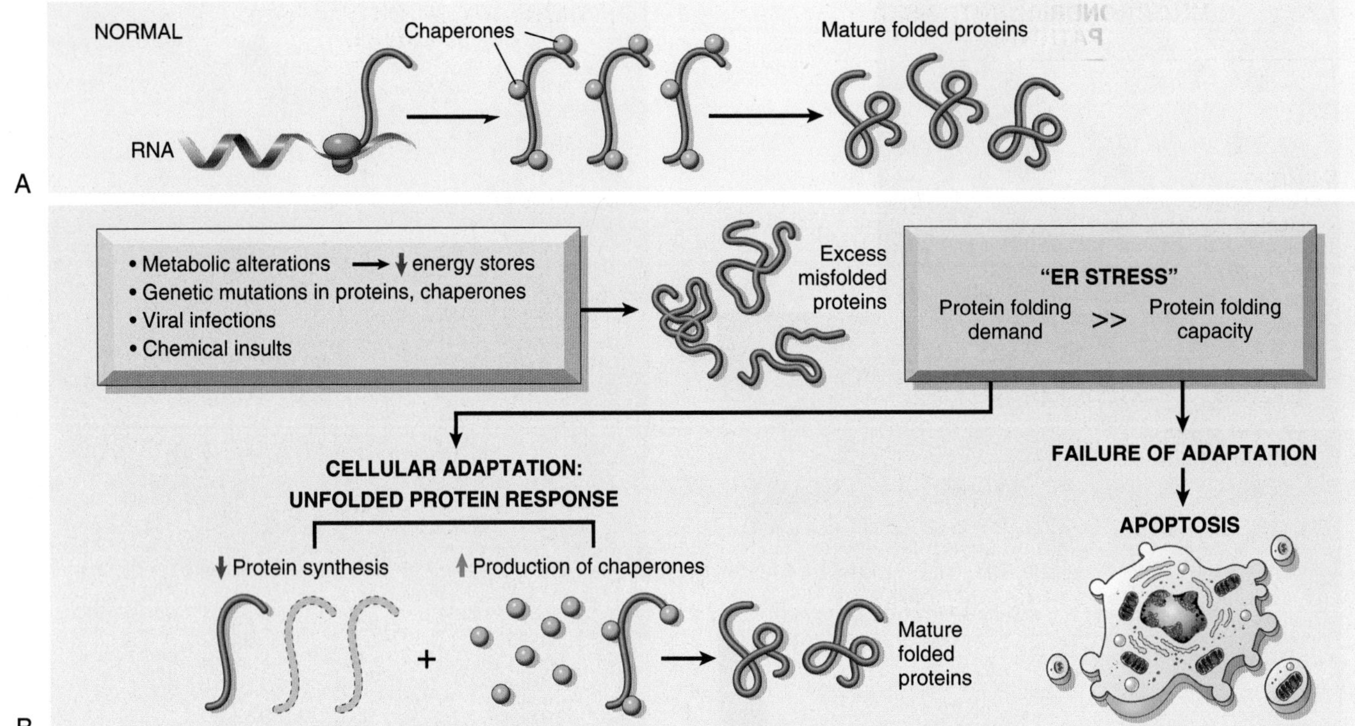

Fig. 2.39 The Unfolded Protein Response, Endoplasmic Stress, and Apoptosis. (A) In normal or healthy cells, the newly made proteins are folded with help from chaperones and then incorporated into the cell or secreted. **(B)** Various stressors can cause endoplasmic reticulum (ER) stress, whereby the cell is challenged to cope with the increased load of misfolded proteins. The accumulation of the protein load initiates the *unfolded protein response* in the ER; if restoration of the protein fails, the cell dies by apoptosis. An example of a disease caused by misfolding of proteins is Alzheimer disease. (From Kumar V, Abbas AK, Aster JC. *Robbins & Cotran pathophysiologic basis of disease*, 10th edition. Philadelphia: Elsevier; 2020:55.)

apoptosis occurs in several neurodegenerative diseases and with ischemic injury, such as with myocardial infarction and stroke, and in the context of virus-infected cells.

Initiation of apoptosis requires tightly regulated cell signaling. Key components involve proteases, enzymes that divide other proteins. Caspases are a family of aspartic acid-specific enzymes that trigger proteolytic activity in response to signals, which induce apoptosis. Specifically, activated caspases cleave other proteins within the system, initiating a series of sequential reactions known as the "suicide" cascade. The cascade results in a rapid and contained cell death. Caspase activation triggers two different but convergent pathways: the *mitochondrial (intrinsic) pathway* and the *death receptor (extrinsic) pathway* (Fig. 2.40). Cells undergoing apoptosis release chemical factors, which recruit phagocytes. The phagocytes quickly engulf cellular remnants, reducing their potential to induce damaging inflammation. Cell death secondary to necrosis is less contained because injured cells swell and burst, spilling their contents into the extracellular spaces, triggering an inflammatory response.

Autophagy

The Greek term autophagy means "eating of self." Autophagy is a "recycling factory" as well as a survival mechanism. It is a self-destructive process that delivers cytoplasmic contents to the lysosome for degradation. Box 2.4 includes terminology used to describe autophagy.

When cells are starved or nutrient deprived, autophagy initiates a "cannibalization response" that digests the cell and recycles the contents. Autophagy can maintain cellular metabolism under conditions of starvation. Under conditions of stress, autophagy removes damaged organelles, thus enhancing the likelihood of survival. Autophagy also has been implicated in physiologic states (e.g., aging), and pathologic processes (e.g., cancer, heart disease, neurodegeneration diseases, inflammation, and infection). The process begins with a cup-shaped, curved membrane known as a *phagophore* (Fig. 2.41). This membrane expands and engulfs intracellular contents—organelles, ribosomes, and proteins—forming a double membrane *autophagosome*. The autophagosome fuses with the lysosome, forming an *autophagolysosome*. Lysosomal acid proteases then degrade the autophagosome into amino acids and other elemental substances. These end-products are transported out of the cytoplasm, where they are subsequently utilized for the synthesis of macromolecules or for fueling metabolism.

The "garbage collecting" and recycling functions characterizing autophagy become less efficient and less discriminating in

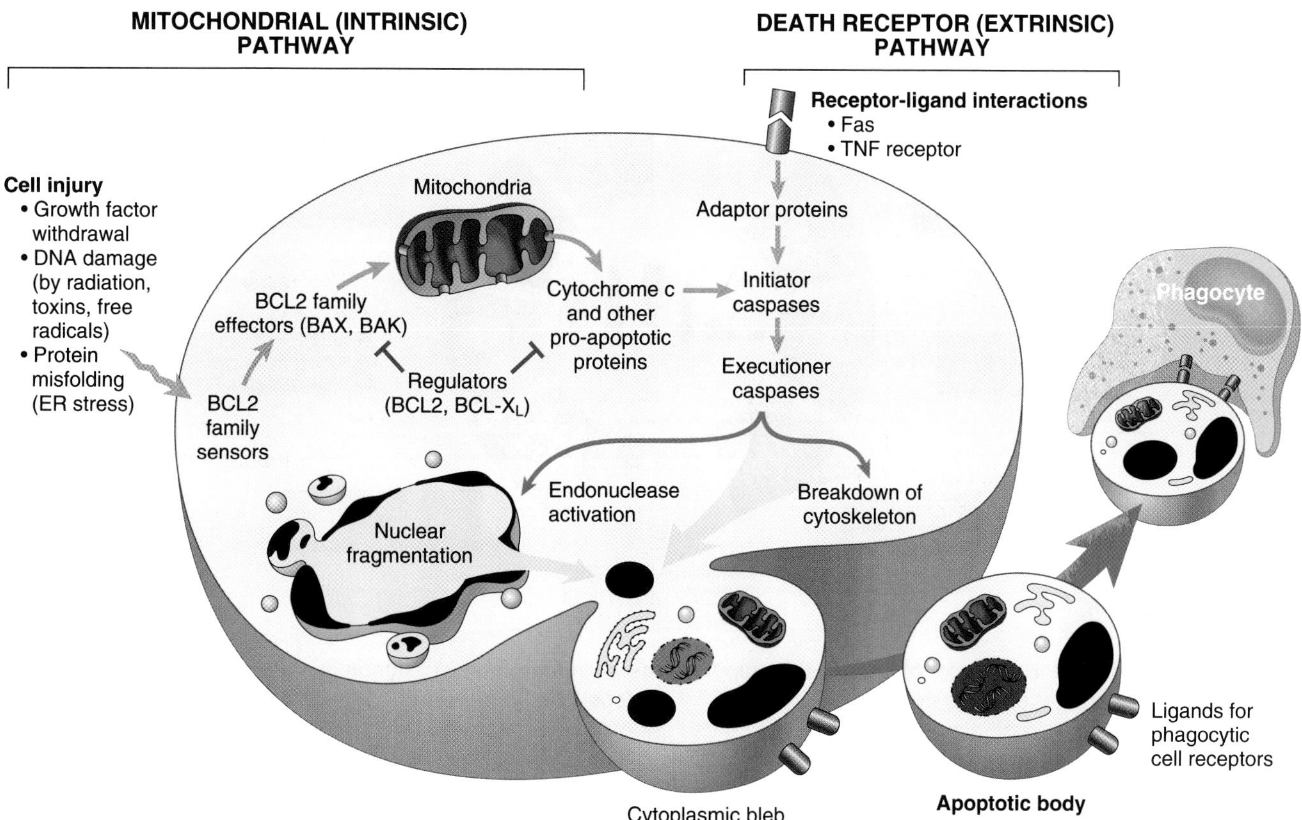

Fig. 2.40 Mechanisms of Apoptosis. Two pathways of apoptosis differ in their induction and regulation, and both culminate in the activation of "executioner" caspases. The induction of apoptosis by the mitochondrial pathway involves BCL2 family, which causes leakage of mitochondrial proteins. The regulation of the death receptor pathway involves the proteases, called caspases. *ER*, Endoplasmic reticulum. (From Kumar V, Abbas AK, Aster JC. *Robbins & Cotran pathophysiologic basis of disease*, 10th edition. Philadelphia: Elsevier; 2020.)

BOX 2.4 The Major Forms of Autophagy

Macroautophagy, the most common term to refer to autophagy, involves the sequestration and transportation of parts (cargo) of the cytosol in an autophagic vacuole (autophagosome).

Microautophagy is the inward invagination of the lysosomal membrane for cargo delivery.

Chaperone-mediated autophagy is the chaperone-dependent proteins that direct cargo across the lysosomal membrane.

aging individuals. Consequently, harmful agents accumulate and cause increasing cell damage as people age. Failure to clear protein products in neurons of the CNS has been linked with dementia. Similarly, failure to clear mitochondria, which generates ROS, can lead to nuclear DNA mutations and cancer. These processes may even partially define normal aging. Enhancing autophagy may serve to decrease the incidence of cancer and prevent the development of certain degenerative diseases.

AGING AND ALTERED CELLULAR AND TISSUE BIOLOGY

Aging is defined as a time-dependent functional decline which is universal and, so far, inevitable. Life span is the period from birth to death, and its study offers insight into the aging process. Aging is associated with a gradual loss of homeostatic mechanisms. It is a complex process involving a multiplicity of factors; however, the underlying causes of aging are conceptualized as the "Hallmarks of Aging." Investigators have focused on genomic instability, telomere attrition, epigenetic alterations, loss of proteostasis or maintenance of protein homeostasis, deregulated nutrient-sensing, mitochondrial dysfunction, cellular senescence, stem cell exhaustion, and altered intercellular communication (Table 2.13). These hallmarks are identifying the differences between the young cell and the old cell (Fig. 2.42). Active investigation includes the study of genetic signatures in humans with exceptional longevity. One area of current research is epigenetic mechanisms that modulate gene expression and the role of intrauterine environment. Lifelong patterns of health, the effects of personality, behavioral patterns, and social support also are thought to be highly relevant.

Pathways that regulate the aging process and associated disease risks include senescence, proteostasis, and changes in metabolism. Senescence is a process leading to permanent proliferative arrest or nondividing state of cells *(replicative senescence)* in response to various stressors. Mechanisms of replicative senescence include progressive telomere shortening or repeated sequences of DNA present at the ends of linear chromosomes that regulate replication of chromosome ends and protect them

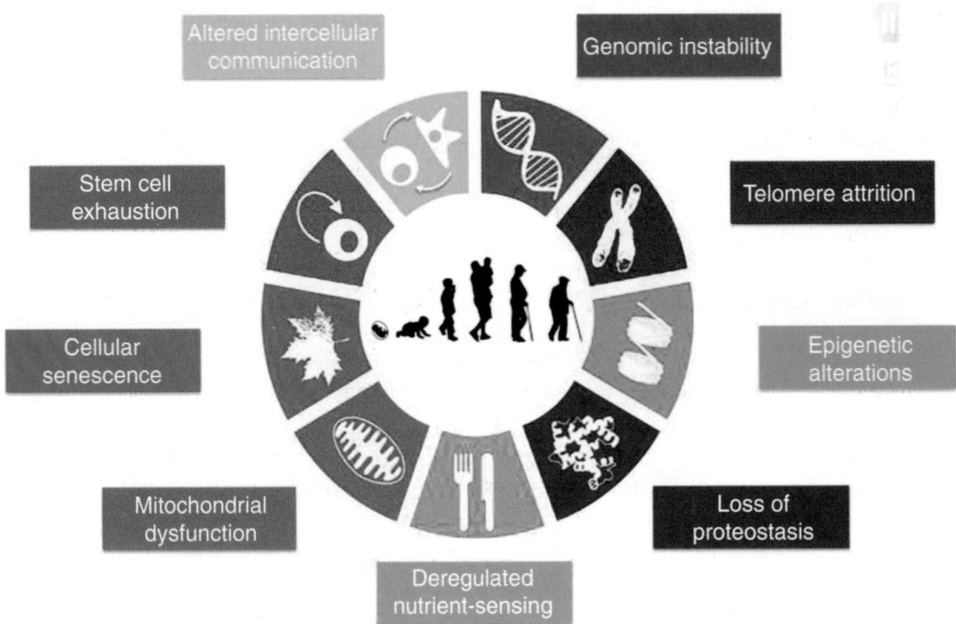

Fig. 2.41 Hallmarks of Aging. Emerging are the hallmarks of aging: genomic instability, telomere attrition, epigenetic alterations, loss of proteostasis, deregulated nutrient-sensing, mitochondrial dysfunction, cellular senescence, stem cell exhaustion, and altered intercellular communication. (From López-Otin C, Blasco MA, Partridge L, et al. The hallmarks of aging. *Cell*, 2013;153(6):1194–1217.)

against fusion and deterioration.[123] The two best-studied mechanisms of senescence are (1) impeding the replicative potential of tissue stem cells (another hallmark of aging, stem cell exhaustion), immune cells (immunosenescence), and stromal cells; and (2) disrupting organ function from release of pro-inflammatory factors (e.g., interleukin 6 [IL-6]and tumornecrosis factor alpha [TNF-α]) by senescent cells.[94,123]

Senescent cells accumulate with time and contribute to tissue dysfunction. The biologic understanding of senescence in humans is limited, but it seems significant because of two factors: (1) senescence causes a loss of tissue-repair capacity because of cell cycle arrest in progenitor cells, and (2) it produces proinflammatory and matrix-degrading molecules in what is known as the *senescence-associated secretory phenotype (SASP)*. Fig. 2.43 shows the benefits and costs of senescence.

Diet is believed to play a significant role in both the development and the prevention of age-related diseases. A major research challenge has been to separate the causes of cell and tissue aging from the changes that characterize it. Understanding the physiology of aging supports public health efforts to promote healthy aging and delay the progression to vulnerability and frailty.

Traditionally, aging has not been considered a disease; rather it has been regarded as a normal process. Disease has been defined as deviation from the normal state secondary to injury or abnormal function. Conceptually this distinction has been clear; however, issues involving cellular injury or damage challenge traditional views. Life span can be altered in animals. But extending life span is not equivalent to delaying aging. For example, death can be prevented through treatment of an acute infection, but the *rate* of aging continues. What is critical is extending a person's *health span*, which results in an increase in life span and a decrease in time spent in a frail state. The passage of time cannot be stopped *(chronologic aging)*, but it may be possible to delay the decline in health, or *biologic aging*. Table 2.14 presents examples of degenerative changes and tissue and systemic aging.

Normal Life Span and Life Expectancy

The maximal life span of humans is 80 to 100 years, and it does not vary significantly among populations. In primitive societies, few individuals reach the maximal life span. However, in societies with improved sanitation, housing, nutrition, and health care, many individuals attain the maximal life span. Life expectancy is the *average* number of years of life remaining at a given age (Box 2.5). Life expectancy in the United States has declined since 2014.[124] Life expectancy in the United States in 1980 was 73.6 years, in 2014 was 78.9 years, and in 2018 was 78.7 years. These trends have been driven by increasing mortality among working-age adults, particularly those of lower socioeconomic status.[125] Although working-age adults with a 4-year college degree have experienced gains in life expectancy, those with a high school diploma have experienced a decline. Differences in longevity are not the same across racial and ethnic groups, with elevated rates of mortality among Black and American Indian adults.[126]

Frailty

Frailty, a common clinical syndrome in older adults, is characterized by overall weakness, decreased stamina, and functional

TABLE 2.13 Hallmarks of Aging

Hallmarks	Characteristics
Genomic Instability	Aging is the accumulation of genetic damage throughout life. Integrity and stability of DNA is constantly challenged by exogenous factors (physical, chemical, biological) and endogenous factors (DNA replication errors reactive oxygen species [ROS], spontaneous hydrolytic factors).
Telomere Attrition	Chromosomal regions, such as telomeres, are susceptible to age-related deterioration. Telomeres are short, repeated sequences of DNA at the ends of linear chromosomes; they enable the complete replication of chromosome ends. Animal models have established links between telomere loss, cellular senescence, and aging.
Epigenetic Alterations	Epigenetic alterations affect all cells and tissues throughout life (see Chapter 6). Epigenetic changes involve DNA methylation patterns, histone changes, and chromatin remodeling. Chromatin modifying proteins (such as SIRT1) are involved in DNA repair, proteostasis, mitochondrial function, nutrient-sensing pathways, and inflammation. Collectively, the epigenome holds promise of improving age-related pathologies and extending healthy lifespan. Resveratrol upregulates SIRT1 activity and has been studied in relation to aging.
Loss of Proteostasis	Impaired protein homeostasis or proteostasis is linked to aging. Proteostasis involves mechanisms of corrected folded proteins (see Chapter 1), heat-shock family of proteins (protect cells under stress, such as different temperatures), and mechanisms for degradation of proteins. Chronic expression of unfolded, misfolded or aggregated proteins contributes to some age-related pathologies (Alzheimer disease, Parkinson disease), cataracts.
Deregulated Nutrient-sensing	Genetic mutations can reduce the function of growth hormone (GH), insulin-like growth factor (IGF-1) receptor, insulin receptor and intracellular effectors such as, Ak strain transforming enzyme (AKT), mammalian target of rapamycin (mTOR), and Forkhead box O proteins (FOXO), all have been linked to longevity. In investigated species, dietary restriction (DR) increases lifespan or health span. Anabolic signaling accelerates aging and decreased nutrient signaling extends longevity.
Mitochondrial Dysfunction	As cells and organisms age, the efficiency of the respiratory chain diminishes, increasing electron leakage and reducing adenosine triphosphate (ATP). Multiple sources of data support increased ROS increases aging, mitochondrial dysfunction, and global cellular damage. Multiple mechanisms causing defective mitochondria include mutations, deletions in mitochondrial DNA (mtDNA), oxidation of mitochondrial proteins, destabilization of the respiratory chain, changes in lipid composition of mitochondrial membranes, fission and fusion events, and defective autophagy. Endurance training and alternate-day-fasting may improve health span.
Cellular Senescence	Cellular senescence is defined as stable arrest of the cell cycle linked to phenotypic changes. Cellular senescence is not a generalized property of all tissues in aged organisms. The accumulation of senescent cells with aging reflects either an increase in the rate of senescent cells and/or a decrease in their clearance because of a decreased immune response. The primary purpose, however, of senescence is to prevent the propagation of damaged cells and to trigger their demise by the immune system. It is possible, therefore, that it plays a protective stress response, for example, as a potent anticancer mechanism. However, the accumulation of senescent cells drives aging and age-related diseases. Senescent cells produce and secrete a complex of factors, collectively known as the **senescent-associated secretory-phenotype (SASP)**.
Stem Cell Exhaustion	The decline in the regenerative potential of tissues is often called stem cell exhaustion. For example, hemopoiesis declines with age resulting in a decrease of adaptive immune cells (immunosenescence), an increased incidence of anemia, and myeloid malignancies. Telomere shortening is also a cause of stem cell decline. From animal studies, a functional attrition of other stem cells has been found in the forebrain, the bone, muscle fibers, and others. An excessive increase in stem cells is also deleterious because it can exhaust stem cell niches. Transplantation of muscle-derived stem cells from young mice to old mice extends lifespan and improves degenerative changes in these mice. Experiments call *parabiosis* ("living beside," a technique that combines two living organisms, such as one young and one old) have demonstrated that the decline in neural and muscle stem cell function in old mice can be reversed by systemic factors from young mice. Stem cell exhaustion is thought to be one of the "key" culprits of aging.
Altered Intracellular Communication	Aging involves changes at the level of intercellular communication, including endocrine, neuroendocrine, or neuronal.
Inflammation	An aging-associated alteration in intercellular communication is "inflammaging," a smoldering pro-inflammatory phenotype that accompanies aging in mammals. Inflammaging results from multiple causes, such as the accumulation of pro-inflammatory tissue damage, a dysfunctional immune system to clear pathogens, dysfunctional host cells, propensity to secrete pro-inflammatory cytokines, enhanced activation of the NF-κB transcription factor, or a defective autophagy response. Importantly, evidence indicates that aging-related changes in one tissue can lead to aging-specific deterioration of other tissues, emphasizing the inter-organ concept, or "contagious aging" of the aging phenotype. The microenvironment is involved, as well as the microbiome.

Data From López-Otin C, Blasco MA, Partridge L, et al. The hallmarks of aging. *Cell*, 2013;153(6):1194–1217; Herranz N, Gil J. Mechanisms and functions of cellular senescence. *Journal of Clinical Investigation*, 2018;128(4):1238–1246; DiLoreto R, Murphy CT. The cell biology of aging. *Molecular Biology of the Cell*, 2015;26(25):4524–4531; Chakravarti D, La Bella KA, DePinho RA. Telomeres: History, health, and hallmarks of aging. *Cell*, 2021;184(2):306–322; Di Micco R, Krizhanovsky V, Baker D, et al. Cellular senescence in ageing: From mechanisms to therapeutic opportunities. *Nature Reviews: Molecular Cell Biology*, 2021;22:75–95.

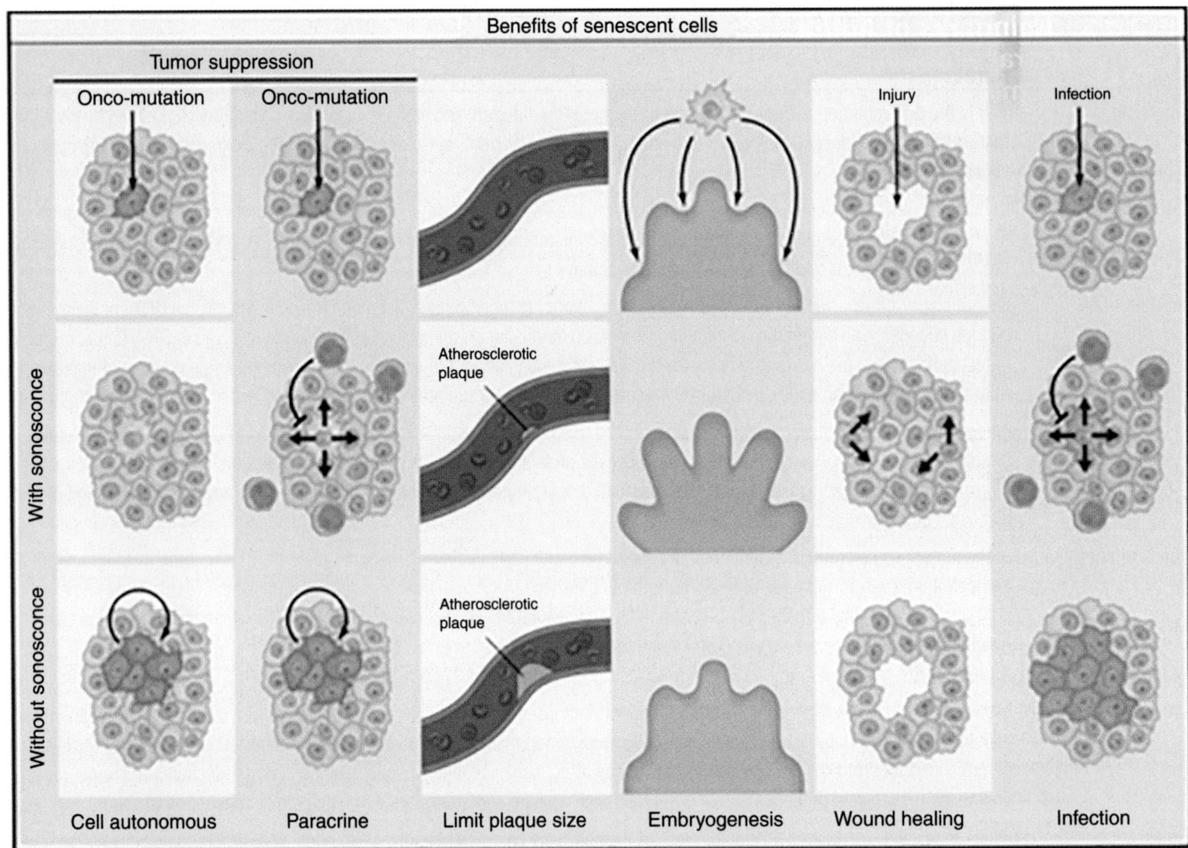

A

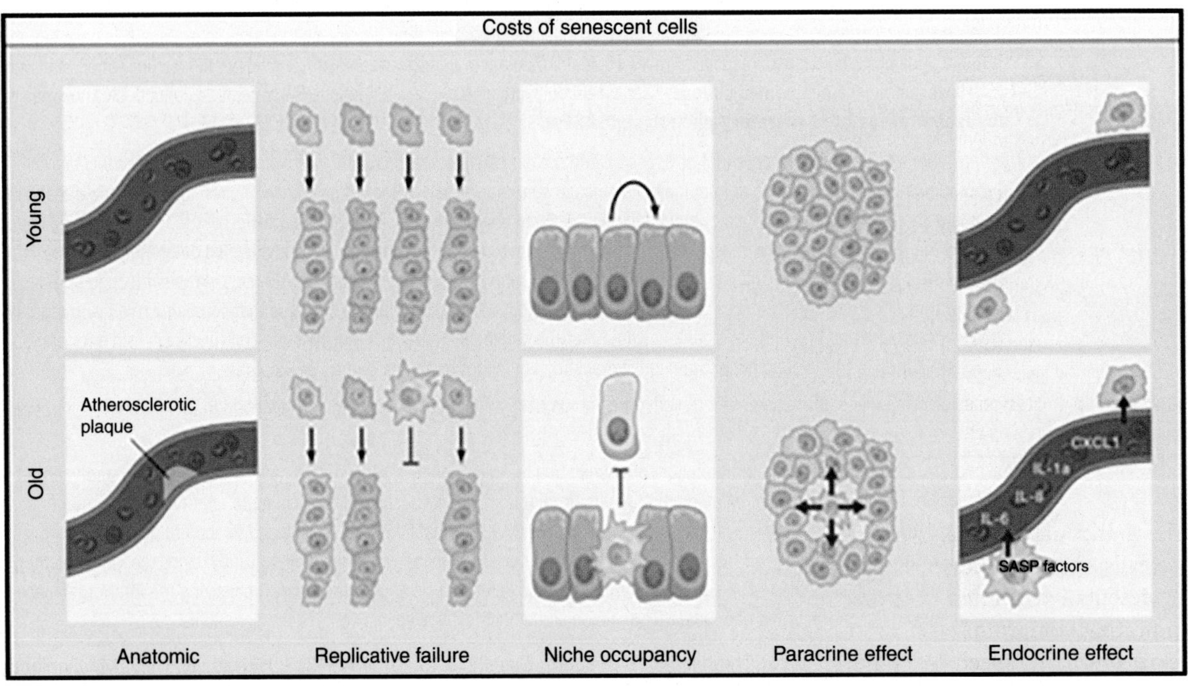

B

Fig. 2.42 Benefits and Costs of Senescence. (A) Senescence allows tumor suppression by boosting local anti-tumor immunity. The activation of the *CDKN2A* locus appears to limit the size of atherosclerotic plaques, thus reducing blood vessel obstruction. Senescence resulting from $p21^{CIP}$ expression during embryogenesis might be required for properties of fetal development. Senescence contributes to wound healing and overall host immunity. **(B)** Accumulation of senescent cells can lead to anatomic lesions such as in atherosclerotic plaque. Loss of replicative capacity of some senescent cells, such as T cells or pancreatic β cells, may result in defects in tissue regeneration. Occupancy of prized "niches" by senescent cells may impair tissue homeostasis. Paracrine and endocrine amplification of pro-inflammatory hormones and enzymes promotes tissue dysfunction locally and at the organismal level (From He S, Sharpless NE. Senescence in health and disease. *Cell*, 2017;169(6);1000–1011.)

TABLE 2.14 Aging: Examples of Degenerative Extracellular Changes and Tissue and Systemic Aging

Degenerative extracellular changes	Binding of collagen; increase in free radicals; alterations of tendons, ligaments, bones, and joints; development of peripheral vascular disease, particularly, arteriosclerosis Extracellular matrix with increased cross-linking, decreased synthesis, and increased degradation of collagen
	Oxidative stress damages cellular function Development of cardiovascular diseases with endothelial cell shifts to proinflammatory, proliferative, and procoagulative state
Tissue and systemic aging	Progressive stiffness or rigidity affects many systems (arterial, pulmonary, musculoskeletal) Peripheral resistance to blood flow Thymus atrophy occurs at puberty, causing a decreased response to T-dependent antigens (foreign proteins), increased formation of autoantibodies and immune complexes, decreasing effectiveness of immune function later in life Reproductive system loss of ova and spermatogenesis decreased in men Responsiveness to hormones decreases in the breast and endometrium Stomach decreases in the rate of emptying and secretion of hormones and hydrochloric acid Muscular atrophy decreases motor tone and contractility Sarcopenia or loss of muscle mass and strength Decrease in height Reduction in circumference of the neck, thighs, and arms; widening of the pelvis; lengthening of the nose and ears Increase in body weight in middle age followed by a decrease in stature, weight, fat-free mass, and body mass As the amount of fat increases, the percentage of total body water decreases. Increased body fat distribution (abdominal) is associated with non-insulin-dependent diabetes and heart disease. Total body potassium concentration decreases

decline. The individual is susceptible to functional and cognitive decline, falls, chronic illnesses, hospitalization, and mortality.[127] This presentation is often described as frailty syndrome. Criteria indicating compromised functioning include low grip strength, slowed walking speed, low physical activity, and unintentional weight loss.[128] The pathophysiology of frailty includes several interrelated physiologic systems (Fig. 2.43). It is complex, with multiple aging mechanisms influenced by genetic factors, epigenetic factors, or both, as well as environmental factors. Frailty also can involve such alterations as osteopenia, cognitive impairment, and anemia. Differences between men and women in presentation include the following: (1) Higher baseline levels of muscle mass in men may be protective against frailty; (2)

BOX 2.5 Life Expectancy Differences Across the United States

- Improved public health strategies and health advances in the United States between the years 1900 and 2000 added about 30 years to life expectancy.
- The increase in life expectancy, however, does not apply to all Americans.
- Women outnumber men in each successive age group from 65 years and older.
- The historic advances in life expectancy resulted in a larger older adult population and, for some, problems of disability, disease, and socioeconomic hardship.
- Although U.S. spending on health care far exceeds that of other countries, rates of life expectancy and key measures of health lag behind those of other high-income countries.
- The National Center for Health Statistics has reported that Americans, on average, have a life expectancy of 78.8 years, a decline from 78.9 in 2014.
- The decline in life expectancy is attributed to rising fatalities from heart disease and stroke; diabetes; drug overdoses; accidents, including unintentional injuries; and other conditions.
- Chronic health problems associated with modifiable risk factors, such as smoking, poor nutrition, overweight, and lack of physical activity, represent 6 of the 10 costliest in terms of health care burden.
- The preventable conditions lead to injuries and diseases and cause soaring medical and labor costs that burden U.S. employers and bankrupt families.
- All these conditions are highly amenable to population-based preventive strategies.
- The current generation of children and young adults in the United States could become the first generation to have shorter life spans, multiple medical conditions, and fewer years of healthy life.

testosterone and growth hormone can provide advantages to men in muscle mass maintenance; however, high testosterone in men may weaken immune response; (3) cortisol is more dysregulated, especially in older women; (4) alterations in immune function and immune responsiveness to sex steroids make men more susceptible to sepsis and infection, and make women more susceptible to chronic inflammatory conditions and loss of muscle mass; (5) chronic inflammation plays a more critical role in the pathophysiology of frailty in females; and (6) lower levels of activity and caloric intake may increase the risk of frailty in women.[129] Sarcopenia and cachexia are common sequelae of aging and also occur secondary to many chronic illnesses.

SOMATIC DEATH

Somatic death is systemic death of the entire body. Unlike the changes that follow cellular death, postmortem change is diffuse and does not involve an inflammatory response. In some instances, postmortem evaluation by autopsy is the only opportunity to macroscopically observe organs and take optimal samples for histological and molecular analyses (see Emerging Science Box: COVID-19 and Postmortem Changes).[130] Within minutes after death, postmortem changes appear, and it becomes readily evident that death has occurred. Upon somatic death, there is complete cessation of respiration and circulation, followed rapidly by a host of other changes. The surface of the skin becomes pale and yellowish, marking the first stage after death known as

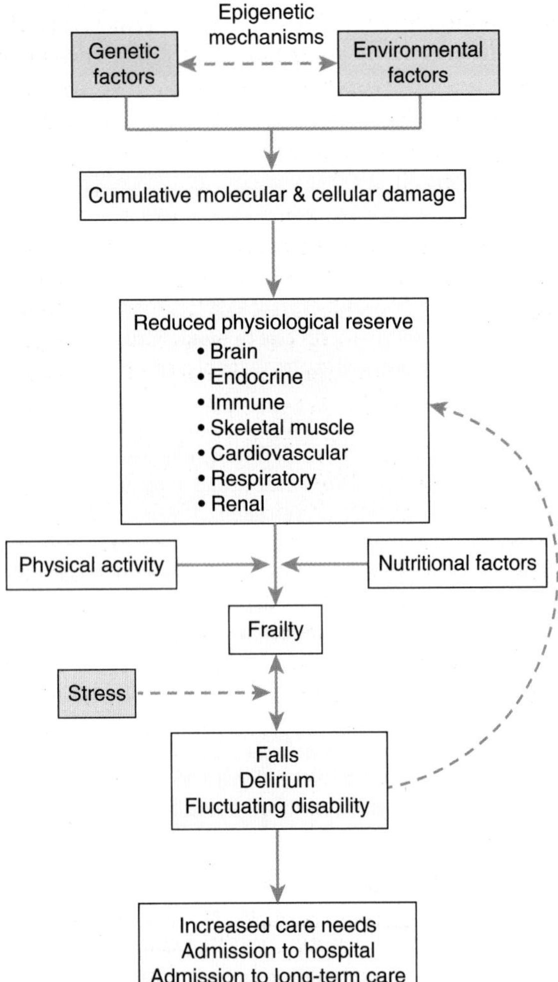

Fig. 2.43 Frailty. Frailty is a disorder of multiple interrelated physiologic systems. A gradual decline progresses with aging, but in frailty this decline becomes accelerated. Homeostatic mechanisms begin to fail, and vulnerability becomes disproportionate to changes in health status after a relatively minor stressor event. (Reprinted with permission from Elsevier. From Clegg A, et al. Frailty in elderly people, *Lancet* 2013;381(9868): 752–762.)

pallor mortis. In instances of death secondary to carbon monoxide poisoning, drowning, or chloroform poisoning, this phenomenon may not be apparent; instead, a lifelike coloration of the cheeks and lips may persist even after death has occurred.[131] Postmortem reduction of body temperature is algor mortis. Immediately after death, body temperature gradually falls and then decreases more rapidly (approximately 1.0°F to 1.5°F/hr.) until body temperature equals environmental temperature.

In cases of death caused by certain infective diseases, body temperature may transiently rise for a short time.

Blood pressure within the retinal vessels decreases, causing muscle tension to decrease and the pupils to become dilated. The face, nose, and chin begin to look "sharp" or "peaked" as blood and fluids drain from these areas. Gravity causes blood to settle in the most dependent, or lowest, tissues, causing a purple discoloration called livor mortis, which appears within half-an-hour to 1 hour of death and becomes fixed within 6 to 8 hours after death. Similarly, muscle stiffening or rigidity begins within a few hours of death, leading to the development of full body rigor mortis.[132] The smaller muscles are usually affected first, particularly the muscles of the jaws. Rigor mortis is caused by acidic compounds accumulating within the muscles due to the breakdown of carbohydrate and the depletion of ATP. This interferes with ATP-dependent detachment of myosin from actin (contractile proteins).[133] The development of rigor mortis is a process of change in the intensity of muscular rigidity over time. Initially, the muscular intensity is weak and affects involuntary muscles first and then voluntary muscles; subsequently, the intensity increases and reaches the maximum; finally, intensity decreases and practically disappears.[132] Rigor mortis develops sequentially, maintaining a steady state for approximately 12 hours, and becomes fully developed, affecting the entire body. Then, it gradually diminishes, and the body becomes flaccid in the

EMERGING SCIENCE BOX

COVID-19 and Postmortem Changes

Since the novel Coronavirus disease 2019 (COVID-19) became pandemic, there has been an abundance of information gained from post-mortem evaluation by autopsy. Approximately 15% of those affected undergo a severe disease and 5%–6% are critical (respiratory failure, and/or multiple organ dysfunction/failure); however, COVID-19 pathogenesis is still not sufficiently understood. Thus, systematic examination is mandatory to comprehend the extent and mechanisms of this novel disease. Autopsy is the only opportunity to macroscopically observe organs and take optimal samples for histological and molecular analyses. Thereby, autopsy is very likely superior to postmortem core needle biopsies. Consequently, several reports have recently demonstrated that autopsy-based examinations generate important insights into the disease manifestations, the mechanisms of organ failure, and the association with viral distribution. Disseminated diffuse alveolar damage at different stages (the histopathological correlate of acute respiratory distress syndrome) was the major histologic finding. Diffuse alveolar damage was detectable in all lobes but appeared unevenly distributed with pronounced manifestation in middle and lower lung fields. Minor neutrophil infiltration was indicative of secondary infection and/or aspiration. Mild lymphocytic myocarditis and signs of epicarditis were detectable. Liver histology showed minimal periportal lymphoplasmacellular infiltration and signs of fibrosis. There was no morphologically detectable pathology in other organs. Specifically, no signs of encephalitis or central nervous system vasculitis were found. At the time of autopsy, severe acute respiratory syndrome coronavirus 2 (SARS-CoV-2) was still detectable in the respiratory tracts of all affected persons. Polymerase chain reaction testing was positive in pleural effusion but negative in all cerebrospinal fluid (CSF) samples.

SARS-CoV-2 preferentially infects cells in the respiratory tract, but its direct affinity for organs other than the lungs remains poorly defined. The highest levels of SARS-CoV-2 copies per cell were detected in the respiratory tract, and lower levels were detected in the kidneys, liver, heart, brain, and blood. These findings indicate a broad organotropism of SARS-CoV-2.

Data from Puelles VG, et al. Multiorgan and renal tropism of SARS-CoV-2. *New England Journal of Medicine*, 2020. doi:10.1056/NEJMc2011400; Schaller T, et al. Postmortem examination of patients with COVID-19. *Journal of the American Medical Association*, 2020. doi: 10.1001/jama.2020.8907.

following 12 to 14 hours. The disappearance of rigor mortis is the same as its order of appearance. The disappearance of rigor mortis denoted by flaccidity of muscles is caused by the action of alkaline liquids produced by putrefaction.[132,134] Putrefaction is the decomposition of the body carried out by microbes. Natural gut bacteria migrate into the blood vessels and spread all over the body while other external microorganisms enter the body through the alimentary canal, respiratory tract, and open wounds. Without the body's natural defense and immune mechanisms, the bacteria continue to replicate, feeding on the proteins and carbohydrates of the blood and body parts. The principal bacterial agent causing putrefaction is the gram-positive, anaerobic, and rod-shaped *Clostridium welchi*.[135] Signs of putrefaction—state of decay with foul-smelling odor—are generally obvious about 24 to 48 hours after death. Putrefaction changes vary depending on the temperature of the environment. The most visible is greenish discoloration of the skin, particularly on the abdomen. The discoloration is from bacteria generating hydrogen sulfide and then reacting with the hemoglobin forming sulfahemoglobin, which stains the surrounding area green. The greenish-blue discoloration seen in superficial blood vessels, which is often visible through the skin, is from putrefaction of erythrocytes, and is known as "marbling" of the skin.[136] Slippage or loosening of the skin from underlying tissues occurs at the same time. After this, swelling or bloating of the body and liquefactive changes occur, sometimes causing opening of the body cavities. At a microscopic level, putrefactive changes are associated with the release of enzymes and lytic dissolution called postmortem autolysis.

Decomposition occurs when the organic matter of the body is broken down into elemental matter and recycled into the earth's biosphere. The body's own enzymes and chemicals drive this process. Putrification may be ongoing simultaneously. Skeletonization, the final stage after death, occurs when the various tissues of the body have degraded and decayed to the point of exposing the skeleton. When all the organic matter of the body is gone, the process is complete, and only disarticulated bones will remain. Depending on the environment surrounding the skeleton, bones can persist for periods lasting from several years to relatively indefinitely. Under rare circumstances, fossilization may occur. At this stage, the bones are infiltrated and replaced with inorganic mineral deposits. If this process transpires, the fossilized bones will have the permanence of rocks, thus accounting for many museum specimens. Fossilization is uncommon and only occurs under select and relatively unusual environmental conditions.

SUMMARY REVIEW

Cellular Adaptation

1. Injury to cells and their surrounding environment, called the *extracellular matrix*, leads to tissue and organ injury. Cellular adaptation is an alteration that enables the cell to maintain a steady state despite adverse conditions.
2. The most significant *adaptive* changes include atrophy, hypertrophy, hyperplasia, and metaplasia. Dysplasia is not a true cellular adaptation but rather atypical hyperplasia.
3. Atrophy is a decrease in cellular size, can affect any organ, and is most common in skeletal muscle, the heart, secondary sex organs, and the brain. Pathologic atrophy occurs as a result of disuse, insufficient blood supply, insufficient hormonal or neural stimulation, and decreased amino acid uptake.
4. Physiologic atrophy occurs with early development; for example, the thymus gland involutes and atrophies.
5. Aging causes brain cells and endocrine-dependent organs, such as the gonads, to become atrophic.
6. Hypertrophy is an increase in the size of cells caused by increased work demands or hormonal stimulation. Hypertrophy can be physiologic or pathologic. Amounts of protein in the plasma membrane, endoplasmic reticulum, microfilaments, and mitochondria are increased.
7. Hyperplasia is an increase in the number of cells caused by an increased rate of cellular division. Compensatory hyperplasia enables certain organs to regenerate. The main mechanism for hyperplasia is the production of hormones or growth factors. Hormonal hyperplasia occurs chiefly in estrogen-dependent organs to replace lost tissue or support new growth, such as during pregnancy.
8. Pathologic hyperplasia is the abnormal proliferation of normal cells in response to excessive hormonal stimulation or the effects of growth factors on target cells.
9. Dysplasia, or atypical hyperplasia, is an abnormal change in the size, shape, and organization of mature tissue cells. Importantly, the term dysplasia is not cancer and may not progress to cancer. Dysplastic tissues that do not involve the entire thickness of the epithelium may be completely reversible.
10. Metaplasia is the reversible replacement of one mature cell type by another, sometimes less differentiated, cell type. It is found in association with tissue damage, repair, and regeneration. Metaplasia develops from reprogramming of local tissue stem cells or colonization by differentiated cell populations from adjacent sites.

Cellular Injury

1. Injury to cells and to the extracellular matrix (ECM) leads to injury of tissues and organs, ultimately determining the structural patterns of disease. Injured cells may recover (reversible injury) or die (irreversible injury).
2. Cellular injury is caused by a lack of oxygen (hypoxia), free radicals, caustic or toxic chemicals, infectious agents, unintentional and intentional injury, inflammatory and immune responses, genetic factors, insufficient nutrients, or physical trauma from many causes. Injurious stimuli cause cell stress.
3. Cell injury can be acute or chronic, and it can be reversible or irreversible. It can involve necrosis, apoptosis, autophagy, accumulation, or pathologic calcification.

4. Four biochemical themes are important to cell injury: (a) depletion of ATP, (b) decreased levels of oxygen and increased levels of oxygen-derived free radicals, (c) increased concentration of intracellular calcium and loss of calcium steady state, and (d) defects in membrane permeability.
5. The sequence of events leading to cell death is commonly decreased ATP production, failure of active transport mechanisms (the Na^+-K^+ pump), cellular swelling, detachment of ribosomes from the endoplasmic reticulum, cessation of protein synthesis, mitochondrial swelling as a result of calcium accumulation, vacuolation, leakage of digestive enzymes from lysosomes, autodigestion of intracellular structures, lysis of the plasma membrane, and death.
6. Injury to cell components includes membrane damage, protein folding defects, mitochondrial compromise, and DNA damage.
7. The initial insult in hypoxic injury is usually ischemia—the cessation of blood flow into vessels that supply the cell with oxygen and nutrients. Hypoxia can induce inflammation, and inflamed lesions can become hypoxic. Hypoxia is a prominent feature encountered in bacterial infections, wounds, cardiovascular defects, and cancer.
8. Restoration of oxygen after ischemic injury can result in reperfusion (reoxygenation) injury. Reperfusion injury results from the generation of highly reactive oxygen intermediates or radicals and promotes proinflammatory neutrophil adhesion to the endothelium.
9. Inherent reactive oxygen species (ROS) from aerobic metabolism play a crucial biologic role, not just in various diseases but also in cellular communication and cell function. ROS reversibly modulates many intracellular signaling pathways. ROS can affect protein functions through several mechanisms, including regulation of protein expression, posttranslational modifications, and alteration of protein stability.
10. Reduction-oxidation- (redox) dependent regulation and the roles of ROS include both normal physiologic and pathologic roles. These expanding roles include proliferation and differentiation, immune function, stem cell self-renewal, tumor progression, autoimmunity, stem cell exhaustion, senescence, and longevity.
11. Cell injury produced by free radicals, particularly ROS, is an important mechanism of cell damage in many conditions, including chemical and radiation injury, ischemia-reperfusion injury, microbial killing by phagocytes, and cellular aging.
12. A significant mechanism of membrane damage is injury caused by free radicals, including oxidative stress. Oxidative stress can activate several intracellular signaling pathways because ROS can modulate enzymes and transcription factors. Free radicals are difficult to control and initiate chain reactions.
13. Sources of oxidants are numerous and include cellular organelles, particularly mitochondria, endoplasmic reticulum, and peroxisomes, NADPH oxidases, and other enzymes.
14. Free radicals can cause (a) lipid peroxidation or the destruction of unsaturated fatty acids, (b) alterations of proteins, protein loss, and protein misfolding, and (c) mutations in DNA.
15. Mitochondria contain their own DNA, called *mitochondrial DNA* (mtDNA), and can encode proteins involved in energy production. mtDNA encodes enzymes involved in oxidative phosphorylation, and mutations affecting these genes exert their damaging effects on organs most dependent on oxidative phosphorylation, such as the CNS, skeletal muscle, cardiac muscle, liver, and kidneys. Emerging is the role mitochondria have in mediating environmental changes and genomic responses.
16. Humans are exposed to thousands of chemicals that have inadequate toxicologic data. Toxicity pathways or cellular response pathways result in adverse health effects when disturbed. Components of these pathways include oxidative stress, heat shock response, DNA damage response, hypoxia, ER stress, mental stress, inflammation, and osmotic stress.
17. The initial insult in chemical and toxic injury is damage or destruction of the plasma membrane. Two general mechanisms include direct toxicity and conversion to toxic intermediates or metabolites. Examples of chemical agents that cause cellular injury include air pollutants, insecticides, herbicides, alcohol, lead, carbon monoxide, ethanol, mercury, opioids (heroin, morphine, prescription drugs for pain), and social or street drugs.
18. Drug overdoses dramatically increased with the COVID-19 pandemic as a contributing factor. The leading cause of poisoning in children is cosmetics and personal care products, cleaning substances, and analgesics. The use of e-cigarettes, or vaping, by adolescents, children, and young adults has become a leading cause of lung injury.
19. Under investigation are the beneficial effects of chemical compounds called *phytochemicals*. Examples of these products include certain fruits and plants, chamomile, silymarin, carrot, ginger root, milk thistle seed, rosemary leaf, turmeric, and others.
20. Globally, snakebite envenoming or poisoning by venom can have significant morbidity and mortality. Global data show 4.5 to 5.4 million people per year get bitten by snakes. Most snakebites in the United States are from pit vipers, with the majority from rattlesnakes. In the United States, about 9000 people per year suffer a snake bite, and 5 deaths occur. Worldwide, 1.8 to 2.7 million develop clinical illness and 81,000 to 138,000 deaths from complications.
21. High-risk groups for snakebite include rural agricultural workers, herders, fishermen, hunters, working children, living in poorly constructed homes, and those with limited education and medical resources. Risks also occur for professional snake handlers, and hiking or walking and stepping on snakes or moving close to them while they are hiding.
22. Snakes have hollow fangs in their anterior mouth and inject venom into subcutaneous tissue. Venom has both fibrinolytic and protein C activation, which can cause

coagulopathy. Certain species can cause neurotoxic effects, including cranial nerve dysfunction, weakness, and paralysis. In total, snakebites can cause various local, hematologic, neurologic, and systemic effects.

23. The world's largest single environmental health risk is air pollution. Air pollution was the fourth leading risk factor for premature death globally, with nearly 12% of all deaths and more than 6.67 million in 2019 alone. Three types of air pollution that impact human health are ambient (outdoor) fine particle pollution, ambient tropospheric ozone, and household air pollution. Air pollution is contamination of the environment by any chemical, physical, or biologic agent that modifies natural characteristics of the atmosphere.
24. Six pollutants as criteria air pollutants: carbon monoxide, lead, nitrogen oxides, photochemical oxidants, ground-level ozone particle pollution or particulate matter, and sulfur oxides. Fine particles or particulate matter $PM_{2.5,}$ pose the greatest risk to health.
25. By reducing air pollution levels, countries can lower the burden of diseases from stroke, heart disease, lung cancer, and chronic and acute respiratory diseases, including asthma. Prompt and sustained health benefits can come from improved air quality.
26. Ground level, or tropospheric, ozone is a highly reactive pollutant that causes adverse effects on human health, food crops, and other vegetation.
27. Indoor air pollution from the use of solid fuels was estimated to cause 2.31 to close to 4 million premature deaths globally.
28. Heavy metals commonly associated with harmful effects in humans include lead, mercury, arsenic, and cadmium. Studies of the involvement of metals in pathophysiology include DNA repair mechanisms, tumor suppressor functions, and interference with signal transduction pathways.
29. Unintentional and intentional injuries are an important health problem in the United States. Injuries include motor vehicle crashes, opioid overdoses, poisonings, sports and recreation-related injuries, firearms, falls, blunt force (tearing, shearing, crushing of tissues), asphyxia (suffocation, strangulation, chemical asphyxiants, drowning), and others, including injury from medical care itself.
30. Injury from microorganisms lies in their ability to survive and proliferate in the human body. Injury depends on the microorganisms' ability to invade and destroy cells, produce toxins, and produce damaging hypersensitivity reactions. In 2020, COVID-19 was the third leading cause of death, following heart disease and cancer.
31. Activation of inflammation and immunity, which occurs after cellular injury or infection, involves powerful biochemicals and proteins capable of damaging normal (uninjured and uninfected) cells.
32. Globally, the direct and indirect impacts of climate change on human health continue to be observed. The direct effects on health include increasing temperatures, which include heat-related mortality and morbidity, increased occurrence and intensity of storms, which increase injury, death, and psychological stressors. Indirect climate change affects health because of altered environmental conditions, such as water quality and quantity, foodborne disease from changing ecosystems intensify food and nutritional security.
33. Climate is changing beyond the range of the recent geological era because levels of carbon dioxide, methane, nitrous oxide, and fluorinated gases called greenhouse gases trap heat in the atmosphere. Wildfires are becoming more common and are projected to worsen with climate change.
34. Genetic disorders injure cells by altering the nucleus and the plasma membrane's structure, shape, receptors, or transport mechanisms.
35. Deprivation of essential nutrients (proteins, carbohydrates, lipids, vitamins) can cause cellular injury by altering cellular structure and function, particularly of transport mechanisms, chromosomes, the nucleus, and DNA. Excessive amounts of other nutrients, for example, carbohydrates, can lead to obesity, changes in insulin utilization, and diabetes.
36. Injurious physical agents include temperature extremes and climate change, changes in atmospheric pressure, ionizing radiation, illumination, mechanical stresses (e.g., repetitive body movements), and noise.

Manifestations of Cellular Injury

1. Manifestations of cellular injury include accumulations of water, lipids, carbohydrates, glycogen, proteins, pigments, hemosiderin, bilirubin, calcium, and urate.
2. Accumulations harm cells by "crowding" the organelles and by causing excessive (and sometimes harmful) metabolites to be produced during their catabolism. The metabolites are released into the cytoplasm or expelled into the extracellular matrix.
3. Cellular swelling, the accumulation of excessive water in the cell, is caused by the failure of transport mechanisms and is a sign of many types of cellular injury.
4. Accumulations of organic substances—lipids, carbohydrates, glycogen, proteins, and pigments—are caused by disorders in which (a) cellular uptake of the substance exceeds the cell's capacity to catabolize (digest) or use it or (b) cellular anabolism (synthesis) of the substance exceeds the cell's capacity to use or secrete it.
5. Calcium salts accumulate in both injured and dead tissues resulting in cellular calcification. Mechanisms include the influx of extracellular calcium in injured mitochondria, and calcium can accumulate in alveoli, gastric epithelium, and renal tubules because of the excretion of acid at these sites, leading to the local production of hydroxyl ions. Damage occurs when calcium salts clump and harden, interfering with normal cellular structure and function.
6. Dystrophic calcification (accumulation of calcium salts) is always a sign of pathologic change because it occurs only in injured or dead cells. Free calcium in the cytosol can cause activation of protein kinases, activation of phospholipases and membrane damage, and damage or disassembly of the cytoskeleton. Metastatic calcification, however, can occur in uninjured cells in individuals with hypercalcemia.

7. Disturbances in urate metabolism can result in hyperuricemia and deposition of sodium urate crystals in tissue, leading to a painful disorder called *gout*.
8. Systemic manifestations of cellular injury include fever, leukocytosis, increased heart rate, pain, and serum elevations of enzymes in the plasma.

Cellular Death

1. Cells die from accidental cell death (ACD) or regulated cell death (RCD). Cell death has historically been classified as necrosis and apoptosis. Necrosis is characterized by rapid loss of the plasma membrane structure, organelle swelling, mitochondrial dysfunction, and the lack of typical features of apoptosis. Apoptosis is known as regulated or programmed cell process by the "dropping off" of cellular fragments called *apoptotic bodies*. Oxidative stress can lead to various types of RCD as well as the antioxidant defenses. Other forms of cell loss include autophagy.
2. The five major types of necrosis are coagulative, liquefactive, caseous, fat, and fibrinoid. Different types of necrosis occur in different tissues.
3. Gangrenous necrosis, or gangrene, is tissue necrosis caused by hypoxia and subsequent bacterial invasion.
4. Autophagy is a recycling factory, a self-destructive process, and a survival mechanism. It degrades cytoplasmic components and organelles in lysosomes and salvages key metabolites to promote metabolic and nutrient homeostasis. Autophagy has a central role in cell homeostasis. It is important in diverse processes and conditions such as development, cell proliferation, remodeling, aging, cancer, heart disease, neurodegenerative diseases, inflammation, infection, metabolic diseases, and cell death.

Aging

1. Aging is a time-dependent functional decline. It is difficult to determine the physiologic (normal) from the pathologic changes of aging. The hallmarks of aging include genomic instability, telomere attrition, epigenetic alterations, loss of proteostasis or maintenance of protein homeostasis, deregulated nutrient-sensing, mitochondrial dysfunction, cellular senescence, stem cell exhaustion, and altered intercellular communication.
2. Senescence is a process of permanent proliferative arrest or nondividing state called replicative senescence. Senescence is important because it causes a loss of tissue-repair capacity, and it produces proinflammatory and matrix-degrading molecules known as the senescence-associated secretory phenotype (SASP).
3. Aging is associated with increased levels of circulating cytokines and proinflammatory markers. There are changes in the immune system with aging known as *inflammaging*. The microbiota plays a fundamental role in the induction and function of the immune system. Diet is believed to have a major influence on both the development and the prevention of age-related diseases.
4. Humans have an inherent maximal life span (80 to 100 years) that is dictated by currently unknown intrinsic mechanisms.
5. Although the maximal life span has not changed significantly over time, the average life span, or life expectancy, has declined since 2014.
6. Frailty is a common clinical syndrome in older adults, leaving a person vulnerable to falls, functional decline, disability, disease, and death. The syndrome is complex, involving oxidative stress, dysregulation of inflammatory cytokines and hormones, malnutrition, physical inactivity, and muscle changes. Women have a higher risk of frailty than men.

Somatic Death

1. Somatic death is death of the entire organism. Postmortem change is diffuse and does not involve the inflammatory response.
2. Manifestations of somatic death are progressive, occurring in a sequenced manner. Death typically begins with the cessation of respiration and circulation and characteristic dilation of the pupils and culminates with the skeletonization of the body. The stages of death are (1) pallor mortis, (2) algor mortis, (3) rigor mortis, (4) livor mortis, (5) putrefaction, (6) decomposition, and (7) skeletonization.
3. Depending on the environment surrounding the bones, a rare eighth stage, fossilization, may occur.

REFERENCES

1. Kumar V, Abbas AK, Aster JC. *Robbins & Cotran Pathophysiologic Basis of Disease*. ed 10, Philadelphia: Elsevier; 2020.
2. Lee P, Chandel NS, Simon MC. Cellular adaptation to hypoxia through hypoxia inducible factors and beyond. *Nat Rev Mol Cell Biol*. 2020;21:268–283. Available at https://doi.org/10.1038/s41580-020-0227-y. (Accessed October 12, 2021).
3. Rogers J, Baker M. Understanding the most commonly billed diagnoses in primary care: atherosclerotic cardiovascular disease. *Nurse Pract*. 2020;45(7):35–41. Available at https://doi.org/10.1097/01.npr.0000669136.88720.65. (Accessed October 12, 2021).
4. Wang ZJ, et al. The effect of intravenous vitamin C infusion on periprocedural myocardial injury for patients undergoing elective percutaneous coronary intervention. *Can J Cardiol*. 2014;30(1):96–101. Available at https://doi.org/10.1016/j.cjca.2013.08.018. (Accessed October 12, 2021).
5. Rodrigo R, Prieto JC, Castillo R. Cardioprotection against ischaemia/reperfusion by vitamins C and E plus n-3 fatty acids: molecular mechanisms and potential clinical applications. *Clin Sci (Lond)*. 2013;124(1):1–15. Available at https://doi.org/10.1042/cs20110663. (Accessed October 12, 2021).
6. Thomas RS, et al. The US Federal Tox21 program: a strategic and operational plan for continued leadership. *ALTEX*. 2018;35(2):163–168. Available at https://doi.org/10.14573/altex.1803011. (Accessed October 12, 2021).
7. Pankaj B, et al. Chapter 12: Major metabolites after degradation of xenobiotics and enzymes involved in these pathways. In: Pankaj B, ed. *Smart bioremediation technologies*. Cambridge, MA: Academic Press; 2019:205–215. Available at https://doi.org/10.1016/B978-0-12-818307-6.00012-3. (Accessed October 11, 2021).

8. Lewis JH. Liver disease caused by anesthetic, chemicals, toxins, and herbal and dietary supplements. In: Feldman M, et al, ed. *Sleisenger and Fordtran's gastrointestinal and liver disease: pathophysiology, diagnosis, management*. ed 11, Philadelphia: Elsevier; 2020:1399–1414.
9. Szabo G, McClain CJ. Alcoholic liver disease. In: Feldman M, et al, ed. *Sleisenger and Fordtran's gastrointestinal and liver disease: pathophysiology, diagnosis, management*. ed 11, Philadelphia: Elsevier; 2020:1336–1353.
10. Shivakumar C, Teob NC, Farrell GC. Liver disease caused by drugs. In: Feldman M, ed. et al, *Sleisenger and Fordtran's gastrointestinal and liver disease: pathophysiology, diagnosis, management*. ed 11, Philadelphia: Elsevier; 2020:1367–1398.
11. Centers for Disease Control and Prevention (CDC), *Overdose deaths accelerating during COVID-19*. Atlanta, GA: CDC; 2020. Page last reviewed: December 18, 2020. Available at https://www.cdc.gov/media/releases/2020/p1218-overdose-deaths-covid-19.html. (Accessed October 11, 2021).
12. Centers for Disease Control and Prevention (CDC) *Drug overdose deaths*. Atlanta, GA: CDC; 2018. Page last reviewed: March 3, 2021. Available at: https://www.cdc.gov/drugoverdose/data/statedeaths.html. (Accessed October 11, 2021).
13. Gummin DD, et al. 2019 Annual Report of the American Association of Poison Control Centers' National Poison Data System (NPDS): 37th Annual Report. *Clin Toxicol (Phila)*. 2020;58(12):1360–1541. Available at https://doi.org/10.1080/15563650.2020.1834219. (Accessed October 11, 2021).
14. American Association of Poison Control Centers (AAPCC). *National poison data system*. Arlington, VA: AAPCC; 2021. Available at https://aapcc.org/national-poison-data-system. (Accessed October 11, 2021).
15. World Health Organization (WHO). *Snakebite envenoming*. Geneva, Switzerland: WHO; 2021. Last modified May 17, 2021. Available at https://www.who.int/news-room/fact-sheets/detail/snakebite-envenoming. (Accessed October 12, 2021).
16. Patel V, Kong EL, Hamilton RJ. *Rattle snake toxicity*. In *StatPearls*. Treasure Island, FL: StatPearls Publishing; 2021. Last updated July 25, 2021. Available at https://www.ncbi.nlm.nih.gov/books/NBK431065/. (Accessed October 12, 2021).
17. World Health Organization (WHO). *Air pollution*. Geneva, Switzerland: WHO; 2021. Available at http://www.who.int/topics/air_pollution/en/. (Accessed October 12, 2021).
18. U.S. Environmental Protection Agency (EPA). *EPA criteria air pollutants*. Washington, DC: EPA; 2021. Last modified August 16, 2021. Available at https://www.epa.gov/criteria-air-pollutants. (Accessed October 12, 2021).
19. World Health Organization (WHO). *Household air pollution and health*. Geneva, Switzerland: WHO; 2021. Last modified: September 22, 2021. Available at https://www.who.int/news-room/fact-sheets/detail/household-air-pollution-and-health. (Accessed October 12, 2021).
20. GDB 2016. Risk Factors Collaborators: Global, regional, and national comparative risk assessment of 84 behavioural, environmental and occupational, and metabolic risks or clusters of risks, 1990–2016: a systematic analysis for the Global Burden of Disease Study 2016. *Lancet*. 2017;390(10100):1345–1422. Available at https://doi.org/10.1016/S0140-6736(17)32366-8. (Accessed October 12, 2021).
21. Health Effects Institute. *State of Global Air 2020. Special report*. Boston, MA: Health Effects Institute; 2020. Available at https://www.stateofglobalair.org/resources. (Accessed October 12, 2021).
22. Occupational Safety and Health Administration (OSHA). *Lead*. Washington, DC: OSHA; 2018. Available at https://www.osha.gov/lead. (Accessed October 12, 2021).
23. Centers for Disease Control and Prevention (CDC). *Lead*. Atlanta, GA: CDC; 2021. Page last reviewed September 24, 2021. Available at https://www.cdc.gov/nceh/lead/. (Accessed October 12, 2021).
24. Council on Environmental Health: Prevention of childhood lead toxicity. *Pediatrics*. 2016;138(1):e20161493. Available at https://doi.org/10.1542/peds.2016-1493. (Accessed October 12, 2021).
25. Nichani WI, et al. Blood lead levels in children after phase-out of leaded gasoline in Bombay, India. *Sci Total Environ*. 2006;363(1–3):95–106. Available at https://doi.org/10.1016/j.scitotenv.2005.06.033. (Accessed October 12, 2021).
26. Luo XS, Yu S, Li XD. Distribution, availability, and sources of trace metals in different particle size fractions of urban soils in Hong Kong: implications for assessing the risk to human health. *Environ Pollut*. 2011;159(5):1317–1326. Available at https://doi.org/10.1016/j.envpol.2011.01.013. (Accessed October 12, 2021).
27. United States Environmental Protection Agency (EPA). *National Ambient Air Quality Standards (NAAQS) for lead (Pb) fact sheets and additional information*. Washington, DC: EPA; 2016. Last updated September 27, 2021. Available at: https://www.epa.gov/lead-air-pollution/national-ambient-air-quality-standards-naaqs-lead-pb-fact-sheets-and-additional. (Accessed October 12, 2021).
28. Center for Disease Control (CDC) *Childhood lead poisoning prevention: blood lead levels in children*. Atlanta, GA: CDC; 2021. Page last reviewed April 5, 2021. Available at https://www.cdc.gov/nceh/lead/prevention/blood-lead-levels.htm. (Accessed October 12, 2021).
29. Neal AP, Guilarte TR. Mechanisms of lead and manganese neurotoxicity. *Toxicol Res*. 2013;2(2):99–114. Available at https://doi.org/10.1039/c2tx20064c. (Accessed October 12, 2021).
30. Centers for Disease Control and Prevention (CDC): Blood lead levels in children aged 1-5 years—United States, 1999-2010. *Morb Mortal Wkly Rep*. 2013;62(13):245–248. Page last updated April 5, 2013. Available at https://www.cdc.gov/mmwr/preview/mmwrhtml/mm6213a3.htm. (Accessed October 12, 2021).
31. Raymond J, Brown MJ. Childhood blood lead levels in children aged <5 years—United States, 2009–2014. *MMWR Surveill Summ*. 2017;66(No. SS-3):1–10. Available at https://doi.org/10.15585/mmwr.ss6603a1. (Accessed October 12, 2021).
32. Halmo L, Nappe TM. *Lead toxicity*. In: *StatPearls*. Treasure Island, FL: StatPearls Publishing; 2021. Last updated July 10, 2021. Available at https://www.ncbi.nlm.nih.gov/books/NBK541097/. (Accessed October 12, 2021).
33. Alarcon WA. Elevated blood lead levels among employed adults — United States, 1994–2013. *MMWR Morb Mortal Wkly Rep*. 2016;63:59–65. Available at https://doi.org/10.15585/mmwr.mm6355a5. (Accessed October 12, 2021).
34. Egan KB, Tsai RJ, Chuke SO. Integrating childhood and adult blood lead surveillance to improve identification and intervention efforts. *J Public Health Manag Pract*. 2019;25:S98–S104. Available at https://doi.org/10.1097/PHH.0000000000000872. (Accessed October 12, 2021).
35. Quail MT. Retained bullet or bullet fragments: a potential source of elevated blood lead levels. *Nursing*. 2018;48(10):15 Available at https://doi.org/10.1097/01.NURSE.0000545014.98790.6e. (Accessed October 12, 2021).
36. Santucci RJ, Scully JR. The pervasive threat of lead (PB) in drinking water: unmasking and pursuing scientific factors that govern lead release. *Proc Natl Acad Sci U S A*.

2020;117(38):23211–23218. Available at https://doi.org/10.1073/pnas.1913749117. (Accessed October 12, 2021).

37. Lassiter MG, et al. Cross–species coherence in effects and modes of action in support of causality determinations in the U S. Environmental Protection Agency's Integrated Science Assessment for Lead. *Toxicology*. 2015;330:19–40. Available at https://doi.org/10.1016/j.tox.2015.01.015. (Accessed October 12, 2021).
38. Wu X, et al. A review of toxicity and mechanisms of individual and mixtures of heavy metals in the environment. *Environ Sci Pollut Res Int*. 2016;23(9):8244–8259. Available at https://doi.org/10.1007/s11356-016-6333-x. (Accessed October 12, 2021).
39. Lanphear BP, et al. Low-level environmental lead exposure and children's intellectual function: an international pooled analysis. *Environ Health Perspect*. 2005;113(7):894–899. Available at https://doi.org/10.1289/ehp.7688. (Accessed October 12, 2021).
40. Zhang N, et al. Early childhood lead exposure and academic achievement: evidence from Detroit public schools, 2008–2010. *Am J Public Health*. 2013;103(3):e72–e77. Available at https://doi.org/10.2105/AJPH.2012.301164. (Accessed October 12, 2021).
41. Centers for Disease Control and Prevention (CDC). *Thimerosal and vaccines*. Atlanta, GA: CDC; 2020. Page last reviewed August 25, 2020. Available at: https://www.cdc.gov/vaccinesafety/concerns/thimerosal/index.html. (Accessed October 12, 2021).
42. United Nations Environment Programme (UNEP). *Global mercury assessment 2013: sources, emissions, releases and environmental transport*. Geneva, Switzerland: UNEP Chemicals Branch; 2013. Available at https://wedocs.unep.org/20.500.11822/7984. (Accessed October 12, 2021.
43. U.S. Food and Drug Administration (FDA). *Food safety for moms-to-be*. Washington, DC: FDA; 2018. Content current as of September 3, 2018. Available at https://www.fda.gov/food/people-risk-foodborne-illness/food-safety-moms-be. (Accessed October 12, 2021).
44. Substance Abuse and Mental Health Services Administration (SAMHSA). *2018 National Survey of Drug Use and Health (NSDUH) Release*. Rockville, MD: SAMHSA; 2018. Available at https://www.samhsa.gov/data/release/2018-national-survey-drug-use-and-health-nsduh-releases. (Accessed October 12, 2021).
45. National Institute of Health (NIH), National Institute of Alcohol Abuse and Alcoholism (NIAAA). *Facts and statistics*. Bethesda, MD: NIH NIAAA; 2021. Last modified June 2021. Available at https://www.niaaa.nih.gov/publications/brochures-and-fact-sheets/alcohol-facts-and-statistics. (Accessed October 12, 2021).
46. Porter WF, Moyer TP. Clinical toxicology. In: Burtis CA, Ashwood ER, eds. *Tietz textbook of clinical chemistry*. ed 4, Philadelphia: WB Saunders Company; 1993:1155–1235.
47. Kamran U, et al. Nutrition in alcohol-related liver disease: physiopathology and management. *World J Gastroenterol*. 2020;26(22):2916–2930. Available at https://doi.org/10.3748/wjg.v26.i22.2916. (Accessed October 12, 2021).
48. Wang SC, et al. Alcohol addiction, gut microbiota, and alcoholism treatment: a review. *Int J Mol Sci*. 2020;21(17):6413 Available at https://doi.org/10.3390/ijms21176413. (Accessed October 12, 2021).
49. Gupta KK, Gupta VK, Shirasaka T. An update on fetal alcohol syndrome—pathogenesis, risks, and treatment. *Alcohol Clin Exp Res*. 2016;40(8):1594–1602. Available at https://doi.org/10.1111/acer.13135. (Accessed October 12, 2021).
50. Jin S, et al. Brain ethanol metabolism by astrocytic ALDH2 drives the behavioral effects of ethanol intoxication. *Nat Metab*. 2021;3:337–351. Available at https://doi.org/10.1038/s42255-021-00357-z. (Accessed October 12, 2021).
51. U.S. Department of Agriculture, U.S. Department of Health and Human Services. *Dietary Guidelines for Americans, 2020-2025*. ed 9, Washington, DC: USDA/USHHS; 2020. Last modified December 2020. Available at https://www.dietaryguidelines.gov/. (Accessed October 12, 2021).
52. Centers for Disease Control and Prevention (CDC) *Dietary guidelines for alcohol*. Atlanta, GA: CDC; 2020. Last reviewed December 29, 2020. Available at https://www.cdc.gov/alcohol/fact-sheets/moderate-drinking.htm. (Accessed October 12, 2021).
53. Julien J, et al. Projected prevalence and mortality associated with alcohol-related liver disease in the USA, 2019–40: a modelling study. *Lancet Public Health*. 2020;5(6):e316–e323. Available at https://doi.org/10.1016/s2468-2667(20)30062-1. (Accessed October 12, 2021).
54. National Cancer Institute (NCI). *Alcohol and cancer risk*. Bethesda, MD: NCI; 2021. Updated July 14, 2021. Available at: https://www.cancer.gov/about-cancer/causes-prevention/risk/alcohol/alcohol-fact-sheet. (Accessed October 12, 2021).
55. Pasala S, Barr T, Messaoudi I. Impact of alcohol abuse on the adaptive immune system. *Alcohol Res*. 2015;37(2):185–197.
56. National Institute on Alcohol Abuse and Alcoholism (NIAAA). *HIV/AIDS*, Bethesda, MD, NIAAA. Available at https://www.niaaa.nih.gov/alcohols-effects-health/special-populations-co-occurring-disorders/hivaids. (Accessed October 12, 2021).
57. Barr T, et al. Opposing effects of alcohol on the immune system. *Prog Neuropsychopharmacol Biol Psychiatry*. 2016;65:242–251. Available at https://doi.org/10.1016/j.pnpbp.2015.09.001. (Accessed October 12, 2021).
58. May PA, et al. Prevalence of fetal alcohol spectrum disorders in 4 US communities. *JAMA*. 2018;319(5):474–482. Available at https://doi.org/10.1001/jama.2017.21896. (Accessed October 12, 2021).
59. Maenner MJ, et al. Prevalence of autism spectrum disorder among children aged 8 years—autism and developmental disabilities monitoring network, 11 sites, United States, 2016. *MMWR Surveill Summ*. 2020;69(No. SS-4):1–12. Available at https://doi.org/10.15585/mmwr.ss6904a1. (Accessed October 12, 2021).
60. Centers for Disease Control and Prevention (CDC). *Fetal alcohol spectrum disorders (FASDs): basics about FASDs*. Atlanta, GA: CDC; 2021. Last modified May 21, 2021. Available at https://www.cdc.gov/ncbddd/fasd/facts.html. (Accessed October 12, 2021).
61. Burd L, et al. Prenatal alcohol exposure, blood alcohol concentrations and alcohol elimination rates for the mother, fetus and newborn. *J Perinatol*. 2012;32(9):652–659. Available at https://doi.org/10.1038/jp.2012.57. (Accessed October 12, 2021).
62. Jarmasz JS, et al. Human brain abnormalities associated with prenatal alcohol exposure and fetal alcohol spectrum disorder. *J Neuropathol Exp Neurol*. 2017;76(9):813–833. Available at https://doi.org/10.1093/jnen/nlx064. (Accessed October 12, 2021).
63. Stoicea N, et al. Current perspectives on the opioid crisis in the US healthcare system: a comprehensive literature review. *Medicine*. 2019;98(20):e15425 Available at https://doi.org/10.1097/MD.0000000000015425. (Accessed October 12, 2021).
64. Centers for Disease Control and Prevention (CDC). *Synthetic opioid overdose data*. Atlanta, GA: CDC; 2021. Last modified 25 March 2021. Available at: https://www.cdc.gov/drugoverdose/deaths/synthetic/index.html. (Accessed October 12, 2021).

65. Centers for Disease Control and Prevention (CDC). *Multiple cause of death, 1999-2019 request: mortality data on CDC WONDER*. Atlanta, GA: CDC; 2020. Available at https://wonder.cdc.gov/controller/datarequest/D77. (Accessed 1 October, 2021).
66. Centers for Disease Control and Prevention (CDC). *NCHS data on drug overdose deaths: NCHS fact sheet, June 2021*. Atlanta, GA: CDC; 2021. Page last reviewed May 17, 2021. Available at: https://www.cdc.gov/nchs/about/factsheets/factsheet-drug-overdose.htm. (Accessed October 12, 2021).
67. Centers for Disease Control and Prevention (CDC). *Underlying cause of death 1999-2019 request: mortality data on CDC WONDER*. Atlanta, GA: CDC; 2020. Available at http://wonder.cdc.gov/ucd-icd10.html. (Accessed October 12, 2021).
68. Centers for Disease Control and Prevention (CDC). *WISQARS™: web-based injury statistics query and reporting system*. Atlanta, GA: CDC; 2020. Available at https://www.cdc.gov/injury/wisqars/index.html. (Accessed October 12, 2021).
69. Centers for Disease Control and Prevention (CDC) *Sexual violence is preventable*. Atlanta, GA: CDC; 2020. Page last reviewed April 19, 2021. Available at https://www.cdc.gov/injury/features/sexual-violence/index.html. (Accessed October 12, 2021).
70. U.S. Department of Justice, Bureau of Justice Statistics. *National Crime Victimization Survey (NCVS)*. Washington, DC: U.S. Department of Justice, Bureau of Justice Statistics; 2019. Latest data available 2019. Available at https://bjs.ojp.gov/data-collection/ncvs. (Accessed October 12, 2021). [Note: The Rape, Abuse & Incest National Network (RAINN) applies a 5-year rolling average to adjust for changes in the year-to-year NCVS survey data.].
71. Rui P, Ashman JJ, Akinseye A. Emergency department visits for injuries sustained during sports and recreational activities by patients aged 5-24 years, 2010-2016. *Natl Health Stat Report*. 2019(133):1–15. Available at https://www.cdc.gov/nchs/data/nhsr/nhsr133-508.pdf. (Accessed October 12, 2021).
72. Xu JQ, et al. Mortality in the United States, 2018. *NCHS Data Brief*. 2020(355):1–8. Available at https://www.cdc.gov/nchs/data/databriefs/db355-h.pdf. (Accessed October 12, 2021).
73. Ahmad FB, et al. Provisional Mortality Data - United States, 2020. *MMWR Morb Mortal Wkly Rep*. 2021;70(14):519–522. Available at https://doi.org/10.15585/mmwr.mm7014e1. (Accessed October 13, 2021).
74. Robertson JJ, Long B. Suffering in silence: medical error and its impact on health care providers. *J Emerg Med*. 2018;54(4):402–409. Available at https://doi.org/10.1016/j.jemermed.2017.12.001. (Accessed October 13, 2021).
75. Center for Disease Control and Prevention (CDC). *Healthcare-associated infections (HAIs)*. Atlanta, GA: CDC; 2020. Page last reviewed December 14, 2017. Available at https://www.cdc.gov/winnablebattles/report/HAIs.html. (Accessed October 13, 2021).
76. Agency for Healthcare Research and Quality (AHRQ) *AHRQ national scorecard on hospital-acquired conditions: Final results for 2014 through 2017*. Rockville, MD: AHRQ; 2020. Content last reviewed July 2020. Available at https://www.ahrq.gov/hai/pfp/index.html. (Accessed October 13, 2021).
77. Rodziewicz TL, Houseman B, Hipskind JE. *Medical error reduction and prevention*. In: *StatPearls*. Treasure Island, FL: StatPearls Publishing; 2021. Last update August 6, 2021. Available at https://www.ncbi.nlm.nih.gov/books/NBK499956/. (Accessed October 13, 2021).
78. World Health Organization (WHO). *Patient safety*. Geneva, Switzerland: WHO; 2019. Last updated 13 September 13, 2019. Available at: https://www.who.int/news-room/fact-sheets/detail/patient-safety. (Accessed 1 October, 2021).
79. Slawomirski L, Auraaen A, Klazinga N. *The economics of patient safety in primary and ambulatory care: flying blind*. Paris: OECD; 2018. Available at https://www.oecd.org/health/health-systems/The-Economics-of-Patient-Safety-in-Primary-and-Ambulatory-Care-April2018.pdf. (Accessed October 13, 2021).
80. de Vries EN, et al. The incidence and nature of in-hospital adverse events: a systematic review. *Qual Saf Health Care*. 2008;17(3):216–223. Available at https://doi.org/10.1136/qshc.2007.023622. (Accessed October 13, 2021).
81. World Health Organization (WHO) *Global Patient Safety Action Plan 2021-2030*. Geneva, Switzerland: WHO; 2021. Available at https://www.who.int/teams/integrated-health-services/patient-safety/policy/global-patient-safety-action-plan. (Accessed October 13, 2021).
82. Lambert ABE, et al. Sleep-related infant suffocation deaths attributable to soft bedding, overlay, and wedging. *Pediatrics*. 2019;143(5):e20183408. Available at https://doi.org/10.1542/peds.2018-3408. (Accessed October 13, 2021).
83. De Boos J. Review article: non-fatal strangulation: hidden injuries, hidden risks. *Emerg Med Australas*. 2019;31(3):302–308. Available at https://doi.org/10.1111/1742-6723.13243. (Accessed October 13, 2021).
84. Center for Disease Control and Prevention (CDC). *Drowning prevention: drowning facts*. Atlanta, GA: CDC; 2021. Page last reviewed June 17, 2021. Available at https://www.cdc.gov/drowning/facts/index.html. (Accessed October 13, 2021).
85. World Health Organization (WHO) *Drowning*. Geneva, Switzerland: WHO; 2021. Published April 27, 2021. Available at https://www.who.int/news-room/fact-sheets/detail/drowning. (Accessed October 13, 2021).
86. Abelairas-Gómez C, et al. Drowning: epidemiology, prevention, pathophysiology, resuscitation, and hospital treatment. *Emergencias*. 2019;31(4):270–280. Available at http://emergencias.portalsemes.org/descargar/el-ahogamiento-epidemiologa-prevencin-fisiopatologa-reanimacin-de-la-vctima-ahogada-y-tratamiento-hospitalario/. (Accessed October 13, 2021).
87. Xu R, et al. Wildfires, global climate change, and human health. *N Engl J Med*. 2020;383(22):2173–2181. Available at https://doi.org/10.1056/NEJMsr2028985. (Accessed October 13, 2021).
88. Finlay SE, et al: Health impacts of wildfires, *PLoS Curr* 4:e4f959951cce2c, 2012. Available at https://www.ncbi.nlm.nih.gov/pmc/articles/PMC3492003/. (Accessed October 13, 2021).
89. Reid CE, et al. Critical review of health impacts of wildfire smoke exposure. *Environ Health Perspect*. 2016;124(9):1334–1343. Available at https://doi.org/10.1289/ehp.1409277. (Accessed October 13, 2021).
90. Black C, et al. Wildfire smoke exposure and human health: significant gaps in research for a growing public health issue. *Environ Toxicol Pharmacol*. 2017;55:186–195. Available at https://doi.org/10.1016/j.etap.2017.08.022. (Accessed October 13, 2021).
91. Vanos JK. Children's health and vulnerability in outdoor microclimates: a comprehensive review. *Environ Int*. 2015;76:1–15. Available at https://doi.org/10.1016/j.envint.2014.11.016. (Accessed October 13, 2021).
92. National Council on Radiation Protection and Measurements (NCRP) *Ionizing radiation exposure of the population of the United States: NCRP Report No. 160*. Bethesda, MD: NCRP; 2015.
93. Venkatesulu BP, et al. Radiation-induced endothelial vascular injury: a review of possible mechanisms. *JACC Basic Transl*

Sci. 2018;3(4):563–572. Available at https://doi.org/10.1016/j.jacbts.2018.01.014. (Accessed October 13, 2021).
94. Coppé JP, et al. The senescence-associated secretory phenotype: the dark side of tumor suppression. *Annu Rev Pathol.* 2010;5(1):99–118. Available at https://doi.org/10.1146/annurev-pathol-121808-102144. (Accessed October 13, 2021).
95. Baselet B, et al. Pathological effects of ionizing radiation: endothelial activation and dysfunction. *Cell Mol Life Sci.* 2019;76(4):699–728. Available at https://doi.org/10.1007/s00018-018-2956-z. (Accessed October 13, 2021).
96. Hall E, Giaccia AJ. Milestones in the radiation sciences. In: Hall E, Giaccia AJ, eds. *Radiobiology for the radiologist.* ed 6, Philadelphia: Lippincott Williams & Wilkins; 2006.
97. Linet S, et al. Cancer risks associated with external radiation from diagnostic imaging procedures. *CA Cancer J Clin.* 2012;62(2):75–100. Available at https://doi.org/10.3322/caac.21132. (Accessed October 13, 2021).
98. Shuryak I, Brenner DJ. Quantitative modeling of multigenerational effects of chronic ionizing radiation using targeted and nontargeted effects. *Sci Rep.* 2021;11:4776. Available at https://doi.org/10.1038/s41598-021-84156-2. (Accessed October 13, 2021).
99. Du Y, et al. Radiation-induced bystander effect can be transmitted through exosomes using miRNAs as effector molecules. *Radiat Res.* 2020;194(1):89–100. Available at https://doi.org/10.1667/RADE-20-00019.1. (Accessed October 13, 2021).
100. Mothersill C, Seymour C. Are epigenetic mechanisms involved in radiation-induced bystander effects? *Front Genet.* 2012;3:74. Available at https://doi.org/10.3389/fgene.2012.00074. (Accessed October 13, 2021).
101. Li Z, et al. Replication stress and FOXM1 drive radiation induced genomic instability and cell transformation. *PLoS One.* 2020;15(11):e0235998 Available at https://doi.org/10.1371/journal.pone.0235998. (Accessed October 13, 2021).
102. Preston DL, et al. Solid cancer incidence in atomic bomb survivors: 1958–1998. *Radiat Res.* 2007;168(1):1–64. Available at https://doi.org/10.1667/RR0763.1. (Accessed October 13, 2021).
103. Yoon I, Slesinger TL. *Radiation exposure in pregnancy.* In *StatPearls.* Treasure Island, FL: StatPearls Publishing; 2021. Updated May 8, 2021. Available at https://www.ncbi.nlm.nih.gov/books/NBK551690/. (Accessed October 13, 2021).
104. Vu L, et al. Evaluation of MRI for the diagnosis of appendicitis during pregnancy when ultrasound is inconclusive. *J Surg Res.* 2009;156(1):145–149. Available at https://doi.org/10.1016/j.jss.2009.03.044. (Accessed October 13, 2021).
105. Authors on behalf of International Commission for Radiological Protection (ICRP). Stewart FA, et al. ICRP publication 118: ICRP statement on tissue reactions and early and late effects of radiation in normal tissues and organs—threshold doses for tissue in a radiation protection context. *Ann ICRP.* 2012;41(1–2):1–322. Available at https://doi.org/10.1016/j.icrp.2012.02.001. (Accessed October 13, 2021).
106. Brenner DJ, Shuryak I, Einstein AJ. Impact of reduced patient life expectancy on potential cancer risks from radiologic imaging. *Radiology.* 2011;261(1):193–198. Available at https://doi.org/10.1148/radiol.11102452. (Accessed October 13, 2021).
107. Cooper JS, Hanson KC. Decompression sickness. In *StatPearls.* Treasure Island, FL: StatPearls Publishing; 2021. Last update July 18, 2021. Available at https://www.ncbi.nlm.nih.gov/books/NBK537264/. (Accessed October 13, 2021).
108. Eichhorn L, Leyk D. Diving medicine in clinical practice. *Dtsch Arztebl Int.* 2015;112(9):147–158. Available at https://doi.org/10.3238/arztebl.2015.0147. (Accessed October 13, 2021).
109. Fahlman A, Dromsky DM. Dehydration effects on the risk of severe decompression sickness in a swine model. *Aviat Space Environ Med.* 2006;77(2):102–106.
110. Lynch JH, Bove AA. Diving medicine: a review of current evidence. *J Am Board Fam Med.* 2009;22(4):399–407. Available at https://doi.org/10.3122/jabfm.2009.04.080099. (Accessed October 13, 2021).
111. National Oceanic and Atmospheric Administration (NOAA), Office of Marine and Aviation Operations (OMAO). *NOAA diving standards and safety manual.* Silver Spring, MD: NOAA; 2020. Available at https://www.omao.noaa.gov/sites/default/files/documents/NDSSM%20Rev%2005%20May%202020.pdf. (Accessed October 13, 2021).
112. Kirkland PJ, et al. Nitrogen narcosis in diving. In *StatPearls.* Treasure Island, FL: StatPearls Publishing; 2021. Last update August 1, 2021. Available at https://www.ncbi.nlm.nih.gov/books/NBK470304/. (Accessed October 13, 2021).
113. Webb JT, Pilmanis AA. Fifty years of decompression sickness research at Brooks AFB, TX: 1960–2010. Aviat Space Environ Med. 2011;82(Suppl):A1–A25. Available at https://doi.org/10.3357/asem.2576.2011. (Accessed October 13, 2021).
114. Prince TS, Thurman J, Huebner K. Acute mountain sickness. In *StatPearls.* Treasure Island, FL: StatPearls Publishing; 2021. Last update July 29, 2021. Available at https://www.ncbi.nlm.nih.gov/books/NBK430716/. (Accessed October 13, 2021).
115. Kurtzman RA, Caruso JL. High altitude illness death investigation. *Acad Forensic Pathol.* 2018;8(1):83–97. Available at https://doi.org/10.23907/2018.006. (Accessed October 13, 2021).
116. Luks AM, et al. Wilderness Medical Society clinical practice guidelines for the prevention and treatment of acute altitude illness: 2019 update. *Wilderness Environ Med.* 2019;30(4S):S3–S18. Available at https://doi.org/10.1016/j.wem.2019.04.006. (Accessed October 13, 2021).
117. Johnson NJ, Luks AM. High-altitude medicine. *Med Clin North Am.* 2016;100(2):357–369. Available at https://doi.org/10.1016/j.mcna.2015.09.002. (Accessed October 13, 2021).
118. Bärtsch P, Swenson ER. Acute high-altitude illnesses. *N Engl J Med.* 2013;368(24):2294–2302. Available at https://doi.org/10.1056/NEJMcp1214870. (Accessed October 13, 2021).
119. Luks AM. Physiology in medicine: a physiologic approach to prevention and treatment of acute high-altitude illnesses. *J Appl Physiol.* 2015;118(5):509–519. Available at https://doi.org/10.1152/japplphysiol.00955.2014. (Accessed October 13, 2021).
120. Davis C, Hackett P. Advances in the prevention and treatment of high-altitude illness. *Emerg Med Clin North Am.* 2017;35(2):241–260. Available at https://doi.org/10.1016/j.emc.2017.01.002. (Accessed October 13, 2021).
121. Stream JO, Grissom CK. Update on high-altitude pulmonary edema: pathogenesis, prevention, and treatment. *Wilderness Environ Med.* 2008;19(4):293–303. Available at https://doi.org/10.1580/07-WEME-REV-173.1. (Accessed October 13, 2021).
122. Tang D, et al. The molecular machinery of regulated cell death. *Cell Res.* 2019;29:347–364. Available at https://doi.org/10.1038/s41422-019-0164-5. (Accessed October 13, 2021).
123. Chakravarti D, LaBella KA, DePinho RA. Telomeres: history, health, and hallmarks of aging. *Cell.* 2021;184(2):306–322.

Available at https://doi.org/10.1016/j.cell.2020.12.028. (Accessed October 13, 2021).

124. Woolf SH, Schoomaker H. Life expectancy and mortality rates in the United States, 1959-2017. *JAMA*. 2019;322(20):1996–2016. Available at https://doi.org/10.1001/jama.2019.16932. (Accessed October 13, 2021).
125. Venkataramani AS, O'Brien R, Tsai AC. Declining life expectancy in the United States: the need for social policy as health policy. *JAMA*. 2021;325(7):621–622. Available at https://doi.org/10.1001/jama.2020.26339. (Accessed October 13, 2021).
126. Sasson I, Hayward MD. Association between educational attainment and causes of death among white and black US adults, 2010-2017. *JAMA*. 2019;322(8):756–763. Available at https://doi.org/10.1001/jama.2019.11330. (Accessed October 13, 2021).
127. Walston J. Frailty research moves beyond risk assessment. *J Gerontol A Biol Sci Med Sci*. 2017;72(7):915–916. Available at https://doi.org/10.1093/gerona/glx085. (Accessed October 13, 2021).
128. Grabovac I, et al. Frailty status predicts all-cause and cause-specific mortality in community dwelling older adults. *J Am Med Dir Assoc*. 2019;20(10):1230–1235. Available at https://doi.org/10.1016/j.jamda.2019.06.007. (Accessed October 13, 2021.
129. Gordon EH, Hubbard RE. Differences in frailty in older men and women. *Med J Aust*. 2020;212(4):183–188. Available at https://doi.org/10.5694/mja2.50466. (Accessed October 13, 2021).
130. Puelles VG, et al. Multiorgan and renal tropism of SARS-CoV-2. *N Engl J Med*. 2020;383:590–592. Available at https://doi.org/10.1056/NEJMc2011400. (Accessed October 13, 2021).
131. Shennan T. *Postmortems and morbid anatomy*. ed 3, *Baltimore*: William Wood; 1935.
132. Kori S. Time since death from rigor mortis: forensic prospective. *J Forensic Sci Crim Investig*. 2018;9(5):555771. Available at https://doi.org/10.19080/JFSCI.2018.09.555771. (Accessed October 13, 2021).
133. Khartade HK, et al. Study of rigor mortis and factors affecting its development for determination of postmortem interval. *Indian J Forensic Med Toxicol*. 2017;11(2):70–74.
134. Dettmeyer RB, Verhoff MA, Schütz HF. *Forensic medicine: fundamentals and perspectives*. Berlin: Springer-Verlag; 2014. Available at https://doi.org/10.1007/978-3-642-38818-7. (Accessed October 13, 2021).
135. Elliott S, Lowe P, Symonds A. The possible influence of micro-organisms and putrefaction in the production of GHB in post-mortem biological fluid. *Forensic Sci Int*. 2004;139(2–3):183–190. Available at https://doi.org/10.1016/j.forsciint.2003.10.018. (Accessed October 13, 2021).
136. Goff ML. Early post-mortem changes and stages of decomposition in exposed cadavers. *Exp Appl Acarol*. 2009;49(1–2):21–36. Available at https://doi.org/10.1007/s10493-009-9284-9. (Accessed October 13, 2021).

3

The Cellular Environment: Fluids and Electrolytes, Acids and Bases

Linda Felver

http://evolve.elsevier.com/Rogers/pathophysiology/

CHAPTER OUTLINE

The cells of the body live in a fluid environment that requires electrolyte and acid-base concentrations to be maintained within a very narrow range. A balance is maintained by an integration of renal, hormonal, neural, and respiratory functions. Changes in electrolyte concentration affect the electrical activity of nerve and muscle cells and cause shifts of fluid from one compartment to another. Fluid fluctuations also affect blood volume and therefore blood pressure. Alterations in acid-base balance disrupt the cellular function of enzyme systems and can cause cell injury. Disturbances in fluid and electrolyte or acid-base balance are common and can be life-threatening. Understanding how alterations occur and the body's ability to compensate or correct the disturbance is important for comprehending many pathophysiologic conditions.

DISTRIBUTION OF BODY FLUIDS

Body fluids are distributed among functional compartments, or spaces, and provide a transport medium for cellular and tissue function. **Intracellular fluid (ICF)** is all the fluid within cells and comprises approximately two-thirds of total body water (TBW). **Extracellular fluid (ECF)** is all the fluid outside the cells and comprises approximately one-third of TBW. ECF includes the interstitial fluid, the intravascular fluid, and the various transcellular fluids. The **interstitial fluid** is the fluid surrounding the cells and found in the spaces between cells but not within the blood vessels. The **intravascular fluid** is the fluid found within blood vessels; it is more commonly known as the blood plasma. The **transcellular fluids**, the smallest component of ECFs, are the fluids contained within epithelial-lined cavities of the body. The major transcellular fluids are summarized in Table 3.1. Other transcellular fluids include pleural, synovial, peritoneal, pericardial, and intraocular fluids.

The sum of fluids within all compartments constitutes the **total body water (TBW)** (Table 3.2). The volume of TBW is usually expressed as a percentage of body weight in kilograms. Average TBW volumes are summarized in Table 3.3.

Although daily fluid intake may fluctuate widely, the body regulates water volume within a relatively narrow range. The primary sources of body water are drinking of fluids, ingestion of water in food, and derivation of water from oxidative metabolism. Most water is lost through renal excretion. Lesser amounts are eliminated through the stool and through vaporization from the skin and lungs. Skin losses of water include visible sweat and insensible (invisible) water loss (Table 3.4). Fluid loss from the body must be replaced daily to maintain normal fluid balance.

The amount of fluid within the various compartments is relatively constant with solutes (e.g., salts) and water being exchanged between compartments to maintain their unique compositions. The percentage of TBW varies with the amount of body fat and age. Fat is hydrophobic (water repelling), and very little water is contained in adipose (fat) cells. Individuals with more body fat have proportionately less TBW and tend to be more susceptible to dehydration.

AGING AND DISTRIBUTION OF BODY FLUIDS

The distribution and amount of TBW change with age (see Table 3.3). In newborn infants, TBW is approximately 70% to 80% of body weight because infants store less fat. In the immediate postnatal period, a physiologic loss of body water occurs, equivalent to approximately 5% of body weight as the infant adjusts to a new environment. Infants are particularly susceptible to significant changes in TBW because of their high metabolic rate and potential for evaporative fluid loss attributable to their greater body surface area in proportion to total body size. Loss of fluids from diarrhea can represent a significant proportion of body weight in infants. Renal mechanisms that regulate fluid and electrolyte conservation may not be mature enough to counter the losses, so dehydration can develop rapidly.

TABLE 3.1 Approximate Concentrations of Electrolytes in Transcellular Fluids

Fluid	Na^+ (mEq/L)	K^+ (mEq/L)	Cl^- (mEq/L)	HCO_3^- (mEq/L)
Saliva	33	20	34	40
Gastric juice[a]	60	9	84	0
Bile	149	5	101	45
Pancreatic juice	141	5	77	92
Ileal fluid	129	11	116	29
Cecal fluid	80	21	48	22
Cerebrospinal fluid	141	3	127	23
Sweat	45	5	58	0

[a]The Cl^- concentration exceeds the Na^+, K^+ concentration by 15 mEq/L in gastric juice. This largely represents the secretions of hydrochloric acid by parietal cells.

During childhood, TBW slowly decreases to 60% to 65% of body weight. At adolescence the percentage of TBW approaches adult proportions, and sex differences begin to appear. Males eventually have a greater percentage of body water as a function of increasing muscle mass. Females have more body fat and less muscle as a function of estrogens and therefore have less body water.

With increasing age, the percentage of TBW declines further still. The decrease is caused in part by an increased amount of fat and a decreased amount of muscle and by a reduced ability to regulate sodium and water balance. With older age, the kidneys become less efficient at conserving sodium and therefore have difficulty concentrating the urine. Insensible water loss through the skin may increase and thirst perception may be impaired. The normal reduction of TBW in older adults becomes clinically important when the body is under physiologic stress, such as development of fever or dehydration; loss of body fluids at such times can be severe and life-threatening.

Water Movement Between ICF and ECF

Water moves between ICF and ECF compartments primarily as a function of osmotic forces. (See Chapter 1.) Water moves freely by diffusion through the lipid bilayer cell membrane and through aquaporins, a family of water channel proteins that provide permeability to water.[1] Sodium is responsible for the osmotic balance of the ECF space and potassium helps maintain the ICF osmotic balance. The osmotic force of ICF proteins and other nondiffusible substances is balanced by the active transport of ions out of the cell. Water crosses cell membranes freely; thus the osmolality of TBW normally is at equilibrium. Under normal conditions, the ICF is not subject to rapid changes in osmolality; however, when the ECF osmolality changes, water moves from one compartment to another until osmotic equilibrium is reestablished.

TABLE 3.2 Distribution of Body Water

Fluid Compartment	% of Body Weight	Volume (L) in Medium Weight Young or Middle-aged Adult Male	VOLUME (L) in Medium Weight Young or Middle-aged Adult Female
Intracellular fluid (ICF) $\frac{2}{3}$ of body water	40	28	24
Extracellular fluid (ECF) $\frac{1}{3}$ of body water	20	14	11
Interstitial $\frac{4}{5}$ of ECF	(15)	(11)	(9)
Intravascular $\frac{1}{5}$ of ECF	(5)	(3)	(2)
Total body water (TBW)	Adult male 58 ± 8% Adult female 48 ± 6%	42	35

The values listed are based on the average total water in the body.

TABLE 3.3 Total Body Water (%) in Relation to Body Weight

Body Build	Newborn (up to 1 month)	Infant (1 month to 1 year)	Child (1–10 years)	Young or Middle-aged Adult Male	Young or Middle-aged Adult Female	Older Adult Male	Older Adult Female
Medium weight	74	60	60	48–50	34	46–48	32–33

Note: The values listed are based on the average total water in the body as a percentage of body weight.
Note: Formulas for calculating estimates of total body water considering sex, age, height, and weight are available at: MD App, Total Body Water (TBW) Calculator; https://www.mdapp.co/total-body-water-tbw-calculator-448/.
Data from Buchkremer F, Segerer S. Body surface area, creatinine excretion rate, and total body water: Reference data for adults in the United States. *Kidney Medicine.* 2021;3(2):312–313; Watson PE, Watson ID, Batt RD. Total body water volumes for adult males and females estimated from simple anthropometric measurements. *The American Journal of Clinical Nutrition*, 1980;33(1):27–39; Hume R, Weyers E. Relationship between total body water and surface area in normal and obese subjects. *Journal of Clinical Pathology.* 1971;24:234–238; Mendley SR, Majkowski NL, Schoeller DA. Validation of estimates of total body water in pediatric dialysis patients by deuterium dilution. *Kidney International.* 2005;67(5):2056-2062.

TABLE 3.4 Normal Water Gains and Losses (70-kg Man)

	Daily Intake (mL)		Daily Output (mL)
Drinking ≈60%	1400–1800	Urine ≈60%	1400–1800
Water in food ≈30%	700–1000	Stool ≈2%	100
Water of oxidation ≈10%	300–400	Skin ≈10%	300–500
		Lungs ≈28%	600–800
Total	2400–3200	**Total**	2400–3200

Water Movement Between Plasma and Interstitial Fluid

The distribution of water and the movement of nutrients and waste products between the plasma in the tissue capillaries and interstitial spaces occurs as a result of changes in hydrostatic pressure and osmotic/oncotic pressure at the arterial and venous ends of the capillary (see Fig. 1.25). Hydrostatic pressure pushes water out of the capillaries; osmotic/oncotic pressure pulls water into the capillaries. Water, sodium, and glucose readily move across the capillary membrane. Under normal conditions, plasma proteins (particularly albumin) do not cross the capillary membrane. They maintain physiologic osmolality by generating oncotic pressure within the plasma.

Filtration refers to fluid movement out of the capillary and into the interstitial space. *Reabsorption* refers to fluid movement into the capillary from the interstitial space. As plasma flows from the arterial to the venous end of the capillary, four forces, sometimes called Starling forces, determine whether the net effect is filtration or reabsorption.

1. Capillary hydrostatic pressure (blood pressure) facilitates the outward movement of water from the capillary to the interstitial space.
2. Capillary (plasma) oncotic pressure osmotically attracts water from the interstitial space back into the capillary.
3. Interstitial hydrostatic pressure facilitates the inward movement of water from the interstitial space into the capillary.
4. Interstitial oncotic pressure osmotically attracts water from the capillary into the interstitial space.

The forces controlling the net movement of fluid across the capillary wall are summarized by these equations:

$$\textit{Net filtration} = (\text{Forces favoring filtration}) - (\text{Forces opposing filtration})$$

$$\textit{Forces favoring filtration} = \text{Capillary hydrostatic pressure and interstitial oncotic pressure}$$

$$\textit{Forces opposing filtration} = \text{Capillary oncotic pressure and interstitial hydrostatic pressure}$$

At the arterial end of the capillary, hydrostatic pressure exceeds capillary oncotic pressure and water moves into the interstitial space (filtration). At the *venous end* of the capillary, oncotic pressure within the capillary exceeds capillary hydrostatic pressure; thus fluids move into the capillary to enter into the circulation (reabsorption). Interstitial hydrostatic pressure promotes the movement of approximately 10% of the interstitial fluid, along with small amounts of protein, into the lymphatic vessels, which is then returned to the systemic circulation. These two systems, the lymphatic and circulatory systems, connect at a location near the left internal jugular vein where the lymphatic thoracic duct joins the left subclavian vein. Because significant amounts of albumin do not normally cross the capillary membrane, interstitial oncotic pressure normally is minimal. Fig. 3.1 illustrates net filtration.

An important factor in capillary filtration of fluid is the integrity of the capillary membrane. Increases in membrane permeability may permit the escape of plasma proteins into the interstitial space. The normal net filtration is altered, with the osmotic movement of water into the interstitial space causing tissue edema.

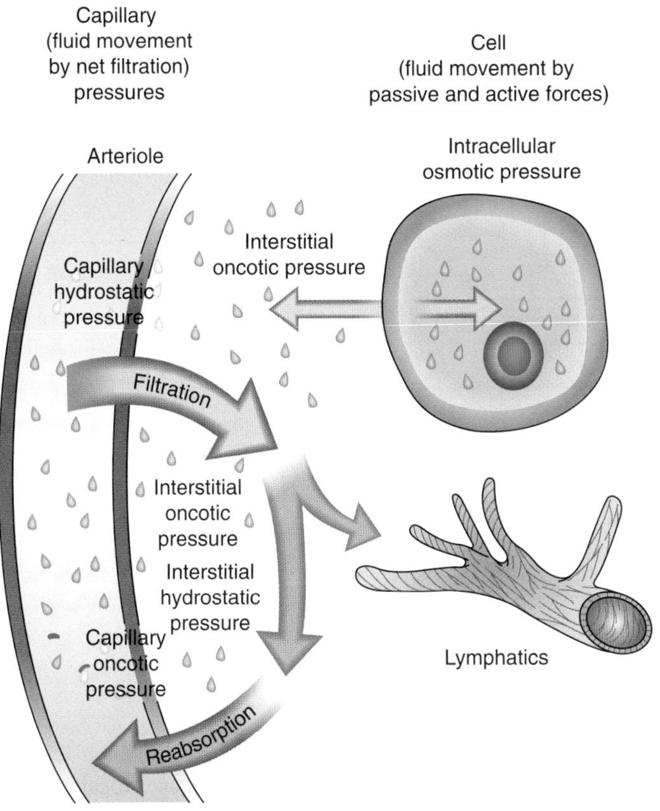

Arterial Capillary Pressures		Venous Capillary Pressures	
Capillary hydrostatic pressure	35 mm Hg	Capillary hydrostatic pressure	18 mm Hg
Interstitial fluid hydrostatic pressure	2 mm Hg	Interstitial fluid hydrostatic pressure	1 mm Hg
Net hydrostatic pressure	**33 mm Hg**	**Net hydrostatic pressure**	**17 mm Hg**
Capillary oncotic pressure	24 mm Hg	Capillary oncotic pressure	25 mm Hg
Interstitial fluid oncotic pressure	0 mm Hg	Interstitial fluid oncotic pressure	0 mm Hg
Net oncotic pressure	**24 mm Hg**	**Net oncotic pressure**	**25 mm Hg**
Net filtration pressure	**+9 mm Hg**	**Net filtration pressure**	**–8 mm Hg**

Fig. 3.1 Capillary Filtration Forces. Water, electrolytes, and small molecules exchange freely between the vascular compartment and the interstitial space at the site of capillaries and small venules. The rate and amount of exchange are driven by the physical forces of hydrostatic and oncotic pressures and the permeability and surface area of the capillary membranes. The two opposing hydrostatic pressures are capillary hydrostatic pressure and interstitial hydrostatic pressure. The two opposing oncotic pressures are capillary oncotic pressure and interstitial oncotic pressure. The *forces that favor filtration* from the capillary are capillary hydrostatic pressure and interstitial oncotic pressure, and the *forces that oppose filtration* are capillary oncotic pressure and interstitial hydrostatic pressure. The sum of these forces is known as *net filtration pressure.* In the example of normal exchange illustrated here, a small amount of fluid moves to the lymph vessels, which accounts for the net filtration difference between the arterial and venous ends of the capillary.

ALTERATIONS IN WATER MOVEMENT

Edema

Edema is the excessive accumulation of fluid within the interstitial spaces. It results from a shift of fluid from the capillaries (intravascular fluid) or lymphatic vessels into the tissues (Fig. 3.2). The four most common mechanisms are:

1. Increased capillary hydrostatic pressure
2. Decreased capillary oncotic pressure
3. Increased capillary membrane permeability
4. Lymph channel obstruction

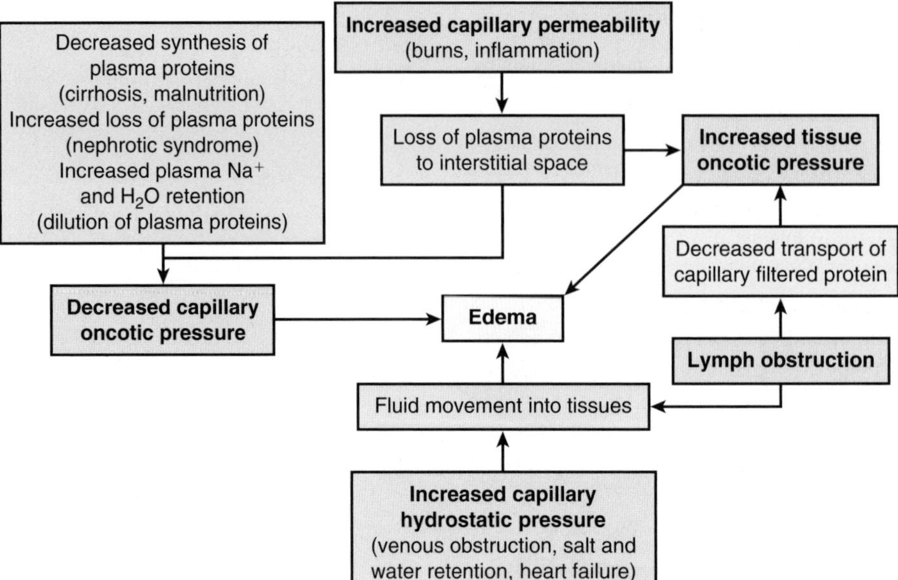

Fig. 3.2 Mechanisms of Edema Formation.

Pathophysiology. Increased capillary hydrostatic pressure results from either venous obstruction or sodium and water retention. Venous obstruction results in an increased hydrostatic pressure behind the obstruction, pushing fluid from the capillaries into the interstitial spaces. Common causes of venous obstruction include thrombophlebitis, blood clots, hepatic venous outflow obstruction, right heart failure, tight clothing around the extremities, and prolonged standing. Excessive sodium and water retention result in edema secondary to plasma volume overload. The overload produces an increased capillary hydrostatic pressure. Common predisposing causes include heart failure, oliguric kidney disease, and cirrhosis of the liver. In these circumstances, the volume of interstitial fluid exceeds the capacity of the lymphatics to return fluid to the vascular system.

Decreased capillary oncotic pressure occurs when plasma proteins, especially albumin, are lost or production is diminished. Decreased synthesis of plasma proteins occurs with severe liver disease or protein malnutrition. Losses of plasma proteins occur with glomerular diseases of the kidney (nephrotic syndrome), hemorrhage, serous drainage from open wounds or burns, and occasionally from protein-losing enteropathies.[2] Decreased oncotic attraction of fluid within the capillary causes more fluid to filter into the interstitial space than is reabsorbed into the systemic circulation through the capillaries. As fluid accumulates within the tissues, edema worsens.

Increased capillary membrane permeability resulting in edema occurs with *inflammation and immune responses.* (Immunity is discussed in Chapters 7, 8, and 9; inflammation is discussed in Chapters 7 and 9.) The increased vessel permeability permits significant amounts of proteins to escape from within blood vessels (the vascular space) into the interstitial space, producing edema. This edema results primarily from interstitial fluid protein accumulation, which increases the oncotic pressure in the interstitial space; localized decreased capillary oncotic pressure may also contribute. These responses are often the result of trauma such as burns or crushing injuries, neoplastic disease, allergic reactions, and infection.

Lymphatic channel obstruction causing edema occurs when the *lymphatic channels are blocked.* The lymphatic system normally absorbs interstitial fluid, along with small amounts of protein. These substances travel through a *one-way system* of progressively larger lymphatic vessels until they are returned to the systemic circulation. When lymphatic channels are blocked or surgically removed, proteins and fluids are not reabsorbed and accumulate in the interstitial space, causing lymphedema. Lymphedema of the arm or leg can occur after surgical removal of axillary or femoral lymph nodes, associated with the surgical treatment of cancer.[3]

Clinical Manifestations. Edema may be localized or generalized. *Localized edema* is usually limited to the site of tissue injury, as in a sprained joint. Local edema can also occur within particular organs, causing for example, vasogenic cerebral edema in the brain, pulmonary edema in the lungs, or laryngeal edema. Edema of specific organs, such as the brain, lung, or larynx, can be life-threatening. *Generalized edema* is manifested by a more uniform distribution of fluid in interstitial spaces throughout the body. *Anasarca* refers to a severe generalized edema. *Dependent edema,* in which fluid accumulates in gravity-dependent areas of the body, might appear in the feet and legs when standing and in the sacral area and buttocks when supine. Dependent edema can be identified by using the fingers to press into edematous fluid in tissues overlying bony prominences. A pit will be left in the skin, hence the term *pitting edema* (Fig. 3.3).

Edema is associated with sudden weight gain, swelling and puffiness, tight-fitting clothes and shoes, and limited movement of affected joints. It usually presents along with symptoms associated with the underlying pathologic condition. Fluid accumulation increases the distance required for nutrients, oxygen, and wastes to move between capillaries and cells in the tissues. Increased tissue pressure also may diminish capillary blood flow, leading to ischemia. Therefore wounds heal more slowly and risk of infection or pressure injury increases.

Fluid accumulation within a body cavity or space is referred to as an *effusion*. Examples include a *pleural effusion* (fluid accumulation in the pleural space) and a *pericardial effusion* (fluid accumulation within the membrane surrounding the heart). Fluid accumulation in the peritoneal cavity is called *ascites*. The region where edema fluid or an effusion accumulates sometimes is referred to as a *third space;* the term *third spacing* is used to refer to the process of this fluid accumulation. Fluid trapped in such spaces is unavailable for metabolic processes or perfusion. Common third spacing situations include ascites, large local interstitial edema, pleural effusion, pericardial effusion, and rapid movement of fluid into the intestinal lumen with an acute intestinal obstruction. Although a person with generalized edema appears swollen because of excess fluid, hypovolemia (decreased intravascular volume) can develop as a result of the fluid sequestering. With severe burns, large amounts of vascular fluid are lost into the interstitial spaces and shock often occurs secondary to the resulting reduced blood volume (see Chapter 48).

Clinically, lymphedema presents differently from edema secondary to fluid accumulation from the capillaries. With edema from capillary sources, the edematous tissue is easily compressed (i.e., pitting edema). By contrast, lymphedema is firm and noncompressible. In severe cases, lymphedema can be profound and causes gross enlargement and distortion of the body parts affected.

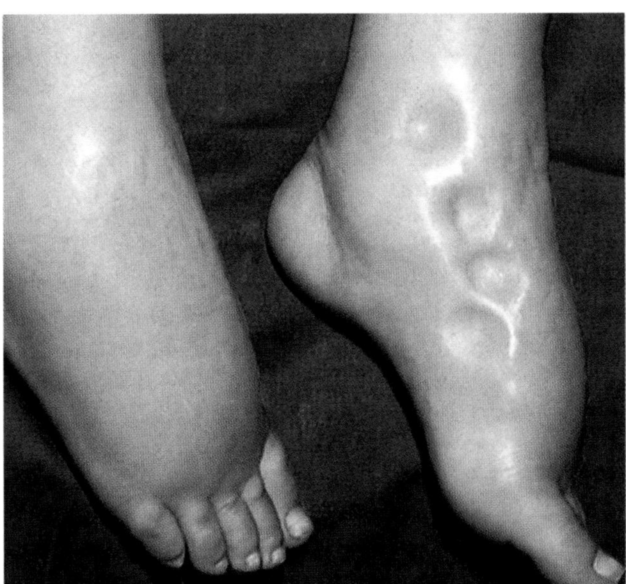

Fig. 3.3 Pitting Edema. (From Bloom A, Ireland J. *Color atlas of diabetes*, 2nd edition. St. Louis: Mosby; 1992.)

Evaluation and Treatment. Medical treatment for edema varies, depending on the underlying conditions that cause fluid retention. Generalized edema often is treated symptomatically, commonly with diuretics. Diuretics may be used until the underlying disorder has been corrected or continued chronically if the underlying disorder persists. In addition to diuretics, symptomatic treatment includes elevating edematous limbs, applying compression stockings, avoiding prolonged standing, and restricting salt intake.

Sodium, Chloride, and Water Balance

The combined influences of the kidneys and hormones have a central role in maintaining sodium and water balance. Because water follows the osmotic gradients established by changes in salt concentration, sodium concentration and water balance are integrally related. The amount of sodium in the ECF is regulated by the renal effects of aldosterone from the adrenal cortex and natriuretic peptides from the heart. Water balance is primarily regulated by the renal response to antidiuretic hormone (ADH; also known as *arginine-vasopressin*) from the posterior pituitary and is discussed in the Water Balance section.

Sodium accounts for 90% of the ECF cations (positively charged ions) (Table 3.5). The *amount* of sodium in the ECF is regulated by renal tubular reabsorption of sodium and water within the kidney in response to neural and hormonal influences. That process is a major regulator of ECF volume. The *concentration* of sodium in the ECF reflects water balance, which is regulated by ADH and is discussed later. Sodium in concert with chloride and bicarbonate, the two major anions (negatively

TABLE 3.5 Representative Distribution of Electrolytes in Body Compartments

	Extracellular Fluid (mEq/L)	Intracellular Fluid (mEq/L)
Cations		
Sodium	142	10
Potassium	5	156
Calcium	5	4
Magnesium	2	26
Total	154	196
Anions		
Bicarbonate	24	12
Chloride	104	4
Phosphate	2	40–95
Proteins	16	54
Other anions	8	31–86
Total	154	196 (average)

Values may vary slightly among different laboratories.

charged ions), influences water distribution by contributing to extracellular osmotic forces. Sodium has an important role in other physiologic functions, including nerve impulse conduction, regulation of acid-base balance, cellular chemical reactions, and transport of substances across the cellular membrane (see Chapter 1).

In general, sodium intake matches sodium excretion. The average dietary intake of sodium ranges from 5 to 6 g/day; the minimal daily requirement of sodium is 500 mg. Sweating depletes sodium and water volume and increases the body's sodium requirement.

Hormonal regulation of sodium (and potassium) balance is mediated by **aldosterone**, a mineralocorticoid (steroid) synthesized and secreted from the adrenal cortex. Aldosterone is a component of the renin-angiotensin-aldosterone system (Fig. 3.4). Aldosterone secretion is influenced by a number of factors, including circulating blood volume, blood pressure, and plasma concentrations of sodium and potassium. When the circulating blood volume or blood pressure is reduced, increased amounts of **renin**, an enzyme secreted by the juxtaglomerular cells of the kidney, are released. More renin also is released when sodium levels in the renal tubules are depressed or there is increased firing of the renal sympathetic nerves. Once released, renin stimulates the formation of **angiotensin I**, an inactive polypeptide from *angiotensinogen*, a substance secreted by the liver. Angiotensin-converting enzyme (ACE), found primarily in pulmonary vessels and to a lesser extent in endothelial and renal epithelial cells, converts angiotensin I to **angiotensin II**, a potent vasoconstrictor. Vasoconstriction elevates blood pressure and restores renal perfusion. Restoring renal perfusion inhibits further release of renin. Angiotensin II also stimulates both the secretion of aldosterone from the adrenal cortex and ADH from the posterior pituitary. Aldosterone promotes sodium and water reabsorption, in addition to the excretion of potassium within the renal tubules. The net effect is to increase blood volume and blood pressure (see Fig. 3.4).

Drugs used for the treatment of hypertension include ACE inhibitors and angiotensin receptor blockers (ARBs). Both of these classes of drugs inhibit the renin-angiotensin-aldosterone system (RAAS) and lower blood pressure.

Natriuretic peptides are hormones primarily produced by the myocardium. Atrial natriuretic peptide (ANP) is produced by the atria. B-type natriuretic peptide (BNP) is produced by the ventricles. Urodilatin (an ANP analogue) is synthesized within the kidney. Natriuretic peptides are released from the heart when the transmural atrial pressure increases (increased volume) or the tension in the left ventricular wall increases, which commonly occurs with heart failure, or when the mean arterial pressure increases (Fig. 3.5). Measurement of BNP is used as a means to assist with the initial diagnosis and management of people with heart failure. Urodilatin is released from distal tubular kidney cells when there is increased arterial pressure and increased renal blood flow. These hormones are natural antagonists to the RAAS; although they are less powerful than aldosterone, they can moderate its physiologic effect on extracellular volume. Natriuretic peptides cause vasodilation and increase renal sodium and water excretion, decreasing blood pressure. Natriuretic peptides sometimes are called a "third factor" in sodium regulation. An increased glomerular filtration rate is considered to be the first factor, and aldosterone is considered to be the second factor.

Chloride (Cl^-) is the major anion in the ECF and provides electroneutrality, particularly in relation to sodium. Chloride

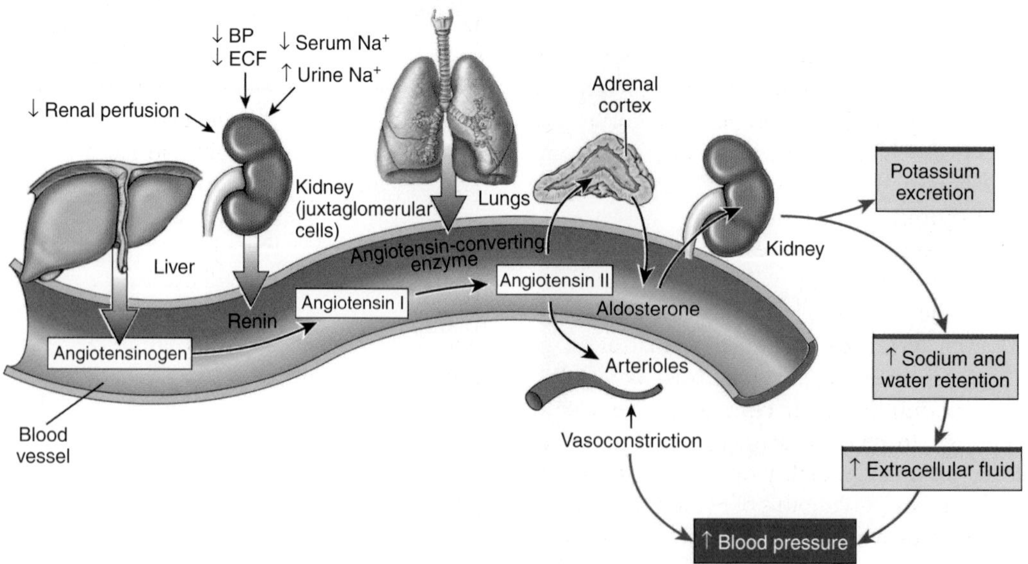

Fig. 3.4 The Renin-Angiotensin-Aldosterone System. *BP*, Blood pressure; *ECF*, extracellular fluid; *Na⁺*, sodium ion. (Modified from Herlihy B, Maebius N. *The human body in health and disease*, 4th edition. Philadelphia: Saunders; 2011. Borrowed from Lewis, et al. *Medical-surgical nursing: Assessment and management of clinical problems*, 9th edition. St. Louis: Mosby; 2014.)

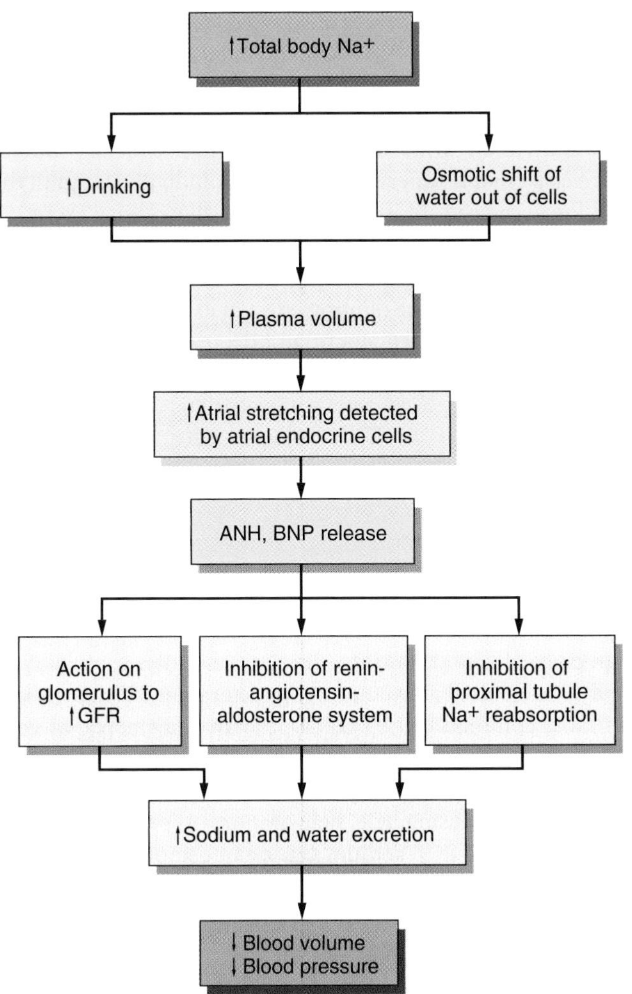

Fig. 3.5 The Natriuretic Peptide System. *ANP*, Atrial natriuretic peptide; *BNP*, brain natriuretic peptide; *GFR*, glomerular filtration rate.

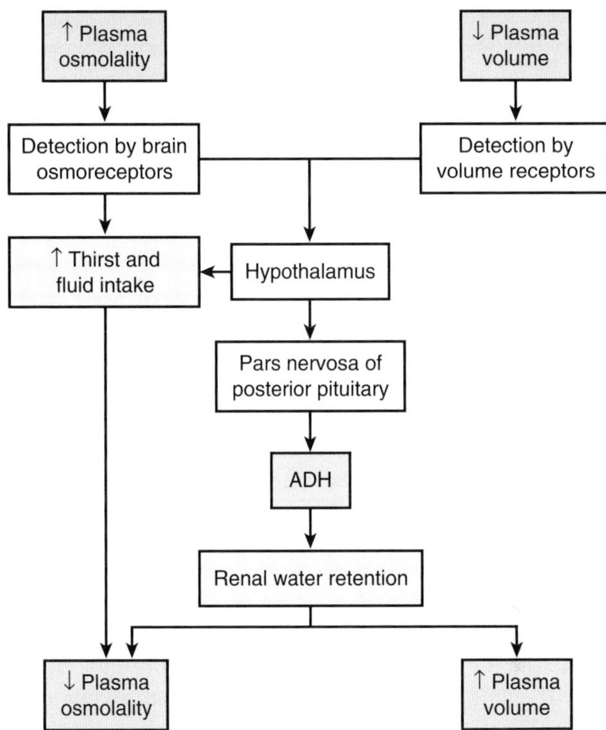

Fig. 3.6 The Antidiuretic Hormone *(ADH)* System.

transport is generally passive, except in the renal tubules, and follows the active transport of sodium so that increases or decreases in chloride concentration are proportional to changes in sodium concentration. Chloride concentration tends to vary inversely with changes in the concentration of bicarbonate (HCO_3^-), the other major ECF anion.

Water balance is regulated by the secretion of ADH, also known as arginine-vasopressin. ADH is synthesized by neurons with cell bodies in the hypothalamus that release ADH from their axon terminals in the posterior pituitary. It is secreted in larger amounts when plasma osmolality increases (the major stimulus) or if circulating blood volume decreases enough to cause a drop in blood pressure (Fig. 3.6). Increased plasma osmolality occurs when there is a decrease in water or an excess amount of sodium in relation to TBW. The increased osmolality stimulates hypothalamic osmoreceptors, which cause increased release of ADH. This hormone increases water reabsorption from the renal distal tubules and collecting ducts into the plasma (see Chapter 37). Stimulation of the hypothalamic osmoreceptors also causes thirst, which stimulates the individual to consume liquids. The net effect of both increased water intake and increased renal reabsorption of water is to decrease plasma osmolality, returning it to a normal status. ADH increases urine concentration and decreases urine volume as less water is excreted into the urine. The restoration of plasma osmolality, blood volume, and blood pressure then reduces ADH secretion back to its baseline level.

With fluid loss secondary to vomiting, diarrhea, or excessive sweating, a decrease in systemic blood volume and blood pressure often follows. Volume-sensitive receptors and baroreceptors, both of which are nerve endings sensitive to changes in blood volume and pressure, also stimulate thirst and the release of ADH, which prompts fluid consumption. The volume receptors are located in the right and left atria and in the thoracic vessels; baroreceptors are found in the aorta, pulmonary arteries, and carotid sinus. When arterial and atrial pressure drops, baroreceptors signal the hypothalamus to release ADH. The reabsorption of water mediated by the renal response to ADH promotes the restoration of plasma volume and blood pressure (see Fig. 3.6). Higher concentrations of ADH stimulate peripheral arterial vasoconstriction, thus increasing arterial blood pressure.

ALTERATIONS IN SODIUM, WATER, AND CHLORIDE BALANCE

Alterations in sodium and water balance are closely related. Serum sodium imbalances occur with gains or losses of body water. Extracellular volume imbalances develop with gains or losses of salt. These alterations can be classified as changes in

TABLE 3.6 Water and Solute Imbalances

Tonicity	Mechanism
Isotonic (isoosmolar) imbalance	Gain or loss of extracellular fluid (ECF) resulting in a concentration equivalent to a 0.9% sodium chloride (salt) solution (normal saline); no shrinking or swelling of cells
Hypertonic (hyperosmolar) imbalance	Imbalance that results in an ECF concentration >0.9% salt solution; that is, water loss or solute gain; cells shrink in a hypertonic fluid
Hypotonic (hypo-osmolar) imbalance	Imbalance that results in an ECF <0.9% salt solution; that is, water gain or solute loss; cells swell in a hypotonic fluid
Formula for calculating Serum osmolarity	(2 × [Na] + [Glu]/18+ BUN/2.8

BUN, Blood serum urea nitrogen (mg/dL); *[Glu]*, serum glucose concentration (mg/dL); *[Na]*, serum sodium concentration (mEq/dL).

tonicity (i.e., the change in the concentration of solutes in relation to the amount of water present).[4] Normal plasma osmolality is 275 to 295 milliosmoles (mOsm)/kg. Solutions are classified as isotonic, hypertonic, or hypotonic as a function of the solute concentration compared with that of normal body cells (Table 3.6 and Fig. 3.7). *Isotonic solutions* have solute concentrations that are equal to that of normal cells; *hypertonic* or *hypotonic* solutions have higher or lower solute concentration, respectively. Changes in tonicity (solute concentration of solutes that cannot cross semipermeable membranes) affect the volume of water within the extracellular compartment, resulting in *isovolemia*, *hypervolemia*, or *hypovolemia* (i.e., normal volume, excess volume, or less than normal volume in the blood, respectively).

Isotonic Alterations

Isotonic alterations are the most common and occur when changes in TBW are accompanied by proportional changes in the concentration of electrolytes. *Isotonic fluid loss* causes hypovolemia. For example, if an individual loses pure plasma or ECF, fluid volume is depleted, but the number and type of electrolytes (e.g., sodium) and the osmolality remain within a normal range (275 to 295 mOsm/kg). Causes include hemorrhage, severe wound drainage, and excessive diaphoresis (sweating). There is loss of extracellular volume with weight loss, dryness of skin and mucous membranes, decreased urine output, increased hematocrit value, and symptoms of hypovolemia. Indicators of hypovolemia include a rapid heart rate and flattened neck veins and can present with a normal or decreased blood pressure. In severe states, hypovolemic shock (severe hypotension) can occur. Isotonic fluids containing electrolytes and glucose are given orally, intravenously (IV) (i.e., 0.9% saline solution or Ringer's lactate [RL] solution), and in some cases, subcutaneously (hypodermoclysis). A variety of isotonic oral fluid replacement solutions are available as beverages and pediatric oral replacement solutions without a prescription.

Isotonic fluid excesses cause hypervolemia. Causes include excessive administration of sodium-containing IV fluids, hypersecretion of aldosterone, the effects of drugs such as prednisone and other corticosteroids (cause renal reabsorption of sodium and water), or oliguric kidney disease. Increased dietary sodium intake causes mild hypervolemia in many individuals , until the resulting decreased aldosterone secretion allows renal excretion of the excess sodium and water. As plasma volume expands, hypervolemia with sudden weight gain develops, because a liter of fluid weighs 1 kg. The diluting effect of excess plasma volume leads to a decreased hematocrit and decreased plasma protein concentration. The neck veins may distend, and the blood pressure increases. Increased capillary hydrostatic pressure leads to edema formation. If the plasma volume is great enough, pulmonary edema and heart failure develop. These presentations may be acute or chronic, depending on the underlying pathophysiology causing the fluid overload. Diuretics are commonly used for treatment.

Hypertonic Alterations

Hypertonic fluid alterations develop when the osmolality of the ECF is elevated above normal (greater than 295 mOsm/kg). The most common causes are hypernatremia (increased concentration of ECF sodium), a deficit of ECF water, or both. In either case the ECF hypertonicity attracts water from the intracellular space, causing ICF dehydration. A primary increase in the amount of ECF sodium causes an osmotic attraction of water and symptoms of *hypervolemia*. In contrast, a hypertonic state caused primarily by loss of electrolyte-free water leads to *hypovolemia* (Table 3.7).

Hypernatremia

Pathophysiology. Hypernatremia occurs when serum sodium levels exceed 145 mEq/L. Increased levels of serum sodium cause hypertonicity. Hypernatremia can be hypovolemic, euvolemic, or hypervolemic, depending on the accompanying ECF water volume. Risk factors include advanced age, impaired mental state, fever, diarrhea, and vomiting.

Hypovolemic hypernatremia occurs when a loss of sodium is accompanied by a relatively greater loss of body water. Causes include use of loop diuretics (diuretics that inhibit sodium and chloride reabsorption in the kidney loop of Henle) or diuretic stages of renal disease in which the kidneys fail to concentrate urine and excrete a large volume of urine, and osmotic diuresis from diabetes mellitus induced hyperglycemia or use of mannitol (an osmotic diuretic).

Isovolemic hypernatremia is the most common and occurs when there is a *loss of electrolyte-free water* with a near normal body sodium concentration. Causes include inadequate water intake; excessive sweating (sweat is hypotonic); fever with hyperventilation and increased water loss from lungs; burns; vomiting; diarrhea; and central or nephrogenic diabetes insipidus (lack of ADH or inadequate renal response to ADH). Infants with severe diarrhea are vulnerable and at increased risk because they cannot communicate thirst. Insufficient water intake occurs particularly in individuals who are comatose, confused, immobilized, or receiving gastric feedings. The term

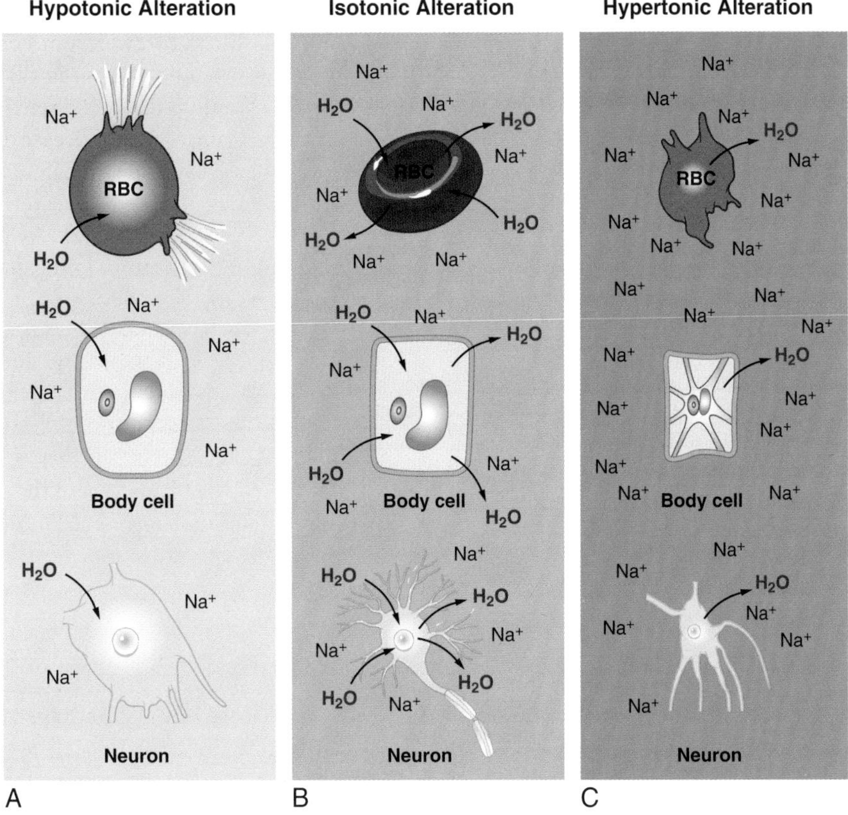

Fig. 3.7 Effects of Alterations in Extracellular Sodium Concentration in RBCs, Body Cells, and Neurons. (A) *Hypotonic Alteration:* Decrease in ECF sodium ion *(Na^+)* concentration (hyponatremia) results in ICF osmotic attraction of water with swelling and potential busting of cells. **(B)** *Isotonic Alteration:* Normal concentration of sodium in the ECF and no change in shifts of fluid in or out of cells. **(C)** *Hypertonic Alteration:* An increase in ECF sodium concentration (hypernatremia) results in osmotic attraction of water out of cells with cell shrinkage. *ECF,* Extracellular fluid; *ICF,* intracellular fluid; *RBC,* red blood cell.

dehydration can refer to water deficit but also is commonly used to indicate both sodium and water loss (isotonic or isoosmolar dehydration) or even hypovolemic hypernatremia. Hypervolemic hypernatremia is rare. It occurs when there is an increase in TBW accompanied by a greater increase in total body sodium, resulting in hypervolemia with elevated serum sodium concentration. One cause is infusion of hypertonic saline solutions in an effort to replace sodium in cases of salt depletion that can occur with renal impairment or heart failure. Other causes include oversecretion of adrenocorticotropic hormone (ACTH) or aldosterone as can occur with Cushing syndrome or adrenal hyperplasia and deliberate ingestion of large amounts of soy sauce or concentrated salt water. High amounts of dietary sodium rarely cause hypervolemic hypernatremia in a healthy individual because the aldosterone and ADH responses allow the kidneys to correct the osmolality. Symptoms of hypervolemic hypernatremia include weight gain, bounding pulse, increased blood pressure, and may include lethargy and other cerebral manifestations of hypernatremia.

Because chloride follows sodium, hyperchloremia (elevation of serum chloride concentration greater than 105 mEq/L) often accompanies hypernatremia. Plasma bicarbonate deficits, as occur in hyperchloremic metabolic acidosis, are discussed later in the chapter. There are no specific symptoms for chloride excess, and treatment is related to management of the underlying disorder.

Clinical Manifestations. Central nervous system signs are the most serious signs of hypernatremia and are related to shrinking of brain cells, brain dehydration, and alterations in membrane potentials. Signs include weakness, lethargy, muscle twitching, and hyperreflexia (hyperactive reflexes). Confusion, coma, and seizures can occur. Hypernatremia with marked water deficit is manifested by signs and symptoms of both intracellular and extracellular dehydration with volume depletion (Box 3.1).

Evaluation and Treatment. Serum sodium levels are greater than 145 mEq/L and urine specific gravity is greater than 1.030, unless the cause is diabetes insipidus. Hematocrit and plasma protein levels will be elevated if there is an accompanying

TABLE 3.7 Causes and Consequences of Hypertonic Imbalances

Causative Factor	Mechanism	ECF Effects	ICF Effects
Increased sodium (hypernatremia)	Excessive hypertonic salt solutions Intravenous hypertonic sodium Saline-induced abortions Select infant formulas Hyperaldosteronism Cushing syndrome	Hypervolemia Weight gain Bounding pulse Increased blood pressure Edema Venous distention Neuromuscular symptoms Muscle weakness	Intracellular dehydration Thirst Fever Decreased urine output Shrinkage of brain cells Confusion Coma Seizures Cerebral hemorrhage
Water deficit	Water deprivation Confusion or coma Inability to communicate Loss of thirst Water loss Watery diarrhea Diabetes insipidus Excessive diuresis Excessive diaphoresis	Hypovolemia Weight loss Weak pulses Postural hypotension Tachycardia	Intracellular dehydration See above
Other factors	Hyperglycemia	Initial dilutional hyponatremia Polyuria Polydipsia Weight loss Hypovolemia Late hypernatremia	Intracellular dehydration See above

ECF, Extracellular fluid; *ICF*, intracellular fluid.

BOX 3.1 Signs and Symptoms of Dehydration

Increased serum sodium concentration	Sunken fontanels in infants
Thirst	Prolonged capillary refill time
Headache	Tachycardia
Sudden weight loss	Weak pulses
Oliguria and concentrated urine	Postural hypotension
Hard stools	Low blood pressure
Decreased skin turgor	Hypovolemic shock
Dry mucous membranes	Lethargy
Decreased sweating and tears	Weakness
Elevated body temperature	Confusion
Soft eyeballs	Coma

water loss. The history, physical examination, and laboratory values provide information about underlying disorders and events. The treatment for isovolemic and hypovolemic hypernatremia is to give oral water or an isotonic salt-free fluid (5% dextrose in water) until the serum sodium concentration returns to normal. Fluid replacement must be given slowly to prevent cerebral edema. Treatment for hypervolemic hypernatremia is to administer loop diuretics. Serum sodium levels need to be closely monitored and the underlying clinical condition managed.

Hypotonic Alterations

Hypotonic fluid imbalances occur when the osmolality of the ECF is less than 275 mOsm/kg. The most common causes are decreased sodium concentration (hyponatremia) or excess of electrolyte-free water (water intoxication). Either problem leads to an intracellular overhydration (cell swelling). When there is a decreased sodium concentration, the osmotic pressure of the ECF decreases; water moves into the cell, where the higher osmotic pressure pulls it in (see Fig. 3.7A). As water leaves the ECF, plasma volume decreases, resulting in symptoms of hypovolemia. When there is electrolyte-free water excess (water intoxication), the ECF volume is elevated, causing symptoms of hypervolemia (Table 3.8). Cerebral and pulmonary edema occurs in conjunction with extreme water intoxication.

Hyponatremia

Pathophysiology. **Hyponatremia** develops when the serum sodium concentration decreases to less than 135 mEq/L. Hyponatremia results from a loss of sodium, inadequate intake of sodium, or dilution of sodium by water excess. Sodium depletion usually causes hypoosmolality with an associated movement of water into cells (see Fig. 3.7A). Cell dysfunction or even membrane rupture may then occur.

Hypovolemic hyponatremia occurs with a loss of total body fluid that involves a greater loss of body sodium *(hypotonic*

TABLE 3.8 **Causes and Consequences of Hypotonic Imbalances**

Causative Factor	Mechanism	ECF Effects	ICF Effects
Decreased sodium (hyponatremia)	Inadequate intake Hypoaldosteronism Excessive diuretic therapy Loop diuretics Thiazides	Extracellular volume contraction and hypovolemia (but may not if there is water excess)	Increased intracellular water; edema Brain cell swelling, irritability, depression, confusion Systemic cellular edema, including weakness, anorexia, nausea, and diarrhea
Water excess	Excessive pure water intake Excessive administration of hypotonic intravenous solutions Drinking water to replace isotonic fluid losses Tap water enemas Psychogenic polydipsia Renal water retention Syndrome of inappropriate secretion of antidiuretic hormone (SIADH)	Extracellular volume expands with hypervolemia (but may not if fluid is trapped in intracellular space)	Edema (see above)
Other factors	Isotonic dehydration treated with intravenous D_5W; glucose in D_5W solution is metabolized to water, contributing to hyponatremia Nephrotic syndrome Cirrhosis Cardiac failure	Hypervolemia or hypovolemia	Edema (see above)

D_5W, Dextrose 5% in water; *ECF*, extracellular fluid; *ICF*, intracellular fluid.

hyponatremia) than body water. The extracellular volume is decreased. Causes include prolonged vomiting, severe diarrhea, inadequate secretion of aldosterone (e.g., adrenal insufficiency), and renal losses from diuretics. ADH will be released to facilitate repletion of blood volume.

Isovolemic hyponatremia occurs when there is loss of sodium without a significant loss of water (pure sodium deficit). Causes can include water retention secondary to syndrome of inappropriate antidiuretic hormone (SIADH; see Chapter 22, which enhances water retention), hypothyroidism, pneumonia, and glucocorticoid deficiency. Inadequate intake of dietary sodium is rare but possible in individuals consuming low-sodium diets, particularly when diuretics are also being used.

Dilutional hypotonic hyponatremia (water intoxication) occurs when there is intake of large amounts of electrolyte-free water or replacement of fluid loss with IV 5% dextrose in water, which dilutes sodium. The glucose is metabolized to carbon dioxide and water, leaving a hypotonic solution with a diluting effect. Excessive sweating stimulates thirst and intake of large amounts of electrolyte-free water, as can occur in endurance athletes. Some individuals with psychogenic disorders develop water intoxication from compulsive water drinking. Other causes can include tap water enemas, aspiration of fresh water from nonfatal drowning, use of selective-serotonin reuptake inhibitors (SSRIs), and SIADH. When the body is functioning normally, it is quite difficult to produce an excess of TBW by water intoxication because water balance is regulated by ADH action on the kidneys.

Hypervolemic hyponatremia occurs when the total body sodium amount is increased and there is excess water. The increased sodium leads to an increase in ECF volume, and the serum sodium concentration is decreased. Causes include heart failure, cirrhosis of the liver, and nephrotic syndrome. Edema typically is present in these cases.

Hypertonic hyponatremia develops with the shift of water from the ICF to the ECF, as occurs with hyperglycemia, hyperlipidemia, and hyperproteinemia. The osmotic fluid shift to the ECF in turn dilutes the concentration of sodium (pseudohyponatremia) and other electrolytes.

Clinical Manifestations. Serum sodium concentration is less than 135 mEq/L, and with severe sodium deficits, the concentration is less than 120 mEq/L. The high concentration of intracellular solutes, compared with the low concentration of extracellular solutes (hyponatremia), causes an osmotic shift of water into the cells, and cell swelling occurs. The decrease in the ECF sodium concentration changes the cell's ability to depolarize and repolarize normally, altering the action potential in neurons and muscle (see Chapter 1). Clinical manifestations are related to impaired nerve conduction and neurologic changes (see Table 3.8). Hyponatremia is a major cause of morbidity and mortality among individuals hospitalized in intensive care units and in older adults.

Nausea and vomiting are more common with less severe hyponatremia (i.e., decreases between 125 and 130 mEq/L). Neurologic symptoms occur with severe hyponatremia (i.e., decreases less than 125 mEq/L or less severe very rapid decreases) and include lethargy, headache, confusion, apprehension, seizures, and coma.[5] Hypovolemic hyponatremia with pure sodium loss is accompanied by loss of ECF with symptoms of hypotension, tachycardia, and decreased urine output.

Hypervolemic hyponatremia is accompanied by weight gain, edema, ascites, and jugular vein distention. Cerebral edema can be a life-threatening complication of hyponatremia caused by increased shifts of fluid to the intracellular space and increased intracranial pressure.

Evaluation and Treatment. Evaluation of hyponatremia includes the history, physical examination, and laboratory tests for serum and urine sodium. In hyponatremic states, serum sodium concentration decreases to less than 135 mEq/L. With pure sodium deficits, the hematocrit and plasma protein levels may be elevated. Urine specific gravity is less than 1.010 when renal function is normal because sodium is maximally conserved. Evaluation of urine sodium concentration and urine osmolality assists with differential diagnosis. High urine sodium level (normal is 40 to 220 mEq/L in 24 hours) and high urine osmolality are associated with cerebral salt wasting syndrome and adrenal insufficiency. Low urine sodium level (30 mEq/L in 24 hours) and high urine osmolality are associated with extrarenal losses, such as vomiting and diarrhea or severe burns, heart failure, or cirrhosis. Serum osmolality is usually decreased, but secondary conditions of hyperlipidemia, hyperglycemia, or hyperproteinemia can increase serum osmolality.

Treatment of hyponatremia depends on the contributing disorder and severity and acuity of sodium loss. Losses of sodium and water volume are calculated from the clinical evaluation, and appropriate solutions then are selected for replacement. Restriction of water intake is required in most cases of dilutional hyponatremia because body sodium levels may be normal or increased even though serum concentrations are low. Hypertonic saline solutions are used cautiously with severe hyponatremia or the presence of symptoms such as seizures. Rapid correction of chronic hyponatremia can lead to osmotic demyelination syndrome with axonal damage in the brain resulting in neurologic disability or death.[6] Arginine-vasopressin (ADH) receptor antagonists (vaptans) are a class of drugs used for the treatment of hypervolemic and isovolemic hyponatremia, particularly with SIADH.[7] Serum sodium concentration must be monitored to prevent overcorrection.

Hypochloremia

Hypochloremia, a low level of serum chloride (less than 97 mEq/L), is rare and usually occurs with hyponatremia or an elevated bicarbonate concentration, as in metabolic alkalosis. Sodium deficit associated with restricted intake, use of diuretics, and vomiting is accompanied by chloride deficiency. Cystic fibrosis is a genetic disease characterized by hypochloremia (see Chapters 36 and 42). In all cases, treatment of the underlying cause is required.

ALTERATIONS IN POTASSIUM, CALCIUM, PHOSPHATE, AND MAGNESIUM BALANCE

Potassium

Potassium (K^+) is the major intracellular electrolyte and is found in most body fluids (see Table 3.5). Total body potassium content is approximately 4000 mEq, with most of it located in the cells. The ICF concentration of K^+ is approximately 150 to 160 mEq/L; the ECF concentration is approximately 3.5 to 5.0 mEq/L. This concentration gradient is maintained by an *active transport system*, the sodium-potassium adenosine triphosphatase pump (Na^+-K^+ ATPase pump) (see Chapter 1). The ratio of ICF K^+ concentration to ECF K^+ concentration is the major determinant of the resting potential of cells, which makes K^+ balance crucial for the transmission and conduction of nerve impulses, maintenance of normal cardiac rhythms, and contraction of skeletal and smooth muscles (Figs. 3.8A and 1.27). Daily dietary intake of potassium is 40 to 150 mEq/day, with an average of 1.5 mEq/kg body weight. Approximately 90% of dietary potassium is absorbed in the gastrointestinal tract and is transported rapidly into the cells after ingestion. The distribution of potassium between the intracellular and ECFs is influenced by several factors. Insulin, epinephrine, and alkalosis all facilitate the shift of potassium into cells. Insulin deficiency, aldosterone deficiency, some types of acidosis, cell lysis, and strenuous exercise promote a shift of potassium out of cells. Glucagon blocks entry of potassium into cells; glucocorticoids promote potassium excretion. Aldosterone promotes renal excretion of K^+ by the distal tubules, accounting for 90% to 95% of K^+ excretion.[8]

As the predominant ICF ion, potassium exerts a major influence on the regulation of ICF osmolality and fluid balance as well as on intracellular electrical neutrality in relation to hydrogen (H^+) and Na^+ levels. Potassium can move out of cells, along with water, with an increased ECF osmolarity.

Insulin contributes to the regulation of plasma potassium levels by stimulating the Na^+-K^+ ATPase pump, thereby promoting the movement of K^+ into liver and muscle cells. Clinically, insulin (usually with dextrose to prevent hypoglycemia) is used to treat severe hyperkalemia. In cases of hyperglycemia, dangerously low levels of plasma potassium can result when insulin is administered to treat elevated glucose levels. Particularly in emergency settings, it is crucial to check potassium levels before administering insulin for hyperglycemia. Monitoring potassium status is a key factor in any diabetes treatment regimen involving the administration of insulin.

In addition to conserving sodium, *aldosterone* regulates the potassium concentration. Aldosterone is secreted from the adrenal cortex in response to increases in plasma potassium concentration or stimulation by angiotensin II, part of the RAAS; it stimulates the secretion of potassium into the urine by the distal renal tubules. Aldosterone also increases the secretion of potassium from the colon and sweat glands.

Although potassium is found in most body fluids, the kidney is the most significant regulator of potassium balance. Potassium is freely filtered by the renal glomerulus; 90% is reabsorbed by the proximal tubule and loop of Henle. In the distal tubules, *principal cells* secrete potassium under the influence of aldosterone, and *intercalated cells* reabsorb potassium. The net effect of secretion and reabsorption determines the amount of potassium excreted from the body. Evidence suggests that the gut also may sense the amount of K^+ ingested and stimulate renal K^+ excretion, independent of aldosterone.[9]

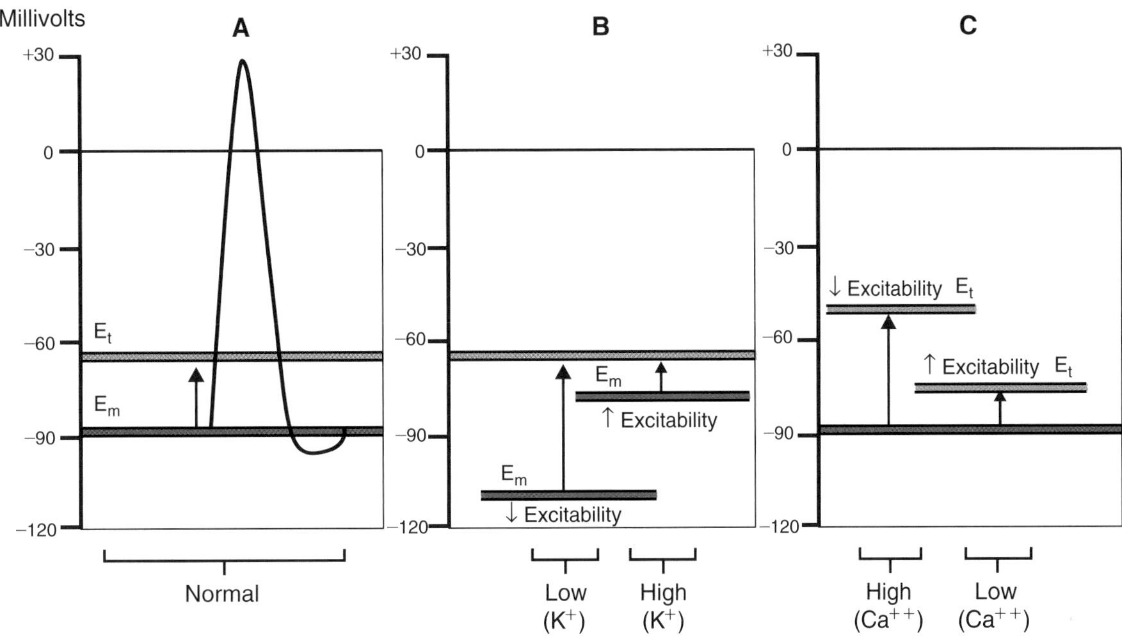

Fig. 3.8 Effects of Potassium (K^+) and Calcium (Ca^{++}) Ions on Membrane Excitability. (A) Normal membrane excitability: Potassium affects the resting membrane potential *(E_m)*, and calcium affects the threshold potential *(E_t)*. **(B)** Effects of potassium ion (K^+) changes on membrane potential. **(C)** Effect of calcium ion (Ca^{++}) on threshold potential. NOTE: *Hyperpolarization* can be caused by either hypokalemia (E_m more negative) or hypercalcemia (E_t less negative)—the distance between E_m and E_t is increased (decreased excitability); and *hypopolarization* can be caused by either mild hyperkalemia (E_m less negative) or hypocalcemia (E_t more negative)—the distance between E_m and E_t is decreased (increased excitability).

The potassium concentration in the distal tubular cells is determined primarily by the plasma concentration of potassium in the *peritubular capillaries.* When plasma potassium concentration increases, potassium is secreted into the urine by the distal tubules, which is facilitated by the action of aldosterone. Decreased levels of plasma potassium result in decreased distal tubular secretion, although approximately 5 to 15 mEq/day will continue to be lost. Changes in the rate of filtrate (urine) flow through the distal tubule also influence the concentration gradient for potassium secretion. When the urine flow rate is high (e.g., with diuretic use), the potassium concentration in the distal tubular urine is lower; more potassium subsequently is secreted into the urine.[10]

Changes in pH (hydrogen ion concentration) also affect the potassium balance. During acute acidosis, hydrogen ions accumulate in the ICF. Unless the anion portion of the acid (e.g., acetoacetate or lactate) has entered the ICF, the accumulated H^+ would create a charge imbalance. To maintain ionic balance, potassium shifts out of the cell and into the ECF. This shift occurs, in part, because of a decrease in the Na^+-K^+ ATPase pump activity and can contribute to hyperkalemia. Decreased ICF potassium also results in decreased potassium secretion by the distal tubular cells, increasing the potential for hyperkalemia. In acute alkalosis, hydrogen ions within the ICF move to the ECF, resulting in a shift of potassium into the cell to maintain ionic balance. This contributes to development of hypokalemia; in addition, potassium secretion increases within the distal tubular cells, which increases the potential for hypokalemia. The management of alterations associated with acid-base imbalances requires concurrent treatment of changes in K^+ concentration.

In summary, renal regulation of potassium includes:

1. The action of aldosterone
2. The concentration gradient for K^+ at the distal tubule and collecting duct
3. The distal tubule flow rate and distal tubule sodium delivery
4. Changes in pH (causing acidosis or alkalosis)

Potassium loss occurs through normal body functions, but without causing hypokalemia, unless the individual has very low dietary potassium intake. Average daily losses of K^+ are as follows:

Location	Daily Loss (mEq/L)
Stool	5–10
Sweat	0–20
Urine	40–120

Potassium adaptation is the ability of the body to adapt to increased levels of K^+ intake over time. A sudden increase in K^+ level may be fatal. If the intake is slow, the kidney can increase the urinary excretion of K^+ and maintain K^+ balance.

Hypokalemia

Pathophysiology. Potassium deficiency, or hypokalemia, develops when the serum K^+ concentration decreases to less than 3.5 mEq/L. Because intracellular and total body stores of

K^+ are difficult to measure, changes in K^+ balance are reflected by the plasma concentration, although not always accurately. In general, lowered serum K^+ level indicates a loss of total body K^+. When K^+ is lost from the ECF, the change in the concentration gradient favors the movement of K^+ from the cell into the ECF. The ICF/ECF concentration ratio is maintained, but the amount of total body K^+ is depleted.

Factors contributing to the development of hypokalemia include a reduced intake of potassium, an increased entry of K^+ into cells, and increased losses of K^+. A dietary deficiency of K^+ may occur in people who have inadequate intake of potassium-rich fruits and vegetables (influenced by fad diets, food insecurity, or lack of transportation to purchase fresh produce), and in individuals with alcoholism or eating disorders. A reduced K^+ intake generally becomes a problem when combined with other causes of K^+ depletion.

ECF hypokalemia can develop without losses of total body K^+. As discussed previously, with some types of acidosis, potassium shifts from the ECF to the ICF in exchange for hydrogen ions to maintain the plasma acid-base balance. In alkalosis, ECF hydrogen moves out of the cell to correct the alkalosis, and K^+ moves into the cell to maintain an ionic balance. Insulin promotes cellular uptake of K^+, and insulin administration can cause an ECF potassium deficit, particularly with the intake of high carbohydrate loads. For this reason, it is crucial to evaluate potassium status in emergency settings when treating a person with diabetes who presents with severe hyperglycemia and/or diabetic ketoacidosis (DKA). Failure to do so before administering IV insulin can result in life-threatening hypokalemia. Treating DKA typically requires administration of supplemental potassium simultaneously with IV insulin and rehydration therapy. With DKA, the overall insulin deficit results in potassium shifts from the ICF to the ECF, due to lack of insulin action on the Na^+-K^+ ATPase pump. A normal serum potassium level usually is maintained; however, potassium excretion through the kidney continues, resulting in a deficit of total body potassium. The deficit becomes clinically evident when insulin treatment and rehydration therapy are initiated. Accordingly, in the treatment of hyperglycemia with or without DKA, the standard of care is potassium supplementation with close monitoring.

Treatment of pernicious anemia with vitamin B_{12} or folate also may precipitate hypokalemia if the formation of new red blood cells causes enough K^+ uptake to effect an extracellular decrease in K^+ concentration. Familial hypokalemic periodic paralysis is a rare genetically transmitted disease that causes K^+ to shift into the intracellular space with episodes of extreme muscle weakness.

Losses of K^+ from body stores are most commonly caused by gastrointestinal and renal disorders. Diarrhea, intestinal drainage tubes, fistulae, excessive ingestion of black licorice, and laxative overuse can all result in hypokalemia. Normally, only 5 to 10 mEq of potassium and approximately 100 mL of water are excreted in the stool each day. With diarrhea, fluid and electrolyte losses can be voluminous, with several liters of fluid and 100 to 200 mEq of K^+ lost per day. Vomiting or continuous nasogastric suction frequently is associated with K^+ depletion. The loss occurs in part because of the K^+ lost from the gastric fluid. However, the loss principally is caused by renal compensation for volume depletion and metabolic alkalosis, which occurs secondary to losses of sodium, chloride, and hydrogen ion. The loss of fluid and sodium stimulates the secretion of aldosterone, which in turn results in renal loss of K^+.

Renal losses of K^+ are related to increased secretion of K^+ by the distal tubule. Predisposing factors include the use of diuretics, excessive aldosterone secretion, an increased distal tubular flow rate, and a low plasma magnesium concentration. Many diuretics inhibit the reabsorption of sodium chloride, resulting in increased urine production. With enhanced fluid excretion, the increased flow through the distal tubule also promotes potassium excretion. If sodium loss is severe, the compensating aldosterone secretion (which causes secondary hyperaldosteronism) may further deplete K^+ stores. Primary hyperaldosteronism with excessive secretion of aldosterone from an adrenal adenoma also causes K^+ wasting. Many kidney diseases impair the kidney's ability to conserve sodium. The decreased sodium reabsorption produces a diuretic effect. As a result, the increased flow through the distal tubule promotes the secretion of K^+. Magnesium deficiency increases loop of Henle and distal potassium secretion, causing secondary hypokalemia.[11] Several medications, including amphotericin B, gentamicin, and nafcillin, cause hypokalemia by increasing the rate of potassium excretion. Rare hereditary defects in renal potassium transport (Bartter and Gitelman syndromes) also can result in hypokalemia (Table 3.9).

Clinical Manifestations. Mild losses of K^+ are usually asymptomatic. With severe hypokalemia (<2.5 mEq/L), neuromuscular excitability decreases, causing skeletal muscle weakness, smooth muscle atony, cardiac dysrhythmias, glucose intolerance, and impaired urinary concentrating ability.

Symptoms occur in proportion to the rate of potassium depletion. The body can accommodate slow losses of potassium. Decreases in the ECF potassium concentration may facilitate a

TABLE 3.9 Causes of Potassium Alterations

Hypokalemia <3.5 mEq/L	Causes
Decreased intake: starvation or eating disorders, inadequate replacement	Intake
Increased renal loss: renal concentrating defect, K^+-losing diuretics, hyperaldosteronism, vomiting, diarrhea, use of specific medications	Loss
Shift from ECF to ICF: metabolic alkalosis, insulin administration, gene mutations in K^+ transport	Cellular shifts
Hyperkalemia >5.0 mEq/L	**Causes**
Excess dietary or intravenous intake	Intake
Decreased renal loss: oliguric renal disease, K^+-sparing diuretics, hypoaldosteronism	Loss
Shift from ICF to ECF: some types of metabolic acidosis, massive cell injury or death	Cellular shifts

ECF, Extracellular fluid; *ICF*, intracellular fluid; K^+, potassium.

shift in potassium away from the intracellular space and into the ICF. This dynamic promotes the return of the potassium concentration gradient toward a more normal status, reducing neuromuscular symptoms. With acute and severe potassium loss, the changes in neuromuscular excitability are more profound. Skeletal muscle weakness initially occurs in the larger muscles of the legs and arms and ultimately affects the diaphragm, compromising ventilation. With severe losses, paralysis and respiratory arrest may occur. Loss of smooth muscle tone may result in a variety of gastrointestinal manifestations, such as constipation, intestinal distention, anorexia, nausea, vomiting, and paralytic ileus (paralysis of the intestinal muscles). Table 3.10 contains a summary of K^+ alterations.

The cardiac effects of hypokalemia are related to changes in membrane excitability. As the ECF potassium concentration decreases, the resting membrane potential becomes more negative (i.e., *hyperpolarized;* e.g., from −90 to −100 millivolts). A hyperpolarized membrane requires a greater stimulus to trigger an action potential (Fig. 3.8B). Potassium also contributes to the repolarization phase of the action potential; hypokalemia delays ventricular repolarization. Consequently, hypokalemia may result in various dysrhythmias, including sinus bradycardia, atrioventricular block, and paroxysmal atrial tachycardia. The characteristic changes in the electrocardiogram (ECG) reflect *delayed ventricular repolarization* with slowed conduction and pacemaker activity. The amplitude of the T wave decreases, the amplitude of the U wave increases, and the ST segment is depressed (Fig. 3.9). In severe states of hypokalemia, P waves peak, the QT interval is prolonged, and T-wave inversions may be seen. Hypokalemia enhances the therapeutic effect of digitalis by slowing the Na^+-K^+ pump and excessively increasing intracellular calcium and sodium concentrations. The risk of digitalis toxicity is increased.

Concurrent alterations in *plasma calcium concentration* also contribute to changes in neuromuscular excitability associated with hypokalemia. Increases in ECF calcium concentration tend to make the threshold potential (E_t) less negative. The result is decreased membrane excitability and potentiation of hyperpolarization, amplifying the neuromuscular effects of hypokalemia (see Fig. 3.8C).

A wide range of metabolic dysfunctions may result from potassium deficiency. Carbohydrate metabolism is affected. Hypokalemia depresses insulin secretion and alters hepatic and skeletal muscle glycogen synthesis. Renal function is impaired

TABLE 3.10 Organ System Manifestations of Potassium Alterations

Organ System	Hypokalemia <3.5 mEq/L	Hyperkalemia >5.0 mEq/L
Cardiovascular	Postural hypotension Dysrhythmias ECG changes (flattened T waves, U waves, ST depression, peaked P wave, prolonged QT interval) Weak, irregular pulse rate Ventricular fibrillation	Dysrhythmias ECG changes (peaked T waves, prolonged PR interval, absent P wave with widened QRS complex) Bradycardia Heart block Cardiac arrest
Nervous	Lethargy Fatigue Confusion Paresthesias Decreased tendon reflexes	Anxiety Tingling Numbness
Gastrointestinal	Nausea and vomiting Decreased motility Distention Decreased bowel sounds Ileus	Nausea and vomiting Early: Diarrhea Early: Colicky pain
Kidney	Inability to concentrate urine Water loss Thirst Kidney damage	Oliguria Kidney damage
Skeletal and smooth muscle	Weakness Flaccid paralysis Respiratory arrest Constipation Bladder dysfunction	Early: hyperactive muscles and reflexes SLate: weakness and flaccid paralysis

ECG, Electrocardiogram.

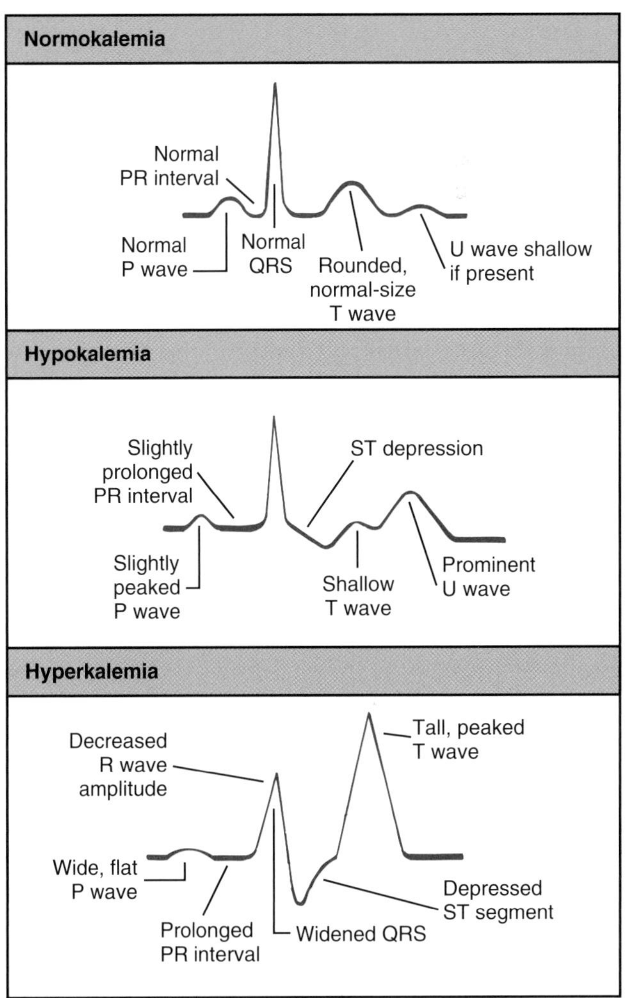

Fig. 3.9 Electrocardiogram Changes With Potassium Imbalance.

by a decreased responsiveness to ADH, resulting in a decreased ability to concentrate urine, causing polyuria (increased urine). Polydipsia (increased thirst) may occur. Chronic potassium deficits lasting more than 1 month may damage renal tissue, with resulting interstitial fibrosis and tubular atrophy.

Evaluation and Treatment. The diagnosis of hypokalemia is based on serum K^+ levels. Hypokalemia can result from disorders associated with potassium loss or from shifts of extracellular potassium into the intracellular space. Treatment involves replacing lost potassium to restore normal levels and correcting the associated fluid and acid-base imbalances. Once these have been corrected, further potassium loss should be prevented by correcting the underlying mechanism. In particular, individuals should be encouraged to eat potassium-rich foods. With normal renal function, the maximal rate of oral replacement is 40 to 80 mEq/day. A maximal safe rate of IV replacement is 20 mEq/h. Potassium is irritating to blood vessels and can result in considerable pain for the individual. Accordingly, IV infusions containing potassium should not exceed 40 mEq/L. Replacement therapy requires close monitoring of the plasma potassium concentration. Hypokalemia concurrent with hypomagnesemia is refractory to treatment until magnesium levels are corrected.

Hyperkalemia

Pathophysiology. Hyperkalemia is defined as an ECF potassium concentration greater than 5.5 mEq/L.[11a] Increases in the total body potassium level are relatively rare, largely because of efficient renal excretion. Acute increases in the serum potassium level are handled quickly through increased renal excretion of potassium, with some uptake also into cells.

Hyperkalemia may be caused by *excessive intake*, a *shift of potassium from the ICF to the ECF*, or *decreased renal excretion*.[12] If renal function is normal, slow and long-term increases in K^+ intake are usually well tolerated through K^+ adaptation. Dietary excesses of potassium are uncommon, but accidental ingestion of potassium salt substitutes can cause toxicity. Acute K^+ loading can exceed renal excretion rates. Use of stored whole blood, administration of IV boluses of penicillin G, or excessive replacement of K^+ can precipitate hyperkalemia, particularly if renal function is impaired. Drugs that decrease renal potassium excretion (e.g., ACE inhibitors, ARBs, potassium-sparing diuretics, and aldosterone antagonists) also may contribute to hyperkalemia.

Potassium shifts from the ICF to the ECF occur when there is a *change in cell membrane permeability* caused by cell hypoxia, some types of acidosis, or insulin deficiency. Hypoxia can lead to hyperkalemia by diminishing the efficiency of cell membrane active transport, resulting in the escape of K^+ to the ECF. Burns, massive crush injuries, and extensive surgeries can cause cell trauma and release of ICF potassium to the ECF. If renal function is sustained, K^+ will be excreted. As cell repair begins, hypokalemia may develop if the excreted K^+ is not replaced.

In states of *acidosis*, hydrogen ions shift into the cells in exchange for ICF potassium, unless the anion portion of the acid also enters cells; therefore hyperkalemia and acidosis often occur together. Insulin promotes cellular entry of K^+; consequently, *insulin deficits*, which occur with conditions such as DKA, are often accompanied by hyperkalemia. Hyperkalemia may result secondary to digitalis toxicity. High levels of digitalis inhibit the Na^+-K^+ ATPase transport pump, allowing potassium to remain outside the cell.

Decreased renal function is commonly associated with hyperkalemia. Oliguria (urine output <30 mL/h) secondary to acute kidney injury or end-stage renal disease typically presents with elevations of serum K^+ concentration. The severity of hyperkalemia is a function of the amount of K^+ intake, the degree of acidosis, and the rate of renal cell damage. *Hypoaldosteronism* can cause decreases in the urinary excretion of K^+. For example, Addison disease, characterized by adrenal cortical insufficiency, often presents with hyperkalemia secondary to decreased aldosterone secretion.

Clinical Manifestations. Symptoms vary with the severity of hyperkalemia. With a mild presentation, increased neuromuscular irritability may manifest as restlessness, intestinal cramping, and diarrhea. Severe hyperkalemia decreases the resting membrane potential from −90 to −70 millivolts, resulting in muscle weakness, loss of muscle tone, and paralysis. In mild states of hyperkalemia, myocardial cell repolarization is more rapid and reflected in the ECG as narrow and taller T waves with a shortened QT interval. Severe hyperkalemia (serum levels ≥6 mEq/L) causes delayed cardiac conduction, preventing repolarization of heart muscle. There is a decrease in conduction velocity, depressed ST segment, prolonged PR interval, and widening of the QRS complex (loss of atrial activity) (see Fig. 3.9). Brady dysrhythmias and delayed conduction are common in hyperkalemia; severe hyperkalemia can cause ventricular fibrillation or cardiac arrest.

Changes in the ratio of intracellular to extracellular K^+ concentration contribute to the clinical presentation of hyperkalemia (see Table 3.9). If extracellular K^+ concentration increases without a significant change in intracellular K^+ concentration, the resting membrane potential becomes more positive (e.g., changes from −90 to −80 millivolts) and the cell membrane is hypopolarized (the inside of the cell becomes less negative or partially depolarized [increased excitability]) (see Fig. 3.8B). With mild elevations in extracellular K^+ concentration, the cell more rapidly repolarizes and becomes more irritable (peaked T waves). An action potential then is initiated more rapidly because the distance between the resting membrane potential and the threshold potential has been decreased. With more severe hyperkalemia, the resting membrane potential approaches or exceeds the threshold potential (wide QRS merging with T wave). In this case the cell is not able to repolarize and therefore does not respond to excitation stimuli. The most serious consequence is cardiac arrest.

Like the effects of hypokalemia, the neuromuscular effects of hyperkalemia are related to the rate of increase in the ECF potassium concentration and the presence of other contributing factors, such as acidosis and calcium balance. Long-term increases in ECF potassium concentration result in shifts of K^+ into the cell because the tendency is to maintain a normal ratio of intracellular/extracellular potassium concentrations. Acute elevations of extracellular K^+ concentration affect neuromuscular irritability because this ratio is disrupted.

Because calcium influences the threshold potential, changes in ECF calcium concentration can augment or override the effects of hyperkalemia. With hypocalcemia the threshold potential becomes more negative, enhancing the neuromuscular effects of hyperkalemia. Hypercalcemia causes the threshold potential to become less negative, counteracting the effects of hyperkalemia on resting membrane potential (see Fig. 3.8C).

Evaluation and Treatment. Hyperkalemia is a common finding in many clinical settings (e.g., renal disease, massive trauma, insulin deficiency, Addison disease, use of potassium salt substitutes, or some types of metabolic acidosis). How rapidly symptoms evolve often is a function of the underlying cause. An ECG will identify conduction abnormalities or dysrhythmias.

Management of hyperkalemia includes both treating the contributing causes and correcting excessive potassium concentration. Normalizing the extracellular potassium concentration can be achieved with a variety of methods; the treatment chosen is related to the cause and severity of the problem. Calcium gluconate can be administered to restore membrane excitability when serum potassium levels are dangerously high. Administration of glucose, which readily stimulates insulin secretion, or administration of glucose and insulin for those with diabetes, facilitates cellular entry of potassium. Renin-angiotensin-aldosterone system inhibitor therapy and use of the newer oral potassium binders optimize therapy. Buffered solutions correct metabolic acidosis and lower serum potassium level. Dialysis effectively removes potassium in cases of renal dysfunction.[13]

Calcium and Phosphate

The total body content of calcium is approximately 1200 g. Most calcium (99%) is located in bone as hydroxyapatite (an inorganic compound that contributes to bone rigidity), and the remainder is in the plasma and body cells. The total fraction of calcium circulating in the blood is small (9.0 to 10.5 mg/dL), and approximately 50% is bound to plasma proteins, primarily albumin. Approximately 40% is in the free or ionized form (5.5 to 5.6 mg/dL). Ionized calcium has the most important physiologic functions. Approximately 20% of ingested calcium is absorbed in the small intestine, primarily in the duodenum.

Calcium ($Ca2+$) is a necessary ion for many fundamental metabolic and cellular processes. In bound form, it is the major cation associated with the structure of bones and teeth. The ionized form serves as an enzymatic cofactor for blood clotting and is required for hormone secretion and the function of cell receptors. Plasma membrane stability, permeability, and repair are directly related to calcium ions, as is the transmission of nerve impulses and the contraction of muscles. Calcium metabolism is linked to phosphate and magnesium metabolism.

Phosphate (HPO_4^-) is found primarily in bone (85%), with smaller amounts found within the intracellular and extracellular spaces. In the plasma, phosphate exists in phospholipids and phosphate esters and as inorganic phosphate, which is the ionized form. The normal serum levels of inorganic phosphate range from 2.5 to 4.5 mg/dL and may be as high as 6.0 to 7.0 mg/dL in infants and young children. Intracellular phosphate has many metabolic forms, including the high-energy structures creatine phosphate and adenosine triphosphate (ATP). Phosphate acts as an intracellular and extracellular anion buffer in the regulation of acid-base balance; in the form of ATP, it provides energy for muscle contraction.

Calcium and phosphate concentrations are rigidly controlled. They are related by the product of calcium and phosphate (HPO_4^-) concentrations, which is a constant (K) [$Ca2+) \times HPO_4^- = K$]. Thus, if the concentration of one ion increases or decreases, that of the other normally increases or decreases.

Calcium and phosphate balance is regulated by three hormones: parathyroid hormone (PTH), vitamin D, and calcitonin. Acting together, these substances determine the amount of dietary calcium and phosphate absorbed from the intestine, the deposition and absorption of calcium and phosphate from bone, and the renal reabsorption and excretion of calcium and phosphate by the kidney.

The parathyroid glands secrete PTH in response to low levels of serum calcium. (The specific actions of PTH in relation to calcium and phosphate are described in Chapter 21.) Parathyroid hormone (PTH) controls levels of ionized calcium and phosphate in the blood and other ECFs. Renal regulation of calcium and phosphate balance requires PTH. PTH stimulates reabsorption of calcium along the distal tubule of the nephron and inhibits phosphate reabsorption by the proximal tubule of the nephron. The net result is an increase in serum calcium concentration and increased urinary excretion of phosphate. Fig. 3.10 summarizes hormonal regulation of calcium.

Another compound important to calcium and phosphate regulation is vitamin D. Vitamin D (cholecalciferol) is a fat-soluble steroid ingested in food or synthesized in the skin in the presence of ultraviolet light. Several steps of activation are required before vitamin D can act on target tissues. The first step occurs in the liver; final activation is in the kidney. The renal activation of vitamin D begins when the serum calcium level

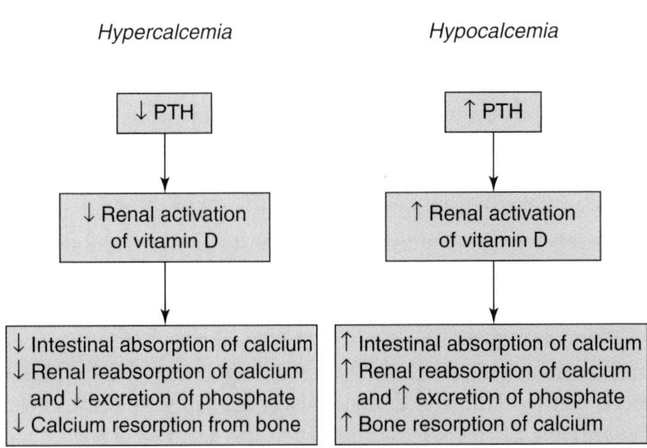

Fig. 3.10 Hormonal Regulation of Calcium Balance. *PTH,* Parathyroid hormone.

decreases and stimulates secretion of PTH. PTH then acts to increase calcium reabsorption and enhance renal excretion of phosphate, producing decreased phosphate levels. The combination of low calcium level and increased PTH secretion causes the renal activation of vitamin D. The activated vitamin D (vitamin D_3—calcitriol) then circulates as a hormone in the plasma and acts to increase absorption of calcium and phosphate in the small intestine, enhance bone calcification, increase renal tubular reabsorption of calcium, and increase excretion of phosphate. When end-stage renal disease occurs, vitamin D is not activated; serum calcium levels decrease; and phosphate levels increase.

As calcium levels increase, an opposite adaptation occurs, leading to suppression of PTH secretion, decreased renal vitamin D activation, decreased intestinal calcium absorption, and increased renal phosphate reabsorption. Calcitonin (produced by C cells of the thyroid gland) decreases calcium levels by inhibiting osteoclastic activity in bone and increasing renal calcium and phosphate excretion.

The fractions of serum calcium that are freely ionized or bound to plasma proteins are influenced by pH. In states of acidosis, levels of ionized calcium increase. When alkalosis develops, with an increase in pH, the amount of protein-bound calcium increases and the physiologically active, ionized calcium level decreases. The decreased concentration of ionized calcium may be great enough to cause symptoms of hypocalcemia, such as tetany.

Hypocalcemia

Pathophysiology. Hypocalcemia occurs when serum total calcium concentrations are less than 9.0 mg/dL and ionized levels are less than 5.5 mg/dL. In general, deficits in calcium are related to inadequate intestinal absorption, decreases in levels of PTH and vitamin D, or deposition of ionized calcium into bone or soft tissue.[14]

Nutritional deficiencies of calcium can occur in the instance of inadequate sources of dairy products or green, leafy vegetables, eating disorders, and malabsorption syndromes (celiac disease or short bowel syndrome). Excessive amounts of dietary phosphorus also bind with calcium in the gastrointestinal tract, so neither mineral is absorbed when such an excess occurs. Removal of the parathyroid glands (e.g., during total thyroidectomy) with the resulting loss of PTH also causes hypocalcemia. Severe hypomagnesemia suppresses PTH secretion, also causing hypocalcemia. Vitamin D deficiency, which can result from inadequate intake or lack of exposure to sunlight, causes decreased intestinal absorption of calcium. Malabsorption of fat, including fat-soluble vitamin D, also may contribute to calcium deficiency. Neoplastic bone metastases may inhibit bone resorption and increase calcium deposition into bone, thereby decreasing serum calcium levels.

Blood transfusions are also a common cause of hypocalcemia because the citrate solution used in storing whole blood binds with calcium and makes it unavailable to the tissues. Pancreatitis causes release of lipases into soft tissue spaces, so the free fatty acids that are formed bind calcium, causing a decrease in the concentration of ionized calcium. Metabolic or respiratory alkalosis causes symptoms of hypocalcemia because the change in pH enhances protein binding of ionized calcium. Hypoalbuminemia lowers total serum calcium levels by decreasing the amount of bound calcium in the plasma.

Clinical Manifestations. Many individuals with chronic hypocalcemia are asymptomatic. The clinical manifestations are a function of severity and rapidity of onset. Severe manifestations are caused by an increase in neuromuscular excitability with partial depolarization of nerves and muscles. As the threshold potential becomes more negative and approaches the resting membrane potential (hypopolarization) (see Fig. 3.8C), a smaller stimulus is required for initiating an action potential. The symptoms include paresthesias around the mouth and in the digits, carpopedal spasm (muscle spasms in the hands and feet), hyperreflexia, seizures, laryngospasm, and anxiety.

Two clinical signs of increased neuromuscular excitability are Chvostek sign and Trousseau sign. *Chvostek sign* is elicited by tapping on the facial nerve over the zygomatic arch. A positive sign is a strong twitch of the nose or lip. *Trousseau sign* is contraction of the hand and fingers when the arterial blood flow in the arm is occluded for 3 to 5 minutes with the use of a blood pressure cuff.

The characteristic ECG change is a prolonged QT interval, indicating prolonged ventricular depolarization and decreased cardiac contractility. Intestinal cramping and hyperactive bowel sounds also may be present because hypocalcemia affects the smooth muscles of the gastrointestinal tract. Table 3.11 contains a summary of the manifestations of calcium level alterations.

Evaluation and Treatment. Serum and ionized calcium, albumin, phosphate, and magnesium levels are evaluated. Further evaluation includes renal function and measurement of PTH and vitamin D. Severe symptoms of hypocalcemia require emergency treatment with IV 10% calcium gluconate, volume repletion, and ECG monitoring. The underlying cause must be identified. Oral calcium replacement should be initiated, and serum calcium levels should be monitored. Decreasing phosphate intake facilitates long-term management of hypocalcemia.

Hypercalcemia

Pathophysiology. Hypercalcemia with total serum calcium concentrations exceeding 10.5 mg/dL (5.2 mEq/L) can be caused by a number of diseases. The most common among these are hyperparathyroidism (which can be associated with thyrotoxicosis); many different types of cancer; sarcoidosis; and vitamin D toxicity. Many malignant tumors produce PTH or PTH-related protein, which causes bone resorption, thus elevating the serum calcium levels. Mild hypomagnesemia also stimulates PTH secretion and increases serum calcium. Sarcoidosis appears to increase vitamin D levels. Prolonged immobilization can also lead to hypercalcemia from enhanced bone resorption and decreased calcium deposition into bone. Acidosis decreases serum binding of calcium to albumin, increasing ionized calcium levels.

Clinical Manifestations. Many symptoms of hypercalcemia are nonspecific and related to severity and rapidity of onset.

TABLE 3.11 **Alterations in Calcium, Phosphate, and Magnesium Levels**

Causes	Manifestations
Hypocalcemia (<8.5 mg/dL)	
Inadequate intestinal absorption, deposition of ionized calcium into bone or soft tissue, blood administration, or decreases in PTH and vitamin D levels; nutritional deficiencies occur with inadequate sources of dairy products or green, leafy vegetables; alkalosis, elevated calcitonin level	Increased neuromuscular excitability; tingling, muscle spasms (particularly in hands, feet, and facial muscles), intestinal cramping, hyperactive bowel sounds; osteoporosis and fractures; severe cases show seizures and tetany; prolonged QT interval, cardiac arrest
Hypercalcemia (>10.5 mg/dL)	
Hyperparathyroidism; secretion of PTH and PTH-related protein from cancer cells; sarcoidosis; excess vitamin D; overuse of calcium-containing antacids	Many nonspecific; fatigue, weakness, lethargy, anorexia, nausea, constipation; impaired renal function, kidney stones; dysrhythmias, bradycardia, cardiac arrest; bone pain, osteoporosis, fractures
Hypophosphatemia (<2.0 mg/dL)	
Intestinal malabsorption related to vitamin D deficiency, overuse of magnesium- and aluminum-containing antacids, long-term alcohol abuse, and malabsorption syndromes; respiratory alkalosis; increased renal excretion of phosphate associated with hyperparathyroidism	Conditions related to reduced capacity for oxygen transport by red blood cells and disturbed energy metabolism; leukocyte and platelet dysfunction; deranged nerve and muscle function; in severe cases, irritability, confusion, numbness, coma, seizures; possibly respiratory failure (because of muscle weakness), cardiomyopathies, bone resorption (leading to rickets or osteomalacia)
Hyperphosphatemia (>4.7 mg/dL)	
Acute or chronic oliguric renal disease with significant loss of glomerular filtration; treatment of metastatic tumors with chemotherapy that releases large amounts of phosphate into serum; long-term use of laxatives or enemas containing phosphates; hypoparathyroidism	Symptoms primarily related to low serum calcium levels (caused by high phosphate levels) similar to symptoms of hypocalcemia; when prolonged, calcification of soft tissues in lungs, kidneys, joints
Hypomagnesemia (<1.5 mEq/L)	
Malnutrition, malabsorption syndromes, alcoholism, urinary losses (renal tubular dysfunction, loop diuretics)	Behavioral changes, irritability, increased reflexes, muscle cramps, ataxia, nystagmus, tetany, seizures, tachycardia, hypotension
Hypermagnesemia (>3.0 mEq/L)	
Usually oliguric renal disease; also excessive intake of magnesium-containing antacids, adrenal insufficiency	Lethargy, drowsiness; loss of deep tendon reflexes; nausea and vomiting; muscle weakness; hypotension; bradycardia; respiratory depression or arrest; heart block, cardiac arrest

PTH, Parathyroid hormone.

Because serum calcium levels are increased, a greater amount of calcium is also contained inside the cells. The threshold potential becomes more positive (hyperpolarized) (e.g., moves from −60 to −50 millivolts) and the cell membrane becomes refractory to depolarization (decreased excitability) and results in a greater difference between threshold potential and resting membrane potential (see Fig. 3.8C). Thus, many of the symptoms are related to loss of cell membrane excitability. Fatigue, weakness, lethargy, anorexia, nausea, and constipation are common.

Mental status changes and confusion may occur. Impaired renal function frequently develops with polyuria or formation of kidney stones from precipitates of calcium salts. A shortened QT segment and depressed widened T waves also may be observed on the ECG, with bradycardia and varying degrees of heart block. Table 3.11 contains a summary of the manifestations of alterations in calcium levels.

Evaluation and Treatment. With elevated serum calcium levels, often a reciprocal decrease in serum phosphate values occurs. Specific diagnostic procedures to identify the contributing pathologic condition are required.

Treatment is related to the severity of symptoms and the underlying disease. When renal function is normal, oral phosphate administration is effective. When acute illness and high calcium levels are present, treatment options include IV administration of large amounts of normal saline to enhance renal excretion of calcium, administration of bisphosphonates in the absence of renal dysfunction, and administration of calcitonin. Bisphosphonates and denosumab are used for malignancy-associated hypercalcemia, and cinacalcet is approved for the reduction of hypercalcemia associated with parathyroid carcinoma.[15] Ultimately, the underlying pathologic condition must be treated.

Hypophosphatemia

Pathophysiology. Hypophosphatemia is a serum phosphate level less than 2.0 mg/dL and is usually an indication of phosphate deficiency. In some conditions, total body phosphate concentration is normal, but serum concentrations are low. The most common causes are intestinal malabsorption and increased renal excretion of phosphate. Inadequate absorption is associated with vitamin D deficiency, use of magnesium- and aluminum-containing antacids (which bind with phosphorus), long-term alcohol abuse, malabsorption syndromes, and refeeding syndromes after starvation. Respiratory alkalosis can cause severe hypophosphatemia because of cellular use of phosphorus for accelerated glycolysis (ATP) formation. Increased renal excretion of phosphorus is associated with hyperparathyroidism. Risk of hypophosphatemia has also been associated with IV iron therapy for treatment of pernicious anemia.[16] Genetic mutations in fibroblast growth factor 23 (FGF23) are associated with decreased renal reabsorption of phosphorus.

Clinical Manifestations. The consequences of phosphate deficiency are not clinically evident until hypophosphatemia is severe, and multiple organ systems can be affected. There is reduced capacity for oxygen transport by red blood cells and disturbed energy metabolism. When phosphate is depleted, erythrocyte 2,3-DPG (diphosphoglycerate) and ATP levels become low and diminish the release of oxygen to the tissues, leading to hypoxia with bradycardia and varying degrees of heart block.

Leukocyte and platelet dysfunctions also are associated with hypophosphatemia. There is a greater risk of infection and blood-clotting impairment, with potential for hemorrhage. Nerve and muscle function can be affected because of derangement in energy metabolism. Muscle weakness may become serious enough to cause respiratory failure, and cardiomyopathies also can develop. Irritability, confusion, numbness, coma, and seizures develop with severe phosphate losses. In response to low phosphate levels, bone resorption occurs and may lead to rickets or osteomalacia. (Table 3.11 contains a summary of the manifestations of phosphate level alterations).

Evaluation and Treatment. To correct the condition, the underlying cause must be identified and treated. The rate and amount of replacement are determined by the cause and presenting symptoms.[17]

Hyperphosphatemia

Pathophysiology. Hyperphosphatemia, or an elevated serum phosphate level of more than 4.7 mg/dL, develops with exogenous or endogenous addition of phosphorus to the ECF or with significant loss of glomerular filtration and chronic kidney disease. Because most phosphate is located in cells, rapid cell destruction associated with treatment of metastatic tumors with chemotherapy can release large amounts of phosphate into the ECF. Long-term use of phosphate-containing enemas or laxatives also may lead to hyperphosphatemia. Hypoparathyroidism can cause elevated phosphate levels by increasing renal tubular reabsorption of phosphate.

High levels of serum phosphate also lower serum calcium levels, and increased amounts of phosphate and calcium are deposited in bone and soft tissues. Serum calcium levels may become low enough to cause symptoms of hypocalcemia, including tetany.

Clinical Manifestations. Symptoms of hyperphosphatemia are related primarily to low serum calcium levels and thus are comparable with symptoms of hypocalcemia. With prolonged hyperphosphatemia, calcification of soft tissues occurs in the lungs, kidneys, and joints. (See Table 3.11 contains a summary of the manifestations of alterations in phosphate concentration.)

Evaluation and Treatment. To correct hyperphosphatemia, the underlying pathologic condition must be identified and treated. Aluminum hydroxide may be administered because it binds phosphate in the gastrointestinal tract and is then eliminated; however, aluminum can be toxic, causing encephalopathy and osteomalacia. Nonaluminum, non–calcium phosphate binders (e.g., lanthanum carbonate or sevelamer) are used but can have serious side effects and are costly.[18] Newer iron-based binders are being evaluated.[19] Dialysis is required for management of end-stage chronic kidney disease.

Magnesium

Magnesium (Mg^{++}) is a major intracellular cation, second to potassium. Approximately 40% to 60% is stored in muscle and bone, with 30% in the cells. A small amount (1%) is in the plasma. Plasma concentration is 1.5 to 3.0 mg/dL with approximately one-third bound to plasma proteins and the rest in ionized form. Regulation of magnesium metabolism is balanced by dietary intake, small intestinal absorption, and renal reabsorption and excretion. Low serum levels cause renal conservation of magnesium. Magnesium is a cofactor in intracellular enzymatic reactions, protein synthesis, and nucleic acid stability. Extracellular magnesium is necessary for normal neuromuscular excitability and nerve conduction. Magnesium improves myocardial metabolism and cell function; influences vascular smooth muscle tone (reduces peripheral vascular resistance and afterload); reduces cardiac dysrhythmias; and improves lipid and glucose metabolism. Magnesium also reduces vulnerability to oxygen-derived free radicals and systemic inflammation, improves human endothelial function, and inhibits platelet function, including platelet aggregation and adhesion.

Magnesium has been shown to counteract vascular calcification by inhibiting hyperphosphatemic-induced crystalline calciprotein particle formation in vascular smooth muscle.[20] Calcium and magnesium often interact in reactions at the intracellular level, with magnesium being an antagonist of calcium. Mg^{++} reduces PTH secretion mainly when a moderate-low calcium concentration is present.

Hypomagnesemia occurs when serum magnesium concentration is less than 1.5 mEq/L and clinical symptoms are present.[11] Malnutrition, malabsorption syndromes, alcoholism, renal tubular dysfunction, metabolic acidosis, use of loop and thiazide diuretics, and prolonged use of proton pump inhibitors can cause magnesium losses. Hypomagnesemia is associated with insulin resistance, diabetes mellitus, left ventricular hypertrophy, systemic inflammation, hypoalbuminemia, and osteoporosis. Because extracellular magnesium inhibits potassium channels, loss of magnesium results in movement of potassium out of the cell, with renal excretion resulting in hypokalemia. Signs and symptoms of hypomagnesemia are often absent and develop with severe losses. Clinical manifestations are similar to those of hypocalcemia. Neuromuscular irritability, positive Chvostek and Trousseau signs, increased reflexes, muscle weakness, ataxia, nystagmus, tetany, seizures, and tachydysrhythmias may be observed. Treatment is intramuscular or IV administration of magnesium sulfate. Magnesium supplementation may be beneficial in the treatment of preeclampsia, migraine, depression, cardiovascular disease, metabolic syndrome, and asthma.[21–23]

Hypermagnesemia, in which magnesium concentration is greater than 3.0 mEq/L, is rare and usually is caused by oliguric renal disease. Magnesium-containing antacids or cathartics can potentiate excess magnesium levels. Excess magnesium concentration inhibits calcium-mediated nerve conduction and depresses skeletal muscle contraction and nerve function. Signs and symptoms include nausea and vomiting, decreased deep tendon reflexes, muscle weakness, hypotension, bradycardia, and respiratory depression. Treatment is avoidance of magnesium-containing substances and removal of magnesium by dialysis.[24] (See Table 3.11 contains a summary of the manifestations of magnesium level alterations.)

ACID-BASE BALANCE

Acid-base balance and hydrogen ion concentration must be regulated within a narrow range for normal body function. Slight changes in amounts of hydrogen ion and pH changes can significantly alter biologic processes in cells and tissues. Hydrogen ions are required to maintain membrane integrity and the speed of enzymatic reactions.[25] Many pathologic conditions disturb acid-base balance, and the degree of severity may be more harmful than the disease process itself.

Hydrogen Ion and pH

The concentration of hydrogen ions in body fluids is very small—approximately 0.0000001 mg/L. This number is expressed as the negative logarithm 10^{-7} mg/L and is indicated on the pH scale as pH 7.0, a neutral status. Values less than 7.0 are more acid. Values more than 7.0 are more alkaline. Accordingly, the pH number indicates the acidity or alkalinity of a solution. The pH scale is logarithmic, not linear, meaning the difference between numbers on the scale is not constant. Each number on the scale is 10 times more acid or more alkaline than the preceding number. Accordingly, a pH of 5 is 10 times more acid than a pH of 6; a pH of 4 is 10 times more acid than a pH of 5 and 100 times more acid than a pH of 6. As the pH changes by one unit from a pH 7 to a pH 6, the H^+ increases 10-fold, making the solution much more acid than a neutral solution with a pH of 7.0. Solutions with an excess of hydrogen ions are acidic in nature; solutions with an excess of hydroxide ions (OH^-) are basic, or alkaline, in nature. In arterial blood, the normal pH range is 7.35 to 7.45, with 7.4 being the midpoint of that normal range. Accordingly, a blood pH less than 7.35 is defined as acidic, and a pH greater than 7.45 is defined as alkaline, or basic (Table 3.12).

TABLE 3.12 pH of Body Fluids

Body Fluid	pH	Factors Affecting pH
Gastric juices	1.0–3.0	Hydrochloric acid production
Urine	5.0–6.0	H^+ ion excretion from waste products
Arterial blood	7.35–7.45	pH is slightly higher because there is less carbonic acid (H_2CO_3)
Venous blood	7.37	pH is slightly lower because there is more carbonic acid
Cerebrospinal fluid	7.32	Decreased bicarbonate and higher carbon dioxide content decrease pH
Pancreatic fluid	7.8–8.0	Contains bicarbonate produced by exocrine cells
Bile	7.0–8.0	Contains bicarbonate
Small intestine fluid	6.5–7.5	Contains alkaline fluid from pancreas, liver, and gallbladder

The average person generates 50 to 100 mEq/day of acid from the metabolism of proteins, carbohydrates, and fats, as well as from loss of alkaline fluids in the stool. To maintain a normal pH, acids must be balanced by base substances within the body. A base is a substance that accepts hydrogen ions; an acid is a substance that donates hydrogen ions. Body acids exist in two forms: volatile acids (substances that can be eliminated as carbon dioxide [CO_2] gas) and nonvolatile acids (substances that can be eliminated only by the kidney). The sole volatile acid formed in the body is carbonic acid (H_2CO_3), a *weak acid*, which means that in body fluids, some of the carbonic acid molecules release their hydrogen ions, but other carbonic molecules do not. In the presence of the enzyme carbonic anhydrase, it readily dissociates into CO_2 and water (H_2O). The CO_2 is eliminated through pulmonary ventilation. The rest of the body acids are nonvolatile acids, such as lactic acid, phosphoric acid, sulfuric acid, acetoacetic acid, and beta-hydroxybutyric acid. A few nonvolatile acids are *strong acids*, meaning they readily release their hydrogen ions; however, most of the nonvolatile acids are weak acids. Nonvolatile acids are secreted into the urine by the renal tubules in amounts of approximately 50 to 100 mEq of hydrogen per day, or approximately 1 mEq/kg of body weight.

Mechanisms to Maintain Normal pH

The body has three mechanisms, or lines of defense, to maintain the acid-base balance: (1) physiologic (chemical) buffer systems (plasma bicarbonate, phosphate, hemoglobin [Hb], and protein), the first line of defense; (2) respiratory acid-base control, the second line of defense; and (3) renal acid-base control, the third line of defense. The physiologic buffers function instantaneously to correct alterations in the acid-base balance. The lungs and the kidneys work in concert to maintain a normal pH. The lungs respond relatively quickly (within seconds to minutes), but the kidneys require more time (hours to days) to bring the system into balance. Although the lungs respond more quickly, mechanisms involving the kidney produce more long-term acid-base balance.

Buffer Systems

Buffer systems resist changes in pH and maintain pH within the normal range. Metabolic processes primarily generate H^+ (acid) ions. Unchecked, these ions would alter the pH of the body. Buffers can absorb excessive H^+ ions (acid) or hydroxide ions (OH^-) (base) to minimize fluctuations in pH. The buffer systems are located in both the ICF and the ECF compartments,

TABLE 3.13 Buffer Systems

Buffer Pairs	Buffer System	pK Values	Reaction	Rate
HCO_3^-/H_2CO_3	Bicarbonate	6.1	$H^+ + HCO_3^- \rightleftarrows H_2O + CO_2$	Instantaneous
Hb^-/HHb	Hemoglobin	7.3	$HHb \rightleftarrows H^+ + Hb^-$	Instantaneous
$HPO_4^-/H_2PO_4^-$	Phosphate	6.8	$HPO_4^- + H^+ \rightleftarrows H_2PO_4^-$	Instantaneous
Pr^-/HPr	Plasma proteins	6.7	$HPr \rightleftarrows H^+ + Pr^-$	Instantaneous
Organs	**Mechanism**			**Rate**
Lungs	Regulates retention or elimination of CO_2 and therefore H_2CO_3 concentration			Minutes to hours
Ionic shifts	Exchange of intracellular potassium and sodium for hydrogen			2–4 hours
Kidneys	Bicarbonate reabsorption and regeneration, ammonia formation, phosphate buffering			Hours to days
Bone	Exchanges of calcium and phosphate, release of carbonate			Hours to days

H^+, Hydrogen ion; HCO_3^-, bicarbonate; H_2CO_3, carbonic acid; *Hb^-*, hemoglobin; *HHb*, hydrogenated hemoglobin; $H_2PO_4^-$, monobasic phosphate; HPO_4^-, dibasic phosphate; *HPr*, hydrogenated protein; *Pr^-*, protein.

and function at different rates (Table 3.13). The most important are the plasma buffer systems, which have two components: carbonic acid–bicarbonate and the protein Hb. The important intracellular buffers are phosphate and protein. Ammonia and phosphate can attach hydrogen ions and are important renal buffers.

Carbonic Acid–Bicarbonate Buffering

Cellular respiration results in the production of CO_2, which combines with water to form carbonic acid (H_2CO_3). H_2CO_3 dissociates, forming one hydrogen (H^+) ion and one bicarbonate ion (HCO_3^-) in the blood. The bicarbonate ion is a base component of the **buffer system**, and the hydrogen ion is the acid component. These reactions are readily reversible, depending on whether an acid or a base environment exists. The reactions can move in one or the other direction to maintain a neutral pH. Accordingly, these reactions can correct for imbalances in pH by releasing hydrogen ions or absorbing hydrogen ions as the need arises. If excess H^+ ions are present, the buffer absorbs these ions. If excess bicarbonate ions are present, the buffer releases H^+ ions. The relationship between bicarbonate (HCO_3^-) and carbonic acid (H_2CO_3) usually is expressed as a ratio. Under normal conditions, the bicarbonate level is approximately 24 mEq/L and the carbonic acid level is approximately 1.2 mEq/L when the arterial CO_2 ($Paco_2$) is 40 mm Hg. Therefore the ratio of bicarbonate to carbonic acid is 20:1 (24/1.2). This ratio maintains a normal pH of 7.40 (Fig. 3.11).

Both the lungs and the kidneys augment the action of the bicarbonate–carbonic acid buffer system. The lungs eliminate CO_2 and water and can increase the amount of CO_2 eliminated by increasing the rate and depth of ventilation. Although the lungs do not respond as rapidly as the physiologic buffering system, they have twice the ability to correct for pH imbalances compared with all the chemical buffering systems combined. Similarly, the kidneys augment the **carbonic acid–bicarbonate buffer** system by reabsorbing or regenerating bicarbonate from CO_2 and water in the renal tubules or excreting hydrogen ions

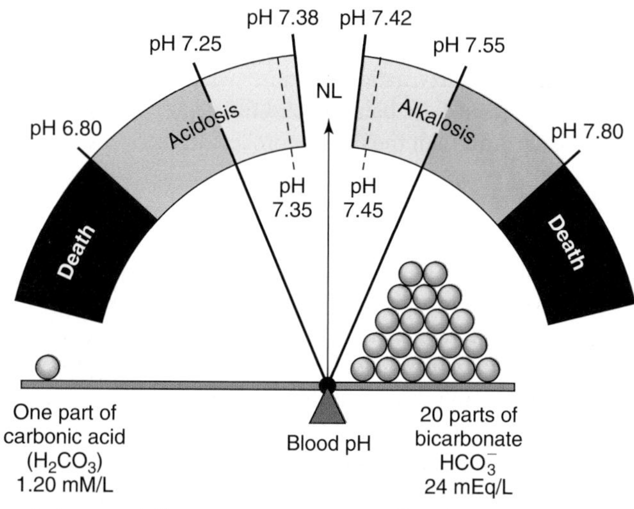

Fig. 3.11 Ratio of Carbonic Acid and Bicarbonate Concentration in Maintaining pH Within Normal Limits. An increase in H_2CO_3 or decrease in HCO_3^- concentration causes acidosis. A decrease in H_2CO_3 or increase in HCO_3^- concentration causes alkalosis. *NL*, Normal. (From Monahan, FD, et al. *Medical-surgical nursing: Health and illness perspectives*, 8th edition. St. Louis: Mosby; 2007.)

into the urine. The renal response takes considerably longer than does the respiratory response. However, the kidneys' ability to regulate and maintain a normal pH is necessary because the kidneys are the only organs that can excrete nonvolatile acids.

The pH ratio equation of 20/1 can be symbolically expressed as follows:

$$pH = 20/1 = \frac{Base}{Acid} \quad or \quad pH = \frac{Renal\ regulation\ (slow)}{Pulmonary\ regulation\ (fast)}$$

Changes in either the numerator or the denominator will change the pH. For example, if the amount of bicarbonate is

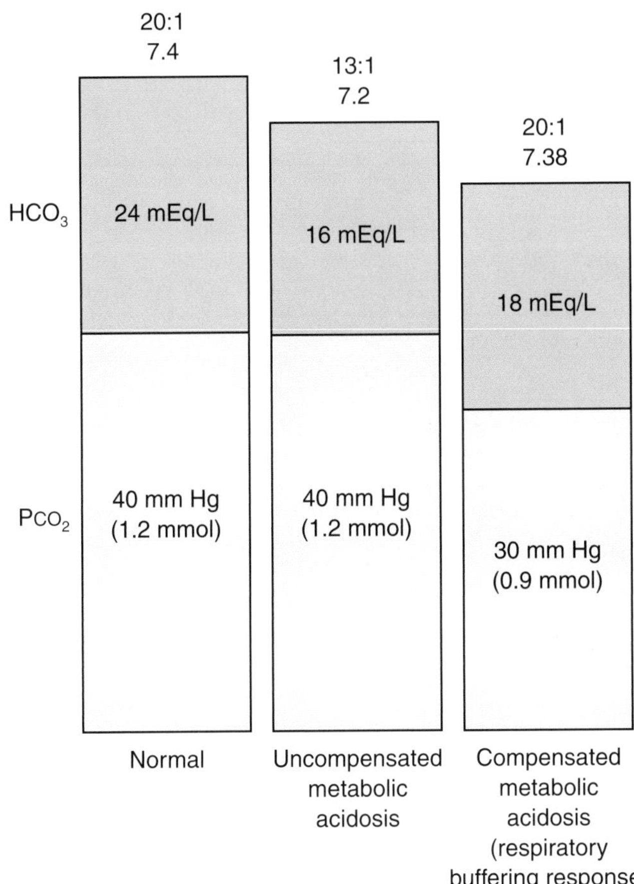

Fig. 3.12 Compensated Maintenance of $[HCO_3^-]/Pco_2$ (H_2CO_3) Ratio in Metabolic Acidosis.

decreased, the pH also decreases, causing a state of acidosis (Fig. 3.12). The pH can be returned to a normal range if the value of the denominator or the amount of carbonic acid also decreases. When a disease process causes an alteration in the bicarbonate/carbonic acid ratio, the kidneys or lungs (i.e., the organ not responsible for causing the alteration) respond to restore the ratio and maintain a normal pH.

Protein Buffering

All proteins can attach or release a hydrogen ion. Most proteins are inside cells; hence protein-based buffering is primarily an intracellular buffer system. Hb in erythrocytes is an excellent blood protein buffer. As the pH increases, Hb loses hydrogen ions, and the reverse happens when the pH decreases. Hb also affects the pH through a different mechanism when it binds CO_2 to form carbaminohemoglobin ($HHbCO_2$). The bound CO_2 is transported to the lungs, where it is released from the body through ventilation. This dynamic is important because CO_2 is a *potential acid*. Unbound CO_2 can react in water to form H_2CO_3, a weak acid. Carbonic acid releases hydrogen ion, lowering the pH. By binding CO_2, the Hb is preventing CO_2 from becoming carbonic acid; it thereby prevents the release of excess H^+ ions into the environment. The pH control system is illustrated in Fig. 3.13.

Respiratory and Renal Buffering

The respiratory system regulates acid-base balance by controlling the rate of ventilation when there is metabolic acidosis or alkalosis. Central chemoreceptors sense increases or decreases in pH and $Paco_2$ When acidemia exists, the respiratory rate increases (eliminating CO_2 and thus reducing carbonic acid concentration) (see Fig. 3.13). When alkalemia occurs, the respiratory rate decreases (retaining CO_2 and increasing carbonic acid concentration).

The renal buffering of H^+ ions requires the use of carbonic anhydrase in renal tubular cells to combine CO_2 and H_2O to form H_2CO_3. The H^+ ion is secreted from the tubular cell and buffered in the lumen by phosphate and ammonia. The bicarbonate is reabsorbed. The end effect is the addition of new bicarbonate to the blood, which contributes to the alkalinity of the plasma, because the hydrogen ion is excreted from the body (Fig. 3.14-1).

Two additional buffer systems are active in the renal tubules, the *phosphate buffer* and the *ammonia buffer*. Once H^+ has reacted with all available, any additional H^+ ions react with either the phosphate or the ammonia buffer systems. The *phosphate buffer* functions both in the renal tubules and in the ICF. The two components of this system, monobasic phosphate (HPO_4^-) and dibasic phosphate ($H_2PO_4^-$), usually function in association with sodium to form a sodium salt. As with any buffer, these components bind or release H^+ to maintain physiologic neutrality (pH 7.40) (Fig. 3.14-2). The *ammonia buffer* functions within the renal tubules. The components for this system are ammonia (NH_3) and ammonium ion (NH_4^+) (Fig. 3.14-3). Both monobasic phosphate and ammonium ion (NH_4^+) are lipid insoluble, preventing them from diffusing back across the tubular cells and into the blood; thus, they are excreted in the urine.

Other Buffers

A cellular ion exchange mechanism is also an important buffering system. The best example is the shift of potassium in exchange for hydrogen during states of acidosis or alkalosis. During acidosis, potassium tends to leave the intracellular space in exchange for hydrogen. The reverse occurs during alkalosis. Although the ionic shifts facilitate buffering, the changes in intracellular or extracellular potassium concentrations may have serious consequences (e.g., hyperkalemia or hypokalemia).

Acid-Base Imbalances

Pathophysiologic changes in the concentration of H^+ ion or base in the blood lead to acid-base imbalances. Acidemia is a state in which the pH of arterial blood is less than 7.35. A systemic increase in hydrogen ion concentration or a loss of base is termed acidosis. Alkalemia is a state in which the pH of arterial blood is greater than 7.45. A systemic decrease in hydrogen ion concentration or an excess of base is termed alkalosis. These changes may be caused by either *respiratory* or *metabolic* processes, or both. If the altered pH occurs secondary to biochemical processes within the body or to renal dysfunction, it

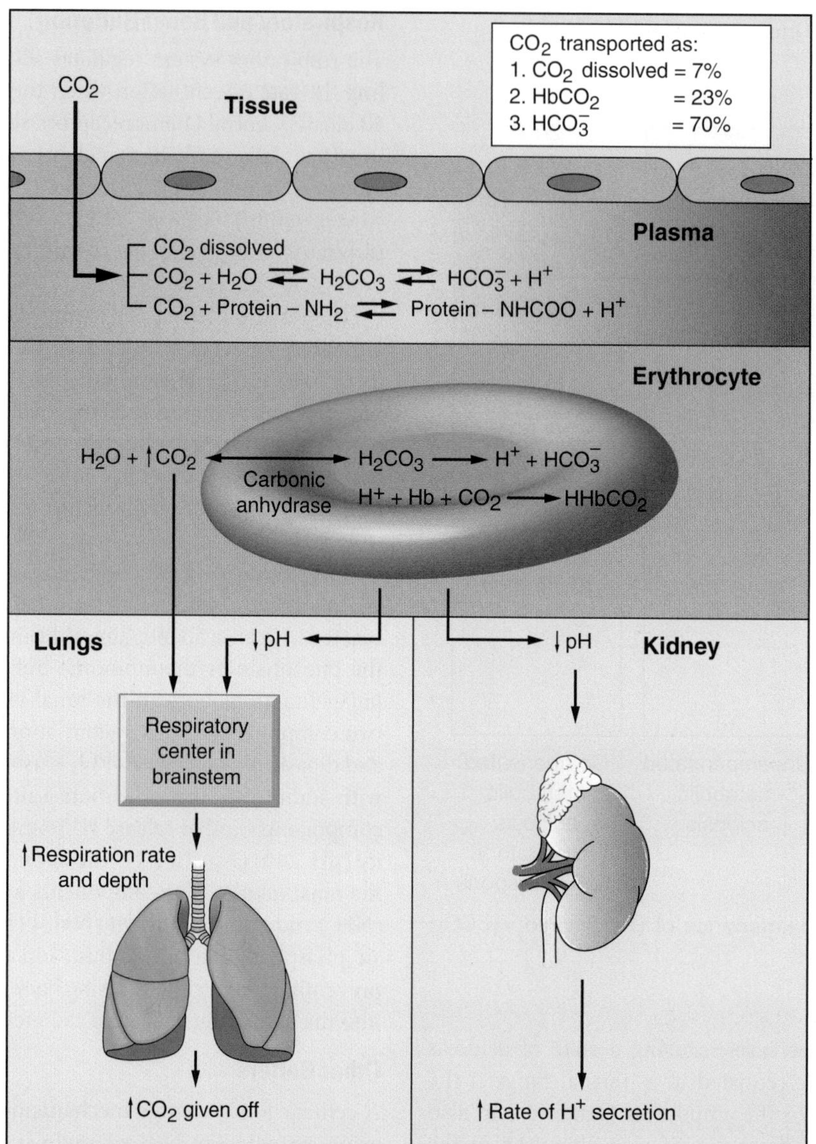

Fig. 3.13 Integration of pH Control Mechanisms. CO_2 is produced in tissue cells and diffuses to plasma, where it is transported as dissolved CO_2, or it combines with water to form carbonic acid (H_2CO_3), or it combines with protein from which hydrogen has been released. Most of the CO_2 diffuses into the red blood cells and combines with water to form H_2CO_3. The H_2CO_3 dissociates to form hydrogen ion (H^+) and bicarbonate (HCO_3^-). Hydrogen ion combines with hemoglobin that has released its oxygen to form hydrogenated hemoglobin (HHb), which buffers the hydrogen ion and makes venous blood slightly more acidic than arterial blood. The increase in H^+ concentration coupled with elevated CO_2 levels results in $HHbCO_2$ and an increase in the respiratory rate (eliminates CO_2) and secretion of H^+ by the kidneys.

is *metabolic*. If the alteration in pH is secondary to an alteration with ventilation, it is *respiratory*. Accordingly, four clinical alterations in the acid-base status can develop: *respiratory acidosis, metabolic acidosis, respiratory alkalosis*, and *metabolic alkalosis*.[25]

Arterial blood gases are measured to determine which of the four alterations is present. This measurement typically includes four parameters: the blood pH, Pao_2 (oxygen), $Paco_2$ (carbon dioxide), and (bicarbonate).[26] The Pao_2 provides information about the person's oxygenation status, but it does not directly provide information about the acid-base status. The blood pH, $Paco_2$, and bicarbonate level, when evaluated together, provide information about whether an individual is experiencing acidosis or alkalosis, and whether the cause is respiratory or metabolic. Fig. 3.15 summarizes the relationships among pH, $Paco_2$, and bicarbonate during different acid-base alterations. Fig. 3.11 summarizes the relationship among pH, the partial pressure of carbon dioxide (respiratory regulation), and the concentration

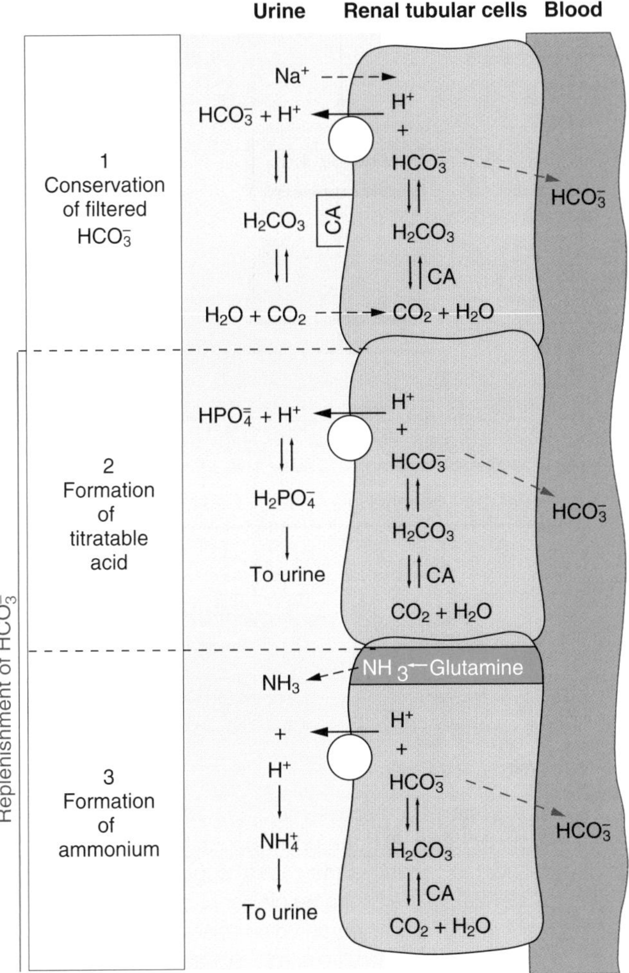

Fig. 3.14 Renal Excretion of Acid. ***1,*** *Conservation of Filtered Bicarbonate.* Filtered bicarbonate (HCO_3^-) combines with secreted hydrogen ion (H^+) to form carbonic acid (H_2CO_3), which then is converted to water (H_2O) and carbon dioxide (CO_2) by carbonic anhydrase (CA); both diffuse into the renal tubular cell. The CO_2 and H_2O combine to form H_2CO_3 in the presence of CA, and the resulting bicarbonate ion (HCO_3^-) is reabsorbed into the blood. ***2,*** *Formation of Titratable Acid.* Hydrogen ion (H^+) is secreted and combines with dibasic phosphate (HPO_4^-) to form monobasic phosphate ($H_2PO_4^-$). The secreted hydrogen ion (H^+) is formed from the dissociation of H_2CO_3, and the remaining HCO_3^- is reabsorbed into the blood. ***3,*** *Formation of Ammonium Ions.* Ammonia (NH_3) is produced from glutamine in the renal tubular cell and diffuses to the urine where it combines with H^+ to form ammonium ion (NH_4^+). Once NH_4^+ has been formed it cannot return to the renal tubular cell (diffusional trapping) and the bicarbonate remaining in the renal tubular cell is reabsorbed into the blood. NOTE: The white circles with the arrows on top represent a renal tubular cell active transport pump.

of bicarbonate (renal regulation) during alkalosis and acidosis. An individual can experience both metabolic and respiratory disorders at the same time. In such cases, the person may have a mixed acid-base alteration.

Renal and respiratory adjustments to *primary* changes in pH are known as compensation. With compensation, a 20:1 ratio may be achieved, but the actual values for HCO_3^- and H_2CO_3 concentrations are not normal (see Fig. 3.12). The respiratory system compensates for changes in pH by increasing or decreasing ventilation, a rapid response occurring within minutes to hours. The renal system compensates by producing more acidic or more alkaline urine, which may take hours to days. Correction occurs when the values for both components of the buffer pair ratio (bicarbonate and carbonic acid) return to normal.

Carbon dioxide is referred to as a *potential acid* because it is readily converted to carbonic acid. Breathing more shallowly and slowly (hypoventilation) causes a retention of CO_2 (hypercapnia), whereas breathing more rapidly and deeply (hyperventilation) blows off CO_2 (hypocapnia). In this manner, the lungs compensate for excess acidity or alkalinity of the blood. The $Paco_2$ and bicarbonate levels provide information on the source of the altered pH and also indicate whether any compensation is ongoing. A low blood pH signals acidosis. If the $Paco_2$ is high, the source of the problem is respiratory (e.g., retained CO_2). Such a scenario might occur with an opioid overdose, in which respirations are depressed and CO_2 is retained. This individual is described as having a primary *respiratory acidosis.* If the pH is low and the $Paco_2$ is normal or low, the acidosis is not caused by respiratory factors. Instead, it is caused by metabolic processes within the body. In this case, the individual is described as having a primary *metabolic acidosis.* An example of a primary metabolic acidosis is an individual experiencing DKA from a lack of insulin secretion or administration. The diabetic individual, lacking insulin, cannot metabolize glucose. The body metabolizes fat stores, and as a result, acid by-products are released into the blood, causing *metabolic acidosis.*

Metabolic Acidosis

Pathophysiology. In metabolic acidosis, the concentration of nonvolatile (non–carbonic) acids increase. Less commonly this condition can result if bicarbonate (base) is lost from the ECF or cannot be regenerated by the kidney (Table 3.14). Metabolic acidosis can occur quickly, as in lactic acidosis secondary to poor perfusion or hypoxemia. It can also occur more slowly, as in oliguric renal disease (failure to excrete acid), ingestion of acid precursors that are metabolized to acids, starvation states (excess production of ketoacids from excess metabolism of fats and proteins), or DKA (excess production of ketoacids from lack of insulin) (see Chapter 22).

The buffer systems manage the excess acid and attempt to maintain the arterial pH within a normal range. Hydrogen ions will move to the intracellular space, and potassium will move to the extracellular space to maintain an ionic balance. Buffering by bicarbonate lowers the serum value of hydrogen ions and increases the previously decreased pH. The respiratory system compensates for a metabolic acidosis as the reduced pH stimulates hyperventilation, lowering the $Paco_2$ and the amount of H_2CO_3 circulating in the blood. The kidneys excrete the excess acid as NH_4^+ and titratable acid ($H_2PO_4^-$). When acidosis is severe, buffers become depleted and cannot compensate for the increasing H^+ load and the pH continues to decrease. The

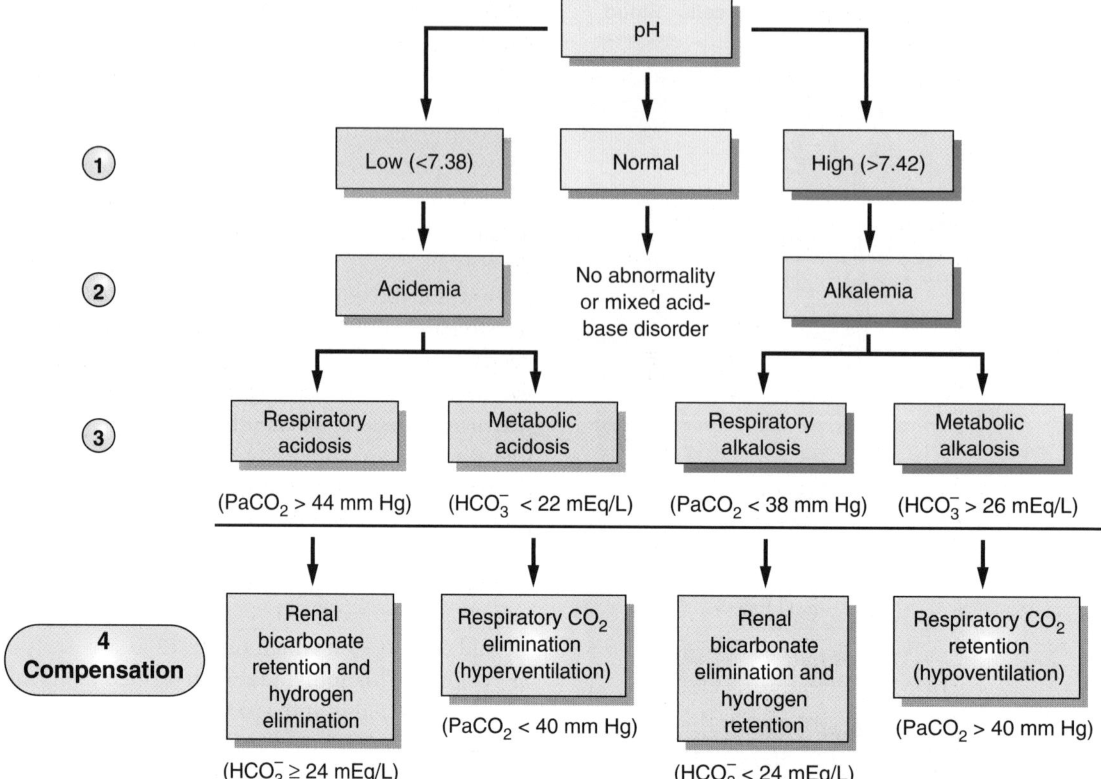

Fig. 3.15 Primary and Compensatory Acid-Base Changes. A systematic approach can be used to interpret the cause of an acid-base imbalance. ***1,*** Is the pH low or high? ***2,*** If the pH is low, there is acidemia; if the pH is high, there is alkalemia. ***3,*** If the pH is low (acidemia), is the cause respiratory (high $Paco_2$) or metabolic (low HCO_3^-)? If the pH is high (alkalemia), is the cause respiratory (low $Paco_2$) or metabolic (high HCO_3^-)? ***4,*** Is there compensation for the primary acid-base disorder? *(a)* HCO_3^- will be ≥24 mEq/L if there is renal compensation for a primary respiratory acidosis; *(b)* $Paco_2$ will be <40 mm Hg if there is respiratory compensation of a primary metabolic acidosis; *(c)* HCO_3^- will ≤24 mEq/L if there is renal compensation for primary respiratory alkalosis; *(d)* $Paco_2$ will be >40 mm Hg if there is respiratory compensation for primary metabolic alkalosis. NOTE: Examine the pH first. Then examine the changes in HCO_3^- and $Paco_2$. HCO_3^- concentration will be elevated when there is primary metabolic alkalosis or renal compensation for primary respiratory acidosis. HCO_3^- concentration will be decreased when there is primary metabolic acidosis or renal compensation for primary respiratory alkalosis. $Paco_2$ will be elevated when there is primary respiratory acidosis or respiratory compensation for primary metabolic alkalosis. $Paco_2$ will be decreased when there is primary respiratory alkalosis or respiratory compensation for metabolic acidosis.

TABLE 3.14 Causes of Metabolic Acidosis

Increased Non–Carbonic Acids (Elevated Anion Gap)	Bicarbonate Loss (Normal Anion Gap)
Increased H+ load—overproduction of acid	Diarrhea
Ketoacidosis (e.g., diabetes mellitus, alcoholic ketoacidosis, starvation)	Ureterosigmoidoscopy Early chronic kidney disease
Lactic acidosis (e.g., shock)	Proximal renal tubule acidosis
Ingestions (e.g., ammonium chloride, ethylene glycol, methanol, salicylates, paraldehyde)	
Decreased H+ excretion	
Acute or chronic oliguric renal disease	
Distal renal tubule acidosis	

ratio of bicarbonate to carbonic acid decreases to less than 20:1 (Fig. 3.16). In states of metabolic acidosis, potassium may be redistributed from the intracellular to the extracellular space and is reabsorbed at the apical membrane of the renal collecting tubule. There is also an increase in the levels of ionized calcium because acidosis decreases the amount of calcium bound to albumin.

The evaluation of the **anion gap** can be helpful when used cautiously to distinguish different factors contributing to metabolic acidosis.[27] Normally, the concentrations of cations and anions in the plasma are equivalent. However, some anions, such as protein, sulfates, phosphates, and organic acids, are not measured in the common laboratory evaluations of the blood. Therefore the normal anion gap represents these unmeasured negative ions (sulfate, phosphate, lactate, ketoacids, albumin). A convenient measure of the anion gap is the difference between

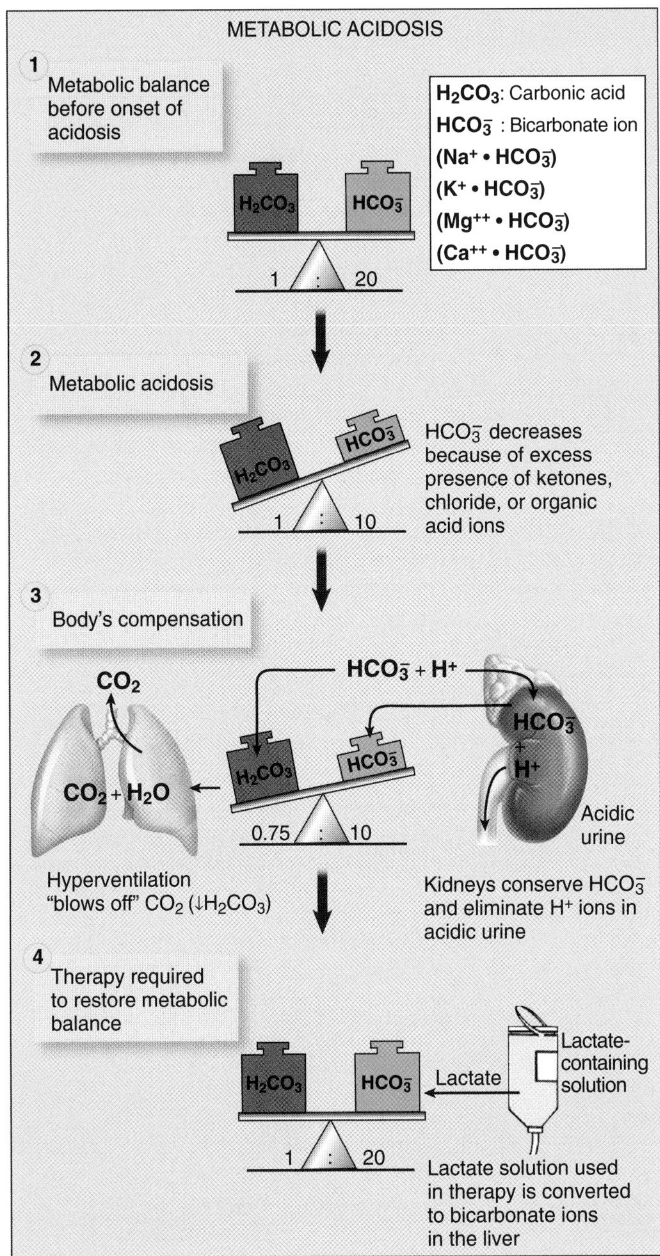

Fig. 3.16 Metabolic Acidosis With Compensation and Correction. See text for abbreviations. (From Patton KT, Thibodeau, GA. *Anatomy & physiology*, 9th edition. St. Louis: Mosby; 2016.)

the sum of Na^+ and K^+ concentrations and the sum of HCO_3^- and Cl^- concentrations, or approximately 10 to 12 mEq/L:

$$\text{Anion gap} = [Na^+(140) + K^+(4.0)] - [HCO_3^-(24) + Cl^-(110)] \\ = 10 - 12 \text{ mEq/L}$$

In metabolic acidosis a normal anion gap is characteristic of conditions related to bicarbonate loss with retention of chloride to maintain an ionic balance. This is called hyperchloremic metabolic acidosis, and it occurs with chronic kidney disease or prolonged diarrhea with bicarbonate loss. An elevated anion gap is characteristic of acidosis associated with accumulation of anions other than chloride (see Table 3.14). With severe pH disturbances, changes in the concentration of serum albumin, which behaves as an anion, can have a significant impact on the anion gap and a correction for this measure can be used in these cases.[28]

Clinical Manifestations. Metabolic acidosis is manifested by changes in the neurologic, respiratory, gastrointestinal, and cardiovascular systems. Early symptoms include headache and lethargy, which progress to confusion and coma in severe acidosis. The respiratory system's efforts to compensate for the increase in metabolic acids result in what are termed *Kussmaul respirations*, a form of hyperventilation in which ventilations are deep and rapid. This represents the body's attempt to increase the pH by expelling carbon dioxide (respiratory compensation), which in turn decreases the carbonic acid concentration. Other symptoms include anorexia, nausea, vomiting, diarrhea, and abdominal discomfort. Death can result in the most severe and prolonged cases, preceded by dysrhythmias and hypotension.

Evaluation and Treatment. The diagnosis of metabolic acidosis is established from the health history, clinical symptoms, and laboratory findings. Arterial blood pH is less than 7.35, and bicarbonate concentration is less than 22 mEq/L. The anion gap can facilitate identifying the specific cause. The oxyhemoglobin curve is shifted to the right (see Fig. 34.16), reducing Hb affinity for oxygen and impairing tissue oxygenation.

The underlying condition must be determined to establish effective treatment with a buffering solution. During severe acidosis (pH $\leq$ 7.1), base administration is required to elevate the pH to a safe level, particularly if there is oliguric renal disease. Accompanying sodium and water deficits must also be corrected.[28] Use of bicarbonate for alkali therapy for treatment of chronic metabolic acidosis can be controversial, and a new drug is currently under investigation as an alternative treatment option (Emerging Science Box: Veverimer for Treatment of Chronic Metabolic Acidosis).

Metabolic Alkalosis

Pathophysiology. Metabolic alkalosis occurs when bicarbonate concentration is increased, usually caused by excessive loss of metabolic acids or, less commonly, by large intake of bicarbonate or substances that are metabolized to bicarbonate. With alkalemia, hydrogen ions are redistributed from the intracellular to the extracellular space and potassium moves to the intracellular space to preserve electroneutrality.[29] When acid loss is caused by vomiting or gastric suctioning, renal compensation is not very effective because loss of chloride (an anion) in hydrochloric acid (HCl) stimulates renal retention of bicarbonate (an anion). The result is known as hypochloremic metabolic alkalosis (Fig. 3.17). Renal compensation is not very effective because the volume depletion and loss of electrolytes stimulate a paradoxical response by the kidneys. The kidneys increase bicarbonate reabsorption to maintain an anionic balance because the ECF chloride concentration is decreased. The resulting excretion of H^+ and reabsorption of bicarbonate prevent correction of the alkalosis.

Hyperaldosteronism also can lead to alkalosis as a result of sodium bicarbonate retention and loss of hydrogen and potassium. Diuretics may produce a mild alkalosis because they

EMERGING SCIENCE BOX

Veverimer for Treatment of Chronic Metabolic Acidosis

Metabolic acidosis is a common and difficult problem to manage among individuals with chronic kidney disease (CKD). As CKD progresses, there is saturation of the body's buffering capacity and net acid excretion decreases to less than net endogenous acid production, resulting in chronic metabolic acidosis. Chronic acidosis causes increased protein catabolism and muscle wasting; loss of bone mineral density and impaired growth in children with increased risk of renal osteodystrophy in adults; and stimulation of inflammation with progression of kidney injury and increased mortality. Daily administration of oral alkali products, such as sodium bicarbonate and sodium citrate, neutralizes endogenously produced and retained acids associated with CKD and maintains serum sodium bicarbonate levels within a normal range. A low-protein, fruit- and vegetable-enriched diet and supplementation with water-soluble vitamins has a similar effect. Both approaches can prevent or decrease the severity of metabolic acidosis in CKD. However, low-protein diets may lead to muscle wasting, and sodium bicarbonate supplements can increase total body carbon dioxide and sodium load with potential for an increased risk for edema, hypertension, and heart failure.

Veverimer is an investigational oral drug with a different approach to treating the chronic metabolic acidosis of CKD. Veverimer is nonabsorbed polymer that selectively binds hydrogen ions and chloride ions in the gastrointestinal tract and removes them in feces. Serum bicarbonate concentration increases and total body acid decreases without administering sodium. There is a presumed equivalent loss of endogenous chloride and therefore no fluid, sodium, or potassium losses with a decrease in serum anion gap. It is proposed that, in individuals with CKD and comorbidities such as peripheral edema, hypertension, cardiovascular disease, or heart failure, treatment with veverimer would be an effective alternative to sodium-based alkali therapies. Additional clinical trials are in progress to evaluate mechanism of action, safety profiles, interaction with colonic bacteria, and its use in other forms of chronic acidosis such as diabetic ketoacidosis. Application for approval by the US Food and Drug Administration is in progress.

Data from Adrogué HJ, et al. Veverimer: An emerging potential treatment option for managing the metabolic acidosis of CKD. *American Journal of Kidney Diseases.* 2020;76(6):861–867; Klaerner G, et al. Mechanism of action of veverimer: A novel, orally administered, nonabsorbed, counterion-free, hydrochloric acid binder under development for the treatment of metabolic acidosis in chronic kidney disease. *Journal of Pharmacology and Experimental Therapeutics.* 2020;375(3):439–450; Mannon EC, et al. Alkali supplementation as a therapeutic in chronic kidney disease: What mediates protection? American Journal of Physiology. *Renal Physiology.* 2020:319(6):F1090–F1104; Patschan D, et al. Chronic metabolic acidosis in chronic kidney disease. *Kidney and Blood Pressure Research.* 2020;45:812–822.

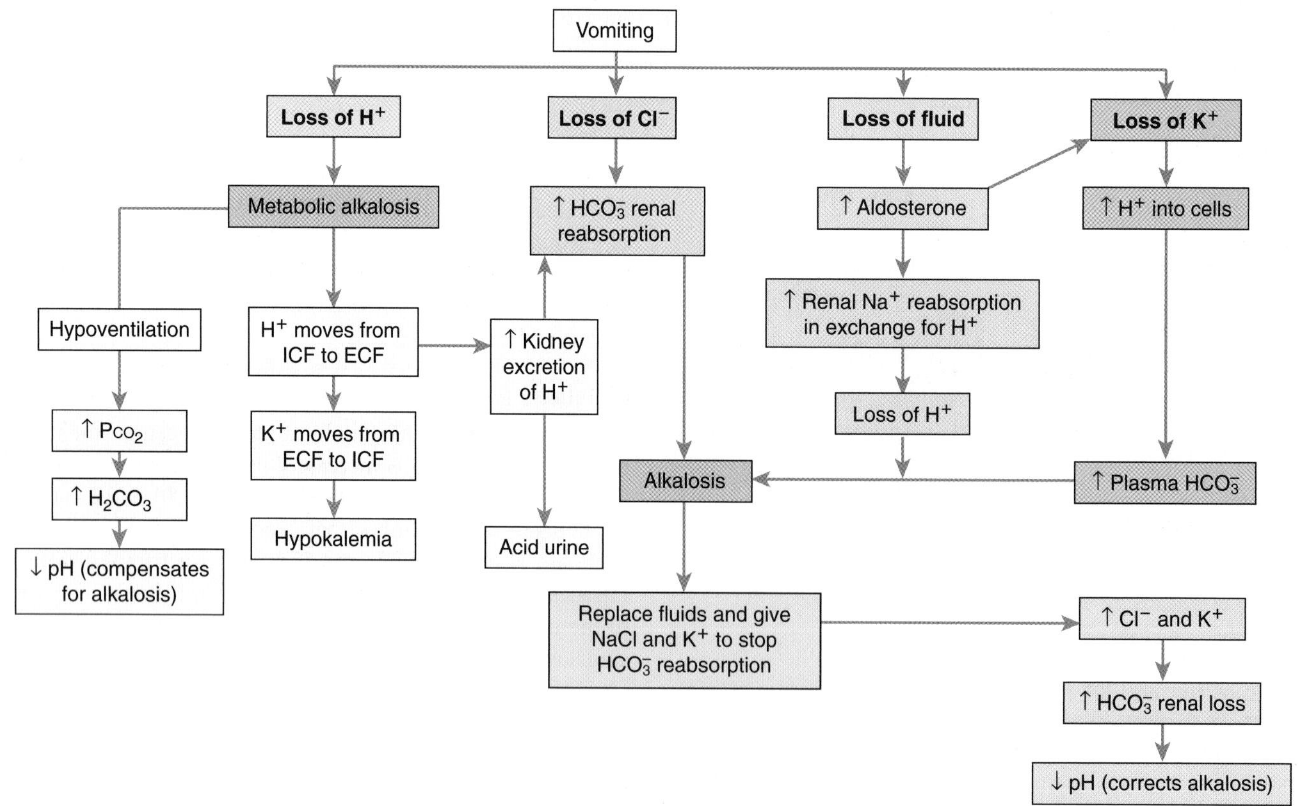

Fig. 3.17 Metabolic Alkalosis With Compensation and Correction. See text for abbreviations. (From Patton KT, Thibodeau, GA. *Anatomy & physiology*, 9th edition. St. Louis: Mosby; 2016.)

promote greater excretion of sodium, potassium, and chloride than of bicarbonate. Overuse of baking soda (sodium bicarbonate) as an antacid also can cause metabolic alkalosis, as can massive blood transfusions, which contain citrate that the liver metabolizes to bicarbonate.

Respiratory compensation for metabolic alkalosis occurs when the elevated pH inhibits the respiratory center. The rate and depth of ventilation are decreased, causing retention of carbon dioxide. The ratio of HCO_3^- concentration to H_2CO_3 concentration is reduced toward normal. Respiratory compensation

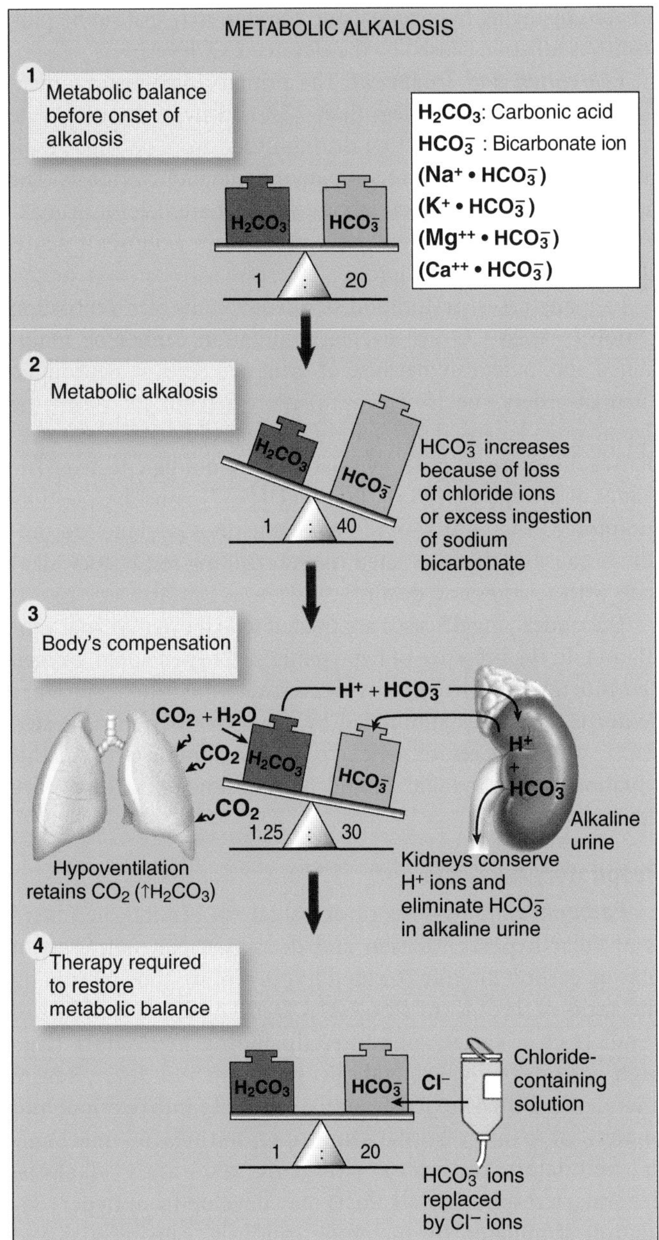

Fig. 3.18 Hypochloremic Metabolic Alkalosis. See text for abbreviations.

is not very efficient because the need for oxygen limits this compensation. Chronic or severe metabolic alkalosis requires therapeutic intervention (Fig. 3.18).

Clinical Manifestations. Because of the many causes of metabolic alkalosis, the symptoms vary. Some common symptoms, such as weakness, muscle cramps, and hyperactive reflexes, are related to volume depletion and electrolyte losses. Because alkalosis increases binding of Ca^{++} to plasma proteins (albumin), ionized calcium concentration decreases, causing excitable cells to become hypopolarized, which initiates an action potential more easily. Paresthesia (especially numbness/tingling of the fingertips and perioral area), tetany, and seizures may develop (see section on Hypocalcemia).

Respirations are slow and shallow to increase carbon dioxide retention. The oxyhemoglobin curve is shifted to the left, decreasing the dissociation of oxyhemoglobin, promoting hypoxemia, and increasing the risk of dysrhythmias (see Fig. 34.16). Atrial tachycardia is a potential problem.

Evaluation and Treatment. The health history provides significant clues to the diagnosis of metabolic alkalosis. The arterial pH is greater than 7.45, and bicarbonate levels exceed 26 mEq/L. With respiratory compensation, the $Paco_2$ increases to greater than 40 mm Hg. With hypochloremic metabolic alkalosis, serum chloride values are less than normal. Serum potassium levels are usually depleted because H^+ is released from the cells in exchange for potassium to help regulate the pH level. The potassium is then secreted from renal distal tubule cells into the urine.

With hypochloremic alkalosis or contraction alkalosis with volume depletion, a sodium chloride solution is required for *correction*. The renal stimulus to increase ECF volume by retaining Na^+ is diminished, and HCO_3^- can be excreted as $NaHCO_3$ in the urine. The administration of potassium corrects alkalosis caused by hyperaldosteronism or hypokalemia. The potassium causes H^+ to move back into the ECF and decreases loss of H^+ from the distal tubule.

Respiratory Acidosis

Pathophysiology. Respiratory acidosis occurs when there is alveolar hypoventilation resulting in hypercapnia (an excess of carbon dioxide in the blood). The arterial carbon dioxide pressure ($Paco_2$) is greater than 45 mm Hg and the pH is less than 7.35 (Fig. 3.19). Decreased alveolar ventilation, in relation to the metabolic production of carbon dioxide, produces an increased concentration of carbonic acid, which results in respiratory acidosis. The common causes include depression of the respiratory center (brainstem trauma, oversedation), paralysis of the respiratory muscles, disorders of the chest wall (kyphoscoliosis, obesity hypoventilation syndrome, flail chest), and disorders of the lung parenchyma (e.g., pneumonitis, pulmonary edema, and chronic obstructive lung disease).

Respiratory acidosis may be acute or chronic. Airway obstruction is the most common cause of acute respiratory acidosis (e.g., acute airway edema and bronchoconstriction from an acute asthma episode, or upper airway angioedema). Acute compensation for respiratory acidosis is not effective because the renal buffer mechanism takes time to function. Furthermore, the protein buffers provide marginal assistance, and HCO_3^- is not a good buffer for its conjugate acid (carbonic acid). Acute uncompensated respiratory acidosis is characterized by decreased arterial pH, elevated $Paco_2$, and normal or slightly increased bicarbonate concentration.

Chronic respiratory acidosis is commonly associated with chronic obstructive pulmonary disease and deformities of the chest wall or neuromuscular disorders. Renal compensation is effective and is established over several days. The acidosis produced from CO_2 retention stimulates the kidney to secrete H^+ ions and regenerate bicarbonate. Serum bicarbonate and $Paco_2$

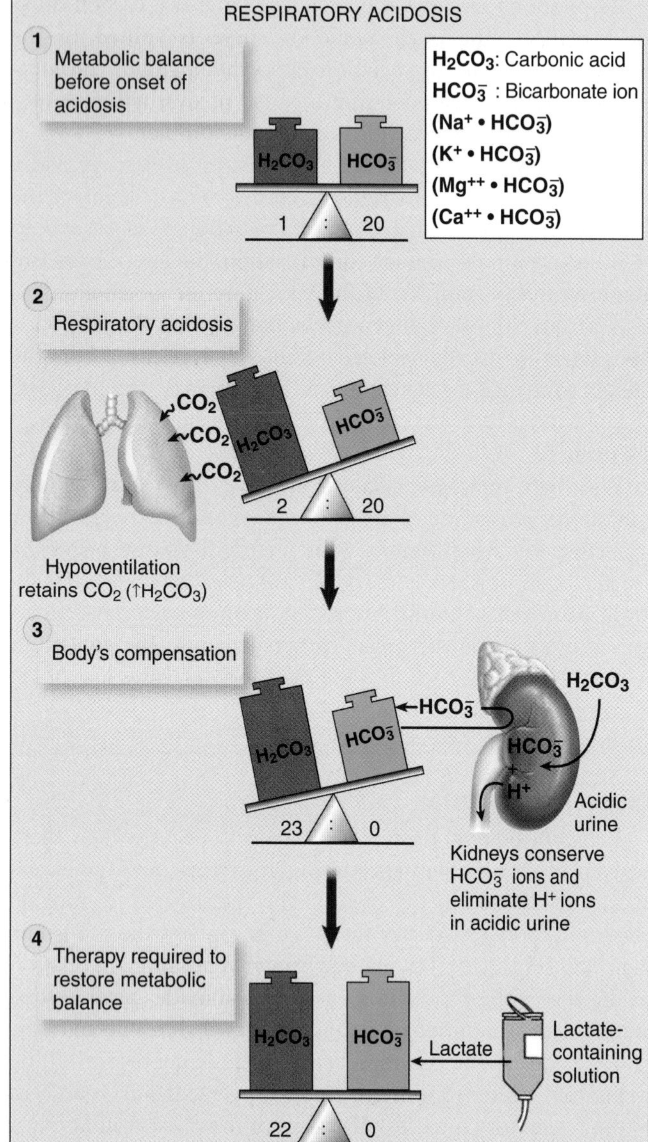

Fig. 3.19 Respiratory Acidosis With Compensation and Correction. See text for abbreviations. (From Patton KT, Thibodeau, GA. *Anatomy & physiology*, 9th edition. St. Louis: Mosby; 2016.)

levels are both elevated, and pH is restored toward normal (see Fig. 3.19).

Clinical Manifestations. The symptoms of respiratory acidosis are related to acuity of onset and severity of $Paco_2$ retention. Initial symptoms include headache, restlessness, blurred vision, and apprehension. Lethargy, muscle twitching, tremors, seizures, and coma may follow. Chronic acidosis causes myocardial depression, dysrhythmias, and hypotension. Neurologic symptoms are caused by a decrease in the pH of cerebrospinal fluid and cerebral vasodilation. CO_2 readily moves into vascular smooth muscle, causing both cerebral and peripheral vasodilation. The respiratory rate may be rapid at first and gradually becomes depressed, because over time, the respiratory center adapts to increasing levels of CO_2. Cyanosis does not occur unless there is an accompanying hypoxemia, and the skin may instead be pink from vasodilation caused by the elevated CO_2 level.

Evaluation and Treatment. The primary diagnostic indicators are an arterial pH less than 7.35 and hypercapnia. Acute respiratory acidosis must be distinguished from chronic respiratory acidosis and any accompanying metabolic acidosis. The health history and clinical laboratory data are helpful in making a determination whether the respiratory acidosis is acute, chronic, or acute on chronic.

In many cases, restoration of adequate alveolar ventilation removes excess CO_2. If alveolar ventilation cannot be maintained spontaneously because of drug overdose or neuromuscular disorders, mechanical ventilation is required. When the hypercapnia is caused by alterations in gas diffusion at the alveolar-capillary membrane, ventilation may not be effective. The values of arterial pH, Pco_2, Po_2, and HCO_3^- must be carefully monitored. The reduction of $Paco_2$ must not be done too rapidly because of the associated risks, including respiratory alkalosis with seizures and death.[30]

The underlying diseases are treated to achieve maximal ventilation. In the presence of hypoxemia and hypercapnia, oxygen can function as a respiratory depressant when the respiratory center is no longer stimulated by the lower pH and elevated $Paco_2$ value. Therefore, when oxygen is administered in this situation, the individual should be monitored for respiratory depression.

Respiratory Alkalosis

Pathophysiology. Respiratory alkalosis occurs when there is alveolar hyperventilation and decreased concentration of plasma carbon dioxide (termed hypocapnia), thus increasing the ratio of HCO_3^- to Pco_2 (H_2CO_3). Hyperventilation can result from a variety of causes, including hypoxemia (e.g., high altitudes); hypermetabolic states such as fever, severe anemia, and thyrotoxicosis; early salicylate intoxication; and anxiety or panic disorder. Improper settings on mechanical ventilators can cause iatrogenic respiratory alkalosis. Secondary respiratory alkalosis may develop from hyperventilation stimulated by metabolic acidosis, causing a mixed acid-base disorder.

The onset of acute respiratory alkalosis occurs within minutes of hyperventilation. Cellular buffers provide immediate response (i.e., protein and shifts of H^+ from ICF to ECF). The H^+ shifts are not very effective if the $Paco_2$ level is significantly decreased. Renal compensation occurs with chronic respiratory alkalosis and is characterized by decreased hydrogen excretion and decreased bicarbonate reabsorption (Fig. 3.20).

Clinical Manifestations. Respiratory alkalosis, like metabolic alkalosis, is irritating to the central and peripheral nervous systems. Symptoms include dizziness, confusion, tingling of extremities (paresthesias), seizures, and coma. Cerebral vasoconstriction reduces the cerebral blood flow. Carpopedal spasm and other symptoms of hypocalcemia are similar to those of metabolic alkalosis. Deep and rapid respirations (tachypnea) are primary symptoms of the disorders that cause respiratory alkalosis.

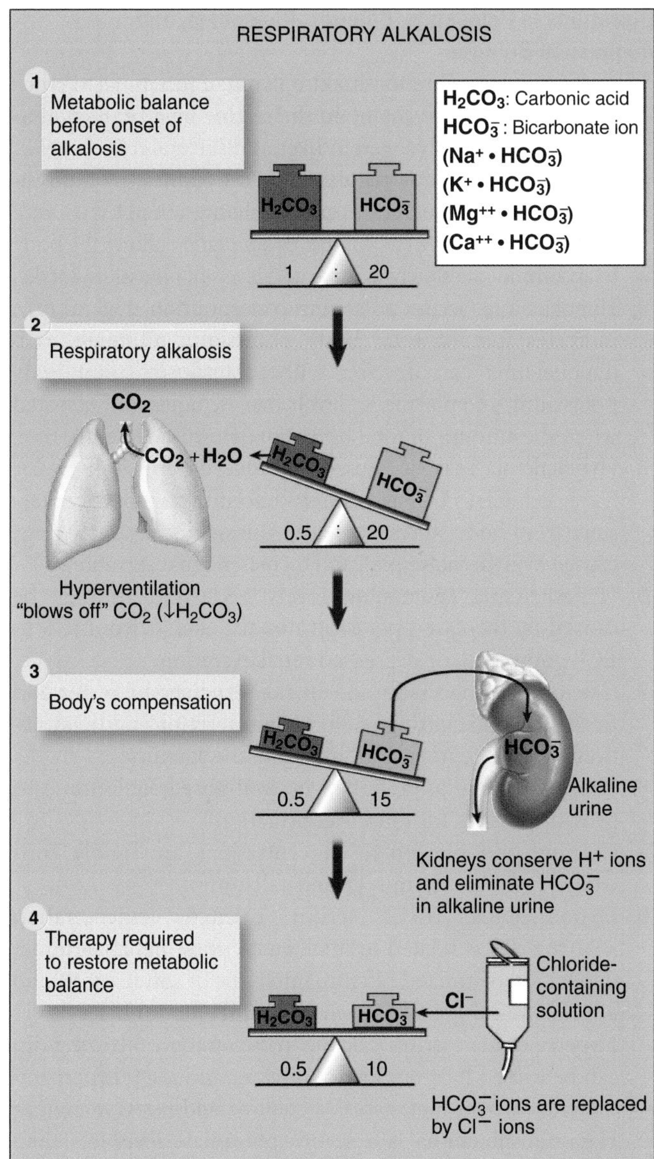

Fig. 3.20 Respiratory Alkalosis With Compensation and Correction. See text for abbreviations. (From Patton KT, Thibodeau, GA. *Anatomy & physiology*, 9th edition. St. Louis: Mosby; 2016.)

Evaluation and Treatment. The underlying disturbance must be identified. The arterial pH is greater than 7.45, and the $Pa{CO_2}$ is less than 38 mm Hg. In acute states, bicarbonate levels are normal. With chronic respiratory alkalosis, a compensatory decrease in the bicarbonate level occurs and the pH is closer to normal.

Treating the underlying disturbance is the most effective treatment. Hypoxemia must be corrected and hypermetabolic states reversed. Symptoms from hyperventilation caused by anxiety or acute pain can be corrected by managing the acute pain, anxiety-reducing conversation, assisting the individual to breathe more slowly while counting, or occasionally by rebreathing from a paper bag, which increases the concentration of inspired CO_2 and reverses the respiratory alkalosis. However, the use of paper bag rebreathing is associated with hypoxemia and can harm individuals with underlying cardiac and respiratory disorders. It may even worsen the situation if the hyperventilation is a compensatory response to a metabolic acidosis.

Mixed Acid-Base Disorders

Mixed acid-base disorders are two or more primary acid-base disorders occurring at the same time. They are more common in hospitalized individuals, often those in critical care with comorbid conditions (i.e., combined metabolic and respiratory disorders or combinations of acute and chronic disorders). For these individuals, the clinical history and analysis of electrolytes, medications, the anion gap, and the osmolality of plasma and urine are informative. The primary disorder is assessed, and then the degree of compensation is evaluated to determine if it is adequate, greater, or lesser than expected. Renal and respiratory compensation rarely returns the pH to normal. Therefore mixed acid-base disorders can have alterations in $Pa{CO_2}$ and/or bicarbonate and a normal pH. Examples of conditions with mixed acid-base disorders include individuals with chronic obstructive pulmonary disease who develop heart failure and are treated with high doses of diuretics, or individuals who have acute kidney injury and vomiting or severe hypoxia with extracellular volume depletion.[31,32]

SUMMARY REVIEW

Distribution of Body Fluids

1. Body fluids are distributed among functional compartments and are classified as ICF or ECF.
2. The sum of all fluids is the TBW, which varies with age and amount of body fat and is higher in infants because they have less body fat. With older age, the percent of TBW decreases as there is loss of muscle and an increase in body fat.
3. Water moves between the ICF and ECF compartments principally by osmosis.
4. Water moves between the plasma and interstitial fluid by osmosis and hydrostatic pressure, which occur across the capillary membrane.
5. Movement across the capillary wall is called *net filtration* and is described according to Starling forces (forces favoring filtration minus forces opposing filtration).

Alterations in Water Movement

1. Edema is the excessive accumulation of fluid within the interstitial spaces.
2. Edema is caused by venous or lymphatic obstruction or increased vascular volume (increases hydrostatic pressure), plasma protein losses, or increased capillary membrane permeability (decreases plasma oncotic pressure).

3. The pathophysiologic process that leads to edema is related to an increase in forces favoring fluid filtration from the capillaries into the tissues.
4. Edema may be localized or generalized and usually is associated with swelling and puffiness, tighter-fitting clothes and shoes, limited movement of the affected area, and, in severe cases, weight gain.
5. An effusion is fluid accumulation within a body cavity or space sometimes called a third space.

Sodium, Chloride, and Water Balance

1. Sodium accounts for 90% of the ECF cations.
2. Sodium balance and water balance are intimately related; chloride levels are generally proportional to changes in sodium levels.
3. Sodium balance is regulated by aldosterone, which increases reabsorption of sodium by the distal tubule of the kidney.
4. Renin and angiotensin are enzymes that promote or inhibit secretion of aldosterone and thus regulate sodium and water balance.
5. ANH is also involved in decreasing renal tubular resorption and promoting urinary excretion of sodium.
6. Water balance is regulated by the sensation of thirst and by the level of ADH, which is initiated by an increase in plasma osmolality or a decrease in circulating blood volume.

Alterations in Sodium, Water, and Chloride Balance

1. Alterations in water balance may be classified as isotonic, hypertonic, or hypotonic.
2. Isotonic alterations occur when changes in TBW are accompanied by proportional changes in concentrations of electrolytes.
3. Hypertonic alterations develop when the osmolality of the ECF is increased to greater than normal, usually because of an increased concentration of ECF sodium or a deficit of ECF water.
4. Hypernatremia occurs when ECF sodium levels exceed 145 mEq/L.
5. Hypernatremia can be hypovolemic, euvolemic, or hypervolemic, depending on the accompanying ECF water volume.
6. Hyperchloremia occurs when ECF chloride exceeds 105 mEq/L and often accompanies hypernatremia.
7. Hypotonic alterations occur when the osmolality of the ECF is less than normal.
8. Hyponatremia occurs when the serum sodium concentration decreases to less than 135 mEq/L and may be caused by inadequate intake of sodium or dilution of the body's sodium level.
9. Water excess is rare but can be caused by compulsive water drinking, decreased urine formation, or the syndrome of inappropriate secretion of ADH.
10. Hyponatremia usually causes movement of water into cells.
11. Hypochloremia is usually the result of hyponatremia or elevated bicarbonate concentrations.

Alterations in Potassium, Calcium, Phosphate, and Magnesium Balance

1. Potassium is the predominant ICF ion; it functions to regulate ICF osmolality, maintain the resting membrane potential, and deposit glycogen in liver and skeletal muscle cells.
2. Potassium balance is regulated by the kidney, by aldosterone and insulin secretion, and by changes in pH.
3. A mechanism known as *potassium adaptation* allows the body to accommodate slowly to increased levels of potassium intake.
4. Hypokalemia (serum potassium concentration <3.5 mEq/L) indicates loss of total body potassium, although ECF hypokalemia can develop without losses of total body potassium, and plasma K^+ levels may be normal or elevated when the amount of total body potassium is depleted.
5. Hypokalemia may be caused by reduced potassium intake, increased ICF to ECF potassium concentration, loss of potassium from body stores, increased aldosterone secretion (e.g., caused by hypernatremia), and increased renal excretion.
6. Hyperkalemia (potassium levels >5.0 mEq/L) may be caused by increased potassium intake, a shift from ICF to ECF potassium, or decreased renal excretion.
7. Calcium is a necessary ion in the structure of bones and teeth, in blood clotting, in hormone secretion and the function of cell receptors, and in membrane stability.
8. Phosphate acts as a buffer in acid-base regulation and provides energy for muscle contraction.
9. Calcium and phosphate concentrations are rigidly controlled by PTH, vitamin D, and calcitonin.
10. Hypocalcemia (total serum calcium concentration <9.0 mg/dL) is related to inadequate intestinal absorption, deposition of ionized calcium into bone or soft tissue, blood administration, or decreased PTH and vitamin D levels.
11. Hypercalcemia (serum calcium concentration >10.5 mg/dL) can be caused by a number of diseases, including hyperparathyroidism, bone metastases, sarcoidosis, and excess vitamin D.
12. Hypophosphatemia is a serum phosphate level less than 2.0 mg/dL and is usually caused by intestinal malabsorption and increased renal excretion of phosphate.
13. Hyperphosphatemia is a serum phosphate level more than 4.7 mg/dL and develops with acute or chronic renal failure with significant loss of glomerular filtration.
14. Magnesium is a major intracellular cation.
15. Magnesium functions in enzymatic reactions and often interacts with calcium at the cellular level.
16. Hypomagnesemia (serum magnesium concentrations <1.5 mEq/L) may be caused by malabsorption syndromes.
17. Hypermagnesemia (serum magnesium concentrations >3.0 mEq/L) is rare and is usually caused by renal failure.

Acid-Base Balance

1. Hydrogen ions, which maintain membrane integrity and the speed of enzymatic reactions, must be concentrated within a narrow range if the body is to function normally.
2. Hydrogen ion concentration is expressed as pH, which represents the negative logarithm of hydrogen ions in solution (e.g., a negative logarithm 10^{-7} mg/L is indicated on the pH

scale as pH 7.0, a neutral status). In arterial blood, the normal pH range is 7.35 to 7.45
3. Different body fluids have different pH values.
4. The renal and respiratory systems, together with the body's buffer systems, are the principal regulators of acid-base balance.
5. Buffers are substances that can absorb excessive acid or base to minimize fluctuations in pH.
6. The principal plasma buffers are bicarbonate, protein (Hb), and phosphate.
7. The lungs and kidneys act to compensate for changes in pH by increasing or decreasing ventilation (increasing or decreasing carbon dioxide in the form of carbonic acid) and by producing more acidic or more alkaline urine.
8. Correction is a process different from compensation; correction occurs when the values for both components of the buffer pair are returned to normal.
9. Acid-base imbalances are caused by changes in the concentration of H^+ in the blood; an increase causes acidosis, and a decrease causes alkalosis.
10. An abnormal increase or decrease in bicarbonate concentration causes metabolic acidosis or metabolic alkalosis; changes in the rate of alveolar ventilation produce respiratory acidosis or respiratory alkalosis.
11. Metabolic acidosis is caused by an increase in the concentrations of non–carbonic acids or by loss of bicarbonate from the ECF.
12. Metabolic alkalosis occurs with an increase in bicarbonate concentration usually caused by loss of metabolic acids from conditions such as vomiting, gastrointestinal suctioning, excessive bicarbonate intake, hyperaldosteronism, and diuretic therapy.
13. Respiratory acidosis occurs with a decrease of alveolar ventilation and an increase in levels of carbon dioxide, or hypercapnia.
14. Respiratory alkalosis occurs with alveolar hyperventilation and excessive reduction of carbon dioxide concentration, or hypocapnia.

REFERENCES

1. Magouliotis DE, et al. Aquaporins in health and disease. *Adv Clin Chem*. 2020;98:149–171.
2. Zhang X, et al. Protein-losing enteropathy as a complication of spontaneous isolated superior mesenteric artery dissection: a case report. *Medicine (Baltimore)*. 2020;99(25):e20580.
3. Manrique OJ, et al: Overview of lymphedema for physicians and other clinicians: a review of fundamental concepts, *Mayo Clin Proc*. Published online August 20, 2020. Available at: https://doi.org/10.1016/j.mayocp.2020.01.006. Accessed 09.07.21.
4. Seay NW, Lehrich RW, Greenberg A. Diagnosis and management of disorders of body tonicity-hyponatremia and hypernatremia: core curriculum 2020. *Am J Kidney Dis*. 2020;75(2):272–286.
5. McDonough AA, Youn JH. Potassium homeostasis: the knowns, the unknowns, and the health benefits. *Physiology (Bethesda)*. 2017;32(2):100–111.
6. Gankam Kengne F, Decaux G. Hyponatremia and the brain. *Kidney Int Rep*. 2017;3(1):24–35.
7. Elliott TL. Electrolytes: potassium disorders. *FP Essent*. 2017;459:21–28.
8. Palmer BF. Regulation of potassium homeostasis. *Clin J Am Soc Nephrol*. 2015;10(6):1050–1060.
9. Youn JH. Gut sensing of potassium intake and its role in potassium homeostasis. *Semin Nephrol*. 2013;33(3):248–256.
10. Zacchia M, et al. Potassium: from physiology to clinical implications. *Kidney Dis (Basel)*. 2016;2(2):72–79.
11. Hansen BA, Bruserud Ø. Hypomagnesemia in critically ill patients. *J Intensive Care*. 2018;6:21.
11a. Hunter RW, Bailey MA. Hyperkalemia: pathophysiology, risk factors and consequences. *Nephrol Dial Transplant*. 2019 Dec 1;34(Suppl 3):iii2–iii11.
12. Sharma S, Hashimi MF, Aggarwal S. Hyperchloremic acidosis. *StatPearls* [Internet]. Treasure Island, FL: StatPearls Publishing; 2021. Updated May 7, 2021. Available at: http://www.ncbi.nlm.nih.gov/books/NBK482340/. Accessed 09.07.21.
13. Palmer BF, et al. Clinical management of hyperkalemia. *Mayo Clin Proc*. 2021;96(3):744–762.
14. Tinawi M. Disorders of calcium metabolism: hypocalcemia and hypercalcemia. *Cureus*. 2021;13(1):e12420.
15. Goldner W. Cancer-related hypercalcemia. *J Oncol Pract*. 2016;12(5):426–432.
16. Bellos I, Frountzas M, Pergialiotis V. Comparative risk of hypophosphatemia following the administration of intravenous iron formulations: a network meta-analysis. *Transfus Med Rev*. 2020;34(3):188–194.
17. Florenzano P, et al. Approach to patients with hypophosphataemia. *Lancet Diabetes Endocrinol*. 2020;8(2):163–174.
18. Carfagna F, et al. Current and potential treatment options for hyperphosphatemia. *Expert Opin Drug Saf*. 2018;17(6):597–607.
19. Ganz T, Bino A, Salusky IB. Mechanism of action and clinical attributes of Auryxia® (ferric citrate). *Drugs*. 2019;79(9):957–968.
20. Ter Braake AD, et al. Calciprotein particle inhibition explains magnesium-mediated protection against vascular calcification. *Nephrol Dial Transplant*. 2020;35(5):765–773.
21. Barbagallo M, Veronese N, Dominguez LJ. Magnesium in aging, health and diseases. *Nutrients*. 2021;13(2):463.
22. Liu M, Dudley SC Jr. Magnesium, oxidative stress, inflammation, and cardiovascular disease. *Antioxidants (Basel)*. 2020;9(10):907.
23. Urits I, et al. Pharmacological options for the treatment of chronic migraine pain. *Best Pract Res Clin Anaesthesiol*. 2020;34(3):383–407.
24. Chang WT, Radin B, McCurdy MT. Calcium, magnesium, and phosphate abnormalities in the emergency department. *Emerg Med Clin North Am*. 2014;32(2):349–366.
25. Quade BN, Parker MD, Occhipinti R. The therapeutic importance of acid-base balance. *Biochem Pharmacol*. 2021;183:114278.
26. Pompey J, Abraham-Settles B. Clarifying the confusion of arterial blood gas analysis: is it compensation or combination? *Am J Nurs*. 2019;119(3):52–56.
27. Matyukhin I, et al. Etiology and management of acute metabolic acidosis: an update. *Kidney Blood Press Res*. 2020;45(4):523–531.
28. Dhondup T, Qian Q. Acid-base and electrolyte disorders in patients with and without chronic kidney disease: an update. *Kidney Dis (Basel)*. 2017;3(4):136–148.
29. Emmett M. Metabolic alkalosis: a brief pathophysiologic review. *Clin J Am Soc Nephrol*. 2020;15(12):1848–1856.
30. Adrogué HJ, Madias NE. Alkali therapy for respiratory acidosis: a medical controversy. *Am J Kidney Dis*. 2020;75(2):265–271.
31. Weyker PD, Pérez XL, Liu KD. Management of acute kidney injury and acid-base balance in the septic patient. *Clin Chest Med*. 2016;37(2):277–288.
32. Bruno CM, Valenti M. Acid-base disorders in patients with chronic obstructive pulmonary disease: a pathophysiological review. *J Biomed Biotechnol*. 2012;2012:915150.

4

Genes and Genetic Diseases

Lynn B. Jorde

http://evolve.elsevier.com/Rogers/pathophysiology/

CHAPTER OUTLINE

Genetics is the study of biologic inheritance. An understanding of genetics is essential to study human, animal, plant, or microbial life. In the 19th century, microscopic studies of cells led scientists to suspect the nucleus of the cell contained the important mechanisms of inheritance. Scientists found chromatin, the substance giving the nucleus a granular appearance, which is observable in nondividing cells. Just before the cell divides, the chromatin condenses to form discrete, dark-staining organelles, which are called chromosomes. (Cell division is discussed in Chapter 1.) With the rediscovery of Mendel's important breeding experiments at the turn of the 20th century, it soon became apparent the chromosomes contained genes, the basic units of inheritance (Fig. 4.1).

The primary constituent of chromatin is deoxyribonucleic acid (DNA). Genes are composed of sequences of DNA. By serving as the blueprints of proteins in the body, genes ultimately influence all aspects of body structure and function. Humans have approximately 20,000 protein-coding genes and at least an additional 9000 to 10,000 genes that encode various types of ribonucleic acid (RNA; see below) that are not translated into proteins. An error in one of these genes often leads to a recognizable genetic disease.

To date, more than 20,000 genetic traits and diseases have been identified and cataloged. As infectious diseases continue to be more effectively controlled, the proportion of beds in pediatric hospitals occupied by children with genetic diseases has risen. In addition to genetic diseases in children, there are many common diseases that primarily affect adults and are now known to have important genetic components, such as hypertension, coronary heart disease, diabetes, and cancer.

Great progress continues to be made in the diagnosis of genetic diseases and in the understanding of genetic mechanisms underlying them. With the huge strides being made in molecular genetics, "gene therapy"—the utilization of normal genes to correct genetic disease—has begun (Fig. 4.2).[1,2]

DNA, RNA, AND PROTEINS: HEREDITY AT THE MOLECULAR LEVEL

Definitions

Composition and Structure of DNA

Genes are composed of DNA, which has three basic components: the five-carbon monosaccharide deoxyribose; a phosphate molecule; and four types of nitrogenous bases. Two of the bases, cytosine and thymine, are single carbon-nitrogen rings called pyrimidines. The other two bases, adenine and guanine, are double carbon-nitrogen rings called purines. The four bases are commonly represented by their first letters: A (adenine), C (cytosine), T (thymine), and G (guanine).

Watson and Crick demonstrated how these molecules are physically assembled as DNA, proposing the double-helix model in which DNA appears like a twisted ladder with chemical bonds as its rungs (Fig. 4.3). The two sides of the ladder consist of deoxyribose and phosphate molecules, united by strong phosphodiester bonds. Projecting from each side of the ladder, at regular intervals, are the nitrogenous bases. The base projecting from one side is bound to the base projecting from

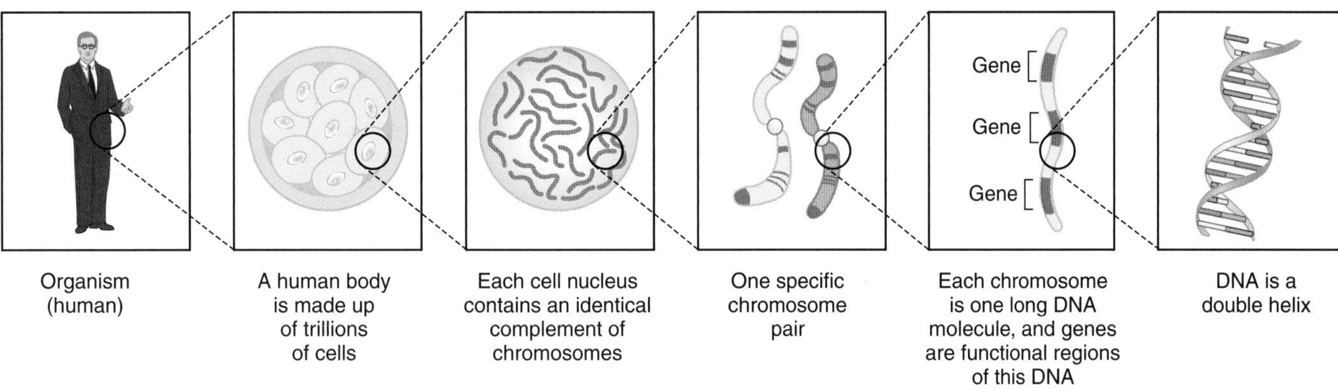

Fig. 4.1 Successive Enlargements from a Human to the Genetic Material.

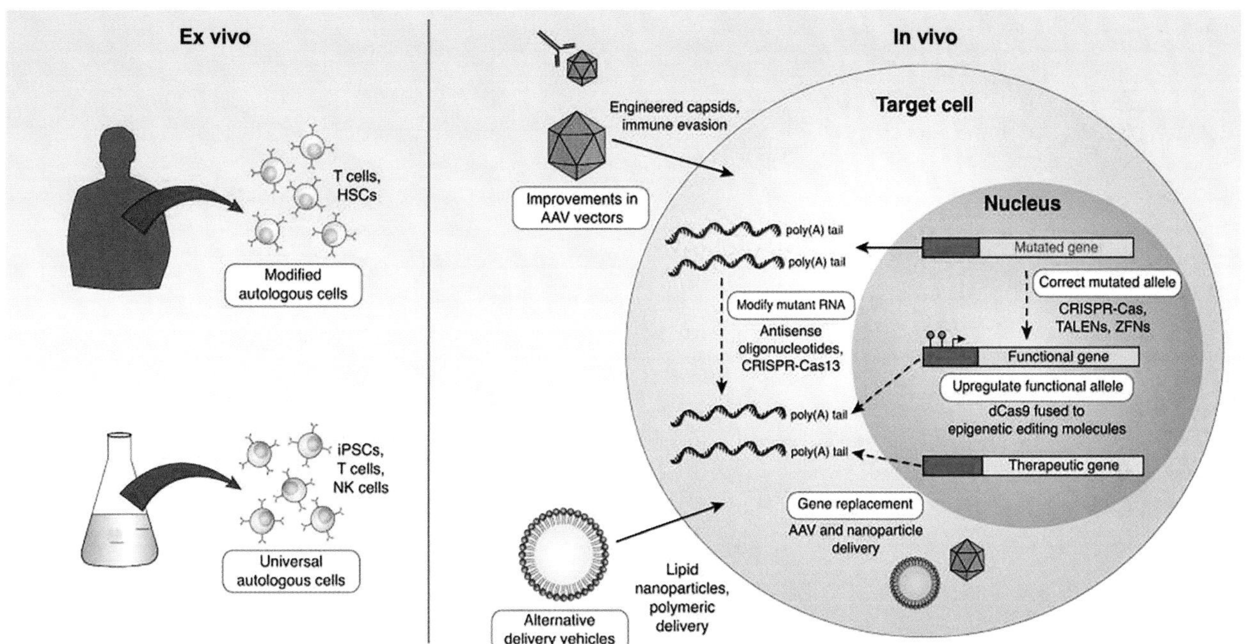

Fig. 4.2 Gene Therapy. Schematic of ex vivo and in vivo gene therapy strategies *(colored blue)* for treating genetic diseases. Ex vivo methods *(left panel)*, autologous cells can be isolated from the person directly and genetically modified to cause a therapeutic effect, Allogenic cells can be produced and readily available "off the shelf". In vivo strategies require targeting of specific cells to achieve a therapeutic gene or correct pathological mechanisms to enable functional gene expression *(dashed arrows)*. (From Bulaklak K, Gersbach CA. The once and future gene therapy. *Nature Communications*, 2020;11(1). doi:10.1038/s41467-020-19505-2.)

the other by a weak hydrogen bond. Therefore, the nitrogenous bases form the rungs of the ladder; adenine pairs with thymine, and guanine pairs with cytosine. Each DNA subunit—consisting of one deoxyribose molecule, one phosphate group, and one base—is called a nucleotide.

DNA as the Genetic Code

DNA directs the synthesis of all the body's proteins. Proteins are composed of one or more polypeptides (intermediate protein compounds), which in turn consist of sequences of amino acids. The body contains 20 different types of amino acids; they are specified by the 4 nitrogenous bases. To specify (code for) 20 different amino acids with only 4 bases, different combinations of bases, occurring in groups of 3 (triplets), are used. These triplets of bases are known as codons. Each codon specifies a single amino acid in a corresponding protein. Because there are 64 (4 times 4 times 4) possible codons but only 20 amino acids, there are many cases in which several codons correspond to the same amino acid.

The genetic code is universal: with a few rare exceptions, all living organisms use precisely the same DNA codes to specify proteins. A notable exception is mitochondria, the cytoplasmic organelles in which cellular respiration takes place (see Chapter 1)—they have their own extranuclear DNA. Several codons of DNA encode different amino acids, compared with the same nuclear DNA codons.

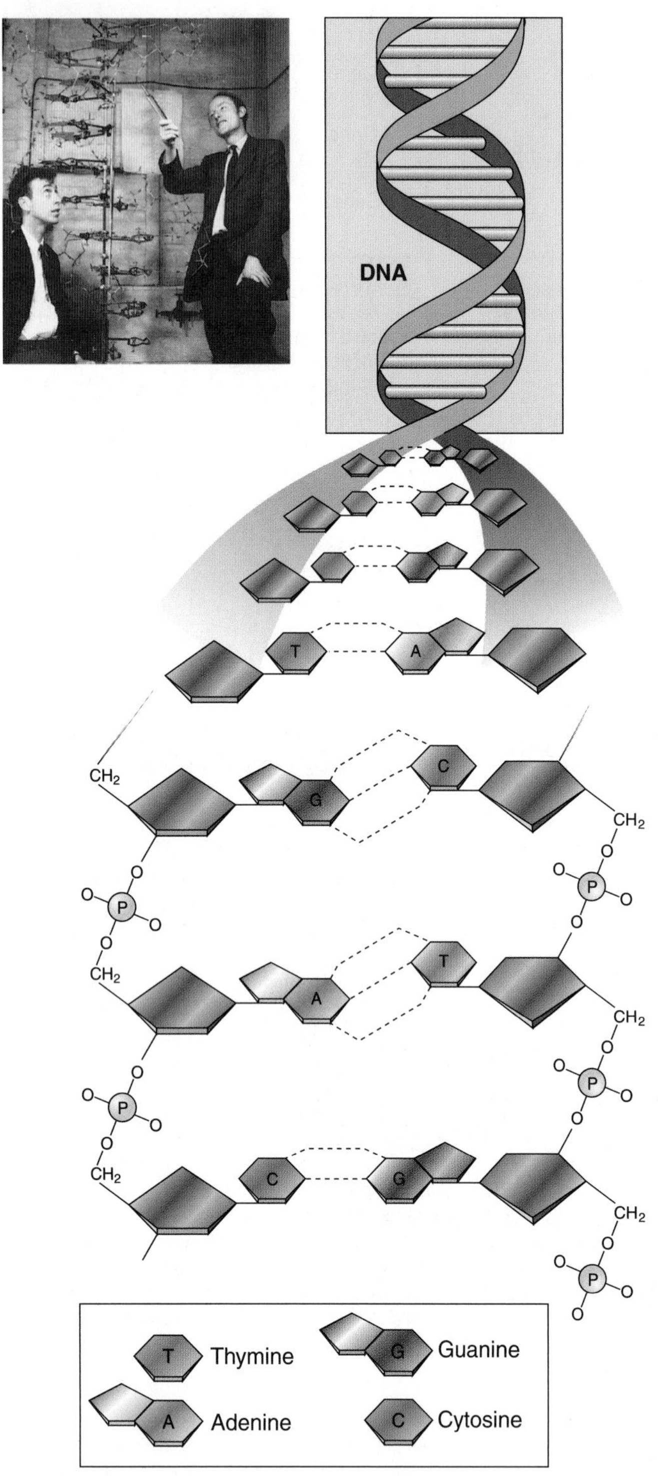

Fig. 4.3 Watson-Crick Model of the DNA Molecule. The DNA structure illustrated here is based on that published by James Watson *(photograph, left)* and Francis Crick *(photograph, right)* in 1953. Note that each side of the DNA molecule consists of alternating sugar and phosphate groups. Each sugar group is bonded to the opposing sugar group by a pair of nitrogenous bases (adenine–thymine or cytosine–guanine). The sequence of these pairs constitutes a genetic code that determines the structure and function of a cell. (Illustration from Herlihy B. *The human body in health and illness*, 5th edition. St. Louis: Saunders; 2015.)

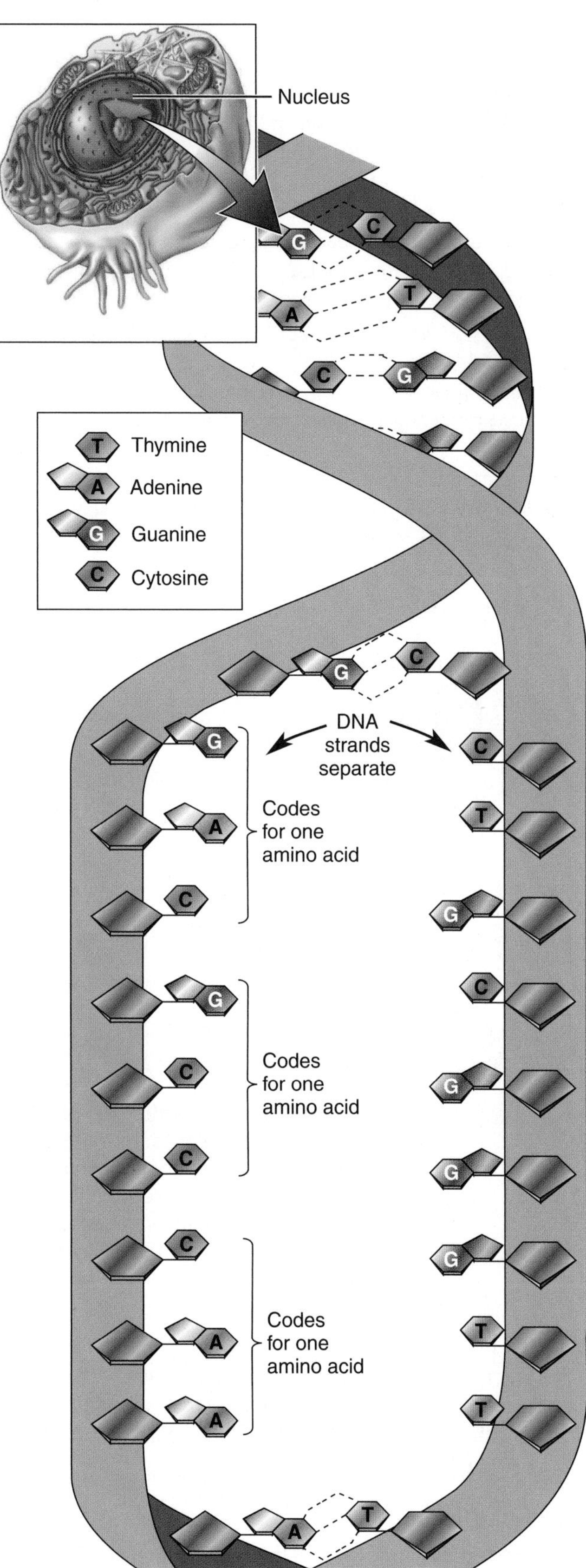

Fig. 4.4 Replication of DNA. The two chains of the double helix separate and each chain serves as the template for a new complementary chain. (From Herlihy B. *The human body in health and illness*, 5th edition. St. Louis: Saunders; 2015.)

Replication of DNA

DNA replication consists of breaking the weak hydrogen bonds between the bases, leaving a single strand with each base unpaired (Fig. 4.4). The consistent pairing of adenine with thymine and of guanine with cytosine, known as complementary base pairing, is the key to accurate replication. The unpaired base attracts a free nucleotide only if the nucleotide has the proper complementary base. When replication is complete, a new double-stranded molecule identical to the original is formed. The single strand is said to be a template, or molecule on which a complementary molecule is built, and is the basis for synthesizing the new double strand.

Several different proteins are involved in DNA replication. The most important of these proteins is an enzyme known as DNA polymerase. This enzyme travels along the single DNA strand, adding the correct nucleotides to the free end of the new strand and checking to ensure that its base is complementary to the template base. This mechanism of DNA proofreading substantially enhances the accuracy of DNA replication (Fig. 4.5).

Mutation

A mutation is any alteration of genetic material. One type of mutation is the base pair substitution, in which one base pair replaces another. This replacement *can* result in a change in the amino acid sequence. However, because of the redundancy of the genetic code, many of these mutations do not change the amino acid sequence and, thus, have no consequence. Such mutations are called silent mutations. Base pair substitutions altering amino acids consist of two basic types: missense mutations, which produce a change (i.e., the "sense") in a single amino acid; and nonsense mutations, which produce one of the three stop codons (UAA, UAG, or UGA; where U is uracil; A is adenine; and G is guanine) in the messenger RNA (mRNA) (Fig. 4.6). Missense mutations (see Fig. 4.6A) produce a single amino acid change, whereas nonsense mutations (see Fig. 4.6B) produce a premature stop codon in the mRNA. Stop codons terminate translation of the polypeptide.

The frameshift mutation involves the insertion or deletion of one or more base pairs of the DNA molecule. As Fig. 4.6C shows, these mutations change the entire "reading frame" of the DNA sequence because the deletion or insertion is not a multiple of three base pairs (the number of base pairs in a codon). Frameshift mutations can thus greatly alter the amino acid sequence and typically cause a premature stop codon. (*In-frame* insertions or deletions, in which a multiple of three bases is inserted or lost, tend to have less severe disease consequences than do frameshift mutations.) Individuals that have non-sense, frame-shift mutations, missense mutations, or gene duplications

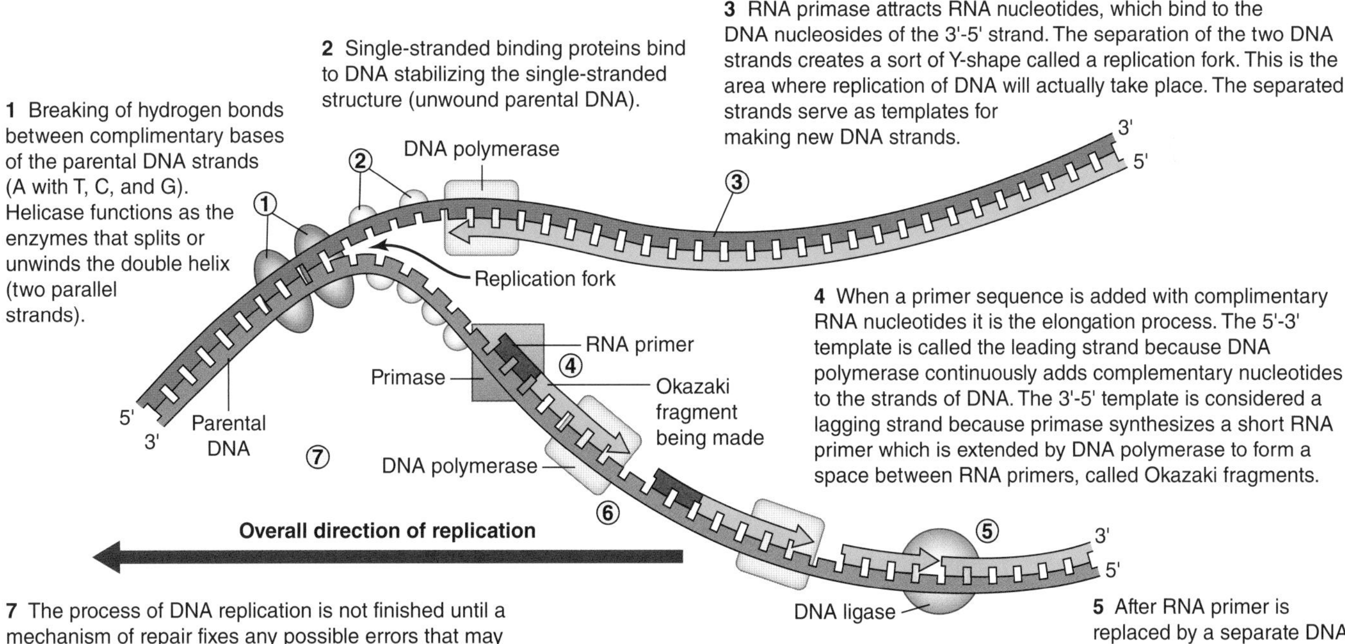

Fig. 4.5 Process of DNA Replication. The hydrogen bonds between the two original strands are broken, allowing the bases in each strand to undergo complementary base pairing with free bases. The process proceeds in the 5′ to 3′ direction on each strand forming two new double strands of DNA.

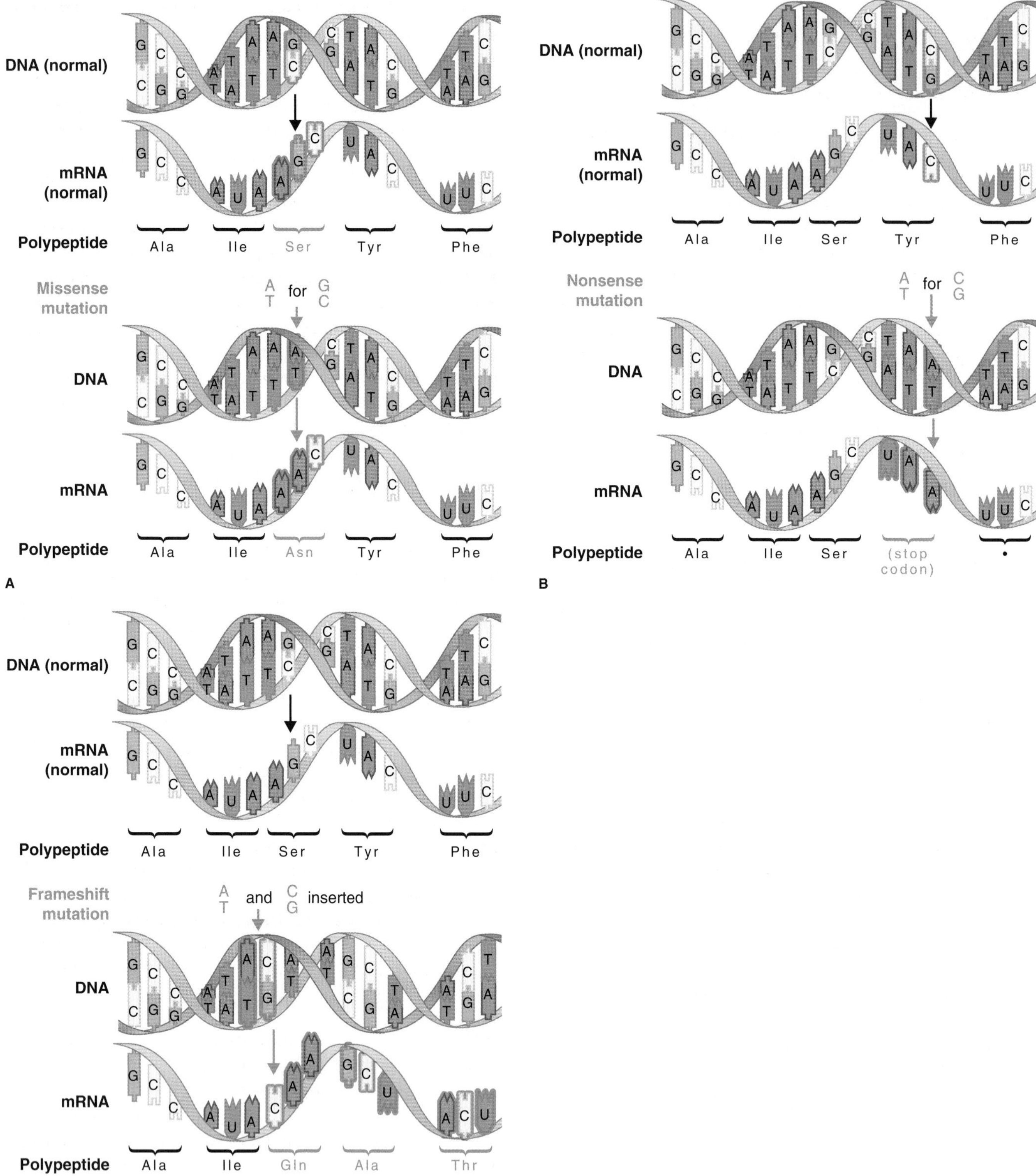

Fig. 4.6 Base Pair Substitution. Missense mutations **(A)** produce a single amino acid change, whereas nonsense mutations **(B)** produce a stop codon in the messenger ribonucleic acid *(mRNA)*. Stop codons terminate translation of the polypeptide. **(C)** Frameshift Mutations. Frameshift mutations result from the addition or deletion of a number of bases that is not a multiple of 3. This mutation alters all of the codons downstream from the site of insertion or deletion. (B and C, From Jorde LB, Carey JC. *Medical genetics*, 4th edition. St. Louis: Mosby; 2010.)

EMERGING SCIENCE BOX

Predictions of Individual Response to Pharmacotherapies Based on Genotype-Phenotype Correlations

Providing individualized pharmacological treatment for disease has been a long-time goal in healthcare, however, this becomes challenging due to the complexity and multivariate genetic components involved. Cytochrome P450 CYP2D6 is the most widely studied polymorphic drug-metabolizing enzyme. The gene encoding the CYP2D6 enzyme is located on chromosome 22. This gene displays a large genetic diversity among human population, including non-sense, frame-shift, and missense mutations and gene duplications. CYP2D6 genetic variation influences the metabolism of numerous drugs, and this marked inter-individual variation in activity can have significant clinical consequences affecting drug efficacy and safety. Individuals with a deficiency of the CYP2D6 enzyme, usually inherited as an autosomal recessive trait, have a decreased ability to metabolize certain drugs (e.g., antidepressants, neuroleptics, some antiarrhythmics, lipophilic β-adrenoceptor blockers, and opioids). However, CYP2D6 activity can range from complete absence to increased activity. The clinical importance of the polymorphism depends on whether the parent compound, metabolite(s), or both are metabolized or formed by CYP2D6, whether one or both are active, and if so, the potency of the active species, as well as the overall contribution of the CYP2D6-dependent pathway to the clearance of the drug. Increased understanding of the mechanisms underlying genotype–phenotype correlations associated with the genetic variability of the CYP2D6 will improve knowledge acquisition on the metabolizing function of CYP2D6. The research conducted on CYP2D6 could provide accurate predictions and implications for individual responses to pharmacological treatments.

Data from Pey AL. Towards accurate genotype-phenotype correlations in the CYP2D6 gene. *Journal of Personalized Medicine*, 2020;10(4):158. doi:10.3390/jpm10040158. PMID: 33049937. PMCID: PMC7711719; Nofziger C, Turner AJ, Sangkuhl K, et al. PharmVar GeneFocus: CYP2D6. *Clinical Pharmacology and Therapeutics*, 2020;107(1):154–170. doi:10.1002/cpt.1643.

may have the complete inability or have an increased ability to metabolize certain drugs (Emerging Science Box: Predictions of Individual Response to Pharmacotherapies Based on Genotype-Phenotype Correlations).

Agents known as mutagens increase the frequency of mutations. Examples include radiation and chemicals, such as nitrogen mustard, vinyl chloride, alkylating agents, formaldehyde, and sodium nitrite. Mutations are rare events. The rate of spontaneous mutations (those occurring in the absence of exposure to known mutagens) in humans is about 10–4 to 10–7 per gene per generation. This rate varies from one gene to another. Some DNA sequences have particularly high mutation rates and are known as mutational hot spots.

From Genes to Proteins

DNA is formed and replicated in the cell nucleus, but protein synthesis takes place in the cytoplasm. The DNA code is transported from nucleus to cytoplasm, and subsequent protein is formed through two basic processes: transcription and translation. These processes are mediated by RNA, which is chemically similar to DNA except the sugar molecule is ribose rather than deoxyribose, and uracil rather than thymine is one of the four bases. The other bases of RNA, as in DNA, are adenine, cytosine, and guanine. Uracil is structurally similar to thymine, so it also can pair with adenine. DNA usually occurs as a double strand, whereas RNA usually occurs as a single strand.

Transcription

Transcription is the process by which RNA is synthesized from a DNA template. Key steps of gene transcription are shown in Fig. 4.7.[3] The result is the formation of mRNA from the base sequence specified by the DNA molecule. Transcription of a gene begins when an enzyme called RNA polymerase binds to a promoter site on the DNA. A promoter site is a sequence of DNA that specifies the beginning of a gene. In addition to RNA polymerase, proteins called transcription factors are involved in the process of converting, or transcribing, DNA into RNA (Fig. 4.8). Transcription factors initiate and regulate the transcription of genes; they are the master regulators of gene expression.[4] The action of transcription factors enables unique expression of each gene in different cell types and during development. Transcription factors bind to DNA sequences called transcription factor binding sites near genes to regulate gene expression via transcription. Transcription factors have DNA-binding domains that give them the ability to bind to specific sequences of DNA called *enhancer* or *promote*r sequences. Certain transcription factors bind to a DNA promoter sequence near the transcription start site and help form the *transcription initiation complex*. Other transcription factors bind to regulatory sequences, such as enhancer sequences, and can either stimulate or repress transcription of the related gene. Regulation of transcription is the most common form of gene control.

Predictive models for 94 human transcription factors demonstrate their utility in genome-wide association studies.[5] Advances in fluorescence microscopy have made it possible to visualize real-time transcription factor dynamics.[6]

The sequence of bases in the mRNA is thus complementary to the template strand, and except for the presence of uracil instead of thymine, the mRNA sequence is identical to that of the other DNA strand. Transcription continues until a termination sequence—codons that act as signals for the termination of protein synthesis—is reached. Then the RNA polymerase detaches from the DNA, and the transcribed mRNA is freed to move out of the nucleus and into the cytoplasm (see Figs. 4.7 and 4.8).

Gene Splicing

When the mRNA is first transcribed from the DNA template, it reflects exactly the base sequence of the DNA. In eukaryotes, many RNA sequences are removed by nuclear enzymes, and the remaining sequences are spliced together to form the functional mRNA that migrates to the cytoplasm. The excised sequences are called introns (intervening sequences), and the sequences that are left to code for proteins are called exons.

Translation

In translation, RNA directs the synthesis of a polypeptide (Fig. 4.9), interacting with transfer RNA (tRNA), a cloverleaf-shaped strand of about 80 nucleotides. The tRNA molecule has a site where an amino acid attaches. The three-nucleotide sequence at the opposite side of the cloverleaf is called the anticodon. It undergoes complementary base pairing

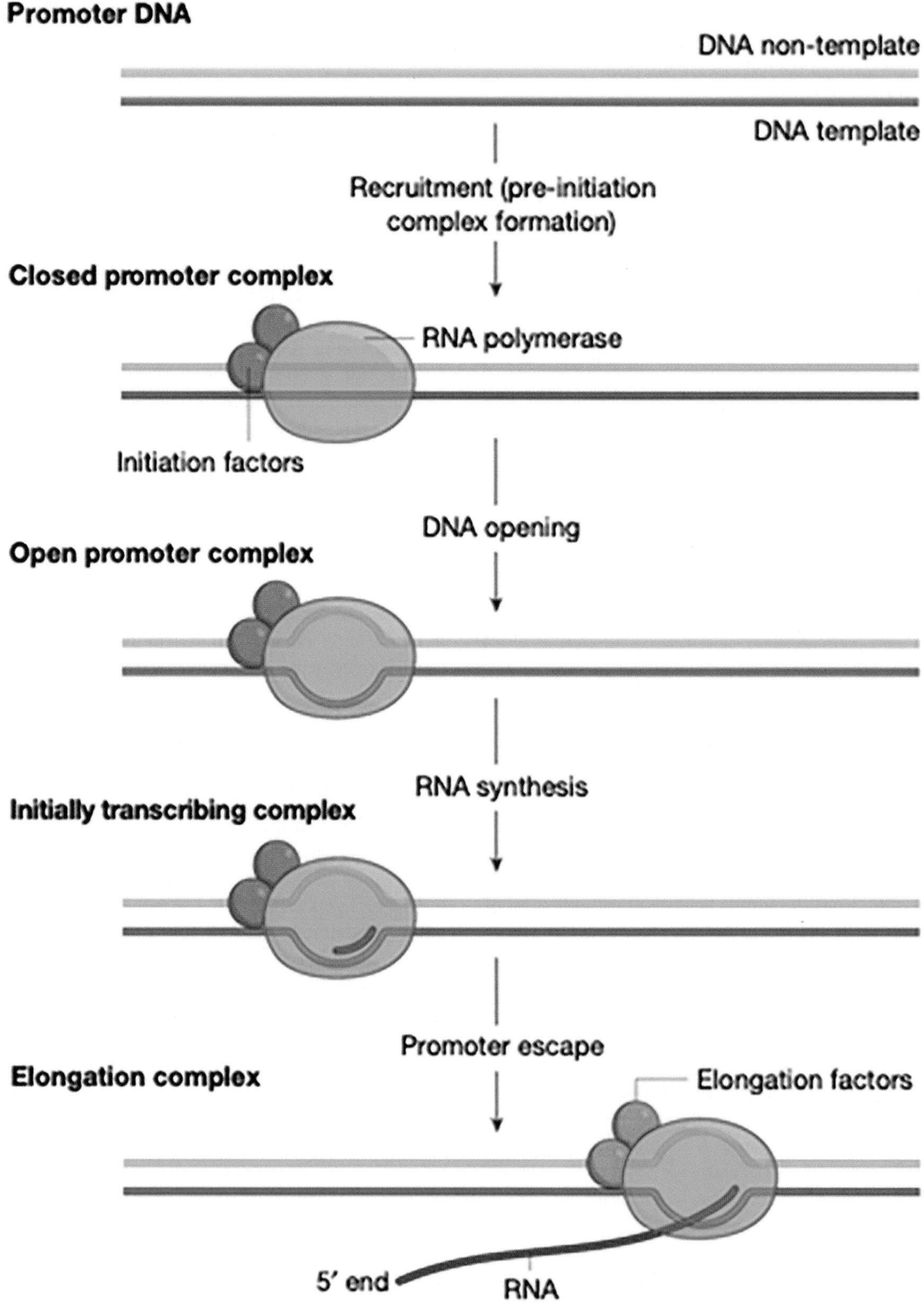

Fig. 4.7 Key Steps of Gene Transcription. The RNA polymerase enzyme associates with transcription initiation factors to recognize promoter DNA and form a pre-initiation complex (PIC). Later DNA opening converts the closed promoter complex to the open promoter complex, which contains the DNA template strand in the polymerase active site. DNA-dependent RNA synthesis subsequently generates an initially transcribing complex. When RNA grows to a certain critical length, the polymerase escapes from the promoter and forms an elongation complex that can bind elongation factors. Eventually, polymerase dissociation from DNA and RNA terminates the transcription cycle (not shown). (From Cramer P. Organization and regulation of gene transcription. *Nature*, 2019;573(7772):45–54. doi:10.1038/s41586-019-1517-4.)

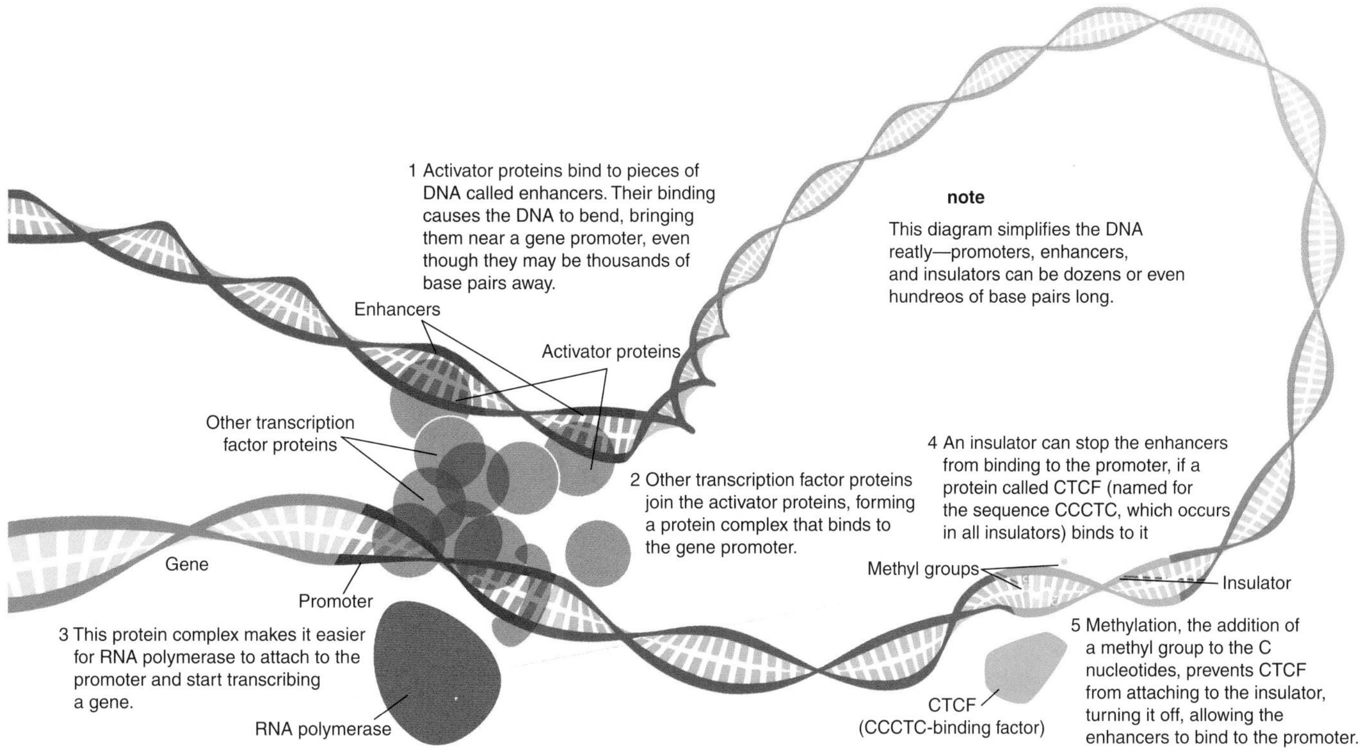

Fig. 4.8 Transcription Factors and Simplified Schematic of Gene Expression. Transcription factors are proteins and bind to specific sites on DNA. They read and interpret the genetic blueprint of the DNA, thereby controlling transcription or the flow of genetic information from DNA to mRNA. Transcription factors are essential for gene expression (e.g., proteins that function as receptors, enzymes, or biomarkers). Not only do transcription factors act downstream from biological stimuli but they can be downstream of signaling cascades promoted by various environmental stimuli (hormones, temperature). Transcription factors can alter gene expression to promote pathophysiology. (From Song K. *Transcription Factors*. Wikimedia Commons; 2012. https://commons.wikimedia.org/wiki/File:Transcription_Factors.svg.)

with an appropriate codon in the mRNA, which specifies the sequence of amino acids through tRNA.

The site of actual protein synthesis is in the ribosome, which consists of approximately equal parts of protein and ribosomal RNA (rRNA). During translation, the ribosome first binds to an initiation site on the mRNA sequence and then binds to its surface so that base pairing can occur between tRNA and mRNA. The ribosome then moves along the mRNA sequence, processing each codon and translating an amino acid by way of the interaction of mRNA and tRNA.

The ribosome provides an enzyme that catalyzes the formation of covalent peptide bonds between the adjacent amino acids, resulting in a growing polypeptide. When the ribosome arrives at a termination signal on the mRNA sequence, translation and polypeptide formation cease; the mRNA, ribosome, and polypeptide separate from one another; and the polypeptide is released into the cytoplasm to perform its required function.

CHROMOSOMES

Human cells can be categorized into gametes (sperm and egg cells) and somatic cells, which include all cells other than gametes. Each somatic cell nucleus has 46 chromosomes in 23 pairs (Fig. 4.10). These are diploid cells, and the individual's father and mother each donate one chromosome per pair. New somatic cells are formed through mitosis and cytokinesis. Gametes are haploid cells: They have only 1 member of each chromosome pair, for a total of 23 chromosomes. Haploid cells are formed from diploid cells by meiosis (Fig. 4.11).

In 22 of the 23 chromosome pairs, the two members of each pair are virtually identical in microscopic appearance: thus, they are homologous (Fig. 4.12B). These 22 chromosome pairs are homologous in both males and females and are termed autosomes. The remaining pair of chromosomes, the sex chromosomes, consists of two homologous X chromosomes in females and a nonhomologous pair, X and Y, in males.

Fig. 4.12A, illustrates a metaphase spread, which is a photograph of the chromosomes as they appear in the nucleus of a somatic cell during metaphase. (Chromosomes are easiest to visualize during this stage of mitosis.) In Fig. 4.12A, the chromosomes are arranged according to size, with the homologous chromosomes paired. The 22 autosomes are numbered according to length, with chromosome 1 being the longest and chromosome 22 the shortest. A karyotype, or karyogram, is an ordered display of chromosomes. Some natural variation in relative chromosome length can be expected from person to person,

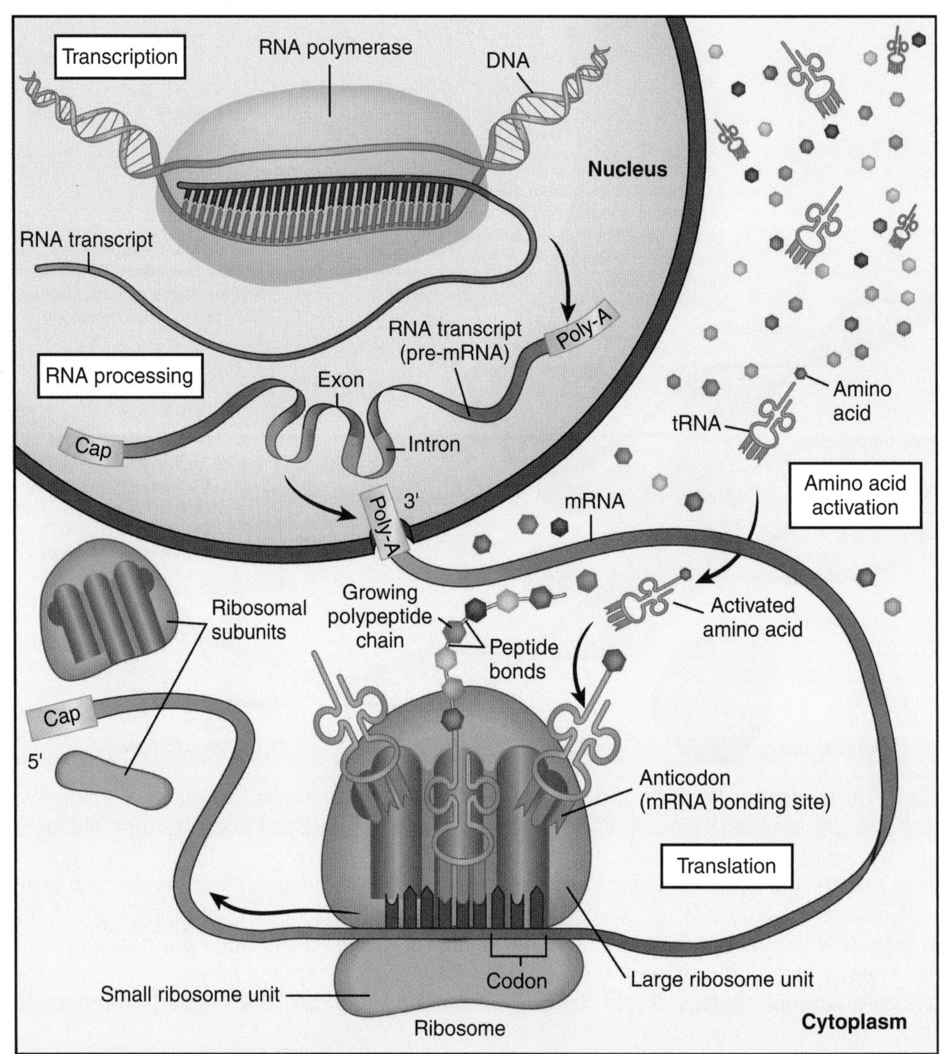

Fig. 4.9 Protein Synthesis. The site of transcription is the nucleus and the site of translation is the cytoplasm. See the text for details.

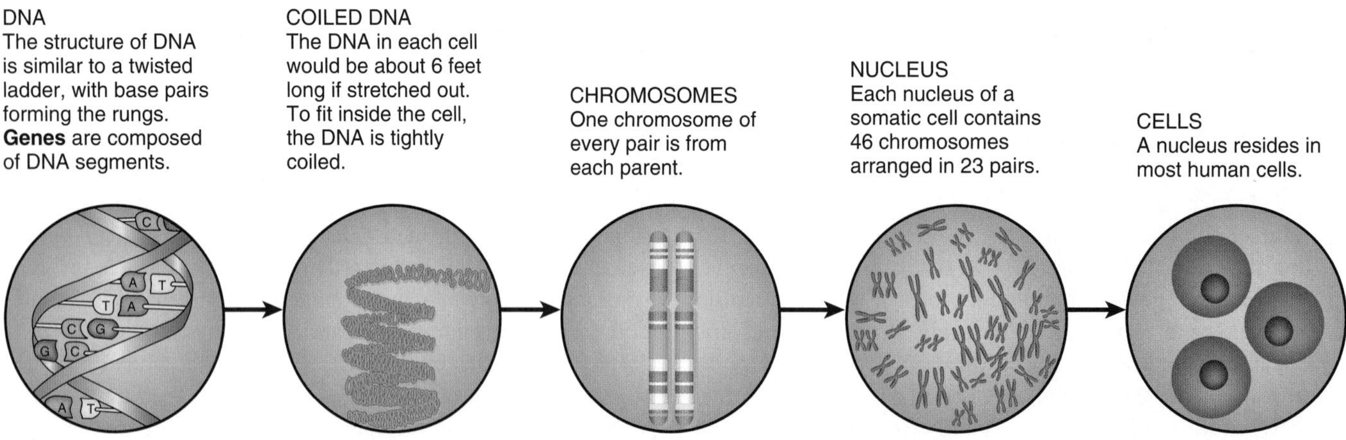

Fig. 4.10 From Molecular Parts to the Whole Somatic Cell.

so it is not always possible to distinguish each chromosome by its length. Therefore, the position of the centromere (region of DNA responsible for movement of the replicated chromosomes into the two daughter cells during mitosis and meiosis) also is used to classify chromosomes (see Figs. 4.12B and 4.13).

The chromosomes in Fig. 4.12 were stained with Giemsa stain, resulting in distinctive chromosome bands. These form various patterns in the different chromosomes so that each chromosome can be distinguished easily. Using banding techniques, researchers can number chromosomes and study individual

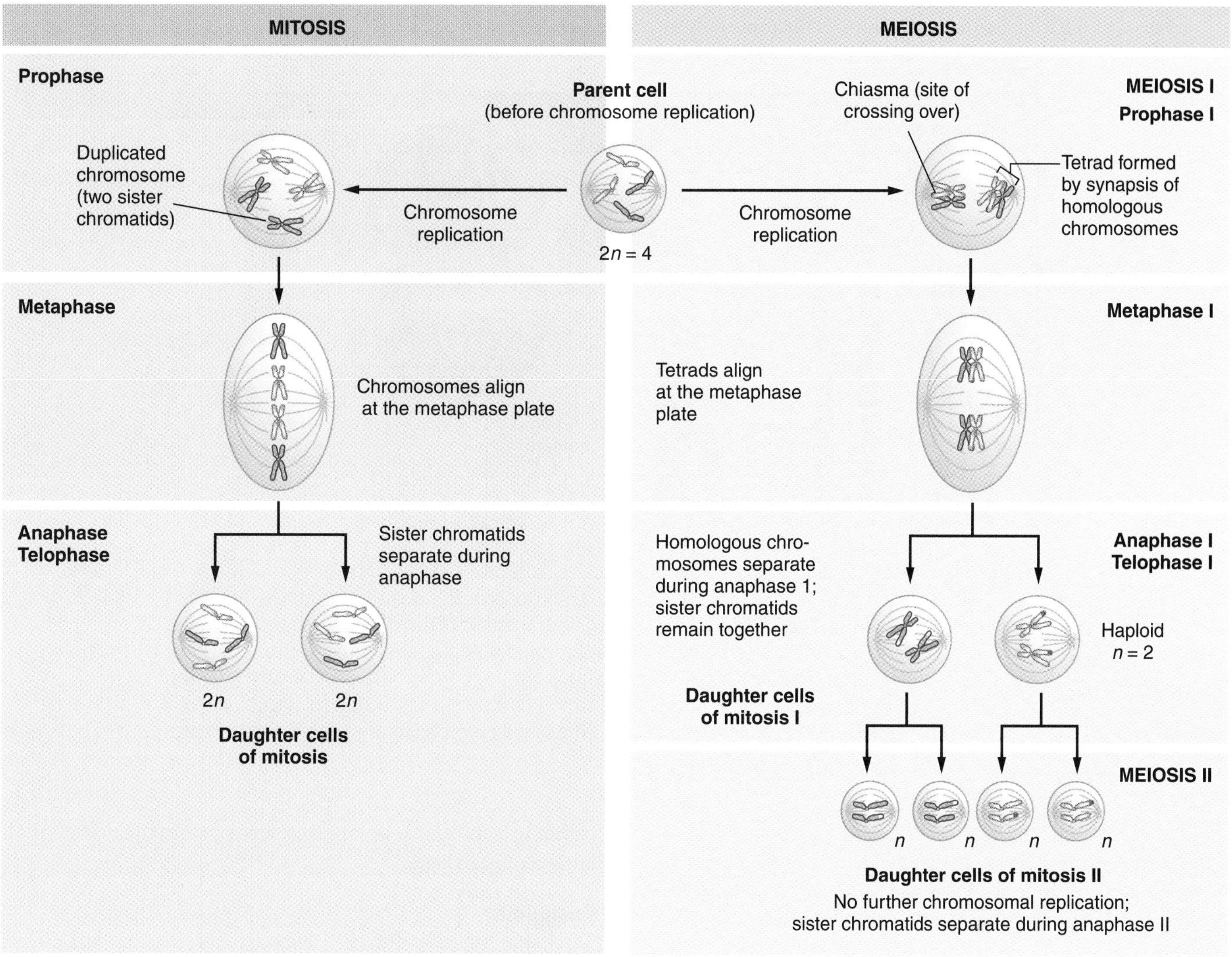

MITOSIS
MEIOSIS
Prophase
Parent cell
(before chromosome replication)
Chiasma (site of crossing over)
MEIOSIS I
Prophase I
Duplicated chromosome (two sister chromatids)
Chromosome replication
2n = 4
Chromosome replication
Tetrad formed by synapsis of homologous chromosomes
Metaphase
Metaphase I
Chromosomes align at the metaphase plate
Tetrads align at the metaphase plate
Anaphase
Telophase
Sister chromatids separate during anaphase
Homologous chromosomes separate during anaphase 1; sister chromatids remain together
Anaphase I
Telophase I
Haploid
n = 2
2n
2n
Daughter cells of mitosis
Daughter cells of mitosis I
MEIOSIS II
n
n
n
n
Daughter cells of mitosis II
No further chromosomal replication; sister chromatids separate during anaphase II

Fig. 4.11 Phases of Meiosis and Comparison to Mitosis. (From Jorde LB, Carey JC. *Medical genetics*, 5th edition. St. Louis: Elsevier; 2016.)

1
2
3
4
5
6
7
8
9
10
11
12
13
14
15
16
17
18
Y
X
19
20
21
22
A
9.2 μm
B
Homologous chromosomes
Homologous chromosomes
Kinetochore
Replication
Centromere
Cohesin proteins
Kinetochores
Sister chromatids
Sister chromatids

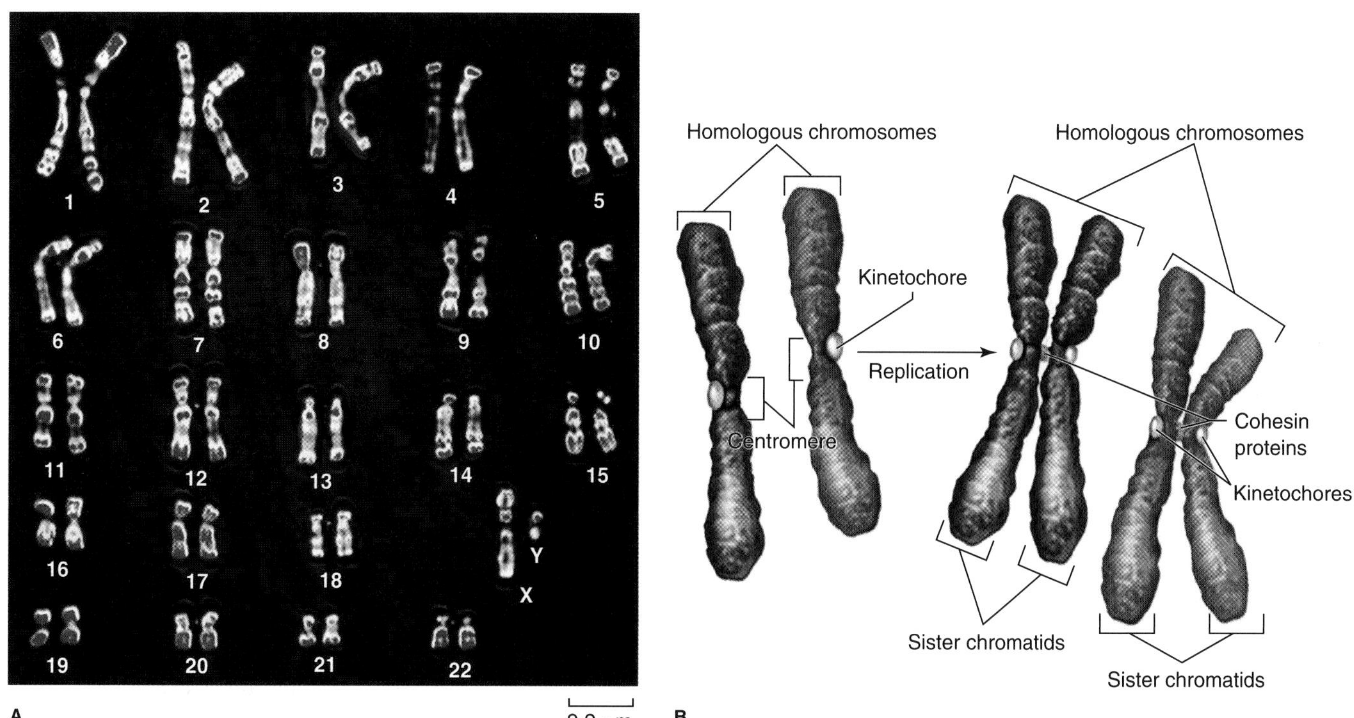

Fig. 4.12 Karyogram of Chromosomes. (A) Human karyogram. (B) Homologous chromosomes and sister chromatids. (From Raven PH, et al. *Biology*, 8th edition. New York: McGraw-Hill, 2008.)

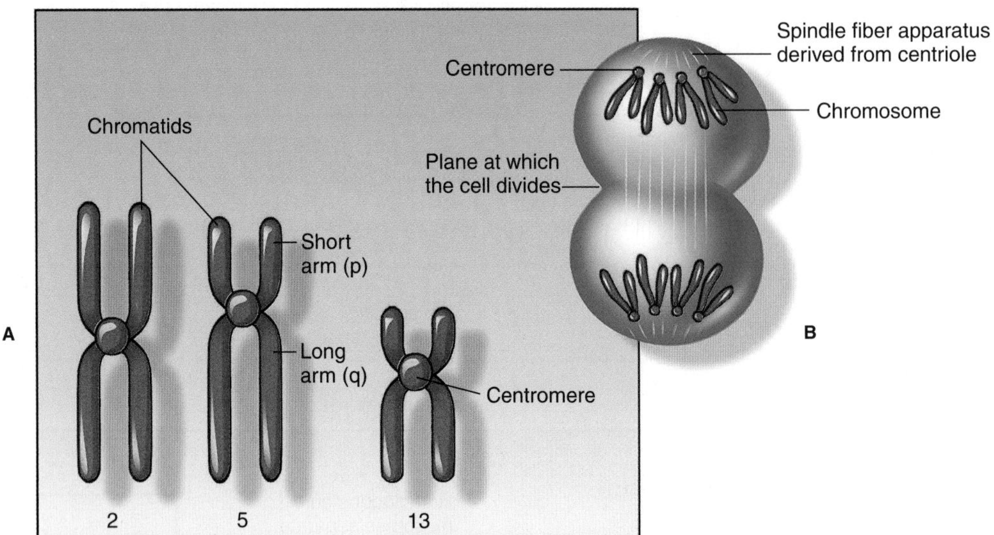

Fig. 4.13 Structure of Chromosomes. (A) Human chromosomes 2, 5, and 13. Each is replicated and consists of two chromatids. Chromosome 2 is a metacentric chromosome because the centromere is close to the middle; chromosome 5 is submetacentric because the centromere is set off from the middle; chromosome 13 is acrocentric because the centromere is at or very near the end. **(B)** During mitosis, the centromere divides and the chromosomes move to opposite poles of the cell. At the time of centromere division, the chromatids are designated as chromosomes.

variations. Missing or duplicated portions of chromosomes, which often result in serious diseases, also are readily identified. More recently, techniques have been devised permitting each chromosome to be visualized with a different color.

Chromosome Aberrations and Associated Diseases

Chromosome abnormalities are the leading known cause of intellectual disability and miscarriage. Estimates indicate that a major chromosome aberration occurs in at least 1 in 12 conceptions. Most of these fetuses do not survive to term; about 50% of all recovered first-trimester spontaneous abortuses have major chromosome aberrations.[7]

The number of live births affected by these abnormalities is significant; approximately 1 in 150 has a major diagnosable chromosome abnormality.[7]

Polyploidy

Cells with a multiple of the normal number of chromosomes are euploid cells (Greek *eu* = good or true). Because normal gametes are haploid and most normal somatic cells are diploid, they are both euploid forms. When a euploid cell has more than the diploid number of chromosomes, it is said to be a polyploid cell. Several types of body tissues, including some liver, bronchial, and epithelial tissues, are normally polyploid. A zygote that has three copies of each chromosome, rather than the usual two, has a form of polyploidy called triploidy. Nearly all triploid fetuses are spontaneously aborted or stillborn. The prevalence of triploidy among live births is approximately 1 in 10,000. Tetraploidy, a condition in which euploid cells have 92 chromosomes, has been found primarily in early abortuses, although occasionally affected infants have been born alive. Like triploid infants, however, they do not survive. Triploidy and tetraploidy are relatively common conditions, accounting for approximately 10% of all known miscarriages.[8]

Aneuploidy

A cell that does not contain a multiple of 23 chromosomes is an aneuploid cell. A cell containing three copies of one chromosome is said to be trisomic (a condition termed trisomy) and is aneuploid. Monosomy, the presence of only one copy of a given chromosome in a diploid cell, is the other common form of aneuploidy. Among the autosomes, monosomy of any chromosome is lethal, but newborns with trisomy of chromosomes 13, 18, 21, or X can survive. This difference illustrates an important principle: *In general, loss of chromosome material has more serious consequences than duplication of chromosome material.*

Aneuploidy of the sex chromosomes is less serious than that of the autosomes. Very little genetic material—only about 50 genes—is located on the Y chromosome. For the X chromosome, inactivation of extra chromosomes (see the X-linked Inheritance section) largely diminishes their effect. A zygote bearing *no* X chromosome, however, will not survive.

Aneuploidy is usually the result of nondisjunction, an error in which homologous chromosomes or sister chromatids fail to separate normally during meiosis or mitosis (Fig. 4.14). Nondisjunction produces some gametes that have two copies of a given chromosome and others that have no copies of the chromosome. When such gametes unite with normal haploid gametes, the resulting zygote is monosomic or trisomic for that chromosome. Occasionally, a cell can be monosomic or trisomic for more than one chromosome.

Autosomal aneuploidy. Trisomy can occur for any chromosome, but fetuses with other trisomies of chromosomes (other than 13, 18, 21, or X) do not survive to term. Trisomy 16, for

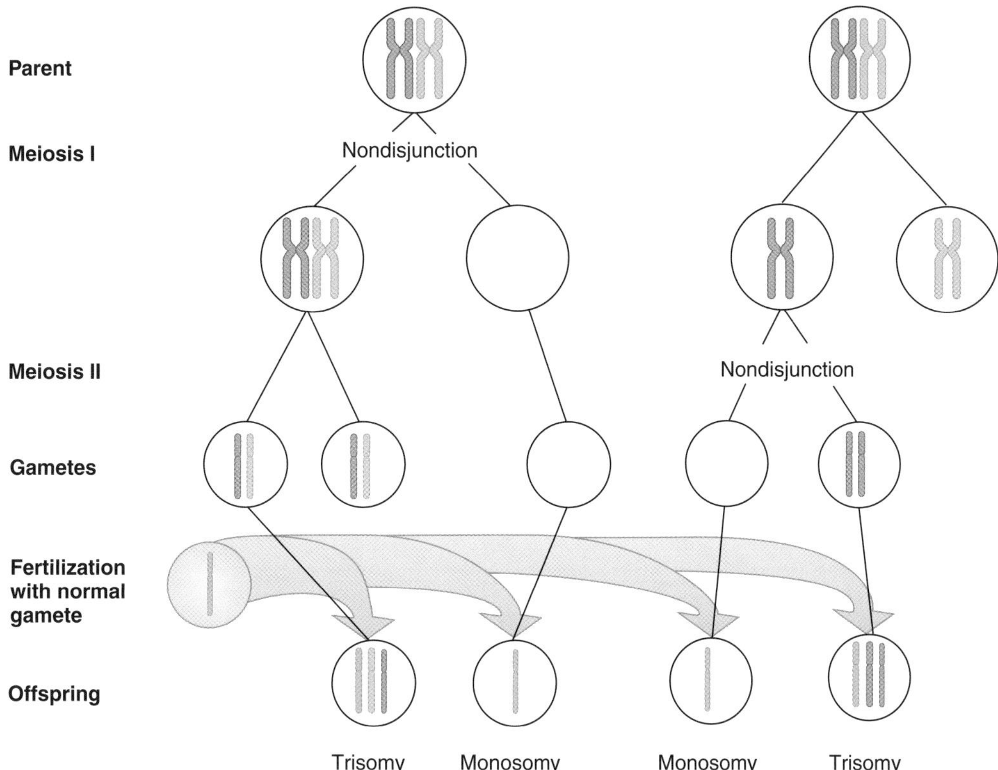

Fig. 4.14 Nondisjunction. Nondisjunction causes aneuploidy when chromosomes or sister chromatids fail to divide properly. (From Jorde LB, Carey JC. *Medical genetics*, 5th edition. St. Louis: Elsevier; 2016.)

example, is the most common trisomy among abortuses, but it is not seen in live births.

Partial trisomy, in which only an extra portion of a chromosome is present in each cell, can occur also. The consequences of partial trisomies are not as severe as those of complete trisomies. Trisomies may occur in only some cells of the body. Individuals affected are said to be chromosomal mosaics, meaning that the body has two or more different cell lines, each of which has a different karyotype. Mosaics are often formed by early mitotic nondisjunction occurring in one embryonic cell but not in others.

The best-known example of aneuploidy in an autosome is trisomy of chromosome 21, which causes Down syndrome (named after J. Langdon Down, who first described the syndrome in 1866). Down syndrome is seen in approximately 1 in 800 to 1 in 1000 live births; its principal features are shown and outlined in Fig. 4.15 and Table 4.1.

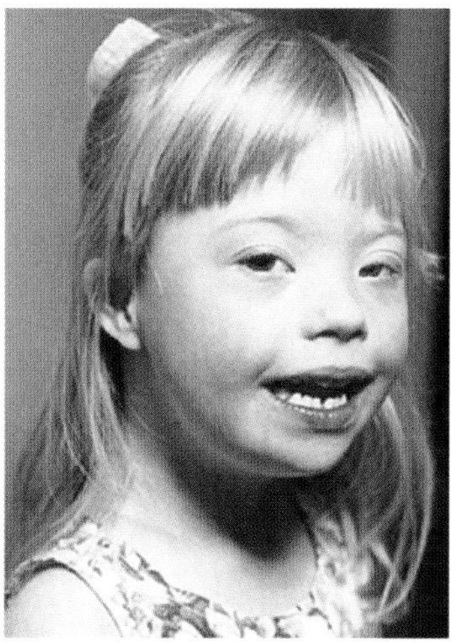

Fig. 4.15 Child with Down Syndrome. (Courtesy Drs. A. Olney and M. MacDonald, University of Nebraska Medical Center, Omaha, Nebraska.)

The risk of having a child with Down syndrome increases greatly with maternal age. As Fig. 4.16 demonstrates, women younger than 30 years of age have a risk ranging from about 1 in 1000 births to 1 in 2000 births. The risk begins to rise substantially after age 35 years and reaches 3% to 5% for women older than 45 years of age. This dramatic increase in risk is caused by the age of maternal egg cells, which are held in an arrested state of prophase I from the time they are formed in the female embryo until they are shed in ovulation. Thus, an egg cell formed by a 45-year-old woman is itself 45 years old. This long-suspended state causes defects to accumulate in the cellular proteins responsible for meiosis, leading to nondisjunction. The risk of Down syndrome, as well as other trisomies, does not increase with paternal age.

Sex chromosome aneuploidy. The incidence of sex chromosome aneuploidies is fairly high. Among live births, about 1 in 500 males and 1 in 900 females have a form of sex chromosome

TABLE 4.1 **Characteristics of Various Chromosome Disorders**

Disease/Disorder	Features
Down Syndrome	
Trisomy of Chromosome 21	
Intelligence quotient (IQ)	Usually ranges from 20 to 70 (intellectual disability)
Male/female findings	Virtually all males are sterile; some females can reproduce
Face	Distinctive: low nasal bridge, epicanthal folds, protruding tongue, low-set ears
Musculoskeletal system	Poor muscle tone (hypotonia), short stature
Systemic disorders	Congenital heart disease (one-third to half of cases), reduced ability to fight respiratory tract infections, increased susceptibility to leukemia—overall reduced survival rate; by age 40 years, usually develop symptoms similar to those of Alzheimer disease
Mortality	About 75% of fetuses with Down syndrome abort spontaneously or are stillborn; 20% of infants die before age 10 years; those who live beyond 10 years have life expectancy of about 60 years
Causative factors	97% caused by nondisjunction during formation of one of parent's gametes or during early embryonic development; 3% result from translocations; in 95% of cases, nondisjunction occurs when mother's egg cell is formed; remainder involve paternal nondisjunction; 1% are mosaics—these have a large number of normal cells, and effects of trisomic cells are attenuated and symptoms are generally less severe
Turner Syndrome	
(45,X) Monosomy of X Chromosome	
IQ	Not considered to be intellectually disabled, although some impairment of spatial and mathematical reasoning ability is found
Male/female findings	Found only in females
Musculoskeletal system	Short stature common, characteristic webbing of neck, widely spaced nipples, reduced carrying angle at elbow
Systemic disorders	Coarctation (narrowing) of aorta, edema of feet in newborns, usually sterile and have gonadal streaks rather than ovaries; streaks are sometimes susceptible to cancer
Mortality	About 15%–20% of spontaneous abortions with chromosome abnormalities have this karyotype, most common single-chromosome aberration; highly lethal during gestation, only about 0.5% of these conceptions survive to term
Causative factors	75% inherit X chromosome from mother, thus caused by meiotic error in father; frequency low compared with other sex chromosome aneuploidies (1:5000 newborn females); 50% have simple monosomy of X chromosome; remainder have more complex abnormalities; combinations of 45, X cells with XX or XY cells common
Klinefelter Syndrome	
(47,XXY) XXY Condition	
IQ	Moderate degree of mental impairment may be present
Male/female findings	Have a male appearance but usually sterile; 50% develop female-like breasts (gynecomastia); occurs in 1:1000 male births
Face	Voice somewhat high pitched
Systemic disorders	Sparse body hair, sterile, small testicles
Causative factors	50% of cases the result of nondisjunction of X chromosomes in mother, frequency rises with increasing maternal age; also involves XXY and XXXY karyotypes with degree of physical and mental impairment increasing with each added X chromosome; mosaicism fairly common with most prevalent combination of XXY and XY cells

aneuploidy. Because these conditions are generally less severe than autosomal aneuploidies, all forms except complete absence of any X chromosome material allow at least some individuals to survive.

One of the most common sex chromosome aneuploidies, affecting about 1 in 1000 newborn females, is trisomy X. Instead of two X chromosomes, these females have three X chromosomes in each cell. Most of these females have no overt physical abnormalities, although sterility, menstrual irregularity, or intellectual disability is sometimes seen. Some females have four X chromosomes, and they are more often intellectually disabled. Those with five or more X chromosomes generally have more severe intellectual disability and various physical defects.

A condition that leads to more serious problems is the presence of a single X chromosome and no homologous X or Y chromosome, so that the individual has a total of 45 chromosomes. The karyotype is usually designated 45,X, and it causes a set of symptoms known as Turner syndrome

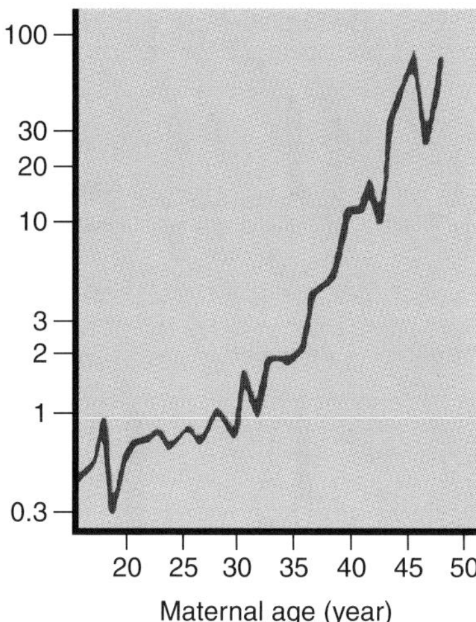

Fig. 4.16 Down Syndrome Increases With Maternal Age. Rate is per 1000 live births related to maternal age.

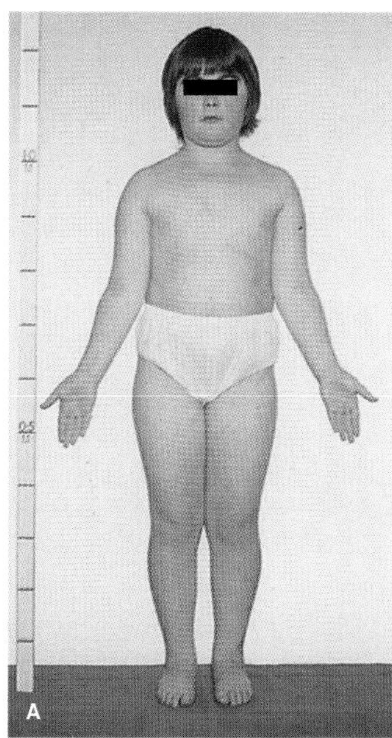

Fig. 4.17 Turner Syndrome. (A) A sex chromosome is missing, and the person's chromosomes are 45,X. Characteristic signs are short stature, female genitalia, webbed neck, shield-like chest with underdeveloped breasts and widely spaced nipples, and imperfectly developed ovaries. (From Patton KT, Thibodeau GA. *Anatomy & physiology*, 8th edition. St. Louis: Mosby; 2013. Courtesy Nancy S. Wexler, PhD, Columbia University.)

(Fig. 4.17; see Table 4.1). Individuals with at least two X chromosomes and one Y chromosome in each cell (47,XXY karyotype) have a disorder known as Klinefelter syndrome (Fig. 4.18; see Table 4.1).

Abnormalities of Chromosome Structure

In addition to the loss or gain of whole chromosomes, parts of chromosomes can be lost or duplicated as gametes are formed, and the arrangement of genes on chromosomes can be altered. Unlike aneuploidy and polyploidy, these changes sometimes have no serious consequences for an individual's health. Some of them can even remain entirely unnoticed, especially when very small pieces of chromosomes are involved. Nevertheless, abnormalities of chromosome structure can also produce serious disease in individuals or their offspring.

During meiosis and mitosis, chromosomes usually maintain their structural integrity, but chromosome breakage occasionally occurs. Mechanisms exist to "heal" these breaks and usually repair them perfectly with no damage to the daughter cell. However, some breaks remain or heal in a way that alters the chromosome's structure. The risk of chromosome breakage increases with exposure to harmful agents called clastogens (e.g., ionizing radiation, viral infections, or some types of chemicals).

Deletions. Broken chromosomes and lost DNA cause deletions (Fig. 4.19). Usually, a gamete with a deletion unites with a normal gamete to form a zygote. The zygote thus has one chromosome with the normal complement of genes and one with some missing genes. Because many genes can be lost in a deletion, serious consequences result, even though one normal chromosome is present. The most often cited example of a disease caused by a chromosomal deletion is the cri du chat syndrome. The term literally means "cry of the cat" and describes the characteristic cry of the affected child. Other symptoms include low birth weight, severe intellectual disability, microcephaly (smaller than normal head size), and heart defects. The disease is caused by a deletion of part of the short arm of chromosome 5.

Duplications. A deficiency of genetic material is more harmful than an excess, so duplications usually have less serious consequences than deletions. For example, a deletion of a region of chromosome 5 causes cri du chat syndrome, but a duplication of the same region causes intellectual disability, but less serious physical defects.

Inversions. An inversion occurs when two breaks take place on a chromosome, followed by the reinsertion of the missing fragment at its original site but in inverted order. Therefore, a chromosome symbolized as ABCDEFG might become ABEDCFG after an inversion.

Unlike deletions and duplications, no loss or gain of genetic material occurs, so inversions are "balanced" alterations of chromosome structure, and they often have no apparent physical effect. Some genes are influenced by neighboring genes, however, and this position effect, a change in a gene's expression caused by its position, sometimes results in physical defects in these persons. Inversions can cause serious problems in the offspring of individuals carrying the inversion because the inversion can lead to duplications and deletions in the chromosomes transmitted to the offspring.

Translocations. The interchange of genetic material between nonhomologous chromosomes is called translocation. A reciprocal translocation occurs when breaks take place in two

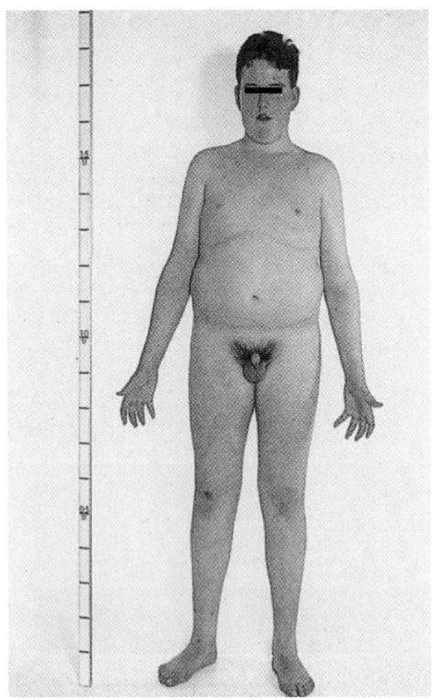

Fig. 4.18 Klinefelter Syndrome. This young man exhibits many characteristics of Klinefelter syndrome: small testes, some development of the breasts, sparse body hair, and long limbs. This syndrome results from the presence of two or more X chromosomes with one Y chromosome (genotypes XXY or XXXY, for example). (From Patton KT, Thibodeau GA. *Anatomy & physiology*, 9th edition. St. Louis: Mosby; 2016. Courtesy Nancy S. Wexler, PhD, Columbia University.)

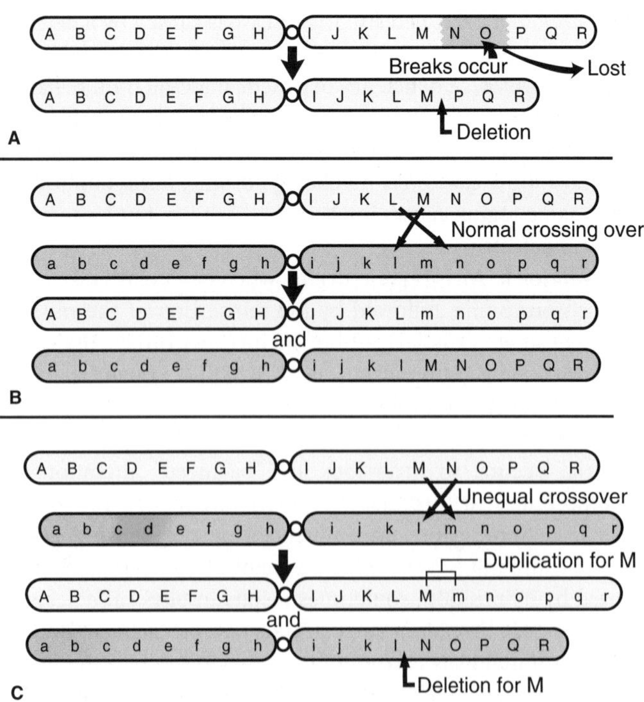

Fig. 4.19 Abnormalities of Chromosome Structure. **(A)** Deletion occurs when a chromosome segment is lost. **(B)** Normal crossing over. (C) The generation of duplication and deletion through unequal crossover.

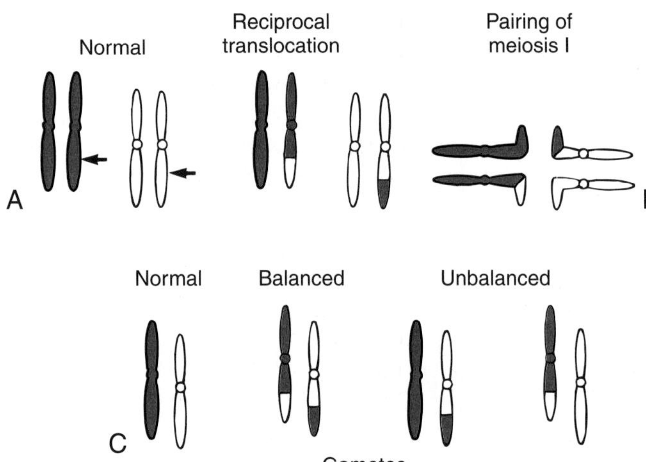

Fig. 4.20 Normal and Abnormal Chromosome Translocation. **(A)** Normal chromosomes and reciprocal translocation. **(B)** Pairing at meiosis. **(C)** Consequences of translocation in gametes; unbalanced gametes result in zygotes that are partially trisomic and partially monosomic and, consequently, develop abnormally.

different chromosomes and the material is exchanged (Fig. 4.20A). As with inversions, the carrier of a reciprocal translocation is usually normal, but his or her offspring can have duplications and deletions.

A second and clinically more important type of translocation is Robertsonian translocation. In this disorder, the long arms of two nonhomologous chromosomes fuse at the centromere, forming a single chromosome. Robertsonian translocations are confined to chromosomes 13, 14, 15, 21, and 22 because the short arms of these chromosomes are very small and contain no essential genetic material. The short arms are usually lost during subsequent cell divisions. Because the carriers of Robertsonian translocations lose no important genetic material, they are unaffected, although they have only 45 chromosomes in each cell. Their offspring, however, may have serious monosomies or trisomies. For example, a common Robertsonian translocation involves the fusion of the long arms of chromosomes 21 and 14. An offspring who inherits a gamete carrying the fused chromosome can receive an extra copy of the long arm of chromosome 21 and develop Down syndrome. Robertsonian translocations are responsible for approximately 3% to 5% of Down syndrome cases. Parents who carry a Robertsonian translocation involving chromosome 21 have an increased risk for producing multiple offspring with Down syndrome.

Fragile sites. Several areas on chromosomes develop distinctive breaks and gaps (observable microscopically) when the cells are cultured. Most of these fragile sites do not appear to be related to disease. However, one fragile site, located on the long arm of the X chromosome, is associated with *fragile X syndrome*. The most important feature of this syndrome is intellectual disability. With a relatively high population prevalence (affecting approximately 1 in 4000 males and 1 in 8000 females), fragile X syndrome is the second most common genetic cause of intellectual disability (after Down syndrome).

In fragile X syndrome, females who inherit the mutation do not necessarily express the disease condition, but they can pass it on to descendants who do express it. Ordinarily, a male who inherits a disease gene on the X chromosome expresses the condition because he has only one X chromosome. An uncommon feature of this disease is that about one-third of carrier females are affected, although less severely than males. Unaffected transmitting males have been shown to have more than about 50 repeated DNA sequences near the beginning of the fragile X gene. These trinucleotide sequences, which consist of CGG sequences duplicated many times, cause fragile X syndrome when the number of copies exceeds 200.[9] The number of these repeats can increase from generation to generation. More than 20 other genetic diseases, including Huntington disease and myotonic dystrophy, also are caused by this mechanism.[10]

ELEMENTS OF FORMAL GENETICS

The mechanisms by which an individual's set of paired chromosomes produces traits are the principles of genetic inheritance. Mendel's work with garden peas first defined these principles. Later geneticists have refined Mendel's work to explain patterns of inheritance for traits and diseases that appear in families.

Analysis of traits that occur with defined, predictable patterns has helped geneticists assemble the pieces of the human gene map. Current research focuses on determining the RNA or protein products of each gene and understanding the way they contribute to disease. Eventually, diseases and defects caused by single genes can be traced and therapies to prevent and treat such diseases can be developed.

Traits caused by single genes are called mendelian traits (after Gregor Mendel). Each gene occupies a position along a chromosome, known as a locus. The genes at a particular locus can have different forms (i.e., they can be composed of different nucleotide sequences) called alleles. A locus that has two or more alleles that each occur with an appreciable frequency in a population is said to be polymorphic (or to have a polymorphism).

Because humans are diploid organisms, each chromosome is represented twice, with one member of the chromosome pair contributed by the father and one by the mother. At a given locus, an individual has one allele whose origin is paternal and one whose origin is maternal. When the two alleles are identical, the individual is homozygous at that locus. When the alleles are not identical, the individual is heterozygous at that locus.

Phenotype and Genotype

The composition of genes at a given locus is known as the genotype. The outward appearance of an individual, which is the result of both genotype and environment, is the phenotype. For example, an infant who is born with an inability to metabolize the amino acid phenylalanine has the single-gene disorder known as phenylketonuria (PKU) and thus has the PKU genotype. If the condition is left untreated, abnormal metabolites of phenylalanine will begin to accumulate in the infant's brain and irreversible intellectual disability will occur. Intellectual disability is thus one aspect of the PKU phenotype. By imposing dietary restrictions to exclude food that contains phenylalanine, however, intellectual disability can be prevented. Foods high in phenylalanine include proteins found in milk, dairy products, meat, fish, chicken, eggs, beans, and nuts. Although the child still has the PKU genotype, a modification of the environment (in this case, the child's diet) produces an outwardly normal phenotype.

Dominance and Recessiveness

In many loci, the effects of one allele mask those of another when the two are found together in a heterozygote. The allele whose effects are observable is said to be dominant. The allele whose effects are hidden is said to be recessive (from the Latin root for "hiding"). Traditionally, for loci having two alleles, the dominant allele is denoted by an uppercase letter and the recessive allele is denoted by a lowercase letter. When one allele is dominant over another, the heterozygote genotype *Aa* has the same phenotype as the dominant homozygote *AA*. For the recessive allele to be expressed, it must exist in the homozygote form, *aa*.

A carrier is an individual who has a disease gene but is phenotypically normal. Many genes for a recessive disease occur in heterozygotes, who carry one copy of the gene but do not express the disease. When recessive genes are lethal in the homozygous state, they are eliminated from the population when they occur in homozygotes. By "hiding" in carriers, however, recessive genes for diseases are passed on to the next generation.

TRANSMISSION OF GENETIC DISEASES

The pattern in which a genetic disease is inherited through generations is termed the mode of inheritance. Knowing the mode of inheritance can reveal much about the disease-causing gene itself, and members of families with the disease can be given reliable genetic counseling.

The known single-gene diseases can be classified into four major modes of inheritance: autosomal dominant, autosomal recessive, X-linked dominant, and X-linked recessive. The first two types involve genes known to occur on the 22 pairs of autosomes. The last two types occur on the X chromosome; very few disease-causing genes occur on the Y chromosome.

The pedigree chart summarizes family relationships and shows which members of a family are affected by a genetic disease (Fig. 4.21). Generally, the pedigree begins with one individual in the family, the proband. This individual is usually the first person in the family diagnosed or seen in a clinic.

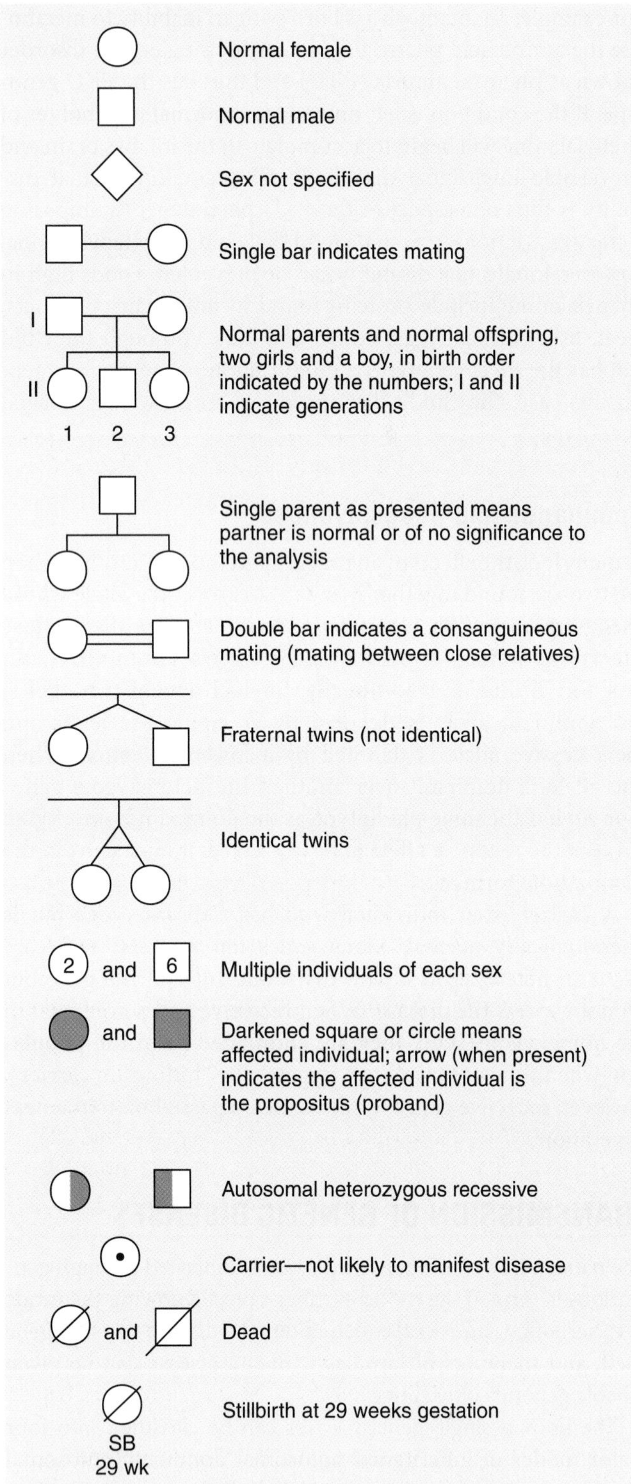

Fig. 4.21 Symbols Commonly Used in Pedigrees. (From Jorde LB, Carey JC. *Medical genetics*, 5th edition. St. Louis: Elsevier; 2016.)

Autosomal Dominant Inheritance

Characteristics of Pedigrees

Diseases caused by autosomal dominant genes are rare, with the most common occurring in fewer than 1 in 500 individuals. Therefore, it is uncommon for two individuals who are both affected by the same autosomal dominant disease to produce offspring together. Fig. 4.22A illustrates this unusual pattern. Affected offspring are usually produced by the union of a normal parent with an affected heterozygous parent. The Punnett square in Fig. 4.22B illustrates this mating. The affected parent can pass either a disease-causing allele or a normal allele to the next generation. On average, half the children will be heterozygous and will express the disease, and half will be normal.

A

Affected parent		Affected parent: D	Affected parent: d
Affected parent	D	DD Homozygous affected (usually rare)	Dd Heterozygous affected
	d	Dd Heterozygous affected	dd Homozygous normal

B

		Normal parent: d	Normal parent: d
Affected parent	D	Dd Heterozygous affected	Dd Heterozygous affected
	d	dd Homozygous normal	dd Homozygous normal

Fig. 4.22 Punnett Square and Autosomal Dominant Traits. **(A)** Punnett square for the mating of two individuals with an autosomal dominant gene. Here both parents are affected by the trait. **(B)** Punnett square for the mating of a normal individual with a carrier for an autosomal dominant gene.

The pedigree in Fig. 4.23 shows the transmission of an autosomal dominant allele. Several important characteristics of this pedigree support the conclusion that the trait is caused by an autosomal dominant gene:

1. The two sexes exhibit the trait in approximately equal proportions; males and females are equally likely to transmit the trait to their offspring.
2. No generations are skipped. If an individual has the trait, one parent must also have it. If neither parent has the trait, none of the children will have it (apart from new mutations, as discussed later).
3. Affected heterozygous individuals transmit the trait to approximately half their children, and because gamete transmission is subject to chance fluctuations, all or none of the children of an affected parent may have the trait. When large numbers of matings of this type are studied, however, the proportion of affected children closely approaches one-half.

Recurrence Risks

Parents at risk for producing children with a genetic disease nearly always ask the question, "What is the *chance* that our child will have this disease?" The probability that an individual

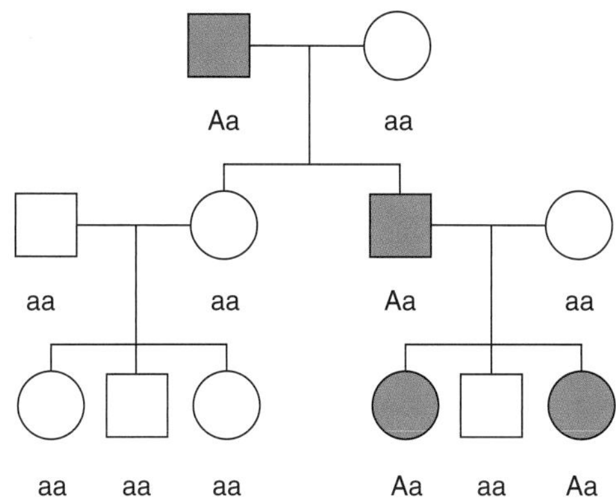

Fig. 4.23 Pedigree Illustrating the Inheritance Pattern of Postaxial Polydactyly, an Autosomal Dominant Disorder. Affected individuals are represented by shading. (From Jorde LB, Carey JC. *Medical genetics*, 5th edition. St. Louis: Elsevier; 2016.)

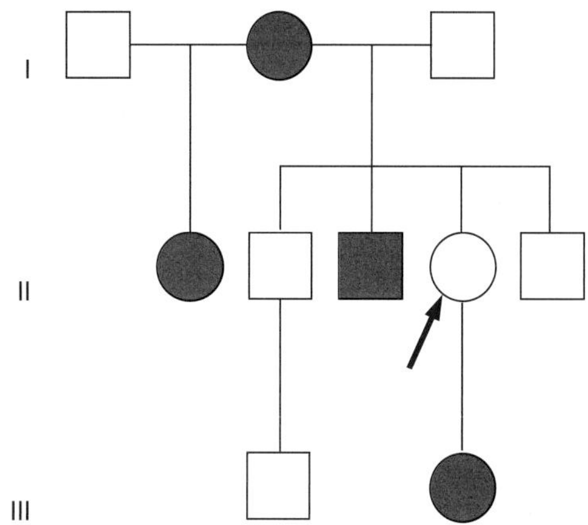

Fig. 4.24 Pedigree for Retinoblastoma Showing Incomplete Penetrance. Female with marked arrow in line II must be heterozygous, but she does not express the trait.

will develop a genetic disease is termed the recurrence risk. When one parent is affected by an autosomal dominant disease (and is a heterozygote) and the other is unaffected, the recurrence risk for each child is one-half.

An important principle is that each birth is an independent event, much like a coin toss. Thus, even though parents may have already had a child with the disease, their recurrence risk remains one-half. Even if they have produced several children, all affected (or all unaffected) by the disease, the law of independence dictates that the probability their next child will have the disease is still one-half. Parents' misunderstanding of this principle is a common problem encountered in genetic counseling.

If a child is born with an autosomal dominant disease and there is no history of the disease in the family, the child is probably the product of a new mutation. The gene transmitted by one of the parents has thus undergone a mutation from a normal allele to a disease-causing allele. The alleles at this locus in most of the parent's other germ cells are still normal. In this situation, the recurrence risk for the parent's subsequent offspring is not greater than that of the general population. The offspring of the affected child, however, will have a recurrence risk of one-half (probability of 0.5). Because these diseases often reduce the potential for reproduction, many autosomal dominant diseases result from new mutations.

Delayed Age of Onset

One of the best-known autosomal dominant diseases is Huntington disease, a neurologic disorder whose main features are progressive dementia and increasingly uncontrollable limb movements (chorea; discussed further in Chapter 17). A key feature of this disease is its delayed age of onset: Symptoms usually are not seen until 40 years of age or later. Thus, those who develop the disease often have borne children before they become aware that they have the disease-causing mutation. If the disease was present at birth, nearly all affected persons would die before reaching the reproductive age, and the occurrence of the disease-causing allele in the population would be much lower. An individual whose parent has the disease has a 50% chance of developing it during middle age. He or she is thus confronted with a torturous question: Should I have children, knowing that there is a 50:50 chance that I may have this disease-causing gene and will pass it to half my children? A DNA test can now be used to determine whether an individual has inherited the trinucleotide repeat mutation that causes Huntington disease.

Penetrance and Expressivity

The penetrance of a trait is the percentage of individuals with a specific genotype who also exhibit the expected phenotype. Incomplete penetrance means individuals who have the disease-causing genotype may not exhibit the disease phenotype at all, even though the genotype and the associated disease may be transmitted to the next generation. A pedigree illustrating the transmission of an autosomal dominant mutation with incomplete penetrance is provided in Fig. 4.24. Retinoblastoma, the most common malignant eye tumor affecting children, typically exhibits incomplete penetrance. About 10% of the individuals who are obligate carriers of the disease-causing mutation (i.e., those who have an affected parent and affected children and therefore must themselves carry the mutation) do not have the disease. The penetrance of the disease-causing genotype is then said to be 90%.

The gene responsible for retinoblastoma is a tumor-suppressor gene. The normal function of its protein product is to regulate the cell cycle, so cells do not divide uncontrollably. When the protein is altered because of a genetic mutation, its tumor-suppressing capacity is lost and a tumor can form (see Chapters 12 and 20).[11]

Expressivity is the extent of variation in phenotype associated with a particular genotype. If the expressivity of a disease is variable, penetrance may be complete, but the severity of the disease can vary greatly. A good example of variable expressivity in an autosomal dominant disease is neurofibromatosis type 1, or von Recklinghausen disease. As in retinoblastoma, the mutations that cause neurofibromatosis type 1 occur in a tumor-suppressor gene.[12] The expression of this disease varies from a few harmless café-au-lait (light brown) spots on the skin to numerous neurofibromas, scoliosis, seizures, gliomas, neuromas, malignant peripheral nerve sheath tumors, hypertension, and learning disorders (Fig. 4.25).

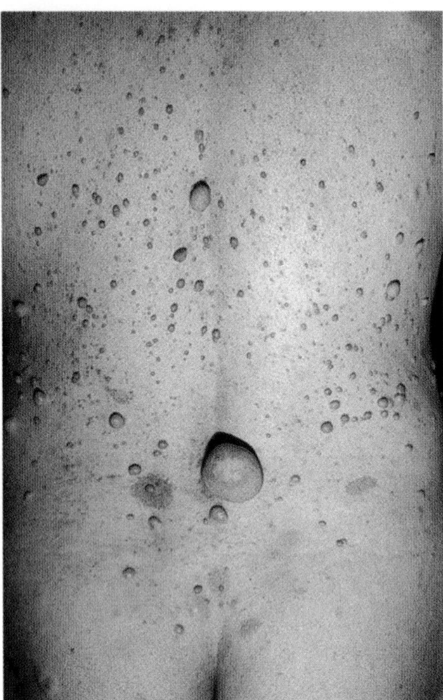

Fig. 4.25 Neurofibromatosis: Tumors. The most common is sessile or pedunculated. Early tumors are soft, dome-shaped papules or nodules that have a distinctive violaceous hue. Most are benign. (From Habif et al. Skin disease: Diagnosis and treatment, 2nd edition. St. Louis: Mosby; 2005.)

Several factors cause variable expressivity. Genes at other loci sometimes modify the expression of a disease-causing gene. Environmental (i.e., nongenetic) factors also can influence expression of a disease-causing gene. Finally, different mutations at a locus can cause variation in severity. For example, a mutation that alters only one amino acid of the factor VIII gene usually produces a mild form of hemophilia A, whereas a "stop" codon (premature termination of translation) usually produces a more severe form of this blood coagulation disorder.

Epigenetics and Genomic Imprinting

Although this chapter focuses on DNA sequence variation and its consequence for disease, there is increasing evidence that the same DNA sequence can produce dramatically different phenotypes because of chemical modifications altering the expression of genes (these modifications are collectively termed epigenetic; see Chapter 6). An important example of such a modification is DNA methylation, the attachment of a methyl group to a cytosine base followed by a guanine base in the DNA sequence (Fig. 4.26). These sequences, which are common near many genes, are termed CpG islands. When the CpG islands located near a gene become heavily methylated, the gene is less likely to be transcribed into mRNA. In other words, the gene becomes transcriptionally inactive. One study showed that identical (monozygotic) twins accumulate different methylation patterns in the DNA sequences of their somatic cells as they age, causing increasing numbers of phenotypic differences. Intriguingly twins with more differences in their lifestyles (e.g., smoking versus nonsmoking) accumulated larger numbers of differences in their methylation patterns. The twins, despite having identical DNA sequences, become more and more different as a result of epigenetic changes, which, in turn, affect the expression of genes (see Fig. 6.8).

Epigenetic alteration of gene activity can have important disease consequences. For example, a major cause of one form of inherited colon cancer (termed *hereditary nonpolyposis colorectal cancer [HNPCC]*) is the methylation of a gene whose protein product repairs damaged DNA. When this gene becomes inactive, damaged DNA accumulates, eventually resulting in colon tumors. Epigenetic changes are also discussed in Chapters 6, 12, and 13.

Approximately 100 human genes are thought to be methylated differently, depending on which parent transmits the gene. This epigenetic modification, characterized by methylation and other changes, is termed genomic imprinting. For each of these genes, one of the parents *imprints* the gene (inactivates it) when it is transmitted to the offspring. An example is the insulin-like growth factor 2 gene *(IGF2)* on chromosome 11, which is transmitted by both parents, but the copy inherited from the mother is normally methylated and inactivated (imprinted). Thus, only one copy of *IGF2* is active in normal individuals. However, the maternal imprint is occasionally lost, resulting in two active copies of *IGF2*. This causes excess fetal growth and contributes to a condition known as *Beckwith-Wiedemann syndrome* (see Chapter 6).

A second example of genomic imprinting is a deletion of part of the long arm of chromosome 15 (15q11–q13), which, when inherited from the father, causes the offspring to manifest a disease known as *Prader-Willi syndrome* (short stature, obesity, hypogonadism). When the same deletion is inherited from the mother, the offspring develop *Angelman syndrome* (intellectual disability, seizures, ataxic gait). The two different phenotypes reflect the fact that different genes are normally active in the maternally and paternally transmitted copies of this region of chromosome 15.

Autosomal Recessive Inheritance

Characteristics of Pedigrees

Like autosomal dominant diseases, diseases caused by autosomal recessive genes are rare in populations, although there can be numerous carriers. Cystic fibrosis, the most common lethal recessive disease in white children, occurs in about 1 in 2500 births. Approximately 1 in 25 whites carries a copy of a mutation that causes cystic fibrosis (see Chapter 36). Carriers are phenotypically unaffected. Some autosomal recessive diseases are characterized by delayed age of onset, incomplete penetrance, and variable expressivity.

Fig. 4.27 shows a pedigree for cystic fibrosis. The gene responsible for cystic fibrosis encodes a chloride ion channel in some epithelial cells. Defective transport of chloride ions leads to a salt imbalance, which results in secretions of abnormally thick, dehydrated mucus. Some digestive organs, particularly the pancreas, become obstructed, causing malnutrition, and the lungs become clogged with mucus, making them highly susceptible to bacterial infections. Death from lung disease or heart failure occurs by age 40 years in about half the individuals with cystic fibrosis.

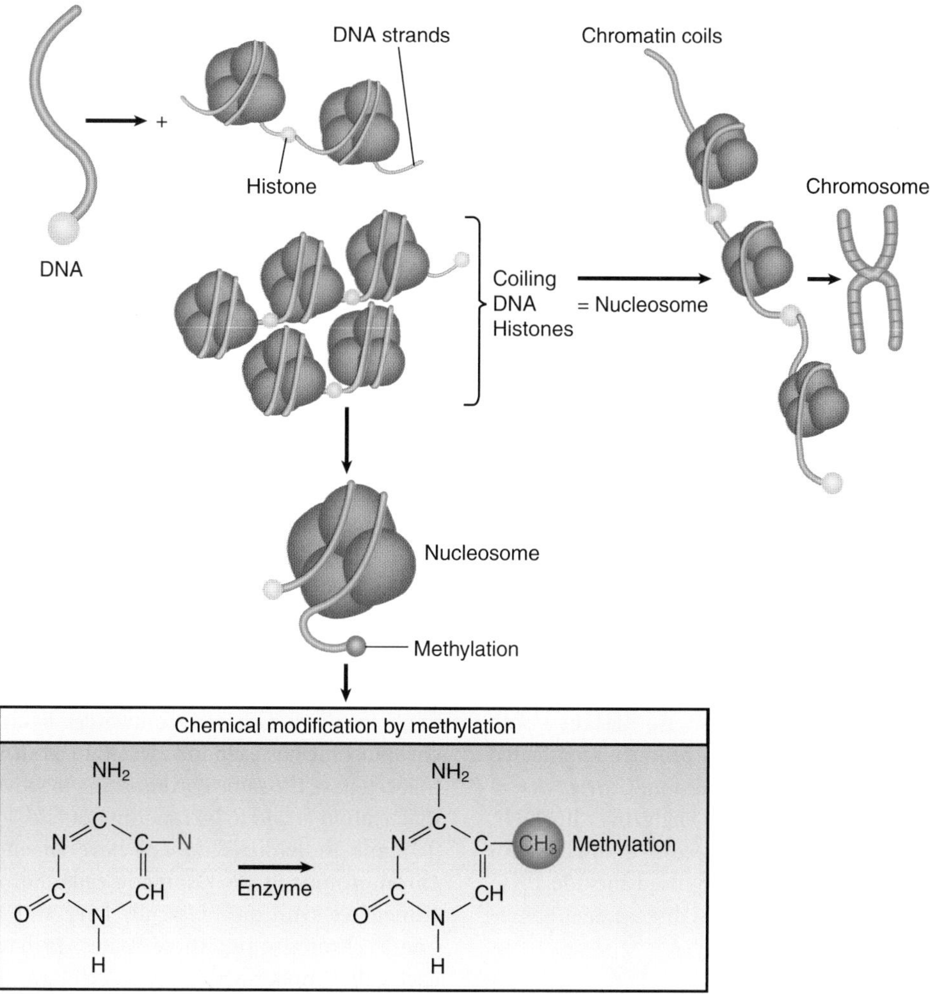

Fig. 4.26 **Epigenetic Modifications.** Because deoxyribonucleic acid (DNA) is a long molecule, it needs packaging to fit in the tiny nucleus. Packaging involves *coiling* of the DNA in a "left-handed" spiral around spools, made of four pairs of proteins individually known as *histones* and collectively termed the *histone octamer*. The entire spool is called a nucleosome (also see Fig. 1.2). Nucleosomes are organized into chromatin, the repeating building blocks of a chromosome. Histone modifications are correlated with methylation, are reversible, and occur at multiple sites. Methylation occurs at the 5 position of cytosine and provides a "footprint" or signature as a unique epigenetic alteration *(red)*. When genes are expressed, chromatin is open or active; however, when chromatin is condensed because of methylation and histone modification, genes are inactivated.

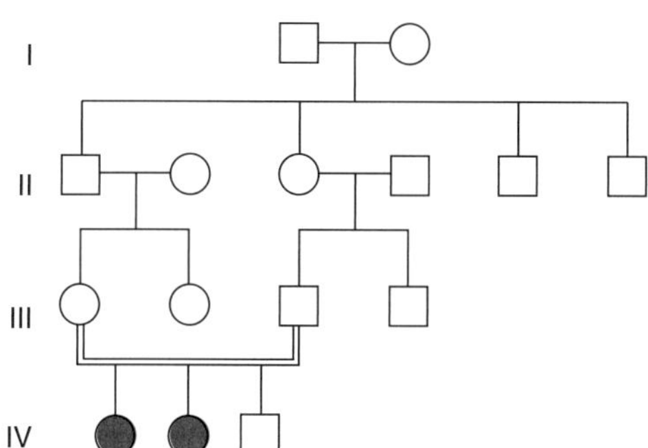

Fig. 4.27 **Pedigree for Cystic Fibrosis.** Cystic fibrosis is an autosomal recessive disorder. The double bar denotes a consanguineous mating. Because cystic fibrosis is relatively common in European populations, most cases do not involve consanguinity.

The important criteria for discerning autosomal recessive inheritance include the following:

1. Males and females are affected in equal proportions.
2. Consanguinity (marriage between related individuals) is sometimes present, especially in cases of rare recessive diseases.
3. The disease may be seen in siblings of affected individuals but usually not in their parents.
4. On average, one-fourth of the offspring of carrier parents will be affected.

Recurrence Risks

In most cases of recessive disease, both parents of affected individuals are heterozygous carriers. On average, one-fourth of their offspring will be normal homozygotes, half will be phenotypically normal carrier heterozygotes, and one-fourth will be

	D	d
D	DD Homozygous normal	Dd Heterozygous carrier
d	Dd Heterozygous carrier	dd Homozygous affected

Fig. 4.28 Punnett Square for the Mating of Heterozygous Carriers Typical of Most Cases of Recessive Disease.

homozygotes with the disease (Fig. 4.28). Thus, the recurrence risk for the offspring of carrier parents is 25%. However, in any given family, there are chance fluctuations.

If two parents have a recessive disease, they each must be homozygous for the disease. Therefore, all their children also must be affected. This distinguishes recessive from dominant inheritance because two parents both affected by a dominant gene are nearly always both heterozygotes, and thus one-fourth of their children will be unaffected.

Because carrier parents usually are unaware that they both carry the same recessive allele, they often produce an affected child before becoming aware of their condition. Carrier detection tests can identify heterozygotes by analyzing the DNA sequence to reveal a mutation. Some recessive diseases for which carrier detection tests are routinely used include PKU, sickle cell disease, cystic fibrosis, Tay-Sachs disease, hemochromatosis, and galactosemia.

Consanguinity

Consanguinity and inbreeding are related concepts. Consanguinity refers to the mating of two related individuals, and the offspring of such mating are said to be *inbred*. Consanguinity is sometimes an important characteristic of pedigrees for recessive diseases because relatives share a certain proportion of genes received from a common ancestor. The proportion of shared genes depends on the closeness of their biologic relationship. Consanguineous mating produces a significant increase in recessive disorders and are seen most often in pedigrees for rare recessive disorders.

X-Linked Inheritance

Some genetic conditions are caused by mutations in genes located on the sex chromosomes, and this mode of inheritance is termed sex linked. Only a few diseases are known to be inherited as X-linked dominant or Y chromosome traits, so only the more common X-linked recessive diseases are discussed here.

Because females receive two X chromosomes, one from the father and one from the mother, they can be homozygous for a disease allele at a given locus, homozygous for the normal allele at the locus, or heterozygous. Males, having only one X chromosome, are hemizygous for genes on this chromosome. If a male inherits a recessive disease gene on the X chromosome, he will be affected by the disease because the Y chromosome does not carry a normal allele to counteract the effects of the disease gene. Because a single copy of an X-linked recessive gene will cause disease in a male, whereas two copies are required for disease expression in females, more males are affected by X-linked recessive diseases than are females.

X Inactivation

In the late 1950s, Mary Lyon proposed that one X chromosome in the somatic cells of females is permanently inactivated, a process termed X inactivation.[13] This proposal, the Lyon hypothesis, explains why most gene products coded by the X chromosome are present in equal amounts in males and females, even though males have only one X chromosome and females have two X chromosomes. This phenomenon is called dosage compensation. The inactivated X chromosomes are observable in many interphase cells as highly condensed intranuclear chromatin bodies, termed Barr bodies (after Barr and Bertram, who discovered them in the late 1940s). Normal females have one Barr body in each somatic cell, whereas normal males have no Barr bodies.

X inactivation occurs very early in embryonic development—approximately 7 to 14 days after fertilization. In each somatic cell, one of the two X chromosomes is inactivated. In some cells, the inactivated X chromosome is the one contributed by the father; in other cells, it is the one contributed by the mother. Once the X chromosome has been inactivated in a cell, all the descendants of that cell have the same chromosome inactivated (Fig. 4.29). Thus, inactivation is said to be random but *fixed*.

Some individuals do not have the normal number of X chromosomes in their somatic cells. For example, males with Klinefelter syndrome typically have two X chromosomes and one Y chromosome. These males do have one Barr body in each cell. Females whose cell nuclei have three X chromosomes have two Barr bodies in each cell, and females whose cell nuclei have four X chromosomes have three Barr bodies in each cell. Females with Turner syndrome have only one X chromosome and no Barr bodies. Thus, the number of Barr bodies is always one less than the number of X chromosomes in the cell. All but one X chromosome are always inactivated.

Persons with abnormal numbers of X chromosomes, such as those with Turner syndrome or Klinefelter syndrome, are not physically normal. This situation presents a puzzle because they presumably have only one active X chromosome, the same as individuals with normal numbers of chromosomes. This is probably because the distal tips of the short and long arms of the X chromosome, as well as several other regions on the chromosome arm, are not inactivated. Thus, X inactivation is also known to be *incomplete*. The inactivated X chromosome DNA is heavily methylated. Inactive X chromosomes can be at least partially reactivated in vitro by administering 5-azacytidine, a demethylating agent.

Sex Determination

The process of sexual differentiation, in which the embryonic gonads become either testes or ovaries, begins during the sixth week of gestation. A key principle of mammalian sex determination is that one copy of the Y chromosome is sufficient to initiate the process of gonadal differentiation that produces a male fetus. The number of X chromosomes does not alter this

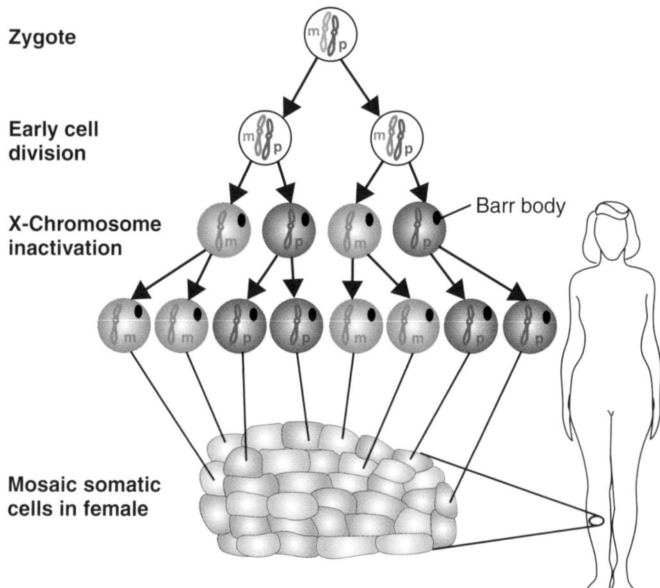

Fig. 4.29 The X Inactivation Process. The maternal *(m)* and paternal *(p)* X chromosomes are both active in the zygote and in early embryonic cells. X inactivation then takes place, resulting in cells having either an active paternal X or an active maternal X. Females are thus X chromosome mosaics, as shown in the tissue sample at the bottom of the page. (From Jorde LB, Carey JC. *Medical genetics*, 5th edition. St. Louis: Elsevier; 2016.)

process. For example, an individual with two X chromosomes and one Y chromosome in each cell is still phenotypically a male. Thus, the Y chromosome contains a gene that begins the process of male gonadal development.

This gene, termed *SRY* (for "sex-determining region on the Y"), has been located on the short arm of the Y chromosome.[14] The *SRY* gene lies just outside the pseudoautosomal region (Fig. 4.30A and B), which pairs with the distal tip of the short arm of the X chromosome during meiosis and exchanges genetic material with it (crossover), just as autosomes do. The DNA sequences of these regions on the X and Y chromosomes are highly similar. The rest of the X and Y chromosomes, however, do not exchange material and are not similar in DNA sequence.

Other genes that contribute to male differentiation are located on other chromosomes. Thus, *SRY* triggers the action of genes on other chromosomes. This concept is supported by the fact that the *SRY* protein product is similar to other proteins known to regulate gene expression.

Occasionally, the crossover between X and Y occurs closer to the centromere than it should, placing the *SRY* gene on the X chromosome after crossover. This variation can result in offspring with an apparently normal XX karyotype but a male phenotype. Such XX males are seen in about 1 in 20,000 live births and resemble males with Klinefelter syndrome. Conversely, it is possible to inherit a Y chromosome that has lost the *SRY* gene (the result of either a crossover error or a deletion of the gene). This situation produces an XY female. Such females have gonadal streaks rather than ovaries and have poorly developed secondary sex characteristics.

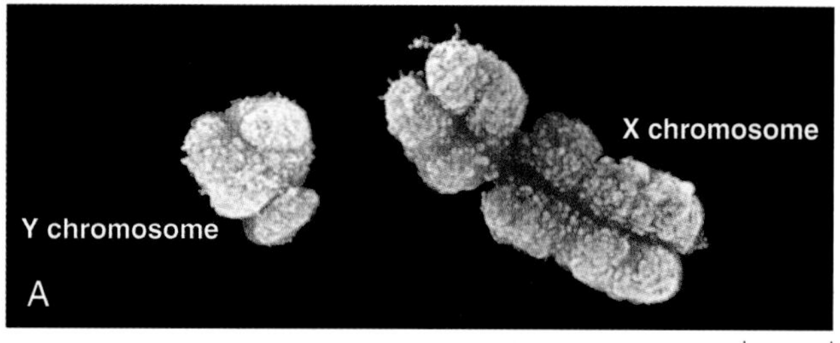

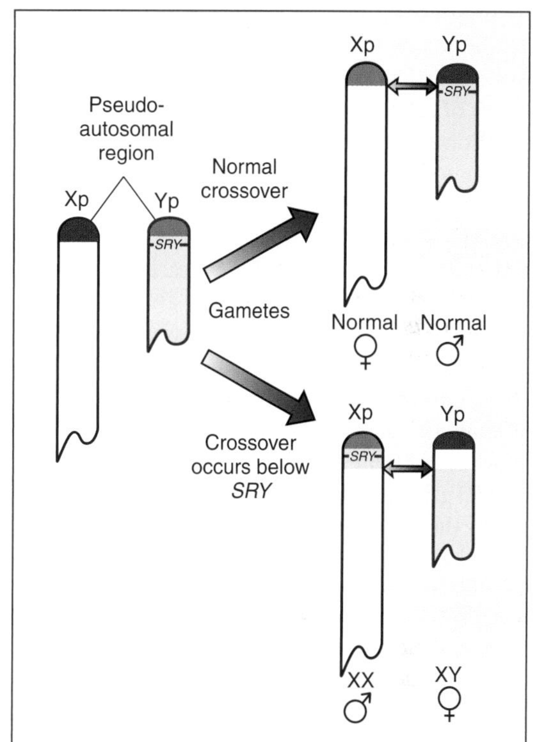

Fig. 4.30 Distal Short Arms of the X and Y Chromosomes Exchange Material During Meiosis in the Male. The region of the Y chromosome in which this crossover occurs is called the *pseudoautosomal region.* The *SRY* gene, which triggers the process leading to male gonadal differentiation, is located just outside the pseudoautosomal region. Occasionally, the crossover occurs on the centromeric side of the *SRY* gene, causing it to lie on an X chromosome instead of a Y chromosome. An offspring receiving this X chromosome will be an XX male, and an offspring receiving the Y chromosome will be an XY female. (A, from Raven PH, et al. *Biology*, 8th edition. New York: McGraw-Hill; 2008. B, From Jorde LB, Carey JC. *Medical genetics*, 5th edition. Philadelphia: Elsevier; 2016.)

Characteristics of Pedigrees

X-linked pedigrees show distinctive modes of inheritance. The most striking characteristic is that females seldom are affected. To express an X-linked recessive trait fully, a female must be homozygous: either both her parents are affected, or her father is affected, and her mother is a carrier. Such matings are rare.

The following are important principles of X-linked recessive inheritance:

1. The trait is seen much more often in males than in females.
2. Because a father can give a son only a Y chromosome, the trait is never transmitted from father to son.

3. The gene can be transmitted through a series of carrier females, causing the appearance of one or more "skipped generations."
4. The gene is passed from an affected father to all his daughters, who, as phenotypically normal carriers, transmit it to approximately half their sons, who are affected.

A relatively common X-linked recessive disorder is Duchenne muscular dystrophy (DMD), which affects approximately 1 in 3500 males. As its name suggests, this disorder is characterized by progressive muscle degeneration. Affected individuals usually are unable to walk by age 10 or 12 years. The disease affects the heart and respiratory muscles, and death caused by respiratory or cardiac failure usually occurs before age 20 years. Identification of the disease-causing gene (on the short arm of the X chromosome) has greatly increased our understanding of the disorder.[15]

The *DMD* gene is the largest gene ever found in humans, spanning more than 2 million DNA bases. It encodes a previously undiscovered muscle protein, termed dystrophin. Extensive study of dystrophin indicates that it plays an essential role in maintaining the structural integrity of muscle cells: it may also help regulate the activity of membrane proteins. When dystrophin is absent, as in DMD, the cell cannot survive, and muscle deterioration ensues. Most cases of DMD are caused by frameshift deletions of portions of the *DMD* gene and thus involve alterations of the amino acids encoded by the DNA following the deletion.

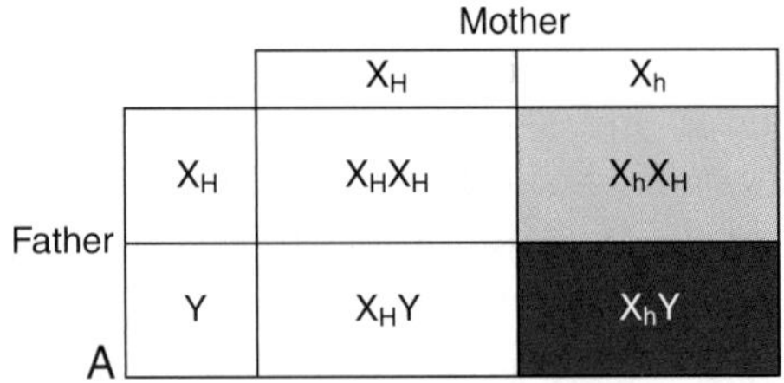

Father \ Mother	X_H	X_H
X_h	X_HX_h	X_HX_h
Y	X_HY	X_HY

B

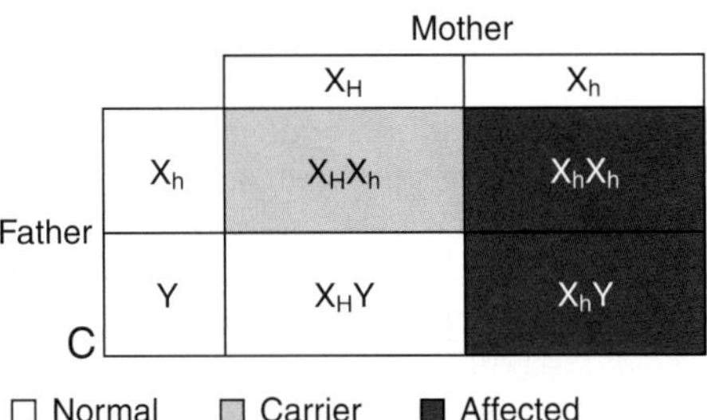

Fig. 4.31 Punnett Square and X-Linked Recessive Traits. (A) Punnett square for the mating of a normal male (X_HY) and a female carrier of an X-linked recessive gene (X_HX_h). **(B)** Punnett square for the mating of a normal female (X_HX_H) with a male affected by an X-linked recessive disease (X_hY). **(C)** Punnett square for the mating of a female who carries an X-linked recessive gene (X_HX_h) with a male who is affected with the disease caused by the gene (X_hY).

Recurrence Risks

The most common mating type involving X-linked recessive genes is the combination of a carrier female and a normal male (Fig. 4.31A). On average, the carrier mother will transmit the disease-causing allele to half her sons (who are affected) and half her daughters (who are carriers).

The other common mating type is an affected father and a normal mother (see Fig. 4.31B). In this situation, all the sons will be normal because the father can transmit only his Y chromosome to them. Because all the daughters must receive the father's X chromosome, they will all be heterozygous carriers. Because the sons *must* receive the Y chromosome and the daughters *must* receive the X chromosome with the disease gene, these are precise outcomes and not probabilities. None of the children will be affected.

The final mating pattern, less common than the other two, involves an affected father and a carrier mother (see Fig. 4.31C). With this pattern, on average, half the daughters will be heterozygous carriers, and half will be homozygous for the disease allele and thus affected. Half the sons will be normal, and half will be affected. Some X-linked recessive diseases, such as DMD, are fatal or incapacitating before the affected individual reaches reproductive age, and therefore, affected fathers are rare.

Sex-Limited and Sex-Influenced Traits

A sex-limited trait can occur in only one sex, often because of anatomic differences. Inherited uterine and testicular defects are two obvious examples. A sex-influenced trait occurs much more often in one sex than in the other. For example, male-pattern baldness occurs in both males and females but is much more common in males. Autosomal dominant breast cancer, which is much more commonly expressed in females than in males, is another example of a sex-influenced trait.

LINKAGE ANALYSIS AND GENE MAPPING

Locating genes on specific regions of chromosomes has been one of the most important goals of human genetics. The location and identification of a gene can tell much about the function of the gene, the interaction of the gene with other genes, and the likelihood that certain individuals will develop a genetic disease.

Classic Pedigree Analysis

During the first meiotic stage, the arms of homologous chromosome pairs intertwine and sometimes exchange portions of their DNA (Fig. 4.32) in a process known as crossover. During crossover, new combinations of alleles can be formed. For example, two loci on a chromosome have alleles *A* and *a* and alleles *B* and *b*. Alleles *A* and *B* are located together on one member of a chromosome pair, and alleles *a* and *b* are located on the other member. The genotype of this individual is denoted as *AB*/*a0b*.

As Fig. 4.32A shows, the allele pairs would be transmitted together when no crossover occurs. However, when crossover occurs (Fig. 4.32B), all four possible pairs of alleles can be transmitted to the offspring. The process of forming such new arrangements of alleles is called recombination. Loci that are located very close to one another are unlikely to experience recombination and are said to demonstrate linkage. The frequency of recombination can be assessed in families and is used to determine the relative positions of loci on chromosomes (the gene map, discussed below).

Complete Human Gene Map: Prospects and Benefits

The major goals of the Human Genome Project were to find the locations of all human genes (the "gene map") and to determine the entire human DNA sequence. These goals have now been accomplished, and the genes responsible for approximately 5000 mendelian conditions have been identified (Fig. 4.33).[7,16]

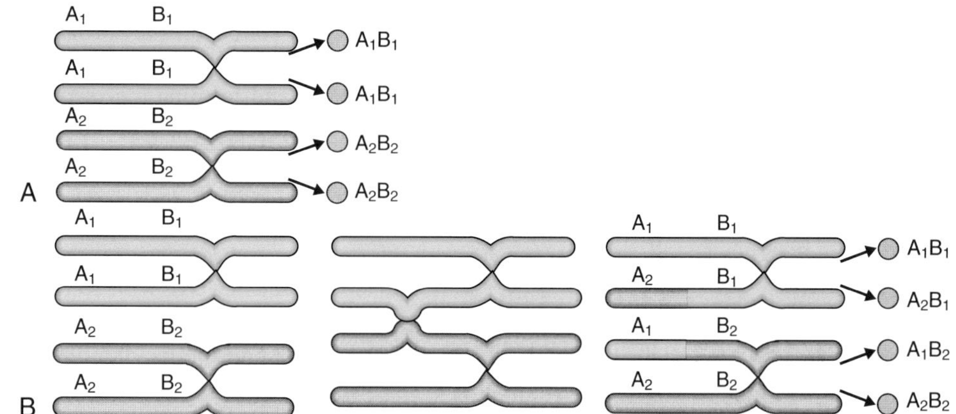

Fig. 4.32 Genetic Results of Crossover. (A) No crossing over. (B) Crossing over with recombination.

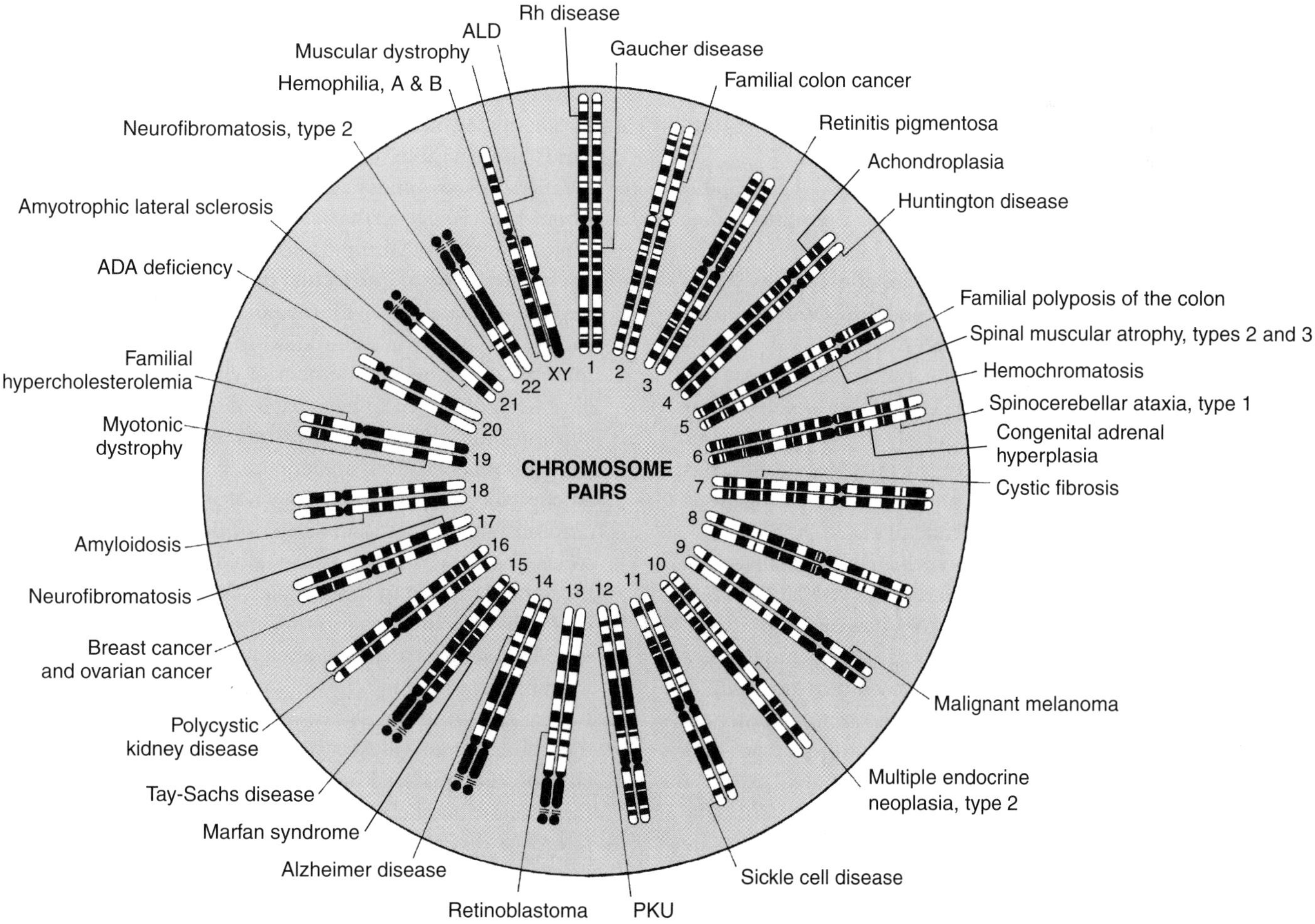

Fig. 4.33 Example of Diseases: A Gene Map. *ADA*, Adenosine deaminase; *ALD*, adrenoleukodystrophy; *PKU*, phenylketonuria.

This has greatly increased our understanding of the mechanisms that underlie many diseases, such as retinoblastoma, cystic fibrosis, neurofibromatosis, and Huntington disease. The project also has led to more accurate diagnosis of these conditions and, in some cases, more effective treatment.[17] DNA sequencing has become much less expensive and more efficient in recent years. Consequently, hundreds of thousands of individuals have now been sequenced, leading, in many cases, to the identification of disease-causing genes.[16]

SUMMARY REVIEW

DNA, RNA, and Proteins: Heredity at the Molecular Level

1. Genes, the basic units of inheritance, are composed of sequences of deoxyribonucleic acid (DNA) and are located on chromosomes.
2. Each subunit of DNA, called a nucleotide, is composed of one deoxyribose, a phosphate molecule, and one of four types of nitrogenous bases. The physical structure of DNA is a double helix. The two strands connect by the nitrogenous bases, with thymine bonding to adenine, and guanine bonding to cytosine.
3. The four DNA bases code for amino acids, which in turn make up proteins. The amino acids are specified by triplet sets of nitrogenous bases in specific orders, called codons. Several codons correspond to the same amino acid in many cases.
4. DNA replication is based on complementary base pairing, in which a single strand of DNA serves as the template for attracting complementary bases that form a new strand of DNA.
5. DNA polymerase is the primary enzyme involved in replication. It adds bases to the new DNA strand and performs "proofreading" functions.
6. A mutation is an alteration of genetic material (e.g., base pair substitution, frameshift mutation). Substances that cause mutations are called mutagens.
7. Mutations are rare events, and the rate of mutations varies from gene to gene. Mutational hot spots are DNA sequences with particularly high mutation rates.
8. Transcription and translation, the two basic processes in which proteins are specified by DNA, both involve ribonucleic acid (RNA). RNA is chemically similar to DNA, but it is single stranded, has a ribose sugar molecule, and has uracil rather than thymine as one of its four nitrogenous bases (uracil pairs with the base adenine).
9. Transcription is the process by which a DNA template synthesizes a RNA, thus forming messenger RNA (mRNA). Proteins called transcription factors are involved in the process of converting—or transcribing—DNA into RNA.
10. Much of the RNA sequence is spliced from the mRNA before the mRNA leaves the nucleus. The excised sequences are called introns, and those that remain to code for proteins are called exons.
11. Translation is the process by which RNA directs the synthesis of polypeptides. This process takes place in the ribosomes, which consist of proteins and ribosomal RNA (rRNA).
12. During translation, mRNA interacts with transfer RNA (tRNA), a molecule that has an attachment site for a specific amino acid and an anticodon, a region that matches up with a three-base codon on the mRNA. The ribosome moves along the mRNA, matching different tRNAs to codons on the mRNA, and forming a growing chain of amino acids called a polypeptide.

Chromosomes

1. Human cells consist of diploid somatic cells (body cells with 23 pairs of chromosomes, 46 total) and haploid gametes (sperm and egg cells with 23 total chromosomes).
2. Humans have 23 pairs of chromosomes. Twenty-two of these pairs are autosomes, ones that appear virtually identical (homologous) between males and females). The remaining pair consists of the sex chromosomes. Females have two homologous X chromosomes as their sex chromosomes; males have an X and a Y chromosome.
3. A karyogram is an ordered display of chromosomes arranged according to length and the location of the centromere. The karyogram is the visual representation of the individual's chromosome karyotype.
4. Various types of stains can be used to make chromosome bands more visible. Chromosome bands can be used to identify chromosomes and identify variations.
5. About 1 in 150 live births has a major diagnosable chromosome abnormality. Chromosome abnormalities are the leading known cause of intellectual disability and miscarriage.
6. Euploid cells are ones with the normal number of chromosomes. Polyploidy is a condition in which a cell has some multiple of the normal number of chromosomes. Humans have been observed to have triploidy (three copies of each chromosome) and tetraploidy (four copies of each chromosome); both conditions are lethal.
7. Aneuploidy is when a cell does not have a multiple of 23 chromosomes; there is an extra or missing single chromosome. Trisomy is a type of aneuploidy in which one chromosome is present in three copies. A partial trisomy is one in which only part of a chromosome is present in three copies. Monosomy is a type of aneuploidy in which one chromosome is present in only one copy.
8. In general, monosomies cause more severe physical defects than do trisomies, illustrating the principle that the loss of chromosome material has more severe consequences than the duplication of chromosome material.
9. Down syndrome, a trisomy of chromosome 21, is the best-known disease caused by a chromosome aberration. It affects 1 in 800 to 1 in 1000 live births.
10. Most aneuploidies of the sex chromosomes have less severe consequences than those of the other chromosomes.

11. The most observed sex chromosome aneuploidies are the 47,XXX karyotype, 45,X karyotype (Turner syndrome), 47,XXY karyotype (Klinefelter syndrome), and 47,XYY karyotype.
12. Abnormalities of chromosome structure include deletions, duplications, inversions, and translocations.

Elements of Formal Genetics

1. Mendelian traits are caused by single genes, each of which occupies a position, or locus, on a chromosome.
2. Alleles are different forms of genes located at the same locus on a chromosome.
3. At any given locus in a somatic cell, an individual has two genes, one from each parent. An individual may be homozygous (alleles are identical) or heterozygous (alleles are different) for a locus.
4. An individual's genotype is his or her genetic makeup, and the phenotype reflects the interaction of genotype and environment.
5. In a heterozygote, a dominant gene's effects mask those of a recessive gene. The recessive gene is expressed only when it is present in two copies.

Transmission of Genetic Diseases

1. Genetic diseases caused by single genes usually follow autosomal dominant, autosomal recessive, X-linked dominant, or X-linked recessive modes of inheritance. Pedigree charts are important tools in the analysis of modes of inheritance.
2. Autosomal dominant inheritance affects males and females equally and the two sexes are equally likely to transmit to their offspring. Skipped generations are not seen in classic autosomal dominant pedigrees. Affected heterozygous individuals transmit the trait to approximately half their children.
3. Recurrence risks specify the probability that future offspring will inherit a genetic disease. For single-gene diseases, recurrence risks remain the same for each offspring, regardless of the number of affected or unaffected offspring.
4. Many genetic diseases have a delayed age of onset: symptoms are not seen until sometime after birth.
5. The penetrance of a trait is the percentage of individuals with a specific genotype who also exhibit the expected phenotype. A gene that is not always expressed phenotypically is said to have incomplete penetrance.
6. Expressivity is the extent of variation in phenotype associated with a particular genotype. If the expressivity of a disease is variable, penetrance may be complete, but the severity of the disease can vary greatly.
7. Epigenetics involves changes, such as the methylation of DNA bases, that do not alter the DNA sequence but can alter the expression of genes.
8. Genomic imprinting, which is associated with methylation, results in differing expression of a disease gene, depending on which parent transmitted the gene.
9. Autosomal recessive inheritance affect males are females in equal proportions. Consanguinity (mating of related individuals) is sometimes present in families with autosomal recessive diseases, and it becomes more prevalent with rarer recessive diseases. The disease may be seen in siblings but not their parents. The recurrence risk for autosomal recessive diseases is 25%.
10. Most commonly, biologic parents of children with autosomal recessive diseases are both heterozygous carriers of the disease gene.
11. Carrier detection tests for autosomal recessive diseases are routinely available.
12. In each normal female somatic cell, one of the two X chromosomes is inactivated early in embryonic development. X inactivation is random, fixed, and incomplete (i.e., only part of the chromosome is inactivated) and involves methylation.
13. Gender is determined embryonically by the presence of the *SRY* gene on the Y chromosome. Embryos that have a Y chromosome (and thus the *SRY* gene) become males, whereas those lacking the Y chromosome become females. When the Y chromosome lacks the *SRY* gene, an XY female can be produced. Similarly, an X chromosome that contains the *SRY* gene can produce an XX male.
14. Sex linked inheritance is caused by mutations in genes on sex chromosomes. X-linked genes are those that are located on the X chromosome. Nearly all known X-linked diseases are caused by X-linked recessive genes.
15. Males are hemizygous for genes on the X chromosome. If a male inherits a recessive disease gene on the X chromosome, he will be affected by the disease because the Y chromosome does not carry a normal allele to counteract the effects.
16. X-linked recessive inheritance produces traits more often in males than in females because males need only one copy of the gene to express the disease. Because a father can give a son only a Y chromosome, biologic fathers cannot pass X-linked genes to their sons. Skipped generations often are seen in X-linked recessive disease pedigrees because the gene can be transmitted through carrier females. The gene is passed from an affected father to his daughters, who transmit to approximately half of their sons.
17. Recurrence risks for X-linked recessive diseases depend on the carrier and affected status of the mother and father.
18. A sex-limited trait is one that occurs only in one sex (gender). A sex-influenced trait is one that occurs more often in one sex than in the other.

Linkage Analysis and Gene Mapping

1. During meiosis I, crossover occurs and can cause recombination of alleles located on the same chromosome. Loci that are located very close to one another are unlikely to experience recombination and are said to demonstrate linkage.
2. The major goals of the Human Genome Project were to find the locations of all human genes (the "gene map") and to determine the entire human DNA sequence. These goals have now been accomplished and the genes responsible for approximately 5000 mendelian conditions have been identified.

REFERENCES

1. Bulaklak K, Gersbach CA. The once and future gene therapy. *Nat Commun*. 2020;11(1):5820.
2. Scholefield J, Harrison PT. Prime editing—an update on the field. *Gene Ther*. 2021;28:396–401.
3. Cramer P. Organization and regulation of gene transcription. *Nature*. 2019;573:45–54.
4. Suter DM. Transcription factors and DNA play hide and seek. *Trends Cell Biol*. 2020;30(6):491–500.
5. Yan J, et al. Systematic analysis of binding of transcription factors to noncoding variants. *Nature*. 2021;591:147–151.
6. Lu F, Lionnet T. Transcription factor dynamics. *Cold Spring Harb Perspect Biol*. 2021;13(11):a040949.
7. Jorde LB, ed. *Medical Genetics*. ed 5, St Louis: Elsevier; 2016.
8. Gardner RJM, Amor DJ. *Gardner and Sutherland's Chromosome Abnormalities and Genetic Counseling*. ed 5, Oxford: Oxford University Press; 2018.
9. Mila M, et al. Fragile X syndrome: an overview and update of the FMR1 gene. *Clin Genet*. 2017;93(2):197–205.
10. Hannan AJ. Tandem repeats mediating genetic plasticity in health and disease. *Nat Rev Genet*. 2018;19(5):286–298.
11. Rahman N. Realizing the promise of cancer predisposition genes. *Nature*. 2014;505(7483):302–308.
12. Kresak JL, Walsh M. Neurofibromatosis: a review of NF1, NF2, and schwannomatosis. *J Pediatr Genet*. 2016;5(2):98–104.
13. Lee JT, Bartolomei MS. X-inactivation, imprinting, and long noncoding RNAs in health and disease. *Cell*. 2013;152(6):1308–1323.
14. Larney C, et al. Switching on sex: transcriptional regulation of the testis-determining gene Sry. *Development*. 2014;141(11):2195–2205.
15. Flanigan KM. The muscular dystrophies. *Semin Neurol*. 2012;32(3):255–263.
16. Boycott KM, et al. International cooperation to enable the diagnosis of all rare genetic diseases. *Am J Hum Genet*. 2017;100(5):695–705.
17. Rehm HL. Evolving health care through personal genomics. *Nat Rev Genet*. 2017;18(4):259–267.

5

Genes, Environment-Lifestyle, and Common Diseases

Lynn B. Jorde

http://evolve.elsevier.com/Rogers/pathophysiology/

CHAPTER OUTLINE

Chapter 4 focuses on diseases that are caused by single genes or by abnormalities of single chromosomes. Much progress has been made in identifying specific mutations that cause these diseases, leading to better risk estimates and, in some cases, more effective treatment of the disease. However, these conditions form only a portion of the total burden of human genetic disease. Most congenital malformations are not caused by single genes or chromosome defects. Many common adult diseases, such as cancer, heart disease, and diabetes, have genetic components, but again they are usually not caused by single genes or by chromosomal abnormalities. These diseases, whose treatment collectively occupies the attention of most healthcare practitioners, are the result of a complex interplay of multiple genetic and environmental factors.

FACTORS INFLUENCING INCIDENCE OF DISEASE IN POPULATIONS

Concepts of Incidence and Prevalence

How common is a given disease, such as diabetes, in a population? Well-established measures are used to answer this question.

The incidence rate is the number of new cases of a disease reported during a specific period (typically 1 year) divided by the number of individuals in the population. The denominator is often expressed as *person-years*. The incidence rate can be contrasted with the prevalence rate, which is the proportion of the population affected by a disease at a specific point in time. Prevalence is thus determined by both the incidence rate and the length of the survival period in affected individuals. For example, the prevalence rate of acquired immunodeficiency syndrome (AIDS) is larger than the yearly incidence rate because most people with AIDS survive for at least several years after diagnosis.

Many diseases vary in prevalence from one population to another. Cystic fibrosis is relatively common among Europeans, occurring approximately once in every 2500 births. In contrast, it is quite rare in Asians, occurring only once in every 90,000 births. Similarly, sickle cell disease affects approximately 1 in 600 American Blacks, but it is seen much less frequently in Whites. Both diseases are single-gene disorders, and they vary among populations because disease-causing mutations are common in different populations. (This is in turn the result of differences in the evolutionary history of these populations.) Nongenetic (environmental) factors have little influence on the current prevalence of these diseases.

The picture often becomes more complex with the common diseases of adulthood. For example, colon cancer was until recently relatively rare in Japan, but it is the second most common cancer in the United States. In contrast, stomach cancer is common in Japan but relatively rare in the United States. These statistics, in themselves, cannot distinguish environmental from genetic influences in the two populations. However, because large numbers of Japanese emigrated first to Hawaii and then to the US mainland, we can observe what happens to the rates of stomach and colon cancer among the migrants. It is important that the Japanese émigrés maintained a genetic identity, marrying largely among themselves. Among first-generation Japanese in Hawaii, the frequency of colon cancer rose severalfold—not yet as high as in the US mainland but higher than that in Japan. Among second-generation Japanese on the US mainland, colon cancer rates rose to 5%, equal to the US average. At the same time, stomach cancer has become relatively rare among Japanese Americans.

These observations strongly indicate an important role for environmental factors in the etiology of cancers of the colon and stomach. In each case, diet is a likely culprit—a high-fat, low-fiber diet in the United States is thought to increase the risk of colon cancer, whereas techniques used to preserve and season the fish commonly eaten in Japan are thought to increase the risk of stomach cancer. It is interesting that the incidence of colon cancer in Japan has increased dramatically during the past several decades as the Japanese population has adopted a more "Western" diet. However, these results do not rule out the potential contribution of genetic factors in common cancers. Genes also play a role in the etiology of colon and other cancers.

Analysis of Risk Factors

The comparison just discussed is one example of the analysis of risk factors (in this case, diet) and their influence on the prevalence of disease in populations. A common measure of the effect of a specific risk factor is the relative risk. This quantity is expressed as a ratio:

$$\frac{\text{Increased rate of the disease among individuals exposed to a risk factor}}{\text{Incidence rate of the disease among individuals not exposed to a risk factor}}$$

A classic example of a relative risk analysis was carried out in a sample of more than 40,000 British physicians to determine the relationship between cigarette smoking and lung cancer. This study compared the incidence of death from lung cancer in physicians who smoked with those who did not. The incidence of death from lung cancer was 1.66 (per 1000 person-years) in heavy smokers (more than 25 cigarettes daily), but it was only 0.07 in the nonsmokers. The ratio of these two incidence rates is 1.66/0.07, which yields a relative risk of 23.7. Thus it is concluded that the risk of dying from lung cancer increased by approximately 24-fold in heavy smokers compared with nonsmokers. Many other studies have obtained similar risk figures.

Although cigarette smoking clearly increases one's risk of developing lung cancer (as well as heart disease, as will be seen later), it is equally clear that *most* smokers do not develop lung cancer. Other lifestyle factors are likely to contribute to one's risk of developing this disease (e.g., exposure to cancer-causing substances in the air, such as asbestos fibers). In addition, differences in genetic background may be involved. Smokers who have variants in genes that are involved in the metabolism of components of tobacco smoke (e.g., *CYP1A1* and *GSTM1*) are at significantly increased risk of developing lung cancer.

Many factors can influence the risk of acquiring a common disease such as cancer, diabetes, or high blood pressure. These include age, gender, diet, amount of exercise, and family history of the disease. Usually, complex interactions occur among these genetic and nongenetic factors. The effects of each factor can be quantified in terms of relative risks. The following discussion demonstrates how genetic and environmental factors contribute to the risk of developing common diseases.

PRINCIPLES OF MULTIFACTORIAL INHERITANCE

Basic Model

Traits in which variation is thought to be caused by the combined effects of multiple genes are polygenic ("many genes"). When environmental factors are also believed to cause variation in the trait, which is usually the case, the term multifactorial trait is used.[1]

Many quantitative traits (those, such as blood pressure, that are measured on a continuous numeric scale) are multifactorial. Because they are caused by the additive effects of many genetic and environmental factors, these traits tend to follow a normal, or bell-shaped, distribution in populations.

An example illustrates this concept. To begin with the simplest case, suppose (unrealistically) that height is determined by a single gene with two alleles, *A* and *a*. Allele *A* tends to make people tall, whereas allele *a* tends to make them short. If there is no dominance at this locus, then the three possible genotypes (*AA, Aa, aa*) will produce three phenotypes: tall, intermediate, and short, respectively. Assume that the gene frequencies of *A* and *a* are each 0.50. When looking at a population of individuals, the height distribution depicted in Fig. 5.1A, will be observed.

Now suppose, a bit more realistically, that height is determined by two loci instead of one. The second locus also has two alleles, *B* (tall) and *b* (short), and they affect height in exactly the same way as alleles *A* and *a*. There are now nine possible genotypes in our population: *aabb, aaBb, aaBB, Aabb, AaBb, AaBB, AAbb, AABb,* and *AABB*. An individual may have zero, one, two, three, or four "tall" alleles, so now five distinct phenotypes are possible (see Fig. 5.1B). Although the height distribution in this fictional population is still not normal compared with an actual population, it approaches a normal distribution more closely than in the single-gene case just described.

From extension of this example, *many* genes and environmental factors influence height, each having a small effect. Then many phenotypes are possible, each differing slightly from the others, and the height distribution of the population approaches the bell-shaped curve shown in Fig. 5.1C.

It should be emphasized that the individual genes underlying a multifactorial trait such as height follow the mendelian principles of segregation and independent assortment, just like any other gene. The only difference is that many of them *act together* to influence the trait. More than 400 genes have now been shown to be associated with variation in human height.

Blood pressure is another example of a multifactorial trait. A correlation exists between parents' blood pressures (systolic and diastolic) and those of their children. The evidence is good that this correlation is partially caused by genes, but blood pressure is

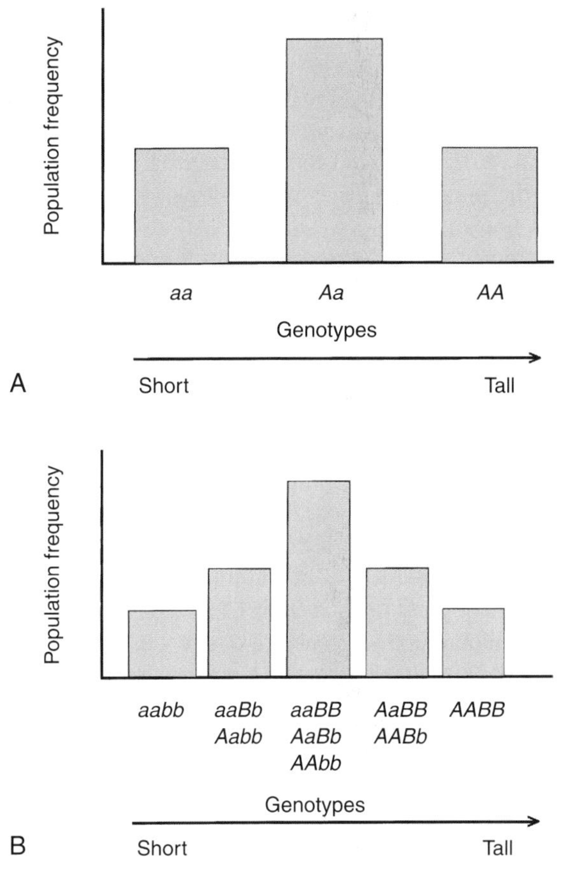

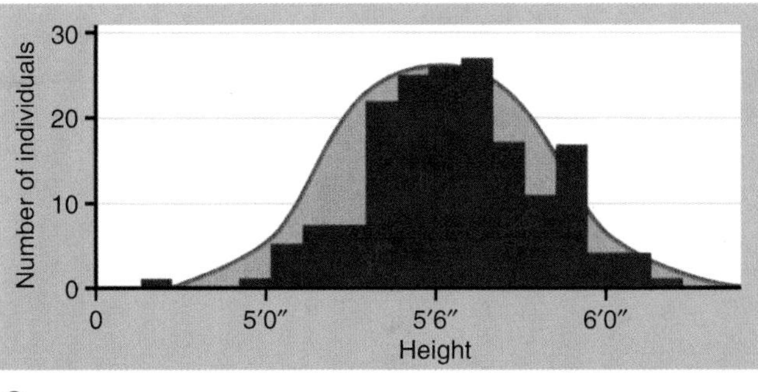

Fig. 5.1 **Distribution of Height.** (A) Distribution of height in a population, assuming that height is controlled by a single locus with genotypes *AA, Aa,* and *aa.* (B) Distribution of height, assuming that height is controlled by two loci. Five distinct genotypes are shown instead of three, and the distribution begins to look more like the normal distribution. (C) Height is portrayed, realistically, as a trait with a continuous statistical distribution. Because many genes contribute to height and tend to segregate independently of one another, the cumulative contribution of different combinations of alleles to height forms a continuous distribution of possible heights, in which the extremes are much rarer than the intermediate values. Variation also can be caused by environmental factors such as nutrition. (A and B, Adapted from Jorde LB, Carey JC, Bamshad MJ. *Medical genetics*, 6th edition. Philadelphia: Elsevier; 2020; C, From Raven PH, et al. *Biology*, 8th edition. New York: McGraw-Hill; 2008.)

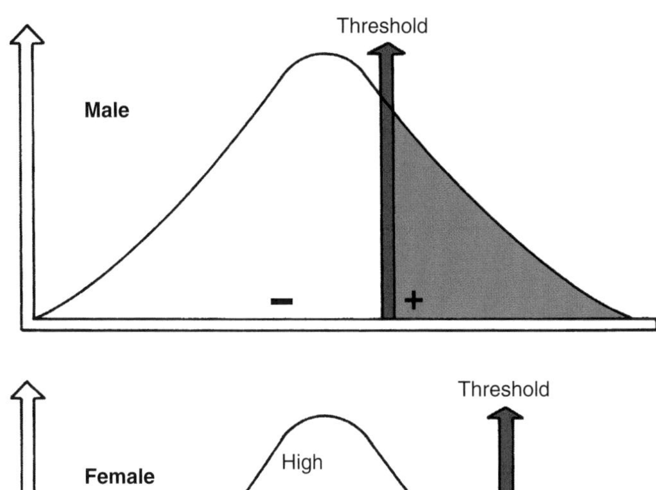

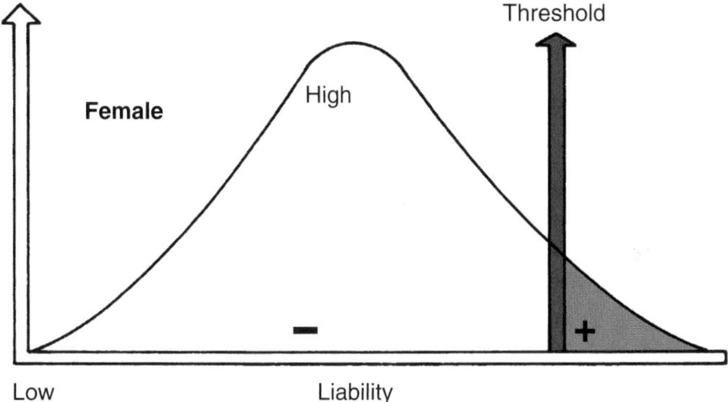

Fig. 5.2 **Threshold of Liability for Pyloric Stenosis in Males and Females.** To be affected with the disease, an individual must exceed the threshold on the liability distribution. This figure shows two thresholds, a lower one for males and a higher one for females (as in pyloric stenosis; see text). (From Jorde LB, Carey JC, Bamshad MJ. *Medical genetics*, 6th edition. Philadelphia: Elsevier; 2020)

also influenced by environmental factors, such as diet, exercise, and stress. Two goals of genetic research are the identification and measurement of the relative roles of genes and environment in the causation of multifactorial diseases.

Threshold Model

Several diseases do not follow the bell-shaped distribution. Instead, they appear to be either present or absent in individuals, yet they do not follow the inheritance patterns expected of single-gene diseases. A commonly used explanation for such diseases is that there is an underlying **liability distribution** for the disease in a population (Fig. 5.2).

Those individuals who are on the "low" end of the distribution have little chance of developing the disease in question (i.e., they have few of the alleles or environmental factors that would cause the disease). Individuals who are closer to the "high" end of the distribution have more of the disease-causing genes and environmental factors and are more likely to develop the disease. For diseases that are either present or absent, it is thought that a **threshold of liability** must be crossed before the disease is expressed. Below the threshold, an individual appears normal; above it, he or she is affected by the disease.

A disease that is thought to correspond to this threshold model is *pyloric stenosis*, a disorder that presents shortly after birth and is caused by a narrowing or obstruction of the pylorus, the area between the stomach and intestine. Chronic vomiting,

TABLE 5.1 Recurrence Risks (%) for Pyloric Stenosis, Subdivided by Genders of Affected Probands and Relatives

	MALE PROBANDS		FEMALE PROBANDS	
Relatives	**London**	**Belfast**	**London**	**Belfast**
Brothers	3.8	9.6	9.2	12.5
Sisters	2.7	3.0	3.8	3.8

NOTE: The risks differ somewhat between the two populations. Data from Carter CO. Genetics of common single malformations. *British Medical Bulletin,* 1976;32(1):21–26.

constipation, weight loss, and imbalance of electrolyte levels result from the condition, but it sometimes resolves spontaneously or can be corrected by surgery. The prevalence of pyloric stenosis is approximately 3 per 1000 live births in Whites. It is much more common in males than females, affecting 1 of 200 males and 1 of 1000 females. It is thought that this difference in prevalence reflects two thresholds in the liability distribution—a lower one in males and a higher one in females (see Fig. 5.2). A lower male threshold implies that fewer disease-causing factors are required to generate the disorder in males.

The liability threshold concept may explain the pattern of recurrence risks for pyloric stenosis seen in Table 5.1. Note that males, having a lower threshold, always have a higher risk than females. However, the sibling recurrence risk also depends on the sex of the proband (i.e., the first affected individual diagnosed in a family). It is higher when the proband is female than when the proband is male. This reflects the concept that females, having a higher liability threshold, must be exposed to more disease-causing factors than males to develop the disease. Thus a family with an affected female must have more genetic and environmental risk factors, producing a higher recurrence risk for pyloric stenosis in future offspring. It would be expected that the highest risk category would be *male* relatives of *female* probands; Table 5.1 shows that this is the case.

A similar pattern has been observed in studies of *autism spectrum disorder*, a behavioral disorder in which the male to female ratio is close to 3:1.[2] As expected for a multifactorial disorder, the recurrence risk for siblings of male probands (6.6) is lower than that of siblings of female probands (10.2).[3] When the sex ratio for a disease is reversed (i.e., more affected females than males), one would expect a higher recurrence risk when the proband is male.

Several other congenital malformations are thought to correspond to this model. They include isolated *cleft lip and/or cleft palate (CL/P), neural tube defects (anencephaly, spina bifida), clubfoot (talipes)*, and some forms of congenital heart disease. In this context, "isolated" means that this is the only observed disease feature (i.e., the feature is not part of a larger constellation of findings, as in CL/P secondary to trisomy 13). In addition, many common adult diseases, such as *hypertension, coronary heart disease* (CHD), *stroke, diabetes mellitus* (types 1 and 2), and *some cancers*, are caused by complex genetic and environmental factors and can thus be considered multifactorial diseases.

Recurrence Risks and Transmission Patterns

Although sibling recurrence risks can be given with confidence for single-gene diseases (e.g., 50% for typical autosomal dominant diseases, 25% for autosomal recessive diseases), the situation is more complicated for multifactorial diseases. This is because the number of genes contributing to the disease is usually not known, the precise allelic constitution of the parents is not known, and the extent of environmental effects can vary substantially. For most multifactorial diseases, **empirical risks** (i.e., risks based on direct observation of data) have been derived. To estimate empirical risks, a large series of families is examined in which one child has developed the disease (the proband). Then the siblings of each proband are surveyed to calculate the percentage of siblings who also have developed the disease. For example, in the United States approximately 3% of siblings of individuals with neural tube defects also have neural tube defects (Box 5.1). Thus the recurrence risk for parents who have had one child with a neural tube defect is 3% in the United States. For conditions such as CL/P that are not lethal or severely debilitating, recurrence risks also can be estimated for the offspring of affected parents. Because each multifactorial disease has different numbers and types of risk factors, empirical recurrence risks vary for each disease.

In contrast to most single-gene diseases, recurrence risks for multifactorial diseases can change substantially from one population to another because gene frequencies as well as environmental factors can differ among populations (note the differences between the London and Belfast populations in Table 5.1).

It is sometimes difficult to distinguish polygenic or multifactorial diseases from single-gene diseases that have reduced penetrance or variable expression. Large data sets and good epidemiologic data are necessary to make the distinction. Several criteria are commonly used to define multifactorial inheritance.

First, *the recurrence risk becomes higher if more than one family member is affected*. For example, the sibling recurrence risk for a *ventricular septal defect* (VSD, a type of congenital heart defect) is 3% if one sibling has been affected by a VSD but increases to approximately 10% if two siblings have been diagnosed with VSDs.[4] The same trend is seen for other multifactorial diseases such as neural tube defects and autism. In contrast, the recurrence risk for single-gene diseases remains the same regardless of the number of affected siblings. It should be emphasized that this increase does not mean that the family's risk has changed. Rather, it means that there is more information about the family's true risk; because they have had two affected children, they are probably located higher on the liability distribution than a family with only one affected child. In other words, they have more risk factors (genetic or environmental) and are more likely to produce an affected child.

Second, *if the expression of the disease in the proband is more severe, the recurrence risk is higher*. This is again consistent with the liability model because a more severe expression indicates that the affected individual is at the extreme tail end of the liability distribution (see Fig. 5.2). His or her relatives are thus at a higher risk for inheriting disease genes. For example,

BOX 5.1 Neural Tube Defects

Neural tube defects (NTDs), which include *anencephaly, spina bifida*, and *encephalocele* (as well as several other less common forms), are one of the most important classes of birth defects, and they are seen in 0.5–2 of 1000 pregnancies. The prevalence of NTDs among different populations varies considerably, with an especially high rate among some northern Chinese populations (as high as 6 or more per 1000 births). The prevalence of NTDs has been decreasing in many parts of the United States and Europe during the past three decades, partly because of dietary changes.

Normally the neural tube closes at approximately the fourth week of gestation. A defect in closure, or a subsequent reopening of the neural tube, results in a neural tube defect. Spina bifida (see Fig. 5.4A) is the most observed NTD and consists of a protrusion of spinal tissue through the vertebral column (the tissue usually includes meninges, spinal cord, and nerve roots). Approximately 75% of individuals with spina bifida have secondary hydrocephalus, which sometimes in turn produces intellectual disability. Paralysis or muscle weakness, lack of sphincter control, and clubfeet are often observed. A study conducted in British Columbia showed that survival rates for people with spina bifida have improved dramatically over the past several decades. Less than 30% of people born between 1952 and 1969 survived to 10 years of age, whereas 65% of those born between 1970 and 1986 survived to this age. Anencephaly (see Fig. 5.4B) is characterized by partial or complete absence of the cranial vault and calvarium and partial or complete absence of the cerebral hemispheres. At least two-thirds of newborns with anencephaly are stillborn; term deliveries do not survive more than a few hours or days.

NTDs are thought to arise from a combination of genetic and environmental factors. In most populations surveyed thus far, empirical recurrence risks for siblings of affected people range from 2% to 5%. Consistent with a multifactorial model, the recurrence risk increases with additional affected siblings. Studies conducted in Great Britain showed that the sibling recurrence risk was approximately 5% when one sibling was affected and 10% when two were affected. A Hungarian study showed that the overall prevalence of NTDs was 1 in 300 births and that the sibling recurrence risks were 3%, 12%, and 25% after one, two, and three affected offspring, respectively. Recurrence risks tend to be slightly lower in populations with lower NTD prevalence rates, as predicted by the multifactorial model. Recurrence risk data support the idea that the major forms of NTDs are caused by similar factors. An anencephalic conception increases the recurrence risk for subsequent spina bifida conceptions, and vice versa.

NTDs can usually be diagnosed prenatally, sometimes by ultrasound and usually by an elevation in α-fetoprotein (AFP) level in the maternal serum or amniotic fluid (see Chapter 20). A spina bifida lesion can be either open or closed (i.e., covered with a layer of skin). Fetuses with open spina bifida are more likely to be detected by AFP assays.

A major epidemiologic finding is that mothers who supplement their diet with folic acid at the time of conception are less likely to produce children with NTDs. This result has been replicated in several different populations and thus appears to be well confirmed. It has been estimated that as many as 50% to 70% of NTDs can be avoided simply by dietary folic acid supplementation. (Traditional prenatal vitamin supplements have little effect because administration does not usually begin until well after the time that the neural tube closes.) It is now recommended that all women of reproductive age supplement their diet with 0.4 mg of folic acid each day; many foods in the United States are supplemented with folic acid. Consequently, average folate levels in US females have doubled, and the incidence of neural tube defects has declined by 30% to 50% in the past decade.

Because mothers would be likely to ingest similar amounts of folic acid from one pregnancy to the next, folic acid deficiency could well account for at least part of the elevated sibling recurrence risk for NTDs. This is an important example of a *nongenetic* factor that contributes to familial clustering of a disease. It is likely that there is genetic variation in response to folic acid, which helps to explain why most mothers with folic acid deficiency do not bear children with NTDs and why some who ingest adequate amounts of folic acid nonetheless bear children with NTDs. To address this issue, researchers are testing for associations between NTDs and variants in several genes whose products (e.g., methylene tetrahydrofolate reductase) are involved in folic acid metabolism.

Data from Copp AJ, Stanier P, Greene ND. Neural tube defects: Recent advances, unsolved questions, and controversies. *Lancet Neurology*, 2013;12(8):799–810; Daly LE, Kirke PN, Molloy A, et al. Folate levels and neural tube defects: implications for prevention. *JAMA*, 1995;274(21):1698–1702.

the occurrence of a bilateral (both sides) CL/P confers a higher recurrence risk on family members than does the occurrence of a unilateral (one side) cleft.

Third, *the recurrence risk is higher if the proband is of the less commonly affected sex* (see the preceding discussion of pyloric stenosis). This is because an affected individual of the less susceptible sex is usually at a more extreme position on the liability distribution.

Fourth, *the recurrence risk for the disease usually decreases rapidly in more remotely related relatives* (Table 5.2). Although the recurrence risk for single-gene diseases decreases by 50% with each degree of relationship (e.g., an autosomal dominant disease has a 50% recurrence risk for siblings, 25% for uncle-nephew relationships, 12.5% for first cousins), it decreases much more quickly for multifactorial diseases. This reflects the fact that many genes and environmental factors must combine to produce a trait. All the necessary risk factors are unlikely to be present in less closely related family members.

Finally, *if the prevalence of the disease in a population is f, the risk for offspring and siblings of probands is approximately* $\sqrt{f}$. This does not hold true for single-gene traits because their recurrence risks are largely independent of population prevalence. It is not an absolute rule for multifactorial traits either, but many such diseases tend to conform to this prediction. Examination of the risks given in Table 5.2 shows that the first three diseases follow the prediction well. However, the observed sibling risk for the fourth disease, infantile autism, is substantially higher than that predicted by $\sqrt{f}$.

TABLE 5.2 Recurrence Risks (%) for First-, Second-, and Third-Degree Relatives

	RISK			
Degree	First Degree	Second Degree	Third Degree	General Population
Cleft lip/palate	4	0.7	0.3	0.1
Clubfoot	2.5	0.5	0.2	0.1
Congenital hip dislocation	5	0.6	0.4	0.2

NATURE AND NURTURE: DISENTANGLING THE EFFECTS OF GENES AND ENVIRONMENT

Family members share genes and a common environment. Family resemblance in traits such as blood pressure reflects both genes (nature) and environment (nurture). For centuries people have debated the relative importance of these two types of factors. It is a mistake, of course, to view them as mutually exclusive. Few traits are influenced only by genes or only by environmental factors. Most are influenced by both. It is useful to try to determine the *relative* influence of genetic and environmental factors (Fig. 5.3). See Emerging Science Box: Polygenic Risk Scores and Disease Prediction for more information on polygenic risk scores and disease prediction. This can lead to a better understanding of disease etiology. It can also help in planning public health strategies. A disease in which the genetic influence is relatively small, such as lung cancer, may be prevented most effectively through emphasis on lifestyle changes (avoidance of tobacco). When a disease has a relatively larger genetic component, as in breast cancer, examination of family history should be emphasized in addition to lifestyle modification. Here, two research strategies are reviewed that often are used to estimate the relative influence of genes and environment: twin studies and adoption studies.

Twin Studies

Twins occur with a frequency of approximately 1 in 100 births in White populations. They are a bit more common in Blacks and a bit less common among Asians. **Monozygotic (MZ, identical) twins** originate when the developing embryo divides to form two separate but identical embryos. Because they are genetically identical, MZ twins are an example of natural clones. **Dizygotic (DZ, fraternal) twins** are the result of a double ovulation followed by the fertilization of each egg by a different sperm. Thus DZ twins are genetically no more similar than siblings. Because two different sperm cells are required to fertilize the two eggs, it is possible for each DZ twin to have a different father. MZ twinning rates are constant across populations, whereas DZ twinning rates vary somewhat. DZ twinning increases with maternal age until approximately 40 years, after which it declines.

Because MZ twins are genetically identical, any differences between them should be caused only by environmental effects.[5] MZ twins should thus resemble one another very closely for traits that are strongly influenced by genes. DZ twins provide a convenient comparison because their environmental differences should be like those of MZ twins but their genetic differences are as great as those between siblings. Twin studies thus usually consist of comparisons between MZ and DZ twins.[6]

If both members of a twin pair share a trait (e.g., a CL), they are said to be **concordant**. If they do not share the trait, they are **discordant**. For a trait determined totally by genes, MZ twins should always be concordant, whereas DZ twins should be concordant less often, because they, like full siblings, share only 50% of their DNA. Concordance rates may differ between opposite-sex DZ twin pairs and same-sex DZ pairs for some traits, such as those that have different frequencies in males and females. For such traits, only same-sex DZ twin pairs should be used when comparing MZ and DZ concordance rates, because MZ twins are necessarily of the same sex.

EMERGING SCIENCE BOX
Polygenic Risk Scores and Disease Prediction

The great majority of DNA variants associated with common diseases have only a small effect on disease risk. Individually, they have little value in predicting disease risk. However, by amalgamating the predicted effects of these variants, it is possible to identify a portion of the population that has a significantly elevated risk of disease. The **polygenic risk score** (also sometimes termed genetic risk score) adds the effects of many disease-associated variants together. For everyone, the number of copies of a disease-associated variant (either 0, 1, or 2) is weighted (multiplied) by the increase in risk associated with the variant (e.g., a variant that increases risk by 5% could have a weight of 0.05, while a variant that increases risk by 10% would have a weight of 0.10). The weighted effects of all disease-associated variants are then added together to yield the risk score for an individual.

As discussed in the text, genetic studies have revealed hundreds of DNA variants associated with nearly every common disease (e.g., heart disease, common cancers, diabetes, psychiatric diseases). Polygenic risk scores have now been estimated for these diseases. Persons with high scores (e.g., top 1%, or top 5%, representing the right tail of the distribution shown in Fig. 5.7) have substantial elevations in disease risk. The increase in risk, which is typically on the order of threefold to fivefold, is like the elevation in risk associated with some single-gene disorders, such as autosomal dominant familial hypercholesterolemia.

Polygenic risk score estimation can be sensitive to the same factors that influence disease identification studies, such as differences in genetic ancestry. Thus a score estimated for one population group (e.g., East Asians) is unlikely to be accurate for another. Before polygenic risk scores are used widely in the clinical setting, it will be important to validate them with extensive follow-up studies. With appropriate evaluation and validation, polygenic risk scores have the potential to identify members of the population who may need earlier or more aggressive screening or intervention. Their use could become an important component of precision medicine.

Data from Khera AV, et al. Genome-wide polygenic scores for common diseases identify individuals with risk equivalent to monogenic mutations. *Nature Genetics*, 2018;50(9):1219–1224. https://doi.org/10.1038/s41588-018-0183-z

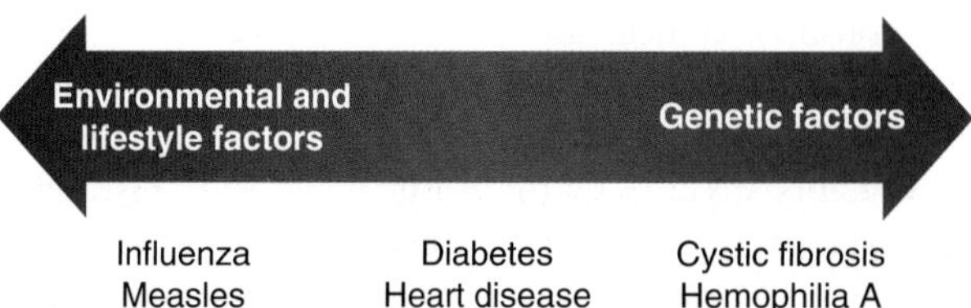

Fig. 5.3 Continuum of Genetic Diseases. Some diseases (e.g., cystic fibrosis) are strongly determined by genes, whereas others (e.g., infectious diseases) are strongly determined by environmental factors. (From Jorde LB, Carey JC, Bamshad MJ. *Medical genetics*, 6th edition. Philadelphia: Elsevier; 2020.)

TABLE 5.3 Concordance Rates in Monozygotic and Dizygotic Twins for Selected Traits and Diseases

	CONCORDANCE RATE		
Trait or Disease	**MZ Twins**	**DZ Twins**	**Heritability**
Affective disorder (bipolar)	0.79	0.24	>1[a]
Affective disorder (unipolar)	0.54	0.19	0.7
Alcoholism	>0.6	<0.3	0.6
Autism	0.92	0	>1
Blood pressure (diastolic)[b]	0.58	0.27	0.62
Blood pressure (systolic)[b]	0.55	0.25	0.6
Body fat percentage[b]	0.73	0.22	>1
Body mass index[b]	0.95	0.53	0.84
Cleft lip/palate	0.38	0.08	0.6
Clubfoot	0.32	0.03	0.58
Dermatoglyphics (finger ridge count)[b]	0.95	0.49	0.92
Diabetes mellitus	0.45–0.96	0.03–0.37	>1
Diabetes mellitus (type 1)	0.55	–	–
Diabetes mellitus (type 2)	0.9	–	–
Epilepsy (idiopathic)	0.69	0.14	>1
Height[b]	0.94	0.44	1
Intelligence quotient (IQ)[b]	0.76	0.51	0.5
Measles	0.95	0.87	0.16
Multiple sclerosis	0.28	0.03	0.5
Myocardial infarction (males)	0.39	0.26	0.26
Myocardial infarction (females)	0.44	0.14	0.6
Schizophrenia	0.47	0.12	0.7
Spina bifida	0.72	0.33	0.78

NOTE: Heritability, which is defined as the proportion of the variation in a trait that is due to genetic factors, can be measured as $2(C_{MZ} - C_{DZ})$, where C_{MZ} and C_{DZ} are the concordance rates for MZ twins and DZ twins, respectively. These figures were compiled from a large variety of sources and represent primarily European and US populations.

DZ, Dizygotic; *MZ*, monozygotic.

[a]Several heritability estimates exceed 1. Because it is impossible for greater than 100% of the variance of a trait to be genetically determined, these values indicate that other factors, such as shared environmental factors, must be operating.

[b]Because these are quantitative traits, correlation coefficients are given rather than concordance rates.

Table 5.3 gives concordance rates for several traits. Note that the concordance rates for contagious diseases such as measles are quite similar in MZ and DZ twins. This is expected because a contagious disease is unlikely to be influenced markedly by genes. In contrast, the concordance rates are quite dissimilar for *schizophrenia* and *bipolar affective disorder*, suggesting a sizable genetic component for these diseases. The MZ correlations for dermatoglyphics (fingerprints), which are determined almost entirely by genes, are close to 1.0.

At one time, twins were thought to provide a perfect "natural laboratory" in which to determine the relative influences of genetics and environment, but several difficulties arose. One of the most important is the assumption that the environments of MZ and DZ twins are equally similar. As one would expect, MZ twins are often treated more similarly than DZ twins. A greater similarity in environment can make MZ twins more concordant for a trait, inflating the apparent influence of genes. In addition, MZ twins may be more likely to seek the same type of environment, further reinforcing environmental similarity. On the other hand, it has been suggested that MZ twins tend to develop personality differences to assert their individuality.

Adoption Studies

Studies of adopted children also are used to estimate the genetic contribution to a multifactorial trait. Children born to parents who have a disease but are then subsequently adopted by parents lacking the disease can be studied to find out whether these children develop the disease. In some cases, such children develop the disease more often than a comparative control population (i.e., adopted children who were born to parents who do *not* have the disease). This provides some evidence that genes may be involved in the causation of the disease, because the adopted children do not share an environment with their affected natural parents. For example, approximately 8% to 10% of adopted children of a schizophrenic parent develop *schizophrenia*, whereas only 1% of adopted children of unaffected parents develop schizophrenia.

As with twin studies, several precautions must be exercised in interpreting the results of adoption studies. First, prenatal environmental influences could have long-lasting effects on an adopted child. Second, children are sometimes adopted after they are several years old, ensuring that some environmental influence would have been imparted by the natural parents. Finally, adoption agencies sometimes try to match the adoptive parents with the natural parents in terms of background, socioeconomic status, and other factors. All these factors could exaggerate the apparent influence of biologic inheritance.[7]

These reservations, as well as those summarized for twin studies, underscore the need for caution in basing conclusions on twin and adoption studies. These approaches do not provide definitive measures of the role of genes in multifactorial disease, nor can they identify specific genes responsible for disease. Instead, they serve a useful purpose in providing a preliminary indication of the extent to which a multifactorial disease may be caused by genetic factors. Sophisticated molecular techniques are being used to identify the specific genes that underlie predisposition to multifactorial diseases.

This discussion should make clear that most common diseases are not the result of either genetics *or* environment. Instead, genetic and nongenetic factors usually interact to influence one's likelihood of developing a common disease. In some cases, a genetic predisposition may interact with an environmental factor to increase the risk of disease acquisition to a much higher level than would either factor acting alone. A

BOX 5.2 α1-Antitrypsin Deficiency: Interaction of Genes and Environment-Lifestyle

α_1-Antitrypsin (AAT) deficiency is one of the most common autosomal recessive disorders among Whites, affecting approximately 1 in 2500 members of this ethnic group. AAT, synthesized primarily in the liver, is a serine protease inhibitor. It does bind trypsin, as its name suggests. However, AAT binds much more strongly to neutrophil elastase, a protease that is produced by neutrophils (a type of leukocyte) in response to infections and irritants. It carries out its binding and inhibitory role primarily in the lower respiratory tract, where it prevents elastase from digesting the alveolar septi of the lung.

Individuals with less than 10%–15% of the normal level of AAT activity will experience significant lung damage and typically develop emphysema during their 30s, 40s, or 50s. In addition, at least 10% develop liver cirrhosis because of the accumulation of variant AAT molecules in the liver; AAT deficiency accounts for nearly 20% of all nonalcoholic liver cirrhosis cases in the United States. An important feature of this disease is that cigarette smokers with AAT deficiency develop emphysema much earlier than do nonsmokers. This is because cigarette smoke irritates lung tissue, increasing secretion of neutrophil elastase. At the same time, it inactivates AAT, so there is also less inhibition of elastase. One study showed that the median age of survival of nonsmokers with AAT deficiency was 62 years, whereas it was only 40 years for smokers with this disease. Because the combination of cigarette smoking (an environmental factor) and the AAT mutation (a genetic factor) produces more severe disease than either factor alone, it is an example of a gene-environment interaction.

Typically, AAT deficiency is tested first by a straightforward assay for reduced serum AAT concentration. Because a variety of conditions can reduce serum AAT level, additional testing, through a type of protein electrophoresis or DNA testing, is carried out to confirm a diagnosis of AAT deficiency. Direct DNA testing became feasible with the identification of *SERPINA1*, the gene that encodes AAT. More than 100 *SERPINA1* mutations have been identified, but only 2 missense variants, labeled the *S* and *Z* alleles, are common and clinically significant. Approximately 95% of cases of AAT deficiency are either *ZZ* homozygotes or *SZ* compound heterozygotes. The latter genotype generally produces less severe disease symptoms. Two large studies have indicated that the risk of developing emphysema among *ZZ* homozygotes is 70% for nonsmokers and 90% for smokers.

Data from Abboud RT, Nelson TN, Jung B, et al. Alpha1-antitrypsin deficiency: A clinical-genetic overview. *Application of Clinical Genetics*, 2011;4:55–65; Stockley RA, Turner AM. α-1-Antitrypsin deficiency: Clinical variability, assessment, and treatment. *Trends in Molecular Medicine*, 2014;20(2):105–115.

good example of a gene-environment interaction is given by α_1-antitrypsin deficiency, a genetic condition that causes pulmonary emphysema and is greatly exacerbated by cigarette smoking (Box 5.2).

GENETICS OF COMMON DISEASES

Some common multifactorial disorders, the congenital malformations, are present at birth. Others, including heart disease, cancer, diabetes, and most psychiatric disorders, are seen primarily in adolescents and adults. Because these disorders are complex, unraveling their genetics is a daunting task. Nonetheless, significant progress is being made.

TABLE 5.4 Prevalence Rates of Common Congenital Malformations in Whites

Disorder	Prevalence Per 1000 Births (Approximate)
Cleft lip/palate	1
Clubfoot	1
Congenital heart defects	4–8
Hydrocephaly	0.5–2.5
Isolated cleft palate	0.4
Neural tube defects	1–3
Pyloric stenosis	3

Congenital Malformations

Congenital diseases are present at birth. Approximately 2% of newborns present with a congenital malformation; most of these are multifactorial in etiology. Table 5.4 lists some more common congenital malformations. Sibling recurrence risks for most of these disorders range from 1% to 5%.

Some congenital malformations, such as CL/P and pyloric stenosis, are relatively easy to repair and thus are not considered to be serious problems. Others, such as neural tube defects, usually have more severe consequences. Although some cases of congenital malformations occur in the absence of any other problems, it is quite common for them to be associated with other disorders. For example, hydrocephaly and clubfoot are often seen secondary to spina bifida, CL/P is often seen in babies with trisomy 13, and congenital heart defects are seen in children with many other disorders, including Down syndrome (Fig. 5.4).

Environmental factors also cause some congenital malformations. An example is thalidomide, a sedative used during pregnancy in the early 1960s. When ingested during early pregnancy, this drug often caused phocomelia (severely shortened limbs) in babies. Maternal exposure to retinoic acid, which is used to treat acne, can cause congenital defects of the heart, ear, and central nervous system. Maternal rubella infection can cause congenital heart defects.

Multifactorial Disorders in the Adult Population

Until quite recently, very little was known about specific genes responsible for common adult diseases. With the more powerful laboratory and analytic techniques now available, this situation is changing. This section reviews recent progress in understanding the genetics of the major common adult diseases.

Coronary Heart Disease

It is well known that CHD is the leading killer of Americans, accounting for approximately 25% of all deaths in the United States. It is caused by *atherosclerosis* (narrowing because of the formation of lipid-laden lesions) of the coronary arteries. This narrowing impedes blood flow to the heart and can eventually result in a *myocardial infarction* (destruction of heart tissue caused by an inadequate supply of oxygen). When

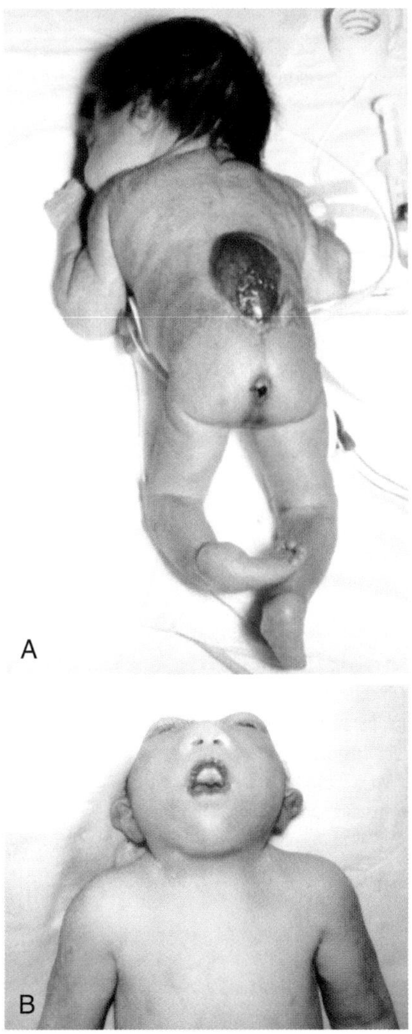

Fig. 5.4 Spina Bifida and Anencephaly. (A) Spina bifida in a newborn. **(B)** Anencephaly, showing the absence of the cranial vault. (From Jones KL, *Smith DM. Smith's recognizable patterns of human malformation*, 6th edition. Philadelphia: Saunders; 2006:705.)

atherosclerosis occurs in arteries supplying blood to the brain, a *stroke* can result. Many risk factors for heart disease have been identified, including obesity, cigarette smoking, hypertension, elevated cholesterol level, and positive family history (usually defined as having one or more affected first-degree relatives). Many studies have examined the role of family history in CHD, and they show that an individual with a positive family history is two to seven times more likely to have heart disease than is an individual with no family history (this would be the relative risk of heart disease because of a positive family history). In general, these studies also show that the risk increases if (1) there are more affected relatives; (2) the affected relative or relatives are female (the less commonly affected sex) rather than male; and (3) the age of onset in the affected relative is early (before 55 years). For example, one study showed that men between the ages of 20 and 39 years had a relative risk of 3 for CHD if they had one affected first-degree relative. The relative risk increased to 13 if two first-degree relatives were affected with CHD before 55 years of age.[8]

What part do genes play in the familial clustering of heart disease? Because of the key role of lipids in atherosclerosis, many studies are focusing on the genetic determination of various lipoproteins.[9]

An important advance in this area has been the identification of several genes that encode the processing of low-density lipoproteins and that, when mutated, can cause *familial hypercholesterolemia* (Box 5.3). Many other genes involved in lipid variation, coagulation, and hypertension have been identified, including several genes encoding apolipoproteins (the protein components of lipoproteins) (Fig. 5.5). Functional analysis of these genes is leading to an increased understanding and eventually more effective treatment of CHD. Xanthomas, which are fatty deposits, are often noted in individuals with familial hypercholesterolemia (Fig. 5.6).[10]

Environmental factors, many of which are easily modified, are also important causes of CHD. Abundant epidemiologic evidence shows that cigarette smoking and obesity increase the risk of CHD, whereas exercise and a diet low in saturated fats decrease the risk. Indeed, the approximate 50% decline in CHD prevalence in the United States during the past 40 years is usually attributed to a decrease in the proportion of adults who smoke cigarettes, a decreased consumption of saturated fats, and an increased emphasis on exercise and a generally healthier lifestyle.

Hypertension

Systemic hypertension, which has a worldwide prevalence of approximately 25% to 30%, is a key risk factor for heart disease, stroke, and kidney disease. Studies of blood pressure correlations within families indicate that approximately 20% to 40% of the variation in both systolic and diastolic blood pressure is caused by genetic factors. The fact that this figure is substantially less than 100% indicates that environmental factors also must be important causes of blood pressure variation. The most important environmental risk factors for hypertension are increased sodium intake, decreased physical activity, psychosocial stress, and obesity (but, as discussed later, the latter factor is itself influenced by both genes and environment).

Blood pressure regulation is a highly complex process that is influenced by many physiologic systems, including various aspects of kidney function (see Chapter 37), cellular ion transport, and heart function (refer to Chapter 31).[11]

Because of this complexity, much research is now focused on specific components that may influence blood pressure variation, such as the renin-angiotensin system (involved in sodium reabsorption and vasoconstriction), vasodilators such as nitric oxide and the kallikrein-kinin system, and ion-transport systems such as adducin and sodium-lithium counter-transport (Fig. 5.7). These individual factors are more likely to be under the control of smaller numbers of genes than is blood pressure itself, simplifying the task of identifying these genes and their role in blood pressure regulation. For example, linkage and association studies have implicated several genes involved in

BOX 5.3 Familial Hypercholesterolemia

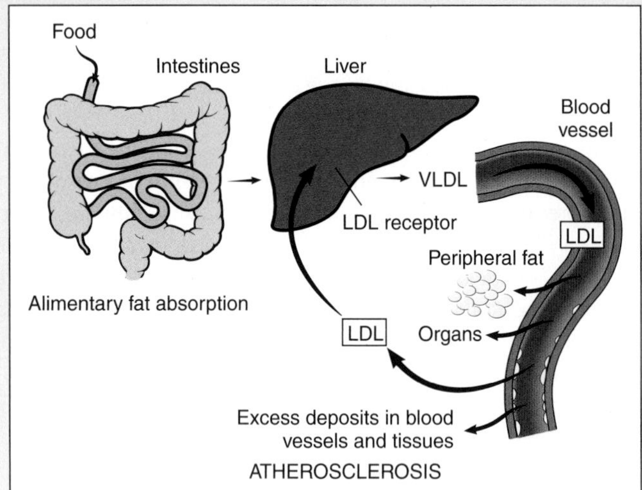

Autosomal dominant familial hypercholesterolemia (FH) is an important cause of heart disease, accounting for approximately 5% of myocardial infarctions in individuals younger than 60 years of age. FH is one of the most common autosomal dominant disorders: in most populations surveyed to date, approximately 1 in 500 people is a heterozygote. Plasma cholesterol levels are approximately twice as high as normal (i.e., approximately 300–400 mg/dL), resulting in substantially accelerated atherosclerosis and distinctive cholesterol deposits in skin and tendons (*xanthomas* [see Fig. 5.6]). Data compiled from five studies showed that approximately 75% of men with FH developed coronary disease, and 50% had a fatal myocardial infarction by 60 years. The corresponding percentages for women were lower (45% and 15%) because women generally develop heart disease at a later age than men.

Consistent with Hardy-Weinberg predictions, approximately 1 in 1 million births is homozygous for the FH gene. Homozygotes are much more severely affected, with cholesterol levels ranging from 600 to 1200 mg/dL. Most experience myocardial infarctions before 20 years of age, and a myocardial infarction at 18 months of age has been reported. If untreated, most FH homozygotes die before 30 years of age.

All cells require cholesterol as a component of their plasma membrane. They can either synthesize their own cholesterol or, preferably, obtain it from the extracellular environment, where it is carried primarily by low-density lipoprotein (LDL). In a process known as *endocytosis*, LDL-bound cholesterol is taken into the cell via LDL receptors on the cell's surface (see Fig. 5.5). FH is most caused by a reduction in the number of functional LDL receptors on cell surfaces. Lacking the normal number of LDL receptors, cellular cholesterol uptake is reduced and circulating cholesterol levels increase.

Much of what we know about endocytosis has been learned through the study of LDL receptors. The process of endocytosis and the processing of LDL in the cell are described in detail in Fig. 5.5 (endocytosis is discussed in Chapter 1). These processes result in a fine-tuned regulation of cholesterol levels within cells, and they influence the level of circulating cholesterol as well.

The identification of the LDL receptor gene in 1984 was critical in understanding exactly how LDL receptor defects cause FH. More than 1000 different mutations, including missense and nonsense substitutions as well as insertions and deletions, have been identified in the LDL receptor gene. These can be grouped into five broad classes according to their effects on the activity of the receptor. Class 1 mutations result in no detectable protein product. Thus heterozygotes would produce only half the normal number of LDL receptors. Class 2 mutations in the LDL receptor gene result in production of the LDL receptor, but it is altered such that it cannot leave the endoplasmic reticulum. It is eventually degraded. Class 3 mutations produce an LDL receptor that can migrate to the cell surface but incapable of normal binding to LDL. Class 4 mutations, which are comparatively rare, produce receptors that are normal except that they do not migrate specifically to coated pits and thus cannot carry LDL into the cell. The final group of mutations, class 5, produces an LDL receptor that cannot dissociate from the LDL particle after entry into the cell. The receptor cannot return to the cell surface and is degraded. Each class of mutations reduces the number of effective LDL receptors, resulting in decreased LDL uptake and hence elevated levels of circulating cholesterol. The number of effective receptors is reduced by approximately half in FH heterozygotes, and homozygotes have virtually no functional LDL receptors.

Understanding the defects that lead to FH has helped to develop effective therapies for the disorder. Dietary reduction of cholesterol (primarily through the reduced intake of saturated fats) has only modest effects on cholesterol levels in FH heterozygotes. Because cholesterol is reabsorbed into the gut and then recycled through the liver (where most cholesterol synthesis takes place), serum cholesterol levels can be reduced by the administration of bile acid–absorbing resins, such as cholestyramine. The absorbed cholesterol is then excreted. It is interesting that reduced recirculation from the gut causes the liver cells to form additional LDL receptors, lowering circulating cholesterol levels. However, the decrease in the concentration of intracellular cholesterol also stimulates cholesterol synthesis by liver cells, so the overall reduction in plasma LDL level is only approximately 15% to 20%. This treatment is much more effective when combined with agents that reduce cholesterol synthesis by inhibiting 3-hydroxy-3-methylglutaryl coenzyme A (HMG-CoA) reductase (the "statin" class of drugs). Decreased synthesis leads to further production of LDL receptors. When these therapies are used in combination, serum cholesterol levels in FH heterozygotes can be reduced to approximately normal levels.

The picture is less encouraging for FH homozygotes. The therapies just discussed can enhance cholesterol elimination and reduce its synthesis, but they are largely ineffective because homozygotes have few or no LDL receptors. Liver transplants, which provide hepatocytes that have normal LDL receptors, have been successful in some cases, but this option is often limited by a lack of donors. Plasma exchange carried out every 1–2 weeks, in combination with drug therapy, can reduce cholesterol levels by approximately 50%. However, this therapy is difficult to continue for long periods. Somatic cell gene therapy, in which hepatocytes carrying normal LDL receptor genes are introduced into the portal circulation, is now being tested. It may eventually prove to be an effective treatment for FH homozygotes.

FH also can be caused by inherited mutations in the gene that encodes apolipoprotein B. In addition, a small number of FH cases are caused by mutations in the gene that encodes PCSK9 (proprotein convertase subtilisin/kexin type 9), an enzyme that plays a key role in degrading LDL receptors. Gain-of-function mutations in the *PCSK9* gene reduce the number of LDL receptors, causing FH. Loss-of-function mutations in this gene can increase the number of LDL receptors, resulting in exceptionally low circulating LDL levels. These findings have led to the development of drugs that inhibit PCSK9 activity, thus lowering LDL cholesterol levels. These drugs, which have been approved for clinical use, can reduce LDL cholesterol levels by approximately 50% in the general population of persons with hypercholesterolemia and produce significant effects even in those who are using statin drugs.

The FH story illustrates how medical research has made important contributions both to our understanding of basic cell biology and to our advances in clinical therapy. The process of receptor-mediated endocytosis, elucidated largely by research on the LDL receptor defects, is of fundamental significance for cellular processes throughout the body. Equally important is that this research, by clarifying how cholesterol synthesis and uptake can be modified, has led to significant improvements in therapy for this important cause of heart disease. The discovery of rare mutations in PCSK9 has led to PCSK9 inhibitor drugs that may benefit millions of persons with high cholesterol levels.

Data from Brautbar A, Leary E, Rasmussen K, et al. Genetics of familial hypercholesterolemia. *Current Atherosclerosis Reports*, 2015;17:491; Roberts R, Davidson MH, Hirsh BJ, et al. Genetics and causality of triglyceride-rich lipoproteins in atherosclerotic cardiovascular disease. *Journal of the American College of Cardiology*, 2014;64(23):2525–2540; Varret MM, Abifadel M, Rabès JP, et al. Genetic heterogeneity of autosomal dominant hypercholesterolemia. *Clinical Genetics*, 2008;73(1):1–13.

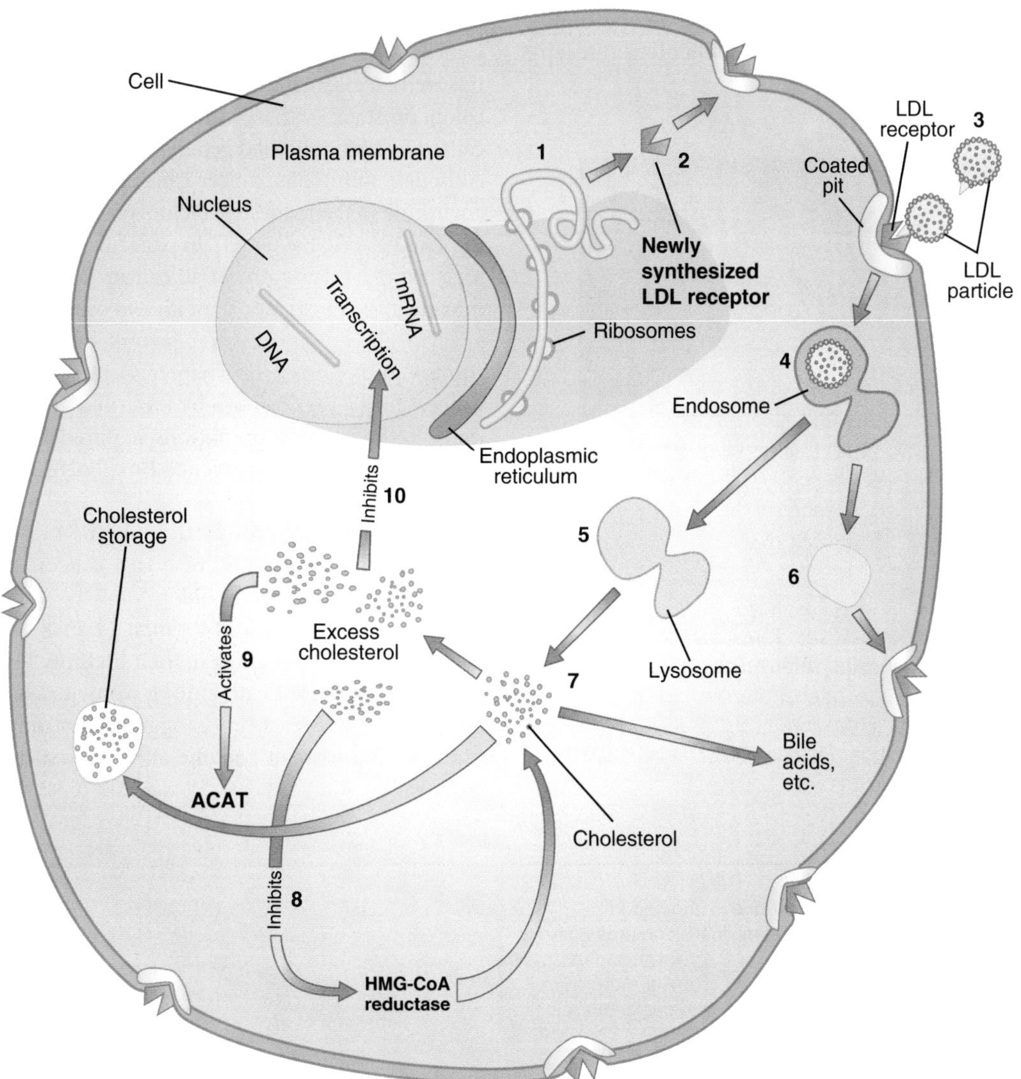

Fig. 5.5 Process of Receptor-Mediated Endocytosis. 1, The low-density lipoprotein *(LDL)* receptors, which are glycoproteins, are synthesized in the endoplasmic reticulum of the cell. *2*, From here, they pass through the Golgi apparatus to the cell surface, where part of the receptor protrudes outside the cell. *3*, The circulating LDL particle is bound by the LDL receptor and localized in cell surface depressions called *coated pits* (so named because they are coated with a protein called *clathrin*). *4*, The coated pit invaginates, bringing the LDL particle inside the cell. *5*, Once inside the cell, the LDL particle is separated from the receptor, taken into a lysosome, and broken down into its constituents by lysosomal enzymes. *6*, The LDL receptor is recirculated to the cell surface to bind another LDL particle (each LDL receptor goes through this cycle approximately once every 10 minutes even if it is not occupied by an LDL particle). *7*, Free cholesterol is released from the lysosome for incorporation into cell membranes or metabolism into bile acids or steroids. Excess cholesterol can be stored in the cell as a cholesterol ester or removed from the cell by associating with high-density lipoprotein *(HDL)*. *8*, As cholesterol levels in the cell rise, cellular cholesterol synthesis is reduced by inhibition of the rate-limiting enzyme 3-hydroxy-3-methylglutaryl coenzyme A *(HMG-CoA)* reductase. *9*, Rising cholesterol levels also increase the activity of acyl coenzyme A (acyl CoA):cholesterol acyltransferase *(ACAT)*, an enzyme that modifies cholesterol for storage as cholesterol esters. *10*, In addition, the number of LDL receptors is decreased by lowering the transcription rate of the LDL receptor gene itself. This decreases cholesterol uptake. (From Jorde LB, Carey JC, Bamshad MJ. *Medical genetics*, 6th edition. Philadelphia: Elsevier; 2020.)

the renin-angiotensin system (e.g., the genes that encode angiotensinogen, angiotensin-converting enzyme, angiotensin receptors) in the causation of hypertension.

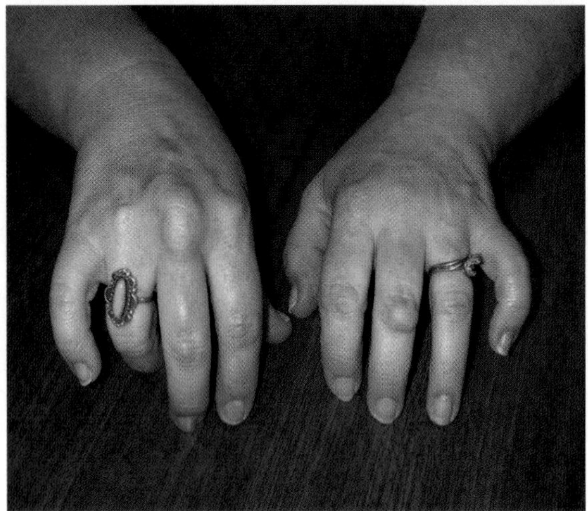

Fig. 5.6 Xanthoma. Fatty deposits, referred to as xanthomas as seen here on the knuckles, are often noted in individuals with familial hypercholesterolemia. (From Jorde LB, Carey JC, Bamshad MJ. *Medical genetics*, 6th edition. Philadelphia: Elsevier; 2020.)

Cancer

Cancer is the second leading cause of death in the United States. It is well established that many major types of cancer (e.g., breast, colon, prostate, ovarian) cluster strongly in families. Clustering is caused by both inherited genes and shared environmental factors. Although numerous cancer-causing genes are being isolated,[12] environmental and lifestyle factors play an important role in causing cancer (see Chapter 13). In particular, tobacco use is estimated to account for one-third of all cancer cases in the United States, making it the most important known cause of cancer.[13]

Typically, environmental factors cause cancer by creating somatic mutations (see Chapter 4) in specific cell types. Thus cancer can be caused both by inherited genetic variants and by noninherited somatic mutations acquired during an individual's lifetime. See Emerging Science Box: Polygenic Risk Scores and Disease Prediction.

Breast cancer. Breast cancer is the most common cancer among women, with 82% of breast cancers diagnosed among women aged 50 years and older.[14]

Approximately 13% of women (1 in 8) will be diagnosed with invasive breast cancer in their lifetime.[14] Formerly the leading cause of cancer death among women, it has been surpassed by lung cancer. Breast cancer aggregates strongly in families; for example, if a woman has one affected first-degree relative, her

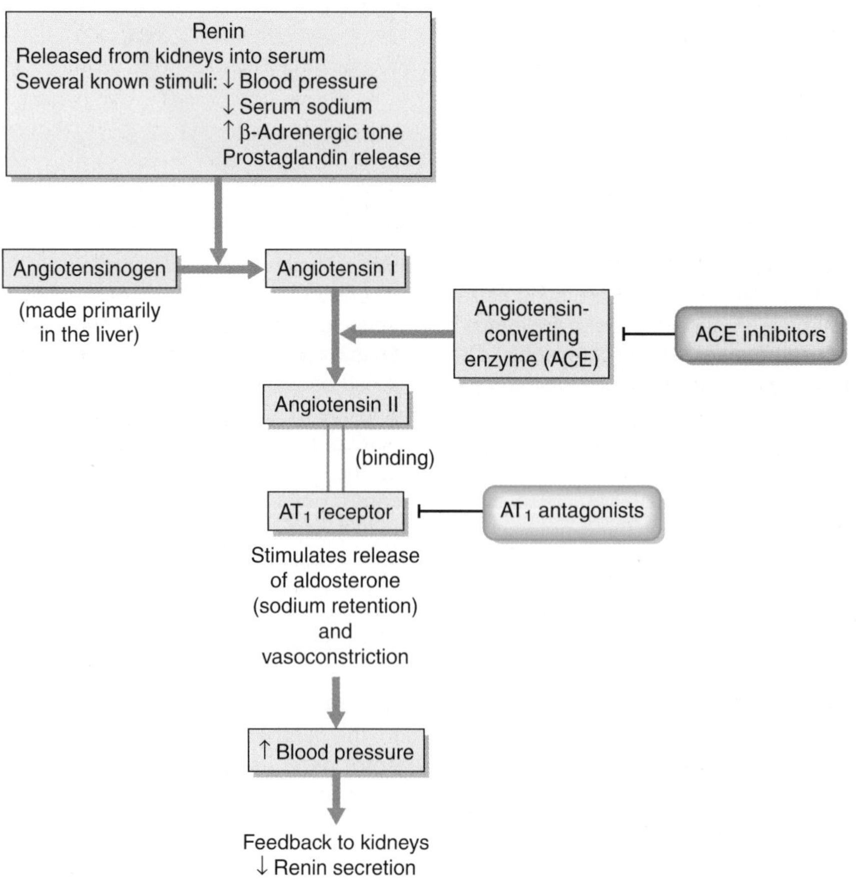

Fig. 5.7 Renin-Angiotensin-Aldosterone System. (Adapted from Khera AV, Chaffin M, Aragam KG, et al., 2018. Nature genetics in Jorde LB, Carey JC, Bamshad MJ. *Medical genetics*, 6th edition. Philadelphia: Elsevier; 2020.)

risk of developing breast cancer doubles. This risk increases further if the age of onset in the affected relative is early and if the cancer is bilateral (tumors in both breasts).

An autosomal dominant form of breast cancer accounts for approximately 5% to 10% of breast cancer cases in the United States.[15] Genes responsible for this form of breast cancer have been identified on chromosomes 17 (*BRCA1*) and 13 (*BRCA2*), and these genes can be tested for inherited cancer-causing mutations.[16,17]

It is reported that women who inherit a mutation in *BRCA1* or *BRCA2* experience a 50% to 80% lifetime risk of developing breast cancer.[15] However, in a seminal paper of more than 8000 unselected cases of breast or ovarian cancer, the average cumulative risk of developing breast cancer with a *BRCA1* mutation was 65%.[18] *BRCA1* mutations also increase the risk of ovarian cancer among women (39%), and they confer a modestly increased risk of prostate and colon cancers.[15] *BRCA2* mutations also confer an increased risk of ovarian cancer (11%).[15] Approximately 5% to 8% of males who inherit a *BRCA2* mutation will develop breast cancer, representing a 100-fold increase over the risk in the general male population.[19] Evaluation of the *BRCA1* and *BRCA2* gene products, which are both involved in deoxyribonucleic acid (DNA) repair, is yielding valuable evidence on the etiology of breast cancer in general.

Although *BRCA1* and *BRCA2* mutations are the most commonly known causes of inherited breast cancer, this disease also can be caused by inherited mutations in several other genes (e.g., *ATM, CDH1, CHEK2, NBN, NF1, PALB2, PTEN, STK11,* and *TP53*).[16] Germline mutations in a tumor-suppressor gene called *PTEN* are responsible for Cowden disease, which is characterized by multiple benign tumors and an increased susceptibility to breast cancer. Despite the significance of these genes, it should be emphasized that more than 90% of breast cancer cases are not inherited as mendelian diseases (also see Chapter 6).

Colorectal cancer. Colorectal cancer is second only to lung cancer in the number of cancer deaths occurring annually in the United States, with approximately 148,000 new cases and 53,000 deaths annually.[20] Approximately 1 in 21 Americans will develop colorectal cancer. Like breast cancer, it clusters in families (in fact, familial clustering of this form of cancer was reported in the medical literature as early as 1881). The risk of colorectal cancer in people with one affected first-degree relative is two to three times higher than that in the general population.

This familial aggregation is caused in part by subsets of colorectal cancer cases that are inherited as single-gene traits. For example, *familial adenomatous polyposis* occurs in approximately 1 in 8000 Whites. The gene responsible for this disorder, *APC*, encodes a tumor suppressor.[21] Importantly, somatic mutations of *APC* are found in at least 85% of all colon tumors. Thus, although inherited *APC* mutations cause rare familial adenomatous polyposis, somatic mutations are involved in the great majority of all common colorectal cancers.

Among hereditary forms of colorectal cancer, the most frequent is *hereditary nonpolyposis colorectal cancer*, which accounts for 3% to 4% of colorectal cancer cases and is caused by mutations in any of six genes.[22,23] Research has shown that all of these genes are involved in the vital process of DNA repair. When this function is compromised, cancer-causing mutations can persist in cells, leading eventually to growth of a tumor.

Other colorectal cancer cases are likely to be caused by a complex interaction of multiple genes. In addition, environmental factors, such as a high-fat, low-fiber diet, are thought to increase the risk of colorectal cancer.

Prostate cancer. Prostate cancer is the second most diagnosed cancer in men (after skin cancer), with approximately 165,000 new cases annually in the United States and a lifetime risk of 11%.[24,25]

Prostate cancer is second only to lung cancer as a cause of cancer death in men, causing more than 30,000 deaths each year. Having an affected first-degree relative increases the risk of developing prostate cancer by a factor of 2 to 3, and the heritability of prostate cancer is estimated to be approximately 40%.

The relatively late age of onset of most prostate cancer cases (median age 72 years) makes genetic analysis especially difficult. However, loss of heterozygosity (see Chapter 12) has been observed in several genomic regions in prostate tumor cells, possibly indicating the presence of genetic alterations in these regions. In addition, genome-wide association studies have identified several dozen polymorphisms associated with prostate cancer risk. Several of these are in chromosome 8q24, which contains polymorphisms associated with several other cancers as well (colon, pancreas, and esophagus). Although the 8q24 region contains no protein-coding genes, it contains enhancer elements that affect expression of the *MYC* oncogene, located approximately 250 kilobytes (kb) from 8q24.[26]

Nongenetic factors for prostate cancer may include a high-fat diet. Because prostate cancer usually progresses slowly and because it can be detected by digital examination and by the prostate-specific antigen (PSA) test, fatal metastasis can usually be prevented.

Cancer gene identification. Recently developed techniques, including large-scale DNA sequencing, have identified hundreds of genes that are mutated in various cancers. Some of these genes contribute directly to a growth advantage in tumors and are considered primary causes of cancer. Approximately 150 such **driver genes** have been described.[12,27] A much larger number of genes undergo somatic mutations during tumorigenesis, but these genes do not directly confer a growth advantage to cells; these are termed **passenger genes**.[27] The gene responsible for retinoblastoma (see Chapter 20), which normally acts as a "brake" on cell division, is an example of a well-known driver gene. The *APC* gene, discussed previously, is another example.

Although many types of cancer, such as retinoblastoma or familial adenomatous polyposis, are relatively rare, study of the causative genes has provided many important insights into the nature of carcinogenesis in general. This can lead to more effective treatment and prevention of all cancers.

Diabetes mellitus. Like the other disorders discussed in this chapter, the etiology of diabetes mellitus is complex and not fully understood (see Chapter 22). Nevertheless, progress is being made in understanding the genetic basis of this disorder, which is a leading cause of blindness, heart disease, and kidney failure.[28,29]

An important advance has been the recognition that diabetes is a heterogeneous group of disorders, all characterized by elevated blood glucose level. The focus here is on the two major types of diabetes: type 1 (insulin-dependent diabetes mellitus [IDDM]) and type 2 (non–insulin-dependent diabetes mellitus [NIDDM]).

Type 1 diabetes. Type 1 diabetes, which is characterized by T-cell infiltration of the pancreas and destruction of the insulin-producing beta cells, usually (although not always) presents before age 40. Individuals with type 1 diabetes must receive exogenous insulin to survive. In addition to T-cell infiltration of the pancreas, autoantibodies are formed against pancreatic cells; the latter can be observed long before clinical symptoms occur. These findings, along with a strong association between type 1 diabetes and the presence of several major histocompatibility complex (MHC) class II alleles, indicate that this is an autoimmune disease. Over the past few decades, the incidence of type 1 diabetes has increased substantially.

Siblings of individuals with type 1 diabetes face a substantial elevation in risk: approximately 6%, as opposed to a risk of approximately 0.3% to 0.5% in the general population. The recurrence risk is also elevated when there is a diabetic parent, although this risk varies with the sex of the affected parent. The risk for offspring of diabetic mothers is only 1% to 3%, whereas it is 4% to 6% for the offspring of diabetic fathers (because type 1 diabetes affects males and females in approximately equal proportions in the general population, this risk difference is inconsistent with the sex-specific threshold model for multifactorial traits). Twin studies show that the empirical risks for identical twins of people with type 1 diabetes range from 30% to 70%. In contrast, the concordance rates for DZ twins are 5% to 10%. The fact that type 1 diabetes is not 100% concordant among identical twins indicates that genetic factors are not solely responsible for the disorder. There is good evidence that specific viral infections contribute to the causation of type 1 diabetes in at least some individuals, possibly by activating an autoimmune response.

The association of specific MHC class II alleles (see Chapter 22) and type 1 diabetes has been studied extensively, and it is estimated that these alleles account for approximately 40% of the familial clustering of type 1 diabetes. Approximately 95% of Whites with type 1 diabetes have the human leukocyte antigen (HLA) (part of the MHC), DR3, and/or DR4 alleles, whereas only approximately 50% of the general White population has either of these alleles. If an affected proband and a sibling are heterozygous for the DR3 and DR4 alleles, the sibling's risk of developing type 1 diabetes is nearly 20% (i.e., approximately 40 times higher than the risk in the general population). In addition, the presence of aspartic acid at position 57 of the HLA DQ chain is strongly associated with resistance to type 1 diabetes. In fact, those who do not have this amino acid at position 57 (and instead are homozygous for a different amino acid) are 100 times more likely to develop type 1 diabetes. The aspartic acid substitution alters the shape of the HLA class II molecule and thus its ability to bind and present peptides to T cells. Altered T-cell recognition may help protect individuals with the aspartic acid substitution from an autoimmune episode.

The insulin gene, which is located on the short arm of chromosome 11, is another logical candidate for type 1 diabetes susceptibility. Polymorphisms within and near this gene have been tested for association with type 1 diabetes. It is estimated that inherited genetic variation in the insulin region accounts for approximately 10% of the familial clustering of type 1 diabetes.

More than 50 additional genes have been shown to be associated with susceptibility to type 1 diabetes. The most significant of these are cytotoxicT-lymphocyte-associatedantigen 4 (CTLA-4), which encodes a protein involved in the regulation of T-cell proliferation, and *PTPN22*, which encodes a lymphoid-specific tyrosine phosphatase that negatively regulates T-cell activation. It is interesting that variation in the latter gene has been associated with several other autoimmune diseases, including systemic lupus erythematosus (SLE), rheumatoid arthritis, and autoimmune thyroid disease.

Type 2 diabetes. Type 2 diabetes accounts for more than 90% of all diabetes cases and affects 10% to 20% of the adult populations of many high-income countries. Several features distinguish it from type 1 diabetes. There is nearly always some endogenous insulin production in people with type 2 diabetes, and the disease can often be treated successfully with dietary modification and/or oral drugs. People with type 2 diabetes suffer from insulin resistance (i.e., their cells have difficulty in using insulin). This disease typically occurs among people older than age 40 and, in contrast to type 1 diabetes, is seen more commonly among the obese. However, the incidence of type 2 diabetes is rising dramatically among adolescents and young adults in developed countries and is strongly correlated with an increased incidence of obesity. Neither MHC associations nor autoantibodies are commonly seen in this form of diabetes. MZ twin concordance rates are substantially higher than those seen in type 1 diabetes, ranging from 70% to 90% (because of age dependence, the concordance rate increases if older subjects are studied). The empirical recurrence risks for first-degree relatives of type 2 diabetes cases are higher than those for type 1, generally ranging from 15% to 40%. The differences between type 1 and type 2 diabetes are summarized in Table 5.5.

Hundreds of studies have been undertaken to identify genes that may contribute to type 2 diabetes susceptibility, and more than 250 genes and more than 400 genomic variants are now known to be associated with risk of this disease.[30] An important risk factor is *TCF7L2*, which encodes a transcription factor involved in the secretion of insulin. A variant of *TCF7L2* is associated with a 50% increased risk of developing type 2 diabetes.[31] A significant association has also been observed between type 2 diabetes and a common allele of the gene that encodes peroxisome proliferator–activated receptor-gamma (PPAR-γ), a nuclear receptor that is involved in adipocyte differentiation and glucose metabolism.[32] This receptor is the target of thiazolidinediones (TZDs), a class of drugs commonly used to increase insulin sensitivity in those with type 2 diabetes. Although the disease-associated allele confers only a 25% increase in the risk of developing type 2 diabetes, it is found in more than 75% of individuals of European descent and thus helps to account for a significant proportion of type 2 diabetes cases. Variation in *KCNJ11*, which encodes a potassium channel necessary for

TABLE 5.5 Comparison of Major Features of Types 1 and 2 Diabetes

Feature	Type 1 Diabetes	Type 2 Diabetes
Age of onset	Usually <40 years	Usually >40 years (except maturity-onset diabetes of the young [MODY])
Insulin production	None	Partial
Insulin resistance	No	Yes
Autoimmunity	Yes	No
Obesity	Not common	Common
Monozygotic (MZ) twin concordance	0.30–0.70	0.35–0.60
Sibling recurrence risk	1%–6%	10%–40%

glucose-stimulated insulin secretion, confers an additional 20% increase in type 2 diabetes susceptibility. The associations between diabetes susceptibility and each of these genes have been widely replicated in multiple populations.

The two most important risk factors for type 2 diabetes are positive family history and obesity; the latter increases insulin resistance. The disease tends to rise in prevalence when populations adopt a diet and exercise pattern typical of US and European populations. Increases have been seen, for example, among Japanese immigrants to the United States and among some native populations of the South Pacific, Australia, and the Americas. Several studies, conducted on male and female subjects, have shown that regular exercise can substantially lower one's risk of developing type 2 diabetes, even among individuals with a family history of the disease. This is partly because exercise reduces obesity. However, even in the absence of weight loss, exercise increases insulin sensitivity and improves glucose tolerance.

Because of the dramatic increase in obesity in the United States and other developed countries, the prevalence of type 2 diabetes is also rising rapidly, and the average age of onset is decreasing (one study estimates that up to one-third of Americans born in the year 2000 will develop type 2 diabetes).[33] A small proportion of type 2 diabetes cases occurs early in life, often before 25 years of age, and typically exhibits autosomal dominant inheritance (unlike most type 2 diabetes cases). This subset is termed *maturity-onset diabetes of the young* (MODY). Studies of MODY pedigrees have shown that approximately half of cases of the disease are caused by mutations in the glucokinase gene. Glucokinase converts glucose to glucose-6-phosphate in the pancreas. In addition to the glucokinase gene, five other genes, all of which are involved in pancreatic development or regulation of insulin levels, have now been shown to be causes of MODY. Currently, 13 MODY genes are known.[34]

Obesity

Obesity is most defined as a body mass index (BMI) greater than 30. (BMI is defined as W/H^2, in which W is weight in kilograms and H is height in meters.) Using this criterion, more than one-third of American adults are obese, and an additional one-third are overweight (BMI greater than 25 but less than 30). The proportion of obese adults and children continues to increase rapidly. Although obesity itself is not a "disease," it is an important risk factor for several common diseases, including heart disease, stroke, type 2 diabetes, and cancers of the prostate, breast, and colon.

As one might expect, there is a strong correlation between obesity in parents and their children. This could easily be ascribed to common environmental effects: parents and children usually share similar dietary and exercise habits. However, there is good evidence for genetic components as well. Four adoption studies each showed that the body weights of adopted individuals correlated significantly with their natural parents' body weights but not with those of their adoptive parents. Twin studies also provide evidence for a genetic effect on body weight, with most studies yielding heritability estimates between 0.60 and 0.80.

Research, aided substantially by mouse models, has shown that many genes each play a role in human obesity. Important among these are the genes that encode leptin (Greek, "thin") and its receptor. The leptin hormone is secreted by adipocytes (fat storage cells) and binds to receptors in the hypothalamus, the site of the body's appetite control center. Cloning of the human leptin gene and its receptor led to optimistic predictions that leptin could be a key to weight loss in humans (without the perceived unpleasantness of dieting and exercise). Although mutations in the human leptin gene and its receptor have been identified in a few humans with severe obesity (BMI >40), they both appear to be extremely rare. Clinical trials using recombinant leptin have demonstrated moderate weight loss in a subset of obese individuals. In addition, leptin participates in important interactions with other components of appetite control, such as neuropeptide Y and α-melanocyte–stimulating hormone and its receptor, the melanocortin-4 receptor (MC4R). Mutations in the gene that encodes MC4R have been found in 3% to 5% of severely obese individuals. Homozygosity for a DNA variant in the *FTO* gene (which is seen in 16% of Whites) has been associated with 40% and 70% increases in the risks of overweight and obesity, respectively. Recent evidence shows that the *FTO* variant is part of an enhancer that binds to the *IRX* gene, which is located 2 million base pairs away from *FTO* and is involved in regulation of fat mass. Identification of these human genes is leading to a better understanding of natural weight control in the human, and it could eventually lead to effective treatments for some cases of obesity.

Alzheimer Disease

Alzheimer disease (AD), which is responsible for 50% to 80% of cases of progressive cognitive impairment (dementia) among older adults, affects approximately 1 in 10 individuals older than 65 years of age and 1 in 3 individuals older than 85 years of age.[35]

Because of the aging of the population, the number of Americans with AD is predicted to increase substantially during the coming decade. AD is characterized by progressive dementia and memory loss and by the formation of amyloid plaques and neurofibrillary tangles in the brain, particularly in the cerebral cortex and hippocampus. The plaques and tangles lead to progressive neuronal loss, and death usually occurs within 7 to 10 years after the first appearance of symptoms.

The risk of developing AD doubles in individuals who have an affected first-degree relative. Although most cases do not appear to be caused by single loci, approximately 10% follow an autosomal dominant mode of transmission. Approximately 5% of AD cases occur before age 65 and are considered early onset; these are much more likely to be an autosomal dominant inheritance.[36] AD is a genetically heterogeneous disorder. Approximately half of early-onset cases can be attributed to mutations in any of three genes, all of which affect amyloid-β deposition.[35] Two of the genes, presenilin 1 *(PSEN1)* and presenilin 2 *(PSEN2)*, are very similar to one another, and their protein products are involved in cleavage of the amyloid-β precursor protein (APP). When APP is not cleaved normally, a long form of it accumulates excessively and is deposited in the brain. This is thought to be a primary cause of AD. Mutations in *PSEN1* typically result in early-onset AD, with the first occurrence of symptoms in the fifth decade of life.

A small number of cases of early-onset AD are caused by mutations of the gene that encodes APP itself, which is located on chromosome 21. These mutations disrupt normal cleavage sites in APP, again leading to the accumulation of the longer protein product. It is interesting that this gene is present in three copies in trisomy 21 individuals, in which the extra gene copy leads to amyloid deposition and the occurrence of AD in those with Down syndrome (see Chapter 4). High-throughput DNA sequencing (techniques allowing the sequencing of massive amounts of DNA at once) studies have revealed an allele in APP that is protective against AD and may help to prevent cognitive decline.

An important risk factor for the more common late-onset form of AD is allelic variation in the apolipoprotein E *(APOE)* locus, which has three major alleles: *ε2*, *ε3*, and *ε4*. Studies conducted in diverse populations have shown that persons who have one copy of the *ε4* allele are at least 2 to 5 times more likely to develop AD, whereas those with two copies of this allele are at least 5 to 10 times more likely to develop AD. The risk varies somewhat by population, with higher *ε4*-associated risks in Europeans and Japanese and relatively lower risks in Hispanics and Blacks. Despite the strong association between *ε4* and AD, approximately half of individuals who develop late-onset AD do not have a copy of the *ε4* allele, and many who are homozygous for *ε4* remain free of AD even at advanced age. The APOE protein product is not involved in cleavage of APP but instead appears to be associated with clearance of amyloid from the brain. Recent large-scale studies have revealed at least 20 additional genes are associated with AD.

Alcoholism

At some point, alcoholism (now formally termed alcohol use disorder) is diagnosed in approximately 10% of adult males and 3% to 5% of adult females in the United States. The national cost of alcoholism, in terms of lost productivity and direct medical costs, is approximately $250 billion per year.[37] More than 100 studies have shown that this disease clusters in families.[38] The risk of developing alcoholism among individuals with one affected parent is three to five times higher than for those with unaffected parents.

Most twin studies have yielded concordance rates for DZ twins less than 30% and concordance rates for MZ twins more than 60%. Adoption studies have shown that the offspring of an alcoholic parent, even when raised by nonalcoholic parents, have a fourfold increased risk of developing the disorder. To control for possible prenatal effects in an alcoholic mother, some studies have included only the offspring of alcoholic fathers. The results have remained the same. One study showed that the offspring of nonalcoholic parents, when reared by alcoholics, did *not* have an increased risk of developing alcoholism. These data argue that there may be genetic variants that predispose some people to alcoholism.

It has long been known that an individual's physiologic response to alcohol can be influenced by variation in the key enzymes responsible for alcohol metabolism: alcohol dehydrogenases (ADHs), which convert ethanol to acetaldehyde; and aldehyde dehydrogenases (ALDHs), which convert acetaldehyde to acetate. An allele of the *ALDH2* gene *(ALDH2*2)* results in excessive accumulation of acetaldehyde and thus in facial flushing, nausea, palpitations, and lightheadedness.[39] Because of these unpleasant effects, individuals who have the *ALDH2*2* allele are much less likely to become alcoholics. This "protective" allele is common in some Asian populations but is rare in other populations.

Several other genes are associated with susceptibility to alcohol addiction, including genes that encode components of gamma-aminobutyric acid (GABA) receptors. This finding is biologically plausible, because the GABA neurotransmitter system inhibits excitatory signals in neurons, exerting a calming effect. Alcohol has been shown to increase GABA release, and allelic variation in GABA receptor genes may modulate this effect.

It should be underscored that genes may increase one's *susceptibility* to alcoholism. Obviously, this is a disease that requires an environmental component, regardless of genetic constitution.

Psychiatric Disorders

The major psychiatric diseases, schizophrenia and bipolar disorder, have been the subjects of numerous genetic studies.[40] Twin, adoption, and family studies have shown that both disorders aggregate in families.

Schizophrenia. *Schizophrenia* is a severe emotional disorder characterized by delusions, hallucinations, retreat from reality, and bizarre, withdrawn, or inappropriate behavior. (Contrary to popular belief, schizophrenia is not a "split personality" disorder.) The estimated heritability of schizophrenia is up to 85%.[41] The risk of schizophrenia among relatives with one schizophrenic proband is eightfold. This increases to 11-fold for relatives with two schizophrenic probands.[42] The lifetime risk for schizophrenia among offspring of one affected parent is approximately 8% to 10%, which is approximately 10 times higher than the risk in the general population.[43]

As one might expect, the empirical risks increase when more relatives are affected. For example, an individual with an affected sibling and an affected parent has a risk approaching 20% and an individual with two affected parents has a risk of nearly 50%. The risks decrease when the affected family member is a second- or third-degree relative. Details are given in

TABLE 5.6 Recurrence Risks for Relatives of Schizophrenic Probands

Relationship to Proband	Recurrence Risk (%)
Monozygotic twin	44.3
Dizygotic twin	12.1
Offspring	9.4
Sibling	7.3
Niece/nephew	2.7
Grandchild	2.8
First cousin	1.6
Spouse	1

NOTE: Figures are based on multiple studies of Western European populations.

Data from McGue M, Gottesman II, Rao DC. The analysis of schizophrenia family data. *Behavioral Genetics*, 1986;16(1):75–87.

Table 5.6. On inspection of Table 5.6, it may seem puzzling that the proportion of schizophrenic probands who have a schizophrenic parent is only approximately 5%, which is substantially lower than the risk for other first-degree relatives (e.g., siblings, affected parents and their offspring). This can be explained by the fact that people with schizophrenia are less likely to marry and produce children than are other individuals. Thus substantial selection against schizophrenia occurs in the population.

Twin and adoption studies also indicate that genetic factors are likely to be involved in schizophrenia. Data pooled from five different twin studies show a 47% concordance rate for MZ twins, compared with a concordance rate of only 12% for DZ twins. When the offspring of a schizophrenic parent are adopted by normal parents, their risk of developing the disease is approximately 10%, which is approximately the same as the risk when raised by a schizophrenic biologic parent. Large-scale genetic studies have revealed more than 200 loci that are associated with risk of schizophrenia. The most significant of these associations implicates complement component genes (*C4A* and *C4B*) located in the MHC region. These genes are expressed in neurons and affect synaptic function and likely contribute to the decline in synaptic structures observed in the brains of persons with schizophrenia. Other schizophrenia-associated genes encode components of the dopaminergic and glutamatergic neuronal signaling pathways. These findings are biologically plausible because the major therapeutic drugs used to treat schizophrenia block dopamine receptors.

Bipolar disorder. *Bipolar disorder*, also known as *manic-depressive disorder*, is a form of psychosis with extreme mood swings and emotional instability. The prevalence for bipolar type I in the United States is approximately 1%, but it rises to 5% to 10% among those with an affected first-degree relative.[44] Twin and family studies show that approximately 60% of the risk for bipolar disorder is attributable to genetic factors, whereas approximately 30% of the risk for unipolar disorder (major depression) is because of genetic factors.[45]

As with schizophrenia, large-scale studies have revealed more than 20 genes associated with susceptibility to bipolar disorder. Some of the best-replicated genetic studies implicate genes that encode voltage-gated calcium and sodium channels.[44] Ion-channel modulating drugs are frequently used as mood stabilizers, lending the genetic results functional plausibility. Many of the genes associated with bipolar disorder also are associated with schizophrenia.

Genetic studies of psychiatric disorders are especially challenging because these disorders are undoubtedly heterogeneous, reflecting the influence of numerous genetic and environmental factors. In addition, definition of the phenotype is not always straightforward, and it may change through time, significantly complicating genetic analysis.

Other Complex Disorders

The disorders discussed in this chapter represent some of the most common multifactorial disorders and those for which significant progress has been made in identifying genes. Many other multifactorial disorders are being studied as well, and in some cases specific susceptibility genes have been identified. These include, for example, Parkinson disease, hearing loss, multiple sclerosis, amyotrophic lateral sclerosis, epilepsy, asthma, inflammatory bowel disease, and some forms of blindness.

Some General Principles and Conclusions

Some general principles can be deduced from the results obtained thus far on the genetics of complex disorders. First, the more strongly inherited forms of complex disorders generally have an earlier age of onset (e.g., breast cancer, AD, heart disease). Often these represent subsets of cases in which there is single-gene inheritance. Second, when laterality is a component, the bilateral forms are more likely to cluster strongly in families (e.g., breast cancer, CL/P). Third, although the sex-specific threshold model fits some of the complex disorders (e.g., pyloric stenosis, CL/P, autism, heart disease), it fails to fit others (e.g., type 1 diabetes).

A tendency exists, particularly among the lay public, to assume that the presence of a genetic component means that the course of a disease cannot be altered. *This is incorrect.* Most of the diseases discussed in this chapter have both genetic and environmental components. Thus lifestyle modification (e.g., diet, exercise, stress reduction) often can reduce risk significantly. Such modification may be especially important for individuals with a family history of a disease because they are likely to develop the disease earlier in life. For example, those with a family history of heart disease can often add many years of productive living with relatively minor lifestyle alterations. By targeting those who can benefit most from intervention, genetics helps to serve the goal of preventive medicine.

In addition, it should be stressed that the identification of a specific genetic lesion can lead to more effective prevention and treatment of the disease. Identification of mutations that cause autosomal dominant breast cancer may enable early screening and prevention of metastasis. Pinpointing a gene responsible for a neurotransmitter defect in a behavioral disorder such as schizophrenia could lead to the development of more effective drug treatments. In some cases, such as those with familial hypercholesterolemia, targeted drug therapy or gene therapy may prove to be useful in treating the disease. It is important for healthcare practitioners to help individuals to understand these facts.

Although the genetics of common disorders is complex and often confusing, the community health effect of these diseases, together with the evidence for hereditary factors in their etiology, demands that genetic studies be pursued. Substantial progress is already being made. The next decade will undoubtedly witness many further advances in the understanding and treatment of these disorders.

SUMMARY REVIEW

Factors Influencing Incidence of Disease in Populations

1. The incidence rate is the number of new cases of a disease reported during a specific period (typically 1 year) divided by the number of individuals in the population.
2. The prevalence rate is the proportion of the population affected by a disease at a specific point in time. This rate and the incidence rate can be used to compare population variations in disease frequency.
3. Relative risk is a common measure of the effect of a specific risk factor. It is expressed as a ratio of the incidence rate of the disease among individuals exposed to a risk factor divided by the incidence of the disease among individuals *not* exposed to a risk factor.
4. Many factors can influence the risk of acquiring a common disease, such as cancer, diabetes, or hypertension. The factors can include age, gender, diet, exercise, and family history of the disease.

Principles of Multifactorial Inheritance

1. Traits in which variation is thought to be caused by the combined effects of multiple genes are polygenic.
2. The term *multifactorial* is used when environmental factors also are believed to cause variation in the trait.
3. Many quantitative traits (e.g., blood pressure) are multifactorial.
4. Because traits are caused by the additive effects of many genetic and environmental factors, they tend to follow a normal or bell-shaped distribution in populations.
5. Those diseases, however, that do not follow a bell-shaped distribution appear to be either present or absent in individuals. They do not follow the inheritance patterns of single-gene disease. Instead, such diseases may follow an underlying liability distribution. It is thought that a threshold of liability must be crossed before the disease is expressed.
6. Examples of diseases that correspond to the liability model include pyloric stenosis, neural tube defects, CL/P, and some forms of congenital heart disease.
7. Many of the common adult diseases, such as hypertension, coronary heart disease, stroke, diabetes mellitus (types 1 and 2), and some cancers, are caused by complex genetic and environmental factors and are thus multifactorial diseases.
8. For most multifactorial diseases, empirical risks (risks based on direct observation of data) have been derived.
9. In contrast to most single-gene diseases, recurrence risks for multifactorial diseases can change significantly from one population to another because gene frequencies, as well as environmental factors, can differ among populations.
10. Several criteria are used to define multifactorial inheritance: (a) the recurrence risk becomes higher if more than one family member is affected; (b) if the expression of the disease in a proband is more severe, the recurrence risk is higher; (c) the recurrence risk is higher if the proband is of the less commonly affected sex; (d) the recurrence risk for the disease usually decreases rapidly in more remotely related relatives; and (e) if the prevalence of the disease in a population is f, the risk for offspring and siblings of probands is approximately $\sqrt{f}$.

Nature and Nurture: Disentangling the Effects of Genes and Environment

1. Family members share genes and a common environment; therefore resemblance in traits, such as high blood pressure, reflects both genetic and environmental factors (nature and nurture, respectively).
2. Few traits are influenced *only* by genes or *only* by environment. Most are influenced by both.
3. When a disease has a relatively larger genetic component, as in breast cancer, examination of family history should be emphasized in addition to lifestyle modification.
4. Two research strategies often are used to estimate the relative influence of genes and environment-lifestyle: twin studies and adoption studies.
5. MZ twins originate when the developing embryo divides to form two separate but identical embryos.
6. DZ twins are the result of a double ovulation followed by the fertilization of each egg by a different sperm.
7. If both members of a twin pair share a trait, they are said to be *concordant*. If they do not share the same trait, they are *discordant*.
8. Studies of adopted children also are used to estimate the genetic contribution to a multifactorial trait.
9. A genetic predisposition may interact with an environmental-lifestyle factor to increase the risk of disease; this is called a *gene-environment interaction*.

Genetics of Common Diseases

1. Congenital diseases are those present at birth. Most of these diseases are multifactorial in etiology.
2. Multifactorial diseases in adults include coronary heart disease, hypertension, breast cancer, colon cancer, diabetes mellitus, obesity, Alzheimer disease, alcoholism, schizophrenia, and bipolar affective disorder.
3. It is incorrect to assume that the presence of a genetic component means that the course of a disease cannot be altered—most diseases have *both* genetic and environmental aspects.

REFERENCES

1. Duarte CW, et al. Multifactorial inheritance and complex diseases. In: Rimoin DL, ed. *Emery and Rimoin's Principles and Practice of Medical Genetics*. ed 6 Philadelphia: Elsevier; 2012.
2. Hodges H, Fealko C, Soares N. Autism spectrum disorder: definition, epidemiology, causes, and clinical evaluation. *Transl Pediatr*. 2020;9(Suppl 1):S55–S65.
3. Hansen SN, et al. Recurrence risk of autism in siblings and cousins: a multi-national, population-based study. *J Am Acad Child Adolesc Psychiatry*. 2019;58:866–875.
4. Clarke A. *Harper's Practical Genetic Counseling*. ed 8, London: Hodder Arnold; 2017.
5. Jansweijer JA, et al. Heritability in genetic heart disease: the role of genetic background. *Open Heart*. 2019;6(1):e000929.
6. Kaprio J, Silventoinen K. Advanced methods in twin studies. *Methods Mol Biol*. 2011;713:143–152.
7. Kendler KS, et al. An extended Swedish national adoption study of bipolar disorder illness and cross-generational familial association with schizophrenia and major depression. *JAMA Psychiatry*. 2020;77(8):814–822.
8. Hunt SC, Williams RR, Barlow GK. A comparison of positive family history definitions for defining risk of future disease. *J Chronic Dis*. 1986;39(10):809–821.
9. Khera AV, Kathiresan S. Genetics of coronary artery disease: discovery, biology and clinical translation. *Nat Rev Genet*. 2017;18:331–344.
10. Jorde LB, Carey JC, Bamshad MJ, eds. *Medical Genetics*. ed 6, Philadelphia: Elsevier; 2020.
11. Ng FL, Warren HR, Caulfield MJ. Hypertension genomics and cardiovascular prevention. *Ann Transl Med*. 2018;6:291.
12. ICGC/TCGA Pan-Cancer Analysis of Whole Genomes Consortium: Pan-cancer analysis of whole genomes. *Nature*. 2020;578(7793):82–93.
13. Gallaway MS, et al. Surveillance for cancers associated with tobacco use—United States, 2010–2014. *MMWR Surveill Summ*. 2018;67(12):1–42.
14. DeSantis CE, et al. Breast cancer statistics, 2019. *CA Cancer J Clin*. 2019;69(6):438–451.
15. Lee A, Moon BI, Kim TH. BRCA1/BRCA2 pathogenic variant breast cancer: treatment and prevention strategies. *Ann Lab Med*. 2020;40(2):114–121.
16. Beitsch PD, et al. Underdiagnosis of hereditary breast cancer: are genetic testing guidelines a tool or an obstacle? *J Clin Oncol*. 2019;37(6):453–460.
17. Shah PD, Nathanson KL. Application of panel-based tests for inherited risk of cancer. *Annu Rev Genomics Hum Genet*. 2017;18:201–227.
18. Antoniou A, et al. Average risks of breast and ovarian cancer associated with BRCA1 or BRCA2 mutations detected in case series unselected for family history: a combined analysis of 22 studies. *Am J Hum Genet*. 2003;72:1117–1130.
19. Gaddam S, et al. Male breast cancer risk assessment and screening recommendations in high-risk men who undergo genetic counseling and multigene panel testing. *Clin Breast Cancer*. 2021;21(1):74–79.
20. American Cancer Society *Cancer Facts & Figures 2020*, Atlanta: American Cancer Society; 2020. Available at https://www.cancer.org/content/dam/cancer-org/research/cancer-facts-and-statistics/annual-cancer-facts-and-figures/2020/cancer-facts-and-figures-2020.pdf. (Accessed September 6, 2021).
21. Valle L, et al. Genetic predisposition to colorectal cancer: syndromes, genes, classification of genetic variants and implications for precision medicine. *J Pathol*. 2018;247:574–588.
22. Mantovani G, et al. Hereditary nonpolyposis colorectal cancer (HNPCC): from diagnosis to surgical management of the main hereditary form of colorectal cancer: a review. *J Surg Res (Houst)*. 2020;3(1):020–030. Available at https://doi.10.26502/jsr.10020051. (Accessed September 6, 2021).
23. Sinicrope FA. Lynch syndrome–associated colorectal cancer. *N Engl J Med*. 2018;379(8):764–773.
24. Siegel RL, Miller KD, Jemal A. Cancer statistics, 2018. *CA Cancer J Clin*. 2018;68(1):7–30.
25. Jain MA, Sapra A. *Cancer prostate screening. StatPearls*. Treasure Island, FL: StatPearls Publishing; 2020. Available at https://www.ncbi.nlm.nih.gov/books/NBK556081/ (Accessed September 6, 2021).
26. Wang Y, et al. MicroRNA-1205, encoded on chromosome 8q24, targets *EGLN3* to induce cell growth and contributes to risk of castration-resistant prostate cancer. *Oncogene*. 2019;38:4820–4834.
27. Bailey MH, et al. Comprehensive characterization of cancer driver genes and mutations. *Cell*. 2018;173:371–385. e18.
28. Langenberg C, Lotta LA. Genomic insights into the causes of type 2 diabetes. *Lancet*. 2018;391:2463–2474.
29. Robertson CC, Rich SS. Genetics of type 1 diabetes. *Curr Opin Genet Dev*. 2018;50:7–16.
30. Meigs JB. The genetic epidemiology of type 2 diabetes: opportunities for health translation. *Curr Diab Rep*. 2019;19:62.
31. Grant SFA. The *TCF7L2* locus: a genetic window into the pathogenesis of type 1 and type 2 diabetes. *Diabetes Care*. 2019;42(9):1624–1629.
32. Ahsan W. The journey of thiazolidinediones as modulators of PPARs for the management of diabetes: a current perspective. *Curr Pharm Des*. 2019;25(23):2540–2554.
33. Boyle JP, et al. Projection of the year 2050 burden of diabetes in the US adult population: dynamic modeling of incidence, mortality, and prediabetes prevalence. *Popul Health Metr*. 2010;8:29.
34. Valkovicova T, et al. Novel insights into genetics and clinics of the HNF1A-MODY. *Endocr Regul*. 2019;53(2):110–134.
35. Di Resta C, Ferrari M. New molecular approaches to Alzheimer's disease. *Clin Biochem*. 2019;72:81–86.
36. Naj AC, Schellenberg GD. Genomic variants, genes, and pathways of Alzheimer's disease: an overview. *Am J Med Genet B Neuropsychiatr Genet*. 2017;174:5–26.
37. Witkiewitz K, Litten RZ, Leggio L. Advances in the science and treatment of alcohol use disorder. *Sci Adv*. 2019;5(9):eaax4043.
38. Reilly MT, et al. Genetic studies of alcohol dependence in the context of the addiction cycle. *Neuropharmacology*. 2017;122:3–21.
39. Carvalho AF, et al. Alcohol use disorders. *Lancet*. 2019;394(10200):781–792.
40. Cross-Disorder Group of the Psychiatric Genomics Consortium Genomic relationships, novel loci, and pleiotropic mechanisms across eight psychiatric disorders. *Cell*. 2019;179:1469–1482. e11.
41. Habtewold TD, et al. Association of schizophrenia polygenic risk score with data-driven cognitive subtypes: a six-year longitudinal study in patients, siblings and controls. *Schizophr Res*. 2020;223:135–147.
42. Lo LE, et al. Risk of schizophrenia in relatives of individuals affected by schizophrenia: a meta-analysis. *Psychiatry Res*. 2020;286:112852.

43. Smeland OB, et al. The polygenic architecture of schizophrenia—rethinking pathogenesis and nosology. *Nat Rev Neurol.* 2020;16(7):366–379.
44. Rowland TA, Marwaha S. Epidemiology and risk factors for bipolar disorder. *Ther Adv Psychopharmacol.* 2018;8(9):251–269.
45. Harrison PJ, Geddes JR, Tunbridge EM. The emerging neurobiology of bipolar disorder. *Trends Neurosci.* 2018;41:18–30.

Epigenetics and Disease

Diane P. Genereux

http://evolve.elsevier.com/Rogers/pathophysiology/

CHAPTER OUTLINE

OVERVIEW OF EPIGENETIC MECHANISMS

Humans exhibit an impressive diversity of physical and behavioral features. Much of this diversity is attributable to genetic variation. Another substantial contributor is "epigenetic" ("upon genetic") modification. Although the specific definition of *epigenetic* remains a topic of discussion among biologists,[1,2] it is generally used to describe nongenetic modifications that are heritable when a somatic cell divides (mitotic inheritance), when gametes are produced (germline inheritance),[3] or both. For the purposes of this chapter, *epigenetics* is defined as the broad set of processes that modulate how a given set of genomic information gives rise to phenotype. Epigenetic mechanisms include chemical modifications to DNA and associated histones, and the production of small RNA molecules. Gene regulation by epigenetic processes can occur at the level of either transcription or translation.

Epigenetic modification is critical for fundamental processes of human development, including the differentiation of embryonic stem cells into specific cell types and the inactivation of one of the two X chromosomes in each cell of a genetic female. Some genes are said to be imprinted, meaning that their epigenetic modifications are always inherited such that it is always the allele from the father or from the mother, that is expressed in the offspring.

A variety of diseases can result from abnormal epigenetic states. Metabolic disease can occur when there is aberrant expression of both copies of a locus that is typically imprinted. Environmental stressors can markedly increase the risk of aberrant epigenetic modification and are strongly associated with some cancers. Because of their increasingly clear role in a wide range of pathologies, abnormal epigenetic states are currently a focus of both preventative efforts and pharmaceutical intervention.

EPIGENETIC MECHANISMS

Currently known epigenetic marks (Fig. 6.1) include:

1. DNA methylation, which occurs through the attachment of a methyl group (CH_3) to C5 of a cytosine. In the somatic cells of adults, methylation typically occurs only at cytosines that are followed by a guanine base-site known as a "CpG dinucleotide" (Fig. 6.2). The fraction of CpG dinucleotides that are methylated is variable across the genome. In human embryonic stem cells, methylation also can occur at cytosines outside of the CpG context. Dense DNA methylation of a given region of DNA is typically coincident with hypoacetylation (decrease of functional group acetyl) of the histone proteins around which the DNA is wound (see "Histone modification" later). Together, DNA methylation and histone hypoacetylation tend to be associated with transcriptional silencing, with the exclusion of transcription factors. Binding of transcription factors is required for production of messenger RNAs (mRNAs), which are then transcribed to form protein (see Chapter 4). Marks that are associated with the exclusion of transcription factors typically indicate suppression of expression of the encoded protein.

   DNA methylation plays a prominent role in both human development and disease. For example, in each cell of a normal human female, one of the two X chromosomes is silenced by dense methylation and associated molecular marks, whereas the other X chromosome is transcriptionally active and largely devoid of methylation (see Chapter 4). Dense methylation is characteristic of regions that are heterochromatic, meaning that the DNA is tightly bound into a condensed state and is not actively transcribed. During gastrulation (early embryonic development), there is epigenetic inactivation of one of the two X chromosomes in each cell of a human female, either the X chromosome inherited from her mother or the X chromosome inherited from her father. The determination of which chromosome is to be silenced occurs at random and independently in each of the cells present at this stage of development; the silent state of that chromosome is inherited by all subsequent copies. If a female's two X chromosomes carry different alleles at a given locus, random X inactivation can lead to somatic mosaicism, wherein the alleles active in two different cells can confer two very different traits. Striking examples include the patchy coloration of calico cats and *anhidrotic ectodermal dysplasia*,[4] a condition characterized by patchy presence and absence of sweat glands in the skin of human females who have one X chromosome bearing a normal allele and one X chromosome bearing a mutant allele at the X-encoded locus. Because of the somatic mosaicism that arises through random inactivation of the X chromosome, females tend to have less severe

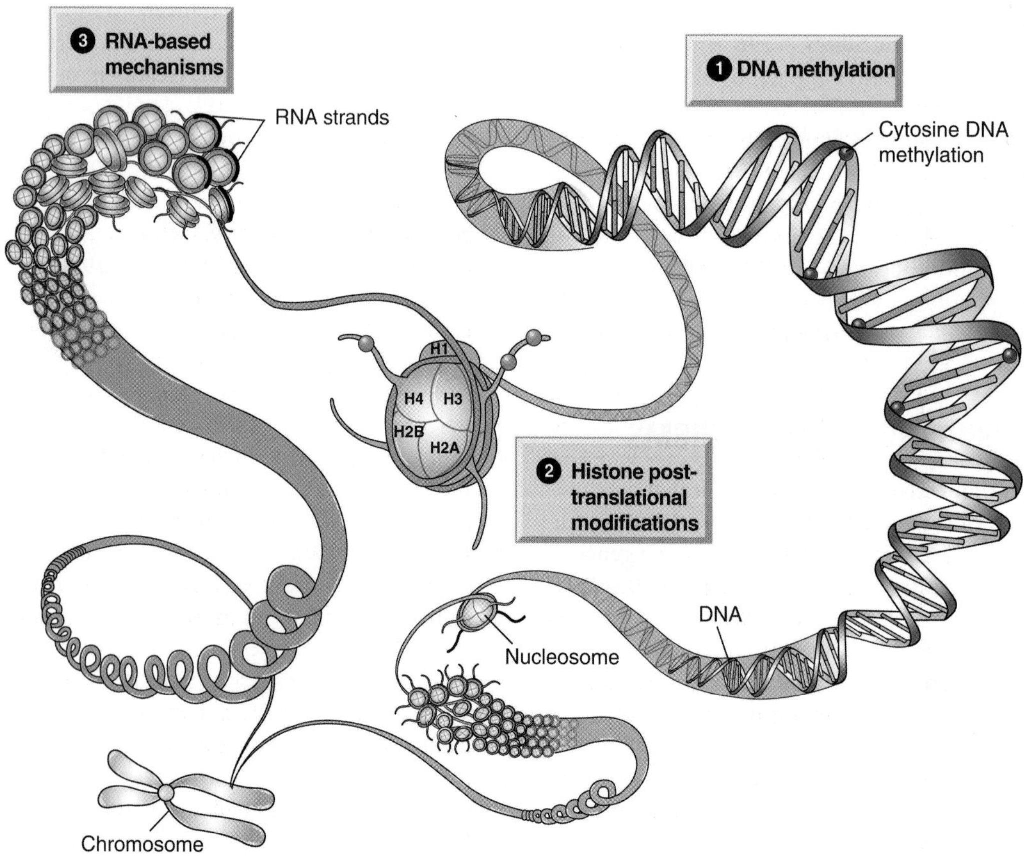

Fig. 6.1 Three Types of Epigenetic Processes. Investigators are studying three epigenetic mechanisms: *(1)* DNA methylation. *(2)* Histone modifications. *(3)* RNA-based mechanisms. See text for discussion.

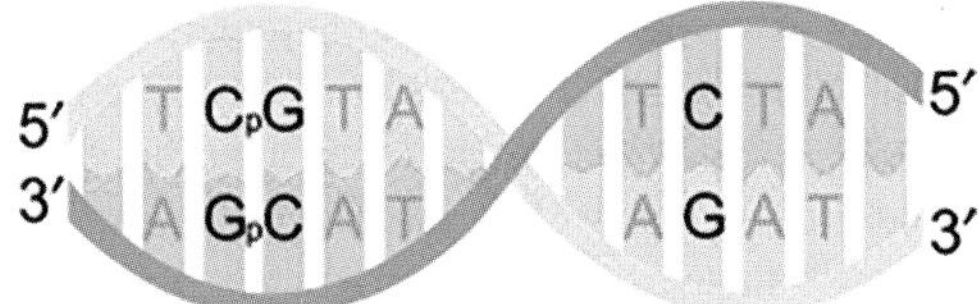

Fig. 6.2 CpG site. A CpG site is the 5′-C-phosphate-G-3′ sequence of nucleotides, shown on one DNA strand *(yellow)*. On the reverse DNA strand *(blue)*, the complementary 5′-CpG-3′ site is shown. A C-G base-pairing between the two strands is also shown *(right)*. (From Moini J, Avgeropoulos NG, Samsam M. Li-Fraumeni syndrome. *Epidemiol Brain Spinal Tumors*. 2021; 367–377. https://doi.org/10.1016/b978-0-12-821736-8.00010-8.)

phenotypes than do males for a variety of X-linked disorders, including color blindness and fragile X syndrome.

Aberrant DNA methylation, either the presence of dense methylation where it is typically absent or absence of methylation where it is typically present, is associated with misregulation of tumor-suppressor genes and oncogenes. Specific alterations to DNA methylation states are a common feature of several human cancers, including those of the colon,[5] breast,[6] and ovaries.[7] Profiling these changes can be useful for cancer diagnosis[8] and for assessing disease prognosis.[9,10] Methods now in development focus on using cell-free DNA and are collected from blood draws to screen individuals for atypical methylation patterns associated with specific cancers. These developments raise the prospect of simultaneous screening for cancers across multiple different tissues (Box 6.1).[11]

BOX 6.1 Cancer of Ovary and Breast Can Arise Through Epigenetic Silencing of Tumor-Suppressor Gene *BRCA1*

Inherited mutations in the coding region of the *BRCA1* and *BRCA2* genes are known to increase risk of breast, ovarian, and prostate cancer. However, such mutations cannot explain all cases of breast cancer. Many families have a high incidence of breast cancer but no known pathogenic variants in the coding regions of the *BRCA1* gene. Researchers sought to identify *epimutations* (errors in epigenetic gene repression) that could potentially account for breast cancer in these families.

Evans et al. used bisulfite sequencing to examine the promoter region of the *BRAC1* or *BRCA2* genes in 49 women who had breast or ovarian cancer but did not have mutations in the coding regions of either gene. Abnormal, dense DNA methylation in the *BRCA1* promoter was found in two of these women. Both women also had a single mutation in the promoter of the gene. Examination of DNA from other women in the families of these women revealed that the point mutation was strongly associated with DNA methylation and transcriptional silencing of the *BRCA1* gene.

In conclusion, point mutations in the promoter region of the *BRCA1* gene can increase the probability of dense methylation. This dense methylation can lead to gene inactivation, indicating that epigenetic mechanisms driven by noncoding mutations can lead to breast cancer through loss of *BRCA1* function.

Data from Evans DGR, van Veen EM, Byers HJ, et al. Inherited BRCA1 epimutation as a novel cause of breast and ovarian cancer. 2018. https://doi.org/10.1101/246934; Evans DGR, van Veen EM, Byers HJ, et al. A dominantly inherited 5′ UTR variant causing methylation-associated silencing of BRCA1 as a cause of breast and ovarian cancer. *Am J Human Genet*. 2018;103:213–220.

2. **DNA hydroxymethylation** is most often observed in cells that are undergoing epigenetic transition. DNA hydroxymethylation differs from DNA methylation, in that it is a hydroxymethyl group, rather than methyl group, that is affixed to the C5 of cytosine. Until recently, considerable uncertainty surrounded the question of how genomic regions, dense in DNA methylation, undergo methylation loss during periods of epigenetic transition. In 2011, Wossidlo et al.[12] found that genome-wide declines in DNA methylation in early murine zygotes occur in concert with genome-wide increases in DNA hydroxymethylation. They also found that this loss of methylation and parallel gain in hydroxymethylation were obliterated in zygotes deficient in the Tet3 enzyme. These results helped to establish that the Tet enzymes can convert DNA methylation into hydroxymethylation. Abnormally low levels of hydroxymethylation in fetal tissue have been linked to neural tube defects[13] and to disease severity in multiple myeloma.[14] Like DNA methylation, DNA hydroxymethylation is under active investigation as a possible target for early detection of cancer using cell-free DNA.[15]
3. **Histone modifications** are chemical changes to the histone proteins around which DNA is coiled and include histone acetylation and deacetylation. **Histones** are proteins that facilitate compaction of genomic DNA by coiling into the nucleus of a cell, much like how a spool helps to organize a long piece of thread for storage in a small space. Chemical modification of histones in a region of DNA can either upregulate or downregulate nearby gene expression by increasing or decreasing the tightness of the interaction between DNA and histones, thus modulating the extent to which DNA is accessible to transcription factors. DNA in association with histones is referred to as "chromatin." At any given time, various regions of chromatin are typically in one of two forms: *euchromatin*, an open state in which most or all nearby genes are transcriptionally active, or *heterochromatin*, a closed state in which most or all nearby genes are transcriptionally inactive.

Chromatin structure plays a critical role in determining the developmental potential of a given cell lineage and can undergo dramatic changes during organismal development. Chromatin states differ substantially between embryonic stem cells, which are poised to give rise to all the different cell types that comprise an individual, and terminally differentiated cells, which are committed to a specific developmental path. The fraction of DNA that is in the heterochromatic state increases as cells differentiate. This is consistent with the decrease in the fraction of the genome that is transcriptionally active when a cell lineage transitions from pluripotency into a terminally differentiated somatic lineage.[16] Mutations in genes that encode histone proteins can render cells refractory to differentiation signals,[17] and specific mutations are useful for assessing disease prognosis in children with aggressive gliomas.[18]

In contrast to most other cell types, including oocytes, sperm cells express not histones but protamines, which are evolutionarily derived from histones. Protamines, encoded by just two genes in the human genome,[19] enable sperm DNA to wind into an even more compact state than does the histone-bound DNA in somatic cells. This tight compaction improves the hydrodynamic features of the sperm head, facilitating its movement. Expression of protamine-encoding gene can be modulated by some dietary factors,[20] hinting at connections between environment and male fertility.

4. Noncoding RNAs (ncRNAs) play an important role in regulating a wide variety of cellular processes, including RNA splicing and DNA replication.[21] Of relevance to gene regulation are the hairpin-shaped microRNAs (miRNAs), which are encoded by DNA sequences of approximately 22 nucleotides, typically within the introns of genes or in noncoding DNA located between genes. In contrast to DNA methylation and histone modification, both of which principally impacted gene expression at the level of transcription, miRNAs typically modulate the stability and translational efficiency of existing mRNAs encoded at other loci. Interaction between miRNAs and mRNAs targeted for degradation is typically mediated by regions of partial sequence complementarity. As a result, miRNAs can at once be specific enough so that they do not bind to *all* the mRNAs in a cell and general enough to regulate many different mRNA sequences. miRNAs also directly modulate translation by impairing ribosomal function. miRNAs regulate diverse signaling pathways; those that stimulate cancer development and progression are called oncomirs. For example, miRNAs have been linked to carcinogenesis because they alter the activity of oncogenes and tumor-suppressor genes.

THREE TYPES OF EPIGENETIC PROCESSES

Epigenetics and Human Development

Each of the cells in the very early embryo has the potential to give rise to a somatic cell of any type. These embryonic stem cells are said to be *totipotent* ("possessing all powers"). A key process in early development is the differential epigenetic modification of specific DNA nucleotide sequences in these embryonic stem cells, which ultimately leads to the differential gene-expression profiles that characterize the various differentiated somatic cell types. These early modifications ensure that specific genes are expressed only in the cells and tissue types in which their gene products typically function (e.g., factor VIII expression primarily in hepatocytes, or dopamine receptor expression in neurons).

Epigenetic modifications that arise during early development ensure that specific genes are expressed only in the cells and tissue types in which their gene products normally function. Only a small percentage of genes, termed housekeeping genes, are ubiquitously expressed across cell types, escaping epigenetic silencing to remain transcriptionally active in all or nearly all cell types. Housekeeping genes include those encoding histones, DNA and RNA polymerases, and ribosomal RNA genes.

How do embryonic stem cells achieve epigenetic states typical of totipotency and can give rise to all the diverse cell types that comprise a fully developed organism? One hypothesis is that early embryogenesis (the 10 or so days just after fertilization) is characterized by rapid fluctuation in genome-wide DNA methylation densities. Fertilization triggers a global loss of DNA methylation at most loci in both the oocyte-contributed and the sperm-contributed genomes. This loss of methylation is accomplished in part by suppression of the DNA methyltransferases, the enzymes that add methyl groups to DNA. Methylation is not directly copied by the DNA replication process. Instead, immediately following replication, the methyltransferases read the pattern of methylation on the parent DNA strand and use that information to determine which daughter-strand cytosines should be methylated. As embryonic cell division proceeds in the absence of DNA methyltransferases, cell division continues, eventually yielding cells that have nearly all their loci in unmethylated, transcriptionally active states. Around the time of implantation in the uterus, the DNA methyltransferases become active again, permitting establishment of the cell lineage–specific marks required for the establishment of organ systems.

Genomic Imprinting

A baby inherits two copies of each autosomal gene: one from its mother and one from its father. For a large subset of these genes, expression is biallelic, meaning that both the maternal and the paternal inherited copies contribute to offspring phenotype. For another, smaller subset of these genes, expression is stochastically monoallelic, meaning that the maternal copy is randomly chosen for inactivation in some somatic cells and the paternal copy is randomly chosen for inactivation in other somatic cells. For a third and smaller subset of autosomes (approximately 1%), either the maternal copy or the paternal copy is imprinted, meaning that either the copy inherited through the sperm or the copy inherited through the egg is inactivated and remains in this inactive state in all of the somatic cells of the individual.[22]

The subset of genes that are subject to imprinting is highly enriched for loci that are relevant to organismal growth. The *genetic conflict hypothesis*[23] was developed as a potential explanation for this pattern. Although both the mother and father benefit genetically from the birth and survival of offspring, their interests are not entirely aligned. Because a mother makes a large physiologic investment in each child, it is in her evolutionary best interest to limit the flow of energetic resources to any given offspring, to maintain her physiologic capacity to bear subsequent children. By contrast, it is in the best interest of the father for his child to extract maximum resources from the mother because his own future fecundity (fertility) is not contingent on the sustained fecundity of the mother. In general, imprinting of maternally inherited genes tends to reduce offspring size, whereas imprinting of paternally inherited genes tends to increase offspring size. One hallmark of imprinting-associated disease is that the phenotype of affected individuals is critically dependent on whether the mutation is inherited from the mother or from the father.

A well-known disease example of imprinting is associated with a deletion of approximately 4 million base (Mb) pairs

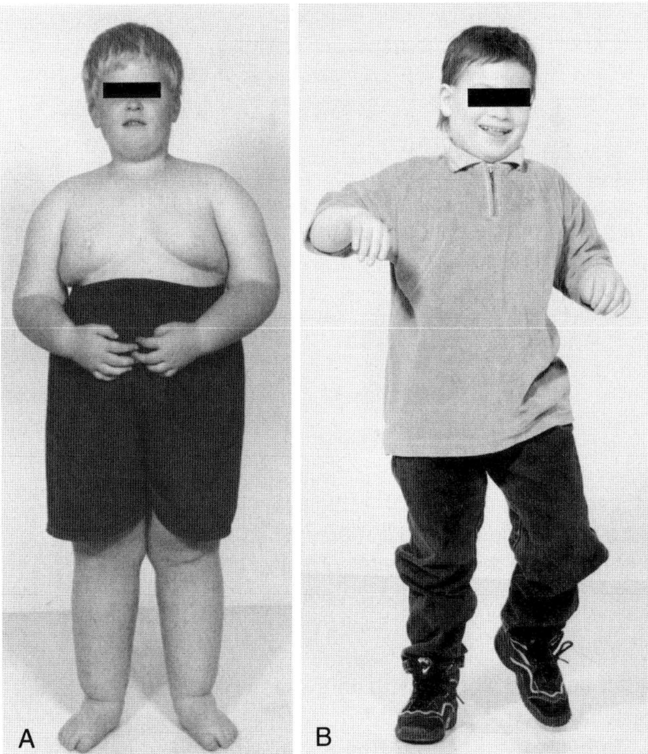

Fig. 6.3 Prader-Willi and Angelman Syndromes. **(A)** A child with Prader-Willi syndrome (truncal obesity, small hands and feet, inverted V-shaped upper lip). **(B)** A child with Angelman syndrome (characteristic posture, ataxic gait, bouts of uncontrolled laughter). (From Jorde LB, Carey JC, Bamshad MJ. *Medical Genetics*. 4th ed. Philadelphia: Mosby; 2010.)

of the long arm of chromosome 15. When this deletion is inherited from the father, the child manifests Prader-Willi syndrome, whose features include short stature, hypotonia, small hands and feet, obesity, mild to moderate intellectual disability, and hypogonadism (Fig. 6.3A). The same 4-Mb deletion, when inherited from the mother, causes Angelman syndrome, which is characterized by severe intellectual disability, seizures, and an ataxic gait (see Fig. 6.3B). These diseases are each observed in approximately 1 of every 10,000 to 30,000 live births; chromosome deletions are responsible for approximately 70% of cases of both diseases.[24] The deletions that cause Prader-Willi and Angelman syndromes are indistinguishable at the DNA sequence level and affect the same group of genes.

Prader-Willi and Angelman Syndromes

For several decades, it was unclear how the same deletion could produce such disparate results in different individuals. Further analysis showed that the 4-Mb deletion (the *critical region*) contains several genes that are normally transcribed only on the copy of chromosome 15 that is inherited from the father.[25]

These genes are transcriptionally inactive (imprinted) on the copy of chromosome 15 inherited from the mother. Similarly, other genes in the critical region are transcriptionally active only on the chromosome copy inherited from the mother and are inactive on the chromosome inherited from the father. Thus several genes in this region are normally active on only one chromosome copy. If the single active copy of one of these genes is lost because of a chromosome deletion, then no gene product is produced resulting in disease.

Prader-Willi Syndrome Pedigrees

Molecular analysis has revealed much about genes in this critical region of chromosome 15.[25] The gene responsible for Angelman syndrome encodes a ligase involved in protein degradation during brain development (consistent with the intellectual disability and ataxia observed in this disorder). In brain tissue, this gene is active only on the chromosome copy inherited from the mother. Consequently, for this gene a maternally transmitted deletion removes the single active copy. Several genes in the critical region are associated with Prader-Willi syndrome, and they are transcribed only on the chromosome transmitted by the father. A paternally transmitted deletion removes the only active copies of these genes producing the features of Prader-Willi syndrome (Fig. 6.4).

Beckwith-Wiedemann Syndrome

Another well-known example of imprinting is Beckwith-Wiedemann syndrome, an overgrowth condition accompanied by an increased predisposition to cancer. Beckwith-Wiedemann syndrome is usually identifiable at birth because of large size for gestational age, neonatal hypoglycemia, a large tongue, creases on the ear lobe, and omphalocele (birth defect of infant intestines). Children with Beckwith-Wiedemann syndrome have an increased risk of developing Wilms tumor or hepatoblastoma. Both tumors can be treated effectively if they are detected early; thus screening at regular intervals is an important part of management.[26] Some children with Beckwith-Wiedemann syndrome also develop asymmetric overgrowth of a limb or one side of the face or trunk (hemihyperplasia) (Fig. 6.5). As with Angelman syndrome, a minority of Beckwith-Wiedemann syndrome cases (approximately 20% to 30%) are caused by the inheritance of two copies of a chromosome from the father and no copy of the chromosome from the mother (uniparental disomy, in this case affecting chromosome 11). Several genes on the short arm of chromosome 11 are imprinted on either the paternally or maternally transmitted chromosome. These genes are found in two separate, differentially methylated regions (DMRs). In DMR1, the gene that encodes insulin-like growth factor 2 *(IGF2)* is inactive on the maternally transmitted chromosome but active on the paternally transmitted chromosome. Thus a normal individual has only one active copy of *IGF2*. When two copies of the paternal chromosome are inherited (i.e., paternal uniparental disomy) or there is loss of imprinting on the maternal copy of *IGF2*, an active *IGF2* gene is present in double dose. These changes produce increased levels of IGF2 during fetal development contributing to the overgrowth features of Beckwith-Wiedemann syndrome. Note that, in contrast to Prader-Willi and Angelman syndromes, which are produced by a missing gene product, Beckwith-Wiedemann syndrome is caused, in part, by overexpression of a gene product.

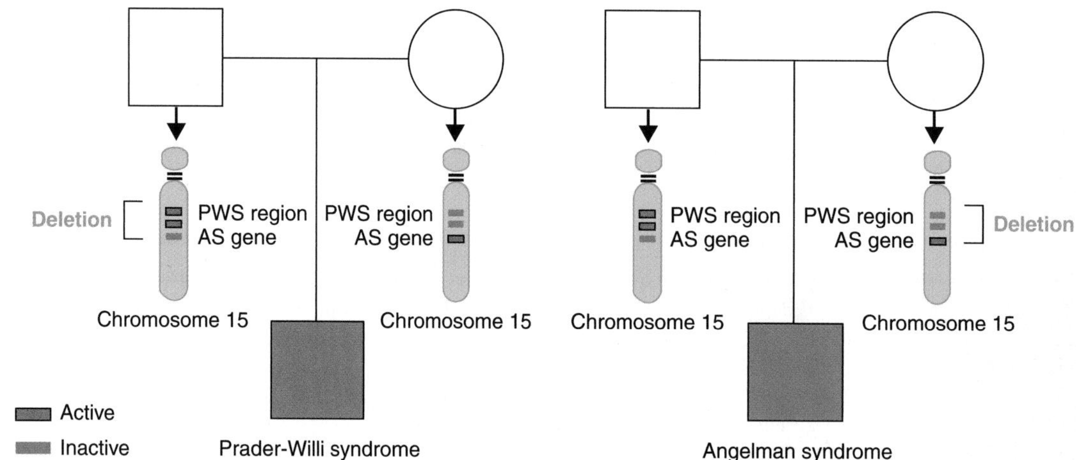

Fig. 6.4 Prader-Willi Syndrome Pedigrees. These pedigrees illustrate the inheritance patterns of Prader-Willi syndrome, which can be caused by a 4-million base pair (Mb) deletion of chromosome 15q when inherited from the father. In contrast, Angelman syndrome can be caused by the same deletion but only when it is inherited from the mother. The reason for this difference is that different genes in this region are normally imprinted (inactivated) in the copies of 15q transmitted by the mother and the father. (From Jorde LB, Carey JC, Bamshad MJ. *Medical Genetics*. 4th ed. Philadelphia; Mosby; 2010.)

Russell-Silver Syndrome

Russell-Silver syndrome is characterized by growth retardation; proportionate short stature; leg length discrepancy; and a small, triangular-shaped face (Fig. 6.6). Approximately one-third of Russell-Silver syndrome cases are caused by imprinting abnormalities of chromosome 11p15.5 that led to downregulation of IGF2 and therefore diminished growth. Another 10% of cases of Russell-Silver syndrome are caused by maternal uniparental disomy. Thus upregulation or extra copies of active IGF2 causes overgrowth in Beckwith-Wiedemann syndrome, whereas downregulation of IGF2 causes the diminished growth seen in Russell-Silver syndrome.[27]

Epigenetics in Development and Mental Health

Several lines of evidence suggest a role for epigenetic abnormalities in disorders of development.

Epigenetics and Ethanol Exposure in Utero

The impact of ethanol exposure in utero on skeletal and neural development was first reported in 1973[28] and led to broad awareness of fetal alcohol syndrome (see Chapter 2). Only recently did population-based and molecular-level studies begin to clarify the epigenetic signals that mediate these impacts via both genome-wide and locus-specific mechanisms. The DNA methylation status of specific CpG sites differs between children with and without fetal alcohol spectrum disorder. The epigenetic impacts of ethanol exposure may extend to adulthood, with large cohort studies indicating changes in global[29] and site-specific methylation[30] as candidate markers of high level of alcohol consumption.

Epigenetics and Mental Health

Several emerging lines of evidence indicate an association between altered epigenetic states and mental health. Methylation profiles at genes associated with social behavior differ between women with anorexia nervosa and normal, age-matched controls.[31]

Individuals with posttraumatic stress disorder (PTSD) are reported to have changes in the methylation states of four cytosines within an immune-regulatory locus,[32] offering a potential explanation for the earlier finding of immune hyperactivation in affected individuals.[33] Many studies indicate an impact of adverse events during childhood on methylation profiles in adulthood (See Emerging Science Box: Parsing Apart Contributions of Genotype and Childhood Adversity to Methylation States in Adulthood).[34] Genomic regions may vary

EMERGING SCIENCE BOX

Parsing Apart Contributions of Genotype and Childhood Adversity to Methylation States in Adulthood

Although some studies have suggested that epigenetic mechanisms may mediate the long-term health effects of adversity in early life (reviewed in Kundakovic and Champagne, 2015), results have been highly variable across studies. Cazmara and colleagues (2021) sought to address these complexities directly by quantifying the relative contributions of genotype and early-life adversity to methylation states in blood and saliva samples taken from individuals of a range of ages. Exposure to childhood adversity was assessed through retrospective surveys. The study finds little evidence of a direct role for childhood adversity in shaping methylation states at any age. However, the authors detected evidence of a role for interactions between genotype and childhood adversity in explaining methylation states later in life. The finding that some genotypes could heighten the potential for adverse experiences early in life will yield epigenetic outcomes could help to explain inconsistent outcomes across studies in which genotype was not measured, or not considered in data analysis.

Data from Czamara D, et al. Combined effects of genotype and childhood adversity shape variability of DNA methylation across age. *Transl Psychiatry.* 2021;11(1):88; Kundakovic M, et al. Early-life experience, epigenetics, and the developing brain. *Neuropsychopharmacology.* 2015;40(1):141–153.

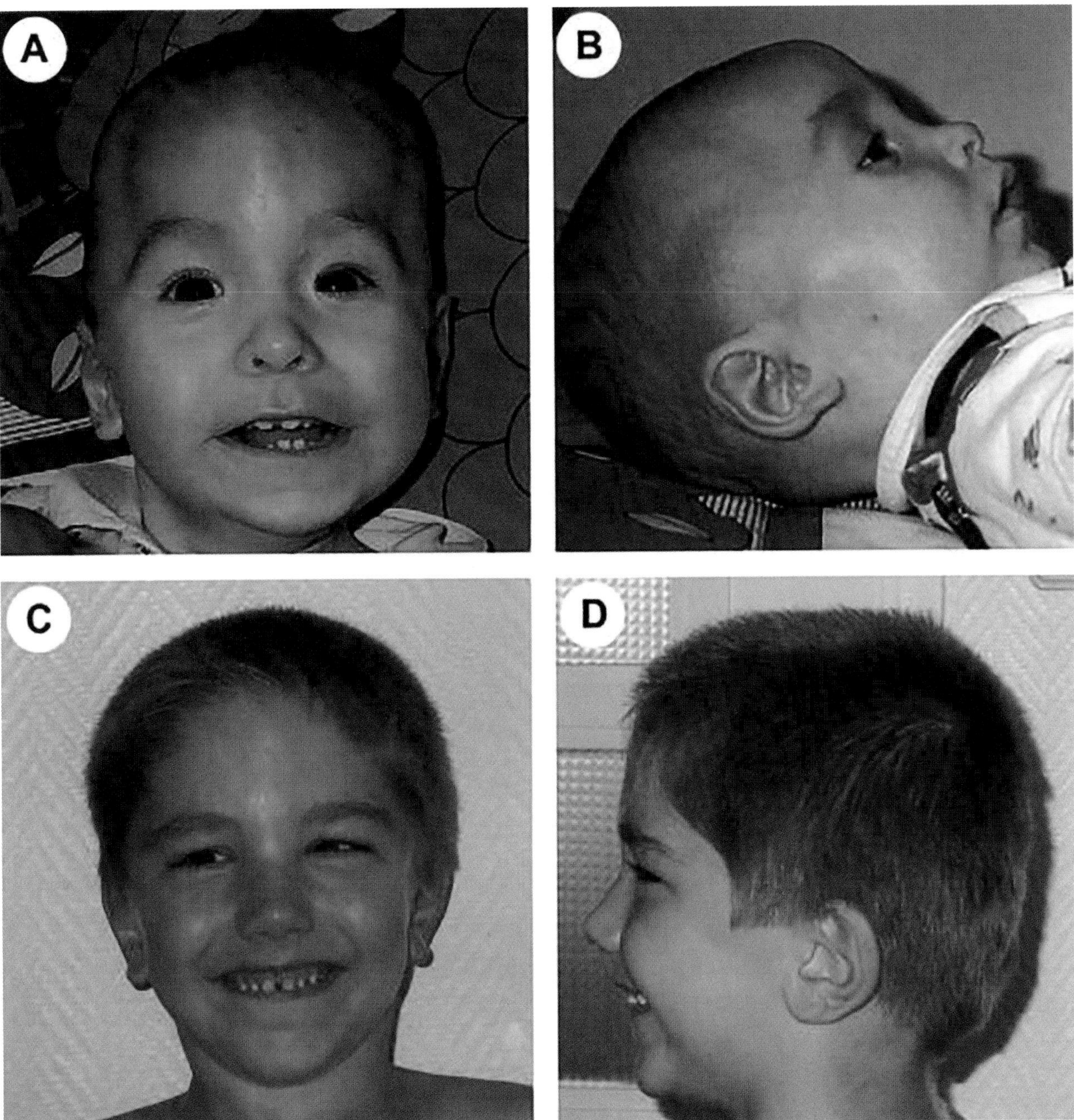

Fig. 6.5 Beckwith-Wiedemann Syndrome. Facial features of individuals with Beckwith-Wiedemann Syndrome (BWS). **A** and **B**, Frontal and lateral views of 1-year-old who had craniostensosis from a 1-bp NSD1 deletion. The Frontal bossing and antimongoloid slant of the palpebral fissure are not typical of BWS. **C** and **D**, Frontal and lateral views of a 4-year-old child with BWS who had a 4-bp NSD1 deletion. (From Baujat G, Rio M, Rossignol S, et al. Paradoxical NSD1 mutations in Beckwith-Wiedemann syndrome and 11p15 anomalies in Sotos syndrome. *Am J Hum Genet.* 2004;74[4]:715–720.)

in the timing of their greatest sensitivity to the environment, with some reports indicating that adversity before age three has the greatest impact.[35] An ongoing challenge for studies linking environment to mental health is to determine whether observed epigenetic alterations play a mechanistic role in the etiology of cognitive syndromes or whether information on this link is considered principally for suggesting biomarkers potentially useful for diagnosis.

Fragile X Syndrome: A Genetic/Epigenetic Syndrome

In some diseases, both genetic and epigenetic factors contribute to the origin of abnormal phenotypes. For example, several abnormal phenotypes can arise in individuals with mutations at the fragile X locus, *FMR1*. The most common genetic abnormality at *FMR1* involves expansion in the number of cytosine-guanine (CG) dinucleotide repeats in the gene promoter. Females who have CG repeats more than the approximate 35

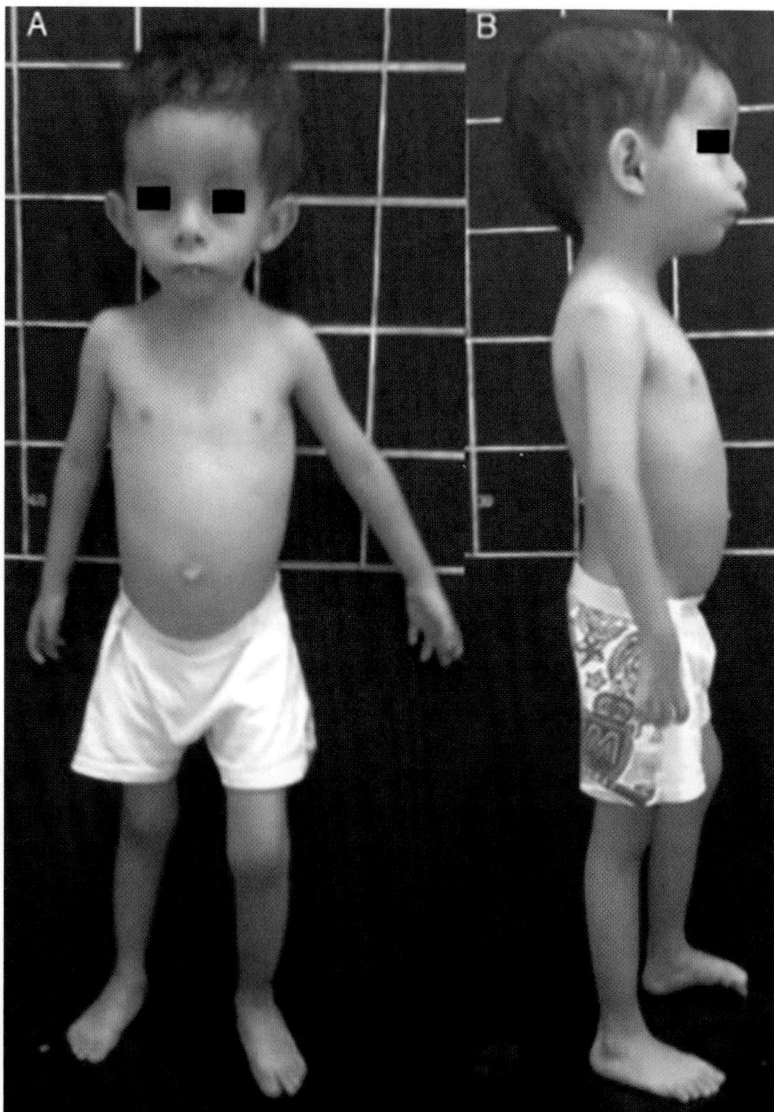

Fig. 6.6 Russell-Silverman Syndrome. Child with Russell-Silverman Syndrome. **A**, Front view. **B**, Lateral view. Note hemihypertrophy with asymmetry, relative macrocephaly, triangular facies, prominent upper jaw, and an undersized lower jaw. (From Galaz-Montoya CI, García-Delgado C, Cervantes-Peredo A, et al. Clinical profile of a cohort of Silver-Russell syndrome patients followed at the Hospital Infantil de México Federico Gómez from 1998 to 2012. *Bol Med Hosp Infant Mex.* 2014;71[4]:218–226.)

that are typical at this locus are at risk for fragile X–associated primary ovarian insufficiency, characterized by an elevated risk of early menopause.[36] Males with moderate expansions are at risk of fragile X tremor ataxia syndrome (FXTAS), characterized by a late-onset intention tremor and mitochondrial dysfunction.[37] Psychiatric phenotypes in the absence of intention tremor have also been reported for males with a premutation allele.[38]

Individuals with 200 repeats are at risk of fragile X syndrome, characterized by reduced IQ and a set of behavioral abnormalities. Fragile X syndrome, which is characterized by cognitive impairment, results from abnormal epigenetic silencing of the *FMR1* locus via accrual of dense methylation within the expanded CG repeat region (Fig. 6.7A); targeted demethylation is sufficient to restore transcriptional activity of the expanded allele in cultured neurons, suggesting a potential therapeutic path. Remarkably, although possession of a large CG repeat in the *FMR1* promoter dramatically increases the probability that an individual will have fragile X syndrome, the disease can be present in males who have the large repeat and absent in their male siblings who have inherited an allele of very similar size.[39] The difference can be explained in part by the observation that acquisition of methylation-based silencing at *FMR1* is stochastic, meaning that the presence of a large repeat increases the probability of the dense promoter methylation that could lead to gene silencing but does not

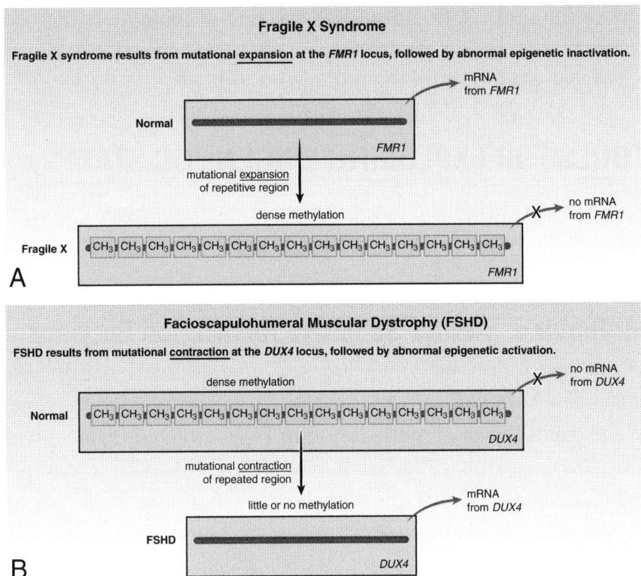

Fig. 6.7 Comparing the Molecular Mechanisms of Fragile X and Facioscapulohumeral Muscular Dystrophy. (A) *FMR1* in normal, expanded permutation, and full-mutation states. (B) *DUX4* in normal and contracted states.

guarantee it. It remains to be seen whether dietary or environmental features can modulate the probability that dense methylation at *FMR1* will accrue in individuals with the full-mutation allele. Facioscapulohumeral muscular dystrophy results from the converse process, wherein mutational contraction of the DUX4 locus results in loss of methylation and aberrant expression (see Fig. 6.7B).

EXPLORING THE MULTIGENERATIONAL PERSISTENCE OF EPIGENETIC STATES

In some cases, epigenetic changes arising during an individual's lifetime may be transmitted through the germline, with the potential to impact gene expression in future generations.

Epigenetics and Nutrition

During the winter of 1943, millions of people in urban areas of the Netherlands suffered starvation conditions because of Nazi blockage of shipments of food from agricultural areas. When researchers sought to investigate how exposure to famine in utero had impacted individuals born in a historically prosperous country, they found individuals who suffered nutritional deprivation in utero were more likely to suffer from obesity and diabetes as adults than individuals in the Netherlands who had not experienced nutritional deprivation during gestation. There also seemed to be a transgenerational impact. The children of individuals who were in utero during the Dutch Hunger Winter were found to be significantly smaller than the children of those not impacted by the blockade. Other data sets reveal elevated risk of cardiovascular and metabolic disease for offspring of individuals exposed during early development to fluctuations in agricultural yields,[40] suggesting an intergenerational effect. More recent studies have

BOX 6.2 Epigenetics Could Explain Correlation Between Birth Month and Body Mass Index

It has long been observed that people conceived during cold times of the year tend to have lower body mass index (BMI) compared with people conceived during warmer times of the year. Sun et al. exposed male and female mice to cold temperatures before mating, then assessed the body mass and gene expression in their offspring. Their findings confirmed data from human populations. Offspring of male mice exposed to cold before mating tend to have larger amounts of brown adipose, a tissue with very high metabolic rate, as well as a lower overall probability of diet-induced obesity. Exposing female mice to cold before mating had no impact on brown adipose or obesity risk in their offspring. Exploration of DNA methylation in the sperm of cold-exposed male mice revealed methylation in the promoters of several genes involved in the production of brown adipose tissue.

In conclusion, the sperm of male mice exposed to cold have reduced methylation in several genes relevant to the development of brown adipose tissue by a yet unknown mechanism. The offspring of these cold-exposed males have higher expression of these genes, resulting in higher amounts of brown adipose tissue, higher metabolic rate, and lowering risk of diet-induced obesity. Future work could focus on potential applications of cold exposure in the treatment or prevention of obesity.

Data from Sun W, Dong H, Becker AS, et al. Cold-induced epigenetic programming of the sperm enhances brown adipose tissue activity in offspring. *Nat Med.* 2018;24(9):1372–1383.

also uncovered a relationship between exposures in utero and metabolic health in adulthood.[41,42]

The specific molecular mechanisms that mediate reported relationships between exposure to famine and disease risk in adulthood or in subsequent generations remain largely unknown. From some animal models, it seems that the IGF2 gene is a possible target of epigenetic modifications arising through nutritional deprivation. Exposure in utero and through lactation to some chemicals (including bisphenol A, a constituent of plastics sometimes used in food preparation and storage) seems to lead to epigenetic modifications similar to those that arise through nutritional deprivation in early life (Box 6.2).[43]

Epigenetics and Maternal Care

Mice and other rodents can exhibit two alternative styles of nursing behavior: frequent arched-back nursing, with a high level of licking and grooming behavior, and a style with infrequent arched-back nursing, with reduced licking and grooming behavior. A number of studies[44] have found that methylation states at the glucocorticoid receptor differ between mice exposed to these two different categories of maternal care. Because the glucocorticoid receptor is involved in a pathway that intensifies fearfulness and response to stress, these findings suggest that alteration to methylation states could help to explain the finding that exposure to stress early in life can modulate behavior in adulthood. These findings also highlight the concept that epigenetic processes can help store information about the environment and that the relevant epigenetic modifications can modulate behavior later in life.

EPIGENETIC CHANGE OVER THE LIFESPAN

Twin Studies Provide Insights on Epigenetic Modification

Identical (monozygotic) twins, whose DNA sequences are essentially the same, offer a unique opportunity to isolate and examine the trajectory of epigenetic change over the lifespan. A recent study found that, as twins age, they exhibit increasingly substantial differences in methylation patterns of the DNA sequences of their somatic cells; these changes are often reflected in increasing numbers of phenotypic differences. Twins with significant lifestyle differences (e.g., smoking versus nonsmoking) tend to accumulate larger numbers of differences in their methylation patterns. These results, along with findings that caloric restriction and other factors known to slow aging can also alter methylation states,[45] suggest that changes in epigenetic patterns may be an important part of the aging process (Fig. 6.8).

The 2013 discovery of a set of approximately 350 CpG sites whose methylation status corresponds closely to an individual's age in years has inspired and enabled study of how specific environmental factors modulate the rate of biologic aging. For example, one recent study uncovered significant effects of vegetable consumption on the body mass index.[46]

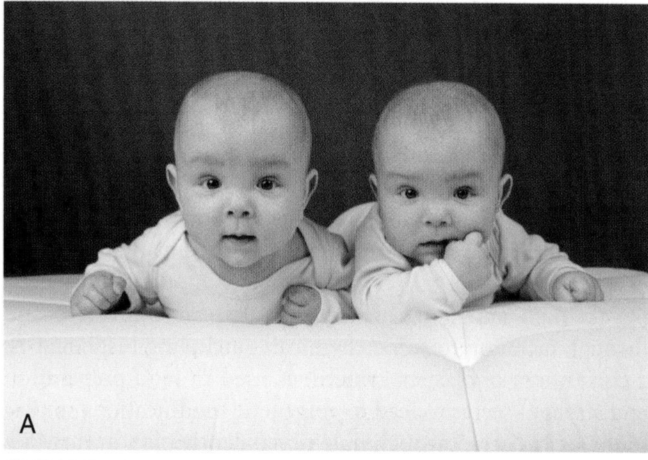

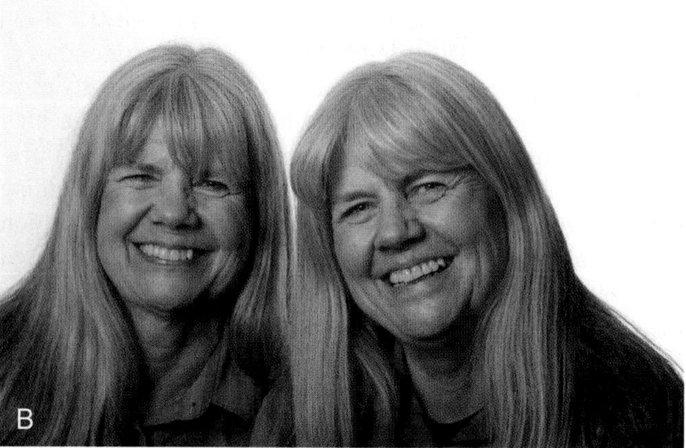

Fig. 6.8 Twins and Aging. **(A)** Twins as babies look very much alike but **(B)** as adults have slight differences in appearance, possibly because of epigenetics. (A, vgm/Shutterstock. B, Stacey Bates/Shutterstock.)

TOOLS FOR EXPLORING EPIGENETIC STATES

Epigenetic information is not encoded DNA sequence. Therefore specialized methods must be used to detect and quantify it.

Detecting DNA Methylation in Populations of Molecules: Methyl-Sensitive Restriction Enzymes

Many restriction enzymes are sensitive to methylation and cleave DNA only at cytosines that are free of methylation. Clues to the overall level of methylation in DNA isolated from a given individual can be gathered by treating DNA with a methyl-sensitive enzyme and then comparing banding patterns for enzyme-treated and non–enzyme-treated samples.[47]

Detecting DNA Methylation in Single Molecules: Bisulfite Conversion

However, it is of interest to gather information about methylation on individual molecules. For example, among males who inherit a full-mutation fragile X allele, there is a strong correlation of the severity of the syndrome to the number of cells in which the fragile X allele is densely methylated.[39] To collect information on the methylation states of individual molecules, DNA can be subjected to bisulfite conversion prior to sequencing. Bisulfite treatment does not alter most nucleotides, including methylated cytosines, but deaminates unmethylated cytosines to uracil (Fig. 6.9).[48] Because uracil complements adenine, not guanine, methylated and unmethylated cytosines can be distinguished in resulting sequence data if the reference nucleotide sequence is known. Either subcloning followed by Sanger sequencing, or next-generation sequencing can then be applied to ascertain the detailed methylation patterns of individual molecules.

Detecting DNA Hydroxymethylation: Fluorescence Resonance Energy Transfer

Efforts to track the early-developmental transition from methylation to hydroxymethylation were initially hampered by the absence of a method to detect relative levels of DNA methylation and DNA hydroxymethylation within individual molecules. The introduction of Tet-assisted pyridine borane sequencing (TAPS) solves this problem. Like bisulfite treatment, TAPS involves a chemical conversion step but follows this step with enzyme-mediated C-to-T transition.

Identifying Histone-Modification States: Chromatin Immunoprecipitation

Information on the identity of DNA-bound proteins can provide important clues as to the activity states of individual regions. The goal of chromatin immunoprecipitation (ChIP) is to ascertain the sequences bound to specific proteins of interest. Broadly, this is achieved in six steps:

1. Crosslink DNA-bound proteins and the specific genomic regions to which they are attached. At this step, binding is

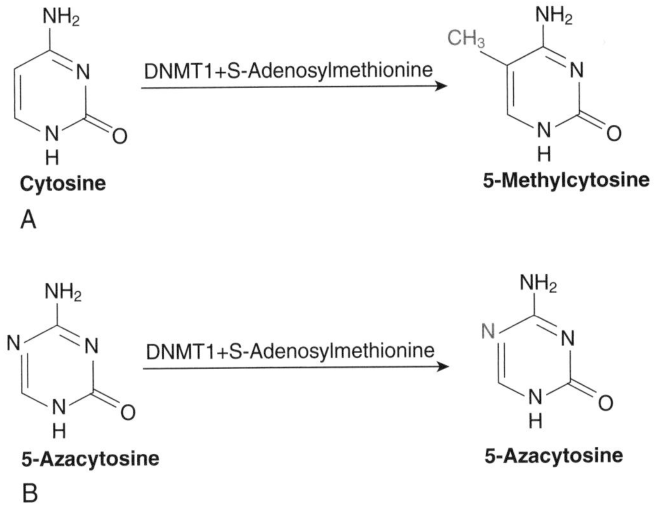

Fig. 6.9 5-Azacytosine as Demethylating Agent. **(A)** Unmethylated cytosines in DNA are typically subject to the addition of methyl groups by DNA methyltransferase 1 (DNMT1), a DNA methyltransferase, using methyl groups supplied by the methyl donor S-adenosylmethionine. **(B)** In 5-azacytosine, the 5′ carbon of cytosine is replaced with a nitrogen. This chemical difference is sufficient both to block the addition of a methyl group and to confer irreversible binding to DNMT1. Incorporation of 5-azacytosine into DNA is therefore sufficient to drive passive loss of methylation from replicating DNA and thus to reactivate hypermethylated loci. 5-Azacytosine, bound to a sugar, can be integrated into DNA and has been administered with some success in treating epigenetic diseases that arise through hypermethylation of individual loci.

not specific, meaning that all proteins, regardless of identity, are crosslinked to DNA.

2. Shear DNA, effectively lysing DNA regions that are not protein bound.
3. Select for proteins of interest, using an antibody specific to the protein of interest.
4. Capture protein-DNA complexes using a secondary antibody that can bind to the first; wash away any remaining, unbound DNA fragments.
5. Remove protein-DNA crosslinks and wash away proteins.
6. Sequence DNA fragments to profile the portion of genome that was bound by the protein of interest.

Detecting DNA Accessibility States: DNAse Hypersensitivity Testing

One of the hallmarks of transcriptionally active regions of the genome is sensitivity to cleavage by DNAses, enzymes that cleave DNA regions that are not protein bound. To identify these regions of active transcription, bulk DNA samples are initially treated with DNAses. Uncut regions can then be mapped to a reference genome sequence, and hypersensitive, transcriptionally active sites can be identified. DNAse hypersensitivity assays enable high-throughput data collection and comparison of chromatin-accessibility profiles across cell types and health and disease states.[49]

Detecting DNA Accessibility States in Single Molecules: Assay for Transposase-Accessible Chromatin

Like DNAse hypersensitivity testing, the recently introduced assay for transposase-accessible chromatin (ATAC-seq) is focused on identifying genomic regions whose "open" states suggest that they could be transcriptionally active.[50] However, in contrast to DNAse assays, under which transcriptionally active states are identified by their overall sensitivity to DNAse cleavage enzyme cleavage, ATAC-seq uses a transpose for which cleavage of accessible sites is followed immediately by specific ligation of a linker that bears barcodes that differ among cells. Genomic regions that have been ligated to adapters can then be isolated, amplified, and sequenced. As expected, chromatin activity states of specific genomic regions tend to be variable across tissues, and consistent across.[51]

Application of single-cell barcodes in ATAC-seq enables comparison of epigenomes across individual cells in a sample.[52] Using single-cell ATAC-seq, one group found that there is an unexpectedly high level of variation among the epigenetic states of individual intestinal lymphoid cells and that this variation is shaped by the microbiome.[53] This approach enables identification and quantification of the relative abundance of different cell types, aiding, for example, in detecting gene-regulatory features of type II diabetes. Single-cell ATAC-seq can also provide high-resolution data on the evolution of epigenomic changes within a tumor.[54]

Detecting Overall Chromatin State on Individual Chromatin Fibers: Fiber-seq

Although bisulfite conversation, DNAse-hypersensitivity assays, and ATAC-seq can each provide invaluable information on genome-wide activity states, each of these methods chemically or enzymatically alters target molecules. The newly introduced Fiber-seq method[55] escapes these limitations by treating chromatin with a methyltransferase that adds methyl groups to adenines within regions of open chromatin. By applying sequencing technologies that can distinguish between methylated and unmethylated adenines, Fiber-seq yields paired, genetic and epigenetic data from individual molecules, raising the prospect for a molecule-level perspective on how somatic mutations impact gene expression.

Publicly Available Resources Enable Exploration of Epigenetic States at Genome Scale

One of the great steps of the genomics era is the emergence of public, online data repositories, for researchers to share their data, and enabling insights that might not be accessible from the work of an individual lab. In the case of epigenetics research, such publicly available datasets have provided unprecedented opportunities to compare epigenomic profiles over developmental time, and between tissues in disparate functional states.

The Encyclopedia of DNA Elements (ENCODE), a project supported by the National Human Genome Research Institute (NHGRI), was founded in 2003 and serves as an ever-growing repository of datasets that, collectively, help to discover drivers of genome activity across cell types and developmental stages. Although the first phases of the project catalogued elements in human cells alone, recent phases have extended assays to model organisms, including mice,[56] offering the potential for features of genome regulation that contribute to unique human traits. One of the strengths of ENCODE is that it imposes a set of standards for data collection and analysis and requires both technical and biologic replication before a dataset can be made fully available to the public, ensuring reliability to a degree unattainable if data were instead collected by a large set of researchers, each imposing their own sets of standards and assumptions. The project has been especially successful in identifying conserved *cis*-regulation elements, genomic regions that control gene expression in humans and DNA sequence more similar across diverse species than expected by chance alone.

The vastness and diversity of the data freely available from ENCODE have enabled deep exploration of many developmental processes. For example, He et al. used ENCODE data to track changes in DNA methylation states within several different organs across embryonic development in mice.[57] In many cases, genomic regions transcriptionally active during embryonic development became epigenetically silenced shortly after birth, pointing to the existence of embryo-specific gene-expression profiles. He et al. also noted that many human diseases are associated with mutations in human homologs of murine regions active during development, underscoring the power of ENCODE data to help uncover the mechanisms of disease phenotypes.[57]

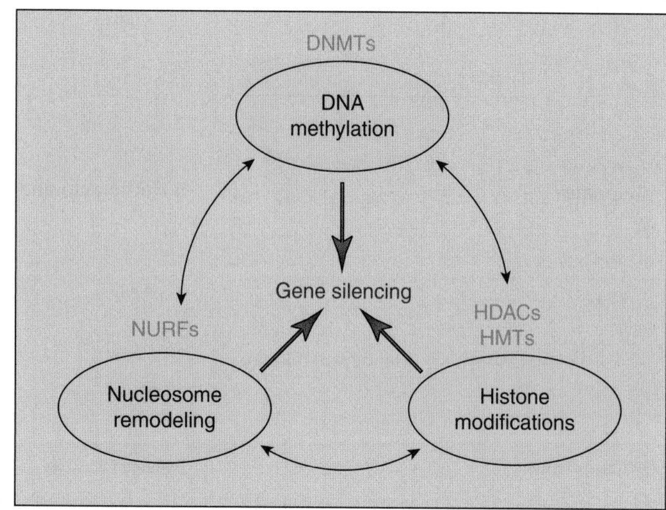

Fig. 6.10 Global Changes in Three Processes Relevant to Cancer. Three processes—DNA cytosine methylation, histone modification, and nucleosomal remodeling—are intimately linked. Alterations in these processes result in permanent silencing of cancer-relevant genes. (From Jones PA, Baylin SB. The epigenomics of cancer. *Cell.* 2007;128[4]:683–692.)

EPIGENETICS AND CANCER

DNA Methylation and Cancer

Some of the most extensive evidence for the association of epigenetic modification with human disease comes from studies of cancer. Almost 30,000 research studies focusing on cancer genomics were published in 2020 alone (Fig. 6.10).[58] Tumor cells often exhibit genome-wide hypomethylation (decreased methylation), which can increase the activity of oncogenes (see Chapter 12). Hypomethylation increases as tumors progress from benign neoplasms to malignancy. In addition, the promoter regions of tumor-suppressor genes are often hypermethylated, which decreases their rate of transcription and their ability to inhibit tumor formation. Hypermethylation of the promoter region of the *RB1* gene is often seen in retinoblastoma[59]; hypermethylation of the *BRCA1* gene is present in some cases of inherited breast cancer[60] (see Box 6.1 for data on epigenetics and breast cancer); and colon cancer cells often have the hypermethylation in the promoter region of the *MLH1* gene that encodes a protein that repairs DNA damage. When *MLH1* becomes inactive, DNA damage accumulates, giving rise to colon tumors.[61,62]

Importantly, the observation of perturbed DNA methylation states in tumors is not, itself, an indication that perturbation in DNA methylation is the proximate cause of cancer. However, as described later, the finding that many tumors have epigenetic abnormalities hints at exciting new opportunities for minimally invasive cancer screening and diagnosis.

Global Epigenomic Alterations and Cancer

A major feature of one form of inherited colon cancer (hereditary nonpolyposis colorectal cancer [HNPCC]) is the methylation of the promoter region of a gene, *MLH1*, whose protein product repairs damaged DNA. Inactivation of *MLH1*, a DNA mismatch repair enzyme, is associated with accrual of DNA damage, another common feature of colon tumors. Abnormal methylation of tumor-suppressor genes also is common in the progression of Barrett esophagus,[63] a condition in which the lining of the esophagus is replaced by cells that have features typically associated with the lower intestinal tract.

Epigenetic Screening for Cancer

The epigenetic abnormalities observed for a given tumor are often a defining feature of the tumor but cannot necessarily be inferred as the cause of disease. Regardless of the connection between the epigenetic abnormality and any cancer, the ability to screen for abnormal epigenetic states raises the possibility that epigenetic screening approaches could complement or even replace existing early-detection methods. In some cases, epigenetic screening could be done using bodily fluids, such as urine or sputum,[64] eliminating the need for the more invasive and costly strategies.

Misregulation of miRNAs in Cancer

Hypermethylation is seen in miRNA genes, which encode small (22 base pair) RNA molecules that bind to the ends of mRNAs, degrading them and preventing their translation. More than 1000 miRNA sequences have been identified in humans, and hypermethylation of specific subgroups of miRNAs is associated with tumorigenesis. When miRNA genes are methylated, their mRNA targets are overexpressed, sometimes leading to cancer.[65]

Emerging Strategies for the Treatment of Epigenetic Disease

Epigenetic modifications are potentially reversible: DNA can be demethylated, histones can be modified to change the transcriptional state of nearby DNA, and miRNA-encoding loci can be upregulated or downregulated. This raises the prospect for treating epigenetic disease with pharmaceutical agents that directly reverse the changes associated with the disease phenotype. In recent years, interventions involving all three types of epigenetic modulators (DNA methylation, histone modification, and miRNAs) have shown considerable promise for the treatment of disease.

DNA Demethylating Agents

5-Azacytidine has been used as a therapeutic drug in the treatment of leukemia and myelodysplastic syndrome.[66] A cytosine analogue, 5-azacytidine, is incorporated into DNA opposite its complementary nucleotide, guanine. Chemical differences between 5-azacytidine and conventional cytosine cause it to achieve irreversible binding to the DNA methyltransferases. As a result, the administration of 5-azacytidine tends to reduce the density of DNA methylation,[67] offering prospects for reversing the aberrant accumulation of methylation at tumor-suppressor loci and even for activating an individual's own immune response against tumor cells.[68] Although 5-azacytidine can be an effective treatment for leukemia, it is effective in only approximately half of individuals. Findings suggest that its benefits of demethylation by 5-azacytidine may be limited to individuals for whom mutations in TET2 have resulted in hypermethylation.[69]

Histone Deacetylase Inhibitors

The activity of the histone deacetylases (HDACs) increases chromatin compaction, decreasing transcriptional activity. In many cases, excessive activity of HDACs results in transcriptional inactivation of tumor-suppressor genes, leading ultimately to the development of tumors. Treatment with HDAC inhibitors, either alone or in combination with other drugs, is a promising strategy for cancer treatment.[70]

miRNA Coding

A major challenge in developing drugs that modify epigenetic alterations is to target only the genes responsible for a specific cancer. Therapeutic approaches that use miRNA offer a potential solution to this problem because treatment can be targeted to individual loci using sequence characteristics of relevant RNA molecules.

EPIGENETICS AND COVID-19

SARS-CoV-2, the virus that has caused the COVID-19 pandemic, depends primarily on two proteins for entry into human cells[71]: the ACE2 receptor and the TMPRSS2 serine protease. Because viral pathogens must enter cells to replicate, there is potential for epigenetic variation among cells, tissues, and individuals, resulting in differential expression of these two proteins, which impacts susceptibility to infection. For example, epigenetic mechanisms modulating ACE2 expression have been proposed to explain variation in COVID-19 susceptibility and severity across age groups (Emerging Science Box: Vaccination History, COVID-19, and Epigenetics).[72]

EPIGENETIC MODIFICATION OF mRNA

Recently, there is renewed focus on yet another layer of epigenetic modification: changes to mRNA molecules.[73] Depending on tissue context, the attachment of methyl groups to the adenines within a given mRNA molecule can variously inhibit its use in protein synthesis or inhibit cellular differentiation. Recent findings indicate that excessive methylation of RNA molecules is a feature of some leukemias, wherein tumors develop from cells that do not proceed along normal differentiation trajectories. These findings suggest that drugs that inhibit aberrant accumulation of methylation on mRNA molecules could offer a promising strategy for treating leukemia.[74] Epigenetic modifications to mRNA are also reported to modulate memory formation[75,76] by impacting the probability that an individual RNA molecule will guide protein synthesis without changing the amino acid sequence of the resulting protein.

FUTURE DIRECTIONS

Epigenetic information is essential to fundamental processes, such as human development and memory formation. Ongoing work is untangling the complex interactions among genetic,

EMERGING SCIENCE BOX

Vaccination History, COVID-19, and Epigenetics

Is there a role for vaccination history and epigenetic mechanisms in protecting against severe COVID-19? The Sars-CoV-2 pandemic has raised several biomedical mysteries. Among them, why do some people suffer severe illness, whereas others experience only mild symptoms or remain asymptomatic? Some emerging studies suggest a potential role for epigenetic mechanisms.

Severe cases of COVID-19 are reported to be less common in individuals who previously received the Bacillus Calmette–Guérin (BCG) vaccine against tuberculosis. In a separate study not focused on COVID-19, de Laval et al. found that both infection with some pathogens and certain vaccinations can leave an enduring impact on chromatin structures in myeloid progenitor cells. Moreover, severe COVID-19 is very rare in children, who typically receive several vaccinations in the first years of life.

Based on these observations, some scientists have proposed that vaccination may provide broad "training" for myeloid cells, priming them to respond effectively to other pathogens, including Sars-CoV-2. The potential value of BCG vaccination in preventing severe COVID-19 and the search for possible epigenetic mediators remains active topics of investigation.

Data from de Laval B, et al. C/EBPβ-dependent epigenetic memory induces trained immunity in hematopoietic stem cells. *Cell Stem Cell*. 2020;26:793–793; Mehta NS, et al. SARS-CoV-2 (COVID-19): what do we know about children? A systematic review. *Clin Infect Dis*. 2020;71:2469–2479; Rivas MN, et al. BCG vaccination history associates with decreased SARS-CoV-2 seroprevalence across a diverse cohort of health care workers. *J Clin Invest*. 131(2):e145157; Mantovani A, et al. Trained innate immunity, epigenetics, and Covid-19. *N Engl J Med*. 2020;383:1078–1080.

epigenetic, and environmental factors in determining human phenotypes and developing new strategies that monitor and modify epigenetic information to diagnose and treat human disease.

REFERENCES

1. Deans C, Maggert KA. What do you mean, "epigenetic"? *Genetics*. 2015;199(4):887.
2. Adrian-Kalchhauser I, et al. Understanding "non-genetic" inheritance: insights from molecular-evolutionary crosstalk. *Trends Ecol Evol*. 2020;35(12):1078–1089.
3. Miska EA, Ferguson-Smith AC. Transgenerational inheritance: models and mechanisms of non–DNA sequence–based inheritance. *Science*. 2016;354(6308):59–63.
4. Anbouba GM, Carmany EP, Natoli JL. The characterization of hypodontia, hypohidrosis, and hypotrichosis associated with X-linked hypohidrotic ectodermal dysplasia: a systematic review. *Am J Med Genet A*. 2020;182(4):831–841.
5. Liang Y, Zhang C, Dai DQ. Identification of differentially expressed genes regulated by methylation in colon cancer based on bioinformatics analysis. *World J Gastroenterol*. 2019;25(26):3392.
6. Matsui S, et al. LATS2 promoter hypermethylation and its effect on gene expression in human breast cancer. *Oncol Lett*. 2018;15(2):2595.
7. Reid BM, Fridley BL. DNA methylation in ovarian cancer susceptibility. *Cancers*. 2021;13(1):108.
8. Jamialahmadi K, et al. A DNA methylation panel for high performance detection of colorectal cancer. *Cancer Genet*. 2021;252-253:64–72.
9. Jung H, et al. DNA methylation loss promotes immune evasion of tumours with high mutation and copy number load. *Nat Commun*. 2019;10(1):4278.
10. Wang Y, et al. Colon cancer-specific diagnostic and prognostic biomarkers based on genome-wide abnormal DNA methylation. *Aging*. 2020;12(22):22626–22655.
11. Taylor WC. Comment on "Sensitive and specific multi-cancer detection and localization using methylation signatures in cell-free DNA" by M.C. Liu et al. *Ann Oncol*. 2020;31(9):1266–1267.
12. Wossidlo M, et al. 5-Hydroxymethylcytosine in the mammalian zygote is linked with epigenetic reprogramming. *Nat Commun*. 2011;2:241.
13. Huang Y, et al. Decreased global DNA hydroxymethylation in neural tube defects: association with polycyclic aromatic hydrocarbons. *Epigenetics*. 2019;14(10):1019–1029.
14. Alberge JB, et al. DNA hydroxymethylation is associated with disease severity and persists at enhancers of oncogenic regions in multiple myeloma. *Clin Epigenet*. 2020;12(1):163.
15. Guler GD, et al. Detection of early stage pancreatic cancer using 5-hydroxymethylcytosine signatures in circulating cell free DNA. *Nat Commun*. 2020;11(1):5270.
16. Schlesinger S, Meshorer E. Open chromatin, epigenetic plasticity, and nuclear organization in pluripotency. *Dev Cell*. 2019;48(2):135–150.
17. Klein BJ, et al. Recognition of cancer mutations in histone H3K36 by epigenetic writers and readers. *Epigenetics*. 2018;13(7): 683–692.
18. Mosaab A, et al. Histone H3K27M mutation overrides histological grading in pediatric gliomas. *Sci Rep*. 2020;10(1):8368.
19. Balhorn R. The protamine family of sperm nuclear proteins. *Genome Biol*. 2007;8(9):227.
20. Bronson R. *The Male Role in Pregnancy Loss And Embryo Implantation Failure*. Springer; 2015.
21. Morillon A. *Long Non-Coding RNA: the Dark Side of the Genome*. Elsevier; 2018.
22. Kravitz SN, Gregg C. New subtypes of allele-specific epigenetic effects: implications for brain development, function and disease. *Curr Opin Neurobiol*. 2019;59:69–78.
23. Haig D, Westoby M. An earlier formulation of the genetic conflict hypothesis of genomic imprinting. *Nat Genet*. 2006;38(3):271.
24. Butler MG, Miller JL, Forster JL. Prader-Willi syndrome — clinical genetics, diagnosis and treatment approaches: an update. *Curr Pediatr Rev*. 2019;15(4):207–244.
25. Horsthemke B, Wagstaff J. Mechanisms of imprinting of the Prader–Willi/Angelman region. *Am J Med Genet A*. 2008;146A(16):2041–2052.
26. Wang KH, et al. Diagnosis and management of Beckwith-Wiedemann syndrome. *Front Pediatr*. 2019;7:562.
27. Wakeling EL, et al. Diagnosis and management of Silver-Russell syndrome: first international consensus statement. *Nat Rev Endocrinol*. 2017;13(2):105–124.
28. Jones KL, Smith DW. Recognition of the fetal alcohol syndrome in early infancy. *Lancet*. 1973;302(7836):999–1001.
29. Friedel E, et al. Impact of long-term alcohol consumption and relapse on genome-wide DNA methylation changes in alcohol-dependent subjects: a longitudinal study. *Alcohol Clin Exp Res*. 2020;44(7):1356–1365.
30. Liang X, et al. DNA methylation signature on phosphatidylethanol, not on self-reported alcohol consumption, predicts hazardous alcohol consumption in two distinct populations. *Mol Psychiatry*. 2021;26:2238–2253.
31. Thaler L, et al. Methylation of the OXTR gene in women with anorexia nervosa: relationship to social behavior. *Eur Eat Disord Rev*. 2020;28(1):79–86.
32. Smith AK, et al. Epigenome-wide meta-analysis of PTSD across 10 military and civilian cohorts identifies methylation changes in AHRR. *Nat Commun*. 2020;11(1):5965.
33. Neigh GN, Ali FF. Co-morbidity of PTSD and immune system dysfunction: opportunities for treatment. *Curr Opin Pharmacol*. 2016;29:104–110.
34. Brown A, Fiori LM, Turecki G. Bridging basic and clinical research in early life adversity, DNA methylation, and major depressive disorder. *Front Genet*. 2019;10:229.
35. Dunn EC, et al. Sensitive periods for the effect of childhood adversity on DNA methylation: results from a prospective, longitudinal study. *Biol Psychiatry*. 2019;85(10):838–849.
36. Fink DA, et al. Fragile X associated primary ovarian insufficiency (FXPOI): case report and literature review. *Front Genet*. 2018; 9:529.
37. Gohel D, et al. The emerging molecular mechanisms for mitochondrial dysfunctions in FXTAS. *Biochim Biophys Acta Mol Basis Dis*. 2020;1866(12):165918.
38. Cabal-Herrera AM, et al. Fragile X associated neuropsychiatric disorders in a male without FXTAS. *Intractable Rare Dis Res*. 2020;9(2):113–118.
39. Stöger R, et al. Epigenetic variation illustrated by DNA methylation patterns of the fragile-X gene FMR1. *Hum Mol Genet*. 1997;6(11):1791–1801.
40. Bygren LO. Intergenerational health responses to adverse and enriched environments. *Annu Rev Public Health*. 2013;34:49–60.
41. Yan S, et al. Prenatal exposure to the Chinese famine and the risk of metabolic syndrome in adulthood across consecutive generations. *Eur J Clin Nutr*. 2020;74(8):1229–1236.

42. Lkhagvadorj K, et al. Prenatal smoke exposure induces persistent methylation and increases nicotine metabolism in the liver of neonatal and adult male offspring. *Epigenetics*. 2020;15(12):1370–1385.
43. Talia C, Connolly L, Fowler PA. The insulin-like growth factor system: a target for endocrine disruptors? *Environ Int*. 2021;147:106311.
44. Provenzi L, et al. Maternal caregiving and DNA methylation in human infants and children: systematic review. *Genes Brain Behav*. 2020;19(3):e12616.
45. Bell CG, et al. DNA methylation aging clocks: challenges and recommendations. *Genome Biol*. 2019;20(1):249.
46. Quach A, et al. Epigenetic clock analysis of diet, exercise, education, and lifestyle factors. *Aging*. 2017;9(2):419.
47. Bird AP, Southern EM. Use of restriction enzymes to study eukaryotic DNA methylation: I. The methylation pattern in ribosomal DNA from Xenopus laevis. *J Mol Biol*. 1978; 118(1):27–47.
48. Frommer M, et al. A genomic sequencing protocol that yields a positive display of 5-methylcytosine residues in individual DNA strands. *Proc Natl Acad Sci U S A*. 1992;89(5):1827–1831.
49. Chen Y, Chen A. Unveiling the gene regulatory landscape in diseases through the identification of DNase I-hypersensitive sites. *Biomed Rep*. 2019;11(3):87–97.
50. Buenrostro JD, et al. ATAC-seq: a method for assaying chromatin accessibility genome-wide. *Curr Protoc Mol Biol*. 2015;109(21). 29.1–21.29.9.
51. Deng Q, et al. Single-cell RNA-seq reveals dynamic, random monoallelic gene expression in mammalian cells. *Science*. 2014;343(6167):193–196.
52. Buenrostro JD, et al. Single-cell chromatin accessibility reveals principles of regulatory variation. *Nature*. 2015;523(7561):486–490.
53. Gury-BenAri M, et al. The spectrum and regulatory landscape of intestinal innate lymphoid cells are shaped by the microbiome. *Cell*. 2016;166(5):1231–1246.
54. Nam AS, Chaligne R, Landau DA. Integrating genetic and non-genetic determinants of cancer evolution by single-cell multi-omics. *Nat Rev Genet*. 2021;22(1):3–18.
55. Stergachis AB, et al. Single-molecule regulatory architectures captured by chromatin fiber sequencing. *Science*. 2020;368(6498):1449–1454.
56. The ENCODE Project Consortium Perspectives on ENCODE. *Nature*. 2020;583(7818):693–698.
57. He Y, et al. Spatiotemporal DNA methylome dynamics of the developing mammalian fetus. *Nature*. 2020;583:752–759.
58. Jusue-Torres I, et al. The 100 most cited papers about cancer epigenetics. *Cureus*. 2020;12(4):e7623.
59. Raizis AM, et al. DNA hypermethylation/boundary control loss identified in retinoblastomas associated with genetic and epigenetic inactivation of the gene promoter. *Epigenetics*. 2021;16(9):940–954.
60. Liang F, et al. Liquiritigenin decreases tumorigenesis by inhibiting DNMT activity and increasing BRCA1 transcriptional activity in triple-negative breast cancer. *Exp Biol Med (Maywood)*. 2021;246(4):459–466.
61. Lynch HT, de la Chapelle A. Hereditary colorectal cancer. *N Engl J Med*. 2003;348:919–932.
62. Pino MS, Chung DC. Microsatellite instability in the management of colorectal cancer. *Expert Rev Gastroenterol Hepatol*. 2011;5(3):385–399.
63. Wani S. *Advances in Barrett's Esophagus, an Issue of Gastrointestinal Endoscopy Clinics*. ed 1 : Elsevier Health Sciences; 2020.
64. Valihrach L, Androvic P, Kubista M. Circulating miRNA analysis for cancer diagnostics and therapy. *Mol Aspects Med*. 2020;72:100825.
65. Zabaleta ME, et al. Effect of polyphenols on HER2-positive breast cancer and related miRNAs: epigenomic regulation. *Food Res Int*. 2020;137:109623.
66. Stahl M, et al. Hypomethylating agents in relapsed and refractory AML: outcomes and their predictors in a large international patient cohort. *Blood Adv*. 2018;2(8):923–932.
67. Christman JK, Schneiderman N, Acs G. Formation of highly stable complexes between 5-azacytosinesubstituted DNA and specific non-histone nuclear proteins. Implications for 5-azacytidine-mediated effects on DNA methylation and gene expression. *J Biol Chem*. 1985;260(7):4059–4068.
68. Ebelt ND, et al. 5-Azacytidine potentiates anti-tumor immunity in a model of pancreatic ductal adenocarcinoma. *Front Immunol*. 2020;11:538.
69. Reilly BM, et al. 5-Azacytidine transiently restores dysregulated erythroid differentiation gene expression in TET2-deficient erythroleukemia cells. *Mol Cancer Res*. 2021;19:451–464.
70. Suraweera A, O'Byrne KJ, Richard DJ. Combination therapy with histone deacetylase inhibitors (HDACi) for the treatment of cancer: achieving the full therapeutic potential of HDACi. *Front Oncol*. 2018;8:92.
71. Hoffmann M, et al. SARS-CoV-2 cell entry depends on ACE2 and TMPRSS2 and is blocked by a clinically proven protease inhibitor. *Cell*. 2020;181(2):271–280,e8.
72. Yildirim Z, Yazar SS, Çetintaş VB. Genetic and epigenetic factors associated with increased severity of Covid-19. *Cell Biol Int*. 2021;45(6):1158–1174.
73. Huang H, Weng H, Chen J. The biogenesis and precise control of RNA mA methylation. *Trends Genet*. 2020;36(1):44–52.
74. Ianniello Z, Paiardini A, Fatica A. N-methyladenosine (mA): a promising new molecular target in acute myeloid leukemia. *Front Oncol*. 2019;9(April):251.
75. Chen J, et al. N6-methyladenosine modifications: interactions with novel RNA-binding proteins and roles in signal transduction. *RNA Biol*. 2019;16(8):991–1000. https://doi.org/10.1080/15476286.2019.1620060.
76. Zhang Z, et al. METTL3-mediated N6-methyladenosine mRNA modification enhances long-term memory consolidation. *Cell Res*. 2018;28:1050–1061. https://doi.org/10.1038/s41422-018-0092-9.

7

Innate Immunity: Inflammation and Wound Healing

Valentina L. Brashers

http://evolve.elsevier.com/Rogers/pathophysiology/

CHAPTER OUTLINE

The human body is continually exposed to a large variety of toxic substances, physical trauma, and infectious agents (viruses, bacteria, fungi, and parasites) that can cause damage to cells and tissues. Damage can also come from within, such as with cancers. In response, the human body has developed a highly sophisticated system of interactive immune defense mechanisms. *Innate immunity* refers to defense mechanisms that are present at birth and provide the initial nonspecific response to invasion and injury. *Adaptive immunity* refers to immunity that develops over the lifetime of the individual and provides long-term protection against specific invaders.

INNATE IMMUNITY

The human body has several ways to protect itself from injury and infection. Innate immunity includes natural barriers and inflammation. Innate barriers form the first line of defense at the body's surfaces. They serve to prevent damage by the environment and thwart infection by pathogenic microorganisms. If these barriers are breached, the second line of defense, the inflammatory response, is activated to protect the body from further injury, fight infection, and promote healing. The third line of defense, adaptive immunity (also known as acquired or specific immunity), is induced through a slower and more specific process and targets particular invaders and diseased tissues for the purpose of eradicating them. Adaptive immunity also involves "memory," which results in a more rapid response during future exposure to the same invader. Comparisons among defense mechanisms are described in Table 7.1.

While these defense mechanisms are essential for maintaining health and preventing disease, uncontrolled or chronic immune activation and inflammation play a role in virtually all diseases, including heart, lung, and kidney diseases; cancer; neurodegenerative disorders; and rheumatologic disease. The information presented in this chapter introduces the components and processes of innate immunity and sets the stage for Chapter 8, which presents an overview of adaptive immunity; Chapter 9, which discusses alterations in immunity; and Chapter 10, which reviews infection. Innate immunity in the newborn and changes associated with aging are reviewed in the Pediatric Considerations and Geriatric Considerations boxes at the end of the chapter.

TABLE 7.1 Overview of Human Defenses

	Innate Immunity		
Characteristics	**Barriers**	**Inflammatory Response**	**Adaptive Immunity**
Level of defense	First line of defense against infection and tissue injury	Second line of defense; occurs as response to tissue injury or infection (inflammatory response)	Third line of defense; initiated when innate immune system signals cells of adaptive immunity
Timing of defense	Constant	Immediate response	Delay between first exposure to antigen and maximal response; immediate against secondary exposure to same antigen
Specificity	Broadly specific	Nonspecific	Response is very specific toward target
Cells	Epithelial cells	Mast cells, granulocytes (neutrophils, eosinophils, basophils), monocytes/ macrophages, natural killer (NK) cells, platelets, endothelial cells	T lymphocytes, B lymphocytes, macrophages, dendritic cells
Memory	No memory involved	No memory involved	Specific immunologic memory by T and B lymphocytes
Active molecules	Defensins, collectins, lactoferrin, bacterial toxins	Activation of complement, clotting factors, kinins, cytokines	Antibodies, complement, cytokines
Protection	Protection includes anatomic barriers (i.e., skin and mucous membranes), cells and secretory molecules (e.g., lysozymes, low pH of stomach and urine), and ciliary activity	Protection includes vascular responses, cellular components (e.g., mast cells, neutrophils, macrophages), secretory molecules or cytokines, and activation of plasma protein systems	Protection includes activated T and B lymphocytes, cytokines, and antibodies

FIRST LINE OF DEFENSE: PHYSICAL AND BIOCHEMICAL BARRIERS AND THE HUMAN MICROBIOME

Innate barriers form the first line of defense at the body's surfaces. These barriers can be physical, mechanical, and biochemical. Surface barriers also house a group of beneficial microorganisms known as the *normal microbiome* that protect us from pathogenic microorganisms.

Physical and Mechanical Barriers

Physical barriers offer considerable protection from tissue damage and infection. These barriers are comprised of tightly associated epithelial cells of the skin and of the linings of the gastrointestinal (GI), genitourinary, and respiratory tracts (Fig. 7.1). When pathogens attempt to penetrate such barriers, they may be removed by mechanical means. For example, microorganisms may be sloughed off with dead skin cells (which are then replaced). Epithelial cells of the upper respiratory tract can trap microorganisms through the production of mucus and remove them through the action of hair-like cilia, which move the mucus upward where it is expelled through coughing or sneezing. Invading microorganisms can be removed from the GI tract through vomiting or defecation and from the urinary tract through urination. Other protective mechanisms of innate barriers include the relatively low temperature present on the skin and the low pH found in the stomach and the vagina, both of which inhibit the growth of pathogenic microorganisms.

Biochemical Barriers

Epithelial surfaces also provide biochemical barriers by synthesizing and secreting substances meant to trap or destroy microorganisms (epithelial-derived chemicals). Mucus, perspiration, saliva, tears, and earwax are all examples of biochemical secretions that can trap and kill potential disease-causing microorganisms. Sebaceous glands in the skin secrete fatty acids and lactic acid, substances which kill bacteria and fungi. These secretions also create an acidic environment on the skin surface (pH 3 to pH 5) which is inhospitable to most bacteria.

Epithelial cell secretions contain antimicrobial peptides, substances that kill or inhibit the growth of disease-causing bacteria, fungi, and viruses. Defensins are antimicrobial peptides produced by neutrophils and epithelial cells that defend against bacterial infection by disrupting bacterial membranes. Collectins are soluble glycoproteins that facilitate the ability of macrophages to recognize and kill pathogenic microorganisms and can activate the complement system (see the Plasma Protein Systems and Inflammation section). They are produced by various organs, including the lungs (e.g., surfactant is a type of collectin).

The Normal Microbiome

The body's surfaces are colonized with an array of microorganisms, called the normal microbiome (previously referred to as

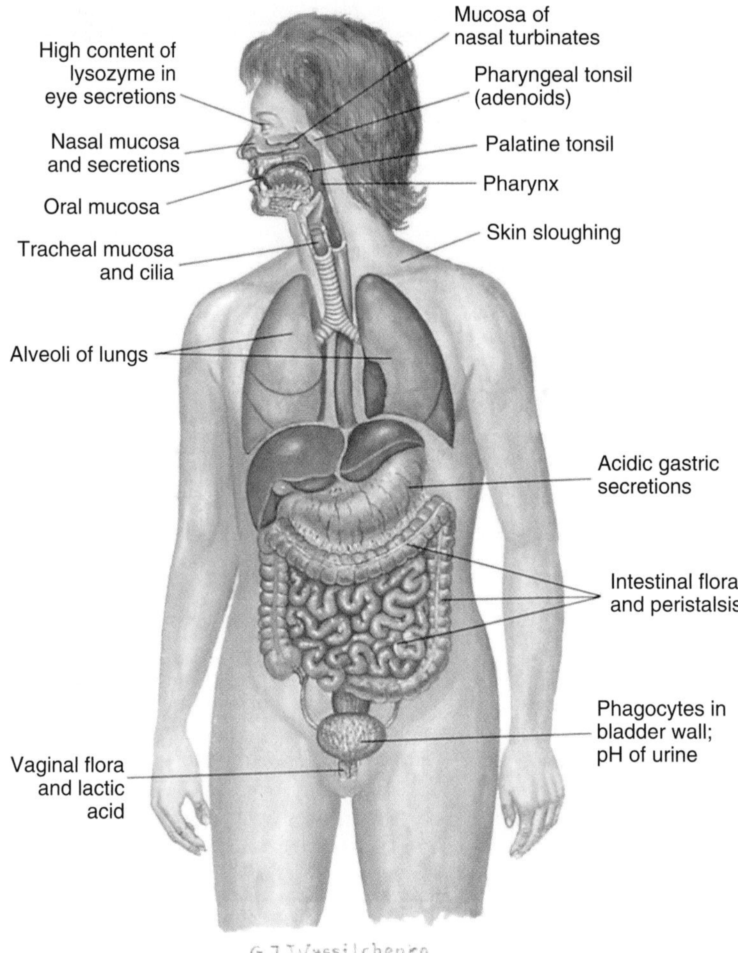

Fig. 7.1 Protection at Body Surfaces. (From Grimes, DE. *Infectious diseases.* St. Louis: Mosby; 1991.)

normal flora). Molecular profiling of these microorganisms has shown that each individual has a unique suite of microbial strains that is acquired early in life, beginning in utero and continuing with exposure to the vaginal microbiome during birth.[1] With subsequent environmental exposures such as diet, antimicrobials, toxins, and animals, the composition of the microbiome diversifies. Changes in the microbial make-up of the infant microbiome can have lifelong impacts on health and disease.[2]

Body surfaces that have their own specialized microbiome include the skin; mucous membranes of the eye, nose, and mouth; upper and lower GI tracts; upper respiratory tract; urethra; and vagina. These surfaces are colonized by a combination of bacteria and fungi unique to the anatomic location and the particular individual (Fig. 7.2).

The microorganisms in the microbiome do not normally cause disease. The normal microbiome benefits the human body in a number of ways, and the human body provides an ideal environment for the microbiome to grow.[3] The interaction between host cells and the microbiome plays an essential role in fostering healthy innate and immune defense systems.[1,4,5]

Mechanisms by which the microbiome contributes to health and immunity include:

1. Produces enzymes which facilitate digestion of fatty acids and large polysaccharides
2. Synthesizes essential metabolites (e.g., vitamins K and B)
3. Releases antibacterial substances that are toxic to pathogenic microorganisms (e.g., ammonia, phenols, and indoles)
4. Competes with pathogens for nutrients and blocks attachment of the pathogens to the epithelium, an obligatory first step in the infectious process
5. Fosters healthy innate and adaptive immunity by inducing protective immune responses to pathogens, while at the same time maintaining regulatory pathways that support immune tolerance of innocuous microorganisms.

The health of the microbiome can be positively or negatively influenced by a wide range of environmental exposures (see Emerging Science Box: The Microbiome and Disease). For example, prolonged treatment with broad-spectrum antibiotics can alter the normal microbiome, decreasing its protective activity and leading to an overgrowth of pathogenic microorganisms. In the intestine, for example, overgrowth of the yeast *Candida albicans* or the bacterium *Clostridioides difficile* (the cause of pseudomembranous colitis) may occur with antibiotic use. Some members of the normal bacterial microbiome are opportunistic pathogens—that is, they are harmless under normal conditions

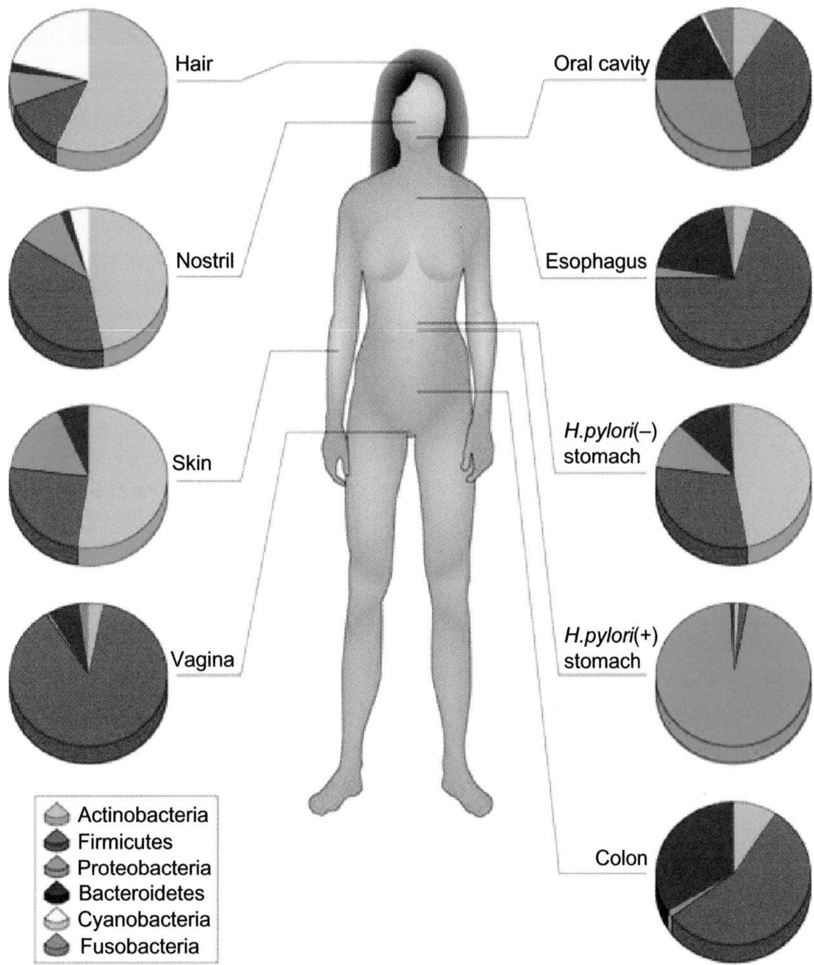

Fig. 7.2 The Human Microbiome. Typical phylum-level composition of the human microbiota that vary at each site (From Cho I, Blaser MJ. The human microbiome: At the interface of health and disease. *Nature Reviews. Genetics*, 2012; 13:260–270.)

but can cause disease in immunocompromised individuals who lack the usual defense mechanisms. For example, *Pseudomonas aeruginosa* is a member of the normal microbiome of the skin, where it produces a toxin that protects the skin from infections caused by pathologic bacteria. With severe burns or critical illnesses in which the integrity of the skin and mucous membranes is compromised, *Pseudomonas* may enter the bloodstream and cause life-threatening systemic infections.

Epidemiologic studies have been used to associate negative changes in the microbiome (dysbiosis) with disease states (see Emerging Science Box: The Microbiome and Disease). Included in the long list of dysbiosis-associated diseases are mental health disorders, obesity, hypertension, heart failure, asthma, emphysema, rheumatologic conditions, diabetes, bowel disease, and cancer. Studies aimed at altering the microbiome for health promotion, disease prevention, and improved responses to treatment are ongoing.[1]

SECOND LINE OF DEFENSE: INFLAMMATION

Inflammation is a protective response that supports recovery from injury and disease. The inflammatory process is activated by virtually any injury to vascularized tissues. Triggers include infection and tissue damage (e.g., ischemia, trauma, chemical injury, foreign bodies, and immune reactions). When pathogen invasion or tissue damage occurs, inflammation is initiated by guardian cells (mast cells, macrophages, and dendritic cells) that are located near epithelial surfaces, in lymph nodes, and near blood vessels. Inflammatory mediators are released, causing both a vascular and a cellular response. The ultimate result of these responses is the migration of leukocytes, platelets, plasma proteins, and other biochemical mediators from the circulation into the nearby damaged tissue, where they can work together to destroy invaders, limit tissue injury, and promote healing. Algorithm 7.1 summarizes the process.

The inflammatory response is characterized by the following:

1. The process occurs in vascularized tissues (i.e., tissues with a blood supply).
2. Activation is rapid (within seconds) after damage occurs.
3. The response includes chemical, vascular, and cellular components.
4. The response is nonspecific—that is, it takes place in approximately the same way regardless of the type of injury (stimulus) and whether or not the same stimulus has occurred in the past.

Inflammation, although producing pain and functional limitations in the affected individual, also results in numerous

EMERGING SCIENCE BOX

The Microbiome and Disease

The postulated mechanisms by which microbiome dysbiosis contributes to the development of disease are numerous and complex. The presence of microorganisms (especially in the gut) modulates both the induction and the suppression of local and systemic immune responses. In return, the host immune system fine-tunes the composition of the microbiome to maintain a beneficial symbiosis. When this symbiosis is altered, both innate and adaptive immunity are negatively impacted. With regard to innate immunity, neutrophils and macrophages engage in a constant "crosstalk" with the microbiome that modulates the inflammatory response. When dysbiosis occurs, these phagocytes become dysregulated leading to a chronic inflammatory state, which in turn can contribute to a large number of diseases. For example, early studies in Alzheimer disease suggest that changes in the microbiome can be linked to neuroinflammation and brain dysfunction. Communication between the microbiome and the body is impacted by environmental influences such as stress and diet. A high-fat diet leads to changes in the gut microbiome which in turn lead to inflammation and increased fat accumulation around viscera which is associated with atherosclerosis and diabetes. Dysbiosis in the gut also can result in the formation of toxic metabolites from food (e.g., phenylalanine) which contribute to cardiovascular disease risk. New studies indicate that the microbiome may be intentionally modulated to improve responses to treatment. For example, there is a great deal of optimism among researchers that altering the gut microbiome will prove an effective way of managing inflammatory bowel disease. Other studies suggest that altering the microbiome can improve the efficacy of hypertensive and psychiatric medications. To date, the most common techniques being used to alter the microbiome include probiotics, prebiotics, and fecal microbial transplantation (FMT).

Data from Araujo DV, et al. Bugs as drugs: The role of microbiome in cancer focusing on immunotherapeutics. *Cancer Treatment Reviews*, 2021; 92:102125; Durack J, et al. The gut microbiome: Relationships with disease and opportunities for therapy. *Journal of Experimental Medicine*, 2019; 216(1):20–40; Lam KN, et al. Precision medicine goes microscopic: Engineering the microbiome to improve drug outcomes. *Cell Host and Microbe*; 26(1):22–34; Na YR, et al. Macrophages in intestinal inflammation and resolution: A potential therapeutic target in IBD. *Nature Reviews Gastroenterology and Hepatology*, 2019; 16(9):531–543; Naqvi S, et al. A cross-talk between gut microbiome, salt and hypertension. *Biomedicine and Pharmacotherapy*, 2021; 134:111156; Proctor LM, et al. The integrative human microbiome project. *Nature*, 2019; 569:641–648; Rackaityte E, et al. The human microbiome in the 21st century. *Nature Communications*, 2020; 11:5256; Yang D, et al. The impact of lung microbiota dysbiosis on inflammation. *Immunology*, 2020; 159(2):156–166; Rajendiran E, et al. Understanding connections and roles of gut microbiome in cardiovascular diseases. *Canadian Journal of Microbiology*, 2021; 67(2): 101–111; Zhang D, et al. Interaction between microbiota and immunity in health and disease. *Cell Research*, 2020; 30:492–506; Zhi C, et al. Connection between gut microbiome and the development of obesity. *European Journal of Clinical Microbiology and Infectious Diseases*; 38(11):1987–1998.

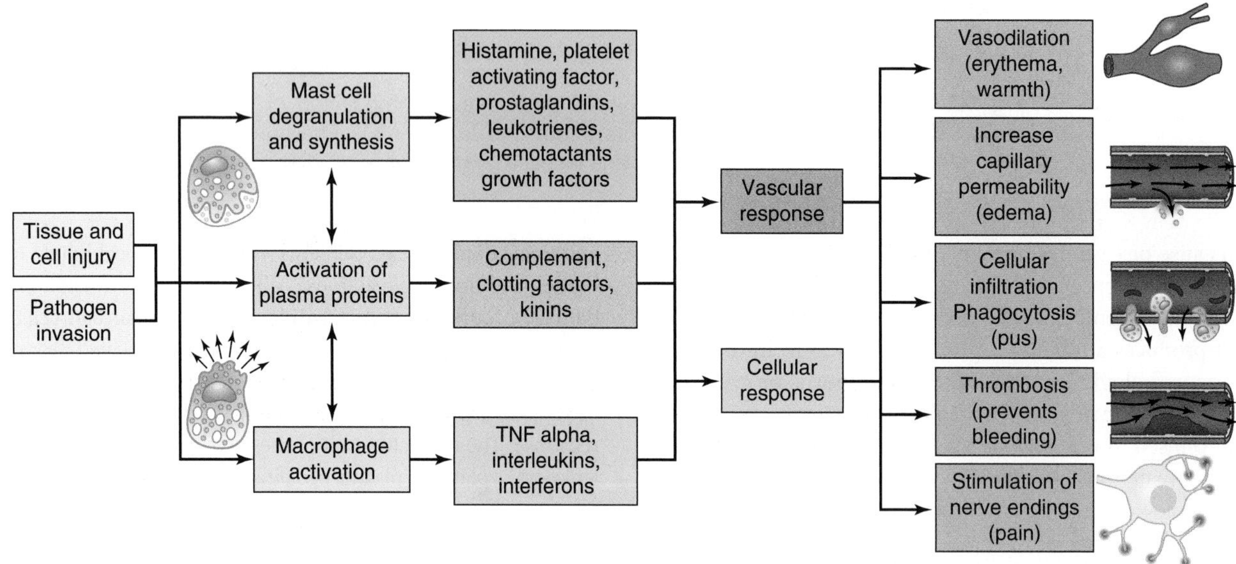

Algorithm 7.1 Acute Inflammatory Response. Inflammation is usually initiated by cellular injury and may be complicated by infection. The inflammatory response involves mast cell degranulation, the activation of three plasma protein systems, and the activation of macrophages that release numerous cytokines. These systems are interdependent so that induction of one (e.g., mast cell degranulation) can result in the induction of the other two. The result is the development of the characteristic microscopic and clinical hallmarks of inflammation. *TNF alpha*, Tumor necrosis factor-alpha.

physiologic benefits. Protective functions of inflammation include the following:

1. *Prevention of infection and further damage caused by invading microorganisms:* Inflammatory exudates dilute the toxins produced by both bacteria and dying cells. The activation of plasma protein systems (e.g., complement and clotting systems) serves to contain and destroy invading microorganisms. The influx of phagocytes (neutrophils and macrophages)

removes toxic cellular debris and pathogenic microorganisms, preventing them from further harming the body.

2. *Preparation of injury for healing and repair:* This involves removal of bacterial microorganisms, dead cells, and other physiologic debris through the epithelial channels and the lymphatic vessels that drain the region. Mechanisms of healing and repair are initiated.
3. *Facilitation of the development of adaptive immunity:* As fluid and cellular debris drain through the lymphatic vessels, lymphoid tissue and lymph nodes, microbial antigens encounter macrophages and lymphocytes concentrated in these areas. Adaptive immunity is initiated and helps fight off invaders and protect the body from future exposures to particular pathogens (see Chapter 8).

Plasma Protein Systems and Inflammation

Plasma protein systems are essential to an effective vascular and cellular inflammatory response (see Algorithm 7.1). There are three plasma protein systems that are especially important to innate immunity: the complement system, the clotting system, and the kinin system (Fig. 7.3). Although each system has a unique role in inflammation, all three systems have many

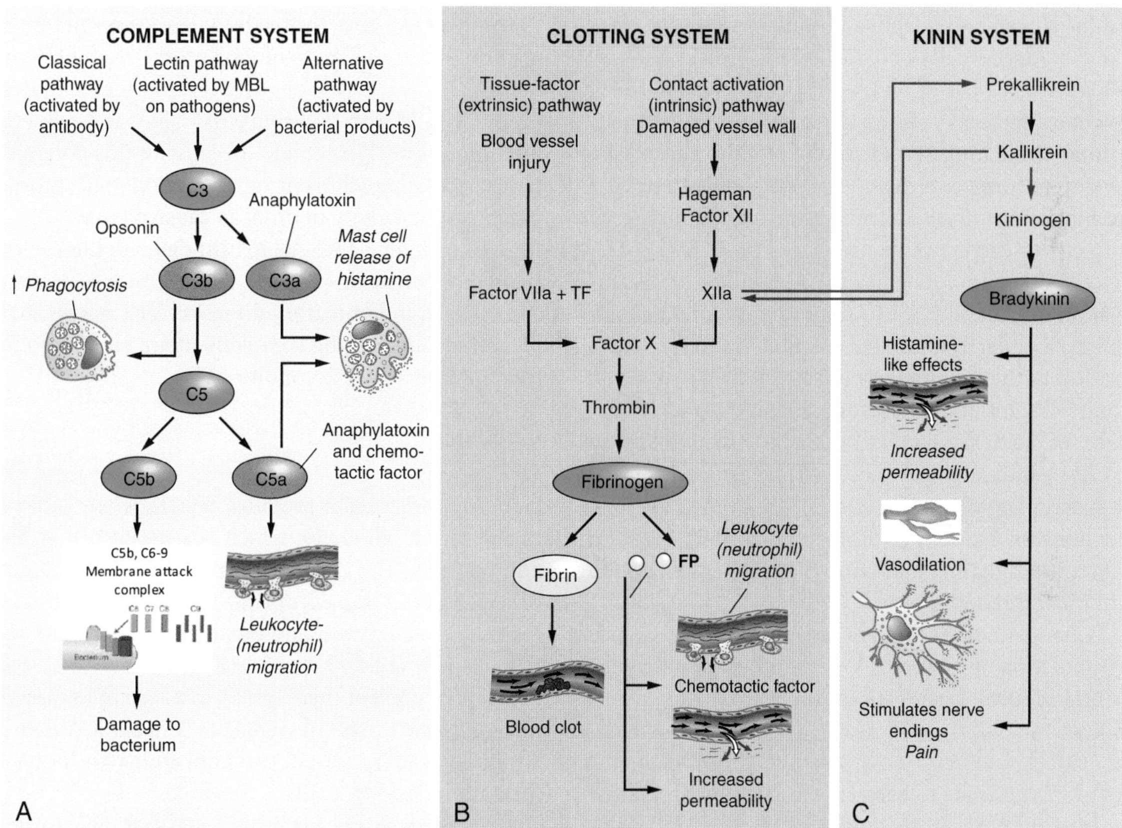

Fig. 7.3 Plasma Protein Systems in Inflammation: Complement, Clotting, and Kinin Systems. Each plasma protein system consists of a family of proteins that are activated in sequence to create potent biologic effects. **(A)** The complement system can be activated by three mechanisms, each of which results in proteolytic activation of C3. The fragments of C3 activation, C3a and C3b, are major components of inflammation. C3a is a potent anaphylatoxin, which induces degranulation of mast cells. C3b can bind to the surface or cells, such as bacteria, and either serve as an opsonin for phagocytosis or proteolytically activate the next component of the complement cascade, C5. The smaller fragment of C5 activation is C5a, a powerful anaphylatoxin, and is also chemotactic for neutrophils, attracting them to the site of inflammation. The larger fragment, C5b, activates the components of the membrane attack complex (C5b–C9), which damage the bacterial membrane and kill the bacteria. **(B)** The clotting system can be activated by the tissue factor (extrinsic) pathway and the contact activation (intrinsic) pathway. All routes of clotting initiation lead to activation of factor X and thrombin. Thrombin is an enzyme that activates fibrinogen to form fibrin and small FPs. Fibrin comes together to form a clot, and the FPs are highly active as chemotactic factors and cause increased vascular permeability. **(C)** Factor XIIa produced by the clotting system can also be activated by kallikrein of the kinin system *(red arrow)*. Prekallikrein is enzymatically converted to kininogen, which activates bradykinin. Bradykinin functions similar to histamine and increases vascular permeability. Bradykinin can also stimulate nerve endings to cause pain. *FP*, Fibrinopeptide; *MBL*, mannose binding lectin; *TF*, tissue factor.

similarities as well. Each system consists of multiple proteins and enzymes usually present in blood as inactive forms. The proteins are activated early in inflammation by enzymes, which circulate as proenzymes until some form of tissue damage triggers the system initiating the sequence. Activation of the first components results in sequential activation of other components of the system, leading to a protective biologic function. This sequential activation is referred to as a cascade, hence the common terminology that references the complement cascade, the clotting cascade, or the kinin cascade.

Complement System

The complement system intensifies or complements the capacity of cells of the innate and adaptive immune systems to clear pathogens and damaged cells and to activate inflammation.[6] Complement consists of a large number of proteins (sometimes called complement factors), which, together, constitute about 10% of the total circulating serum protein. Activation of the complement system initiates a cascade of proteolytic steps that result in the formation of several substances that can destroy pathogens directly or can eradicate pathogens through enhancing the activity of other components of the immune response.

The activation of C3 and C5, two important components of the complement cascade, results in the creation of several potent molecules critical to the immune response:

1. C3b—along with antibodies, serves as opsonins which coat the surface of bacteria increasing their susceptibility to phagocytosis by inflammatory cells (i.e., phagocytes [neutrophils and macrophages]).
2. C5a—functions as a chemotactic factor which serves as a form of chemical signaling that causes leukocytes to move to the area of inflammation.
3. C3a and C5a—sometimes called anaphylatoxins, induce rapid degranulation of mast cells to release histamine, a substance which induces vasodilation and increased capillary permeability.
4. Membrane attack complex (MAC)—composed of elements C6 through C9 and leads to bacterial destruction and tissue injury by creating pores in the outer membranes of cells or bacteria. These pores facilitate the infusion of water into the cells culminating in cellular death.

Three major pathways or cascades control the activation of complement (see Fig. 7.3A): the classical pathway, the alternative pathway, and the lectin pathway. The classical pathway is activated by antibodies, which are components of the adaptive immune system. Antibodies bind to antigens, which are typically proteins or carbohydrates produced by infectious microorganisms. Such antibodies activate the first complement component, C1, which, in turn, leads to the sequential activation of other components of the complement cascade, specifically C3 and C5, triggering inflammation.

The alternative pathway is activated directly by substances found on the surface of infectious microorganisms. These substances would include lipopolysaccharides (endotoxins) found on bacterial membranes and carbohydrates (zymosan) found on yeast cell walls. This pathway uses unique proteins (factor B, factor D, and properdin) to form a complex that sequentially activates the complement proteins C3 and C5. At this point, the process converges with the classical pathway. The alternative pathway provides a mechanism whereby the complement system can be activated in the absence of antibodies.

The lectin pathway, like the alternative pathway, is independent of antibodies and is activated by several plasma proteins, particularly mannose-binding lectin (MBL). MBL binds to bacterial polysaccharides that contain the carbohydrate mannose and activates the complement cascade. Infectious agents that do not activate the alternative pathway may still be susceptible to the complement system through the lectin pathway.

In summary, the complement pathway or cascade is a sequential series of cellular events that serve as defense mechanisms for the body. It can be activated by at least three different pathways, resulting in one or more of four protective functions: *opsonization* (C3b), *anaphylatoxic activity* from mast cell degranulation (C3a, C5a), *leukocyte chemotaxis* (C5a), and *cell lysis* (C5b–C9; membrane attack complex). Because of this potent defense system, successful pathogens must develop mechanisms that resist complement activity in order to cause disease.[7]

While highly beneficial to host defense, the complement system can contribute to tissue damage in a wide range of acute and chronic inflammatory diseases (see Chapter 9). New therapies aimed at blocking complement are proving to be beneficial for a number of these conditions.[8]

Clotting

The clotting system (also known as the coagulation system) is a group of plasma proteins, which, when activated sequentially, form a blood clot which is a meshwork of fibrin strands and platelets. The clotting system can be activated by a variety of substances released during tissue injury or infection, such as collagen, enzymes, and bacterial toxins. Clots serve to plug damaged vessels and stop bleeding (hemostasis), trap microorganisms to prevent their spread to adjacent tissues, and provide a framework for future repair and healing. When the wall of a blood vessel is injured, two converging pathways lead to clot formation (see Fig. 7.3B):

1. The tissue factor (extrinsic) pathway is activated by tissue factor (TF), also called tissue thromboplastin, a substance released by damaged endothelial cells of the blood vessels. It reacts with activated factor VII (VIIa).
2. The contact activation (intrinsic) pathway is activated when vessel wall damage causes negatively charged subendothelial substances to come into contact with Hageman factor (factor XII) found in plasma.

Both pathways converge at factor X and thrombin. Thrombin activates fibrinogen to form fibrin. Fibrin, in turn, comes together to form a fibrin clot. The purposes of the fibrin clot are to:

1. Stop bleeding.
2. Help prevent the spread of inflammation and infection.
3. Keep the invader near the site of injury, thus maximizing the access of inflammatory cells and proteins.
4. Initiate the formation of two fibrinopeptides (A and B) that are released during the formation of fibrin and are chemotactic for neutrophils and increase vascular permeability.
5. Provide a framework for repair and healing.[9]

Platelets also play a crucial role in inflammation, including the secretion of immunoregulatory cytokines and the ability to bind infectious pathogens.[10] Additional details concerning the clotting system are discussed in Chapter 28.

Kinin System

The third plasma protein system, the kinin system (see Fig. 7.3C), interacts closely with the clotting system. Both the clotting and kinin systems can be initiated through activation of Hageman factor (factor XII), which, in turn, results in the formation of factor XIIa, also known as *prekallikrein activator*. Factor XIIa activates *prekallikrein*, the first component of the kinin system. The next product in the cascade is kallikrein, followed by *kininogen*, a precursor molecule, and then bradykinin, the final product of the kinin system. Bradykinin causes dilation of blood vessels. Bradykinin also acts in concert with prostaglandins to induce pain, trigger smooth muscle cell contraction (i.e., bronchoconstriction), and increase vascular permeability.

Control and Interaction of Plasma Protein Systems

The three plasma protein systems are highly interactive. The activation of one system results in the production of a large number of biologically active substances that activate other systems. Tight regulation of these processes is essential for two reasons. First, the inflammatory process is critical for an individual's survival; therefore, efficient activation must occur regardless of the cause of tissue injury. The interaction among the three systems means that the entire inflammatory response may be activated regardless of which system initially triggers the sequence. Second, the biochemical mediators released during the inflammatory response are potent and potentially harmful to the individual. Their actions must be controlled and confined to injured or infected tissues.

Multiple mechanisms are available to regulate the plasma protein systems, activating or inactivating the reactions to maintain balance, and contain the inflammatory response. Plasma entering the tissues during inflammation contains enzymes that destroy the mediators of inflammation and downregulate the inflammatory response. These enzymes include protease inhibitors (e.g., C1-inhibitor) and carboxypeptidase, which inhibit the complement system; and kininase and histaminase, which inhibit the kinin system. The formation of clots activates a fibrinolytic system. This system serves to limit the size of the clot and degrade the clot after bleeding has ceased. In this system thrombin activates plasminogen, forming the enzyme plasmin, which degrades the fibrin polymers in clots and has been implicated in a wide range of inflammatory diseases.[11] Defects in these mechanisms can be genetic or acquired. For example, a genetic defect in the protease C1 inhibitor (C1-inh) results in hereditary angioedema, a self-limiting edema of cutaneous and mucosal layers. Acquired defects in plasminogen activation and control, which is seen in severe infection, can result in widespread clotting.[12]

Initial Cellular Responders in Inflammation

Mast cells and macrophages can be thought of as guardian cells and are the primary cellular initiators of the inflammatory response (see Algorithm 7.1). Also present are dendritic cells which are a specialized type of macrophage that connects the innate and adaptive immune responses. These three types of cells reside near epithelial tissues, blood vessels, and lymphatics. They are equipped with receptors that allow them to detect pathogens and the cellular products of tissue damage (Algorithm 7.2).

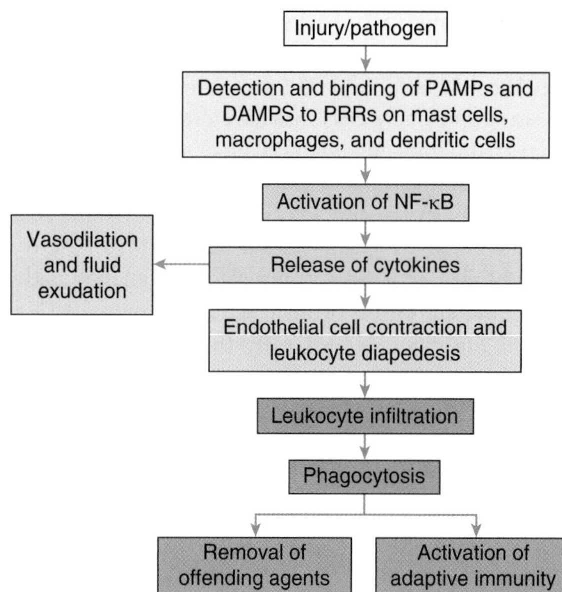

Algorithm 7.2 Overview of the Sequence of Events in the Acute Inflammatory Response. As a result of tissue injury or pathogen invasion, pattern recognition receptors *(PRRs)* on mast cells, macrophages, and dendritic cells are activated by binding to pathogen-associated molecular patterns *(PAMPs)* or damage-associated molecular patterns *(DAMPs)*. This leads to activation of NF-κB and the release of multiple cytokines that initiate vascular and cellular responses that work to bring immune cells to the area of injury/invasion, remove offending agents, activate adaptive immunity, and prepare the tissues for healing.

Cellular Receptors

Mast cells, macrophages, and dendritic cells have evolved a set of receptors referred to as pattern recognition receptors (PRRs) (Table 7.2). PRRs are generally expressed on cells in tissues near the body's surfaces (skin, respiratory tract, GI tract, genitourinary tract), where they monitor the environment for products of cellular damage and infectious microorganisms. PRRs can also be found on mucosal epithelial cells, neutrophils, and some lymphocytes. PRRs recognize two types of molecular patterns:

1. Pathogen-associated molecular patterns (PAMPs), which are molecules expressed by infectious agents either found on their surface or released as soluble molecules.
2. Damage-associated molecular patterns (DAMPs), which are products of cellular damage. Accordingly, cells of the innate immune system can respond to both sterile tissue damage (DAMPs) and septic tissue damage (PAMPs and DAMPs). It is estimated that at least 100 different PRRs are found on innate immune cells, rendering them capable of recognizing more than 1000 different molecules.

An important group of PRRs are Toll-like receptors (TLRs), which recognize a large variety of PAMPs located on the surface of microorganisms (e.g., bacterial lipopolysaccharide, peptidoglycans, lipoproteins, yeast zymosan, flagellin, bacterial or viral nucleic acid, and viral coat proteins). TLRs are expressed on the surface of many cells that have direct and early contact with potential pathogens. Such cells include mucosal epithelial cells, mast cells, macrophages, dendritic cells, neutrophils, and lymphocytes. TLRs also are activated by oxidative stress, tissue injury, and damaged cellular contents (DAMPs). Activation of TLRs initiates a cascade of intracellular signaling pathways leading to the activation of nuclear factor-[kappa]B (NF-κB) in the cell nucleus.[13] NF-κB activation results in increased transcription and subsequent release of numerous inflammatory cytokines. Among these are tumor necrosis factor (TNF), interleukins, and interferons (IFNs) which play key roles in the inflammatory process, activation of the adaptive immune response, and the destruction of many pathogenic microorganisms (these cytokines are discussed in detail later in this chapter). Pathophysiologic changes in TLR stimulation and NF-κB activation have been implicated in numerous conditions such as neuroinflammation, heart disease, and cancer[13] (see Emerging Science Box: The Role of Toll-like Receptors [TLRs] and Nuclear Factor-kappaB [NF-κB] in Disease).[13]

TABLE 7.2 Pattern Recognition Receptors

Receptors	Number of Receptors	What They Recognize	Where They Are Found
Toll-like receptors (TLRs)	10	PAMPs and DAMPs	Outer membrane of innate immune cells especially macrophages and dendritic cells
NOD-like receptors and NLR receptors	~22	PAMPs and DAMPs	Cytoplasm of innate immune cells
Scavenger receptors (including C-type lectin receptors (CLRs)	12	PAMPs, DAMPS, Cell membrane phospholipids	Outer membrane of phagocytes
Complement and Cytokine receptors[a]	Multiple	C3a, C3b, C5a, TNF-α, interleukins, interferons, chemotactic factors, prostaglandins, platelet activating factor, IL-10, TGF-β	Outer membrane of innate immune cells, platelets, epithelial cells, vascular smooth muscle

[a]Complement and cytokine receptors are not true pattern recognition receptors but are essential for innate immune cell function
DAMP, Damage-associated molecular patterns; *IL-10*, interleukin-10; *NOD*, nucleotide oligomerization domain-like receptors; *NRL*, nucleotide-binding-like receptors; *PAMP*, pathogen-associated molecular patterns; *TGF-β*, transforming growth factor-beta; *TNF-α*, tumor necrosis factor-alpha).

EMERGING SCIENCE BOX

The Role of Toll-like Receptors (TLRs) and Nuclear Factor-kappaB (NF-κB) in Disease

TLRs play a key role in the detection of invasion and tissue injury by immune cells. These receptors bind to a wide range of molecular patterns from pathogens (PAMPs) and damaged host cells (DAMPs). The subsequent steps in intracellular signaling and activation of NF-κB lead to the production of cytokines that are central to the inflammatory response and initiation of adaptive immunity. However, an uncontrolled inflammatory response may lead to a host of deleterious effects on cells and tissues. Changes in TLR binding and excessive NF-κB activity have been associated with a large number of inflammatory diseases affecting virtually every organ in the body. TLRs may detect byproducts of other pathophysiologic conditions leading to an exaggerated or misdirected immune response. For example, TLR binding to advanced glycation end-products (AGEs) produced in diabetes leads to widespread inflammatory injury to vascular tissues. Exaggerated NF-κB activation is linked to sepsis as well as acute and chronic diseases of the cardiovascular, neurologic, pulmonary, gastrointestinal, and renal systems. NF-κB activation is modulated by the nuclear peroxisome proliferator-activated receptor (PPAR) family which consists of three types of PPAR receptors (PPAR-α, β, and γ). These receptors are located on macrophages and lymphocytes as well as other tissues. Activation of PPAR pathways prevents excessive inflammation and tissue damage. Therapeutically, PPAR receptors are activated by nonsteroidal anti-inflammatory drugs (NSAIDs), thus reducing inflammatory symptoms. Other PPAR agonists that are currently in use include fibrates (treat dyslipidemia) and thiazolidinediones (treat diabetes). However, these medications have significant side effects. Dozens of new PPAR agonists to treat a wide range of conditions including biliary cirrhosis, Alzheimer disease, heart disease, renal disease, inflammatory bowel disease, gout, cancer, and eye diseases are currently in clinical trials. Other therapeutic interventions that seek to modulate TLR and NF-κB activation are being explored.

Data from Christofides A, et al. The role of peroxisome proliferator-activated receptors (PPAR) in immune responses. *Metabolism: Clinical and Experimental,* 2021; 114:154338; Fiordelisi A, et al. NF-kappaB is a key player in the crosstalk between inflammation and cardiovascular diseases. *International Journal of Molecular Sciences,* 2019; 20(7):1599; Dhillon B, et al. The evolving role of TRAFs in mediating inflammatory responses. *Frontiers in Immunology,* 2019; 10:104; Holm LJ, et al. PPARs and the development of type 1 diabetes. *PPAR Research,* 2020; 6198628; Korbecki J, et al. Self-regulation of the inflammatory response by peroxisome proliferator-activated receptors. *Inflammation Research,* 2019; 68(6):443–458; McCarthy CG, et al. Paying the toll for inflammation. *Hypertension,* 2019; 73(3):514–521; Mussbacher M, et al. Cell type-specific roles of NF-kappaBI linking inflammation and thrombosis. *Frontiers in Immunology,* 2019; 10:85; Rai RC. Host inflammatory responses to intracellular invaders: Review study. *Life Sciences,* 2020; 240:117084; Teissier T, et al. The receptor for advanced glycation end-products (RAGE) is an important pattern recognition receptor (PRR) for inflammaging. *Biogerontology,* 2019; 20(3):279–301; Yu H, et al. Targeting NF-κB pathway for the therapy of diseases: Mechanism and clinical study. *Signal Transduction and Targeted Therapy,* 2020; 5:209.

Nucleotide-binding-like receptors (NLRs) (including nucleotide oligomerization domain–like [NOD-like] receptors) are cytoplasmic (intracellular) receptors in lymphocytes, macrophages, and dendritic cells. At least 23 NLRs have been identified in humans. They recognize intracellular microorganisms and damaged cells and initiate the production of proinflammatory mediators. NLRs also detect cells that are forming inflammasomes, which are large cytoplasmic complexes that activate cytokines. Inflammasomes are implicated in a wide variety of diseases including Coronavirus Disease 2019 (COVID-19) inflammatory lung damage.[14]

Scavenger receptors are membrane receptors primarily expressed on macrophages and are categorized into 12 classes.[15] They have multiple functions including the recognition and subsequent phagocytosis of bacterial pathogens and damaged cells. They also recognize soluble lipoproteins, such as high-density lipoprotein (HDL), low-density lipoprotein (LDL), and oxidized LDL, and have been implicated in atherosclerotic vascular diseases.[16] C-type lectin receptors (CLRs) are a type of scavenger receptor that binds to both PAMPs and DAMPs. There are many types of CLRs, such as macrophage mannose, Dectin 1 and 2, and mannose-binding lectin receptors. They are particularly important in recognizing fungal antigens and subsequent activation of innate immune cells.

Complement and cytokine receptors are found on many cells involved in the immune response, as well as on some epithelial cells. These are not true PRRs but are essential to innate immune cell function. Complement receptors recognize several fragments produced through activation of the complement system, particularly C3a, C5a, and C3b. This results in chemotaxis and activation of innate immune cells. Cytokine receptors recognize both proinflammatory and anti-inflammatory cytokines (these cytokines are discussed later in this chapter).

Mast Cells

Mast cells are significant and potent activators of the inflammatory response. They have abundant granules containing biochemical mediators, which are released in instances of pathogen invasion and tissue injury (Fig. 7.4). Mast cells are activated by PAMPs and DAMPs binding to PRRs, as well as by direct physical, chemical, and thermal injury. They also can be activated by components of the complement cascade and by immunoglobulin E (IgE) antibodies produced in allergies (see Chapter 9). Located in connective tissue and close to vessels, they can be found near the body's surfaces (skin, GI, and respiratory tract linings). A variety of stimuli associated with tissue injury can induce inflammation by triggering the release of potent soluble substances from mast cells. These substances are released in two ways:

1. *Degranulation*—release of preformed contents of mast cell granules
2. *Synthesis*—the new production and release of mediators in response to a stimulus

Degranulation. Mast cells release biochemical mediators from their granules into the surrounding tissues within seconds of a stimulus. Substances within the granules include histamine, chemotactic factors, and cytokines. Their effects occur immediately.

Histamine is a small-molecular-weight molecule with potent effects on many other cells, particularly those that control the circulation. Histamine binds to *histamine receptors* (H1, H2, H3, and H4 receptors) on various cell surfaces. The binding of histamine to the *H1 receptor* is proinflammatory (Fig. 7.5). This causes a rapid, temporary constriction of smooth muscle, along with dilation of the postcapillary venules. The net result of these two effects is increased blood flow within the microvasculature. H1 receptor binding also causes increased vascular permeability secondary to the retraction of endothelial cells lining the capillaries (opening the tight junctions between them), and increased leukocyte adherence to the endothelial walls. The H1 receptor also is present on smooth muscle cells within the bronchi. H1 stimulation results in bronchial smooth muscle contraction and bronchoconstriction often seen in asthma. Antihistamines are drugs that block the binding of histamine to the H1 receptor, resulting in decreased vascular effects. *H4 receptors* are highly expressed on mast cells where their stimulation is proinflammatory by promoting histamine and cytokine generation, and H4 receptor blockers are being developed in an effort to better treat many allergic and inflammatory disorders.[17] The role of histamine receptors and hypersensitivity is discussed in Chapter 9.

In contrast, histamine binding to the *H2 receptor* is generally anti-inflammatory because it results in the suppression of leukocyte function. Both H1 and H2 receptors are often present on the same immune cells where they may act in an antagonistic fashion. For example, stimulation of H1 receptors on neutrophils results in an augmentation of neutrophil chemotaxis, whereas stimulation of the H2 receptor results in its inhibition. The H2 receptor also is abundant on parietal cells of the stomach mucosa, where stimulation induces the secretion of gastric acid as part of the normal physiology of the stomach. *H3 receptors* inhibit the release of histamine and other neurotransmitters on neurons in the central nervous system. They are involved in blood–brain barrier function, and non-inflammatory processes including cognition, sleep, and regulation of food intake.[18] Research into the role of H3 receptors in health and disease are revealing potential uses treating neurodegeneration (Alzheimer and Parkinson disease), migraine, narcolepsy, and control of eating in obesity.[19]

Mast cell granules also contain chemotactic factors (chemokines). Chemotaxis is directional movement of cells along a chemical gradient formed by a chemotactic factor. Two important factors are neutrophil chemotactic factor (NCF) and eosinophil chemotactic factor of anaphylaxis (ECF-A). Neutrophils are the predominant cells that destroy bacteria in inflammation. Eosinophils help regulate the inflammatory response. Both cells are discussed in more detail later in this chapter.

Synthesis of mediators. Activated mast cells initiate synthesis of other mediators of inflammation. These mediators include leukotrienes, prostaglandins, platelet-activating factor and growth factors (see Fig. 7.4B).

1. Leukotrienes (slow-reacting substances of anaphylaxis [SRS-A]) are products of arachidonic acid. Arachidonic acid is released from mast cell membranes by intracellular phospholipase A2 which acts on membrane phospholipids. Leukotrienes are produced from arachidonic acid by the

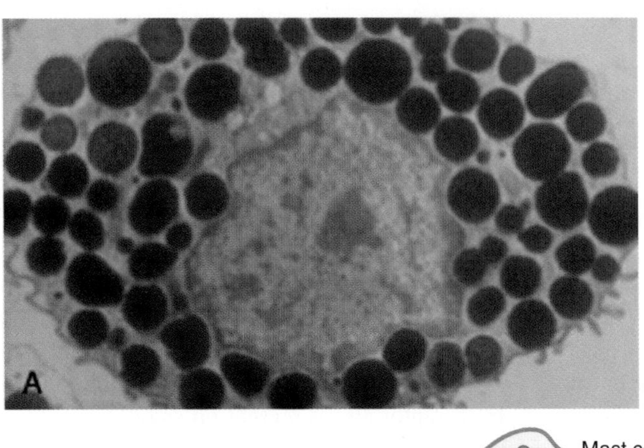

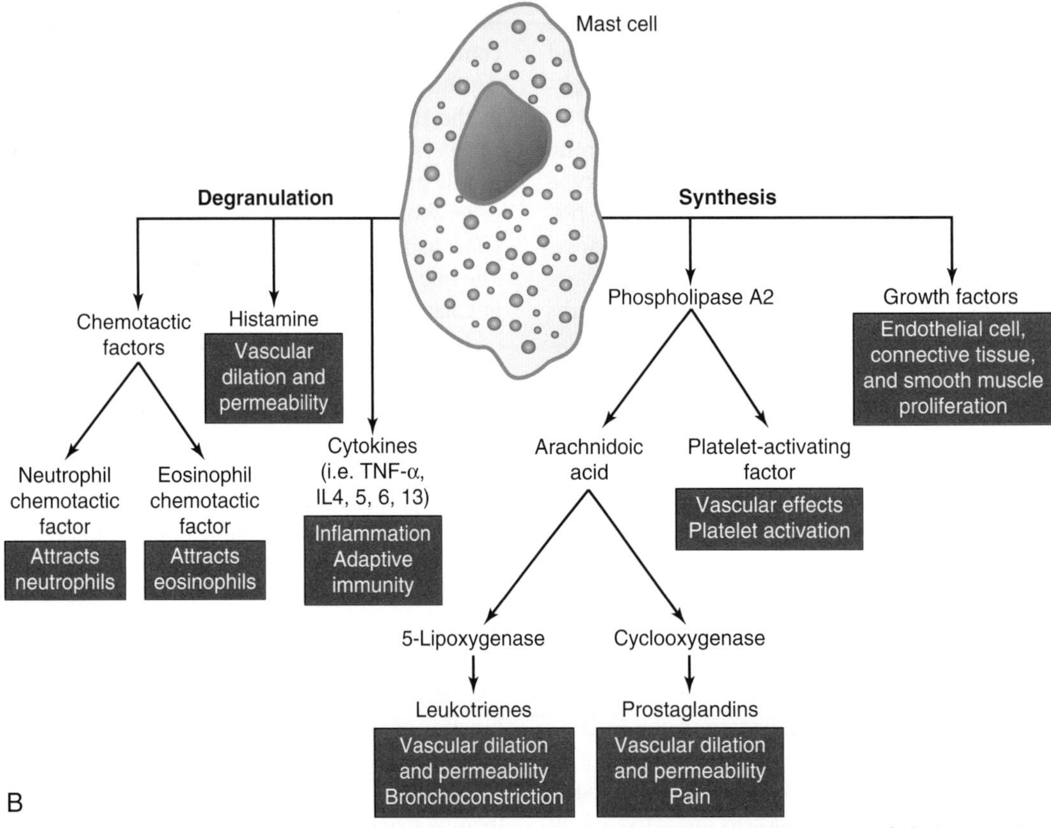

Fig. 7.4 Mast Cell Degranulation and Synthesis of Inflammatory Mediators. (A) Colorized photomicrograph of mast cell; dense granules contain biologically active substances. Among these are histamine, which is a major initiator of vascular changes, and a variety of chemotactic factors. **(B)** Mast cell degranulation *(left)* and synthesis *(right)*. Histamine and other biologically active substances are released immediately after stimulation of mast cells. Long-term responses are mediated by the synthesis and release of products of phospholipase A metabolism (leukotrienes, prostaglandins, and platelet-activating factor) and growth factors that promote tissue proliferation. *IL*, Interleukin; *TNF-α*, tumor necrosis factor-alpha. (A, From Roitt IM, Brostoff J, Male DK. *Immunology*, 3rd edition. St. Louis: Mosby, 1993.)

action of *lipoxygenase* and consist of several different subtypes (Fig. 7.6) Leukotrienes induce smooth muscle contraction (especially bronchoconstriction) and increased vascular permeability. Leukotrienes appear to be important in the later stages of the inflammatory response because they stimulate slower and more prolonged inflammatory responses than does the rapid-acting histamine.

2. Prostaglandins also are products of arachidonic acid. They cause increased vascular permeability, neutrophil chemotaxis, and pain. Pain results from the direct effects on nerves. Prostaglandins are long-chain, unsaturated fatty acids produced by the action of cyclooxygenase (COX). COX exists in two different forms: COX-1, which produces prostaglandins that activate platelets and protect the stomach lining, and COX-2, which activates prostaglandins associated with inflammation (see Fig. 7.6). Aspirin, acetaminophen, and nonsteroidal anti-inflammatory drugs (NSAIDs) inhibit COX-1 and/or COX-2. They suppress inflammation and

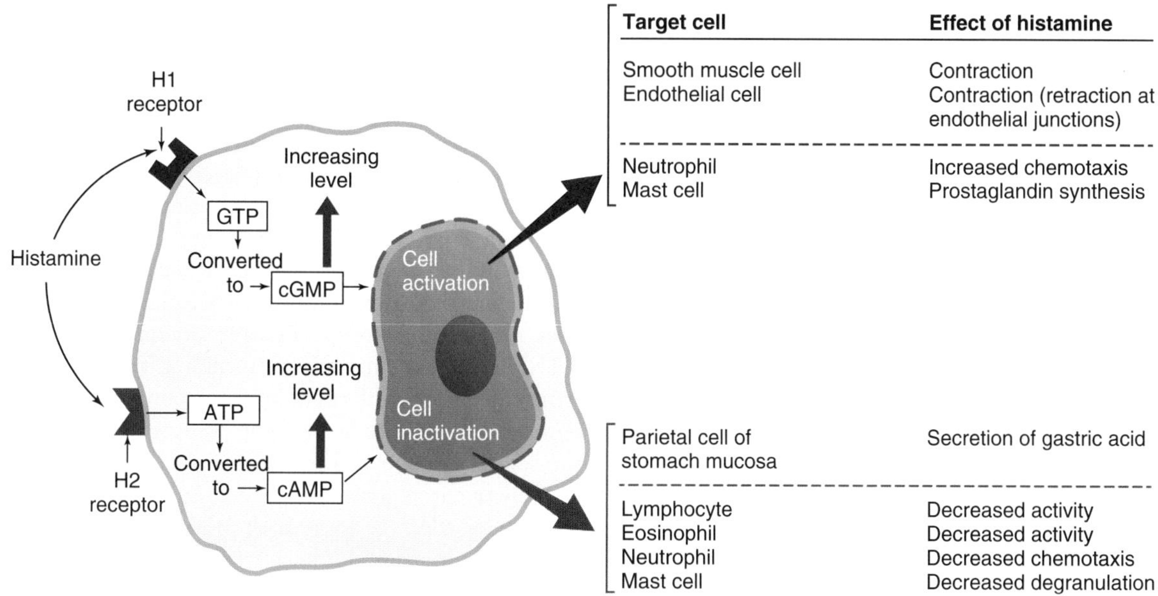

Fig. 7.5 Effects of Histamine Through H1 and H2 Receptors. The effects depend on *(1)* the density and affinity of H1 or H2 receptors on the target cell and *(2)* the identity of the target cell. *ATP*, Adenosine triphosphate; *cAMP*, cyclic adenosine monophosphate; *cGMP*, cyclic guanosine monophosphate; *GTP*, guanosine triphosphate.

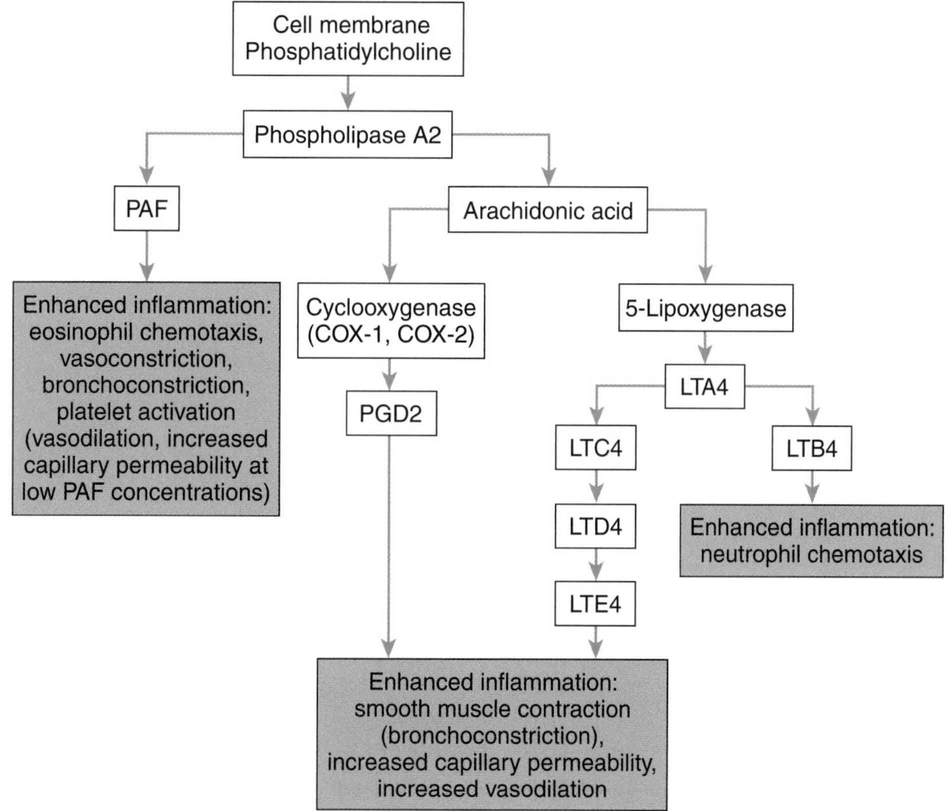

Fig. 7.6 Production of Lipid Vasoactive Substances by Mast Cells. *LTA4, LTC4, LTD4, LTE4, LTB4*, Various leukotriene molecules; *PAF*, platelet-activating factor; *PGD2*, prostaglandin D2.

improve symptoms but have associated side effects. NSAIDs can cause GI tract bleeding, hypertension, renal dysfunction, and cardiovascular disease especially in older individuals who take them regularly for underlying conditions such as osteoarthritis.[20]

3. Platelet-activating factor (PAF) molecules are produced by neutrophils, monocytes, endothelial cells, mast cells, and platelets. The biologic activity of PAF is similar to that of leukotrienes. It causes increased vascular permeability, leukocyte adhesion to endothelial cells, and platelet activation (see Fig. 7.6).

4. Growth factors synthesized and released by mast cells include vascular endothelial growth factor (VEGF) which promotes endothelial cell proliferation, and platelet-derived growth factor (PDGF) which promotes connective tissue and smooth muscle proliferation (see Fig. 7.4B). These growth factors contribute to wound healing.

Macrophages

Macrophages are derived from circulating monocytes. As with other blood cell types, monocytes are produced in bone marrow and enter into the circulation. They migrate to tissues throughout the body where they transform to macrophages. These **tissue macrophages** have many different names depending on where they are located, including Kupffer cells (liver), alveolar macrophages (lungs), and microglia (brain) (see Table 28.3). Tissue macrophages are important initial mediators of the inflammatory response.

Macrophages and dendritic cells have an abundance of PRRs on their surface that can recognize a wide range of pathogens and molecules released from damaged tissues. PRR receptor binding to PAMPs and DAMPs results in intracellular communication leading to activation of NF-κB and the subsequent release of proinflammatory chemokines and cytokines. Chemokines (a type of cytokine) are members of a family of low-molecular-weight peptides that function primarily to induce leukocyte chemotaxis. They facilitate the movement of phagocytes from the blood stream through the vessel wall into the area of injury. Cytokines constitute a family of intercellular signaling molecules that are secreted, bind to specific membrane receptors, and regulate innate and adaptive immunity. Macrophages release both *proinflammatory* and *antiinflammatory* cytokines (Fig. 7.7). The most important proinflammatory cytokines secreted by macrophages are tumor necrosis factor-alpha (TNF-α), interleukins, and IFNs.

Tumor necrosis factor-alpha. Tumor necrosis factor-alpha (TNF-α) is secreted primarily by activated macrophages, but is also released by mast cells, neutrophils, and lymphocytes. When PRRs on the surface of macrophages bind to PAMPs or DAMPs, NF-κB is activated and TNF-α is one of the most important proinflammatory cytokines that is then produced. It plays a role in promoting the innate response to virtually any injury or infection including chemotaxis and adherence of neutrophils, phagocytosis, and inflammatory and adaptive immune cell proliferation.[21] TNF-α has systemic effects, including the induction of fever, increased liver synthesis of inflammation-related serum proteins (acute phase proteins), muscle wasting (cachexia), and intravascular thrombosis. These effects can be deleterious in cases of severe or chronic infection and cancer. TNF-α contributes to the damaging effects of severe acute inflammatory conditions such as sepsis and to many chronic inflammatory diseases.

Interleukins. Interleukins (ILs) are produced predominantly by macrophages and lymphocytes in response to stimulation of PRRs or by cytokines secreted by other immune cells. More than 30 interleukins have been identified. Their effects include the following:

1. Regulation of cell adhesion molecules (CAMs), which are proteins that facilitate leukocyte binding with other cells or with the extracellular matrix
2. Attraction of leukocytes to a site of inflammation (chemotaxis)
3. Induction, proliferation, and maturation of leukocytes in bone marrow
4. General enhancement or suppression of inflammation and the adaptive immune response

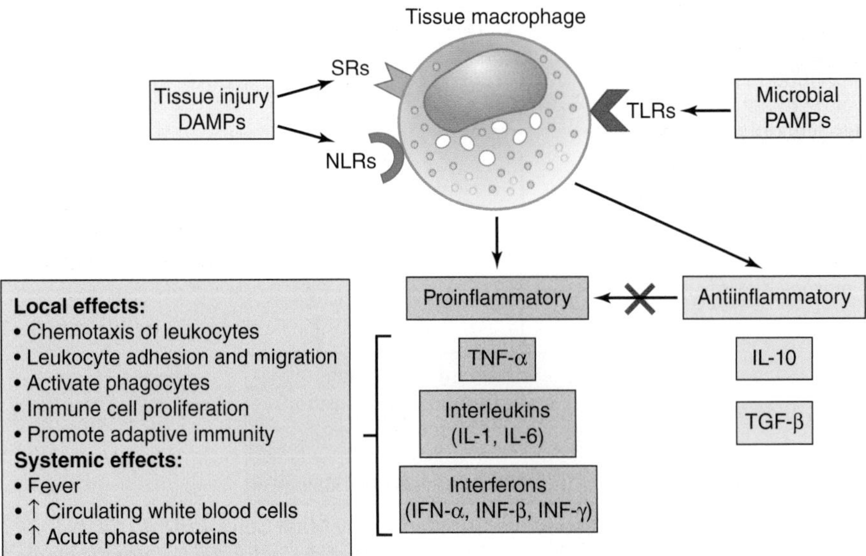

Fig. 7.7 Tissue Macrophage-Derived Cytokines. When stimulated by pathogen invasion or tissue injury, macrophages release proinflammatory cytokines that have a wide range of local and systemic effects. Antiinflammatory cytokines are also released which limit the effects on inflammation. *DAMPs*, Damage-associated molecular patterns; *IFN*, interferon; *IL*, interleukin; *NLRs*, nucleotide-binding-like receptors; *PAMPs*, pathogen-associated molecular patterns; *SRs*, scavenger receptors; *TLRs*, Toll-like receptors; *TNF-α*, tumor necrosis factor alpha.

Two major proinflammatory interleukins are interleukin-1 (IL-1) and interleukin-6 (IL-6). IL-1 is produced mainly by macrophages and activates monocytes, other macrophages, and lymphocytes, thereby enhancing both innate and adaptive immunity. It also acts as a growth factor for many cells. IL-1 is an endogenous pyrogen (fever-causing cytokine) which reacts with receptors on cells of the hypothalamus resulting in increased body temperature. IL-6 is produced by macrophages, lymphocytes, fibroblasts, and other cells. IL-6 directly induces hepatocytes in the liver to produce many of the proteins needed for inflammation (acute phase proteins). IL-6 also stimulates growth and differentiation of blood cells in the bone marrow and the growth of fibroblasts required for wound healing. IL-1 and IL-6 play important roles in numerous inflammatory diseases and infections, and monoclonal antibodies that block these cytokines are used to treat many of them. For example, in severe COVID-19 infection, blockade of IL-1 and IL-6 resulted in decreased mortality.[22]

Interferons. Interferons (IFNs) are members of a family of cytokines that protect against viral infections and modulate the immune response. They are considered essential components of both innate and adaptive immunity. Type I IFNs (primarily IFN-α, IFN-β) are produced and released by virally infected cells. These IFNs do not kill viruses; rather they induce antiviral proteins in neighboring healthy cells. Type II IFN (IFN-γ) is produced primarily by lymphocytes. It activates macrophages and increases their capacity to detect and process invaders and abnormal cells so that they can be removed by the adaptive immune system.

Antiinflammatory cytokines. Some cytokines are antiinflammatory and diminish and control the inflammatory response. Two of the most important are IL-10 and TGF-β. Interleukin-10 (IL-10) is primarily produced by lymphocytes. It suppresses the activation and proliferation of other lymphocytes and limits the production of proinflammatory cytokines by macrophages. The result is a downregulation of both the inflammatory and the adaptive immune responses. Recent evidence suggests that IL-10 also may have proinflammatory effects in certain severe conditions such as Crohn disease and COVID-19.[23] Transforming growth factor-beta (TGF-β) is produced by many cells in response to inflammation. Its primary role in immunity is to suppress the activity of lymphocytes and downregulate the production of proinflammatory cytokines by macrophages.

Dendritic Cells

Dendritic cells can be considered a specialized type of macrophage derived from a common precursor stem cell in the bone marrow. Some, like macrophages, differentiate from circulating monocytes. They provide one of the major links between the innate and adaptive immune responses. They are located in tissues that have contact with the outside environment, e.g. the gut, respiratory tract, and skin. Like tissue macrophages, they recognize invaders with PRRs and phagocytose them. They are different from tissue macrophages in that they migrate from the tissues through lymphatic vessels to lymph nodes, where they present antigens from the phagocytosed invaders to T lymphocytes resulting in an adaptive immune response (see Chapter 8). Dendritic cells produce many of the same cytokines as macrophages.

The Vascular Response in Inflammation

After initiation by the plasma protein systems, mast cells, tissue macrophages, and dendritic cells, the inflammatory response has an almost immediate effect on blood vessels (see Algorithm 7.1). Inflammatory changes in the microcirculation (arterioles, capillaries, and venules) surrounding the site of an injury happen within seconds. They include the following processes:

1. Hemostasis (coagulation): Injury to blood vessels initiates the clotting cascade and activates platelets. Clotting slows blood flow, walls off injury, and provides a meshwork for healing.
2. Vasodilation: Arteriole and venule dilation increase the diameter of blood vessels, the volume of blood delivered to the injured site, and slows the velocity of blood flow. This action allows more time for the movement of fluids, chemicals, and cells into surrounding tissues, resulting in erythema (redness) and warmth in the area of injury.
3. Increased vascular permeability: Blood vessels become porous, secondary to retraction of endothelial cells, thus opening vascular tight junctions and enlarging the spaces between these cells. This results in exudation (the leaking of fluid and cells from vessels) and edema (tissue swelling from fluid leakage) of the area surrounding the injury.
4. Leukocyte cell adhesion: Leukocytes adhere to the inner walls of vessels, where they migrate through the enlarged spaces between endothelial cells and into the surrounding tissue (diapedesis). Accordingly, there is an influx of phagocytes (neutrophils and macrophages) to the injured tissue, where they target invaders and damaged cells.

Together, these vascular changes deliver leukocytes (particularly neutrophils and macrophages), plasma proteins, and other biochemical mediators to the site of injury. Chemical mediators activate pain fibers. Tissue injury, pain, and swelling contribute to loss of function.

Lymphatic vessels, which drain the extravascular fluid to lymph nodes, may become secondarily inflamed. The resulting lymphangitis (inflammation of lymph vessels) or lymphadenitis (inflammation of nodes) can present as enlarged and painful lymph nodes. For example, in an individual with a sore throat, the infected and inflamed pharynx can result in enlarged and painful lymph nodes, which are readily palpable in the neck region.

The Cellular Response in Inflammation

Once the inflammatory response has been initiated by plasma proteins, mast cells, tissue macrophages, and dendritic cells, other leukocytes move out of the blood vessels and travel quickly to the area of invasion or injury. Neutrophils are the most important phagocyte in the cellular response in inflammation and arrive early at the scene in large numbers where they begin the process of removing microorganisms and cellular debris. Monocyte-derived macrophages play an essential role in removing debris and initiating the healing process. Both of these cell types function primarily through the process of phagocytosis.

Neutrophils

The neutrophil, or polymorphonuclear neutrophil (PMN), is a granulocyte named for its characteristic staining pattern as well as its multilobed nucleus. Neutrophils circulate in the blood in large numbers and are attracted to the area of injury by chemotactic factors, such as mast cell cytokines, chemokines, and complement. Neutrophils are the predominant phagocytes in early inflammation, arriving at the inflammatory site within 6 to 12 hours after the initial injury. The primary role of the neutrophil is to phagocytize pathogenic microbes and remove cellular debris and dead cells from lesions. The neutrophil is a mature cell incapable of division and is sensitive to the acidic environment found at inflammatory sites. Accordingly, it is short-lived and rapidly becomes a component of the purulent exudate (pus) removed from the body through the epithelium or drained from the infected site through the lymphatic system. They are present in sterile lesions, which drain "sterile pus," as well as in septic (nonsterile) lesions found in bacterial infections.

In addition to phagocytosis, neutrophils can form neutrophil extracellular traps (NETs) which are crucial in attacking pathogens. NETs are formed of material from cell nucleus breakdown (chromatin and histones) and neutrophil granules which contribute numerous enzymes that can degrade microorganisms. These enzymes include neutrophil elastase, myeloperoxidase, matrix metalloproteinases, and others.[24] NET formation usually leads to the destruction of the neutrophil. NETs may also contribute to tissue damage and autoimmune diseases.[25]

Monocyte-Derived Macrophages

Monocyte-derived macrophages are also essential phagocytes in inflammation. They begin appearing at the inflammatory site as soon as 24 hours after the initial neutrophil infiltration but do not arrive in large numbers until 3 to 7 days later. They are attracted by chemotactic factors released by the neutrophils that are already present at the site. Macrophage activation results in two subpopulations, M1 and M2 macrophages, each with specialized functions. *M1 macrophages* are proinflammatory and have bactericidal activity, promote adaptive immunity, and can attack cancer cells.[26] *M2 macrophages* are primarily involved in tissue healing and repair. Macrophages can survive and divide in the acidic environment of the inflammatory site and so are capable of conducting prolonged phagocytosis of microorganisms and damaged cells. They play an essential role in removing debris and promoting the formation of new blood vessels (angiogenesis) and secretion of growth factors that prepare the tissue for healing.[27]

Phagocytosis

Phagocytosis is the ingestion of microbes, foreign particles, or cell fragments. The two most important cells for phagocytizing pathogens or damaged cells are neutrophils and macrophages. Inflammatory cytokines and chemokines serve to activate these cells and through chemotactic factors cause them to move toward the area of injury. These cytokines also open the tight junctions between endothelial cells, creating spaces between them. Additionally, inflammation induces endothelial nitric oxide synthase (iNOS), increasing the amount of nitric oxide (NO) production. Effects of NO in inflammation include vasodilation and changes in inflammatory cell function.[28]

The first step in the migration of phagocytes to the area of invasion or injury starts when endothelial cells, monocytes, and neutrophils begin expressing new CAMs on their surfaces. The most important CAMs related to vascular inflammation are selectins, integrins, and intracellular adhesion molecules (ICAMs). These CAMs increase the adhesion, or stickiness, between phagocytes and endothelial cells in the walls of the capillaries. At first, the phagocytes roll down the endothelial surface. This is followed by tight binding to the endothelium in a process called margination, or pavementing (Fig. 7.8A). Other adhesion molecules such as platelet endothelial cell adhesion molecules (PECAMs) then are expressed leading to diapedesis or **emigration** of the cells through the openings between endothelial cells. The leukocytes digest the basement membrane and migrate into the surrounding tissues.[29] Monoclonal antibodies that block adhesion molecules are used to reduce inflammation in a variety of conditions including cancer (see Chapter 9).[30]

Once inside the connective tissue in the perivascular space, phagocytes migrate to the inflammatory site by means of chemotaxis. They detect chemotactic factors (chemokines) in the environment through chemoreceptors on their plasma membranes and migrate in the direction of highest concentration (see Fig. 7.8A). The most important chemotactic factors include bacterial products, complement fragments C3a and C5a, and chemokines. Neutrophils also respond to chemotactic factors released from mast cells (NCF). Monocyte-derived macrophages are attracted to monocyte chemotactic factor (MCF) that has already been released by neutrophils at the site of injury.

Phagocytosis at the inflammatory site involves four steps (see Fig. 7.8C):

1. Recognition and adherence of the phagocyte to its target through PRRs
2. Engulfment (ingestion or endocytosis) and formation of phagosomes
3. Fusion of the phagosome with lysosomal granules within the phagocyte
4. Destruction of the target

Most phagocytes can trap and engulf pathogens using their PRRs which recognize PAMPs on the microorganisms (see Fig. 7.8B). However, some pathogens such as encapsulated bacteria (see Chapter 10) are more difficult to engulf. Opsonization greatly enhances adherence of the phagocyte to the target microorganism or cell. Opsonins that coat the target bacteria or cell act as a "glue" tightening the affinity between the phagocyte and the target, making phagocytosis more effective. The most efficient opsonins are C3b of the complement system and antibodies produced during the adaptive immune response.

Engulfment (endocytosis) is a process whereby the microorganism is drawn into the interior of a phagocytic cell. Engulfment is carried out by small pseudopods that extend from the plasma membrane of the phagocyte to surround the target, forming an intracellular phagocytic vacuole, or phagosome. Upon formation of a phagosome, the lysosomes (containing destructive enzymes) converge, fuse with the phagosome, and discharge their contents to create a phagolysosome. Destruction of the target takes place within the phagolysosome. Destruction is accomplished by both oxygen-dependent and oxygen-independent mechanisms.

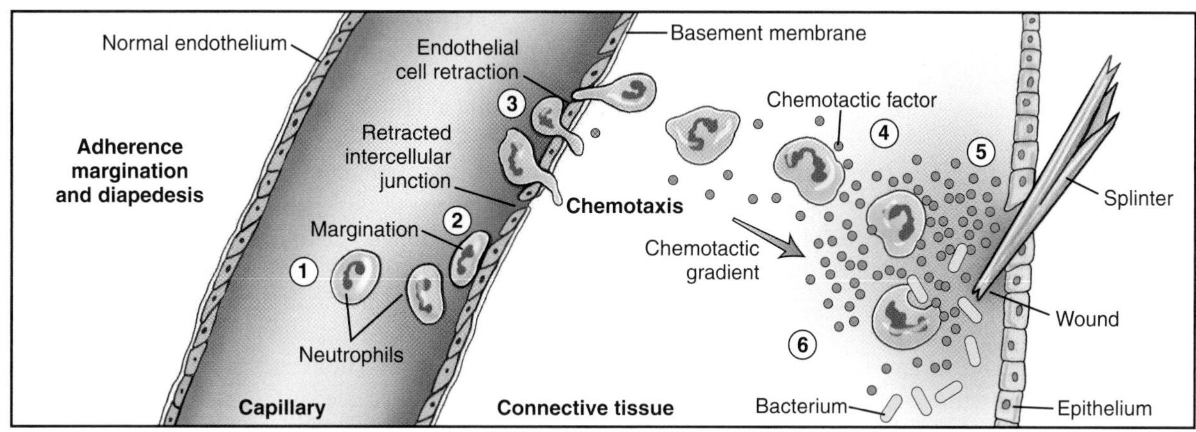

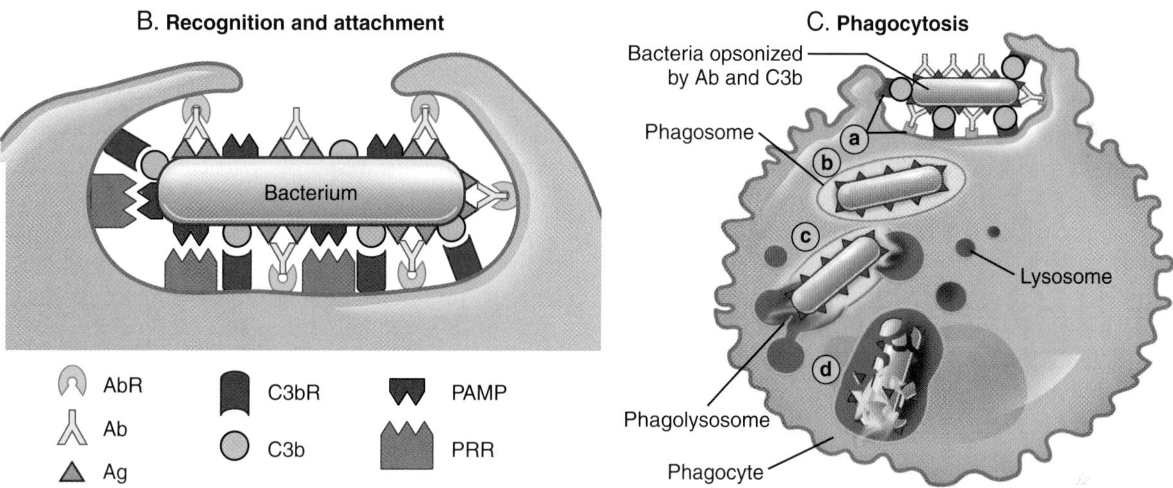

Fig. 7.8 Process of Phagocytosis. The process that results in phagocytosis is characterized by three interrelated steps: adherence and diapedesis, tissue invasion by chemotaxis, and phagocytosis. **(A) Tissue damage**. *Adherence, margination, and diapedesis*: The primary phagocyte in the blood is the neutrophil, which usually moves freely within the vessel *(1)*. At sites of inflammation, neutrophils and endothelial cells respond to inflammatory cytokines by expressing adhesion molecules (selectins, integrins, and ICAMs). This causes the neutrophils to progressively develop increased adherence to the endothelium, leading to accumulation along the vessel wall (margination or pavementing) *(2)*. At sites of endothelial cell retraction, other adhesion molecules such as PECAMs allow the neutrophil to move through the vessel wall by means of diapedesis *(3)*. *Chemotaxis:* In the tissues, the neutrophil detects chemotactic factor gradients through surface receptors *(4)* and migrates toward higher concentrations of the factors *(5)*. The high concentration of chemotactic factors at the site of inflammation immobilizes the neutrophil *(6)*. **(B) Recognition and attachment**. Specific receptors are expressed on the surface of phagocytes that facilitate recognition and attachment to ligands found on the surface of target invaders such as bacteria. **(C) Phagocytosis**. ***(a)*** Antibodies and complement serve to opsonize the surface of microorganisms which are then more easily recognized and bound to the surface of a phagocyte. ***(b)*** The microorganism is engulfed (ingested) into a phagocytic vacuole, or phagosome. ***(c)*** Lysosomes fuse with the phagosome, resulting in the formation of a phagolysosome. ***(d)*** The microorganism is killed and digested. *Ab*, Antibody; *AbR*, antibody receptor; *Ag*, antigen; *C3b*, complement component C3b; *C3bR*, complement C3b receptor; *PAMP*, pathogen-associated molecular pattern; *PRR*, pattern recognition receptor.

Oxygen-dependent killing mechanisms result from the production of toxic oxygen species (e.g., hydrogen peroxide, singlet oxygen, or hydroxyl radicals). Phagocytosis is accompanied by a burst of oxygen uptake by the phagocyte. Chemical mediators and other reactive oxygen species are highly damaging to bacteria.

Oxygen-independent mechanisms of microbial killing include (1) the acidic pH (3.5 to 4.0) of the phagolysosome, (2) cationic proteins that bind to and damage target cell membranes, (3) enzymatic attack of the microorganism's cell wall by lysozyme and other enzymes, and (4) inhibition of bacterial growth by lactoferrin binding of iron (iron is essential for bacterial growth).

Throughout the process, these toxic substances are isolated within membrane-bound vesicles. This isolation protects the phagocyte from harm secondary to the phagocyte's own enzymes.

Several bacteria are resistant to destruction by phagocytes and can survive inside macrophages. Microorganisms, such as *Mycobacterium tuberculosis* (tuberculosis), *Mycobacterium leprae* (leprosy), *Salmonella typhi* (typhoid fever), *Brucella abortus* (brucellosis), and *Listeria monocytogenes* (listeriosis), can remain dormant or multiply inside the phagolysosomes of macrophages.[31]

In addition to removing pathogens and damaged cells, phagocytes (especially macrophages) are responsible for removing cells that have completed their normal life cycle. For example, white blood cells and erythrocytes are programmed to live for only weeks or months. These dead cells number in the billions per day and must be recognized and removed from the body via phagocytosis.[32] Phagocytosis of a red blood cell is illustrated in Fig. 7.9.

Dying phagocytes can cause tissue damage at the site of inflammation. When a phagocyte dies at an inflammatory site, it frequently lyses (breaks open), releasing its enzymatic contents into the tissue. These enzymes can cause inflammation-associated tissue destruction. The destructive effects of enzymes released by dying phagocytes are minimized by natural inhibitors found in blood. Examples of such inhibitors would include catalase, which breaks down hydrogen peroxide, and alpha1-antitrypsin (α1-antitrypsin), a protease inhibitor produced by the liver. An inherited deficiency of α_1-antitrypsin, a disease known as alpha-1 antitrypsin deficiency, results in pulmonary emphysema secondary to chronic lung inflammation, even in nonsmokers (see Chapter 35).[33]

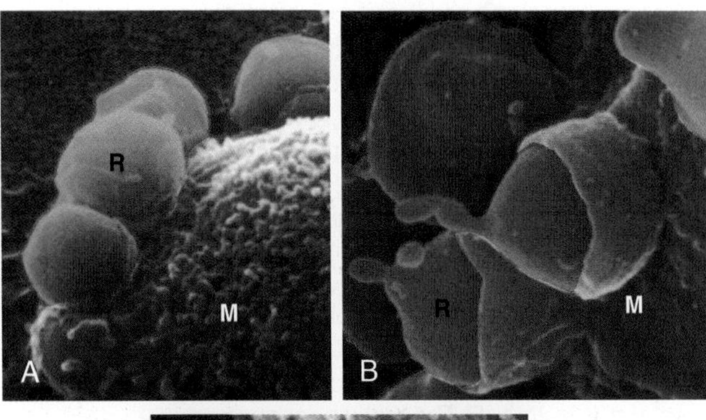

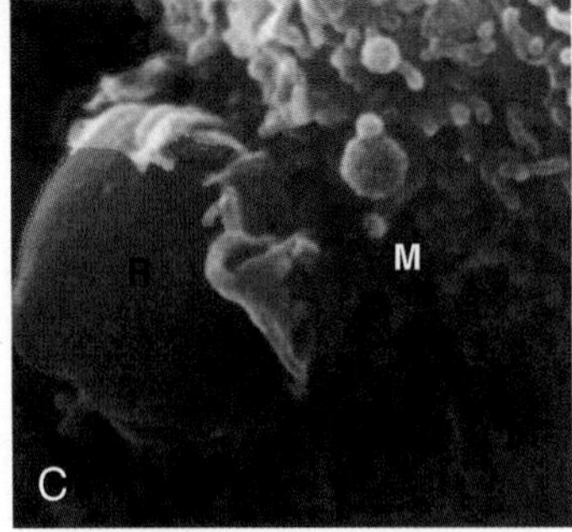

Fig. 7.9 Steps in Phagocytosis. This scanning electron micrograph shows the progressive steps in phagocytosis. **(A)** Red blood cells *(R)* attach to the surface of a macrophage *(M)*. **(B)** Part of the macrophage *(M)* membrane starts to enclose the red cell *(R)*. **(C)** The red blood cells are almost totally engulfed by the macrophage. (From King DW, Fenoglio CM, Lefwitch JH. *General pathology: Principles and dynamics.* Philadelphia: Lea & Febiger; 1983.)

Other Cells of Inflammation

Another type of innate immune cell is the eosinophil. Although eosinophils are only mildly phagocytic, they serve as the body's primary defense against *parasites* and regulate *vascular mediators* released from mast cells. Lysosomal granules within the eosinophil contain enzymes that degrade vasoactive substances from mast cells, thus limiting and controlling the vascular effects of inflammation. Eosinophils also are important components of allergic conditions and can contribute to tissue damage; these effects are discussed in Chapter 9.

The basophil is the least prevalent granulocyte in the blood. It is similar to mast cells with respect to the contents of its granules. Basophilic granules also contain heparin, a naturally occurring anticoagulation product. Basophils release histamine which, as discussed previously, has potent vasoactive properties. Basophils are an important source of cytokines involved in the adaptive immune response, particularly responses associated with allergies and asthma.

Lymphocytes, another type of leukocyte, initiate specific, protective immune responses against pathogens and cancer. B lymphocytes produce antibodies, and T lymphocytes regulate other immune cells and kill viruses and cancer cells (see Chapter 8). Natural killer (NK) cells, a type of lymphocyte, eliminate virally infected and cancerous cells. NK cells have inhibitory and activating receptors that allow differentiation between infected or tumor cells and normal cells. If the NK cell binds to a target cell through activating receptors, it produces several cytokines and toxic molecules, which, in turn, kill the target cell. Innate lymphoid cells (ILCs) also are derived from lymphocyte precursors that reside near mucosal surfaces. There are three major groups of ILCs (ILC1s, ILC2s, and ILC3s) which contribute in different ways to preventing pathogen invasion and activating both the innate and adaptive immune responses (see Chapter 8).[34]

Acute and Chronic Inflammation

Inflammation can be divided into two phases: acute inflammation and chronic inflammation (Algorithm 7.3). The acute inflammatory response is self-limiting; it continues only until the threat to the body is eliminated. The process usually takes 8 to 10 days from onset of injury to healing. If the acute inflammatory response proves inadequate or does not resolve appropriately, chronic inflammation may develop and persist for weeks or months. The characteristics of the acute inflammatory response differ from those of a chronic response. Each phase involves different biochemical mediators and cells, all of which function in a coordinated manner. Depending on the successful containment of tissue damage and infection, both the acute and chronic phases may eventually lead to healing.

Manifestations of Local and Systemic Acute Inflammation

The cells and plasma protein systems involved in the inflammatory response interact to produce the characteristic changes of inflammation, whether local or systemic. They also determine the duration of inflammation, either acute or chronic.

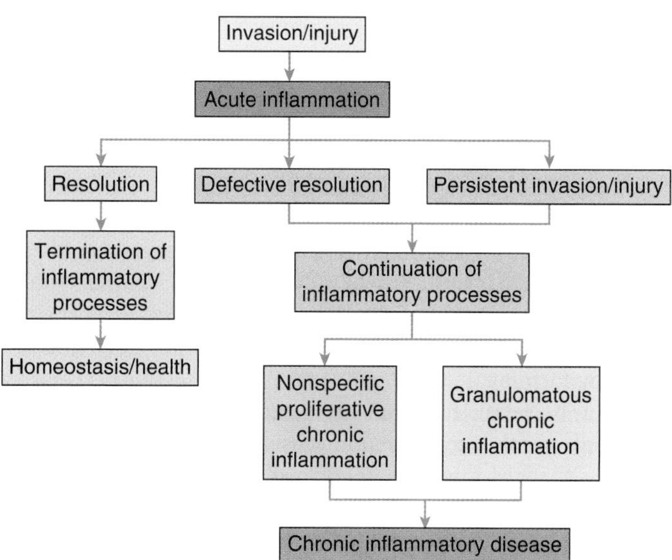

Algorithm 7.3 Chronic Inflammatory Response. The acute inflammatory response to invasion or injury usually leads to resolution of the inciting event, reduction of inflammatory cytokines and cells, and restoration of tissue homeostasis and health. However, defects in the resolution process or persistent invasion and injury lead to chronic inflammatory damage to tissues and resultant disease.

The classic or cardinal signs of the acute local inflammatory response were described in the first century by a Roman named Celsus. They include the following:

1. Rubor (redness, erythema)
2. Calor (heat)
3. Tumor (swelling)
4. Dolor (pain)
5. Functio laesa (loss of function)

Inflammatory exudates result from increased vascular permeability and the leakage of fluid into tissues. Exudates vary in composition, depending on the stage of inflammation, and, to a lesser extent, the triggering event. In early or mild inflammation, the exudate may be a serous exudate (watery) with very few plasma proteins or leukocytes (e.g., fluid in a blister). In more severe or advanced inflammation, the exudate may be a fibrinous exudate (thick and clotted) (e.g., the fluid exudates in the lungs of an individual with pericarditis). A purulent exudate (pus) is the accumulation of a large number of leukocytes, as occurs in bacterial infections (e.g., sputum in persons with pneumonia). A purulent exudate can also occur within walled-off lesions, known as cysts or abscesses. When bleeding occurs, the exudate is filled with erythrocytes and is described as a hemorrhagic exudate.

Systemic manifestations of acute inflammation include three primary systemic changes: fever, leukocytosis (a transient increase in the levels of circulating leukocytes), and increased levels of circulating plasma proteins. It is important to realize that individuals who are immunocompromised (e.g., those taking corticosteroids, chemotherapy agents, and antirejection medications) may not demonstrate these clinical manifestations, making it difficult to recognize acute infection or tissue injury.

Fever

Fever is partially induced by specific cytokines (e.g., TNF-α and IL-1) released from neutrophils and macrophages. These cytokines are known as endogenous pyrogens to differentiate them from pathogen-produced exogenous pyrogens (e.g., endotoxins produced by some bacteria). Pyrogens act directly on the hypothalamus, the portion of the brain which controls the body's thermostat. A fever can be beneficial, as many microorganisms are sensitive to small increases in body temperature. For example, the microorganisms causing syphilis or gonococcal urethritis are highly sensitive to small increases in body temperature. However, fever may have harmful side effects when it enhances the body's susceptibility to endotoxins associated with severe bacterial infections.

Leukocytosis

Leukocytosis is an increase in the number of circulating white blood cells beyond the upper limit of normal (11,000/mL^3 in adults) (see Chapter 29). Inflammation stimulates the proliferation and release of granulocyte and monocyte precursors in bone marrow. The cells migrate into the systemic circulation resulting in both an increase in the total number of circulating leukocytes and an increased ratio of immature to mature cell forms. In particular, increased numbers of immature neutrophil forms such as band cells, metamyelocytes, and (rarely) myelocytes are released from the marrow into blood causing an abnormal complete blood count (CBC), a common laboratory analysis of blood cells. The differential count is a measure of the ratio or proportion of each of the various blood cell types circulating in the blood. An increase in the total number of white blood cells in combination with an abnormal differential count is a clue that there may be an ongoing infection.

Plasma Protein Synthesis

The hepatic synthesis of many plasma proteins is increased during inflammation. These proteins, which can be either proinflammatory or anti-inflammatory in nature, are referred to as acute-phase reactants (proteins). Acute-phase reactants reach maximal circulating levels within 10 to 40 hours after the onset of inflammation.

Laboratory tests that measure levels of acute-phase reactants are available. For example, an increase in blood levels of the acute-phase reactants fibrinogen is associated with an increased adhesiveness of erythrocytes. Erythrocytes adhere to one another under these circumstances, forming large clumps that are buoyant and slow to settle to the bottom of a test tube of blood. This results in an increased value for the laboratory test referred to as erythrocyte sedimentation rate (ESR) or, as it is more commonly known, the "sed rate." Although this increased ESR is a nonspecific reaction, persons found to have an elevated ESR will likely have an inflammatory process going on somewhere within the body. Another common laboratory measure of inflammation is the C-reactive protein (CRP), a laboratory measurement which also is increased during an inflammatory response. CRP is used to look for subclinical inflammation in individuals at risk for heart disease and to estimate the severity of certain infectious and autoimmune diseases.[35]

Chronic Inflammation

In its simplest terms, the difference between acute and chronic inflammation is duration. Chronic inflammation is slow, long-term inflammation lasting for prolonged periods of several months to years. It is characterized by low-grade persistent inflammatory changes that result in collateral damage to tissues.[36] Virtually all chronic diseases are characterized by a component of chronic inflammation. Although the cause of defective resolution and a persistent inflammatory response is often unknown, some common conditions associated with chronic inflammation include increasing age, cardiac and neurologic disorders, malignancy, autoimmune disorders, and chronic infection.

Chronic inflammation is most often thought to be preceded by an unsuccessful acute inflammatory response, although that initial insult may not have been recognized (see Algorithm 7.3). For example, if bacterial contamination or foreign objects (dirt, wood splinter, silica, glass, etc.) persist in a wound, the inflammatory response will be prolonged. Some microorganisms are resistant to killing by the acute inflammatory response or may produce toxins which damage tissue and cause persistent inflammation, even after the original microorganism is killed. Chronic inflammation also can occur as a result of defective resolution of acute inflammation, due to an inability to appropriately dampen the innate immune response.[37] Trained immunity in which innate immune cells remain hyperreactive to inflammatory stimuli may also play a role (see Emerging Science Box: Understanding the Causes of Chronic Inflammatory Disease).[38]

There are two major types of chronic inflammation (Fig. 7.10). *Nonspecific proliferative chronic inflammation* is characterized by the infiltration of lymphocytes and macrophages followed by a proliferation of fibroblasts, connective tissue, and epithelial cells. This often leads to scar or polyp formation. *Granulomatous chronic inflammation* occurs when macrophages and eosinophils attempt to wall off and isolate a foreign body or an infected area by forming a granuloma (Fig. 7.11). Infections caused by certain bacteria (tuberculosis, listeriosis, brucellosis), fungi (histoplasmosis, coccidioidomycosis), and parasites (leishmaniasis, schistosomiasis, toxoplasmosis) commonly result in granuloma formation. Many autoimmune conditions also are associated with granulomatous tissue changes.[39]

Granuloma formation is mediated by TNF-α and other proinflammatory cytokines. Macrophages are called to the area of persistent inflammation, where some differentiate into large epithelioid cells, which specialize in taking up debris and other small particles. Other macrophages fuse into multinucleated giant cells, which are active phagocytes, which can engulf particles larger than those that can be engulfed by a single

EMERGING SCIENCE BOX

Understanding the Causes of Chronic Inflammatory Disease

Chronic inflammatory diseases such as myocardial infarction, stroke, cancer, diabetes, kidney failure, and autoimmune conditions cause more than half of all deaths in the world today. Although the cause of the persistent inflammatory response is often unknown, the most common triggers of chronic inflammation include chronic infections, physical inactivity, disrupted sleep, poor diet, obesity, microbiome dysbiosis, psychological stress, social isolation, and exposure to environmental toxins such as air pollutants (especially particulate matter), chemicals, and tobacco smoking. In addition, there is increasing evidence that maternal health during pregnancy can have a profound effect on the developing fetal immune system that may increase the risk for chronic inflammatory diseases later in life. Lack of adequate resolution of the acute inflammatory response is considered the primary underlying cause of chronic inflammation. Recent studies implicate trained immunity of the innate immune system in the development of chronic inflammatory conditions. Trained immunity describes the process by which innate immune cells are epigenetically and metabolically reprogrammed to remain hyperresponsive even after brief stimulation. For example, microorganisms and oxidized LDL are capable of inducing memory in macrophages. Trained immunity is thought to provide some protection against infectious diseases, but it can also contribute to chronic inflammation and the development of chronic inflammatory diseases such as atherosclerosis. Chronic inflammation in older individuals is thought to result in part from cellular senescence called inflammaging, a condition which is characterized by DNA damage, decreased cell proliferation, and increased secretion of pro-inflammatory cytokines. Many lifestyle changes recommended for specific chronic inflammatory disorders such as heart disease, cancer, and diabetes are thought to positively impact underlying inflammatory processes. For example, skeletal muscle releases small proteins called myokines during exercise which systemically reduces inflammation. A better understanding of how inflammation becomes chronic is leading to emerging ideas about how to better manage inflammatory conditions and prevent many common diseases.

Data from Anderton H, et al. Cell death in chronic inflammation: Breaking the cycle to treat rheumatic disease. *Nature Reviews Rheumatology,* 2020; 16:496–513; Bondy SC, et al. Attenuation of acute and chronic inflammation using compounds derived from plants. *Experimental Biology and Medicine,* 2021; 246(4):406–413; Furman D, et al. Chronic inflammation in the etiology of disease across the life span. *Nature Medicine,* 2019; 25:1822–1832; GBD 2017 Causes of Death Collaborators. Global, regional, and national age-sex-specific mortality for 282 causes of death in 195 countries and territories, 1980–2017: A systematic analysis for the Global Burden of Disease Study 2017. *Lancet,* 2018; 392:1736–1788; Fleming TP, et al. Origins of lifetime health around the time of conception: causes and consequences. *Lancet,* 2018; 391:1842–1852; Fullerton JN, et al. Resolution of inflammation: A new therapeutic frontier. *Nature Reviews. Drug Discovery,* 2016; 15:551–567; Gomarasca M, et al. Myokines: The endocrine coupling of skeletal muscle and bone. *Advances in Clinical Chemistry,* 2020; 94:155–218; Michels N, et al. Chronic inflammation towards cancer incidence: A systematic review and meta-analysis of epidemiological studies. *Critical Reviews in Oncology-Hematology,* 2021; 157:103177; Netea MG. Therapeutic targeting of trained immunity. *Nature Reviews. Drug Discovery,* 2019; 18(7):553–566; Suzuki K. Chronic inflammation as an immunological abnormality and effectiveness of exercise. *Biomolecules,* 2019; 9(6):223; Tercan H, et al. Trained immunity: long-term adaptation in innate immune responses. *Arteriosclerosis, Thrombosis and Vascular Biology,* 2021; 41:55–61; Tsai DH, et al. Effects of short- and long-term exposures to particulate matter on inflammatory marker levels in the general population. *Environmental Science and Pollution Research International,* 2019; 26(19):19697–19704.

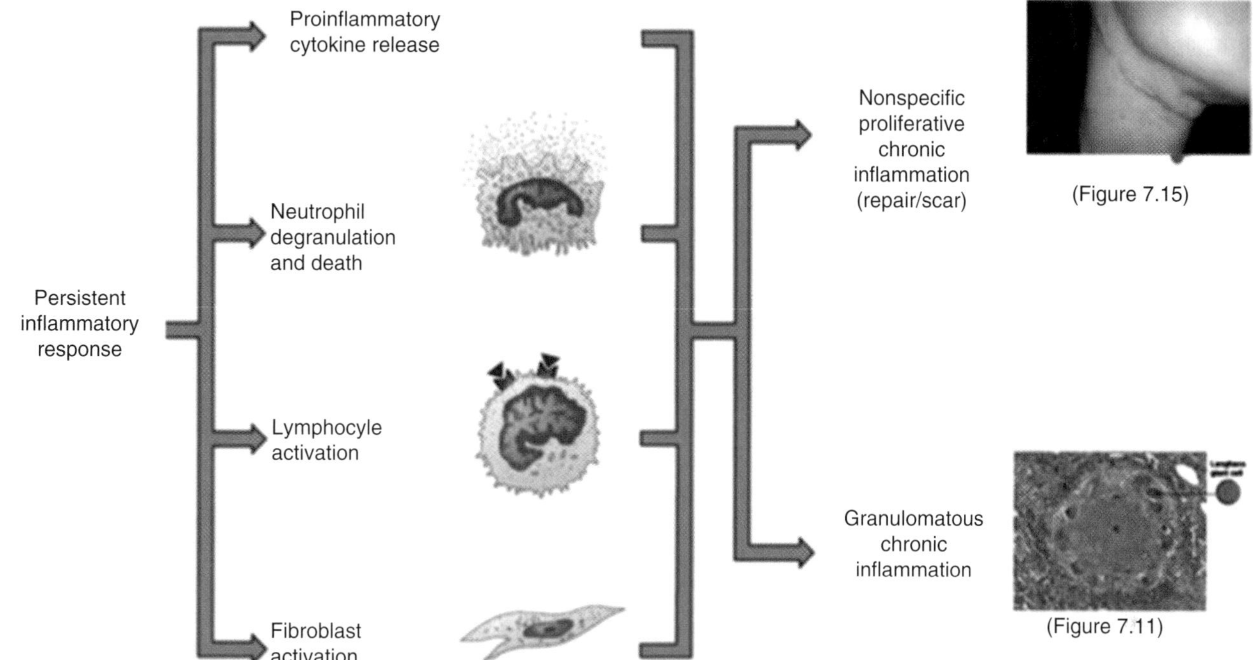

Fig. 7. 10 Types of Chronic Inflammation. Chronic inflammation is characterized by the persistence of many of the processes of acute inflammation. In addition, large amounts of neutrophil degranulation and death, the activation of lymphocytes, and the concurrent activation of fibroblasts result in the release of mediators that induce the infiltration of more lymphocytes and monocytes/macrophages leading to two types of chronic inflammatory outcomes.

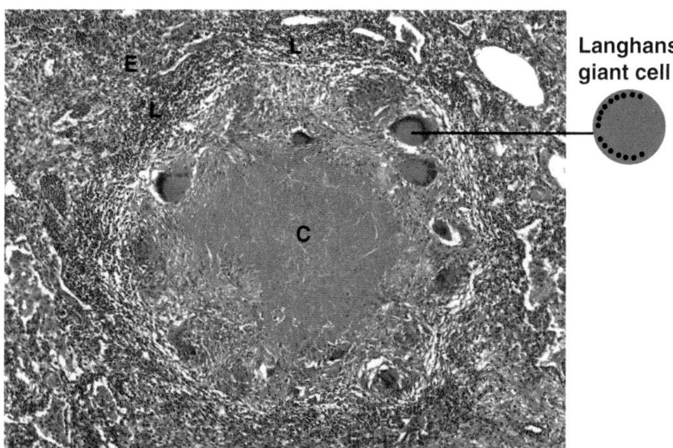

Fig. 7.11 Tuberculous Granuloma. A central area of amorphous caseous necrosis *(C)* is surrounded by a zone of lymphocytes *(L)* and enlarged epithelioid macrophage cells *(E)*. Activated macrophages frequently fuse to form multinucleated cells (Langerhans giant cells). In tuberculoid granulomas the nuclei of the giant cells move to the cellular margins in a horseshoe-like formation. (From Kumar V, Abbas AK, Aster JC. *Robbins basic pathology*, 9th edition. Philadelphia: Saunders; 2013.)

macrophage. These two types of specialized cells form the center of the granuloma and are surrounded by lymphocytes. The granuloma itself is often encapsulated by fibrous deposits of collagen. It may become cartilaginous or even calcified by deposits of calcium carbonate and calcium phosphate.

The classic granuloma associated with tuberculosis is characterized by a wall of lymphocytes and epithelioid cells surrounding the mycobacteria. Death of cells within the granuloma results in the release of acids and enzymatic lysosomal contents from dead phagocytes forming a cheese-like proteinaceous center which consists of decaying tissue (caseous necrosis). In this inhospitable environment, the cellular debris is broken down into its basic constituents, forming a clear fluid within the granuloma (liquefaction necrosis). Eventually, this fluid diffuses out, leaving a hollow, thick-walled structure that has replaced normal tissue, resulting in the reduced lung function seen with tuberculosis infections.

WOUND HEALING

The most favorable outcome of inflammation is healing with a return to normal structure and function. Some destroyed tissues are capable of regeneration, a process where damaged tissue is replaced with healthy tissue of the original type. Regeneration occurs within the epithelia of the skin and intestines as well as in some organs, notably the liver. This restoration is an example of effective resolution of the acute inflammatory response.

Regeneration does not always follow inflammation and may not be possible when extensive damage has occurred and at sites where the original tissue is not capable of complete restoration of normal tissue structure. Where resolution is not possible, tissue repair occurs. Repair refers to the replacement of destroyed tissue with scar tissue. Scar tissue is composed primarily of collagen, a substance which fills in the lesion and restores tissue integrity and strength but cannot carry out the physiologic functions of the tissue it has replaced, resulting in loss of function.

A clean incision, such as a paper cut or a sutured surgical wound, heals primarily through the process of primary intention. Because this type of wound has minimal tissue loss and close apposition of the wound edges, healing can occur quickly (Fig. 7.12).

Other wounds do not heal as readily. Healing of an open wound, such as a severe burn, requires a great deal of tissue replacement. In these cases, healing occurs through secondary intention (see Fig. 7.12). Healing by either primary or secondary intention may occur at different rates for different types of tissue injury.

Epidermal wounds that heal by secondary intention are not completely restored by healing. At best, repaired tissue regains 80% of its original tensile strength. In fibrous connective tissue, such as joints and ligaments, normal healing results in replacement of the original tissue with new tissue which does not exactly replicate the structure or function of the original. Some tissues heal without replacement of any functional cells as those cells are not capable of replication. For example, damage resulting from myocardial infarction heals with fibrous scar tissue rather than with cardiac muscle. Accordingly, cardiac function is not restored completely and the individual surviving the infarction will have varying amounts of impaired myocardial contractility and cardiac function depending on the size of the scar.

Wound healing occurs in four overlapping phases or stages: (1) *hemostasis (coagulation)*, (2) *inflammation*, (3) *proliferation with new tissue formation*, and (4) *remodeling and maturation* (Fig. 7.13).

Phase I: Hemostasis (Coagulation)

Tissue injury damages capillaries and blood vessels and causes bleeding into the wound. Damage to blood vessels causes immediate vasoconstriction followed by vasodilation and initiates the coagulation cascade and activation of platelets. The fibrin mesh of the blood clot acts as a scaffold for cells that participate in healing. Platelets contribute to clot formation. As the platelets degranulate, they release factors which cause increased capillary permeability and promote growth factors which initiate proliferation in undamaged cells. In addition to activation of clotting, there is activation of complement and kinins.

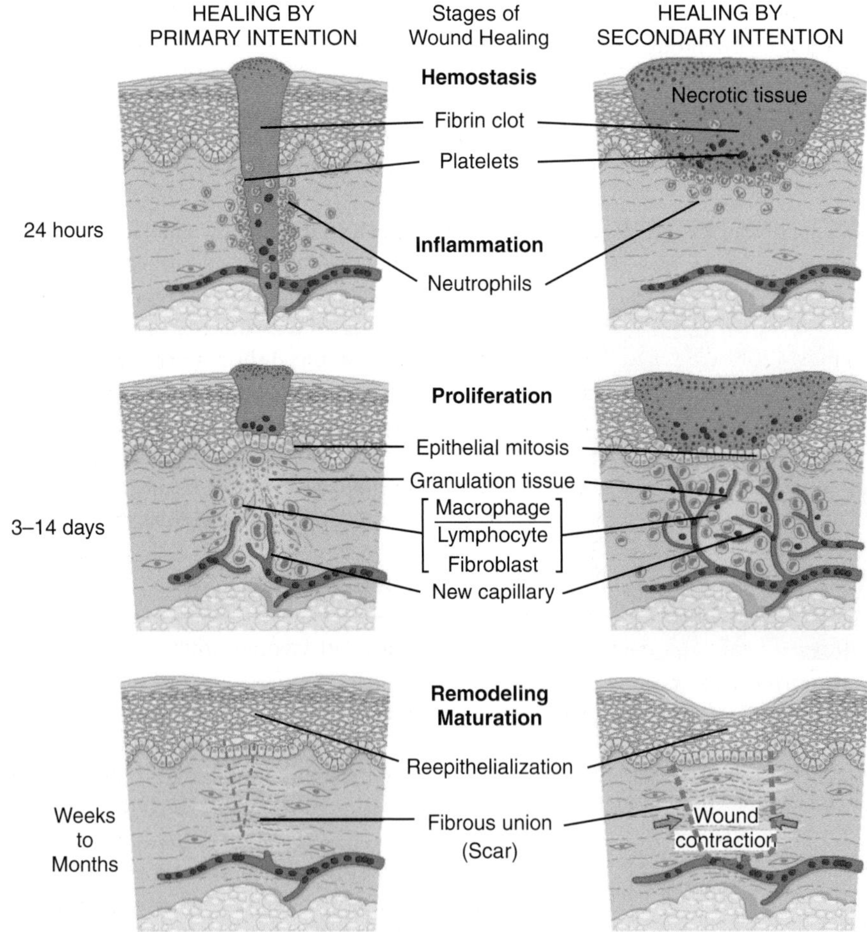

Fig. 7.12 Wound Healing by Primary and Secondary Intention and Stages of Wound Healing. Phases of wound healing (coagulation, inflammation, proliferation/ tissue formation, remodeling, and maturation) and steps in wound healing by primary intention *(left)* and secondary intention *(right)*. Note the large amounts of granulation tissue and wound contraction in healing by secondary intention. (From Roberts JR, Custalow CB. *Roberts and Hedges' clinical procedures in emergency medicine,* 6th edition. Philadelphia: Elsevier/Saunders; 2013.)

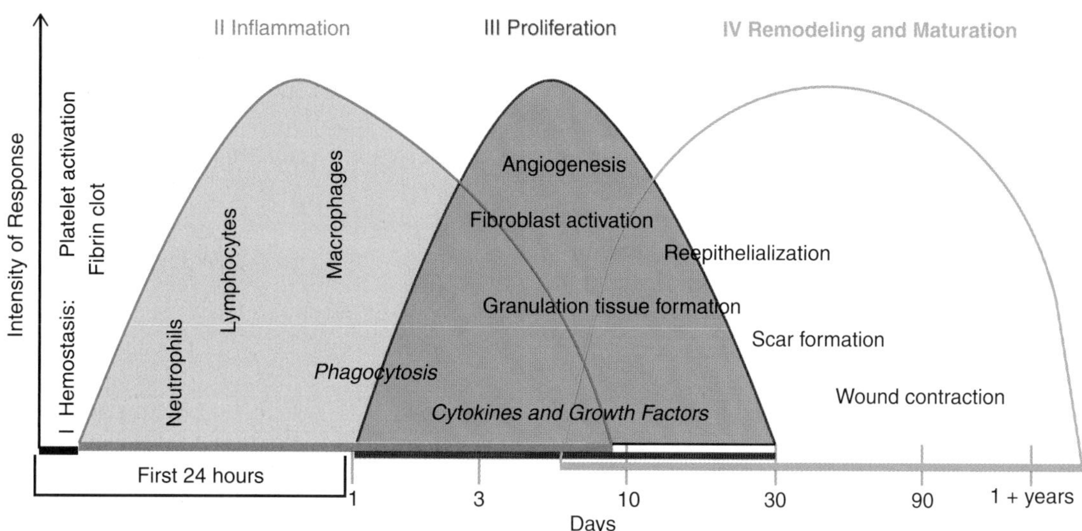

Fig. 7.13 Phases of Wound Healing and Time Course.

Phase II: Inflammation

The inflammatory phase begins within minutes. As has been described in detail previously, macrophages and mast cells release numerous vasoactive cytokines that increase blood flow to the wound and bring needed cells and proteins to the area of injury. DAMPs and chemokines released by injured cells recruit and activate inflammatory cells, especially neutrophils.[40] Neutrophils infiltrate the area of injury and initiate the process of clearing the wound of debris and bacteria. Lymphocytes initiate an adaptive immune response.

Phase III: Proliferation and New Tissue Formation

The proliferative phase begins 3 to 4 days after the injury and continues for as long as 2 weeks. The wound is sealed, and the fibrin clot is replaced by normal tissue or scar tissue during this phase. The proliferative phase is characterized by an invasion of macrophages. During this phase, both monocyte-derived and tissue macrophages are stimulated by a variety of cytokines to become M2 macrophages.[41] They clear debris, release numerous growth factors, recruit fibroblasts, and promote collagen synthesis and angiogenesis. Angiogenesis describes the process of the formation of new blood vessels and is one of the most important steps in wound healing. When blood vessels are injured, growth factors such as VGEF and PDGF secreted by M2 macrophages cause endothelial cells to sprout new capillaries. This brings nutrients and oxygen to the healing wound.[40]

The cleanup of the lesion, which also involves dissolution of fibrin clots (or scabs), is called debridement. After debridement, the remaining debris is drained away by blood and lymphatic vessels and the vascular dilation and permeability associated with early inflammation are reversed, thus preparing the lesion for either regeneration or repair. An important role for macrophages during this phase is the engulfment of neutrophils *(efferocytosis)* to clear them and promote resolution of inflammation.[40]

As wound healing progresses, granulation tissue grows into the wound from surrounding healthy connective tissue. It consists of invasive cells, new lymphatic vessels, and new capillaries, all derived from the analogous structures found in the surrounding healthy tissue. These components lend a red and granular appearance to the newly formed granulation tissue. Capillary buds sprout from vascular endothelial cells around the wound and extend into the débrided areas. Loops form when the young capillaries join (anastomose). The loops are more fragile and permeable than mature vessels, resulting in leakage of erythrocytes and neutrophils. The erythrocytes are phagocytosed by macrophages, and the neutrophils assist in further debridement of the inflammatory lesion. Many of the new capillaries differentiate into larger vessels as repair continues, promoting influx of nutrients and removal of metabolic wastes. New lymphatic vessels also grow into the granulation tissue by a similar process.

Epithelialization is the process by which epithelial stem cells proliferate and grow into the wound from surrounding healthy tissue. Epithelial cells migrate under the clot or scab using matrix metalloproteinases to unravel the collagen. The migrating epithelial cells connect with similar cells from all sides of the wound and seal it. The epithelial cells remain active, undergoing differentiation to give rise to the various epidermal layers. Epithelialization of a skin wound can be hastened if the wound is kept moist, preventing the fibrin clot from becoming a scab.

Fibroblasts are important cells during healing because they secrete collagen and other connective tissue proteins. Fibroblasts deposit connective tissue proteins in debrided areas, about 6 days after they have entered a lesion. Collagen is the most abundant protein in the body. It contains high concentrations of the amino acids glycine, proline, and lysine, many of which are enzymatically modified during the healing process. Additionally, wound healing requires iron, ascorbic acid (vitamin C), and molecular oxygen (O_2). The absence of any of these components results in impaired wound healing. As healing progresses, collagen molecules form collagen fibrils which further modify to form collagen fibers. The complete process takes several months.

In granulation tissue, some fibroblasts transition into myofibroblasts, specialized cells responsible for wound contraction. Myofibroblasts have features of both smooth muscle cells and fibroblasts. Wound contraction occurs as extensions from the plasma membrane of myofibroblasts establish connections between neighboring cells. They anchor themselves to the wound bed then contract their fibers so as to exert tension on the neighboring cells. Wound contraction is necessary for closure of all wounds, especially those that heal by secondary intention. Contraction is noticeable 6 to 12 days after injury.

Phase IV: Remodeling and Maturation

Tissue remodeling and maturation are a process that begins several weeks after injury. Tissue regeneration and wound contraction continue in this phase during which there is a continuation of cellular differentiation, scar formation, and scar remodeling. The fibroblast is the major cell involved in tissue remodeling, where it functions to deposit collagen into an organized matrix. For wounds that heal by scarring, scar tissue is remodeled, and capillaries disappear, resulting in an avascular scar. Within 2 to 3 weeks after maturation has begun, the scar tissue has gained about two-thirds of its eventual maximal strength, which may be less than the strength prior to injury.

Dysfunctional Wound Healing

Dysfunctional wound healing and impaired epithelialization may occur during any phase of the healing process. The causes of dysfunctional wound healing include ischemia; excessive bleeding; excessive fibrin deposition; a predisposing disorder, such as diabetes mellitus; obesity; wound infection; inadequate nutrition; use of certain drugs; and tobacco smoking as well as history of keloid formation.

Ischemic (oxygen-deprived) *tissue* is susceptible to cellular death and infection, which prolongs inflammation and delays healing. Ischemia (both acute following injury as well as chronic) reduces energy production and impairs collagen synthesis as well as the tensile strength of regenerating connective tissue.

Excessive bleeding delays healing. Large clots increase the amount of space that granulation tissue must fill. Clots also serve as mechanical barriers to oxygen diffusion further amplified by tissue ischemia. Accumulated blood is an excellent growth medium for bacteria. Bacteria predispose the wound to infection and prolong inflammation through increased exudation and pus formation. Under normal conditions, vessels dilate, delivering inflammatory cells, nutrients, and oxygen to the site of injury. Decreased blood volume, associated with bleeding, inhibits inflammation secondary to vessel constriction.

Excessive fibrin deposition is detrimental to healing. Fibrin released in response to injury must eventually be reabsorbed to prevent the formation of fibrous adhesions. Adhesions that form in the pleural, pericardial, or abdominal cavities can bind together, forming fibrous bands. Such bands distort, impinge on, or strangulate the affected organs. An adhesion, so formed, may bind an organ to an adjacent organ resulting in both pain and/or impaired organ function (Fig. 7.14).

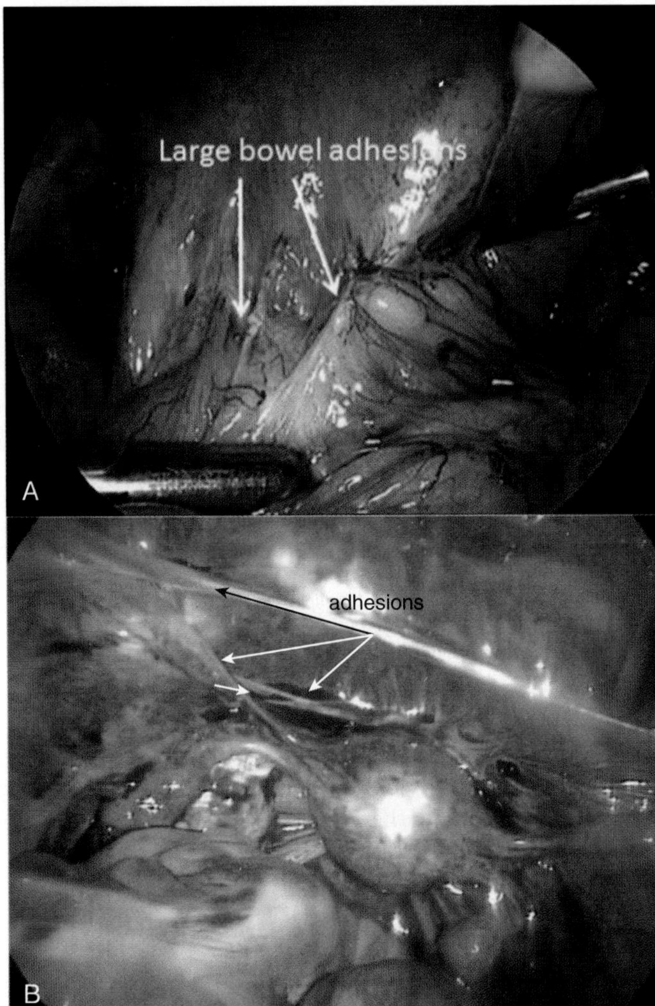

Fig. 7.14 Fibrous Adhesions. Large bowel adhesion **(A)**. Uterine adhesion **(B)** and adhesions that extend from the liver to the inner lining (peritoneum) of the abdominal wall. (A, From Lee ETC, Wong FWS. Small bowel obstruction from barbed suture following laparoscopic myomectomy—A case report. *International Journal of Surgery Case Reports,* 2015; 16:146–149. https://doi.org/10.1016/j.ijscr.2015.09.039; B, From Burke C. Surgical adhesions: Implications for women's health: Part one of a two-part series. *Nursing for Women's Health,* 2012; 16(Supplement 1): S3–S11. https://doi.org/10.1111/j.1751-486X.2012.01707.x)

Obesity delays wound healing through impairing leukocyte function, which, in turn, predisposes the wound to infection, decreased growth factor production, and increases in proinflammatory cytokines. Additionally, there is a dysregulation of collagen synthesis and a decrease in angiogenesis.

Persons with *diabetes* are at risk for prolonged wound healing and wound infection, especially if they have persistent hyperglycemia. The causes of poor wound healing in diabetes are multifactorial and complex. Ischemia, hyperglycemia, infection, and decreased immune function all play a role [42] (see Emerging Science Box: Mechanisms of Impaired Wound Healing in Diabetes).

EMERGING SCIENCE BOX

Mechanisms of Impaired Wound Healing in Diabetes

Diabetes is a complex metabolic disease that affects millions of people in the United States and worldwide. Many of these individuals will suffer from chronic wounds such as diabetic foot ulcers. The mechanisms that contribute to impaired wound healing in diabetes are the result of defects in immune function, cellular metabolism, and tissue integrity. The insulin resistance of persons with diabetes results in deficient glucose transport into many of the key cells involved in wound healing such as mast cells, macrophages, neutrophils, fibroblasts, lymphocytes, and epithelial cells. Cells require glucose to produce energy for physiologic functioning. Furthermore, hyperglycemia in diabetes suppresses macrophage function and prevents them from becoming effective M2 macrophages. Wounds in an individual with diabetes tend to be ischemic because of the prevalence of small-vessel diseases and impaired blood flow, along with glycosylation of hemoglobin that reduces oxygen release into tissues. Hypoxia-induced changes in nuclear function (e.g., microRNAs) reduce cellular proliferation and angiogenesis. The combination of these many factors results in a persistent pro-inflammatory state, decreased release of growth factors, increased risk for infection, and impairment of cellular and tissue function at every step in the healing process. While there are numerous treatment modalities in use and in development, good nutrition, exercise, and maintenance of normoglycemia remain central to improving wound healing in diabetes.

Data from Kalan LR, et al. The role of the microbiome in nonhealing diabetic wounds. *Annals of the New York Academy of Sciences*, 2019; 1435(1):79–92; Knipper JA, et al. Diabetes impedes the epigenetic switch of macrophages into repair mode. *Immunity*, 2019; 51(2):199–201; Morey M, et al. Hyperglycemia acts in synergy with hypoxia to maintain the pro-inflammatory phenotype of macrophages. *PLoS ONE [Electronic Resource]*, 2019; 14(8):e0220577; Moura J, et al. Immune aging in diabetes and its implications in wound healing. *Clinical Immunology*, 2019; 200:43–54; Ozdemir D, et al. MicroRNAs in diabetic wound healing: Pathophysiology and therapeutic opportunities. *Trends in Cardiovascular Medicine*, 2019; 29(3):131–137; Patel S, et al. Mechanistic insight into diabetic wounds: Pathogenesis, molecular targets and treatment strategies to pace wound healing. *Biomedicine and Pharmacotherapy*, 2019; 112:108615; Williams R, et al. Laser capture microdissection on surgical tissues to identify aberrant gene expression in impaired wound healing in type 2 diabetes. *Journal of Visualized Experiments*, 2021; 167.

Wound infection is caused by the infiltration of pathogens into the injured or compromised tissues. Infection is promoted by the necrotic debris, low oxygen tension, and a decreased host immune response. Biofilms may form within the wound and prevent healing.[43] Biofilms are accumulations of microbes that adhere to the wound surface and secrete a matrix of polysaccharides that protect the pathogens from the immune response and from antibiotics (see Chapter 10). Such pathogens damage cells, stimulate the continued release of inflammatory mediators, consume nutrients, and delay wound healing.[43]

Optimal *nutrition* is important during all phases of healing because of the increased metabolic needs of the affected tissues. Hypoproteinemia with decreased levels of amino acids, such as arginine and glutamine, impairs fibroblast proliferation and collagen synthesis.[44] Prolonged lack of vitamins A and C, which are cofactors required for collagen synthesis, results in poorly formed connective tissue and significantly impaired healing. Other cofactors for collagen synthesis include iron, zinc, manganese, and copper. Accordingly, malnutrition results in an increased risk for wound infection, delayed healing, and reduced wound tensile strength.

Medications associated with delayed or dysfunctional wound healing include antineoplastic (anticancer) agents, NSAIDs, and steroids. Antineoplastic agents slow cell division and inhibit angiogenesis. NSAIDs suppress acute inflammation and inhibit prostaglandin production, resulting in delayed wound healing, especially healing involving bone tissue.[45] Corticosteroids (e.g., prednisone) disrupt wound healing by preventing macrophages from migrating to the site of injury and through inhibiting the release of both collagenase and plasminogen activator. Steroids also inhibit fibroblast migration into the wound during the proliferative phase, thus delaying epithelialization.

Toxic agents in *tobacco smoke* (carbon monoxide and hydrogen cyanide) delay wound healing. Nicotine is a potent vasoconstrictor that compromises wound healing by predisposing the tissue to ischemia and infection.

Dysfunctional collagen synthesis may involve excessive production of collagen, leading to a hypertrophic scar or keloid. Myofibroblasts release growth factors and inflammatory cytokines and contribute to excessive tissue contraction and extracellular matrix deposition.[46] A hypertrophic scar is raised but remains within the original boundaries of the wound. It tends to regress over time (Fig. 7.15A). A keloid is a raised scar that extends beyond the original boundaries of the wound, invading surrounding tissue. Keloids are fibrous lesions and are often characterized by pruritis, pain, and psychological discomfort.[40] They are likely to recur after surgical removal and treatment is often ineffective (see Fig. 7.15B). A familial tendency to keloid formation has been observed, with a greater incidence in persons with darker skin pigmentation, especially African Americans.

Wound Disruption

Even after the healing process has occurred, wounds can be disrupted in a variety of ways that may reverse the healing process or negatively impact function. These complications are more likely if wound healing was dysfunctional.

Dehiscence

A potential complication of wounds that are closed with sutures is dehiscence, a scenario where the wound pulls apart at the suture line. Dehiscence generally occurs 5 to 12 days after suturing, at a time when collagen synthesis is at its peak. Approximately half of dehiscence occurrences are associated with wound infection. Other instances result from suture rupture caused by excessive strain. Adipose tissue is difficult to suture, increasing the risk of dehiscence in individuals who are obese. Wound dehiscence is usually heralded by increased serous drainage from the wound; there often is a perception by the individual that "something gave way." Prompt surgical attention is required.

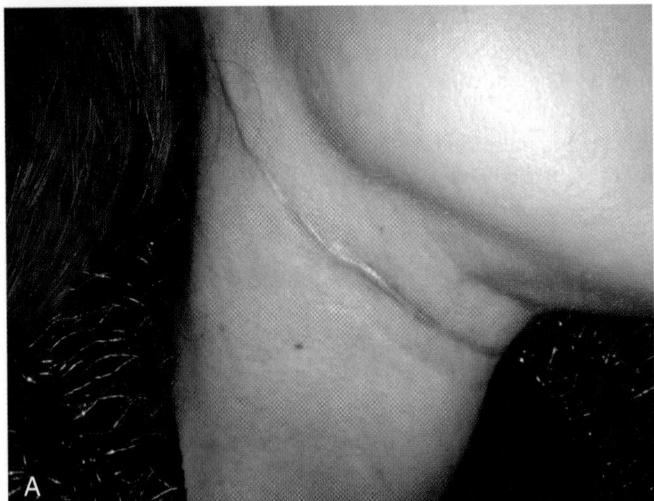

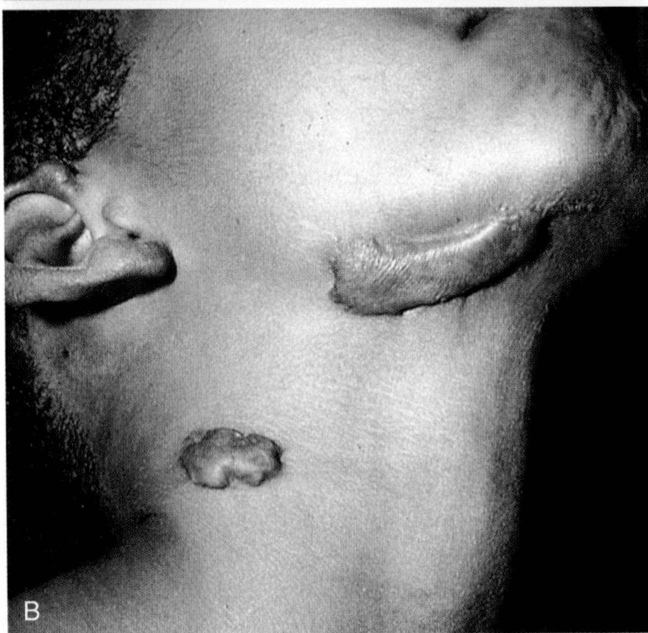

Fig. 7.15 Hypertrophic Scar and Keloid Scar Formation. Hypertrophic scar **(A)** and keloid scar **(B)** caused by excessive synthesis of collagen at suture sites. (A, From Flint PW, Haughey B, Lund V, et al. *Cummings otolaryngology: Head and neck surgery,* 6th edition. Philadelphia: Mosby; 2015; B, From Damjanov I, Linder J. *Anderson's pathology,* 10th edition. St. Louis: Mosby; 1996.)

Contracture

Wound contraction, necessary for healing, may become excessive where it results in an anatomic deformity or contracture of scar tissue. Burns of the skin are especially prone to contracture, particularly at joints with a resultant loss of joint function. Internal contractures include duodenal strictures, caused by dysfunctional healing of a peptic ulcer; esophageal strictures, caused by chemical burns, such as lye ingestion; or abdominal adhesions, caused by surgery, infection, or radiation. Contracture may occur in cirrhosis of the liver, where constricted vascular flow contributes to the development of portal hypertension and esophageal varices. Proper positioning, range-of-motion exercises, compression, and surgery are among the strategies used to prevent or treat skin contractures. Internal contractures, such as those caused by fibrous adhesions between loops of bowel, cause pain or result in a loss of function and are released with surgery.

GERIATRIC CONSIDERATIONS

Innate Immunity in the Elderly

Immunity decreases with aging in a process called immunosenescence. Weakened innate antimicrobial responses put the elderly at increased risk for infection. Several cellular components of innate immunity are deficient in number (e.g., tissue macrophages) or have diminished activity (e.g., neutrophil chemotaxis, degranulation, and phagocytosis). One explanation for this diminished inflammatory cellular activity is an age-related decrease in expression and function of several, if not all, TLRs. NF-κB function is disordered, and there is decreased expression of adhesion molecules on immune cells. In addition, telomere dysfunction leads to immune cell senescence and death.

Paradoxically, elderly individuals are at increased risk for unopposed tissue inflammation called inflammaging. Levels of pro-inflammatory cytokines (e.g., TNF-α, IFN-γ, and IL-1) are elevated, along with higher levels of reactive oxygen species (oxidative stress). These factors contribute to the increased risk for chronic inflammatory diseases (e.g., heart disease and diabetes) that occurs with aging.

Other factors affect immunity and wound healing in the elderly. Because of impaired sensation or mobility and physiologic changes in the skin, older adults are at increased risk for sustaining various wounds. With aging, subcutaneous fat is lost, diminishing a layer of protection. Aging also alters the tissue microenvironment and macrophage function with changes in wound healing angiogenesis and fibrosis. Collagen fibers become thicker and a certain percentage of elastin is lost, further contributing to loss of protection. The regenerative capability of the skin is maintained with aging, but the epidermis undergoes age-associated changes that include atrophy of the underlying capillaries. The consequent decrease of perfusion makes older adults more susceptible than younger people to the adverse effects of hypoxia in the wound bed. Finally, aging fibroblasts may have a slower rate of proliferation, and therefore wound healing is attenuated.

Data from Fülöp T, Larbi A, Witkowski JM. Human inflammaging. *Gerontology,* 2019; 65:495–504; Duong L, Radley HG, Lee B, et al. Macrophage function in the elderly and impact on injury repair and cancer. *Immunity and Ageing,* 2021; 18:4; Fuentes E, Fuentes M, Alarcón M, et al. Immune system dysfunction in the elderly. Anais da Academia Brasileira de Ciências, 2017; 89(1):285–299; Bailey KL, Smith LM, Heires AJ, et al. Aging leads to dysfunctional innate immune responses to TLR2 and TLR4 agonists. *Aging Clinical and Experimental Research,* 2019; 31(9):1185–1193; Weyand CM, Goronzy JJ. Aging of the immune system. Mechanisms and therapeutic targets. *Annals of the American Thoracic Society,* 2018; 13(S5): S422–S428; Zuo L, Prather ER, Stetskiv M, et al. Inflammaging and oxidative stress in human diseases: From molecular mechanisms to novel treatments. *International Journal of Molecular Sciences,* 2019; 20(18):4472.

PEDIATRIC CONSIDERATIONS

Innate Immunity in the Newborn Child

Neonates have transiently depressed immune function. In newborns, the innate immune response is limited in several ways. Complement levels are diminished. Neutrophils and monocytes are incapable of efficient chemotaxis due to decreased ability to express adhesion molecules and impaired margination and diapedesis. Furthermore, these phagocytes exhibit diminished expression of PRRs on their cell surfaces and have impaired ability to destroy microorganisms within phagolysosomes. As a result of these transient innate immune deficiencies, newborns are predisposed to infection, especially cutaneous abscesses caused by staphylococci or cutaneous candidiasis. In addition, newborns are predisposed to develop severe overwhelming sepsis and meningitis when infected by bacteria against which there are no circulating maternal antibodies. Factors that can enhance neonatal immunity include the establishment of a healthy gut microbiome through vaginal delivery and feeding via breast milk whenever possible.

Data from Collins A, Weitkamp JH, Wynn JL. Why are preterm newborns at increased risk of infection? *Archives of Disease in Childhood. Fetal and Neonatal Edition,* 2018; 103(4):F391–F394; Kumar SK, Bhat BV. Distinct mechanisms of the newborn innate immunity. *Immunology Letters,* 2016; 173:42–54; Tsafaras GP, Ntonsi P, Xanthou G. Advantages and limitations of the neonatal immune system. *Frontiers in Pediatrics,* 2020; 8:5; Yu JC, Khodadadi H, Malik A, et al. Innate immunity of neonates and infants. *Frontiers in Immunology,* 2018; 9:1759.

SUMMARY REVIEW

Human Defense Mechanisms

1. Innate defenses are the first line of defense, are present at birth, and include the surface barriers skin and mucous membranes.
2. Inflammation is the second line of defense and is activated with injury or infectious disease.
3. Adaptive (acquired) immunity is the third line of defense, is specific to particular antigens, and has memory.

Innate Immunity

1. There are three layers of human defense: physiologic barriers, the inflammatory response, and adaptive (acquired) immunity.
2. Physical barriers are the first lines of defense functioning to prevent damage to the individual and thwart the entrance of pathogens. These barriers include the skin and mucous membranes.
3. Antibacterial peptides are found in mucous secretions, perspiration, saliva, tears, and other secretions. They provide a biochemical barrier against pathogenic microorganisms.
4. The skin, mucous membranes, and the lining of the gastrointestinal (GI) tract are colonized by commensal or mutualistic microorganisms called the microbiome. These microorganisms provide protection by releasing biochemical compounds which facilitate immune responses and prevent colonization by pathogens. Within the gut, they also facilitate digestion in the GI tract.
5. The second line of defense is the *inflammatory response*, a rapid and nonspecific protective response to cellular injury resulting from any cause. It can occur only in vascularized tissues.
6. Inflammation is mediated by three key plasma protein systems: the complement system, the clotting system, and the kinin system. The components of all three systems are a series of inactive proteins which are activated sequentially in the presence of tissue injury.
7. The complement system can be activated by antigen–antibody reactions (through the classical pathway) or by other products, especially bacterial polysaccharides (through the lectin pathway or the alternative pathway). The lectin and alternative pathways do not require antibody activation to recruit phagocytes, activate mast cells, and destroy pathogens.
8. The most biologically potent products of the complement system are C3b (opsonin), C3a (anaphylatoxin), and C5a (anaphylatoxin, chemotactic factor).
9. The clotting system stops bleeding, localizes microorganisms, and provides a meshwork for repair and healing.
10. Bradykinin is the most important product of the kinin system and causes vascular permeability, smooth muscle contraction, and pain.
11. Control of inflammation regulates inflammatory cells and enzymes and localizes the inflammatory response to the area of injury or infection.
12. Carboxypeptidase, histaminase, kinase, and C1 inhibitor are inactivating enzymes. The fibrinolytic system and plasmin facilitate clot degradation after bleeding is stopped.
13. Mast cells and macrophages are the most important cells for initiating the inflammatory response.
14. These cells express plasma membrane pattern recognition receptors (PRRs) which recognize molecules produced by infectious microorganisms. These molecules include pathogen-associated molecular patterns (PAMPs) and damage-associated molecular patterns (DAMPs). Toll-like receptors (TLRs) are transmembrane receptors and nucleotide-binding-like receptors (NLR-like), and nucleotide oligomerization domain-like (NOD-like) receptors are cytoplasmic receptors. They are expressed by many inflammatory cells and recognize both PAMPs and DAMPs. Upon recognition, they promote the release of cytokines and inflammatory mediators, which, in turn, eliminate damaged cells and protect against invasion by microbes.

15. Mast cells are near epithelial surfaces and capillaries. Mast cells initiate inflammation by releasing biochemical mediators (histamine and chemotactic factors) from cytoplasmic granules. They also synthesize other mediators (prostaglandins, leukotrienes, and platelet-activating factor [PAF]) in response to stimuli. Basophils, found in blood, function in a manner that is similar to mast cells.
16. Histamine is the major vasoactive amine released from mast cells. It increases vascular permeability through dilation of capillaries and retraction of endothelial cells lining the capillaries.
17. Tissue macrophages use PRRs to identify microorganisms and molecules from damaged tissue, and then secrete many biochemical mediators (cytokines), which are responsible for activating other cells and regulating the inflammatory response. These cytokines include TNF-α, interleukins, interferons, and other molecules.
18. TNF-α is produced when PRR binding sends intracellular messengers to the nucleus of the macrophage which activates NF-κB. TNF-α has multiple pro-inflammatory effects including vascular effects, chemotaxis, cellular proliferation, and systemic inflammatory changes.
19. Interleukins are produced primarily by lymphocytes and macrophages. They activate the growth and differentiation of leukocytes and contribute to systemic inflammatory changes such as fever.
20. The most important proinflammatory interleukins are interleukin-1 (IL-1) and interleukin-6.
21. Interferons are produced by cells that are infected by viruses. Once released from infected cells, interferons can stimulate neighboring healthy cells to produce substances that prevent viral infection.
22. There are also anti-inflammatory cytokines such as TGF-β and IL-10 which downregulate the inflammatory response.
23. The vascular responses to inflammation are vasodilation, increased capillary permeability, and an accumulation of fluid and cells at the inflammatory site.
24. The cellular response to inflammation includes neutrophils, monocyte-derived macrophages, and other inflammatory cells.
25. The endothelial cells lining the circulatory system (vascular endothelium) regulate circulating components of the inflammatory system, maintaining normal blood flow. During inflammation, the endothelium expresses receptors that stimulate leukocytes to exit the vessel. The endothelial cell body also retracts to allow fluid to pass into the tissues.
26. The polymorphonuclear neutrophil (PMN), the predominant phagocytic cell in the early inflammation, exits the circulation, through retracted endothelial junctions, by diapedesis. On exiting, it moves to the inflammatory site by chemotaxis.
27. The monocyte-derived macrophage, the predominant cell in the late inflammatory response, is highly phagocytic. Additionally, it is responsive to cytokines, which promote wound healing.
28. Phagocytosis is a multistep cellular process, which usually results in the destruction of pathogens and foreign debris. The steps include recognition and attachment, engulfment, formation of a phagosome, formation of a phagolysosome, and eventual destruction of the pathogen or foreign debris. Phagocytic cells engulf microorganisms, enclosing them within phagocytic vacuoles (phagolysosomes). The vacuoles contain toxins (especially metabolites of oxygen) and/or enzymes that kill and digest the microorganisms.
29. Opsonins are molecules which enhance phagocytosis by coating the antigen. This activity results in a stronger attraction between the microorganism and the phagocyte ("marking" the organism). It also enhances the affinity with which the phagocyte binds to the microorganism. Examples include antibodies and the complement component C3b.
30. Eosinophils release products that control the inflammatory response, and they are the principal cells that destroy parasitic organisms.
31. Other cells of innate immunity include dendritic cells which function as messengers between the innate and acquired (adaptive) immune systems, NK cells which detect certain invaders and cancer cells, and innate lymphoid cells which modulate many aspects of innate immunity.

Acute and Chronic Inflammation

1. *Acute inflammation* is self-limiting and usually resolves within 8 to 10 days.
2. *Local* manifestations of inflammation include the classic signs of redness, heat, swelling, pain, and loss of function. They are the result of vascular changes associated with the inflammatory process, including vasodilation and increased capillary permeability.
3. The principal *systemic effects* of inflammation are fever, leukocytosis (increased levels of circulating leukocytes), and an increase in plasma proteins, primarily the acute-phase reactants, IL-1, and IL-6.
4. *Chronic inflammation* is the persistence of the inflammatory response often contributing to tissue damage.
5. Chronic inflammation is characterized by a dense infiltration of lymphocytes and macrophages. It can take two forms, nonspecific proliferative chronic inflammation and granulomatous chronic inflammation.
6. Nonspecific proliferative chronic inflammation occurs when the acute inflammatory response fails to eliminate the invader/injury or there is dysfunctional resolution of the acute inflammatory response.
7. *Granuloma* formation is a process wherein the body walls off and isolates certain infectious microorganisms or foreign bodies that could not be removed by acute inflammation. It serves to protect the body from further tissue damage.
8. Both forms of chronic inflammation can contribute to tissue dysfunction and organ damage and are the major causes of chronic disease.

Wound Healing

1. *Resolution* (regeneration) is the return of tissue to nearly normal structure and function. *Repair* is healing by scar tissue formation.
2. Resolution occurs when little tissue has been lost or where the injured tissue is capable of regeneration. This type of healing is called *healing by primary intention.*

3. Tissues that have sustained extensive damage or tissue types that are incapable of regeneration heal by repair, a process which results in the formation of a scar. This process is called *healing by secondary intention.*
4. Wound healing occurs in four overlapping phases; hemostasis, inflammation, proliferation with new tissue formation, and remodeling or maturation. Each of these phases is characterized by the complex interaction of multiple cells including platelets, neutrophils, macrophages fibroblasts, endothelial cells, and epithelial cells.
5. Dysfunctional wound healing can be secondary to ischemia, excessive bleeding, excessive fibrin deposition, predisposing disorders (e.g., diabetes mellitus), wound infection, inadequate nutrients, use of NSAIDs and steroids, or altered collagen synthesis.
6. *Dehiscence* is a disruption where the wound pulls apart at the suture line.
7. A *contracture* is a structural deformity caused by the excessive shortening of collagen in scar tissue.

Pediatric and Geriatric Considerations

1. Neonates often have transiently depressed inflammatory function, particularly decreased phagocyte chemotaxis and killing of microorganisms and limited complement activity.
2. Aging impairs the immune system due to a process called immunosenescence which causes impairment of cellular function in both immunity and wound healing.
3. Impaired wound healing in the aging population is multifactorial and includes changes in innate immunity, cellular metabolism, and tissue integrity.
4. The elderly are also at risk for excessive and disordered innate immune responses called inflammaging that contribute to many chronic diseases.

REFERENCES

1. Zheng D, Liwinski T, Elinav E. Interaction between microbiota and immunity in health and disease. *Cell Res.* 2020;30:492–506.
2. Durack J, Lynch SV. The gut microbiome: relationships with disease and opportunities for therapy. *J Exp Med.* 2019;216(1):20–40.
3. Dominguez-Bello MG, et al. Role of the microbiome in human development. *Gut.* 2019;68(6):1108–1114.
4. Ahern PP, Maloy KJ. Understanding immune-microbiota interactions in the intestine. *Immunology.* 2020;159(1):4–14.
5. Ganal-Vonarburg SC, Duerr CU. The interaction of intestinal microbiota and innate lymphoid cells in health and disease throughout life. *Immunology.* 2020;159(1):39–51.
6. Kumar V. The complement system, toll-like receptors and inflammasomes in host defense: three musketeers' one target. *Int Rev Immunol.* 2019;38(4):131–156.
7. Ermert D, Ram S, Laabei M. The hijackers guide to escaping complement: lessons learned from pathogens. *Mol Immunol.* 2019;114:49–61.
8. Mastellos DC, Ricklin D, Lambris JD. Clinical promise of next-generation complement therapeutics. *Nat Rev Drug Discov.* 2019;18(9):707–729.
9. Luyendyk JP, Schoenecker JG, Flick MJ. The multifaceted role of fibrinogen in tissue injury and inflammation. *Blood.* 2019;133(6):511–520.
10. Chen Y, et al. Role of platelet biomarkers in inflammatory response. *Biomark Res.* 2020;8:28.
11. Baker SK, Strickland S. A critical role for plasminogen in inflammation. *J Exp Med.* 2020;217(4):e20191865.
12. Shahzad K, et al. Cell biology of activated protein C. *Curr Opin Hematol.* 2019;26(1):41–50.
13. Yu H, et al. Targeting NF-κB pathway for the therapy of diseases: mechanism and clinical study. *Signal Transduct Target Ther.* 2020;5:209.
14. Rodrigues TS, et al. Inflammasomes are activated in response to SARS-CoV-2 infection and are associated with COVID-19 severity in patients. *J Exp Med.* 2021;218(3):e20201707.
15. PrabhuDas MR, et al. A Consensus definitive classification of scavenger receptors and their roles in health and disease. *J Immunol.* 2017;198(10):3775–3789.
16. Santiago-Fernández C, et al. Overexpression of scavenger receptor and infiltration of macrophage in epicardial adipose tissue of patients with ischemic heart disease and diabetes. *J Transl Med.* 2019;17:95.
17. Schirmer B, Neumann D. The function of the histamine H4 receptor in inflammatory and inflammation associated diseases of the gut. *Int. J. Mol. Sci.* 2021;22:6116.
18. Schlicker E, Kathmann M. Role of the histamine H3 receptor in the central nervous system. *Handb Exp Pharmacol.* 2017;241:277–299.
19. Ghamari N, et al. Histamine H3 receptor antagonists/inverse agonists: Where do they go? *Pharmacol Ther.* 2019;200:69–84.
20. Cooper C, et al. Safety of oral non-selective non-steroidal anti-inflammatory drugs in osteoarthritis: What does the literature say? *Drugs Aging.* 2019;36(Suppl 1):15–24.
21. Dostert C, et al. The TNF family of ligands and receptors: communication modules in the immune system and beyond. *Physiol Rev.* 2019;99:115–160.
22. Cavalli G, et al. Interleukin-1 and interleukin-6 inhibition compared with standard management in patients with COVID-19 and hyperinflammation: a cohort study. *Lancet Rheumatol.* 2021;3(4):e253–e261.
23. Lu L, et al. A potential role of interleukin 10 in COVID-19 pathogenesis. *Trends Immunol.* 2021;42(1):3–5.
24. Song W, et al. Neutrophil extracellular traps tied to rheumatoid arthritis: points to ponder. *Front Immunol.* 2021;11:3668.
25. Niedźwiedzka-Rystwej P, et al. "In sickness and in health"—how neutrophil extracellular trap (NET) works in infections, selected diseases and pregnancy. *J Inflamm.* 2019;16:15.
26. Ley K. M1 means kill; M2 means heal. *J Immunol.* 2017;199(7):2191–2193.
27. Lee KY. M1 and M2 polarization of macrophages: a mini-review. *Med Biol Sci Eng.* 2019;2(1):1–5. https://doi.org/10.30579/mbse.2019.2.1.1.
28. Cooke JP. Inflammation and its role in regeneration and repair. *Circ Res.* 2019;124(8):1166–1168.
29. Filippi MD. Neutrophil transendothelial migration: updates and new perspectives. *Blood.* 2019;133(20):2149–2158.
30. Gires O, et al. Expression and function of epithelial cell adhesion molecule EpCAM: Where are we after 40 years? *Cancer Metastasis Rev.* 2020;39:969–987.
31. Thakur A, Mikkelsen H, Jungersen G. Intracellular pathogens: host immunity and microbial persistence strategies. *J Immunol Res.* 2019;2019:1356540.
32. Lemke G. How macrophages deal with death. *Nat Rev Immunol.* 2019;19:539–549.

33. Strange C. Alpha-1 antitrypsin deficiency associated COPD. *Clin Chest Med*. 2020;41(3):339–345.
34. Ebihara T. Dichotomous regulation of acquired immunity by innate lymphoid cells. *Cells*. 2020;9(5):1193.
35. Lapic I, et al. Erythrocyte sedimentation rate and C-reactive protein in acute inflammation. *Am J Clin Pathol*. 2020;153(1):14–29.
36. Furman D, et al. Chronic inflammation in the etiology of disease across the life span. *Nat Med*. 2019;25:1822–1832.
37. Feehan KT, Gilroy DW. Is resolution the end of inflammation? *Trends Mol Med*. 2019;25(3):198–214.
38. Tercan H, et al. Trained immunity: long-term adaptation in innate immune responses. *Arterioscler Thromb Vasc Biol*. 2021;41:55–61.
39. Ariyaratne A, Finney CAM. Eosinophils and macrophages within the Th2-induced granuloma: balancing killing and healing in a tight space. *Infect Immun*. 2019;87(10):e00127–19.
40. Rodrigues M, et al. Wound healing: a cellular perspective. *Physiol Rev*. 2019;99(1):665–706.
41. Kim SY, Nair MG. Macrophages in wound healing: activation and plasticity. *Immunol Cell Biol*. 2019;97(3):258–267.
42. Patel S, et al. Mechanistic insight into diabetic wounds: pathogenesis, molecular targets and treatment strategies to pace wound healing. *Biomed Pharmacother*. 2019;112:108615.
43. Goldberg SR, Diegelmann RF. What makes wounds chronic. *Surg Clin North Am*. 2020;100(4):681–693.
44. Barchitta M, et al. Nutrition and wound healing: An overview focusing on the beneficial effects of curcumin. *Int J Mol Sci*. 2019;20:1119.
45. Wheatley BM, et al. Effect of NSAIDs on bone healing rates: a meta-analysis. *J Am Acad Orthop Surg*. 2019;27(7):e330–e336.
46. Lingzhi Z, Meirong L, Xiaobing F. Biological approaches for hypertrophic scars. *Int Wound J*. 2020;17(2):405–418.

8

Adaptive Immunity

Valentina L. Brashers

http://evolve.elsevier.com/Rogers/pathophysiology/

CHAPTER OUTLINE

The third line of defense in the human body is adaptive (acquired) immunity, often called the immune response or immunity. Adaptive immunity consists of lymphocytes (Fig. 8.1) and serum proteins called *antibodies*. Once external barriers have been compromised, and inflammation has been activated (innate immunity; see Chapter 7), the adaptive immune response is mobilized. Inflammation is the "first responder" that contains the initial injury and slows the spread of infection, whereas adaptive immunity *slowly* augments the initial defenses and promotes processes against reinfection.

OVERVIEW OF ADAPTIVE IMMUNITY

Inflammation and adaptive immunity differ in several key ways. First, the components of innate immunity and inflammation are activated immediately after tissue damage. Adaptive immunity is *inducible;* the effectors of the immune response, lymphocytes, and antibodies, do not preexist in large numbers but are produced in response to infection or other abnormal molecules. Thus, adaptive immunity develops more slowly than inflammation.

Second, the inflammatory response is similar regardless of differences in the cause of tissue damage or whether the inflammatory site is sterile or contaminated with infectious microorganisms. The adaptive immune response is exquisitely *specific*. For example, the lymphocytes and antibodies induced in response to infection are extremely specific to the particular strain of the infecting microbe.

Third, the residual mediators of inflammation must be removed quickly to limit damage to surrounding healthy tissue and allow healing. The effectors of the adaptive immune response are *long-lived* and systemic, providing long-term protection against specific invaders.

Finally, the inflammatory responses to both recurrent tissue damage and infection are identical. The adaptive immune response has *memory*. For example, if reinfected with the same microbe, the adaptive immune system immediately produces protective lymphocytes and antibodies, thus providing long-term protection against infection.

Despite the differences, the innate and adaptive immune systems are highly interactive and complementary. Many components of innate resistance are necessary for the development of the adaptive immune response. Conversely, products of the adaptive immune response activate components of innate resistance. Thus, both systems are essential for complete protection against infectious disease.

The mechanisms underlying the adaptive immune response will be discussed in this chapter. As with Chapter 7, a complete description of all the important components and processes of an effective immune response would require far more space than available. Therefore, this chapter will focus on the basic concepts and the most important, or well-studied, mediators of the adaptive immune response.

The adaptive immune response has its own vocabulary. Antigens are the molecular targets of antibodies and lymphocytes. Antigens are generally small molecules (usually within proteins, carbohydrates, or lipids) found on the surface of microbes, infected cells, or abnormal tissues (this definition is expanded with immunologic diseases discussed in Chapter 9).

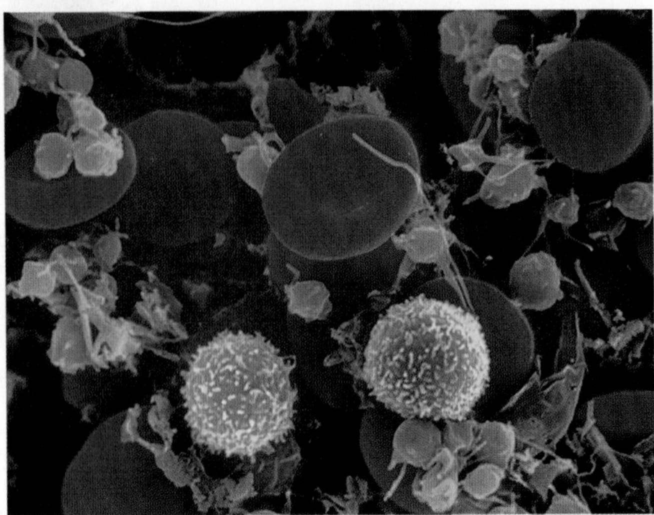

Fig. 8.1 Lymphocytes. A scanning electron micrograph showing lymphocytes (*yellow*, like cotton candy), red blood cells, and platelets. (Copyright Dennis Kunkel Microscopy, Inc.)

In the fetus and throughout life, lymphocytes undergo extensive differentiation. Some lymphoid stem cells enter the thymus and differentiate into T lymphocytes (T cells, *T* refers to thymus-derived). In contrast, others enter specific regions of the bone marrow and differentiate into B lymphocytes (B cells, *B* refers to bone marrow derived) (Fig. 8.2). Each type of cell develops cell surface proteins that identify them as T or B cells. Both B and T cells also develop cell surface antigen receptors. These receptors are remarkable because an individual lymphocyte is programmed to recognize only one specific antigen. It is estimated that before birth, each individual has produced a population of lymphocytes capable of recognizing as many as 10^{16} different antigens. This is called the generation of clonal diversity and refers to the process by which the extensive diversity of antigen receptors on B and T cells is established. During this process, self-reactive lymphocytes are also created but are then removed from the body via clonal deletion.

B and T lymphocytes leaving the primary lymphoid organs (bone marrow and thymus) are immunocompetent (able to respond to antigens) but have not been exposed to antigen and thus are naïve. These cells enter the blood and lymphatic vessels and migrate to the systemic immune system's secondary lymphoid organs (e.g., lymph nodes, spleen) (Fig. 8.3A). Some take up residence in B cell and T cell-rich areas of those organs. Lymph nodes contain high concentrations of naïve B cells within follicles in the cortex and naïve T cells more centrally in the paracortex (Fig. 8.3B). Other lymphocytes reenter the circulation where approximately 60% to 70% of circulating lymphocytes are immunocompetent T cells, and 10% to 20% are immunocompetent B cells.

Induction of the adaptive immune response begins when exposure to an antigen occurs. This process begins with recognizing invaders by specialized antigen-presenting cells (APCs) (macrophages, dendritic cells, and B cells), which then *process* and *present* the antigen to lymphocytes. Thus begins a symphony of cellular interactions referred to as clonal selection involving:

- Intercellular communication through specific antigen receptors along with intercellular adhesion and costimulatory molecules
- Production and response to multiple cytokines
- Activation and regulation of the immune response by **T helper cells [Th cells]**
- Proliferation (clonal expansion) and differentiation of immunocompetent B and T cells into highly specialized effector cells (B cells developing into plasma cells that become factories to produce antibodies and T cells developing into T cytotoxic (Tc) cells that can identify and kill a target cell.)
- Suppression of inappropriate immune responses (T regulatory cells [Treg cells])
- Differentiation of T and B cells into very long-lived memory cells that exist for decades or, in some cases, for the life of the individual
- Activation of memory cells if a second exposure occurs with the same antigen

Antibodies circulate in the blood and defend against extracellular antigens, such as microbes and microbial toxins. This is referred to as *humoral immune response* or humoral immunity. T cytotoxic cells (Tc cells) defend against intracellular pathogens (e.g., viruses) and abnormal cells, such as cancer cells. This is referred to as *cell-mediated immunity* or cellular immunity.

ANTIGENS

The term antigen describes a molecule that can *bind with* antibodies or antigen receptors on B and T cells. Self-antigens are molecules found on healthy host cells. Non-self or foreign antigens are molecules that are generally not found on host cells. The healthy adaptive immune system can distinguish between self- and non-self antigens. When that ability is lost, autoimmune or hypersensitivity diseases can arise (see Chapter 9).

Exogenous antigens are extracellular non-self antigens that enter the body and circulate in blood and lymph. Common non-self exogenous antigens include infectious agents, allergens, and chemical agents (including some medications). Endogenous antigens are intracellular non-self antigens that have been generated when the cell has become abnormal because of injury, infection (e.g., viruses), or mutation of its DNA as occurs in cancer.

The ability of an antigen to induce an immune response is frequently related to the size of the antigen. In general, large molecules (those >10,000 daltons), such as proteins and polysaccharides, are the most immunogenic antigens. Many low-molecular-weight molecules can function as haptens; they are too small to induce an immune response by themselves but become immunogenic after combining with larger molecules that function as carriers for the hapten. For example, the widely used anticoagulant drug heparin can serve as a hapten by binding to a protein called platelet factor 4 (PF4) on the surface of platelets. When this occurs, antibodies may be produced that attack the heparin+PF4 complex and can destroy the platelets resulting in a common condition called *heparin-induced thrombocytopenia*. Similar conditions will be discussed in Chapter 9.

Lymphocytes of adaptive immunity have highly specialized receptors for antigens. This specificity means that most antigens will activate a relatively small number of cells. In contrast, a group

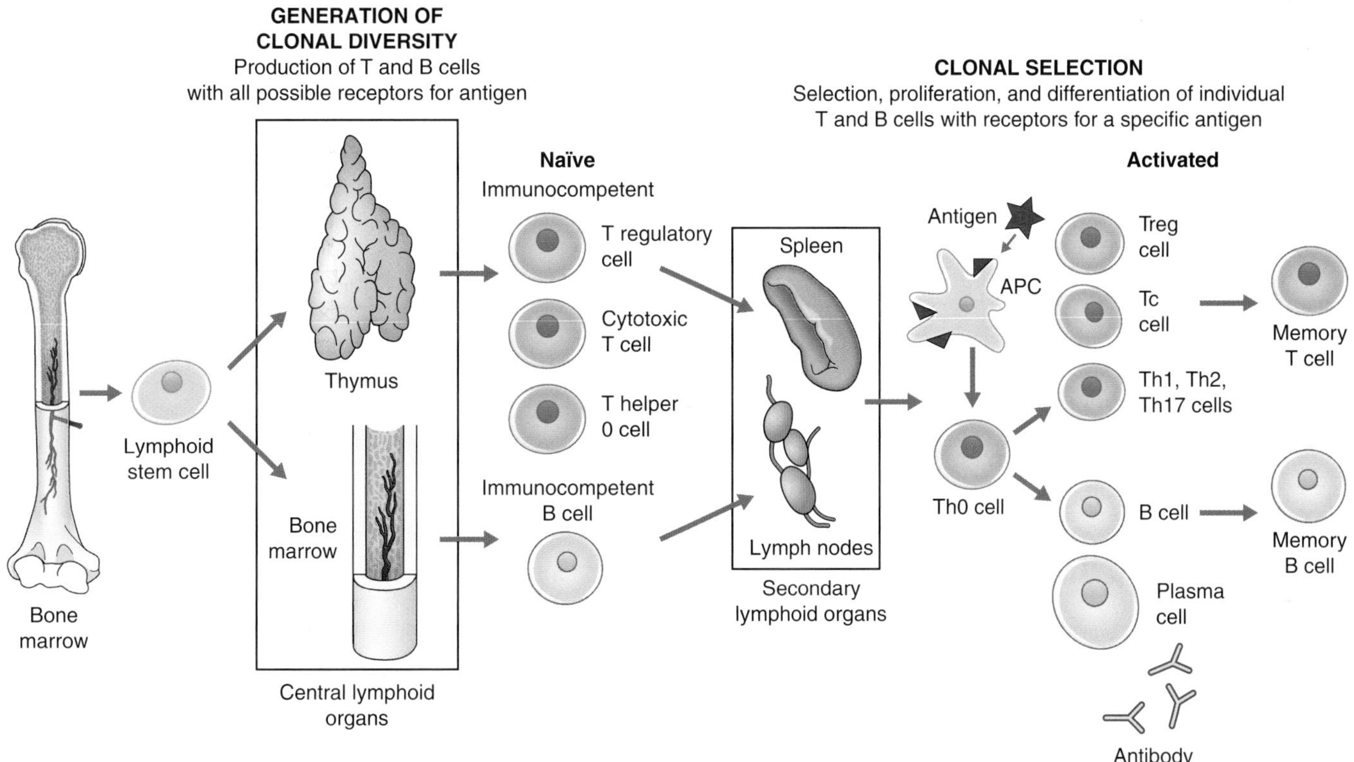

Fig. 8.2 Overview of the Adaptive Immune Response. Lymphoid stem cells from the bone marrow migrate to the central lymphoid organs (the thymus or regions of bone marrow). Cells that travel to the thymus undergo a series of differentiation stages resulting in several types of T cells (T helper [Th], T cytotoxic cells [Tc], and T regulatory cells [Treg]) each with its own unique antigen receptor (clonal diversity). B cells also undergo additional differentiation and gain an antigen-specific receptor in the bone marrow. These cells are "naïve," meaning that they have not yet encountered antigen. The cells enter the circulation and migrate to the secondary lymphoid organs (e.g., spleen and lymph nodes), where they establish residence in B and T cell-rich areas. When these cells are presented with a foreign antigen, they become activated and undergo additional cellular proliferation and differentiation (clonal selection). Th0 cells differentiate into three subtypes of cytokine-producing cells (Th1, Th2, Th17) that contribute to the further differentiation of Tc, Treg, and B cells. The result is an active cellular immunity or humoral immunity, or both. Cellular immunity is mediated by *effector* Tc cells that can kill targets. Treg cells regulate the immune response. Humoral immunity is conducted by B cells that have recognized antigen and differentiated into plasma cells that make antibodies to that antigen. Both T and B cells make memory cells that can produce a more rapid adaptive immune response to a second challenge with the same antigen.

of microbial molecules called superantigens (SAGs) can activate a large population of immune cells resulting in the overproduction of immune cytokines. The result can be severe disease and even shock and death. Some examples of SAGs are the bacterial toxins produced by *Staphylococcus aureus and Streptococcus pyogenes* (SAGs that cause toxic shock syndrome and food poisoning).

LYMPHOCYTE DEVELOPMENT

The primary cells involved in the adaptive immune response are T and B lymphocytes. T and B lymphocytes recognize antigens from invaders and abnormal tissues, differentiate into effector cells, and provide memory.

Development of B Lymphocytes

Lymphocyte stem cells destined to become B cells circulate through the specialized regions of bone marrow (the primary [central] lymphoid organs for B cells), where they are exposed to hormones and cytokines that induce proliferation and differentiation into B cells. As the stem cell begins to mature, it progressively develops a variety of necessary surface markers essential for the further differentiation and proliferation of the B cell. The next stage in development is the formation of the B-cell receptor (BCR) (Algorithm 8.1).

The B-cell receptor (BCR) is a complex of cell surface-bound antibodies and other molecules involved in intracellular signaling (Fig. 8.4). Its role is to recognize an antigen and

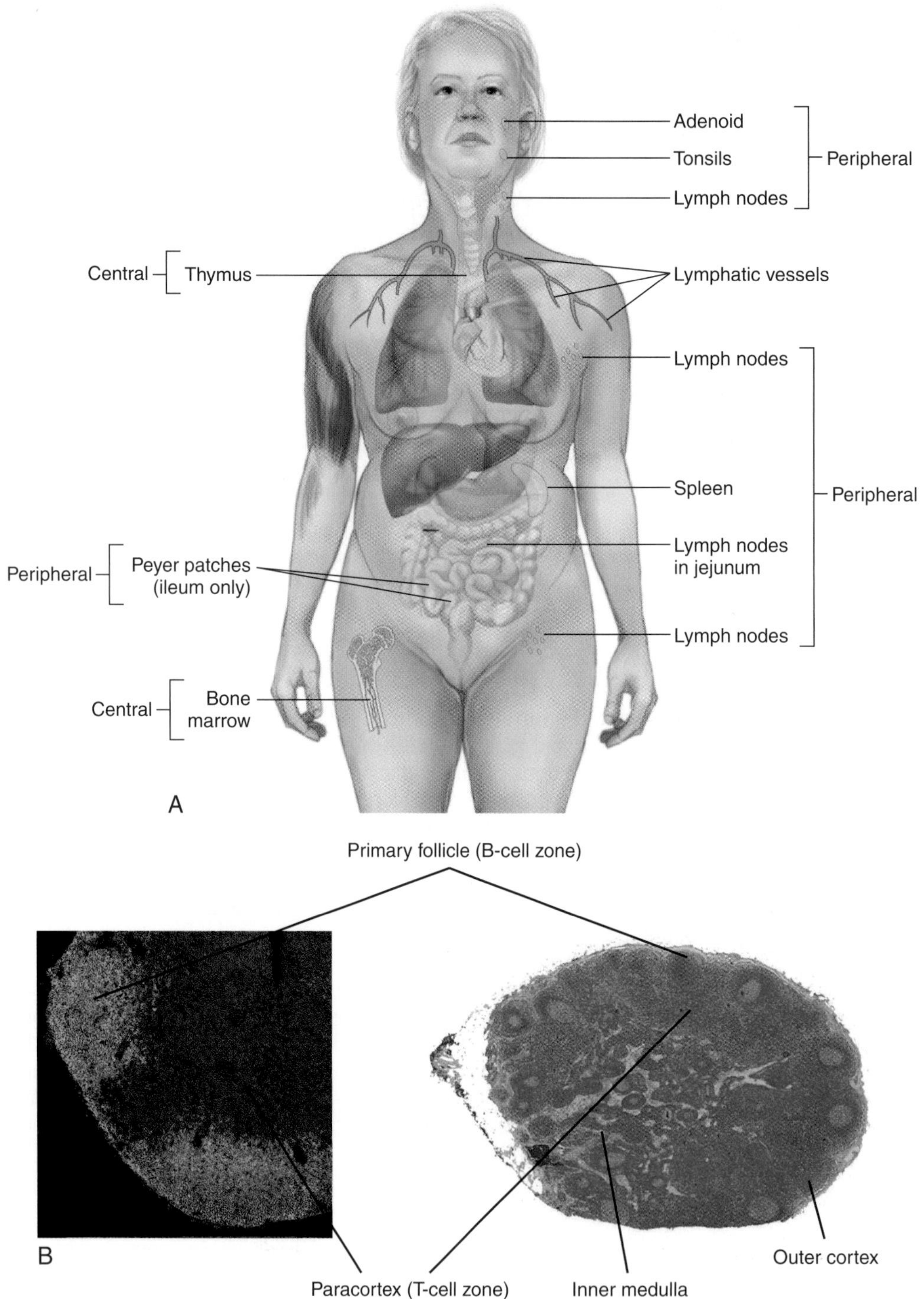

Fig. 8.3 Primary and Secondary Lymphoid Tissues. (A) Immature lymphocytes migrate through central (primary) lymphoid tissues: the bone marrow (central lymphoid tissue for B lymphocytes) and the thymus (central lymphoid tissue for T lymphocytes). Mature lymphocytes later reside in the T and B lymphocyte–rich areas of the peripheral (secondary) lymphoid tissues. **(B)** Lymph nodes contain numerous B cells within cortical follicles and T cells within the paracortex. The lymph node medulla contains blood and lymphatic vessels.

communicate that information to the cell's nucleus. The BCRs in immunocompetent cells are membrane-associated immunoglobulin M (mIgM) with or without IgD (mIgD) antibodies with identical antigen-specificities.

The enormous repertoire of BCR specificities (clonal diversity) is made possible by rearranging existing deoxyribonucleic acid (DNA) during B cell development in the primary lymphoid organs, a process known as somatic recombination. Multiple loci

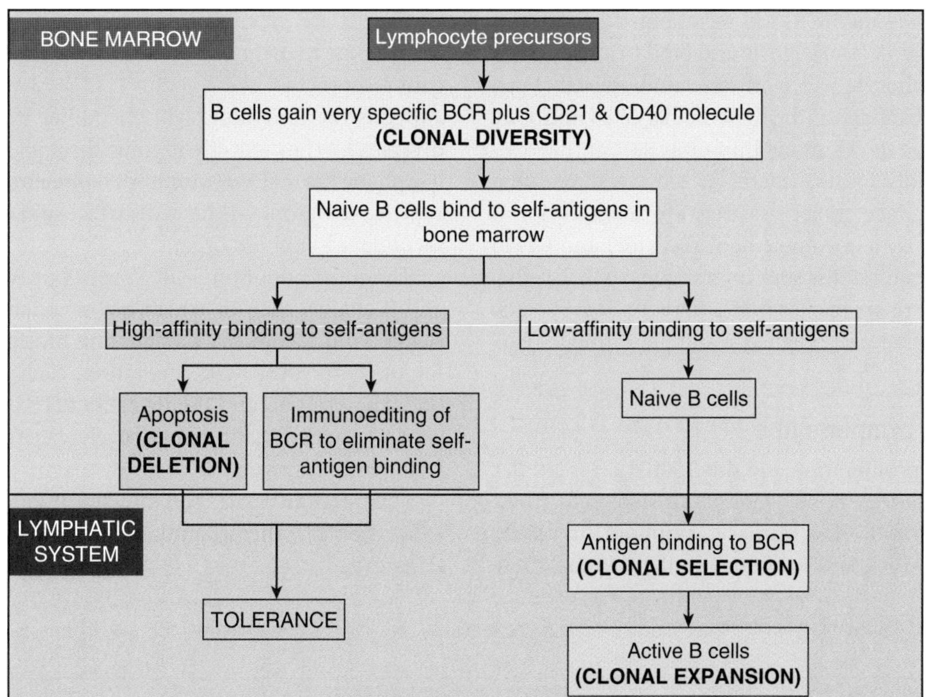

Algorithm 8.1 Steps in B-Cell Development. Lymphocyte precursor cells that remain in the bone marrow each gain a very specific B-cell receptor (BCR) that can recognize a single antigen. The generation of millions of different lymphocytes, each with its own specific BCR, is called *clonal diversity*. These naïve B cells bind with self-antigens in the bone marrow. If they bind with high affinity to self-antigens, they either undergo apoptosis *(clonal deletion)* or undergo a process called immunoediting in which their BCRs are changed so that they no longer recognize self-antigens. This results in tolerance. If the B cells bind with only low affinity to self-antigens, then they move into the lymphatic system. If they encounter antigen to which they can bind their BCR *(clonal selection)*, they mature and proliferate to active B cells *(clonal expansion)*.

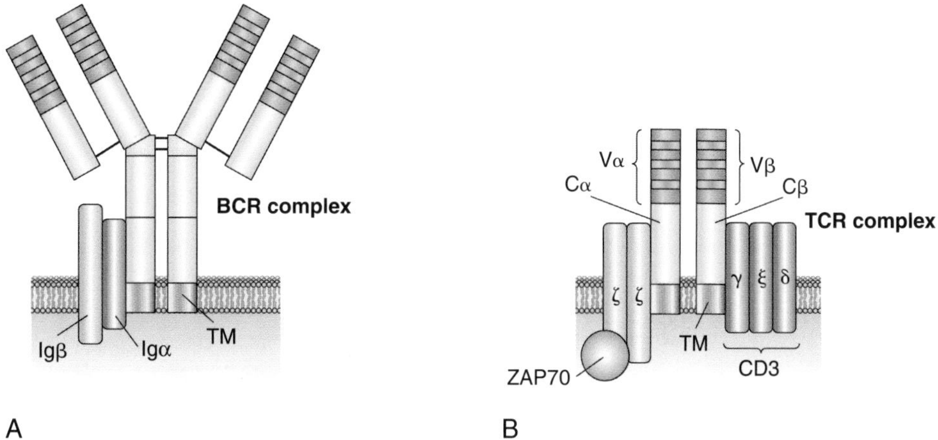

Fig. 8.4 B-cell Antigen Receptor and T-cell Antigen Receptor. (A) The antigen receptor on the surface of B cells (B-cell receptor *[BCR]* complex) is a monomeric (single) antibody with a structure similar to that of circulating antibody, with an additional transmembrane region *(TM)* that anchors the molecule to the cell surface. The active BCR complex contains molecules (*Igα* and *Igβ*) responsible for intracellular signaling after the receptor has bound antigen. **(B)** The T-cell receptor *(TCR)* consists of an α- and a β-chain joined by a disulfide bond. Each chain consists of a constant region (*Cα* and *Cβ*) and a variable region (*Vα* and *Vβ*). Each variable region contains CDRs and FRs in a structure similar to that of antibody. The active TCR is associated with several molecules that are responsible for intracellular signaling after antigen binding. These include the CD3, which is a complex of γ (gamma), ε (epsilon); and δ (delta) subunits and a complex of two ζ (zeta) molecules. The ζ molecules are attached to a cytoplasmic protein kinase *(ZAP70)* that is critical to intracellular signaling.

in the DNA that encode for BCRs are recombined to generate receptors that collectively can recognize and bind to any possible antigen. A single lymphocyte will synthesize antibodies that can recognize the identical antigen as the BCR on that cell. (Antibody synthesis is discussed in the Humoral Immunity section.)

B-cell differentiation is also characterized by developing various important surface molecules that are markers for B cells. These include CD21 (a complement receptor) and CD40 (adhesion molecule required for later interactions with T cells). The designation "CD" refers to cluster of differentiation, specific cell-surface proteins that are assigned a unique number (e.g., CD21 and CD40).

Development of T Lymphocytes

The process of T-cell proliferation and differentiation is similar to that for B cells (Algorithm 8.2). Lymphoid stem cells travel from the bone marrow to the primary lymphoid organ for T-cell development, which is the thymus. In the thymus, these stem cells are exposed to thymic hormones and the cytokine interleukin 7 (IL-7) and are driven to undergo cell division and gain receptors (T-cell receptors [TCRs]) against the diversity of antigens the individual will encounter throughout life (clonal diversity).[1] They exit the thymus through the blood vessels and lymphatics as mature (immunocompetent) T cells with antigen-specific receptors on the cell surface and establish residence in secondary lymphoid organs.

The most common TCR consists of two protein chains, α- and β-chains, each of which has a variable region, a constant region, and a complex of signaling molecules called CD3 (see Fig. 8.4). As with BCR generation, each T cell expresses only one type of TCR, and the diversity of TCRs generated through somatic recombination collectively can recognize and bind to any possible antigen.

Differentiation of T cells in the thymus also results in the expression of other essential surface molecules. Initially, proteins called CD4 and CD8 are concurrently expressed on the

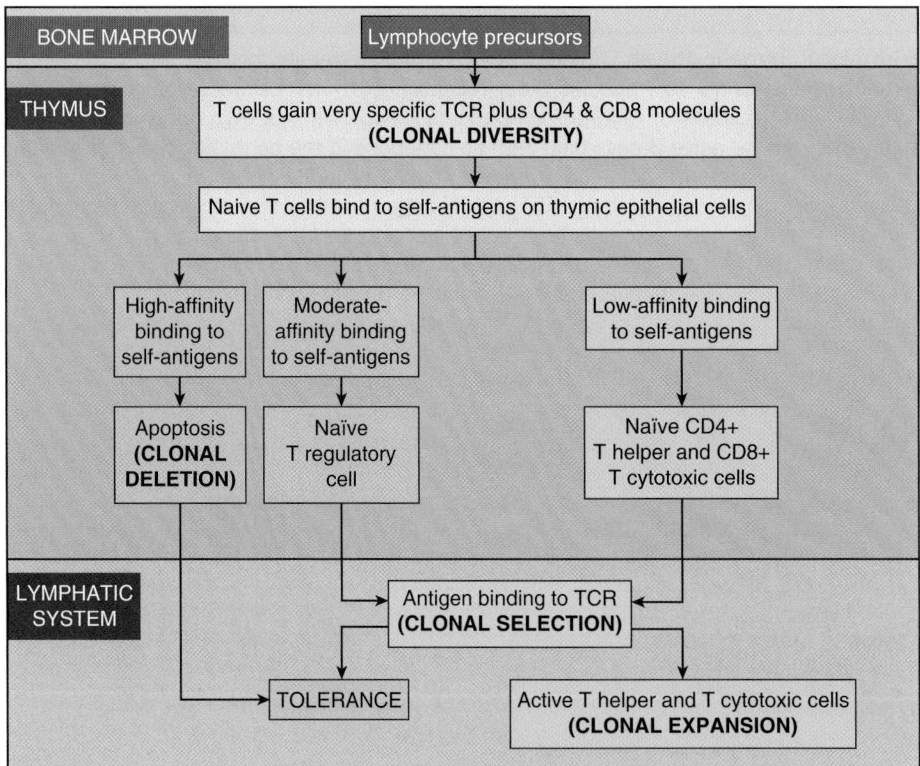

Algorithm 8.2 Steps in T-Cell Development. When lymphocyte precursor cells from the bone marrow travel to the thymus, they each gain a very specific T-cell receptor *(TCR)* that can recognize a single antigen (clonal diversity). T cells at this stage also gain both a CD4 and a CD8 molecule on their surface. These naïve T cells bind to self-antigens presented by thymic epithelial cells. If they bind tightly (high affinity), this indicates that they can attack the host's own tissues, and most are eliminated through apoptotic cell death (clonal deletion). A few of these T cells lose their CD8 molecule, gain a CD25 molecule, and become T regulatory cells. The clonal deletion of T cells or the induction of T regulatory cells results in immune system tolerance to self-antigens. If the naïve T cells instead bind with only low affinity to self-antigens, they either lose their CD8 molecule and become $CD4^+$ T helper cells or lose their CD4 molecule and become $CD8^+$ T cytotoxic cells. These naïve T cells then move into the lymphatic system where, if they encounter antigen recognized by their TCRs, they are clonally selected to proliferate and become active immune cells (clonal expansion).

developing cells. As the cells mature, they retain either the CD4 molecule or the CD8 molecule, but not both. Those that retain the CD4 molecule develop into Th cells, whereas those that retain the CD8 molecule become T cytotoxic (Tc) cells. Approximately 60% of immunocompetent T cells in the circulation express CD4, and 40% express CD8. A much smaller number of T cells express CD4 and CD25 and become T regulatory cells (Treg). The functions of Th, Tc, and Treg cells are discussed later in this chapter

As described in Chapter 7, innate lymphoid cells (ILCs) also are derived from lymphoid precursors and resemble T helper cells in their function but do not have TCRs and instead respond to nonspecific tissue injury. These cells are found near mucosal barriers and are organized into three major groups of ILCs (ILC1s, ILC2s, and ILC3s). Broadly, ILC1s promote cellular immunity, ILC2s promote humoral immunity, and ILC3s enhance epithelial barriers.[2]

Clonal Diversity, Clonal Deletion, Clonal Selection, and Clonal Expansion

As described previously in this chapter, clonal diversity occurs during the production of B cells and T cells in the primary lymphoid organs (Table 8.1). This process begins before birth and continues throughout life. Each B cell and T cell develops its own specific BCR or TCR, which can recognize only one antigen; yet taken together, the total population of lymphocytes can recognize almost any foreign antigen found in the environment that will be encountered throughout life. It is estimated that B and T cells can collectively recognize more than 10^{16} different antigenic determinants. Because there are so many potential antigens for which a single type of lymphocyte receptor is created, the body cannot sustain adequate numbers of all of the many millions of lymphocytes that might be needed.[3] Thus, the adaptive immune system is inducible, i.e., once an antigen is encountered by a particular lymphocyte (clonal selection), then many copies of that same lymphocyte are generated in order to adequately respond to that antigen (clonal expansion) (see Table 8.1). The lymphocytes that are produced move into the circulation as immunocompetent cells and migrate to the circulation and secondary lymphoid organs where they can provide a specific and long-lasting defense. This process takes time, so the adaptive immune response is slower than the innate immune response.

Tolerance refers to the ability of the adaptive immune system to remove or suppress adaptive immune responses to self-antigens or innocuous non-self-antigens (see Table 8.1). A lack of tolerance to self-antigens results in a wide range of disorders called autoimmune or hypersensitivity disorders. The process of generating tolerance occurs both centrally during the development of B and T lymphocytes or peripherally through activation of a specialized kind of T lymphocyte called a T reg. Central tolerance is achieved within the bone marrow for B lymphocytes and within the thymus for T lymphocytes. In both cases, developing lymphocytes that bind with high affinity to self-antigens within these organs are either killed (clonal deletion) or altered in such a way that they no longer will attack host tissues (see Algorithms 8.1 and 8.2). It is estimated that greater than 90% of developing B and T cells are eliminated in this way. Self-reactive B cells may instead undergo a change in the structure of their antigen receptors (BCRs) in a process called *immunoediting*, which renders them harmless to the host. Self-reactive T cells that bind to self-antigens in the thymus with moderate affinity do not undergo clonal deletion but rather gain other surface molecules and become T regulatory cells (Treg) that suppress the adaptive immune response and therefore prevent autoimmunity.[4] Treg cells can also be induced from circulating Th cells in response to excessive inflammation and autoimmunity in a process known as peripheral tolerance. Both types of Treg cells produce very high levels of immunosuppressive cytokines TGF-β and IL-10, which decrease T-cell activity. Enhancement of Treg activity

TABLE 8.1 Generation of Clonal Diversity, Clonal Deletion, Clonal Selection & Expansion

	Clonal Diversity	Clonal Deletion	Clonal Selection and Expansion
Purpose?	To produce large numbers of T and B lymphocytes with maximum diversity of antigen receptors	To remove self-reactive T and B lymphocytes	Select, expand, and differentiate clones of T and B cells against specific antigen
When does it occur?	In the fetus and throughout life	In the fetus and throughout life	Primarily after birth and throughout life
Where does it occur?	Central lymphoid organs: thymus for T cells, bone marrow for B cells	Central lymphoid organs: thymus for T cells, bone marrow for B cells	Peripheral lymphoid organs, including lymph nodes, spleen, and other lymphoid tissues
Is foreign antigen involved?	No	No	Yes, antigen determines which clones of cells will be selected
What tissues, hormones, or cytokines are involved?	Thymic hormones, IL-7, others	Thymic epithelial cells	Many cytokines produced by Th cells and APCs
Final product?	Immunocompetent T and B cells that can react with antigen but have not seen antigen (naïve) and migrate to secondary lymphoid organs	Promotes tolerance and prevents autoimmunity	Plasma cells that produce antibody, effector T cells that help (Th cells), kill targets (Tc cells) or regulate immune responses (Treg cells); memory B and T cells

APCs, Antigen-presenting cells; *IL*, interleukin; *Tc*, T cytotoxic cells; *Th*, T helper cells; *Treg cells*, T regulatory cells.

is an emerging approach to the management of autoimmune diseases (see Chapter 9).[5,6]

INDUCTION OF THE IMMUNE RESPONSE

Induction of the adaptive immune response involves a complex interaction among antigen-presenting cells (APCs), lymphocytes, and cytokines. Most cells of the immune system cannot react directly with antigens. To initiate an effective immune response, most antigens must be *processed* and *presented* to the immune cells in a specific manner.

Antigen-Presenting Cells

Antigen presenting cells (APCs) are responsible for processing antigens and presenting them on their surface so that T lymphocytes can recognize them. The three major types of APCs are macrophages, dendritic cells, and B cells. Macrophages are phagocytes that are derived from circulating monocytes and reside in tissues, especially near epithelial surfaces. They detect both pathogen-associated molecular patterns (PAMPs) and damage-associated molecular patterns (DAMPs) using their surface pattern recognition receptors (PRRs) (see Chapter 7). Dendritic cells are a specialized type of macrophage. There are three major types of dendritic cells: conventional, follicular, and plasmacytoid. Conventional dendritic cells are vital to adaptive immune responses because once they have recognized and phagocytosed antigens, they are capable of migrating to secondary lymph tissues (especially lymph nodes), where they can present those antigens to areas of highly concentrated lymphocytes (Fig. 8.5).[7] Follicular and plasmacytoid dendritic cells secrete multiple cytokines that influence B cell development. B lymphocytes are not phagocytes but can detect antigen with their surface receptors (BCRs) and endocytose BCR/antigen complexes.

Antigen Processing

Extracellular exogenous antigens that enter the body and circulate in blood and lymph are detected by macrophages and dendritic cells via their PRRs and are phagocytosed (see Chapter 7). Once the exogenous antigen is inside an APC, a complex series of intracellular processes leads to the enzymatic fragmentation of the antigen followed by assembly of an antigen molecule complex that is presented on the surface of the APC (Fig. 8.6). B cells recognize and capture exogenous antigens using their BCRs, endocytose BCR/antigen complexes, and then process them so the antigens can be presented on the surfaces of the B cells. Endogenous antigens generated when a cell has become infected by an intracellular microorganism (e.g., viruses) or

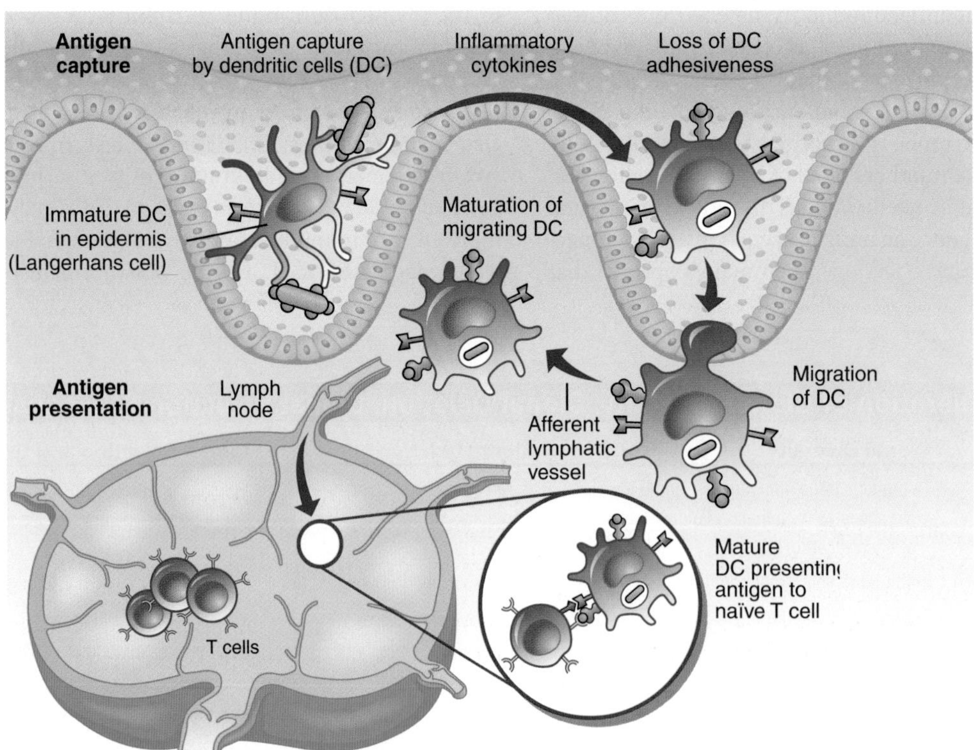

Fig. 8.5 The Role of the Dendritic Cell in Capturing Antigen. Immature dendritic cells in the tissues encounter a phagocytose antigen, resulting in the production of inflammatory cytokines and a loss of adhesive interactions with neighboring cells. The maturing dendritic cell migrates through the lymphatic vessels to a regional lymph node, presenting the antigen to immunocompetent T cells to initiate the clonal selection process. (Redrawn from Kumar V, Abbas A, Fausto N. Robbins & Cotran pathologic basis of disease, 8th edition. Philadelphia: Saunders; 2010. McCance K, Huether S. Pathophysiology, 8th edition. St. Louis: Elsevier; 2019.

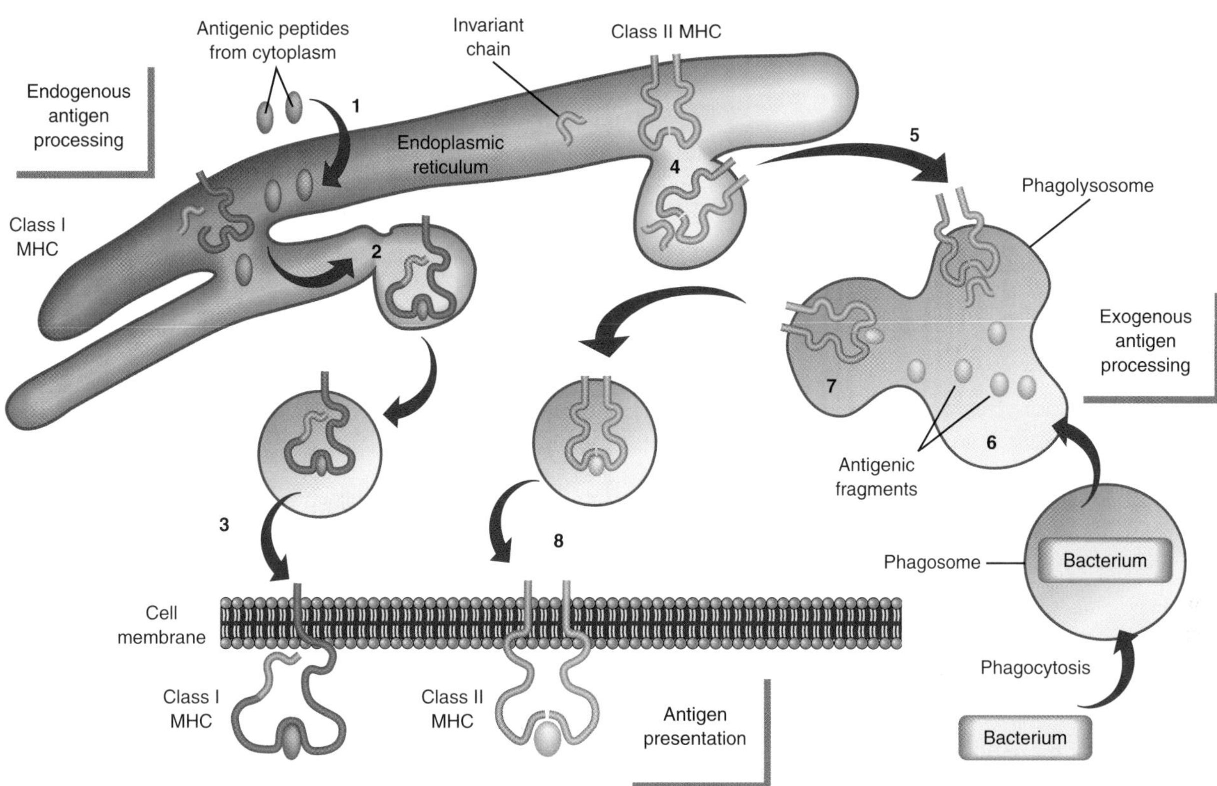

Fig. 8.6 Antigen Processing. ***(1)*** Endogenous antigens (viruses, cancer) are transported into the endoplasmic reticulum (ER) where major histocompatibility complex (MHC) molecules are being assembled. ***(2)*** Endogenous antigen fragments bind to the α-chains of the MHC class I molecule. ***(3)*** The antigen/MHC class I complex is transported to the cell surface where it is presented to T cells. ***(4)*** The α- and β-chains of the MHC class II molecules are also being assembled in the ER. ***(5)*** The MHC class II molecule is transported to phagolysosomes where ***(6)*** exogenous antigenic fragments have been produced by phagocytosis. ***(7)*** The antigen fragments bind to the MHC class II molecule and ***(8)*** the antigen/MHC class II complex is transported to the cell surface where it is presented to T cells.

mutation of its DNA (like occurs in cancer) also undergo antigen processing.

Antigen Presentation

Antigen processing results in the presentation of antigens on the surface of APCs and abnormal cells by molecules of the major histocompatibility complex (MHC) (see Fig. 8.6). MHC molecules in humans also are called human leukocyte antigens (HLAs) when they are identified for organ transplantation (see Chapter 9). MHC molecules are glycoproteins found on the surface of all human cells except red blood cells. They are divided into two general classes, class I and class II, based on their molecular structure, distribution among cell populations, and function in antigen presentation. MHC I molecules are found on all nucleated cells. They are composed of a large alpha (α) chain along with a smaller chain called β_2-microglobulin that are coded for by gene complexes on chromosome 6 (HLA-A, HLA-B, HLA-C) (Fig. 8.7). MHC II molecules are found only on APCs and are composed of a different type of α- and β-chains that are coded for by another set of genes on chromosome 6 (HLA-DR, HLA-DP, HLA-DQ). In healthy tissues, these molecules identify cells as self, i.e., immune cells recognize MHC molecules on healthy host cells and do not attack them. Deleterious changes in the structure of MHC molecules can lead to autoimmune disorders and vulnerability to cancer and infection.[8,9] MHC genes are highly polymorphic; therefore, no two individuals (except identical twins) will have a complete set of identical MHC molecules. Transplantation of one person's cells into another person will result in an adaptive immune attack on the foreign tissue (rejection) (see Chapter 9).

Because APCs have both MHC II and MHC I molecules on their surface, they can present antigens on both types of MHC molecules. In essence, antigen processing and presentation result in the creation of an antigen/MHC complex on the surface of the APC that makes it appear to T cells as foreign. T cells can only recognize antigens that are presented in this way. Antigens presented on MHC II molecules are recognized and bound by T helper cells, whereas antigens presented on MHC I molecules are recognized and bound by Tc cells.[10] B cells that have captured exogenous antigens preferentially present them on their MHC II molecules, thus primarily activating T helper cells. Because only APCs have MHC class II molecules, all other nucleated cells that have undergone intracellular

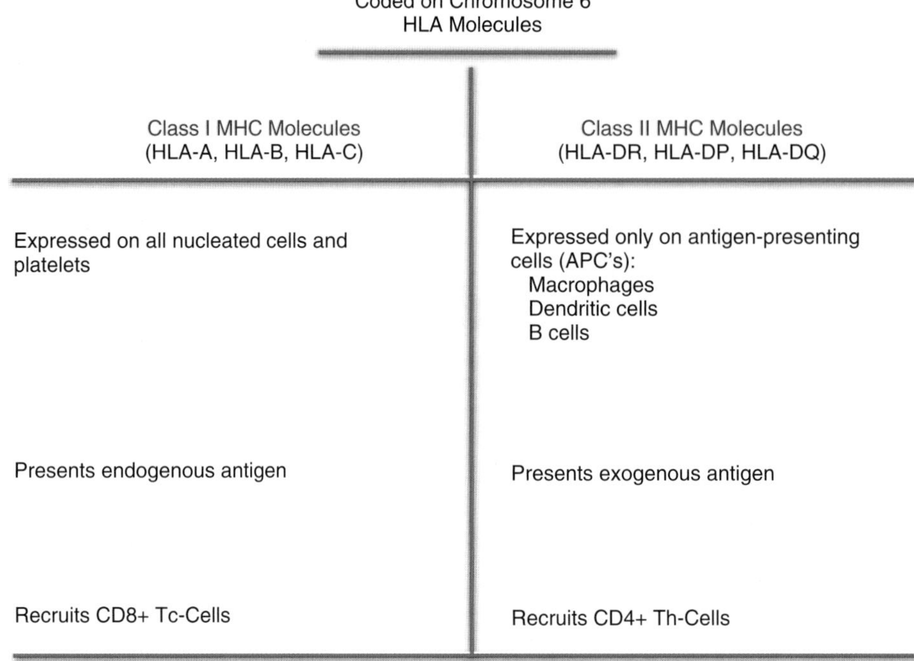

Fig. 8.7 Antigen-Presenting Molecules. *HLA-A, HLA-B, HLS-C,* isotypes of class I MCH molecules; *HLA-DR, HLA-DP, HLA-DQ,* isotypes of class II MCH molecules.

infection or DNA mutation can only present antigen on MHC I molecules.

CD1 molecules on APCs also present antigen to immune cells. These molecules specialize in presenting lipid antigens found on some pathogens, particularly with bacteria of the *Mycobacterium* spp. (e.g., *Mycobacterium tuberculosis*).

In summary, the terms antigen processing and antigen presentation refer to how exogenous and endogenous antigens are cut up into small antigenic fragments and then presented to Tc cells (MCH I) or Th cells (MCH II). This interaction among APCs and subpopulations of T cells facilitates immune responses. When cells present antigen on MHC I, the primary response is the destruction of the presenting cell by Tc cells. When cells present antigen on MCH II Th cells are activated which modulate many elements of the adaptive immune response. Th cells support the differentiation of B cells into more effective antibody-producing cells (plasma cells). Th cells also promote Tc cell proliferation and function. Defects in any aspect of this cellular collaboration will lead to defects in cell-mediated immunity, humoral immunity, or both, depending on the specific defect (see Chapter 9).[11]

T-Helper Cells

To induce an optimal cellular or humoral immune response, APCs must present antigens to Th cells. When Th cells are first activated by antigen binding, they are often called Th0 cells. Depending on the antigen and signals from the APC, the Th0 cell further differentiates into three subtypes: T helper 1 (Th1), T helper 2 (Th2), and T helper 17 (Th17). Some Th cells become Treg cells.

T Helper Cell Activation

After an APC presents antigen held by the MHC class II molecules, activation of the Th0 cell requires six steps (Fig. 8.8):

1. The presented antigen is recognized and bound by the TCR on the Th0 cell.
2. Intercellular antigen binding is strengthened by the binding of the CD4 on the Th0 cell with the β_2 region of the MHC class II molecule.
3. The cytoplasmic portions of the TCR and CD4 molecules interact to activate intracellular signaling pathways.
4. Intercellular communication between the APC and Th cell through adhesion molecules and co-stimulatory signals further activates the Th0 cell, the most critical being the B7 protein on the APC and CD28 on the Th cell.
5. Interleukin-1 (IL-1) and interleukin-12 (IL-12) are secreted by the APC and provide additional signals to the Th0 cell.
6. IL-2 is secreted by the Th0 cell and acts in an autocrine (self-stimulating) fashion to induce further maturation and proliferation of the Th cell. Without IL-2 production, the Th0 cell cannot efficiently mature into a functional helper cell.

T Helper Cell Function

Th cells are necessary for the development of most humoral and cellular immune responses. To provide effective immunity, activated Th0 cells undergo differentiation into one of several subsets: Th1, Th2, Th17, or Treg. (Fig. 8.9). The subset created in the greatest numbers depends on the intercellular communication from the APC to the Th0 cell (through interleukins and costimulatory molecules) and the predominant cytokines in the immediate environment. These subsets have different functions: Th1 cells

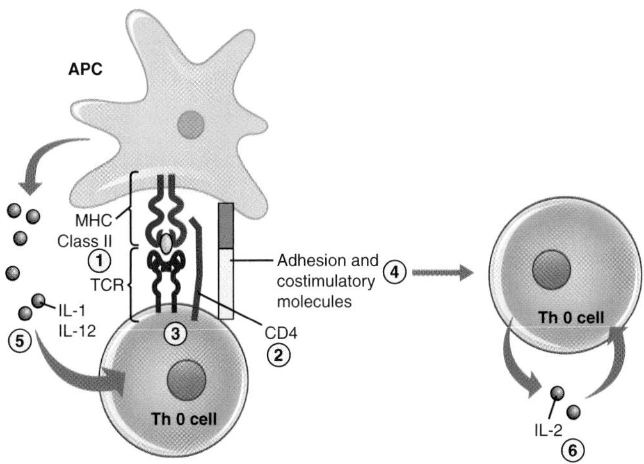

Fig. 8.8 T helper (Th) Cell Activation. Once an antigen-presenting cell *(APC)* presents antigen on its major histocompatibility class II *(MHC II)* molecules, activation of a T helper 0 *(Th0)* cell requires six steps: ***(1)*** Binding of the T cell receptor *(TCR)* on the Th0 cell to the presented antigen; ***(2)*** Binding of the CD4 molecule on the Th0 cell to the β2 region of the MHC II molecule; ***(3)*** Activation of intracellular signaling pathways within the Th0 cell; ***(4)*** Intercellular adhesion and costimulatory molecules such as B7 on the APC and CD 28 on the Th0 cell provide intercellular communication; ***(5)*** Interleukins 1 and 12 (*IL-1* and *IL-12*) are secreted by the APC and provide additional signals to the Th0 cell; ***(6)*** Interleukin 2 (IL-2) is secreted by the Th0 cell and provides autocrine stimulation to induce further maturation and proliferation of the Th cell.

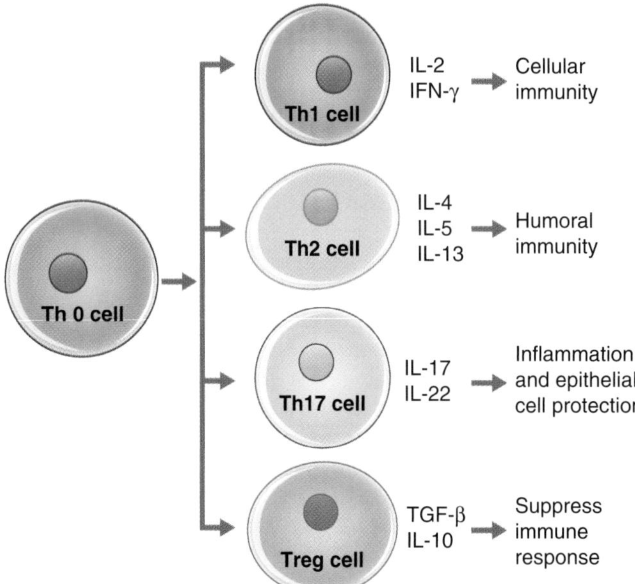

Fig. 8.9 Development of T helper (Th) Cell Subsets. Once T helper 0 *(Th0)* cells are activated, they undergo differentiation to become *Th1, Th2, Th17,* and T regulatory *(Treg)* cells. These Th subtypes are crucial to the development of effective cellular and humoral immune responses. Intercellular communication between the antigen-presenting cell and the Th0 cell and cytokines produced by the innate and adaptive immune systems determine which of the four subtypes will be created in the greatest numbers. Th1 cells secrete interferon-gamma *(IFN-γ)*, which promotes macrophage phagocytosis of invaders, and *IL-2*, which promotes differentiation of T-cytotoxic (Tc) cells leading to cellular immunity. Th2 cells produce *IL-4* and *IL-13*, which favor B-cell differentiation and humoral immunity. Th2 cells also produce *IL-5*, which stimulates eosinophils, a process important in fighting parasites and in causing allergic disease. Th17 cells produce *IL-17* which stimulates cells of the innate immune system, thus increasing inflammation, and *IL-22*, which promotes epithelial cell protection. Treg cells produce immunosuppressive cytokines such as transforming growth factor-beta *(TGF-β)* and *IL-10*, which prevent the immune response from being excessive.

preferentially support cell-mediated immunity, Th2 cells support humoral immunity, and Th17 cells support innate immunity and epithelial cell protection against invasion. Many antigens will produce excellent humoral and cell-mediated responses simultaneously. Treg cells secrete cytokines that suppress the immune system and promote tolerance (discussed previously in this chapter).

Th1 cells. Th1 cells produce interferon-γ (IFN-γ). IFN-γ strongly activates macrophages to be better phagocytes. Th1 cells also produce IL-2, which supports the proliferation and activation of Tc cells. These processes promote the phagocytosis and cytotoxic killing of infected, cancerous, or damaged cells. In other words, Th1 cells primarily support cellular immunity.

Th2 cells. Th2 cells differentiate when extracellular antigens are presented by the APC, especially under the influence of IL-4 produced by other activated immune cells. Th2 cells support B cells proliferation and differentiation through IL-4 production, thus promoting humoral immunity. IL-13 produced by Th2 cells also supports humoral immunity. IL-5 also is produced by Th2 cells and promotes eosinophil proliferation and activation.

Th17 cells. Th17 cells primarily produce the cytokine IL-17. IL-17 stimulates the innate immune system and plays a crucial role in autoimmune disorders (see Emerging Science Box: IL-17 in Health and Disease). The presence of IL-17 causes an inflammatory reaction that is stronger and more prolonged than that provided by innate immune responses alone.[12] Th17 cells also produce IL-22 which helps maintain the integrity of epithelial barriers through the production of antimicrobial substances (defensins—see Chapter 7) and by promoting the repair of damaged epithelia.[13]

HUMORAL IMMUNITY

When a B cell matures in response to antigen exposure, it becomes a plasma cell capable of producing antibodies. These antibodies conduct the humoral immune response. The terms antibody and immunoglobulin (Ig) are frequently used interchangeably. However, the term *antibody* is used more frequently in health care settings.

B-Cell Activation

Cellular interactions between B cells and other components of adaptive immunity are required to produce an effective antibody response. B cells express surface immunoglobulin molecules that comprise the BCR (see Fig. 8.4). Unlike the TCR, which can only recognize processed and presented antigens, the BCRs on B cells can react with soluble antigens that have not been processed. When B cells bind to antigen, they can be activated to become antibody-producing plasma cells in two significant

EMERGING SCIENCE BOX

IL-17 in Health and Disease

The cytokine IL-17 has many protective functions and is responsible for a wide range of inflammatory and autoimmune conditions. IL-17 is a family of 6 proteins (IL-17A—IL17F), of which IL-17A is most often linked to disease. In addition to T helper 17 (Th17) cells, IL-17A is produced by some T cytotoxic cells, natural killer cells, and innate lymphoid cells. IL-17A binds to receptors on innate immune cells such as neutrophils and macrophages and activates Nuclear Factor KappaB (NF-κB), which in turn induces the production of multiple proinflammatory cytokines (e.g., TNF-α, and IL-1), chemokines, and proteases. This effect is synergistic with other cytokines of the innate immune response and contributes to neutrophil and macrophage activation and function. Thus IL-17A is important to immune defense and wound healing. Unfortunately, IL-17A also has been shown to contribute to a wide range of conditions, including inflammatory rheumatologic, neurogenerative, pulmonary, cardiovascular, and ophthalmologic disorders, as well as cancer and other conditions as broad-ranging as periodontitis, type 1 diabetes, obesity, and pregnancy loss. Therapeutic blockade of IL-17A by monoclonal antibodies (e.g., secukinumab and Ixekizumab) effectively treats psoriasis, psoriatic arthritis, and ankylosing spondylitis; however, results have not been as promising for other IL-17-related conditions. Of increasing interest for new therapies is the discovery that Th17 cells can be induced by anti-inflammatory cytokines such as Transforming Growth Factor- Beta (TGF-β) to become Treg 17 cells that suppress the inflammatory response. IL-17F is also being recognized as a major contributor to chronic inflammatory diseases and monoclonal antibodies such as bimekizumab are being developed that can block both IL-17A and IL-17F.

Data from Chang SH. T helper 17 (Th17) cells and interleukin-17 (IL-17) in cancer. *Archives of Pharmacal Research*, 2019;42(7):549–559; Deng J, et al. Inflammasome activation and Th17 responses. *Molecular Immunology*, 107:142–164; Gorczynski RM. IL-17 Signaling in the tumor microenvironment. *Advances in Experimental Medicine and Biology*, 2020;1240:47–58; Kamali AN, et al. A role for Th1-like Th17 cells in the pathogenesis of inflammatory and autoimmune disorders. *Molecular Immunology*, 2019;105:107–115; McGeachy MJ, et al. The IL-17 Family of Cytokines in Health and Disease. *Immunity*, 2019;50(4):892–906; Ruiz de Morales JMG, et al. Critical role of interleukin (IL)-17 in inflammatory and immune disorders: An updated review of the evidence focusing in controversies. *Autoimmunity Reviews*, 2020;19(1):102429; Singh B, et al. Novel regulatory Th17 cells and regulatory B cells in modulating autoimmune diseases. *Cellular Immunology*, 2019;339:29–32; Yeremenko N. Out of the shadow of interleukin-17A: the role of interleukin-17F and other interleukin-17 family cytokines in spondyloarthritis. *Current Opinion in Rheumatology*, 2021;33(4), 333–340.

ways: (1) coactivation with Th cells by processing and presenting antigen (Fig. 8.10), or (2) through a T cell-independent mechanism (Fig. 8.11).

Coactivation of B cells and Th cells is a multistep process. B cells preferentially present processed antigen on their MHC class II molecules and therefore activate Th cells.[14] The subsequent steps in Th0 cell are similar to those that occur when antigen is presented by APCs (see Fig. 8.8) in which the TCR binds to antigen, the CD4 on the Th0 cell binds to the MHC II molecule on the B cell, and there is intercellular communication via costimulatory molecules. The primary costimulatory molecules involved in Th cell and B cell coactivation are CD40 ligand on the Th cell and CD40 on the B cell (see Fig. 8.10). The Th0 cell is induced to become a Th2 cell, which secretes the Th2 cytokines,

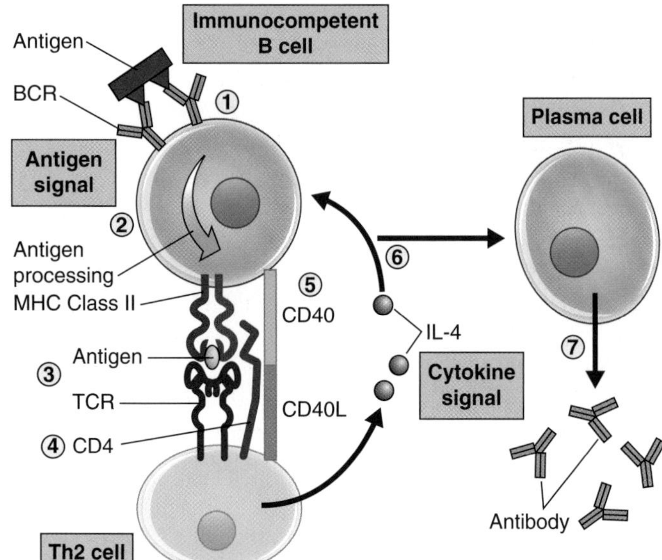

Fig. 8.10 B-Cell Activation. Immunocompetent B cells undergo proliferation and differentiation into antibody-secreting plasma cells. Multiple signals are necessary ***(1)***. The B cell itself can directly bind soluble antigen through the B-cell receptor *(BCR)* and act as an antigen-processing cell. Antigen is internalized, processed ***(2)***, and presented to the T-cell receptor *(TCR)* on a T-helper 2 *(Th2)* cell by a major histocompatibility complex *(MHC)* II molecule ***(3)***. The CD4 molecule on the Th2 cell binds to the MHCII molecule on the B cell ***(4)***. The CD40 molecule on the B cell binds to the CD40 ligand (CD40L) on the Th2 cell providing a costimulatory signal between the cells ***(5)***. The Th2 cell cytokines provide a cytokine signal (e.g., interleukin-4 [IL-4]) that reacts with the B cell ***(6)***. The B cell differentiates into plasma cells that secrete antibody specific to the antigen ***(7)***.

especially IL-4. IL-4 promotes B-cell proliferation and maturation into plasma cells. Plasma cells are activated B cells that produce antibodies capable of detecting the identical antigen as was bound by the BCR.

Although most antigens require B cells to interact with Th cells, a few antigens can bypass the need for cellular interactions and directly stimulate B-cell maturation and proliferation. These are called *T cell-independent antigens* (see Fig. 8.11). These antigens are mostly bacterial products that are large and can cross-link several BCRs. T cell-independent antigens usually induce plasma cells to secrete only IgM.

Molecular Structure and Classes of Antibodies

An antibody molecule consists of four polypeptide chains: two identical light (L) chains and two identical heavy (H) chains. The light and heavy chains are held together by noncovalent bonds and covalent disulfide linkages. There are three parts to an antibody molecule (Fig. 8.12). Two identical fragments can bind antigen and are termed antigen-binding fragments (Fab). The third fragment is termed the crystalline fragment (Fc).

The Fab portions contain the recognition sites (receptors) for antigens and confer the molecule's specificity toward a particular antigen. The Fab portion on the antibody is sometimes referred to as the antigen-binding site or paratope. Its specificity for a particular antigen corresponds to the BCR on the B cell that produced the antibody. Because antigens are relatively small, a large molecule (e.g., protein, polysaccharide, nucleic acid) usually contains multiple and diverse antigens. The specific area of the antigen recognized by a particular antibody is called its antigenic determinant, or epitope. The antigen fits into the antigen-binding site of the antibody with the specificity of a key into a lock and is held there by noncovalent chemical interactions.

The antibody class is determined by the different amino acid sequences in the heavy chains that make up the Fc portion of the antibody. The Fc portion is responsible for most of the biologic functions of antibodies. There are five classes of antibodies (IgG, IgA, IgM, IgE, and IgD) characterized by differences in structure and function (Fig. 8.13). Both IgG and IgA have subclasses.

IgG is the most abundant antibody class, constituting 80% to 85% of the antibodies in the blood and accounting for most of the protective activity against infections. During pregnancy, maternal IgG is transported across the placenta and protects the newborn child during the first 6 months of life.

IgM is the largest antibody and usually exists as a pentamer (a molecule consisting of five identical smaller molecules) that is stabilized by a J chain. It is the first antibody produced during the initial, or primary, response to antigens. IgM is usually

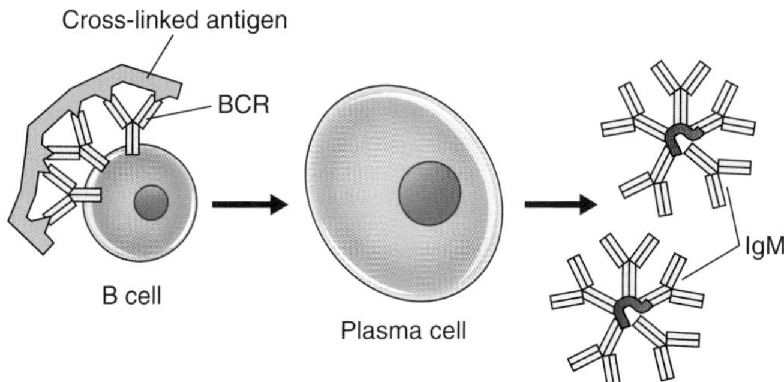

Fig. 8.11 Activation of a B Cell by a T Cell–Independent Antigen. Antigens that can cross-link several B-cell receptors *(BCRs)* can directly induce the B cell to become an antibody-producing plasma cell. Because T-helper 2 cells do not participate, class switch does not occur, and the resultant antibody response is immunoglobulin M *(IgM)*.

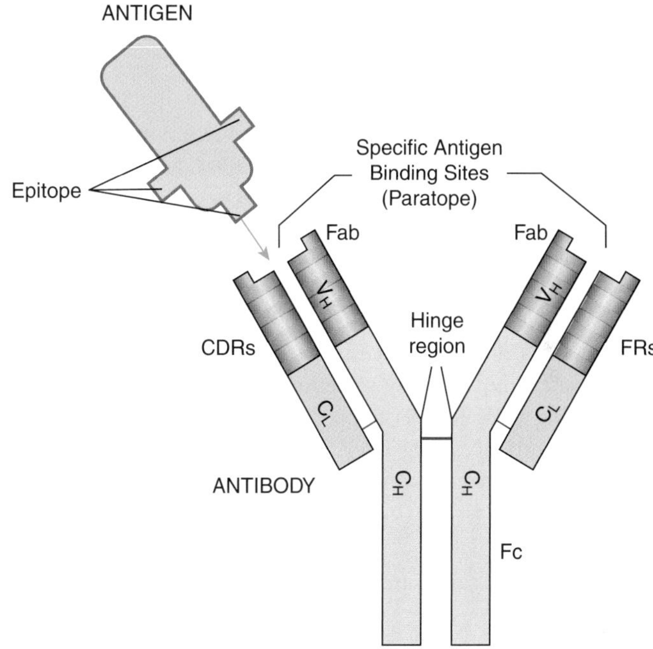

Fig. 8.12 Structure of Antibodies. *CDRs*, Complementary determining regions; C_H, constant region heavy chain; C_L, constant region light chain; *Fab*, fragment antigen binding; *Fc*, crystalline fragment; *FRs*, framework regions V_H, variable region heavy chain; V_L, variable region light chain;. *Red lines* are disulfide linkages.

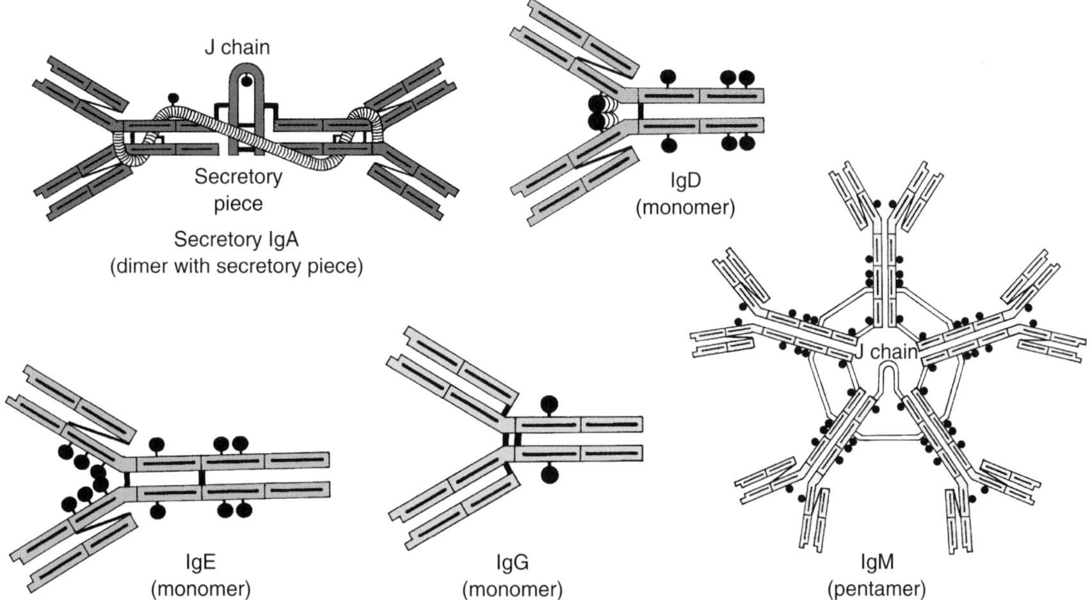

Fig. 8.13 Classes of Antibodies Secretory immunoglobulin A (IgA), IgD, IgE, IgG, and IgM. The *black circles* attached to each molecule represent carbohydrate residues.

synthesized early in neonatal life but may be increased as a response to infection in utero. mIgM serves as part of the BCR complex on B cells.

IgA is found in blood and bodily secretions as secretory IgA (subclass IgA2). Secretory IgA is a *dimer* consisting of two IgA2 molecules held together through a J chain and secretory piece. The secretory piece is attached to dimeric IgA during transportation through mucosal epithelial cells to protect against degradation by enzymes also found in secretions.

IgD functions as a part of the BCR antigen receptor on the surface of early B cells (mIgD).

IgE is normally at low concentrations in the circulation. It has specialized functions to mediate many common allergic responses (see Chapter 9) and defense against parasitic infections.

A significant component of B-cell maturation is class switch, which changes antibody production from one class to another (e.g., IgM to IgG). Antibody diversification through this process is essential for the immune system to produce protective humoral responses. B cells proliferate during the clonal selection process and develop into antibody-secreting plasma cells, which begin by secreting IgM. The plasma cell then can change the class of antibody it produces to IgG, IgA, or IgE. The antigenic specificity of the antibody remains unchanged. Thus, a B cell may produce a population of plasma cells capable of producing many different classes of antibodies against the same antigen. The type of antibody produced is under the control of Th cytokines. For instance, when the Th2 cytokines IL-4 and IL-13 are secreted in high amounts, they preferentially stimulate a class switch to IgE secretion.

Function of Antibodies

The chief function of antibodies is to protect against infection. The mechanism can be either *direct* (through the action of antibody alone) or *indirect* (requiring activation of other components of the innate immune response) (Fig. 8.14). Directly, antibodies can affect infectious agents or their toxic products by neutralization (inactivating or blocking the binding of antigens to receptors). For instance, the influenza virus must attach to specific receptors on respiratory tract epithelial cells, and *Neisseria gonorrhoeae* (causes gonorrhea) must attach to specific sites on urogenital epithelial cells. Antibodies may protect the host by covering sites on the microorganism needed for attachment, thereby preventing infection. Vaccination with inactivated or attenuated (weakened) viruses can prevent many viral infections by inducing neutralizing antibody production. Antibodies can also protect against infection through agglutination (clumping insoluble particles in suspension)

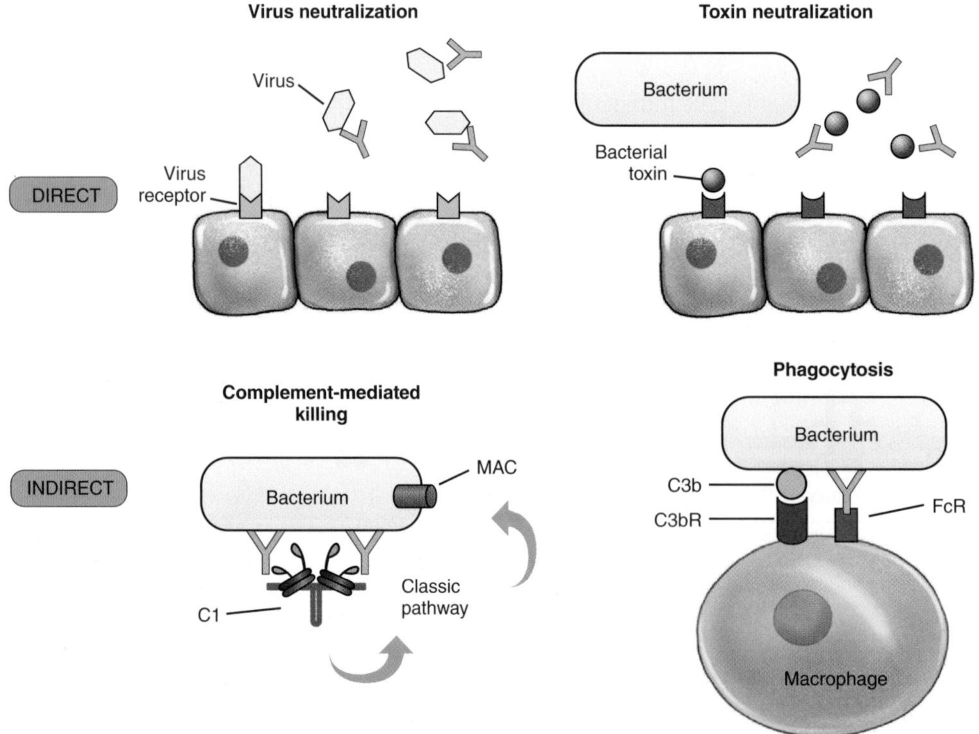

Fig. 8.14 Direct and Indirect Functions of Antibody. Protective activities of antibodies can be direct (through the action of antibody alone) or indirect (requiring activation of other components of the innate immune response, usually through the Fc region). *Direct* means include neutralizing viruses or bacterial toxins before they bind to receptors on the surface of the host's cells. *Indirect* means include activation of the classical complement pathway through C1, resulting in the formation of the membrane attack complex *(MAC)*, or increased phagocytosis of bacteria opsonized with antibody and complement components bound to appropriate surface receptors (*FcR* and *C3bR*), resulting in antibody-dependent cellular cytotoxicity (ADCC).

or precipitation (making a soluble antigen into an insoluble precipitate).

Some bacteria secrete toxins that harm individuals. For instance, bacterial toxins cause the symptoms of tetanus or diphtheria. Most toxins are proteins that bind to surface molecules on cells and damage those cells. Protective antibodies produced against the toxin, known as antitoxins, can bind to the toxins, prevent interaction with host cells, and neutralize their biologic effects.

Indirectly, antibodies activate components of innate immunity, including complement and phagocytes (see Fig. 8.14). Through the classical pathway, complement component C1 is activated by binding simultaneously to the Fc regions of two adjacent antibodies bound to a microbe, resulting in activation of the entire cascade and ultimate killing of the microbe by the complement membrane attack complex (see Chapter 7). In addition, phagocytic cells express receptors that bind the Fc portion of antibody; thus, antibody is an opsonin that facilitates phagocytosis of bacteria. IgM is the best complement-activating antibody, and IgG is the best opsonin. The process by which antibodies opsonize and connect antigens to phagocytic cells is called antibody-dependent cellular cytotoxicity (ADCC).

Immunoglobulin E

If IL-4 levels are moderate, B cells are stimulated to become plasma cells that secrete IgG. In individuals with parasitic infection or allergies, high levels of IL-4 result in plasma cell production of IgE. IgE is a special class of antibody that protects the individual from infection by large parasitic worms (helminths). When large multicellular parasites invade mucosal tissues, IgG, IgM, and IgA bind to the surface of parasites and activate both complement and ADCC. This response, however, does not significantly damage parasites. IgE initiates an inflammatory reaction that provides a more effective response to parasitic infection. Mast cells in the tissues have Fc epsilon receptors that bind the Fc portion of IgE molecules to the mast cell surface. Soluble antigen molecules from the parasite bind to the Fab portion of these IgE antibodies resulting in mast cell degranulation. Eosinophil chemotactic factor of anaphylaxis (ECF-A) is released from the mast cells and attracts eosinophils from the circulation. Eosinophils contain granules whose contents include major basic protein, eosinophil cationic protein, eosinophil peroxidase, and eosinophil neurotoxin, each of which can damage infectious worms. Thus, elevated levels of IgE are commonly found in parasitic infection. The steps of this process are presented in Fig. 8.15.

When IgE is produced against relatively innocuous environmental antigens, it is also the primary cause of common allergies (e.g., hay fever, dust allergies, bee stings). Monoclonal antibodies are used to block the functions of IgE in individuals who have a severe allergy. The role of IgE in allergies is discussed in Chapter 9.

IgE is also capable of activating ADCC. Recent studies suggest that it may be possible to use IgE-mediated ADCC to increase the effectiveness of immune cells that invade tumors but are otherwise unable to detect and kill the cancer cells.[15]

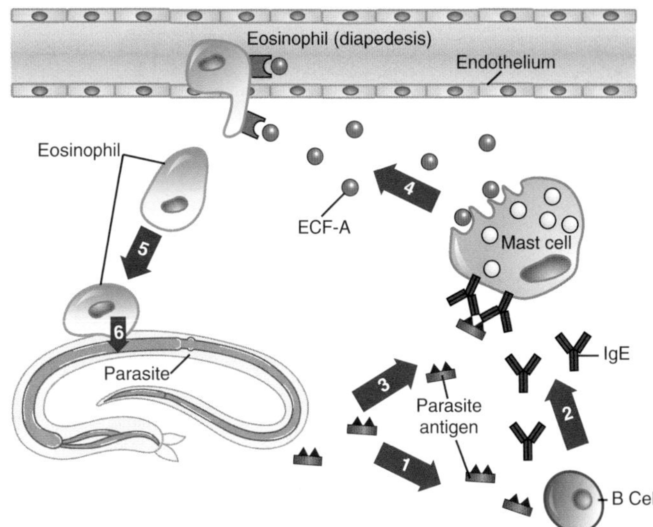

Fig. 8.15 Immunoglobulin E Function. ***(1)*** Soluble antigens from a parasitic infection cause production of immunoglobulin E *(IgE)* antibody by B cells. ***(2)*** Secreted IgE binds to IgE-specific receptors on the mast cell. ***(3)*** Additional soluble parasite antigen cross-links the IgE on the mast cell surface, ***(4)*** leading to mast cell degranulation and release of many proinflammatory products, including eosinophil chemotactic factor of anaphylaxis (ECF-A). ***(5)*** ECF-A attracts eosinophils from the circulation. ***(6)*** The eosinophil attaches to the parasite's surface and releases potent lysosomal enzymes that damage microorganisms.

Secretory Immune System

Immunocompetent lymphocytes migrate among secondary lymphoid organs and tissue as part of the systemic immune system. Another partially independent immune system protects the external surfaces of the body through lacrimal and salivary glands and a network of lymphoid tissues residing in the breasts, bronchi, intestines, and genitourinary tract known as mucosal-associated lymphoid tissues (MALTs). This system is called the secretory (mucosal) immune system (Fig. 8.16). Plasma cells in those sites secrete antibodies in bodily secretions, such as tears, sweat, saliva, mucus, and breast milk, to prevent pathogenic microorganisms from infecting and penetrating the body's surfaces.

IgA is the dominant secretory immunoglobulin, although IgM and IgG also are present in secretions. The primary role of IgA is to prevent the attachment and invasion of pathogens through mucosal membranes, such as those of the gastrointestinal, pulmonary, and genitourinary tracts. Dimeric IgA antibodies are produced by plasma cells in the mucosa. Mucosal epithelium expresses a cell surface receptor that binds and internalizes IgA. The IgA, along with the epithelial receptor, is secreted as secretory IgA (sIgA). This sIgA protects against a variety of pathogens as well as helps to maintain a healthy microbiome in the gut.[16]

The lymphoid tissues of the secretory immune system are connected; thus, many foreign antigens in a mother's gastrointestinal tract (e.g., polio virus) induce the secretion of specific antibodies into breast milk. Colostral antibodies (i.e., those found in the colostrum of breast milk) may protect the nursing newborn against infectious disease agents that enter through the infant's gastrointestinal tract. Although colostral antibodies provide the newborn with passive immunity against

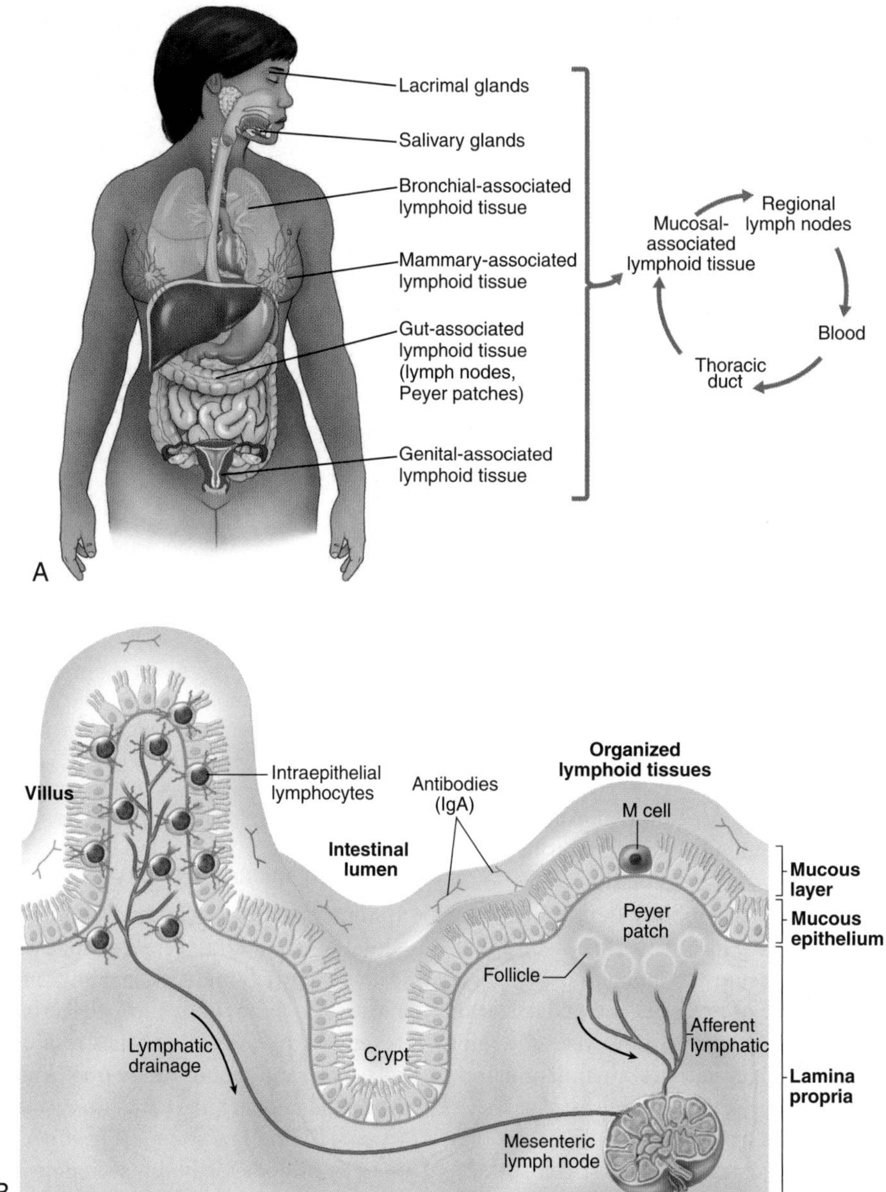

Fig. 8.16 Secretory Immune System. (A) Lymphocytes from the mucosal-associated lymphoid tissues (MALTs) circulate throughout the body in a pattern separate from other lymphocytes. For example, lymphocytes from the gut-associated lymphoid tissue circulate through the regional lymph nodes, the thoracic duct, and the blood and return to other MALTs rather than to lymphoid tissue of the systemic immune system. **(B)** Lymphoid tissue associated with mucous membranes is referred to as MALT.

gastrointestinal infections, they do not provide systemic immunity because the transport of these antibodies across the newborn's gut into the bloodstream is discontinued after the first 24 hours of life. Maternal antibodies that pass across the placenta into the fetus before birth provide passive systemic immunity.

Primary and Secondary Humoral Immune Responses

The immune response to antigen has classically been divided into two phases—primary and secondary responses. Although these two phases occur in cellular immune responses, this process is most easily demonstrated by measuring concentrations of circulating antibodies over time (Fig. 8.17). After a single initial exposure to most antigens, there is a latent period, or lag phase, during which clonal selection occurs. After approximately 5 to 7 days, IgM antibody is detected in the circulation. This is the primary immune response, typically characterized by IgM's initial production followed by IgG production against the same antigen. The quantity of IgG may be about equal to or less than the amount of IgM. The amount of antibody in a serum sample is frequently referred to as the titer; a higher titer indicates more antibodies. If no further exposure to the antigen occurs, the circulating antibody is catabolized (broken down), and titers fall. The individual's immune system, however, has been primed.

A second challenge by the same antigen results in the secondary immune response, characterized by the more rapid production of a larger amount of antibody compared with the primary response. The rapidity of the secondary immune response is the result of memory cells that are already differentiated. IgM may be transiently produced in the secondary response, but IgG production is increased considerably, making it the predominant antibody class. Natural infection (e.g., rubella) may result in measurable levels of protective IgG for the individual's life. Some vaccines (e.g., polio) also may produce extremely long-lived protection, although many vaccines require boosters at specified intervals.

Clinical Uses of Antibodies

Antibodies have many protective, diagnostic, and therapeutic uses in clinical settings (Table 8.2).[17] Because the secondary immune response takes time to develop, individuals with recent or potential exposure to a serious infectious agent may benefit from administering preformed antibody in a process termed passive immunity (passive acquired immunity). Examples include individuals exposed to an infectious agent without preexisting vaccine-induced immunity (e.g., hepatitis A virus or severe acute respiratory syndrome coronavirus 2 [SARS-CoV-2]). Antibodies also may be measured in the blood in individuals suspected of having an acute, chronic, or past infection (e.g., hepatitis B). The measurement of circulating antibody is also useful in diagnosing cancer, allergies, and autoimmune diseases (see Chapters 9 and 12). Passive treatment with antibodies is available for only a few infections (e.g., respiratory syncytial virus infection and SARS-CoV-2). However, it is now a common procedure to administer monoclonal antibodies to treat a wide variety of neoplastic, allergic, and autoimmune conditions (see Emerging Science Box: Monoclonal Antibodies).[18]

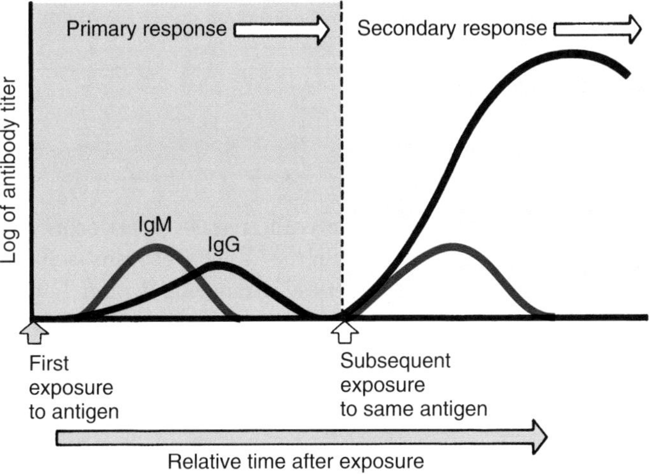

Fig. 8.17 Primary and Secondary Immune Responses. The initial administration of antigen induces a primary response during which immunoglobulin M *(IgM)* is initially produced, followed by immunoglobulin G *(IgG)*. Another administration of the antigen induces the secondary response in which IgM is transiently produced, and larger amounts of IgG are produced over a longer period.

CELL-MEDIATED IMMUNITY

Cell-mediated immunity (or cellular immunity) is conducted primarily by Tc cells. Natural killer cells and phagocytes (macrophages and neutrophils) also play a role. Cellular immunity most often destroys the target cell.

T-Cytotoxic Cells

Tc cells are activated when their TCRs detect foreign intracellular antigens presented on MHC I molecules. They attack infected and damaged cells and destroy them.

T Cytotoxic Cell Activation

The differentiation of immunocompetent T cells into effector Tc cells requires similar intercellular communications as described for Th cells. The Tc cell TCR recognizes antigen presented by MHC class I molecules on the surface of the APC and virus-infected or cancerous cells (Fig. 8.18). The Tc cell CD8 binds to the MHC class I molecule, which initiates cytoplasmic signaling pathways that promote differentiation of the Tc cell. L-2 produced by Th1 cells and other cytokines activate receptors on the Tc cells resulting in proliferation and further differentiation into active Tc cells.[3]

T Cytotoxic Cell Function

Tc cells are responsible for the cell-mediated destruction of abnormal cells, such as tumor cells or cells infected with viruses (Fig. 8.19). Tc cells form tight connections to the target cell through the action of adhesion molecules (integrins). Attachment to a target cell activates Tc killing mechanisms. The

TABLE 8.2 Clinical Uses of Antibodies

Antigen	Protection	Diagnosis	Therapy
Infectious agents	Passive immunization (e.g., for exposure to hepatitis A)	Measure circulating antibodies to diagnose acute, chronic, or past infection (e.g., diagnosis of hepatitis B infection—see Chapter 42)	Passive treatment with antibody to treat infection (e.g., SARS-CoV-2)
Cancers	No clear example	Measure circulating antigens and antibodies (e.g., to tailor immunotherapy against certain cancers—see Chapter 12)	Immunotherapy (e.g., administration of monoclonal antibodies against cancer antigens and immune checkpoints—see Chapter 12)
Environmental substances	No clear example	Measure circulating antibody (e.g., measure IgE levels to certain allergens—see Chapter 9)	Immunotherapy (e.g., administration of monoclonal antibodies to IgE in severe allergy—see Chapter 9)
Self-antigens	No clear example	Measure circulating antibody against self-antigen for diagnosis of autoimmune disease (see Chapter 9)	Immunotherapy (e.g., administration of monoclonal antibodies to block platelet adhesion and rheumatologic autoimmunity—see Chapter 9)

IgA, Immunoglobulin A; *IgE*, Immunoglobulin E; *PSA*, Prostate-specific antigen; *SARS-CoV-2*, severe respiratory syncytial virus infection.

EMERGING SCIENCE BOX

Monoclonal Antibodies

Monoclonal antibodies (mAb) are produced in the laboratory from one B cell that has been cloned; thus, all the antibodies produced are of the same class, specificity, and function. The advantages of monoclonal antibodies are that (1) a single antibody of known antigenic specificity is generated rather than a mixture of different antibodies; (2) monoclonal antibodies have a single, constant binding affinity; (3) monoclonal antibodies can be diluted to a constant titer (concentration in fluid) because the actual antibody concentration is known; and (4) the antibody can be easily purified. mAbs have been created and used to develop extremely specific and sensitive laboratory tests (e.g., home and laboratory pregnancy tests) and therapies. The therapeutic uses of mAbs have expanded exponentially over the past decade. The generic names of these drugs are usually easy to recognize because most end in the letters mAb. Current treatment options using mAbs are available for a wide variety of inflammatory, autoimmune, neurologic, vascular, and clotting disorders such as collagen vascular diseases (e.g., rheumatoid arthritis and systemic lupus erythematosus), asthma and allergy, inflammatory bowel disease, multiple sclerosis, migraine, atherosclerosis, and transplant rejection. One of the most exciting groups of mAbs in use today are those that block the ability of cancer cells to turn off immune cells that are trying to attack them (checkpoint inhibitors—see Chapter 12). Among the newest uses being explored for mAb is the treatment of anti-microbial resistant infections. Many more uses of mAb are being explored.

Data from Chahine EB, et al. Ibalizumab: The first monoclonal antibody for the treatment of HIV-1 infection. *Annals of Pharmacotherapy*, 2021;55(2): 230–239; Cruz-Teran C, et al. Challenges and opportunities for antiviral monoclonal antibodies as COVID-19 therapy. *Advanced Drug Delivery Reviews*, 2021;169:100–117; Dibo M, et al. Antibody therapy for the control of viral diseases: An update. *Current Pharmaceutical Biotechnology*, 2019;20(13): 1108–1121; Ghahremanloo A, et al. Recent advances in the clinical development of immune checkpoint blockade therapy. *Cellular Oncology*, 2019;42(5):609–626; McConnell MJ. Where are we with monoclonal antibodies for multidrug-resistant infections? *Drug Discovery Today*, 2019;24(5): 1132–1138; Marin-Acevedo JA, et al. Next generation of immune checkpoint inhibitors and beyond. *Journal of Hematology and Oncology 14*, 45; Kaplon, H., Reichert J.M. Antibodies to watch in 2021. *mAbs*, 2021;13(1):1860476; Pelfrene E, et al. Monoclonal antibodies as anti-infective products: a promising future? *Clinical Microbiology and Infection*, 2019;25(1):60–64; Schmid AS, et al. Advances in antibody engineering for rheumatic diseases. *Nature Reviews Rheumatology*, 2019;15(4):197–207; Sivaccumar J, et al. Monoclonal antibodies: A prospective and retrospective view. *Current Medicinal Chemistry*, 2021;28(3): 435–471; Tsumoto K, et al. Future perspectives of therapeutic monoclonal antibodies. *Immunotherapy*, 2019;11(2):119–127; Yoo SM, et al. Targets of monoclonal antibodies for immunological diseases. *Archives of Pharmacal Research*, 2019;42(4):293–304.

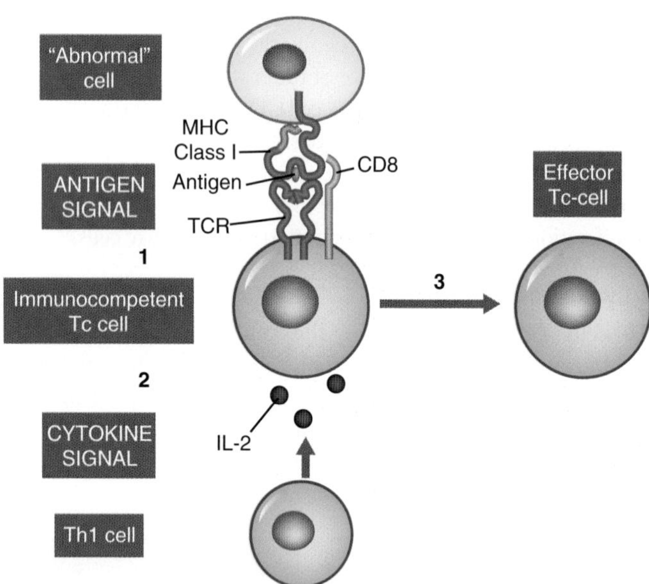

Fig. 8.18 T-Cytotoxic (Tc)-Cell Activation. The immunocompetent Tc cell can react with antigen but cannot yet kill target cells. During clonal selection, this cell reacts with antigen presented by major histocompatibility complex class I (MHC I) molecules on the surface of a virally infected or cancerous *abnormal* cell. ***(1)*** The antigen–MHC I complex is recognized simultaneously by the T-cell receptor *(TCR)*, which binds to antigen, and CD8, which binds to the MHC I molecule. ***(2)*** A separate signal is provided by cytokines, particularly IL-2 from T-helper 1 *(Th1)* cells. ***(3)*** In response to these signals, the Tc cell develops into an effector Tc cell with the ability to kill abnormal cells.

primary Tc killing mechanism is the release of perforins and granzymes from granules within the Tc cell. Perforins facilitate granzyme entry into the target cell. Granzyme B from Tc cells activates intracellular caspases in the target cell, which induces apoptosis. Tc cells also express a surface protein called Fas ligand. This protein binds to a receptor on the surface of the target cell, leading to caspase-mediated apoptosis. Cells that have undergone apoptosis are phagocytosed and removed from the body. Tc cells that have killed a target cell can detach and go on to kill other cells.

Natural Killer Cells

Natural killer (NK) cells are a special group of lymphoid cells that are important components of both innate and adaptive immunity. They are similar to T cells but lack antigen-specific receptors. Instead, they express various cell surface activation receptors (see Fig. 8.19), which identify protein changes on the surface of cells infected with viruses or that have become cancerous. After attachment, the NK cell kills its target like that of Tc cells. Unlike Tc cells, NK cells lack CD8, and binding to MHC class I molecules results in the inactivation of the NK cell. Thus, if MHC class I antigen presentation has occurred, Tc cells provide the target cell killing. But in some instances, a virus-infected or cancerous cell will "protect" itself from Tc cells by downregulating MHC class I molecule expression. In these instances, the lack of MHC class I inhibition allows NK cells to become activated and kill the target cell. Modified NK cells are being used in a variety of approaches to cancer

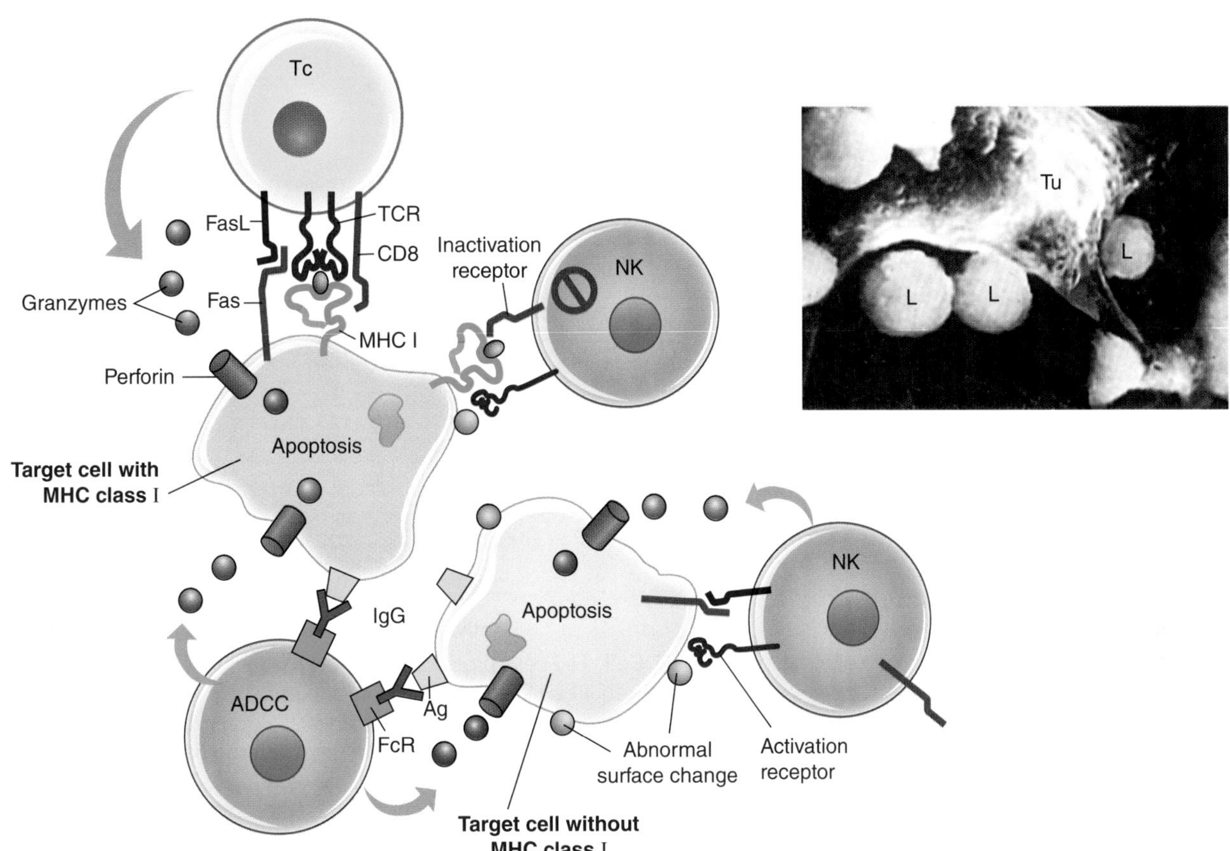

Fig. 8.19 Cellular Killing Mechanisms. Several cells can kill abnormal (e.g., virally infected, cancerous) target cells. T-cytotoxic *(Tc)* cells recognized endogenous antigen presented by major histocompatibility complex *(MHC)* class I molecules *(cell on upper left)*. The intercellular interaction is enhanced through a variety of costimulatory adhesion molecules (not shown). The Tc cell mobilizes multiple killing mechanisms that induce apoptosis of the target cell. Tc cells contain granules that empty their contents into the target cell. These substances include perforin, which creates pores in the target cell, and granzymes which enter through these pores and induce apoptosis. Tc cells also provide stimulation of Fas molecules on the target cell surface by Fas ligand *(FasL)* on the Tc cell, which also induces apoptosis. Natural killer *(NK)* cells use the same mechanisms to kill target cells but do so through activation of non-MHC-dependent receptors that recognize abnormal surface changes on damaged, cancerous, or infected cells (*cell on bottom right*). NK cells specifically kill cancer cells that have down-regulated expression of surface MHC class I molecules. Target cells that express MHC class I molecules inactivate NK cells through various inactivation receptors *(cell on upper right)*. Several cells, including macrophages and NK cells, can kill by antibody-dependent cell-mediated cytotoxicity *(ADCC)*. IgG antibody binds to foreign antigen on the target cell. Cells involved in ADCC *(cell on lower left)* bind IgG through Fc receptors *(FcRs)* and initiate killing. The insert is a scanning electron microscopic view of Tc cells *(L)* attacking a much larger tumor cell *(Tu)*. (*Insert* from Abbas A, Lichtman A. *Cellular and molecular immunology*, 5th edition. Philadelphia: Saunders; 2003.)

immunotherapy.[19,20] NK cells and some macrophages can also specifically target abnormal cells by linking to antibodies that are bound to foreign antigens on these cells. NK cells express Fc receptors for IgG. If antigens on the infected or cancerous cell bind IgG, the NK cell can attach through Fc receptors and activate its standard killing mechanisms via ADCC (see Fig. 8.19).[21]

Macrophages

In addition to their vital roles in initiating innate and adaptive immune responses, macrophages are important effector cells of cell-mediated immunity. After binding to the presented antigen, Th1 cells adhere loosely to macrophages resulting in intercellular communication via costimulatory molecules such as CD40 and CD40 ligand (CD40L) (Fig. 8.20). The Th1 cells secrete interferon-γ (IFN-γ). IFN-γ induces the macrophages to become M1 macrophages which release proinflammatory cytokines and kill infected cells within their phagolysosomes (described in Chapter 7). Activated M1 macrophages also can contribute to a wide range of autoimmune conditions through a process called *delayed hypersensitivity*. (see Chapter 9)

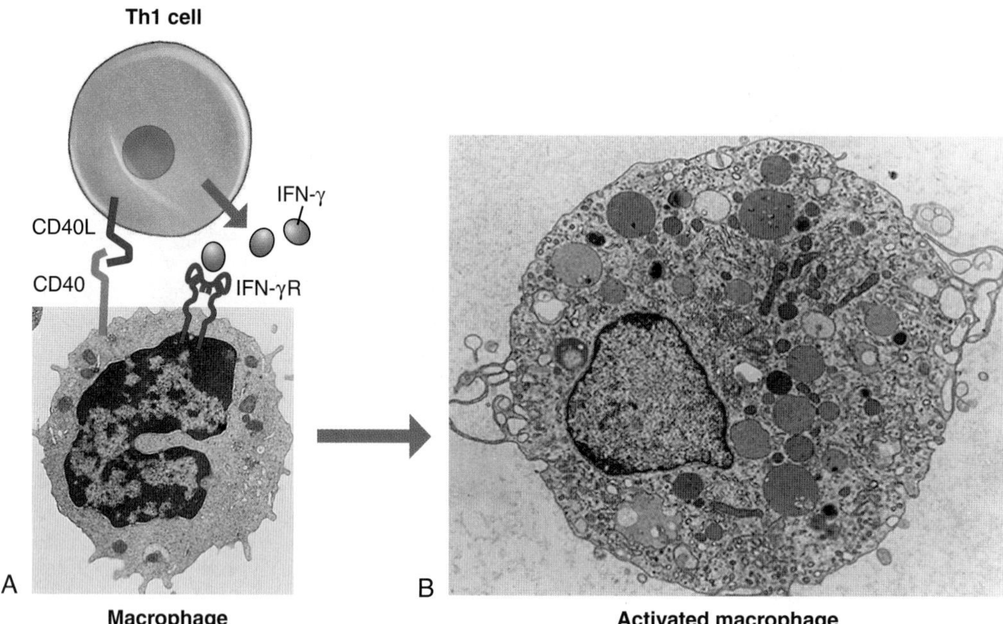

Fig. 8.20 Activation of a Macrophage by a T Cell. *Th1* cells produce cytokines that activate macrophages. Optimal macrophage activation also requires close contact among the cells, mediated by a variety of costimulatory molecules expressed on the surface of each cell (CD40L and CD40 shown here). *CD40L*, CD40 ligand; *IFN-γ*, interferon-gamma; *IFN-γR*, receptor for interferon-gamma. (Micrograph in [A] courtesy Dr. Noel Weidner, Department of Pathology, University of California, San Diego. [B] From Fawcett DW. Bloom and Fawcett: *A textbook of histology*, 12th edition. New York: Chapman & Hall; 1994. With kind permission of Springer Science and Business Media.)

IMMUNOLOGIC MEMORY

During the activation (clonal selection) process, both B cells and T cells differentiate and proliferate into a large population of long-lived memory cells. Memory cells remain inactive until subsequent exposure to the same antigen. Upon re-exposure, these memory cells do not require the multiple cellular activation steps described previously and will therefore rapidly become new plasma cells or effector T cells. The establishment and maintenance of immunologic memory is complex and essential to host defenses (see Emerging Science Box: Immunologic Memory).[22]

EMERGING SCIENCE BOX

Immunologic Memory

Memory B and T cells can facilitate the generation of large numbers of effector Th, Tc, and antibody-producing plasma cells. This immunologic memory of the adaptive immune system is crucial to gaining more rapid and effective immune responses upon secondary exposures to invasion and injury. The processes that underlie immunologic memory are highly complex. For example, it is now known that there are several different types of T memory cells (T effector memory cells, T central memory cells, tissue T resident memory cells, and T stem cell memory cells). B-cell immunologic memory is also similarly complex, including the presence of different B memory cell morphologies (e.g., T-bet+ B cells) and long-lived effector plasma cells. Furthermore, these cells undergo multiple structural and functional adaptations over time (e.g., plasticity, priming, and exhaustion). The epigenetic and metabolic changes that control when and how these memory cells are maintained and activated are still being explored. To further complicate these processes, it is now known that cells of innate immunity such as monocytes, macrophages, natural killer cells, and innate lymphoid cells are also capable of immunologic memory. After exposure to an invader or injury, these cells undergo long-term changes in their metabolism and epigenetic programming, which changes their responses to secondary exposures. This type of innate immunologic memory is called "trained immunity." Cutting-edge research is exploring techniques to modulate both adaptive and trained immunologic memory to achieve a better balance between immune attack and tolerance to antigens. Therapeutic uses could include down-regulation of these processes for conditions characterized by excessive immunity such as autoimmune disorders or enhancement of these processes for conditions driven by inadequate immunity such as cancer and chronic infections.

Data from Dan JM, et al. Immunological memory to SARS-CoV-2 assessed for up to 8 months after infection. *Science*, 2021;371(6529):eabf4063; Dominguez-Andres J, et al. Induction of innate immune memory: The role of cellular metabolism. *Current Opinion in Immunology*, 2019;56:10–16; Ionescu L, et al. Memory B Cells and Long-lived Plasma Cells. *Transplantation*, 2019;103(5):890–898; Kavazović I, et al. Eomes broadens the scope of CD8 T-cell memory by inhibiting apoptosis in cells of low affinity. *PLoS Biology*, 2020;18(3):e3000648; Jarjour NN, et al. T cell memory: Understanding COVID-19. *Immunity*, 2021;54(1):14–18; Knox JJ, et al. T-bet+ memory B cells: Generation, function, and fate. *Immunological Reviews*, 2019;288(1):149–160; Mulder WJM, et al. Adaptation and memory in immune responses. *Nature Immunology*, 2019;20(7):783–792; Nguyen QP, et al. Origins of CD4+ circulating and tissue-resident memory T-cells. *Immunology*, 2019;157(1):3–12; Quast I, et al. B cell memory: Understanding COVID-19. *Immunity*, 2021;54(2):205–210; Rodriguez RM, et al. Therapeutic epigenetic reprogramming of trained immunity in myeloid cells. *Trends in Immunology*, 2019;40(1):66–80.

PEDIATRIC CONSIDERATIONS

Mechanisms of Self-Defense in the Newborn Child

The average human infant is immunologically immature at birth. Healthy development of the neonatal immune system is essential to long-term health. Although cell-mediated immunologic capabilities begin developing early in gestation and probably are entirely functional at birth, phagocytic activity, antibody production, and complement activity are clearly deficient. In the last trimester, the fetus appears capable of producing a primary immune response (almost entirely IgM) to in utero infections (e.g., cytomegalovirus, rubella virus, and *Toxoplasma gondii*) but is unable to produce a significant IgG response. Although some IgA can be detected, the capacity to produce IgA is underdeveloped.

To protect the child against infectious agents both in utero and during the first few postnatal months, a system of active transport facilitates the passage of maternal antibodies into the fetal circulation (Fig. 8.21). In the placenta, maternal and fetal blood are separated by a layer of specialized multinucleate cells termed *syncytiotrophoblasts*. Immunoglobulins are too large to diffuse across this cellular layer, so the trophoblastic cells actively transport immunoglobulins from the maternal to the fetal circulation. Active transport of maternal IgG is mediated by surface receptors specific to the Fc portion of free IgG but not for IgM, IgE, or IgA. In addition to antibodies, maternal cytokines and cells are transferred in utero and influence the fetal immune system. Maternal vaccination has been promoted as a way of increasing the amount of antibody transferred to the fetus to protect the child after birth. This has decreased the antibody titers after newborn vaccination, but cellular immunity in the infant remains intact.

At birth, total IgG levels in the umbilical cord are near adult levels (Fig. 8.22). When the source of maternal antibodies is severed at birth, antibody titers in the newborn begin to drop as the maternal antibody is catabolized. Thus, antibody titers drop rapidly as the neonate's production of IgG is beginning to rise. The rate of catabolism is usually more rapid than the production rate so that the total immunoglobulin levels reach a minimum at 5–6 months in the typical child, occasionally causing transient hypogammaglobulinemia (insufficient quantities of circulating immunoglobulins). Many normal infants experience recurrent mild respiratory tract infections at this age.

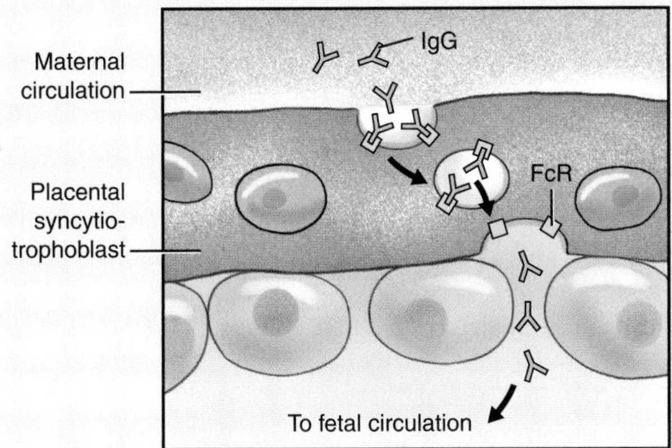

Fig. 8.21 Transport of IgG Across the Syncytiotrophoblast. The human placenta is covered with a specialized multinucleated cell, the syncytiotrophoblast. Transport of maternal immunoglobulin G (IgG) across the syncytiotrophoblast and into the fetal circulation is an active process. Maternal IgG binds to Fc receptors on the surface of the syncytiotrophoblast and is internalized by the process of endocytosis. Receptors on the syncytiotrophoblast are specific for the Fc portion of IgG and do not bind other classes of immunoglobulins. Interaction of IgG with Fc receptors protects the antibody from lysosomal digestion during transport of the vacuole across the cell (i.e., transcytosis). On the fetal side of the syncytiotrophoblast, IgG is released by exocytosis (see Chapter 1). (From McCance K, Huether S. *Pathophysiology*, 8th edition. St. Louis: Elsevier; 2019.)

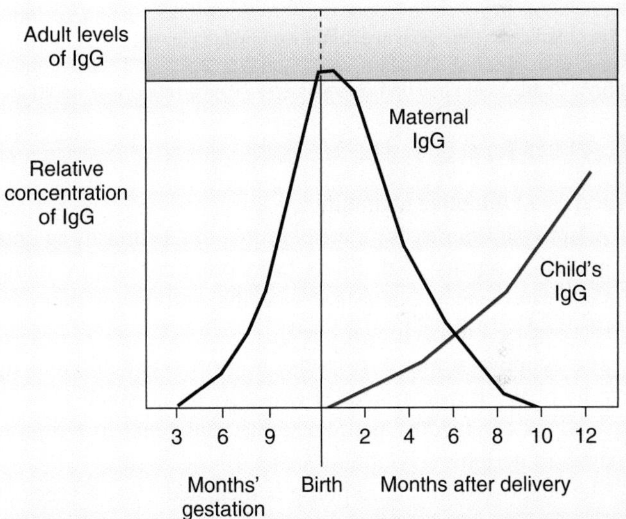

Fig. 8.22 Antibody Levels in Umbilical Cord Blood and Neonatal Circulation. Early in gestation, maternal IgG begins crossing the placenta and enters the fetal circulation. At birth, the fetal circulation may contain nearly adult levels of IgG, which is almost exclusively from the maternal source. The fetal immune system can produce IgM and small amounts of IgA before birth (not shown). After delivery, maternal IgG is rapidly catabolized, and neonatal IgG production increases. (From McCance K, Huether S. *Pathophysiology*, 8th edition. St. Louis: Elsevier; 2019.)

Data from Albrecht M, Pagenkemper M, Wiessner C, et al. Infant immunity against viral infections is advanced by the placentadependent vertical transfer of maternal antibodies. *Vaccine*, 2021;S0264-410X(20)31629–7; Albrecht M, Arck PC. Vertically transferred immunity in neonates: Mothers, mechanisms and mediators. *Frontiers in Immunology*, 2020;11:555; Jennewein MF, Abu-Raya B, Jiang Y, et al. Transfer of maternal immunity and programming of the newborn immune system. *Seminars in Immunopathology*, 2017;39:605–613; Orije MRP, Maertens K, Corbiere V, et al. The effect of maternal antibodies on the cellular immune response after infant vaccination: a review. *Vaccine*, 2020;38:20–28; Zazara DE, Arck PC. Developmental origin and sex-specific risk for infections and immune diseases later in life. *Seminars in Immunopathology*, 2019;41:137–151.

GERIATRIC CONSIDERATIONS

Aging and Immune Function

Adaptive immune function decreases with age due to changes in both lymphocyte function and relative lymphocyte populations due to a process called *immunosenescence*. These changes render the older individual more susceptible to infectious disease and cancer and less able to respond to vaccination. The ability to respond to new antigens diminishes as the number of peripheral naïve T and B cells declines. The thymus, where T cells begin their development, reaches its maximum size at sexual maturity, and then undergoes involution until the thymus is only 15% of its maximum size by middle age. A decrease in thymic activity is accompanied by decreased production of thymic hormones, and the capacity to mediate T-cell differentiation decreases with this atrophy. The capacity for Th cells to produce IL-2 declines, yet there is a shift in the populations of T-cell subtypes, with Tc cells significantly outnumbering Th cells. This dysfunction is coupled with increased T cell senescence and exhaustion. B-cell function is altered with age, as shown by decreases in specific antibody production in response to antigenic challenge. A decline in the number of circulating memory B cells is also observed. In the elderly, there is an increase in a subset of B cells called *age-associated B cells (ABCs)*. ABCs are paradoxically associated with the increased presentation of antigen, the release of cytokines, and secretion of antibodies; however, a significant proportion of these antibodies are autoantibodies and contribute to autoimmune disease. The combined effects of T and B lymphocyte dysfunction increase the risk for disease in the elderly. In addition, immune responses to vaccination are diminished, rendering older individuals more vulnerable to infections such as influenza and SARS-CoV-2 even in vaccinated individuals. In addition to these direct effects of aging on the adaptive immune system, the development of comorbidities in the elderly influences the immune response. Cardiovascular, pulmonary, renal, and hepatic diseases are associated with immune dysfunction, especially prevalent in the elderly.

Data from Bartleson JM, Radenkovic D, Covarrubias A.J, et al. SARS-CoV-2, COVID-19 and the aging immune system. *Nature Aging*, 2021;1:769–782; Dodig S, Čepelak I, Pavić I. Hallmarks of senescence and aging. *Biochemia Medica*, 2019;29(3):030501; Dugan HL, Henry C, Wilson PC. Aging and influenza vaccine-induced immunity. *Cellular Immunology*, 2020;348:103998; Dunn-Walters DK, Stewart AT, Sinclair EL, et al. Age-related changes in B cells relevant to vaccine responses. *Interdisciplinary Topics in Gerontology and Geriatrics*, 2020;43:56–72; Kwetkat A, Heppner HJ. Comorbidities in the elderly and their possible influence on vaccine response. *Interdisciplinary Topics in Gerontology and Geriatrics*, 2020;43:73–85; Ma S, Wang C, Mao X, et al. B cell dysfunction associated with aging and autoimmune diseases. *Frontiers in Immunology*, 2019;10:318; Wong GC, Strickland MC, Larbi A. Changes in t cell homeostasis and vaccine responses in old age. *Interdisciplinary Topics in Gerontology and Geriatrics*, 2020;43:36–55.

SUMMARY REVIEW

Overview of Adaptive Immunity

1. Adaptive immunity is a state of protection, primarily against infectious agents, that differs from inflammation by being slower to develop, being more specific, and having memory that makes it much longer lived.
2. The adaptive immune response is most often initiated by cells of the innate system. These cells process and present portions of invading pathogens (i.e., antigens) to lymphocytes in peripheral lymphoid tissue.
3. The adaptive immune response is mediated by two types of lymphocytes—B lymphocytes and T lymphocytes. Each has distinct functions. B cells are responsible for humoral immunity that is mediated by circulating antibodies, whereas T cells are responsible for cell-mediated immunity, in which they kill targets directly or stimulate the activity of other leukocytes.
4. B and T lymphocytes leaving the primary lymphoid organs are immunocompetent but have not been exposed to antigen, thus are naïve.
5. Clonal selection with cellular proliferation and further differentiation of T and B cells into active effort cells of the adaptive immune system is initiated when exposure to an antigen occurs.

Antigens

1. Antigens are molecules that bind and react with components of the immune response, such as antibodies and receptors on B and T cells.
2. Common antigens include infectious agents, allergens, chemical agents, and abnormal molecules on the surface of cells.
3. Large molecules, such as proteins, polysaccharides, and nucleic acids, are most immunogenic. Thus, molecular size is a crucial factor for antigen immunogenicity.
4. Haptens are antigens too small to be immunogens by themselves but become immunogenic after combining with larger molecules.
5. The antigenic determinant, or epitope, is the precise chemical structure with which an antibody or B-cell/T-cell receptor (BCR/TCR) reacts.
6. Self-antigens are antigens on an individual's own cells. The individual's immune system does not usually recognize self-antigens as immunogenic, a condition known as *tolerance*.

Lymphocyte Development

1. The generation of clonal diversity results in the production of B and T lymphocytes with receptors against millions of antigens that possibly will be encountered in an individual's lifetime occurs in the fetus in the primary lymphoid organs: the thymus for T cells and portions of bone marrow for B cells.
2. The generation of clonal diversity is the differentiation of lymphoid stem cells into B and T lymphocytes with specific BCRs and TCRs, respectively.
3. The enormous repertoire of BCR specificities is made possible by rearranging existing deoxyribonucleic acid (DNA) during B-cell development in the primary lymphoid organs, a process called *somatic recombination*.
4. Somatic rearrangement of the antibody variable regions will frequently result in a BCR that recognizes the individual's own antigens, which may result in attack on "self" antigens expressed on various tissue and organs. Many of these "autoreactive" B cells are eliminated in the bone marrow. Most of the developing B cells undergo apoptosis. This entire process is referred to as clonal deletion or central tolerance.

5. Treg cells are a diverse group of T cells that control the immune response, usually suppressing the response and maintaining tolerance against self-antigens. Treg cells produce very high levels of immunosuppressive cytokines, which induce tolerance.
6. The process of T-cell proliferation and differentiation is similar to that for B cells. The primary lymphoid organ for T-cell development is the thymus. Lymphoid stem cells travel through the thymus, where they gain a TCR, and receptors become immunocompetent. Self-reactive T cells undergo clonal deletion.
7. Proteins called *CD4* and *CD8* are expressed on the developing T cells. As the cell matures, it retains either the CD4 molecule or the CD8 molecule but not both. Eventually, CD4 cells develop into T-helper cells (Th cells), and CD 8 cells become T-cytotoxic cells (Tc cells). Other mature T cells include T-regulatory cells (Treg cells) and memory cells.
8. The generation of clonal diversity concludes when immunocompetent T and B cells migrate from the primary lymphoid organs into the circulation and secondary lymphoid organs to await antigen.

Induction of the Adaptive Immune Response

1. The induction of an immune response, or clonal selection, begins when antigen enters the individual's body and interacts with antigen-presenting cells (APCs) (e.g., dendritic cells, macrophages, and B cells).
2. To induce an optimal cellular or humoral immune response, APCs must present antigens to Th cells. Antigen is processed in the APCs and presented on the cell surface by molecules of the major histocompatibility complex (MHC). The particular MHC molecule (class I or class II) that presents antigen determines which cell will respond to that antigen. Th cells require that the antigen be presented in a complex with MHC class II molecules. MHC class II molecules are found only on APCs. Tc cells require that the antigen be presented by MHC class I molecules.
3. The T cell binds to the presented antigen through the TCR and accessory molecules: CD4 or CD8. CD4 is found on Th cells and reacts specifically with MHC class II. CD8 is found on Tc cells and reacts specifically with MHC class I.
4. Further differentiation of these Th0 cells results in the formation of Th1 cells, which help Tc cells respond to antigen; Th2 cells, which help B cells develop into plasma cells; and Th17 cells, which help activate macrophages.

Humoral Immunity (Antibodies)

1. The humoral immune response consists of molecules (antibodies) produced by B cells. B cells are lymphocytes. B cells can detect antigen with their BCR molecules and differentiate into APCs that interact closely with Th cells.
2. Th cell activation by B cells results in the production of IL-4, which, along with costimulatory molecules CD40 and CD40L, activate the B cell to become an antibody-producing plasma cell.
3. B cells can also be activated to become antibody-producing plasma cells through a T-cell independent process.
4. A typical antibody molecule is constructed of two identical heavy chains and two identical light chains (either κ or λ) and has two Fab portions that bind antigen and an Fc portion that interacts with complement or receptors on cells.
5. Antibodies are plasma glycoproteins that can be classified by chemical structure and biologic activity as immunoglobulin G (IgG), IgM, IgA, IgE, or IgD.
6. The protective effects of antibodies may be *direct* through the action of antibody alone or *indirect*, requiring activation of other components of the innate immune response.
7. IgE is a special class of antibody produced against environmental antigens that are the primary cause of common allergies. It also protects the individual from infection by large parasitic worms (helminths).
8. The secretory immune system protects the external surfaces of the body through the secretion of antibodies in bodily secretions, such as tears, sweat, saliva, mucus, and breast milk. IgA is the dominant secretory immunoglobulin.

Cell-Mediated Immunity

1. The cells of cell-mediated immunity include Tc cells, NK cells, and macrophages. These cells kill damaged, cancerous, or infected cells,
2. Tc cells bind with antigen presented on the MHC I molecule on an APC. This, along with IL-2 from Th cells, activates the Tc cell.
3. Tc cell attachment to a target cell activates multiple killing mechanisms through which the target cell is induced to undergo apoptosis.
4. Natural killer (NK) cells are a special group of lymphoid cells that express various cell surface activation receptors that identify protein changes on the surface of cells infected with viruses or that have become cancerous. After attachment, the NK cell kills its target like that of Tc cells.
5. Macrophages are activated by interferon-γ (IFN-γ). From Th1 cells. Activated M1 macrophages secrete proinflammatory cytokines and kill infected cells within their phagolysosomes.

Immunologic Memory

1. When T and B cells are activated, they make long-lived copies of themselves called memory cells.
2. Upon re-exposure, these memory cells will rapidly become new plasma cells or effector T cells

Pediatric Considerations: Age-Related Factors Affecting Mechanisms of Self-Defense in the Newborn Child

1. Neonates often have a transiently depressed inflammatory function, particularly neutrophil chemotaxis and alternative complement pathway activity.
2. The T cell-independent immune response is adequate in the fetus and neonate, but the T cell-dependent immune response develops slowly during the first 6 months of life.
3. Maternal IgG antibodies are transported across the placenta into the fetal blood and protect the neonate for the first 6 months, after which they are replaced by the child's own antibodies.

Geriatric Considerations: Age-Related Factors Affecting Mechanisms of Self-Defense in the Elderly

1. Elderly persons are at risk for impaired wound healing, usually because of chronic illnesses.
2. T-cell function declines, and the relative kind of T cells produced is altered in elderly persons.
3. Elderly individuals also develop impaired humoral immunity and are at risk for increased levels of circulating autoantibodies (antibodies against self-antigens).

REFERENCES

1. Mahe E, Pugh T, Kamel-Reid S. T cell clonality assessment: past, present and future. *J Clin Pathol.* 2018;71(3):195–200.
2. Panda SK, Colonna M. Innate lymphoid cells in mucosal immunity. *Front Immunol.* 2019;10:861.
3. Kavazovic I, Polic B, Wensveen FM. Cheating the hunger games; mechanisms controlling clonal diversity of CD8 effector and memory populations. *Front Immunol.* 2018;9:2831.
4. Grover P, Goel PN., Greene MI. Regulatory T cells: Regulation of identity and function. *Front Immunol.* 2021;12:4061.
5. Kumar P, et al. Restoring self-tolerance in autoimmune diseases by enhancing regulatory T-cells. *Cell Immunol.* 2019;339:41–49.
6. Mukhatayev Z, et al. Engineered antigen-specific regulatory T cells for autoimmune skin conditions. *Autoimmun Rev.* 2021;20(3):102761.
7. Ugur M, Mueller SN. T cell and dendritic cell interactions in lymphoid organs: more than just being in the right place at the right time. *Immunol Rev.* 2019;289(1):115–128.
8. D'Alicandro V, et al. Role of genetic variations on MHC class I antigen-processing genes in human cancer and viral-mediated diseases. *Mol Immunol.* 2019;113:11–15.
9. Jongsma MLM, Guarda G, Spaapen RM. The regulatory network behind MHC class I expression. *Mol Immunol.* 2019;113:16–21.
10. Jurewicz MM, Stern LJ. Class II MHC antigen processing in immune tolerance and inflammation. *Immunogenetics.* 2019;71(3):171–187.
11. Lees JR. Targeting antigen presentation in autoimmunity. *Cell Immunol.* 2019;339:4–9.
12. Ruiz de Morales JMG, et al. Critical role of interleukin (IL)-17 in inflammatory and immune disorders: an updated review of the evidence focusing in controversies. *Autoimmun Rev.* 2020;19(1):102429.
13. Kier ME, et al. The role of IL-22 in intestinal health and disease. *J Exp Med.* 2020;217(3):e20192195.
14. Cyster JG, Allen CDC. B cell responses: cell interaction dynamics and decisions. *Cell.* 2019;177(3):524–540.
15. McCraw AJ, et al. Insights from IgE immune surveillance in allergy and cancer for anti-tumour IgE treatments. *Cancers (Basel).* 2021; 13(17):4460.
16. Catanzaro JR, et al. IgA-deficient humans exhibit gut microbiota dysbiosis despite secretion of compensatory IgM. *Nat Sci Rep.* 2019;9:13574.
17. Posner J, et al. Monoclonal antibodies: past, present and future. *Handb Exp Pharmacol.* 2019;260:81–141.
18. Sivaccumar J, et al. Monoclonal antibodies: a prospective and retrospective view. *Curr Med Chem.* 2021;28(3):435–471.
19. Tanaka J. Recent advances in chimeric antigen receptor natural killer cell therapy for overcoming intractable hematological malignancies. *Hematol Oncol.* 2021;39(1):11–19.
20. Zhang C, Hu Y, Shi C. Targeting natural killer cells for tumor immunotherapy. *Front Immunol.* 2020;11:60.
21. Temming AR, et al. Functional attributes of antibodies, effector cells, and target cells affecting NK cell–mediated antibody-dependent cellular cytotoxicity. *J Immunol.* 2019;203(12):3126–3135.
22. Kavazović I, et al. Eomes broadens the scope of CD8 T-cell memory by inhibiting apoptosis in cells of low affinity. *PLoS Biol.* 2020;18(3):e3000648.

Alterations in Immunity

Valentina L. Brashers

http://evolve.elsevier.com/Rogers/pathophysiology/

CHAPTER OUTLINE

Innate and adaptive immunity serve to fight infection, remove diseased tissue, and promote healing. The innate immune system reacts quickly to virtually any form of injury or invasion primarily through the activation of inflammation. Adaptive immunity is a slower protective response system designed to recognize and remove antigens expressed by disease causing agents and to provide long-term immunity. These defensive systems are fine-tuned networks, but they are not perfect. There are two major categories of immune dysfunction: (1) excessive or misdirected responses, and (2) inadequate responses (immunocompromise) (Algorithm 9.1).

Excessive or misdirected innate immunity is the cause of tissue damage in most acute and chronic diseases. For example, chronic inflammation of the blood vessels leads to atherosclerosis and heart disease. In chronic obstructive lung disease (COPD), inflammation destroys the architecture of lung tissue. An excessive innate immune response also can lead to systemic complications of acute injury or infection. In the case of severe infection, an uncontrolled systemic inflammatory response can lead to septic shock, failure of multiple organs, and death (see Chapter 48). Excessive inflammation like that seen in coronavirus disease 2019 (COVID-19) infection (see Chapter 10) results in overwhelming lung injury and respiratory failure.[1]

Excessive or misdirected adaptive immune responses result in what are called hypersensitivity reactions. These reactions may be (1) exaggerated against noninfectious environmental substances (allergy); (2) misdirected against the body's own cells (autoimmunity); or (3) directed against beneficial foreign issues, such as transfusions or transplants (alloimmunity). Several of these inappropriate responses can be serious or life-threatening.

Immune responses that are insufficient to protect the host against pathogens and abnormal or foreign cells (immune deficiency) may be the result of inherited or acquired immune defects. Immunocompromise often is caused by therapies aimed at treating other conditions such as cancer. This chapter will describe the mechanisms of hypersensitivity reactions with examples of allergy, autoimmunity, and alloimmunity. This will be followed by a summary of selected inherited and acquired immune deficiency diseases. Many other autoimmune and immune deficiency diseases are covered in detail in later chapters in this textbook.

HYPERSENSITIVITY REACTIONS

A hypersensitivity reaction is an altered immunologic response to an antigen that results in disease or damage to the individual. Hypersensitivity reactions can be classified by the immunologic mechanism that causes disease. These mechanisms have been divided into four distinct types: *type I* (immunoglobulin E [IgE]-mediated reactions), *type II* (tissue-specific reactions), *type III* (immune complex–mediated reactions), and *type IV* (cell-mediated reactions) (Table 9.1). The four mechanisms are interrelated, and in most hypersensitivity reactions, several mechanisms can be functioning simultaneously or sequentially.

Immunologic Mechanisms of Hypersensitivity Reactions

Although the inflammatory responses of the innate immune system cause much of the tissue damage associated with hypersensitivity reactions, the mechanisms that initiate inflammation and tissue damage involve misdirected or excessive responses of the adaptive immune system. Hypersensitivity reactions are complicated, but an understanding of these mechanisms is essential to providing appropriate management of the many disorders that result from them.

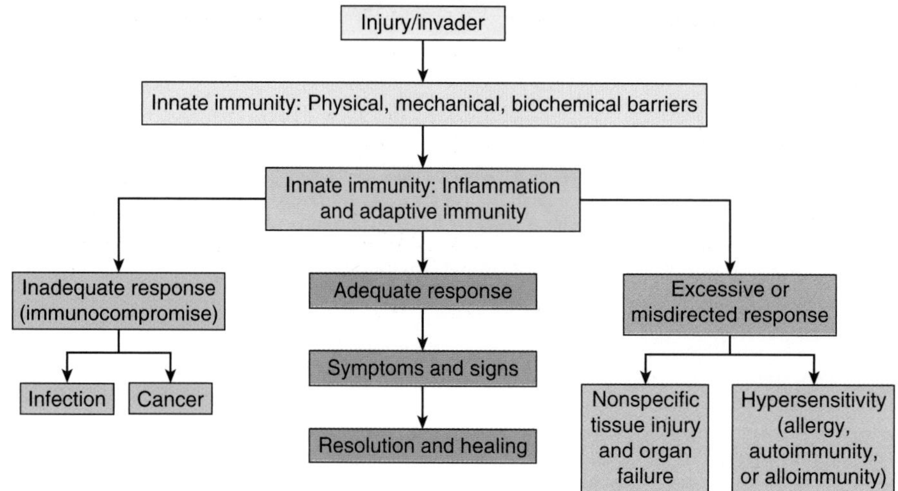

Algorithm 9.1 Overview of Immune Responses. Innate and adaptive immune defense mechanisms function to fight infection, remove diseased tissue, and promote healing. An adequate immune response often causes symptoms and signs such as pain, swelling, and redness but leads to resolution of injury and healing. However, immune responses may be excessive or misdirected, resulting in tissue injury which can be nonspecific or related to hypersensitivity reactions (e.g., allergy, autoimmunity, and alloimmunity). Immune responses may also be inadequate and result in systemic immunocompromise that may lead to overwhelming infection or cancer.

TABLE 9.1 Immunologic Mechanisms of Hypersensitivity Reactions

Type	Name	Mechanism of Hypersensitivity	Clinical Examples
I	Immunoglobulin E (IgE)-mediated reaction	T helper 2 cells produce high levels of interleukin-4, leading to B-cell activation and subsequent plasma cell production of IgE antibody. IgE binds to mast cell receptors resulting in their immediate degranulation and release of histamine, leukotrienes, and other inflammatory mediators.	Allergic rhinitis, Asthma, Anaphylaxis
II	Tissue-specific reaction	Altered self-antigens on tissues are bound by autoantibodies resulting in tissue destruction by complement, macrophages, neutrophils, or natural killer cells. Some autoantibodies bind to hormone or neurotransmitter receptors causing decreased or increased receptor activation.	Autoimmune hemolytic anemia, Heparin-induced thrombocytopenia, Graves disease, Myasthenia gravis
III	Immune complex–mediated reaction	Antibodies are formed to circulating antigens resulting in the formation of immune complexes that deposit in tissues. These immune complexes activate complement and neutrophils resulting in tissue destruction.	Systemic lupus erythematosus, Raynaud phenomenon
IV	Cell-mediated reaction	T helper 1 cells produce interferon gamma resulting in the activation of macrophages and T cytotoxic cells that attack the target cell through the release of destructive enzymes. In some cases, destruction of an invader is not possible, and granuloma formation walls it off from the rest of the body	Contact sensitivity to poison ivy and latex, Mycobacterial infection

Type I: IgE-Mediated Hypersensitivity Reactions

Type I hypersensitivity reactions are mediated by antigen-specific IgE and the products of tissue mast cells (Fig. 9.1). Most common allergic reactions are type I reactions against environmental antigens (e.g., pollen, bee venom, nuts, medications). Individuals who are genetically predisposed to this type of hypersensitivity generate an inappropriate IgE-mediated response to what would otherwise be an innocuous exposure. Most commonly, the term *allergy* indicates IgE-mediated reactions. However, some allergic reactions can be caused by other adaptive immune mechanisms, and IgE can contribute to some autoimmune and alloimmune diseases.

Mechanisms of type I, IgE-mediated hypersensitivity reactions. Type I hypersensitivity reactions require *sensitization* against a particular environmental antigen (allergen) that results in a primary immune response. The response occurs when the immune system first encounters an antigen (primary exposure) and forms antigen-specific memory B cells and T cells (immunologic memory). Disease symptoms appear after secondary exposure to the offending antigen when memory cells are rapidly activated against the same antigen (see Chapter 8). These reactions occur within minutes to a few hours after exposure to antigen and are termed immediate hypersensitivity reactions.

When allergens enter the body of a genetically predisposed individual, they are detected by dendritic cells and B cells, then undergo antigen processing and presentation (Fig. 9.1A). T helper (Th) cells are activated to produce large amounts of the Th2 cytokines, especially interleukin (IL)-4, IL-5, and IL-13. High levels of IL-4 and IL-13 cause B cells to proliferate and become plasma cells that produce antigen-specific IgE. IL-5 recruits and activates eosinophils, which contain granules full of enzymes that are especially damaging to the respiratory system (see Chapter 36). Other interleukins such as IL-9 and IL-33 also play a role in exacerbating type I hypersensitivity reactions.[2,3]

IgE has a relatively short life span in blood because it rapidly binds to Fc receptors (antibody receptors) on mast cells. The Fc receptors on mast cells specifically bind IgE that has not previously interacted with antigen. After a large amount of IgE has bound to the mast cells, an individual is considered *sensitized*. When there is a secondary or reexposure of a sensitized individual to the allergen, the IgE antibodies signal the mast cells to degranulate and release mediators.

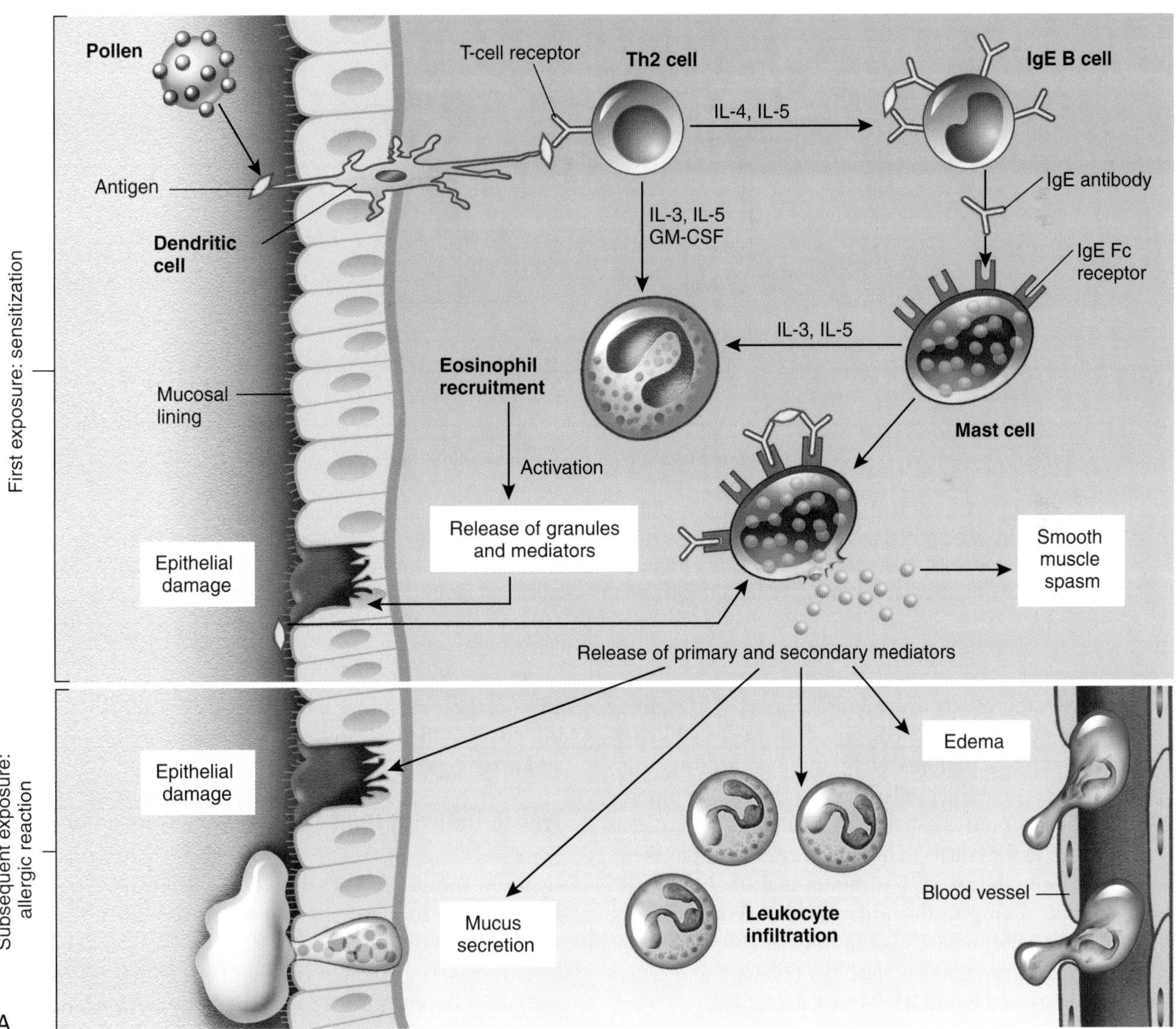

Fig. 9.1 Mechanism of Type I, Immunoglobulin E (IgE)-Mediated Reactions. (A) Th2 cells are activated by antigen-presenting dendritic cells to produce cytokines, including IL-4 and IL-5. IL-5 attracts and promotes the survival of eosinophils. High levels of IL-4 induce B cells to class-switch to IgE-producing plasma cells. The IgE coats the surface of the mast cell by binding with IgE-specific Fc receptors on the mast cell's plasma membrane (sensitization). Further exposure to the same allergen cross-links the surface-bound IgE and activates signals from the cytoplasmic portion of the IgE Fc receptors. These signals initiate two parallel and interdependent processes: mast cell degranulation and discharge of preformed mediators (e.g., histamine, chemotactic factors) and production of newly formed mediators such as leukotrienes and prostaglandins. Type I hypersensitivity reactions have two well-defined phases. On first exposure, there is an initial phase characterized by vasodilation, vascular leakage, and, depending on the location, smooth muscle spasm. Eosinophils contribute to mucosal epithelial cell damage. Subsequent exposures are characterized by infiltration of tissues with more eosinophils and with other inflammatory leukocytes resulting in prolonged epithelial cell damage and mucus secretion.

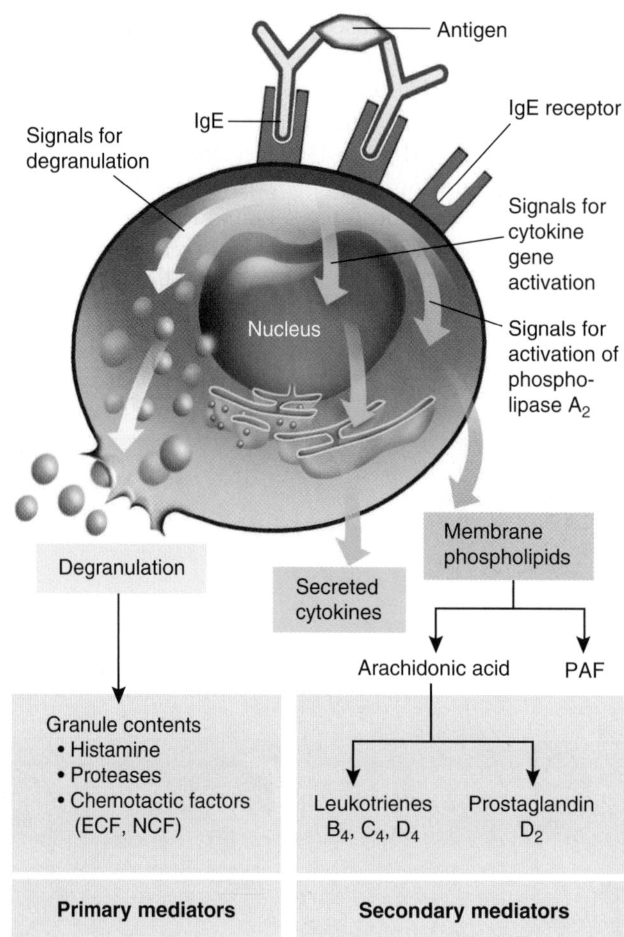

Fig. 9.1, cont'd (B) Activation of mast cells leading to degranulation of preformed mediators (primary mediators) and synthesis of newly formed (de novo) mediators (secondary mediators). *ECF*, Eosinophilic chemotactic factor; *Fc*, fragment crystallizable; *Ig*, immunoglobulin; *IL*, interleukin; *NCF*, neutrophil chemotactic factor; *PAF*, platelet-activating factor; *Th*, T helper.

Mast cells release a variety of cytokines (Fig. 9.1B). Histamine is the most potent preformed mediator of IgE-mediated hypersensitivity. Histamine acts immediately (within 15 to 30 minutes) and affects several key target cells. The tissues most commonly affected by type I responses contain large numbers of mast cells and are sensitive to the effects of histamine released from them. These tissues are found in the gastrointestinal tract, skin, and respiratory tract. Acting through histamine 1 (H1) receptors, histamine contracts bronchial smooth muscles (bronchial constriction), increases vascular permeability (edema), and causes vasodilation (increased blood flow) (see Chapter 7).

Mast cells also synthesize secondary mediators, such as leukotrienes, prostaglandins, and platelet activating factor, which act more slowly (within hours) and have effects similar to that of histamine (see Fig. 9.1B). These newly formed mediators also attract other immune cells (e.g., eosinophils, neutrophils, basophils, monocytes), activate kinins, and initiate the complement cascade with release of the anaphylatoxins C3a, C4a, and C5a (see Chapter 7). These mediators are responsible for a late phase reaction that sets in 2 to 24 hours later even without additional exposure to antigen and may last for several days. The overall effect of these cytokines is inflammation of affected tissues leading to vasodilation, mucous secretion, bronchoconstriction, and tissue injury.

Type II: Tissue-Specific Hypersensitivity Reactions

Type II hypersensitivities are generally immune reactions against a specific cell or tissue. Cells express a variety of antigens on their surfaces, some of which are called tissue-specific antigens because they are expressed on the membranes of only certain cells. For example, platelets have groups of antigens that are found on no other cells of the body. Environmental antigens (e.g., drugs or their metabolites) may bind to the plasma membranes of specific cells and function as haptens, making them targets of type II reactions. The three general mechanisms by which type II hypersensitivity reactions can affect cells are complement mediated lysis, antibody-dependent cellular cytotoxicity, and antireceptor antibodies (Fig. 9.2). Each mechanism begins with antibody binding to tissue-specific antigens or antigens present on particular tissues. The symptoms of many type II diseases are determined by which tissue or organ expresses the particular antigen.

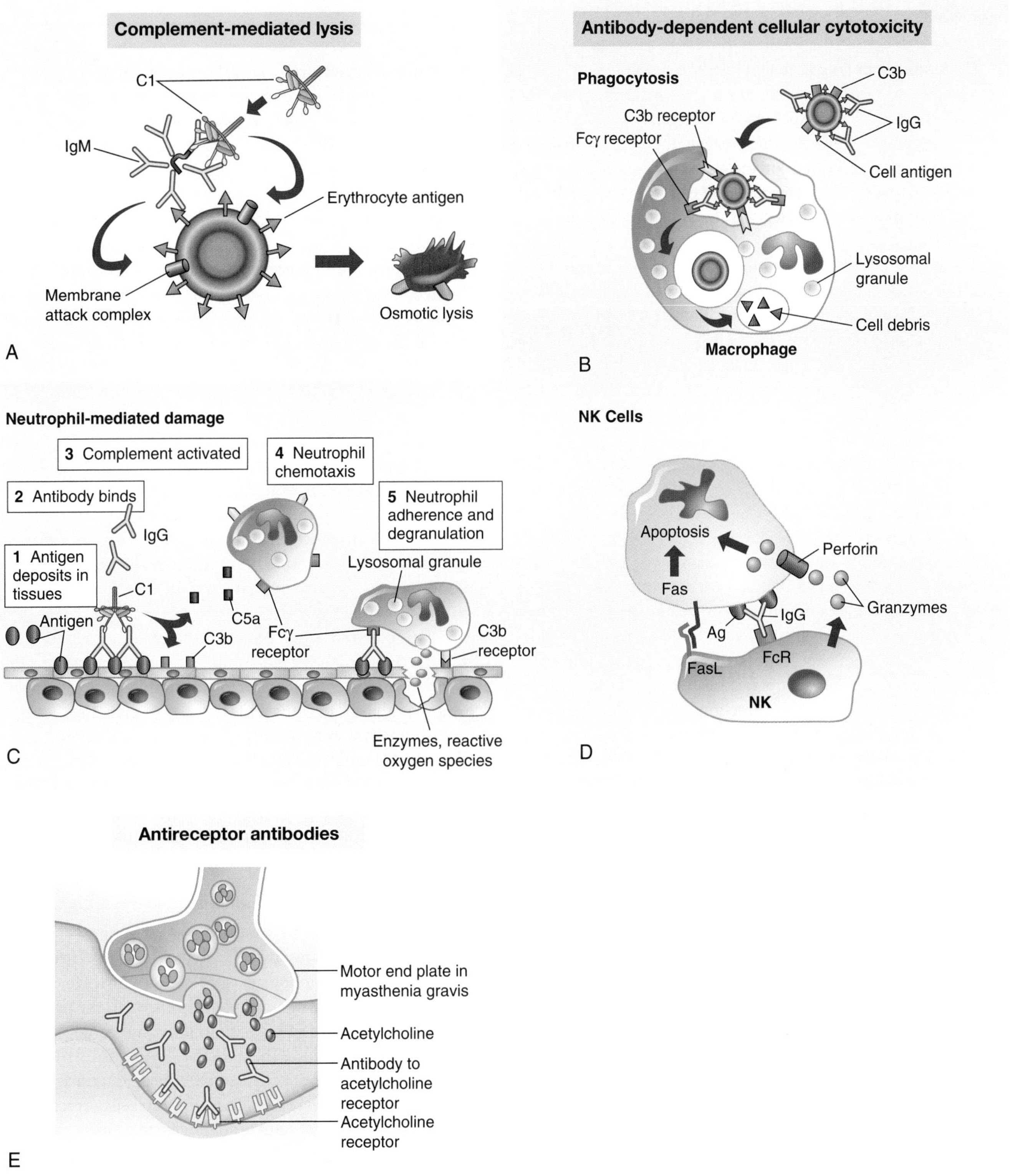

Complement-mediated lysis

C1

IgM

Erythrocyte antigen

Membrane attack complex

Osmotic lysis

A

Antibody-dependent cellular cytotoxicity

Phagocytosis

C3b

C3b receptor

IgG

Fcγ receptor

Cell antigen

Lysosomal granule

Cell debris

Macrophage

B

Neutrophil-mediated damage

3 Complement activated

4 Neutrophil chemotaxis

2 Antibody binds

5 Neutrophil adherence and degranulation

IgG

1 Antigen deposits in tissues

C1

Lysosomal granule

C5a

Antigen

C3b

Fcγ receptor

C3b receptor

Enzymes, reactive oxygen species

C

NK Cells

Apoptosis

Perforin

Fas

Granzymes

IgG

Ag

FcR

FasL

NK

D

Antireceptor antibodies

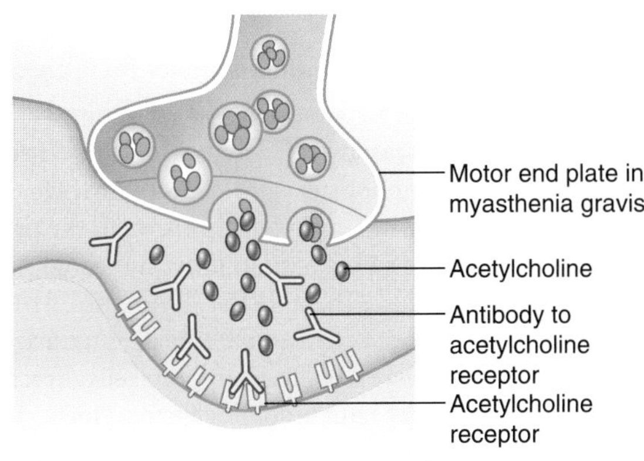

E

Fig. 9.2 Mechanisms of Type II, Tissue-Specific Reactions. Antigens on the target cell bind with antibody and are destroyed or prevented from functioning by one of three mechanisms: *Complement-mediated lysis* **(A)** Complement binding to autoantibodies on a target cell (an erythrocyte target is illustrated here) results in destruction of the cell by the complement membrane attack complex. *Antibody-dependent cellular cytotoxicity* occurs through three processes: **(B)** Clearance (phagocytosis) by macrophages in the tissue; **(C)** Neutrophil-mediated immune destruction; **(D)** Apoptosis of target cells by natural killer (NK) cells by the release of granzymes and perforin and by the interactions of Fas ligand. *Antireceptor antibodies* **(E)** Modulation or blocking of the normal function of receptors by antireceptor antibody. This example of mechanism depicts myasthenia gravis in which acetylcholine receptor antibodies block acetylcholine from attaching to its receptors on the motor end plates of skeletal muscle, thereby impairing neuromuscular transmission and causing muscle weakness. *C1*, Complement component C1; *C3b*, complement fragment produced from C3, which acts as an opsonin; *C5a*, complement fragment produced from C5, which acts as a chemotactic factor for neutrophils; *Fcγ receptor*, cellular receptor for the Fc portion of IgG; *FcR*, Fc receptor.

Mechanisms of type II, tissue-specific reactions.

(1) *Complement-mediated lysis* occurs when antibodies (IgM or IgG) bound to tissue-specific antigens cause activation of the complement cascade through the classical pathway (Fig. 9.2A). Formation of the membrane attack complex (C5-9) damages the membrane and results in lysis of the cell. For example, erythrocytes are destroyed by complement-mediated lysis in individuals who have received mismatched transfused blood cells (see the section on Alloimmunity).

(2) *Antibody-dependent cell-mediated cytotoxicity (ADCC)* (Fig. 9.2B–D) occurs when antibodies bound to tissue-specific antigens activate macrophages, neutrophils, and natural killer (NK) cells, which attack the target cells. When antibodies activate complement, there is the deposition of C3b on the target cell surface. Receptors on macrophages and neutrophils recognize and bind these opsonins (antibody plus C3b) and increase phagocytosis of the target cell (see Fig. 9.2B). Toxic products produced by neutrophils (lysozymes and toxic oxygen radicals) also cause tissue damage (Fig. 9.2C). ADCC also involves NK cells (Fig. 9.2D). Antibodies on the target cell are recognized by Fc receptors on NK cells, which release toxic substances that destroy the target cell. Examples of ADCC include autoimmune conditions in which autoantibodies are made against antigens on platelets or red blood cells causing them to be removed by phagocytes in the spleen.

(3) *Antireceptor antibodies* do not destroy the target cell but rather cause the cell to malfunction (Fig. 9.2E). These autoantibodies change the function of the target receptor by blocking, overstimulating, or destroying it. For example, in Graves disease, autoantibodies called thyroid-stimulating immunoglobulins (TSIs) bind to and activate receptors for thyroid-stimulating hormone (TSH) on thyroid gland cells. TSH normally stimulates thyroid hormone secretion but is under the control of feedback mechanisms. When TSIs bind to the TSH receptors, they stimulate the thyroid cells to overproduce thyroxine, thus producing symptoms of hyperthyroidism (see Chapter 22).

Type III: Immune Complex–Mediated Hypersensitivity Reactions

Type III hypersensitivity disease reactions are caused by antigen-antibody (immune) complexes that are formed in the circulation and are deposited in vessel walls or other tissues (Fig. 9.3). The primary difference between type II and type III mechanisms is that in type II hypersensitivity, antibody binds to antigen on the cell surface, whereas in type III, antibody binds to soluble antigen that was released into blood or body fluids.

Mechanisms of type III, immune-mediated hypersensitivity reactions. When antibodies bind to circulating antigens, immune complexes are then deposited in vascular tissues. Type III reactions are not organ specific and most commonly result in a vasculitis in the skin, kidney, or lungs. The harmful effects of immune complex deposition are caused by complement activation and by neutrophils attempting to phagocytose the immune complexes. During the attempted phagocytosis, large quantities of lysosomal enzymes are released into the inflammatory site instead of into phagolysosomes. The attraction of neutrophils and the subsequent release of lysosomal enzymes cause most of the resulting tissue damage. Two prototypic models of type III hypersensitivity help to explain the variety of diseases in this category. Serum sickness is a model of systemic type III hypersensitivities, and the *Arthus reaction* is a model of localized or cutaneous reactions.

Serum sickness–type reactions are caused by the formation of immune complexes in the blood and their subsequent generalized deposition in target tissues. A form of serum sickness is Raynaud phenomenon, a condition caused by the temperature-dependent deposition of immune complexes in the capillary beds of the peripheral circulation. Certain immune complexes precipitate at temperatures less than normal body temperature, particularly in the tips of the fingers, toes, and nose, and are called cryoglobulins. The precipitates block the circulation and cause localized pallor and numbness, followed by cyanosis (a bluish tinge resulting from oxygen deprivation) and eventually gangrene if the circulation is not restored.

Arthus reaction is vasculitis caused by repeated local exposure to an antigen that reacts with preformed antibody and forms immune complexes in the walls of the local blood vessels. Symptoms of Arthus reaction begin within 1 hour of exposure and peak 6 to 12 hours later. The lesions are characterized by a typical inflammatory reaction, with increased vascular permeability, an accumulation of neutrophils, edema, hemorrhage, clotting, and tissue damage. For example, gluten-sensitive enteropathy (celiac disease) follows ingestion of antigen, usually gluten from wheat products (see Chapter 42). Allergic alveolitis (farmer lung disease, pigeon breeder disease) is Arthus-like acute hemorrhagic inflammation of the air sacs (alveoli) of the lungs, resulting from inhalation of fungal antigens, usually particles from moldy hay or pigeon feces (see Chapter 35).

Type IV: Cell-Mediated Hypersensitivity Reactions

Types I, II, and III hypersensitivity reactions are mediated by antibodies, whereas type IV hypersensitivity reactions are mediated by T lymphocytes and do not involve antibodies (Fig. 9.4). Type IV mechanisms occur through the presentation of antigens on major histocompatibility molecules (MHCs) to T cells. Th cells produce Th1 and Th17 cytokines. Th1 and Th17 cytokines recruit and activate macrophages and cytotoxic T lymphocytes (Tc cells) (see Chapter 8). Tc cells directly kill target cells. Macrophages release soluble factors, such as lysosomal enzymes and toxic reactive oxygen species. Together, these responses cause tissue damage. The response is delayed, occurring 24 to 72 hours after antigen reexposure, compared with an immediate type I reaction, which occurs within minutes. The response is delayed because of the time it takes for sensitized T cells to travel to the site of antigen reexposure and the time needed to produce cytokines that activate other cells including macrophages (delayed hypersensitivity).

In some cases, Tc cells and macrophages cannot kill or remove the offending agent. In these cases, they surround and contain the invader through the formation of a *granuloma* (see Chapter 7). The formation of multiple granulomas can lead to tissue damage and organ dysfunction.

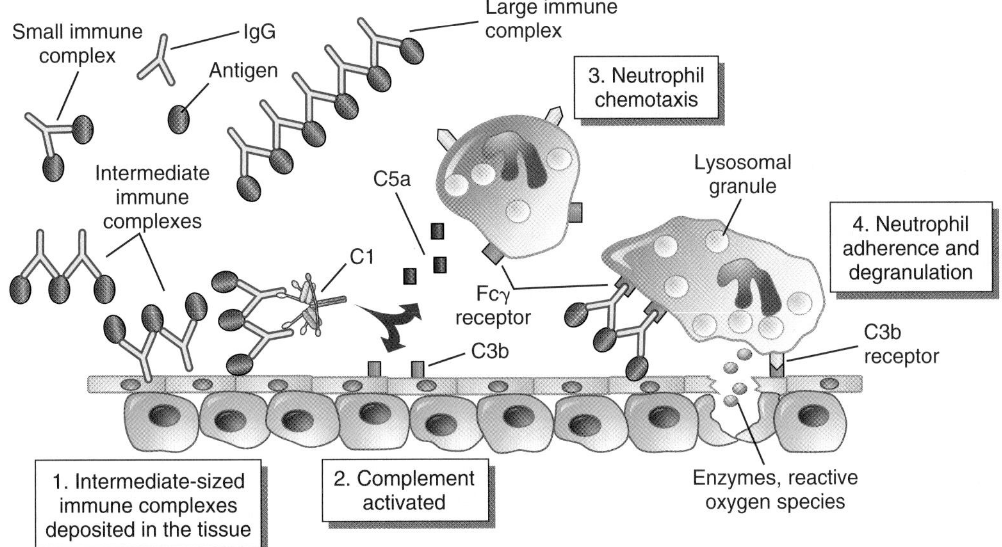

Fig. 9.3 Mechanism of Type III, Immune Complex–Mediated Reactions. Immune complexes form in the blood from circulating antigen and antibody. Both small and large immune complexes are removed successfully from the circulation and do not cause tissue damage. Intermediate-sized complexes are deposited in certain target tissues in which the circulation is slow or filtration of blood occurs. The complexes activate the complement cascade through C1 and generate fragments, including C5a and C3b. C5a is chemotactic for neutrophils, which migrate into the inflamed area and attach to the IgG and C3b in the immune complexes. The neutrophils attempt unsuccessfully to phagocytose the tissue and, in the process, release a variety of degradative enzymes that destroy the healthy tissues. Fcγ receptor is the cellular receptor for the Fc portion of immunoglobulin G.

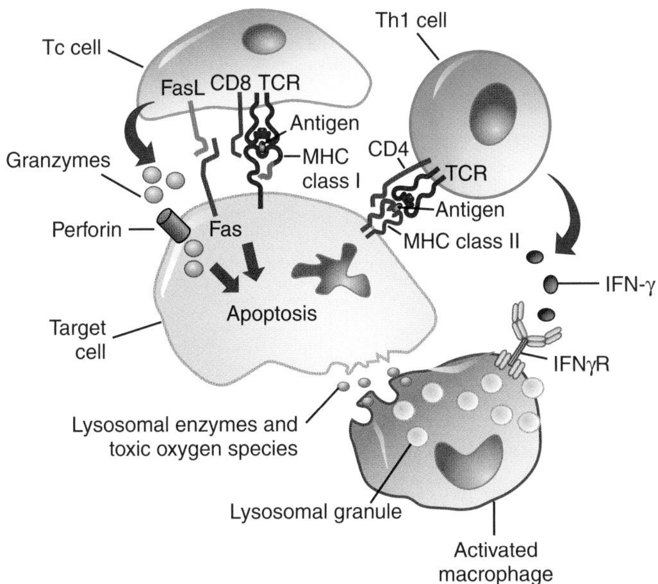

Fig. 9.4 Mechanism of Type IV, Cell-Mediated Reactions. Antigens from target cells stimulate T cells to differentiate into T cytotoxic cells (Tc cells), which have direct cytotoxic activity through release of granzymes or the induction of apoptosis via Fas and Fas ligand binding. T helper cells (Th1) cells produce lymphokines (especially interferon-γ) that activate macrophages through specific receptors (e.g., IFN-γ receptor). The macrophages can attach to targets and release enzymes and reactive oxygen species that are responsible for most of the tissue destruction. *FasL*, Fas ligand; *IFN-γ*, interferon-γ; *IFN-γR*, interferon-γ receptor; *MCH*, major histocompatibility complex; *TCR*, T cell receptor.

Mechanisms of type IV cell-mediated hypersensitivity reactions. Clinical examples of type IV hypersensitivity reactions include graft rejection, reaction on the skin test for tuberculosis, and allergic reactions resulting from skin contact with some substances, such as poison ivy and metals. A type IV component also may be present in many autoimmune diseases. For example, T cells against type II collagen (a protein present in joint tissues) contribute to the destruction of joints in rheumatoid arthritis, and T cells against an antigen on the surface of pancreatic beta cells (the cell that normally produces insulin) are responsible for beta-cell destruction in insulin-dependent (type 1) diabetes mellitus.

In 1891, Ehrlich was the first to thoroughly describe type IV hypersensitivity reaction in the skin, leading to the development of a diagnostic skin test for tuberculosis. The reaction follows an intradermal injection of tuberculin antigen (purified protein derivative [PPD]) into an individual who has latent or active tuberculosis and is therefore sensitized (has developed adaptive immune cells against tuberculosis antigen). After 24 to 72 hours the reaction site becomes infiltrated with T lymphocytes and macrophages, resulting in a clear hard center (induration) and a reddish surrounding area (erythema). The reaction is referred to as a positive skin test result (i.e., positive PPD) for tuberculosis infection.

Allergic type IV reactions are elicited by some environmental antigens that are haptens and become immunogenic after binding to larger (carrier) proteins in the individual. In allergic contact dermatitis, the carrier protein is in the skin. The best-known example is the reaction to poison ivy (Fig. 9.5). The

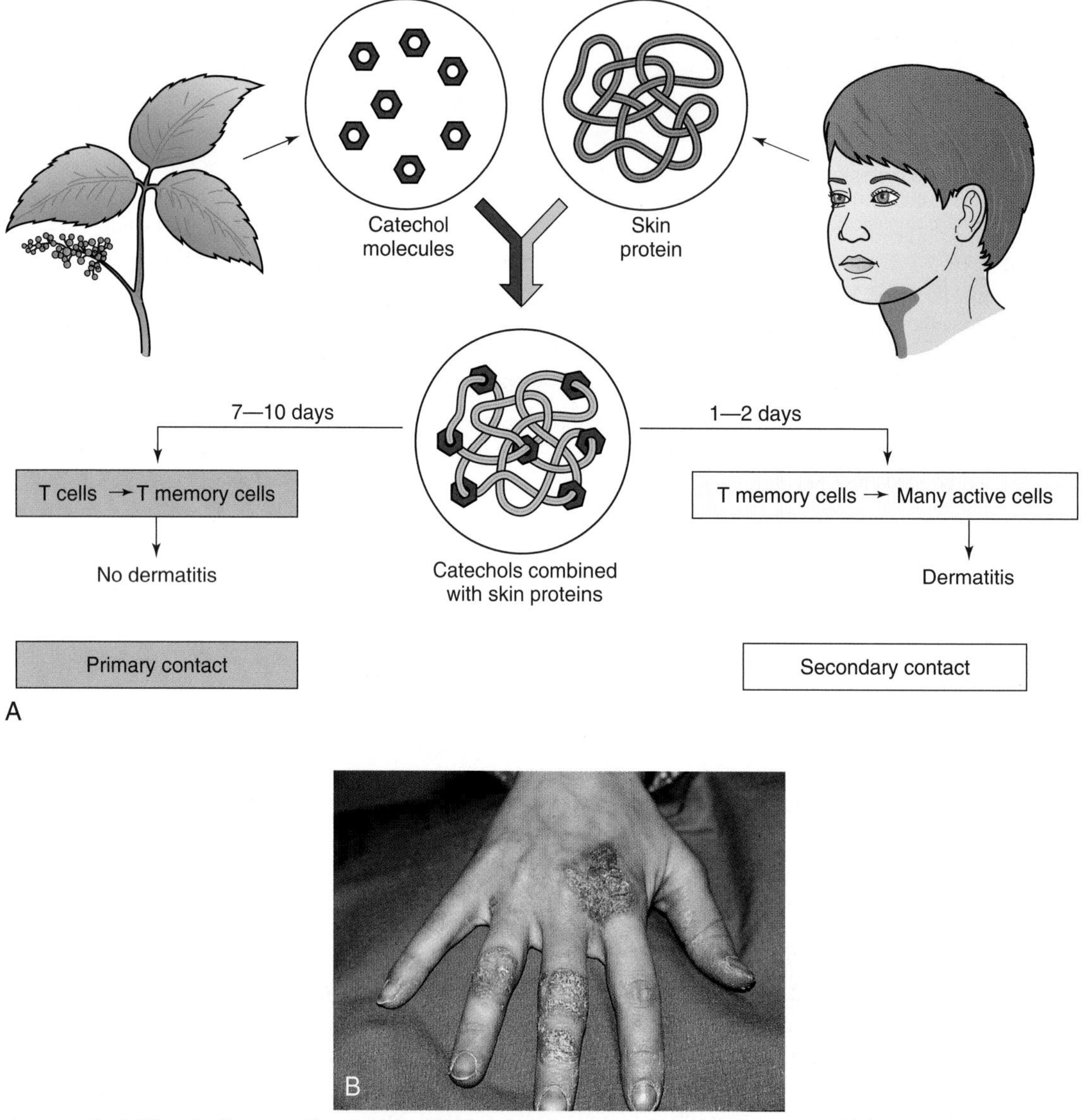

Fig. 9.5 Development of Allergic Contact Dermatitis. (A) The development of type IV hypersensitivity to poison ivy. The first (primary) contact with allergen sensitizes (produces reactive T cells) the individual but does not produce a rash (dermatitis). Secondary contact activates a type IV cell-mediated reaction that causes dermatitis. **(B)** Contact dermatitis caused by a delayed hypersensitivity reaction leading to vesicles and scaling at the sites of contact. From Damjanov I, Linder J. *Anderson's pathology,* 10th edition. St. Louis: Mosby; 1996.

antigen is a plant catechol, urushiol, which reacts with normal skin proteins and evokes a cell-mediated immune response. Skin reactions to industrial chemicals, cosmetics, detergents, clothing, food, metals, and topical medicines (e.g., penicillin) are elicited by the same mechanism. Contact dermatitis consists of lesions only at the site of contact with the allergen, as in metal allergy to jewelry.

Antigenic Targets of Hypersensitivity Reactions

The four types of hypersensitivity reactions contribute to tissue damage and clinical diseases in a variety of ways. Often, several mechanisms of hypersensitivity are active at the same time. The three major types of hypersensitivity disorders are allergy, autoimmunity, and alloimmunity. The mechanisms that initiate the onset of hypersensitivity reactions are not completely understood. It is generally accepted that genetic and environmental agents are contributing factors.

Allergy

Allergy (atopy) refers to hypersensitivity to environmental antigens. These can include medicines, natural products (e.g., pollens, bee stings), infectious agents, and any other antigen that is not naturally found in the individual. Allergies are the most common hypersensitivity reactions. The majority of allergies are type I IgE-mediated reactions. These reactions usually lead to relatively mild symptoms such as rhinitis and sneezing. However, in some individuals, these reactions can be excessive and life-threatening (anaphylaxis). Antigens that cause allergic responses are called allergens. Typical allergens include pollens (e.g., ragweed), molds and fungi (e.g., *Penicillium chrysogenum*), foods (e.g., milk, eggs, fish), animals (e.g., cat dander, dog dander), cigarette smoke, and components of house dust (e.g., fecal pellets of house mites). The most common forms of atopic disease are allergic rhinitis, bronchial asthma, anaphylaxis, and atopic dermatitis (eczema).

Genetic predisposition and environmental factors. Genes and environment interact in complex ways in individuals with type I hypersensitivity.[4] Certain individuals are genetically predisposed to develop type I IgE-mediated hypersensitivity and are called *atopic*. In families in which one parent has an allergy, allergies develop in approximately 40% of the offspring. If both parents have allergies, the incidence in the offspring may be as high as 80%. Atopic individuals tend to produce higher quantities of IgE and to have more Fc receptors for IgE on their mast cells. The airways and the skin of atopic individuals are also more responsive to a wide variety of both specific and nonspecific stimuli than are the airways and skin of individuals who are not atopic. Multiple genes have been associated with the atopic state, including polymorphisms in a large variety of cytokines that regulate IgE synthesis (e.g., IL-4, IL-13) and cellular receptors.

The environment has a significant impact on allergic disease. Diet, medications, and comorbidities impact the microbiome and the health of the adaptive immune system (see Emerging Science Box: The Microbiome and Food Allergy).[5] In genetically predisposed individuals, exposure to large quantities of allergens and irritants in the environment can trigger symptoms. The role of infection in allergic disease is complex and may be protective or may render organ systems such as the respiratory tract more vulnerable to allergic symptoms.

Clinical symptoms of allergy. The clinical manifestations of allergy are attributable mostly to the biologic effects of histamine. Tissues most commonly affected contain large numbers of mast cells and are sensitive to the effects of histamine released from them. These tissues are found in the gastrointestinal tract, skin, and upper and lower respiratory tracts (Fig. 9.6). The particular symptoms frequently reflect the main portal of entry for the allergen. For instance, pollens and other airborne allergens usually cause respiratory symptoms.

Effects of allergens on the mucosa of the eyes, nose, and respiratory tract include conjunctivitis (inflammation of the membranes covering the front of the eye and the lining the eyelids), rhinitis (inflammation of the mucous membranes of the nose), and asthma (constriction and swelling of the bronchi). Symptoms of all these conditions are caused by vasodilation, hypersecretion of mucus, edema, and swelling of the mucosa. Because the mucous membranes lining the respiratory tract (accessory sinuses, nasopharynx, and upper and lower respiratory tracts) are continuous, they are all adversely affected. The degree to which each is affected determines the symptoms of the disease. One of the most common type I reactions is asthma. It is presented in detail in Chapter 35. The central problem in asthma is obstruction of the large and small airways (bronchi) of the lower respiratory tract by bronchospasm (constriction of smooth muscle in airway walls), edema, and thick secretions. This leads to ventilatory insufficiency, wheezing, and difficult or labored breathing.

Urticaria, or hives, is a dermal (skin) manifestation of type I allergic reactions (see Fig. 9.6). The underlying mechanism is the localized release of histamine and increased vascular permeability, resulting in limited areas of edema. Urticaria is characterized by white fluid-filled blisters (wheals) surrounded by areas of redness (flares). The wheal and flare reaction is usually accompanied by itching. Not all urticarial symptoms are caused by allergic (immunologic) reactions. Some, termed nonimmunologic urticaria, result from exposure to cold temperatures, emotional stress, medications, systemic diseases, hyperthyroidism, or malignancies (e.g., lymphomas).

EMERGING SCIENCE BOX

The Microbiome and Food Allergy

Last year, 6.5% of US children were reported to have a food allergy. Among the most common are allergies to nuts, peanuts, and shellfish. The mechanisms underlying food allergies remain unclear; however, several studies have found that dysbiosis in gut microbiome plays an important role. Within the gastrointestinal tract, finely tuned mechanisms enable nutrients to be broken down and absorbed without causing an immune reaction to food antigens. Gut microorganisms may modify food antigens thus increasing or reducing their immunogenicity. They also influence the effectiveness of intestinal barriers to antigens and infectious agents. A healthy gut microbiome induces tolerance to food antigens through several mechanisms including the differentiation of T cells into T regulatory cells. Dysbiosis of the gut microbiome has been linked to activation of B cells and the production of immunoglobulin E antibodies in atopic individuals. Environmental factors that have been associated with gut microbiome dysbiosis and food allergy include a low-fiber/high-fat diet, antibiotics, lack of breastfeeding, and medications. A maternal diet rich in fruits and vegetables, fish, vitamin D-rich foods is associated with a healthier microbiome and a lower risk of allergic disease in their offspring. Dietary changes for children (including the early introduction of foods like peanuts) and adults as well as the use of prebiotics or probiotics are being evaluated to assess their impact on the gut microbiome and the incidence of fool allergies.

Data from CDC National Center for Health Statistics. https://www.cdc.gov/nchs/fastats/allergies.htm; Berni Canani R, et al. Gut Microbiome as Target for Innovative Strategies Against Food Allergy. *Frontiers in Immunology*, 2019;10:191; Caminero A, et al. Mechanisms by which gut microorganisms influence food sensitivities. *Nature Reviews Gastroenterology and Hepatology*, 2019;16(1):7–18; Chernikova D, et al. Prevention of allergy with diverse and healthy microbiota: an update. *Current Opinion in Pediatrics*, 2019;31(3):418–425; Einstein M. The microbial ambassadors of the immune system. *Nature*, 2020; 588:S11–S13; Koidl L, et al. (2021) The clinical implications of the microbiome in the development of allergy diseases. Expert Rev. *Clin. Immunol.* 17(2),115–126; Lopez-Santamarina, A., et al (2021). Probiotics as a possible strategy for the prevention and treatment of allergies. Foods 10(4), 701; Shu SA, et al. Microbiota and food allergy. *Clinical Reviews in Allergy and Immunology*, 2019;57(1):83–97; Zhao W, et al. The gut microbiome in food allergy. *Annals of Allergy, Asthma, and Immunology*, 2019;122(3):276–282; Zheng D, et al. Interaction between microbiota and immunity in health and disease. *Cell Research*, 2020;30:492–506.

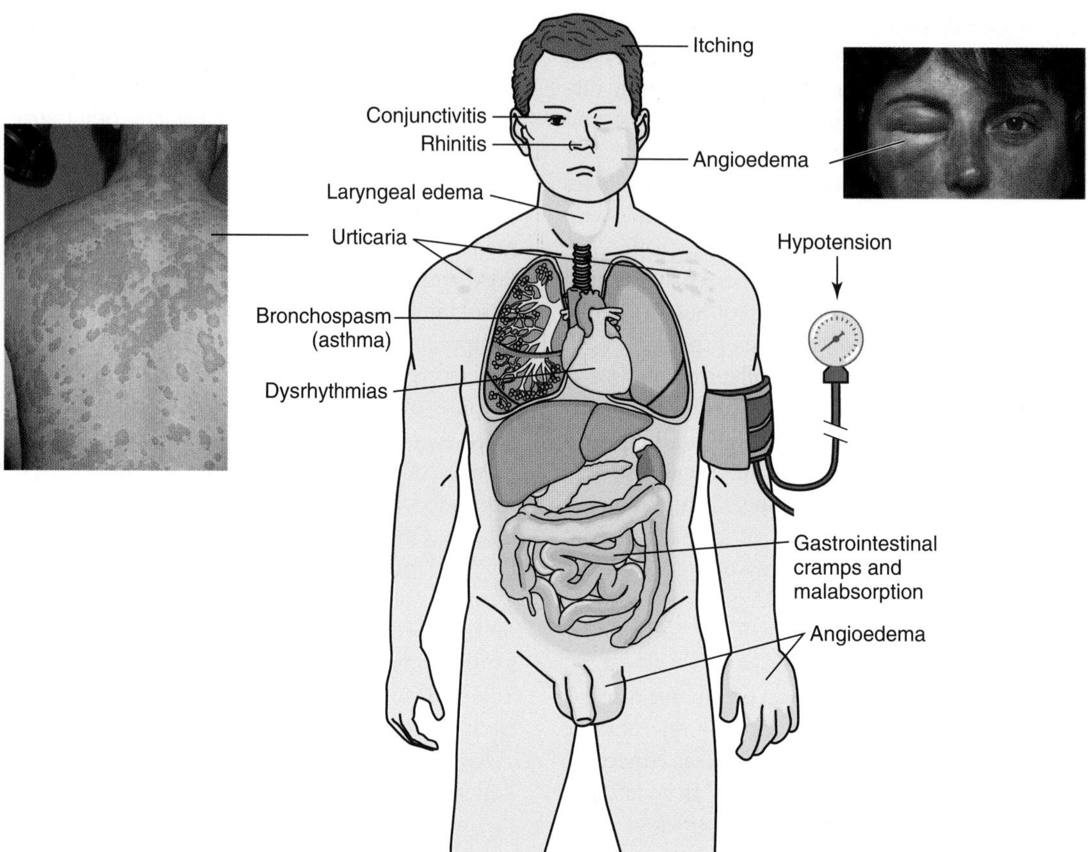

Fig. 9.6 Type I Hypersensitivity Reactions. Manifestations of allergic reactions as a result of type I hypersensitivity include pruritus, angioedema (swelling caused by exudation), edema of the larynx, urticaria (hives), bronchospasm (constriction of airways in the lungs), hypotension (low blood pressure), and dysrhythmias (irregular heartbeat) because of anaphylactic shock, and gastrointestinal cramping caused by inflammation of the gastrointestinal mucosa. Photographic inserts show a diffuse allergy-like eye and skin reaction on an individual. The skin lesions have raised edges and develop within minutes or hours, with resolution occurring after about 12 hours. (*Inserts* from Male D, Brostoff J, Roth D, et al. *Immunology*, 8th edition. St. Louis: Mosby; 2013.)

Gastrointestinal allergies are caused primarily by allergens that enter through the mouth—usually foods or medicines. When food is the allergen, the active immunogen may be a product of food breakdown by digestive enzymes. Acute symptoms usually occur rapidly (frequently within minutes) and include vomiting, diarrhea, or abdominal pain. Prolonged or recurrent reactions may result in malabsorption or protein-losing enteropathy. Systemic symptoms may range from urticaria to life-threatening anaphylactic reactions. The most common food allergies are tree nuts, peanuts, milk, shellfish, and fish. The prevalence of food allergies is estimated at 3% to 10% of adults and 8% of children worldwide.[6] The most rapid and severe allergic reaction is anaphylaxis. Anaphylaxis occurs within minutes of reexposure to the antigen and can be either systemic (generalized) or cutaneous (localized). Symptoms of systemic anaphylaxis include pruritus, erythema, vomiting, abdominal cramps, diarrhea, and breathing difficulties, and the most severe reactions may include contraction of bronchial smooth muscle, edema of the throat, and decreased blood pressure that can lead to shock and death (see Chapter 48). Examples of systemic anaphylaxis are allergic reactions to antibiotics, bee stings, or peanuts.

Diagnosis and management of allergic reactions. Several tests are available to diagnose allergic reactions, including skin tests and measurement of IgE in the blood. Reactivity to a particular allergen may be tested by controlled administration of small doses of the suspected allergen or injection of an allergen into (intradermal) or onto (epicutaneous or prick test) the skin. If the individual is allergic to a particular allergen, a local wheal and flare reaction may occur within a few minutes at the site of injection. A variety of immunoassays can be used can detect IgE antibodies in serum. These assays can be used to measure circulating levels of total IgE, or circulating levels of specific IgE antibodies against selected allergens.

If possible, avoidance of the allergen is the best method to limit allergic responses. Clinical desensitization to allergens can be achieved in some individuals. Minute quantities of the allergen are injected in increasing doses over a prolonged period. The procedure may reduce the severity of the allergic reaction in the treated individual.

Some type I allergic responses can be controlled by blocking histamine receptors with antihistamines. The effects of allergy on the respiratory system may require bronchodilators or medications that block leukotrienes (see Chapter 35). The most effective medications for allergic disease are the corticosteroids, which can be given by local administration (e.g., inhalers or topical ointments) or systemically to decrease tissue inflammation. For individuals with severe allergy, monoclonal antibodies that block IgE may be required (omalizumab). Other monoclonal antibodies that block IL-4 (dupilamab) and IL-5 (mepolizumab) are now available. In anaphylaxis, systemic administration of sympathomimetic medications such as epinephrine may be required to support the respiratory and cardiovascular systems (see Chapter 48).

Autoimmunity

Autoimmunity occurs when the immune system reacts against self-antigens to such a degree that autoantibodies or autoreactive T cells damage the individual's tissues. It is the result of a disturbance in the immunologic *tolerance* of self-antigens (see Chapter 8). This breakdown in tolerance is believed to occur in a genetically predisposed individual when there is some initiating event. Most often, the initiating event is unrecognized but is hypothesized to be an environmental factor such as infection or toxins, or some change in neurologic, endocrine, and/or immune status.

It is well established that autoimmune diseases can be familial. In familial cases, affected family members may not all have the same disease but rather may develop different autoimmune disorders. However, most autoimmune diseases appear as isolated events without a positive family history, and susceptibility for developing such diseases appears to be linked to a combination of multiple genes and multifactorial. Genetic associations with particular autoimmune diseases have been identified for a variety of major histocompatibility complex (MHC) genes (see Chapter 8). Some associations are strong; others are more tenuous. Autoimmunity may result from changes in the way MHC molecules present antigen. These changes may cause an inappropriate or exaggerated response to environmental antigens such as microorganisms. A large variety of non-MHC genes also have been identified as risk factors for the development of specific autoimmune diseases. Most of these genes encode for inflammatory cytokines or costimulatory molecules found on the cell surface.

Tolerance is a state of immunologic control so that the individuals do not make a detrimental immune response against their own cells and tissues. *Central tolerance* occurs when autoreactive lymphocytes are either eliminated or suppressed in the primary lymphoid organs during differentiation of immature T or B lymphocytes (see Algorithms 8.1 and 8.2). *Peripheral tolerance* is maintained in the secondary lymphoid organs through the action of T regulatory (Treg) lymphocytes (see Chapter 8). Many autoimmune diseases display defects in either the number or the function of Treg cells in peripheral blood (see Emerging Science Box: T regulatory Cells and Autoimmunity).[7] In addition to Treg cells, dendritic cell processing and presentation of antigen are critical for the adaptive immune system to differentiate between self- and nonself-antigens. Defects in dendritic cell interaction with T cells have been linked to autoimmunity.[8]

In the vast majority of autoimmune diseases, the nature of the initiating event that results in a breakdown of tolerance is unclear. One of the most studied of these potential initiating events is the role of foreign antigens from infectious microorganisms causing molecular mimicry. Some antigens of infectious agents so closely resemble (mimic) a particular self-antigen that antibodies or T cells produced to protect against the infection also recognize the self-antigen as foreign (cross-reactive antibody or T cell). One example is rheumatic heart disease that may occur after a group A streptococcal sore throat. In this example, the M protein and group A carbohydrate in the streptococcal bacterial capsule mimic normal antigens in the heart valves resulting in the production of antibodies and T cells that damage the valves. Most potential associations between infection and autoimmunity are much less clear. For example, many researchers believe that there is a link between viral or bacterial infection and the onset of type 1 diabetes.[9] The link between infectious microorganisms and autoimmune disease continues to be investigated.

EMERGING SCIENCE BOX

T Regulatory Cells and Autoimmunity

T regulatory cells (Tregs) are important for the induction and maintenance of peripheral tolerance and are key in preventing excessive immune responses and autoimmunity. It is believed that autoimmunity arises, at least in part, from a lack of peripheral tolerance associated with reduced Treg numbers or failure in their function. Tregs are differentiated in the thymus when T precursor cells bind to self-antigens. Most of these self-reactive T cells will be clonally deleted, but some will instead be induced to become Treg which then migrate to the periphery. In addition, Tregs can be induced from T helper (Th) cells already in the periphery under inflammatory conditions. When Tregs recognize antigens, they release immunosuppressive cytokines such as interleukin (IL)-10 and transforming growth factor-beta (TGF-β). Recent studies have shown that Treg cells can be "unstable," meaning they have the ability to transform into other types of T cells under certain conditions (Treg plasticity). In autoimmune diseases, Tregs may become Th1, Th2, or Th17 cells, which promote cell-mediated and humoral immunity and inflammation rather than suppress it. These findings have led to the exploration of treatments for autoimmune diseases in which activated T cells that are attacking tissues are therapeutically induced to transform into Tregs, thus halting immune-mediated tissue damage. Tregs produced in the laboratory have been infused into individuals with severe autoimmune conditions such as graft-versus-host disease with promising results. These kinds of treatments might provide adequate tolerance without the use of immunosuppressive drugs that increase the risk of infection and cancer. Another potential use for Treg therapies is the prevention and management of transplant rejection in which Tregs would provide antigen-specific tolerance to the graft tissues without the need for systemic immunosuppression.

Data from Ferreira LMR, et al. Next-generation regulatory T cell therapy. *Nature Reviews. Drug Discovery,* 2019;18(10):749–769; Goschl L, et al. Treg cells in autoimmunity: From identification to Treg-based therapies. *Seminars In Immunopathology,* 2019;41(3):301–314; Kumar P, et al. Restoring selftolerance in autoimmune diseases by enhancing regulatory T-cells. *Cellular Immunology,* 2019;339:41–49; Mohr A, et al. The role of FOXP3+ regulatory T cells in human autoimmune and inflammatory diseases. *Clinical and Experimental Immunology,* 2019;197(1):24–35; Mukhatayev Z, et al. Engineered antigen-specific regulatory T cells for autoimmune skin conditions. Autoimmunity Reviews, 2021;20(3):102761; Romano M, et al. Past, present, and future of regulatory T cell therapy in transplantation and autoimmunity. *Frontiers in Immunology,* 2019;10:43; Serra P, et al. Antigen-specific therapeutic approaches for autoimmunity. Nature Biotechnology, 2019;37(3):238–251.

Women are far more likely to develop autoimmune disease than are men. Many theories have been proposed to explain this prevalence of autoimmunity in women. Many of the genes that code for immune function reside on the X chromosome. Although having two X chromosomes is protective against X-linked disorders (see Chapter 4), it has been proposed that hormonal changes during the life of a female individual may cause skewed activation of immune genes on X chromosomes.[10,11] Another hypothesis to explain the prevalence of autoimmunity in women is that a gene called VGLL3, which is more active in female than male skin cells, is overexpressed in women with autoimmune disease. This gene influences the function of several other genes involved in immune control.[12]

These kinds of initiating and contributing factors result in adaptive immune responses that are misdirected toward self-antigens. Self-directed immune responses often include a combination of hypersensitivity mechanisms II, II, and IV. The innate system is also activated with inflammatory damage to tissues.

Examples of Autoimmune Diseases

Many clinical disorders are associated with autoimmunity and are collectively referred to as autoimmune diseases. Table 9.2 provides a list of a few of the many autoimmune diseases. Many of these and other autoimmune disorders will be discussed in later chapters of this textbook. In this chapter, we will discuss only two representative examples, heparin-induced thrombocytopenia (HIT) and systemic lupus erythematosus (SLE).

Autoimmune disease: Heparin-induced thrombocytopenia. Heparin-induced thrombocytopenia (HIT) is a common complication associated with the use of the anticoagulant drug heparin (see Chapter 29). Heparin serves as a hapten and forms molecular complexes with the tissue-specific platelet antigen called platelet factor 4 (PF4). These hapten/antigen complexes are then attacked by autoantibodies causing type II hypersensitivity. When these autoantibodies bind to the surface of platelets, they cause two problems. The first is that they destroy platelets, leading to thrombocytopenia and bleeding. The second is that the destroyed platelets release particles that activate thrombin, forming clots that can block blood vessels (thrombosis).[13]

Approximately 2% of individuals treated with heparin will develop clinically significant HIT.[14] To diagnose HIT, laboratory tests are done to document thrombocytopenia and/or thrombosis and to look for the presence of the autoantibodies. Management requires stopping heparin therapy and, if anticoagulation is still needed, substituting with a nonheparin anticoagulant.[13]

Autoimmune disease: Systemic lupus erythematosus. Systemic lupus erythematosus (SLE) is one of the most common, complex, and serious of the autoimmune disorders. It can affect any organ in the body. SLE is characterized by the production of a large variety of antibodies (autoantibodies) against self-antigens, including nucleic acids, erythrocytes, coagulation proteins, phospholipids, lymphocytes, platelets, and many other self-components. The most characteristic autoantibodies are against nucleic acids (e.g., single-stranded deoxyribonucleic acid [ssDNA], double-stranded DNA [dsDNS]), histones, ribonucleoproteins, and other nuclear materials. The blood normally contains many of these products of cellular turnover and breakdown. In SLE, autoantibodies react with the circulating antigen and form circulating immune complexes. The deposition of circulating DNA/anti-DNA complexes in the kidneys can cause severe kidney inflammation (Fig. 9.7). Similar reactions can occur in other systems, such as the brain, heart, spleen, lung, gastrointestinal tract, peritoneum, and skin. Thus many of the symptoms of SLE result from a type III hypersensitivity reaction and affect many systems. Other symptoms are related to type II hypersensitivity reactions and include destruction of red blood cells (anemia), lymphocytes (lymphopenia), and platelets (thrombocytopenia).

SLE, like most autoimmune diseases, occurs more often in women (approximately a 9:1 predominance of females), especially in the 20- to 40-year-old age group.[15] Blacks are affected more often compared with Whites (approximately an eightfold increased risk). Several genes have been identified that are associated with an increased risk for SLE, including changes in MHC molecular structure.[16,17] Environmental triggers (e.g., ultraviolet radiation exposure, smoking, medications, viruses such as Epstein-Barr virus [EBV], low vitamin D levels, environmental pollutants) and hormonal changes interplay with genetic predisposition in disease development and activity.[18] As in many autoimmune conditions, microbiome dysbiosis is thought to negatively impact adaptive immune responses in SLE.[19]

As with other autoimmune diseases, clinical manifestations of SLE may wax and wane; the individual may go through periods of remission and be relatively disease free until the onset of a *flare* (exacerbated disease activity). Clinical manifestations of SLE depend on organ systems involvement, including skin (rashes and photosensitivity), eyes (keratoconjunctivitis, scleritis, uveitis retinopathy), mucus membranes (ulcers), joints (arthralgias), linings of the viscera (serositis, pleuritis), kidney (proteinuria), blood (anemia), gut (abdominal pain, vasculitis, hepatobiliary disease), and the neurologic system (seizures or psychosis).[20] Lupus nephritis is common and carries a high risk for end-stage renal failure. Cardiovascular disease is common.[21] Fever also may be present. Classification of SLE is based on the type and severity of organ system damage along with measurement of antibodies and complement levels.[22]

Laboratory diagnosis is usually based on a positive antinuclear antibody (ANA) screening test. This is a very sensitive test, but a substantial number of false-positive results occur in healthy individuals and those with other diseases. Detection of ANAs is usually followed by one or more specific tests (e.g., antibodies against Smith antigen [Sm], and dsDNA).[20] Further diagnostic testing may be indicated such as urinalysis and serum C reactive protein and complement levels.

There is no cure for SLE or most other autoimmune diseases. Fatalities resulting from SLE are usually related to infection, organ failure, or cardiovascular disease. The goals of treatment are to control symptoms and prevent further damage by suppressing the autoimmune response. Ultraviolet light may initiate flares, and protection from sun exposure is helpful. Nonsteroidal

TABLE 9.2 **Examples of Autoimmune Diseases**

System Disease	Organ or Tissue	Probable Self-Antigen
Endocrine System		
Hyperthyroidism (Graves disease)	Thyroid gland	Receptors for thyroid-stimulating hormone
Hashimoto hypothyroidism	Thyroid gland	Thyroid cell surface antigens, thyroglobulin
Insulin-dependent diabetes	Pancreas	Islet cells, insulin, insulin receptors on pancreatic cells
Addison disease	Adrenal gland	Surface antigens on steroid-producing cells; microsomal antigens
Male infertility	Testis	Surface antigens on spermatozoa
Skin		
Pemphigus vulgaris	Skin	Intercellular substances in stratified squamous epithelium
Bullous pemphigoid	Skin	Basement membrane
Vitiligo	Skin	Surface antigens on melanocytes (melanin-producing cells)
Neuromuscular Tissue		
Multiple sclerosis	Neural tissue	Surface antigens of nerve cells
Myasthenia gravis	Neuromuscular junction	Acetylcholine receptors; striations of skeletal and cardiac muscle
Rheumatic heart disease	Heart	Cardiac tissue antigens that cross-react with group A streptococcal antigen
Cardiomyopathy	Heart	Cardiac muscle
Gastrointestinal System		
Ulcerative colitis	Colon	Mucosal cells
Pernicious anemia	Stomach	Surface antigens of parietal cells; intrinsic factor
Primary biliary cirrhosis	Liver	Cells of bile duct
Chronic active hepatitis	Liver	Surface antigens of hepatocytes, nuclei, microsomes, smooth muscle
Eye		
Sjögren syndrome	Lacrimal gland	Antigens of lacrimal gland, salivary gland, thyroid, and nuclei of cells
Connective Tissue		
Ankylosing spondylitis	Joints	Sacroiliac and spinal apophyseal joint
Rheumatoid arthritis	Joints	Collagen, immunoglobulin G (IgG)
Systemic lupus erythematosus	Multiple sites	Numerous antigens in nuclei, organelles, and extracellular matrix
Renal System		
Immune complex glomerulonephritis	Kidney	Numerous immune complexes deposited in glomerular vessels
Goodpasture syndrome	Kidney	Glomerular basement membrane
Hematologic System		
Idiopathic neutropenia	Neutrophil	Surface antigens on polymorphonuclear neutrophils
Idiopathic lymphopenia	Lymphocytes	Surface antigens on lymphocytes
Autoimmune hemolytic anemia	Erythrocytes	Surface antigens on erythrocytes
Autoimmune thrombocytopenic purpura	Platelets	Surface antigens on platelets
Respiratory System		
Goodpasture syndrome	Lung	Septal membrane of alveolus

antiinflammatory drugs (NSAIDs), such as ibuprofen, reduce inflammation and relieve pain. Hydroxychloroquine is the preferred treatment for individuals with stable disease. Corticosteroids are often prescribed for flares and more serious active disease. Immunosuppressive drugs, (e.g., methotrexate, cyclophosphamide, azathioprine, tacrolimus, or mycophenolate mofetil) are used to treat severe symptoms. Immunotherapies focused on B-cell depletion (e.g., belimumab, rituximab) are used in selected individuals.[23] Many new biologic agents, such as anifrolumab (anti–type I interferon receptor antibody) and ustekinumab (antibody against IL-12/23 [p40]), are in clinical trials.[24]

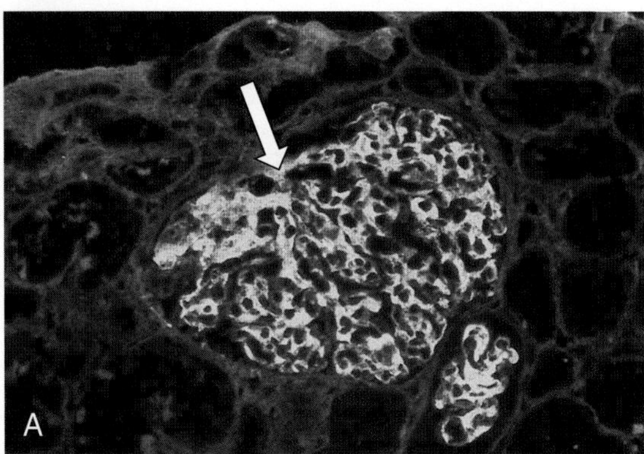

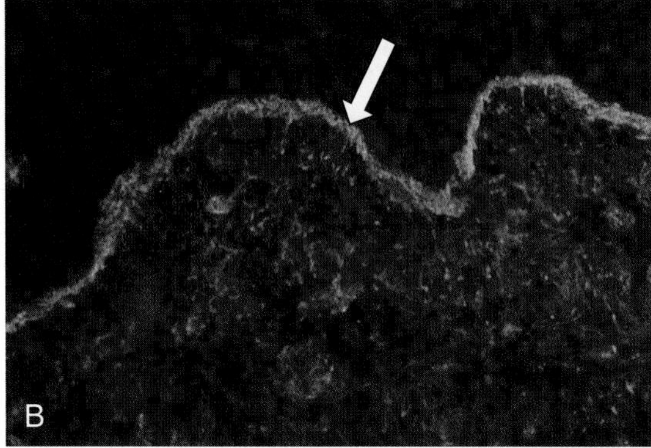

Fig. 9.7 Deposition of Immunoglobulin G (IgG) in the Kidney and Skin of Individuals With Lupus. These photographs of tissue were obtained from individuals with lupus and stained with fluorescent anti-IgG. **(A)** Section from a kidney showing a glomerulus with deposits of IgG (*arrow*, indicating bright areas of staining). **(B)** Section of the skin showing deposition of IgG along the dermal-epidermal junction (*arrow*, indicating bright green staining). A courtesy Dr. Helmut Rennke, Department of Pathology, Brigham and Women's Hospital, Boston; B courtesy Dr. Richard Sontheimer, Department of Dermatology, University of Texas Southwestern Medical School, Dallas.

Alloimmunity

Alloimmunity (isoimmunity) occurs when the immune system of one individual produces an immunologic reaction against tissues of another individual. Alloantigens (isoantigens) are nonself-antigens from members of the same species. No two individuals have exactly the same antigens on their tissues; therefore the introduction of one individual's tissues and cells into another will result in a strong immune response to the foreign antigens. Alloimmunity can be observed during immunologic reactions to blood transfusions, fetal tissues, or transplanted tissue.

Alloimmune disease: Transfusion reactions. Red blood cells (erythrocytes) express several important surface antigens, which are known collectively as the blood group antigens and can be targets of alloimmune reactions. More than 80 different red blood cell antigens are grouped into several dozen blood group systems. The most important of these, because they provoke the strongest humoral alloimmune response, are the ABO and Rh systems.

The ABO blood group consists of two major carbohydrate antigens, labeled A and B (Fig. 9.8), that are expressed on virtually all cells. These are codominant so that both A and B can be simultaneously expressed, resulting in an individual having any one of four different blood types. The erythrocytes of blood type A express the type A carbohydrate antigen, those with blood type B express the B antigen, those with blood type AB express both A and B antigens on the same cell, and those of blood type O express neither the A nor the B antigen. A person with type A blood also has circulating antibodies to the B carbohydrate antigen. If this person receives blood from a type AB or B individual, a severe transfusion reaction occurs, and the transfused erythrocytes are destroyed by agglutination or complement-mediated lysis. Similarly, a type B individual (whose blood contains anti-A antibodies) cannot receive blood from a type A or AB donor. Type O individuals, who have neither antigen but have both anti-A and anti-B antibodies, cannot accept blood from any of the other three types. These naturally occurring antibodies, called isohemagglutinins, are IgM antibodies developed early in life because of the presence of similar antigens expressed on naturally occurring bacteria in the intestinal tract.

Harmful transfusion reactions can be prevented by complete and careful ABO matching between donor and recipient. Because individuals with type O blood lack both types of antigens, they are considered universal donors—that is, anyone can accept their red blood cells. Similarly, type AB individuals are considered universal recipients because they lack both anti-A and anti-B antibodies and can be transfused with any ABO blood type.

Alloimmune disease: Hemolytic disease of the fetus and newborn. Hemolytic disease of the fetus and newborn (HDFN) (also known as erythroblastosis fetalis) is a condition in which maternal blood antigens do not match those of the fetus. This disorder usually results from incompatibility between maternal and fetal red blood cell (erythrocyte) Rho(D) antigens. The Rh blood group is a group of antigens expressed on red blood cells. This is the most diverse group of red blood cell antigens, consisting of at least 45 separate antigens, although only one is considered of major importance: the D antigen. Individuals who express the D antigen on their red blood cells are Rh positive, whereas individuals who do not express the D antigen are Rh negative. Approximately 85% of North Americans are Rh positive. Rh-negative individuals make IgG antibody to the D antigen (anti-D) if exposed to Rh-positive erythrocytes. In an Rh-negative mother whose fetus is Rh-positive, antibodies from the mother cross the placenta and attack fetal erythrocytes. The attack induces severe anemia in the fetus (erythroblastosis fetalis) or in the newborn (erythroblastosis neonatorum). With each successive pregnancy with an Rh-positive fetus, the mother's immune system makes anti-D antibodies faster and in greater amounts. Diagnosis involves measurement of maternal antibodies and fetal testing. Prenatal and postnatal management may include intrauterine transfusions, exchange transfusions, intravenous immunoglobulin (IVIG), or plasmapheresis.[25] The occurrence of this particular form of the disease has decreased dramatically because of the use of prophylactic anti-D immunoglobulin (i.e., RhoGAM). Administration of anti-D antibody within a few days of exposure to RhD-positive erythrocytes prevents sensitization against the D antigen (see Chapter 30).

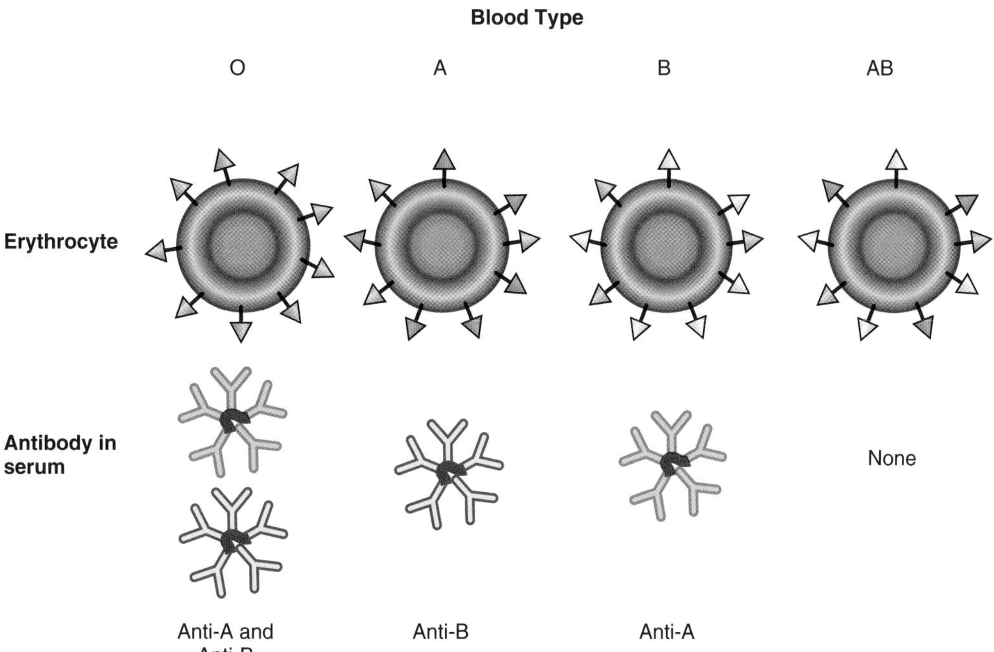

Fig. 9.8 ABO Blood Types. This figure shows the relationship of antigens and antibodies associated with the ABO blood groups. The surfaces of erythrocytes of individuals with blood group O have a core carbohydrate that is present on cells of all ABO blood groups (H antigen, depicted in *blue*). The sera of blood group O individuals contain immunoglobulin M (IgM) antibodies against both A and B carbohydrates. In individuals of the blood group A, some of the H antigens have been modified into A antigens (depicted in *green*). The sera of these individuals have IgM antibodies against the B antigen. In individuals with blood group B, some of the H antigens have been modified into B antigens (depicted in *yellow*). These individuals have IgM antibodies against the A antigen in their sera. In individuals of the blood group AB, some of the H antigens have been modified into both the A and B antigens. These individuals do not have antibody to either A or B antigens.

Alloimmune disease: Transplant rejection. Molecules of the major histocompatibility complex (MHC) were discussed in Chapter 8 as antigen-presenting molecules (see Figs. 8.6 and 8.7). MHC molecules also are a major target of transplant rejection. The human MHC molecules are also referred to as human leukocyte antigens (HLAs), especially in the context of transplantation. The different MHC genetic loci are identified as class I: HLA-A, HLA-B, and HLA-C, and class II: HLA-DR, HLA-DQ, and HLA-DP (Fig. 9.9). Humans have two copies of each MHC locus (one inherited from each parent) that are codominant so that molecules encoded by each parent's genes are expressed on the surface of every cell, except erythrocytes. The tremendous number of possible alleles that can be expressed throughout the population makes it highly unlikely that any two unrelated individuals will have the same HLA antigens. This diversity of HLA molecules becomes clinically relevant during organ transplantation. The recipient of a transplant will mount an immune response against the foreign HLA antigens on the donor tissue, resulting in rejection. To minimize the chance of tissue rejection, the donor and recipient are tissue-typed to identify differences in HLA antigens prior to transplantation. The more similar the two individuals are in their HLA tissue type, the more likely it is that transplantation will be successful. The chance of finding a reasonably close match among siblings is much higher than the general population, and, clearly, the most successful transplants would be between identical twins because they are nearly identical genetically.

When donor tissue is transplanted into a recipient, the recipient's T cells recognize alloantigens in two different ways: (1) *direct* recognition of foreign HLA antigens, and (2) *indirect* recognition of donor peptides that are presented on recipient antigen-presenting cells (see Algorithm 9.1). Both processes result in the widespread activation and proliferation of Th cells. Th cells differentiate into several subtypes that produce numerous cytokines, including IL-2 and interferon (IFN)-γ (Th1 cells), IL-4 (Th2 cells), and IL-17 (Th17 cells) (see Chapter 8). These cytokines activate T cytotoxic cells, macrophages, NK cells, and B cells such that there is an intense cell-mediated and humoral attack on the graft tissue.

Transplant rejection may be classified as hyperacute, acute, or chronic, depending on the amount of time that elapses between transplantation and rejection and the mechanisms by which rejection occurs. Hyperacute rejection is immediate and rare. Hyperacute rejection occurs because of the presence of preexisting antibodies (type II hypersensitivity) to HLA antigens on the vascular endothelial cells in the grafted tissue. These preexisting antigens are usually found in individuals who have received multiple blood transfusions or previous transplants. When the

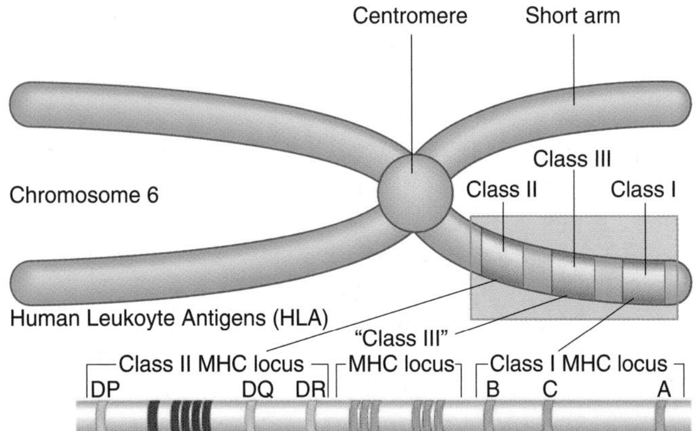

Fig. 9.9 Human Leukocyte Antigens (HLAs). The major histocompatibility complex *(MHC)* is located on the short arm of chromosome 6 and contains genes (genetic loci) that code for class I antigens (found mostly on nucleated cells), class II antigens (found mostly on dendritic cells, macrophages and B lymphocytes), and class III proteins (i.e., complement proteins and cytokines). From Peakman M, Vergani D. *Basic and clinical immunology*, 2nd edition. London: Churchill Livingstone; 2009 and Abbas AK, Lichtman AH, Pillai S. *Basic immunology*, 4th edition. St. Louis: Elsevier; 2014.

circulation is reestablished to the grafted area, the graft may immediately turn white (the so-called white graft) instead of a normal pink color. Hyperacute rejection can be avoided by testing the recipient for preexisting antibodies prior to transplantation.

Acute rejection occurs within days to months after transplantation. This type of rejection occurs when the recipient develops an immune response against unmatched HLA antigens after transplantation. Both humoral and cell-mediated immune responses play a role (Algorithm 9.2). Direct and indirect recognition of alloantigens result in release of Th1, Th2, and Th17 cytokines. Alloantibodies are formed to graft blood vessels (type II hypersensitivity) which then activate complement, resulting in necrosis of graft vessels (vasculitis). Tc cells and macrophages are activated, resulting in direct lysis of graft cells and disruption of tissue architecture; this leads to graft dysfunction and destruction (type IV hypersensitivity). NK cells and other components of innate immunity also play a role. The release of IL-2 is of particular importance in acute rejection; thus several antirejection medications target IL-2 synthesis or receptors (e.g., cyclosporin, tacrolimus, basiliximab). Other antirejection medications deplete T- and B-cell numbers, metabolism, and function (e.g., mycophenolate mofetil, rituximab, prednisone, azathioprine, belatacept), or block inflammatory cytokines such

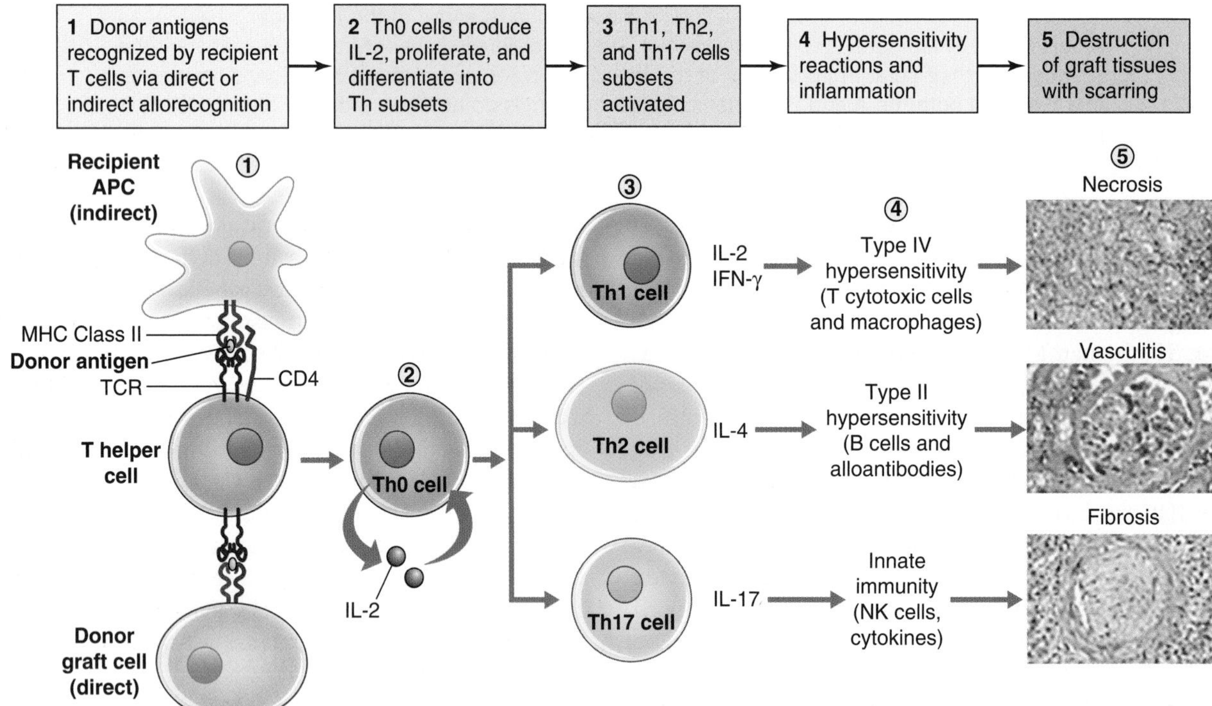

Algorithm 9.2 Acute Graft Rejection. Acute graft rejection occurs days to months after transplantation. Recipient T helper (Th) cells recognize graft human leukocyte antigens (direct allorecognition) or donor antigens presented on recipient antigen-presenting cells (indirect allorecognition). These cells then secrete IL-2, proliferate, and differentiate into Th1, Th2, or Th17 cells. Th1 cells secrete IL-2 and IFN-γ which activate T cytotoxic cells and macrophages which participate in type IV hypersensitivity (cell-mediated immunity). Th2 cells secrete IL-4 which activate B cells to become alloantibody-producing plasma cells. Th17 cells secrete IL-17 which stimulates inflammation. These processes result in necrosis of graft cells, vasculitis of graft blood vessels, and fibrosis (scarring) of graft tissue. The end result is dysfunction and death of the transplanted organ. *IFN-γ*, Interferon-gamma; *IL*, interleukin; *MHC*, major histocompatability complex; *Th*, T helper; *TCR*, T cell receptor.

as IL-6 (e.g., tocilizumab). New methods for achieving graft tolerance include adoptive transfer of donor and recipient Treg cells and myeloid-derived suppressor cells.[26,27] Studies are exploring the potential for modifying the epigenetic profiles of immune cells and the use of messenger RNA (mRNA) in the prevention of graft rejection.[28] The choice of immunosuppressive medications is based on the type of organ being transplanted and the potential for recipient toxicity.

Chronic rejection may occur after a period of months or years of normal function. It is characterized by slow, progressive organ failure. Chronic rejection occurs most often in recipients who were poorly matched to their donor, have comorbidities (e.g., diabetes, hypertension), received a graft that was in poor condition or was damaged during the transplantation procedure, or have required treatment for multiple acute rejection episodes.

Chronic rejection involves several mechanisms. A cell-mediated (type IV hypersensitivty) reaction against minor histocompatibility antigens on the grafted tissue contributes to persistent Tc-cell and phagocyte activation. Th17 cytokines trigger chronic inflammation. There also is binding of alloantibodies to donor graft MHC molecules, resulting in complement activation and tissue destruction (late antibody-mediated rejection).[29] These processes are subacute and slowly progressive, leading to graft fibrosis (scarring), dysfunction, and tissue death. Once chronic rejection is well established, there are few effective treatments, and it may be necessary to replace the graft with a new transplanted organ.

DEFICIENCIES IN IMMUNITY

Immune deficiency is the failure of the immune or inflammatory response to function normally, resulting in increased susceptibility to infections and cancer. Primary (congenital) immune deficiency is caused by a genetic defect, whereas secondary (acquired) immune deficiency is caused by another condition, such as cancer, infection, or normal physiologic changes, such as aging. Acquired forms of immune deficiency are far more common than the congenital forms.

Initial Clinical Presentation

The clinical hallmark of immune deficiency is a tendency to develop unusual or recurrent, severe infections. The most severe primary immune deficiencies develop in children 2 years of age and younger. Potential immune deficiencies should be considered if the individual has experienced severe, documented bouts of pneumonia, otitis media, sinusitis (sinus infection), bronchitis, septicemia (blood infection), meningitis, or infections with opportunistic microorganisms (e.g., *Pneumocystis jiroveci*). Infections are generally recurrent, and multiple simultaneous infections are common. Invasive fungal infections are rare in healthy individuals and strongly indicate a defective immune system. Children frequently present with failure to thrive because of diarrhea and other chronic symptoms. A familial history of immune deficiency may be found in some types of primary deficiency.

The type of recurrent infections may indicate the type of immune defect. Deficiencies in T-cell immune responses are associated with recurrent infections caused by certain viruses (e.g., varicella zoster, cytomegalovirus [CMV]), fungi, yeasts (e.g., *Candida, Histoplasma*), or atypical microorganisms (e.g., *P. jiroveci*). B-cell deficiencies and phagocyte deficiencies are suggested if the individual has documented, recurrent infections with microorganisms that require opsonization (e.g., encapsulated bacteria, such as *Pneumococcus*) or those with viruses against which humoral immunity is normally effective (e.g., rubella virus). Some complement deficiencies resemble defects in antibody or phagocyte function, but others are associated with disseminated infections with bacteria of the genus *Neisseria* (*Neisseria meningitides* and *Neisseria gonorrhoeae*).

Primary (Congenital) Immune Deficiencies

Most primary immune deficiencies are the result of *single gene defects*. To date, 430 gene mutations are associated with immunodeficiency disorders.[30] In general, the mutations are sporadic and not inherited: a family history exists in only approximately 25% of individuals. The sporadic mutations occur before birth, but the onset of symptoms may be early or later, depending on the particular syndrome. In some instances, symptoms of immune deficiency appear within the first 2 years of life. Other immune deficiencies are slowly progressive, with the onset of symptoms appearing in the second or third decade of life.

The prevalence of primary immune deficiency diseases globally varies dramatically from country to country, and data are complicated by differences in diagnostic and reporting methods. The prevalence of diagnosed primary immune deficiency in North America is approximately 5 cases per 100,000 individuals; however, it is estimated that as many as 70% of cases are undiagnosed.[31] Many are subtle with minor deficiencies, but several result in major defects and lead to recurrent life-threatening infections. Sex distribution is approximately even, although some specific diseases have a male or female predominance. Primary immune deficiencies are classified into 10 groups, based on the principal component of the immune or inflammatory systems that is defective.[30] Of these 10 groups, the most common disorders are included within combined immunodeficiencies (affecting both cellular and humoral immunity). These disorders may also be associated with syndromic features. The other classification groups include predominantly antibody deficiencies, diseases of immune dysregulation, defects in phagocyte number or function, defects in innate immunity, autoinflammatory disorders, complement defects, bone marrow failure, and phenocopies of inborn errors of immunity.[30] To provide a better understanding of the diversity and severity of primary immune deficiencies, a few select examples of each category will be discussed.

Combined Deficiencies

Combined deficiencies include the most life-threatening disorders and result from defects that directly affect the development of both T and B lymphocytes. The severity of each disorder depends on the degree to which B and T cells are affected.

Combined deficiencies wthout nonimmunologic abnormalities. Severe combined immunodeficiencies (SCIDs) are the most common combined deficiency without nonimmunologic abnormalities. Most often, it is inherited in an autosomal recessive pattern, or it may be X-linked.[32] There are at least 20 different forms of SCID, depending on how the underlying genetic defect affects lymphocyte development and function. T-cell differentiation is defective, and, depending on the type of SCID, B cells and NK cells also are affected.[32] Most individuals with SCIDs have few detectable lymphocytes or NK cells in the circulation and secondary lymphoid organs (spleen, lymph nodes). Immunoglobulin levels, especially IgM and IgA, are absent or greatly reduced. The most severe form of SCID is due to *reticular dysgenesis* in which a common stem cell fails to develop into mature immune cells. Most children with this form of SCID die in utero or soon after birth.

Several forms of SCID are caused by autosomal recessive enzymatic defects that result in the accumulation of toxic metabolites, and rapidly dividing cells, such as lymphocytes, are especially sensitive. For instance, deficiency of adenosine deaminase (ADA deficiency) results in the accumulation of toxic purines. Enzyme replacement therapy is available for this form of SCID.[33] X-linked SCID results from a common defect in important IL receptors needed for lymphocyte maturation (e.g., IL-2, IL-4, IL-7, and others). Recent reports demonstrate the remarkable effectiveness of gene therapy in which a lentivirus is used as a vector to insert a normal copy of the IL-2 receptor (IL-2R) gene into a person's own hematopoietic stem cells.[34]

Even if nearly adequate numbers of B and T cells are produced, their cooperation may be defective. Bare lymphocyte syndrome is the form of SCID characterized by the inability of lymphocytes and macrophages to produce MHC class I or class II molecules. Without MHC molecules, antigen presentation and intercellular cooperation cannot occur effectively. Children with this deficiency develop serious, life-threatening infections and usually die before age 5 years.

A SCID newborn screening test is available and has been in use in the United States since 2008. After an abnormal screening, additional testing is needed to determine which type of SCID is present.[35] This approach has resulted in prompt treatment and higher survival rates and is now performed for all newborns in the United States. Hematopoietic stem cell transplantation is the standard treatment for infants with SCID; unfortunately, it is not universally effective and can be associated with serious complications such as graft-versus-host disease (GVHD). New gene therapies are emerging for several forms of SCID.[36]

Combined deficiencies with nonimmunologic abnormalities. Wiskott-Aldrich syndrome (WAS), an X-linked disorder characterized by the clinical triad of low platelet count (thrombocytopenia), eczema, and recurrent infections, is a condition in which IgM antibody production is greatly depressed. WAS results from a mutation of the *WAS* gene which causes defects in the WAS protein (WASP). WASP is required for normal differentiation of B cells and several other hematopoietic cell types. For example, defective WASP affects the actin cytoskeleton, which is important for platelet function. Immunodeficiencies include reduced antibody responses against antigens that primarily elicit an IgM response, such as polysaccharide antigens from bacterial cell walls (e.g., *Pseudomonas aeruginosa, Streptococcus pneumoniae, Haemophilus influenzae*). Defective WASP also impacts neutrophil migration and function. Clinical manifestations include bleeding, eczematous rash, and recurrent infections (e.g., otitis media, pneumonia, herpes simplex, CMV). Autoimmune conditions (e.g., hemolytic anemia) are also common. Management includes IVIG or subcutaneous immunoglobulin (SQIG), stem cell transplantation, and gene therapy.[37]

Chromosome 22q11.2 deletion syndrome (DiGeorge syndrome or velocardiofacial syndrome) is another combined immunodeficiency with syndromic features. Chromosome 22q11.2 deletion is the most common microdeletion genetic syndrome in humans.[38] This mutation is associated with a wide spectrum of phenotypes even within families. The deletion of a particular gene, T-box transcription factor 1 (TBX1), is thought to be responsible for many of the syndrome's characteristic signs and symptoms. The TBX1 gene provides instructions for making a protein called T-box 1. The T-box 1 protein is necessary for the development of muscles and bones of the face and neck, aorta, and the thymus and parathyroid glands.[39] In most cases, hypoplasia of the thymus results in greatly decreased T-cell numbers and function. Immunocompromise with susceptibility to infection is complicated by a shift in Th-cell function to Th2 predominance resulting in allergies, as well as a reduction in Treg function resulting in autoimmune disorders. Cardiac and endocrine problems are also common. Defective development of the third and fourth pharyngeal pouches during embryonic development results in thymic defects and the absence of the parathyroid gland (causing inability to regulate calcium concentration). Low blood calcium levels cause the development of tetany or involuntary rigid muscular contraction. This syndrome frequently is associated with abnormal development of facial features that are controlled by the same embryonic pouches; these include low-set ears, fish-shaped mouth, and other altered features (Fig. 9.10). Loss of this gene may also contribute to behavioral problems such as schizophrenia and bipolar disorder. Dopaminergic neurons are also affected, leading to an increased risk for development of Parkinson disease later in life.[40] Management includes monitoring and intervention for hypoparathyroidism, heart defects, facial abnormalities, infections, and neurologic complications. No specific treatment for the underlying condition is currently available.

Predominantly Antibody Deficiencies

Predominantly antibody deficiencies result from defects in B-cell maturation or function and are the most common of immune deficiencies. T-cell immune responses are not affected in pure B-lymphocyte deficiencies. The results are lower levels of circulating immunoglobulins (hypogammaglobulinemia) or occasionally totally or nearly absent immunoglobulins (agammaglobulinemia).

Common variable immune deficiency. Common variable immunodeficiency (CVID) is the most common symptomatic primary immune deficiency, affecting up to 1 in 10,000 individuals.[41] There are two peak ages of onset, one before the age of 10 and another between 30 and 40 years of age. As the name

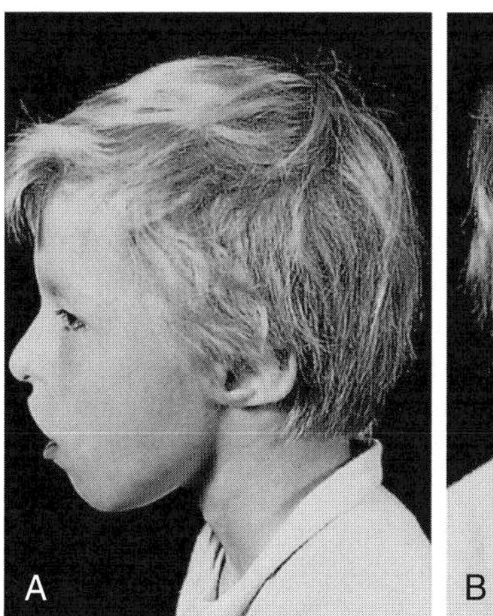

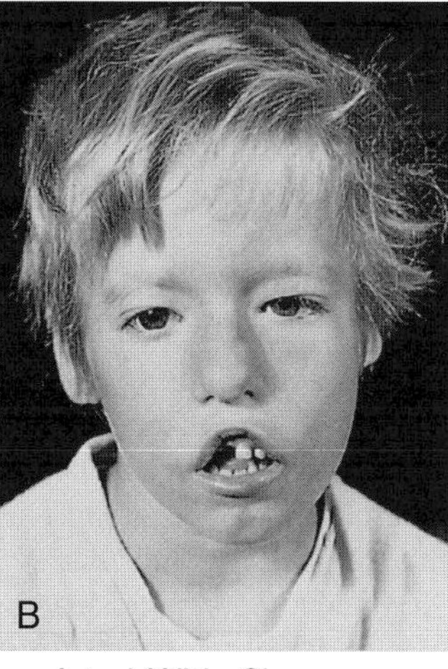

Fig. 9.10 Facial Anomalies Associated With Chromosome 22q11.2 deletion syndrome (DiGeorge Syndrome). Note the wide-set eyes **(B)**, low-set ears **(A and B)**, shortened structure of the upper lip **(B)**, and underdeveloped chin **(A and B)**. From Male D, Brostoff J, Roth D, et al. *Immunology*, 8th edition. St. Louis: Mosby; 2013.

implies, the presentation is very heterogeneous. It is characterized by hypogammaglobulinemia, but the particular class of antibody that is decreased varies. Although B-cell numbers are normal, most individuals have low amounts of IgG, which may or may not be accompanied by decreased levels of IgA and IgM. Multiple genetic defects in terminal differentiation of B lymphocytes may account for this condition, although the pathogenesis remains poorly understood.[42] Failure to produce sufficient immunoglobulins results in recurrent infections in 90% of individuals with CVID. Pneumonia caused by *S. pneumoniae* or *H. influenzae*, and infections with adenovirus, CMV, and varicella zoster are common.[41] Secondary complications include arthritis (infectious and noninfectious), gastrointestinal symptoms (malabsorption, chronic diarrhea), autoimmune disease (anemia, thrombocytopenia, endocrine diseases), and cancer (of the lymphoid system, skin, and gastrointestinal tract).[43] Interstitial lung disease is a significant cause of morbidity and mortality in CVID and is believed to be the result of dysregulated B-cell function.[44] Because of the heterogeneity of clinical features, diagnosis is difficult and may be delayed for several years. The advent of new diagnostic techniques will likely improve outcomes.[42]

Selective IgA deficiency. Some defects may involve a particular class of antibody, such as selective IgA deficiency, in which only IgA is suppressed. It is the most prevalent of the selective antibody deficiencies and is defined as a decreased serum IgA level lower than 7 mg/dL in individuals older than 4 years with normal levels of IgM and IgG in serum and exclusion of other causes of hypogammaglobulinemia. Selective IgA deficiency occurs in 1 in 700 to 1 in 400 individuals, and familial inheritance occurs in approximately 20% of cases. There is an increased incidence of common variable immune deficiency and transient hypogammaglobulinemia of infancy among family members of those with selective IgA deficiency. It results from defects in the process of IgA class switch, production and secretion of IgA, and long-term survival of IgA-switched memory B cells and plasma cells.[45] Many individuals are asymptomatic, although others have a history of recurring sinus, joint, and pulmonary infections.[41] Some have gastrointestinal infection such as chronic intestinal candidiasis (infection with *C. albicans*). Complications of IgA deficiency include severe allergic disease and autoimmune diseases. Some individuals are at risk for life-threatening allergic reactions when they receive blood products that contain some IgA. This is thought to be due to IgG (or possibly IgE) anti-IgA antibodies, which may be found in some IgA-deficient individuals. Management includes treatment of infections and allergic reactions, but no specific treatment for this immunodeficiency is currently available.

IgG subclass deficiency. Deficiencies in certain subclasses of antibody, particularly IgG2 (IgG subclass deficiency), may result from a defect in switch to a particular subclass constant region. A reduced level of IgG2 results in an inability to adequately attack polysaccharide antigens on the surface of encapsulated bacteria. Low levels of IgG2 therefore are responsible for recurrent risk for pneumonias caused by these bacteria. Management with IVIG reduces the number of infections.[46]

Bruton agammaglobulinemia. Bruton agammaglobulinemia (X-linked agammaglobulinemia) is caused by blocked development of mature B cells in bone marrow. It results from mutations of genes responsible for the synthesis of Bruton tyrosine kinase (BTK). An absence of BTK causes absent precursor B-cell differentiation in the bone marrow and severe B-cell deficiency (<2%).[47] There is an associated inability to generate plasma cells and antibodies of all classes (panhypogammaglobulinemia). B-lineage cells in all organs are affected resulting in reduced sizes of lymph nodes and tonsils. Encapsulated bacterial infections are common. Nearly 85% of affected individuals develop infections early in life including otitis media, skin infection, sepsis, sinusitis, acute gastroenteritis, cervical lymphadenitis, epididymitis, meningitis, osteomyelitis, urinary tract infection, and encephalitis. Treatment consists of replacement immunoglobulin and prophylactic antibiotics to prevent infections.

Immune Dysregulation

Primary immunodeficiencies categorized as immune dysregulation include disorders specific to Tc and NK cell function. This group of conditions is also characterized by autoimmune conditions as a result of alterations in tolerance.

Perforin deficiency results from a mutation in the perforin gene, the product of which is an important component of cellular killing by Tc and NK cells. Several other perforin deficiencies result from mutations in secretory vesicle function, including fusion with the cell membrane and other aspects of the process.

Chédiak-Higashi syndrome results from a defect in the movement of intracellular cytoplasmic granules and is caused by an autosomal recessive mutation in the lysosomal trafficking regulator (LYST) gene. Dysregulation of LYST function results in defects in lysosomal biogenesis.[48] As a result of these defects, the granules remain in the cytoplasm and form large aggregates that are readily apparent microscopically. Leukocytes from individuals with Chédiak-Higashi syndrome have decreased chemotaxis, granular fusion, and bacterial killing. Platelet granules also may be affected, resulting in prolonged bleeding, and partial albinism can occur because of defects in melanocyte granules. Affected children develop recurrent infections of the skin, respiratory tract, and mucous membranes, especially with gram-positive bacteria.

Autoimmune conditions associated with primary immunodeficiencies caused by immune dysregulation may result from abnormalities in Treg function. For example, mutations in IL-10 or its receptor IL-10R suppress the production or response to IL-10 (an immunosuppressive cytokine from Treg cells), resulting in excessive inflammation and an increased risk for early-onset inflammatory bowel disease, or recurrent respiratory disease. Lymphoproliferative disorders (adenopathy, splenomegaly, colitis) may also occur.[30]

Phagocyte Defects: Number, Function or Both

Phagocyte defects include inadequate numbers of phagocytes (e.g., severe congenital neutropenia) or defects in phagocyte function. These defects result in recurrent infections caused by a wide range of microorganisms that can infect lungs, skin, bones, and other organs.

Congenital neutropenia results from the inheritance of a large range of autosomal dominant, recessive, or X-linked mutations that result in lack of neutrophil maturation and function. Without adequate neutrophils, the innate immune response is severely impacted, particularly with regard to defense against microorganisms. Congenital neutropenia results in recurrent bacterial infections commensurate with the absolute count of neutrophil granulocytes in the circulation.[49] It is associated with several syndromic conditions, including oculocutaneous albinism, metabolic diseases, and bone marrow failure syndromes. Approximately 20% of people with severe congenital neutropenia develop certain cancerous conditions of the blood, particularly myelodysplastic syndrome or leukemia. Management includes in injections of granulocyte colony-stimulating factor and, in severe cases, bone marrow transplantation.

Primary autoimmune neutropenia (chronic benign neutropenia of childhood) is an idiopathic self-limiting condition affecting infants and toddlers. In most cases, mild to moderate decreases in neutrophil numbers resolve by early childhood without intervention. However, Black children have a 3.5 higher risk of having persistent neutropenia and may require treatment with granulocyte colony-stimulating factor.[50]

Chronic granulomatous disease (CGD) is a severe defect in the myeloperoxidase–hydrogen peroxide system (NADPH oxidase system)—a major means of bacterial destruction within the phagolysosome (see Chapter 7). Deficient production of hydrogen peroxide and other oxygen products needed for phagocytic killing results in recurrent severe pneumonias; tumor-like granulomata in the lungs, skin, and bones; and other infections with some opportunistic microorganisms, such as *Staphylococcus aureus, Serratia marcescens*, and *Aspergillus* species. These infections are characterized by recurrent episodes of cutaneous and organ abscess, pneumonia, and osteomyelitis. CGD is also associated with other phagocytic defects, including decreased Toll-like receptor (TLR) recognition of pathogens, inability to form neutrophil extracellular traps, and hyperinflammatory states (see Chapter 7).[51]

Defects in Innate Immunity

Some immune deficiencies are characterized by a defect in the capacity to produce an immune response against a particular antigen. Innate immune cytokines such as interferons and ILs may be affected. Depending on the specific defect, there can be increased susceptibility to infection by mycobacteria, (e.g., tuberculosis), viruses (e.g., herpes simplex), bacteria, or fungi.[30] In chronic mucocutaneous candidiasis, interaction between the Th17 lymphocytes and macrophages is ineffective related to a specific infectious agent, *Candida albicans*. Thus the macrophage cannot be activated, and these individuals usually have mild to extremely severe recurrent *Candida* infections involving the mucous membranes and skin. Other defects in innate immunity include defects in TLRs and NK cells resulting in susceptibility to infections with mycobacteria, salmonella, and viruses (EBV, herpes, influenza viruses).

Autoinflammatory Disorders

Autoinflammatory disorders are characterized by abnormally high levels of inflammation secondary to mutations in genes that control inflammasome activation or in defects in cellular receptors of cytokines designed to decrease inflammation. These disorders are frequently related to diminished control of infections of epithelial surfaces. Vasculitis, inflammatory lung disorders, arthritis, inflammatory bowel disease, SLE, and other autoimmune conditions are common.[30]

Complement Deficiencies

Many complement deficiencies have been described. Every component of the complement cascade (see Chapter 7) may be affected.[30] C3 deficiency is the most severe defect because of its central role in the complement cascade. Loss of C3b results in an inability to opsonize, causing recurrent life-threatening infections with encapsulated bacteria (e.g., *H. influenzae* and *S. pneumoniae*) at an early age. Deficiencies of any of the terminal components of the complement cascade (C5, C6, C7, C8, or C9 deficiencies) are associated with increased infections with only one group of bacteria—those of the genus *Neisseria* (*N. meningitides* or *N. gonorrhoeae*). *Neisseria* species usually cause localized infections (meningitis or gonorrhea), but terminal pathway defects result in a very high risk for systemic infections with atypical strains of these microorganisms. Management includes prompt treatment for infection. No specific treatments for complement deficiency are currently available.

Bone Marrow Failure

Some primary immune deficiencies result in failure of the bone marrow to produce hematopoietic cells, including those necessary for immune defense. One of the best described examples is Fanconi anemia. There are 22 different mutations that can cause Fanconi anemia (A-W); most are inherited in an autosomal recessive pattern.[30] These mutations result in dysfunction of some of the proteins involved in DNA replication, causing bone marrow failure. Severe anemia and life-threatening infections result. It is also associated with a significant risk of cancer.[52] Allogenic hematopoietic stem cell transplantation is curative for the bone marrow failure; however, those with malignant transformation prior to transplantation have a high rate of toxicity and transplant-related death.[53] Stem cell transplantation with lentiviral-mediated gene corrections is emerging as a potential cure for this condition.[54]

Phenocopies of Inborn Errors of Immunity

This group of conditions includes a wide variety of somatic mutations affecting T- or B-cell function, or the production of autoantibodies to inflammatory cytokines.[30] These abnormalities cause lymphoid changes such as splenomegaly and lymphadenopathy or may be associated with infections by mycobacteria, fungi, or staphylococci.

Evaluation of Those With Primary Immune Deficiency

The evaluation of primary immune deficiencies relies on next-generation sequencing methodology (exomes and genomes). These techniques have greatly improved genetic diagnosis with resulting improvements in care and genetic counseling.[55] In addition to genetic analysis, other evaluations include a complete blood count (CBC) with a differential. The CBC provides information on the numbers of red blood cells, white blood cells, and platelets, and the differential indicates the quantities of lymphocytes, granulocytes, and monocytes in blood. Quantitative determination of immunoglobulins (IgG, IgM, IgA) is a screening test for antibody production, and an assay for total complement (total hemolytic complement, CH_{50}) is useful if a complement defect is suspected.

Therapies for Primary Immune Deficiencies

The rapidly increasing knowledge of genetic, cellular, and molecular mechanisms that characterize primary immune deficiencies has fueled research into therapies aimed at specific immune defects.[56] As has been noted previously, some primary immune deficiencies can be successfully treated by replacing the missing component of the immune system. For example, individuals with B-cell deficiencies that cause hypogammaglobulinemia or agammaglobulinemia are usually treated by administration of IVIG, antibody-rich fractions prepared from plasma pooled from large numbers of donors. Administration of IVIG replaces the individual's antibodies temporarily; these antibodies have a half-life of 3 to 4 weeks. Thus individuals must be treated repeatedly to maintain a protective level of antibodies in blood.

Bone marrow transplants containing hematopoietic stem cells have been routinely used to treat SCID, WAS, and other primary immunodeficiencies.[57] However, individuals with SCID are at risk for graft-versus-host disease (GVHD). This occurs if T cells in a transplanted graft (e.g., transfused blood, bone marrow transplants) are mature and therefore capable of cell-mediated immunity against the recipient's HLA. The primary targets for GVHD are the skin (e.g., rash, loss or increase of pigment, thickening of skin), liver (e.g., damage to bile duct, hepatomegaly), mouth (e.g., dry mouth, ulcers, infections), eyes (e.g., burning, irritation, dryness), and gastrointestinal tract (e.g., severe diarrhea), and the disease may lead to death from infections. The risk of GVHD can be diminished by removing mature T cells from tissue used to treat individuals with immune deficiencies. Mesenchymal stem cells (MSCs) are present in all adult tissues and may be useful in treating GVHD. MSCs have potent immunosuppressive properties. Several clinical trials have demonstrated complete suppression of GVHD in a large number of recipients of MSCs.[58]

Gene therapy involves the use of viral vectors to transfer healthy genes into stem cells that are then transplanted into affected individuals. This approach provides long-term replacement of specific immune factors. Gene therapy has become safer and more effective since new viral vectors (e.g., lentiviruses) are being used. Trials have verified immune reconstitution in individuals with ADA deficiency, X-linked SCID, CGD, WAS, and Fanconi anemia, and numerous clinical trials are underway for this form of treatment.[34,36,57,59,60]

Secondary (Acquired) Immune Deficiencies

Secondary, or acquired, immune and inflammatory deficiencies are far more common than primary deficiencies. These deficiencies are complications of other physiologic or pathophysiologic conditions (Box 9.1). Although secondary deficiencies are common, many are not clinically relevant. In many cases, the degree of the immune deficiency is relatively minor and without any apparent increased susceptibility to infection. Alternatively, the immune system may be substantially suppressed but only for a short duration, thus minimizing the incidence of clinically relevant infections. However, some secondary immune deficiencies (e.g., acquired immunodeficiency syndrome [AIDS] or immunosuppression by cancer) are severe and may result in recurrent life-threatening infections. Management usually consists of supportive care, prompt treatment of infections, and reversal of the underlying immu nocompromising condition if possible.

Psychological Stress

The relationship between emotional stress and depressed immune function is an area of intense research, and the mechanisms linking them are now beginning to be understood. Many lymphoid organs are innervated and can be affected by nerve stimulation. In addition, lymphocytes have receptors for many hormones (e.g., sex hormones, neurotransmitters, and neuropeptides) and can respond to changing levels of these chemicals with increased or decreased function. For instance, stress-induced catecholamines affect the expression of adhesion molecules and the movement of lymphocytes among lymphoid organs. (Further discussion of the effects of stress on susceptibility to disease is the subject of Chapter 11.)

BOX 9.1 Some Conditions Known to Be Associated With Acquired Immunodeficiencies

Normal Physiologic Conditions
Pregnancy
Infancy
Aging

Psychological Stress
Emotional trauma
Eating disorders

Dietary Insufficiencies
Malnutrition caused by insufficient intake of large categories of nutrients, such as protein or calories
Insufficient intake of specific nutrients, such as vitamins, iron, or zinc

Infections
Congenital infections, such as rubella, cytomegalovirus, hepatitis B
Acquired infections, such as acquired immunodeficiency syndrome (AIDS)

Malignancies
Malignancies of lymphoid tissues, such as Hodgkin disease, acute or chronic leukemia, or myeloma
Malignancies of nonlymphoid tissues, such as sarcomas and carcinomas

Physical Trauma
Burns

Medical Treatments
Stress caused by surgery
Anesthesia
Immunosuppressive treatment with corticosteroids or antirejection drugs
Splenectomy
Cancer treatment with cytotoxic drugs or ionizing radiation

Other Diseases or Genetic Syndromes
Diabetes
Alcoholic cirrhosis
Sickle cell disease
Systemic lupus erythematosus (SLE)
Chromosome abnormalities, such as trisomy 21

Physical Trauma

Major trauma results in a systemic inflammatory response that is paralleled by a compensatory antiinflammatory response syndrome (CARS). This results in a period of critical illness in during which there is persistent inflammatory and immunosuppressive responses.[61] Although the innate immune system is overactive, the adaptive immune system is suppressed. Antigen presentation by macrophages is reduced. Neutrophils and NK cells demonstrate decreased phagocytosis, cytokine production, and cytotoxic activity, as well as elevated rates of apoptosis.[62] Treg activity is increased. This immune suppression is associated with poor wound healing, infection, and multiple organ dysfunction.

Dietary Insufficiencies

Nutritional status can have a profound effect on immune function, and malnutrition is the predominant cause of secondary immune deficiencies worldwide. Severe deficits in protein or calorie (protein-calorie malnutrition) intake lead to immune deficiencies. Marasmus (deficiency in calories) and kwashiorkor (deficiency in protein but adequate calories) have similar outcomes. T cell–rich areas of primary (thymus) and secondary lymphoid tissue are greatly affected, resulting in impaired T-cell function. Antibody levels are normal, but neutrophil function (chemotaxis, phagocytosis, bacterial killing), complement levels, and NK activity are impaired, resulting in infections with microorganisms that are normally destroyed by opsonization and phagocytosis. Deficiencies in specific nutritional components such as zinc and vitamins may also contribute to T- and B-cell dysfunction. In hospitalized individuals with malnutrition, modifications in the gut microbiota and decreased functioning of the gut mucosal immune system result in increased nosocomial infections and mortality.[63]

Chronic Diseases

Chronic diseases of the cardiovascular, gastrointestinal, endocrine, and renal systems are commonly complicated by a secondary immune suppression. For example, diabetes results in altered glucose metabolism and suppresses many aspects of the immune and inflammatory responses, including phagocytosis and chemotaxis, and lymphocyte proliferation.[64] Diminished T-cell memory for pathogens, impaired B-cell function, low levels of complement, and glycation of circulating antibodies are also found in those with uncontrolled diabetes.[65] Chronic heart failure is associated with poor nutrition, chronic inflammation, and adaptive immune dysfunction. Inflammatory bowel diseases, such as Crohn disease, ulcerative colitis, celiac disease, gastrointestinal infections, and cancer of the gastrointestinal tract are associated with decreased circulating levels of immunoglobulins.

Malignancies

Virtually all malignancies are complicated by immunosuppression, either through the effect of the disease itself on the body's defense mechanisms or as the result of treatment. Cancers cause both chronic inflammation and suppression of the adaptive immune system. For example, chronic inflammation releases growth factors such as vascular endothelial growth factor which causes the growth of new blood vessels (angiogenesis). At the same time, immunosuppressive macrophages and Treg cells are activated thus reducing the adaptive immune response to the tumor. Cancer cells are capable of protecting themselves by directly suppressing T lymphocytes that seek to destroy cancer cells (see Chapter 12). Cancer cells release metabolites and create a microenvironmental acidosis that hinder immune cell metabolism, proliferation, and functioning.[66] Late-stage malignancies result in generalized deficiency of the immune response and greatly increased susceptibility to developing life-threatening infections. Mechanisms include malnutrition, replacement of bone marrow by cancer cells, decreased NK and T lymphocyte function, and the release of soluble immunosuppressive chemicals. In fact, many people with malignancies die as a result of infections rather than of the direct effects of the tumor. Some malignancies (e.g., lymphomas, leukemias, plasmacytomas) present with an early and specific immune depression through a direct effect on B cells.

Immunosuppressive treatments

The list of medications that affect the immune response is ever increasing and includes anesthetics, analgesics, antithyroid medications, anticonvulsants, antihistamines, antimicrobial agents, antilymphocyte antibodies, and tranquilizers. The most profound immunosuppressive treatments are those that are intentionally used to suppress the immune system to manage immune-mediated disease, to treat malignancy, or to prevent rejection of transplanted tissues.

Corticosteroids are intentionally used to control hypersensitivity diseases (especially autoimmune disease) or to prevent rejection of transplants. They predominantly inhibit T-cell function, prevent lymphocyte proliferation, inhibit production of critical cytokines, and suppress monocyte/macrophage functions. These effects greatly increase an individual's susceptibility to infection.

Many drugs and other treatments such as radiation that are used to treat cancer (e.g., chemotherapeutic agents, irradiation) are not specific for cancer cells but are designed to attack cells at susceptible stages in their cell cycles. They attack rapidly proliferating cells, thus killing immune cells as well as malignant cells. Depending on the dose of chemotherapy and/or irradiation administered, the entire immune system may be depleted.

Antirejection drugs are used to prevent immune-mediated rejection of transplanted tissue. Although more targeted treatments are becoming available, most antirejection regimens cause generalized immune suppression and increase the likelihood of infection and cancer.[67] A careful therapeutic balance must be maintained between protecting the graft and preventing these complications.

Infections

Many infectious microorganisms successfully invade the human body using mechanisms for fighting off specific immune/inflammatory responses against themselves (discussed in Chapter 10). However, some infectious agents more broadly suppress the immune response. HIV is one of the few microorganisms that directly attacks the central processes involved in the development of an immune response (discussed in detail in Chapter 10). It infects and destroys CD4$^+$ Th cells, which are necessary to provide help for the maturation of both plasma cells and Tc cells. Therefore HIV suppresses the immune response against itself and secondarily creates a generalized immune deficiency by suppressing the development of immune responses against other pathogens and opportunistic microorganisms.

Severe acute respiratory syndrome coronavirus 2 (SARS-CoV-2) infection has been shown to decrease innate immune responses, including the production of interferon, which can contribute to a lack of adequate initiation of adaptive immunity.[67,68] Decreased innate immune responses to the virus have been linked to an increase in asymptomatic COVID-19, as well as an increase in severity in those with progressive disease.[69] T-cell activation may be delayed, leading to decreased early symptoms, but can contribute to morbidity and mortality.[70] Lymph nodes from individuals with COVID-19 were found to have a loss of germinal centers, and those remaining contained only one-third of normal T- and B-cell numbers.[67]

Several other viruses (e.g., measles; hepatitis B; and herpes viruses, such as EBV, CMV, and herpes simplex viruses) may suppress various components of the immune response. Measles virus can infect both B and T cells and macrophages. Infection may result in a transient lymphopenia and a suppressed T-cell response. Acute infections with herpes viruses also may transiently suppress the immune system. EBV not only infects B cells, but it also may suppress both CD4$^+$ and CD8$^+$ T cells and NK cells, although immunosuppression is generally not severe. Many viruses produce molecules similar in function to IL-10 that further contribute to immunosuppression. CMV infects mucosal epithelium and can infect macrophages where antigen processing and presentation may be impaired. Tumor viruses such as human papillomavirus (HPV) help to create a tumor microenvironment in which cancer cells are free to grow.[71]

Some fungal infections may suppress the immune response. In disseminated *C. albicans* infections, T-cell responses and neutrophil chemotaxis are suppressed to various degrees. Similar immunosuppression may be observed in individuals with disseminated histoplasmosis (infections with *Histoplasma capsulatum*). The most severe form of acute malaria (caused by the parasite *Plasmodium falciparum*) suppresses specific antibody responses against protein and polysaccharide antigens by dysregulation of CD4$^+$ T-cell function and decreased IL-2 production.

SUMMARY REVIEW

Hypersensitivity: Allergy, Autoimmunity, and Alloimmunity

1. Inappropriate immune responses are exaggerated misdirected responses innocuous environmental antigens (allergy), the host's own tissues (autoimmunity), or beneficial foreign tissues (alloimmunity); or insufficient responses to protect the host (immune deficiency).
2. Allergy, autoimmunity, and alloimmunity are collectively known as hypersensitivity reactions.
3. Mechanisms of hypersensitivity are classified as type I (IgE-mediated) reactions, type II (tissue-specific) reactions, type III (immune complex–mediated) reactions, and type IV (cell-mediated) reactions.
4. Hypersensitivity reactions can be immediate (developing within minutes to a few hours) or delayed (developing within several hours or days).
5. Allergens are antigens that cause allergic responses.
6. Type I (IgE-mediated) hypersensitivity reactions are mediated through the binding of IgE to Fc receptors on mast cells and cross-linking of IgE by antigens that bind to the Fab portions of IgE. Cross-linking causes mast cell degranulation and the release of histamine (the most potent mediator) and other inflammatory substances.
7. Histamine, acting through the H1 receptor, contracts bronchial smooth muscles, causing bronchial constriction;

increases vascular permeability, causing edema; and increases blood flow into the affected area, causing vasodilation. Histamine with H2 receptors results in increased gastric acid secretion and a decrease of histamine released from mast cells and basophils.

8. Type II (tissue-specific) hypersensitivity reactions are caused by five possible mechanisms: complement-mediated lysis, opsonization and phagocytosis, neutrophil-mediated tissue damage, antibody-dependent cell-mediated cytotoxicity, and modulation of cellular function.
9. Type III (immune complex–mediated) hypersensitivity reactions are caused by the formation of immune complexes that are deposited in target tissues, where they activate the complement cascade, generating chemotactic fragments that attract neutrophils into the inflammatory site. Neutrophils release lysosomal enzymes that result in tissue damage.
10. Immune complex disease can be a systemic reaction, such as serum sickness, or a localized response, such as the Arthus reaction.
11. Type IV (cell-mediated) hypersensitivity reactions are caused by cytotoxic T lymphocytes (Tc cells), lymphokine-producing Th1 cells and activated macrophages.
12. Typical allergens include pollen, molds and fungi, certain foods (milk, eggs, fish, peanuts), animals, certain drugs, cigarette smoke, and house dust.
13. Clinical manifestations of allergic reactions usually are confined to the areas of initial intake or contact with the allergen. Ingested allergens induce gastrointestinal symptoms, airborne allergens induce respiratory tract or skin manifestations, and contact allergens induce allergic responses at the site of contact.
14. Autoimmune diseases originate from the coincidence of an initiating event in a genetically predisposed individual leading to an autoimmune mechanism that affects specific target tissues or cells. Central tolerance develops during the embryonic period. Peripheral tolerance is maintained in secondary lymphoid organs by regulatory T lymphocytes or antigen-presenting dendritic cells.
15. Heparin-induced thrombocytopenia is a condition in which heparin molecules attach to proteins in the surface of platelets resulting in the formation of autoantibodies that destroy platelets (bleeding) and promote clotting (thrombosis).
16. Systemic lupus erythematosus (SLE) is a chronic, multisystem, inflammatory disease and is one of the most serious of the autoimmune disorders. SLE is characterized by the production of a large variety of autoantibodies.
17. Alloimmunity is the immune system's reaction against antigens on the tissues of other members of the same species.
18. Alloimmune disorders include transient neonatal disease, in which the maternal immune system becomes sensitized against antigens expressed by the fetus; transplant rejection; and transfusion reactions, in which the immune system of the recipient of an organ transplant or blood transfusion reacts against foreign antigens on the donor's cells.
19. Red blood cell antigens may be the targets of autoimmune or alloimmune reactions. The most important of these, because they provoke the strongest humoral immune response, are the ABO and Rh systems.
20. Antigens on fetal red blood cells (Rh) can cause maternal antibodies to cross the placenta and cause severe anemia in the fetus.
21. Hyperacute graft rejection (preexisting antibody) is immediate and rare, acute rejection is both antibody and cell mediated and occurs days to months after transplantation, and chronic rejection is caused by inflammatory damage to endothelial cells as a result of a weak cell-mediated reaction.

Deficiencies in Immunity

1. Disorders resulting from immune deficiency are the clinical sequelae of impaired function of components of the immune or inflammatory response, phagocytes, or complement.
2. Immune deficiency is the failure of mechanisms of self-defense to function in their normal capacity.
3. Immune deficiencies are either congenital (primary) or acquired (secondary). Primary immune deficiencies are caused by genetic defects that disrupt lymphocyte development, whereas secondary immune deficiencies are secondary to disease or other physiologic alterations.
4. The clinical hallmark of immune deficiency is a propensity to unusual or recurrent severe infections. The type of infection usually reflects the immune system defect.
5. The most common infections in individuals with defects of the cell-mediated immune response are fungal and viral, whereas infections in individuals with defects of the humoral immune response or complement function are primarily bacterial.
6. Severe combined immunodeficiency is a total lack of T-cell function and a severe (either partial or total) lack of B-cell function. Other combined defects may result from deficiencies in antigen-presenting molecules (bare lymphocyte syndrome) or cytoskeletal proteins (WAS).
7. Chromosome 22q11.2 deletion syndrome (DiGeorge syndrome) is characterized by complete or partial lack of the thymus (resulting in depressed T-cell immunity) and the parathyroid glands (resulting in hypocalcemia) and the presence of cardiac anomalies.
8. Defects in B-cell function are diverse, ranging from a complete lack of the human bursal equivalent function, the lymphoid organs required for B-cell maturation (as in Bruton agammaglobulinemia), to deficiencies in a single class of immunoglobulins (e.g., selective IgA deficiency).
9. Defects in phagocyte function, which include insufficient numbers of phagocytes or defects of chemotaxis, phagocytosis, or killing, can result in recurrent life-threatening infections such as septicemia and disseminated pyogenic lesions.
10. Immune dysregulation disorders are characterized by abnormally high levels of inflammation secondary to mutations in control of inflammasome activation or in defects in cellular receptors of cytokines designed to decrease inflammation. These disorders are frequently related to diminished control of infections of epithelial surfaces.

11. Almost any portion of the complement cascade may be defective. The most severe defect is C3 deficiency, which results in recurrent life-threatening bacterial infections. Defects in proteins of the membrane attack complex usually result in unusual, disseminated infections with bacteria of the *Neisseria* spp.
12. Bone marrow failure and somatic mutations in immune genes may also result in severe primary immunodeficiency states.
13. Primary immune deficiencies may sometimes be treated by replacement therapy. Deficient antibody production is treated by replacement of missing immunoglobulins with commercial gamma-globulin preparations. Lymphocyte deficiencies are treated with the replacement of host lymphocytes with bone marrow and stem cell transplants and gene therapies when available.
14. Acquired immunodeficiencies are caused by superimposed conditions, such as aging, malnutrition, infections, malignancies, physical or psychological trauma, environmental factors, some medical treatments, or other diseases chronic disease, or infections.

REFERENCES

1. Gustine JN, Jones D. Immunopathology of hyperinflammation in COVID-19. *Am J Pathol.* 2021;191:4–17.
2. Angkasekwinai P. Th9 cells in allergic disease. *Curr Allergy Asthma Rep.* 2019;19(5):29.
3. Johansson K, McSorley HJ. Interleukin-33 in the developing lung—roles in asthma and infection. *Pediatr Allergy Immunol.* 2019;30(5):503–510.
4. Acevedo N, et al. Perinatal and early-life nutrition, epigenetics, and allergy. *Nutrients.* 2021;13(3):724.
5. Peroni DG, et al. Microbiome composition and its impact on the development of allergic diseases. *Front Immunol.* 2020;11:700.
6. Messina M, Venter C. Recent surveys on food allergy prevalence. *Nutr Today.* 2020;55(1):22–29.
7. Mukhatayev Z, et al. Engineered antigen-specific regulatory T cells for autoimmune skin conditions. *Autoimmun Rev.* 2021;20(3):102761.
8. Morante-Palacios O, et al. Tolerogenic dendritic cells in autoimmunity and inflammatory disease. *Trends Immunol.* 2021;42(1):P59–P75.
9. Roep BO. A viral link for type 1 diabetes. *Nat Med.* 2019;25: 1816–1818.
10. Desai MK, Brinton RD. Autoimmune disease in women: endocrine transition and risk across the lifespan. *Front Endocrinol (Lausanne).* 2019;10:265.
11. Mousavi MJ, Mahmoudi M, Ghotloo S. Escape from X chromosome inactivation and female bias of autoimmune diseases. *Mol Med.* 2020;26(1):127.
12. Billi AC, et al. The female-biased factor VGLL3 drives cutaneous and systemic autoimmunity. *JCI Insight.* 2019;4(8):e127291.
13. Marchetti M, et al. Heparin-induced thrombocytopenia: a review of new concepts in pathogenesis, diagnosis, and management. *J Clin Med.* 2021;10(4):683.
14. Farley S, et al. Prevalence and overtesting of true heparin-induced thrombocytopenia in a 591-bed tertiary care, teaching hospital. *J Intensive Care Med.* 2019;34(6):464–471.
15. Nusbaum JS, et al. Sex differences in systemic lupus erythematosus: epidemiology, clinical considerations, and disease pathogenesis. *Mayo Clin Proc.* 2020;95(2):384–394.
16. Javinani A, et al. Exploring the etiopathogenesis of systemic lupus erythematosus: a genetic perspective. *Immunogenetics.* 2019;71(4):283–297.
17. Rosetti F, de la Cruz A, Crispin JC. Gene-function studies in systemic lupus erythematosus. *Curr Opin Rheumatol.* 2019;31(2):185–192.
18. Durcan L, O'Dwyer T, Petri M. Management strategies and future directions for systemic lupus erythematosus in adults. *Lancet.* 2019;393:2332–2343.
19. Kim JW, et al. Recent advances in our understanding of the link between the intestinal microbiota and systemic lupus erythematosus. *Int J Mol Sci.* 2019;20(19):4871.
20. Kiriakidou M, Ching CL. Systemic lupus erythematosus. *Ann Intern Med.* 2020;172(11):ITC81–ITC96.
21. Lu X, et al. Patients with systemic lupus erythematosus face a high risk of cardiovascular disease: a systematic review and meta-analysis. *Int Immunopharmacol.* 2021;94:107466.
22. Aringer M, et al. European League Against Rheumatism/American College of Rheumatology classification criteria for systemic lupus erythematosus. *Arthritis Rheumatol.* 2019;71:1400–1412.
23. Singh JA, Shah NP, Mudano AS. Belimumab for systemic lupus erythematosus. *Cochrane Database Syst Rev.* 2021;2(2):CD010668.
24. Tanaka Y. State-of-the-art treatment of systemic lupus erythematosus. *Int J Rheum Dis.* 2020;23(4):465–471.
25. Jackson ME, Baker JM. Hemolytic disease of the fetus and newborn: historical and current state. *Clin Lab Med.* 2021;41(1):133–151.
26. Raffin C, Vo LT, Bluestone JA. Treg cell-based therapies: challenges and perspectives. *Nat Rev Immunol.* 2020;20(3):158–172.
27. Vandermeulen M, et al. Mesenchymal stromal cells in solid organ transplantation. *Transplantation.* 2020;104:923–936.
28. Vasco M, et al. Clinical epigenetics and acute/chronic rejection in solid organ transplantation: an update. *Transplant Rev (Orlando).* 2021;35(2):100609.
29. Bohmig GA, et al. The therapeutic challenge of late antibody-mediated kidney allograft rejection. *Transpl Int.* 2019;32(8): 775–788.
30. Tangye SG, et al. Human inborn errors of immunity: 2019 Update on the classification from the International Union of Immunological Societies Expert Committee. *J Clin Immunol.* 2020;40:24.
31. Abolhassani H, et al. Global systematic review of primary immunodeficiency registries. *Expert Rev Clin Immunol.* 2020;16(7):717–732.
32. Kumrah R, et al. Genetics of severe combined immunodeficiency. *Genes Dis.* 2020;7:52–61.
33. Kohn DB, et al. Consensus approach for the management of severe combined immune deficiency caused by adenosine deaminase deficiency. *J Allergy Clin Immunol.* 2019;143(3):852–863.
34. Mamcarz E, et al. Lentiviral gene therapy combined with low-dose busulfan in infants with SCID-X1. *N Engl J Med.* 2019;380:1525–1534.
35. Chong HJ, Maurer S, Heimall J. What to do with an abnormal newborn screen for severe combined immune deficiency. *Immunol Allergy Clin North Am.* 2019;39(4):535–546.
36. Houghton BC, Booth C. Gene therapy for primary immunodeficiency. *Hemasphere.* 2021;5(1):e509.

37. Ferrua F, et al. Lentiviral haemopoietic stem/progenitor cell gene therapy for treatment of Wiskott-Aldrich syndrome: interim results of a non-randomised, open-label, phase 1/2 clinical study. *Lancet Haematol.* 2019;6(5):e239–e253.
38. Sullivan KE. Chromosome 22q11.2 deletion syndrome and DiGeorge syndrome. *Immunol Rev.* 2019;287:186–201.
39. Du Q, de la Morena MT, van Oers NSC. The genetics and epigenetics of 22q11.2 deletion syndrome. *Front Genet.* 2020;10:1365.
40. Inoue H. Dopaminergic neurons in chromosome 22q11.2 deletion syndrome. *EBioMedicine.* 2021;63:103180.
41. Demirdag YY, Gupta S. Update on infections in primary antibody deficiencies. *Front Immunol.* 2021;12:634181.
42. Callery EL, et al. New approach to investigate common variable immunodeficiency patients using spectrochemical analysis of blood. *Sci Rep.* 2019;9:7239.
43. Le Saos-Patrinos C, et al. Functions of Tfh cells in common variable immunodeficiency. *Front Immunol.* 2020;11:6.
44. Matson EM, et al. B cell dysregulation in common variable immunodeficiency interstitial lung disease. *Front Immunol.* 2021;11:3842.
45. Bagheri Y, et al. The heterogeneous pathogenesis of selective immunoglobulin A deficiency. *Int Arch Allergy Immunol.* 2019;179:231–245.
46. Khokar A, Gupta S. Clinical and immunological features of 78 adult patients with primary selective IgG subclass deficiencies. *Arch Immunol Ther Exp.* 2019;67:325–334.
47. Lougaris V, et al. Long-term follow-up of 168 patients with X-linked agammaglobulinemia reveals increased morbidity and mortality. *J Allergy Clin Immunol.* 2020;146(2):429–437.
48. Sharma P, et al. Chediak-Higashi syndrome: a review of the past, present, and future. *Drug Discov Today Dis Models.* 2020;31: 31–36.
49. Spoor J, Farajifard H, Rezaei N. Congenital neutropenia and primary immunodeficiency diseases. *Crit Rev Oncol Hematol.* 2019;133:149–162.
50. Nagalapuram V, et al. Outcomes of isolated neutropenia referred to pediatric hematology-oncology clinic. *Pediatrics.* 2020;146(4):e20193637.
51. Anjani G, et al. Recent advances in chronic granulomatous disease. *Genes Dis.* 2020;7(1):84–92.
52. Liu W, et al. Fanconi anemia pathway as a prospective target for cancer intervention. *Cell Biosci.* 2020;10:39.
53. Giardino S, et al. Outcome of patients with Fanconi anemia developing myelodysplasia and acute leukemia who received allogeneic hematopoietic stem cell transplantation: a retrospective analysis on behalf of EBMT group. *Am J Hematol.* 2020;95: 809–816.
54. Shafqat S, et al. Role of gene therapy in Fanconi anemia: A systematic and literature review with future directions, *Hematology/Oncology and Stem Cell Therapy.* 2021;14(4):290–301.
55. Ziegler JB, Ballow M. Primary immunodeficiency: new approaches in genetic diagnosis, and constructing targeted therapies. *J Allergy Clin Immunol Pract.* 2019;7(3):839–841.
56. Leiding JW, Forbes LR. Mechanism-based precision therapy for the treatment of primary immunodeficiency and primary immunodysregulatory diseases. *J Allergy Clin Immunol Pract.* 2019;7(3):761–773.
57. Lankester AC, et al. EBMT/ESID inborn errors working party guidelines for hematopoietic stem cell transplantation for inborn errors of immunity. *Bone Marrow Transplant.* 2021;56:2052–2062.
58. Zhao L, et al. The role of mesenchymal stem cells in hematopoietic stem cell transplantation: prevention and treatment of graft-versus-host disease. *Stem Cell Res Ther.* 2019;10:182.
59. Cavazzana M, et al. Gene therapy targeting haematopoietic stem cells for inherited diseases: progress and challenges. *Nat Rev Drug Discov.* 2019;18(6):447–462.
60. Kohn LA, Kohn DB. Gene therapies for primary immune deficiencies. *Front Immunol.* 2021;12:451.
61. Brakenridge SC, et al. Distinct immunologic endotypes are associated with clinical trajectory after severe blunt trauma and hemorrhagic shock. *J Trauma Acute Care Surg.* 2021;90(2):257–267.
62. Mortaz E, et al. Does neutrophil phenotype predict the survival of trauma patients? *Front Immunol.* 2019;10:2122.
63. Quiroz-Olguín G, et al: The effect of enteral stimulation on the immune response of the intestinal mucosa and its application in nutritional support, *Eur J Clin Nutr.* 2021;75:1533–1539.
64. Toniolo A, et al. The diabetes pandemic and associated infections: suggestions for clinical microbiology. *Rev Med Microbiol.* 2019;30:1–17.
65. Pal R, Banerjee M. Are people with uncontrolled diabetes mellitus at high risk of reinfections with COVID-19? *Prim Care Diabetes.* 2021;15(1):18–20.
66. Xia L, Oyang L, Lin J, et al. The cancer metabolic reprogramming and immune response. *Mol Cancer.* 2021;20:28.
67. Carvalho T, Krammer F, Iwasaki A. The first 12 months of COVID-19: a timeline of immunological insights. *Nat Rev Immunol.* 2021;21(4):245–256.
68. Galani IE, et al. Untuned antiviral immunity in COVID-19 revealed by temporal type I/III interferon patterns and flu comparison. *Nat Immunol.* 2021;22:32–40.
69. Brodin P. Immune determinants of COVID-19 disease presentation and severity. *Nat Med.* 2021;27:28–33.
70. Sette A, Crotty S. Adaptive immunity to SARS-CoV-2 and COVID-19. *Cell.* 2021;184(4):861–880.
71. Achraf A, et al. Tumor immunity and immunotherapy for HPV-related cancers. *Cancer Discovery.* 2021;11(8):1896–1912.

10

Infection

Valentina L. Brashers

http://evolve.elsevier.com/Rogers/pathophysiology/

CHAPTER OUTLINE

Modern health care has shown great progress in preventing and treating infectious diseases. However, infectious disease continues to be a threat to human health because of the emergence of previously unknown infections, the reemergence and spread of old infections that were thought to be under control, and the development of infectious agents that are resistant to multiple antibiotics. Deadly infections are not confined to developing nations, as the Coronavirus Disease 2019 (COVID-19) pandemic has made clear in recent years. Diseases, such as chronic hepatitis, human immunodeficiency virus (HIV) infection, bacterial and viral pneumonia, and foodborne infections remain major challenges in the United States. Most deaths related to infections occur in individuals whose immune systems are compromised (young children, the elderly, and those with chronic disease). The concepts and processes of infection are presented in this chapter. Specific infections are presented in Part Two of the book with the organ system chapters (i.e., infections that occur in the cardiovascular, pulmonary, genitourinary tract, gastrointestinal tract, and skin).

MICROORGANISMS AND HUMANS: A DYNAMIC RELATIONSHIP

For many microorganisms, the human body is a hospitable site in which to grow and flourish because of sufficient nutrients and appropriate conditions of temperature and moisture. Only a small number of microorganisms are capable of causing disease. The relationship between humans and microorganisms is summarized in Box 10.1. Both host-related and microorganism-related factors influence the ability of microorganisms to become pathogenic and cause infection. The multiple layers of defense against pathogens are described in detail in Chapters 7 and 8 and are summarized in Algorithm 10.1.

Infectious diseases are caused by pathogenic microorganisms. There are many factors that influence the capacity of a microorganism to infect humans and cause disease. These factors include:

Communicability: The ability to spread from one individual to others and cause disease (e.g., severe acute respiratory coronavirus 2 [SARS-CoV-2], influenza, and measles viruses spread very easily; HIV is of lower communicability)
Immunogenicity: The ability to induce an immune response
Infectivity: The ability to invade and multiply in the host
Mechanism of action: How the microorganism damages tissue
Pathogenicity: The ability to produce disease—success depends on communicability, infectivity, extent of tissue damage, and virulence
Portal of entry: The route by which a microorganism infects the host (e.g., direct contact, inhalation, ingestion, or bites of an animal or insect)
Toxigenicity: The ability to produce soluble toxins or endotoxins, factors that greatly influence the degree of virulence
Virulence: The capacity to cause severe disease; for example, measles virus is of low virulence; rabies virus is highly virulent
ID50: The estimated number of organisms or virus particles required to produce infection in 50% of a population

The symbiotic microorganisms that make up the normal human microbiome (the resident microorganisms found in different parts of the body, including the skin, mouth,

BOX 10.1 Relationships Between Humans and Microorganisms

Symbiosis: Benefits only the human; no harm to the microorganism
Mutualism: Benefits the human and the microorganism
Commensalism: Benefits only the microorganism; no harm to the human
Pathogenicity: Benefits the microorganism; harms the human
Opportunism: A situation in which benign microorganisms become pathogenic because of decreased human host resistance, increase in numbers, or translocation to other body sites.

gastrointestinal tract, respiratory tract, and genital tract [see Chapter 7]) produce antibacterial factors that prevent pathogenic microorganisms from being able to colonize tissues, multiply, and invade.[1] Physical barriers (e.g., skin and lining of respiratory, intestinal and genital tracts) and the complex interaction of the microbiome and inflammatory and immune systems maintain this important relationship between host and resident microorganisms. When microorganisms in the microbiome cause infection because protective barriers are breached or defensive systems are weakened, they are referred to as *opportunistic microorganisms*. For example, alterations in the microbiome by antibiotics may allow local overgrowth of opportunistic microorganisms that can cause disease (e.g., *Clostridioides difficile, Candida albicans*). Individuals with primary or secondary immune deficiencies also may become infected with opportunistic microorganisms.

The Process of Infection

The process of infection includes encounter (contact) and transmission, colonization, invasion, dissemination, and cellular or tissue damage by the pathogenic microorganisms. There are several different ways that an individual can encounter or come in contact with microorganisms. *Endogenous microorganisms* are already present in the body and part of the normal microbiome. *Exogenous microorganisms* are transmitted from an external source (e.g., contaminated water, food, or from another human, animals or insects).

Transmission of microorganisms can occur in several different ways:

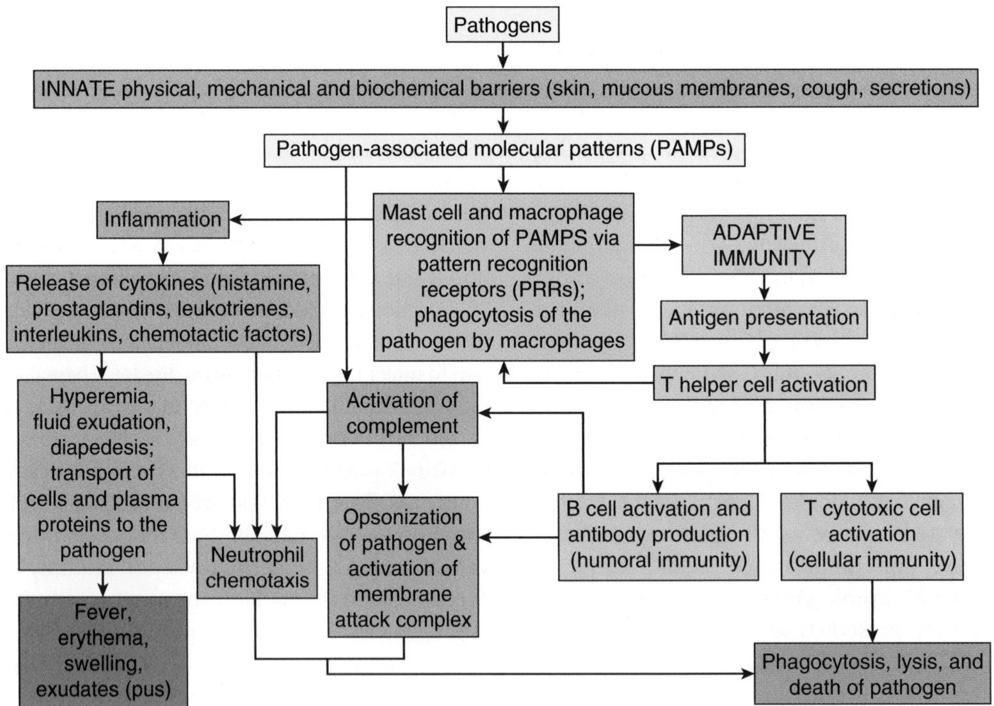

Algorithm 10.1 Host Defenses Against Pathogens. If pathogens breach the physical, mechanical, and biochemical barriers of innate immunity, mast cells and macrophages recognize pathogen-associated molecular patterns *(PAMPs)* via their pattern recognition receptors *(PRRs)*. The complement plasma protein system is activated by pathogen molecules via the alternative pathway. An inflammatory response is initiated during which numerous cytokines are released. Chemotactic factors call neutrophils to the area of invasion. The inflammatory vascular response (hyperemia, fluid exudation, and diapedesis of inflammatory cells) facilitates the transport of complement and cells to the area of invasion, as well as causes the symptoms and signs of infection. The adaptive immune system is activated and pathogen antigens are presented to Th cells. Th cells release a host of cytokines that activate B cells and T cytotoxic cells and contribute to further macrophage activation. Antibody production by B cells (plasma cells) activates complement via the classic pathway. Complement and antibodies work together to opsonize the pathogens and facilitate phagocytosis by neutrophils. In addition, the complement membrane attack complex directly lyses pathogens, and T cytotoxic cells are activated to kill intracellular pathogens.

Direct transmission occurs through direct contact with infections of another individual, such as the skin lesions of impetigo (*Staphylococcus aureus*) and STIs (see Chapter 27).

Indirect transmission: Occurs from contact with fomites, or from respiratory, fecal oral, or vector-borne transmission.

Fomites are inanimate objects that can become contaminated with infectious agents and serve as a mechanism for transfer between hosts (e.g., towels, toys, contact lenses). This is a common mechanism for the transmission of many types of infections and is the primary reason why frequent handwashing is an essential component of infection control.

Respiratory transmission may occur by means of several mechanisms. Coughing or sneezing creates a mist that can be inhaled from the air for considerable time. This mechanism readily transmits many viral diseases, including the common cold, influenza, and COVID-19. Infected individuals also may produce airborne droplets that settle on environmental surfaces. Other microorganisms such as fungi may be airborne by circulating air that carries microorganisms picked up from the soil, dried droppings, or other sites.

Fecal-oral transmission occurs when contaminated food or water is ingested. Examples include *Salmonella* (salmonella food poisoning), cholera, hepatitis A virus, *Giardia lamblia*, and many others that cause minor or major gastrointestinal diseases.

Vector-borne transmission most commonly occurs when an infectious agent undergoes part of its life cycle within an insect that feeds off the blood of infected animals or humans. The microorganism is then transmitted to other individuals through bites or stings (e.g, malaria [*Plasmodium* spp.]; Lyme disease [*Borrelia burgdorferi*]).

Horizontal transmission from one person to another through exposure to blood and body fluids (e.g., HIV, *Neisseria gonorrhoeae*); or zoonotic infections directly transmitted from animals (e.g., giardiasis, toxoplasmosis).

Vertical transmission from mother to child across the placenta (e.g., *Listeria monocytogenes*, cytomegalovirus [CMV]), during delivery from the birth canal (e.g., group B *Streptococcus, Escherichia coli, Chlamydia trachomatis*), or from breast milk (e.g., *S. aureus*).

Colonization is the ability of a pathogenic microorganism to survive and multiply on or within the human environment. *Adherence* is a part of the colonization process and helps protect the microorganism from removal by mechanical or other nonspecific forces, such as coughing of respiratory mucus. Adherence occurs between receptors on the microorganism and on the surface of cells. The specificity of these receptors results in localization of an infectious agent to particular sites, such as the confinement of common cold viruses to the respiratory tract.

Invasion or **penetration** is the ability of pathogens to cross surface barriers, including the skin and mucous membranes. This may involve penetration (e.g., mosquito bite) or a break in the integrity of the barrier (e.g., trauma). Normal protective barriers are described in Chapter 7. Other microorganisms are able to invade directly into cells.

Dissemination or spread of infection can occur by direct extension through surrounding tissue or through the blood or lymphatic vessels. **Tissue damage** or cellular alterations can occur directly by lysis caused during replication of the microorganism or the production of toxins, or indirectly as a result of an immune response with inflammation, swelling, scarring, or necrosis. The ability to damage tissues enhances the pathogenicity of the organism.

Stages of Infection

The clinical process of infection occurs in the following four distinct stages:

Incubation period: The period from initial exposure to the infectious agent and the onset of the first symptoms; during this time, the microorganisms have entered the individual, undergone initial colonization, and begun multiplying but are at insufficient numbers to cause symptoms. This period may last from several hours to years. The time between exposure and symptoms is often termed *clinical latency*. With some infections (e.g., HIV and varicella zoster infection), there is an acute symptomatic phase, followed by a latency period that can last months or even years.

Prodromal stage: The occurrence of initial symptoms, which are often mild and include a feeling of discomfort and tiredness; pathogens continue to multiply during this stage.

Invasion or acute illness period: The pathogen is multiplying rapidly, invading farther and affecting the tissues at the site of initial colonization as well as other areas; the immune and inflammatory responses have been triggered; symptoms may be specifically related to the pathogen or to the inflammatory response.

Convalescence: In most instances, the individual's immune and inflammatory systems successfully remove the infectious agent and symptoms decline; alternatively, the disease may be fatal or enter a latency phase with resolution of symptoms until pathogen reactivation at a later time.

Some infections are contagious well before symptoms begin. For example, during HIV infection, there is an acute phase where the individual may have very mild, non-specific symptoms, but the infection is very contagious. In other infections, such as hepatitis B, some individuals never develop symptoms yet can spread the infection to others. Many infections are contagious during all stages of infection, even well into convalescence.

INFECTIOUS DISEASE

Infectious disease may occur as isolated or recurrent events within individuals or populations. They sometimes are classified by their prevalence and spread within the community:

Endemic: Diseases with relatively high but constant rates of infection in a particular population. Many tropical infections are endemic to countries in the tropics.

Epidemic: The number of new infections in a particular population greatly exceeds the number usually observed

Pandemic: An epidemic that spreads over a large area, such as a continent or worldwide

Microorganisms are classified based on different morphologic characteristics and life cycles. However, groups of disease-causing microorganisms share many properties related to clinical disease, processes of infection, and evasion of human protective systems. Classes of pathogenic microorganisms and their characteristics are summarized in Table 10.1 and discussed in detail in the following sections.

Bacterial Infection

Bacteria are prokaryotes (lack a discrete nucleus), are relatively small, and are a common cause of disease (Fig. 10.1A). They can be aerobic or anaerobic and motile or immotile. Spherical bacteria are called *cocci*, rod-like forms are called *bacilli*, and spiral forms are termed *spirochetes*. Gram staining differentiates the microorganisms as gram-positive or gram-negative bacteria. Gram-positive bacteria have teichoic acid and peptidoglycan in their outer membranes, whereas gram-negative bacteria have lipopolysaccharide (LPS) in their outer membranes (Fig. 10.1B). LPS also is known as *endotoxin*. Gram-positive bacteria appear dark purple on Gram stain, whereas gram-negative appear light pink on Gram staining (Fig. 10.1C and D).

Bacteria can survive in an extracellular or intracellular environment. Extracellular bacteria use virulence mechanisms to proliferate in the body fluids of the extracellular environment. Intracellular bacteria can enter and survive in cells (including immune, epithelial, and endothelial cells). Intracellular microbes can persist for long periods (e.g., *C. trachomatis, Mycobacterium tuberculosis*, and *Mycobacterium leprae*) and cause disease by disrupting cellular structure and function.

Examples of human diseases caused by specific bacteria are listed in Table 10.2. **Bacteremia** occurs when bacteria are present in the blood. **Sepsis**, or **septicemia**, occurs when bacteria are growing in the blood and release large amounts of toxins causing clinical symptoms and signs.

Mechanisms of Bacterial Invasion and Tissue Damage

Virulence factors that help bacteria cause infection include:

Pili (fimbria): Hair-like projections that express adhesion molecules to attach to cells and invade tissue and to connect one bacterium to another (Fig. 10.2)

Flagella: A rotary structure that provides motility and expresses adhesion molecules (see Fig. 10.1A)

Toxins: Poisonous substances that cause injury, such as exotoxins (direct injury), endotoxins (indirect injury)

Enzymes: Proteins that promote tissue invasion (e.g., proteases and lipases)

Capsules: An outer covering of the cell wall that prevents phagocytosis and resists host immunity

Biofilms: A matrix excreted by bacteria that protects them from immune cells and antibiotics

Many bacteria use toxins as virulence factors, including exotoxins and endotoxins. **Exotoxins** are secreted molecules, mostly protein enzymes. They directly injure cells by damaging cell membranes or by entering cells and changing their function. One of the most poisonous exotoxins is botulinum neurotoxin produced by *Clostridium botulinum*, which causes paralysis and respiratory compromise. Different strains of *S. aureus* are capable of producing a wide array of diseases, many of which result from exotoxins (Fig. 10.3). Some damage the cell membrane and others cause blood clots (coagulase); break down clots; cause separation of the epidermis, resulting in scalded skin syndrome (exfoliative toxins); secrete enzymes, which degrade lipids on the skin surface and facilitate abscess formation (lipases); produce enterotoxins, which cause food poisoning; or produce superantigens (a type of exotoxin), which stimulate a profound immune response.

Another type of toxin is endotoxin. Unlike secreted exotoxins, **endotoxin** (also called lipopolysaccharide) is contained in the cell walls of gram-negative bacteria and is released during lysis (or destruction) of the bacteria (see Fig. 10.1B). The innermost part of LPS, lipid A, is made of polysaccharides and fatty acids and is responsible for the substance's toxic effects. Endotoxin also may be released during bacterial growth or during treatment with antibiotics. At low levels, endotoxin initiates an effective innate immune response, including activation of inflammatory cells and complement (Fig. 10.4) (see Chapter 7). As the infection progresses, increasing amounts of endotoxin

TABLE 10.1 Classes of Microorganisms Infectious to Humans

Class	Size	Site of Reproduction	Example
Virus	20–300 nm	Intracellular	Human immunodeficiency virus, hepatitis A and B, chicken pox, measles, SARS-CoV-2
Bacteria	0.8–15 mcg	Skin	Staphylococcal wound infection
		Mucous membranes	Cholera
		Extracellular	Streptococcal pneumonia
			Mycoplasma pneumonia
		Intracellular	Tuberculosis, chlamydiasis
Fungi	2–200 mcg	Skin	Tinea pedis (athlete's foot)
		Mucous membranes	Candidiasis (e.g., thrush)
		Extracellular	Sporotrichosis
		Intracellular	Histoplasmosis
Protozoa	1–50 mm	Mucosal	Giardiasis
		Extracellular	African trypanosomiasis (sleeping sickness)
Helminths	3 mm to 10 m	Intracellular	Trichinosis
		Extracellular	Filariasis

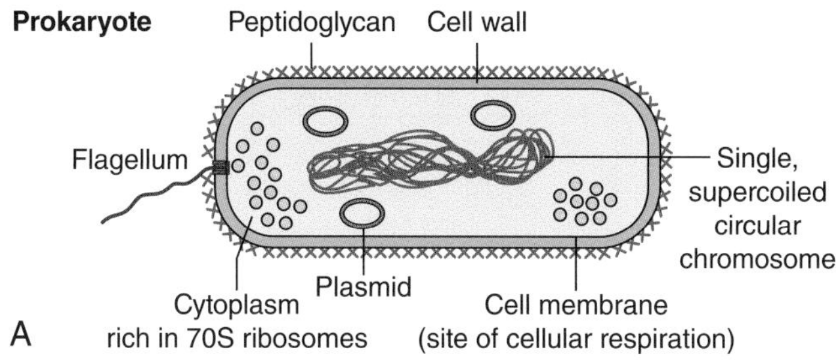

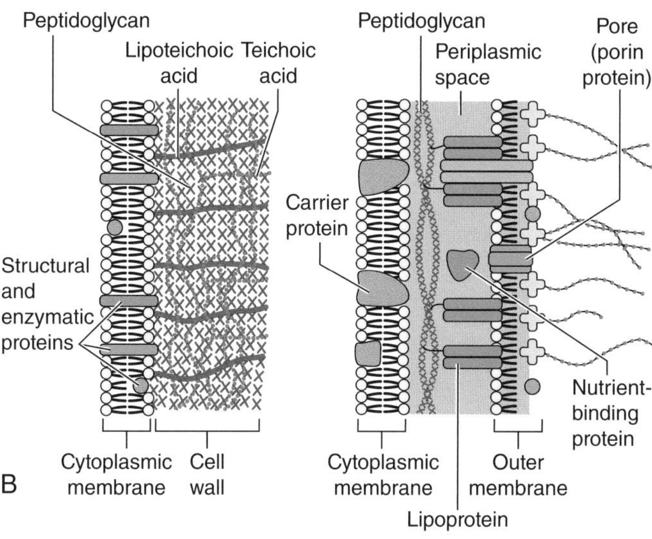

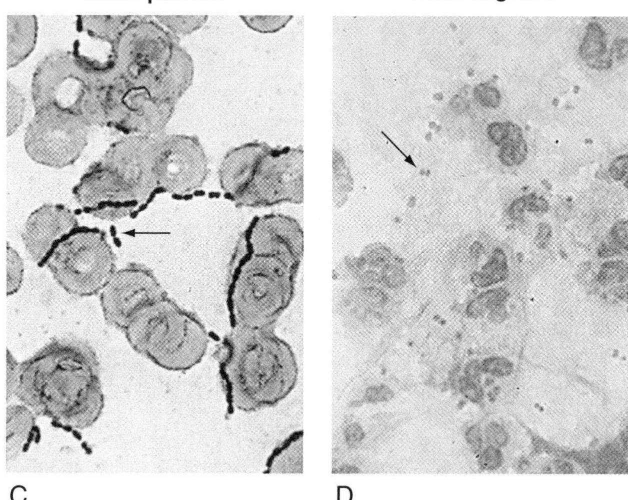

Fig. 10.1 General Structure of Bacteria. **(A)** Major features of prokaryotes. Unlike a human cell, a prokaryote does not have nuclei and endoplasmic reticulum. Instead, it has a single chromosome and a cytoplasm rich in small ribosomes. A prokaryote also lacks mitochondria but has a complex cell membrane in which cellular respiration and energy production occurs. **(B)** Comparison of gram-positive and gram-negative bacterial cell walls. A gram-positive bacterium has a thick peptidoglycan layer that contains teichoic and lipoteichoic acids. A gram-negative bacterium has a thin peptidoglycan layer and an outer membrane that contains lipopolysaccharide, phospholipids, and proteins. The periplasmic space between the cytoplasmic and outer membranes contains transport, degradative, and cell wall synthetic proteins. **(C)** Example of a gram-positive (darkly stained microorganisms, *arrow*) group A *Streptococcus*. This microorganism consists of cocci that frequently form chains. **(D)** Example of a gram-negative (pink microorganisms, *arrow*) *Neisseria meningitidis* in cerebrospinal fluid. Neisseria form complexes of two cocci (diplococci). (A and B, From Murray PR, Rosenthal KS, Pfaller MA. *Medical microbiology*, 7th edition. Philadelphia: Saunders; 2013; C and D, From Murray PR, Rosenthal KS, Kobayashi GS, et al. *Medical microbiology*, 4th edition. St. Louis: Mosby; 2002.)

stimulate the release of inflammatory mediators such as tumor necrosis factor-α (TNF-α) interleukin- 1 (IL-1), IL-6, IL-8, nitric oxide, and platelet activating factor that produce fever and cause the local and systemic effects of inflammation (see Fig. 10.4). Once in the blood in high quantities, endotoxins cause the release of toxic levels of these cytokines that promote vasodilation (reduces blood pressure), decrease oxygen delivery to tissues, and may result in endotoxic shock (septic shock) (see Fig. 10.4) (see Chapter 48). Endotoxins also can activate the coagulation cascade, leading to the syndrome of disseminated (or diffuse) intravascular coagulation (see Chapter 29).

In addition to toxins, bacteria can release enzymes that promote infection and damage tissues and organs. Some of the most important bacterial enzymes are proteases, lipases, deoxyribonucleases (DNases), and hyaluronidase. These enzymes are not specific for any particular cell or cell receptor but facilitate spread of the microorganism by weakening the surrounding connective tissue to allow invasion. For example, kinases (e.g., streptokinase and staphylokinase) activate plasminogen to digest large clots that interfere with bacterial spread. In contrast, many staphylococcus species produce coagulase, an enzyme that produces clotting around the bacterium as a way of protecting itself. Many enzymes also will digest membranes of tissue cells leading to lysis and release of nutrients that are useful to the microorganisms.

While bacterial toxins and enzymes contribute to tissue injury, much of the damage caused by infections is secondary to the inflammatory and immune responses. Infectious microorganisms routinely initiate an immune and inflammatory response, including infiltrates of phagocytic cells and a wide variety of T cells, production of antibodies, and activation of plasma systems (complement, clotting) (see Chapters 7, 8, and 9). Cytokines and chemokines secreted by inflammatory and immune cells are designed to inhibit the proliferation and spread of infectious agents; however, most also are damaging to the surrounding tissue.

Bacterial Evasion of Immune and Inflammatory Defenses

In order for bacteria to invade, replicate, and cause disease, they must evade the inflammatory and immune defense mechanisms (see Algorithm 10.1). For example, some microorganisms produce proteases that digest components of the plasma systems (complement, clotting, fibrinolysis),

TABLE 10.2 Examples of Common Bacterial Infections

Primary Site of Infection	Bacteria	Staining Characteristic	Disease (Primary)
Upper respiratory tract	*Corynebacterium diphtheriae*	Gram +	Diphtheria
	Streptococcus pyogenes (group A)	Gram +	Streptococcal pharyngitis
Lower respiratory tract	*Streptococcus pneumoniae*	Gram +	Pneumococcal pneumonia
	Mycoplasma pneumoniae	Immunofluorescent stain	Atypical pneumonia
	Chlamydophila pneumophila	Immunofluorescent stain	Atypical pneumonia
	Bordetella pertussis	Gram −	Whooping cough
	Legionella pneumophila	Gram −	Legionella pneumonia
	Mycobacterium tuberculosis	Ziehl–Neelsen stain	Tuberculosis
	Pseudomonas aeruginosa	Gram −	Pseudomonas pneumonia
Gastrointestinal tract	*Clostridium difficile*	Gram +	Pseudomembranous colitis
	Helicobacter pylori	Gram −	Gastritis and upper gastrointestinal ulcers
	Vibrio cholerae	Gram −	Infectious diarrhea
	Salmonella typhi	Gram −	Infectious diarrhea
	Clostridium botulinum	Gram +	Food poisoning
	Campylobacter jejuni	Gram −	Food poisoning
Urinary tract	*Escherichia coli*	Gram −	Cystitis and pyelonephritis
	Klebsiella pneumoniae	Gram −	Cystitis and pyelonephritis
	Proteus mirabilis	Gram −	Cystitis and pyelonephritis
Sexually transmitted infections	*Chlamydia trachomatis*	Immunofluorescent stain	Pelvic inflammatory disease
	Neisseria gonorrhoeae	Gram −	Gonorrhea
	Treponema pallidum	Gram −	Syphilis
Skin and wound infections	*Staphylococcus aureus*	Gram +	Cellulitis, wound and medical device infections
	Staphylococcus epidermidis	Gram +	Wound and medical device infections
	S. pyogenes	Gram +	Impetigo, erysipelas, cellulitis, fasciitis
Meninges	*Neisseria meningitidis*	Gram −	Meningitis
	Hemophilus influenza	Gram −	Meningitis
	Listeria monocytogenes	Gram +	Meningitis
Zoonotic infections	*Borrelia burgdorfer*	Gram −	Lyme disease
	Rickettsia rickettsii	Gram −	Rocky Mountain Spotted Fever

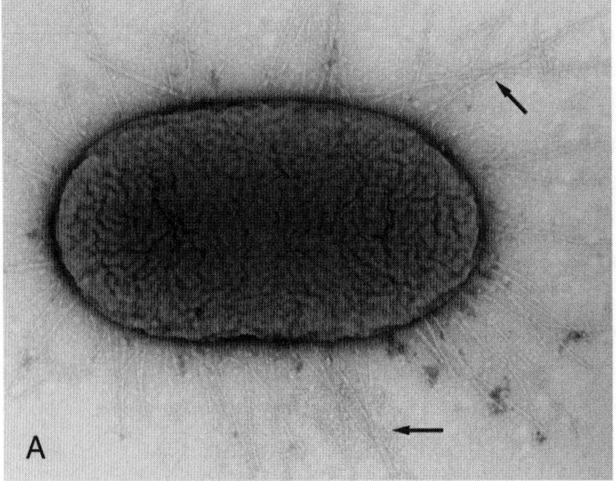

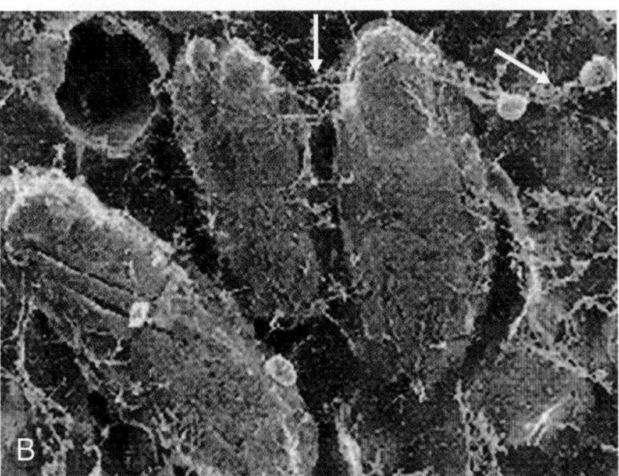

Fig. 10.2 Attachment of *Escherichia coli* Through Pili. (A) Transmission electron micrograph showing pili *(arrows)* of pathogenic *E. coli.* **(B)** Scanning electron micrograph of *E. coli (orange)* attached by pili *(arrows)* to bladder epithelium *(blue)*. (A, Courtesy Eric Buckles and Paula J. Fernandes; B, Modified from Wein A, Kavoussi LR, Novick AC, et al. *Campbell-Walsh urology*, 9th edition. Philadelphia: Saunders; 2007.)

immunoglobulins, cytokines, and antimicrobial peptides. Others produce leukocidins that lyse phagocytes. Table 10.3 provides other examples of mechanisms used by pathogens to resist the immune system.

Antiphagocytic capsules are expressed by most bacterial pathogens involved in pneumonia and meningitis (Fig. 10.5). **Capsules** are mostly polysaccharide, although proteins also may be capsular components. Encapsulated bacteria are

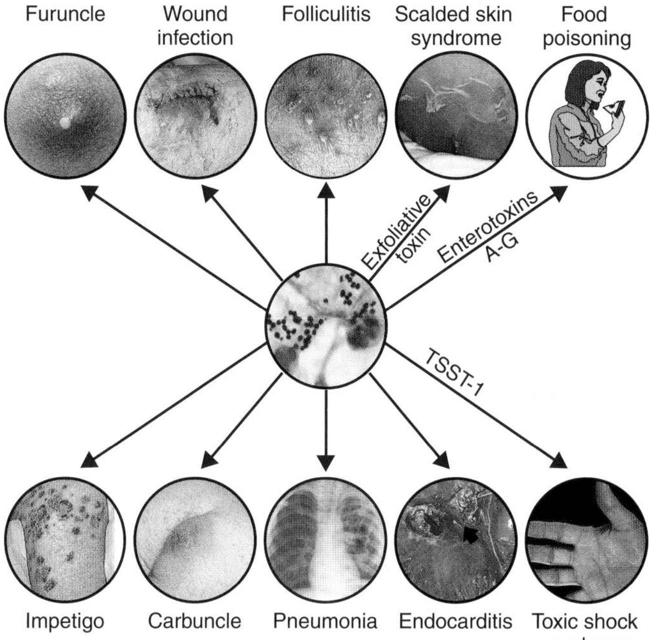

Fig. 10.3 ***Staphylococcus aureus*** **Infections.** Different strains of *S. aureus* (gram-positive cocci) cause a variety of infections in different organ systems. The center photograph shows *S. aureus* in sputum from an individual with pneumonia. The particular infection may depend on the toxin produced: exfoliative toxin (scalded skin syndrome), enterotoxins A–G (food poisoning), or toxic shock syndrome toxin-1 (TSST-1). Toxic shock syndrome, carbuncle, impetigo, and wound infection photos: From Cohen J, Powderly WG. *Infectious diseases*, 3rd edition. St. Louis: Mosby; 2010. Folliculitis photo: From Goldman L, Ausiello D. *Cecil medicine*, 24th edition. Philadelphia: Saunders; 2012. Center photo and photos of food poisoning and endocarditis: From Kumar V, Abbas AK, Aster JC, et al. *Robbins and Cotran pathologic basis of disease*, 8th edition. Philadelphia: Saunders; 2010. Furuncle photo: From Long S, Pickering LK, Prober CG. *Principles and practice of pediatric infectious diseases*, 4th edition. Philadelphia: Saunders; 2012. Scalded skin syndrome and pneumonia photos: From Mandell G, Bennett JE, Dolin R. *Principles and practice of infectious diseases*, 7th edition. Philadelphia: Churchill Livingstone; 2010.

difficult for macrophages and neutrophils to phagocytose until they are opsonized by complement and antibodies, thus delaying the immune response to these microorganisms.[2] Examples include the thick polysaccharide covering of pneumococci *(S. pneumoniae)* and *Neisseria meningitidis*, the waxy capsule surrounding the tubercle bacillus *(M. tuberculosis)*, and the polysaccharide "slime" capsule of *Pseudomonas aeruginosa.*

Many bacteria are capable of developing increased virulence, antibiotic resistance, and other adaptive factors through a process called horizontal gene transfer. Bacteria can share segments of genetic material through bacteriophages or plasmids.[3] Bacteriophages are viruses that infect bacteria and can inject genetic material from one bacterium into another during their infectious process. Plasmids are small circular DNA molecules within bacteria that exist outside of chromosomes and can move from one microorganism to another through a process called conjugation. Conjugation is the process by which two bacteria fuse together via pili (see Fig. 10.2). Horizontal gene transfer occurs within and across species of bacteria and can create hybrid bacteria that demonstrate improved ability to infect and replicate, and to resist treatment.[3,4]

Another way microorganism overcome host defenses is by the formation of biofilms (Fig. 10.6). Biofilms consist of mixed species of microorganisms, including bacteria and fungi, immersed in a highly organized extracellular matrix of polysaccharides, nucleic acids, and proteins produced by the microorganisms. These biofilms become a multicellular community within a protective structure providing protection from external threats, including host defense mechanisms and antimicrobial treatment, making them difficult to eradicate. For example, there is increasing evidence that biofilm bacteria can skew T helper (Th) cell responses such that the immune response is unable to clear the bacteria.[5] Biofilms form on implanted medical devices (e.g., catheters, pacemakers, implanted heart valves, prosthetic joints, dentures). This type of biofilm most commonly is caused by *Staphylococcus epidermidis* and *S. aureus*, although biofilms formed by fungi and other bacteria such as *P. aeruginosa* may also occur.[6,7] Biofilms also occur on teeth, as well as on epithelial surfaces (e.g., persistent nasopharyngeal colonization with staphylococci; otitis media; diabetes-associated foot ulcers; infected burns; or pneumonia associated with cystic fibrosis). *C. difficile* forms biofilms in the gut, making gastrointestinal infection by this bacterium difficult to treat.[8] Biofilms are associated with chronic infections, especially in wounds where they contribute to poor wound healing.[9,10] Of great concern is the recognition that horizontal transfer of antibiotic resistance genes between bacterial is facilitated within biofilms.[11] Bacteria may be released from the surface of biofilms, potentially resulting in distant infections.

Viral Infection

Viral diseases are common and range in severity from the common cold to the acquired immunodeficiency syndrome (AIDS). Examples of human diseases caused by specific viruses are listed in Table 10.4 Viruses are extremely simple microorganisms that do not possess any of the metabolic organelles found in prokaryotes (e.g., bacteria) or eukaryotes (e.g., human cells). Viral replication depends on their ability to infect a permissive host cell. The basic viral structure (virion) consists of nucleic acid protected by a protein shell, the capsid. The viral genome can be double-stranded deoxyribonucleic acid (dsDNA), single-stranded DNA (ssDNA), double-stranded ribonucleic acid RNA (dsRNA), or single-stranded RNA (ssRNA). Many viruses also are surrounded by a protective envelope, which contains the viral proteins needed for attachment to host cells. Viruses also contain enzymes that drive viral replication. Viral pathogens directly destroy or damage cells as part of their replication in infected cells. Transmission is usually from one infected individual to an uninfected individual by aerosols of respiratory tract fluids, contact with infected blood or contaminated surfaces, sexual

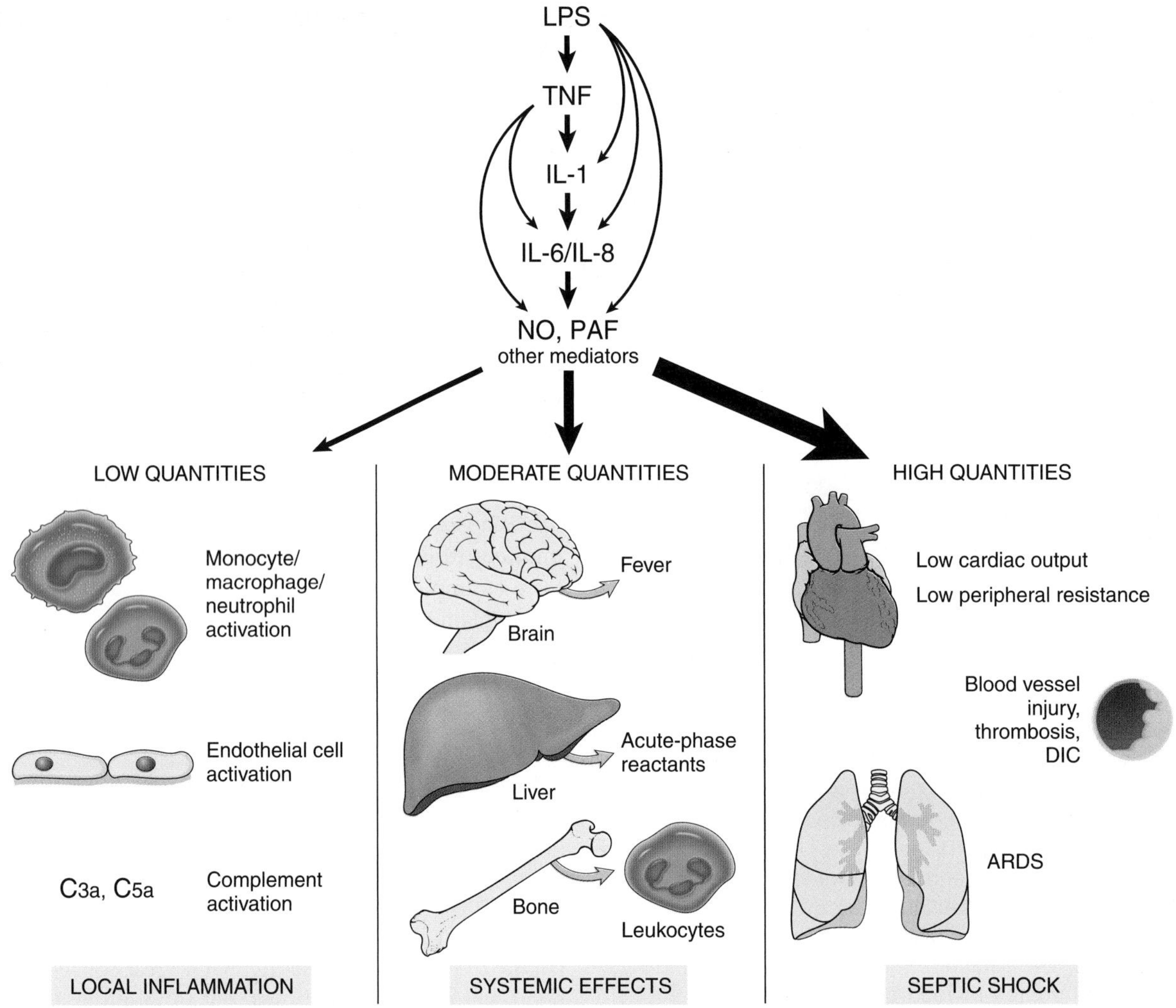

Fig. 10.4 The Many Effects of Lipopolysaccharide. Bacterial endotoxin lipopolysaccharide *(LPS)* activates almost every aspect of inflammation. The release of LPS from gram-negative bacteria triggers successive waves of cytokine production, including tumor necrosis factor *(TNF)*, interleukin-1 *(IL-1)*, interleukin-6 *(IL-6)*, and interleukin-8 *(IL-8)*, and secondary mediators of inflammation, such as nitric oxide *(NO)* and platelet-activating factor *(PAF)*. At low levels of LPS the effect is local. Moderate levels of LPS cause more systemic inflammatory responses. High levels of LPS may lead to septic shock and death. *ARDS*, Acute respiratory distress syndrome; *DIC*, disseminated intravascular coagulation. (From Kumar V, Abbas A, Fausto N. *Robbins & Cotran pathologic basis of disease*, 7th edition. Philadelphia: Saunders; 2005; Modified from Abbas AK, Lichtman AH, Pober JS. *Cellular and molecular immunology*, 4th edition. Philadelphia: WB Saunders; 2000.)

contact, transmission from an animal reservoir (zoonotic infection), or through a vector, such as mosquitoes.

Viruses are obligatory intracellular microbes. Although classes of viruses differ in the ways they reproduce, they share common replicative steps (Fig. 10.7):

1. *Recognition* and *attachment* allow the virus to bind to a specific receptor on the target cell. The specificity of the virus-receptor attachment dictates the range of host cells that a particular virus will infect. Therefore, clinical symptoms reflect the damage to the specific type of infected cells (e.g., hepatitis A causes symptoms of liver failure; HIV infection results in destruction of CD4+ T cells and immunodeficiency).
2. *Penetration* into the cell most commonly occurs by endocytosis or membrane fusion.
3. *Uncoating* is the release of viral nucleic acid (genome) from the viral capsid by viral or host enzymes.
4. *Replication* is the synthesis of new DNA or RNA strands and messenger RNA (mRNA). Most DNA viruses (except poxviruses) replicate their genome in the nucleus where they use the host's transcriptase enzymes to produce messenger RNA (mRNA). Most RNA viruses (except influenza and HIV) replicate in the cytoplasm and directly make mRNA using viral polymerases.
5. *Translation* results in viral structural protein synthesis in the host cell endoplasmic reticulum and Golgi apparatus.
6. *Assembly* is the formation of new virions.
7. *Release* or shedding of new virions is by lysis of the cell, exocytosis of the viral particle, or budding from the cell

TABLE 10.3 Examples of Mechanisms Used by Pathogens to Resist the Immune System

Mechanisms	Effect on Immunity	Example of Specific Microorganisms
Destroy or Block Component of Immune System		
Produce toxins	Kills phagocyte or interferes with chemotaxis Prevents phagocytosis by inhibiting fusion between phagosome and lysosomal granules	*Staphylococcus* *Streptococcus* *Mycobacterium tuberculosis*
Produce antioxidants (e.g., catalase, superoxide dismutase) Produce protease to digest immunoglobulin A (IgA)	Prevents killing by oxygen-dependent mechanisms Promotes bacterial attachment	*Mycobacterium* sp. *Salmonella typhi* *Neisseria gonorrhoeae* (urinary tract infection), *Haemophilus influenzae*, and *Streptococcus pneumoniae* (pneumonia)
Produce surface molecules that mimic Fc receptors and bind antibody	Prevents activation of complement system Prevents antibody functioning as opsonin	*Staphylococcus* Herpes simplex virus
Mimic Self-Antigens		
Produce surface antigens (e.g., M protein, red blood cell antigens) that are similar to self-antigens	Pathogen resembles individual's own tissue; in some individuals, antibodies can be formed against self-antigen, leading to hypersensitivity disease (e.g., antibody to M protein also reacts with cardiac tissue, causing rheumatic heart disease; antibody to red blood cell antigens can cause anemia)	Group A *Streptococcus* (M protein) *Mycoplasma pneumoniae* (red cell antigens)
Change Antigenic Profile		
Undergo mutation of antigens or activate genes that change surface molecules	Immune response delayed because of failure to recognize new antigen	Influenza virus Human immunodeficiency virus (HIV) Some parasites

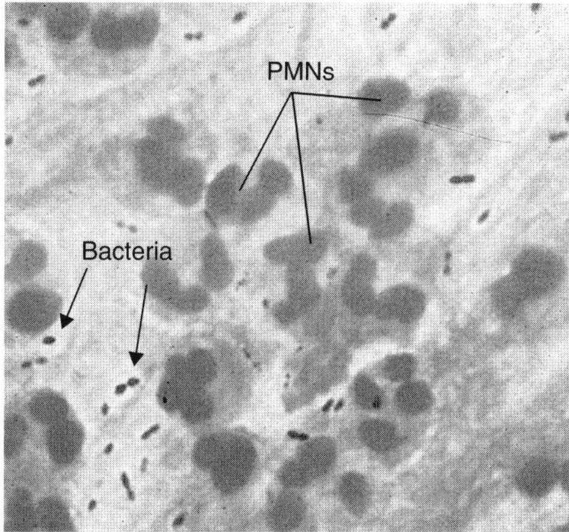

Fig. 10.5 Bacterial Capsules. Bacterial Capsule. Gram stain of a sputum sample from an individual with pneumococcal pneumonia (×1000 magnification). The sputum is rich in polymorphonuclear *(PMN)* cells and slightly elongated, gram-positive cocci (*Streptococcus pneumoniae*). Clear areas *(arrows)* around the bacteria indicate capsules. (Modified from Mandell G, Bennett J, Dolin R. *Principles and practice of infectious diseases,* 7th edition. Philadelphia: Churchill Livingstone; 2010.)

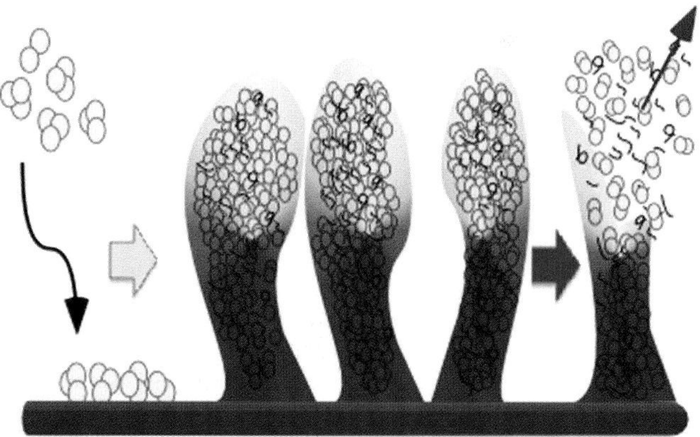

Fig. 10.6 Biofilm Development. Biofilm formation occurs in three main steps: **(1)** microorganisms attach to an epithelial surface or medical device; **(2)** they proliferate and form the protective biofilm structure; and **(3)** they can detach and spread to other surfaces or the bloodstream. (From Joo HS, Otto M. Molecular basis of in vivo biofilm formation by bacterial pathogens. *Chemistry and Biology*, 2012;19(12):1503–1513.)

membrane. A select group of viruses (e.g., HIV, herpesviruses, coronaviruses) retain a portion of the cell's plasma membrane when they bud from the surface of an infected cell providing added protection from immune processes.

Mechanisms of Viral Invasion and Tissue Damage

The effects of a virus on an infected cell vary greatly and often result in destruction of the cell. These destructive processes can include cessation of DNA, RNA, and protein synthesis

TABLE 10.4 Examples of Human Diseases Caused by Specific Viruses

Baltimore Classification	Family	Virus	Envelope	Main Route of Transmission	Disease
dsDNA	Adenoviruses	Adenovirus	No	Droplet contact	Acute febrile pharyngitis
	Herpesviruses	Herpes simplex virus type 1 (HSV-1)	Yes	Direct contact with saliva or lesions	Lesions in mouth, pharynx, conjunctivitis
		Herpes simplex virus type 2 (HSV-2)	Yes	Sexually, contact with lesions during birth	Sores on labia, meningitis in children
		Herpes simplex virus type 8 (HSV-8)	Yes	Sexually, body fluids	Kaposi sarcoma
		Epstein-Barr virus (EBV)	Yes	Saliva	Mononucleosis, Burkitt lymphoma
		Cytomegalovirus (CMV)	Yes	Body fluids, mother's milk, transplacental	Mononucleosis, congenital infection
		Varicella-zoster virus (VZV)	Yes	Droplet contact	Chickenpox, shingles
ssDNA	Papovaviruses	Human papillomavirus (HPV)	No	Direct contact	Warts, cervical carcinoma
dsRNA	Reoviruses	Rotavirus	No	Fecal–oral	Severe diarrhea
ssRNA+	Picornaviruses	Coxsackievirus	No	Fecal–oral, droplet contact	Nonspecific febrile illness, conjunctivitis, meningitis
		Hepatitis A virus	No	Fecal–oral	Acute hepatitis
		Poliovirus	No	Fecal–oral	Poliomyelitis
		Rhinovirus	No	Droplet contact	Common cold
	Flaviviruses	Hepatitis C virus	Yes	Blood, sexually	Acute or chronic hepatitis, hepatocellular carcinoma
		Yellow fever virus	Yes	Mosquito vector	Yellow fever
		Dengue virus	Yes	Mosquito vector	Dengue fever
		West Nile virus	Yes	Mosquito vector	Meningitis, encephalitis
	Togaviruses	Rubella virus	Yes	Droplet contact, transplacental	Acute or congenital rubella
	Coronaviruses	SARS-CoV-1, SARS-CoV-2	Yes	Droplets in aerosol or direct contact	Severe respiratory tract disease
	Caliciviruses	Norovirus	No	Fecal–oral	Gastroenteritis
ssRNA–	Orthomyxoviruses	Influenza virus	Yes	Droplet contact	Influenza
	Paramyxoviruses	Measles virus	Yes	Droplet contact	Measles
		Mumps virus	Yes	Droplet contact	Mumps
		Parainfluenza virus	Yes	Droplet contact	Croup, pneumonia, common cold
		Respiratory syncytial virus (RSV)	Yes	Droplet contact, hand-to-mouth	Pneumonia, influenza-like syndrome
	Rhabdoviruses	Rabies virus	Yes	Animal bite, droplet contact	Rabies
	Bunyaviruses	Hantavirus	Yes	Aerosolized animal fecal material	Viral hemorrhagic fever
	Filoviruses	Ebola virus	Yes	Direct contact with body fluids	Viral hemorrhagic fever
		Marburg virus	Yes	Direct contact with body fluids	Viral hemorrhagic fever
	Arenavirus	Lassa virus	Yes	Aerosolized animal fecal material	Viral hemorrhagic fever
ssRNA+ with RT	Retroviruses	HIV	Yes	Sexually, blood products	AIDS
dsDNA with RT	Hepadnaviruses	Hepatitis B virus	Yes	All body fluids	Acute or chronic hepatitis, hepatocellular carcinoma

AIDS, Acquired immunodeficiency syndrome; *DNA*, deoxyribonucleic acid; *ds*, double-stranded; *HIV*, human immunodeficiency virus; *RNA*, ribonucleic acid; *RT*, reverse transcriptase; *SARS*, severe acute respiratory syndrome; *ss*, single-stranded.

(e.g., herpesvirus); disruption of lysosomal membranes resulting in release of digestive lysosomal enzymes that can kill the cell (e.g., herpesvirus); fusion of host cells producing multinucleated giant cells (e.g., respiratory syncytial virus [RSV]); and alteration of the antigenic properties of the infected cell, causing the individual's immune system to attack the cell as if it were foreign (e.g., hepatitis B virus). Alternatively, there are viruses that cause transformation of host cells into cancerous cells, resulting in uninhibited and unregulated growth (e.g., human papillomavirus [HPV]; Epstein-Barr virus [EBV]), or promote secondary bacterial infection in tissues damaged by viruses (e.g., RSV and influenza viruses).

Viruses rarely produce toxins or other destructive products that cause tissue damage, and the severity of clinical symptoms is

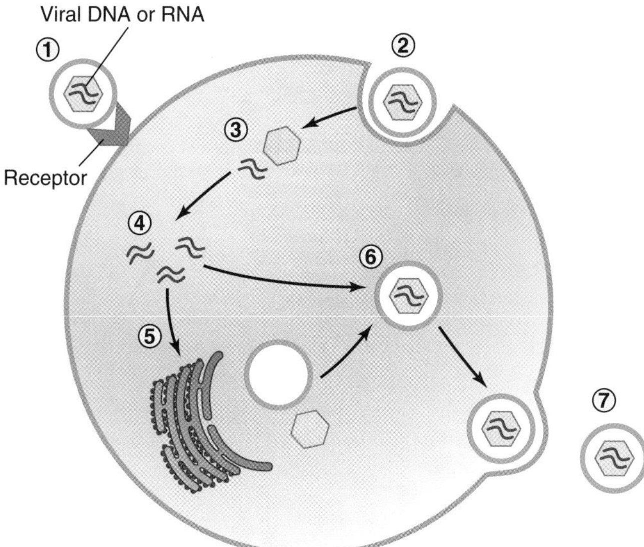

Fig. 10.7 Stages of Viral Infection of a Host Cell. Viral life cycle includes several steps. ***(1)*** Recognition and attachment of the virus to a host receptor or cell wall molecule. ***(2)*** Penetration into the host cell by fusion or endocytosis. ***(3)*** Uncoating of the viral genome within the cell cytoplasm. ***(4)*** Replication of the viral genome using host or viral transcriptases and polymerases. ***(5)*** Translation with viral structural protein synthesis in the host cell endoplasmic reticulum and Golgi apparatus. ***(6)*** Assembly of the virus. ***(7)*** Release of the virus by budding or exocytosis, or by lysis of the host cell.

most often secondary to the level of inflammatory and immune cytokines produced in response to the infected cells. In most cases, the symptoms of viral infection (e.g., fever, aches, nausea) are generally mild, caused by the individual's own inflammatory response to infection, and usually resolve in a relatively short time. However, more severe local cellular effects may result from destruction of infected cells by lymphocytes. For example, the dermal and ocular lesions of herpes simplex virus infection result from T cell–mediated cytotoxicity of epithelial cells. Hepatitis B causes immune-mediated destruction of infected liver cells causing liver failure and cirrhosis. Many viruses induce excessive production of proinflammatory cytokines and reactive oxygen species, all of which contribute to tissue damage. Severe systemic illness also can occur in viral infection resulting in significant morbidity and mortality (e.g., influenza pneumonia; COVID-19).

Viral Evasion of Immune and Inflammatory Defenses

Some viruses bypass intracellular defenses and hide within cells and away from normal inflammatory or immune responses in a process called *viral latency* (e.g., varicella zoster virus, HPV, and HIV). Varicella zoster virus (which causes chickenpox) will enter a latency phase and spread from mucosal and epidermal sites to remain dormant in the dorsal root ganglion. Later in life and in response to stimuli, such as stress, hormonal changes, or disease, the virus may exit latency and enter a productive cycle causing herpes zoster (shingles) or postherpetic neuralgia.

Viruses also can elude the immune system by making small changes to the genes that produce viral surface antigens, a process known as **antigenic variation**. **Antigenic drift** is a minor form of antigenic variation and results from mutations in the viral genome. For example, antigenic drift can lead to changes in the surface hemagglutinin (HA) and neuraminidase (NA) proteins that allow the influenza virus to attach to human cells. HA and NA also serve as specific antigens that can be detected by the adaptive immune system and allow the production of virus-specific antibodies. Vaccine protection gained from the previous year's infection does not necessarily protect against influenza in the following year because the HA and NA antigens undergo yearly change via antigenic drift.[12] A virus may undergo a sudden major antigenic variation known as **antigenic shift** (Fig. 10.8). Two or more different viruses combine to form a new strain having a mixture of surface antigens of the two or more original strains. For example, influenza A can infect humans, birds, and pigs. Antigenic shift occurs in pigs coinfected by a human and an avian strain of influenza. The genome is segmented into portions that undergo recombination during which the virus obtains a new HA or NA antigen. When an antigenic shift occurs, previous protection by vaccination may not exist, resulting in a major pandemic (an epidemic that spreads over a large area, such as a continent or worldwide) and much more severe disease. Such an event occurred in 2009 with the emergence of H1N1 influenza ("swine flu"). In an effort to improve vaccine effectiveness in the face of antigenic drift and antigenic shift, new methods for creating vaccines such as computationally optimized broadly reactive antigen (COBRA) and mRNA technologies have been developed.[13,14]

Human Immunodeficiency Virus and Acquired Immunodeficiency Syndrome

The **human immunodeficiency virus (HIV)** is the cause of a severe secondary immune deficiency called **acquired immunodeficiency syndrome (AIDS)**. AIDS is responsible for millions of deaths worldwide, with sub-Saharan Africa suffering the highest number of deaths. At the end of 2020, it is estimated that globally there were an estimated 37.7 million people living with HIV, over two thirds of whom are in the WHO African Region.[15] Despite these staggering numbers, the incidence and mortality of HIV has declined around the world due to increasing availability of diagnostic and treatment options. In the United States, there are over 1 million Americans who are living with HIV, and 36,801 new cases were diagnosed in 2019.[16] Although new infection rates are declining or stable in most racial and ethnic groups, the incidences of new infections increased by over 30% in American Indian and Alaska Native populations between 2015 and 2019.[16]

There are two types of HIV: HIV-1 (the most common [95% of HIV infections]) and HIV-2 (less common and less infectious). The discussion in this chapter is confined to HIV-1 and will be referred to as "HIV." There are four genotypes of HIV: M (Main), N (Non-M), O (Outlier), and P.[17] Most HIV is of the M genotype, which is further is divided into nine clades (subtypes), designated A–D, F–H, J, and K.[18] Different regions of the world have a predominance of one or more types of HIV. Globally, HIV clade C is the most prevalent, comprising 46% of global infections, and is the dominant subtype in Southern

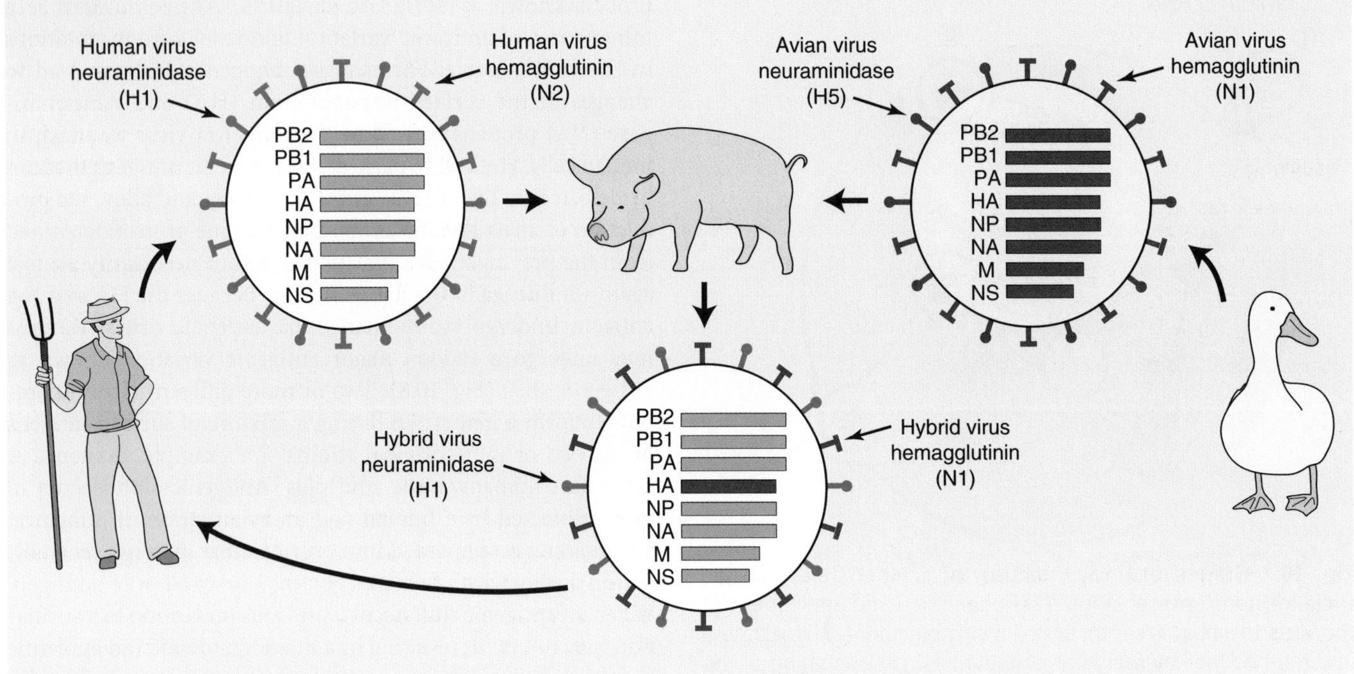

Fig. 10.8 Antigenic Shifts in Influenza Virus. Antigenic shifts occur when viruses from two different species combine to create a new virus. In this figure, a human influenza virus *(blue)* and an avian influenza virus *(red)* coinfect a species that is permissive for both. Each virus contains single-stranded RNA that codes for eight important viral components including hemagglutinin *(HA)* and neuraminidase *(NA)* which are important for viral attachment to host cells. Different strains of influenza virus are designated by the molecular components of HA and NA—in this case the human virus is H1N2 and the avian virus is H5N1. When these viruses coinfect the permissive host (pig), their RNA strands mix, thus producing a hybrid virus, H1N1. This hybrid virus may cause more serious infection because there is likely to be less residual human immunity that normally provides partial protection against more common influenza infections.

Africa and India. It is postulated that this high prevalence is due to the fact that subtype C has a lower replication capacity and is associated with a slower disease progression allowing more asymptomatic individuals to spread the disease before they know they are infected.[17] HIV clade B is the most common subtype in the United States, Western Europe, and Central and South America.

Transmission of HIV. The most common route of transmission worldwide is through heterosexual activity. However, in the United States almost 70% of new HIV infections occur among gay and bisexual men.[19] Other routes of transmission include blood or blood products, intravenous drug use, and maternal–child transmission before or during birth. Worldwide, women constitute more than half of those living with HIV/AIDS. Hundreds of thousands of cases of HIV/AIDS have been reported in children who contracted the virus from their mothers across the placenta, through contact with infected blood during delivery, or through the milk during breastfeeding.

Host genetic factors influence the transmission of HIV. Individuals with certain gene polymorphisms of their CXCR4 or CCR5 coreceptor molecules (see HIV Replication) are less likely to become infected.[17] In fact, individuals who are homozygous for the Δ32 mutation of the CCR5 coreceptor are immune to the virus. Other host factors that influence the transmission of HIV are related the viral load of the source of the infection and to the effectiveness of immune function in the exposed individual.

HIV replication. HIV is a member of a family of viruses called *retroviruses*. HIV carries its genetic information in the form of two identical copies of ssRNA contained in a capsid constructed of viral capsid protein p24. The capsid is encased in an envelope. The envelope displays glycoprotein 120 (gp120) on its surface connected to a transmembrane glycoprotein 41 (gp41) (Fig. 10.9). The genome of HIV codes for its structure (e.g., *gag, env*) as well as the viral enzymes reverse transcriptase, integrase, and protease *(pol, int, pro)*. Some HIV genes code for proteins that affect host immune responses to the virus (e.g., *nef*).[20] Other HIV genes code for infectivity, replicative rates, viral assembly, and release *(tat, tax, rex, rev, vif, vpu, vpr)*.

After transmission from one person to another, HIV replication begins with attachment to the target cell (Fig. 10.10). The virus first attaches to macrophages and to dendritic cells, which then carry the virus into the lymph nodes where it can infect its primary target cell, the Th lymphocyte (see Chapter 8). For both dendritic cells and Th cells, the process of viral attachment

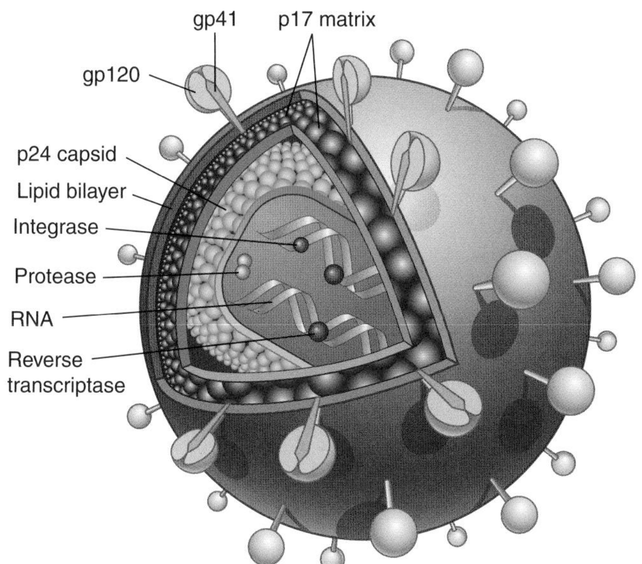

Fig. 10.9 Human Immunodeficiency Virus-1 (HIV-1) Structure. The HIV-1 virion consists of a core of two identical strands of viral ribonucleic acid *(RNA)* molecules of viral enzymes (reverse transcriptase [RT], protease [PR], integrase [IN]) enveloped in a core capsid structure consisting primarily of the structural viral protein p24. The capsid is further encased in a matrix consisting primarily of viral protein p17. The outer surface is an envelope consisting of the plasma membrane of the cell from which the virus budded (lipid bilayer) and two viral glycoproteins: a transmembrane glycoprotein, gp41, and a noncovalently attached surface glycoprotein, gp120 (site of viral attachment). (Modified from Kumar V, Abbas AK, Fausto N, et al. *Robbins and Cotran pathologic basis of disease*, 10th edition. Philadelphia: Saunders; 2021.)

begins with the binding of gp120 to CD4 molecules present on the surface of these cells. Further viral attachment requires binding to chemokine coreceptors. The coreceptor on macrophages and dendritic cells is CCR5. On Th cells, the coreceptor is CXCR4. Fusion of the virus to the cellular membrane requires that the gp120/CD4 molecule complex undergoes conformational changes that allow the transmembrane gp41 to fuse with the target cell. At this point, the viral envelope and the cellular membrane are fully fused and the viral capsid is released into the target cell cytoplasm. A group of antiretroviral medications are used to block these steps in viral attachment and fusion (see Fig. 10.10). Once the virus has been released into the target cell cytoplasm, the viral enzyme HIV reverse transcriptase converts RNA into dsDNA. Using a second viral enzyme, HIV integrase, the new DNA is inserted into the infected cell's genetic material. If the cell is activated, transcription and translation of the viral information are initiated, resulting in the production of a long strand of viral components which is then processed by the viral enzyme HIV protease. Antiretroviral medications have been developed that prevent the action of all three HIV enzymes (see Fig. 10.10). Assembly of the virus occurs at the host cell plasma membrane.

The final step in the HIV lifecycle is the formation and release of new virions. As the virus buds, it takes some of the host cell membrane with it, making the virus less vulnerable to adaptive immune attack. Host cell membrane proteins that have been incorporated into the viral envelope are biologically active and can impact infectivity and viral pathogenesis.[21] Viruses that have budded from one host cell then travel through the body to infect other host cells. There is mounting evidence that direct intercellular transmission of HIV also occurs when infected cells are phagocytosed by healthy immune cells, or through the uptake of extracellular vesicles (exosomes) released by infected cells.[22,23] This cell-to-cell transmission of virus may play an important role in HIV infecting Th memory cells that form reservoirs for latent HIV infection.

HIV pathogenesis. Macrophages and dendritic cells are the first cells to be infected with HIV after exposure. Infected dendritic cells travel to the lymph node where the virus can infect numerous Th cells (Algorithm 10.2). Rapid HIV replication leads to a burst of virus into the bloodstream (viremia) and is often associated with flu-like symptoms (acute HIV). As more and more circulating Th cells become infected, they become the primary factories for further HIV replication. HIV also preferentially infects Th cells in gut lymphoid tissues.[24] T cytotoxic (Tc) cells become activated and kill virally infected Th cells in the circulation and in the gut (see Algorithm 10.2). In fact, Tc memory cells for HIV come to reside permanently in the gut and provide a sustained immune response to infected Th cells in intestinal lymphoid tissue.[25] While the killing of infected Th cells is essential for suppressing HIV replication, this process causes the destruction of billions of Th cells each day. The bone marrow is capable of producing large numbers of Th cells to replace those that are killed; thus, Th cell numbers remain relatively stable for some years in the untreated individual. However, later in the course of infection, the ability of the bone marrow to generate healthy Th cells diminishes, and there is a decline in both circulating and gut Th cells resulting in systemic immunocompromise and AIDS (Fig. 10.11). HIV also infects bone marrow precursor cells, hastening the decline in Th cell numbers (see Algorithm 10.2). HIV infects Th memory cells and can remain latent as a provirus in those cells for years. Many of these viral reservoir cells are located in mucosal tissues and the gut.[26] When infected memory cells are activated by exposure to new infections, reactivation of HIV replication leads to new bursts of viremia and accelerated Th cell infection (see Algorithm 10.2).[27] HIV can also infect macrophages and dendritic cells in the central nervous system, liver, adipose tissue, skin, and genital tract.[28] These cells also serve as a reservoir for latent HIV infection.

The effects of HIV on the body extend beyond immune suppression. Chronic inflammation, recurrent opportunistic infections, and changes in the gut microbiome contribute to long-term effects on organ function. For example, HIV infection can impact alveolar cells and alter the production of surfactant proteins contributing to chronic lung disease.[29] Metabolic perturbations in Th cells and macrophages (immunometabolism) such as changes in glycolysis, fatty acid oxidation, and amino acid metabolism, persist despite therapy.[30] Direct viral toxicity to the gut mucosa leads to translocation of bacterial products

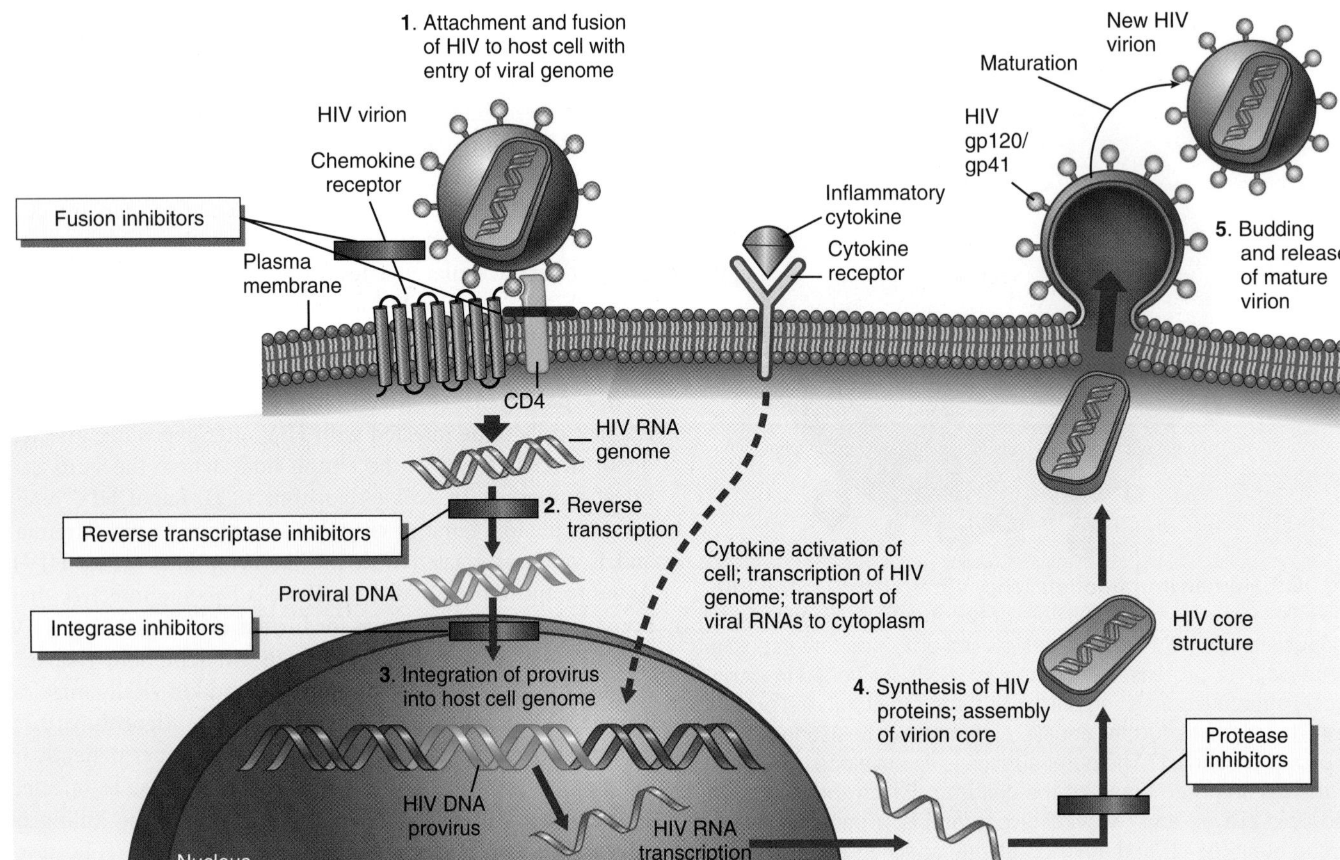

Fig. 10.10 Human Immunodeficiency Virus-1 (HIV-1) Life Cycle and Sites of Drug Intervention. The HIV virion consists of a core of two identical strands of viral ribonucleic acid *(RNA)* enveloped in a protein capsid with viral glycoproteins gp41 and gp120 on its surface (envelope). ***(1)*** HIV infection begins when a virion attaches to CD4 and the chemokine co-receptor CCR5 on macrophages or dendritic cells, and to CD4 and the chemokine co-receptor CXCR4 on T-helper cells. Conformational changes in the gp120/CD4 complex allow for fusion of the virus to the cell membrane and entry into a cell where it uncoats. ***(2)*** The viral enzyme reverse transcriptase causes reverse transcription of viral RNA into deoxyribonucleic acid *[DNA]*. ***(3)*** The viral enzyme integrase inserts the DNA into the host cell chromosomes. When the host cell is activated by cytokines, viral mRNA travels into the cytoplasm. ***(4)*** Translation results in synthesis of HIV proteins, which are then divided into viral components by the viral enzyme protease. ***(5)*** The virus reassembles and buds from the cell. The HIV life cycle is susceptible to blockage at several sites (see the text for further information), including attachment and fusion inhibitors, reverse transcriptase inhibitors, integrase inhibitors, and protease inhibitors. Modified from Kumar V, Abbas AK, Fausto N, et al. *Robbins and Cotran pathologic basis of disease*, 10th edition. Philadelphia: Saunders; 2021.

from the intestines into the blood stream. These antigens, along with associated changes in the gut microbiome (dysbiosis) contribute systemic chronic inflammation.[31] People living with HIV demonstrate epigenetic age acceleration and carry an increased burden of age-related comorbidities (cardiovascular disease, cancer, cognitive impairment, osteoporosis, and frailty) hypothesized to be the result of immunosenescence and chronic inflammation that persist despite successful treatment.[32]

Clinical manifestations of HIV infection. According to the CDC, there are three stages of HIV infection:

1. Acute HIV begins 2 to 4 weeks after infection and is associated with flu-like symptoms or may be asymptomatic. It is during this time that the virus initially infects long-lived cells such as Th memory cells and the central nervous system.[33] Viral titers in the blood are high and the individual is highly contagious. Viral antigens can be measured in the blood during this stage.
2. Clinical latency (chronic HIV infection) is the period during which the virus continues to replicate, but the bone marrow is able to replace infected cells and immune defenses decline very slowly. This period may last for 10 to 11 years in untreated individuals or may last for decades if antiretroviral therapy (ART) is successful in keeping viral titers low. Individuals are often asymptomatic or have low level infections such as thrush. Some individuals fail to achieve latency and progress quickly and are known as rapid progressors. A

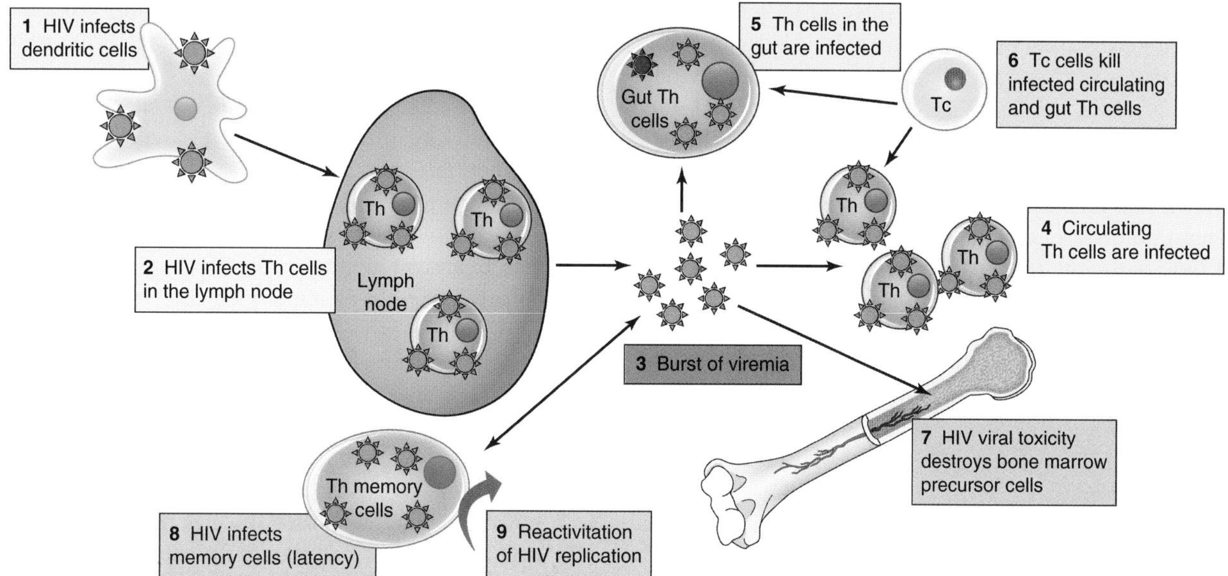

Algorithm 10.2 Pathogenesis of Human Immunodeficiency Virus Infection (HIV). ***(1)*** Dendritic cells that populate mucosal surfaces are often the first cells to be infected with HIV. ***(2)*** Infected dendritic cells travel to the lymph node where the virus can infect numerous T helper (Th cells). ***(3)*** Viral replication occurs at a rapid rate, resulting in a burst of viremia. ***(4)*** Circulating Th cells are infected, greatly accelerating HIV replication. ***(5)*** HIV infects gut Th cells. ***(6)*** T cytotoxic (Tc) cells kill virally infected Th cells leading to a decline in circulating and gut Th cells. ***(7)*** HIV infects bone marrow precursor cells, hastening the decline in immunity. ***(8)*** HIV infects Th memory cells and can remain latent in those cells for years. ***(9)*** Memory cell reactivation by exposure to pathogens results in reactivation of HIV replication.

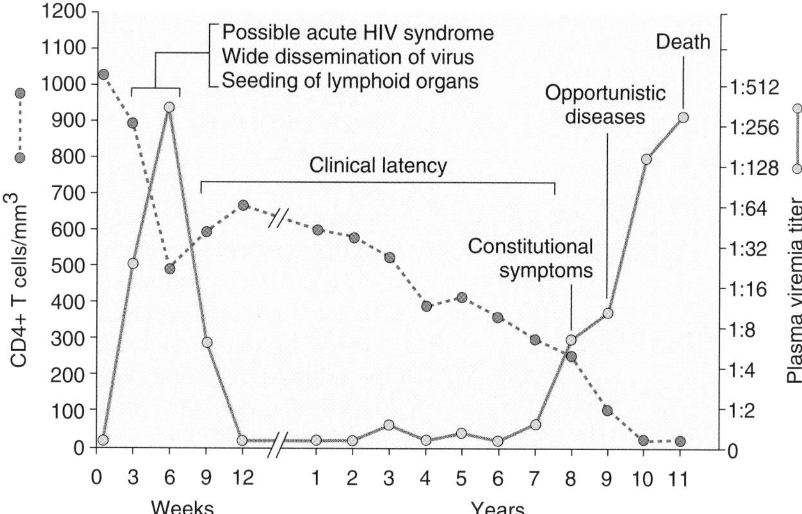

Fig. 10.11 Typical Progression From Human Immunodeficiency Virus *(HIV)* Infection to Acquired Immunodeficiency Syndrome (AIDS) in Untreated Persons. Clinical progression begins within weeks after infection; the person may experience symptoms of acute HIV syndrome. During this early period, the virus progressively infects T cells and other cells and spreads to the lymphoid organs, with a sharp decrease in the number of circulating CD4+ T cells. During a period of clinical latency, the virus replicates and T-cell destruction continues, although the person is generally asymptomatic. The individual may develop HIV-related disease (constitutional symptoms)—a variety of symptoms of acute viral infection that do not involve opportunistic infections or malignancies. When the number of CD4+ cells is critically suppressed, the individual becomes susceptible to a variety of opportunistic infections and cancers with a diagnosis of AIDS. The length of time for progression from HIV infection to AIDS may vary considerably from person to person. (Redrawn from Fauci AS, Lane HC. Human immunodeficiency virus disease: AIDS and related conditions. In A. S. Fauci, E. Braunwald, K. J. Isselbacher, et al. [Eds.]. *Harrison's principles of internal medicine*, 14th edition. New York: McGraw-Hill; Saunders; 1998.)

more rapid progression in a newly infected individual may be correlated with a high source partner viral load at the time of transmission. A small number of HIV-infected individuals remain in clinical latency for an extended period and are known as long-term nonprogressors (LTNPs), although most of these individuals eventually develop symptoms without treatment. Elite controllers are HIV infected individuals in whom no disease progression can be detected for a very long time despite not receiving antiretroviral treatment. In fact, some maintain undetectable levels of virus and stable immunologic parameters for more than 25 years after infection. Low viral replication rates and highly effective immune responses have been documented in these individuals.[34]

3. **Acquired immunodeficiency syndrome (AIDS)** occurs when significant immune compromise develops. This is defined when Th cell numbers decline below 200 cells/mm or when opportunistic infections or certain cancers occur (Box 10.2). The rate at which AIDS progresses is related to the rate in decline of Th cells and the rate of increase in serum viral titers (see Fig. 10.11). Clinical manifestations include the signs and symptoms related to AIDS-defining infections, cancers, and neurologic (neuroinflammation; encephalopathy) or metabolic (wasting) complications (Fig. 10.12). Side-effects from antiviral medications are also common.

BOX 10.2 AIDS-Defining Opportunistic Infections and Neoplasms

Infections

Protozoal and Helminthic Infections

Cryptosporidiosis or isosporiasis (enteritis)
Pneumocystosis (pneumonia or disseminated infection)
Toxoplasmosis (pneumonia or CNS infection)

Fungal Infections

Candidiasis (esophageal, tracheal, or pulmonary)
Coccidioidomycosis (disseminated)
Cryptococcosis (CNS infection)
Histoplasmosis (disseminated)

Bacterial Infections

Mycobacteriosis ("atypical," e.g., *Mycobacterium avium-intracellulare*, disseminated or extrapulmonary
Mycobacterium tuberculosis, disseminated or extrapulmonary)
Nocardiosis (pneumonia, meningitis, disseminated)
Salmonella infections (septicemia, recurrent)

Viral Infections

Cytomegalovirus (pulmonary, intestinal, retinitis, or CNS)
Herpes simplex virus (localized or disseminated)
Progressive multifocal leukoencephalopathy
Varicella-zoster virus (localized or disseminated)

Neoplasms

Invasive cancer of the uterine cervix
Kaposi sarcoma
Non-Hodgkin lymphomas (Burkitt, immunoblastic)
Primary lymphoma of brain

AIDS, Acquired immunodeficiency syndrome; *CNS*, Central nervous system; *HIV*, human immunodeficiency virus.

From Kumar V, Abbas AK, Fausto N, et al. *Robbins and Cotran pathologic basis of disease*, 10th edition. Philadelphia: Saunders; 2021.

Diagnosis and management of HIV infection. In 2021, the World Health Organization (WHO) released new guidelines on HIV prevention, testing, treatment, service delivery and monitoring.[35] These guidelines provide guidance on management of HIV along the continuum of care including prevention, testing, ARV regimens, treatment monitoring, the management of comorbidities, palliative care and pain management. Current CDC recommendations indicate that screening for HIV infection in all health care settings should be performed routinely for all persons 13 to 64 years of age after the individual is notified orally or in writing that testing will be performed unless the individual declines (known as *opt-out screening*). Screening also is recommended for men who have sex with men (MSM), pregnant women, and those with other sexually transmitted diseases (STDs) or tuberculosis (TB).[36] The CDC also recommends that clinicians screen asymptomatic sexually active MSM at least annually.[37]

HIV is diagnosed by the simultaneous measurement of both antibodies against HIV and HIV antigens in blood. If positive, these tests are confirmed by HIV DNA (nucleic acid tests [NATs]). The amount of virus in the blood (viral load) and the Th cell count are used to determine what is called the "set point," which describes the severity of infection and the level of risk for rapid progression to AIDS.

HIV prevention includes avoidance of HIV risk behaviors (e.g., unprotected sex, needle-sharing), adherence to antiretroviral treatment by infected individuals, and pre- and post-exposure prophylaxis with antiretroviral medications.[38] Advances in pre-exposure prophylaxis are emerging, including long-acting formulations of ART (cabotegravir) and insertable vaginal rings that release ART over 30 days. Monoclonal antibody treatment to prevent HIV is also being explored.[39] While vaccine development remains challenging, reports are emerging from early trials that describe the development of promising new vaccines.[40]

HIV/AIDS treatment guidelines are published by the National Institutes of Health (NIH) and are revised frequently as new antiretroviral medications are approved.[41] ART should be initiated as soon as possible after HIV infection is diagnosed. Approved HIV medications are classified by mechanism of action: **chemokine receptor inhibitors** (CCR5 antagonist prevents viral attachment), **HIV fusion inhibitors** (prevent CD4-gp 120 conformational changes during binding), **reverse transcriptase inhibitors** (nucleoside and nonnucleoside inhibitors of reverse transcriptase), **HIV integrase inhibitors** (inhibitors of viral integration into host genome), and **HIV protease inhibitors** (inhibitors of the proteases HIV uses for assembly of new virus) (see Fig. 8.12). The current regimen for the treatment of HIV infection is a combination of drugs, termed **antiretroviral therapy (ART)**. Current ART protocols indicate that individuals who are being treated for the first time should be given a combination of two synergist drugs from different classes.[41] Specific regimens (e.g., timing of drug administration, doses, drug combinations) are adapted on the basis of the age of the individual, secondary clinical symptoms (renal or hepatic insufficiency), CD4+ T-cell levels, viral load, presence

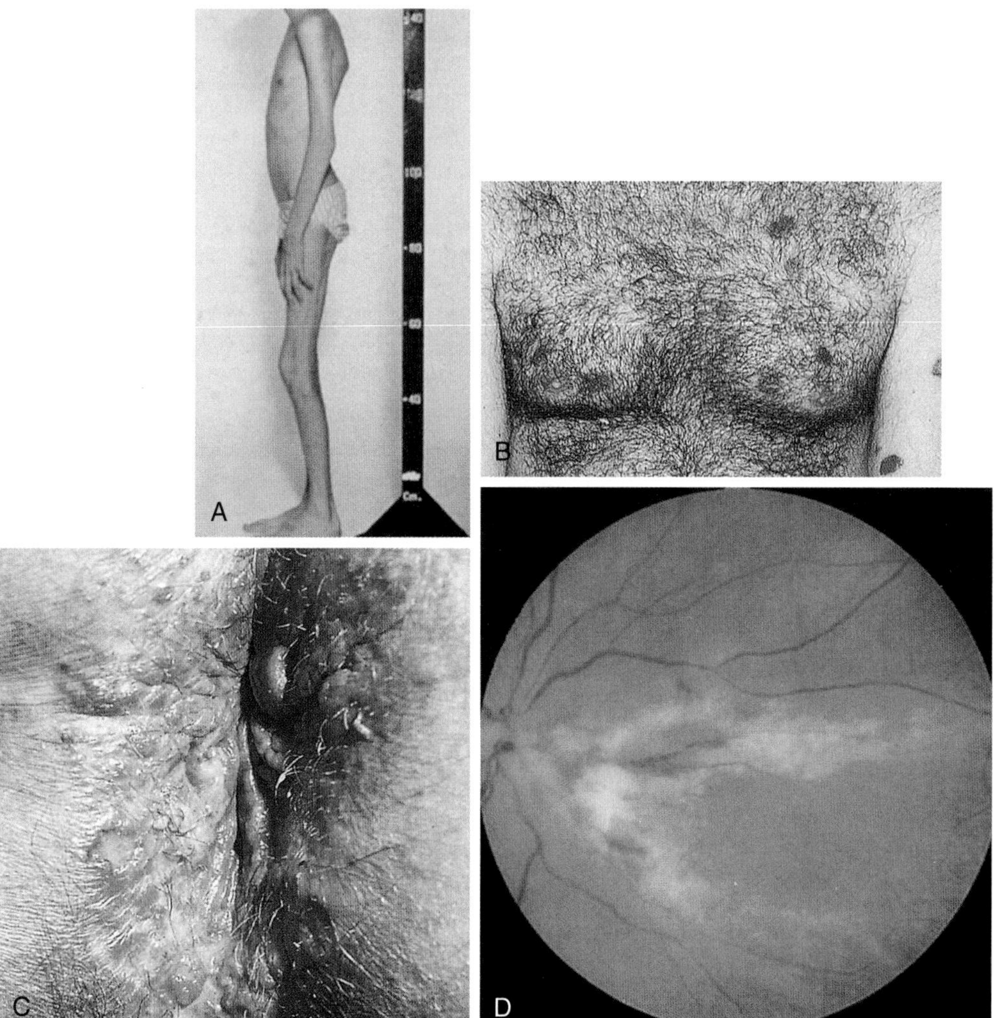

Fig. 10.12 Clinical Symptoms of Acquired Immunodeficiency Syndrome (AIDS). (A) Severe weight loss and anorexia. **(B)** Kaposi sarcoma lesions. **(C)** Perianal lesions of herpes simplex infection. **(D)** Deterioration of vision from cytomegalovirus retinitis leading to areas of infection, which can lead to blindness. (A and D, From Taylor PK. *Diagnostic picture tests in sexually transmitted diseases*. London: Mosby; 1995; B and C, From Morse SA, et al. [Eds]. *Atlas of sexually transmitted diseases and AIDS*, 4th edition. London: Saunders; 2011.)

of coinfections, preexisting cardiac risk factors, past history of treatment failure, ART drug resistance, and other parameters. Significant side effects from ART may occur and can result in reduced adherence with recurrence of disease progression and viral infectivity in some individuals. In January 2021, a long-acting formulation (cabotegravir and rilpivirine) given once per month via intramuscular injection was FDA approved with the goal of increasing adherence to treatment.[42]

The prevalence of HIV variants resistant to antiretroviral therapies is increasing. Resistance testing in an individual prior to starting ART is done routinely. Resistant strains may be found even in individuals when they are first diagnosed with HIV infection.[43] In 2018, the U.S. Food and Drug Administration (FDA) approved the first humanized monoclonal antibody called iblaizumab-uiyk for the treatment of multidrug-resistant HIV. This antibody blocks the conformational change of gp120 required for viral fusion with host cells and has been found to be effective in lowering HIV titers and improving immune function.[44] Several new drugs are in clinical trials including new monoclonal antibody treatments.[45] Unfortunately, drug therapy for HIV is not curative because the virus incorporates into the genetic material of the host, particularly CD4+ T memory cells. Additionally, HIV may persist in organs where the antiviral drugs are not as effective, such as the central nervous system (CNS). Therefore, ART must continue for the lifetime of the individual. Many new HIV treatments are being explored in an attempt to eliminate persistent HIV infection (see Emerging Science Box: Future Treatments for HIV Infection).

In spite of the challenges, progress in global treatment outcomes for HIV and AIDS has been substantial. By the end of 2020, globally 73% of adults and 54% of children living with HIV were receiving lifelong ART. Between 2000 and 2019, new HIV infections fell by 39% and HIV-related deaths fell by 51%, with 15.3 million lives saved due to ART.[15]

EMERGING SCIENCE BOX

Future Treatments for HIV Infection

Anti-retroviral therapies (ARTs) for HIV/AIDS can effectively suppress virus replication in active T helper (Th) cells, and infected individuals can lead relatively healthy lives so long as treatment continues. However, ART is not curative, and if discontinued, there is a rapid re-emergence of virus from latent provirus reservoirs such as T memory cells. Numerous approaches designed to eliminate HIV from these reservoirs are currently under investigation. One approach is the use of bone marrow transplantation with CCR5 and CXCR4-modified hematopoietic stem cells. To date, two HIV infected individuals who underwent allogeneic bone marrow transplantation for other conditions received lymphoid stem cells that lacked the CCR5 chemokine co-receptor needed for HIV fusion with macrophage and dendritic cell membranes. HIV that cannot enter host cells cannot replicate and, therefore, are not able to cause infection. It is believed that these two individuals have been cured of their HIV infection. However, bone marrow transplantation is associated with significant morbidity and mortality, therefore is unlikely to become a feasible approach to treating HIV infection in the near future. Another approach involves improving immune responses to HIV through genetic modification of T cytotoxic (Tc) cells. This can be accomplished through the use of viral vectors or nanotechnology to insert DNA into host Tc cells. The goal is the formation of new chimeric antigen receptors on Tc cells that can better recognize the virus (CAR-T Cell therapy). Because HIV mutates rapidly to evade the antigen-specific receptors on native Tc cells, CAR-T cell therapy includes the creation of numerous receptors that can recognize multiple HIV antigens. CAR-T cell approaches can also be used to alter the CD4 molecule on T helper cells, potentially rendering them resistant to HIV gp120 binding. A recent B cells are also targeted by emerging gene therapies. Vectored passive immunity is the delivery of synthetic genes that code for protective antibodies or antiviral proteins. Vectors such as attenuated viruses and plasmids deliver genetic material that produces neutralizing antibodies or antibodies capable of mediating antibody-dependent cellular cytotoxicity for HIV infected cells. Yet another approach is called "Shock and Kill" in which latency-reversing agents (e.g., histone deacetylases, protein kinase modulators) are used to reactivate latent HIV. As HIV begins to replicate, immunotherapies, and aggressive antiviral treatment are introduced to kill the newly- exposed viruses. A major barrier is that current methods that reactivate HIV also promote global T-cell activation, which can result in a life-threatening complication known as cytokine release syndrome. "Lock and Block" strategies involve the use of latency-promoting agents that prevent HIV transcription (e.g. tat inhibitors, epigenetic methylating agents) or damage the HIV genome (use of CRISPER/Cas9 s gene editing), thus keeping HIV in a provirus state. To date, neither shock and kill nor lock and block have been found to be adequately safe or effective in humans, but studies continue. Finally, there are ongoing efforts to create more effective monoclonal broadly neutralizing antibodies (bNAbs) that could prevent cell-to-cell transmission of HIV and better recognize and kill infected cells that contain latent virus.

Data from Ahlenstiel CL, et al. Delivery of gene therapy to resting immune cells for an HIV cure. *Current Opinion in HIV & AIDS*, 2019;14(2):129–136; Cornu TI, et al. HIV Gene Therapy: An Update. *Human Gene Therapy*, 2021;32(1-2):52–65; Dashto A, et al. Broadly neutralizing antibodies against HIV: Back to blood. *Trends in Molecular Medicine*, 2019;25(3):228–240; Deeks SG, et al. Research priorities for an HIV cure: International AIDS Society Global Scientific Strategy 2021. *Nat Med*, Epub Dec 2021, available at https://doi.org/10.1038/s41591-021-01590-5; Gupta RK, et al. Evidence for HIV-1 cure after CCR5Δ32/Δ32 allogeneic haemopoietic stem-cell transplantation 30 months post analytical treatment interruption: A case report. *The Lancet HIV*, 2020;7:e340–e347; Hu J, et al. Coreceptor-based hematopoietic stem cell gene therapy for HIV disease. *Current Stem Cell Research and Therapy*, 2019;14(7):591–597; Jilg N, et al. On the road to a HIV cure: Moving beyond Berlin and London. *Infectious Disease Clinics of North America*, 2019;33(3):857–868; Pauza CD, et al. Advances in cell and gene therapy for HIV disease: It is good to be specific. *Current Opinion in HIV and AIDS*, 2021;16(2):83–87; Liu B, et al. Broadly neutralizing antibody–derived CAR T cells reduce viral reservoir in individuals infected with HIV-1. *J Clin Invest*, 2021;131(19):e150211; Richard J, et al. Across functional boundaries: Making nonneutralizing antibodies to neutralize HIV-1 and mediate Fc-mediated effector killing of infected cells. *mBio*, 2021;12(5):e01405–2; and Tuyishime M, et al. Engineering antibody-based molecules for HIV treatment and cure. *Current Opinion in HIV and AIDS*, 2020;15(5):290–299.

Severe Acute Respiratory Syndrome Coronavirus -2 and Coronavirus Disease 2019

An outbreak of pneumonia in Wuhan, China in December 2019 led to the identification of the severe acute respiratory syndrome coronavirus -2 (SARS-CoV-2). The virus has distinctive spikes on its surface making it look like a solar corona, thus its name (Fig. 10.13A). It is postulated that the virus originated in bats and may have been transferred to humans through exposure to an unidentified animal vector.[46] Genomic studies have identified related coronaviruses in bats in China, Cambodia, Thailand, and Laos.[47] A global pandemic called coronavirus disease-2019 (COVID-19) ensued, with human-to-human transmission resulting in hundreds of millions of cases worldwide and millions of deaths. According to the World Health Organization, the United States leads the world in the number of coronavirus cases and deaths, followed by India and Brazil.[48] Although this is the third major coronavirus-related serious illness to appear in the last 20 years (SARS in 2003 and Middle Eastern respiratory syndrome [MERS] in 2012), it is by far the most widespread.

Transmission. SARS-CoV-2 has been detected at the highest levels in human sputum, pharyngeal swabs, and feces. It is transmitted most easily between infected persons via droplets released during cough, sneezing, or talking.[49] It is believed that transmission of the virus from infected individuals who remain completely asymptomatic is relatively rare; however, presymptomatic transmission is thought to be a major contributor to the spread of SARS-CoV-2.[50] During the 3 to 7 days between infection and symptoms, shedding of virus can be high from the respiratory tract, but infected individuals do not realize they are ill. Viral shedding peaks during early symptomatic illness (3-5 days after symptom onset) and declines below that which is readily transmissible approximately 5 to 7 days after the onset of symptoms in most individuals.[51]

The risk of transmission is greatest in indoor environments with poor ventilation and close contact (less than 6 ft) with infected individuals. Although the virus can be detected on nonporous surfaces for days to weeks, transmission of the virus from surfaces to hands and then to mouth, nose, or eyes is inefficient, and the risk of developing infection from contacting infected surfaces (fomites) is believed to be less than 1 in 10,000 exposures.[49] Viral mutations have led to the emergence of variants that have increased infectivity. These variants include the B.1.1.7 (alpha) variant that emerged in the United Kingdom, the B.1.1.351 (beta) variant that emerged in South Africa, and the B.1.1.33 (P.1) variant that emerged in Brazil. In 2021, two new variants emerged. The B.1.617.2 (delta) variant and the B.1.1.529 (omicron) variants have been found to have increased infectivity compared to previous forms of the virus and have been the cause of surges in new infections worldwide.[52,53] More new variants are emerging.

Pathogenesis. SARS-CoV-2 is a β coronavirus that consists of ssRNA and four major structural proteins: the spike (S) protein, nucleocapsid (N) protein, membrane (M) protein, and the envelope (E) protein (Fig. 10.13B).

Infection begins as the virus targets nasal and bronchial epithelial cells and pneumocytes. Other cells susceptible to infection include intestinal, cardiac, olfactory, bile duct, testicular, thyroid, pancreatic, adrenal, and pituitary cells.[54] The steps in the viral life cycle are the same as for many other viruses: (1) attachment; (2) fusion; (3) uncoating; (4) replication of the viral genome; (5) viral structural synthesis in the endoplasmic reticulum and golgi apparatus; (6) assembly; and (7) release (see Fig. 10.7).[55] Attachment of the virus occurs via its spike protein. The SARS-CoV-2 spike is a transmembrane glycoprotein composed of a receptor-binding domain and two subunits (S1 and S2). During attachment, the receptor-binding portion of the spike protein binds with high affinity to the membrane-bound form of angiotensin-converting enzyme 2 (ACE2) on human cells. ACE2 is highly expressed in lung, brain, and fat, and to a lesser extent in heart, kidney, pancreas, and intestine.[56] After attachment, the ACE 2 receptor and the S1 and S2 spike protein subunits undergo structural rearrangement. A transmembrane serine protease expressed on the target cell causes cleavage of the S protein subunits, stabilizing viral fusion with the host cell. SARS-CoV-2 is unusual in that it has a *furin cleavage site* at the S1/S2 boundary. Scientists are looking to this site as a potential target for antiviral drug therapy.[55] Following fusion, replication of the virus begins.

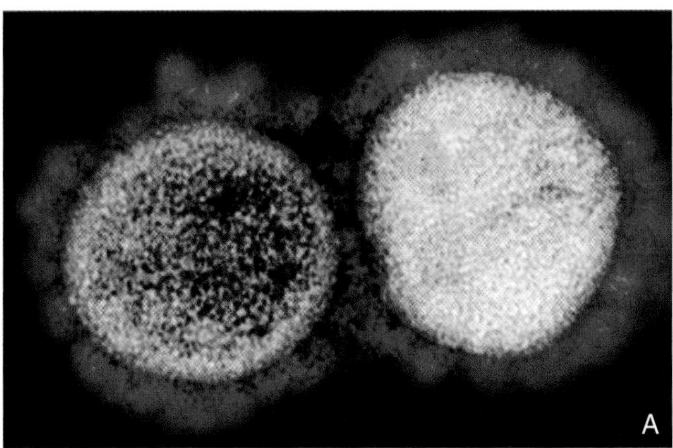

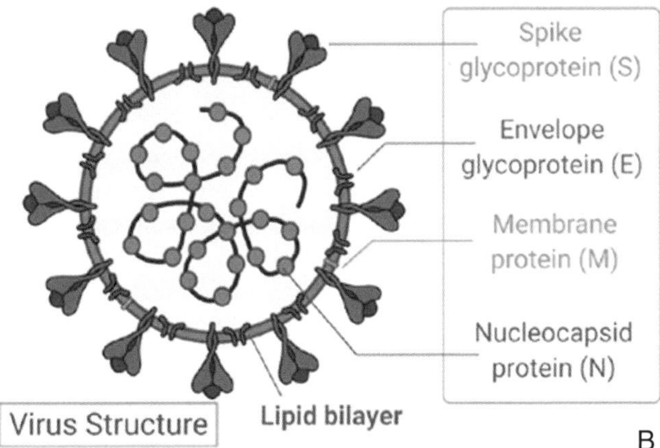

Fig. 10.13 Structure of SAR-CoV-2e. (A) Transmission electron micrograph of SARS-CoV-2 virus particles, isolated from an individual. Image captured and color-enhanced at the NIAID Integrated Research Facility (IRF) in Fort Detrick, Maryland. **(B)** SARS-CoV-2 contains 4 major structureal proteins. A, (From Jha NK, Jeyaraman M, Rachamalla M, et al. Current understanding of novel coronavirus: Molecular pathogenesis, diagnosis, and treatment approaches. *Immuno* 2021;1:30–66. https://www.mdpi.com/2673-5601/1/1/4.)

The pathophysiologic mechanisms of acute COVID-19 include endothelial damage and microvascular injury, immune system dysregulation with stimulation of a hyperinflammatory state, hypercoagulability with resultant thromboses, and maladaptation of the ACE2 pathway.[54] It primarily is the host response, rather than the virulence of the virus, that determines the progression and severity of COVID-19.[57] There is evidence that the virus can evade the triggering of early innate responses, especially the release of type I and type III interferons.[56] This allows for unopposed viral replication and slows the initiation of the adaptive immune response. Once infection is established, a powerful inflammatory response is initiated, sometimes progressing to a "cytokine storm" in which numerous interleukins (Il-1, IL-6, IL-8, IL-17), TNFα, and other inflammatory cytokines are produced at high levels.[56] This hyperinflammatory response causes increased permeability of vascular and epithelial membranes, edema, and tissue necrosis, especially in lung tissue.[54] As the disease progresses, neutrophil and natural killer cell dysfunction develops, and the virus is effective in killing T cells—which can result in a profound lymphopenia.[57]

Multiple organs may be affected, most commonly severe inflammation of lung tissue resulting in an acute respiratory distress syndrome (ARDS)-like condition (see Chapter 35). In addition, the hyperinflammatory response causes endothelial injury, microangiopathic changes, and platelet activation, giving rise to a hypercoagulable state that resembles disseminated intravascular coagulation (DIC) but is characterized by clotting without bleeding.[54] The virus causes inflammatory and immune changes in the myocardium, contributing to cardiomyocyte death. Neuroinflammation is common with damage to both the brain parenchyma and cerebral vasculature. Acute kidney injury may occur, especially in critically ill individuals, resulting in COVID-19-associated nephropathy (COVAN) characterized by acute tubular necrosis, which is followed by glomerulosclerosis in some persons.

Clinical Manifestations. The average incubation period for COVID-19 is thought to be approximately 6 days from exposure to symptoms onset. It is estimated that about 25%

of all cases remain asymptomatic.[58] Most infected individuals have only mild symptoms; however, elderly individuals and those with underlying medical conditions—such as cardiovascular disease, diabetes, and cancer—are at risk for severe disease and death. Many organ systems may be affected (Fig. 10.14). The most common symptoms are fever, cough, shortness of breath, myalgias, and fatigue. Loss of smell and taste is also common (see Chapter 16 Emerging Science Box: Loss of Taste and Smell in SARS-CoV-2-Positive Patients). Some individuals also exhibit non-respiratory symptoms resulting from neurologic, cardiac, endocrine, hepatic and renal injury. Thrombotic complications are common and are linked to an increased risk for stroke and venous thromboembolism. Respiratory failure and septic shock are the primary causes of mortality. Most individuals recover within 3 to 4 weeks after infection. However, it is estimated that nearly one-third of affected persons have persistent symptoms lasting for many weeks and even months. This prolonged syndrome is called post-acute COVID-19 or "long COVID" (see Emerging Science Box: Post-Acute COVID-19).

Evaluation and Treatment. Testing for COVID-19 is indicated for individuals with appropriate symptoms, known exposures, or who are required to be tested for community or employment purposes. Two types of viral tests are used: nucleic

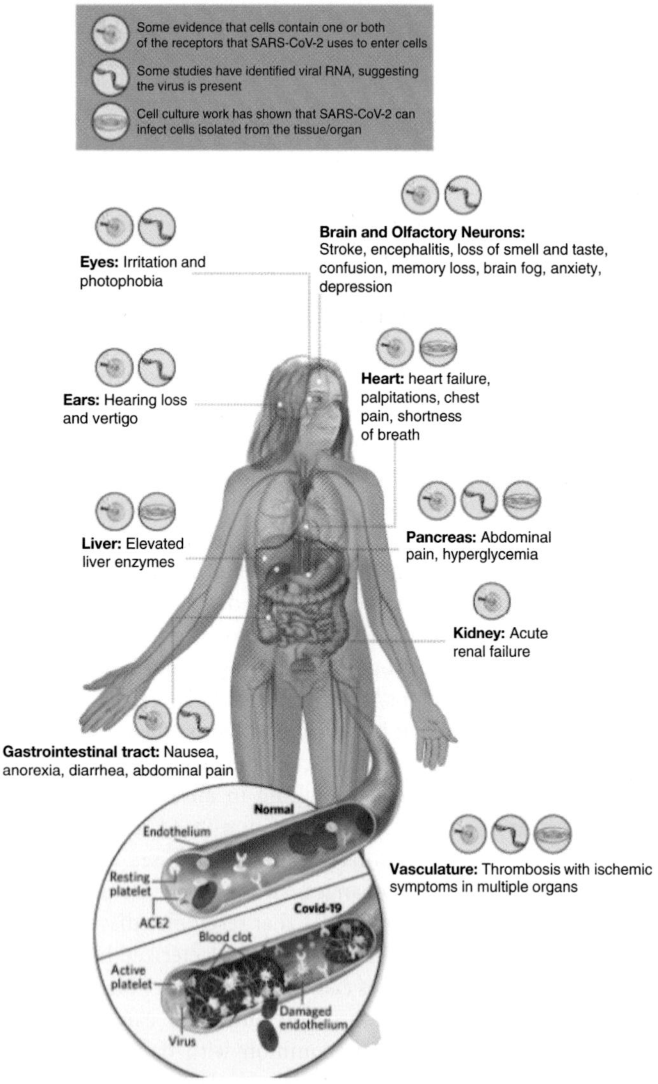

Fig. 10.14 Clinical Manifestations of Acute COVID 19. Acute Covid-19 affects multiple organs in the body, including the neurologic, cardiac, renal, gastrointestinal, and endocrine systems. Widespread thrombosis can result in ischemic damage to multiple organs. (Adapted from The Scientist. SARS-CoV-2's Wide-Ranging Effects on the Body. September 2021. https://www.the-scientist.com/features/sars-cov-2-s-wide-ranging-effects-on-the-body-69109.)

EMERGING SCIENCE BOX

Post-Acute COVID-19

Post-acute COVID-19 (long COVID; long haulers) is considered the continuation of COVID-19 symptoms or complications after 3–4 weeks post-acute infection, although a consensus definition remains to be developed. It is estimated that nearly half of those infected with SARS-CoV-2 develop some post-acute symptoms within 12 months after the acute infection. It can occur in those after hospital discharge and in individuals who suffered only mild-moderate acute illness. Continued viral toxicity, microvascular injury, immune system dysregulation, and persistent hyperinflammatory state. Underlying comorbidities, deconditioning, and recurrent infections also may play a role. Fatigue and dyspnea are the most common persistent symptoms, occurring in 50%–75% of individuals at 2–3 months, and persisting 6 months after acute illness in approximately 25% of individuals. Dyspnea is attributed to a reduction in diffusion capacity in the lung, with approximately 50% of individuals in one study having persistent ground-glass abnormalities seen on high-resolution computed tomography of the chest at 6 months. Neuorolgic disorders constitute the second most common sequelae. Persistent neuroinflammation is associated with cognitive and behavioral changes, with many individuals complaining of decreased memory and ability to concentrate. Muscular weakness, joint pain, anxiety, hair loss, and sleep disturbances also are common. The risk of thromboembolic events is also increased. Overall quality of life measures are significantly reduced. Compounding these symptoms are the potential sequelae of critical illness that occur in those hospitalized for COVID-19, including worsening abnormalities in physical, cognitive and psychiatric health after critical illness. Experts currently recommend that all individuals with acute COVID-19 be screened for symptoms and respiratory, psychiatric and thromboembolic sequelae at 4–6 weeks and again at 12 weeks after discharge, with the initiation of appropriate diagnostic and holistic therapeutic interventions when indicated.

Data from Chopra V, et al. Sixty-day outcomes among patients hospitalized with COVID-19. *Annals of Internal Medicine*, 2020; https://doi.org/10.7326/M20-5661. Epub ahead of print; Goff D, et al. Short-term and long-term rates of postacute sequelae of SARS-CoV-2 infection: A systematic review. *JAMA Netw Open*, 2021;4(10):e2128568; Huang C, et al. 6-month consequences of COVID-19 in patients discharged from hospital: a cohort study. *Lancet*, 2021;397(10270):220–232; Moreno-Pérez O, et al. Post-acute COVID-19 syndrome. Incidence and risk factors: A Mediterranean cohort study. *Journal of Infection*, 2021;82(3):378–383; Nalbandian A, et al. Post-acute COVID-19 syndrome. *Nature Medicine*, 2021;27:601–615. https://doi.org/10.1038/s41591-021-01283-z; Rando HM, et al. Challenges in defining Long COVID: Striking differences across literature, electronic health records, and patient-reported information. *medRxiv* [Preprint], 2021; 2021.03.20.21253896. https://doi.org/10.1101/2021.03.20.21253896; and Wildwing T, et al. The neurological symptoms of COVID-19: A systematic overview of systematic reviews, comparison with other neurological conditions and implications for healthcare services. *Therapeutic Advances in Chronic Disease*, 2021;28:12. 2040622320976979.

acid amplification tests (NAATs) and antigen tests. Serologic tests can confirm the presence of the virus in the nasopharynx and sputum and can detect the development of antibodies after infection. Laboratory findings include decreased lymphocytes in the blood, elevated levels of inflammatory cytokines and D-dimer, and bilateral lung infiltrates on computed tomography.

For individuals with mild to moderate COVID-19 who do not require hospitalization, NIH guidelines recommend the use of monoclonal antibodies that target the spike protein of the virus including bamlanivimab plus etesevimab or casirivimab plus imdevimab or sotrovimab to reduce the risk for disease progression.[59] Management guidelines for severe acute COVID-19 recommend isolation, oxygen, mechanical ventilation if needed, and anticoagulation. The antiviral remdesivir is used to decrease the time to recovery for hospitalized individuals. Dexamethasone is recommended for those requiring supplemental oxygen. NIH guidelines also recommend the administration of monoclonal antibodies that block inflammatory cytokines (e.g. janus kinase and IL-6) including baricitinib or tocilizumab or sarilumab for the treatment severe disease.[59] Additionally, several different blood-derived products and immunomodulators are under investigation for the management of COVID-19 including immune sera (convalescent serum).[60] Oral medications such as molnupiravir have been found to reduce the risk of hospitalization if taken early in the course of symptomatic infection.[61] The list of potential therapies is growing as new discoveries are made.

Several different vaccines have been developed globally to prevent SARS-CoV-2 infection. Two of these use an mRNA backbone carrying the spike protein sequence and are created in the laboratory. These mRNA constructs use the host cells' own translation machinery to make harmless pieces of viral spike proteins that elicit an immune response to the virus. These two vaccines have been found to have over 95% efficacy in preventing infection, and so far appear to be effective against SARS-CoV-2 variants.[62] Other vaccines use more conventional technologies such as adenovirus vector vaccines. It is still unknown whether prolonged immunity to the virus can be achieved, and booster immunizations are recommended. The effectiveness of all of these vaccines will need to be retested as new variants emerge.

Fungal Infection

Fungi are relatively large eukaryotic microorganisms with thick walls that have one of two basic structures: single-celled yeasts (spheres) or multicellular molds (filaments or hyphae) (Fig. 10.15). Some fungi can exist in either form called **dimorphic fungi**. They usually reproduce by simple division or budding. The cell walls of fungi are rigid and multilayered and composed of polysaccharides different from the peptidoglycans of bacteria. The lack of

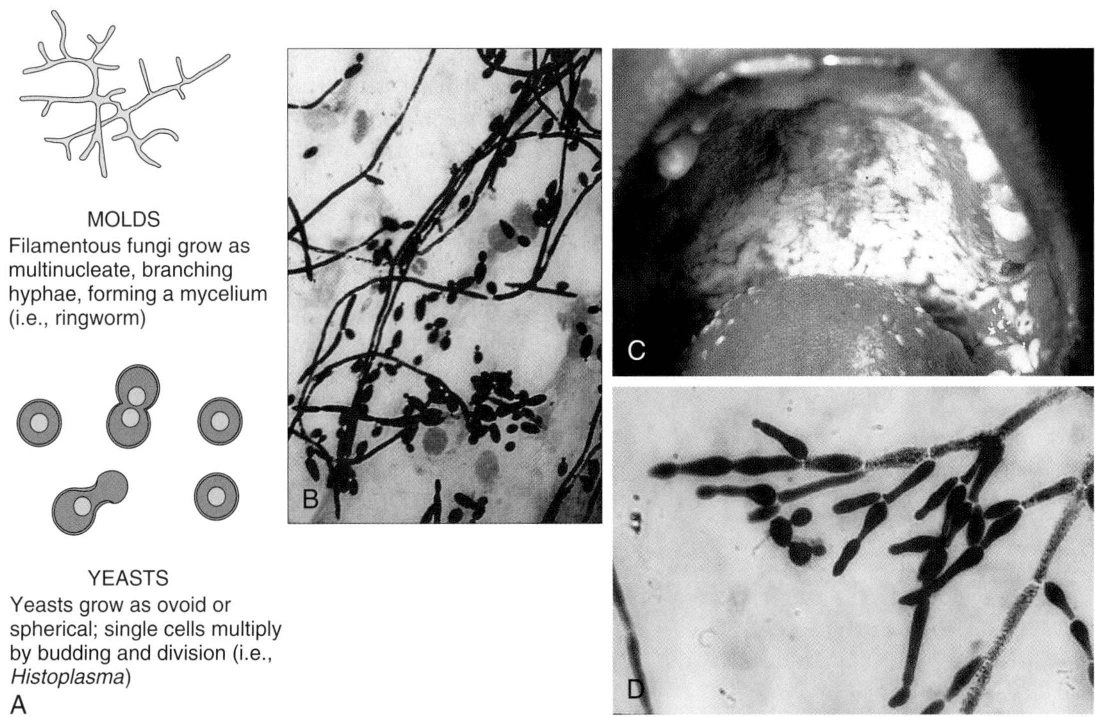

Fig. 10.15 Morphology of Fungi. (A) Fungi may occur in either mold or yeast forms, or they may be dimorphic. **(B)** Photograph showing *Candida albicans* with both the mycelial and the yeast forms. **(C)** Oral infection with *C. albicans* (candidiasis, i.e., thrush). **(D)** Gram staining of sputum showing that clinical isolates of *C. albicans* present as chains of elongated budding yeasts (×1000). (A and B, From Goering R, et al. *Mims' medical microbiology*, 5th edition. London: Saunders; 2013. C, From McPherson R, Pincus M. *Henry's clinical diagnosis and management by laboratory methods*, 22nd edition. Philadelphia: Saunders; 2012; D, Courtesy Dr. Stephen Raffanti.)

TABLE 10.5 Examples of Human Diseases Caused by Fungi

Primary Site of Infection	Fungus	Disease (Primary)	Symptoms
Superficial (no tissue invasion, little inflammation)	*Malassezia furfur*	Tinea versicolor, seborrheic dermatitis, dandruff	Red rash on body
Cutaneous (no tissue invasion, inflammatory response)	*Trichophyton mentagrophytes; Trichophyton rubrum*	Tinea pedis; Tinea cruris	Scaling, rash, fissures, pruritus
	Candida albicans	Cutaneous candidiasis	Pruritic lesions in skin, mucous membranes
Subcutaneous (tissue invasion)	*Sporothrix schenckii*	Sporotrichosis	Ulcers or abscesses on skin and other organ systems
Systemic (dimorphic; causes disease in healthy individuals)	*Coccidioides immitis*	Coccidioidomycosis	Valley fever, flulike symptoms
	Histoplasma capsulatum	Histoplasmosis	Flu-like symptoms, disseminates to lungs and other organs
	Blastomyces dermatitidis	Blastomycosis	Flulike symptoms, chest pains
Systemic (opportunistic)	*Aspergillus fumigatus, Aspergillus flavus*	Aspergillosis	Invasive to lungs and other organs
	Pneumocystis jirovecii	Pneumocystis pneumonia (PJP)	Pneumonia
	Cryptococcus neoformans	Cryptococcosis	Pneumonia-like illness, skin lesions, disseminates to brain, meningitis
	Candidia albicans	Systemic candidiasis	Sepsis, endocarditis, meningitis

peptidoglycans allows fungi to resist the action of bacterial cell wall inhibitors, such as penicillin and cephalosporin. Molds are aerobic and yeasts are facultative anaerobes, which can adapt to anaerobic conditions.

Phagocytes and T lymphocytes are important in controlling fungi. There is increasing evidence that the phagocytes of the innate immune system are capable of trained innate immunity toward fungi, thus serious fungal infection is most common in individuals who have a compromised innate immune system (see Chapter 9).[63] Low white blood cell counts promote fungal infection, and infection control is particularly important for individuals who are immunosuppressed because of diseases such as cancer or AIDS, or because of treatment with immunosuppressive drugs such as chemotherapeutic agents, transplant rejection medications, or corticosteroids.

By mechanisms similar to those described for bacteria, pathogenic fungal infections damage tissue directly by secretion of enzymes and indirectly by initiation of an inflammatory response. Several toxins secreted by molds in the environment cause disease without fungal infection. Mycotoxins are produced by molds that grow on nuts, beans, and grains. Ingestion of these toxins affect muscle coordination, causes tremors, and may be fatal. Other fungal toxins may cause cancer, for example aflatoxins produced by some *Aspergillus* species are especially carcinogenic.

Infections caused by fungi are called **mycoses**. Common pathogenic fungi are summarized in Table 10.5. Mycoses can be superficial, deep, or opportunistic. Superficial mycoses occur on or near skin or mucous membranes and usually produce mild and superficial disease. Fungi that invade the skin, hair, or nails are known as dermatophytes. The diseases they produce are called tineas (ringworm), for example, tinea capitis (scalp), tinea pedis (feet), and tinea cruris (groin). Chapter 46 discusses the various skin disorders caused by fungi.

C. albicans is the most common cause of fungal infections in humans. It is an opportunistic yeast that is a commensal inhabitant in the normal microbiome of many healthy individuals, residing in the skin, gastrointestinal tract, mouth, and vagina. *C. albicans* is normally under the control of local defense mechanisms, including members of the microbiome that produce antifungal agents. In healthy individuals, antibiotic therapy can negatively impact the microbiome causing overgrowth of Candida, resulting in localized infection, such as vaginitis or oropharyngeal infection (thrush).

In immunocompromised individuals (particularly those with diminished levels of neutrophils [neutropenia]), disseminated infection may occur. *C. albicans* is the most common fungal species to cause infection in people with cancer (particularly acute leukemia and other hematologic cancers), transplantation (bone marrow and solid organ), and HIV/AIDS. Invasive candidiasis is the fourth most common healthcare-associated bloodstream infection and is commonly associated with iatrogenic immunocompromise, critical illness, and the use of indwelling catheters and intravenous lines in intensive care units (ICUs).[64] Prophylaxis with antifungal agents for individuals with hematologic disease or undergoing stem cell transplantation reduces the risk for invasive infection.[65] Disseminated candidiasis may involve deep infections of several internal organs, including abscesses in the kidney, brain, liver, and heart, and is characterized by persistent or recurrent fever, shock-like symptoms (hypotension, tachycardia), and DIC. The mortality rate among individuals with septic or disseminated candidiasis is about 30%. Diagnosis of candidiasis requires culture of the organisms and serologic tests. Management requires systemic antifungal medications and supportive measures. Unfortunately, most systemic antifungal drugs are associated with significant toxicity and resistance.[66] A new species of Candida *(Candida auris)* emerged in Asia in 2009 and has since spread across five continents. Multidrug-resistant strains have been identified with increased mortality (30% to 60%) in healthcare settings.[67]

In individuals with or without immunocompromise, an important fungal pathogen is *Aspergillus fumigatus*. Aspergillosis of the lungs and sinuses causes an allergic disease that results in asthma-like symptoms. In some individuals, *Aspergillus* can form a fungus ball in the lung known as an aspergilloma. It can also cause a systemic illness called invasive pulmonary aspergillosis (IPA), which can occur in up to 15% of individuals who are being treated for lung disease in the ICU.[68] It also commonly affects individuals with cystic fibrosis. Aspergillosis has emerged as an important and serious complication of COVID-19.[69] Invasive aspergillosis requires systemic antifungal treatment. Strains resistant to antifungal treatment are increasing in prevalence.[70]

Another very important fungal pathogen in immunocompromised individuals is *Pneumocystis jerovicii* (previously *Pneumocystis carinii*). Pneumocystis pneumonia occurs most commonly in individuals with iatrogenic immunocompromise (antirejection medications, corticosteroids, cancer treatment), AIDS, autoimmune disorders, and critical illness including COVID-19. It can also complicate chronic lung disease. Human host-to-host transmission occurs via inhalation of spores and the fungus is tropic for lung tissue.[71] It can cause serious respiratory compromise, and mortality rates are high in those individuals who require hospitalization.[72] Diagnosis relies on silver staining and serologic testing of expectorated sputum or of lung tissue obtained at biopsy. *P. jirovecii* is resistant to amphotericin B and other antifungals (azoles).[71] Treatment consists of trimethoprim/sulfamethoxazole or alternative antimicrobials for those individuals who are intolerant of sulfa-containing antibiotics. At-risk individuals may receive chemoprophylaxis to prevent *P. jirovecii* pneumonia, especially those whose respiratory tracts are already colonized with this microorganism.[73]

Parasitic Infection

Parasitic microorganisms establish a relationship in which the parasite benefits at the expense of the other species. Parasites range from a unicellular protozoan to large worms. Parasitic worms (helminths) include intestinal and tissue nematodes (e.g., hookworm, roundworm), flukes (e.g., liver fluke, lung fluke), and tapeworms. A protozoan is a eukaryotic, unicellular microorganism with a nucleus and cytoplasm. Pathogenic protozoa include sporozoan (e.g., *Plasmodium falciparum* which causes malaria), amebae (e.g., *Entamoeba histolytica*, which causes amoebic dysentery), and flagellates (e.g., *G. lamblia*, which causes diarrhea). Important parasites of humans are listed in Table 10.6.

Water and food can be contaminated with protozoal parasites (e.g., *E. histolytica*, *G. lamblia*). Many protozoan parasites are transmitted through vectors. Important vectors for parasites include the tsetse fly, sand fleas, and mosquitoes. The tsetse fly can transmit the parasites *Trypanosoma cruzi* (causes Chagas disease and *Trypanosoma brucei* (causes sleeping sickness). Sand fleas can carry *Leishmania* species from infected dogs to people causing skin sores, infection of viscera, and the mucosa of the nose, mouth and throat (Leishmaniasis). The Zika virus is transmitted by mosquitoes and causes fever, rash, headache, conjunctivitis, and musculoskeletal discomfort. Of greatest concern is that it can be passed from a pregnant mother to her fetus and cause birth defects. Transmission of *Plasmodium* is through the bite of an infected female *Anopheles* mosquito, in which the parasite grows in the salivary gland.

There are several types of *Plasmodium* species that can cause malaria (Fig. 10.16). The most common is *P. falciparum*. *Plasmodium* replication occurs in erythrocytes and results in the release of additional parasites that infect other erythrocytes. Periodic (48 to 72 hours) lysis of the erythrocytes results in anemia and induction of cytokines (e.g., TNF-β, interferon-gamma [IFN-γ], IL-1) that provoke fever, chills, sweating, headache, muscle pains, and vomiting. Most of the tissue damage caused by parasites is secondary to the release of enzymes that help invasion by destroying surrounding extracellular matrix and tissue. Profound anemia and pulmonary edema may occur. Neurologic complications may result from infected red blood cells adhering to endothelium in capillaries of the brain. Left untreated, malaria can result in serious illness and death. Antimalarial drugs are effective in many individuals, but relapses and antimicrobial

TABLE 10.6 Examples of Human Diseases Caused by Parasites

Category	Subgroup	Species	Disease	Organs Affected/Symptoms
Protozoa	Ameboid	*Entamoeba histolytica*	Amebiasis	Dysentery, liver abscess
	Flagellate	*Giardia lamblia*	Giardiasis	Diarrhea
		Trichomonas vaginalis	Trichomoniasis	Inflammation of reproductive organs
		Trypanosoma cruzi, *Trypanosoma brucei*	Chagas disease: African sleeping sickness	Generalized, blood and lymph nodes, progressing to cardiac and central nervous system
	Ciliate	*Balantidium coli*	Balantidiasis	Small intestines, invasion of colon, diarrhea
	Sporozoa (nonmotile)	*Cryptosporidium parvum*	Cryptosporidiosis	Intestine, diarrhea
		Plasmodium spp.	Malaria	Blood, liver
		Toxoplasma gondii	Toxoplasmosis	Intestine, eyes, blood, heart, liver
Helminths	Flukes (trematodes)	*Fasciola hepatica*	Fasciolosis	Liver destruction
		Schistosoma mansoni	Schistosomiasis	Blood, diarrhea, bladder, generalized symptoms
	Tapeworms (cestodes)	*Taenia solium*	Pork tapeworm	Encysts in muscle, brain, liver
	Roundworms (nematodes)	*Ascaris lumbricoides*	Ascariasis	Intestinal obstruction, bile duct obstruction
		Necator americanus (hookworm)	Hookworm disease	Intestinal parasite
		Trichinella spiralis	Trichinosis	Intestine, diarrhea, muscle, CNS, death
		Enterobius vermicularis (pinworm)	Pinworm infection	Intestines

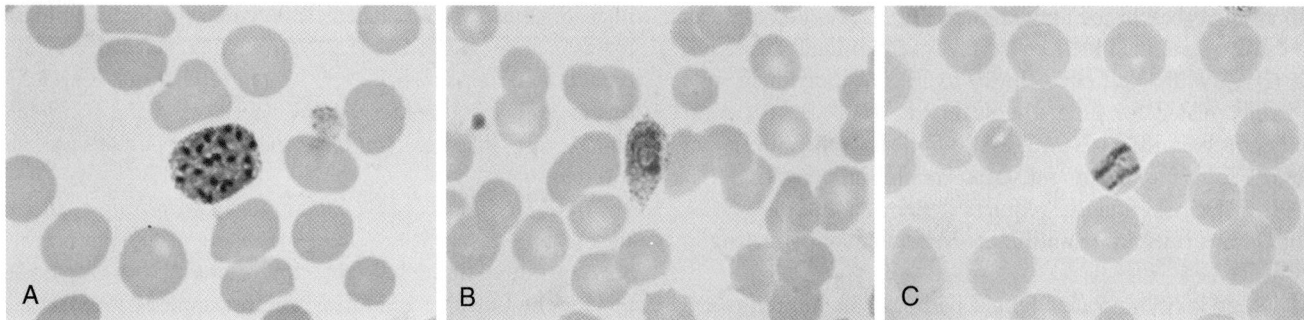

Fig. 10.16 Malaria. Malaria Giemsa-stained smears. **(A)** *Plasmodium vivax* schizont. **(B)** *Plasmodium ovale* trophozoite. **(C)** Characteristic band from trophozoite of *Plasmodium malariae* containing intracellular pigment hemozoin. (From Kliegman R, et al. *Nelson textbook of pediatrics*, 20th edition. St. Louis: Saunders; 2016.)

resistance are common.[74] The world's first malaria vaccine, called Mosquirix, was endorsed by the WHO in fall 2021. It has an efficacy of about 50 percent against severe malaria in the first year. Although protection drops rapidly over the 3 years after full inoculation, it is estimated that in high prevalence areas it could prevent 116, 480 cases of clinical malaria and 484 deaths per 100,000 children vaccinated.[75] Malaria diagnosis and treatment is guided by the 2021 World Health Organization Guidelines.[76] Diagnosis rests on recognition of likely exposures, symptoms, and parasitological testing. Rapid diagnostic tests are available. Individuals who present with symptoms of malaria and a positive parasitological test but with no features of severe malaria are treated with a 3-day course of artemisinin-based combination therapy, whereas recurrent or severe malaria requires multiple medications and more prolonged treatment regimens.[76]

The most common parasitic infections in the United States are *Toxoplasma gondii* and *Trichomonas vaginalis. T. gondii* can be found colonizing up to 30% to 50% of non-immunocompromised asymptomatic individuals.[77] The innate immune system is primarily responsible for keeping the organism in check in healthy individuals. Toxoplasmosis occurs in immunocompromised individuals such as those with AIDS or hematologic malignancies. It typically results in central nervous system infection including encephalitis and abscesses.[78] Ocular infections can occur in infants. Treatment with combinations of antimicrobials that block the folate pathway of parasite metabolism is indicated, but may be associated with significant serious adverse outcomes.[77] *T. vaginalis* is a common sexually transmitted infection (see Chapter 27). It causes genitourinary infections is linked to an increased risk for premature delivery for pregnant women.

ANTIBIOTIC/ANTIMICROBIAL RESISTANCE

Some antibacterial antibiotics are *bactericidal* (kill the microorganism), whereas others are *bacteriostatic* (inhibit growth until the microorganism is destroyed by the individual's own protective mechanisms). The mechanisms of action of most antibiotics are (1) inhibition of the function or production of the cell wall/membrane, (2) prevention of protein synthesis, (3) blockage of DNA replication, or (4) interference with folic acid metabolism (Table 10.7). Because viruses use the enzymes of the host's cells, there has been less success in developing antivirals.

TABLE 10.7 Mechanisms of Action of Commonly-Used Antimicrobials

Mechanism of Action	Agents
Inhibits synthesis of cell wall	Penicillins, cephalosporins, monobactams, carbapenems, vancomycin, bacitracin, cycloserine, fosfomycin
Cell membrane inhibitors	Amphotericin, ketoconazole, polymycin
Damages cytoplasmic membrane	Polymyxins, polyene antifungals, imidazoles
Alters metabolism of nucleic acid	Quinolones, rifampin, nitrofurans, nitroimidazoles
Inhibits protein synthesis	Aminoglycosides, tetracyclines, chloramphenicol, macrolides, clindamycin, spectinomycin
Inhibits folic acid synthesis (needed for protein synthesis)	Sulfonamides, trimethoprim
Alters energy metabolism	Trimethoprim, dapsone, isoniazid

Adapted from Visovsky CG, Zambroski CH, Holser S. *Introduction to clinical pharmacology*, 9th edition. St. Louis: Elsevier; 2019.

Antibiotic-resistant infections to one or multiple antibiotics are growing in number and severity.[79,80]. The CDC's publication "Antibiotic Resistance Threats in the United States, 2019 (2019 AR Threats Report)" states that more than 2.8 million antibiotic-resistant infections occur in the United States each year and more than 35,000 people die as a result. This report lists 18 pathogens sorted into "Urgent Threats," "Serious Threats," and "Concerning Threats."[81] Much of this resistance results from of a combination of factors such as antibiotic overuse, lack of compliance, antimicrobial use in agriculture, and the development of new strains of pathogens.[82]

Many infections once considered routine and easily treatable are now resistant to most currently available antibiotics. Important examples include **methicillin-resistant S. aureus [MRSA]** and *Streptococcus pneumoniae*, which causes pneumonia, meningitis, and acute otitis media (middle ear infection). Of interest, additionally, there are major increases in resistant *Enterococcus* (sepsis, wound infection, urinary tract infection), *P. aeruginosa* (burn infection, sepsis), and *M. tuberculosis*

(tuberculosis). Antimicrobial-resistant strains of fungi and parasites are also increasing.

Microbes can use various mechanisms to resist or inactivate antibiotics (Fig. 10.17). The type of antibiotic affected by these resistance mechanisms is primarily determined by how the drug enters the microorganism or its mechanisms of action. For example, an enzyme called *beta-lactamase*, which is produced by most *S. aureus* species, prevents the action of penicillin on the microorganismal cell wall. Other antibiotics, such as fluoroquinolones and macrolides, are rendered ineffective by multiple resistance mechanisms. Many potential new approaches to antimicrobial resistance are being explored. Examples include antimicrobial peptides, monoclonal antibodies, bacteriophages, stem cells, liposomes, and new vaccines.[83]

VACCINES AND PROTECTION AGAINST INFECTION

Active Immunization

Recovery from an infection generally results in the strongest resistance to a future infection with the same microbe. Vaccines are biologic preparations of antigens that, when administered, stimulate production of protective antibodies or cellular immunity against a specific pathogen without causing potentially life-threatening disease. There are several types of vaccines. Some use live-attenuated (rendered unable to cause disease) or inactivated (killed) microorganisms (e.g., measles, influenza). Others use portions of the microbe and are called subunit, recombinant, peptide, polysaccharide, capsid, or conjugate vaccines (e.g., Hepatitis B, Pneumococcus). Toxoid vaccines use parts of the microbial toxin (e.g., diphtheria, tetanus). Recently, nucleic acid vaccines that include pieces of pathogen DNA or RNA are being developed, often using a recombinant vector vaccine to expose the individual's immune system to the pathogen (e.g., Zika, SARS-CoV-2). Most recently, mRNA vaccines for COVID-19 have been developed and have been shown to have high levels of efficacy.[62] This type of vaccine has been in development for decades and are expected to be developed for many other infectious (including HIV) and non-infectious diseases such as cancer.[84]

The purpose of vaccination is to induce long-lasting protective immune responses under safe conditions. The primary immune response from vaccination is generally short lived; therefore, booster injections are used to push the immune response through multiple secondary responses that result in large numbers of memory cells and sustained protective levels of antibody or T cells, or both (see Chapter 8). In the United States the CDC provides updated vaccine schedules, which are available at www.cdc.gov/vaccines/schedules/index.html.

Passive Immunotherapy

Passive immunotherapy is a form of countermeasure against pathogens in which preformed antibodies are given to the

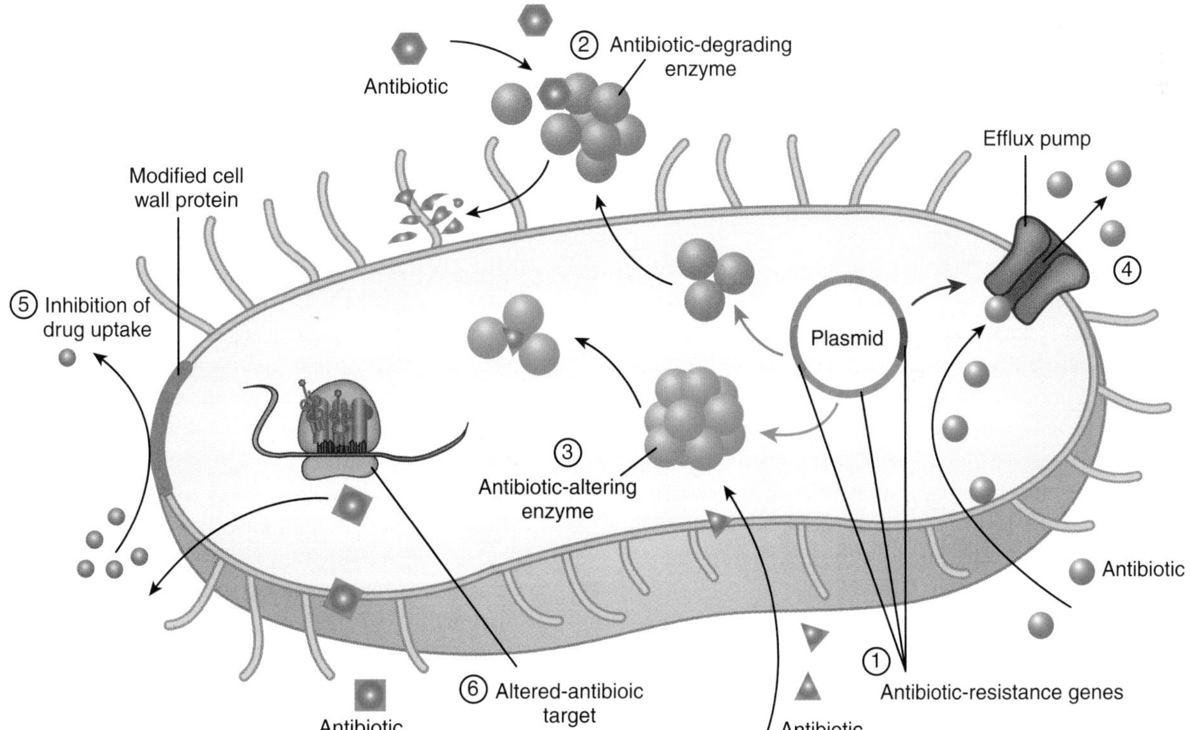

Fig. 10.17 Mechanisms of Antibiotic Resistance. Mechanisms of antibiotic resistance include the following: ***(1)*** Resistance genes that are spread within the bacterial community by horizontal gene transfer to other generations of microbes. ***(2)*** Antibiotics are degraded by enzymes released from the microbe. ***(3)*** Antibiotics are altered by enzymes within the microbe. ***(4)*** Antibiotics are ejected from inside the microbe by efflux pumps in the cell membrane. ***(5)***The cell wall can be modified to prevent antibiotic binding or uptake. ***(6)*** Modification of the cellular target of the antibiotic.

individual. Passive immunotherapy with human immunoglobulin has been approved for several infections, including hepatitis A and hepatitis B. Treatment of potential rabies infection after a bite combines passive and active immunization. Individuals who have been bitten receive passive immunization with monoclonal antibody to slow further viral proliferation, followed by active immunization via multiple injections with a killed viral vaccine to induce greater protective immunity. Monoclonal antibodies are now being used as prophylaxis to protect high risk individuals from certain infections (e.g., RSV, Ebola).[85] Monoclonal antibodies are also used to treat individuals infected with SARS-CoV-2.[59] With the increase in antibiotic-resistant microorganisms, the development of new vaccines for old diseases is needed.

SUMMARY REVIEW

Microorganisms and Humans: A Dynamic Relationship

1. Infectious disease is a significant cause of morbidity and mortality in the United States and worldwide.
2. Pathogens have unique characteristics that influence their ability to overcome body defense mechanisms and cause disease.
3. The process of infection includes encounter and transmission, colonization, invasion, dissemination, and cellular or tissue damage by the pathogenic microorganisms.
4. There are four distinct stages of infection: incubation period, prodromal stage, invasion or acute illness stage, and convalescence.

Infectious Disease

1. Bacteria have virulence factors that promote their ability to cause infection and cell injury, including pili, flagella, capsules, enzymes, competition for iron, and toxins.
2. Bacteria produce exotoxins or endotoxins. Exotoxins are enzymes that can damage the plasma membranes of host cells or can inactivate enzymes critical to protein synthesis, and endotoxins activate the inflammatory response and produce fever.
3. Septicemia results from the proliferation of bacteria in blood. Toxins released by bloodborne bacteria cause the release of vasoactive enzymes that increase the permeability of blood vessels. Leakage from vessels causes hypotension that can result in septic shock.
4. Viruses are intracellular parasites. They enter host cells and use their metabolic processes to proliferate and cause disease.
5. Viral replication includes seven steps: recognition and attachment, penetration, uncoating, replication, translation, assembly, and release.
6. Viruses that have invaded host cells may decrease protein synthesis; disrupt lysosomal membranes; form inclusion bodies, where synthesis of viral nucleic acids is occurring; fuse with host cells to produce giant cells; alter antigenic properties of the host cell; transform host cells into cancerous cells; and promote bacterial infection.
7. Viruses can elude the immune system by making small changes to the genes that produce viral surface antigens, a process known as *antigenic variation*.
8. SARS-Cov-2 is a novel coronavirus that emerged in fall 2019 causing a severe respiratory illness pandemic in 2020. New and emerging viral infections pose global threats.
9. HIV is a blood-borne pathogen present in body fluids with typical routes of transmission: blood or blood products, intravenous drug abuse, heterosexual and homosexual activity, and maternal-child transmission before or during birth.
10. The primary surface receptor on HIV is the envelope glycoprotein gp120, which binds to the CD4 molecule found mostly on the surface of T-helper cells. Viral binding with chemokine coreceptors CXCR4 on T helper cells and CCR5 on macrophages and dendritic cells is essential for viral fusion to the target cell membrane.
11. HIV is a member of the retrovirus family, which carries genetic information in the form of RNA. An enzyme, reverse transcriptase (RT), converts RNA into a double-stranded DNA. Another enzyme, an integrase, inserts the new DNA into the infected cell's genetic material. On activation, translation of the viral information may be initiated, forming new virions, resulting in lysis and death of the infected cell, and shedding infectious HIV particles.
12. HIV infects macrophages, dendritic cells, and circulating Th cells. It also infects T helper cells in the gut. T helper memory cells serve as reservoirs for HIV infection that persist for life, even in those who are treated with antiretroviral drugs.
13. The major immunologic finding in AIDS is a decrease in the number of CD4+ Th cells resulting in decreasing immune competence.
14. AIDS is characterized by immunocompromise and the development of opportunistic infections and cancers.
15. The COVID-19 pandemic is caused by infection with SARS-CoV-2 which has caused serious illness and death for millions of people worldwide.
16. SARS-CoV-2 is spread primarily by respiratory droplets produced when infected individuals cough, sneeze, or talk.
17. SARS-CoV-2 attaches to respiratory epithelial cells via its spike protein. Upon entering the cell, it sets of an immunologic response that can escalate to a cytokine storm which may cause severe lung disease and death.
18. Diseases caused by fungi are called *mycoses*, and fungi occur in two forms: yeasts (spheres) and molds (filaments or hyphae).
19. Dermatophytes are fungi that infect skin, hair, and nails with diseases, such as ringworm and athlete's foot.
20. *Candida albicans* is the most common cause of fungal infections in humans. Other important fungal pathogens include *Aspergillus fumigatus* and *Pneumocystis jiroveci*.
21. Parasitic microorganisms range from unicellular protozoa to large worms. Although less common in the United States, parasites and protozoa are common causes of infection worldwide.

22. Parasitic and protozoal infections are rarely transmitted from human to human. Infection mainly spreads through vectors (e.g., through mosquito bites) or through contaminated water.
23. *Plasmodium falciparum* is the most common cause of malaria.
24. *Toxoplasma gondii* and *Trichomonas vaginalis* are the two most common parasitic infections in the United States.

Antibiotic/Antimicrobial Resistance

Pathogens can use various mechanisms to resist the effects of antibiotics, including transmission of resistance genes to new generations of bacteria, enzyme degradation of the antibiotic, ejection of the antibiotic from the pathogen, modification of the cell wall to prevent binding or uptake of the antibiotic, or modification of the target of the antibiotic.

Vaccines and Protection Against Infection

1. Vaccines are biologic preparations of antigens that, when administered, stimulate production of protective antibodies or cellular immunity against a specific pathogen.
2. Passive immunotherapy is the administration of preformed antibodies for protection against a specific pathogen, such as hepatitis A and B or rabies.

REFERENCES

1. Stacy A, et al. Infection trains the host for microbiota-enhanced resistance to pathogens. *Cell.* 2021;184(3):615–627.
2. Hsieh SA, Allen PM:. Immunomodulatory roles of polysaccharide capsules in the intestine. *Front Immunol.* 2020;11:690.
3. Redondo-Salvo S, et al. Pathways for horizontal gene transfer in bacteria revealed by a global map of their plasmids. *Nat Commun.* 2020;11:3602.
4. Power JJ, et al. Adaptive evolution of hybrid bacteria by horizontal gene transfer. *Proc Natl Acad Sci U S A.* 2021;118(10). e2007873118.
5. Gonzalez JF, Hahn MM, Gunn JS. Chronic biofilm-based infections: skewing of the immune response. *Pathog Dis.* 2018;76:fty023.
6. Wi YM, Patel R. Understanding biofilms and novel approaches to the diagnosis, prevention, and treatment of medical device-associated infections. *Infect Dis Clin North Am.* 2018;32:915–929.
7. Wibowo D, Rehm BHA. Pseudomonas aeruginosa biofilms. *Int J Mol Sci.* 2020;21(22):8671.
8. Frost LR, et al. Clostridioides difficile biofilms: a mechanism of persistence in the gut? *PLoS Pathog.* 2021;17(3):e1009348.
9. Versey Z, et al. Biofilm-innate immune interface: Contribution to chronic wound formation. *Front Immunol.* 2021;12:1067.
10. Gajula B, Munnamgi S, Basu S. How bacterial biofilms affect chronic wound healing: a narrative review. *Int J Surg Glob Health.* 2020;3(2):e16.
11. Bowler P, Murphy C, Wolcott R. Biofilm exacerbates antibiotic resistance: Is this a current oversight in antimicrobial stewardship? *Antimicrob Resist Infection Control.* 2020;9:162.
12. Tenforde MW, et al. Effect of Antigenic drift on influenza vaccine effectiveness in the United States—2019–2020. *Clin Infect Dis.* 2021;2021:ciaa1884.
13. Allen JD, Ross TM. Next generation methodology for updating HA vaccines against emerging human seasonal influenza A(H3N2) viruses. *Sci Rep.* 2021;11:4554.
14. Wang Z, et al. mRNA vaccine-elicited antibodies to SARS-CoV-2 and circulating variants. *Nature 2021.* 2021;592(7855):616–622.
15. World Health Organization (WHO): HIV/AIDS fact sheets, Geneva, Switzerland: WHO. Available at: https://www.who.int/news-room/fact-sheets/detail/hiv-aids. Accessed 11.12.2021.
16. Centers for Disease Control and Prevention (CDC): HIV statistics, Atlanta, GA: CDC. Available at: https://www.cdc.gov/hiv/statistics/index.html. Accessed 11.12.2021.
17. Gartner MJ, et al. Understanding the mechanisms driving the spread of subtype C HIV-1. *EBioMedicine.* 2020;53:102682.
18. Nicholas B, Pontiano K, Deogratius S. HIV subtype diversity worldwide. *Curr Opin HIV AIDS.* 2019;14(3):153–160.
19. Centers for Disease Control and Prevention (CDC): HIV in the United States and dependent areas, Atlanta, GA: CDC. Available at https://www.cdc.gov/hiv/statistics/overview/ataglance.html. Accessed 11.12.2021.
20. Kwon Y, et al. Structural basis of CD4 downregulation by HIV-1 Nef. *Nat Struct Mol Biol.* 2020;27:822–828.
21. Burnie J, Guzzo C. The incorporation of host proteins into the external HIV-1 envelope. *Viruses.* 2019;11(1):85.
22. Pedro KD, Henderson AJ, Agosto LM. Mechanisms of HIV-1 cell-to-cell transmission and the establishment of the latent reservoir. *Virus Res.* 2019;265:115–121.
23. Rezaie J, et al. The versatile role of exosomes in human retroviral infections: from immunopathogenesis to clinical application. *Cell Biosci.* 2021;11(1):19.
24. Cicala C, Arthos J, Fauci AS. Role of T-cell trafficking in the pathogenesis of HIV disease. *Curr Opin HIV AIDS.* 2019;14(2):115–120.
25. Buggert M, Japp AS, Betts MR. Everything in its right place: resident memory CD8+ T cell immunosurveillance of HIV infection. *Curr Opin HIV AIDS.* 2019;14(2):93–99.
26. Shacklett BL, Ferre AL, Kiniry BE. Tissue issues: mucosal T-cell responses in HIV-1 infection. *Curr Opin HIV AIDS.* 2019;14(2):100–107.
27. Bruner KM, Cohn LB. HIV-1 reservoir dynamics in CD4+ T cells. *Curr Opin HIV AIDS.* 2019;14(2):108–114.
28. Sadowski I, Hashemi FB. Strategies to eradicate HIV from infected patients: elimination of latent provirus reservoirs. *Cell Mol Life Sci.* 2019;76(18):3583–3600.
29. Cribbs SK, Crothers K, Morris A. Pathogenesis of HIV-related lung disease: immunity, infection, and inflammation. *Physiol Rev.* 2020;100:603–632.
30. Sáez-Cirión A, Sereti I. Immunometabolism and HIV-1 pathogenesis: food for thought. *Nat Rev Immunol.* 2021;21:5–19.
31. Huerta L. Editorial: Anti-infective 2020: HIV—from pathogenesis to treatment. *Curr Opin Pharmacol.* 2020;54:x–xii.
32. Esteban-Cantos A, et al. Epigenetic age acceleration changes 2 years after antiretroviral therapy initiation in adults with HIV: a substudy of the NEAT001/ANRS143 randomised trial. *Lancet HIV.* 2021;8(4):e197–e205.
33. Subra C, Trautmann L. Role of T lymphocytes in HIV neuropathogenesis. *Curr HIV/AIDS Rep.* 2019;16(3):236–243.
34. Casado C, et al. Permanent control of HIV-1 pathogenesis in exceptional elite controllers: a model of spontaneous cure. *Sci Rep.* 2020;10:1902.
35. World Health Organization (WHO): Consolidated guidelines on HIV prevention, testing, treatment, service delivery and monitoring: recommendations for a public health approach. 2021. Available at https://www.who.int/publications/i/item/9789240031593. Accessed 24.10.21.

36. Branson BM, et al. Revised recommendations for HIV testing of adults, adolescents, and pregnant women in health-care settings. *MMWR Recomm Rep*. 2006;55(RR-14):1–17. Available at: https://www.cdc.gov/mmwr/preview/mmwrhtml/rr5514a1.htm. Accessed 24.10.21.
37. DiNenno EA, Prejean J, Irwin K, et al. Recommendations for HIV screening of gay, bisexual, and other men who have sex with men — United States, 2017. *MMWR Morb Mortal Wkly Rep*. 2017;66:830–832. Available at: https://doi.org/10.15585/mmwr.mm6631a3. Accessed 11.12.2021.
38. Centers for Disease Control and Prevention (CDC): HIV risk and prevention, Atlanta, GA: CDC. Available at https://www.cdc.gov/hiv/risk/index.html. Accessed 24.10.21.
39. HIV.gov: Final HIV prevention and treatment research highlights from the 2021 Conference on Retroviruses and Opportunistic Infections (CROI). Available at: https://www.hiv.gov/blog/final-hiv-prevention-treatment-research-highlights-croi-2021-video. Accessed 11.12.2021.
40. Hargrave A, Mustafa AS, Hanif A, Tunio JH, Hanif SNM. Current status of HIV-1 vaccines. *Vaccines*. 2021;9(9):1026.
41. Clinical Info HIV.gov: Clinical guidelines for HIV/AIDS. Available at https://clinicalinfo.hiv.gov/en/guidelines. Accessed 11.12.2021.
42. Orkin C, et al. Long-acting cabotegravir plus rilpivirine for treatment in adults with HIV-1 infection: 96-week results of the randomised, open-label, phase 3 FLAIR study. *Lancet HIV*. 2021;8(4):e185–e196.
43. Maeda K, et al. Discovery and development of anti-HIV therapeutic agents: progress towards improved HIV medication. *Curr Top Med Chem*. 2019;19(18):1621–1649.
44. Chahine EB, Durham SH. Ibalizumab: the first monoclonal antibody for the treatment of HIV-1 infection. *Ann Pharmacother*. 2021;55(2):230–239.
45. Richard J, Nguyen DN, Tolbert WD, Casser R, Ding S, et al. Across functional boundaries: Making nonneutralizing antibodies to neutralize HIV-1 and mediate Fc-mediated effector killing of infected cells. *mBio*. 2021;12(5):e01405–2.
46. Holmes EC, Goldstein SA, Rasmussen AL, Robertson DL, Crits-Christoph A, et al. The origins of SARS-CoV-2: A critical review. *Cell*. 2021;184(19):4848–4856.
47. Wacharapluesadee S, Tan CW, Maneeorn P, et al. Evidence for SARS-CoV-2 related coronaviruses circulating in bats and pangolins in Southeast Asia. *Nat Commun*. 2021;12:972.
48. World Health Organization (WHO): WHO coronavirus (COVID-19) dashboard, Geneva, Switzerland: WHO. Available at: https://covid19.who.int/. Accessed 11.12.2021.
49. Centers for Disease Control and Prevention (CDC): Science brief: SARS-CoV-2 and surface (fomite) transmission for indoor community environments, Atlanta, GA: CDC. Available at: https://www.cdc.gov/coronavirus/2019-ncov/more/science-and-research/surface-transmission.html. Accessed 11.12.2021.
50. Bender JK, Brandl M, Höhle M, Buchholz U, Zeitlmann N. Analysis of asymptomatic and presymptomatic transmission in SARS-CoV-2 outbreak, Germany, 2020. *Emerg Infect Dis*. 2021 Apr [cited 10/15/21].
51. Wiersinga WJ, et al. Pathophysiology, transmission, diagnosis, and treatment of coronavirus disease 2019 (COVID-19): a review. *JAMA*. 2020;324(8):782–793.
52. Mlcochova P, Kemp SA, Dhar MS, et al. SARS-CoV-2 B.1.617.2 Delta variant replication and immune evasion. 2021;599: 114–119.
53. Center for Disease Control and Prevention Morbidity and Mortality Weekly Report: SARS-CoV-2 B.1.1.529 (Omicron) Variant — United States, December 1–8, 2021. Available at: https://www.cdc.gov/mmwr/volumes/70/wr/mm7050e1.htm?s_cid=mm7050e1_w. Accessed 11.12.21
54. Osuchowski MF, Winkler MS, Skirecki T, Cajander S, Shankar-Hari M, et al. The COVID-19 puzzle: deciphering pathophysiology and phenotypes of a new disease entity. *Lancet Respir Med*. 2021;9: 622–642.
55. Ratre YK, et al. Molecular mechanism, diagnosis, and potential treatment for novel coronavirus (COVID-19): a current literature review and perspective. *3 Biotech*. 2021;11(2):94.
56. Marik PE, Iglesias J, Varon J, Kory P. A scoping review of the pathophysiology of COVID-19. *International Journal of Immunopathology and Pharmacology*. 2021;35:1–16.
57. Schultze JL, Aschenbrenner AC. COVID-19 and the human innate immune system. *Cell*. 2021;184(7):1671–1692.
58. Alene M, Yismaw L, Assemie MA, Ketema DB, Mengist B, Kassie B, et al. Magnitude of asymptomatic COVID-19 cases throughout the course of infection: A systematic review and meta-analysis. *PLoS ONE*. 2021;16(3):e0249090.
59. National Institutes of Health (NIH): COVID 19 treatment guidelines. Clinical Management, Bethesda, MD: NIH. Available at: https://www.covid19treatmentguidelines.nih.gov/. Accessed 11.12.2021.
60. Katz LM. (A little) clarity on convalescent plasma for COVID-19. *N Engl J Med*. 2021;384:666–668.
61. Kabinger F, Stiller C, Schmitzová J, et al. Mechanism of molnupiravir-induced SARS-CoV-2 mutagenesis. *Nat Struct Mol Biol*. 2021;28:740–746.
62. Bernal JL, Andrews N, Gower C, Gallagher E, Simmons R, Thelwall S, et al. Effectiveness of Covid-19 vaccines against the B.1.617.2 (delta) variant. *N Engl J Med*. 2021;385:585–594.
63. Quintin J. Fungal mediated innate immune memory, what have we learned? *Semin Cell Dev Biol*. 2019;89:71–77.
64. Bassetti M, et al. Diagnosis and treatment of candidemia in the intensive care unit. *Semin Respir Crit Care Med*. 2019;40(4):524–539.
65. Wang J, et al. Comparison of antifungal prophylaxis drugs in patients with hematological disease or undergoing hematopoietic stem cell transplantation: a systematic review and network meta-analysis. *JAMA Netw Open*. 2020;3(10):e2017652.
66. Nicola AM, et al. Antifungal drugs: new insights in research & development. *Pharmacol Ther*. 2019;195:21–38.
67. De Carolis E, et al. Are we ready for nosocomial Candida auris infections? Rapid identification and antifungal resistance detection using MALDI-TOF mass spectrometry may be the answer. *Front Cell Infect Microbiol*. 2021;11:172.
68. Tudesq JJ, et al. Invasive pulmonary aspergillosis in nonimmuno-compromised hosts. *Semin Respir Crit Care Med*. 2019;40(4): 540–547.
69. Salmanton-García J, et al. COVID-19–associated pulmonary aspergillosis, March–August 2020. *Emerg Infect Dis*. 2021;27(4): 1077–1086.
70. Guegan H, et al. Azole resistance in Aspergillus fumigatus: a five-year follow up experience in a tertiary hospital with a special focus on cystic fibrosis. *Front Cell Infect Microbiol*. 2021;10:929.
71. Nevez G, Hauser PM, Le Gal S. Pneumocystis jirovecii. *Trends Microbiol*. 2020;28(12):1034–1035.
72. Cilloniz C, et al. Pneumocystis pneumonia in the twenty-first century: HIV-infected versus HIV-uninfected patients. *Expert Rev Anti Infect Ther*. 2019;17(10):787–801.
73. Le Gal S, et al. The shift from pulmonary colonization to Pneumocystis pneumonia. *Med Mycol*. 2021;59(5):510–513.

74. Capela R, Moreira R, Lopes F. An overview of drug resistance in protozoal diseases. *Int J Mol Sci*. 2019;20(22):5748.
75. Laurens MB. RTS,S/AS01 vaccine (Mosquirix™): an overview. *Human Vaccines & Immunotherapeutics*. 2020;16(3):480–489.
76. World Health Organization (WHO): WHO guidelines for malaria, Geneva, Switzerland: WHO. Available at: https://www.who.int/publications/i/item/WHO-UCN-GMP-2021.01. Accessed 14.12.21.
77. Shammaa AM, Powell TG, Benmerzouga I. Adverse outcomes associated with the treatment of Toxoplasma infections. *Sci Rep*. 2021;11:1035.
78. Garcia HH, Nath A, Del Brutto OH. Parasitic infections of the nervous system. *Semin Neurol*. 2019;39(3):358–368.
79. Centers for Disease Control and Prevention (CDC): Antibiotic/antimicrobial resistance (AR / AMR), Atlanta, GA: CDC. Available at: https://www.cdc.gov/drugresistance/index.html. Accessed 14.12.21.
80. Centers for Disease Control and Prevention (CDC): Emerging infectious diseases. Antimicrobial resistance spotlight, Atlanta, GA: CDC. Available at: https://wwwnc.cdc.gov/eid/spotlight/antimicrobial-resistance. Accessed 14.12.21.
81. Centers for Disease Control and Prevention (CDC): Antibiotic / antimicrobial resistance (AR / AMR). Biggest threats and data. 2019 AR threats report, Atlanta, GA: CDC. https://www.cdc.gov/drugresistance/biggest-threats.html. Accessed 14.12.21.
82. Yagnik D, Ward M, Shah AJ. Antibacterial apple cider vinegar eradicates methicillin resistant Staphylococcus aureus and resistant Escherichia coli. *Sci Rep*. 2021;11:1854.
83. Rello J, Parisella FR, Perez A. Alternatives to antibiotics in an era of difficult-to-treat resistance: new insights. *Expert Rev Clin Pharmacol*. 2019;12(7):635–642.
84. Pardi N. mRNA Innovates the vaccine field. *Vaccines*. 2021;9(5):486.
85. Wang XY, Wang B, Wen YM. From therapeutic antibodies to immune complex vaccines. *NPJ Vaccines*. 2019;4:2.

11

Stress and Disease

Lorey K. Takahashi

http://evolve.elsevier.com/Rogers/pathophysiology/

CHAPTER OUTLINE

Stress is broadly defined as a perceived or anticipated threat that disrupts a person's well-being, or homeostasis, and exceeds the individual's capacity to meet the demands. The demands can be physical in nature (e.g., exposure cold temperatures, moving heavy equipment) or psychological (e.g., rush to meet exam deadlines, attempting to complete multiple job assignments). In everyday life, the term *stress* is commonly used to describe negative thoughts and uncontrolled feelings. Experiences that cannot be easily reconciled and threaten one's sense of security are considered stressful, and the random and constant external and internal challenges are called stressors.[1,2] Stressful events perceived as especially threatening, chaotic, and chronic are personal, such as loss of a family member, loss of job security, cancer diagnosis, physical abuse, social neglect, or feelings of social discrimination. The National Institute of Mental Health further defines *stress* in terms of how the brain responds to a demand by activating the neuroendocrine hypothalamic-pituitary-adrenal (HPA) system, including the autonomic nervous system (ANS) and the immune system (IS). Importantly, chronic stress-induced activation of these physiologic systems has the potential to compromise recovery from stress and predispose the individual to engage in a wide range of unhealthy coping strategies, such as foregoing sleep, eating high-calorie comfort foods, and withdrawing from physical activity. Continued engagement in these unhealthy behavioral activities is linked to a number of serious illnesses, such as hypertension, depression, diabetes, and obesity. This chapter discusses the role played by the body and brain in relation to psychosocial and emotional stressors that promote the onset and progression of human diseases.

BACKGROUND AND GENERAL CONCEPTS OF STRESS

Early Years of Stress Biology

Walter B. Cannon used the term *stress* in both a physiologic and a psychological sense as early as 1914 and coined the term *fight-or-flight response* to describe the body's preparation to deal with threat.[3] He applied the engineering concepts of stress and strain in a physiologic context and believed that emotional stimuli also were capable of causing stress. The physiologic reactions to stress included increased heart rate and blood supply of oxygen and glucose to muscles and the brain, elevated respiration, dilation of pupils, and inhibition of gastric secretions. It should be noted the "fight-or-flight" response involving the brain's perception of threat and rapid release of hormones is adaptive in protection from harm. Only when we overreact and cannot reconcile chronic threats will we become susceptible to the development of physical and mental disorders.

The concept of stress was further advanced by Hans Selye and discussed in terms of a chemical or physical change (i.e., physiologic stress, in response either to the external environment or within the body itself).[4] Physiologic stress involves (1) enlargement of the adrenal gland, (2) decreased lymphocyte levels in blood from damage to lymphatic structures of the IS, and (3) development of bleeding ulcers in the stomach and duodenal lining. Selye concluded that physiologic stress will impair the ability of the organism to resist future stressors and represented the hallmark pattern of a nonspecific stress response that was labeled general adaptation syndrome (GAS).

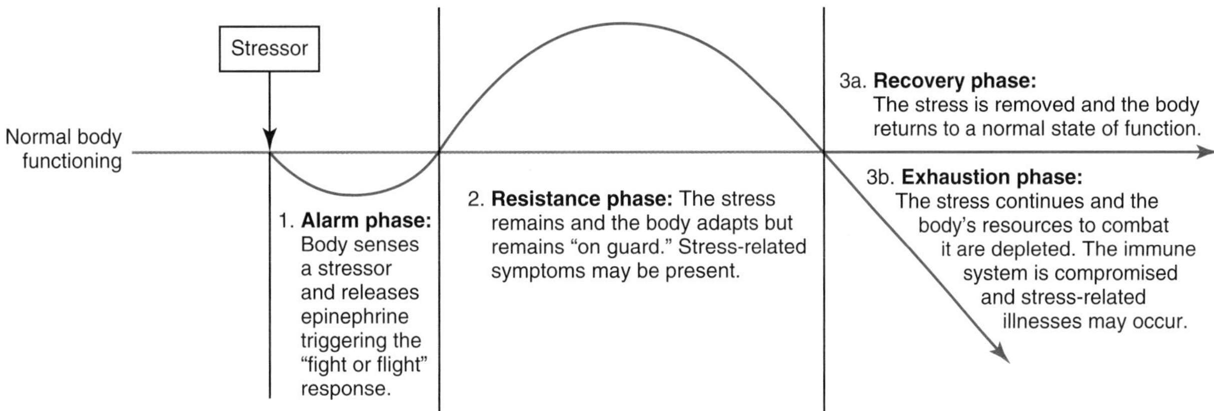

Fig. 11.1 The General Adaptation Syndrome. Hans Selye describes three phases of the body's physiologic response to stress that involve the alarm phase, the resistance phase, and the exhaustion stage. (From Bonewit-West K, Hunt S. *Today's medical assistant*, 4th edition. St. Louis: Elsevier; 2021.)

GAS involves three successive stages: the alarm, the resistance or adaptation, and the exhaustion stages. The alarm stage is the emergency reaction that prepares the body to fight or flee from threat. This stage involves the secretion of hormones and catecholamines (CAs) to support physiologic/metabolic activity (Figs. 11.1 and 11.2) and boosts the IS to thwart infection and disease. The ensuing resistance or adaptation stage requires continued mobilization of the body's resources, such as cortisol and adrenaline, to cope and overcome a sustained challenge. However, prolonged use of these resources may weaken the IS and increase the risk of developing diseases. The exhaustion stage (currently described as allostatic overload; discussed later) occurs when the body's physiologic resources are depleted and the IS no longer is able to cope with the stressor. The body now becomes vulnerable to psychosomatic and physical diseases, and mental disorders (diseases of adaptation). That is, when stress continues unabated, body organs, such as the heart and kidney, may no longer function normally, and disease may develop followed by premature death.

More recent studies have shown that a number of psychological factors, such as the degree of discomfort, unpleasantness, or suddenness of an unanticipated stimulus, are capable of activating the stress response. In fact, psychological stressors are as effective as physical stressors in activating adrenal hormone secretion. Psychological stressors can elicit a reactive or anticipatory stress response. For example, a routine medical examination involving no physical stressor may, nonetheless, elicit a reactive physiologic response, such as accelerated heart rate and dry mouth. Anticipatory responses can be generated by the fear of a potential encounter with a dangerous, unconditioned stimulus (e.g., a predator) or in conditioned situations when a person learns that a specific event is associated with an aversive outcome. A child with a history of parental abuse may show a physiologic stress response in anticipation of further abuse when that parent enters the room. Another well-known example of a conditioned emotional response is the recall of intense fear memories in posttraumatic stress disorder (PTSD). Military veterans and survivors of extreme natural disasters, car accidents, physical assaults, or rape show intense conditioned fear and debilitating responses that are triggered by sounds, odors, visual images, or other stimuli associated with the traumatic event.

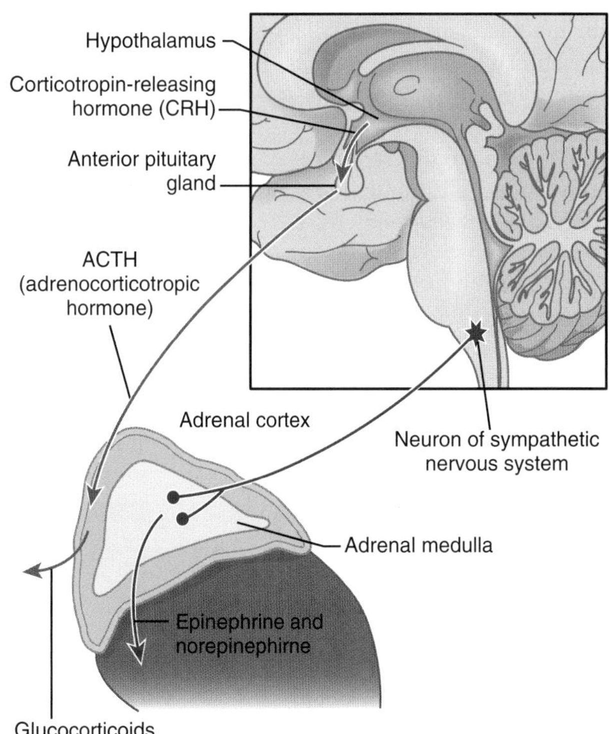

Fig. 11.2 The Alarm Reaction. The alarm reaction includes increased secretion of glucocorticoids (cortisol) by the adrenal cortex and increased secretion of epinephrine and small amounts of norepinephrine from the adrenal medulla. *ACTH,* Adrenocorticotropic hormone. (Adapted from Patton KT, Thibodeau GA. *Anatomy & physiology*, 9th edition. St. Louis: Mosby; 2016.)

It should be noted not all stress has negative health consequences. Eustress is a term to describe positive stress. For example, getting a new job, buying a new house, and meeting new friends are stressful situations that generate excitement, induce motivation, and focus energy to become successful. The challenge to gain self-control and self-esteem is considered positive stress.

Modern Overview of Stress: Allostasis and Allostatic Overload

The emerging link between stress and disease became the basis of the concept of allostasis, introduced by Sterling and Eyer (Fig. 11.3).[5] This concept refers to "stability through change" and differs from the "fixed homeostasis model" in which physiologic regulation revolves around a narrow set point range. For example, after exposure to a challenging stressor, heighted physiologic secretion of stress hormones (e.g., cortisol) is expected to return to basal levels. By contrast, allostasis involves a dynamic adaptation with the brain continuously monitoring many parameters in anticipation of what the HPA and the ANS system must do to meet future challenges. In other words, the brain modulates neurophysiologic systems in anticipation of future stressful situations and continuously adjusts its normal operating range (e.g., hormone secretion) rather than returning to basal hormone levels. Different parts of the brain's limbic system respond to different types of stress (see Fig. 11.3).[6] This adaptive strategy is thought to support coping with an unpredictable stressful environment.

Physiologic and Behavioral Stress Responses

Allostatic load is an index of the cumulative wear and tear on the body caused by repeated activation of multiple physiologic systems over time in response to environmental demands in an effort to maintain internal equilibrium.[7] Chronic activation of regulatory systems has the potential to tax the body and brain and lead to the emergence of diseases and disorders. Allostatic overload is the term used to describe chronic overactivation of adaptive regulatory physiologic systems that may lead to pathophysiology and onset of disease.[1,2] Situations that can contribute to allostatic overload include exposure to frequent stressors that cause repeated physiologic arousal, lack of adaptation to stressors, inability to shut off the stress response, and an allostatic response that is not sufficient to deal with the stressor.[7] In short, frequent and longer exposures to stress accelerate the wear and tear on the body and brain.

Allostasis and allostatic overload are highly individualized. An event or situation considered normal in one person may be stressful to another as a result of genetic, environmental (or both), or experiential factors. For example, some studies have shown that low socioeconomic status (SES), ethnicity, gender dysphoria, sexual orientation, and aging are associated with high levels of allostatic load.[7] The brain plays a key role in perceiving stress and determines when we have reached allostatic overload. Thus psychological or uncontrollable stress is increasingly recognized both as a precipitating factor for some diseases as well as a contributor that worsens symptoms in behavioral (e.g., anxiety), physiologic (e.g., chronic pain, asthma), or metabolic disorders (e.g., obesity, type 2 diabetes).[1,2] In addition, stress disrupts the biologic process of sleep and growth and reproductive functions. In the United States, chronic exposure to toxic, allostatic overload is a contributing factor underlying early mortality.[8] The susceptibility to stress varies from person to person, and factors related to susceptibility include coping style, type of personality, social support, mental health, immune function, and other factors.[9] Examples of stress-related diseases and conditions can be found in Table 11.1.

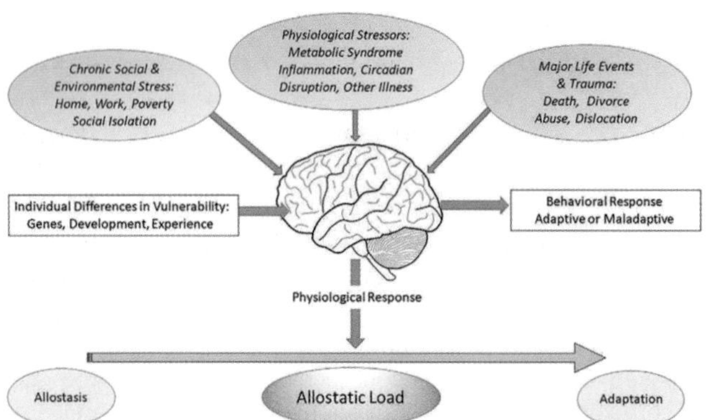

Fig. 11.3 Physiologic and Behavioral Stress Responses and Allostatic Load. The brain is a primary organ that perceives and responds to what is stressful to an individual. The major function of cortisol and other mediators of allostasis is to promote adaptation. However, overuse and/or dysregulation among the mediators of allostasis lead to allostatic load (or overload) and accelerate disease processes such as cardiovascular disease, diabetes, and affective disorders. Three limbic brain regions are noted. (From McEwen BS, Akil H. Revisiting the stress concept: Implications for affective disorders. *Journal of Neuroscience Research*, 2020;40(1):12–21.)

THE STRESS SYSTEMS

The perception or anticipation of a threat activates three major physiologic stress systems: the HPA axis; the sympathetic nervous system (SNS); and the IS. Acute activation of these stress-related systems modulates a broad range of mediators on the body and brain to protect and meet the physiologic and behavioral demands of the stressor to facilitate recovery (Fig. 11.4). For example, stress-induced activation of the SNS and the HPA axis triggers the release of hormones (e.g., epinephrine, cortisol), which rapidly mobilizes resources necessary to prepare the body and brain for "fight-or-flight" responses to threat. In addition, both stress systems send signals to the IS to release cytokines, the mediators of inflammatory processes, such as interleukin-1 (IL-1), IL-6, and tumor necrosis factor-α (TNF-α).[10] The acute release of these sympathetic, neuroendocrine, and immune mediators has profound effects on supporting immune functions, adaptive behavior, physiologic actions, cognitive ability, and mental health.[11,12]

Adaptive Roles of Stress Systems

Allostatic overload occurs when these protective physiologic regulatory systems are taxed by chronic, persistent exposure to

TABLE 11.1 **Examples of Stress-Related Diseases and Conditions**

Target Organ or System	Disease or Condition	Target Organ or System	Disease or Condition
Cardiovascular system	Coronary artery disease Hypertension Stroke Disturbances of heart rhythm	Gastrointestinal system	Ulcer Irritable bowel syndrome Diarrhea Nausea and vomiting Ulcerative colitis
Muscle	Tension headaches Muscle contraction backache	Genitourinary system	Diuresis Impotence Frigidity
Connective tissues	Rheumatoid arthritis (autoimmune disease) Related inflammatory diseases of connective tissue	Skin	Eczema Neurodermatitis Acne
Pulmonary system	Asthma (hypersensitivity reaction) Hay fever (hypersensitivity reactions)	Endocrine system	Type 2 diabetes mellitus Amenorrhea
Immune system	Immunosuppression or deficiency Autoimmune diseases	Central nervous system	Fatigue and lethargy Type A behavior Overeating Depression Insomnia

threat and no longer able to adapt to the demands of the current and new stressors. Key physiologic changes involved in allostatic overload include exaggerated secretion of adrenal cortisol, CAs from the SNS, and proinflammatory cytokines that may initiate gene expression changes with widespread effects on neurobiologic structures and processes (Fig. 11.5). Brain regions, including the hippocampus, amygdala, and prefrontal cortex, may undergo structural remodeling that alters connections between brain cells and consequently influences both the structure and function of brain circuits underlying adaptive behavioral, cognitive, and physiologic responses. Brain alterations may impact our ability to process information that promote beneficial coping strategies and instead increase the risk of developing mental illness and cognitive impairments.[6] Becoming "stressed out," or allostatic overload, may lead to sleep deprivation; elevated evening cortisol secretion; heightened insulin and blood glucose levels; increased blood pressure; reduced parasympathetic activity; increased levels of proinflammatory cytokines; and increased secretion of the hormone ghrelin (primarily by cells of the stomach and pancreas), which promotes appetite. To summarize, allostatic overload points to the damaging effects of chronic stress on mediating many disease processes.

Regulation of the Hypothalamic-Pituitary-Adrenal Axis

An essential feature of the stress hormone system is the regulation of the hypothalamic-pituitary-adrenal (HPA) axis (Fig. 11.6). Stress activates the hypothalamus to secrete corticotropin-releasing hormone (CRH), which binds to receptors on anterior pituitary cells, which, in turn, produce adrenocorticotropic hormone (ACTH). ACTH is then released into the bloodstream and transported to the adrenal glands located on the top of the kidneys. After binding to receptors on the cortex of the adrenal glands, the glucocorticoid (GC) hormone, primarily cortisol, is released and reaches all tissues, including the brain.[6,13]

A key aspect of the HPA axis is the negative feedback loops that inhibit further secretion of cortisol. Feedback loops between cortical and subcortical regions work together to return cortisol to allostatic levels that prevent cellular damage in the brain. Understanding the links between stress and HPA cortisol secretion are beginning to offer many insights into stress-related illnesses and health outcomes. Notably, stressors can exert lasting effects on an organism's physiology and on the HPA axis through GC signaling that activates the mineralocorticoid receptor and the glucocorticoid receptor (GR). Stressor characteristics, including stressor duration, intensity, type, and context, have the potential to alter the regulation of the HPA axis and secretion of GCs.[6] Dysregulation of the HPA axis can be programmed in an age- and sex-dependent manner; these programming effects are linked with susceptibility to psychiatric and age-related diseases in both human studies and animal models. Furthermore, human and animal research shows that stress and GCs may induce long-lasting alterations in epigenetic modifications and changes in DNA methylation.[14,15]

Physiologic Effects of Cortisol

Cortisol reacts with numerous intracellular GRs (Table 11.2) to exert diverse biologic actions (see Chapter 21). Cortisol regulates many functions, including arousal, cognition, mood, sleep, metabolism, maintenance of cardiovascular tone, the immune and antiinflammatory responses, and growth and reproduction.

Cortisol plays a key role in mobilizing substances needed for cellular metabolism and stimulates gluconeogenesis or the formation of glucose from noncarbohydrate sources, such as

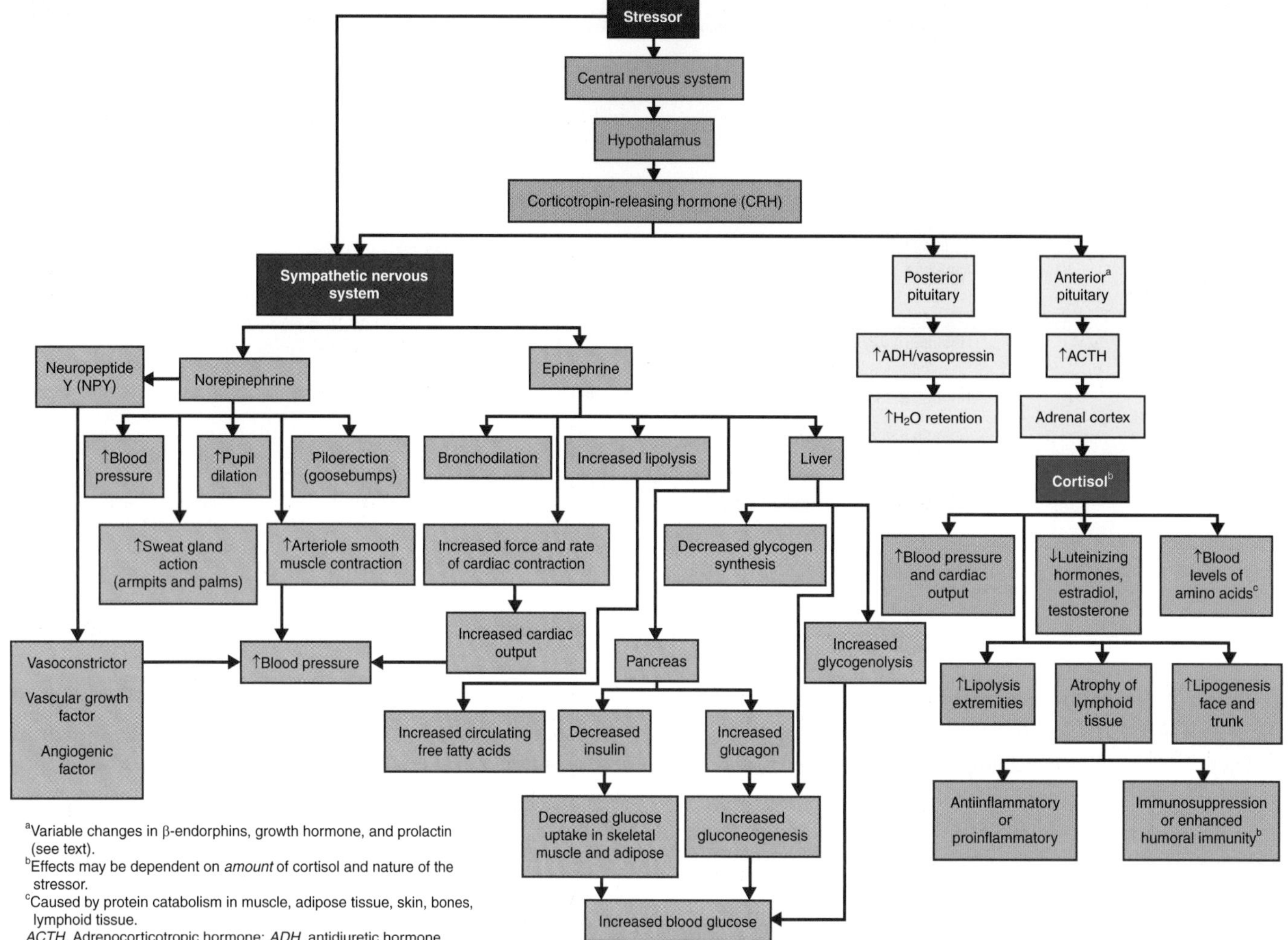

[a]Variable changes in β-endorphins, growth hormone, and prolactin (see text).
[b]Effects may be dependent on *amount* of cortisol and nature of the stressor.
[c]Caused by protein catabolism in muscle, adipose tissue, skin, bones, lymphoid tissue.
ACTH, Adrenocorticotropic hormone; *ADH*, antidiuretic hormone.

Fig. 11.4 The Stress Response. Stress activates the brain, endocrine, and immune systems to defend the individual from threat. Stress-induced physiologic responses involve the sympathetic nervous system and the hypothalamic-pituitary-adrenal (HPA) axis. The sympathetic nervous system is responsible for rapid fight-or-flight responses. Through the release of catecholamines, namely epinephrine and norepinephrine, a cascade of events occurs to prepare the body for rapid mobilization and metabolic changes, including heart rate acceleration, dilation of pupils and bronchi, liver glucose release, and other adaptive functions. Systemic vasoconstriction and elevated blood pressure are accompanied by vasodilation and increased blood flow through arteries that supply striated muscle. Engagement of the HPA system and secretion of cortisol plays key roles in supporting the diverse effects of catecholamines, suppression of the immune-inflammatory response, delayed wound healing, and modulation of the reproductive hormone system. The physiologic responses to stress have significance in the clinical setting as chronic stress and the accompanying pathophysiology can lead to a wide range of disease and disorders in the body and brain.

amino acids or free fatty acids in the liver. In addition, cortisol enhances the elevation of blood glucose levels that is promoted by other hormones, such as epinephrine, glucagon, and growth hormone. The effects of cortisol are considered to be permissive for the actions of other hormones. Cortisol also inhibits the uptake and oxidation of glucose by many body cells. Overall, the cortisol-induced increase in carbohydrate metabolism serves to energize the body to cope with the stressor.

Cortisol has anabolic effects on protein metabolism by increasing the rate of protein synthesis and ribonucleic acid (RNA) in the liver, and this effect is countered by cortisol's catabolic effect on protein stores in other tissues. Protein catabolism acts to increase levels of circulating amino acids; therefore chronic exposure to excess cortisol can severely deplete protein stores in muscle, bone, connective tissue, and skin.

Another important adaptive function of acute stress-induced cortisol secretion is to induce an antiinflammatory state to contain an inflammatory immune response. Cortisol also promotes resolution and repair by facilitating the actions of the GR, namely, the transcription of genetic material (through

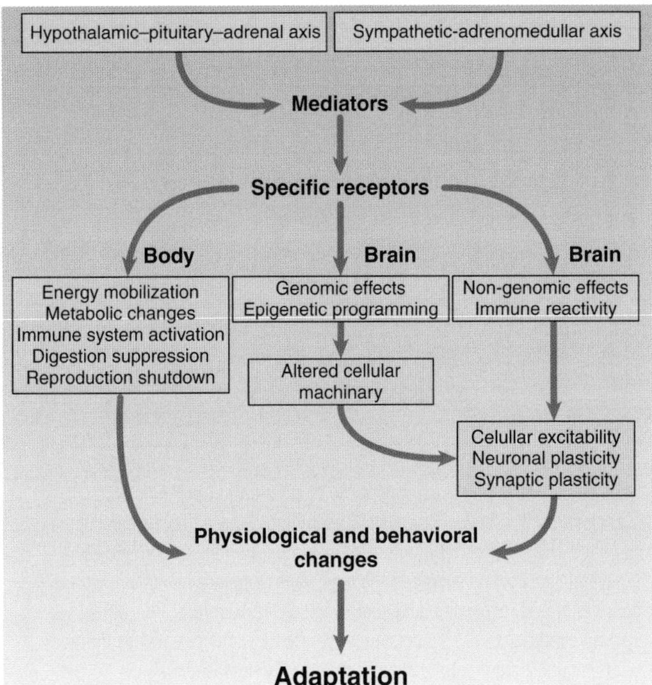

Fig. 11.5 Adaptive Roles of Stress Systems. In response to stress, the hypothalamus activates the pituitary and adrenal cortex to secrete the glucocorticoid hormone cortisol. The hypothalamus also activates the sympathetic nervous system to release the catecholamines epinephrine and norepinephrine from the adrenal medulla and from nerve endings in the periphery. Together, the glucocorticoids and catecholamines prepare the body and brain for action and protect and keep the individual from harm with the accompanying activation of the immune system. See text for further details. (Adapted from Godoy LD, Rossignoli MT, Delfino-Pereira P, et al. A comprehensive overview on stress neurobiology: basic concepts and clinical implications. *Frontiers in Behavioral Neuroscience*, 2018;12:127.)

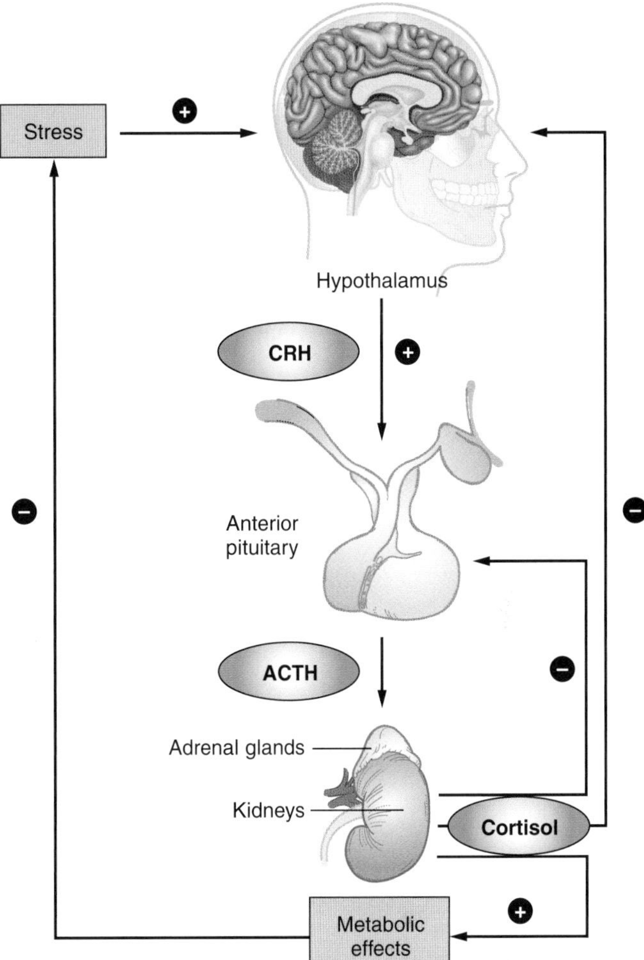

Fig. 11.6 Hypothalamic-Pituitary-Adrenal Axis. The response to stress begins in the brain. The hypothalamus is the control center in the brain for many hormones, including corticotropin-releasing hormone *(CRH)*, adrenocorticotropic hormone *(ACTH)*, and glucocorticoids (cortisol).

deoxyribonucleic acid [DNA] binding) within leukocytes. Because GRs are widely expressed, they influence virtually all immune cells. The adaptiveness or destructiveness of cortisol-induced effects may depend on the intensity, type, and duration of the stressor; the tissue involved; and the subsequent concentration and length of cortisol exposure.

Pathophysiologic Effects of Chronic Cortisol

Dysregulation of the HPA axis, especially chronic elevation of cortisol, is linked to a wide variety of disorders, including obesity, sleep deprivation, lipid abnormalities, hypertension, diabetes, atherosclerosis, and loss of bone density.[16] High HPA axis reactivity to stress, along with increased peripheral tissue sensitivity to GCs, is associated with the severity of coronary artery disease. Heightened stress-induced cortisol levels also promote gastric secretion in the stomach and intestines, potentially causing gastric ulcers, which may account for the gastrointestinal ulceration observed by Selye. Furthermore, GCs contribute to the development of metabolic syndrome and the pathogenesis of obesity by directly causing insulin resistance and influencing genetic variations that predispose to obesity.[17,18]

Chronic stress-induced secretion of GCs stimulates food intake and increases fat storage. As obesity develops, inflammatory cytokine levels increase, as do lipoproteins and free fatty acids (Fig. 11.7). The resulting low-grade inflammation is associated with an increased risk for diabetes, heart disease, cancer, disability, and early death (see Chapter 23).

In the brain, GCs bind to hippocampal GRs and may lead to temporary dendritic shrinkage and loss of spines, and chronic elevations in GCs may initiate cell death and inhibit neurogenesis.[19] Because GRs support the HPA negative feedback effects of cortisol, chronic stress-induced disruption of hippocampal GRs may compromise the negative feedback system and facilitate excess GC secretion. This elevated, stress-induced increase in cortisol is linked to suppressed synaptic function, reduced neuroplasticity, and neural damage.[6] Chronic stress in the medial prefrontal cortex may shrink the dendrites, which may induce cognitive rigidity or inflexibility. Furthermore, the effects of chronic stress on the prefrontal cortex are linked to age-related loss of resilience, impaired memory, and impairment in fear memory extinction.[20]

TABLE 11.2 Physiologic Effects of Cortisol

Functions Affected	Physiologic Effects
Carbohydrate and lipid metabolism	Diminishes peripheral uptake and utilization of glucose; promotes gluconeogenesis in liver metabolism cells; enhances gluconeogenic response to other hormones; promotes lipolysis in adipose tissue
Protein metabolism	Increases protein synthesis in liver and decreases protein synthesis (including immunoglobulin synthesis) in muscle, lymphoid tissue, adipose tissue, skin, and bone; increases plasma level of amino acids; stimulates deamination in liver
Antiinflammatory effects (systemic effects)	High levels of cortisol used in drug therapy suppress inflammatory response and inhibit proinflammatory activity of many growth factors and cytokines; however, over time some individuals may develop tolerance to glucocorticoids, causing an increased susceptibility to both inflammatory and autoimmune diseases
Proinflammatory effects (possible local effects)	Cortisol levels released during stress response may increase proinflammatory effects
Lipid metabolism	Lipolysis in extremities and lipogenesis in face and trunk
Immune effects	*Treatment* levels of glucocorticoids are immunosuppressive; thus they are valuable agents used in numerous diseases/conditions; T cell or innate immune system is particularly affected by these larger doses of glucocorticoids, with suppression of T helper cell 1 (Th1) function or innate immunity; *stress* can cause a different pattern of immune response; these nontherapeutic levels can suppress innate (Th1) and increase adaptive (Th2) immunity—the so-called Th2 shift; several factors influence this complex physiology and include long-term adaptations, reproductive hormones (i.e., overall, androgens suppress and estrogens stimulate immune responses), defects of the hypothalamic-pituitary-adrenal axis, histamine-generated responses, and acute versus chronic stress; thus stress seems to cause a Th2 shift *systemically*, whereas *locally*, under certain conditions, it can induce proinflammatory activities and by these mechanisms may influence onset or course of infections, autoimmune/inflammatory, allergic, and neoplastic diseases
Digestive function	Promotes gastric secretion
Urinary function	Enhances excretion of calcium
Connective tissue function	Decreases proliferation of fibroblasts in connective tissue (thus delaying healing)
Muscle function	Maintains normal contractility and maximal work output for skeletal and cardiac muscle
Bone function	Decreases bone formation
Vascular system/ myocardial function	Maintains normal blood pressure; permits increased responsiveness of arterioles to constrictive action of adrenergic stimulation; optimizes myocardial performance
Central nervous system function	Somehow modulates perceptual and emotional functioning; essential for normal arousal and initiation of daytime activity
Possible synergism with estrogen in pregnancy?	May suppress maternal immune system to prevent rejection of fetus

Notably, not all stress-related disorders are associated with elevated cortisol levels. Posttraumatic stress disorder (PTSD), involving exposure to a life-threatening trauma, induces a unique neurobiologic alteration in the HPA axis. For example, some people with PTSD are reported to show low urinary cortisol levels. The reduction in cortisol may reflect an adaptation of the body to protect itself from the deleterious effects of chronic, elevated GC secretion. However, GR sensitivity is increased and feedback to the HPA may be altered.[21] In other brain regions such the amygdala, animal models show that acute stressors cause an increase in spine density and chronic stress leads to the expansion of dendrites in anxiety and in PTSD-like behavior. In addition, prolonged stress in the orbitofrontal cortex expands dendrites, which increases startle and vigilance. Other studies have shown that high GC levels during critical illness and trauma may help to prevent the development of PTSD.[22] The physiologic effects of other hormones, organs, and tissues involved in the stress response are summarized in Table 11.3.

The Autonomic Nervous System

Sympathetic and Parasympathetic Nervous Systems

Activation of the SNS induces rapid release of catecholamines (CAs), particularly norepinephrine, especially from sympathetic nerve terminals, and epinephrine, from the medulla of the adrenal gland. Sympathetic nerves also contain nonadrenergic mediators that amplify or antagonize the effects of adrenal CAs. CAs work in concert with the ANS to regulate the cardiovascular, pulmonary, hepatic, skeletal muscle, and ISs.

The parasympathetic system balances the SNS and thus also influences adaptation or maladaptation to stressful events. The parasympathetic system generally opposes the sympathetic

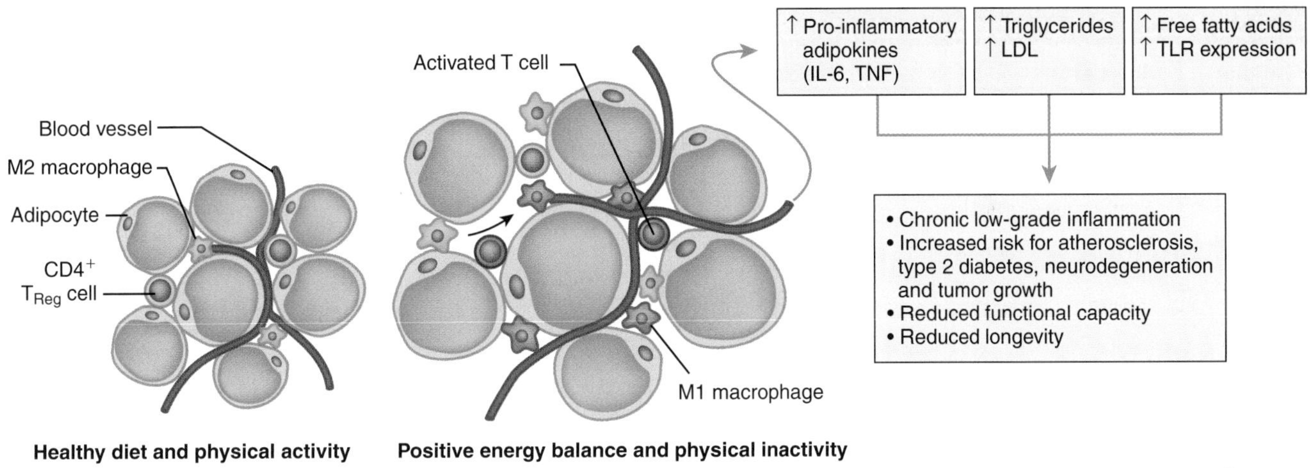

Fig. 11.7 Obesity: Adipocytes and Inflammation. People who consume a healthy diet and engage in physical activity have small adipocytes accompanied by antiinflammatory immune cells (e.g., M2-type macrophages and CD4+ T regulatory *[Treg]* cells). In contrast, positive energy balance and physical inactivity increases adipose tissue size with proinflammatory M1 macrophages that release proinflammatory adipokines (e.g., tumor necrosis factor *[TNF]*, interleukin-6 *[IL-6]*, C-reactive protein). Levels of triglycerides, low density lipoprotein (LDL), and free fatty acids are elevated, along with increased expression of toll-like receptors (TLR) on the surface of inflammatory cells. This low-grade inflammatory state accompanied by sedentary behavior, as well as stress, poor diet, etc., increases the risk of developing insulin resistance, colon cancer, breast cancer, atherosclerosis, depression, and neurodegeneration (e.g., Parkinson disease, Alzheimer disease). Notably, regular engagement in physical activity has anti-inflammatory effects that lessen the onset of many disease conditions. (From Gleeson M, Bishop NC, Stensel DJ, et al. The anti-inflammatory effects of exercise: Mechanisms and implications for the prevention and treatment of disease. *Nature reviews. Immunology,* 2011;11(9):607–615.)

system; for example, the parasympathetic nervous system slows the heart rate. The parasympathetic system also has antiinflammatory effects.

CAs stimulate two major classes of receptors: α-adrenergic receptors (α1 and α2) and β-adrenergic receptors (β1 and β2). Table 11.4 summarizes the actions of the two subclasses of adrenergic receptors. (A discussion of receptors can be found in Chapters 1, 15, and 21.) Epinephrine binds with and activates both α and β receptors, whereas norepinephrine binds primarily with α receptors.

Epinephrine in the liver and skeletal muscles is rapidly metabolized. Epinephrine influences cardiac action by enhancing myocardial contractility (inotropic effect), increasing heart rate (chronotropic effect), and increasing venous return to the heart, ultimately increasing both cardiac output and blood pressure. Epinephrine dilates blood vessels to allow greater oxygenation to skeletal muscles and also mobilizes free fatty acids and cholesterol.

CAs cannot cross the blood-brain barrier (BBB) and are synthesized and secreted in the brain to promote arousal, increase vigilance, facilitate anxiety, and other emotional responses.

Pathophysiologic Effects of Catecholamines

CA secretion increases proinflammatory cytokine production, which elevates heart rate and blood pressure and impairs wound healing. Chronic stress-induced release in norepinephrine contributes to the production of inflammatory leukocytes that adhere to vessel walls and promote the development of *plaque* (see Chapter 32).[23] Proteases released from these inflammatory leukocytes increase the risk of myocardial infarction and stroke by weakening the fibrous cap of the plaque, which can promote plaque rupture. In addition to a stress-induced risk of cardiovascular disease, the effects of stress on elevated inflammatory cytokine production also influence the onset of depression and autoimmune disorders and may facilitate functional decline that leads to frailty, disability, and untimely death. Stress-induced excessive levels of inflammatory cytokines during infection or inflammatory illness may activate a collection of nonspecific symptoms (e.g., fever, elevated HPA hormone secretion, loss of appetite, and loss of interests in physical and social activities) called the "sickness syndrome."[24] Finally, stress-induced CAs may promote tumor development by modulating the microenvironment.[25]

Role of the Immune System

The immune, nervous, and endocrine systems communicate through similar (and highly complex) pathways using hormones, neurotransmitters, neuropeptides, and immune cell products. Various components of IS responses are affected by neuroendocrine-produced factors involved in the stress reaction. Several pathways regulate communication among these systems (Fig. 11.8). The human gut microbiome also plays a role in stress and physiologic processes related to the immune response (see Emerging Science Box: The Gut Microbiota in Stress, Inflammation, and Disease).

Effects of Acute and Chronic Stress on the Immune System

Stress-induced secretion of HPA hormones and CAs by the sympathetic branch of the ANS directly influences the IS. Immune cells have receptors for ACTH, CRH, endorphins, norepinephrine, growth hormone, steroids, and other products of the stress response. In addition, cholinergic, adrenergic, and peptidergic

TABLE 11.3 Other Hormones that Influence the Stress Response

Hormone	Source	Action
β-Endorphins (endogenous opiates)	Pituitary and hypothalamus	• Activates endorphin (opiate) receptors on peripheral sensory nerves, leading to pain relief or analgesia • Hemorrhage increases levels to inhibit blood pressure or delay compensatory changes that would increase blood pressure
Growth hormone (GH, somatotropin)	Anterior pituitary gland	• Affects protein, lipid, and carbohydrate metabolism • Counters effects of insulin • Involved in tissue repair • May participate in growth and function of immune system • Levels increase after variety of stressful stimuli (cardiac catheterization, electroshock therapy, gastroscopy, surgery, fever, physical exercise) • Increased levels associated with psychological stimuli (taking examinations, viewing violent or sexually arousing films, participating in certain psychological performance tests) • Prolonged stress (chronic stress) suppresses growth hormone
Prolactin	Anterior pituitary gland; numerous extrapituitary tissue sites	• Increases in response to many stressful stimuli (including such procedures as gastroscopy, proctoscopy, pelvic examination, and surgery); increased for in situ breast cancer • Requires more intense stimuli than those leading to increases in catecholamine or cortisol levels • Levels show little change after exercise
Oxytocin	Hypothalamus	• Promotes bonding and social attachment • In animals associated with reduced hypothalamic-pituitary-adrenal (HPA) activation levels and reduced anxiety
Testosterone	Leydig cells in testes	• Regulates male secondary sex characteristics and libido • Levels decrease after stressful stimuli (anesthesia, surgery, marathon running, mountain climbing) • Decreased by psychological stimuli; however, some data indicate that psychological stress associated with competition (e.g., pistol shooting) increases both testosterone and cortisol levels, especially in athletes older than 45 years of age • Markedly reduced in individuals with respiratory failure, burns, and congestive heart failure • Decreased levels occur during aging and are associated with lowered cortisol responsiveness to stress-induced inflammation
Estrogen	Ovaries	• Works in concert with oxytocin, exerting calming effect during stressful situations
Melatonin	Produced by pineal gland	• Increases during stress response; release is suppressed by light and increased in dark; receptors have been identified on lymphoid cells, possibly higher density of receptors on T cells than on B cells; suppression of lymphocyte function by trauma was reversed by melatonin
Somatostatin (SOM)	Produced by sensory nerve terminals found in and released from lymphoid cells and hypothalamus	• Natural killer (NK) cell function and immunoglobulin synthesis decreased by SOM; growth hormone secretion decreased by SOM
Vasoactive intestinal peptide (VIP)	Found in neurons of central nervous system (CNS) and in peripheral nerves	• VIP increases during stress; VIP-containing nerves are located in both primary and secondary lymphoid tissues, around blood vessels, and in gastrointestinal tract; VIP receptors are on both T and B cells; VIP may influence lymphocyte maturation; cytokine production by T cells is modified by VIP; B-cell and antibody production is influenced by VIP
Calcitonin gene–related peptide (CGRP)	Found in spinal cord motor neurons and in sensory neurons near dendritic cells of skin and in primary and secondary lymphoid tissues	• CGRP receptors are present on T and B lymphocytes; thus it is likely that CGRP can modulate immune function; CGRP may enhance acute inflammatory response because it is vasodilator; maturation of immune B lymphocytes is inhibited by CGRP; interleukin-1 is inhibited by CGRP, which is important for activation of T cells; it has been shown to interfere with lymphocyte activation
Neuropeptide Y (NPY)	Present in neurons of CNS and in neurons throughout body; colocalized in nerve terminals in lymphatic tissues with norepinephrine	• Lymphocytes have receptors for NPY and thus may modulate their function; several lines of evidence suggest that NPY is neurotransmitter and neurohormone involved in stress response; increased levels of NPY occur in plasma in response to severe or prolonged stress; may be responsible for stress-induced regional vasoconstriction (splanchnic, coronary, and cerebral); may also increase platelet aggregation. May be important in preventing depression.
Substance P (SP)	Produced by neuropeptide classified as tachykinin (increases heart rate subsequent to lowering blood pressure) found in brain, as well as nerves innervating secondary lymphoid tissues	• SP increases in response to stress; receptors for SP are found on membranes of both T and B cells, mononuclear phagocytic cells, and mast cells; proinflammatory activity induces release of histamine from mast cells during stress response; causes smooth muscle contraction, causes macrophages and T cells to release cytokines, and increases antibody production

TABLE 11.4 Physiologic Effects of Catecholamines

Organ/Tissue	Process or Result
Brain	Increased blood flow; increased glucose metabolism
Cardiovascular system	Increased rate and force of contraction Peripheral vasoconstriction
Pulmonary system	Bronchodilation
Skeletal muscle	Increased glycogenolysis Increased contraction Increased dilation of muscle vasculature Decreased glucose uptake and utilization (decreases insulin release)
Liver	Increased glucose production Increased glycogenolysis
Adipose tissue	Increased lipolysis Decreased glucose uptake
Skin	Decreased blood flow
Gastrointestinal and genitourinary tracts	Decreased protein synthesis Decreased smooth muscle contraction Increased renin release Increased gastrointestinal sphincter tone
Lymphoid tissue	Acute as well as chronic stress inhibits several components of innate immunity, particularly decreasing natural killer cells
Macrophages	Inhibit and stimulate macrophage activity Depends on availability of type 1/proinflammatory cytokines, presence or absence of antigenic stressors, and peripheral corticotropin-releasing hormone (CRH)

Some of these responses require glucocorticoids (e.g., cortisol) for maximal activity (see text for explanation).
Data from Elenkov IJ, Chrousos GP. Stress hormones, proinflammatory and antiinflammatory cytokines, and autoimmunity. *Annals of the New York Academy of Sciences*, 2002;966:290–303; Granner DK. Hormones of the adrenal medulla. In Murray RK, et al., eds. *Harper's biochemistry*, 25th edition. New York: McGraw-Hill; 2000.

nerves innervate lymphoid organs, such as the thymus, spleen, lymph nodes, and bone marrow. Exposure to stress increases endogenous opiate secretion, which can modulate immune cell function.[26]

Lymphocytes also produce ACTH and endorphins in small amounts that influence the immune response in an autocrine (same cell stimulation) or paracrine (cell to cell) manner in ongoing immune and memory cytotoxic responses. The T-cell growth factor IL-2 can upregulate pituitary ACTH. Immune-derived cytokines have direct and indirect effects on HPA and adrenal cell functions. Thus the IS has an adaptive role as a signal organ to alert other systems of internally threatening stimuli (e.g., pathogens, infection, tissue damage, tumor cells). The release of immune inflammatory mediators (e.g., IL-6, TNF-β, interferon [IFN]) is triggered by bacterial or viral infections, cancer, tissue injury, and other stressors, which, in turn, initiate a stress response through the HPA pathway. Enhanced systemic production of these cytokines also induces other central nervous system (CNS) and behavior changes during an acute inflammatory infectious episode.

It is important to recognize that inflammation is considered to be beneficial in the short term by destroying pathogens and facilitating the healing process. However, chronic low-grade systemic inflammation characterized by prolonged secretion of proinflammatory cytokines is associated with cardiovascular disease, osteoporosis, arthritis, type 2 diabetes mellitus, chronic obstructive pulmonary disease (COPD), and diseases associated with aging (Fig. 11.9). Prolonged severe stress may lead to enlargement of the adrenal gland with simultaneous involution of the thymus and lymph nodes. Chronic stress secretion of GCs impacts many immune cell functions, including decreased natural killer (NK) cell and T-cell cytotoxicity and impaired β-cell function. Thus prolonged secretion of cortisol is an important mechanism underlying stress-related immune structure alterations, suppression of the immune response, and chronic inflammation.[27]

The elevation in inflammation levels also stems from chronic stimulation of the SNS and the gradual downregulation of key antiinflammatory pathways, such as the HPA axis and the parasympathetic nervous system. Studies show that psychosocial stress-induced modulation of lymphoid and myeloid cells and chronic inflammation by cytokines, such as IL-6, are implicated in cancer progression, metastasis, and recurrence.

Stress-induced SNS release of CAs and activation of β-adrenergic receptor (β-AR) are implicated in primary tumor growth and metastasis and colonization of tumors in distant tissues.[25,28] For example, inflammatory factors such as IL-6 are regulated by β-AR signaling and increase in circulation after stressor exposure. IL-6 and associated gene polymorphisms of IL-6 are prognostic indicators of tumor progression, metastasis,

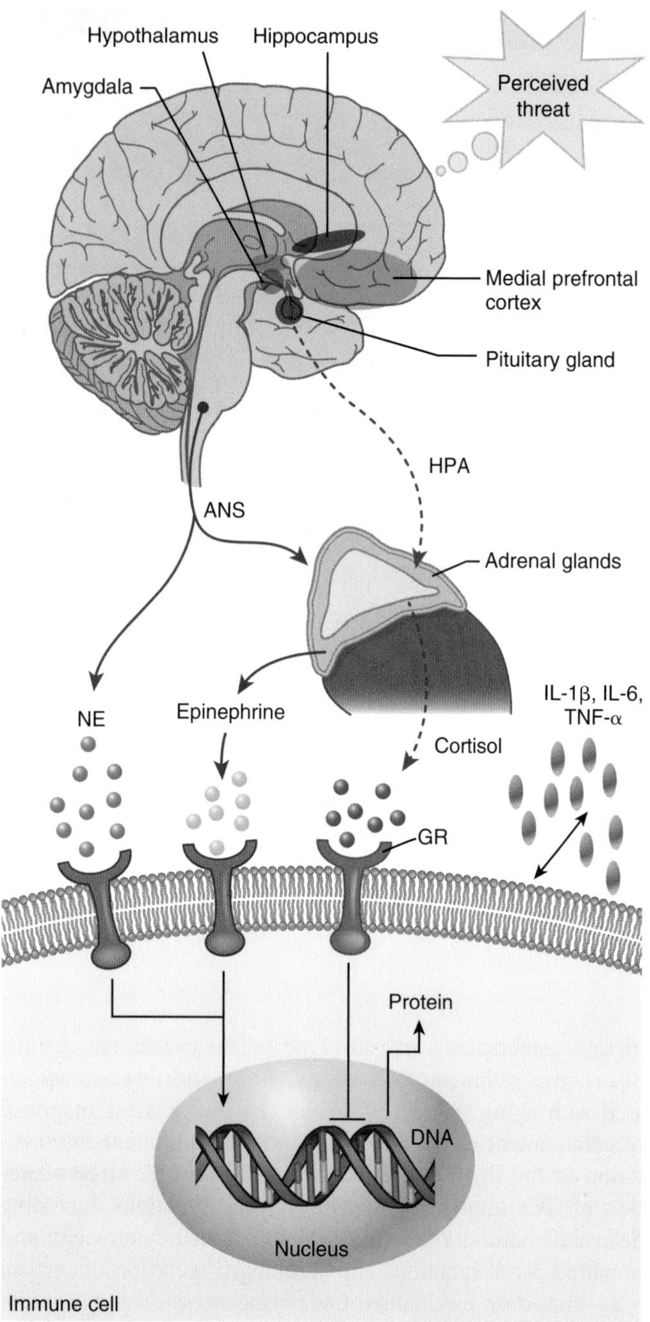

Fig. 11.8 Neurophysiologic Pathways Linking Perceived Threat to Inflammation. Neurophysiologic pathways linking stress or threat-related neural activity in the amygdala, medial prefrontal cortex, and hippocampus with the hypothalamic-pituitary-adrenal *(HPA)* axis, the autonomic nervous system *(ANS)*, and immune cells that increase inflammation. Threat perception activates the HPA axis, leading to increased release of the glucocorticoid hormone cortisol from the adrenal glands *(broken lines)*. In addition, activation of the sympathetic arm of the ANS leads to increased release of the catecholamine epinephrine and norepinephrine *(solid lines)*. Cortisol and catecholamines bind to receptors on immune cells to increase synthesis and release of cytokines, including interleukin-1β *(IL-1β)*, interleukin-6 *(IL-6)*, and tumor necrosis factor-α *(TNF-α)*, which serve adaptive roles in protecting the body from disease. However, when chronic stress-induced cortisol secretion occurs, the glucocorticoid receptor *(GR)* becomes downregulated and limits the antiinflammatory effects of cortisol. In addition, the expression of proinflammatory genes is increasingly expressed that heighten the secretion of proinflammatory cytokines. Altogether these effects ultimately lead to elevated inflammation that increases the risk of disease. (From O'Donovan A, Slavichc GM, Epela ES, et al. Exaggerated neurobiological sensitivity to threat as a mechanism linking anxiety with increased risk for diseases of aging. *Neuroscience and Biobehavioral Reviews*, 2013;37:96–108.)

and survival in human cancers. Peripheral immune cells which are responsive to β-AR signaling and secrete IL-6 and other regulatory factors reside within and around the tumor microenvironment and can promote or prevent malignant disease.[29] Inflammatory cell recruitment into the primary tumor microenvironment may serve as a biomarker for early detection of disease progression or serve as a prognostic indicator of therapeutic success and resolution of disease.

Microglia activation in the brain is an important component of neuroinflammation. Microglia are resident immune cells in the brain. If injury or infection occurs, the microglia play an active protective role in protecting the brain tissues. Microglia also are involved in the pruning and maintenance of synapses,

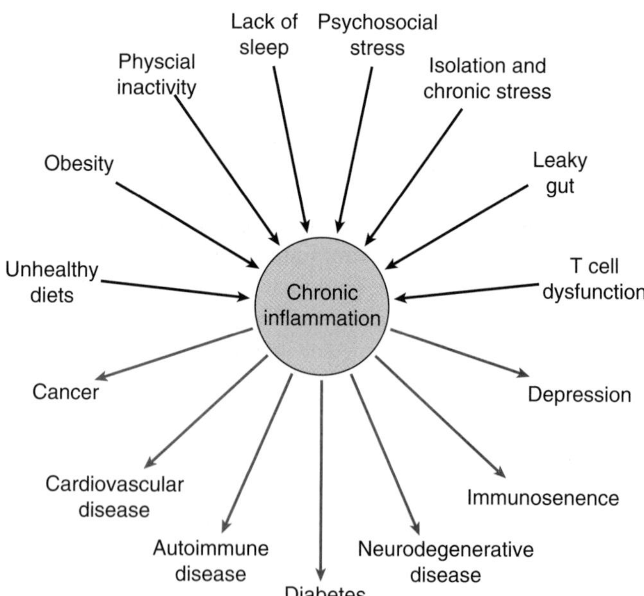

Fig. 11.9 The Broad Negative Health Effects of Inflammation on the Body and Brain. Numerous factors, including unhealthy diets, obesity, physical inactivity, lack of sleep, stress, social isolation, leaky gut, and T-cell dysfunction, contribute to a chronic inflammatory state. Currently, chronic inflammation is recognized as a common underlying condition leading to pathology and a diverse set of illnesses, such as autoimmune disease, cancer, cardiovascular disease, neurodegenerative disease, diabetes, immunosenescence, and depression.

EMERGING SCIENCE BOX

The Gut Microbiota in Stress, Inflammation, and Disease

The human gut microbiota consists of trillions of bacteria and plays an important role in physiologic processes, including interactions with the host immune system and the brain. In addition, it plays a role in stress by modulating the intestinal barrier permeability and the gut-brain axis signaling through the vagal nerve, inflammatory molecules, endocrine molecules, and microbial metabolites.

A stable gut microbiota promotes normal gut physiology and contributes to appropriate physiologic functions along the microbiota-brain-gut axis to maintain the healthy status of the individual (see Figure below). Conversely, intestinal dysbiosis, or the imbalance in the gut microbial community, adversely impacts gut physiology leading to inappropriate brain-gut axis signaling and the progression to disease states. Examples of intestinal dysbiosis include *Clostridioides difficile* infection (infectious disease), inflammatory bowel disease (intestinal immune-mediated disease), obesity (metabolic disease), colorectal cancer, and autism spectrum disorder (neuropsychiatric disorder).

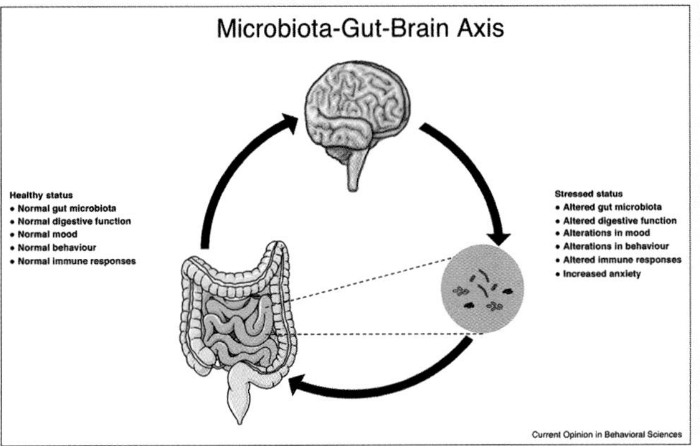

(Figure from Hollins SL, et al. Stress, microbiota, and immunity. *Current Opinion in Behavioral Sciences*, 2019;28:66–71. ISSN 2352–1546. https://doi.org/10.1016/j.cobeha.2019.01.015.)

The gut microbiota signals the brain through a number of pathways including regulating immune activity and proinflammatory cytokines that stimulate the hypothalamic-pituitary-adrenal (HPA) axis to produce corticotropin-releasing hormone (CRH), adrenocorticotropic hormone (ACTH), and cortisol. The gut microbiota also can directly impact central nervous system (CNS) immune activity through release of short-chain fatty acids (SCFAs), such as propionate, butyrate, and acetate, as well as tryptophan metabolites including kynurenic acid and quinolinic acid. Neuronal and spinal pathways, particularly afferent signaling from the vagus nerve, are critical in mediating the effect of the gut microbiota on brain function and behavior.

Good bacteria probiotics act to stabilize digestive pH, reduce inflammation, and increase neuroprotective molecules, such as brain-derived neurotrophic factor (BDNF). Impaired microbiota dysbiosis can induce neuroinflammation and reduce the expression of BDNF and N-methyl-D-aspartate receptor (NMDA) receptors, leading to cognitive impairment, mood disorders, and higher levels of amyloid beta formation.

A study in mice reported that stress worsens inflammation in the colon and the composition of the microbiome changes. Levels of SCFAs, which play a major role in maintaining normal gut and immune function by regulating colonic motility, blood flow, and gastrointestinal pH, were found to decrease when stress and the expression of the receptors also changed. Furthermore, when mice were stressed and infected with *Citrobacter rodentium*, a gram-negative bacterium that causes mild/moderate inflammation in the descending colon, colonic expression of the SCFA receptor GPR41 was positively associated with inflammatory cytokines and colonic histopathology scores. The results show that stress altered the microbiome, which in turn increased the level of colonic inflammation. This mouse model may have relevance to irritable bowel disease in humans.

Other research on the effects of stress on the gut lining examines how increased intestinal permeability plays a role in chronic diseases, such as celiac and Crohn disease. When the gut lining is compromised *(leaky gut)*, partially digested foods, bacteria, and toxins now penetrate the barrier and leak into the body and blood stream to trigger inflammation.

Another relevant study examined the effects social stress or marital discord on inflammatory markers associated with the leaky gut. They found that men and women who engage in hostile behavior toward each other had high serum levels of lipopolysaccharide-binding protein (LPB), which indicates the presence of bacteria in the blood. The leaky gut LPB was even greater in participants who were particularly hostile to their spouse and with a history of depression or another mood disorder. Furthermore, a strong relationship was found between LPB and C-reactive protein, a primary marker of inflammation. Individuals with the highest LBP had 79% higher levels of C-reactive protein compared to people who were not in hostile marital relationships. Of note, depressed people also may have a history of cardiovascular disease, metabolic syndrome, and/or diabetes. The results now demonstrate a link between marital discord and the leaky gut pathway leading to a proinflammatory state with implications on mental and physical health.

Data from Bear T, et al. The microbiome-gut-brain axis and resilience to developing anxiety or depression under stress. *Microorganisms*. 2021;9(4):723; Cryan JF, et al. Mind-altering microorganisms: The impact of the gut microbiota on brain and behavior. *Nature reviews. Neuroscience*, 2012;13:701–712; Dubinski P, et al. The influence of gut microbiota on the cardiovascular system under conditions of obesity and chronic stress. *Curr Hypertens Rep.* 2021;23:31; Kiecolt-Glaser JK, et al. Marital distress, depression, and a leaky gut: Translocation of bacterial endotoxin as a pathway to inflammation. *Psychoneuroendocrinology*, 2018;98:52–60; Kho ZY, et al. The human gut microbiome—A potential controller of wellness and disease. *Frontiers in Microbiology*, 2018;9:1835; Maltz RM, et al. Social stress affects colonic inflammation, the gut microbiome, and short-chain fatty acid levels and receptors. *Journal of Pediatric Gastroenterology and Nutrition*, 2019;68:533–540; Ma T, et al. Probiotic consumption relieved human stress and anxiety symptoms possibly via modulating the neuroactive potential of the gut microbiota. *Neurobiology of Stress*. 2021;14:100294; Miller AH, et al. Inflammation and its discontents: The role of cytokines in the pathophysiology of major depression. *Biological Psychiatry*, 2009;65:732–741.

trafficking of neurotransmitters, and phagocytosis or the removal of cell fragments and damaged cells. However, excessive stress and microglia activation that increase cytokine production may compromise the tightly controlled BBB and allow cytokines and leukocytes to enter the brain from the periphery.

The resultant inability to control inflammatory cells in the brain has the potential to impair adaptive brain functions. Stress-induced inflammation by microglia disrupts corticoamygdala and corticobasal ganglia neural circuits that balance positive and negative states, and predisposes people to negative thinking and to engage in self-medicating behaviors such as smoking, drug use, and consumption of high-fat diets. Repetitive negative thinking has been linked to the development of dementia (see Emerging Science Box: Repetitive

Negative Thinking is a Risk Factor for Alzheimer Disease). Depression has been linked to stress-induced inflammation.[11,12,30] This link may explain the high prevalence of depression in association with other chronic inflammatory conditions such as heart disease (see Emerging Science Box: Stress and Inflammation Are Causal Factors Linking Heart Disease with Depression).

EMERGING SCIENCE BOX

Repetitive Negative Thinking Is a Risk Factor for Alzheimer Disease

A recent observational study reported that repetitive negative thinking (RNT) is a potential risk factor for dementia. RNT is defined as a cognitive process that involves persistent worrying and ruminating thoughts. Previous research showed that depression and anxiety are risk factors for dementia and people diagnosed with depression and anxiety exhibit chronic negative thinking. However, the precise relationship between RNT and dementia was not clear. The current study demonstrated that people with high levels of RNT experiences were more likely to show both decline in global cognition and episodic memory within a 4-year period and aggregation of amyloid and tau deposits, the neuropathologic markers of Alzheimer disease.

The researchers suggest that RNT elevates stress factors such as high blood pressure which can contribute to onset of amyloid and tau deposition. In addition, the researchers propose that behavioral interventions known to reduce RNT, such as mindfulness therapy could be used to investigate its benefits on decreasing cognitive deficits and neuropathologic markers of Alzheimer disease.

Data from Marchant NL, et al. Repetitive negative thinking is associated with amyloid, tau, and cognitive decline. *Alzheimer's and Dementia,* 2020;16(7):1054–1064. https://doi.org/10.1002/alz.12116.

EMERGING SCIENCE BOX

Stress and Inflammation are Causal Factors Linking Heart Disease with Depression

The association between heart disease and stress-induced depression is well known, but the underlying basis of these illnesses is unclear. Are people with heart disease more likely to develop depression, or are depressed people more likely to show an increased risk of heart disease? Are there similar genetic or environmental factors in people who develop heart disease and depression?

A recent study involving 367,703 unrelated, middle-aged participants of European ancestry found that the link between the two disorders could not be explained entirely by genetic factors. That is, a genetic risk score strongly associated with heart disease was not associated with depression. Instead, a Mendelian randomization analyses showed that triglycerides, interleukin-6 (IL-6), and C-reactive protein (CRP) were found in high levels in people with both heart disease and depression. IL-6 and CRP are both inflammation-related proteins occurring in response to various damaging stimuli, including smoking, infection, and stress. The findings suggest that stress-induced inflammation, a common biologic mechanism occurring in both the cardiovascular system and brain, is a causal risk factor linking comorbidity in depression and heart disease.

Data from Khandaker GM, et al. Shared mechanisms between coronary heart disease and depression: Findings from a large UK general population-based cohort. *Molecular Psychiatry,* 2020;25:1477–1486.

THE IMPACT OF CHRONIC STRESS ACROSS THE LIFE SPAN

The deleterious effects of chronic stress can foster pathophysiologic changes that impact health and disease across the life span. These negative effects may begin before birth and extend into the aging process later in life.

Negative Effects of Chronic Stress at an Early Age

Human brain development begins from the fetal period to the neonatal period, infancy, childhood, adolescence, and early adulthood. Throughout this developmental time span, the brain is undergoing a host of critical changes, such as cell proliferation, cell migration, differentiation, and eventual synaptic maturation, and neuronal connections and functioning. These dynamic changes in the development of stress-responsive systems and brain structures, including the amygdala, hippocampus, and prefrontal cortex, can be significantly impacted by the effects of early stress. Changes in these systems may induce pathophysiologic, cognitive, motivational, emotional, and genetic alterations that become embedded and thus impact health and the risk of disease later in life.[19,31]

Many epidemiologic studies show that stress in women during pregnancy has the potential to adversely affect the early development of a child.[15] Prenatal stress also increases the incidence of spontaneous abortions, fetal malformations, and preterm birth and impairs the intellectual, language, and emotional development of a child. Other studies reported increased propensity to acquire cardiovascular and metabolic disorders in later life.[18] Prenatal stress is a predicator of low birth weight associated with a higher risk of depression during adolescence and adulthood.

Activation of the HPA axis and release of cortisol is suggested to be a major source mediating the negative effects of maternal stress on the fetus. High levels of stress-induced maternal cortisol secretion could cross the placental barrier and enter the fetus to alter brain development and the HPA axis.[31] Convincing data point to high maternal cortisol, a key biomarker of stress, during pregnancy with low birth weight. The consequences of cortisol-induced low birth weight have extended to disease risk in later life, including overweight/obesity, cardiovascular conditions (e.g., hypertension), and behavioral disorders attributed to altered brain structures and epigenetic modifications (i.e., changes in gene expression). Allostatic overload of elevated GC secretion in early life potentially compromises the well-being of the individual throughout life.

The fetus exposed to elevated levels of proinflammatory cytokines also is at risk of developing a range of neurodevelopmental disorders. Excessive exposure to proinflammatory cytokines has the potential to alter brain morphology in the prenatal period, which compromises cognitive functioning in late life. An example is maternal obesity during gestation, which produces an inflammatory state linked to offspring neurodevelopmental alterations that predict insulin resistance, an elevated body mass index (BMI), and increased risk of attention-deficit/hyperactivity disorder.[32]

The caregiving environment is believed to support and protect the child and buffer the potential effects of stress on altering the development of stress systems. However, allostatic overload or a chronic proinflammatory state induced by psychosocial stress in early life may promote dysregulation of the HPA and ANS and predispose an individual to show increased hypervigilance to threat, poor emotional regulation, and increased health risk behaviors (e.g., poor dietary choices, risky behaviors). Childhood trauma involving physical, sexual, and emotional abuse or neglect is associated with psychiatric illnesses, including depression, anxiety, and PTSD, and with health problems, such as rheumatoid arthritis, cardiovascular disease, metabolic syndrome, and cancer. Studies have reported that exposure to childhood trauma was associated with elevated baseline levels of peripheral C-reactive protein (CRP), TNF-α, and the cytokine IL-6 in adulthood.[33,34] This chronic inflammatory state may be the culprit contributing to the development of both physical and mental disorders observed in adults exposed to childhood trauma.

A well-documented risk factor linked to chronic stress and poor health is low SES.[35] Families with low SES are exposed to a host of stressors, such as financial unpredictability, household chaos and violence, noisy neighborhood environment, and disruption of family routines, all of which contribute to an increase in stress for both parents and children. Socioeconomically disadvantaged young children exhibit elevated levels of cortisol and mental illness. Children living in lower-SES households and from racial/ethnic minorities also are at risk of age-related diseases widely linked to cardiometabolic morbidity and mortality.[36] Chronic childhood adversity–induced activation of the HPA axis affects GC metabolism and immune function, which predispose individuals to chronic inflammation, as indicated by elevations in IL-6, the proinflammatory CRP; fibrinogen; and other biomarkers associated with cardiometabolic disease.[34] Of further interest, people living below the poverty level and have low education exhibit CRP levels nearly twice the value in those living above the poverty level. Early life adversity and associated stress impacts brain development. For example, people who suffered from maltreatment in childhood show greater amygdala reactivity to threat. In addition, functional connectivity is altered between brain areas (i.e., amygdala) responsible for threat detection and connective brain areas (prefrontal cortex) responsible for cognitive regulation and coping to threat responses.[37] Childhood poverty is linked with deficits in executive function through stress-related structural changes in the prefrontal cortex.[38] Impairments in executive functioning may compromise the ability to manage psychosocial functions including social relationships, emotions, and ability to cope with stress. As a result, these cognitive impairments increase the risk for developing the symptoms of anxiety, depression, and other health-related problems.[39]

Depending on the temporal developmental periods when the child is exposed to stress, brain development may occur in different ways that affect cognitive and mental health issues. Exposure to negative stressful experiences, such as illness or parental separation, occurring from age 0 to 5 years was associated with faster maturation of the prefrontal cortex and amygdala during puberty. These parts of the brain are responsible for personality expression, decision-making, moderating social behavior, and expressing emotions. Thus, although early-life stress accelerates brain maturation during adolescence, the rapidly maturing brain may compromise the effects of adaptive developmental plasticity, which may lead to subsequent mental and physical disorders.

Telomeres are DNA-based caps located at the end of chromosomes. These end-caps protect genetic information and degradation during cell division. Telomeres shorten during repeated cell divisions over time and are an indication of biologic aging. Stress has a major influence on telomere shortening that can begin in utero by increasing early telomere damage. Maternal stress during pregnancy and childhood adversity are reported to impact telomere length during the periods of exposure as well as later in life.[40,41] Children who experienced cumulative exposures to violence, poverty, and traumatic life events showed significantly more telomere erosion prior to puberty, even after adjusting for confounding factors.[42]

Another consequence of childhood stress is an accelerated increase in BMI.[43] Stress triggers the secretion of the neurohormone ghrelin, which increases appetite, food-seeking behavior, and food-associated reward. Children exposed to chronic stress also are deficient in leptin, a hormone involved in the regulation of energy balance. The imbalance in physiologic factors that normally regulate body weight likely contributes to the onset of obesity in children. Exposure to maternal stress also may increase the risk of childhood overweight/obesity, which may be caused by epigenetic modifications (i.e., DNA methylations cause changes in gene expression).[44] In summary, exposure to early stress disrupts a number or adaptive regulatory systems in the body and brain which increases risk of disease in later life.

Negative Effects of Chronic Stress in Adolescents and Adults

Social or personal stress occurring at a later age may produce a different developmental trajectory. From age 14 to 17 years, adolescents who were ridiculed or disliked by their peers showed reduced gray matter volume in different parts of the brain, including the prefrontal cortex and the hippocampus, which is responsible for memory. In addition, gray matter volume of the anterior cingulate was reduced and may be related to the higher incidence in antisocial traits reported at these ages. Callous, unemotional behavior occurring at this time may be linked to the future development of psychopathy.[45]

Stress-induced developmental alterations in these neural circuits may sensitize the individual to thoughts or situations as threatening and increase the activation of stress systems and their negative consequences. Stress-induced structural changes in the prefrontal cortex may impair working memory, executive function, attention, self-awareness, and inhibitory or impulse control. Overtime, the growing child may be less likely to develop cognitive, behavioral, and self-regulatory control of emotions that enable them to manage and adapt to stress.

In adults, telomere shortening or attrition linked to biologic aging can be accelerated by a number of conditions associated with stress-induced inflammation. Adults who experienced childhood adversity or allostatic load exhibited higher inflammatory markers (IL-6, TNF-α) and shorter telomere length.[40] Shorter telomere length found in white blood cells reflects an increased risk of aging-related morbidity and mortality. Research showed that adults with telomeres in the shortest category had 25% greater early risk of death compared with those in the longest telomere category.[46]

A clear example of the effects of chronic psychosocial stress in adults is burnout, a syndrome associated with a number of negative consequences to workers' well-being and health. Uncontrolled work stress is a significant predictor of adverse physical consequences, including hypercholesterolemia, type 2 diabetes, coronary heart disease, and hospitalization caused by a cardiovascular disorder, musculoskeletal pain, changes in pain experiences, prolonged fatigue, headaches, gastrointestinal issues, respiratory problems, severe injuries, and early mortality at age younger than 45 years. Potential mechanisms contributing to burnout include dysregulation of the HPA axis and ANS, which are accompanied by impaired immune function and inflammation.[47] These interrelated stress systems increase the risk of adopting poor health choices (e.g., smoking, lack of physical activity and sleep, bad eating habits) that make the individual vulnerable to infectious disease, such as flu-like illnesses, the common cold, and gastroenteritis.

Similar to burnout, social isolation and loneliness are becoming increasingly common in older people who are living longer and with reduced social interactions. Loneliness is associated with chronic stress that activates the hypothalamic-pituitary-adrenocortical axis and the SNS. Prolonged activation of these stress systems leads to GC resistance and compromises the IS to protect the body and brain, which increases the risk of many health issues, including heart disease, high blood pressure, diabetes, and dementia. Furthermore, loneliness increases the risks of morbidity and mortality similar to cardiovascular disease, smoking, obesity, depression, and cognitive decline. The World Health Organization recognizes the importance of social connections, and research points to a growing epidemic of loneliness in many countries, which can have serious health and economic effects in the years to come.[48,49]

COPING AND INTERVENTION STRATEGIES

Coping is the process of managing stressful challenges that impact the individual's resources.[50] Coping responses may be adaptive or maladaptive, and the extent to which an individual responds to distress using effective positive coping strategies will determine the degree of successful moderation of the stress challenge (Fig. 11.10). Personality characteristics, such as academic achievement, motivation, optimism, and aggression are associated with differences in appraisal and response to stressors. These personality characteristics may facilitate or impede the efficacy of interventions for preventing disease and managing illness in a clinical setting.

Staying on the Good Side of the Stress Spectrum

Maladaptive coping responses to stressors, such as increased smoking, decreased exercise and sleep, and poor diets provide an important pathway through which stressors influence the risk of disease. Constant disturbances of the sleep-wake cycle observed in many stressed people may exacerbate the pathophysiologic status of some individuals. Sleep deprivation and circadian disruption, even in young otherwise healthy individuals, have detrimental influences on respiratory and IS function. Sleep deprivation has been shown to cause chronic inflammation and is associated with diseases such as diabetes and atherosclerosis.[51]

Altered immune function, depression, hypertension, and many other disorders have been linked to repressive coping behaviors toward emotions and stress.[52] School teachers who devote long hours without reward and are unable to disengage from work-related tasks also are found to have lower innate immune responses. Coping strategies are especially beneficial when they are problem-focused and receive social support. Effective interventions may result in greater stress resilience and improved psychological and physiologic outcomes.

Other important factors, such as social support and development of self-esteem, may mitigate the adverse effects of stress and confer resilience. Furthermore, the social environment may alter genes (i.e., epigenetics) which are expressed or suppressed to promote adaptation to stress or disease. For example, research in animals showed that maternal protective caregiving behavior may turn on genes that efficiently regulate the HPA stress response in offspring. The effects of the parental rearing environment found in animals also may extend to the human caregiving situation where children reared by highly attentive mothers showed lower stress-induced cortisol secretion to an inoculation procedure at the doctor's office than offspring of less-attentive mothers. Different parental rearing styles may impact how the developing child responds and copes to stress.[53]

Social support also can be beneficial for adults with limited education on how to care for themselves and for children who require caregiving attention. Teaching adults how to engage the child with problem-solving skills, planning, and emotional self-regulation in positive interactions offers a way to alleviate potential negative health effects of stress on the adult and child family members.

Effects of Exercise

Coping behaviors, such as regular physical activity, can significantly enhance mental well-being and lessen symptoms of depression and anxiety as effectively as psychotherapy.[54–56] The beneficial effects of exercise are found at all age groups—from adolescents to the elderly. Stress-induced imbalances in brain neurotransmitters are noted in people with depression, which is associated with negative emotions, such as increased anger, confusion, fatigue, tension, and reduced vigor. Animal and human studies further indicate that maternal exercise during pregnancy has the potential to strengthen the cardiac autonomic control of the fetus that could reduce the prevalence of age-related diseases and lead to an increase in quality of life and life span.

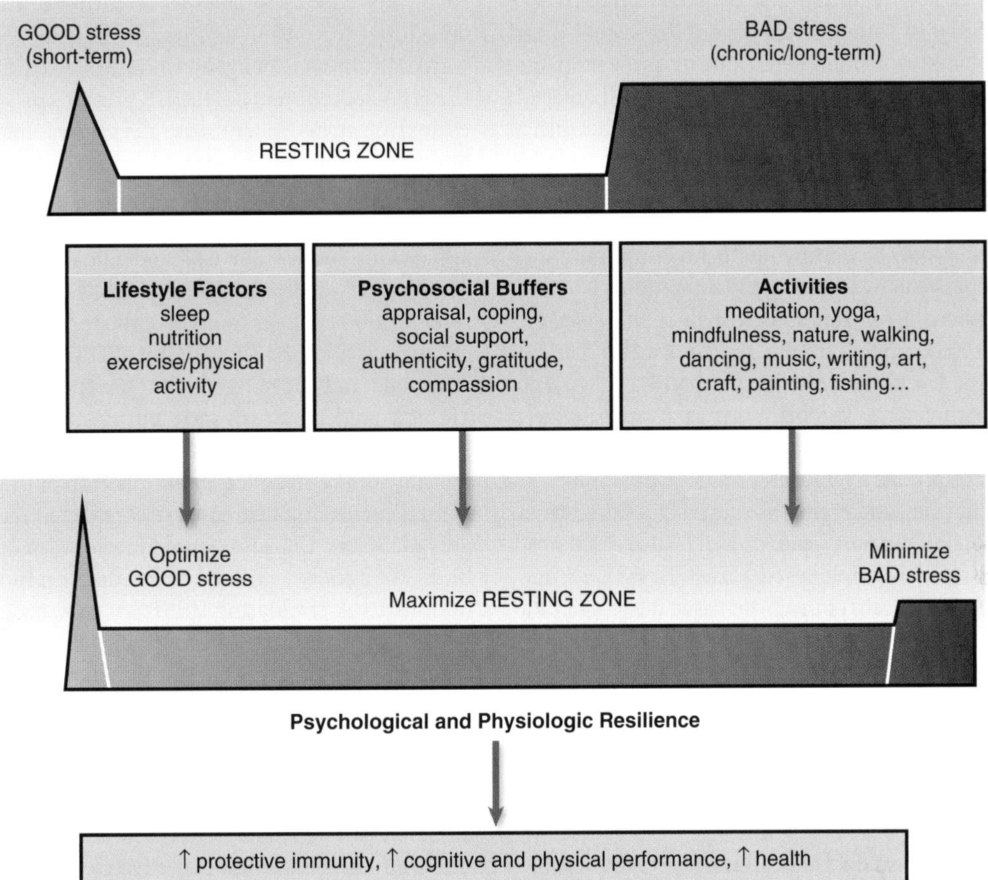

Fig. 11.10 Staying on the Good Side of the Stress Spectrum. GOOD stress is shown on the left of the spectrum and involves a rapid biologic response to the stressor, followed by a rapid shutdown of the response upon cessation of the stressor. These responses support physiologic conditions that are likely to enhance protective immunity, cognitive and physical performance, and overall health. BAD stress, represented on the right of the spectrum, involves exposure to chronic or long-term biologic changes that are likely to result in dysregulation or suppression of immune function, a decrease in cognitive and physical performance, and an increased likelihood of disease. Short- and/or long-term stress is generally superimposed on a psychophysiologic RESTING ZONE of low/no stress that also represents a state of health maintenance/restoration. To maintain health, one needs to optimize GOOD stress, maximize the RESTING ZONE, and minimize BAD stress. Achieving psychological and physiologic resilience involves a multipronged approach. Sleep of good quality and duration that helps one to feel rested in the morning, a moderate and healthy diet, and consistent and moderate exercise or physical activity are three LIFESTYLE FACTORS that are likely to enable one to stay on the "good" side of the stress spectrum. Effective appraisal and coping mechanisms, genuine gratitude, social support, and compassion toward others and oneself are likely to provide PSYCHOSOCIAL BUFFERS against bad stress and enable one to stay on the "good" side of the stress spectrum. In addition, depending on individual preferences, ACTIVITIES, such as meditation, yoga, being in nature, exercise/physical activity, music, art, craft, dance, or fishing, painting, may reduce BAD stress, extend the RESTING ZONE, and optimize GOOD stress. Such personal activities are likely to involve different strokes for different folks and need not always be meditative or reflective in nature. (Adapted from Dhabhar FS, McEwen BS. Bidirectional effects of stress on immune function: Possible explanations for salubrious as well as harmful effects. In: Ader R, ed. *Psychoneuroimmunology*. Vol. IV. San Diego: Elsevier; 2007.)

Impairments in serotonin neurotransmission are linked to depression, which can be treated with selective serotonin reuptake inhibitors (SSRIs) in some cases. This antidepressant drug increases the availability of brain serotonin by preventing its reuptake in the synapse. Blood levels of serotonin are increased in aerobic exercise.[57] Increases in serotonin are correlated with a decrease in depression.

The positive effects of exercise on depression also may occur as a result of the ability of exercise to reduce inflammation.[58] Thus physical exercise may be improving the neuroimmune status observed in depression by reducing inflammation.

Another major benefit of exercise is to reduce the development of obesity, a major public health problem in the United States and across the world. Because people exposed to chronic stress often seek high-calorie comfort foods as a way to alleviate stress, they are at risk to develop obesity and diabetes, heart disease, metabolic disorders, liver disease, cancer, inflammatory disorders, mental illnesses, and premature death. Obesity leads to a chronic low-grade inflammatory state caused by increased production of proinflammatory cytokines (e.g., IL-1, IL-6, IL-17, and TNF) from adipocytes (fat cells) in adipose tissue (see Fig. 11.7). Coping with stress and obesity through exercise has the potential to reduce adipose tissue, attenuate serum proinflammatory cytokine levels, and create an antiinflammatory environment. The interplay between obesity, inflammation, and depression may be mediated through diet and exercise through the loss of adipose tissue and the restoration of adaptive immune and behavioral functions.[55,59]

Finally, another positive effect of exercise, especially aerobic exercise, is to enhance cognitive and brain functions. Exercise increases brain metabolism and brain structure and synaptic proteins, such as brain-derived neurotrophic factor (BDNF). Exercise-related BDNF levels have been linked to improvements in memory and hippocampal volumes.[60] Because the role of stress is linked to the development of cognitive and mental disorders, such as anxiety and depression, the positive effects of aerobic exercise on improving cognitive functions may be related to brain functions that are not compromised by stress.

Mindfulness Therapy

One type of cognitive therapy that is gaining increasing attention for the treatment of stress-related disorders is mindfulness therapy, which involves the personal monitoring of current experiences with acceptance; it is thought to dampen psychological and physiologic stress reactions, thereby limiting the cumulative impact of allostatic load or stress on health. Mindfulness therapy, such as mindfulness-based stress reduction (MBSR), is effective in coping with various medical conditions, including chronic pain and depression, and attenuating the negative perception of stress. MBSR has been shown to reduce stress, anxiety, and depression among nurses.[61] Mindfulness training in adults with attention-deficit/hyperactivity disorder also improves neurocognitive deficits, such as attention deficit, and enhances emotional regulation and quality of life.

Mindfulness is believed to improve health by modulating[62] the HPA secretion of cortisol, a primary product of the neuroendocrine stress system, with pervasive effects throughout the body and brain. As discussed earlier, chronic stress-induced secretion of cortisol is involved in a wide range of mental and physiologic health functions. A major role of mindfulness appears to reduce cortisol and allostatic load.[62] The neural mechanisms or stress systems linked to mindfulness training interventions appear to involve the top-down prefrontal cortical regions that modulate connected neural sites, such as the amygdala and the subgenual anterior cingulate cortex, which are activated by stress and contribute to stress reactions. In stressed adults, mindfulness was found to increase the resting state of the stress-regulatory region of the dorsolateral prefrontal cortex and decreases stress-related regions between the amygdala and the subgenual anterior cingulate cortex. These brain changes were linked to a reduction in stress biomarkers (i.e., cortisol, circulating IL-6).[63]

Although the majority of mindfulness interventions have focused on adults, recent research has begun to examine the beneficial effects of mindfulness on at-risk children and adolescents.[64,65] These studies demonstrate that children and adolescents participating in mindfulness training showed improvement in their sleep and self-esteem, greater well-being, and reduction in depression and anxiety. These outcomes of mindfulness classes appear effective in mitigating the toxic effects of stress in youth. The intervention of mindfulness beginning at a young age has the potential to teach valuable coping skills in at-risk children that may lower their long-term burden of disease in adulthood.

In summary, the current understanding of the role of stress in modulating the complex interplay between the brain and the body is beginning to offer promising avenues of effective interventions for health and disease. Alterations in biomarkers of stress systems (e.g., cortisol, norepinephrine, proinflammatory cytokines) are revealing insights into potential targets to address their causal basis in disease and mental disorders. However, treatments for many stress-related diseases will likely continue to be a major challenge. The young exposed to stress may have already undergone neuroanatomic, physiologic, and cognitive changes that are different from those in people exposed to stress in adulthood. The specific biologic changes induced by the length of stress exposure, the nature of the stressor, and the age, sex, and genetic makeup of individual are a few of a number of factors that complicate the treatment of this disease. The dynamic nature of stress on the individual and the subsequent occurrence of chronic diseases may require early stress reduction interventions that prevent or reduce the toxic effects of stress on the body and the brain.

SUMMARY REVIEW

Background and General Concepts of Stress

1. Stress is broadly defined as a perceived or anticipated threat that activates stress-related systems in the body and the brain (the stress response).
2. The term *fight-or-flight response* was coined by Walter Cannon to describe how the brain's perception of threat and rapid physiologic responses prepares the body to deal with threat.
3. Cannon's view was further developed by Hans Selye in 1946 by demonstrating that internal or external stressors could result in adrenal gland enlargement, immune alterations (increased leukocytes), and gastrointestinal manifestations (ulcers). These global physiologic responses, characterized by Selye, were labeled general adaptation syndrome (GAS).
4. GAS occurs in three stages: the alarm stage; the stage of resistance or adaptation; and the stage of exhaustion. The latter stage is now referred to as *allostatic overload*. Diseases of adaptation develop if the stage of resistance or adaptation does not restore homeostasis. Although important, this approach is now thought to be greatly oversimplified.
5. Stress research continued into the mid-1950s to show that psychological stressors are as effective as physical stressors in activating adrenal gland hormone secretion. Psychological stressors can be anticipatory and triggered by expectations of an upcoming negative event or can be reactive to a stressor. Both of these psychological stressors are capable of eliciting a physiologic stress response.
6. The emerging link between stress and disease became the basis for the concept of allostasis (stability through change; monitoring the environment for adaptive response). This allostasis concept differs from a "fixed homeostasis model" (i.e., stress-induced heightened physiologic responses eventually returning to a narrow step point range) by involving a dynamic adaptation of the brain to constantly adjust its physiologic operating range to meet future anticipated demands. In other words, returning stress-induced hormone levels to prestress levels may not be the most adaptive strategy to cope with impending stressful encounters.
7. Chronic activation of regulatory stress systems has the potential to tax the body and the brain and lead to the emergence of diseases and disorders. In allostatic overload, chronic overactivation of adaptive regulatory physiologic systems may lead to pathophysiology and onset of disease.

The Stress Systems

1. The perception or anticipation of threat activates three major physiologic stress systems: (1) the hypothalamic–pituitary–adrenal (HPA) axis, (2) the sympathetic nervous system (SNS), and (3) the immune system (IS). Acute stress-induced activation of these stress systems modulates a broad range of mediators in the body and the brain to protect and meet the physiologic and behavioral demands of the stressor to facilitate recovery.
2. Key physiologic changes involved in allostatic overload include exaggerated or chronic secretion of adrenal cortisol, catecholamines from the sympathetic nervous system, and proinflammatory cytokines that may initiate gene expression changes with widespread effects on the body, and neurobiologic structures and processes.
3. Becoming "stressed out" by allostatic overload may lead to sleep deprivation, heightened insulin and blood glucose levels, increased blood pressure, and reduced parasympathetic activity. These physiologic consequences are often linked to insomnia, depression, chronic pain and fatigue syndromes, obesity, metabolic syndrome, essential hypertension, type 2 diabetes, atherosclerosis and its cardiovascular consequences, osteoporosis, and autoimmune inflammatory and allergic disorders.
4. Activation of the HPA system involves sequential secretion of corticotropin-releasing hormone from the hypothalamus, which stimulates receptors in the anterior pituitary to secrete adrenocorticotropic hormone (ACTH), which, in turn, stimulates the adrenal cortex to secrete the glucocorticoid cortisol.
5. Cortisol secretion induced by acute stress binds to glucocorticoid receptors to activate diverse biologic actions throughout the body and the brain. The many adaptive functions include, but are not limited to, arousal, cognition, mood, metabolism, maintenance of cardiovascular tone, and effects on the immune system.
6. Cortisol's main effects involve metabolic processing by mobilizes glucose, amino acids, lipids, and fatty acids and delivers them to the bloodstream. As an example, anabolic effects of cortisol increase the rate of protein synthesis in the liver, whereas the catabolic effects of cortisol increase levels of amino acids, ultimately depleting protein stores in muscle, bone, skin, and connective tissue.
7. Chronic dysregulation of the HPA axis, especially abnormal elevated secretion of cortisol, is linked to a wide variety of disorders, including obesity, metabolic syndrome, sleep deprivation, lipid abnormalities, coronary heart disease, diabetes, atherosclerosis, and loss of bone density. In the brain, chronic glucocorticoid secretion may lead to cognitive impairments and emotional disorders, such as depression. For example, depression is accompanied by shrinkage of the hippocampus and the prefrontal cortex.
8. Activation of the autonomic nervous system (ANS) consists of sympathetic stimulation of the adrenal medulla and nerve endings to rapidly secrete catecholamines (norepinephrine, epinephrine).
9. Epinephrine exerts its chief effects on the cardiovascular system by increasing cardiac output and blood flow to the heart, brain, and skeletal muscles by dilating vessels that supply these organs. It also dilates the airways, thereby increasing delivery of oxygen to the bloodstream. Norepinephrine and epinephrine contribute to arteriolar vasoconstriction to other parts of the body raising blood pressure.

10. The parasympathetic nervous system balances or restrains the sympathetic system, resulting in slowed heart rates and antiinflammatory effects. During prolonged stress (allostatic overload), the parasympathetic system becomes less effective in opposing the sympathetic system.
11. Acute stress-induced secretion of HPA hormones and catecholamines (CAs) directly influences the immune system, which plays an adaptive role as a signal organ to alert other systems from internally threatening stimuli (e.g., infection, tissue damage, tumor cells). The release of immune inflammatory mediators (e.g., interleukin-6 [IL-6], tumor necrosis factor-β [TNF-β], interferon [IFN]) serves to protect the body from bacterial or viral infections, cancer, tissue injury, and other stressors.
12. Chronic stress induced by prolonged, intrusive, and/or negative thoughts may lead to pathophysiology of the immune system. Persistent secretion of proinflammatory cytokines and inflammation is linked to cardiovascular disease, osteoporosis, arthritis, type 2 diabetes mellitus, chronic obstructive pulmonary disease (COPD), and other diseases associated with aging.
13. Clear examples of the adverse effects of chronic psychosocial stress are burnout, a syndrome associated with a number of negative impacts on workers' well-being and health, as well as loneliness and social isolation. Mechanisms contributing to the effects of psychosocial stress include dysregulation of the HPA axis and the ANS which are accompanied by impaired immune function and inflammation.

Chronic Stress at an Early Age Increases the Risk of Developing Long-Lasting Pathophysiologic Alterations Linked to Poor Health and to Disease

1. Children exposed to prenatal or postnatal stressors increase the risk of developing long-lasting pathophysiologic alterations linked to poor health and to disease.
2. High levels of stress-induced maternal cortisol secretion could cross the placental barrier and enter the fetus to cause low birth weight and increase the risk of disease in later life, including obesity, cardiovascular conditions (e.g., hypertension), and behavioral disorders (e.g., depression and attention-deficit/hyperactivity disorder).
3. Early exposure to psychosocial stressors (e.g., parental, sexual, or emotional abuse, low socioeconomic status [SES] or poverty) are linked to the development of dysregulated HPA and ANS leading to a chronic proinflammatory state that increases the risk of disease.
4. Early life stressors may impair brain systems that govern executive functions involved in attention, self-awareness, impulse control behavior that regulate emotions, and adaptive coping behavior.

Negative Effects of Stress on Telomere Length, Aging, and Disease

1. Telomeres are deoxyribonucleic acid (DNA)–based caps located at the end of chromosomes to protect genetic information and degradation during cell division.
2. Telomere shortening or attrition is linked to biologic aging and can be accelerated by a number of conditions associated with inflammation and oxidative stress. Shorter telomere length found in white blood cells reflects an increased risk of aging-related morbidity and mortality and is associated with a range of conditions in people with obesity, smoking, type 2 diabetes, and low SES.
3. Stress has a major role on telomere shortening that can begin in utero by increasing early telomere damage, inflammation, and greater rate of leukocyte division.
4. Studies showed that childhood psychosocial stress predicts telomere erosion and increased risk of developing depression and metabolic disorders.

Coping and Intervention Strategies

1. Coping styles affect the ability of a person to handle stress. Personality characteristics, such as academic achievement, motivation, and optimism, increase the likelihood of successfully dealing with stress. In addition, people who engage in coping strategies that receive social support develop greater stress resilience and improved psychological and physiologic outcomes.
2. Maladaptive coping responses to stress, such as increased smoking, decreased exercise and sleep, and poor diets, are likely to alter adaptive immune functions and increase susceptibility to disease.
3. Engagement in exercise as a means of coping with stress has beneficial effects at all ages. Exercise has the potential to rebalance neurotransmitter effects that were altered by stress. Exercise also may improve the neuroimmune status (i.e., inflammation) by inhibiting the secretion of proinflammatory cytokines. Exercise increases brain metabolism that improves cognitive functions that could be compromised by chronic exposure to stress.
4. Another major benefit of exercise is to reduce obesity, a major contributor of the pathophysiology of diabetes, heart disease, metabolic disorders, liver disease, cancer, inflammatory disorders, mental illnesses, and premature death. Coping with stress and obesity by exercising reduces adipose tissue, attenuates serum proinflammatory cytokine levels, and creates an antiinflammatory environment.
5. Mindfulness therapy is increasingly used to reduce the chronic impact of allostatic load on health. This therapy involves monitoring current experiences with acceptance and is effective in coping with various medical conditions, including chronic pain, depression, and attenuating the negative perception of stress.
6. Mindfulness appears to improve health by modulating the stress-induced secretion of cortisol by the HPA and by dampening brain regions activated by stress that facilitate a range of stress reactions.
7. In children and adolescents experiencing chronic stress, mindfulness training can result in improvement in sleep, self-esteem, well-being, and reduction in depression and anxiety. Mindfulness teaches valuable coping skills that potentially reduce the likelihood of at-risk children developing chronic diseases in adulthood.

REFERENCES

1. McEwen BS. Brain on stress: how the social environment gets under the skin. *Proc Natl Acad Sci U S A*. 2012;109:17180–17185.
2. Chrousos GP. Stress and disorders of the stress system. *Nat Rev Endocrinol*. 2009;5:374–381.
3. Cannon WB, Bringer CAL, Fritz R. Experimental hyperthyroidism. *Am J Physiol*. 1914;36:363.
4. Selye H. The general adaptation syndrome and the diseases of adaptation. *J Clin Endocrinol*. 1946;6:117–230.
5. Sterling P, Eyer J. Allostasis: a new paradigm to explain arousal pathology. In: Fisher S, Reason J, eds. *Handbook of life stress, cognition, and health*. New York: John Wiley and Son; 1988:629–649.
6. McEwen BS, Akil H. Revisiting the stress concept: implications for affective disorders. *J Neurosci*. 2020;40(1):12–21.
7. Guidi J, et al. Allostatic load and its impact on health: a systematic review. *Psychother Psychosom*. 2021;90:11–27.
8. Akinyemiju T, et al. Association of allostatic load with all-cause and cancer mortality by race and body mass index in the REGARDS cohort. *Cancers*. 2020;12(6):1695.
9. Salleh MR. Life event, stress and illness. *Malays J Med Sci*. 2008; 15(4):9–18.
10. Kiecolt-Glaser JK, et al. Psychoneuroimmunology: psychological influences on immune function and health. *J Consult Clin Psychol*. 2002;70(3):537–547.
11. Maydych V. The interplay between stress, inflammation, and emotional attention: relevance for depression. *Front Neurosci*. 2019;13:384.
12. Pedraz-Petrozzi B, Neumann E, Sammer G. Pro-inflammatory markers and fatigue in patients with depression: a case-control study. *Sci Rep*. 2020;10:9494.
13. Chrousos GP, Kino T. Glucocorticoid signaling in the cell: expanding clinical complications to complex human behavioral and somatic disorders. *Ann N Y Acad Sci*. 2009;1179:153–166.
14. Wiechmann T, et al. Identification of dynamic glucocorticoid-induced methylation changes at the FKBP5 locus. *Clin Epigenet*. 2019;11:83.
15. Krontira A, Cruceanu C, Binder EB. Long lasting impact of early-life stress and adversity. *Trends Neurosci*. 2020;43(6):394–405.
16. McEwen BS. Neurobiological and systemic effects of chronic stress. *Chronic Stress*. 2017;1:1–11.
17. Balsevich G, et al. Stress and glucocorticoid modulation of feeding and metabolism. *Neurobiol Stress*. 2019;11:100171.
18. Eberle C, et al. Impact of maternal prenatal stress by glucocorticoids on metabolic and cardiovascular outcomes in their offspring: a systematic scoping review. *PLoS One*. 2021;16(1):e0245386.
19. Provençal N, et al. Glucocorticoid exposure during hippocampal neurogenesis primes future stress response by inducing changes in DNA methylation. *Proc Natl Acad Sci U S A*. 2020;117(38): 23280–23285.
20. McEwen BS, Nasca C, Gray JD. Stress effects on neuronal structure: hippocampus, amygdala, and prefrontal cortex. *Neuropsychopharmacology*. 2016;41(1):3–23.
21. Somvanshi PR, et al. Role of enhanced glucocorticoid receptor sensitivity in inflammation in PTSD: insights from computational model for circadian-neuroendocrine-immune interactions. *Am J Physiol Endocrinol Metab*. 2020;319(1):E48–E66.
22. Hill AR, Spencer-Segal JL. Glucocorticoids and the brain after critical illness. *Endocrinology*. 2021;162(3):bqaa242.
23. Yao BC, et al. Chronic stress: a critical risk factor for atherosclerosis. *J Int Med Res*. 2019;47(4):1429–1440.
24. Konsman JP. So many faces, phases, and facets, sickness behavior beyond disciplines. *Front Psychiatry*. 2021;12:630331.
25. Hanns P, et al. Stress and catecholamines modulate the bone marrow microenvironment to promote tumorigenesis. *Cell Stress*. 2019;3(7):221–235.
26. Eisenstein TK. The role of opioid receptors in immune system function. *Front Immunol*. 2019;10:2904.
27. Furman D, et al. Chronic inflammation in the etiology of disease across the life span. *Nat Med*. 2019;25:1822–1832.
28. Dai S, et al. Chronic stress promotes cancer development. *Front Oncol*. 2020;10:1492.
29. Hirano T. IL-6 in inflammation, autoimmunity and cancer. *Int Immunol*. 2021;33(3):127–148.
30. Kokkosis A, Valais K, Tsirka SE. Depression mediated by inflammatory responses to chronic stress. *FASEB J*. 2020;34(S1):1 Supplement: Experimental Biology 2020 Meeting Abstracts April 2020. https://doi.org/10.1096/fasebj.2020.34.s1.02479.
31. van den Heuvel MI, et al. Maternal stress during pregnancy alters fetal cortico-cerebellar connectivity in utero and increases child sleep problems after birth. *Sci Rep*. 2021;11:2228.
32. Kong L, et al. Relationship of prenatal maternal obesity and diabetes to offspring neurodevelopmental and psychiatric disorders: a narrative review. *Int J Obes*. 2020;44:1981–2000.
33. Baumeister D, et al. Childhood trauma and adulthood inflammation: a meta-analysis of peripheral C-reactive protein, interleukin-6 and tumour necrosis factor-α. *Mol Psychiatry*. 2016;21:642–649.
34. Rasmussen LJH, et al. Association of adverse experiences and exposure to violence in childhood and adolescence with inflammatory burden in young people. *JAMA Pediatr*. 2020;174(1):38–47.
35. Humphreys KL, Zeanah CH. Deviations from the expectable environment in early childhood and emerging psychopathology. *Neuropsychopharmacology*. 2015;40(1):154–170.
36. Danese A, McEwen BS. Adverse childhood experiences, allostasis, allostatic load, and age-related disease. *Physiol Behav*. 2012;106:29–39.
37. Teicher MH, et al. The effects of childhood maltreatment on brain structure, function and connectivity. *Nat Rev Neurosci*. 2016;17:652–666.
38. Blair C, Raver CC. Poverty, stress, and brain development: new directions for prevention and intervention. *Acad Pediatr*. 2016;16(3 Suppl):S30–S36.
39. Compas BE, et al. Neurocognitive deficits in children with chronic health conditions. *Am Psychol*. 2017;72:326–338.
40. Gorenjak V, et al. Telomere length determinants in childhood. *Clin Chem Lab Med*. 2020;58:162–177.
41. Verner G, et al. Maternal psychological resilience during pregnancy and newborn telomere length: a prospective study. *Am J Psychiatry*. 2021;178(2):183–192.
42. Rentscher KE, Carroll JE, Mitchell C. Psychosocial stressors and telomere length: a current review of the science. *Annu Rev Public Health*. 2020;41:223–245.
43. Wall MM, et al. Childhood psychosocial challenges and risk for obesity in U.S. men and women. *Transl Psychiatry*. 2019;9:16.
44. Jiang S, et al. Epigenetic modifications in stress response genes associated with childhood trauma. *Front Psychiatry*. 2019;10:808.
45. Tyborowska A, et al. Early-life and pubertal stress differentially modulate grey matter development in human adolescents. *Sci Rep*. 2018;8:9201.
46. Weischer M, et al. Short telomere length, myocardial infarction, ischemic heart disease, and early death. *Arterioscler Thromb Vasc Biol*. 2012;32:822–829.

47. Sara JD, et al. Association between work-related stress and coronary heart disease: a review of prospective studies through the job strain, effort-reward balance, and organizational justice models. *J Am Heart Assoc*. 2018;7(9):e008073.
48. Perissinotto C, et al. A practical approach to assessing and mitigating loneliness and isolation in older adults. *J Am Geriatr Soc*. 2019;67:657–662.
49. Cacioppo S, et al. Toward a neurology of loneliness. *Psychol Bull*. 2014;140:1464–1504.
50. Folkman S, Lazarus RS. The relationship between coping and emotion: implications for theory and research. *Soc Sci Med*. 1988;26(3):309–317.
51. Besedovsky L, Lange T, Haack M. The sleep-immune crosstalk in health and disease. *Physiol Rev*. 2019;99(3):1325–1380.
52. Patel J, Patel P. Consequences of repression of emotion: physical health, mental health and general well being. *Int J Psychother Pract Res*. 2019;1(3):16–21.
53. Loman MM, Gunnar MR. Early experience and the development of stress reactivity and regulation in children. *Neurosci Biobehav Rev*. 2010;34:867–876.
54. Gordon BR, et al. Resistance exercise training for anxiety and worry symptoms among young adults: a randomized controlled trial. *Sci Rep*. 2020;10:17548.
55. Mikkelsen K, et al. Exercise and mental health. *Maturitas*. 2017;106:48–56.
56. Pascoe M, et al. Physical activity and exercise in youth mental health promotion: a scoping review. *BMJ Open Sport Exerc Med*. 2020;6:e000677.
57. Yabut JM, et al. Emerging roles for serotonin in regulating metabolism: new implications for an ancient molecule. *Endocr Rev*. 2019;40(4):1092–1107.
58. Nieman DC, Wentz LM. The compelling link between physical activity and the body's defense system. *J Sport Health Sci*. 2019;8(3):201–217.
59. Patsalos O, et al. Diet, obesity, and depression: A systematic review. *J Pers Med*. 2021;11(3):176.
60. Miranda M, et al. Brain-derived neurotrophic factor: a key molecule for memory in the healthy and the pathological brain. *Front Cell Neurosci*. 2019;13:363.
61. Ghawadra SF, et al. The effect of mindfulness-based training on stress, anxiety, depression and job satisfaction among ward nurses: a randomized control trial. *J Nurs Manag*. 2020;28(5):1088–1097.
62. Nicastro R, et al. Mindfulness training for adults with attention-deficit/hyperactivity disorder: Implementation of mindful awareness practices in a French-speaking attention-deficit/hyperactivity disorder unit. *JACM*. 2021;27(2):179–183.
63. Reive C. The biological measurements of mindfulness-based stress reduction: a systematic review. *Explore (NY)*. 2019;15(4):295–307.
64. Razza R, et al. The benefits of mindfulness for promoting resilience among at-risk adolescents: Results from the inner strength teen program. *ECNU Review of Education*. 2021:1–23.
65. Dunning DL, et al. Research Review: The effects of mindfulness-based interventions on cognition and mental health in children and adolescents – a meta-analysis of randomized controlled trials. *J Child Psychol Psychiatry*. 2019;60(3):244–258.

12

Cancer Biology

Kathryn L. McCance

http://evolve.elsevier.com/Rogers/pathophysiology/

OUTLINE

Cancer is a leading cause of suffering and death in the developed world. Intensive research has led to a significantly enhanced understanding of this complex and frightening disease. Experts now know that cancer is a collection of more than 100 different diseases, each caused by a specific and often unique age-related accumulation of genetic and epigenetic alterations. Environment, heredity, and behavior interact to modify the risk of developing cancer and the response to treatment. Improvements in treatment strategies and supportive care, coupled with new, often individualized therapies based on advances of the basic pathophysiology of malignancy, have contributed to an increasing number of effective options for these diverse, often lethal disorders collectively called *cancer*.

CANCER TERMINOLOGY AND CHARACTERISTICS

Cancer is a collection of related diseases. The National Cancer Institute (NCI) of the National Institutes of Health (NIH) defines cancer as diseases in which "some of the body's cells begin to divide without stopping and spread into surrounding tissues."[1] The term *cancer* comes from the Latin translation of the Greek word for crab, *karkinoma*, which the physician Hippocrates used to describe the appendage-like projections extending from tumors into adjacent tissue. The word tumor originally referred to any swelling that is caused by inflammation but is now generally reserved for describing a new growth, or neoplasm. Neoplasms result from an abnormal growth following uncontrolled proliferation serving no physiologic purpose. Not all tumors or neoplasms, however, are cancer. The term cancer refers to a *malignant* tumor and is not used to refer to *benign growths*, such as lipomas or hypertrophy of an organ.

Tumor Classification and Nomenclature

The careful evaluation of each cancer is important for many reasons. Different cancers will have different causes, different rates and patterns of progression, and different responses to treatment. The classification starts with knowing the tissue and organ of origin, the extent of distribution to other sites, and the microscopic appearance of the lesion. Increasingly, it also includes a detailed description of the critical genetic changes in the cancer.

Benign and Malignant

Tumors can be benign or malignant (cancerous). Benign tumors are usually encapsulated with connective tissue and contain fairly well-differentiated cells and well-organized surrounding supportive tissue called stroma (Fig. 12.1). They retain recognizable normal tissue structure and do not invade beyond their capsule, nor do they spread to regional lymph nodes or distant locations. Mitotic cells are rarely present during microscopic analysis. Benign tumors are generally named according to the tissues from which they arise with the suffix "-oma," which indicates a tumor or mass. For example, a benign tumor of the smooth muscle of the uterus is a *leiomyoma*, and a benign tumor of fat cells is a *lipoma*. Benign tumors can become extremely large and, depending on their location in the body, can cause morbidity or be life-threatening. For example, a benign meningioma at the base of the skull may cause symptoms by compressing adjacent normal brain tissue. Other benign tumors of endocrine organs can produce hormones, sometimes excessively.

Some tumors initially described as benign can progress to cancer and then are referred to as malignant tumors, which are distinguished from benign tumors by more rapid growth rates and specific microscopic alterations, including loss of differentiation and absence of normal tissue organization (Fig. 12.2). One of the microscopic hallmarks of cancer cells is anaplasia, the loss of cellular differentiation. Malignant cells are also pleomorphic, with marked variability of size and shape. They often have large darkly stained nuclei, and mitotic cells are common. Malignant tumors may have a substantial amount of stroma, but it is disorganized, with loss of normal tissue structure. Malignant tumors lack a capsule and grow to invade nearby blood vessels, lymphatics, and surrounding structures. The most important and most deadly characteristic of malignant tumors is their ability to spread far beyond the tissue of origin, a process known as *metastasis*.

Unlike benign tumors, which are named related to the tissue of origin, cancers generally are named according to the cell type from which they originate. Cancers arising in epithelial tissue are called carcinomas, and if they arise from or ductal or glandular structures are named adenocarcinomas. Hence a malignant tumor arising from breast glandular tissue is a mammary adenocarcinoma; an example of a benign breast tumor is a fibroadenoma. Cancers arising from mesenchymal tissue (including connective tissue, muscle, and bone) usually have the suffix sarcoma. For example, malignant cancers of skeletal muscle are known as *rhabdomyosarcomas*. Cancers of lymphatic tissue are called lymphomas, whereas cancers of blood-forming cells are called leukemias. However, many cancers, such as Hodgkin disease and Ewing sarcoma, are named for historical reasons that do not follow this nomenclature convention.

Carcinoma In Situ

Carcinoma in situ (CIS) refers to preinvasive epithelial tumors of glandular or squamous cell origin. Cancers develop incrementally as they accumulate specific genetic lesions. Careful surveillance for cancer often detects abnormal growths in epithelial tissues that have atypical cells and an increased proliferation rate compared with normal surrounding tissues. These early-stage cancers are localized to the epithelium and have not penetrated the local basement membrane or invaded the surrounding stroma. Based on these characteristics, they are not

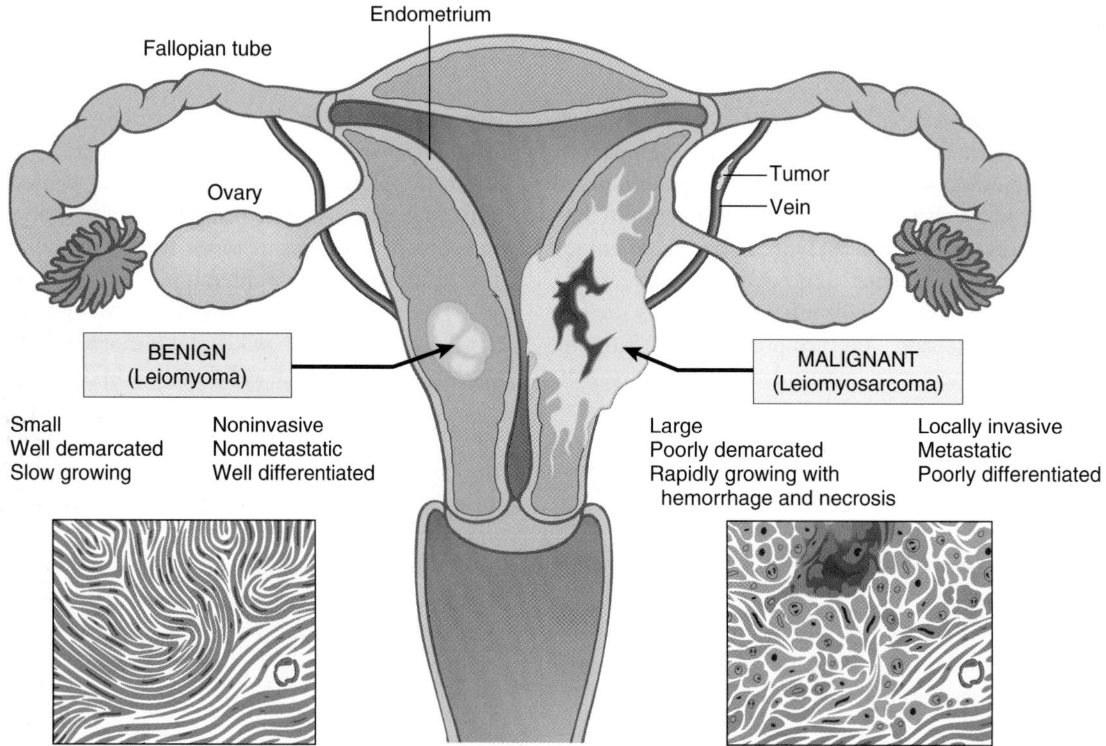

Fig. 12.1 **Comparison Between a Benign Tumor and a Malignant Tumor of the Same Origin.** (From Kumar V, Abbas AK, Aster JC. *Robbins and Cotran pathologic basis of disease*, 10th edition. Philadelphia: Saunders; 2021.)

malignant though they are called CIS. CIS occurs in several sites, including the cervix, skin, oral cavity, esophagus, and bronchus. In glandular epithelium, in situ lesions occur in the stomach, endometrium, breast, and large bowel. In the breast, ductal carcinoma in situ (DCIS) fills the mammary ducts but has not progressed to local tissue invasion. DCIS lesions are readily treatable; however, the optimal therapeutic approach is controversial. CIS lesions can have one of the following three fates: (1) they can remain stable for a long time, (2) they can progress to invasive and metastatic cancers, or (3) they can

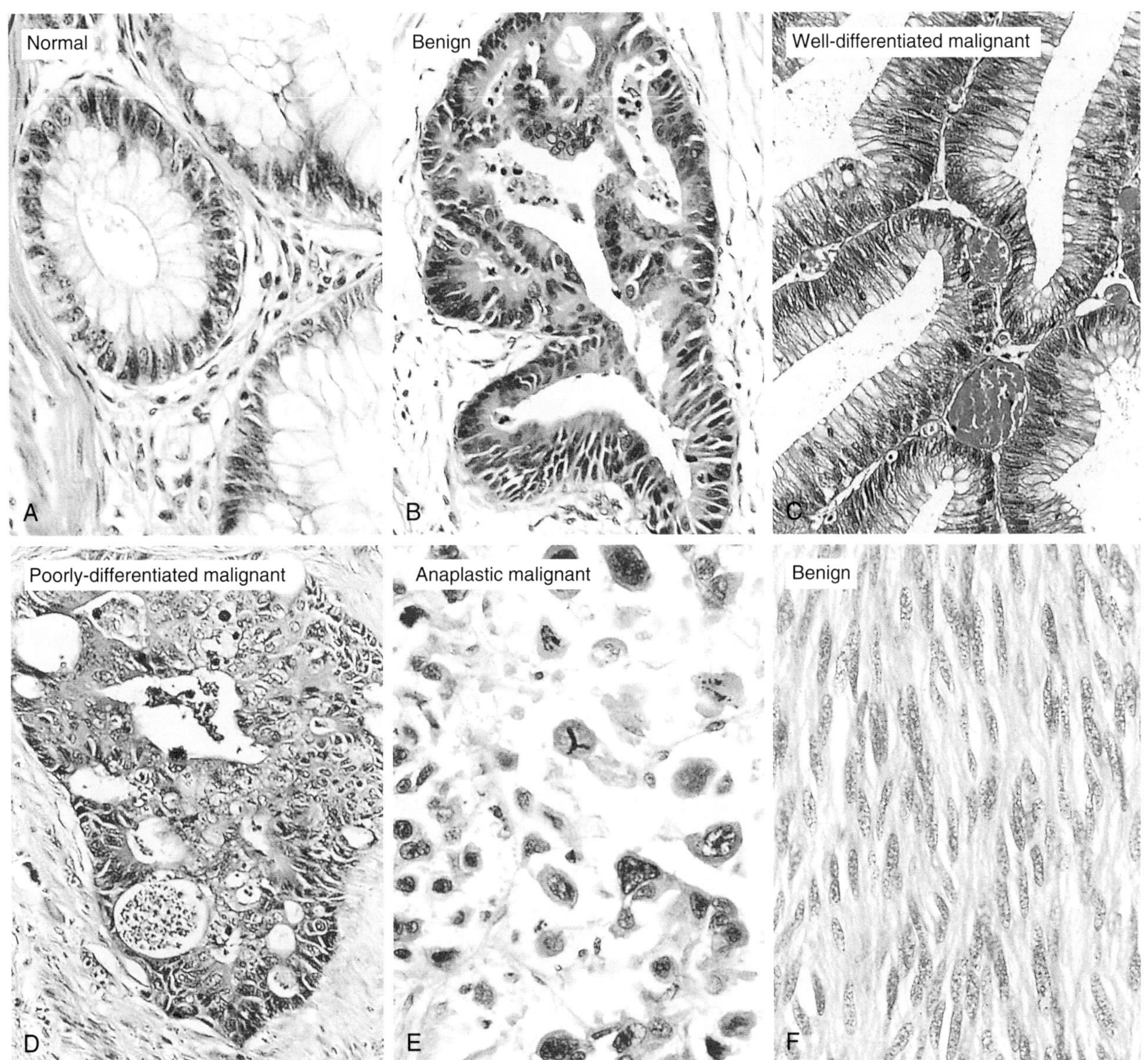

Fig. 12.2 Loss of Cellular and Tissue Differentiation During the Development of Cancer. The cells of a benign neoplasm **(B)** resemble those of the normal colonic epithelium **(A)** in that they are columnar and have an orderly arrangement. Loss of some degree of differentiation is evident in that the neoplastic cells do not show much mucin vacuolization. Cells of the well-differentiated malignant neoplasm **(C)** of the colon have a haphazard arrangement, and although gland lumina are formed, they are architecturally abnormal and irregular. Nuclei vary in shape and size, especially when compared with those illustrated in A. Cells in the poorly differentiated malignant neoplasm **(D)** have an even more haphazard arrangement, with very poor formation of gland lumina. Nuclei show greater variation in shape and size compared with the well-differentiated malignant neoplasm in C. Cells in anaplastic malignant neoplasms **(E)** bear no relation to the normal epithelium with no recognizable gland formation. Tremendous variation is found in the size of cells and their nuclei, with very intense staining (hyperchromatic nuclei). Not knowing the site of origin would make it impossible to classify this tumor by microscopic appearance alone. Well-differentiated tumors often resemble their cell of origin, as shown in the example of a benign tumor of smooth muscles **(F)**. (From Stevens A, Lowe J. *Pathology*, 2nd edition. London: Mosby; 2000.)

regress and disappear. CIS can vary from low-grade to high-grade dysplasia, with the high-grade lesions having the highest likelihood of becoming invasive cancers. The time that such preinvasive lesions remain in situ before becoming invasive is unknown. Some carcinomas of the cervix appear as preinvasive lesions in situ for several years before they progress to invasive carcinoma and metastatic tumors (Fig. 12.3). Knowing the best treatment for low-grade CIS lesions is challenging because the proportion that progress to cancer versus the proportion that will never cause clinical problems is usually not known. Although most persons prefer removal of any CIS as opposed to "watchful waiting," this topic continues to be a source of great debate.

THE BIOLOGY OF CANCER CELLS

In two seminal publications, Douglas Hanahan and Robert Weinberg[2,3] described what they considered the hallmarks of cancer. Both articles stimulated considerable discussion and, especially, debate. The original publication contained six hallmarks, but with time and new research findings, increased to eight hallmarks and two traits that enable cancer progression. Their analysis remains the leading overview of why a cell is malignant. The following discussion is organized in the context of those 10 hallmarks/enablers (Fig. 12.4). Two fundamental concepts are the foundation for understanding the biology of cancer: (1) cancer is a complex disease, and (2) the microenvironment of a tumor is a heterogeneous mixture of cells, both cancerous and benign.

Cancer is a disease of cumulative genetic changes during aging. The fraction of individuals who develop cancer increases dramatically with age. Genetic changes involve mutational and epigenetic mechanisms. *Mutation* means an alteration in the DNA sequence affecting expression or function of a gene (Fig. 12.5; also see Chapter 4). Mutations include point mutations or a small-scale change in DNA, the alteration of one or more nucleotide base pairs. This type of change can have profound effects on the activity of resultant proteins. Chromosome translocations are large changes in chromosome structure in which a piece of one chromosome is translocated to another chromosome. Gene amplification is the result of repeated duplication of a region of a chromosome. Instead of the normal two copies of a

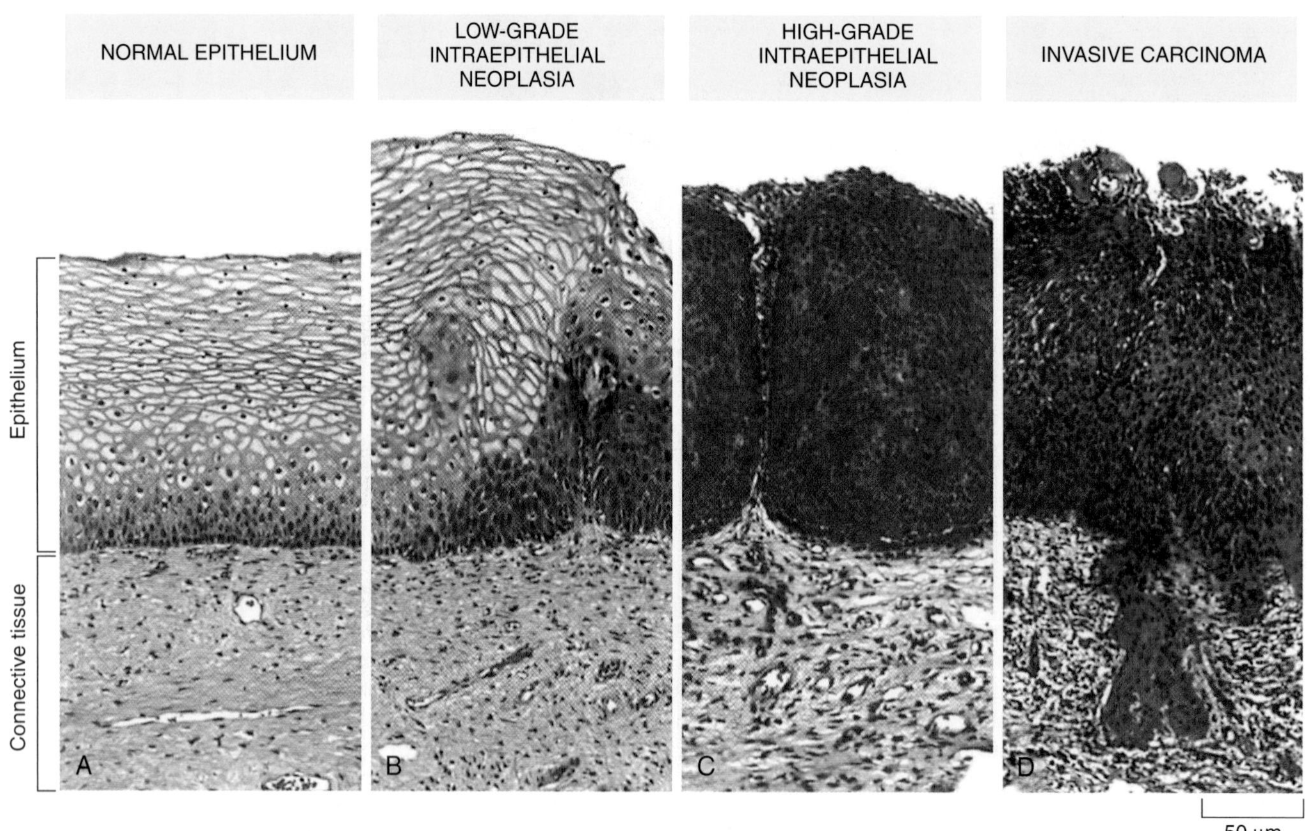

Fig. 12.3 Progression from Normal to Neoplasm in the Uterine Cervix. A sequence of cellular and tissue changes progressing from low-grade to high-grade intraepithelial neoplasms (also called *carcinoma in situ*), and then to invasive cancer is seen often in the development of cancer. In this example of the early stages of cervical neoplastic changes, the presence of anaplastic cells and the loss of normal tissue architecture signify the development of cancer. The high rate of cell division and the presence of local mutagens and inflammatory mediators all contribute to the accumulation of genetic abnormalities that lead to cancer. (From Alberts B, Johnson A, Lewis J, et al. *Molecular biology of the cell*, 5th edition. New York: Garland; 2002.)

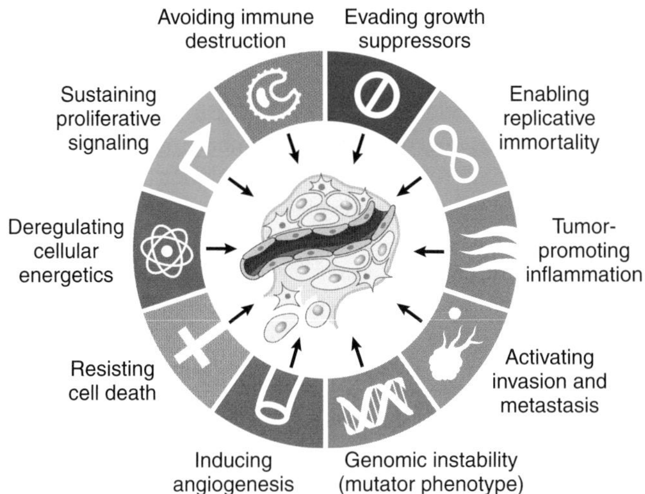

Fig. 12.4 Hallmarks of Cancer. Adapted from Hanahan D, Weinberg RA. Hallmarks of cancer: The next generation. *Cell*, 2011;144(5):646–674. Found in Kumar V, et al. *Robbins and Cotran pathologic basis of disease*, 10th edition, Philadelphia: Elsevier; 2021.

gene, tens or even hundreds of copies are present. Epigenetic effects can alter gene expression indirectly and include DNA methylation, histone acetylation, or altered expression of non-coding RNA (see Chapter 6).[4] Driver mutations "drive" the progression of cancer. There are over 100 different driver mutations, although some are more critical than others, and a small number of these are present in an individual cancer. Not all mutations in cancer contribute to the malignant phenotype. Some are just random events, called passenger mutations, and are just along for the ride. After a critical number of driver mutations has occurred, a cell becomes cancerous. Unfortunately, the cancer cell has a selective advantage over its neighbors; its progeny can accumulate faster than its nonmutant neighbors. This advantage is known as clonal proliferation or clonal expansion (Fig.12.6). As a clone with mutations proliferates, it may become an early-stage tumor, for example, a CIS or a benign colonic polyp.

The increasingly rapid cell division and impaired DNA repair mechanisms of cancer cells result in a continuing accumulation of mutations throughout the progression to the most aggressive metastatic lesion. Thus, malignant transformation, the process

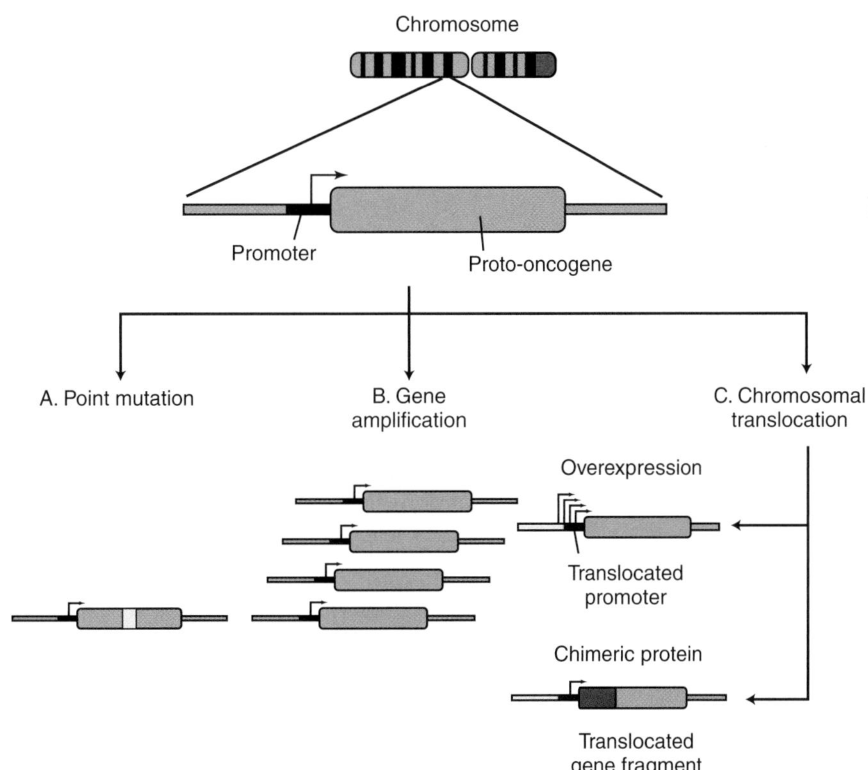

Fig. 12.5 Oncogene Activation Mechanisms. Cellular genes may become cancerous oncogenes as a result of **(A)** point mutations that alter one or a few nucleotide base pairs, causing the production of a protein that is activated as a result of the altered sequence (e.g., *ras*), **(B)** amplification of the cellular gene, resulting in higher levels of protein expression (e.g., N-myc in neuroblastoma), or **(C)** chromosomal translocations that either lead to the juxtaposition of a strong promoter, causing increased protein expression (c-myc in Burkitt lymphoma), or produce a novel fusion protein that is derived from gene fragments normally present on different chromosomes (BCR-ABL in chronic myeloid leukemia). (From Haber DA. Molecular genetics of cancer. In *ACP Medicine*. Danbury, CT: WebMD; 2004.)

by which a normal cell becomes a cancer cell, is directed by progressive accumulation of genetic changes that alter the basic nature of the cell and drive it to malignancy. The process of tumor development involves cancer cells with a heritable change that confers a survival advantage on them, enabling them to out-compete their neighbors. Each cancer cell may develop its own set of mutations resulting in a genomically *heterogeneous* mixture of cancer cells with subsets that have accumulated more and more mutations that increase the cell's malignant potential, while other subsets of cancer cells that do not accumulate a critical set of mutations eventually lose the competition and die.[5] The degree of intratumor mutational heterogeneity may vary considerably among tumors. For instance, melanomas have a rather high degree of genetic homogeneity, whereas pancreatic cancers are more heterogeneous and appear to arise from independent mutational events in the pancreas.

The processes occurring during the development of cancer are, in many ways, analogous to wound healing (see Chapter 7). The initial proliferation of cancer cells and enlargement of the tumor elicit the synthesis of proinflammatory mediators by the cancer cells and adjacent nonmalignant cells. As with wound healing, mediators recruit inflammatory/immune cells (primarily T lymphocytes and macrophages, but also B cells and neutrophils) and cells normally associated with tissue repair (fibroblasts, adipocytes, mesenchymal stem cells, endothelial cells, and pericytes). These cells form the stroma (tumor microenvironment) that surrounds and infiltrates the tumor (Fig. 12.7).[6] In some conditions, stromal cells may make up 90% of the tumor mass. Extensive paracrine signaling among the stromal and cancer cells affects both populations; cancer cells increase proliferation and become more heterogeneous during tumor growth, and several populations of stromal cells undergo evolution to phenotypes that promote cancer progression and metastatic potential. Intratumoral genetic heterogeneity or diversity arises from ongoing proliferation and mutation.[7] Tumor-associated endothelial cells, fibroblasts, and inflammatory cells develop different and distinct gene expression profiles with unique cell surface molecules and patterns of secreted molecules. During this process, many cancer cells die, but the surviving cells are more aggressive, and many take on a metastatic phenotype.[7] Because continuing somatic mutations may be random, cancer cells in different regions of the tumor may be genetically diverse. Additionally, a population of cancer stem cells may arise, the origin of which is still unclear. Many of the hallmarks of cancer are consequences of *cancer-stromal interactions* (discussed later in the chapter).

Several of the hallmarks/enablers are primarily genomic alterations that initiate and maintain development of cancer. These will be discussed first and include sustained proliferative signaling, evading growth suppression, genomic instability, and replicative immortality (see Fig. 12.4). Other hallmarks/enablers are secondary to genomic change and include inducing angiogenesis and reprogramming energy metabolism. A third group,

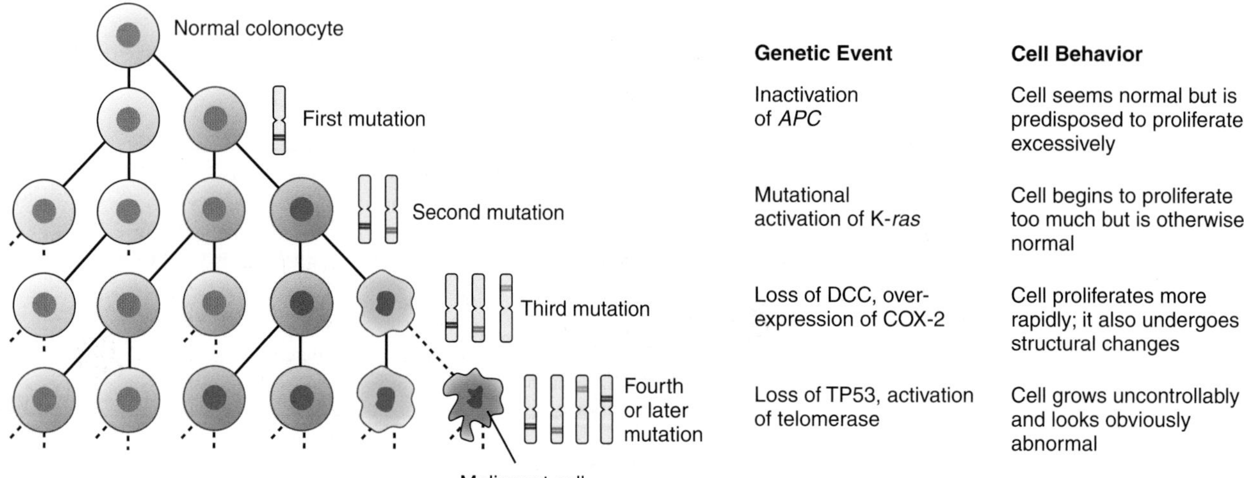

Fig. 12.6 Clonal Proliferation Model of Neoplastic Progression in the Colon. During clonal proliferation, progressively altered populations of colon cells (colonocytes) arise over time. As genetic and epigenetic changes occur, different subclones (indicated by different color cells) coexist for a time. Clones that grow the fastest out-compete other clones, producing even more malignant, and abnormal-appearing, growths. The sequential accumulation of mutations has been well studied in the progression from a normal colon cell to a benign intestinal polyp to a malignant colon cancer. One of the earliest mutations in colon cancer is loss of the tumor-suppressor gene *APC*. Additional mutations (often in the oncogene *RAS*), activation of COX-2, and loss of the tumor suppressors *DCC* and TP53 occur as the lesion progresses from a benign polyp to an invasive carcinoma. *APC*, Adenomatous polyposis coli; *COX-2*, cyclooxygenase-2; *DCC*, deleted in colon cancer; TP53, *p53* gene. (Modified from Mendelsohn I, et al. *The molecular basis of cancer*, 2nd edition. Philadelphia: Saunders; 2001; and Kumar V, et al. *Basic pathology*, 6th edition. Philadelphia: Saunders; 1997.)

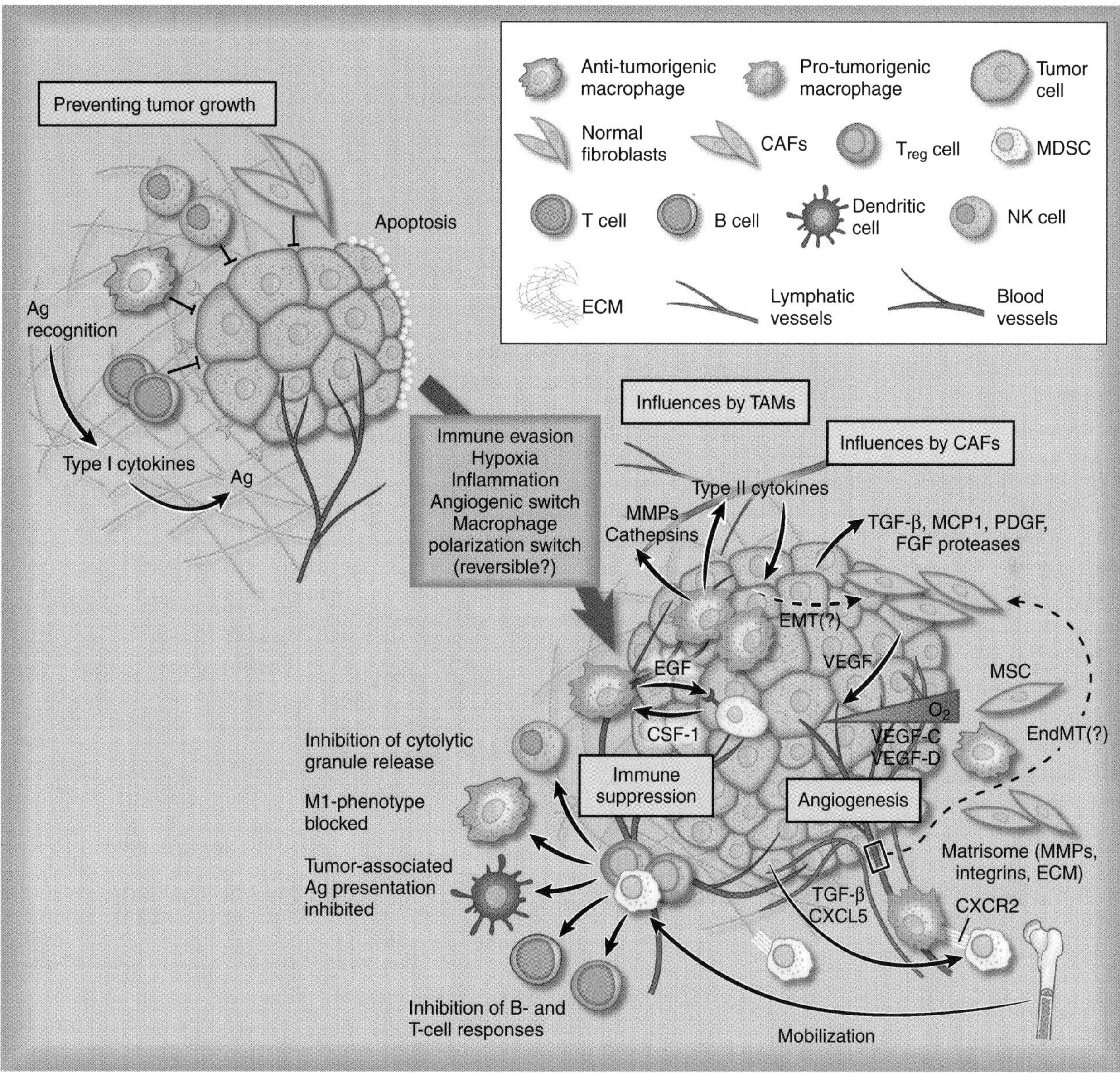

Fig. 12.7 Cancers Live in a Complex Microenvironment. Cancer cells express tumor-specific antigens that ideally can be recognized by cells of the immune system and inflammatory systems (natural killer cells, antitumor M1 macrophages, T-cytotoxic cells) and destroyed by apoptosis or undergo growth suppression by type I cytokines. However, successful cancers produce a variety of cytokines and chemokines that are chemoattractants for stromal cells that infiltrate the tumor and undergo change to pro-tumor phenotypes. These include tumor-associated M2 macrophages *(TAMs)*, cancer-associated fibroblasts *(CAFs)*, mesenchymal stem cells *(MSCs)*, and immune suppressor cells of T-cell origin (T-regulatory cells) and myeloid origin (myeloid-derived suppressor cells). Through multiple receptor-mediated interactions between other stromal cells and the cancer cells, the stromal cells, as well as the cancer cells, collectively produce a battery of additional cytokines (e.g., TGF-β, type II cytokines), chemokines (e.g., CXCL5), growth factors (e.g., VEGF, EGF, CSF-1, FGF, PDGF), and proteases (e.g., MMPs) and secrete components of the extracellular matrix *(ECM)*. The stromal reaction promotes tumor progression, including new blood vessel growth (angiogenesis), tumor cell proliferation and differentiation, suppression of immune rejection and tumor cell apoptosis, invasion, and commitment to metastasis. *CAF*, Cancer-associated fibroblast; *CSF-1*, colony-stimulating factor-1; *CXCL5*, C-X-C motif chemokine 5; *EGF*, epidermal growth factor; *FGF*, fibroblast growth factor; *MMP*, matrix metalloproteinase; *MSC*, mesenchymal stem cell; *NK*, natural killer cell; *PDGF*, platelet-derived growth factor; *TAM*, tumor-associated macrophage; *TGF-β*, tumor growth factor-beta; T_{reg}, T-regulatory cell; *VEGF*, vascular endothelial cell growth factor. (Modified from Quail DF, Joyce JA. Microenvironmental regulation of tumor progression and metastasis. *Nature Medicine*, 2013;19(11):1423–1437.)

tumor resistance to destruction by the host's protective mechanisms, includes resistance to apoptotic cell death, tumor-promoting inflammation, and avoiding immune destruction. The last hallmark is the culmination of the previous nine: activating invasion and metastasis.

Genomic Hallmarks

Sustained Proliferative Signaling

The first and prime hallmark of cancer is uncontrolled cellular proliferation. Normal cells generally only enter proliferative phases in response to growth factors that bind to specific receptors on the cell surface. The cytoplasmic components of the receptors send signaling molecules that activate intracellular pathways leading to induction/activation of regulatory factors affecting DNA synthesis, entrance into the cell cycle, and changes in expression of other genes related to cell metabolism for optimal growth (Fig. 12.8). One example is initiation of proliferation by epidermal growth factor (EGF). EGF binds and cross-links two EGF receptors on the cell surface.[8] The cytoplasmic portions of the receptors are tyrosine kinases that attach phosphorus to tyrosine in neighboring proteins, including each other (autophosphorylation). Phosphorylation allows a bridging protein to link the EGF receptors to plasma membrane–associated inactive RAS. RAS is an acronym for "rat sarcoma," where it was found originally. EGF receptor activation and linkage by the bridging protein activates RAS via the replacement of guanine diphosphate (GDP) with guanine triphosphate (GTP). Activated RAS then initiates signaling pathways such as the mitogen-activated protein kinase (MAPK) pathway and the phosphatidylinosityl-3-kinase (PI3K) pathway. These signaling pathways phosphorylate other cytoplasmic proteins and affect activity and nuclear localization of transcription factors, such as myelocytomatosis viral oncogene homolog (MYC), that govern the transcription of cell cycle regulators, such as cyclins, and entrance into cellular proliferation. PI3K also activates AK strain transforming (Akt) kinases and mammalian target of rapamycin (mTOR) proteins, which contribute to cell proliferation and growth. Proliferation can be discontinued through this pathway by decreased levels of growth factors in the environment or inactivation of signaling pathway components. These signaling pathways are inactivated by GTPase-activating proteins (GAPs), which inactivate RAS, and by phosphatase and tensin homologue (PTEN), which inactivates PI3K (see Fig.12.8).

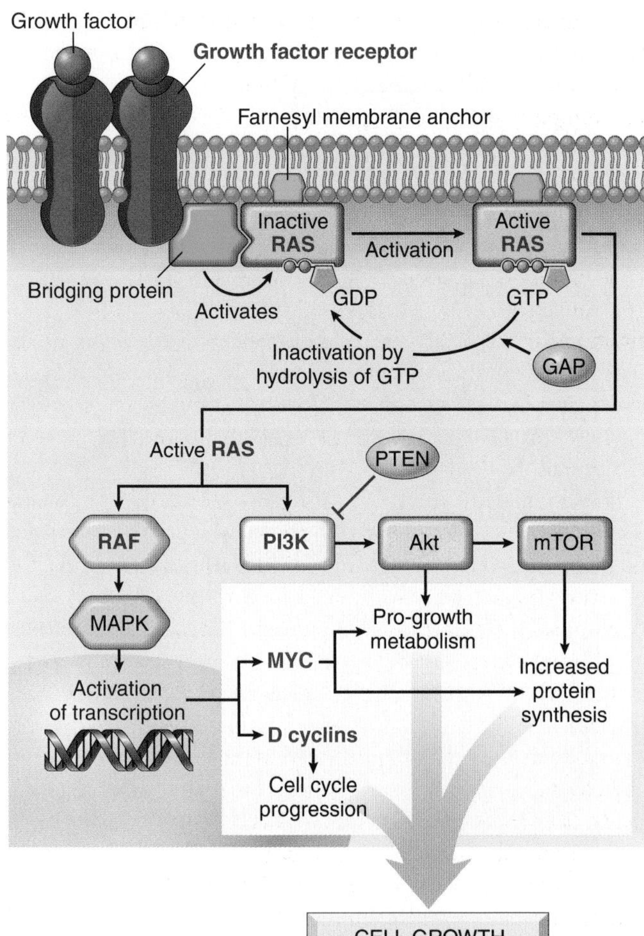

Fig. 12.8 Growth Factor Signaling Pathways in Cancer. Growth factor receptors, RAS, PI3K, MYC, and D cyclins are oncoproteins that are activated by mutations in various cancers. GTPase-activating proteins (GAPs) apply brakes to RAS activation, and phosphatase and tensin homologue (PTEN) serves the same function for PI3K. *Akt,* AK strain transforming kinases; *GDP,* guanosine diphosphate; *GTP,* guanosine triphosphate; *MAPK,* mitogen-activated protein kinase; *PI3K,* phosphatidylinositide-3-kinase; *mTOR* mammalian target of rapamycin. (From Kumar V, et al. *Robbins and Cotran pathologic basis of disease*, 10th edition, Philadelphia: Elsevier; 2021.)

The genes that encode components of receptor-mediated pathways designed to regulate normal cellular proliferation are collectively called proto-oncogenes. Cancerous cells characteristically express mutated or overexpressed proto-oncogenes, which are called oncogenes. Oncogenes are independent of normal regulatory mechanisms; thus, the cell is driven into a state of unregulated expression of proliferation signals and uncontrolled cell growth. Oncogenes can affect any portion of the growth factor pathways, such as described for EGF. For instance, most growth factors originate from neighboring cells, but some cancers acquire the ability to secrete growth factors that stimulate their own growth, a process known as autocrine stimulation. As described later in this chapter, noncancerous stromal cells within a tumor are frequently modified to benefit the cancer. In some instances, stromal cells produce excessive growth factors that drive the proliferation of cancer cells. Other cancers increase the expression of growth factor receptors (GFRs); for example, in breast cancer, production of the human epidermal growth factor receptor 2 (HER2), also known as the epidermal growth factor receptor gene (ERBB2), is upregulated and is hyperresponsive to low levels of EGF. Some breast and lung cancers are treated by inhibitors of HER2 and other EGF receptors that block this pathway.[9]

Oncogenes may lead to constant activation of the signal cascade from the cell surface receptor to the nucleus. Up to a third of all cancers have an activating mutation in the RAS gene resulting in a continuous cell growth signal even when growth factors are missing (see Fig. 12.8). Other mutations in the EGF receptor pathway include excessive proliferation signaling by hyperactivation of the PI3 kinase.

Several types of genetic events can activate oncogenes. A point mutation that is frequently observed in lung cancer results in continuous activation of the EGF receptor tyrosine kinase. A point mutation in the *RAS* gene converts it from a regulated proto-oncogene to an unregulated oncogene. Activating point mutations in *RAS* are found in many cancers, especially pancreatic and colorectal cancer. Specialized tests, such as direct DNA sequencing, can detect such point mutations in clinical samples, and new treatments are being developed that target cells with RAS mutations.[10]

Translocations can activate oncogenes by one of two distinct mechanisms (Fig. 12.9). First, a translocation can cause excess and inappropriate production of a proliferation factor. One of the best examples is the t(8;14) translocation found in many Burkitt lymphomas; t(8;14) designates a chromosome that has a piece of chromosome 8 fused to a piece of chromosome 14 (see Chapter 29). Burkitt lymphoma is an aggressive cancer of B lymphocytes. The MYC proto-oncogene found on chromosome 8 is normally activated at low levels in proliferating lymphocytes and is inactivated in mature lymphocytes. If the t(8;14) translocation occurs, the *MYC* gene is aberrantly placed under the control of a B-cell immunoglobulin gene *(IG)* present on chromosome 14. The *IG* gene is very active in maturing B lymphocytes. The t(8;14) translocation alters the control of *MYC;* its normal low-level expression is switched to high levels, as directed by an *IG* gene promoter. Hyperproduction of MYC protein drives proliferation and blocks differentiation.

Second, chromosome translocations can lead to production of novel proteins with growth-promoting properties. In chronic myeloid leukemia (CML), a specific chromosome translocation is almost always present (see Fig. 12.9). This translocation, t(9;22), was first identified in association with CML in Philadelphia in 1960 and is often referred to as the Philadelphia chromosome. Translocation fuses two chromosomes in the middle of two different genes: *BCR* (breakpoint cluster region gene) on chromosome 9 and *ABL* (Abelson gene) on chromosome 22. The result is production of a BCR-ABL fusion protein containing the first half of BCR and the second half of ABL (a nonreceptor tyrosine kinase). BCR-ABL is an unregulated protein tyrosine kinase that promotes growth of myeloid cells. Imatinib, a drug that specifically targets this tyrosine kinase, represents the first successful chemotherapy targeted against the product of a specific oncogenic mutation.[9] Imatinib and related tyrosine kinase inhibitors (TKIs) are highly effective in the treatment of CML and, because of their specificity, lack the toxic side effects noted with nonspecific anticancer drugs. However, imatinib is not effective in cancers that do not have the t(9;22) translocation or related mutations. In modern personalized cancer therapy, knowledge of the specific genetic alteration can dictate the optimal drugs for the individual.

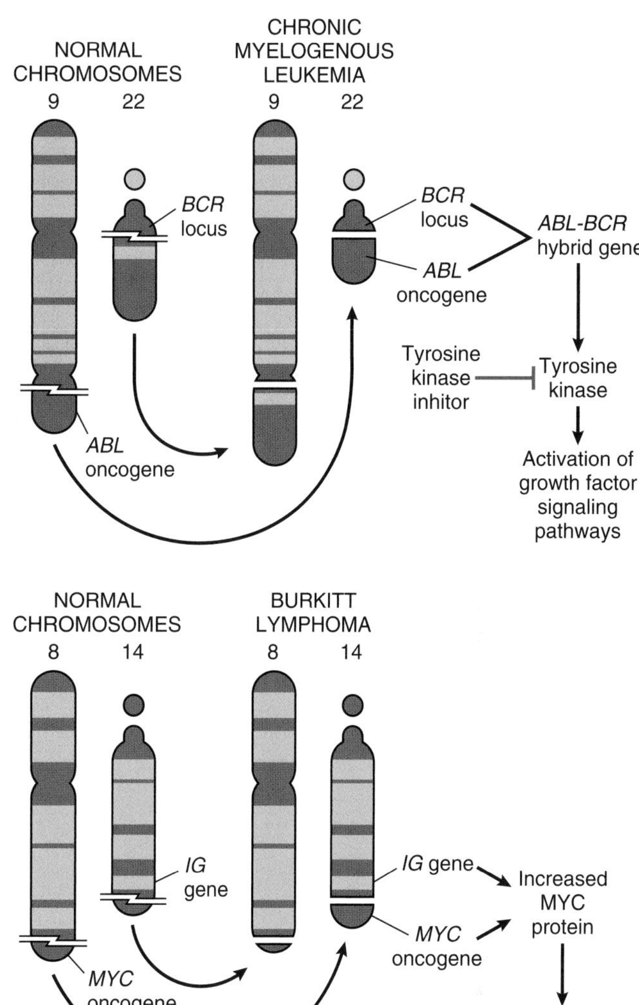

Fig. 12.9 Examples of Chromosomal Translocations and Associated Oncogenes. See text for further explanation. (From Kumar V, et al. *Robbins and Cotran pathologic basis of disease,* 10th edition, Philadelphia: Elsevier; 2021.)

Oncogenes also may be activated by gene amplification (Fig. 12.10). Gene amplification results in increased expression of an oncogene, or in some cases drug resistance genes. The N-MYC oncogene, a member of the MYC family, is amplified in 25% of childhood neuroblastomas and confers a poor prognosis. The HER2 gene *(ERBB2)* is amplified in 20% of breast cancers.

Evading Growth Suppressors

Uncontrolled cancer cell proliferation also is related to inactivation of tumor-suppressor genes. Tumor-suppressor genes normally regulate the cell cycle, inhibit proliferation resulting from growth signals, stop cell division when cells are damaged, and prevent mutations. Therefore, they also have been referred to as *anti-oncogenes.* Whereas oncogenes are activated in cancers,

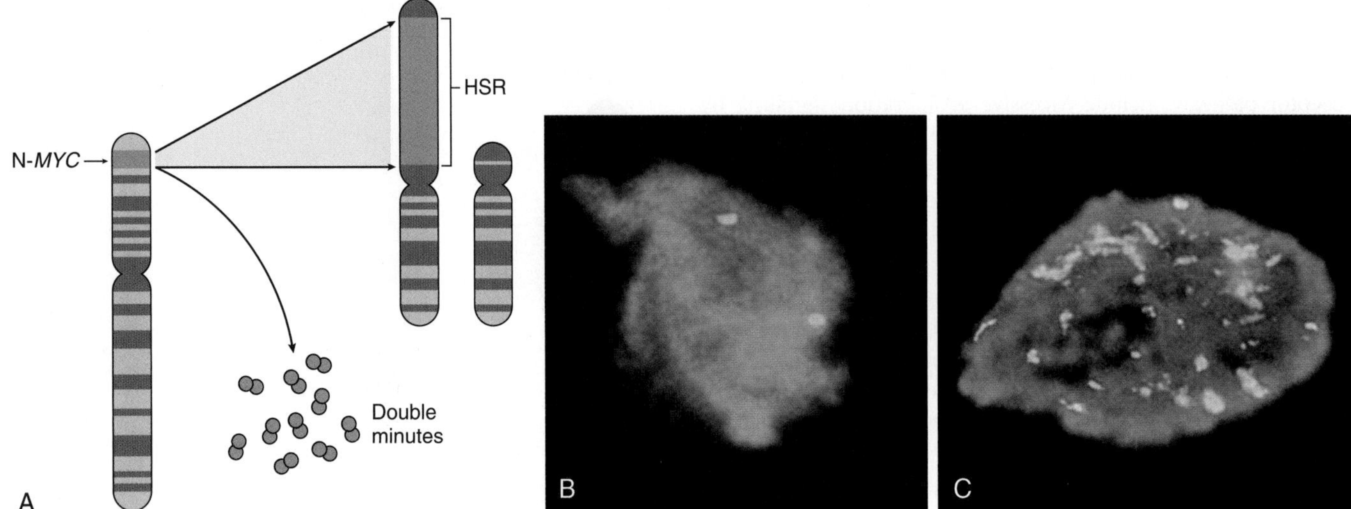

Fig. 12.10 N-Myc Gene Amplification in Neuroblastoma. (A) The N-Myc gene is present on chromosome 2, becomes amplified, and is seen either as extra chromosomal double minutes or as a chromosomal homologous staining region. The N-Myc gene is detected in human neuroblastoma cells using a technique called FISH (fluorescent in situ hybridization). **(B)** A single pair of N-Myc genes is detected in normal cells and in low-grade neuroblastoma. **(C)** Multiple, amplified copies of the N-Myc gene are detected in some cases of neuroblastoma. Amplification of the N-Myc gene is strongly associated with a poor prognosis in childhood neuroblastoma. (A, From Kumar V, et al. *Robbins and Cotran pathologic basis of disease*, 10th edition, Philadelphia: Elsevier; 2021; B and C, Courtesy Arthur R. Brothman, PhD, FACMG, University of Utah School of Medicine, Salt Lake City, UT.)

TABLE 12.1 Comparison of Cancer Gene Types

Gene Type	Normal Function	Mutation Effect
Caretaker	DNA and chromosome stability	Chromosome instability and increased rates of mutation
Dominant oncogenes[a]	Encode proteins that promote growth (e.g., growth factors)	Overexpression or amplification causes gain of function
Tumor suppressors (recessive oncogenes)	Encode proteins that inhibit proliferation and prevent or repair mutations	Requires loss of function of both alleles to increase cancer risk

[a]Nonmutant state referred to as proto-oncogene.

tumor suppressors must be *inactivated* to allow cancer to occur (Table 12.1 and Fig. 12.11). A single genetic event can activate an oncogene because it can act in a dominant manner in the cell. However, we have two copies of each tumor-suppressor gene, one from each parent. Both copies must be inactivated; thus, two mutations are necessary (homozygous mutations, also called loss of heterozygosity).

The most mutated gene in many human cancers is the p53 tumor-suppressor gene (TP53). *TP53* missense mutations are the most common mutation in human cancers.[11] The protein p53 acts as a tumor suppressor, which means it regulates cell division by restricting cells from growing and dividing too fast or in an uncontrolled way; thus, it is called the *guardian of the genome*.[12] The p53 protein is in the nucleus of cells in the body and attaches directly to DNA. When DNA becomes damaged by such agents as toxic chemicals, radiation, or ultraviolet (UV) rays, the protein plays a critical role in whether the DNA will be repaired or the damaged cell with die from apoptosis.[12] If the DNA can be repaired, p53 activates other genes, caretaker genes, for repair. If the DNA cannot be repaired, p53 prevents the cell from dividing and signals it to undergo apoptosis.[12] From all these roles of p53, it assists in the prevention of tumors (Fig. 12.12). Many types of cellular stress (e.g., anoxia, oncogene expression, nuclear damage) produce intracellular signals (e.g., levels of nucleotides and glucose, degree of oxygenation, DNA damage, and other indicators of cellular abnormalities) detectable by p53. Typically, p53 is in an inactive complex with inhibitor molecules. Stress activates kinases that phosphorylate p53 into an active suppressor of cell division and activator of caretaker genes. Caretaker genes encode proteins involved in repairing damaged DNA, such as occurs with errors in DNA replication and mutations caused by numerous stressors. The p53 tumor suppressor protein is a DNA transcriptional regulator[13] and importantly, controls initiation of cellular senescence (cease dividing) or apoptosis and

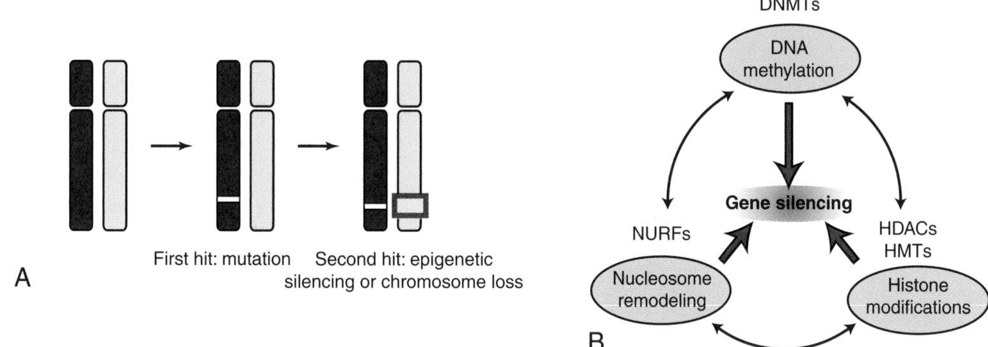

Fig. 12.11 Silencing Tumor-Suppressor Genes by Epigenetic Alterations. Tumor-suppressor genes can be turned off by a variety of mechanisms. **(A)** In this example, the first hit is a point mutation in a tumor-suppressor gene *(white box)*, followed by either epigenetic silencing or chromosome loss of the second allele *(red box)*. **(B)** Genes can normally be silenced by a variety of interacting processes including DNA methylation, histone modifications, nucleosome remodeling, and microRNAs (not shown). Several cellular enzymes contribute to these modifications, including DNA methyltransferases *(DNMTs)*, histone deacetylases *(HDACs)*, histone methyltransferases *(HMTs)*, and complex nucleosomal remodeling factors *(NURFs)*. Gene silencing is essential for normal development and differentiation. (B, Adapted from Jones PA, Baylin SB. The epigenomics of cancer. *Cell*, 2007;128:683–692.)

suppresses cell division until DNA repair is complete or other effects of stress are corrected. If not corrected, the cell enters senescence or apoptosis, thus preventing further DNA damage and mutations. Cellular senescence has been shown to exhibit both a tumor suppressor and an oncogenic effect.[14] Senescence can promote cancer development by altering the cellular environment through a senescence-associated secretory phenotype (SASP).[15] Early-stage senescence may protect cells from cancer transformation, but prolonged senescence often promotes cancer development.[15] Aberrant redox signaling assists senescence and carcinogenesis.[14] Loss of function of *TP53* or caretaker genes leads to increased mutation rates and cancer. *TP53* mutations in many cancers are linked to a poor prognosis.[13] Li-Fraumeni syndrome is a very rare inheritable loss-of-function mutation in *TP53* in one allele resulting in a 25-fold increase of developing malignancy at an early age (<50 years of age). These malignancies may include breast cancer, brain tumors, acute leukemia, soft tissue sarcomas, bone sarcoma, and adrenal cortical carcinoma.

Because inactivation of tumor-suppressor genes requires at least two mutations (one in each allele), a single germ cell mutation (sperm or egg) results in the transmission of cancer-causing genes from one generation to the next, producing families with a high risk for specific cancers. These inherited mutations that predispose to cancer are almost invariably in tumor-suppressor genes because only a single additional mutation in any other cell (somatic cell mutation) is needed to inactivate completely the tumor-suppressor gene (Table 12.2). Another way that tumor suppressor-genes can be inactivated is through epigenetic silencing or modulation of gene function (see Fig. 12.11 and Chapters 4, 6, and 13). Many cancers have increased methylation of DNA in the promoter region of tumor-suppressor genes. They also have associated changes in the modification of histones in the chromatin, often correlated with methylation of DNA. These changes alter the promoter regions of genes, leading to their silencing or altered gene expression.

An example of increased risk for cancer that can be inherited is the familial form of retinoblastoma. The retinoblastoma (*RB1*) gene resides on chromosome 13, in a region referred to as q14 (13q14). *RB1* gene provides instructions for a protein called pRB.[16] It is responsible for monitoring antigrowth cellular signals and blocking activation of the growth/division phase in the cell cycle; thus *RB1* is a tumor suppressor gene and mutations in RB1 lead to persistent cell growth.[17] Most individuals with RB mutations have a subtle mutation, such as a point mutation, in one allele. The RB gene in the other chromosome may be inactivated through loss of the 13q14 region or epigenetic mechanisms. In the inherited form of retinoblastoma, a mutation in one *RB* allele is inherited so that only one additional mutation in the normal allele leads to cancer (see Table 12.2). RB is mutated in childhood retinoblastoma, and in some lung, breast, bladder, bone cancers (osteosarcoma), leukemias, and melanoma as well.[16] Approximately 40% of children with retinoblastoma have the inheritable form and most will develop tumors in both eyes (bilateral retinoblastoma) and are at increased risk for a second primary cancer, such as a sarcoma or malignant melanoma.[18]

Other familial cancers with inheritable mutations in tumor-suppressor genes include Wilms tumor, a childhood cancer of the kidney (*WT1* gene), neurofibromatosis (*NF1* gene), and familial polyposis coli or adenomas of the colon (*APC* gene). Characterization of cancer-causing genes and other genetic factors

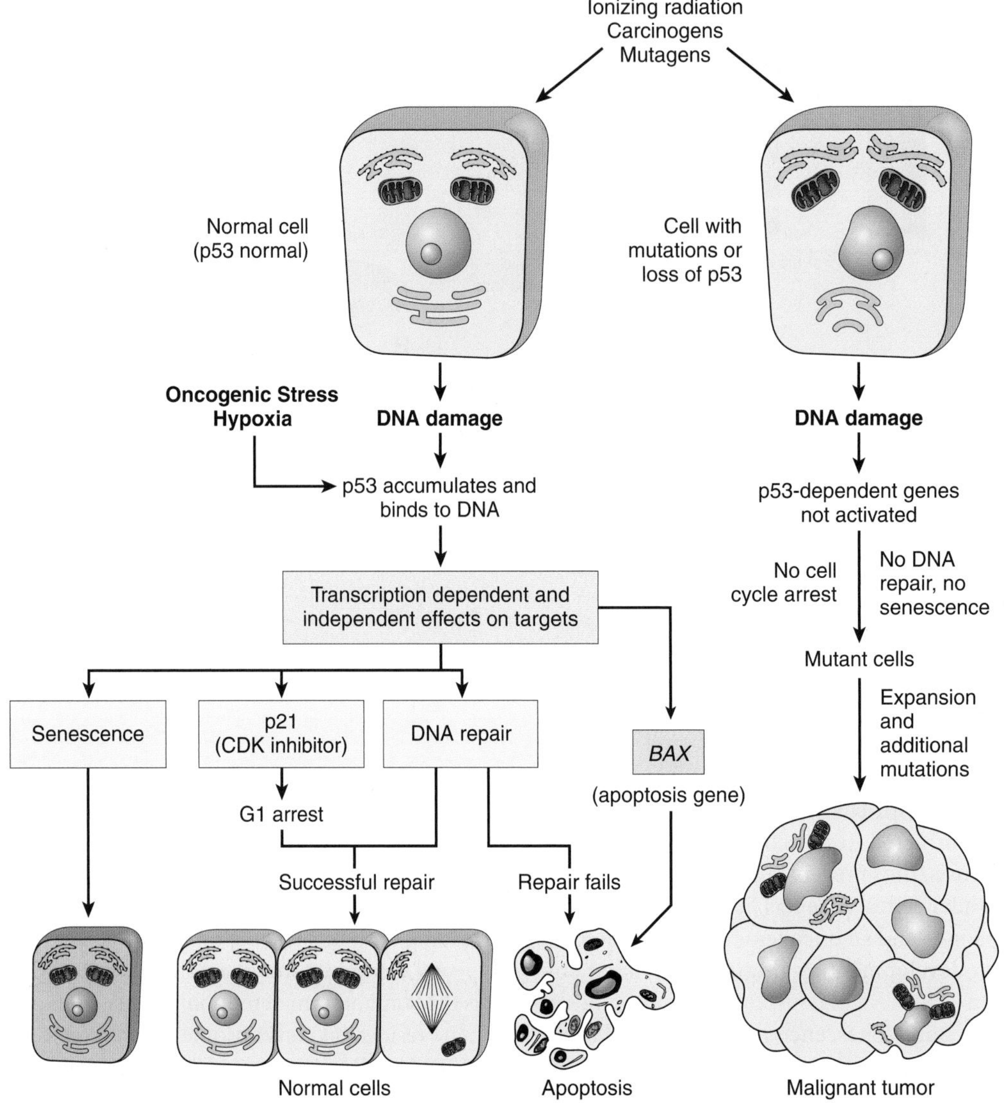

Fig. 12.12 The Role and Network of p53. (A) The Role of p53 in Maintaining the Integrity of the Genome. Activation of normal p53 by DNA-damaging agents or by hypoxia leads to cell cycle arrest in G_1 by up-regulation of the cell cycle inhibitor p21 and induction of DNA repair transcriptional up-regulation of the cyclin-dependent kinase inhibitor *CDKN1A* (encoding the cyclin-dependent kinase inhibitor p21) and the *GADD45* genes. Successful repair of DNA allows cells to proceed with the cell cycle. If DNA repair fails, *p53* triggers either apoptosis or senescence. In cells with loss or mutation of the *p53* gene, DNA damage does not induce cell cycle arrest or DNA repair, and genetically damaged cells proliferate, giving rise eventually to malignant neoplasms. (From Kumar V, et al. *Robbins and Cotran pathologic basis of disease*, 10th edition, Philadelphia: Elsevier; 2021.)

Continued

helps identify individuals prone to developing cancer and contributes to understanding of sporadic cancers. Individuals known to carry mutations in tumor-suppressor genes are offered targeted cancer screening to facilitate early cancer detection and therapy.

Genomic Instability

Genomic instability is an increased tendency of alterations—mutability—in the genome during the life cycle of cells. Inherited and acquired mutations in caretaker genes that protect the integrity of the genome and DNA repair increase the level of genomic instability and risk for developing cancer.[19] Acquired mutations in "guardians of the genome," such as *TP53*, that detect DNA damage and activate repair mechanisms result in genomic instability and an increasing accumulation of mutations. Xeroderma pigmentosum is a defect in the repair of DNA pyrimidine dimers created by UV light

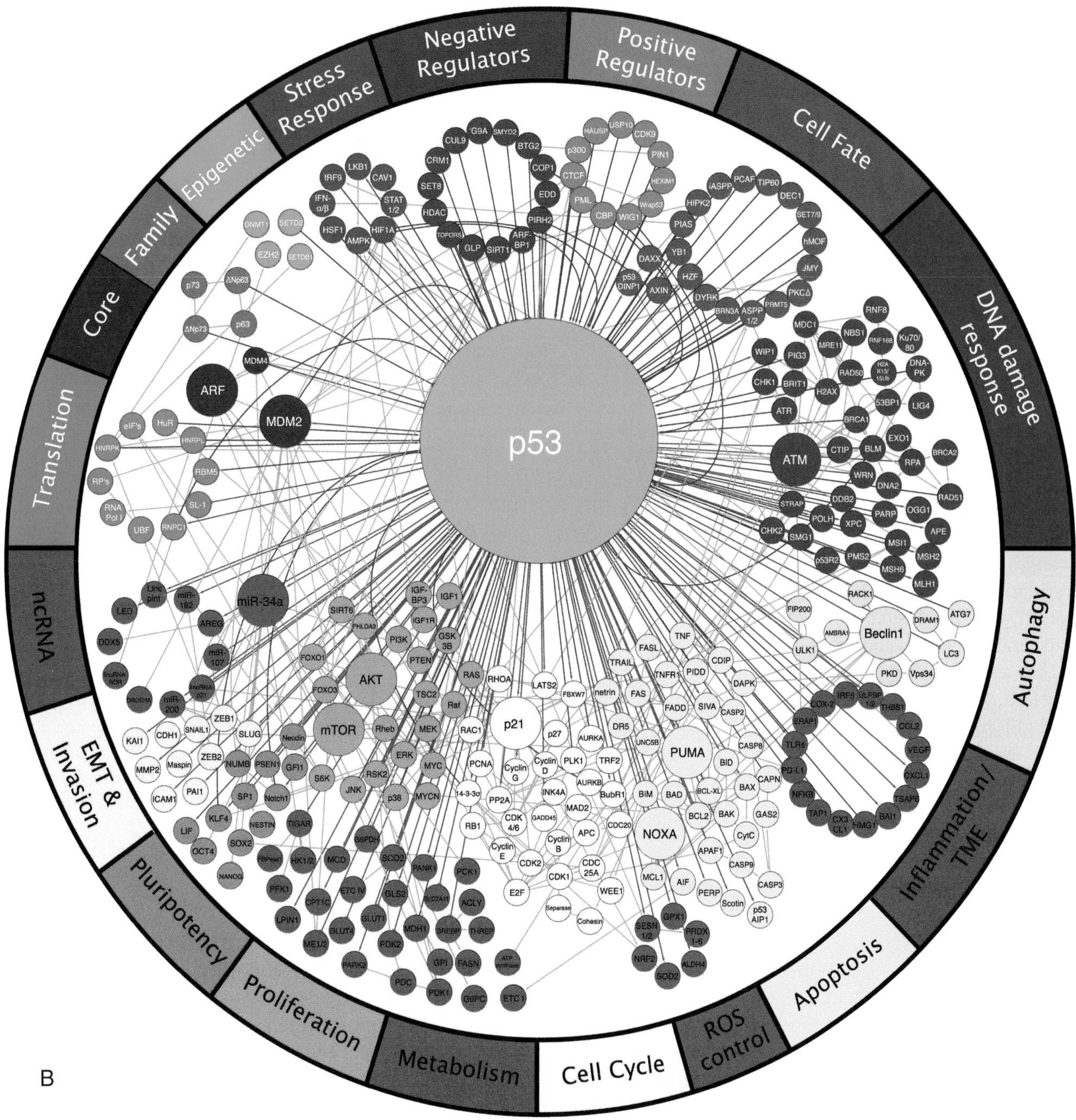

Fig. 12.12, cont'd **(B)** The p53 network is large and it controls many biological processes. Each node or circle represents a gene, and each line represents an interaction. Direct p53 inputs are indicated as blue lines and direct p53 outputs as red lines. P53 controls effector processes by activating multiple target genes. Although not shown here, the pathways are highly interconnected, and interactions are positive, negative, or modifying. (Adapted from Data from Kastenhuber ER, Lowe SW. Putting p53 in context. *Cell*, 2017;170:1062–1078.)

that increases the risk for skin cancers. Hereditary nonpolyposis colorectal cancer results from an inherited defect in repairing DNA base pair mismatches that occur occasionally during DNA replication. Affected individuals have an increased rate of small insertions and deletions in DNA, leading to a high rate of colon and other cancers. Some inherited mutations threaten the integrity of entire chromosomes. Bloom syndrome, caused by mutations in a DNA helicase, presents with an increased risk of several forms of cancer, and those with Fanconi aplastic anemia, caused by loss of function for repairing DNA double-strand breaks, have a particularly increased risk of acute myelogenous

TABLE 12.2 Some Familial Cancer Syndromes Caused by Loss of Tumor-Suppressor Gene Function

Syndrome	Gene
Retinoblastoma	*RB1*
Li-Fraumeni syndrome	*p53* (TP53)
Familial melanoma	*p16^{INK4a} (CDKN2A)*
Neurofibromatosis	*Neurofibromin (NF1)*
Familial adenomatous polyps	*APC*
Breast cancer	*BRCA1*

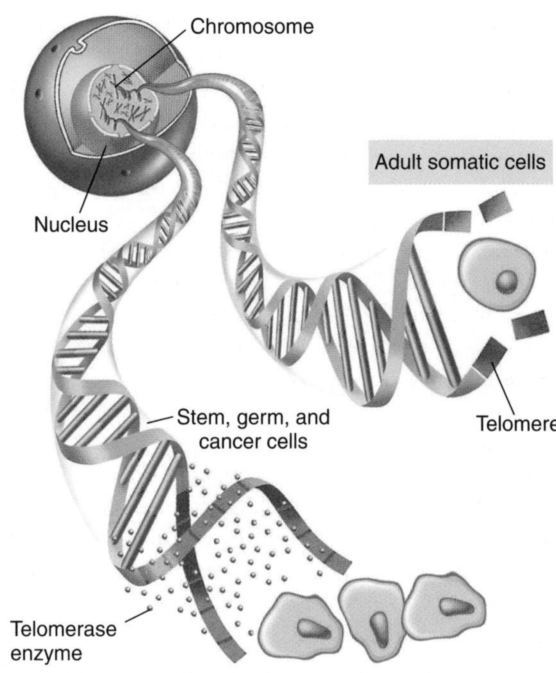

Fig. 12.13 Control of Immortality: Telomeres and Telomerase. Normal adult somatic cells cannot divide indefinitely because the ends of their chromosomes are capped by telomeres. In the absence of the telomerase enzyme, telomeres become progressively shorter with each division until, when they are critically short, they signal to the cell to stop dividing. In germ cells, adult stem cells, and cancer cells, the telomerase gene is "switched on," producing an enzyme that rebuilds the telomeres. Thus, like germ cells, the cancer cell becomes immortal and able to divide indefinitely without losing its telomeres.

leukemia. These examples are autosomal recessive disorders in which affected individuals demonstrate marked chromosomal instability. Genomic instability also may result from increased epigenetic silencing or modulation of gene function discussed earlier (see Chapter 6).

Changes in gene regulation can affect not just single genes, but also entire intracellular signaling networks. Gene expression networks can be regulated by changes in microRNAs (miRNAs or miRs) and other non–coding RNAs (ncRNAs). miRNAs regulate gene expression by binding to target messenger RNA, thereby leading to repression or promotion of DNA translation. Through this process, miRNAs regulate cell differentiation, proliferation, apoptosis, autophagy, and stem cell maintenance.[20] miRNAs can be divided into those that promote cancer (oncogenic miRNAs or oncomirs), and those that prevent cancer (tumor suppressor miRNAs). Oncomirs promote multiple cancer pathways, including genomic instability, methylation patterns, immune dysfunction, tumor microenvironment, and drug resistance.[20]

Mutations in *BRCA1* and *BRCA2* (breast cancer 1 and 2, early-onset genes) are important clinically. Both are tumor-suppressors and caretaker genes that repair double-stranded DNA breaks. Inherited harmful mutations in *BRCA1* or *BRCA2* can occur from either a mother or father. Either gene with a high-risk mutation greatly increases the risk for a variety of tumors, especially breast cancer in both women and men, and ovarian or prostate cancers.[21] From a seminal paper, the average cumulative risk of developing breast cancer by age 70 years with a *BRCA1* mutation was 65%, and ovarian cancer was 39%.[22] The corresponding estimates for *BRCA2* mutation were 45% for breast cancer and 11% for ovarian cancer.[22] At-risk women are currently offered enhanced screening, prophylactic (risk-reducing) surgery, and chemoprevention.

In addition to specific gene mutations and abnormal epigenetic silencing, chromosome instability (CIN) also appears to be increased in malignant cells, resulting in a high rate of chromosome loss, as well as loss of heterozygosity and chromosome amplification. The underlying mechanism of this instability is not clear but may be caused by malfunctions in the cellular machinery that regulates chromosome segregation at mitosis. CIN has been associated with resistance to cancer therapies in many cancers.[23]

Enabling Replication Immortality

A hallmark of cancer cells is their immortality; they seem to have an unlimited life span and will continue to divide for years under appropriate laboratory conditions. One of the most commonly used laboratory cell lines, HeLa cells, was derived from a cervical cancer specimen obtained in 1951 that continues to grow and divide in laboratories worldwide. Most normal cells are not immortal and can divide only a limited number of times (known as the *Hayflick limit*) before they either enter senescence (cease dividing) or enter crisis (apoptosis) and die. One major block to unlimited cell division (i.e., immortality) is the size of a specialized structure called the *telomere*. Telomeres are protective ends, or caps, of repeating hexanucleotides (six nucleotide units) on each chromosome and are placed and maintained by a specialized enzyme called telomerase (see Fig. 12.13). Telomerase is usually active only in germ cells (in ovaries and testes) and in stem cells. All other cells of the body lack telomerase activity. Thus, when non–germ cells begin to proliferate abnormally, their telomere caps shorten with each cell division. Short telomeres usually signal the cell to cease cell division. If the telomeres become critically small, the chromosomes become unstable and fragment, and the cells die.

Cancer cells are very heterogeneous, and many cells die as the cancer develops. When they reach a critical age, most cancer cells reactivate telomerase to restore and maintain their telomeres, thereby allowing continuous division. Telomerase not only maintains telomere length, but it also affects DNA replication, cellular apoptosis, tumorigenesis, and resistance to therapy by cancer cells, including those of breast and cervical origin.[24] The trigger for re-expression of telomerase activity remains unclear; however, evidence is emerging that promotor mutations, genomic rearrangements, and epigenetic dysregulation of telomerase reverse transcriptase (TERT) are core steps.[24] Cancer cells move closer to immortality by upregulating telomerase and downregulating tumor suppressor genes. Telomerase activity is restored in about 90% of cancers and is an attractive therapeutic target.[25]

Cancer stem cells (CSCs) are a subpopulation of tumor cells that have replication immortality. They arise from tissue resident stem cells or develop from transformed differentiated cells. Transformation from differentiated cells into CSCs occurs through the activation of oncogenes, inactivation of tumor suppressor genes, and re-expression of telomerase.[26] CSCs can change their appearance and function in response to the tumor microenvironment such that they drive cancer progression, serving as the cellular seeds for both tumor growth, metastases, and disease recurrence[27] (See section Activating Invasion and Metastasis). CSCs exist in a variety of tumor types such as leukemia, brain, breast, lung, and gastrointestinal (GI) cancers. Detection of CSCs is conducted via identification of surface protein markers and metabolic/functional properties. They often are highly resistant to traditional forms of cancer treatment. New therapies that target CSCs are being developed.[28]

Cellular Adaptations

Inducing Angiogenesis

An important component of wound healing is the process of establishing new blood vessels within the tissue undergoing repair (called neovascularization or angiogenesis). Access to a blood supply also is obligatory for the growth and spread of cancer. Without a blood supply to deliver oxygen and nutrients, growth of a tumor is limited to about a millimeter in diameter.

Angiogenic factors and angiogenic inhibitors typically control development of new vessels. In cancerous tumors, several mechanisms increase and maintain secretion of angiogenic factors by the cancer cells and prevent release of angiogenic inhibitors. Hypoxia-inducible factor-1α (HIF-1α), an oxygen-sensitive transcription factor, is a primary regulator of angiogenesis in normal tissue; HIF-1α is stabilized under hypoxic conditions and induces expression of pro-angiogenic factors, such as vascular endothelial growth factor (VEGF) and basic fibroblast growth factor (bFGF).[29] Inactivation of tumor-suppressor genes (e.g., *p53*) or increased expression of oncogenes (e.g., *HER2*) leads to increased expression of HIF-1α–regulated angiogenic factors and increased vascularization. Increased expression of HIF-1α also is related to increased resistance to chemotherapy, increased tumor cell glycolysis, increased metastasis, and a poor prognosis. These effects may likely occur through an autocrine mechanism by which VEGF activates tumor-associated VEGF receptors.

Other routes of angiogenic factor induction include mutations in cancer oncogenes (e.g., *RAS*, *MYC*) that increase transcription of VEGF by cancer cells. Most cells in the tumor microenvironment also secrete VEGF, including tumor-infiltrating monocytes, endothelial cells, adipocytes, and cancer-associated fibroblasts. Endogenous angiogenesis inhibitors, such as thrombospondin-1 (TSP-1), typically bind to cellular surface receptors on inflammatory cells and negatively regulate angiogenesis in wound healing and tissue remodeling. The expression of angiogenesis inhibitors is under the control of p53, which is suppressed in cancer cells, thus diminishing the control of stromal inflammatory cell secretion of angiogenic factors.

Cancer cells and stromal cells may increase production of matrix metalloproteinases (MMPs) (e.g., MMP-9) (Fig. 12.14).[30] MMPs are zinc-dependent proteases that digest the surrounding extracellular matrix (ECM). The ECM contains stored latent (inactive) forms of some angiogenic factors (e.g., bFGF, transforming growth factor-beta [TGF-β]). MMPs activate the stored forms into functional angiogenic factors.

The vessels formed within tumors differ from those in healthy tissue. They originate from endothelial sprouting from existing capillaries and irregular branching, rather than regular branching seen in healthy tissue. The interendothelial cell contact is less tight, so the vessels are more porous and prone to hemorrhage and allow passage of tumor cells into the vascular system. Another form of angiogenesis in tumors is called vasculogenic mimicry. Tumor cells form tubular structures like blood vessels that contain erythrocytes. These tubular tissues can attach to blood vessels to form a vascular network.[31]

Angiogenic inhibitors targeting VEGF signaling have been used to inhibit angiogenesis and diminish tumor growth.[32] Unfortunately, anti-VEGF therapies have not improved survival of individuals as much as was expected due to therapy resistance.[33,34] For example, tumors may use alternative growth factors other than VEGF to activate angiogenesis or may revert to other ways of securing blood flow. New therapies to block angiogenesis are being explored.[33,35]

Reprogramming Energy Metabolism

Cancer cells live in a distinct environment from normal cells and have different nutritional requirements from nonproliferating cells (Box 12.1). The successful cancer cell divides rapidly, with the consequent requirement for the building blocks to construct new cells. Nonmalignant cells in the presence of adequate oxygen normally generate adenosine triphosphate (ATP) by mitochondrial oxidative phosphorylation (OXPHOS), generating 36 ATP molecules from each glucose molecule that is broken down to water and carbon dioxide. In the absence of sufficient oxygen (hypoxia), normal cells perform glycolysis, or the breakdown of glucose by enzymes (anaerobic glycolysis), generating only two ATP molecules per molecule of glucose with lactic acid and pyruvate as by-products.

Energy metabolism in cancer cells has received renewed attention and is deemed as important as other hallmark characteristics, such as sustained angiogenesis. In the 1920s, the emerging distinction between normal cells and cancer cells was first reported by Otto Warburg, termed the *Warburg effect*. The

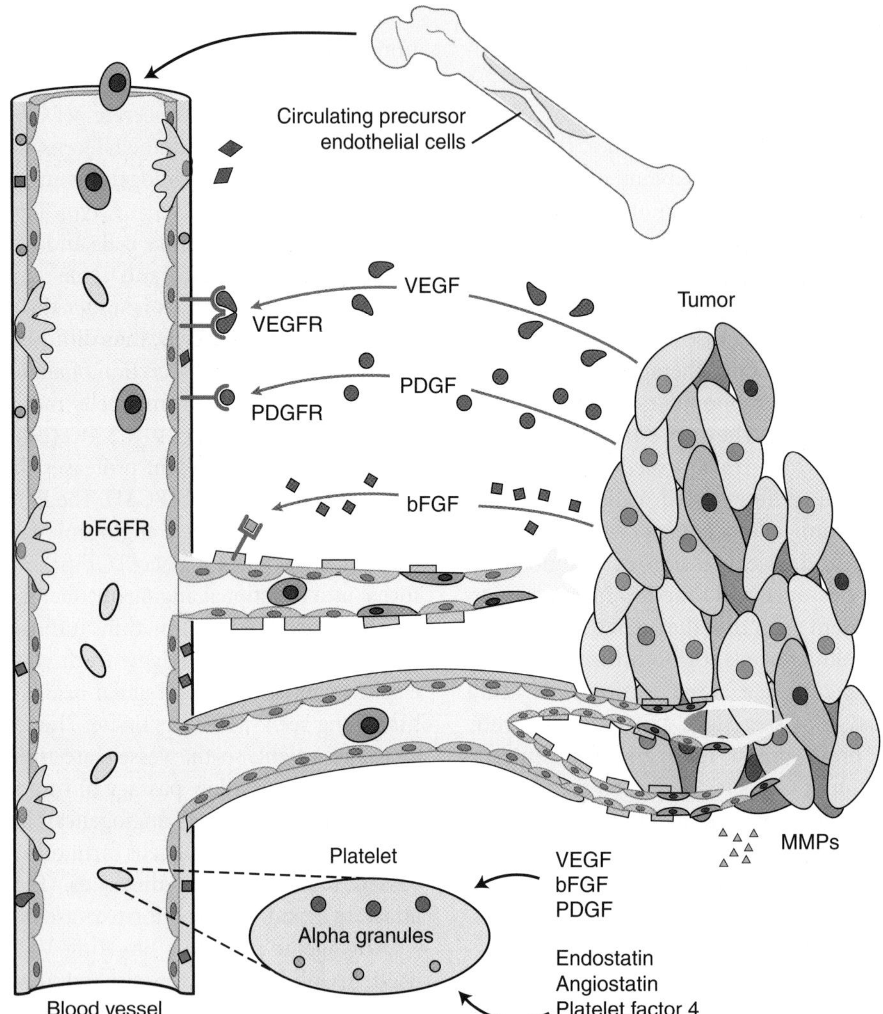

Fig. 12.14 Tumor-Induced Angiogenesis. Malignant tumors secrete angiogenic factors and tissue-remodeling matrix metalloproteinases *(MMPs)* that actively induce formation of new blood vessels. New blood vessels are formed from both local endothelial cells and circulating precursor cells recruited from the bone marrow. Circulating platelets can also release regulatory proteins into the tumor. *bFGF* and *bFGFR*, Basic fibroblast growth factor and its receptor, respectively; *PDGF* and *PDGFR*, platelet-derived growth factor and its receptor, respectively; *VEGF* and *VEGFR*, vascular endothelial growth factor and its receptor, respectively. (Adapted from Folkman J. Angiogenesis: An organizing principle for drug discovery? *Nature Review Drug Discovery*, 2007;6(4):273–286.)

Warburg effect suggests that even in the presence of sufficient oxygen, cancer cells prefer to produce ATP through glycolysis instead of OXPHOS (Fig. 12.15).[9] Thus, the Warburg Effect is the use of glycolysis under normal oxygen conditions, hence the name aerobic glycolysis.[36] Although aerobic glycolysis was postulated to arise from cancer-specific mitochondrial dysfunction, it is now apparent that this is a highly regulated and beneficial adaptation for cancer cells. The shift from OXPHOS to glycolysis allows lactate and other products of glycolysis to be used for the more efficient production of lipids, nucleosides, amino acids, and other molecular building blocks needed for rapid cell growth. Recent work, however, challenges the Warburg Effect because mitochondrial OXPHOS still contributes to overall ATP generation under normal conditions for certain cancer cells and reduces significantly in hypoxic environments. Perhaps more significantly, the Warburg Effect does not focus on the metabolic interactions between cancer cells and other components of the microenvironment.[37,38] Ongoing investigations involve glucose, amino acids, and possibly lactate dehydrogenase and their importance in cancer metabolism.

A new model, the reverse Warburg effect, may play a role in certain cancers.[39] Cancer cells may continue using the OXPHOS to generate large amounts of ATP. However, they also may manipulate the cancer-associated fibroblasts (CAFs) (see Fig. 12.18) perhaps by inducing oxidative stress to undergo aerobic glycolysis and secrete metabolites (e.g., lactate, pyruvate) that the cancer cells can use in the citric acid cycle (Krebs cycle) to feed OXPHOS and produce ATP.

BOX 12.1 Cancer Metabolism

Reprogrammed metabolism is a hallmark of cancer. Reprogramming describes usual metabolic pathways that are enhanced or suppressed in tumor cells compared to benign tissues because of cancer mutations and/or other factors. Tumors reprogram pathways of nutrient obtainment and metabolism to meet the energetic, biosynthetic, and redox needs of tumor cells. An explosion of research in cancer metabolism is highlighting core principals. Cancer metabolic reprogramming has profound effects on gene expression, cellular differentiation, and the tumor microenvironment. Metabolic hallmarks of cancer metabolism include:

1. deregulated uptake of glucose and amino acids
2. grasping or opportunistic modes of nutrient acquisition
3. use of glycolysis/tricarboxylic acid (TCA) cycle intermediates for synthesis and nicotinamide adenine dinucleotide phosphate (NADPH) production
4. increased demand for nitrogen
5. alterations in metabolic-driven gene regulation and
6. metabolic interactions with microenvironment.

Most tumors display several of these hallmarks, but few display all six.

Understanding tumor metabolism is essential for determining treatment. Tumor cells adapt to nutrient-limited environments by inducing gene expression that secures adequate nutrients to sustain their metabolic demands. For example, acute lymphoblastic leukemia (ALL) cells are sensitive to the amino acid asparagine biosynthesis. ALL cells are responsive to asparagine depletion thus the use of the asparagine depletion enzyme L-asparaginase

Data from DeBerardins RJ, Chandel NS. Fundamentals of cancer metabolism. *Sci Adv.* 2016;2[5]:e1600200; Pavlova NN, Thompson CB. The Emerging Hallmarks of Cancer Metabolism. *Cell Metab.* 2016;23(1):27– 47.

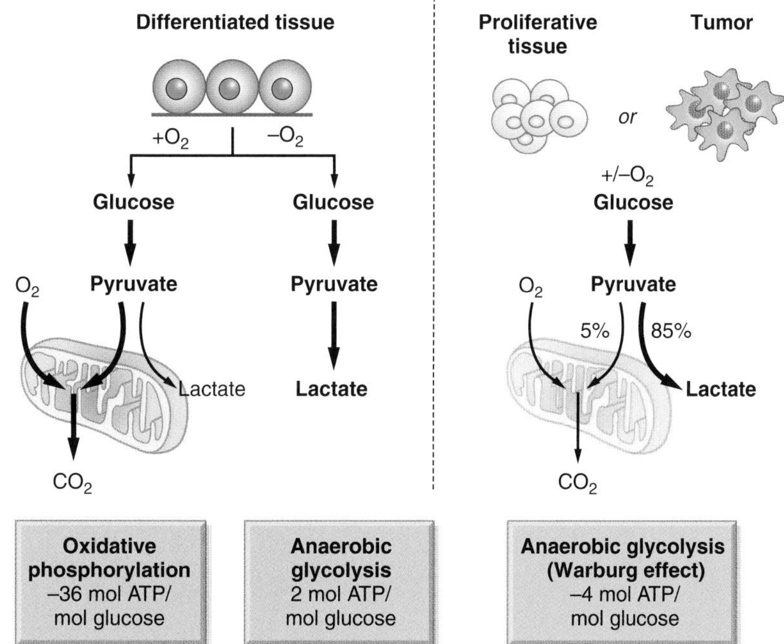

Fig. 12.15 Cancers Have Altered Metabolism. Normal tissues use oxidative phosphorylation (OXPHOS) to turn glucose into CO_2 and energy (in the form of ATP). Cancers take a different approach; even in the presence of oxygen, usually they do not use OXPHOS. Instead, they consume large quantities of glucose to make cellular building blocks, supporting rapid proliferation. *ATP,* Adenosine triphosphate. (From Van der Heiden MG, Cantley LC, Thompson CB. Understanding the Warburg effect: The metabolic requirements of cell proliferation. *Science,* 2009;324: 1029–1033.)

A recent finding is that the mammalian/mechanistic target of rapamycin complex 1 (mTORC1) is a significant nutrient sensor and regulator of cellular metabolic processes.[40]

Clinically, the high glucose utilization of a cancer can be exploited for its detection. 18F-Fluorodeoxyglucose (FDG) is incorporated into cells in the same way as glucose, with two key differences. Because it is missing a key hydroxyl group, it cannot be broken down by glycolysis, and thus FDG accumulates in cells. Because it is tagged with F^{18}, it can be imaged by a positron emission tomography (PET) scan. Small metastatic tumor masses that are consuming huge amounts of glucose can readily be detected with this imaging method (Fig. 12.16).

Resistance to Destruction

Resisting Apoptotic Cell Death

Programmed cell death (apoptosis) is a mechanism by which individual cells can self-destruct under conditions of tissue remodeling or as a protection against aberrant cell growth that may lead to malignancy. Two pathways may trigger apoptosis.

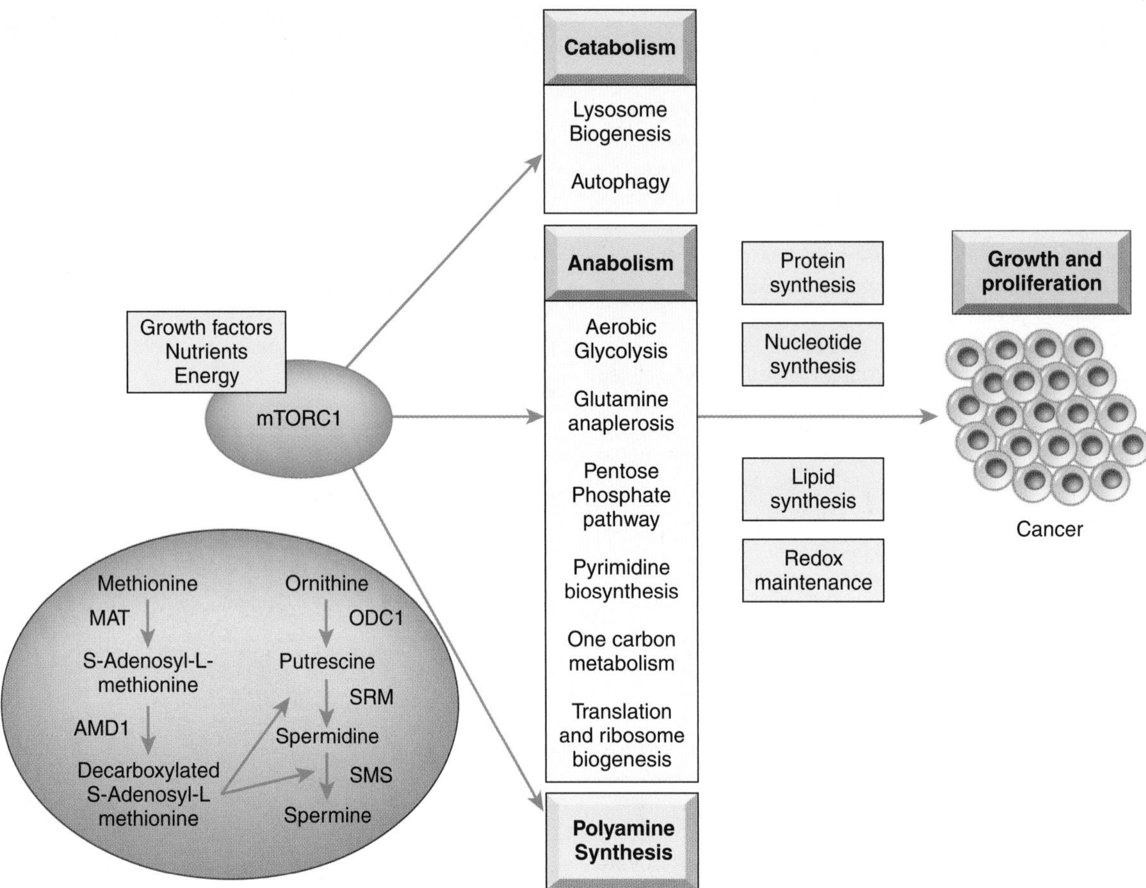

Fig. 12.16 Intense Glucose Requirement Aids in Diagnosis of Metastatic Non–Small Cell Lung Cancer. This 54-year-old woman had a non–small cell lung cancer resected from the left upper lobe. Five years later, these studies were obtained. The positron emission tomography (PET) scan using 18-fluorodeoxyglucose (FDG) shows metastatic lesions in the brain, right shoulder, and mediastinal and cervical lymph nodes, as well as in the liver, left pelvis, and proximal femur. *PET whole-body image* ***(left)****:* Representative coronal image from the whole-body FDG-PET/CT–fused image of the same person ***(right)***. The fused image consists of the computed tomography (CT) image with the metabolic information superimposed in color. The pattern of spread is most likely from the primary tumor to the large mediastinal lymph nodes, followed by lymphatic spread to cervical nodes. Blood-borne dissemination produced the bone, brain, and liver metastases. Normally, only the heart, brain, and bladder show a strong signal in PET scans. (Images courtesy John Hoffman, MD, Huntsman Cancer Institute, Salt Lake.)

The intrinsic pathway (mitochondrial pathway) monitors cellular stress. Cellular stress may include DNA damage, genomic instability, aberrant proliferation, loss of adhesion to ECM or to adjacent cells, and other causes and characteristics of abnormal cellular physiology. The extrinsic pathway is activated through a plasma membrane receptor complex linked to intracellular activators of apoptosis (known as the *death receptor*) (see Chapter 2) (Fig. 12.17).

Apoptotic pathways are dysregulated in most cancers. Most commonly, loss-of-function mutations to the *TP53* gene suppress activation of apoptosis during DNA damage. The balance between pro- and anti-apoptotic molecules also can be affected by overexpression of anti-apoptotic molecules or diminished expression of anti-apoptotic molecules resulting from mutations. By whatever mechanism, or combination of mechanisms, successful cancers suppressed apoptotic pathways and increased resistance to cell death.

Tumor-Promoting Inflammation

The relationship between a cancer and the inflammatory system is complex. The inflammatory response contributes to the onset of cancer, and cancer is a cause of chronic systemic and local inflammation. Tumors can manipulate the inflammatory process in their local tumor microenvironment to benefit tumor progression and spread.[41] Cancer also causes systemic perturbations in both innate and adaptive immune processes that reduce the body's ability to fight the cancer (see Evading Immune Destruction section).

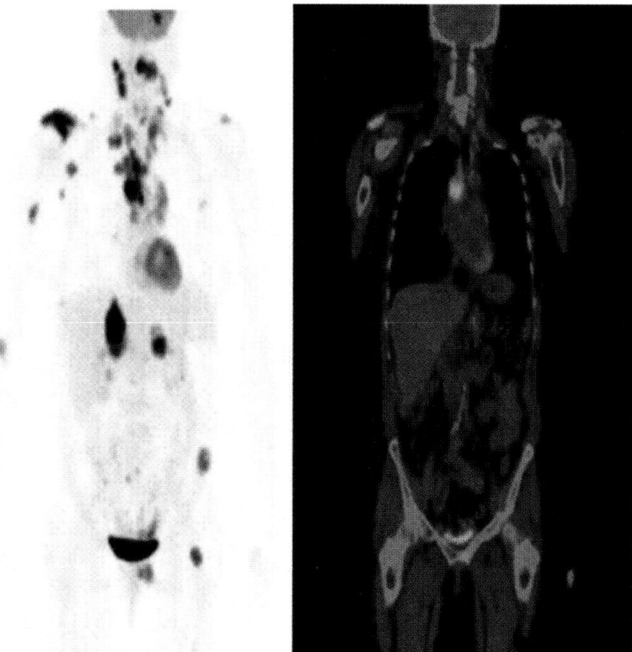

Fig. 12.17 Extrinsic and Intrinsic Pathways of Apoptosis and Mechanisms Used by Tumor Cells to Evade Cell Death. ***(1)*** Loss of p53 through mutation leading to reduced function of proapoptotic factors, such as BAX. ***(2)*** Reduced egress of cytochrome *c* from mitochondria as a result of up-regulation of antiapoptotic factors, such as BCL-2. ***(3)*** Loss of apoptotic peptidase-activating factor 1 *(APAF-1)*. ***(4)*** Upregulation of inhibitors of apoptosis *(IAP)*. ***(5)*** Reduced CD 95. ***(6)*** Inactivation of death domain signaling complex (FADD). (From Kumar V, Abbas AK, Aster JC. *Robbins and Cotran pathologic basis of disease*, 9th edition. Philadelphia: Saunders; 2015.)

Chronic inflammation has been recognized for close to 150 years as being an important factor in the development of cancer. Chronic inflammations may result from many causes, for example, solar irradiation, asbestos exposure (mesothelioma), pancreatitis, and infection (Table 12.3). Additionally, some organs appear to be more susceptible to the oncogenic effects of chronic inflammation (e.g., the GI tract, prostate, thyroid gland). Individuals who have suffered with ulcerative colitis for 11 years or more have up to a 30-fold increase in the risk of developing colon cancer. Chronic viral hepatitis caused by hepatitis B virus (HBV) or hepatitis C virus (HCV) infection markedly increases the risk of liver cancer.

A specific example is the association between gastric inflammation induced by infection with the bacterium *Helicobacter pylori (H. pylori)* and the risk for gastric cancer. *H. pylori* is a bacterium that infects more than half of the world's population. Chronic infection with *H. pylori* is a significant cause of peptic ulcer disease and is strongly associated with gastric carcinoma, a leading cause of cancer deaths worldwide (see Chapter 41). It also is associated with a less common cancer, gastric mucosa-associated lymphoid tissue (MALT) lymphomas. *H. pylori* infection is often acquired in childhood and disproportionately affects lower socioeconomic classes. Although most infections are asymptomatic, prolonged chronic inflammation, oxidative stress, and stimulation of GFRs may lead to increased gastric acid secretion, atrophic gastritis, and duodenal ulcers, or benign cellular proliferation that in 1% to 2% of individuals progress to dysplastic changes and finally gastric adenocarcinoma.[42]

TABLE 12.3 Chronic Inflammatory Conditions and Infectious Agents Associated With Neoplasms

Inflammatory Conditions	Associated Neoplasm(s)
Inflammatory Conditions	
Asbestosis, silicosis	Mesothelioma, lung carcinoma
Bronchitis	Lung carcinoma
Cystitis, bladder inflammation	Bladder carcinoma
Gingivitis, lichen planus	Oral squamous cell carcinoma
Inflammatory bowel disease, Crohn disease, chronic ulcerative colitis	Colorectal carcinoma
Lichen sclerosus	Vulvar squamous cell carcinoma
Chronic pancreatitis, hereditary pancreatitis	Pancreatic carcinoma
Reflux esophagitis, Barrett esophagus	Esophageal carcinoma
Sialadenitis	Salivary gland carcinoma
Sjögren syndrome, Hashimoto thyroiditis	MALT lymphoma
Skin inflammation	Melanoma
Infectious Agent (Nonviral)	
Helicobacter pylori	Gastric adenocarcinoma, MALT lymphoma
Chronic bacterial cholecystitis	Gallbladder cancer
Schistosomiasis	Bladder, liver, rectal carcinoma; follicular lymphoma of spleen
Liver flukes	Cholangiocarcinoma
Infectious Agent (Viral)	
Human immunodeficiency virus type 1 (HIV-1)	Non-Hodgkin lymphoma, squamous cell carcinomas, Kaposi sarcoma
Hepatitis B and hepatitis C	Hepatocellular carcinoma
Epstein-Barr virus	B-cell non-Hodgkin lymphoma, Burkitt lymphoma, nasopharyngeal carcinoma
Kaposi sarcoma-associated herpesvirus (KSHV/HHV8)	Kaposi sarcoma
Human papilloma virus (HPV)-16, -18, -31, others	Cervical, anogenital warts
Human T-cell lymphotropic virus 1 (HTLV-1) Merkel cell polyomavirus	Adult T-cell leukemia/lymphoma Merkel cell carcinoma a rare skin cancer

MALT, Mucosa-associated lymphoid tissue.
Modified from Kuper H, Adami HO, Trichopoulos D. Infections as a major preventable cause of human cancer. *Journal of Internal Medicine*, 2000;248(3):171–183. American Society for Microbiology. *The 7 Viruses That Cause Human Cancers* (see Table 12.3). Washington, DC: The American Society for Microbiology; 2019.

H. pylori infection can both directly and indirectly produce genetic and epigenetic changes in cells of infected stomachs, including mutations in *TP53* and alterations in the methylation of specific genes. Eradication of *H. pylori* from infected individuals before the development of dysplasia may prevent the development of cancer. However, there is no expert consensus on the value of population screening and treatment strategies. The MALT lymphomas associated with chronic *H. pylori* infections may depend on chronic inflammation and antigenic stimulation associated with infections, and therefore treatment with antibiotics may be useful even in cases of early lymphoma.[43]

Once cells with malignant phenotypes have developed, additional complex interactions occur between the tumor and the surrounding stroma and cells of the immune and inflammatory systems. Cancers disrupt the environment, initiate or enhance inflammation, and recruit local and distant cells (macrophages, lymphocytes, and other cellular components of inflammation). The acute inflammatory response is initially designed to eliminate infection but evolves to initiate and direct the healing process (see Chapter 7). Successful tumors appear capable of manipulating cells of the inflammatory response from a rejection response towards the phenotypes associated with wound healing and tissue regeneration; a process that includes induction in the damaged tissue of cellular proliferation, neovascularization, and local immune suppression.[41] These activities benefit cancer progression and increase resistance to chemotherapeutic agents.

One of the key cells that promote tumor survival is the tumor-associated macrophage (TAM). Tumors commonly produce cytokines and chemokines that are chemotactic factors for monocytes/macrophages (e.g., colony-stimulating factor-1 [CSF1; also known as *macrophage colony–stimulating factor* or *M-CSF*], the chemokine ligand 2 [CCL2; also known as *monocyte chemotactic protein-1* or *MCP-1*]). Levels of CCL2 in human breast cancer and cancers of the esophagus are related to the degree of macrophage infiltration and progression of the tumor. Most tumors have large numbers of TAMs, whose presence frequently correlates with a worse prognosis.[44] Thus, monocytes are attracted from the blood and into the tumor, where they mature into macrophages. Monocytes can differentiate into several macrophage phenotypes (sometimes known as *plasticity* and *versatility*), depending on the conditions in the microenvironment. The classic proinflammatory macrophage (M1) is the primary macrophage in the acute inflammatory response and is responsible for removal and destruction of infectious agents. During healing, however, a different phenotype (M2) produces anti-inflammatory mediators to suppress ongoing inflammation and induce cellular proliferation, angiogenesis, and wound healing. TAMs appear to phenotypically mimic the M2 phenotype.

TAMs have diminished cytotoxic response and release a variety of immunosuppressive cytokines that block T-cytotoxic cell and natural killer (NK)-cell functions and promote tumor growth and spread.[44] TAMs secrete cellular growth factors (e.g., TGF-β and fibroblast growth factor-2 [FGF-2]) that favor tumor cell proliferation, angiogenesis, and tissue remodeling, similar to their activities in wound healing. They also secrete angiogenesis factors (e.g., VEGF) that induce neovascularization and matrix metalloproteinases (MMPs) that degrade intercellular matrix.[44] The overall effect is increased tumor growth, invasion of the blood vessels, increased oxygen to the tumor, and invasion through the degraded matrix into the local tissue.

Cancer-associated fibroblasts (CAFs) synthesize the ECM that surrounds and permeates the tumor (Fig. 12.18). Cytokines and growth factors stored in the matrix, as well as growth factors, metalloproteases, proteoglycans, and other molecules secreted by CAFs, contribute greatly to cancer progression, local spread, and metastasis (see Fig. 12.18.; Box 12.2: Cancer Associated Fibroblasts: Critical Facts).[45,46] Box 12.2 lists critical facts about the role and function of CAFs in cancer biology and tumor behavior. It is important to understand the significant roles of CAFs in clinical therapy. Several studies have documented how the number of CAFs or their function is linked to outcomes.[47–49] Much investigative activity is ongoing, with several clinical trials involving CAF-targeting agents in combination with existing therapies.[46] New methods are being developed to target fibroblasts specifically such as fibroblast activation protein (FAP) ligands coupled with cytotoxic drugs.[50] Clinical benefit might require targeting of CAF subtypes or reprogramming of CAFs to a normal fibroblast or an antitumorigenic CAF phenotype. Importantly, this requires the defining of CAF subtypes and their interrelationships.[46] The heterogeneity of CAFs, their functions, and possible changeability pose a challenge for the field, with preclinical studies suggesting that the non-specific targeting or deletion of stromal fibroblasts may not increase tumor control.[51,52] An example of making CAFs more normal is provided by the targeting of the vitamin D receptor in pancreatic cancer. Treatment with a vitamin D receptor ligand caused activated *stellate cells* (stellate cells are quiescent fibroblasts) to revert to a quiescent state and reduced disease aggressiveness.[53,54]

Viruses and Cancer

Several viruses have been associated with human cancer; human papillomavirus (HPV), Epstein-Barr virus (EBV; also known as HHV4), Kaposi sarcoma herpesvirus (KSHV; also known as HHV8), hepatitis B and C viruses (HBV, HCV), and Merkel cell polyomavirus are associated with about 12% to 20% of all human cancers worldwide (see Table 12.3).[55] Cancer of the cervix and hepatocellular carcinoma account for approximately 80% of virus-linked cancer cases.

Virtually all cervical cancer is caused by infection with specific types of HPV, which infects basal skin cells and commonly causes warts. There are more than 120 HPV types, but only about 40 can infect human mucosal tissue, and only a few (HPV-16, -18, -31, and -45) are associated with the highest risk for developing cervical, anogenital, and penile cancer. Most HPV infection is handled effectively and rapidly by the immune system and does not cause cancer. Cancer is more common in people with prolonged infection with HPV (a decade or more), during which the viral DNA becomes integrated into the genomic DNA of the infected basal cell of the cervix and directs the persistent production of viral oncogenes. (see Chapter 25 and Box 27.5 for current CDC guidelines on HPV vaccine).

Chronic hepatitis B infections are common in parts of Asia and Sub-Saharan Africa and confer a 200-fold increased risk of

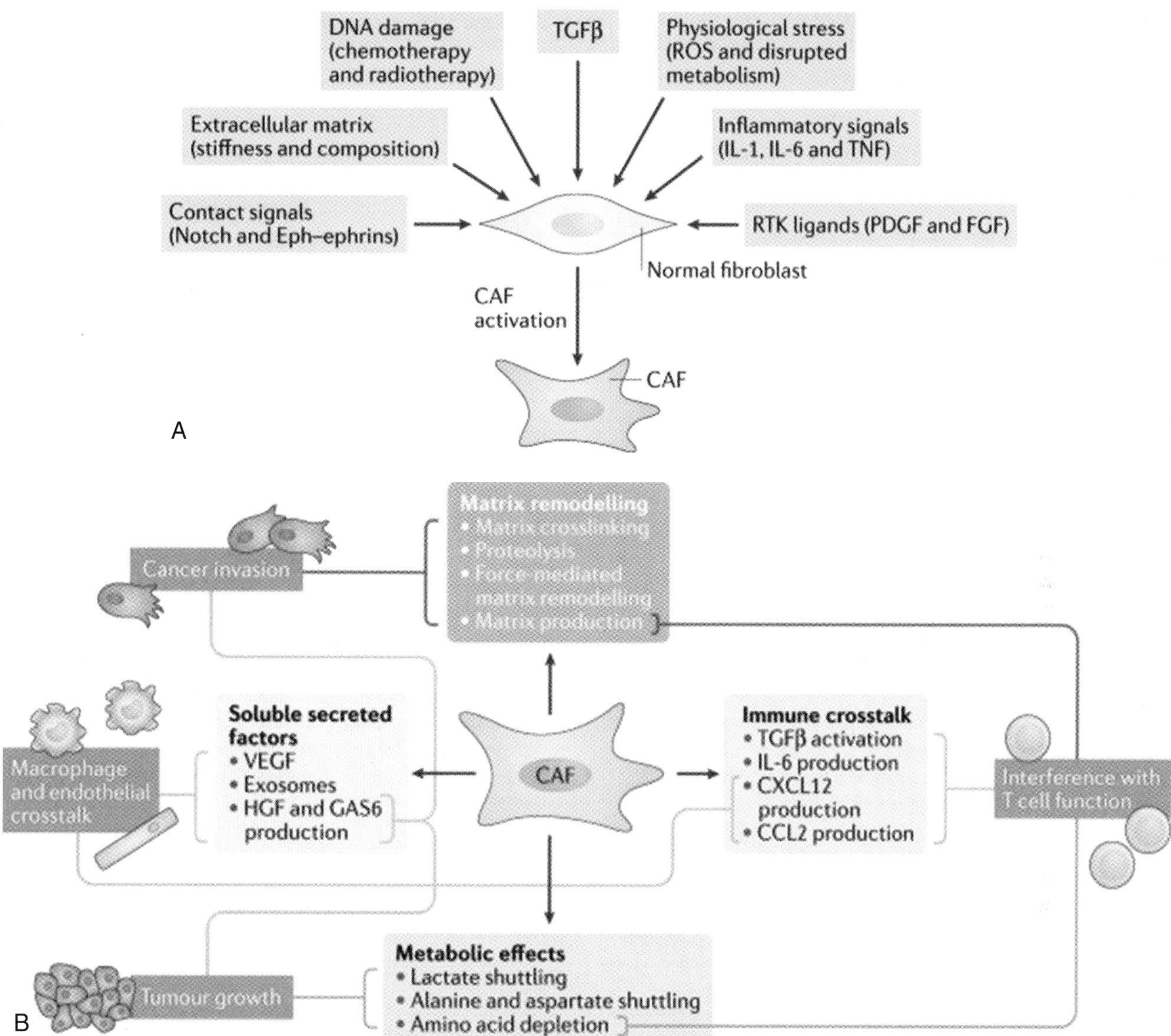

Fig. 12.18 Cancer Associated Fibroblasts. **(A)** Depicts several mechanisms of cancer associated fibroblast *(CAF)* activation. **(B)** Summary of CAF functions and corresponding mechanisms. *FGF,* Fibroblast growth factor; *HGF,* hepatocyte growth factor; *IL,* interleukin; *PDGF,* platelet-derived growth factor; *ROS,* reactive oxygen species; *TGF-β,* transforming growth factor-beta; *TNF,* tumor necrosis factor; *VEGF,* vascular endothelial growth factor. (Data from Sahai E, Astsaturov I, Cukierman E, et al. A framework for advancing our understanding of cancer-associated fibroblasts. *Nature Reviews.* Cancer, 2020;20:174–186.)

developing liver cancer. Chronic hepatitis C infections have become increasingly recognized in Western countries. Up to 80% of liver cancer cases worldwide are associated with chronic hepatitis caused either by HBV or by HCV. About 60% of HBV-infected persons are unaware of their infection.[56] The initial infection with hepatitis B or C is not associated with cancer; instead, it is acquisition of a chronic viral hepatitis that markedly increases cancer risk. In both cases, it appears that a lifetime of chronic liver inflammation predisposes to the development of hepatocellular carcinoma. Widespread use of the HBV vaccine is expected to significantly decrease the incidence of chronic hepatitis B and hence hepatocellular carcinoma (see Chapter 41). So far, there is no vaccine for HCV;[57] however, effective treatment of chronic infection is available and can prevent the development of hepatocellular carcinoma.[58]

For most other human tumor viruses, immunoprophylaxis is not yet available. EBV and HHV8 are members of the Herpesviridae family. More than 90% of adults have been infected with EBV, usually as children and without symptoms. EBV infection during adolescence may cause infectious mononucleosis. The virus infects B lymphocytes, stimulates their limited proliferation, and usually becomes latent throughout their lives. If the individual is immunosuppressed because of human immunodeficiency virus (HIV) infection or because of drugs given for an organ transplant, persistent EBV infection can lead to the development of B-cell lymphomas. EBV infection also is associated with Burkitt lymphoma in areas of endemic malaria

BOX 12.2 Cancer Associated Fibroblasts: Critical Facts

- In normal development and physiology, fibroblasts are the main producers of connective tissue extracellular matrix (ECM)
- Their function changes with age
- Fibroblasts play a key role in tissue repair and are activated following tissue damage
- During wound healing they can produce transforming growth factor β (TGFβ)
- Following tissue injury, they crosstalk with adjacent epithelia and influence epithelial stem cell behavior
- Fibroblasts promote angiogenesis via vascular endothelial growth factor A (VEGA)
- They coordinate the function of the immune system via the production of chemokines and cytokines
- They play a functional role within the immune system; fibroblastic reticular cells (FRCs) within lymph nodes generate ECM conduits for the movement of potential antigens and serve migration "highways" for leukocytes
- Fibroblasts promote immune tolerance by the expression and presentation or normally tissue-restricted antigens
- Emerging is complex crosstalk between fibroblastic cells and epithelial cells in exocrine organs (such as, stellate cells are a distinctive type of fibroblast found in the liver and pancreas, they store lipid droplets and specific derivatives of retinoic acid
- Activation and quiescence of stellate cells is regulated by the vitamin D receptor, and deletion of which leads to spontaneous liver and pancreas fibrosis.
- Stellate cells play a broad role in metabolic homeostasis
- Fibroblasts play key roles in communicating with many other cell types in normal tissue homeostasis as well as repair
- Cancer associated CAFs may be the most effective cell within the tumor microenvironment at depositing and remodeling the ECM
- CAFs contribute to increased stiffness of tumor tissue and this triggers pro-survival and proproliferation signaling in cancer cells
- Increased mechanical stress can collapse blood vessels, leading to hypoxia, promoting more aggressive cancer phenotypes, and reducing drug delivery.
- Altered tissue mechanics may play a role in cancer development and premalignant disease; this is evidenced by the links between mammographic density and breast cancer incidence
- CAFs are a substantial source of growth factors, cytokines, and exosomes which, can promote tumor growth and regulate therapy responses. For example, fibroblast growth factor (FGF5), leukemia inhibitory factor (LIF), growth arrest-specific protein 6 (GAS6), TGF β, hepatocyte growth factor (HGF) promotes invasion and proliferative behavior in cancer cells.
- CAFs via cytokines and chemokines act on leukocytes, including CD+8 T cells, regulatory T (Treg) and macrophages, with both immunosuppressive and immunopromoting outcomes.
- Consensus from recent work is that the predominant effect of CAFs is immunosuppressive with IL-6, CXC-chemokine 9 (CXCL9) and TGFβ having well-established roles in reducing T cell responses.
- Antigen cross presentation by CAFs has been recently observed, and this may lead to CD+4 T cell activation and suppression of CD+8 T cells
- IL-6 may promote immunosuppression via systemic effects on metabolism
- Interference with the action of CXCL12 produced by CAFs promotes T cell mediated tumor control and targeting focal adhesion kinase (FAK) in cancer cells concomitantly reduces stromal fibroblast activation and the development of an immunosuppressive environment
- CAFs and cancer cells exchange metabolites and amino acids, which is an additional avenue by which stromal fibroblasts, interact with tumor cells
- Autophagy in stromal fibroblasts can generate alanine, which is used by pancreatic ductal adenocarcinoma (PDAC) cells to fuel the tricarboxylic acid (TCA) cycle.
- Metabolic dysregulation of CAFs is linked to altered immunoregulation, possibly through IL-6 production or depletion of immunomodulating amino acids.
- Both conventional DNA damaging chemotherapy and radiotherapy can trigger changes in CAF biology and fibrosis is a common late side effect of radiotherapy. Conventional chemotherapies, radiotherapy and target agents can promote the generation of CAFs, modulate their function, and lead to therapy resistance
- An appealing clinical strategy is to make CAFs more "normal," such as, targeting of the vitamin D receptor in pancreatic cancer. Treatment with vitamin D receptor ligand caused activated stellate cells (stellate cells are quiescent fibroblasts) to revert to a more quiescent state and reduced disease aggressiveness

Data from Sahai E, Astsaturov I, Werb ZA. Framework for advancing our understanding of cancer-associated fibroblasts. *Nature Reviews*. Cancer, 2020;20:174–186; A complete list of all references for this box are found in this review article.

and with nasopharyngeal carcinoma, a cancer endemic in Chinese populations in Southeast Asia. HHV8 is linked to the development of Kaposi sarcoma, a cancer that was once seen primarily in older men but now occurs in a markedly more virulent form in immunosuppressed individuals, especially those with acquired immunodeficiency syndrome (AIDS). HHV8 also has been linked to several rare lymphomas. Human T-cell lymphotropic virus type 1 (HTLV-1) is an oncogenic retrovirus linked to the development of adult T-cell leukemia and lymphoma (ATLL). HTLV is transmitted vertically (that is, inherited by children from infected parents) and horizontally (e.g., by breastfeeding, sexual intercourse, blood transfusions, and exposure to infected needles). Infection with HTLV may be asymptomatic, and only a small fraction of infected individuals progress to ATLL, often many years after acquiring the virus. Immunization has proven beneficial in preventing viral-induced cancers. Merkel cell polyomavirus is associated with a rare skin cancer or Merkle cell carcinoma.

Evading Immune Destruction

Based on the processes of adaptive immunity, cancer cells are abnormal and should be recognized and removed from the body (see Chapter 8). The *immune surveillance hypothesis* predicts that most developing malignancies are suppressed by an efficient immune response against antigens found on cancer cells. Tumor-specific antigens are found only on cancer cells and include antigens from oncogenic viruses and altered glycoproteins and glycolipids (neoantigens). When present, tumor-specific antigens are processed by the tumor cell and presented on the cell surface by major histocompatibility complex (MHC) class I molecules and are targets of CD8+ T-cytotoxic cells (Tc cells) (Fig. 12.19) (see Chapter 8). NK cells recognize altered cell surface glycoproteins and glycolipids (see Chapter 7). Thus, cancer cells should be recognized as foreign and destroyed by the immune system. There is evidence to support the immune surveillance hypothesis, primarily based on the observance that individuals who are

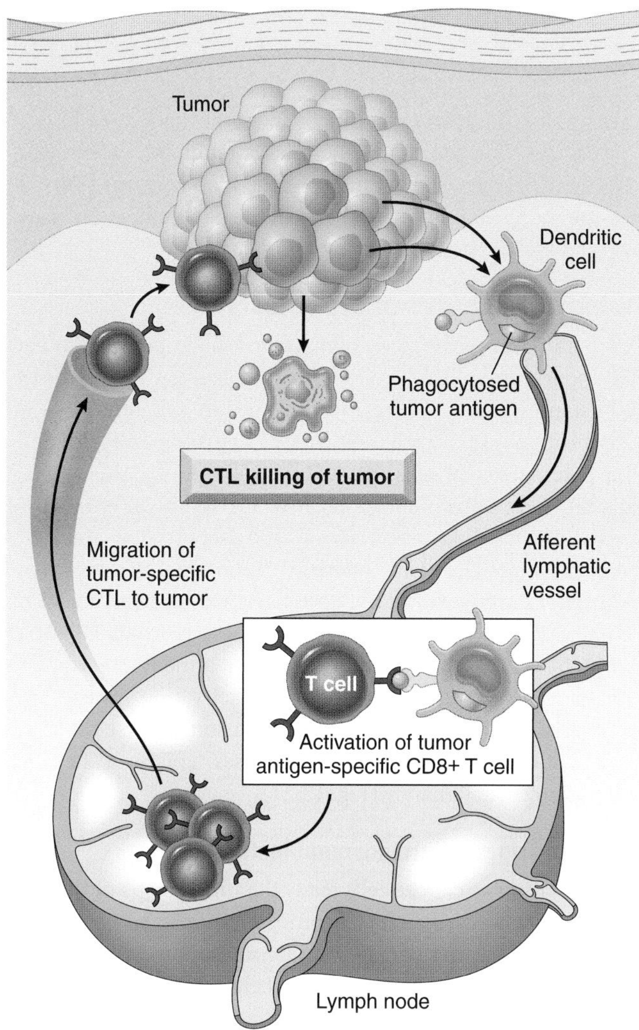

Fig. 12.19 Tumor Antigens and Induction of CD8+ Cytotoxic T cell Response. Dendritic cells and macrophages in the tumor microenvironment ingest tumor cells or released tumor antigens and migrate to draining lymph nodes. Here, they present the antigens in the context of major histocompatibility complex (MHC) class II molecules and from the process called *cross-presentation*, from MHC class I molecules, enabling the tumor antigens to be recognized by naive CD8+ cytotoxic T lymphocytes *(CTLs)*. CTLs have the ability to kill tumor cells. (From Kumar et al., 2021 modified from Abbas AK, Lichtman AH. *Cellular and molecular immunology*, 8th edition. Philadelphia: Elsevier; 2017.)

significantly immunosuppressed (e.g., after organ transplantation) have an increased risk for cancers of the skin, head and neck, lung, liver, and colon as well as lymphomas and leukemias. However, the incidence of these cancers in immunocompromised individuals is less than would be predicted if immune surveillance is highly effective. This discrepancy is the result of cancer cells having developed multiple mechanisms to evade the immune system including (1) absence of tumor-specific antigens, (2) lack of appropriate antigen processing and presentation and (3) production of immunosuppressive factors and activation of inhibitory molecules on immune cells (Fig. 12.20). As cancer cells proliferate, clonal development of immune-resistant variants arises. The link between these escape mechanisms and current cancer treatment is discussed in detail later in this chapter.

Although some cancer cells do express tumor-specific antigens that can be recognized by the immune system, most cancer cells do not, and those that do most often present antigens that are undetectable by the immune system (see Fig. 12.20).[59] These cells can hide or mutate their surface antigens so that Tc and NK cells cannot recognize them. Tumor vaccination is a form of cancer treatment used to make the cancer cells antigenically detectable by the immune system.[60]

Even if the adaptive immune system is activated in the presence of a cancer, tumors are able to produce immunosuppressive factors that suppress or subvert the immune response (see Fig. 12.20). For example, many tumors have an abundance of tumor-infiltrating lymphocytes (TILs). Although the immune cells frequently found in tumors were once thought to be futile attempts at an antitumor response; instead, it appears that cancers actively recruit an immune and stromal response to assist in remodeling of tissues, formation of new blood vessels, and

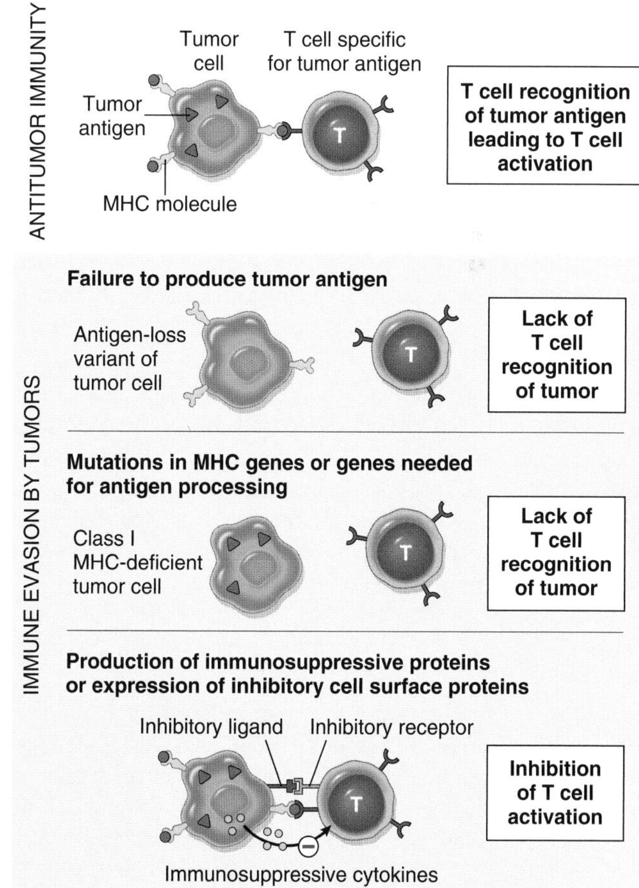

Fig. 12.20 Mechanisms by Which Tumor Cells Evade the Immune System. Tumors may evade the immune response by losing expression of antigens or major histocompatibility complex *(MHC)* molecules or by producing immunosuppressive cytokines or ligands for inhibitory receptors on T cells. (From Kumar V, et al. *Robbins and Cotran pathologic basis of disease*, 10th edition. Philadelphia: Elsevier; 2021.)

promotion of metastasis. The predominant TILs are T-regulatory (Treg) cells.[41] Treg cells are CD4+ cells that differentiate under the control of specific cytokines, primarily TGF-β (see Chapter 8). The role of Treg cells during wound healing is to control or limit the immune response to protect the host's own tissues against autoimmune reactions. Their role in tumors is manipulated to prevent a destructive antitumor immune response and provide cytokines that facilitate tumor cell proliferation and spread.[61] Treg cells and TAMs, as well as other stromal cells, produce very high levels of TGF-β and interleukin-10 (IL-10). IL-10 is an immunosuppressive cytokine, which generally decreases T-helper cell 1 (Th1) and Th2 activity, suppresses antigen recognition and cell proliferation by Th cells, and suppresses the capacity of CD8+ T-cytotoxic (Tcyto) cells to recognize, proliferate, and kill tumor cells. The goal of current immunotherapy regimens is to reverse this relationship and facilitate T-cell–mediated cancer cell death (discussed later in this chapter). The release of immunosuppressive factors into the tumor microenvironment also increases resistance of the tumor to chemotherapy and radiotherapy. Increased levels of Treg cells in blood and lymph nodes and infiltrating the tumor correlate with poor outcomes in breast and GI tumors. In advanced non–small cell lung cancer, an elevated ratio of Treg to Tcyto cells is related to a poor response to platinum-based chemotherapy. Immunosuppressive cytokines additionally lower the cancer cell's sensitivity to immune-mediated death (see Fig. 12.19). Adoptive T cell transfer is a cancer treatment in which lymphocytes are removed from the affected individual and activated or modified so that when they are reinfused, they attack the tumor.[62]

Immune cells have surface molecules whose purpose is to activate (co-stimulatory factors) or suppress (co-inhibitory factors) immune responses to antigens (see Chapter 8). Co-inhibitory molecules are often called immune *checkpoints*. Cancer cells may suppress T cells by binding to immune checkpoints, causing the lymphocyte to turn off its attack (see Fig. 12.20). An example is the checkpoint programed cell death receptor 1 (PD-1) binding with programmed cell death ligand-1 (PDL-1). Checkpoint inhibitors are a group of immunotherapy drugs that block this interaction, thus reactivating the immune cell to attack the tumor (see Immunotherapy section)[63]

With increasing heterogeneity of cells within the tumor, subpopulations of antigen-negative cancer cell variants may selectively outgrow more immune-sensitive cells. Variants may suppress the production of particular antigens or suppress levels of antigen-presenting MHC class I. Other cytokines appear to increase the cancer cells' resistance to apoptosis. For example, the Th2 cytokine IL-4 increases the resistance of thyroid cancer to chemotherapy; IL-6 produced by Th cells, adipocytes, and fibroblasts activates survival pathways in breast cancer leading to resistance to radiotherapy; and adipocytes enhance the transcription of the anti-apoptotic factor Bcl-2 in leukemia cells. Current chemotherapeutic regimens seek to kill as many cancer cells as possible so that there is less likelihood for the development of more resistant variants; however, toxicity of these treatments limits their effectiveness.

ACTIVATING INVASION AND METASTASIS

Metastasis is the spread of cancer cells from the site of the original tumor to distant tissues and organs through the body. Metastasis is a defining characteristic of cancer and is the main cause of death from cancer. The process of metastases requires cancer cells to leave their primary site, circulate in the bloodstream, withstand pressure in the blood vessels, thrive in the new cellular surroundings, and escape "destruction" by immune cells.[64–66]

Biologic Processes of Metastasis

New paradigms in the study of metastasis have identified molecular underpinnings of the dissemination process.[64] An improved understanding of how the invading tumor cell interacts with other proteins and cells has elucidated new biological principles by which metastatic cells regulate their mobility and plasticity.[64] Unfortunately, communications with the tumor microenvironment allow invading cancer cells to conquer stromal challenges, settle, and colonize.[64] Characteristics are driven by genetics and epigenetic changes within the tumor cell itself and its microenvironment.[64] It is critical to understand these mechanisms of the metastatic process to develop successful treatment interventions. Hanahan and Weinberg identify that "activating invasion and metastasis" is a hallmark of cancer.[3] Invasion of close tissue and seeding at distant sites to form metastases remains a "key" feature of cancer malignancy (Fig. 12.21).

The Main Trigger: Chromosomal Instability

Dissemination of cancer cells leads the initial steps of the invasion-metastasis cascade.[67] Chromosomal instability becomes the "trigger" causing constant and continuous errors in chromosome segregation during mitosis (Fig. 12.22). Abnormalities in chromosome segregation cause the rupture of micronuclei and the secretion of genomic DNA into the surrounding cytosol. This cytosolic DNA then activates sensing pathways such as cyclic GMP-AMP synthase-stimulator of interferon (IFN genes) and downstream nuclear factor κ-light chain-enhancer of activated B (NF-κB) signaling.[68]

Investigators suggest that the nature of the primary seeding cancer cell determines the various and different metastatic properties aligned with growth and response to therapy.[69]

Both in vivo and in vitro studies show that metastatic cancer cells migrate individually.[70] In humans, however, it is believed that seeding requires the joint action of a cluster of tumor cells moving together,[71] which now highlights epithelial-mesenchymal transition (EMT).

Epithelial-Mesenchymal Transition (EMT)

EMT is the developmental (transdifferentiation) process whereby transformed epithelial cells lose their cell polarity and cell-cell adhesion, and gain the ability to invade, resist stress, and disseminate. Usually, epithelial cells are immobile and tightly bound to each other by tight junctions, gap junctions, and adherens junctions and to the neighboring EMC.[72] EMT is a reversible biochemical process that permits a specific epithelial cell to attain a mesenchymal phenotype, such as a stem cell, which is critical for cancer progression and

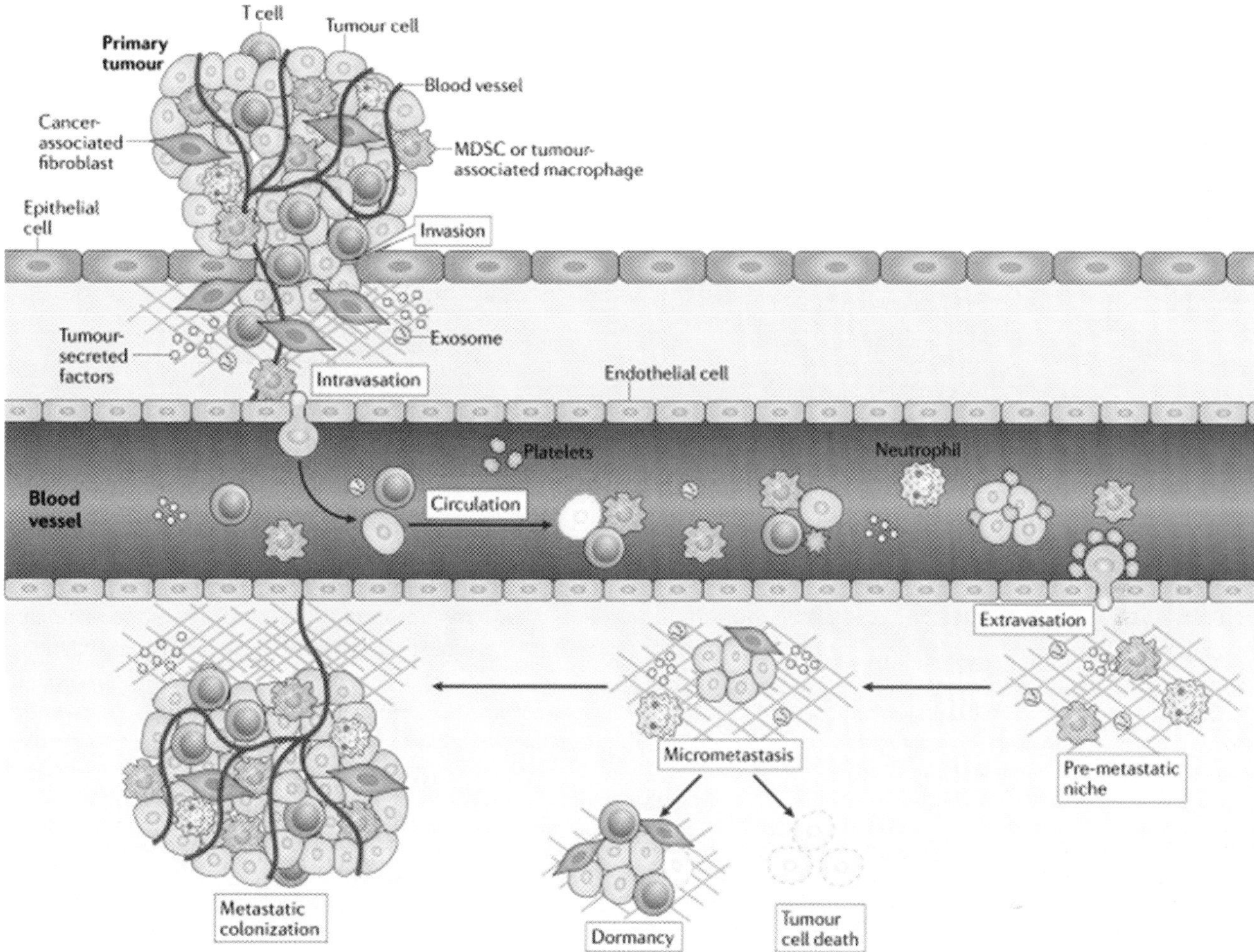

Fig. 12.21 Metastasis. Metastasis is complex with many steps. The key steps of metastasis include invasion, intravasation, circulation, extravasation, and colonization. (From Anderson RL, Balasas T, Callaghan J, et al. A framework for the development of effective antimetastatic agents. *Nature Reviews. Clinical Oncology*, 2019;16:185–204. https://doi.org/10.1038/s41571-018-0134-8.)

metastasis (Fig. 12.23). Thus, EMT involves profound morphological and phenotypic changes to a cell. From the study of using a mouse model of breast cancer, the determinant of metastasis is the availability of asparagine synthetase, a metabolic enzyme.[73] Decreasing the level of asparagine through L-asparaginase treatment through dietary restriction decreased metastatic spread. Thus, asparagine availability promoted EMT. It is now known that the EMT program is a spectrum of *transitional stages* between the epithelial and mesenchymal phenotypes and not full-epithelial and full-mesenchymal phenotypes.[74] The transition is assisted by growth factors and signaling pathways. A spontaneous EMT in primary tumor cells shifts between different intermediate states with different invasive, metastatic, and differentiation characteristics.[75] Importantly, tumor cells that express a mix of epithelial and mesenchymal phenotypes are more effective in circulating, colonization at the secondary site, and the development of metastasis.[75] The various stages possess diverse cellular characteristics, chromatin landscapes, and gene expression signatures that are regulated by common and distinct transcription factors and signaling pathways. The various EMT stages are present in varied microenvironments and are in contact with diverse stromal cells.[75] For example, tumor cells with the most marked mesenchymal phenotype proliferate near endothelial cell and inflammatory cells.[75] These metastatic cells release large quantities of chemokines and proteins to attract immune cells and stimulate angiogenesis, thereby promoting the development of a unique inflammatory and very vascularized niche.[75] CAFs can also drive and direct cancer cell migration though fibronectin alignment.[76] The triggers for EMT in cancer cells include hypoxia, metabolic stressors, and matrix stiffness.[77,78] Transcription factors are programmed to repress epithelial genes and activate mesenchymal genes.[79] Epigenetic and posttranslational modulators also play a crucial role in controlling the EMT process.[74]

Despite these associations between cancer metastasis and EMT, controversy remains as to whether EMT plays a key role in cancer metastasis and resistance to chemotherapy.[79–81] For example, research in pancreatic and lung cancers reveals that EMT might not be essential for metastasis but it does contribute to chemoresistance.[80,82] Much more evidence is needed on this important issue.

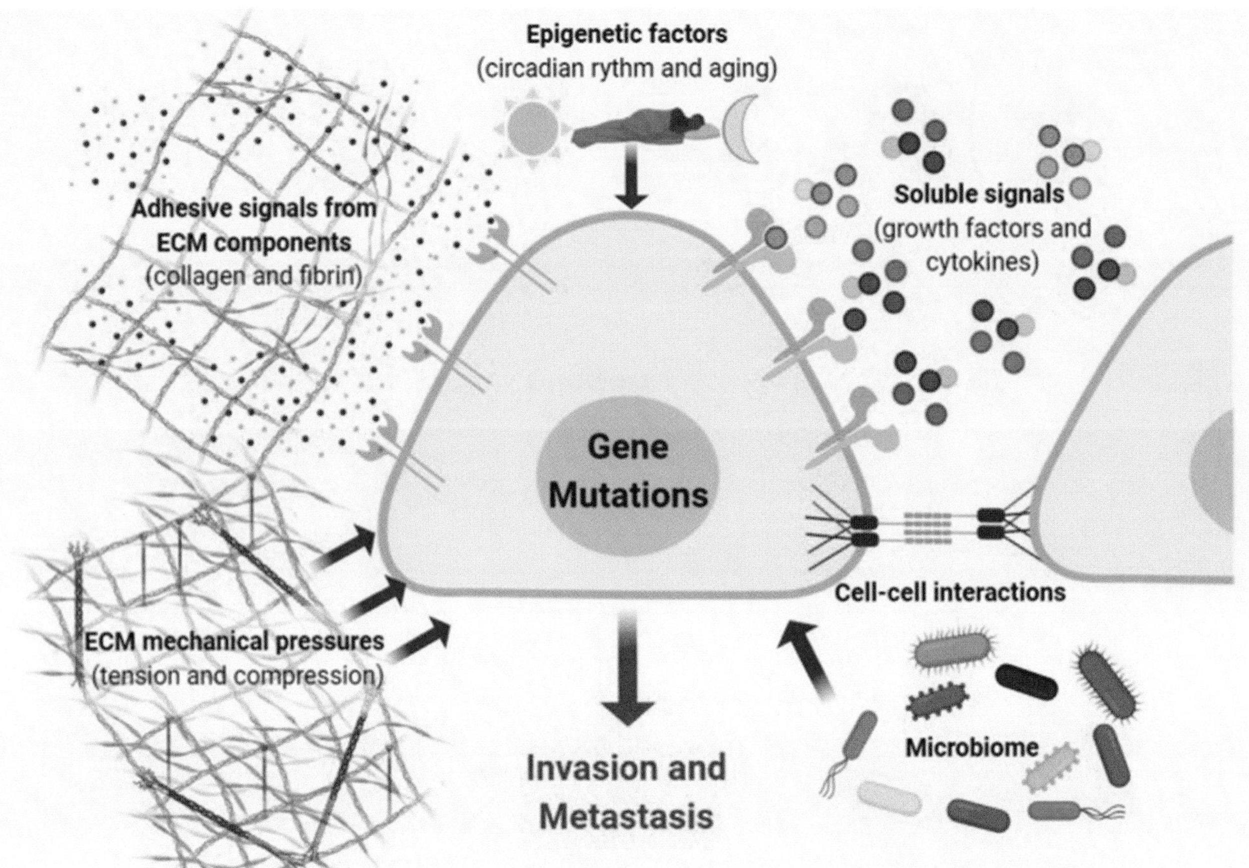

Fig. 12.22 Determinants of Metastases. Invasion and metastasis is triggered by epigenetic factors induced by environmental stimuli, such as aging, circadian disruptions, and many others; adhesive signals from the extracellular matrix *(ECM)* constituents, such as collagen and fibrin; ECM mechanical pressures, including tension and compression; cell-interactions; soluble signals, such as growth factors and cytokines; and the intratumoral microbiota. (Data from Fares J, Fares MY, Khachfe HH, et al. Molecular principles of metastasis: a hallmark of cancer revisited. *Signal Transduction Target Therapy,* 2020;5:28.)

Although the initiation of metastasis may involve EMT, mesenchymal-epithelial transition (MET) is necessary for metastatic progression.[64] E-selectin in the bone vasculature induces MET and WNT (signaling pathway) activation in cancer cells to drive metastatic tumor development.[83]

Metastatic Cells and Genetics

Various metastatic cells possess different genetic and epigenetic or phenotypic changes, which differentially drive tumor progression, metastasis, and drug resistance.[84] A "metastatic genetic signature" is suggested because hundreds of genes are reported associated with invasive potential.[85–87] Predominant genes somatically altered in metastatic cells include TP53, CDKN2A, PTEN, PIK3CA, and RB1.[88,89] Germline pathogenic variants were present in 12.2% of cases, and 75% were associated with DNA repair defects.[88]

Markers that predict metastatic progression have shown that advanced cancers arise from many different cell types, which significantly affects the eventual genetic and epigenetic alterations that promote metastasis.[90] These differences help explain why some cancer cells respond to treatment and others do not. It is critical to understand intertumoral heterogeneity because it can reveal the mechanisms of metastatic progression and how the cell type of origin is related to tumor development.[64] Nonetheless, the cytotoxic immune signature and the presence of lymphatic vessels plays an essential role in cancer metastasis (see Immune Environment at the Primary Site and Metastasis).

Metabolic Metabolism of Metastatic Cells

Genetic expression is affected by oxygen homeostasis in the tumor microenvironment.[91] Hypoxia-inducible factors (HIF) enable cancer cells to adapt to their environment by modulating angiogenesis, EMT, invasion, metastasis, and energy metabolism.[3,64] HIF signaling drives the secretion of lysyl oxidase (LOX). LOX-like proteins, and exosomes, develop a pro-metastatic environment in the lungs and bones of individuals with breast cancer.[77,92] Hypoxic factors and other factors are associated with tumor aggressiveness and resistance to therapy.[93] Tumors with more extensive hypoxia and anoxic areas exhibit higher rates of metastasis and a poor prognosis.[64] Metabolic

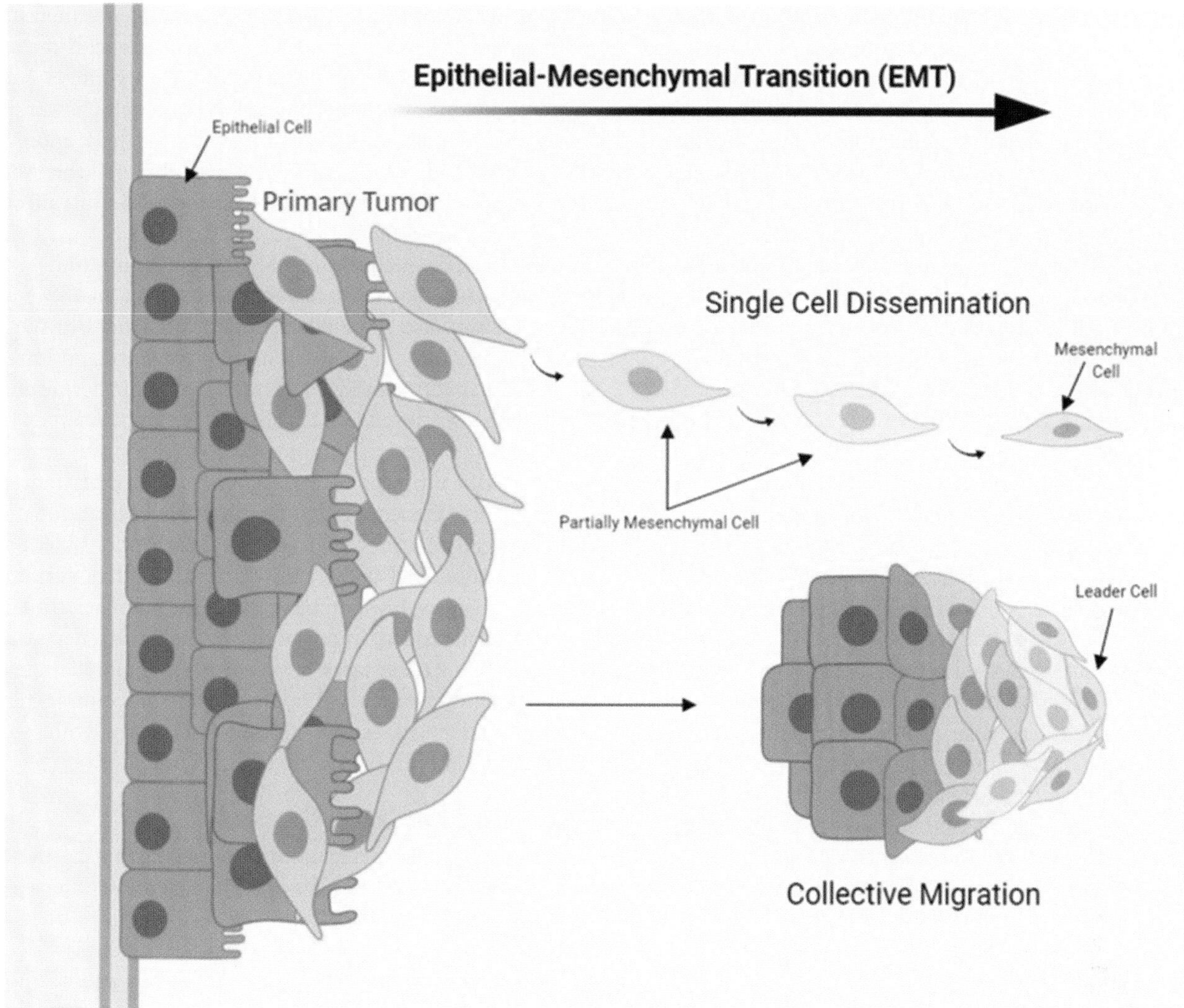

Fig. 12.23 Epithelial-Mesenchymal Transition (EMT). EMT occurs through either single cell dissemination or collective migration. The process has several transition stages between the initial epithelial cell and the invasive mesenchymal cell. (Data from Fares J, Fares MY, Khachfe HH, et al. Molecular principles of metastasis: a hallmark of cancer revisited. *Signal Transduction Target Therapy*, 2020;5:28. doi: 10.1038/s41392-020-0134-x, 2020.)

differences among cancer cells lead to differences in metastatic behavior, and metastatic cells depend on mono-carboxylate transporter 1 (MCT1) to handle oxidative stress.[64] Highly metastatic cells have increased levels of MCT1 and inhibition of MCT1 decreases their metastatic potential.[94] Changes in ATP/ADP and ATP/AMP ratios promote metastatic behavior.[95]

Priming the Premetastatic Niche

Invading cancer cells require a permissive environment before metastasis can be established. This environment is achieved through the active priming of secondary sites by the primary tumor. The host microenvironment called the premetastatic niche (PMN) is primed by the primary tumor even before the initiation of metastasis.[96] The development of PMN is a multistep process that involves secretory factors and extracellular vesicles that cause vascular leakage, ECM remodeling, and immunosuppression in the secondary sites, thus promoting the ability of cancer cells to successfully establish metastasis.[96] Amazingly, high-definition microscopes have obtained images of cancer cells sharing biological material with less malignant cells, making these cells more malignant.[97] Tumor cells release vesicles that carry messenger RNA transcribed from genes that are involved in cell migration and metastasis, which are then received by cells in the PMN.[97] Once a non-cancerous cell engulfs these vesicles they start to migrate faster.[97] The transferred genes enhance the ability of cells to invade other organs.[97] Metastatic characteristics are transferred through extracellular vesicle exchange.[97]

Extracellular vesicles called exosomes transfer invasion-promoting factors from the primary tumor, such as miRNAs, to tumorigenic cancer cells.[98–100] For example, miR-10b is carried and released by exosomes driving metastatic properties in breast cancer cells.[101] Exosomes secrete EMT inducers that stimulate EMT progression in host epithelial cells, enabling them to invade and metastasize.[102–107] Additionally, exosomes can assist remodeling the ECM by communicating with fibroblasts, stromal cells, and endothelial cells to degrade components such as collagen, laminin, and fibronectin.[108] ECM altered by exosomes exhibits increased stromal cell proliferation, cancer cell migration and survival, and tumor cell resistance to apoptotic signals. These changes plus effects of growth factors and chemokines, leads to the formation of a new microenvironment for cancer cells, immune cells, and other stromal elements, known as the PMN,[109–112] where metastatic cells may arrest, extravasate, and later colonize.[113–115] Exosomes drive cancer cell organotropism or metastatic bias toward certain organs. The preference originates from exosome eagerness or avidity for specific host cells.[102] Exosome proteomic expression of bone cancer revealed different integrin patterns and specific integrins (α6β4 and α6β1) were associated with lung metastasis and αvβ5 was associated with liver metastasis.[116] Targeting integrins decreased exosome uptake and lung and liver metastasis.[116] Various membrane proteins and lipids associated with ECM properties and adhesion influence the specific targeting of exosomes to their specific host cells.[116–120]

Exosome-mediated metastasis is not just dependent upon tumor-released exosomes. For example, astrocyte-derived exosomes mediate the intercellular transfer of miRNAs that target the PTEN tumor suppressor gene to metastatic cancer cells, advancing invasion and brain metastasis.[121] This leads to increased secretion of CCL2, which recruits myeloid cells, increasing the outgrowth of brain metastatic cells and reducing the effect of apoptotic signaling.[121] Inhibition of astrocytic exosome release prevents PTEN loss and inhibits brain metastasis.[121]

Epigenetic Factors in Metastasis

Chromatin and associated epigenetic mechanisms stabilize gene expression, cellular states, and appropriate responses to developmental or environmental cues.[122] Genetic, environmental, and metabolic conditions influence chromatin to become permissive or "plastic" states. Chromatin alterations can induce cells to gain oncogenic characteristics. Researchers are studying the specific effects of epigenetic *plasticity* when *permissive* chromatin induces oncogenic expression to promote metastatic development.[122] Approximately 50% of human cancers have mutations in chromatin proteins.[123,124] Malignant cells exhibit epigenetic changes such as genome-wide alterations in DNA methylation, chromatin structures, and regulatory element activities. Also, many tumors exhibit altered developmental programs indicative of differentiation block or epigenetic reprogramming.[125–127] The overriding premise is that specific genetic, environmental, and metabolic stimuli disrupt the homeostatic balance of chromatin, causing it to become either aberrantly restrictive or aberrantly permissive. Thus, chromatin is switchable. Such stimuli may act in a pre-malignant cell to promote tumor initiation and in a malignant cell to accelerate tumor evolution and adaptation.[122] This model is critical to understand as it can explain *diverse* oncogenic stimuli whose effects are mediated through chromatin aberrations. The pervasiveness of such stimuli suggests that epigenetic defects contribute to *diverse* aspects of cancer biology and may, in fact, satisfy every hallmark of cancer.[2,3]

One example of how epigenetics may influence metastasis is with cutaneous melanoma. Older individuals with melanoma exhibit different patterns of metastasis than younger cohorts. Older individuals with melanoma tend to develop fewer metastases in proximal sentinel lymph nodes but have more distal metastases and worse survival than that of the younger cohorts.[128] Aging is a process (often stated as stimuli) affected by chromatin and epigenetic processes, such as DNA methylation. Aging also is characterized by alterations in immunity and the motility of immune cells leading to changes in the immune microenvironment. Age-related physical changes in the ECM inhibit or promote tumor cell motility, invasion, and metastasis.[64] From in vitro studies, increased lymphatic permeability of endothelial membranes was shown to be the reason as lymph nodes of older cohorts exhibited less ECM complexity in comparison with those of younger cohorts with metastatic melanoma.[128,129] Further study revealed that hyaluronan and proteoglycan link protein 1 (*HAPLN1*) is responsible for controlling endothelial permeability.[128,129] These data suggest age-related changes in tumor phenotype (epigenetics) drive lymphatic metastasis. Importantly, the biological effects of aging on patterns of metastases have not been explored sufficiently and has significant clinical implications. For example, regional lymphatic metastases are treated frequently with surgery, whereas distant metastases are often incurable.[128]

Microbiome and Cancer Metastasis

Bacteria have been detected in tumors constituting the *tumor microbiome*.[64] Microbes have been reported to confer vulnerability to specific cancers; however, no links have been established to patient outcome or survival.[130] Bacteria selectively translocate to tumors rich in vascular vessels and chemotactic pressures. Anaerobic and facultative bacteria survive well in hypoxic tumor microenvironments.[131,132]

Tumoral bacteria are metabolically active and can change the chemical structure of chemotherapeutic agents affecting the response to treatment.[133,134] For example, gammaproteobacteria in pancreatic tumors confer resistance to gemcitabine, a common drug used in GI cancers.[133–136] Fap2 protein of Fusobacterium prevents the activation of NK cells, protecting the tumor cells of adenocarcinoma cell lines.[137] Some bacteria stimulate antitumoral immunity; others cause immunosuppression, contributing to the response of immunotherapy.[131,138,278–282]

Circadian Cycle and Dietary Effects on Tumorigenesis

Importantly, the circadian clock controls a wide spectrum of processes in cellular physiology through metabolic and gene expression pathways. It has been associated with cancer initiation and progression.[64] Epidemiological studies of night-shift workers, meal timing, and exposure to light have linked circadian patterns to tumorigenesis,[139–145] revealing that an active epigenetic mechanism may be responsible for genome alterations.[64]

Alterations in transcription complexes and cellular metabolism drive cancer progression by affecting cancer cell interactions with the microenvironment.[146] The MYC oncogene plays a role in cyclical metabolism in osteosarcoma cells resulting in increased consumption of glucose and glutamine.[147] Several circadian regulating genes have been linked to MYC expression.[64]

Diet has also been shown to impact cancer metastasis. Some of these dietary effects may be related to changes in the microbiome. Other effects are more direct. For example, as stated previously, asparagine is an important promotor of metastasis, and researchers have found that removing asparagine from the diet of mice reduced breast cancer metastases.[73] CD36+ metastasis-initiating cells rely on palmitic acid, a dietary lipid, to promote metastasis and blocking CD36+ inhibits metastatic ability.[148] These and other emerging data suggest that diet affects the metastatic potential of metastasis-initiating cells.[149]

Invasive Cancer Cells: Remodeling the Extracellular Matrix

The extracellular matrix (ECM) is a scaffold, the interstitial matrix forms porous three-dimensional networks around cells that interconnect cells in the stroma and can connect to the basement membrane (see Chapter 1). Tissues are dynamically shaped by bidirectional communication between resident cells and the ECM through cell-matrix interactions and ECM remodeling.[150] The interstitial matrix assures the structural integrity of tissues and organs and modulates cellular processes such as cell differentiation and migration.[150] The interstitial matrix is composed of collagens, fibronectin, and elastin. Amount and composition of the interstitial matrix vary between tissue types, between microenvironments within the same tissue and can be remodeled in response to stress or trauma such as wound repair or tissue regeneration.[151] In cancer, remodeling of the interstitial ECM causes a broad range of biophysical and biochemical changes affecting cell signaling, ECM stiffness, cell migration, and tumor progression.[152] Contrastingly, the basement membrane is more stable, sheetlike, dense, and lines the basal surface of, for example, epithelial and endothelial cells, surrounds muscle cells and adipocytes, and separates tissues into different, well-organized compartments.[150] Binding of cells to the basement membrane is critical for establishing cell polarity (see Fig. 1.12D) and crucial for several developmental processes and maintenance of tissue homeostasis.[153]

Remodeling of the basement membrane is required for cancer cells to invade stromal tissue and become a malignant tumor.[154] Changes in the ECM are a result of different remodeling mechanisms that can be divided into four major processes: (1) ECM deposition, which refers to changing the abundance and composition of ECM components, which affect biochemical and mechanical ECM properties; (2) chemical modification at the post-translational level, which alters biochemical and structural properties of the ECM; (3) proteolytic degradation from ECM-degrading enzymes called *matrikines* are released to remodel the ECM, re-establish an appropriate functional meshwork, and maintain tissue homeostasis; and (4) force-mediated physical remodeling, which affects ECM organization by aligning ECM fibers and opening up passages for cell migration.[150] It comes as no surprise that ECM remodeling becomes dysregulated in pathologic conditions such as inflammatory diseases, tissue fibrosis, and cancer.[155]Cancer cells and tumor-associated stromal cells modify all four ECM remodeling mechanisms, hijacking the normal matrix into a cancer-supporting matrix or niche that actively contributes to the pathology of the tumor (Fig. 12.24).

Tumor cells themselves show altered expression of ECM components, such as collagens I and III and ECM-modifying enzymes such as LOX and LOX-like proteins (see Fig. 12.24A). In healthy tissue and tumors, the key producers of ECM in the interstitial matrix are fibroblasts, specifically when activated and transformed to myofibroblasts. Chondrocytes and osteoblasts are also important depending on the context and tissue.[156] Myofibroblasts have a combined phenotypic characteristic of fibroblasts and smooth muscle cells; they secrete ECM and exert contractile functions allowing mechanical alterations of the geography of the ECM.[150] Activation of myofibroblasts is triggered by inflammation resulting in the secretion of TGF-β.[157]

Sustained inflammatory stimuli and subsequent TGF-β secretion by immune cells, such as macrophages and tumor cells can produce deregulated, hyperproliferative and overactive myofibroblasts that are the major offender in pathologic conditions such as fibrosis and cancer.[158] Tumor-derived activation factors induce the differentiation of stromal cells towards CAFs, which function as myofibroblasts and remodel the ECM to support tumor growth.[45,158–160]

An important step in invasion is the disassembly of the ECM and its constituents through enzymes such as MMPs.[161] MMPs have a significant role in cell proliferation, immune response, angiogenesis, and survival.[154,158,162] They are associated with poor prognosis.[163,164] Remodeling of the ECM by cancer cells drives cancer growth.[64] ECM is complex, and numerous specific cells and matrikines engage in invasion and metastasis.

Autophagy and Cancer Cell Invasion

Autophagy is a self-degradative or catabolic process that targets cellular contents to the lysosomal compartment for degradation (see Chapter 2).[165] Autophagy is initiated by the advancement of several cancers to metastasis. In vivo studies reveal that autophagy participates in modulating tumor cell motility and invasion, cancer stem viability and differentiation, resistance to anoikis (apoptosis in cells upon loss of attachment to the ECM), EMT, metastatic cell dormancy, and escape from immune surveillance at the primary site (Fig. 12.25).[165] Many attributes of these autophagy-dependent changes during acquisition of invasiveness possibly contribute to the ability of disseminating cells to intravasate, survive, and migrate in the circulation before extravasating at secondary sites. Autophagy, at the secondary site, is required to maintain tumor cells in a dormant state, probably through its ability to promote quiescence and a stem cell phenotype linked to tumor cell survival and drug resistance.[165] From laboratory studies, inhibition of autophagy significantly reduced tumor cell invasion.[64,166]

Neurons and Metastasis

How nerves emerge in the tumor microenvironment and just what their function is have always been mysteries. Recently, investigators found neural progenitors from the central nervous system that express doublecortin infiltrate in prostate tumors and metastases.[167] These progenitors initiate neurogenesis

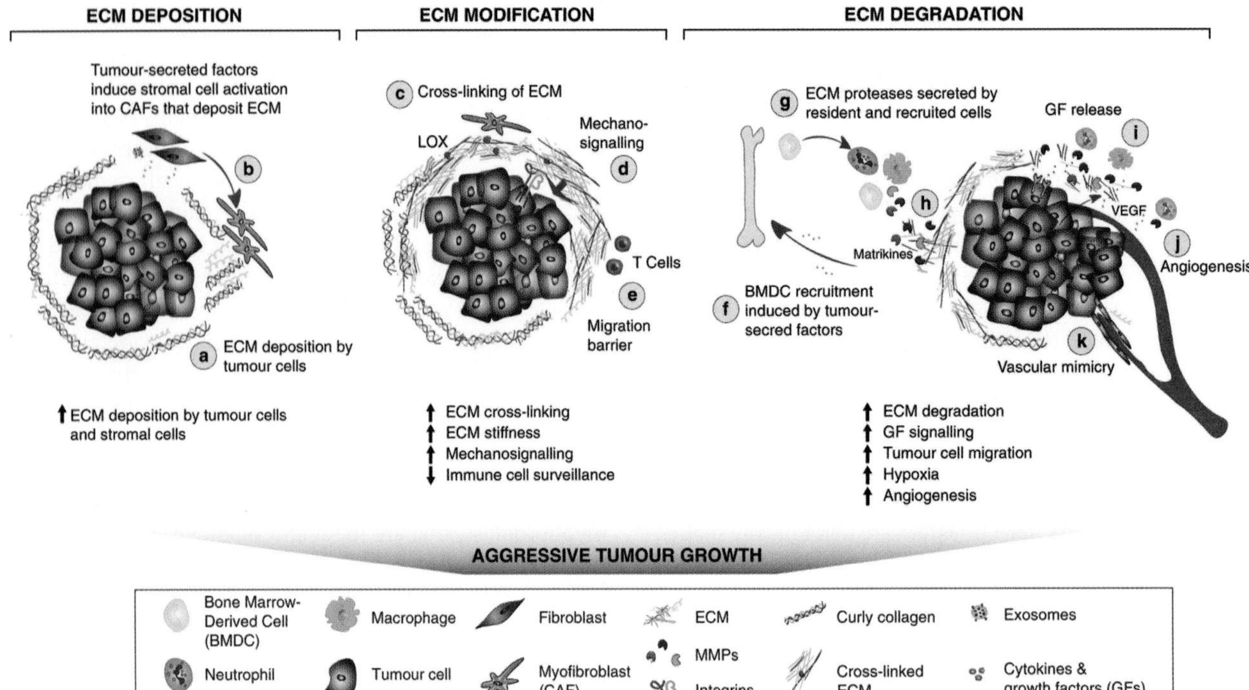

Fig. 12.24 Extracellular Matrix Remodeling in the Primary Tumor. (**a and b**) Tumor-derived factors activate stromal cells which differentiate into cancer-associated fibroblasts *(CAFs)*, which leads to the secretion and deposition of large amounts of extracellular matrix *(ECM)* constituents along with the cancer cells. **(c)** ECM-modifying enzymes such as lysyl oxidase *(LOX)* expressed by tumor cells and CAFs cross-link and align collagen fibers, which increases matrix stiffness around the tumor and **(d)** the formation of a physical barrier to evade immune surveillance by T-cells. **(e)** Increased matrix stiffness promotes the interaction between ECM constituents and cell-surface receptors on tumor cells that triggers mechanosignaling mediated by integrins. **(f)** In order to sustain a tumorigenic microenvironment, tumor cells and resident immune cells secrete cytokines, chemokines, and growth factors (GFs), which differentiate and recruit bone marrow-derived cells (BMDCs). **(g)** The BMDCs, CAFs and tumor cells secrete ECM-degrading proteases, including MMPs, which are cell surface-bound (e.g., MT1-MMP) or secreted (e.g., MMP-9). **(h)** Proteolytic ECM degradation generates bioactive matrikines and **(i)** releases matrix-bound GFs. These factors induce pro-tumorigenic ECM signaling that promotes tumor proliferation, migration, invasion, and angiogenesis. **(j)** Altogether the changes to the ECM create a hypoxic environment. Neutrophils secrete potent MMP-9 that degrades ECM and releases matrix-bound VEGF that forms a concentration gradient for new angiogenic sprouting. **(k)** Stimulated by dense ECM, the tumor cells can gain endothelial-like functions and mimic the vasculature that connects to blood vessels. (Data from Winkler J, Abisoye-Ogunniyan A, Metcalf KJ, et al. Concepts of extracellular matrix remodelling in tumour progression and metastasis. *Nature Communications*, 2020;11:5120. https://doi.org/10.1038/s41467-020-18794-x.)

(neurons produced from neural stem cells).[168] Importantly, nerve fibers in the tumor microenvironment regulate cancer initiation and dissemination, mandating much further research on targeting doublecortin-expressing neurons for treatment.

Immune Environment at the Primary Site and Metastasis

The immune environment surrounding the tumor plays a significant role in dictating the metastatic potential of the disseminating cells.[64] An investigation of about 800 people with colorectal cancer compared people with whose tumors were metastatic with those whose tumors were not.[169] Both groups had analogous mutation patterns in cancer genes; but tumors that had fewer cytotoxic T cells had metastasized.[169] The invasive ends of the spread tumor cells had reduced densities of lymphatic vessels that transport immune cells.[169] These changes contribute to metastasis and suggest immunotherapies that augment T-cell responses can stop metastasis in people with early-stage cancer.[170] Silencing the IFN regulatory factor (Irf)-7 pathway contributes to metastatic cells escape from immune surveillance.[171] Restoration of Irf7 in tumor cells or administration of IFN decreased bone metastases and enhanced longer survival time.[171] Irf7-driven suppression of metastasis depends on IFN signaling to host immune cells.[170,171] More research on suppression of metastases is key for increasing survival.

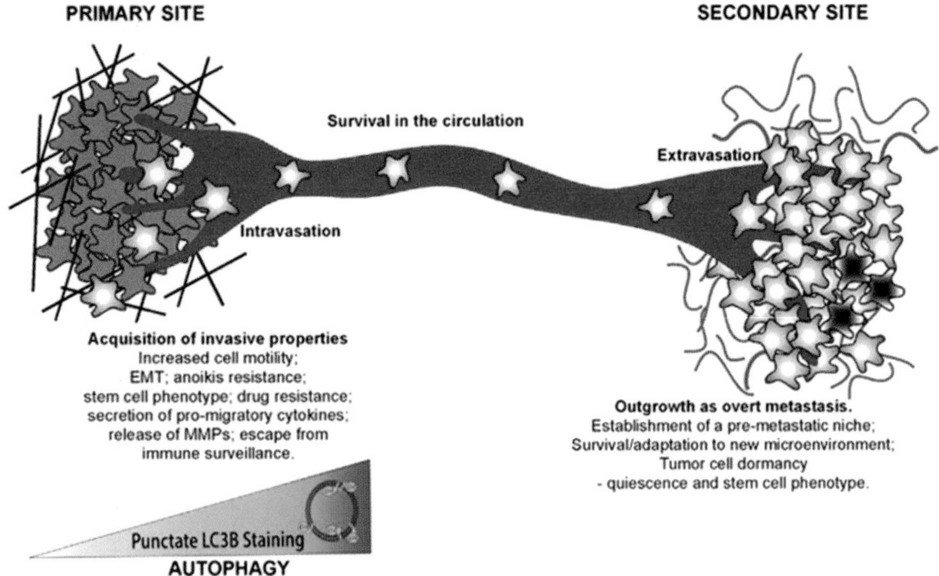

Fig. 12.25 **Autophagy in the Metastatic Cascade.** Autophagy increases as tumor cells progress to invasion, which is linked to increased cell motility, epithelial-mesenchymal transition *(EMT)*, a stem cell phenotype, secretion of pro-migratory factors, release of matrix metalloproteinases *(MMPs)*, drug resistance, and escape from immune surveillance at the primary site in some tumors. Many of these autophagy-linked properties during acquisition of invasiveness possibly contribute to the ability of disseminating tumor cells to intravasate, survive and migrate in the circulation before extravasating at secondary site. At the secondary site, autophagy is required to maintain tumor cells in a dormant state, which is linked to tumor cell survival, and drug resistance. (Data from Mowers EE, Sharfin MN, MacLeod KF. Autophagy in cancer metastasis. *Oncogene*, 2017;36:1619–1630.)

Surgical Intervention and Metastatic Dissemination

Sometimes disseminated cancer cells survive and can invade even after the removal of the primary tumor.[64] For example, individuals with pancreatic ductal adenocarcinoma often develop liver metastases following surgical excision of the primary tumor.[64,172] Metastasis may arise from dormant disseminated cancer cells that avoid elimination by the immune system and are present at the time of surgery.[172] Studies of mouse models and tissue samples from individuals with pancreatic ductal adenocarcinoma showed dormant disseminated cancer cells do not express a cell surface molecule or phenotype that triggers T-cell-mediated attacks.[172] This phenotype is associated with their inability to relieve endoplasmic reticulum stress (refers to various stressors) (Fig. 12.26 and Chapter 2).[172] Once the stress is resolved, disseminated cells start multiplying and invading tissue to form metastases.[172]

Another mechanism for promoting metastatic dissemination is anesthetics during surgery.[64] Murine models of breast cancer, sevoflurane led to significantly increased lung metastasis compared with that of propofol.[173] Sevoflurane increased IL-6, which led to the signal transducer and activation of transcription (STAT)-3 and subsequent infiltration of myeloid cells into the lung.[173]

Intravasation

Intravasation, or the movement of cancer cells through the lumen of the vasculature, is mediated both actively and passively, depending on the tumor type, microenvironment, and vasculature.[174–176] An in vitro model shows that the endothelium poses a barrier to tumor cell intravasation and is regulated by factors in the tumor microenvironment.[177] In vitro models using live-cell fluorescence reveal a mitosis-mediated mechanism where tumor cells located along the vessel periphery disrupt the vessel endothelium from cell division and detach into the circulation.[178] Tissue itself imposes mechanical pressures on invading tumor cells during intravasation.[179] Disruptive is nuclear squeezing on integrity of the nucleus, which causes genomic rearrangement increasing the metastatic potential.[179]

Almost every step of cancer progression involves integrins or critical cellular adhesion receptors.[180] Altered integrin expression is common in tumors, and they have roles in supporting oncogenic signals, such as oncogenic GFR signaling.[180] Importantly, integrins regulate the colonization process by easing anchorage-independent survival of circulating tumor cells (CTCs). Metastatic cells use E-cadherin in metastatic sites to detach, disseminate, and seed, thereby promoting metastatic cell survival and block apoptosis.[181] Inhibiting E-cadherin in metastatic cancer cells may be an essential treatment strategy that needs much more research.[181]

Circulation

CTCs need help to survive the vasculature. Survival of tumor cells in the circulation is challenging. Interactions between CTCs and the microenvironmental components of circulation

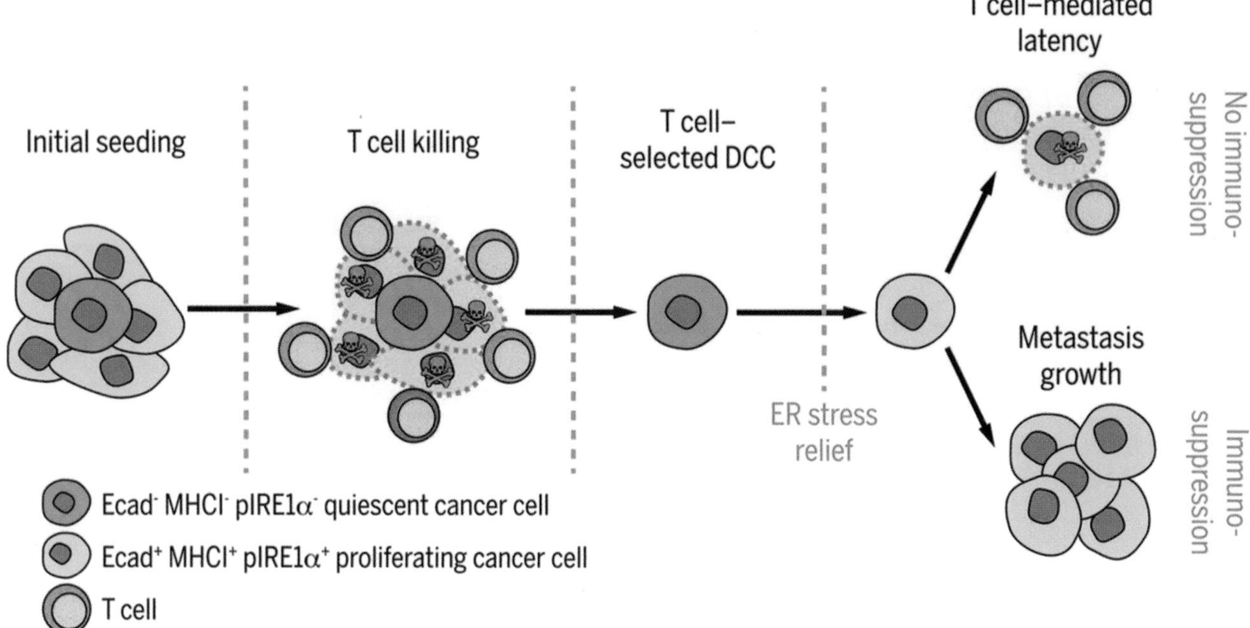

Fig. 12.26 Unresolved Endoplasmic Reticulum *(ER)* Stress Allows Disseminated Cancer Cells to Escape the T cell Response. Quiescent cancer cells that have unresolved ER stress lack expression of MHCI. With this phenotype they avoid killing by T cells and become latent disseminated cancer cells *(DCCs)*. Resolution of ER stress allows DCCs to regain proliferative abilities and then grow as metastases, only if the T cell response is disrupted, because they regain MHCI. *Ecad*, E-cadherin; *MHCI*, major histocompatibility complex class I. (Data from Pommier A, Anaparthy N, Memos N, et al. Unresolved endoplasmic reticulum stress engenders immune-resistant, latent pancreatic cancer metastases. *Science*, 2018;360:6394, eaa04908.)

determine survival and the ability of CTCs to extravasate in distant places.[182–184]

Circulating tumor cells interaction with immune cells. Most CTCs circulate as single cells and others as clusters (Fig. 12.27). Circulating clusters appear to be "hardier" and more likely to form metastases.[185] Clusters not only involve invading cancer cells but contain stromal cells and immune components from the original microenvironment that contribute to the heterogeneity of the cluster and augment its survival.[185–189] Neutrophils increase the chances of CTCs survival because they suppress leukocyte activation. Additionally, the interaction of CTCs with platelets leads to the formation of a "shield" coating the cancer cells that prevents CTC detection by immune cells and provides the structure to withstand the physical stresses of circulation.[190–192] The dissemination of CTCs is supported by very close association with activated platelets and macrophages.[193] Data show that CTCs form aggregates that sustain adhesion to the endothelium and contribute to metastasis.[190] A CTC-immune cell association was found in 70 women with advanced breast cancer.[194] The leukocytes that showed the greatest interaction were neutrophils, suggesting that neutrophil clustering with CTCs increases their metastatic potential.[194] Women with advanced breast cancer who had CTC-neutrophil clusters experienced faster metastatic advancement.[194] Mice studies showed CTCs from both CTC-neutrophil clusters and others that had not been part of clusters were injected into blood vessels had an increased number of metastases. From this remarkable study, the eradication of neutrophils from mice with breast tumors, the number of CTC-neutrophil clusters was significantly decreased (KLM add to Breast Cancer section).[200] Furthermore, these mice had delayed metastases in the lungs when compared with those mice with breast tumors that did not have their neutrophils removed.[194] Thus, the complex interaction between cancer cells and leukocytes promotes metastasis because metastatic cells possess sugar on their cell surface that binds to galectin-3.[195] Galectin-3 increases the ability of cells to colonize by interacting with mobilized leukocytes.[195]

Despite these findings, questions remain. Challenging these data are studies suggesting that an increase in megakaryocytes provide some measure of protection against metastasis.[196] Other data suggest that neutrophils may inhibit metastasis.[67,197] Further study about the interactions of CTCs with immune cells is ongoing.

Fighting against vascular forces and mechanical pressure. CTCs can sense and respond to tissue mechanics and initiate brief or lasting tissue alterations, including compression and deformation, ECM stiffening, protein unfolding, proteolytic remodeling, and clogging or obstructing transitions.[198] Distant metastases are dependent on CTCs flow through the vasculature, locating, and depositing at distant sites.[199] Easy passage of CTCs through the bloodstream is interrupted when their adhesive properties become greater than the shear forces imposed by the blood flow.[199] Thus, regions with low hemodynamic flow are the regions where most CTCs stabilize and engage with

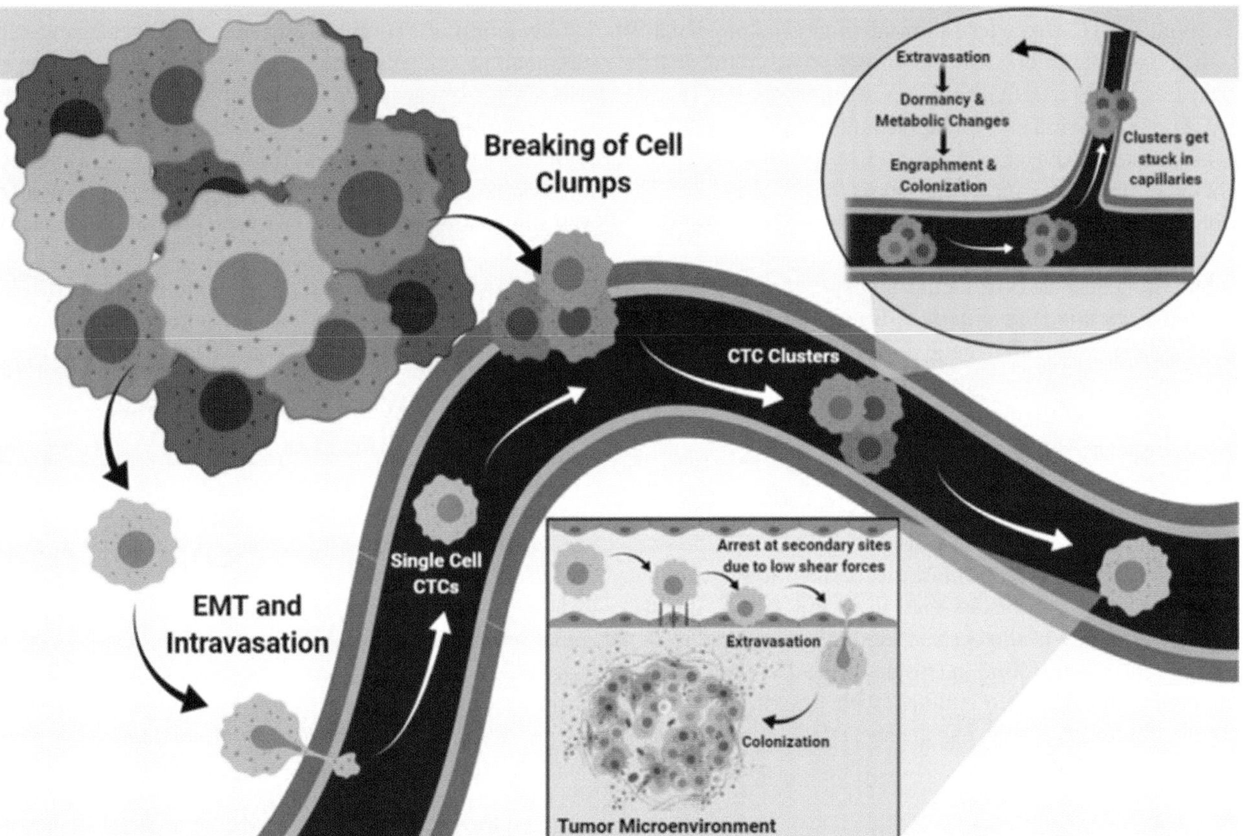

Fig. 12.27 How Cancer Cells Circulate. Cancer cells circulate as single cells or in clusters. After arrest at secondary sites or getting stuck in tiny capillaries, circulating cancer cells *(CTCs)* extravasate and colonize their new home or niche. Some cells become dormant as an adaptive mechanism to the new stressful environment. (Data From Fares J, Fares MY, Khachfe HH, et al. Molecular principles of metastasis: a hallmark of cancer revisited. *Signal Transduction Target Therapy*, 2020;5:28.)

endothelial cells. It is here in these regions that single CTCs might form intravascular clusters. CTCs that are fixed in the microvasculature are fragmented by the flow of blood allowing immune-derived molecules to promote extravasation and develop metastases from the surviving CTCs. This hypothesis was tested in 100 individuals with brain metastases, and the results showed that these metastases formed in those regions with low cerebral blood flow.[199] Thus, shear forces are important in hematogenous metastasis and determinations of the CTCs final resting site.[64]

Release of chemokines and cytokines assist circulating tumor cells. Chemokines and complement components direct tumor cells through the vasculature.[200,201] Obese mice induce granulocyte macrophage colony-stimulating factor and cytokines such as IL-5, lead to lung neutrophilia and assist in breast cancer metastasis.[202] Crowded cancer cells boost the production of IL-6 and IL-8, two immune molecules that stimulate biochemical pathways and assist tumor migration.[203] Importantly, in mouse models, blocking of IL-6 and IL-8 receptors decreased metastasis at lymph nodes, lungs, and liver compared with the control group.[203] Further data revealed that metastatic tumors induce the release of IL-1β, which induces gamma delta (γδ) T cells to release IL-17. IL-17 suppresses the cytotoxic CD+8 T lymphocytes and therefore promotes metastasis. Also, the loss of *TP53* in cancer cells causes the secretion of WNT ligands that produce IL-1β causing metastatic neutrophilic inflammation (see previous discussion on *TP53*).[204]

Routes of tumor cell circulation. Most now accept that CTCs use or even exploit and survive in the bloodstream during metastasis.[199,205] CTCs also cause distant metastases through the lymphatic circulation.[206–208] The *sequential progression model* is the basis for excision of tumor-draining lymph nodes during surgery.[206] Metastatic tumor cells travel from a primary site to a distant site directly through the bloodstream or through a lymph node close to the primary tumor site.[209] Not completely clear are the biological mechanisms by which tumor cells survive and grow within lymph nodes. In vitro studies show cancer cells shift to fatty acid oxidation to survive the lymph node microenvironment.[209] The yas-associated protein (YAP) transcription factor facilitated the shift to fatty acid oxidation and importantly, inhibition of fatty acid oxidation or YAP blocked lymph node metastasis in mice.[209] Overall, the metabolic achievements need much more research.

Diagnosing cancer from the circulation. Laboratory enrichment of CTCs improved their classification and tumor identification.[210] CTC characterization identifies the molecular aspects of metastatic tumors. An emerging approach is the analysis of cell-free DNA (cfDNA).[211] cfDNA identifies the heterogeneity of CTCs in individuals with high counts of CTCs, and this helps with clinical management. Also, cfDNA profiling tracks the subclonal traits of cancer metastasis.[212] As such, liquid biopsy of CTCs and/or cfDNA in the bloodstream may have the potential to augment current understanding of cancer metastasis (see Emerging Science Box: Liquid Biopsy).[210]

Targeting circulating tumor cells. Advancements in the field of CTC detection assays offers hope for future successful applications.[64] In fact, a paradigm shift is occurring in the field. For example, a photoacoustic method for direct use in individuals with melanoma has been developed, enabling the detection of very low numbers of CTCs in vivo and their destruction with laser pulses.[213] This amazing advancement reflects the therapeutic potential of such patient-centered approaches. In addition, with DNA methylation profiles more clearly identifying tumor phenotypes among CTC clusters than from single cells, it can add another key target to the destruction of CTCs. These phenotypic differences were found in clusters instead of single cells from patients and in vitro studies with breast cancer.[214] Importantly, tumor cell clustering shapes DNA methylation to enable metastasis seeding.[214]

Extravasation

Critical in the metastatic process is the ability of CTCs to adhere and extravasate through endothelial cells and colonize the premetastatic niche (PMN).[215] When CTCs arrest in capillaries, they either extravasate by transendothelial migration or grow in the vessel itself before extravasation and colonization of the PMN.[216–219]

How Do Circulating Tumor Cells Extravasate?

In small capillaries CTCs become trapped leading to either rupture or extravasation. Organs with highly permeable sinusoidal vessels exhibit a high rate of metastasis, such as liver and bone.[64] Other organs require genetic and molecular changes to be able to extravasate among tight barriers and basement membranes.

> **EMERGING SCIENCE BOX**
>
> ***Liquid Biopsy Enters the Clinic***
>
> Studies of disseminated tumor cells in bone marrow and circulating tumor cells in peripheral blood have provided major insights into cancer biology and metastasis. Advances in the detection and characterization of circulating tumor DNA (ctDNA) have enabled the introduction of liquid biopsy assays into clinical practice.The FDA has approved single gene assays, and more recently, multigene assays to detect genetic alterations in plasma cell-free (cfDNA). These approvals are for personswith advanced-stage cancer. The next goal is likely to be the systemic treatment of persons with "ctDNA relapse," a term introduced for ctDNA detection prior to imaging-detected relapse after intention to cure for early-stage disease. In the future, after more rigorous research, applications are for screening and diagnosis.
>
> Data from Ignatiadis M, Sledge GW, Jeffrey SS. Liquid Biopsy enters the clinic-implementation issues and future challenges. *Nature Reviews. Clinical Oncology*, 2021;18:297–312.

Extravasation is a complex process. It involves ligand-receptor interactions, chemokines, and circulating non-tumor cells.[175,220,221] Integrins are once again very important; they help to determine the location for extravasation and colonization.[180] Many have reported that extravasation occurs in a similar fashion to leukocyte transendothelial migration.[175,222,223] Recently, it was shown that cancer cells induce programmed necrosis of endothelial cells, driving metastatic cells to extravasate. Specific treatments, such as the receptor-interacting serine/threonine-protein kinase, and others reduced endothelial necrosis and metastatic extravasation.[224]

Circulating Tumor Cells Target Specific Sites

It appears that most cancers metastasize to specific target organs, a process called metastatic organotropism. Breast cancer research has supported this process, and researchers have defined the genetic basis for cancer colonization in distant sites.[225] Importantly, the host microenvironment and the ensuing adaptive process that invading cancer cells undergo play a role in extravasation and colonization at specific sites.[226] For example, breast cancer metastasizes most frequently to the bone, often after long latency, suggesting that metastatic seeds are resistant to therapy and can regrow. Metastasis to bone is a common characteristic of many cancers including breast, prostate, lung, thyroid and kidney.[227] Metastatic organotropism is illustrated in Fig. 12.28.

A mechanism between the bone osteogenic niche and cancer cells is the influx of calcium, which promotes the progression of bone metastasis.[228] Women with postpartum breast cancer are at increased risk for liver metastasis.[229] The identification of the "weaning-induced liver involution," with its established metastatic microenvironment, accounts in part for the poorer prognosis of women with postpartum breast cancer.[229]

Colonization

To establish metastatic tumors at distant sites, extravasated CTCs must locate, exploit, and modify the structural and metabolic features of secondary sites. Circulating cells face harsh conditions after extravasation at the distant site.[230]

Colonizing Cells and Stromal Challenges

Formation of the PMN, where the tumor cells colonize and grow depends on signaling from various tumor secreted derived factors and bone marrow-derived factors.[72,92,231,232] Importantly, exosomes play a major role (discussed earlier).[232] Like breast cancer, these results apply to pancreatic cancer, whereby exosomes initiated PMN formation in the liver.[115] Optimal colonization depends on cancer-cell host interactions. For example, hepatocytes control myeloid cell accumulation and fibrosis within the liver and increase the susceptibility of the liver to metastatic colonization.[64] From murine models, hepatocytes induce IL-6-mediated STAT3 signaling and increase secretion of serum amyloid A1 and A2 (SAA). Inhibition of IL-6-STAT3-SAA signaling prevents the formation of a PMN and inhibits liver metastasis.[233] These important findings need more research.

Formation of a vascular network is critical for optimal colonization. Vascular mimicry is a process where tumors create

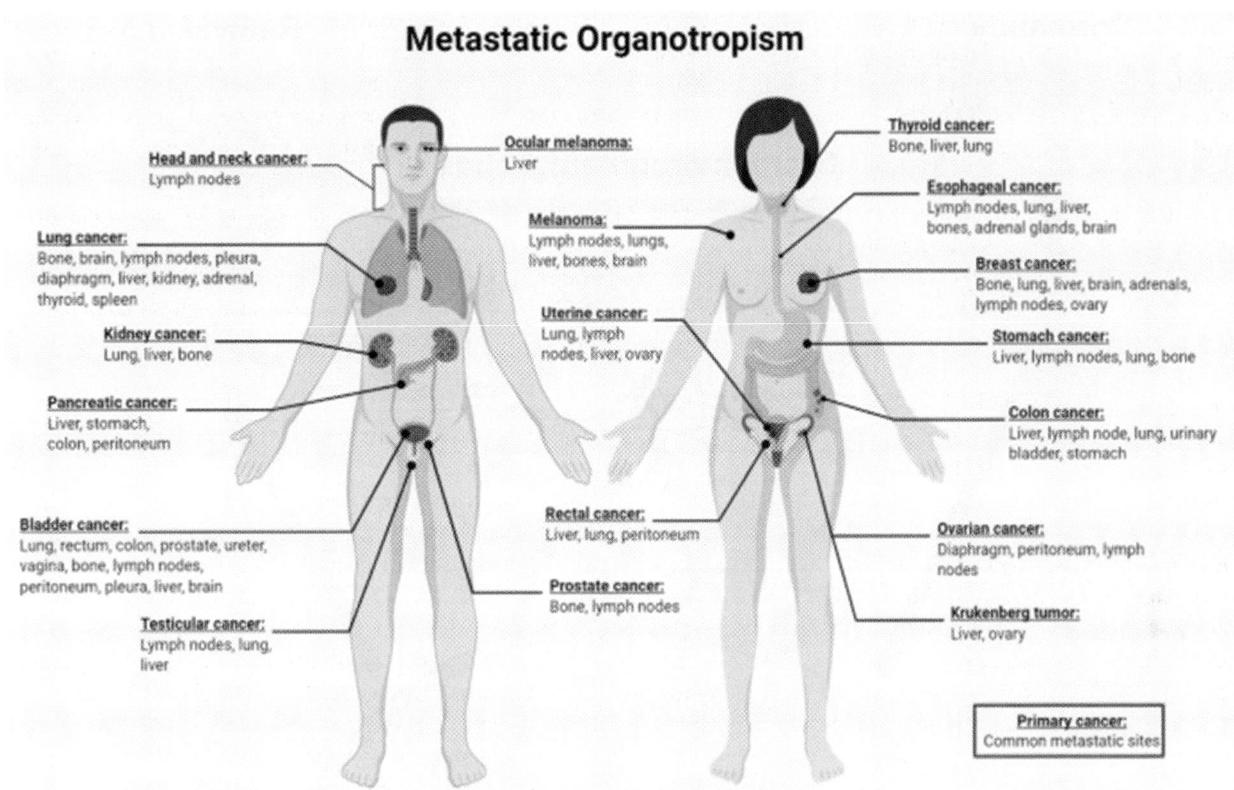

Fig. 12.28 Metastatic Organotropism. Clinical data suggest most cancers metastasize to specific organs, a process known as metastatic organotropism. (Data from Fares J, Fares MY, Khachfe HH., et al. Molecular principles of metastasis: A hallmark of cancer revisited. *Signal Transduction Target Therapy*, 2020;5:28.)

their own channels for fluid transport that drives the ability of some breast cancer cells to contribute to distant metastases through the expression of *SERPINE2* and *SLPI*.[234] These two genes are increased in women with breast cancer lung metastases, suggesting their role in metastatic progression.[234]

Colonizing cancer cells use signaling from neuronal pathways for growth and adjustment to new sites. For example, proximity of breast cancer cells to neuronal synapses enables cancer cells to hijack *N*-methyl-D-aspartate receptor signaling to promote brain metastasis.[235] Metastatic cancer cells use cancer-cell astrocyte gap junctions to transfer cGAMP to astrocytes activating IFN genes and producing inflammatory cytokines which supports tumor growth and chemoresistance.[236]

Sleeping or Dormant Cancer Cells

Cancer dormancy is a rest phase in cancer progression that occurs during the primary tumor formation phase or after invasion into secondary sites.[237] Metastatic dormancy occurs because of the delayed adjustment of disseminating cells to their secondary niches or sites affecting single invading cells or cancer clusters after circulation.[238] These dormant cancer cells (DCCs) are rarely detectable with current diagnostic approaches.[239]

The details of dormancy are emerging, but dormancy is not completely understood. DCCs are present long after the primary tumor has been removed and are thought to be responsible for late relapses.[238] Dormancy involves quiescence and angiogenic dormancy, whereby a balance is attained between dividing and dying cancer cells. Immune-mediated dormancy is when the tumor mass is preserved by immune cell cytotoxicity.[71,240]

Regulation of tumor cell dormancy is dependent on communication or reciprocal crosstalk between the environment and transcriptional programs (Fig. 12.29).[241] Much evidence supports the notion that extracellular signal-regulated kinase (ERK) activation has a determinant role in whether cancer cells will proliferate or enter the phase of dormancy.[239] Proliferating cancer cells exhibit essential ERK activation, which permits cell cycle phase transition and cell division.[242,243] During ERK-induced proliferation, a high level of p38 mitogen-activated protein kinase (p38) activity functions as an inhibitory regulator of ERK and prevents cell proliferation by inducing cell cycle arrest or triggering senescence and apoptosis.[239] In vivo studies visualized ERK and p38 MAPK activities providing direct evidence of p38/ERK activity as an indicator of DCCs in various cancers, including breast, prostate, melanoma, and fibrosarcoma.[239,244] Importantly, many pharmacological and genetic interventions that change the balance of p38/ERK activity in favor of ERK broke in vivo dormancy and induced cancer growth.[239] Overall, the genetic and signaling pathways that regulate cancer cell dormancy and future reactivation involve intracellular signaling, extracellular signaling, and induction signals derived from the bone marrow niche.[64]

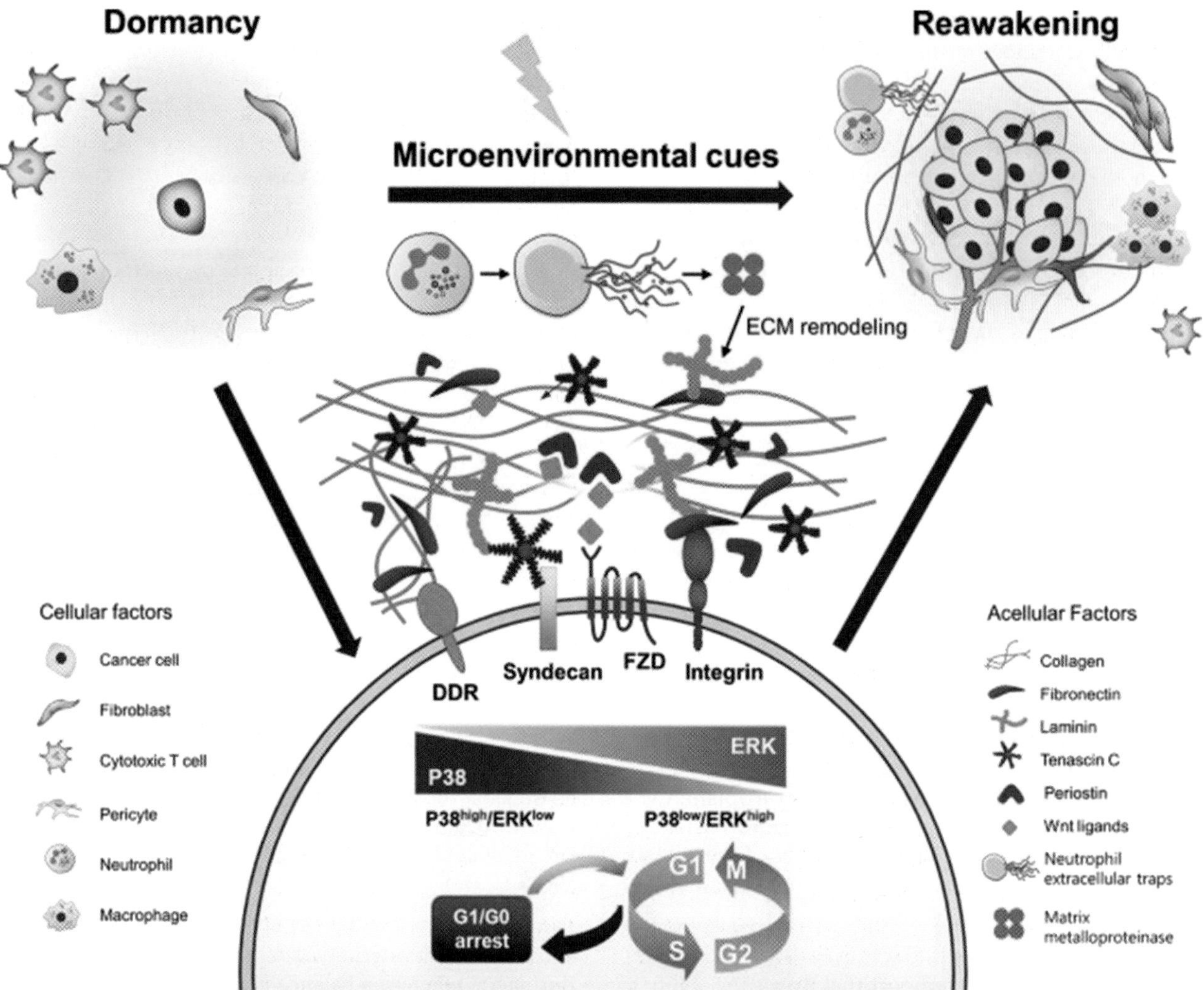

Fig. 12.29 Cancer Cells Become Dormant to Escape Immune Attack. After cancer cells reach a new location, these dormant cancer cells *(DCCs)* receive signals from the surrounding tissue and gain the ability to re-enter the cell cycle. Chronic inflammation can reactive DCCs, triggering tumor development. Critical signaling pathways involved in DCC reactivation are being investigated which, may help to fight this leading cause of death from cancer. *DDR*, Discoidin domain receptor; *ECM*, extracellular matrix; *FZD*, frizzled. (Data from Park SY, Nam JS. The force awakens: Metastatic dormant cancer cells. *Experimental and Molecular Medicine*, 2020;52:569–581.)

As discussed earlier, chronic inflammation is involved in cancer development (see Table 12.3), yet not all individuals who have experienced chronic inflammatory diseases eventually develop cancer.[239] In situ carcinoma lesions can be found without chronic inflammation. This observation has caused debate about the cause-effect relationship between chronic inflammation and cancer.[239] One explanation about this conflicting evidence is that reawakening DCCs could be a critical factor for cancer development from chronic inflammation.[239] For example, chronic inflammation supports angiogenesis, which disrupts cancer dormancy by supplying sufficient oxygen and nutrients and advances cancer growth.[245] Also, there is a robust correlation between inflammation and recurrence of cancer, including recurrence of endometrial,[246] oral,[247] and breast cancer.[248,249] In vitro studies show that escape of cancer from dormancy can be induced by the inflammatory cytokine interferon-gamma (IFN-γ).[238] Further support of this hypothesis has been shown with the correlation between the high levels of serum inflammatory cytokines and cancer recurrence.[238] From a cohort of 734 individuals with breast cancer, high levels of circulating acute phase proteins (APPs) were positively correlated with distant recurrence.[250] C-reactive protein (CRP) and IL-6, other markers of inflammation, have shown their potential as posttreatment prognostic factors for predicting the risk of cancer recurrence and death.[239] Altogether, these data support the hypothesis that inflammation can be the DCC reawakening factor and can function as a cancer-promoting factor.[239] Chronic inflammation can induce epigenetic alterations and DNA mutations in tumor suppressor genes, thus promoting carcinogenesis.[239]

A growing body of evidence indicates the potential of CD4 and CD8 T cells in maintaining cancer dormancy.[251,252] Studies are indicating that DCCs can escape anticancer immunity and survive for an extended time.[239] Neutrophils are gaining attention because of their DCC-reawakening activity.[239] Exposure to tobacco smoke or the nasal instillation of polysaccharide induced chronic lung inflammation and converted DCCs to aggressively growing cancer cells and metastasis. From this process, neutrophils governed the DCC reawakening through the formation of neutrophil extracellular traps (NETs), which are scaffolds of chromatin released into the extracellular space.[253] Treatment with antibodies against NET-remodeled laminin prevented the DCCs from awakening and reduced metastasis.[239] In summary, the existence of DCCs has led to the emergence of therapy resistance because critically, the cells may resume growth, increasing the risk of unleashing lethal metastatic outbreaks even after a long latency period of months to years.[239]

Plasticity of Cancer Cells and Tumor Progression

Plasticity is the ability of cancer cells to dynamically switch between a differentiated state with limited tumorigenic potential and an undifferentiated or cancer stem-like state, required for long-term tumor growth.[64] Unfortunately, cancer cell plasticity facilitates the development of therapy resistance and malignant progression.[64] The hope is that cancer cell plasticity may be treatable. Researchers have forced the trans differentiation of EMT-derived breast cancer cells into adipocytes by using MEK inhibitors and rosiglitazone, an antidiabetic drug, and inhibited the metastatic cascade.[254]

Cell plasticity directly contributes to tumor heterogeneity and is critical for malignant tumor progression and therapy challenges. For example, breast cancer reveals a mutational spectrum or tumor heterogeneity and tumor cell plasticity. Glucocorticoids have been used to treat individuals with cancer complication. The progression of breast cancer is initiated by increasing stress hormone and glucocorticoid levels, which activates secondary site glucocorticoid receptors, increases cancer colonization, and decreases survival rates.[255] The activation of the glucocorticoid receptor increases heterogeneity and metastasis, which suggests caution when treating with glucocorticoid therapy.[255]

Recent data reveal questions about treating with cytotoxic chemotherapy for invasive breast cancer. Despite the exhibited effectiveness of cytotoxic chemotherapy in treating invasive breast cancer, studies have shown that the treatment has pro-metastatic effects.[64,256] From mice studies, paclitaxel and doxorubicin trigger the production of tumor-derived extracellular vesicles in models of chemoresistant breast cancer.[256] The vesicles facilitate colonization of tumors in metastatic sites in the lungs.[64,256]

Treatment Strategies to Target Metastasis

Metastasis suppressors inhibit cancer growth and proliferation at the metastatic site but do not affect the primary tumor.[257] Specifically, they target oncogenic pathways and proteins involved in invasion and subsequent metastatic colonization.[64] In the last decade, a significant number of metastasis suppressors have been identified, most notably miRNAs.[257–261]

Numerous investigators are studying and exploring strategies that target pathways in the metastatic cascade.[64] The seeding of cancer cells can be targeted by inhibiting intratumoral interactions, intercellular interactions through ECM adhesion molecules, EMT, the release of proteases and intravasation.[64] Mounting evidence of the majority of approved cancer drugs, including TKIs, systemic cytotoxic therapies (chemotherapy) and antibody-drug conjugates (ADCs), reveals they do not have a durable impact with metastatic disease often because of therapeutic resistance.[262,263]

Metastatic cancers may be approached through a biomarker-driven strategy that validates single-agent or combination of agents depending fully on the molecular makeup of individual tumors.[263] Concurrent depletion of immune-suppressive factors and tumor-intrinsic targeting will be a central paradigm to improve survival (also see the section on Immunotherapy).[263] Combinational therapies with specific mechanisms of action will be critical to preventing metastasis-associated resistance and promoting durable responses.[263]

A priority is the importance of lifestyle and diagnostic factors in reducing cancer mortality.[263] Obesity is becoming a critical etiologic driver of cancer and initiation of metastasis[202] (also see Chapter 23). Worldwide, other preventable risk factors are a major cause of cancer (also see Chapter 13). For those cancers with a slow onset of metastasis, improved diagnostic, and early detection efforts will clearly improve survival.[263] Finally, prevention, early diagnosis and treatment methods must be comprehensively optimized to reduce cancer mortality.[263]

CLINICAL MANIFESTATIONS OF CANCER

The clinical manifestations of cancer are numerous and depend on the localization and type of tumor, and some are apparent before actual diagnosis of a malignancy. Generally, the variety and intensity of symptoms will increase as the malignancy progresses.

Paraneoplastic Syndromes

Paraneoplastic syndromes are rare disorders with complex clinical manifestations that are triggered by a cancer but are not caused by direct local effects of the tumor mass. In paraneoplastic syndromes, malignant cells do not cause symptoms related to metastasis, but they generate autoantibodies, cytokines, hormones, or peptides that affect may organ systems.[264] Most cases of paraneoplastic syndrome exhibit immunologic mechanisms; however, there are also non-immunologic mechanisms of paraneoplastic syndrome.[264] A number of cancers trigger an antibody response that attacks the nervous system, causing a variety of neurologic disorders that can precede other symptoms of cancer by months. An example of a non-immunologic mechanism is carcinoid tumors that release substances, including serotonin, into the bloodstream causing flushing, diarrhea, wheezing, and rapid heartbeat.

Although infrequent, paraneoplastic syndromes are significant because they may be the earliest symptom of an unknown cancer and, in affected individuals, can be serious, often irreversible, and sometimes life-threatening. Table 12.4 presents the classifications of paraneoplastic syndromes. Other clinical manifestations of cancer are summarized in Box 12.3. Factors

TABLE 12.4 **Paraneoplastic Syndromes**

Clinical Syndromes	Major Forms of Underlying Cancer	Causal Mechanism
Endocrinopathies		
Cushing syndrome	Small cell carcinoma of lung Pancreatic carcinoma Neural tumors	ACTH or ACTH-like substance
Syndrome of inappropriate antidiuretic hormone (SIADH) secretion	Small cell carcinoma of lung Intracranial neoplasms	Antidiuretic hormone or atrial natriuretic hormones
Hypercalcemia	Squamous cell carcinoma of lung Breast carcinoma Renal carcinoma Adult T-cell leukemia/lymphoma	Parathyroid hormone-related protein (PTHRP), TGF-α, TNF, IL-1
Hypoglycemia	Ovarian carcinoma Fibrosarcoma Other mesenchymal sarcomas	Insulin or insulin-like substance
Polycythemia	Renal carcinoma Cerebellar hemangioma Hepatocellular carcinoma	Erythropoietin
Osteomalacia	Phosphaturic mesenchymal tumor	FGF-23
Nerve and Muscle Syndromes		
Myasthenia	Bronchogenic carcinoma Thymic neoplasms	Immunologic
Disorders of the central and peripheral nervous systems	Breast carcinoma	
Dermatologic Disorders		
Acanthosis nigricans	Gastric carcinoma Lung carcinoma Uterine carcinoma	Immunologic; secretion of epidermal growth factor
Dermatomyositis	Bronchogenic carcinoma Breast carcinoma	Immunologic
Osseous, Articular, and Soft Tissue Changes		
Hypertrophic osteoarthropathy and clubbing of the fingers	Bronchogenic carcinoma Thymic neoplasms	Unknown
Vascular and Hematologic Changes		
Venous thrombosis (Trousseau phenomenon)	Pancreatic carcinoma Bronchogenic carcinoma Other cancers	Tumor products (mucins that activate clotting)
Disseminated intravascular coagulation	Acute promyelocytic leukemia Prostatic carcinoma	Tumor products that activate clotting
Nonbacterial thrombotic endocarditis	Advanced cancers	Hypercoagulability
Red cell aplasia	Thymic neoplasms	Unknown
Others		
Nephrotic syndrome	Various cancers	Tumor antigens, immune complexes

ACTH, Adrenocorticotropic hormone; *FGF-23*, fibroblast growth factor-23; *IL*, interleukin; *TGF*, transforming growth factor; *TNF*, tumor necrosis factor.

From Kumar V, et al. *Robbins & Cotran pathologic basis of disease*, 10th edition. Philadelphia: Elsevier; 2021. Table 7.11, p. 329.

predisposing individuals with cancer to infection are contained in Table 12.5.

Molecular Mechanisms of Cachexia

Cachexia is a complex metabolic syndrome associated with basic illness and is characterized by the loss of muscle with or without loss of fat mass (Fig. 12.30).[265] Cachexia is observed in many medical conditions, including cancer, AIDS, chronic obstructive pulmonary disease, multiple sclerosis, chronic heart failure, tuberculosis, familial amyloid polyneuropathy, mercury poisoning, and hormonal deficiency.[265] Cancer cachexia is characterized by systemic inflammation, negative protein and

BOX 12.3 Common Side Effects of Cancer and Cancer Therapy

Anemia: Commonly associated with malignancy, with 20% of persons diagnosed with cancer having hemoglobin concentrations less than 9 g/dL (normal value = 15 g/dL). Mechanisms of anemia include chronic bleeding (resulting in iron deficiency), severe malnutrition, cytotoxic chemotherapy, and malignancy in blood-forming organs. Chronic bleeding and iron deficiency can accompany colorectal or genitourinary malignancy. Iron also is malabsorbed in individuals with gastric, pancreatic, or upper intestinal cancer.

Bone Density Loss: Osteoporosis, or less severe osteopenia, may occur secondary to hormone treatment, such as used for breast cancer and prostate cancer, or in individuals treated with steroids.

Cachexia: A syndrome that includes many symptoms including anorexia, early satiety (filling), weight loss, anemia, asthenia (marked weakness), taste alterations, and altered protein, lipid, and carbohydrate metabolism. It is the most severe form of malnutrition associated with cancer and results in wasting, emaciation, and decreased quality of life. Cytokines and metabolites from the tumor may contribute to cachexia.

Cardiac and Pulmonary Damage: Chemotherapy and localized radiation can damage the heart and lungs, resulting in increased risk for heart failure and decreased pulmonary function.

Fatigue: Severe fatigue is the most frequently reported and persistent symptom of cancer and cancer treatment, particularly chemotherapy. Suggested causes include sleep disturbances, chronic inflammation, anemia, depression, level of activity, nutritional status, and other environmental and physical factors.

Gastrointestinal (GI) Tract: Rapidly proliferating cells of the GI tract are particularly sensitive to radiation and chemotherapy, leading to oral ulcers (stomatitis), malabsorption, and diarrhea, as well as increased risk for infection from the individual's own microbiome.

Hair Loss (Alopecia) and Skin: Some chemotherapy generally affects hair follicles, whereas radiation is more localized. It is usually temporary, although hair may regrow with a different texture initially. Decreased renewal rates of the epidermal layers in the skin may lead to skin breakdown and dryness, altering the normal barrier protection against infection. Radiation therapy may cause skin erythema (redness) and contribute to breakdown.

Infection: The most significant cause of complications and death in people with malignant disease is infection. Immune suppression, lymphopenia, and granulocytopenia may result from the underlying cancer or secondary to treatment increasing the risk of serious microbial (bacterial and fungal) infections. (Factors that predispose individuals with cancer to infection are summarized in Table 12.5.) The prevalence of hospital-acquired (nosocomial) infections increases because of indwelling medical devices, inadequate wound care, and the introduction of microorganisms from visitors and other individuals.

Infertility: Male or female infertility may be secondary to the cancer, surgical treatment, or treatment with chemotherapy or radiation. Many infertility clinics will freeze sperm, eggs, or embryos before initiation of therapy.

Leukopenia and Thrombocytopenia: Causes can include many chemotherapeutic drugs and radiation therapy because they are toxic to the bone marrow, often causing granulocytopenia and thrombocytopenia. Thrombocytopenia is a major cause of hemorrhage in people with cancer and is often treated with platelet transfusions.

Lymphedema: Accumulation of fluid in the tissues results from damage to the lymphatic system from lymphoid cancer or metastatic disease, surgery, or radiation treatment.

Pain: Pain may occur during the early stages of malignant disease but intensifies with disease progression. Direct pressure, obstruction, invasion of a sensitive structure, stretching of visceral surfaces, tissue destruction, infection, and inflammation all can cause pain. Chronic pain may result from nerve damage secondary to surgery, chemotherapy, or radiation.

TABLE 12.5 Factors Predisposing Individuals with Cancer to Infection

Factor	Basis
Age	Many common malignancies occur mostly in older age. Immunologic functions decline with age. General debility reduces immunocompetence. Immobility predisposes to infection. Far-advanced cancer often results in immobility and general debility that worsen with age. Elderly persons are predisposed to nutritional inadequacies. Malnutrition impairs immunocompetence.
Tumor	Nutritional derangements can result. Sites and circumstances favorable to growth of microorganisms (obstruction, serous or blood effusion, ulceration) can be created. Far-advanced disease predisposes individuals to debility and immobility. Humoral or cellular immune defects may result. Metastasis to bone marrow may cause leukopenia or other defects in immunity.
Leukemias	Inadequate granulocyte production can occur (e.g., neutropenia, impaired phagocytosis). Thrombocytopenia (bleeding) can occur. Late effect: chronic lung disease from *Pneumocystis carinii* pneumonia can develop during therapy.
Lymphomas and other mononuclear phagocyte malignancies	Humoral and cellular immune defects (anergy, altered immunoglobulin production) result. Late effect: splenectomy in children can cause increased susceptibility to infection.
Surgical treatment	Invasive procedure interrupts first lines of defense. Radical nature of surgery (removal of large blocks of tissue in lengthy procedures) causes hemorrhage, decreased tissue perfusion, creation of dead spaces, and tissue necrosis. Procedure may be "dirty" surgery (bowel, infected, or contaminated areas). Persons for surgery are often older and at poor risk. Long preoperative hospitalization often precedes surgery. They may have received previous adrenocorticosteroid therapy, and they may have infections at sites remote from the operative area. Nutritional derangements (especially important in head and neck surgery) may result. Lymph node dissection may predispose an individual to local infection and impair containment to area. Gynecologic surgery may result in fistulae. Lung surgery may cause bronchopleural fistulae. Debility and immobility may result.

Data from Donovan MI, Girton SF. *Cancer care nursing*, 2nd edition. New York: Appleton-Century-Crofts; 1984; and Murphy GP, et al. *Clinical oncology*, 2nd edition. New York: American Cancer Society; 1994.

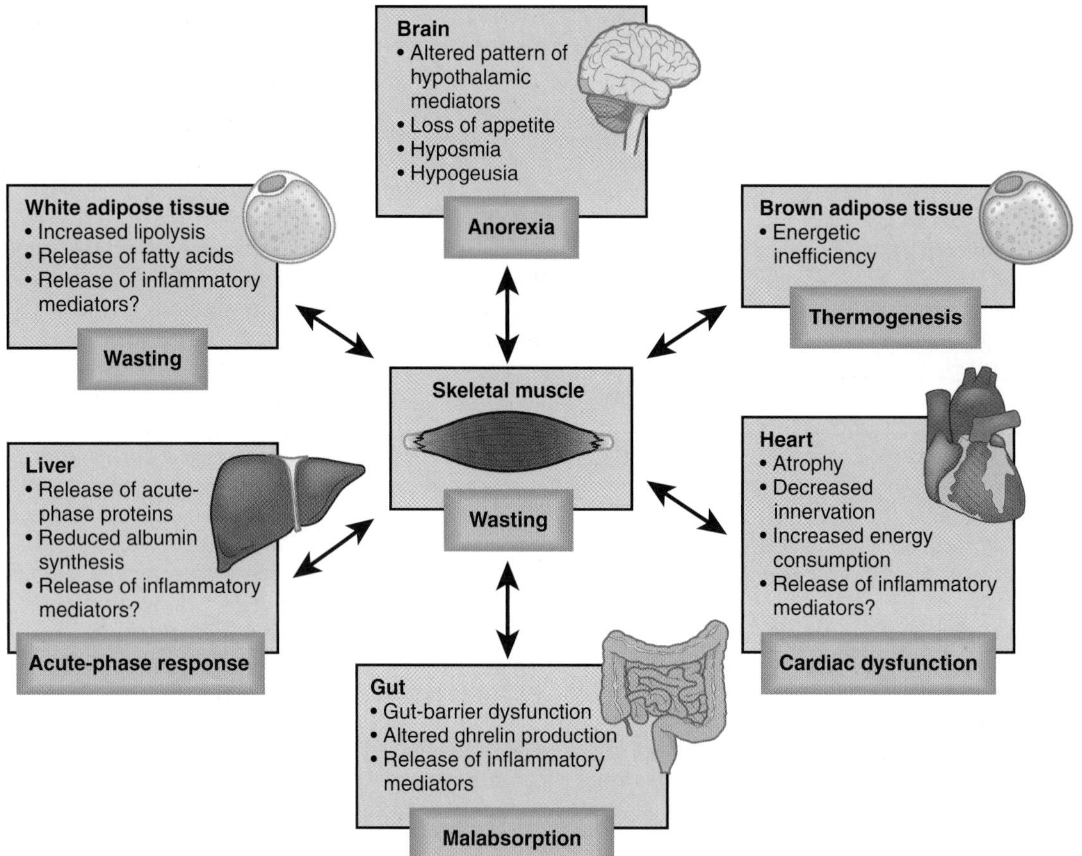

Fig. 12.30 Cachexia: A Multiorgan Syndrome. Loss of skeletal muscle and adipose tissue are major contributors to cachexia. But many other organs have a role in the cachexia syndrome, and the wasting that takes place in muscle may be dependent on alterations in these other organs or tissues. Changes in hypothalamic function and activation of brown adipose tissue, as well as alterations in liver and heart function, also are involved in the syndrome. Recent studies support a role for gut microbiota in cancer cachexia and the possibility of a gut–microbiota–skeletal muscle relationship. Recent data suggest that the conversion of white adipose tissue to brown adipose tissue is triggered by both humoral inflammatory mediators, such as interleukin-6, and tumor-derived compounds, such as parathyroid hormone–related protein. (From Bindels LB, Delzenne NM. Muscle wasting: The gut microbiota as a new therapeutic target? *International Journal of Biochemistry and Cell Biology*, 2013;45:2186–2190; Bindels LB, Beck R, Schakman O, et al. Restoring specific lactobacilli levels decreases inflammation and muscle atrophy markers in an acute leukemia mouse model. *PLoS One*, 2012;7(6):e37971.)

energy balance, and loss of lean body mass with or without wasting of adipose tissue.[266] Clinically, cachexia affects 50% to 80% of people with cancer, is represented by substantial weight loss, and may account for up to 20% of cancer deaths.[267] The most obvious symptom of cancer cachexia is the loss of skeletal muscle mass and cardiac muscle wasting, while other visceral organs may maintain muscle mass. Although management of advanced cancers usually does not reverse cachexia, treatment of earlier cancers can reverse the cachexia syndrome.[265] Because individuals receiving total parenteral nutrition still lose weight, increased resting energy expenditure may be the cause of the wasting syndrome.

Multiple mechanisms are involved in the development and progression of cachexia, including anorexia, decreased secretion of anabolic hormones, inflammation, decreased physical activity, and altered metabolic responses with abnormalities in protein, lipid, and carbohydrate metabolism (see Fig.12.30).[265] Investigators are studying the role of both mitochondria and sarcoplasmic reticulum (SR) in muscle function and the relationship to cachexia. Muscle weakness and fatigue are related to loss of myofibrillar proteins in muscle cells (Fig. 12.31). Contributing further to muscle wasting are an increase in apoptosis and an impaired capacity for regeneration. Many signaling pathways are involved in protein turnover, leading to the wasting process, and are activated by inflammatory mediators including cytokines, myostatin, and tumor-derived factors. In addition to muscle wasting, miRNAs may be involved in stimulating the breakdown of adipose tissue. In cancer cachexia, skeletal muscle loss includes significant loss of white adipose tissue (WAT). The WAT loss is thought to be caused by (1) increased lipolysis, (2) decreased activity of lipoprotein lipase (LPL), and (3) decreased new or de novo lipogenesis in adipose tissue. Data

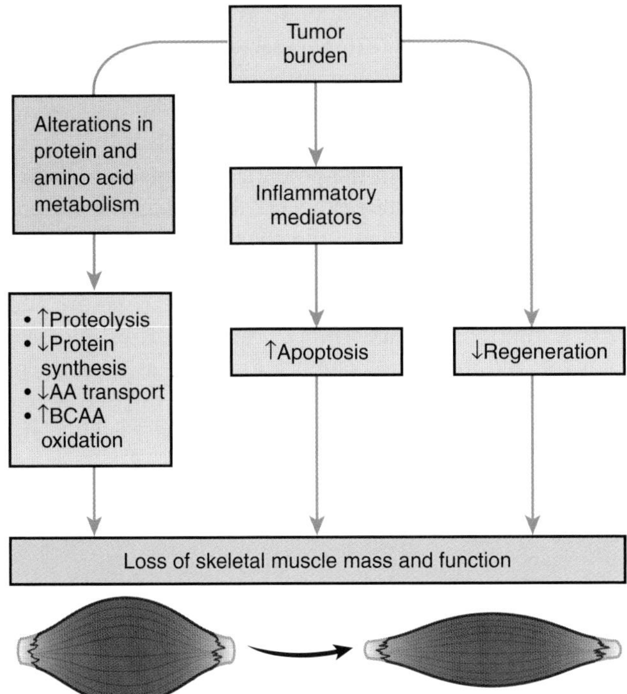

Fig. 12.31 Wasting of Skeletal Muscle. Inflammation plays a significant role in muscle wasting and is linked to alterations in protein and amino acid metabolism, activation of muscle cell apoptosis, and decreased regeneration. *AA*, amino acids; *BCAA*, branched-chain amino acids. (Adapted from Argilés JM, Busquets S, Stemmler B, et al. Cancer cachexia: Understanding the molecular basis. *Nature Reviews. Cancer,* 2014;14(11):754–762.)

show that WAT cells undergo a "browning" process during cancer cachexia where they change to beige cells called *BAT-like cells.* Browning is associated with increased thermogenesis. Tumor-derived compounds, such as IL-6 (which also may be released by immune cells) and parathyroid hormone–related protein (PTHRP), may be the drivers of thermogenesis.

An unusual and frustrating component of cancer care is the person's early satiety, or a sense of being full after only a few mouthfuls of food. Brain mediators are involved in the regulation of food intake and include appetite, satiation, taste, and smell of food. Therefore, the brain is an important organ in anorexia and consequently altered energy balance. Both the orexigenic (appetite-stimulating) and anorexigenic (appetite-suppressing) brain pathways are profoundly altered. (Cytokines are discussed in detail in Chapters 6 and 7.)

DIAGNOSIS AND STAGING OF CANCER

Histologic Staging

Cancer can be discovered in many ways: after screening tests, from routine exams, and after investigation of symptoms. The symptoms a cancer produces are as diverse as the types of cancer. The location of the cancer can determine symptoms by physical pressure, obstruction, and loss of normal function, or a cancer can cause problems far away from its source by pressing on nerves or secreting bioactive compounds. Whatever the initial complaint, once the diagnosis is suspected and a tumor has been identified, the tumor tissue must be obtained to establish a definitive diagnosis and correctly classify the disease. Various methods of obtaining tissue are described in Table 12.6. and Emerging Science Box describes the liquid biopsy. Once tissue is obtained, it is examined microscopically by the pathologist for the histologic hallmarks of cancer detailed in the beginning of this chapter. The classification of the cancer can be further facilitated by a variety of clinically available tests, including immunohistochemical stains, flow cytometry, electron microscopy, chromosome analysis, and genetic studies.

If the diagnosis of cancer is established, it is critical to determine if the cancer has spread, known as the *stage of the cancer.* Cancer staging initially involves determining the size of the tumor, the degree to which it has invaded locally, and the extent to which it has spread (metastasized). Specific molecular tests are increasingly being used in staging. Diverse schemes are used for staging different tumors. In general, a four-stage system is used, with CIS regarded as a special case. Cancer confined to the organ of origin is stage 1; cancer that is invasive locally is stage 2; cancer that has spread to regional structures, such as lymph nodes, is stage 3; and cancer that has spread to distant sites (e.g., a liver cancer that has spread to a lung or a prostate cancer that has spread to bone) is stage 4. One common scheme for standardizing staging is the World Health Organization's TNM system: *T* indicates tumor spread, *N* indicates node involvement, and *M* indicates the presence of distant metastasis (see Fig. 12.28). The prognosis generally worsens with increasing tumor size, lymph node involvement, and metastasis. Staging also may alter the choice of therapy; more aggressive therapy is delivered to more invasive disease.

Tumor Markers

During surveillance or diagnosis of cancer, as well as following therapy, specific biochemical markers of tumors have proven to

TABLE 12.6 Obtaining Tissue—The Biopsy

Procedure	Purpose	Example
Excisional biopsy	Complete removal, usually with a margin of normal tissue	Full resection (e.g., mastectomy, partial colectomy)
Incisional biopsy	Removal of a portion of a lesion	Lymph node biopsy, muscle mass biopsy
Core needle biopsy	Often performed with direct vision, or guided with ultrasound or computed tomography (CT)	Needle biopsy of prostate or liver mass
Fine-needle aspiration	Obtains dissociated cells for cytologic study but does not preserve tissue structure	Thyroid, breast mass
Exfoliative cytology	Cells shed from the surface, for example, from cervix, sputum (lung), or urine	Brushings from lung or colon endoscopy

be helpful. These tumor markers are substances produced by both benign and malignant cells that are either present in or on tumor cells or found in blood, spinal fluid, or urine. Some tumor markers have been known for many decades. Tumor markers include hormones, enzymes, genes, antigens, and antibodies (Table 12.7). For example, the tumor-associated antigen carcinoembryonic antigen (CEA) is released from colon cancer. If the tumor marker itself has biologic activity, then it can cause symptoms, such as those described in Table 12.7. For example, the adrenal medulla normally secretes the catecholamine epinephrine (adrenaline). Benign tumors of the adrenal medulla (pheochromocytoma) can produce catecholamines (e.g., adrenaline) in vast excess, leading to rapid pulse rate, high blood pressure, diaphoresis (i.e., sweating), and tremors. Detection of elevated blood or urine levels of catecholamines helps confirm the diagnosis, and treatment of the disease relieves the symptoms. Tumor markers can be used in three ways: (1) to screen and identify individuals at high risk for cancer; (2) to help diagnose the specific type of tumor in individuals with clinical manifestations relating to their tumor, as in adrenal tumors or enlarged liver or prostate; and (3) to follow the clinical course of a tumor.

To date, no tumor marker has proven satisfactory to screen populations of healthy individuals for cancer. Testing large populations will always detect a few normal individuals with test results at the high end of the normal distribution (the "false positives"), which can lead to expensive and invasive additional tests and unnecessary concern. Similarly, some individuals with disease will have test results in the normal range ("false negatives"). More importantly, some nonmalignant conditions can produce tumor markers. The presence of an elevated tumor marker, therefore, may suggest a specific diagnosis, but it is not used alone as a definitive diagnostic test. For instance, prostate tumors secrete *prostate specific antigen (PSA)* into the blood. But enthusiasm has waned for routine testing for PSA levels, and now the US Preventive Services Task Force (USPSTF) recommends that clinicians inform men ages 55 to 69 years about the potential benefits and harms of PSA screening for prostate cancer.[268] Screening offers a small potential benefit of reducing the chance of dying of prostate cancer. Many men, however, will experience harm from screening, including false-positive results that require additional testing and possible biopsy, overdiagnosis and overtreatment, and treatment complications such as incontinence and erectile dysfunction. Clinicians should not screen men who do not express a preference for screening.[268] Falling levels of PSA after radiation or surgical therapy may indicate successful treatment for prostate cancer, and a later rise may indicate a recurrence. Identification of ideal sensitive and specific tumor markers that are elevated early during common cancers remains a high priority because the early detection of cancer often improves the treatment outcome.

Classification of Tumors: Immunohistochemical and Genetic Analysis

Because knowledge about the cellular and molecular alterations in individual cancers can influence the choices of therapy, it becomes increasingly important for clinicians to accurately classify each cancer. The classification, and hence the treatment decisions, of cancers was originally based on gross and light microscopic appearance and is now commonly accompanied by immunohistochemical analysis of protein expression.

TABLE 12.7 Examples of Tumor Markers in Body Fluids

Marker Name	Nature	Type of Tumor
Adrenocorticotropic hormone (ACTH)	Peptide hormone	Pituitary adenomas
Alpha fetoprotein (AFP)	70-kDa protein	Hepatic, germ cell
Beta-2-microglobulin (β2 M)	11-kDa protein	Multiple myeloma, CLL
Beta-human chorionic gonadotropin (β-hCG)	Glycopeptide hormone β-chain	Germ cell, choriocarcinoma
CA15-3/CA27-29	Large MW glycoproteins	Breast
CA-125	Large MW glycoprotein	Ovary
CA19-9	201-kDa glycoprotein	Pancreas, gallbladder, bile duct, gastric
Calcitonin	3.4-kDa polypeptide hormone	Thyroid
Carcinoembryonic antigen (CEA)	200-kDa glycoprotein	GI, pancreas, lung, breast, etc.
Catecholamines	Epinephrine and precursors	Pheochromocytoma (adrenal medulla)
CD20	33–36-kDa glycosylated phosphoprotein	Non-Hodgkin lymphoma
Chromogranin A (CgA)	48-kDa protein	Neuroendocrine
Homovanillic acid/vanillylmandelic acid (HVA/VMA)	Catecholamine metabolites	Neuroblastoma
Prostate-specific antigen (PSA)	33-kDa glycoprotein	Prostate
Urinary Bence-Jones protein	Ig light chain	Multiple myeloma

CLL, Chronic lymphocytic leukemia; *GI*, gastrointestinal; *Ig*, immunoglobulin; *kDa*, kilodalton(s); *MW*, molecular weight.

Increasingly, this is supplemented by a more extensive genetic analysis of the tumors. The range of genetic analysis is expanding rapidly. In a research setting and increasingly in clinical settings, global gene expression and mutation analysis can be measured using polymerase chain reaction (PCR), microarray, or advanced DNA sequencing technology. These analyses can be used to classify tumors more precisely and may predict the most effective therapy. This detailed analysis of each tumor is a form of personalized medicine that offers therapy based on a very detailed knowledge of the characteristics of each individual's specific cancer. This enhanced molecular characterization subdivides cancers into therapeutically and prognostically relevant smaller groups. As an example, breast cancers can now be subclassified into over four types (luminal A, luminal B, basal-like, and others) based on their expression of specific markers, such as estrogen receptor, *HER2/Neu*, and other specific genes and proteins. Each subtype has a different response to therapy and a different prognosis.

TREATMENT OF CANCER

Until late in the last century the mainstays of cancer therapy have been surgery, chemotherapy, and radiation therapy. These approaches have been highly successful for certain types of cancer but have many limitations. Evidence has long been emerging that the immune system, in particular T cells, is capable of waging war on cancer tissue—Immunotherapy.[269,270] Immunotherapy has now established itself as a pillar of cancer care from the metastatic stage to the adjuvant and neoadjuvant settings in many cancer types.[270] From almost miraculous results to current pitfalls and limitations of checkpoint immunotherapy, novel research in the fields of personalized cancer vaccines, autoimmunity, the microbiome, the tumor microenvironment and metabolomics is aiming to solve those challenges.[270] Current immunotherapeutic approaches are being developed and tested to address the complexity of cancer pathogenesis, immune destruction, and precise cancer targeting (see further discussion under Immunotherapy).[269]

Cancer therapy is in a process of rapid evolution. Armed with a clearer understanding that cancer is in fact multiple diseases that share general hallmarks/enablers, and that the specific mechanisms underlying each hallmark may vary considerably among cancers (e.g., the large variety of oncogenes that may be used to differentiate cancers), modern cancer therapy is reaching a stage where complete genetic analysis of an individual cancer may determine the appropriate combination of therapies. Thus, effective therapy may include a combination of reagents targeting several hallmarks and under constant modification to target the evolving cancer cells.

Classic Approaches

Surgery

Surgery plays many roles in the care of individuals with cancer. The multiple approaches to obtaining tissue for diagnosis have been discussed. Surgery is often the definitive treatment of cancers that do not spread beyond the limits of surgical excision. It also is indicated for the relief of symptoms, for instance, those caused by tumor mass obstruction. In selected high-risk diseases, surgery plays a role in the prevention of cancer. For example, individuals with familial adenomatous polyposis because of germline mutations of the *APC* gene have close to a 100% lifetime risk of colon cancer, so a prophylactic colectomy is indicated. Similarly, women with *BRCA1/2* mutations have a markedly increased risk of breast and ovarian cancer, and often choose prophylactic mastectomy or bilateral salpingo-oophorectomy (removal of ovaries and fallopian tubes), or both.

Key principles apply specifically to cancer surgery, including obtaining adequate surgical margins during a resection to prevent local recurrences, placing needle tracks and biopsy incision scars (that may be contaminated with cancer cells) carefully so they can be removed in subsequent incisions, avoiding the spread of cancer cells during surgical procedures through careful technique, and paying attention to obtaining adequate tissue specimens during biopsies so that the pathologist can be confident of the diagnosis. Additionally, the surgeon provides critical staging information by inspection, sampling, and removal of local and regional lymph nodes during procedures.

Radiation Therapy

Radiation therapy is used to kill cancer cells while minimizing damage to normal structures. Ionizing radiation damages cells by imparting enough energy to cause molecular damage, especially to DNA. The damage may be lethal, in which the cell is killed by radiation; potentially lethal, in which the cell is so severely affected by radiation that modifications in its environment will cause it to die; or sublethal, in which the cell can subsequently repair itself. Cellular compartments with rapidly renewing cells are, in general, more radiosensitive. Effective cell killing by radiation also requires good local delivery of oxygen, something not always present in large cancers. Radiation produces slow changes in most cancers and irreversible changes in normal tissues as well. Because of these irreversible changes, each tissue has a maximum lifetime dose of radiation it can tolerate. Radiation is well suited to treat localized disease in areas that are hard to reach surgically, for example, in the brain and pelvis. Several radiation delivery methods are available, with external beam being the most common. Radiation sources, such as small ^{125}I-labeled capsules (also called *seeds*), can also be temporarily placed into body cavities, a delivery method termed brachytherapy. Brachytherapy is useful in the treatment of cervical, prostate, and head and neck cancers.

Chemotherapy

The era of modern chemotherapy began with the observation in World War II that mustard gas exposure caused suppression of the bone marrow. Related compounds, such as nitrogen mustard and cyclophosphamide, were then tested and produced clinical responses in hematologic malignancies, including lymphomas. Also in the late 1940s, based on the remarkable clinical observation that the vitamin folic acid could *increase* leukemia growth, antifolate drugs were developed (leading ultimately to methotrexate) that produced remissions in previously untreatable leukemia.

All chemotherapeutic agents take advantage of specific vulnerabilities in target cancer cells. Antimetabolites, such as methotrexate and L-asparaginase, block normal growth pathways in all cells, but leukemia and other cancer cells are exquisitely sensitive to folic acid and asparagine deprivation, whereas nonmalignant cells are far less sensitive. Similarly, some cancer cells are highly sensitive to DNA-damaging agents, such as cyclophosphamide and anthracyclines, because of the oncogenic mutations that accelerate the cell cycle and DNA synthesis. Cellular checkpoints prevent normal cells treated with microtubule-directed drugs, such as vincristine and the taxanes, from undergoing mitosis, whereas cancer cells treated with these agents lack normal checkpoints, continue through mitosis, and undergo mitotic catastrophe (see Chapter 1).

Single chemotherapeutic agents often shrink cancers, but these drugs given alone rarely provide a cure. Increasing evidence of the majority of approved cancer drugs, including TKIs, systemic cytotoxic therapies (chemotherapy) and ADCs, reveals they do not have a durable impact with metastatic disease often because of therapeutic resistance.[262,263] Hence chemotherapy drugs are usually given in combinations designed to attack a cancer from many different weaknesses at the same time and to limit the dose and, therefore, the toxicity of any single agent.

Chemotherapy can be used for several distinct purposes. Induction chemotherapy seeks to cause shrinkage or disappearance of tumors. In Hodgkin lymphoma, for example, chemotherapy alone can be used in some cases to cure the disease. In other settings, chemotherapy may shrink the tumor and improve symptoms without ultimately providing a cure. Adjuvant chemotherapy is given after surgical excision of a cancer with the goal of eliminating micrometastases. Neoadjuvant chemotherapy is given before localized (surgical or radiation) treatment of a cancer. As with induction chemotherapy, the effectiveness, or lack thereof, of neoadjuvant therapy can be measured (for example, with follow-up scans). Neoadjuvant therapy can shrink a cancer so that surgery may spare more normal tissue. For example, in the bone cancer osteogenic sarcoma, neoadjuvant therapy often converts a large tumor mass into a much smaller mass, allowing the surgeon to perform a limb-sparing excision rather than an amputation.

A major complication of chemotherapy is death of rapidly dividing cells that are not cancerous, such as those of the bone marrow. Hematopoietic growth factors also have been used to counter the effects of chemotherapy on bone marrow cells.

Immunotherapy

Cancer immunotherapy has been transformational in the care of persons with cancer, providing significant improvements for both survival and quality of life.[270] The field of cancer immunotherapy has a long history, and since the 1950s, the quest has been characterized by promises and frustrations. Yet, in the twentieth century, cancer immunotherapy made significant advances with the advent of new technology and even a Nobel Prize in Physiology or Medicine to Drs. Allison and Honjo.[269,270] The expression of unique antigens on cancer cells that can be targeted by T cells has driven the quest for effective therapies to initiate an immune response, boost a currently inadequate immune response, or convert a tumor-protective immune response to a destructive one.[271] The recent discovery of T cell immune checkpoints, such as cytotoxic T lymphocyte antigen 4 (CTLA-4) and programmed cell death 1 (PD-1), moved the field of immuno-oncology into its current era. The challenge is harnessing immune signals that maintain a fine balance between immune surveillance against foreign pathogens or abnormal cells and autoimmunity. Blocking T cell surface receptors results in increased autoimmunity that induces an immune response against tumors but can also enhance the chance of powerful autoimmune reactions.[270]

Immune Checkpoint Inhibitors

Various immune system components protect the host against primary tumor development, enhance tumor escape from immune mechanisms, or both. The process of orchestrating tumor immunogenicity or reducing antitumor immune responses is tightly regulated by immune checkpoints. These checkpoints are immune-cell surface receptors regulating either the activation or the inhibition of immune responses.[270] On the one hand, activation of the immune system is the desired outcome, but on the other hand, it is responsible for autoimmunity.[270] CTLA4 blocking antibodies (α-CTLA4), especially when bound to an Fc receptor (FcR) on an antigen-presenting cell (APC), can promote antibody-dependent cellular cytotoxicity (ADCC) (see Chapter 8). PD1 engages with its specific ligand (PDL1 or PDL2) to decrease activation. Blocking of the PD1 axis through the administration of an anti-PD1 (or anti-PDL1 or anti-PDL2) antibody prevents this inhibitory interaction and releases antitumoral T lymphocyte activity by increasing T cell activation and proliferation. The process is further supported by promoting formation of memory cells. The result is the release of cytolytic mediators, such as perforin and granzyme, causing increased tumor killing.[269]

Immune checkpoint inhibitor (ICI) therapies are now indicated in numerous cancer types.[269] Clinical trials are assessing the potential of other inhibitory or agonistic checkpoints to affect clinical outcomes.[270] The checkpoints are not equal in their outcomes; for example, the agonistic OX40 antibody has modest clinical activity, but the CD28 antibody resulted in a severe immune reaction called cytokine syndrome even at very sub-therapeutic doses (see Chapter 10).[270] Critical is finding the right combination of ICIs hence, requiring ongoing clinical trials. Recently, a meta-analysis reported a fatality rate of up to 1 person in every 77 treated using an ICI combination.[272] Immunotherapies are limited by their immune-related adverse events (irAEs). For specific irAEs, such as immune-related myocarditis, the mortality rate is as high as 50% in treated individuals.[273] Numerous predictors of irAEs have been proposed and will need prospective research validation. Promising results of single-agent PD-1 inhibitor varies from almost non-existent in pancreatic cancer and microsatellite-stable colonic adenocarcinoma, to an average of 15% to 30% in most other tumor types, but an impressive 50% to 80% in melanoma, Hodgkin lymphoma, squamous-cell carcinoma of the skin, and Merkle cell carcinoma.[270] Dedicated scientists and clinicians are mobilized to achieve a higher response rate without increasing autoimmunity.

One logical approach has been to combine an ICI with another therapy that can sensitize the host's immune system to the tumor in advance.[270] Recent studies have shown that using a person's own cancer cells to develop a vaccine (personalized neo-antigen-base tumor specific vaccines) holds great promise.[270]

Vaccines

Tumor cell vaccines were one of the first attempts at immunotherapy for cancer and have been extremely effective in protecting individuals against infective agents. Two categories of vaccines are prophylactic and therapeutic. Prophylactic vaccines against hepatitis B and HPV have been important in reducing the incidence of hepatocellular carcinoma and cervical cancer, respectively.[269,274]

Therapeutic vaccines aim to harness the immune system to rid disease-causing cells that are cancerous.[274] The research required is rigorous, and requires data points longitudinally, numerous tumor vaccines are in phase II and phase III trials but have yet to receive FDA approval.[269] Hematologic malignancies have a common antigen that is uniformly expressed on the surface of all malignant cells, making it possible to target therapies with chimeric antigen receptor T cells (CAR T cell) (Box 12.4). CAR T cells are engineered with *chimeric* (artificially derived from two different genes) antigen receptors. Solid tumors,

BOX 12.4 Engineering T Cells for Better Anticancer Killing and Chimeric Antigen Receptor T Cells

The specificity and function of T-cytotoxic cells (Tc cells) is controlled by three signals: (1) the T-cell receptor (TCR) that binds antigen and is associated with a complex of transmembrane signaling molecules (CD3); (2) the transmembrane co-receptor CD8 that binds to class I major histocompatibility complex (MHC) that is presenting antigen, resulting in proximity of CD3 with the intracellular portion of CD8 leading to activation of a signaling molecule; and (3) transmembrane accessory molecules, such as CD28, that bind to ligands on the target cell surface and provide an additional activation signal (see Fig. A). Cancers have developed multiple mechanisms for escaping the cytotoxic effects of Tc cells, among which are suppression of antigen presentation, reduction of CD3 expression, and inhibition of the CD28 signal by expression of soluble CTLA-4, which competes for binding to the CD28 ligand. Thus recognition of cancer-associated antigens by the Tc cell may be completely suppressed.

A variety of approaches have been designed to bypass suppression of the TCR. Initial attempts included cloning Tc cells expressing high-affinity TCRs for tumor antigen. However, suppression of antigen presentation by the tumor prevented recognition by these Tc cells. This has led to a unique approach of engineering T cells with chimeric antigen receptors (CAR T cells). Early success with these novel cells has led to further sophisticated approaches to constructing more complex CARs.

The process involves collection of circulating white blood cells from the blood of an individual with cancer using leukapheresis. The lymphocytes are enriched, induced to proliferate, and transfected by a virus containing the genetically engineered CAR. The CAR T cells are cloned in bulk, verified for expression of the CAR, and cryopreserved. When used, the cells are thawed and infused into the individual with cancer.

The CAR receptors are V_H and V_L regions cloned from monoclonal antibodies and inserted in tandem into the *CAR* gene. Because tumors suppress MHC presented antigen, the CAR receptors are designed against other surface molecules that do not require presentation. The *CAR* gene also contains information for hydrophobic transmembrane regions, followed by genetic information for costimulatory signals. Initially the costimulatory signals included the cytoplasmic portions of CD28 and CD3, but more recently developed CARs include multiple costimulatory signaling peptides. Thus binding of the receptor to a cancer-related molecule activates linked intracellular signaling peptides, such as CD3, CD28, and others, contained sequentially in the *CAR* gene. (Fig. B)

Targets for CAR T cells have included CD19, CD20, and CD22 on hematologic cancers and HER2, EGFR, and others on solid tumors. The most notable success has been treatment of CD19-positive B-cell malignancies. CD19 is expressed on cancer cells at a very high level related to normal B cells. Infusion of CAR T cells has led to remissions of greater than 80% of people with ALL and about 50% of those with CLL. Success against solid tumors has been less spectacular.

The next generation of CAR T cells is in development. These include the addition of more costimulatory signals, simultaneous expression of two CAR molecules on the T cell (both targeted to the same cancer-related molecule, but one CAR providing a strong TCR-like signal and the second providing a costimulatory signal), CARs directed to apoptosis-inducing molecules or cytokine receptors, and the use of engineered allogeneic T cells. The use of allogeneic T cells would accelerate treatment by circumventing the current 2- to 3-week process of preparing CAR T cells from the individual's own cells.

ALL, Acute lymphocytic leukemia; *CLL*, chronic lymphocytic leukemia.

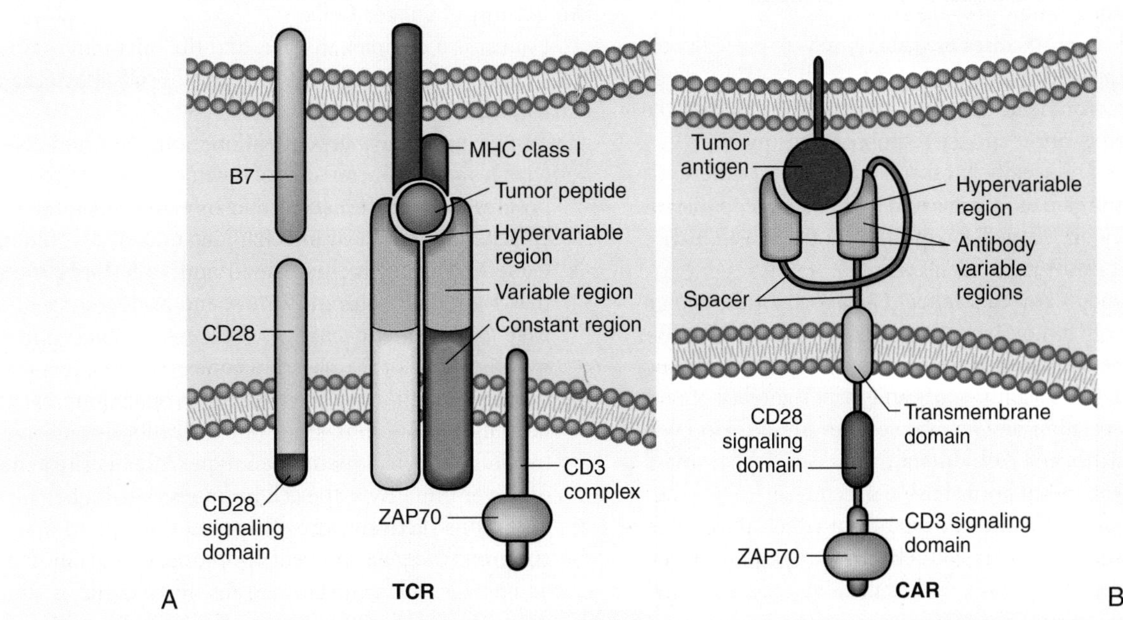

Data from Fesnak AD, June CH, Levine BL. Engineered T cells: The promise and challenges of cancer immunotherapy. *Nature Reviews*. Cancer, 2016;16(9):566–581; Lim WA, June CH. The principles of engineering immune cells to treat cancer. *Cell*, 2017;168(4):724–740; Sadelain M. Chimeric antigen receptors: Driving immunology towards synthetic biology. *Current Opinion in Immunology*, 2016;41:68–76.

however, either lack such an antigen or undergo mutations when exposed to therapeutic interventions like monoclonal antibodies.[270] Bioinformatics is guiding precision immuno-oncology to identify personal neoantigens for targeting.[270] Efficacy for the optimal vaccine relies on the selection of a target antigen for delivering a personalized vaccine. Using a person's own cancer cells to develop a vaccine and then to combine this approach with another immunotherapy, like ICI, is evolving.

The host microbiome plays a significant role in the efficacy of vaccine immune responses, promotion of carcinogenesis, efficacy and toxicity of anticancer treatments, such as ICIs.[270] The tumor microenvironment has a critical role in the modulation of anticancer immune responses. From research findings the term "immune contexture" has been proposed and validated with tumors classified by their tumor microenvironment and include four categories (hot, excluded, immunosuppressed, and cold). There is ongoing work to convert "cold" tumors with a strong expression of mesenchymal and collagen barriers that impede migration of tumor-infiltrating lymphocytes to the tumor bed.[270] Thus, research is progressing on the transformation of "cold" tumors into fertile "hot" tumors that are much more responsive to ICIs. Hot tumors are characterized by the accumulation of proinflammatory cytokines and T cell infiltration.[275]

TARGETED DISRUPTION OF CANCER

As discussed previously, cancers appear to share a variety of hallmarks that contribute to the malignant phenotype. Recent molecular and genetic analyses of groups of cancer can classify an individual's cancer by the spectrum of mutations underlying the cancer phenotype.

Tumor growth and progression are dependent on a variety of mutations leading to expression of oncogenes, inactivation of tumor-suppressor molecules, and interactions with inflammatory cells in the tumor microenvironment. These interactions foster angiogenesis, resistance to apoptosis and immune-mediated cancer cell death, altered tumor cell metabolism, and metastasis. An efficacious therapeutic approach, therefore, may be a combination of drugs highly targeted to cancer hallmarks.[276]

The NCI describes the many different targeted therapies approved for use in cancer treatment.[277] Cancer-targeting agents include those that inactivate oncogenes, block angiogenesis, and affect cancer cell metabolism. Monoclonal antibodies are available that induce apoptosis in tumor-infiltrating cells such as TAM, Treg cells, and tumor endothelium. Additionally, specific antagonists may neutralize the effects of cytokines, chemokines, and other tumor-enhancing mediators produced in the tumor microenvironment. These are usually in the form of monoclonal antibodies, which are available against tumor necrosis factor-α (TNF-α), VEGF, HER-2, and other ligands and their receptors. Such highly specific targeting would minimize secondary toxic effects. Information on the prevention of cancer by altering and eliminating high-risk lifestyle behaviors is contained in Chapter 13.

SUMMARY REVIEW

Cancer Terminology and Characteristics

1. Cancer is a leading cause of suffering and death in the developed world. Intensive research is defining this collection of related complex diseases. It is a disease in which abnormal cells divide uncontrollably, invade, and metastasize to other tissues. A tumor is a new growth, or neoplasm.
2. Cancer is more than 100 diseases, each caused by a specific and often unique age-related accumulation of genetic and epigenetic alterations. Environment, behavior, and heredity modify the risk of developing cancer and the response to treatment.
3. Benign tumors are usually encapsulated and well differentiated with well-organized stroma and do not spread to distant locations. They are named for the tissues from which they arise. Benign tumors are noncancerous.
4. Malignant tumors are cancerous. Compared with benign tumors, malignant tumors have more rapid growth rates, specific microscopic alterations (anaplasia, or loss of differentiation, and pleomorphism, or variability in size and shape), absence of normal tissue organization, and no capsule. They invade blood vessels and lymphatics and have distant metastases. The stroma is disorganized with loss of normal tissue structure.
5. Cancers are named for the cell type from which they originate. Carcinomas arise from epithelial tissue, lymphomas are cancers of lymphatic tissue, and leukemias are cancers of blood-forming cells.
6. Carcinoma in situ (CIS) refers to noninvasive epithelial tumors of glandular or squamous cell origin. These early–stage cancers are localized to the epithelium and have not penetrated the local basement membrane.

The Biology of Cancer Cells

1. Cancer is a complex disease, and the microenvironment of a tumor is a heterogenous mixture of cells, both cancerous and benign.
2. Tumor initiation is dependent on mutational and epigenetic changes and characteristics of the microenvironment. Tumor progression is governed further by more genetic mutations, epigenetic alterations, and changing microenvironment.
3. Genetic changes include small and large DNA mutations that alter genes, chromosomes, and non–coding RNAs, as well as epigenetic changes because of altered chemical modifications of DNA and histones.
4. Driver mutations "drive" the progression of cancer. Passenger mutations are random events that do not contribute to the malignant phenotype. After a critical number of driver mutations, the cell becomes cancerous.
5. Mutations activate growth-promotion pathways, block antigrowth signals, prevent apoptosis, stimulate telomerase and new blood vessel growth, and allow tissue invasion and distant metastasis.

6. Each cancer cell may develop its own set of mutations resulting in a genomically heterogeneous mixture of cancer cells with subsets that have accumulated more and more mutations. Intratumoral genetic heterogeneity or diversity arises from ongoing proliferation and mutation and can lead to therapy resistance.
7. The processes that occur during the development of cancer are analogous to wound healing. The proliferation of cancer cells and enlargement of the tumor elicit synthesis of proinflammatory mediators by the cancer cells and adjacent nonmalignant cells.
8. Like wound healing, mediators recruit inflammatory/immune cells and cells normally associated with tissue repair. These cells form the stroma (tumor microenvironment) that surrounds and infiltrates the tumor.
9. Hallmarks of cancer that are primarily genomic alterations include sustained proliferative signaling, evading growth suppression, genomic instability, and replicative immortality.
10. Other hallmarks secondary to genomic change include induction of angiogenesis and reprogramming energy metabolism. A third group, tumor resistance to destruction by the host's protective mechanisms, include resistance to apoptotic cell death, tumor-promoting inflammation, avoiding immune destruction, and the last hallmark activating invasion and metastasis.
11. Many of the hallmarks of cancer are consequences of cancer-stromal interactions.
12. Normal cells only enter proliferative phases in response to growth factors. Cancerous cells characteristically express mutated or overexpressed proto-oncogenes, referred to as oncogenes, which are independent of normal regulatory mechanisms and signal uncontrolled sustained proliferation. Genetic translocation alters the MYC proto-oncogene and hyperproduction of MYC protein drives proliferation and blocks differentiation.
13. Some oncogenes, such as *RAS*, result from point mutations. Other oncogenes can result from genetic translocations. Genetic translocation alters the MYC proto-oncogene and hyperproduction of MYC protein drives proliferation and blocks differentiation.
14. Translocation can cause excess and inappropriate production of a proliferation factor, such as with Burkitt lymphoma. Translocations can also lead to production of novel proteins with growth-promoting properties, as is seen with the Philadelphia chromosome in chronic myeloid leukemias (CMLs).
15. Tumor-suppressor genes normally regulate cell cycle, but they must be inactivated in cancer cells by mutations to each allele, one from each parent.
16. The most mutated gene in a wide variety of human cancers is the p53 tumor-suppressor gene *(TP53)*. The protein, p53 acts as a tumor suppressor, thus it regulates cell division by restricting cells from growing and dividing too fast or in an uncontrolled way the "guardian of the genome." The *p53* is in the nucleus and attaches directly to DNA. If DNA is damaged by such agents or stressors as toxic chemicals, radiation or ultraviolet radiation and others the protein plays a critical role in whether DNA is repaired, or the damaged cells undergo apoptosis. If the DNA can be repaired, p53 activates other genes or caretaker genes, for repair. If the DNA cannot be repaired, p53 prevents the cell from dividing and signals it to undergo apoptosis.
17. The p53 controls initiation of senescence (cease dividing), which has been shown to exhibit both a tumor suppressor and an oncogenic effect.
18. Cellular senescence can promote cancer development by altering the cellular environment through a senescence-associated secretory phenotype (SASP).
19. The retinoblastoma gene1 *(RB1)*, a tumor suppressor gene is mutated in childhood retinoblastoma and in some lung, breast, bladder, bone cancers, leukemias, and melanoma.
20. Genomic instability refers to an increased tendency of mutations in the genome during the life cycle of cells. Genomic instability in inherited and acquired mutations in caretaker genes increase the level of genomic instability and risk for developing cancer. Genomic instability may result from increased epigenetic silencing or modulation of gene function.
21. Changes in gene regulation can affect entire networks of signaling, not just single genes. Gene expression networks can be regulated by changes in microRNAs (miRNAs or miRs) and other non–coding RNAs (ncRNAs).
22. Oncomirs or oncogenic miRNAs promote multiple cancer pathways.
23. In addition to specific gene mutations and abnormal epigenetic silencing, chromosome instability (CIN) also appears to be increased in malignant cells, resulting in a high rate of chromosome loss, as well as loss of heterozygosity and chromosome amplification.
24. Cancer cells are immortal. When they reach a critical age, most cancer cells re-activate telomerase to restore and maintain their telomeres, thereby allowing cancer cells to divide repeatedly. Cancer cells move closer to immortality by upregulating telomerase and downregulating tumor suppressor genes.
25. Telomerase also affects DNA replication, cellular apoptosis, tumorigenesis, and resistance to therapy.
26. Cancer stem cells (CSCs) are a subpopulation of tumor cells that have replication immortality. They arise from tissue resident stem cells or develop from transformed differentiated cells. Transformation from differentiated cells into CSCs occurs through the activation of oncogenes, inactivation of tumor suppressor genes, and re-expression of telomerase.
27. CSCs can change their appearance and function in response to the tumor microenvironment such that they drive cancer progression, serving as the cellular seeds for tumor growth, metastases, and disease recurrence.
28. Access to the vascular system is essential for tumor growth. Cancerous tumors maintain secretion of angiogenic factors and prevent the release of angiogenic inhibitors, which stimulates new blood vessel growth (called neovascularization or angiogenesis).

29. The vessels formed within tumors originate from endothelial sprouting from existing capillaries and irregular branching, rather than regular branching seen in healthy tissue. The vessels are also more porous and prone to hemorrhage and allow passage of tumor cells into the vascular system.
30. Another form of angiogenesis in tumors is called vasculogenic mimicry. Tumor cells form tubular structures like blood vessels that contain erythrocytes. These tubular tissues can attach to blood vessels to form a vascular network.
31. Cancer cells can reprogram energy metabolism. The successful cancer cell divides rapidly, with the consequent requirement for the building blocks of new cells, such as ATP. Many cancer genes encourage aerobic glycolysis instead of oxidative phosphorylation, which allows for a more efficient production of molecular building blocks needed for rapid growth.
32. Oncogenes can drive metabolic reprogramming, enabling cancer cells to (1) maintain deregulated proliferation, (2) withstand challenges associated with oxygen and nutrient limitations, (3) maintain a dedifferentiated state with associated alterations in gene expression, and (4) corrupt the surrounding microenvironment to assist tumor growth and dissemination.
33. In cancer, defects in the intrinsic or extrinsic cell death pathways, or both, provide resistance to apoptotic cell death.
34. The inflammatory response contributes to the onset of cancer, and cancer is a cause of chronic systemic and local inflammation. Tumors can manipulate the inflammatory process in their local tumor microenvironment to benefit tumor progression and spread.
35. Cancer also causes systemic perturbations in both innate and adaptive immune processes that reduce the body's ability to fight the cancer.
36. Some conditions of chronic inflammation increase the risk of developing cancer. A prime example is the association between gastric cancer and infection with *Helicobacter pylori*.
37. One of the key cells that promotes tumor survival is the tumor-associated macrophage (TAM). Most tumors have large numbers of TAMs, whose presence may correlate with a worse prognosis.
38. Cancer-associated fibroblasts (CAFs) contribute greatly to cancer progression, local spread, and metastasis. Studies have documented how the number of CAFs, or their function is linked to outcomes. The heterogeneity of CAFs, their functions and possible changeability, pose a challenge for the field,
39. Several viruses are associated with cancer and include human papillomavirus (HPV), Epstein-Barr virus (EBV; also known as HHV4), Kaposi sarcoma herpesvirus (KSHV; also known as HHV8), hepatitis B and C viruses (HBV, HCV), and Merkel cell polyomavirus. Cancer of the cervix and hepatocellular carcinoma account for approximately 80% of virus-linked cancer cases.
40. Although some cancer cells do express tumor-specific antigens that can be recognized by the immune system, most cancer cells do not, and those that do, most often present antigens that are undetectable by the immune system. Cancer cells have developed multiple mechanisms to evade the immune system. As cancer cells proliferate, clonal development of immune-resistant variants arises.
41. Immune cells have surface molecules whose purpose is to activate (co-stimulatory factors) or suppress (co-inhibitory factors) immune responses to antigens. Co-inhibitory molecules are often called immune *checkpoints*. Cancer cells may suppress T cells by binding to immune checkpoints, causing the lymphocyte to turn off its attack. Checkpoint inhibitors are a group of immunotherapy drugs that block this interaction, thus reactivating the immune cell to attack the tumor.
42. The role of the immune system in protecting against cancer has been clearly documented against oncogenic viruses. Antibodies induced by vaccines against oncogenic viruses, such as human papillomavirus (HPV) and hepatitis B virus (HBV), protect against initial infection and development of cervical and liver tumors, respectively.

Activating Invasion and Metastasis

1. New paradigms in the study of metastasis have identified molecular underpinnings of the dissemination process.
2. Improved understanding of how the invading tumor cell interacts with other proteins and cells has elucidated new biological principles by which metastatic cells regulate their mobility and plasticity.
3. Communications with the tumor microenvironment allows invading cancer cells to conquer stromal challenges, settle, and colonize. Characteristics are driven by genetics and epigenetic changes within the tumor cell itself and its microenvironment.
4. Hanahan and Weinberg identify that "activating invasion and metastasis" is a hallmark of cancer. Understanding these mechanisms of the metastatic process is critical to develop successful treatment interventions.
5. Dissemination of cancer cells leads the initial steps of the invasion-metastasis cascade. Chromosomal instability becomes the "trigger" causing constant and continuous errors in chromosome segregation during mitosis.
6. Investigators suggest that the nature of the primary seeding cancer cell determines the various and different metastatic properties aligned with growth and response to therapy.
7. Seeding may require the joint action of a cluster of tumor cells moving together.
8. EMT is the developmental (transdifferentiation) process whereby transformed epithelial cells lose their cell polarity and cell-cell adhesion, and gain the ability to invade, resist stress, and disseminate. The triggers for EMT in cancer cells include hypoxia, metabolic stressors, and matrix stiffness.
9. Research in pancreatic and lung cancers reveals that EMT might not be essential for metastasis, but it does contribute to chemoresistance.

10. Although the initiation of metastasis may involve EMT, mesenchymal-epithelial transition (MET) is necessary for metastatic progression.
11. Various metastatic cells possess different genetic and epigenetic or phenotypic changes, which differentially drive tumor progression, metastasis, and drug resistance.
12. Genetic expression is affected by oxygen homeostasis in the tumor microenvironment.
13. Hypoxia-inducible factors (HIFs) enable cancer cells to adapt to their environment by modulating angiogenesis, EMT, invasion, metastasis, and energy metabolism.
14. Metastatic characteristics are transferred through extracellular vesicle exchange. Extracellular vesicles called exosomes transfer invasion-promoting factors from the primary tumor, such as miRNAs, to tumorigenic cancer cells. Exosomes secrete EMT inducers that stimulate EMT progression in host epithelial cells, enabling them to invade and metastasize.
15. ECM altered by exosomes exhibits increased stromal cell proliferation, cancer cell migration and survival, and tumor cell resistance to apoptotic signals. These changes plus effects of growth factors and chemokines, lead to the formation of a new microenvironment for cancer cells, immune cells, and other stromal elements, known as the PMN.
16. Age-related physical changes in the ECM inhibit or promote tumor cell motility, invasion, and metastasis.
17. The circadian clock controls a wide spectrum of processes in cellular physiology through metabolic and gene expression pathways. It has been associated with cancer initiation and progression.
18. Diet has been shown to impact cancer metastasis. Some of these dietary effects may be related to changes in the microbiome. Other effects are more direct. For example, asparagine is an important promotor of metastasis, and researchers have found that removing asparagine from the diet of mice reduced breast cancer metastases.
19. In cancer, remodeling of the interstitial ECM causes a broad range of biophysical and biochemical changes affecting cell signaling, ECM stiffness, cell migration, and tumor progression.
20. Binding of cells to the basement membrane is critical for establishing cell polarity, and crucial for several developmental processes and maintenance of tissue homeostasis. Remodeling of the basement membrane is required for cancer cells to invade stromal tissue and become a malignant tumor.
21. Tumor-derived activation factors induce the differentiation of stromal cells towards CAFs, which function as myofibroblasts and remodel the ECM to support tumor growth. ECM is complex, and numerous specific cells and matrikines engage in invasion and metastasis.
22. The immune environment surrounding the tumor plays a significant role in dictating the metastatic potential of the disseminating cells.
23. Intravasation, or the movement of cancer cells through the lumen of the vasculature, is mediated both actively and passively depending on the tumor type, microenvironment, and vasculature.
24. Importantly, integrins regulate the colonization process by easing anchorage-independent survival of circulating tumor cells (CTCs). Metastatic cells use E-cadherin in metastatic sites to detach, disseminate, and seed, thereby promoting metastatic cell survival and block apoptosis.
25. Interactions between CTCs and the microenvironmental components of circulation determine survival and the ability of CTCs to extravasate in distant places. The dissemination of CTCs is supported by very close association with activated platelets and macrophages. The leukocytes that showed the greatest interaction were neutrophils, their role in metastasis is not yet clear. The complex interaction between cancer cells and leukocytes promotes metastasis because metastatic cells possess sugar on their cell surface that binds to galectin-3. Galectin-3 increases the ability of cells to colonize by interacting with mobilized leukocytes.
26. In mouse models, blocking of IL-6 and IL-8 receptors decreased metastasis at lymph nodes, lungs, and liver.
27. CTCs use, exploit, and survive in the bloodstream during metastasis and cause distant metastases also through the lymphatic circulation. CTC characterization identifies the molecular aspects of metastatic tumors.
28. Cell-free DNA (cfDNA) identifies the heterogeneity of CTCs in those with high counts of CTCs. Liquid biopsy of CTCs and /or cfDNA in the bloodstream may have the potential to increase understanding of metastasis. A photoacoustic method for direct use in persons with melanoma enables the detection of very low numbers of CTCs in vivo and their destruction with laser pulses. Additionally, DNA methylation profiles more clearly identify tumor phenotypes among CTC clusters than from single cells.
29. Critical in the metastatic process is the ability of CTCs to adhere and extravasate through endothelial cells and colonize the premetastatic niche (PMN).
30. Extravasation is a complex process. It involves ligand-receptor interactions, chemokines, and circulating non-tumor cells. Integrins are once again very important. They help to determine the location for extravasation and colonization. Cancer cells induce programmed necrosis of endothelial cells, driving metastatic cells to extravasate.
31. Most cancers metastasize to specific target organs, a process called metastatic organotropism. The host microenvironment and the ensuing adaptive process that invading cancer cells undergo play a role in extravasation and colonization at specific sites.
32. Formation of the PMN, where the tumor cells colonize and grow, depends on signaling from various tumor secreted derived factors and bone marrow-derived factors. Exosomes play a significant role. Formation of a vascular network is critical for optimal colonization.
33. Vascular mimicry where tumors create their own channels for fluid transport drives the ability of some breast cancer cells to contribute to distant metastases through the expression of *SERPINE2* and *SLPI*.

34. Colonizing cancer cells use signaling from neuronal pathways for growth and adjustment to new sites.
35. Cancer dormancy is a rest phase in cancer progression that occurs during the primary tumor formation phase or after invasion into secondary sites. Metastatic dormancy occurs because of the delayed adjustment of disseminating cells to their secondary niches or sites affecting single invading cells or cancer clusters after circulation. These dormant cancer cells (DCCs) are rarely detectable with current diagnostic approaches. Much evidence supports the notion that extracellular signal-regulated kinase (ERK) activation has a determinant role in whether cancer cells will proliferate or enter the phase of dormancy. Reawakening DCCs could be a critical factor for cancer development from chronic inflammation. Chronic inflammation can induce epigenetic alterations and DNA mutations in tumor suppressor genes, thus promoting carcinogenesis. Existence of DCCs has led to the emergence of therapy resistance because the cells may resume growth, increasing the risk of unleashing lethal metastatic outbreaks even after a long latency period of months to years.
36. In the last decade a significant number of metastasis suppressors have been identified, most notably miRNAs. Metastatic cancers may be approached through a biomarker-driven strategy that validates single-agent or combination of agents depending fully on the molecular makeup of individual tumors.
37. A priority is the importance of lifestyle and diagnostic factors in reducing cancer mortality. Obesity is becoming a critical etiologic driver of cancer and initiation of metastasis. Worldwide, other preventable risk factors are a significant cause of cancer.

Clinical Manifestations of Cancer

1. Paraneoplastic syndromes are rare disorders with complex clinical manifestations that are triggered by a cancer but are not caused by direct local effects of the tumor mass. Malignant cells do not cause symptoms related to metastasis, but they generate autoantibodies, cytokines, hormones, or peptides that affect may organ systems.
2. Common side effects of cancer and cancer therapy include anemia, bone density loss, cachexia, cardiac and pulmonary damage, fatigue, gastrointestinal issues, hair loss and skin conditions, infection, infertility, leukopenia and thrombocytopenia, lymphedema, and pain.
3. Anemia associated with cancer usually occurs because of malnutrition, chronic bleeding and resultant iron deficiency, chemotherapy, radiation, and malignancies in the blood-forming organs.
4. Cachexia is a complex metabolic syndrome associated with basic illness and is characterized by the loss of muscle with or without loss of fat mass. Cancer cachexia is characterized by systemic inflammation, negative protein and energy balance, and loss of lean body mass with or without wasting of adipose tissue. Multiple mechanisms are involved in the development and progression of cachexia including anorexia, decreased secretion of anabolic hormones, inflammation, decreased physical activity, and altered metabolic responses with abnormalities in protein, lipid, and carbohydrate metabolism. Profoundly altered are both appetite-stimulating and appetite-suppressing brain pathways.
5. Fatigue is the most frequently reported symptom of cancer and cancer treatment.
6. The gastrointestinal tract relies on rapidly growing cells to provide an absorptive surface for nutrients. Both chemotherapy and radiation therapy may cause decreased cell turnover, thereby leading to oral ulcers (stomatitis), malabsorption, and diarrhea.
7. Alopecia (hair loss) results from chemotherapy effects on hair follicles. Alopecia is usually temporary, although hair may initially regrow with a different texture. Not all chemotherapeutic agents cause alopecia. Decreased renewal rates of the epidermal layers in the skin may lead to skin breakdown and dryness, altering the normal barrier protection against infection.
8. Infection is a significant cause of complications and death. Immune suppression, lymphopenia, and granulocytopenia may result from the underlying cancer or secondary to treatment increasing the risk of serious microbial infections.
9. Leukopenia and thrombocytopenia are usually a result of chemotherapy (which is toxic to bone marrow) or radiation (which kills circulating leukocytes). Thrombocytopenia is a major cause of hemorrhage in people with cancer.
10. Pain is generally associated with the late stages of cancer. It can be caused by pressure, obstruction, invasion of a structure sensitive to pain, stretching, tissue destruction, and inflammation.

Diagnosis and Staging of Cancer

1. Tumor tissue is obtained to establish a definitive diagnosis and correctly classify the disease. Once tissue is obtained, it is examined microscopically by the pathologist for the histologic hallmarks of cancer. Cancer classification is established by a variety of tests including immunohistochemical stains, flow cytometry, electron microscopy, chromosome analysis, and genetic studies.
2. Tumor staging involves the size of the tumor, the degree to which it has locally invaded, and the extent to which it has spread. One common scheme for staging is the T (tumor spread), N (node involvement), and M (metastasis) system.
3. Tumor markers are substances (i.e., hormones, enzymes, genes, antigens, antibodies) found in cancer cells and in blood, spinal fluid, or urine. They are used to screen and identify individuals at high risk for cancer, to help diagnose specific types of tumors, and to follow the clinical course of cancer. To date, no tumor marker has proven satisfactory to screen populations of healthy individuals for cancer.
4. Cancer is treated routinely with surgery, radiation therapy, chemotherapy, and combinations of these modalities. Immunotherapy has now established itself as a pillar of cancer care from the metastatic stage to the adjuvant and

neoadjuvant settings in many cancer types. Cancer therapy is rapidly evolving, and genetic analysis may help determine appropriate therapies.

5. Surgical therapy is used for nonmetastatic disease (in which cure is possible by removing the tumor) and as a palliative measure to alleviate symptoms.
6. Ionizing radiation causes cell damage; therefore, the goal of radiation therapy is to damage the tumor without causing excessive toxicity or damage to no diseased structures.
7. The theoretic basis of chemotherapy is the vulnerability of tumor cells in various stages of the cell cycle. Modern chemotherapy uses combinations of drugs with different targets and different toxicities.
8. Increasing evidence of most approved cancer drugs, including tyrosine kinase inhibitors (TKIs), systemic cytotoxic therapies (chemotherapy) and antibody-drug conjugates (ADCs), reveals they do not have a durable impact with metastatic disease often because of therapeutic resistance.
9. Induction chemotherapy seeks to cause shrinkage or disappearance of tumors. Adjuvant chemotherapy is given after surgical excision of a cancer with the goal of eliminating micrometastases. Neoadjuvant chemotherapy is given before localized (surgical or radiation) treatment of a cancer to shrink a cancer so that surgery may spare more normal tissue.
10. The recent discovery of T cell immune checkpoints, such as cytotoxic T lymphocyte antigen 4 (CTLA-4) and programmed cell death 1 (PD-1), moved the field of immuno-oncology into its current era. The challenge is harnessing immune signals that maintain a fine balance between immune surveillance against foreign pathogens or abnormal cells and autoimmunity. Immunotherapy attempts to modify the immune system from a cancer-protective state to a destructive condition. Dedicated scientists and clinicians are mobilized to achieve a higher response rate without increasing autoimmunity.

REFERENCES

1. National Cancer Institute (NCI): *Fact sheet: what is cancer?* Bethesda, MD, 2021, NCI. Updated May 5, 2021. Available at: https://www.cancer.gov/about-cancer/understanding/what-is-cancer. (Accessed August 6, 2021).
2. Hanahan D, Weinberg RA. Hallmarks of cancer. *Cell.* 2000;100(1):57–70.
3. Hanahan D, Weinberg RA. Hallmarks of cancer: the next generation. *Cell.* 2011;144(5):646–674.
4. Bradner JE, Hnisz D, Young RA. Transcriptional addition in cancer. *Cell.* 2017;168(4):629–643.
5. McGranahan N, Swanton C. Clonal heterogeneity and tumor evolution: past, present, and the future. *Cell.* 2017;168(4):613–628.
6. Hanahan D, Coussens LM. Accessories to the crime: functions of cells recruited to the tumor microenvironment. *Cancer Cell.* 2012;21(3):309–322.
7. Marusyk A, Janiszewska M, Polyak K. Intratumoral heterogeneity: the Rosetta Stone of therapy resistance. *Cancer Cell.* 2020;37(4): 471–484.
8. Hsu JL, Hung M-C. The role of HER2 EGFR, and other receptor tyrosine kinases in breast cancer. *Cancer Metastasis Rev.* 2016; 35(4):575–588.
9. Cohen P, Cross D, Jänne PA. Kinase drug discovery 20 years after imatinib: progress and future directions. *Nat Rev Drug Discov.* 2021;20(7):551–569.
10. Liu M, et al. Selective killing of cancer cells harboring mutant RAS by concomitant inhibition of NADPH oxidase and glutathione biosynthesis. *Cell Death Dis.* 2021;12:189.
11. Baugh E, et al. Why are there hotspot mutations in the *TP53* gene in human cancers?,. *Cell Death Differ.* 2018;25:154–160.
12. MedlinePlus: TP53 gene. Bethesda, MD, 2021, U.S. National Library of Medicine. Available at: https://medlineplus.gov/genetics/gene/tp53/. (Accessed August 6, 2021).
13. Kastenhuber ER, Lowe SW. Putting p53 in context. *Cell.* 2017; 170(6):1062–1078.
14. Ramu D, et al. Cellular senescence: silent operator and therapeutic target in cancer. *IUBMB Life.* 2021;73(3):530–542.
15. Zeng S, Shen WH, Liu L. *Cancer Transl Med.* 2018;4(3):70–74.
16. MedlinePlus: RB1 gene, Bethesda, MD, 2020, U.S. National Library of Medicine. Available at: https://medlineplus.gov/genetics/gene/rb1/. (Accessed August 6, 2021).
17. Davies HR, et al. Whole-genome sequencing of retinoblastoma reveals the diversity of rearrangements disrupting RB1 and uncovers a treatment-related mutational signature. *Cancers (Basel).* 2021;13(4):754.
18. Gregersen PA, et al. Incidence and mortality of second primary cancers in Danish patients with retinoblastoma, 1943-2013. *JAMA Netw Open.* 2020;3(10). e2022126.
19. Tubbs A, Nussenzweig A. Endogenous DNA damage as a source of genomic instability in cancer. *Cell.* 2017;168(4):644–656.
20. Chen D, et al: Roles of miRNA dysregulation in the pathogenesis of multiple myeloma, Cancer Gene Ther. Online ahead of print: January 5, 2021. Available at: https://doi.org/10.1038/s41417-020-00291-4. (Accessed August 6, 2021).
21. Nielsen FC, van Overeem Hansen T, Sorensen CS. Hereditary breast and ovarian cancer: new genes in confined pathways. *Nat Rev Cancer.* 2016;16(9):599–612.
22. Antoniou A, et al. Average risks of breast and ovarian cancer associated with BRCA1 or BRCA2 mutations detected in case series unselected for family history: a combined analysis of 22 studies. *Am J Hum Genet.* 2003;72:1117–1130.
23. Salgueiro L, et al. Acquisition of chromosome instability is a mechanism to evade oncogene addiction. *EMBO Mol Med.* 2020; 12:e1094.
24. Dogan F, Forsyth NR. Telomerase regulation: a role for epigenetics. *Cancers (Basel).* 2021;13(6):1213.
25. Guterres AN, Villanueva J. Targeting telomerase for cancer therapy. *Oncogene.* 2020;39:5811–5824.
26. Walcher L, et al. Cancer stem cells—origins and biomarkers: perspectives for targeted personalized therapies. *Front Immunol.* 2020;11:1280.
27. Lambert AW, Weinberg RA. Linking EMT programmes to normal and neoplastic epithelial stem cells. *Nat Rev Cancer.* 2021;21:325–338.
28. Chu DT, et al. Recent progress of stem cell therapy in cancer treatment: molecular mechanisms and potential applications. *Cells.* 2020;9(3):563.
29. Nakazawa MS, Keith B, Simon MC. Oxygen availability and metabolic adaptations. *Nat Rev Cancer.* 2016;16(10):663673.
30. Jackson HW, et al. TIMPs: versatile extracellular regulators in cancer. *Nat Rev Cancer.* 2017;17(1):38–53.

31. Jiang X, et al. The role of microenvironment in tumor angiogenesis. *J Exp Clin Cancer Res*. 2020;39:204.
32. Madu CO, et al. Angiogenesis in breast cancer progression, diagnosis, and treatment. *J Cancer*. 2020;11(15):4474–4494.
33. Lopes-Coelho F, et al. Anti-angiogenic therapy: current challenges and future perspectives. *Int J Mol Sci*. 2021;22:3765.
34. Eelen G, et al. Basic and therapeutic aspects of angiogenesis updated. *Circ Res*. 2020;127(2):310–329.
35. Alsaab HO, et al. Nanomaterials for antiangiogenic therapies for cancer: a promising tool for personalized medicine. *Int J Mol Sci*. 2021;22(4):1631.
36. Vander Heiden MG, DeBerardinis RJ. Understanding the intersections between metabolism and cancer biology. *Cell*. 2017;168(4):657–669.
37. Flores A. Increased lactate dehydrogenase activity is dispensable in squamous carcinoma cells of origin. *Nat Commun*. 2019;10(1):91.
38. Pavlova NN, Thompson CB. The emerging hallmarks of cancer metabolism. *Cell Metab*. 2016;23(1):27–47.
39. Martinez-Outschoorn UE, et al. Cancer metabolism: a therapeutic perspective. *Nat Rev Clin Oncol*. 2017;14(1):11–31.
40. Kim LC, Cook RS, Chen J. mTORC1 and mTORC2 in cancer and the tumor microenvironment. *Oncogene*. 2017;36(16):2191–2201.
41. Hiam-Galvez KJ, Allen BM, Spitzer MH. Systemic immunity in cancer. *Nat Rev Cancer*. 2021;21(6):345–359.
42. Piscione M, et al. Eradication of *Helicobacter pylori* and gastric cancer: a controversial relationship. *Front Microbiol*. 2021;12:630852.
43. Kuo SH, et al. First-line antibiotic therapy in *Helicobacter pylori*-negative low-grade gastric mucosa-associated lymphoid tissue lymphoma. *Sci Rep*. 2017;7:14333.
44. Zhu S, et al. Tumor-associated macrophages: role in tumorigenesis and immunotherapy implications. *J Cancer*. 2021;12(1):54–64.
45. Kalluri R. The biology and function of fibroblasts in cancer. *Nat Rev Cancer*. 2016;16(9):582–598.
46. Sahai E, et al. A framework for advancing our understanding of cancer-associated fibroblasts. *Nat Rev Cancer*. 2020;20:174–186.
47. Calon A, et al. Stromal gene expression defines poor-prognosis subtypes in colorectal cancer. *Nat Genet*. 2015;47:320–329.
48. Guinney J, et al. The consensus molecular subtypes of colorectal cancer. *Nat Med*. 2015;21:1350–1356.
49. Franco-Barraza J, et al. Matrix-regulated integrin alphavbeta5 maintains alpha5beta1-dependent desmoplastic traits prognostic of neoplastic recurrence. *eLife*. 2017;6:e206000.
50. Kim MG, et al. Selective activation of anticancer chemotherapy by cancer-associated fibroblasts in the tumor microenvironment. *J Natl Cancer Inst*. 2017;109(1). djw186.
51. Rhim AD, et al. Stromal elements act to restrain, rather than support, pancreatic ductal adenocarcinoma. *Cancer Cell*. 2014;25:735–747.
52. Özdemir BC, et al. Depletion of carcinoma-associated fibroblasts and fibrosis induced immunosuppression and accelerates pancreas cancer with reduced survival. *Cancer Cell*. 2014;25(6):719–734.
53. Sherman MH, et al. Vitamin D receptor-mediated stromal reprogramming suppresses pancreatitis and enhances pancreatic cancer therapy. *Cell*. 2014;159:80–93.
54. Hah N, et al. Targeting transcriptional and epigenetic reprogramming in stromal cells in fibrosis and cancer. *Cold Spring Harb Symp Quant Biol*. 2015;80:249–255.
55. American Society for Microbiology (ASM). The 7 viruses that cause human cancers. Washington, DC, 2021, ASM. https://asm.org/Articles/2019/January/The-Seven-Viruses-that-Cause-Human-Cancers. (Accessed August 6, 2021.)
56. Abara WE, et al. Hepatitis B vaccination, screening, and linkage to care: best practice advice from the American College of Physicians and the Centers for Disease Control and Prevention. *Ann Intern Med*. 2017;167(11):794–804.
57. Centers for Disease Control and Prevention (CDC) *Hepatitis C questions and answers for the public. Atlanta*. GA: CDC; 2020. https://www.cdc.gov/hepatitis/hcv/cfaq.htm. (Accessed August 6, 2021).
58. Kalidindi Y, et al. Association of direct-acting antiviral treatment with mortality among Medicare beneficiaries with hepatitis C. *JAMA Netw Open*. 2020;3(7):e2011055.
59. Apavaloaei A, et al. The origin and immune recognition of tumor-specific antigens. *Cancers (Basel)*. 2020;12(9):2607.
60. Jou J, et al. The changing landscape of therapeutic cancer vaccines—novel platforms and neoantigen identification. *Clin Cancer Res*. 2021;27(3):689–703.
61. Togashi Y, Shitara K, Nishikawa H. Regulatory T cells in cancer immunosuppression—implications for anticancer therapy. *Nat Rev Clin Oncol*. 2019;16:356–371.
62. Albinger N, Hartmann J, Ullrich E. Current status and perspective of CAR-T and CAR-NK cell therapy trials in Germany. *Gene Ther*. March 22, 2021. https://doi.org/10.1038/s41434-021-00246-w. Published online before print (Accessed August 6, 2021).
63. Marin-Acevedo JA, Kimbrough EO, Lou Y. Next generation of immune checkpoint inhibitors and beyond. *J Hematol Oncol*. 2021;14:45.
64. Fares J, et al. Molecular principles of metastasis: a hallmark of cancer revisited. *Curr Signal Transduct Ther*. 2020;5:28. https://doi.org/10.1038/s41392-020-0134-x. (Accessed August 6, 2021.)
65. Maitra A. Molecular envoys pave the way for pancreatic cancer to invade the liver. *Nature*. 2019;567:181–182.
66. Massague J, Obenauf AC. Metastatic colonization by circulating tumour cells. *Nature*. 2016;529:298–306.
67. Lambert AW, Pattabiraman DR, Weinberg RA. Emerging biological principles of metastasis. *Cell*. 2017;168:670–691.
68. Bakhoun SF, et al. Chromosomal instability drives metastasis through a cytosolic DNA response. *Nature*. 2018;553:467–472.
69. Tabassum DP, Polyak K. Tumorigenesis: it takes a village. *Nat Rev Cancer*. 2015;15:473–483.
70. Clark AG, Vignjevic DM. Modes of cancer cell invasion and the role of the microenvironment. *Curr Opin Cell Biol*. 2015;36:13–22.
71. Cheung KJ, Ewald AJ. A collective route to metastasis: seeding by tumor cell clusters. *Science*. 2016;352:167–169.
72. Fouad YA, Aanei C. Revisiting the hallmarks of cancer. *Am J Cancer Res*. 2017;7:1016–1036.
73. Knott SRV, et al. Asparagine bioavailability governs metastasis in a model of breast cancer. *Nature*. 2018;554:378–381.
74. Nieto MA, et al: EMT: 2016, Cell 166(1):21–45, 2016.
75. Pastushenko I, et al. Identification of the tumour transition states occurring during EMT. *Nature*. 2018;556:463.
76. Erdogan B, et al. Cancer associated fibroblasts promote directional cancer cell migration by aligning fibronectin. *J Cell Biol*. 2016;216:3799–3816.
77. Rankin EB, Giaccia AJ. Hypoxic control of metastasis. *Science*. 2016;352:175–180.
78. Lamouille S, Xu J, Derynck R. Molecular mechanisms of epithelial-mesenchymal transition. *Nat Rev Mol Cell Biol*. 2014;15:178–196.
79. De Craene B, Berx G. Regulatory networks defining EMT during cancer initiation and progression. *Nat Rev Cancer*. 2013;13:97–110.

80. Fischer KR, et al. Epithelial-to mesenchymal transition is not required for lung metastasis but contributes to chemoresistance. *Nature*. 2015;527:472–476.
81. Diepenbruck M, Christofori G. Epithelial-mesenchymal transition (EMT) and metastasis: yes, no, maybe? *Curr Opin Cell Biol*. 2016;43:7–13.
82. Zheng XF, et al. Epithelial-to-mesenchymal transition is dispensable for metastasis but induces chemoresistance in pancreatic cancer. *Nature*. 2015;527:525.
83. Esposito M, et al. Bone vascular niche E-selectin induces mesenchymal-epithelial transition and Wnt activation in cancer cells to promote bone metastasis. *Nat Cell Biol*. 2019;21(5): 627–639.
84. Lawson DA, et al. Tumour heterogeneity and metastasis at single-cell resolution. *Nat. Cell Biol*. 2018;20:1349–1360.
85. van't Veer LJ, et al. Gene expression profiling predicts clinical outcome of breast cancer. *Nature*. 2002;415(6871): 530–536.
86. Ramaswamy S, et al. A molecular signature of metastasis in primary solid tumors. *Nat Genet*. 2003;33:49–54.
87. Hunter K, Welch DR, Liu ET. Genetic background is an important determinant of metastatic potential. *Nat Genet*. 2003;34(1):23–24. author reply 25.
88. Robinson DR, et al. Integrative clinical genomics of metastatic cancer. *Nature*. 2017;548:297–303.
89. Birkbak NJ, McGranahan N. Cancer genome evolutionary trajectories in metastasis. *Cancer Cell*. 2020;37:8–19.
90. Yang D, et al. Intertumoral heterogeneity in SCLC is influenced by the cell type of origin. *Cancer Discov*. 2018;8:1316–1331.
91. Carnero A, Lleonart M. The hypoxic microenvironment: a determinant of cancer stem cell evolution. *Bioessays*. 2016;38(Suppl 1):S65–S74.
92. Salvador F, et al. Lysyl oxidase-like protein LOXL2 promotes lung metastasis of breast cancer. *Cancer Res*. 2017;77(21): 5846–5859.
93. Semenza GL. Oxygen sensing, hypoxia-inducible factors, and disease pathophysiology. *Annu Rev Pathol*. 2014;9:47–71.
94. Tasdogan A, et al. Metabolic heterogeneity confers differences in melanoma metastatic potential. *Nature*. 2020;577:115–120.
95. Papalazarou V, et al. The creatine–phosphagen system is mechanoresponsive in pancreatic adenocarcinoma and fuels invasion and metastasis. *Nat Metab*. 2020;2:62–80.
96. Peinado H, et al. Pre-metastatic niches: organ-specific homes for metastases. *Nat Rev Cancer*. 2017;17:302–317.
97. Zomer A, et al. In vivo imaging reveals extracellular vesicle-mediated phenocopying of metastatic behavior. *Cell*. 2015;161:1046–1057.
98. Weidle UH, et al. The multiple roles of exosomes in metastasis. *Cancer Genomics Proteomics*. 2017;14:1–15.
99. Tickner JA, et al. Functions and therapeutic roles of exosomes in cancer. *Front Oncol*. 2014;4:127.
100. Harris DA, et al. Exosomes released from breast cancer carcinomas stimulate cell movement. *PLoS One*. 2015;10:e0117495.
101. Singh R, et al. Exosome-mediated transfer of miR-10b promotes cell invasion in breast cancer. *Mol Cancer*. 2014;13:256.
102. Syn N, et al. Exosome-mediated metastasis: from epithelial-mesenchymal transition to escape from immunosurveillance. *Trends Pharm Sci*. 2016;37:606–617.
103. Aga M, et al. Exosomal HIF1alpha supports invasive potential of nasopharyngeal carcinoma-associated LMP1-positive exosomes. *Oncogene*. 2014;33:4613–4622.
104. You Y, et al. Matrix metalloproteinase 13-containing exosomes promote nasopharyngeal carcinoma metastasis. *Cancer Sci*. 2015;106:1669–1677.
105. Franzen CA, et al. Urothelial cells undergo epithelial-to-mesenchymal transition after exposure to muscle invasive bladder cancer exosomes. *Oncogenesis*. 2015;4:e163.
106. Jeppesen DK, et al. Quantitative proteomics of fractionated membrane and lumen exosome proteins from isogenic metastatic and nonmetastatic bladder cancer cells reveal differential expression of EMT factors. *Proteomics*. 2014;14:699–712.
107. Escrevente C, et al. Interaction and uptake of exosomes by ovarian cancer cells. *BMC Cancer*. 2011;11:108.
108. Tarbe N, et al. Identification of rat pancreatic carcinoma genes associated with lymphogenous metastasis. *Anticancer Res*. 2002;22:2015–2027.
109. Mu W, Rana S, Zoller M. Host matrix modulation by tumor exosomes promotes motility and invasiveness. *Neoplasia*. 2013;15:875–887.
110. Fabbri M, et al. MicroRNAs bind to Toll-like receptors to induce prometastatic inflammatory response. *Proc Natl Acad Sci U S A*. 2012;109:E2110–E2116.
111. Ye S-b, et al. Tumor-derived exosomes promote tumor progression and T-cell dysfunction through the regulation of enriched exosomal microRNAs in human nasopharyngeal carcinoma. *Oncotarget*. 2014;5:5439.
112. Clayton A, et al. Cancer exosomes express CD39 and CD73, which suppress T cells through adenosine production. *J Immunol*. 2011;187:676–683.
113. Peinado H, et al. Melanoma exosomes educate bone marrow progenitor cells toward a pro-metastatic phenotype through MET. *Nat Med*. 2012;18:883.
114. Hood JL, San RS, Wickline SA. Exosomes released by melanoma cells prepare sentinel lymph nodes for tumor metastasis. *Cancer Res*. 2011;71:3792–3801.
115. Costa-Silva B, et al. Pancreatic cancer exosomes initiate pre-metastatic niche formation in the liver. *Nat Cell Biol*. 2015;17:816–826.
116. Hoshino A, et al. Tumour exosome integrins determine organotropic metastasis. *Nature*. 2015;527:329–335.
117. Yue S, et al. The tetraspanins CD151 and Tspan8 are essential exosome components for the crosstalk between cancer initiating cells and their surrounding. *Oncotarget*. 2015;6:2366.
118. Luga V, et al. Exosomes mediate stromal mobilization of autocrine Wnt-PCP signaling in breast cancer cell migration. *Cell*. 2012;151:1542–1556.
119. Smyth TJ, et al. Examination of the specificity of tumor cell derived exosomes with tumor cells in vitro. *Biochim Biophys Acta*. 2014 1838:2954–2965.
120. Zoller M. Tetraspanins: push and pull in suppressing and promoting metastasis. *Nat Rev Cancer*. 2009;9:40–55.
121. Zhang L, et al. Microenvironment-induced PTEN loss by exosomal microRNA primes brain metastasis outgrowth. *Nature*. 2015;527:100–104.
122. Flavahan WA, Gaskell E, Bernstein BE. Epigenetic plasticity and the hallmarks of cancer. *Science*. 2017;357(6348). eaaal2380.
123. You JS, Jones PA. Cancer genetics and epigenetics: two sides of the same coin? *Cancer Cell*. 2012;22:9–20.
124. Shen H, Laird PW. Interplay between the cancer genome and epigenome. *Cell*. 2013;153:38–55.
125. Laugesen A, Helin K. Chromatin repressive complexes in stem cells, development , and cancer. *Cell Stem Cell*. 2014;14:735–751.

126. Suva ML, Riggi N, Berstein BE. Epigenetic reprogramming in cancer. *Science*. 2013;339:1567–1570.
127. Kim J, Orkin SH. Embryonic stem-cell specific signatures in cancer: insights into genomic regulatory networks and implications for medicine. *Genome Med*. 2011;3:75.
128. Ecker BL, et al. Age-related changes in HAPLN1 increase lymphatic permeability and affect routes of melanoma metastasis. *Cancer Discov*. 2019;9(1):82–95.
129. Kaur A, et al. Remodeling of the collagen matrix in aging skin promotes melanoma metastasis and effects immune cell motility. *Cancer Discov*. 2019;9(1):64–81.
130. Helmink BA, et al. The microbiome, cancer, and cancer therapy. *Nat Med*. 2019;25:377–388.
131. Pushalkar S, et al. The pancreatic cancer microbiome promotes oncogenesis by induction of innate and adaptive immune suppression. *Cancer Disc*. 2018;8:403–416.
132. Cronin M, et al. Orally administered bifidobacteria as vehicles for delivery of agents to systemic tumors. *Mol Ther*. 2010;18: 1397–1407.
133. Panebianco C, Andriulli A, Pazienza V. Pharmacomicrobiomics: exploiting the drug-microbiota interactions in anticancer therapies. *Microbiome*. 2018;6:92.
134. Lehouritis P, et al. Local bacteria affect the efficacy of chemotherapeutic drugs. *Sci Rep*. 2015;5:14554.
135. Geller LT, et al. Potential role of intratumor bacteria in mediating tumor resistance to the chemotherapeutic drug gemcitabine. *Science*. 2017;357:1156–1160.
136. Alexander JL, et al. Gut microbiota modulation of chemotherapy efficacy and toxicity. *Nat Rev Gastroenterol Hepatol*. 2017;14:356–365.
137. Gur C, et al. Binding of the Fap2 protein of *Fusobacterium nucleatum* to human inhibitory receptor TIGIT protects tumors from immune attack. *Immunity*. 2015;42:344–355.
138. Zheng JH, et al. Two-step enhanced cancer immunotherapy with engineered *Salmonella typhimurium* secreting heterologous flagellin. *Sci Transl Med*. 2017;9(376). eaak9537.
139. Lie J-AS, Roessink J, Kjaerheim K:. Breast cancer and night work among Norwegian nurses. *Cancer Causes Control*. 2006;17: 39–44.
140. Papantoniou K, et al. Night shift work, chronotype and prostate cancer risk in the MCC-Spain case-control study. *Int J Cancer*. 2015;137(5):1147–1157.
141. Schernhammer ES, et al. Rotating night shifts and risk of breast cancer in women participating in the Nurses' Health Study. *J Natl Cancer Inst*. 2001;93:1563–1568.
142. Knutsson A, et al. Breast cancer among shift workers: results of the WOLF longitudinal cohort study. *Scand J Work Environ Health*. 2013;39:170–177.
143. Straif K, et al. Carcinogenicity of shift-work, painting, and fire-fighting. *Lancet Oncol*. 2007;8:1065–1066.
144. Kakizaki M, et al. Sleep duration and the risk of prostate cancer: the Ohsaki Cohort Study. *Br J Cancer*. 2008;99:176–178.
145. Srour B, et al. Circadian nutritional behaviours and cancer risk: new insights from the NutriNet-santé prospective cohort study: disclaimers. *Int J Cancer*. 2018;143:2369–2379.
146. Masri S, Sassone-Corsi P. The emerging link between cancer, metabolism, and circadian rhythms. *Nat Med*. 2018;24: 1795–1803.
147. Altman BJ, et al. MYC disrupts the circadian clock and metabolism in cancer cells. *Cell Metab*. 2015;22:1009–1019.
148. Pascual G, et al. Targeting metastasis-initiating cells through the fatty acid receptor CD36. *Nature*. 2017;541:41–45.
149. Steck SE, Murphy EA. Dietary patterns and cancer risk. *Nat Rev Cancer*. 2020;20:125–138.
150. Winkler J, et al. Concepts of extracellular matrix remodelling in tumour progression and metastasis. *Nat Commun*. 2020;11:5120.
151. Mouw JK, Ou G, Weaver VM. Extracellular matrix assembly: a multiscale deconstruction. *Nat Rev Mol Cell Biol*. 2014;15: 771–785.
152. Egeblad M, Rasch MG, Weaver VM. Dynamic interplay between the collagen scaffold and tumor evolution. *Curr Opin Cell Biol*. 2010;22:697–706.
153. Jayadev R, Sherwood DR. Basement membranes. *Curr Biol*. 2017;27:R207–R211.
154. Kessenbrock K, Plaks V, Werb Z. Matrix metalloproteinases: regulators of the tumor microenvironment. *Cell*. 2010;141:52–67.
155. Cox TR, Erler JT. Remodeling and homeostasis of the extracellular matrix: implications for fibrotic diseases and cancer. *Dis Model Mech*. 2011;4:165–178.
156. Hinz B, et al. Recent developments in myofibroblast biology: paradigms for connective tissue remodeling. *Am J Pathol*. 2012;180:1340–1355.
157. Dooley S, ten Dijke P. TGF-β in progression of liver disease. *Cell Tissue Res*. 2012;347:245–256.
158. Barbazán J, Matic Vignjevic D. Cancer associated fibroblasts: is the force the path to the dark side? *Curr Opin Cell Biol*. 2019;56:71–79.
159. Orimo A, et al. Stromal fibroblasts present in invasive human breast carcinomas promote tumor growth and angiogenesis through elevated SDF-1/CXCL12 secretion. *Cell*. 2005;121: 335–348.
160. Ishii G, Ochiai A, Neri S. Phenotypic and functional heterogeneity of cancer-associated fibroblast within the tumor microenvironment. *Adv Drug Deliv Rev*. 2016;99:186–196.
161. Curren S, Murray GI. Matrix metalloproteinases : molecular aspects of their roles in tumour invasion and metastasis. *Eur J Cancer*. 2000;36:1621–1630.
162. Shuman Moss LA, Jensen-Taubman S, Stetler-Stevenson WG. Matrix metalloproteinases changing roles in tumor progression and metastasis. *Am J Pathol*. 2012;181:1895–1899.
163. Egeblad M, Werb Z. New functions for the matrix metalloproteinases in cancer progression. *Nat Rev Cancer*. 2002;2:161–174.
164. Hadler-Olsen E, Winberg JO, Uhlin-Hansen L. Matrix metalloproteinases in cancer: their value as diagnostic and prognostic markers and therapeutic ta-gets. *Tumor Biol*. 2013;34:2041–2051.
165. Mowers EE, Sharfin MN, MacLeod KF. Autophagy in cancer metastasis. *Oncogene*. 2017;36:1619–1630.
166. Macintosh RL, et al. Inhibition of autophagy impairs tumor cell invasion in an organotypic model. *Cell Cycle*. 2012;11:2022–2029.
167. Mauffrey P, et al. Progenitors from the central nervous system drive neurogenesis in cancer. *Nature*. 2019;569:672–678.
168. Fares J, et al. Neurogenesis in the adult hippocampus: history, regulation, and prospective roles. *Int J Neurosci*. 2019;129:598–611.
169. Mlecnik B, et al. The tumor microenvironment and Immunoscore are critical determinants of dissemination to distant metastasis. *Sci Transl Med*. 2016;8(327):327ra26.
170. Fares J, Fares MY, Fares Y. Immune checkpoint inhibitors: advances and impact in neuro-oncology. *Surg Neurol Int*. 2019;10:9.
171. Bidwell BN, et al. Silencing of Irf7 pathways in breast cancer cells promotes bone metastasis through immune escape. *Nat Med*. 2012;18:1224–1231.

172. Pommier A, et al. Unresolved endoplasmic reticulum stress engenders immune-resistant, latent pancreatic cancer metastases. *Science*. 2018;360:1202.
173. Li R, Huang Y, Lin J. Distinct effects of general anesthetics on lung metastasis mediated by IL-6/JAK/STAT3 pathway in mouse models. *Nat Commun*. 2020;11:642.
174. Fouad YA, Aanei C. Revisiting the hallmarks of cancer. *Am J Cancer Res*. 2017;7:1016–1036.
175. Reymond N, d'Agua BB, Ridley AJ. Crossing the endothelial barrier during metastasis. *Nat Rev Cancer*. 2013;13:858–870.
176. Bockhorn M, Jain RK, Munn LL. Active versus passive mechanisms in metastasis: do cancer cells crawl into vessels, or are they pushed? *Lancet Oncol*. 2007;8:444–448.
177. Zervantonakis IK, et al. Three-dimensional microfluidic model for tumor cell intravasation and endothelial barrier function. *Proc Natl Acad Sci U S A*. 2012;109:13515–13520.
178. Wong AD, Searson PC. Mitosis-mediated intravasation in a tissue-engineered tumor-microvessel platform. *Cancer Res*. 2017;77:6453–6461.
179. Denais CM, et al. Nuclear envelope rupture and repair during cancer cell migration. *Science*. 2016;352:353–358.
180. Hamidi H, Ivaska J. Every step of the way: integrins in cancer progression and metastasis. *Nat Rev Cancer*. 2018;18:532–547.
181. Padmanaban V, et al. E-cadherin is required for metastasis in multiple models of breast cancer. *Nature*. 2019;573(7774): 439–444.
182. Pantel K, Speicher MR. The biology of circulating tumor cells. *Oncogene*. 2016;35:1216–1224.
183. Gao H, et al. The BMP inhibitor Coco reactivates breast cancer cells at lung metastatic sites. *Cell*. 2012;150:764–779.
184. Lu X, et al. VCAM-1 promotes osteolytic expansion of indolent bone micrometastasis of breast cancer by engaging alpha4beta1-positive osteoclast progenitors. *Cancer Cell*. 2011;20:701–714.
185. Aceto N, et al. Circulating tumor cell clusters are oligoclonal precursors of breast cancer metastasis. *Cell*. 2014;158:1110–1122.
186. Zhang Y, et al. VN-NDP: a neighbor discovery protocol based on virtual nodes in mobile WSNs. *Sensors (Basel)*. 2019;19(21): 4739.
187. Yu M, et al. Circulating breast tumor cells exhibit dynamic changes in epithelial and mesenchymal composition. *Science*. 2013;339:580–584.
188. Ankrum JA, Ong JF, Karp JM. Mesenchymal stem cells: immune evasive, not immune privileged. *Nat Biotechnol*. 2014;32:252.
189. Duda DG, et al. Malignant cells facilitate lung metastasis by bringing their own soil. *Proc Natl Acad Sci U S A*. 2010;107: 21677–21682.
190. Gay LJ, Felding-Habermann B. Contribution of platelets to tumour metastasis. *Nat Rev Cancer*. 2011;11:123–134.
191. Placke T, et al. Platelet-derived MHC class I confers a pseudonormal phenotype to cancer cells that subverts the antitumor reactivity of natural killer immune cells. *Cancer Res*. 2012;72:440–448.
192. Hu C, et al. Thrombocytosis is a significant indictor of hypercoagulability, prognosis and recurrence in gastric cancer. *Exp Ther Med*. 2014;8:125–132.
193. Smith HA, Kang Y. The metastasis-promoting roles of tumor-associated immune cells. *J Mol Med (Berl)*. 2013;91:411–429.
194. Szczerba BM, et al. Neutrophils escort circulating tumour cells to enable cell cycle progression. *Nature*. 2019;566:553.
195. Perrotta RM, et al. Reprogramming the tumor metastasis cascade by targeting galectin-driven networks. *Biochem J*. 2021;478(3):597–617.
196. Jackson W, et al. Role of megakaryocytes in breast cancer metastasis to bone. *Cancer Res*. 2017;77:1942–1954.
197. Granot Z, et al. Tumor entrained neutrophils inhibit seeding in the premetastatic lung. *Cancer Cell*. 2011;20:300–314.
198. van Helvert S, Storm C, Friedl P. Mechanoreciprocity in cell migration. *Nat Cell Biol*. 2018;20:8–20.
199. Follain G, et al. Hemodynamic forces tune the arrest, adhesion, and extravasation of circulating tumor cells. *Dev Cell*. 2018;45 33–52.e12.
200. Boire A, et al. Complement component 3 adapts the cerebrospinal fluid for leptomeningeal metastasis. *Cell*. 2017;168:1101.
201. Bonecchi R, et al. Chemokines and chemokine receptors: an overview. *Front Biosci (Landmark Ed)*. 2009;14:540–551.
202. Quail DF, et al. Obesity alters the lung myeloid cell landscape to enhance breast cancer metastasis through IL5 and GM-CSF. *Nat Cell Biol*. 2017;19:974.
203. Jayatilaka H, et al. Synergistic IL-6 and IL-8 paracrine signalling pathway infers a strategy to inhibit tumour cell migration. *Nat Commun*. 2017;8:15584.
204. Wellenstein MD, et al. Loss of p53 triggers WNT-dependent systemic inflammation to drive breast cancer metastasis. *Nature*. 2019;572:538–542.
205. Headley MB, et al. Visualization of immediate immune responses to pioneer metastatic cells in the lung. *Nature*. 2016;531: 513–517.
206. Naxerova K, et al. Origins of lymphatic and distant metastases in human colorectal cancer. *Science*. 2017;357:55–60.
207. Brown M, et al. Lymph node blood vessels provide exit routes for metastatic tumor cell dissemination in mice. *Science*. 2018;359:1408–1411.
208. Pereira ER, et al. Lymph node metastases can invade local blood vessels, exit the node, and colonize distant organs in mice. *Science*. 2018;359:1403–1407.
209. Lee CK, et al. Tumor metastasis to lymph nodes requires YAP-dependent metabolic adaptation. *Science*. 2019;363:644.
210. Joosse SA, Gorges TM, Pantel K. Biology, detection, and clinical implications of circulating tumor cells. *EMBO Mol Med*. 2015;7:1–11.
211. Fares J, et al. Diagnostic clinical trials in breast cancer brain metastases: barriers and innovations. *Clin Breast Cancer*. 2019;19:383–391.
212. Abbosh C, et al. Phylogenetic ctDNA analysis depicts early-stage lung cancer evolution. *Nature*. 2017;545:446.
213. Galanzha EI, et al. In vivo liquid biopsy using Cytophone platform for photoacoustic detection of circulating tumor cells in patients with melanoma. *Sci Transl Med*. 2019;11 eaat5857.
214. Gkountela S, et al. Circulating tumor cell clustering shapes DNA methylation to enable metastasis seeding. *Cell*. 2019;176:98.
215. Strilic B, Offermanns S. Intravascular survival and extravasation of tumor cells. *Cancer Cell*. 2017;32:282–293.
216. Leong HS, et al. Invadopodia are required for cancer cell extravasation and are a therapeutic target for metastasis. *Cell Rep*. 2014;8:1558–1570.
217. Stoletov K, et al. Visualizing extravasation dynamics of metastatic tumor cells. *J Cell Sci*. 2010;123:2332–2341.
218. Schumacher D, et al. Platelet-derived nucleotides promote tumor-cell transendothelial migration and metastasis via P2Y2 receptor. *Cancer Cell*. 2013;24:130–137.
219. Raskov H, et al. Premetastatic niches, exosomes and circulating tumor cells: early mechanisms of tumor dissemination and the relation to surgery. *Int J Cancer*. 2020;146(12):3244–3255.

220. Alix-Panabieres C, Pantel K. Clinical applications of circulating tumor cells and circulating tumor DNA as liquid biopsy. *Cancer Discov*. 2016;6:479–491.
221. Stegner D, Dutting S, Nieswandt B. : Mechanistic explanation for platelet contribution to cancer metastasis. *Thromb Res*. 2014;133(Suppl 2):S149–S157.
222. Labelle M, Hynes RO. The initial hours of metastasis: the importance of cooperative host-tumor cell interactions during hematogenous dissemination. *Cancer Discov*. 2012;2:1091–1099.
223. Joyce JA, Pollard JW. Microenvironmental regulation of metastasis. *Nat Rev Cancer*. 2009;9:239–252.
224. Strilic B, et al. Tumour-cell-induced endothelial cell necroptosis via death receptor 6 promotes metastasis. *Nature*. 2016;536:215–218.
225. Nguyen DX, Massague J. Genetic determinants of cancer metastasis. *Nat Rev Genet*. 2007;8:341–352.
226. Croucher PI, McDonald MM, Martin TJ. Bone metastasis: the importance of the neighborhood. *Nat Rev Cancer*. 2016;16: 373–386.
227. Kreps LM, Addison CL. Targeting intercellular communication in the bone microenvironment to prevent disseminated tumor cell escape from dormancy and bone metastatic tumor growth. *Int J Mol Sci*. 2021;22(6):2911.
228. Wang H, et al. The osteogenic niche is a calcium reservoir of bone micrometastases and confers unexpected therapeutic vulnerability. *Cancer Cell*. 2018;34:823.
229. Goddard ET, et al. The rodent liver undergoes weaning-induced involution and supports breast cancer metastasis. *Cancer Discov*. 2017;7:177–187.
230. Valastyan S, Weinberg RA. Tumor metastasis: molecular insights and evolving paradigms. *Cell*. 2011;147:275–292.
231. Psaila B, et al. Priming the 'soil' for breast cancer metastasis: the pre-metastatic niche. *Breast Dis*. 2006;26:65–74.
232. Peinado H, Lavotshkin S, Lyden D. The secreted factors responsible for pre-metastatic niche formation: old sayings and new thoughts. *Semin Cancer Biol*. 2011;21:139–146.
233. Lee JW, et al. Hepatocytes direct the formation of a pro-metastatic niche in the liver. *Nature*. 2019;567:249–252.
234. Wagenblast E, et al. A model of breast cancer heterogeneity reveals vascular mimicry as a driver of metastasis. *Nature*. 2015;520:358–362.
235. Zeng Q, et al. Synaptic proximity enables NMDAR signalling to promote brain metastasis. *Nature*. 2019;573:526–531.
236. Chen Q, et al. Carcinoma-astrocyte gap junctions promote brain metastasis by cGAMP transfer. *Nature*. 2016;533:493–498.
237. Gomis RR, Gawrzak S. Tumor cell dormancy. *Mol Oncol*. 2017;11:62–78.
238. Giancotti FG. Mechanisms governing metastatic dormancy and reactivation. *Cell*. 2013;155:750–764.
239. Park SY, Nam JS. The force awakens: metastatic dormant cancer cells. *Exp Mol Med*. 2020;52:569–581.
240. Sosa MS, Bragado P, Aguirre-Ghiso JA. Mechanisms of disseminated cancer cell dormancy: an awakening field. *Nat Rev Cancer*. 2014;14:611–622.
241. Sosa MS, Bernstein E, Aguirre-Ghiso JA. Epigenetic regulation of cancer dormancy as a plasticity mechanism for metastasis initiation. In: Yuzhuo Wang Y, Crea F, eds. *Tumor dormancy and recurrence, Totowa, NJ.* : Humana Press; 2017:1–16.
242. Chambard J, et al. ERK implication in cell cycle regulation. *Biochim Biophys Acta*. 1773;1299–1310:2007.
243. Mebratu Y, Tesfaigzi Y. How ERK1/2 activation controls cell proliferation and cell death: Is subcellular localization the answer? *Cell Cycle*. 2009;8:1168–1175.
244. Aguirre-Ghiso JA, et al. ERKMAPK activity as a determinant of tumor growth and dormancy; regulation by p38SAPK. *Cancer Res*. 2003;63:1684–1695.
245. Teng MW, et al. Immune-mediated dormancy: an equilibrium with cancer. *J Leukoc Biol*. 2008;84:988–993.
246. Machida H, et al. Significance of monocyte counts at recurrence on survival outcome of women with endometrial cancer. *Int J Gynecol Cancer*. 2017;27:302–310.
247. Okubo M, et al. M2-polarized macrophages contribute to neovasculogenesis, leading to relapse of oral cancer following radiation. *Sci Rep*. 2016;6:27548.
248. Bowers LW, et al. NSAID use reduces breast cancer recurrence in overweight and obese women: role of prostaglandin–aromatase interactions. *Cancer Res*. 2014;74:4446–4457.
249. Hughes R, et al. Perivascular M2 macrophages stimulate tumor relapse after chemotherapy. *Cancer Res*. 2015;75:3479–3491.
250. Cole SW. Chronic inflammation and breast cancer recurrence. *J Clin Oncol*. 2009;27:3418.
251. Linde N, Fluegen G, Aguirre-Ghiso J. The relationship between dormant cancer cells and their microenvironment. *Adv Cancer Res*. 2016;132:45–71.
252. Wang H, et al. Immune checkpoint blockade and CAR-T cell therapy in hematologic malignancies. *J Hematol Oncol*. 2019;12:59.
253. Albrengues J, et al. Neutrophil extracellular traps produced during inflammation awaken dormant cancer cells in mice. *Science*. 2018;361 eaao4227.
254. Ishay-Ronen D, et al. Gain fat-lose metastasis: converting invasive breast cancer cells into adipocytes inhibits cancer metastasis. *Cancer Cell*. 2019;35:17.
255. Obradovic MMS, et al. Glucocorticoids promote breast cancer metastasis. *Nature*. 2019;567:540–544.
256. Keklikoglou I, et al. Chemotherapy elicits pro-metastatic extracellular vesicles in breast cancer models. *Nat Cell Biol*. 2019;21:190.
257. Khan I, Steeg PS. Metastasis suppressors: functional pathways. *Lab Invest*. 2018;98:198–210.
258. Li M, Cai O, Tan S. LOXL1-AS1 drives the progression of gastric cancer via regulating miR-142-5p/PIK3CA axis. *Onco Targets Ther*. 2019;12:11345–11357.
259. Wang X, et al. Identification of FOXN4 as a tumor suppressor of breast carcinogenesis via the activation of TP53 and deactivation of Notch signaling. *Gene*. 2020;722:144057.
260. Yu M, et al. miR-10b downregulated by DNA methylation acts as a tumor suppressor in HPV-positive cervical cancer via targeting Tiam1. *Cell Physiol Biochem*. 2018;51:1763–1777.
261. Duan S, et al. MicroRNA-135a-3p is downregulated and serves as a tumour suppressor in ovarian cancer by targeting CCR2. *Biomed Pharmacother*. 2018;107:712–720.
262. Ma B, Wells A, Clark AM. The pan-therapuetic resistance of disseminated tumor cells: role of phenotypic plasticity and the metastatic microenvironment. *Semin Cancer Biol*. 2020;60:138–147.
263. Esposito M, Ganesan S, Kang Y. Emerging strategies for treating metastasis. *Nat Cancer*. 2021;2:258–270.
264. Thapa B, Ramphul K: Paraneoplastic syndromes. In StatPearls [Internet], Treasure Island, FL, 2021, StatPearls Publishing. Available at: https://www.ncbi.nlm.nih.gov/books/NBK507890/. (Accessed August 6, 2021).
265. Aoyagi T, et al. Cancer cachexia, mechanism and treatment. *World J Gastrointest Oncol*. 2015;7(4):17–29.
266. Fearon K, et al. Definition and classification of cancer cachexia: an international consensus. *Lancet Ocncol*. 2011;12:489–495.
267. Argilés JM, et al. Cancer cachexia: understanding the molecular basis. *Nat Rev Cancer*. 2014;14(11):754–762.

268. US Preventive Services Task Force (USPSTF): Prostate cancer screening, *2018*. Rockville, MD, 2018, USPSTF. Available at: https;//www.uspreventiveservicestaskforce.org/uspstf/recommendation/prostate-cancer-screening. (Accessed August 6, 2021).
269. Waldman AD, Fritz Lenardo MJ. A guide to immunotherapy: from T cell basic science to clinical practice. *Nat Rev Immunol.* 2020;20:651–668.
270. Esfahani K, et al. A review of cancer immunotherapy: from the past, to the present, to the future. *Curr Oncol.* 2020;27(Suppl2):S87–S97.
271. Schumacher TN, Hacohen N. Neoantigens encoded in the cancer genome. *Curr Opin Immunol.* 2016;41(4):98–103.
272. Wang DY, et al. Fatal toxic effects associated with immune checkpoint inhibitors: a systematic review and meta-analysis. *JAMA Oncol.* 2018;4:1721–1728.
273. Moslehi JJ, et al. Increased reporting of fatal immune checkpoint inhibitor– associated myocarditis. *Lancet.* 2018;391:933.
274. Guo C, et al. Therapeutic cancer vaccines: past, present, and future. *Adv Cancer Res.* 2013;119:421–475.
275. Duan Q, et al. Turning cold into hot: firing up the tumor microenvironment. *Trends Cancer.* 2020;6(7):605–618.
276. Hanahan D. Rethinking the war on cancer. *Lancet.* 2014;383(9916):558–563.
277. National Cancer Institute (NCI): Targeted cancer therapies. Bethesda, MD, 2021, NCI. Updated July 12, 2021. Available at: https://www.cancer.gov/about-cancer/treatment/types/targeted-therapies/targeted-therapies-fact-sheet. (Accessed August 6, 2021).
278. Kim OY, et al. Bacterial outer membrane vesicles suppress tumor by interferon-gamma-mediated antitumor response. *Nat Commun.* 2017;8:626.
279. Panda A, et al. Immune activation and benefit from avelumab in EBV-positive gastric cancer. *J Natl Cancer Inst.* 2018;110(3):316–320.
280. Host KM, et al. Kaposi's sarcoma-associated herpesvirus increases PD-L1 and proinflammatory cytokine expression in human monocytes. *mBio.* 2017;8 e00917–e00917.
281. Smola S. Immunopathogenesis of HPV-associated cancers and prospects for immunotherapy. *Viruses.* 2017;9(9):254.
282. Thiele Orberg E, et al. The myeloid immune signature of enterotoxigenic Bacteroides fragilis-induced murine colon tumorigenesis. *Mucosal Immunol.* 2017;10:421–433.

13

Cancer Epidemiology

Devra Davis, Kathryn L. McCance, and Valentina L. Brashers

http://evolve.elsevier.com/Rogers/pathophysiology/

CHAPTER OUTLINE

Cancer develops from complex interactions between genes and the environment, including epigenetics, environmental-lifestyle factors, altered metabolism and biologic processes, and exposure to carcinogens (cancer-causing chemical or physical agents (Fig. 13.1).[1–3] According to the World Health Organization (WHO), the causes of specific cancers, aside from those tied with smoking and asbestos and other workplace exposures, are not fully understood.[3] Because the National Cancer Institute estimates that about 10% or fewer of all cancers arise from inherited germ-line mutations, many forms of cancer are preventable.[4]

Contributing factors include high risk activities[5–7] (see Fig. 13.1) such as

- Lifestyle choices, such as smoking, alcohol intake, and diet
- Obesity and lack of physical exercise
- Certain mold, bacterial, and viral infections, parasites, and predisposing sexual practices
- Environmental exposures, including exposure to sunlight; natural and medical ionizing radiation; non-ionizing radiation (NIR); and/or air, water and soil carcinogens, or those in household, pharmaceutical and recreational drugs, personal care products
- Occupational exposures to chemical and physical carcinogens
- Certain prescribed drugs and other hormones, and illicit medications
- Socioeconomic, racial, geographic, and ethnic factors that affect exposures, risk, and detection and treatment

Estimates of the contributions of environmental and occupational factors to cancer development vary considerably and are difficult to calculate. As of 2011, the International Agency for Research on Cancer (IARC) identified more than 100 chemicals, occupations, physical agents, biologic agents and pharmaceuticals, and other agents as human carcinogens.[5] Table 13.1 lists risk factors classified by cancer site within the body based on epidemiological evidence.

INCIDENCE, MORTALITY TRENDS, AND RACE

According to a 2021 report by GLOBOCAN, 1 in 5 people worldwide will develop cancer in their lifetime, and 1 in 8 men and 1 in 11 women will die from the disease.[8] An estimated 19.3 million new cancer cases and 10 million cancer deaths were reported worldwide in 2020 (Fig. 13.2). For the first time, female breast cancer has surpassed lung cancer as the most commonly diagnosed cancer in the world, primarily because of increases in low- and middle-income countries. Lung cancer is the most commonly diagnosed cancer in men, and for both sexes it is the leading cause of cancer death in the world. Prostate cancer is the second most common cancer in men. Other common cancers worldwide arise from the gastrointestinal (GI) tract including colorectum, stomach, and liver cancers.[8]

In the United States, there will be an expected 1.9 million cases of cancer in 2021 and over 600,000 cancer deaths (these estimates exclude basal cell and squamous cell skin cancers).[9] Breast cancer accounts for 30% of all cancer cases and 15% of cancer deaths in

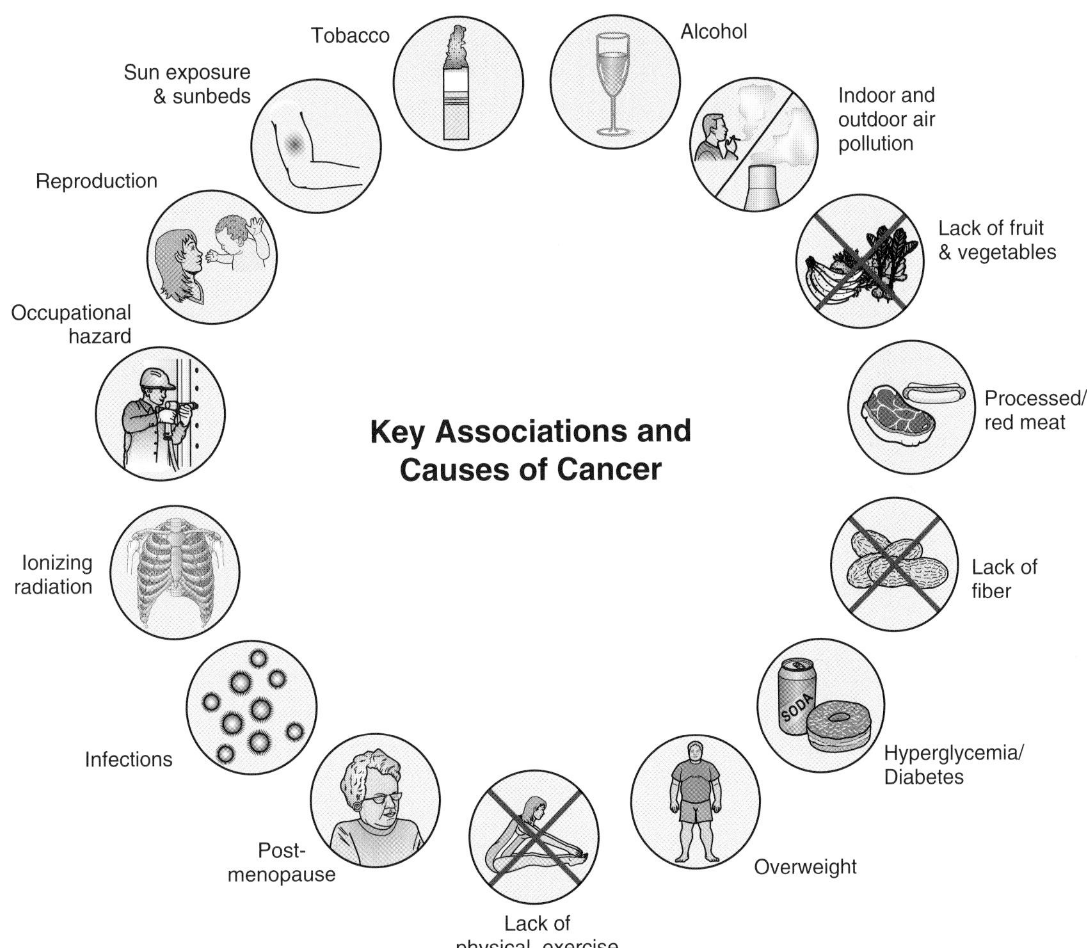

Fig. 13.1 Key Associations and Causes of Cancer. Tobacco, diet and alcohol, obesity, pollution, lack of physical activity, hormones, infections, ionizing radiation, occupational hazards, reproductive factors, and ultraviolet light are key factors for cancer. Although diet is key and known to affect cancer risk, determining specific dietary factors has been very difficult and is emerging.

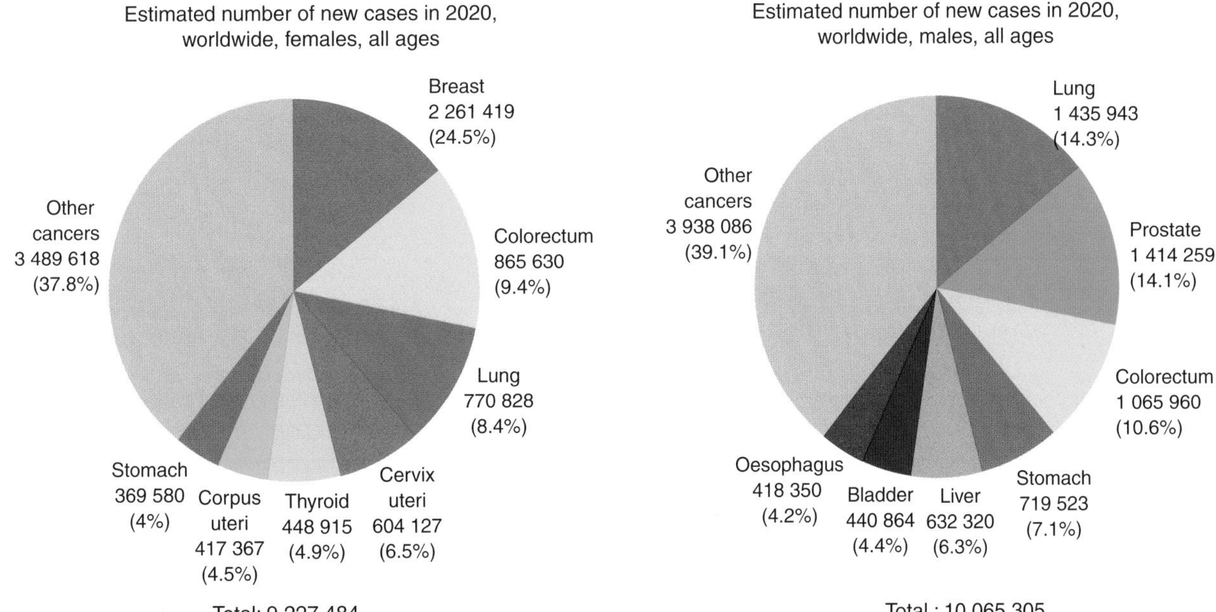

Fig. 13.2 Global Cancer Incidence. (New global cancer data from Globocan 2020.)

TABLE 13.1 **List of Classifications by Cancer Sites With *Sufficient* or *Limited* Evidence in Humans[a]**

Cancer Site	Carcinogenic Agents With *Sufficient Evidence* in Humans	Agents With *Limited Evidence* in Humans
Lip, Oral Cavity, and Pharynx		
Lip		Hydrochlorothiazide Solar radiation
Oral cavity	Alcoholic beverages Betel quid with tobacco Betel quid without tobacco Human papillomavirus type 16 Tobacco, smokeless Tobacco smoking	Human papillomavirus type 18
Salivary gland	X-radiation, γ-radiation	Radioiodines, including iodine-131
Tonsil	Human papillomavirus type 16	
Pharynx	Alcoholic beverages Betel quid with tobacco Human papillomavirus type 16 Tobacco smoking	Asbestos (all forms) Opium (consumption of) Printing processes Tobacco smoke, secondhand
Nasopharynx	Epstein-Barr virus Formaldehyde Salted fish, Chinese style Tobacco smoking Wood dust	
Digestive tract, upper	Acetaldehyde associated with consumption of alcoholic beverages	
Digestive Organs		
Esophagus	Acetaldehyde associated with consumption of alcoholic beverages Alcoholic beverages Betel quid with tobacco Betel quid without tobacco Tobacco, smokeless Tobacco smoking X-radiation, γ-radiation	Dry cleaning Opium (consumption of) Pickled vegetables (traditional Asian) Rubber production industry Very hot beverages (squamous cell carcinoma)
Stomach	*Helicobacter pylori* Rubber production industry Tobacco smoking X-radiation, γ-radiation	Asbestos (all forms) Epstein-Barr virus Lead compounds, inorganic Nitrate or nitrite (ingested) under conditions that result in endogenous nitrosation Opium (consumption of) Pickled vegetables (traditional Asian) Processed meat (consumption of) Salted fish (Chinese style)
Colon and rectum	Alcoholic beverages Processed meat (consumption of) Tobacco smoking X-radiation, γ-radiation	Asbestos (all forms) Night shift work Red meat (consumption of) *Schistosoma japonicum*
Anus	Human immunodeficiency virus type 1 Human papillomavirus type 16	Human papillomavirus types 18, 33
Liver and bile duct	Aflatoxins Alcoholic beverages *Clonorchis sinensis* 1,2-Dichloropropane Estrogen-progestogen contraceptives Hepatitis B virus Hepatitis C virus *Opisthorchis viverrini* Plutonium Thorium-232 and its decay products Tobacco smoking (in smokers and in smokers' children) Vinyl chloride	Androgenic (anabolic) steroids Arsenic and inorganic arsenic compounds Betel quid without tobacco Dichlorodiphenyltrichloroethane (DDT) Dichloromethane (Methylene chloride) Human immunodeficiency virus type 1 *S. japonicum* Trichloroethylene X-radiation, γ-radiation

TABLE 13.1 List of Classifications by Cancer Sites With *Sufficient* or *Limited* Evidence in Humans[a]–Cont'd

Cancer Site	Carcinogenic Agents With *Sufficient Evidence* in Humans	Agents With *Limited Evidence* in Humans
Gallbladder	Thorium-232 and its decay products	
Pancreas	Tobacco, smokeless Tobacco smoking	Alcoholic beverages Opium (consumption of) Red meat (consumption of) Thorium-232 and its decay products X-radiation, γ-radiation
Digestive tract, unspecified		Radioiodines, including iodine-131
Respiratory Organs		
Nasal cavity and paranasal sinus	Isopropyl alcohol production Leather dust Nickel compounds Radium-226 and its decay products Radium-228 and its decay products Tobacco smoking Wood dust	Carpentry and joinery Chromium (VI) compounds Formaldehyde Textile manufacturing
Larynx	Acid mists, strong inorganic Alcoholic beverages Asbestos (all forms) Opium (consumption of) Tobacco smoking	Human papillomavirus type 16 Rubber production industry Sulfur mustard Tobacco smoke, secondhand
Lung	Acheson process, occupational exposures associated with Aluminum production Arsenic and inorganic arsenic compounds Asbestos (all forms) Beryllium and beryllium compounds Bis(chloromethyl) ether; chloromethyl methyl ether (technical grade) Cadmium and cadmium compounds Chromium (VI) compounds Coal, indoor emissions from household combustion Coal gasification Coal-tar pitch Coke production Engine exhaust, diesel Hematite mining (underground) Iron and steel founding MOPP (vincristine-prednisone-nitrogen mustard-procarbazine mixture) Nickel compounds Opium (consumption of) Outdoor air pollution Painting Particulate matter in outdoor air polution Plutonium Radon-222 and its decay products Rubber production industry Silica dust, crystalline Soot Sulfur mustard Tobacco smoke, secondhand Tobacco smoking Welding fumes X-radiation, γ-radiation	Acid mists, strong inorganic Art glass, glass containers, and pressed ware (manufacture of) Benzene Biomass fuel (primarily wood), indoor emissions from household combustion of Bitumens, occupational exposure to oxidized bitumens and their emissions during roofing Bitumens, occupational exposure to hard bitumens and their emissions during mastic asphalt work Carbon electrode manufacture α-Chlorinated toluenes and benzyl chloride (combined exposures) Cobalt metal with tungsten carbide Creosotes Diazinon Fibrous silicon carbide Frying, emissions from high temperature Hydrazine Insecticides, nonarsenical, occupational exposures in spraying and application Printing processes 2,3,7,8-Tetrachlorodibenzo-*para*-dioxin

(Continued)

TABLE 13.1 List of Classifications by Cancer Sites With *Sufficient* or *Limited* Evidence in Humans[a]–Cont'd

Cancer Site	Carcinogenic Agents With *Sufficient Evidence* in Humans	Agents With *Limited Evidence* in Humans
Bone, Skin, Mesothelium, Endothelium, and Soft Tissue		
Bone	Plutonium Radium-224 and its decay products Radium-226 and its decay products Radium-228 and its decay products X-radiation, γ-radiation	Radioiodines, including iodine-131
Skin (melanoma)	Solar radiation Ultraviolet-emitting tanning devices Polychlorinated biphenyls	
Skin (other malignant neoplasms)	Arsenic and inorganic arsenic compounds Azathioprine Coal-tar distillation Coal-tar pitch Cyclosporine Methoxypsoralen plus ultraviolet A Mineral oils, untreated or mildly treated Shale oils Solar radiation Soot X-radiation, γ-radiation	Creosotes Human immunodeficiency virus type 1 Human papillomavirus types 5 and 8 (in individuals with *epidermodysplasia verruciformis*) Hydrochlorothiazide Merkel cell polyomavirus (MCV) Nitrogen mustard Petroleum refining, occupational exposures Ultraviolet-emitting tanning devices
Mesothelium (pleura and peritoneum)	Asbestos (all forms) Erionite Fluoro-edenitePainting	
Endothelium (Kaposi sarcoma)	Human immunodeficiency virus type 1 Kaposi sarcoma herpes virus	
Soft tissue		Polychlorophenols or their sodium salts (combined exposures) Radioiodines, including iodine-131 2,3,7,8-Tetrachlorodibenzo-*para*-dioxin
Breast and Female Genital Organs		
Breast	Alcoholic beverages Diethylstilbestrol Estrogen-progestogen contraceptives Estrogen-progestogen menopausal therapy X-radiation, γ-radiation	Dieldrin Digoxin Estrogen menopausal therapy Ethylene oxide Night shift work Polychlorinated biphenyls Tobacco smoking
Vulva	Human papillomavirus 16	Human immunodeficiency virus type 1 Human papillomavirus types 18, 33
Vagina	Diethylstilbestrol (exposure in utero)Human papillomavirus type 16	Human immunodeficiency virus type 1
Uterine cervix	Diethylstilbestrol (exposure in utero) Estrogen-progestogen contraceptives Human immunodeficiency virus type 1 Human papillomavirus types 16, 18, 31, 33, 35, 39, 45, 51, 52, 56, 58, 59 Tobacco smoking	Human papillomavirus types 26, 53, 66, 67, 68, 70, 73, 82
Endometrium	Estrogen menopausal therapy Estrogen-progestogen menopausal therapy Tamoxifen	Diethylstilbestrol
Ovary	Asbestos (all forms) Estrogen menopausal therapy Tobacco smoking	Talc-based body powder (perineal use) X-radiation, γ-radiation

TABLE 13.1 List of Classifications by Cancer Sites With *Sufficient* or *Limited* Evidence in Humans[a]–Cont'd

Cancer Site	Carcinogenic Agents With *Sufficient Evidence* in Humans	Agents With *Limited Evidence* in Humans
Male Genital Organs		
Penis	Human papillomavirus type 16	Human immunodeficiency virus type 1 Human papillomavirus type 18
Prostrate		Androgenic (anabolic) steroids Arsenic and inorganic arsenic compounds Cadmium and cadmium compounds Firefighters, occupational exposure Malathion Night shift work Red meat (consumption of) Rubber production industry Thorium-232 and its decay products X-radiation, γ-radiation
Testis		DDT Diethylstilbestrol (exposure in utero) *N,N*-Dimethylformamide Firefighters, occupational exposure Perfluorooctanoic acid
Urinary Tract		
Kidney	Tobacco smoking Trichloroethylene X-radiation, γ-radiation	Arsenic and inorganic arsenic compounds Cadmium and cadmium compounds Perfluorooctanoic acid Printing processes Welding fumes
Renal pelvis and ureter	Aristolochic acids, plants containing Phenacetin, analgesic mixtures containingTobacco smoking	Aristolochic acids
Urinary bladder	Aluminum production 4-Aminobiphenyl Arsenic and inorganic arsenic compounds Auramine production Benzidine Chlornaphazine Cyclophosphamide Magenta production 2-Naphthylamine Opium (consumption of) Painting Rubber production industry *Schistosoma haematobium* Tobacco smoking *ortho*-Toluidine X-radiation, γ-radiation	4-Chloro-*ortho*-toluidine Coal-tar pitch Dry cleaning Engine exhaust, diesel Hairdressers and barbers, occupational exposure 2-Mercaptobenzothiazole Pioglitazone Printing processes Soot Tetrachloroethylene Textile manufacturing
Eye, Brain, and Central Nervous System		
Eye	Human immunodeficiency virus type 1 Ultraviolet emissions from welding Ultraviolet-emitting tanning devices	Solar radiation
Brain and central nervous system	X-radiation, γ-radiation	Radiofrequency electromagnetic fields (including from wireless phones)
Endocrine Glands		
Thyroid	Radioiodines, including iodine-131 X-radiation, γ-radiation	

(Continued)

TABLE 13.1 List of Classifications by Cancer Sites With *Sufficient* or *Limited* Evidence in Humans[a]–Cont'd

Cancer Site	Carcinogenic Agents With *Sufficient Evidence* in Humans	Agents With *Limited Evidence* in Humans
Lymphoid, Hematopoietic, and Related Tissue		
Leukemia and/or lymphoma	Azathioprine	Benzene[b]
	Benzene[b]	Bischloroethyl nitrosourea (BCNU)
	Busulfan	Chloramphenicol
	1,3-Butadiene	DDT
	Chlorambucil	Diazinon
	Cyclophosphamide	Dichloromethane (methylene chloride)
	Cyclosporine	Ethylene oxide
	Epstein-Barr virus	Etoposide
	Etoposide with cisplatin and bleomycin	Firefighters, occupational exposure
	Fission products, including strontium-90	Glyphosate
	Formaldehyde	Hepatitis B virus
	H. pylori	Magnetic fields, extremely low frequency (childhood leukemia)
	Hepatitis C virus	Malaria (caused by infection with *Plasmodium falciparum* in holoendemic areas)
	Human immunodeficiency virus type 1	Malathion
	Human T-cell lymphotropic virus type 1	Mitoxantrone
	Kaposi sarcoma herpesvirus	Nitrogen mustard
	Lindane	Painting (childhood leukemia from maternal exposure)
	Melphalan	Petroleum refining, occupational exposures
	MOPP (vincristine-prednisone-nitrogen mustard-procarbazine mixture)	Polychlorinated biphenyls
	Pentachlorophenol	Polychlorophenols or their sodium salts (combined exposures)
	Phosphorus-32	Radioiodines, including iodine-131
	Rubber production industry	Radon-222 and its decay products
	Semustine (methyl-CCNU)	Styrene
	Thiotepa	Teniposide
	Thorium-23 and its decay products	2,3,7,8-Tetrachlorodibenzo-*para*-dioxin
	Tobacco smoking	Tobacco smoking (childhood leukemia in smokers' children)
	Treosulfan	Trichloroethylene
	X-radiation, γ-radiation	
Multiple or Unspecific Sites		
Multiple sites (unspecified)	Cyclosporine	Chlorophenoxy herbicides
	Fission products, including strontium-90	Plutonium
	X-radiation, γ-radiation (exposure in utero)	
All cancer sites (combined)	2,3,7,8-Tetrachlorodibenzo-*para*-dioxin	

[a]This table does not include factors not covered in the *IARC Monographs*, notably genetic traits, reproductive status, and some nutritional factors.
[b]For benzene, the evidence in humans is sufficient for acute non-lymphocytic leukemia, including acute myeloid leukemia; and the evidence in humans is limited for non-Hodgkin lymphoma, chronic lymphoid leukemia, multiple myeloma, chronic myeloid leukemia, and acute myeloid leukemia in children.
Adapted from Cogliano VJ, Baan R, Straif K, et al. Preventable exposures associated with human cancers. *Journal of the National Cancer Institute*, 2011;103:1–13. http://jnci.oxfordjournals.org/content/early/2011/12/11/jnci.djr483.short?rss=1.

US women, while prostate cancer accounts for 26% of all cancer cases and 11% of cancer deaths in US men. Lung cancer continues to constitute the second highest percentage of new cancer cases (12% to 13%) and the highest number of cancer deaths (22%) in both men and women. Colorectal cancer is the third most common cause of both cancer incidence and cancer deaths in US women and men, and when all major digestive cancer types are combined (colorectal, stomach, esophagus, liver, and pancreas), overall mortality rates exceed that for lung cancer.[9]

The generation in which an individual is born affects the incidence of cancer diagnosis. The concept of generational risk (GR) has been advanced to allow analysis of changes in risk that reflect the impact of a specified time (birth cohort) on cancer risk. Despite the decline in overall cancer mortality rates, adults are experiencing increased incidence of cancers that are not associated with tobacco or screening relative to their parents.[10,11]

For example, white men born in the 1940s had twice as much cancer overall as those born in 1888 through 1897, and the same birth cohort was shown to have more than twice as much cancer not linked to smoking. Comparing the same birth cohorts, women had 50% more cancers overall and 30% more non-smoking related cancers.[11] Steady reductions in colorectal cancer incidence in younger persons occurred between 1969 and 1995; however, recent rates surpassed historical levels and are the highest ever recorded in birth cohorts after 1990. Those born in the United States in the 1990s have a doubled risk of colon cancer (GR = 2) and a fourfold increase in rectal cancer (GR = 4) by the time they reach age 24, as compared to those born six decades ago.[12] Related factors contributing to the increase in colorectal cancer include Western and sugary diet, gut microbiome changes, sedentary lifestyle, smoking, and heavy alcohol consumption.[13] Exposures to non-ionizing radiation (NIR) from cellphones, as well as increased use of pediatric computed tomography (CT) scans and obesity, are additional possible contributing causes for colorectal cancer increases in the younger generation. Studies of colon cells in animals indicate sensitive carcinogenic responses to both NIR and ionizing radiation (IR), while modeling studies note that absorption of microwave radiation into the lower abdomen can be considerable.[12] Despite these increases in incidence, overall US cancer death rates have decreased 31% since 1991, with a notable decline in lung cancer deaths. Unfortunately, the rate of decline in cancer-rated mortality has slowed for prostate, breast, and colorectal cancer since 2018.[9]

Significant racial disparities exist for cancer patterns. For black and brown Americans, the risk of death from some types of cancer is often higher than for whites, especially at younger ages. For example, although fewer black women are diagnosed with breast cancer, they have a higher mortality rate. Significant racial disparities also are evident for cervical and prostate cancers. The American Cancer Society reports that blacks have the highest mortality rate and shortest survival of any racial and ethnic group in the United States for most cancers. Differences in access to care and treatment, employment in high-risk occupations, residential exposure to hazardous wastes, lack of access to quality nutrition, and other factors may account for the disparities (Box 13.1). Since 1990, the overall cancer mortality rate has declined faster in blacks than whites for both males and females, largely because of more rapid declines in blacks for lung, colorectal, and prostate cancers.[14,15]

GENETICS, EPIGENETICS, TUMOR MICROENVIRONMENT, AND CELLULAR SIGNALING IN CANCER

Cancer development is a complex process that results from gene mutations, epigenetic and environmental factors, the tumor microenvironment, and changes in both intra- and intercellular signaling (see Chapter 12). This chapter emphasizes the complex interaction between these processes and the environment/lifestyle exposures that influence them.

Genetics and Epigenetics

Gene mutations can be either inherited or acquired. Inherited gene mutations *(germline mutations)* are rare and are passed to the next generation by a parent's sperm or egg. Acquired mutations are more common than inherited mutations and cause most cancers. They occur when the healthy genes, with which we are born, lose the ability to function properly in direct cell signaling and repair, especially during periods of growth. Gene mutations that are acquired after birth are called *somatic mutations*. Somatic mutations occur from exposures to oxidizing agents that directly affect deoxyribonucleic acid (DNA). However, most acquired changes in gene function are not due to direct damage to DNA, but rather are a consequence of the complex effects that lifestyle and environmental exposures have on epigenetic patterns (Fig. 13.3). Epigenetics describes the chemical modulation of gene functions that control cell replication and other cell processes (see Chapter 6). Lifestyle factors, carcinogens, and occupational exposures alter epigenetic patterns, and therefore, may increase susceptibility to cancer (Fig. 13.4A). Epigenetic modifications have many different causes and may take several forms without directly damaging DNA by affecting the production of messenger RNA that directs the translation of proteins (see Fig. 13.4B).

Tumor Microenvironment

At the cellular level, inflammatory, hormonal, and metabolic systems can contribute to a tumor microenvironment that supports growth and metastasis (see Chapter 12). Systemic chronic inflammation is proposed to be the primary cause of most diseases including cancer.[16,17] The inflammatory process leads to the infiltration of inflammatory cells and cytokines into the tissue microenvironment (stroma). Chronic inflammation can *precede* and *initiate* cancer changes (e.g., inflammation-induced colon cancer) and can *promote or exacerbate* chronic processes (e.g., colonic polyposis) that may progress to cancer. When malignant transformation develops, tumor cells continually interact with surrounding stromal cells and, importantly, the infiltrated immune and inflammatory cells (see Chapter 12).

Many environmental and lifestyle factors impact the inflammatory process and may influence cancer development. For example, some nutritional factors such as deficiencies in vitamin D or excesses in refined sugars can induce inflammation. Other environmental factors are significant for lung and respiratory tract cancers where proinflammatory factors include viruses, inhaled tobacco smoke, asbestos fibers, numerous air pollutants, airborne pesticides, radon gas, and industrial sources.[18,19] Such exposures vary greatly with socioeconomics and other factors and influence the degree to which tumors grow, spread, or both. For example, mortality from melanoma is highest in Danish persons from the lowest socioeconomic classes with the lowest educational attainment.[20] In the United States, significant disparities exist between cancer mortality and morbidity for white, brown, and black Americans.[14,15]

Cellular Signaling

Cells must use intracellular communication pathways to connect the messages received from the extracellular environment to the cells' control machinery, which is localized mainly in the DNA (see Chapter 1). Many chronic diseases are formed because of malfunction or dysregulation of these intracellular

BOX 13.1 Race: A Social Construction

Race alone is a social construction. Despite years of assumptions that genetic distinctions can consistently be found that differentiate black, brown, and white Americans, aside from sickle cell trait and other relatively rare genetic anomalies, no uniform differences have been identified. Racial groups are not genetically homogenous. African-derived groups in North America incorporated a large proportion of European and some Native American genes. There is more heterogeneity *within* black and brown ethnic groups than *between* these groups and whites. Although it is well accepted that ancestral alleles can affect disease rates, susceptibility, and medication efficacy, these alleles do not fall along any racial categories. Specifically, admixture and migration have produced broad variation so that race categories are in no way comparable to genetic ancestry.

There is growing recognition that the tendency to deem race a biological fact may cause clinicians to employ racial signifiers as clinically meaningful without full examination or understanding of their complex origins and significance. This problem appears especially acute with respect to the assumptions with which health care providers of any race treat black and brown women. For example, there has long been the assumption that Americans of African descent retain more salt than those of European ancestry, thus contributing to the higher prevalence of hypertension in blacks. This assumption was based on the hypothesis that survival during the slave trade in the 17th through 19th centuries resulted in black Americans having greater capacity to retain salt, a claim that has been widely disputed. Chrysant and colleagues found no significant differences in variations between blood pressure and salt by race, age, sex, or body weight. Stark evidence of racial, economic, and ethnic disparities in cancer outcomes exist.

Academic, governmental, and non-governmental organizations are devoting more resources to elucidating the role of "epigenetics" in the development of common forms of cancer, including the metabolome and the microbiome which can modify expressions of our inherited genomes. Nonetheless, there is vastly more research on genomic mechanisms than on the social factors underlying health. In light of, it is important to develop strategies to address these determinants. Improving efficiencies in health care cannot suffice if the demand for care is also not reduced through primary preventive strategies.

Female Breast Cancer Incidence (2012–2016) and Mortality (2013–2017 Rates by Race/Ethnicity, United States. In 2018, while fewer blacks than whites developed breast cancer, blacks were 50% more likely to die of the disease. AIAN, American Indian/Alaska Native; API, Asian/Pacific Islander; NHB, non-Hispanic black; NHW, non-Hispanic white. (From: DeSantis CE, Ma J, Gaudet MM, et al. Breast cancer statistics. *Cancer Journal for Clinicians,* 2019;69(6), 438–451.)

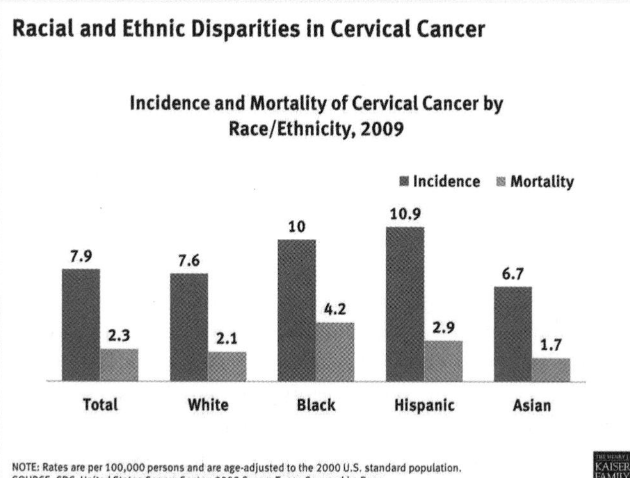

Patterns of Incidence and Mortality of Cervical Cancer Vary with Race and Ethnicity (From Henry, J. Kaiser Family Foundation. https://www.kff.org/womens-health-policy/slide/racial-and-ethnic-disparities-in-cervical-cancer/)

Data from: Ashley-Koch A, Yang Q, Olney RS. Sickle hemoglobin (Hb S) allele and sickle cell disease: A HuGE review. *American Journal of Epidemiology*, 2000;151(9):839–845; Chrysant SG, Weir MR, Weder AB, et al. There are no racial, age, sex, or weight differences in the effect of salt on blood pressure in salt-sensitive hypertensive patients. *Archives of Internal Medicine*, 1997;157(21):2489–2494; Lujan HL, DiCarlo SE. The "African gene" theory: It is time to stop teaching and promoting the slavery hypertension hypothesis. *Advances in Physiology Education*, 2018;42(3):412–416; Kurtz TW, DiCarlo SE, Morris Jr RC. Logical issues with the pressure natriuresis theory of chronic hypertension. *American Journal of Hypertension*, 2016;29(12):1325–133; Kurtz TW, DiCarlo SE, Pravenec M, et al. The pivotal role of renal vasodysfunction in salt sensitivity and the initiation of salt-induced hypertension. *Current Opinion in Nephrology and Hypertension*, 2018;27(2):83–92; Tang H, Coram M, Wang P, et al. Reconstructing genetic ancestry blocks in admixed individuals. *American Journal of Human Genetics*, 2006;79(1):1–12; Tsai J, Ucik L, Baldwin N, et al. Race matters? Examining and rethinking race portrayal in preclinical medical education. *Academic Medicine*, 2016;91(7):916–920.

communication pathways. Internal factors such as dysregulated hormonal systems (see Fig. 13.1) and abnormal glucose or lipid metabolism affect cellular communication and play a significant role in the development of many common diseases, including type 2 diabetes, neurological disorders, and cancer.

External factors also play a critical role in cancer development. Humans are constantly exposed to a variety of compounds termed xenobiotics (the Greek word xenos means "foreign"; bios means "life") that include toxic, mutagenic, and carcinogenic chemicals that contribute to inflammation and can affect

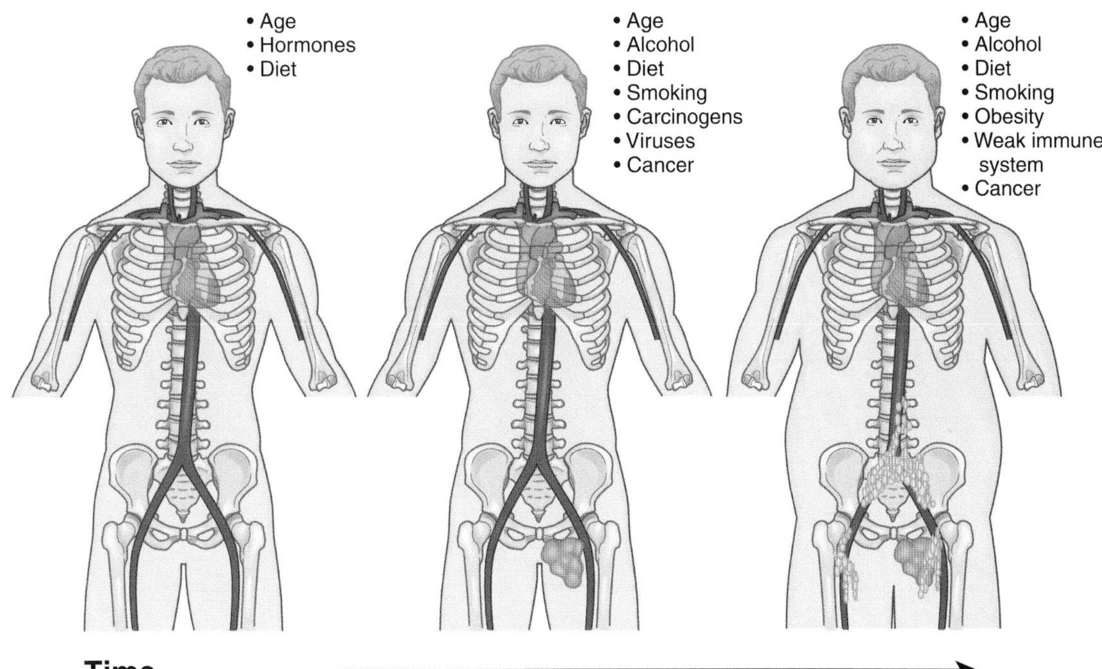

Fig. 13.3 Environmental Factors and Genetic, Epigenetic, and Other Host Factors. Over time, a person's internal genetic makeup persistently interacts with external or environmental factors. Environmental factors (e.g., diet, smoking, alcohol use, hormones [including xenoestrogens], certain viruses, chemical carcinogens) collectively interact with internal epigenetic factors and genetic mutations to destabilize normal biologic factors including immune factors for balancing growth and maturation. (Adapted from NCI. *Understanding Cancer Series: Cancer: Inside and Outside Factors.* Washington, DC: National Cancer Institute, National Institutes of Health; 2007.)

cellular communication. Examples of xenobiotic stimuli include xenoestrogens[21] and other synthetic hormonal growth factors.

Increasingly, several agents that modulate intracellular communication (e.g., antioxidants melatonin and epigallocatechin gallate [EGCG] and antiangiogenic and topoisomerase inhibitors) are being explored as therapeutic drugs that can reduce inflammation and potentially prevent cancer development. Unfortunately, many such agents have been found to have serious side effects and adverse consequences. For example, while the use of EGCG in adults induces cell death in acute myelogenous leukemia, it is contraindicated during pregnancy as prenatal exposure has been linked with neonatal leukemia.[22,23] It is possible that drugs that affect the tissue microenvironment and cell signaling will be tapped to repair precancerous conditions or to avoid or diminish adverse radiation effects of both IR and NIR, especially in electro-hypersensitive individuals.

IN UTERO AND EARLY LIFE CONDITIONS

It is widely accepted that a long latency period precedes the onset of most adult cancers. Accumulating data suggest early life events, including prenatal factors, influence later susceptibility to cancer and certain other chronic diseases. The timing of exposure and dose-rate of potential carcinogens can be critically important. Exposures that take place during gestation and early childhood may have greater impacts than those that take place later in life. Developmental plasticity is the degree to which an organism's development is contingent on external cues from its environment. *Plasticity* refers to the ability of genes to organize physiologically or structurally in response to environmental conditions during fetal development. Specifically, the *developmental origins hypothesis* postulates that nutrition and other environmental factors affect cellular pathways during gestation, enabling a single genotype to produce a broad range of adult phenotypes.

Maternal nutrition and other environment factors wield significant biologic influences and are therefore more thoroughly evaluated. Persistent epigenetic adaptations, occurring early in development, are believed to be associated with increased susceptibility to cancer and other adult-onset chronic diseases. During *in utero* development, factors such as undernutrition and exposure to toxins and alcohol result in decreased immunity and increased vulnerability to multiple diseases including cancer in adulthood.[24,25] It is estimated that up to 5% of all school-aged children have some form of fetal alcohol syndrome (FASD) that affects multiple health and psychological outcomes.[26]

One of the best examples of early life events that trigger future cancer is *in utero* exposure to diethylstilbestrol (DES), a synthetic estrogen. Originally synthesized and used in Nazi Germany as a hormone that fattened cattle and pigs,[27] DES was

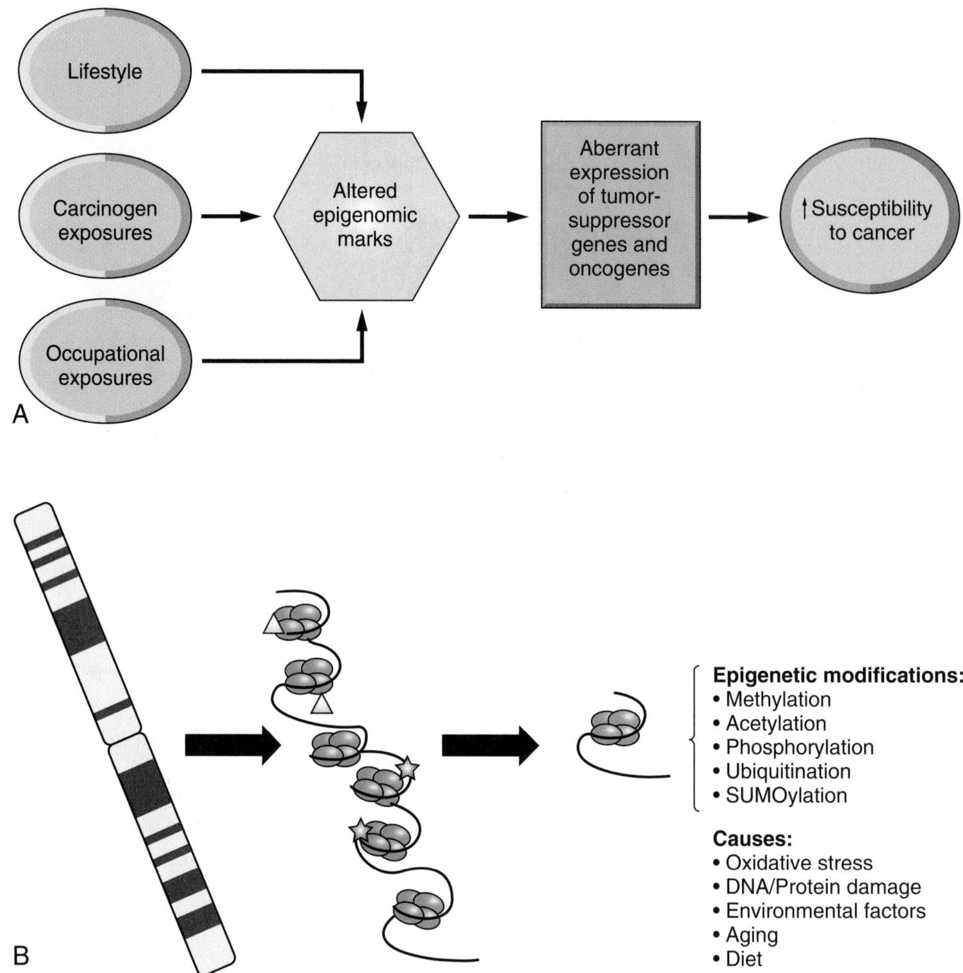

Fig. 13.4 Epigenetic Modulation and Modifications. (A) Overview of the potential role of epigenetic modulation by dietary and other environmental factors in cancer development. **(B)** Epigenetic modulation model according to current knowledge. The different types of chemical modifications, such as methylation or acetylation, of promoter regions and/or other regulatory DNA sequences outside the gene can have a severe impact on gene transcription and translation and a resultant high modulation of gene expression and product (protein) functionality. (B, Adapted from Nowsheen S, Aziz K, Tran PT, et al. Epigenetic inactivation of DNA repair in breast cancer. *Cancer Letters*, 2014;342(2):213–222.)

prescribed between 1938 and 1971 to avert miscarriage, premature birth, and abnormal bleeding. In 1971, an astute clinician reported an unusual cluster of rare cancers of the vagina (adenocarcinoma) in a group of young teens who had been exposed to DES during gestation.[28] The same clinician showed that the drug did *not* prevent miscarriage. Subsequent monitoring of exposed cohorts found that DES exposure in utero increases the risk of female reproductive tract cancer and of male reproductive impairment throughout childbearing years. Daughters of women who took DES during pregnancy have an increased risk of breast cancer before age 40. A recent meta-analysis demonstrated that prenatally exposed males have a threefold increase in testicular cancer risk.[29]

Evidence is increasing that adverse environmental exposures can affect the genes and epigenetic patterns of reproductive cells in both men and women that are then transmitted to their offspring during conception.[17] For example, maternal smoking during pregnancy has been shown to alter the epigenome of children into adolescence, and has been linked to an increased risk for childhood cancer including retinoblastoma and brain tumors.[30,31] Men who have had preconception exposures to smoking, air pollution, IR, heavy metals, pesticides, and compounds such as bisphenol A, DES, and dioxin have been found to have altered DNA epigenetic methylation patterns in their sperm. As a result, evidence shows that their offspring are more likely to suffer from male-mediated developmental toxicity in the form of spontaneous abortion, low birth weight, developmental delays, and childhood cancer.[32]

Bisphenol A (BPA) and several other endocrine disrupting chemicals (EDCs) (such as those found in pesticides, flame retardants, nonstick coatings) serve as obesogens, agents that stimulate embryonic development of adipose tissue. When exposed to alcohol or other adipose-stimulating agents later in life, prenatally programmed stem cells manufacture more

TABLE 13.2 Differences Between Multigenerational and Transgenerational Phenotypes

Phenotype	Exposure	Definition
Multigenerational	Direct	Simultaneous exposure of multiple generations to an environmental factor
Transgenerational	Initial germline exposure (ancestral)	Transgenerational phenotype is transmitted to future generations via germline inheritance

TABLE 13.3 Somatic Versus Germ Cell Inheritance

Cell Type	Biologic Response
Somatic cells	Critical for adult-onset disease in exposed individual; not transmitted to future generations as transgenerational effect
Germ cells	Allows transmission between generations; promotes transgenerational phenotype

adipocytes and permanently alter germline epigenome in both males and females, enhancing development of obesity across generations.[33] Obesity is a well-recognized risk factor for cancer and is discussed later in this chapter.

In summary, fetal programming influences developmental origins of health and disease. It also may help explain epigenetic transgenerational effects (Tables 13.2 and 13.3).

ENVIRONMENTAL-LIFESTYLE FACTORS

Tobacco Use

Smoking remains an important preventable cause of death globally. Smoking causes cancer, heart disease, stroke, lung diseases, diabetes, and chronic obstructive pulmonary disease (COPD) along with many other systemic disorders (Fig. 13.5). Worldwide, tobacco use and secondhand smoke exposure cause more than 8 million deaths per year.[34] More than 16 million Americans are living with a disease caused by smoking. Cigarette smoking accounts for more than 480,000 deaths each year, including more than 41,000 deaths resulting from secondhand smoke.[35]

The risks associated with smoking are greatest in persons who begin to smoke when young and continue throughout life; however, tobacco smoking is pandemic and affects all ages. Thousands of young people start smoking cigarettes every day.[35] Although rates of smoking in high school students have plummeted, possibly reflecting anti-smoking programs directed at this age group, more young adults are beginning to smoke now than previously. The risks of smoking-related cancer are now equal in men and women.

Secondhand smoke, also called environmental tobacco smoke (ETS), consists of *sidestream smoke* (smoke from the burning end of a cigarette, cigar, or pipe) and *mainstream smoke* (smoke exhaled directly by the smoker). More than 7000 chemicals have been identified in tobacco smoke; hundreds are toxic and can cause cancer in animals, and about 70 are known to cause cancer in humans.[36,37] During 2011 through 2012, about 58 million nonsmokers in the United States were exposed to secondhand smoke.[34]

Smoking tobacco causes cancer in over 15 organ sites and affects nearly every organ of the body:[36,38]

- Cancers of the lung and upper respiratory tract (oral cavity, pharynx, larynx, nasal cavity, paranasal sinuses)
- Cancers of the digestive tract (esophagus, stomach, liver, and colorectum)
- Cancers of the lower urinary tract (renal pelvis, penis, and bladder)
- Cancers of the kidney, pancreas, cervix, and uterus
- Myeloid leukemia

Non-cigarette tobacco use also is hazardous. Cigar or pipe smoking is strongly related to cancers of the oral cavity, oropharynx, hypopharynx, larynx, esophagus, and lung. Cigar smokers who inhale are prone to develop coronary heart disease and COPD. Pipe smokers have an increased risk of cancers of the lung, lip, throat, esophagus, larynx, pancreas, and colon and rectum. Smokeless tobacco is associated with oral cavity, esophageal, and pancreatic cancers.

Electronic cigarettes (e-cigarettes) come in many shapes and sizes, have a battery, a heating element, and a place to hold liquid containing nicotine, flavorings, and other chemicals. Among the more insidious forms of e-cigarettes are those that look like USB drives, highlighters, or pens so they cannot readily be detected in schoolbags. These electronic nicotine delivery systems feature a range of flavors, such as bubble gum, popcorn, peppermint candy, and butterscotch, all tailored to appeal to younger users. In 2020, nearly 20% of high school students and nearly 5% of middle school students reported current e-cigarette use.[39] E-cigarettes produce a sidestream aerosol that contains more heavy metals than cigarette smoke because of the use of metal coils. They also contain cancer-causing volatile aromatic hydrocarbons, flavoring (diacetyl), and other toxic agents, including nicotine, and ultrafine particles that can be inhaled deeply in the lungs. The smallest of these inhaled particles cross through the lung into the blood. A popular E-cigarette device, called *JUUL*, is shaped like a USB flash drive. The nicotine liquid refills are called pods. Pods come in many flavors, such as cool cucumber, fruit medley, mango, and mint. All *JUUL* e–cigarettes have a high level of nicotine; according to the manufacturer, a single *JUUL* contains as much nicotine as a pack of 20 regular cigarettes. Serious illness and death have occurred in some users of e-cigarettes, possibly due to contaminated fluids such as polyethylene glycol ethers (see Chapter 35).[40]

Tobacco smoke and vapors from e-cigarettes are a type of xenobiotic that can affect genes, the tumor microenvironment, and cell signaling.[41] As with other carcinogens, exposure to tobacco smoke is associated with tissue inflammation and release of toxic oxygen radicals (Fig. 13.6). Resulting mutations and epigenetic changes in key cell cycle genes promote tumor

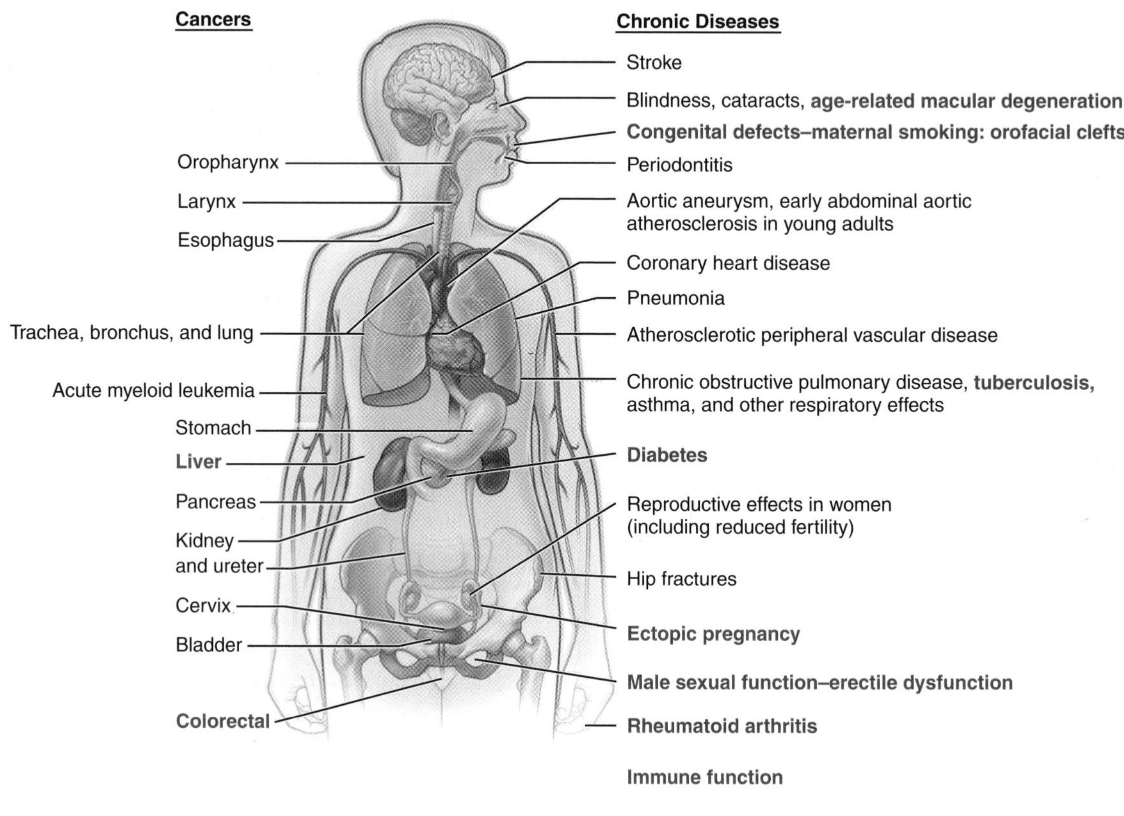

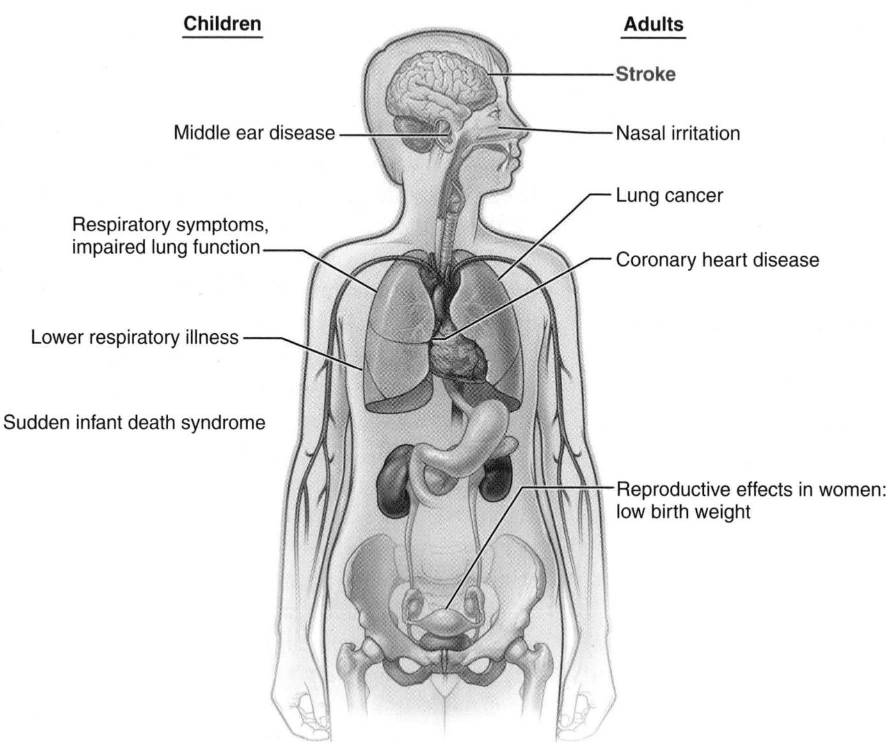

Fig. 13.5 The Health Consequences Linked to Smoking. NOTE: The conditions in red are new diseases that have been causally linked to smoking. See text for discussion. Stroke is a new disease causally linked to secondhand smoke. (Reproduced from the World Cancer Research Fund/American Institute for Cancer Research. *Diet, Nutrition, Physical Activity and Cancer: A Global Perspective*. Continuous Update Project Expert Report; 2018. dietandcancerreport.org.)

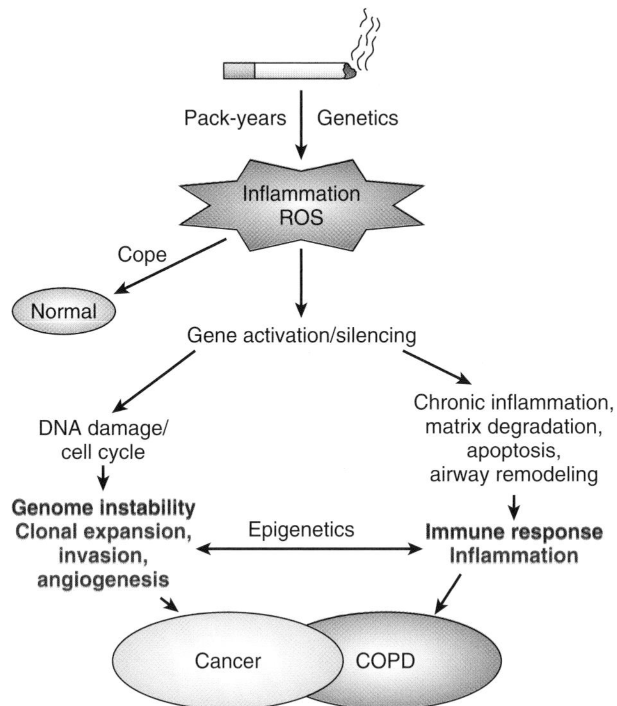

Fig. 13.6 Working Model of Carcinogenesis by Cigarette Smoke. The main inducer of both lung cancer and chronic obstructive pulmonary disease *(COPD)* is cigarette smoke. Nonsmokers may develop these diseases caused by other environmental or genetic/epigenetic factors. Cigarette smoke induces an inflammatory response and causes an increase in reactive oxygen species *(ROS)*, causing oxidative stress. Oxidative stress is a risk factor for many diseases because it can alter many cellular proteins. A combination of immune-inflammatory signals and epigenetic events may increase the risk for individuals with COPD developing lung cancer. (From Adcock IM, Caramori G, Barnes PJ. Chronic obstructive pulmonary disease and lung cancer: New molecular insights. *Respiration*, 2011;81(4):265–284.)

initiation and growth. Inflammation also contributes to a tumor microenvironment that further supports cancer development and spread. These effects may occur not only in the lungs, but throughout the body. Individuals with COPD are at increased risk for lung cancer due to increased inflammation and oxidative stress.[42] The mechanisms of cancer development are described in detail in Chapter 12.

Diet and Nutrition, Obesity, Alcohol Consumption, and Physical Activity: Impacts on Cancer

Diet and nutrition, weight, and activity level all influence risks for the development of specific types of cancers (Fig. 13.7).[17] Everyday choices and lifelong habits matter and impact the risk of developing cancer.

Diet and Nutrition

Researchers targeting associations between diet and nutrition with disease face a variety of challenges, including the difficulty in accurate measurement of specific nutrients, food types, and dietary patterns. Cancer is a disease with long latencies and may depend as much or more on diet in early life as on adult eating practices. Therefore, understanding decades of old dietary patterns is critical to interpreting cancer risks in older adults. Nutrigenomics is the study of the effects of nutrition on genomics, epigenomics, transcription factors (transcriptomics), proteomics, and metabolic factors (metabolomics) and the ways that modifying any one of these factors influences cancer risk (Fig. 13.8). Fig. 3.9 shows cell functions thought to be influenced by diet, weight, and activity level. The impact of diet, nutrition, physical activity and other environmental exposures on the cancer process is illustrated in Fig. 3.10.

The advocacy of specific dietary recommendations, such as those of the Mediterranean diet (MD), is becoming more common as studies indicate that the MD reduces mortality from several chronic diseases, including cancer, cardiovascular, and neurodegenerative diseases.[43] Culture and geographic location influence patterns of physical activity and diet and play a significant role in health and disease. For example, the incidence of colorectal cancer differs fivefold in various geographic regions and is believed to be tied to differences in the consumption of red or processed meat, fiber, and alcohol. As persons migrate from South Asian areas with lower rates of breast, colorectal, and prostate cancer to western zones, their cancer risks rise, particularly when migrating individuals adopt the so-called Western diet and more sedentary lifestyle. Japan has seen a rapid increase in the incidence of colorectal cancer with the westernization of its diet. However, recent changes in colorectal cancer in younger adults are unlikely to reflect dietary factors alone and may be linked to increased uses of CT scans and NIR from cellphones kept close to the body for hours daily.[12]

As described previously, gene expression is influenced by epigenetic processes, such as DNA methylation or acetylation (addition of an acetyl group) (see Chapters 4, 6, and 12). Dietary sources of methyl groups, including folate, methionine, betaine, serine, and choline, are potential modulators of DNA methylation (Fig. 13.11). The European Prospective Investigation into Cancer and Nutrition (EPIC) found that individuals with high plasma concentrations of methionine, choline, and betaine may be at reduced risk for colorectal cancer.[44] Other examples of epigenetic changes and diet are presented in Box 13.2.

Nutritional factors play an important role in cancer development, growth, and responsiveness to treatment. Bioactive xenobiotics found in food have a profound effect on cell differentiation, including the differentiation of cancer stem cells. Cancer stem cells utilize several developmental mechanisms for self-renewal; these mechanisms appear to be fundamental to the initiation, recurrence, and regression or apoptosis of tumors (see Chapter 12). Even if chemotherapy or radiation eliminates cancer cells, it is only when cancer stem cells are destroyed that a full recovery is achievable. Repopulation with radioresistant or chemo-resistant stem cells may significantly contribute to therapy resistance. Evidence from both drug and bioactive food constituents shows that nutritional factors substantially affect cancer stem cell self-renewal capabilities; for example, retinoic acid may promote differentiation of breast cancer stem cells.

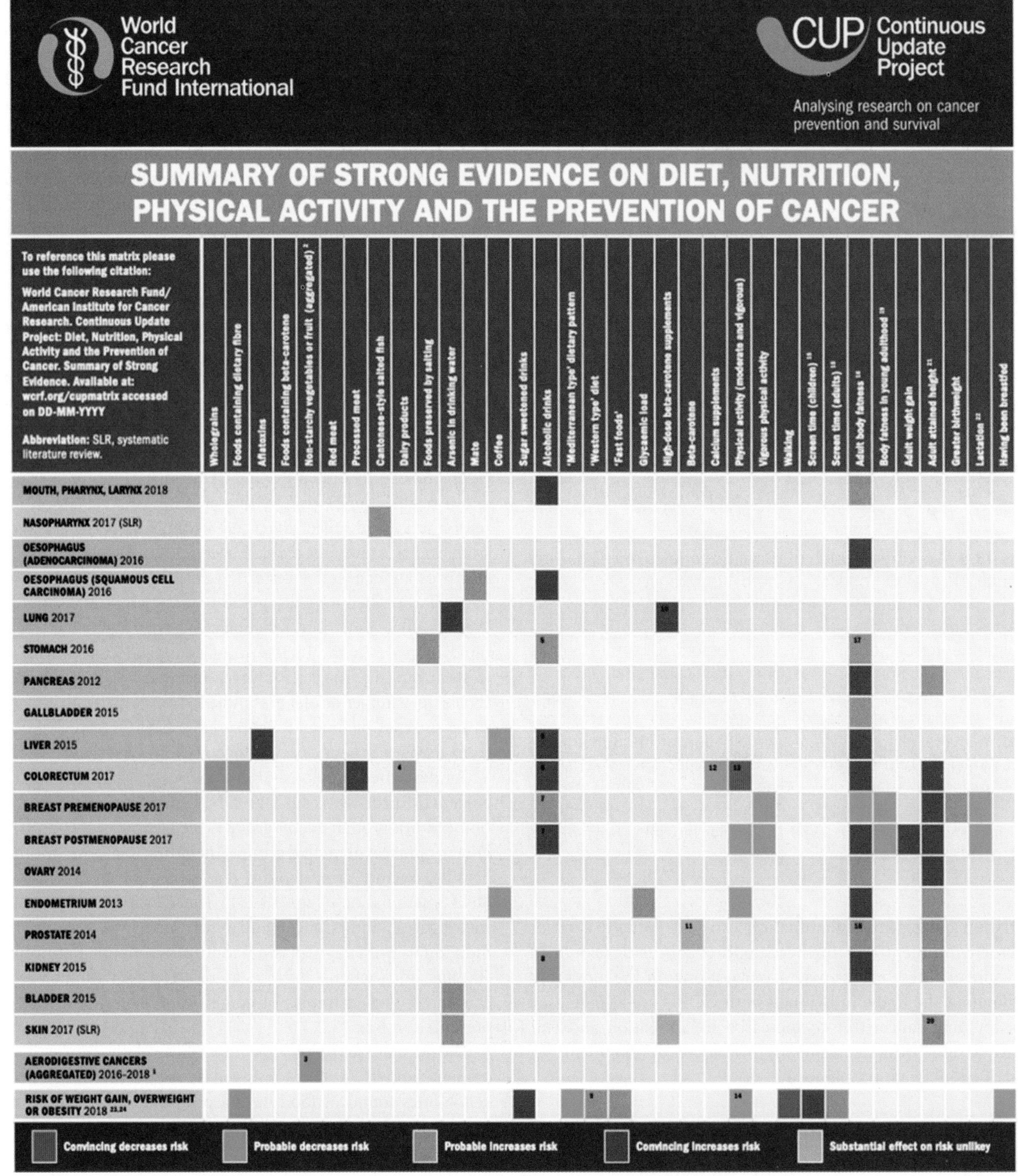

Fig. 13.7 Summary of Strong Evidence on Diet, Nutrition, Physical Activity, and Prevention of Cancer. (This material has been reproduced from the World Cancer Research Fund/American Institute for Cancer Research. Diet, Nutrition, Physical Activity and Cancer: a Global Perspective. Continuous Update Project Expert Report 2018. Available at dietandcancerreport.org.)

Increased consumption of specific food compounds, including vitamin A and D, genistein, green tea, epigallocatechin, sulforaphane, theanine, curcumin, choline, and possibly many others, may suppress cancer stem renewal.[45,46] The relationship between diet and cancer is of such great interest that an entire scientific journal is dedicated to the topic (Nutrition and Cancer).

A variety of food constituents also influence the cell cycle and DNA repair (Fig. 13.12). Observational studies suggest that

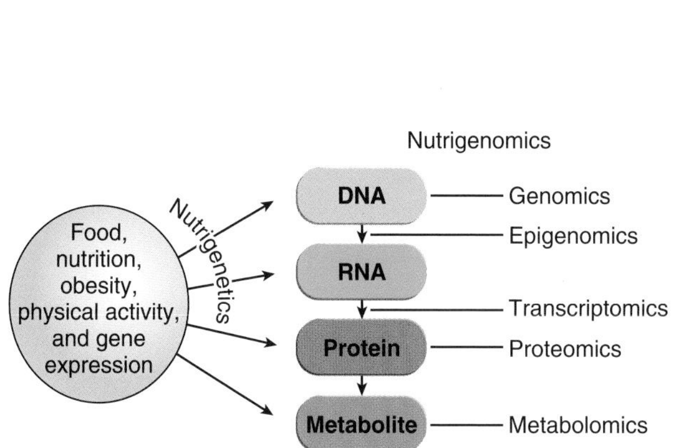

Fig. 13.8 Basis for the Study of Food, Nutrition, Obesity, Physical Activity, and the Cancer Process. The genetic message in the DNA code is translated to RNA, and then into protein synthesis, and so determines metabolic processes. Research methods, called "-omics," address these different stages. (Adapted from World Cancer Research Fund/American Institute for Cancer Research. *Food, Nutrition, Physical Activity, and the Prevention of Cancer: A Global Perspective*. Washington, DC: AICR; 2007.)

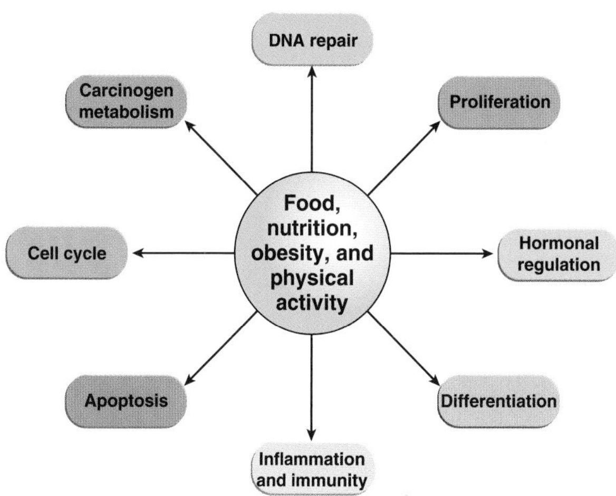

Fig. 13.9 Food, Nutrition, Obesity, Physical Activity, and Cellular Processes Linked to Cancer. Food, nutrition, and physical activity can influence fundamental processes shown here, which may promote or inhibit cancer development and progression. (This material has been reproduced from the World Cancer Research Fund/American Institute for Cancer Research. Food, Nutrition, Physical Activity, and the Prevention of Cancer: a Global Perspective. Washington DC: AICR, 2007.)

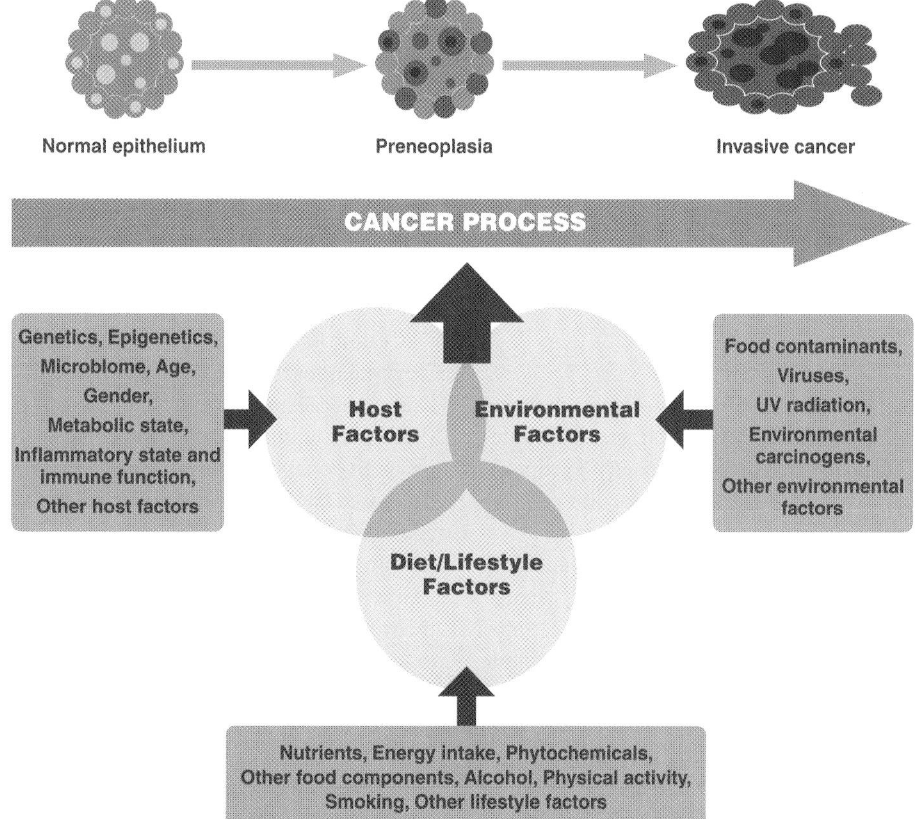

Fig. 13.10 Diet, Nutrition, Physical Activity and Other Environmental Exposures Affect the Cancer Process. It can take many years for a normal cell to transform into invasive cancer cells. Carcinogenesis involves a complex interaction of diet, nutrition, physical activity, and other lifestyle and environmental factors with host factors that are related to inheritance, prior experience, and epigenetic changes. With time, the accumulated genetic damage and impairment of function, for example, DNA repair processes with aging, can all lead to carcinogenesis. Thus critical to this process are everyday lifestyle choices and exposures. (This material has been reproduced from the World Cancer Research Fund/American Institute for Cancer Research. Diet, Nutrition, Physical Activity and Cancer: a Global Perspective. Continuous Update Project Expert Report 2018. Available at dietandcancerreport.org.)

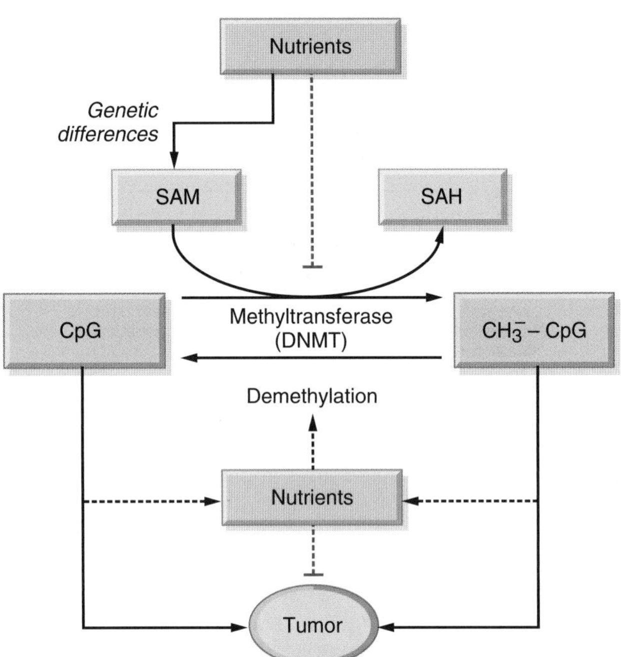

Fig. 13.11 Dietary Factors, DNA Methylation, and Cancer. Certain dietary factors may supply methyl groups (+CH_3) that can be donated through *S*-adenosylmethionine *(SAM)* to many acceptors in the cell (DNA, proteins, lipids, and metabolites). Donation and removal (demethylation) are affected by numerous enzymes, including DNA methyltransferase *(DNMT)*. Increased DNMT activity occurs in many tumor cells. Hypermethylation can inhibit or silence tumor-suppressor genes (see Chapter 12, and DNA methylation inhibitors as anticancer agents can block DNMT, thus reactivating tumor-suppressor genes. DNA hypomethylation can reactivate and mutate genes, including cancer-causing oncogenes. *SAH, S*-Adenosylhomocysteine; *CH_3*, methyl group; *CpG site*, cytosine (C) lies next to guanine (G).

BOX 13.2 Examples of Epigenetic Changes and Diet

- B vitamins (B_2, B_6, B_{12}) are modulators of DNA methylation
- Periconceptual maternal supplementation with 400 mcg of folic acid per day was associated with methylation in the offspring
- From the Waterland study, methylation effects were similar in all tissues examined. These data suggest that the methylation mechanism may alter stem cells early in embryogenesis before tissue differentiation and persist throughout life
- Severe folate deficiency, which increases the risk of hepatocellular cancer, induces hypomethylation of the *p53* tumor suppressor gene
- There is strong evidence for the epigenetic effects of organosulfur compounds from garlic and of isothiocyanates from cruciferous vegetables
- Sulforaphane from cruciferous vegetables can act as a histone deacetylase inhibitor to maintain DNA stability or modify transcription
- The potential role of dietary polyphenols, such as curcumin, resveratrol, genistein, epigallocatechin gallate (EGCG), and indole-3-carbinol, may promote antiproliferation and proapoptosis through epigenetic regulation of microRNAs (miRNAs).
- Natural agents in cancer therapies are being investigated in clinical trials

Data from World Cancer Research Fund/American Institute from Cancer Research. *Food, Nutrition, Physical Activity, and the Prevention of Cancer: A Global Perspective.* Washington, DC; 2007; AICR and World Cancer Research Fund/American Institute for Cancer Research. *Diet, Nutrition, Physical Activity and Cancer: A Global Perspective.* Continuous Update Project Report; 2018. dietandcancerreport.org.

malnutrition can reduce the capacity of DNA to repair damage. Healthy adults consuming kiwifruit, cooked carrots, or supplemental coenzyme Q_{10} improve DNA repair capacity. Lycopene, a plant-based antioxidant, may reduce the risk for lung cancer by preventing DNA damage and improving DNA repair.[47]

Humans are constantly exposed to a variety of xenobiotics that include toxic, mutagenic, and carcinogenic chemicals. Many xenobiotics are chemicals found in medications. A surprising number of widely used pharmaceuticals, including popular agents such as gabapentin, azopyrimidine, hydrochlorothiazide, and paroxetine, can also increase cancer risk. Common pharmaceutical agents linked to cancer are listed in Box 13.3. Most xenobiotics are transported in the blood by lipoproteins and penetrate lipid membranes. The body has two main defense systems for counteracting these effects: (1) detoxification enzymes that work through the liver and (2) antioxidant systems (see Chapter 2). When a compound is absorbed through the GI tract, it enters the hepatic circulation through the portal vein. The liver metabolizes dietary or pharmaceutical xenobiotics that are orally ingested through the *first pass effect* that can metabolize and thereby prevent many potentially carcinogenic agents from entering the body. Although the liver is the main site of detoxification, this process occurs to a lesser extent at other sites (i.e., extrahepatic detoxification). Many foods, such as isothiocyanates from cruciferous vegetables, induce detoxification enzymes that enhance the efficiency and degree of detoxification of xenobiotics and thus can serve a protective role in metabolizing carcinogens.

Certain enzymes (glutathione-*S*-transferases [GSH]) are "enzyme housekeepers" that play essential roles in the metabolism of environmental carcinogens and reactive oxygen species (ROS). Individuals who have absent or reduced levels of these protective enzymes may be at higher risk for cancers because of a decreased capacity to effectively neutralize carcinogens by metabolic transformation into less toxic forms. For example, there are fungi that form on certain crops such as peanuts and some grains that produce carcinogenic aflatoxin. The production of this toxin can be counteracted by ascorbate, n-acetylcysteine, or other nutritional components that affect the production of GSH. Activated in the liver, aflatoxins produce adducts with N-7 guanine-DNA that can trigger the formation of malignant cells. Individuals lacking protective enzymes or having lower levels of those enzymes are at higher risk for developing colon, liver, and other types of cancer.

The EPIC trial, which included 478,040 people from 10 countries, reported convincing data linking colon cancer to consumption of meats that contain nitrites, nitrates, or other preservatives in products such as bacon, sausages, bratwursts, frankfurters, and other nitrite-containing meats.[48] The resulting *N*-nitroso compounds increase nitrogenous residues in the colon that can cause DNA damage that increases cancer risk.

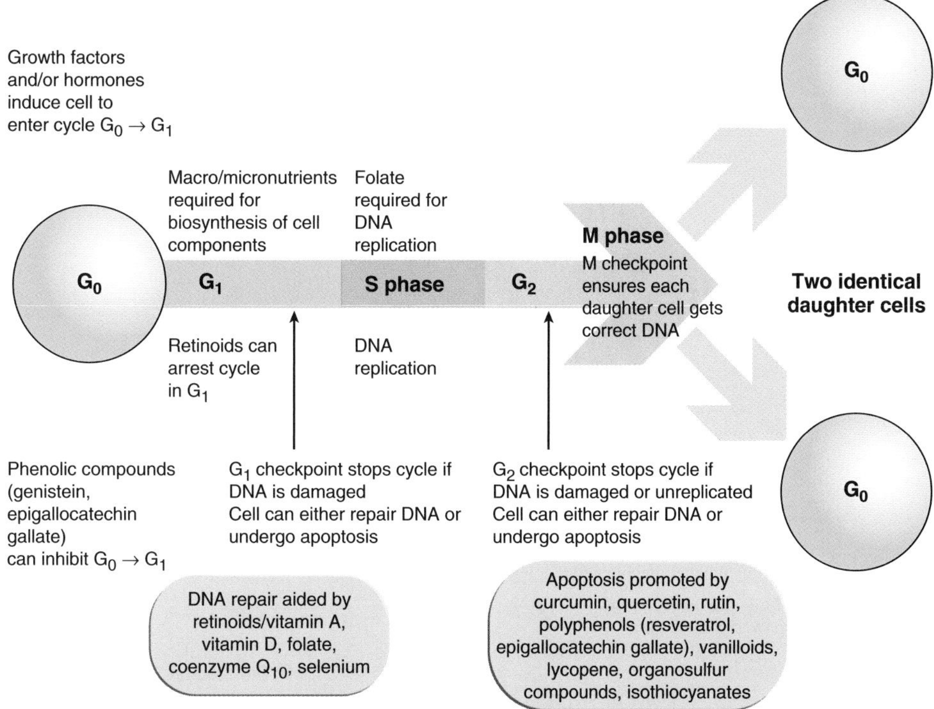

Fig. 13.12 Cell Cycle and Nutrition Regulation. Nutrition may influence the regulation of the normal cell cycle, which ensures correct DNA replication. G_0 represents the resting phase, G_1 the growth and preparation of the chromosome for replication, S the synthesis of DNA, G_2 the preparation of the cell for division, and M mitosis. (Adapted from World Cancer Research Fund/ American Institute for Cancer Research. *Food, Nutrition, Physical Activity, and the Prevention of Cancer: A Global Perspective.* Washington, DC: AICR; 2007.)

BOX 13.3 Common Pharmaceutical Agents Associated With Increased Cancer Risk

Fluoxetine and paroxetine with testicular cancer
Hydrochlorothiazide with renal and lip cancer
Hyoscyamine with non-Hodgkin lymphoma
Nifedipine with lip cancer
Nortriptyline with esophageal and hepatic cancer
Oxazepam with lung cancer
Sulindac with gallbladder cancer and leukemia

Data from https://www.mdlinx.com/article/common-prescription-drugs-you-didn-t-know-could-cause-cancer/5Ts67N8oKAP5GEVMderxUq.

Observational and experimental studies indicate that supplementation with chlorophyllin, vitamin A, and other antioxidants may reduce the risk of cancer development.

Metabolic reactions that impact cancer development include pro-carcinogenic processes, as well as protective reactions. Other products of normal metabolism produced in adipose tissue (hormones, inflammatory mediators, adipokines) can contribute to tumor microenvironment. Furthermore, microorganisms in the digestive tract (gut microbiome, see Chapter 7) play an important role in the metabolism of food and produce many small molecules that may impact cancer development.[49] Some reactions activate dietary compounds to form potential carcinogens as with aflatoxin. Other metabolic processes, such as ingested antioxidants, can inactivate ingested carcinogenic components thus preventing DNA damage. Red meat and its preservatives have been the subject of considerable scrutiny. A high intake of red meat may result in the synthesis of higher levels of heme iron, a substance known to activate oxidative stress and inflammation in the colon. Additionally, meat may have certain thermoresistant oncogenic bovine viruses (e.g., polyoma-papilloma) or single-stranded DNA viruses. Cooking meats at high temperatures (pan frying or grilling) may pose additional hazards because it results in the formation of highly mutagenic heterocyclic amines (HCAs) and polycyclic aromatic hydrocarbons (PAHs), both identified as carcinogens in laboratory animals. Future research is needed to define robust biomarkers of cancer risk.

Obesity

Obesity constitutes a special form of poor nutrition that is epidemic over the past 20 years in most developed countries, including the United States, and in urban areas of many rapidly developing countries. The Lancet Commission on the epidemic of obesity, malnutrition, and climate change has documented global patterns where several countries simultaneously have both increased rates of obesity as well as problems of underweight. Over 40% of US adults are obese, affecting nearly half of non-Hispanic Blacks (see Chapter 23).[50] The prevalence of obesity in children has increased significantly in the past decade such that now nearly one in five US children are obese.[51] Worldwide, it is estimated that nearly 2 billion adults are overweight, and of these over 650 million are obese.[52] Criteria for overweight status and obesity are based on the body mass index (BMI) (see Chapter 23).

Obesity constitutes a significant setback to improvements in other areas of health during the past century. Numerous serious chronic health conditions are linked to obesity and physical inactivity, including diabetes, cardiovascular disease, and 13 distinct forms of cancer (liver, advanced prostate, ovarian, gallbladder, kidney, colorectal, esophageal [adenocarcinoma], postmenopausal breast, pancreatic, endometrial, stomach [cardia], multiple myeloma, and meningioma) (Fig. 13.13). The accelerating, long-term costs of obesity for both the individual and society underlie the urgency to accelerate progress in prevention and treatment. IARC has established a preventive relationship between the absence of excess weight and the risk of cancer in humans.

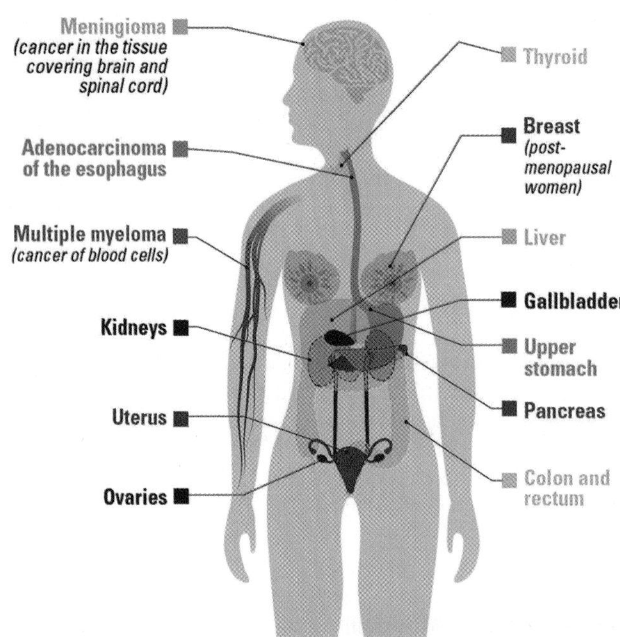

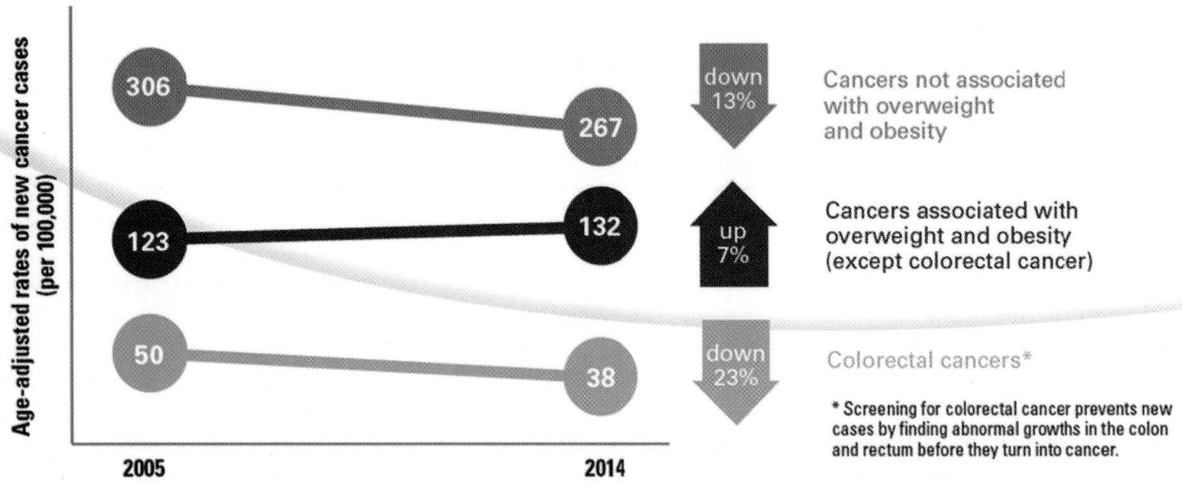

Fig. 13.13 Overweight and Obesity and Increased Risk for 13 Cancers. (A) Cancers associated with overweight and obesity are meningioma, adenocarcinoma of the esophagus, multiple myeloma, kidneys, uterus, ovaries, thyroid, breast (post-menopausal, liver, gallbladder upper stomach, pancreas, colon and rectum; **(B)** Although most cancers associated with overweight and obesity increased, other cancers decreased from 2005 to 2014. (From CDC Cancer and obesity. *Overweight and Obesity Are Associated With Cancer Vital Signs Centers for Disease Control and Prevention US Department of Health &Human Services.* US Cancer Statistics; 2017.)

Obesity has been linked mechanistically to both an increase in cancer risk and cancer progression. Because tumor growth is regulated by interactions between tumor cells and their tissue microenvironment, stromal compartments rich in adipose tissue can promote the development of tumor cells. During cancer progression, cancer-associated adipocytes (CAAs) undergo both structural and functional alterations that create a favorable micro-environment for increased cellular invasiveness and aggression (Fig. 13.14A). Cancer cells alter adipocytes through lipolysis and delipidation leading to CAAs that produce abnormal amounts of adipocyte-derived cytokines (increased leptin and decreased adiponectin), as well as release inflammatory cytokines and protease enzymes. The adipokine leptin increases inflammation and is associated with stromal effects that promote cancer cell proliferation, metabolism, angiogenesis, and invasion.[53] In obese individuals, changes in glucose and lipid metabolism are found in the tumor microenvironment as well as systemically. Obesity causes dysfunctional adipose tissue to produce increased levels of insulin–like growth factor 1 (IGF-1), sex hormones, and adipokines that contribute to obesity-related metabolic changes such as insulin resistance, hyperglycemia, dyslipidemia, hypoxia, and chronic inflammation (see Fig. 13.14B). As described previously, inflammation is an important contributor to both tumor initiation and progression. Excess adipose tissue can become reservoirs of lipophilic organochlorines and other fat-seeking toxic agents that can enhance proinflammatory mediators, which attract macrophages and cancer-associated fibroblasts, all of which are tumor-promoters. Additionally, the associated insulin resistance and hypoxia can trigger compensatory angiogenesis, thus providing an energy reservoir for any embedded cancer cells. Type 2 diabetes, elevated insulin levels, and altered insulin signaling pathways in obese individuals have been linked to cancer risk and progression as well as resistance to cancer therapies.[54]

Increasing BMI is related to less favorable outcomes for cancer recurrence, survival, and comorbidities (e.g., cardiovascular disease, diabetes, wound healing). Survivors of childhood cancers appear to have an increased risk of developing obesity, diabetes, thyroid cancer, and other cancers throughout the aging process.[55]

Alcohol Consumption

Alcohol is classified by IARC as a human carcinogen and is known to increase circulating unbound hormones as well as obesity. Overall, there are strong data linking alcohol with cancers of the mouth, pharynx, larynx, esophagus, liver, colorectum, and breast (in both males and females) (Table 13.4).[56] The evidence does not support any "safe limit" of intake. The deleterious effects come from the ethanol content and are not affected by the type of drink consumed.

Gene variations among alcohol users may increase the likelihood of alcohol-related toxicities. For example, genes that encode for ethanol metabolism affect the ability of the body to convert acetaldehyde to acetate. Acetaldehyde is the most toxic metabolite of alcohol and is the chief cause of alcohol-related carcinogenesis. Other toxic effects of alcohol result from the induction of cytochrome P-450 2E1 (genetic variant CYP2E1) leading to the generation of ROS and oxidative stress.[57] Some factors that can enhance the carcinogenicity of ethanol include an increase in pro-carcinogens (e.g., nitrosamines from preserved meats) and viral co-factors, such as hepatitis, that weaken the capacity of the liver to induce protective enzymes. Such changes predispose the individual to enzyme and metabolic dysfunction, as well as structural abnormalities (e.g., altered mucosal integrity). Associated nutritional deficiencies in cancer-protective agents, such as retinol, retinyl esters, folic acid, and other vitamins also contribute to tumor initiation and progression. For example, deficiencies in folate cause epigenetic changes in DNA methylation that promote tumor cell proliferation.[58]

Physical Activity

Regular exercise is reported to decrease the risk of breast cancer, colon cancer (men), and endometrial cancer independent of weight changes. Data are showing the vital importance of regular exercise in the primary and secondary prevention of several other chronic diseases, including cardiovascular disease, hypertension, diabetes, obesity, depression, osteoporosis, and premature death.[17,59] Millions of deaths in the United States are attributable to physical inactivity.[60] In a recent study, those with high levels of sedentary behavior were found to have a 28% to 44% increased risk of colon cancer, an 8% to 17% increased risk for breast cancer, and a 28% to 36% risk for endometrial cancer.[61] Several biologic mechanisms have been proposed to account for the protective effect of exercise against many forms of cancer, including

- Decreasing insulin and IGF levels
- Decreasing obesity
- Increasing free radical scavenger systems
- Altering inflammatory mediators
- Decreasing levels of circulating unbound sex hormones and metabolic hormones
- Improving immune function
- Decreasing oncogenes
- Enhancing cytochrome P-450 and thereby modifying carcinogen activation
- Increasing gut motility and excretion of carcinogens
- Increasing antitumor effects from the release of myokines or proteins from contracting muscles (see Emerging Science Box: Exercise and Anticancer Effects of Myokines)

Many questions remain unanswered concerning the ideal frequency, intensity, and duration of exercise. According to the US Department of Health and Human Services, significant health benefits are achieved when adults engage weekly in at least 150 minutes (2 hours and 30 minutes) to 300 minutes (5 hours) of moderate-intensity aerobic physical activity, 75 minutes (1 hour and 15 minutes) to 150 minutes (2 hours and 30 minutes) of vigorous-intensity aerobic physical activity, or an equivalent combination of moderate- and vigorous-intensity activity.[62] The guidelines recommend at least 60 minutes of physical activity everyday (mostly moderate- or vigorous-intensity aerobic) for children and adolescents. Being physically active after a cancer diagnosis is linked to improved quality of life and increased survival for several cancer types. A Cochrane review found that aerobic exercise

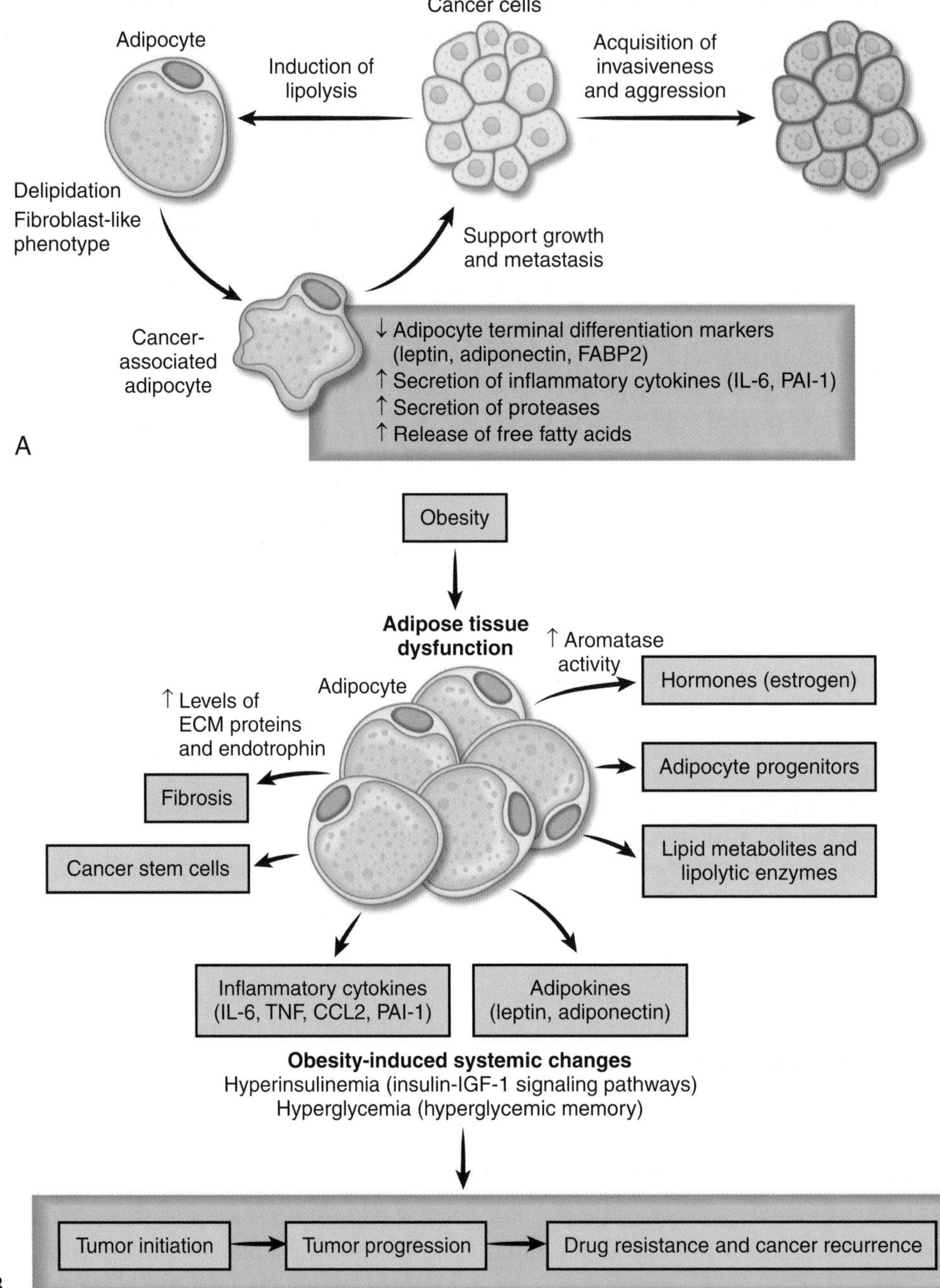

Fig. 13.14 Structural and Functional Changes in Adipocytes and Interaction With the Microenvironment Contribute to Cancer Progression and Metastases: A Working Model. **(A)** Signaling interactions occur between cancer cells and cancer-associated adipocytes. This interaction within the tumor microenvironment creates a place or *niche* permissive for cancer growth. Cancer cells stimulate the breakdown of lipids in adipocytes, leading to *delipidation* and the emergence of a fibroblast-like phenotype in adipocytes. The continuing alterations are associated with functional changes in the cells and include increased secretion of inflammatory mediators (cytokines) and proteases, and increased release of free fatty acids. All of these changes can support tumor growth and invasiveness. **(B)** Obesity leads to excessive levels of proinflammatory cytokines, sex hormones, lipid metabolites, and altered adipokines. The altered adipose tissue becomes a source of various extracellular matrix proteins, cancer stem cells, and cancer-associated adipokines. Collectively these alterations contribute to tumor initiation, growth, and recurrence. The systemic metabolic changes of obesity—hyperinsulinemia and hyperglycemia—can further contribute to a tumor-permissive environment. *CCL2*, Chemokine ligand 2; *ECM*, extracellular matrix; *FABP2*, fatty acid–binding protein 2; *IGF*, insulin-like growth factor; *IL*, interleukin; *TNF*, tumor necrosis factor. (Adapted from Park J, Morley TS, Kim M, et al. Obesity and cancer—Mechanisms underlying tumour progression and recurrence. *Nature Reviews Endocrinology* 2014;10(8):455–465.)

was beneficial for adults with cancer-related fatigue both during and after cancer treatment.[63] Another Cochrane review found exercise in children with cancer associated with improved body composition, flexibility, and cardiorespiratory fitness.[64]

Air Pollution

The US Environmental Protection Agency, WHO, the Institute for Health Metrics and Evaluation (IHME) of the University of Washington, and others report that long-term exposure to air pollution increases morbidity from respiratory disease, lung cancer, and bronchitis, as well as a wide range of other chronic diseases. Air pollution also shortens life expectancy from cardiovascular disease, respiratory disease, lung cancer, and possibly neurodegenerative diseases and other forms of cancer.[65] Worldwide, air pollution is the fifth leading cause of death, and is the leading known environmental cause of death.[66,67] Indoor

TABLE 13.4 Alcoholic Drinks and Risk of Cancer[a]

	DECREASES RISK		INCREASES RISK	
	Exposure	Cancer Site	Exposure	Cancer Site
Convincing			Alcoholic drinks	Mouth, pharynx and larynx, esophagus Colorectum (men)[b] Breast (premenopause and postmenopause)
Probable			Alcoholic drinks	Liver[c] Colorectum (women)[b]
Limited—suggestive				
Substantial effect on risk unlikely	Alcoholic drinks (adverse effect): kidney[d]			

[a]In the judgment of the Panel (WCRF/AICR), the factors listed modify the risk of cancer. Judgments are graded according to the strength of the evidence.
[b]The judgments for men and women are different because there are fewer data for women. Increased risk is only apparent above a threshold of 30 g/day of ethanol for both sexes.
[c]Cirrhosis is an essential precursor of liver cancer caused by alcohol. The International Agency for Research on Cancer has graded alcohol as a class 1 carcinogen for liver cancer. Alcohol alone only causes cirrhosis in the presence of other factors.
[d]The evidence was sufficient to judge that alcoholic drinks are unlikely to have an adverse effect on the risk of kidney cancer; it was inadequate to draw a conclusion regarding the protective effect.
Adapted from World Cancer Research Fund/American Institute for Cancer Research (WCRF/AICR). *Second Expert Report: Food, Nutrition, Physical Activity, and the Prevention of Cancer: A Global Perspective*. London: Author.

EMERGING SCIENCE BOX

Exercise and Anticancer Effects of Myokines

A newly identified anticancer mechanism of exercise is the release of proteins called myokines into the bloodstream. Myokines have beneficial effects, such as increasing insulin sensitivity of many systems (see first figure below). Additionally, myokines can induce apoptosis in breast cancer and colon cancer cells. Other investigators have found antitumorigenic effects of another myokine, interleukin-6 (IL-6), from working muscles. Epinephrine from the adrenal glands also increases mobilization of natural killer (NK) cells, which migrate into tumors and destroy tumor cells (see second figure below).

Biological Roles of Myokines

Only a few myokines have been allocated to specific function in humans. The biological roles of myokines include, for example, effects on cognition, lipid and glucose metabolism, browning of white fat, bone formation, endothelial cell function, hypertrophy, skin structure, and tumor growth.

Data from Laurens C, Bergouignan A, Moro C. Exercise-released myokines in the control of energy metabolism. *Frontiers in Physiology*, 2020;11:91. DOI: 10.3389/fphys.2020.00091; Severinsen MCK, Pedersen BK. Muscle–organ crosstalk: the emerging roles of myokines. *Endocr Rev.* 2020;41(4):594–609.; Son JS, Chae SA, Testroet ED, et al. Exercise-induced myokines: A brief review of controversial issues of this decade. *Expert Review of Endocrinology and Metabolism*, 2018;13(1):51–58.

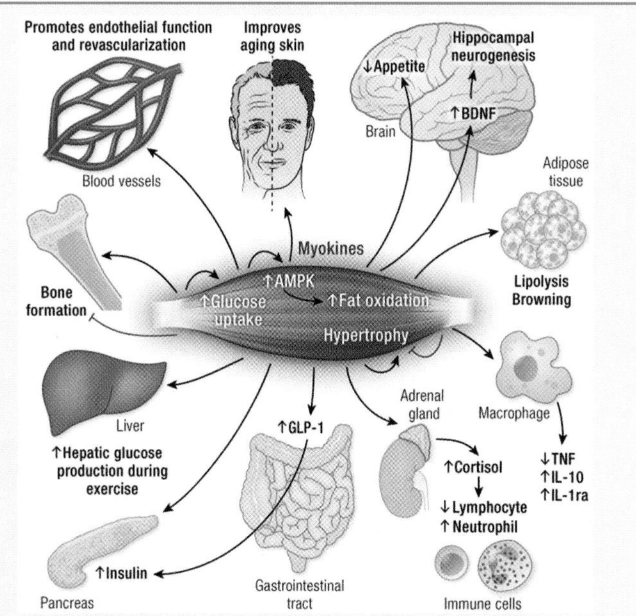

(From Severinsen M, Pedersen BK. Muscle-organ crosstalk: The emerging roles of myokines. *Endocrine Reviews*, 2020;41(4):594–609. https://doi.org/10.1210/endrev/bnaa016.)

(Continued)

EMERGING SCIENCE BOX

Exercise and Anticancer Effects of Myokines—Cont'd

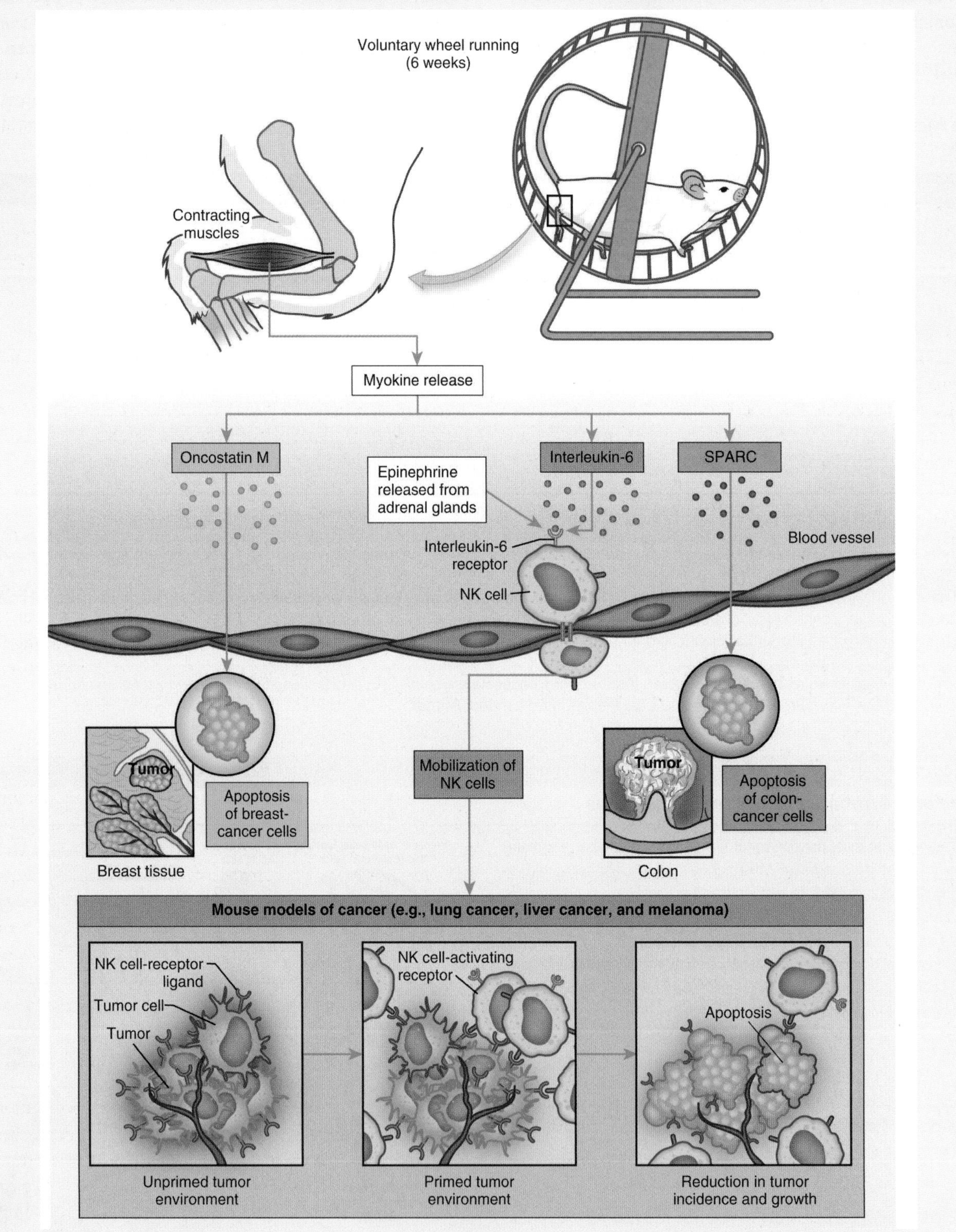

Antitumor Effects of Myokines (Adapted from Lucia A, Ramírez M. (2016). Muscling in on cancer. *New England Journal of Medicine*, 2016;375(9):892–894; Pedersen L, Idorn M, Olofsson GH, et al. Voluntary running suppresses tumor growth through epinephrine-and IL-6-dependent NK cell mobilization and redistribution. *Cell Metabolism*, 2016;23(3):554–562.)

air pollution from burning coal, charcoal, wood, dung, or other biomass also poses a significant health burden.

IARC has concluded that outdoor air pollution is carcinogenic to humans (IARC Group 1) and causes lung cancer.[68] A recent systematic review found that leukemia is also linked to air pollution exposure.[69] Specific constituents of polluted air are highly mutagenic and carcinogenic.[70] Outdoor air pollution consists of fine particulates, gases of nitrogen and sulfur, heavy metals, volatile organic compounds, and combustion exhausts that form ozone in the presence of sunlight. It is the only carcinogen in IARC Group 1 that is a mixture of components, some of which exhibit high toxicity and carcinogenic potential when isolated, whereas other components do not. Studies of this mixture sometimes reveal no effects compared to the effects caused by toxic compounds tested individually. Thus, the mechanism of carcinogenicity induced by air pollution is a mixture of multiple cellular responses, revealing synergies and antagonisms between components.[71]

Some of the compounds in air pollution are classified by the IARC as carcinogens including benzo[a]pyrene and benzo[a]anthracene. IARC classifies diesel engine exhaust as carcinogenic with sufficient evidence that it is linked to an increased risk of lung cancer and an association with bladder cancer. The most significant association, however, between air pollution and cancer involves exposures to particulate matter (PM) (see Chapter 2). PM is a mixture of extremely small particles, including heavy metals and liquid droplets, that are a complex mix of acids (nitrates and sulfates), organic chemicals, metals, and soil or dust particles. PM varies in size categorized as PM_{10} (particles with an aerodynamic diameter equal to or less than 10 µm), $PM_{2.5}$ (particles with an aerodynamic diameter equal to or less than 2.5 µm), and ultrafine particles (Fig. 13.15). The size of the particles determines where they are distributed in the respiratory tract, with large particles deposited in upper airways, while fine particles are deposited in deeper airways.

The mechanisms of adverse effects of PM include (1) oxidative stress, (2) ROS generation, (3) DNA oxidative damage, (4) mutagenicity, (5) stimulation of proinflammatory factors, and (6) induction of senescence. $PM_{2.5}$ or smaller particles are easily absorbed by the lungs Within the blood, these tiny particles are phagocytosed by macrophages and neutrophils that release tissue-damaging inflammatory mediators. PM causes pulmonary inflammation, which leads to oxidative stress and oxidation of DNA, sustained cellular proliferation, and tissue remodeling progressing to fibrosis and tumor development. $PM_{2.5}$ inhalation has an antiapoptotic effect that sustains cell division in damaged cells, induces angiogenesis, and activates invasion and metastasis of cancer cells.[71]

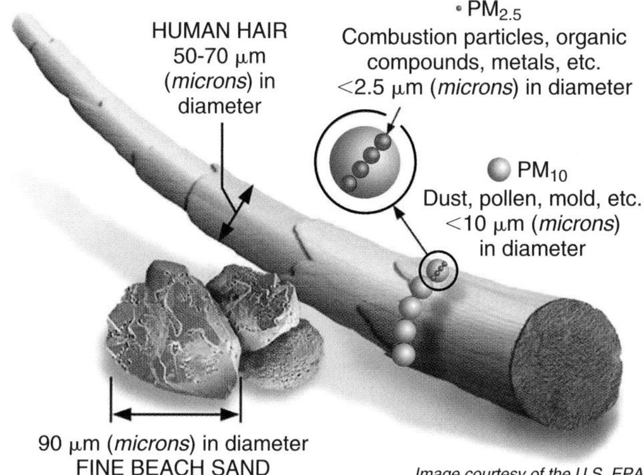

Fig. 13.15 Particle Sizes and Pollution. (From Environmental Protection Agency. *Particulate Matter Updated March 18, 2013.* Washington, DC: Author; 2013.)

Levels of ozone, another common outdoor air pollutant, are rising around the world in both higher income and lower/middle income regions contributing to about 365,000 annual deaths from chronic lung disease and lung cancer. Over 70% of these deaths occurred in India and China. In the United States, it is estimated that there were 12,800 deaths in 2019 attributable to ozone exposure.[66]

Living close to petrochemical and other industries is a recognized cancer risk factor in India, Brazil, China, and the United States. *Cancer Alley* is the term used to depict an array of historically black and brown and impoverished small factory towns situated on an 85-mile stretch of industrial plants along the banks of the Mississippi River that extends from New Orleans to Baton Rouge. Similar phenomena can be found in many rapidly industrializing zones across the globe, where the economically and ethnically disadvantaged incur far greater burdens of pollution and poor health. In India, up to half of all lung cancer occurs in non-smokers and is believed to reflect levels of both indoor (from cooking fuels) and outdoor air pollution that are without historic precedence.

Levels of pollutants, such as cigarette smoke and fuel byproducts, can easily become concentrated indoors. Both active and passive smoking (secondhand smoke) and fuel combustion lead to the formation of ROS and damaging free radicals. These byproducts can remain airborne for weeks, inducing cell death (apoptosis) in the lungs, promoting inflammation, and increasing biochemical markers known to increase DNA damage and the risk of cancer. Non-smokers in some regions in China and India have high levels of lung cancer from exposures to cooking fumes, as well as domestic coal byproducts that can produce indoor particulate levels many times greater than outdoor pollution or tobacco smoke.[72]

Another significant indoor air pollutant is radon gas, which is considered the leading indoor cause of lung cancer in non-smokers in the United States.[73,74] Radon is a natural radioactive decay product of uranium that can become trapped indoors after it is released from rock and soil. Exposure levels are greater in underground mines as compared to houses. Radon gas in the air breaks down into tiny radioactive elements that are inhaled directly into the lungs or attach to small dust particles that are then inhaled and lodge in the bronchi. Here, they can give off radiation that damages lung cells and may eventually lead to lung cancer. Non-smokers with polymorphisms of genes for DNA-repair are most susceptible to developing radon-associated lung cancer.[75] Houses with carcinogenic radon hazards can be identified by testing basements when doors and windows are kept closed. If levels are above 4 μg/dL, the Environmental Protection Agency advises that they should be mitigated.

Ionizing Radiation

Much of the knowledge of the effects of IR on human cancer has stemmed from observations of cancer patterns in survivors of the Hiroshima and Nagasaki atomic bombs from 1945 who were exposed over the dose range from 20 to 250 centigray (cGy), which includes low linear energy transfer (LET) radiation, like that from x-rays or γ-rays. Other evidence is derived from groups exposed to IR for medical reasons or various occupational exposures (Table 13.5). Within the first decade after the bombings in Japan, increased risks of acute leukemia were evident in children as were increased frequencies of thyroid and breast carcinomas. Other cancers later added to the list include lung, stomach, colon, esophageal, urinary tract cancers, and multiple myeloma. At Nagasaki and Hiroshima, the leukemia incidence in individuals 15 years or younger reached its peak 6 to 7 years after the explosions and has declined steadily since 1952. Those 45 years or older at the time of exposure had a longer latent period of 20 years before developing acute leukemia.

Age at the time of exposure is one of the main determinants of the type of radiation-induced cancer that is likely to develop. Susceptibility to cell damage is a function of the rate of cell replication; thus radiation exposures at early ages are the most carcinogenic. Sensitivity to radiation decreases until maturity but increases again at older ages when exposures can promote previously tumor-initiated cells and immune systems are more compromised.[76] Studies of Japanese atomic bomb survivors and Oak Ridge Y-12 uranium-processing plant workers suggest that this bimodal distribution indicates that radiation risks from early age exposures are related to *initiation* of cancer processes; whereas radiation exposures at later ages are mostly associated with the *promotion* of preexisting premalignant cells or exposures to chemical or physical agents that function as co-carcinogens.[77,78]

Human exposure to IR includes environmental emissions (e.g., radon), as well as diagnostic or therapeutic medical exposures (x-rays, CT scans, radioisotopes), and other radioactive sources. Studies of the childhood cohort treated with radiation to the skull to treat tinea capitis (ringworm) also show increased risks of brain cancer later in life along with elevations in thyroid cancer risk.[79,80] More recent pooled analyses reaffirm a linear relationship between dose and increased risk of thyroid cancer. This association persisted greater than 45 years after exposure, was greater at younger age of exposures, and was similar by sex and number of treatments.[81] Radiation-induced damage depends not only on dose, fractionation, and mechanism of the radiation delivery but also on critical indices of vulnerability that affect inherent repair mechanisms of the organism.

Radiation health risks involve not only neoplastic diseases but also cardiovascular disease. Cardiac and blood vessel damage causes fibrosis of the heart and blood vessels resulting in increased risk for coronary artery disease, valvular disease, cardiomyopathy, arrhythmias, and pericardial disease.[82] Other risks from IR even at low doses include somatic mutations and tissue alterations that contribute to other diseases, such as respiratory diseases, birth defects, and eye maladies, and may affect future generations. Fetal radiation exposure increases the risk for growth restriction, major malformations, death, and postnatal development of cancer.[83] In 2009, the National Council on Radiation Protection and Measurements (NCRP) reported Americans were exposed to more than seven times as much IR from medical procedures as compared with the 1980s (see Emerging Science Box: Increasing Use of Computed Tomography Scans and Risks).[84] In another study, the use of CT scans increased by 7.8% per year between 1996 and 2010 resulting in a doubling of the average per-person dose of radiation exposure for study subjects during that period.[85] In an effort to reduce pediatric exposure, the concept of "as low as reasonably achievable (ALARA)" levels of radiation from diagnostic or therapeutic procedures was introduced in the 1980s. An international program called "Image Gently" has since been successful in reducing unnecessary radiation exposure to children.[86]

TABLE 13.5 Cancer Associated With Exposure to Ionizing Radiation

Cancer Type	AB	AS	PM	TC	TH	RP	UM	RD
Leukemia	X	X			X			X
Thyroid	X			X				
Breast	X		X					
Lung	X	X			X		X	
Bone						X		
Stomach	X	X						
Esophagus	X	X						
Lymphoma	X	X						X
Brain			X				X	
Liver				X				
Skin				X			X	X

AB, Atomic bomb survivors; *AS*, ankylosing spondylitis individuals; *PM*, postpartum mastitis individuals; *RD*, radiologists; *RP*, radium dial painters; *TC*, tinea capitis individuals; *TH*, individuals receiving Thorotrast; *UM*, underground miners.

Data from Jones JA, et al. Ionizing radiation as a carcinogen. In: McQueen E, ed. *CA comprehensive toxicology*, 2nd edition. St Louis: Elsevier; 2010.

Radiation-Induced Cancer

IR is a potent mutagen and carcinogen. It can penetrate cells and tissues, depositing random energy within tissues in the form of ionizations (e.g., excitation or removal of an electron from the target atom). Such ionization can lead to irreversible or indirect damage secondary to the formation of water-based free radicals (radiolysis). The *general* characteristics of IR-induced carcinogenesis are well established. Research over the past two decades has focused on *specific* cellular and molecular mechanisms which impact cancer development and other chronic illnesses. Considerations include dose-response relationships for mutations, chromosome aberrations, cell transformation, and both genetic and epigenetic expression that vary with host

EMERGING SCIENCE BOX

Increasing Use of Computed Tomography Scans and Risks

An analysis of computed tomography (CT) patterns by radiology researchers at Columbia University confirmed that the sevenfold increase in both diagnostic and therapeutic radiation from CT scans in the past 4 decades has contributed to major increases in cancer risks especially for those exposed as children. Where adult CT scanners are not adjusted to smaller bodies, infants can incur up to 4000 chest x-rays from a single whole-body CT scan. Based on data from Japanese survivors of atomic bombs, the authors estimated that 1.5% to 2.0% of all cancers in the United States in the next decades might be attributable to CT radiation. The researchers also note that pediatric, young adult, and adult CT scans are sometimes ordered excessively and repeated unnecessarily because of defensive medicine. Finally, they advocate three ways to reduce radiation exposures: (1) reduce radiation doses in individual studies (i.e., use modern scanners adjusted to smaller bodies), (2) whenever possible substitute ultrasonography with magnetic resonance imaging (MRI) for CT, and (3) order CT scans only when absolutely necessary. The NCRP reports that most radiation exposures today are because of diagnostic procedures. In 2006, 67 million CT scans (compared with 3 million in 1980), 18 million nuclear medicine procedures, 17 million interventional fluoroscopy procedures, and 18 million nuclear medicine procedures were performed in the United States. Davis calculated that a single, unadjusted pediatric head CT can be equivalent to as many as 4000 chest x-rays.

Progress is being made in reducing pediatric CT procedures as a result of major educational efforts to promote awareness that as many as a third of CT scans are medically unnecessary and that the highest 25% of doses can be substantially reduced. If both these radiation-reducing strategies are undertaken, it is estimated that 62% of projected radiation-induced cancers could be averted in the next two decades.

Median Effective Radiation Dose for Each Type of Computed Tomography Study

Anatomic Area, Study Type	Median (mSv)	Range (mSv)	Dose Equivalent (No. of Chest X-rays)
Head and Neck			
Routine head	2	0.3–6	30
Routine neck	4	0.7–9	55
Suspected stroke	14	4–56	199
Unadjusted pediatric head	240	70-400	4000
Chest			
Chest, no contrast	8	2–24	117
Chest, with contrast	8	2–19	119
Suspected pulmonary embolus	10	2–30	137
Coronary angiogram	22	7–39	309
Abdomen-Pelvis			
Routine abdomen-pelvis, no contrast	15	3–43	220
Routine abdomen-pelvis, with contrast	16	4–45	234
Multiphase abdomen-pelvis	31	6–90	442
Suspected aneurysm or dissection	24	4–68	347

Data from Brenner DJ, et al. Computed tomography—An increasing source of radiation exposure. *New England Journal of Medicine*, 2007;357(22):2277–2284; Brett AS. *Journal Watch*, 2008;28(1):3; Davis DL. Secret history of the war on cancer. New York, NY: Basic Books; 2007:413; Food and Drug Administration. *What Are the Radiation Risks from CT?* Silver Spring, MD: Author; 2017; Food and Drug Administration Public Health Notification. *Reducing Radiation Risk from Computed Tomography for Pediatric and Small Adult Patients.* Silver Spring, MD: Radiology tool box recommendations; 2001. https://jamanetwork.com/journals/jamapediatrics/fullarticle/1696279. Accessed January 10, 2022; Society for Pediatric Radiology and National Cancer Institute. *Radiation & Pediatric Computed Tomography.* Summer 2002. cancer.gov/cancertopics/causes/radiation-risks-pediatric-CT. Accessed January 10, 2022.

conditions. Other important areas of investigation include effects on the microenvironment and nontargeted cells, which are the biologic effects that occur in nonirradiated bystander cells.

IR is a potent DNA-damaging agent causing cross-linking, nucleotide base damage, and single- or double-strand DNA breaks thus disrupting cellular regulation processes leading to carcinogenesis. The double-strand break (DSB) (Fig. 13.16) is considered one hallmark lesion. This type of DNA damage commonly can be repaired by the *nonhomologous end joining (NHEJ) pathway* that efficiently joins broken ends of DNA. However, repair errors can occur and increase with age and malnutrition. Irradiated human cells that are unable to execute the NHEJ pathway are extremely vulnerable to large-scale mutations and chromosomal aberrations.[87]

Although evidence suggests that interindividual differences in radiation responses may be attributed to certain genes and epigenetic conditions (see Chapter 6, Epigenetics and Disease), IR can activate oncogenes, resulting in uncontrolled cell growth (see Chapter 12). Several sensitive tumor-suppressor genes have been identified that are deactivated by IR and promote carcinogenesis after low doses of radiation. For example, IR has been shown to disrupt the p53 gene, which is the most commonly mutated gene in human cancers and is responsible for DNA repair and for inducing apoptosis in irreparably damaged cells (see Chapter 12). In women with breast cancer who have an inherited mutation in the p53 gene at one allele, treatment with radiation can induce mutations in the other p53 allele leading to enhanced carcinogenesis in cells that survive the treatment.[88] Gene expression can change as a function of radiation dose, timing, and type of exposure.[89]

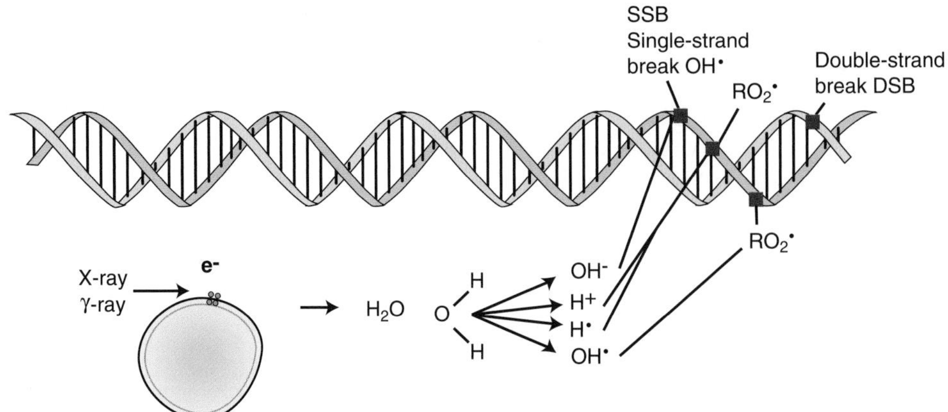

Fig. 13.16 Free Radicals. Free radicals formed by water nearby and around DNA cause indirect effects. These free radicals have a short life as single free radicals. Oxygen can modify the reaction, enabling longer lifetimes of oxidative free radicals.

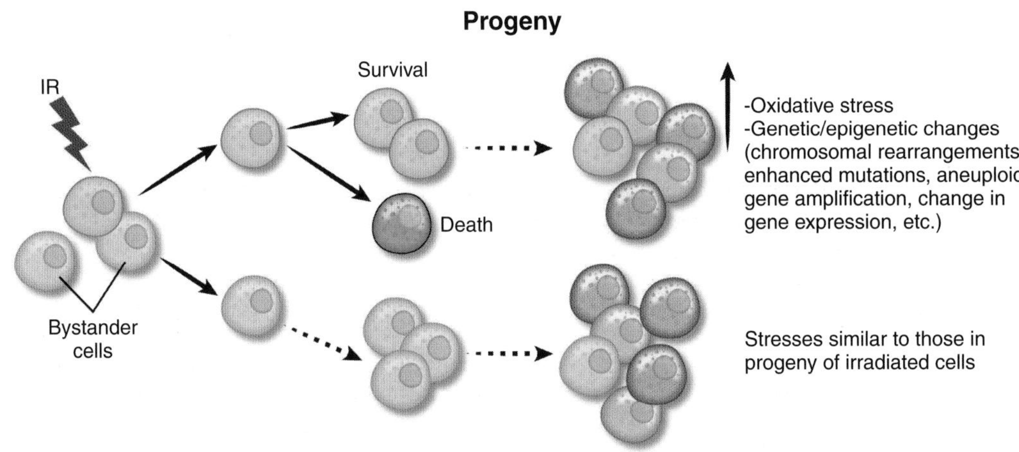

Fig. 13.17 Radiation: Targeted and Nontargeted or Bystander Effects. Signaling from cells exposed to irradiation causes stressful effects, including oxidative stress, to those cells not directly irradiated (called *bystander cells*) and their progeny. These induced effects may be similar to those reported in the progeny of irradiated cells. (Adapted from Azzam EI, Jay-Gerin JP, Pain D. Ionizing radiation-induced metabolic oxidative stress and prolonged cell injury. *Cancer Letters*, 2012;327(1–2):48–60.)

Nontargeted Effects

Nontargeted effects (NTEs) occur in cells not directly traversed by a radiation particle but in the vicinity of a cell that has been exposed or has received signals (cell-to-cell communication) from irradiated cells. Contradicting a long-held assumption that direct exposures are required to produce aberrant responses, it is now understood that cells can participate in the final damage response even though they are not directly exposed. In addition, cells that are the progeny of irradiated cells may express a high level of gene mutations, cell lethality, and chromosomal aberration. These deleterious effects, stemming from previous generations of irradiated cells, constitute genomic instability that may contribute to secondary cancers and can lead to effects in nearby cells, termed bystander cells.[90]

Radiation-induced bystander effects (RIBEs) can occur in cells not directly exposed to IR and show heritable changes that include DNA damage, mutations, chromosomal aberrations, chromosomal instability, senescence, apoptosis, and oncogenic transformation.[91,92] Both DSBs and apoptotic cell death can be induced by bystander effects, supporting a signaling role between the irradiated cells (the targeted cells) and nonirradiated cells (the nontargeted or bystander cells) (Fig. 13.17). Emerging data indicate the importance of exosomes mediating microRNA transfer and the cellular communication between

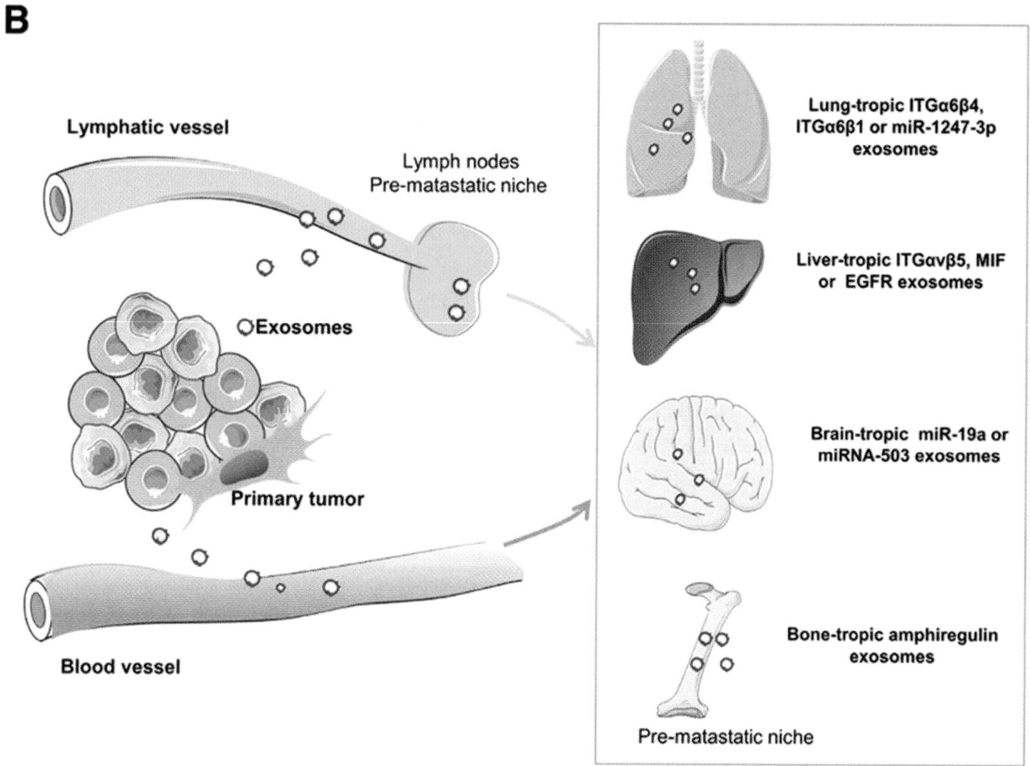

Fig. 13.18 Exosomes in Cancer. **(A)** Exosomes are vesicles that carry cargo. Tumor-derived exosomes can be released into extracellular sites. These vesicles carry oncoproteins and nucleic acids that induce different signaling pathways and activation of different immune cells. This communication can promote a cancer-favorable inflammatory microenvironment that promotes metastatic initiation and progression. Tumor derived exosomes are involved in the epithelial-to-mesenchymal transition (EMT), angiogenesis, increase of vascular permeability, alteration of the immune system, transformation of recipient cells and reprogramming of energy metabolism. **(B)** Exosomes are involved in organotropic metastasis (see Chapter 12). (From Wu M, Wang G, Hu W, et al. Emerging roles and therapeutic value of exosomes in cancer metastasis. *Mol Cancer.* 2019;18[1]. https://doi.org/10.1186/s12943-019-0964-8.)

the directly irradiated cells and the nonirradiated cells (see Chapters 1,12 and Fig. 13.18).[93] Investigators reported that cell-free chromatin (cfCh) particles released from dying cells can integrate into genomes of surrounding healthy cells to induce DNA damage and inflammation.[94]

Numerous intercellular and intracellular signaling pathways are implicated in the bystander response, and these effects have been shown to be transmitted to cell descendants. Importantly, exosome communication is being studied for the capacity to induce a favorable inflammatory microenvironment that promotes cancer cell metastasis.[95–97] In contrast, therapeutic interference with specific signaling pathways may result in genome stabilization and the generation of novel therapeutics.

These bystander effects, demonstrated in vivo, reflect an ongoing inflammatory response (oxidative stress response) to the initial radiation-induced injury (see Emerging Science Box: Paradigm Shift? Responses to Ionizing Radiation Mediated by Inflammatory Mechanisms).

Acute, Latent, and Microenvironmental Effects

IR causes both acute and persistent effects. Acute exposure to IR can cause damage to multiple organ systems, especially those with highly proliferative cells, such as the hematopoietic and reproductive systems, the skin, and the GI system. Investigators have postulated that radiation's carcinogenic potential persists as a direct result of nontargeted radiation effects, which are known to alter cell signaling and induce changes in the microenvironment. Investigators report the brain's innate immune system is especially vulnerable to cranial irradiation, especially at young ages when the skull is thin and neurons poorly myelinated. The radiation alters the microenvironment and induces the recruitment of macrophages, which infiltrate the region. With improvements in pediatric cancer survival, the long-term risks of a second cancer developing from radiation or chemotherapeutic treatments become increasingly important.

Radiation-induced cancer in humans has latent periods, usually 5 to 10 years, but latency for some radiation-related

EMERGING SCIENCE BOX

A Paradigm Shift? Responses to Ionizing Radiation Mediated by Inflammatory Mechanisms

Many observations have not been supportive of the conventional paradigm of biologic responses to ionizing radiation (IR). The conventional paradigm is that the consequences of exposure to IR have been attributed solely to mutational DNA damage or cell death induced in irradiated cells at the time of exposure. The challenges to this paradigm come from three types of published data: (1) **abscopal**, or "out-of-field," effects, where radiation treatment to one local area of the body results in an antitumor effect distant to the radiation site; (2) detection of plasma factors in vivo (clastogenic [or capable of chromosome damage] factors) that can affect the survival and function of irradiated cells; and (3) effects in non-irradiated cells that are in the vicinity of irradiated cells (bystander effects) or in the descendants of irradiated cells several generations after the initial radiation exposure (genomic instability). These nontargeted effects are different than the targeted effects that arise in cells upon immediate deposition of energy at the time of radiation exposure. The nontargeted effects arise as a result of intracellular signaling and appear to represent a genotype-dependent balance (and various epigenetic influences) of toxic factors and cellular responses that can involve both oxidative stress and inflammatory type processes (see Fig. 13.17). The continuous activation and increase in endogenous and exogenous ROS damages the body's antioxidant system, stimulates more ROS, and forms a cascade of amplified inflammatory responses which eventually leads to cell death. The interconnected network of inflammatory and immune response pathways activated by IR include (1) cytokines, growth factors, adhesion molecules, (2), DNA damage, ER stress, ROS/RNS, hypoxia (3) inflammasomes, (4) cell death and senescence and (5) coagulation and fibrinolysis.

Recently, an increasing number of studies have been focusing on the underlying mechanisms involved in hematopoietic stem cell (HSC) fate after radiation exposure. The mechanisms include DNA damage response (DDR), including DNA-damage repair, cell cycle arrest, apoptosis and senescence, or bone marrow (BM) microenvironmental effects. Exposure to radiation not only causes acute myelosuppression but can lead to long-term residual hematopoietic problems because of the induction of HSC senescence. Caution is required from extrapolation of animal studies to humans. ROS, reactive oxygen species; RNS, reactive nitrogen species. ROS, reactive oxygen species; RNS, reactive nitrogen species.

Data from Azzam EI, et al. Ionizing radiation-induced metabolic oxidative stress and prolonged cell injury. *Cancer Letters*, 2012;327(1–2):48–60; Mukherjee D, et al. Responses to ionizing radiation mediated by inflammatory mechanisms. *Journal of Pathology*, 2014;232(3):289–299; Dong S, et al. *Radiation Medicine and Protection*, 2020;1:179–185; Wang Y, et al. Hematopoietic stem cell senescence and long-term bone marrow injury. *Cell Cycle*, 2006;5(1):35– 38; Dong S, et. al. Oxidative stress: a critical hint in ionizing radiation induced pyroptosis. *Radiat Med Prot.* 2020;1:179-185. Wang Y, et al. Total body irradiation selectively induces murine hematopoietic stem cell senescence. *Blood*, 2006;107(1):358–366; Green DE, et al. Consequences of irradiation on bone and marrow phenotypes, and its relation to disruption of hematopoietic precursors. *Bone*, 2014;63:87–94; Lumniczky K, et al. Low dose ionizing radiation effects on the immune system. *Environment International*, 2021;149:106212; McKelvey KJ, et al. Radiation, inflammation and the immune response in cancer. *Mammalian Genome*, 2018;29(11):843–865.

tumors can span decades. British investigators have reported that for solid tumors, except brain tumors, radiation-related excess risk begins to appear about 5 years after exposure in therapeutically irradiated groups. For leukemia, it appears within 5 years of exposure.[98] Using US Surveillance Epidemiology and End Results (SEER) data, the estimated excess of secondary cancers that could be related to radiotherapy is about 8%.[99] Data from the United Kingdom, which included diagnostic procedures but excluded therapeutic irradiation, yielded an estimation of 15%.[98]

Low Dose and Dose Rate

Recent events, including the 2011 Fukushima and Chernobyl nuclear accidents, terrorist attacks, and exposure to radiation from medical procedures, have increased the need to identify risks from low-level IR exposures. Because reliable surveillance of large populations cannot easily be accomplished, simulation models also may provide reasonable approximations that employ theoretic models to estimate response curves (Box 13.4).

Non-Ionizing Radiation and Electromagnetic Radiation

NIR includes electromagnetic radiation and differs from IR in the way it acts on materials like air, water, and living tissue. NIR includes the spectrum of ultraviolet (UV), visible light, infrared (IR), microwave (MW), radio frequency (RF), and extremely low frequency (ELF) (Box 13.5). NIR is found in a wide range of occupational settings and can pose a health risk to potentially exposed workers if not adequately controlled.

Electromagnetic radiation (EM or EMR) is produced by coupled electric and magnetic fields that propagate as waves through materials and air. Its frequency range is usually defined from radio waves (10 kHz and above, such as AM broadcasts), through microwaves (1 to 10 GHz) up to visible light, and beyond to diagnostic x-rays and even gamma rays originating in deep space (see Box 13.5). EMR originating in the UV part of the spectrum and above can interact with materials leading to the direct ionization of atoms and molecules. Health risks associated with the non-ionizing part of the spectrum (termed electromagnetic fields [EMFs]) have been a concern for many decades. The impact of EMR on human health or the physical environment has not been fully assessed. In addition, with competing priorities (convenience, financial interest, and health necessity) and the limited availability of independent research on the topic, a consensus on the risks and benefits of different types of EMR exposure may be difficult to achieve. Safety standards vary significantly among countries. The National Institute of Environmental Health Sciences Electric and Magnetic Fields Working Group and the Environmental Protection Agency have recommended that low-frequency EMFs be classified as possible carcinogens.

Recent research has addressed low-intensity or low power fields and radiofrequency radiation (RFR, also termed *microwave radiation*) from devices such as phones, broadcast antennas, Wi-Fi, security monitors, baby monitors, wireless charging stations, routers, antennas, and others. Typically, these emissions are in the frequency range of 10^8 to 10^{10} Hz. Exposure to electric and magnetic fields is widespread. Electric fields are blocked by or weakened by walls and other objects, but

BOX 13.4 Theoretical Models to Understand Low-Dose Radiation

Several models include the linear no-threshold (LNT) relationship, in which any dose, including very low doses, has the potential to cause mutations (see A). Another model, the linear-quadratic relationship, proposes there is a risk mathematical term that is directly proportional to the dose (linear term) and another term proportional to the square of the dose (quadratic term) (see B). The threshold model proposes a threshold dose below which radiation may not cause cancer in humans (see C). Proponents of this model argue that such thresholds are derived, for example, from the ability to repair damage caused by lower doses of radiation. There is some evidence that low doses may actually produce a higher level of risk per unit of dose, which is called the *supralinear hypothesis* (see D). E, Stochastic or random probability is a major model for understanding low-dose radiation. Currently, the shape of the response curve for the low-dose region is unknown.

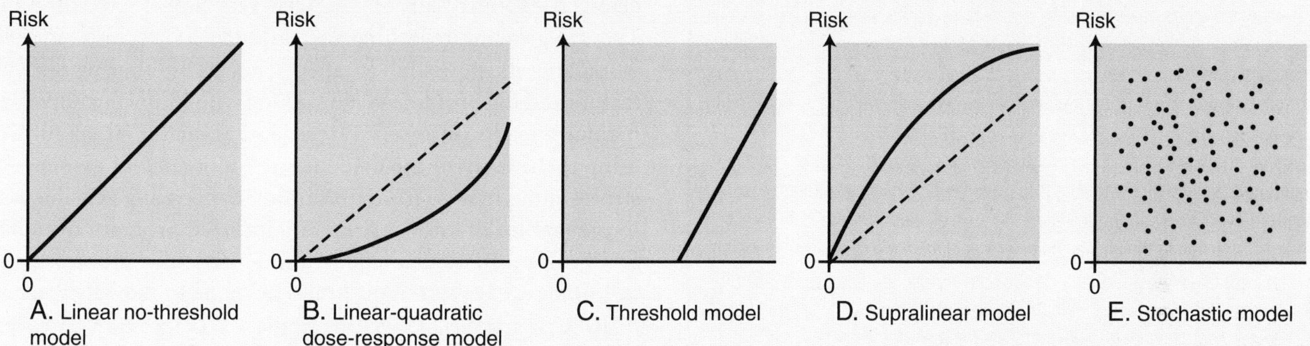

Theoretic Models for Estimating Risk of Low-Dose Ionizing Radiation. Collective population dose is expressed as a person-rem (roentgen equivalent, man). Estimating a collective dose then enables an application of a "constant risk factor" to obtain a statistical estimate of the number of additional cancers (above background radiation) from that exposure. These computations apply to low doses–low dose rates only (A). Many propose the best fit is the linear no-threshold (LNT) model (B). The most common alternative to the LNT model is the linear-quadratic model. The quadratic term is the square of the dose. The linear term is equal to zero (C). The threshold model is a threshold below which there is *no* increase in cancer risk. Proponents of this model argue that because some toxic chemicals/materials exhibit such thresholds, radiation must also have a threshold. Their arguments are related to repair of the radiation damage caused by lower doses of radiation (D). Some evidence exists that low levels of radiation produce a higher level of risk per unit dose, which is called the supralinear model. The stochastic model describes effects that are random, and the events cannot be predicted (E). (Adapted from Makhijani A, Smith B, Thorne MC. Science for the vulnerable: Setting radiation and multiple exposure environmental health standards to protect those at most risk. Takoma Park, MD: Institute for Energy and Environmental Research; 2006.)

BOX 13.5 Terms Used for Non-Ionizing Radiation and Electromagnetic Radiation

Non-Ionizing Radiation=NIR
Electromagnetic Radiation=EMR(EM)
Radiofrequency Radiation=RFR (RF)
Radiofrequency Electromagnetic Radiation=RF-EMR
Ultraviolet=UV
Infrared Radiation=IR
Microwave=MW
Extremely low frequency=ELF

From Flores-McLaughlin J, Runnells J, Gaza, R. Overview of non-ionizing radiation safety operations on the International Space Station. *Journal of Space Safety Engineering*, 2017;4(2):6–63. doi:10.1016/j.jsse.2017.02.007. ISSN 2468-8967. http://www.sciencedirect.com/science/article/pii/S2468896717300204.

magnetic fields are not. EMFs affect cardiac and neural functioning. The most common sources of radiofrequency electromagnetic radiation (RF-EMR) are wireless telecommunication devices and equipment, including cell phones, smart meters, and portable wireless devices (laptop computers and tablets). It is projected that 50 billion wireless radiating devices will be connected through the Internet of Things (IoT) in the next few years. Exposures to microwave or radiofrequency-radiation EMF associated with increased human brain cancers led to its classification as a possible cause of cancer by the IARC in 2011. Studies published since then have strengthened the evidence.[100] The most extensively studied public exposure to microwave radiation is from use of wireless telephones (mobile and cordless). Other exposures include occupational and military settings and sources from the general environment where few studies have been done. Recent studies from the National Toxicology Program (NTP) exposing rodents in their 2-year lifetimes to the same levels of RFR humans can receive in 70 years, resulted in what independent peer-reviewers deemed "clear evidence" of tumors in tissues surrounding the nerves in the hearts (schwannomas) of male rats, "some evidence" of glioma, "some evidence" of an association with tumors in the

BOX 13.6 Cell Phone Radiation and Children's Health: What Parents Need to Know

Use text messaging when possible and use cell phones in speaker mode or with the use of hands-free kits.
When talking on the cell phone, try holding it an inch or more away from the head.
Make only short or essential calls on cell phones.
Avoid carrying your phone against the body, such as in a pocket, sock, or bra; cell phonemanufacturers cannot guarantee that the amount of radiation absorbed will be at a safe level.
Do not talk on the phone or text while driving; this increases the risk of automobile crashes.
Exercise caution when using a phone or texting while walking or performing other activities; "distracted walking" injuries also are on the rise.
If you plan to watch a movie on your device, download it first, then switch to airplane mode while watching it to avoid unnecessary radiation exposure.
Keep an eye on signal strength (i.e., how many bars); the weaker your cell signal, the harder the phone has to work and the more radiation it gives off; it is better to wait until there is a stronger signal before using the device.
Avoid making calls in cars, elevators, trains, and buses; the cell phone works harder to get a signal through metal, so the power level increases.
Remember that cell phones are not toys or teething items.

Data from *American Academy of Pediatrics*; June 13, 2016. Available at http://www.healthychildren.org.

adrenal glands of male rats, hyperplasia, and DNA damage in multiple organs in rats and mice.[101,102] The report also noted statistically significant increases in tumors found in other organs at one or more of the exposure levels studied, including the brain, prostate gland, pituitary gland, adrenal gland, liver, and pancreas. Potential mechanisms underlying these findings included genotoxicity, effects on immune function, gene and protein expression, DNA repair mechanisms, cell signaling, oxidative stress, decreased melatonin, and apoptosis. Long-term exposure to elevated magnetic fields may lead to increased free radical concentrations, which are associated with aging, cancers, and neurodegenerative diseases. The NTP studies took more than 10 years to complete and are the most comprehensive assessment to date of health effects in animals exposed to RFR.

Children are now spending up to 9 hours a day with wireless radiating devices that are often held much closer to young bodies than manufacturers advise. The effects of exposure may be compounded because of increased vulnerability of young, rapidly growing cells to radiation and children's longer lifetime use of cell phones. In response to the NTP study discussed earlier, the American Academy of Pediatrics issued specific recommendations to reduce wireless cell phone exposure (Box 13.6). Chapter 14 discusses cancer in children. Low intensity NIR exposure in children can damage DNA, induce cancer, and impair reproductive health.[103] Senior investigators have noted that 13 epidemiological studies published since 2011 associate mobile phone use with increased tumors. Nine studies specifically report increased risk of brain cancer from mobile phone use, and four case-control studies report increased risk of vestibular nerve tumors from mobile phone use.[101]

As is evident from the atomic bomb survivors' studies, cancers that stem from environmental exposure to radiation can take four decades to be evident in the general population. With the unprecedented demand for computer-based schooling and pandemic-fueled increases in uses of all wireless radiating devices, the intensity and frequency of RFR exposures has changed exponentially in the past year alone. Controversies also are growing regarding the untested 5 G technology network and its potential to affect cancer by altering growth factors and the immune system, along with important environmental impacts on insects, trees, and animals. When considering the totality of the evidence at hand, current evidence is strong enough to go from precaution concerning possible risk to prevention of known risks. A concerted program of public and health professional education is needed to promote safer technology. Every attempt should be made to reduce exposure to RFR in schools, as well as homes.[101] Lingering controversies exist about how best to set standards for RFR. The Federal Communications Commission (FCC) relies on 24-year-old scientific evidence and insists that only thermal effects are to be avoided, dismissing findings from the NTP. Many authorities dispute this FCC determination noting that it relies heavily on the International Commission on Non-ionizing Radiation Protection (ICNIRP), a small, self-appointed, self-monitored group with no independent oversight. "In adopting ICNIRP positions of a group of 13 scientists, many of whom have close ties to industry, the agency ignores the fact that the majority, including several hundred experts in the fields of bioelectromagnetics and related matters, strongly dissent from the conclusions of ICNIRP."[104]

Ultraviolet Radiation

Ultraviolet (UV) radiation is produced naturally from sunlight and artificially from electric lights, black lights, and tanning lamps. UV radiation is divided into three major wavelengths: UVA, UVB, and UVC radiation. Most of the UV radiation received on earth is UVA; some is UVB. UVA radiation is weaker than UVB but penetrates more deeply into the skin and is more constant throughout the year regardless of weather conditions. UVB primarily affects the outer layer of the skin. UVC radiation effects do not increase health risks as much as UVB radiation. UV radiation also can be important to health as it promotes the synthesis of di-hydroxy vitamin D metabolism in the liver, which is essential for the absorption of calcium and phosphorus from food for bone development. Skin color greatly influences natural metabolism. The WHO generally recommends 5 to 15 minutes of sun exposure two to three times a week, but darker skinned people may require more. Overexposure, however, can result in acute and chronic health effects, including melanoma and other forms of cancer of the skin and eyes, as well as impacts on the immune system.

There are three main types of skin cancer (see Chapter 46):

- Basal cell carcinoma (BCC): cancer in the lower part of the epidermis or outer layer of the skin
- Squamous cell carcinoma (SCC): cancer in the flat cells that form the surface of the skin
- Melanoma: cancer that forms in melanocytes (i.e., pigment cells)

In the United States, skin cancer is the most commonly diagnosed malignancy; however, the actual number of non-melanoma skin cancers is unknown because they are not reported to cancer registries. BCC commonly occurs on the head and neck. SCC typically occurs on sun-exposed areas of the skin, including the forehead, nose, ears, lower lip, and dorsa of the hand. The incidence of BCC and SCC is strongly correlated with lifetime sunlight exposure (i.e., photocarcinogenesis). Specific patterns of sunlight exposure, intermittent or chronic, confer different host effects. Intense intermittent recreational sun exposure has been associated with melanoma and BCC. Chronic occupational sun exposure has been associated with SCC. Tanning bed exposure is associated with an increased risk of all forms of skin cancer, with higher risks when exposure took place at younger ages.[105] Other skin cancer risk factors include IR, use of photosensitive medications (e.g. tetracycline, thiazide diuretics, and retinoids), immunosuppression, and genetic factors.[106] In general, skin cancers have a higher incidence among people with a light or fair skin tone, but they can occur in anyone, including those who do not usually burn from exposure to sunlight. The pathogenesis of non-melanoma skin cancers involves specific gene mutations, epigenetic alterations, oxidative stress, inflammation, and reduced immune surveillance (see Chapter 46 for a more complete discussion of skin cancers).[106]

In 2021, the estimated number of new cases of melanoma of the skin will be 106,110 with an estimated 7180 deaths.[107] Melanoma can occur at many sites, many of which are not usually exposed to sunlight. *Intermittent acute* sun exposure causing sunburn early in life is associated with an increased risk of melanoma. Germline mutations have been identified in melanoma cells, as well as numerous somatic mutations that include several different types of oncogenes and tumor suppressor genes (see Chapter 12).[108] Low levels of melanin in white skin result in significant vulnerability to UV-mediated genetic alterations and a higher risk of melanoma formation, especially in persons with fair, freckled skin or immune deficiencies.[109] Although rare in people with dark skin, melanoma may be found under the fingernails or toenails or on the palms of the hands and soles of the feet.

The US Preventive Services Task Force (USPSTF) concludes that the current evidence is insufficient to justify screening for early detection of skin cancer. Moreover, the risks of overdiagnosis and overtreatment appear considerable relative to the benefits of annual visual skin examination by a clinician to screen for skin cancer in asymptomatic adults.[110] White men and women are more likely to die of melanoma than any other group. Risk factors vary for different types of skin cancer. Box 13.7 identifies the main risk factors for skin cancers.

Infection, Sexual and Reproductive Behavior

Infections with certain viruses, bacteria, and parasites are important contributors to or co-factors for cancer worldwide. The number of cases varies widely by region, with less developed areas having three times more infection-related cancers than more developed countries.[111] Among the more notable infections contributing to new cancer cases are *Helicobacter pylori (H. pylori)*, human papillomavirus (HPV), hepatitis B virus (HBV), hepatitis C virus (HCV), and Epstein–Barr virus (EBV). *H. pylori* contributes to about 75% of stomach cancers. HPV, HBV, and HCV infect the liver and together account for the preponderance of liver cancer cases (see Chapter 41). EBV is linked to nasopharyngeal carcinoma, Hodgkin lymphoma, diffuse large B-cell lymphoma (DLBCL), Burkitt lymphoma, EBV-associated malignant B-cell lymphoma, other lymphomas, and gastric adenocarcinoma.

HPV is the most common sexually transmitted virus in the United States and accounts for more than half of the total infection-attributable cancers in women worldwide. When detected through regular screening at an early stage, cervical cancer is treatable and curable. However, many national screening programs fail to reach poor women; sex-workers; black, brown, and native Americans; and those who are marginalized in society.[112]

Many sexually active women and men will be infected with HPV at some point in their lifetime, and some repeatedly. Although the main mode of HPV transmission is sexual contact, HPV can be contracted through contact with contaminated fomites, fingers, and mouth, as well as vertical transfer to infants at birth.[113] HPVs are a group of more than 200 related viruses, and at least 13 are cancer causing. *Low-risk HPVs* are not associated with cancer but can cause skin warts, called *condylomata acuminata*. *High-risk*, or oncogenic. HPV types 16 and 18 are responsible for most cancers. Most high-risk HPV infections cause cytologic abnormalities or abnormal cell changes that regress spontaneously. According to the National Cancer Institute, most HPV infections will be suppressed by an individual's immune system.[114] Persistence of infection with high-risk HPV is a precursor to the development of cervical intraepithelial neoplasia (CIN)

BOX 13.7 Common Risk Factors for Skin Cancers

Lighter natural skin color
Family history of skin cancer
A personal history of skin cancer
Exposure to sun through work and play
History of sunburns, especially early in life
History of indoor tanning
Skin that burns, reddens easily, or becomes painful in the sun
Freckles
Blue or green eyes
Blonde or red hair
Certain types of moles and a large number of moles
Higher coffee intake was associated with a modest decrease in melanoma (large cohort study)

(see Chapter 25), lesions, and invasive cervical cancers. HPV infection also has been identified as a definite carcinogen for several other types of cancer: penis, vulvar, vaginal, anal, and some oropharyngeal cancers (OPCs). Half of the OPCs most commonly linked to HPV-16 include the base of the tongue, tonsils, and pharynx. The incidence of HPV-associated OPC has increased during the past 20 years, especially among men, and may reflect persistent chronic inflammation. Co-factors that may increase the risk of developing cancer following a high-risk HPV infection include alcohol, smoking, decreased immunity, having many children (cervical cancer), long-term oral contraceptive use (cervical cancer), poor oral hygiene (OPC), and chronic inflammation.

Current guidelines recommend that sexually active women should have a Pap test every 3 years beginning at age 21 to 29. Women 30 to 65 years of age may receive Pap testing with HPV screening every 5 years (preferred) or Pap testing alone every 3 years. After age 65, Pap testing and HPV screening are no longer recommended for women with previous normal testing results since the risk of new malignancy is low. Women who had a hysterectomy with removal of the uterine cervix for a noncancerous condition also do not need Pap smears or HPV testing the rest of their lives. Currently, although the HPV vaccine does reduce the risk for cervical cancer, it does not change the frequency or need for Pap and HPV testing (see Chapters 25 and 27).

Other Viruses and Microorganisms

The relationship between viruses, bacteria, and cancer is discussed in Chapter 12. Human herpesvirus type 8 is linked to Kaposi sarcoma, and human T-cell lymphotropic virus type 1 is linked to leukemia and lymphoma. Other microorganisms involved in carcinogenesis include parasites such as *Opisthorchis viverrini* (bile duct cancer) and *Schistosoma haematobium* (bladder cancer). Their specific roles in carcinogenesis are thought to be related to functioning as cofactors or as direct carcinogens, or both.

Environmental and Occupational Hazards as Carcinogens

According to the Center for Disease Control Agency for Toxic Substances and Disease Registry, there are tens of thousands of synthetic chemicals that are widely used in the United States, of which only a fraction have been tested for their health effects.[115] Despite the 1976 US Toxic Substances Control Act and the 2016 Frank R. Lautenberg Chemical Safety for the 21st Century Act, widespread and low-level exposure to multiple toxic chemicals occurs every day in air, soil, food, water, household products, toys, personal care products, workplaces, and homes. Several hundred chemicals have been found to be carcinogens in controlled studies of experimental animals. According to IARC and the NTP, experimental chemical carcinogens should be regarded as potentially carcinogenic in humans. Table 13.1 provides a summary of a limited number of chemicals for which IARC judges there to be sufficient or limited evidence in humans by cancer site. A simplified overview of the Occupational Safety and Health Administration (OSHA) listing of carcinogenic factors is presented in Table 13.6.

Chemical carcinogenesis can arise from genotoxic and nongenotoxic or epigenetic mechanisms (Fig. 13.19). Genotoxic mechanisms create genetic damage directly and nongenotoxic mechanisms (inflammation, immunosuppression, ROS, receptor activation, epigenetic silencing) alter signal transduction and the reduce the potential for repair of damage.

A substantial percentage of cancers of the upper respiratory passages, lung, bladder, and peritoneum are attributed to occupational factors; however, the contributing role of smoking is often not easily evaluated in studies of workplace cancer. Millions of US workers, and even more of those in rapidly developing regions that lack regulatory controls, are regularly exposed to substances tested as carcinogens in animal studies. It has been estimated that 4% of all cancer deaths and 12.5% of all lung cancer deaths are caused by workplace exposures to carcinogens.[116] Some groups of workers are especially vulnerable and face much higher risks, such as those working with aromatic hydrocarbons, butadiene, and some pesticides. For close to a century, it has been known that textile industry workers can be continuously exposed to different kinds of carcinogenic chemicals (dyes, solvents, fiber dusts, others) and face greater cancer risks as a result.[117]

One notable occupational cause of cancer is asbestos, a heat-resistant, fibrous silicate mineral found in cementitious products, plaster, flooring, house siding, or woven into fabrics and fire-resistant and insulating materials, such as brake linings and vehicle components such as clutches. Asbestos increases the risk of mesothelioma and lung cancer (see Chapter 35), and is implicated in ovarian and other cancers as well (see Chapter 35). Noncancerous disorders related to asbestos exposures include pleural plaques, diffuse pleural thickening, and pulmonary fibrosis. These asbestos-related disorders (ARDs) represent a significant occupational and public health concern. In Western Europe, because of the long latency of disease onset, the epidemic of mesothelioma in building workers born after 1940 did not become apparent until the 1990s. Building materials containing asbestos have been banned in most developed countries, but such materials are still used in many developing countries, where the incidence of cases of ARDs is rising. No exposure to asbestos is without risk.

For nearly a century, carcinoma of the bladder has been linked with the manufacture of dyes, rubber, paint, and aromatic amines, especially β-naphthylamine and benzidine. Benzene inhalation is linked to leukemia in shoemakers and in workers employed in the rubber cement, explosives, and dye-manufacture industries. Other notable occupational hazards include heavy metals (high-nickel alloy, chromium VI compounds, inorganic arsenic), silica, PAHs, sulfuric acid, and chloromethyl ether. Disentangling data related to lung cancer, air pollution, and occupational risks is challenging, especially in combination with risk factors, such as active and passive smoking, other environmental factors, and genetic polymorphisms at multiple loci.

TABLE 13.6 Overview of Occupational Safety and Health Administration-Relevant Carcinogenic Factors

Group	Example
Chemicals	
Gases	Vinyl chloride Formaldehyde
Liquids, volatile	Trichloroethylene Tetrachloroethylene Methylchloride Styrene Benzene Xylene
Liquids, nonvolatile	Metalworking fluids Mineral oils Hair dyes
Solids, dust	Silica Wood dust Talc containing asbestiform fibers
Solids, fibers	Asbestos Man-made mineral fibers, for example, ceramic fibers
Solids	Lead Nickel compounds Chromium VI compounds Arsenic Beryllium Cadmium Carbon black Bitumen
Fumes, smoke	Welding fumes Diesel emissions Coal tar fumes Bitumen fumes Fire, combustion emissions PAHs Tobacco smoke
Mixtures	Solvents
Pesticides	
Halogenated organic compounds	DDT Ethylene dibromide
Others	Amitrole
Pharmaceuticals	
Antineoplastic drugs	MOPP (Mustargen, oncovin, procarbazine, and prednisone, a combination chemotherapy regimen used to treat Hodgkin disease) and other combined chemotherapies, including alkylating agents
Anesthetics	There is evidence from in vitro experiments that isoflurane increases cancer cells' potential to grow and migrate
Emerging Factors	
Air pollution and fine particulate matter	Emissions from motor vehicles, industrial processes, power generation, and other sources polluting the ambient air
Endocrine-disrupting compounds	Certain pesticides Certain flame retardants
Biologic Factors	
Bacteria	*Helicobacter pylori*
Viruses	Hepatitis B Hepatitis C
Mycotoxin-producing fungi	Bulk handling of agricultural foodstuffs (nuts, grain, maize, coffee), animal-feed production, brewing/malting, waste management, composting, food production, working with indoor molds, horticulture
Aspergillus flavus, A. parasiticus	Aflatoxin (A1)
Penicillium griseofulvum	Griseofulvin (IARC group 2B)
A. ochraceus, A. carbonarius, P. verrucosum	Ochratoxin A (group 2B)
A. versicolor, Emericella nidulans, Chaetomium spp., A. flavus, A. parasiticus	Sterigmatocystin (group 2B)
Fusarium spp.	Fumonisin B1 (group 2B)
Physical Factors	
Ionizing radiation	Radon X-rays
Ultraviolet radiation (UVR)	Solar radiation Artificial UVR
Ergonomics	Sedentary work
Other	
Work organization	Shift work that involves circadian disruptionStatic workProlonged sitting and standing
Lifestyle factors	Stress-related obesity, smoking, drinking, drug consumption
Combinations of Various Factors	
Chemicals and radiation	Methoxsalen and UVA radiation Some chemicals, called *promoters*, can increase the cancer-causing ability of UVR. Conversely, UVR can act as a promoter and increase the cancer-causing ability of some chemicals, particularly coal tar and pitch.
Work organization and chemicals	Shift work and solvents

DDT, Dichlorodiphenyltrichloroethane; *IARC*, International Agency for Research on Cancer; *PSHs*, polycyclic aromatic hydrocarbons; *UVA*, ultraviolet A.
Data from European Agency for Safety and Health at Work. *Exposure to Carcinogens and Work-related Cancer: A Review of Assessment Methods European Risk Observatory Report*. Luxembourg: European Agency for Safety and Health at Work Eu-OSHA. http://europa.eu.OSHA, Occupational Safety and Health Administration.

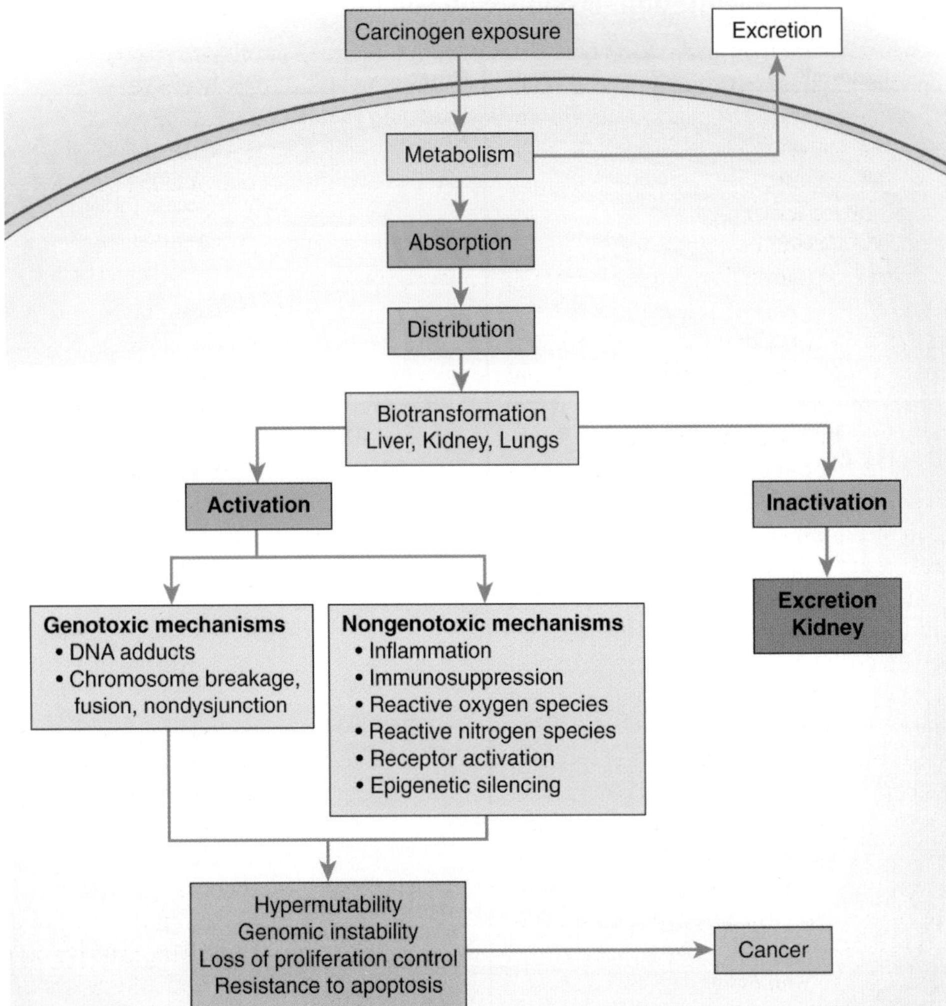

Fig. 13.19 Mechanisms of Chemical Carcinogenesis. Cellular internalization of chemical carcinogens results in metabolic products that are either excreted or retained by the cell. Within the cell, carcinogens or their metabolic products can directly or indirectly affect the regulation and expression of genes involved in cell cycle control, DNA repair, cell differentiation, or apoptosis. Some chemical carcinogens act by *genotoxic* mechanisms, such as DNA adducts, chromosomal breakage, fusion, deletion, missegregation, and nondisjunction. Other carcinogens act by *nongenotoxic* mechanisms, such as induction of inflammation, immunosuppression, formation of reactive oxygen species (oxidative stress), activation of receptors, and epigenetic mechanisms, such as silencing. Both genotoxic and nongenotoxic mechanisms can alter signal transduction pathways that result in many features of cancer cells (Adapted from Luch A. Nature and nurture–Lessons from chemical carcinogenesis. *Nature Reviews: Cancer*, 2005;5(2):113–125.)

SUMMARY REVIEW

Genetics, Epigenetics, and Tissue

1. Cancer arises from a complicated and interacting web of multiple etiologies, with fewer than 10% of all cases stemming from inherited germline factors. All cancer develops when the healthy genes with which we are born lose their ability to enhance DNA repair, direct proteins to induce cell death at appropriate times, or promote beneficial cell signaling. Avoiding high-risk behaviors and exposure to carcinogens can prevent many types of cancers.
2. Risk factors for cancer include lifestyle behaviors (smoking, alcohol intake, diet), lack of physical exercise and obesity, certain infections, environmental factors (exposure to sunlight, ionizing or non-ionizing radiation as well as drinking water contaminants), occupational exposure to carcinogens,

and certain medications or common contaminants in pharmaceuticals that can turn on malignant processes through chromosome rearrangements or other processes.
3. Cancers are caused by interactions between environmental-lifestyle factors and inherited or acquired genetic/epigenetic factors. Contributing factors include weaker immune systems, variations in detoxifying enzymes or DNA repair genes, differences in hormone levels, and metabolic factors such as disordered glucose and lipid metabolism.
4. Cancer-causing factors are influenced by the surrounding microenvironment or stroma. Once malignant phenotypes have developed, complex interactions occur between the tumor, the surrounding stroma, and cells of the immune and inflammatory systems.
5. Globally, cancer is reported to remain a major cause of morbidity and mortality in the coming decades in both developed and developing regions.
6. For the first time, female breast cancer has surpassed lung cancer as the most commonly diagnosed cancer in the world, primarily because of increases in low- and middle-income countries. Lung cancer is the most commonly diagnosed cancer in men, and for both sexes it is the leading cause of cancer death in the world. Prostate cancer is the second most common cancer in men. Other common cancers worldwide arise from the gastrointestinal tract including colorectum, stomach, and liver cancers. Despite these increases in incidence, overall US cancer death rates have decreased 31% since 1991, especially due to a decline in lung cancer deaths. The rate of decline in cancer-rated mortality has slowed for prostate, breast, and colorectal cancer since 2018.
7. Increased Generational Risk (GR) is evident in trends in cancer not related to smoking or diagnostic ascertainment, with persons born after 1940 experiencing up to twice as much cancer as those born earlier. Explanations for increases in specific subtypes of non-smoking related cancer need to be sought.
8. Race, ethnicity, and social class are major determinants of the risk of developing and dying of cancer around the world, reflecting largely socioeconomic factors that affect access to care, good nutrition, workplace, and environmental exposures.

In Utero and Early Life Conditions

1. Emerging data suggest prenatal and early life events influence later susceptibility to cancer and other chronic diseases.
2. Developmental plasticity is the degree to which an organism's development is contingent on its environment. Plasticity refers to the ability of genes to organize physiologically or structurally in response to environmental conditions during fetal development.
3. The developmental origins hypothesis suggests that nutrition and other environmental factors affect cellular pathways during gestation, enabling a single genotype to affect a broad range of adult phenotypes. Maternal nutrition, as well as environment factors, are proposed as significant biological influences.
4. Undernutrition in utero is linked to increased heart disease, metabolic disorders, and possibly breast cancer decades later. Deficiencies that occur in the first trimester are far more influential than those that take place in the last trimester in affecting disease outcome in adulthood.

Environmental-Lifestyle Factors

Tobacco Use

1. Cigarette smoking is carcinogenic and the most important known avoidable cause of cancer that is controlled by individual behaviors. Tobacco smoking causes cancer in more than 15 organ sites, and exposure to secondhand smoke and parental smoking causes cancer in children and in other nonsmokers. The risk is greatest in those who begin to smoke when young and continue throughout life. Smoking is, however, a pandemic affecting all ages.
2. Worldwide, tobacco use causes more than 7 million deaths per year.
3. Environmental tobacco smoke (i.e., secondhand smoke) is a cause of stroke; increases the risk of death in people with cancer and cancer survivors as well as those with macular degeneration, tuberculosis, ectopic pregnancy, and diabetes mellitus. Secondhand smoke exposure increases inflammation, impairs immunity, and is a cause of rheumatoid arthritis.
4. Smoking tobacco is linked to cancers of the lung, upper aerodigestive tract, stomach, lower urinary tract, kidney, pancreas, cervix, uterus, and myeloid leukemia. Recently added to the list of smoking-related cancers are liver and colorectal cancer. Smoking causes even more deaths from respiratory, vascular, and other diseases than from cancer.
5. Cigar or pipe smoking is related to cancers of the oral cavity, oropharynx, hypopharynx, larynx, esophagus, and lung. Pipe smokers have an increased risk of cancers of lung, lip, throat, esophagus, larynx, pancreas, and colon and rectum.
6. Electronic cigarettes can contain harmful, highly-addictive, and potentially cancer-causing substances and have been extensively marketed to young teens and are targeted by public health authorities as potential gateways to tobacco smoking.

Diet

1. The influence of diet on cancer development is complicated. Cancer risks in older adults may depend as much or more on diet in early life as on current eating practices.
2. Nutrigenomics is the study of the effects of nutrition on the phenotypic variability of individuals based on genomic differences.
3. Nutrition, obesity, alcohol consumption, and physical activity all influence risks for cancer development and can interact synergistically.
4. As a tool for preventive medicine aimed at reducing disease, dietary recommendations, such as the Mediterranean diet, are becoming more widespread.

5. The importance of diet has been illustrated by data showing changes in cancer risk among migrants that move from countries with low-cancer risk to those with high-cancer risk countries. With geographic migration, particularly with the adoption of the Western diet, cancer risks approximate those of the new region within a generation.
6. Bioactive components have a profound effect on differentiation, potentially including differentiation of cancer stem cells. Intake of a broad range of specific food compounds may suppress cancer stem renewal.
7. A variety of food compounds may serve as antioxidants and influence cell signaling and DNA repair.
8. Xenobiotics can be toxic, mutagenic, and carcinogenic chemicals that humans are constantly exposed to. The body has several immunological systems for counteracting these effects, including enhanced production of Natural Killer cells and other anticarcinogens. Many foods enhance the efficiency and degree of detoxification of xenobiotics and thus serve a protective role in metabolizing carcinogens.
9. Diets high in red meat or processed meat may lead to increased risks of colorectal cancer. Meats containing nitrites, nitrates, or other preservatives can leave residues in the colon that cause DNA damage.
10. Obesity is an epidemic in both developed and developing countries. Obesity is a form of poor nutrition or overnutrition, that impacts energy balance, cancer risk, cancer recurrence, and survival.
11. Obesity is a risk factor for 13 cancers: liver, advanced prostate, ovarian, gallbladder, kidney, colorectal, esophageal, breast (postmenopausal), pancreatic, endometrial, meningioma, multiple myeloma, and stomach.
12. Understanding the mechanisms of obesity-associated cancer risks is evolving and varies by type of tumor and distribution of body fat. Emerging data point to three main factors: (1) insulin-insulin-like growth factor (IGF-1) axis, (2) sex hormones, and (3) adipokines.
13. Metabolic changes in adipose tissue from obesity result in several alterations and include insulin resistance, hyperglycemia, dyslipidemia, hypoxia, and chronic inflammation. Tumor growth is regulated by interactions between tumor cells and their tissue microenvironment, so stromal compartments that are rich in adipose tissue can promote the development of tumor cells.
14. Alcohol is classified as a human carcinogen. Strong data link alcohol with cancers of the mouth, pharynx, larynx, esophagus, liver, colorectum, and breast.
15. Evidence does not show any safe limit of alcohol and the health effects are from ethanol regardless of the type of drink.
16. Alcohol-related carcinogenesis involves acetaldehyde, reactive oxygen species (ROS), pro-carcinogen activation, cellular regeneration, nutritional deficiencies, and enzyme and metabolic dysfunction.
17. Physical activity, independent of weight changes, reduces the risk for breast cancer, colon cancer (in men), and endometrial cancer.
18. Biologic mechanisms for the protective effects of physical activity include decreasing insulin and IGF levels, decreasing obesity, increasing free radical scavenger systems, altering inflammatory mediators, decreasing levels of circulating unbound sex hormones and metabolic hormones, improving immune function, decreasing oncogenes, enhancing cytochrome P-450 activity (thus modifying carcinogen activation), increasing gut motility, and increasing release of myokines (proteins from contracting muscles with antitumor effects).
19. Many unanswered questions remain regarding frequency of exercise, intensity, and duration.
20. Recent data encourage 150 minutes of moderate-intensity aerobic or 75 minutes of vigorous-intensity aerobic physical activity each week for adults. Children and adolescents should get at least 60 minutes of physical activity daily.

Air Pollution

1. Air pollution, indoor and outdoor, is the leading environmental cause of death worldwide. Long-term exposure to air pollution increases mortality and morbidity and shortens life expectancy from cardiovascular, respiratory disease, and lung cancer.
2. There is a significant association between increased rates of lung cancer and exposure to particulate matter, a mixture of small particles and liquid droplets. Primary particles are emitted directly from a source, for example, construction sites, unpaved roads, fields, or smokestacks. Secondary particles are emitted from power plants, industries, and automobiles.
3. Diesel exhaust is carcinogenic and causes lung cancer. Acute exposure to diesel exhaust that contains particles is linked to lung, throat, and eye irritations; asthma attacks; and myocardial ischemia.
4. The mechanisms of adverse effects of particulate matter include (1) oxidative stress, (2) ROS generation, (3) DNA oxidative damage, (4) mutagenicity, (5) stimulation of proinflammatory factors, and (6) induction of senescence.
5. Fine particle pollution also is linked to (1) premature death in people with heart or lung disease, (2) nonfatal heart attacks, (3) irregular heartbeat, (4) aggravated asthma, (5) decreased lung function, and (6) respiratory symptoms.
6. Indoor air pollution is generally considered worse than outdoor pollution. Sources of indoor air pollution include tobacco smoke, heating and cooking combustion sources, radon, and coal use.

Ionizing Radiation

1. Much of the knowledge of the effects of ionizing radiation on human cancer has come from Hiroshima and Nagasaki atomic bomb exposures, particularly the Life Span Study. Other evidence is from exposure to radiation for medical reasons, underground miners, and other occupational exposures. Human exposure includes emissions from the environment, x-rays, CT scans, radioisotopes, and other radioactive sources.
2. Atomic bomb exposures in Japan caused acute leukemias and increased frequencies of thyroid, breast, lung, stomach,

colon, esophageal, and brain, urinary tract cancers and multiple myeloma.
3. Excess relative risks (ERRs) for radiation-induced cancers at a given age are much higher for individuals exposed during childhood or over age 40.
4. The bimodal age distribution of radiation-induced cancer risk means that radiation exposure in early ages is related to initiation of cancer processes, whereas exposure in later ages is associated with promotion of pre-existing premalignant cells.
5. Other health risks from radiation include cardiovascular and neurodegenerative effects and somatic mutations that may contribute to other diseases. These effects may manifest years after radiation exposure.
6. There is concern about the increased IR exposure from medical procedures, particularly CT scans.
7. IR is a potent mutagen and carcinogen; it can penetrate cells and tissues and deposit energy in tissues at random in the form of ionizations.
8. IR affects DNA by causing cross-linking, nucleotide base damage, and single- and double-strand DNA breaks. Disrupted cellular regulation processes can lead to carcinogenesis. The double-strand break is considered the hallmark lesion associated with IR.
9. It is now known that radiation may induce genomic instability to the progeny of the directly irradiated cells over many generations of cell divisions and can affect so-called bystander cells. Investigators are studying genomic instability as it may contribute to secondary cancers.
10. The risks from low-dose radiation are difficult to calculate because they require monitoring of large populations, and this is not regularly done.

Ultraviolet Radiation

1. Ultraviolet (UV) radiation comes from sunlight, electric lights, black lights, and tanning lamps. Most of the UV radiation received on earth is UVA and some UVB. UVA radiation is weaker than UVB, but UVA penetrates more deeply into the skin and is more constant throughout the year despite the weather.
2. The incidence of basal cell carcinoma (BCC) and squamous cell carcinoma (SCC) is strongly correlated with lifetime sunlight exposure. Intense intermittent recreational sun exposure has been associated with melanoma and BCC. Chronic occupational sun exposure has been associated with SCC. Tanning bed use has been associated with an increased risk of BCC, especially in women.
3. Skin cancer risk factors include cumulative sun exposure (the additive effects of intermittent sun exposure, chronic sun exposure, or both), ionizing radiation, chronic arsenic ingestion and other chemical exposures, immunosuppression, and genetic factors.
4. The pathogenesis of nonmelanoma skin cancers involves specific gene mutations, epigenetic alterations, oxidative stress, inflammation, and reduced immune surveillance.

Electromagnetic Radiation

1. EMR occurs in the form of magnetic and electric fields, and varies with power, frequency, polarity, information content, wave form, and other variables. Exposures are widespread and growing exponentially in recent years, especially for toddlers and young children who must rely on wireless devices for education during the pandemic. Wireless telecommunication devices (e.g., cell phones, wireless laptops, smart meters) are the most common sources of radiofrequency electromagnetic radiation (RF-EMR).
2. Competing priorities (convenience, financial interest, and health necessity) may make a consensus on the risk/benefit ratio of EMR difficult to achieve.
3. Low-frequency electromagnetic fields (EMFs) and higher-frequency EMFs (from cellphones and other wireless transmitting devices) have been classified as possible carcinogens by several expert groups, including the EPA, and the IARC of the WHO in 2011. More recently, experimental and epidemiological evidence amassed in the past decade reveal that EMF/RF constitutes a known cause of cancer in humans.
4. Importantly, exposures from numerous wireless transmitting devices have expanded dramatically, especially for children.
5. Children are a main concern since the effects of exposure may be compounded because of their increased vulnerability to both IR and NIR/EMF radiation, their immature immune systems, thinner skulls, and immature nervous systems and their longer use of cell phones and other wireless transmitting devices throughout their lifetimes.
6. Exposures from the proposed 5 G system are poorly understood but involve beam-forming from closely placed antennas that will also send and receive 3 G and 4 G frequencies to connect billions of existing devices; the millions of new antennas that are needed for this system have not been adequately evaluated for impacts on public health or the environment according to the US Government Accountability Office, 2020, and the European Union, 2020.

Infection, Sexual and Reproductive Behavior

1. Infection with certain viruses, bacteria, and parasites are an important contributor to cancer worldwide. The most notable infections implicated in new cancer cases include Epstein-Barr virus (EBV), *Helicobacter pylori*, hepatitis B and C viruses (HBV and HCV), and human papillomavirus (HPV).
2. *H. pylori* is the cause of about 75% of stomach cancers. EBV is linked to nasopharyngeal carcinoma, Hodgkin lymphoma, diffuse large B-cell lymphoma, Burkitt lymphoma, EBV-associated malignant B-cell lymphoma, other lymphomas, and gastric adenocarcinoma. HBV and HCV infect the liver and together account for the large majority of liver cancer cases.
3. HPV is the most common sexually transmitted virus in the United States and accounts for more than half of the total infection-attributable cancers in women worldwide. HPV types 16 and 18 are responsible for the majority of cancers. Persistence of infection with high-risk HPV is a prerequisite for the development of cervical intraepithelial neoplasia, lesions, and invasive cancer.
4. HPV infection has been identified as a definite carcinogen for several types of cancer: cervical, penis, vulvar, vaginal,

anal, and some oropharyngeal (including the base of the tongue, tonsils, and pharynx).
5. The incidence of HPV-associated oropharyngeal cancer has increased during the past 20 years, especially among men.
6. Biologic factors that may interact with HPV infection to increase cancer risk include smoking, decreased immunity, having many children, long-term oral contraceptive use, poor oral hygiene and nutrition, and chronic inflammation.
7. HPV may be transmitted by genital contact (oral, touching, or sexual intercourse). The possible modes of transmission in children are controversial; however, it is thought that newborn babies can be exposed to cervical HPV infection from the mother.
8. Although the HPV vaccine reduces the risk for cervical cancer, women should still get Pap tests and HPV screening at regular intervals.

Other Viruses and Microorganisms

1. Human herpes virus type 8 and HIV-AIDs are linked to Kaposi sarcoma, and human T-cell lymphotropic virus type 1 is linked to leukemia and lymphoma.
2. Microorganisms involved in carcinogenesis include parasites such as *Opisthorchis viverrini* (bile duct cancer) and *Schistosoma haematobium* (bladder cancer).

Chemicals and Occupational Hazards as Carcinogens

1. Synthetic chemicals are widely used in the United States, of which only a fraction have been tested for their health.
2. Exposure to chemicals occurs from air, soil, food, water, personal care products, toys, household products, medications, workplaces, and homes
3. A large number of chemicals are known carcinogens in experimental animals, and it is suspected that most of these are potentially carcinogenic in humans. When adequately tested, all agents known to cause cancer in humans also produce it in experimental animals when adequately evaluated.
4. Chemical carcinogenesis involves genotoxic mechanisms (create genetic damage) and nongenotoxic mechanisms (alter signal transduction).
5. A substantial percentage of cancers of the upper respiratory passages, lung, bladder, and peritoneum are attributed to occupational factors. Notable occupational hazards include dyes, rubber, paint, aromatic amines, benzol, heavy metals, silica, polycyclic aromatic hydrocarbons, sulfuric acid, and chloromethyl ether. Asbestos is linked to an epidemic of mesothelioma and asbestos usage has been banned in most developed countries.

REFERENCES

1. Clapp RW, et al. Environmental and occupational causes of cancer: a call to act on what we know. *Biomed Pharmacother.* 2007;61(10):631–639.
2. Clapp RW, et al. Environmental and occupational causes of cancer; new evidence 2005-2007. *Rev Environ Health.* 2008;23(1):1–37.
3. World Health Organization (WHO) *World cancer report 2014.* Geneva, Switzerland: Agency for Research on Cancer, World Health Organization; 2014.
4. PDQ® Cancer Genetics Editorial Board *PDQ cancer genetics overview.* Bethesda, MD: National Cancer Institute; 2021. Updated July 6, 2021. Available at https://www.cancer.gov/about-cancer/causes-prevention/genetics/overview-pdq. (Accessed January 2, 2022).
5. Cogliano VJ, et al. Preventable exposures associated with human cancers. *J Natl Cancer Inst.* 2011;103(24):1827–1839.
6. Institute of Medicine (IOM): *Rebuilding the unity of health and the environment: a new vision of environmental health for the 21st century. Workshop summary.* Washington, DC: National Academy Press; 2001.
7. National Toxicology Program. 15th Report on carcinogens. Washington, D.C: US Department of Health and Human Services; 2021 (Accessed January 10, 2022).
8. Union for International Cancer Control (UICC). *World Health Organization (WHO), International Agency for Research on Cancer (IARC): GLOBOCAN 2020.* Geneva, Switzerland: New Global Cancer Data; 2020. Updated February 15, 2021. Available at https://www.uicc.org/news/globocan-2020-new-global-cancer-data. (Accessed January 2, 2022).
9. Siegel RL, et al. Cancer statistics 2021. *CA Cancer J Clin.* 2021;70(1):7–33.
10. Han YY, et al. Generational risks for cancers not related to tobacco, screening, or treatment in the United States. *Cancer.* 2010;116(4):940–948.
11. Davis DL, Dinse GE, Hoel DG. Decreasing cardiovascular disease and increasing cancer among whites in the United States from 1973 through 1987. Good news and bad news. *JAMA.* 1994;271(6):431–437.
12. Davis DL, et al. Increased generational risk of colon and rectal cancer in recent birth cohorts under age 40—the hypothetical role of radiofrequency radiation from cell phones. *Ann Gastroenterol Dig Disord.* 2020;3(1):9–16.
13. Zimmer K. There's a troubling rise in colorectal cancer among young adults. *The Scientist.* August 26, 2019. Available at https://www.the-scientist.com/news-opinion/theres-a-troubling-rise-in-colorectal-cancer-among-young-adults--66354. (Accessed January 2, 2022).
14. American Cancer Society (ACS). *Cancer facts & figures for African Americans 2019–2021.* Atlanta, GA: ACS; Available at https://www.cancer.org/research/cancer-facts-statistics/cancer-facts-figures-for-african-americans.html (Accessed January 1, 2022).
15. DeSantis CE, et al. Cancer statistics for African Americans. *CA Cancer J Clin.* 2019;69(3):211–233.
16. Davis DL, Pilarcik AM, Miller AB. Increased generational risk of colon and rectal cancer in recent birth cohorts under age 40—the hypothetical role of radiofrequency radiation from cell phones. *Ann Gastroenterol Dig Disord.* 2020;3(1):9–16.
17. Furman D, Campisi J, Verdin E, et al. Chronic inflammation in the etiology of disease across the life span. *Nat Med.* 2019;25:1822–1832.
18. International Agency for Research on Cancer (IARC). *Special report: policy—a review of human carcinogens—part C: metals, arsenic, dusts, and fibres.* Lyon, France: IARC; 2012. Available at http://monographs.iarc.fr/ENG/Monographs/vol100C/index.php. (Accessed January 2, 2022).
19. Straif K, et al. A review of human carcinogens—part C: metals, arsenic, dusts, and fibres. *Lancet Oncol.* 2009;10(5):453–454.

20. Steding-Jessen M, et al. Regional and socioeconomic variation in survival of melanoma patients in Denmark. *Dan Med J.* 2019;66(11):A5572.
21. Davis D, et al. Medical hypothesis: xenoestrogens as preventable causes of breast cancer. *Environ Health Perspect.* 1993;101(5):372–377.
22. Paolini M, Sapone A, Valgimigli L. Avoidance of bioflavonoid supplements during pregnancy: a pathway to infant leukemia? *Mutat Res.* 2003;527:99–101.
23. Hachul ACL, et al. Effect of the consumption of green tea extract during pregnancy and lactation on metabolism of mothers and 28d-old offspring. *Sci Rep.* 2018;8:1869.
24. Forgie AJ, et al. The impact of maternal and early life malnutrition on health: a diet-microbe perspective. *BMC Med.* 2020;18:135.
25. Pullar J, et al. The impact of maternal nutrition on offspring's risk of non-communicable diseases in adulthood: a systematic review. *J Glob Health.* 2019;9(2):020405.
26. National Institutes of Health (NIH) *New releases, Study of first-graders shows fetal alcohol spectrum disorders prevalent in US communities.* Bethesda, MD: NIH; 2018. Available at https://www.nih.gov/news-events/news-releases/study-first-graders-shows-fetal-alcohol-spectrum-disorders-prevalent-us-communities. (Accessed January 2, 2022).
27. Davis DL. *The secret history of the war on cancer.* New York, NY: Basic Books; 2007.
28. Herbst AL, Ulfelder H, Poskanzer DC. Adenocarcinoma of the vagina. Association of maternal stilbestrol therapy with tumor appearance in young women. *N Engl J Med.* 1971;284(15):878–881.
29. Hom M, et al. Systematic review and meta-analysis of testicular germ cell tumors following in utero exposure to diethylstilbestrol. *JNCI Cancer Spectr.* 2019;3(3):pkz045.
30. Heck JE, et al. Smoking in pregnancy and risk of cancer among young children: A population based study. *Int J Cancer.* 2016;139(3):613–616.
31. Rauschert S, et al. Maternal smoking during pregnancy induces persistent epigenetic changes into adolescence, independent of postnatal smoke exposure and is associated with cardiometabolic risk. *Front Genet.* 2019;10:770.
32. Anderson D, Schmid TE, Baumgartner A. Male-mediated developmental toxicity. *Asian J Androl.* 2014;16(1):81–88.
33. Egusquiza RJ, Blumberg B. Environmental obesogens and their impact on susceptibility to obesity: new mechanisms and chemicals. *Endocrinology.* 2020;161(3):bqaa024.
34. World Health Organization (WHO): *Tobacco: key facts.* Geneva, Switzerland: WHO; 2021. Available at https://www.who.int/news-room/fact-sheets/detail/tobacco. (Accessed January 2, 2022).
35. Centers for Disease Control and Prevention (CDC): *Smoking and tobacco use: fast facts and fact sheets*, Atlanta, GA, Office on Smoking and Health, National Center for Chronic Disease Prevention and Health Promotion, CDC. Available at https://www.cdc.gov/tobacco/data_statistics/fact_sheets/index.htm. (Accessed January 2, 2022).
36. US Department of Health and Human Services *The health consequences of smoking—50 years of progress. A report of the Surgeon General. Executive summary.* Atlanta, GA: US Department of Health and Human Services, Centers for Disease Control and Prevention, National Center for Chronic Disease Prevention and Health Promotion, Office on Smoking and Health; 2014. Available at https://www.hhs.gov/sites/default/files/consequences-smoking-exec-summary.pdf. (Accessed January 2, 2022).
37. Singhavi H, Ahluwalia JS, Stepanov I, Gupta PC, Gota V, Chaturvedi P, Khariwala SS. Tobacco carcinogen research to aid understanding of cancer risk and influence policy. *Laryngoscope investigative otolaryngology.* 2018;3(5):372–376.
38. Lushniak BD. A historic moment: the 50th anniversary of the first Surgeon General's Report on smoking and health. *Public Health Rep.* 2014;129(1):5–6.
39. Wang TW, et al. E-cigarette use among middle and high school students—United States, 2020. *MMWR Morb Mortal Wkly Rep.* 2020;69:1310–1312.
40. Hage R, Fretz V, Schuurmans MM. Electronic cigarettes and vaping associated pulmonary illness (VAPI): a narrative review. *Pulmonology.* 2020;26(5):291–3030.
41. Ma Y, Li MD. Establishment of a strong link between smoking and cancer pathogenesis through DNA methylation analysis. *Sci Rep.* 2017;7(1):1811.
42. Caramori G, et al. Molecular links between COPD and lung cancer: new targets for drug discovery? *Expert Opin Ther Targets.* 2019;23(6):539–553.
43. Serra-Majem L, et al. Benefits of the Mediterranean diet: epidemiological and molecular aspects. *Mol Aspects Med.* 2019;67:1–55.
44. Nitter M, et al. Plasma methionine, choline, betaine, and dimethylglycine, in relation to colorectal cancer risk in the European Prospective Investigation into Cancer and Nutrition (EPIC). *Ann Oncol.* 2014;25(8):1609–1615.
45. Kim YS, et al. Cancer stem cells: potential target for bioactive food components. *J Nutr Biochem.* 2012;23:691–698.
46. Strekalova E, et al. S-adenosylmethionine biosynthesis is a targetable metabolic vulnerability of cancer stem cells. *Breast Cancer Res Treat.* 2019;175(1):39–50.
47. Mustra Rakic J, Wang XD. Role of lycopene in smoke-promoted chronic obstructive pulmonary disease and lung carcinogenesis. *Arch Biochem Biophys.* 2020;689:108439.
48. Aykan NF. Red meat and colorectal cancer. *Oncol Rev.* 2015;9(1):288.
49. Smith CJ, Perfetti TA. Exposure to chemicals formed from natural processes is ubiquitous. *Toxicol Res Appl.* 2020;4:1–15.
50. Hales CM, et al. *Prevalence of obesity and severe obesity among adults: United States, 2017–2018. NCHS data brief, no 360.* Hyattsville, MD: National Center for Health; 2020. Available at https://www.cdc.gov/nchs/products/databriefs/db360.htm. (Accessed January 2, 2022).
51. Centers for Disease Control and Prevention (CDC). *Division of Nutrition, Physical Activity, and Obesity, National Center for Chronic Disease Prevention and Health Promotion: Childhood obesity facts.* Atlanta, GA: CDC; 2021. Available at https://www.cdc.gov/obesity/data/childhood.html. (Accessed January 2, 2022).
52. World Health Organization (WHO). *Obesity and overweight.* Geneva, Switzerland: WHO; 2021. Available at https://www.who.int/news-room/fact-sheets/detail/obesity-and-overweight. (Accessed January 2, 2022).
53. Barone I, et al. The weight of obesity in breast cancer progression and metastasis: clinical and molecular perspectives. *Semin Cancer Biol.* 2020;60:274–284.
54. Gallagher EJ, LeRoith D. Hyperinsulinaemia in cancer. *Nat Rev Cancer.* 2020;20(11):629–644.

55. Mostoufi-Moab S, et al. Endocrine abnormalities in aging survivors of childhood cancer: a report from the Childhood Cancer Survivor Study. *J Clin Oncol.* 2016;34(27):3240–3247.
56. American Cancer Society (ACS). *Alcohol and cancer.* Atlanta, GA: ACS; 2020. Available at https://www.cancer.org/cancer/cancer-causes/diet-physical-activity/alcohol-use-and-cancer.html. (Accessed January 2, 2022).
57. Ratna A, Mandrekar P. Alcohol and cancer: mechanisms and therapies. *Biomolecules.* 2017;7(3):61.
58. Sharma J, Krupenko SA. Folate pathways mediating the effects of ethanol in tumorigenesis. *Chem Biol Interact.* 2020;324: 109091.
59. Pedersen BK. The physiology of optimizing health with a focus on exercise as medicine. *Annu Rev Physiol.* 2019;81:607–627.
60. Lee IM, et al. Annual deaths attributable to physical inactivity: whither the missing 2 million? *Lancet.* 2013;381(9871):992–993.
61. Jochem C, Wallmann-Sperlich B, Leitzmann MF. The influence of sedentary behavior on cancer risk: epidemiologic evidence and potential molecular mechanisms. *Curr Nutr Rep.* 2019;8(3):167–174.
62. US Department of Health and Human Services (USDHHS) *Physical activity guidelines for Americans.* 2nd edition Washington, DC: USDHHS; 2018. Available at https://health.gov/sites/default/files/2019-09/Physical_Activity_Guidelines_2nd_edition.pdf. (Accessed January 2, 2022).
63. Cramp F, Byron-Daniel J. Exercise for the management of cancer-related fatigue in adults. *Cochrane Database Syst Rev.* 2012;11:CD006145.
64. Braam KI, et al. Physical exercise training interventions for children and young adults during and after treatment for childhood cancer. *Cochrane Database Syst Rev.* 2016;3(3):CD008796.
65. Cohen AJ, et al. Estimates and 25-year trends of the global burden of disease attributable to ambient air pollution: an analysis of data from the Global Burden of Diseases Study 2015. *Lancet.* 2017;389(10082):1907–1918.
66. Health Effects Institute *State of global air 2020. Special report.* Boston, MA: Health Effects Institute; 2020. https://www.stateofglobalair.org/. Accessed January 10, 2022.
67. Tong S. Air pollution and disease burden. *Lancet Planet Health.* 2019;3(2):E49–E50.
68. IARC Working Group on the Evaluation of Carcinogenic Risks to Humans: Outdoor air pollution. *IARC Monogr Eval Carcinog Risks Hum.* 2016;109:9–444.
69. Pourvakhshoori N, et al. The association between air pollution and cancers: controversial evidence of a systematic review. *Environ Sci Pollut Res Int.* 2020;27(31):38491–38500.
70. Loomis D, et al. The carcinogenicity of outdoor air pollution. *Lancet Oncol.* 2013;14:1262–1263.
71. Santibanez-Andrade M, et al. Deciphering the code between air pollution and disease: the effect of particulate matter on cancer hallmarks. *Int J Mol Sci.* 2019;21(1):136.
72. Mu L, et al. Indoor air pollution and risk of lung cancer among Chinese female non-smokers. *Cancer Causes Control.* 2013;24(3):439–450.
73. Environmental Protection Agency (EPA). *Health risk of radon.* Washington, DC: EPA; 2018. Available at https://www.epa.gov/radon/health-risk-radon. (Accessed January 10, 2022).
74. Lorenzo-Gonzalez M, et al. Radon exposure: a major cause of lung cancer. *Expert Rev Respir Med.* 2019;13(9): 839–850.
75. Lorenzo-Gonzalez M, et al. Residential radon, genetic polymorphisms in DNA damage and repair-related. *Lung Cancer.* 2019;135:10–15.
76. Hernandez L, et al. Aging and radiation: bad companions. *Aging Cell.* 2015;14(2):153–161.
77. Preston DL, et al. Studies of mortality of atomic bomb survivors. Report 13: solid cancer and noncancer disease mortality: 1950–1997. *Radiat Res.* 2003;160:381–407.
78. Richardson DB, Wing S. Greater sensitivity to ionizing radiation at older age: follow-up of workers at Oak Ridge National Laboratory through 1990. *Int J Epidemiol.* 1999;28:428–436.
79. Sadetzki S, et al. Long-term follow-up for brain tumor development after childhood exposure to ionizing radiation for tinea capitis. *Radiat Res.* 2005;163(4):424–432.
80. Sadetzki S, et al. Risk of thyroid cancer after childhood exposure to ionizing radiation for tinea capitis. *J Clin Endocrinol Metab.* 2006;91(12):4798–4804.
81. Lubin JH, et al. Thyroid cancer following childhood low-dose radiation exposure: a pooled analysis of nine cohorts. *J Clin Endocrinol Metab.* 2017;102(7):2575–2583.
82. Belzile-Dugas E, Eisenberg MJ. Radiation-induced cardiovascular disease: Review of an underrecognized pathology. *J Am Heart Assoc.* 2021;10:e0211686.
83. Centers for Disease Control and Prevention (CDC). *Radiation and pregnancy: a fact sheet for clinicians.* Atlanta, GA: National Center for Environmental Health (NCEH), Emergency Management, Radiation, and Chemical Branch, CDC; 2020. Available at https://www.cdc.gov/nceh/radiation/emergencies/prenatalphysician.htm. (Accessed January 10, 2022).
84. National Council on Radiation Protection and Measurements (NCRP). *Ionizing radiation exposure of the population of the United States. Report No. 160.* Bethesda, MD: NCRP; 2009.
85. Smith-Bindman R, et al. Use of diagnostic imaging studies and associated radiation exposure for patients enrolled in large integrated health care system, 1996-2010. *JAMA.* 2012;307(22):2400–2409.
86. Applegate KE, Cost NG. Image Gently: A campaign to reduce children's and Adolescents' risk for cancer during adulthood. *J Adolesc Health* 2013;52(5):S93-S97.
87. Chang H, et al. Non-homologous DNA end joining and alternative pathways to double-strand break repair. *Nat Rev Mol Cell Biol.* 2017;18:495–506.
88. Ghaleb A, Yallowitz A, Marchenko N. Irradiation induces p53 loss of heterozygosity in breast cancer expressing mutant p53. *Commun Biol.* 2019;2:436.
89. Jones JA, et al. Ionizing radiation as a carcinogen. In: McQueen CA, ed. *Comprehensive toxicology.* ed 3 St Louis: Elsevier; 2018.
90. Li Z, et al. Replication stress and FOXM1 drive radiation induced genomic instability and cell transformation. *PLoS One.* 2020;15(11):e0235998.
91. Bazalytska SV, Persidsky Y, Romanenko AM. Molecular mechanisms of initiation of carcinogenesis in the testis. *Exp Oncol.* 2019;41(3):224–234.
92. Widel M. Radiation induced bystander effect: from in vitro studies to clinical application. *Int J Med Phys Clin Eng Radiat Oncol.* 2016;5(1):1–17. Available at http://doi.org/10.4236/ijmpcero.2016.51001. (Accessed January 10, 2022).
93. Du Y, et al. Radiation-induced bystander effect can be transmitted through exosomes using miRNAs as effector molecules. *Radiat Res.* 2020;194(1):89–100.

94. Mittra I, et al. Cell-free chromatin from dying cancer cells integrate into genomes of bystander healthy cells to induce DNA damage and inflammation. *Cell Death Discov*. 2017;3:17015.
95. Rajagopal C, Harikumar KB. The origins and functions of exosomes in cancer. *Front Oncol*. 2018;8:66.
96. Wu M, et al. Emerging roles and therapeutic value of exosomes in cancer metastasis. *Mol Cancer*. 2019;18(1):53.
97. Dai J, et al. Exosomes: key players in cancer and potential therapeutic strategy. *Signal Transduct Target Ther*. 2020;5 (1):145.
98. Parkin DM, Darby SC. Cancers in 2010 attributable to ionising radiation exposure in the UK. *Br J Cancer*. 2011;105(Suppl 2):S57–S65.
99. Berrington de Gonzalez A, et al. Proportion of second cancers attributable to radiotherapy treatment in adults: a prospective cohort study in the US SEER cancer registries. *Lancet Oncol*. 2011;12(4):353–360.
100. Vienne-Jumeau A, Tafani C, Ricard D. Environmental risk factors of primary brain tumors: a review. *Rev Neurol (Paris)*. 2019;175(10):664–678.
101. Miller AB, et al. Cancer epidemiology update, following the 2011 IARC evaluation of radiofrequency electromagnetic fields (Monograph 102). *Environ Res*. 2018;167:673–683.
102. National Toxicology Program (NTP) *Cell phone radio frequency radiation*. Research Triangle Park, NC: NTP; 2020. Last updated December 10, 2020. Available at https://ntp.niehs.nih.gov/whatwestudy/topics/cellphones/index.html?utm_source=direct&utm_medium=prod&utm_campaign=ntpgolinks&utm_term=cellphone. (Accessed January 10, 2022).
103. Belpomme D, et al. Thermal and non-thermal health effects of low intensity non-ionizing radiation: an international perspective. *Environ Pollut*. 2018;242(Part A):643–658.
104. Ben Ishai PB et al: Proposed FCC changes to measuring and evaluating human exposure to radiofrequency electromagnetic fields and wireless power transfer devices are flawed: need for biologically-based standards (ET Docket No. 19–226; FCC 19–126; FRS 16618). Available at https://ecfsapi.fcc.gov/file/1061621406508/FCC%20Submission%2019-226%20Environmental%20Health%20Trust.pdf. (Accessed January 10, 2022).
105. Gandini S, et al. Epidemiological evidence of carcinogenicity of sunbed use and of efficacy of preventive measures. *J Eur Acad Dermatol Venereol*. 2019;33(Suppl 2):57–62.
106. Fania L, et al. Basal cell carcinoma: from pathophysiology to novel therapeutic approaches. *Biomedicines*. 2020;8(11):449.
107. American Cancer Society (ACS) *Cancer facts & figures 2021*. Atlanta, GA: ACS; 2021. https://www.cancer.org/research/cancer-facts-statistics/all-cancer-facts-figures/cancer-facts-figures-2021.html. Accessed January 10, 2022.
108. Ticha I, et al. A comprehensive evaluation of pathogenic mutations in primary cutaneous melanomas, including the identification of novel loss-of-function variants. *Sci Rep*. 2019;9:17050.
109. Abbas K, Qadir MI, Anwar S. The role of melanin in skin cancer. *Crit Rev Eukaryot Gene Expr*. 2019;29(1):17–24.
110. US Preventive Services Task Force (USPSTF). Screening for skin cancer: US Preventive Services Task Force recommendation statement. *JAMA*. 2016;316(4):429–435.
111. de Martel C, et al. Global burden of cancers attributable to infections in 2008: a review and synthetic analysis. *Lancet Oncol*. 2012;13(6):607–615.
112. Perehudoff K, et al. Universal cervical cancer control through a right to health lens: refocusing national policy and programmes on underserved women. *BMC Int Health Hum Rights*. 2020;20(1):21.
113. Petca A, et al. Non-sexual HPV transmission and role of vaccination for a better future (Review). *Exp Ther Med*. 2020;20(6):186.
114. National Cancer Institute (NCI). *Pap and HPV testing*. Bethesda, MD: NCI; 2019. Available at https://www.cancer.gov/types/cervical/pap-hpv-testing-fact-sheet. (Accessed January 10, 2022).
115. Center for Disease Control and Prevention (CDC). Agency for Toxic Substances and Disease Registry (ATSDR) *Toxic chemicals portal*. Atlanta, GA: CDC, ATSDR; 2021. Available at https://www.atsdr.cdc.gov/substances/index.asp. (Accessed January 10, 2022).
116. Takala J. Eliminating occupational cancer. *Ind Health*. 2015;53(4):307–309. Available at: https://doi.org/10.2486/indhealth.53-307. (Accessed January 10, 2022).
117. Singh Z, Chadha P. Textile industry and occupational cancer. *J Occup Med Toxicol*. 2016;11:39.

14

Cancer in Children and Adolescents

Lauri A. Linder

http://evolve.elsevier.com/Rogers/pathophysiology/

CHAPTER OUTLINE

Although cancer in children and adolescents is rare, it is the leading cause of death resulting from disease in this age group.[1] Five-year survival rates among children and adolescents with cancer have dramatically improved from 59% in the 1960s to nearly 85% today.[2] Factors leading to improved cure rates include combination chemotherapy; multimodal treatment for children with solid tumors; targeted therapies, including immunotherapy; and participation in multisite clinical trials.

INCIDENCE AND TYPES OF CHILDHOOD CANCER

More than 16,500 children and adolescents 19 years of age and younger are anticipated to be diagnosed with cancer in the United States in 2020.[3] The overall incidence of childhood and adolescent cancer is 18.7 per 100,000 (Fig. 14.1).[4] Childhood cancer demonstrates a bimodal distribution, with peaks among children <5 years of age and adolescents 15 to 19 years of age. In the United States, childhood cancer is also slightly more common in boys than in girls. The male/female ratio for childhood cancers is 1.2:1.0.[4] In the United States, cancer is more common in white children relative to other racial groups (Table 14.1); however, incidences can vary across racial/ethnic groups.[3] For example, the overall incidence of acute lymphocytic leukemia (ALL) is 1.6 times greater among white children than black children, yet the overall incidence of leukemia is greatest among Hispanic children.[4]

Although death rates from childhood and adolescent cancers are declining, approximately 1,730 cancer-related deaths among children and adolescents in the United States are anticipated in 2020.[3] Childhood cancer-related deaths are most frequently attributed to brain tumors followed by leukemias; however, survival further varies based on cancer type and age at diagnosis.[3] Between 2013 and 2017, the cancer-related death rates among children and adolescents, from birth to age 19 years, were 2.5 per 100,000 for males and 2.0 per 100,000 for females.[4] By comparison, the cancer-related mortality rate in adults was 183.9 per 100,000 in 2017.[5]

Childhood cancers differ greatly from those in adults in relation to the site and type of the malignancy, as well as the role of environmental exposures. The most common types of cancer among adults include prostate, breast, lung, and colon cancers. Many adult cancers have associated lifestyle factors that could theoretically be avoided, thereby preventing the development of cancer, such as smoking and exposure to the sun.

Among children up to 14 years of age, leukemias and brain tumors account for 61% of childhood cancers; solid tumors, such as neuroblastoma and soft tissue or bone sarcomas, are less common.[3] Lymphomas (including Hodgkin and non-Hodgkin subtypes) are the most common type of cancer among adolescents (15 to 19 years of age). Leukemia, thyroid carcinoma, brain tumors, and germ cell tumors also are among the most common adolescent cancers.[2,3,6] Although very few environmental factors have been linked to pediatric and adolescent malignancies, more data are emerging that the developing child may be affected by both maternal and paternal exposures before conception, exposures in utero, and the contents of breast milk. These exposures may result in epigenetic changes, creating an increased vulnerability to the development of childhood cancer.[7–9]

Most childhood cancers originate from the mesodermal germ layer. This layer develops into connective tissue, bone, cartilage, muscle, blood, blood vessels, gonads, kidney, and the lymphatic system (Fig. 14.2). As a result, the most common childhood cancers include leukemias, sarcomas, and embryonic tumors. In general, childhood cancers are fast-growing, resulting in a relatively short latency period—that is, the time from the initial exposure to the onset of symptoms. Additionally, childhood and adolescent cancers tend to be fast growing, with 80% having distant spread (metastases) at diagnosis.

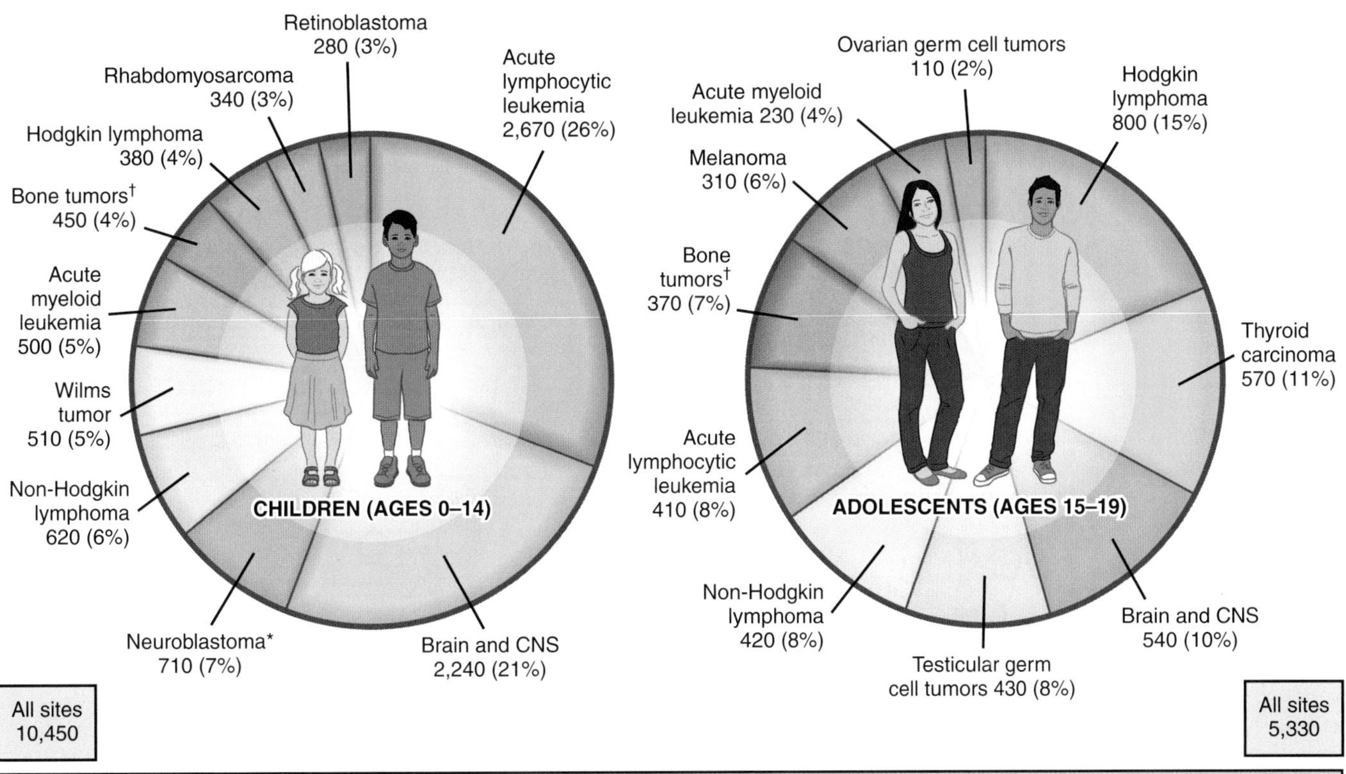

Fig. 14.1 Estimated Cases for Childhood and Adolescent Cancers, United States, 2014. (Data from American Cancer Society, Atlanta, GA, 2014.)

TABLE 14.1 Childhood Age-Adjusted Cancer Incidence Rates for Children Younger Than 19 Years of Age by Primary Site, Race, and Ethnicity, United States[a]

Cancer Site	Non-Hispanic White	Non-Hispanic Black	Asian/Pacific Islander	American Indian/ Alaska Native	Hispanic
All cancer sites combined	18.5	14.6	15.3	9.7	17.1
Brain and other nervous systems	5.9	3.7	3.4		4.5
Leukemia	5.5	3.8	4.3		6.5
Lymphoma	3.1	2.4	2.1		2.7
Other	6.5	4.1	4.3		5.3

[a]Rates are per 100,000 persons and are age-adjusted to the 2000 US standard population (19 age groups—Census P25-1130).
Data from National Cancer Institute. Surveillance Epidemiology and End Results Program. *SEER Cancer Statistics Review 1975-2017*. https://seer.cancer.gov/csr/1975_2017/browse_csr.php?sectionSEL=28&pageSEL=sect_28_zfig.03#table1; https://seer.cancer.gov/csr/1975_2017/browse_csr.php?sectionSEL=28&pageSEL=sect_28_table.02. Accessed December 16, 2021.

Childhood cancers are often diagnosed during peak times of physical growth and maturation and are likely influenced by altered cellular regulatory mechanisms at given times in the child or adolescent's development. These underlying processes associated with growth and development likely account for the bimodal distribution in their incidence, with peak incidences among children age <6 years and then again during adolescence.

The distribution of cancer types also changes during childhood and adolescence. Leukemia is the most common

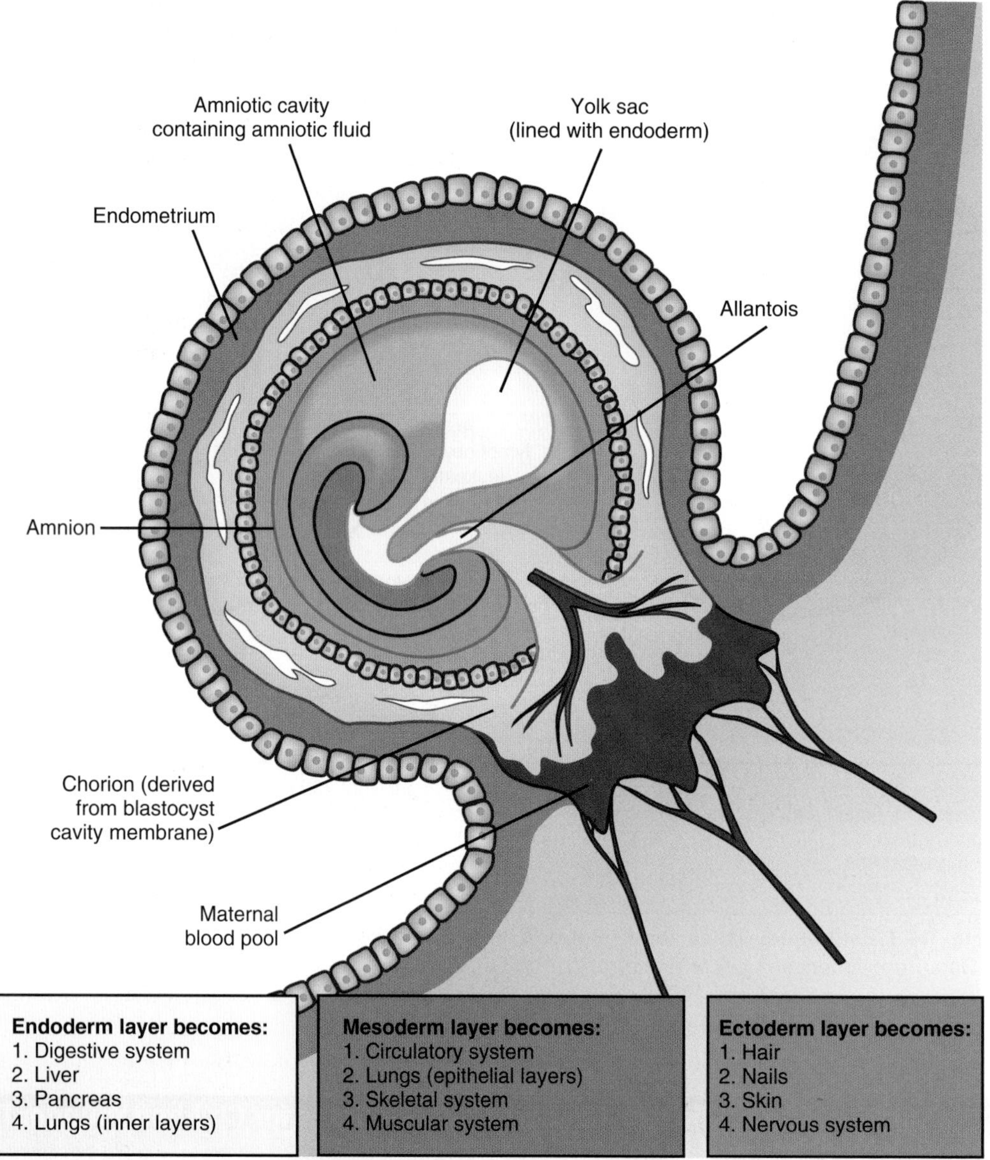

Fig. 14.2 Mesodermal Germ Layer.

malignancy in children, with most cases occurring in children between 2 and 5 years of age. The most common type of leukemia is ALL, which represents approximately 75% of all childhood and nearly half of all adolescent leukemia cases.[3] Although the presenting signs of the various types of leukemia may be similar, the treatment and response to treatment of childhood leukemias vary greatly (see Chapter 30).

Central nervous system (CNS) tumors are the most common types of solid tumors in children and account for 26% of all childhood cancers and 20% of adolescent cancers[3] (see Chapter 20). The peak incidence of these tumors is among children age <15 years; however, the incidence of specific subtypes of brain and CNS tumors varies across childhood and adolescence. Not all brain tumors are diagnosed malignant by histologic studies; however, even a benign tumor can have devastating effects, depending on the anatomic location. The treatment for brain tumors in children often presents difficulties because therapies, such as radiation, may have debilitating effects on the developing brain, particularly in children younger than 3 years of age.

Lymphomas, both Hodgkin and non-Hodgkin types, are the third most common type of childhood cancer. Lymphoma is rare in children age <5 years. It occurs most frequently in children and adolescents 10 years of age and older; however, the incidence of the subtypes differs across the lifespan (see Chapter 13).

Embryonal tumors begin during intrauterine life. These tumors contain abnormal cells that appear to be immature embryonic tissue; they are unable to mature or differentiate into fully developed cells. Embryonal tumors are most often diagnosed early in life, usually before the child is 5 years of age. They are rare in older children, adolescents, and adults. The names of these tumors often include the root term *blast* (e.g., neuroblastoma, retinoblastoma), which indicates the embryonal stage of development of the involved cells.

TABLE 14.2 Childhood Age-Adjusted Invasive Cancer Incidence Rates by Primary Site and Age, United States[a]

Site	Birth to 14 Years	Birth to 19 Years
All sites	16.0	18.1
Leukemia (all types)	5.3	4.8
Acute lymphocytic leukemia	4.1	3.4
Brain and other nervous system	3.2	3.1
Soft tissue	1.1	1.1
Kidney and renal	0.8	0.7
Bones and joints	0.7	0.9
Non-Hodgkin lymphoma	1.0	1.4
Hodgkin lymphoma	0.6	1.1

[a]Rates are per 100,000 persons and are age-adjusted to the 2000 US standard population (19 age groups—Census P25-1130).
Data from National Cancer Institute. Age-adjusted SEER Cancer Incidence Rates, 1975–2017 by primary cancer site and year of diagnosis. https://seer.cancer.gov/csr/1975_2017/browse_csr.php?sectionSEL=28&pageSEL=sect_28_table.02

Rhabdomyosarcoma is the most common soft tissue sarcoma of childhood. This tumor has a bimodal age distribution. Two-thirds of cases occur in children age <6 years, and one-third occur in children and adolescents 10 years of age and older. The two most common types of bone tumors are osteosarcoma and Ewing sarcoma. These cancers are more likely to occur in adolescents age ≥15 years (Table 14.2).

Although sarcomas, leukemias, and lymphomas are cancers observed in childhood, they also occur in adults. Most adult cancers develop from epithelial tissue and are therefore carcinomas. Because carcinomas most often result from environmental exposures to carcinogens, they rarely occur in children. A long period (up to decades) of exposure is required until the development of carcinoma. The incidence of carcinomas increases between ages 15 and 19 years. Carcinoma is the most common cancer tissue type observed after adolescence.[3]

ETIOLOGY

The causes of cancer in children are largely unknown. A few environmental factors can predispose a child to cancer; however, causal factors have not been established for most childhood cancers. A number of host factors, many of which are genetic risk factors or congenital conditions, have been implicated in the development of childhood cancer (Table 14.3). The interaction of many factors most likely produces cancer, a concept referred to as multiple causation or multifactorial etiology. According to this premise, cancer develops because of the predisposing characteristics of the person and the interaction with environmental factors.

Most children who are diagnosed with cancer do not have known predisposing environmental or host factors. Because of their relatively short latency period, most childhood cancers do not lend themselves to early cancer warning signs. The American Cancer Society's seven warning signs are less relevant for children. These warning signs describe manifestations of environmentally caused carcinomas that are much more common among adults. Efforts to establish early population-based screening strategies for childhood cancers have not been effective. Children with a family history of cancer and who are known to have mutations associated with cancer, such as those involving the *TP53* gene, however, will receive additional screening.[10–12]

A multiple causation model is useful when the results of epidemiologic studies are interpreted. For example, laboratory and epidemiologic studies may indicate that exposure to a certain chemical or ionizing radiation can cause leukemia, but not all children exposed to that chemical will develop leukemia. Additional studies will be needed to determine what other factors, including underlying genetic risk factors, must interact with chemical exposure to cause the disease.

Genetic and Genomic Factors

Acquired or inherited mutations in individual genes may contribute to the development of cancer in children and adolescents. In general, children who develop cancer have a greater frequency of mutations in germline cancer predisposition genes compared with children who do not develop cancer.[13–15] Genes associated with childhood cancers also tend to differ from those associated with adult cancers.[16,17]

Mutations in proto-oncogenes, tumor-suppressor, and mismatch repair genes are associated with the development of childhood cancer (see Chapter 12). Proto-oncogenes code for proteins that help regulate normal cell growth and differentiation. If mutated, proto-oncogenes become oncogenes that help to turn normal cells into cancer cells. Changes produced by specific oncogenes cause the cell cycle to become dysregulated. An example of an oncogene identified in pediatric cancer is *MYCN*, which is involved in neuroblastoma and glioblastoma. Tumor-suppressor genes are protective genes that normally suppress cancer cell proliferation but have lost their suppressor function. When both copies of a tumor-suppressor gene acquire mutations, normal cell function is lost, and cancer can develop. Some childhood and adolescent cancers identified with tumor-suppressor genes include leukemia, osteosarcoma, rhabdomyosarcoma, retinoblastoma, and Wilms tumor.[18] Mismatch repair genes recognize and repair errors in the DNA base sequence that can arise during DNA replication and recombination. Mismatch repair genes also repair some types of DNA damage. Mutations in both alleles of a mismatch repair gene are associated with a distinct phenotype termed constitutional mismatch repair deficiency syndrome (CMMMRD). Children affected with CMMRD, a highly penetrant cancer predisposition syndrome, can develop highly aggressive cancers, including lymphoma, leukemia, and sarcoma.[19]

An underlying single gene, multifactorial, and chromosomal conditions may increase a child's risk for the development of childhood cancer. Fanconi anemia and Bloom syndrome are single-gene autosomal recessive conditions that are risk factors for the development of cancer. Fanconi anemia results in altered DNA repair, and many affected individuals develop acute myelogenous leukemia. Bloom syndrome results in chromosomal fragility leading to increased mutations. It is associated with a spectrum of cancers, including leukemias, lymphomas, and carcinomas.

TABLE 14.3 Congenital Factors Associated With Childhood Cancer

Syndrome	Associated Childhood Cancer
Chromosome Alterations	
Down syndrome	Acute leukemia
13q syndrome	Retinoblastoma
Chromosome Instability	
Ataxia-telangiectasia	Lymphoma
Bloom syndrome	Acute leukemia, lymphoma, Wilms tumor
Fanconi anemia	Acute myelogenous leukemia, myelodysplastic syndrome, hepatic tumors
Hereditary Syndromes	
Beckwith-Wiedemann syndrome	Wilms tumor, sarcoma, brain tumors, neuroblastoma, hepatoblastoma
Neurofibromatosis type I	Brain tumor, sarcomas, neuroblastomas, Wilms tumor, nonlymphocytic leukemia
Neurofibromatosis type II	Meningioma (malignant or benign), acoustic neuroma/schwannoma, gliomas, ependymomas
Tuberous sclerosis	Glial tumors
Li-Fraumeni syndrome	Sarcoma, adrenocortical carcinoma
Von Hippel-Lindau disease	Cerebellar hemangioblastoma, retinal angioma, renal cell carcinoma, pheochromocytomas
Ataxia-telangiectasia	Leukemia, lymphoma, brain tumors
Gorlin syndrome	Medulloblastoma, skin tumors
Immunodeficiency Disorders	
Congenital	
Agammaglobulinemia	Lymphoma, leukemia, brain tumors
Immunoglobulin A (IgA) deficiency	Lymphoma, leukemia, brain tumors
Wiskott-Aldrich syndrome	Leukemia, lymphoma
Acquired	
Aplastic anemia	Leukemia
Human immunodeficiency virus/Acquired immunodeficiency syndrome (HIV/AIDS)	Non-Hodgkin lymphoma, leiomyosarcoma
Organ transplantation	Leukemia, lymphoma
Congenital Malformation Syndromes	
Aniridia, hemihypertrophy, hamartoma, genitourinary anomalies	Wilms tumor
Cryptorchidism	Testicular tumor
Gonadal dysgenesis	Gonadoblastoma
Family Susceptibility	
Twin or sibling with leukemia	Leukemia

Li-Fraumeni syndrome (LFS) is an autosomal dominant disorder involving mutations in the tumor protein p53 *(TP53)* gene, a tumor-suppressor gene on the short arm of chromosome 17. For individuals carrying a TP53 mutation, the risk of developing cancer as a child or adult is significantly higher than that seen in the unaffected population. Children and adults in these families are at risk for soft tissue sarcoma, breast cancer, leukemia, osteosarcoma, melanoma, and cancer of the colon, pancreas, adrenal cortex, and brain. Individuals with LFS are also at increased risk for developing multiple primary cancers.[10,20]

Retinoblastoma, a malignant embryonal tumor of the eye, results from deletions in the long arm of chromosome 13, which is the locus for the *RB1* gene, a tumor-suppressor gene. Deletions may occur as germline or acquired mutations. Germline deletions are associated with familial retinoblastoma, whereas acquired deletions are associated with sporadic cases (see Chapter 20).

An increased familial risk has been observed in some pediatric cancers. Although the majority of pediatric cancers are not genetically transmitted as single-gene disorders, shared genetic and environmental risk factors may contribute to an increased familial risk. A child who has a sibling with leukemia has a risk for the development of leukemia that is 2 to 4 times greater than that for children with healthy siblings. The occurrence of leukemia in monozygous twins is estimated as being as high as 25%. Although susceptibility gene loci have been identified for ALL, they explain only a relatively small portion of the familial risk for recurrence of ALL among siblings. Additional currently unidentified genetic loci are likely to contribute to the additional familial risk.[21,22] The heritability of adult cancers across the lifespan also is increased among both monozygotic and dizygotic twins.[23,24]

Chromosomal abnormalities also may contribute to the development of childhood cancer. These may include abnormalities in the number (e.g., aneuploidy) or in the structure (e.g., deletions, amplifications, translocations, and fragility) of chromosomes (see Chapter 4). Abnormalities may occur within the affected cancer cells as a result of malignant transformation.

A chromosomal translocation results from the rearrangement of two nonhomologous chromosomes. Translocations may result in the creation of a fusion gene, in which the two previously separate gene regions unite. Two fusion genes associated with ALL in children are the *BCR-ABL* gene, resulting from a translocation between chromosomes 9 and 22, and the *TEL-AML1* gene, resulting from a translocation between chromosomes 12 and 21.

Translocations, or the exchange of chromosomal material between nonhomologous chromosomes, also are associated with childhood and adolescent cancers. A well-known chromosomal translocation is the Philadelphia chromosome, which involves chromosomes 9 and 22. The Philadelphia chromosome results in the production of the BCR-Abl fusion protein, which accelerates cell division and inhibits DNA repair. It is commonly found in chronic myelogenous leukemia and some cases of acute lymphoblastic leukemias.[25] Chromosomal translocations also are commonly observed in sarcomas.

Chromosomal abnormalities associated with cancer development may also be present in congenital syndromes. One of the more recognized syndromes is trisomy 21 (Down syndrome), which is the most common genetic condition associated with the development of acute leukemia. Children with Down syndrome have a 10- to 20-fold increased risk of developing acute lymphoblastic and myelogenous leukemias and a higher risk of developing acute megakaryocytic leukemia.[26] The risk is highest in early childhood, and the age distribution for developing ALL among children with Down syndrome is similar to that of children without Down syndrome. The risk of leukemia also is increased for children with congenital malformations involving the circulatory system.[27]

Several other syndromes associated with specific congenital malformations are associated with a higher incidence of cancer development. The mechanisms associated with cancer development, however, are not fully understood.

Wilms tumor, a malignant tumor of the kidney, may occur in combination with other congenital anomalies, including aniridia or congenital absence of the iris of the eye, ambiguous genitalia, and intellectual disability (WAGR syndrome). WAGR syndrome is caused by a mutation on the short arm of chromosome 11. This region includes the Wilms tumor gene *(WT1)* as well as the *PAX6* gene that is associated with ocular development. Wilms tumor also is associated with neurofibromatosis and Beckwith-Wiedemann syndrome, a condition associated with hemihypertrophy (muscular overgrowth of half of the body and/or face).[28] Most cases of Wilms tumor, however, do not occur in children with underlying congenital syndromes. Approximately 17% of children with Wilms tumor have identifiable malformations and congenital predisposition syndromes.[29] This subset of children is likely to receive additional early cancer screening.

Children with congenital anomalies not associated with a known chromosomal syndrome may also have an increased risk of developing childhood cancer. Compared with healthy children, children with ventricular septal defects have a 10 times greater risk of developing hepatoblastoma.[30] Population-based studies indicate that children with CNS birth defects have a 10 to 20 times increased risk of developing some types of brain tumors.[31] Additionally, the siblings of children with congenital malformations involving the central nervous system, eye, ear, face, or neck are at an increased risk for cancer compared with the siblings of unaffected children.[32]

Cancers in children and adolescents are associated with fewer genetic mutations compared with adult cancers; however, efforts to understand the scope of predisposing mutations in pediatric cancer are ongoing. Recent studies have identified a greater frequency of germline mutations in cancer predisposition genes among children and adolescents with cancer compared with individuals who do not have cancer. More than one-half of the children and adolescents with germline mutations did not have a family history of cancer[13,14] (see Emerging Sciences Box: Cancer Predisposition Genes and Pediatric Cancer).

Mutations in individual genes also may result in epigenetic modifications that, in turn, increase an individual's vulnerability to cancer. For example, mutations in genes encoding histone proteins can decrease the expression of other genes without changing the sequence of these genes. This subsequent decreased gene expression can alter cell differentiation, leading to cancer development. Such epigenetic changes are being investigated in relation to the development of diffuse intrinsic pontine glioma (DIPG), an incurable brain tumor, as well as sarcomas.[33,34]

Environmental Factors

Although many adult cancers are associated with exposure to environmental agents, few childhood tumors share a similar strong association. Because of the lengthy latency period required between exposure and development of cancer, early exposure to carcinogens is presumed not to result in cancer until the child is an adult. To date, exposures to high-dose and high-dose-rate ionizing radiation have been established as risk factors for childhood leukemia.[35,36] Multiple other possible environmental risk factors for childhood cancer have been explored. Results of these studies have been mixed, and no definitive causal pathway for childhood cancer has been determined (Box 14.1).

Prenatal Exposure

Prenatal exposure to some drugs and to ionizing radiation has been linked to childhood cancers. The most well-described drug is diethylstilbestrol (DES), which was prescribed by physicians to prevent recurrent spontaneous abortion. In 1971, DES

EMERGING SCIENCE BOX

Cancer Predisposition Genes and Pediatric Cancer

Recent studies using advanced genome sequencing techniques have provided additional insight into the prevalence of germline genetic mutations that may predispose children and adolescents to cancer. In a US-based study, germline mutations have been identified in 565 genes associated with cancer development in 1120 children and adolescents with cancer and 966 individuals who did not have cancer.[1] The investigators found that 8.5% of individuals with cancer had a mutation associated with cancer development compared with only 1.1% of the individuals who did not have cancer. Mutations most frequently occurred in the TP53 gene, a gene involved in regulating cell division and preventing tumor formation. Other frequently affected genes were APC and BRCA2. The majority of children and adolescents with mutations in cancer predisposition genes did not have a family history of cancer. In a cohort study of 40 children and their parents in the Netherlands, investigators identified germline mutations that were the likely cause of cancer in 8 (20%) individuals.[2] They also identified additional genes that are likely associated with cancer predisposition.

Germline mutations in cancer-causing genes also have implications for survivors of childhood cancer. As survival rates increase, the number of individuals at risk for developing secondary cancers also increases. A recent US-based study identified mutations in 156 cancer predisposition genes among 11.8% of 2,450 childhood cancer survivors.[3] Variants in cancer predisposition genes were most prevalent among survivors of central nervous system tumors. The most frequently mutated genes included RB1, NF1, and BRCA2.

The results of these studies will guide additional epidemiologic studies, as well as studies investigating mechanisms of cancer development in children and adolescents across the cancer care continuum. Identifying the presence of these mutations also may help guide treatment, as well as genetic testing and counseling of other family members.

Data from Zhang J, et al. Germline mutations in predisposition genes in pediatric cancer. *New England Journal of Medicine*, 2015;373(24):2336–2346; Diets IJ, et al. High yield of pathogenic germline mutations causative or likely causative of the cancer phenotype in selected children with cancer. *Clinical Cancer Research*, 2018;24(7):1594–1603; Wilson CL, et al. Estimated number of adult survivors of childhood cancer in the United States with cancer-predisposing germline variants. *Pediatric Blood Cancer*, 2020;67(2):e28047.

BOX 14.1 Factors That May Contribute to the Development of Childhood and Adolescent Cancers

- Genetic, genomic, and epigenetic factors
- Diet
- Immune function
- Occupational exposure
- Ionizing radiation
- Hormonal variations
- Viral illnesses
- Individual characteristics, such as the biologic, social, and physical environments

was identified as a transplacental chemical carcinogen because adenocarcinomas of the vagina and cervix occurred in a small percentage of the daughters of women who took DES. No other studies have identified other drugs taken by pregnant women that may cause cancer in their children. Since then, other studies have attempted to identify drugs taken by pregnant women that may cause cancer in their offspring, but no other drugs have been found. In 2006, the Office of the US Surgeon General suggested evidence of a causal relationship among childhood leukemia, lymphoma, and brain tumors related to prenatal or postnatal environmental tobacco smoke exposure.

Current evidence suggests that an increased risk of childhood leukemia is associated with low levels of exposure to antenatal x-rays.[12,36] An association between antenatal x-ray exposure and childhood brain tumors has not been established. Other current areas of research include exploring epigenetic modifications resulting from prenatal exposures and their role in future cancer development.

Recent meta-analyses have suggested associations between parental exposure to pesticides and other potential environmental toxins before or during pregnancy and subsequent development of childhood cancer.[37,38] The strongest associations have been identified in relation to maternal exposure. Recent studies indicate that the risk of leukemia, lymphoma, and neuroblastoma is increased when the mother is exposed to pesticides in the prenatal period.[38–40] Maternal occupational benzene exposure has been associated with an increased risk of acute lymphoblastic leukemia.[41] Maternal exposure to hair dyes and occupational chemical exposure was associated with an increased risk of leukemia and neuroblastoma.[41–43]

The role of paternal exposure is less clearly defined. However, recent prospective analyses from the International Childhood Cancer Cohort Consortium indicated that paternal exposure to pesticides was associated with an increased risk of acute myelogenous leukemia but not acute lymphoblastic leukemia or central nervous system tumors.[44] In contrast, another study using more detailed exposure-related information identified an association between acute lymphoblastic leukemia and paternal, but not maternal, occupational exposure to pesticides.[45]

In contrast, however, a meta-analysis of 1426 cases of neuroblastoma failed to show an association between paternal occupational exposure to pesticides and the development of disease.[46]

Parental occupational exposure to livestock has also been a recent focus of investigation. A recent case control from Denmark spanning nearly 50 years identified an association between paternal exposure and germ cell tumors as well as maternal exposure and subsequent astrocytomas.[47]

Childhood Exposure

Childhood exposures to ionizing radiation, drugs, electromagnetic fields, or viruses have been associated with the risk of cancer. Although high doses of ionizing radiation are established risk factors for the development of childhood cancer,[48] evidence is emerging about the role of lower doses as well as additional variables that may further convey an increased risk. Retrospective studies have shown a significant correlation between radiation-induced malignancies and either radiotherapy (cancer treatment) or radiation exposure from diagnostic imaging[49,50] (see Emerging Sciences Box: Risks from CT Imaging Scans and Pediatric Cancer). A case-control study of more than 1000 children in Finland with leukemia who were less than 15 years of age

EMERGING SCIENCE BOX

Risks from CT Imaging Scans and Pediatric Cancer

Computed tomography (CT) is the largest contributor to medical radiation exposure in the US population. CT exposures represent only about 12% of diagnostic radiologic procedures in large hospitals; however, it accounts for almost 49% of the US population's collective radiation dose from all medical x-ray examinations.

Concern about the risk of cancer in children associated with radiation exposure from CT is increasing. Epidemiologic studies have shown that children are more sensitive to radiation compared to adults. Because children have a longer life expectancy compared with adults, the window of opportunity to express radiation damage is increased. Children also may receive a higher radiation dose than necessary if the CT setting is not adjusted for their smaller size. The absolute cancer risks associated with CT, however, are very small. Lifetime risks of cancer because of CT exposures have been estimated by using projection models based on atomic bomb survivors. These risks are about 1 case of cancer for every 1000 people scanned, with a maximal incidence of about 1 case of cancer for every 500 people. A recent meta-analysis of seven studies that included 1,180,987 children identified a 1.32-fold greater risk of subsequent cancer development among children exposed to CT compared with those who were not exposed to CT.

The benefits of properly performed and clinically justified CT examinations should always outweigh the risks for an individual child. Key strategies to minimize radiation exposure include: (1) performing only necessary CT scans, (2) adjusting exposure parameters for children, and (3) using lower resolution scans when appropriate to the clinical decision to be made.

Future population-based studies should evaluate the changes in childhood cancers attributable to medical imaging scans as institutions adopt practices to reduce radiation from CT scans. Future studies should also include longer follow-up periods as well as provide additional detail regarding underlying genetic conditions that may provide insights into mechanisms by which CT exposure may contribute to increased cancer risk.

Data from Huang R, et al. Radiation exposure associated with computed tomography in childhood and the subsequent risk of cancer: A meta-analysis of cohort studies. *Dose Response*, 2020;18(2):1559325820923828; National Cancer Institute, National Institutes of Health. NCI Radiation Risks and Pediatric Computed Tomography (CT): A Guide for Health Care Workers. Bethesda, MD: National Cancer Institute; 2012. https://www.cancer.gov/about-cancer/causes-prevention/risk/radiation/pediatric-ct-scans. Accessed August 16, 2020.

did not demonstrate an overall association of childhood leukemia with background gamma radiation.[51] This study did, however, demonstrate an increased risk of leukemia in relation to increasing radiation dose among children between 2 and 7 years of age. Additionally, this study identified a positive association between leukemia with high hyperdiploid features and radiation dose. A similar increased risk was not identified for leukemia with other genetic features. Few studies have followed children for a long enough period of time to determine whether the risk of cancer remains increased in adulthood, although current studies with more rigorous methodology are assessing this risk.

In addition to the drug and environmental agents that are known to cause cancer in adults and therefore also are risks for exposure during childhood, a few drugs may particularly increase cancer risk during childhood (Table 14.4). Exposures during childhood to unspecified residential pesticides and insecticides have been associated with childhood leukemia.[52]

TABLE 14.4 Drugs That May Increase Risk of Childhood Cancer

Drug Class	Uses	Cancer Risk
Anabolic androgenic steroids	Stimulate bone growth and appetite; induce puberty; increase muscle mass and physical strength	Hepatocellular carcinoma Brain tumors
Epipodophyllotoxin and anthracycline chemotherapy agents	Cancer treatment	Leukemia
Immunosuppressive agents	Prevent organ rejection following transplantation surgery	Lymphoma

In contrast, some exposures may be protective against childhood cancer. Current research suggests that early exposure to common infections may help "prime" the immune system, thereby protecting the child against acute lymphoblastic leukemia.[53]

Multiple other possible environmental risk factors for childhood cancer have been explored. The relationship between childhood cancer and exposure to radon[54–56] and electromagnetic fields has been the focus of many international epidemiologic studies, yet no conclusive evidence has been observed. A review of studies from 1997 to 2013 indicated that magnetic field exposure may be associated with an increased incidence of childhood leukemia[57]; however, the reported risk associated with exposure to magnetic fields and the development of childhood leukemia has been decreasing over the past 20 years.[58] In 2007, a task group of scientific experts convened by the World Health Organization (WHO) reported that it could not confirm the existence of any health consequences from exposure to low-level magnetic fields[59] (see Emerging Sciences Box: Magnetic Fields and Development of Pediatric Cancer).

The strongest association between viruses and the development of cancer in children has been seen in cases of the Epstein-Barr virus (EBV) infection, which is linked to endemic Burkitt lymphoma, nasopharyngeal carcinoma, and Hodgkin disease. Children with acquired immunodeficiency syndrome (AIDS) have an increased risk of developing non-Hodgkin lymphoma and Kaposi sarcoma. The use of highly active antiretroviral therapy (HAART) in the developed world has dramatically reduced the incidence of AIDS-related malignancies.

PROGNOSIS

Nearly 85% of children and adolescents diagnosed with cancer are cured. Mortality rates have declined from 6.5 per 100,000 in 1969 to 2.3 per 100,000 in 2015, largely because of advances in treatment and increased participation in clinical trials.[60]

Factors leading to these improved cure rates include the use of combination chemotherapy, multimodal treatment, advances in biotherapy, and improvements in nursing and supportive care. The development of research centers for comprehensive childhood cancer treatment, cooperation among treatment institutions, and the development of cooperative study groups facilitate refinements in treatment protocols and data sharing,

EMERGING SCIENCE BOX

Magnetic Fields and Development of Pediatric Cancer

The role of magnetic fields has been an ongoing area of concern as an environmental exposure that in relation to cancer development. Exposure to extremely low to mid-frequency magnetic fields is common, and common sources include electric power lines, computers, mobile phones, radio waves, and microwaves. These types of magnetic fields are non-ionizing and do not directly damage DNA.

The World Health Organization (WHO) identified a better understanding of health risks, including cancer, and exposure to low-frequency magnetic fields as a research priority in 2007. A recent meta-analysis evaluated nine case-control studies, representing eight different countries, conducted between 1997 and 2013 and involving 11,699 cases of children with leukemia and 13,194 controls. This meta-analysis identified an increased risk of childhood leukemia associated with high levels of magnetic field exposure ($\geq 0.4\ \mu T$). For additional perspective, <1% of the children in these studies experienced this level of exposure. The WHO has estimated that only about 1% to 4% of children worldwide live in conditions that exceed 0.4 μT.

Ongoing research is needed because any environmental factor may require many years of exposure to cause disease. Additionally, an association between a given factor and childhood cancer does not establish causality. Research is needed to better understand the relationships between exposures to extremely low- and low-frequency magnetic fields and other potential causative factors associated with childhood cancers. Research also is needed to identify potential mechanisms by which these types of magnetic fields, including the dose and duration of exposure, may contribute to the development of childhood cancer.

Data from National Cancer Institute. Electromagnetic fields and cancer; 2020. https://www.cancer.gov/about-cancer/causes-prevention/risk/radiation/electromagnetic-fields-fact-sheet. Accessed August 16, 2020; World Health Organization. Fact sheet: electromagnetic fields and public health: exposure to extremely low frequency fields; 2020. www.who.int/peh-emf/publications/facts/fs322/en/. Accessed August 16, 2020; Zhao L, et al. Magnetic fields exposure and childhood leukemia risk: A meta-analysis based on 11,699 cases and 13,194 controls. *Leukemia Research*, 2014;38(3):269–274.

which further contribute to improved survival rates. Currently, clinical trials are being conducted by the Children's Oncology Group (COG) at more than 175 hospitals across the United States and are funded by the National Cancer Institute through CureSearch for Children's Cancer.

Although survival rates for adolescents have lagged behind those for children less than 15 years of age, recent data from the Centers for Disease Control and Prevention's National Center for Health Statistics are encouraging. These data indicate that, since 2000, 5-year survival rates for adolescents and young adults have aligned with those for younger children.[61]

Even with these improvements, adolescents remain vulnerable to poorer outcomes relative to younger children. A particular area of concern is lower rates of participation in clinical trials among adolescents relative to younger children. Because many adolescents are transitioning to adult providers for primary care services, they may be referred to an adult cancer center rather than a pediatric center at the time of diagnosis. If adolescents are treated in adult cancer centers, a clinical trial may not be available. Some clinical trials that are available to adults may not be open to adolescents younger than 18 years of age even if their disease biology is similar to that of adult disease,[61] and fewer trials are available for young adolescents. The National Cancer Institute (NCI) and pediatric and adult cooperative groups sponsored by the NCI have launched a national initiative to increase the numbers of adolescents and young adults participating in clinical trials.

Childhood cancer survivors have a greater risk of developing a second cancer later in life. This risk may be associated with a variety of factors, including specific types of chemotherapy, as well as radiation to certain areas of the body. Genetic factors and the type of primary cancer also influence the risk of a second cancer. For example, children with a history of familial retinoblastoma are at increased risk of osteosarcoma developing later in life.

Because childhood cancer is viewed as a chronic disease instead of a fatal illness, treatment includes attention to the quality of life and symptom management. Even children whose cancers cannot be cured can experience improved quality of life with palliative care. Children and adolescents whose cancers are regarded as cured continue to face residual and late effects of their treatment. These late effects are more significant in children than in adults because children receive their treatment at a time when they are still physically immature and growing. Many late effects of cancer treatment need further study. Common late effects include physical impairments, reproductive dysfunction, soft tissue and bone atrophy, learning disabilities, secondary cancers, and psychological sequelae. Priorities for future research include learning about the genetic and genomic consequences of treatment, such as telomere shortening, and their associated consequences on survivor health and well-being.[62] A referral to genetic services is appropriate for families of children whose cancer is known to be transmitted genetically (e.g., retinoblastoma, LFS).

SUMMARY REVIEW

Incidence and Types of Childhood Cancers

1. Cancer in children and adolescents is rare, but it is still the leading cause of death from disease in this population.
2. Leukemia is the most common type of cancer among children less than 14 years of age. Tumors involving the brain or central nervous system are the second most common type of childhood cancer.
3. The most common cancers among adolescents (15 to 19 years of age) are Hodgkin and non-Hodgkin lymphoma, leukemia, germ cell tumors (particularly testicular), CNS tumors, thyroid cancer, and sarcomas.

Etiology

1. The interaction of many factors most likely produces cancer in children and adolescents, a concept referred to as multiple causation or multifactorial etiology.
2. Mutations in proto-oncogenes, tumor-suppressor genes, and mismatch repair genes have been associated with childhood and adolescent malignancies.

3. Risk factors associated with the development of childhood cancer include inherited and acquired genetic and genomic changes, nutrition and diet, immune function, occupational exposure, hormonal variations, and viral illnesses, as well as other individual characteristics, such as biologic, social, or physical environments.
4. Children with Down syndrome have an increased risk for the development of leukemia.
5. Childhood exposure to ionizing radiation, drugs, or viruses has been associated with the risk of developing cancer.

Prognosis

1. Nearly 85% of children and adolescents diagnosed with cancer are cured.
2. Childhood cancer survivors have a greater risk of developing a second cancer during their lifetime compared with the general population.
3. Reasons for improved survival among children and adolescents with cancer include research aimed at identifying less toxic treatments with fewer long-term side effects.
4. Young children are particularly prone to long-term sequelae of cancer therapy. The development of more effective, targeted therapies with fewer side effects is imperative.

REFERENCES

1. Heron M. Deaths: leading causes for 2018. *Natl Vital Stat Rep.* 2021;70(4):1–115. Available at https://www.cdc.gov/nchs/data/nvsr/nvsr70/nvsr70-04-508.pdf. (Accessed 08.08.21).
2. American Cancer Society. *Cancer in children*, 2021. Available at https://www.cancer.org/cancer/cancer-in-children.html. (Accessed 08.08.21).
3. Siegel RL, Miller KD, Jemal A. Cancer statistics, 2020. *CA Cancer J Clin.* 2020;70(1):7–30.
4. Howlader N, ed. *SEER Cancer Statistics Review, 1975-2018.* Bethesda, MD: National Cancer Institute; 2021. (Based on November 2020 SEER data submission, posted to the SEER website, April 15, 2021). Available at https://seer.cancer.gov/csr/1975_2018/. (Accessed 08.08.21).
5. Kochanek KD, et al. Deaths: final data for 2017. *Natl Vital Stat Rep.* 2019;68(9):1–77. Available at https://stacks.cdc.gov/view/cdc/79486. (Accessed 08.08.21).
6. National Cancer Institute (NCI): *Adolescents and young adults with cancer*, Bethesda, MD, 2018, NCI. Available at http://www.cancer.gov/cancertopics/aya/types. (Accessed 08.08.21).
7. Ghantous A, et al. Characterizing the epigenome as a key component of the fetal exposome in evaluating in utero exposures and childhood cancer risk. *Mutagenesis.* 2015;30:733–742.
8. Timms JA, et al. DNA methylation as a potent mediator of environmental risks in the development of childhood acute lymphoblastic leukemia. *Epigenomics.* 2016;8(4):519–536.
9. Braun JM, Messerlian C, Hauser R. Fathers matter: why it's time to consider the impact of paternal environmental exposures on children's health. *Curr Epidemiol Rep.* 2017;4(1):46–55.
10. Kratz CP, et al. Cancer screening recommendations for individuals with Li-Fraumeni syndrome. *Clin Cancer Res.* 2017;23(11):e38–e45.
11. Ballinger ML, et al. Baseline surveillance in Li-Fraumeni syndrome using whole-body magnetic resonance imaging: a meta-analysis. *JAMA Oncol.* 2017;3(12):1634–1639.
12. Tak CR, et al. Cost-effectiveness of early cancer surveillance for patients with Li-Fraumeni syndrome. *Pediatr Blood Cancer.* 2019;66(5):e27629.
13. Zhang J, et al. Germline mutations in predisposition genes in pediatric cancer. *N Engl J Med.* 2015;373(24):2336–2346.
14. Diets IJ, et al. High yield of pathogenic germline mutations causative or likely causative of the cancer phenotype in selected children with cancer. *Clin Cancer Res.* 2018;24(7):1594–1603.
15. Gröbner SN, et al. The landscape of genomic alterations across childhood cancers. *Nature.* 2018;555(7696):321–327.
16. Ma X, et al. Pan-cancer genome and transcriptome analyses of 1,699 paediatric leukemias and solid tumors. *Nature.* 2018;555(7696):371–376.
17. Sweet-Cordero EA, Biegel JA. The genomic landscape of pediatric cancers: implications for diagnosis and treatment. *Science.* 2019;363(6432):1170–1175.
18. Potter JW, Jones KB, Barrott JJ: Sarcoma—the standard-bearer in cancer discovery, *Crit Rev Oncol Hematol* 126:1–5.
19. Tabori U, et al. Clinical management and tumor surveillance recommendations of inherited mismatch repair deficiency in childhood. *Clin Cancer Res.* 2017;23(11):e32–e37.
20. Mai PL, et al. Risks of first and subsequent cancers among TP53 mutation carriers in the National Cancer Institute Li-Fraumeni syndrome cohort. *Cancer.* 2016;122(23):3673–3681.
21. Churchman ML, et al. Germline genetic IKZF1 variation and predisposition to childhood acute lymphoblastic leukemia. *Cancer Cell.* 2018;33(5):937–948.
22. Vijayakrishnan J, et al. Genome-wide association study identifies susceptibility loci for B-cell childhood acute lymphoblastic leukemia. *Nat Commun.* 2018;9(1):1340.
23. Graff RE, et al. Familial risk and heritability of colorectal cancer in the Nordic twin study of cancer. *Clin Gastroenterol Hepatol.* 2017;15(8):1256–1264.
24. Mucci LA, et al. Familial risk and heritability of cancer among twins in Nordic countries. *JAMA.* 2016;315(1):68–76.
25. Boer JM, et al. Tyrosine kinase fusion genes in pediatric BCR-ABL1-like acute lymphoblastic leukemia. *Oncotarget.* 2017;8(3):4618–4628.
26. Lee P, et al. The biology, pathogenesis and clinical aspects of acute lymphoblastic leukemia in children with Down syndrome. *Leukemia.* 2016;30(9):1816–1823.
27. Mandalenakis Z, et al. Risk of cancer among children and young adults with congenital heart disease compared with healthy controls. *JAMA Netw Open.* 2019;2(7):e196762.
28. MacFarland SP, et al. Diagnosis of Beckwith-Wiedeman syndrome in children presenting with Wilms tumor. *Pediatr Blood Cancer.* 2018;65(10):e27296.
29. D'Angelo P, et al. Factors possibly affecting prognosis in children with Wilms' tumor diagnosed before 24 months of age: a report from the Associazione Italiana Ematologia Oncologia Pediatrica (AIEOP) Wilms Tumor Working Group. *Pediatr Blood Cancer.* 2017;64(12):e26644.
30. Schraw JM, et al: *A population-based assessment of cancer risk among children with non-chromosomal birth defects in 10 million live births*, Abstract LB-161, presented at the American Association for Cancer Research Annual Meeting, April 14–18, 2018, Chicago, IL. Available at https://www.abstractsonline.com/pp8/#!/4562/presentation/10867. (Accessed 08.08.21).
31. Johnson KJ, et al: Pediatric cancer risk in association with birth defects: a systematic review, *PLoS One* 12(7):e0181246
32. Sun Y, et al. Cancer risk in siblings of children with congenital malformations. *Cancer Epidemiol.* 2016;44(1):59–64.

33. Castel D, et al. Transcriptomic and epigenetic profiling of 'diffuse midline gliomas, H3 K27M-mutant' discriminate two subgroups based on the type of histone H3 mutated and not supratentorial or infratentorial location. *Acta Neuropathol Commun.* 2018;6(1):117.
34. Chaiyawat P, et al. Expression patterns of class I histone deacetylases in osteosarcoma: a novel protnostic marker with potential therapeutic implications. *Mod Pathol.* 2018;31(2):264–274.
35. Hsu WL, et al. The incidence of leukemia, lymphoma, and multiple myeloma among atomic bomb survivors: 1950-2001. *Radiat Res.* 2013;179(3):361–382.
36. Kendall GM, et al. Childhood cancer research in Oxford III: the work of CCRG on ionizing radiation. *Br J Cancer.* 2018;119(6): 771–778.
37. Van Maele-Fabry G, et al. Childhood leukaemia and parental occupational exposure to pesticides: a systematic review and meta-analysis. *Cancer Causes Control.* 2010;21(6):787–809.
38. Bailey HD, et al. Parental occupational pesticide exposure and the risk of childhood leukemia in the offspring: findings from the Childhood Leukemia International Consortium. *Int J Cancer.* 2014;135(9):2157–2172.
39. Ferri GM, et al. Maternal exposure to pesticides, paternal occupation in the army/police force, and CYP2D6*4 polymorphism in the etiology of childhood acute leukemia. *J Pediatr Hematol Oncol.* 2018;40(4):e207–e214.
40. Rios P, et al. Maternal use of household pesticides during pregnancy and risk of neuroblastoma in offspring. A pooled analysis of the ESTELLE and ESCALE French studies (SFCE). *Cancer Causes Control.* 2017;28(10):1125–1132.
41. Heck JE, et al. Parental occupational exposure to benzene and the risk of childhood and adolescent acute lymphoblastic leukemia: a population-based study. *Occup Environ Med.* 2019;76(8): 527–529.
42. Couto AC, et al. Pregnancy, maternal exposure to hair dyes and hair straightening cosmetics, and early age leukemia. *Chem Biol Interact.* 2013;205(1):46–52.
43. Parodi S, et al. Risk of neuroblastoma, maternal characteristics and perinatal exposures: the SETIL study. *Cancer Epidemiol.* 2014; 38(6):686–694.
44. Patel DM, et al. Parental occupational exposure to pesticides, animals and organic dust and risk of childhood leukemia and central nervous system tumors: findings from the International Childhood Cancer Cohort Consortium (I4C). *Int J Cancer.* 2020; 146(4):943–952.
45. Gunier RB, et al. A task-based assessment of parental occupational exposure to pesticides and childhood acute lymphoblastic leukemia. *Environ Res.* 2017;156:57–62.
46. Moore A, Enquobahrie DA. Paternal occupational exposure to pesticides and risk of neuroblastoma among children: a meta-analysis. *Cancer Causes Control.* 2011;22(11):1529–1536.
47. Hall C, et al. Occupational livestock or animal dust exposure and offspring cancer risk in Denmark, 1968-2016. *Int Arch Occup Environ Health.* 2020;93(5):659–668.
48. Hsu WL, et al. The incidence of leukemia, lymphoma, and multiple myeloma among atomic bomb survivors: 1950-2001. *Radiat Res.* 2013;179(3):361–382.
49. Huang R, et al. Radiation exposure associated with computed tomography in childhood and the subsequent risk of cancer: a meta-analysis of cohort studies. *Dose Response.* 2020;18(2). 1559325820923828.
50. National Cancer Institute (NCI) *NCI radiation risks and pediatric computed tomography (CT): a guide for health care workers.* Bethesda, MD: NCI; 2012. Reviewed September 4, 2018. Available at https://www.cancer.gov/about-cancer/causes-prevention/risk/radiation/pediatric-ct-scans. (Accessed 08.08.21).
51. Nikkilä A, et al. Background radiation and childhood cancer: a nationwide register-based case-control study. *Int J Cancer.* 2016; 139(9):1975–1982.
52. van Maele-Fabry Household exposure to pesticides and risk of leukemia in children and adolescents: Updated systematic review and meta-analysis. *Int J Hyg Environ Health.* 2019;222(1):49–67.
53. Gröbner SN, et al. The landscape of genomic alterations across childhood cancers. *Nature.* 2018;555(7696):321–327.
54. Nikkila A, et al. Predicting residential radon concentrations in Finland: model development, validation, and application to childhood leukemia. *Scand J Work Environ Health.* 2020;46(3): 278–292.
55. Chen J, Xie L. Domestic radon exposure and childhood leukaemia and lymphoma: a population-based study in Canada. *Radiat Prot Dosimetry.* 2019;184(3-4):486–492.
56. Berlivet J. Ecological association between residential natural background radiation exposure and the rate of childhood central nervous system tumors in France, 2000-2012. *J Environ Radioact.* 2020;211:106071.
57. Zhao L, et al. Magnetic fields exposure and childhood leukemia risk: a meta-analysis based on 11,699 cases and 13,194 controls. *Leuk Res.* 2014;38(3):269–274.
58. Swanson J, et al. Changes over time in the reported risk for childhood leukaemia and magnetic fields. *J Radiol Prot.* 2019; 39(2):470–488.
59. World Health Organization (WHO) *Electromagnetic fields and public health: exposure to extremely low frequency fields.* Geneva, Switzerland: WHO; 2007. Available at https://www.who.int/teams/environment-climate-change-and-health/radiation-and-health/non-ionizing/elff. (Accessed 08.08.21).
60. National Cancer Institute (NCI) *Cancer in children and adolescents.* Bethesda, MD: NCI; 2018. Available at https://www.cancer.gov/types/childhood-cancers/child-adolescent-cancers-fact-sheet. (Accessed 08.08.21).
61. Close AG, et al. Adolescent and young adult oncology—past, present, and future. *CA Cancer J Clin.* 2019;69(6):485–496.
62. Song N, et al. Shortened leukocyte telomere length associates with an increased prevalence of chronic health conditions among survivors of childhood cancer: a report from the St. Jude lifetime cohort. *Clin Cancer Res.* 2020;26(10):2362–2371.

15

Structure and Function of the Neurologic System

Karen C. Turner

http://evolve.elsevier.com/Rogers/pathophysiology/

CHAPTER OUTLINE

The human nervous system is a remarkable structure responsible for decision-making, the body's ability to interact with the environment, and the regulation and control of activities involving our internal organs, muscles, and glands. It is a network composed of complex structures that transmit electrical and chemical signals between the brain and the body's many organs and tissues. This chapter provides a basic overview of the structure and function of the nervous system and supports the understanding of nervous system pathophysiology in the following chapters.

OVERVIEW AND ORGANIZATION OF THE NERVOUS SYSTEM

Although the nervous system functions as a unified whole, structures and functions have been divided here to facilitate understanding. Structurally, the nervous system is divided into the central nervous system and the peripheral nervous system (Fig. 15.1). The central nervous system (CNS) consists of the brain and spinal cord, enclosed within the protective cranial vault and vertebrae, respectively. The peripheral nervous system (PNS) is composed of the cranial nerves, which project from the brain, and the spinal nerves, which project from the spinal cord. Cranial nerves can be viewed as modified spinal nerves. Cranial nerves control motor and sensory functions similarly to spinal nerves and have specialized sensory tasks, such as smell, taste, sight, and hearing (see section on Peripheral Nervous System). PNS pathways are differentiated into afferent pathways (ascending pathways), which carry sensory impulses toward the CNS, and efferent pathways (descending pathways), which innervate skeletal muscle or effector organs by transmitting motor impulses away from the CNS. Most peripheral nerves carry a combination of both afferent and efferent pathways.

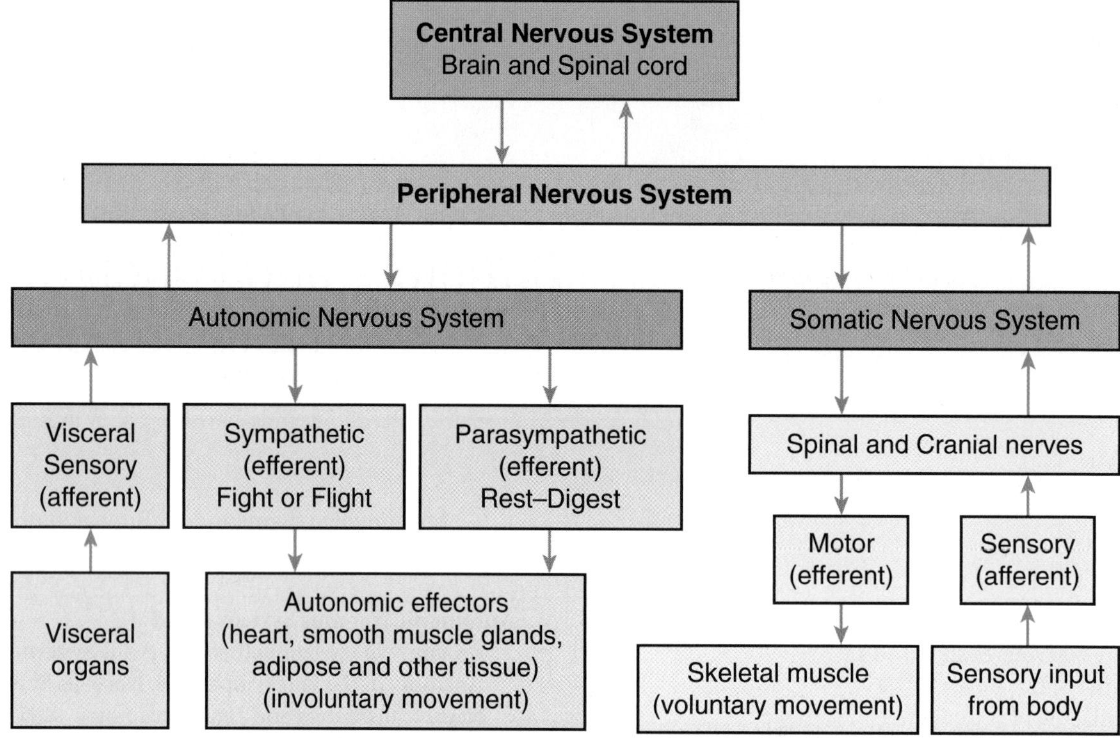

Fig. 15.1 Organization of the Nervous System.

Functionally, the PNS can be divided into the somatic nervous system and the autonomic nervous system. The somatic nervous system consists of pathways that regulate voluntary motor control (e.g., skeletal muscle). The autonomic nervous system (ANS) is involved in regulating the body's internal environment (viscera) through the involuntary control of organ systems. The ANS is further divided into sympathetic and parasympathetic divisions. Organs innervated by specific components of the nervous system are called effector organs.

CELLS OF THE NERVOUS SYSTEM

Two basic types of cells constitute nervous tissue: neurons and supporting nonneuronal neuroglial cells. The neuron is the primary cell of the nervous system. It is an electrically excitable cell, which transmits and receives information. Neuroglial cells provide structural support, protection, and nutrition for the neurons and facilitate neurotransmission. Neuroglial cells include astrocytes, microglia, and oligodendrocytes in the CNS; and Schwann (neurilemma) and satellite cells (a type of Schwann cell) in the PNS.

Neurons

Working alone or in units, neurons detect environmental changes and initiate body responses to maintain a dynamic steady state. Neuronal size and structure vary markedly, and each neuron is adapted to perform specialized functions. The cellular constituents of neurons include microtubules (transport substances within the cell), neurofibrils (very thin supportive fibers that extend throughout the neuron), microfilaments (proteins thought to be involved in the transport of cellular products), and Nissl substances (endoplasmic reticulum and ribosomes involved in protein synthesis). Although most neurons are nondividing cells, some neurons continue to divide after birth; for example, olfactory neurons in the nose continue to divide throughout life.

A neuron (Fig. 15.2) has three components: a cell body (soma), the dendrites (thin branching fibers of the cell), and the axons. Cell bodies for most neurons, even those extending axons into peripheral nerves, are located within the CNS. Dense collections of cell bodies in the CNS are called **nuclei**. Those in the PNS usually are found in groups called ganglia (or plexuses—a group of relay nerves). The dendrites are extensions that carry nerve impulses *toward* the cell body. The **dendritic zone** is the receptive portion of a neuron that receives a stimulus. Axons are long, conductive projections that carry nerve impulses *away* from the cell body. The axon hillock is the cone-shaped process where the axon leaves the cell body. The first part of the axon hillock has the lowest threshold for stimulation, so action potentials begin there.

A typical neuron has only one axon, which may be wrapped with a myelin sheath—a membrane made of a lipid material called myelin. In the CNS, myelin is produced by oligodendrocytes. Regions of the brain and spinal cord with a high level of myelination constitute the white matter, whereas regions lacking significant myelination (typically primarily composed of cell bodies) are gray matter. In the PNS, myelin is produced by Schwann cells. The myelin sheaths are interrupted at regular intervals by the nodes of Ranvier. Nutrient exchange is not possible through the myelin sheath, although it can occur

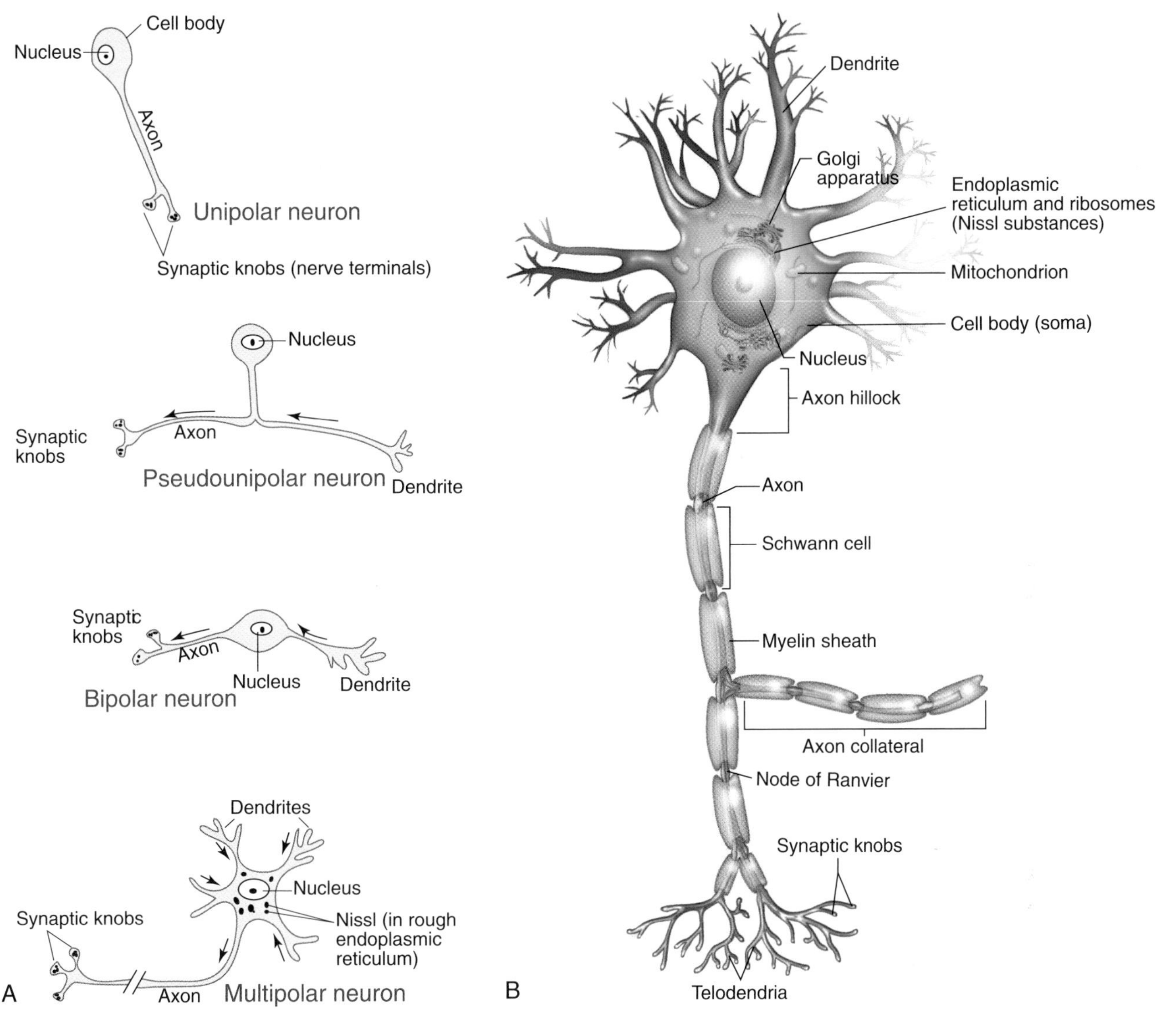

Fig. 15.2 Neuron Structure. (A) Structural classifications of neurons based on the number of processes: unipolar, pseudopolar, bipolar, and multipolar. **(B)** Typical multipolar neuron: Peripheral nervous system neuron with multiple extensions from the cell body. (A, From Watson C, Kirkcaldie M, Paxinos G. *The brain*. London: Academic Press; 2011. B, Modified from Patton KT, Thibodeau GA, Douglas MM. *Essentials of anatomy & physiology*. St. Louis: Mosby; 2012.)

at the nodes of Ranvier. Axons can branch at the nodes of Ranvier, forming axon collaterals. Axons end with telodendria, branches that terminate with synaptic knobs, which are used in neurotransmission.

Where there is myelin, the velocity of nerve impulses increases. Myelin acts as an insulator that allows an action potential to leap between segments rather than flowing along the entire length of the membrane, yielding the increased velocity. This mechanism is referred to as **saltatory conduction**. Disorders of the myelin sheath (demyelinating diseases), such as multiple sclerosis, Guillain-Barré syndrome, and Charcot-Marie-Tooth disease, demonstrate the important role myelin plays in nerve conduction (see Chapter 17). Conduction velocities depend not only on the myelin coating but also on the diameter of the axon. Larger axons transmit impulses at a faster rate.

Neurons are structurally classified based on the number of processes (projections) extending from the cell body (see Fig. 15.2A). There are four basic types of cell configuration: (1) unipolar, (2) pseudounipolar, (3) bipolar, and (4) multipolar. **Unipolar neurons** have one process, an axon, which branches shortly after leaving the cell body. One example is found in the retina. **Pseudounipolar neurons** (*unipolar*) have one axon process and one dendrite process, but the dendrite and axon are fused near the cell body, and the axon then extends into the CNS. This configuration is typical of sensory neurons in both cranial and spinal nerves. **Bipolar neurons** have two distinct processes (one axon and one dendrite) arising directly from the cell body. This type of neuron connects the rod and cone cells of the retina. **Multipolar neurons** are the most common and have multiple processes capable of extensive branching. A motor neuron is typically multipolar.

Functionally, there are three types of neurons (their typical configuration is noted in parentheses): (1) sensory (mostly pseudounipolar), (2) associational (multipolar), and (3) motor (multipolar). **Sensory neurons** are afferent neurons, carrying impulses from peripheral sensory receptors to the CNS. **Associational neurons (interneurons)** transmit impulses from neuron to neuron, sensory to motor neurons. They are located solely within the CNS. **Motor neurons** are efferent neurons, transmitting impulses from the CNS to an effector (i.e., skeletal muscle or organs). In skeletal muscle, the end processes form a **neuromuscular (myoneural) junction** (see Fig. 15.14 and the Spinal Cord section later in the chapter).

Neuroglia

Neuroglia ("nerve glue") is the general classification of nonneuronal cells that support the nervous system's neurons. They comprise approximately 50% of the total brain and spinal cord volume. Neuroglia are present in both the CNS and PNS. **Astrocytes, oligodendroglia (oligodendrocytes), ependymal cells**, and **microglia** are found in the CNS; **Schwann cells, nonmyelinating Schwann cells**, and **satellite glial cells** are found in the PNS (Fig. 15.3) (Emerging Science Box: Schwann Cells). The different types of neuroglia serve different functions (Table 15.1).

EMERGING SCIENCE BOX

Schwann Cells

Schwann cells (SCs) are peripheral neuroglial cells derived from the neural crest. They are the most common cell type in the peripheral nervous system. There are several subtypes in addition to the myelin-forming cells. These include non–myelin-forming autonomic nervous system cells, perisynaptic cells, and perineuronal satellite cells of the dorsal root ganglia and of the autonomic ganglia. SCs are important for the maintenance of normal nervous system function, repair of neural injury, immune modulation, and upregulation of pain. Myelin-forming SCs form spirals of compact myelin lamellae in both small and large neurons. Increasing layers of lamellae increase the speed of salutatory conduction. These cells also can recognize antigen and be the target of autoimmune responses as occur with Guillain-Barré syndrome. Most neural cells in the peripheral nervous system are unmyelinated, and SCs in these nerves, as well as the dorsal root and sympathetic and parasympathetic ganglia, provide an axonal sheath but do not form myelin. With peripheral nerve injury, perineuronal satellite cells can up-regulate nerve growth factor and other molecules important to peripheral chronic pain syndromes. At the neuromuscular junction (NMJ), nonmyelinating SCs function to facilitate neurotransmission and repair damage. Transplant of SCs and use of exogenous neurotrophic factors are in the preclinical stage of evaluation.

Data from Armati PJ, et al. An update on Schwann cell biology—Immunomodulation, neural regulation and other surprises. *Journal of the Neurological Sciences*, 2013;333(1–2):68–72; Armati PJ, et al. Clinical implications of Schwann cell biology. *Journal of the Peripheral Nerve System*, 2014;19(1):14–23; Jones S, et al. Advances and future applications of augmented peripheral nerve regeneration. *International Journal of Molecular Sciences*, 2016;17(9):1494; Monk KR, et al. New insights on Schwann cell development. *Glia*, 2015;63(8):1376–1393; Namgung U. The role of Schwann cell-axon interaction in peripheral nerve regeneration. *Cells Tissues Organs*, 2014;200(1):6–12.

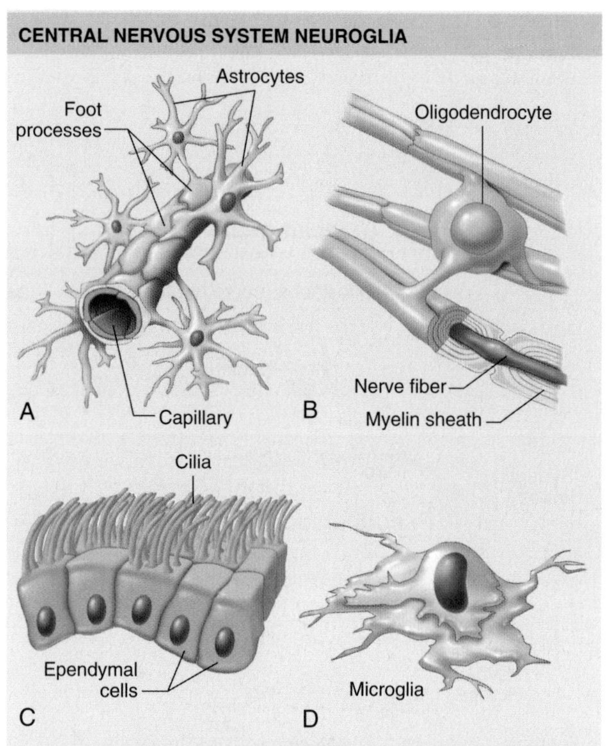

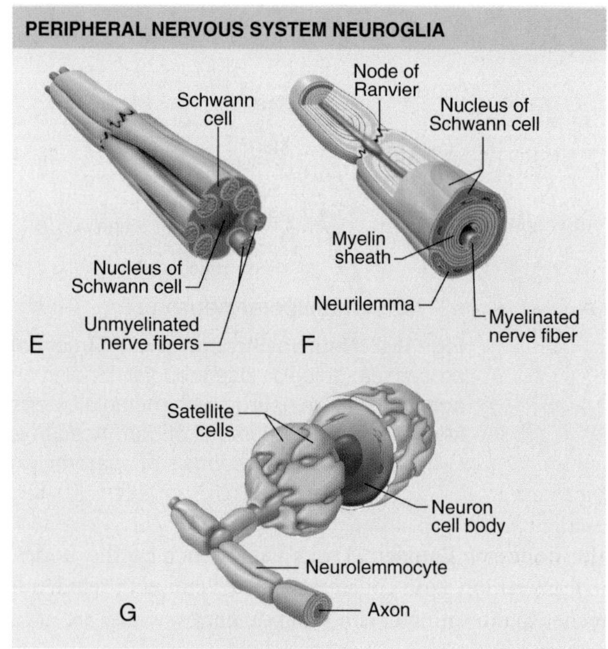

Fig. 15.3 Types of Neuroglial Cells. Neuroglia of the central nervous system (CNS): **(A)** Astrocytes attached to the outside of a capillary blood vessel in the brain. **(B)** An oligodendrocyte with processes that wrap around nerve fibers in the CNS to form myelin sheaths. **(C)** Ciliated ependymal cells forming a sheet that usually lines fluid cavities in the brain. **(D)** A phagocytic microglial cell. Neuroglia of the peripheral nervous system (PNS): **(E)** A Schwann cell supporting a bundle of nerve fibers in the PNS. **(F)** Another type of Schwann cell encircling a peripheral nerve fiber to form a thick myelin sheath. **(G)** Satellite cells, another type of Schwann cell, surround and support cell bodies of neurons in the PNS. (From Patton KT, Thibodeau GA, Douglas MM. *Essentials of anatomy & physiology*. St. Louis: Mosby; 2012.)

TABLE 15.1 Support Cells of the Nervous System

Cell Type	Primary Functions
Central Nervous System	
Astrocytes	Form specialized contacts between neuronal surfaces and blood vessels Provide rapid transport for nutrients and metabolites Thought to form an essential component of blood-brain barrier Appear to be scar-forming cells of CNS, which may be foci for seizures Appear to work with neurons in processing information and memory storage
Oligodendroglia (oligodendrocytes)	Formation of myelin sheath in CNS
Microglia	Responsible for clearing cellular debris (phagocytic properties) and the key immune cell in the CNS
Ependymal cells	Serve as a lining for ventricles and choroid plexuses involved in production of cerebrospinal fluid
Peripheral Nervous System	
Schwann cells	Formation of myelin sheath in PNS Direct axonal regrowth and functional recovery in PNS
Nonmyelinating Schwann cells	Provide neuronal metabolic support and regeneration in PNS
Satellite glial cells	Surround sensory, sympathetic, and parasympathetic nerve cell bodies and ganglia to provide protection and promote cellular communication (similar to astrocytes in CNS)

CNS, Central nervous system; *PNS*, peripheral nervous system.

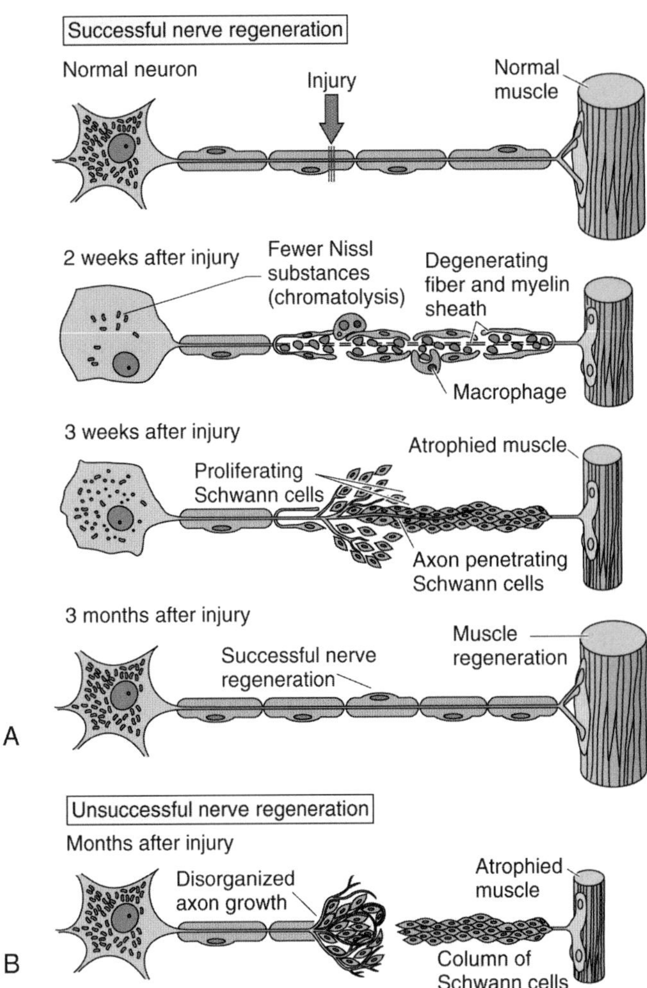

Fig. 15.4 Peripheral Nerve Regeneration Following Injury. (A) In successful nerve regeneration, Schwann cells detach from the axons, proliferate, and, with recruited macrophages, help clear cellular and myelin debris. A damaged motor axon can regrow to its distal connection only if the neurilemma remains intact (to form a guiding tunnel) and if scar tissue does not block its pathway. **(B)** Unsuccessful nerve regeneration results in the neuron remaining cut off from the effector organ. (From Gartner LP. *Textbook of histology*, 4th edition. Philadelphia: Elsevier; 2017.)

Nerve Injury and Regeneration

Mature nerve cells do not divide; therefore, injury can cause permanent loss of function. Wallerian degeneration occurs in the distal axon when an axon is severed, the portion cut off from the cell body, within hours of the injury. The morphologic and biochemical changes that occur in the distal axon include: (1) a characteristic swelling within the portion of the axon distal to the cut; (2) neurofilaments hypertrophy; (3) shrinkage and fragmentation of the myelin sheath; and (4) axon degeneration, and disappearance. The myelin sheaths reform into Schwann cells that align in a column between the severed part of the axon and the effector organ (Fig. 15.4B).

At the proximal end of the injured axon, similar changes occur but only back to the next node of Ranvier. The cell body responds to trauma by swelling and dying by chromatolysis (dispersing the Nissl substance) or apoptosis. During the repair process, the cell increases protein synthesis and mitochondrial activity. Days to weeks after injury, new terminal sprouts project from the proximal segment and may enter the remaining Schwann cell pathway. (Fig. 15.4A contains a more detailed representation of these events.)

This process is very slow (about 1 mm/day) and is limited to myelinated fibers in the PNS. The regeneration of axonal constituents in the CNS is limited by an increased incidence of glial scar formation (gliosis) and the different nature of myelin formed by the oligodendrocyte.

Nerve regeneration depends on many factors, such as the location of the injury, the type of injury, the presence of inflammatory responses, and the process of scarring. The closer the injury is to the nerve's cell body, the greater chance that the nerve cell will die and not regenerate. A crushing injury allows for fuller recovery compared with a cut injury. Crushed nerves sometimes recover fully, whereas cut nerves often form connective tissue scars that block or slow regenerating axonal branches. Peripheral nerves injured close to the spinal cord recover poorly and slowly because of the long distance between the cell body and the peripheral termination of the axon.[1]

NERVE IMPULSE

Neurons generate and conduct electrical and chemical impulses by selectively changing the electrical potential of the plasma membrane and influencing other nearby neurons by releasing chemicals (neurotransmitters). An unexcited neuron maintains a resting membrane potential. When the membrane potential is sufficiently raised, an action potential is generated, and the nerve impulse then flows to all parts of the neuron. The action potential response occurs only when the stimulus is strong enough; the membrane remains unexcited if it is too weak. This property is termed the *all-or-none response* (see Chapter 1 for a discussion of electrical impulse conduction).

Synapses

Neurons are not physically contiguous with one another. The region between adjacent neurons is called a synapse (Fig. 15.5). The neurons that conduct a nerve impulse are named according to whether they relay impulses toward (presynaptic neurons) or away from (postsynaptic neurons) the synapse. The synapse is composed of a bulbous end of the presynaptic neuron (synaptic knob) that is separated from the postsynaptic neuron by a gap called the synaptic cleft. Four basic types of connections occur in regions of contact between the presynaptic and postsynaptic neurons. These are between axons (axo-axonic), from axon to cell body (axo-somatic), from axon to dendrite (axo-dendritic), and from dendrite to dendrite (dendro-dendritic).

Impulses are transmitted across the synapse by chemical and electrical conduction (only chemical conduction is discussed here. Chapter 1 contains information on electrical conduction [see Fig.1.31].) When an impulse originates in a presynaptic neuron, the impulse reaches the vesicles, where chemicals (neurotransmitters) are stored in the synaptic bouton. Once released from the vesicles, the neurotransmitters diffuse across the synaptic cleft and bind to specific neurotransmitter (protein) receptor sites on the plasma membrane of the postsynaptic neuron, relaying the impulse (see Fig. 15.5). Brain synapses can change in strength and number throughout life, and this is known as synaptic plasticity or neuroplasticity.

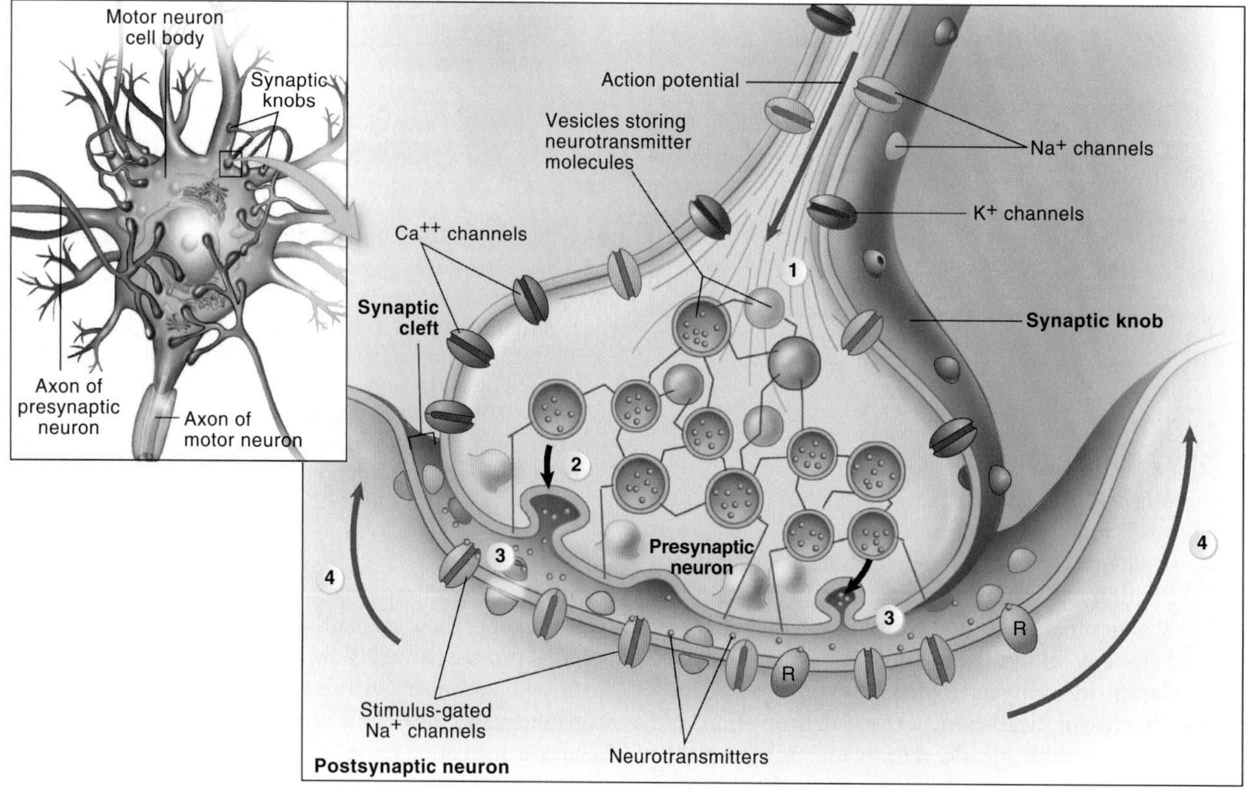

Fig 15.5 Neuronal Transmission and Synaptic Cleft. Details illustrate the synaptic bouton (knob) of a presynaptic neuron, the plasma membrane of a postsynaptic neuron, and a synaptic cleft. At **step 1**, the action potential arrives at the synaptic bouton. At **step 2**, the rapid exocytosis of neurotransmitter molecules from vesicles in the knob occurs. At **step 3**, neurotransmitter diffuses into the synaptic cleft and binds to receptor molecules *(R)* in the plasma membrane of the postsynaptic neuron. The postsynaptic receptors directly or indirectly trigger the opening of stimulus gated ion channels, initiating a local potential in the postsynaptic neuron. At **step 4**, the local potential may move toward the axon, where an action potential may begin. (Adapted from Patton KT. *Anatomy & physiology,* 10th edition. St. Louis: Mosby; 2019.)

Neurotransmitters

Neurotransmitters are chemicals synthesized in the neuron and localized in the presynaptic terminal (synaptic bouton). Neurotransmitters are released into the synaptic cleft in response to the arrival of an electrical impulse and bind to a receptor site (binding site) on the postsynaptic membrane of another neuron or effector, where they affect ion channels (see Fig. 15.5). Each neurotransmitter is removed by a specific mechanism from its site of action. Neurons can synthesize more than one neurotransmitter, and postsynaptic membranes can contain more than one type of transmitter-specific receptor. Many substances are neurotransmitters, including norepinephrine, acetylcholine, dopamine, histamine, and serotonin. Many of these transmitters have more than one function. Neuromodulators are chemical messengers released from a neuron in the CNS or the PNS, and this affects a group of neurons that have receptors for that messenger. They may have excitatory or inhibitory effects. Neurotransmitter and neuromodulator substances are summarized in Table 15.2.

Because the neurotransmitter is normally stored on one side of the synaptic cleft, and the receptor sites are on the other side, chemical synapses operate in one direction. Therefore, action

TABLE 15.2 Substances That Are Neurotransmitters or Neuromodulators

Substance	Location	Effect	Clinical Example
Acetylcholine	Many parts of the brain, spinal cord, neuromuscular junction of skeletal muscle, and many ANS synapses	Excitatory or inhibitory	Alzheimer disease (a type of dementia) is associated with a decrease in the number of acetylcholine-secreting neurons. Muscle weakness caused by myasthenia gravis results from an autoimmune response to acetylcholine receptors on the postsynaptic terminal.
Monoamines			
Norepinephrine	Many areas of the brain and spinal cord; also in some ANS synapses	Excitatory or inhibitory	CNS: Sleep-wake cycles and mood. Cocaine and amphetamines[a] result in overstimulation of postsynaptic neurons. PNS: Sympathetic nerve transmission.
Serotonin	Many areas of the brain and spinal cord	Generally inhibitory	Is involved with mood, anxiety, and sleep induction. Levels of serotonin are elevated in schizophrenia (delusions, hallucinations, withdrawal).
Dopamine	Some areas of the brain and ANS synapses	Generally excitatory	Parkinson disease (depression of voluntary motor control) results from destruction of dopamine-secreting neurons. Drugs used to increase dopamine can induce vomiting and hallucinations.
Histamine	Posterior hypothalamus	Excitatory (H1 and H2 receptors) and inhibitory (H3 receptors)	There is no clear indication of histamine-associated pathologic conditions. Histamine is involved with arousal and attention and links to other brain transmitter systems.
Amino Acids			
Gamma-aminobutyric acid (GABA)	Most neurons of the CNS have GABA receptors	Majority of postsynaptic inhibition in the brain	Drugs that increase GABA function have been used to treat epilepsy by inhibiting excessive discharge of neurons.
Glycine	Spinal cord	Most postsynaptic inhibition in the spinal cord	Glycine receptors are inhibited by strychnine.
Glutamate and aspartate	Widespread in brain and spinal cord	Excitatory	Drugs that block glutamate or aspartate, such as riluzole, are used to treat amyotrophic lateral sclerosis. These drugs might prevent overexcitation from seizures and neural degeneration.
Neuropeptides			
Endorphins and enkephalins	Widely distributed in the CNS and PNS	Generally inhibitory	Morphine and heroin bind to endorphin and enkephalin receptors on presynaptic neurons and reduce pain by blocking the release of neurotransmitters.
Substance P	Spinal cord, brain, and sensory neurons associated with pain, GI tract	Generally excitatory	Substance P is a neurotransmitter involved in pain transmission pathways. Blocking release of substance P by morphine reduces pain.
Vasoactive intestinal peptide	Gastrointestinal tract	Generally excitatory	Stimulates secretion, vasodilation, and smooth muscle relaxation (vasodilation, sphincter relaxation).

[a]Increase the release and block the reuptake of norepinephrine.
ANS, Autonomic nervous system; *CNS*, central nervous system; *GI*, gastrointestinal; *PNS*, peripheral nervous system.
From Mtui E, Gruener G, Dockery P. *Fitzgerald's clinical neuroanatomy and neuroscience*, 7th edition. Philadelphia: Elsevier; 2016.

potentials are transmitted along a multineuronal pathway in one direction. The binding of the neurotransmitter at the receptor site changes the permeability of the postsynaptic neuron and, consequently, its membrane potential. Two possible scenarios can occur:

1. The postsynaptic neuron may be excited (depolarized), called excitatory postsynaptic potentials (EPSPs). If the EPSP reaches the threshold potential, an action potential is initiated.
2. The postsynaptic neuron's plasma membrane may be inhibited (hyperpolarized), called inhibitory postsynaptic potentials (IPSPs). This makes the membrane less likely to reach the threshold potential, meaning the action potential is inhibited.

Chapter 1 reviews electrical impulses and membrane potentials.

Usually, a single EPSP cannot induce a neuron's action potential and the nerve impulse propagation. Whether this occurs, depends on the number and frequency of potentials the postsynaptic neuron receives—a concept known as summation. Temporal summation (time relationship) refers to the effects of successive, rapid impulses received from a single neuron at the same synapse. Spatial summation (spacing effect) is the combined effects of impulses from several neurons onto a single neuron simultaneously. Facilitation refers to the effect of EPSP on the plasma membrane potential. The plasma membrane is *facilitated* when summation brings the membrane closer to the threshold potential and decreases the stimulus required to induce an action potential. The effect that a chemical neurotransmitter has on the plasma membrane potential depends on the balance of these effects. The mechanisms of convergence (many neurons firing and converging on one neuron), divergence (one neuron firing and diverging on many neurons), summation, and facilitation allow for the integrative processes of the nervous system.

CENTRAL NERVOUS SYSTEM

Brain

The brain is a functionally integrated circuit of millions of neurons with different genomes, structures, molecular composition, networks, and connections. It weighs approximately 3 pounds and receives 15% to 20% of the total cardiac output. The brain enables a person to reason, function intellectually, express personality and mood and perceive and interact with the environment.

The cerebrum is the largest part of the brain and contains both gray matter and white matter. The three primary embryonic vesicles (structural divisions) of the brain are (1) the forebrain (prosencephalon), (2) the midbrain (mesencephalon), and (3) the hindbrain (rhombencephalon). These three vesicles then develop further into the secondary vesicles and their structures, which are summarized in Table 15.3 and Fig. 15.6. The midbrain, medulla, and pons comprise the brainstem, which connects the brain's hemispheres, cerebellum, and spinal cord. A collection of nerve cell bodies (nuclei) within the brainstem makes up the reticular formation. The reticular formation is a large network of diffuse nuclei that connect the brainstem to the cortex and control vital reflexes, such as cardiovascular function and respiration. It is essential for maintaining wakefulness and attention and is referred to as the reticular activating system (Fig. 15.7). Some nuclei within the reticular formation support specific motor movements, such as balance and posture.

Divisions of the brain are associated with different functions but attributing specific functions to definite brain regions is not entirely accurate. However, functional specificity is very useful for localizing pathologic conditions in various nervous system regions for clinical considerations. Brodmann areas are used to correlate functional activities to many regions of the cerebral

TABLE 15.3 Divisions of the Central Nervous System

Primary Brain Vesicles	Secondary Vesicles	Structures in Secondary Vesicles
Forebrain (prosencephalon)	Telencephalon	Cerebral hemispheres Cerebral cortex Basal ganglia
	Diencephalon	Epithalamus Thalamus Hypothalamus Subthalamus
Midbrain (mesencephalon)	Mesencephalon	Tectum (corpora quadrigemina) Superior and inferior colliculi Tegmentum Red nucleus Substantia nigra Cerebral peduncles
Hindbrain (rhombencephalon)	Metencephalon	Cerebellum Pons
	Myelencephalon	Medulla oblongata
Spinal cord	Spinal cord	Spinal cord

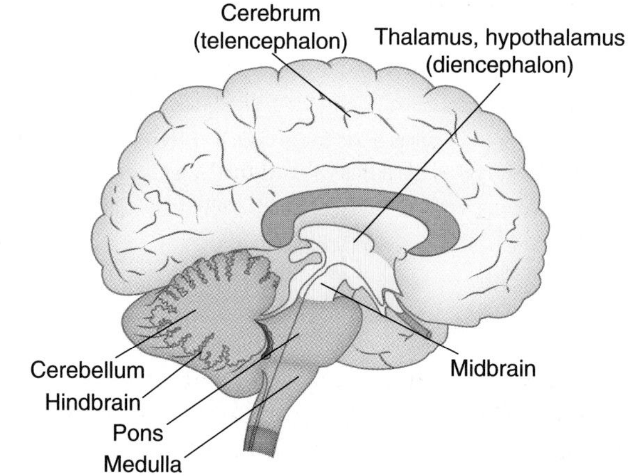

Fig. 15.6 Structural Divisions of the Brain. (From Standring S. *Gray's anatomy: The anatomical basis of clinical practice*, 40th edition. Philadelphia: Elsevier; 2008.)

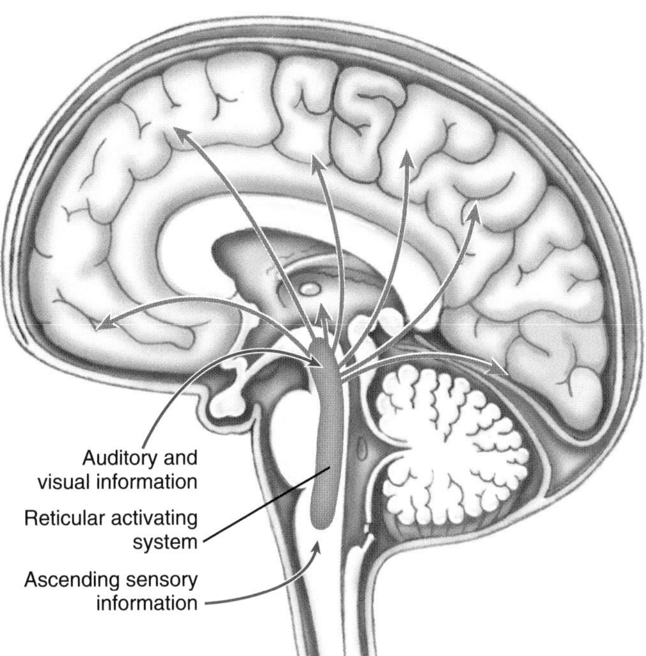

Fig. 15.7 Reticular Activating System. The reticular activating system consists of nuclei in the brainstem reticular formation plus fibers that conduct sensory information to the nuclei and fibers that conduct from the nuclei to widespread areas of the cerebral cortex. Functioning of the reticular activating system is essential for consciousness.

cortex.[2] Fig. 15.8C illustrates these regions and describes some of the areas. The mapping of brain networks is also helpful in discovering how varying parts of the brain are interconnected when performing a specific function (see Emerging Science: Brain Networks).

Forebrain

Telencephalon. The telencephalon (cerebral hemispheres) consists of the cerebral cortex (the largest portion of the brain) and the basal ganglia (composed of several *nuclei*). The surface of the cerebral cortex is covered with convolutions called *gyri* (see Fig. 15.8A), which greatly increase the cortical surface area and the number of neurons. Grooves between adjacent gyrus are termed sulci; deeper grooves are fissures. The cerebral cortex contains an outer layer of cell bodies of neurons called gray matter, which is organized into columns perpendicular to the surface that receive, integrate, store, and transmit information. The cerebral cortex is located in the frontal, parietal, temporal, and occipital lobes. White matter lies beneath the cerebral cortex and is composed of myelinated nerve fibers (axons).

Lobes. The two cerebral hemispheres are separated by a deep groove known as the longitudinal fissure (see Fig. 15.10B). The surface of each hemisphere is divided into lobes named after the region of the skull under which each lobe lies: frontal, parietal, occipital, and temporal lobes.

The posterior margin of the frontal lobe is on the central sulcus (fissure of Rolando), and it borders inferiorly on the lateral sulcus (Sylvian fissure, lateral fissure) (see Fig. 15.8A).

EMERGING SCIENCE

Brain Networks

The architecture and integrated function of neural nodes, networks, and interconnected pathways within the brain are being mapped in the advancing field of human connectomics. Imaging techniques are combined with mathematical and computational models to produce visual representations of brain networks.

The figure below provides an illustration of brain connectivity showing interconnecting cortical pathways using diffusion tensor imaging tracking technology (the imaging of diffusion of water in tissue). Such mapping of the brain contributes to an understanding of the commonalities and individual differences of the normally functioning brain and changes associated with aging and disease (i.e., degenerative brain disease, epilepsy, schizophrenia, and brain tumors).

The Human Connectome Project (HCP) began in 2010 with funding from the National Institutes of Health and sought to collect high-quality images from a wide variety of subjects that would be shared openly. HCP processed images to minimize blurring that often occurs with scans due to head movements, which makes the images produced of exceptionally high quality. They have also provided numerous neuroimaging software and informatic tools for free use. The HCP data has been used in more than 140 studies thus far and will hopefully accelerate progress in understanding the healthy and diseased brain.

Data from Filippi M, et al. Assessment of system dysfunction in the brain through MRI-based connectomics, *Lancet Neurology*. 2013;12(12):1189–1199; Glasser MF, et al. The human connectome project's neuroimaging approach. *Nature Neuroscience*, 2016;19(9):1175–1187.

The prefrontal area is responsible for goal-oriented behavior (e.g., ability to concentrate), short-term or recall memory, the elaboration of thought, and inhibition of the limbic areas of the CNS. The premotor area (Brodmann area 6) (see Fig. 15.8C) is involved in programming motor movements. This area contains the cell bodies that form part of the basal ganglia system. The frontal eye fields (the lower portion of Brodmann area 8), which control eye movements, are located on the middle frontal gyrus.

The primary motor area (Brodmann area 4) is located along the precentral gyrus forming the primary voluntary motor area. It has a specific correspondence between a body region and an area in the brain (somatotopic organization) that is often referred to as a *homunculus* (little man) (Fig. 15.9). Electrical stimulation of specific areas of this cortex causes specific muscles of the body to move. For example, stimulation of Brodmann area 4 in the medial longitudinal fissure affects the lower limb and foot, whereas stimulation of the superior lateral surface of the precentral gyrus affects the torso and arm, the middle third of the hand, and the lower third of the face and mouth/throat. The axons traveling from the cell bodies in and on either side of this gyrus project fibers (axons) that form the pyramidal system. This system includes the corticobulbar tract that synapses in the brainstem and provides voluntary control of muscles in the head and neck and the corticospinal tracts that descend into the spinal cord and provide voluntary control of muscles throughout the body. Cerebral impulses control function on the opposite side of the body, a phenomenon called *contralateral control* (see Fig. 15.15 later in the chapter). The Broca speech area is on the inferior frontal gyrus (Brodmann areas 44, 45). It is usually on the left hemisphere and is responsible for the motor aspects of speech. Damage to this area, commonly as a result of a cerebrovascular accident (stroke), results in the inability to

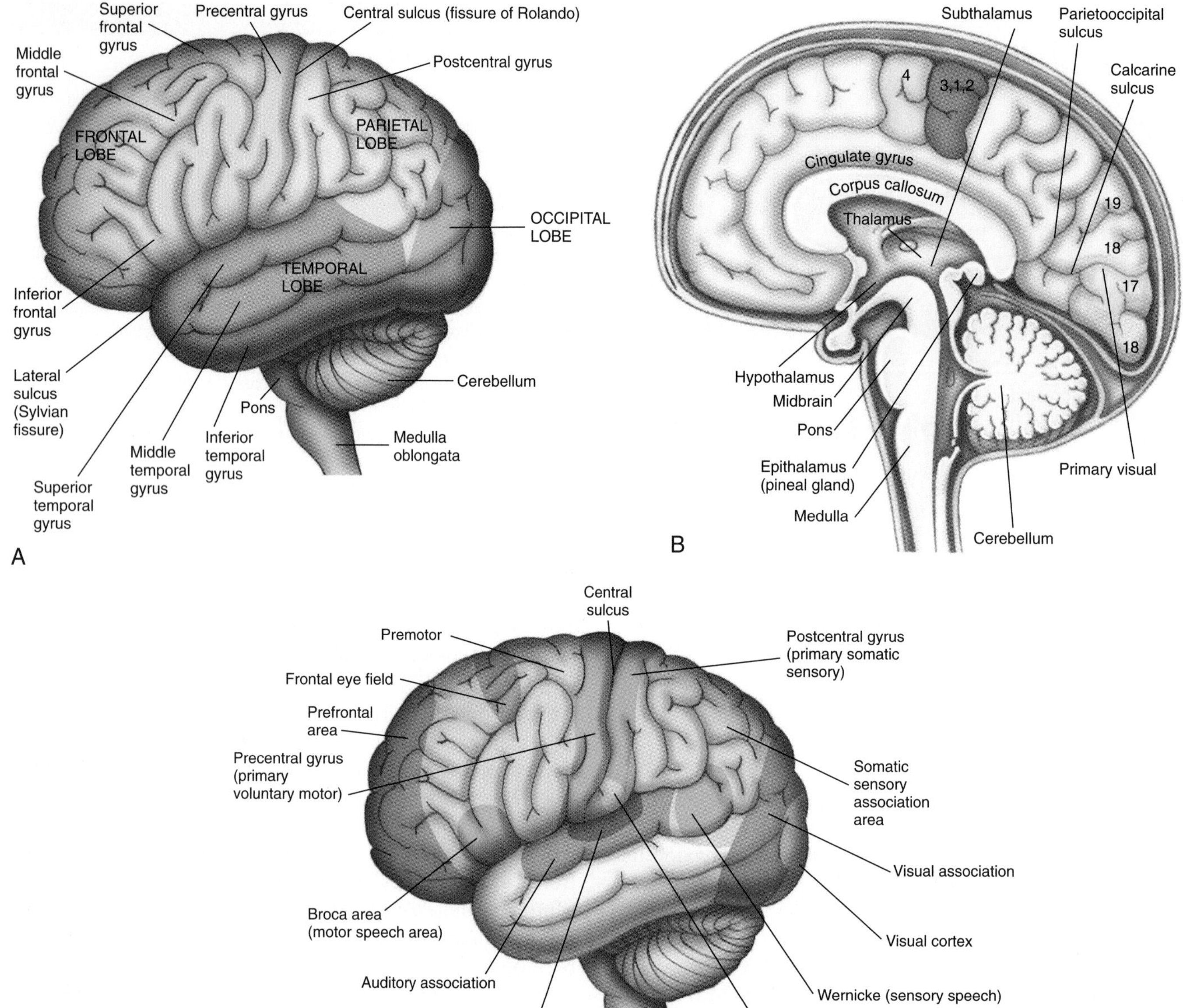

Fig. 15.8 The Cerebral Hemispheres. (A) Left hemisphere of cerebrum, lateral view. **(B)** Functional areas of the cerebral cortex, midsagittal view. **(C)** Functional areas of the cerebral cortex, lateral view.

form words or at least some difficulty in forming words (expressive aphasia) (see Chapter 17).

The parietal lobe lies within the borders of the central, parietooccipital, and lateral sulci. This lobe contains the major area for somatic sensory input, located primarily along the postcentral gyrus (Brodmann areas 3, 1, 2) (see Fig. 15.8), which is adjacent to the primary motor area precentral gyrus. Communication between the motor and sensory areas (and among other regions in the cortex) is provided by association fibers. Much of this region is involved in sensory association (storage, analysis, and interpretation of stimuli). Fig. 15.9 shows the distribution of functions associated with both the primary motor area and the primary sensory area of the cerebral cortex.

The occipital lobe lies caudal to the parietooccipital sulcus and is superior to the cerebellum. The primary visual cortex (Brodmann area 17) is located in this region and receives input from the retinas. Much of the remainder of this lobe is involved in visual association (Brodmann areas 18, 19). The temporal lobe lies inferior to the lateral fissure and is composed of the superior, middle, and inferior temporal gyri. The primary auditory cortex (Brodmann area 41) and related association area (Brodmann area 42) lie deep within the lateral sulcus on the superior temporal gyrus. The Wernicke area (posterior portion of Brodmann area 22) and adjacent portions of the parietal lobe constitute a *sensory speech area*. This area is responsible for reception and interpretation of speech, and dysfunction may result in receptive aphasia or dysphasia.

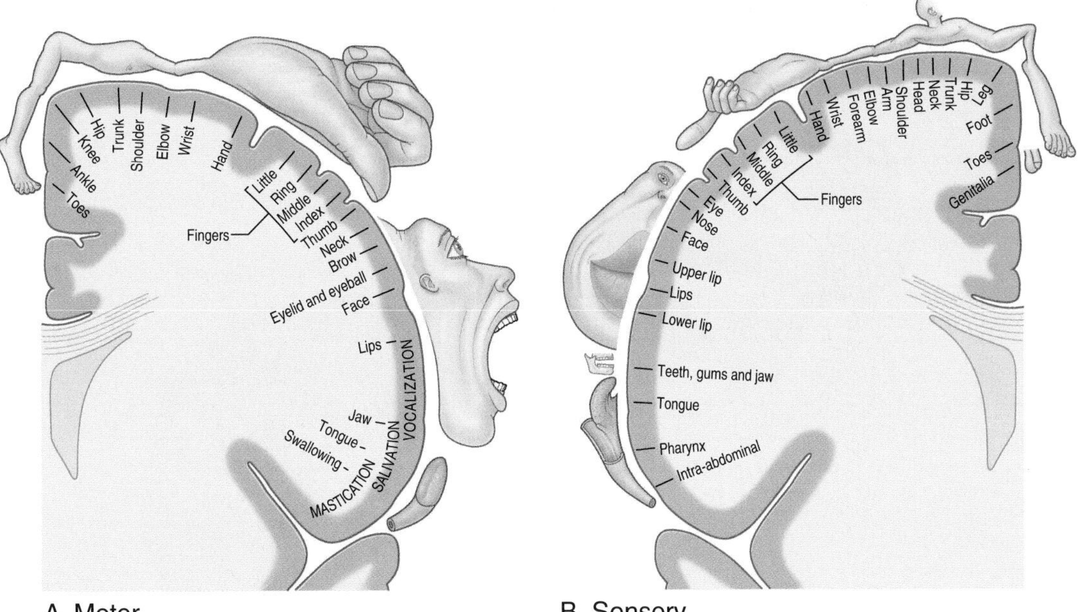

Fig. 15.9 Primary Somatic Sensory (A) and Motor (B) Areas of the Cortex. (A) The motor homunculus shows proportional somatotopic representation in the main motor area. **(B)** The sensory homunculus shows proportional somatotopic representation in the somaesthetic cortex. (From Standring S. *Gray's Anatomy*. 40th edition. Edinburgh: Churchill Livingstone; 2008.)

The temporal lobe also is involved in memory consolidation and smell.

Another lobe, the insula (insular lobe), lies hidden from view in the lateral sulci between each hemisphere's temporal and frontal lobes. The insula processes sensory and emotional information and routes the information to other areas of the brain. Lying directly beneath the longitudinal fissure is a mass of white matter pathways called the corpus callosum (transverse or commissural fibers). This structure connects the two cerebral hemispheres through sensory and motor contralateral projection of axons and is essential in coordinating activities between hemispheres (see Fig. 15.8B).

Basal ganglia. Inside the cerebrum are numerous tracts (white matter) and nuclei (gray matter). The major subcortical nuclei are called the basal ganglia (basal nuclei) system. The basal ganglia system is a group of nuclei that includes the caudate nucleus, putamen, and globus pallidus (Fig. 15.10). The putamen and the globus pallidus together are called the lentiform nucleus (because they are shaped like a lentil). The caudate nucleus, putamen, and nucleus accumbens together are called the striatum. Functionally, the substantia nigra is a component of the basal ganglia. It synthesizes dopamine, a neurotransmitter and precursor of norepinephrine. The basal ganglia nuclei are important for voluntary movement and cognitive and emotional functions (i.e., the nucleus accumbens has pleasure and reward functions).

The internal capsule is a thick layer of white matter in which axons of afferent (sensory) and efferent (motor) pathways pass to and from the cerebral cortex through the center of the cerebral hemispheres and between the caudate and lentiform nuclei (see Fig. 15.10B). The basal ganglia, plus their direct and indirect interconnections with the thalamus, premotor cortex, red nucleus, reticular formation, and spinal cord, have been considered part of the extrapyramidal system. The extrapyramidal system is part of the motor control system that causes involuntary reflexes and coordinated movement and stabilizes motor control. Parkinson disease and Huntington disease are characterized by disruption of the extrapyramidal system and various involuntary or exaggerated motor movements (see Chapter 17).

Limbic system. The limbic system is a group of interconnected structures between the telencephalon and diencephalon and surrounding the corpus callosum. It comprises the amygdala, hippocampus, fornix, hypothalamus, and related autonomic nuclei (see Fig. 15.10A). It is an extension or modification of the olfactory system and influences the autonomic and endocrine systems. Its principal effects are involved in primitive behavioral responses, visceral reaction to emotion, motivation, mood, feeding behaviors, biologic rhythms, and the sense of smell. The limbic system mediates emotion and long-term memory through connections in the prefrontal cortex (limbic cortex).

Diencephalon. The diencephalon (interbrain) is surrounded by the cerebrum and sits on top of the brainstem. It controls vital functions and visceral activities and is closely associated with those of the limbic system. The diencephalon has four divisions: epithalamus, thalamus, hypothalamus, and subthalamus (see Table 15.3 and Fig. 15.8). The epithalamus forms the roof of the third ventricle (a brain cavity) and composes the most superior portion of the diencephalon.

The thalamus is the largest component of the diencephalon, and it borders and surrounds the third ventricle. It is a major integrating center for afferent impulses to the cerebral cortex.

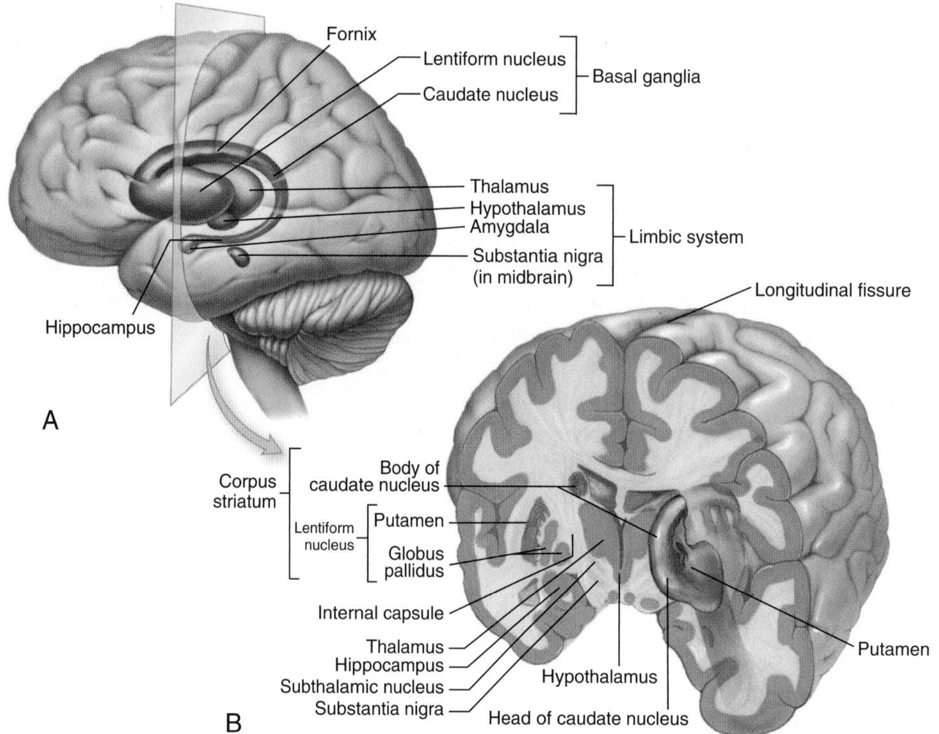

Fig. 15.10 Basal Ganglia. **(A)** The basal ganglia seen through the cortex of the left cerebral hemisphere. **(B)** The basal ganglia seen in a frontal (coronal) section of the brain. The nucleus accumbens is not visible in this figure; it lies between the caudate nucleus and putamen. (From Patton KT, Thibodeau GA. *Anatomy & Physiology*. 9th edition. St. Louis: Mosby; 2016.)

Various sensations are perceived at this level, but cortical processing is required for interpretation. The thalamus also serves as a relay center for information from the basal ganglia and cerebellum to the appropriate motor area.

The hypothalamus forms the base of the diencephalon. The hypothalamus functions to (1) maintain a constant internal environment and (2) implement behavioral patterns. Integrative centers control ANS function, regulate body temperature and endocrine function, and adjust emotional expression. The hypothalamus exerts its influence through the endocrine system and neural pathways (Box 15.1). The subthalamus flanks the hypothalamus laterally. It serves as an important basal ganglia center for motor activities.

BOX 15.1 Functions of the Hypothalamus

- Visceral and somatic responses
- Affectual responses
- Hormone synthesis
- Sympathetic and parasympathetic activity
- Temperature regulation
- Fluid balance
- Appetite and feeding responses
- Physical expression of emotions
- Sexual behavior
- Pleasure-punishment centers
- Level of arousal or wakefulness

Midbrain

Mesencephalon. The midbrain (mesencephalon) is composed of the tectum (corpora quadrigemina [forms roof of the midbrain]), the tegmentum, and the cerebral peduncles. The tectum includes two pairs of superior colliculi and two pairs of inferior colliculi. The superior colliculi are involved with voluntary and involuntary visual-motor movements (e.g., the ability of the eyes to track moving objects in the visual field). The inferior colliculi accomplish similar motor activities but involve movements affecting the auditory system (e.g., positioning the head to improve hearing). The tegmentum (the floor of the midbrain) is composed of the red nucleus and substantia nigra. The red nucleus receives ascending sensory information from the cerebellum and projects a minor motor pathway, the rubrospinal tract, to the cervical spinal cord. The substantia nigra synthesizes dopamine. The cerebral peduncles of the anterior midbrain are made up of efferent fibers of the corticospinal, corticobulbar, and corticopontocerebellar tracts (tracts that link the cortex to the brainstem).

Other notable structures of this region are the nuclei of the third and fourth cranial nerves. The cerebral aqueduct (aqueduct of Sylvius), which carries cerebrospinal fluid (CSF), also traverses this structure. Obstruction of this aqueduct is often the cause of hydrocephalus.

Hindbrain

Metencephalon. The major structures of the metencephalon are the cerebellum and the pons. The cerebellum (see Fig. 15.8) is composed of two lobes of gray matter and white matter, and its cortical surface is convoluted, similar to the surface of the cerebrum. It also is divided by a central fissure into the right and left lobes connected by the vermis.

The cerebellum is responsible for reflexive, involuntary fine-tuning of motor control and maintaining balance and posture through extensive neural connections with the medulla (through the inferior cerebellar peduncle) and the midbrain (through the superior cerebellar peduncle). The two hemispheres are connected to the pons by the middle cerebellar peduncles. These connections allow extensive sampling of visual, vestibular, and proprioceptive data from other regions of the CNS and periphery. The cerebellum has *ipsilateral control* (same side) of the body, in contrast to the cerebral cortex, which has contralateral control of the body.

The pons (bridge) is easily recognized by its bulging appearance below the midbrain and above the medulla. Primarily it transmits information from the cerebellum to the brainstem and between the two cerebellar hemispheres. The nuclei of the fifth through eighth cranial nerves are located in this structure.

Myelencephalon. The myelencephalon usually is called the *medulla oblongata* and forms the lowest portion of the brainstem. Reflex activities, such as heart rate, respiration, blood pressure, coughing, sneezing, swallowing, and vomiting, are controlled in this area. The nuclei of cranial nerves IX through XII are located in this region.

A major portion of the descending motor pathways (i.e., corticospinal tracts) cross to the other side, or decussate, at the medulla (see Fig. 15.15 later in the chapter). These pathways, together with other areas of decussation in the CNS, are the basis for the phenomenon of contralateral control when cerebral impulses control function on the opposite side of the body. Sleep–wake rhythms also are processed by neural influences from lower brain centers and are associated with a complex group of diffuse structures and functions (see Chapter 16), including the reticular activating system (cells that receive collateral signals from the afferent sensory pathways and project the signals to the higher brain centers, thus controlling CNS activity) (see Fig. 15.7).

Spinal Cord

The spinal cord is the portion of the CNS that lies within the vertebral canal and is surrounded and protected by the vertebral column. The spinal cord has many functions, including connecting the brain and the body through a long nerve cable, somatic and autonomic reflexes, motor pattern control, and sensory and motor modulation. The spinal cord originates in the medulla oblongata and ends at the first or second lumbar vertebra level in adults (Fig. 15.11A). The end of the spinal cord, the conus medullaris, is cone-shaped. Spinal nerves continue from the end of the spinal cord and form a nerve bundle called the cauda equine. The filament anchor from the conus medullaris to the coccyx is the filum terminale. The coverings of the spinal cord are illustrated in Fig. 15.11C.

Grossly, the spinal cord is divided into vertebral sections (8 cervical, 12 thoracic, 5 lumbar, 5 sacral, and 1 coccygeal) that correspond to paired nerves (see Fig. 15.11A). A cross section of the spinal cord (Fig. 15.12) is characterized by a butterfly-shaped inner core of gray matter (containing nerve cell bodies). The central canal is filled with CSF, lies in the center of this region, and extends through the spinal cord from its origin in the fourth ventricle. The gray matter of the spinal cord is divided into three regions and displays specific functional characteristics. These regions include the posterior horn, the lateral horn, and the anterior horn. The posterior horn, or dorsal horn, is composed primarily of interneurons and axons from sensory neurons whose cell bodies lie in the dorsal root ganglion. At the tip of the posterior horn is the substantia gelatinosa, a structure involved in pain transmission (see Chapter 16). The lateral horn contains cell bodies involved with the ANS. The anterior horn, or ventral horn, contains the nerve cell bodies for efferent pathways that leave the spinal cord by way of spinal nerves.

Surrounding the gray matter is white matter, which forms ascending and descending pathways called spinal tracts. Spinal tracts are named to denote their beginning and ending points. For example, the spinothalamic tract (see Fig. 15.12) carries sensory nerve impulses from the spinal cord to the thalamus in the diencephalon. Numerous spinal tracts are grouped into columns according to their location within the white matter. These include the anterior columns, lateral columns, and **posterior columns** (see Fig. 15.12).

Neural circuits in the spinal cord, when activated, display specific sets of motor responses. Reflex arcs form basic units that respond to stimuli and provide protective circuitry for motor output. Structures needed for a reflex arc are a receptor, an afferent (sensory) neuron, an efferent (motor) neuron, and an effector muscle or gland. A simple reflex arc (e.g., knee-jerk reflex) may contain only two neurons (Fig. 15.13). Interneurons are usually present and provide a link between sensory and motor neurons. The motor effects of reflex arcs generally occur before the event is perceived in the brain's higher centers. Much internal environmental regulation is mediated by the ANS's reflex activity (e.g., cardiac muscle and smooth muscle contraction/relaxation and glandular responses).

Afferent pathways transmit sensory information from peripheral receptors toward the cerebrum. The pathways terminate in the cerebral or cerebellar cortex or both. Efferent pathways primarily relay information away from the cerebrum to the brainstem or spinal cord. Upper motor neurons (i.e., corticospinal and corticobulbar tracts) are completely contained within the CNS. Their primary roles are controlling fine motor movement and influencing/modifying spinal reflex arcs and circuits. Generally, upper motor neurons form synapses with interneurons, forming synapses with lower motor neurons that project into the periphery. Lower motor neurons directly influence muscles. Their cell bodies lie in the brainstem and spinal cord's gray matter, but their processes extend out of the CNS and into the PNS. Destruction of upper motor neurons usually results in initial paralysis followed within days or weeks by partial recovery, whereas destruction of the *lower motor neurons*

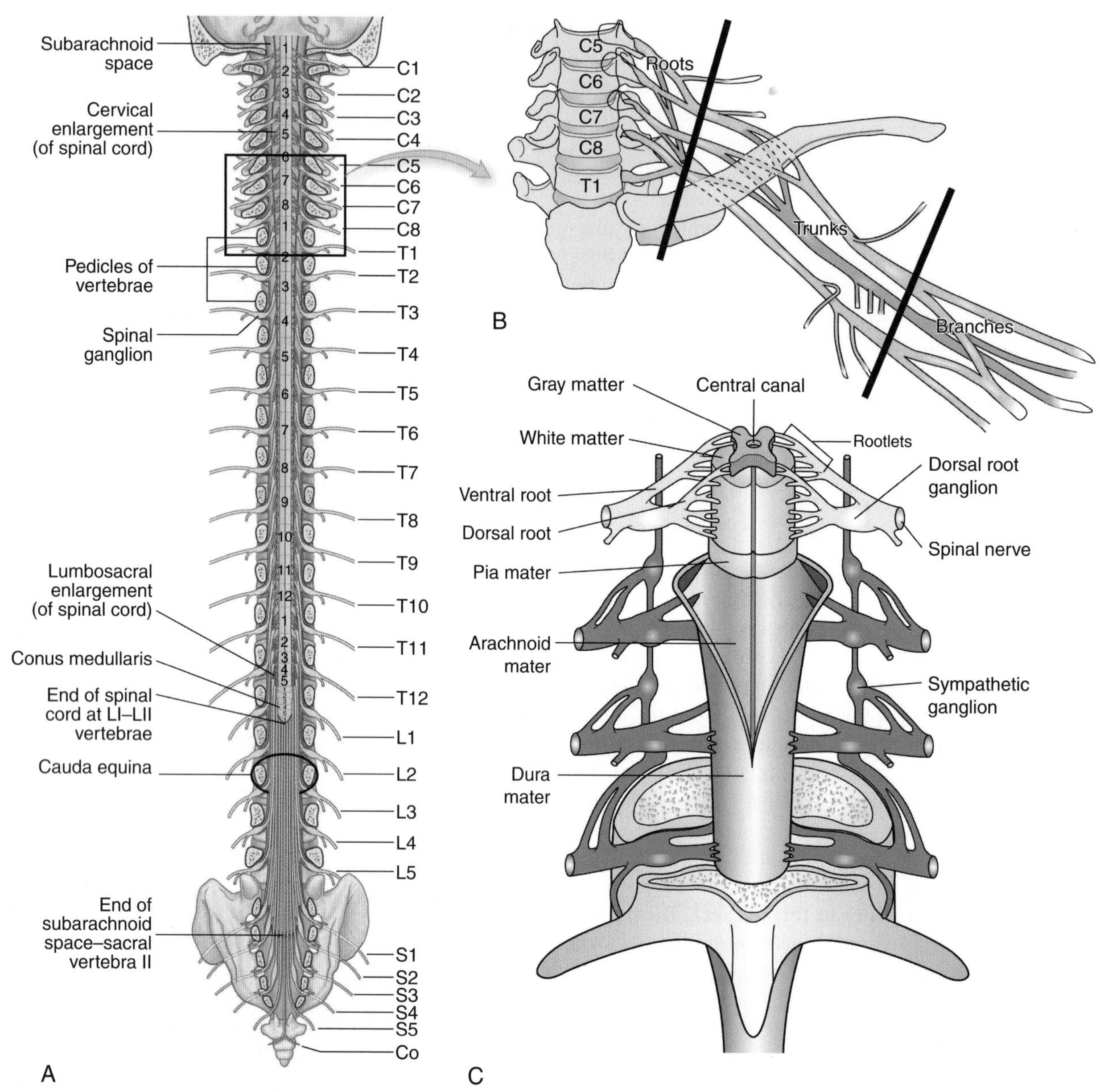

Fig. 15.11 Vertebral Canal, Spinal Cord, and Spinal Nerves. **(A)** Spinal cord and nerve root; cranial through sacral nerve distributions. **(B)** Enlarged schematic of the brachial plexus is shown. The general schematic of a spinal nerve can be compared to a tree with roots, trunks, and branches. **(C)** Coverings of the spinal cord. The dura mater is shown in purple. Note how it extends to cover the spinal nerve roots and nerves. The arachnoid mater is highlighted in pink and the pia mater in orange. (A, From Drake R, Gray H, Vogl W, et al. *Gray's anatomy for students*, 3rd edition. London: Churchill Livingstone; 2015. B, From Tu YK, Chung KC. *Practical management of pediatric and adult brachial plexus palsies*. London: Saunders; 2012. C, From Patton KT, Thibodeau GA. *Structure and function of the body*, 15th edition. St. Louis: Mosby; 2016.)

leads to paralysis unless peripheral nerve damage is followed by nerve regeneration and recovery (see Fig. 15.4). Differences in injury to upper and lower motor neurons are presented in Chapter 17.

Nerve impulses regulate muscle activity (i.e., stimulation and contraction). Motor neurons innervate one or more muscle cells, forming motor units, consisting of a neuron and the skeletal muscles it stimulates. The junction between the axon of the motor neuron and the plasma membrane of the muscle cell is called the neuromuscular (myoneural) junction (Fig. 15.14). (Injury to motor neurons is discussed in Chapter 17.)

Motor Pathways

Clinically relevant motor pathways are the lateral corticospinal (connects motor cortex with anterior horn cells in the spinal cord) and pyramidal tracts (connects the motor cortex with the medullary pyramids and descend to synapse with lower motor neurons of several cranial nerves in the brain stem or

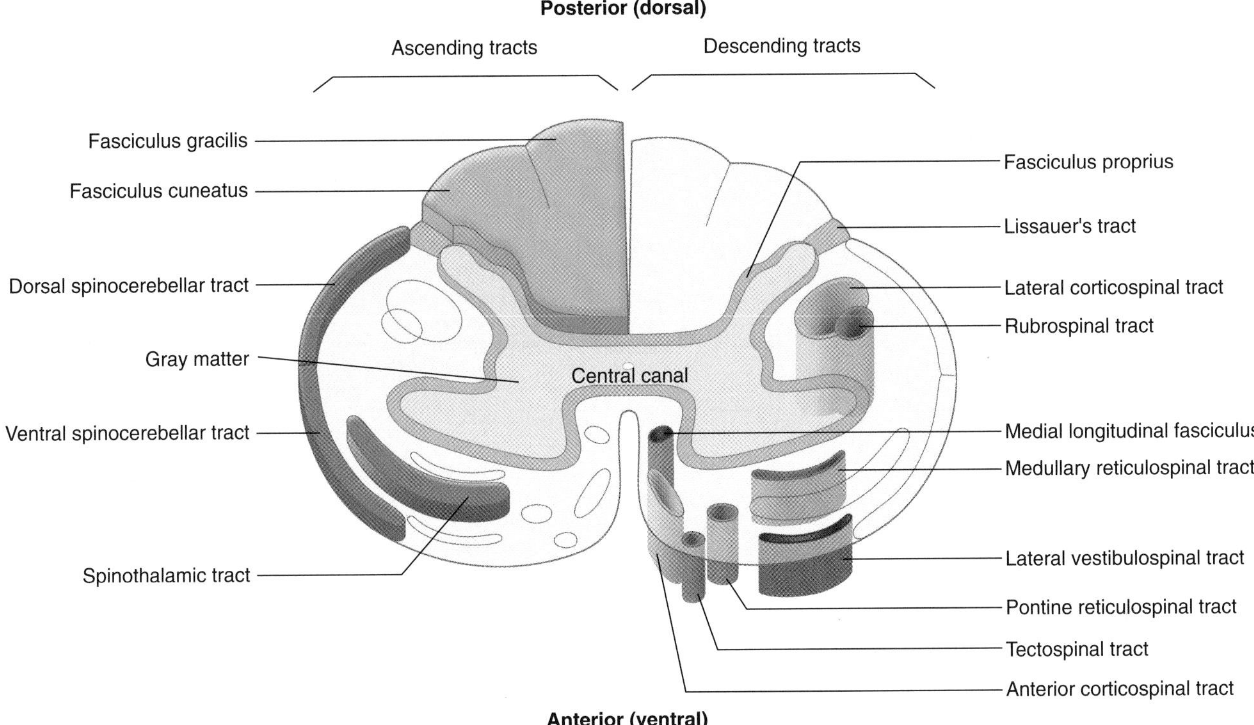

Fig. 15.12 The Spinal Cord. All ascending *(sensory)* and descending *(motor)* tracts are present bilaterally. In this figure, ascending tracts are emphasized on the left side, and descending tracts are emphasized on the right side. The location of the Lissauer tract and the fasciculus proprius (which contain both ascending and descending fibers) are also shown. (From Crossman AR, Neary D. *Neuroanatomy: An illustrated colour text*, 4th edition. London: Churchill Livingstone; 2015.)

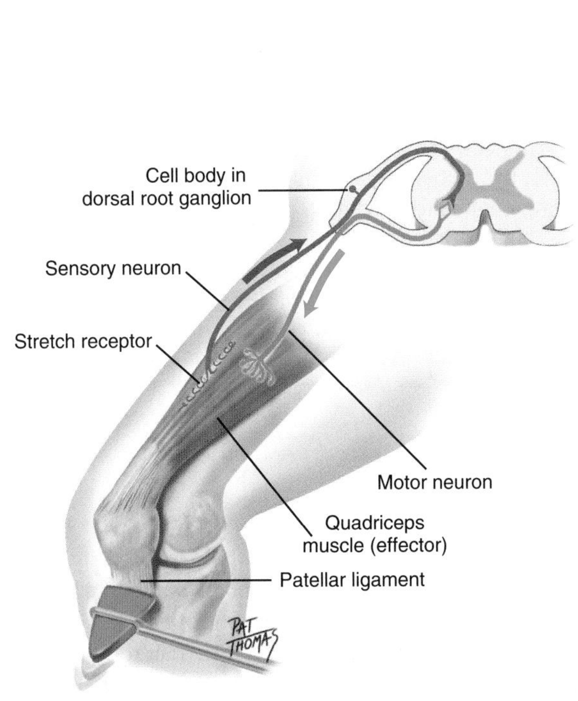

Fig. 15.13 Cross-Section of Spinal Cord Showing Simple Reflex Arc. (From Jarvis C. *Physical examination & health assessment*, 7th edition. St. Louis: Saunders; 2016.)

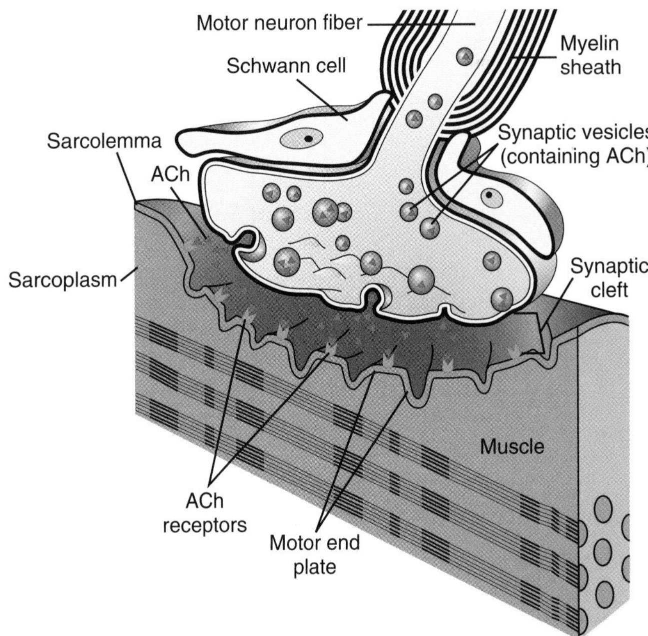

Fig. 15.14 Normal Neuromuscular Junction. This figure shows how the distal end of a motor neuron fiber forms a synapse, or "chemical junction," with an adjacent muscle fiber. Neurotransmitters (specifically, acetylcholine *[ACh]*) are released from the neuron's synaptic vesicles and diffuse across the synaptic cleft. There they stimulate receptors in the motor end-plate region of the sarcolemma. (From Damjanov I. *Pathology for the health professions*, 4th edition. St. Louis: Saunders; 2012.)

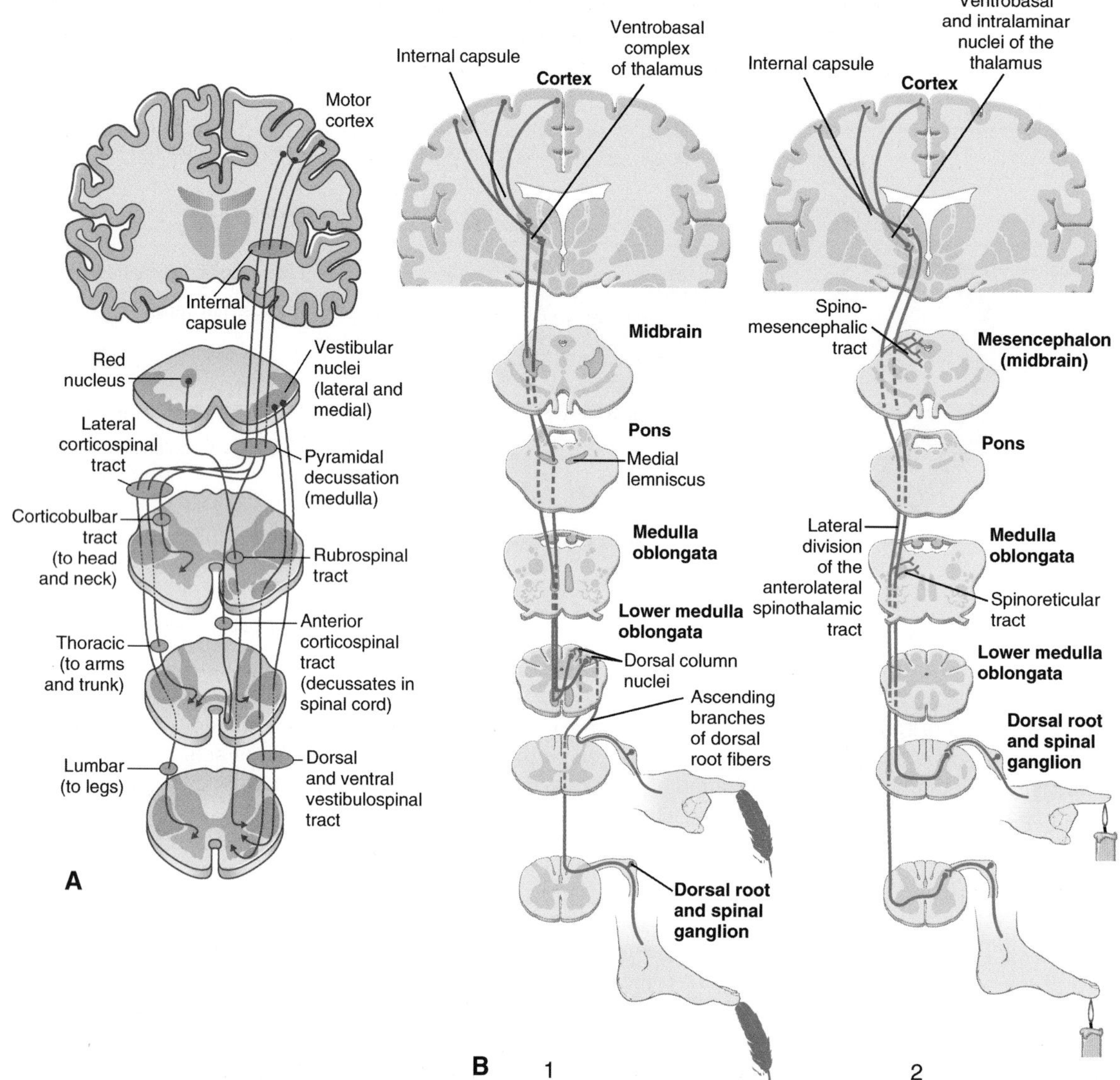

Fig. 15.15 Examples of Somatic Motor and Sensory Pathways. (A) Motor tracts. The pyramidal pathway through the lateral corticospinal tract and the extrapyramidal pathways through the rubrospinal, reticulospinal, and vestibulospinal tracts. Note that the pathways from the motor cortex cross over to the opposite side of the body, demonstrating contralateral control. **(B)** Sensory tracts. **1,** The dorsal column-medial lemniscal pathway for transmitting critical types of tactile signals: touch/proprioception. Note the lateral corticospinal tract decussation; the point where it crosses to the other side is in the lower medulla. **2,** Anterior and lateral divisions of the anterolateral spinothalamic sensory tract: pain/temperature. Note the decussation is in the spinal cord. (A, From Compston A, Lassmann H, McDonald I. *McAlpine's multiple sclerosis*, 4th edition. London: Churchill Livingstone; 2006. B, From Hall JE. *Guyton and Hall textbook of medical physiology*, 13th edition. Philadelphia: Saunders; 2016.)

spinal cord); and the extrapyramidal reticulospinal, vestibulospinal, and rubrospinal tracts. The corticospinal and corticobulbar pathways are essentially the same tract and consist of a two-neuron chain (Fig. 15.15). The cell bodies (upper motor neurons) originate in and around the precentral gyrus; pass through the corona radiata (connects motor and sensory pathways) of the cerebrum, the internal capsule, middle three-fifths of the cerebral pedunculus, pons, and pyramid; and decussate (cross contralaterally) in the medulla oblongata and form the lateral corticospinal tract of the spinal cord (see Figs. 15.12 and 15.15A) and thus control the opposite side of the body. The **corticobulbar tract axons** synapse on motor cranial nuclei within the brainstem that control the face, head, and neck muscles. The lateral corticospinal tract axons leave the tract to go to specific interneurons or motor neurons in the anterior horn. The **lateral corticospinal tract** has the same somatotopic organization as the body (see Figs. 15.9 and 15.15A). These lower motor neurons project through nerves to specific muscles.

The extrapyramidal tracts are involved in precise motor movements. The reticulospinal tract arises in the reticular formation of the medulla or pons (see Fig. 15.12) and modulates motor movement by inhibiting and exciting spinal activity. The vestibulospinal tract arises from a vestibular nucleus in the pons and causes the extensor muscles of the body to rapidly contract, most dramatically witnessed when a person starts to fall backward. The rubrospinal tract originates in the red nucleus, decussates, and terminates in the cervical spinal cord. It is important for muscle movement and fine muscle control in the upper extremities.

Sensory Pathways

The three clinically important spinal afferent pathways are the posterior column, anterior spinothalamic tract, and lateral spinothalamic tract (see Figs. 15.12 and 15.15B). The posterior (dorsal) column (fasciculus gracilis and fasciculus cuneatus) carries fine-touch sensation, two-point discrimination, and proprioceptive information (i.e., epicritic information). The posterior column is formed by a three-neuron chain. The first neuron of the chain is the primary afferent neuron. It also is the sensory neuron of the reflex arc. After entering the spinal cord, it sends its axon ipsilaterally (on the same side) up the spinal cord to a specific part of the posterior column and synapses in the three posterior column nuclei in the medulla oblongata. For example, a basketball player who is above 6 feet tall has primary afferent neurons that could be 6 feet long, running from the great toe up to the medulla oblongata. The axon of the second-order neuron crosses contralaterally in the medial lemniscus and ascends in the medulla and pons to synapse with a specific nucleus of the thalamus. The third-order neuron, originating in the thalamus, continues the tract into the internal capsule, corona radiata, and postcentral gyrus (Brodmann areas 3, 1, 2) (see Fig. 15.8, and 15.15B).

The **anterior** and lateral spinothalamic tracts are responsible for vague touch sensation and pain and temperature perception, respectively (see Figs. 15.12 and 15.15; see Chapter 16). These modalities are referred to as protopathic. These tracts also form a three-neuron chain. However, their primary afferent neurons synapse in the posterior horn of the spinal cord is not just at the level they enter the intervertebral foramen but in several spinal segments above and below their point of entry. This is an example of divergence. The axons of the second-order neurons in the posterior horn cross to the contralateral side in the spinal cord in the lateral column, ascend to the same thalamic nucleus as the posterior column pathway, and continue with the posterior column pathway to the postcentral gyrus.

Protective Structures

Cranium

The cranial vault encloses and protects the brain and its associated structures. The bony cranium comprises eight bones (frontal, two parietal, two temporal, ethmoid, sphenoid, and occipital). The galea aponeurotica, a thick, fibrous band of tissue overlying the cranium between the frontal and occipital muscles, affords added protection to the skull. The subgaleal space has venous connections with the dural sinuses. If there is increased intracranial pressure, blood can be shunted to the space, thus reducing pressure in the intracranial cavity. The subgaleal space is also a common site for wound drains after intracranial surgery.

The floor of the cranial vault is irregular and contains many foramina (openings) for cranial nerves, blood vessels, and the spinal cord to exit. The cranial floor is divided into three fossae (depressions). The frontal lobes lie in the anterior fossa, the temporal lobes and base of the diencephalon lie in the middle fossa (temporal fossa), and the cerebellum lies in the posterior fossa. These terms are commonly used anatomic landmarks to describe the location of intracranial lesions.

Meninges

Surrounding the brain and spinal cord are three protective membranes: the dura mater, the arachnoid, and the pia mater. Collectively they are called the meninges (Fig. 15.16C). The dura mater (meaning literally "hard mother") is composed of two layers, with the venous sinuses formed between them. The outermost layer forms the periosteum (endosteal layer) of the skull. The inner dura (meningeal layer) is responsible for forming rigid membranes that support and separate various brain structures. One of these membranes, the falx cerebri, dips between the two cerebral hemispheres along the longitudinal fissure. The falx cerebri is anchored anteriorly to the base of the brain at the crista galli of the ethmoid bone. The tentorium cerebelli, a common landmark, is a membrane that separates the cerebellum below from the cerebral structures above. Internal to the dura mater is the location of the arachnoid, a spongy, web-like structure that loosely follows the contours of the cerebral structures.

The subdural space lies between the dura and arachnoid. Many small bridging veins that have little structural support traverse the subdural space. Their disruption results in a subdural hematoma (see Chapter 18). The subarachnoid space lies between the arachnoid and the pia mater and contains CSF (see Fig. 15.16C). Unlike the dura mater and the arachnoid, the delicate pia mater adheres to the brain and spinal cord contours. It provides support for blood vessels serving brain tissue. The choroid plexuses, which are structures that produce CSF, arise from the pia membrane.

The spinal cord is anchored to the vertebrae by extension of the meninges (see Fig. 15.11C). The meninges continue beyond the end of the spinal cord (at vertebrae levels L1 and L2) to the lower portion of the sacrum. CSF within the subarachnoid space also circulates down to the large lumbar cistern, extending from the second lumbar vertebra to the second sacral vertebra. Cisterns are expanded areas of the subarachnoid space. The cerebellomedullary cistern (cisterna magna) and the pontine cistern are two other important cisterns.

The meninges form potential and real spaces important to understanding functional and pathologic mechanisms. For example, between the dura mater and skull lies a potential space termed the extradural space (also called the epidural space) (see Fig. 15.16C). The arterial supply to the meninges consists of blood vessels that lie within grooves in the skull. A skull fracture can sever one of these vessels and produce an epidural hematoma.

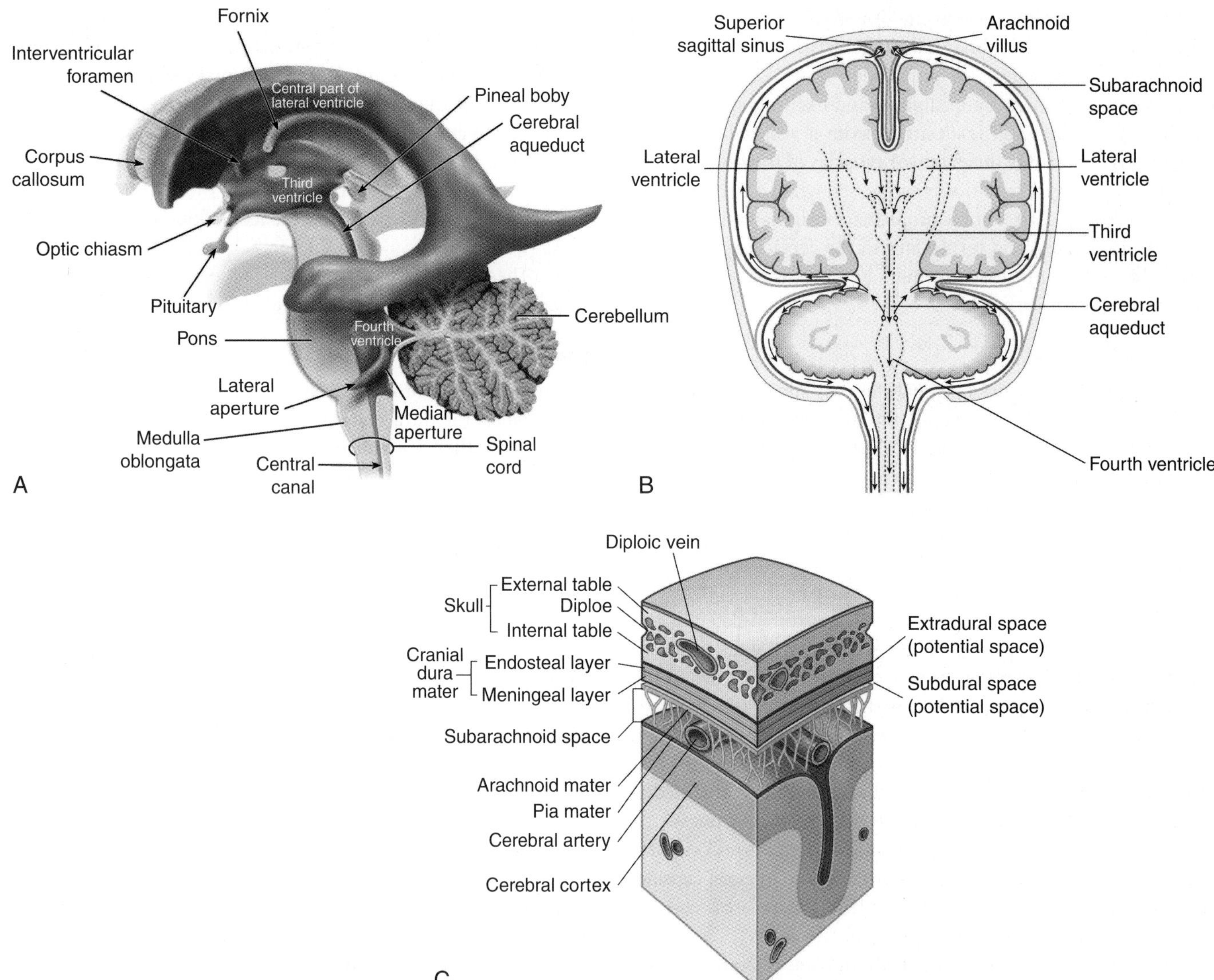

Fig. 15.16 Flow of Cerebrospinal Fluid and Meninges of the Brain. (A) Ventricles highlighted in blue within a translucent brain in a left lateral view. **(B)** Flow of cerebral spinal fluid. The fluid produced by filtration of blood by the choroid plexus of each ventricle flows inferiorly through the lateral ventricles, interventricular foramen, third ventricle, cerebral aqueduct, fourth ventricle, and subarachnoid space to the blood. **(C)** Meninges of the brain in relation to cerebrospinal fluid and venous blood flow. (A and B, From Waugh A, Grant A. *Ross and Wilson anatomy and physiology in health and illness*, 12th edition. London: Churchill Livingstone; 2012. C, From Drake RL, Gray H, Vogl W, et al. *Gray's anatomy for students*, 3rd edition. London: Churchill Livingstone; 2015.)

Cerebrospinal Fluid and the Ventricular System

Cerebrospinal fluid (CSF) is a clear, colorless fluid similar to blood plasma and interstitial fluid. The intracranial and spinal cord structures float in CSF and are thereby partially protected from jolts and blows. The buoyant properties of the CSF also prevent the brain from tugging on meninges, nerve roots, and blood vessels. (Constituents of CSF are listed in Table 15.4.) Between 125 and 150 mL of CSF is circulating within the ventricles (small cavities) and subarachnoid space at any given time. Approximately 600 mL of CSF is produced daily.

Ependymal cells in the choroid plexuses of the lateral, third, and fourth ventricles produce the major portion of CSF. (Ventricles are illustrated in Fig. 15.16A.) These plexuses are characterized by a rich network of blood vessels supplied by the pia mater and lie close to the ependymal cells of the ventricles. The tight junctions of the choroid blood vessel provide a limiting barrier between CSF and blood, which functions similarly to the blood-brain barrier (see the Blood-Brain Barrier section).

CSF exerts pressure within the brain and the spinal cord. When a person is supine, CSF pressure is about 80 to 180 mm of water pressure or approximately 5 to 14 mm of mercury pressure, but doubles when the person moves to the upright position. CSF flow results from the pressure gradient between the arterial system and the CSF-filled cavities. Beginning in the lateral ventricles,

TABLE 15.4 Composition of Cerebrospinal Fluid

Constituent	Normal Value
Sodium (Na^+)	148 mM
Potassium (K^+)	2.9 mM
Chloride (Cl^-)	125 mM
Bicarbonate (HCO3−)	22.9 mM
Glucose (fasting)	50–75 mg/dL (60% of serum glucose)
pH	7.3
Protein	15–45 mg/dL
Albumin	80%
Globulin	6%–10%
Blood cells	
White (lymphocyte)	0–6/mm^3
Red	0

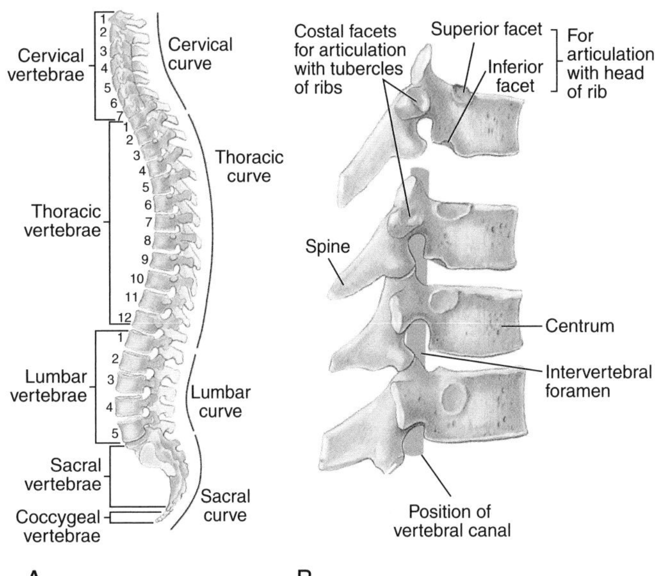

Fig. 15.17 Vertebral Column. (A) The normal curves and regions of the vertebral column. The vertebrae in each region are numbered. **(B)** Lateral view of several vertebrae showing how they articulate. (From Solomon E. *Introduction to human anatomy and physiology*, 4th edition. St. Louis: Saunders; 2016.)

the CSF flows through the interventricular foramen (foramen of Monro) into the third ventricle and then passes through the cerebral aqueduct (aqueduct of Sylvius) into the fourth ventricle (see Fig. 15.16B). The CSF may pass through the fourth ventricle, through the paired lateral apertures (foramen of Luschka), or the median aperture (foramen of Magendie) before communicating with the subarachnoid spaces of the brain and spinal cord. CSF is produced continually but does not accumulate. Instead, it is reabsorbed into the venous circulation through the arachnoid villi. The arachnoid villi protrude from the arachnoid space through the dura mater and lie within the blood flow of the venous sinuses (see Fig. 15.16B). CSF is reabsorbed through a pressure gradient between the arachnoid villi and the cerebral venous sinuses. The villi function as one-way valves directing CSF outflow into the blood but preventing blood flow into the subarachnoid space. Thus, CSF is formed from blood, and after circulating throughout the CNS, it returns to blood.

Vertebral Column

The vertebral column (Fig. 15.17) is composed of 33 vertebrae: 7 cervical, 12 thoracic, 5 lumbar, 5 fused sacral, and 4 fused coccygeal. Between each vertebra (except for the fused sacral and coccygeal vertebrae) is an intervertebral disk (Fig. 15.18). At the center of the intervertebral disk is the nucleus pulposus, a pulpy mass of elastic fibers. The intervertebral disk absorbs shocks, preventing damage to the vertebrae. The intervertebral disk is also a common source of back problems. If too much stress is applied to the vertebral column, the disk contents may rupture and protrude into the spinal canal, causing spinal cord compression or nerve roots. The disks can also degenerate.

BLOOD SUPPLY

Blood Supply to the Brain

The brain receives approximately 20% of the cardiac output or 800 to 1000 mL of blood flow per minute. Cerebral blood flow is autoregulated to maintain a stable flow during fluctuating perfusion pressures. Carbon dioxide is a primary regulator of blood flow within the CNS. It is a potent vasodilator, and its effects ensure an adequate blood supply.

The brain derives its arterial supply from the internal carotid arteries and the vertebral arteries (Fig. 15.19). The internal carotid arteries supply a proportionately greater amount of blood flow. They originate at the common carotid arteries, enter the cranium through the base of the skull, and pass through the cavernous sinus. After forming some small branches, these arteries divide into the anterior and middle cerebral arteries (Fig. 15.20). The vertebral arteries originate at the subclavian arteries and pass through the transverse foramina of the cervical vertebrae, entering the cranium through the foramen magnum. They join at the junction of the pons and medulla to form the basilar artery (see Fig. 15.20). The basilar artery divides at the level of the midbrain to form paired posterior cerebral arteries.

Three major paired arteries perfuse the cerebellum and brainstem: the posterior inferior cerebellar artery, the anterior inferior cerebellar artery, and the superior cerebellar arteries. They originate from the basilar artery. The basilar artery also gives rise to small pontine arteries. The large arteries on the surface of the brain and their branches are called superficial arteries (conducting arteries). Small branches that project into the brain are termed projecting arteries (nutrient arteries).

The circle of Willis (see Fig. 15.20B) provides an alternative route for blood flow when one of the contributing arteries is obstructed (collateral blood flow). The circle of Willis is formed by the posterior cerebral arteries, posterior communicating arteries, internal carotid arteries, anterior cerebral

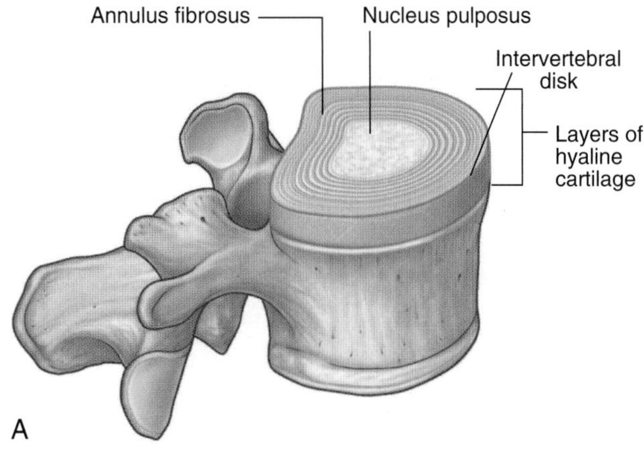

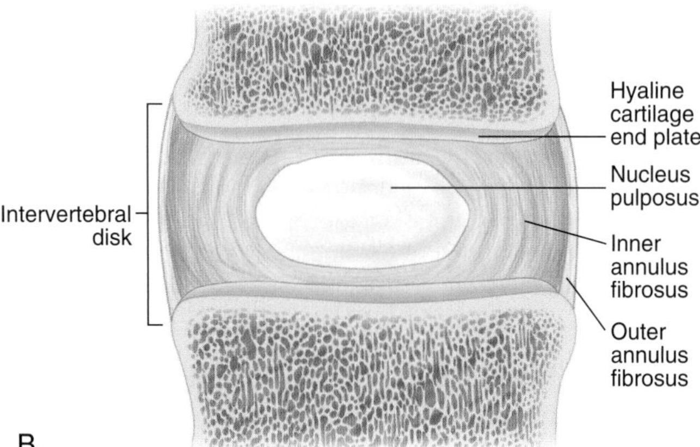

Fig. 15.18 Intervertebral Disk. (A) Sagittal view of vertebra and intervertebral disk. **(B)** Lateral view of several vertebrae showing how they articulate. (A, From Drake R, Vogl AW, Mitchell AWM. *Gray's anatomy for students*, 3rd edition. London: Churchill Livingstone; 2015. B, From Lawry GV, Kreder HJ, Hawker G, Jerome, D. *Fam's musculoskeletal examination and joint injection techniques*, 2nd edition. Philadelphia: Mosby; 2010.)

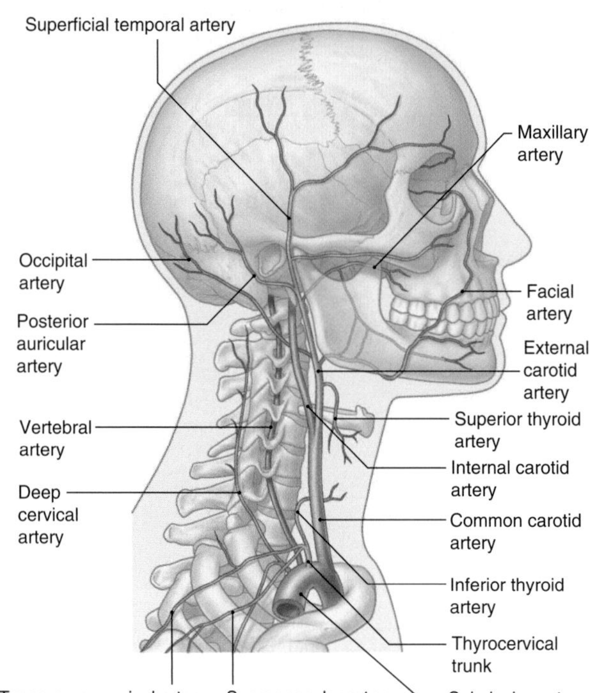

Fig. 15.19 Major Arteries of the Head and Neck. (From Moses KP. *Atlas of clinical gross anatomy*, 2nd edition. Philadelphia: Saunders; 2013.)

arteries, and anterior communicating arteries. The anterior cerebral, middle cerebral, and posterior cerebral arteries leave the circle of Willis and extend to various brain structures, serving their associated brain territories. The border zone is the area between the major arterial territories. (Table 15.5 and Fig. 15.21 describe the structures served, the functional relationships, and the pathologic considerations related to occlusion of cerebral arteries.)

Cerebral venous drainage does not parallel its arterial supply, whereas the venous drainage of the brainstem and cerebellum does parallel the arterial supply of these structures. The cerebral veins are classified as superficial and deep veins. The veins drain into venous plexuses and dural sinuses (formed between the dural layers) and eventually join the internal jugular veins at the skull base (Fig. 15.22). Adequacy of venous outflow can significantly affect intracranial pressure. For example, when individuals with a head injury turn or let their heads fall to the side, the action partially occludes venous return, and intracranial pressure can increase because of decreased flow through the jugular veins.

Blood-Brain Barrier

The blood-brain barrier (BBB) describes cellular structures that selectively inhibit certain potentially harmful substances in the blood from entering the interstitial spaces of the brain or CSF, thus allowing neurons to function normally. Endothelial cells in brain capillaries with their intracellular tight junctions are the site of the BBB (Fig. 15.23). Supporting cells include astrocytes, pericytes, and microglia.[3] Some substances, including glucose, lipid-soluble molecules, electrolytes, and chemicals, can cross into and out of the brain facilitated by transport molecules. This has substantial implications for drug therapy because certain antibiotics and chemotherapeutic drugs show a greater propensity than others to cross this barrier. Breakdown of the BBB can contribute to brain invasion by toxic molecules or pathogens promoting neuroinflammation and neurodegeneration. The epithelium of the choroid plexus and the arachnoid membrane also provide barrier functions.[4]

Blood Supply to the Spinal Cord

The spinal cord derives its blood supply from branches of the vertebral arteries and from branches from various regions of the aorta. The anterior spinal artery and the paired posterior spinal arteries branch from the vertebral artery at the base of the cranium and descend alongside the spinal cord. Arterial branches from vessels exterior to the spinal cord follow the spinal nerve through the intervertebral foramina, pass through the dura, and divide into the anterior and posterior radicular arteries (Fig. 15.24).

The radicular arteries eventually connect to the spinal arteries. Branches from the radicular and spinal arteries form

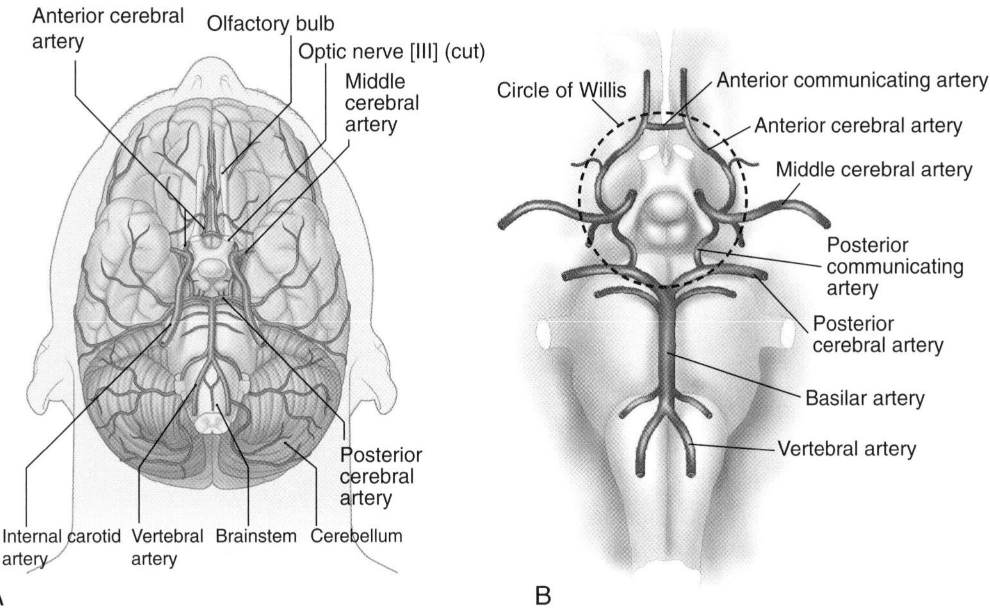

Fig. 15.20 Arteries at the Base of the Brain. (A) View of the arteries at the base of the brain. **(B)** Circle of Willis. The arteries that compose the circle of Willis are the two anterior cerebral arteries, joined to each other by the anterior communicating artery and two short segments of the internal carotids, off of which the posterior communicating arteries connect to the posterior cerebral arteries. (A, From Moses KP. *Atlas of clinical gross anatomy*, 2nd edition. Philadelphia: Saunders; 2013. B, From Hagen-Ansert S. *Textbook of diagnostic sonography*, 7th edition. St. Louis: Mosby; 2012.)

TABLE 15.5 Arterial Systems Supplying the Brain

Arterial Origin	Structures Served	Conditions Caused by Occlusion
Anterior cerebral artery	Basal ganglia; corpus callosum; medial surface of cerebral hemispheres; superior surface of frontal and parietal lobes	Hemiplegia on contralateral side of body, greater in lower than in upper extremities
Middle cerebral artery	Frontal lobe; parietal lobe; temporal lobe (primarily cortical surfaces)	Aphasia in dominant hemisphere and contralateral hemiplegia (see Chapter 17)
Posterior cerebral artery	Part of diencephalon (thalamus, hypothalamus) and temporal lobe; occipital lobe	Visual loss; sensory loss; contralateral hemiplegia if cerebral peduncle affected

plexuses whose branches penetrate the spinal cord, supplying the deeper tissues. Venous drainage parallels the arterial supply closely and drains into venous sinuses located between the dura and periosteum of the vertebrae.

PERIPHERAL NERVOUS SYSTEM

The peripheral nervous system (PNS) includes the nerves outside the CNS (see Fig. 15.1). The somatic nervous system is the part of the PNS that controls voluntary muscle movement (efferent nerves) and sensory information (afferent nerves). The cranial and spinal nerves, including their branches and ganglia, constitute the PNS. The spinal nerves originate in the spinal cord. The cranial nerves originate in the brain and pass out of the skull. A peripheral nerve is composed of individual axons/dendrites, with most wrapped in a myelin sheath. These individual fibers are arranged in bundles called *fascicles* (Fig. 15.25B). The coverings provide structural support, a blood supply, and interstitial compartments necessary to deliver essential electrolytes to support nerve impulse conduction.

The 31 pairs of spinal nerves derive their names from the vertebral level from which they exit: 8 cervical, 12 thoracic, 5 lumbar, 5 sacral, and 1 coccygeal. The first cervical nerve exits above the first cervical vertebra, and the rest of the spinal nerves exit below their corresponding vertebrae. From the thoracic region (and inferiorly), nerves correspond to the vertebral level above their exit (see Fig. 15.11).

Spinal nerves contain both sensory and motor neurons and are called mixed nerves. Their structure can be compared to that of a tree with roots, trunk, and branches (see Fig. 15.11B). They arise as rootlets that combine into *roots* lateral to anterior and posterior horns of the spinal cord. These two spinal nerve roots converge in the region of the intervertebral foramen to form the spinal nerve *trunk*. Shortly after converging, the spinal nerve divides into anterior and posterior rami *(branches)*.

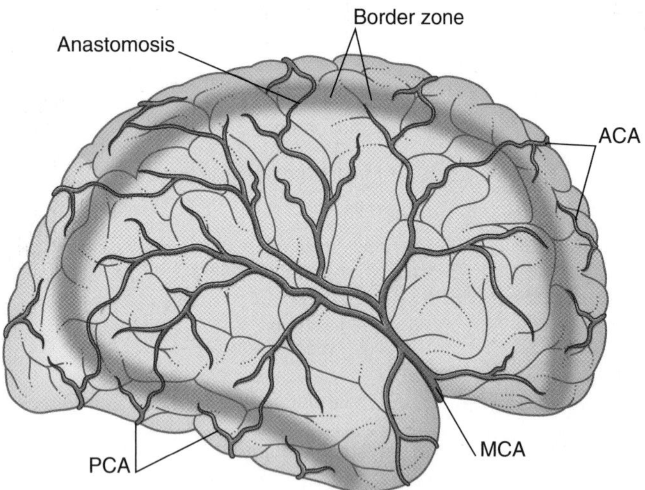

Fig. 15.21 Areas of the Brain Affected by Occlusion of the Anterior, Middle, and Posterior Cerebral Artery Branches. *ACA*, Gray area affected by occlusion of branches of anterior cerebral artery; *MCA*, pink area affected by occlusion of branches of middle cerebral artery; *PCA*, orange area affected by occlusion of branches of posterior cerebral artery. Occlusions can occur in the cortical or deep areas of the border zone. (From Mtui E, Gruener G, Fitzgerald MJT. *Clinical neuroanatomy and neuroscience*, 6th edition. Philadelphia: Saunders; 2012.)

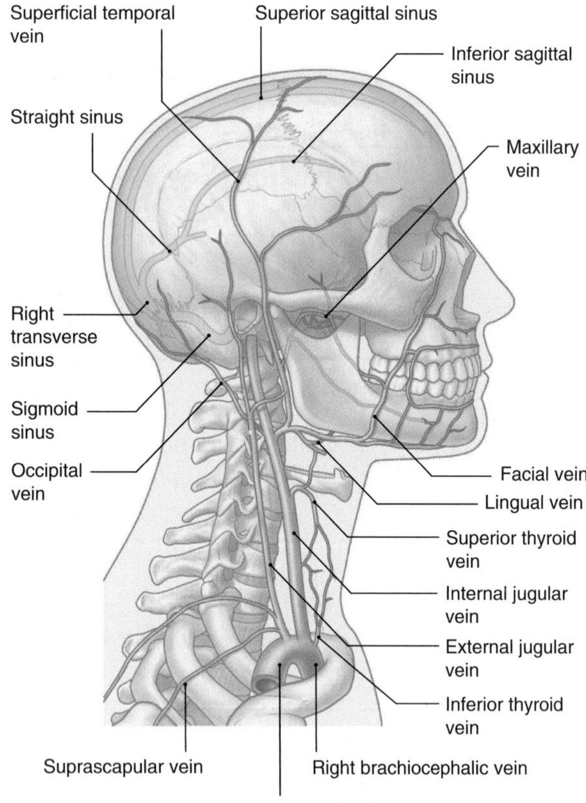

Fig. 15.22 Veins of the Head and Neck. Deep veins and dural sinuses are projected on the skull. Note two superficial veins in the face are tributaries that send blood through emissary veins in the skull foramen into deep veins inside the skull, terminating in the internal jugular vein. (From Moses KP. *Atlas of clinical gross anatomy*, 2nd edition. Philadelphia: Saunders; 2013.)

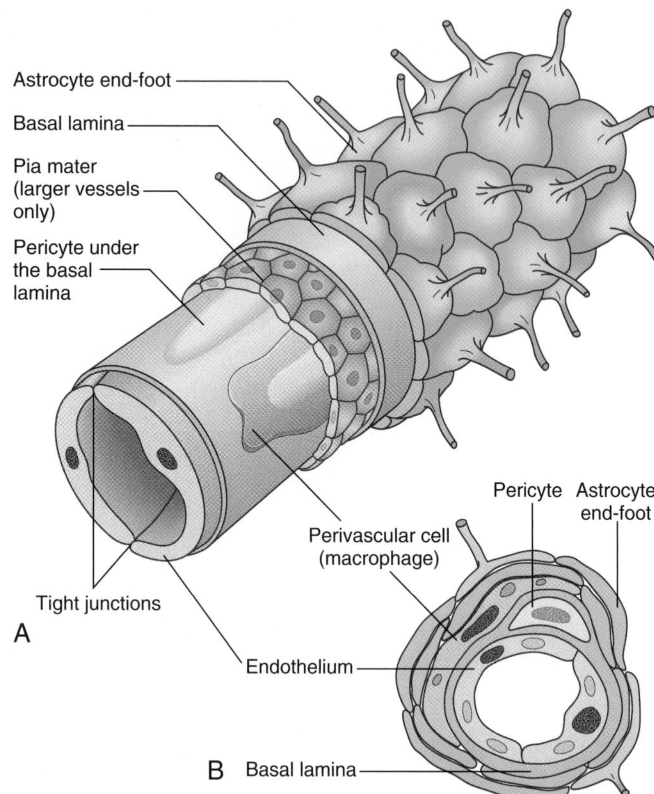

Fig. 15.23 Blood-Brain Barrier. (A) Cellular structure of brain capillary. Endothelial cell membranes with tight junctions create a physical barrier between capillary blood and the brain, restricting movement of bacteria or neurotoxic substances. The pia mater is present only in larger vessels. **(B)** Cross-section. (From Standring S. *Gray's anatomy*, 41st edition. London: Elsevier; 2016.)

The anterior rami (except the thoracic) initially form **plexuses** (networks of nerve fibers), branching into the peripheral nerves. Instead of forming plexuses, the thoracic nerves pass through the thorax's intercostal spaces and innervate regions.

The main spinal nerve plexuses innervate the skin and the underlying muscles of the limbs. The **brachial plexus**, for example, is formed by the last four cervical nerves (C5 to C8) and the first thoracic nerve (T1) (see Fig. 15.11B). The brachial plexus innervates the nerves of the arm, wrist, and hand.

The posterior rami of each spinal nerve, with their many processes, are distributed to a specific area in the body. Sensory signals thus arise from specific sites associated with a specific spinal cord segment. Specific areas of cutaneous (skin) innervation at these spinal cord segments are called **dermatomes** (Fig. 15.25C). The dermatomes of various spinal nerves are distributed in a fairly regular pattern, although adjacent regions between dermatomes can be innervated by more than one spinal nerve.

Like spinal nerves, **cranial nerves** are categorized as peripheral nerves. Most of these are mixed nerves (like the spinal nerves), although some are purely sensory or purely motor. Cranial nerves connect to nuclei in the brain and brainstem (see Fig. 15.25A). Table 15.6 describes the cranial nerves and how to test them.

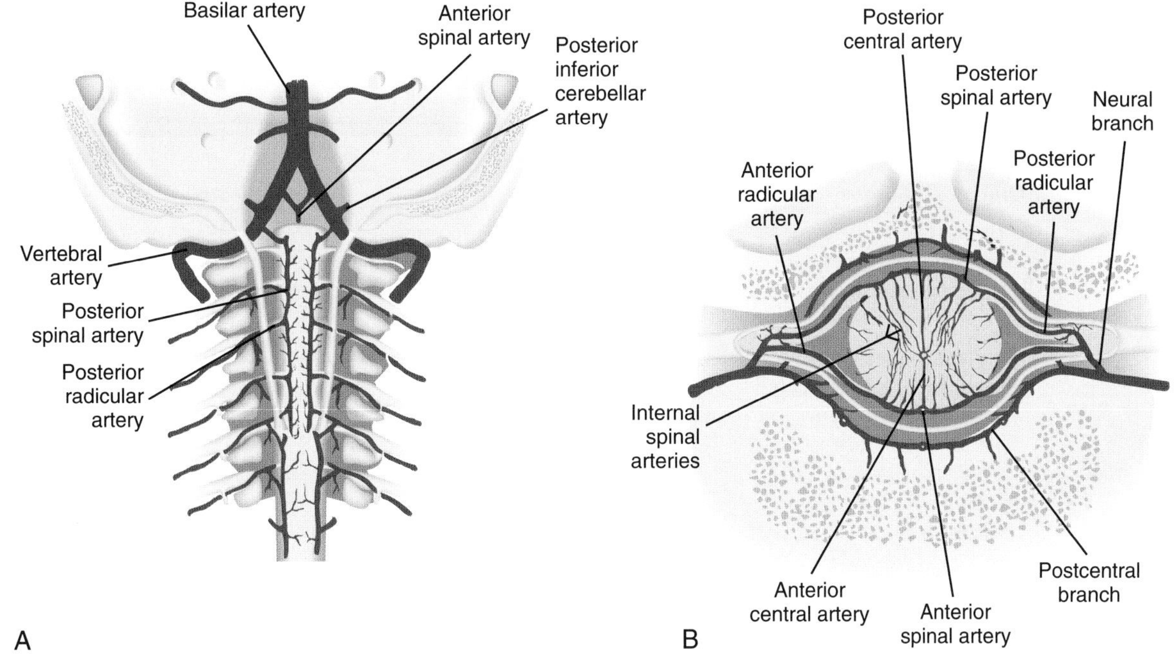

Fig. 15.24 Arteries of the Spinal Cord. (A) Arteries of cervical cord exposed from the rear. **(B)** Arteries of spinal cord diagrammatically shown in horizontal section. (Redrawn from Rudy EB, eds. *Advanced neurological and neurosurgical nursing*. St. Louis: Mosby; 1984.)

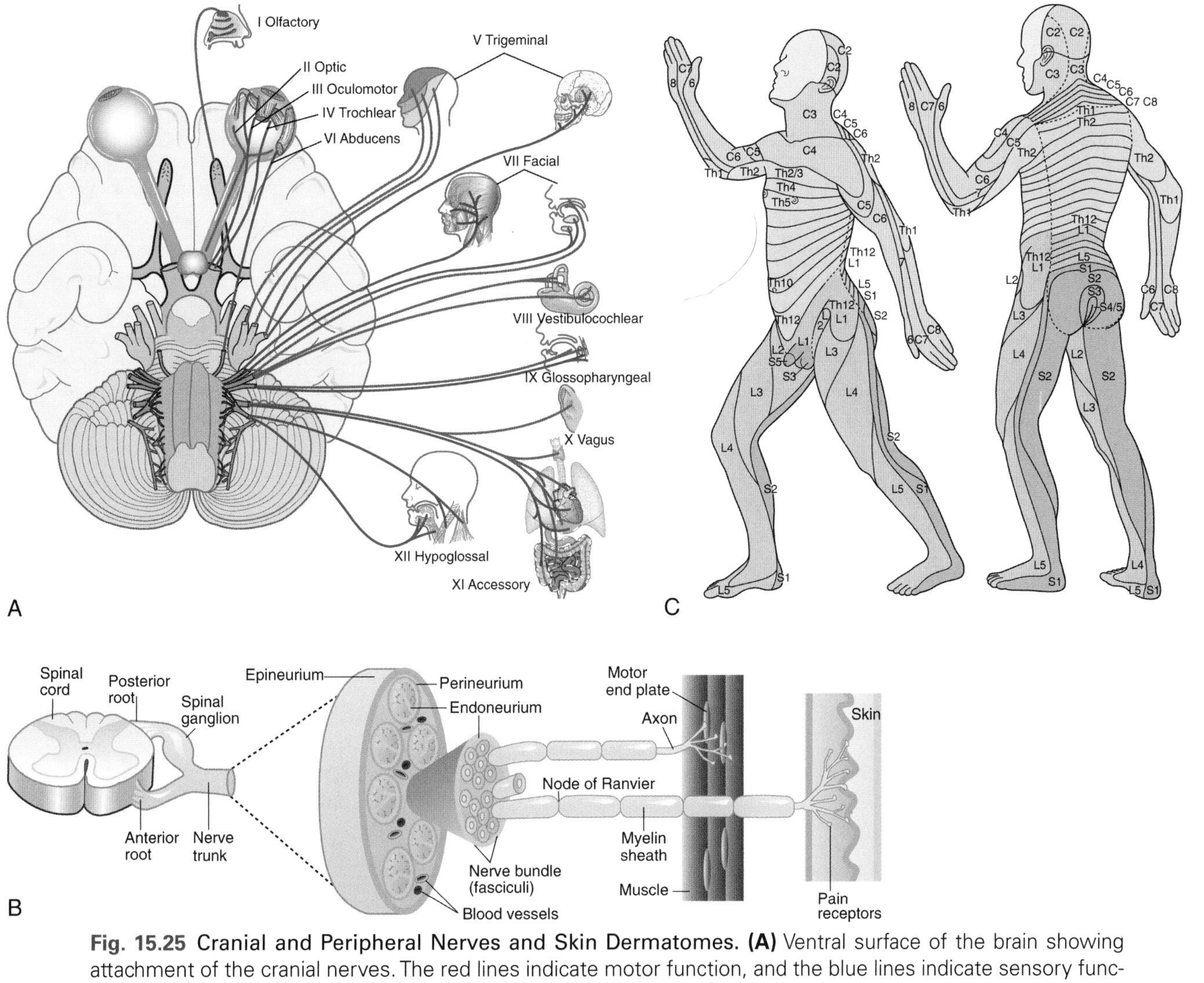

Fig. 15.25 Cranial and Peripheral Nerves and Skin Dermatomes. (A) Ventral surface of the brain showing attachment of the cranial nerves. The red lines indicate motor function, and the blue lines indicate sensory function. **(B)** Peripheral nerve trunk and coverings. **(C)** Dermatome map, anterolateral view *(left)*, and posterolateral view *(right)*. (A, From Applegate E. *The anatomy and physiology learning system*, 4th edition. St. Louis: Saunders; 2011. C, From Salvo SG. *Mosby's pathology for massage therapists*, 3rd edition. St. Louis: Mosby; 2014.)

TABLE 15.6 The Cranial Nerves

Number and Name	Origin and Course	Function	How Tested
I. Olfactory	Fibers arise from nasal olfactory epithelium and form synapses with olfactory bulbs that transmit impulses to temporal lobe	Purely sensory; carries impulses for sense of smell	Person is asked to sniff aromatic substances, such as oil of cloves and vanilla, and to identify them
II. Optic	Fibers arise from retina of eye to form optic nerve, which passes through sphenoid bone; two optic nerves then form optic chiasma (with partial crossover of fibers) and eventually end in occipital cortex	Purely sensory; carries impulses for vision	Vision and visual field tested with an eye chart and by testing point at which person first sees an object (finger) moving into visual field; inside of eye is viewed with ophthalmoscope to observe blood vessels of eye interior
III. Oculomotor	Fibers emerge from midbrain and exit from skull, and extend to eye	Contains motor fibers to inferior oblique and to superior, inferior, and medial rectus extraocular muscles that direct eyeball; levator muscles of eyelid; smooth muscles of iris and ciliary body; and proprioception (sensory) to brain from extraocular muscles	Pupils examined for size, shape, and equality; pupillary reflex tested with a penlight (pupils should constrict when illuminated); ability to follow moving objects
IV. Trochlear	Fibers emerge from posterior midbrain and exit from skull to run to eye	Proprioceptor and motor fibers for superior oblique muscle of eye (extraocular muscle)	Tested in common with cranial nerve III relative to ability to follow moving objects
V. Trigeminal	Fibers emerge from pons and form three divisions that exit from skull and run to face and cranial dura mater	Both motor and sensory for face; conducts sensory impulses from mouth, nose, surface of eye, and dura mater; also contains motor fibers that stimulate chewing muscles	Sensations of pain, touch, and temperature tested with safety pin and hot and cold objects; corneal reflex tested with a wisp of cotton; motor branch tested by asking subject to clench teeth, open mouth against resistance, and move jaw from side to side
VI. Abducens	Fibers leave inferior pons and exit from skull, and extend to eye	Contains motor fibers to lateral rectus muscle and proprioceptor fibers from same muscle to brain	Tested in common with cranial nerve III relative to ability to move each eye laterally
VII. Facial	Fibers leave pons and travel through temporal bone and extend to face	Mixed: (1) supplies motor fibers to muscles of facial expression and to lacrimal and salivary glands, and (2) carries sensory fibers from taste buds of anterior part of tongue	Anterior two-thirds of tongue tested for ability to taste sweet (sugar), salty, sour (vinegar), and bitter (quinine) substances; symmetry of face checked; subject asked to close eyes, smile, whistle, and so on; tearing tested with ammonia fumes
VIII. Vestibulocochlear (acoustic)	Fibers run from inner ear (hearing and equilibrium receptors in temporal bone) to enter brainstem just below pons	Purely sensory; vestibular branch transmits impulses for sense of equilibrium; cochlear branch transmits impulses for sense of hearing	Hearing checked by air and bone conduction by use of a tuning fork; vestibular tests: Bárány and caloric tests
IX. Glossopharyngeal	Fibers emerge from midbrain and leave skull and extend to pharynx, salivary glands, and tongue	Mixed: (1) motor fibers serve pharynx (throat) and salivary glands, and (2) sensory fibers carry impulses from pharynx, posterior tongue (taste buds), and pressure receptors of carotid artery	Gag and swallow reflexes checked; subject asked to speak and cough; posterior one-third of tongue may be tested for taste
X. Vagus	Fibers emerge from medulla, pass through skull, and descend through neck region into thorax and abdominal region	Fibers carry sensory and motor impulses for pharynx; a large part of this nerve is parasympathetic motor fibers, which supply smooth muscles of abdominal organs; receives sensory impulses from viscera	Same as for cranial nerve IX (IX and X are tested in common) because they both serve muscles of the throat
XI. Spinal accessory	Fibers arise from medulla and superior spinal cord and extend to muscles of neck and back	Provides sensory and motor fibers for sternocleidomastoid and trapezius muscles and muscles of soft palate, pharynx, and larynx	Sternocleidomastoid and trapezius muscles checked for strength by asking subject to rotate head and shrug shoulders against resistance
XII. Hypoglossal	Fibers arise from medulla and exit from skull, and extend to tongue	Carries motor fibers to muscles of tongue and sensory impulses from tongue to brain	Subject asked to stick out tongue, and any position abnormalities are noted

AUTONOMIC NERVOUS SYSTEM

The autonomic nervous system (ANS) coordinates and maintains a steady state among body organs and regulates cardiac muscle, smooth muscle, and the body's glands.[5] This system is considered an involuntary system because one generally cannot *will* these functions to happen. Components of the ANS are located in both the CNS and the PNS, but the ANS is considered to be part of the efferent division of the PNS. The ANS is separated both structurally and functionally into two divisions: (1) the sympathetic nervous system and (2) the parasympathetic nervous system (Fig. 15.26). The effects of these two divisions are usually antagonistic, which means one stimulates an effector and one inhibits an effector. In this way, an effector, such as the heart or the blood vessels, can be precisely controlled. Many neurons of the ANS travel in the spinal nerves and certain cranial nerves. The widespread activity of this system indicates that its components are distributed all over the body. The peripheral autonomic nerves carry mainly efferent fibers, and that will be the emphasis here. The *visceral* or *enteric autonomic nervous system* controls the gastrointestinal tract's sensory and motor function and operates independently of the brain and spinal cord.

The CNS has cardiovascular and respiratory centers in the reticular formation and the sympathetic and parasympathetic areas in the hypothalamus. CNS pathways interconnect all these areas and project to autonomic areas in the brain stem and spinal cord. Both divisions of the ANS are composed of autonomic nerves, ganglia, and plexuses. These structures, in turn, are made up of efferent (motor) autonomic neurons that conduct impulses away from the brainstem or spinal cord and down to the autonomic effectors. The efferent component of the ANS is a two-neuron system. Preganglionic neurons (myelinated) conduct impulses from the brainstem or spinal cord to an autonomic ganglion, where they synapse with a postganglionic neuron. Postganglionic neurons (unmyelinated) conduct impulses away from the ganglion to the effector (Fig. 15.27). This arrangement contrasts with the efferent somatic nervous system, where a single motor neuron travels from the CNS to the innervated structure without passing through the ganglia (see Fig. 15.27D).

Anatomy of the Sympathetic Nervous System

The sympathetic nervous system mobilizes energy stores in times of need (e.g., in the "fight or flight" or stress response) (see Chapter 11 and Fig. 11.2). The sympathetic division is innervated by cell bodies located from the first thoracic (T1) through the second lumbar (L2) regions of the spinal cord and therefore is called the thoracolumbar division (see Fig. 15.26). The preganglionic axons of the sympathetic division form synapses shortly after leaving the spinal cord in the sympathetic (paravertebral) ganglia (see Fig. 15.27A). These preganglionic axons travel in several different ways: (1) directly synapsing with postganglionic neurons in the sympathetic chain ganglion at their level; (2) by traveling up the sympathetic chain ganglia; (3) by traveling down the sympathetic chain ganglion before forming synapses with a higher or lower postganglionic neuron; or (4) by traveling through the sympathetic chain ganglion to synapse with collateral ganglia (i.e., the splanchnic nerves, which lead to collateral ganglia on the front of the aorta). The collateral ganglia are named according to the branches of the aorta nearest them, namely the celiac, superior mesenteric, and inferior mesenteric ganglia (see Fig. 15.26). Postganglionic neurons leave the collateral ganglia and innervate the viscera below the diaphragm.

Preganglionic sympathetic neurons that innervate the adrenal medulla also travel in the splanchnic nerves and *do not* synapse before reaching the gland (see Figs. 15.26 and 15.27B). The secretory cells in the adrenal medulla are considered modified postganglionic neurons. Because preganglionic sympathetic fibers are all myelinated, travel to the adrenal medulla is quick, and innervation causes the rapid release of epinephrine and norepinephrine, which are mediators of the fight-or-flight response (see Chapter 11).

Anatomy of the Parasympathetic Nervous System

The parasympathetic nervous system conserves and restores energy when a person is at rest. The nerve cell bodies of this division are located in the cranial nerve nuclei and the sacral region of the spinal cord and therefore constitute the craniosacral division. Unlike the sympathetic branch, the preganglionic fibers in the parasympathetic division are longer and travel close to the organs they innervate before forming synapses with the relatively short postganglionic neurons (see Fig. 15.26). Parasympathetic nerves arising from nuclei in the brainstem travel to the viscera of the head, thorax, and abdomen within cranial nerves—including the oculomotor (III), facial (VII), glossopharyngeal (IX), and vagus (X) nerves.

Preganglionic parasympathetic nerves that originate from the sacral region of the spinal cord run either separately or together with some spinal nerves. The preganglionic axons unite to form the pelvic splanchnic nerve, which innervates the viscera of the pelvic cavity. These preganglionic axons synapse with postganglionic neurons in terminal ganglia located close to the organs they innervate.

Similar to the spinal nerves, the autonomic nerves also form plexuses. These are networks of nerves that have both parasympathetic and sympathetic neurons. They are usually located near the organs they innervate. Examples include the celiac (solar) plexus (contains the celiac ganglia and innervates many abdominal and pelvic organs), the cardiac plexus (innervates the heart), and Meissner and Auerbach plexuses (innervate the gastrointestinal tract).

Neurotransmitters and Neuroreceptors

Sympathetic preganglionic fibers and parasympathetic preganglionic and postganglionic fibers release acetylcholine—the same neurotransmitter released by somatic efferent neurons (see Fig. 15.27). These fibers are characterized by cholinergic transmission. Most postganglionic sympathetic fibers release norepinephrine (noradrenaline) and thus are considered to function by adrenergic transmission. A few postganglionic sympathetic fibers, such as those that innervate the sweat glands, release acetylcholine.

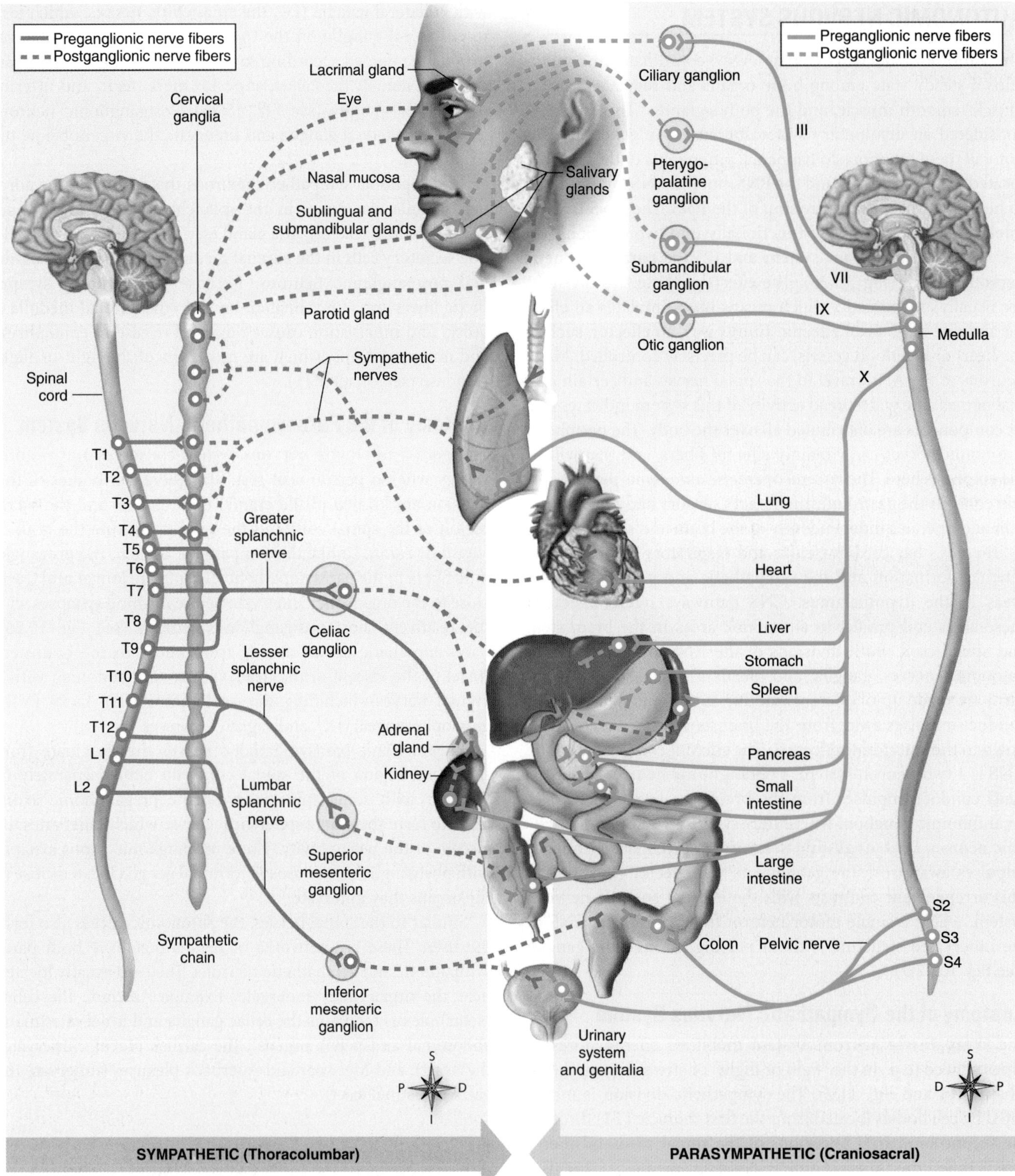

Fig. 15.26 Sympathetic and Parasympathetic Divisions of the Autonomic Nervous System. Preganglionic neuron cell bodies are located in the brainstem and sacral cord segments (parasympathetic or "craniosacral" division) and thoracic and upper lumbar cord segments (sympathetic or "thoracolumbar" division). The axons of these neurons synapse with postganglionic neurons, which innervate smooth muscle, cardiac muscle, and glands of the body. The postganglionic neuron cell bodies may be located in distinct autonomic ganglia *(represented by circles)* or very near the wall of the innervated visceral organ. Note that sympathetic fibers provide the only innervation to peripheral effectors (sweat glands, arrector pili muscles, adipose tissue, and blood vessels). (From Patton KA. *Anatomy & physiology*, 10th edition. St. Louis: Elsevier; 2019.)

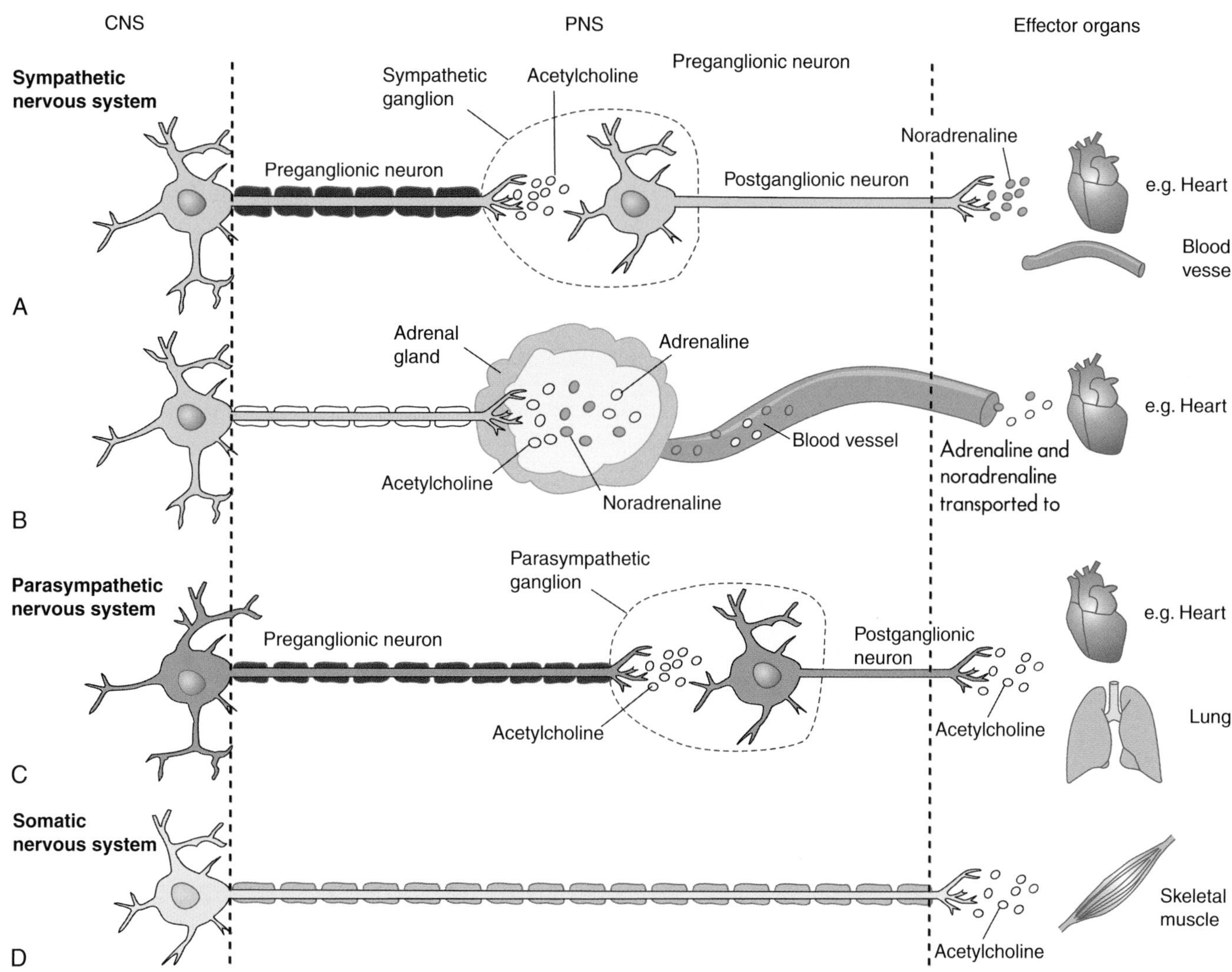

Fig. 15.27 Comparison of Neurotransmitters and Receptors Between the Sympathetic and Parasympathetic Nervous Systems. Although not part of the autonomic nervous system, the somatic nervous system is included because of its similarity for comparison. In each case, the cell body of the first neuron is located in the central nervous system. (From Craft J, Gordon C, Huether SE, et al. *Understanding pathophysiology, Australian adaptation*, 2nd edition. Marrickville, Australia: Elsevier Australia; 2015.)

The action of catecholamines (adrenalin, noradrenaline, dopamine) varies with the type of neuroreceptor stimulated. Catecholamines are also released by the adrenal medulla gland, which physiologically and biochemically resembles the sympathetic nervous system. Two types of adrenergic receptors exist, α and β. Cells of the effector organs may have one or both types of adrenergic receptors. α-Adrenergic receptors have been further subdivided according to the action produced. α_1-Adrenergic activity is associated mostly with excitation or stimulation; α_2-adrenergic activity is associated with relaxation or inhibition. Most of the α-adrenergic receptors on effector organs belong to the α_1 class. β-Adrenergic receptors are classified as β_1-adrenergic receptors (which facilitate increased heart rate and contractility and cause the release of renin from the kidney) and β_2-adrenergic receptors (which facilitate all remaining effects attributed to β receptors).[6] Norepinephrine stimulates all α_1 and β_1 receptors and only certain β_2 receptors. The primary response from norepinephrine, however, is stimulation of α_1-adrenergic receptors that cause vasoconstriction. Epinephrine strongly stimulates all four types of receptors and induces general vasodilation because of the predominance of β receptors in muscle vasculatures. (Table 15.7 summarizes the effects of neuroreceptors on their effector organs.)

Functions of the Autonomic Nervous System

Many body organs are innervated by both the sympathetic and parasympathetic nervous systems. The two divisions often cause opposite responses; for example, sympathetic stimulation of the stomach causes decreased peristalsis, whereas parasympathetic stimulation of the intestine increases peristalsis. In general,

TABLE 15.7 Actions of Autonomic Nervous System Neuroreceptors

Effector Organ or Tissue	Adrenergic Receptors	Adrenergic Effects	Cholinergic Effects
Eye, iris			
Radial muscle	α_1	Dilation	—
Sphincter muscle	—	—	Constriction
Eye, ciliary muscle	β_2	Relaxation for far vision	Contraction for near vision
Lacrimal glands	α_1	Secretion	Secretion
Nasopharyngeal glands	—	—	Secretion
Salivary glands	α_1	Secretion of potassium and water	Secretion of potassium and water
	β	Secretion of amylase	—
Heart			
Sinoatrial (SA) node	β_1, β_2	Increase heart rate	Decrease heart rate; vagus arrest
Atrial	β_1, β_2	Increase contractility and conduction velocity	Decrease contractility; shorten action potential duration
Atrioventricular (AV) junction	β_1, β_2	Increase automaticity and propagation velocity	Decrease automaticity and propagation velocity
Purkinje system	β_1, β_2	Increase automaticity and propagation velocity	—
Ventricles	β_1, β_2	Increase contractility	Slight decrease in contraction
Arterioles			
Coronary	α_1, α_2, β_2	Constriction, dilation	Dilation
Skin and mucosa	α_1, α_2	Constriction	Dilation
Skeletal muscle	α, β_2	Dilation, constriction	Dilation
Cerebral	α_1	Constriction (slight)	Dilation
Pulmonary	α_1, β_2	Constriction, dilation	Dilation
Mesenteric	α_1	Constriction	Dilation
Renal	α_1, β_1, β_2	Constriction, dilation	Dilation
Salivary glands	α_1, α_2	Constriction	Dilation
Veins, systemic	α_1, α_2, β_2	Constriction, dilation	—
Lung			
Bronchial muscle	α_2	Relaxation	Contraction
Bronchial glands	α_1, β_2	Decrease secretion; increase secretion	Stimulation
Stomach			
Motility	α_1, α_2, β_1, β_2	Decrease (usually)	Increase
Sphincters	α_1	Contraction (usually)	Relaxation (usually)
Secretion	α_2	Inhibition	Stimulation
Liver	α_1, β_2	Glycogenolysis and gluconeogenesis	—
Gallbladder and ducts	β_2	Relaxation	Contraction
Pancreas			
Acini	α	Decrease secretion	Secretion

TABLE 15.7 Actions of Autonomic Nervous System Neuroreceptors–Cont'd

Effector Organ or Tissue	Adrenergic Receptors	Adrenergic Effects	Cholinergic Effects
Islet cells	α_2, β_2	Decrease secretion; increase secretion	—
Intestine			
Motility and tone	α_1, α_2, β_1, β_2	Decrease	Increase
Sphincters	α_1	Contraction	Relaxation (usually)
Secretion	α_2	Inhibition	Stimulation
Adrenal medulla	—	Secretion of epinephrine and norepinephrine	
Kidney			
Renin secretion	α_1, β_1	Decrease; increase	—
Ureter			
Motility and tone	β_1	Increase	Increase (?)
Urinary bladder			
Detrusor	β_2	Relaxation	Contraction
Trigone and sphincter	α_1	Contraction	Relaxation
Sex organs, male	α_1	Ejaculation	Erection
Skin			
Pilomotor muscles	α_1	Contraction	—
Sweat glands	α_1	Localized secretion	—
Fat cells	α_2, β_1, β_2, β_3	Inhibition of lipolysis; stimulation of lipolysis	—
Pineal gland	β	Melatonin synthesis	—

Modified from Brunton LL, Chabner B, Knollmann BC, eds. *Goodman & Gilman's pharmacological basis of therapeutics*, 12th edition. New York: McGraw-Hill; 2010; Dowd FJ, Yagiela JA, Johnson B, et al. *Pharmacology and therapeutics for dentistry*, 6th edition. St. Louis: Mosby; 2011.

sympathetic stimulation promotes responses for the protection of the individual. For example, sympathetic activity increases blood glucose levels and temperature and increases heart rate and blood pressure. In emergency situations, a generalized and widespread discharge of the sympathetic system occurs and is known as the "fight or flight" reflex or acute stress response (see Chapter 11). This is accomplished by an increased firing frequency of sympathetic fibers and by activation of sympathetic fibers normally silent and at rest (fibers to the sweat glands, pilomotor muscles, and the adrenal medulla, as well as vasodilator fibers to muscle). Regulation of vasomotor tone is considered the single most important function of the sympathetic nervous system. (Fig. 15.28 illustrates some of the most important functions of the sympathetic nervous system.)

Increased parasympathetic activity promotes rest and tranquility and is characterized by reduced heart rate and enhanced visceral functions concerned with digestion. Stimulation of the vagus nerve (cranial nerve X) in the gastrointestinal tract increases peristalsis and secretion, as well as the relaxation of sphincters. Activation of parasympathetic fibers in the head, provided by cranial nerves III, VII, and IX, causes pupil constriction, tear secretion, and increased salivary secretion. Stimulation of the sacral division of the parasympathetic system contracts the urinary bladder and facilitates the process of penile erection.

The parasympathetic system lacks the generalized and widespread response of the sympathetic system. Specific parasympathetic fibers are activated to regulate particular functions. Although the actions of the parasympathetic and sympathetic systems are usually antagonistic, there are exceptions. Peripheral vascular resistance, for example, is increased dramatically by sympathetic activation but is not altered appreciably by activity of the parasympathetic system. Most blood vessels involved in the control of blood pressure are innervated by sympathetic nerves. To decrease blood pressure, therefore, it is more important to block or paralyze the continuous (tonic) discharge of the sympathetic system than to promote parasympathetic activity.

The CNS mechanisms involved in the aging process are extremely complex, and many questions have yet to be answered. *Geriatric Considerations: Aging & the Nervous System* summarizes the structural, cellular, cerebrovascular, and functional changes that occur in the nervous system with aging.

GERIATRIC CONSIDERATIONS

Aging and the Nervous System

Structural Changes with Aging
Decreased brain weight and size, particularly frontal regions
Increase in ventricular volume
Fibrosis and thickening of the meninges
Narrowing of gyri and widening of sulci
Increase in size of ventricles

Cellular Changes with Aging
Decrease in number of neurons not consistently related to changes in mental function
Decreased myelin
Lipofuscin deposition (a pigment resulting from cellular autodigestion)
Decreased number of dendritic processes and synaptic connections
Intracellular neurofibrillary tangles; significant accumulation in cortex associated with Alzheimer dementia
Imbalance in amount and distribution of neurotransmitters
Decrease in glucose metabolism

Cerebrovascular Changes with Aging
Arterial atherosclerosis (may cause infarcts and scars)
Increased permeability of blood-brain barrier
Decreased vascular density

Functional Changes with Aging
Decreased tendon reflexes
Progressive deficit in taste and smell
Decreased vibratory sense
Decrease in accommodation and color vision
Decrease in neuromuscular control with change in gait and posture
Sleep disturbances
Memory impairments
Cognitive alterations associated with chronic disease
Functional changes and nervous system aging have significant individual variation

Data from Chételat G, Landeau B, Salmon E, et al. Relationships between brain metabolism decrease in normal aging and changes in structural and functional connectivity. *NeuroImage*, 2013;76:167–177; Fjell AM, Walhovd KB. Structural brain changes in aging: Courses, causes and cognitive consequences. *Nature Reviews Neuroscience*, 2010;21(3):187–221; Fjell AM, McEvoy L, Holland D, et al. What is normal in normal aging? Effects of aging, amyloid and Alzheimer's disease on the cerebral cortex and the hippocampus. *Progress in Neurobiology*, 2014;117:20–40; Xekardaki A, Kövari E, Gold G, et al. Neuropathological changes in aging brain. *Advances in Experimental Medicine and Biology*, 2015;821:11–17.

TESTS OF NERVOUS SYSTEM STRUCTURE AND FUNCTION

Skull and Spine Roentgenograms

Roentgenograms (x-ray films) of the skull or spine from multiple angles (views) are used primarily to localize bony defects, bone density, erosion, or calcified structures. The pineal gland in older people becomes calcified and is useful as an internal brain landmark. Probably the most commonly used radiologic studies are x-ray films.

Computed Tomography

Computed tomography (CT) creates two-dimensional reconstructions from multiple radiologic images (x-rays) using computer-assisted analysis. It can demonstrate fine distinctions in shape, size, and densities of a variety of tissues based on differential absorption of x-rays. CT imaging is a noninvasive procedure used in evaluating cranial and spinal structures and hemorrhages, tumors, and distortions in the brain caused by pressure differences. A variety of contrast media are also commonly used in conjunction with this procedure to enhance the delineation of selected structures. Spiral or helical CT uses a multidetector scanner mounted on a rotating gantry to provide several axial images of a large continuous anatomic area in a matter of seconds. Helical CT angiography uses contrast media for the detection of aneurysms or ruptured aneurysms.

Magnetic Resonance Imaging

Magnetic resonance imaging (MRI) uses a static magnetic field, instead of x-rays, to orient physiologic atomic particles. Disruption of this orientation by excitation of the particles using serial radiofrequency pulsations provides the image data. The specific tissue reaction is computer-analyzed to give an image with much better spatial resolution than that provided by CT. The MRI also reconstructs images in three angles at right angles (i.e., axial, sagittal, coronal). MRI is reported to have none of the adverse effects associated with radiation examinations. Magnetic resonance spectroscopy (MRS) can be completed simultaneously as a standard MRI by analyzing the chemical composition of proton (hydrogen) or phosphorous-based molecules and is useful for differentiating the chemical composition and function of various regions of the brain. Functional MRI (fMRI) detects changes in blood oxygenation and flow and can produce maps showing the parts of the brain that are functioning during a mental process. Diffusion tensor imaging (DTI) is an MRI technique that quantifies the size and direction of white matter tracts by measuring asymmetries in the magnitude and direction of the diffusion of water molecules. Color coding and fiber tracking (tractography) add detail.

Magnetic Resonance Angiography

Magnetic resonance angiography (MRA) uses special imaging techniques to visualize blood vessels in great detail. MRA can be used in conjunction with cerebral angiography to detect and localize pathologic lesions of the circulatory system of the brain, particularly the arterial system. In some cases, contrast agents are used.

Positron-Emission Tomography Scan

The positron-emission tomography (PET) scan uses CT imaging to detect the emission of positive electrons from trace amounts of radioactive substances injected into the bloodstream or administered as inhaled gases. With radioactive

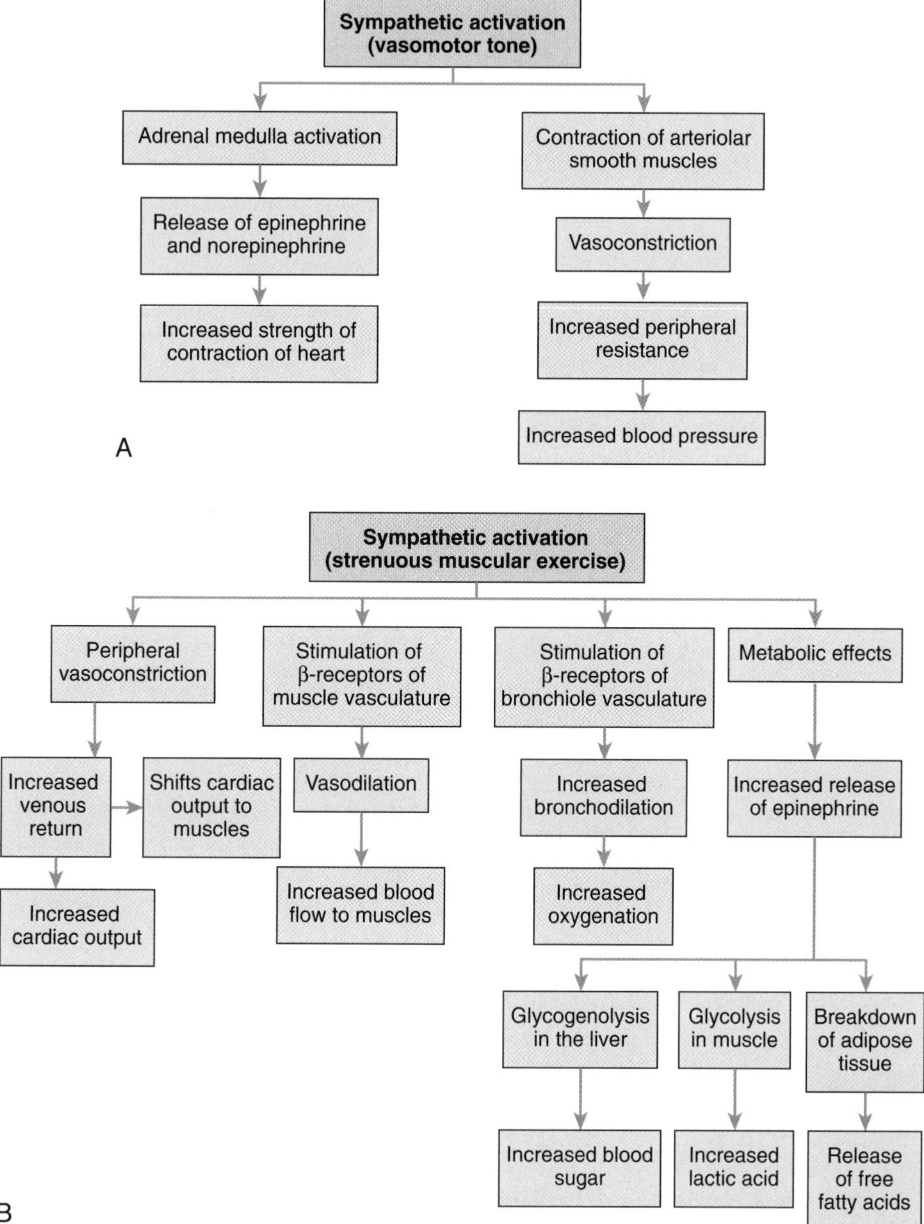

Fig. 15.28 Examples of Important Functions of the Sympathetic Nervous System. **(A)** Regulation of vasomotor tone. **(B)** Regulation of strenuous muscular exercise ("fight-or-flight" or stress response). (See also Chapter 11 and Fig. 11.2 for more detail on the stress response.)

decay, radioactive substances emit a positron. As they are distributed in tissues, they display characteristic patterns that indicate physiologic and metabolic processes, for example, glucose and oxygen uptake, cerebral blood flow, neural and neurotransmitter function, and the effects of drugs. As a research tool, PET is being used to visualize the specific brain sites involved in the processing of information in the brain.

Single Photon Emission Computed Tomography

Single photon emission computed tomography (SPECT) uses radiotracers with longer half-lives than those used in PET scans. CT creates images after radionuclide substances (technetium [^{99m}Tc]) have been introduced into the bloodstream. For example, visualization of tissue uptake of the radioactive agent indicates blood-brain barrier integrity (increased uptake of the agent indicates disruption). This scanning technique also can identify abnormalities in blood-flow dynamics and cellular metabolic function. The brain scan is particularly helpful in detecting abnormal vascularity resulting from neoplasms, abscesses, and vascular lesions.

Cerebral Angiography

Cerebral angiography is a radiologic technique that demonstrates cerebrovascular blood flow. The introduction of a small catheter commonly performs this technique into the femoral artery. The catheter is then passed to the level of the cerebral circulation and through the aorta, and a contrast dye is injected. Serial x-ray films are then taken. These films demonstrate the flow of the dye through the cerebral vasculature and provide information on the patency, location, size, and flow pattern of the vessels. Another technique used in cerebral angiography is the retrograde (reverse flow) injection of the dye through catheterization of a brachial, axillary, subclavian, or femoral vein.

Echoencephalography (Ultrasound)

Echoencephalography, or ultrasound, is a safe, noninvasive procedure using sound waves deflected at differing rates, depending on the density of the tissue. Information is processed and displayed on an oscilloscope screen. It is useful primarily in detecting structural characteristics of intracranial space-occupying mass lesions and the determination of ventricular dimensions, especially in newborns where open fontanelles provide good acoustic windows.

Electroencephalography

The electroencephalograph (EEG) is a recording of electrical impulses arising from the brain's cortical surface that are detected by scalp electrodes. The recording of brain wave patterns is analyzed for alterations or localization (or both) of specific electrical activity. This test is especially useful in detecting and localizing foci that initiate seizure activity. It is also an important technique in the assessment of encephalopathy (altered mental status). Complete absence of electrical activity is seen in individuals who are legally "brain dead."

Magnetoencephalography

Magnetoencephalography (MEG) is a specialized imaging technique used to measure magnetic fields induced by electrical activity in the brain. Electrical activity in the brain, such as that detected by EEG, induces an orthogonally oriented magnetic field. MEG uses multiple sensors that allow vectoring and ultimately localization of the origin of the electrical activity that generated the field. The use of MEG has the advantage over EEG in that the induced magnetic field is not significantly dispersed by passing through the skull and soft tissues of the scalp. Co-registration of MEG and MRI data allow precise localization of the electrical focus for seizure onset.

Evoked Potentials

Evoked potentials (EPs) are a method of detecting electrical brain activity that results from a stimulus—primarily auditory, visual, or peripheral sensory. Electrical activity is computer-formatted to display changes in trends. The primary uses of EPs include perioperative detection of sensory pathway integrity and disease- or drug-related sensory dysfunction.

Cerebrospinal Fluid Analysis

CSF generally is obtained from the lumbar or cisternal subarachnoid space using a hollow needle that allows passive flow. The lumbar puncture is performed most often at the L3–L4 interspace (below the level of the spinal cord at L1–L2). Cisternal puncture is performed by inserting a needle into the cerebellomedullary cistern using an approach from the back of the neck in the region of the foramen magnum. CSF pressure is commonly measured during these procedures. The CSF can also be analyzed for gross characteristics and constituents (color, blood cells, electrolytes, and protein) and cultured for microorganisms.

SUMMARY REVIEW

Overview and Organization of the Nervous System

1. The nervous system divisions have been categorized as either structural (central nervous system [CNS] and peripheral nervous system [PNS]) or functional (somatic nervous system and autonomic nervous system [ANS]).
2. The CNS is contained within the brain and spinal cord.
3. The PNS is composed of cranial and spinal nerves, which carry impulses toward the CNS (afferent—sensory) and away from the CNS (efferent—motor) to and from target organs or skeletal muscle.
4. The somatic nervous system consists of pathways regulating voluntary motor control.

The ANS is involved in the involuntary control of organ systems. The ANS is divided into sympathetic and parasympathetic divisions.

Cells of the Nervous System

1. The neuron and neuroglial cells (nonnerve cells) make up nervous tissue. The neuron is specialized to transmit and receive electrical and chemical impulses, whereas the neuroglial cell provides supportive and maintenance functions.
2. The neuron is composed of a cell body, dendrite(s), and an axon. A myelin sheath around selected axons forms insulation that allows faster nerve impulse conduction, referred to as saltatory conduction.
3. The neuron is further divided into unipolar, pseudounipolar, bipolar, and multipolar categories, according to its structure and particular mechanics of impulse transmission. Functionally, the neuron can be sensory, associational, and motor.
4. Neuroglial cells ("nerve glue") support the CNS and comprise approximately half of the total brain and spinal cord volume.
5. Nerve injury usually leads to the degeneration of the portion cut off from the cell body, called Wallerian degeneration. The part of the axon connected to the cell body can undergo slow regeneration depending on the type and location of the injury.

The Nerve Impulse

1. The region between adjacent neurons is the synapse, and the region between the neuron and muscle is the neuromuscular junction.

2. Neurotransmitters are responsible for chemical conduction across the synapse, and the nerve impulse is regulated predominantly by a balance of inhibitory postsynaptic potentials (IPSPs) and excitatory postsynaptic potentials (EPSPs), temporal and spatial summation, and convergence and divergence.

The Central Nervous System

1. The cerebrum is the largest part of the brain and contains gray matter and white matter. The cerebral cortex is the brain's outer layer and contains only gray matter arranged in folds, composed mostly of cell bodies.
2. The brain is contained within the cranial vault and is divided into three distinct regions: (1) forebrain, (2) hindbrain, and (3) midbrain.
3. The forebrain includes the *telencephalon* (the two cerebral hemispheres) and allows conscious perception of internal and external stimuli, thought and memory processes, and voluntary control of skeletal muscles. The deep portion of the forebrain is termed the *diencephalon* and processes incoming sensory data. The center for the voluntary control of skeletal muscle movements is located along the precentral gyrus in the frontal lobe, whereas the center for perception is along the postcentral gyrus in the parietal lobe. The Broca area (inferior frontal gyrus—motor function) and the Wernicke area (superior temporal gyrus—sensory function) are major speech centers.
4. The midbrain is primarily a relay center for motor and sensory tracts and a center for auditory and visual reflexes.
5. The hindbrain allows sampling and comparison of sensory data received from the periphery and motor impulses of the cerebral hemispheres for coordination and refinement of skeletal muscle movement.
6. The spinal cord contains most of the nerve fibers that connect the brain with the periphery. The corticospinal tracts are descending pyramidal (motor) pathways from the motor cortex. The rubrospinal and reticulospinal tracts are descending extrapyramidal tracts that coordinate movement. The anterior, posterior, and lateral spinothalamic tracts carry sensory information to the brainstem and thalamus, where information is relayed to the sensory cortex. Reflex arcs are sensory and motor circuits completed in the spinal cord and influenced by the higher centers in the brain.
7. The CNS is protected by the bony cranium, meninges (dura mater, arachnoid, membrane, and pia mater), cerebrospinal fluid (CSF), and vertebral column. CSF is formed from blood components in the choroid plexuses of the ventricles and is reabsorbed in the arachnoid villi (located in the dural venous sinuses) after circulating through the brain and subarachnoid space.
8. The paired carotid and vertebral arteries supply blood to the brain and connect to form the circle of Willis. The major branches projecting from the circle of Willis are the anterior, middle, and posterior cerebral arteries. Drainage of blood from the brain is accomplished through the venous sinuses and jugular veins.
9. The blood-brain barrier is provided by tight junctions between the cells of brain capillary endothelial cells and surrounding supporting cells.
10. Blood supply to the spinal cord originates from the vertebral arteries and branches arising from the aorta.

The Peripheral Nervous System

1. The cranial and spinal nerves constitute the PNS. The PNS relays information from the CNS to muscle and effector organs through cranial and spinal nerve tracts arranged in fascicles (multiple fascicles bound together form the peripheral nerve).

The Autonomic Nervous System

1. The ANS is responsible for maintaining a steady state in the internal environment. Two opposing systems make up the ANS: (1) the sympathetic nervous system (thoracolumbar division) responds to stress by mobilizing energy stores and prepares the body to defend itself, and (2) the parasympathetic nervous system (craniosacral division) conserves energy and the body's resources. Both systems function, more or less, at the same time. The enteric autonomic nervous system controls the function of the gastrointestinal tract.

Tests of Nervous System Structure and Function

1. Tests of nervous system structure and function include x-ray films, CT, MRI and MRA, PET, SPECT, cerebral angiography, echoencephalography, electroencephalography, magnetoencephalography, EPs, and analysis of CSF.

REFERENCES

1. Sulaiman W, Gordon T. Neurobiology of peripheral nerve injury. *regeneration, and functional recovery: from bench top research to bedside application, Ochsner J*. 2013;13(1):100–108.
2. Vanderah T, Gould D. *Nolte's the human brain: an introduction to its functional anatomy*. ed 8 St Louis: Elsevier; 2021.
3. Daneman R, Prat A. The blood-brain barrier. *Cold Spring Harb Perspect Biol*. 2015;7(1):a020412.
4. Serlin Y, et al. Anatomy and physiology of the blood-brain barrier. *Semin Cell Dev Biol*. 2015;38:2–6.
5. Karemaker JM. An introduction into autonomic nervous function. *Physiol Meas*. 2017;38(5):R89–R118.
6. Siegel R, et al. *Basic neurochemistry: molecular, cellular, and medical aspects*. ed 8 Philadelphia: Academic Press; 2012.

16

Pain, Temperature Regulation, Sleep, and Sensory Function

Jodi A. Allen

http://evolve.elsevier.com/Rogers/pathophysiology/

CHAPTER OUTLINE

Alterations in sensory function may involve dysfunctions of the general or the special senses. Dysfunctions of the general senses include chronic pain, abnormal temperature regulation, and tactile or proprioceptive dysfunction. Pain is a unique sensory experience that, although universally described as unpleasant, is nonetheless essential to an individual's survival. Pain provides protection by signaling the presence of disease or injury. Like pain, variations in temperature can signal disease. Fever is a common manifestation of dysfunction and is often the first symptom observed in an infectious or inflammatory condition.

Sleep is a normal cyclic process that restores the body's energy and maintains normal function. Sleep is so essential to physiologic and psychologic function that sleep deprivation causes a wide range of clinical manifestations. Prolonged deprivation or disruption of sleep ultimately leads to serious dysfunction.

The special senses of vision, hearing, touch, smell, and taste are the means by which individuals perceive stimuli that are essential for interacting with the environment. Special sensory receptors are connected to specific areas of the brain through the afferent pathways of the peripheral and central nervous system (CNS). Each of the special senses thus involves a connected system of organs and tissues that receives stimuli and sends sensory messages to areas of the CNS, where they are processed and guide behavior. Dysfunctions of the special senses include visual, auditory, olfactory, and gustatory (taste).

PAIN

Pain is one of the body's most important adaptive and protective mechanisms. It is a complex experience comprised of dynamic interactions among physical, cognitive, spiritual, emotional, and environmental factors and cannot be characterized as only a response to injury. McCaffery defined pain as "whatever the experiencing person says it is, existing whenever he says it does."[1] The International Association for the Study of Pain and the American Pain Society defined pain as "an unpleasant sensory and emotional experience associated with actual or potential tissue damage or described in terms of such damage."[2] A more recent proposal for the definition of pain is "pain is a mutually recognizable somatic experience that reflects a person's apprehension of threat to their bodily or existential integrity."[3] Acute pain is protective and promotes withdrawal from painful stimuli, allows the injured part to heal, and teaches avoidance of painful stimuli.

Neuroanatomy of Pain

Three parts of the nervous system are responsible for the sensation, perception, and response to pain:

1. The *afferent pathways*, which begin in the peripheral nervous system (PNS), travel to the spinal gate in the dorsal horn, and then ascend to areas in the diencephalon (thalamus, epithalamus, and hypothalamus) and cortex.

2. The *interpretive centers* located in the subcortical and cortical networks, brainstem, midbrain, diencephalon, and cerebral cortex.
3. The *efferent pathways* that descend from the central nervous system (CNS) back to the dorsal horn of the spinal cord.

The processing of potentially harmful (noxious) stimuli through a normally functioning nervous system is called nociception. Nociceptors, or pain receptors, are free nerve endings in the afferent peripheral nervous system. When they are stimulated, they cause nociceptive pain. The cell bodies of nociceptors are located in the dorsal root ganglia (DRG) for the body and in the trigeminal ganglion for the face. Nociceptors have a peripheral and central axonal branch that innervates their target organ and the spinal cord, respectively. Nociceptors are unevenly distributed throughout the body, so the relative sensitivity to pain differs according to their location (Table 16.1). Nociceptors respond to different types of noxious stimuli: mechanical (pressure or mechanical distortion), thermal (extreme temperatures), or chemical (acids or chemicals of inflammation, such as bradykinin, histamine, leukotrienes, or prostaglandins). Nociception involves four phases: transduction, transmission, perception, and modulation.[4]

TABLE 16.1 Stimuli That Activate Nociceptors (Pain Receptors)

Location of Receptor	Provoking Stimuli
Skin	Pricking, cutting, crushing, burning, freezing
Gastrointestinal tract	Engorged or inflamed mucosa, distention or spasm of smooth muscle, traction on mesenteric attachment
Skeletal muscle	Ischemia, injuries of connective tissue sheaths, necrosis, hemorrhage, prolonged contraction, injection of irritating solutions
Joints	Synovial membrane inflammation
Arteries	Piercing, inflammation
Head	Traction, inflammation, or displacement of arteries, meningeal structures, and sinuses; prolonged muscle contraction
Heart	Ischemia and inflammation
Bone	Periosteal injury: fractures, tumor, inflammation

Pain transduction is the process of converting a painful stimulus into an electrical signal that is transmitted to the CNS. Transduction begins when nociceptors are activated by a painful stimulus (physical, chemical, or thermal), causing ion channels (sodium, potassium, calcium) on nociceptors to open, creating electrical impulses that travel through axons of two primary types of nociceptors that are transmitted to the spinal cord, brainstem, thalamus, and cortex (see Fig. 15.15).[5] The two primary types of nociceptors are A-delta (Aδ) fibers and C fibers. Aδ fibers are larger myelinated fibers that rapidly transmit sharp, well-localized "fast" pain sensations, such as intense heat or a pinprick to the skin. Activation of these fibers causes a spinal reflex withdrawal of the affected body part from the stimulus, before a pain sensation is perceived. C fibers are the most numerous, are smaller, unmyelinated, and are located in muscle, tendons, body organs, and the skin. They slowly transmit dull, aching, or burning sensations that are poorly localized and often constant.

Pain transmission is the conduction of pain impulses along the Aδ and C fibers (primary-order neurons) into the dorsal horn of the spinal cord (Fig. 16.1). Here they form synapses with excitatory

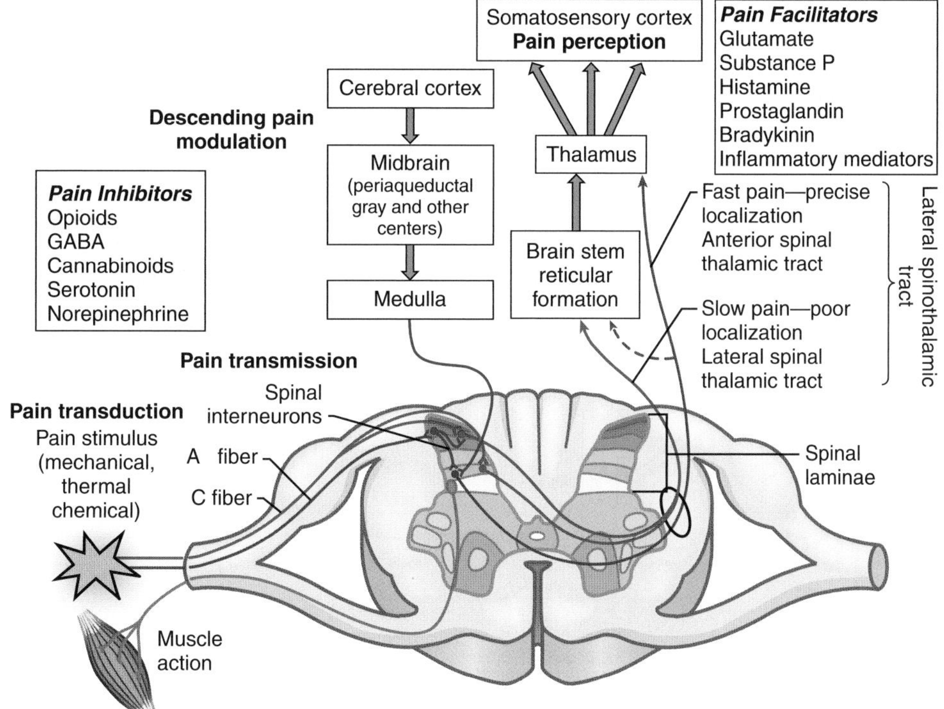

Fig. 16.1 Transmission of Pain Sensations. The Aδ and C fibers synapse in the laminae of the dorsal horn, cross over to the contralateral spinothalamic tract, and then ascend to synapse in the midbrain through the neospinothalamic and paleospinothalamic tracts. Impulses are then conducted to the sensory cortex. Descending pain inhibition is initiated in the cerebral cortex or from the midbrain and medulla.

or inhibitory interneurons (second-order neurons) in the substantia gelatinosa of the dorsal horn. The impulses then synapse with projection neurons (third-order neurons), cross the midline of the spinal cord, and ascend to the brain through two lateral spinothalamic tracts (Fig. 16.2). The anterior spinal thalamic tract carries fast impulses for acute sharp pain. The lateral spinothalamic tract carries slow impulses for dull or chronic pain. The fast, sharp pain is perceived first, followed by dull, throbbing pain. These tracts connect to the reticular formation, hypothalamus, thalamus (the major relay station of sensory information), and limbic system. The impulses are then projected to the somatosensory cortex for interpretation of the location and intensity of the pain (Fig. 16.3), and to other areas of the brain for an integrated response to pain.

Pain perception is the conscious awareness of pain, which occurs primarily in the reticular and limbic systems and the cerebral cortex. Interpretation of pain is influenced by many factors, including genetics, cultural preferences, sex roles, age, level of health, and past pain experiences. Three systems interact to produce the perception of pain.[6]

The sensory-discriminative system is mediated by the somatosensory cortex and is responsible for identifying the presence, character, location, and intensity of pain. The affective-motivational system determines an individual's conditioned avoidance behaviors and emotional responses to pain. It is mediated through the reticular formation, limbic system, and brainstem. The cognitive-evaluative system overlies the individual's learned behavior concerning the experience of pain and therefore can modulate perception of pain. It is mediated through the cerebral cortex. The integration of these three systems is referred to as the "pain matrix"[7] or networks of cerebral connectivity.

Pain threshold and tolerance are subjective phenomena that influence an individual's perception of pain. They can be influenced by genetics, sex, cultural perceptions, expectations, role socialization, physical and mental health, and age (Table 16.2A).

Pain threshold is defined as the lowest intensity of pain that a person can recognize.[2] Intense pain at one location may increase the threshold in another location. For example, a person with severe pain in one knee is more likely to experience less intense chronic back pain (this is called perceptual dominance). Because of perceptual dominance, pain at one site may mask other painful areas. Stress, excessive physical exertion, acupuncture, sexual activity, and other factors can increase the levels of circulating neuromodulators, thereby raising the pain threshold.

Pain tolerance is defined as the greatest intensity of pain that a person can endure.[2] It varies greatly among people and in the same person over time because of the body's ability to

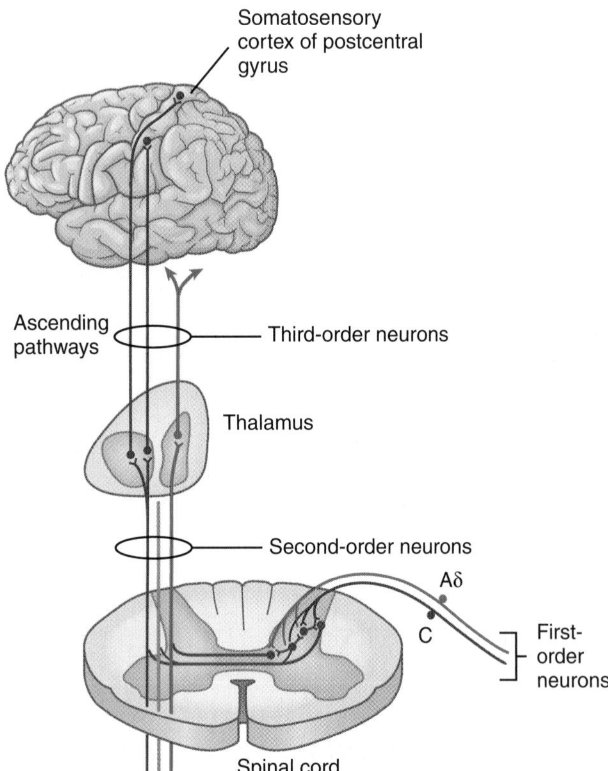

Fig. 16.2 Nociception Pathways. Aδ and C fibers comprise the primary, first-order sensory afferents coming into the gate at the dorsal horn of the spinal cord. Second-order neurons cross the cord ("decussate") and ascend to the thalamus as part of the spinothalamic tract. Third-order afferents project to higher brain centers of the limbic system, the frontal cortex, and the primary sensory cortex of the postcentral gyrus of the parietal lobe.

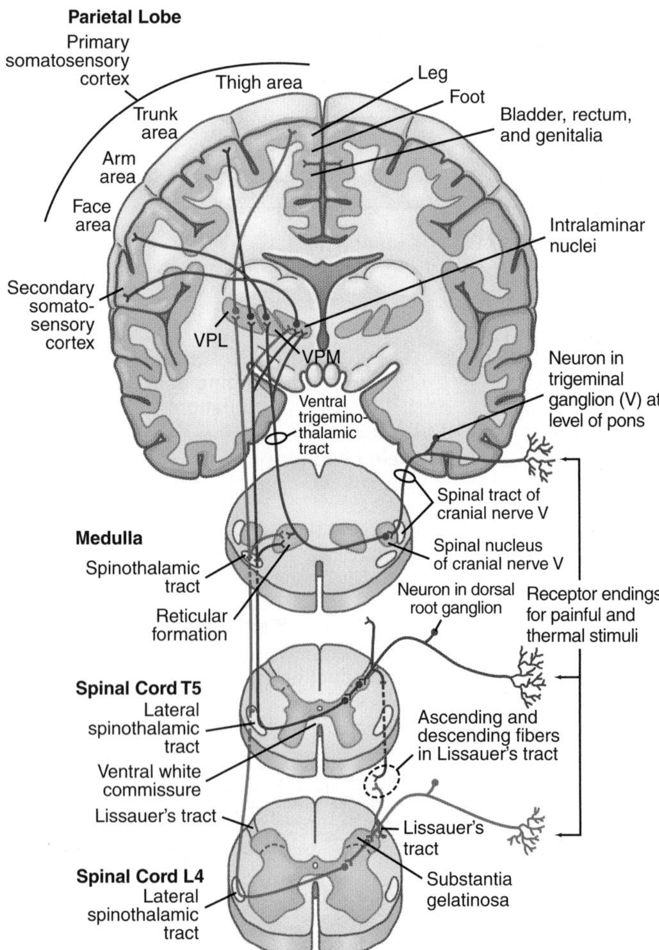

Fig. 16.3 Central Nervous System Pathways That Mediate the Sensations of Pain and Temperature. *VPL*, Ventral posterior lateral thalamic nuclei; *VPM*, ventral posterior medial thalamic nuclei.

Table 16.2A Pain Perception in Infants, Children, and Older Adult Persons

	Infants	Children	Older Adult Persons
Pain threshold	Painful neonatal experiences increase pain sensitivity (lower threshold); pain may be increased with future procedures.	Lower or same as adults.	Individual responses may vary but pain threshold may be elevated.
Physiologic symptoms	Increased heart rate, blood pressure, and respiratory rate; flushing or pallor, sweating, and decreased oxygen saturation.	Same as infants; nausea and vomiting	Same as infants and children; may be decreased in individuals with cognitive impairment.
Behavioral responses	Facial overexpression with furrowed eyebrows and exaggerated eye closure, vertical bulge and furrows in forehead between brows, broadened nasal root, body rigidity, loud crying, angular, square-shaped mouth, chin quiver, sleep disorders, resistance, flailing, and shifting the painful part of the body away from touch.	Individual responses vary. May exhibit verbal or physical aggression, crying, guarding, or defending the body part exposed to pain.	Individual responses vary and may be influenced by presence of painful chronic diseases and decline in renal, intestinal, hepatic, cardiovascular, and neurologic function. Older adults with cognitive impairment may demonstrate changes in behavior (e.g., combative, withdrawn, or increased confusion).

Data from Anand KJS. Defining pain in newborns: need for a uniform taxonomy? *Acta Paediatr.* 2017;106(9):1438–1444; Lautenbacher S, et al. Age changes in pain perception: A systematic-review and meta-analysis of age effects on pain and tolerance thresholds. *Neurosci Biobehav Rev.* 2017;75:104–113; Tracy B, Sean Morrison R. Pain management in older adults. *Clin Ther.* 2013;35(11):1659–1668; Walker SM. Neonatal pain. *Paediatr Anaesth.* 2014;24(1):39–48.

PEDIATRIC CONSIDERATIONS

Pain Perception of Infants and Children

Infants and children have the anatomic and functional ability to perceive pain. However, in the pediatric population, pain is frequently under-recognized and inadequately treated.

Pain pathways and cortical and subcortical centers for pain perception, as well as neurochemicals associated with pain transmission and modulation, are functional in preterm and newborn infants. Alterations in biological factors (e.g., peripheral and central somatosensory function and modulation, brain structure and connectivity) and psychosocial factors (e.g., gender, coping style, mood, and parental response) that influence pain have been identified in children and young adults born very preterm or extremely preterm.[8]

Repetitive, painful experiences and prolonged exposure to analgesic drugs in preterm infants may permanently alter developing synaptic and neuronal pain-processing networks, causing irreversible hypersensitivity to pain with subsequent injury. Alterations occur in both the excitatory and inhibitory pathways in the spinal cord and descending inhibitory processing from the brainstem. When children are not sufficiently treated for pain, stress hormones are released into their systems, resulting in increased catabolism, immunosuppression, and hemodynamic instability.[9]

Facial overexpression with furrowed eyebrows and exaggerated eye closure, body rigidity, loud crying, sleep disorders, resistance, and shifting the painful part of the body away from touch are the most consistent expressions of pain in infants.[9] There may be finger clenching, writhing, back arching, and head banging.

Toddlers in pain may exhibit verbal or physical aggression and crying, or may guard or defend the body part exposed to pain. Children, like adults, have highly individual responses to pain. Any behavioral and physiologic indicators of pain must be carefully and accurately assessed and adequately treated for

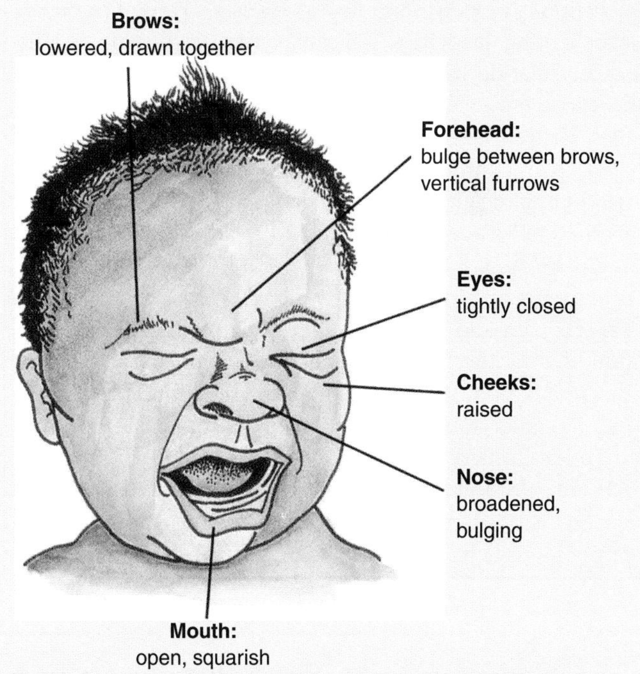

Painful Facial Expression of Infants. (From Hockenberry MJ. *Wong' s Nursing Care of Infants and Children.* 7th ed. St Louis: Mosby; 2003.)

children of all ages. Physiologic responses in all age groups may include increases in heart rate, blood pressure, and respiratory rate; flushing or pallor; sweating; and decreased oxygen saturation.

Assessment of pain includes a thorough pain history received from the child and/or parent, exploring the pain quality, characteristics, location, onset, duration, aggravating

PEDIATRIC CONSIDERATIONS—CONT'D

and alleviating factors, and impact on function. The measurement of pain severity should be done routinely using a developmentally appropriate validated tool. Commonly used tools are listed in Table 16.2B with specified age ranges for the tool.

There are biological and psychosocial factors that influence the perception and severity of pain. Alterations in biological factors, such as peripheral and central somatosensory function, pain modulation, brain structure, and connectivity, have been identified in children and young adults born very preterm or extremely preterm and play a role in pain. There are also psychosocial factors such as gender, coping style, mood, and parental response that influence pain.[8]

GERIATRIC CONSIDERATIONS

Aging and Pain

Pain in the older adult population is highly prevalent and is a complex issue to both identify and treat. Some older adults have an increased pain threshold while others have a decreased pain tolerance; both factors play a role in the identification and treatment of pain.[10,11] It is important to assess the presence of pain in elderly persons with cognitive decline, as it is often neglected, underreported, underestimated, misdiagnosed, and not adequately treated.[12] Inadequate assessment of pain or lack of proper pain management is associated with adverse outcomes including depression, anxiety, sleep disturbances, and mood changes, which often lead to significant suffering, disability, and social isolation with greater costs and burden to the health care system.[10] Chronic and somatic pain have been shown to negatively affect the degree of frailty.[13] The most frequent pain conditions in older adults are chronic unspecified joint pain, chronic back pain, and chronic neck pain.[12] Pain must be accurately treated in relation to its effect on cognitive function, coexisting disease, drug interactions, other reactions to treatment, and an individual's ability to express pain and maintain safety. Treatment is often compounded by the high prevalence of polypharmacy within this population. Pharmacotherapies used for pain management in older adults are usually only partially effective and are often limited by side effects.[10] Older adults prescribed pharmacological treatment must be monitored carefully for any alterations in cognition, liver and renal function, physiological changes, and possible drug interactions.[12]

Table 16.2B Pediatric Pain Assessment Tools

Pain Assessment Tool	Age Range
Revised Premature Infant Pain Profile (PIPP-R)[1]	Less than 28 weeks to greater than 36 weeks gestational age
Revised Face Legs Activity Cry and Consolability (r-FLACC) scale[2]	2 months to 7 years of age
Faces Pain Scale—Revised (FPS-R)[3]	4 years of age and older
Children and Infants Postoperative Pain Scale (CHIPPS)[4] [*Paediatr Anaesth.* 2000;10(3): 303–318.]	Under 5 years of age
Numerical Rating Scale (NRS)[5]	8 years of age and older

[1]Stevens BJ, Gibbins S, Yamada J, et al. The premature infant pain profile-revised (PIPP-R). *Clin J Pain.* 2014;30(3):238–243.
[2]Malviya S, Voepel-Lewis T, Burke C, et al. The revised FLACC observational pain tool: improved reliability and validity for pain assessment in children with cognitive impairment. *Pediatr Anesth.* 2006;16(3):258–265.
[3]Hicks CL, von Baeyer CL, Spafford PA, et al. The faces pain scale-revised: toward a common metric in pediatric pain measurement. *Pain.* 2001;93(2):173–183.
[4]Büttner W, Finke W. Analysis of behavioural and physiological parameters for the assessment of postoperative analgesic demand in newborns, infants and young children: a comprehensive report on 7 consecutive studies. *Paediatr Anaesth.* 2000;10(3):303–318.
[5]Breivik H, Borchgrevink PC, Allen SM, et al. Assessment of pain. *Br J Anaesth.* 2008;101(1):17–24.
Data from Zieliński J, Morawska-Kochman M, Zatoński T. Pain assessment and management in children in the postoperative period: a review of the most commonly used postoperative pain assessment tools, new diagnostic methods and the latest guidelines for postoperative pain therapy in children. *Adv Clin Exp Med.* 2020;29(3):365–374. doi:10.17219/acem/112600. PMID: 32129952.

respond differently to noxious stimuli. Pain tolerance generally *decreases* with repeated exposure to pain, fatigue, anger, boredom, apprehension, and sleep deprivation and may *increase* with alcohol consumption, persistent use of opioid medications, hypnosis, distracting activities, and strong beliefs or faith.

Pain Modulation

Pain modulation involves many different facilitatory and inhibitory mechanisms that increase or decrease the transmission of pain signals throughout the nervous system. Mechanisms include neurotransmitters and central and spinal pathways. Depending on the mechanism, modulation can occur before, during, or after pain is perceived.[14] Analgesic drugs, anesthesia, and nonpharmacologic interventions such as transcutaneous nerve stimulation, acupuncture, hypnosis, and physical therapies are examples of strategies for enhancing pain modulation.

Neurotransmitters of Pain Modulation

A wide variety of neurotransmitters act to modulate control over transmission of pain impulses in the periphery, spinal cord, and brain. The peripheral triggering mechanisms that initiate release of excitatory neurotransmitters include tissue injury (prostaglandins, histamine, bradykinin) and chronic inflammatory lesions (lymphokines). Glutamate, aspartate, substance P, and calcitonin are common excitatory neurotransmitters in the brain and spinal cord. These substances sensitize nociceptors by reducing the activation threshold, leading to increased responsiveness of nociceptors.

Inhibitory neurotransmitters in the CNS include gamma-aminobutyric acid (GABA) and glycine. Norepinephrine and 5-hydroxytryptamine (serotonin) contribute to pain inhibition in the CNS but can excite peripheral nerves.

Endogenous opioids are a family of morphine-like neuropeptides that inhibit transmission of pain impulses in the periphery, spinal cord, and brain by binding with specific opioid receptors (mu [μ], kappa [κ], and delta [δ]) on neurons. They inhibit ion channels, preventing the release of excitatory neurotransmitters, such as substance P and glutamate, in the dorsal horn. In the midbrain they influence descending inhibitory pathways (Fig. 16.4).[15] In peripheral inflamed tissue, opioids are produced and released from immune cells and activate opioid receptors on sensory nerve terminals.[16] Opioid receptors are widely distributed throughout the body and are responsible for general sensations of well-being and modulation of many physiologic processes, including control of respiratory and cardiovascular functions, stress and immune responses, gastrointestinal function, reproduction, and neuroendocrine control.[17,18]

Enkephalins are the most prevalent of the natural opioids and bind to δ opioid receptors. Endorphins (endogenous morphine) are produced in the brain. The best-studied endorphin is β-endorphin, which binds to μ receptors and is purported to produce the greatest sense of exhilaration as well as substantial natural pain relief. Dynorphins are the most potent of the endogenous opioids, binding strongly with κ receptors to impede pain signals. Paradoxically, they play a role in neuropathic pain and in mood disorders and drug addiction. Endomorphins bind with μ receptors and have potent analgesic effects. Nociceptin/orphanin FQ is an opioid that *induces* pain or hyperalgesia but does not interact with opioid receptors. The nociceptin receptor is widely distributed throughout the PNS and CNS and is associated with numerous biological functions, including immune regulation, mood, feeding, muscle contractility, heart rate, and emotion.

Synthetic and natural opiates have pharmacologic actions similar to morphine and bind as direct agonists to the opioid receptors. Morphine has a 50 times higher affinity for μ receptors in comparison with other opioids. Naloxone is the only clinically used opioid receptor antagonist, with a higher affinity for the μ receptors than for the other receptors.

Endocannabinoids are synthesized from phospholipids and are classified as eicosanoids. They activate cannabinoid CB_1 (primarily in the CNS) and CB_2 receptors (primarily in immune tissue [e.g., the spleen]) to modulate pain and other functions, including memory, appetite, immune function, sleep, stress response, thermoregulation, and addiction. CB_1 receptors decrease pain transmission by inhibiting release of excitatory neurotransmitters in the spinal dorsal horn, periaqueductal gray (PAG; the gray matter surrounding the cerebral aqueduct), thalamus, rostral ventromedial medulla (RVM), and amygdala. Cannabis (marijuana) produces a resin containing cannabinoids. Cannabinoids are analgesic in humans, but

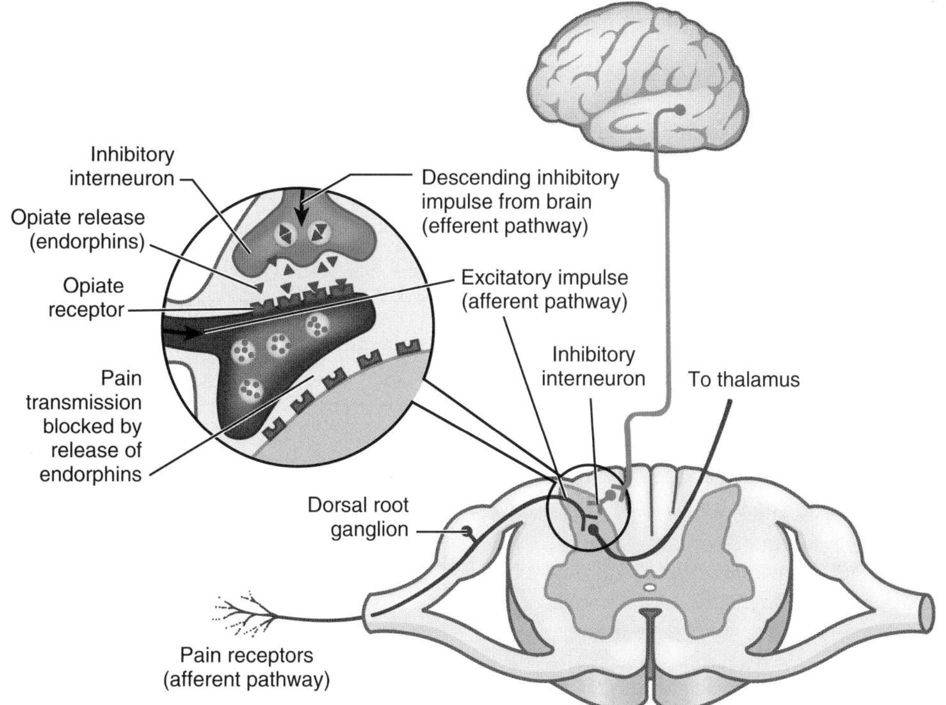

Fig. 16.4 Descending Pathway and Endorphin Response. In this figure, a descending inhibitory impulse is transmitted from the brain to an inhibitory interneuron in the dorsal horn, stimulating the release of endorphin. The endorphin activates a μ opioid receptor and results in inhibition of pain transmission to ascending pathways.

their use is limited by their psychoactive and addictive properties. Work is in progress to develop cannabinoid receptor agonists that do not have addictive side effects.[19,20]

Pathways of Modulation

Descending inhibitory and facilitatory pathways inhibit or facilitate pain. Inhibitory pathways can activate opioid receptors and inhibit release of excitatory neurotransmitters, facilitate release of inhibitory neurotransmitters, or stimulate inhibitory interneurons. Afferent stimulation of particularly the ventromedial medulla and PAG in the midbrain stimulates efferent pathways, which inhibit ascending pain signals at the dorsal horn. The RVM stimulates descending pathways that facilitate or inhibit pain in the dorsal horn.

Segmental pain inhibition occurs when A-beta (Aβ) fibers (large myelinated fibers that transmit touch and vibration sensations) are stimulated and the impulses arrive at the same spinal level or segment as impulses from Aδ or C fibers. They stimulate an inhibitory interneuron and decrease pain transmission. An example is rubbing an area that has been injured to relieve pain.

Diffuse noxious inhibitory control (DNIC) is an endogenous inhibitory pain system that involves a spinal-medullary-spinal pathway. Pain is relieved when two noxious or painful stimuli occur at the same time from different sites (pain inhibiting pain). The efficacy of DNIC is evaluated clinically by testing subjective responses to pain using conditioned pain modulation (CPM). A CPM test uses a consistent protocol to deliver a measurable test pain stimulus at one site before and during or after the application of a measurable conditioning pain stimulus at a comparable site (e.g., the arms). A subjective pain intensity rating scale (i.e., 1 to 10) is used to measure intensity of pain at both sites. The conditioning pain stimulus is expected to affect the pain experience of the test stimulus. Use of CPM assessments can be helpful in determining an individual's endogenous pain inhibitory capacity and for managing acute or chronic pain.[21,22] Expectancy-related cortical activation (placebo effect [beneficial expectations] or nocebo effect [adverse expectations]) can exert control over analgesic systems to attenuate or intensify pain.[23] In other words, cognitive expectations can cause real, measurable physiologic effects that share some of the same descending pain pathways as the pain modulatory systems (see Emerging Science Box: Pain Management With Pharmacogenics).

EMERGING SCIENCE BOX

Pain Management With Pharmacogenics

Pain management has been challenging in light of the United States public health crisis related to use of opioid drugs. Opiate misuse, abuse, and overdose has led to a forced reduction of opioid use for the treatment of pain. Pain is well known for its subjectivity and variability among individuals, creating challenges in development of successful treatment regimens. An emerging approach is the use of pharmacogenics, the study of genetic variants that influence the effects of a drug, to guide clinicians in the development of individualized pain management plans. Pharmacogenics focuses on individual genes, specifically CYP2D6. CYP2D6 is highly polymorphic and is involved in the metabolism of 25% of all drugs currently used in clinical practice. Many commonly used opioids are metabolized by CYP2D6 and their metabolic rate is dependent on the CYP2D6 polymorphism of the individual. Understanding specific gene alleles of individuals will identify ultra-rapid metabolizers, extensive metabolizers, intermediate metabolizers, and poor metabolizers, which would allow for person-specific dosing to limit the potential for opiate misuse, abuse, or overdose. DNA is obtained via buccal swab and analyzed in a pain-related gene panel. While this gene panel is not yet FDA approved, investigative studies have identified improved pain control with safe opioid administration when clinicians are able to tailor the pain management plan to the pharmacogenomics of each person. Pharmacogenomics can also identify potentially opioid-vulnerable individuals who can then be provided with opioid alternative treatments for their pain.

Data from Hockings JK, et al. Pharmacogenomics: an evolving clinical tool for precision medicine. *Cleve Clin J Med.* 2020;87(2):91–99; Kaye AD, et al. Update on the pharmacogenomics of pain management. *Pharmgenomics Pers Med.* 2019;12:125–143; LaPietra MA, et al. A country in crisis: opioid sparing solutions for acute pain management. *Mo Med.* 2019;116(2):140–145.

Clinical Descriptions of Pain

Pain can be described in a variety of ways. Due to the complex nature of pain, many terms overlap, and more than one description is often used. The broad categories of pain are summarized in Box 16.1.

BOX 16.1 Categories of Pain

I. Neurophysiologic Pain
- A. Nociceptive pain
  1. Somatic (e.g., skin, muscle, bone)
  2. Visceral (e.g., intestine, liver, stomach)
  3. Referred
- B. Neuropathic (non-nociceptive)
  1. Central pain (lesion in brain or spinal cord)
  2. Peripheral pain (lesion in peripheral nervous system)

II. Neurogenic Pain
- A. Neuralgia (pain in the distribution of a nerve)
- B. Constant
  1. Sympathetically independent
  2. Sympathetically dependent

III. Temporal Pain (Time Related, Duration)
- A. Acute pain
  1. Somatic
  2. Visceral
  3. Referred
- B. Chronic (pain lasting longer than 3 months)

IV. Pain Location
- A. Abdominal pain
- B. Chest pain
- C. Headache
- D. Low back pain
- E. Orofacial pain
- F. Pelvic pain

V. Etiologic Pain
- A. Cancer pain
- B. Dental pain
- C. Inflammatory pain
- D. Ischemic pain
- E. Vascular pain

Adapted from Mersky H. Taxonomy and classification of chronic pain syndromes. In: Benzon HT, et al, eds. *Practical Management of Pain.* 5th ed. St Louis: Mosby; 2014:13–18.

Some of the most common clinical pain presentations are summarized here.

Acute pain (nociceptive pain) is a normal protective mechanism that alerts the individual to a condition or experience that is immediately harmful to the body and mobilizes the individual to take prompt action to relieve it. Acute pain is transient, usually lasting seconds to days, sometimes up to 3 months. It begins suddenly and is relieved after the chemical mediators (usually related to inflammation) that stimulate pain receptors are removed. Stimulation of the autonomic nervous system results in physical manifestations, including increased heart rate, hypertension, diaphoresis, and dilated pupils. Anxiety related to the pain experience, including its cause, treatment, and prognosis, is common, as is the hope of recovery and expectation of limited duration.

Acute pain arises from cutaneous, deep somatic, or visceral structures and can be classified as (1) somatic, (2) visceral, or (3) referred. Somatic pain arises from the skin (i.e., from an abrasion or a laceration), joints (pain from arthritis or injured tendons), and muscles (strain from overuse or muscle injury). It is either sharp and well localized (especially fast pain carried by Aδ fibers) or dull, aching, throbbing, and poorly localized, as seen in polymodal unmyelinated C fiber transmissions. Visceral pain is transmitted by C fibers and refers to pain in internal organs and the lining of body cavities. It tends to be poorly localized with an aching, gnawing, throbbing, or intermittent cramping quality. It is carried by sympathetic fibers and is associated with nausea and vomiting, hypotension, and, in some cases, shock. Visceral pain often radiates (spreads away from the actual site of the pain) or is referred. Examples of conditions that cause visceral pain include gallstones, pancreatitis, kidney stones, bowel obstruction, appendicitis, and bladder infection. Referred pain is felt in an area removed or distant from its point of origin—the area of referred pain is supplied by the same spinal segment as the actual site of pain. Referred pain can be acute or chronic. Impulses from many cutaneous and visceral neurons converge on the same ascending neuron, and the brain cannot distinguish between the different sources of pain. Because the skin has more receptors, the painful sensation is experienced at the referred site instead of at the site of origin. Referred pain can be acute or chronic. For example, the pain of pancreatitis may be felt in the right shoulder or scapula, or pain from the heart may be referred to the left shoulder or arm. Fig. 16.5 illustrates common areas of referred pain and their associated sites of origin.

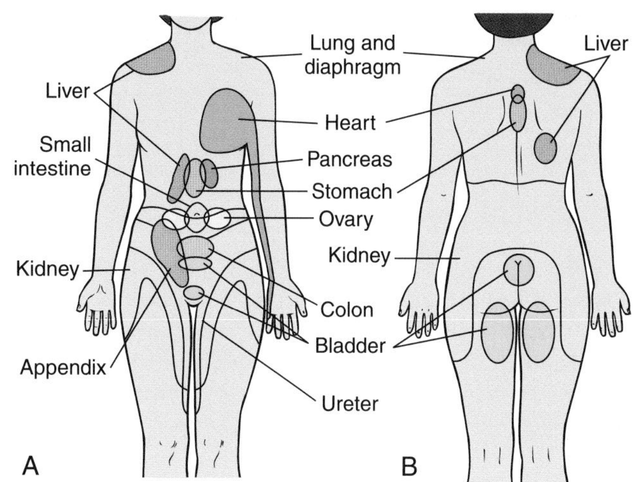

Fig. 16.5 Sites of Referred Pain. **(A)** Anterior view. **(B)** Posterior view.

Chronic or persistent pain has been defined as lasting for more than 3 to 6 months in adults and is pain lasting well beyond the expected normal healing time. It varies with the type of injury, is different among age groups, and produces varietal levels of disability.[24]

Chronic or persistent pain serves no purpose, is poorly understood, and causes suffering. It often appears to be out of proportion to any observable tissue injury. It may be ongoing (e.g., low back pain) or intermittent (e.g., migraine headaches). Changes in the PNS and CNS that cause dysregulation of nociception and pain modulation processes (peripheral and central sensitization) are thought to lead to chronic pain (see the discussion of neuropathic pain later in this section).

Neuroimaging studies have demonstrated brain changes in individuals with chronic pain, which may lead to cognitive deficits and decreased ability to cope with pain.[25,26] These negative manifestations of chronic pain are thought to be due, in part, to the stress of coping with continuous pain and may be reversible when pain is controlled. Because it is not yet possible to predict when acute pain will develop into chronic pain, early treatment of acute pain is encouraged. Comparison of acute and chronic pain is summarized in Table 16.3.

Physiologic responses to intermittent chronic pain are similar to those for acute pain, whereas persistent pain allows for physiologic adaptation, producing a normal heart rate and blood pressure. This leads many to mistakenly conclude that people with chronic pain are malingering because they do not appear to be in pain. As chronic pain progresses, certain behavioral and psychologic changes often emerge, including depression, difficulty eating and sleeping, preoccupation with the pain, and avoidance of pain-provoking stimuli.[27] The desire to relieve pain and the need to hide it become conflicting drives for those with chronic pain, who fear being labeled complainers.[28] Chronic pain is perceived as meaningless and is often associated with a sense of hopelessness as more time elapses; no relief seems possible. Some of the chronic pain syndromes are listed in Table 16.4. Chronic pain associated with specific organ systems is discussed in later chapters.

Neuropathic pain is chronic pain initiated or caused by a primary lesion or dysfunction in the somatosensory nervous system and leads to long-term changes in pain pathway structures (neuroplasticity) and abnormal processing of sensory information. There is amplification of pain without stimulation by injury or inflammation. Neuropathic pain is often described as burning, shooting, shock-like, or tingling. It is characterized by increased sensitivity to painful or nonpainful stimuli with hyperalgesia, allodynia (the induction of pain by normally nonpainful stimuli), and the development of spontaneous pain.[29] Neuropathic pain is classified as either peripheral or central and is associated with central and peripheral sensitization. Peripheral neuropathic pain is caused by peripheral nerve lesions. Peripheral sensitization is an increase in the sensitivity and excitability of primary sensory neurons and cells in the DRG. Examples include nerve entrapment, diabetic neuropathy, and chronic pancreatitis.

TABLE 16.3 Comparison of Acute and Chronic Pain

Characteristic	Acute Pain	Chronic Pain
Experience	An event	A situation; state of existence
Source	External agent or internal disease, injury, or inflammation	Unknown; if known, treatment is prolonged or ineffective
Onset	Usually sudden	May be sudden or develop insidiously
Duration	Transient (up to 3 months); usually of short durationResolves with treatment and healing	Prolonged (months to years); lasts beyond expected normal healing time
Pain identification	Painful and nonpainful areas generally well identified	Painful and nonpainful areas less easily differentiated; change in sensations becomes more difficult to evaluate
Clinical signs	Typical response pattern with more visible signs Anxiety and emotional distress common	Response patterns vary; fewer overt signs (adaptation) Can interfere with sleep, productivity, and quality of life
Significance	Significant (informs person something is wrong); protective	Person looks for significance and meaning; serves no useful purpose
Pattern	Self-limiting or readily corrected	Continuous or intermittent; intensity may vary or remain constant
Course	Suffering usually decreases over time	Suffering usually increases over time
Actions	Leads to actions to relieve pain	Leads to actions to modify pain experience
Prognosis	Likelihood of eventual complete relief	Complete relief usually not possible

TABLE 16.4 Common Chronic Pain Syndromes

Condition	Description
Persistent low back pain	Most common chronic pain condition Results from poor muscle tone, inactivity, muscle strain, or sudden, vigorous exercise
Myofascial pain syndromes	Pain results from muscle spasm, tenderness, stiffness, or injury to muscle and fascia with peripheral and central sensitization Examples include myositis, fibrositis, myalgia, fibromyalgia, and muscle strain Trigger points—small hypersensitive regions in muscle or connective tissues that, when stimulated, produce pain in a specific area As disorder progresses, pain becomes increasingly generalized
Chronic postoperative pain	Persistent pain that can occur with disruption or cutting of sensory nerves; examples include post-thoracotomy, postmastectomy; risk factors may include preexisting pain and genetic susceptibility
Cancer pain	Attributed to advance of disease, treatment, or coexisting disease entities
Deafferentation pain	Pain because of alteration of sensory input into central nervous system is caused by damage to peripheral nerves Common types include severe burning pain triggered by various stimuli, such as cold, light touch, or sound, and complex regional pain syndromes (occur after peripheral nerve injury and are characterized by continuous, severe, burning pain associated with vasomotor changes and muscle wasting)
Hyperalgesia	Increased sensitivity and decreased pain threshold to tactile and painful stimuli Pain is diffuse, modified by fatigue and emotion, and mixed with other sensations May result from chronic irritation of central nervous system areas
Hemiagnosia	Loss of ability to identify source of pain on one side of body Painful stimuli on that side produce discomfort, anxiety, moaning, agitation, and distress but no attempt to withdraw from stimulus Associated with stroke
Phantom limb pain	Pain experienced in amputated limb after stump has completely healed; may be immediate or occur months later; associated with preamputation pain, acute postoperative pain Exact cause is unknown, thought to originate in brain; can be influenced by emotions/sympathetic stimulation
Complex regional pain syndrome	Chronic pain is usually associated with limb injury, surgery, or fractures Characterized by autonomic and neuroinflammatory features and pain out of proportion to expected pain

Central neuropathic pain is caused by a lesion or dysfunction in the brain or spinal cord. A progressive repeated stimulation of group C neurons (known as *wind-up*) in the dorsal horn leads to central sensitization, an increased sensitivity of central pain signaling neurons. This results in pathologic changes in the CNS that cause chronic pain. Examples include brain or spinal cord trauma, tumors, vascular lesions, multiple sclerosis, Parkinson disease, postherpetic neuralgia, and phantom limb pain.

The following mechanisms have been implicated in the cause of neuropathic pain[30]:

- Changes in sensitivity of neurons—lower threshold with peripheral and central sensitization
- Spontaneous impulses from regenerating peripheral nerves
- Alterations in the DRG and spinothalamic tract in response to peripheral nerve injury (i.e., deafferentation pain—loss of pain-related afferent information to the brain)
- Loss of pain inhibition and stimulation of pain facilitation by excitatory neurotransmitters in the dorsal horn (e.g., release of glutamate)
- Loss of descending inhibitory pain modulation
- Hyperexcitable spinal interneurons stimulated by Aβ fibers (nonpainful stimulation of pain)
- Release of nociceptive inflammatory cytokines, chemokines, and growth factors by activated glial cells
- Structural and functional alterations in brain processing neural networks

Because of the complexity of the causes of neuropathic pain syndromes, they are difficult to treat. Multimodal therapy is often needed, including nondrug treatment.[31]

An Overview of Chronic Pain Syndromes

Myofascial pain syndrome (MPS) is a regional pain syndrome associated with injury to muscle, fascia, and tendons and includes myositis, fibrositis, myofibrositis, myalgia, (see Chapter 44 for fibromyalgia), and muscle strain. MPS involves myofascial trigger points within a taut band of skeletal muscle ("muscle knots"). Compression of the trigger point causes a local twitch response (a small, quick contraction of muscle fibers) accompanied by referral of pain, motor dysfunction, and autonomic responses (e.g., flushing, diaphoresis, temperature changes). The symptoms often occur in association with poor muscle tone, inactivity, repeated muscle or tendon strain, sudden vigorous exercise, or muscle overuse. The pathophysiology is not clearly known. The pain may be the result of peripheral and central sensitization with low-threshold mechanosensitive afferents projecting to sensitized dorsal horn neurons. There may be neuroaxonal degeneration with alterations in neuromuscular transmission (e.g., extra leakage of acetylcholine at the neuromuscular junction induces persistent contraction) or muscle energy consumption that exceeds energy supply.[32] During the early stages of the disorder the pain is localized, but as the disorder progresses, it becomes deep, aching, and more generalized. Chronic postoperative pain is pain that persists for at least 3 months after surgery, after ruling out any other possible causes, such as infection, tumor recurrence, or pain arising from pre-existing conditions. The types of pain can include nerve injury, complex regional pain syndrome, phantom limb pain, chronic donor site pain, post-thoracotomy pain syndrome, post-mastectomy pain syndrome, joint arthroplasty pain, and postsurgical abdominal and pelvic pain. Nerve injury and inflammation may induce plastic changes in the PNS and CNS contributing to peripheral and central nerve sensitization with allodynia and hypersensitivity. There may also be alterations in descending inhibitory pathways. Psychological factors, including anxiety and depression, also influence the occurrence of postoperative pain. Multimodal approaches to analgesia are needed for pain management including adequate management of preoperative pain and postoperative management of acute pain.[33–35] Cancer pain is often chronic, and the causes are multifactorial and related to site and type of cancer, extent of disease, treatment modalities, age, and access to care.[36] Cancers generate and secrete mediators that sensitize and activate primary afferent nociceptors in the area of the tumor, resulting in neurochemical reorganization of the spinal cord, which contributes to spontaneous activity and enhanced pain responsiveness. Increasing pressure of a growing tumor on nerve endings, tissue destruction, inflammatory mediators, distention of visceral surfaces, obstruction of ducts and intestine, pathologic fractures, chemotherapy, radiation therapy, surgical procedures, and opioid-induced hyperalgesia also promote pain. These processes lead to both nociceptive and neuropathic pain.[37] Therapeutic approaches to the management of cancer pain have advanced significantly in recent years, particularly in palliative care and hospice programs. Frequent assessment of pain, management of breakthrough pain, and implementation of individualized interdisciplinary therapeutic strategies (including pharmacotherapeutic, anesthetic, neurosurgical, psychologic, and rehabilitative techniques along with frequent evaluations) are essential to optimal cancer pain management. Research is in progress to evaluate the effects of different opioid receptors on tumor growth and suppression and will assist in selecting the optimum drugs for pain treatment.[38] Poststroke pain syndromes can be acute but often occur up to 6 months after stroke and become chronic. Both nociceptive and neuropathic mechanisms of pain can be involved. Pain can include central poststroke pain or be secondary to spasticity, headache, shoulder pain, and complex region pain syndrome (see below). Central poststroke pain is pain and sensory abnormalities that manifest in the body parts that correspond to the area of the brain that have been injured by the cerebrovascular lesion. Hyperalgesia, dysesthesias, allodynia, spontaneous pain, and other sensory deficits are common.

There may be hyperexcitation in the damaged sensory pathways, damage to the central inhibitory pathways, or a combination of the two, making it difficult to differentiate from other causes of pain.[39]

Phantom limb pain (PLP) is pain that an individual feels in the amputated limb, usually distally (hands and feet) after the stump has completely healed (1 to 3 months after amputation). PLP is differentiated from *residual limb pain*, which is pain originating from the actual site of the amputated limb and can be associated with infection and neuroma formation. Both types of pain can occur at the same time. PLP can be intermittent or severe and occasional or constant, throbbing, stabbing, burning, or cramping. Both peripheral and central mechanisms of pain contribute to phantom limb pain. There is injury to peripheral nerves with increased excitability. Changes in pain processing in both the brain and spinal cord are known to occur.[40] Nonpainful phantom limb sensations occur in almost all amputees, but the sensations usually fade with time. Chronic regional pain syndrome type II can also be a component of PLP.

Complex regional pain syndrome (CRPS) is chronic neuropathic pain usually associated with limb injury. Two forms are described: complex regional pain syndrome-I (CRPS-I) (previously termed reflex sympathetic dystrophy syndrome) associated with injury but no apparent nerve injury; and complex regional pain syndrome-II (CRPS-II) (previously termed causalgia) with evidence of nerve injury. The symptoms of both forms are similar. CRPS is distinguished from other chronic pain disorders by signs of autonomic and inflammatory changes in the pain region of the injured nerve. There are *autonomic symptoms*: changes in skin color, temperature, and sweating and alterations in hair and nail growth for the affected limb; *motor symptoms*: tremor or weakness may be present; and *sensory symptoms*: hypersensitivity, hyperalgesia, and allodynia. CRPS is further distinguished as "warm CRPS," associated with a warm, red, and edematous extremity; and "cold CRPS," associated with a cold, dusky, and sweaty extremity. Peripheral and central sensitization contribute to the pain syndrome, but the mechanisms are unknown. A combination of injury and the presence of inflammatory cytokines and neuropeptides may lead to peripheral nociceptive sensitization and physiologic change in pain transmission and in autonomic and motor systems.[41]

TEMPERATURE REGULATION

Human thermoregulation is achieved through precise balancing of heat production, heat conservation, and heat loss The normal range of body temperature is considered to be 36.2°C to 37.7°C (96.2°F to 99.4°F) overall, but a person's individual body parts will vary in temperature. Body temperature rarely exceeds 41°C (105.8°F). The extremities are generally cooler than the trunk, and the temperature at the core of the body (as measured by rectal temperature) is generally 0.5°C higher than the surface temperature (as measured by oral temperature). Internal temperature varies in response to activity, environmental temperature, and daily fluctuation (circadian rhythm). Oral temperatures fluctuate within 0.2°C to 0.5°C during a 24-hour period. Women tend to have wider fluctuations that follow the menstrual cycle, with a sharp rise in temperature just before ovulation. The daily fluctuating temperature in both sexes peaks around 6 p.m. and is at its lowest during sleep. Maintenance of body temperature within the normal range is necessary for life.

Control of Body Temperature

Temperature regulation (thermoregulation) is mediated primarily by the hypothalamus and endocrine system. Peripheral thermoreceptors in the skin, liver, and skeletal muscle (unmyelinated C fibers and thinly myelinatewd Aδ fibers) and central thermoreceptors in the hypothalamus, spinal cord, viscera, and great veins provide the hypothalamus with information about body temperatures. If these temperatures are low or high, the hypothalamus triggers heat production and heat conservation or heat loss mechanisms.[42]

Body heat is produced by the chemical reactions of metabolism and skeletal muscle tone and contraction. The heat-producing mechanism (chemical or non-shivering thermogenesis) begins with hypothalamic thyrotropin-releasing hormone (TRH); it stimulates the anterior pituitary to release thyroid-stimulating hormone (TSH), which acts on the thyroid gland and stimulates the release of thyroxine. Thyroxine then acts on the adrenal medulla, causing the release of epinephrine into the bloodstream. Epinephrine causes cutaneous vasoconstriction, stimulates glycolysis, and increases metabolic rate, thus increasing body heat. Norepinephrine and thyroxine activate brown fat thermogenesis where energy is released as heat (non-shivering thermogenesis) instead of as adenosine triphosphate (ATP). Heat is distributed by the circulatory system.

The hypothalamus also triggers heat conservation by stimulating the sympathetic nervous system and results in increased skeletal muscle tone, initiating the shivering response and producing vasoconstriction. Sympathetic stimulation also constricts peripheral blood vessels and redistributes blood flow. Centrally warmed blood is shunted away from the periphery to the core of the body, where heat can be retained. This involuntary mechanism takes advantage of the insulating layers of the skin and subcutaneous fat to protect the core temperature. The hypothalamus relays information to the cerebral cortex about cold, and voluntary responses result. Individuals typically bundle up, keep moving, or curl up in a ball. These types of voluntary physical activities provide insulation, increase skeletal muscle activity, and decrease the amount of skin surface available for heat loss through radiation, convection, and conduction.

The hypothalamus responds to warmer core and peripheral temperatures by reversing the same mechanisms resulting in heat loss. Heat loss is achieved through (1) radiation, (2) conduction, (3) convection, (4) vasodilation, (5) evaporation (sweating), (6) decreased muscle tone, (7) increased respiration, (8) voluntary measures, and (9) adaptation to warmer climates (i.e., increasing or decreasing the volume of sweat). Table 16.5 summarizes further information about heat production and loss.

Temperature Regulation in Infants and Older Adult Persons

Infants (particularly low-birth-weight infants) and older adult persons require special attention to maintenance of body temperature. Term infants produce sufficient body heat, primarily through metabolism of brown fat, but cannot conserve heat produced because of their small body size, greater ratio of body surface to body weight, and inability to shiver. Infants also have little subcutaneous fat and thus are not as well insulated as adults. Children also have a greater ratio of body surface to body weight, lower sweating rate, higher peripheral blood flow in the heat, and a greater extent of vasoconstriction in the cold than adults. They can acclimatize to changes in environmental temperatures but do so at a lower rate than adults.

Older adult persons respond poorly to environmental temperature extremes because of their slowed blood circulation, structural and functional skin changes, overall decreased heat-producing activities, and the presence of disease (i.e., congestive heart failure, chronic lung disease, diabetes mellitus, or peripheral vascular disease). Cold stress in older adults also decreases coronary perfusion.[43] In addition, older adult persons have a decreased shivering response (delayed onset and decreased effectiveness), slowed metabolic rate, decreased vasoconstrictor response, diminished or absent ability to sweat, decreased peripheral sensation, desynchronized circadian rhythm, decreased perception of heat and cold, decreased thirst, decreased nutritional reserves, decreased brown adipose tissue, and decreased shivering response.[44,45]

TABLE 16.5 Mechanisms of Heat Production and Heat Loss

Condition	Description
Heat Production	
Chemical reactions of metabolism	Occur during ingestion and metabolism of food and while maintaining body at rest (basal metabolism); occur in body core (e.g., liver)
Skeletal muscle contraction	Gradual increase in muscle tone or rapid muscle oscillations (shivering)
Nonshivering thermogenesis	Epinephrine is released and produces rapid, transient increase in heat production by raising basal metabolic rate; quick, brief effect that counters heat lost through conduction and convection; involves brown adipose tissue, which decreases markedly in older adults; thyroid hormone increases metabolism
Heat Loss	
Radiation	Heat loss through electromagnetic waves emanating from surfaces with temperature higher than surrounding air
Conduction	Heat loss by direct molecule-to-molecule transfer from one surface to another, so that warmer surface loses heat to cooler surface
Convection	Transfer of heat through currents of gases or liquids; exchanges warmer air at body's surface with cooler air in surrounding space
Vasodilation	Diverts core-warmed blood to surface of body, with heat transferred by conduction to skin surface and from there to surrounding environment; occurs in response to autonomic stimulation under control of hypothalamus
Evaporation	Body water evaporates from surface of skin and linings of mucous membranes; major source of heat reduction connected with increased sweating in warmer surroundings
Decreased muscle tone	Exhausted feeling caused by moderately reduced muscle tone and curtailed voluntary muscle activity
Increased respiration	Air is exchanged with environment through normal process; minimal effect
Voluntary mechanisms	"Stretching out" and "slowing down" in response to high body temperatures; increasing body surface area available for heat loss; dressing in light-colored, loose-fitting garments
Adaptation to warmer climates	Gradual process beginning with lassitude, weakness, and faintness; proceeding through increased sweating, lowered sodium content, decreased heart rate, and increased stroke volume and extracellular fluid volume; and terminating in improved warm weather functioning and decreased symptoms of heat intolerance (work output, endurance, and coordination increase; subjective feelings of discomfort decrease)

Pathogenesis of Fever

Fever (febrile response) is a temporary resetting of the hypothalamic thermostat to a higher level in response to exogenous or endogenous pyrogens. Exogenous pyrogens (endotoxins produced by pathogens; see Chapter 10) stimulate the release of inflammatory endogenous pyrogens from phagocytic cells (primarily macrophages), including Prostaglandin E2 (PGE_2), tumor necrosis factor-α (TNF-α), interleukin-1 (IL-1), interleukin-6 (IL-6), and interferon γ (IFNγ). These pyrogenic cytokines raise the thermal set point by acting on the hypothalamus to induce an integrated endocrine, autonomic nervous system, and behavioral response and also initiate the acute phase response (described below). The hypothalamic set point for temperature regulation is elevated, signaling an increase in heat production and conservation. Peripheral vasoconstriction shunts blood from the skin to the body core. Epinephrine release increases metabolic rate and muscle tone. Decreased release of vasopressin (anti-diuretic hormone) reduces the volume of body fluid to be heated. The individual feels colder, dresses more warmly, decreases body surface area by curling up, and may go to bed in an effort to get warm. Symptoms of lassitude and anorexia are common and may be related to energy conservation to support the increased metabolic demands of fever. Body temperature is maintained at the new level until the fever "breaks," when the set point begins to return to normal with decreased heat production and increased heat reduction mechanisms. The individual feels very warm, dons cooler clothes, throws off the covers, and stretches out. Once the body has returned to a normal temperature, the individual feels more comfortable and the hypothalamus adjusts thermoregulatory mechanisms to maintain the new temperature (Fig. 16.6).

An acute phase response (see Chapter 7) is a defensive reaction to control pathogens that occurs when pyrogenic and other cytokines are released in response to infection and inflammation. Protective proteins such as C-reactive protein, fibrinogen, and ferritin are produced. Other proteins such as albumin, transferrin, and transthyretin are reduced. Neutrophils numbers are increased. In addition to fever, other symptoms occur, including anorexia, fatigue, malaise, somnolence, and loss of concentration. At the cellular level, inflammatory pyrogenic cytokines promote muscle catabolism and hyperglycemia (gluconeogenesis, glycogenolysis, and insulin resistance) by stimulating release of adrenocorticotropic hormone (ACTH) and glucocorticoids to support glucose-consuming cells.[46]

During inflammation and fever, cryogens modulate the duration and intensity of the febrile response. Antipyretic cytokines such as arginine vasopressin (AVP), melanocyte-stimulating hormone

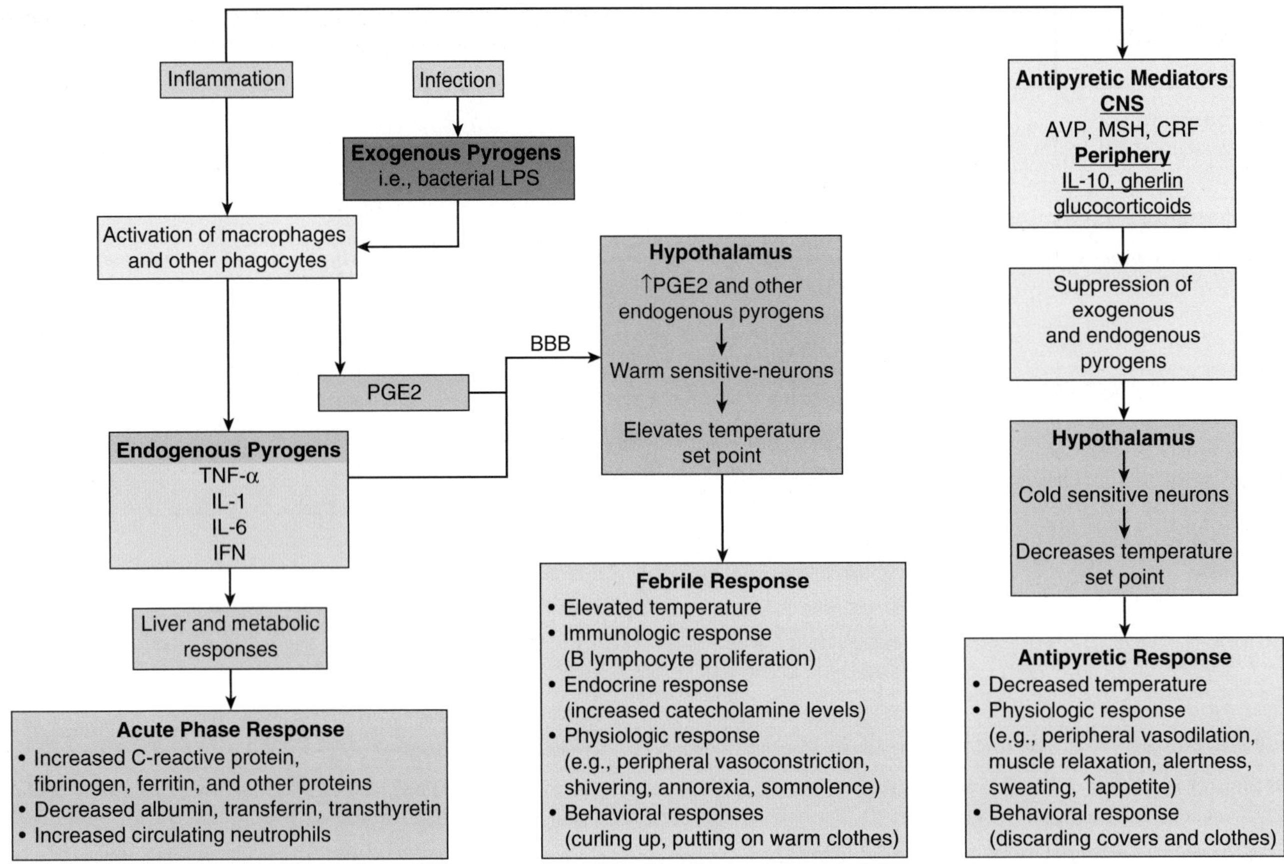

Fig. 16.6 Modulation of Fever and Acute Phase Response. Infection and inflammation initiate the release of exogenous pyrogens from pathogens and endogenous pyrogens from macrophages and other immune cells. Endogenous pyrogens and PGE_2 act on the hypothalamus to elevate the temperature set point and initiate fever and the acute phase response. Fever is modulated by antipyretic mediators (cryogens) from both the CNS and periphery which suppress the febrile response and prevent damage from excessively high temperatures. *BBB*, Blood brain barrier; *AVP*, arginine vasopressin; *CRP*, C-reactive protein; *IFN*, interferon; *IL*, interleukin-1, interleukin-6; *MCH*, melanocortin; *PGE_2*, prostaglandin E_2; *TNF-α*, tumor necrosis factor-alpha.

(MSH), and corticotropin-releasing factor (CRF) are released from the brain, and systemic anti-inflammatory mediators (e.g., IL-10, ghrelin, glucocorticoids) are released from the periphery. These mediators act as endogenous cryogens or antipyretics to decrease the thermal set point in the hypothalamus (see Fig. 16.6).[47] This antipyretic effect constitutes a negative-feedback loop for temperature control and prevents lethal effects of uncontrolled temperature elevation. When this antipyretic effect is ineffective or the physiologic response to fever is dangerous to organ system function, antipyretic medications (e.g., aspirin, acetaminophen, or ibuprofen) may be given to suppress PGE_2 and fever.

Febrile seizures may occur in children with temperatures greater than 38°C (100.4°F) without CNS infection, hypoglycemia, or electrolyte disorders. The seizures are caused by systemic infection with the release of inflammatory cytokines that cross the blood-brain barrier and stimulate neuronal hyperexcitability, triggering the seizure.[48] Febrile seizures are more predominant in boys before age 5 years, and genetic factors contribute to susceptibility. Simple febrile seizures are generally brief and self-limiting, lasting less than 5 minutes and without recurrence. Complex febrile seizures last more than 15 minutes with focal neurologic signs (e.g., one side of body involved, stiff neck) and recur within 24 hours. Although in most instances there appear to be no long-term effects on the child, a small percentage of children may develop epilepsy.[49] Prolonged febrile seizures are associated with the development of temporal lobe epilepsy in children and are probably associated with functional changes in neurons and neural networks. Treatment includes antipyretic and/or antiepileptic drugs.[50]

Fever of unknown origin (FUO) is a body temperature of greater than 38.3°C (101°F) for longer than 3 weeks' duration that remains undiagnosed after 3 days of hospital investigation, three outpatient visits, or 1 week of ambulatory investigation. The clinical categories of FUO include infectious, rheumatic/inflammatory, neoplastic, HIV-associated, and miscellaneous and undiagnosed disorders.[51]

BOX 16.2 Effects of Fever at the Extremes of Age

Older Adult Persons

Subtle or atypical responses to infectious fever are often accompanied by dehydration, and in severe systemic infection there may be no fever. Symptoms can include feeling cold or warm, having strange body sensations, headache, vivid dreams, and hallucinations.

Severe systemic infections may cause alternating hypothermia and high fever in a 24 h period.

Infants and Children

Infected babies may not develop infectious fever in the first few days of life.

Young infants (less than 60–90 days of age) often present with fever and no other symptoms, making differential diagnosis difficult.

Children develop higher temperatures than adults for relatively minor infections, and any skin vasoconstriction can lead to a rapid increase in body temperature.

Febrile seizures before age 5 years are more common and can be related to an autosomal dominant polygenic inheritance.

Severe systemic infections may cause alternating hypothermia and high fever in a 24 h period, the same as elderly adults.

Benefits of Fever

Moderate fever helps the body respond to infectious processes through several mechanisms.[52,53]

1. Raising of body temperature kills many pathogens and adversely affects their growth and replication.
2. Higher body temperatures decrease serum levels of iron, zinc, and copper—minerals needed for bacterial replication.
3. Increased temperature causes lysosomal breakdown and autodestruction of cells, preventing viral replication in infected cells.
4. Heat increases lymphocytic transformation and motility of polymorphonuclear neutrophils, facilitating the immune response.
5. Phagocytosis is enhanced, and production of antiviral interferon is augmented.

Suppression of fever with antipyrogenic medications can be effective but should be used with caution.[54]

Infection and fever responses in older adult persons and children may vary from those in normal adults. Box 16.2 lists the principal features associated with fever at these extremes of age.[45,55]

Disorders of Temperature Regulation

Hyperthermia

Hyperthermia is elevation of the body temperature without an increase in the hypothalamic set point. Hyperthermia can produce nerve damage, coagulation of cell proteins, and death. At 41°C (105.8°F), nerve damage produces convulsions in the adult. Death results at 43°C (109.4°F). Hyperthermia may be therapeutic, accidental, or associated with stroke or head trauma. Prevention of hyperthermia in stroke and head trauma assists in limiting brain injury.[56]

Therapeutic hyperthermia is a form of local, regional, or whole-body hyperthermia used to destroy pathologic microorganisms or tumor cells by facilitating the host's natural immune process or tumor blood flow or activate drugs.[57,58]

The forms of accidental hyperthermia are summarized as follows.[59]

1. Heat cramps—severe, spasmodic cramps in the abdomen and extremities that follow prolonged sweating and associated sodium loss. Usually occur in those not accustomed to heat or those performing strenuous work in very warm climates. Fever, rapid pulse rate, and increased blood pressure accompany the cramps. Treatment includes administration of oral dilute salt solutions.
2. Heat exhaustion—results from prolonged high core or environmental temperatures that cause profound vasodilation and profuse sweating, leading to dehydration, decreased plasma volumes, hypotension, decreased cardiac output, and tachycardia. Symptoms include weakness, dizziness, confusion, nausea, and fainting. Treatment includes administration of oral or parenteral dilute salt solution.
3. Heat stroke—a potentially lethal condition associated with multiorgan failure. Heat stroke can be caused by exertion, by overexposure to environmental heat, or from impaired physiologic mechanisms for heat loss. With very high core temperatures (>40°C [104°F]), there is cell injury and loss of body heat regulation. Symptoms include high core temperature, absence of sweating, rapid pulse rate, confusion, agitation, and coma. The increase in skin blood flow requirements decreases intestinal blood flow and increases intestinal membrane permeability. Increased circulating endotoxin, release of inflammatory mediators, and hypovolemia promote coagulation with microvascular thrombosis leading to multiorgan system and neuronal dysfunction. Complications include cerebral edema, degeneration of the CNS, swollen dendrites, renal tubular necrosis, and hepatic failure with delirium, coma, and eventually death if treatment is not undertaken. There is controversy about whether there is failure of the hypothalamic thermoregulatory center during the acute phase of recovery.[60,61]
4. Malignant hyperthermia—a potentially lethal hypermetabolic complication of a rare autosomal dominant inherited muscle disorder that may be triggered by inhaled halogenated anesthetics and depolarizing muscle relaxants.[62] The syndrome involves uncontrolled release of calcium from muscle cells with hypermetabolism, uncoordinated muscle contractions, increased muscle work, increased oxygen consumption, hypercarbia, and a raised level of lactic acid production. Acidosis develops, and body temperature rises, with resulting tachypnea, tachycardia, cardiac dysrhythmias, hypotension, decreased cardiac output, and cardiac arrest. Signs resemble those of coma—unconsciousness, absent reflexes, fixed pupils, apnea, and occasionally a flat electroencephalogram. Oliguria and anuria are common. It is most common in children and adolescents. Treatment includes withdrawal of the provoking agent, oxygen therapy, body cooling therapy, administration of drugs that inhibit calcium release from muscle (dantrolene), treatment of arrhythmias, and maintenance of urine output.

Hypothermia

Hypothermia (core body temperature less than 35°C [95°F]) produces depression of the CNS and respiratory system, vasoconstriction, alterations in microcirculation and coagulation, and ischemic tissue damage. Hypothermia may be accidental or therapeutic (Box 16.3). Most tissues can tolerate low temperatures in controlled situations, such as surgery. However, in severe hypothermia, ice crystals form on the inside of the cell, causing cells to rupture and die. Tissue hypothermia slows cell metabolism, increases the blood viscosity, slows microcirculatory blood flow, facilitates blood coagulation, and stimulates profound vasoconstriction (also see Frostbite, Chapter 46).

Trauma and Temperature

Major body trauma can affect temperature regulation through various mechanisms. Damage to the CNS, release of inflammatory mediators, increased intracranial pressure, or intracranial bleeding typically produces a body temperature of greater than 39°C (102.2°F), generally higher than infectious fever. This sustained noninfectious fever, often referred to as a central fever or neurogenic fever, appears with or without bradycardia. A central fever does not induce sweating and is very resistant to antipyretic therapy.[63] Other traumatic mechanisms that produce temperature alterations include accidental injuries, hemorrhagic shock, major surgery, and thermal burns. The severity and type of alteration (hyperthermia or hypothermia) vary with the severity of the cause and the body system affected.

Accidental Hypothermia. Accidental hypothermia is generally the result of sudden immersion in cold water or prolonged exposure to cold environments. At particular risk for accidental hypothermia are infants and older adults, because thermoregulatory mechanisms are immature or altered in these two groups. Also at risk are individuals with conditions that diminish the ability to generate heat. Such conditions include hypothyroidism, hypopituitarism, decreased liver function, malnutrition, Parkinson disease, and rheumatoid arthritis. Other risk factors include chronic increased vasodilation and decreased thermoregulatory control caused by cerebral injuries, ketoacidosis, uremia, and drug overdoses. In acute hypothermia, peripheral vasoconstriction shunts blood away from the cooler skin to the core in an effort to decrease heat loss, which produces peripheral tissue ischemia. Intermittent reperfusion of the extremities (the Lewis phenomenon) helps preserve peripheral oxygenation. Intermittent peripheral perfusion continues until core temperatures drop dramatically.

The hypothalamic center stimulates shivering in an effort to increase heat production. Severe shivering occurs at core temperatures of 35°C (95°F) and continues until core temperature

BOX 16.3 Defining Characteristics of Hypothermia

Accidental Hypothermia

The unintentional decrease in core temperature to less than 35°C (95°F) results from sudden immersion in cold water, prolonged exposure to cold environments, diseases that diminish the ability to generate heat, or altered thermoregulatory mechanisms. It is most common among young and older adult persons.

Factors That Increase Risk

1. Hypothyroidism
2. Hypopituitarism
3. Malnutrition and muscle wasting
4. Parkinson disease
5. Rheumatoid arthritis
6. Chronic increased vasodilation
7. Failure of thermoregulatory control resulting from cerebral injury, ketoacidosis, uremia, sepsis, and drug overdose

Response Mechanisms

1. Peripheral vasoconstriction—shunts blood away from cooler skin to core to decrease heat loss and produces peripheral tissue ischemia
2. Intermittent reperfusion of extremities (Lewis phenomenon) helps preserve peripheral oxygenation until core temperature drops dramatically
3. Hypothalamic center induces shivering; thinking becomes sluggish, and coordination is depressed
4. Stupor; heart rate and respiratory rate decline; cardiac output diminishes; metabolic rate falls; acidosis; eventual ventricular fibrillation and asystole occur at 30°C (86°F) and lower

Treatment

1. Most changes are reversible with rewarming
2. Core temperature greater than 30°C (86°F)—active rewarming (external)
3. Core temperature less than 30°C (86°F) or with severe cardiovascular problems—active core rewarming (internal)

Targeted Temperature Management (Therapeutic Hypothermia)

Used to slow metabolism, prevent hypoxia and ischemic injury, and provide neuroprotection after cardiac arrest, during surgery (e.g., limb reimplantation), for treatment of neonatal encephalopathy, or to prevent fever or maintain normothermia. Studies are in progress to evaluate outcomes of hypothermia for management of neurologic injury.

Effects and Cautions

1. Stresses the heart, leading to ventricular fibrillation and cardiac arrest (may be desired outcome in open heart surgery when heart must be stopped)
2. Shivering increases metabolic rate, oxygen consumption, heart and respiratory rate, and exhausts liver glycogen stores.
3. Decreases insulin secretion, increases insulin resistance leading to hyperglycemia
4. Surface cooling may cause burns, frostbite, and fat necrosis
5. Immunosuppression with increased infection risk
6. Slows drug distribution, hepatic metabolism, and renal clearance of drug metabolites

From Willmore R. Cardiac arrest secondary to accidental hypothermia: the physiology leading to hypothermic arrest. *Air Med J.* 2020;39(2):133–136; Rasmussen TP, Bullis TC, Girotra S. Targeted temperature management for treatment of cardiac arrest. *Curr Treat Options Cardiovasc Med.* 2020;22(11):39. doi:10.1007/s11936-020-00846-6; McAdams RM, Berube MW. Emerging therapies and management for neonatal encephalopathy-controversies and current approaches. *J Perinatol.* 2021; Wu L, Wu D, Yang T, et al. Hypothermic neuroprotection against acute ischemic stroke: the 2019 update. *J Cereb Blood Flow Metab.* 2020;40(3):461–481.

(measure by esophageal probe) drops to about 30° to 32°C (86° to 89.6°F). Prolonged shivering can lead to exhaustion of liver glycogen stores. Thinking becomes sluggish and coordination is decreased at 34°C (93.2°F). As hypothermia deepens, paradoxical undressing may occur as hypothalamic control of vasoconstriction is lost and vasodilation occurs with loss of core heat to the periphery. The hypothermic individual therefore feels suddenly warm and begins to remove clothing.

At 30°C (86°F), the individual becomes stuporous, heart rate and respiratory rate decline, and cardiac output is diminished. Cerebral blood flow is decreased. Metabolic rate declines, further decreasing core temperature. Sinus node depression occurs with slowing of conduction through the atrioventricular node. In severe hypothermia (core temperature of 26° to 28°C [78.8° to 82.4°F]), pulse and respirations may be undetectable and require resuscitation. Acidosis is moderate to severe. Coagulopathy, ventricular fibrillation, and asystole are common.[117] Surface cooling may cause frostbite and fat necrosis.

If hypothermia is mild, passive rewarming may be sufficient. If core temperature is greater than 30°C (86°F), active rewarming also may be required. Active rewarming uses warm-water baths, warm blankets, heating pads, and warm oral fluids when the individual is fully alert. Core rewarming may be accomplished through administration of warm intravenous (IV) solutions, warm gastric lavage, warm peritoneal lavage, inhalation of warmed gases, and, in extreme cases, exchange transfusions, warming blood in a pump oxygenator circuit, and mediastinal lavage.

Rewarming generally should proceed no faster than a few degrees per hour. Short-term complications of rewarming include acidosis, rewarming shock, and dysrhythmias. Long-term complications include congestive heart failure, hepatic and renal failure, abnormal erythropoiesis, myocardial infarction, pancreatitis, and neurologic dysfunctions.

Therapeutic Hypothermia. Therapeutic hypothermia is used to slow metabolism and preserve ischemic tissue after brain trauma or during brain surgery, after cardiac arrest, and in neonatal hypoxic encephalopathy. Hypothermia protects the brain by reduction in metabolic rate, ATP consumption, oxidative stress, and the critical threshold for oxygen delivery; modulation of excitotoxic neurotransmitters and calcium antagonism; preservation of protein synthesis and the blood-brain barrier; decreased edema formation; and modulation of the inflammatory response.

SLEEP

Sleep is an active multiphase process that provides restorative functions and promotes memory consolidation. Complex neural circuits, interacting hormones, and neurotransmitters involving the hypothalamus, thalamus, brainstem, and cortex control the timing of the sleep-wake cycle and coordinate this cycle with circadian rhythms (24-hour rhythm cycles).[64] Normal sleep has two primary phases that can be documented by electroencephalogram (EEG), a test that detects electrical activity in your brain: rapid eye movement (REM) sleep (20% to 25% of sleep time) and slow-wave (non-REM) sleep. Non-REM sleep is further divided into three stages (N1, N2, N3) from light to deep sleep. REM cycles do not typically start to occur until about 90 minutes into sleep. Four to six cycles of REM and non-REM sleep occur each night in an adult. Sleep duration and sleep architecture do not mature in children until after adolescence.[65] The hypothalamus is a major sleep center, and the hypocretins (orexins), acetylcholine, and glutamate are neuropeptides secreted by the hypothalamus that promote wakefulness. Prostaglandin D_2, adenosine, melatonin, serotonin, L-tryptophan, GABA, and growth factors promote sleep. The pontine reticular formation is primarily responsible for generating REM sleep, and projections from the thalamocortical network produce non-REM sleep.[66]

Rapid eye movement (REM) sleep is initiated by *REM-on* and *REM-off* neurons in the pons and mesencephalon. REM sleep occurs about every 90 minutes beginning 1 to 2 hours after non-REM sleep begins. This sleep is known as *paradoxical sleep* because the EEG pattern is similar to that of the normal awake pattern and the brain is very active with dreaming. REM and non-REM sleep alternate throughout the night, with lengthening intervals of REM sleep and fewer intervals of deeper stages of non-REM sleep toward morning. The changes associated with REM sleep include increased parasympathetic activity and variable sympathetic activity associated with rapid eye movement; muscle relaxation; loss of temperature regulation; altered heart rate, blood pressure, and respiration; penile erection in men and clitoral engorgement in women; release of steroids; and many memorable and often bizarre dreams. Respiratory control appears largely independent of metabolic requirements and oxygen variation. Loss of normal voluntary muscle control in the tongue and upper pharynx may produce respiratory obstruction which, in turn, can precipitate apneic events. Cerebral blood flow increases.

Non-REM sleep accounts for 75% to 80% of sleep time in adults and is initiated when inhibitory signals are released from the hypothalamus. Sympathetic tone is decreased and parasympathetic activity is increased during non-REM sleep, creating a state of reduced activity. The basal metabolic rate falls by 10% to 15%; temperature decreases 0.5°C to 1°C (0.9°F to 1.8°F); heart rate, respiration, blood pressure, and muscle tone decrease; and knee jerk reflexes are absent. Pupils are constricted. During the various stages, cerebral blood flow to the brain decreases and growth hormone is released, with corticosteroid and catecholamine levels depressed. Non-REM sleep is associated with memory consolidation during slow wave sleep.[67] Box 16.4 summarizes sleep characteristics in infants, children, and older adult persons.

Sleep Disorders

Because classification of sleep disorders is complex, a system has been established by the American Academy of Sleep Medicine and includes seven major categories: (1) insomnia, (2) sleep-related breathing disorders, (3) central disorders of hypersomnolence, (4) circadian rhythm sleep-wake disorders, (5) parasomnias, (6) sleep-related movement disorders, and (7) other sleep disorders.[68] The most common disorders are summarized here.

BOX 16.4 Sleep Characteristics of Infants, Children, and Older Adult Persons

Infants

- Infants sleep 10–16 h/day: 50% REM (active) sleep, 25% non-REM (inactive) sleep.
- Infant sleep cycles are 50–60 min in length; 10–45 min of REM sleep accompanied by movement of the arms, legs, and facial muscles followed by about 20 min of non-REM sleep.
- At 1 year, REM and non-REM sleep cycles are about equal in length and infants sleep through the night with about two naps per day.

Children

- Children assume an adult sleep pattern between 3 and 5 years and sleep about 9–10 h per night.
- Inadequate sleep in adolescents is associated with obesity, depression, and poor academic performance.

Older Adult Persons

- Total sleep time is decreased with a longer time to fall asleep and poorer-quality sleep.
- Total time in slow-wave and final phase of non-REM sleep decreases by 15%–30%.
- Increases in stage 1 and 2 non-REM sleep, attributable to an increased number of spontaneous arousals.
- Older adult individuals tend to go to sleep earlier in the evening and wake earlier in the morning because of a phase advance in their normal circadian sleep cycle.
- Alterations in sleep patterns occur about 10 years later in women than in men.
- Sleep disorders are more likely in older adults and increase risks of morbidity, mortality, and changes in cognitive function.

non-REM, Non-rapid eye movement; *REM*, rapid eye movement.
From Gulia KK, Kumar VM. Sleep disorders in the elderly: a growing challenge. *Psychogeriatrics.* 2018;18(3):155–165; Owens J. Adolescent sleep working group; committee on adolescence. Insufficient sleep in adolescents and young adults: an update on causes and consequences. *Pediatrics.* 2014;134(3):e921–e932; Scullin MK, Bliwise DL. Sleep, cognition, and normal aging: integrating a half century of multidisciplinary research. *Perspect Psychol Sci.* 2015;10(1):97–137.

Common Dyssomnias

Insomnia is the inability to fall or stay asleep; it is accompanied by fatigue, malaise, and difficulty with performance during wakefulness and may be mild, moderate, or severe. It may be transient, lasting a few days or months (primary insomnia), and related to travel across time zones or caused by acute stress, or very commonly inadequate "sleep hygiene." Sleep hygiene simply refers to behavioral and environmental practices that are intended to promote better-quality sleep (e.g., avoiding all-nighters and caffeine late in the evening). Chronic insomnia lasts at least 3 months and can be idiopathic, start at an early age, and be associated with drug or alcohol abuse, chronic pain disorders, chronic depression, the use of certain drugs, obesity, aging, genetics, and environmental factors that result in hyperarousal.[69]

Obstructive sleep apnea syndrome (OSAS) is the most commonly diagnosed sleep disorder and occurs in all age groups. However, the incidence of OSAS increases with age beyond 60 years. Major risk factors include obesity, male sex, older age, and postmenopausal status (not on hormone therapy) in women, craniofacial anomalies, and increased size of tonsillar and adenoid tissue.[70] OSAS results from partial or total upper airway obstruction to airflow recurring during sleep with continuous respiratory efforts made against a closed airway. It is often accompanied by excessive loud snoring, gasping, and multiple apneic episodes that last 10 seconds or longer. *Central sleep apnea* is the temporary absence or diminution of ventilatory effort during sleep with decreased sensitivity to carbon dioxide and oxygen tensions, and decreased airway dilator muscle activation. It may be associated with heart failure, neurologic disease, high altitude, or narcotic medications. *Obesity hypoventilation syndrome* is a combination of obesity (body mass index $\geq 30\,kg \cdot m^{-2}$), daytime hypercapnia (arterial carbon dioxide tension $\geq 45\,mmHg$), and sleep disordered breathing not caused by other disorders of hypoventilation. It may be related to leptin resistance because leptin also is a strong respiratory stimulant. The periodic breathing eventually produces arousal, which interrupts the sleep cycle, reducing total sleep time and producing sleep and REM deprivation. Sleep apnea produces hypercapnia and low oxygen saturation and if left untreated, eventually leads to polycythemia, pulmonary hypertension, systemic hypertension, stroke, right-sided congestive heart failure, dysrhythmias, liver congestion, cyanosis, and peripheral edema.

Hypersomnia (excessive daytime sleepiness) is associated with OSAS. Individuals may fall asleep while driving a car, working, or even while conversing, with significant safety concerns.[71] Sleep deprivation also can result in impaired mood and cognitive function characterized by impairments of attention, episodic memory, working memory, and executive functions (i.e., decision-making ability).

Polysomnography and home sleep testing are used to diagnose OSAS, in addition to the history and physical examination. Treatments include use of continuous positive airway pressure (CPAP) and dental devices, surgery of the upper airway, hypoglossal nerve stimulation in selected individuals, and management of obesity.[72] Adenotonsillar hypertrophy is the major cause of obstructive sleep apnea in children, and obesity increases the risk. Tonsillectomy with or without adenoidectomy is the treatment of choice.[73]

Narcolepsy is a primary hypersomnia with disruption in REM sleep-wake cycles characterized by hallucinations, sleep paralysis, excessive daytime sleepiness, and, rarely, cataplexy (brief spells of muscle weakness). Narcolepsy is usually sporadic or can occur in families. Type I narcolepsy (narcolepsy with cataplexy) is associated with immune-mediated T-cell destruction of hypocretin (orexin)-secreting cells in the hypothalamus. Orexins stimulate wakefulness. Type II narcolepsy (narcolepsy without cataplexy) is less severe and associated with normal levels of orexins (hypocretins). The cause is unknown.[74]

Circadian rhythm sleep disorders are common disorders of the 24-hour sleep-wake schedule with disruption in the timing of sleep. They involve difficulty falling asleep, waking up during the sleep cycle, or waking up too early and being unable to fall back to sleep. These disorders can result from extrinsic causes, such as rapid time zone changes (or jet-lag syndrome), alternating the sleep schedule (rotating work shifts) involving 3 hours or more in sleep time, or changing the total sleep time from day to day. Common types of these disorders include advanced sleep phase disorder (early evening sleeping, e.g., 6:00 pm and early morning waking, e.g., 3:00 to 5:00 am), or delayed sleep phase disorder (late night sleeping, e.g., at 2:00 am and late morning or afternoon waking). A circadian rhythm sleep disorder known as shift work sleep disorder affects many shift workers who rotate or swing long shifts (such as nurses), particularly between the hours of 2200 (10 PM) and 0600 (6 AM). Jet lag disorder is a disturbance in the circadian rhythm from crossing time zones more rapidly than the circadian system can keep pace. Eastward travel is more difficult than westward travel because it is easier to delay sleep than to advance sleep.

The disruption of circadian rhythms may cause problems in the short term, such as cognitive deficits, poor vigilance, difficulty concentrating, and inadequate performance of psychomotor tasks. However, long-term health consequences of shift work sleep disorder may be quite serious and include depression/anxiety, increased risk for cardiovascular disease, and increased all-cause mortality. Sleep cycle phenotype also has a genetic basis and influences the timing and cycles of sleep and can affect advances or delays in sleep-wake times (see Emerging Science Box: Shift Work Disorder).[75]

Common Parasomnias

Parasomnias are unusual behaviors occurring during non-REM stage 3 (slow-wave) sleep (disorders of arousal) and REM-related sleep behavior disorder.[76] Non-REM sleep behaviors are associated with an inability to maintain deep sleep and an increased number of arousals. Behaviors include sleepwalking, having night terrors, rearranging furniture, eating food, exhibiting sleep sex or violent behavior, and having restless leg syndrome. REM sleep behavior disorder (RBD) is manifested by loss of REM paralysis, leading to potentially injurious dream enactment. Nonmotor symptoms are nonspecific and include olfactory dysfunction, abnormal color vision, autonomic dysfunction, excessive daytime sleepiness, depression, and cognitive impairment. RBD is a common prodromal non-motor manifestation of Parkinson disease.[77]

Two dysfunctions of sleep (somnambulism and night terrors) are common in children and may be related to CNS immaturity. Somnambulism (sleepwalking) is a non-REM parasomnia disorder primarily of childhood and appears to resolve within a few years. Sleepwalking is therefore not associated with dreaming, and the child has no memory of the event on awakening. Sleepwalking in adults is often associated with sleep-disordered breathing. Night terrors are characterized by sudden apparent arousals in which the child expresses intense fear or emotion. However, the child is not awake and can be difficult to arouse. Once awakened, the child has no memory of the night terror event. Night terrors are not associated with dreams. Although this problem occurs most often in children, adults also may experience it with corresponding daytime anxiety.

EMERGING SCIENCE BOX

Shift Work Disorder

Shift work disorder coincides with a deviation between the light-dark cycle and the human activity-rest cycle. The circadian system works to ensure the body functions as a well-tuned clock. Within the hypothalamus, the suprachiasmatic nucleus (SCN) coordinates 24 h physiological rhythms. When aligned appropriately with the environment, the SCN promotes sleep and anabolic functions at night and wakefulness and catabolic functions during the day. The internal rhythm of the SCN becomes askew with shift work. There has already been strong evidence that links shift work with negative health outcomes, specifically cardiovascular disease and metabolic disorders. Emerging science has shown the biological consequences of shift work based on estimation of DNA methylation (DNAm), an epigenetic age estimator, which represents the aging process. Individuals with higher than usual DNAm compared with their chronological age have been termed "age-accelerated" which increases risk for age-related disease processes (i.e., stroke, cardiovascular disease, cancer, and death). Shift work and epigenetic age has most notably been associated with women who work more than 10 years, specifically involving night shifts. The estimated epigenetic age is 3 years older than those who have never worked shifts.

Data from Moreno CRC, et al. Working time society consensus statements: evidence-based effects of shift work on physical and mental health. *Ind Health.* 2019;57(2):139–157; White AJ, et al. Shift work, DNA methylation and epigenetic age. *Int J Epidemiol.* 2019;48(5):1536–1544.

Restless Leg Syndrome

Restless legs syndrome (RLS)/Willis Ekbom disease is a common sensorimotor disorder associated with unpleasant sensations (prickling, tingling, crawling) and nonvolitional periodic leg movements that occurs at rest and is worse in the evening or at night. There is a compelling urge to move the legs for relief, with a significant effect on sleep and quality of life. The disorder is more common in women, during pregnancy, in older adults, and in individuals with iron deficiency. RLS has a familial tendency, although no monogenetic cause has been found. RLS is associated with a circadian fluctuation of dopamine in the substantia nigra. Iron is a cofactor in dopamine production, and some individuals respond to iron administration as well as low-dose dopamine agonists. Diagnostic and treatment guidelines have been established to assist with disease management.[78]

THE SPECIAL SENSES

Vision

The eyes are complex sense organs responsible for vision. Within a protective casing, each eye has receptors, a lens system for focusing light on the receptors, and a system of nerves for conducting impulses from the receptors to the brain. Visual dysfunction may be caused by abnormal ocular movements or alterations in visual acuity, refraction, color vision, or accommodation. Visual dysfunction also may be the secondary effect of another neurologic disorder.

The Eye

The wall of the eye consists of three layers: (1) sclera, (2) choroid, and (3) retina (Fig. 16.7). The sclera is the thick, white,

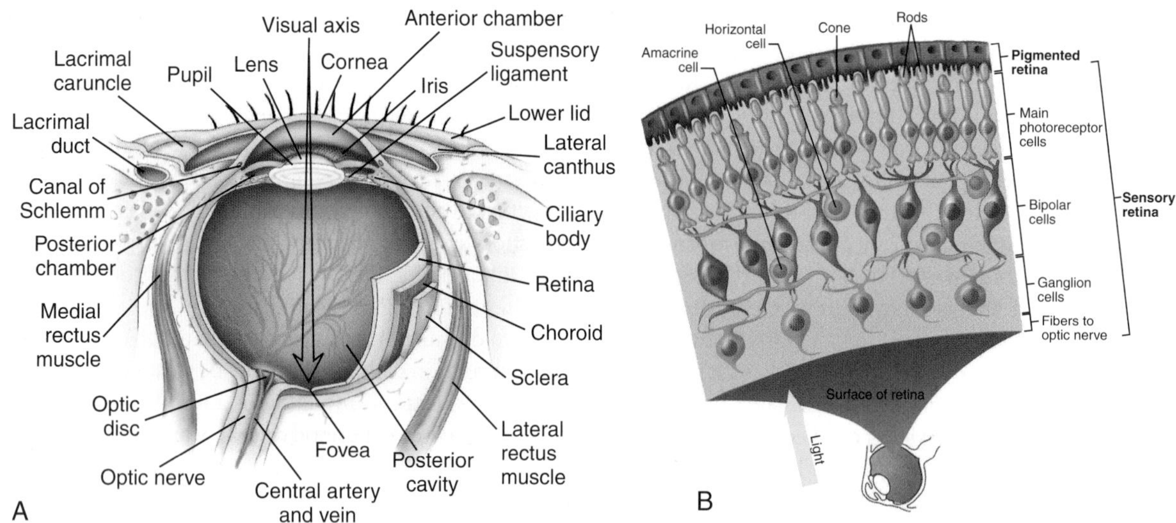

Fig. 16.7 (A) Internal anatomy of the eye. **(B)** The retina. (A, Adapted from Patton KT, Thibodeau GA. *Structure & function of the human body.* 13th ed. St Louis: Mosby; 2008. B, From Patton KT, Thibodeau GA. *The human body in health & disease,* 7th ed, St Louis: Mosby; 2018.)

outermost layer. It becomes transparent at the cornea—the portion of the sclera in the central anterior region that allows light to enter the eye. The choroid is the deeply pigmented middle layer that prevents light from scattering inside the eye. The iris, part of the choroid, has a round opening, the pupil, through which light passes. Smooth muscle fibers control the size of the pupil so that it adjusts to bright light or dim light and to close or distant vision.

The retina is the innermost layer of the eye and contains millions of rods and cones—special photoreceptors that convert light energy into nerve impulses (see Fig. 16.7B). Rods mediate peripheral and dim light vision, do not mediate color, and are densest at the periphery. Cones are color and detail receptors, and densest in the center of the retina. There are no photoreceptors where the optic nerve leaves the eyeball; this creates the optic disc, or blind spot. Lateral to each optic disc is the macula lutea, the area of most distinct vision, and in the center is the fovea centralis, a tiny area that contains only cones and provides the greatest visual acuity (see Fig. 16.7).

Nerve impulses pass through the optic nerves (second cranial nerve) to the optic chiasm (Fig. 16.8). The nerves from the inner (nasal) halves of the retinas cross to the opposite side and join fibers from the outer (temporal) halves of the retinas to form the optic tracts (see Fig. 16.8). The fibers of the optic tracts synapse in the dorsal lateral geniculate nucleus and pass by way of the optic radiation (or geniculocalcarine tract) to the primary visual cortex in the occipital lobe of the brain. Some fibers terminate in the suprachiasmatic nucleus (SCN) of the hypothalamus (located above the optic chiasm) and are involved in circadian regulation of the sleep-wake cycle. Light entering the eye is focused on the retina by the **lens**—a flexible, biconvex, crystal-like structure. The flexibility of the lens allows a change in curvature with contraction of the ciliary muscles, called *accommodation,* and allows the eye to focus on objects at different distances. The eye has two segments divided by the lens: the anterior and posterior segments. The anterior segment has two chambers. The anterior chamber lies between the cornea and the iris; the posterior chamber lies between the iris and the lens. Aqueous humor fills the anterior segment and helps maintain pressure inside the eye, as well as provide nutrients to the lens and cornea. Aqueous humor is secreted by the ciliary processes in the posterior chamber, flows through the pupil into the anterior chamber and drains though the trabecular meshwork, and is absorbed by endothelial cells in the canal of Schlemm. It then passes into the venous circulation. If drainage is blocked, intraocular pressure increases, causing glaucoma. The posterior segment extends from the back of the lens to the retinae and is filled with a gel-like substance called vitreous humor that cannot regenerate. Vitreous humor maintains intraocular pressure and prevents the eyeball from collapsing inward.

Blood supply to the eye is provided by branches of the ophthalmic artery. The ciliary artery and its branches provide blood to the anterior eye and the layers of the eye wall. The central retinal artery provides blood to the inner retinal surface, and the choroid supplies nutrients to the outer surface of the retina. Six extrinsic eye muscles allow gross eye movements and permit eyes to follow a moving object (Fig. 16.9).

Visual Dysfunction

Alterations in ocular movements. Abnormal ocular movements result from oculomotor, trochlear, or abducens cranial nerve dysfunction (see Table 15.6). The three types of eye movement disorders are (1) strabismus, (2) nystagmus, and (3) paralysis of individual extraocular muscles.

In strabismus, one eye deviates from the other when the person is looking at an object. This is caused by a weak or hypertonic muscle in one eye. The deviation may be upward, downward, inward (esotropia), or outward (exotropia). Strabismus in children requires early intervention to prevent amblyopia (reduced

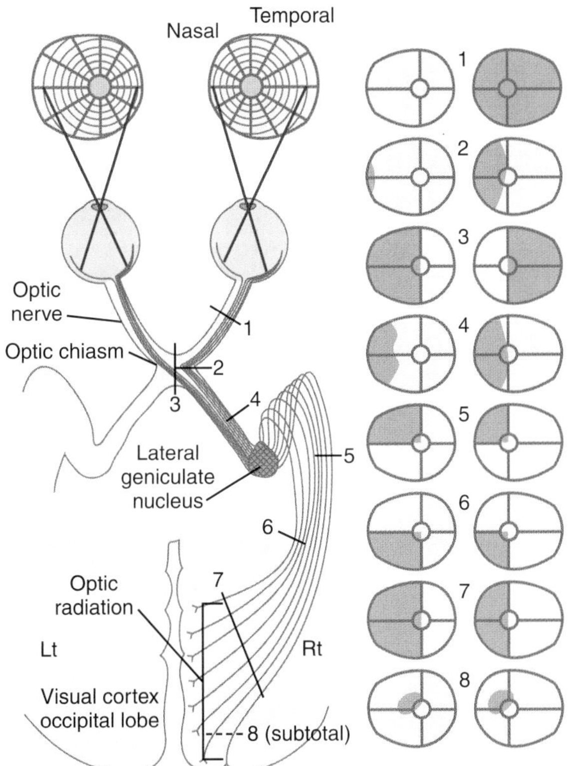

Fig. 16.8 Visual Pathways and Defects. *1,* Optic nerve: blindness. *2,* Lateral optic chiasm: grossly incongruous, incomplete (contralateral) homonymous hemianopsia. *3,* Central optic chiasm: bitemporal hemianopsia. *4,* Optic tract: incongruous, incomplete homonymous hemianopsia. *5,* Temporal loop of the optic radiation: congruous partial or complete (contralateral) homonymous superior quadrantanopia. *6,* Parietal *(superior)* projection of the optic radiation: congruous partial or complete homonymous inferior quadrantanopia. *7,* Complete parieto-occipital interruption of the optic radiation: complete congruous homonymous hemianopsia with psychophysical shift of the foveal point, often sparing central vision and resulting in "macular sparing." *8,* Incomplete (subtotal) damage to the visual cortex: congruous homonymous scotomas, usually encroaching at least acutely on central vision. (From Goldman C, ed. *Goldman's Cecil Medicine.* 24th ed. Vol 2. Philadelphia: Saunders; 2012.)

vision in the affected eye caused by cerebral blockage of the visual stimuli). The primary symptom of strabismus is diplopia (double vision). Causes include neuromuscular disorders of the eye muscle, diseases involving the cerebral hemispheres, or thyroid disease.

Nystagmus is an involuntary unilateral or bilateral rapid, rhythmic oscillatory movement of the eyes. It may be present at rest or when the eye moves. Pendular nystagmus is characterized by a regular back and forth movement of the eyes with only slow phases. In jerk nystagmus, one phase of the eye movement is faster than the other. Nystagmus may be caused by imbalanced reflex activity of the inner ear, vestibular nuclei, cerebellum, medial longitudinal fascicle, or nuclei of the oculomotor, trochlear, and abducens cranial nerves (see Table 15.6 and Fig. 15.25). Drugs, retinal disease, diseases involving the cervical cord, stroke syndromes, brain tumors, and brain trauma also may produce nystagmus.[79]

Paralysis or loss of neuromuscular coordination of specific extraocular muscles may cause limited abduction, abnormal closure of the eyelid, ptosis (drooping of the eyelid), or diplopia (double vision) as a result of unopposed muscle activity. Trauma or pressure in the area of the cranial nerves or diseases such as diabetes mellitus and myasthenia gravis also paralyze specific extraocular muscles.

Alterations in visual acuity. Visual acuity is the ability to see objects in sharp detail. With advancing age, the lens of the eye becomes less flexible and adjusts slowly, and there is altered refraction of light by the cornea and lens. Thus visual acuity declines with age. Table 16.6 contains a summary of changes in the eye caused by aging. Specific causes of visual acuity changes are (1) amblyopia, (2) scotoma (blind spot in visual field), (3) cataracts, (4) papilledema, (5) dark adaptation, (6) glaucoma, (7) retinal detachment, and (8) macular degeneration (Table 16.7).

A cataract is a cloudy or opaque area in the ocular lens and leads to visual loss when located on the visual axis (see Fig. 16.7). It is the leading cause of blindness in the world. The incidence of cataracts increases with age as lens proteins break down, leading to opacification. Cataracts develop because of alterations of metabolism and transport of nutrients within the lens. Although the most common form of cataract is degenerative, cataracts also may occur congenitally or as a result of infection, radiation, trauma, drugs, or diabetes mellitus. Cataracts cause decreased visual acuity, blurred vision, glare, and decreased color perception. Cataracts are treated by removal of the entire lens and replacement with an intraocular artificial lens.

Glaucomas are the second leading cause of blindness and are characterized by intraocular pressures greater than 12 to 20 mm Hg with death of retinal ganglion cells and their axons and irreversible loss of central and sometimes peripheral vision. There is a strong genetic tendency with higher prevalence among Black Americans. Chronic use of corticosteroids or drugs with anticholinergic properties can predispose to glaucoma. The two primary types of age-related glaucoma are differentiated by the configuration of the anterior chamber drainage angle and the location of where aqueous humor is obstructed from exiting the eye (Fig. 16.10).[80]

1. *Open angle.* This type of glaucoma is the most common and is characterized by outflow obstruction of aqueous humor at the trabecular meshwork or canal of Schlemm, even though there is adequate space for drainage. Often this is an inherited disease and is a leading cause of blindness with few preliminary symptoms. Obstruction results in high intraocular pressures with compression of the optic nerve head, which can cause blindness within hours or days. With *normal tension glaucoma* there may be neurodegeneration of the optic nerve head that leads to loss of vision without elevated intraocular pressures.
2. *Angle closure* or *narrow angle.* In this type of glaucoma there is displacement of the iris toward the cornea with obstruction of

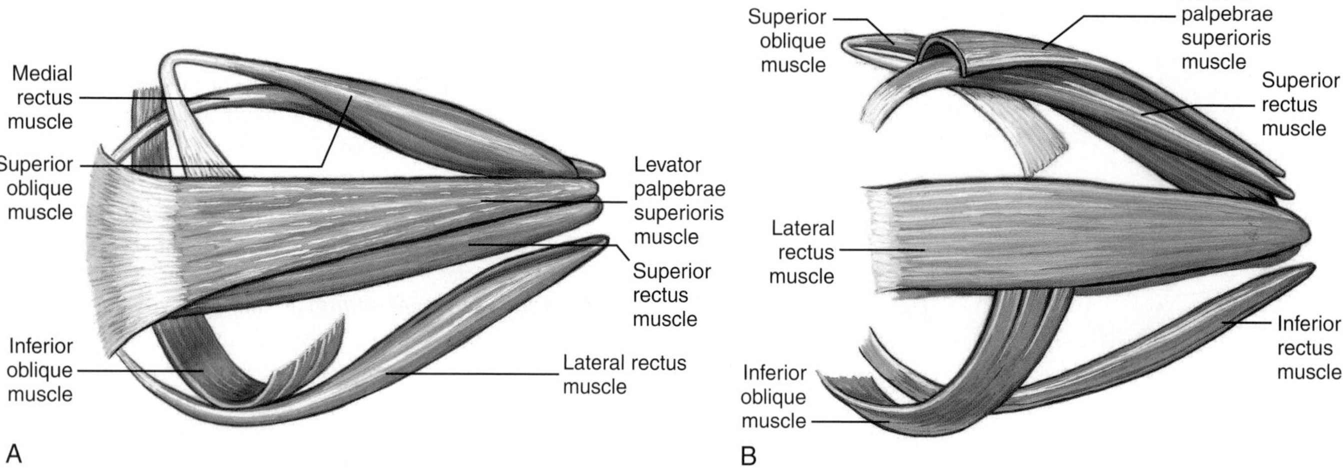

Fig. 16.9 Extrinsic Muscles of the Right Eye. **(A)** Superior view. **(B)** Lateral view. (From Dutton JJ. *Atlas of Clinical and Surgical Orbital Anatomy*. 2nd ed. Philadelphia: Saunders; 2011.)

TABLE 16.6 Changes in the Eye Caused by Aging

Structure	Change	Consequence
Cornea	Thicker and less curved Formation of gray ring at edge of cornea (arcus senilis)	Increase in astigmatism Not detrimental to vision
Anterior chamber	Decrease in size and volume caused by thickening of lens	Occasionally exerts pressure on Schlemm canal and may lead to increased intraocular pressure and glaucoma
Lens	Increase in opacity	Decrease in refraction with increased light scattering (blurring) and decreased color vision (green and blue); can lead to cataracts
Ciliary muscles	Reduction in pupil diameter, atrophy of radial dilation muscles	Persistent constriction (senile miosis); decrease in critical flicker frequency[a]
Retina	Reduction in number of rods at periphery, loss of rods and associated nerve cells	Increase in minimum amount of light necessary to see an object
Macula	Atrophy (age-related macular degeneration)	Loss of vision
Vitreous	Liquefaction of vitreous and decrease in gel volume	Posterior vitreous detachment causing "floaters;" risk for retinal detachment

[a]The rate at which consecutive visual stimuli can be presented and still be perceived as separate.

the trabecular meshwork and obstruction of outflow of aqueous humor from the anterior chamber; it may occur acutely with a sudden rise in intraocular pressure, causing pain and visual disturbances, and will need immediate treatment.

Congenital closure glaucoma is a rare disease associated with congenital malformations and other genetic anomalies. There is a defect in the development of the drainage angle formed by the cornea and iris. Aqueous humor cannot flow out normally. The intraocular pressure increases and leads to optic nerve damage. The disease is usually diagnosed by one year of age.

Glaucoma is often treated with pharmaceutical eyedrops to reduce secretion or increase absorption of aqueous humor. Angle closure glaucoma is a medical emergency. Surgical therapies are available to open the spaces of the trabeculae to control intraocular pressure.

Age-related macular degeneration (AMD) is a severe and irreversible loss of vision and a major cause of blindness in older individuals. Hypertension, cigarette smoking, diabetes mellitus, and a family history of AMD are risk factors. The degeneration usually occurs after the age of 60 years. The cause of AMD is unknown and complex because of the many components of eye structure, genetic diversity, and variable environmental factors. There are two forms: dry or non-neovascular (atrophic) and wet or exudative (neovascular). The *dry form* is more common and is slowly progressive with accumulation of drusen (waste products from photoreceptors) in the macula, choriocapillary loss, accumulation of lipofuscin (a lysosomal pigmented residue) in the retinae, and atrophy, leading to permanent central vision loss. Early symptoms include limited night vision and difficulty reading. The *wet form* includes abnormal choroidal blood vessel growth within the macula (neovascularization), leakage of blood or serum, retinal tears or detachment, fibrovascular scarring, loss of photoreceptors, and more severe and rapid loss of central vision.[81] There are no approved treatments for dry AMD. Daily high doses of vitamins C and E, beta-carotene, and the minerals zinc and copper—called the AREDS formulation—can help slow the progression of dry AMD.[82] Treatment of wet AMD includes anti–vascular endothelial growth factor (anti-VEGF) intraocular injection to provide an anti-angiogenesis effect. New

TABLE 16.7 Causes of Visual Acuity Changes

Disorder	Description
Amblyopia	Reduced or dimmed vision; cause unknown Associated with strabismus Accompanies such diseases as diabetes mellitus, renal failure, and malaria and use of drugs such as alcohol and tobacco
Scotoma	Circumscribed defect of central field of vision Often associated with retrobulbar neuritis and multiple sclerosis, compression of optic nerve by tumor, inflammation of optic nerve, pernicious anemia, methyl alcohol poisoning, and use of tobacco
Cataract	Cloudy or opaque area in ocular lens—the leading cause of blindness Incidence increases with age because most commonly a result of degeneration; other causes are congenital
Papilledema	Edema and inflammation of optic nerve where it enters eyeball Caused by obstruction of venous return from retina by one of three main sources: increased intracranial pressure, retrobulbar neuritis, or changes in retinal blood vessels
Dark adaptation	With age, eye does not adapt as readily to dark Also, changes in quantity and quality of rhodopsin are causative; vitamin A deficiencies can produce this at any age
Glaucoma	Increased intraocular pressures (>12–20 mm Hg) Loss of acuity results from pressure on optic nerve, which blocks flow of nutrients to optic nerve fibers, leading to their death; second leading cause of blindness
Retinal detachment	Tear or break in retina with accumulation of fluid and separation from underlying tissue; seen as floaters, flashes of light, or a curtain over visual field; risks include extreme myopia, diabetic retinopathy, sickle cell disease

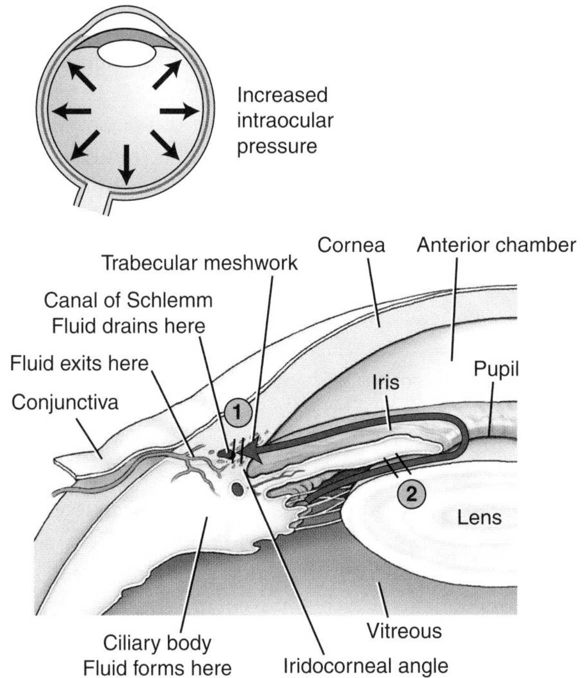

Fig. 16.10 Glaucoma. *1*, Open-angle glaucoma. The obstruction to aqueous humor flow lies in the trabecular meshwork near canal of Schlemm, *2*, Closed-angle glaucoma. The iris presses against the lens, blocking aqueous flow into the anterior chamber.

treatments are being evaluated including anti-VEGF antibodies, stem cell, and gene therapy.[81]

Retinal detachment is a common cause of visual impairment and blindness. Risk factors include retinal holes and vitreoretinal traction. Fluid (exudate, hemorrhage, or liquid vitreous) separates the retinal pigment epithelium from the photoreceptors in the neuroepithelium (see Fig. 16.7). The separation deprives the outer retina of oxygen and nutrients because the diffusion distance is increased. Communication is also disrupted between the pigment epithelium and photoreceptors. There is retinal degeneration and fibrosis with loss of vision. Rhegmatogenous retinal detachment (full-thickness retinal breaks caused by vitreoretinal traction) is the most common form of retinal detachment. Causes include intracapsular cataract extraction, severe myopia, age-related lattice degeneration, vitreoretinal traction, and trauma. Contraction of fibrous membranes can cause tractional separation of the retinal layers as occurs in proliferative diabetic retinopathy. Symptoms include dark floaters or squiggly lines in the field of vision; flashes of light; or a dark curtain or shadow on the sides or center of the visual field. Retinal detachment is a medical emergency. Treatment involves immediate surgical retinal reattachment.[83]

Alterations in accommodation. Accommodation refers to changes in the shape of the lens and allows for a change of focus from distant to near images. Accommodation is mediated through the oculomotor nerve. Pressure, inflammation, age, and disease of the oculomotor nerve may alter accommodation, causing diplopia, blurred vision, and headache.

Loss of accommodation with advancing age is termed presbyopia, a condition in which the ocular lens becomes larger, firmer, and less elastic. The major symptom is reduced near vision, causing the individual to hold reading material at arm's length. Treatment includes corrective forward, contact, and intraocular lenses, corneal inlays, or laser refractive surgery for monovision.[84]

Alterations in refraction. Alterations in refraction are the most common visual problem. Causes include irregularities of the corneal curvature, the focusing power of the lens, and the

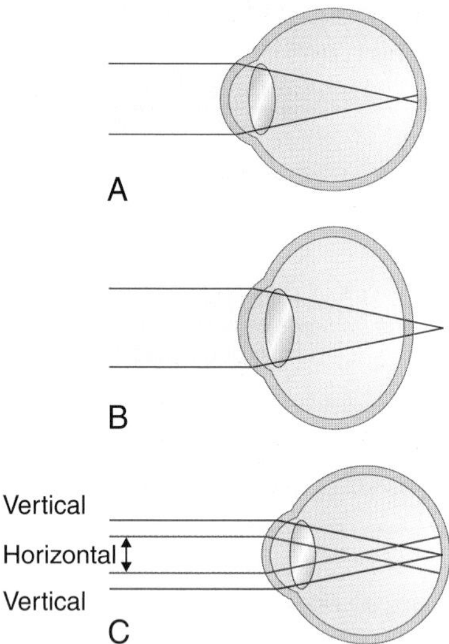

Fig. 16.11 Alterations in Refraction. **(A)** Myopic eye. Parallel rays of light are brought to a focus in front of the retina. **(B)** Hyperopic eye. Parallel rays of light come to a focus behind the retina in the unaccommodative eye. (C) Simple myopic astigmatism. The vertical bundle of rays is focused on the retina; the horizontal rays are focused in front of the retina. (From Stein HA, et al. *The Ophthalmic Assistant: A Text for Allied and Associated Ophthalmic Personnel*. 9th ed. Philadelphia: Saunders; 2013.)

length of the eye. The major symptoms of refraction alterations are blurred vision and headache. Three types of refraction alterations are as follows (Fig. 16.11):

Myopia—nearsightedness: The eyeball is lengthened, and light rays are focused in front of the retina when the person is looking at a distant object causing blurry vision. A concave lens is needed for correction. There is increased risk for retinal detachment, cataract formation, and glaucoma.

Hyperopia—farsightedness: the axis of the eyeball is too short and light rays are focused behind the retina when a person is looking at a near object and vision is blurry. A convex lens is needed for correction.

Astigmatism—unequal curvature of the cornea: Light rays enter the eye at two points and do not come to a single focus on the retina and cause blurry vision. Astigmatism may coexist with myopia, hyperopia, or presbyopia. Corrective lenses or laser surgery provide correction.

Alterations in color vision. Normal sensitivity to color diminishes with age because of the progressive yellowing of the lens that occurs with aging. All colors become less intense, although color discrimination for blue and green is greatly affected. Color vision deteriorates more rapidly for individuals with diabetes mellitus than for the general population because diabetic neuropathy can also affect photoreceptors.

Abnormal color vision also may be caused by color blindness and is an X-linked genetic trait.[85] Congenital color blindness affects 6% to 8% of the male population and about 0.5% of the female population. Mutations in the genes coding for wavelength sensitivity of retinal cone photopigments leads to color blindness. Although many forms of color blindness exist, most commonly the affected individual cannot distinguish red from green rather than yellow from blue. In the most severe form (achromatopsia) individuals see only shades of gray, black, and white. Acquired color vision deficiency occurs with ocular, neurologic, or systemic disease.

Neurologic disorders causing visual dysfunction. Various neurologic disorders may cause visual dysfunction including stroke, traumatic brain injury, tumors, and neurodegenerative diseases. Vision may be disrupted at many points along the visual pathway, causing a variety of defects in fields of vision.[86] Visual changes do not always cause defects or blindness in the entire visual field; hemianopia is the term that describes defective vision in half of a visual field. Fig. 16.8 illustrates areas along the visual pathway that may be damaged and the associated visual changes. Because of the anatomy of the optic nerves, injury to the optic nerve causes ipsilateral (same side) blindness but a normal contralateral (opposite side) visual field. Injury to the optic chiasm (the X-shaped crossing of the optic nerves), often caused by atherosclerotic ischemia or external compression from trauma or aneurysm, can cause a variety of defects, depending on the location of injury. These defects vary because at the optic chiasm, nerve fibers from the medial half of each retina separate from the lateral half and enter the opposite optic tract.

Because of the normal structure of the visual pathways, destruction of one optic tract causes homonymous hemianopsia (complete loss of vision in the inner half of one eye and the outer half of the other). Thus, if an injury to the left optic tract occurs, the individual is blind in the right eye's medial (inner) field and the left eye's lateral (outer) field. If the compression of the optic tract is asymmetric, an incongruous (or uneven) homonymous defect results. Injury to one optic radiation (an ocular pathway in the internal capsule, temporal lobe, or occipital lobe) also causes a homonymous (same field) defect. A major injury in the optic radiation causes homonymous hemianopsia. A lesser injury may cause an upper quadrant homonymous defect. Generally the defects are the same size in both eyes. When the homonymous hemianopsia is caused by an occipital lobe lesion, the area of hemianopsia is split. Although visual acuity may remain unimpaired, reading is difficult because of the inability to group words.

Papilledema is edema of the optic nerve at its point of entrance into the eyeball. Papilledema is caused by increased intracranial pressure (e.g., brain tumors, intracranial hemorrhage, hydrocephalus, or cerebral edema). The subarachnoid space of the brain is continuous with the optic nerve sheath. As cerebrospinal fluid (CSF) pressure increases, the pressure is transmitted to the optic nerve and the optic nerve sheath compresses the nerve and impedes axoplasmic transport. This leads to accumulation of axoplasmic substances at the level of the lamina cribrosa (a mesh-like structure in the sclera where the retinal nerves exit the eye and form the optic nerve), resulting in the characteristic swelling of the optic disc. Obliteration of the physiologic cup (a bright area normally located in the center of the optic disc) follows. Later the optic disc becomes raised above the level of the surrounding retina, and the margins become blurred and indistinct. With severe swelling, hemorrhage and patches of white exudate (caused by nerve infarcts) surround the disc margins. The edematous nerves compress the small retinal veins, causing venous stasis and engorgement. Headache is common and there may be no visual changes, blurred vision, or constriction of visual fields.[87]

External Eye Structure and Disorders

Protective external eye structures include the eyelids (palpebrae), conjunctivae, and lacrimal apparatus. The eyelids control the amount of light reaching the eyes, and the conjunctiva lines the eyelids. Tears released from the lacrimal apparatus bathe the surface of the eye and prevent friction, maintain hydration, and wash out foreign bodies and other irritants (Fig. 16.12).

Infection and inflammatory responses are the most common conditions affecting the supporting structures of the eyes. Blepharitis is an inflammation of the eyelids caused by *Staphylococcus* or seborrheic dermatitis. A hordeolum (stye) is an infection (usually staphylococcal) of the sebaceous glands of the eyelids, usually centered near an eyelash. A chalazion is a noninfectious lipogranuloma of the Meibomian (oil-secreting) gland that often occurs in association with a hordeolum and appears as a deep nodule within the eyelid. These conditions present with redness, swelling, and tenderness and are treated symptomatically. Entropion is a common eyelid malposition in which the lid margin turns inward against the eyeball. In ectropion, the eyelid turns outward away from the eye. Trichiasis is abnormally positioned eyelashes that grow back toward the eye. There are both surgical and nonsurgical treatments to reposition the lid margin. There are both surgical and nonsurgical treatments to reposition the lid margin.

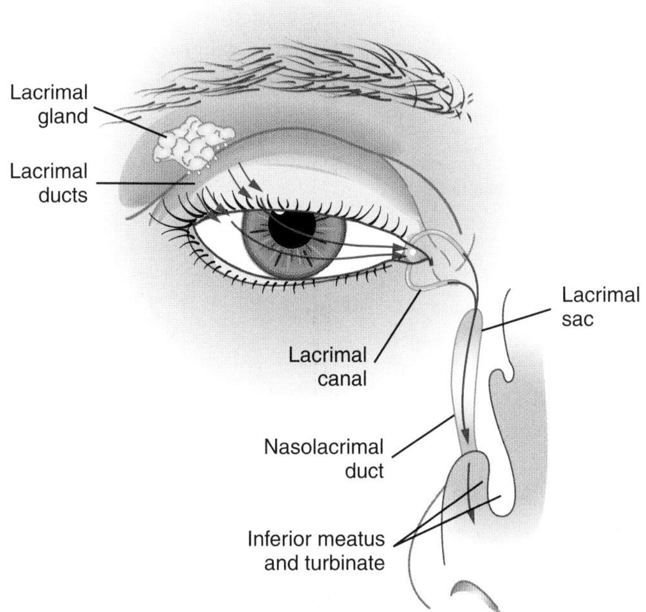

Fig. 16.12 Lacrimal Apparatus. Fluid produced by lacrimal glands (tears) streams across the eye surface, enters the canals, and then passes through the nasolacrimal duct to enter the nose. (From Applegate E. *The Anatomy and Physiology Learning System*. 4th ed. St Louis: Saunders; 2011.)

Conjunctivitis is an inflammation of the conjunctiva (mucous membrane covering the front part of the eyeball) caused by viruses (most common), bacteria, allergies, or chemical irritants. Conjunctivitis can be acute, recurrent, or chronic and can be associated with systemic disease.[88]

Acute bacterial conjunctivitis (pinkeye) is highly contagious and often caused by *Staphylococcus, Haemophilus, Streptococcus pneumoniae*, and *Moraxella catarrhalis*, although other bacteria may be involved (Fig. 16.13). In children younger than 6 years, *Haemophilus* infection often leads to otitis media (conjunctivitis-otitis syndrome). Bilateral matting of the eyelids, gluing of eyelashes on awakening, lack of itching, and no previous history of conjunctivitis are predictors of bacterial conjunctivitis and differentiate it from viral conjunctivitis. Preventing the spread of the microorganism with meticulous hand washing and use of separate towels is important. The disease is also treated with topical antibiotics.

Viral conjunctivitis is caused by an adenovirus and is very contagious. Symptoms include edema, watering, redness, petechial hemorrhages of the conjunctiva, and photophobia. Treatment is usually symptomatic and can include antihistamines and cold compresses.

Allergic conjunctivitis is associated with a variety of antigens, including pollens. Chronic conjunctivitis results from any persistent conjunctivitis lasting more than 4 weeks. Trachoma (chlamydial conjunctivitis) is caused by *Chlamydia trachomatis* and often is associated with poor hygiene and leads to corneal scarring. It is the leading cause of preventable blindness in the world and is treated with azithromycin.[89]

Keratitis is an infection of the cornea caused by bacteria, viruses, fungus, or parasites. Bacterial infections can cause corneal ulceration, and type 1 herpes simplex virus can involve both the cornea and the conjunctiva. *Acanthamoeba* keratitis

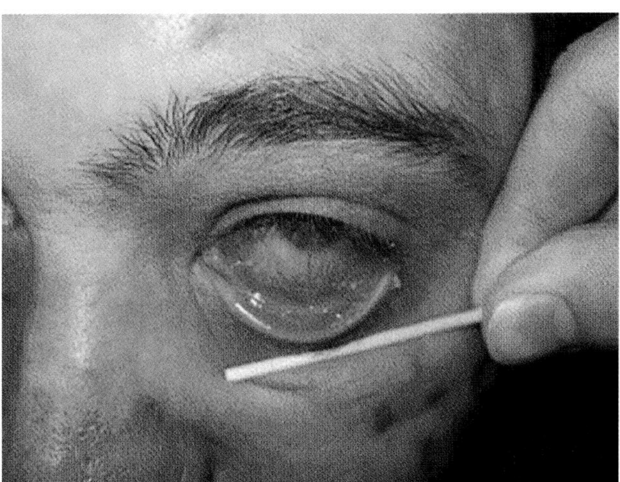

Fig. 16.13 Bacterial Conjunctivitis. Staphylococcal conjunctivitis of the left eye with mild erythema and inflammatory edema of the eyelids. Purulent exudate can be seen at the lateral canthus. (From Durkin SR, et al. Recurrent staphylococcal conjunctivitis associated with facial impetigo contagiosa. *Am J Ophthalmol*. 2006;141(1):189–190. https://doi.org/10.1016/j.ajo.2005.07.079.)

can occur from contact lens wear because of poor hygiene. Fungal infections are most common in tropical and subtropical climates. Severe ulcerations with residual scarring require corneal transplantation.[90]

Hearing

The Normal Ear

The ear is divided into three areas: (1) the external ear, involved only with hearing; (2) the middle ear, involved only with hearing; and (3) the inner ear, involved with both hearing and equilibrium.

The external ear is composed of the pinna (auricle), which is the visible portion of the ear, and the external auditory canal, a tube that leads to the middle ear (Fig. 16.14). The external auditory canal is surrounded by the bones of the cranium. The opening (meatus) of the canal is just above the mastoid process. The air-filled sinuses, called mastoid air cells, of the mastoid process promote conductivity of sound between the external and the middle ear. The tympanic membrane separates the external ear from the middle ear. Sound waves entering the external auditory canal hit the tympanic membrane (eardrum) and cause it to vibrate.

The middle ear is composed of the tympanic cavity, a small chamber in the temporal bone. Three ossicles (small bones known as the malleus [hammer], incus [anvil], and stapes [stirrup]) transmit the vibration of the tympanic membrane to the inner ear. When the tympanic membrane moves, the malleus moves with it and transfers the vibration to the incus, which passes it on to the stapes. The stapes presses against the oval window, a small membrane of the inner ear. The movement of the oval window promotes movement of the round window and sets the fluids of the inner ear in motion (Fig. 16.15).

The eustachian (pharyngotympanic) tube connects the middle ear with the thorax. Normally flat and closed, the eustachian tube opens briefly when a person swallows or yawns, and it equalizes the pressure in the middle ear with atmospheric pressure. Equalized pressure permits the tympanic membrane to vibrate freely. Through the eustachian tube the mucosa of the middle ear is continuous with the mucosal lining of the throat.

The inner ear is a system of osseous labyrinths (bony, mazelike chambers) filled with a fluid, the perilymph. The bony labyrinth is divided into the cochlea, the vestibule, and the semicircular canals (see Fig. 16.15). Suspended in the perilymph is the endolymph-filled membranous labyrinth that basically follows the shape of the bony labyrinth.

Within the cochlea is the organ of Corti, which contains hair cells (hearing receptors). Sound waves that reach the cochlea through vibrations of the tympanic membrane, ossicles, and oval window set the cochlear fluids into motion. Receptor cells on the basilar membrane are stimulated when their hairs are bent or pulled by fluid movement. Once stimulated, hair cells transmit impulses along the cochlear nerve (a division of the vestibulocochlear nerve) to the auditory cortex of the temporal lobe in the brain (see Fig. 16.15 and view an animation at www.youtube.com/watch?v=46aNGGNPm7s). This is where interpretation of the sound occurs.

The semicircular canals and vestibule of the inner ear contain equilibrium receptors. In the semicircular canals the dynamic equilibrium receptors respond to changes in direction of movement. Within each semicircular canal is the crista ampullaris, a receptor region composed of a tuft of hair cells covered by a gelatinous cupula. When the head is rotated, the endolymph in the canal lags behind and moves in the direction opposite to the head's movement. The hair cells are stimulated, and impulses are transmitted through the vestibular nerve (a division of the vestibulocochlear nerve) to the cerebellum.

The vestibule in the inner ear contains maculae—receptors essential to the body's sense of static equilibrium. As the head moves, otoliths (small pieces of calcium salts) move in a gel-like

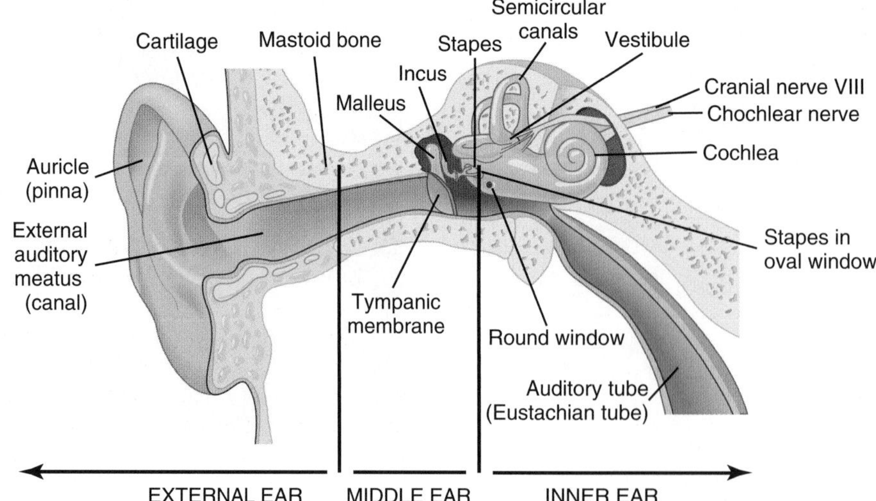

Fig. 16.14 External, Middle, and Inner Ears. (Anatomic structures are not drawn to scale.) (From Applegate E. *The Anatomy and Physiology Learning System*. 4th ed. St Louis: Saunders; 2011.)

material in response to changes in the pull of gravity. The otoliths pull on the gel, which in turn pulls on the hair cells in the maculae. Nerve impulses in the hair cells are triggered and transmitted to the brain (see Fig. 16.15). Thus the ear not only permits the hearing of a large range of sounds but also assists with maintaining balance through the sensitive equilibrium receptors.

Auditory Dysfunction

Between 5% and 10% of the general population have impaired hearing, and it is the most common sensory defect. The major categories of auditory dysfunction are conductive hearing loss, sensorineural hearing loss, mixed hearing loss, and functional hearing loss. Hearing loss may range from mild to profound. Auditory changes caused by aging are common and incremental (see the box Geriatric Considerations: Aging and Changes in Hearing).

Conductive hearing loss. A conductive hearing loss occurs when physical anomalies in the outer or middle ear impair conduction of sound from the outer to the inner ear. Conditions that commonly cause a conductive hearing loss include impacted cerumen, foreign bodies lodged in the ear canal, benign tumors of the middle ear, carcinoma of the external auditory canal or middle ear, eustachian tube dysfunction, otitis media, acute viral otitis media, chronic suppurative otitis media, cholesteatoma (accumulation of keratinized epithelium), and otosclerosis.

GERIATRIC CONSIDERATIONS

Aging and Changes in Hearing[a]

Changes in Structure	Changes in Function
Cochlear hair cell degeneration	Inability to hear high-frequency sounds (presbycusis, sensorineural loss); interferes with understanding speech; hearing may be lost in both ears at different times
Loss of auditory neurons in spiral ganglia of organ of Corti	Inability to hear high-frequency sounds (presbycusis, sensorineural loss); interferes with understanding speech; hearing may be lost in both ears at different times
Degeneration of basilar (cochlear) conductive membrane of cochlea	Inability to hear at all frequencies but more pronounced at higher frequencies (cochlear conductive loss)
Decreased vascularity of cochlea	Equal loss of hearing at all frequencies (strial loss); inability to disseminate localization of sound
Loss of cortical auditory neurons	Equal loss of hearing at all frequencies (strial loss); inability to disseminate localization of sound

[a]Hearing loss affects about 50% of individuals older than 60 years and 80% of individuals 85 years or older. Hearing loss is associated with declining cognitive function; changes in perception, comprehension, and memory; impaired communication; and reduced quality of life. Causal mechanisms are not clearly known. Data from Jayakody DMP, Friedland PL, Martins RN, et al. Impact of aging on the auditory system and related cognitive functions: a narrative review. *Front Neurosci.* 2018;12:125; Wu PZ, Liberman LD, Bennett K, et al. Primary neural degeneration in the human cochlea: evidence for hidden hearing loss in the aging Ear. *Neuroscience.* 2019;407:8–20.

Symptoms of conductive hearing loss include diminished hearing and a soft speaking voice. A soft speaking voice is often used because the individual hears his or her voice, conducted by bone, as loud.

Sensorineural hearing loss. A sensorineural hearing loss is caused by impairment of the organ of Corti or its central connections to the auditory cortex. The loss may occur gradually or suddenly. Conditions causing sensorineural loss include congenital and hereditary factors, noise exposure, aging, Ménière disease, ototoxicity, systemic disease (syphilis, Paget disease, collagen diseases, diabetes mellitus),

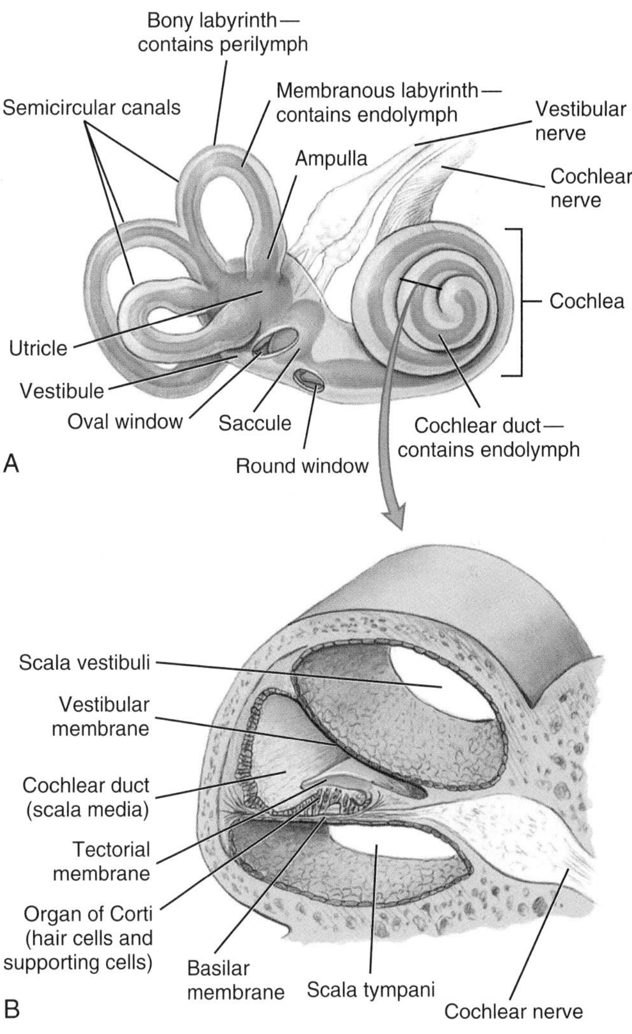

Fig. 16.15 The Inner Ear. (A) The bony labyrinth *(tan)* is the hard outer wall of the entire inner ear and includes the semicircular canals, vestibule, and cochlea. Within the bony labyrinth is the membranous labyrinth *(purple)*, which is surrounded by perilymph and filled with endolymph. Each ampulla in the vestibule contains a crista ampullaris that detects changes in head position and sends sensory impulses through the vestibular nerve to the brain. **(B)** Section of the membranous cochlea. Hair cells in the organ of Corti detect sound and send the information through the cochlear nerve. The vestibular and cochlear nerves join to form the eighth cranial nerve. (From Applegate E. *The Anatomy and Physiology Learning System.* 4th ed. St Louis: Saunders.)

neoplasms, and autoimmune processes. Congenital and neonatal sensorineural hearing loss may be caused by maternal rubella, ototoxic drugs, prematurity, traumatic delivery, erythroblastosis fetalis, bacterial meningitis, and congenital hereditary malfunction. Diagnosis is often made when delayed speech development is noted. Sudden-onset bilateral sensorineural hearing loss can be associated with stroke or trauma and is a medical emergency.[91]

Presbycusis is the most common form of sensorineural hearing loss in older adults and is usually bilateral and symmetric. Its cause may be atrophy of the basal end of the organ of Corti, loss of auditory receptors, changes in vascularity, or stiffening of the basilar membranes. Drug ototoxicities (drugs that cause destruction of auditory function) have been observed after exposure to various chemicals; for example, antibiotics such as aminoglycosides (streptomycin, neomycin, gentamicin), and vancomycin; diuretics such as ethacrynic acid and furosemide; and chemicals such as salicylate, quinine, carbon monoxide, nitrogen mustard, arsenic, mercury, gold, tobacco, and alcohol. In most instances, the drugs and chemicals listed initially cause tinnitus (ringing in the ear) followed by a progressive high-tone sensorineural hearing loss that is permanent. With presbycusis there is loss of sound clarity related to cochlear impairment and hearing loss at high frequencies.[92]

Mixed and functional hearing loss. A mixed hearing loss is caused by a combination of conductive and sensorineural losses. With functional hearing loss, which is rare, the individual does not respond to voice and appears not to hear. It is thought to be caused by emotional or psychologic factors.

Ménière disease. Ménière disease (endolymphatic hydrops) is an episodic chronic disorder of the middle ear with an unknown etiology that can be unilateral or bilateral and with variable presentations. The most likely cause is excessive endolymph and pressure in the membranous labyrinth that disrupts both vestibular and hearing functions. There are four symptoms: recurring episodes of vertigo (often accompanied by severe nausea and vomiting), hearing loss, ringing in the ears (tinnitus), and a feeling of fullness in the ear. Treatment is symptomatic with medical management or surgical management when medications fail.[93]

Ear Infections

Otitis Externa. Otitis externa is the most common inflammation of the outer ear and may be acute or chronic, infectious or noninfectious. Risk factors include swimming with ear plugs, chronic dermatitis, and irritants such as hair spray or hair dyes. The most common origins of acute infections are bacterial microorganisms including *Pseudomonas aeruginosa, Staphylococcus aureus*, and, less commonly, *Escherichia coli*. Fungal infections are less common. Infection usually follows prolonged exposure to moisture (swimmer's ear). The earliest symptoms are inflammation with pruritus, swelling, and clear drainage, progressing to purulent drainage with obstruction of the canal. Tenderness and pain with earlobe retraction accompany inflammation. Acidifying solutions are used for early treatment and prevention. Topical antimicrobials and steroids usually provide effective treatment for later stages of disease. Chronic infections are more often related to allergy or skin disorders. Malignant otitis externa is a very rare serious complication of the spread of otitis externa into the mastoid and/or temporal bone causing osteomyelitis. It presents with headache and otalgia. Diagnosis requires advanced imaging, and treatment requires intravenous antibiotics.[94]

Otitis media. Otitis media (OM) is a common infection of infants and children. Most children have one episode by 3 years of age. The most common pathogens are *Streptococcus pneumoniae, Haemophilus influenzae*, and *Moraxella catarrhalis*. Respiratory viruses have also been associated with OM.[95] Predisposing factors include allergy, sinusitis, submucosal cleft palate, adenoidal hypertrophy, eustachian tube dysfunction, and immune deficiency. Breast-feeding is a protective factor. Recurrent acute otitis media may be genetically determined.[96]

Acute otitis media (AOM) is associated with ear pain, fever, irritability, inflamed tympanic membrane, fluid in the middle ear, and holding or tugging at the ear. The appearance of the tympanic membrane progresses from erythema to opaqueness with bulging as fluid accumulates. There is an increasing prevalence of AOM caused by penicillin-resistant microorganisms. Otitis media with effusion (OME) is the presence of fluid in the middle ear without symptoms of acute infection (Fig. 16.16). Treatment includes symptom management, particularly of pain, with watchful waiting, antimicrobial therapy for severe illness, and placement of tympanostomy tubes when there is persistent bilateral effusion and significant hearing loss (chronic suppurative otitis media). Complications include mastoiditis, brain abscess, meningitis, and chronic otitis media with hearing loss. Persistent middle ear effusions may affect speech, language, and cognitive abilities. Multivalent vaccines for influenza result in modest prevention of acute otitis media.[97,98]

Olfaction and Taste

Olfaction (smell) is a function of cranial nerve I and part of cranial nerve V. Taste (gustation) is a function of multiple nerves in the tongue, soft palate, uvula, pharynx, and upper esophagus innervated by cranial nerves VII and IX. Both cranial nerves are influenced by hormones within the sensory cells. Dysfunctions of smell and taste may occur separately or jointly. The strong relationship between smell and taste creates the sensation of flavor. If either sensation is impaired, the perception of flavor is altered. Olfactory structures are illustrated in Fig. 16.17.

Olfactory cells, located in the olfactory epithelium, are the receptor cells for smell. Seven different primary classes of olfactory stimulants have been identified: (1) camphoraceous, (2) musky, (3) floral, (4) peppermint, (5) ethereal, (6) pungent, and (7) putrid. Olfaction is important for detection of hazards in the environment, generating feelings of pleasure, promoting adequate nutrition, influencing sexuality, and maintenance of mood.[99]

Olfactory dysfunctions include hyposmia, anosmia, hallucinations, and parosmia. Hyposmia is the impaired sense of smell, and anosmia is the complete loss of smell. Both conditions are associated with aging, neurodegenerative and nasal/sinus disorders, and head trauma. When hyposmia or anosmia occurs bilaterally, it is usually the result of rhinitis (inflammation of nasal

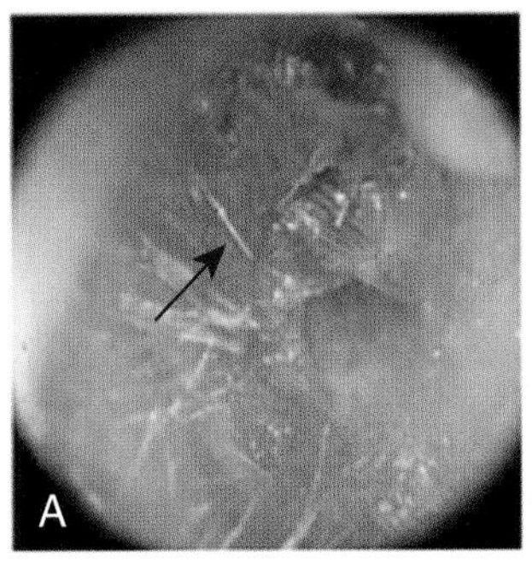

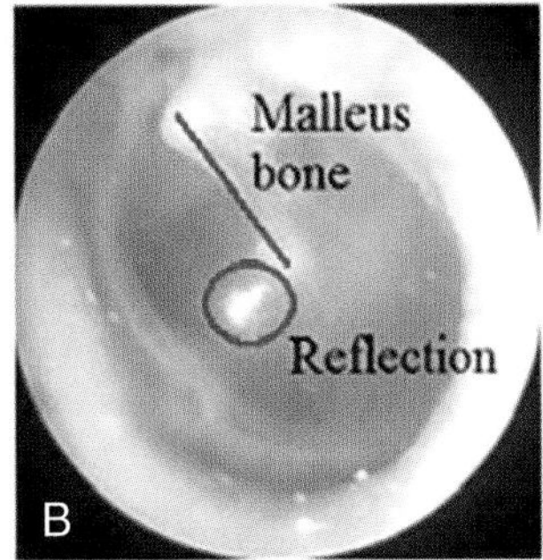

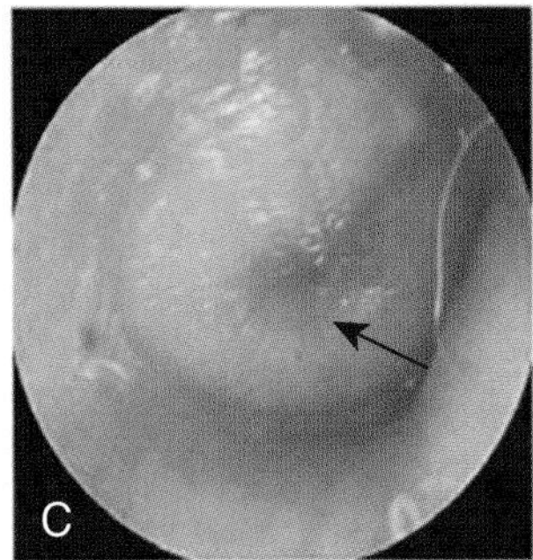

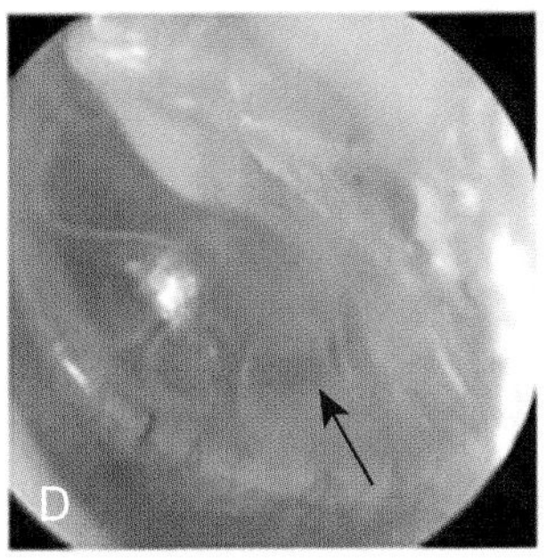

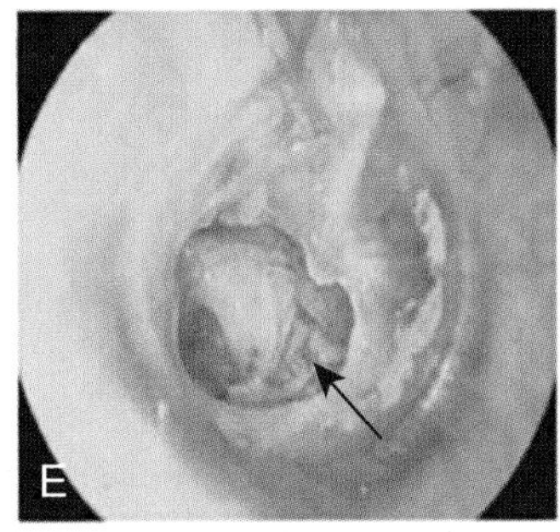

Fig. 16.16 Otitis Media. (A) Obstructing wax or foreign bodies in external ear canal *(see arrow)* precluding visualization of the TM to establish an OM diagnosis. **(B)** A normal TM *(n-TM)* showing a semitransparent pearly white TM, triangular-shaped light reflex, and malleus bone clearly visible (red ring and line, respectively). **(C)** Acute otitis media showing a bulging TM with red color *(see arrow)*. **(D)** Otitis media with effusion *(see arrow)* showing a retracted TM and fluid in the middle ear *(see arrow)*. **(E)** Chronic suppurative otitis media showing a TM perforation *(see arrow)*. *TM*, Tympanic membrane. (From Myburgh HC, et al. Otitis media diagnosis for developing countries using tympanic membrane image-analysis. *EBioMedicine*. 2016;5:156–160. https://www.sciencedirect.com/science/article/pii/S2352396416300500.)

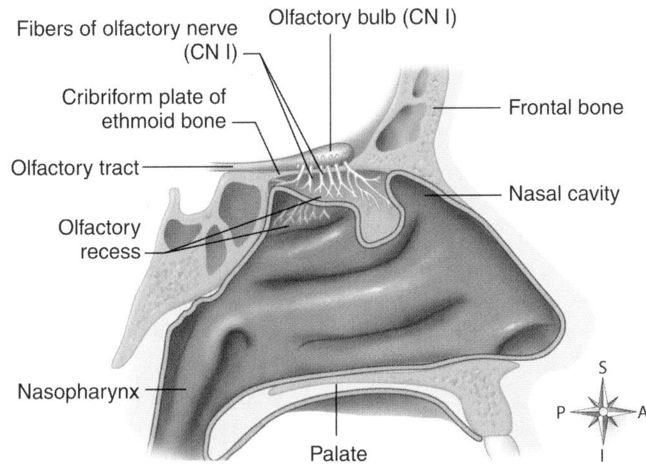

Fig. 16.17 Olfaction. Midsagittal section of the nasal area shows the location of major olfactory sensory structures. (From Patton KT, Thibodeau GA, Douglas MM. *Essentials of Anatomy & Physiology*. St Louis: Mosby; 2012.)

mucosa), sinusitis, nasal polyps, or excessive smoking. Unilateral hyposmia or anosmia may indicate compression of one olfactory bulb (a bulb-like portion of the olfactory nerves) or nerve tract (olfactory nerve pathway), possibly by tumor or head trauma. Olfactory hallucinations arise from hyperactivity in cortical neurons and involve smelling odors that are not really present. They are associated with temporal lobe seizures and rarely with schizophrenia. Parosmia, an abnormal or perverted sense of smell, may occur with severe depression and in Parkinson and Alzheimer disease.[100] Sensitivity to odors declines steadily with aging. (See the box Geriatric Considerations: Aging and Changes in Olfaction and Taste for a summary of changes in olfaction and taste with aging.)

The primary sensations of taste are (1) sour, (2) salty, (3) sweet, (4) bitter, and (5) umami (savory taste of glutamate). Taste buds (fungiform, foliate, and circumvallate) sensitive to each of the primary sensations are located in specific areas of the tongue and are continuously renewing: sweet near the tip, salty on frontal sides, sour on the posterior sides, bitter on the very back, and umami overall surface of tongue. Taste receptors also are found on airway smooth muscle, bladder, breast cancer cells, ovarian cancer cells, and neuroblastoma (bitter) and in the gastrointestinal tract (bitter and sweet). Their function is not for taste. In the lung they stimulate bronchodilation and in the gastrointestinal tract they may participate in metabolic and digestive regulation. These receptors are being evaluated as targets for diagnosis and treatment.[101,102]

GERIATRIC CONSIDERATIONS

Aging and Changes in Olfaction and Taste

- Decline in sensitivity to odors, usually after age 80, occurs.
- Loss of olfaction may diminish appetite, taste, and food selection and may affect nutrition.
- Inability to smell toxic fumes or gases can pose a safety hazard.
- Decline in taste sensitivity is more gradual than decline in sense of smell. Sensitivity to sweetness is maintained and sensitivity to saltiness declines.
- Higher concentrations of flavors required to stimulate taste.
- Taste may be influenced by decreased salivary secretion.

Olfactory and Taste Dysfunctions

Olfactory dysfunctions include the following:

1. **Hyposmia**—impaired sense of smell
2. **Anosmia**—complete loss of sense of smell
3. **Olfactory hallucinations**—smelling odors that are not really present
4. **Parosmia**—abnormal or perverted sense of smell

The sense of taste can be impaired by injury, medications, oral infections, or aging. A change in taste may be attributed to impaired smell associated with injury near the hippocampus.

Hypogeusia is a decrease in taste sensation, whereas **ageusia** is an absence of the sense of taste. These disorders result from cranial nerve injuries and can be specific to the area of the tongue innervated. Dysgeusia is a perversion of taste in which substances possess an unpleasant flavor (i.e., metallic). Ageusia affecting the entire tongue may follow head injury. Hypogeusia and ageusia occur with viral respiratory and oral infections. Autoimmune disease (e.g., systemic lupus erythematosus) and cancer chemotherapy alter taste sensitivity. Damage to the glossopharyngeal nerve (cranial nerve IX, which innervates the posterior one-third of the tongue) causes the loss of the ability to detect bitterness. This loss occurs because the receptors for bitter are located on the base of the tongue. Damage to the facial nerve (cranial nerve VII, which innervates the anterior two-thirds of the tongue) causes loss of the ability to detect sour, sweet, and salty tastes. Only bitter tastes can be detected. These losses occur because sour, sweet, and salt receptors are located on the anterior portion of the tongue.[103] Alterations in taste may compromise adequate nutrition or cause anorexia. Variations in taste and smell are important early manifestations of SARS-CoV-2 viral infection (see Emerging Science Box: Loss of Taste and Smell in SARS-CoV-2-Positive Persons).[104]

SOMATOSENSORY FUNCTION

Touch

The sensation of touch involves four afferent fiber types that mediate tactile sensation and there may be an additional sensory nerve that transmits pleasurable touch.[105] Receptors sensitive to touch are present in the skin with high densities in the fingers and lips. Meissner and Pacinian corpuscles sense movement across the skin and vibration, respectively.

EMERGING SCIENCE BOX

Loss of Taste and Smell in SARS-CoV-2-Positive Persons

The coronavirus SARS-CoV-2 or COVID-19 became a global viral pandemic in March 2020. Based on early research, a typical clinical presentation was known to include fever, cough and/or difficulty breathing, headache, and diarrhea. Early in the disease progression, an atypical presentation was identified in Europe including anosmia and ageusia. While many viral infections can lead to some degree of hyposmia, this symptom is concomitant with rhinorrhea. Similarly, ageusia is a common side effect of nasal obstruction often linked with viral infections. In those who are SARS-CoV-2-positive, anosmia has been present, but unassociated with rhinorrhea and ageusia has been present, but unassociated with nasal obstruction. Preliminary research also identified a predominantly slow resolution to anosmia and ageusia in SARS-CoV-2-positive individuals. The SARS-CoV-2 virus has been shown to infect the salivary glands and gingival mucosa and has been correlated with loss of taste. Additionally, the virus infects the supporting cells in the olfactory epithelium rather than the sensory neurons. Damage to these cells could affect the olfactory bulb and impair neuronal signaling for taste. Cells at these sites express angiotensin-converting enzyme 2 (ACE2) receptors and cell surface transmembrane serine protease 2 (TMPRSS2), both of which are critical for viral entry.

Data from Brann DH, et al. Non-neuronal expression of SARS-CoV-2 entry genes in the olfactory system suggests mechanisms underlying COVID-19-associated anosmia. *Sci. Adv.* 2020;6:eabc5801; Huang N, et al. SARS-CoV-2 infection of the oral cavity and saliva. *Nat Med.* 2021. Based on the emerging science of COVID-19 studies, sudden loss of taste (ageusia) and loss of smell (anosmia) have been listed as important symptoms in the identification of active SARS-CoV-2 infection; Mastrangelo A, et al. Smell and taste disorders in COVID-19: from pathogenesis to clinical features and outcomes. *Neurosci Lett.* 2021;748:135694.

Merkel disks sense sustained light touch, and Ruffini endings respond to deep sustained pressure, stretch, and joint position. Specific sensory input is carried to the higher levels of the CNS by the dorsal column of the spinal cord and the anterior spinothalamic tract.

The cutaneous senses develop before birth, but structural growth continues into early adulthood. Then a gradual decline occurs, with loss in tactile discrimination with advancing age. Abnormal tactile perception may be caused by alterations at any level of the nervous system, from the receptor to the cerebral cortex. Factors that interrupt or impair reception, transmission, perception, or interpretation of touch—including trauma, tumor, infection, metabolic changes, vascular changes, and degenerative diseases—may cause tactile dysfunction. In addition, most tactile sensations evoke affective responses that determine whether the sensation is unpleasant, pleasant, or neutral. With aging, touch sensitivity declines and gentle touch becomes more pleasant. There is a decline in skin elasticity and tactile receptors and changes in central somatotropic organization.[106]

Proprioception

Proprioception is the awareness of the position of the body and its parts. It depends on impulses from the inner ear and from receptors in joints and ligaments. Sensory data are transmitted to higher centers, primarily through the dorsal columns and the spinocerebellar tracts, with some data passing through the medial lemnisci and thalamic radiations to the cortex. These stimuli are necessary for the coordination of movements, the grading of muscular contraction, and the maintenance of equilibrium.

As with tactile dysfunction, any factor that interrupts or impairs the reception, transmission, perception, or interpretation of proprioceptive stimuli also alters proprioception and increases the risk for falls and injury. A progressive loss of proprioception has been reported in older adult persons with an increased risk for falls and injury.[107] Two common causes are vestibular dysfunction and neuropathy.

Specific vestibular dysfunctions are vestibular nystagmus and vertigo. Vestibular nystagmus is the constant, involuntary movement of the eyeball and develops when the semicircular canal system is overstimulated. Vertigo is the sensation of spinning that occurs with inflammation of the semicircular canals in the ear. The individual may feel either that he or she is moving in space or that the world is revolving. Vertigo often causes loss of balance, and nystagmus may occur. Ménière disease can cause loss of proprioception during an acute attack, so that standing or walking is impossible.

Peripheral neuropathies also can cause proprioceptive dysfunction. They may be caused by several conditions and commonly are associated with renal disease and diabetes mellitus. Although the exact sequence of events is unknown, neuropathies cause a diminished or absent sense of body position or position of body parts. Gait changes often occur.

SUMMARY REVIEW

Pain

1. Pain (nociception) is a complex, sensory experience involving emotion, cognition, and motivation. Acute pain is protective, promoting withdrawal from painful stimuli.
2. Three portions of the nervous system are responsible for the sensation, perception, and response to pain: (1) the afferent pathways, (2) the interpretive centers in the central nervous system, and (3) the efferent pathways.
3. Nociception involves four phases: transduction, transmission, perception, and modulation.
4. Pain transduction begins when nociceptors (pain receptors) are activated by noxious stimulants. There are two types of nociceptors: myelinated Aδ fibers transmit sharp, "fast" pain; smaller, unmyelinated C fibers more slowly transmit dull, less localized pain.
5. Pain transmission is the conduction of pain impulses along the nociceptors into the spinal cord and eventually to the brain.
6. Pain perception is the conscious awareness of pain. It occurs with the integration of three systems. The sensory-discriminative system (mediated by the somatosensory cortex) identifies the location and intensity of pain. The affective-motivational system (mediated by the reticular formation, limbic system, and brain stem) controls emotional and affective responses to pain. The cognitive-evaluative system (mediated by the cortex) coordinates the meaning and experience of pain.
7. Pain threshold is the lowest intensity of pain that a person can recognize. Pain tolerance is the greatest level of pain that an individual is prepared to tolerate. Both are subjective and influenced by many factors.
8. Pediatric pain considerations
9. Geriatric pain considerations
10. Pain modulation facilitates or inhibits the transmission of pain signals throughout the nervous system. Neuromodulators of pain include substances that (1) stimulate pain nociceptors (e.g., prostaglandins, bradykinins, lymphokines, substance P, glutamate) and (2) suppress pain (e.g., GABA, endogenous opioids, endocannabinoids). Some substances excite peripheral nerves but inhibit central nerves (e.g., serotonin, norepinephrine).
11. Endogenous opioids inhibit pain transmission and include enkephalins, endorphins, dynorphins, and endomorphins. They are produced in the central nervous system and by immune cells.
12. Descending inhibitory and facilitatory pathways and nuclei inhibit or facilitate pain. Efferent pathways from the ventromedial medulla and PAG inhibit pain impulses at the dorsal horn. The RVM stimulates efferent pathways that facilitate or inhibit pain in the dorsal horn.
13. Segmental pain inhibition occurs when impulses from Aβ fibers (touch and vibration sensations) arrive at the same spinal level as impulses from Aδ or C fibers.
14. DNIC occurs when pain signals from two different sites are transmitted simultaneously and inhibit pain through a spinal-medullary-spinal pathway. Conditioned pain modulation uses a test pain stimulus and a conditioning pain stimulus with subjective measures of pain intensity to evaluate the efficacy of DNIC responses.
15. Because of the complex nature of pain, classifications of pain often overlap, and more than one description is often used.
16. Acute pain is a signal to the person of a harmful stimulus and may be (1) somatic (skin, joints, muscles), (2) visceral (inner organs, body cavities), or (3) referred (present in an area distant from its origin). The area of referred pain is supplied by the same spinal segment as the actual site of pain.
17. Chronic pain is pain lasting well beyond the expected normal healing time and may be ongoing (e.g., low back pain) or intermittent (e.g., migraine headaches). Psychologic, behavioral, and physiologic responses to chronic pain include depression, sleep disorders, preoccupation with pain, lifestyle changes, and physiologic adaptation.
18. Neuropathic pain is chronic pain with increased sensitivity to painful or nonpainful stimuli and results from abnormal processing of pain information in the peripheral or central nervous system.

19. Chronic pain syndromes include myofascial pain, chronic postoperative pain, cancer pain, post-stroke pain, phantom limb pain, and complex regional pain syndrome. These syndromes are complex, often involve both nociceptive and neuropathic pain mechanisms, and are difficult to treat.

Temperature Regulation

1. Temperature regulation (thermoregulation) is achieved through precise balancing of heat production, heat conservation, and heat loss. Body temperature is maintained in a range around 37°C (98.6°F).
2. Temperature regulation is mediated by the hypothalamus and endocrine system through peripheral thermoreceptors in the skin, liver, and skeletal muscle and central thermoreceptors in the hypothalamus, spinal cord, viscera, and great veins.
3. Heat is produced through chemical reactions of metabolism and skeletal muscle contraction. Heat is distributed by the circulatory system.
4. Heat is lost through radiation, conduction, convection, vasodilation, decreased muscle tone, evaporation of sweat, increased respiration, voluntary mechanisms, and adaptation to warmer climates.
5. Heat conservation is accomplished through vasoconstriction and voluntary mechanisms.
6. Infants do not conserve heat well because of their greater body surface/mass ratio and decreased amounts of subcutaneous fat. Older adult persons have poor responses to environmental temperature extremes as a result of slowed blood circulation, structural and functional changes in the skin, and overall decrease in heat-producing activities.
7. Fever involves the temporary "resetting of the hypothalamic thermostat" to a higher level. When the fever breaks, the set point returns to normal. Fever is triggered by the release of exogenous pyrogens from bacteria or the release of endogenous pyrogens (cytokines) from phagocytic cells.
8. Fever kills many pathogens and decreases serum levels of iron, zinc, and copper that are needed for bacterial replication.
9. The acute phase response is a defensive reaction to infection or injury that includes an inflammatory response, fever, and the production of immune cytokines and proteins that support the immune system in eliminating pathogens.
10. Endogenous cryogens are antipyretic substances that diminish fever and control the febrile response.
11. Febrile seizures occur in children with temperatures greater than 38°C (100.4°F) without CNS infection, hypoglycemia, or electrolyte disorders. They are usually brief and without recurrence.
12. Fever of unknown origin is a body temperature greater than 38.3°C (101°F) for longer than 3 weeks that remains undiagnosed after 3 days of investigation.
13. Fever production aids responses to infectious processes. Higher temperatures kill many microorganisms, promote immune responses, and decrease serum levels of iron, zinc, and copper, which are needed for bacterial replication.
14. Hyperthermia (marked warming of core temperature) can produce nerve damage, coagulation of cell proteins, and death. Therapeutic hyperthermia may be used to promote natural immune processes or promote tumor blood flow. Forms of accidental hyperthermia include heat cramps, heat exhaustion, heat stroke, and malignant hyperthermia. Heat stroke and malignant hyperthermia are potentially lethal.
15. Hypothermia (marked cooling of core temperature) slows the rate of cell metabolism, increases the viscosity of the blood, slows blood flow through the microcirculation, facilitates blood coagulation, and stimulates profound vasoconstriction. Hypothermia may be accidental or therapeutic.
16. Major body trauma can affect temperature regulation by damaging the CNS or causing inflammation, increased intracranial pressure, or intracranial bleeding. It results in a sustained, noninfectious fever called central fever.

Sleep

1. Sleep is an active process that provides restorative functions and promotes memory consolidation. Sleep is divided into REM and non-REM stages, each of which has its own series of stages. While asleep, an individual progresses through REM and non-REM (slow wave) sleep multiple times in a predictable cycle.
2. REM sleep is controlled by mechanisms in the pons and mesencephalon. It is known as paradoxical sleep because the EEG pattern is similar to that of an awake person. The brain is very active with dreaming.
3. Non-REM sleep is controlled by release of inhibitory signals from the hypothalamus and accounts for 75% to 80% of sleep time. The body is in a state of reduced activity.
4. The sleep patterns of the newborn and young child vary from those of the adult in total sleep time, cycle length, and percentage of time spent in each sleep cycle. Older adult persons experience a total decrease in sleep time.
5. The restorative, reparative, and growth processes occur during slow-wave (non-REM) sleep. Sleep deprivation can cause profound changes in personality and functioning.
6. Sleep disorders include (1) dyssomnias, which are disorders of initiating or maintaining sleep (i.e., insomnia, obstructive sleep apnea syndrome, hypersomnia, or disorders of the sleep-wake schedule) and (2) parasomnias, which are unusual behaviors during sleep (i.e., sleepwalking or night terrors and restless leg syndrome).

The Special Senses

1. The special senses include vision, hearing, olfaction, and taste.
2. The eyes are responsible for vision. The wall of the eye has three layers: sclera, choroid, and retina. The retina contains millions of baroreceptors known as rods and cones that receive light through the lens and then convey signals to the optic nerve and subsequently to the visual cortex of the brain.
3. The eye is filled with vitreous and aqueous humor, which prevent it from collapsing.
4. The major alterations in ocular movement include strabismus, nystagmus, and paralysis of the extraocular muscles.

5. Alterations in visual acuity (the ability to see objects in sharp detail) can be caused by amblyopia, scotoma, cataracts, papilledema, dark adaptation, glaucoma, retinal detachment, and macular degeneration. Visual acuity decreases with age due to structural eye changes.
6. A cataract is a cloudy or opaque area in the ocular lens and leads to visual loss when located on the visual axis. Cataracts are the leading cause of blindness in the world.
7. Glaucoma is characterized by intraocular pressure with death of retinal ganglion cells and their axons. Open angle, angle closure or narrow angle, and congenital closure are the various forms, with angle closure glaucoma being a medical emergency.
8. Age-related macular degeneration is irreversible loss of vision with atrophic (dry) or neovascular (wet) forms.
9. Retinal detachment is a separation of the retinal pigment epithelium from the photoreceptors in the neuroepithelium with loss of vision.
10. Alterations in accommodation (changes in lens shape that changes focus from distant to near images) develop with increased intraocular pressure, inflammation, age, and disease of the oculomotor nerve. Presbyopia is loss of accommodation caused by loss of elasticity of the lens with aging.
11. Alterations in refraction, including myopia, hyperopia, and astigmatism, are the most common visual disorders.
12. Alterations in color vision can be related to yellowing of the lens with aging and color blindness, an inherited trait.
13. Trauma or disease of the optic nerve pathways can cause defects or blindness in the entire visual field or in half of the visual field (hemianopia).
14. The eyelids, conjunctivae, and lacrimal apparatus protect the eye externally. Infections are the most common disorders; they include blepharitis, conjunctivitis, chalazion, and hordeolum.
15. Blepharitis is an inflammation of the eyelid; a hordeolum (stye) is an infection of the eyelid's sebaceous gland; and a chalazion is an infection of the eyelid's Meibomian gland.
16. Conjunctivitis is an inflammation of the conjunctiva, and can be acute or chronic, bacterial, viral, or allergic. Redness, edema, pain, and lacrimation are common symptoms. Trachoma (chlamydial conjunctivitis) is the leading cause of preventable blindness in the world and is associated with poor hygiene.
17. Keratitis is a bacterial or viral infection of the cornea that can lead to corneal ulceration.
18. The ears are responsible for hearing. The ear is composed of external, middle, and inner structures.
19. The external ear structures are the pinna, auditory canal, and tympanic membrane. The external ear is only involved in hearing.
20. The middle ear is composed of the tympanic cavity (containing three bones: the malleus, the incus, and the stapes), oval window, eustachian tube, and fluid. These transmit sound vibrations to the inner ear. The middle ear is only involved in hearing.
21. The inner ear is involved in both hearing and equilibrium. It includes the bony and membranous labyrinths that transmit sound waves through the cochlea and to the cochlear nerve and ultimately to the brain. The semicircular canals and vestibule help maintain balance through the equilibrium receptors.
22. Impaired hearing is the most common sensory defect, occurring in 5% to 10% of the general population.
23. Hearing loss can be classified as conductive, sensorineural, mixed, or functional.
24. Conductive hearing loss occurs when sound waves cannot be conducted through the middle ear.
25. Sensorineural hearing loss develops with impairment of the organ of Corti or its central connections. Presbycusis is the most common form of sensorineural hearing loss in older adults.
26. A combination of conductive and sensorineural loss is mixed hearing loss. Loss of hearing with no known organic cause is functional hearing loss.
27. Ménière disease is a disorder of the middle ear that affects hearing and balance.
28. Otitis externa is an infection of the outer ear associated with prolonged exposure to moisture.
29. Otitis media is an infection of the middle ear that is common in children. Accumulation of fluid (effusion) behind the tympanic membrane is a common finding.
30. Olfaction (smell) is a function of cranial nerve I and part of cranial nerve V. Taste (gustation) is a function of multiple nerves in the tongue, soft palate, uvula, pharynx, and upper esophagus innervated by cranial nerves VII and IX.
31. The perception of flavor is altered if olfaction or taste dysfunctions occur. Sensitivity to odor and taste decreases with aging.
32. Hyposmia is an impaired sense of smell, and anosmia is the complete loss of the sense of smell.
33. Hypogeusia is a decrease in taste sensation, and ageusia is the absence of the sense of taste.

Somatosensory Function

1. The sensation of touch is a function of receptors present in the skin, and the sensory response is conducted to the brain through the dorsal column and anterior spinothalamic tract.
2. Alterations in touch can result from alterations at any level of the nervous system.
3. Proprioception is the awareness of the position and location of the body and its parts. Proprioceptors are located in the inner ear, joints, and ligaments. Proprioceptive stimuli are necessary for balance, coordinated movement, and grading of muscular contraction.
4. Disorders of proprioception can occur at any level of the nervous system and result in impaired balance and lack of coordinated movement. Vestibular nystagmus is the constant, involuntary movement of the eyeball and develops when the semicircular canal system is overstimulated. Vertigo is the sensation of spinning that occurs with inflammation of the semicircular canals in the ear.

REFERENCES

1. McCaffery M. *Nursing Practice Theories Related to Cognition, Bodily Pain and Man-Environment Interactions*. Los Angeles, CA: University of California at Los Angeles Students' Store; 1968.
2. International Association for the Study of Pain (IASP) *IASP Pain Terminology. Definition of Pain*. Washington, DC: IASP; 2017. Last updated December 14, 2017. Available at https://www.iasp-pain.org/Education/Content.aspx?ItemNumber=1698#Pain. (Accessed August 11, 2021).
3. Cohen M, Quintner J, van Rysewyk S. Reconsidering the International Association for the Study of Pain definition of pain. *Pain Rep*. 2018;3(2):e634.
4. Lee GI, Neumeister MW. Pain: pathways and physiology. *Clin Plast Surg*. 2020;47(2):173–180.
5. Yam MF, et al. General pathways of pain sensation and the major neurotransmitters involved in pain regulation. *Int J Mol Sci*. 2018;19(8):2164.
6. Thompson JM, Neugebauer V. Cortico-limbic pain mechanisms. *Neurosci Lett*. 2019;702:15–23.
7. Frediani F, Bussone G. When does the brain choose pain? *Neurol Sci*. 2019;40(Suppl 1):27–29.
8. Walker SM. Long-term effects of neonatal pain. *Semin Fetal Neonatal Med*. 2019;24(4):101005.
9. Zieliński J, Morawska-Kochman M, Zatoński T. Pain assessment and management in children in the postoperative period: a review of the most commonly used postoperative pain assessment tools, new diagnostic methods and the latest guidelines for postoperative pain therapy in children. *Adv Clin Exp Med*. 2020;29(3):365–374.
10. Domenichiello AF, Ramsden CE. The silent epidemic of chronic pain in older adults. *Prog Neuropsychopharmacol Biol Psychiatry*. 2019;93:284–290.
11. Schwan J, Sclafani J, Tawfik VL. Chronic pain management in the elderly. *Anesthesiol Clin*. 2019;37(3):547–560.
12. Cravello L, et al. Chronic pain in the elderly with cognitive decline: a narrative review. *Pain Ther*. 2019;8(1):53–65.
13. Ardoino I, et al. Pain and frailty in hospitalized older adults. *Pain Ther*. 2020;9(2):727–740.
14. Khan A, Khan S, Kim YS. Insight into pain modulation nociceptors sensitization and therapeutic targets. *Curr Drug Targets*. 2019;20(7):775–788.
15. Berna C, et al. Opioid-independent and opioid-mediated modes of pain modulation. *J Neurosci*. 2018;38(42):9047–9058.
16. Liu JA, Yu J, Cheung CW. Immune actions on the peripheral nervous system in pain. *Int J Mol Sci*. 2021;22(3):1448.
17. Wenzel JM, Cheer JF. Endocannabinoid regulation of reward and reinforcement through interaction with dopamine and endogenous opioid signaling. *Neuropsychopharmacology*. 2018;43(1):103–115.
18. Gibula-Tarlowska E, Kotlinska JH. Crosstalk between opioid and anti-opioid systems: an overview and its possible therapeutic significance. *Biomolecules*. 2020;10(10):1376.
19. Saldaña-Shumaker SL, Grenning AJ, Cunningham CW. Modern approaches to the development of synthetic cannabinoid receptor probes. *Pharmacol Biochem Behav*. 2021;203:173119.
20. Sholler DJ, et al. Therapeutic potential and safety considerations for the clinical use of synthetic cannabinoids. *Pharmacol Biochem Behav*. 2020;199:173059.
21. Ramaswamy S, Wodehouse T. Conditioned pain modulation—a comprehensive review. *Neurophysiol Clin*. 2020;51(3):197–208.
22. Lockwood S, Dickenson AH. What goes up must come down: insights from studies on descending controls acting on spinal pain processing. *J Neural Transm (Vienna)*. 2020;127(4):541–549.
23. Benedetti F, Piedimonte A. The neurobiological underpinnings of placebo and nocebo effects. *Semin Arthritis Rheum*. 2019;49(3S):S18–S21.
24. Rostami K, Zadeh SH, Rakhshan M. Chronic pain: a concept analysis. *Electronic Journal of General Medicine*. 2019;16(2):em130. Available at https://doi.org/10.29333/ejgm/94098. (Accessed August 11, 2021).
25. Xu X, Huang Y. Objective pain assessment: a key for the management of chronic pain. *F1000Res*. 2020;9 F1000 Faculty Rev-35.
26. Filippi M, Messina R. The chronic migraine brain: what have we learned from neuroimaging? *Front Neurol*. 2020;10:1356.
27. Ong WY, Stohler CS, Herr DR. Role of the prefrontal cortex in pain processing. *Mol Neurobiol*. 2019;56(2):1137–1166.
28. Paul-Savoie E, et al. The impact of pain invisibility on patient-centered care and empathetic attitude in chronic pain management. *Pain Res Manag*. 2018;2018:6375713.
29. Wang S, et al. Roles of TRPV1 and TRPA1 in spontaneous pain from inflamed masseter muscle. *Neuroscience*. 2018;384:290–299.
30. Colloca L, et al. Neuropathic pain. *Nat Rev Dis Primers*. 2017;3:17002.
31. Bates D, et al. A comprehensive algorithm for management of neuropathic pain. *Pain Med*. 2019;20(Suppl 1):S2–S12.
32. Urits I, et al. Treatment and management of myofascial pain syndrome. *Best Pract Res Clin Anaesthesiol*. 2020;34(3):427–448.
33. Lopes A, Menezes MS, Moreira de Barros GA: Chronic postoperative pain: ubiquitous and scarcely appraised—narrative review, *Braz J Anesthesiol*. 2021;71(6):649–655. ISSN 0104-0014. https://doi.org/10.1016/j.bjane.2020.10.014. (Accessed April 10, 2022).
34. Fregoso G, et al. Transition from acute to chronic pain: evaluating risk for chronic postsurgical pain. *Pain Physician*. 2019;22(5):479–488.
35. Gulur P, Nelli A. Persistent postoperative pain: mechanisms and modulators. *Curr Opin Anaesthesiol*. 2019;32(5):668–673.
36. Russo MM, Sundaramurthi T. An overview of cancer pain: epidemiology and pathophysiology. *Semin Oncol Nurs*. 2019;35(3):223–228.
37. Caraceni A, Shkodra M. Cancer pain assessment and classification. *Cancers (Basel)*. 2019;11(4):510.
38. Carli M, et al. Opioid receptors beyond pain control: the role in cancer pathology and the debated importance of their pharmacological modulation. *Pharmacol Res*. 2020;159:104938.
39. Wan L, et al. Epoxyeicosatrienoic acids: emerging therapeutic agents for central post-stroke pain. *Pharmacol Res*. 2020;159:104923.
40. Candido Santos L, et al. Intracortical Inhibition in the affected hemisphere in limb amputation. *Front Neurol*. 2020;11:720.
41. Neumeister MW, Romanelli MR. Complex regional pain syndrome. *Clin Plast Surg*. 2020;47(2):305–310.
42. Romanovsky AA. The thermoregulation system and how it works. *Handb Clin Neurol*. 2018;156:3–43.
43. Gao Z, et al. Altered coronary vascular control during cold stress in healthy older adults. *Am J Physiol Heart Circ Physiol*. 2012;302(1):H312–H318.
44. Millyard A, et al. Impairments to thermoregulation in the elderly during heat exposure events. *Gerontol Geriatr Med*. 2020;6 2333721420932432.

45. Székely M, Garai J. Thermoregulation and age. *Handb Clin Neurol*. 2018;156:377–395.
46. Watson J, et al. Use of multiple inflammatory marker tests in primary care: using Clinical Practice Research Datalink to evaluate accuracy. *Br J Gen Pract*. 2019;69(684):e462–e469.
47. Prajitha N, Athira SS, Mohanan PV. Comprehensive biology of antipyretic pathways. *Cytokine*. 2019;116:120–127.
48. Mosili P, et al. The pathogenesis of fever-induced febrile seizures and its current state. *Neurosci Insights*. 2020;15 2633105520956973.
49. Smith DK, Sadler KP, Benedum M. Febrile seizures: risks, evaluation, and prognosis. *Am Fam Physician*. 2019;99(7):445–450.
50. Laino D, Mencaroni E, Esposito S. Management of pediatric febrile seizures. *Int J Environ Res Public Health*. 2018;15(10):2232.
51. Wright WF, Auwaerter PG. Fever and fever of unknown origin: review, recent advances, and lingering dogma. *Open Forum Infect Dis*. 2020;7(5). ofaa132.
52. Wrotek S, et al. Let fever do its job: the meaning of fever in the pandemic era. *Evol Med Public Health*. 2020;9(1):26–35.
53. Belon L, et al. Effect of a fever in viral infections—the 'Goldilocks' phenomenon? *World J Clin Cases*. 2021;9(2):296–307.
54. Ludwig J, McWhinnie H. Antipyretic drugs in patients with fever and infection: literature review. *Br J Nurs*. 2019;28(10):610–618.
55. Palladino L, Woll C, Aronson PL. Evaluation and management of the febrile young infant in the emergency department. *Pediatr Emerg Med Pract*. 2019;16(7):1–24.
56. Wang H, et al. Thermal regulation of the brain—an anatomical and physiological review for clinical neuroscientists. *Front Neurosci*. 2016;9:528.
57. Datta NR, et al. Integrating loco-regional hyperthermia into the current oncology practice: SWOT and TOWS analyses. *Front Oncol*. 2020;10:819.
58. Ibelli T, Templeton S, Levi-Polyachenko N. Progress on utilizing hyperthermia for mitigating bacterial infections. *Int J Hyperthermia*. 2018;34(2):144–156.
59. Lipman GS, et al. Wilderness Medical Society clinical practice guidelines for the prevention and treatment of heat illness: 2019 update. *Wilderness Environ Med*. 2019;30(4S):S33–S46.
60. Laitano O, et al. Controversies in exertional heat stroke diagnosis, prevention, and treatment. *J Appl Physiol (1985)*. 2019;127(5):1338–1348.
61. Shimada T, et al. Analysis of clinical symptoms and brain MRI of heat stroke: 2 case reports and a literature review. *J Stroke Cerebrovasc Dis*. 2020;29(2):104511.
62. McCamish J. Malignant hyperthermia knowledge. *Dissector*. 2019;46(4):22–26.
63. Goyal K, Garg N, Bithal P. Central fever: a challenging clinical entity in neurocritical care. *Journal of Neurocritical Care*. 2020;13(1):19–31. Available at https://doi.org/10.18700/jnc.190090. (Accessed August 11, 2021).
64. Serin Y, Acar Tek N. Effect of circadian rhythm on metabolic processes and the regulation of energy balance. *Ann Nutr Metab*. 2019;74(4):322–330.
65. Agostini A, Centofanti S. Normal sleep in children and adolescence. *Child Adolesc Psychiatr Clin N Am*. 2021;30(1):1–14.
66. Schwartz WJ, Klerman EB. Circadian neurobiology and the physiologic regulation of sleep and wakefulness. *Neurol Clin*. 2019;37(3):475–486.
67. Klinzing JG, Niethard N, Born J. Mechanisms of systems memory consolidation during sleep. *Nat Neurosci*. 2019;22(10):1598–1610.
68. Sateia MJ. International classification of sleep disorders—third edition: highlights and modifications. *Chest*. 2014;146(5): 1387–1394.
69. Bollu PC, Kaur H. Sleep medicine: insomnia and sleep. *Mo Med*. 2019;116(1):68–75.
70. Rundo JV. Obstructive sleep apnea basics. *Cleve Clin J Med*. 2019;86(9 Suppl 1):2–9.
71. Garbarino S, et al. Obstructive sleep apnea with or without excessive daytime sleepiness: clinical and experimental data-driven phenotyping. *Front Neurol*. 2018;9:505.
72. Gottlieb DJ, Punjabi NM. Diagnosis and management of obstructive sleep apnea: a review. *JAMA*. 2020;323(14): 1389–1400.
73. Bitners AC, Arens R. Evaluation and management of children with obstructive sleep apnea syndrome. *Lung*. 2020;198(2): 257–270.
74. Mahoney CE, et al. The neurobiological basis of narcolepsy. *Nat Rev Neurosci*. 2019;20(2):83–93.
75. Ruan W, Yuan X, Eltzschig HK. Circadian rhythm as a therapeutic target. *Nat Rev Drug Discov*. 2021;20:287–307.
76. Singh S, et al. Parasomnias: a comprehensive review. *Cureus*. 2018;10(12):e3807.
77. Yang Z, et al. Molecular mechanisms underlying reciprocal interactions between sleep disorders and Parkinson's disease. *Front Neurosci*. 2021;14:592989.
78. Memon MD, et al. Unraveling the mysteries of restless leg syndrome. *Cureus*. 2020;12(10):e10951.
79. Eggers SDZ, et al. Classification of vestibular signs and examination techniques: nystagmus and nystagmus-like movements. *J Vestib Res*. 2019;29(2-3):57–87.
80. Stein JD, Khawaja AP, Weizer JS. Glaucoma in adults—screening, diagnosis, and management: a review. *JAMA*. 2021;325(2): 164–174.
81. Hadziahmetovic M, Malek G. Age-related macular degeneration revisited: from pathology and cellular stress to potential therapies. *Front Cell Dev Biol*. 2021;8:612812.
82. Evans JR, Lawrenson JG. Antioxidant vitamin and mineral supplements for slowing the progression of age-related macular degeneration. *Cochrane Database Syst Rev*. 2017;7(7):CD000254.
83. Sultan ZN, et al. Rhegmatogenous retinal detachment: a review of current practice in diagnosis and management. *BMJ Open Ophthalmol*. 2020;5(1):e000474.
84. Kollbaum PS, Bradley A. Correction of presbyopia: old problems with old (and new) solutions. *Clin Exp Optom*. 2020;103(1):21–30.
85. Isherwood ZJ, et al. Plasticity in perception: insights from color vision deficiencies. *Fac Rev*. 2020;9:8.
86. Raffin E, Salamanca-Giron RF, Hummel FC. Perspectives: hemianopia—toward novel treatment options based on oscillatory activity? *Neurorehabil Neural Repair*. 2020;34(1):13–25.
87. Thurtell MJ, Kawasaki A. Update in the management of idiopathic intracranial hypertension. *Neurol Clin*. 2021;39(1):147–161.
88. Azari AA, Arabi A. Conjunctivitis: a systematic review. *J Ophthalmic Vis Res*. 2020;15(3):372–395.
89. West SK. Milestones in the fight to eliminate trachoma. *Ophthalmic Physiol Opt*. 2020;40(2):66–74.
90. Ting DSJ, et al. Infectious keratitis: an update on epidemiology, causative microorganisms, risk factors, and antimicrobial resistance. *Eye (Lond)*. 2021;35:1084–1101.
91. Newsted D, et al. Approach to hearing loss. *Can Fam Physician*. 2020;66(11):803–809.

92. Cunningham LL, Tucci DL. Hearing loss in adults. *N Engl J Med.* 2017;377(25):2465–2473.
93. Christopher LH, Wilkinson EP. Meniere's disease: Medical management, rationale for vestibular preservation and suggested protocol in medical failure. *Am J Otolaryngol.* 2021;42(1):102817.
94. Szmuilowicz J, Young R. Infections of the ear. *Emerg Med Clin North Am.* 2019;37(1):1–9.
95. Thornton RB, et al. Panel 7—Pathogenesis of otitis media—a review of the literature between 2015 and 2019. *Int J Pediatr Otorhinolaryngol.* 2020;130(Suppl 1):109838.
96. Mittal R, et al. Recent perspectives on gene-microbe interactions determining predisposition to otitis media. *Front Genet.* 2019;10:1230.
97. Gaddey HL, Wright MT, Nelson TN. Otitis media: rapid evidence review. *Am Fam Physician.* 2019;100(6):350–356.
98. Brennan-Jones CG, et al. Topical antibiotics for chronic suppurative otitis media. *Cochrane Database Syst Rev.* 2020;1(1):CD013051.
99. Patel RM, Pinto JM. Olfaction: anatomy, physiology, and disease. *Clin Anat.* 2014;27(1):54–60.
100. Attems J, Walker L, Jellinger KA. Olfactory bulb involvement in neurodegenerative diseases. *Acta Neuropathol.* 2014;127(4): 459–475.
101. Jeruzal-Świątecka J, Fendler W, Pietruszewska W. Clinical role of extraoral bitter taste receptors. *Int J Mol Sci.* 2020;21(14):5156.
102. Nayak AP, Villalba D, Deshpande DA. Bitter taste receptors: an answer to comprehensive asthma control? *Curr Allergy Asthma Rep.* 2019;19(10):48.
103. Risso D, Drayna D, Morini G. Alteration, reduction and taste loss: main causes and potential implications on dietary habits. *Nutrients.* 2020;12(11):3284.
104. Lutz M, et al. Considerations for the development of innovative foods to improve nutrition in older adults. *Nutrients.* 2019;11(6):1275.
105. Glatte P, et al. Architecture of the cutaneous autonomic nervous system. *Front Neurol.* 2019;10:970.
106. McIntyre S, et al. The effects of ageing on tactile function in the human nervous system. *Neuroscience.* 2021;464:53–58.
107. Ferlinc A, et al. The importance and role of proprioception in the elderly: a short review. *Mater Sociomed.* 2019;31(3):219–221.

17

Alterations in Cognitive Systems, Cerebral Hemodynamics, and Motor Function

Kaveri Roy and Sue E. Huether

http://evolve.elsevier.com/Rogers/pathophysiology/

CHAPTER OUTLINE

Intellectual and behavioral functions are achieved by integrated processes of cognitive systems, sensory systems, and motor systems. The purpose of this chapter is to present the concepts and processes of these alterations as an approach to understanding the manifestation of neurologic dysfunction that can occur with disease or injury. Some specific diseases are also presented in this chapter (Parkinson disease [PD], Huntington disease [HD], and amyotrophic lateral sclerosis [ALS]) because they fit best here. The manifestations for specific central and peripheral nervous system disorders are presented in Chapter 18 (brain and spinal cord injury, stroke, seizure, and headache syndromes). Alterations in sensory function and sleep were presented in Chapter 16 (pain, temperature regulation, sleep, and the special senses—vision, hearing, touch, and proprioception).

The neural systems are structures that build, support, facilitate, and organize sensorimotor input and output.[1] The neural systems essential to cognitive function are (1) attentional systems that provide arousal and maintenance of attention over time, (2) memory and language systems by which information is communicated, and (3) affective or emotive systems that mediate mood, emotion, and intention. These core systems are fundamental to the processes of abstract thinking and reasoning. The products of abstraction and reasoning are organized and made operational through the executive attentional networks. The normal functioning of these systems manifests through the motor system in a behavioral array viewed by others as being appropriate to human activity and successful living.

ALTERATIONS IN COGNITIVE SYSTEMS

Consciousness is a state of awareness both of oneself and of the environment and a set of responses to that environment. Consciousness has two distinct components: arousal (state of wakefulness or alertness) and awareness (content of thought). Arousal is mediated by the reticular activating system, which regulates aspects of attention and information processing and maintains consciousness (see Fig. 15.7). Cognitive cerebral functions require a functioning reticular activating system (RAS). Awareness encompasses all cognitive functions and is mediated by attentional systems, memory systems, language systems, and executive systems.

Alterations in Arousal

Alterations in level of arousal may be caused by structural, metabolic, or psychogenic (functional) disorders.

Pathophysiology. Structural alterations in arousal are divided according to the original location of the pathologic condition: supratentorial (above the tentorium cerebelli—membrane), infratentorial (subtentorial, below the tentorium cerebelli—membrane) (see Figs. 15.17 and 17.17), extracerebral (outside the brain tissue), and intracerebral (within the brain tissue). Causes include infection, vascular alterations, neoplasms, traumatic injury, congenital alterations, degenerative changes, polygenic traits, and metabolic disorders.

Supratentorial disorders (above the tentorium cerebelli) produce changes in arousal by either diffuse or localized dysfunction. Diffuse dysfunction may be caused by disease processes affecting the cerebral cortex or the underlying subcortical white matter (e.g., encephalitis). Disorders outside the brain but within the cranial vault (extracerebral) also can produce diffuse dysfunction, including neoplasms, closed-head trauma with subsequent bleeding (i.e., subdural hematoma or subarachnoid hemorrhage), and subdural empyema (accumulation of pus). Disorders within the brain substance (intracerebral)—bleeding, infarcts, emboli, and tumors—function primarily as masses. Such localized destructive processes directly impair function of the thalamic or hypothalamic activating systems or secondarily compress these structures in a process of expansion or herniation.

Infratentorial disorders (below the tentorium cerebelli) produce a decline in arousal by (1) direct destruction or compression of the RAS and its pathways (e.g., accumulations of blood or pus, neoplasms, and demyelinating disorders), or (2) the brainstem (midbrain, pons, and medulla) may be destroyed either by direct invasion or by indirect impairment of its blood supply. The most common cause of direct destruction is cerebrovascular disease. Demyelinating diseases, neoplasms, granulomas, abscesses, and head injury also may cause brainstem destruction by tissue compression. This compression may occur because of (1) direct pressure on the pons and midbrain, producing ischemia and edema of the neurons of the RAS; (2) upward herniation of the cerebellum through the tentorial notch, thus compressing the upper midbrain and diencephalon; or (3) downward herniation of the cerebellum through the foramen magnum, compressing and displacing the medulla oblongata.

Metabolic alterations in arousal produce a decline in arousal by alterations in delivery of energy substrates as occurs with hypoxia, electrolyte disturbances, hypoglycemia, or hyperglycemia. Examples of systemic diseases that eventually produce nervous system disorders include liver or renal failure that cause alterations in neuronal excitability because of failure to metabolize or eliminate drugs and toxins. Hypothyroidism and adrenal insufficiency may be associated with alterations in arousal (e.g., myxedema coma and adrenal crisis) and are medical emergencies (see Chapter 22).

Psychogenic alterations in arousal (unresponsiveness), although uncommon, may signal general psychiatric disorders (see Chapter 19). Despite apparent unconsciousness, the person is physiologically awake, and the neurologic examination reflects normal responses.

Clinical Manifestations and Evaluation. Five patterns of neurologic function are critical to the evaluation process: (1) level of consciousness, (2) pattern of breathing, (3) pupillary reaction, (4) oculomotor responses, and (5) motor responses. Patterns of clinical manifestations help determine the extent of brain dysfunction and serve as indices for identifying increasing or decreasing central nervous system (CNS) function. Distinctions are made between metabolic and structurally induced manifestations (Table 17.1). The types of manifestations suggest the mechanisms of the altered arousal state (Table 17.2).

Patterns of Neurologic Function

Level of consciousness is the most critical clinical index of nervous system function, with changes indicating either improvement or deterioration of the individual's condition. A person who is alert and oriented to self, others, place, and time is functioning at the highest level of consciousness, which implies full use of all the person's cognitive capacities. From this normal alert state, levels of consciousness diminish in stages from

TABLE 17.1 Clinical Manifestations of Metabolic and Structural Causes of Altered Arousal

Manifestation	Metabolically Induced	Structurally Induced
Blink to threat (cranial nerves II, VII)	Equal	Asymmetric
Optic discs (cranial nerve II)	Flat, good pulsation	Papilledema
Extraocular movement (cranial nerves III, IV, VI)	Roving eye movements; normal doll's eyes and calorics	Gaze paresis, nerve III palsy, medial longitudinal fasciculus (MLF) syndrome (internuclear ophthalmoplegia)
Pupils (cranial nerves II, III)	Equal and reactive; may be large (e.g., atropine), pinpoint (e.g., opiates), or midposition and fixed (e.g., glutethimide [Doriden])	Asymmetric and/or nonreactive; may be midposition (midbrain injury), pinpoint (pons injury), large (tectal injury)
Corneal reflex (cranial nerves V, VII)	Symmetric response	Asymmetric response
Grimace to pain (cranial nerve VII)	Symmetric response	Asymmetric response
Motor function movement	Symmetric	Asymmetric
Muscle tone	Symmetric	Paratonic, spastic, flaccid, especially if asymmetric
Posture	Symmetric	Decorticate, especially if symmetric; decerebrate, especially if asymmetric
Deep tendon reflexes	Symmetric	Asymmetric
Babinski sign	Absent or symmetric response	Present
Sensation	Symmetric	Asymmetric

TABLE 17.2 Differential Characteristics of Disorders Causing Altered Arousal

Mechanism	Manifestations
Supratentorial mass lesions compressing or displacing diencephalons or brainstem	Initiating signs usually of focal cerebral dysfunction Signs of dysfunction progress rostral to caudal Neurologic signs at any given time point to one anatomic area (e.g., diencephalon, mesencephalon, medulla) Motor signs often asymmetric
Infratentorial mass or destruction, causing coma	History of preceding brainstem dysfunction or sudden onset of coma Localizing brainstem signs precede or accompany onset of coma and always include oculovestibular abnormality Cranial nerve palsies; usually manifest as "bizarre" respiratory patterns that appear at onset
Metabolic coma Exogenous toxins (e.g., drugs, carbon monoxide, heavy metals, pesticides) Endogenous toxins (organ system failure)	Confusion and stupor commonly precede motor signs Motor signs usually are symmetric Pupillary reactions usually are preserved Asterixis, myoclonus, tremor, and seizures are common Acid-base imbalance with hyperventilation or hypoventilation is common
Psychiatric unresponsiveness	Lids close actively Pupils reactive or dilated (cycloplegics) Oculocephalic reflexes are unpredictable; oculovestibular reflexes are physiologic (nystagmus is present) Motor tone is inconsistent or normal Eupnea or hyperventilation is usual No pathologic reflexes are present Electroencephalogram (EEG) is normal

TABLE 17.3 Levels of Altered Consciousness

State	Definition
Confusion	Loss of ability to think rapidly and clearly; impaired judgment and decision making; difficulty following instructions
Disorientation	Beginning loss of consciousness; disorientation to time followed by disorientation to place and impaired memory; lost last is recognition of self
Lethargy	Limited spontaneous movement or speech; easy arousal with normal speech or touch; may not be oriented to time, place, or person
Obtundation	Mild to moderate reduction in arousal (awakeness) with limited response to the environment; falls asleep unless stimulated verbally or tactilely; answers questions with minimum response
Stupor	A condition of deep sleep or unresponsiveness from which the person may be aroused or caused to open eyes only by vigorous and repeated stimulation; response is often withdrawal or grabbing at stimulus
Light coma	Associated with purposeful movement on stimulation
Coma	No verbal response to the external environment or to any stimuli; noxious stimuli such as deep pain or suctioning yields motor movement
Deep coma	Associated with unresponsiveness or no response to any stimulus

confusion and disorientation (can occur simultaneously) to coma, each of which is clinically defined (Table 17.3). Guidelines are available to assist with the evaluation of prolonged disorders of consciousness.[2]

Patterns of breathing help evaluate the level of brain dysfunction and coma. Rate, rhythm, and pattern should be evaluated. Breathing patterns can be categorized as hemispheric or brainstem (Table 17.4 and Fig. 17.1).

With normal breathing, a neural center in the forebrain (cerebrum) produces a rhythmic breathing pattern. When consciousness decreases, lower brainstem centers regulate the breathing pattern by responding only to changes in $PaCO_2$ levels. This pattern is called ***posthyperventilation apnea (PHVA)***.

Cheyne-Stokes respiration is an abnormal rhythm of ventilation (periodic breathing) with alternating periods of hyperventilation and apnea (crescendo-decrescendo pattern). In the damaged brain, higher levels of $PaCO_2$ are required to stimulate ventilation, and increases in $PaCO_2$ lead to tachypnea. The $PaCO_2$ level then decreases to below normal and breathing stops (apnea) until the carbon dioxide reaccumulates and again stimulates tachypnea (see Fig. 17.1). In cases of opiate or sedative drug overdose, the respiratory center is depressed, and the rate of breathing gradually decreases until respiratory failure occurs.

Central neurogenic hyperventilation is a respiratory pattern of sustained hyperventilation caused by a lesion that stimulates the respiratory center in the central pons. Apneustic respirations have prolonged inspiratory phase and a short expiratory phase caused by injury to the pons or upper medulla. ***Cluster (Biots) respirations*** are characterized by periods or clusters of rapid respirations of near equal depth resulting from trauma or compression to the medulla near the pontine junction or from chronic opioid abuse. ***Ataxic respirations*** are variable respirations with irregular prolonged periods of apnea associated with damage to the medulla (see Fig. 17.1).

TABLE 17.4 Patterns of Breathing

Breathing Pattern	Description	Location of Injury
Hemispheric Breathing Patterns		
Normal	After a period of hyperventilation that lowers the arterial carbon dioxide pressure ($Paco_2$), the individual continues to breathe regularly but with a reduced depth.	Response of the nervous system to an external stressor—not associated with injury to the central nervous system (CNS)
Posthyperventilation apnea	Respirations stop after hyperventilation has lowered the $Paco_2$ level below normal. Rhythmic breathing returns when the $Paco_2$ level returns to normal. (Usually, an intact cerebral cortex will trigger breathing within 10 s regardless of $Paco_2$.)	Associated with diffuse bilateral metabolic or structural disease of the cerebrum
Cheyne-Stokes respirations	Breathing pattern has a smooth increase (crescendo) in the rate and depth of breathing (hyperpnea), which peaks and is followed by a gradual smooth decrease (decrescendo) in the rate and depth of breathing to the point of apnea when the cycle repeats itself. The hyperpneic phase lasts longer than the apneic phase (represents an amplitude change).	Bilateral dysfunction of the deep cerebral or diencephalic structures; seen with supratentorial injury and metabolically induced coma states unrelated to neurologic dysfunction; may see also in congestive heart failure (CHF)
Brainstem Breathing Patterns		
Central reflex hyperpnea (central neurogenic hyperventilation)	A sustained deep rapid but regular pattern (hyperpnea) occurs, with a decreased $Paco_2$ and a corresponding increase in pH and increased Po_2.	May result from CNS damage or disease that involves the lower midbrain and upper pons; seen after increased intracranial pressure and blunt head trauma
Apneusis	A prolonged inspiratory cramp (a pause at full inspiration) occurs. A common variant of this is a brief end-inspiratory pause of 2 or 3 s, often alternating with an end-expiratory pause.	Indicates damage to the respiratory control mechanism located at the pontine level; most commonly associated with pontine infarction but documented with hypoglycemia, anoxia, and meningitis
Cluster (Biot) breathing	A cluster of breaths has a disordered sequence with irregular pauses between breaths.	Dysfunction in the lower pontine and high medullary areas
Ataxic breathing	Completely irregular breathing occurs, with random shallow and deep breaths and irregular pauses. Often the rate is slow.	Originates from a primary dysfunction of the medulla
Gasping breathing pattern (agonal gasps)	A pattern of deep "all-or-none" breaths is accompanied by a slow respiratory rate.	Indicative of a failing medullary respiratory center

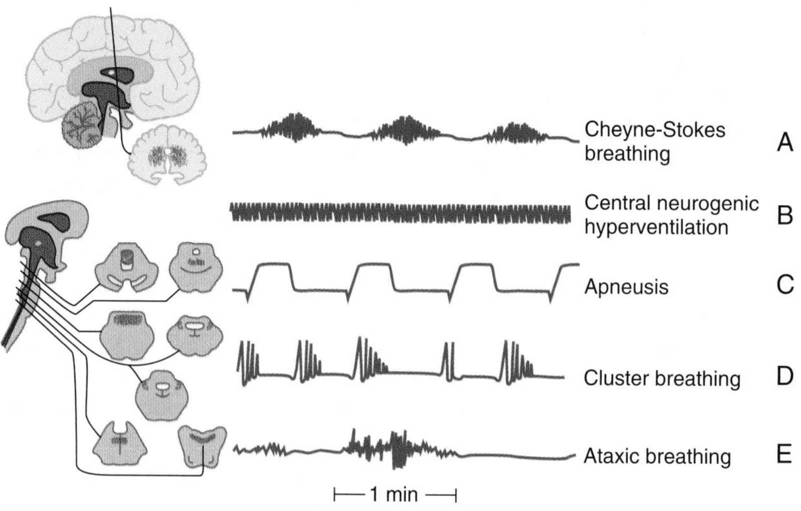

Fig. 17.1 Abnormal Respiratory Patterns With Corresponding Level of Central Nervous System Injuries. **(A)** Cheyne-Stokes respiration is seen with metabolic injury and lesions in the forebrain and diencephalon. **(B)** Central neurogenic hyperventilation is most commonly seen with metabolic encephalopathies (lesion of midbrain, pons, or medulla). **(C)** Apneustic breathing (inspiratory pauses) is seen in persons with bilateral pontine lesions. **(D)** Cluster (Biots) breathing and ataxic breathing are seen in lesions at the pontine medullary junction. **(E)** Ataxic breathing occurs when the medullary ventral respiratory nuclei are injured. (From Urden LD, et al. *Critical care nursing: Diagnosis and management*, 6th edition. St. Louis: Mosby; 2010.)

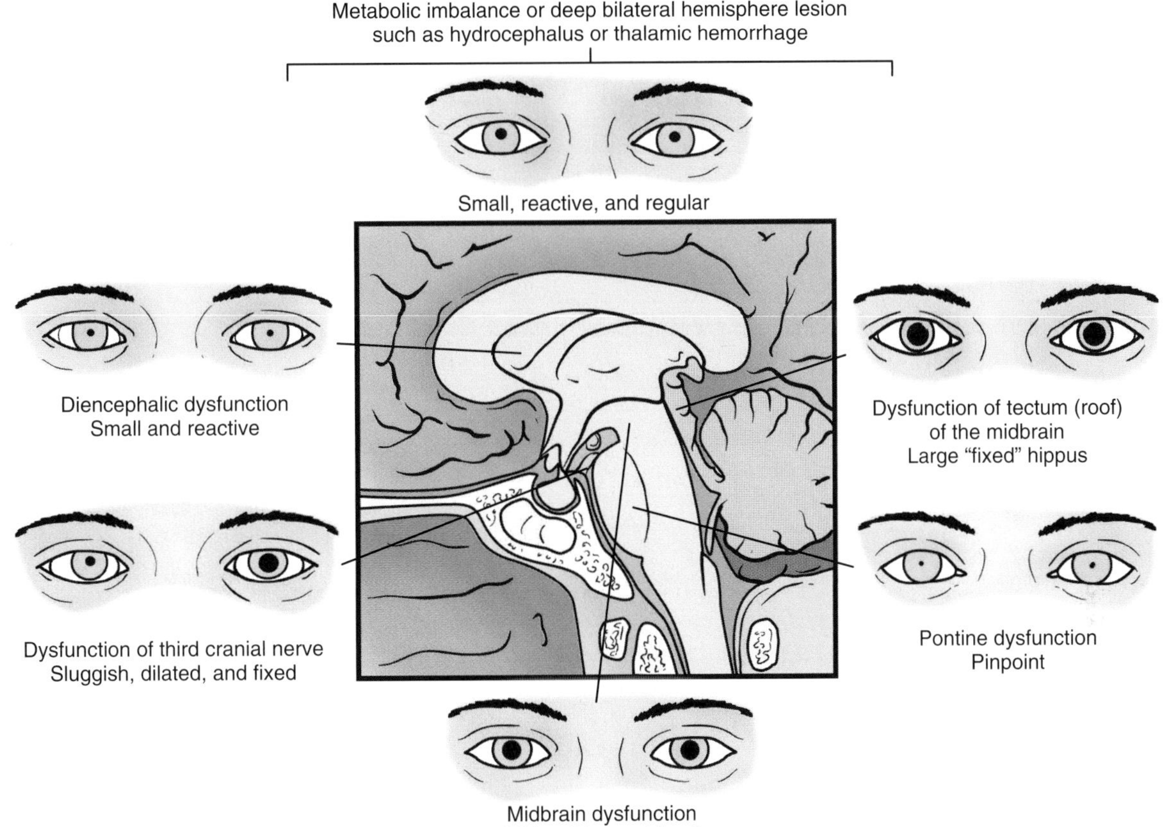

Fig. 17.2 Appearance of Pupils at Different Levels of Consciousness.

Pupillary changes indicate the presence and level of brainstem dysfunction because brainstem areas that control arousal are adjacent to areas that control the pupils (Fig. 17.2). For example, severe ischemia and hypoxia usually produce dilated, fixed pupils. Hypothermia may cause fixed pupils. Some drugs affect pupils and must be considered in evaluating individuals in comatose states. Large doses of atropine and scopolamine (drugs that block parasympathetic stimulation) fully dilate and fix pupils. Doses of sedatives (e.g., glutethimide) in sufficient amounts to produce coma cause the pupils to become midposition or moderately dilated, unequal, and commonly fixed to light. Opiates (which stimulate the parasympathetic nervous system) cause pinpoint pupils.

Oculomotor responses are resting, spontaneous, and reflexive eye movements. They change at various levels of brain dysfunction in comatose individuals (Table 17.5). Persons with metabolically induced coma, except in cases of barbiturate-hypnotic and phenytoin (Dilantin) poisoning, generally retain ocular reflexes, even when other signs of brainstem damage, such as central neurogenic hyperventilation, are present.

The presence of brisk oculocephalic reflexes and roving eye movements, as well as the failure to elicit nystagmus with instillation of cold or warm water into the external ear canal, indicates a decrease in consciousness (loss of cortical influence) but an intact brainstem (Figs. 17.3 and 17.4).

Destructive or compressive injury to the brainstem causes specific abnormalities of the oculocephalic and oculovestibular reflexes. For example, a skewed deviation, in which one eye diverges downward and the other looks upward, indicates brainstem dysfunction. Destructive or compressive disease processes that involve an oculomotor nucleus or nerve cause the involved eye to deviate outward, producing a resting dysconjugate lateral position of the eyes (each eye diverges laterally). Unilateral abducens paralysis (paralysis of cranial nerve VI) results in an upward deviation of the ipsilateral eye. With bilateral abducens paralysis, the eyes come together (converge). Reflexive eye movements may be suppressed by drugs, most commonly phenytoin, tricyclics, and barbiturates. Occasionally alcohol, phenothiazines, and diazepam may alter reflex eye movements.

Assessment of motor responses helps to evaluate the level of brain dysfunction and determine the side of the brain that is maximally damaged. The pattern of response noted may be (1) purposeful (a defensive or withdrawal movement of limbs to noxious stimuli); (2) inappropriate, or not purposeful (generalized motor movement, posturing, grimacing, or groaning); or (3) not present (unresponsive, no motor response). Purposeful movement requires an intact corticospinal system. Nonpurposeful movement is evidence of severe dysfunction of the corticospinal system.

Motor signs indicating loss of cortical inhibition are commonly associated with decreased consciousness and include primitive reflexes and rigidity (paratonia). Primitive reflexes include grasping, reflex sucking (tapping on lips stimulates sucking), snout reflex (tapping of closed lips at midlines causes pursing of lips), and palmomental reflex (stroking palm causes twitch of chin muscle), all of which are normal in the newborn

TABLE 17.5 Changes in Oculomotor Responses

State	Resting and Spontaneous Eye Movements	Reflexive Eye Movements
Full consciousness	Eyes at rest, still (cortical gaze centers inhibit spontaneous roving eye movements)	Eyes move as the head turns Oculocephalic responses not elicited or inconsistently elicited (frontal gaze centers inhibit brainstem reflexes that fix gaze straight ahead) Oculovestibular (caloric) stimulation produces nystagmus
Cortical dysfunction or disruption of efferent pathways	Conjugate, horizontal, roving eye movements may well be present (cortical gaze centers no longer inhibit these brainstem-generated roving eye movements)	Gaze fixed straight ahead regardless of head position—positive doll's eyes reaction (normal oculocephalic reflexes are no longer inhibited by frontal gaze centers)
Diffuse anoxic damage to cortex	"Ocular dipping"—slow, dysrhythmic downward movement followed by faster, upward movement	Nystagmus is no longer induced by caloric stimulation (normally, a cold-water stimulus produces deviation of the eyes opposite the irrigated ear; a warm-water stimulus deviates the eyes to the same [ipsilateral] side) With an injury that depresses cortical gaze center function, the eyes (and often the entire head) deviate or appear to look toward the side of the injured hemisphere With an injury that irritates (stimulates) the neurons of the cortical gaze center, the eyes (and often the entire head) deviate away from the injured hemisphere (all fibers from the frontal gaze centers decussate and therefore control the function of the contralateral pontine gaze center, which moves the eyes in the ipsilateral direction)
Mesencephalon dysfunction	Roving eye movements cease, and the eyes become immobile and directed ahead (roving eye movements require an intact brainstem) Eyes may turn down and inward	Oculovestibular reflexes become inconsistent and abnormal Loss of Bell phenomenon (upward deviation of eyes on stimulation) (requires intact eye movement pathways from the mesencephalon to pons)
Pontine dysfunction	Loss of spontaneous blinking (requires an intact pons) "Ocular bobbing"—brisk, conjugate, downward movement of eyes with loss of horizontal eye movements	

but disappear in infancy (Fig. 17.5). Abnormal flexor and extensor responses in the upper and lower extremities are defined in Table 17.6 and illustrated in Fig. 17.6.

Vomiting, yawning, and hiccups are complex reflex-like motor responses that are integrated by neural mechanisms in the lower brainstem. These responses may be produced by compression or diseases involving tissues of the medulla oblongata (e.g., infection, neoplasm, infarct, or other more benign stimuli to the vagal nerve). Most CNS disorders produce nausea and vomiting. Vomiting without nausea indicates direct involvement of the central neural mechanism (or pyloric obstruction). Vomiting often accompanies CNS injuries that (1) involve the vestibular nuclei or its immediate projections, particularly when double vision (diplopia) also is present; (2) impinge directly on the floor of the fourth ventricle; or (3) produce brainstem compression secondary to increased intracranial pressure (IICP).

Complications of Alterations in Arousal

Complications of alterations in arousal fall into two categories: *extent of disability (morbidity)* and *mortality*. The outcomes depend on the cause and extent of brain damage and the duration of coma. Some individuals may recover consciousness and an original level of function, some may have permanent disability, and some may never regain consciousness and experience neurologic death. Two forms of neurologic death—brain death and cerebral death—result from severe pathologic conditions and are associated with irreversible coma. Other possible outcomes are a vegetative state (VS), a minimally conscious state (MCS), or locked-in syndrome. The extent of disability has four subcategories: recovery of consciousness, residual cognitive function, psychologic function, and vocational function. Technological advances in imaging, including functional magnetic resonance imaging (MRI) and positron emission tomography (PET), have provided new opportunities for assessing cognition and detecting consciousness for individuals in a prolonged coma.[3]

Brain death (total brain death) occurs when brain damage is so extensive that it can never recover (irreversible) and cannot maintain the body's internal homeostasis. State laws define brain death as irreversible cessation of function of the entire brain, including the brainstem and cerebellum. On postmortem examination, the brain is autolyzing (self-digesting) or already autolyzed. Brain death has occurred when there is no evidence of brain function for an extended period.[4] The abnormality of brain function must result from structural or known metabolic disease and must *not* be caused by a depressant drug, alcohol poisoning, or hypothermia. An isoelectric, or flat, electroencephalogram (EEG) (electrocerebral silence) for 6 to 12 hours in a person who is not hypothermic and has not ingested depressant drugs indicates brain death. The clinical criteria used to determine brain death are noted in Box 17.1. A task force for determination of brain death in children recommended the same criteria as for adults but with a longer observation period.[5,6]

Cerebral death or irreversible coma is death of the cerebral hemispheres exclusive of the brainstem and cerebellum. Brain damage is permanent, and the individual is unable to ever respond behaviorally in any significant way to the environment. The brainstem may continue to maintain internal homeostasis (i.e., body temperature, cardiovascular functions, respirations, and metabolic functions). The survivor of cerebral death may remain in a coma or emerge into a persistent VS or a MCS. In coma, the eyes are usually closed with no eye opening. The person does not follow commands, speak, or have voluntary movement (Table 17.7).

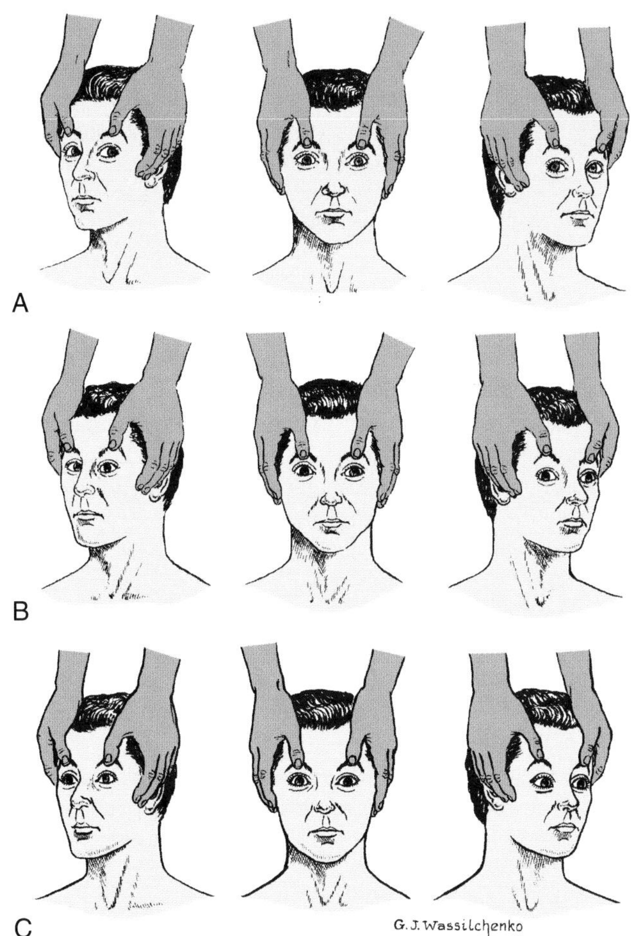

Fig. 17.3 Test for Oculocephalic Reflex Response (Doll's Eyes Phenomenon). **(A)** Normal response—eyes turn together to side opposite from turn of head. **(B)** Abnormal response—eyes do not turn in conjugate manner. **(C)** Absent response—eyes do not turn as head position changes. (A and C, From Rudy EB. *Advanced neurological and neurosurgical nursing*. St. Louis: Mosby; 1984.)

A persistent VS, or unresponsive wakefulness syndrome, is complete unawareness of the self or surrounding environment and complete loss of cognitive function. The individual does not speak any comprehensible words or follow commands.[7] Sleep-wake cycles are present, eyes open spontaneously, and blood pressure and breathing are maintained without support. Brainstem reflexes (pupillary, oculocephalic, chewing, swallowing) are intact but cerebral function is lost. There may be random hand, extremity, or head movements. There is bowel and bladder incontinence. Recovery is unlikely if the state persists for 12 months.

In a MCS, individuals may follow simple commands; manipulate objects; gesture or give yes/no responses; have intelligible speech; and have movements, such as blinking or smiling, that

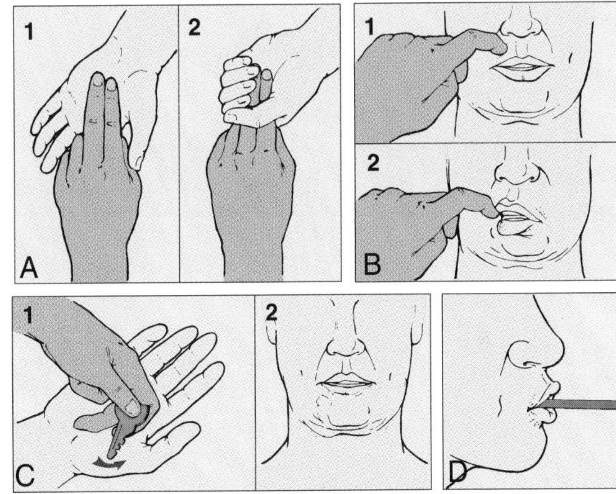

Fig. 17.5 Pathologic Reflexes. **(A)** Primitive reflexes include grasping. (A1) Absent grasp; (A2) Grasp present. **(B)** Reflex sucking (tapping on lips stimulates sucking). (B1) Absent reflex. (B2) Reflex present. **(C)** Palmomental reflex. (C1) Stroking palm causes (C2) twitch of chin muscle. **(D)** Snout reflex (tapping of closed lips at midlines causes pursing of lips). (D1) Absent reflex. (D2) Reflex present.

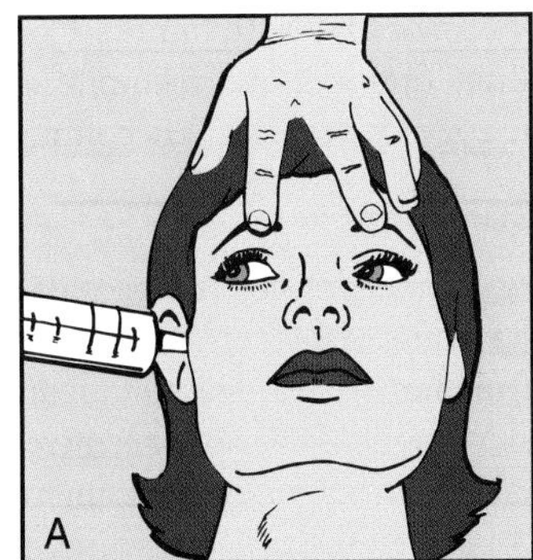

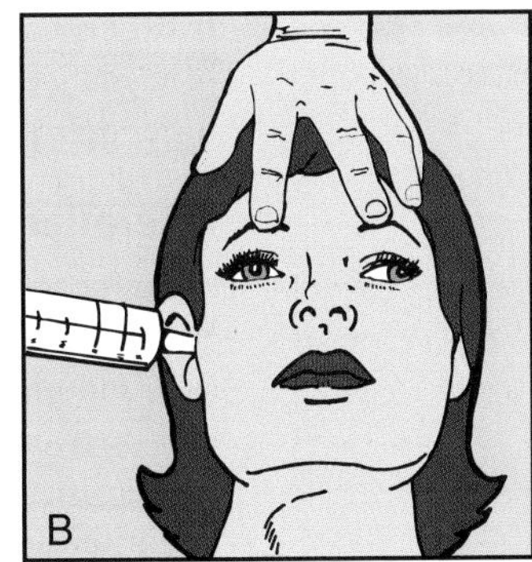

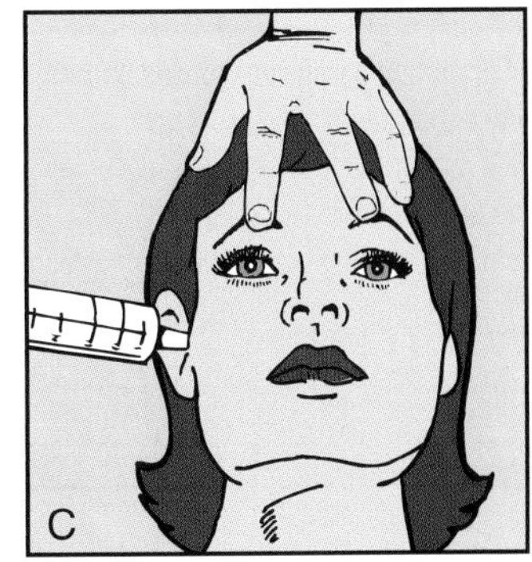

Fig. 17.4 Test for Oculovestibular Reflex (Caloric Ice-Water Test). **(A)** Normal response—conjugate eye movements. **(B)** Abnormal response—dysconjugate or asymmetric eye movements. **(C)** Absent response—no eye movements.

TABLE 17.6 Abnormal Motor Responses With Decreased Responsiveness

Motor Response	Description of Motor Responses	Location of Injury
Decorticate posturing/rigidity: upper extremity flexion, lower extremity extension (see Fig. 17.6)	Slowly developing flexion of the arm, wrist, and fingers with abduction in the upper extremity and extension, internal rotation, and plantar flexion of the lower extremity	Hemispheric damage above midbrain releasing medullary and pontine reticulospinal systems
Decerebrate posturing/rigidity: upper and lower extremity extensor responses (see Fig. 17.)	Opisthotonos (hyperextension of the vertebral column) with clenching of the teeth; extension, abduction, and hyperpronation of the arms; and extension of the lower extremities	Associated with severe damage involving midbrain or upper pons
	In acute brain injury, shivering and hyperpnea may accompany unelicited recurrent decerebrate spasms	Acute brain injury may cause limb extension regardless of location
Extensor responses in the upper extremities accompanied by flexion in the lower extremities		Pons
Flaccid state with little or no motor response to stimuli		Lower pons and upper medulla

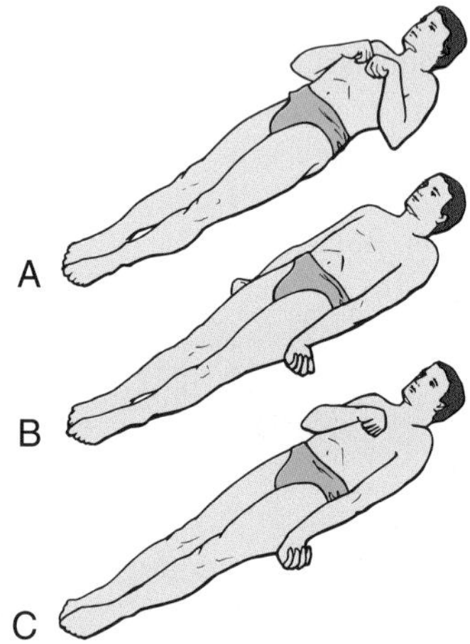

Fig. 17.6 Decorticate and Decerebrate Responses. **(A)** *Decorticate response (flexor posturing):* bilateral flexion of elbows and wrists with shoulder adduction in upper extremities. Extension, internal rotation of lower extremities (lesions above the midbrain). **(B)** *Decerebrate response (extensor posturing):* all four extremities in rigid extension, internal rotation of shoulders with hyperpronation of forearms (midbrain lesions). **(C)** *Decorticate response on right side of body and decerebrate response on left side of body:* the most pronounced response differences are in the upper body. (From Rudy EB. *Advanced neurological and neurosurgical nursing*. St. Louis: Mosby; 1984.)

BOX 17.1 Criteria for Brain Death

1. Completion of all appropriate diagnostic and therapeutic procedures with no possibility of brain function recovery
2. Unresponsive coma (no motor or reflex movements)
3. No spontaneous respiration (apnea)
4. No brainstem functions (ocular responses to head turning or caloric stimulation; dilated, fixed pupils; no gag or corneal reflex [see Figs. 17.3 and 17.4])
5. Isoelectric (flat) EEG (electrocerebral silence)
6. Persistence of these signs for an appropriate observation period

EEG, Electroencephalogram.
Summarized from Wijdicks EF, Varelas PN, Gronseth GS, et al. Evidence-based guideline update: Determining brain death in adults: Report of the Quality Standards Subcommittee of the American Academy of Neurology. *Neurology*, 2010;74(23):1911–1918

occur in a meaningful relationship to the eliciting stimulus and are not attributable to reflexive activity.[8]

With locked-in syndrome (ventral pontine syndrome), there is complete paralysis of voluntary muscles apart from vertical gaze and upper eyelid movement. Content of thought and level of arousal are intact, but the efferent pathways are disrupted (injury at the base of the pons with the reticular formation intact, often caused by basilar artery occlusion).[9] The individual cannot communicate either through speech or through body movement but is fully conscious with intact cognitive function. The upper cranial nerves (I to IV) often are preserved so that the person possesses vertical eye movement and blinking as a means of communication.

Akinetic mutism (AM) is a rare neurobehavioral state characterized by a severe loss of motivation to move or inability to voluntarily initiate goal-directed motor responses (akinetic), including speech (mutism), gestures, and facial expression. Generally, these individuals are alert, orient to external stimuli, and can follow the examiner with their eyes but do not initiate other voluntary activity or movement. This is not attributable to decreased wakefulness, motor weakness, or paralysis but rather a lack of "willfulness" to do so. The neuropathology is different when compared with the VS and locked-in syndrome and involves damage to frontal-subcortical structures involved in the translation of a motivational stimulus to a behavioral response. It may occur with cerebrovascular disease, obstructive hydrocephalus, or be associated with tumors. Combined deficits of vigilance, detection, and working memory accompanied by other deficits of the cognitive systems are common.[10]

Alterations in Awareness

Awareness (content of thought) encompasses all cognitive functions, including awareness of self, environment, affective states (i.e., moods), and memory. Awareness is mediated by all the core networks under the guidance of executive attention networks, including selective attention and memory. Executive attention networks involve abstract reasoning, planning, decision making, judgment, error correction, and self-control. Each attentional function is a network of interconnected brain circuits and not localized to a single brain area.

TABLE 17.7 Comparative Clinical Features of Alterations in Levels of Arousal

Diagnosis	Arousal	Awareness	Communication
Coma	Eyes do not open spontaneously or in response to stimulation	No evidence of perception, communication ability, only reflexes and postural responses	None
Persistent vegetative state	Eyes open spontaneously; no visual tracking; sleep-wake cycle resumes or state of chronic wakefulness; arousal often sluggish	No evidence of cognitive function or purposeful motor activity	None
Akinetic mutism	Eyes open spontaneously; normal sleep-wake cycle; arousal level is normal	Visual tracking present; little or no following of commands	Little or no volitional speech or movement
Minimally conscious state	Eyes open spontaneously; normal to abnormal sleep-wake cycle; arousal level ranges from obtunded to normal	Inconsistent evidence of perception, communication ability, or purposeful motor activity; visual tracking often intact	Inconsistent verbalization and gesturing
Locked-in syndrome	Full arousal; sleep-wake cycle present; quadriplegic	Perceptions and emotions intact	Cannot speak or move muscles except vertical eye movement and blinking

Data from Giacino JT, Ashwal S, Childs N, et al. The minimally conscious state: Definition and diagnostic criteria. *Neurology*, 2002;58(3):349–353; Owen AM. Disorders of consciousness. *Annals of the New York Academy of Sciences*, 2008;1125:225–238.

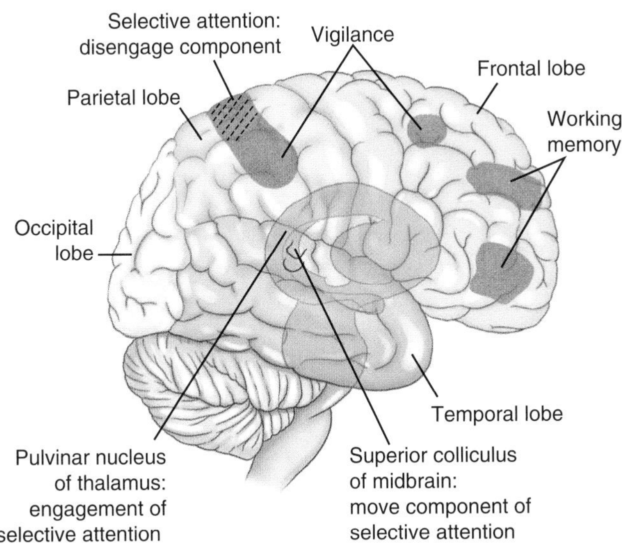

Fig. 17.7 Right cortical, subcortical, and brainstem areas of the brain—mediating cognitive functions. (From Boss BJ, Wilkerson R. Communication: Language and pragmatics. In: Hoeman SP, ed. *Rehabilitation nursing: Prevention, intervention, & outcomes*, 4th ed. St. Louis: Mosby; 2008:508.)

Selective attention (orienting) refers to the ability to select specific information to be processed from available, competing environmental and internal stimuli and to focus on that stimulus (i.e., to concentrate on a specific task without being distracted) to guide behavior. *Selective visual (spatial) attention* is the ability to select objects/events from multiple visual stimuli (location and movement in visual space) and process them to complete a task. *Selective auditory* or *hearing attention* is the ability to select or filter specific sounds and process them to complete a task. Multiple areas of the brain are involved in selective attention, including cortical areas, thalamic nuclei, and the limbic system. Frontal and parietal regions of the right hemisphere contribute to selective attention. The engagement component (identifying the target of attention) is mediated by the pulvinar nucleus of the thalamus and regulates cortical synchrony (Fig. 17.7).[11] The disengagement mechanism (shifting attention to a new target and re-engaging on the new target) is mediated by the right parietal lobe. The motor consequences of attention are mediated by the superior colliculus for visual orienting and spatial attention.[12]

Selective attention deficits can be temporary, permanent, or progressive. Disorders associated with selective attention deficits include seizure activity, parietal lobe contusions, subdural hematomas, stroke, gliomas or metastatic tumor, late Alzheimer dementia, frontotemporal dementia (FTD), and psychotic disorders. Disorders of selective attention related to visual orienting behavior are produced by disease that involves portions of the midbrain. Disease affecting the superior colliculi manifests as a slowness in orienting attention. Parietal lobe disease may produce *unilateral neglect syndrome*, which is failure to report, respond, or orient to visual, auditory, or tactile stimuli that are presented contralateral to a brain lesion, provided this failure is not explained by primary sensory or motor disorders. For example, an individual with neglect following a right hemisphere lesion may fail to recognize a left limb, read from the left side of a book, ignore the food on the left side of the plate, remain unaware of numerals on the left side of a clock, or have an abnormal rightward shift in head and eye position. The person can recognize individual sensory input from the ipsilateral side (the side with the hemispheric lesion) when asked but ignores (i.e., neglects, extinguishes) the sensory input from the contralateral side when stimulated from both sides. This phenomenon is called *extinction*.[13] The entire complex of sensory inattentiveness, loss of recognition of one's own body parts, and extinction, sometimes referred to as *neglect syndrome*, is common after stroke, generally in the right hemisphere.[14]

Memory is the recording, retention, and retrieval of information. Two types of long-term memory exist: declarative and nondeclarative (Fig. 17.8).[168]

Declarative memory (conscious or explicit) involves the learning and remembrance of *episodic memories* (personal history and the where, what, and when of events and experiences) and *semantic memories* (facts and information). Declarative

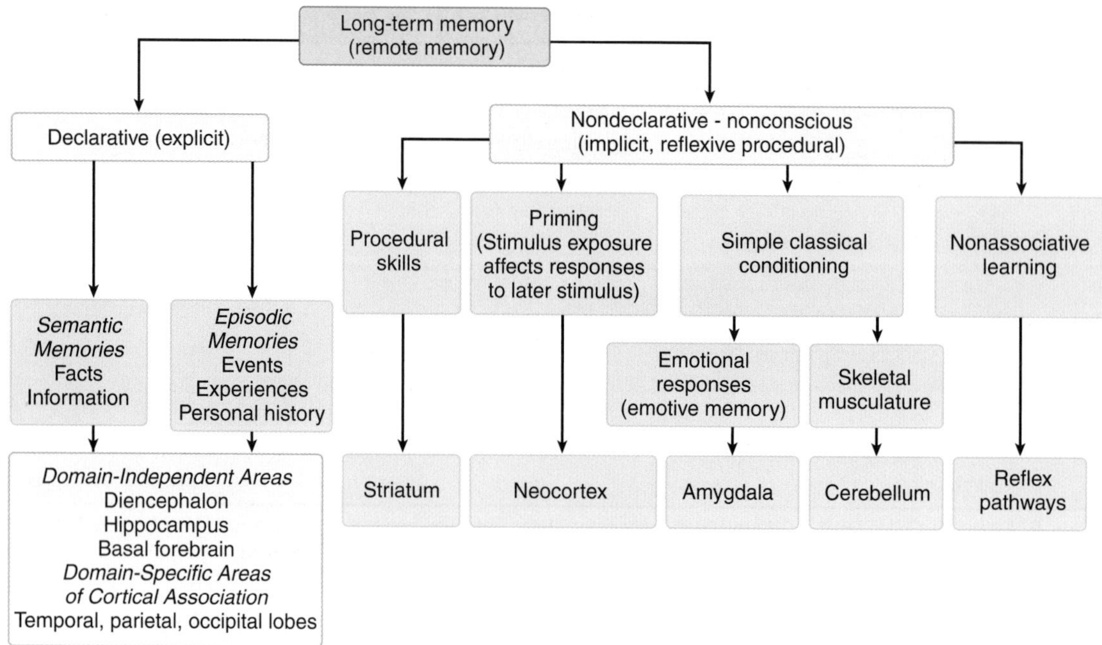

Fig. 17.8 Types of Memory and Associated Brain Systems. (From Miller RD, et al. *Miller's anesthesia*, 7th edition. Philadelphia: Churchill Livingstone; 2010.)

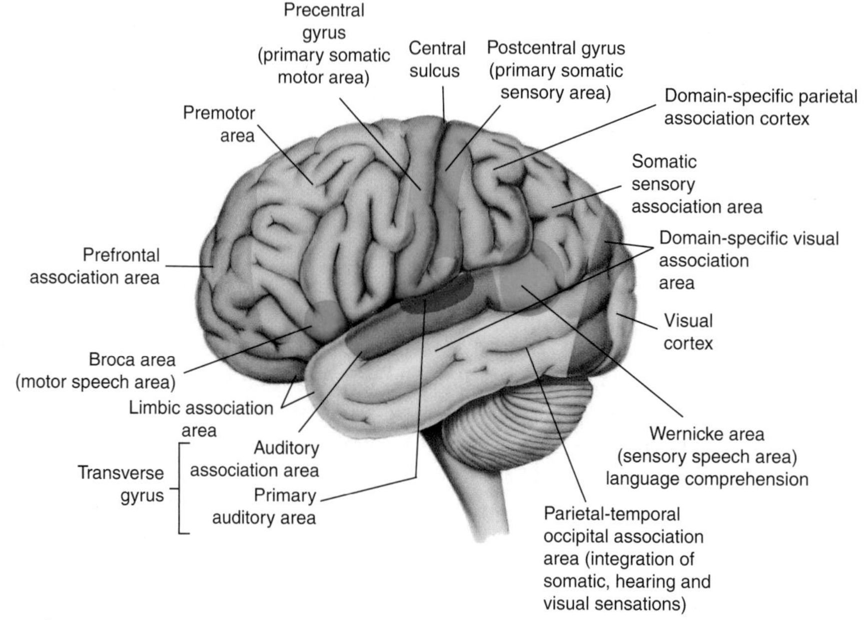

Fig. 17.9 Cortical Areas of the Left (Dominant) Hemisphere. (Adapted from Patton KT, Thibodeau GA. *The human body in health & disease*, 7th edition. St. Louis: Elsevier; 2018.)

memory is mediated by domain-specific cortical areas of the association areas. This includes (1) areas of the temporal, parietal, and occipital lobes (Fig. 17.9), where long-term memories are thought to be stored; and (2) domain-independent areas of the medial temporal lobe (e.g., hippocampus), the diencephalon (thalamic structures and hypothalamus), and the basal forebrain (located ventral to the striatum and produces acetylcholine) (Fig. 17.10), where it is thought distinct, domain-specific features of an experience are related or bound.[168]

Nondeclarative memory (nonconscious), also called *reflexive, procedural, or implicit memory*, is the memory for actions, behaviors (habits), skills, and outcomes.[168] It is not a language memory but a motor memory. Nondeclarative memory involves the construction of the motor pattern so that the action, behavior, or skill becomes increasingly automatic. The striatum of the basal ganglia supports this learning across trials (stimulus-response learning), as well as probabilistic classification learning, which supports outcome prediction. All skills and

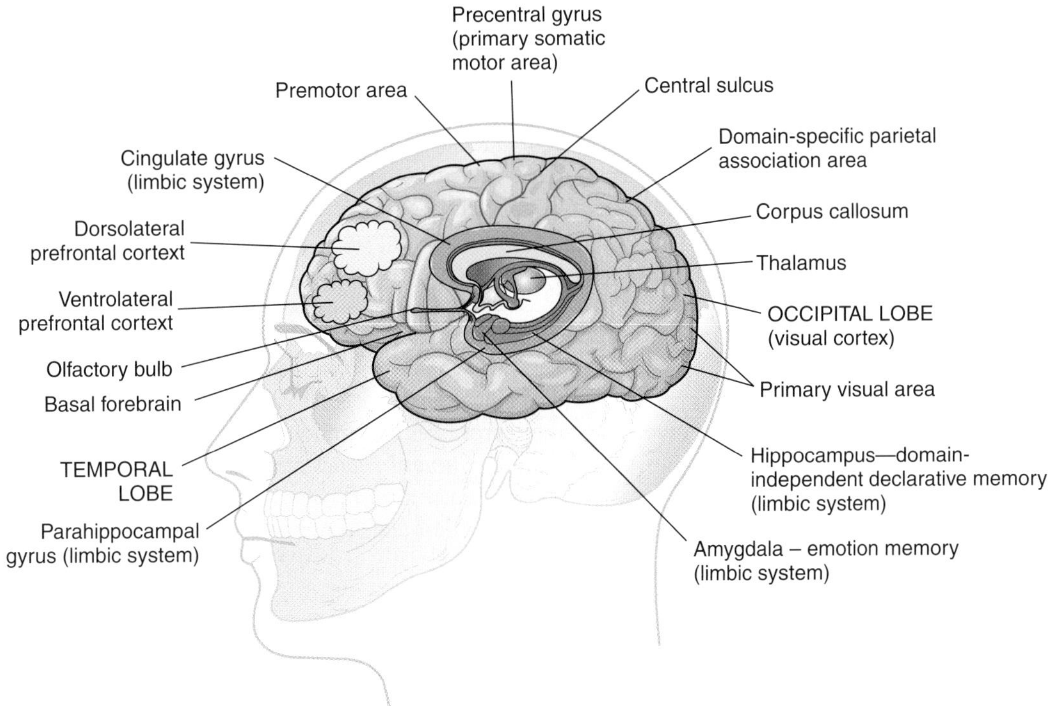

Fig. 17.10 Midline Cortical and Deep Areas of the Cerebral Hemisphere.

habits are stored in this memory network.[15] *Cerebellar memory* is involved in working memory (short term memory), in addition to motor coordination and nonmotor functions of cognition, emotion, and learning.[16] *Emotional memory* is mediated by the amygdala (located on the inner surface of the temporal lobe) (see Fig. 17.10) and other neural networks. The amygdala attaches positive (e.g., pleasure) or negative (e.g., fear) dispositions to stimuli in the absence of conscious recollection of the circumstances of the emotional experience.[17]

Amnesia is the loss of memory and can be mild or severe. Two types of amnesia are retrograde amnesia and anterograde amnesia. The person experiencing retrograde amnesia has difficulty retrieving past personal history memories or past factual memories. In anterograde amnesia, new personal or factual memories cannot be formed, but memories of the distant past are retained and retrieved. These are disorders of domain-independent declarative memory networks, and the hippocampus and other temporal lobe structures often are involved. These memory disorders may be temporary (e.g., after a seizure) or permanent (e.g., after severe head injury or in Alzheimer disease [AD]). There may be only the memory disorder, or the memory disorder may be associated with other cognitive disorders. Global amnesia is a combination of anterograde and retrograde amnesia and involves the hippocampus. *Transient global amnesia* has a sudden onset, lasts less than 24 hours, and occurs in the absence of other neurological signs or symptoms. The causal mechanisms are not clear, but it can be associated with migraine headache, vagal stimulation, and cerebrovascular ischemia.[18] *Permanent global amnesia* is rare and associated with damage to the hippocampus.[19] *Domain-specific declarative memory loss* can manifest as agnosias (agnosias are in the section on Data Processing Deficits).

Image processing is a higher level of memory function and includes the ability to use sensory data and language to form concepts, assign meaning, and make abstractions. Alterations in image processing include an inability to form concepts and generalizations or to reason. Thinking is very concrete. These memory disorders may be temporary (e.g., after a seizure or postconcussive states) or permanent (e.g., after severe head injury, severe stroke, or in AD). There may be only the memory disorder, or the memory disorder may be associated with other cognitive disorders.

The prefrontal areas mediate several cognitive functions, called *executive attention functions* (planning, problem solving, goal setting). The *vigilance system* provides the person with the ability to maintain a sustained state of alertness or concentration for searching and scanning activities and involves the right frontal areas and the locus ceruleus (LC) (located in the rostral pons) (see Fig. 17.7). Through the neurotransmitter norepinephrine from the LC, the speed of the orienting (selective attention) network is increased, and the detection function of the anterior cingulate gyrus (see Fig. 17.10) is decreased.

Detection is the recognition of the object's identity and the realization that the object fulfills a desired goal (e.g., target selection among competing, complex contingencies). There is conscious execution of an instruction, ensuring that the instructions are followed. The anterior cingulate cortex inhibits automatic responses so that a less routine response can be given. The basal ganglia and cingulate, as well as other frontal areas, function in color, motion, and form detection.

The anterior cingulate plus the ventrolateral and dorsolateral prefrontal cortex (see Fig. 17.10) are involved in the representations of information in the absence of a stimulus, such as spatial position of visual events in memory when the event is removed from view. Working memory (short-term or recent memory) gives the person control over information processing (see Fig. 17.7). These temporary storage areas permit the brain to maintain or discard a limited amount of information (e.g., to retrieve instructions, such as strings or patterns of words or colors) and other information (e.g., strings of digits) needed to maintain a current stream of thought, resist distraction, and perform an immediate task. When attention is diverted, long-term memory is required to complete the task.[168]

Isolated (pure) vigilance deficit, detection deficit, and working memory deficits are uncommon and involve focal lesions of the prefrontal cortex. Whether these losses are temporary or permanent depends on the cause and severity of injury.[20,21]

Executive attention deficits include the inability to maintain sustained attention and a working memory deficit. Sustained attention deficit is an inability to plan, set goals, and recognize when an object meets a goal. A working memory deficit is an inability to focus and remember instructions and information needed to guide behavior and complete a single task. Executive attention deficits may be temporary, progressive, or permanent.[22]

Pathophysiology. Very generally, the primary pathophysiologic mechanisms that operate in disorders of awareness are (1) direct destruction because of ischemia and hypoxia or indirect destruction because of compression and (2) the effects of toxins, inflammation, and chemicals, or metabolic derangement, including processes related to dementia. The pathophysiologic processes are summarized in Fig. 17.11.

Clinical Manifestations. Clinical manifestations of selective attention deficits, memory deficits, and executive attention function deficits are presented in Table 17.8.

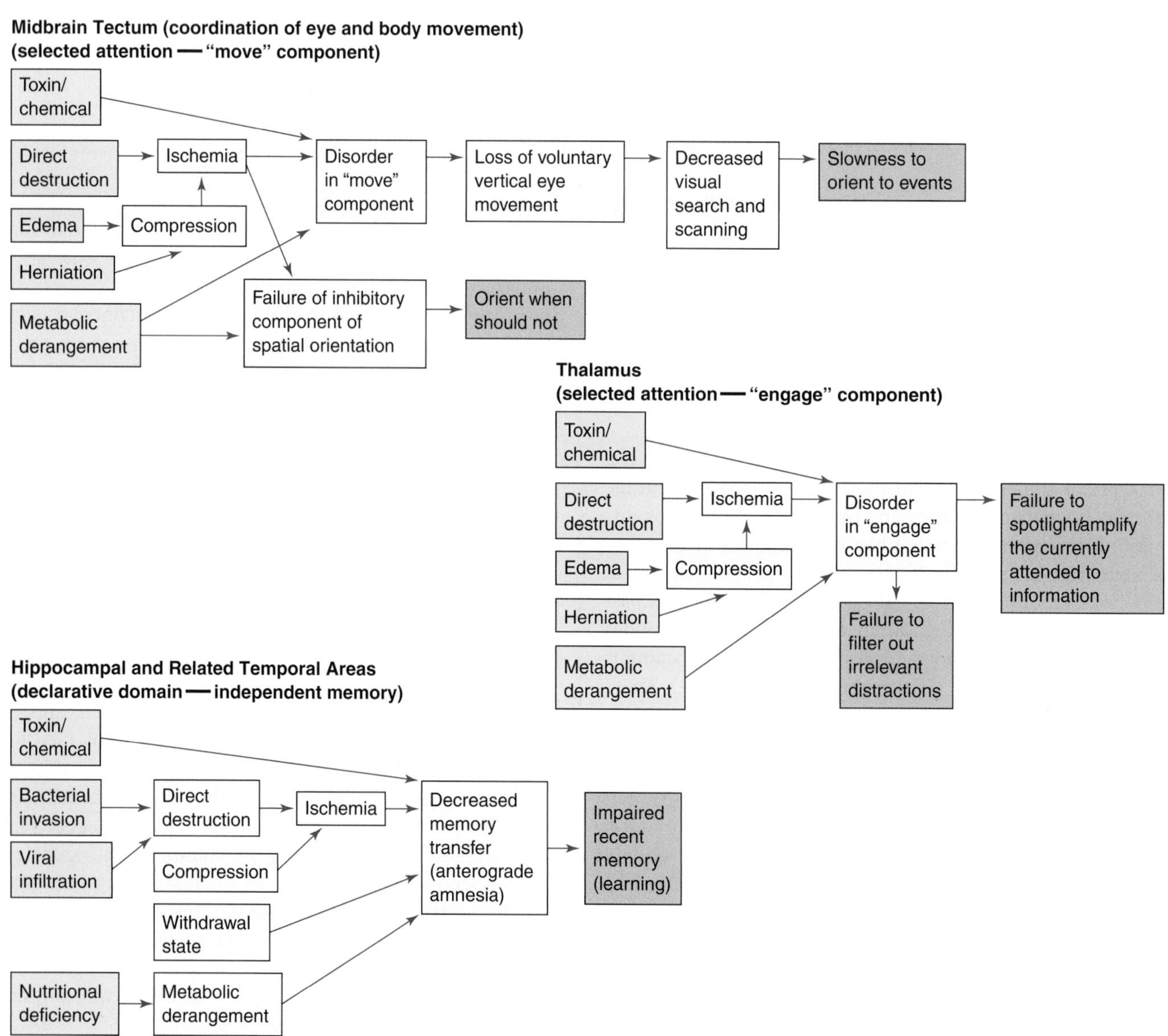

Fig. 17.11 Cognitive Network Deficits. General pathophysiologic mechanisms underlying cognitive network deficits.

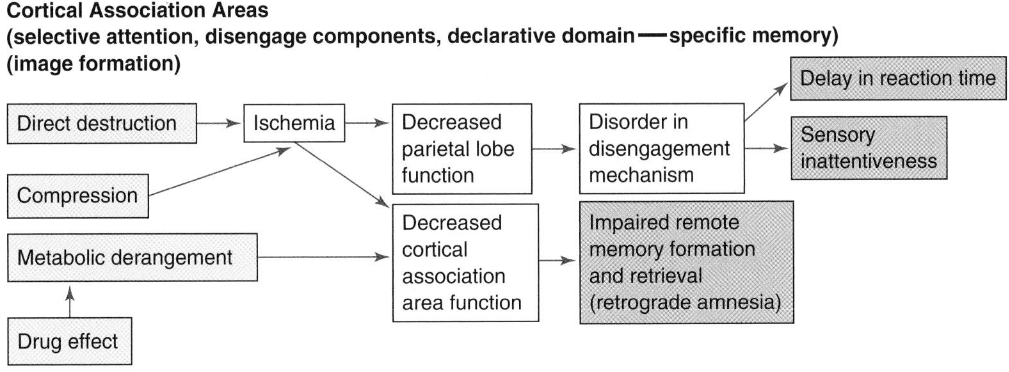

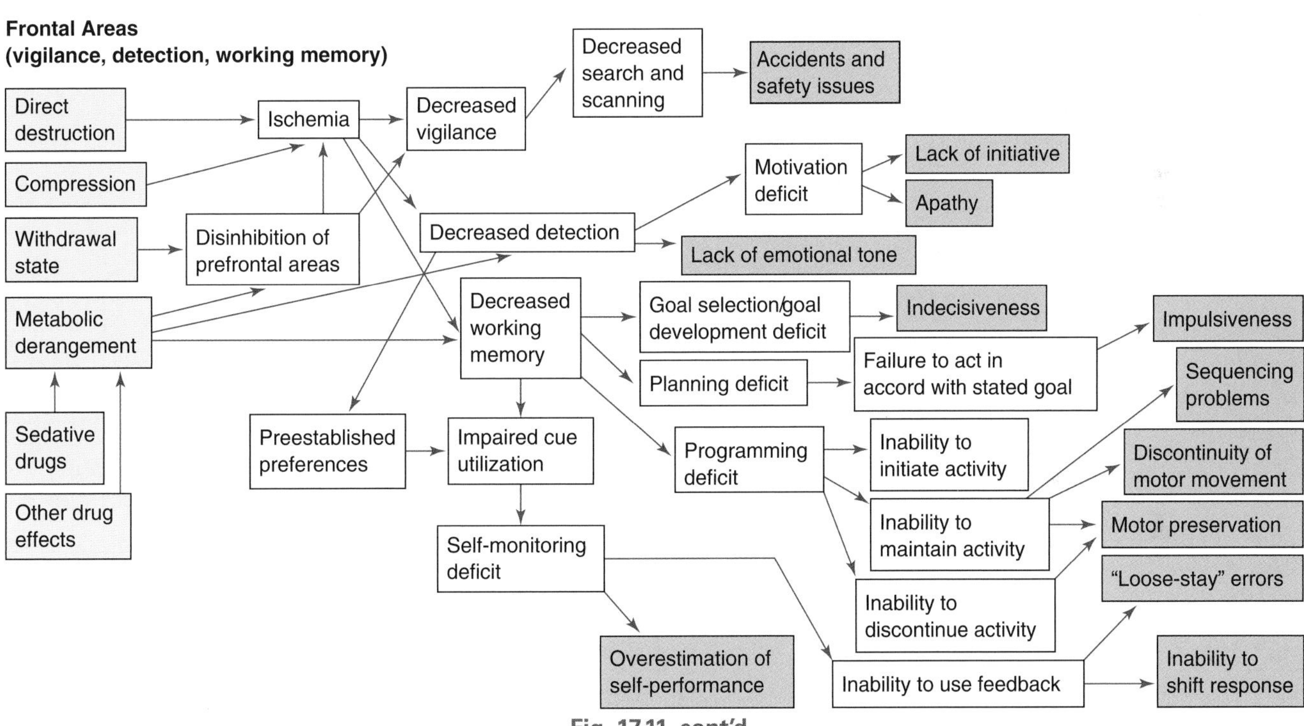

Fig. 17.11, cont'd

Evaluation and Treatment. Immediate medical management is directed at diagnosing the cause and treating reversible factors. Rehabilitative measures for cognitive system deficits generally are either compensatory or restorative in nature and have been greatly facilitated by computer technology and other electronic-assisted devices. Approaches based on behavioral techniques tend to be compensatory, whereas process-oriented approaches are restorative.

Selective attention and executive attention deficits masquerade as other cognitive deficits. Differential diagnosis of other cognitive deficits is blocked, and learning potential is largely obscured by the presence of an attention deficit. Therefore, diagnosis and treatment of attention deficits are fundamental.

Data Processing Deficits

Data processing deficits are problems associated with recognizing and processing sensory information and include agnosia, aphasia, and acute confusional states (ACSs).

Agnosia

Agnosia is a defect of pattern recognition—a failure to recognize the form and nature of objects by one or more of the senses. Agnosia can be tactile, visual, or auditory. For example, an individual may be unable to identify a safety pin by touching it with a hand but able to name it when looking at it. Agnosia may be as minimal as a finger agnosia (failure to identify by name the fingers of one's hand) or more extensive, such as a color agnosia.

Agnosia is produced by damage to the primary sensory area or in the interpretive areas of the cerebral cortex (parietal, temporo-occipital areas—Broca area and Wernicke area) (see Fig. 17.9). The symptoms of agnosia vary according to the location of the damage. The types of agnosia and the associated areas most involved with each are presented in Table 17.9. Although agnosia is commonly associated with cerebrovascular accidents, it may arise from any pathologic process that injures these specific areas of the brain (e.g., encephalitis, tumors, PD, trauma, or toxins).[23]

TABLE 17.8 Clinical Manifestations of Cognitive Network Deficits

Deficit	Clinical Signs	Symptoms
Attention		
Selective attention (orienting)	Inability to focus attention; decreased eye, head, and body movements associated with focusing on the stimuli; decreased search and scanning; faulty orientation to stimuli causing safety problems	Person reports inability to focus attention, failure to perceive objects and other stimuli (history of injuries, falls, and safety problems)
Memory (Long Term, Remote)		
Domain-independent declarative	*Left hemisphere:* disorientation to time, situation, place, name, person (verbal identification); impaired language memory (e.g., names of objects); impaired semantic memory *Right hemisphere:* disorientation to self, person (visual), place (visual); impaired episodic memory (personal history); impaired emotional memory *Either or both hemispheres:* confusion; behavioral change	Person reports disorientation, confusion, "not listening," "not remembering"; reports by others of person being disoriented, not able to remember, not able to learn new information
Domain-specific declarative	*Left hemisphere:* inability to retrieve personal history, past medical history; unaware of recent current events *Right hemisphere:* inability to recognize persons, places, objects, music, etc., from the past	Person reports remote memory problems; others report that person cannot recall formerly known information
Image processing (semantic processing)	Inability to categorize (identify similarities and differences), sort; inability to form concepts; inability to analyze relationships; misinterpretation; inability to interpret proverbs Inability to perform deductive reasoning (convergent reasoning); inability to perform inductive reasoning (divergent reasoning); inability to abstract; concrete reasoning demonstrated; delusions	Reports by others of frequent misinterpretation of data; failure to conceptualize or generalize information Reports by others of predominantly concrete thinking; lack of understanding of everyday situations, healthcare regimens, delusional thinking
Executive Attention Deficits		
Vigilance	Failure to search and scan environment	Person reports accidents, safety issues
Detection	Lack of initiative (anergy); lack of ambition; lack of motivation; flat affect; no awareness of feelings; appears depressed, apathetic, and emotionless; fails to appreciate deficit; disinterested in appearance; lacks concern about childish or crude behavior	Reports by others of laziness or apathy, flat affect or lack of emotional expression, failing to exhibit or be aware of feelings
Mild	Responds to immediate environment but no new ideas; grooming and social graces are lacking	Reports by others of lack of ambition, motivation, or initiative; failure to carry out adult tasks; lack of social graces and new ideas
Severe	Motionless, lack of responding to even internal cues; does not respond to physical needs; does not interact with surroundings Inability to use feedback regarding behavior; failure to recognize omissions and errors in self-care, speech, writing, and arithmetic; impaired cue utilization; overestimation of performance Failure to shift response set; failure to change behavior when conditions change; cue utilization may be impaired	Reports by others of failure to groom or toilet self, unawareness of surroundings and own physical needs Reports by others of not changing behavior when requested; unawareness of limitations; does not recognize and correct errors in dressing, grooming, toileting, eating; fails to recognize speech and arithmetic errors; careless speech Reports by others of failure to use feedback; inability to incorporate feedback (does not correct when feedback is given)
Working memory (recent memory, short-term memory)	Inability to set goals or form goals; indecisiveness Failure to make plans; inability to produce a complete line of reasoning; inability to make up a story; appears impulsive Failure to initiate behavior; failure to maintain behavior; failure to discontinue behavior; slowness to alternate response for the next step; motor perseveration	Reports by others of failure to set goals, indecisiveness Reports by others of failure to plan, impulsiveness, "does not think things through" Reports by others of not knowing where to begin, inability to carry out sequential acts (maintain a behavior), inability to cease a behavior

Aphasia

Aphasia is typically an acquired impairment of comprehension or production of language with impaired written or verbal communication. The terms aphasia and dysphasia are often used interchangeably; the term aphasia is used here.[24] Aphasia results from dysfunction in the left cerebral hemisphere (e.g., Broca area [inferior frontal gyrus] and Wernicke area [superior temporal gyrus]) and the subcortical and cortical connecting networks (see Fig. 15.8B and C). Aphasias are commonly associated with a cerebrovascular accident involving the middle cerebral artery or one of its many branches (see Fig. 15.21). Language disorders, however, may arise from a variety of

TABLE 17.9 Types of Agnosia (Concept Disorders)

Type of Agnosia	Definition	Location of Injury
Tactile agnosia (astereognosis)	Inability to recognize objects by touch	Parietal lobe
Spatial agnosia	Incapacity to find one's way around familiar places; disturbance of perception of space (disorders of [1] topographic [extrapersonal] orientation or [2] topographic and geographic memory [construction])	Parietal lobe
Gerstmann syndrome	Inability to write; loss of ability to do mathematics; inability to identify one's own or another's fingers; inability to make the distinction between the right and left side of the body.	Left angular gyrus (parietal lobe)
Finger agnosia (digital agnosia)	Inability to identify the names of one's fingers	
Right-left confusion	Inability to distinguish right from left	
Agraphia	Inability to write	
Acalculia	Inability to perform mathematic calculations	
Visual agnosia		
Object agnosia	Inability to recognize objects and pictures	Temporo-occipital area
Prosopagnosia	Inability to recognize faces	Temporo-occipital lobe, ventromedial region
Color agnosia	Inability to understand colors as qualities of objects; faulty color concepts and inability to evoke color images in the absence of color blindness; specific types: (1) "hue" problem, (2) color anomia (cannot name color)	Inferior occipital cortex in left hemisphere
Body image agnosias (may be spatial)		
Anosognosia	Ignorance or denial of existence of the disease	Right parietal lobe
Autotopagnosia	Loss of ability to identify the body, in whole or in part, or to recognize relationships among various parts	Right parietal lobe
Word blindness (alexia/dyslexia)	Inability to recognize written symbols	Left parietotemporal region
Auditory agnosia (pure word deafness)	Inability to recognize speech sounds	Superior temporal area
Amusia (music deafness)	Loss of capacity to recognize tones and melodies	Right superior temporal area

injuries and diseases, including vascular, neoplastic, traumatic, degenerative, metabolic, or infectious causes. Most language disorders result from acute processes or a chronic residual deficit of the acute process.

Aphasias have been classified anatomically (e.g., Wernicke or Broca area aphasias) or functionally as disorders of fluency (quality and content of speech). Aphasia associated with the frontal lobe, also known as *Broca or motor aphasia*, involves loss of ability to produce spoken or written language with slow or difficult speech. The speech that is produced is dysfluent and agrammatic. Verbal comprehension is usually present. Aphasia is differentiated from *dysarthria*, in which words cannot be articulated clearly because of cranial nerve damage or muscle impairment. Aphasia that is known as *Wernicke or sensory* involves an inability to understand written or spoken language. Speech is fluent, flowing at a normal rate, but words and phrases have no meaning (fluent dysphasia). Language deficits can be comprehensive; motor language deficits can be accompanied by deficits in comprehension, and comprehension deficits can be accompanied by motor deficits in language. For this reason, it can be misleading to classify aphasia as being expressive or receptive.[25]

Anomic aphasia is a sensory aphasia distinguished by difficulty finding words and naming a person or object. It is the most common symptom of cerebrovascular-related aphasia. Circumlocution, or describing an object as a way of trying to name something, is common in anomic aphasia. Auditory comprehension is present in conductive aphasia, but there is impaired verbatim repetition. Naming also can be impaired. The person recognizes the errors and tries to correct them. Speech is fluent, but words and sounds may be transposed. Damage is typically in the left hemisphere to networks that connect Broca and Wernicke areas. Anomic aphasias can also result from AD and other neurodegenerative diseases. Transcortical aphasias are rare and can be motor, sensory, or mixed. They involve areas of the brain that connect to the language centers. Anomic aphasia resulting from right hemisphere damage is rare as well.

Global aphasia is the most severe aphasia and involves both motor and sensory aphasia. The individual is non-fluent or mute; cannot read or write; and has impaired comprehension, naming, reading, and writing. Global aphasia is usually associated with a cerebrovascular accident involving the middle cerebral artery. Table 17.10 compares types of aphasia, and Table 17.11 illustrates some of the language disturbances. Pure aphasias are rare and are often mixed, making diagnosis difficult. Most types of aphasia improve with speech rehabilitation; however, if the cause is progressive disease (e.g., AD), improvement is not expected. Maintenance and quality of life are typically the treatment goals for progressive disease.

TABLE 17.10 Major Types of Aphasia

Type	Expression	Verbal Comprehension	Repetition	Reading Comprehension	Writing	Location of Lesion	Cause of Lesion
Expressive							
Broca, nonfluent or motor aphasia	Cannot find words, difficulty writing	Relatively intact	Impaired	Variable	Impaired	Left posteroinferior frontal lobe (Broca area)	Occlusion of one or several branches of left middle cerebral artery supplying inferior frontal gyrus
Transcortical motor, nonfluent aphasia	Halting speech	Intact	Intact	Impaired	Impaired	Anterior superior frontal lobe	Occlusion at the border zone between two arterial territories
Receptive							
Wernicke, receptive fluent or sensory aphasia	Meaningless verbal language, inappropriate words or unable to monitor language for correctness so errors are not recognized Intonation, accent, cadence, rhythm, and articulation normal	Impaired; disturbance in understanding all language	Impaired	Impaired	Impaired	Left posterosuperior temporal lobe (Wernicke area)	Occlusion of inferior division of left middle cerebral artery
Conductive aphasia	Difficulty repeating words, phrases spoken to them; naming is impaired	Intact	Severely impaired	Variable	Variable	Inferior and posterior temporal lobe; parietotemporal junction	Occlusion in distributions of left middle cerebral artery
Anomic aphasia	Hesitancy, difficulty recalling names, objects, or numbers	Intact	Impaired	Variable	Intact except for anomia	Left temporoparietal zones; arcuate fasciculus	Diffuse left hemisphere brain disease
Transcortical sensory, fluent aphasia	Repeats words and phrases spoken to them	Poor	Intact	Impaired	Impaired	Posterior temporal lobe	Occlusion at the border zone between two cerebral arterial territories
Other							
Transcortical mixed motor and sensory, nonfluent	Repeats words and phrases spoken to them	Impaired	Intact	Impaired	Impaired	Left cerebral hemisphere; spares the perisylvian cortex	Occlusion at the border zone between two cerebral arterial territories
Global or nonfluent; summation of motor and sensory aphasia	Mute	Impaired	Impaired	Impaired	Impaired	Large areas of the left cortex and subcortical regions	Occlusion of left middle cerebral artery of left internal carotid artery, tumors, other mass lesions, hemorrhage, embolic occlusion of ascending parietal or posterior temporal branch of middle cerebral artery

TABLE 17.11 Examples of Aphasia

Disorder	Example
Wernicke/Fluent/Sensory Aphasia	
Verbal paraphasia	*Question:* What did the car do? *Person:* The car would spit sweetly down the road. (The car sped swiftly down the road.)
Literal paraphasia	*Request:* Say "persistence is essential to success." *Person:* Mesastence is instans to success.
Neologism	*Question:* What do you call this? (Pointing to a plant.) *Person:* It's a logper.
Anomic aphasia (circumlocution example)	*Question:* What do you call this? (Pointing to a plant.) *Person:* Something that grows. *Person:* It's ... Or *Question:* What did you do this morning? *Person:* Reading. *Question:* Were you reading a book or newspaper? *Person:* One of those.
Broca or Motor Aphasia	
Telegraphic style	*Question:* Where is your daughter? *Person:* New Orleans ... home ... Monday.

From Boss BJ. Dysphasia, dyspraxia, and dysarthria: Distinguishing features, Part I. *Journal of Neurosurgical Nursing*, 1984;16(3):151–160.

Acute Confusional States

Delirium (also known as acute confusional states or acute organic brain syndromes) are disorders of awareness, may be transient (acute) or persistent (chronic), and have either a sudden or a gradual onset. Delirium can be considered as a type of ACS, but for this discussion, ACSs, acute organic brain syndrome, and delirium are synonymous. Hospitalized older individuals are at greatest risk for delirium.[26,27]

Pathophysiology. Delirium or ACSs arise from disruption of a widely distributed neural network (see Figs. 17.7 and 17.10) and involve alterations in cognitive function, emotion, perception, and consciousness. Delirium symptoms typically develop over hours to days. The pathogenesis of delirium is not well understood. Many risk factors are associated with delirium; they are summarized in Table 17.12. There does not seem to be a single mechanism to explain the sensory and processing dysfunction of the brain during delirium. The etiological factors leading to delirium appear to be an alteration in neurotransmitter availability and function, as well as a failure in the function of neuronal networks that integrate and process sensory information and motor response. The System Integration Failure Hypothesis (SIFH) connects the pathology of the network dysconnectivity and dysfunction. The hypothesis integrates five pathological precipitants of delirium (neuronal aging, neuroinflammation, oxidative stress, neuroendocrine dysregulation, and circadian dysregulation) and proposes that all these factors are linked and have a role in causing delirium.[28]

Neuronal aging causes increased astrocyte and microglial activity, resulting in brain inflammation and neurodegenerative disease. Proinflammatory cytokines and reactive oxygen species (ROS) are produced, causing chronic inflammation. As part of the inflammatory process, leukocytes cause increased permeability of the blood-brain barrier, increasing edema and promoting neuronal apoptosis. The consequences are a lack of perfusion and brain ischemia.

TABLE 17.12 Risk Factors for Delirium

Premorbid Factors	Precipitating Factors	Hospital Factors
Advanced age Comorbidities—chronic disease Frailty Low educational level Visual/hearing impairment Alcohol/illicit drug use Poor nutrition Depression Dementia History of delirium	*Surgical stress:* cardiovascular, major abdominal, aortic, joint, brain, and emergency surgeries; anesthesia	Pain, infection, immobility, metabolic disorders, prolonged ileus, invasive devices, blood transfusion. Immobility, fall risk Sensory overload or deprivation Prolonged length of stay Lack of family communication
	Severe Medical Illness: Unplanned admission Dehydration Electrolyte imbalance Febrile illness Acute kidney injury Liver dysfunction Thyroid dysfunction Uncontrolled diabetes mellitus Heart failure Seizures Stroke Alcohol/drug withdrawal Failure of non-invasive ventilation	*Treatment Related* Opioids, benzodiazepines, anticholinergics, polypharmacy Sleep deprivation Day-night disorientation Deep sedation Physical restraints Ventilation exceeding 96 h

Data from Wilson JE, Mart MF, Cunningham C, et al. Delirium. *Nature Reviews: Disease Primers*, 2020;6(1):90; Bellelli G, Brathwaite JS, Mazzola P. Delirium: A marker of vulnerability in older people. *Frontiers in Aging Neuroscience*, 2021;13:626127.

Chronic inflammatory processes go on to produce oxidative stress. Oxidative stress causes damage to the brain by the formation of ROS. ROS damages myelin sheaths and increases injury to cerebral tissues. This can lead to cognitive decline and potentially irreversible or persistent delirium. Oxidative stress can also cause a failure in oxidative metabolism, which leads to failure of ionic pumps and thus an alteration in the release of neurotransmitters (e.g., glutamate, dopamine, acetylcholine, serotonin, and gamma-aminobutyric acid).

Physiological stress may result in neuroendocrine dysfunction. Continued stressors can cause high glucocorticoid levels. Chronic sleep deprivation, or circadian rhythm dysregulation, is considered a physiological stressor, which increases proinflammatory cytokines and cortisol levels, leading to cognitive alterations and delirium. With increased and prolonged exposure, glucocorticoids may affect neuronal function and cause neuronal injury and death.

Most metabolic disturbances (e.g., hypoglycemia, thyroid disorders, liver, or kidney disease) that produce delirium interfere with neuronal metabolism or synaptic transmission. Many drugs and toxins also interfere with neurotransmission function at the synapse.

Clinical Manifestations. There are four different types of delirium: hyperactive, hypoactive, mixed, and terminal. Delirium causes deficits in five different areas of brain function: cognitive deficits, attentional deficits, circadian rhythm dysfunction, emotional dysregulation, and psychomotor dysregulation. *Hyperactive delirium* manifests as restlessness, irritability, insomnia, tremulousness, hallucinations, or delusions. In a fully developed delirium state, the individual is completely inattentive, and perceptions are grossly altered, with extensive misperception and misinterpretation. The person appears distressed and often perplexed; conversation is incoherent. Frank tremor and high levels of restless movement are common. Violent behavior may be present. The individual cannot sleep, is flushed, and has dilated pupils, a rapid pulse rate (tachycardia), elevated temperature, and profuse sweating (diaphoresis).

Excited delirium syndrome (ExDS), also known as *agitated delirium*, is a type of hyperactive delirium that can lead to sudden death. Its symptoms include altered mental status, combativeness, aggressiveness, tolerance to significant pain, rapid breathing, sweating, severe agitation, elevated temperature, noncompliance, or poor awareness of direction from police or medical personnel, inability to become fatigued, unusual or superhuman strength, and inappropriate clothing for the current environment. Hypoglycemia, thyroid storm, certain kinds of seizures, cocaine, methamphetamine intoxication, and/or catecholamine-induced fatal arrhythmias are associated with ExDS.[29]

Hypoactive delirium is the most common form of delirium. It is associated with underactivity and may occur in individuals who have fevers or metabolic disorders (e.g., chronic liver or kidney failure), are under the influence of CNS depressants or are postoperative. The individual exhibits decreased mental function, specifically alertness, attention span, accurate perception, interpretation of the environment, and reaction to the environment. Forgetfulness, confusion, and apathy are prominent; speech may be slow, and the individual dozes frequently. Hypoactive delirium can be mistaken for depression or dementia, including AD (Table 17.13). It has the highest rate of mortality, as it is often undiagnosed, and treatment is delayed.[30]

Mixed delirium is a combination of both hyperactive and hypoactive delirium, fluctuating from one to the other. Delirium resolves suddenly or gradually in 2 to 3 days, although delirium states occasionally persist for weeks.

Terminal delirium, also known as *terminal restlessness* or *terminal agitation*, is often seen in individuals during the final stages of dying. Metabolic dysfunction, common at the end of life as organs shut down, and neurotransmitter abnormalities are thought to be a major cause. Onset is often preceded by physical, emotional, or spiritual distress, anxiety, restlessness, and agitation. Hallucinations may also be seen (e.g., talking to someone who is not present). Terminal delirium is not reversible, but symptoms may come and go during the actively dying period. It is important to rule out all other causes of delirium prior to a diagnosis of terminal delirium.[31,32]

TABLE 17.13 Comparison of Delirium and Dementia

Feature	Delirium	Dementia
Age	Usually older	Usually older
Onset	Acute—common during hospitalization	Usually insidious; acute in some cases of strokes/trauma
Associated conditions	Urinary tract infection, thyroid disorders, hypoxia, hypoglycemia, toxicity, fluid-electrolyte imbalance, renal insufficiency, trauma, multiple medications	May have no other conditions Brain trauma
Course	Fluctuating; remits with treatment	Chronic slow decline, usually starts with memory loss
Duration	Hours to weeks	Months to years
Attention	Impaired	Intact early; often impaired late
Sleep-wake cycle	Disrupted	Usually normal or fragmented
Alertness	Impaired	Normal
Orientation	Impaired	Intact early; impaired late
Behavior	Agitated, withdrawn/depressed	Intact early
Speech	Incoherent, rapid/slowed	Word-finding problems
Thoughts	Disorganized, delusions	Impoverished
Perceptions	Hallucinations/illusions	Usually intact early

Adapted from Caplan JP, Rabinowitz T. An approach to the patient with cognitive impairment: Delirium and dementia. *Medical Clinics of North America*, 2010;94(6):1103–1116, ix.

Evaluation and Treatment. An ACS is an acute medical problem. The initial goal is to establish that the individual's confusion arises from delirium and to identify the cause and contributing factors. Hypoactive delirium will need to be differentiated from depression or an underlying dementia. A complete history and physical examination, as well as laboratory tests including an electrocardiogram and bloodwork, urine, cerebral spinal fluid (CSF), and imaging studies are needed. Several assessment scales are available to guide evaluation.[33–35]

Once the cause is established, treatment is directed at addressing the underlying condition. Delirium can be preventable and reversible in some individuals with management of risk factors and early intervention. Assessing pain management, hydration, nutrition, sleep maintenance, hygiene, and toileting may prevent or treat the delirium. Drugs that may be contributing to or causing the condition are discontinued unless the problem is the result of drug withdrawal. Nonpharmacologic measures should be utilized initially to treat the delirium. Measures such as turning the lights low, minimizing noise, playing soothing music, and orientation to surroundings may reduce agitation and anxiety. If the individual is agitated, verbal de-escalation techniques and validating their reality instead of trying to reorient them may help to decrease their agitation and promote a feeling of calmness.

Pharmacologic (i.e., antipsychotics) interventions may be implemented once the underlying cause of delirium has been determined and all reversible causes have been ruled out. Typically, this route is only for individuals who display agitated forms of delirium. Though there is no approved medication for delirium, drugs such as risperidone, olanzapine, quetiapine, and haloperidol can be used with caution. If these pharmacological measures are used, initial drug doses should be low and slowly titrated up.[36] If the individual has terminal delirium with severe refractory agitation, palliative sedation may be considered.[37]

Dementia

Dementia is an acquired deterioration and a progressive failure of many cerebral functions that includes impairment of intellectual processes with decreasing abilities in the areas of orientation, memory, language, judgment, and decision making. Because of declining intellectual ability, the individual may exhibit alterations in behavior, for example, agitation, wandering, and aggression.[38]

Dementias can be classified according to etiologic factors (e.g., genetics, trauma, tumors, vascular disorders, infections) and to associated clinical and laboratory signs. Dementing processes also have been grouped as cortical, subcortical, or both. Box 17.2 lists the potentially reversible and irreversible causes of dementia. AD is the most common cause followed by vascular dementia, then dementia with Lewy bodies (i.e., Parkinsonian dementia [see section on PD]), and FTD. Parkinsonian and Lewy body (intracellular inclusions with high concentrations and abnormal folding of alpha-synuclein and other proteins) dementia can be difficult to diagnose, and AD and vascular disease can appear concurrently. When different types of dementia occur concurrently, it is classified as a mixed dementia.[39] In people younger than 60 years, FTD rivals AD in terms of frequency.[40]

Pathophysiology. Mechanisms leading to dementia include neuron degeneration, compression of brain tissue, atherosclerosis of cerebral vessels, and brain trauma. Genetic predisposition (Table 17.14) is associated with the neurodegenerative diseases, including AD, FTD, HD (see section on HD), and PDs (see section on PD) leading to abnormal protein accumulation within neurons and other vulnerable parts of the brain. CNS infections, including the human immunodeficiency virus (HIV) and prions in Creutzfeldt-Jakob disease (CJD) (see Table 17.14 and Box 17.3), also lead to nerve cell degeneration and brain atrophy. The neuropathology associated with HIV and HIV associated neurocognitive disorder (HAND) is presented in Chapter 18.

Clinical Manifestations. Clinical manifestations of the major dementias are presented in Table 17.15.

BOX 17.2 Causes of Dementia

Potentially Reversible Causes of Dementia

Infection
Encephalitis
Meningitis
Neurosyphilis

Normal Pressure Hydrocephalus

Chronic Subdural Hematoma

Nutritional Deficiencies
Vitamin B_1 (thiamine) deficiency
Vitamin B_{12} (cobalamin) deficiency
Nicotinic acid deficiency (pellagra)

Side Effects of Medications
Anticholinergics
Antihypertensives
Antihistamines

Chronic Intoxications
Alcohol[a]
Sedatives

Metabolic Disorders
Thyroid abnormalities
Addison disease
Cushing disease
Chronic hepatic encephalopathy
Renal failure with uremia

Central Nervous System Disorders
Frontal and temporal lobe tumors
Depression
Hydrocephalus
Cerebral vasculitis
Neurosarcoidosis
Pseudodementia

Irreversible Causes of Dementia

Neurodegenerative Disorders
Alzheimer disease[a]
Dementia with Lewy bodies
Frontotemporal dementia
Pick disease
Huntington disease
Parkinson disease

Vascular Disease
Vascular dementia[a]
Multi-infarct brain lesions
Focal infarct brain lesion
Binswanger disease (a rare diffuse white matter disease caused by arteriosclerosis and thromboembolism affecting the blood vessels that supply the white-matter, basal ganglia, and thalamus)
Amyloid angiopathy

Infection
Creutzfeldt-Jakob disease (CJD)
Postencephalitic dementia
HIV-associated dementia

Evaluation and Treatment. Establishing the cause of dementia may be complicated, and individuals with clinical manifestations of dementia should be evaluated with laboratory and neuropsychologic testing to identify underlying conditions that may be treatable. Controlling associated risk factors such as head injury, diabetes, hypertension, hyperlipidemia, obesity, smoking, air pollution, and exposure to environmental toxins, as well as treating depression and avoiding excessive alcohol intake, may cause less neuronal damage and help to prevent dementia.

Increasing or maintaining cognitive reserve (brain resilience) is an important component of dementia prevention. Studies have found that individuals with untreated hearing loss, lower levels of education, and social isolation have a higher risk of dementia. Treating hearing loss, staying mentally active, and having a social network are also ways to reduce the risk of dementia. Individuals with dementia are known to go through an initial stage called mild cognitive impairment (MCI). MCI causes cognitive changes that can be noticed, but these changes are not serious enough to affect activities of daily living. Though individuals with MCI are at higher risk for dementia, not everyone

TABLE 17.14 The Most Common Molecular Mechanisms and Genes Associated With Degenerative Dementia

Dementia	Molecular Mechanism	Causal Genes (Chromosome)	Susceptibility Genes (Chromosome)	Pathology
Alzheimer disease (familial)	Amyloid beta protein Phosphorylated tau protein	*Early onset: autosomal dominant:* <2% carry these mutations APP (21), *PSEN1 (14), PSEN2* (1) (most mutations are in *PSEN1)*	*Late onset: risk gene apoE4* (19) *CUGBP2* (10p)	Amyloid plaques, neurofibrillary tangles; neuronal and synaptic loss in the brain
Creutzfeldt-Jakob disease (hereditary form)	PrP^{SC} proteins type 1 and 2	Prion (20) (up to 15% of cases carry these dominant mutations)	*PRNP* codon 129 homozygosity for methionine or valine	Tau inclusions, spongiform changes, gliosis
Dementia with Lewy bodies	Alpha-synuclein	Very rare alpha-synuclein (4) (dominant)	Unknown	Alpha-synuclein inclusions (Lewy bodies)
Behavioral variant frontotemporal dementia	Microtubule-associated protein tau (MAPT) Progranulin (PGRN)	Tau exon and intron mutation (17) (about 10% of familial cases) *PGRN* (17) (10% of familial cases)	Tau haplotypes *(H1* and *H2)*	Tau inclusions, Pick bodies, neurofibrillary tangles
Huntington disease (autosomal dominant)	Huntingtin protein (polyglutamine)	*Autosomal dominant:* *HD-IT15* (4) (trinucleotide repeat expansion)	None known	Neuronal degeneration, astrogliosis
Parkinson disease Dementia	*Autosomal dominant:* Alpha-synuclein Leucine-rich repeat kinase 2 *Autosomal recessive:* Parkin (juvenile onset) DJ-1 protein PTEN-induced putative kinase 1	*Autosomal dominant:* *SNCA-PARK1* (4) *LRRK2-PARK8* (12) *Autosomal recessive:* *PARK2* (4) oncogene DJ-1 *(PARK7)* *PINK1 (PARK6)*	*GBA* (glucosidase beta acid) *SNCAIP* (alpha-synuclein interacting protein) *NR4A2* (orphan nuclear receptor) *UCH-L1 (PARK5)* ubiquitin C-terminal hydrolase Other low-risk genes	Neuronal degeneration, alpha-synuclein inclusions (Lewy bodies), gliosis; neuronal degeneration

APP, Amyloid precursor protein; *PRNP,* pr ion protein; *PrP^{SC}*, prion protein scrapie form; *PSEN,* presenilin; *PTEN,* phosphatase and tensin homolog.

BOX 17.3 Creutzfeldt-Jakob Disease

Creutzfeldt-Jakob disease (CJD) is a progressive, fatal, dementing neurologic illness caused by an infectious protein known as a *prion.* Prions are composed of misfolded prion proteins and can self-replicate and cause spongiform encephalopathy (numerous small vacuoles within the grey matter). The incidence is about 1 in 2 million population per year. Most cases are sporadic, and about 10% of cases are associated with mutations in the prion protein gene. Diagnosis is made by clinical evaluation, magnetic resonance imaging, and electroencephalography. Spinal fluid analysis shows the presence of 14-3-3 protein or human prion protein (PrP^{Sc}), and it also may be detected in olfactory epithelium, blood, and/or urine samples. Definitive diagnosis is made at autopsy. There may be years before onset of symptoms, which include rapidly progressive dementia and at least two of the four following features: myoclonus, visual disturbance or cerebellar ataxia, motor signs, and akinetic mutism. The disease is fatal in an average of 8 months from onset of symptoms, and there is no treatment. Tissue from persons with prion disease must not be transplanted. Animal forms of prion disease include scrapie in sheep; chronic wasting disease in deer, elk, and moose; and bovine spongiform encephalopathy (BSE) in cows. BSE can be transmitted to humans by consumption of infected meat and is known as *new variant Creutzfeldt-Jakob disease.*

Data from Uttley L, Carroll C, Wong R, et al. Creutzfeldt-Jakob disease: A systematic review of global incidence, prevalence, infectivity, and incubation. *Lancet Infectious Diseases*, 2020;20(1):e2–e10; Will RG, Ironside JW. Sporadic and infectious human prion diseases. *Cold Spring Harbor Perspectives in Medicine*, 2017;7(1):a024364.

with MCI progresses to dementia.[41–43] Unfortunately, no specific cure exists for most progressive dementias. Therapy is directed at maintaining and maximizing use of the remaining capacities, restoring functions if possible, and accommodating to lost abilities. Educating the family and caregivers on the progressive nature of the disease process and ways to assist the individual physically and mentally is essential.

Alzheimer disease. AD also known as *Alzheimer type dementia (ATD)* is the leading cause of severe cognitive and behavioral dysfunction in older adults. An estimated 6.2 million Americans have AD, and two-thirds of these individuals are women.[44] However, the estimated number of Americans with dementia is thought to be much higher. Individuals with MCI are at a higher risk of developing AD. With better diagnostic tools, such as imaging and biomarkers, individuals with MCI related to AD will be included in the prevalence numbers. The greatest risk factors associated with AD are age and family history. Modifiable risk factors for dementia have been discussed previously (see previous section on Dementia). Fig. 17.12 summarizes the risk factors and pathogenesis of AD.

Pathophysiology. The exact cause of AD is unknown. However, studies are ongoing to classify the genetic variations. Genome-wide association studies have identified numerous single nucleotide variations for late-onset AD. Epigenetic mechanisms are

TABLE 17.15 Clinical Differentiation of the Major Degenerative Dementias

Disease	Mental Status	Neurobehavior	Neurologic Examination
Alzheimer disease	Memory loss, disorientation to place and time, loss of facial recognition	Initially normal; progressive cognitive, language, abstraction, and judgment impairment	Initially normal
Dementia with Lewy body (Lewy body dementia)	Initially affects concentration and attention, then memory or cognition loss but unpredictable levels of ability, attention, or alertness; delirium prone	Visual hallucinations, depression, sleep disorder, delusions, transient loss of consciousness	Parkinsonism Changes in walking or movement may present first
Frontotemporal disorders/ degeneration/ dementia	*PPA variant* Language loss (difficulty with word finding and object knowledge), talking less and speech becoming hesitant, or loss of understanding of language, which may precede memory loss; spares drawing	*Behavioral variant FTD* Apathy, loss of empathy or sympathy, increased inappropriate social conduct, loss of judgment and reasoning, hyperorality, euphoria, depression	Caused by CBD and PSP variants
Huntington disease	Anxiety and depression	Apathy, loss of interest early; impaired cognition, judgment, and memory occur later	Chorea, bradykinesia, dystonia
Vascular dementia	Frontal/executive, cognitive slowing; memory can be intact	Often but not always sudden, usually within 3 months of a stroke; variable; apathy, falls, focal weakness, delusions, anxiety	Usually motor slowing, spasticity; can be normal or may have symptom improvement with stroke recovery

CBD, Corticobasal (cortex and basal ganglia) degeneration; *FTD*, frontotemporal dementia; *PPA*, primary progressive aphasia; *PSP*, progressive supranuclear palsy.

Data from Bott NT, Radke A, Stephens ML, et al. Frontotemporal dementia: Diagnosis, deficits and management. *Neurodegenerative Disease Management*, 2014;4(6):439–454; Darrow MD. A practical approach to dementia in the outpatient primary care setting. *Primary Care*, 2015;42(2):195–204; Hugo J, Ganguli M. Dementia and cognitive impairment: epidemiology, diagnosis, and treatment. *Clinical Geriatric Medicine*, 2014;30(3):421–442; Nordberg A. Dementia in 2014. Towards early diagnosis in Alzheimer disease. *Nature Reviews: Neurology*, 2015;11(2):69–70.

associated with the pathology of AD, but the mechanisms are yet to be determined.

Early-onset AD (EOAD) accounts for 5% to 10% of cases of AD. Early-onset AD can be familial (FAD) or sporadic. The cause of sporadic EOAD is unknown. FAD represents about 10% to 15% of early-onset AD and is an autosomal dominant disease.[45] FAD has been linked to three causal genes with mutations on chromosome 21, although the mechanism of how they cause disease is not clear. The mutations result in the dysregulation of amyloid precursor protein (APP) processing and leads to alterations of folding and concentration of the derived amyloid beta protein. The consequence is the formation of amyloid plaque in the brain. The three gene mutations are:

1. *APP* gene mutation—abnormal APP. Normally APP is a transmembrane protein; processing of APP generates amyloid beta-protein, which is important for synapse formation, synaptic plasticity, increased release of acetylcholine, nicotinic acetylcholine receptor activation, and memory formation. Mutations change the structure and result in accumulation of beta-amyloid.[46,47]
2. *PSEN1* gene mutation (more common and found in more severe disease)—abnormal presenilin 1 protein (more than 200 mutations have been described)—PSEN 1 protein normally functions as a protease to cleave APP, generating amyloid-beta protein of varying lengths. Either loss or gain of function may alter amyloid beta production and accumulation and cause FAD.[48]
3. *PSEN2* gene—abnormal presenilin 2 protein (19 reported mutations)—PSEN2 protein is also a protease that cleaves APP, and mutation leads to alterations in amyloid-beta structure and aggregation.

Apolipoprotein E gene-allele 4 *(APOE4)* on chromosome 19 is also found. APOE4 protein helps to carry cholesterol and other lipids in the bloodstream, and the gene mutation is associated with alterations in lipid metabolism and interference with amyloid-beta protein clearance from the brain. The amyloid-beta protein is processed into neurotoxic fragments found in the plaques in the brain of people with AD.[49] Chromosome 21 is also involved in Down syndrome (Trisomy 21); as such, individuals with Down syndrome have a high incidence of EOAD. Many individuals with Down syndrome develop AD by age 40 and have clinical manifestations of the disease before age 65. EOAD has an atypical clinical presentation (headaches, seizures, hyperreflexia), a faster rate of deterioration, delayed diagnosis, and a higher mortality rate. Traumatic brain injury is a common risk factor for those with EOAD; however, other associated risks, such as diabetes, cerebrovascular disease, and obesity, are not as common.[50]

Sporadic late-onset AD is the most common type of AD and does not have a specific genetic association; however, the cellular pathology is the same as that for gene-associated early- and late-onset AD. The main genetic risk for late-onset AD is related to age and *APO4E*.[51]

Pathologic alterations in the brain in both early- and late-onset AD include accumulation of extracellular neuritic plaques containing a core of abnormally folded beta amyloid proteins, intraneuronal neurofibrillary tangles consisting of hyper-phosphorylated tau proteins, and degeneration of basal forebrain

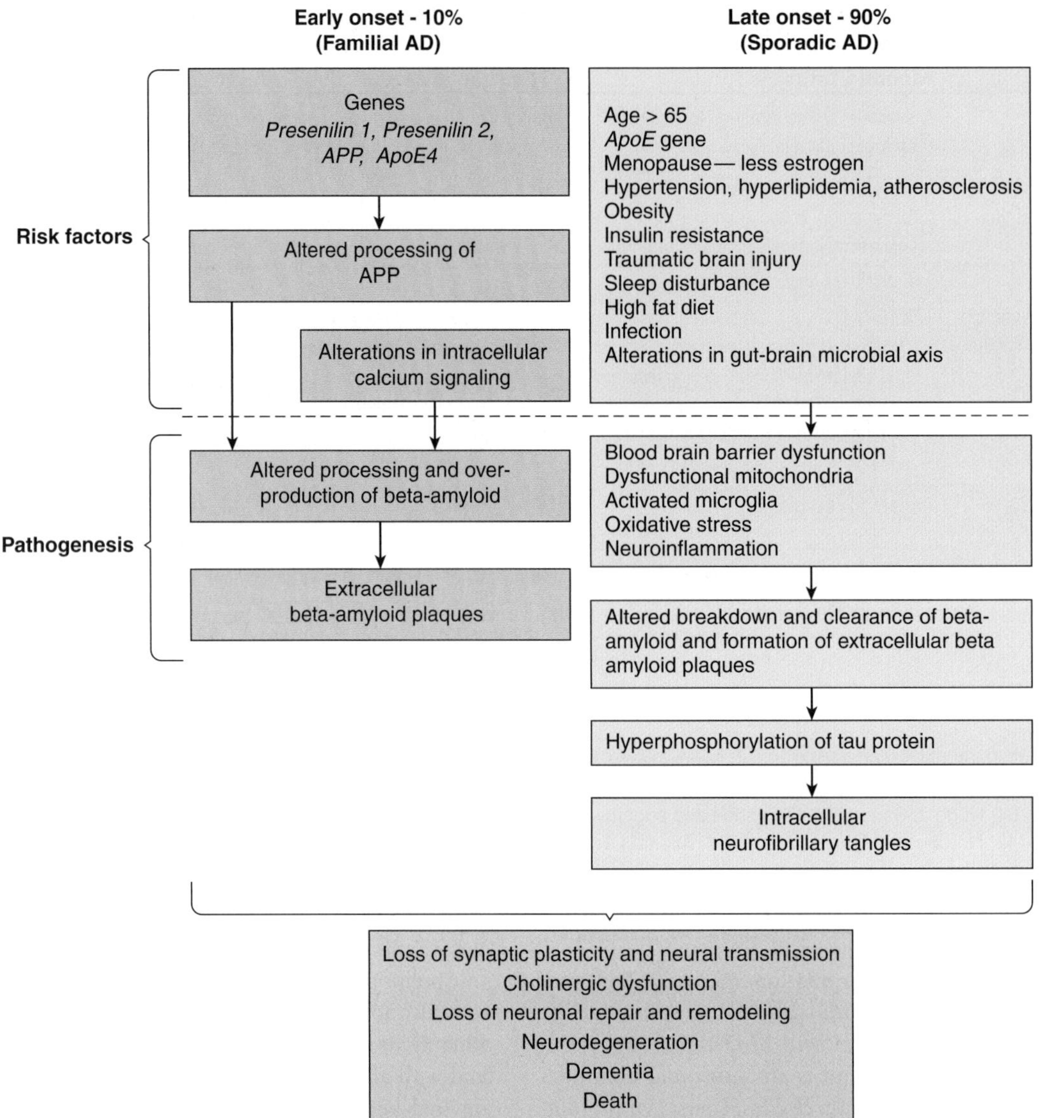

Fig. 17.12 Proposed Risk Factors and Pathogenesis of Alzheimer Disease. *AD*, Alzheimer disease; *ApoE*, apolipoprotein E; *APP*, amyloid precursor protein. (Data from Ganguly U, Kaur U, Chakrabarti SS et al. Oxidative stress, neuroinflammation, and nadph oxidase: Implications in the pathogenesis and treatment of Alzheimer's disease. *Oxidative Medicine and Cellular Longevity*, 2021;2021:7086512; Tini G, Scagliola R, Monacelli F et al. Alzheimer's disease and cardiovascular disease: A particular association. *Cardiology Research and Practice*, 2020;2020:2617970; Knopman DS, Amieva H, Petersen RC et al. Alzheimer disease. *Nature Reviews: Disease Primers*, 2021;7(1):33; Neuner SM, Tcw J, Goate AM. Genetic architecture of Alzheimer's disease. *Neurobiology of Disease*, 2020;143:104976; Edwards Iii GA, Gamez N, Escobedo G Jr, et al. Modifiable risk factors for Alzheimer's disease. *Frontiers in Aging Neuroscience*, 2019;11:146.)

cholinergic neurons with loss of acetylcholine. Failure to process and clear APP results in the accumulation of toxic fragments of amyloid-beta protein that leads to formation of diffuse neuritic plaques, disruption of nerve impulse transmission, and death of neurons. Amyloid-beta protein is also deposited in the smooth muscle of cerebral arteries, causing an amyloid angiopathy and chronic brain hypoperfusion, contributing to neurodegeneration. In some cases, differentiating AD from vascular dementia may be difficult (see next section) (Fig. 17.13).[52] However, the role of amyloid-beta protein in the diagnosis of AD is controversial as individuals without clinical manifestations of dementia have amyloid-beta plaques like individuals with dementia and individuals with other neurodegenerative diseases. There is also a hypothesis that amyloid-beta proteins may play a protective role in herpes-induced AD. There are different forms of amyloid-beta proteins and it is not yet clear which forms are the most pathological and by what mechanism they cause dementia.[53]

The tau protein (a microtubule-binding protein) in neurons becomes hyperphosphorylated, detached from microtubules, and forms an insoluble intracellular filament called a neurofibrillary tangle. Tangles are flame-shaped (Fig. 17.14) and have been implicated in neuronal death by blocking transport of essential nutrients into the neuron. The spread of tau protein in the brain has four different distinct variants associated with AD

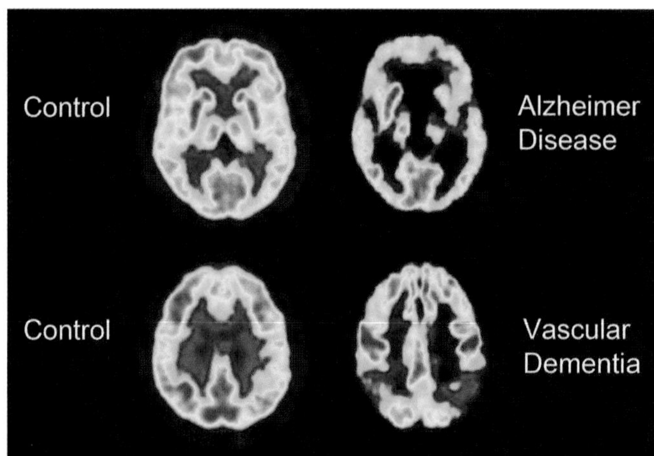

Fig. 17.13 PET scan comparison of Alzheimer disease (AD) and vascular dementia (VD; tracer added to glucose). Clinically, the severity of dementia was comparable. However, the pattern of pathologic changes differentiated these two diseases: in AD there is hypometabolism bilateral in the parieto-temporal cortex and to a lesser degree in the frontal association areas, whereas the primary cortical regions are spared; in VD there are patchy metabolic defects in the frontal lobe, basal ganglia, and thalamus. (From Heiss WD, Zimmermann-Meinzingen S. PET imaging in the differential diagnosis of vascular dementia. *Journal of Neurological Sciences*, 2012:322(1–2):268–273.)

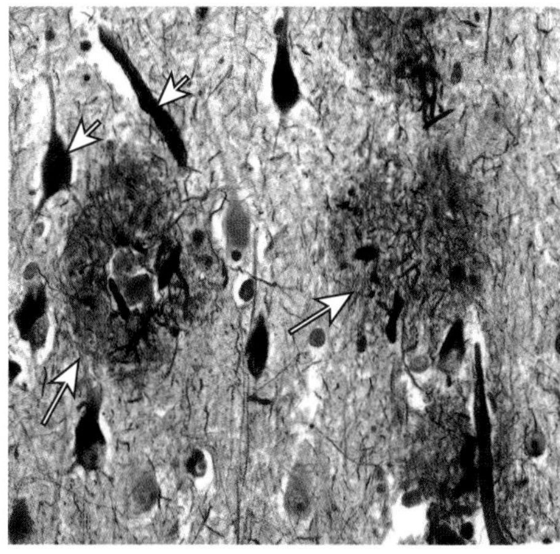

Fig. 17.14 Major Histopathologic Changes in Alzheimer Disease. Amyloid-beta protein deposits (plaques) *(long arrows)* and neurofibrillary tangles *(short arrows)*. (From Kumar V, Abbas AK, Aster J. *Robbins basic pathology*, 9th edition. Philadelphia: Saunders; 2013.)

symptoms (Box 17.4). Identifying tau variants within individuals with AD may lead to a better understanding of prognoses and clinical symptoms. Because different variants may respond differently to treatment, the goal is to have variant-specific interventions to reduce the accumulation of tau protein in the brain.[54]

Neuritic plaques and neurofibrillary tangles are more concentrated in the cerebral cortex and hippocampus (important for memory). The loss of neurons results in brain atrophy with decreases in weight and volume. The sulci widen, and the gyri thin, especially in the frontal and temporal lobes, and the ventricles enlarge to fill the space (Fig. 17.15). Loss of synapses, acetylcholine, and other neurotransmitters contributes to the decline of memory and attention and the loss of other cognitive functions associated with AD.

Aging and injury may result in systemic changes and inflammation that contribute to the development and progression of AD. Misfolded and aggregated amyloid-beta and tau proteins trigger immune responses with activation of microglia and release of cytokines leading to neuroinflammation and oxidative stress, decreased oxygen and glucose transport, molecular changes in vascular smooth muscle and the blood-brain barrier, and mitochondrial defects that alter cell metabolism and processing of proteins that lead to neuronal cell death.[55–57]

BOX 17.4 Variants of Tau Protein Distribution and Symptoms of Alzheimer Disease

Variant one (33%)—affects the temporal lobe and causes memory impairment.

Variant two (18%)—spreads in the cerebral cortex and causes problems with executive function but does not affect memory as much as variant one.

Variant three (30%)—causes the accumulation of tau protein in the visual cortex. Individuals with this variant have difficulties with orientation and distinguishing shapes, distance, location, and movement.

Variant four (19%)—spreads in an asymmetrical fashion in the left side of the brain and affects language abilities.

Data from: Vogel JW, Young AL, Oxtoby NP, et al. Four distinct trajectories of tau deposition identified in Alzheimer's disease. *Nature Medicine*, 2021;27(5):871–881.

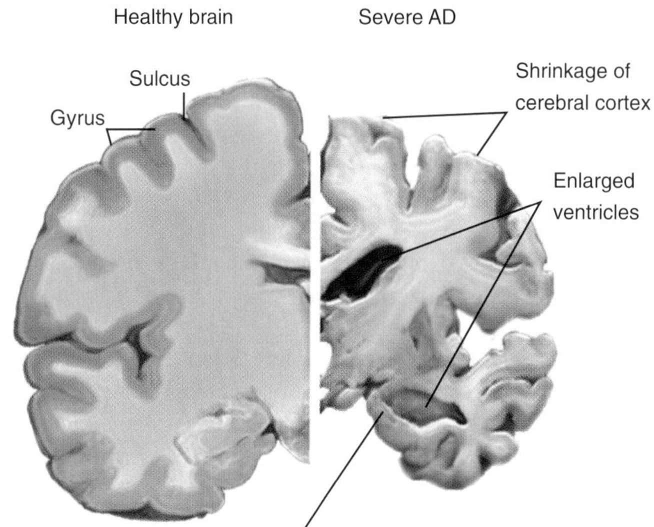

Fig. 17.15 Comparison of Normal and Alzheimer Brain. The brain decreases in volume and weight, the sulci widen, and the gyri thin, especially in the temporal and frontal lobes. The ventricles enlarge to fill the space. *AD*, Alzheimer disease. (From National Institute on Aging Scientific Images, Brain images. Available at https://www.nia.nih.gov/alzheimers/scientific-images.)

Infectious factors have also been associated with increased rates of AD. Herpes simplex virus-1 (HSV-1) and its viral DNA has been found within the amyloid plaques of persons diagnosed with AD. As HSV-1 has an extremely high prevalence rate in all populations, the correlation between AD and HSV-1 is significant. In many individuals, the HSV-1 virus becomes latent within neuronal cells, and antibodies are produced against the virus; however, if an individual is immunocompromised, HSV-1 can become reactivated. This reactivated viral replication can cause inflammation and damage to neuronal cells, leading to AD. Human immunodeficiency viral infection (HIV) has also been associated with AD as the virus causes increased production of amyloid-beta proteins and decreased ability to clear these proteins. The Epstein-Barr virus, varicella zoster virus, spirochetes, and *Chlamydia pneumoniae* have also been linked to neuronal damage and cell death leading to AD.[58,59] In women, estrogen decline during the menopausal transition can promote a systemic inflammatory state contributing to neurodegenerative disease.[60] Sleep deprivation and sleep apnea can influence expression and development of AD.[61,62] Recently, it has been suggested that there is bidirectional neural, hormonal, and immunological signaling along the gut-brain microbial axis. Alterations in the gut microbiome (dysbiosis) have been hypothesized to lead to brain dysfunction and AD. These alterations can be caused by aging, dietary patterns, lifestyle, and infection.[63,64] (See Emerging Science Box: The Oral and Gut Microbiome and Alzheimer Disease.)

Clinical Manifestations. AD has a long preclinical and prodromal course, and pathophysiologic changes can occur decades before the appearance of the clinical dementia syndrome. The disease progresses from mild, short-term memory deficits to total loss of cognition and executive functions. Initial clinical manifestations are insidious and often attributed to forgetfulness, emotions, or other illness. The individual becomes progressively more forgetful over time, particularly in relation to recent events. Memory loss increases as the disorder advances, and the person becomes disoriented, confused, and loses the ability to concentrate. Abstraction, problem solving, and judgment gradually deteriorate with failure in mathematic calculation ability, language, and visuospatial orientation. Dyspraxia may appear.

Mental status changes induce behavioral changes, including irritability, agitation, and restlessness. Mood changes result from the deterioration in cognition. The person may become anxious, depressed, hostile, emotionally labile, and prone to mood swings. Motor changes may occur if the posterior frontal lobes are involved, causing rigidity and flexion posturing. Weight loss can be significant in the later stages of AD due to difficulty swallowing, aspiration, and decreased appetite. Skin breakdown and pressure ulcers are commonly seen in the later stages of AD as well. Great variability in age of onset, intensity and sequence of symptoms, and location and extent of brain abnormalities is common. Stages for the progression of AD are summarized in Table 17.16.

Once an individual reaches end-stage dementia, they are often unable to ambulate or communicate and need assistance with all the activities of daily living. Death typically occurs from AD-related sequelae, such as aspiration pneumonia and sepsis.

Evaluation and Treatment. The clinical diagnosis of AD is made by ruling out other causes and utilizing the criteria that have been developed to assist in making a diagnosis.[65] A definitive diagnosis can only be made at autopsy. The clinical history, including mental status examinations (mini–mental status examination, clock drawing, and geriatric depression scale), cerebrospinal fluid analysis, brain imaging of structure, blood flow and metabolism, and the course of the illness (which may span 5 years or more) is used to assess progression of the disease. Genetic susceptibility tests for *PSEN1, PSEN2*, and *APP* are used to screen for EOAD.[66]

Progress has been made in identifying imaging and biochemical markers to assist with risk assessment, early diagnosis, and evaluation of progression of Alzheimer-type and other neurodegenerative causes of dementia. A CT or MRI may show cortical and asymmetric hippocampal atrophy, both signs of AD. PET imaging can diagnose early-AD by showing accumulations of amyloid and hyperphosphorylated tau proteins. CSF

EMERGING SCIENCE BOX

The Oral and Gut Microbiome and Alzheimer Disease

Chronic periodontitis is thought to be one of the major factors linking the gut microbiome to Alzheimer disease (AD) as individuals with periodontitis have greater memory decline among individuals with mild cognitive impairment. It is thought that toxic substances released by *Porphyromonas gingivalis*, and other gram-negative bacteria associated with periodontal disease, damage the blood-brain barrier, and promote neuroinflammation, amyloid deposition, and Tau protein phosphorylation, contributing to cognitive decline. Bacteria may also enter the bloodstream via dental procedures, including root canals and extractions, cross the damaged blood-brain barrier (BBB) and directly injure nerve tissue. With periodontal disease, large quantities of bacteria are swallowed. These pathogens initiate an inflammatory response within the gut, releasing proinflammatory cytokines. The inflammatory response increases intestinal permeability, releasing pathogens and proinflammatory mediators into the bloodstream. Systemic inflammation then occurs, which causes the BBB to leak, allowing pathogens, inflammatory mediators, and leukocytes to enter the brain, leading to neuroinflammation, neurodegeneration, and cell death. Probiotics, fecal transplantation, antibiotic use. and diet are being explored as ways to restore a healthy intestinal flora and slow down AD progression.

Data from Seaks CE, et al. Infectious hypothesis of Alzheimer disease. *PLoS Pathogens*, 2020;12;16(11):e1008596. https://www.ncbi.nlm.nih.gov/pmc/articles/PMC7660461/; Narengaowa W, et al. The oral-gut-brain AXIS: The influence of microbes in Alzheimer's disease. *Frontiers in Cellular Neurosciences*, 2021;15:633735; De la Fuente M. The role of the microbiota-gut-brain axis in the health and illness condition: A focus on Alzheimer's disease. *Journal of Alzheimers Disease*, 2021. doi: 10.3233/JAD-201587. Epub ahead of print. PMID: 33935086; Shabbir U, et al. Crosstalk between gut and brain in Alzheimer's disease: The role of gut microbiota modulation strategies. *Nutrients*, 2021;13(2):690; Shabbir U, Arshad MS, Sameen A, et al. Crosstalk between gut and brain in Alzheimer's disease: The role of gut microbiota modulation strategies. *Nutrients*, 2021;13(2):690; Ide M, et al. Periodontitis and cognitive decline in Alzheimer's disease. *PLoS One*. 2016;11(3):e0151081.

TABLE 17.16 **Progression of Alzheimer Disease**

Stage	Mild Cognitive Impairment	Early Stage	Middle Stage	Late Stage	End Stage
Cognitive	Mild memory loss, particularly for recent event (episodic memory) and new information (semantic memory)	Measurable short-term memory loss; difficulty planning; disorientation to location	Significant forgetfulness; easy to get lost; may dress inappropriately; may hallucinate	Little cognitive ability; language not clear; personality change; does not recognize family members; wandering; repetitive behavior	No significant cognitive function; loss of word speech
Functional	Possibly depression (vs. apathy); mild anxiety	Mild IADL problems	IADL-dependent; some ADL problems	ADL-dependent; incontinent; difficulty eating	Nonambulatory/ bedbound; unable to eat

ADL, Activities of daily living; *IADL*, instrumental activities of daily living.
Adapted from National Conference of Gerontological Nurse Practitioners and the National Gerontological Nursing Association. *Counseling Points* 2008;1(1):6.

EMERGING SCIENCE BOX

Aducanumab for the Treatment of Alzheimer Disease

In June 2021, the first anti-amyloid medication produced by Biogen and called aducanumab (Aduhelm) was granted Fast Track designation by the Food and Drug Administration (FDA). Aducanumab is a monoclonal antibody that reduces aggregated beta amyloid in the brain and is used specifically for the treatment of Alzheimer disease (AD). It is the first new medication in a decade to be approved for individuals with AD and the only medication that is purported to reverse the damage of beta amyloid and cognitive decline of affected individuals. Results of the drug have been mixed, and the FDA decision to approve it also came with the recommendation to continue Phase III clinical trials to verify the efficacy of this medication. US Food and Drug Administration. FDA news release: FDA Grants Accelerated Approval for Alzheimer's Drug, June 7, 2021. Available at https://www.fda.gov/news-events/press-announcements/fda-grants-accelerated-approval-alzheimers-drug.

Data from Petch J, et al. Aducanumab for Alzheimer's disease: The never-ending story that nurses should know. *Nursing Open*, 2021;8(4):1524–1526; Knopman DS, et al. Failure to demonstrate efficacy of aducanumab: An analysis of the EMERGE and ENGAGE trials as reported by Biogen, December 2019. *Alzheimers Dementia*, 2021;17(4):696–701; Alexander GC, et al. Evaluation of aducanumab for Alzheimer disease: Scientific evidence and regulatory review involving efficacy, safety, and futility. *JAMA*, 2021;325(17):1717–1718; Srivastava S, et al. Alzheimer's disease and its treatment by different approaches: A review. *European Journal of Medicinal Chemistry*, 2021;216:113320.

biomarkers that indicate AD are low amyloid levels and high tau levels. Serum biomarker levels of amyloid protein can also indicate AD.[67] More recently, flotillin-1, a protein found in the plasma membrane of neurons within the amygdala, hippocampus, and isocortex of individuals with AD, has been identified as a promising serum and CSF biomarker. Low levels of flotillin-1 would indicate an AD diagnosis.[68]

AD currently has no cure. Therefore, treatment is directed at using devices to compensate for impaired cognitive function, such as memory aids, maintaining unimpaired cognitive functions, and maintaining or improving the general state of hygiene, nutrition, and health. Though healthy diet and exercise are recommended, randomized clinical trials have not shown that specific diets or supplements have a role in arresting the pathogenesis of dementia. Nonpharmacological interventions, such as providing specialized caregiver-patient dyad care plans and multidisciplinary care (social work, physical therapy, occupational therapy, speech and language therapy, caregiver support groups, and palliative and hospice care), have been effective in maintaining patient-caregiver quality of life.

Unfortunately, there are few pharmacotherapy options available to treat AD, and those available are largely ineffective at slowing the long-term progression of AD. Cholinesterase inhibitors (ChE-Is) are used in mild to moderate AD cases. Preserving acetylcholine in the brain is thought to delay neurofibrillary degeneration and death of neurons.[69] An *N*-methyl-*D*-aspartate (NMDA) receptor antagonist blocks glutamate activity and may provide symptom relief in moderate to severe AD. Excess glutamate is excitotoxic by allowing excess calcium to enter cells, causing cell death. NMDA receptor antagonists are thought to stabilize synaptic transmission and are neuroprotective.[70]

Currently, combination drug trials with disease-modifying and symptomatic therapies are being conducted. Add-on trials are being conducted with new medications that target amyloid proteins, tau proteins, or neuroinflammation while continuing standard treatment with ChE-Is or NMDA receptor antagonists. Combination therapies with symptomatic medications (targeting cognition, agitation, and seizures) include utilization of a 5-HT receptor antagonist, MAO-B inhibitor, anticonvulsants, melatonin, and glutamate modulators.[71] Anti-amyloid drugs targeting amyloid-beta and small molecules that can cross the blood-brain barrier as well as stem cell therapy are under investigation (see Emerging Science Box: Aducanumab for the Treatment of Alzheimer Disease).

Vascular cognitive impairment (vascular dementia). Vascular cognitive impairment (vascular dementia) is a progressive disease and the second most common cause of dementia following AD (10% to 20% of cases). The specific pathogenesis of vascular dementia is not clearly known, but it is caused by reduced brain blood flow.[72] The pathology can be variable, including carotid artery stenosis, intracranial atherosclerotic small vessel disease, multiple ischemic infarcts, and hemorrhages that occur in different parts of the brain. The chronic hypoperfusion is associated with increased blood-brain barrier permeability, neuronal dysfunction and death, loss of white matter, and brain atrophy (see Fig. 17.13). Risk factors are the same as those for cerebrovascular disease: hypercholesterolemia, hypertension, diabetes, coronary artery disease, obesity, older age, physical inactivity, diet, and depression.[73,74]

There is no typical presentation for vascular dementia. The disease can be difficult to differentiate clinically from AD, and the symptoms can be much more variable. The diseases often coexist as a mixed dementia. Loss of executive function, decreased cognitive speed, and loss of information processing often occur first. Brain imaging provides the most definitive diagnosis. Prevention by reducing cardiovascular risk factors is a key strategy in stopping or slowing progression to vascular dementia. Treatment is mainly supportive and consists of multidisciplinary care.[75]

Frontotemporal dementia. FTD, previously known as *Pick disease*, is a form of dementia and a degenerative disease of the frontal lobes. The specific mechanism of pathogenesis is unknown; however, there is a familial association with an age of onset less than 60 years and an estimated lifetime risk of 1 in 742. Most cases involve mutations of genes encoding tau protein, progranulin, and chromosome 9.[76] Three distinct clinical syndromes or variants have been described depending on the site of atrophy: frontal variant affecting behavior (loss of social function), personality progressive nonfluent aphasia, and semantic dementia (loss of meaning of words). Individuals with FTD may have a genetic predisposition to developing ALS or PD. MRI neuroimaging can identify grey matter atrophy and white matter abnormalities within the frontal and temporal lobes. Currently, there are no identified serum or CSF biomarkers or specific disease-modifying treatments. Supportive multidisciplinary care is recommended.[77,78]

ALTERATIONS IN CEREBRAL HEMODYNAMICS

An injured brain reacts with structural, chemical, and pathophysiologic changes. Primary brain injury is the original trauma, and secondary brain injury (see Chapter 18) is a consequence of alterations in cerebral blood flow, intracranial pressure (ICP), oxygen delivery, and inflammation. Several relevant features of cerebral hemodynamics relate to cerebral oxygenation (Box 17.5).

Alterations in cerebral blood flow may be related to three injury states: inadequate cerebral perfusion, normal cerebral perfusion but with an elevated ICP, and excessive cerebral blood volume (CBV—hyperemia). Treatments for these injury states are directed at improving or maintaining cerebral perfusion pressure (CPP) and controlling ICP. Target values for relevant cerebral blood flow parameters are presented in Table 17.17.

BOX 17.5 Cerebral Hemodynamics

Cerebral blood flow (CBF) to the brain is normally maintained at a rate that matches local metabolic needs of the brain. CBF to gray matter is about 3 to 4 times greater than that to white matter because of the increased metabolic activity.

Cerebral perfusion pressure (CPP) (70–90 mm Hg) is the pressure required to perfuse the cells of the brain.

Cerebral blood volume (CBV) is the amount of blood in the intracranial vault at a given time.

Cerebral blood oxygenation is measured by oxygen saturation in the internal jugular vein.

Intracranial pressure (ICP) is normally 1–15 mm Hg, or 60–180 cm H_2O.

TABLE 17.17 Therapeutic Management Goals for Individuals With Altered Cerebral Hemodynamics

Clinical Parameter	Target Value
Central perfusion pressure	>70 mm Hg
Intracranial pressure	<20 mm Hg
Arterial CO_2 pressure ($Paco_2$)	35 mm Hg
Mean arterial pressure	90 mm Hg
Temperature	34°C–36°C (93.2°F–96.8 °F)
Pulmonary capillary wedge pressure	10–15 mm Hg

Increased Intracranial Pressure

ICP normally is 5 to 15 mm Hg, or 60 to 180 mm H_2O. IICP, or intracranial hypertension, is generally defined as ICP greater than 20 to 25 mm Hg and may result from an increase in intracranial content (as occurs with tumor growth), edema, excess CSF, or hemorrhage. It necessitates an equal reduction in volume of the other cranial contents. The most readily displaced content is CSF. If ICP remains high after CSF displacement out of the cranial vault, CBV and blood flow are altered.

There are four progressive stages of IICP. In *stage 1 of intracranial hypertension*, vasoconstriction and external compression of the venous system occur to further decrease the ICP. Thus, during the first stage of IICP, the ICP may not change because of effective compensatory mechanisms, and there may be few symptoms (Fig. 17.16). Small increases in volume, however, cause an increase in pressure, and the pressure may take longer to return to baseline. This can be detected with ICP monitoring.

In *stage 2 of intracranial hypertension*, there is continued expansion of intracranial contents. The resulting IICP may exceed the brain's compensatory capacity to adjust. The pressure begins to compromise neuronal oxygenation, and systemic arterial vasoconstriction occurs to elevate the systemic blood pressure sufficiently to overcome the IICP. Clinical manifestations at this stage are usually subtle and transient, including episodes of confusion, restlessness, drowsiness, and slight pupillary and breathing changes (see Fig. 17.16). Interventions at this stage reduce ICP and promote better clinical outcomes.

In *stage 3 of intracranial hypertension*, the ICP begins to approach arterial pressure, the brain tissues begin to experience hypoxia and hypercapnia, and the individual's condition rapidly

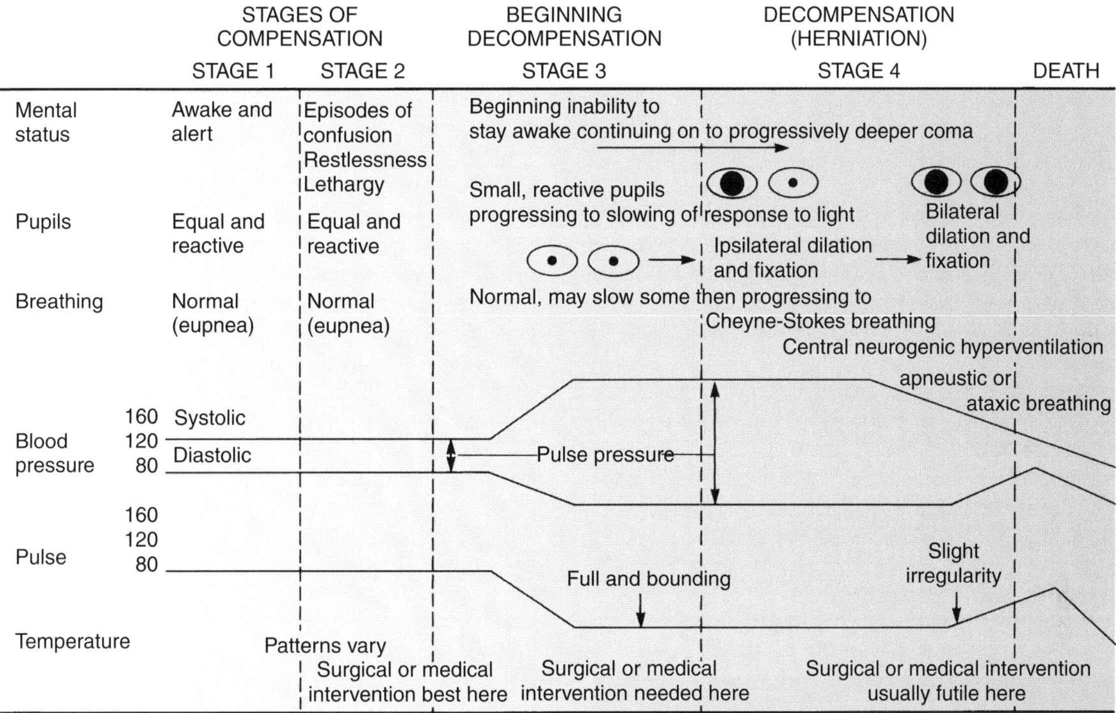

Fig. 17.16 Clinical Correlates of Compensated and Uncompensated Phases of Intracranial Hypertension. (From Beare PG, Myers JL. *Principles and practice of adult health nursing*, 3rd edition. St. Louis: Mosby; 1998.)

deteriorates. Clinical manifestations include decreasing levels of arousal or central neurogenic hyperventilation, widened pulse pressure, bradycardia, and pupils that become small and sluggish (see Fig. 17.16).

Dramatic, sustained rises in ICP are not seen until all compensatory mechanisms have been exhausted. Then, dramatic rises in ICP occur over a very short period. Autoregulation, the compensatory alteration in the diameter of the intracranial blood vessels designed to maintain a constant blood flow during changes in CPP, is lost with progressively IICP. Accumulating carbon dioxide may still cause vasodilation locally, but without autoregulation, this vasodilation causes the hydrostatic (blood) pressure in the vessels to drop and blood volume to increase. The increasing pressure may exceed venous pressure and obstruct venous outflow. The brain volume is thus further enhanced, and ICP continues to rise. Small increases in volume cause dramatic increases in ICP, and the pressure takes much longer to return to baseline. As the ICP begins to approach systemic blood pressure, CPP falls, and cerebral perfusion slows dramatically. The brain tissues experience severe hypoxia, hypercapnia, and acidosis, all of which cause cerebrovascular vasodilation.

In *stage 4 of intracranial hypertension*, brain tissue shifts (herniates) from the compartment of greater pressure to a compartment of lesser pressure. IICP in one compartment of the cranial vault is not evenly distributed throughout the other vault compartments (see Figs. 17.16 and 17.17). With this shift in brain tissue, the herniating brain tissue's blood supply is compromised, causing further ischemia and hypoxia in the herniating tissues. The volume of content within the lower pressure compartment increases, exerting pressure on the brain tissue that normally occupies that compartment and impairing its blood supply. For example, herniation into the brainstem impairs the vital cardiovascular and respiratory regulatory centers and can cause death. Obstructive hydrocephalus, a blockage that prevents the flow of CSF in the brain, may develop. The herniation process markedly and rapidly increases ICP. Mean systolic arterial pressure

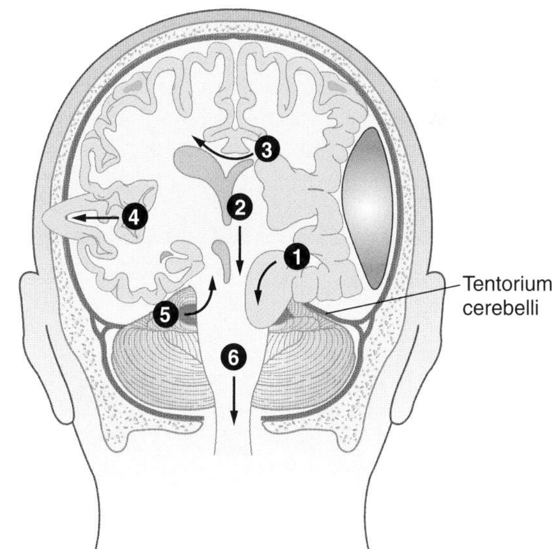

Fig. 17.17 Brain Herniation. Herniations can occur both above and below the tentorium cerebelli. *Supratentorial: 1*, uncal (transtentorial); *2*, central; *3*, cingulate; *4*, transcalvarial (external herniation through an opening in the skull). *Infratentorial: 5*, upward herniation of cerebellum; *6*, cerebellar tonsil moves down through foramen magnum.

BOX 17.6 Brain Herniation Syndromes

Supratentorial Herniation

1. *Uncal herniation.* This occurs when the uncus or hippocampal gyrus, or both, shifts from the middle fossa through the tentorial notch into the posterior fossa, compressing the ipsilateral third cranial nerve, the contralateral third cranial nerve, and the mesencephalon. Uncal herniation generally is caused by an expanding mass in the lateral region of the middle fossa. The classic manifestations of uncal herniation are a decreasing level of consciousness, pupils that become sluggish before fixing and dilating (first the ipsilateral, then the contralateral pupil), Cheyne-Stokes respirations (which later shift to central neurogenic hyperventilation), and the appearance of decorticate and then decerebrate posturing.
2. *Central herniation.* This is the straight downward shift of the diencephalon through the tentorial notch. It may be caused by injuries or masses located around the outer perimeter of the frontal, parietal, or occipital lobes; extracerebral injuries around the central apex (top) of the cranium; bilaterally positioned injuries or masses; and unilateral cingulate gyrus herniation. The individual rapidly becomes unconscious; moves from Cheyne-Stokes respirations to apnea; develops small, reactive pupils and then dilated, fixed pupils; and passes from decortication to decerebration.
3. *Cingulate gyrus herniation.* This occurs when the cingulate gyrus shifts under the falx cerebri. Little is known about its clinical manifestations.
4. *Transcalvarial herniation.* The brain shifts through a skull fracture or a surgical opening in the skull. This type of external herniation may occur during a craniectomy—surgery in which a flap of skull is removed, preventing the piece of skull from being replaced.

Infratentorial Herniation

The most common syndrome is *cerebellar tonsillar herniation.* The cerebellar tonsil shifts down through the foramen magnum because of increased pressure within the posterior fossa. The clinical manifestations are a stiff arched neck, paresthesias in the shoulder area, decreased consciousness, respiratory abnormalities, and pulse rate variations. Occasionally the force produces an *upward transtentorial* herniation of a cerebellar tonsil or the lower brainstem. There is increased intracranial pressure with compression of the ascending arousal system and loss of consciousness. If the cerebral aqueduct is compressed, there can be obstructive hydrocephalus. Cerebellar ischemia may occur from compression of the superior cerebellar artery (see Fig. 17.17).

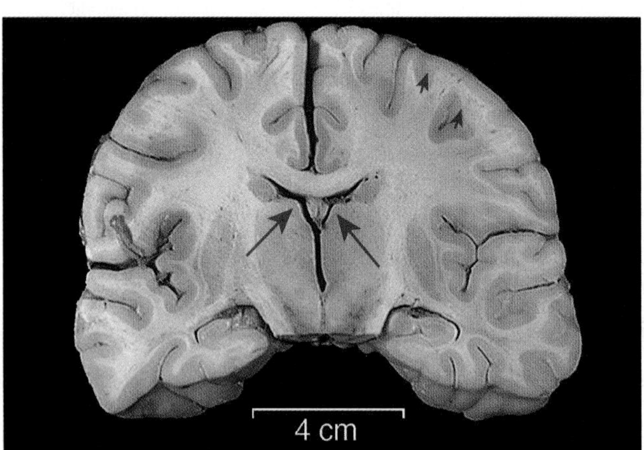

Fig. 17.18 Brain Edema. This coronal section of cerebrum demonstrates marked compression in the lateral ventricles *(long arrows)* and flattening of gyri *(short arrows)* from extensive bilateral cerebral edema. Edema increases intracranial pressure, leading to herniation. (From Klatt EC. *Robbins and Cotran atlas of pathology*, 2nd edition. Philadelphia: Saunders; 2010.)

soon equals ICP, and cerebral blood flow ceases at this point. The types of herniation syndromes are outlined in Box 17.6.

Cerebral Edema

Cerebral edema is an increase in the fluid content of brain tissue (Fig. 17.18). The result is increased extracellular or intracellular tissue volume. It occurs after brain insult from trauma, inflammation, infection, toxicity, hemorrhage, tumor, ischemia, infarction, or hypoxia. The harmful effects of cerebral edema are caused by the distortion of blood vessels, the displacement of brain tissues, IICP, and the eventual herniation of brain tissue to a different brain compartment.

There are three types of cerebral edema: (1) vasogenic edema, (2) cytotoxic (metabolic) edema, and (3) interstitial edema. Vasogenic edema is clinically the most common form. It is caused by the increased permeability of the capillaries (inflammatory response) that form the blood-brain barrier. Consequently, plasma proteins leak into the extracellular spaces, drawing water to them, and increasing the water content of brain parenchyma. Vasogenic edema begins in the area of injury and spreads with fluid accumulating in the white matter of the ipsilateral side because the parallel myelinated fibers separate more easily. Edema promotes formation of more edema because of ischemia from the IICP.

Clinical manifestations of vasogenic edema include focal neurologic deficits, disturbances of consciousness, and a severe increase in ICP. Vasogenic edema resolves by slow diffusion of fluid back into the blood stream.

In cytotoxic (metabolic) edema, toxic factors directly affect the cellular elements of the brain parenchyma (neuronal, glial, and endothelial cells), causing failure of the active transport systems. The most common cause is ischemia/hypoxia. The blood-brain barrier is not disrupted. The cells lose their potassium and gain larger amounts of sodium because of failure of cell membrane ion pumps. Water follows by osmosis into the cell so that the cells swell (intracellular edema). Cytotoxic edema occurs principally in the gray matter and may lead to increased vasogenic edema because of the loss of endothelial tight junctions.

Interstitial edema is seen most often with noncommunicating or obstructive hydrocephalus (see following section and Chapter 20). The edema is caused by increased CSF volume and transependymal movement of CSF from the ventricles into the extracellular spaces of the brain tissues. The brain fluid volume thus is increased predominantly around the ventricles. The hydrostatic pressure within the white matter increases, and the size of the white matter is reduced because of the rapid disappearance of myelin lipids.

Treatment of cerebral edema is directed at decreasing IICP. Treatment can include the use of oxygen, osmotherapy (e.g., mannitol), diuretics, the placement of a CSF drain tube, and maintenance of systemic blood pressure with fluid management.

Steroids (dexamethasone) may be used to treat edema associated with brain tumors. Work is in progress to identify drug treatments that prevent cerebral edema before perfusion is compromised.[79]

Hydrocephalus

The term hydrocephalus refers to various conditions characterized by an excess of fluid within the cerebral ventricles, subarachnoid space, or both (see Fig. 20.8). Hydrocephalus occurs because of interference with CSF flow caused by increased fluid production, obstruction within the ventricular system, or defective reabsorption of the fluid. A tumor of the choroid plexus may, in rare instances, cause overproduction of CSF (Fig. 17.19). Hydrocephalus may develop from infancy through adulthood.

Types of Hydrocephalus

Noncommunicating hydrocephalus (obstructive) *(internal or intraventricular hydrocephalus)* is caused by obstruction within the ventricular system and occurs more often in children (see Chapter 20). Impaired absorption of CSF from the subarachnoid space occurs when an obstructive process disrupts the flow of CSF through the subarachnoid space. The fluid is prevented from reaching the convex portion of the cerebrum where the

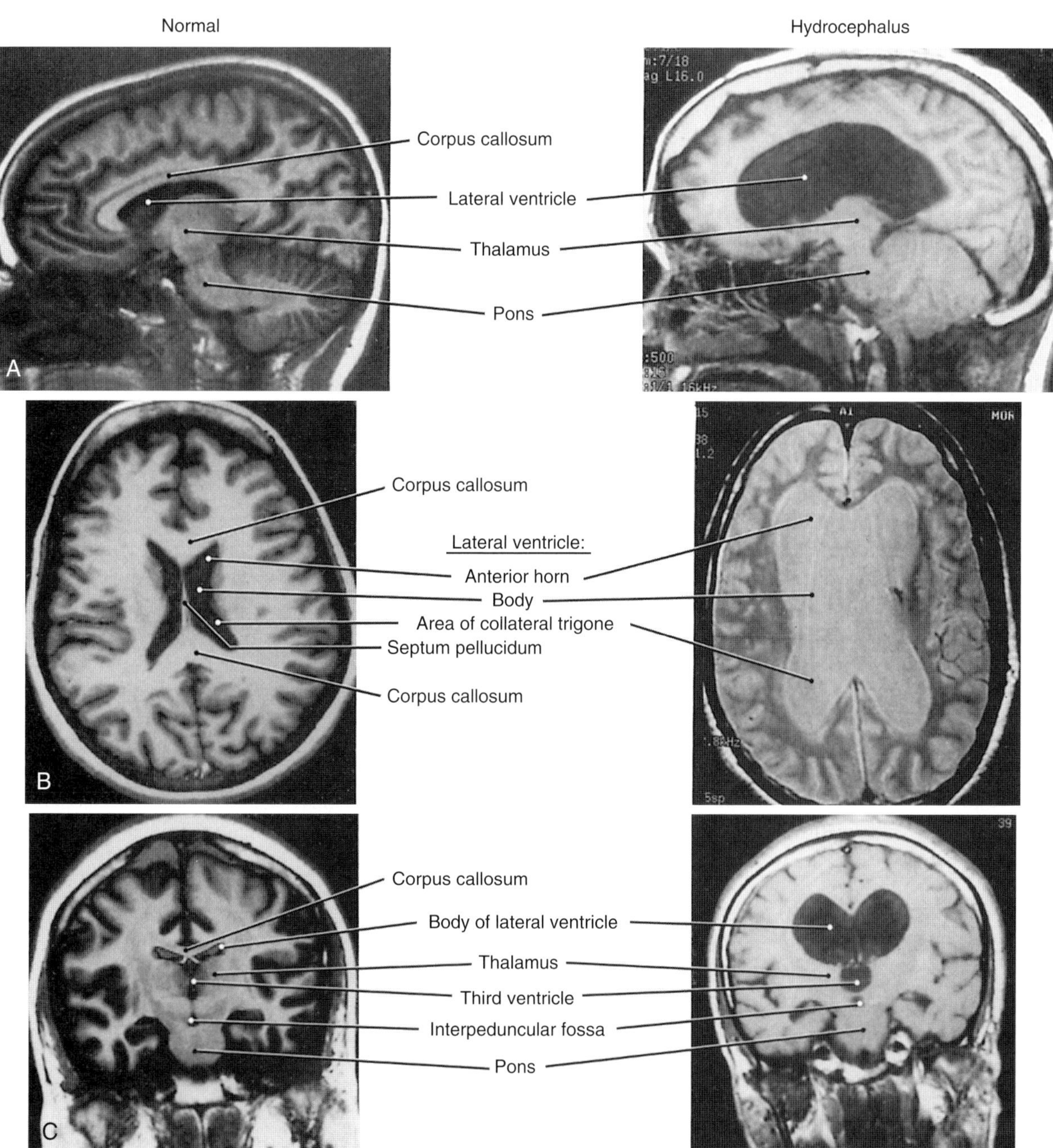

Fig. 17.19 Comparison of Normal and Hydrocephalic Brains. (A) Sagittal; **(B)** axial; and **(C)** coronal planes as seen in magnetic resonance imaging (MRI). (From Haines DE, ed. *Fundamental neuroscience for basic and clinical applications*, 4th edition. Philadelphia: Saunders; 2013.)

arachnoid granulations are located. There is dilation of the ventricular system proximal to the obstruction.

Communicating hydrocephalus (nonobstructive) *(extraventricular)* results from impaired reabsorption of CSF in the absence of obstruction between the ventricles and subarachnoid space. The most common causes of communicating hydrocephalus are subarachnoid hemorrhage, developmental malformation, head injury, neoplasm, inflammation (e.g., meningitis), scar tissue formation, high venous pressure in the sagittal sinus, and increased CSF secretion by the choroid plexus. It occurs more commonly in adults.

Normal-pressure hydrocephalus (NPH) is the dilation of the ventricles without increased pressure. It is a slowly developing form of communicating hydrocephalus that is often idiopathic and occurs mostly after age 65. Age-related impairment of meningeal lymphatic CSF drainage and glymphatic fluid exchange between CSF and interstitial fluid may contribute to the pathogenesis of idiopathic NPH.[80] The ventricles are enlarged, and the CSF pressure is minimally elevated. This form of hydrocephalus can also occur secondarily as a complication of head injury, subarachnoid hemorrhage, or can be associated with a benign external hydrocephalus (enlarged frontal subarachnoid spaces) in infancy.[81] Acute hydrocephalus may develop within several hours in persons who have sustained head injuries and is also known as traumatic hydrocephalus (see Subarachnoid Hemorrhage in Chapter 18). Acute hydrocephalus contributes significantly to IICP.

Pathophysiology. The obstruction of CSF flow associated with hydrocephalus produces increased pressure and dilation of the ventricles proximal to the obstruction. The increased pressure and dilation cause atrophy of the cerebral cortex and degeneration of the white matter tracts. Selective preservation of gray matter occurs. When excess CSF fills a defect caused by atrophy, a degenerative disorder, or a surgical excision, this fluid is not under pressure; therefore, atrophy and degenerative changes are not induced. This is known as hydrocephalus ex vacuo.

Clinical Manifestations. Most cases of hydrocephalus develop gradually and insidiously over time. Symptoms can include dizziness, headaches, nausea, vomiting, gait disturbances, change in personality, and seizures. Acute hydrocephalus presents with signs of rapidly developing IICP. The person rapidly deteriorates into a deep coma if not promptly treated. NPH has a long-term presentation and develops slowly over time. A triad of symptoms, including declining memory with loss of cognitive function; unsteady, broad-based gait; and urinary urgency and incontinence from detrusor overactivity, are common and make diagnosis difficult to differentiate from other causes of dementia. Additional clinical manifestations are apathy, inattentiveness, and indifference to self, family, and the environment.[82]

Evaluation and Treatment. A diagnosis of hydrocephalus is made based on clinical history, physical examination, CT scan, MRI, and evaluation of CSF dynamic parameters. A radioisotopic cisternogram may be performed to diagnose NPH. Hydrocephalus can be treated by surgery to resect cysts, neoplasms, or hematomas or by ventricular bypass into the normal intracranial channel or into an extracranial compartment using a shunting procedure, one of the three most common neurosurgical procedures. Excision or coagulation of the choroid plexus is occasionally needed when a papilloma is present. In NPH, reduction in CSF is achieved through diuresis or placement of a ventriculoperitoneal shunt.[83]

ALTERATIONS IN NEUROMOTOR FUNCTION

Movements are complex patterns of activity controlled by the cerebral cortex, upper motor neurons of the pyramidal system, lower motor neurons (LMNs) (including the cranial and spinal nerves and gamma motor neurons) originating in the spinal cord and terminating at the myoneural junction (see section on Neuromuscular Junction), and the extrapyramidal system (EPS) (basal ganglia, thalamus, reticular formation, and cerebellum). Dysfunction in any of these areas can cause motor dysfunction. Alterations in motor function are associated with changes in muscle tone, muscle movement, and complex motor performance. Some types of diseases and disorders have concurrent alterations in cognitive, sensory, and autonomic nervous system function.

Upper and Lower Motor Neuron Syndromes

Upper Motor Neuron Syndromes

Upper motor neurons are nerves that travel in the pyramidal tract, divide into the corticobulbar and corticospinal tracts, and synapse on LMNs in the brainstem (cranial nerves) or lateral and anterior spinal cord (peripheral nerves). They carry the signals for voluntary motor movement. Upper motor neuron syndromes are the result of injury to pyramidal pathways that descend from the motor cortex (Figs. 17.20, 17.21, and 15.15). Upper motor neuron injury may be in the cerebral cortex, subcortical white matter, internal capsule, brainstem, or spinal cord but above the anterior horn cell. Injury may be caused by trauma, stroke, tumor, or infection (see Chapter 18). The injury causes the upper motor neuron signs and symptoms that are summarized in Table 17.18.

Upper motor neuron paresis is partial paralysis with incomplete loss of muscle power, whereas paralysis is complete loss of motor function. Different terms are used to describe the location of paralysis (Box 17.7). Upper motor neuron injury causes clinical manifestations that reflect muscle overactivity (spasticity and clonus) and loss of descending inhibitory control on LMNs. There is great variation in symptomology, depending on extent of injury, the suddenness of onset, and the age of the individual.

If the pyramidal system is interrupted above the level of the pons, the hand and arm muscles are significantly affected. Paralysis rarely involves all the muscles on one side of the body even when the hemiplegia results from complete damage to the internal capsule. Bilateral movements, such as those of the eye, jaw, and larynx, are affected only slightly, if at all. The antigravity muscles of the legs are predominately influenced. Because of their bilateral control, trunk muscles are much less affected. Spasticity is common, although rigidity occasionally occurs. Most often, passive range of motion causes the "clasp-knife" phenomenon or reflex (increased tone/resistance when rapidly flexing a limb joint with sudden relaxation) by activating stretch

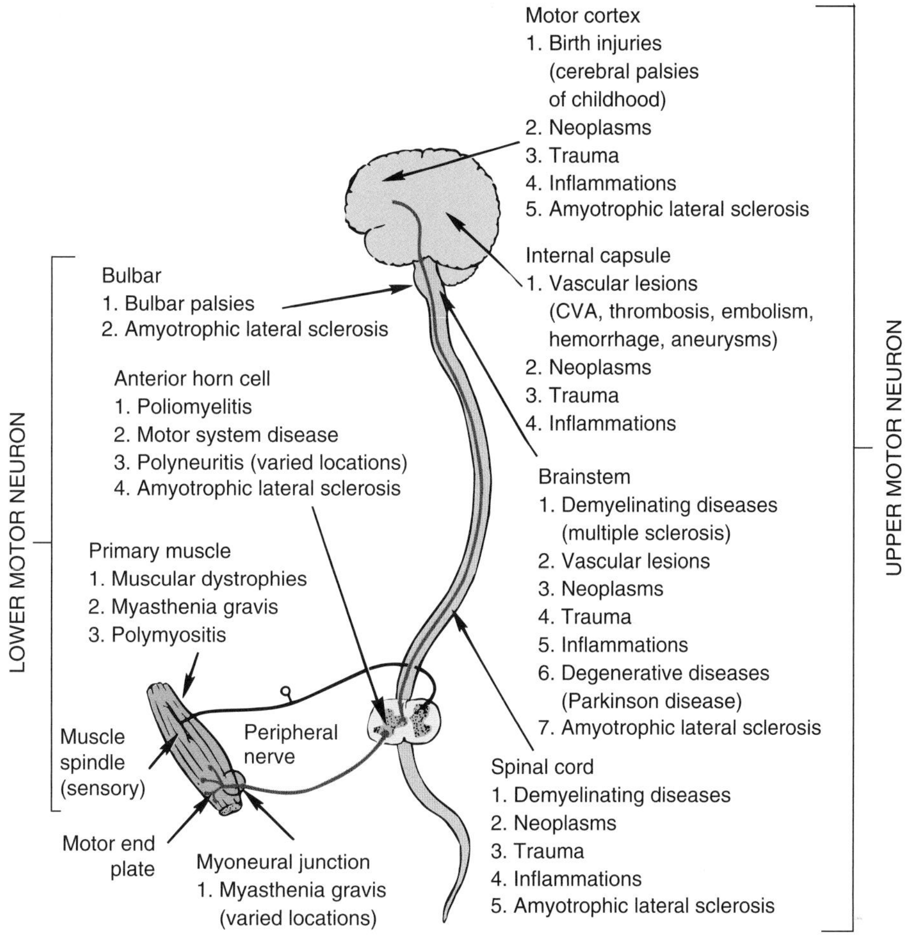

Fig. 17.20 Disturbances in Motor Function. Disturbances in motor function are classified pathologically along upper and lower motor neuron structures. It should be noted that neoplasms occur at more than one site in an upper motor neuron *(above right)*. A few pathologic conditions, such as amyotrophic lateral sclerosis, involve upper and lower motor neuron structures. Other lesion sites include myoneural junctions and primary muscles, making it possible to classify conditions as neuromuscular and muscular, respectively. *CVA*, Cerebrovascular accident.

receptors in the muscle spindles and Golgi tendon organ. (Muscle function is discussed in Chapter 43.) The Babinski sign is present (an abnormal plantar reflex-stroking the sole of the foot causes extension of the big toe rather than the normal dorsiflexion and fanning of the other toes). The presence of the Babinski sign is normal in infants prior to maturation of the corticospinal tracts. Dysphagia and dysarthria are associated with damage to the corticobulbar tract. Interruption of the pyramidal tract below the pons results in spinal shock (see Chapter 18) with complete flaccid paralysis, absence of reflexes, and marked disturbances of bowel and bladder function.

Lower Motor Neuron Syndromes

Lower (primary, alpha) motor neurons are the large motor neurons that arise from nuclei in the anterior (ventral) horn of the spinal cord and the motor nuclei of the brainstem. They receive input from upper motor neurons, sensory neurons, and interneurons and extend as peripheral nerves to the myoneural junction. The axons from the nerve cell bodies directly innervate extrafusal fibers of skeletal muscles through the anterior spinal roots or cranial nerves (Fig. 17.22) and cause skeletal muscle contraction. Damage to alpha motor neurons (the cell body or the axon and surrounding myelin) results in symptoms called LMN syndromes.[84] The symptoms result from impairment of voluntary and involuntary movement, usually without sensory impairment (see Table 17.18). The symptoms include flaccid paresis or paralysis, hypotonia, hyporeflexia or areflexia, muscle atrophy, fasciculations, and fibrillations. The paresis and paralysis associated with anterior horn cell injury are segmental, but because each muscle is supplied by two or more spinal nerve roots, the segmental character of the weakness may be difficult to recognize. The cause of LMN syndromes can be sporadic or hereditary. Polio, facial (Bell) palsy (Box 17.8), and spinal muscular atrophy (rare inherited diseases of anterior horn cells) are examples of LMN diseases. The degree of paralysis or paresis is proportional to the number of LMNs affected. If only some of the motor units that supply a muscle are affected, only partial paralysis or paresis results. If all the motor units are affected, complete paralysis results. Other clinical manifestations also are proportional to the degree of dysfunction, but the precise manifestations depend on the location of the dysfunction in the motor unit and in the CNS.

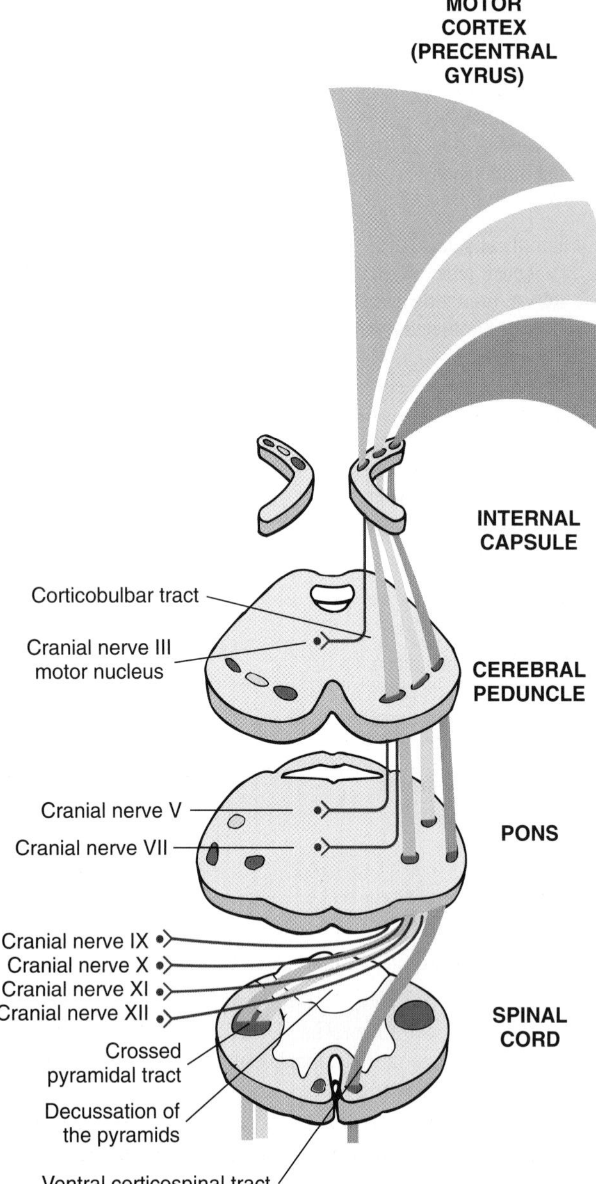

Fig. 17.21 Structures of the Upper Motor Neuron, or Pyramidal, System. Pyramidal system fibers are shown to originate primarily in the cells in the precentral gyrus of the motor cortex; to converge at the internal capsule; to descend to form the central third of the cerebral peduncle; to descend further through the pons, where small fibers supply cranial nerve motor nuclei along the way; to form pyramids at the medulla, where most of the fibers decussate; and then to continue to descend in the lateral column of the white matter of the spinal cord. A few fibers descend without crossing at the medulla level.

Gamma neurons (fusimotor neurons) are small and innervate muscle spindles (proprioceptors), the striated portions of intrafusal muscle fibers. The cell body is in the anterior gray column of the spinal cord and is dependent on input from the muscle spindle (arriving through an afferent limb rising to the cord). Gamma neurons maintain an appropriate level of tension on the muscle spindle receptor and maintain sensitivity of the muscle to the stretch reflex, maintain muscle tone, and protect the muscle from injury. They do not cause movement of a joint; dysfunction

TABLE 17.18 Upper and Lower Motor Neuron Syndromes Signs and Symptoms

Upper Motor Neuron (Pyramidal Cells—Motor Cortex)	Lower Motor Neuron (Cranial Nerve Nuclei—Brainstem; Ventral Horn—Spinal Cord)
Muscle groups are affected	Individual muscles may be affected
Mild weakness (paresis)	Mild weakness (paresis)
Spastic paralysis	Flaccid paralysis
Minimal disuse muscle atrophy	Marked muscle atrophy
No fasciculations	Fasciculations
Hyperreflexia, increased muscle stretch reflexes (clasp-knife spasticity; resistance to passive flexion that releases abruptly to allow easy flexion)	Hyporeflexia, decreased muscle stretch reflexes
Clonus may be present	Clonus not present
Hypertonia, spasticity	Hypotonia, flaccidity
Pathologic reflexes (Babinski and Hoffmann signs, loss of abdominal reflexes)	No Babinski sign
Often initial impairment of only skilled movements	Asymmetric and may involve one limb only in beginning to become generalized as disease progresses

BOX 17.7 Upper Motor Neuron Paralysis

Hemiparesis/hemiplegia is paresis/paralysis of the upper and lower extremities on one side.

Diplegia is paralysis of corresponding parts of both sides of the body as a result of cerebral hemisphere injuries.

Paraparesis/paraplegia is weakness/paralysis of the lower extremities as a result of lower spinal cord injury.

Quadriparesis/quadriplegia is paresis/paralysis of all four extremities as a result of upper spinal cord injury (spinal cord injury is discussed in Chapter 18).

in this sensory-motor system (the gamma loop or alpha-gamma loop) (see Fig. 17.22) impairs tone and reduces the tendon reflexes, causing hyporeflexia. The muscles become susceptible to damage from hyperextensibility because the normal protective mechanisms that prevent muscle fiber injury are impaired, as seen in Ehler-Danlos syndrome. The degree of muscle tone loss and the loss of tendon reflexes are proportional to the dysfunction in these reflex motor units. Generally, the alpha and gamma motor neuron systems are equally affected. Therefore, the muscle is hypotonic or atonic and is accompanied by hyporeflexia or areflexia (loss of tendon reflexes) and flaccid paresis/paralysis.

Denervated muscles (i.e., muscles that have lost their nervous system input) atrophy over weeks to months, mostly from disuse, and demonstrate fasciculations (spontaneous action potentials that cause muscle rippling or quivering under the skin). Occasionally, denervated muscles will cramp. Fibrillation is an

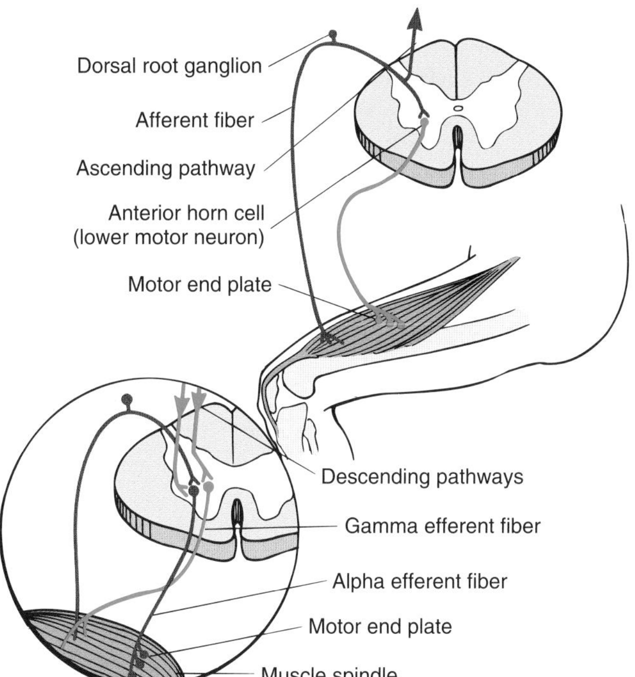

Fig. 17.22 Component Structure of a Lower Motor Neuron, Including Motor (Efferent) and Sensory (Afferent) Elements. *Top*, Anterior horn cell (in anterior gray column of spinal cord and its axon), terminating in motor end plate as it innervates extrafusal muscle fibers in the quadriceps muscle. *Detailed enlargement:* Sensory and motor elements of the gamma loop system. The gamma efferent fiber is shown innervating the polar, or end, region of the muscle spindle (sensory receptor of skeletal muscle). Contraction of muscle spindle fibers stretches the central portion of the spindle and causes the afferent spindle fiber to transmit the impulse centrally to the cord. Muscle spindle afferent fibers in turn synapse on the anterior horn cell and are transmitted by way of gamma efferent fibers to skeletal (extrafusal) muscle, causing it to contract. Muscle spindle discharge is interrupted by active contraction of extrafusal muscle fibers.

isolated contraction of a single muscle fiber because of metabolic changes in denervated muscle and is not clinically visible.

Several brainstem syndromes involve damage to one or more of the cranial nerve nuclei. These are called *cranial nerve palsies* (e.g., oculomotor nerve and facial nerve palsies) and may be caused by vascular occlusion, tumor, aneurysm, tuberculosis, or hemorrhage. Cranial nerve palsies may cause complete or partial paralysis of the areas innervated by the affected nerve.

The anterior horn cells and the motor nuclei of the cranial nerves may be affected secondarily in many severe pathologic processes that primarily involve the peripheral nerves. The condition may extend proximally to affect the nerve roots or rootlets and the motor neurons themselves, a process commonly seen, for example, in Guillain-Barré syndrome (GBS) (see Chapter 18). If enough motor neurons are destroyed, permanent loss of motor function results because regeneration of the damaged axons requires a living neuronal cell body.

A group of degenerative disorders principally cause progressive motor cell atrophy.[85] One of these disorders is progressive spinal muscular atrophy, an LMN disease in which degenerated anterior horn cells of the spinal cord are the affected motor neurons. This disorder occurs in adults and closely resembles the familial progressive muscular atrophies that occur in infants and children and are considered inherited metabolic disorders (see Chapter 45). If the motor nuclei of the cranial nerves are affected instead of the anterior horn cells, the disorder is labeled progressive bulbar palsy (a variant of ALS), so named because the myelencephalon (medulla and upper cranial nerves) originally was called the *bulb*, and a degenerative process causes a progressively more serious condition. When any LMN syndrome involves the cranial nerves that arise from the bulb (i.e., cranial nerves IX, X, and XII), the dysfunction is called a bulbar palsy.

The clinical manifestations of bulbar palsy include paresis or paralysis of the jaw, face, pharynx, and tongue musculature. Articulation is affected, especially articulation of the lingual *(r, n, l)*, labial *(b, m, p, f)*, dental *(d, t)*, and palatal *(k, g)* consonants. Modulation is impaired, making the voice rasping or nasal. Pharyngeal reflexes are diminished or lost. Palate and vocal cord movement during phonation is impaired, and chewing and swallowing are affected. The facial muscles are weak, and the face appears to droop. The jaw jerk reflex is decreased. Atrophy eventually becomes apparent, as do fasciculations. All these manifestations become progressively worse, leading to aspiration, malnutrition, possible dehydration, and an inability to communicate verbally.

BOX 17.8 Bell Palsy

Bell palsy is the most common paralysis of the seventh cranial (facial) nerve. The etiology of Bell palsy remains unknown, and diagnosis remains one of exclusion. There is usually an inflammatory reaction compressing the facial nerve in the fallopian (facial) canal of the middle ear, particularly in the narrowest labyrinthine segment, followed by demyelinating neural change. The most distressing symptoms are unilateral facial weakness and inability to smile or whistle. Bell palsy may be caused by reactivation of herpesviruses in cranial nerve VII (facial) geniculate ganglia or an autoimmune response. The signs usually have an acute onset (within 72 h). Herpes simplex type 1 has been detected in up to 78% of cases and herpes zoster in 30% of cases. Severe pain with facial palsy and a vesicular rash in the ear or mouth suggest herpes zoster infection. Ramsay Hunt syndrome (herpes zoster oticus) is rare, but complete recovery is less than 50%. Recovery from Bell palsy is usually complete within 4 months to 1 year and may not require treatment. Both disorders may be treated with antivirals, corticosteroids, or both, and physiotherapy. Facial nerve decompression is considered for complete facial nerve paralysis. Treatment should be individualized according to severity of symptoms.

Data from Zhang W, Xu L, Luo T, et al. The etiology of Bell's palsy: A review. *Journal of Neurology*, 2020;267(7):1896–1905; Lee SY, Seong J, Kim YH. Clinical implication of facial nerve decompression in complete bell's palsy: A systematic review and meta-analysis. *Clinical and Experimental Otorhinolaryngology*, 2019;12(4):348–359.

Extrapyramidal Motor Syndromes

The EPS encompasses all the motor pathways except the upper and LMNs. The EPS primarily controls fine motor and involuntary/automatic movement, complex coordinated movements, postural control, and locomotion. The EPS modulates voluntary motility through tonic inhibition or facilitation. Several regions of the brain are involved, including parts of the cerebral cortex, the cerebellum, thalamus, reticular formation, and nuclei of the basal ganglia. These regions project subcortical tracts and terminate in the spinal cord providing a complex motor control system. Symptoms of alterations of involuntary movement include tremors, spasms, inability to maintain posture, hypotonia, weakness, slowness of movement, and impairment of voluntary movements. There may also be impairment of cognitive functions, including memory and affective disorders such as depression. Alterations in EPS function are primarily related to neurodegenerative diseases (i.e., PD, ALS, and HD) and involve selective components of the system.

Two types of motor dysfunction comprise the extrapyramidal motor syndromes: (1) the basal ganglia motor syndromes and (2) the cerebellar motor syndromes. The cerebellum and basal ganglia are interconnected and communicate with the motor cortex, thalamus, and sensory pathways to control voluntary movement. Their pathways synapse on LMNs. Unlike pyramidal or upper motor syndromes, extrapyramidal motor syndromes result in movement or posture disturbance without significant paralysis, along with other distinctive symptoms (Table 17.19). These syndromes are associated with neurodegenerative diseases.[86]

Basal ganglia motor syndromes are movement disorders that involve either a paucity or an excess of involuntary movements: hypotonic/hyperkinetic (e.g., chorea [irregular intervals of successive jerk-like contractions] associated with HD) or hypertonic/hypokinetic (e.g., bradykinesia/akinesia associated with PD) syndromes.[87] Stress and nervous tension typically worsen the symptoms, whereas relaxation improves motor performance. Akinesia may occur despite normal strength. Involuntary hyperkinetic movements include resting tremor, chorea, ballism (rhythmic writhing movements of the proximal limbs), athetosis (slow continuous involuntary rolling writhing movement often in the hand), and dystonia (a sudden sustained contraction). They can be associated with brain trauma, stroke, tumors, infection, metabolic disorders, multiple sclerosis (MS), progressive supranuclear palsy, HD, and medication side effects.

Basal ganglia motor syndromes also are characterized by hypotonia and alterations in posture. Rigidity, together with the cogwheel phenomenon, is present in all muscle groups but is most prominent in those that maintain flexed position (as seen in PD). Postural abnormalities result from the loss of normal postural reflexes. Dysfunctional equilibrium results from the loss of postural stability.

Cerebellar motor syndromes involve the cerebellum and may result in (1) acute loss of muscle tone; (2) difficulty with coordination of goal-directed voluntary movements such as gait (ataxia) or purposeful arm movements; (3) minor degrees of muscle weakness (slurred speech, difficulty swallowing, altered eye movements), tendency toward fatigue, and impairment of associated movements; (4) intention tremor (occurs at the end of a purposeful movement, such as pushing a button) and essential tremor (most common and occurs involuntarily and manifests as a rhythmic shaking of the body); and (5) disorders of equilibrium and posture. These syndromes are associated with hereditary ataxias, stroke, brain trauma, MS, or tumors; systemic disorders (toxin exposure, celiac disease, heat stroke); or are idiopathic. Cerebellar effects can be ipsilateral (primarily affecting the same side of the body), so damage to the right cerebellum generally causes symptoms on the right side of the body. Predominant symptoms depend on the area and extent of damage within the cerebellum (Table 17.20).[88]

TABLE 17.19 Pyramidal Versus Extrapyramidal Motor Syndromes

Manifestations	Pyramidal Motor Syndrome	Extrapyramidal Motor Syndrome
Unilateral movement	Paralysis of voluntary movement	Little or no paralysis of voluntary movement
Tendon reflexes	Increased tendon reflexes	Normal or slightly increased tendon reflexes
Babinski sign	Present	Absent
Involuntary movements	Absence of involuntary movements	Presence of tremor, chorea, athetosis, or dystonia
Muscle tone	Spasticity in muscles (e.g., clasp-knife phenomenon)	Plastic (equal throughout movement) rigidity, or intermittent (generalized but predominantly in flexors of limbs and trunk) rigidity (cogwheel rigidity); Bradykinesia
	Hypertonia present in flexors of arms and extensors of legs	Hypotonia, weakness, and gait disturbance in cerebellar disease

TABLE 17.20 Cerebellar Motor Syndromes

Anatomic Location of Dysfunction	Characteristics
Rostral vermis (so-called *anterior lobe*)	Ataxia of stance and gait with varying degrees of instability of the trunk and ataxia of legs; anteroposterior body sway; presence of Romberg sign
Caudal vermis (including flocculonodular lobe)	Truncal, postural, and gait ataxia; omnidirectional body sway; Romberg negative; tendency to fall; saccadic slow pursuit, nystagmus; inability to suppress vestibulo-ocular reflex (doll's eyes)
Cerebellar hemisphere (neocerebellar syndrome)	Severe disturbance in ipsilateral limb movements; hypotonia in acute situation; dysmetria (extremity overshooting its target); decomposition of movement; kinetic tremor, past-pointing; deviation of gait; dysarthria
Pancerebellum (combines all other syndromes)	Ataxia of trunk and bilateral limbs; ataxia of gait and stance; dysarthria; oculomotor disturbance

Data from McGee S. *Evidence-based physical diagnosis*, 4th edition. St. Louis: Elsevier; 2018; Timmann D, Diener HC. Coordination and ataxia. In: Goetz GC, ed. *Textbook of clinical neurology*. St. Louis: Saunders; 2007.

Alterations in Complex Motor Performance

The alterations in complex motor performance include disorders of posture (stance), disorders of gait and balance, and disorders of expression. They primarily involve alterations of coordinating functions between the extrapyramidal and pyramidal motor systems.

Disorders of Posture (Stance)

An inequality of tone in muscle groups because of a loss of normal postural reflexes results in a posturing of limbs. Many reflex systems govern tone and posture, but the most important factor in posture control is the stretch reflex, in which extensor (antigravity) muscles stretching, causes increased extensor tone and inhibited flexor tone. Four types of postural disorders are described: (1) dystonic posture, (2) decerebrate posture, (3) basal ganglion posture, and (4) senile posture. Equilibrium and balance are disrupted when postural disorders are present.

Dystonia is the maintenance of an abnormal posture through excessive muscular contractions. Dystonia can affect any muscle and occur at any age. When muscular contractions are sustained for several seconds, they are called dystonic movements. When contractions last for longer periods, they are called dystonic postures, such as in torticollis. Dystonic postures may last for weeks, causing permanent fixed contractures. Dystonia has been associated with basal ganglia abnormality, but the exact pathophysiologic mechanisms are unknown. Botulinum toxin injection is an effective treatment for some types of dystonia (Box 17.9).

One dystonic posture is decorticate posture (striatal posture or upper motor neuron dysfunction posture), which may be unilateral or bilateral in occurrence. Decorticate posture (also known as antigravity posture, hemiplegic posture, or flexor posturing) is characterized by upper extremities that are flexed at the elbows and held close to the body and by lower extremities that are externally rotated and extended (see Fig. 17.6). Decorticate posture/response is believed to occur with injury to the midbrain when the brainstem is not inhibited by the motor function of the cerebral cortex. Upper motor neuron posture is more commonly described as the arm flexed at the elbow with a wristdrop; the leg inadequately bent at the knee, the hip excessively circumducted, and the presence of a footdrop.

Decerebrate posture (decerebrate rigidity, extensor posturing) refers to increased tone in extensor muscles and trunk muscles with active tonic neck reflexes. When the head is in a neutral position, all four limbs are rigidly extended (see Fig. 17.6). The decerebrate posture is caused by severe injury to the brain and brainstem, resulting in overstimulation of the postural righting and vestibular reflexes. Decerebrate posturing is also caused by reversible metabolic disorders including electrolyte disorders (e.g., hyponatremia, hypocalcemia), hypoglycemia, and encephalitis.

Basal ganglion posture refers to a stooped, hyperflexed posture with a narrow-based, short-stepped gait. This postural abnormality results from the loss of normal postural reflexes and not from defects in proprioceptive, labyrinthine, or visual function. Dysfunctional equilibrium results when the individual loses stability and cannot make the appropriate postural adjustment to tilting or loss of balance, falling instead. Dysfunctional righting is the inability to right oneself when changing from a lying or crouching to a standing position or when rolling from the supine to the lateral or prone position. Dysfunctional postural fixation is the involuntary flexion of the head and neck, causing the person difficulty in maintaining an upright trunk position while standing or walking. Basal ganglion dysfunction, with loss of dopaminergic and cholinergic neurons, accounts for this posture and is commonly associated with PD (see PD section).

BOX 17.9 Treatment of Dystonia

Treatment of dystonia is individually determined. Botulinum toxin injection, both A and B, is effective in relieving cervical dystonia (spasmodic torticollis) symptoms in adults and is an effective treatment for focal dystonia and pain. Other drugs (benzodiazepines, gamma-aminobutyric acid [GABA] inhibitors, atypical anticonvulsants, dopaminergic agonists and antagonists), surgical interventions (deep brain stimulation and ablative therapies) or physical therapies can provide symptom relief.

Data from Jinnah HA. Medical and surgical treatments for dystonia. *Neurologic Clinics*, 2020;38(2):325–348. Lizarraga KJ, Al-Shorafat D, Fox S. Update on current and emerging therapies for dystonia. *Neurodegenerative Disease Management*, 2019;9(3):135–147.

Disorders of Gait and Balance

Performance of gait and maintenance of balance are coordinated by vision, the vestibular system, the frontal lobes, basal ganglia, and cerebellum. Four predominant types of gait associated with neurologic disorders are (1) upper motor neuron dysfunction gait, (2) cerebellar (ataxic) gait, (3) basal ganglion gait, and (4) frontal lobe ataxic gait. As with posture, equilibrium and balance are affected with gait disturbances.[89] Several upper motor neuron gaits exist. With mild forms, the individual may have footdrop, fatigue, hip pain, and leg pain. A spastic gait, which is associated with unilateral injury, is manifested by a shuffling gait with the leg extended and held stiff, causing a scraping over the floor surface. The leg swings improperly around the body rather than being appropriately lifted and placed. The foot may drag on the ground, and the person tends to fall to the affected side. A scissors gait is associated with bilateral injury and spasticity. The legs are adducted, causing them to touch each other. As the person walks, the legs are still swung around the body but then cross in front of each other because of adduction. Injury to the pyramidal system accounts for these gaits (e.g., stroke, cerebral palsy, MS, and spinal cord tumor).

A cerebellar gait is wide based with the feet apart and often turned outward or inward for greater stability. The pelvis is held stiff, and the individual staggers and cannot walk a straight line. There is decreased walking speed and stride length and difficulty with balance. Cerebellar dysfunction with loss of coordination accounts for this particular gait.[90]

A basal ganglion gait is a wide-based gait in which the person walks with small steps and a decreased arm swing. The head and body are flexed, and the arms are semiflexed and abducted, whereas the legs are flexed and rigid in more advanced states. Basal ganglion dysfunction accounts for this gait and is associated with PD.

A frontal lobe ataxic gait is wide based with increased body sway and falls, loss of control of truncal motion, gait ignition failure, start hesitation, shuffling, and freezing. The gait is associated with frontal lobe damage or dementia. The pattern may change as the frontal disease progresses. The slowness of walking, lack of heel-shin or upper limb ataxia, dysarthria, or nystagmus distinguishes the wide stance from cerebellar gait ataxia.

Gait disorders are often accompanied by balance, coordination, and sensory dysfunction that further alter mobility and increase risk for falls. Assessment and intervention strategies are important for prevention of injury.

Disorders of Expression

Disorders of expression involve motor aspects of communication and include (1) pseudobulbar affect (PBA), also known as pathological laughing or crying, (2) aprosody, and (3) dyspraxias and apraxias. PBA is a disinhibition phenomenon of inappropriate episodes of exaggerated uncontrollable laughter, crying, or both, without an apparent motivational stimulus and incongruent with mood or feeling. It occurs with various neurologic diseases including stroke, tumors, ALS, PD, traumatic brain injury, and epilepsy. The exact pathophysiology is not known, but it is associated with loss of descending control of brainstem centers (i.e., cortico-pontine-cerebellar pathway) that control emotional expression with decreases in serotonin and dopamine and increases in glutamate.[91,92]

Aprosody is the loss of voice modulation (pitch, speed, emphasis, emotion). Receptive aprosody involves an inability to *understand* emotion in speech and facial expression, whereas expressive aprosody involves the inability to *express* emotion in speech and facial expression. Work is in progress to identify the neural pathways linked to aprosody, including hemispheric lateralization and the amygdala.[93,94]

Dyspraxia is the partial inability and apraxia is the complete inability to perform purposeful or skilled motor acts in the absence of paralysis, sensory loss, abnormal posture and tone, abnormal involuntary movement, incoordination, or inattentiveness. There is a disconnect between movement and the purpose of the movement.[95] These are disorders of learned skilled movements (e.g., arm and hand movement [eating], standing and turning around, blowing out a candle, and using tools). Dyspraxias/apraxias may result from any pathologic process that disrupts the cortical areas necessary for the conceptualization and execution of a complex motor act, primarily in the motor-dominant left hemisphere.[96] Subtypes of dyspraxias/apraxias are associated with different locations of brain injury and include both dorsal and ventral pathways.[96] Numerous neurologic disorders can be associated with apraxia. including vascular disorders, particularly stroke, trauma, tumor, and degenerative disorders (PD and dementia), infections, and metabolic disorders. Both motor and sensory neural networks play a role in the planning and execution of skilled movements. True dyspraxias/apraxias occur when the connecting pathways between the left and right cortical areas are interrupted, causing language-motor and motor representation disconnections between the hemispheres.

Alterations in Muscle Tone

Normal muscle tone involves a slight resistance to passive movement. The resistance is smooth, constant, and even throughout the range of motion. The alterations of muscle tone and their characteristics and causes are presented in Table 17.21.

Hypotonia

In hypotonia (decreased muscle tone), passive movement of a muscle occurs with little or no resistance. Hypotonia is commonly a symptom of LMN damage with loss of reflexes. It is thought to be caused by decreased muscle spindle activity secondary to decreased excitability of alpha motor neurons. Hypotonia contributes to ataxia and intention tremor in cerebellar damage and manifests with minimal weakness and normal or slightly exaggerated reflexes. A pure pyramidal tract injury (very rare) produces hypotonia and weakness. Hypotonia, often described as flaccidity (a state in which the muscle may be moved rapidly without resistance), occurs when nerve impulses necessary for muscle tone are lost, such as in spinal cord injury or cerebrovascular accident.

Individuals with hypotonia report that they tire easily (asthenia) or are weak. They may have difficulty rising from a sitting position, sitting down without using arm support, or walking up and down stairs, as well as an inability to stand on their toes. Because of their weakness, accident proneness during locomotion and self-care activities is common. The joints become hyperflexible, so people with hypotonia may be able to assume positions that require extreme joint mobility. The joints may appear loose. The muscle mass atrophies because of decreased neural input entering the motor unit. Muscle cells are gradually replaced by connective tissue and fat. The muscles are flabby on palpation and are flat in appearance. Fasciculations may be present in some cases.

Hypertonia

Hypertonia is increased muscle tone. With passive movement of a muscle, there is resistance to stretch. Hypertonia is caused by upper motor neuron damage with loss of inhibitory control of LMNs (see the section on Upper Motor Neuron Syndromes). The four types of hypertonia are spasticity (usually corticospinal in origin with overactivation of alpha motor neurons), paratonia (gegenhalten), dystonia, and rigidity (usually extrapyramidal in origin). Four types of rigidity are described: plastic or lead-pipe, cogwheel, gamma (independent of stretch reflex pathways), and alpha (dependent on stretch reflex pathways) (see Table 17.21).

Spasticity results from hyperexcitability of the stretch reflexes (overactivation of the alpha motor neurons) and is associated with damage to upper motor neurons (motor, premotor, and supplementary motor areas, as well as the lateral corticospinal tract) (Fig. 17.23). Spasticity is accompanied by increased deep tendon reflexes (hyperreflexia) and the spread of reflexes (clonus).

Paratonia (gegenhalten) is resistance to passive movement that increases with velocity of movement. Dystonia is increased involuntary muscle contractions, manifested as sustained,

TABLE 17.21 Alterations in Muscle Tone

Alterations	Characteristics	Cause
Hypotonia	Passive movement of a muscle mass with little or no resistance Muscles may be moved rapidly without resistance	Thought to be caused by decreased muscle spindle activity as a result of decreased excitability of alpha motor neurons (e.g., muscular dystrophy, cerebral palsy)
Flaccidity	Associated with limp, atrophied muscles, and paralysis	Occurs typically when nerve impulses necessary for muscle tone are lost
Hypertonia	Increased muscle resistance to passive movement May be associated with paralysis May be accompanied by muscle hypertrophy	Results when upper motor neuron damage results in loss of inhibitory control of lower motor neurons (e.g., stroke, brain tumors, multiple sclerosis)
Spasticity	A gradual increase in tone, causing increased resistance until tone suddenly diminishes, which results in clasp-knife phenomenon; increased deep tendon reflexes (hyperreflexia); clonus (spread of reflexes)	Damage to upper motor neurons with excitability of alpha motor neurons to any input because of absence of descending inhibition of pyramidal systems (e.g., multiple sclerosis, brain trauma, cerebral palsy)
Paratonia (gegenhalten)	Resistance to passive movement, which varies in direct proportion to force applied	Exact mechanism unclear; associated with frontal lobe injury (e.g., progressive Alzheimer dementia)
Dystonia	Sustained involuntary muscle contraction with twisting movement	Produced by slow muscular contraction; lack of reciprocal inhibition of muscle (e.g., neuroleptic drug side effects, meningitis)
Rigidity	Muscle resistance to passive movement of a rigid limb that is uniform in both flexion and extension throughout the motion	Occurs as a result of constant, involuntary contraction of muscle—usually involves extrapyramidal tracts (e.g., Parkinson disease)
Plastic or lead-pipe rigidity	Increased muscular tone relatively independent of degree of force used in passive movement; does not vary throughout the passive movement	Associated with basal ganglion damage (e.g., Parkinson disease)
Cogwheel rigidity	Uniform resistance may be interrupted by a series of brief jerks, resulting in movements much like a ratchet, "cogwheel" phenomenon	Associated with basal ganglion damage
Gamma rigidity	Characterized by extensor posturing (decerebrate rigidity)	Loss of excitation of extensor inhibitory areas by cerebral cortex decreasing inhibition of alpha and gamma motor neurons
Alpha rigidity	Impaired relaxation characterized by extensor rigidity of skeletal muscle after contraction	Loss of cerebellum input to lateral vestibular nuclei

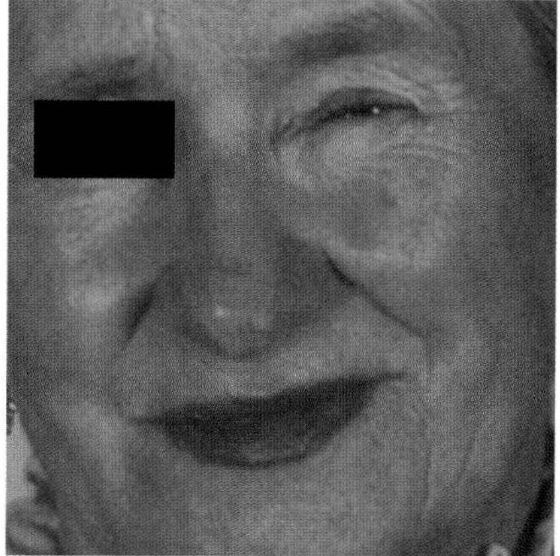

Fig. 17.23 Left-Sided Hemifacial Spasm. (From Perkin GD. *Mosby's color atlas and text of neurology*. London: Mosby-Wolfe; 1998.)

involuntary twisting movements. It is caused by slow muscle contraction and may be caused by a failure of reciprocal inhibition of muscles in close proximity (Figs. 17.24 and 17.25). Impairment of several levels of sensorimotor integration between the cortex, cerebellum, basal ganglia, and thalamus contribute to dystonia and hyperkinetic movement.[97]

Rigidity produced by tonic reflex activity mediated by gamma motor neurons may be continuous or intermittent. The involved muscles are firm and tense; the increase in muscle movement is even and uniform throughout the range of passive movement. Four types of rigidity are described: plastic or lead pipe, cogwheel, gamma, and alpha (see Table 17.21).

Individuals with hypertonia may tire easily (asthenia) or are weak. Passive movement and active movement are equally affected, except in paratonia, in which more active than passive movement is possible. As a result of hypertonia and weakness, accident proneness during locomotion and self-care activities is common.

With these disorders, muscles may atrophy because of decreased use. However, hypertrophy occasionally occurs from overstimulation of muscle fibers. Overstimulation occurs when the motor unit reflex arc remains intact and functioning but is not inhibited by higher centers. The loss of inhibition and the constant state of excitation cause continual muscle contraction, resulting in enlargement of the muscle mass and the development of firm muscles (Fig. 17.26).

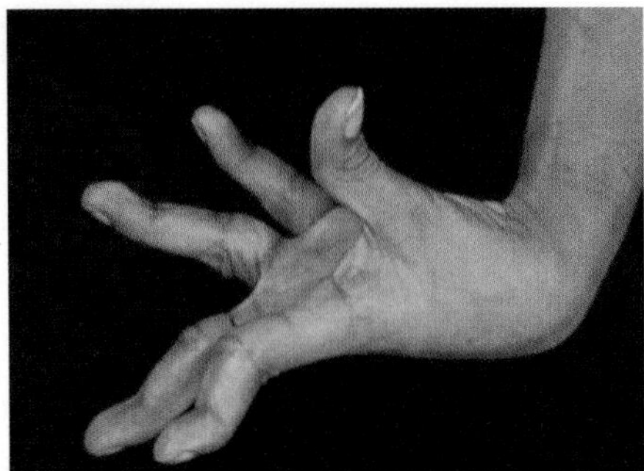

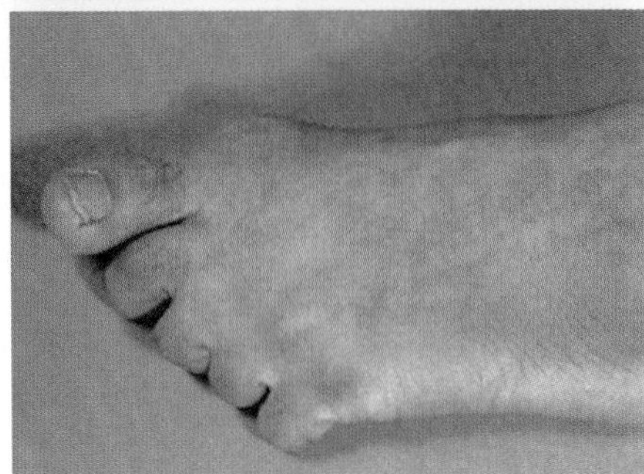

Fig. 17.24 Dystonic Posturing of the Hand and Foot. (From Perkin GD. *Mosby's color atlas and text of neurology*. London: Mosby-Wolfe; 1998.)

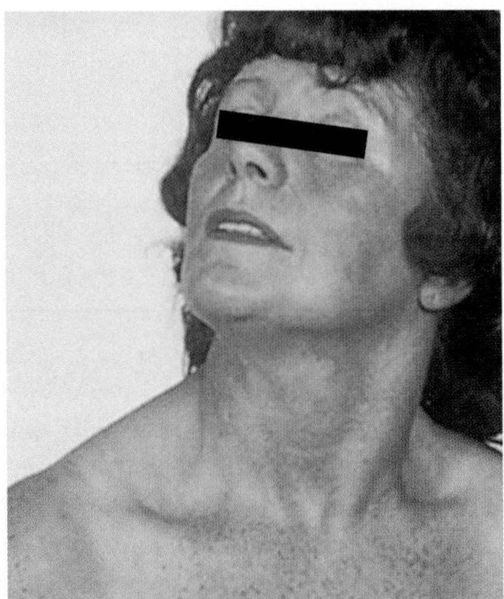

Fig. 17.25 Spasmodic Torticollis. A characteristic head posture related to muscle spasticity, often involving the sternocleidomastoid muscle. (From Perkin GD, et al. *Atlas of clinical neurology*, 3rd edition. Philadelphia: Saunders; 2011.)

Alterations in Muscle Movement

Movement requires a change in the contractile state of muscles. Abnormal movements may occur when a variety of CNS dysfunctions alter muscular innervation. *Dopamine*, a neurotransmitter, has a role in several movement disorders. Some movement disorders (e.g., the akinesias) result from too little dopaminergic activity, whereas others (e.g., chorea, ballism, and tardive dyskinesia) result from too much dopaminergic activity. Still, others are not related primarily to dopamine function. Movement disorders are not associated necessarily with mass, strength, or tone but are neurologic dysfunctions with either an excess of movement or a lack of voluntary movement. Muscle strength is quantitatively evaluated on a scale of 0 to 4+ or 0 to 5, in which 4+ or 5 is normal, and 0 indicates an inability to move against gravity (Table 17.22).

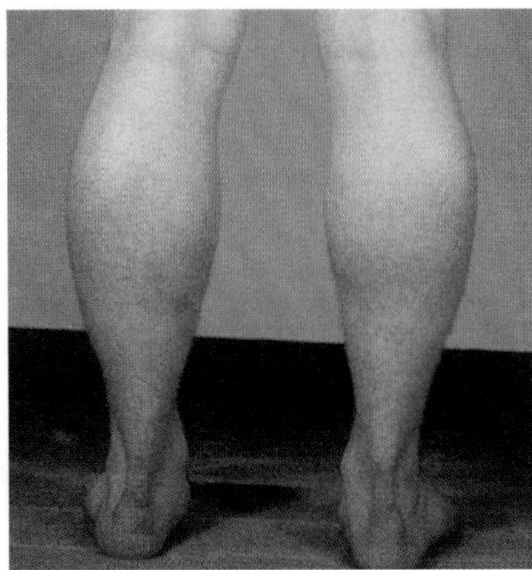

Fig. 17.26 Pseudohypertrophy of the Calf Muscles. (From Perkin GD, et al. *Atlas of clinical neurology*, 3rd edition. Philadelphia: Saunders, 2011.)

TABLE 17.22 United Kingdom Medical Research Council Classification of Muscle Power

Grade	Definition
0	Total paralysis—no muscle contraction
1	Flicker of contraction—no joint movement
2	Movement with gravity eliminated
3	Movement against gravity but not resistance
4	Movement against resistance but incomplete
5	Normal power against resistance

Data from Vanhoutte EK, Faber CG, van Nes SI, et al. Modifying the Medical Research Council grading system through Rasch analyses. *Brain*, 2012;135(Pt 5):1639–1649.

Hypokinesia

Hypokinesia, bradykinesia, and akinesia are terms that represent a deficit of voluntary movement with loss of associated movement. PD symptoms are the hallmark of a lack of voluntary movement. Hypokinesia (decreased movement) is decreased amplitude of voluntary movement despite preserved consciousness and normal peripheral nerve and muscle function. Types of hypokinesia include akinesia, bradykinesia, and loss of associated movement.

Akinesia is a decrease in voluntary and associated movements. It is related to dysfunction of the basal ganglia and substantia nigra (SN) and is caused by either a deficiency of dopamine or a defect of the postsynaptic dopamine receptors. Bradykinesia is slowness of voluntary movements. All voluntary movements become slow, labored, and deliberate with difficulty in (1) initiating movements, (2) continuing movements smoothly, and (3) performing synchronous (at the same time)

EMERGING SCIENCE BOX

Tourette Syndrome

There is growing evidence that Tourette syndrome (TS, also known as Tourette Disorder) occurs worldwide and has common features across all races and cultures. The hallmark features of TS are the presence of involuntary motor tics (sudden, rapid, repetitive, nonrhythmic movements) and vocal–phonic tics (unintentional uttering of sounds). The tics may be either simple, involving only an individual muscle group (e.g., eye blinking or grunting), or complex, requiring coordinated movement of muscle groups (e.g., head banging or repeating of another person's words) and may be preceded by an aura. Sensory tics involve unpleasant sensations in the face, head, and neck areas. Probably underdiagnosed, the onset of TS is typically between the ages of 2 and 15 years, with the tics lessening in adulthood. The syndrome has a complex multifactorial etiology with undetermined genetic, environmental, immune, and hormonal factors. The pathophysiology of TS is unclear and currently under study. There is evidence of cortico-striato-thalamocortical dysfunction and, in some cases, altered dopaminergic neurotransmission and abnormalities in brain gamma-aminobutyric acid (loss of inhibition). The criteria for diagnosis include the occurrence of two or more motor tics *and* at least 1 vocal tic (usually every day), have been present for at least a year, started before age 18 years, and not due to taking medicine or other drugs or due to having another medical condition that can cause tics. TS is often diagnosed in association with anxiety, depression, attention-deficit/hyperactivity disorder (ADHD), and obsessive-compulsive disorder. Habit reversal therapy addressing the urge to move is the most common behavioral therapy. However, the efficacy of all behavioral therapies needs further investigation. Pharmacologic treatments target symptoms and can have significant side effects. Deep brain stimulation has also been used to treat refractory symptoms of TS in selected individuals with some success.

Data from American Psychiatric Association. DSM-5 Task Force. Diagnostic and Statistical Manual of Mental Disorders: DSM-5. 5th ed. Washington, DC: American Psychiatric Association; 2013; Seideman MF, et al. A review of the current treatment of tourette syndrome. *J Pediatr Pharmacol Ther*. 2020;25(5):401–412; Martino D, et al. The 5 Pillars in Tourette syndrome deep brain stimulation patient selection: present and future. *Neurology*. 2021;96(14):664–676.

and consecutive tasks. Both akinesia and bradykinesia involve a delay in the time it takes to start to perform a movement.

In hypokinesia there is loss of associated movement. The normal, habitually associated movements that provide skill, grace, and balance to voluntary movements are lost. Decreased associated movements accompanying emotional expression cause an expressionless face, a statue-like posture, absence of speech inflection, and absence of spontaneous gestures. Decreased associated movements accompanying locomotion cause reduction in arm and shoulder movements, hip swinging, and rotary motion of the cervical spine.

Hyperkinesia

Hyperkinesia is excessive, purposeless movement. Within this category are several specific dysfunctions, including tremors (Table 17.23). Also included under the general category of hyperkinesia are *dyskinesias* and abnormal involuntary movements. HD symptoms are the hallmark of hyperkinesia.

Dyskinesias

Paroxysmal dyskinesias are abnormal, involuntary movements that occur as spasms. The type of dyskinesia varies depending on the specific disorder. There is no loss of consciousness with this disorder.

Tardive dyskinesia (slow onset dyskinesia) is the involuntary movement of the face, trunk, and extremities. Although the condition occurs occasionally in individuals with PD, it usually occurs as a side effect of prolonged dopamine-receptor blocking agents, including antipsychotic drug therapy.[98] The antipsychotic drugs cause denervation hypersensitivity, thereby mimicking the effect of excessive dopamine. The most common symptom of tardive dyskinesia is rapid, repetitive, stereotypic movements, such as continual chewing with intermittent protrusions of the tongue, lip smacking, and facial grimacing.

Other movement disorders in this category are (1) complex repetitive movements, including automatism (unconscious behavior), stereotypy (ritualistic behavior such as rocking), complex tics, such as Tourette syndrome (see Emerging Science Box: Tourette Syndrome), compulsions, perseverations, and mannerisms; (2) excessive reactions to certain stimuli; and (3) paroxysmal excessive activity, including cataplexy and excessive startle reaction.

CHRONIC DISEASES AND DISORDERS INVOLVING MOTOR FUNCTION

There are several chronic progressive diseases (PD, ALS, HD) in adults that primarily involve alterations in motor function with neurodegeneration. Additionally, there are diseases that primarily involve myelin degeneration (MS and Guillain Barré syndrome) or the myoneural junction (myasthenia gravis (MG). These diseases may involve the sensory and autonomic nervous systems with nonmotor symptoms, including decline of cognitive function. The pathogenesis varies, but they are commonly influenced by gene mutations, gene-to-environment interaction, or epigenetic expression. Most have a subtle onset, may progress rapidly or slowly, and/or with a pattern of remission and exacerbation of symptoms. The etiology may be unknown, and there is no cure. Early diagnosis, prevention of disease progression, and maintenance of function and quality of life are the aims of treatment and management. Table 17.24 summarizes the features of the most common of these diseases.

Chronic Progressive Motor Diseases of the Central Nervous System

Parkinson Disease

PD is a complex motor disorder accompanied by systemic nonmotor and neurologic symptoms. Etiologic classification includes primary parkinsonism and secondary parkinsonism. The onset of primary PD usually begins after 40 years of age, with the incidence increasing after 60 years. It is estimated there will be 1,238,000 cases by 2030 compared to 930,000

TABLE 17.23 **Types of Hyperkinesia Syndromes**

Type	Characteristics	Causes
Chorea[a]	Nonrepetitive muscular contractions, usually of the extremities of the face; random pattern of irregular, involuntary rapid contractions of groups of muscles; disappears with sleep, decreases with resting; increases with emotional stress and attempted voluntary movement	Associated with excess concentration of or a supersensitivity to dopamine within basal ganglia
Athetosis[a]	Disorder of distal-muscle postural fixation; slow, twisting, sinuous, irregular movements most obvious in the distal extremities, more rhythmic than choreiform movements and always much slower; movements accompany characteristic hand posture; slowly fluctuating grimaces	Occurs most commonly as a result of injury to the putamen of the basal ganglion; exact pathophysiologic mechanism is not known
Ballism	Disorder of proximal-muscle postural fixation with wild flinging movement of the limbs; movement is severe and stereotyped, usually lateral; does not lessen with sleep; ballism is most common on one side of the body, a condition termed *hemiballism*	Results from injury to the subthalamic nucleus (one of the nuclei that comprise the basal ganglia); thought to be caused by reduced inhibitory influence in the nucleus, a release phenomenon; hemiballism results from injury to the contralateral subthalamic nucleus
Hyperactivity	State of prolonged, generalized, increased activity that is largely involuntary but may be subject to some voluntary control; not highly stereotyped but rather manifests as continual changes in total body posture or in excessive performance of some simple activity, such as pacing under inappropriate circumstances	May be caused by frontal and reticular activating system injury
Wandering	Tendency to wander without regard for environment	"Release" phenomenon; associated with bilateral injury to globus pallidus or putamen
Akathisia	Special type of hyperactivity; mild compulsion to move (usually more localized to legs); severe frenzied motion possible; movements are partly voluntary and may be transiently suppressed; carrying out the movement brings a sense of relief; a frequent complication of antipsychotic drugs	Dopaminergic transmission may be involved
Tremor at rest	Rhythmic, oscillating movement affecting one or more body parts	Caused by regular contraction of opposing groups of muscles
Parkinsonian tremor	Regular, rhythmic, slow flexion-extension contraction; involves principally the metacarpophalangeal and wrist joints; alternating movements between thumb and index finger described as "pill rolling"; disappears during voluntary movement	Loss of inhibitory influence of dopamine in the basal ganglia, causing instability of basal ganglia feedback circuit within the cerebral cortex
Postural Tremor		
Asterixis (tremor of hepatic encephalopathy)	Irregular flapping movement of the hands accentuated by outstretching arms	Caused by transient inhibition of muscles that maintain posture; thought to be related to accumulation of products normally detoxified by the liver
Metabolic	Rapid, rhythmic tremor affecting fingers, lips, and tongue; accentuated by extending the body part; enhanced physiologic tremor	Occurs in conditions associated with disturbed metabolism or toxicity, as in thyrotoxicosis (hyperthyroidism), alcoholism, and chronic use of barbiturates, amphetamines, lithium, amitriptyline (Elavil); exact mechanism responsible unknown
Essential (familial)	Tremor of fingers, hands, and feet; absent at rest but accentuated by extension of body part, prolonged muscular activity, and stress	Not associated with any other neurologic abnormalities; cause unknown
Intentional Tremor		
Cerebellar	Tremor initiated by movement, maximal toward end of movement	Occurs in disease of the dentate nucleus (one of the deep cerebellar nuclei responsible for efferent output) and the superior cerebellar peduncle (a stalklike structure connected to the pons); caused by errors in feedback from the periphery and errors in preprogramming goal-directed movement
Rubral	Rhythmic tremor of limbs that originates proximally by movement	Results from lesions involving the dentatorubrothalamic tract (a spinothalamic tract connecting the red nucleus in the reticular formation and the dentate nucleus in the cerebellum)
Myoclonus	Series of shocklike, nonpatterned contractions of a portion of a muscle, entire muscle, or group of muscles that cause throwing movements of a limb; usually appear at random but frequently triggered by sudden startle; do not disappear during sleep	Associated with an irritable nervous system and spontaneous discharge of neurons; structures associated with myoclonus include the cerebral cortex, cerebellum, reticular formation, and spinal cord

[a]Choreoathetosis involves chorea and athetosis; precise pathophysiology unknown.

TABLE 17.24 Comparative Features of Progressive Diseases Involving Motor Function

	Parkinson Disease	Amyotrophic Lateral Sclerosis	Huntington Disease	Multiple Sclerosis	Myasthenia Gravis
Age at onset	40 years, peak in 60s	40 years, peak in 50s	40–50 years	20–40 years	20–40 years
Pathophysiology	Genetic predisposition. Degeneration of basal ganglia (corpus striatum, globus pallidus, subthalamic nucleus, substantia nigra) Loss of dopaminergic-pigmented neurons in substantia nigra	Genetic predisposition. Diffuse degeneration of upper and lower motor neurons Scarring of corticospinal tract in lateral column of spinal cord.	Genetic predisposition. Depletion of GABA in basal ganglia, frontal cortex	Probable gene-environment interaction. Diffuse autoimmune destruction of myelin with glial scar formation involving brain, spinal cord, and optic nerve. Involves neuroimmune inflammation of motor, sensory and autonomic nerves	Probable gene-environment interaction. Autoimmune formation of antibodies to AchR and MuSK neuromuscular junction receptors (see Fig. 17.37).
Clinical Manifestations	MOTOR: Resting tremor, rigidity (cogwheel, lead pipe), bradykinesia-akinesia, postural instability, slow shuffling gait, fixed facial expression, drooling, NONMOTOR: hyponosmia, fatigue, pain, autonomic dysfunction, sleep fragmentation, depression, dementia with or without psychosis.	MOTOR: Initial onset of cramping or weakness that affects a limb, incoordination, slurring of speech, difficulty swallowing. UMN SYNDROME: Spastic paresis progressing to paralysis and associated with spasticity and muscle atrophy secondary to disuse. Spasticity manifest with clasp knife phenomenon; hyperactive reflexes; Babinski and Hoffman sign; absent abdominal and cremasteric reflexes. Dementia may develop later in the disease. LOWER MOTOR NEURON SYNDROME: Flaccid paresis with weakness of individual muscles, progressing to paralysis, associated with hypotonia and primary muscle atrophy. Hypotonia manifested by (1) decreased resistance to passive movement, (2) hypoactive or absent deep tendon reflexes, (3) absent abdominal and cremasteric reflexes, (4) absent Babinski sign. Primary atrophy is manifested by 1. severe, irreversible muscle wasting 2. fasciculations with fibrillations prominent feature 3. specific EMG findings. Metabolic changes include 1. thinning of the skin, 2. thickening of the nails, 3. loss of body hair, 4. decreased sweating	MOTOR: Chorea, dystonia NONMOTOR: Difficulty concentrating Delusions Depression Dementia	Variable depending on location, type and extent of nerve involvement—focal or diffuse onset: Visual impairment, nystagmus, dysarthria, difficulty walking or moving arms, numbness and tingling, bowel and bladder disturbances	Involvement of different muscle groups: extraocular eye muscles (diplopia, ocular palsies, ptosis); facial (drooping, loss of expression); difficulty chewing and swallowing, drooling, change in speech pattern. Remissions may occur for months or years. Exacerbations have occurred with use of immune check point inhibitors for cancer treatment.

Continued

TABLE 17.24 Comparative Features of Progressive Diseases Involving Motor Function—cont'd

	Parkinson Disease	Amyotrophic Lateral Sclerosis	Huntington Disease	Multiple Sclerosis	Myasthenia Gravis
Diagnosis	Family history Clinical presentation Genetic testing Single-photon emission computerized tomography (SPECT) scan, dopamine transporter scan (DaTscan), MRI, CT to rule out other neurological disorders	Family history Clinical presentation Genetic testing MRI, CT, EMG to rule out other neurological disorders	Family history Clinical presentation Genetic testing MRI, CT to rule out other neurological disorders	Family history Clinical presentation Spinal tap for abnormal antibodies MRI to identify areas of lesions Evoked potentials to measure conduction time	Clinical presentation Blood screening for antibodies Electromyography to evaluate muscle function Tensilon testing, Ice test, EMG
Treatment	• No curative treatment • Dopaminergic drugs • Treatment of associated symptoms	• No curative treatment • Riluzole, an antiglutamate, prolongs life for months. • Maintain quality of life; Involve family in care	• No curative treatment • Treatment of associated symptoms	No curative treatment Ocrelizumab for primary progressive multiple sclerosis Corticosteroids to reduce acute inflammation Other oral and injectable drugs are available to modify disease progression and suppress immune response for relapsing-remitting multiple sclerosis.	No curative treatment Pyridostigmine to increase acetylcholine and improve muscle strength Corticosteroids and immunosuppressants (i.e., azathioprine, mycophenolate mofetil) to suppress immune response. Intravenous immunoglobulin or plasmapheresis to deplete serum autoantibodies Eculizumab for refractory disease

AchR, Acetylcholine receptor; *CT*, computerized tomography scan; *EMG*, electromyography; *GABA*, gamma-aminobutyric acid; *LMN*, Lower motor neiuron; *MRI*, Magnetic resonance imaging; *MuSK*, muscle-specific kinase; *UMN*, Upper motor neuron.

BOX 17.10 Primary and Secondary Causes of Parkinsonism

Primary Parkinsonism

Sporadic (idiopathic); most common form
Genetic: autosomal dominant; autosomal recessive
Phenotype may be influenced by gene-environment interactions

Secondary Parkinsonism

Neurodegenerative disorders (sporadic or genetic)
- Disorders associated with alpha-synuclein pathology
  - Multiple system atrophies (glial and neuronal inclusions)
    - Nigrostriatal degeneration
    - Olivopontocerebellar atrophy
    - Multiple system atrophy (Shy-Drager syndrome)
    - Motor neuron disease with Parkinson disease (PD) features
  - Dementia with Lewy bodies (cortical and brainstem neuronal inclusions)

Disorders associated with primary tau pathology ("tauopathies")
- Progressive supranuclear palsy
- Corticobasal degeneration
- Frontotemporal dementia

Disorders associated with primary amyloid pathology ("amyloidopathies")
- Alzheimer disease with parkinsonism

Genetically mediated disorders with occasional parkinsonian features
- Wilson disease
- Hallervorden-Spatz disease
- Chédiak-Higashi syndrome
- SCA-3 spinocerebellar ataxia
- X-linked dystonia-parkinsonism *(DYT3)*
- Fragile X permutation associated with ataxia-tremor-parkinsonism syndrome
- Huntington disease (Westphal variant)
- Prion disease
- Rett syndrome

Miscellaneous acquired conditions
- Vascular parkinsonism: atherosclerosis, amyloid angiopathy
- Normal pressure hydrocephalus
- Catatonia
- Cerebral palsy

Repeated head trauma ("dementia pugilistica" with parkinsonian features)

Infectious and postinfectious diseases
- Postencephalitic Parkinson disease
- Creutzfeldt-Jakob disease
- Neurosyphilis

Metabolic conditions
- Hypoparathyroidism or pseudohypoparathyroidism with basal ganglia calcifications
- Nonwilsonian hepatolenticular degeneration

Multiple sclerosis

Neoplastic disease

Drugs
- Neuroleptics (typical antipsychotics)
- Selected atypical antipsychotics
- Antiemetics (e.g., prochlorperazine, metoclopramide)
- Dopamine-depleting agents (reserpine, tetrabenazine)
- α-Methyldopa
- Lithium carbonate
- Valproic acid
- Fluoxetine

Toxins
- 1-Methyl-1,2,4,6-tetrahydropyridine (MPTP)
- Manganese
- Cyanide
- Methanol
- Carbon monoxide
- Carbon disulfide
- Hexane
- Pesticides (i.e., paraquat, rotenone)

Data from Checkoway H, Nielsen SS, Racette BA. Environmental exposures and risks for Parkinson's disease. In: Aschner M, ed. *Environmental factors in neurodevelopmental and neurodegenerative disorders.* Amsterdam: Academic Press; 2015:253–265; Fahn S, Jankovic J, Hallett M. Atypical parkinsonism, parkinsonism-plus syndromes, and secondary parkinsonian disorders. In: Fahn S, Jankovic J, Hallett M, eds. *Principles and practice of movement disorders*, 2nd edition. Philadelphia: Saunders; 2011:197–240; Singer HS, et al., eds. *Movement disorders in childhood*, 2nd edition. Amsterdam: Academic Press; 2016:301–316.

cases in 2020 across North America.[99] Men are much more likely to have PD than women. The familial form represents about 3% to 5% of PD; most cases are sporadic or idiopathic. Secondary parkinsonism is caused by other neurodegenerative diseases and acquired disorders (head trauma, infection, neoplasm, atherosclerosis, toxins, and drug intoxication). Drug-induced parkinsonism, caused by neuroleptics, antiemetics, and antihypertensives, is the most common secondary form and is usually reversible. Box 17.10 summarizes the numerous diseases and contributing factors associated with parkinsonism.

Pathophysiology. The pathogenesis of primary PD is unknown. Several gene mutations have been identified, including those associated with Lewy body (inclusions with high concentrations and abnormal folding of alpha-synuclein and other proteins) dementia. The most significant are listed in Table 17.14, and epigenetic interactions are probable causes of neurodegeneration in PD.[100] Potential environmental risk factors include exposure to pesticides, herbicides, chlorinated solvents, and heavy metals and head injury. The hallmark pathologic features of PD are loss of dopaminergic pigmented neurons in the SN pars compacta with dopaminergic deficiency in the putamen portion of the striatum (the striatum includes the putamen and caudate nucleus) (Fig. 17.27). Dopamine loss in other brain areas, including the brainstem, thalamus, and cortex, also occurs. The primary pathology is degeneration of the basal ganglia (corpus striatum, globus pallidus, subthalamic nucleus, and SN) (Fig. 17.28) with formation of Lewy bodies in the SN and dorsal striatum.

It has been proposed that there is cell-to-cell pathogenic transmission of alpha synuclein through tunneling nanotubes, which induces the formation of Lewy bodies. This transmission is thought to move from the olfactory bulb and from gut axons traveling via the vagus nerve, to the upper brainstem, and to the cortex.[101] Recent studies of the gut microbiome indicate that gut dysbiosis is a cause of synucleinopathies and neuroinflammation, contributing to early manifestations of subtle motor and gastrointestinal symptoms, such as constipation.[102]

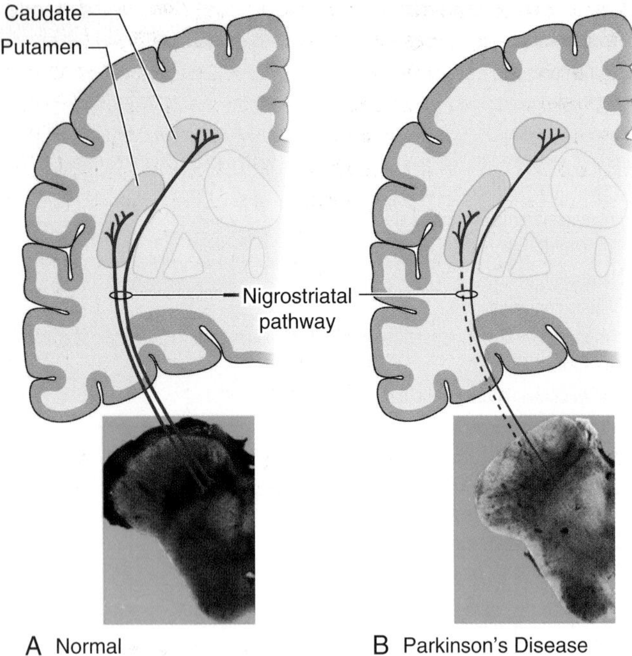

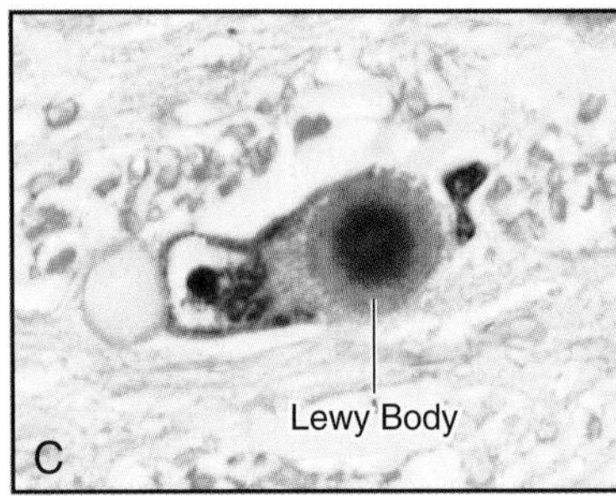

Fig. 17.27 Pathogenesis of Parkinson Disease. (A) Diagram of the normal nigrostriatal pathway projecting from cell bodies in the substantia nigra pars compacta (SNpc) *(photo)*. These neurons project *(thick solid red lines)* to the basal ganglia and synapse in the striatum to the putamen and caudate nucleus. **(B)** There is marked loss of pigmented dopaminergic neurons *(photo)* that project to the putamen *(thin dashed red line)* and a much more modest loss of those that project to the caudate *(thin red solid line)* in the diseased nigrostriatal pathway. Decreased neurotransmission to other neural centers, including the thalamus, primary motor cortex, sensory association areas, and other nerve centers occurs as the disease advances (not shown in this figure). **(C)** A Lewy body stained for alpha synuclein from a dopaminergic neuron in the SNpc. (Diagram from parts A and B and C (Lewy Body) are from Dauer W, Przedbprski S. Parkinson's disease: Mechanisms and models. *Neuron*, 2003;39(6);889–909, Figure. 1. The photos with the green background in Parts A and B are from Cross SS. *Underwood's pathology, a clinical approach*, 7th edition. Livingston: Churchill; 2019. ISBN 978-0-7020-7211-6 [main edition], Figure 26.29.)

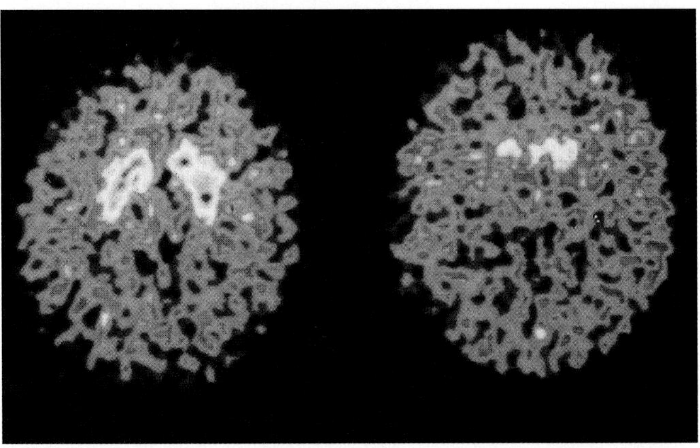

Fig. 17.28 Reduced Fluorodopa in Parkinson Disease. Positron-emission tomography scan showing reduced fluorodopa (a radiotracer) uptake in the striatal basal ganglia consistent with neurodegeneration *(right)* compared with a normal control *(left)*. (From Perkin GD; Miller, DC; Lane, R; Patel, MC; Hochberg, FH. *Atlas of clinical neurology*, 3rd edition. Philadelphia: Saunders; 2011.)

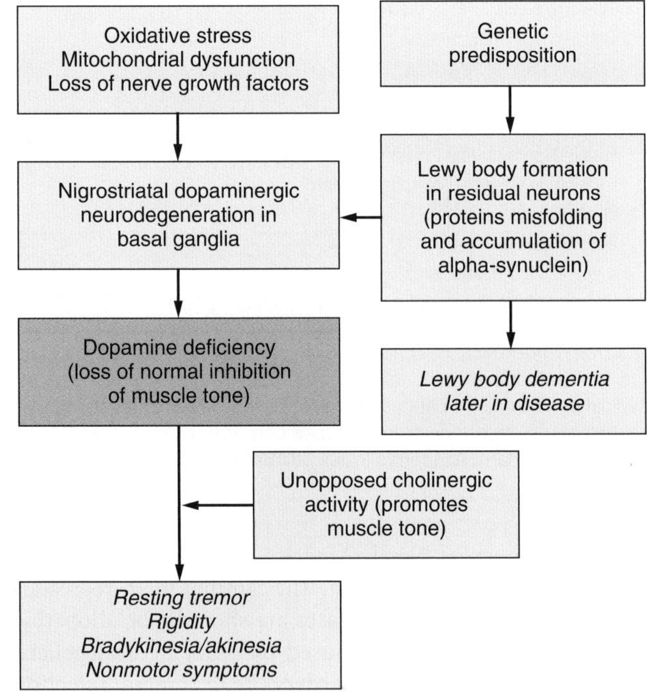

Fig. 17.29 Pathophysiology of Parkinson Disease.

Degeneration of the locus coeruleus (LC), which contains noradrenergic neurons, also occurs in PD. Norepinephrine is thought to be neuroprotective, and loss of LC neurons may be associated with a worsening of disease progression and the behavioral symptoms of PD.[103] Other molecular events thought to be associated with the neurodegeneration of PD include neuroinflammation and mitochondrial oxidative stress.[104] The resulting depletion of dopamine (inhibitory) and relative excess of cholinergic (excitatory) activity in the feedback circuit are manifested by hypertonia (tremor and rigidity) and episodes of akinesia (freezing of movement), producing a syndrome of abnormal movements called parkinsonism (Parkinson syndrome, parkinsonian syndrome, paralysis agitans) (Fig. 17.29). Neuroimaging shows degeneration of dopaminergic neurons preceding the onset of motor symptoms by as long as 3 to 6 years. Dementia may develop over decades with infiltration of Lewy bodies and plaque formation, like AD. Loss of cholinergic subcortical input into the cortex is also associated with nonmotor symptoms of PD.

Clinical Manifestations. The classic manifestations of PD are resting tremor (decreases with voluntary movement), muscular rigidity, bradykinesia/akinesia (slowness of movement and freezing, postural instability and difficulty maintaining balance, dysarthria, and dysphagia). Nonmotor symptoms may precede motor symptoms by up to 20 years.[105] The symptoms may develop alone or in combination, but as the disease progresses, all are usually present. There is no true paralysis. Onset of symptoms is insidious, and symptoms appear after a significant loss of pigmented nigral neurons and striatal dopamine. The symptoms are always bilateral but usually involve one side early in the illness. Because the onset is insidious, the beginning of symptoms is difficult to document; symptoms may evolve and progress over a period of years. Reflex status, sensory status, and mental status usually are normal early in the disease.

Postural abnormalities (flexed, forward leaning), difficulty walking, and weakness develop (i.e., dragging one leg) as neurodegeneration progresses (Fig. 17.30). Disorders of equilibrium result from postural abnormalities. The person with PD is unable to make the appropriate postural adjustment to tilting or falling and falls like a post when starting to tilt. The short, accelerating steps of the person with PD are an attempt to maintain an upright position while walking. Individuals also are unable to right themselves when changing from a reclining or crouching position to a standing position. Speech may be slurred.

Nonmotor symptoms are common. Sleep disorders and excessive daytime sleepiness are commonly experienced. Sensory disturbances (pain and impaired smell and vision), urinary urgency, difficulty concentrating, depression, apathy, and hallucinations are some of the nonmotor symptoms of PD. Autonomic nervous system changes (i.e., alterations in blood pressure, heart rhythm, temperature control, digestion, bladder function, and sexual function) often begin early in the disease process and contribute to nonmotor symptoms. They are summarized in Table 17.25.

Progressive cognitive impairment and dementia are more common in persons older than 70 years with alterations in executive function (concept formation, planning, abstraction, calculations, and judgment) and memory and visuospatial (complex perceptual discrimination and spatial orientation) deficits. Lewy bodies are distributed diffusely within many neurons, causing a Lewy body dementia.[106] Mental status may be further compromised by the side effects of the medication taken to control symptoms. A proposed progression of PD symptoms is summarized in Fig. 17.31.

Evaluation and Treatment. There is no diagnostic marker for sporadic PD, and definitive diagnosis is made by postmortem examination of neural tissue revealing the loss of nigrostriatal dopaminergic neurons and the presence of Lewy bodies within neurons. The clinical diagnosis of PD is based on the history and presenting features of the disease. Causes of secondary parkinsonism are first excluded. Specific gene panels and imaging studies are evolving for early diagnosis and for identifying early

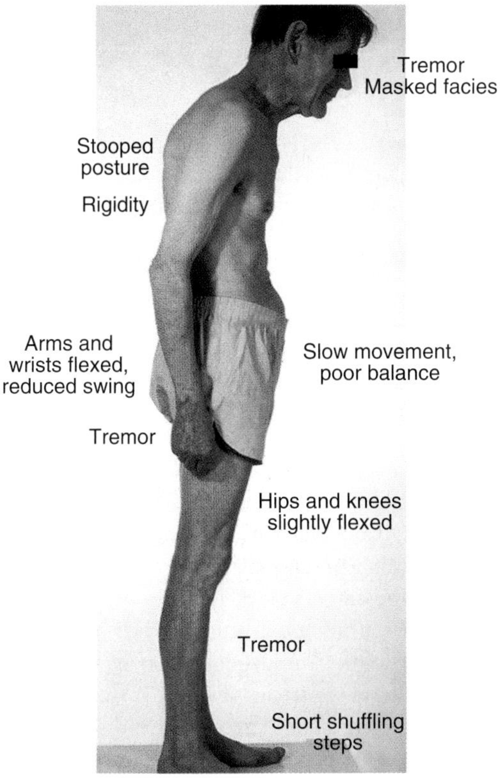

Fig. 17.30 Stooped Posture of Parkinson Disease. (From Perkin DG, et al. *Mosby's color atlas and text of neurology*, 2nd edition. London: Mosby; 2002.)

TABLE 17.25 Non-Motor Signs and Symptoms in Parkinson Disease

Function	Symptoms
Cardiovascular (>80%)	Orthostatic hypotension Supine hypertension Postprandial hypertension "Nondipping" blood pressure[a]
Gastrointestinal	Hypersalivation (>50%) Dysphagia (11%–81%) Gastroparesis (70%–100%) Constipation (20%–70%) Difficult defecation (77%) SIBO (20%–69%)
Thermoregulation	Hyperhidrosis (nocturnal sweating) hypohidrosis
Ocular	Pupillary supersensitivity Tear abnormality
Urinary (27%–85%)	Nocturia, frequency, incontinence
Sexual	Erectile dysfunction/ejaculation abnormality (>50%)

[a]Absence of nocturnal decrease "dip" in blood pressure (compared to mean systolic BP).

SIBO, Small intestine bacterial overgrowth.

Data from Chen Z, Li G, Liu J. Autonomic dysfunction in Parkinson's disease: Implications for pathophysiology, diagnosis, and treatment. *Neurobiology Disease*, 2020;134:104700.

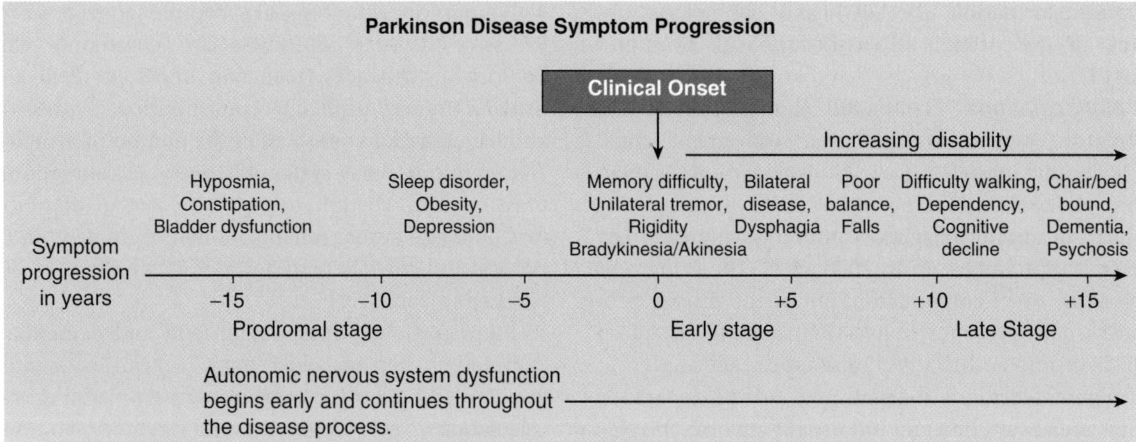

Fig. 17.31 Parkinson Disease Symptom Progression. The progression of Parkinson disease symptoms from onset to death is shown as linear over a period of 30 years, but there is considerable individual variability and likely increasing disability in later years of the disease. Motor and non-motor symptoms are present. (Data from Hawkes CH, Del Tredici K, Braak H. A timeline for Parkinson's disease. *Parkinsonism and Related Disorders*, 2010;16(2):79–84; Tolosa E, Garrido A, Scholz SW, et al. Challenges in the diagnosis of Parkinson's disease. *Lancet Neurology*, 2021;20(5):385–397.)

stages of structural and functional areas of brain changes.[107] Prodromal nonmotor symptoms of PD can precede motor symptoms (constipation, loss of smell, and sleep disorders), and their identification may assist early diagnosis and guide disease-modifying strategies. Biomarkers are being tested for early identification of prodromal disease.[108] Imaging techniques are being developed for identifying early stages of the disease and structural and functional areas of brain changes.[107]

Treatment of PD is symptomatic, with drug therapy to protect or restore striatal dopamine levels and decrease akinesia and manage nonmotor symptoms. Levodopa is first-line treatment and is generally well tolerated. ChE-Is may be helpful for MCI or dementia.[109] Deep brain stimulation (i.e., subthalamic neurostimulation) is replacing surgery to treat persons unresponsive to drug therapy. Implants of stem cells and fetal cells, as well as gene therapy and immunotherapy, are strategies for future treatments.[110,111] Nonmotor symptoms and general immobility are special problems requiring interdisciplinary efforts to improve functional status.[112]

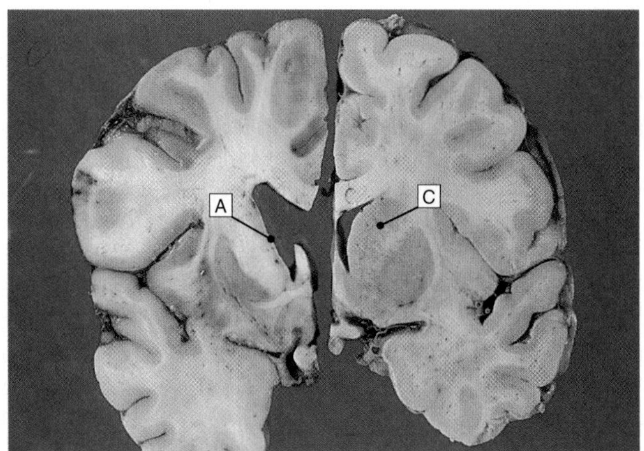

Fig. 17.32 Huntington Disease. On the right is a normal brain with a normal caudate *(C)*; on the left is a brain from an individual with Huntington disease showing severe atrophy of the caudate *(A)* and an enlarged lateral ventricle. (From Stevens A, Lowe J, Scott I. *Core pathology*, 3rd edition. London: Mosby; 2009.)

Huntington Disease

HD, also known as ***chorea***, is a relatively rare, hereditary, degenerative hyperkinetic movement disorder diffusely involving the basal ganglia and cerebral cortex. The onset of HD is usually between 25 and 45 years of age, when the trait may already have been passed to the person's children. The disease may progress for 10 to 25 years. The disorder has a prevalence rate of approximately 5 to 10 per 100,000 persons, occurs in all races, and rates vary in different regions across the world.[113]

Pathophysiology. HD is inherited from one or both parents who have the autosomal dominant trait with high penetrance. The genetic defect of HD is on the short arm of chromosome 4. There is an abnormally long polyglutamine tract in the huntingtin (HTT) protein with abnormal folding that is toxic to neurons caused by a cytosine-adenine-guanine (CAG) trinucleotide repeat expansion (40 to 70 repeats instead of 9 to 34). Age of symptom onset is related to the length of the repeat sequences and mechanisms of toxicity. Repeat lengths greater than 60 cause the juvenile form of the disease. Individuals with fewer CAG repeats develop disease symptoms when they are older and have a slower disease progression. Fathers, but not mothers, with high normal alleles do not develop HD but are at risk of transmitting potentially penetrant HD alleles (≥36) to their offspring, who can develop HD.[114]

The principal pathologic feature of HD is severe degeneration of the striatum. The degeneration of the basal ganglia leaves enlarged lateral ventricles (Fig. 17.32), and there is widespread degeneration in late stages of the disease. Expression of the *huntingtin* gene produces tangles of protein that collect in brain cells and chains of glutamine on the abnormal molecules that adhere to each other. The mechanism of neuronal death is unknown. The excitotoxic theory of striatal and cortical degeneration proposes that the mutated HTT protein produces excitotoxic pathways mediated by glutamate function that also induce concomitant dysregulation of dopaminergic function. Lysosomal autophagy is disrupted, resulting in accumulation of misfolded proteins. The HTT protein also alters cellular organelles, including mitochondrial function, axon transport, and synapses. Apoptotic pathways may be activated and cause neuronal death. Neurotrophic factors also may be depleted, and oxidative stress and inflammation likely contribute to loss of neurons and neurodegeneration.[115]

Clinical Manifestations. Symptoms of HD progress slowly through three stages. During the early stage, there are few symptoms, as there is adaptation to the slowly accumulating amounts of the HTT protein. During the middle stage, there are progressive motor symptoms, including involuntary fragmentary movements, such as chorea, athetosis, and ballism (see Table 17.23). Chorea, the most common type of abnormal movement, begins in the face and arms, eventually affecting the entire body. There is emotional lability and progressive dysfunction of intellectual and thought processes that may precede motor symptoms. Cognitive deficits include loss of working memory and reduced capacity to plan, organize, and sequence. Thinking is slow, and apathy is present. Any one of these features may mark the onset of the disease. Restlessness, disinhibition, and irritability are common. Euphoria or depression may be present. During late stages, chorea decreases and is replaced by rigidity, dystonia, and bradykinesia (Parkinsonian symptoms). The individual may be unable to talk, is bedridden, and requires help with all activities of daily living.[116]

Evaluation and Treatment. The diagnosis of HD is based on family history, clinical presentation of the disorder, and genetic testing. Neuroradiologic abnormalities can be demonstrated up to 15 years before clinical symptoms. No known treatment is effective in halting the degeneration or progression of symptoms, and the disease is fatal. Efforts are underway to identify biomarkers for early diagnosis and to monitor disease progression and treatment effectiveness. Symptomatic drug therapies are available, and HTT protein lowering therapies are being developed.[117]

Amyotrophic Lateral Sclerosis

ALS (also known as *motor neuron disease or* ***Lou Gehrig disease***) is a severe degenerative disorder with loss of lower and upper motor neurons resulting in progressive muscle weakness, paralysis, and death. *Amyotrophic* (without muscle nutrition and progressive muscle wasting) refers to the LMN component of the syndrome. *Lateral sclerosis*, scarring of the spinal cord, refers to the upper motor neuron component of the syndrome. Other brain systems become involved as the disease progresses, including cortical projections to subcortical structures leading to extra-motor deficits such as cognitive-behavioral disturbances, impaired ocular movements, and extrapyramidal alterations.[118] Thus, ALS is a multimodal systemic disorder, and currently, there are no biomarkers for predicting the onset and course of the disease.[119]

ALS may begin at any time from the fourth decade of life; its median age of onset is between 51 and 66 years of age, with about 5.2 cases per 100,000 persons in the United States. The prevalence is higher in individuals who are assigned male at birth. The prevalence of ALS is also much higher in individuals who are White compared to other ethnic groups.[120] Most cases of ALS are sporadic or simplex cases (an individual with ALS with no other familial occurrence of the disease). A subset (about 10% to 20%) has the familial form with four common genetic mutations in C9ORF72 (chromosome 9 open reading frame 72), superoxide dismutase *(SODI)*, and fused in sarcoma *(FUS)* that contribute to the neurotoxicity of proteins affecting motor neurons. Mutated TAR RNA-binding protein 43 (*TDP-43*-important for RNA processing and synthesis of cell proteins) is a major constituent of the toxic ubiquitinated protein inclusions found in motor neurons and glial cells. More than 30 ALS-associated genes have been identified, adding to the complexity of the disease. Onset is earlier in individuals with familial ALS.[121] Genetic testing is available for familial ALS.

Pathophysiology. The cause of ALS is unknown. Risk factors for ALS include age, male sex, and familial history. Environmental risk factors including smoking, BMI, and exercise; occupational and environmental exposures to toxins, head injuries, and viral infections are being examined. Nucleocytoplasmic transport defects, dysfunctional RNA metabolism, protein aggregation, impaired DNA repair, mitochondrial dysfunction and oxidative stress, impaired axonal transport, vesicular transport deficits, neuroinflammation, glutamate excitotoxicity, and oligodendrocyte dysfunction are some of the pathogenic mechanisms being investigated.[122] The principal pathologic feature of ALS is degeneration and death of upper and LMNs, including the neuromuscular junction (NMJ). Cortical hyperexcitability is an important early mechanism in the pathology of ALS, especially when evaluating neurodegeneration and disease progression. The mechanisms leading to enhanced neuronal intrinsic excitability and changes in excitatory and inhibitory synaptic activity are starting to be understood. Initially, ALS was thought to originate in the LMNs at the myoneuronal junction from pathologic activation of complement proteins and was erroneously classified as a neuromuscular disease. The disease then advanced from LMNs to the CNS. This process was called the dying back hypothesis. However, with advances in neuroimaging, the dying forward hypothesis is now widely accepted. The dying forward hypothesis states that ALS originates in the cortical motor neurons and mediate anterograde motor neuron degeneration due to glutamate excitotoxicity and accumulation of TDP-43, and advances to LMNs (Fig. 17.33). ALS is also now known to be a neurodegenerative disease, not a neuromuscular disease, that causes multisystem dysfunction.[123–125]

The accumulation of microscopic protein aggregates (e.g., *TDP-43* proteinopathy) in neurons and glia associated with degeneration of the primary motor cortex and motor cortex-spinal cord axis varies by cell pattern and genotype and may have implications for targeted therapy.[126] However, the source of neurotoxic molecules leading to neurodegeneration is still not clearly understood.[127] As the disease progresses, there is a decrease in large motor neurons in the spinal cord, brainstem, and cerebral cortex (premotor and motor areas) with ongoing degeneration in the remaining motor neurons. The nuclei of

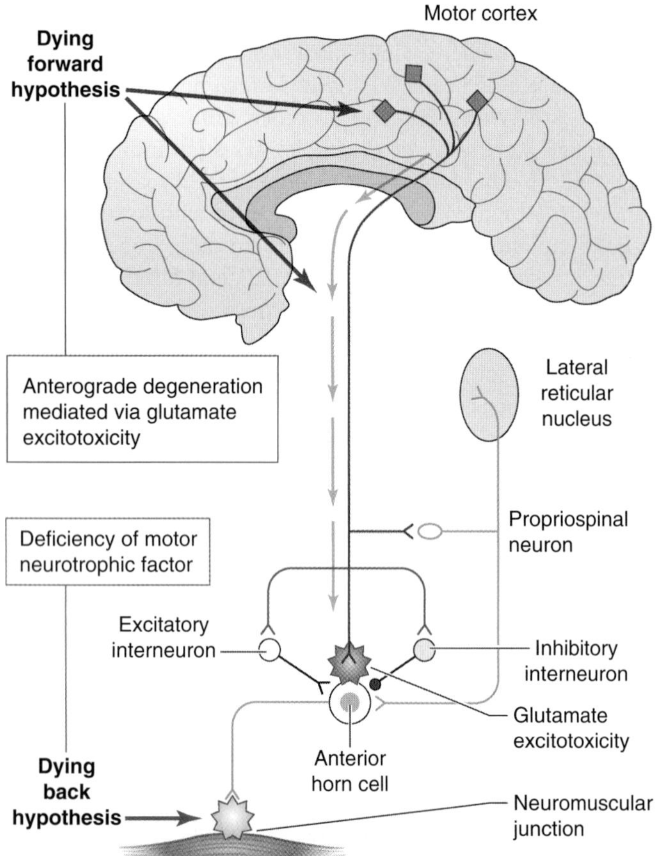

Fig. 17.33 The dying forward *(red arrows)* and dying back hypotheses *(blue arrow)* of amyotrophic lateral sclerosis pathogenesis. *NMJ,* Neuromuscular junction. (Reprinted with permission from Elsevier (From Kiernan MC, Vucic S, Cheah BC, et al. Amyotrophic lateral sclerosis. *The Lancet* 2011; 377(9769), 942–955. https://doi.org/10.1016/s0140-6736(10)61156-7.)

cranial nerves III, IV, and VI usually are not involved. Death of the motor neuron results in axonal degeneration and secondary demyelination with glial proliferation and sclerosis (scarring) along the corticospinal tract. However, there also is widespread neural degeneration of nonmotor neurons in the spinal cord and motor cortices, as well as in the premotor, sensory, and temporal cortices. Altered astrocyte function, activated microglia, and edema are seen to occur. Metabolic dysfunction is also common, causing weight loss, hypermetabolism, and hyperlipidemia, all of which suggest that ALS is a systemic disease. Hypermetabolism may also be associated with increased mitochondrial energy production, leading to large amounts of cytotoxic oxygen reactive species.[128] LMN degeneration denervates motor units. Adjacent, still-viable LMNs attempt to compensate by distal intramuscular sprouting, reinnervation, and enlargement of motor units.

Clinical Manifestations. Presentation of symptoms can be variable among individuals because of the numerous genes and multiple systems involved. The initial onset of ALS can be subtle, with cramping or weakness that affects a limb, incoordination, slurring of speech, and difficulty swallowing. About 70% to 75% of individuals have spinal ALS, with focal muscle weakness beginning in the arms and legs and progressing to muscle wasting and atrophy, spasticity, and loss of manual dexterity and gait (Fig. 17.34). The other 25% to 30% of individuals with ALS experience bulbar onset, with symptoms such as dysarthria, dysphagia, and dysphonia. Bulbar onset disease has a more rapid and progressive course. No associated sensory or autonomic symptoms are present. Muscle weakness in ALS exhibits the following characteristics:

1. Paresis usually begins in a single muscle group.
2. Corresponding muscle groups are asymmetrically affected in a mottled distribution.
3. Gradual involvement occurs in all striated muscles, except extraocular and heart muscles, and progresses to paralysis with no remissions.
4. Flaccid and spastic paresis may coexist in a single muscle group; flaccid paresis may mask spasticity, which is usually mild.
5. Urethral and anal sphincter weakness is uncommon.

The LMN syndrome of flaccid paresis consists of weakness of individual muscles, progressing to paralysis, associated with hypotonia and primary muscle atrophy (i.e., atrophy caused by denervation). Hypotonia is manifested by (1) decreased resistance to passive movement, (2) hypoactive or absent deep tendon reflexes, (3) absent abdominal and cremasteric reflexes, and (4) absent Babinski sign. Primary atrophy is manifested by (1) severe, irreversible muscular wasting; (2) fasciculations and fibrillation; (3) metabolically related changes in the skin and appendages; and (4) specific electromyographic (EMG) findings. Metabolic changes include: (1) thinning of the skin, (2) thickening of the nails, (3) loss of body hair, and (4) decreased perspiration.

The upper motor neuron syndrome of spastic paresis consists of weakness of movement patterns, progressing to paralysis, associated with spasticity, and, in some cases, atrophy secondary to disuse. Spasticity is manifested by (1) clasp-knife phenomenon, evident with passive movement; (2) hyperactive deep tendon reflexes and clonus with severe spasticity; (3) absent abdominal and cremasteric reflexes; and (4) presence of Babinski sign. A subset of individuals also demonstrates extrapyramidal symptoms with difficulty initiating gait and postural instability.[129]

The coexistence of FTD dementia and ALS has been demonstrated and has been found to be related to common gene mutations. Cognitive impairment due to FTD occurs in around 50% of ALS (spinal and bulbar onset) individuals and can cause executive dysfunction, behavior changes, and language deficits.[130,131] A summary of upper and lower motor and extramotor signs and symptoms is presented in Table 17.26.

Evaluation and Treatment. The diagnosis of ALS is based predominantly on medical history and physical examination with no evidence of other neuromuscular disorders. Transcranial magnetic stimulation, electromyography, and muscle biopsy results can verify cortical hyperexcitability, LMN degeneration, and denervation. Imaging studies and cerebrospinal fluid biomarkers can assist in making the diagnosis. Neurofilament light chains, found in the cerebrospinal fluid after motor neuron damage, may be a promising biomarker and prognostic tool as it correlates with disease severity.[132]

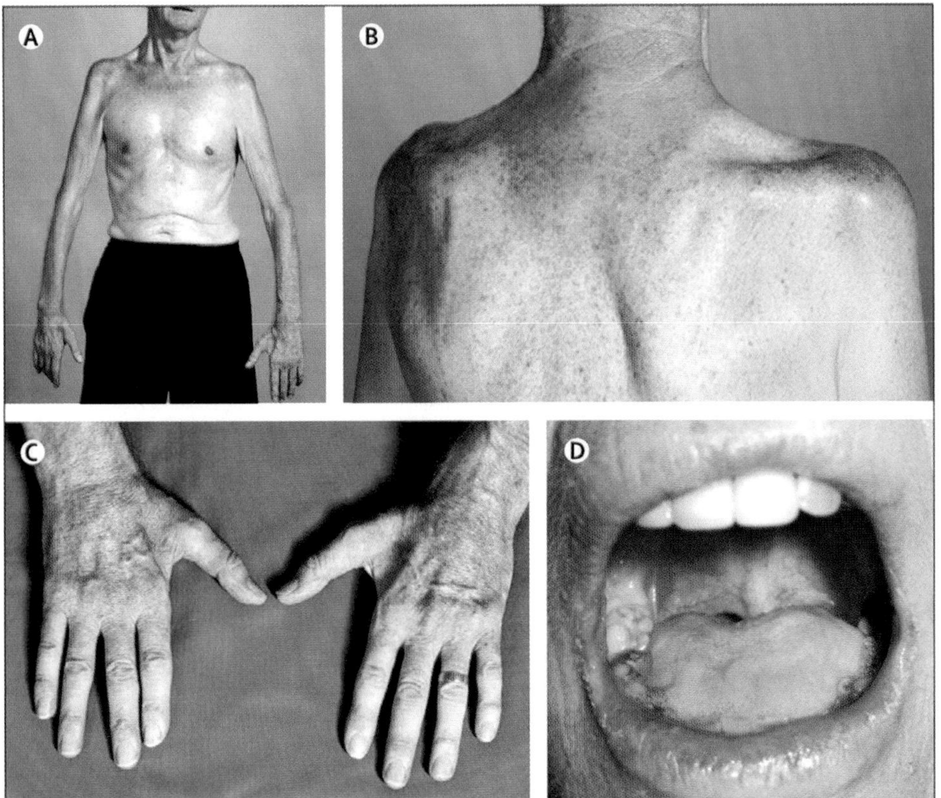

Fig. 17.34 Muscle Wasting and Amyotrophic Lateral Sclerosis. (A) Symmetrical upper limb wasting results in an inability to lift arms against gravity ("man-in-the-barrel" or flail-arm variant amyotrophic lateral sclerosis [ALS]). **(B)** Wasting of supraspinatus and infraspinatus muscles, as well as substantial loss of deltoid muscle. The glenohumeral joint becomes prominent, and prone to subluxation. **(C)** Disproportionate wasting of the thenar muscles combined with the first dorsal interossei, the so-called "split-hand," is a typical feature in ALS. **(D)** Substantial wasting of the tongue muscles in bulbar-onset ALS. Note the absence of palatal elevation present on vocalization. Difficulty with mouth opening and dysphagia might require supplementary feeding through a percutaneous endoscopic gastrostomy. (Reprinted with permission from Elsevier (From Kiernan MC, Vucic S, Cheah BC, et al. Amyotrophic lateral sclerosis. *The Lancet* 2011; 377(9769), 942–955. https://doi.org/10.1016/s0140-6736(10)61156-7.)

Riluzole (Rilutek), an antiglutamate, was the first drug approved by the Food and Drug Administration (FDA) for treatment of ALS. It is an oral medication and prolongs life for about 3 months. The mechanism of action is a decreased uptake of glutamate and neuromuscular excitation. In 2017, the FDA approved a second treatment, Edaravone (Radicava), to treat ALS. Edaravone is an antioxidant and free radical scavenger thought to reduce oxidative stress and neuronal death. It is administered intravenously and delays progression of the disease. Dextromethorphan-Quinidine (Neudexta) is an FDA-approved symptom management drug that helps bulbar symptoms, such as swallowing, hypersalivation, and speaking. Clinical trials are in progress for evaluation of gene therapy, immunotherapy, and targeted drug therapy.[133–135] Supportive and rehabilitation management is directed at relief of symptoms, prevention of complications, maintenance of maximal function, and maintenance of optimal quality of life. Special problems requiring preventive and symptomatic management are communication difficulties caused by dysmasesis and dysphonia, salivation problems with either thick saliva or excessively thin saliva (sialorrhea), and dyspnea caused by diaphragmatic and intercostal weakness. Ventilatory issues become prominent. Mobility and safety needs related to ambulation and activities of daily living must also be addressed. Psychologic support of the affected individual and the family is extremely important in this disorder. ALS is fatal from respiratory failure, usually within 2 to 5 years of diagnosis. A small percentage of individuals live 5 years or longer.[136]

Demyelinating Disorders

Demyelinating disorders are the result of damage to the myelin nerve sheath and affect neural transmission. They can occur in either the central (i.e., MS) or the peripheral (i.e., GBS) nervous system. Contributing factors include genetics, infections, autoimmune reactions, environmental toxins, and unknown factors.

Multiple Sclerosis

MS is a chronic immune-mediated inflammatory disease involving degeneration of CNS myelin, scarring (sclerosis or plaque formation), and loss of axons. MS is caused by an autoimmune response to self or microbial antigens in genetically susceptible individuals. The etiology of MS is unknown. The onset of MS is usually between 20 and 40 years of age and is more common in women. Men may have a more severe progressive course.

TABLE 17.26 Clinical Signs and Symptoms of Amyotrophic Lateral Sclerosis

Spinal Onset	Bulbar Onset
Upper Motor Neuron	*Upper Motor Neuron*
Weakness and slow movement	Slow speech
Spasticity and loss of dexterity	Hyperactive reflexes
Babinski sign	Palmomental reflex
Hoffman sign	Jaw jerk reflex
Lower Motor Neuron	*Lower Motor Neuron*
Weakness	Facial weakness
Muscle atrophy	Low palatal elevation
Fasciculations	Dysarthria Tongue fasciculations Tongue atrophy
EXTRAPYRAMIDAL SIGNS Tremors, akinesia Postural disturbances Gait difficulty Rigidity	
EXTRA-MOTOR SIGNS Pain Fatigue Paresthesias Depression	
FRONTO-TEMPORAL DEMENTIA Personality change Behavioral abnormalities Language dysfunction Memory impairment	

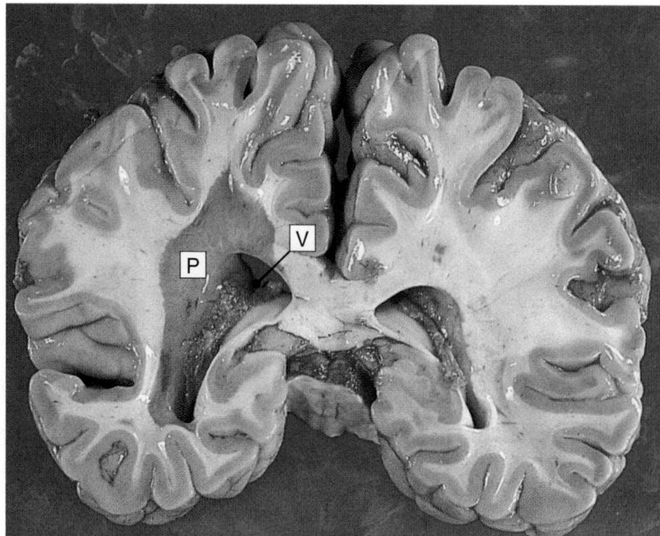

Fig. 17.35 Multiple Sclerosis (Gross). Seen here in periventricular white matter is a large "plaque" *(P)* of demyelination that has a sharp border with adjacent normal white matter. Such plaques have a gray-tan appearance and are typically associated with the clinical appearance of transient or progressive loss of neurologic function in multiple sclerosis (MS). Because MS is often multifocal, and the lesions appear in various white matter locations in the central nervous system over time, the clinical course and findings can be quite varied. *V*, ventricle. (From Stevens A, Lowe J, Scott, IS. *Core pathology*, 3rd edition. London: Mosby; 2009.)

The prevalence rate is higher in northern latitudes and areas with lack of sun exposure. Inconclusive risk factors that may be involved include a gene-environment interaction including factors such as smoking, vitamin D deficiency, obesity, and Epstein-Barr virus infection.[137,138] Life expectancy is not greatly altered by MS, and the disease course often extends over 30 years.

Pathophysiology. MS is a diffuse and progressive CNS autoimmune inflammatory disease that affects white and gray matter throughout the brain and spinal cord. There are multiple focal areas of myelin loss within the CNS called *plaques.* The plaques form when autoreactive T cells and B cells cross the blood–brain barrier into the brain and spinal cord. T cells recognize myelin as autoantigens and attack it. B cells produce myelin-specific antibodies, which are recognized by glial cells (macrophages). Activated glial cells engulf the antibodies, damaging the myelin. These attacks on myelin leave patches disrupting neurotransmission. With resolution of inflammation (a period of remission), the injury leaves a glial scar or sclerosis, the classic lesion of MS (Fig. 17.35). During early stages oligodendrocytes (myelin-producing cells) repair myelin. With progressive attacks, oligodendrocytes are also injured and lost. The loss of oligodendrocytes prevents remyelination, and over time the injury is irreversible with loss of axons (Fig. 17.36). Loss of myelin disrupts nerve conduction, leading to symptom presentation. There is at least partial myelin repair during relapse of symptoms. Ultimately there is death of neurons and brain atrophy in the most progressive forms of the disease. *Spinal MS* can occur concurrently with or independently of brain lesions. The multifocal, multistage features of MS lesions produce symptoms that are multiple and variable. Thus, inflammation, demyelination, myelin repair, loss of oligodendrocytes, and scar formation distinguish MS from other demyelinating disorders of the CNS.[139]

Clinical Manifestations. The onset, duration, and severity of symptoms are different for each person and depend on the location and extent of disease. A *clinically isolated syndrome* of neurologic symptoms that lasts 24 hours or less may initially occur. It can be related to inflammation and demyelination but may never progress to develop into MS. There is no evidence of previous episodes of demyelination. Work is in progress to identify the prodromal symptoms of MS more specifically.[140]

MS develops when symptoms last more than 24 hours; occur in the absence of fever, infection, or encephalopathy; and are caused by inflammation and demyelination in the CNS. The subtypes of MS are based on the clinical course and are summarized in Table 17.27. The most common initial symptoms of MS are paresthesia of the face, trunk, or limbs; weakness; impaired gait; or urinary incontinence, indicating diffuse CNS involvement. Monofocal symptoms are caused by a single lesion and include optic neuritis, spinal cord syndrome, and brainstem and cerebellar syndromes. *Optic neuritis* is a common presentation in one eye with progressive blurring of vision and pain

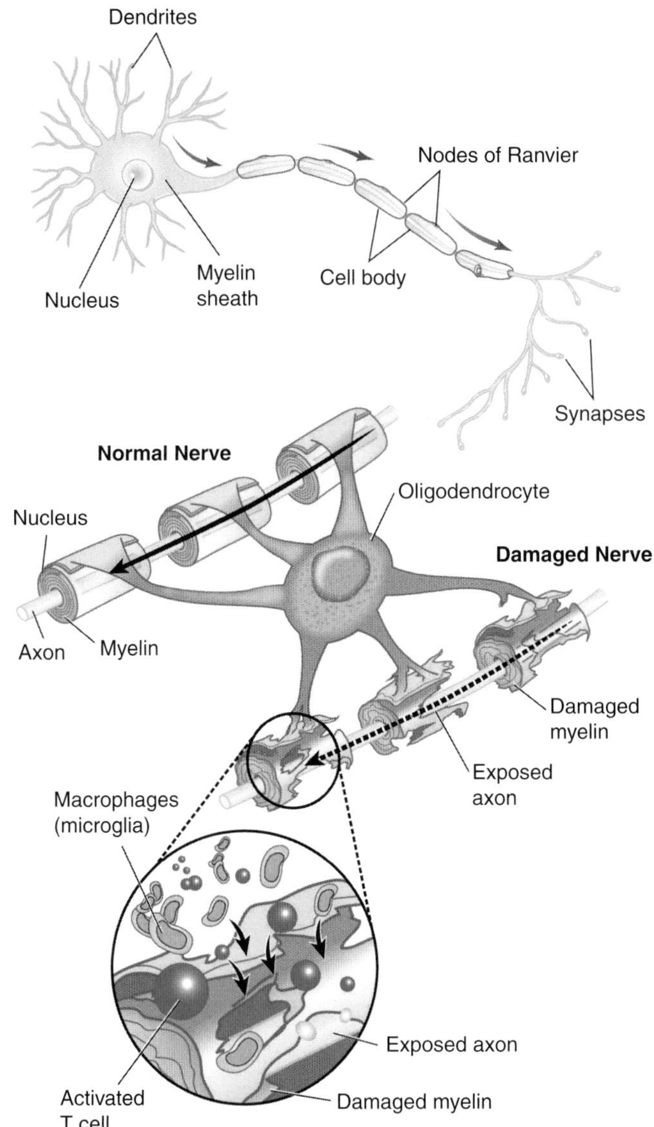

Fig. 17.36 Pathogenesis of Multiple Sclerosis.

with eye movement. *Spinal cord syndrome* is common and can involve both sensory and motor tracks starting on one side and progressing to the other. *Brainstem syndromes* can involve facial sensory loss or weakness, vertigo, or double vision. *Cerebellar syndromes* demonstrate lack of coordination, intention tremor, gait instability, ataxia, and nystagmus.

Lesions in the cerebrum present as hemifacial weakness, pain, and motor impairments. Cognitive deficits, including memory and attention problems, are common later in the disease, as well as emotional liability psychiatric disorders, depression, and dementia. Most persons present with a remitting-relapsing course and without treatment transition to the progressive types with insidious neurologic decline that occurs over years. After years of disease, 50% of individuals appear to have established syndromes of multifocal involvement.

Disease exacerbations (also known as *relapses* or *flares*) are the temporary occurrence or worsening of symptoms. The symptoms may be mild or serious, may last for several days or weeks, and may be followed by progressive symptoms, including paresthesia, difficulty speaking, ataxia, or visual changes. The mechanism of these exacerbations is related to delayed or blocked conduction caused by inflammation and demyelination. Various events can occur immediately before the exacerbation of symptoms and are regarded as precipitating factors or triggers, including trauma, emotional stress, and pregnancy. Painful sensory events, spastic paralysis, and bowel and bladder incontinence are common with spinal involvement.

Recovery from symptoms during remissions is caused by down-regulation of inflammation and the restoration of axonal function, either by remyelination, the resolution of inflammation, or the restoration of conduction to demyelinated axons. Pregnancy does not appear to alter the course of MS. Symptoms improve in some cases and may be related to the immune tolerance that develops during pregnancy.[141] There are no specific markers for early detection of disease or disability progression.[142] Disability progression is evaluated by the Expanded Disability Status Scale and components of the MS Functional Composite (timed 25-foot walk, 9-hole peg test, low-contrast visual acuity, symbol digit modalities test).[143,144]

Evaluation and Treatment. There is no single test available to diagnose or rule out MS. Diagnostic criteria include history, clinical examination, CSF findings, and evoked potentials in combination with MRI (most sensitive test for detecting demyelinated plaque, disease progression [new lesions], and treatment response).[145,146] Clinical symptoms include neurologic findings not attributable to another diagnosis with two or more episodes lasting at least 24 hours and occurring at least 1 month apart. Persistently elevated levels of CSF immunoglobulin G (IgG) are found in about two-thirds of individuals with MS, and oligoclonal IgG bands on electrophoresis are found in more than 90% of individuals with MS. Evoked potential studies aid diagnosis by detecting decreased conduction velocity in visual, auditory, and somatosensory pathways. The 2017 revisions of the McDonald criteria are used to guide diagnosis.[145]

The treatment goal in MS is prevention of exacerbations, prevention of permanent neurologic damage, and control of symptoms. Disease-modifying drugs are initiated with diagnosis and include corticosteroids, immunosuppressants, and immune system modulators.[147] Continuous monitoring is important because of the increased risk for infection when taking these drugs. Plasma exchange may be used in persons who do not respond to steroids. Drugs are also available for symptom control. Supportive care includes participation in a regular exercise program, cessation of smoking, and avoidance of overwork, extreme fatigue, and heat exposure. The administration of vitamin D to prevent disease progression has found no therapeutic effect, and further clinical trials are needed.[148] New treatments are becoming available, including stem cell transplantation and monoclonal antibodies.[149,150]

Guillain-Barré Syndrome

GBS is a rare demyelinating disorder caused by a humoral (antibody) and cell-mediated immunologic reaction directed at the peripheral nerves. There is a demyelinating subtype known as acute inflammatory demyelinating polyneuropathy

TABLE 17.27 **Types of Multiple Sclerosis**

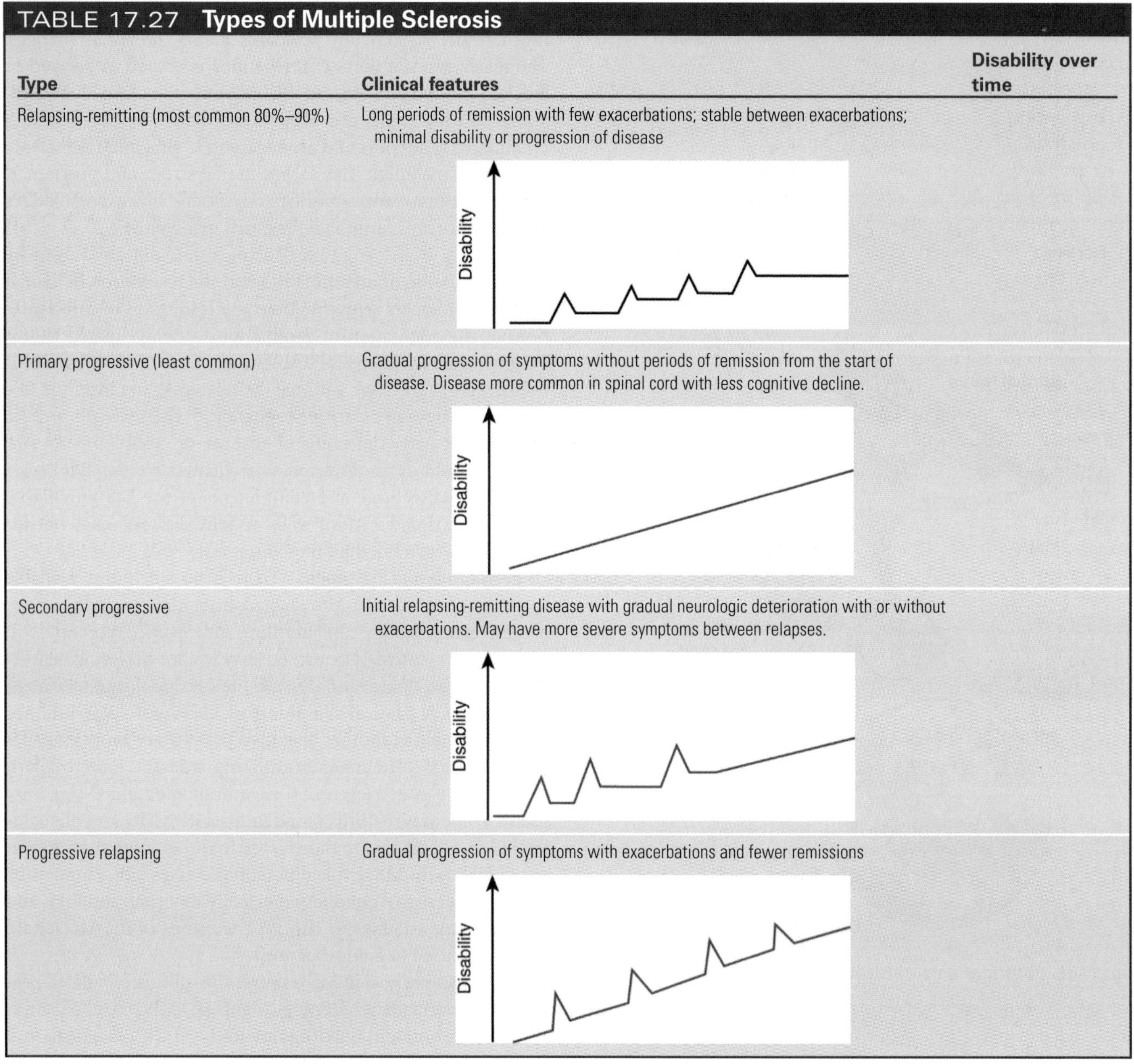

Type	Clinical features	Disability over time
Relapsing-remitting (most common 80%–90%)	Long periods of remission with few exacerbations; stable between exacerbations; minimal disability or progression of disease	
Primary progressive (least common)	Gradual progression of symptoms without periods of remission from the start of disease. Disease more common in spinal cord with less cognitive decline.	
Secondary progressive	Initial relapsing-remitting disease with gradual neurologic deterioration with or without exacerbations. May have more severe symptoms between relapses.	
Progressive relapsing	Gradual progression of symptoms with exacerbations and fewer remissions	

ADIP and an axonal subtype known as acute motor axonal neuropathy (AMAN—absence of sensory involvement). GBS usually occurs within 4 weeks after a respiratory tract or gastrointestinal infection and has been associated with surgery, immunization, immune check point inhibitors, and infections, including *Campylobacter jejuni*, the Zika virus, and the severe acute respiratory syndrome coronavirus 2 (SARS-CoV-2).[151] In axonal forms of GBS, it is proposed that molecular mimicry of pathogen-borne antigens (i.e., *C. jejuni*) leads to the generation of cross-reactive antibodies that target axonal gangliosides at nodes of Ranvier, activate complement, and disrupt nerve conduction in peripheral motor nerves.[152] Supportive diagnostic studies include evaluation of blood serum, cerebrospinal fluid, and electromyography.[153]

The clinical manifestations can vary from tingling and weakness to ascending flaccid paralysis starting in the legs and progressing to complete quadriplegia, respiratory insufficiency, and autonomic nervous system instability (low blood pressure and arrhythmias). Diagnostic criteria include progressive weakness of more than two limbs, areflexia, and progression for no more than 4 weeks. Intravenous immunoglobulin or plasmapheresis is used during the acute phase with respiratory support as needed, followed by aggressive rehabilitation. Targeted immunotherapy to human complement is under investigation. Recovery occurs within weeks to months or up to 2 years. Approximately 20% of individuals have residual weakness.[153]

Neuromuscular Junction Disorders

Motor function requires the transmission of the nerve impulse at the NMJ with the release of adequate amounts of neurotransmitter from the presynaptic terminals of the axon and effective binding of the released transmitter to the receptors on the membranes of muscle cells (see Fig. 15.14). Alterations in the amount or function of the neurotransmitter or the receptors affects motor function.

Neuromuscular junction disorders (NMJDs), whose pathogenesis is caused by autoantibodies, include MG and the rare pre-synaptic Lambert-Eaton myasthenic syndrome. In addition, there are rare inherited (congenital) myasthenic syndromes that result from mutations in different key proteins for the postsynaptic nicotinic acetylcholine receptor, ion channels, and motor end plates at the NMJ. Details related to those disorders are not included here.

Myasthenia Gravis

MG is an acquired chronic autoimmune disease mediated by antibodies against the acetylcholine receptor (AChR) at the postsynaptic membrane of the NMJ. About 14 to 40 per 100,000 people in the United States have the disease. It is more common in women at ages 20 to 30 years and more common in men over 60 years.[154]

MG is associated with an increased incidence of thymomas and other autoimmune diseases, including systemic lupus erythematosus, rheumatoid arthritis, polymyositis, and thyrotoxicosis. (Autoimmune mechanisms are discussed in Chapter 9.) About 27% of family members have autoimmune diseases. The etiology of MG is unknown, and the disease is usually sporadic. Some persons have genetic susceptibility related to variants in AchR genes, as well as the major histocompatibility genes, and they can present with varying clinical phenotypes.[155]

Presynaptic autoimmune diseases are rare and include Lambert-Eaton myasthenic syndrome. There are autoantibodies to calcium channels on presynaptic nerve terminals, which presents with more leg and arm weakness and is commonly associated with small-cell lung carcinoma (Fig. 17.37).[156]

Pathophysiology. MG is a T cell-dependent, B-cell mediated autoimmune disease (type II hypersensitivity) caused by IgG antibodies against nicotinic acetylcholine receptors (AchR) (80%–90% of cases) in the postsynaptic membrane at the NMJ. The autoantibodies destroy the AchR receptor sites through antibody-mediated complement activation and formation of membrane attack complex or block Ach attachment to the membrane receptor. The consequence is diminished transmission of nerve impulses across the NMJ (see Fig. 17.37). Muscle depolarization is incomplete or unsuccessful and leads to muscle weakness. The cause of this autosensitization is unknown. Thymic abnormalities are common with hyperplasia of germinal centers, where T cells interact with B cells to produce antibodies. There is breakdown in self-tolerance leading to immune-mediated destruction of the AChR. This is more common in women with early-onset disease. About 10% to 20% of individuals with MG develop thymoma, and about 30% of individuals with thymoma develop MG.[157,158]

In some types of MG, antibodies are directed against other components of the NMJ. About 10% to 15% of individuals with MG do not have AchR antibodies on testing but have MuSK antibodies (an IgG4 subtype). This is now subtyped as MuSK antibody–associated MG, which is not complement-mediated.

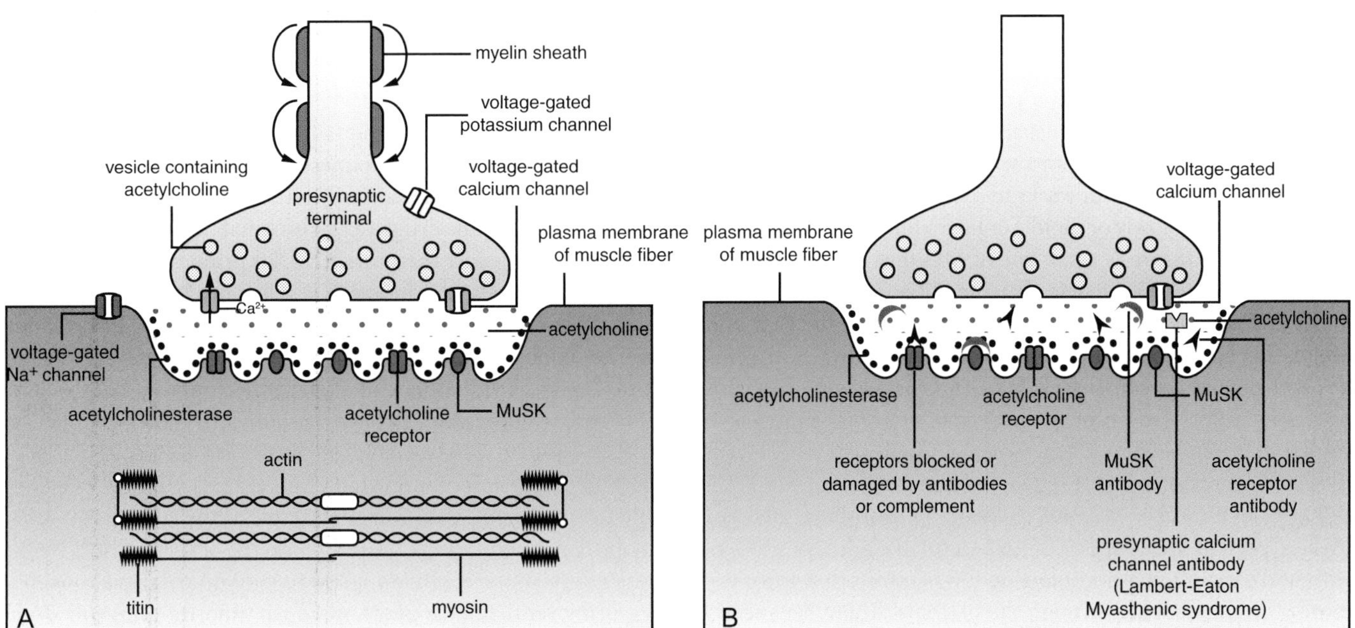

Fig. 17.37 Antibodies and Myasthenia Gravis. Schematic diagrams of **(A)** a normal neuromuscular junction illustrating locations of the presynaptic vesicles, acetylcholine within the synapse, and the postsynaptic acetylcholine receptors, as well as **(B)** a neuromuscular junction affected by myasthenia gravis, with antibodies that interfere with the binding or structure, or both, of the acetylcholine receptors and muscle-specific kinase (MuSK). (Note that antibodies to both proteins are not typically present in the same individual, though this phenomenon has been reported on occasion.) Presynaptic calcium channel antibodies occur with Lambert-Eaton myasthenic syndrome. (From Darras BT, et al. *Neuromuscular disorders of infancy, childhood, and adolescence*, 2nd edition. London: Academic Press; 2015.)

It is more common in females in their 40 s and affects individuals of equatorial nations and African descent. Other subgroups of antibodies include lipoprotein-related protein 4 (LRP4), or agrin, a component of MuSK receptor function.[159]

Clinical Manifestations. The onset of *generalized AchR myasthenia* is insidious and may develop over several years. Early-onset MG is more common in women at ages 20 to 40 years of age. Late-onset MG is more common in men older than 60 years. The hallmark clinical manifestation is fatigable muscle weakness, which may involve ocular, bulbar (muscles of the eyes, face, mouth, throat, and neck), respiratory, and limb muscles. The variable distribution of ACh receptor sites, number of and different isoforms of antibodies, or the presence of thymoma determine when and which muscle groups are affected first. The extraocular eye muscles and the levator muscles of the eyelid are most affected as they have a small number of AchR.

Manifestations include diplopia, ptosis, and ocular palsies. The muscles of facial expression, mastication, swallowing, and speech are the next most involved. The results are facial droop and an expressionless face; difficulty chewing and swallowing, which are associated with dietary changes and weight loss; drooling; episodes of choking and aspiration; and a nasal, low volume but high-pitched monotonous speech pattern. The muscles of the neck, shoulder girdle, and hip flexors are less frequently affected, but muscle fatigue is common after exercise, and there can be progressive weakness. The respiratory muscles of the diaphragm and chest wall become weak, with impaired ventilation. Impairment in deep breathing and coughing predisposes the individual to atelectasis and congestion. Clinical manifestations may also appear during pregnancy, during the postpartum period, or in conjunction with the administration of certain anesthetic agents.

The progression of MG varies. The clinical manifestations of MG involve remissions and exacerbation of different types: relapsing-remitting, primary progressive, secondary progressive, and progressive-relapsing. It usually appears first as a mild case that spontaneously remits, with a series of relapses and symptom-free intervals ranging from weeks to months. Over time, the disease can progress slowly or rapidly or take a fulminating course.[160]

Ocular myasthenia is a subtype of MG that may occur with milder forms of MG. Ocular myasthenia is more common in males and with a late onset. Weakness of the eye muscles and eyelids is characteristic and may include swallowing difficulties and slurred speech as well.[161] *Juvenile MG* is very rare and occurs in children younger than 18 years of age. The disease is similar to generalized AchR myasthenia, usually less severe, and is treated aggressively to prevent long-term progression and disability.[162] In *transient neonatal myasthenia*, transitory signs of MG are present in about 10% to 15% of infants born to mothers with MG. Myasthenia immunoglobulin is transferred from the mother to the neonate through the placenta. There is generalized hypotonia, respiratory distress, and poor sucking in addition to extraocular muscle weakness. The signs appear 1 to 3 days after birth and persist for a few days to a few weeks.[163]

MuSK antibody type MG often involves severe swallowing and breathing (bulbar) problems. Clinical manifestations may first appear during pregnancy, during the postpartum period, or in conjunction with the administration of certain anesthetic agents. The progression of MG varies, appearing first as a mild case that spontaneously remits with a series of relapses and symptom-free intervals ranging from weeks to months. Over time, the disease can progress, and all muscles are weak.[164]

Myasthenic crisis occurs when severe muscle weakness causes extreme quadriparesis or quadriplegia, respiratory insufficiency with shortness of breath and a markedly decreased tidal volume and vital capacity, and extreme difficulty in swallowing. The individual in myasthenic crisis is in danger of respiratory arrest. Cholinergic crisis is a result of overstimulation of nicotinic and muscarinic receptors at neuromuscular junctions, usually seondary to the inhibition of acetylcholinesterase. A cholinergic crisis may result from cholinergic drug toxicity, with increased intestinal motility, episodes of diarrhea, and complaints of intestinal cramping, bradycardia, pupillary constriction, increased salivation, and diaphoresis. The clinical picture resembles that of myasthenic crisis, but the weakness occurs 30 to 60 minutes after taking anticholinergic medication. The clinical manifestations are caused by the smooth muscle hyperactivity secondary to excessive accumulation of Ach at the NMJs and excessive parasympathetic-like activity. As in myasthenic crisis, the individual is in danger of respiratory arrest.

Drugs that worsen symptoms include chloroquine, quinine, quinidine, procainamide, and botulinum toxin; aminoglycoside, fluoroquinolones, erythromycin antibiotics, neuromuscular blocking agents (pancuronium, D-tubocurarine), and immune checkpoint inhibitors.[156]

Evaluation and Treatment. The diagnosis of MG is made based on history and physical findings of weakness and muscle fatigability. Detection of AchR, MuSK, and the LRP4 antibodies is diagnostic of MG and defines MG subtypes. Results of EMG studies (rapid nerve stimulation and single-fiber electromyography) can aid diagnosis in seronegative individuals. Mediastinal CT and MRI help determine whether a thymoma is present.[165]

Treatment of MG is individualized and based on the MG subgroup symptoms. Acetylcholinesterase inhibitors (pyridostigmine—prevents degradation of Ach), corticosteroids and other immunosuppressant drugs (e.g., rituximab, chimeric monoclonal antibody against the protein CD20 primarily found on the surface of B cells, azathioprine, cyclosporine, mycophenolate mofetil) are used to treat MG and myasthenic crisis. Intravenous immunoglobulin and plasmapheresis may be lifesaving during myasthenic crisis, before and after thymectomy, and at the start of immunosuppressant therapy. For individuals with cholinergic crisis, treatment is to withhold anticholinesterase drugs (i.e., acetylcholinesterase inhibitors and cholinesterase inhibitors), then initiate treatment with anticholinergic drugs. However, anticholinergic medications do not block the severe muscle weakness effects associated with a severe cholinergic crisis, possibly requiring ventilatory support. At which time, the anticholinergic drugs are generally discontinued until the individual improves.

Thymectomy is the treatment of choice for a thymoma and those with anti-AChR antibodies because this terminates the production of self-reactive T cells and B cells that produce the antibodies. Current treatments for MG have improved prognosis, including in those individuals who have ocular myasthenia. Guidelines are available to guide the management of MG.[166] Several clinical trials are in progress to identify predictive biomarkers, evaluate targeted therapies, including complement and antigen specific T and B cells inhibitors, and vaccines to protect the AchR.[167]

Botulism

Botulism poisoning results from the botulinum neurotoxin released from *Clostridium botulinum*. The toxin inhibits the release of ACh at the myoneural junction and causes flaccid paralysis, including respiratory paralysis and death. Other forms include *C. botulinum*—contaminated wounds, infant and adult intestinal botulism released from spores that grow in the intestine after eating contaminated food, and iatrogenic botulism from accidental overdose of botulinum toxin. The endospores are resilient and resistant to heat. All forms are life-threatening and require emergency treatment. Treatments include supportive care with mechanical ventilation and antitoxin.

SUMMARY REVIEW

Alterations in Cognitive Systems

1. Three systems support cognitive function: attentional systems, memory and language systems, and affective or emotive systems.
2. Full consciousness is an awareness of oneself and the environment and includes an ability to respond to external stimuli with a wide variety of responses.
3. Consciousness has two components: arousal (state of awakeness) and awareness (content of thought).
4. Alterations in level of arousal may be caused by structural, metabolic, or psychogenic disorders.
5. Levels of consciousness can diminish in stages from alert and oriented to confusion and coma.
6. An alteration in breathing pattern and level of coma reflects the level of hemispheric and brainstem dysfunction.
7. Pupillary changes reflect changes in level of brainstem function, drug action, and response to hypoxia and ischemia.
8. Abnormal eye movements, including nystagmus and divergent gaze, reflect alterations in brainstem function.
9. Level of brain dysfunction manifests by changes in generalized motor responses or the presence of no responses.
10. Loss of cortical inhibition associated with decreased consciousness includes abnormal flexor and extensor movements.
11. Brain death represents irreversible total brain damage, including an inability to maintain cardiac, respiratory, and other vital functions. Cerebral death or irreversible coma is death of the cerebral hemispheres exclusive of the brainstem and cerebellum.
12. Arousal returns in the vegetative state and minimally conscious state, but content of thought is absent or markedly reduced, respectively.
13. With locked-in syndrome (ventral pontine syndrome) content of thought and level of arousal are intact, but the efferent pathways are disrupted with complete paralysis.
14. Akinetic mutism is a neurobehavioral state characterized by a severe loss of motivation to move or inability to voluntarily initiate motor responses, or both.
15. Alterations in awareness encompass all cognitive functions, including awareness, selective attention, and memory.
16. With a deficit in selective attention, mediated by the brainstem, the parietal lobe structures, and the pulvinar nucleus of the thalamus, the individual cannot focus on selective stimuli (visual and/or auditory or tactile) and thus neglects those stimuli, causing a neglect syndrome.
17. Memory is the recording, retention, and retrieval of information. Declarative memory is remembrance of personal history, events, experiences, facts, and information. Nondeclarative memory is a motor memory for actions, behaviors, skills, and outcomes. Emotional memory attaches positive or negative qualities to a memory.
18. Amnesia can be retrograde (loss of past memories) or anterograde (retention of old memories but an inability to form new ones). Global amnesia is a combination of both.
19. Frontal areas mediate vigilance, detection, and working memory (temporary storage of information). With a vigilance deficit, the person cannot maintain search and scanning activities. With a detection deficit, the person is unmotivated and unable to use feedback. With executive attention deficits there is working memory deficit and an inability to plan, remember instructions, and complete a task.
20. Data processing deficits are problems associated with recognizing and processing sensory information and include agnosias, aphasia, and acute confusional states.
21. Agnosias are a defect of recognition and may be tactile, visual, or auditory. They are caused by dysfunction in the primary sensory area or the interpretive areas of the cerebral cortex.
22. Aphasia is an impairment of comprehension or production of language. Aphasia may be motor (speaking or writing) or sensory (understanding spoken or written language).
23. Anomic sensory aphasia is an inability to name objects, people, or qualities.
24. Transcortical aphasias can be motor, sensory, or mixed, and are rare.
25. Global aphasia involves anterior and posterior speech areas, with both motor and sensory aphasia.
26. Delirium or acute confusional states are characterized chiefly by alterations in cognitive function, perception, and consciousness, and are associated with neuronal aging, neuroinflammation, oxidative stress, neuroendocrine dysregulation, and circadian dysregulation.
27. There are four types of delirium: hyperactive, hypoactive, mixed, and terminal.
28. Dementia is an acquired impairment of intellectual function, memory, and language with alteration in behavior and can be caused by genetic predisposition, trauma, vascular disease, infection, and progressive neurodegeneration.
29. Alzheimer disease is the most common chronic, irreversible dementia with accumulations of amyloid-beta and tau protein neurofibrillary tangles in the brain. Less common forms include vascular and frontotemporal dementia.

Alterations in Cerebral Hemodynamics

1. Cerebral perfusion pressure is a determinant for cerebral blood flow and oxygenation.
2. An injured brain may experience cerebral hypoperfusion, normal cerebral blood flow but with increased intracranial pressure or cerebral hyperemia.
3. Increased intracranial pressure may result from edema, excess cerebral spinal fluid, hemorrhage, or tumor growth. When intracranial pressure approaches arterial pressure, hypoxia and hypercapnia produce brain damage.
4. Cerebral edema is an increase in the fluid content of the brain resulting from infection, inflammation, hemorrhage, tumor, ischemia, infarct, or hypoxia.
5. The shifting or herniation of brain tissue from one compartment to another disrupts the blood flow of both compartments and damages brain tissue.
6. Supratentorial herniation involves temporal lobe and hippocampal gyrus shifting from the middle fossa to the posterior fossa; transtentorial herniation with a downward shift of the diencephalon through the tentorial notch; and shifting of the cingulate gyrus herniation under the falx.
7. The most common infratentorial herniation is a shift of the cerebellar tonsils through the foramen magnum.
8. Hydrocephalus comprises a variety of disorders characterized by an excess of fluid within the cranial ventricles, subarachnoid space, or both. Hydrocephalus occurs because of interference with cerebral spinal fluid flow caused by increased fluid production or obstruction within the ventricular system or by defective reabsorption of the fluid.

Alterations in Neuromotor Function

1. Motor neuron diseases result from progressive degeneration of upper or lower motor neurons in the cortex, brainstem, or spinal cord.
2. Motor movements are controlled by the pyramidal system (upper motor neurons), lower motor neurons, the extrapyramidal system, and the myoneural junction.
3. An upper motor neuron syndrome is characterized by spastic paresis or paralysis, hypertonia, hyperreflexia, and spasticity from interruption of the pyramidal system.
4. Interruption of the pyramidal tract below the pons results in spinal shock with complete flaccid paralysis, absence of reflexes, and marked disturbances of bowel and bladder function.
5. Lower motor neuron syndromes manifest with impaired voluntary and involuntary movements, usually without sensory impairment and flaccid paralysis, muscle atrophy, fasciculations, and fibrillations.
6. Partial paralysis occurs with only partial loss of alpha motor neurons, and total paralysis is complete loss of alpha motor neurons. Loss of gamma motor neurons impairs muscle tone and decreases deep tendon reflexes.
7. Nuclear palsies involve damage to the cranial nerve nuclei.
8. Bulbar palsies involve cranial nerves IX, X, and XII.
9. Extrapyramidal motor syndromes include basal ganglia and cerebellar motor syndromes and result in alterations of fine motor control with disturbances in posture, balance, and loss of smooth, coordinated movement. They are commonly associated with degenerative diseases of the central nervous system.
10. Basal ganglia disorders manifest with alterations in muscle tone and posture, including rigidity, involuntary movements, and loss of postural reflexes.
11. Cerebellar motor syndromes result in loss of muscle tone, difficulty with coordination, and disorders of equilibrium and gait.
12. Alterations in complex motor performance include disorders of posture (stance), disorders of gait, and disorders of expression.
13. Disorders of posture include dystonic posture, decerebrate posture, basal ganglion posture, and senile posture.
14. Disorders of gait include upper motor neuron gaits (spastic and scissors), cerebellar gait, basal ganglion gait, and frontal lobe ataxic gait.
15. Disorders of expression include hypermimesis and hypomimesis.
16. Dyspraxia is the partial inability and apraxia is the complete inability to perform purposeful or skilled motor acts.
17. Hypotonia and hypertonia are the main categories of altered muscle tone.
18. Hypotonia is decreased muscle tone with flaccidity and loss of reflexes and commonly is a symptom of lower motor neuron damage.
19. Hypertonia is increased muscle tone, and there are four types: spasticity, paratonia (gegenhalten), dystonia, and rigidity.
20. Alteration in muscle movement includes hypokinesia (slow movement), hyperkinesia (excessive movement), and dyskinesias (abnormal voluntary movement including Tourette syndrome).
21. Types of hypokinesia include akinesia, bradykinesia, and loss of associated movements.
22. Hyperkinesias include chorea, athetosis, ballism, akathisia, tremor, and myoclonus.

Chronic Diseases and Disorders Involving Motor Function

1. Parkinson disease is a common degenerative disorder of the basal ganglia (corpus striatum) involving degeneration of the dopamine-secreting nigrostriatal pathway resulting in overactivity by the subthalamic nucleus, causing tremor, rigidity, and bradykinesia. Involvement of the limbic system causes emotional lability. Progressive dementia may be associated with Lewy body formation and advanced stages of the disease. Most cases are sporadic and associated with head trauma, infection, neoplasm, atherosclerosis, toxins, or drug intoxication. Less than 5% have a familial or genetic cause.
2. Parkinson disease nonmotor symptoms are commonly associated with disruption of the autonomic nervous system and include unstable blood pressure, arrhythmias, and alteration in temperature control, digestion, bladder function, and sexual function.
3. Huntington disease (chorea) is a rare hereditary irreversible disease involving the basal ganglia and frontal cerebral

cortex. The *huntingtin* gene produces tangles of protein that collect in brain cells and chains of glutamine on the abnormal molecules that adhere to each other. There is a depletion of neurons that secrete gamma-aminobutyric acid (an inhibitory neurotransmitter) that causes involuntary, fragmentary movements accompanied by emotional lability and progressive dementia.

4. Amyotrophic lateral sclerosis is a disease of upper and lower motor neurons. The pathogenesis of amyotrophic lateral sclerosis is not fully known; however, motor neuron degeneration occurs as well as degeneration of the nonmotor neurons in the cortices and spinal cord. *Lateral sclerosis*, or scarring of the spinal cord, refers to the upper motor neuron component of the syndrome. Most cases are sporadic, and 10% to 20% are familial. Clinical manifestations of amyotrophic lateral sclerosis may include weakness in all muscles that may begin in a single muscle group, slurring of speech, and difficulty swallowing. Flaccid paresis progressing to paralysis is characteristic of the lower motor neuron syndrome.
5. The demyelinating disorders include multiple sclerosis and Guillain Barré syndrome.
6. Multiple sclerosis is a chronic inflammatory disease involving degeneration of central nervous system myelin in genetically susceptible individuals and is more common in women. The cause is unknown. Autoreactive T and B cells recognize myelin autoantigens and produce myelin-specific antibodies, triggering inflammatory demyelination with loss of oligodendrocytes, and plaque formation, leading to disruption of nerve conduction throughout the brain and spinal cord and, over time, loss of neurons.
7. The clinical manifestations of multiple sclerosis involve remissions and exacerbation of different types: relapsing-remitting, primary progressive, secondary progressive, and progressive-relapsing. Optico-spinal multiple sclerosis involves the optic nerve and cranial nerves III through XII. Spinal multiple sclerosis primarily involves the spinal tracts and dorsal column with spastic paresis and bowel and bladder dysfunction. Cerebellar multiple sclerosis manifests with motor ataxia and weakness.
8. Guillain-Barré syndrome is a rare demyelinating disorder caused by an antibody and cell-mediated immunologic reaction directed against peripheral nerves that causes weakness or paralysis and can have irreversible effects. It usually occurs 4 weeks after a respiratory or gastrointestinal infection (e.g., *Campylobacter jejuni* and Zika virus), and molecury mimicry of pathogen-borne antigens has been proposed as a theory of pathogenesis. Different subtypes have been identified, and clinical manifestations depend on the subtype.
9. Disorders of the myoneural junction include myasthenia gravis, Lambert-Eaton syndrome, and botulism.
10. Myasthenia gravis results from a defect in nerve impulse transmission at the neuromuscular junction with generalized, ocular, or neonatal subtypes. Autoantibodies, complement deposits, and membrane attack complex destroy the acetylcholine receptor sites, causing decreased transmission of nerve impulses, leading to muscle weakness, including ocular and systemic muscles. There can be childhood and adult onset.
11. Lambert-Eaton myasthenic syndrome is related to autoantibodies to calcium channels on presynaptic nerve terminals and presents with leg and arm weakness.
12. Botulism is poisoning by botulinum toxin released by *Clostridium botulinum* that acts by inhibiting release of Ach at the myoneural junction, causing life-threatening flaccid paralysis.

REFERENCES

1. Quiroga LFC, Moreno WA. Chapter 5. Neurobiological computation and neural networks. In: Munish Puri M, ed. *Artificial neural network for drug design, delivery and disposition.* Waltham, MA: Academic Press; 2016:103–120. https://doi.org/10.1016/B978-0-12-801559-9.00005-3. (Accessed October 15, 2021).
2. Giacino JT, et al. Practice guideline update recommendations summary: disorders of consciousness: Report of the Guideline Development, Dissemination, and Implementation Subcommittee of the American Academy of Neurology; the American Congress of Rehabilitation Medicine; and the National Institute on Disability, Independent Living, and Rehabilitation Research. *Neurology*. 2018;91(10):450–460.
3. Jain R, Ramakrishnan AG. Electrophysiological and neuroimaging studies—during resting state and sensory stimulation in disorders of consciousness: a review. *Front Neurosci.* 2020;14: 555093.
4. Greer DM, et al. Determination of brain death/death by neurologic criteria: the World Brain Death Project. *JAMA*. 2020;324(11): 1078–1097.
5. Nakagawa TA, et al. Guidelines for the determination of brain death in infants and children: an update of the 1987 task force recommendations. *Crit Care Med.* 2011;39(9):2139–2155.
6. Martin SD, Porter MB. Performing the brain death examination and the declaration of pediatric brain death. *J Pediatr Intensive Care*. 2017;6(4):229–233.
7. Bender A, et al. Persistent vegetative state and minimally conscious state: a systematic review and meta-analysis of diagnostic procedures. *Dtsch Arztebl Int.* 2015;112(14):235–242.
8. Picolas C. Is the "minimally conscious state" patient minimally self-aware? *Front Psychol.* 2020;11:539665.
9. Buchman SL, Merkler AE. Basilar artery occlusion: diagnosis and acute treatment. *Curr Treat Options Neurol.* 2019;21(10):45.
10. Arnts H, et al. On the pathophysiology and treatment of akinetic mutism. *Neurosci Biobehav Rev.* 2020;112:270–278.
11. Bourgeois A, et al. Pulvino-cortical interaction: an integrative role in the control of attention. *Neurosci Biobehav Rev.* 2020;111: 104–113.
12. Veale R, Hafed ZM, Yoshida M. How is visual salience computed in the brain? Insights from behaviour, neurobiology and modelling. *Philos Trans R Soc Lond B Biol Sci.* 2017;372(1714): 20160113.
13. Langer KG, Piechowski-Jozwiak B, Bogousslavsky J. Hemineglect and attentional dysfunction. *Front Neurol Neurosci.* 2019;44:89–99.
14. Rode G, et al. Semiology of neglect: an update. *Ann Phys Rehabil Med.* 2017;60(3):177–185.

15. Lisman J, Sternberg EJ. Habit and nonhabit systems for unconscious and conscious behavior: implications for multitasking. *J Cogn Neurosci.* 2013;25(2):273–283.
16. Marvel CL, Morgan OP, Kronemer SI. How the motor system integrates with working memory. *Neurosci Biobehav Rev.* 2019;102:184–194.
17. Saha R., et al: Intra-amygdala metaplasticity modulation of fear extinction learning, *Eur J Neurosci.* Online ahead of print December 11, 2020. Available at https://doi.org/10.1111/ejn.15080. (Accessed October 16, 2021).
18. Alessandro L, et al. Acute amnestic syndromes. *J Neurol Sci.* 2020;413:116781.
19. Szabo K. Hippocampal stroke. *Front Neurol Neurosci.* 2014;34:150–156.
20. Kirova AM, Bays RB, Lagalwar S. Working memory and executive function decline across normal aging, mild cognitive impairment, and Alzheimer's disease. *Biomed Res Int.* 2015;2015:748212.
21. Matthews BR. Memory dysfunction, *Continuum (Minneap Minn)* 21 (3 Behavioral Neurology and Neuropsychiatry). 2015;613–626.
22. Cohen RA, Marsiske MM, Smith GE. Neuropsychology of aging. *Handb Clin Neurol.* 2019;167:149–180.
23. Perrotta G. Agnosia: definition, clinical contexts, neurobiological profiles and clinical treatments. *Arch Gerontol Geriatr Res.* 2020;5(1):031–035.
24. Worrall L, et al. Let's call it "aphasia": rationales for eliminating the term "dysphasia". *Int J Stroke.* 2016;11(8):848–851.
25. O'Sullivan M, Brownsett S, Copland D. Language and language disorders: neuroscience to clinical practice. *Pract Neurol.* 2019;19(5):380–388.
26. Janssen TL, et al. Prevention of postoperative delirium in elderly patients planned for elective surgery: systematic review and meta-analysis. *Clin Interv Aging.* 2019;14:1095–1117.
27. Oh ST, Park JY. Postoperative delirium. *Korean J Anesthesiol.* 2019;72(1):4–12.
28. Maldonado JR. Delirium pathophysiology: an updated hypothesis of the etiology of acute brain failure. *Int J Geriatr Psychiatry.* 2018;33(11):1428–1457.
29. Strömmer EMF, et al. The role of restraint in fatal excited delirium: a research synthesis and pooled analysis. *Forensic Sci Med Pathol.* 2020;16(4):680–692.
30. Menser C, Smith H. Emergence agitation and delirium: considerations for epidemiology and routine monitoring in pediatric patients. *Local Reg Anesth.* 2020;13:73–83.
31. Albert RH. End-of-life care: managing common symptoms. *Am Fam Physician.* 2017;95(6):356–361.
32. Agar M, Bush SH. Delirium at the end of life. *Med Clin North Am.* 2020;104(3):491–501.
33. Pagad S, et al. Delirium in cardiac intensive care unit. *Cureus.* 2020;12(8):e10096.
34. Stokholm J, et al. Delirium assessment in acute stroke: a systematic review and meta-analysis of incidence, assessment tools, and assessment frequencies. *J Cent Nerv Syst Dis.* 2019;11 1179573519897083.
35. Shenvi C, et al. Managing delirium and agitation in the older emergency department patient: the ADEPT tool. *Ann Emerg Med.* 2020;75(2):136–145.
36. Lee S, Angel C, Han JH. Succinct approach to delirium in the emergency department. *Curr Emerg Hosp Med Rep.* 2021;9:11–18.
37. Sutherland M, et al. Improving the management of terminal delirium at the end of life. *Asia Pac J Oncol Nurs.* 2020;7(4):389–395.
38. Livingston G, et al. Dementia prevention, intervention, and care: 2020 report of the Lancet Commission. *Lancet.* 2020;396(10248):413–446.
39. Iadecola C, et al. Vascular cognitive impairment and dementia: JACC Scientific Expert Panel. *J Am Coll Cardiol.* 2019;73(25):3326–3344.
40. Elahi FM, Miller BL. A clinicopathological approach to the diagnosis of dementia. *Nat Rev Neurol.* 2017;13(8):457–476.
41. Petersen RC, et al. Practice guideline update summary: mild cognitive impairment: Report of the Guideline Development, Dissemination, and Implementation Subcommittee of the American Academy of Neurology. *Neurology.* 2018;90 (3):126–135.
42. Baumgart M, et al. Summary of the evidence on modifiable risk factors for cognitive decline and dementia: a population-based perspective. *Alzheimers Dement.* 2015;11(6):718–726.
43. Litke R, et al. Modifiable risk factors in Alzheimer Disease and related dementias: a review. *Clin Ther.* 2021;43(6):953–965.
44. Alzheimer's Association 2021 Alzheimer's disease facts and figures. *Alzheimers Dement.* 2021;17(3):327–406.
45. Ayodele T, et al. Early-onset Alzheimer's disease: what is missing in research? *Curr Neurol Neurosci Rep.* 2021;21(2):4.
46. Morley JE, et al. What is the physiological function of amyloid-beta protein? *J Nutr Health Aging.* 2019;23:225–226.
47. D'Argenio V, Sarnataro D. New insights into the molecular bases of familial Alzheimer's disease. *J Pers Med.* 2020;10(2):26.
48. Kelleher 3rd RJ, Shen J. Presenilin-1 mutations and Alzheimer's disease. *Proc Natl Acad Sci U S A.* 2017;114(4):629–631.
49. Armstrong R. Risk factors for Alzheimer's disease. *Folia Neuropathol.* 2019;57(2):87–105.
50. Mendez MF. Early-onset Alzheimer disease and its variants. *Continuum (Minneap Minn).* 2019;25(1):34–51.
51. Rabinovici GD. Late-onset Alzheimer disease. *Continuum (Minneap Minn).* 2019;25(1):14–33.
52. Greenberg SM, et al. Cerebral amyloid angiopathy and Alzheimer disease—one peptide, two pathways. *Nat Rev Neurol.* 2020;16(1):30–42.
53. Dubois B, et al. Clinical diagnosis of Alzheimer's disease: recommendations of the International Working Group. *Lancet Neurol.* 2021;20(6):484–496.
54. Vogel JW, et al. Four distinct trajectories of tau deposition identified in Alzheimer's disease. *Nat Med.* 2021;27(5):871–881.
55. Newcombe EA, et al. Inflammation: the link between comorbidities, genetics, and Alzheimer's disease. *J Neuroinflammation.* 2018;15(1):276.
56. Bolós M, Perea JR, Avila J. Alzheimer's disease as an inflammatory disease. *Biomol Concepts.* 2017;8(1):37–43.
57. Gonzalez B, et al. Tau spread, apolipoprotein E, inflammation, and more: rapidly evolving basic science in Alzheimer disease. *Neurol Clin.* 2017;35(2):175–190.
58. Yu H, Wu J. Amyloid-β: a double agent in Alzheimer's disease? *Biomed Pharmacother.* 2021;139:111575.
59. Long JM, Holtzman DM. Alzheimer disease: an update on pathobiology and treatment strategies. *Cell.* 2019;179(2):312–339. Available at https://doi.org/10.1016/j.cell.2019.09.001. (Accessed October 16, 2021).
60. McCarthy M, Raval AP. The peri-menopause in a woman's life: a systemic inflammatory phase that enables later neurodegenerative disease. *J Neuroinflammation.* 2020;17(1):317.
61. Owen JE, et al. Alzheimer's disease neuropathology in the hippocampus and brainstem of people with obstructive sleep apnea. *Sleep.* 2021;44(3):zsaa195.

62. Shokri-Kojori E, et al. β-Amyloid accumulation in the human brain after one night of sleep deprivation. *Proc Natl Acad Sci U S A.* 2018;115(17):4483–4488.
63. Doifode T, et al. The impact of the microbiota-gut-brain axis on Alzheimer's disease pathophysiology. *Pharmacol Res.* 2021;164: 105314.
64. Qian XH, et al. Inflammatory pathways in Alzheimer's disease mediated by gut microbiota. *Ageing Res Rev.* 2021;68:101317.
65. Fink HA, et al. *Diagnosis and Treatment of Clinical Alzheimer's-type Dementia: a Systematic Review.* Rockville, MD: Agency for Healthcare Research and Quality; 2020. Report No.: 20-EHC003. Comparative Effectiveness Review, No. 223. Available at https://www.ncbi.nlm.nih.gov/books/NBK556556/. (Accessed October 16, 2021).
66. Atri A. The Alzheimer's disease clinical spectrum: diagnosis and management. *Med Clin North Am.* 2019;103(2):263–293.
67. Arvanitakis Z, Shah RC, Bennett DA. Diagnosis and management of dementia: review. *JAMA.* 2019;322(16):1589–1599.
68. Angelopoulou E, et al. Flotillin: a promising biomarker for Alzheimer's disease. *J Pers Med.* 2020;10(2):20.
69. Hampel H, et al. The cholinergic system in the pathophysiology and treatment of Alzheimer's disease. *Brain.* 2018;141(7):1917–1933. Available at https://doi.org/10.1093/brain/awy132. (Accessed October 16, 2021).
70. Liu J, et al. The role of NMDA receptors in Alzheimer's disease. *Front Neurosci.* 2019;13:43 Available at https://doi.org/10.3389/fnins.2019.00043. (Accessed October 16, 2021).
71. Cummings JL, Tong G, Ballard C. Treatment combinations for Alzheimer's disease: current and future pharmacotherapy options. *J Alzheimers Dis.* 2019;67(3):779–794.
72. Duong MT, et al. Cholesterol, atherosclerosis, and APOE in vascular contributions to cognitive impairment and dementia (VCID): potential mechanisms and therapy. *Front Aging Neurosci.* 2021;13:647990.
73. Vinciguerra L, et al. Update on the neurobiology of vascular cognitive impairment: from lab to clinic. *Int J Mol Sci.* 2020;21(8):2977.
74. Cipollini V, Troili F, Giubilei F. Emerging biomarkers in vascular cognitive impairment and dementia: from pathophysiological pathways to clinical application. *Int J Mol Sci.* 2019;20(11):2812.
75. Graff-Radford J. Vascular cognitive impairment. *Continuum (Minneap Minn).* 2019;25(1):147–164.
76. Greaves CV, Rohrer JD. An update on genetic frontotemporal dementia. *J Neurol.* 2019;266(8):2075–2086.
77. Devenney EM, Ahmed RM, Hodges JR. Frontotemporal dementia. *Handb Clin Neurol.* 2019;167:279–299.
78. Young JJ, et al. Frontotemporal dementia: latest evidence and clinical implications. *Ther Adv Psychopharmacol.* 2018;8(1):33–48.
79. Stokum JA, et al. Emerging pharmacological treatments for cerebral edema: evidence from clinical studies. *Annu Rev Pharmacol Toxicol.* 2020;60:291–309.
80. Yamada S, Ishikawa M, Nozaki K. Exploring mechanisms of ventricular enlargement in idiopathic normal pressure hydrocephalus: a role of cerebrospinal fluid dynamics and motile cilia. *Fluids Barriers CNS.* 2021;18(1):20.
81. Daou B, et al. Revisiting secondary normal pressure hydrocephalus: does it exist? A review. *Neurosurg Focus.* 2016;41(3):E6.
82. Gavrilov GV, et al. Idiopathic normal pressure hydrocephalus (Hakim-Adams Syndrome): clinical symptoms, diagnosis and treatment. *Psychiatr Danub.* 2019;31(Suppl 5):737–744.
83. Liew BS, et al. Current updates on idiopathic normal pressure hydrocephalus. *Asian J Neurosurg.* 2019;14(3):648–656.
84. Garg N, et al. Differentiating lower motor neuron syndromes. *J Neurol Neurosurg Psychiatry.* 2017;88(6):474–483.
85. National Institute of Neurological Disorder and Stroke (NINDS). *Spinal Muscular Atrophy Fact Sheet.* Bethesda, MD: NINDS; 2020. Date last modified August 10, 2020. Available at https://www.ninds.nih.gov/Disorders/Patient-Caregiver-Education/Fact-Sheets/Spinal-Muscular-Atrophy-Fact-Sheet. (Accessed October 16, 2021).
86. Frey KA. Molecular imaging of extrapyramidal movement disorders. *Semin Nucl Med.* 2017;47(1):18–30.
87. Fazl A, Fleisher J. Anatomy, physiology, and clinical syndromes of the basal ganglia: a brief review. *Semin Pediatr Neurol.* 2018;25:2–9.
88. Manto M. Cerebellar motor syndrome from children to the elderly. *Handb Clin Neurol.* 2018;154:151–166.
89. Ronthal M. Gait disorders and falls in the elderly. *Med Clin North Am.* 2019;103(2):203–213.
90. Manto M, et al. Cerebellar ataxias: an update. *Curr Opin Neurol.* 2020;33(1):150–160.
91. Finegan E, et al. Pathological crying and laughing in motor neuron disease: pathobiology, screening, intervention. *Front Neurol.* 2019;10:260.
92. Nguyen L, Matsumoto RR. The psychopharmacology of pseudobulbar affect. *Handb Clin Neurol.* 2019;165:243–251.
93. Liebenthal E, Silbersweig DA, Stern E. The language, tone and prosody of emotions: neural substrates and dynamics of spoken-word emotion perception. *Front Neurosci.* 2016;10:506.
94. Carota A, Bogousslavsky J. Minor hemisphere major syndromes. *Front Neurol Neurosci.* 2018;41:1–13.
95. Baumard J, Le Gall D. The challenge of apraxia: toward an operational definition? *Cortex.* 2021;141:66–80.
96. Hallett M, et al. Human brain connectivity: clinical applications for clinical neurophysiology. *Clin Neurophysiol.* 2020;131(7):1621–1651.
97. Brüggemann N. Contemporary functional neuroanatomy and pathophysiology of dystonia. *J Neural Transm (Vienna).* 2021;128(4):499–508.
98. Truong DD, Frei K. Setting the record straight: the nosology of tardive syndromes. *Parkinsonism Relat Disord.* 2019;59: 146–150.
99. Marras C, et al. Prevalence of Parkinson's disease across North America. *NPJ Parkinsons Dis.* 2018;4:21.
100. Marras C, Canning CG, Goldman SM. Environment, lifestyle, and Parkinson's disease: implications for prevention in the next decade. *Mov Disord.* 2019;34(6):801–811.
101. Choi YR, Park SJ, Park SM. Molecular events underlying the cell-to-cell transmission of α-synuclein, *FEBS J.* Online ahead of print December 17, 2020. Available at https://doi.org/10.1111/febs.15674. (Accessed October 16, 2021).
102. Kakoty V, et al. The gut-brain connection in the pathogenicity of Parkinson disease: putative role of autophagy. *Neurosci Lett.* 2021;753:135865.
103. Paredes-Rodriguez E, et al. The noradrenergic system in Parkinson's disease. *Front Pharmacol.* 2020;11:435.
104. Bloem BR, Okun MS, Klein C. Parkinson's disease. *Lancet.* 2021;397(10291):2284–2303.
105. Fereshtehnejad SM, et al. Evolution of prodromal Parkinson's disease and dementia with Lewy bodies: a prospective study. *Brain.* 2019;142(7):2051–2067.
106. Sanford AM. Lewy body dementia. *Clin Geriatr Med.* 2018;34(4):603–615.

107. Lauretani F, et al. Imaging the functional neuroanatomy of Parkinson's disease: clinical applications and future directions. *Int J Environ Res Public Health*. 2021;18(5):2356.
108. Tolosa E, et al. Challenges in the diagnosis of Parkinson's disease. *Lancet Neurol*. 2021;20(5):385–397.
109. Sun C, Armstrong MJ. Treatment of Parkinson's disease with cognitive impairment: current approaches and future directions. *Behav Sci (Basel)*. 2021;11(4):54.
110. Stoker TB, Barker RA. Recent developments in the treatment of Parkinson's disease. *F1000Res*. 2020;9 F1000 Faculty Rev-862.
111. Barbuti PA, et al. Recent advances in the development of stem-cell-derived dopaminergic neuronal transplant therapies for Parkinson's disease. *Mov Disord*. 2021;36(8):1772–1780.
112. Church FC. Treatment options for motor and non-motor symptoms of Parkinson's disease. *Biomolecules*. 2021;11(4):612.
113. Rawlins MD, et al. The prevalence of Huntington's disease. *Neuroepidemiology*. 2016;46(2):144–153.
114. Kremer B, et al. Sex-dependent mechanisms for expansions and contractions of the CAG repeat on affected Huntington disease chromosome. *Am J Hum Genet*. 1995;57(2):343–350.
115. Gatto EM, et al. Huntington disease: advances in the understanding of its mechanisms. *Clin Park Relat Disord*. 2020;3:10056 Available at https://doi.org/10.1016/j.prdoa.2020.100056. (Accessed October 16, 2021).
116. Reilmann R. Parkinsonism in Huntington's disease. *Int Rev Neurobiol*. 2019;149:299–306.
117. Dash D, Mestre TA. Therapeutic update on Huntington's disease: symptomatic treatments and emerging disease-modifying therapies. *Neurotherapeutics*. 2020;17(4):1645–1659.
118. Verde F, et al. The multisystem degeneration amyotrophic lateral sclerosis—neuropathological staging and clinical translation. *Arch Ital Biol*. 2017;155(4):118–130.
119. De Marchi F, et al. Cognitive dysfunction in amyotrophic lateral sclerosis: can we predict it? *Neurol Sci*. 2021;42(6):2211–2222.
120. Longinetti E, Fang F. Epidemiology of amyotrophic lateral sclerosis: an update of recent literature. *Curr Opin Neurol*. 2019;32(5):771–776.
121. Siddique N, Siddique T. Amyotrophic lateral sclerosis overview. In: Adam MP, ed. *GeneReviews®*. Seattle, WA: University of Washington; 1993-2021. Updated October 3, 2019. Available at https://www.ncbi.nlm.nih.gov/books/NBK1450/. (Accessed October 16, 2021).
122. Obrador E, et al. Oxidative stress, neuroinflammation and mitochondria in the pathophysiology of amyotrophic lateral sclerosis. *Antioxidants (Basel)*. 2020;9(9):901.
123. Eisen A. The dying forward hypothesis of ALS: tracing its history. *Brain Sci*. 2021;11(3):300.
124. Pradhan J, Bellingham MC. Neurophysiological mechanisms underlying cortical hyper-excitability in amyotrophic lateral sclerosis: a review. *Brain Sci*. 2021;11(5):549.
125. van den Bos MAJ, et al. Pathophysiology and diagnosis of ALS: insights from advances in neurophysiological techniques. *Int J Mol Sci*. 2019;20(11):2818.
126. Nolan M, et al. Quantitative patterns of motor cortex proteinopathy across ALS genotypes. *Acta Neuropathol Commun*. 2020;8(1):98.
127. Ng Kee Kwong KC, et al. 40 years of CSF toxicity studies in ALS: what have we learnt about ALS pathophysiology? *Front Mol Neurosci*. 2021;14:647895.
128. Grad LI, et al. Clinical spectrum of amyotrophic lateral sclerosis (ALS). *Cold Spring Harb Perspect Med*. 2017;7(8):a024117.
129. Feron M, et al. Extrapyramidal deficits in ALS: a combined biomechanical and neuroimaging study. *J Neurol*. 2018;265(9):2125–2136.
130. van Es MA, et al. Amyotrophic lateral sclerosis. *Lancet*. 2017;390(10107):2084–2098.
131. Masrori P, Van Damme P. Amyotrophic lateral sclerosis: a clinical review. *Eur J Neurol*. 2020;27(10):1918–1929.
132. Dreger M, et al. Cerebrospinal fluid neurofilament light chain (NfL) predicts disease aggressiveness in amyotrophic lateral sclerosis: an application of the D50 disease progression model. *Front Neurosci*. 2021;15:651651.
133. Amyotrophic lateral sclerosis: ClinicalTrials.gov. Available at https://clinicaltrials.gov/ct2/results?cond=Amyotrophic+Lateral+Sclerosis+AND+%22Amyotrophic+Lateral+Sclerosis%22. (Accessed October 16, 2021).
134. Amado DA, Davidson BL. Gene therapy for ALS: a review, *Mol Ther*. Online ahead of print April 8, 2021. Available at https://doi.org/10.1016/j.ymthe.2021.04.008. (Accessed October 16, 2021).
135. Gittings LM, Sattler R. Recent advances in understanding amyotrophic lateral sclerosis and emerging therapies. *Fac Rev*. 2020;9:12.
136. Chen JJ. Overview of current and emerging therapies for amyotrophic lateral sclerosis. *Am J Manag Care*. 2020;26(9 Suppl): S191–S197.
137. Angeloni B, et al. A case of double standard: sex differences in multiple sclerosis risk factors. *Int J Mol Sci*. 2021;22(7):3696.
138. Nourbakhsh B, Mowry EM. Multiple sclerosis risk factors and pathogenesis. *Continuum (Minneap Minn)*. 2019;25(3): 596–610.
139. Lassmann H. Multiple sclerosis pathology. *Cold Spring Harb Perspect Med*. 2018;8(3):a028936.
140. Makhani N, Tremlett H. The multiple sclerosis prodrome. *Nat Rev Neurol*. 2021;17:515–521.
141. Vukusic S, et al. Pregnancy with multiple sclerosis. *Rev Neurol (Paris)*. 2021;177(3):180–194.
142. Meca-Lallana V, et al. Deciphering multiple sclerosis progression. *Front Neurol*. 2021;12:608491.
143. Fischer JS, et al. The multiple sclerosis functional composite measure (MSFC): an integrated approach to MS clinical outcome assessment. *Mult Scler*. 1999;5(4):244–250.
144. Kurtzke JF. Rating neurologic impairment in multiple sclerosis: an expanded disability status scale (EDSS). *Neurology*. 1983;33(11):1444–1452.
145. Thompson AJ, et al. Diagnosis of multiple sclerosis: 2017 revisions of the McDonald criteria. *Lancet Neurol*. 2018;17(2): 162–173.
146. Wattjes MP, et al. 2021 MAGNIMS-CMSC-NAIMS consensus recommendations on the use of MRI in patients with multiple sclerosis. *Lancet Neurol*. 2021;20(8):653–670.
147. McGinley MP, Goldschmidt CH, Rae-Grant AD. Diagnosis and treatment of multiple sclerosis: a review. *JAMA*. 2021;325(8): 765–779.
148. Boltjes R, et al. Vitamin D supplementation in multiple sclerosis: an expert opinion based on the review of current evidence. *Expert Rev Neurother*. 2021;21(6):715–725.
149. Boffa G, et al. Long-term clinical outcomes of hematopoietic stem cell transplantation in multiple sclerosis. *Neurology*. 2021;96(8):e1215–e1226.
150. Simpson A, Mowry EM, Newsome SD. Early aggressive treatment approaches for multiple sclerosis. *Curr Treat Options Neurol*. 2021;23(7):19 Available at https://doi.org/10.1007/s11940-021-00677-1. (Accessed October 16, 2021).

151. Canavero I, et al. Guillain Barrè syndrome and myelitis associated with SARS-CoV-2 infection. *Neurosci Lett.* 2021;759: 136040.
152. Shahrizaila N, Lehmann HC, Kuwabara S. Guillain-Barré syndrome. *Lancet.* 2021;397(10280):1214–1228.
153. Leonhard SE, et al. Diagnosis and management of Guillain-Barré syndrome in ten steps. *Nat Rev Neurol.* 2019;15(11):671–683.
154. National Organization for Rare Disorders (NORD). *Myasthenia Gravis.* Danbury, CT: NORD; 2021. Available at https://rarediseases.org/rare-diseases/myasthenia-gravis/. (Accessed October 16, 2021).
155. Green JD, et al. Epidemiological evidence for a hereditary contribution to myasthenia gravis: a retrospective cohort study of patients from North America. *BMJ Open.* 2020;10(9):e037909.
156. Bodkin C, Pascuzzi RM. Update in the management of myasthenia gravis and Lambert-Eaton myasthenic syndrome. *Neurol Clin.* 2021;39(1):133–146.
157. Gilhus NE, et al. Myasthenia gravis—autoantibody characteristics and their implications for therapy. *Nat Rev Neurol.* 2016;12(5): 259–268.
158. Bernard C, et al. Thymoma associated with autoimmune diseases: 85 cases and literature review. *Autoimmun Rev.* 2016;15(1):82–92.
159. Gilhus NE. Myasthenia gravis. *N Engl J Med.* 2016;375(26): 2570–2581.
160. Dresser L, et al. Myasthenia gravis: epidemiology, pathophysiology and clinical manifestations. *J Clin Med.* 2021;10(11):2235.
161. Melson AT, McClelland CM, Lee MS. Ocular myasthenia gravis: updates on an elusive target. *Curr Opin Neurol.* 2020;33(1):55–61.
162. O'Connell K, Ramdas S, Palace J. Management of juvenile myasthenia gravis. *Front Neurol.* 2020;11:743.
163. Kaler J, et al. Neuromuscular junction disorders and floppy infant syndrome: a comprehensive review. *Cureus.* 2020;12(2):e6922.
164. Cao M, Koneczny I, Vincent A. Myasthenia gravis with antibodies against muscle specific kinase: an update on clinical features, pathophysiology and treatment. *Front Mol Neurosci.* 2020;13:159.
165. Rousseff RT. Diagnosis of myasthenia gravis. *J Clin Med.* 2021;10(8):1736.
166. Narayanaswami P, et al. International Consensus Guidance for Management of Myasthenia Gravis: 2020 update. *Neurology.* 2021;96(3):114–122.
167. Myasthenia Gravis Foundation of America (MGFA). *Clinical Trials.* Westborough, MA: MGFA; 2021. Available at https://myasthenia.org/Research/Clinical-Trials. (Accessed October 16, 2021).
168. Squire LR, Dede AJ. Conscious and unconscious memory systems. *Cold Spring Harb Perspect Biol.* 2015;7(3):a021667.

18

Alterations of the Brain, Spinal Cord, and Peripheral Nerves

Jan Powers and Kathleen E. Hubner

http://evolve.elsevier.com/Rogers/pathophysiology/

CHAPTER OUTLINE

Alterations in central nervous system (CNS) function are caused by traumatic injury, vascular disorders, tumor growth, infectious and inflammatory processes, and metabolic derangements, including nutritional deficiencies and drugs or chemicals. Alterations in peripheral nervous system function involve the nerve roots, nerve plexus, the peripheral nerves, or the neuromuscular junction. Disorders related to demyelinating diseases and the neuromuscular junction were presented in Chapter 17.

CENTRAL NERVOUS SYSTEM DISORDERS

Traumatic Brain and Spinal Cord Injury

Traumatic Brain Injury

Traumatic brain injury (TBI) is an alteration in brain function or other evidence of brain pathology caused by an external force. Approximately 1.7 million cases of TBI occur in the United States each year. An estimated 13.5 million individuals live with a disability due to TBI in the United States alone, with nearly 61,000 deaths related to TBI in 2019.[1] Those who survive a TBI may have long-term effects with cognitive function, motor function, and behavior changes.[2] The leading causes of TBI-related deaths are due to suicide, unintentional falls, and motor vehicle crashes. The leading causes of nonfatal TBI in the United States arise from falls, motor vehicle–related injuries, and strikes or blows to the head from or against an object (17%), such as sports injuries. The most common causes of TBI for children and older adults are unintentional falls. Males have the highest incidence in all age groups.

In recent years, individuals with TBI have shown improved survival. This is attributed to advancements in safety measures (e.g., passive seat restraints, air bags, protective head gear), reduced transport time to hospitals or trauma centers, improved on-scene medical management, imaging of brain injury, prevention and management of secondary brain injury, and a better understanding of all degrees of brain injury severity.

TBI can be classified as primary or secondary injuries. Primary brain injury is caused by a direct impact. The injury can be a focal brain injury, affecting only one area of the brain, or a diffuse brain injury, involving more than one area of the brain. Both types of injury can be associated with the same initiating event. Blunt trauma may result in both focal and diffuse brain injuries, and they usually occur at the same time (Table 18.1). Focal brain injury and diffuse brain injuries each account for approximately half of all injuries. However, focal brain injury accounts for more than two-thirds of head injury deaths. Secondary injury is an indirect consequence of the primary injury. It includes systemic and brain tissue responses with a cascade of cellular and molecular cerebral events involving the inflammatory response to injury (Fig. 18.1 and see Table 18.1). TBI can be mild, moderate, or severe (Table 18.2). The Glasgow Coma Scale (GCS) is commonly used to grade severity of injury (Table 18.3). Most TBIs are mild.

Primary brain injury

Focal brain injury. Focal brain injury can be caused by closed (blunt) trauma or open (penetrating) trauma. Closed trauma or injury is more common and involves either the head striking a hard surface (e.g., motor vehicle accidents or falls), a rapidly moving object striking the head (e.g., a baseball or a falling object), or by blast waves (e.g., an explosion or a tornado). A linear skull fracture or simple break or "crack" in the skull may occur. The dura remains intact, and brain tissues are not exposed to the environment. Open head trauma or injury

TABLE 18.1 Classification of Brain Injuries

Type of Injury	
Primary Brain Injury	
Focal Brain Injury	Localized injury from impact
Closed injury	Blunt trauma
• Coup	Injury is directly below site of forceful impact
• Contrecoup	Injury is on opposite side of brain from site of forceful impact
• Epidural (extradural) hematoma	Vehicular accidents, minor falls, sporting accidents
• Subdural hematoma	Forceful impact: vehicular accidents or falls, especially in elderly persons or persons with chronic alcohol abuse
• Contusions	Bleeding caused by forceful impact, usually vehicular accidents or long-distance falls
Open injury	Penetrating trauma: missiles (bullets) or sharp projectiles (knives, ice picks, axes, screwdrivers)
• Compound fracture	Objects strike head with great force or head strikes object forcefully; temporal blows, occipital blows, upward impact of cervical vertebrae (basilar skull fracture)
Diffuse Brain Injury	
Concussion	May or may not have loss of consciousness with no visible changes on brain imaging
Diffuse axonal injury (can occur with focal injury)	Traumatic shearing forces; tearing of axons from twisting and rotational forces with injury over widespread brain areas; moving head strikes hard, unyielding surface or moving object strikes stationary head; torsional head motion without impact
Subarachnoid hemorrhage	Shearing forces tear small bridging blood vessels with bleeding into the subarachnoid space
Secondary Brain Injury	
Systemic processes	Hypotension, hypoxia, ischemia, anemia, hypercapnia, and hypocapnia
Intracerebral processes	Inflammation, cerebral edema, increased intracranial pressure (IICP), brain herniation, decreased cerebral perfusion pressure, ischemia
Cellular processes	Release of excitatory neurotransmitters (glutamate); failure of cell ion pumps, mitochondrial failure; disruption of blood brain barrier, cell death

TABLE 18.2 Comparison of Mild Traumatic Brain Injury With Moderate and Severe Traumatic Brain Injury

Variable	Mild TBI (Concussion)	Moderate and Severe TBI
Clinical definition	Loss of consciousness lasting <30 minutes, any alteration of consciousness, or post-traumatic amnesia lasting <24 h; some definitions include Glasgow Coma Scale score of 13–15	Loss of consciousness lasting ≥30 min to prolonged coma, posttraumatic amnesia lasting ≥24 h up to permanently, or Glasgow Coma score as low as 3
Focal neurologic signs	Usually none or transient	Frequently present
Neuroimaging with CT or MRI	Usually negative	Diagnostic
Natural History	Full recovery is usual; there is lack of consensus on the natural history of concussion and postconcussive symptoms	Natural history and recovery are directly related to the severity of the injury and functional neuroanatomy
Predictors of persistent symptoms or disability	Psychological factors (e.g., depression, anxiety, or PTSD), compensation and litigation, and negative expectations and beliefs are the strongest risk factors	Directly related to injury characteristics
Neurocognitive testing	Often inconclusive beyond the period of acute injury	Essential and valuable component of ongoing clinical care
Neuronal-cell damage	Metabolic and ionic processes caused by axonal twisting or stretching; these can lead to secondary disconnection	Combination of cellular disruption directly related to injury and metabolic, vascular, and ionic processes

CT, Computed tomography; *MRI*, magnetic resonance imaging; *PTSD*, posttraumatic stress disorder; *TBI*, traumatic brain injury.

Adapted from Hoge CW, Goldberg HM, Castro CA. Care of war veterans with mild traumatic brain injury--flawed perspectives. *New England Journal of Medicine*, 2009; 360(16):1588–1591. https://www.aans.org/en/Patients/Neurosurgical-Conditions-and-Treatments/Traumatic-Brain-Injury

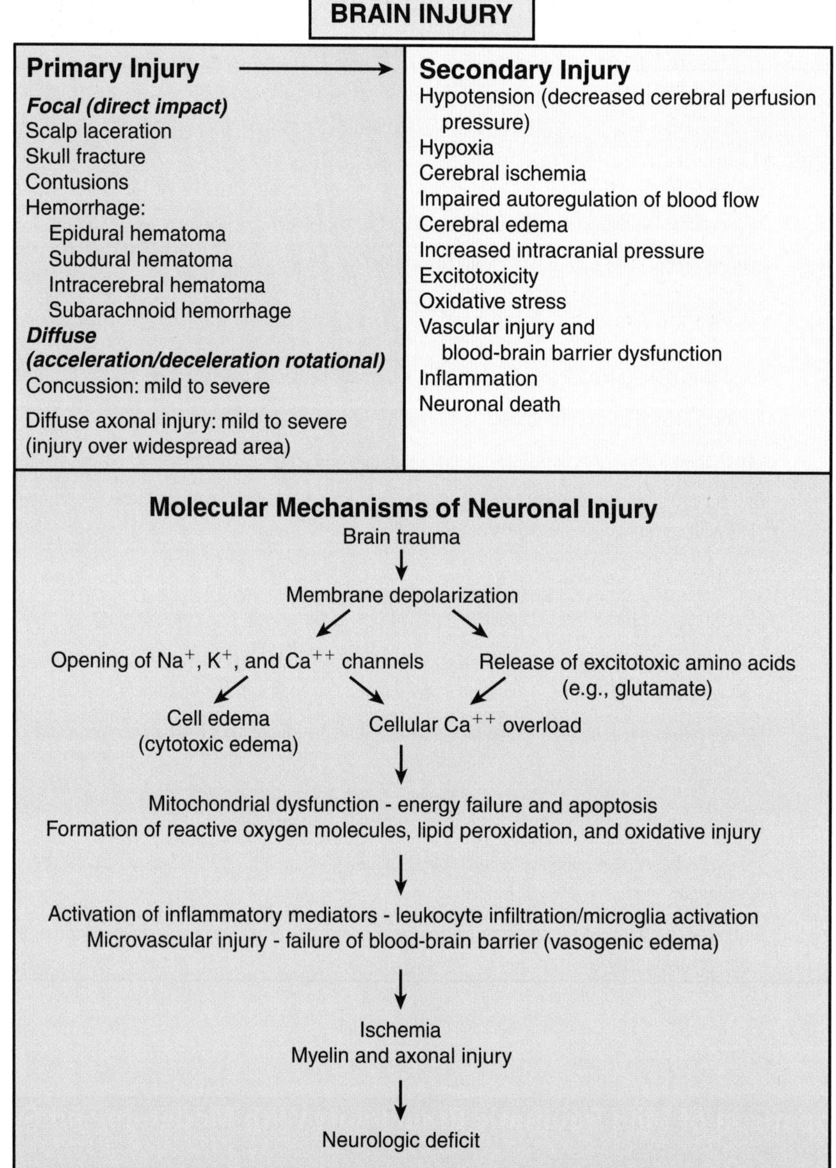

Fig. 18.1 Pathophysiology of Brain Injury Use.

TABLE 18.3 Glasgow Coma Scale[a]

Score[b]	Best Eye Response Score (4)	Best Verbal Response Score (5)	Best Motor Response Score (6)
1	No eye opening	No verbal response	No motor response
2	Eye opening to pain	Incomprehensible sounds	Extension to pain
3	Eye opening to verbal command	Inappropriate words	Flexion to pain
4	Eyes open spontaneously	Confused	Withdrawal from pain
5	NA	Oriented	Localizing pain
6	NA	NA	Obeys commands

[a]The GCS is scored between 3 and 15, with 3 being the worst and 15 the best. It is composed of the sum of three parameters: Best Eye Response (E), Best Verbal Response (V), and Best Motor Response (M). Mild Brain Injury = 13 or higher; Moderate Brain Injury = 9 to 12; Severe Brain Injury = 8 or lower.

[b]It is important to break the scoring report into its components (e.g., E3V3M5 = GCS 11). A total score is meaningless without this information. Age affects the GCS. Elderly individuals with a traumatic brain injury (TBI) have higher (better) GCS scores than younger individuals with a TBI of similar anatomic severity.

NA, Not applicable. Data from Teasdale G, Jennett B. Assessment of coma and impaired consciousness. A practical scale. *Lancet,* 1974;2:81–84; Salottolo K, Levy AS, Slone DS, et al. The effect of age on Glasgow Coma Scale score in patients with traumatic brain injury. *Journal of the American Medical Association Surgery,* 2014;149(7):727–734.

involves a skull fracture, and a break in the dura results in exposure of the cranial contents to the environment. Skull fractures include compound fracture or perforated fracture and linear, comminuted, and basilar skull fracture (BSF; in the cranial vault or at the base of the skull). Focal brain injuries include contusions and hematomas. Types of hematomas include subdural hematomas (SDHs), epidural hematomas (EDHs), and intracerebral hemorrhage (ICH).

Closed head injuries are specific, grossly observable skull and brain lesions that occur in a precise location. Of blunt trauma injuries, 75% to 90% are mild. Injury to the cranial vault, vessels, and supporting structures can produce more severe damage, including contusions and epidural, subdural, subarachnoid, and ICHs. The dura mater remains intact, and brain tissues are not exposed to the environment. The smaller the area of impact, the more severe the injury because of the concentration of force. The injury may be a coup injury (injury at site of impact) or a contrecoup injury (injury from brain rebounding and hitting the opposite side of skull or forces being transmitted through the cerebrospinal fluid [CSF]) (Fig. 18.2). Compression of the skull at the point of impact produces contusions or brain bruising from blood leaking from an injured vessel (Fig. 18.3). The

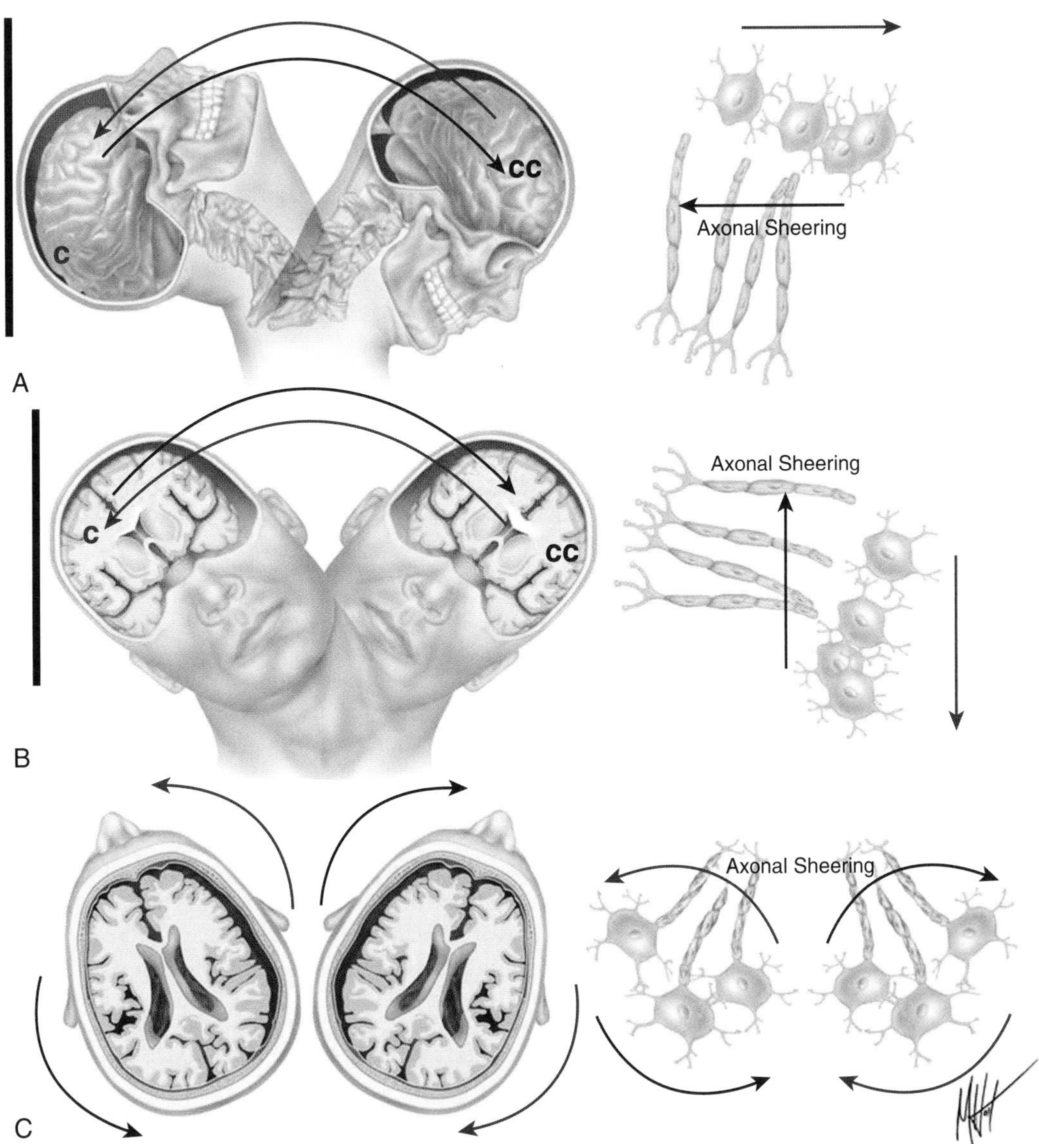

Fig. 18.2 Coup and Contrecoup Focal Injury With Acceleration/Deceleration Axonal Shearing. (A) Sagittal force causing coup *(c)* the site of impact, and contrecoup injury *(cc)*. **(B)** Lateral force causing coup *(c)* and contrecoup *(cc)* injury. **(C)** Axial or rotational injury with shearing of axons, particularly at base of brain. Acceleration/deceleration axonal shearing injury occurs throughout the brain (*red and blue directional arrows* in all three images). (Borrowed from Pascual JM, Preito R. Surgical management of severe closed head injury in adults. In: Quinones-Hinojosa A, eds. *Schmidek and Sweet operative neurosurgical techniques*, 6th ed, vol 2. Philadelphia: Saunders; 2012:1513–1538. Originally redrawn from Adams JH. Brain damage in fatal non-missile head injury in man. In: Braakman R, eds. *Handbook of clinical neurology, head injury*, Vol 13. Gennarelli TA, Thibault LE, Adams JH, et al. Diffuse axonal injury and traumatic coma in the primate. *Annals of Neurology*, 1982;12:564–574.)

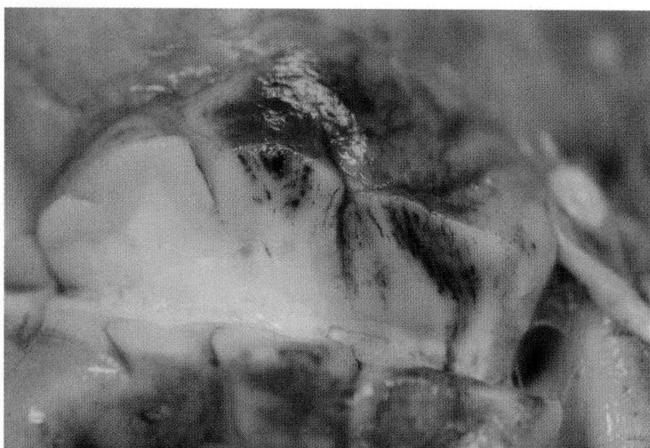

Fig. 18.3 Cerebral Contusion. Close-up view of a contused brain region with characteristic streak-like, densely arranged hemorrhages in the cortex (cut surface here). Such lesions represent "bruises" on the surface of the brain caused by violent contact between the delicate brain parenchyma and the hard inner surface of the skull. (From Pollak S, Saukko P. Blunt Injury, Forensic Medicine/Causes of Death, Encyclopedia of Forensic Sciences. London: Academic Press; 2013.)

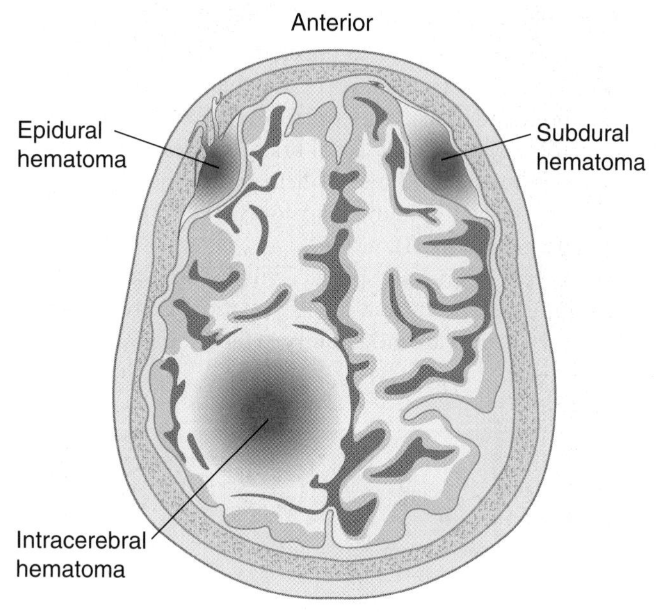

Fig. 18.4 Brain Hematomas.

severity of contusion varies with the amount of energy transmitted by the skull to underlying brain tissue. Contusions occur most commonly in the frontal lobes, the temporal lobes, and at the frontotemporal junction. Injuries in these areas cause changes in attention, memory, intellectual function, affect, emotion, and behavior. Less commonly, contusions occur in the parietal and occipital lobes. Focal cerebral contusions are usually superficial, involving just the brain gyri. Hemorrhagic contusions may coalesce into a large confluent intracranial hematoma.

A contusion may be evidenced by immediate loss of consciousness (generally no longer than 5 minutes), loss of reflexes, transient cessation of respiration, brief period of bradycardia, and decrease in blood pressure (lasting 30 seconds to a few minutes). Vital signs may stabilize to normal values in a few seconds; reflexes then return, and the person regains consciousness over minutes to days. With more severe injury, residual deficits may persist, and some persons never regain a full level of consciousness.

Evaluation is based on the results of the health history, level of consciousness according to the GCS (see Table 18.3), outcomes of imaging studies, and assessment of vital parameters (e.g., intracranial pressure [ICP] and electroencephalogram [EEG]). Large contusions and lacerations with hemorrhage may be surgically excised. Treatment is otherwise directed at controlling ICP, neuroprotection, and managing symptoms.

Brain edema forms around and in damaged neural tissues, contributing to increasing ICP (see Chapter 17). Increased ICP (IICP) occurs when one or more of the contents of the cranial vault—brain tissue, CSF, and blood—increases in volume, because the cranial vault itself is a rigid, fixed compartment. Multiple hemorrhages, edema, infarction, and necrosis can occur within the contused areas. The maximal effects of these injuries peak 18 to 36 hours after severe head injury.

A hematoma is a blood clot within the brain or on its surface. Hematomas include epidural, subdural, and intracerebral locations (Fig. 18.4). An epidural (extradural) hematoma (EDH) is bleeding between the dura mater and the skull. This is often the result of an arterial bleed. The most common site of injury is the temporal fossa as a result of injury to the middle meningeal artery and less commonly to the meningeal vein or dural sinus (Fig. 18.5). It represents 1% to 2% of major head injuries and occurs in all age groups but most commonly in those 20 to 40 years old. An EDH can result in brain herniation (see Fig. 18.5).

Classic presentation of individuals with temporal EDHs involves loss of consciousness at initial injury, a period of lucidity, and then loss of consciousness again. If a vein is bleeding (a slower bleed), one-third of those affected then become lucid for a few minutes to a few days. As the hematoma accumulates, a headache of increasing severity, vomiting, drowsiness, confusion, and seizure occur. The expanding hematoma causes temporal lobe herniation, and the level of consciousness is rapidly lost, with ipsilateral pupillary dilation and contralateral hemiparesis. Imaging usually is needed to diagnose EDH. The prognosis is good if intervention is initiated before bilateral dilation of the pupils occurs. EDHs are medical emergencies requiring evaluation, monitoring, and surgical evacuation of the hematoma.[3]

A subdural hematoma (SDH) is bleeding between the dura mater and the arachnoid membrane covering the brain and is caused by tearing of veins (Fig. 18.6). It is the most common cause of a traumatic intracranial mass lesion, occurring in approximately 10% to 20% of individuals. Nontraumatic SDH can rarely develop in association with anticoagulant therapy or vascular malformations. *Acute SDHs* develop rapidly, commonly within hours. *Subacute SDHs* develop more slowly, often over 48 hours to 2 weeks. *Chronic SDHs* develop over weeks to months. These SDHs act like expanding masses, increasing ICP that eventually compresses the bleeding vessels. If untreated,

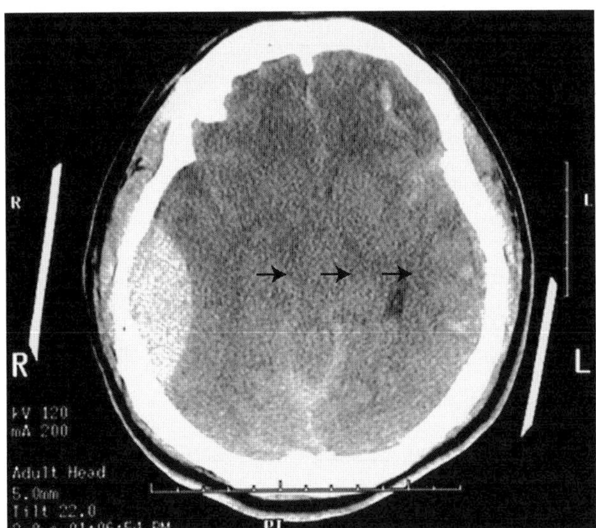

Fig. 18.5 Epidural Hematoma, CT Image. Note the large right epidural hematoma with a lens-shaped outline as the smooth dura becomes indented against the underlying cortex on the right lateral aspect of the cerebrum. The epidural hematoma is confined within an area bounded by cranial sutures where the dura is firmly adherent to the skull. Note the mass effect with effacement of the lateral ventricles and the shift of midline to the left *(arrows)*. In this case the individual fell from a height and struck the right side of his head, severing the middle meningeal artery. This epidural hematoma collected within hours. *CT,* Computed tomography. (From Klatt EC. *Robbins and Cotran atlas of pathology,* 3rd edition. Philadelphia: Saunders, 2015.)

brain herniation can result. With a chronic SDH, the existing subdural space gradually fills with blood. A vascular membrane forms around the hematoma in approximately 2 weeks (Fig. 18.7). Further enlargement may take place.

In acute, rapidly developing SDHs, the expanding clots directly compress the brain. As the ICP rises, bleeding veins are compressed, thus bleeding can be self-limiting. Cerebral compression and displacement of brain tissue can cause temporal lobe herniation.

An acute SDH classically begins with headache, drowsiness, restlessness, or agitation, slowed cognition, and confusion. These symptoms are related to brain shifting or distortion, followed by IICP and low cerebral perfusion pressure. The symptoms worsen over time and progress to loss of consciousness, respiratory pattern changes, and pupillary dilation (i.e., the symptoms of temporal lobe herniation). Homonymous hemianopia (loss of vision in either the right or the left field [see Fig. 16.8]), dysconjugate gaze, and gaze palsies also may occur. Severity of injury is measured using the GCS, ICP monitoring, and brain imaging. In general, clinical deterioration, a clot thickness greater than 10 mm, a midline shift greater than 5 mm, GCS score decreased by 2 or more points from injury to hospital admission, or individuals presenting with pupillary abnormalities are suggested as critical parameters for surgery to remove the clot.[4,5] Of those individuals affected by chronic SDHs, 80% have chronic headaches and tenderness over the hematoma on palpation. Most persons appear to have a progressive dementia with generalized rigidity (paratonia). Chronic SDHs are more

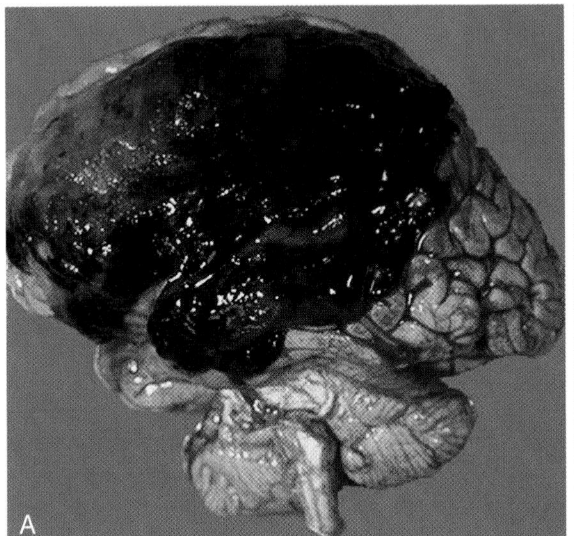

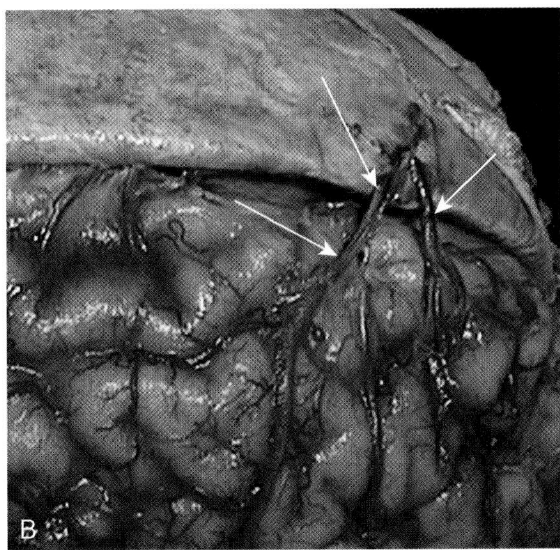

Fig. 18.6 Subdural Hematoma and Bridging Veins. A large subdural hematoma **(A)** is seen in the frontoparietal region. A subdural hematoma forms after head trauma that severs the bridging veins from dura to brain, shown in the right panel **(B)**, where the dura has been folded back to reveal the normal appearance of the bridging veins that extend across to the superior aspect of the cerebral hemispheres. Older adults and the very young are at greater risk because their cerebral veins are more vulnerable to injury. Because the bleeding is venous, blood collects over hours to weeks, with variable onset of symptoms. Because the blood collects beneath the dura, a subdural hematoma can be seen to cross the region of cranial sutures. (From Klatt EC. *Robbins and Cotran atlas of pathology,* 3rd edition. Philadelphia: Saunders, 2015.)

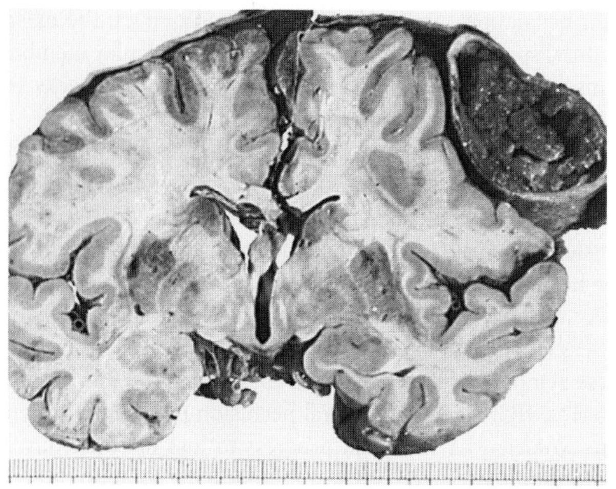

Fig. 18.7 Chronic Subdural Hematoma. Compression of underlying brain and lateral ventricle. Note the capsule around the hematoma. (From Kissane JM, eds. *Anderson's pathology,* 9th edition. St. Louis: Mosby; 1993.)

common in the elderly, resulting from a slow bleed caused by the decrease in brain size (atrophy), which pulls veins from the dura. With brain atrophy, the bleeding may not be recognized right away because there is room within the cranial vault for blood to accumulate before causing IICP. Chronic SDHs require clot evacuation.[6]

Intracerebral (hemorrhage) hematomas (ICHs) (bleeding within the brain tissue) occur in 2% to 3% of persons with head injuries. The hematomas may be single or multiple and are associated with contusions. Most hematomas are located in the frontal and temporal lobes but may occur in the hemispheric deep white matter. Penetrating injury or shearing forces traumatize small blood vessels. The ICH then acts as an expanding mass, increasing the ICP, compressing brain tissues, and causing edema (Fig. 18.8). Delayed ICHs may appear 3 to 10 days after the head injury. ICHs also can occur with non-TBI, such as hemorrhagic stroke.

ICHs cause a decreasing level of consciousness. However, in the case of coma or a confusion state from other injuries, the cause of this increasing unresponsiveness can be difficult to detect. Contralateral hemiplegia also may develop, and, as the ICP rises, temporal lobe herniation may occur. In delayed ICH, the presentation is similar to that of a hypertensive brain hemorrhage—sudden, rapidly progressive decreased level of consciousness with pupillary dilation, breathing pattern changes, hemiplegia, and bilateral positive Babinski reflexes (stroking the lateral side of the sole of the foot causes extension of the big toe—moves up—with fanning of the other toes).

The history and physical examination help to establish the diagnosis, and imaging confirms it. Surgical evacuation of a hematoma is performed, considering clinical signs and symptoms, size, and location of the hematoma, and associated comorbid conditions. Otherwise, treatment is directed at reducing the ICP and allowing the hematoma to reabsorb slowly.[7,8]

Skull Fractures: Linear skull fractures or simple breaks or "cracks" in the skull may accompany TBIs. The dura mater

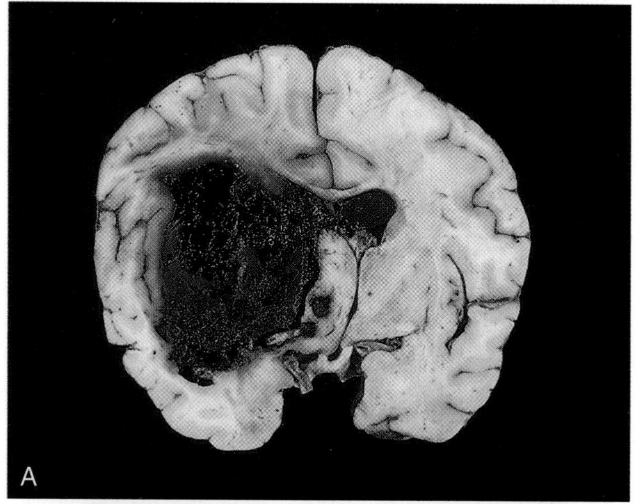

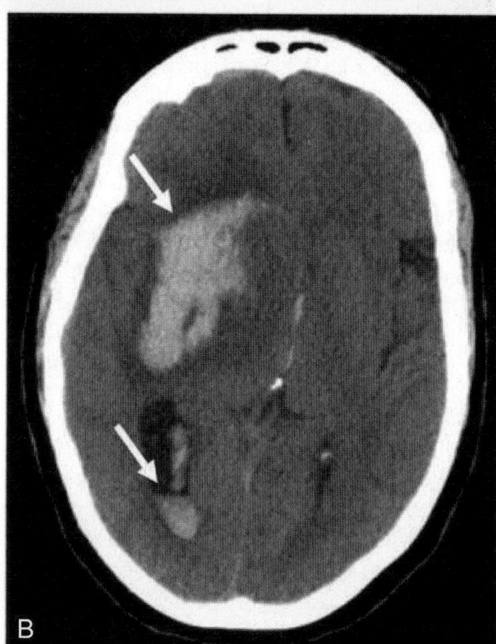

Fig. 18.8 (A) Acute intracerebral hemorrhage. A fresh hematoma has disrupted and expanded the left cerebral hemisphere, causing the midline structures to shift to the right. Uncontrolled hypertension is an important cause of this catastrophic lesion. **(B)** Head computed tomography (CT) scan of intracerebral hemorrhage. Note that the acute hemorrhage appears hyperdense *(white)* on the CT scan. (From Kumar V, Cotran RS, *Robbins SL. Robbins basic pathology,* 7th edition. Philadelphia: Saunders; 2003.)

remains intact. Open brain injury (trauma that penetrates the dura mater) occurs with penetrating trauma or skull fracture. A break in the dura results in exposure of the cranial contents to the environment. Penetration of the dura mater produces both focal and diffuse injuries. An open brain injury can originate from compound skull fractures and missile injuries (e.g., bullets, rocks, shell fragments, knives, and blunt instruments). An open compound skull fracture involves a communication between the cranial contents and the environment and should be investigated whenever lacerations of the scalp, tympanic membrane, sinuses, eye, or mucous membranes are present.

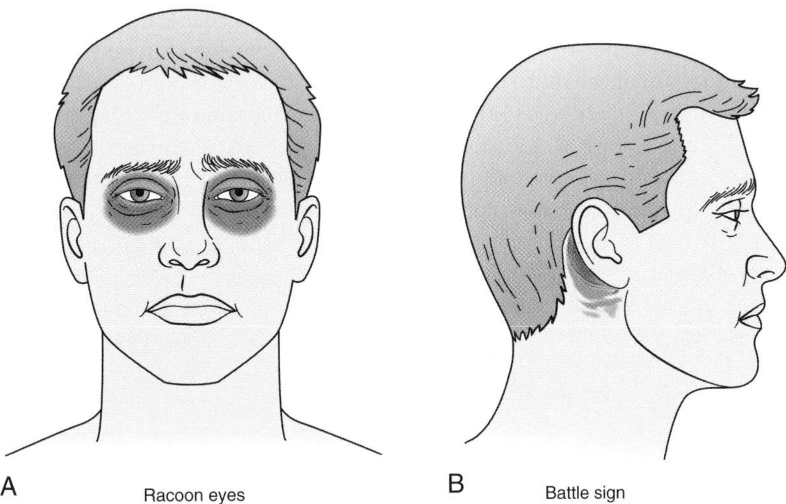

Fig. 18.9 Signs of Basilar Skull Fracture. (A) Raccoon eyes: from leakage of blood from anterior fossa into periorbital tissues. **(B)** Battle Sign: from postauricular hematoma. (From Magee DJ, Manske RC: *Orthopedic physical assessment*, 7th ed. St. Louis, 2021, Elsevier.)

Depressed skull fractures will cause pressure on the brain tissue. These injuries can be associated with environmental debris and are prone to infection. They require prompt débridement and cleaning to prevent infection.[9]

Fractures may involve the cranial vault or the base of the skull. BSFs are problematic because they can cause injury to nerves, arteries, or other structures. If the fracture extends into the sinuses or involves the cribriform plate (BSF), cranial nerve damage and leakage of CSF from the nose or ears may occur.[10] The mechanisms of open brain trauma are crush injury, penetrating injuries, lacerations, and stretch injury (blood vessels and nerves damaged without direct contact as a result of stretching). The tangential injury is to the coverings and the brain (scalp and brain lacerations) and may also include skull fractures as well as meningeal or cerebral lacerations from projectiles and debris driven into the brain.

Most persons lose consciousness with open brain injury. The depth and duration of the coma are related to the location of injury, extent of damage, and amount of bleeding. Open brain injury often requires débridement of the traumatized tissues to prevent infection and to remove blood clots, thereby reducing ICP. The ICP also is managed with dehydrating agents, osmotic diuretics, or a combination of these drugs. Broad-spectrum antibiotics are administered to prevent infection.

A compound fracture may be diagnosed through physical examination, skull x-ray films, or both. BSF is determined based on clinical findings, such as spinal fluid leaking from the ear or nose. Classic signs of periorbital ecchymosis (raccoon eyes) or ecchymosis over the mastoid bone (battle sign) are often noted on assessment for individuals with BSF (Fig. 18.9). Skull x-rays often do not display the fracture, although intracranial air (pneumocephalus) or air in the sinuses on imaging is indirect evidence of a BSF. Bed rest and close observation for meningitis and other complications are prescribed for a BSF.

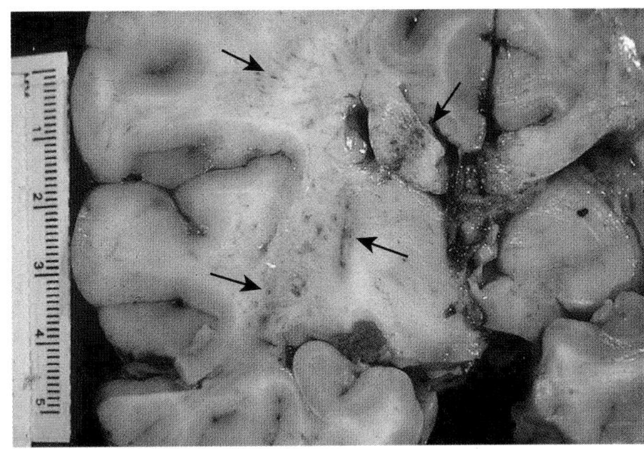

Fig. 18.10 Diffuse Axonal Injury. Gross photograph demonstrating characteristic hemorrhage lesions within the corpus callosum. (Courtesy Walter Kemp, MD, Department of Pathology, University of Texas Southwestern Medical School, Dallas. From Kumar V, Cotran RS, Robbins SL. *Robbins basic pathology*, 7th edition. Philadelphia: Saunders; 2003.)

Diffuse brain injury. TBIs can produce microscopic changes that do not appear on computed tomography (CT) scans and are scattered throughout the brain. This category of injuries, called diffuse brain injury, may occur with or without an associated mass lesion. The most common diffuse brain injury is diffuse axonal injury (DAI) caused by shearing forces (see section later) (Fig. 18.10). Another diffuse injury with TBI is subarachnoid hemorrhage (SAH). SAH is bleeding into the subarachnoid space; this is often caused by aneurysm rupture (see section on Hemorrhagic Stroke). However, SAH can also occur after TBI when shearing forces tear small bridging blood vessels with bleeding into the subarachnoid space. The bleeding appears as diffuse blood spread thinly over the brain. Most cases of SAH associated with head trauma are mild. Severe traumatic SAH can result in hydrocephalus from damage to arachnoid granulations and mechanical blockage to the flow of CSF.[11]

Diffuse axonal injury (DAI), also known as traumatic axonal injury or multifocal axonal injury, involves widespread areas of the brain and occurs with all severities of brain injury. DAI results from mechanical effects of high levels of acceleration and deceleration injury, such as whiplash, or rotational forces that cause shearing and stretch of delicate axonal fibers and white matter tracts that project to or from the cerebral cortex (see Fig. 18.2). The most severe axonal injuries are more peripheral to the brainstem.[12] If enough axons are harmed in this way, the ability of nerve cells to communicate with each other may be lost or greatly impaired, possibly leaving an individual with behavioral, cognitive, and physical changes and severe disabilities. Pathophysiologically, axonal damage can be seen only with an electron microscope at postmortem examination and involves numerous axons, either alone or in conjunction with actual tissue tears. Advanced imaging techniques assist in defining areas of injury. DAI is often not visible on CT imaging but may be seen as diffuse punctate hemorrhages in areas where axons and small blood vessels are torn. More damaged axons are visible 12 hours to several days after the initial injury. The severity of diffuse injury correlates with how much shearing force was applied to the brainstem.

DAI is not associated with intracranial hypertension immediately after injury; however, acute brain swelling, caused by vasodilation, increased intravascular blood flow within the brain, and increased cerebral blood volume, is seen often and can result in hypoxic-ischemic injury and death. DAI may induce long-term neurodegenerative processes. These changes may continue for years after injury, with the development of chronic traumatic encephalopathy (CTE) and Alzheimer disease–like pathologic changes.[13]

Secondary brain injury. Secondary brain injury is an indirect result of primary brain injury, including trauma and stroke syndromes. It occurs as a consequence of primary injury, a cascade of cerebral and molecular events initiated at the time of trauma and lasts for hours to days. Both systemic and cerebral processes are contributing factors. Systemic processes include hypotension, hypoxia, anemia, ischemia, hypercapnia, and hypocapnia. Cerebral contributions include inflammation, cerebral edema, IICP, microthrombosis, decreased cerebral perfusion pressure, cerebral ischemia, and brain herniation. Molecular mechanisms include excitotoxicity (excessive stimulation by excitatory neurotransmitters, such as glutamate), potassium efflux, calcium influx, spreading waves of depolarization, mitochondrial dysfunction, oxidative stress, the secretion of inflammatory cytokines and chemokines, apoptosis, blood brain barrier disruption, and neuronal death.

Cerebrovascular autoregulation (constriction or dilation in response to increases or decreases in cerebral perfusion pressure) is also impaired after brain injury and may be transient or persistent with alterations in CO_2 reactivity (e.g., CO_2 vasodilation). Vasospasm commonly occurs, contributing to brain hypoperfusion and ischemia. The vasospasm is caused by chronic depolarization of vascular smooth muscle, release of endothelin (vasoconstrictor), and decreased availability of nitric oxide (vasodilator). The molecular mechanisms of secondary brain injury are summarized in Fig. 18.1.[14,15]

The management of secondary brain injury is related to prevention of hypoxia and maintenance of cerebral perfusion pressure. Management includes removal of hematomas and treatment of hypotension, hypoxemia, anemia, cerebral edema, ICP, fluid and electrolyte balance, body temperature, ventilation, and nutrition. The development of neuroprotective agents, particularly antiinflammatory agents, is in progress but challenging to develop because of the complexity of multiple interacting secondary injury cascades.[16] Supportive treatments also are important. Nutrition management has emerged as critically important in the care of individuals with severe brain injury and should be initiated within the first 24 hours after injury.[17] Long-term recovery and mortality can be influenced by systemic complications, such as pneumonia, fever, infections, and immobility, that contribute to further brain injury and delays in repair and recovery

Categories of traumatic brain injury. Several categories of TBI exist and are presented here as mild, moderate, and severe. Concussion is the mildest form of TBI and occurs when a head injury causes a sudden change in mental status. More than 50% of the US population participates in sports, and there are approximately 3.8 million concussions each year.[18] The severity of TBI commonly considers the duration of loss of consciousness, the GCS score, posttraumatic amnesia, and brain imaging results.[14]

Mild traumatic brain injury is characterized by immediate but transitory clinical manifestations. There may be no loss of consciousness, or loss of consciousness may last less than 30 minutes. Most blunt trauma injuries cause mild concussion. The GCS score is 13 to 15. The initial confusional state lasts for 1 to several minutes, possibly with amnesia for events preceding the trauma (retrograde amnesia). Persons may experience headache, nausea, vomiting, impaired ability to concentrate, and difficulty sleeping for up to a few days.

Moderate traumatic brain injury is any loss of consciousness lasting more than 30 minutes and up to 6 hours. The GCS score is 9 to 12. A BSF may be present, but there is no brainstem injury; however, there may be transitory decerebration or decortication (see Fig. 17.6). The person is often confused and experiences posttraumatic amnesia that lasts for more than 24 hours. There may be permanent deficits in selective attention, vigilance, detection, working memory, data processing, vision or perception, and language, as well as mood and affect changes ranging from mild to severe. Brain imaging is abnormal.

Severe traumatic brain injury is loss of consciousness lasting more than 6 hours. The GCS is 3 to 8. Frequently there are associated signs of brainstem damage, including changes in pupillary reaction, cardiac and respiratory symptoms, decorticate or decerebrate posturing (see Fig. 17.6), and abnormal reflexes. Brain imaging is abnormal. IICP appears 4 to 6 days after injury. Pulmonary complications occur frequently, with profound sensorimotor and cognitive system deficits. Severely compromised coordinated movements and verbal and written communication, inability to learn and reason, and inability to modulate behavior also are evident. Individuals will require intensive care unit (ICU) care, intubation/mechanical ventilation, and vigilant care to prevent IICP. Severe injury causes permanent neurologic deficits, and some individuals remain in a vegetative state or die as a result of brain injury or secondary complications.

The goal of treating TBI is to maintain cerebral perfusion and oxygenation and promote neuroprotection. Implementation of management guidelines for TBI decreases death and improves neurologic outcome. Corticosteroids increase mortality with acute TBI and, consequently, should not be used.[19]

Complications of Traumatic Brain Injury

Many complications are associated with TBI and are related to the severity of injury and the parts of the brain that are affected. Altered states of consciousness can range from confusion to deep coma (see Table 17.3). Cognitive deficits, hydrocephalus, sensory-motor disorders (including pain, paresis, and paralysis), and loss of coordination may be present. Three of the most common posttraumatic brain syndromes are summarized as follows.

Postconcussion syndrome occurs with mild TBI. Symptoms are nonspecific and include headache (most common), dizziness, fatigue, nervousness or anxiety, irritability, insomnia, depression, inability to concentrate, and forgetfulness; they may last for weeks to months after a mild concussion. Treatment entails reassurance and symptomatic relief in addition to 24 hours of close observation after the concussion in the event bleeding or swelling in the brain occurs. Symptoms requiring further evaluation and treatment include drowsiness or confusion, nausea or vomiting, severe headache, memory deficit, seizures, drainage of cerebrospinal fluid from the ear or nose, weakness, or loss of feeling in the extremities, asymmetry of the pupils, and double vision. Guidelines for the management of pediatric and adult concussion are available.[20–23] Guidelines have been published for the management of sports-related concussion.[24]

Posttraumatic seizures (epilepsy) occur in approximately 10% to 20% of TBIs, with the highest risk among open brain injuries. Seizures can occur early, within days, and up to 2 to 5 years or longer after the trauma. Causal mechanisms are poorly understood, but they are associated with both focal and diffuse brain injury that creates epileptogenic foci with seizures and epilepsy. Seizure prevention using drugs, such as phenytoin, is initiated for moderate to severe TBI at the time of injury and continued for the first week. Continued antiseizure treatments are used only if seizures occur.[25]

Chronic traumatic encephalopathy (CTE) (previously called *dementia pugilistica*) is a progressive dementing disease that develops with repeated brain injury associated with sporting events, blast injuries in soldiers, or work-related head trauma. Tau neurofibrillary tangles are present in the brain. CTE is associated with violent behaviors, loss of control, depression, suicide, memory loss, and cognitive change that lasts at least 12 months. Research is in progress to discover the mechanistic link between neurotrauma and CTE. It is diagnosed from history, clinical evaluation, and at autopsy.[26]

Spinal Cord and Vertebral Injury

A spinal cord injury (SCI) is damage to the nerves within the bony protection of the spinal canal. The nerves can be severed, bruised, stretched, or crushed. The most common cause is trauma from vehicular accidents, falls, diving, violence, and sports injuries. SCI results in the loss of the ability to send and receive messages from the brain to the body's system that controls sensory, motor, and autonomic function. Each year 17,900 persons experience serious SCI, and 78% of new SCI cases are male. The average age at injury is 43 years. Motor vehicle crashes are the leading cause of injury, followed by falls and then violence, other events, and sports activities.[27] Elderly people are particularly at risk for trauma that results in serious SCI because of preexisting degenerative vertebral disorders.

Pathophysiology. Primary spinal cord injury occurs with the initial mechanical trauma and immediate tissue destruction. Injuries to the cord are summarized in Table 18.4. Primary SCI may be complete or incomplete. With complete transection, there is loss of movement and sensation below the site of injury. Spinal

TABLE 18.4 Spinal Cord Injuries

Injury	Description
Cord concussion	Results in temporary disruption of cord-mediated functions
Cord contusion	Bruising of neural tissue causes swelling and temporary loss of cord-mediated functions
Cord compression	Pressure on cord causes ischemia to tissues; must be relieved (decompressed) to prevent permanent damage to spinal cord
Laceration and shearing	Tearing of neural tissues of spinal cord; may be reversible if only slight damage sustained by neural tissues; may result in permanent loss of cord-mediated functions if spinal tracts are disrupted
Transection	Severing of spinal cord causes permanent loss of function
• Complete	All tracts in spinal cord are completely disrupted; all cord-mediated functions below transection are completely and permanently lost
• Incomplete	Some tracts in spinal cord remain intact, together with functions mediated by these tracts; has potential for recovery, although function is temporarily lost
• Preserved sensation only	Some demonstrable sensation below level of injury
• Preserved motor nonfunctional	Preserved motor function without useful purpose; sensory function may or may not be preserved
• Preserved motor functional	Preserved voluntary motor function that is functionally useful
Hemorrhage	Bleeding into neural tissue as a result of blood vessel damage; usually no major loss of function
Damage or obstruction of spinal blood supply	Causes local ischemia

injury can also occur if an injured spine is not adequately immobilized immediately following injury. Primary spinal cord injury can occur in the absence of vertebral fracture or dislocation and is related to longitudinal stretching of the cord with or without flexion or extension of the vertebral column, or both. The stretching causes altered axon transport, edema, myelin degeneration, and retrograde or wallerian neural degeneration (see Chapter 15).

Secondary spinal cord injury is a complex pathophysiologic cascade of vascular, cellular, and biochemical events that begins within a few minutes after injury and continues for weeks. Secondary injury includes hemorrhages, inflammation, edema, ischemia, free radical formation, and apoptosis/necrosis. Hemorrhages develop in the central gray matter, and edema develops in the white matter, impairing the microcirculation of the cord. The hemorrhages and edema are followed by loss of vascular autoregulation, vasospasm and vascular occlusion, reduced perfusion, and development of ischemic areas, which are maximal at the level of injury and two cord segments above and below it. Cord swelling increases the individual's degree of dysfunction, making it difficult to distinguish functions permanently lost from those temporarily impaired. In the cervical region at C1 to C4, cord swelling may be life threatening because cardiovascular and respiratory control functions can be lost. Diaphragm function may be impaired because phrenic nerves exit at C3 to C5. Excitotoxicity (excessive stimulation by excitatory neurotransmitters, such as glutamate), intracellular calcium overload, oxidative damage, and cell death occur similarly to those previously described for TBI. Spared neurons continue to be chronically injured, with death of oligodendrocytes and myelin degeneration, axonal disruption, glial scarring, cystic cavitation, and release of inhibitory mediators. The process presents a physical and chemical barrier to regeneration.[28]

Vertebral injuries result from acceleration, deceleration, or deformation forces occurring at impact. These forces cause vertebral fractures, dislocations, and penetration of bone fragments that can cause compression to the tissues, pull or exert traction (tension) on the tissues, or cause shearing of tissues so they slide into one another (Figs. 18.11–18.14). Vertebral injuries can be classified as (1) simple fracture—a single break usually affecting transverse or spinous processes; (2) compressed (wedged) vertebral fracture—vertebral body compressed anteriorly; (3) comminuted (burst) fracture—vertebral body shattered into several fragments; and (4) dislocation.

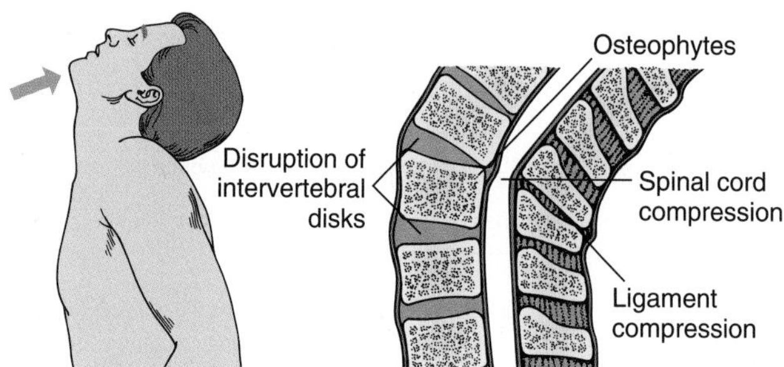

Fig. 18.11 Hyperextension Injuries of the Spine. Hyperextension injuries of the spine can result in fracture or nonfracture injuries with spinal cord damage.

The vertebrae fracture readily with both direct and indirect trauma. When the supporting ligaments are torn, the vertebrae move out of alignment, and dislocations occur. A horizontal force moves the vertebrae straight forward; if the individual is in a flexed position at the time of injury, the vertebrae are then angulated. Flexion and extension injuries may result in dislocations and subluxation of the vertebrae. (Bone, ligament, and joint injuries are presented in Table 18.5).

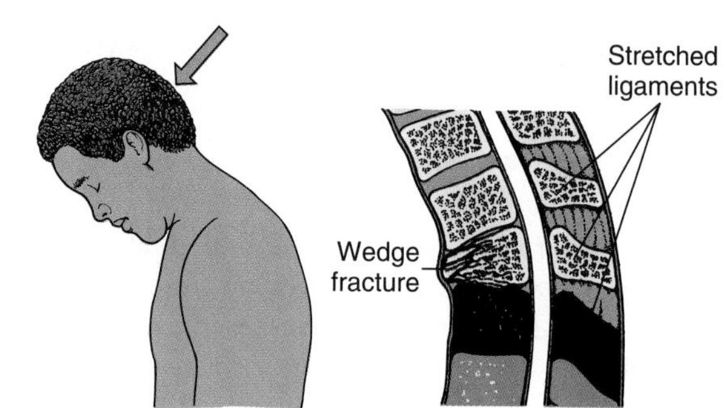

Fig. 18.12 Flexion Injury of the Spine. Hyperflexion produces translation (subluxation) of vertebrae that compromises the central canal and compresses spinal cord parenchyma or vascular structures.

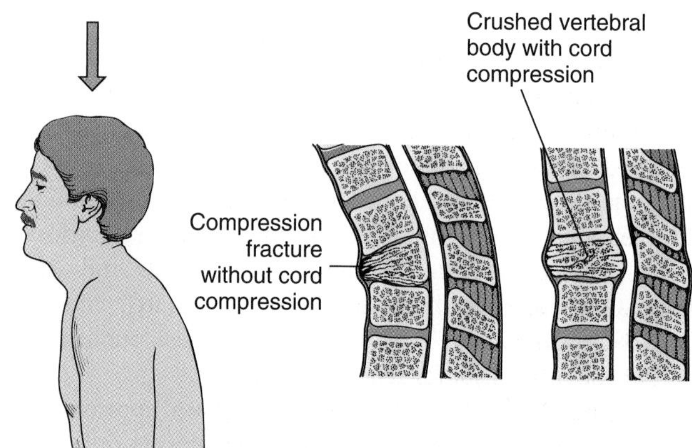

Fig. 18.13 Axial Compression Injuries of the Spine. In axial compression injuries of the spine, the spinal cord is contused directly by retropulsion of bone or disk material into the spinal canal.

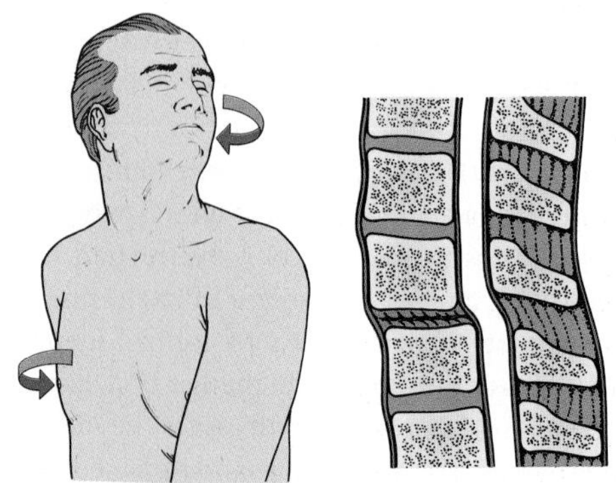

Fig. 18.14 Flexion-Rotation Injuries of the Spine.

TABLE 18.5 Mechanisms of Vertebral Injury Involving Bone, Ligaments, and Joints

Mechanism of Injury	Location of Vertebral Injury	Forces of Injury	Location of Injury
Hyperextension	Fracture and dislocation of posterior elements, such as spinous processes, transverse processes, laminae, pedicles, or posterior ligaments	Results from forces of acceleration/deceleration and sudden reduction in anteroposterior diameter of spinal cord	Cervical area
Hyperflexion	Fracture or dislocation of vertebral bodies, disks, or ligaments	Results from sudden and excessive force that propels neck forward or causes an exaggerated lateral movement of neck to one side	Cervical area
Vertical compression (axial loading)	Shattering fractures	Results from a force applied along an axis from top of cranium through vertebral bodies	T12 to L2
Rotational forces (flexion-rotation)	Rupture support ligaments in addition to producing fractures	Add shearing force to acceleration forces	Cervical area

Vertebral body fractures may not involve cord damage. Vertebral injuries in adults occur most often at vertebrae C1 to C2 (cervical), C4 to C7 (cervical), and T10 (thoracic) to L2 (lumbar) (see Fig. 15.11), the most mobile portions of the vertebral column. The spinal cord also occupies most of the vertebral canal in the cervical and lumbar regions, so it can be easily injured in these locations. Functioning after SCI depends on type and level of injury (Tables 18.6 and 18.7).

Clinical Manifestations/Complications. Spinal shock is the temporary loss of spinal cord functions below the lesion. Spinal shock develops immediately after injury because of loss of continuous tonic discharge from the brain or brainstem and inhibition of central descending impulses that control and modulate spinal cord neurons. It is caused by cord hemorrhage, edema, or anatomic transection. Normal activity of spinal cord cells at and below the level of injury ceases, with complete loss of reflex function, flaccid paralysis, absence of sensation, loss of bladder and rectal control, transient drop in blood pressure, bradycardia, and poor venous circulation. The condition also results in disturbed thermal control because the sympathetic nervous system is damaged. The hypothalamus cannot regulate body heat through vasoconstriction and increased metabolism; therefore the individual assumes the temperature of the air (poikilothermia). Spinal shock can progress for several hours but generally lasts 2 to 3 days. It terminates with the reappearance of bulbocavernosus reflex activity, hyperreflexia, spasticity, and reflex emptying of the bladder, all of which may take weeks to months. Table 18.8 summarizes the clinical manifestations of SCI.

Neurogenic shock, also called *vasogenic shock*, occurs with cervical or upper thoracic cord injury above T6 and may be seen in addition to spinal shock. Neurogenic shock is a serious, life-threatening condition. It occurs as a result of loss of sympathetic tone, through loss of supraspinal control and unopposed parasympathetic tone mediated by the intact vagus nerve. Neurogenic shock causes widespread dilation of blood vessels with severe hypotension, bradycardia, and failure of body temperature regulation with hypothermia (see Chapter 48).

Neurogenic shock may be complicated by hypovolemic or cardiogenic shock if there is concurrent blood loss or heart failure (see Chapters 32 and 48). Loss of motor and sensory function depends on the extent and level of injury. Paralysis of the lower half of the body with both legs involved is termed *paraplegia*. Paralysis involving all four extremities is termed *quadriplegia* (tetraplegia). In complete quadriplegia, the level of injury is above C6 and all upper extremity function is lost.

TABLE 18.6 Level of Injury: American Spinal Injury Association Scale

A = no motor control, no sensation
B = no motor control, some sensation
C = some motor function
D = motor function incomplete with more function below lesion area
E = normal

TABLE 18.7 Level of Injury Outcomes

C1–C3	Limited movement of head and neck.
C3–C4	Usually has head and neck control. Individuals at C4 level may shrug their shoulders.
C5	Typically has head and neck control, can shrug shoulder, and has shoulder control. Can bend his/her elbows and turn palms face up.
C6	Has movement in head, neck, shoulders, arms, and wrists. Can shrug shoulders, bend elbows, turn palms up and down, and extend wrists.
C7	Has similar movement as an individual with C6, with added ability to straighten his/her elbows.
T1	Has added strength and precision of fingers that result in limited or natural hand function.
T2–T6	Has normal motor function in head, neck, shoulders, arms, hands, and fingers. Has increased use of rib and chest muscles, or trunk control.
T7–T12	Has added motor function from increased abdominal control.
L1–L5	Has additional return of motor movement in the hips and knees.
S1–S5	Depending on level of injury, there are various degrees of return of voluntary bladder, bowel, and sexual functions.

Reference: https://www.sci-info-pages.com/spinal-cord-injury-functional-goals/.

TABLE 18.8 **Clinical Manifestations of Spinal Cord Injury**

Stage	Manifestations
Spinal Shock Stage	
Complete spinal cord transection	Loss of motor function 1. Quadriplegia with injuries of cervical spinal cord 2. Paraplegia with injuries of thoracic spinal cord Muscle flaccidity Loss of all reflexes below level of injury Loss of pain, temperature, touch, pressure, and proprioception below level of injury Pain at site of injury caused by zone of hyperesthesia above injury Atonic bladder and bowel Paralytic ileus with abdominal distention Loss of vasomotor tone in lower body parts; low and unstable blood pressure Loss of perspiration below level of injury Loss or extreme depression of genital reflexes, such as penile erection and bulbocavernosus reflex Dry and pale skin; possible ulceration over bony prominences Respiratory impairment
Partial spinal cord transection	Asymmetric flaccid motor paralysis below level of injury Asymmetric reflex loss Preservation of some sensation below level of injury Vasomotor instability less severe than that seen with complete cord transection Bowel and bladder impairment less severe than that seen with complete cord transection Preservation of ability to perspire in some portions of body below level of injury *Brown-Séquard syndrome* (associated with penetrating injuries, hyperextension and flexion, locked facets, and compression fractures) 1. Ipsilateral paralysis or paresis below level of injury 2. Ipsilateral loss of touch, pressure, vibration, and position sense below level of injury 3. Contralateral loss of pain and temperature sensations below level of injury *Cauda equina syndrome* (compression of nerve roots below L1 caused by fracture and dislocation of spine or large posterocentral intervertebral disk herniation) 1. Lower extremity motor deficits 2. Variable sensorimotor dysfunction (i.e., saddle anesthesia) 3. Variable reflex dysfunction in lower extremities 4. Neurogenic bladder or bowel, and sexual dysfunction
Heightened Reflex Activity Stage	
	Emergence of Babinski reflexes Hyperactive ankle and knee reflexes Reflex urinary incontinence and defecation Episodes of hypertension Defective heat-induced sweating Development of extensor reflexes, first in muscles of hip and thigh, later in leg

In incomplete quadriplegia, function at or above C6 is preserved, leaving the shoulder, upper arm, and some forearm muscle control intact. The initial clinical manifestations associated with acute SCI are related to the spinal shock described earlier and include (1) rapid development of flaccid paralysis below the level of injury, (2) loss of sensations in the lower extremities and possibly lower trunk (depending on the level of injury), and (3) loss of spinal and autonomic reflexes below the level of injury. The duration of this areflexic state is highly variable. In most persons, reflex activity returns in approximately a week. Return of spinal neuron excitability occurs slowly. First to return is the bulbocavernosus reflex (indicative of intact S2 to S4 spinal reflex arcs).[29] Depending on the degree of damage, either of the following can occur: (1) motor, sensory, reflex, and autonomic functions return to normal, or (2) autonomic neural activity in the isolated segment develops. Spasticity is common, with hyperreflexia, clonus, and painful muscle spasms. Sometimes after several months, episodes of autonomic hyperreflexia occur.

Autonomic hyperreflexia (dysreflexia) is a severe, life-threatening complication associated with a SCI at level T6 or above, where descending inhibition is blocked resulting in autonomic nervous system dysregulation. Autonomic hyperreflexia occurs because descending inhibition is blocked (Fig. 18.15). It may occur after spinal shock resolves and be a recurrent complication. Characteristics include paroxysmal hypertension (up to 300 mm Hg, systolic), a pounding headache, blurred vision, sweating above the level of the lesion, with flushing of the skin, nasal congestion, nausea, piloerection caused by pilomotor spasm, and bradycardia (30 to 40 beats/min). The symptoms

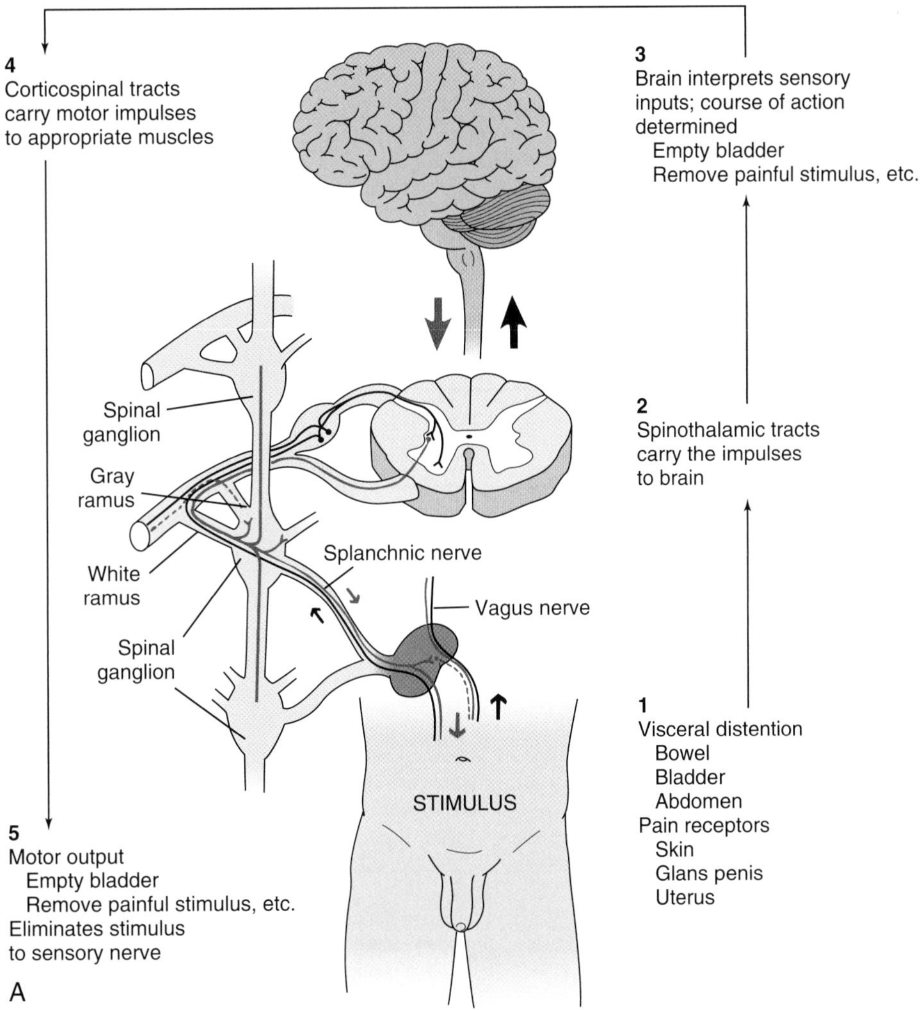

Fig. 18.15 Autonomic Hyperreflexia. **(A)** Normal response pathway.

may develop singly or in combination. The condition can cause serious complications (stroke, seizures, myocardial ischemia, and death) and requires immediate treatment.

In autonomic hyperreflexia, sensory receptors below the level of the cord lesion are stimulated. The intact autonomic nervous system reflexively responds with an arteriolar spasm that increases blood pressure. Baroreceptors in the cerebral vessels, the carotid sinus, and the aorta sense the hypertension and stimulate the parasympathetic system. The heart rate decreases, but the visceral and peripheral vessels do not dilate because efferent impulses cannot pass through the cord, and there is loss of blood pressure regulation.

The most common trigger is a distended bladder or rectum (constipation); however, any sensory stimulation (i.e., skin or pain receptors) can elicit autonomic hyperreflexia (tight clothing or shoes). The primary intervention is to locate and remediate the source causing the autonomic dysreflexia. (e.g., emptying of the bladder or bowel and elevating the head of the bed). Drug therapy may be required to lower blood pressure and reduce complications. Bladder, bowel, and skin care management are important preventive strategies. Education of the individual and family regarding triggers and acute management is important, as is wearing a medic alert tag.[30]

Evaluation and Treatment. Diagnosis of SCI is based on physical examination and imaging studies. Initial treatment should be focused on determination of the extent of the injury. For a suspected or confirmed vertebral fracture or dislocation, regardless of the presence or absence of SCI, the immediate intervention is immobilization of the spine to prevent further injury. Decompression and surgical fixation may be necessary. Neurogenic shock must be differentiated from other kinds of shock (e.g., hypovolemic shock). Blood pressure control, lung function, nutrition, skin integrity, prevention of pressure ulcers, pain management, and bladder and bowel management must be addressed because all systems and organs are affected below the level of neurologic injury. Early intervention and rehabilitation provide the most hope to preserve the cord, prevent irreversible damage, and prevent long term complications The American Spinal Injury International standards for neurologic classification of SCI is a starting evaluation for predicting outcomes after SCI.[31,32] Neuroprotective, neuroregenerative, and neuroplastic strategies are under clinical investigation.[33–37]

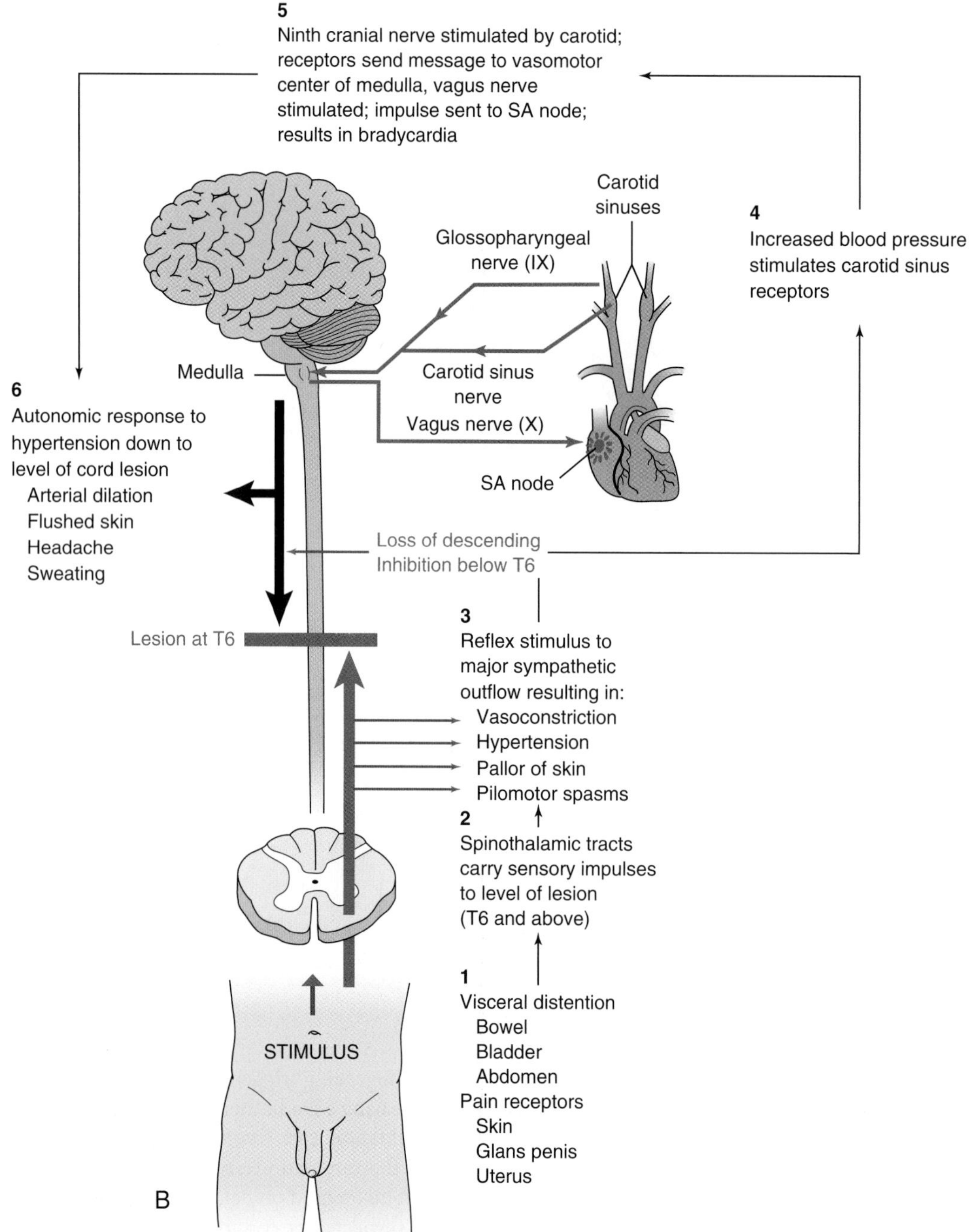

Fig. 18.15, cont'd (B) Autonomic hyperreflexia pathway. *SA*, Sinoatrial. (Modified from Rudy EB. *Advanced neurological and neurosurgical nursing*. St. Louis: Mosby; 1984.)

Degenerative Disorders of the Spine

Low Back Pain

Low back pain (LBP) affects the area between the lower rib cage and gluteal muscles and often radiates into the thighs. Approximately 80% of the population experiences LBP at some time during their lives, and approximately 25% of the adult population in the United States has experienced LBP in the past 3 months.[38] LBP is the leading global cause of years lived with disability.[39]

The burdens of disability include psychological, financial, occupational, and social effects on the person and family members. Risk factors include occupations that require repetitive lifting in the forward bent-and-twisted position, exposure to vibrations caused by vehicles or industrial machinery, obesity, osteoporosis, and cigarette smoking.

Pathophysiology. Most cases of LBP are idiopathic or nonspecific, and no precise diagnosis is possible. Acute LBP (lasting less than 4 weeks) is often associated with muscle or ligament strain and is more common in individuals younger than 50 years

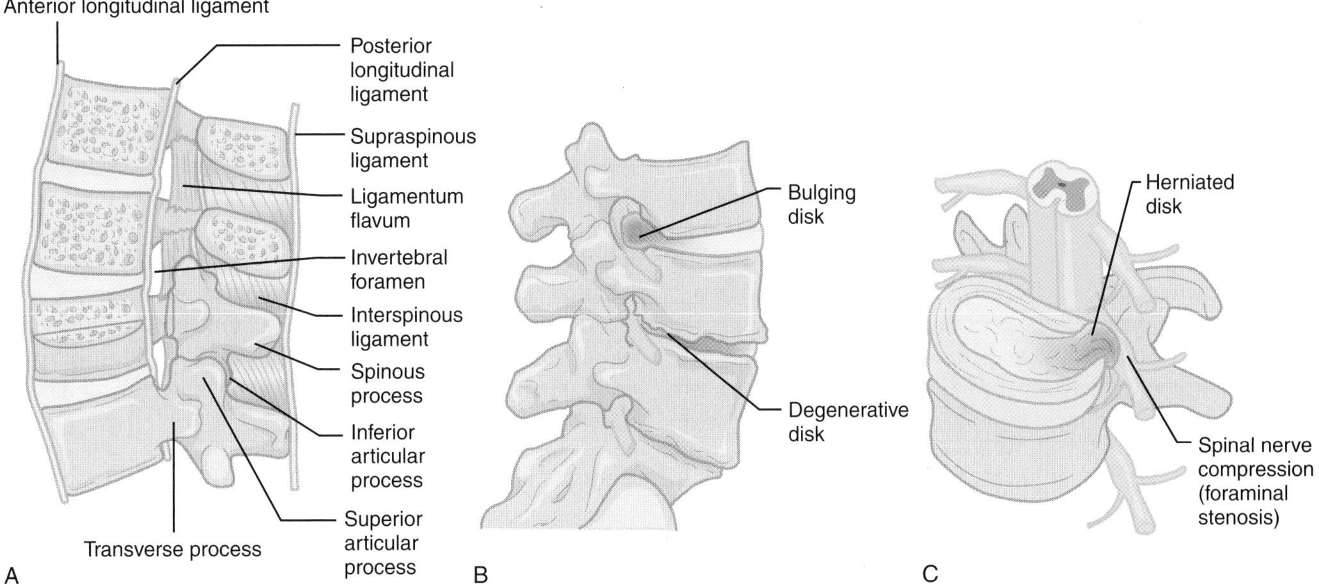

Fig. 18.16 Spinal Ligaments, Degenerating Disk, and Herniated Disk. **(A)** Ligaments of the spine. **(B)** Bulging disk with spinal nerve compression and degenerative disk showing collapse of vertebral body. **(C)** Herniated disk with spinal nerve compression.

of age without a history of cancer. The interspinous bursae can be a source of pain, particularly in the lumbar vertebrae. The ligaments of the spine are supplied with pain receptors, and all these ligaments are vulnerable to traumatic tears (sprains) and fracture. Chronic LBP is also related to inflammation and the development of peripheral and central neuropathic pain (Fig. 18.16A).[40]

Common causes of chronic LBP (greater than 3 months duration) include spondylolysis (vertebral stress fracture), spondylolisthesis (vertebra slides forward or slips in relation to a vertebra below), spinal osteochondrosis (abnormal bone growth), spinal stenosis, degenerative disk disease (DDD), and lumbar disk herniation (see Fig. 18.16). Other causes include tension caused by tumors or disk prolapse, bursitis, synovitis, spinal immobility, inflammation caused by infection (as in osteomyelitis), and pain referred from viscera or the posterior peritoneum. Systemic causes of LBP include bone diseases, such as osteoporosis or osteomalacia, and hyperparathyroidism. Anatomically, LBP must originate from innervated structures, but deep pain is widely referred and varies. The nucleus pulposus has no intrinsic innervation, but when extruded or herniated through a prolapsed disk, it irritates the spinal nerve and associated structures and causes pain referred to the segmental area (see Fig. 18.16C).

Clinical Manifestations. Some individuals with acute LBP have pain along the distribution of a lumbar nerve root (radicular pain), most commonly involving the sciatic nerve (sciatica). Sciatica is often accompanied by neurosensory and motor deficits, such as tingling, numbness, and weakness in various parts of the leg and foot. Chronic LBP may be associated with progressive motor or sensory deficits, cauda equina syndrome (new-onset bowel or bladder incontinence or urinary retention, loss of anal sphincter tone, and saddle anesthesia), a history of cancer metastasis to bone, and suspected spinal infection.

Evaluation and Treatment. Diagnosis of LBP is based on the history and physical examination. Imaging and nerve conduction studies are obtained with severe neurologic deficit or serious underlying disease ("red flags"), including progressive or rapid motor or sensory loss (e.g., saddle anesthesia), new urinary retention or overflow incontinence, history of cancer, recent invasive spinal procedure, and significant trauma relative to age.[41] The straight leg raise test (Lasegue test) assesses sciatic pain (radiating pain from the buttocks to the leg) due to lumbosacral nerve root irritation. Diagnosis and treatment guidelines are available to plan therapy.[42] Most individuals with acute LBP benefit from a nonspecific short-term treatment regimen with return to normal activities, avoiding bed rest, nonsteroidal antiinflammatory drugs, muscle relaxants, exercises, physical therapy, and education.[43] Surgical treatments, specifically discectomy and spinal fusions, are used for individuals not responding to medical management or for emergency management of cauda equina syndrome. Individuals with chronic LBP may benefit from antiinflammatory and muscle relaxant medications, exercise programs, massage, topical heat, spinal manipulation, acupuncture, cognitive-behavioral therapies, and interdisciplinary care. There is scant evidence for efficacy of opioids for chronic LBP but a high risk for addiction. The complexity of causes contributes to the difficulty in defining pathogenesis and clearly defining the most effective therapies.[44,45]

Degenerative Joint Disease

Spondylolysis. Spondylolysis is a structural defect (degeneration, fracture, or developmental defect) in the pars interarticularis of the vertebral arch (the joining of the vertebral body to the posterior structures). The lumbar spine at L5 is affected most often. Mechanical pressure may cause an anterior or posterior displacement of the deficient vertebra (spondylolisthesis).

Heredity plays a significant role, and spondylolysis is associated with an increased incidence of other congenital spinal defects. As a result of torsional and rotational stress, "microfractures" can occur at the affected site and eventually cause dissolution of the pars interarticularis. Segmental instability causes tension on the facet joint capsules and ligaments. There is compensatory muscle spasm related to the instability, and there may be central or foraminal stenosis that generates radicular pain and recurrent LBP.[46]

Cervical spondylolysis is facet hypertrophy and disk degeneration with narrowing in the cervical spine predominantly at C5 to C6 and C6 to C7.[47] It may present as a cervical radiculopathy or a cervical myelopathy. Clinical manifestations of cervical radiculopathy include neck or occipital pain as well as pain in the medial aspects of the scapula, shoulder, or arm. Sensory symptoms, such as tingling or numbness, follow a dermatomal pattern; weakness follows the pattern of innervation of the affected nerve root. Occipital or suboccipital headache is another symptom. Cervical myelopathy can also cause difficulty walking, altered sensation in the feet, and sphincter disturbances (occurs late).

Spondylolisthesis. Spondylolisthesis is an osseous defect of the pars interarticularis and allows a vertebra to slide anteriorly in relation to the vertebra below. The problem is prevalent among athletes related to repetitive stress.[48] Degenerative lumbar spondylolisthesis is a common cause of LBP. Commonly there is involvement of L5 to S1. Spondylolisthesis is graded from 1 to 4 based on the percentage of slip that occurs. Grades 1 and 2 have symptoms of pain in the lower back and buttocks, muscle spasms in the lower back and legs, and tightened hamstrings. Conservative management includes exercise, back bracing, pain medications, epidural steroid injections, transforaminal injections, and physical therapy. Vertebral slippage in grades 3 and 4 usually requires surgical intervention.[49]

Spinal stenosis. Spinal stenosis is a narrowing of the spinal canal that causes pressure on the spinal nerves or cord. It can be congenital or acquired (more common) and is associated with trauma or arthritis. Spinal stenosis is categorized by the area of the spine affected: cervical, thoracic (less common), or lumbar. Acquired conditions include a bulging disk, facet hypertrophy, or a thick, ossified posterior longitudinal ligament (more common in the cervical spins). Symptoms are related to the area of the spine affected and can produce pain; numbness; and tingling in the neck, hands, arms, or legs, with weakness and difficulty walking. Surgical decompression is recommended for those with chronic symptoms and those who do not respond to medical management.[50]

Degenerative Spine Disease

Degenerative disk disease. Degenerative disk disease (DDD) is common in individuals 30 years of age and older. It is, in part, a process of normal aging as a response to continuous vertical compression of the spine (axial loading). DDD includes a genetic component, involving genes that code for spinal cartilage. The combination of environmental interactions and genetic predisposition increases susceptibility to lumbar disk disease by disrupting normal building and maintenance of proteoglycans with inflammation and physical compression of the intervertebral disk matrix.[51] The annulus (outer fibrous ring) can tear, and the disk can herniate, pinching nerves or placing strain on the spine. Fibrocartilage replaces the gelatinous proteoglycans of the nucleus pulposus as the disk changes with age. There may be shrinkage of the nucleus pulposus that produces prolapse or folding of the annulus with secondary osteophyte formation at the margins of the adjacent vertebral body. The pathologic findings in DDD include disk protrusion, spondylolysis and/or subluxation (spondylolisthesis), degeneration of vertebrae, spinal stenosis, and compression of nerves. Lumbar disk disease commonly affects adults at some point in their lives. However, only a small percentage of people with DDD have any functional incapacity because of pain.

Herniated Intervertebral Disk

Herniation of an intervertebral disk is a displacement of the nucleus pulposus or annulus fibrosus beyond the intervertebral disk space (see Fig. 18.16C). Rupture of an intervertebral disk usually is caused by trauma, DDD, or both. Risk factors are weight-bearing sports, light weightlifting, and certain work activities, such as repeated lifting. Men are affected more often than women, with the highest incidence in the 30- to 50-year age group. Most commonly affected are the lumbosacral disks L4 to L5 and L5 to S1 (Fig. 18.17). Disk herniation occasionally occurs in the cervical area, usually at C5 to C6 and C6 to C7. Herniations at the thoracic level are extremely rare.

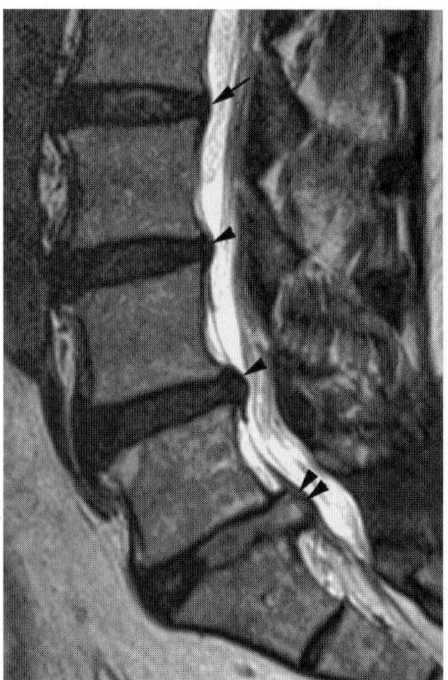

Fig. 18.17 Disc Bulge, Protrusion, and Herniation. Magnetic resonance imaging of lumbar spine. Sagittal T2-weighted image demonstrates examples for all stages of disk pathology. Viewing from rostral to caudal, a disk bulge *(arrow)*, a small and more prominent protrusion *(arrowheads)*, and a herniation *(double arrowhead)* are seen. (From Daroff RB, et al. *Bradley's neurology in clinical practice*. Philadelphia: Saunders; 2012.)

The herniation may occur immediately, within a few hours, or months to years after injury.

Pathophysiology. In a herniated disk, the ligament and posterior capsule of the disk are usually torn, allowing the nucleus pulposus to extrude and compress the nerve root. The vascular supply may be compromised and cause inflammatory changes in the nerve root (radiculitis). Occasionally, the injury tears the entire disk loose, causing the disk capsule and nucleus pulposus to protrude onto the nerve root or compress the spinal cord.

Clinical Manifestations. The location and size of the herniation into the spinal canal, together with the amount of space in the canal, determine the clinical manifestations associated with the injury (Fig. 18.18A). Compression or inflammation, or both, of a spinal nerve resulting from disk herniation follows a dermatomal distribution called radiculopathy (see Fig. 18.18B). A herniated disk in the lumbosacral area is associated with pain that radiates along the sciatic nerve course over the buttock and into the calf or ankle. The pain occurs with straining, including coughing and sneezing, and usually on straight leg raising. Other clinical manifestations include limited range of motion of the lumbar spine; tenderness on palpation in the sciatic notch and along the sciatic nerve; impaired pain, temperature, and touch sensations in the L4 to L5 or L5 to S1 dermatomes of the leg and foot; decreased or absent ankle jerk reflex; and mild weakness of the foot. More rarely, there is development of cauda equina syndrome (see Table 18.8).

With the herniation of a lower cervical disk, paresthesia (sensation of tingling, numbness, or burning) and pain are present in the upper arm, forearm, and hand along the affected nerve root distribution. Neck motion and straining, including coughing and sneezing, may increase neck and nerve root pain. Neck range of motion is diminished. Slight weakness and atrophy of biceps or triceps muscles may occur; the biceps or triceps reflex may decrease. Occasionally, signs of both corticospinal and sensory tract impairments appear, including motor weakness of the lower extremities, sensory disturbances in the lower extremities, and presence of a Babinski reflex.

Evaluation and Treatment. Diagnosis of a herniated intervertebral disk is made through the history and physical examination, imaging, electromyography, and nerve conduction studies. Evidence-based practice guidelines have been published to guide treatment options.[52,53] Most herniated disks heal spontaneously over time and do not require surgery. Physical therapy, interventional modalities such as intradiscal therapies, and epidural injections can relieve pain. Discectomy, fusion, or artificial disc replacement are surgical

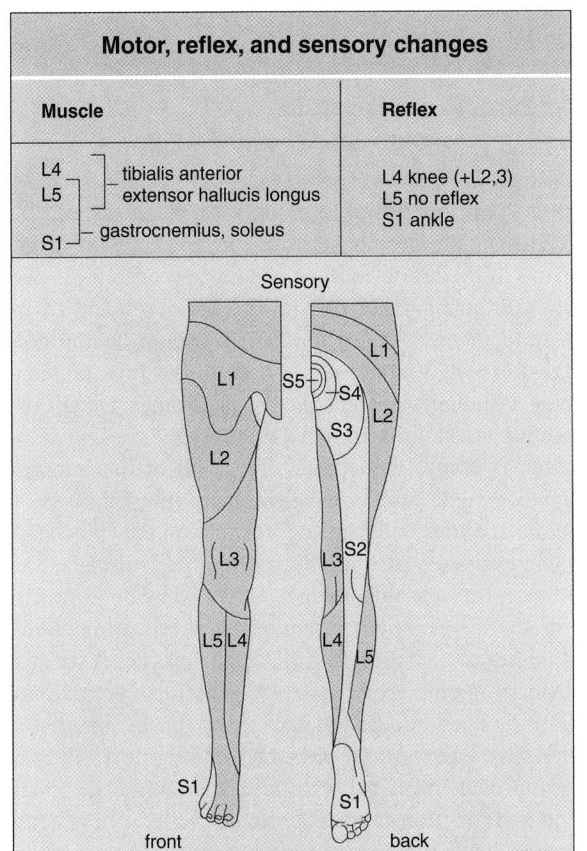

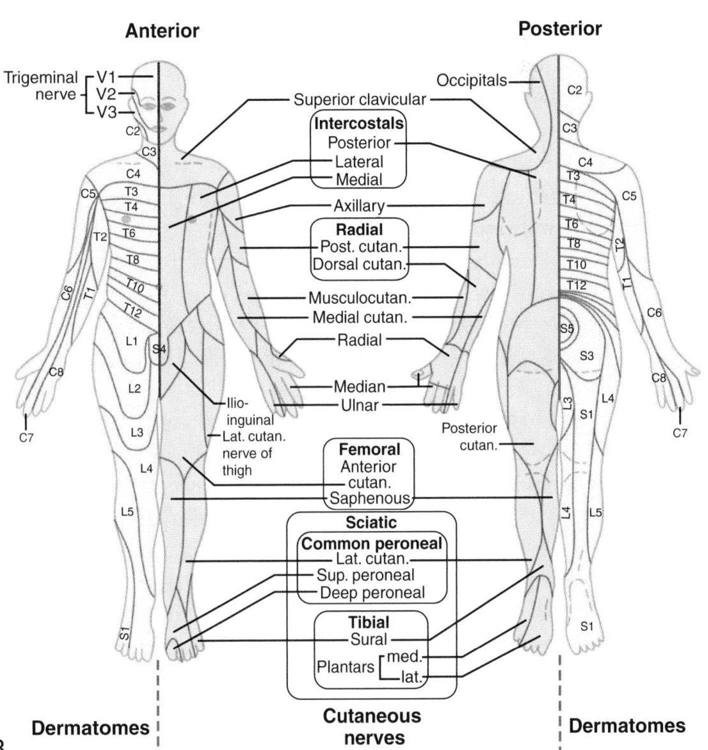

Fig. 18.18 Dermatomes Associated With Muscle, Reflex, and Sensory Changes. (A) Clinical features of herniated nucleus pulposus. **(B)** Sites of radicular pain associated with sensory nerve distribution of skin dermatomes. (Redrawn from Patton HD, et al, eds. *Introduction to basic neurology*. Philadelphia: WB Saunders; 1976. Borrowed from Canale ST, Beaty JH. *Campbell's operative orthopaedics*, 12th edition. St. Louis: Mosby; 2013.)

options if there is evidence of severe compression (weakness or decreased deep tendon, bladder, or bowel reflexes) or if a conservative approach is unsuccessful. Cauda equina syndrome rarely develops and requires emergency surgical evaluation and long-term follow-up.[54]

Seizure Disorders and Epilepsy

Seizure disorders represent a manifestation of disease and not a specific disease entity. A seizure is a sudden, transient disruption in brain electrical function caused by abnormal excessive discharges of cortical neurons. Epilepsy is a cause of seizures and a disease of the brain. Epilepsy is defined using the following criteria: (1) at least two unprovoked seizures occurring more than 24 hours apart; (2) one unprovoked (or reflex) seizure that has at least a 60% risk of recurrence after two unprovoked seizures, occurring over the next 10 years; and (3) diagnosis of an epilepsy syndrome.[55]

An epilepsy syndrome is defined as a characteristic seizure associated with abnormal findings on EEG and magnetic resonance imaging (MRI), that occur together in a recognizable pattern (considerations would be age, time of day, triggers, and type of seizures). There are many of these syndromes; they are rare and often occur in children (e.g., childhood absence epilepsy and juvenile myoclonic epilepsy) (see Chapter 20).[56] Epilepsy was estimated to have affected approximately 3 million adults and 470,000 children in the United States in 2015.[57]

TABLE 18.9 Structural/Metabolic Causes of Recurrent Seizures in Adults

Age at Onset	Probable Cause
Young adults (18–35 years)	Alcohol or drug withdrawal (e.g., barbiturates, benzodiazepines) Brain tumor Idiopathic Illicit drug use (e.g., cocaine, amphetamines) Posttraumatic brain injury Perinatal insults
Older adults (>35 years)	Alcohol or drug withdrawal (e.g., barbiturates, benzodiazepines) Brain tumor Cerebrovascular disease (e.g., stroke, aneurysm, arteriovenous malformations) CNS degenerative diseases (e.g., Alzheimer disease, multiple sclerosis) Major depression Idiopathic Metabolic disorders (e.g., uremia, hepatic failure, electrolyte abnormalities, hypoglycemia) Posttraumatic brain injury

CNS, Central nervous system.
Data from Daroff RB, et al. *Bradley's neurology in clinical practice*, 7th edition. Philadelphia: Elsevier.

Conditions Associated With Seizure Disorders

Any disorder that alters the neuronal environment may cause seizure activity. Conditions that may produce a seizure are metabolic disorders, congenital malformations, genetic predisposition, perinatal injury, postnatal trauma, myoclonic syndromes, infection, brain tumor, vascular disease, drug or alcohol abuse, and toxins. The mechanisms resulting in seizure activity can include stimulation of CNS excitatory pathways, inhibition of inhibitory pathways within the CNS, or withdrawal of long-term CNS depressants.[58] The onset of seizures also may indicate the presence of an ongoing primary neurologic disease. Metabolic and structural causes of recurrent seizures in adults are summarized in Table 18.9. The cause of seizures is often unknown.

The threshold for seizures may be lowered by hypoglycemia; fatigue or lack of sleep; emotional or physical stress; fever; large amounts of water ingestion (hyponatremia); constipation; use of antipsychotic drugs (i.e., chlorpromazine and clozapine), especially when combined with alcohol; or hyperventilation (respiratory alkalosis). Some environmental stimuli, such as blinking lights, a poorly adjusted television screen, loud noises, certain music, certain odors, or merely being startled, have been known to initiate a seizure. Women with epilepsy may have increased seizure activity associated with menses. The patterns include perimenstrual (C1 pattern), at ovulation (C2 pattern), and during the luteal phase (C3 pattern). Patterns C1 and C3 are associated with low progesterone levels with reduced sensitivity to inhibitor neurotransmitters. Pattern C2 is associated with a surge in estrogen, but the mechanism is unknown.[59]

Types of Seizures and Epilepsies

Seizures and epilepsies can be classified in different ways, and the International League Against Epilepsy (ILAE) 2017 classification is commonly used to assist with diagnosis and treatment.[56] The classification of seizures considers: (1) the origin of the seizure in the brain (focal or generalized onset); (2) degree of awareness during the seizure (awareness of self and environment); and (3) level of body movement (motor or nonmotor). The classification of epilepsies considers the type of seizures occurring with epilepsy and epilepsy syndromes. Details of the classification are summarized in Table 18.10.

Pathophysiology. Epilepsy is the result of the interaction of complex genetic mutations with environmental effects that cause abnormalities in synaptic transmission, an imbalance in the brain's excitatory and inhibitory neurotransmitters, alterations of receptors and ion channels activated by neurotransmitters,[60] or the development of abnormal nerve connections or loss of nerves after injury. The ILAE has proposed six groups for categorizing etiology of epilepsy: genetic, structural, metabolic, immune, infectious, and unknown. These categories may be interrelated and continue to be revised (Fig. 18.19).

A group of neurons may exhibit a paroxysmal depolarization shift and function as an epileptogenic focus. These neurons are hyperexcitable and are more easily activated by hyperthermia, hypoxia, hypoglycemia, hypernatremia and hyponatremia (more common), hypocalcemia, hypomagnesemia, repeated sensory stimulation, and certain sleep phases. Epileptogenic neurons fire more frequently and with greater amplitude. When the intensity reaches a threshold point, cortical excitation

TABLE 18.10 Classification of Seizures and Epilepsies

Seizure Type	Description of Seizure Event
Focal seizures (previously partial seizures)	Seizures originating in one area of the brain; an aura is common Motor Tonic: stiffening of body muscles with falling; loss of consciousness; can occur in sleep; more common in infants and children Atonic: sudden, brief loss of muscle tone with falling (drop attacks); usually no loss of consciousness Myoclonic: sudden brief shock-like jerks or twitches of the arms and/or legs; may drop things; no impairment of consciousness; frequently occurs shortly after awakening Tonic-clonic: Abrupt loss of consciousness, body stiffening (tonic) and then shaking (clonic); may begin with sudden cry, sometimes loss of bladder control, or biting of tongue; usually lasts ~2 min, followed by a period of confusion, agitation, and fatigue; headaches and soreness are common afterward Hyperkinetic: bimanual or bipedal motor activity such as kicking and thrashing, clapping and rubbing of both hands, hugging, sometimes with sexual automatisms and autonomic changes with or without preserved awareness Nonmotor Sensory: numbness, tingling or burning sensation, flashing lights, auditory experiences Cognitive: aphasia, hallucination, memory or attention impairment Emotional or affective: fear, agitation, anger, crying, laughing, paranoia Autonomic: blushing, pallor, increased or decreased heart rate, hyperventilation or hypoventilation, nausea
Without loss of awareness	Recall, responsiveness, and consciousness are intact
Impaired awareness (also known as *complex focal seizure*)	Loss of consciousness or awareness; vague or dream-like state
Unknown	Unable to determine awareness or onset
Focal to bilateral tonic-clonic seizure	Begins in one part of brain (focal seizure) and spreads to both sides of brain followed by generalized tonic-clonic seizure; loss of consciousness
Generalized seizures	Seizures originating in both sides of the brain simultaneously with loss of consciousness: *Motor:* tonic-clonic, tonic, atonic, clonic, myoclonic, myoclonic-atonic, clonic-tonic-clonic (see above descriptions); *Nonmotor* (absence seizures): typical, atypical myoclonic, eyelid myoclonia
Epileptic spasms (formerly known as *infantile spasms*)	Episodes of sudden flexion or extension involving neck, trunk, and extremities; clinical manifestations range from subtle head nods to violent body contractions (jackknife seizures); onset between 3 and 12 months of age; may occur after infancy, may be idiopathic, genetic, result of metabolic disease, or in response to CNS insult; spasms occur in clusters of 5–150 times per day; EEG shows large-amplitude, chaotic, and disorganized pattern called "hypsarrhythmia"
EPILEPSY SEIZURE TYPES	Focal, generalized, combined focal and generalized, unknown
Epilepsy Syndromes (examples)	
Childhood absence epilepsy syndrome	Wide variety of abnormal activity occurring many times a day, including rhythmic eye movements, a blank stare with lack of awareness, rhythmic chewing, swimming movements; episodes last 10–20 s and end suddenly followed by normal activity. Child may not be aware seizure activity occurred. Seizures develop between 4 and 8 years of age and may disappear during adolescence.
Lennox-Gastaut syndrome	Epileptic syndrome with onset in early childhood, 1–5 years of age; includes various generalized seizures (tonic-clonic, atonic [drop attacks], akinetic, absence, and myoclonic); EEG has characteristic "slow spike and wave" pattern; results in intellectual disability and delayed psychomotor developments
Juvenile myoclonic epilepsy	Generalized epilepsy syndrome with onset in adolescence; multifocal myoclonus; seizures often occur early in morning, aggravated by lack of sleep or after excessive alcohol intake; occasional generalized convulsions; requires long-term medication treatment
Unclassified epileptic seizures	Etiology remains unknown; seizures do not have distinct clinical and EEG features
Pseudoseizures	Nonepileptic phenomena that look like epileptic seizures; diagnosis often requires video-EEG monitoring to capture spells, and determine that EEG is normal during clinical events; frequently occurs in setting of child abuse
Status Epilepticus	A condition resulting either from the failure of the mechanisms responsible for seizure termination or from the initiation of mechanisms which lead to abnormally prolonged seizures (more than 5 min). It is a condition that can have long-term consequences including neuronal death, neuronal injury, and alteration of neuronal networks, depending on the type and duration of seizures.

CNS, Central nervous system; *EEG*, electroencephalogram.

Data from Sarmast ST, Abdullahi AM, Jahan N. Current classification of seizures and epilepsies: Scope, limitations and recommendations for future action. *Cureus*, 2020;12(9):e10549.

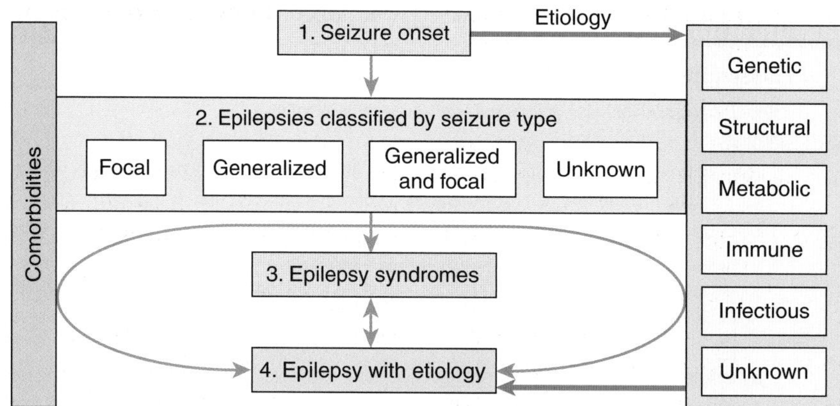

Fig. 18.19 Framework for Classification of Epilepsy. (From Scheffer IE, French J, Hirsch E, et al. Classification of the epilepsies: New concepts for discussion and debate—Special report of the ILAE Classification Task Force of the Commission for Classification and Terminology. *Epilepsia Open*, 2016;1(1–2):37–44.)

spreads. Excitation of the subcortical, thalamic, and brainstem areas corresponds to the tonic phase (muscle contraction with increased muscle tone) and is associated with loss of consciousness. The clonic phase (alternating contraction and relaxation of muscles) begins when inhibitory neurons in the cortex, anterior thalamus, and basal ganglia react to the cortical excitation. The seizure discharge is interrupted, producing intermittent muscle contractions that gradually decrease and finally cease. The epileptogenic neurons are exhausted.

During seizure activity, oxygen is consumed at a high rate—approximately 60% greater than normal. Although cerebral blood flow also increases, oxygen is rapidly depleted along with glucose, and lactate accumulates in brain tissue. Continued, severe seizure activity has the potential for progressive hypoxic brain injury and irreversible damage. In addition, if a seizure focus in the brain is active for a prolonged period, a mirror focus may develop in contralateral normal tissue and cause seizure activity, particularly with focal (i.e., temporal or frontal lobe) epilepsy.

With status epilepticus, the individual may still be in a postictal state (a state that follows an epileptic seizure and returns to baseline) when the next seizure begins. Status epilepticus most often results from abrupt discontinuation of antiseizure medications but also may occur in untreated or inadequately treated persons with seizure disorders. The situation is a medical emergency because of the resulting cerebral hypoxia. Intellectual disability, dementia, other brain damage, and even death are serious threats. There is also a high risk for aspiration to occur.

Clinical Manifestations. The phases associated with a seizure are summarized in Table 18.11. Two types of symptoms signal the preictal phase of a generalized tonic-clonic seizure: prodroma, early manifestations occurring hours to days before a seizure that may include anxiety, depression, or inability to think clearly; and a focal seizure or aura that immediately precedes the onset of a generalized tonic-clonic seizure. Both may become familiar warning signs to the person experiencing recurrent generalized seizures that may enable the person to prevent injuries during the seizure. The ictus is the episode of the epileptic seizure with tonic-clonic activity. Relaxation of urinary and bowel sphincters may occur, leading to bladder and bowel incontinence. Airway maintenance needs to be ensured.

TABLE 18.11 Terminology Used to Describe Phases of a Seizure

Term	Definition
Prodroma	Early clinical manifestations, such as malaise, headache, or a sense of depression, that may occur hours to a few days before the onset of a seizure
Aura	A focal seizure experienced as a peculiar sensation preceding the onset of a generalized seizure or complex partial seizure that may take the form of gustatory, visual, or auditory experience; a feeling of dizziness or numbness; or just "a funny feeling"
Ictus	The episode of the seizure
• Tonic phase	A state of muscle contraction in which there is excessive muscle tone
• Clonic phase	A state of alternating contraction and relaxation of muscles
Postictal state	The period immediately following the cessation of seizure activity

Status epilepticus in adults is defined as: (1) a state of continuous tonic-clonic seizures lasting more than 5 minutes, (2) rapidly recurring seizures before the person has fully regained consciousness from the preceding seizure, or (3) a single seizure lasting more than 30 minutes. It is a condition requiring prompt diagnosis and treatment because of the resulting cerebral hypoxia. Long-term consequences can include neuronal death, neuronal injury, and alteration of neuronal networks.

The postictal state follows an epileptic seizure and can include signs of headache, confusion, aphasia, memory loss, and paralysis that may last hours or a day or two. Deep sleep also is common. Sudden unexpected death during the postictal state is uncommon and is more prevalent with nocturnal, generalized tonic-clonic seizures and treatment failure.[61,62]

Evaluation and Treatment. A thorough health history is a critical aspect of diagnosing a seizure disorder and establishing the cause and onset. Details include subjective sensations, altered consciousness, motor signs, behavioral changes, and the environmental setting.[63] The health history is supplemented by the physical examination and laboratory tests of blood and urine (blood glucose, serum calcium, blood urea nitrogen, urine sodium, and creatinine clearance) to identify any systemic diseases known to have seizures as a clinical manifestation. Brain imaging and CSF examination are useful for identifying any neurologic diseases associated with seizures. The EEG is useful in assessing the type of seizure and may help to determine its focus. Combined EEG and functional MRI (fMRI) can be used to identify neural networks involved in epileptic activity. Differentiating a generalized epilepsy from a focal epilepsy is vital to treatment and prognosis.[64,65]

Treatment for a seizure disorder is first to correct or control its cause, if possible. If this is not possible, the primary means of management is the judicious administration of antiseizure medications to reduce neuron firing. Antiseizure drugs (e.g., diazepam, gabapentin, phenytoin) can enhance gamma-aminobutyric acid (GABA), which mediates inhibitory activity or inhibit glutamate activity by inhibiting glutamate synthesis, by blocking voltage-gated sodium channels at glutamatergic nerve terminals, or by reducing calcium conduction. The therapeutic goal is complete suppression of seizure activity without intolerable side effects of the drug or drug resistance. Dietary treatments (e.g., ketogenic diet or caloric restriction) are effective for some individuals.[66] Surgical interventions (e.g., laser ablation therapy) requires mapping of the seizure onset zone and can improve seizure control and quality of life in people with drug-resistant epilepsy.[67] Neuromodulation (e.g., vagus nerve, trigeminal nerve, or deep brain stimulation) can reduce seizure frequency in some persons with drug-resistant or surgery-resistant seizures.[68] See Emerging Science Box: Ketogenic Diet and Seizure Management in Chapter 20.

Cerebrovascular Disorders

Cerebrovascular disease (CVD) is any abnormality of the brain caused by a pathologic process in the blood vessels. CVD is the most frequently occurring neurologic disorder and frequently requires hospitalization. Included in this category are lesions of the vessel wall (e.g., aneurysm or malformations), occlusion of the vessel lumen by thrombus or embolus, rupture of the vessel, and alteration in blood quality, such as increased blood viscosity.

The brain abnormalities induced by CVD are either (1) ischemia with or without infarction (death of brain tissues) or (2) hemorrhage. The common clinical manifestation of CVD is a cerebrovascular accident (CVA) or stroke. The symptoms occur suddenly and are focal (i.e., slurred speech, difficulty swallowing, limb weakness, or paralysis). In its mildest form, a CVA is so minimal that it is almost unnoticed. In its most severe form, hemiplegia, coma, and death result.

Cerebrovascular Accidents (Stroke Syndromes)

Cerebrovascular accidents (CVAs; stroke syndromes) are the leading cause of disability; they are the third leading cause of death in women and the fifth leading cause of death in men in the United States. Of all strokes, 87% are ischemic and 13% are hemorrhagic (intracerebral 10% and subarachnoid 3%). Approximately 25% of strokes are recurrent strokes. Although hemorrhagic strokes are less common, they account for approximately 40% of stroke-related deaths. Approximately 75% of CVAs occur among those older than 65 years. The incidence is approximately twice as high in Black Americans than in White Americans. Smoking, hypertension, diabetes mellitus, atrial fibrillation, and prior stroke increase the risk for recurrent stroke.[69] Transient ischemic attacks (TIAs) may precede a stroke. CVAs are classified pathophysiologically as ischemic or hemorrhagic strokes. If there is no identifiable cause of an ischemic stroke, it is classified as *undetermined* or *cryptogenic*. Risk factors for stroke are summarized in Box 18.1.

Transient ischemic attacks (TIAs) are episodes of neurologic dysfunction resulting from temporary arterial obstruction of brain blood flow. These episodes last less than 24 hours and do

BOX 18.1 Risk Factors for Stroke

- Poorly controlled or uncontrolled arterial hypertension
- Smoking, which increases the risk of stroke by 2–4 times
- Insulin resistance and diabetes mellitus
- Atrial fibrillation
- Polycythemia (excess red blood cells) and thrombocythemia (excess platelets)
- High total cholesterol or low high-density lipoprotein (HDL) cholesterol, elevated lipoprotein-a

Carotid Artery Disease

- Congestive heart disease, valvular disease, peripheral vascular disease

Chronic Kidney Disease

- Hyperhomocysteinemia
- Sickle cell disease
- Postmenopausal hormone therapy
- High sodium intake >2300 mg; low potassium intake <4700 mg
- Obesity
- Obstructive sleep apnea
- Depression
- *Chlamydia pneumoniae* infection
- Physical inactivity
- Family history of ischemic stroke
- Black American
- Female

Data from: Forouzanfar MH, Alexander L, Anderson HR, et al. Global, regional, and national comparative risk assessment of 79 behavioural, environmental and occupational, and metabolic risks or clusters of risks in 188 countries, 1990–2013: A systematic analysis for the global burden of disease study 2013. *Lancet*, 2015;386:2287–2323. American Stroke Association: Stroke Risk Factors. https://www.stroke.org/en/about-stroke/stroke-risk-factors. Accessed March 4, 2022.

not show evidence of acute infarction on brain imaging.[70] The clinical manifestations of a TIA can include hemiparesis, numbness, sudden confusion, loss of balance, loss of vision, speech disturbances, or a sudden severe headache. Approximately 9% to 17% of individuals experiencing a TIA will have a stroke within 3 months.[71]

Acute Ischemic stroke. Acute ischemic stroke (AIS) occurs when there is sudden neurologic dysfunction caused by focal brain ischemia lasting more than 24 hours or with evidence of acute infarction on brain imaging, irrespective of symptom duration. AIS can be further divided into disabling (major) AIS and nondisabling (minor) AIS, based on the severity of presenting neurologic deficits.[70]

Thrombotic strokes (cerebral thrombosis) arise from arterial obstruction caused by thrombus formation in arteries supplying the brain or intracranial vessels. Conditions causing increased coagulation (e.g., dehydration) or inadequate cerebral perfusion (e.g., hypotension or prolonged vasoconstriction from malignant hypertension) increase the risk of thrombosis. Cerebral thrombosis develops most often from atherosclerosis and inflammatory disease processes that damage arterial walls. It may take as long as 20 to 30 years for obstruction to develop at the branches and curvatures found in the cerebral circulation (see Chapter 32 for a discussion of atherogenesis). The smooth stenotic area can degenerate, forming an ulcerated area of the vessel wall. Platelets and fibrin adhere to the damaged wall, and a clot forms, gradually occluding the artery. Thrombotic strokes also occur when parts of the clot detach, travel upstream, and obstruct blood flow, causing acute ischemia.

Embolic stroke involves fragments that break from a thrombus formed outside the brain, usually in the heart, aorta, or common carotid artery. Other sources of embolism include fat, air, tumor, bacterial clumps, and foreign bodies. The embolus usually involves small brain vessels and obstructs at a bifurcation or other point of narrowing, thus causing ischemia. An embolus may plug the lumen entirely and remain in place or shatter into fragments and become part of the vessel's blood flow. Risk factors for an embolic stroke include atrial fibrillation, left ventricular aneurysm or thrombus, left atrial thrombus, recent myocardial infarction, bacterial endocarditis, rheumatic valve disease, mechanical valvular prosthesis, atrial septal defects, patent foramen ovale, and primary intracardiac tumors. In persons who experience an embolic stroke, a recurrent stroke usually follows because the source of emboli continues to exist. Embolization is usually in the distribution of the middle cerebral artery (see Fig. 15.20). Ischemic strokes in children are associated with congenital heart disease, cerebral arteriovenous malformations (AVMs), and sickle cell disease (see Chapter 20).

Lacunar strokes (lacunar infarcts or small vessel disease) are usually caused by occlusion of a single, deep perforating artery that supplies a small penetrating subcortical vessel, causing ischemic lesions (0.5 to 15 mm) or lacunes deep in the brain (i.e., thalamus or basal ganglia) but not in the cortex. They account for approximately 25% of ischemic strokes, with a 20% recurrence rate, and are associated with cerebral small vessel disease and untreated hypertension. The small area of brain infarction is called a *lacune*. Because of the location and small area of infarction, they may manifest as pure motor or sensory deficits. They may also be silent and are found in approximately 20% to50% of older adults.[72]

Hypoperfusion, or hemodynamic stroke, is associated with *systemic* hypoperfusion caused by cardiac failure, pulmonary embolism, or bleeding that results in inadequate blood supply to the brain. Stroke may occur more readily if there is carotid artery occlusion. Symptoms are usually bilateral and diffuse.

Pathophysiology. Cerebral infarction results when an area of the brain loses its blood supply because of vascular occlusion. Causes include (1) acute vascular occlusion (e.g., embolus or thrombi), (2) gradual vessel occlusion (e.g., atheroma), and (3) partial occlusion of stenotic vessels. Cerebral thrombi and cerebral emboli most commonly produce occlusion, but atherosclerosis and hypertension are the dominant underlying processes.

There is a central core of irreversible ischemia and necrosis within a cerebral infarction. The central core is surrounded by a zone or rim of borderline hypoxic tissue known as the penumbra or ischemic penumbra. Hypoxia in the penumbra is not severe enough to result in structural damage. Prompt restoration of perfusion in the penumbra by injection of thrombolytic agents promotes perfusion and may prevent necrosis and loss of neurologic function. The window of opportunity for protecting the penumbra is approximately 3 hours.

Cerebral infarctions are ischemic or hemorrhagic. In *ischemic infarcts*, the affected area becomes pale and softens 6 to 12 hours after the occlusion. Necrosis, swelling around the insult, and mushy disintegration appear by 48 to 72 hours after infarction. There is infiltration of macrophages and phagocytosis of necrotic tissue. The necrosis resolves by approximately the second week, ultimately leaving a cavity surrounded by glial scarring.

Hemorrhagic transformation of an ischemic stroke is bleeding that occurs into the infarcted area through leaking vessels. Hemorrhagic transformation may be exacerbated by thrombolytic therapy and occurs more commonly with massive ischemic infarction. Unfortunately, reperfusion can compromise recovery by accelerating the sequence of secondary metabolically damaging events, including release of calcium, neuroexcitation (release of glutamate), inflammation, and oxidative stress (reperfusion injury) (see Chapter 2).

Clinical Manifestations. Clinical manifestations of thrombotic and embolic stroke vary, depending on the artery obstructed. Different sites of obstruction create different occlusion syndromes and are summarized in Table 18.12. Contralateral sensory and motor manifestations occur on the opposite side of the body from the location of the brain lesion because motor tracts originate in the cortex and most cross over in the medulla. Sensory tracts originate in the periphery and cross over in the spinal cord. Ipsilateral manifestations occur on the same side as the brain lesion but are rare in stroke syndromes.

Evaluation and Treatment. Diagnosis and treatment should be done as soon as possible. Time of the initiating event and medical and medication history, particularly anticoagulants, can guide therapy. Imaging is critical to diagnose stroke, to exclude hemorrhage or large established infarcts, and to identify potentially treatable large vessel occlusion. Treatment of

TABLE 18.12 Signs and Symptoms of Stroke Involving Major Cerebral Vessels

Cerebral Vessel	Signs and Symptoms
Anterior cerebral artery (ACA)	Contralateral leg more than arm weakness (hemiparesis) and minimal numbness; akinetic mutism (inability to move or speak) and incontinence if bilateral vessel involvement; acute confusional state if nondominant hemisphere
Middle cerebral artery (MCA)	Contralateral upper limb more than leg weakness (hemiparesis) and numbness, ipsilateral hemianopsia and aphasia if stroke in dominant hemisphere
Posterior cerebral artery (PCA)	Contralateral weakness and dizziness, hemianopsia and ataxia, alexia without agraphia (can write but not read), altered memory, visual agnosia, cortical blindness with bilateral hemisphere involvement.
Basilar artery	Difficulty breathing, ataxia (impaired balance and coordination), tremor, diplopia, nystagmus (involuntary, rapid eye movement), dysphagia, dysarthria, vomiting, amnesia, coma
Cerebellar artery	Ataxia, vertigo, headache, nausea and vomiting, slurred speech.

Data from Micieli A, Joundi R, Khosravani H, et al. Stroke syndromes: The code Stroke Handbook. In Micieli A, Joundi R, Gladstone DF, eds. *Approach to the acute stroke patient*. London: Academic Press; 2020.

ischemic stroke is focused on (1) restoring brain perfusion in a time frame that does not contribute to reperfusion injury, (2) counteracting ischemic pathways, (3) lowering cerebral metabolic demand so that the susceptible brain tissue is protected against impaired perfusion, (4) preventing recurrent ischemic events, and (5) promoting tissue restoration. Intravenous reperfusion therapy using tissue-type plasminogen activator (tPA) is given within 3 and up to 4.5 hours of onset of symptoms. Other strategies include endovascular intra-arterial thrombolysis, thrombectomy, and placement of removable stents. Guidelines are available for the early management of AIS.[73,74]

Supportive management is given to control cerebral edema and IICP and to provide neuroprotection. Arresting the disease process and preventing recurrent stroke by control of risk factors is critical, and antiplatelet therapy may be instituted. Guidelines are available for the prevention of stroke risk in women.[75] Rehabilitation is indicated for ischemic strokes, and recovery of function is often possible. Neuroprotective and neuroregenerative strategies are under investigation.[76–79]

Hemorrhagic stroke occurs within the brain tissue. Spontaneous hemorrhages can occur in intracerebral locations or in the subarachnoid or subdural spaces.

The primary cause of intracerebral hemorrhagic stroke is chronic hypertension. Other causes include amyloid angiopathy (accumulation of β amyloid in walls of leptomeningeal vessels and cortical capillaries in the brain), tumors, coagulation disorders, trauma, or illicit drug use, particularly cocaine. Hypertensive causes of hemorrhagic stroke involve primarily smaller arteries and arterioles that have been damaged by chronic hypertension. Microaneurysms in these smaller vessels may precipitate the bleeding. Prevention or control of hypertension reduces the incidence of hemorrhagic stroke.

Subarachnoid hemorrhage (hematoma) (SAH) is associated with ruptured aneurysms, AVMs, or brain trauma. *Subdural hemorrhage* (hematoma) is usually associated with brain trauma (see the Traumatic Brain Injury section).

Pathophysiology. Brain damage occurring with hemorrhagic stroke is categorized into primary and secondary brain injury. Primary injury is the result of blood vessel rupture and the mass effect of bleeding into the brain tissue and hematoma formation. The most common sites for hypertensive hemorrhages are in the deeper parts of the brain: the basal ganglia, thalamus, pons, and caudate nucleus. Adjacent brain tissue is deformed, compressed, and displaced. This causes ischemia, edema, IICP, and necrosis. The expanding mass effect can cause brain stem herniation. Rupture or seepage of blood into the ventricular system often occurs, and hydrocephalus can develop due to microscopic blood obstruction of the CSF outflow tracts at the arachnoid granulations and adhesion formation within the ventricles.[80] Maximal cerebral edema develops in approximately 72 hours and takes approximately 2 weeks to subside. Secondary injury is the cascade of cellular and molecular changes initiated by the primary injury. Complement releases membrane attack complex, promoting edema and red blood cell lysis. Activation of microglia/macrophages and leukocyte infiltration stimulates release of inflammatory cytokines and an inflammatory reaction in surrounding brain tissue that appears rapidly and peaks in several days. Oxidative stress and excitotoxicity contribute to cell injury and death. Blood components including thrombin and iron from hemoglobin breakdown products also promote secondary injury (Fig. 18.20).[81] Most persons survive an initial ischemic stroke unless there is massive cerebral edema, which is nearly always fatal. The cerebral hemorrhage resolves through reabsorption. Macrophages and astrocytes clear blood from the area and a cavity forms, surrounded by a dense scar after reabsorption of the blood.

Clinical Manifestations. The clinical manifestations of hemorrhagic stroke are similar to those for ischemic stroke and depend on the location and size of the bleeding. Symptoms can occur suddenly and with activity. Once a deep unresponsive state occurs, the person rarely survives. The immediate prognosis is grave; however, if the person survives, recovery of function is often possible.

It is difficult to differentiate ischemic from hemorrhagic stroke based on symptoms. Individuals experiencing intracranial hemorrhage from a ruptured or leaking aneurysm have one of three sets of symptoms: (1) onset of an excruciating generalized headache with an almost immediate lapse into an unresponsive state; (2) headache but with consciousness maintained and there may be seizures, nausea, and vomiting; and (3) sudden lapse into unconsciousness. If the hemorrhage is confined to the subarachnoid space, there may be no local signs. If bleeding

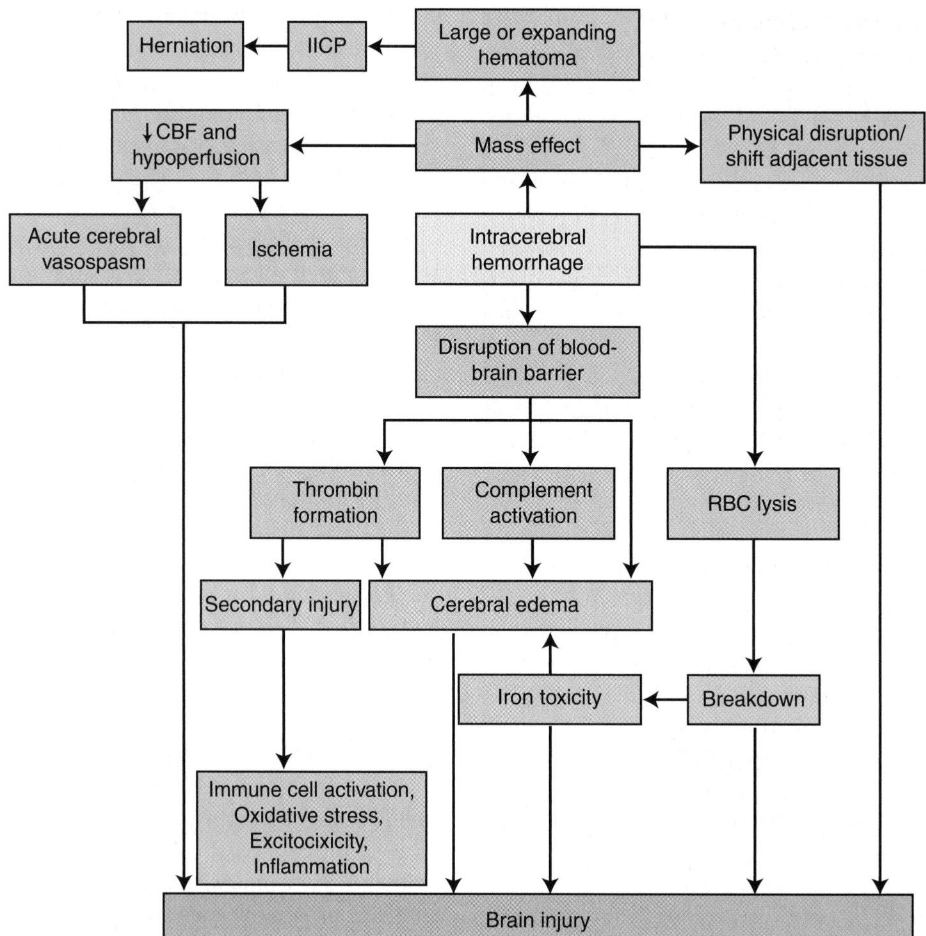

Fig. 18.20 Injury Mechanisms Promoted by Intracerebral Hemorrhage. Hemorrhages can induce neuronal injury through mass effect, particularly in large hematomas that can cause increased intracranial pressure and herniation. Hemorrhages may also cause tissue damage through cerebral edema and secondary "neurotoxic" mechanisms caused by activation of the coagulation cascade, complement, microglia, oxidative stress, neurotoxicity, and inflammation. Not all potential interactions are shown (e.g., thrombin may potentiate iron-induced injury; the complement and inflammatory systems overlap; and several factors contribute to cerebral edema). *CBF*, Cerebral blood flow; *IICP*, increased intracranial pressure; *RBC*, red blood cell. (Data from Dasari R, Bonsack F, Sukumari-Ramesh S. Brain injury and repair after intracerebral hemorrhage: The role of microglia and brain-infiltrating macrophages. *Neurochemistry International*, 2021;142:104923; O'Carroll CB, Brown BL, Freeman WD. Intracerebral hemorrhage: A common yet disproportionately deadly stroke subtype. *Mayo Clinic Proceedings*, 2021;96(6):1639–1654.)

spreads into the brain tissue, hemiparesis/paralysis, dysphasia, or homonymous hemianopia (visual field loss on the same side of both eyes) may be present. Warning signs of an impending aneurysm rupture include headache, transient unilateral weakness, transient numbness and tingling, and transient speech disturbance. However, such warning signs are often absent.

Evaluation and Treatment. Diagnosis of hemorrhagic stroke considers the health history, clinical presentation, laboratory tests, and neuroimaging procedures (CT and MRI). Treatment needs to be initiated within 3 to 4 hours of symptom onset for reversibility of brain ischemia. Treatment of intracranial bleeding, regardless of the cause, focuses on stopping or reducing the bleeding; controlling blood pressure, edema, and IICP; preventing rebleeding; and preventing vasospasm. Surgical treatments, including endovascular approaches, are options for ruptured aneurysms, vascular malformations, and SAH. New minimally invasive surgical techniques for intracranial hematoma evacuation have been developed.[82] Clinical guidelines for the management of spontaneous ICH have been published by the American Heart Association/American Stroke Association.[83] Efforts are in progress to control the mass effects of the hematoma and to suppress secondary cell injury.[84] Care in multidisciplinary stroke rehabilitation units with effective interprofessional communication appears to be most effective at reducing disability, dependency, and length of hospital stay for all stroke syndromes.[85–87]

Intracranial aneurysm. An intracranial aneurysm is a dilation or ballooning of an arterial vessel from a weakness in the vessel wall. Risk factors include arteriosclerosis, congenital abnormality, cocaine use, trauma, cigarette smoking, or family history. The size may vary from 2 mm to 2 or 3 cm. Most aneurysms are located at bifurcations in or near the circle of Willis, in the vertebrobasilar arteries, or within the carotid system, where there is higher wall shear stress (frictional force of blood against the endothelium of a blood vessel) and flow turbulence (see Fig. 18.20). Aneurysms may be single, but, in some instances, more than one is present. In these instances, the aneurysms may be unilateral or bilateral. The peak incidence of rupture occurs in persons 50 to 59 years of age, with the incidence in postmenopausal women slightly higher than that in men.

Pathophysiology. No single pathologic mechanism exists. Aneurysm development is attributed to hemodynamic and wall shear stress and flow turbulence, particularly at bifurcations, such as in or near the circle of Willis, in the vertebrobasilar arteries, or within the carotid artery system (see Fig. 18.20). They are a symptom of underlying hemodynamic stress, and inflammation leads to loss of vessel wall integrity. Hypertension and certain connective tissue disorders in which there are abnormalities in the extracellular matrix exacerbate aneurysm formation.[88] Aneurysms rupture through thin areas of blood vessels, often at bifurcation sites. There is hemorrhage into the subarachnoid space that spreads rapidly, producing localized changes in the cerebral cortex and focal irritation of nerves and arteries. Bleeding ceases when a fibrin-platelet plug forms at the point of rupture and as a result of compression. Blood undergoes reabsorption through arachnoid villi, usually within 3 weeks.

Aneurysms may be classified on the basis of their shape. *Saccular aneurysms (berry aneurysms)* are the most common (in approximately 2% of the population) and can result from congenital abnormalities in the tunica media (middle layer) of the arterial wall and wall weakening related to atherosclerosis and hypertension. The sac gradually grows over time. A saccular aneurysm may be (1) round with a narrow stalk connecting it to the parent artery, (2) broad-based without a stalk, or (3) cylindrical (Figs. 18.21 and 18.22). The highest incidence of rupturing or bleeding (SAH) is among persons 20 to 50 years of age.

Fusiform aneurysms (giant aneurysms) are less common, occur as a result of diffuse arteriosclerotic changes, and are found most commonly in the basilar arteries or terminal portions of the internal carotid arteries (see Fig. 18.21). They act as space-occupying lesions.

Clinical Manifestations. Aneurysms often are asymptomatic, and their presence is unknown until discovered incidentally or at autopsy. Clinical manifestations include sudden severe headache or dizziness and cranial nerve compression, but the signs vary, depending on the location and size of the aneurysm. Cranial nerves III, IV, V, and VI (see Table 15.6) are affected most often. Unfortunately, the most common first indication of the presence of an aneurysm is an acute SAH, ICH, or combined SAH-ICH.

Evaluation and Treatment. Diagnosis before a bleeding episode is made through arteriography. Intracranial aneurysms may be found incidentally during CT or MRI imaging for other conditions. After a subarachnoid or ICH, a tentative diagnosis of an aneurysm is based on clinical manifestations, history, and imaging. Treatments for intracranial aneurysm are individualized, and there are both medical (e.g., control of hypertension and vasospasm) and surgical (e.g., placement of endovascular coils) options. Modifiable risk factors include smoking, alcohol use, and hypertension.[88,89]

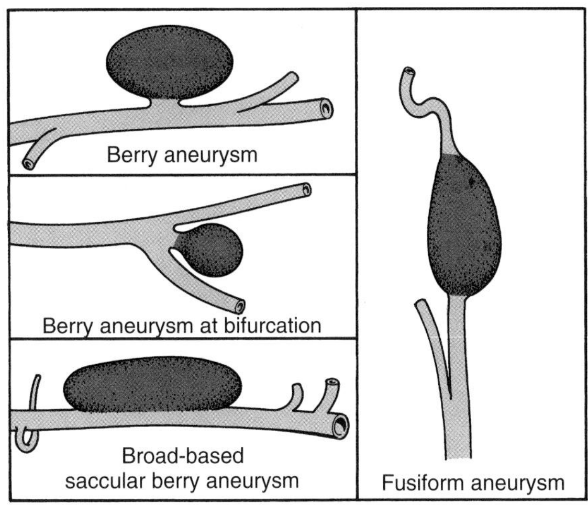

Fig. 18.21 Types of Aneurysms.

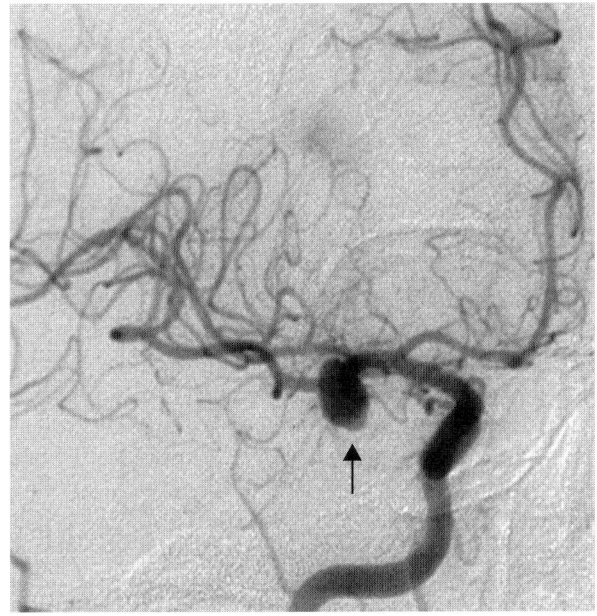

Fig. 18.22 Angiogram of a Berry Aneurysm. In this contrast-enhanced lateral view, a portion of the cerebral arterial circulation can be seen as a berry aneurysm *(arrow)* involving the middle cerebral artery of the circle of Willis at the base of the brain. (From Klatt EC. *Robbins and Cotran atlas of pathology*, 3rd edition. Philadelphia: Saunders, 2015.)

Subarachnoid hemorrhage. Subarachnoid hemorrhage (SAH) is the escape of blood from a defective or injured vessel into the subarachnoid space (Fig. 18.23). Individuals at risk for an SAH are those with intracranial aneurysm, intracranial AVM (see the next section), hypertension, and a family history of SAH and those who have sustained head injuries. SAHs often recur, especially from a ruptured intracranial aneurysm. SAH is associated with approximately 2% to 7% of all strokes and 85% of ruptured intracranial aneurysms.[90]

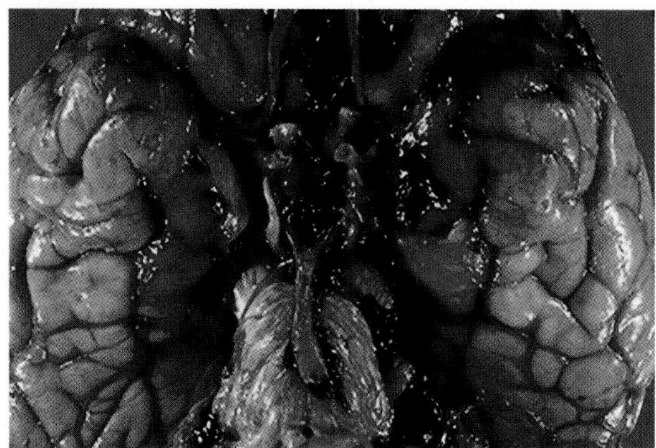

Fig. 18.23 Subarachnoid Hemorrhage, Gross. Subarachnoid hemorrhage resulting from rupture of a berry aneurysm. (From Klatt EC. *Robbins and Cotran atlas of pathology*, 3rd edition. Philadelphia: Saunders; 2015.)

TABLE 18.13 Subarachnoid Hemorrhage Classification Scale

Category	Description
Grade I	Neurologic status intact; mild headache, slight nuchal rigidity
Grade II	Neurologic deficit evidenced by cranial nerve involvement; moderate to severe headache with more pronounced meningeal signs (e.g., photophobia, nuchal rigidity)
Grade III	Drowsiness and confusion with or without focal neurologic deficits; pronounced meningeal signs
Grade IV	Stuporous with pronounced neurologic deficits (e.g., hemiparesis, dysphasia); nuchal rigidity
Grade V	Deep coma state with decerebrate posturing and other brainstem functioning

From Tateshima S, Duckwiler G. Vascular diseases of the nervous system. In Daroff RB, et al, eds. *Bradley's neurology in clinical practice*. Philadelphia: Saunders; 2012.

Pathophysiology. When a vessel is leaking, blood oozes into the subarachnoid space. When a vessel tears, blood under pressure is pumped into the subarachnoid space. Autoregulation of blood flow is impaired, and there is a compensatory increase in systolic blood pressure. The expanding hematoma acts like a space-occupying lesion and expands intracranial volume. There is compression and displacement of brain tissue with IICP, decreased perfusion pressure and cerebral blood flow, blood-brain barrier breakdown, brain edema, inflammation, and cell death. Secondary brain injury can occur as described for TBI and hemorrhagic stroke. In addition, the escaped blood coats nerve roots, clogs arachnoid granulations impairing CSF reabsorption, and obstructs foramina (passages) within the ventricular system impairing CSF circulation. Ultimately, granulation tissue is formed. There may be meningeal scarring with impairment of CSF reabsorption and secondary hydrocephalus. Mortality in SAH is approximately 50% at 1 month.

Delayed cerebral ischemia is a syndrome of progressive neurologic deterioration (i.e., development of hemiparesis or aphasia) associated with cerebral artery vasospasm and decreased perfusion. It occurs in 3 to 14 days after an SAH in approximately 50% of cases and is a significant cause of morbidity and mortality. The mechanism of vasospasm is not completely understood. Proposed mechanism includes microthrombi formation from endothelial damage, the loss of autoregulation of blood flow, cortical spreading depolarization, nitric oxide (a vasodilator) deficiency, increased endothelin-1 (a vasoconstrictor), inflammation-mediated oxidative stress with damage to smooth muscle, and upregulation of apoptotic pathways. Vasospasm with microthrombosis causes decreased cerebral perfusion with extension of ischemic injury and increased risk of death. It is difficult to manage, and there are serious side effects of various preventive and treatment options. New diagnostic and treatment strategies are emerging.[88,91]

Clinical Manifestations. Early manifestations associated with leaking vessels are episodic and include headache, changes in mental status or level of consciousness, nausea or vomiting, and focal neurologic defects (weakness or paralysis, loss of sensation, aphasia). A ruptured vessel causes a sudden, throbbing, "explosive" headache that develops in seconds, accompanied by nausea and vomiting, visual disturbances, motor deficits, and loss of consciousness related to a dramatic rise in ICP. Meningeal irritation and inflammation often occur, causing neck stiffness (nuchal rigidity), photophobia, blurred vision, irritability, restlessness, and low-grade fever.[92] A positive Kernig sign (straightening the knee with the hip and knee in a flexed position produces pain in the back and neck regions) and a positive Brudzinski sign (passive flexion of the neck produces neck pain and increased rigidity) may appear. No localizing signs are present if the bleeding is confined completely to the subarachnoid space. However, they may develop if there is delayed cerebral ischemia.

The Hunt and Hess SAH grading system is commonly used and is based on the description of the clinical manifestations (Table 18.13).[93] Rebleeding is a significant risk with a high mortality (up to 70%). The period of greatest risk is during the first 72 hours and up to 2 weeks after the initial episode of bleeding. Rebleeding is manifested by a sudden increase in blood pressure and ICP, along with a deteriorating neurologic status.

Seizures occur in 25% of persons with an SAH, and hydrocephalus after a bleeding episode occurs in 20% of cases. Hypothalamic dysfunction, manifested by salt wasting, hyponatremia, and electrocardiograph (ECG) changes, is common.

Evaluation and Treatment. Aneurysmal SAH is a neurologic emergency. The diagnosis of an SAH is based on the clinical presentation, imaging, and cerebrospinal fluid evaluation. Treatment is directed at controlling systemic blood pressure, ICP, vasospasm, fluid volume; improving cerebral perfusion pressure; preventing ischemia and hypoxia of neural tissues; and avoiding rebleeding episodes. Surgical intervention is common.[88]

Vascular malformation. Vascular malformations are rare congenital vascular lesions. An arteriovenous malformation (AVM) is a mass of dilated vessels between the arterial and venous systems (arteriovenous fistula) that lacks a muscularis layer and an intervening capillary bed. AVMs may occur in any part of the brain and vary in size from a few millimeters to large

TABLE 18.14 **Characteristics of Common Headaches**

	MIGRAINE		Cluster Headache/	
	Without Aura	**With Aura (25%–30%)**	**Proximal Hemicrania**	**Tension-Type Headache**
Age of onset	Childhood, adolescence, or young adulthood	Childhood, adolescence, or young adulthood	Young adulthood, middle age	Young adulthood, middle age
Sex	Higher in females	Higher in females	Male	Not sex specific
Family history of headaches	Yes	Yes	No	Yes
Onset and evolution	Slow to rapid	Slow to rapid	Rapid	Slow to rapid
Time course	Episodic	Episodic	Clusters in time	Episodic, may become constant
Quality	Usually throbbing	Usually throbbing	Steady	Steady
Location	Variable, unilateral to bilateral	Variable, unilateral to bilateral	Orbit, temple, cheek	Variable
Associated features	Prodrome, vomiting	Aura: visual, sensory, language, and motor disturbanceProdrome, vomiting	Lacrimation, rhinorrhea, Horner syndrome	None

malformations. They occur equally in males and females and, occasionally, in families. Although AVMs are usually present at birth, symptoms exhibit a delayed age of onset and commonly occur before 30 years of age.

Pathophysiology. AVMs have abnormal blood vessel structure with abnormally thin walls. There is direct shunting of arterial blood into the venous vasculature without the dissipation of the arterial blood pressure. One or several arteries may feed the AVM. Over time, they become tortuous and dilated, with an increased risk for rupture. With moderate to large AVMs, sufficient blood is shunted into the malformation to deprive surrounding tissue of adequate blood perfusion.

Clinical Manifestations. Twenty percent of persons with an AVM have a characteristic chronic, nondescript headache, although some experience migraine. Approximately 50% of persons experience seizures. The other 50% experience an ICH, SAH, or subdural hemorrhage with progressive neurologic deficits. Bleeding from an AVM into the subarachnoid space causes symptoms identical to those associated with a ruptured aneurysm. If bleeding occurs in the brain tissue, focal signs that develop resemble a stroke that is progressing in severity. Ten percent of persons experience hemiparesis or other focal signs. At times, noncommunicating hydrocephalus (see Chapter 17) develops with a large AVM that extends into the ventricular lining. Some AVMs never cause symptoms.

Evaluation and Treatment. A systolic bruit over the carotid artery in the neck, the mastoid process, or the eyeball in a young person is almost always diagnostic of an AVM. Confirming diagnosis is made by imaging. There is no established medical therapy. Treatment options include evaluation of risk factors, continuing observation with follow-up imaging, direct surgical excision, endovascular embolization, or stereotactic radiosurgery.[94,95]

Primary Headache Syndromes

Headache is a common neurologic disorder and is usually a benign symptom. However, it can be associated with serious disease, such as brain tumor, meningitis, or CVD. The headache syndromes discussed here are the chronic, recurring type not associated with structural abnormalities, systemic disease, or trauma and include migraine, cluster, and tension headaches. Characteristics of the major types of headache syndromes are summarized in Table 18.14.

Migraine

Migraine is an episodic or chronic neurologic disorder. Migraine is broadly classified as (1) *migraine with aura* with visual, sensory, or motor symptoms, (2) *migraine without aura* (most common), and (3) *chronic migraine.* Migraine is diagnosed using the International Headache Society diagnostic criteria: at least five attacks of a headache lasting 4 to 72 hours with at least two of the following four characteristics (1) unilateral location, (2) pulsating quality, (3) moderate or severe pain intensity, and (4) aggravation by or causing avoidance of routine physical activity; during headache at least one of the following: (1) nausea and/or vomiting, (2) photophobia and phonophobia; and not accounted for by another headache diagnosis.[96] Migraine occurs in 18% of women, 6% of men, and 10% of children in the United States. It is more common in those 18 to 44 years of age. There often is a family history of migraine.[97] In susceptible women, migraine occurs most frequently before and during menstruation. The cyclic withdrawal of estrogen and fluctuating levels of estrogen are associated with migraine.[98]

Migraine is caused by a combination of multiple genetic and environmental factors. Migraine may be precipitated by triggers that decrease the threshold for a migraine. Triggers can be genetic or associated with fatigue, oversleeping, missed meals, overexertion, weather change, stress or relaxation from stress, hormonal changes (menstrual periods), excess afferent stimulation (bright lights, strong smells), and chemicals (alcohol or nitrates).[99]

Pathophysiology. The pathophysiologic basis for migraine is complex and not clearly established. There is no identifiable pathology, but there is activation of the trigeminovascular system and associated changes in brain metabolism and blood flow. Current theories include neurologic, vascular, hormonal, and neurotransmitter components. Migraine aura is associated with cortical spreading depression (CSD). CSD is a spontaneous self-propagating wave of glial and neuronal depolarization, starting in the occipital region and spreading across the cortex, resulting in hyperactivity. CSD initiates the release of excitatory neurotransmitters that activate the trigeminal vascular system (afferent projections from cranial nerve V), stimulating vasodilation of dural blood vessels, activation of inflammation, peripheral and central sensitization of pain receptors (hypersensitivity to pain), and activation of areas of the brainstem and forebrain that modulate pain and prodromal symptoms. Release of inflammatory mediators with sterile meningeal inflammation, edema of blood vessels, and release of neurotransmitters may be important components of migraine pain.

Clinical Manifestations. The clinical phases of a migraine attack are as follows:[100]

1. *Premonitory phase:* Up to one-third of persons have premonitory symptoms hours to days before the onset of the aura or headache. These symptoms may include fatigue, irritability, loss of concentration, stiff neck, and food cravings. There is increased blood flow to the hypothalamic region of the brain.
2. *Migraine aura:* Up to one-third of persons have aura symptoms at least some of the time that may last up to 1 hour. Symptoms can be visual, sensory, or motor and may be associated with CSD.
3. *Headache phase:* Throbbing pain usually begins on one side and spreads to include the entire head. Headache may be accompanied by fatigue, nausea, and vomiting or dizziness. There may be hypersensitivity to anything touching the head. There is activation of the trigeminovascular system and release of inflammatory mediators (e.g., calcitonin gene-related peptide [CGRP], substance P, vasoinhibitory peptide, and pituitary adenylate cyclase-activating polypeptide [PACAP]) with meningeal inflammation, vasodilation, and pain. The inflammatory mediators are targets for emerging treatments.[101] Symptoms may last from 4 to 72 hours (usually about a day).
4. *Recovery (postdrome) phase:* Irritability, fatigue, or depression may take hours or days to resolve. The recovery phase may be associated with continued activation of the brain stem.

Evaluation and Treatment. The diagnosis of migraine is made from the medical history and physical examination. The differential diagnosis is confirmed by imaging and EEG. The management of migraine includes avoidance of triggers (e.g., darkening the room, applying ice). Sleeping can provide some relief with the onset of acute migraine. Pharmacologic management for the treatment and prevention of migraine is available, including 5-hydroxytryptamine agonists, triptans, and CGRP antagonists. Treatment guidelines are available.[102,103] Several neuromodulation therapies are available for the prevention and treatment of migraine.[104,105]

Chronic migraines usually begin as episodic migraines that increase in frequency over time. Chronic migraine occurs at least 15 days in a month (can occur daily or on a near-daily basis) for more than 3 months.[96] Chronic migraines are associated with overuse of analgesic migraine medications (sometimes called *rebound headaches*), obesity, and caffeine overuse. Treatment is similar to that for episodic migraine, and onabotulinumtoxin A is an effective treatment for chronic migraine.[106]

Cluster Headache

Cluster headaches are one of a group of disorders referred to as *trigeminal autonomic cephalalgias* (headaches involving the autonomic division of the trigeminal nerve). They occur in one side of the head (proximal hemicranias) primarily in men between 20 and 50 years of age. The headache attack usually begins without warning. The pain may alternate sides with each headache episode and is severe, stabbing, and throbbing. These uncommon headaches occur in clusters (up to 8 attacks per day) and last for minutes to hours for a period of days, followed by a long period of spontaneous remission. Cluster headache has an episodic and a chronic form with extreme pain intensity and short duration. If the cluster of attacks occurs more frequently without sustained spontaneous remission, the condition is classified as *chronic cluster headaches* (10% to 20% of cases) (see Table 18.14). Triggers include caffeine, alcohol, and smoking.

Pathophysiology and Clinical Manifestations. The trigeminovascular system is activated with release of pain-producing vasoactive peptides and neuroinflammation similar to migraine. Trigeminal-autonomic reflex activation occurs, characterized by sympathetic underactivity and parasympathetic activation. There is unilateral trigeminal distribution of severe pain with ipsilateral autonomic manifestations, including tearing and ptosis of the eye on the affected side, and congestion of the nasal mucosa. Pain often is referred to the midface and teeth. Because of the circadian and rhythmic cycles of headache attacks, hypothalamic dysfunction may be an associated factor.[107]

Treatment. Prophylactic drugs (e.g., verapamil, lithium, melatonin, and topiramate) are used to treat cluster headache, and avoidance of triggers also is important. (See Emerging Science Box: Melatonin and the Central Nervous System.) Acute attacks are managed with oxygen inhalation and sumatriptan. New treatments are under investigation.[108]

Tension-Type Headache

Tension-type headache (TTH) is the most common type of recurrent primary headache. The average age of onset is during the second decade of life. Anxiety and depression are common comorbidities. Individuals with migraine headaches frequently have TTH. The headaches are bilateral and mild with a sensation of a tight band or pressure around the head with gradual onset of pain. *Episodic TTH* occurs less than 15 days per month and may last for several hours or several days. It is not aggravated by physical activity and may be triggered by sleep disorders (insomnia). *Chronic TTH* (CTTH) evolves from episodic TTH and represents a headache that occurs at least 15 days per month for at least 3 months.

Pathophysiology. Both central and peripheral mechanisms operate in causing tension headache. It is not a vascular headache. The peripheral sensitization of myofascial nociceptors may contribute to muscular hypersensitivity and the development of episodic TTH. Pericranial muscle tenderness may develop from the activation of peripheral nociceptors around the blood vessels in striated muscle, tendon insertions, and fascia. A myofascial trigger point is associated with CTTH and is a hyperirritable point associated with a taut band of skeletal muscle that is painful on compression and

EMERGING SCIENCE BOX

Melatonin and the Central Nervous System

Melatonin is a hormone synthesized and secreted primarily at night by the pineal gland and other tissues, including the retina, immune cells, and gastrointestinal tract, and is found in most other organs. The rhythm of pineal secretion is generated by the suprachiasmatic nuclei (SCN) of the hypothalamus and entrained (a pattern or rhythm) to the dark phase of the light/dark cycle; dark stimulates secretion, and light inhibits secretion. The extrapineal sources of melatonin have less of an effect on the rhythm functions of melatonin. Melatonin is synthesized from tryptophan taken up from the circulation and transformed to serotonin and converted into melatonin, and tryptophan deficiency is a cause of low melatonin levels. It is rapidly metabolized by the liver, is excreted in the urine, and has a low level of toxicity even at high doses. The secretion of melatonin declines with aging. Melatonin is lipid and water soluble and readily crosses cell membranes, including the blood-brain barrier, and is present in all bodily fluids. There are three melatonin receptors. M1 and M2 are transmembrane receptors, and M3 is an intracellular receptor. The function of the melatonin receptors in the brain is the regulation of circadian rhythms and sleep. In addition to its chronobiotic functions, melatonin can also activate or suppress the immune system and stimulate or suppress inflammation depending on different physiologic conditions.

Activation of the immune system and the protective inflammatory response can be beneficial in defense against pathogens, including bacterial and viral infections, and meningitis, including the neuroinflammatory effects of SARS CoV-2 infection. In the nervous system, melatonin is cytoprotective and acts as a free radical scavenger and has antioxidant functions by activating antioxidant enzymes (e.g., glutathione peroxidase, superoxide dismutase, and catalase). Melatonin suppresses the secretion of inflammatory cytokines, such as interferon-γ and tumor necrosis factor-α, and increases the amounts of antiinflammatory cytokines interleukin (IL)-4 and IL-10. There is also downregulation of the proinflammatory mediators cyclooxygenase-2 and inducible nitric oxide synthetase. Many of the neurodegenerative diseases, including Alzheimer disease (AD) and Parkinson disease (PD), have low levels of melatonin and are associated with sleep disorders and neuroinflammation. Melatonin is lower in AD individuals than in age-matched controls. A meta-analysis suggests that night time melatonin treatment for greater than 12 weeks may be effective for improvement of cognitive functioning in individuals with mild AD than those with moderate AD. Sleep disturbances are common in AD and may contribute to decreased clearance of beta amyloid. Thus the use of melatonin for the improvement in sleep is a consideration for treatment in early AD. In addition to the management of sleep disorders in PD, it is proposed that melatonin may be neuroprotective and delay disease progression, prevent assembly of α-synuclein proteins, prevent oxidant damage to neurons, maintain normal mitochondrial function, and promote glymphatic elimination of toxic products. Some studies have shown melatonin to be proinflammatory and to have a detrimental effect in multiple sclerosis and rheumatoid arthritis.

Melatonin has been shown to exert neuroprotective effects, but the timing of administration, dosage, and outcome measures in humans need more research. Clinical trials with large sample sizes and standardized methodologies are needed to more effectively guide the use of melatonin in the treatment and prevention of neurodegenerative diseases. Currently there are several studies in progress for the use of melatonin in AD, PD, Huntington disease, multiple sclerosis, and Covid-19.

Data from Bonmati-Carrion MA, et al. Melatonin and cancer: A polyhedral network where the source matters. *Antioxidants (Basel).* 2021;10(2):210; Ostrin LA. Ocular and systemic melatonin and the influence of light exposure. *Clin Exp Optom.* 2019;102(2):99–108; Acuña-Castroviejo D, et al. Extrapineal melatonin: Sources, regulation, and potential functions. *Cell Mol Life Sci.* 2014;71(16):2997–3025; Bubenik GA, et al. Melatonin and aging: Prospects for human treatment. *J Physiol Pharmacol,* 2011;62(1):13–19; Claustrat B, et al. Melatonin: Physiological effects in humans. *Neurochirurgie.* 2015;61(2–3):77–84; Hardeland R. Aging, melatonin, and the pro- and anti-inflammatory networks. *Int J Mol Sci.* 2019;20(5):1223; Chitimus DM, et al. Melatonin's impact on antioxidative and anti-inflammatory reprogramming in homeostasis and disease. *Biomolecules.* 2020;10(9):1211; Zhang D, et al. The potentials of melatonin in the prevention and treatment of bacterial meningitis disease. *Molecules.* 2021;26(5):1419; He F, et al. Bacteriostatic potential of melatonin: Therapeutic standing and mechanistic insights. *Front Immunol.* 2021;12:683879; Wongchitrat P, et al. Role of melatonin on virus-induced neuropathogenesis-A concomitant therapeutic strategy to understand SARS-CoV-2 Infection. *Antioxidants (Basel).* 2021;10(1):47; Cross KM, et al. Melatonin in early treatment for COVID-19: A narrative review of current evidence and possible efficacy. *Endocr Pract.* 2021 S1530–891X(21)01079-X; Claustrat B, et al. Melatonin: Physiological effects in humans. *Neurochirurgie.* 2015;61(2–3):77–84; Rodriguez C, et al. Regulation of antioxidant enzymes: A significant role for melatonin. *J Pineal Res.* 2004;36:1–9; Manchester LC, et al. Melatonin: An ancient molecule that makes oxygen metabolically tolerable. *J Pineal Res.* 2015;59(4):403–419; Chen D, et al. Cellular mechanisms of melatonin: Insight from neurodegenerative diseases. *Biomolecules.* 2020;10(8):1158; Hardeland R. Aging, melatonin, and the pro- and anti-inflammatory networks. *Int J Mol Sci.* 2019;20(5):1223; Cardinali DP. Melatonin: Clinical perspectives in neurodegeneration. *Frontiers in Endocrinology (Lausanne).* 2019;10:480; Wu YH, et al. The human pineal gland and melatonin in aging and Alzheimer's disease. *J Pineal Res.* 2005;38(3):145–152; Cordone S, et al. Sleep and β-Amyloid deposition in Alzheimer disease: Insights on mechanisms and possible innovative treatments. *Front Pharmacol.* 2019;10:695; Sumsuzzman DM, et al. Neurocognitive effects of melatonin treatment in healthy adults and individuals with Alzheimer's disease and insomnia: A systematic review and meta-analysis of randomized controlled trials. *Neurosci Biobehav Rev.* 2021;127:459–473; Shukla M, et al. Mechanisms of melatonin in alleviating Alzheimer's disease. *Curr Neuropharmacol.* 2017;15(7):1010–1031; Pérez-Lloret S, et al. Melatonin as a chronobiotic and cytoprotective agent in Parkinson's disease. *Front Pharmacol.* 2021;12:650597; Carrillo-Vico A, et al. A review of the multiple actions of melatonin on the immune system. *Endocrine.* 2005;27(2):189–200; Hardeland R. Aging, melatonin, and the pro- and anti-inflammatory networks. *Int J Mol Sci.* 2019;20(5):1223; U.S. National Library of Medicine. *Clinical Trials.* https://clinicaltrials.gov/. Accessed August 11, 2021.

stretch. Chronic myofascial pain can induce central sensitization (see Chapter 16) with increased central excitability and decreased central pain inhibition.[109]

Evaluation and Treatment. TTH are diagnosed based on the history, pattern of headache, and palpation of pericranial muscles. Other causes of headache need to be ruled out. Mild TTHs are treated with nonsteroidal antiinflammatory drugs. CTTHs are best managed with a tricyclic antidepressant (e.g., amitriptyline) and behavioral and relaxation therapy. Long-term use of analgesics or other drugs, such as muscle relaxants, antihistamines, tranquilizers, caffeine, and ergot alkaloids, should be avoided.[110]

INFECTION AND INFLAMMATION OF THE CENTRAL NERVOUS SYSTEM

The CNS may be infected by bacteria, viruses, fungi, parasites, and mycobacteria. The invading organisms enter the nervous system either by spreading through arterial blood vessels or by directly invading the nervous tissue from another site of infection. Neurologic infections produce disease by several mechanisms: direct neuronal or glial infection, mass lesion formation, inflammation with subsequent edema, interruption of CSF pathways, neuronal or vascular damage, and secretion of neurotoxins. An immune process may initiate an inflammatory reaction. Signs and symptoms are produced because of (1) interference with the function of the nervous system tissue being invaded or compressed or (2) the inflammatory response produced by the body in response to infection. The cardinal signs of CNS infection are fever, head or spine pain, altered mental state, and focal neurologic dysfunction (See Emerging Science Box: SARS-CoV-2 Infection and Neurologic Manifestations.[111])

Meningitis

Meningitis is inflammation of the brain or spinal cord. Infectious meningitis may be caused by bacteria, viruses, fungi, parasites, or toxins. The infection may be acute, subacute, or chronic, with the pathophysiology, clinical manifestations, and treatment differing for each type of microorganism and any accompanying conditions.

Bacterial Meningitis

Bacterial meningitis is primarily an infection of the pia mater and arachnoid villi, the subarachnoid space, the ventricular system, and the CSF. *Streptococcus pneumoniae* (pneumococcus), *Haemophilus influenzae* type b (Hib), and *Neisseria meningitides* (meningococcus) are the most common pathogens in adults. With pneumococcal meningitis, young persons and those more than 40 years of age are mostly affected with outbreaks in dormitories or military bases. Predisposing conditions are otitis or sinusitis (25%), immunocompromised status (16%), and pneumonia (12%).[112,113] The disease is spread by respiratory droplets and contact with contaminated saliva or respiratory tract secretions (kissing, coughing, sneezing, or sharing utensils, food, and drink). Carriers of the meningococcal bacteria do not develop meningitis but may pass it on to others.

Pathophysiology. Meningococci and pneumococci are inhaled and attach to epithelial cells in the nasopharynx, where they cross the mucosal barrier, enter the bloodstream, travel to cerebral blood vessels, cross the blood-brain barrier, and infect the meninges (Fig. 18.24). With bacterial infection, large numbers of neutrophils are recruited to the subarachnoid space. Release of cytotoxic inflammatory agents and bacterial toxins

EMERGING SCIENCE BOX

SARS-CoV-2 Infection and Neurologic Manifestations

Neuroinvasion of the SARS-CoV-2 into the nervous system may include entry through the olfactory epithelium across the cribriform plate to the olfactory bulb; via infected leukocytes that cross the blood-brain barrier; via the blood stream by infecting endothelium and crossing the vascular endothelium; and via the cranial nerves by transsynapic transport (i.e., via the vagus nerve from the gastrointestinal tract). Once in the brain, SARS-CoV-2 may spread through the ACE2 receptor, through other facilitator receptors, or by adsorptive uptake by neurons and glial cells. Neurologic manifestations may also be related to the secondary immune-mediated cytokine storm associated with a systemic hyperinflammatory state that develops in severe cases. The consequences can include increased blood-brain barrier permeability with cerebral edema and an immune driven hypercoagulable state promoting thrombosis and stroke.

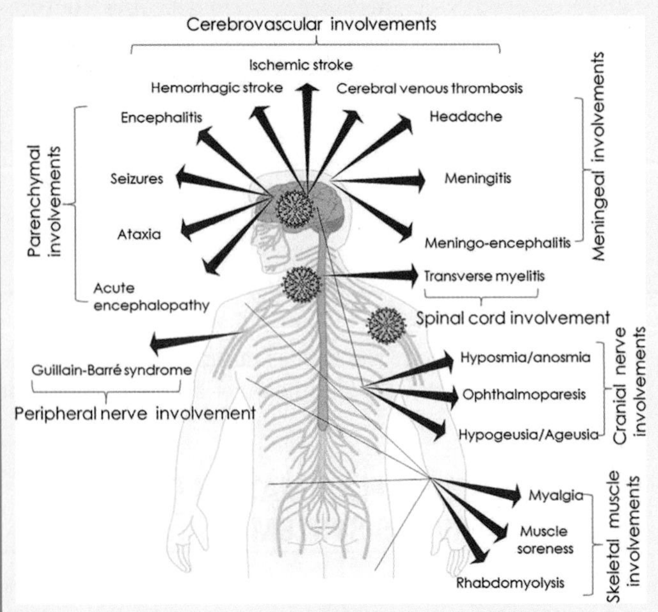

The most common neurologic symptoms are loss of taste and smell, headaches, nausea and vomiting, dizziness, and muscle pain. More severe neurologic manifestations, including ischemic and hemorrhagic strokes, encephalitis, and impaired consciousness, have been associated with more severe disease and older individuals with comorbid conditions, including hypertension, diabetes, and higher levels of C-reactive protein. Guillain-Barré syndrome–type symptoms have also been reported (e.g., hyporeflexia, areflexia, and paraesthesias).

Parkinsonian symptoms have developed in some cases of severe disease, with reduced function of the nigrostriatal dopamine system and positive response to dopaminergic treatment. The figure summarizes the diverse neurologic manifestations among individuals with Covid-19 disease. Research regarding the mechanisms of neuroinvasion, development of treatment, and prevention of long-term consequences continues.

Data from Dewanjee S, et al. Emerging COVID- 19 neurological manifestations: Present outlook and potential neurological challenges in COVID-19 pandemic. *Mol Neurobiol*, 2021:1–22. doi:10.1007/ s12035-021-02450-6. Epub ahead of print; Data from McQuaid C, et al. SARS-CoV-2: Is there neuroinvasion? *Fluids Barriers CNS*, 2021;18(1):32. https://doi.org/10.1186/s12987-021-00267-y; Data from McQuaid C, et al. SARS-CoV-2: Is there neuroinvasion? *Fluids Barriers CNS*, 2021;18(1):32. https://doi.org/10.1186/s12987-021-00267-y; Ellul MA, et al. Neurological associations of COVID-19. *Lancet Neurol*. 2020;19(9):767–783; Ellul MA, et al. Neurological associations of COVID-19. *Lancet Neurol*. 2020;19(9):767–783; Bass DI, et al. The impact of the COVID-19 pandemic on cerebrovascular disease. *Semin Vasc Surg*. 2021;34(2):20–27; Bass DI, et al. The impact of the COVID-19 pandemic on cerebrovascular disease. *Semin Vasc Surg*. 2021;34(2):20–27; Johansson A, et al. Neurological manifestations of COVID-19: A comprehensive literature review and discussion of mechanisms. *J Neuroimmunol*. 2021;358:577658; Johansson A, et al. Neurological manifestations of COVID-19: A comprehensive literature review and discussion of mechanisms. *J Neuroimmunol*. 2021;358:577658; Brundin P, et al. Is COVID-19 a perfect storm for Parkinson's disease? *Trends Neurosci*. 2020;43(12):931–933. Brundin P, et al. Is COVID-19 a perfect storm for Parkinson's disease? *Trends Neurosci*. 2020;43(12):931–933.

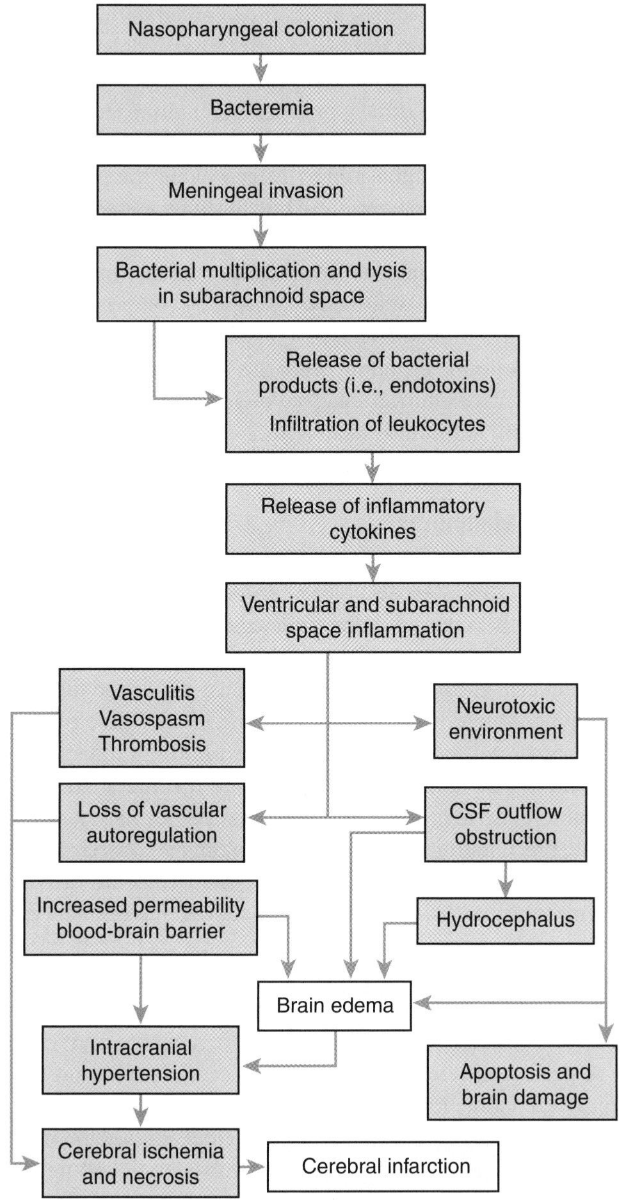

Fig. 18.24 Pathogenesis of Meningitis. (Adapted from Cohen J, Powderly WG. *Infectious diseases*, 2nd edition. Mosby: Edinburgh; 2004.)

alter the blood-brain barrier, causing cerebral edema and damaging brain tissue. The inflammatory exudate thickens the CSF and interferes with normal CSF flow around the brain and spinal cord, possibly obstructing arachnoid villi and producing hydrocephalus. Meningeal cells become edematous, and the combined exudate and edematous cells increase ICP. Engorged blood vessels and thrombi can disrupt blood flow, causing further injury.

Clinical Manifestations. The clinical manifestations of bacterial meningitis can be grouped into infectious signs, meningeal signs, and neurologic signs. The clinical manifestations of systemic infection include fever, tachycardia, and chills. The clinical manifestations of meningeal irritation are a severe throbbing headache, severe photophobia, nuchal rigidity, and positive Kernig and Brudzinski signs (Fig. 18.25). The neurologic signs include a decrease in consciousness, cranial nerve palsies, focal neurologic deficits (e.g., hemiparesis/hemiplegia and ataxia), and seizures. Often there is projectile vomiting. Papilledema develops, as the ICP increases, causing delirium, and may progress to unconsciousness and death. With meningococcal meningitis, a petechial or purpuric rash covers the skin and mucous membranes. A rare complication is acute infectious purpura fulminans. It is caused by bacterial endotoxin and inflammatory cytokines and can cause sepsis. This is a rapidly progressive syndrome of hemorrhagic infarction of the skin and disseminated intravascular coagulation that can lead to multiple organ failure, ischemic necrosis of digits and limbs with amputation required, and death.

Evaluation and Treatment. Rapid diagnosis, antibiotic administration, and supportive treatment are important to prevent morbidity and mortality from bacterial meningitis. Diagnosis is based on physical examination, blood cultures, and the results of nasopharyngeal smear and antigen tests. CSF analysis and cultures are required for differential diagnosis. Serious complications, including septic shock, disseminated intravascular coagulation, purpura fulminans, limb damage, and multiple organ failure, require intensive multidisciplinary care. Long-term neurologic complications include seizures, hearing and vision loss, and neuromotor disability. More subtle effects such as cognitive impairment and memory and behavior changes are often overlooked and

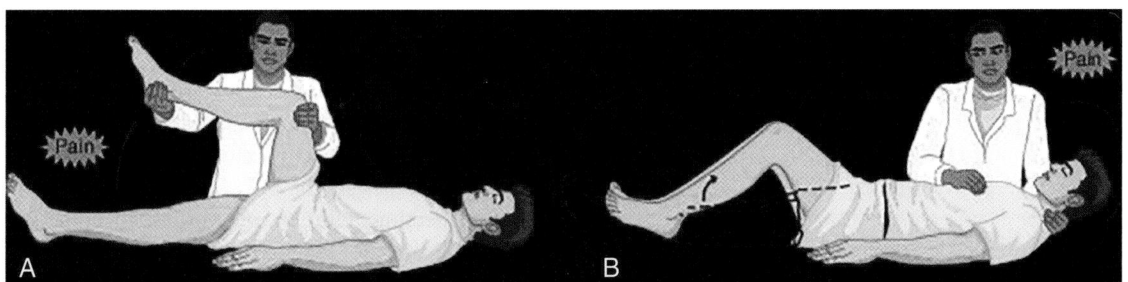

Fig. 18.25 Bacterial Meningitis and Clinical Signs. (A) Kernig sign, supine position with hip flexed 90 degrees. Knees cannot be fully extended. **(B)** Brudzinski Sign, neck rigidity causes flexion of both legs and thighs with passive flexion of the neck.

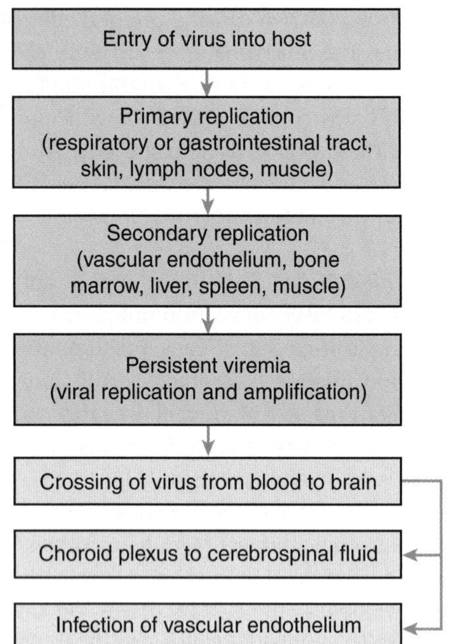

Fig. 18.26 Hematogenous Spread of Viral Pathogens to the Central Nervous System. (Adapted from Cohen J, Powderly WG. *Infectious diseases.* Mosby: Edinburgh, 2007.)

can have detrimental effects on school and work performance.[114] Vaccinations are available to prevent meningococcal, pneumococcal, and *H. influenzae* meningitis.[115]

Viral Meningitis

Viral meningitis (aseptic meningitis) is thought to be limited to the meninges. An identifiable bacterium cannot be found in the CSF. The term aseptic is used to differentiate meningeal inflammation that is caused by pathogens other than pus-producing bacteria. The most common viruses are enteroviral viruses (echovirus, coxsackievirus, and nonparalytic poliomyelitis), arboviruses, and herpes simplex type 1 and 2. Viruses enter the nervous system by crossing the blood-brain barrier, by direct spread along peripheral nerves, through transsynaptic transmission, through the choroid plexus epithelium, or from infected immune cell that cross into the brain (Fig. 18.26).[116] The immune response leads to release of inflammatory cytokines with increased permeability of the blood-brain barrier and entry of circulating immunoglobulins that combat the virus. The clinical manifestations of viral meningitis are similar to those of bacterial meningitis but milder. Viral meningitis is managed pharmacologically with antipyretics, antiemetics, analgesics, and antiviral drugs.[117]

Fungal Meningitis

Fungal meningitis is a chronic, much less common condition than bacterial or viral meningitis. The most common fungal infections of the nervous system are histoplasmosis, cryptococcosis, coccidioidomycosis, mucormycosis, candidiasis, and aspergillosis. Fungal meningitis develops insidiously, usually over days or weeks. The infection most often occurs in persons with impaired immune responses or alterations in normal body flora. Cryptococcal meningitis remains a leading cause of death in human immunodeficiency virus (HIV)–infected persons in resource-limited settings.[118] Fungi enter the nervous system by transcellular or paracellular migration across endothelial cells or by transport inside phagocytes.[119] Fungi in the nervous system usually produce a granulomatous reaction, forming granulomata or gelatinous masses in the meninges at the base of the brain. Fungi also may extend along the perivascular sites in the subarachnoid space and into the brain tissue, producing arteritis with thrombosis, infarction, and communicating hydrocephalus. Meningeal fibrosis develops later in the inflammatory process. Cranial nerve dysfunction, caused by compression, often results from the granulomata and fibrosis. The first manifestations are often nonspecific including headache, fever, convulsions, weakness, progressive confusion, changed mental status, and focal neurologic deficits. Antifungal treatments are microorganism specific and effective. Surgery can remove granulomas and abscesses.[120]

Tubercular Meningitis

Tubercular meningitis is a common and serious form of CNS tuberculosis (TB), especially in immunosuppressed persons or those with acquired immunodeficiency syndrome (AIDS). Mycobacteria are acquired through inhalation of aerosolized droplet nuclei. The bacteria enter the brain as described for fungal meningitis. Miliary tubercles form in the brain. These tubercles can rupture, and the bacteria are released into the subarachnoid space and are disseminated to the CSF and meninges. The bacteria promote meningeal inflammation and the formation of thick exudate precipitating the signs and symptoms of tubercular meningitis. Cerebral ischemia and infarction can occur from vasculitis.

Symptoms are nonspecific and may develop over many days, making early diagnosis difficult. Symptoms include headache, low-grade fever, nausea and vomiting, irritability, difficulty sleeping, and fatigue and increase to confusion, stiff neck, significant behavioral changes, and seizures. Hydrocephalus and cranial nerve palsies or cerebral infarcts may occur. There is no single clinical guideline for the diagnosis of tubercular meningitis. Diagnosis includes the medical history, clinical assessment, CSF investigations and neuroimaging, mycobacterial culture, and molecular testing (nucleic acid amplification testing).[121] Recovery rate is 90% with early diagnosis and treatment with appropriate anti-TB therapy. Treatment is difficult in resource-poor countries, and multidrug-resistant TB is emerging as a global threat.[122,123]

Encephalitis

Encephalitis is an acute inflammation of the brain, usually of viral origin. The most common forms are infectious, autoimmune, and postinfectious.[124] Herpes simplex type 1 is the most common sporadic cause of infectious encephalitis. Viruses infect specific cell types in the CNS, as shown in Fig. 18.27. Referred to as infectious viral encephalitides, encephalitis may occur as a complication of systemic viral diseases, such as herpes simplex type 1, rabies, or mononucleosis, or it may arise after recovery from viral infections, such as rubella, varicella, rubeola, or yellow fever. Encephalitis also may follow vaccination with a live, attenuated virus vaccine if the vaccine has an encephalitis component (e.g., measles, mumps, and rubella). Typhus, trichinosis, malaria, and schistosomiasis also are associated with encephalitis.

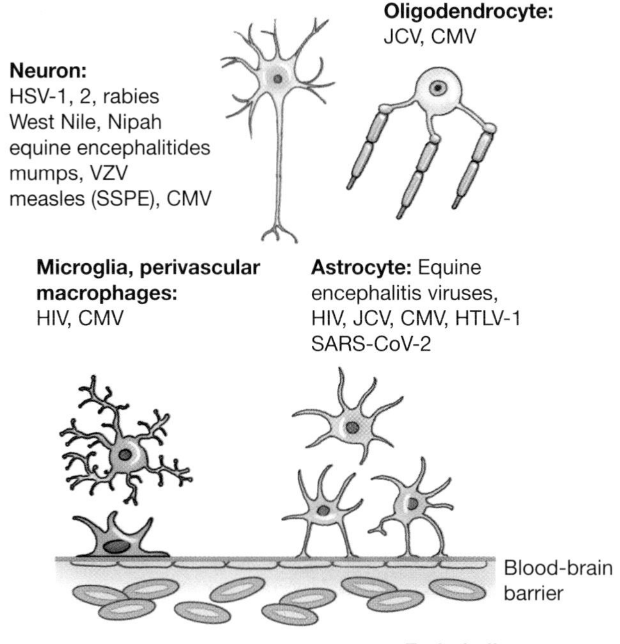

Fig. 18.27 Viral Infection of Specific Cells in the Central Nervous System (CNS). Viruses infect specific cell types within the CNS, depending on the particular properties of the virus together with individual cell membrane proteins expressed on permissive cell types. Normally the brain is protected from circulating pathogens and toxins by the blood-brain barrier. *CMV*, Cytomegalovirus; *HIV*, human immunodeficiency virus; *HSV*, herpes simplex virus; *HTLV-1*, human T-cell lymphotropic virus (causes T-cell leukemia); *JCV*, John Cunningham virus (a polyomavirus causing progressive multifocal leukoencephalopathy); *SARS-CoV-2;* severe acute respiratory syndrome-related coronavirus-2; *SSPE*, subacute sclerosing panencephalitis; *VZV*, varicella-zoster virus. (Adapted from Power C, Noorbakhsh G. Central nervous system viral infections: Clinical aspects and pathogenic mechanisms. In: Gilman S, eds. *Neurobiology of disease. Burlington*, MA: Elsevier; 2007:488.)

With the exception of California viral encephalitis, which is endemic, the arthropod-borne (flies, mosquitoes, and ticks) encephalitides occur in epidemics, varying in geographic and seasonal incidence. West Nile virus (WNV) encephalitis is the most common, and Eastern equine encephalitis is the most serious but least common of the encephalitides.

West Nile Virus

West Nile virus (WNV), a *Flavivirus* transmitted predominantly by the *Culex* mosquito, is the most common cause of epidemic meningoencephalitis in North America and the leading cause of arboviral encephalitis in the United States. Humans and horses, as well as other mammals, are incidental hosts. Birds and mosquitoes are life cycle hosts, and the greatest amount of virus is carried by mosquitoes in early fall. WNV also can be transmitted through blood transfusions and organ transplants.

The human incubation period is 2 to 14 days. Most individuals develop no symptoms. Approximately 20% of those infected have mild symptoms that last 4 to 6 days and generally include fever, headache, myalgia, skin rash, and lymphadenopathy. This is known as West Nile fever. Less than 1% of affected persons develop severe illness, but it is the most frequent of the neuroinvasive infections. Identifiable risk factors are advanced age, immunocompromise, diabetes, hypertension, and pregnancy. The virus crosses the blood-brain barrier and reproduces in neurons. Abnormalities can develop in the thalamus, basal ganglia, cerebellum, hippocampus, spinal cord, dorsal root ganglia, and peripheral motor neuron. Manifestations can include headache, disorientation, stupor, coma, seizures, and movement disorders, including tremor, ataxia, extrapyramidal signs, and paralysis, and are related to the infected areas of the brain. West Nile meningitis is characterized by meningeal signs of severe headache, high fever, and nuchal rigidity. Myelitis and polyradiculitis also may be present. Both severe and mild cases can have long-term neurologic sequelae after recovery, including memory loss, depression, fatigue, generalized or limb weakness, and tremors. These disease features are similar to those encountered in neurodegenerative diseases such as Alzheimer disease and Parkinson disease.[125]

Diagnosis is made if WNV RNA is found in blood or other body fluids or immunoglobulin M (IgM) for the virus is found in serum or cerebrospinal fluid. A rapid test became available in 2007. Plaque reduction neutralization assay (PRNA) is the confirmatory test. Treatment is supportive care. No West Nile vaccine has been developed for humans. Environmental control and prevention of mosquito bites are the best protections. Since 2003, all blood banks use blood-screening tests for WNV. There is a vaccine for horses, but there is not an approved vaccine for humans.[126,127]

Pathophysiology. Viruses gain access to the CNS through the bloodstream, olfactory bulb, or choroid plexus or from peripheral nerves. With *herpes simplex type-1 encephalitis*, the virus may enter the CNS with primary infection or reactivation of the latent virus. In some cases, the viral strain responsible for encephalitis is different from the strain that causes herpetic skin lesions in the same person, indicating the possibility of primary CNS infection.[128] *Autoimmune encephalitis* develops when antibodies form against cell surface antigens, synaptic antigens, and/or intraneuronal antigens on specific neural cells in different parts of the brain. With paraneoplastic neurologic syndromes, there is an underlying cancer, and the autoantibodies (also known as onconeural antibodies) are markers for cytotoxic T cells, which attack the antibodies and disrupt synaptic nerve transmission or destroy the nerve. Virus-induced autoantibody generation against cell surface antigens seems to be a widespread mechanism. Examples include *N*-methyl-D-aspartate receptor (NMDAR) antibodies following herpes simplex type-1 encephalitis. Anti-NMDAR encephalitis and other cell surface antigens are also associated with underlying malignancies. Loss of the NMDAR results in excitotoxicity from excess levels of glutamate.[129,130]

Meningeal involvement is present in all encephalitides. The various encephalitides may cause widespread nerve cell degeneration. Edema, necrosis with or without hemorrhage, and IICP develop.

Clinical Manifestations. Encephalitis ranges from a mild infectious disease to a life-threatening disorder. Mild symptoms include malaise, headache, body aches, nausea, and vomiting. Dramatic clinical manifestations include fever, difficulty with word finding, seizure activity, cranial nerve palsies, paresis and paralysis, involuntary movement, abnormal reflexes, and delirium or confusion progressing to unconsciousness. Signs of marked ICP may be present. The clinical manifestation of autoimmune encephalitis can be acute or subacute and vary with the type of antigen and brain region involved. Deficits of memory and cognition, altered level of consciousness, behavioral and psychiatric symptoms, autonomic disturbances, movement disorders, and seizures are possible manifestations.

Evaluation and Treatment. Diagnosis is made by the history and clinical presentation, aided by CSF examination and culture, serologic studies, white blood cell count, CT scan, or MRI. Empiric treatment is specific to the type of virus and may include antiviral agents, antibiotics, and steroids. Herpes encephalitis is treated with antiviral agents, such as acyclovir. Measures to control the ICP are paramount. Autoimmune encephalitis may be treated with immunotherapy, plasmapheresis, and/or steroids and removal of tumor. When the antibodies are removed (e.g., plasmapheresis or intravenous immunoglobulin), symptoms will improve. Chronic antibody exposure results in neuronal death and irreversible neurologic deficit.[131,132]

Brain or Spinal Cord Abscess

Abscesses are localized collections of pus within the parenchyma of the brain or spinal cord and are rare. Immunosuppressed persons are particularly at risk.

Brain abscesses are classified as epidural, subdural, or intracerebral. *Epidural brain abscesses* (empyemas) are associated with osteomyelitis in a cranial bone. *Subdural brain abscesses* (empyemas) arise from a sinus infection or a vascular source. *Intracerebral brain abscesses* arise from a vascular source. Spinal cord abscesses are very rare and classified as epidural or intramedullary (within the spinal cord). Epidural spinal abscesses usually originate as osteomyelitis in a vertebra; the infection then spreads into the epidural space. (Osteomyelitis is discussed in Chapter 44.)

Pathophysiology. Microorganisms gain entrance to the CNS by direct extension or distribution along the wall of a vein (e.g., trauma, mastoiditis, sinusitis, or dental infection). Infective emboli carry organisms from distant sites such as the heart, lungs, pelvic organs, skin, tonsils, abscessed teeth, osteomyelitis (except for cranial bones), and dirty needles.[133] Illegal drug users who share needles are at risk, as are immunosuppressed persons. For example, *Toxoplasma gondii* is producing an ever-increasing number of CNS abscesses in persons with AIDS. Streptococci, staphylococci, and *Bacteroides* sp., often combined with anaerobes, are the most common bacteria that cause abscesses; however, yeast and fungi also may be involved.

Brain abscesses progress from localized inflammation to a necrotic core with the formation of a connective tissue capsule, usually within 14 days or longer.[134] Existing abscesses also tend to spread and form daughter abscesses.

Clinical Manifestations. Early manifestations include low-grade fever, headache (most common symptom), nausea and vomiting, neck pain and stiffness, confusion, drowsiness, sensory deficits, and communication deficits. Later manifestations are associated with an expanding mass and IICP and include decreased attention span, memory deficits, decreased visual acuity and narrowed visual fields, papilledema, ocular palsy, ataxia, dementia, and seizures. The development of symptoms may be very insidious, often making an abscess difficult to diagnose.

Extradural brain abscesses are associated with localized pain, purulent drainage from the nasal passages or auditory canal, fever, localized tenderness, and neck stiffness. Clinical manifestations of spinal cord abscesses have four stages: (1) spinal aching, (2) severe root pain, accompanied by spasms of the back muscles and limited vertebral movement, (3) weakness caused by progressive cord compression, and (4) paralysis.

Evaluation and Treatment. The diagnosis is suggested by clinical features and confirmed by imaging studies. The primary source of infection should be identified and treated. Antibiotics are usually indicated, often in conjunction with corticosteroid therapy to treat the cerebral edema. The ICP and/or hydrocephalus may have to be managed.[135] Cerebral abscesses are considered a neurosurgical emergency. Spinal cord abscesses are treated with surgical decompression or aspiration, antibiotic therapy, and supportive therapy.

Neurologic Complications of Human Immunodeficiency Virus

Neurologic complications of HIV remain common but are milder due to widespread use of combination antiretroviral therapy (ART). The mechanism of neural involvement includes (1) direct effects of HIV (e.g., neurocognitive impairment), (2) immunocompromise secondary to uncontrolled HIV infection (e.g., opportunistic infections), (3) aberrant immune responses in the setting of ART initiation (e.g., immune reconstitution inflammatory syndrome [IRIS]), and (4) adverse effects of ART (e.g., peripheral neuropathy).

The most common neurologic complication associated with HIV is HIV-associated neurocognitive disorder (HAND), a range of disorders that includes mild neurocognitive disorder and HIV-associated dementia, which is rare. Combined antiretroviral therapy (cART) with more efficient CNS drug penetration has reduced the prevalence and improved survival for individuals with HAND. Milder forms of the disease may persist because of longer life and the ability of the virus to survive within brain tissue in some individuals.

The HIV virus can enter the brain after 1 to 2 weeks of systemic infection. Persistent CNS infection and inflammation probably contribute to the development of HAND, which affects approximately 50% of HIV-infected individuals.[136] Various mechanisms have been proposed for HIV transfer into the brain. HIV-infected monocytes (cell-associated virus) or CD4+ T lymphocytes may pass through the brain-blood barrier. The monocytes mature into macrophages and release cytokines, increasing the permeability of the brain-blood barrier and causing the infiltration of more infected monocytes. Cell-free HIV (virus floating free in plasma) may also pass through the brain-blood barrier. Infected CD4+ T lymphocytes may transfer into the brain and come in contact with macrophages, leading to cell fusion and transfer of viruses to macrophages. The cause of the neuronal damage is thought to occur through two proposed mechanisms, the direct and indirect mechanisms. The direct mechanism suggests that monocytes and other infected cells release the virus, causing viral proteins to bind to neurons directly, causing neuronal damage and death. The indirect mechanism suggests that infected and uninfected monocytes, astrocytes, and microglia mount an inflammatory response against the virus, which causes neuronal damage and death. The infected cells serve as a reservoir for the virus.[137] Neuroinflammation leads to neurodegeneration. The symptoms are similar to other forms of dementia, including cognitive slowing, poor concentration, and memory difficulty. Motor signs can include difficulty speaking, progressive loss of balance, gait disturbances, or paralysis. Diagnosis is difficult during early stages of manifestations and requires neurocognitive testing. CSF analysis and imaging help to establish the diagnosis. HIV antiretroviral treatment improves survival for individuals with severe HAND but does not reverse the impairment. Differentiating HAND from Alzheimer disease and other neurodegenerative disorders can be difficult as the HIV-infected population reaches older ages.[138] Treatment with cART has prevented the most severe forms of HAND, but the less severe forms now predominate. There is no specific treatment.

PERIPHERAL NERVOUS SYSTEM DISORDERS

The peripheral nervous system is composed of motor anterior horn cell fibers, sensory dorsal root ganglia fibers, and peripheral autonomic ganglia and their axons. Acute or chronic disease processes, inflammation, or trauma may injure these peripheral nerves and cause neuropathy. Neuropathic pain is reviewed in Chapter 15.

Peripheral Neuropathies

Peripheral neuropathies occur outside the brain or spinal cord and are diseases or injuries to peripheral nerves (Table 18.15).[139] The injury may affect distinct anatomic areas of the axon, or the spinal nerves may be injured at the roots, at the plexus before peripheral nerve formation, or at the peripheral nerves themselves. Autonomic nerve fibers may be injured as they travel in certain cranial nerves or emerge through the ventral root and plexuses to pass through the peripheral nerves of the body. When myelin is damaged, nerve conduction is delayed or stopped. When the cell body, axon, or ganglia are injured, there is loss of function.

Neuropathies can be acquired, inherited (rare), or idiopathic. Focal nerve injuries involve mononeuropathies and radiculopathies. Mononeuropathies affect a single peripheral nerve (e.g., a sensory or motor neuropathy). Multiple mononeuropathies (multiplex) involve two or more individual nerves in different areas and can be difficult to distinguish from a polyneuropathy. Autonomic neuropathies involve the autonomic nervous system (innervation of the heart, blood vessels, intestine, bladder, sweat glands and pupils). Radiculopathies are disorders of spinal nerve roots as they enter (sensory) or exit (motor) the spine (see Fig 15.13). Cervical and lumbar nerve roots are more commonly affected, and pain is the major symptom. *Radiculitis* (radiculoneuritis) refers to an inflammation of the spinal nerve roots. One (focal) or more roots may be affected. An acute intervertebral disk prolapse (herniated disk), degenerative spondyloarthropathies, or a benign tumor are causes of root compression. Polyneuropathy is generalized involvement of peripheral nerves that is usually bilateral and symmetric and can involve motor, sensory, and autonomic nerves simultaneously. Pathologic processes that cause neuropathies include autoimmune disorders, inflammation, infection, decreased blood flow, compression, damage to supporting connective or

TABLE 18.15 Types of Peripheral Neuropathies

Type	Cause	Example
Mononeuropathy Motor: weakness, paralysis Sensory: numbness, pain	Trauma, compression, infection, inflammation, tumor	Sciatica, carpel tunnel syndrome, radial nerve palsy, facial palsy
Multiple mononeuropathies (multiplex) Motor: weakness, paralysis Sensory: numbness, pain Patchy distribution involving two or more nerves	Metabolic (hyperglycemia, toxins), connective tissue (autoimmune mechanisms) or vascular (hypoxemia) disorders	Usually associated with systemic disease: diabetes mellitus, vasculitis, lupus erythematosus; radiculopathies (spinal nerve roots), and nerve plexus injury
Autonomic neuropathy Affects sympathetic and parasympathetic nerve fibers	Usually associated with systemic disease (i.e., diabetes mellitus, vasculitis, lupus erythematosus)	Alterations in heart rate, blood pressure (dizziness, fainting), bladder function (incontinence or urinary retention), gastrointestinal function (diarrhea or constipation), or thermal regulation
Radiculopathy Affects sensory, motor, and nerves	Nerve root compression from vertebral disease or injury or disc herniation	Degenerative spondyloarthropathy; cervical or lumbar disc herniation
Polyneuropathy Affects sensory, motor and autonomic nerves simultaneously in a symmetric distribution	Systemic metabolic, toxic, autoimmune and infectious diseases	Hyperglycemia, uremia, alcoholism, chemotherapy, Guillain-Barré syndrome, human immunodeficiency virus (HIV) infection

bone tissue, trauma, metabolic disorders (e.g., diabetes mellitus and nutritional deficiencies), toxins (e.g., alcoholism and industrial chemicals) drugs, and tumors.

Pathophysiology. Although distinct pathophysiologic processes are recognized in neuropathy, these are not disease specific and may exist simultaneously in any one neuropathy. Pathologic processes that may be present include *wallerian degeneration*, in which the axon and myelin distal to the site of axonal interruption degenerate (see Chapter 15). This type of degeneration is characteristic of a traumatic nerve injury in which the nerve is severed. *Axonal degeneration* is caused by metabolic failure within an axon or vascular ischemia. In axonal degeneration, distal degeneration of the axon occurs first and is followed by degeneration of the myelin and the axis cylinder. This results in "stocking and glove" sensory or motor symptoms. In *demyelinating neuropathies*, the axon may be spared and only the myelin degenerates. Electromyography, nerve conduction studies, and imaging can assist in differentiating axonal from demyelination neuropathies.[140,141]

Clinical Manifestations. When the axons are affected, muscle strength, muscle tone, and muscle mass also are affected. Whole muscles or groups of muscles are paretic or paralyzed, and the muscles of the feet and legs often are affected first and more severely than the hands and arms. These long, large axons are thought to (1) be more vulnerable to injury because of their size and length, (2) have more Schwann cells available to be injured, and (3) exhibit a "dying back" phenomenon caused by difficulty of the nerve cell body in maintaining the terminal portion of the axon.

Tone and the deep tendon reflexes in the affected muscles generally are decreased, and atrophy is distributed according to the peripheral nerves involved. Fasciculation may be present, especially with associated ventral root or motor neuron changes, or both, as in Guillain-Barré syndrome (see Chapter 17) and diabetic neuropathy (see Chapter 22). Mild fatigue may be experienced. A few disorders, notably Guillain-Barré syndrome, produce a pattern of paresis and paralysis that involves all limbs, the trunk, and the neck (see Chapter 17). Ataxia of gait or limb may arise from the loss of position and vibratory sensations (i.e., proprioceptive sensory loss) and may be enhanced by motor weakness. Diseases that involve spinal roots typically produce local pain; pain on local percussion; pain and paresthesia in the sensory root distribution (called radicular pain and radicular paresthesia (e.g., cervical root pain causes pain in the arm; see Fig. 15.11); increased pain with movement, stretching of the root, and maneuvers that transiently increase CSF pressure; sensory loss in a radicular pattern; and spasms of the muscles surrounding the vertebral column (e.g., paravertebral muscle spasms).

Reflex-mediated autonomic nervous system functions, such as sweating, pupillary size, bladder, gastric, intestinal, and cardiovascular function, may be affected (see Fig. 15.25). Neuropathies associated with autonomic disturbances include diabetes mellitus, alcoholism and related nutritional neuropathies, amyloidosis, and Guillain-Barré syndrome. In many chronic polyneuropathies, the feet, hands, and spine become deformed.

Evaluation and Treatment. The diagnostic work-up to determine the cause of a neuropathy is often extensive and involves a detailed history and physical examination, laboratory evaluations of serum and CSF, electromyelography, nerve conduction studies, and imaging.[140,141] Early diagnosis and treatment before irreversible neuronal cell damage ensues are of paramount importance. Although axonal regrowth and recovery of function may take months, many neuropathies can be reversed. The therapeutic management is directed at elimination of the cause, control of diseases such as diabetes mellitus, and prevention of further nerve damage.

Nerve plexus injuries involve the nerve plexus distal to the spinal roots but proximal to the formation of the peripheral nerves. Such injuries may be caused by trauma, compression (entrapment), or infiltration, or they may be iatrogenic and caused by positioning during surgery or by an intramuscular injection. Clinical manifestations include motor weakness, muscle atrophy, and sensory loss in affected areas. Paralysis can occur with complete plexus lesions.

The diagnosis is made based on history and clinical manifestations. Therapeutic treatment is directed at removal of the cause, surgical repair and approximation of nervous tissue, nerve transfers, growth factors, prevention of further injury, control of discomfort, prevention of complications, and rehabilitation when appropriate.[142]

TUMORS OF THE CENTRAL NERVOUS SYSTEM

CNS tumors include both brain and spinal cord tumors. Primary CNS tumors had an estimated 24,530 new cases and 18,600 deaths in the United States in 2021.[143] The incidence of CNS tumors increases to age 70 years and then decreases. From 2013 to 2017, CNS tumors were the most common group of tumors occurring in children ages 0 to 14 years.[144] Approximately 70% to 75% of all intracranial tumors in children are located infratentorially (see Chapter 20), and in adults, 70% are located supratentorially. Peripheral nerve tumors are rare in children and more common in adults. Carcinogenesis is discussed in Chapter 12, pituitary tumors are discussed in Chapter 22, and cerebral tumors in children are discussed in Chapter 20.

Brain Tumors

Tumors within the cranium can be either primary or metastatic. *Primary (intracerebral) brain tumors* originate from brain substance, including neuroglia, neurons, cells of blood vessels, and connective tissue. *Extracerebral tumors* originate outside substances of the brain and include meningiomas, acoustic nerve tumors, and tumors of the pituitary and pineal glands. *Metastatic (secondary) brain tumors* are the most prevalent and arise in organ systems outside the brain and spread to the brain. Sites of intracranial tumors are illustrated in Fig. 18.28.

Local effects of cranial tumors are caused by the destructive action of the tumor itself on a particular site in the brain and by compression, causing decreased cerebral blood flow. For example, frontal lobe tumors might cause personality changes, weakness, or dysphasia; parietal lobe tumors might cause numbness, hemineglect or spatial disorientation, difficulty speaking, reading, or writing; tumors involving the temporal lobe might involve memory loss or seizures; tumors involving the optic radiation

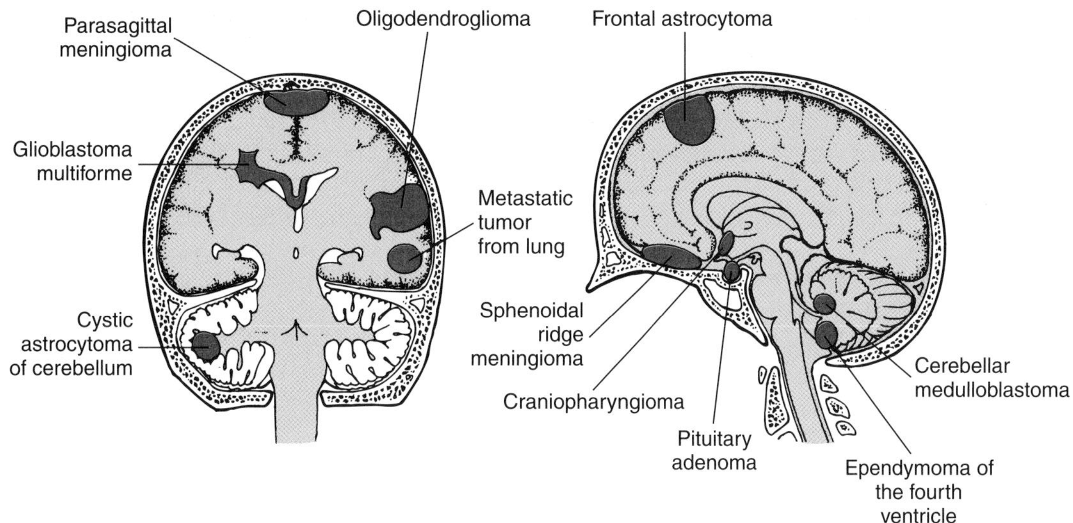

Fig. 18.28 Common Sites of Intracranial Tumors.

might cause visual field defects; and cerebellar tumors might cause gait disturbances, loss of coordination, and dizziness.

Generalized effects result from IICP caused by invasion of the tumor, obstruction of the ventricular system, hemorrhages in and around the tumor, compression of nerve tissue, and cerebral edema. Manifestations include headache, seizures, visual disturbances, unstable gait, nausea and vomiting, and cranial nerve dysfunction.

Intracranial brain tumors do not metastasize as readily as tumors in other organs because there are no lymphatic channels within the brain substance. If metastasis does occur, it is usually through seeding of cerebral blood or CSF during cranial surgery or through artificial shunts.

Primary Brain (Intracerebral) Tumors

Primary brain (intracerebral) tumors, also called gliomas (cells that support brain neurons), include astrocytomas, oligodendrogliomas, glioblastomas (the most common malignant brain tumor), and ependymomas. Other CNS tumors include meningiomas (the most common adult brain tumor), nerve sheath tumors (schwannomas), and neurofibromas.[145] Medulloblastomas primarily occur in children. Brain tumors account for nearly 2% of all cancers in the United States.[143] The etiology for primary brain tumors is not clearly known. Ionizing radiation is the only known environmental risk factor.

Treatment for brain tumors is complex because of interindividual variability, intratumoral heterogeneity, and impediment of drug delivery across the blood-brain barrier. Surgical removal of tumor tissue is difficult because of invasiveness of the tumor. Advances now allow profiling of genomic, epigenomic, transcriptomic, proteomic, and metabolomic changes in brain tumors. Efforts are in progress to individualize treatment to the specific characteristics of the tumor.[146] Treatments currently include surgical or radiosurgical excision or surgical decompression if total excision is not possible. Surgical resection allows histologic and molecular diagnosis to guide further treatment. Chemotherapy (temozolomide), radiation therapy (RT), or their combination, targeted molecular therapies, and alternating electrical field therapy may be used. Treatments for grade IV tumors have not produced long-term survival, and there is often recurrence. The blood-brain barrier is an obstacle to the delivery of chemotherapeutic agents. New methods are in progress for penetration of this barrier, including nanoparticle drug carriers, photodynamic strategies, gene therapy, monoclonal antibodies, and focused ultrasound combined with microbubbles. (Cancer treatment is discussed in Chapter 12).[147–149]

Astrocytoma. Astrocytomas are the most common glioma (approximately 75% of all tumors of the brain and spinal cord). The World Health Organization (WHO) divides astrocytomas into four grades based on histopathologic characteristics or phenotypes: cellular density, atypia, mitotic activity, microvascular proliferation, and necrosis. In addition, molecular characteristics (genetic driver mutations) have been identified to differentiate tumor types (Table 18.16). Molecular characteristics of gliomas include mutation of the isocitrate dehydrogenase 1 *(IDH1)* gene, and, less commonly, mutation of the related *IDH2* gene identified in the vast majority of WHO grades II and III astrocytic and oligodendroglial gliomas. Silencing of the *MGMT* gene (methylated-DNA-protein-cysteine methyltransferase, a DNA repair enzyme) is found in astrocytomas. Mutant epidermal growth factor vIII (EGFRvIII) amplification is found in most subtype gliomas. Chromosome 1p and 19q deletions are associated with oligodendrogliomas, and gliomas may arise from cancer-initiating resident stem cells. Identifying these molecular signatures is guiding tumor-specific individualized therapy.[150,151]

These tumors may occur anywhere in the brain or spinal cord and are generally located in the cerebrum, hypothalamus, or pons. Low-grade astrocytomas tend to be located laterally or supratentorially in adults and in a midline or near-midline position in children (Fig. 18.29).

Headache (caused by pressure on blood vessels and meninges) and subtle neurobehavioral changes may be early signs. Other neurologic symptoms evolve slowly, and IICP occurs late in the tumor's course. Onset of a focal seizure disorder between

TABLE 18.16 **Grades of Astrocytomas Edited**

Grade[a]	Selected Types Diffuse Astrocytic and Oligodendroglial	Description	Characteristics
I	Pilocytic astrocytoma	Common in children and young adults and people with neurofibromatosis type 1 or with *BRAF-KIAA* fusion gene mutation; common in cerebellum	Least malignant, well differentiated; grows slowly; frequently cystic, near-normal microscopic appearance, noninfiltrating
II	Diffuse astrocytoma, IDH mutant (fibrillary, gemistocytic, protoplasmic) Oligodendroglioma, IDH mutant and 1p/19q codeleted	Common in young adults; more common in cerebrum but can occur in any part of brain	Cytological atypia; grows slowly; infiltrates to adjacent tissue; may be malignant or nonmalignant; may recur at higher grade
III	Anaplastic astrocytoma, IDH mutant Anaplastic oligodendroglioma, *IDH* mutant and 1p/19q codeleted	Common in young adults	Anaplasia and mitotic activity, malignant—diffusely infiltrates adjacent tissue; slow growing, frequently recurs at higher grade
IV	Glioblastoma, *IDH- wildtype*, Diffuse midline glioma, *H3k27M*-mutant	Common in older adults, particularly men Predominant in cerebral hemispheres Predominant in brain stem glioma in children	Anaplasia, mitotic activity with microvascular proliferation, and/or necrosis, reproduce rapidly and are very aggressive malignant tumors

[a]World Health Organization grading system for central nervous system tumors.
1p/19q, Combined loss of the short arm chromosome 1p and the long arm of chromosome 19q (inactivation of tumor suppressor gene); *H3k27M*, histone mutation—substitution of lysine amino acid at position 27 with methionine; *IDH*, isocitrate dehydrogenase (a rate-limiting enzyme in the Krebs cycle that plays an important role in energy metabolism); *wildtype*, no genetic mutation or not otherwise specified.
Data from Gupta A, Dwivedi T. A simplified overview of World Health Organization Classification Update of Central Nervous System Tumors 2016. *J Neurosci Rural Pract*, 2017;8(4):629–641.

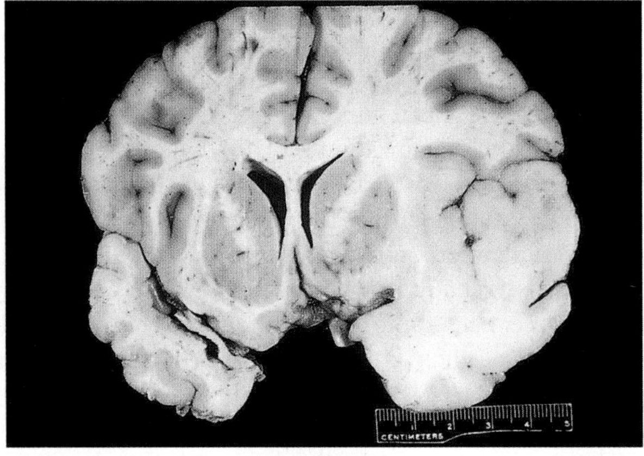

Fig. 18.29 Astrocytoma.

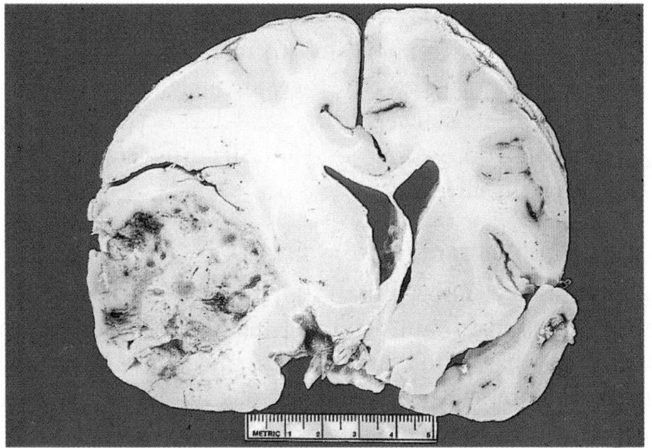

Fig. 18.30 Glioblastoma.

the second and sixth decades of life suggests an astrocytoma. Low-grade astrocytomas are treated with surgery or by external radiation. Approximately 50% of persons survive 5 years when surgery is followed by RT.

Grades III and IV astrocytomas are found predominantly in the frontal lobes and cerebral hemispheres, although they may occur in the brainstem, cerebellum, and spinal cord. Men are twice as likely to have astrocytomas as women; in the 15- to 34-year-old age group, they are the third most common brain cancer, whereas in the 35- to 54-year-old age group they are the fourth most common.

A grade IV astrocytoma, known as glioblastoma, is the most lethal and common type of primary brain tumor (Fig. 18.30). They are highly vascular and extensively irregular and infiltrative, making them difficult to remove surgically. Fifty percent of glioblastomas are bilateral or at least occupy more than one lobe at the time of death. The typical clinical presentation for a glioblastoma is that of diffuse, nonspecific clinical signs, such as headache, irritability, memory loss, and "personality changes," that progress to more clear-cut manifestations of IICP, including headache on position change, papilledema, vomiting, or seizure activity. Symptoms may progress to include definite focal signs, such as hemiparesis, dysphasia, dyspraxia, cranial nerve palsies, and visual field deficits. Survival at 5 years for grades III and IV astrocytomas is approximately 5% to 10%.

Higher-grade astrocytomas are diagnosed using MRI. 18F-fluorodeoxyglucose positron emission tomography is currently the most common imaging diagnostic tracer for glioblastoma diagnosis and assessment of early therapeutic responses.

These tumors are treated surgically and with radiotherapy and chemotherapy (temozolomide). Recurrence is common, and survival time is less than 5 years for grade III tumors and less than 2 years for grade IV tumors. Bevacizumab is a vascular endothelial growth factor monoclonal antibody that suppresses angiogenesis and blocks the blood supply to the tumor. It has been approved for the treatment of recurrent glioblastoma in the United States and Canada but should not be used prior to entry into a clinical trial because most clinical trials exclude its use.[152] Specificity of treatment is advancing with the development of vaccines, cell therapy (T cells and antibodies), reshaping of the tumor microenvironment (e.g., transforming growth factor [TGF]-β inhibition), RNA-based therapies, immune checkpoint inhibitors, and modified polio virus. (Cancer treatment is discussed in Chapter 12.)

Oligodendroglioma. Oligodendrogliomas constitute approximately 2% of all primary brain tumors and approximately 10% of all gliomas. They are typically slow-growing, low-grade tumors (grade II). Most oligodendrogliomas are macroscopically indistinguishable from other gliomas, but they often contain mineral deposits, have cysts and areas of bleeding, and carry genetic signatures (*IDH1* or *IDH2* and codeletion of 1p/19q) (see Table 18.16). Histologically they are described as having "fried egg" cells and "chicken-wire" vasculature.[153] Most are found in the frontal and temporal lobes, often in the deep white matter, but they can be found in other parts of the brain and spinal cord. They are slow growing, and malignant degeneration occurs in approximately one-third of affected persons. These tumors are then known as *anaplastic oligodendrogliomas* (grade III).

More than 50% of individuals experience a focal or generalized seizure as the first clinical manifestation. Only half of those with an oligodendroglioma have IICP at the time of diagnosis and surgery, and only one-third develop focal manifestations. Treatment includes surgery, radiotherapy, and chemotherapy or combination therapy, with approximately 74% survival at 5 years.[154,155]

Ependymoma. Ependymomas are nonencapsulated gliomas that arise from ependymal cells (Fig. 18.31). They are rare in adults, usually occurring in the spinal cord. However, in children, ependymomas are typically located in the supratentorial brain or posterior fossa. They constitute approximately 1.6% of all primary brain tumors in adults and approximately 9% of childhood brain and spinal cord tumors.[156] Several molecular subgroups have been identified, and they are guiding the understanding of tumor biology and targeted therapies.[157] Approximately 70% of these tumors occur in the fourth ventricle, with others found in the third and lateral ventricles and posterior portion of the spinal cord. Approximately 40% of infratentorial (cerebellum) ependymomas occur in children younger than 10 years. Cerebral (supratentorial) ependymomas occur at all ages but are more common in children and are WHO grade II or grade III (anaplastic ependymoma). DNA methylation and gene expression profiling has become available to classify these tumors and is used to guide treatment.[158] Fourth ventricle or posterior fossa ependymomas present with difficulty in balance, unsteady gait, uncoordinated muscle movement, and difficulty with fine motor movement. CT scan and MRI imaging are completed for diagnosis. The clinical manifestations of a lateral and third ventricle ependymoma that involves the cerebral hemispheres are seizures, visual changes, and hemiparesis. Blockage of the CSF pathway produces hydrocephalus and presents with headache, nausea, and vomiting. Spinal cord ependymomas cause back pain, lower extremity weakness, and/or bowel and bladder dysfunction. The interval between first manifestations and surgery may be as short as 4 weeks or as long as 7 or 8 years. Ependymomas are treated with surgery, radiotherapy, and chemotherapy. Overall, approximately 80% to 90% of persons survive 5 years, and survival is related to tumor recurrence presence of anaplastic histology and gene profile.[159]

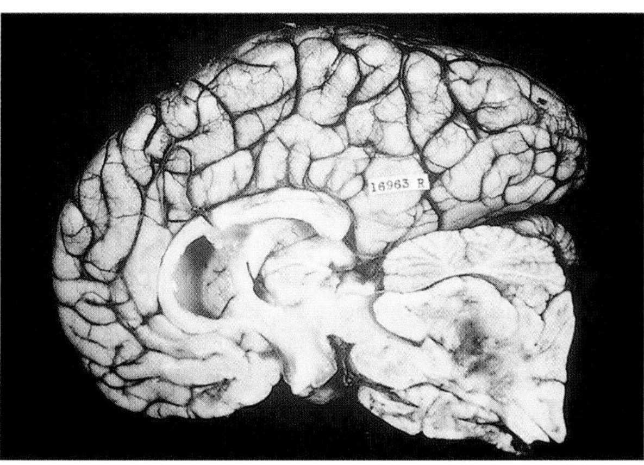

Fig. 18.31 Ependymoma.

Primary Extracerebral Tumors

Meningioma. Meningiomas are the most common intracranial tumor and constitute approximately a third of all intracranial tumors and are usually benign and slow growing. Most occur in adults aged 65 years or older.[154] Predisposing factors include neurofibromatosis (NF) type 2 (NF2; see Nerve Sheath Tumors), ionizing radiation exposure after a several-decade latency period, and obesity.[160] Formation of benign meningiomas has been linked to *NF2* gene mutation, chromosome 22q12–2 loss, and *DAL-1* loss on chromosome 18. Atypical and anaplastic meningiomas have been linked to additional gene alterations involving other multiple chromosomes. They are resistant to treatment.[161] These tumors usually originate from the arachnoidal (meningeal) cells in the pia mater and the trabeculae and septae of the subarachnoid space. There are three grades of tumor: grade I benign meningioma (>80%), grade II atypical meningioma (15% to 20%), and grade III anaplastic meningioma (1.0% to 3.0%)

Meningiomas are commonly located within in the olfactory grooves, on the wings of the sphenoid bone (at the base of the skull), in the tuberculum sellae (next to the sella turcica), on the superior surface of the cerebellum, and in the cerebellopontine angle and spinal cord (Fig. 18.32). Rarely, they can involve the optic nerve sheath, with loss of visual acuity. The cause of meningiomas is unknown.

A meningioma is sharply circumscribed and adapts to the shape it occupies. It may extend to the dural surface and

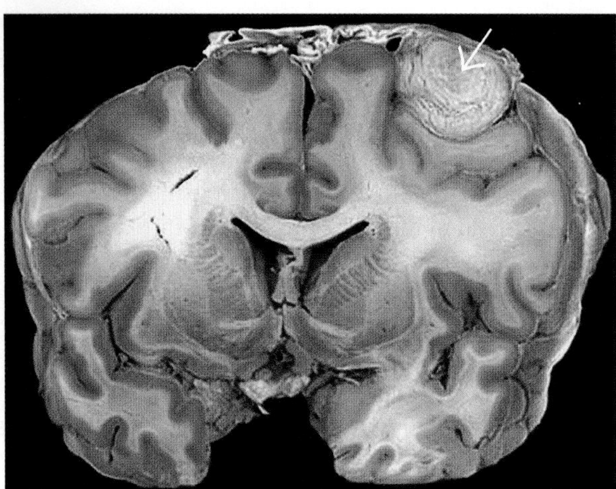

Fig. 18.32 Meningioma.

erode the cranial bones or produce an osteoblastic reaction. Meningiomas are slow growing, and clinical manifestations occur when they reach a certain size and begin to press on the brain tissue. Focal seizures are often the first manifestation, and IICP is less common than with gliomas because they are slow growing. Other symptoms are related to the site of tumor location. Diagnosis is made using MRI, contrast-enhanced CT, or both. The primary treatment is surgical resection, radiotherapy, and rarely chemotherapy.[162] The recurrence rate is higher with higher-grade tumors.[163]

Nerve sheath tumors. Neurofibromas (benign nerve sheath tumors) are a group of autosomal dominant disorders of the nervous system. They may be inherited or develop sporadically as a spontaneous mutation. They include neurofibromatosis type 1 (NF1), previously known as von Recklinghausen disease, and NF2. The two types are also known as *peripheral* and *central NF*, respectively. Schwannomatosis, also known as NF3, is very rare. It is characterized by multiple schwannomas in the absence of bilateral vestibular schwannomas, and approximately 15% are inherited with mutation in the *MARCB1 or LZTR1* genes (tumor suppressor genes). The primary symptom is chronic pain. Diagnostic criteria are available for all three types of neurofibromas.[164]

Neurofibromatosis type 1 (NF1) is the most prevalent, with an incidence of approximately 1 in 3500 people. *Neurofibromin 1* is a gene that encodes the protein neurofibromin, a tumor suppressor (prevents cells from growing and dividing too rapidly), primarily in adult neurons. Mutations of *neurofibromin 1* cause multiple cutaneous neurofibromas, cutaneous light brown macular lesions (café au lait spots and freckles). Less commonly, there are bone and soft tissue tumors. Gliomas may develop in some cases.[165] Inactivation of the *neurofibromin 1* gene results in loss of function of neurofibromin in Schwann cells (produce the myelin sheath around axons) and promotes tumorigenesis (neurofibromas). Cognitive and learning disabilities are present in approximately 50% of affected individuals.[166]

Neurofibromatosis type 2 (NF2) is rare and occurs in approximately 1 in 40,000 to 60,000 people. The *neurofibromin 2 (NF2)* gene product is neurofibromin 2 or merlin, a tumor-suppressor protein that inhibits cell growth. Mutations promote development of CNS tumors, particularly schwannomas, although other tumor types can occur (meningiomas, ependymomas, astrocytomas, and neurofibromas). Schwannomas of the vestibular nerves present with hearing loss and deafness, loss of balance, and dizziness. Schwannomas also may develop in other cranial, spinal, and peripheral nerves. In these cases, cutaneous signs of flesh colored skin flaps and muscle wasting occur.

Genetic testing is available for the management of families susceptible to neurofibromas, and prenatal diagnosis is possible. Diagnosis is based on clinical manifestations and neuroimaging studies. Surgery is the major treatment, and tumors may regrow. Targeted therapy has been used with some success, and several agents are in clinical trials.[164] Individuals with NF2 have extensive morbidity and reduced life expectancy, particularly with early age of onset. Genetically tailored drugs are likely to provide personalized therapy for both devastating conditions.

Metastatic brain tumors. Metastatic brain tumors from systemic cancers are 10 times more common than primary brain tumors, and approximately 20% to 40% of persons with cancer have metastasis to the brain.[167] Mechanisms of metastasis are presented in Chapter 12. Common primary sites include the lung, breast, and skin (e.g., melanomas). Metastasis to the brain is thought to be through vascular channels, although some cancer cells may travel along nerves or through the lymphatics.[168] The cancer cells tend to localize to the cerebral hemispheres, where there is the greatest blood flow.[169]

Metastatic brain tumors produce signs resembling those of glioblastomas, although several unusual syndromes do exist. Carcinomatous (metastatic cancer) encephalopathy causes headache, nervousness, depression, trembling, confusion, forgetfulness, and gait disorder. In carcinomatosis of the cerebellum, headache, dizziness, and ataxia are found. Carcinomatosis of the craniospinal meninges (also called *carcinomatous meningitis*) manifests with headache, confusion, and symptoms of cranial or spinal nerve root dysfunction. Diagnosis is made from clinical signs and imaging. Metastatic brain tumors carry a poor prognosis. Treatment is guided by the pathology of the original tumor; the number, size, and location of the brain metastasis; and prior cancer treatments. Treatment options include various combinations of surgery, radiotherapy, targeted agents, and immunotherapy.[170,171] Survival time is approximately 1 year.

Spinal Cord Tumors

Primary spinal cord tumors are rare and represent approximately 2% of CNS tumors. They may be extramedullary extradural, intradural extramedullary, or intradural intramedullary. Intramedullary tumors are least common and originate within the neural tissues of the spinal cord. They are primarily gliomas (astrocytomas, ependymomas, hemangioblastomas). Gliomas are difficult to resect completely, and radiotherapy is required. Spinal ependymomas may be completely resected and are more common in adults. Extramedullary tumors originate from tissues outside the spinal cord. Extramedullary tumors are either peripheral nerve sheath tumors (neurofibromas or schwannomas) or meningiomas. Neurofibromas are generally found in the thoracic and lumbar region, whereas meningiomas are more evenly distributed through the spine. Complete resection of these tumors can be curative.

Metastatic spinal cord tumors are usually carcinomas (i.e., from breast, lung, or prostate cancer), lymphomas, or myelomas. Their location is often extradural, the cancer having proliferated to the spine through direct extension from tumors of the vertebral structures or from extraspinal sources extending through the interventricular foramen or bloodstream.

Pathophysiology. Intramedullary spinal cord tumors produce dysfunction by both invasion and compression. Extramedullary spinal cord tumors produce dysfunction by compressing adjacent tissue, not by direct invasion. Metastases from spinal cord tumors occur from direct extension or seeding through the CSF or bloodstream.

Clinical Manifestations. An acute onset of clinical manifestations suggests a vascular occlusion of vessels supplying the spinal cord, whereas gradual and progressive symptoms suggest compression. The compressive syndrome (sensorimotor syndrome) involves both the anterior and the posterior spinal tracts, and motor function and sensory function are affected as the tumor grows. Pain is usually a presenting symptom.

The irritative syndrome (radicular syndrome) combines the clinical manifestations of a cord compression with radicular pain that occurs in the sensory root distribution and indicates root irritation. The segmental manifestations include segmental sensory changes, such as paresthesia and impaired pain and touch perception; motor disturbances, including cramps, atrophy, fasciculations, and decreased or absent deep tendon reflexes; and continuous spinal pain.

Evaluation and Treatment. The diagnosis of a spinal cord tumor is made through imaging techniques, CT-guided needle biopsy, or open biopsy. Involvement of specific cord segments is established. Any metastases also are identified. Treatment varies, depending on the nature of the tumor and the person's clinical status, but surgery is essential for all spinal cord tumors. Targeted immunotherapies and image-guided RT are improving survival.[172]

SUMMARY REVIEW

Central Nervous System Disorders

Traumatic Brain Injury

1. TBI is an alteration in brain function caused by an external force. The most common causes of TBI are falls, unintentional blunt trauma, and motor vehicle accidents. TBI is classified as primary or secondary.
2. Primary brain injury is caused by direct impact and involves neural injury, primary glial injury, and vascular responses. Primary brain injuries can be focal (involving only one area of the brain) or diffuse (involving more than one area of the brain).
3. Secondary injury is an indirect consequence of the primary injury.
4. Severity of TBI is graded using the GCS.
5. Causes of focal brain injury include closed (blunt) trauma or open (penetrating) trauma.
6. Closed trauma is more common and involves the head striking a surface or an object striking the head. These injuries include contusion, EDH, SDH, and ICH. Injury may be caused by coup or contrecoup injury or both.
7. A contusion (bruising of the brain) is caused from blood leaking from an injured vessel.
8. Head trauma can result in a hematoma. Hematomas can be classified as an EDH (accumulation of blood above the dura mater), SDH (blood between the dura mater and arachnoid membrane), or ICH (bleeding into the brain).
9. Open brain injury involves a skull fracture with exposure of the cranial vault to the environment and may result from compound skull fractures and missile injuries. Open brain injury can produce both focal and diffuse injuries.
10. DAI results from mechanical forces of acceleration, deceleration, and rotation that cause stretching and shearing of axons and can only be seen microscopically. The injury can be mild, moderate, or severe.
11. Secondary brain injury develops from systemic and intracranial responses to primary brain trauma that result in further brain injury and neuronal death (i.e., trauma or stroke).
12. Categories of TBI are mild, moderate, and severe and are based on the GCS, duration of loss of consciousness, posttraumatic amnesia, and brain imaging results.
13. Complications of TBI include postconcussion syndrome, posttraumatic seizures, and CTE.

Spinal Cord and Vertebral Injury

1. Spinal cord and vertebral injury involve damage to neural tissues by compressing tissue, pulling, or exerting tension on tissue, or shearing tissues so that they slide into one another. Vertebral fracture occurs with direct or indirect trauma.
2. SCI involves primary and secondary injury similar to the processes of TBI. Primary SCI involves damage to vertebral or neural tissues from shearing, compression, or traction forces. Secondary SCI is related to edema, ischemia, excitotoxicity, inflammation, oxidative damage, and activation of necrotic and apoptotic cell death and begins within minutes after injury and continues for weeks.
3. SCI may cause spinal shock with temporary cessation of all motor, sensory, reflex, and autonomic functions below the lesion. Spinal shock generally lasts 2 to 3 days.
4. Neurogenic shock (vasogenic shock) is caused by loss of sympathetic nerve activity and occurs with cervical or upper thoracic cord injury (above T6) and can occur concurrently with spinal shock. Symptoms include vasodilation, hypotension, bradycardia, and loss of temperature control.
5. Loss of motor and sensory function depends on the extent and level of injury. Paralysis of the lower half of the body with both legs involved is called paraplegia. Paralysis involving all four extremities is called quadriplegia.

6. Return of spinal neuron excitability occurs slowly. Spasticity and hyperreflexia are common. Reflex activity can return in 1 to 2 weeks in most people with acute SCI.
7. Autonomic hyperreflexia (dysreflexia) is a severe, life-threatening complication associated with a SCI at level T6 or above where descending inhibition is blocked resulting in autonomic nervous system dysregulation. Autonomic hyperreflexia requires emergency medical management.

Degenerative Disorders of the Spine

1. Degenerative disorders of the spine include LBP, degenerative joint disease, and herniated intervertebral disk.
2. LBP is pain between the lower rib cage and gluteal muscles and often radiates into the thigh. Common causes of chronic LBP include DDD, disk prolapse, tumor, bursitis, synovitis, osteoporosis, hyperparathyroidism, fracture, inflammation, and sprain. Other causes are tension, inflammation, referred pain, and bone diseases.
3. Degenerative joint disease includes DDD, spondylolysis, spondylolisthesis, spinal stenosis, spinal osteochondrosis, and lumbar disk herniation.
4. Spondylolysis is a structural defect of the spine with displacement of the vertebra.
5. Spondylolisthesis involves forward slippage of the vertebra and can include a crack or fracture of the pars interarticularis, usually at the L5 to S1 vertebrae.
6. Spinal stenosis is a narrowing of the spinal canal that causes pressure on the spinal nerves or cord.
7. DDD is an alteration in intervertebral disk tissue and can be related to normal aging, inflammation, and compression.
8. Herniation of an intervertebral disk is a protrusion of part of the nucleus pulposus. Herniation most commonly affects the lumbosacral disks (L5 to S1 and L4 to L5). The extruded pulposus compresses the nerve root, causing pain that radiates along the sciatic nerve course.

Seizure and Epilepsy

1. Seizures represent abnormal, excessive hypersynchronous discharges of cortical neurons with transient alterations in brain function.
2. Epilepsy is a cause of seizures and a disease of the brain. The criterion for epilepsy includes at least two unprovoked seizures occurring more than 24 hours apart and one unprovoked seizure after two unprovoked seizures, occurring over the next 10 years and a diagnosis of an epilepsy syndrome.
3. Seizures may be focal or generalized. The categories of seizures include genetic, structural, metabolic, immune, infectious, and unknown.

Cerebrovascular Disease

1. CVD is the most frequently occurring neurologic disorder and is any abnormality of the brain caused by a pathologic process in the blood vessels The brain abnormalities seen with CVD are either ischemia (with or without infarction) or hemorrhage.
2. CVAs (stroke syndromes) are a common clinical manifestation of CVD. Strokes are classified pathophysiologically as ischemic or hemorrhagic (intracranial hemorrhage).
3. TIAs are temporary decreases in brain blood flow with an increased risk of stroke.
4. Ischemic stroke occurs when there is obstruction to arterial blood flow to the brain from thrombus formation (thrombotic stroke), an embolus (embolic stroke), or hypoperfusion related to decreased blood volume or heart failure (hemodynamic stroke). The inadequate blood supply results in ischemia and can progress to infarction.
5. Lacunar strokes are caused by ischemia from occlusion of a small vessel deep in the brain.
6. Hemorrhagic strokes occur within brain tissue (intracerebral) or in the subarachnoid or subdural space. The primary cause of intracerebral hemorrhagic stroke is chronic hypertension.
7. Intracranial aneurysms result from defects in the vascular wall and are classified based on form and shape. They are often asymptomatic, but the signs vary depending on the location and size of the aneurysm. They are a cause of SAH.
8. An SAH occurs when blood escapes from defective or injured vasculature into the subarachnoid space. When a vessel tears, blood under pressure is pumped into the subarachnoid space. The blood produces an inflammatory reaction in these tissues and IICP.
9. An AVM is a mass of dilated blood vessels. Although sometimes present at birth, AVM exhibits a delayed age of onset with symptoms ranging from headache and dementia to seizures and ICH or SAH. Vasospasm and delayed cerebral ischemia are serious complications.

Primary Headache Syndromes

1. Headache is a common neurologic disorder and is usually a benign symptom. Chronic recurring headaches include migraine, cluster, and tension headaches.
2. Migraine headache is an episodic headache lasting 4 to 72 hours that can be associated with triggers and may have an aura associated with a CSD that alters cortical blood flow. Pain is related to overactivity in the trigeminal vascular system.
3. Cluster headaches are a group of disorders known as trigeminal autonomic cephalalgias and occur primarily in men. They occur in clusters over a period of days, with extreme pain intensity and short duration, and are associated with trigeminal nerve activation.
4. TTH is the most common recurrent headache. Episodic-type headaches involve a peripheral pain mechanism, and the chronic type involves a central pain mechanism and may be related to hypersensitivity of pain fibers from the trigeminal nerve.

Infection and Inflammation of the Central Nervous System

1. Infection and inflammation of the CNS can be caused by bacteria, viruses, fungi, parasites, and mycobacteria.
2. Meningitis is inflammation of the brain or spinal cord and is classified as bacterial (i.e., meningococci), aseptic (viral or nonpurulent), or fungal. Bacterial meningitis primarily is an infection of the pia mater, the arachnoid, and the fluid of the

subarachnoid space. Viral (aseptic) meningitis is thought to be limited to the meninges. Fungal meningitis is a chronic, less common type of meningitis.
3. Encephalitis is an acute inflammation of the brain, usually of viral origin. The most common forms are caused by bites of mosquitos, ticks, or flies and by and herpes simplex type 1. Meningeal involvement appears in all encephalitides. Herpes encephalitis is treated with antiviral agents.
4. WNV is the most common cause of epidemic meningoencephalitis in North America and the leading cause of arboviral encephalitis in the United States.
5. Brain or spinal cord abscesses often originate from infections outside the CNS. Microorganisms gain access to the CNS from adjacent sites or spread along the wall of a vein. Brain abscesses progress from localized inflammation to a necrotic core with the formation of a connective tissue capsule, usually within 14 days or longer.
6. The common neurologic complication of AIDS is HAND, a range of disorders that includes mild neurocognitive disorder and HIV-associated dementia. The onset of clinical manifestations includes neurocognitive impairment, behavioral disturbance, and motor abnormalities.

Peripheral Nervous System and Neuromuscular Junction Disorders

1. Acute or chronic disease processes, inflammation, or trauma may injure these peripheral nerves and cause neuropathy.
2. Injury to peripheral nerves by disease processes, inflammation, or trauma can cause a neuropathy. Neuropathies can be mononeuropathies (affecting a single nerve), multiple mononeuropathies (involving two or more individual nerves), polyneuropathy (generalized involvement of peripheral nerves), or autonomic neuropathies (involving the nervous system).
3. Radiculopathies are disorders of spinal nerve roots as they enter (sensory) or exit (motor) the spine

Tumors of the Central Nervous System

1. Tumors within the cranium can be primary intracerebral, primary extracerebral, or metastatic (secondary).
2. Primary intracerebral tumors originate from brain substance and include astrocytomas, oligodendrogliomas, glioblastoma multiforme, and ependymomas.
3. Extracerebral tumors originate outside of the substances of the brain and include meningiomas and nerve sheath tumors.
4. Metastatic tumors arise in organ systems outside the brain and spread to the brain. Common primary sites include lung, breast, skin, kidney, and colorectal areas.
5. Brain tumors cause local and generalized manifestations. Manifestations include headache, seizures, visual disturbances, unstable gain, and cranial nerve dysfunction.
6. Spinal cord tumors are classified as intramedullary tumors (within the neural tissues) or extramedullary tumors (outside the spinal cord). Metastatic spinal cord tumors are usually carcinomas, lymphomas, or myelomas.
7. Intramedullary spinal cord tumors produce dysfunction by both invasion and compression. Extramedullary spinal cord tumors produce dysfunction by compression of adjacent tissue, not by direct invasion.

REFERENCES

1. Centers for Disease Control and Prevention (CDC). *National Center for Health Statistics: mortality data on CDC WONDER*. Atlanta, GA: CDC; 2020. Page last reviewed December 22, 2020. Available at https://wonder.cdc.gov/mcd.html. (Accessed October 17, 2021).
2. Centers for Disease Control and Prevention (CDC). *Traumatic Brain Injury & Concussion: TBI Data*. Atlanta, GA: CDC; 2020. Page last reviewed May 11, 2021. Available at https://www.cdc.gov/traumaticbraininjury/data/index.html. (Accessed October 17, 2021).
3. Zakaria Z, et al. Extradural haematoma—to evacuate or not? Revisiting treatment guidelines. *Clin Neurol Neurosurg*. 2013;115(8):1201–1205.
4. Shin DS, Hwang SC. Neurocritical management of traumatic acute subdural hematomas. *Korean J Neurotrauma*. 2020;16(2):113–125.
5. Adams H, Kolias AG, Hutchinson PJ. The role of surgical intervention in traumatic brain injury. *Neurosurg Clin N Am*. 2016;27(4):519–528.
6. Feghali J, Yang W, Huang J. Updates in chronic subdural hematoma: epidemiology, etiology, pathogenesis, treatment, and outcome. *World Neurosurg*. 2020;141:339–345.
7. Kobata H. Diagnosis and treatment of traumatic cerebrovascular injury: pitfalls in the management of neurotrauma. *Neurol Med Chir (Tokyo)*. 2017;57(8):410–417.
8. Quiñones-Ossa GA, et al. The puzzle of spontaneous versus traumatic intracranial hemorrhages. *Egypt J Neurosurg*. 2020;35:13.
9. Stein SC. The evolution of modern treatment for depressed skull fractures. *World Neurosurg*. 2019;121:186–192.
10. American Association of Neurological Surgeons (AANS). *Traumatic Brain Injury*. Rolling Meadows, IL: AANS; 2020. Last edited February 3, 2020. Available at https://www.aans.org/en/Patients/Neurosurgical-Conditions-and-Treatments/Traumatic-Brain-Injury. (Accessed October 17, 2021).
11. Chen S, et al. Hydrocephalus after subarachnoid hemorrhage: pathophysiology, diagnosis, and treatment. *Biomed Res Int*. 2017;2017:8584753.
12. Bruggeman GF, et al. Traumatic axonal injury (TAI): definitions, pathophysiology, and imaging-a narrative review. *Acta Neurochir (Wien)*. 2021;163(1):31–44.
13. Graham NSN, et al. Diffuse axonal injury predicts neurodegeneration after moderate-severe traumatic brain injury. *Brain*. 2020;143(12):3685–3698.
14. Capizzi A, Woo J, Verduzco-Gutierrez M. Traumatic brain injury: an overview of epidemiology, pathophysiology, and medical management. *Med Clin North Am*. 2020;104(2):213–238.
15. Soldozy S, et al. Cortical spreading depression in the setting of traumatic brain injury. *World Neurosurg*. 2020;134:50–57.
16. Crupi R, et al. Management of traumatic brain injury: from present to future. *Antioxidants (Basel)*. 2020;9(4):297.
17. Kurtz P, Rocha EEM. Nutrition therapy, glucose control, and brain metabolism in traumatic brain injury: a multimodal monitoring approach. *Front Neurosci*. 2020;14:190.
18. Mullally WJ. Concussion. *Am J Med*. 2017;130(8):885–892.

19. Edwards P, et al. Final results of MRC CRASH, a randomised placebo-controlled trial of intravenous corticosteroid in adults with head injury-outcomes at 6 months. *Lancet.* 2005;365(9475):1957–1959.
20. Lumba-Brown A, et al. Centers for Disease Control and Prevention guideline on the diagnosis and management of mild traumatic brain injury among children. *JAMA Pediatr.* 2018;172(11):e182853 Published correction appears in *JAMA Pediatr* 172(11):1104, 2018].
21. Centers for Disease Control and Prevention (CDC). *Traumatic brain injury and concussion: updated mild traumatic brain injury guideline for adults.* Atlanta, GA: CDC; 2021. Page last reviewed May 11, 2021. Available at https://www.cdc.gov/traumaticbraininjury/mtbi_guideline.html. (Accessed October 17, 2021).
22. Ontario Neurotrauma Foundation (ONF). *Guideline for Concussion/Mild Traumatic Brain Injury & Prolonged Symptoms, third edition, Adults (18+years of age), May 2018.* Toronto, ON, Canada: ONF; 2018. Available at https://braininjuryguidelines.org/concussion/fileadmin/pdf/Concussion_guideline_3rd_edition_final.pdf. (Accessed October 18, 2021).
23. Kim K, Priefer R. Evaluation of current post-concussion protocols. *Biomed Pharmacother.* 2020;129:110406.
24. McCrory P, et al. Consensus statement on concussion in sport—the 5(th) International Conference on Concussion in Sport held in Berlin, October 2016. *Br J Sports Med.* 2017;51(11):838–847. Available at https://doi.org/10.1136/bjsports-2017-097699. (Accessed October 18, 2021).
25. Sharma S, et al. Neuropathophysiological mechanisms and treatment strategies for post-traumatic epilepsy. *Front Mol Neurosci.* 2021;14:612073.
26. Pierre K, et al. Chronic traumatic encephalopathy: update on current clinical diagnosis and management. *Biomedicines.* 2021;9(4):415.
27. National Spinal Cord Injury Statistical Center. *Spinal cord Injury Facts and Figures at a Glance.* Birmingham, AL: University of Alabama at Birmingham; 2021. Available at https://www.nscisc.uab.edu/Public/Facts%20and%20Figures%20-%202021.pdf. (Accessed October 18, 2021).
28. Eli I, Lerner DP, Ghogawala Z. Acute traumatic spinal cord injury. *Neurol Clin.* 2021;39(2):471–488.
29. Previnaire JG. The importance of the bulbocavernosus reflex. *Spinal Cord Ser Cases.* 2018;4:2.
30. Krassioukov A, Stillman M, Beck LA. A primary care provider's guide to autonomic dysfunction following spinal cord injury. *Top Spinal Cord Inj Rehabil.* 2020;26(2):123–127.
31. Chay W, Kirshblum S. Predicting outcomes after spinal cord injury. *Phys Med Rehabil Clin N Am.* 2020;31(3):331–343.
32. American Spinal Injury Association (ASIA) *International Standards for Neurological Classification of spinal Cord Injury (ISNCSCI).* Richmond, VA: ASIA; 2019.
33. Vedantam A, Levi AD. Hypothermia for acute spinal cord injury. *Neurosurg Clin N Am.* 2021;32(3):377–387.
34. Torregrossa F, Sallì M, Grasso G. Emerging therapeutic strategies for traumatic spinal cord injury. *World Neurosurg.* 2020;140:591–601.
35. Mneimneh AT, Mehanna MM. Collagen-based scaffolds: an auspicious tool to support repair, recovery, and regeneration post spinal cord injury. *Int J Pharm.* 2021;601:120559.
36. Srivastava E, Singh A, Kumar A. Spinal cord regeneration: a brief overview of the present scenario and a sneak peek into the future. *Biotechnol J.* 2021;16:e2100167.
37. Pizzolato C, et al. Non-invasive approaches to functional recovery after spinal cord injury: therapeutic targets and multimodal device interventions. *Exp Neurol.* 2021;339:113612.
38. Deyo RA, Mirza SK, Martin BI. Back pain prevalence and visit rates: estimates from U.S. national surveys, 2002. *Spine (Phila Pa 1976).* 2006;31(23):2724–2727.
39. Wu A, et al. Global low back pain prevalence and years lived with disability from 1990 to 2017: estimates from the Global Burden of Disease Study 2017. *Ann Transl Med.* 2020;8(6):299.
40. Li W, et al. Peripheral and central pathological mechanisms of chronic low back pain: a narrative review. *J Pain Res.* 2021;14:1483–1494.
41. Johnson SM, Shah LM. Imaging of acute low back pain. *Radiol Clin North Am.* 2019;57(2):397–413.
42. Kreiner DS, et al. Guideline summary review: an evidence-based clinical guideline for the diagnosis and treatment of low back pain. *Spine J.* 2020;20(7):998–1024.
43. Gianola S, et al: Effectiveness of treatments for acute and subacute mechanical non-specific low back pain: a systematic review with network meta-analysis, *Br J Sports Med* Online ahead of print April 13, 2021. Available at https://doi.org/10.1136/bjsports-2020-103596. (Accessed October 18, 2021).
44. Koumtouzoua S, Higgins S. Evaluating and managing the patient with back pain. *Med Clin North Am.* 2021;105(1):1–17.
45. Will JS, Bury DC, Miller JA. Mechanical low back pain. *Am Fam Physician.* 2018;98(7):421–428.
46. García-Ramos CL, et al. Degenerative spondylolisthesis I: general principles. *Acta Ortop Mex.* 2020;34(5):324–328.
47. Jiang SD, Jiang LS, Dai LY. Degenerative cervical spondylolisthesis: a systematic review. *Int Orthop.* 2011;35(6):869–875.
48. Chung CC, Shimer AL. Lumbosacral spondylolysis and spondylolisthesis. *Clin Sports Med.* 2021;40(3):471–490.
49. Chan AK, et al. Summary of guidelines for the treatment of lumbar spondylolisthesis. *Neurosurg Clin N Am.* 2019;30(3):353–364.
50. Aljuboori Z, Boakye M. The natural history of cervical spondylotic myelopathy and ossification of the posterior longitudinal ligament: a review article. *Cureus.* 2019;11(7):e5074.
51. Kos N, Gradisnik L, Velnar T. A brief review of the degenerative intervertebral disc disease. *Med Arch.* 2019;73(6):421–424. Available at https://doi.org/10.5455/medarh.2019.73.421-424. (Accessed October 18, 2021).
52. North American Spine Society (NASS). *Evidence-Based Clinical Guidelines for Diagnosis and Treatment of Lumbar Disc Herniation with Radiculopathy.* Burr Ridge, IL: NASS; 2012. Available at http://content.guidelinecentral.com/guideline/get/pdf/3473. (Accessed October 18, 2021).
53. Deyo RA, Mirza SK. Clinical practice. Herniated lumbar intervertebral disk. *N Engl J Med.* 2016;374(18):1763–1772.
54. Todd NV, Dickson RA. Standards of care in cauda equina syndrome. *Br J Neurosurg.* 2016;30(5):518–522.
55. Fisher RS, et al. A practical clinical definition of epilepsy. *Epilepsia.* 2014;55:475–482.
56. Sarmast ST, Abdullahi AM, Jahan N. Current classification of seizures and epilepsies: scope, limitations and recommendations for future action. *Cureus.* 2020;12(9):e10549.
57. Centers for Disease Control and Prevention (CDC). *Epilepsy data and statistics.* Atlanta, GA: CDC; 2020. Page last reviewed September 30, 2020. Available at https://www.cdc.gov/epilepsy/data/index.html. (Accessed October 18, 2021).

58. Phillips HN, Tormoehlen L. Toxin-induced seizures. *Neurol Clin.* 2020;38(4):867–879.
59. Maguire MJ, Nevitt SJ. Treatments for seizures in catamenial (menstrual-related) epilepsy. *Cochrane Database Syst Rev.* 2019;10(10):CD013225.
60. Akyuz E, et al. Revisiting the role of neurotransmitters in epilepsy: an updated review. *Life Sci.* 2021;265:118826.
61. Maguire MJ, et al. Treatments for the prevention of sudden unexpected death in epilepsy (SUDEP). *Cochrane Database Syst Rev.* 2020;4(4):CD011792.
62. Ryvlin P, Rheims S, Lhatoo SD. Risks and predictive biomarkers of sudden unexpected death in epilepsy patient. *Curr Opin Neurol.* 2019;32(2):205–212.
63. McGonigal A. Semiology and epileptic networks. *Neurosurg Clin N Am.* 2020;31(3):373–385.
64. International League Against Epilepsy (ILAE). *EpilepsyDiagnosis.org.* Flower Mound, TX: ILAE; 2020. Last updated March 30, 2020. Available at https://www.epilepsydiagnosis.org. (Accessed October 18, 2021).
65. Milligan TA. Epilepsy: a clinical overview. *Am J Med.* 2021;134(7):840–847. Available at https://doi.org/10.1016/j.amjmed.2021.01.038. (Accessed October 18, 2021).
66. Rudy L, et al. Anticonvulsant mechanisms of the ketogenic diet and caloric restriction. *Epilepsy Res.* 2020;168:106499.
67. Ayoubian L, Tadel F, David O. Epileptogenicity mapping: a quantitative approach to identify the seizure onset. *Neurosurg Clin N Am.* 2020;31(3):449–457.
68. Sisterson ND, Kokkinos V. Neuromodulation of epilepsy networks. *Neurosurg Clin N Am.* 2020;31(3):459–470.
69. Kolmos M, Christoffersen L, Kruuse C. Recurrent ischemic stroke—a systematic review and meta-analysis. *J Stroke Cerebrovasc Dis.* 2021;30(8):105935.
70. Easton JD, et al. Definition and evaluation of transient ischemic attack: a scientific statement for healthcare professionals from the American Heart Association/American Stroke Association Stroke Council; Council on Cardiovascular Surgery and Anesthesia; Council on Cardiovascular Radiology and Intervention; Council on Cardiovascular Nursing; and the Interdisciplinary Council on Peripheral Vascular Disease: the American Academy of Neurology affirms the value of this statement as an educational tool for neurologists. *Stroke.* 2009;40(6):2276–2293.
71. Gupta HV, et al. Transient ischemic attacks: predictability of future ischemic stroke or transient ischemic attack events. *Ther Clin Risk Manag.* 2014;10:27–35.
72. Regenhardt RW, et al. Advances in understanding the pathophysiology of lacunar stroke: a review. *JAMA Neurol.* 2018;75(10):1273–1281.
73. Zubair AS, Sheth KN. Emergency care of patients with acute ischemic stroke. *Neurol Clin.* 2021;39(2):391–404.
74. Powers WJ, et al. Guidelines for the early management of patients with acute ischemic stroke: a guideline for healthcare professionals from the American Heart Association/American Stroke Association. *Stroke.* 2018;49(3):e46–e110.
75. Bushnell C, et al. Guidelines for the prevention of stroke in women: a statement for healthcare professionals from the American Heart Association/American Stroke Association. *Stroke.* 2014;45(5):1545–1588. Available at https://doi.org/10.1161/01.str.0000442009.06663.48. (Accessed October 18, 2021). [Erratum in *Stroke* 45(5):e95, 2014. Erratum in *Stroke* 45(10);e214, 2014.].
76. Matei N, Camara J, Zhang JH. The next step in the treatment of stroke. *Front Neurol.* 2021;11:582605.
77. Correa-Paz C, et al. New approaches in nanomedicine for ischemic stroke. *Pharmaceutics.* 2021;13(5):757.
78. Gauberti M, Martinez de Lizarrondo S, Vivien D. Thrombolytic strategies for ischemic stroke in the thrombectomy era. *J Thromb Haemost.* 2021;19(7):1618–1628.
79. Singh M, et al. Application of stem cells in stroke: a multifactorial approach. *Front Neurosci.* 2020;14:473.
80. Kuo LT, Huang AP. The Pathogenesis of hydrocephalus following aneurysmal subarachnoid hemorrhage. *Int J Mol Sci.* 2021;22(9):5050.
81. O'Carroll CB, Brown BL, Freeman WD. Intracerebral hemorrhage: a common yet disproportionately deadly stroke subtype. *Mayo Clin Proc.* 2021;96(6):1639–1654.
82. Hannah TC, Kellner R, Kellner CP. Minimally invasive intracerebral hemorrhage evacuation techniques: a review. *Diagnostics (Basel).* 2021;11(3):576.
83. Hemphill 3rd JC, et al. Guidelines for the management of spontaneous intracerebral hemorrhage: a guideline for healthcare professionals from the American Heart Association/American Stroke Association. *Stroke.* 2015;46(7):2032–2060.
84. Zhao W, et al. Treatment of intracerebral hemorrhage: current approaches and future directions. *J Neurol Sci.* 2020;416:117020.
85. Langhorne P, Bernhardt J, Kwakkel G. Stroke rehabilitation. *Lancet.* 2011;377(9778):1693–1702.
86. Kushner DS, Strasser DC. Stroke inpatient rehabilitation team conferences: leadership and structure improve patient outcomes. *J Stroke Cerebrovasc Dis.* 2020;29(4):104622.
87. Le Danseur M. Stroke rehabilitation. *Crit Care Nurs Clin North Am.* 2020;32(1):97–108.
88. Tawk RG, et al. Diagnosis and treatment of unruptured intracranial aneurysms and aneurysmal subarachnoid hemorrhage. *Mayo Clin Proc.* 2021;96(7):1970–2000.
89. Etminan N, Dörfler A, Steinmetz H. Unruptured intracranial aneurysms—pathogenesis and individualized management. *Dtsch Arztebl Int.* 2020;117(14):235–242.
90. Etminan N, et al. Worldwide incidence of aneurysmal subarachnoid hemorrhage according to region, time period, blood pressure, and smoking prevalence in the population: a systematic review and meta-analysis. *JAMA Neurol.* 2019;76:588–597.
91. Daou BJ, et al. Clinical and experimental aspects of aneurysmal subarachnoid hemorrhage. *CNS Neurosci Ther.* 2019;25(10):1096–1112. Available at https://doi.org/10.1111/cns.13222. (Accessed October 18, 2021).
92. Chung DY, Abdalkader M, Nguyen TN. Aneurysmal subarachnoid hemorrhage. *Neurol Clin.* 2021;39(2):419–442.
93. Cavanaugh SJ, Gordon VL. Grading scales used in the management of aneurismal subarachnoid hemorrhage: a critical review. *J Neurosci Nurs.* 2002;34:288–295.
94. Ruigrok YM. Management of unruptured cerebral aneurysms and arteriovenous malformations. *Continuum (Minneap Minn).* 2020;26(2):478–498.
95. Shaligram SS, et al. Risk factors for hemorrhage of brain arteriovenous malformation. *CNS Neurosci Ther.* 2019;25(10):1085–1095.
96. Headache Classification Committee of the International Headache Society (IHS). The International Classification of Headache Disorders, 3rd edition. *Cephalalgia.* 2018; 38(1):1–211.
97. Migraine Research Foundation. Migraine fact sheet. Available at http://www.migraineresearchfoundation.org/fact-sheet.html. (Accessed October 18, 2021).

98. Reddy N, et al. The complex relationship between estrogen and migraines: a scoping review. *Syst Rev*. 2021;10(1):72.
99. Kesserwani H. Migraine triggers: an overview of the pharmacology, biochemistry, atmospherics, and their effects on neural networks. *Cureus*. 2021;13(4):e14243.
100. Khan J, et al. Genetics, pathophysiology, diagnosis, treatment, management, and prevention of migraine. *Biomed Pharmacother*. 2021;139:111557.
101. Charles A. The pathophysiology of migraine: implications for clinical management. *Lancet Neurol*. 2019;17(2):174–182.
102. Omaer A, et al: Calcitonin gene-related peptide (CGRP) antagonists: a comprehensive review of safety, efficacy and prescribing information, *J Clin Pharm Ther* Published online ahead of print July 12, 2021. Available at https://doi.org/10.1111/jcpt.13445. (Accessed October 18, 2021).
103. Marmura MJ, Silberstein SD, Schwedt TJ. The acute treatment of migraine in adults: the American Headache Society evidence assessment of migraine pharmacotherapies. *Headache*. 2015;55(1):3–20.
104. Moisset X, et al. Neuromodulation techniques for acute and preventive migraine treatment: a systematic review and meta-analysis of randomized controlled trials. *J Headache Pain*. 2020;21(1):142.
105. Ashina M, et al. Migraine: integrated approaches to clinical management and emerging treatments. *Lancet*. 2021;397(10283):1505–1518.
106. Gribbin CL, Dani KA, Tyagi A. Chronic migraine: an update on diagnosis and management. *Neurol India*. 2021;69(Supplement):S67–S75.
107. Cheema S, Matharu M. Cluster headache: what's new? *Neurol India*. 2021;69(Supplement):S124–S134.
108. Wei DY, Goadsby PJ. Cluster headache pathophysiology—insights from current and emerging treatments. *Nat Rev Neurol*. 2021;17(5):308–324.
109. Bhoi SK, Jha M, Chowdhury D. Advances in the understanding of pathophysiology of TTH and its management. *Neurol India*. 2021;69(Supplement):S116–S123.
110. Ashina S, et al. Tension-type headache. *Nat Rev Dis Primers*. 2021;7(1):24.
111. Hasbun R, Tunkel AR. Chapter 86. Approach to the patient with central nervous system infection. In: Bennett J, Dolin R, Blaser MJ, eds. *Mandell, Douglas and Bennett's Principles and Practice of Infectious Disease*. ed 9 : Elsevier; 2020:1186.
112. Thigpen MC, et al. Emerging infections programs network. Bacterial meningitis in the United States, 1998-2007. *N Engl J Med*. 2011;364(21):2016–2025.
113. van de Beek D, et al. Clinical features and prognostic factors in adults with bacterial meningitis. *N Engl J Med*. 2004;351(18):1849–1859.
114. Schiess N, Groce NE, Dua T. The impact and burden of neurological sequelae following bacterial meningitis: a narrative review. *Microorganisms*. 2021;9(5):900.
115. Centers for Disease Control and Prevention (CDC). *Vaccine Information Statements (VISs): Current VISs*. Atlanta, GA: CDC; 2021. Page last reviewed October 15, 2021. Available at https://www.cdc.gov/vaccines/hcp/vis/current-vis.html. (Accessed October 18, 2021).
116. Kakooza-Mwesige A, Tshala-Katumbay D, Juliano SL. Viral infections of the central nervous system in Africa. *Brain Res Bull*. 2019;145:2–17.
117. Kohil A, et al. Viral meningitis: an overview. *Arch Virol*. 2021;166(2):335–345.
118. Bloch KC, Bailin SS. Update on fungal infections of the central nervous system: emerging pathogens and emerging diagnostics. *Curr Opin Infect Dis*. 2019;32(3):277–284.
119. Liu Y, et al. Mechanisms of *Candida albicans* trafficking to the brain. *PLoS Pathog*. 2011;7(10):e1002305.
120. Góralska K, Blaszkowska J, Dzikowiec M. Neuroinfections caused by fungi. *Infection*. 2018;46(4):443–459.
121. Manyelo CM, et al. Tuberculous meningitis: pathogenesis, immune responses, diagnostic challenges, and the potential of biomarker-based approaches. *J Clin Microbiol*. 2021;59(3). e01771-20, Available at https://doi.org/10.1128/JCM.01771-20. (Accessed October 18, 2021).
122. van Toorn R, Solomons R. Update on the diagnosis and management of tuberculous meningitis in children. *Semin Pediatr Neurol*. 2014;21(1):12–18.
123. Katrak SM. Central nervous system tuberculosis. *J Neurol Sci*. 2021;421:117278.
124. Venkatesan A, Murphy OC. Viral encephalitis. *Neurol Clin*. 2018;36(4):705–724.
125. Vittor AY, et al. West Nile virus-induced neurologic sequelae-relationship to neurodegenerative cascades and dementias. *Curr Trop Med Rep*. 2020;7(1):25–36.
126. Centers for Disease Control and Prevention (CDC). *West Nile Virus, Information for Health Care Providers*. Atlanta, GA: CDC; 2018. Page last reviewed December 10, 2018. Available at https://www.cdc.gov/westnile/healthcareproviders/index.html. (Accessed October 18, 2021).
127. Ronca SE, Ruff JC, Murray KO. A 20-year historical review of West Nile virus since its initial emergence in North America: has west nile virus become a neglected tropical disease? *PLoS Negl Trop Dis*. 2021;15(5):e0009190.
128. Bradshaw MJ, Venkatesan A. Herpes simplex virus-1 encephalitis in adults: pathophysiology, diagnosis, and management. *Neurotherapeutics*. 2016;13(3):493–508.
129. Dutra LA, et al. Autoimmune encephalitis: a review of diagnosis and treatment. *Arq Neuropsiquiatr*. 2018;76(1):41–49.
130. Alexopoulos H, Dalakas MC. The immunobiology of autoimmune encephalitides. *J Autoimmun*. 2019;104:102339.
131. Uy CE, Binks S, Irani SR. Autoimmune encephalitis: clinical spectrum and management. *Pract Neurol*. 2021;21(5):412–423.
132. Lancaster E. The diagnosis and treatment of autoimmune encephalitis. *J Clin Neurol*. 2016;12(1):1–13.
133. De Andres Crespo M, McKinnon C, Halliday J. What you need to know about brain abscesses. *Br J Hosp Med (Lond)*. 2020;81(8):1–7.
134. Brouwer MC, et al. Brain abscess. *N Engl J Med*. 2014;371(5):447–456.
135. Alvis Miranda H, et al. Brain abscess: current management. *J Neurosci Rural Pract*. 2013;4(Suppl 1):S67–S81.
136. Smail RC, Brew BJ. HIV-associated neurocognitive disorder. *Handb Clin Neurol*. 2018;152:75–97.
137. Rojas-Celis V, et al. New challenges of HIV-1 infection: how HIV-1 attacks and resides in the central nervous system. *Cells*. 2019;8(10):1245.
138. Milanini B, Valcour V. Differentiating HIV-associated neurocognitive disorders from Alzheimer's disease: an emerging issue in geriatric neuroHIV. *Curr HIV/AIDS Rep*. 2017;14(4):123–132.
139. Hanewinckel R, Ikram MA, Van Doorn PA. Peripheral neuropathies. *Handb Clin Neurol*. 2016;138:263–282.
140. Siao P, Kaku M. A clinician's approach to peripheral neuropathy. *Semin Neurol*. 2019;39(5):519–530.
141. Robblee J, Katzberg H. Distinguishing radiculopathies from mononeuropathies. *Front Neurol*. 2016;7:111.
142. Rubin DI. Brachial and lumbosacral plexopathies: a review. *Clin Neurophysiol Pract*. 2020;5:173–193.

143. American Cancer Society. *Cancer Facts & Figures 2021*. Atlanta, GA: American Cancer Society; 2021. Available at https://www.cancer.org/research/cancer-facts-statistics/all-cancer-facts-figures/cancer-facts-figures-2021.html. (Accessed October 18, 2021).
144. American Brain Tumor Association. *Brain Tumor Education*. Chicago, IL: American Brain Tumor Association; 2020. Available at https://www.abta.org/about-brain-tumors/brain-tumor-education/. (Accessed October 18, 2021).
145. Ostrom QT, et al. CBTRUS statistical report: primary brain and other central nervous system tumors diagnosed in the United States in 2012–2016. *Neuro Oncol*. 2019;21(Suppl 5):v1–v100.
146. Park JH, et al. A systems approach to brain tumor treatment. *Cancers (Basel)*. 2021;13(13):3152.
147. Nguyen HM, et al. Pathogenetic features and current management of glioblastoma. *Cancers (Basel)*. 2021;13(4):856.
148. Hsu JF, et al. Nanotechnology and nanocarrier-based drug delivery as the potential therapeutic strategy for glioblastoma multiforme: an update. *Cancers (Basel)*. 2021;13(2):195.
149. Wu SK, et al. Focused ultrasound and microbubbles-mediated drug delivery to brain tumor. *Pharmaceutics*. 2020;13(1):15.
150. Gupta A, Dwivedi T. A simplified overview of World Health Organization classification update of central nervous system tumors 2016. *J Neurosci Rural Pract*. 2017;8(4):629–641. Available at https://doi.org/10.4103/jnrp.jnrp_168_17. (Accessed October 18, 2021).
151. Mirchia K, Richardson TE. Beyond IDH-mutation: emerging molecular diagnostic and prognostic features in adult diffuse gliomas. *Cancers (Basel)*. 2020;12(7):1817.
152. Wen PY, et al. Glioblastoma in adults: a Society for Neuro-Oncology (SNO) and European Society of Neuro-Oncology (EANO) consensus review on current management and future directions. *Neuro Oncol*. 2020;22(8):1073–1113.
153. Louis DN, et al. The 2016 World Health Organization classification of tumors of the central nervous system: a summary. *Acta Neuropathol*. 2016;131(6):803–820.
154. Ostrom QT, et al. CBTRUS statistical report: primary brain and other central nervous system tumors diagnosed in the United States in 2010–2014. *Neuro Oncol*. 2017;19(suppl_5):v1–v88.
155. Fogh SE, et al. Neuro-oncology practice clinical debate: early treatment or observation for patients with newly diagnosed oligodendroglioma and small-volume residual disease. *Neurooncol Pract*. 2020;8(1):11–17.
156. Ostrom QT, et al. CBTRUS statistical report: primary brain and other central nervous system tumors diagnosed in the United States in 2013–2017. *Neuro Oncol*. 2020;22(suppl_1):iv1–iv96.
157. Mack SC, Taylor MD. Put away your microscopes: the ependymoma molecular era has begun. *Curr Opin Oncol*. 2017;29(6):443–447.
158. Seo SH, et al. An insight into pathophysiological features and therapeutic advances on ependymoma. *Cancers (Basel)*. 2021;13(13):3221.
159. National Cancer Institute (NCI). *PDQ® Pediatric Treatment Editorial Board: PDQ Childhood Ependymoma Treatment*. Bethesda, MD: NCI; 2021. Updated February 9, 2021. Available at https://www.cancer.gov/types/brain/hp/child-ependymoma-treatment-pdq. (Accessed October 18, 2021).
160. Takahashi H, et al. Mendelian randomization provides support for obesity as a risk factor for meningioma. *Sci Rep*. 2019;9(1):309.
161. Ogasawara C, Philbrick BD, Adamson DC. Meningioma: a review of epidemiology, pathology, diagnosis, treatment, and future directions. *Biomedicines*. 2021;9(3):319.
162. Goldbrunner R, et al. EANO guidelines for the diagnosis and treatment of meningiomas. *Lancet Oncol*. 2016;17(9):e383–e391.
163. Huntoon K, Toland AMS, Dahiya S. Meningioma: a review of clinicopathological and molecular aspects. *Front Oncol*. 2020;10:579599.
164. Tamura R. Current understanding of neurofibromatosis type 1, 2, and schwannomatosis. *Int J Mol Sci*. 2021;22(11):5850.
165. Costa AA, Gutmann DH. Brain tumors in neurofibromatosis type 1. *Neurooncol Adv*. 2019;1(1):vdz040.
166. Vogel AC, Gutmann DH, Morris SM. Neurodevelopmental disorders in children with neurofibromatosis type 1. *Dev Med Child Neurol*. 2017;59(11):1112–1116.
167. Ostrom QT, Wright CH, Barnholtz-Sloan JS. Brain metastases: epidemiology. *Handb Clin Neurol*. 2018;149:27–42.
168. Lah TT, Novak M, Breznik B. Brain malignancies: glioblastoma and brain metastases. *Semin Cancer Biol*. 2020;60:262–273.
169. Pekmezci M, Perry A. Neuropathology of brain metastases. *Surg Neurol Int*. 2013;4(Suppl 4):S245–S255.
170. Kotecha R, et al. Recent advances in managing brain metastasis. *F1000Res*. 2018;7(F1000 Faculty Rev-1772).
171. Mitchell DK, et al: Brain metastases: an update on the multi-disciplinary approach of clinical management, *Neurochirurgie*. Online ahead of print April 14, 2021. Available at https://doi.org/10.1016/j.neuchi.2021.04.001. (Accessed October 18, 2021).
172. Hussain I, et al. Surgical management of intramedullary spinal cord tumors. *Neurosurg Clin N Am*. 2020;31(2):237–249.

19

Neurobiology of Schizophrenia, Mood Disorders, Anxiety Disorders, Posttraumatic Stress Disorder, and Obsessive-Compulsive Disorder

Lorey K. Takahashi

http://evolve.elsevier.com/Rogers/pathophysiology/

CHAPTER OUTLINE

Mental illnesses are common and found in different cultures and across the socioeconomic spectrum. When left untreated, the consequences can be devastating. This chapter introduces the neurobiology of schizophrenia, mood disorders, posttraumatic stress disorder, obsessive-compulsive disorder, and some anxiety disorders. The etiology and pathophysiology of mental illnesses are diverse and complex. Diagnostic criteria are constantly being updated to more precisely diagnose and effectively treat the disorders. Every mental disorder manifests a range of symptoms that vary in intensity. Symptom variations likely reflect individual differences in pathologic brain structures and functions, which affect treatment. The onset and progression of mental disorders, which may originate in early life, point to the challenge in understanding how gene expression and environmental risk factors interact to disrupt adaptive brain functions.

The use of visual and quantitative structural and functional neuroimaging techniques provides insight into the pathophysiologic basis of mental disorders. In schizophrenia, neuroanatomic, functional, and neurochemical alterations associated with this debilitating illness have uncovered abnormal brain regions along with a host of candidate genes that confer risk. Similarly, in mood and anxiety disorders, brain scans are revealing structural and functional abnormalities. Notably, many brain regions implicated in normal cognitive and emotional processing are found in schizophrenia, mood, and anxiety disorders. The future lies in unraveling how the highly interconnected brain structures modulated by neurotransmitters, neuropeptides, enzymes, and hormones operate in normal to abnormal mental states.

Knowledge of the pathophysiology associated with a specific mental illness has guided the development of new psychopharmacologic medications with fewer side effects. However, some individuals with mental disorders do not respond to current medications or may relapse after a period of treatment. The use of psychotherapies alone or as an adjunct to pharmacotherapy also may be effective in treating some disorders by making the person aware of potential environmental factors that trigger stress and the onset of the illness. Learning to cope with these triggers offers hope for alleviating psychiatric symptoms or attenuating pathophysiologic functions.

SCHIZOPHRENIA

Schizophrenia is a serious psychiatric illness that strikes 1% of the world's population. The illness is equally prevalent in males and females and emerges in young adults during the late teens and early twenties, with a slightly earlier onset in males than in females. Emil Kraeplin first described schizophrenia as "dementia praecox" in 1883.[1] Later, Eugen Bleuler, in 1911 coined the term schizophrenia to describe a cluster of symptoms characterized by thought disorders, or the discontinuity among thoughts, emotions, and behaviors,[2] which reflect a break in reality or splitting of the cognitive from the emotional side of one's personality. An individual with schizophrenia may exhibit a feeling of happiness when recollecting a terrible event or emotional indifference when describing a joyful occasion. Today, schizophrenia is characterized by positive and negative symptoms. Positive symptoms include auditory hallucinations; visual hallucinations; olfactory, tactile, and gustatory hallucinations; and paranoid or grandiose delusions. Negative symptoms include anhedonia, avolition, alogia, flattened affect, and cognitive deficits that have devastating effects on the individual and the individual's family.

Genetic Predisposition

Etiology and Pathophysiology. Schizophrenia is a heritable disorder. In monozygotic twins, the concordance rate varies from 30% to 50%. This variability may stem from different diagnostic criteria and methodologic or sampling differences across studies. In dizygotic twins and siblings, the concordance rate decreases to 12%, which is still considerably higher than the 1% figure found in the general population.

Nonetheless, schizophrenia is not a simple genetic disorder in which inherited disease alleles will always lead to illness. Schizophrenia likely involves several genes located on different chromosomes and differs from mendelian disorders, in which genes are fully penetrant and recognized as the primary cause of disease (e.g., genes for Huntington disease). As indicated by the 50% concordance rate in monozygotic twins, the genes for schizophrenia show reduced penetrance, resulting in individuals who carry the disease genes without manifesting the illness.

Studies searching for candidate genes associated with schizophrenia have begun to use genome-wide association studies, to identify a number of genes including dysbindin, neuroregulin 1, and disrupted-in-schizophrenia-1 (DISC1). However, the traits of schizophrenia are complex, and candidate genes have not always been directly implicated in the disease.[3] Thus, variability in biological and phenotypic traits among individuals who manifest the illness complicates the understanding of specific genetic underpinnings of schizophrenia.

Prenatal and perinatal vulnerability factors. Because the concordance rate of schizophrenia in monozygotic twins is never 100% as in mendelian disorders, environmental factors likely play an important role in increasing or decreasing the risk of developing the disorder. A leading hypothesis suggests that early environmental factors interfere with genetically programmed neural developmental alterations that eventually compromise normal brain structures and functions.[4]

An early brain defect may remain silent and not dramatically affect the individual until subsequent development requires adaptive use of brain structures.[5] Several hypothesized early environmental factors that may alter brain development and increase the risk of developing schizophrenia include exposure to prenatal infection, prenatal nutritional deficiencies, perinatal complications (such as birth defects and neonatal hypoxia), and upbringing in an urban environment.[6,7]

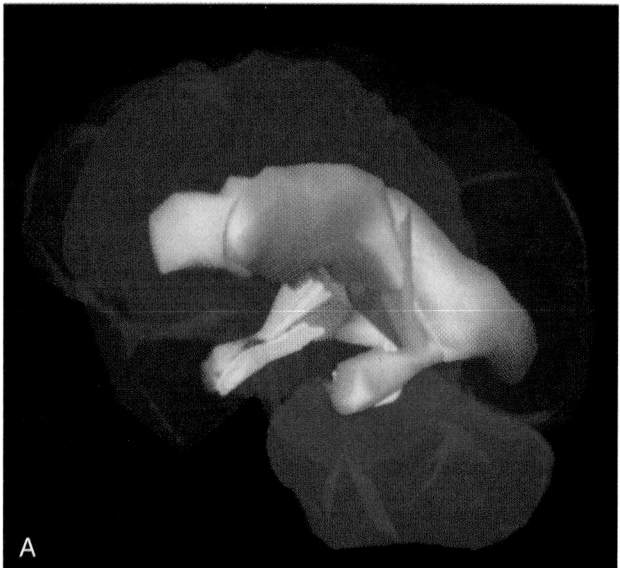

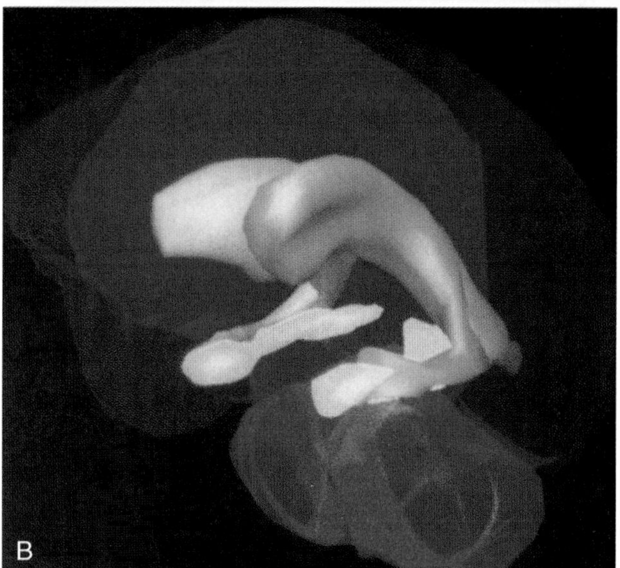

Fig. 19.1 Magnetic Resonance Imaging Comparison of Normal Brain and Brain With Schizophrenia. Three-dimensional magnetic resonance imaging reconstructions showing (A) the cerebral ventricles *(gray regions)* and hippocampus *(yellow regions)* of an individual with schizophrenia, and (B) those of a healthy individual. Note the enlarged cerebral ventricles and reduced hippocampal volume of the brain of the schizophrenic individual. (From Gershon ES, Rieder RO. Major disorders of mind and brain. *Scientific American*, 1992;267:128. Original illustrations by Nancy C. Andreason, University of Iowa.)

Neuroanatomic and Functional Abnormalities

Neuroanatomic alterations. Advanced neuroimaging techniques have revealed structural brain abnormalities in schizophrenia.[8,9] A consistent finding is the enlargement of the lateral and third ventricles and the widening of frontocortical fissures and sulci (Fig. 19.1). Generally, individuals with schizophrenia and cerebral vascular enlargement exhibit cognitive impairment, negative symptoms, and respond poorly to treatment. Other studies reported a reduction in the thalamus and temporal lobe areas (e.g., amygdala, hippocampus, and parahippocampal gyrus).[10] A reduction in thalamus size may disrupt neurotransmission between the frontal cortex and primary sensory and motor areas. Hippocampal volume loss in the first years of the illness is another consistent finding, and hippocampal volume reduction accelerates in individuals with schizophrenia older than 50 years of age.[11] This hippocampal atrophy is strongly associated with global cognitive and socio-occupational functional impairments, which also may reflect a fronto-hippocampal disconnection in socio-cognitive processing.

The amygdala plays a central role in the social brain emotional processing network.[12] Abnormal amygdala connectivity

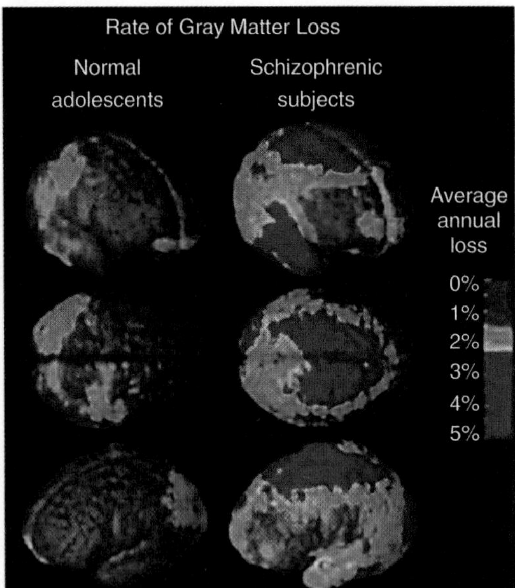

Fig. 19.2 Accelerated Gray Matter Loss in Brains of Early-onset Schizophrenic Adolescents. Annual gray matter loss ranging from 2% to 5% was found in 13- to 18-year-old schizophrenics—compared with age-matched healthy adolescents. (From Thompson PM, Vidal C, Giedd JN, et al. Mapping adolescent brain change reveals dynamic wave of accelerated gray matter loss in very early-onset schizophrenia. *Proceedings of the National Academy of Sciences of the United States of America*, 2001;98:11650.)

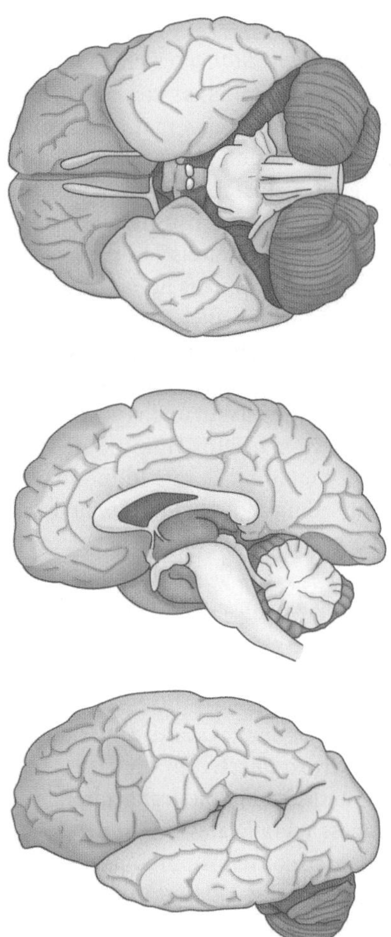

Fig. 19.3 The Prefrontal Cortex. The prefrontal cortex consists of a dorsolateral *(blue)* and an orbitofrontal *(green)* region.

is widely reported in schizophrenia and hypothesized to represent the basis underlying pronounced difficulties for individuals with schizophrenia to make appropriate social judgments as found in tests of facial identity, affect recognition, and in emotional processing.[13] Reported amygdala abnormalities in schizophrenia include reduced volume[10] and abnormal functional activation patterns for social and emotion processing.[14] The emergence of abnormal amygdala projections to brain regions such as the hippocampus during late adolescence and young adulthood may be linked to the onset of schizophrenia.

Brain imaging studies in adolescents with early-onset schizophrenia reveal progressive loss of cortical gray matter in temporal lobes, somatosensory and motor cortices, and the dorsolateral cortex (Fig. 19.2). Of clinical concern is the loss of cortical tissue, which is evident by the time the individual seeks treatment and continues throughout the course of the illness despite the use of antipsychotic medication.[15] The progressive loss in frontal lobe volume is accompanied by increased severity of negative symptoms and further reductions in cognitive functioning. These results highlight the ineffectiveness of current medications for schizophrenia to attenuate or reverse the loss of frontal brain tissue.

Brain abnormalities in schizophrenia are believed to originate in the prenatal period of cell proliferation, myelination, receptor functions, and migration. For example, Reelin, an extracellular matrix protein involved in neuronal migration during development and in synaptic function during adulthood, is reduced in the prefrontal cortex and hippocampus of individuals with schizophrenia.[16] Neuregulin-1 (Nrg1) may also alter brain development in schizophrenia. Nrg1 is widely distributed in the frontal cortex, midbrain, and cerebellum and is involved in regulating myelination, neuronal migration, and neurotransmitter receptor functions.[16,17] Deficits in these processes may impair executive functions such as attention and **working memory** as noted in schizophrenia. Working memory involves the brief storage and use of information to complete cognitive tasks such as language comprehension, learning, and reasoning.

Pathophysiologic changes in the dorsal prefrontal cortex are believed to contribute to the production of negative symptoms in schizophrenia (Fig. 19.3). In particular, the **dorsolateral prefrontal cortex (DLPFC)** (Brodmann areas 9, 10, 46, and 47) is intricately involved in the initiation and maintenance of goal-directed activities and in solving cognitive problems related to working memory. Blood flow and metabolism normally increase in the DLPFC during working memory processing but not in schizophrenics, who also perform poorly in tests of working memory. Thus, the DLPFC appears to be hypoactive in schizophrenia.

Neurotransmitter alterations. The onset of schizophrenia was initially hypothesized to stem from abnormally high concentrations of the brain neurotransmitter dopamine. This **dopamine hypothesis** of schizophrenia was proposed on the basis of pharmacologic studies showing that antipsychotic drugs were potent blockers of brain dopamine receptors. A strong positive correlation was found between the clinical potencies of first-generation antipsychotic drugs (e.g., chlorpromazine, fluphenazine, and haloperidol) and their affinity for the dopamine D_2 receptor. In addition, drugs at high doses that dramatically increased dopaminergic transmission—such as levodopa (L-dopa), cocaine, and amphetamine—produced schizophrenic-like psychosis, which was reversed by dopamine blockers.

A current view of the dopamine hypothesis of schizophrenia is that brain dopamine pathways are altered in different ways (Fig. 19.4). For example, the negative symptoms and cognitive alterations in schizophrenia are proposed to result from reduced dopaminergic neurotransmission in the mesocortical dopamine pathway.[18] This hypodopaminergic transmission in the prefrontal cortex contrasts with the hypothesized hyperdopaminergic secretion in mesolimbic brain regions that may contribute to the production of positive schizophrenia symptoms. The mesolimbic dopamine pathway innervates temporal lobe structures including the hippocampal formation and amygdala, as well as the nucleus accumbens and anterior cingulate cortex.

Another neurotransmitter system that may underlie the pathogenesis of schizophrenia is the excitatory neurotransmitter glutamate and its actions on the *N*-methyl-D-aspartate (NMDA) receptor subtype. The **glutamate hypothesis** of schizophrenia proposes that the underactivation of glutamate receptors contributes to schizophrenia.[19] In schizophrenia, glutamate concentrations in the cerebrospinal fluid (CSF) are reduced along with a decrease in cortical glutamate synthesis. Furthermore, in unaffected individuals, blocking the glutamate NMDA receptor with antagonists, such as phencyclidine (PCP)

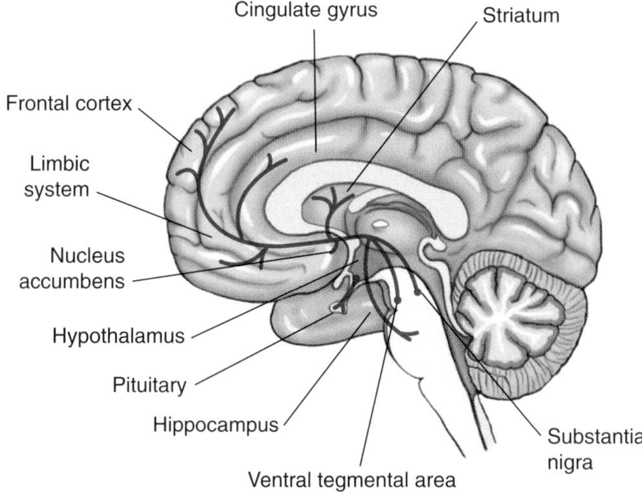

Fig. 19.4 The Dopamine System. Dopamine cell bodies are located in the substantia nigra, where they project to the stratum (nigrostriatal pathway); and in the ventral tegmental area, where they project to the frontal and cingulate cortex (mesocortical pathway), the striatum, the hippocampus, and other limbic structures (mesolimbic pathway). Dopamine nuclei are also located in the hypothalamus and project to the pituitary.

and ketamine, facilitates the positive and negative symptoms of schizophrenia. PCP users report auditory hallucinations and disorientation and may become violent from their delusions. In monkeys, chronic PCP treatment impairs cognitive performance in a test associated with prefrontal cortical damage.[20]

Clinical Manifestations. The symptoms of schizophrenia are currently divided into three broad categories of positive, negative, and cognitive symptoms (Box 19.1). *Positive symptoms* frequently occur during a **psychotic episode**, when an individual loses touch with reality and experiences something that should be absent (e.g., hallucinations). *Negative symptoms* are characterized by disruptions in normal emotional states and expressions. *Cognitive symptoms* are fairly common and involve problems with thought processes that severely impair the ability to perform routine daily tasks that involve attention, planning, and social skills. According to the 5th edition of the *Diagnostic and Statistical Manual of Mental Disorders (DSM-5)*,[21] the diagnosis of schizophrenia begins by eliminating other mental disorders and symptoms not caused by substance abuse, medication, or medical condition. The individual will then be diagnosed with schizophrenia when at least two of the following symptoms (1) delusions, (2) hallucinations, (3) disorganized speech, (4) disorganized or catatonic behavior, and (5) negative symptoms are experienced most of the time during a 1-month-period with some disturbance present over 6 months. In addition, one of the symptoms must be delusions, hallucinations, or disorganized speech.

Psychotic Dimension

Psychotic dimension refers to hallucinations and delusions and reflects a person's confusion or loss of touch with the external world. Hallucinations and delusions are classified as positive symptoms and are the most common in schizophrenia.

Hallucinations. A **hallucination** is a perception experienced without external stimulation of the sense organs. Sensory hallucinations can be auditory, tactile, visual, gustatory, and olfactory. For example, the individual with schizophrenia may hear voices, experience touch or electrical sensations, report images of animate and inanimate objects, or complain of unpleasant tastes and odors. These hallucinations may occur alone or together.

Delusions. A **delusion** is a persistent belief contrary to the educational and cultural background of the individual. Delusions may involve grandiose, nihilistic, persecutory, somatic, sexual, and religious themes. Paranoid beliefs are common and may involve spying, conspiracy, persecution, and ridicule. Delusions also may be referential in that particular stimuli or events become highly personalized, such as believing a television talk show host is directing information specifically at them.

Disorganized Behavior

Disorganized behavior includes disorganized speech and disorganized or bizarre behavior. Incongruity of affect is another dimension of disorganized behavior.

Disorganized speech. A common form of disorganized speech is **formal thought disorder**, which involves fluent

BOX 19.1 Major Symptoms of Schizophrenia

Positive Symptoms

Hallucinations
Auditory
Olfactory
Somatic-tactile
Visual
Voices commenting
Voices conversing

Delusions
Delusions of being controlled
Delusions of mind reading
Delusions of reference
Grandiosity
Guilt
Persecutory
Religious
Somatic
Thought broadcasting
Thought insertion
Thought withdrawal

Positive Formal Thought Disorder
Circumstantiality
Derailment
Distractible speech
Illogicality
Incoherence
Pressure of speech
Tangentiality

Bizarre Behavior
Aggressive, agitated
Clothing, appearance
Repetitive, stereotyped
Social, sexual behavior

Negative Symptoms

Affective Flattening
Affective nonresponsivity
Decreased spontaneous movements
Inappropriate affect
Lack of vocal inflections
Paucity of expressive gestures
Poor eye contact
Unchanging facial expression

Alogia
Blocking
Increase in response latency
Poverty of speech
Poverty of speech content

Anhedonia-Asociality
Few recreational interests
Few social relationships
Impaired intimacy
Little sexual interest

Attention
Social inattentiveness
Inattentiveness during testing

Avolition-Apathy
Impaired personal hygiene
Lack of persistence
Physical anergia

Cognitive Symptoms
Inability to understand information and make proper decision to complete a task
Difficulty paying attention
Problems with working memory or the inability to use recently learned information
Lack of insight

speech that is difficult to comprehend. The speech often moves from one topic to another unexpectedly (loose associations) and illogically, and the person becomes easily distracted when talking.

Another form of disorganized speech is called poverty of content. Here, the use of vocabularies to convey information is severely hindered despite a fair amount of spoken words. For instance, the same phrases are used repeatedly throughout a conversation.

Disorganized behavior. Disorganized (or bizarre) behavior is the conceptual equivalent of disorganized speech. The individual has difficulty engaging in goal-directed activities. Repetitive (e.g., stereotyped rocking) or aimless behavior and poor personal hygiene are exhibited. Another feature is the incongruity of affect or the manifestation of inappropriate situational affect as exemplified by hostility without provocation or child-like silliness in sober situations.

Negative Dimensions

Negative dimensions reflect a deficit in normal functioning and are characterized by affective flattening, anhedonia, alogia (poverty of speech), and avolition. Affective flattening is the near absence of emotional or facial expressions throughout a conversation or in different situations. In anhedonia, individuals are unable to experience emotions such as pleasure or pain and report a sense of detachment from the environment. Alogia is the absence of spontaneous speech production for the purpose of answering questions or expressing oneself. Avolition is a deficit in spontaneous or goal-directed behavior, such as completing simple daily tasks.

Treatment. The use of chlorpromazine in the mid-1950s dramatically altered the treatment of schizophrenia, which previously required extensive institutional hospitalization. The drug was especially effective in reducing positive symptoms such as hallucinations and delusions, as well as thought disorders and hyperactivity. The mechanism of action of chlorpromazine and similar first-generation antipsychotic drugs, such as haloperidol, stem from their ability to block dopaminergic neurotransmission. These first-generation antipsychotics have relative affinities for the dopamine D_2 receptor but may also block histamine-1, muscarinic-1, and alpha-1 receptors.

Antipsychotics that block the D_2 receptor are not without notable neurologic side effects. Parkinsonism (e.g., tremor, shuffling gait, stooped posture, and masked face) are prominent side effects that resemble Parkinson disease, a disorder associated with degeneration of dopamine cell bodies in the substantia nigra that project to the striatum. Another related side effect of conventional antipsychotics that develops in 15% to 30% of individuals with schizophrenia after several months or years of treatment is a condition called tardive dyskinesia.[22] This condition is characterized by delayed onset, irregular, involuntary movements of the tongue, mouth, face, limbs, and trunk. Movements can present as choreiform and/or athetoid. Choreiform movements are characterized as jerky and dance-like. Athetoid movements present as slow, writhing, and snake-like. Other side effects may include sedation, hypotension, akathisia (motor restlessness), constipation, weight gain, amenorrhea, and, less frequently, hepatotoxicity and electrocardiographic changes.

Although the majority of individuals with schizophrenia obtained some positive symptom relief from the first-generation or conventional antipsychotics, approximately, 20% failed to respond to D_2-blocking drugs (Table 19.1), especially those with pronounced symptoms of apathy, disorientation, and social withdrawal. Due to the limitations of the first generation

TABLE 19.1 Medications Used in the Treatment of Schizophrenia

Generic Name	Brand Name
Conventional Antipsychotics	
Chlorpromazine	Thorazine
Fluphenazine	Prolixin
Haloperidol	Haldol
Perphenazine	Trilafon
Pimozide	Orap
Prochlorperazine	Compazine
Thioridazine	Mellaril
Thiothixene	Navane
Trifluoperazine	Stelazine
Second-Generation Atypical Antipsychotics	
Aripiprazole	Abilify
Clozapine	Clozaril
Loxapine	Loxitane
Lurasidone	Latuda
Molindone	Moban
Olanzapine	Zyprexa
Paliperidone	Invega
Quetiapine	Seroquel
Risperidone	Risperdal
Ziprasidone	Geodon

of antipsychotic medications, a second generation of drugs was developed that became known as *atypical antipsychotic drugs*.[23] Atypical antipsychotics also were shown to have superior efficacy in reducing not only the positive but also the negative symptoms in comparison with conventional antipsychotics. For example, clozapine improves some cognitive functions (such as verbal fluency, verbal learning, and memory) and some physical functions (such as psychomotor speed). In addition, the notable neurologic side effects that accompany the use of conventional antipsychotics were diminished.

Unlike conventional antipsychotics (first generation), atypical drugs (second generation) have activity at multiple receptor sites. For example, clozapine has much lower binding affinity for the D_2 receptors but also binds to D_1, D_3, D_4, and D_5 receptors and serotonin (5-hydroxytryptamine, i.e., HT_2, 5-HT_6, 5-HT_7); norepinephrine; and cholinergic and histamine receptors. Risperidone and ziprasidone have higher affinities for blocking 5-HT_2 than D_2 receptors. The higher 5-HT_2/D_2-receptor binding ratio of atypical antipsychotics in comparison with conventional drugs may reflect a normalization of serotonin-dopamine interactions leading to a decreased risk for neurologic side effects observed with D_2-receptor blockade alone.

Atypical antipsychotics are not without adverse effects; tardive dyskinesia occurs in 7%[22] of individuals, and neurologic side effects do occur. However, the most notable are the metabolic abnormalities including regulation of glucose and lipid levels and weight gain. For example, long-term clozapine or olanzapine treatment increases body weight gain, which becomes a risk factor for diabetes and cardiovascular disease. Individuals with schizophrenia treated with clozapine also are required to consent to ongoing lab monitoring due to the risk of developing agranulocytosis, a potentially lethal blood disorder involving the loss of white blood cells and a compromised immune system.

In conjunction with antipsychotic medication, psychosocial therapy can facilitate the management of schizophrenia. Psychosocial relationships assist the individual in developing coping strategies and in identifying stressors and relapse symptoms. Cognitive-behavioral therapy (CBT), a talking therapy that initiates cognitive and behavioral change based on an individualized reappraisal of the person's faulty beliefs, is effective in supporting individuals with schizophrenia who have been stabilized with antipsychotic medications.[24] An important benefit of psychosocial and family support is the encouragement of adherence with antipsychotic medication that requires both consistency and time before the emergence of clinical efficacy.

MOOD DISORDERS: DEPRESSION AND BIPOLAR DISORDER

Mood refers to a sustained emotional state as opposed to brief emotional feelings, which are termed *affective states*. Healthy individuals are normally capable of experiencing a variety of affective states including euphoria, joy, surprise, fear, sadness, anxiety, and depression. When emotional states, such as sadness, become chronic and uncontrollable, individuals may be diagnosed with a mood disorder called *depression*. The two major classifications of mood disorder are (1) unipolar or major depressive disorder, also known as *major depression* or *clinical depression*; and (2) bipolar disorder, which is further classified into bipolar I and bipolar II disorders. Major (unipolar) depressive disorder consists of depressed mood, loss of interest/pleasure, changes in activity, guilt/worthlessness, death/suicide, fatigue/loss of energy, decreased concentration, and changes in sleep, appetite, or weight. In addition, two new specifiers were added in *DSM-5*. One specifier with mixed symptoms allows for the occurrence of manic symptoms as part of the diagnosis in depressed individuals who do not meet the criteria for a manic episode. Another specifier with anxious distress was added because anxiety may affect treatment choices for major depressive disorder. A manic episode consists of elevated, expansive, and irritable mood, as well as changes in energy and activity levels. In bipolar I disorder, the individual experiences at least one manic episode that may be preceded or followed by hypomanic or major depressive episodes. Mania symptoms may significantly impair the individual, trigger psychosis, and require hospitalization. In bipolar II disorder, the individual experiences one major depressive episode for at least 2 weeks and at least one hypomanic episode for at least 4 days. Box 19.2

BOX 19.2 Major Symptoms of Depression and Mania

Symptoms of Depression[a]

Depressed or irritable mood
Loss of interests and pleasure
Significant (>5%) weight gain or loss in a month
Insomnia or hypersomnia
Psychomotor agitation or retardation
Fatigue or loss of energy
Feelings of worthlessness or excessive guilt
Poor concentration or indecisiveness
Recent thoughts of death or suicide

Symptoms of Manic Episode[b]

Elevated mood
Irritable mood
Inflated self-esteem
Decreased need for sleep
Excessive talking
Racing/crowded thoughts
Distractibility
Increase in goal-directed activity
Excessive risky activities

[a]Five or more of the symptoms are present in a 2-week period and at least one of the symptoms is either depressed mood or loss of interests or pleasure.

[b]Three or more symptoms (four if the mood is only irritable) during a distinct period of abnormally and persistently elevated, expansive, or irritable mood occurring for at least 1 week.

presents the major criteria of major depression and bipolar disorder according to the American Psychiatric Association's *DSM-5*.[21] Major (unipolar) depressive disorder is the most common mood disorder and the leading cause of disability in the United States and throughout the world.[25]

Unipolar depression appears in all age groups including young children. In the United States, the lifetime prevalence rate is 16.2% of the population with a twofold greater risk in women than men after adolescence. In children and adolescents, 2% to 6% suffer from depression. The prevalence of bipolar disorder ranges from 3% to 5% in the general population. Bipolar I disorder occurs equally in men and women in comparison with bipolar II disorder, which afflicts more women than men. When left untreated, a number of depressed and bipolar individuals are at risk of developing a host of medical illnesses, including cardiovascular disease, obesity, diabetes, and thyroid disease.

Genetic Predisposition and Environmental Influences

Etiology and Pathophysiology. Family and twin studies indicate a strong basis for mood disorders. Concordance rates for bipolar disorder ranged up to 62% and 42% for monozygotic and dizygotic twins, respectively.[26] Concordance rates of 62% and 28% for unipolar disorder were reported in monozygotic and dizygotic twins, respectively. Even among adoptees with a biological family history of mood disorders, the incidence of developing major depression or manic-depressive illness is higher than among control adoptees. The strong tendency for mood disorders to run in families has encouraged a search for the abnormal gene or genes. Interestingly, loci on chromosomes 18 and 22 have been linked to both bipolar disorder and schizophrenia. Bipolar individuals, who may exhibit psychotic behavior, have deficits in reelin expression linked to genetic loci, located on chromosome 22, which confers susceptibility to schizophrenia (see the preceding section on Schizophrenia). However, the large variation in clinical symptoms suggests that developmental and environmental factors are as important as genetic factors in contributing to the etiology of mood disorders.

Neurochemical Dysregulation

Modern theories of mood disorders began with the important observations that drugs, such as imipramine, elevated norepinephrine levels within the synapse and reduced depression, whereas drugs that depleted monoamine levels (e.g., reserpine) increased depression. These studies led to the dominant **monoamine hypothesis of depression**, in which a deficit in the concentration of brain norepinephrine, dopamine, and/or serotonin is the underlying cause of depression, in contrast to mania, which results from elevated concentrations of monoamines. Three major classes of antidepressant drugs were initially developed and included monoamine oxidase inhibitors (MAOIs), tricyclic antidepressants (TCAs), and selective serotonin reuptake inhibitors (SSRIs). These antidepressants shared the common property, albeit through different mechanisms, that increasing monoamine neurotransmitter levels within the synapse is the basis for their antidepressant effects (Fig. 19.5).

Additional support for the monoamine hypothesis of depression came from studies showing a reduction of monoamine metabolites in the CSF of depressed people. Other work demonstrated that dietary depletion of tryptophan, the precursor of serotonin synthesis, or alpha-methylparatyrosine (AMPT), a drug that inhibits dopamine and norepinephrine synthesis, produced a rapid return to depression in individuals successfully treated with antidepressants.[27]

Neuroendocrine Dysregulation

Stress and hypothalamic-pituitary-adrenal system dysregulation. The hypothalamic-pituitary-adrenal (HPA) system plays an essential role in an individual's ability to cope with stress (see Chapter 11). However, chronic stress-induced activation of the HPA system and elevated glucocorticoid secretion are found in a large percentage (30% to 70%) of people with major depression, suggesting that mechanisms responsible for increased HPA hormone secretion contribute to the pathophysiology of depression.[28]

Notably, antidepressant drugs effective in normalizing the HPA system are associated with a good clinical response, whereas persistent dysregulation of the HPA system is related to continued depression or relapse. Psychosocial stress-induced activation of the immune system increases secretion of proinflammatory cytokines, such as interleukin-1α (IL-1α) and IL-β, tumor necrosis factor-alpha (TNF-α), and IL-6, which modulates signaling pathways throughout the periphery and brain and

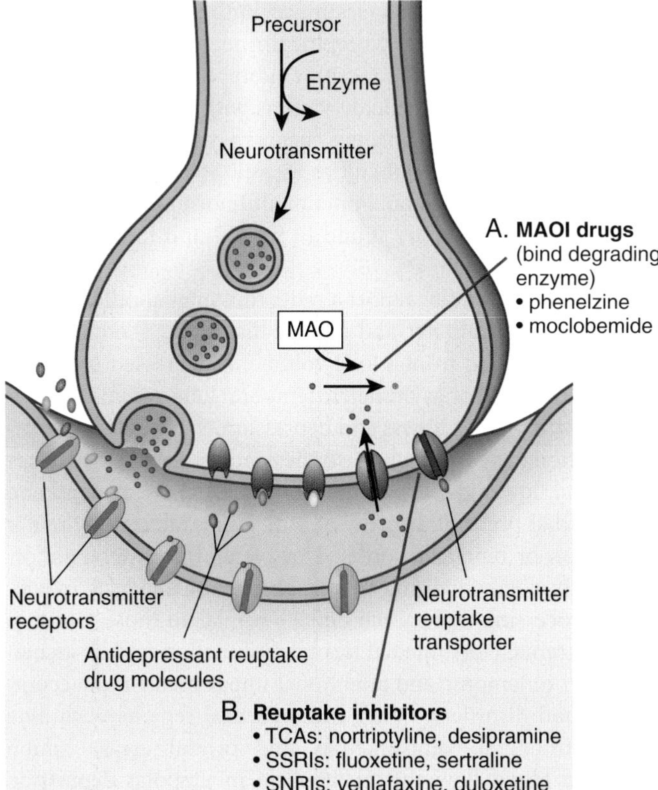

Fig. 19.5 Schematic Diagrams Showing the Sites of Actions of Antidepressants and Their Effects on Neurotransmitter Levels. (A) Monoamine oxidase inhibitors *(MAOIs)* act by blocking the enzyme that normally degrades neurotransmitters, such as norepinephrine and serotonin increasing their presynaptic concentration. **(B)** The tricyclic antidepressants *(TCAs)*, selective serotonin reuptake inhibitors *(SSRIs)*, and serotonin-norepinephrine reuptake inhibitors *(SNRIs)* act by reducing the uptake of neurotransmitters from the synapse, which leads to increased neurotransmitter levels.

augments further secretion of HPA hormones and monoamine metabolism. See the Emerging Science Box: Genetic Basis of Anxiety and Depression for further insight on the genetic links between anxiety and depression.

Evidence suggests that inflammation is another risk factor that triggers the onset of depression. For example, a study involving 73,131 Danish individuals from the general population reported elevated levels of C-reactive protein, a commonly used marker of inflammatory disease, was associated with increased risk of psychologic distress and depression.[29] Another study reported that depressed people treated with antidepressants, a combination of antidepressants and psychotherapy, or psychotherapy alone initially exhibited elevated cytokine levels that returned to normal levels after recovery from depression.[30]

Although there are currently no known effective anti-inflammatory treatments for depression, two omega-3 polyunsaturated fatty acids (PUFAs), eicosapentaenoic acid (EPA) and docosahexaenoic acid (DHA), may have anti-inflammatory effects that could reduce depression. A study examined whether the breakdown of EPA and DHA and some of their metabolites (known as lipid mediators) are able to protect the brain from the harmful effects of inflammation.[31] The research showed that in vitro human hippocampal cells pretreated with EPA or DHA before exposure to proinflammatory cytokines prevented increased cell death and a reduction in neurogenesis. Of clinical relevance, individuals with major depression and were administered high doses of EPA or DHA for 12 weeks, exhibited higher levels of lipid metabolites in their plasma that correlated with less severe symptoms of depression. The investigators note that plasma concentrations of EPA and DHA found in the study are unlikely to be achieved with the typical consumption of food rich in omega-3 fatty acids. Rather, therapeutic doses that reach high omega-3 PUFA levels may be required to produce the beneficial effects of reducing depression.

Increasing evidence from animal models of stress-induced depression shows that depression-like behavior is accompanied by atrophy of neurons in the hippocampus, a reduction in the development of new hippocampal neurons (i.e., neurogenesis), and a deficit in hippocampal brain-derived neurotrophic factor (BDNF) levels.[32] Consistent with animal studies, human postmortem work indicates low hippocampal BDNF levels in depression. Because the growth factor BDNF supports the survival of neurons and facilitates neurogenesis from hippocampal stem cells, a neurotrophic hypothesis of depression has been proposed as an extension of the monoamine hypothesis of depression to broadly account for the pathophysiologic basis of depression. That is, stress-induced depression and the accompanying reduction in levels of monoamines are caused by deficits in neurogenesis and BDNF levels. Of clinical relevance, administration of antidepressants to animals reverses the depression-like state and increases the development of neurogenesis and BDNF levels.

EMERGING SCIENCE BOX

Genetic Basis of Anxiety and Depression

Large-scale genome-wide association studies offer insight into the genetic basis of anxiety and depression. A large genome-wide association study found genetic links between anxiety and major depressive disorder. Over 199,000 participants were sampled to identify genetic risk variants near genes in people with anxiety. Of further relevance, the researchers found significant genetic overlap between anxiety and depression. One finding was the *SATB1* gene, a major regulator of multiple genes that modulates the expression of the Corticotropin Releasing Hormone (*CRH*) gene. The CRH neuropeptide plays a major role in the activation of the hypothalamic-pituitary-adrenal axis and the expression of stress and emotional fear and anxiety responses. Individuals with increased secretion of CRH may be at greater risk of developing anxiety disorders and depression. The study found another gene called ESR1, which encodes for several receptors for estrogen. The association between ESR1 and anxiety may have relevance in understanding sex differences in stress-related anxiety disorders such as post-traumatic stress disorder, which is more prevalent in females. The comorbidity and the genetic overlap between disorders offer new insights and molecular targets to better understand the basis of serious mental illnesses.

Data from Levey DF, et al. Reproducible genetic risk Loci for anxiety: Results from-200,000 participants in the Million Veteran Program. *American Journal of Psychiatry*, 2020;177:223–232.

Hypothalamic-pituitary-thyroid system dysregulation. Alterations in thyroid function and mental illnesses, particularly major depression and anxiety disorders, have long been recognized. People with hyperthyroidism often manifest symptoms of dysphoria, anxiety, irritability, emotional lability, and cognitive impairments. On the other hand, individuals with severe hypothyroid exhibit features of major depression, apathy, psychomotor slowing, and dementia.[33] Notably, although thyroid dysfunction may be linked to symptoms of depression and anxiety, people diagnosed with primary depression generally have normal thyroid function.[34] The causal mechanisms or basis underlying altered thyroid secretion and depression remain to be determined.

Neuroanatomic and Functional Abnormalities

The dorsal and median raphe nuclei, located in the central gray matter of the caudal mesencephalon and rostral pons, contain a large group of serotonin-synthesizing neurons that project extensively to all regions of the cortex, basal ganglia, limbic system, hypothalamus, cerebellum, and brainstem (Fig. 19.6). Postmortem and/or brain imaging studies of depressed individuals revealed a widespread decrease in serotonin 5-HT_{1A} receptor subtype binding in the frontal, temporal, and limbic cortex as well as serotonin transporter binding in the cerebral cortex and hippocampus. Mood disorders in some individuals may reflect a dysfunctional raphe-serotonin system, which normally modulates homeostasis, emotionality, and tolerance to aversive experiences.

A group of norepinephrine-containing cells, located in the locus ceruleus of the rostral pons, project to vast areas of the forebrain, brainstem, and spinal cord (Fig. 19.7). The locus ceruleus–norepinephrine system is implicated in global psychologic processes including attention, vigilance, and orientation to novel, aversive, or threatening stimuli. Activation of the locus ceruleus–norepinephrine system is also capable of inhibiting the raphe-serotonin system, suggesting an indirect role in modulating serotonin functions. Norepinephrine receptor alterations (e.g., α- and β-adrenergic receptor subtypes) are found in the frontal cortex of some suicide victims with major depression. Alterations in norepinephrine systems may be linked to attention or concentration difficulties as well as sleep and arousal disturbances in depression. Functional abnormalities associated with mood disorders are found in frontal and limbic regions such as the amygdala.[35,36]

Postmortem studies report a reduction in glial cell numbers in people with unipolar and bipolar disorders. There are also reports of reduced frontal lobe volume in depressed individuals and decreased or asymmetric temporal lobe volume in individuals with bipolar illness and depression.

Functional neuroimaging studies indicate decreased cerebral blood flow and glucose metabolism in the dorsolateral and dorsomedial prefrontal cortex of individuals affected by major depression or bipolar disorder. Dorsolateral prefrontal abnormalities in depression may be responsible for the delay in cognitive processing and speech deficits similar to those found in schizophrenia. Dorsomedial frontal dysfunction may be associated with mnemonic and attentional impairments that accompany mood disorders. Other frontocortical regions, including the ventrolateral, ventromedial, and orbital areas, exhibit increased blood flow and metabolism in unipolar depression (Fig. 19.8). These frontal brain areas have extensive interconnections with the amygdala, especially in the right, and are positively related to negative affect in depressed individuals. These functional changes in brain activity begin to normalize with successful antidepressant treatments, suggesting they are state rather than trait related.

Hippocampal volume reduction in major depression is a widely reported finding, especially in individuals with a history of recurrent major depression.[37]

Similar to the hippocampus, the amygdala is reduced in volume after experiencing a number of major depressive episodes, and in individuals with a family history of depression, albeit enlarged in the first episode of depression.[38] The cumulative

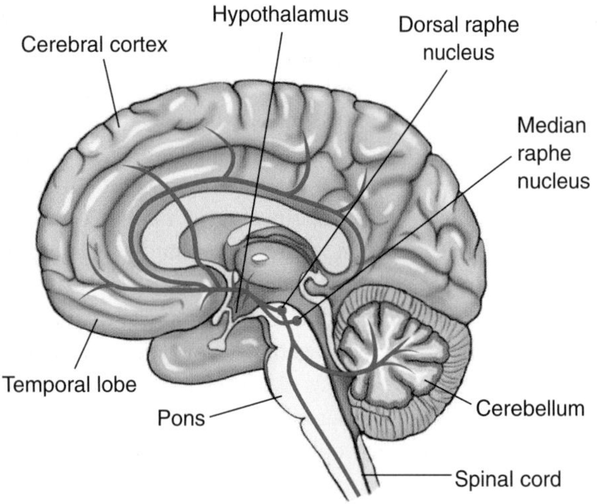

Fig. 19.6 The Serotonin System. Serotonin neurons are located in the brainstem raphe nuclei. They project diffusely to all regions of the cortex, temporolimbic regions, hypothalamus, basal ganglia, cerebellum, the brainstem, and spinal cord.

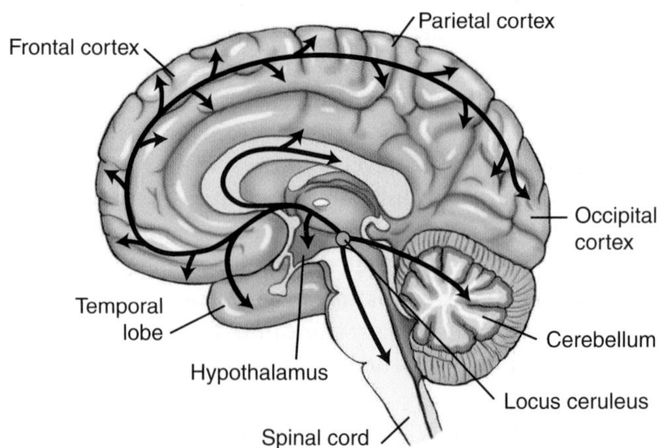

Fig. 19.7 The norepinephrine system. The norepinephrine cell bodies originate in the locus ceruleus and project throughout the brain, including the hypothalamus, the temporal lobe, the entire cortex, the cerebellum, and spinal cord.

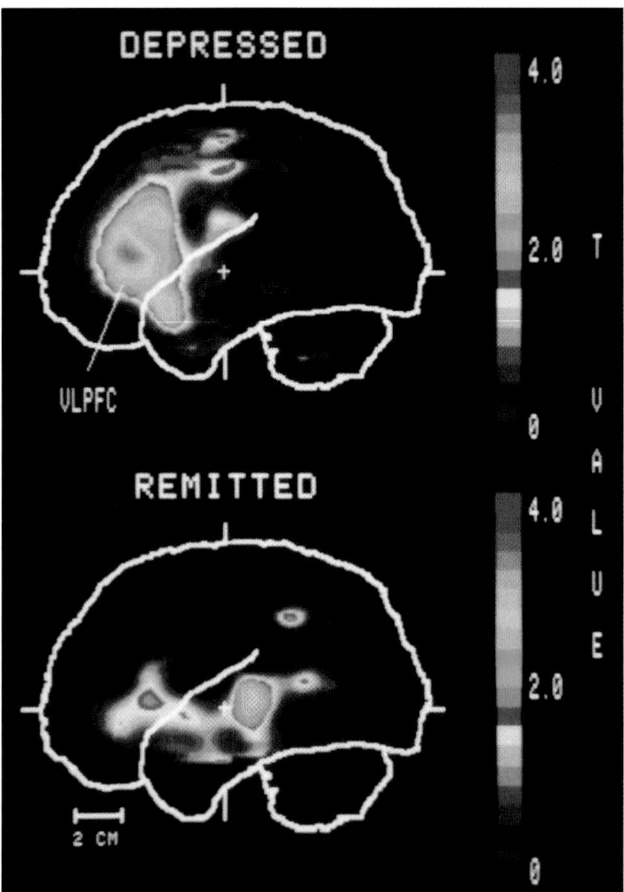

Fig. 19.8 Positron-Emission Tomography (PET). PET comparison of brain activity in depression and in remittance. PET scan showing increased activity in the left prefrontal cortex in a depressed person but not in the remitted person. *VLPFC*, Ventrolateral prefrontal cortex. (From Drevets WC, Videen TO, Price JL, et al. A functional anatomical study of unipolar depression. *Journal of Neuroscience*, 1992;12:3628. Copyright ©1992 by the Society for Neuroscience.)

effects of stress may be responsible for a reduction in hippocampal and amygdala volume. MRI studies showed an increased volume of the amygdala in bipolar illness and larger lateral ventricles in people suffering multiple bipolar episodes compared to those with only a single episode or healthy controls.[39] Ventricular enlargement suggests progressive brain tissue loss resulting from multiple bipolar episodes.

The glutamate system. Because of the delayed onset of action of current antidepressants and poor remission rates, investigators are constantly searching for new drugs with novel mechanisms of actions. An emerging body of evidence suggests that elevated cortical levels of glutamate, the major excitatory neurotransmitter in the central nervous system, may be involved in the pathophysiology of major depression. A potential promising target is the glutamate NMDA receptor. At nontoxic doses, the glutamate receptor antagonist ketamine was found in animal models to rapidly increase synaptic density and signaling in cortical neurons. Of clinical relevance, ketamine is reported to be effective in inducing rapid but transient antidepressant effects in treatment-resistant depressed individuals.[40,41] Investigators have begun to study the possibility of extending the antidepressant effects of ketamine by administrating rapamycin, the mechanistic target of rapamycin complex 1 (mTORC1 inhibitor), to refractory depression individuals prior to ketamine infusion. Individuals with depression treated with rapamycin before ketamine administration continued to show a clinical antidepressant response after two weeks (41%), with 29% in full remission compared to 13% response and 7% remission in the placebo followed by ketamine group. Rapamycin is an immunosuppressant and the results suggest rapamycin may prolong the antidepressant effects of ketamine by protecting newly made synapses and may restore the impaired cellular functions in depressed people.[42]

Recently, esketamine (Spravato), a rapidly acting glutamate receptor antagonist drug, similar to ketamine, was approved by the FDA in a nasal spray form for treatment-resistant depression and works to reduce the symptoms of depression within hours. By blocking the NMDA receptor, esketamine increases glutamate release acting on dendritic spines compromised by stress and depression in brain circuits involved in the regulation of mood. Although the beneficial effects of esketamine are the rapid effects of antidepressant activity, the effects of long-term treatment are still unknown and some side effects of esketamine are reported to include sedation, dizziness, dissociation reactions, and increased blood pressure.[43,44]

Depression

Clinical Manifestations. Major depression is characterized by unremitting feelings of sadness and despair (see Box 19.2). The dysphoric mood or intensely painful mood is accompanied frequently by insomnia, loss of appetite and body weight, and reduced interest in pleasurable activities and interpersonal relationships. Sleep disturbances may include difficulty in initially falling asleep and awakening in the middle of the night, lying awake for several hours with an inability to subsequently fall asleep. Individuals may have reduced motor activity and suffer marked fatigue. Others complain of restlessness and agitation. Feelings of worthlessness and guilt are common, and pessimistic or negative outcomes are often perceived even in routine situations. The ability to function (e.g., work) and concentrate is greatly diminished. Depressive episodes may occur or recur suddenly or gradually and continue from a few weeks to months, and 20% may exhibit a chronic form of depression.

Suicidal risk increases in depression. Factors such as living alone or being divorced, having a prior history of drug abuse or suicide attempt, or having depression at midlife or older ages contribute to suicide in 10% to 15% of depressed individuals.

Bipolar Disorder: Mania

Individuals with mania experience elevated levels of euphoria and self-esteem and feelings of grandiosity. Energy levels are greatly enhanced even after only a few hours of sleep each night. The increased energy, however, does not lead to organized plans and thoughts. The individual may show poor judgment in spending money, may become hypersexual, or may make poor business commitments. Other hallmarks of mania are excessive, rapid, loud, and pressured speech. The individual with mania frequently skips from one topic of conversation to another and is easily distracted both when speaking and when performing tasks. Approximately 50% of manic individuals develop psychotic symptoms, such as delusions or hallucinations, which require hospitalization. The onset and termination of manic symptoms (see Box 19.2) are usually abrupt and may last for a few days or months followed by depression. The risk of recurrence of bipolar disorder is high, especially without immediate treatment.

Depression

Treatment. Approximately 80% of depressed persons will respond to antidepressant drugs such as MAOIs, TCAs, and SSRIs (Table 19.2); psychotherapy; or a combination of both treatment modalities. Although SSRIs have become the standard first-line treatment for major depression, the initial selection of an antidepressant often includes an assessment of the person's symptoms and age as well as the side effects, safety, cost, and convenience of the prescribed medication. For example, medications that produce sedation may be helpful for the treatment of sleep disturbances. Approximately 50% of depressed individuals may not show a favorable response during initial treatment to an antidepressant drug, and 10% to 20% may continue to exhibit symptoms after 2 years. Individuals who are nonresponsive to a specific antidepressant during a 2-month period may be given another antidepressant medication. Atypical antidepressants, such as nefazodone, trazodone, and mirtazapine, presumably produce their clinical effects by blocking specific receptors (e.g., 5-HT_{2A}). A new generation of antidepressants that selectively block serotonin and norepinephrine reuptake is available in the United States (e.g., venlafaxine) and Europe (i.e., milnacipran, reboxetine).

In bipolar depression, antidepressant medications may lead to cycle acceleration or induction of mania. However, SSRIs and bupropion may be less likely to induce these effects than MAOIs or TCAs.

A number of side effects are reported with MAOIs, TCAs, and SSRIs. Commonly reported side effects of MAOIs include sedation or agitation, insomnia, dry mouth, impotence, and weight gain. MAOIs also may induce acute and heightened elevations in blood pressure (e.g., hypertensive crisis) after intake of tyramine-rich foods, such as aged cheeses, sour cream, pods of broad beans, pickled herring, liver, canned figs, raisins, and avocados. In addition, MAOI interactions with TCAs, SSRIs, stimulants, and over-the-counter flu medications are dangerous and should be avoided. Because of these adverse side effect issues, MAOIs are used less often than other antidepressants.

TCAs may produce sedation, insomnia, orthostatic hypotension, seizures, and weight gain. Some TCAs have moderate anticholinergic side effects, including constipation, urinary hesitancy or retention, dry mouth, blurred vision, and memory impairment. These side effects may be an issue when considering TCA treatment of older adults, in which case, the TCAs desipramine and nortriptyline may be preferred because

TABLE 19.2 FDA-Approved Medications Used in the Treatment of Depression and Anxiety Disorders

Generic Name	Brand Name
Monoamine Oxidase Inhibitors	
Isocarboxazid	Marplan
Phenelzine	Nardil
Tranylcypromine	Parnate
Selegiline	Emsam
Tricyclics	
Amitriptyline	Elavil, Endep, Levate
Amoxapine	Asendin
Clomipramine	Anafranil
Desipramine	Norpramin, Pertofrane
Doxepin	Adapin, Sinequan
Imipramine	Tofranil
Maprotiline	Ludiomil
Nortriptyline	Aventyl, Pamelor
Protriptyline	Vivactil
Trimipramine	Surmontil
Selective Serotonin Reuptake Inhibitors	
Citalopram	Celexa
Escitalopram	Lexapro
Fluoxetine	Prozac
Fluvoxamine	Luvox
Paroxetine	Paxil
Sertraline	Zoloft
Serotonin and Norepinephrine Reuptake Inhibitors	
Desvenlafaxine	Pristiq
Duloxetine	Cymbalta
Levomilnacipran	Fetzima
Venlafaxine	Effexor, Effexor XR
Serotonin Reuptake Inhibitor and 5-HT_{1A} Receptor Partial Agonist	
Vilazodone	Viibryd
Norepinephrine and Specific Serotonergic Modulator	
Mirtazapine	Remeron
Norepinephrine–Dopamine Reuptake Inhibitor	
Bupropion	Wellbutrin, Zyban
Serotonin Modulator	
Nefazodone	Serzone
Trazodone	Desyrel, Oleptro
Vortioxetine	Trintellix
Non-competitive *N*-methyl-D-aspartate (NMDA) receptor antagonist	
Esketamine	Spravato

of their reduced anticholinergic, cardiovascular, and sedating effects.

Common side effects of SSRIs include sleep disturbances (e.g., insomnia) and nausea. However, agitation, allergic skin reactions, dry mouth, anxiety, altered appetite, and sexual dysfunction have been reported. Unlike MAOIs and TCAs, SSRIs do not have pronounced effects on the cardiovascular or cholinergic systems. SSRIs are potent inhibitors of cytochrome P-450 isoenzymes, which are involved in drug metabolism. Therefore, SSRIs may lead to dangerous elevations in blood concentrations of other psychiatric medications when taken together. SSRIs should not be taken with MAOIs or immediately after discontinuing MAOI treatment. A serotonin syndrome characterized by excitement or autonomic hyperactivity, abdominal pain, rigidity, and hyperthermia may develop, leading to coma or death.

Side effects of atypical antidepressants may include sedation, dry mouth, weight gain, and constipation. Nefazodone and trazodone have been associated with hepatic toxicity. Venlafaxine and reboxetine lack many of the serious side effects associated with TCAs; however, sweating, dry mouth, and some sedation may occur. Adjunctive therapy with atypical antipsychotics, such as aripiprazole and brexpiprazole, has been FDA approved for treatment-resistant depression. Electroconvulsive therapy (ECT) may be used when individuals fail to respond to antidepressants or when they are severely depressed, pregnant, suicidal, or psychotic. ECT effectively alleviates depressive symptoms in about 50% to 80% of individuals, who may then begin to respond to antidepressant medications. Recent work suggests that ECT increases the volume of the hippocampus and amygdala, brain structures linked to emotion, mood, and cognitive functions.[43,45] Individuals with depression with relatively small hippocampal volumes were most likely to show hippocampal volume increases and improved clinical response after ECT. Neurotrophic processes activated by ECT, including neurogenesis, may underlie these structural changes and clinical benefits.

Deep brain stimulation (DBS) is another treatment showing promise to alleviate major depression in individuals resistant to current antidepressant medications, ECT, and psychotherapy.[46,47] The treatment involves implanting electrodes during neurosurgery into brain regions such as the subcallosal cingulate gyrus (SCG [Brodmann area 25 and parts of 24 and 32]) and the nucleus accumbens.[48] This SCG region was targeted because abnormal SCG brain activity, a suggested pathophysiologic cause of major depression, is reversed by effective antidepressant treatment. A 3- to 6-year follow-up study of 20 treatment-resistant depressed individuals who received DBS in the SCG found that more than half eventually returned to work and improved their quality of life.[49] Preliminary work with DBS in the nucleus accumbens, a region involved in rewarding experiences, was shown to reverse treatment-resistant depression in people unresponsive to pharmacotherapy, psychotherapy, and ECT. Pathophysiology in the nucleus accumbens may be linked to impairments in reward processing and underlie the anhedonic symptom of depression. Preclinical studies suggest that the mechanism responsible for reversing the anhedonic state of depression is caused by the rapid increase in monoamine release in the prefrontal cortical areas following DBS stimulation in the nucleus accumbens.[50]

Another therapy for treatment-resistant depression is transcranial magnetic stimulation (TMS). This FDA-approved treatment involves noninvasive focal brain stimulation—unlike DBS, which requires neurosurgery, or ECT seizure induction. The procedure uses an electromagnetic coil to create a magnetic field that passes from the scalp to the brain, where the electrical current flow stimulates neurons. Daily repeated left prefrontal TMS was shown to induce acute antidepressant effects with few side effects and remission in 30% to 40% of individuals with depression.[51]

A weakness of many antidepressant treatments is that, even among individuals who receive the gold standard of antidepressant pharmacotherapy with psychotherapy, at least 50% of people who recover from a first episode of depression will, nonetheless, experience another one or more depression episodes in their lifetime. The recurrence rate of depression increases to approximately 80% in those with a history of two episodes.[52] One contributing factor for relapse is the failure of individuals to continue with their treatment plan by stopping their therapy sessions or drug medications. Another related factor is low social support and perceived loneliness. Studies reported low social support predicts poor response to depression treatment, early drop-out, and heightened risk of relapse.[53,54] Interventions aimed at increasing social interactions may prove to be valuable in reducing depression symptoms and relapse (Box 19.3).[55]

Bipolar Disorder

FDA-approved treatments are available for bipolar disorders.[56] Individuals with bipolar I disorder are treated with lithium and in some cases with SSRIs. Several medications are also used, including anticonvulsants (e.g., carbamazepine, valproate, gabapentin, lamotrigine, or topiramate). Many individuals with bipolar disorder are currently prescribed second-generation antipsychotics (e.g., clozapine, risperidone, ziprasidone, quetiapine) in an outpatient setting. However, the comparative effectiveness of mood stabilizers and antidepressants compared to second-generation antipsychotics in individuals with bipolar disorder remains unknown.[57] As in depression, ECT is administered when manic individuals fail to respond to medication, are pregnant, or have cardiovascular disease.

Increasing evidence reveals that pharmacotherapy alone is not effective in preventing the recurrences of bipolar disorder. Randomized clinical trials are beginning to show that bipolar persons treated with medication may benefit when exposed to various forms of psychotherapy. Here, pharmacotherapy and psychosocial interventions reduce episode recurrences and promote symptom management strategies and coping skills. Furthermore, individuals with bipolar disorder are more likely to continue the combined treatments when conducted in family or group formats or when brief psychoeducation is used, as opposed to formalized versions of individual psychoeducation in an outpatient setting.[58]

The treatment of bipolar II in children has raised concerns because of complications with its diagnosis. For example,

BOX 19.3 Comprehensive Treatment of Risk Factors May Promote Resilience and Rapid Recovery From Depression

Environmental stressors and genetic predisposition

	Depression risk factors	Therapeutic intervention	Resilience protective factors
Cognitive/behavioral	Weak executive function: weak coping self-efficiency; negative attention bias; cognitive inflexibility	Cognitive behavioral therapy with cognitive reappraisal; positive emotion exercises, coping skill development, and training; well-being therapy	Strong executive function; high coping self-efficacy; positive emotions; realistic optimism; cognitive flexibility
Emotion regulation	Weak regulation (e.g., anhedonia; slow stress recovery)	Mindfulness; training; antidepressant medications	Strong regulation (e.g., delay gratification; rapid stress recovery)
Social	Weak social skills; minimal social network; no resilient role models	Social emotional training; network support treatment	Strong social skills; diverse social network; resilient role models
Physical health	Sleep deprivation; poor cardiovascular fitness; poor nutrition; obesity	Teach sleep hygiene; exercise regimen; improve diet	Strong sleep habits; physically fit; good nutrition
Neurobiology	Dysregulated HPA axis and SNS in response to stress; attenuated prefontal cortical executive function and stress-induced limbic system hyperactivity	Neural circuit training; novel medications (corticotropin-releasing factor, NPY, GABA, glutamate)	Effective regulation of HPA axis and SNS in response to stress; robust prefrontal cortical executive function and capacity to regulate limbic reactivity to stress

(From Southwick SM, Charney DS. The science of resilience: implications for the prevention and treatment of depression. *Science.* 2012;338(6103):79–82.)

Genetic and environmental factors, such as uncontrollable stress, interact to increase the risk of developing major depression. These factors interact in complex ways that are not fully understood to dysregulate neurobiologic systems that compromise adaptive cognitive, emotional, social, and physiologic/health functions. For example, exaggerated stress-induced arousal of sympathetic and neuroendocrine systems may be due, in part, to genetic polymorphisms in serotonin, endocrine, and neuropeptide systems. However, the extent to which a genetic predisposition contributes to severe depression also may arise from the individual's inability to cope with stressors, inexperience in exhibiting flexible psychosocial and emotional skills, and lack of physical health, among others. Identifying and addressing these varied genetic and cognitive/behavioral/socioemotional/health risk factors of depression may open new doors to effective treatment. In particular, combined treatments or behavioral programs that promote resilience, the ability to recover from adversity—such as cognitive-behavioral therapy; social support; and improved diet, sleep, and exercise used in conjunction with current or novel drug medications that lessen or reverse the neuropathophysiology associated with heightened activation of stress systems—may quickly lead to remission. Although in its early stages, the development of comprehensive resilience programs holds promise not only for treating depressed individuals but also for proactively serving to diminish or prevent the risk of acquiring stress-related disorders.

GABA, Gamma-aminobutyric acid; *HPA*, hypothalamic pituitary adrenal axis; *NPY*, neuropeptide Y; *SNS*, sympathetic nervous system.
Data from Karatsoreos IN, McEwen BS. Psychobiological allostasis: Resistance, resilience and vulnerability. *Trends in Cognitive Science*, 2011;15(12):576–584; Southwick SM, Charney DS. The science of resilience: Implications for the prevention and treatment of depression. *Science*, 2012;338(6103):79–82.

bipolar II and attention-deficit/hyperactivity disorder (ADHD) share the common features of elevated behavioral activity levels, excessive talking, restlessness, and distractibility. Misdiagnosing bipolar II as ADHD has negative consequences for treatment because the stimulant drugs Ritalin and Adderall, which are frequently used to treat ADHD, will potentially exacerbate the symptoms of a child with bipolar II disorder. On the other hand, when ADHD is misdiagnosed as bipolar disorder, the child may begin an ineffective treatment regimen. To reduce misdiagnosis of children with bipolar and other similar symptomatic characteristics, such as ADHD as well as conduct disorder and oppositional defiant disorder, the *DSM-5*[21] now includes a category called *disruptive mood dysregulation disorder*. This diagnosis will be used to describe a young child (6 to 10 years of age) who exhibits only some of the symptoms of bipolar II, such as frequent temper outbursts, irritability, and bad moods. This category is hoped to exclude children from being diagnosed with bipolar disorder and reduce possible unwarranted treatment with strong medications.[59]

ANXIETY DISORDERS

Fear and anxiety are normal feelings expressed in threatening or harmful situations. The symptoms may include arousal, tenseness, and increased autonomic activity such as heart rate, blood pressure, and respiration. In addition, individuals often engage in protective behavioral responses such as flight or avoidance. These physiologic and behavioral responses allowed humans to adapt and cope under a variety of situational challenges. However, when fear and anxiety become too intense and undermine the ability to function on a daily basis, the individual may develop an anxiety disorder. Anxiety disorders are the most prevalent psychiatric illness, occurring in approximately 10% to 30% of the general population. Notably, many individuals with anxiety disorders also exhibit symptoms of major depression, and the high comorbidity of anxiety disorders and depression suggests a common neural pathophysiologic basis linking these two illnesses. Nonetheless, a single gene is unlikely to be a major factor linking the occurrence of complex disorders such as depression and anxiety. A recent study identified 509 genes in depression and anxiety. Of interest, nearly 40% of the variation in a neurotic personality correlate strongly with self-doubt, anxiety, and depression and overlap with genes found in people with comorbid conditions of anxiety disorders and major depression. Connecting a number of genes to symptoms of anxiety and depression may offer a broader insight into the shared genetic risk factors and biological mechanisms between psychiatric disorders.[60] This section presents an overview of several anxiety disorders, including panic disorder (PD), social anxiety disorder (SAD), generalized anxiety disorder (GAD), and posttraumatic stress disorder, which in *DSM-5* is listed in the chapter on trauma- and stressor-related disorders.[21]

Panic Disorder

PD consists of multiple disabling panic attacks and is characterized by intense autonomic arousal involving a wide variety of symptoms, including lightheadedness, a rapid heart rate (tachycardia), difficulty breathing, chest discomfort, generalized sweating, general weakness, trembling, abdominal distress, and chills or hot flashes. Between panic attacks, the individual often worries about future panic attacks and fear of losing control and dying. Symptoms originally occur spontaneously and vary in length from several minutes to an hour.

A notable complication of panic disorder is the development of agoraphobia or phobic avoidance of places or situations where escape or help is not readily available. The agoraphobic individual will avoid being away from home, standing in line or in a crowd, or traveling in a train, plane, or automobile. Severely agoraphobic individuals become housebound.

Etiology and Pathophysiology. Genetic factors play a major role in PD. The risk is nearly 20% among first-degree relatives, and the prevalence of PD is about 1.5% in men and up to 3.0% in women with no family history of the illness. Some studies suggest that the cholecystokinin (CCK) receptor gene on chromosome 11p may be linked to PD.[61]

The etiology of PD is not known, but the ability to elicit physical symptoms of panic attacks by chemicals, called *panicogens*, provides insight into its pathophysiology. Panic-prone individuals respond to panicogens that include carbon dioxide, caffeine, CCK, sodium lactate, and adrenergic receptor agonists, such as yohimbine. Carbon dioxide and sodium lactate, two well-studied panicogens, alter brain pH balance that panic-prone people are sensitive in detecting. Brain pH chemosensors are located in the brainstem medulla and pons, the midbrain serotonergic raphe neurons, the hypothalamus, and the amygdala. Heightened pH sensitivity in the amygdala may play a key role in generating fearful perceptions and activating the cerebral cortex and neural circuits in the temporal lobe and brainstem, which further facilitates the production of panic symptoms (see Figs. 19.7 and 19.9).[62] Exaggerated activation of physiologic and behavioral arousal stemming from the noradrenergic locus ceruleus neurons also may enhance the symptoms of panic. Thus, panic-prone individuals appear especially sensitive in detecting pH alterations in brain sites that modulate fear and arousal.

PD also may involve the GABA-benzodiazepine (BZ) receptor system. BZ increases the $GABA_A$ ion channel response to GABA, thereby elevating chloride ion influx and producing a neuronal inhibitory effect. Brain imaging work reveals a reduction in BZ receptor binding in brain regions including the hippocampus, insular, and prefrontal cortex.[63] Drugs that block the BZ receptor are reported to increase panic attacks and feelings of anxiety, suggesting that an alteration in inhibitory neuromodulation contributes to PD.

Treatment. Up to 80% of individuals affected by PD respond to CBT and antidepressant drugs, either separately or in combination. In CBT, the individual learns that the physical symptoms are not fatal and attempts to exert control over the anxiety and panic. For example, breathing exercises to control hyperventilation serve to lessen the intense physiologic symptoms of panic, such as elevated heart and respiration rates. Another benefit of CBT is awareness of adherence with drug medications.

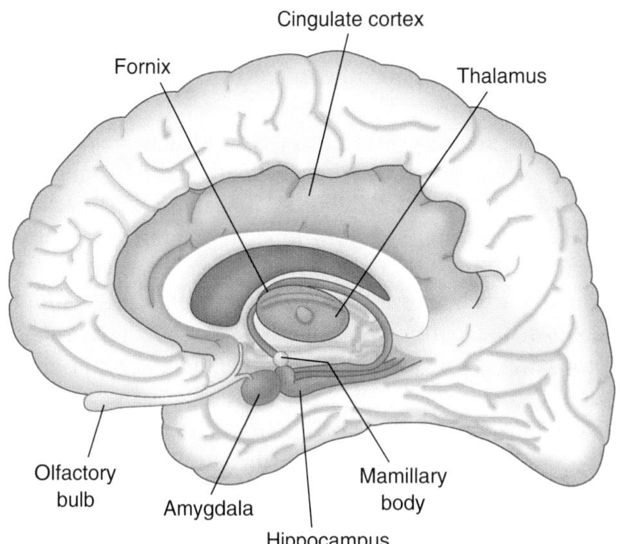

Fig. 19.9 The Lsimbic System. Structures of the limbic system play important roles in emotion, learning, and memory. Pathophysiology in limbic structures is frequently found in mental disorders.

However, for individuals with mild agoraphobia, CBT alone may be effective.

Antidepressants such as SSRIs are considered first-line medications for PD. Among the SSRIs, paroxetine and sertraline have received FDA approval specifically for PD. Venlafaxine, a serotonin-norepinephrine reuptake blocker, also is effective.

BZs, such as alprazolam and clonazepam, are other medications for treating PD. These medications also serve as an adjunct or augmentation therapy for individuals who do not fully respond to SSRIs. Short-term effects of BZs include sedation, ataxia, and cognitive impairments. Long-term BZ treatment may lead to potential physiologic and psychologic dependence. Abrupt BZ withdrawal induces a withdrawal syndrome of heightened reemergence of anxiety, insomnia, photophobia, and diarrhea. A gradual reduction in BZ medication or adjunct CBT may reduce the reliance and withdrawal symptoms of BZs.

Social Anxiety Disorder

SAD, also known as *social phobia*, is characterized by fear and avoidance of social situations. For example, the anxious person may feel very uncomfortable having a conversation or interacting with others and very conscious of being scrutinized and humiliated or rejected by others. A person diagnosed with SAD suffers significant distress or impairment that interferes with ordinary routines in everyday social settings, at work or at school.[21] Epidemiologic surveys indicate that SAD is one of the most common psychiatric disorders with 12-month and lifetime prevalence rates of 6.8% and 12.1%, respectively.[64] The onset of SAD often occurs during adolescence.[65] As with adults, children with SAD exhibit fear of speaking, reading, and eating in public; going to parties; speaking to authority figures; and engaging in informal social interactions.

Etiology and Pathophysiology. A prominent finding from brain imaging work with SAD people is the increased activity found in limbic and frontal cortical areas. Exposure to facial expressions of threat, which individuals with hypersensitive SAD are likely to perceive as extreme dislike, rejection, or criticism, often implicates the amygdala and its connections to other brain regions. Heightened anxiety in SAD may arise from deficits in an inhibitory tone from prefrontal cortical areas to the amygdala resulting in increased amygdala activation and a fear bias in threat-related processing.[66] Support of abnormal signaling comes from work showing decreased white matter connectivity between the amygdala and orbitofrontal cortex.[67]

Neuroimaging studies have also implicated neurotransmitter systems. One study in individuals with SAD noted altered serotonergic neurotransmission,[68] which may be caused by a reduction in the serotonin 5-HT1A-binding protein in the amygdala, anterior cingulate, and insula. Another study found a reduction in GABA in the thalamus of individuals with SAD.[69] Impaired GABAergic function may contribute to amygdala hyperactivity observed in SAD.

The neuropeptide oxytocin (OXT) has attracted considerable research attention. OXT is produced in the hypothalamic paraventricular and supraoptic nuclei and secreted by the posterior pituitary gland. OXT is well known to be secreted during childbirth and lactation. In addition, an increasing body of work indicates that OXT secretion has antianxiety effects by reducing HPA activation; promoting social, attachment, and maternal behavior; and increasing empathy and trust.

Of relevance to SAD, OXT plasma levels are reduced in individuals with SAD before and after playing a trust game, which normally increases OXT levels and promotes cooperation and reciprocation in control groups.[70] The reduction in OXT may account for the amygdala hyperactivity accompanied by excessive social avoidance and fear in SAD.[71] Indeed, intranasal OXT administration is reported to attenuate amygdala reactivity to threatening facial expressions,[72] perhaps by promoting GABAergic inhibition in the amygdala.[73]

Intranasal OXT also improves self-reported speech performance compared with placebo.[74] The oxytocin system is further implicated in SAD on a genetic level. An OXT receptor single nucleotide polymorphism was found to be associated with negative emotionality[75] and moral judgments.[76] On the basis of these studies, the OXT system is a promising target to potentially develop treatments for SAD and disorders related to social dysfunctioning, such as autism.[77]

Treatment. The antidepressant SSRIs that include fluoxetine, paroxetine, sertraline, and fluvoxamine along with the serotonin-norepinephrine reuptake inhibitor (SNRI) venlafaxine are considered first-line pharmacotherapies for SAD. These medications shared similar efficacy profiles and are approved by the FDA for treatment of SAD. However, drug-related side effects, such as agitation and sexual dysfunction, can be distressing for some individuals with SAD. Also, discontinuation of medication increases the risk for relapse. One study reported that 60% of indviduals with SAD relapsed after discontinuation of sertraline treatment.[78] Alternatives to SSRI and SNRI treatments may include psychologic or cognitive and group behavioral therapies.[79,80] Individuals with SAD are reported to respond well to CBT compared to placebo. The choice between pharmacotherapy and CBT may depend on the person's preference and access to treatment. Of note, psychologic interventions at the end of acute drug treatment appear beneficial in continuing to alleviate the symptoms of SAD and may lower the side effects of long-term drug treatment.

Generalized Anxiety Disorder

Excessive and persistent worries are the hallmarks of GAD. The individual worries about life events such as marital relationships, job performance, health, money, or social status. The lifetime prevalence rates of GAD range from 4.1% to 6.6%, with somewhat higher rates in women than in men. GAD usually emerges in the early twenties but can occur in childhood. Six major symptoms of GAD have been identified and include restlessness, muscle tension, irritability, being easily fatigued, difficulty concentrating, and difficulty sleeping. The individual startles easily and frequently suffers from depression and panic attacks. The severity of symptoms fluctuates over time and may be linked to the changing nature of stress. Although GAD tends to be chronic, the symptoms may lessen with age. A frequent complication of GAD is substance abuse, which may result from self-medication with alcohol or drugs to relieve anxiety symptoms.

Etiology and Pathophysiology. Female twin studies suggest a concordance rate of 30%, but disease genes linked to specific chromosomes have yet to be identified. Abnormalities in the norepinephrine and serotonin systems were reported in GAD.[81] For example, there is a reduction in α_2-adrenergic receptor binding, a decrease in serotonin levels in CSF, and reduced platelet binding of paroxetine, an SSRI. Another reported alteration in GAD is a reduction of BZ binding in the left temporal hemisphere.[82] Two functional magnetic resonance imaging (fMRI) studies have revealed alterations in specific brain regions in adults and adolescents with GAD. One study in GAD adults showed that increased anticipatory anxiety was associated with elevated cingulate cortex activity, and both the heightened anxiety and cingulate cortex activation were reduced after 8 weeks of treatment with the SNRI venlafaxine.[83] This study suggests that a decrease in pathophysiologic cingulate cortex activity is a predictor of GAD treatment efficacy. In children and adolescents with GAD, brief exposure to masked angry faces induced heightened right amygdala activation, which correlated positively with the severity of anxiety.[84] This study underscores the role of abnormal amygdala activity in attentional bias or vigilance to threats in GAD.

Treatment. GAD is diagnosed when a person spends at least 6 months worrying excessively and engages in at least three of the six major symptoms.[21] SNRIs, such as venlafaxine or the SSRIs paroxetine and escitalopram, have become first-line therapeutics for managing GAD. These medications may produce relief of GAD symptoms within 1 week and are effective in treating comorbid symptoms of depression. Buspirone, which has an affinity for serotonin receptors (5-HT_{1A}), is another treatment option, although the onset of clinical efficacy may take 2 weeks. The primary side effects of buspirone, which lessen over time, include dizziness, headaches, nausea, and mild nervousness. GAD nonresponders to SNRIs or buspirone may be treated with BZs. However, because GAD tends to be chronic, and comorbid with depression or other anxiety disorders,[85] BZs are usually limited to short-term use and uncomplicated cases of GAD. In addition to drug therapy, behavioral therapy is used to acquire relaxation techniques that control anxiety.

POSTTRAUMATIC STRESS DISORDER

Exposure to a terrifying or life-threatening event may produce posttraumatic stress disorder (PTSD).[86,87] Although the disorder was initially described in combat situations and called "shell shock," "war neurosis," or "traumatic neurosis," PTSD does not develop only from exposure to traumatic experiences in the battlefield. PTSD may develop after exposure to threat of death, serious injury, or sexual violation. The disorder may develop within hours of the traumatic experience or after several months or years. The *DMS-5* criteria for PTSD list four diagnostic clusters described as re-experiencing, avoidance, negative cognitions and mood, and arousal. *Re-experiencing* refers to spontaneous recollection of the traumatic event, recurrent nightmares, flashbacks, or other intense or chronic psychologic distress. *Avoidance* refers to distressing memories, feelings, or external reminders of the traumatic event. *Negative cognitions and mood* may occur from a persistent and distorted sense of blame of self or others, from estrangement from others or diminished interest in activities, or from an inability to remember key aspects of the event. *Arousal* is marked by aggressive, reckless, or self-destructive behavior, sleep disturbances, hypervigilance, or related problems. The "flight" or "fight" behavioral aspects also are associated with the arousing nature of PTSD.

The lifetime prevalence rate of PTSD is 7% to 8%. In men, PTSD is usually found among combat veterans, whereas PTSD in women is often related to rape or assault. Abused children also may develop PTSD. Individuals with a history of psychiatric illness (major depression and panic disorder) or those lacking strong social support appear more sensitive to the effects of traumatic stress.

Etiology and Pathophysiology. The primary etiology of PTSD is exposure to a terrifying life-threatening event and likely involves stress-induced alterations in several neural structures and neurotransmitter systems. The amygdala and prefrontal cortex are highly involved in the pathophysiology of PTSD because these brain structures normally play important roles in how fearful memories are stored, retrieved, and extinguished. Individuals with PTSD who are exposed to trauma-related stimuli generally exhibit increased activity in the amygdala and diminished activity in prefrontal cortical areas. Persistent dysregulation of this fear-based memory system may underlie chronic PTSD—that is, the failure of prefrontal cortical inhibition to control amygdala-induced activation of fear compromises the extinction of fear memory.[88] Structural brain imaging studies show that combat-exposed PTSD victims also have a smaller hippocampus, a brain structure involved in endocrine functions and memory formation. Pediatric PTSD studies reveal a more generalized effect of trauma on reducing total brain volume. Other brain sites exhibiting increased activity in PTSD are the dorsal anterior cingulate cortex and insula, albeit similar findings were reported in other anxiety disorders (e.g., GAD, obsessive-compulsive disorder).[89]

A recent study reported PTSD is linked to neurodegeneration by cortical thinning, cellular aging, and a shorter-than-expected lifespan. Increased neurodegeneration and thinning in the brain occurred in the right lateral orbitofrontal cortex and right posterior cingulate cortex, which are brain areas associated with the regulation of emotions and threats; such neurodegenerative effects are also found in depression and cognitive impairments.[90]

Treatment. Chronic PTSD lasting for years may occur in 30% of diagnosed individuals. Paroxetine and sertraline are considered first-line SSRI medications for chronic PTSD because of their tendency to lessen the recurrent nightmares and flashbacks and to treat the high accompanying prevalence of depression and substance abuse. Other antidepressants, such as the TCAs (amitriptyline and imipramine), have moderate effects and are second-line drugs; drugs such as nefazodone and bupropion may provide benefits. BZs should be avoided as they have been found to be clinically ineffective for PTSD treatment and are associated with increased risks such as severity of PTSD symptoms, aggression, depression, and substance use.[91] Individuals with PTSD may undergo psychotherapy or exposure therapy that re-exposes them to controlled situations that elicit the fear responses. However, some individuals with PTSD are unable to tolerate the fear re-experiencing event. See the Emerging Science Box: Chronic Post-traumatic Stress Disorder Treatment for investigatory treatment options.

OBSESSIVE-COMPULSIVE DISORDER

Obsessive-compulsive disorder (OCD) is a chronic, disabling illness characterized by the two core symptoms of obsessions and compulsions. Obsessions are recurrent, intrusive thoughts or impulses that provoke intense anxiety that leads the individual to perform compulsive repetitive behavioral acts to alleviate the anxiety activated by the obsessions. Although *DSM-5* no longer classifies OCD as an anxiety disorder,[21] obsessions are associated with significant distress and compulsions that are consciously performed to reduce the obsession-related anxiety. OCD is a time-consuming illness that significantly impairs a range of everyday functions, such as social relationships, job performance, and academic success.

Examples of obsessions may include preoccupation with contamination, doubting, religious or sexual themes, or the belief that a negative outcome will occur if a specific act is not performed. Compulsions are ritualized acts such as washing, cleaning, checking, counting, organizing, and repeating specific thoughts or prayers. Performing the compulsions may provide temporary relief of the anxiety but also reinforces the dysfunctional thoughts and neural circuits that underlie the negative obsessions that generate the compulsive anxiety.

The lifetime prevalence rates of OCD range from 2% to 3% with a slightly higher onset in males during childhood or adolescence. In many cases, the OCD individual also is diagnosed with major depression, PD, or GAD.[92–94]

Among children with OCD, common comorbid disorders include Tourette syndrome, oppositional defiant disorder, ADHD, and depression;[95] 30% to 50% of adults report experiencing OCD in childhood.[96]

Etiology and Pathophysiology. Family and twin studies demonstrate that OCD involves polygenetic and environmental risk factors.[97] First-degree relatives of affected adults also are at increased risk (4.6%) of Tourette syndrome and tics in comparison with control relatives (1%). Thus, OCD and Tourette syndrome may share common genes and pathophysiology.

Functional brain imaging studies have identified a pathologic brain circuit consisting of increased metabolism in the anterior thalamus, orbitofrontal cortex, dorsal anterior cingulate cortex, and especially in the basal ganglia (Fig. 19.10) subregions of the caudate and putamen.[93,94] Abnormalities in caudate volume in OCD also are found using structural neuroimaging techniques. This neural circuit is activated in OCD people by symptom provocation and reduced by effective pharmacotherapy or psychotherapy. Some studies suggest that genes affecting the serotonergic, dopaminergic, and glutamate systems may contribute to the pathophysiologic basis of this OCD neural circuit.[95] One particular abnormality in the neural circuit of OCD is the dorsal anterior cingulate cortex (dACC). Several functional neuroimaging studies reported hyperactivity of the dACC in OCD people compared to controls. Furthermore, electrophysiologic

EMERGING SCIENCE BOX

Chronic Posttraumatic Stress Disorder Treatment

A treatment that rapidly reduces the symptoms of chronic posttraumatic stress disorder (PTSD) is currently under investigation. A recent randomized control trial found that repeated intravenous ketamine administration over 2 weeks in people with chronic PTSD significantly and rapidly reduced the symptoms of PTSD in 24 hours and continued over a median of 27.5 days. In addition to an improvement in PTSD symptoms which included intrusive thoughts, avoidance, and negative alterations in cognition and mood, comorbid depressive symptom severity was also significantly reduced compared to midazolam treated groups. Midazolam is a BZ used in this study as psychoactive anxiolytic control drug and found to temporarily reduced symptoms of anxiety in only a few people with PTSD. Esketamine, the s-enantiomer of ketamine, was approved by the FDA for intranasal use for people with treatment-resistant depression. Whether the easy intranasal application of esketamine produces the same beneficial effects of ketamine for chronic PTSD and comorbid depression remains to be determined.

Data from Feder A, et al. A randomized controlled trial of repeated ketamine administration for chronic posttraumatic stress disorder. *American Journal of Psychiatry*, 2021;178:193–202.

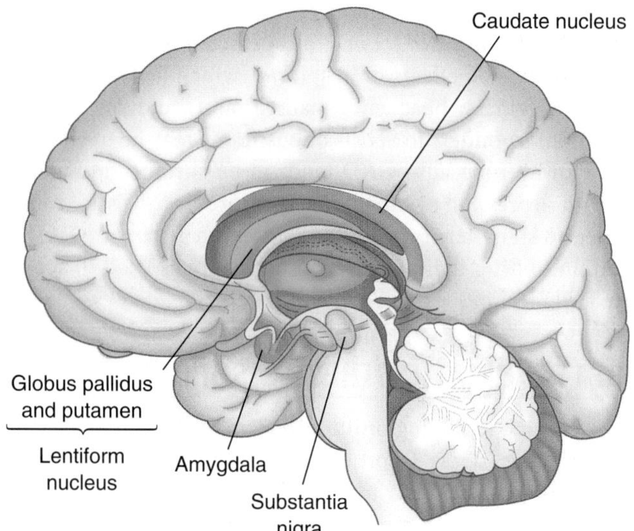

Fig. 19.10 Basal Ganglion. Structures of the basal ganglion, which include the caudate nucleus, putamen, globus pallidus, and substantia nigra, are important in movement.

studies showed altered biomarkers of cognitive control in the dACC. The dACC is hypothesized to be a key center that receives negative emotional and reinforcing information and integrates that information to direct motivated behavior.[98,99]

Treatment. SSRIs, including fluoxetine, fluvoxamine, paroxetine, escitalopram, and sertraline, are the first drugs of choice for OCD.[100] Approximately 70% to 80% of OCD individuals show a partial positive response that may be further improved by other medications. For example, clonazepam, a BZ, is found to improve the effects of fluoxetine and clomipramine therapy. The TCA clomipramine is also used if SSRIs are not effective or are not tolerated by the individual with OCD. The therapeutic effects of SSRIs and clomipramine may be the result of blocking serotonin reuptake and increasing serotonin availability in the brain of individuals with OCD.

Antipsychotic drugs (e.g., aripiprazole, haloperidol, risperidone, or quetiapine) in combination with SSRIs also are effective, especially in comorbid OCD and tic disorders. Here, the normalization of dysfunctional serotonin and dopamine brain systems in OCD may underlie the therapeutic effects of SSRIs and dopamine receptor-related drugs.[101,102]

Psychotherapy involves verbal interactions between a therapist and the individual to overcome the mental disorder. Several types of psychotherapy are available, but CBT and response preventive therapy are effective in treating OCD. CBT is a problem-focused, goal-directed, and time-limited treatment of the abnormal learned obsessions and compulsive actions. Response prevention therapy involves exposure to cues that elicit distress followed by preventing the individual from engaging in compulsive rituals for at least an hour or until the anxiety subsides. CBT employing response prevention therapy is found to produce long-term symptom remission.[103]

Because of the chronic nature of OCD, treatment in adults may involve pharmacotherapy, psychotherapy, a combination of pharmacotherapy and psychotherapy, brain modulation, or invasive brain methods.[104] In children, the American Academy of Child and Adolescent Psychiatry (AACAP)[105] recommends a combination of SSRI and CBT for those with moderate or severe OCD. However, recent meta-analysis studies find no strong evidence for the superiority of SSRI and CBT combination treatment in comparison to CBT alone for children with OCD.[106,107]

In people with severe OCD who are resistant to pharmaco- or psychotherapy, ECT and TMS may be used to provide some relief of OCD symptoms. Although the FDA recently approved TMS for severe treatment-resistant OCD, its long-term efficacy requires further studies.[108] An alternative, promising treatment for OCD is DBS, which also is used for intractable depression.[109] DBS in the anterior limb of internal capsule, striatum/ventral capsule, nucleus accumbens, subthalamic nucleus, and inferior thalamic peduncle is effective in alleviating some OCD symptoms.[110,111]

Stimulating these brain regions may be reducing abnormal neuronal firing in the neuroanatomic circuitry linked to OCD. The long-term treatment effects of DBS are still under investigation.

Another invasive treatment for individuals with severe treatment-resistant OCD is neurosurgery. One focus of neurosurgery is to disconnect the basal ganglia from the frontal cortex.[112] Dorsal anterior cingulotomy also is used in the treatment of refractory OCD.[113] Neurosurgery offers significant relief of obsessions and compulsions in nearly 50% of treatment-resistant OCD individuals.

SUMMARY REVIEW

Schizophrenia

1. Schizophrenia is characterized by thought disorders that reflect discontinuity between emotion, thought, behavior, and cognition.
2. Symptoms of schizophrenia are classified into positive, negative, and cognitive categories. Positive symptoms include hallucinations, delusions, formal thought disorder, and bizarre behavior. Negative symptoms include flattened affect, alogia, anhedonia, attention deficits, and apathy. Cognitive symptoms are the inability to perform daily tasks requiring attention and planning.
3. Schizophrenia has a strong genetic predisposition but environmental factors (e.g., viral infection, nutritional deficiencies, prenatal birth complications, urban upbringing) may interfere with genetically programmed neural development to alter brain structure and function.
4. Brain imaging studies reveal structural brain abnormalities including an enlargement of the cerebral ventricles and widening of the fissures and sulci in the frontal cortex. In addition, there is a reduction in the volumes of both the thalamus, which may disrupt communication among cortical brain regions, and the temporal lobe, which may be responsible for the manifestations of positive symptoms.
5. In schizophrenia, the frontal lobe shows a progressive loss in volume and a worsening of negative symptoms despite the use of antipsychotic medications. Blood flow and metabolism are reduced in the dorsolateral prefrontal cortex, compromising the ability to engage in goal-directed and cognitive problem-solving behavior.
6. Neurochemical abnormalities in dopamine and glutamate systems are found in schizophrenia.
7. The first generation of antipsychotic drugs blocks the dopamine D_2 receptor. The second generation, called atypical antipsychotics, blocks not only D_2 receptors but also dopamine, serotonin, and other neurotransmitter receptors. Antipsychotic medications are not always effective in treating the negative symptoms of schizophrenia. Talk therapies are used to improve medication adherence and to encourage coping strategies.

Mood Disorders: Depression and Bipolar Disorder

1. Major depression and bipolar disorder are two common mood disorders. Major depression is characterized by an intense and sustained unpleasant state of sadness and hopelessness. In bipolar disorder, individuals show recurrent patterns of depression and mania, the latter characterized by extreme levels of energy and euphoria.
2. Environmental triggers such as psychosocial stress appear to facilitate the onset of depression in individuals with a genetic vulnerability.
3. A reduction in brain monoamine neurotransmission is linked to depression, whereas an elevated monoamine level is associated with mania.
4. Exposure to uncontrollable stress elevates secretion of the stress hormone cortisol, which increases both the secretion of proinflammatory cytokines and the risk of developing depression. Abnormalities involving thyroid hormones also are found in depression.
5. Stress-induced depression is accompanied by deficits in brain-derived neurotrophic factor (BDNF) and neurogenesis in the hippocampus. In animal models, stress-induced depression-like behavior and the accompanying deficits in hippocampal BDNF and neurogenesis are reversed by antidepressant treatment.
6. The frontal lobe and limbic system volumes are reduced in major depression and bipolar illness. In addition, blood flow is altered in prefrontal and limbic brain regions that include the amygdala, a structure implicated in emotional behavior.
7. Pharmacotherapy involves the use of monoamine oxidase inhibitors (MAOIs), tricyclic antidepressants (TCAs), selective serotonin reuptake inhibitors (SSRIs), and atypical antipsychotics. Manic and bipolar individuals are treated with lithium, mood stabilizers, and atypical antipsychotic medications. Severely depressed and manic people may be administered electroconvulsive therapy (ECT). Deep brain stimulation is another promising treatment for intractable depression.

Anxiety Disorders

1. When normal fear and anxiety mental states persist and become uncontrollable, an individual may develop an anxiety disorder. Panic disorder (PD), social anxiety disorder (SAD), and generalized anxiety disorder (GAD) are examples of uncontrollable fear and anxiety states that require medical attention.
2. Panic disorder consists of panic attacks characterized by intense autonomic arousal that occurs spontaneously and is accompanied by symptoms including lightheadedness, tachycardia, and difficulty breathing. In addition, the intense occurrence of autonomic responses is accompanied by heightened fear and anxiety that often continue between panic attacks.
3. Panic-prone people are sensitive in detecting pH alterations in the amygdala, a brain structure that modulates fear. An activated amygdala recruits the cerebral cortex and neural circuits in the temporal lobe and brainstem, which may further exacerbate symptoms of panic.
4. A reduction in benzodiazepine (BZ) receptor binding in brain regions, including the hippocampus, insula, and prefrontal cortex, also may contribute to the pathophysiology of panic disorder.
5. Panic disorder is generally treatable with cognitive-behavioral therapy (CBT) and antidepressants such as TCAs and SSRIs. BZs are used as an adjunct or augmentation therapy for individuals who are nonresponsive to SSRIs or TCAs.
6. Social anxiety disorder is a common anxiety disorder that often emerges in adolescence and is characterized by fear and avoidance of social situations. SAD people are very sensitive in being evaluated and embarrassed or rejected by others.
7. Neuroimaging studies in SAD people are revealing abnormal connections between the prefrontal cortex and the amygdala.
8. The neuropeptide oxytocin (OXT) promotes social behavior, empathy, and trust. Secretion of OXT is reduced in SAD people, and a single nucleotide polymorphism of an OXT receptor gene is found to be altered in SAD, both of which suggest that OXT plays a major role in the pathophysiology of SAD.
9. SAD treatment may involve SSRI or serotonin-norepinephrine reuptake inhibitor (SNRI) drug or cognitive therapies.
10. GAD is characterized by excessive and persistent worries about life events. Individuals exhibit varying levels of motor disturbances, irritability, and fatigue that may be linked to fluctuations in psychosocial stress. Many GAD individuals manifest symptoms of depression.
11. Pathophysiologic changes in the cingulate cortex and amygdala may have prominent roles in stimulating anticipatory anxiety and attentional bias to threats in people with GAD.
12. Treatment of GAD usually involves a combination of behavioral therapy and drug medications, especially 5-HT/norepinephrine reuptake inhibitors.

Post-traumatic Stress Disorder

1. Posttraumatic stress disorder (PTSD) develops after exposure to a life-threatening or traumatic experience. Individuals experience recurring thoughts and flashbacks and nightmares of the terrifying event.
2. In PTSD, structural and/or functional alterations exist in the amygdala, prefrontal cortex, and hippocampus, which likely contribute to dysfunction in an emotional fear memory system.
3. Treatment of chronic PTSD is difficult and may involve psychotherapy and SSRI pharmacotherapy. Esketamine, a recently FDA-approved drug for treatment-resistant PTSD appears promising in rapidly alleviating the chronic symptoms of PTSD.

Obsessive-Compulsive Disorder

1. Obsessive-compulsive disorder (OCD) is a chronic illness characterized by irrational obsessions and ritualized acts that impair normal functioning and cause severe distress. It is a chronic disabling illness.

2. OCD is a time-consuming illness, which significantly impairs everyday functions, such as social relationships, job performance, and academic success. Examples of obsessions include preoccupation with doubting, religious or sexual themes, or the belief that a negative outcome will occur if a specific act is not performed.
3. A pathophysiologic brain circuit consisting of the anterior thalamus, orbitofrontal cortex, dorsal anterior cingulate cortex, and especially in the basal ganglia subregions of the caudate and putamen is involved in OCD.
4. OCD requires long-term treatment that may include psychotherapy and pharmacotherapy. In OCD people who are resistant these treatments, electroconvulsive therapy and transcranial magnetic stimulation may be used. People with severe OCD may require neurosurgery to disconnect regions of pathophysiologic brain circuit to provide relief of OCD symptoms. DBS may be another option for uncontrollable OCD.

REFERENCES

1. Kraeplin E. *Dementia praecox and paraphrenia*. Huntington, NY: Robert Krieger; 1971. Barclay RM, translator. Facsimile of 1919 edition.
2. Bleuler E. *Dementia praecox or the group of schizophrenias*. New York, NY: International Universities Press; 1950. Zinkin J, translator.
3. Johnson EC, et al. No evidence that schizophrenia candidate genes are more associated with schizophrenia than noncandidate genes. *Biol Psychiatry*. 2017;82:702–708.
4. Lewis DA, Levitt P. Schizophrenia as a disorder of neurodevelopment. *Annu Rev Neurosci*. 2002;25:409–432.
5. Marenco S, Weinberger DR. The neurodevelopmental hypothesis of schizophrenia: following a trail of evidence from cradle to grave. *Dev Psychopathol*. 2000;12(3):501–527.
6. Réthelyi JM, Benkovits J, Bitter I. Genes and environments in schizophrenia: the different pieces of a manifold puzzle. *Neurosci Biobehav Rev*. 2013;37:2424–2437.
7. Allswede DM, et al. Cytokine concentrations throughout pregnancy and risk for psychosis in adult offspring: a longitudinal case-control study. *Lancet Psychiatry*. 2020;7(3):254–261.
8. Berman KF, Meyer-Lindenberg A. Functional brain imaging studies in schizophrenia. In: Charney DS, Nestler EJ, eds. *Neurobiology of mental illness*. ed 2 New York: Oxford; 2004.
9. Shenton LD, et al. A review of MRI findings in schizophrenia. *Schizophr Res*. 2001;49(1–2):1–52.
10. Ross CA, et al. Neurobiology of schizophrenia. *Neuron*. 2006;52(1):139–153.
11. Pujol N, et al. Hippocampal abnormalities and age in chronic schizophrenia: morphometric study across the adult lifespan. *Br J Psychiatry*. 2014;250:369–375.
12. Bickart KC, Dickerson BC, Barrett LF. The amygdala as a hub in brain networks that support social life. *Neuropsychologia*. 2014;63:235–248.
13. Mukherjee P, et al. Altered amygdala connectivity within the social brain in schizophrenia. *Schizophr Bull*. 2014;40:152–160.
14. Aleman A, Kahn RS. Strange feelings: do amygdala abnormalities dysregulate the emotional brain in schizophrenia? *Prog Neurobiol*. 2005;77:283–298.
15. Costa E, et al. Dendritic spine hypoplasticity and downregulation of reelin and GABAergic tone in schizophrenia vulnerability. *Neurobiol Dis*. 2001;8(5):723–742.
16. Shi L, Bergson CM. Neuregulin 1: an intriguing therapeutic target for neurodevelopmental disorder. *Transl Psychiatry*. 2020;10:190.
17. Fatemi SH, Earle JA, McMenomy T. Reduction in reelin immunoreactivity in hippocampus of subjects with schizophrenia, bipolar disorder and major depression. *Mol Psychiatry*. 2000;5(6):654–663.
18. Duncan GE, Sheitman BB, Lieberman JA. An integrated view of pathophysiological models of schizophrenia. *Brain Res Brain Res Rev*. 1999;29(2–3):250–264.
19. Coyle JT, Tsai G, Goff D. Converging evidence of NMDA receptor hypofunction in the pathophysiology of schizophrenia. *Ann N Y Acad Sci*. 2003;1003:318–327.
20. Jentsch JD, et al. Enduring cognitive deficits and cortical dopamine dysfunction in monkeys after long-term administration of phencyclidine. *Science*. 1997;277:953–955.
21. American Psychiatric Association (APA) *Diagnostic and statistical manual of mental disorders (DSM-5)*. ed 5 Washington DC: APA; 2013.
22. Carbon M, et al. Tardive dyskinesia risk with first and second generation antipsychotics in comparative randomized controlled trials: a meta analysis. *World Psychiatry*. 2018;17(3):330–340.
23. Tamminga CA. Principles of the pharmacotherapy of schizophrenia. In: Charney DS, Nestler EJ, eds. *Neurobiology of mental illness*. ed 2, New York: Oxford; 2004.
24. Tai S, Turkington D. The evolution of cognitive behavior therapy for schizophrenia: current practice and recent developments. *Schizophr Bull*. 2009;35(5):865–873.
25. World Health Organization (WHO) *Depression*. Geneva: WHO; 2021. Available at https://www.who.int/health-topics/depression#tab=tab_1. (Accessed October 18, 2021).
26. Shih RA, Belmonte PL, Zandi PP. A review of the evidence from family, twin and adoption studies for a genetic contribution to adult psychiatric disorders. *Int Rev Psychiatry*. 2004;16:260–283.
27. Heninger GR, et al. The revised monoamine theory of depression: a modulatory role for monoamines, based on new findings from monoamine depletion experiments in humans. *Pharmacopsychiatry*. 1996;29(1):2–11.
28. Holsboer F. The corticosteroid receptor hypothesis of depression. *Neuropsychopharmacology*. 2000;23:477.
29. Wium-Andersen MK, et al. Elevated C-reactive protein levels, psychological distress, and depression in 73131 individuals. *JAMA Psychiatry*. 2013;70:176–184.
30. Dahl J, et al. The plasma levels of various cytokines are increased during ongoing depression and are reduced to normal levels after recovery. *Psychoneuroendocrinology*. 2014;45:77–86.
31. Borsini A, et al: Omega-3 polyunsaturated fatty acids protect inflammation through production of LOX and CYT450 lipid mediators: relevance for major depression and for human hippocampal neurogenesis, *Mol Psychiatry*. Published online ahead of print June 16, 2021. Available at https://doi.org/10.1038/s41380-021-01160-8. (Accessed October 18, 2021).
32. Masi G, Brovedani P. The hippocampus, neurotrophic factors and depression. Possible implications for the pharmacotherapy of depression. *CNS Drugs*. 2012;25(11):913–931.
33. Bauer M, et al. The thyroid-brain interaction in thyroid disorders and mood disorders. *J Neuroendocrinol*. 2008;20:1101–1114.
34. Hage MP, Azar ST. The link between thyroid function and depression. *J Thyroid Res*. 2012;2012:590648.

35. Drevets WC. Prefrontal cortical-amygdalar metabolism in major depression. *Ann N Y Acad Sci.* 1999;877:614–637.
36. Rajkowska G. Depression: what we can learn from postmortem studies. *Neuroscientist.* 2003;9(4):273–284.
37. Frodl T, O'Keane V. How does the brain deal with cumulative stress? A review with focus on developmental stress, HPA axis function and hippocampal structure in humans. *Neurobiol Dis.* 2013;52:24–37.
38. Saleh K, et al. Impact of family history and depression on amygdala volume. *Psychiatry Res.* 2012;203:24–30.
39. Maletic C, Raison C. Integrative neurobiology of bipolar disorder. *Front Psychiatry.* 2014;5:99.
40. Duman RS, Aghajanian GK. Synaptic dysfunction in depression: potential therapeutic targets. *Science.* 2012;338:68–72.
41. Newport DJ, et al. Ketamine and other NMDA antagonists: early clinical trials and possible mechanisms in depression. *Am J Psychiatry.* 2015;172:950–966.
42. Abdallah CG, et al. Modulation of the antidepressant effects of ketamine by the mTORC1 inhibitor rapamycin. *Neuropsychopharmacology.* 2020;45:990–997.
43. Kryst J, Kawalec P, Pilc A. Efficacy and safety of intranasal esketamine for the treatment of major depressive disorder. *Expert Opin Pharmacother.* 2020;21:9–20.
44. Krystal JH, Charney DS, Duman RS. A new rapid-acting antidepressant. *Cell.* 2020;181:7.
45. Whittington CJ, et al. Selective serotonin reuptake inhibitors in childhood depression: systematic review of published versus unpublished data. *Lancet.* 2004;363(9418):1341–1345.
46. Joshi SH, et al. Structural plasticity of the hippocampus and amygdala induced by electroconvulsive therapy in major depression. *Biol Psychiatry.* 2016;79:282–292.
47. Goodman WK, Alterman RL. Deep brain stimulation for intractable psychiatric disorders. *Annu Rev Med.* 2012;63:511–524.
48. Hamani C, et al. The subcallosal cingulate gyrus in the context of major depression. *Biol Psychiatry.* 2011;69:301–308.
49. Kennedy SH, et al. Deep brain stimulation for treatment-resistant depression: follow-up after 3 to 6 years. *Am J Psychiatry.* 2011; 168:502–510.
50. van Dijk A, et al. Deep brain stimulation of the accumbens increases dopamine, serotonin, and noradrenaline in the prefrontal cortex. *J Neurochem.* 2012;123:897–903.
51. George MS, Taylor JJ, Short EB. The expanding evidence base for rTMS treatment of depression. *Curr Opin Psychiatry.* 2013;26:13–18.
52. Boland RJ, Keller MB. The course of depression. In: Davis KL, ed. *Neuropsychopharmacology: the fifth generation of progress.* Philadelphia: Lippincott Williams & Wilkins; 2002.
53. Backs-Dermott BJ, Dobson KS, Jones SL. An evaluation of an integrated model of relapse in depression. *J Affect Disord.* 2010;124(1–2):60–67.
54. Trivedi MH, et al. What moderator characteristics are associated with better prognosis for depression? *Neuropsychiatr Dis Treat.* 2005;1(1):51–57.
55. Cruwys T, et al. Social group memberships protect against future depression, alleviate depression symptoms and prevent depression relapse. *Soc Sci Med.* 2013;98:179–186.
56. Goldberg JF. What psychotherapists should know about pharmacotherapies for bipolar disorder. *J Clin Psychol.* 2007;63(5):475–490.
57. Rhee TG, et al. 20-year trends in the pharmacologic treatment of bipolar disorder by psychiatrist in outpatient care settings. *Am J Psychiatry.* 2020;177:706–715.
58. Miklowitz DJ, et al. Adjunctive psychotherapy for bipolar disorder. A systematic review and component network meta-analysis. *JAMA Psychiatry.* 2020;78:141–150.
59. Parens E, Johnston J. Controversies concerning the diagnosis and treatment of bipolar disorder in children. *Child Adolesc Psychiatry Ment Health.* 2010;4:9.
60. Thorp JG, et al: Symptom-level modelling unravels the shared genetic architecture of anxiety and depression, Nat Hum Behav. Published online ahead of print April 15, 2021. Available at https://doi.org/10.1038/s41562-021-01094-9. (Accessed October 18, 2021).
61. Kennedy JL, et al. Investigation of cholecystokinin system genes in panic disorder. *Mol Psychiatry.* 1999;4(3):284.
62. Wemmie JA. Neurobiology of panic and pH chemosensation in the brain. *Dialogues Clin Neurosci.* 2011;13:475–483.
63. Malizia AL, et al. Decreased brain GABAA-benzodiazepine receptor binding in panic disorder. *Arch Gen Psychiatry.* 1998;55(8):715–720.
64. Kessler RC, et al. Lifetime prevalence and age-of-onset distributions of DSM-IV disorders in the National Comorbidity Survey Replication. *Arch Gen Psychiatry.* 2005;62:593–602.
65. Wittchen HU, Fehm L. Epidemiology, patterns of comorbidity, and associated disabilities of social phobia. *Psychiatr Clin North Am.* 2001;24:617–641.
66. Akirav I, Maroun M. The role of the medial prefrontal cortex-amygdala circuit in stress effects on the extinction of fear. *Neural Plast.* 2007 30873, 2007.
67. Fouche J-P, et al. Recent advances in the brain imaging of social anxiety disorder. *Hum Psychopharmacol.* 2013;28:102–105.
68. Lanzenberger RR, et al. Reduced serotonin-1A receptor binding in social anxiety disorder. *Biol Psychiatry.* 2007;61:1081–1089.
69. Pollack MH, et al. High-field MRS study of GABA, glutamate and glutamine in social anxiety disorder: response to treatment with levetiracetam. *Prog Neuropsychopharmacol Biol Psychiatry.* 2008;32:739–743.
70. Hoge EA, et al. Plasma oxytocin immunoreactive products and response to trust in patients with social anxiety disorder. *Depress Anxiety.* 2012;29:924–930.
71. Gorka SM, et al. Oxytocin modulation of amygdala functional connectivity to fearful faces in generalized social anxiety disorder. *Neuropsychopharmacology.* 2015;40:278–286.
72. Domes G, et al. Oxytocin attenuates amygdala responses to emotional faces regardless of valence. *Biol Psychiatry.* 2007;62:1187–1190.
73. Huber D, Veinante P, Stoop R. Vasopressin and oxytocin excite distinct neuronal populations in the central amygdala. *Science.* 2005;308:245–248.
74. Guastella A-J, et al. A randomized controlled trial of intranasal oxytocin as an adjunct to exposure therapy for social anxiety disorder. *Psychoneuroendocrinology.* 2009;34:917–923.
75. Montag C, et al. Interaction of 5-HTTLPR and a variation on the oxytocin receptor gene influences negative emotionality. *Biol Psychiatry.* 2011;69:601–603.
76. Walter NT, et al. Ignorance is no excuse: moral judgments are influenced by a genetic variation on the oxytocin receptor gene. *Brain Cogn.* 2012;78:268–273.
77. Meyer-Lindenberg A, et al. Oxytocin and vasopressin in the human brain: social neuropeptides for translational medicine. *Nat Rev Neurosci.* 2011;12:524–538.
78. Koen N, Stein DJ. Pharmacotherapy of anxiety disorders: a critical review. *Dialogues Clin Neurosci.* 2011;13:423–437.

79. Barkowski S, et al. Efficacy of group psychotherapy for social anxiety disorder: a meta-analysis of randomized-controlled trials. *J Anxiety Disord*. 2016;39:44–64.
80. Mayo-Wilson E, et al. Psychological and pharmacological interventions for social anxiety disorder in adults: a systematic review and network meta-analysis. *Lancet Psychiatry*. 2014;1:368–376.
81. Jetty PV, et al. Neurobiology of generalized anxiety disorder. *Psychiatr Clin North Am*. 2001;24(1):75.
82. Tiihonen J, et al. Cerebral benzodiazepine receptor binding and distribution in generalized anxiety disorder. *Mol Psychiatry*. 1997;2(6):463–471.
83. Nitschke JB, et al. Anticipatory activation in the amygdala and anterior cingulate in generalized anxiety disorder and prediction of treatment response. *Am J Psychiatry*. 2009;166:302–310.
84. Monk CS, et al. Ventrolateral prefrontal cortex activation and attentional bias in response to angry faces in adolescents with generalized anxiety disorder. *Am J Psychiatry*. 2006;163:1091–1097.
85. Bruce SE. Infrequency of "pure" GAD: impact of psychiatric comorbidity on clinical course. *Depress Anxiety*. 2001;14(4):219–225.
86. Charney DS, et al. Psychobiologic mechanisms of posttraumatic stress disorder. *Arch Gen Psychiatry*. 1993;50(4):294–305.
87. Southwick SM, et al. Neurotransmitter alterations in PTSD: catecholamines and serotonin. *Semin Clin Neuropsychiatry*. 1999;4(4):242–248.
88. Bremner JD, et al. Structural and functional plasticity of the human brain in posttraumatic stress disorder. *Prog Brain Res*. 2008;167:171–186.
89. Shin LM, Liberzon I. The neurocircuitry of fear, stress, and anxiety disorders. *Neuropsychopharmacology*. 2010;35(1):169–191.
90. Katrinli S, et al. Evaluating the impact of trauma and PTSD on epigenetic prediction of lifespan and neural integrity. *Neuropsychopharmacology*. 2020;45:1609–1616.
91. Guina J, et al. Benzodiazepines for PTSD: a systematic review and meta analysis. *J Psychiatr Pract*. 2015;21(4):281–303. Available at https://doi.org/10.1097/pra.0000000000000091. (Accessed October 18, 2021).
92. Fireman B, et al. The prevalence of clinically recognized obsessive-compulsive disorder in a large health maintenance organization. *Am J Psychiatry*. 2001;158(11):1904–1910.
93. Rauch SL, et al. Probing striato-thalamic function in obsessive-compulsive disorder and Tourette syndrome using neuroimaging methods. *Adv Neurol*. 2001;85:207–224.
94. Rosenberg DR, et al. Brain anatomy and chemistry may predict treatment response in paediatric obsessive-compulsive disorder. *Int J Neuropsychopharmacol*. 2001;4:179–190.
95. Geller DA, et al. Fluoxetine treatment for obsessive-compulsive disorder in children and adolescents: a placebo-controlled clinical trial. *J Am Acad Child Adolesc Psychiatry*. 2001;40:773–779.
96. Rasmussen SA. Epidemiology of obsessive compulsive disorder. *J Clin Psychiatry*. 1990;51(Suppl):10–13.
97. Pauls DL, et al. Obsessive-compulsive disorder: an integrative genetic and neurobiological perspective. *Nat Rev Neurosci*. 2014;15:410–424.
98. McGovern RA, Sheth SA. Role of the dorsal anterior cingulate cortex in obsessive-compulsive disorder: converging evidence from cognitive neuroscience and psychiatric neurosurgery. *J Neurosurg*. 2017;126(1):132–147.
99. Shackman AJ, et al. The integration of negative affect, pain and cognitive control in the cingulate cortex. *Nat Rev Neurosci*. 2011;12:154–167.
100. Ahmari SE, Simpson HB. Neurobiology and treatment of OCD. In: Charney DS, ed. *Neurobiology of mental illness*. ed 4 New York: Oxford University Press; 2013:646–661.
101. Komossa K, et al. Second-generation antipsychotics for obsessive compulsive disorder. *Cochrane Database Syst Rev*. 2010;12:CD008121. Available at https://doi.org/10.1002/14651858.cd008121.pub2. (Accessed October 18, 2021).
102. Pampaloni I, Tyagi H, Drummond L. Augmentation in profound, SRI refractory OCD: is aripiprazole superior to other dopamine blockers? *Eur Psychiatry*. 2017;41(S1):S322–S324. Available at https://doi.org/10.1016/j.eurpsy.2017.02.246. (Accessed October 18, 2021).
103. McKay D, et al. Efficacy of cognitive-behavioral therapy for obsessive-compulsive disorder. *Psychiatry Res*. 2015;227:104–113.
104. Koran LM, et al. Practice guideline for the treatment of patients with obsessive-compulsive disorder. *Am J Psychiatry*. 2007;164(7 Suppl):5–53.
105. American Academy of Child and Adolescent Psychiatry (AACAP) Practice parameter for the assessment and treatment of children and adolescents with obsessive-compulsive disorder. *J Am Acad Child Adolesc Psychiatry*. 2012;51:98–113.
106. Ivarsson T, et al. The place of and evidence for serotonin reuptake inhibitors (SRIs) for obsessive compulsive disorder (OCD) in children and adolescents: views based on a systematic review and meta-analysis. *Psychiatry Res*. 2015;227:93–103.
107. Öst L-G, et al. Cognitive behavioral and pharmacological treatments of OCD in children: a systematic review and meta-analysis. *J Anxiety Disord*. 2016;43:58–69.
108. Goodman WK, Storch EA, Sheth SA. Harmonizing the neurobiology and treatment of obsessive-compulsive disorder. *Am J Psychiatry*. 2012;178:17–29.
109. Goodman WK, Alterman RL. Deep brain stimulation for intractable psychiatric disorders. *Annu Rev Med*. 2012;63:511–524.
110. de Koning PP, et al. Current status of deep brain stimulation for obsessive-compulsive disorder: a clinical review of different targets. *Curr Psychiatry Rep*. 2011;13:274–282.
111. Holtzheimer PE, Mayberg HS. Deep brain stimulation for psychiatric disorders. *Annu Rev Neurosci*. 2011;34:289–307.
112. Greenberg BD, Murphy DL, Rasmussen SA. Neuroanatomically based approaches to obsessive-compulsive disorder. *Psychiatr Clin North Am*. 2000;23(3):671–686.
113. Schlösser RGM, et al. Fronto-cingulate effective connectivity in obsessive compulsive disorder: a study with fMRI and dynamic causal modeling. *Hum Brain Mapp*. 2010;31:1834–1850.

20

Alterations of Neurologic Function in Children

John Ruge

http://evolve.elsevier.com/Rogers/pathophysiology/

CHAPTER OUTLINE

Neurologic disorders in children can occur from infancy through adolescence and include congenital malformations, genetic defects in metabolism, brain injuries, infection, tumors, and other disorders that affect neurologic function.

DEVELOPMENT OF THE NERVOUS SYSTEM IN CHILDREN

The nervous system develops from the embryonic ectoderm through a complex, sequential process. A neural tube starts to form 2 and one-half weeks from conception and "zippers shut" by 4 weeks. The spinal cord, spine, brain, and skull form from this neural tube. By approximately day 175, the brain has developed into all of its parts (Fig. 20.1A–C). The brain continues the formation of network connections and synapses from birth to many years postnatally. Many different events happen simultaneously, and critical periods must pass uninterrupted if the vulnerable fetus is to develop normally. Genetic and environmental factors (e.g., nutrition, hormones, oxygen levels, toxins, alcohol, drugs, maternal infections, maternal disease) can have a significant effect on neural development.[1,2]

The growth and development of the brain occur rapidly from the third month of gestation through the first year of life, reflecting the proliferation of neurons and glial cells. Although basically all of the neurons that an individual will ever have are present at birth, development of skills, such as walking, talking, and thinking, depends on these cells making correct connections with other cells and on myelination of the axons making those connections. The head is the fastest-growing body part during infancy. One-half of postnatal brain growth is achieved by the first year and is 90% complete by age 6 years. The cortex thickens with maturation, and the sulci deepen as a result of rapid expansion of the surface area of the brain. Cerebral blood flow and oxygen consumption during these years are approximately twice those of the adult brain.

The bones of the infant's skull are separated at the suture lines, forming two fontanelles, or "soft spots": one diamond-shaped anterior fontanelle and one triangular-shaped posterior fontanelle. The sutures allow for expansion of the rapidly growing brain. The sutures remain open, allowing for brain and skull growth into early and mid-adulthood. The posterior fontanelle may be open until 2 to 3 months of age; the anterior fontanelle normally does not fully close until 18 months of age (Fig. 20.2). Head growth almost always reflects brain growth. Monitoring the fontanelles and careful measurement and plotting of the head circumference on standardized growth charts are essential elements of the pediatric examination.

Because of the immaturity of much of the human forebrain at birth, neurologic examination of the infant detects mostly reflex responses that require an intact spinal cord and brainstem. A maturing brain tends to inhibit most reflexes, so as the brain matures, reflexes of infancy are normally lost. Persistent infantile reflexes can indicate developmental delay or a central nervous system (CNS) lesion. Absence of expected reflex responses at the appropriate age indicates general depression of central or peripheral motor functions. Asymmetric responses may indicate lesions in the motor cortex or peripheral nerves or may occur with fractures of bones after traumatic delivery or postnatal injury (Table 20.1).

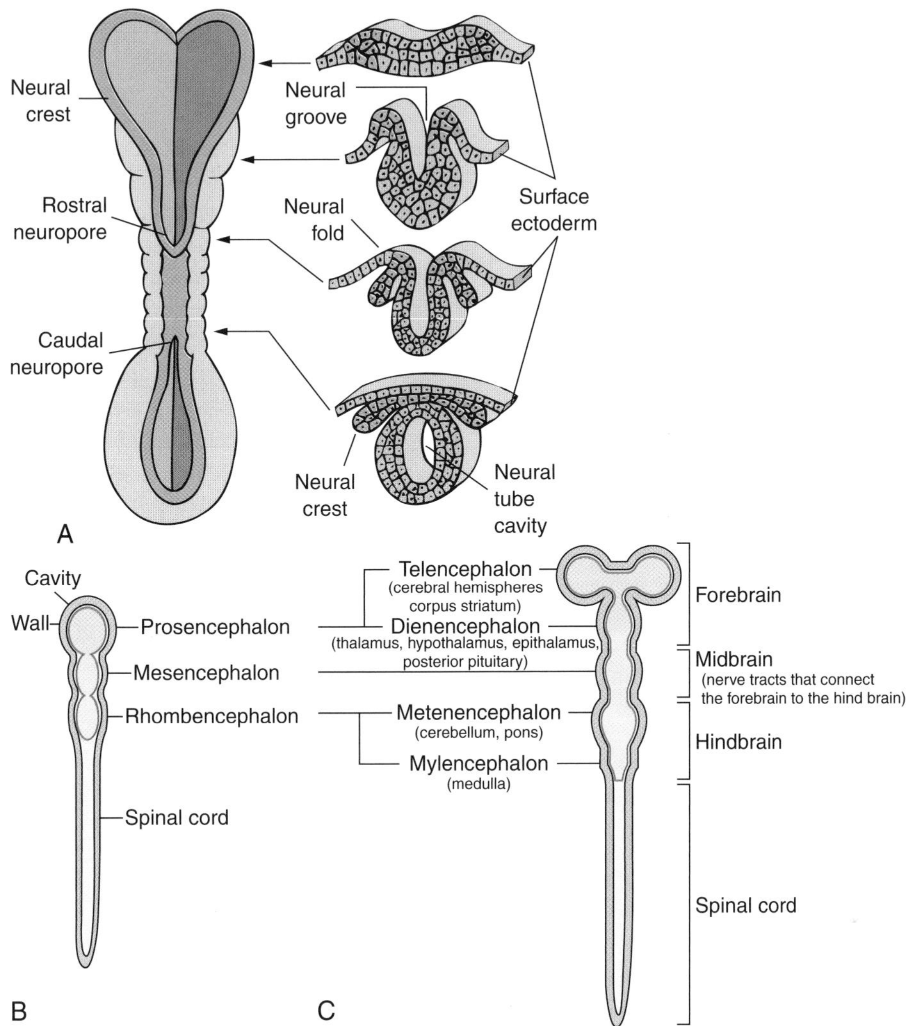

Fig. 20.1 Development of the Brain and Spinal Cord. (A) Neural tube at 3 weeks' gestation. Neural folds have begun to fuse at the cervical level of the future spinal cord. *Right,* Cross sections of the neural tube at four different levels; at any given level the embryonic central nervous system goes through a series of stages resembling these four cross sections. Total length of neural tube at this time is approximately 2.5 mm. **(B)** The anterior part of the neural tube enlarges to form the 3 primary vesicles of the brain. The narrow posterior part forms the spinal cord. **(C)** Primary and secondary vesicles develop into various parts of the brain.

STRUCTURAL MALFORMATIONS

Malformations of the CNS affect approximately 5 to 10 children per 1000 births. CNS malformations are responsible for 75% of fetal deaths and 40% of deaths during the first year of life. CNS malformations account for 33% of all apparent congenital malformations, and 90% of CNS malformations are defects of neural tube closure.

Defects of Neural Tube Closure

Neural tube defects (NTDs) are an arrest of the normal development of the brain and spinal cord during the first month of embryonic development. They occur in approximately 3000 pregnancies in the United States each year, although there are significant regional prevalence variations.[3] Fetal death often occurs in the more severe forms, thereby reducing the actual prevalence of neural defects at birth.

TABLE 20.1 Reflexes of Infancy

Reflex	Age of Appearance	Age at Which Reflex Should No Longer Be Obtainable
Moro	Birth	3 months
Stepping	Birth	6 weeks
Sucking	Birth	4 months awake 7 months asleep
Rooting	Birth	4 months awake 7 months asleep
Palmar grasp	Birth	6 months
Plantar grasp	Birth	10 months
Tonic neck	2 months	5 months
Neck righting	4–6 months	24 months
Landau	3 months	24 months
Parachute reaction	9 months	Persists indefinitely

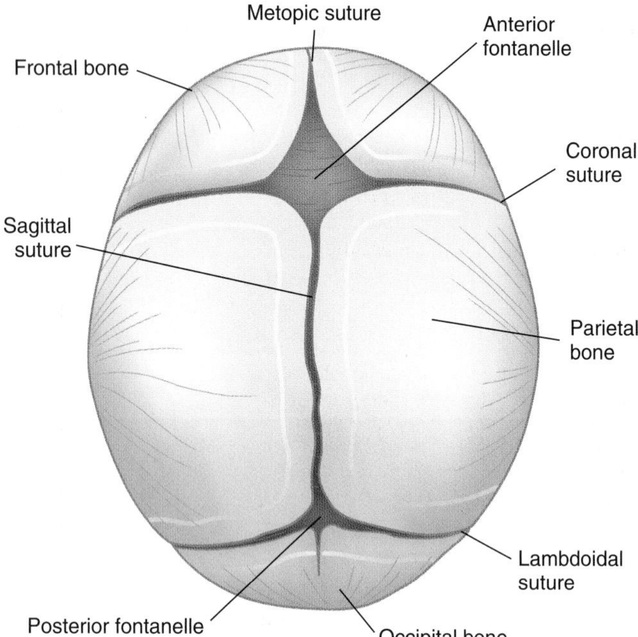

Fig. 20.2 Cranial Sutures and Fontanelles in Infancy. Fibrous union of the suture lines and interlocking of the serrated edges occurs by 6 months; solid union requires approximately 12 years. (Head growth charts are available from the Centers for Disease Control and Prevention at www.cdc.gov/nchs/data/series/sr_11/sr11_246.pdf).

The cause of NTDs is believed to be multifactorial (a combination of genes and environment). No single gene has been found to cause NTDs. Folic acid deficiency during preconception and early stages of pregnancy increases the risk for NTDs, and supplementation (400 mcg of folic acid per day) ensures adequate folate status. In 1996 the United States mandated folate fortification in many foods, and since that time NTDs have decreased by 20% to 30%. Guidelines are available for folic acid supplementation for women at high risk for NTDs.[4] Other risk factors include a previous NTD pregnancy, maternal diabetes or obesity, use of anticonvulsant drugs (particularly valproic acid), and maternal hyperthermia.[5] Defects of neural tube closure are divided into two categories: (1) anterior midline defects (ventral induction) and (2) posterior defects (dorsal induction). Anterior midline defects may cause brain and face abnormalities, with the most extreme form being cyclopia, in which the child has a single midline orbit and eye with a protruding nose-like proboscis above the orbit. Anencephaly (*an*, "without"; *enkephalos*, "brain") and encephalocele are also anterior midline defects. Spina bifida (split spine) is the most common NTD. Vertebrae fail to close in spina bifida, and the defect includes meningocele, myelomeningocele, and spina bifida occulta. Disorders of embryonic neural development are summarized in Fig. 20.3.

Anencephaly is an anomaly in which the soft, bony component of the skull and part of the brain are missing. This disorder occurs in approximately 1 in 4600 births in the United States each year.[6] These infants are stillborn or die within a few days after birth. The pathologic mechanism is unknown. Diagnosis is often made prenatally by using ultrasound or evaluating the maternal serum alpha fetoprotein (AFP).

Encephalocele refers to a herniation or protrusion of the brain and meninges through a defect in the skull, resulting in a sac-like structure. The incidence is approximately 1 in 10,500 live births in the United States each year.[7] Encephalocele treatment involves surgical closure of the skull opening. The complexity of the surgery depends on the location and content of the defect. Often several surgeries may be needed with variable long-term neurologic sequelae.

Meningocele is a sac-like cyst of meninges filled with spinal fluid and is a mild form of spina bifida (Fig. 20.4). It develops during the first 4 weeks of pregnancy when the neural tube fails to close completely and is the rarest type of spina bifida. The cystic dilation of meninges protrudes through the vertebral defect but does not involve the spinal cord or nerve roots and may produce no neurologic deficit or symptoms. Meningoceles occur most commonly in the lumbar spine.

Myelomeningocele (meningomyelocele; spina bifida cystica) is a hernial protrusion of a sac-like cyst (containing meninges, spinal fluid, and a portion of the spinal cord with its nerves) through a defect in the posterior arch of a vertebra. It is most commonly located as a sac on the lumbar and lumbosacral regions, the last regions of the neural tube to close. Myelomeningocele is one of the most common and severe developmental anomalies of the nervous system, with an incidence of approximately 1 per 4000 live births.[8] It accounts for 75% of all spina bifida cases.

Meningocele and myelomeningoceles are evident at birth as a pronounced skin defect on the infant's back (see Fig. 20.4). The bony prominences of the unfused neural arches can be palpated at the lateral border of the defect. The defect usually is covered by a transparent membrane that may have neural tissue attached to its inner surface. This membrane may be intact at birth or may leak cerebrospinal fluid (CSF), thereby increasing the risks of infection and neuronal damage. The spinal cord and nerve roots are malformed below the level of the lesion, resulting in loss of motor, sensory, reflex, and autonomic functions. A brief neurologic examination concentrating on motor function in the legs, reflexes, and sphincter tone is usually sufficient to determine the level above which spinal cord and nerve root function is preserved (Table 20.2). This is useful to predict if the child will ambulate, require bladder catheterization, or be at high risk for developing scoliosis (see Chapter 45).

Hydrocephalus occurs in 85% of infants with myelomeningocele.[9] Seizures also occur in 30% of those with myelomeningoceles. Visual and perceptual problems, including ocular palsies, astigmatism, and visuoperceptual deficits, are common. Motor and sensory functions below the level of the lesions are altered. *These* problems *should not* worsen as the child grows. If a neurologic decline is identified in a child with spina bifida, the cause needs to be investigated.

Myelomeningoceles are almost always associated with the Chiari II malformation.[9] This is a complex malformation of the brainstem and cerebellum in which the cerebellar tonsils are displaced downward through the foramen magnum and into the cervical spinal canal. The upper medulla and lower pons are

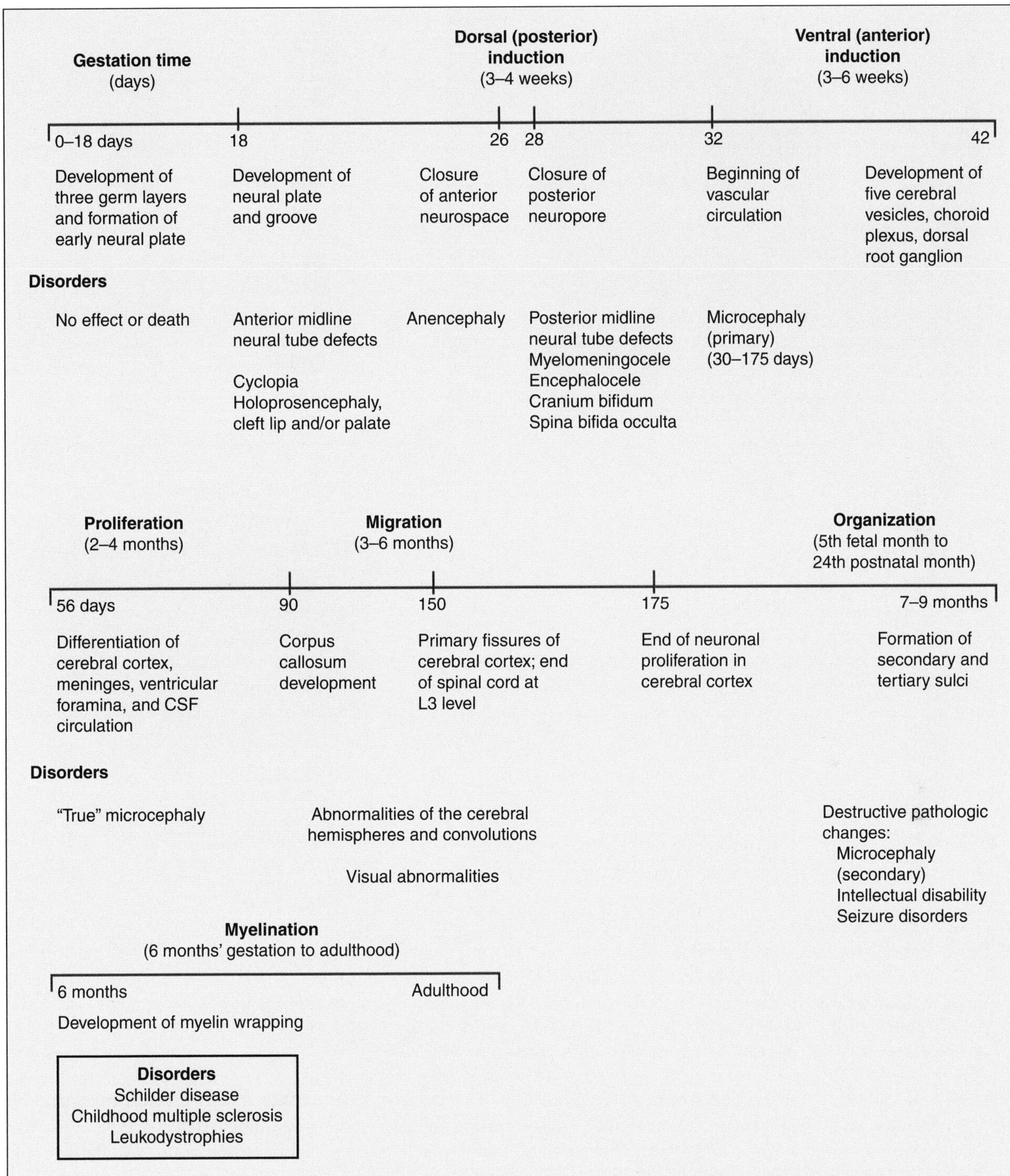

Fig. 20.3 Disorders Associated With Specific Stages of Embryonic Development. *CSF*, Cerebrospinal fluid.

TABLE 20.2 Functional Alterations in Myelomeningocele Related to Level of Lesion

Level of Lesion	Functional Implications
Thoracic	Flaccid paralysis of lower extremities; variable weakness in abdominal trunk musculature; high thoracic level may mean respiratory compromise; absence of bowel and bladder control
High lumbar	Voluntary hip flexion and adduction; flaccid paralysis of knees, ankles, and feet; may walk with extensive braces and crutches; absence of bowel and bladder control
Mid lumbar	Strong hip flexion and adduction; fair knee extension; flaccid paralysis of ankles and feet; absence of bowel and bladder control
Low lumbar	Strong hip flexion, extension, and adduction and knee extension; weak ankle and toe mobility; may have limited bowel and bladder function
Sacral	Normal function of lower extremities; normal bowel and bladder function

Modified from Sandler AD. Children with spina bifida: Key clinical issues. *Pediatric Clinics of North America*, 2010;57(4):879–892.

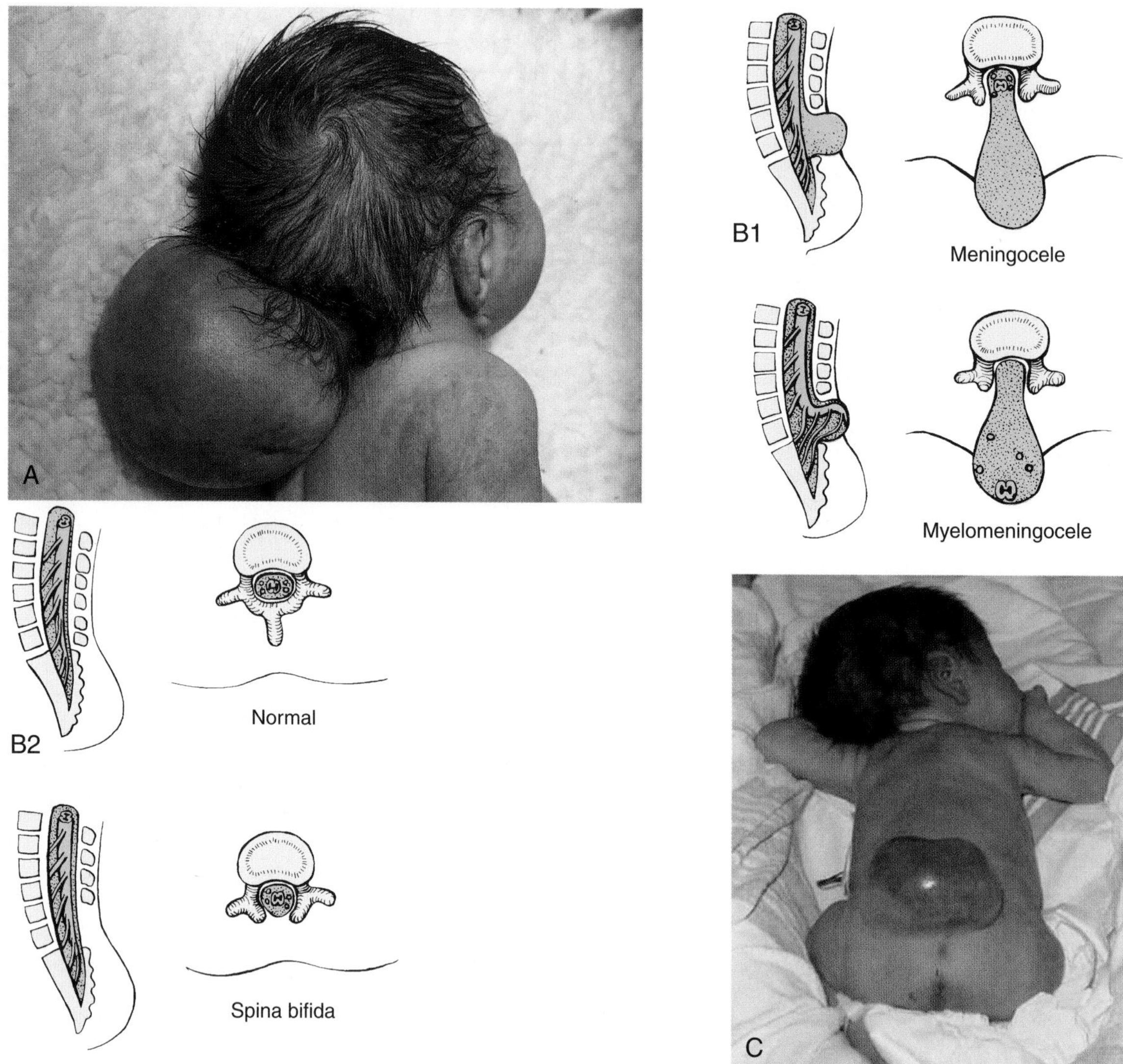

Fig. 20.4 (A) Meningoencephalocele of the Occipital Region. **(B1)** Meningocele, Myelomeningocele. **(B2)** Normal Spine, Spina Bifida. **(C)** Myelomeningocele with an Intact Sac. (From Hockenberry MJ, Wilson D. *Wong's nursing care of infants and children*. 10th ed. St Louis: Mosby; 2015.). (A from (From GilbertBarness: Potter's pathology of the fetus, infant and child, ed 2, Philadelphia: Mosby 2007, B from Hockenberry MJ, Wilson D. *Wong's nursing care of infants and children*, 10th edition. St. Louis: Mosby; 2015.)

elongated and thin, and the medulla is also displaced downward and sometimes has a "kink" (Fig. 20.5). The Chiari II malformation is associated with hydrocephalus from pressure that blocks the flow of CSF. The Chiari II malformation is also associated with syringomyelia, an abnormality resulting from CSF migrating into the center of the spinal cord forming a pocket or cyst (syrinx) that can expand and cause pressure on the spinal cord, resulting in bowel, bladder, sensory, and motor dysfunction. The incidence of Chiari II malformation is reduced in those children operated on in utero for myelomeningocele.

Other types of Chiari malformations are not associated with spina bifida. In type I Chiari malformation the cerebellar tonsils protrude into the foramen magnum and the brainstem is not involved. Type I Chiari is the most common of all Chiari malformations and may be asymptomatic or symptomatic (e.g., neck pain, dizziness, difficulty with gait and swallowing), sometimes requiring neurosurgical intervention. In type III, the brainstem or cerebellum extends into a high cervical myelomeningocele and can cause serious neurologic defects. Type IV is characterized by lack of cerebellar development (cerebellar hypoplasia).

Most cases of meningocele and myelomeningocele are diagnosed prenatally by a combination of maternal serologic testing (AFP) and prenatal ultrasound. In these cases, the fetus is usually delivered by elective cesarean section to minimize trauma during labor. Surgical repair is critical and can be performed by in utero fetal surgery or during the first 72 hours of life.[10] It is possible for a defect to occur without any visible exposure of meninges or neural tissue, and the term spina bifida occulta is then used. The defect is common and occurs to some degree in 10% to 25% of infants. Spina bifida occulta usually causes no neurologic dysfunction because the spinal cord and spinal nerves are normal. A sacral dimple on examination of a newborn infant can be associated with spina bifida occulta and should be further evaluated. Any midline skin abnormality such as a hairy tuft,

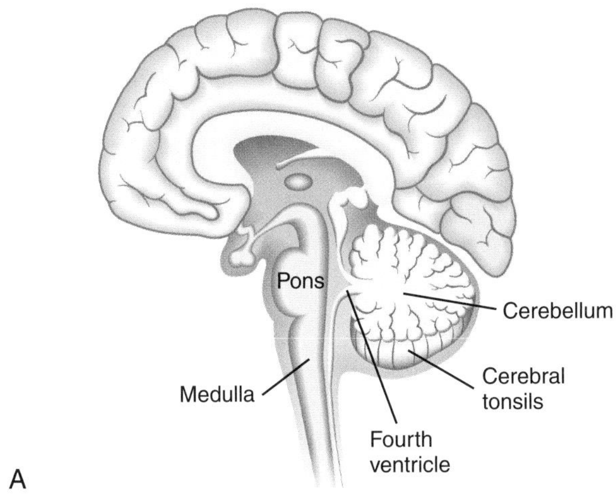

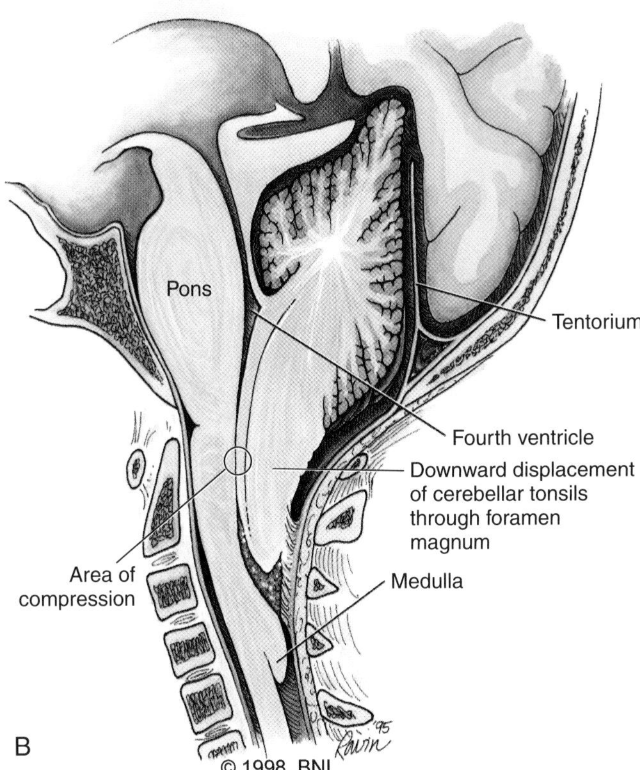

Fig. 20.5 Normal Brain and Arnold-Chiari II Malformation. **(A)** Diagram of a normal brain. **(B)** Diagram of an Arnold-Chiari II malformation, showing downward displacement of the cerebellar tonsils and medulla through the foramen magnum causing, compression and obstruction of cerebrospinal fluid flow. (B, Modified from Barrow Neurological Institute of St Joseph's Hospital and Medical Center. Reprinted with permission.)

hemangioma type lesion, or unusual dimple may indicate underlying spinal pathology and should be evaluated. Tethered cord syndrome may develop after surgical correction for myelomeningocele. The cord becomes abnormally attached or tethered in the lumbar cistern as a result of scar tissue as the cord ascends in the vertebral canal with growth.[11] Although radiographically almost all persons affected by myelomeningocele will appear to be tethered, only those with symptoms or new neurologic decline warrant further investigation, and prompt neurosurgical release of the tethering is appropriate. Special attention should be given to children whose myelomeningocele was corrected in utero, because their risks of spinal cord retethering is increased (see Emerging Science Box: In Utero Myelomeningocele Surgery).

Craniosynostosis

Skull malformations range from minor, insignificant defects to major defects that are incompatible with life. Craniosynostosis (craniostenosis) is the premature closure of one or more of the cranial sutures (sagittal, coronal, lambdoid, metopic) during the first 18 to 20 months of the infant's life. The incidence of craniosynostosis is approximately 1 per 2500 live births.[12] Males are affected twice as often as females. Fusion of a cranial suture prevents growth of the skull perpendicular to the suture line, resulting in an asymmetric shape of the skull. The general term *plagiocephaly*, meaning "misshapen skull," is used to describe deformities that result from craniosynostosis or from asymmetric head posture (positional). When a single coronal suture fuses prematurely, the head is flattened on that side in front. When the sagittal suture fuses prematurely, the head is elongated in the

EMERGING SCIENCE BOX

In Utero Myelomeningocele Surgery

Operating on a fetus in utero with spina bifida reduces the risk of developing hydrocephalus and Chiarimalformation and may improve motor function. This can have a very positive impact for the child in terms quality of life. Prenatal repair of myelomeningocele continues to evolve since first reported by Bruner and Tulipan in 1997. Typically after myelomeningocele has been confirmed and the mother is 18 years of age or older and between 19 and 25.9 weeks' gestation, the surgery is performed either endoscopically or by small open hysterotomy. Candidates for this surgery are typically screened very carefully, and the spinal defect must be below thoracic level 1. Maternal and fetal risks are increasingly being reduced with further experience. Preterm delivery remains a significant problem such that this operation is best performed by an experienced team with delivery by cesarean section. The child may have increased risk of retethering and intraspinal dermoid cysts. Long-term evaluation of neurologic function and quality of life are ongoing.

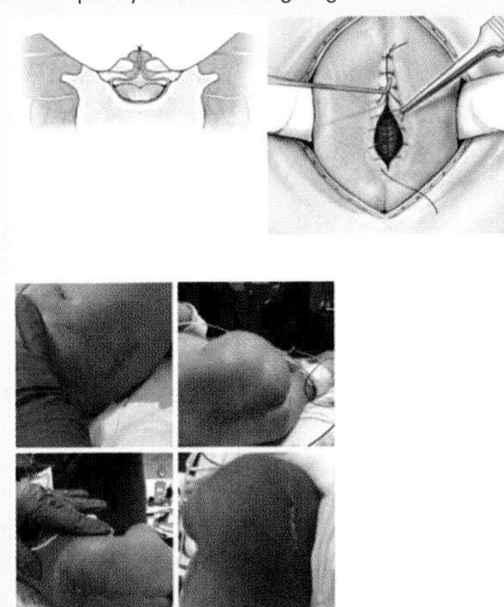

Data from: Bruner JP, et al. Endoscopic coverage of fetalopen myelomeingocelein utero. *Am J ObstetGynecol.*1997;176:256–257:; Eggink AJ, et al. Neural tube anomalies: An update on the pathophysiology and prevention. In: *Fetal therapy: Scientific basis and critical appraisal of clinical benefits*, Cambridge: Cambridge University Press. January 2, 2020:449–455; Dewan MC, et al. Fetal surgery for spina bifida. *Journal of Neurosurgery. Pediatrics*, August 1, 2019;24(2):105–114.

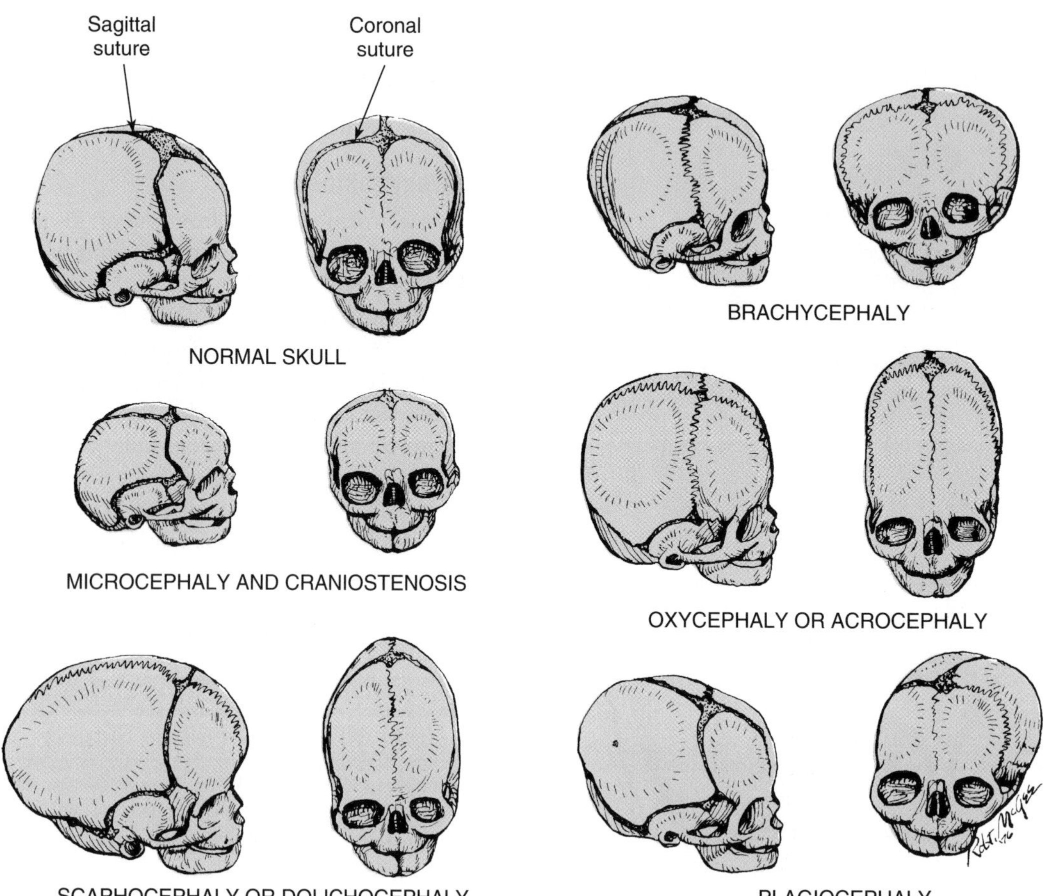

Fig. 20.6 Normal and Abnormal Head Configurations. *Normal skull:* The bones are separated by membranous seams until the sutures gradually close. *Microcephaly and craniostenosis:* In microcephaly, the head circumference is more than 2 standard deviations below the mean for age, gender, race, and gestation, reflecting a small brain. Craniosynostosis is premature closure of the sutures. *Scaphocephaly or dolichocephaly* (frequency 56%): Premature closure of the sagittal suture, resulting in restricted lateral growth. *Brachycephaly:* Premature closure of the coronal suture, resulting in excessive lateral growth. *Oxycephaly or acrocephaly* (frequency 5.8% to 12%): Premature closure of all coronal and sagittal sutures, resulting in accelerated upward growth and a small head circumference. *Plagiocephaly* (frequency 13%): Unilateral premature closure of the coronal suture, resulting in asymmetric growth. (From Hockenberry MJ, Wilson D. *Wong's nursing care of infants and children*, 10th edition. St. Louis: Mosby; 2015.)

anteroposterior direction (known as scaphocephaly). Single suture craniosynostosis requires early surgical intervention because it is not just a cosmetic issue. When multiple sutures fuse prematurely, surgical intervention is necessary. Brain growth may be restricted, and surgical repair may prevent neurologic dysfunction (Fig. 20.6). *Syndromic craniosynostosis* involves deformities in other systems (i.e., the heart, limbs, and CNS).

Malformations of Brain Development

Reduced proliferation or accelerated apoptosis (programmed cell death) of brain cells causes congenital microcephaly (microencephaly—small brain). Increased proliferation of brain cells causes megalencephaly (macrencephaly—abnormally large brain). Both disorders are rare. Diagnosis is made by clinical history, family history, and brain imaging.[13,14]

Microcephaly (small head) is associated with a defect in brain growth as a whole (see Fig. 20.6). Cranial size is significantly below average for the infant's age, gender, race, and gestation. The small size of the skull reflects a small brain (microencephaly), which is caused by reduced proliferation or accelerated apoptosis. *True (primary) microcephaly* is usually caused by an autosomal recessive genetic or chromosomal defect. *Secondary (acquired) microcephaly* is associated with various causes, such as intrauterine infection (including emergence of the Zika virus)[15]; trauma; metabolic disorders; maternal anorexia experienced during the third trimester of pregnancy; in utero exposure to alcohol, toxins, or certain medications; and the presence of other genetic syndromes. Children with microcephaly are usually developmentally delayed. Microcephaly can be familial and, if so, can be associated with normal development.

Cortical dysplasias (malformations) are defects in brain development and related to failure of embryonic neurons to migrate to the right places in the brain. These disorders may range from a small area of abnormal tissue to an entire brain that is smooth and without the normal configuration of gyri and sulci, known as *lissencephaly* (Fig. 20.7), or a brain that has too many small gyri (folds), known as *polymicrogyria*. There is a

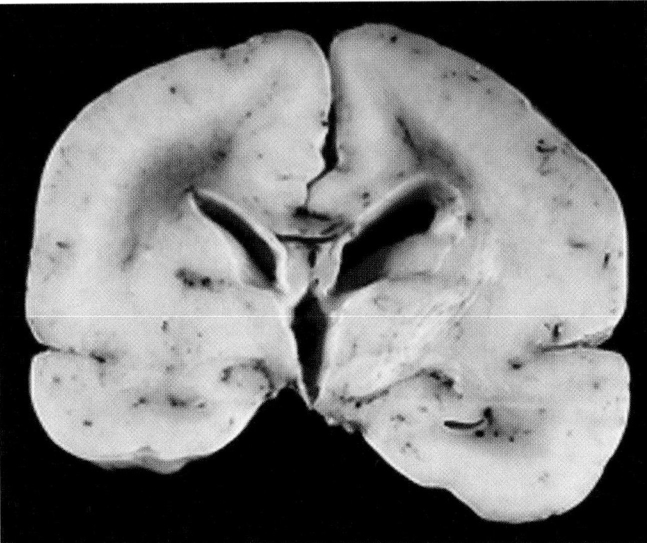

Fig. 20.7 Lissencephaly. The absence of cortical gyri defines this abnormality, seen here in the brain from a full-term infant. (From Kumar V, et al. *Robbins & Cotran pathologic basis of disease*, 8th edition. Philadelphia: Saunders; 2010.)

specific genetic defect for some of these disorders; others are multifactorial or acquired (e.g., intrauterine trauma or infection). Cortical dysplasias increase the risk for seizures that are difficult to control and cause developmental delay and motor dysfunction. Genetic testing assesses risk in other family members and guides therapy.[16,17] Congenital hydrocephalus is present at birth and characterized by increased CSF pressure and enlargement of the ventricles. The overall incidence of hydrocephalus is approximately 1 to 2 per 1000 live births.[18] Hydrocephalus may be caused by blockage within the ventricular system where the CSF flows, an imbalance in the production of CSF, or a reduced reabsorption of CSF. The increased pressure within the ventricular system dilates the ventricles and pushes and compresses the brain tissue against the skull cavity (Fig. 20.8A and B). When hydrocephalus develops before fusion of the cranial sutures, the skull can expand to accommodate this additional space-occupying volume and preserve neuronal function (Types of hydrocephalus are discussed in Chapter 17).

Congenital hydrocephalus may cause fetal death in utero, or the increased head circumference may require cesarean delivery of the infant. Symptoms depend directly on the cause and rate of hydrocephalus development. When there is separation of the cranial sutures, a resonant note sounds when the skull is tapped, a manifestation called the Macewen sign, or "cracked pot" sign. The eyes may assume a staring expression, *unable to look upwards*, with sclera visible above the cornea, called *sunsetting* (see Fig. 20.8D). Treatment outcomes are variable. Cognitive impairment in children with hydrocephalus is often related to associated brain malformations or episodes of shunt failure or infection. Approximately 40% to 65% of children with uncomplicated congenital hydrocephalus complete schooling and are employed when treated successfully with shunting or endoscopic third ventriculostomy with or without choroid plexus cauterization.[19–21]

The Dandy-Walker malformation (DWM) is a congenital defect of the cerebellum characterized by a large posterior fossa cyst that communicates with the fourth ventricle, cerebellar hypoplasia, and macrocephaly. DWM is commonly associated with hydrocephalus. Other causes of obstructions within the ventricular system that can result in hydrocephalus include brain tumors, cysts, trauma, arteriovenous malformations, blood clots, infections, and the Chiari malformations (Emerging Science Box: Gene Therapy for Pediatric Neurologic Conditions).

EMERGING SCIENCE BOX

Gene Therapy for Pediatric Neurologic Conditions

Much has been learned from studies and trials from the 1980's and 1990's. Due to the high risk of germ line gene therapy, where changes made to correct the genetic variants of the reproductive cells would be passed on to offspring, only somatic gene therapies are under trial. Somatic gene therapy involves either in vivo or ex vivo introduction of genetic material into cells in the body or those harvested, altered and then placed back into the body. Three pediatric FDA approved therapies exist at this time for spinal muscular atrophy, B-cell acute lymphoblastic leukemia and a specific retinal dystrophy. Many other trials are underway and being developed due to the great promise this therapy has for certain genetic neurologic conditions. A recent search of the National Cancer Institute website for gene therapy or gene transfer yields 10 trials for CNS childhood tumors, 13 trials for pediatric neurologic disorders including Duchenne muscular dystrophy, Hunter Syndrome, gangliosidosis, Danon disease and others. Currently the Clinical Trials.gov web site lists 45 studies involving children receiving or being evaluated for the outcomes of gene therapy for specific diseases or conditions (Accesses April 20, 2021, Available at https://clinicaltrials.gov/ct2/results?cond=Pediatric+ALL&term=+gene+therapy&cntry=&state=&city=&dist=&Search=Search&recrs=a&recrs=b&age=0).

In 2012 a revolutionary new gene editing technique called CRISPR (clusters of regularly interspaced short palindromic [*reads the same in both directions*] repeats [*sequences of nucleotides*]) was first introduced. This technique allows for precise gene editing by inserting a cut or break in the DNA and allowing a cell's natural DNA repair mechanisms to introduce the desired changes. Gene editing is being investigated for neurologic disorders such as genetic blindness, muscular dystrophy, Huntington disease. cancer, blood disorders, cystic fibrosis and other medical conditions that may likely benefit from CRISPR.

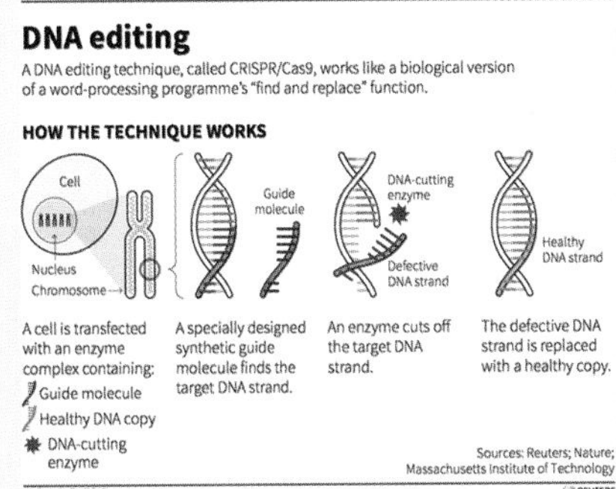

Data from U.S. Food and Drug Administration News Release: FDA approves innovative gene therapy to treat pediatric patients with spinal muscular atrophy, a rare disease and leading genetic cause of infant mortality, May 24, 2019 Available at https://www.fda.gov/news-events/press-announcements/fda-approves-innovative-gene-therapy-treat-pediatric-patients-spinal-muscular-atrophy-rare-disease; Safarzadeh Kozani P, et al. Novel antigens of CAR T cell therapy: New roads; old destination. *Transl Oncol.* 2021 Apr 13;14(7):101079. Ameri H. Prospect of retinal gene therapy following commercialization of voretigene neparvovec-rzyl for retinal dystrophy mediated by RPE65 mutation. *J Curr Ophthalmol.* 2018 Feb 16;30(1):1–2. Sharma G, et al. CRISPR-Cas9: A Preclinical and Clinical Perspective for the Treatment of Human Diseases. *Mol Ther.* 2021 Feb 3;29(2):571–586.

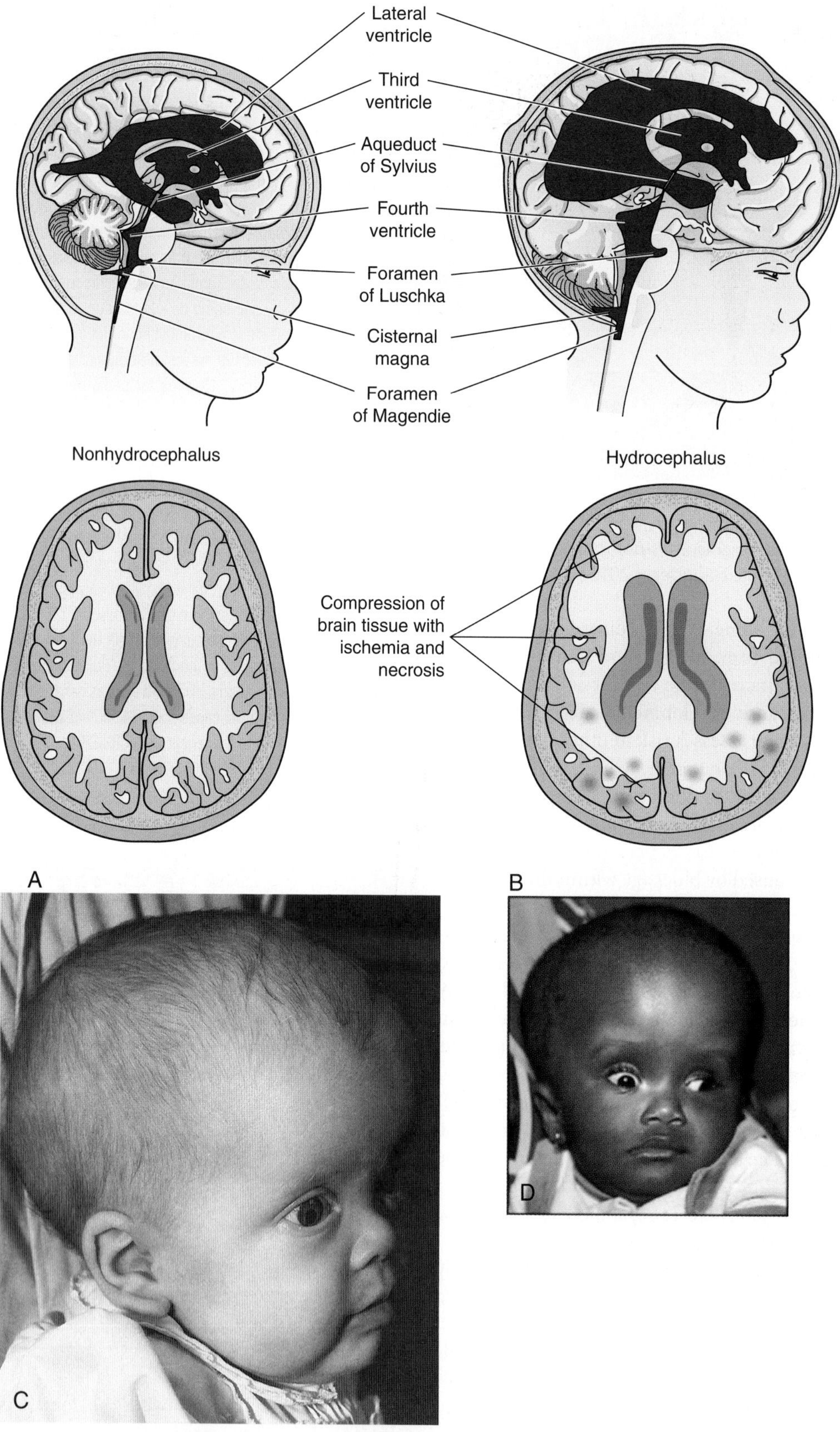

Fig. 20.8 Hydrocephalus. Fluid accumulation in the brain because of blockage in the flow of cerebrospinal fluid (CSF). **(A)** Patent cerebrospinal fluid circulation. **(B)** Enlarged lateral and third ventricles caused by obstruction of circulation of CSF—stenosis of aqueduct of Sylvius. **(C)** Child with enlarged head caused by hydrocephalus. **(D)** Congenital hydrocephalus with sunsetting of the eyes. (C, From McLaurin DC. *Pediatric neurosurgery*, 2nd edition. Philadelphia: Saunders; 1989. D, From Lissauer T, ed. *Illustrated textbook of paediatrics*, 5th edition. Elsevier; 2018.)

ALTERATIONS IN FUNCTION: ENCEPHALOPATHIES

Encephalopathy, meaning brain pathology, is a general category that includes a number of syndromes and diseases (see Chapter 18). These disorders may be acute or chronic, as well as static or progressive. Some common neurologic disorders with a genetic basis are summarized in Table 20.3.

Static (Nonprogressive) Encephalopathies

Static or nonprogressive encephalopathy describes a neurologic condition caused by a fixed lesion without active and ongoing disease. Causes include brain malformations or brain injury that may occur during gestation or birth or at any time during childhood. The degree of neurologic impairment is directly related to the extent of the injury or malformation and the stage of development at the time of injury. Anoxia, trauma, and infections are the most common causes of injury to the nervous system in the perinatal period. Infections, metabolic disturbances (acquired or genetic), trauma, toxins, and vascular disease may injure the nervous system in the postnatal period.[22]

Cerebral palsy is a disorder of movement, muscle tone, or posture that is caused by injury or abnormal development in the immature brain, before, during, or after birth up to 1 year of age. Cerebral palsy is one of the most common crippling disorders of childhood, affecting nearly 764,000 children in the United States alone. Although the exact incidence is unknown, studies suggest that the prevalence is approximately 1 in 345 children in the United States.[23]

Risk factors include prenatal or perinatal cerebral hypoxia, hemorrhage, infection, genetic abnormalities, or low birth weight (Table 20.4). Cerebral palsy can be classified on the basis of neurologic signs and motor symptoms, with the major types being spasticity, dystonia, ataxia, or a combination of these symptoms (mixed). Diplegia, hemiplegia, or tetraplegia may be present.

Pyramidal/spastic cerebral palsy is the most common. It results from damage to corticospinal pathways (upper motor neurons) and is associated with increased muscle tone, persistent primitive reflexes, hyperactive deep tendon reflexes, clonus, rigidity of the extremities, scoliosis, and contractures. Extrapyramidal/nonspastic cerebral palsy is less common and is caused by damage to cells in the basal ganglia or cerebellum and includes two subtypes: dystonic and ataxic. Dystonic (dyskinetic) cerebral palsy is associated with injury to the basal ganglia with extreme difficulty in fine motor coordination and purposeful movements. Movements are stiff, uncontrolled, and abrupt. Ataxic cerebral palsy is caused by damage to the cerebellum, with alterations in coordination and movement. There is a broad-based gait in an attempt to maintain balance, and tremor is common with intentional movements. A child may have symptoms of each of these cerebral palsy types, which leads to a mixed disorder.[24]

Children with cerebral palsy often have associated neurologic disorders, such as seizures and intellectual impairment ranging from mild to severe. Other complications include visual impairment, communication disorders, respiratory problems, bowel and bladder problems, and orthopedic disabilities, such as hip pain or dislocation, balance problems, or hand dysfunction.[25]

Inherited Metabolic Disorders of the Central Nervous System

A large number of inherited metabolic disorders have been identified, typically leading to diffuse brain dysfunction. Early diagnosis and treatment are vital if these infants are to survive without severe neurologic problems. Newborn metabolic screening for 28 metabolic conditions (in most states) has led to most of these children being identified before symptoms develop. Inborn errors of metabolism are present at birth, and most cause disturbances of the nervous system, although they may not manifest until childhood or even adulthood. Defects in amino acid and lipid metabolism are among the most common and are presented here.

Defects in Amino Acid Metabolism

Defects in amino acid metabolism are caused by genetic defects resulting in lack of a normal protein and absence of enzymatic activity. The defects include (1) those in which the transport of an amino acid is impaired; (2) those involving an enzyme or cofactor deficiency; and (3) those encompassing certain chemical components, such as branched-chain or sulfur-containing amino acids.

Phenylketonuria. Phenylketonuria (PKU) is an example of an inborn error of metabolism characterized by phenylalanine hydroxylase deficiency and the inability of the body to convert the essential amino acid phenylalanine to tyrosine (Fig. 20.9). PKU is an autosomal recessive inborn error of metabolism characterized by mutations of the phenylalanine hydroxylase *(PAH)* gene. PKU has an incidence of 1 per 10,000 to 15,000 live births in the United States.[19]

Most natural food proteins contain approximately 15% phenylalanine, an essential amino acid. Phenylalanine hydroxylase controls the conversion of this essential amino acid to tyrosine in the liver. The body uses tyrosine in the biosynthesis of proteins, melanin, thyroxine, and the catecholamines in the brain and adrenal medulla. Phenylalanine hydroxylase deficiency causes an accumulation of phenylalanine in the serum. Elevated phenylalanine levels result in developmental abnormalities of the cerebral cortical layers, defective myelination, and cystic degeneration of the gray and white matter. Unfortunately, brain damage occurs before the metabolites can be detected in the urine, and damage continues as long as phenylalanine levels remain high. Nonselective newborn screening is used to detect PKU in the United States and in more than 30 other countries. Treatment, consisting of reduction of dietary phenylalanine (PKU diet), is effective and allows for normal development. Mutations in the *PAH* gene are by far the most common cause of PKU, although there are other types of PKU. In one such variation, there is impaired synthesis of cofactors (e.g., tetrahydrobiopterin [BH_4]), which contributes to elevated levels of phenylalanine. Individuals with impaired synthesis of BH_4 have a positive response when sapropterin, a synthetic form of BH_4, is included in their treatment.[20]

Defects in Lipid Metabolism

Disorders of lipid metabolism are termed lysosomal storage diseases because each disorder in this group can be traced to a

TABLE 20.3 Selected Neurological Disorders With a Genetic Basis

Syndrome/ Disorders	Currently Known Genetic Components	Pathophysiology	Major Neurologic Features
Angelman syndrome	Microdeletion on chromosome 15 leading to loss of function of the *UBE3A* gene (ubiquitin protein ligase); can be acquired from mother	Protein, important in degradation of proteins in the brain	Little to no verbal language, intellectual disability, seizure disorder, sleep disorder, movement/balance disorder
Batten disease	Autosomal recessive; mutation of the *CLN3* gene (ceroid-lipofuscinosis, neuronal 3) (chromosome 16)	Lysosomal storage defect resulting in abnormal storage of cerebral lipofuscins	Develops normally until 6 months to 2 years of age when progressive brain disease becomes apparent; seizures, intellectual disability, blindness, and death
Branched-chain ketoaciduria (maple syrup urine disease)	Autosomal recessive; most common type is classic caused by mutation of the *BCKDHA* gene (2-oxoisovalerate dehydrogenase subunit alpha, a mitochondrial enzyme) (chromosome 19)	All types result in inability to metabolize three amino acids; these acids accumulate and are toxic at high levels	Intellectual disability, seizures, and death; treatable with early diagnosis
Cri du chat syndrome	Autosomal dominant; deletion on the short arm of chromosome 5 (also called *5p minus syndrome*)	Deletion of multiple genes responsible for phenotype; evidence that deletion of telomerase reverse transcriptase gene contributes to phenotype	High-pitched cry; intellectual disability, microcephaly, low birth weight, failure to thrive; widely spaced eyes (ocular hypertelorism), unusually small jaw (micrognathia)
Lesch-Nyhan syndrome	X-linked recessive; mutation of the *HPRT* gene (hypoxanthine phosphoribosyltransferase 1)	Metabolism disturbance of purines; excessive production of uric acid	Intellectual disability, progressive neurologic disorder, compulsively bitten lips and fingers; self-mutilating
Neurofibromatosis (NF)	Autosomal dominant	Variable expressivity	Multiple café au lait spots, neurofibromas, learning disability, seizure disorder
NF1 (von Recklinghausen disease)	Mutation of the *NF1* gene (neurofibromin) (chromosome 17)	A large, complex protein; this protein may act as a switch to regulate cell growth; mutation may lessen or inhibit the normal output of this protein and allow irregular cell growth that may lead to tumor development	Increased risk for nerve sheath tumors and brain tumors
NF2 (bilateral acoustic NF)	Autosomal dominant: mutation of either the *NF2* gene (merlin; moesin-ezrin-radixin-like protein or schwannomin) (chromosome 22)	A tumor-suppressor protein (merlin or schwannomin)	Multiple tumors (schwannomas) on cranial and spinal nerves, acoustic neuromas, hearing loss
Progressive myoclonic epilepsy (Unverricht-Lundborg disease)	Autosomal recessive; mutation *CSTB* gene (cystatin B, a cysteine protease inhibitor) (chromosome 21)	This protein regulates enzymes that break down other proteins	Onset at age 6–15 years, severe incapacitating stimulus-sensitive progressive myoclonus, tonic-clonic epileptic seizures, and characteristic abnormalities on electroencephalogram; also may develop other neurologic symptoms such as ataxia, incoordination, and dysarthria
Lafora disease	Autosomal recessive; mutation of the *EMP2A* gene (epilepsy, progressive myoclonus type 2A or laforin) and *EMP2B* gene (malin) (chromosome 6)	Concentric amyloid (Lafora) bodies found in neurons, liver, skin, bone, and muscle; defects in protein degradation and clearance	Grand mal seizures and/or myoclonus at about age 15; rapid and severe motor and coordination impairments, rapid mental deterioration, often with psychotic features; survival is short, less than 10 years after onset
Rett syndrome	X-linked dominant; appears to occur only in girls; defective *MECP2* gene (methyl CpG binding protein 2) (X-chromosome)	Protein involved in regulation of gene expression; defects in this gene allow other genes to be expressed at inappropriate times in development	Progressive neurologic disorder; develops normally in first year of life, then loss of mental capacity and motor skills begins; loss of purposeful hand movements; stereotypical hand wringing and flapping
Tay-Sachs disease	Autosomal recessive; mutation of the *HEXA* gene (chromosome 15)	Caused by a deficiency of hexosaminidase, an enzyme, which results in accumulation of a material that damages the brain	Failure to thrive, blindness, seizures, progressive paralysis; usually death by age 4
Tuberous sclerosis	Autosomal dominant; mutation of either the *TSC1* gene (hamartin) (chromosome 9) or the *TSC2* gene (tuberin) (chromosome 16)	These proteins act as tumor growth suppressors	Develops in early childhood; seizures, intellectual disability, skin and eye lesions; multiple benign tumors in brain and other vital organs

TABLE 20.4 Cerebral Palsy: Predisposing Factors and Known Causes

Risk Factors	Associated Causes
Prenatal	
Maternal	Metabolic diseases
	Nutritional deficiencies (e.g., anemia)
	Twin or multiple births
	Bleeding
	Toxemia
	Blood incompatibilities
	Exposure to radiation
	Infection (e.g., rubella, toxoplasmosis, cytomegalic inclusion disease)
	Premature labor
Prematurity	Asphyxia leading to cerebral hemorrhage
Genetic factors	Absence of corpus callosum, aqueductal stenosis, cerebellar hypoplasia
Congenital anomalies of the brain	Unknown causes not evident on clinical examination
Perinatal	Anesthesia or analgesia during labor and delivery
	Mechanical trauma or hypoxia during delivery
	Immaturity at birth
	Metabolic disorders (e.g., hyperbilirubinemia, hypoglycemia, amino acid disorders, hyperosmolality)
	Electrolyte disturbances (e.g., hypernatremia, hypoglycemia)
Postnatal	Head trauma
	Infections (e.g., meningitis, encephalitis)
	Cerebrovascular accidents
	Toxicosis
	Environmental toxins (e.g., lead ingestion, methyl mercury ingestion from contaminated fish)

missing lysosomal enzyme needed for the breakdown and recycling of many cellular products. Lysosomal storage disorders include more than 50 known genetic disorders. The incidence of lysosomal storage disorders is approximately 1 in 5000 live births.[21] These disorders cause an excessive accumulation of a particular cell product, occurring in the brain, liver, spleen, bone, and lung and thus involving several organ systems; these disorders often are highly debilitating and cause progressive physical and neurologic disability. In general, these disorders are not included in newborn screening. Some of these disorders may be treated with enzyme replacement therapy.[26] Perhaps the best known of the lysosomal storage disorders is GM_2 gangliosidosis (Tay-Sachs disease), an autosomal recessive disorder caused by deficiency of the lysosomal enzyme hexosaminidase A (HexA), an enzyme that degrades GM_2 gangliosides (fatty acids) within nerve cell lysosomes. Eighty percent of individuals diagnosed are of Jewish ancestry, although sporadic cases appear in the non-Jewish population. Onset of this disease usually occurs when the infant is 4 to 6 months old. Symptoms of

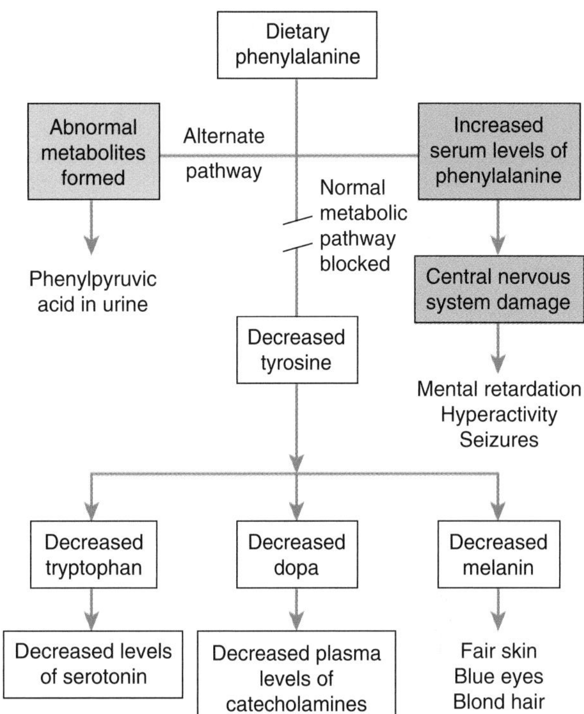

Fig. 20.9 Metabolic Error and Consequences in Phenylketonuria. (From Hockenberry MJ, Wilson D. *Wong's nursing care of infants and children*, 10th edition. St. Louis: Mosby; 2015.)

Tay-Sachs include an exaggerated startle response to loud noise, seizures, developmental regression, dementia, and blindness. Death from this disease is almost universal and occurs by 5 years of age. Screening for carriers of the gene defect concomitant with counseling to prevent disease transmission is possible.[27]

Intoxications of the Central Nervous System

Drug-induced encephalopathies must always be considered a possibility in the child with unexplained neurologic changes. Such encephalopathies may result from accidental ingestion, therapeutic overdose, intentional overdose, or ingestion of environmental toxins. There were 37.7/1000 children younger than 6 years of age with poison exposures in 2018. Approximately 44.2% of all poison exposures occurred in children younger than 6 years of age, with the highest incidence being 1- and 2-year-old children. The most commonly ingested poisons in children younger than 6 years are cosmetics and personal care products, cleaning substances, and over-the-counter analgesics and other medications (Table 20.5).[28]

Lead poisoning results in high blood levels of lead. If lead poisoning is untreated, lead encephalopathy results and is responsible for serious and irreversible neurologic damage. Those at greatest risk are children ages 2 to 3 years and children prone to the practice of pica—the habitual, purposeful, and compulsive ingestion of nonfood substances, such as clay, soil, and paint chips or paint dust. Lead intoxication also may occur from chronic exposure to lead in cosmetics, inhalation of gasoline vapors, and ingestion of airborne lead.[29] Fetal neurotoxicity occurs with maternal lead exposure, particularly during the first trimester.[30] Details related to lead intoxication are described in Chapter 2. Refer to Fig. 20.10 for a summary of toxic lead effects.

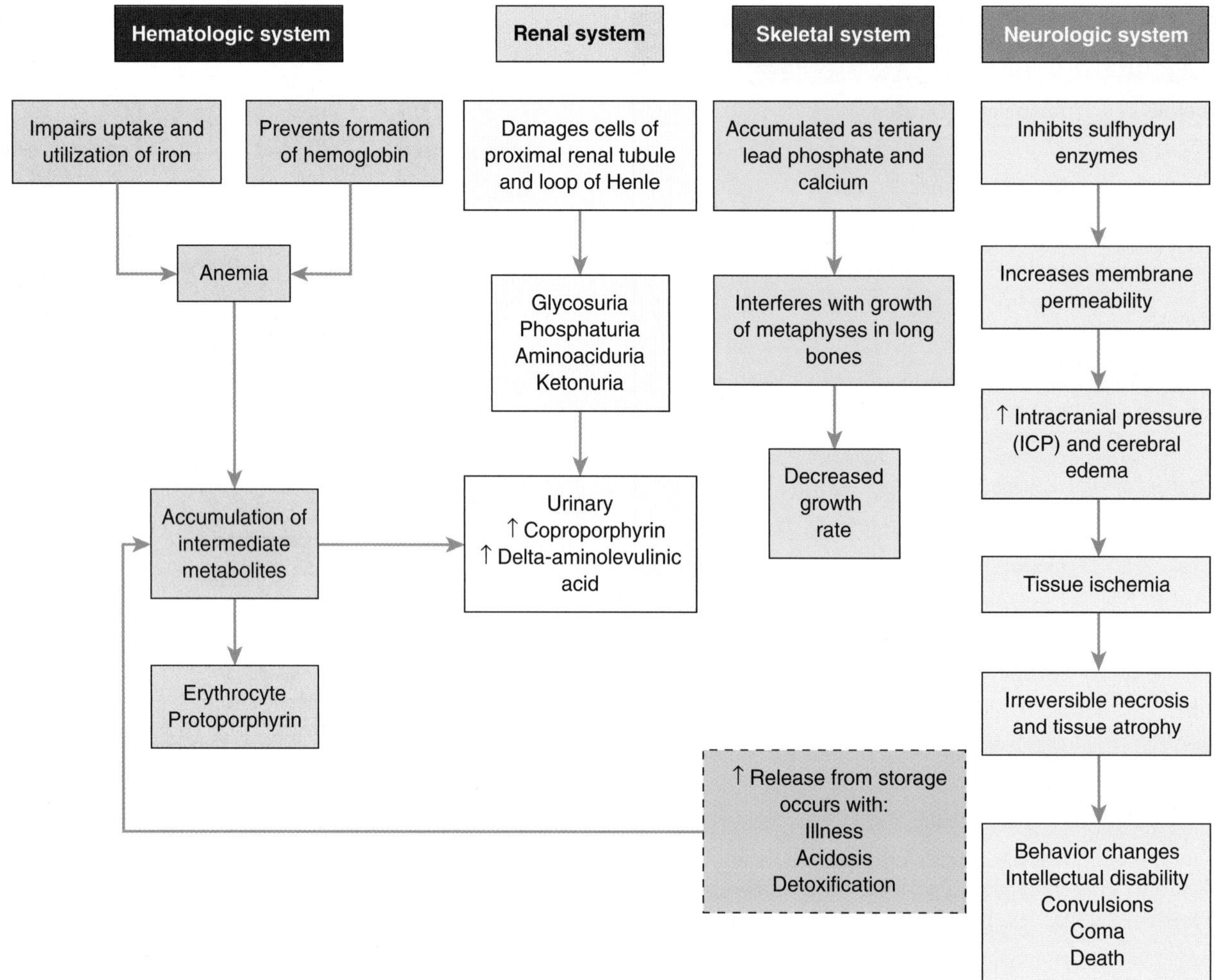

Fig. 20.10 Systemic Effects of Increased Lead Absorption in Children.

Infections of the Central Nervous System

Meningitis is an infection of the meninges and subarachnoid space of the brain and spinal cord. Encephalitis is inflammation within the brain. In many infections of the meninges, encephalitis also is present and the term *meningoencephalitis* is used. The origin of such inflammation and acute encephalopathy can be caused by bacteria, viruses, or other microorganisms. Aseptic meningitis has no evidence of bacterial infection but may be associated with viral infection, systemic disease, or drugs.

Bacterial meningitis. Acute bacterial meningitis is one of the most serious infections to which infants and children are susceptible. The introduction of conjugate vaccines against *Haemophilus influenzae* type B, *Streptococcus pneumoniae*, and *Neisseria meningitidis* (meningococcus) has decreased the incidence of bacterial meningitis.[31] Vaccines for serogroup B *N. meningitidis* are now available.[32]

Group B *Streptococcus* causes lethal meningitis and sepsis in neonates; it is transmitted to the child from the mother's birth canal and is the most common cause of meningitis in newborns. *S. pneumoniae* is the most common microorganism in children 1 to 23 months of age. Staphylococcal or streptococcal meningitis can occur in children of any age but shows a predilection for children who have had neurosurgery, skull fracture, or a complication of systemic bacterial infection. Infections that originate in the middle ear, sinuses, or mastoid cells also may lead to *S. pneumoniae* infection in children. Children with sickle cell disease or who have had a splenectomy are particularly at high risk for infection.

Escherichia coli and group B beta-hemolytic streptococci are the most common causes of meningitis in the newborn period. The second most common microorganism causing bacterial meningitis, particularly in children younger than 4 years, is *N. meningitidis* (meningococcus) and it has the potential to occur in epidemics. Approximately 2% to 5% of healthy children are carriers of *N. meningitidis*. Because the incidence of *N. meningitidis* infection increases in adolescence and with crowded environments, such as in dormitories and among military personnel, it is recommended that all individuals 11 to 12 years of age receive two immunizations against this pathogen. Teens and young adults (16 through 23 year olds) also may be vaccinated with a serogroup B meningococcal vaccine.[33]

Pathophysiology. Pathogens enter the nervous system by direct extension from a contiguous source (e.g., paranasal sinuses or mastoid cells) or, more commonly, by hematogenous spread (e.g., infective endocarditis, pneumonia, neurosurgical procedures, severe burns). Pathogens then cross the

TABLE 20.5 Common Poisons

Pharmacologic Agents	Heavy Metals	Miscellaneous Agents
Analgesics (acetaminophen, salicylates)	Lead Acute Chronic	Cosmetics and personal care products
Topical preparations	Mercury	Household cleaning substances
Antihistamines	Thallium	Alcohols Ethyl, isopropyl, methyl
Vitamins/dietary supplements/ herbs/homeopathic	Arsenic	Pesticides Organophosphates Chlorinated hydrocarbons
Gastrointestinal preparationsCardiovascular drugsSleeping medications	Cadmium	Mushrooms
Antidepressants		Venoms Snake bite Tick paralysis
Stimulants/street drugs Barbiturates Amphetamines		Ethylene glycol
Sedatives/hypnotics/antipsychotic Pain medications/opioids		Aliphatic hydrocarbons Gasoline, kerosene, lamp oil

blood-brain barrier, enter the CSF, and multiply. Bacterial toxins increase cerebrovascular permeability, causing alterations in blood flow and edema. Increased intracranial pressure (ICP) may be increased further by obstruction to the CSF circulation. Herniation of the brainstem causes death.

Clinical manifestations. Acute bacterial meningitis often is preceded by an upper respiratory tract or a gastrointestinal infection. Inflammation leads to the general symptoms of fever, headache, vomiting, and irritability and the CNS symptoms of photophobia, nuchal and spinal rigidity, decreased level of consciousness, and seizures. Irritation of the meninges and spinal roots causes pain and resistance to neck flexion (nuchal rigidity), a positive Kernig sign (resistance to knee extension in the supine position with the hips and knees flexed against the body), and a positive Brudzinski sign (flexion of the knees and hips when the neck is flexed forward rapidly). With severe meningeal irritation the child may demonstrate opisthotonic posturing (rigid arching of the back with the head extended). Infants may have bulging fontanelles. Meningococcal meningitis can produce a characteristic petechial rash.

Viral meningitis may result from a direct infection caused by a virus, or it may be secondary to disease, such as measles, mumps, herpes, or leukemia. The hallmark of viral meningitis, or aseptic meningitis, is a mononuclear response in the CSF and the presence of normal glucose levels. The clinical manifestations are similar to those in bacterial meningitis, although usually milder.

Evaluation and treatment. A definitive diagnosis is made by examination of CSF obtained from a lumbar puncture and by CSF and blood cultures. The principles of treatment are similar to those followed for adults (see Chapter 18) and are based on the culture results in which the causative microorganism is identified. Empirical antibiotic therapy should be initiated and continued until CSF cultures are negative or changed if the empirical therapy is not correct for the bacteria cultured from the CSF. Bacterial lysis induced by antibiotics can cause subarachnoid inflammation; the severity may be reduced with corticosteroid treatment. The factors that influence outcomes are the age of the child (mortality is highest in infants younger than 1 year), the infective microorganisms (the lowest mortality is in meningococcal meningitis and the highest in meningitis caused by gram-negative enteric microorganisms), and the duration and extent of inflammation before treatment. Approximately 8% of children with *H. influenzae* meningitis die; 35% of the survivors have serious and permanent sensory or motor dysfunction caused by pressure on the peripheral nerves during the early phases of the illness. Approximately 5% of the children who survive meningitis have hearing deficits; 15% to 30% have cerebral damage, hydrocephalus, motor deficits, or sensory impairments.

Viral encephalitis in children is similar to viral encephalitis in adults (see Chapter 18, and Fig. 18.28) and can be difficult to distinguish from viral meningitis. Viruses are obligate intracellular pathogens which can directly invade the brain, causing inflammation. Postinfectious encephalitis can develop as a result of an autoimmune response. Inflammatory and autoimmune causes of encephalitis may be treatable if identified early in an individual's course of illness.[34] (Encephalopathy resulting from infection with the human immunodeficiency virus [HIV] is discussed in Chapters 9 and 18.)

CEREBROVASCULAR DISEASE IN CHILDREN

Perinatal Stroke

Perinatal stroke is defined as stroke occurring from 28 weeks' gestation to 28 days postnatal.[35] Perinatal arterial ischemic stroke is estimated at 1 in 4000 live births and is a leading cause of perinatal brain injury, cerebral palsy, and lifelong disability. Although a cause for perinatal stroke is usually not found, clotting abnormalities may make the child prone to further vascular events. Up to 80% are ischemic with the remainder secondary to hemorrhage or cerebral sinovenous thrombosis (CSVT).

Childhood Stroke

Childhood stroke occurs in 1.3 to 1.6 per 100,000 children per year and may be divided into two categories: ischemic and hemorrhagic.[35,36] According to the Center for Disease Control and Prevention, cerebrovascular disease (stroke) is one of the 10 leading causes of death in children and adolescents from 1 to 24 years of age. Ischemic (occlusive) stroke in children may result from embolism, Cerebral sinovenous thrombosis (CSVT), or congenital or iatrogenic narrowing of vessels, leading to decreased flow of blood and oxygen to areas of the brain. Although rare, it is more common than hemorrhagic stroke. Children with arterial ischemic stroke do not have the typical adult risk factors of atherosclerosis and hypertension. Many children with acute ischemic stroke have no identifiable risk factors.[35] Arteriopathies, cardiac anomalies, sickle cell disease, infections, head and neck disorders, systemic conditions, and prothrombic states are the common disorders associated with arterial ischemic stroke.[35]

Hemorrhagic stroke is most commonly caused by bleeding from congenital cerebral arteriovenous malformations and is rare in children younger than 19 years. Intraventricular hemorrhage associated with premature birth is related to immature blood vessels and unstable blood pressure. There is a high risk of developing posthemorrhagic hydrocephalus in very low birth weight (<1000 g) preterm infants with increased risk of developmental disabilities.[37]

The clinical presentation of stroke varies according to the vessels involved and the age of the individual. Symptoms include hemiplegia, weakness, seizures, headaches, high fever, nuchal rigidity, hemianopia, sensory changes, facial palsy, and temporary aphasia. Obtaining a thorough history of evolving symptoms and risk factors is important for diagnosis. Laboratory studies may be indicated. Neuroimaging studies assist in determining the extent of the disease. Surgery is an option for treatment, and anticoagulants and antithrombotics may be used in selected cases.

Moyamoya disease is a rare, chronic, progressive vascular stenosis of the circle of Willis of unknown etiology. There is obstruction of arterial flow to the brain and the development of small basal arterial collateral vessels that vascularize the hypoperfused brain distal to the occluded vessels.[38] Moyamoya means a *puff of smoke* in Japanese and represents the appearance of these small vessels on cerebral angiography. The disease is most common in East Asia and is associated with genetic factors, particularly those associated with vascular growth factors. These children often present with transient ischemic attacks (TIAs) because the new vessels fail to provide adequate perfusions.[39] Diagnosis is made by cerebral angiography, and the most effective treatment is surgical revascularization.

EPILEPSY AND SEIZURE DISORDERS IN CHILDREN

The incidence of epilepsy varies greatly with age, geographic location, and study design. Approximately 470,000 children in the United States had epilepsy in 2015.[40] Seizures are the abnormal discharge of electrical activity within the brain. When a sufficient number of neurons become overexcited, they discharge abnormally, which sometimes results in clinical manifestations (seizures) with alterations in motor function, sensation, autonomic function, behavior, and consciousness. The manifestations depend on the site and spread of abnormal electrical activity within the brain. If a child has more than *two* unprovoked seizures more than 24 hours apart, that child is said to have epilepsy, although there are a few exceptions—one example being febrile seizures (see Chapter 16). Seizures may result from diseases that are primarily neurologic (CNS) or are systemic and affect CNS function secondarily (e.g., diabetes). Seizures can be caused by structural abnormalities of the brain, hypoxia, intracranial hemorrhage, CNS infection, traumatic injury, electrolyte imbalance, or inborn metabolic disturbances (see Chapter 18). Febrile Seizures are benign and the most common type of childhood seizure. Seizures are sometimes clearly familial. Often the cause of epilepsy is unknown and presumed to have a genetic basis. (Table 18.10 summarizes the classification of seizures.)

Antiepileptic drugs (AEDs) stabilize ion channels and neurotransmitters and are effective in treating seizures in 70% of persons. The 30% of individuals with medication-refractory epilepsy are increasingly effectively treated with other modalities. A ketogenic diet with high-fat and low-carbohydrate consumption replaces energy metabolism with ketone bodies instead of glucose and appears to increase the seizure threshold.[41] Neuromodulation (e.g., vagus nerve stimulation) can be effective to suppress epileptogenic activity.[42] Surgery to remove epileptic brain areas or disconnect eliptogenic pathways can reduce seizure activity.[43]

Epileptic spasms (also known as infantile spasms) are rare, severe types of seizures associated with electroencephalogram (EEG) abnormalities and varying clinical manifestations. The cause can be related to underlying brain abnormalities such as intrauterine stroke, cortical dysplasias, or tuberous sclerosis (a benign tumor), whereas others may be caused by mutations in one of several genes. Clinical manifestations of the resulting spasms may range from subtle head nods to violent body contractions, commonly referred to as *jackknife seizures*. Onset of infantile spasms usually is during infancy or early childhood. An EEG will display a classic hypsarrhythmic pattern on a slow, disorganized chaotic background. After infantile spasms begin, there is usually a typical clinical course. The "spasms" usually occur in clusters and transpire 5 to 150 times per day. They are commonly worse when the infant is waking up or falling asleep. Once begun, the seizure activity increases in intensity and severity over time. Invariably, a loss of developmental milestones and disability is associated with this syndrome. Treatment is the administration of adrenocorticotrophic hormone, vigabatrin (particularly for children with tuberous sclerosis), and corticosteroids. Surgery is an option when pharmacologic treatment has failed.[44]

CHILDHOOD TUMORS

Brain Tumors

Brain tumors are the most common solid tumor, are the second most common primary neoplasm in children (after leukemia), and can be benign or malignant.[45,53] They are the leading cause of cancer-related death in children, and the 5-year survival is approximately 74%, varying significantly by tumor type. Primary brain tumors arise from brain tissue and do not metastasize outside the brain. The cause of brain tumors is unknown, although genetic, environmental, and immune factors have been investigated. Exposure to radiation therapy has been the only environmental factor consistently related to the development of brain tumors.[46,53]

Brain tumors can arise from any CNS cell, and tumors are classified by cell type *and molecular markers*. The most common tumors are embryonal tumors, including medulloblastoma, atypical medulloblastoma, atypical teratoid rhabdoid tumors,

CNS primitive neuroectodermal tumors, and high-grade gliomas, including glioblastomas, diffuse pontine gliomas, and other malignant astrocytomas. Other tumor types are less common, including low-grade astrocytomas (especially pilocytic astrocytomas), neuronal and mixed neuronal-glial tumors, and ependymal tumors (ependymomas). Brain tumors in children are often located in the posterior fossa (Fig. 20.11). The types and characteristics of the more common childhood brain tumors are summarized in Table 20.6.

Signs and symptoms of brain tumors in children vary from generalized and vague to localized and related specifically to an anatomic area. Signs of elevated ICP may occur, including headache, vomiting, lethargy, and irritability. If a young child complains of repeated and worsening headache, a thorough investigation should take place because headache is an uncommon complaint in young children. Headache caused by elevated ICP usually is worse in the morning and gradually improves during the day, when the child is upright and venous drainage is enhanced. The frequency of headache and other symptoms increases as the tumor grows. Irritability or possible apathy and increased somnolence also may result. Like headache, vomiting occurs more commonly in the morning. Often it is *not* preceded by nausea and may become projectile, differing from a gastrointestinal disturbance in that the child may be ready to eat immediately after vomiting. Persistent headaches with vomiting in a child should be evaluated promptly. Other signs and symptoms include increased head circumference with bulging fontanelles in the child younger than 2 years, cranial nerve palsies, and papilledema (Box 20.1).

Localized findings relate to the degree of disturbance in physiologic functioning in the area where the tumor is located. The majority of pediatric brain tumors involve the cerebellum, brain stem, and fourth ventricle affecting all pediatric age groups. Children with infratentorial tumors (posterior fossa) exhibit localized signs of impaired coordination and balance, including ataxia, gait difficulties, truncal ataxia, and loss of balance. Supratentorial tumors of the cerebral hemispheres are more common in children younger than 3 years of age.[46] Most pediatric brain tumors require surgical resection. Aggressive radiation and chemotherapy are required for high-grade tumors, although radiation therapy is rarely offered to children younger than 4 years of age, due to significant long-term side effects. Advances are being made in areas of immunotherapy and targeted molecular therapy (see Emerging Science Box: The New Evolving Classification System for Pediatric Brain Tumors).[47]

Embryonal Tumors

Neuroblastoma

Neuroblastoma is an embryonal tumor originating from neural crest tissues of the sympathetic nervous system outside the CNS. It is the most common cancer in infants younger than 1 year of age. Although it accounts for only approximately 6% of pediatric malignancies (approximately 800 new cases per year),

BOX 20.1 Clinical Manifestations of Brain Tumors

Headache
Recurrent and progressive
In frontal or occipital area
Worse on arising; pain lessens during the day
Intensified by lowering head and straining, such as when defecating, coughing, sneezing

Vomiting
With or without nausea or feeding
Progressively more projectile
More severe in morning
Relieved by moving and changing position

Neuromuscular Changes
Incoordination or clumsiness
Loss of balance (use of wide-based stance, falling, tripping, banging into objects)
Poor fine motor control
Weakness
Hyporeflexia or hyperreflexia
Positive Babinski sign
Spasticity
Paralysis

Behavioral Changes
Irritability
Decreased appetite
Failure to thrive
Fatigue (frequent naps)
Lethargy
Coma
Bizarre behavior (staring, automatic movements)

Cranial Nerve Neuropathy
Cranial nerve involvement varies according to tumor location. The most common signs are:
Head tilt
Visual defects (nystagmus, diplopia, strabismus, episodic "graying out" of vision, and visual field defects)

Vital Sign Disturbances
Decreased pulse and respiratory rates
Increased blood pressure
Decreased pulse pressure
Hypothermia or hyperthermia

Other Signs
Seizures
Cranial enlargement[a]
Tense, bulging fontanelle at rest[a]
Separating suture[a]
Nuchal rigidity
Papilledema (edema of optic nerve)

[a]Present only in infants and young children.
From Hockenberry MN. *Wong's essentials of pediatric nursing*, 7th edition. St. Louis: Mosby; 2007.

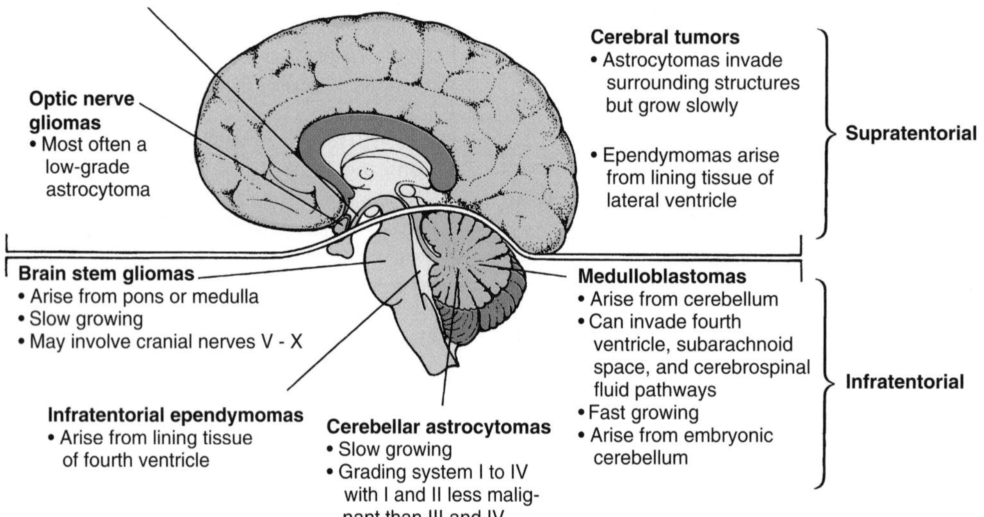

Fig. 20.11 Location of Brain Tumors in Children. (From Ostrom QT, et al. *Neuro-Oncology*, 2017;19(suppl_5):v1-v88.)

TABLE 20.6 More Common Brain Tumors in Children

Type	Characteristics	Treatment
Astrocytoma	Arises from astrocytes, often in cerebellum or lateral cerebral hemisphere Slow growing, solid or cystic Often very large before diagnosed Varies in degree of malignancy	*Cerebellar astrocytoma* Surgery can be curative for juvenile pilocytic astrocytomas Radiation, chemotherapy, and newer targeted therapies can play important role in improving outcome.
Medulloblastoma (neuroectodermal tumor)	Often located in cerebellum, extending into fourth ventricle and spinal fluid pathway Can extend outside central nervous system Rapidly growing malignant tumor	Treatment is age and tumor type dependent Surgery, important to not only reopen cerebrospinal fluid pathways but also to improve outcome Radiation as primary treatment; may include spinal radiation Chemotherapy often helpful in conjunction with craniospinal radiation Targeted therapies for molecular subgroups are in development
Ependymoma	Arises from ependymal cells lining ventricles Circumscribed, solid, nodular tumors	Tumor possibly indolent for many years Surgery resection highly correlated with outcome. Radiation for palliation (current controversy over whether local or craniospinal radiation is best) Chemotherapy used for recurrent disease but with disappointing results Targeted therapies for molecular subgroups are in development
Brainstem glioma	Arises from pons Numerous cell types Compresses cranial nerves V through X	Surgery, resection rarely possible Radiation, primarily palliative treatment Chemotherapy not yet proven beneficial New protocols and agents being studied

neuroblastoma causes approximately 15% of cancer deaths in children.[48] More than with any other cancer, neuroblastoma has been associated with spontaneous remission, commonly in infants. Prognosis is worse for children older than 2 years of age with disseminated disease. Although familial tendency has been noted in individual cases, a nonfamilial or sporadic pattern is found in most children with neuroblastoma. Familial cases of neuroblastoma are considered to have an autosomal dominant pattern of inheritance (mechanisms of inheritance are discussed in Chapter 4).

The most common location of neuroblastoma is in the retroperitoneal region, most often in the adrenal medulla. The tumor is evident as an abdominal mass and may cause anorexia, bowel and bladder alteration, and sometimes spinal cord compression.

EMERGING SCIENCE BOX

The New Evolving Classification System for Pediatric Brain Tumors

Ongoing advances in molecular biology are revolutionizing how we categorize and treat pediatric brain tumors. Brain tumors have historically been categorized by what the cells look like under the microscope. Tumor cells from one person may look like another person's tumor cells but behave very differently and react differently to treatment. The emerging new classification system relies less on how the cells look and more on how they behave and what molecular pathways have been altered to make the cell a tumor. Some low-grade gliomas have significant alterations in the BRAF gene, allowing for targeted therapies incorporating MEK inhibitors. The most common pediatric brain tumor medulloblastoma is now categorized into 4 separate types. Each category has a different prognosis. The most favorable group is the WNT (Wingless/Integrated). Trials using no radiation or reduced dose radiation are underway for that group. Ependymomas have nine recognized subsets.

Understanding the molecular make up of each tumor can open new treatment options as more targeted therapies become available. Even the most highly malignant tumors such as diffuse intrinsic pontine glioma (DPG) may warrant biopsy to understand molecular make up and potential new treatment options.

Data from Pollack IF, et al. Childhood brain tumors: Current management, biological insights, and future directions. *Journal of Neurosurgery. Pediatrics*, 23:261–273.

The second most common location of neuroblastoma is the mediastinum (15% of cases), where the tumor may cause dyspnea or infection related to airway obstruction. Rarely, neuroblastoma may arise from the cervical sympathetic ganglion.

A number of systemic signs and symptoms are characteristic of neuroblastoma, including weight loss, irritability, fatigue, and fever. Intractable diarrhea occurs in some children and is caused by tumor secretion of a hormone called *vasoactive intestinal polypeptide (VIP)*. Most children with neuroblastoma have increased amounts of catecholamines and associated metabolites in their urine (e.g., urinary vanillylmandelic acid [VMA] and homovanillic acid [HVA]). High levels of urinary catecholamines and serum ferritin are associated with a poor prognosis. Immunotherapeutic treatments are undergoing continuing investigation and hold promise for good outcomes without toxicity.[49]

Retinoblastoma

Retinoblastoma (RB) is the most common intraocular congenital eye tumor of young children that originates in the retina of one or both eyes (Fig. 20.12A and B). Two forms of RB are exhibited: inherited and acquired. Both forms of the disease are a consequence of loss of function of the RB gene *(RB1)*. The inherited form of the disease generally is diagnosed during the first year of life. The acquired disease is diagnosed before the age of 5 in 90% of the cases.[50] Approximately 40% of RBs are inherited as an autosomal dominant trait with incomplete penetrance (see Fig. 4.24). The remaining 60% are acquired somatic mutations. The "two-hit" hypothesis explains the occurrence of both hereditary and acquired forms of the disease.[51] This hypothesis predicts that two separate transforming events or "hits" must occur in a normal retinoblast cell to cause the cancer. Furthermore, it proposes that in the inherited form, the first hit or mutation occurs in the germ cell (inherited from either parent), and the mutation is contained in every cell of the child's body. Only a second, random mutation in a retinoblast cell is needed to transform that cell into cancer. Multiple tumors are observed in the inherited form because these second mutations are likely to occur in several of the approximately 1 to 2 million retinoblast cells. In contrast, the acquired form of RB requires two *independent* hits or mutations to occur in the same somatic cell (after the egg is fertilized) for the transformation to cancer. This is much less likely to happen. Fig. 20.13 illustrates the "two-hit" model for these two patterns of mutation. Epigenetic mechanisms (i.e., inactivating the gene without changing its DNA sequence) also play a role in dysregulation of the tumor suppressor and oncogenic pathways of RB, and they may become markers for difficult to diagnose tumors.[52] The primary sign of RB is leukocoria, a white pupillary reflex (white reflex) also called *cat's eye reflex*, which is caused by the mass behind the lens (see Fig. 20.12B). This easy to identify sign can be missed. Other signs and symptoms include strabismus; a red, painful eye; and limited vision.

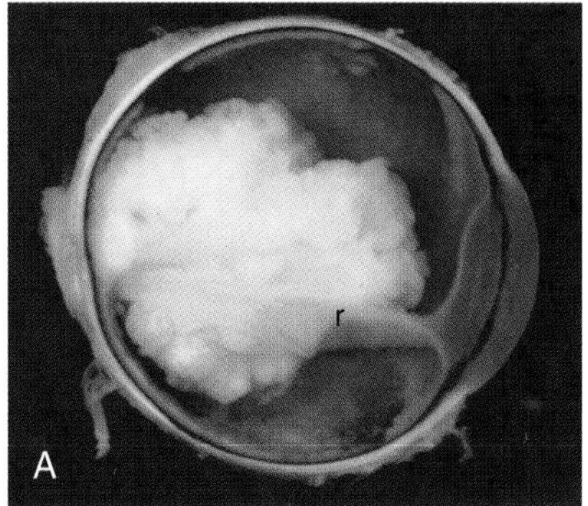

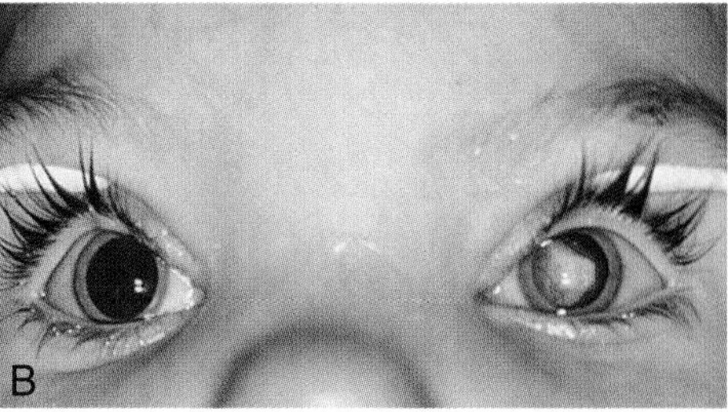

Fig. 20.12 Retinoblastoma. **(A)** Presence of white mass surrounding the detached retina *(r)*. **(B)** The tumor occupies a large portion of the inside of the eye globe. (A, From Roberts F. Macroscopic techniques for ophthalmic tumor specimens. *Seminars in Diagnostic Pathology*, 2016;33(3):114–121. B, From Damjanov I. *Pathology for the health professions*, 3rd edition. St. Louis: Saunders; 2006. Courtesy Dr. Walter Richardson and Dr. Jamsheed Khan, Kansas City, KS.)

Because RB is a treatable tumor, dual priorities are saving the child's life and restoring useful vision. The prognosis for most children with RB is excellent, with a greater than 90% long-term survival.

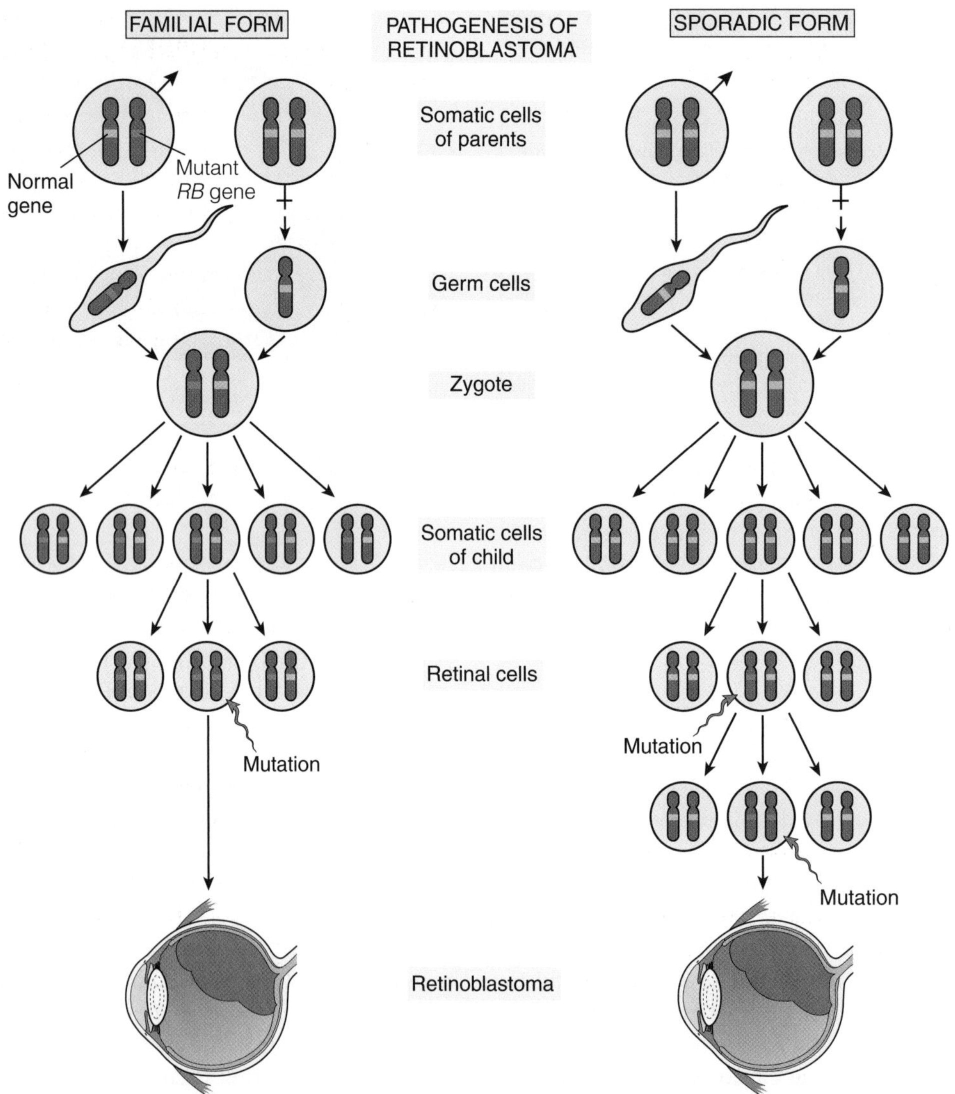

Fig. 20.13 The Two-Mutation Model of Retinoblastoma Development. In inherited retinoblastoma, the first mutation is transmitted through the germline of an affected parent. The second mutation occurs somatically in a retinal cell, leading to development of the tumor. In sporadic retinoblastoma, development of a tumor requires two somatic mutations.

SUMMARY REVIEW

Development of the Nervous System in Children

1. Growth and development of the brain occur most rapidly during fetal development and during the first year of life.
2. The bones of the skull are joined by sutures, and the wide, membranous junctions of the sutures (known as *fontanelles*) allow for brain growth and close by 18 months of age *typically*.
3. At birth, the forebrain is immature, so neurologic examination is primarily of reflex responses that require an intact spinal cord and brainstem.

Structural Malformations

1. Neural tube defects (NTDs) are an arrest of the normal development of the brain and spinal cord during the first month of embryonic development. Risk factors include folic acid deficiency, previous NTD pregnancy, maternal diabetes or obesity, use of anticonvulsants, and maternal hyperthermia.
2. Spina bifida (failure of vertebral closure) is the most common NTD and includes meningocele (a sac-like meningeal cyst of spinal fluid that protrudes through a vertebral defect), myelomeningocele (like a meningocele that also contains a portion of the spinal cord with its nerves), and spina bifida occulta.
3. Premature closure of the cranial sutures causes craniosynostosis, resulting in an asymmetric skull shape. If multiple sutures fuse prematurely, brain growth may be restricted.
4. Microencephaly is a defect in brain cell proliferation that leads to a small brain, small skull, and usually developmental delays.

5. Cortical dysplasias are defects in brain development caused by defects in neuronal cell migration and subsequent abnormalities in connection between cells.
6. Congenital hydrocephalus, characterized by increased cerebrospinal fluid (CSF) pressure, results from impaired absorption or blockage of circulation of CSF and rarely overproduction of CSF. Dandy-Walker deformity, which is commonly associated with hydrocephalus, is associated with cystic dilation of the fourth ventricle and aqueductal compression.

Alterations in Function: Encephalopathies

1. Static (nonprogressive) encephalopathies (e.g., cerebral palsy and epilepsy) are disorders of the brain caused by a fixed lesion without active and ongoing disease. They can occur during gestation, birth, or childhood and can be caused by endogenous or exogenous factors.
2. Cerebral palsy (CP) can be caused by prenatal or perinatal cerebral hypoxia or perinatal trauma, with symptoms of motor dysfunction (including increased muscle tone, increased reflexes, and loss of fine motor coordination), mental retardation, seizure disorders, or developmental disabilities. CP can be extrapyramidal/nonspastic or pyramidal/spastic.
3. Inherited metabolic disorders that damage the nervous system include defects in amino acid metabolism (phenylketonuria) and lysosomal storage defects (GM_2 gangliosidosis/Tay-Sachs disease) and result in abnormal behavior, seizures, and deficient psychomotor development.
4. Seizure disorders are abnormal discharges of electrical activity within the brain. They are associated with numerous nervous system disorders and more often are a generalized rather than a partial type of seizure.
5. Accidental ingestion, therapeutic overdose, intentional overdose, or ingestion of environmental toxins, such as in lead poisoning, can cause serious neurologic damage.
6. Bacterial meningitis is commonly caused by *Neisseria meningitidis* or *Streptococcus pneumoniae* and may result from respiratory tract or gastrointestinal infections; symptoms include fever, headaches, photophobia, seizures, rigidity, and stupor.
7. Viral meningitis may result from direct infection or be secondary to a systemic viral infection (e.g., measles, mumps, herpes, or leukemia).

Cerebrovascular Disease in Children

1. Perinatal arterial ischemic stroke is a leading cause of perinatal brain injury, cerebral palsy, and lifelong disability.
2. Ischemic (occlusive) stroke is rare in children but can occur from embolism, sickle cell disease, cerebral arteriopathies, and cardiac anomalies.
3. Hemorrhagic stroke can occur in association with immature blood vessel associated with prematurity or cerebral arteriovenous malformations.
4. Moyamoya is a rare, progressive vascular stenosis of the circle of Willis that obstructs arterial blood flow to the brain and is associated with transient ischemic attacks.

Epilepsy and Seizure Disorders in Children

1. Seizures are abnormal discharges of electrical activity within the brain. Epilepsy is the occurrence of more than two unprovoked seizures separated by over 24 hours.
2. Seizures can be caused by structural abnormalities of the brain, hypoxia, intracranial hemorrhage, CNS infection, traumatic injury, electrolyte imbalance, or inborn metabolic disturbances.
3. Epileptic spasms (infantile spasms) are a rare severe type of seizure associated with brain injury that occur in clusters of 10 to 150 spasms affecting the whole body or just the arms and legs.

Childhood Brain Tumors

1. Brain tumors are the second most common type of childhood cancer and are the leading cause of cancer related death in children.
2. Symptoms of brain tumors may be generalized or localized. The most common general symptoms are the result of increased intracranial pressure and include headache, irritability, vomiting, somnolence, and bulging of fontanelles.
3. Localized findings relate to the degree of disturbance in physiologic functioning in the area where the tumor is located. Localized signs of infratentorial tumors in the cerebellum include impaired coordination and balance.
4. Neuroblastoma is an embryonal tumor of the sympathetic nervous system and can be located anywhere there is sympathetic nervous tissue. Symptoms include weight loss, irritability, fatigue, fever, and intractable diarrhea. Neuroblastoma has been associated with spontaneous remission in infants.
5. Retinoblastoma is a congenital eye tumor that has two forms: inherited and acquired; both are related to loss of function of the *RB* gene.

REFERENCES

1. Kling PJ. Iron nutrition, erythrocytes, and erythropoietin in the NICU: erythropoietic and neuroprotective effects. *Neoreviews.* 2020;21(2):e80–e88.
2. Eggink AJ, Steegers-Theunissen RP. Neural tube anomalies: an update on the pathophysiology and prevention. In: Kilby MD, Johnson A, Oepkes D, eds. *Fetal therapy: scientific basis and critical appraisal of clinical benefits.* ed 2 Cambridge, UK: Cambridge University Press; 2020:449–455.
3. Centers for Disease Control and Prevention (CDC) Page last reviewed *Folic acid & neural tube defects: data & statistics.* Atlanta, GA: CDC; November 9, 2017. Available at www.cdc.gov/ncbddd/birthdefectscount/data.html. (Accessed August 21, 2021).
4. US Preventive Service Task Force (USPSTF) *Folic acid to prevent neural tube defects: preventive medication.* Rockville, MD: USPSTF; 2017. Released January 10, 2017. Current as of April 2021. Available at https://www.uspreventiveservicestaskforce.org/uspstf/recommendation/folic-acid-for-the-prevention-of-neural-tube-defects-preventive-medication#fullrecommendationstart. (Accessed August 21, 2021).
5. Avagliano L, et al. Overview on neural tube defects: from development to physical characteristics. *Birth Defects Res.* 2019;111(19):1455–1467.

6. National Center on Birth Defects and Developmental Disabilities, Centers for Disease Control and Prevention (CDC) *Facts about anencephaly*. Atlanta, GA: CDC; 2020. Page last reviewed December 28, 2020. Available at https://www.cdc.gov/ncbddd/birthdefects/anencephaly.html. (Accessed August 21, 2021).
7. National Center on Birth Defects and Developmental Disabilities, Centers for Disease Control and Prevention (CDC) *Facts about encephalocele*. Atlanta, GA: CDC; 2020. Page last reviewed December 28, 2020. Available at https://www.cdc.gov/ncbddd/birthdefects/encephalocele.html. (Accessed August 21, 2021).
8. Kliegman RM, et al. ed. *Nelson textbook of pediatrics*. ed 21 : Elsevier; 2020.
9. Tamburrini G, et al. Myelomeningocele: the management of the associated hydrocephalus. *Childs Nerv Syst*. 2013;29(9):1569–1579.
10. Yamashiro KJ, Galganski LA, Hirose S. Fetal myelomeningocele repair. *Semin Pediatr Surg*. 2019;28(4):150823.
11. Ferreira Furtado LM, et al. Tethered cord syndrome after myelomeningocele repair: a literature update. *Cureus*. 2020;12(10):e10949.
12. National Center on Birth Defects and Developmental Disabilities, Centers for Disease Control and Prevention (CDC) *Facts about craniosynostosis*. Atlanta, GA: CDC; 2020. Page last reviewed October 23, 2020. Available at https://www.cdc.gov/ncbddd/birthdefects/craniosynostosis.html. (Accessed August 21, 2021).
13. Alvarado-Socarras JL, et al. Congenital microcephaly: a diagnostic challenge during Zika epidemics. *Travel Med Infect Dis*. 2018;23:14–20.
14. Pavone P, et al. Clinical review on megalencephaly: a large brain as a possible sign of cerebral impairment. *Medicine (Baltimore)*. 2017;96(26):e6814.
15. Antoniou E, et al. Zika virus and the risk of developing microcephaly in infants: a systematic review. *Int J Environ Res Public Health*. 2020;17(11):3806.
16. Severino M, et al. Definitions and classification of malformations of cortical development: practical guidelines. *Brain*. 2020;143(10):2874–2894.
17. Romero DM, Bahi-Buisson N, Francis F. Genetics and mechanisms leading to human cortical malformations. *Semin Cell Dev Biol*. 2018;76:33–75.
18. National Institutes of Health (NIH), National Institute of Neurological Disorders and Stroke *Hydrocephalus fact sheet*. Bethesda, MD: NIH; 2020. Last modified May 13, 2020. Available at https://www.ninds.nih.gov/Disorders/Patient-Caregiver-Education/Fact-Sheets/Hydrocephalus-Fact-Sheet. (Accessed August 21, 2021).
19. National Institutes of Health (NIH), Genetics Home Reference *Phenylketonuria*. Bethesda, MD: NIH; 2020. Page last updated April 7, 2021. Page last reviewed October 1, 2017. Available at https://ghr.nlm.nih.gov/condition/phenylketonuria#resources. (Accessed August 21, 2021).
20. Waisbren S, et al. Long-term preservation of intellectual functioning in sapropterin-treated infants and young children with phenylketonuria: a seven-year analysis. *Mol Genet Metab*. 2021;132(2):119–127.
21. National Organization for Rare Disorders (NORD) *Lysosomal storage disorders*. Danbury, CT: NORD; 2006. Available at https://rarediseases.org/rare-diseases/lysosomal-storage-disorders/. (Accessed August 21, 2021).
22. Ikeudenta BA, Rutkofsky IH. Unmasking the enigma of cerebral palsy: a traditional review. *Cureus*. 2020;12(10):e11004.
23. National Center on Birth Defects and Developmental Disabilities, Centers for Disease Control and Prevention (CDC) *Data and statistics for cerebral palsy*. Atlanta, GA: CDC; 2020. Page last reviewed December 31, 2020. Available at https://www.cdc.gov/ncbddd/cp/data.html. (Accessed August 21, 2021).
24. Patel DR, et al. Cerebral palsy in children: a clinical overview. *Transl Pediatr*. 2020;9(Suppl 1):S125–S135.
25. Vitrikas K, Dalton H, Breish D. Cerebral palsy: an overview. *Am Fam Physician*. 2020;101(4):213–220.
26. Parenti G, Medina DL, Ballabio A. The rapidly evolving view of lysosomal storage diseases. *EMBO Mol Med*. 2021;13(2):e12836.
27. Leal AF, et al. GM2 gangliosidoses: clinical features, pathophysiological aspects, and current therapies. *Int J Mol Sci*. 2020;21(17):6213.
28. National Poison Control Center *Poison statistics national data 2019*. Washington, DC: National Poison Control Center; 2019. Available at https://www.poison.org/poison-statistics-national. (Accessed August 21, 2021).
29. Egendorf SP, et al. Soil toxicants that potentially affect children's health. *Curr Probl Pediatr Adolesc Health Care*. 2020;50(1):100741.
30. American College of Obstetricians and Gynecologists (ACOG) Exposure to toxic environmental agents Committee Opinion No. 575. *Fertil Steril*. 2013;100(4):931–934.
31. Ladomenou F, et al. Conjugate vaccines dramatically reshaped the epidemiology of bacterial meningitis in a well-defined child population. *Acta Paediatr*. 2020;109(2):368–374.
32. Beeslaar J, et al. Clinical data supporting a 2-dose schedule of MenB-FHbp, a bivalent meningococcal serogroup B vaccine, in adolescents and young adults. *Vaccine*. 2018;36(28):4004–4013.
33. Centers for Disease Control and Prevention (CDC), National Center for Immunization and Respiratory Diseases *Vaccines and preventable diseases: meningococcal vaccination*. Atlanta, GA: CDC; 2019. Page last reviewed July 26, 2019. Available at https://www.cdc.gov/vaccines/vpd/mening/index.html. (Accessed August 21, 2021).
34. Erickson TA, et al. Infectious and autoimmune causes of encephalitis in children. *Pediatrics*. 2020;145(6):e20192543.
35. Kupferman JC, et al. Hypertension and childhood stroke. *Pediatr Nephrol*. 2021;36:809–823.
36. Heron M. Deaths: leading causes for 2017. *Natl Vital Stat Rep*. 2019;68:1–77.
37. Gilard V, et al. Intraventricular hemorrhage in very preterm infants: a comprehensive review. *J Clin Med*. 2020;9(8):2447.
38. Fang YC, et al. Pathological circulating factors in moyamoya disease. *Int J Mol Sci*. 2021;22(4):1696.
39. Ferriero DM, et al. Management of stroke in neonates and children: a scientific statement from the American Heart Association/American Stroke Association. *Stroke*. 2019;50: e51–e96.
40. Zack MM, Kobau R. National and state estimates of the numbers of adults and children with active epilepsy—United States, 2015. *MMWR Morb Mortal Wkly Rep*. 2017;66(31): 821–825. 2017.
41. Rudy L, et al. Anticonvulsant mechanisms of the ketogenic diet and caloric restriction. *Epilepsy Res*. 2020;168:106499.
42. Davis P, Gaitanis J. Neuromodulation for the treatment of epilepsy: a review of current approaches and future directions. *Clin Ther*. 2020;42(7):1140–1154.
43. Madaan P, Gupta A, Gulati S: Pediatric epilepsy surgery: indications and evaluation, *Indian J Pediatr*. Published online before print March 19, 2021. Available at https://doi.org/10.1007/s12098-021-03668-x. (Accessed August 21, 2021).
44. Pavone P, et al. West syndrome: a comprehensive review. *Neurol Sci*. 2020;41(12):3547–3562.

45. Central Brain Tumor Registry of the United States: *2020 CBTRUS fact sheet*. Available at https://cbtrus.org/cbtrus-fact-sheet-2020/. (Accessed August 21, 2021).
46. Kerleroux B, et al. Posterior fossa tumors in children: radiological tips & tricks in the age of genomic tumor classification and advance MR technology. *J Neuroradiol*. 2020;47(1):46–53.
47. Wu WT, et al. New era of immunotherapy in pediatric brain tumors: chimeric antigen receptor T-cell therapy. *Int J Mol Sci*. 2021;22(5):2404.
48. American Cancer Society (ACS) *Key statistics about neuroblastoma*. Atlanta, GA: ACS; 2020. Last revised April 28, 2021. Accessed April 13, 2021. Available at http://www.cancer.org/cancer/neuroblastoma/detailedguide/neuroblastoma-key-statistics. (Accessed August 21, 2021).
49. Morandi F, et al. Immunotherapeutic strategies for neuroblastoma: present, past and future. *Vaccines (Basel)*. 2021;9(1):43.
50. Mehyar M, et al. Impact of RB1 gene mutation type in retinoblastoma patients on clinical presentation and management outcome. *Hematol Oncol Stem Cell Ther*. 2020;13(3):152–159.
51. Berry JL, et al. The RB1 story: characterization and cloning of the first tumor suppressor gene. *Genes (Basel)*. 2019;10(11):879.
52. Sun J, et al. Biomarkers in retinoblastoma. *Int J Ophthalmol*. 2020;13(2):325–341.
53. American Cancer Society (ACS) *Risk factors for brain and spinal cord tumors in children*. Atlanta, GA: ACS; 2018. Last revised June 20, 2018. Available at https://www.cancer.org/cancer/brain-spinal-cord-tumors-children/causes-risks-prevention/risk-factors.html. (Accessed August 21, 2021).

21

Mechanisms of Hormonal Regulation

Karen C. Turner and Valentina L. Brashers

http://evolve.elsevier.com/Rogers/pathophysiology/

CHAPTER OUTLINE

The endocrine system is composed of various glands located throughout the body (Fig. 21.1). These glands can synthesize and release special chemical messengers called *hormones*. The endocrine, nervous, and immune systems work together to regulate responses to internal and external environments. The endocrine system has five general functions: (1) differentiation of the reproductive and central nervous systems in the developing fetus; (2) stimulation of sequential growth and development during childhood and adolescence; (3) coordination of the male and female reproductive systems, which makes sexual reproduction possible; (4) maintenance of an optimal internal environment throughout life; and (5) initiation of corrective and adaptive responses when emergency demands occur. Hormones convey specific regulatory information among cells and organs and are integrated with the nervous system to maintain communication and control. The mechanisms of communication and control occur within a cell *(autocrine)*, between local cells *(paracrine)*, and between cells located remotely from each other *(endocrine)*.

MECHANISMS OF HORMONAL REGULATION

Endocrine glands respond to specific signals by synthesizing and releasing hormones into circulation, which then trigger intracellular responses. All hormones share certain general characteristics:

1. Hormones have specific rates and rhythms of secretion. Three basic patterns of secretion are (a) diurnal patterns, (b) pulsatile and cyclic patterns, and (c) patterns that depend on levels of circulating substrates (e.g., calcium, sodium, potassium, or the hormones themselves).
2. Hormones operate within feedback systems, either negative or positive, to maintain an optimal internal environment.
3. Hormones affect only target cells with specific receptors for the hormone and then act on these cells to initiate specific cell functions or activities.
4. Steroid hormones are either excreted directly by the kidneys or metabolized (conjugated) by the liver, which inactivates them and renders the hormone more water soluble for renal excretion. Peptide hormones are catabolized by circulating enzymes and eliminated in the feces or urine.

Hormones may be classified according to structure, gland of origin, effects, or chemical composition. (Table 21.1 categorizes known hormones based on structure.) The mechanisms of action and secretion of hormones represent an extremely complex system of integrated hormonal and neural responses.

Regulation of Hormone Release

Hormones are released to respond to an altered cellular environment or to maintain the level of another hormone or substance. One or more of the following mechanisms regulates hormone release: (1) chemical factors (such as blood glucose or calcium levels), (2) endocrine factors (a hormone from one endocrine gland controlling another endocrine gland), and (3) neural control.

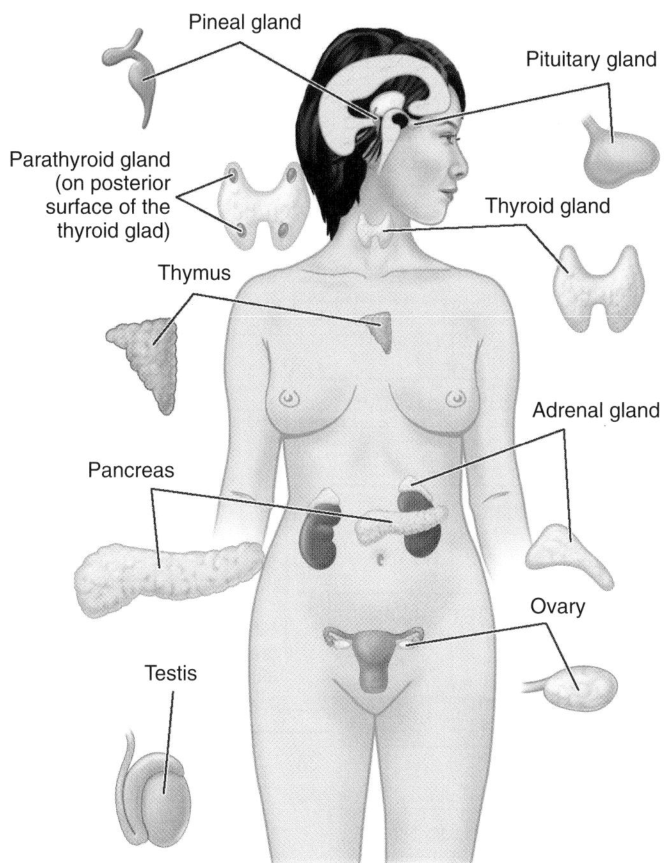

Fig. 21.1 Major Endocrine Glands. (From Applegate E. *The anatomy and physiology learning system*, 4th edition. St. Louis: Saunders; 2011.)

For example, insulin is secreted by the (1) chemical stimulation of increased plasma glucose levels, (2) the hormone cortisol from the adrenal cortex, and (3) direct stimulation of the insulin-secreting cells of the pancreas by the autonomic nervous system, which is a form of neural control.

Feedback systems provide precise monitoring and control of the cellular environment. Both negative- and positive-feedback systems are important for maintaining hormone levels within physiologic ranges. Positive feedback occurs when a neural, chemical, or endocrine response increases the synthesis and secretion of a hormone. Negative feedback, which is more common, occurs when a changing chemical, neural, or endocrine response to a stimulus decreases the synthesis and secretion of a hormone. Fig. 21.2A illustrates both positive and negative feedback within the hypothalamus-pituitary axis and the thyroid gland. Positive feedback occurs when thyrotropin-releasing hormone (TRH) is released from the hypothalamus in response to low thyroid hormone levels. TRH stimulates the secretion of thyroid-stimulating hormone (TSH), which then stimulates the synthesis and secretion of the thyroid hormones thyroxine (T_4) and triiodothyronine (T_3). Negative feedback occurs when increasing levels of T_4 and T_3 feedback on the pituitary and hypothalamus inhibit TRH and TSH synthesis and decrease the synthesis and production of thyroid hormones. Fig. 21.2B illustrates a more complex model for feedback mechanisms across the hormonal system. The lack of positive or negative feedback on hormonal release often results in pathologic changes in hormone production (see Chapter 22).

TABLE 21.1 Structural Categories of Hormones

Structural Category	Examples
Water Soluble	
Peptides	Growth hormone Insulin Leptin Parathyroid hormone Prolactin
Glycoproteins	Follicle-stimulating hormone Luteinizing hormone Thyroid-stimulating hormone
Polypeptides	Adrenocorticotropic hormone Antidiuretic hormone Calcitonin Endorphins Glucagon Hypothalamic hormones Lipotropins Melanocyte-stimulating hormone Oxytocin Somatostatin Thymosin Thyrotropin-releasing hormone
Amines	Epinephrine Norepinephrine
Lipid Soluble	
Thyroxine (an amine but lipid soluble)	Both thyroxine (T_4) and triiodothyronine (T_3)
Steroids (cholesterol is a precursor for all steroids)	Estrogens Glucocorticoids (cortisol) Mineralocorticoids (aldosterone) Progestins (progesterone) Testosterone
Derivatives of arachidonic acid (autocrine or paracrine action)	Leukotrienes Prostacyclins Prostaglandins Thromboxanes

Hormone Transport

Once hormones are released into the circulatory system, they are distributed throughout the body. The protein (peptide) hormones (see Table 21.1) are water soluble and generally circulate in free (unbound) forms. Water-soluble hormones generally have a half-life of seconds to minutes because they are catabolized by circulating enzymes. For example, insulin has a half-life of 3 to 5 minutes and is catabolized by insulinases. Lipid-soluble hormones (see Table 21.1), such as cortisol and adrenal androgens, are transported bound to a water-soluble carrier or transport protein and can remain in the blood for hours to days. Only free hormones (those not bound to a carrier protein) can signal

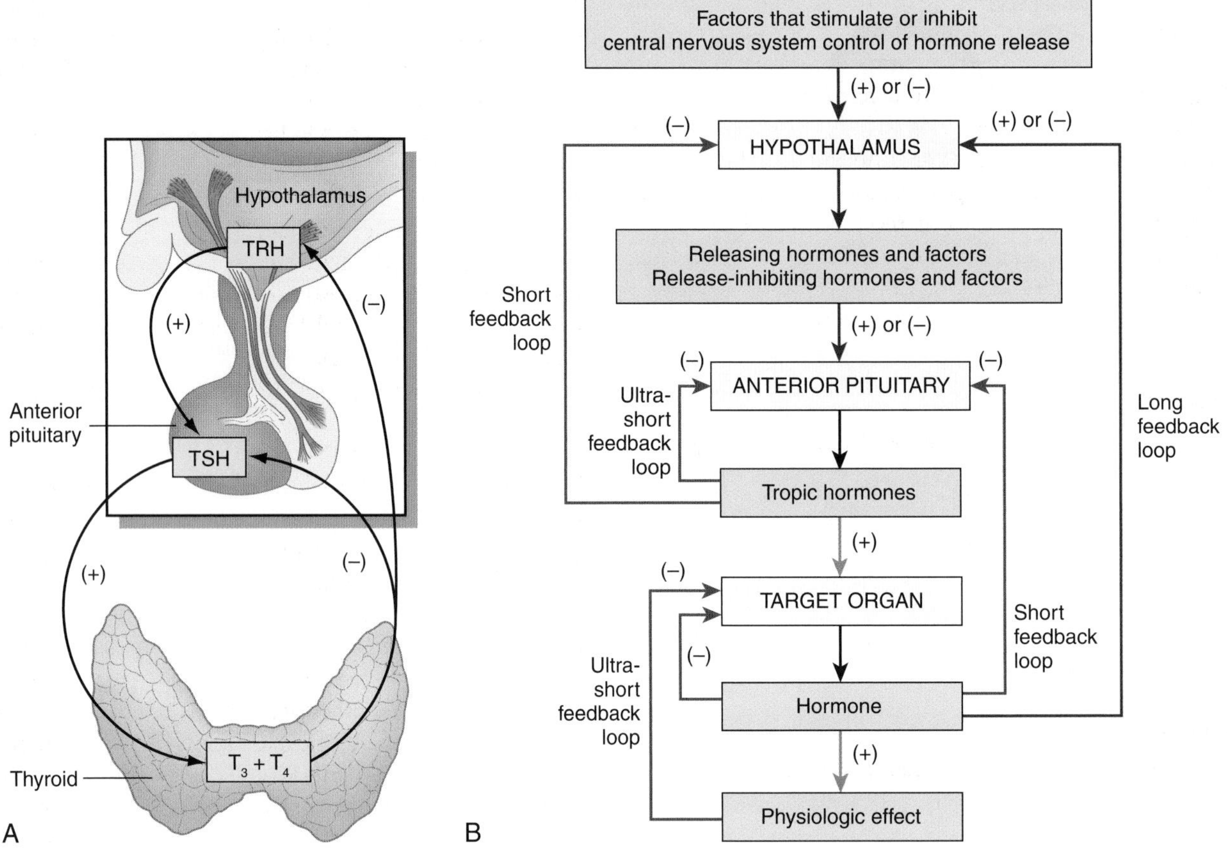

Fig. 21.2 Feedback Loops. (A) Endocrine feedback loops for the thyroid gland: *TRH*, Thyroid-releasing hormone; *TSH*, thyroid-stimulating hormone; T_3, triiodothyronine; T_4, tetraiodothyronine (thyroxine). **(B)** General model for feedback mechanisms in the regulation of hormone secretion., Negative feedback regulation (−) is possible at three levels: target organ (ultrashort feedback), anterior pituitary (short feedback), and hypothalamus (long feedback).

a target cell. At the cell membrane, lipid-soluble hormones dissociate from their carrier protein and diffuse into the cell. Because there is equilibrium between the concentrations of free hormones and hormones bound to plasma proteins, a significant change in the concentration of binding (carrier) proteins can affect the concentration of free hormones in the plasma. For example, malnutrition and liver disease can lower the serum levels of the carrier protein albumin, causing a decrease in the lipid-soluble hormones thyroxine, cortisol, and aldosterone. (Mechanisms of hormone binding are discussed in Chapter 1.) Free hormone levels can be measured using a variety of measurement techniques, including radioimmunoassay (RIA), enzyme-linked immunosorbent assay (ELISA), or bioassay.

Hormone Receptors

Although a hormone is distributed throughout the body, only those cells with appropriate receptors for that hormone, termed target cells, are affected. Target cell response depends on blood levels of the hormone, the concentration of target cell receptors, and affinity of the receptor for the hormone. Hormone receptors of the target cell have two main functions: (1) to recognize and bind specifically and with high affinity (sensitivity) to their particular hormones, and (2) to initiate a signal to appropriate intracellular effectors.

The sensitivity of the target cell to a particular hormone is related to the total number of receptors per cell or the affinity of the receptors for the hormone: the more receptors or the higher the affinity of the receptors, the more sensitive the cell to the stimulating effects of the hormone. Low concentrations of hormone increase the number or affinity of receptors per cell; this is called up-regulation (Fig. 21.3A). High concentrations of hormone decrease the number or affinity of receptors; this is called down-regulation (Fig. 21.3B). Thus, the cell can adjust its sensitivity to the concentration of the signaling hormone. The receptors on the plasma membrane are continuously synthesized and degraded, so that changes in receptor concentration or affinity may occur within hours. Various physiochemical conditions can affect both the receptor number and the affinity of the hormone for its receptor. Some of these physiochemical conditions are the fluidity and structure of the plasma membrane, pH, temperature, ion concentration, diet, and the presence of other chemicals (e.g., drugs). Finally, mutations may affect receptor number or structure. For example, mutations in TSH receptors can lead to resistance to thyroid hormone and can contribute to defective thyroid hormone production.[1]

Hormone receptors may be located in the plasma membrane or in the intracellular compartment of the target cell (Fig. 21.4).

Water-soluble hormones (peptide or nonsteroid hormones), which include the protein hormones and the catecholamines, have a high molecular weight and cannot diffuse across the cell membrane. They interact or bind with receptors located in or on the cell membrane and activate a second messenger to mediate short-acting responses. Lipid-soluble hormones (steroid hormones) diffuse freely across the plasma and nuclear membranes and bind with cytosolic or nuclear receptors, although receptors for some lipid-soluble hormones are located in or near the plasma membrane and facilitate rapid (non-genomic) effects.[2]

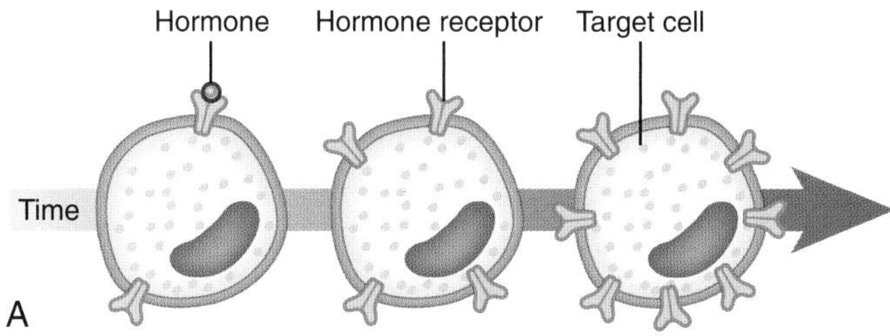

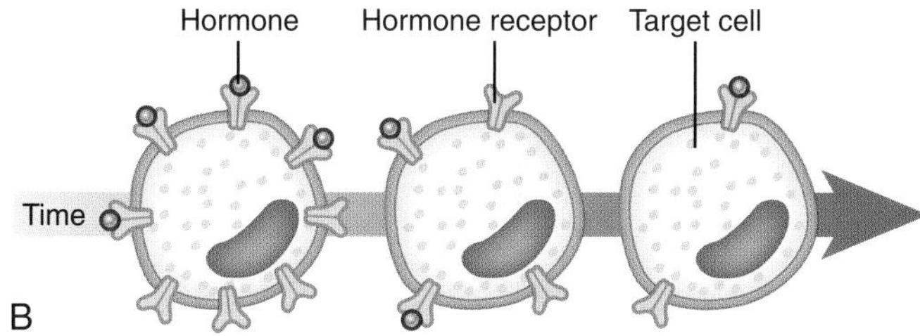

Fig. 21.3 Regulation of Target Cell Sensitivity. **(A)** Low hormone level and up-regulation, or an increase in the number of receptors. **(B)** High hormone level and down-regulation, or a decrease in the number of receptors.

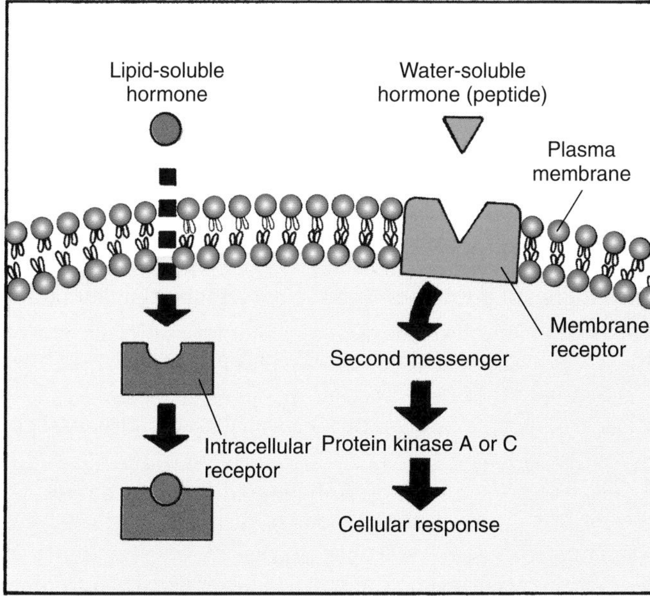

Fig. 21.4 Hormone Binding at Target Cell.

Water-Soluble Hormone Receptors

Water-soluble hormone binding with plasma membrane receptors initiates a complex cascade of intracellular effects. In this cascade, the hormone is termed the first messenger. The hormone-receptor interaction initiates a signal that generates a small molecule inside the cell, called the second messenger. The second messenger conveys the signal from the receptor to the cytoplasm and nucleus of the cell and mediates the effect of the hormone on the target cell. Second messengers include cyclic adenosine monophosphate (cAMP), cyclic guanosine monophosphate (cGMP), calcium, inositol triphosphate (IP_3), and the tyrosine kinase system (Table 21.2).

The second messenger cAMP increases when first messengers from the anterior pituitary gland, such as adrenocorticotropic hormone (ACTH) and TSH, bind to a cell membrane receptor. Increased levels of intracellular cAMP activate protein kinases, leading to activation or deactivation of intracellular enzymes (Fig. 21.5). cGMP also functions as a second messenger following receptor binding of first messengers (e.g., atrial natriuretic peptide and nitric oxide). These hormones and signaling molecules play crucial roles in cardiovascular and pulmonary health and disease. Drugs, such as phosphodiesterase inhibitors that sustain the action of cGMP are used in the treatment of erectile dysfunction and are being explored for the treatment of vascular and pulmonary hypertension and cognitive dysfunction.[3,4]

The second messenger IP_3 is increased in response to angiotensin II and antidiuretic hormone (ADH) receptor binding and triggers a release of intracellular calcium. This leads to the formation of the calcium-calmodulin complex, which mediates the effects of calcium on intracellular activities that are crucial for cell metabolism, growth, and smooth muscle contraction.

TABLE 21.2 Second Messengers Identified for Specific Hormones

Second Messenger	Associated Hormones
Cyclic AMP	Adrenocorticotropic hormone (ACTH) Luteinizing hormone (LH) Human chorionic gonadotropin (hCG) Follicle-stimulating hormone (FSH) Thyroid-stimulating hormone (TSH) Antidiuretic hormone (ADH) Thyrotropin-releasing hormone (TRH) Parathyroid hormone (PTH) Glucagon
Cyclic GMP	Atrial natriuretic peptide
Calcium and IP_3	Angiotensin II Gonadotropin-releasing hormone (GnRH) Antidiuretic hormone (ADH) Luteinizing hormone–releasing hormone (LHRH)
Tyrosine kinases	Insulin Growth hormone Leptin Prolactin

AMP, Adenosine monophosphate; *GMP*, guanosine monophosphate; *IP_3*, inositol triphosphate.

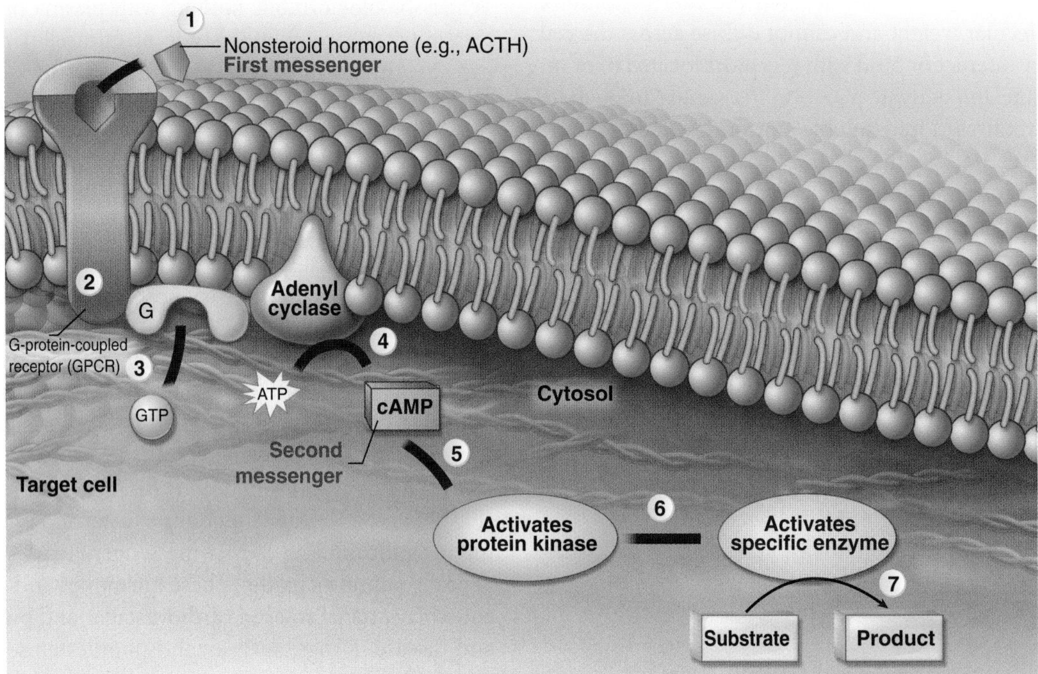

Fig. 21.5 Examples of First- and Second-Messenger Signaling. A water-soluble (nonsteroid) hormone acts as a first messenger and binds to a fixed receptor of the target cell *(1)*. The hormone-receptor complex activates the G protein *(2)*. The activated G protein *(G)* reacts with guanosine triphosphate *(GTP)*, which in turn activates the membrane-bound enzyme adenylyl cyclase *(3)*. Adenylyl cyclase catalyzes the conversion of adenosine triphosphate *(ATP)* to cyclic adenosine monophosphate (*cAMP;* second messenger) *(4)*. cAMP activates protein kinase *(5)*. Protein kinases activate specific intracellular enzymes *(6)*. These activated enzymes then influence specific cellular reactions and metabolic pathways, thus producing the target cell's response to the hormone *(7)*. *ACTH,* Adrenocorticotropic hormone. (From Patton KT, Thibodeau GA. *Anatomy & physiology,* 9th edition. St. Louis: Mosby; 2016.)

Some hormone first messengers, such as insulin, growth hormone (GH), and prolactin, bind to surface receptors that directly activate second messengers of the tyrosine kinase family. These tyrosine kinases include the Janus family of tyrosine kinases (JAK) and signal transducers and activators of transcription (STAT). They regulate a wide range of intracellular processes that contribute to cellular metabolism, immunity, growth, apoptosis, and oncogenesis. They can be targeted for inhibition in treatments aimed at moderating immune-mediated responses, as in rheumatoid arthritis and cancer.[5,6]

Lipid-Soluble Hormone Receptors

With the exception of thyroid hormones, the lipid-soluble hormones are synthesized from cholesterol (giving rise to the term "steroid") (see Table 21.1). Receptors for lipid-soluble hormones are in the cytosol and nucleus, and directly modulate gene expression without complex second messengers (Fig. 21.6). Because these are relatively small, lipophilic, hydrophobic molecules, lipid-soluble hormones can cross the lipid plasma membrane by simple diffusion (see Chapter 1). They bind with cytosolic or nuclear receptors, which keeps them from diffusing back out of the cell. The effects of lipid-soluble hormones on cytosol and nuclear receptors can take hours to days. However, lipid hormone receptors for estrogen, thyroid hormone, and aldosterone are located in the plasma membrane and are associated with rapid responses (seconds or minutes) (see Fig. 21.6). These receptors, when activated, have primarily intracellular nongenomic (membrane-initiated steroid signaling) effects. Through crosstalk, nongenomic responses and gene transcription modulate each other, allowing cells to adapt rapidly to environmental changes.[7,8]

Hormone Effects

The binding of hormones with their receptors stimulates three general types of effects by:

1. Acting on preexisting channel-forming proteins to alter membrane channel permeability
2. Activating preexisting proteins through a second-messenger system
3. Activating genes to cause protein synthesis (genomic effects)

Hormones affect target cells directly or permissively. Direct effects are the obvious changes in cell function that specifically result from stimulation by a particular hormone. Permissive effects are less obvious hormone-induced changes

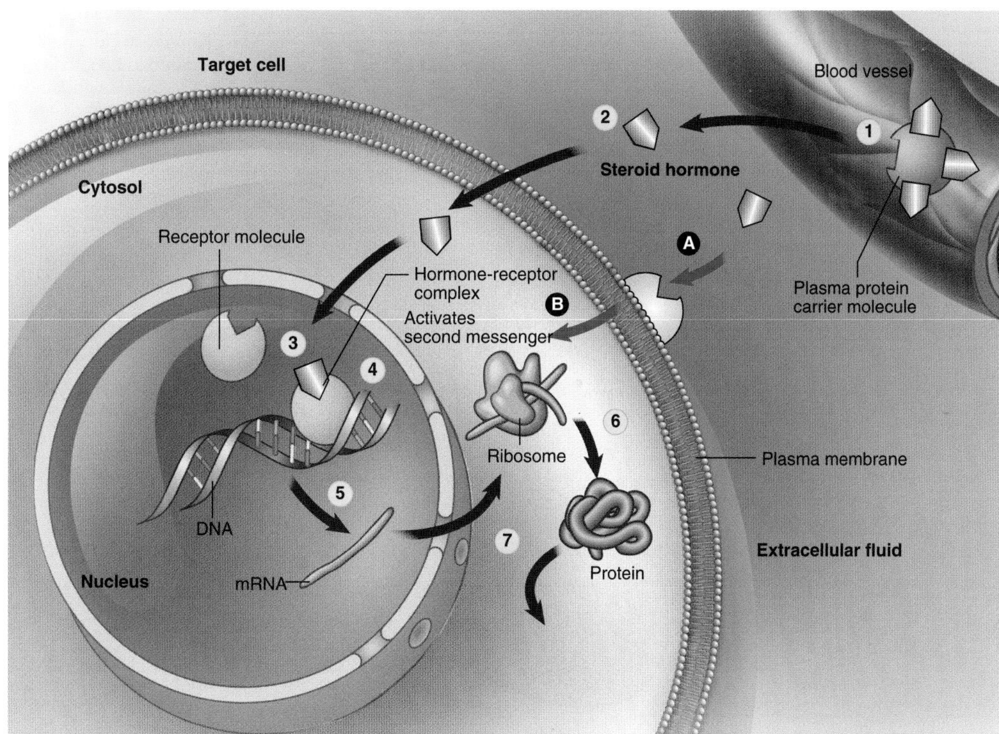

Fig. 21.6 Steroid Hormone Mechanism. Lipid-soluble steroid hormone molecules detach from the carrier protein *(1)* and pass through the plasma membrane *(2)*. Hormone molecules then diffuse into the nucleus, where they bind to a receptor to form a hormone-receptor complex *(3)*. This complex then binds to a specific site on a deoxyribonucleic acid *(DNA)* molecule *(4)*, triggering transcription of the genetic information encoded there *(5)*. The resulting messenger ribonucleic acid *(mRNA)* molecule moves to the cytosol, where it associates with a ribosome, initiating synthesis of a new protein *(6)*. This new protein—usually an enzyme or channel protein—produces specific effects on the target cell *(7)*. The classic genomic action is typically slow *(red arrows)*. Steroids also may exact rapid effects *(green arrows)* by binding to receptors on the plasma membrane ***(A)*** and activating an intercellular second messenger ***(B)***. (From Patton KT, Thibodeau GA. *Anatomy & physiology*, 9th edition. St. Louis: Mosby; 2016.)

that facilitate the maximal response or functioning of a cell and require the presence of another hormone. For example, thyroid hormone has a direct effect on lipid metabolism, causing increased concentration of serum fatty acids and a permissive effect on epinephrine by increasing the number of adrenergic receptors.

STRUCTURE AND FUNCTION OF THE ENDOCRINE GLANDS

Hypothalamic–Pituitary System

The hypothalamic–pituitary axis (HPA) forms the structural and functional basis for central integration of the neurologic and endocrine systems, creating what is called the *neuroendocrine system*. The HPA produces several hormones that affect a number of diverse body functions (Fig. 21.7), including thyroid, adrenal, and reproductive functions.

Hypothalamus

The hypothalamus is located at the base of the brain. It is connected to the pituitary gland by the infundibulum (pituitary stalk) (Fig. 21.8). The hypothalamus is connected to the anterior pituitary through hypophysial portal blood vessels (Fig. 21.9) and to the posterior pituitary via a nerve tract referred to as the *hypothalamohypophysial tract* (Fig. 21.10). These connections are vital to the functioning of the hypothalamic–pituitary system. The hypothalamus contains special neurosecretory cells that synthesize and secrete the hypothalamic-releasing hormones that regulate the release of hormones from the anterior pituitary. In addition, these cells synthesize the hormones ADH (also called *vasopressin*) and oxytocin, which are stored and released from the posterior pituitary gland. ADH and oxytocin travel to the posterior pituitary by way of the hypothalamohypophysial nerve tract. Releasing and inhibitory hormones are synthesized in the hypothalamus and are secreted into the portal blood vessels, through which they travel to their target tissues within the anterior pituitary and control the release of tropic hormones. These releasing/inhibitory hormones from the hypothalamus include prolactin-inhibiting hormone (PIH), prolactin-releasing hormone (PRH), TRH, gonadotropin-releasing hormone (GnRH), hypothalamic somatostatin, growth hormone-releasing hormone (GHRH), corticotropin-releasing hormone (CRH), and substance P. These hormones are summarized in Table 21.3.

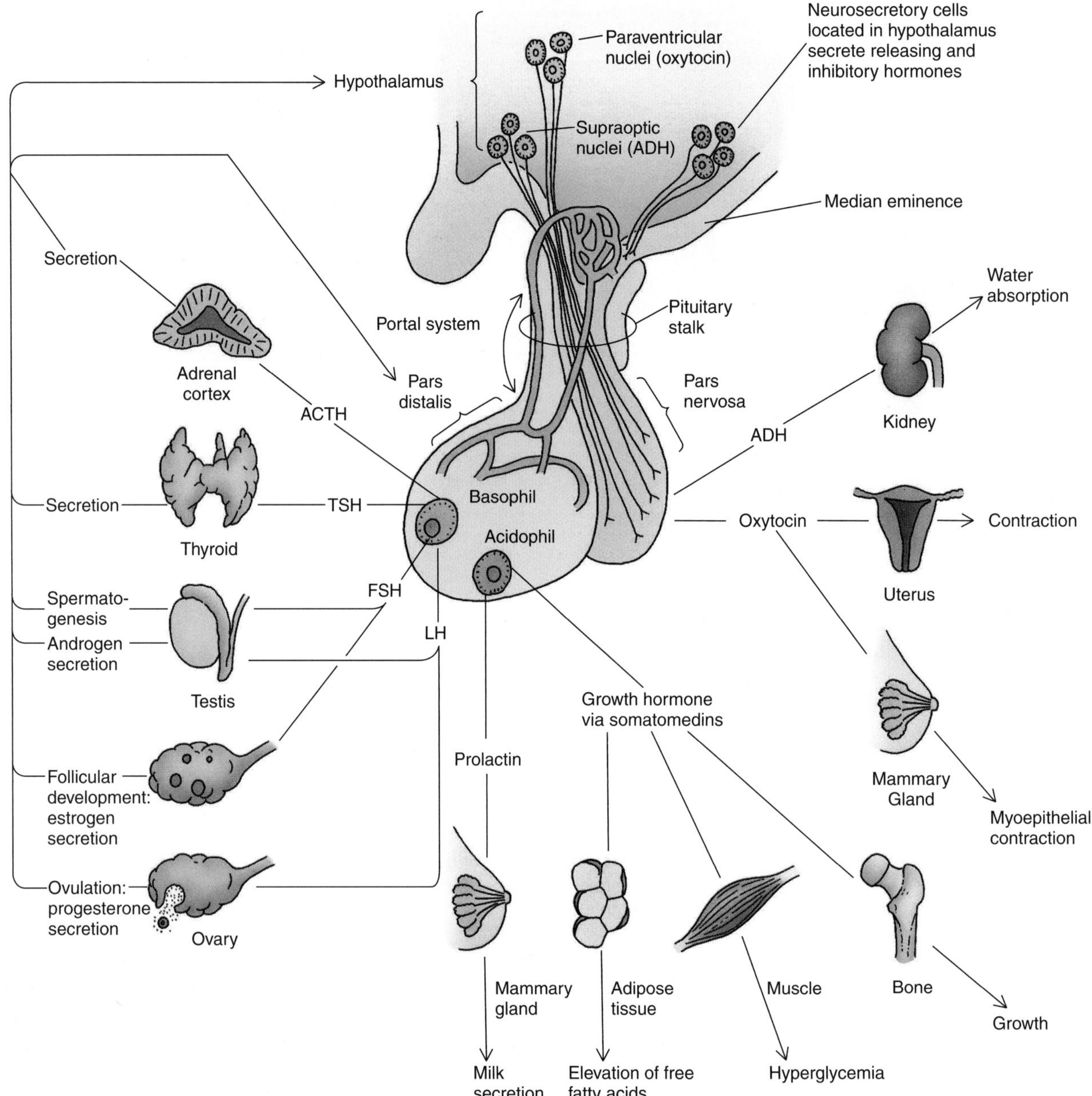

Fig. 21.7 The Hypothalamic-Pituitary Axis and Its Target Organs. *ACTH*, Adrenocorticotropic hormone; *ADH*, antidiuretic hormone; *FSH*, follicle-stimulating hormone; *LH*, luteinizing hormone; *TSH*, thyroid-stimulating hormone. (From Gartner LP, Hiatt JL. *Color textbook of histology*, 3rd edition. Philadelphia: Saunders; 2007.)

Pituitary Gland

The pituitary gland is located in the sella turcica (a saddle-shaped depression of the sphenoid bone at the base of the skull). It weighs approximately 0.5 g, except during pregnancy, when its weight increases by about 30%. It is composed of two distinctly different lobes: (1) the anterior pituitary, or adenohypophysis, and (2) the posterior pituitary, or neurohypophysis (see Fig. 21.8). These two lobes differ in their embryonic origins, cell types, and functional relationship to the hypothalamus.

Anterior Pituitary

The anterior pituitary (adenohypophysis) accounts for 75% of the total weight of the pituitary gland and is composed of three regions: (1) the pars distalis, (2) the pars tuberalis, and (3) the pars intermedia. The pars distalis is the major component of the anterior pituitary and is the source of the anterior pituitary hormones. The pars tuberalis is a thin layer of cells on the anterior and lateral portions of the pituitary stalk. The pars intermedia lies between the two and secretes melanocyte-stimulating hormone in the fetus. In the adult, the distinct pars intermedia

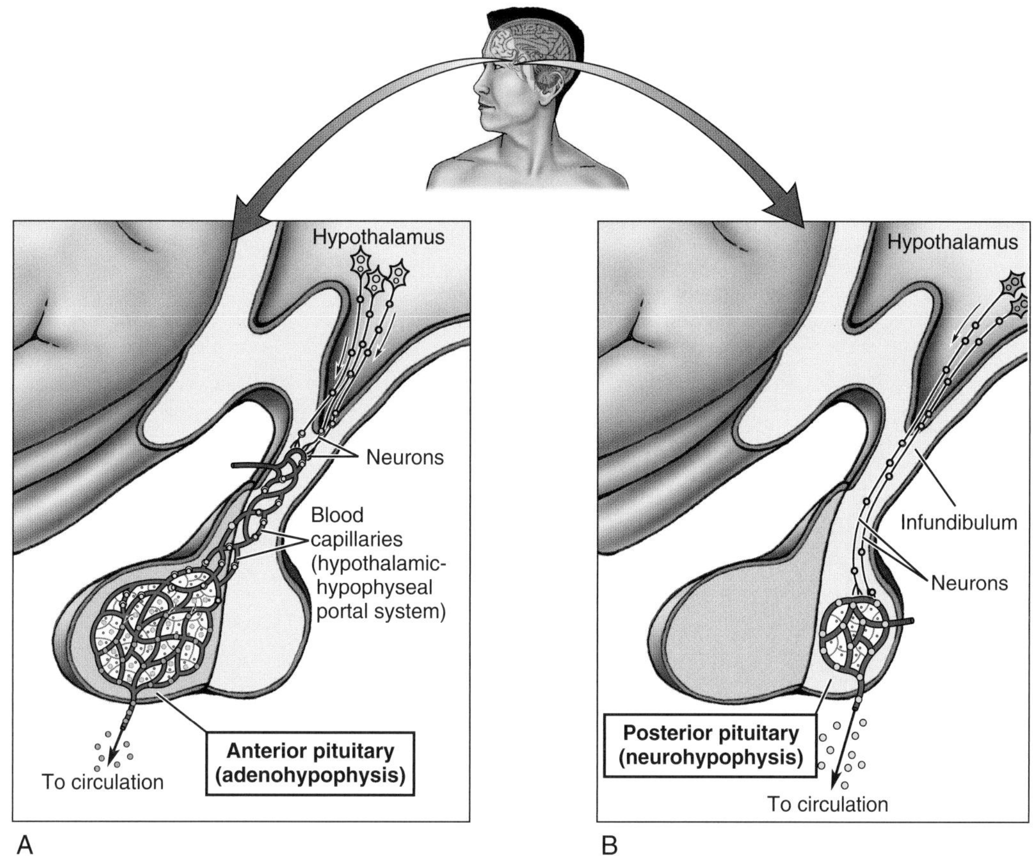

Fig. 21.8 Pituitary Gland. The pituitary gland sits within the sella turcica of the sphenoid bone of the skull. **(A)** Relationship of the hypothalamus to the anterior pituitary gland. **(B)** Relationship of the hypothalamus to the posterior pituitary gland. (From Herlihy B. *The human body in health and illness*, 5th edition. St. Louis: Saunders; 2015.)

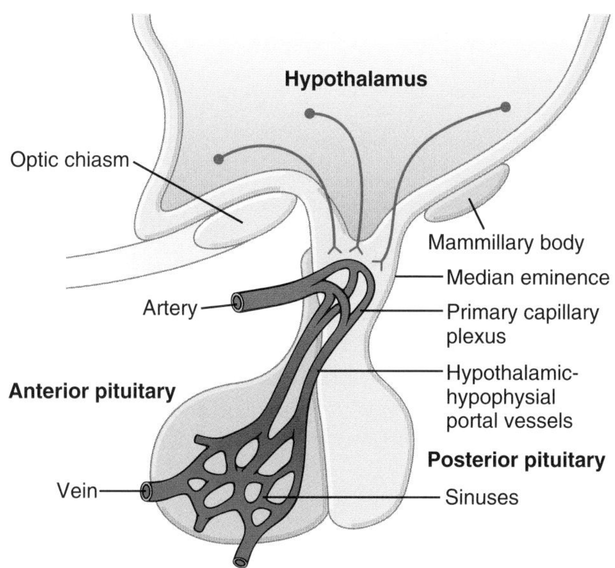

Fig. 21.9 Hypophysial Portal System. (From Hall JE. *Guyton and Hall textbook of medical physiology*, 13th edition. Philadelphia: Saunders; 2016.)

disappears, and the individual cells are distributed diffusely throughout the pars distalis and pars nervosa (neural lobe) of the posterior pituitary.

The anterior pituitary is composed of two main cell types: (1) the chromophobes, which appear to be nonsecretory, and (2) the chromophils, which are the secretory cells of the adenohypophysis. The chromophils are subdivided into seven secretory cell types, and each cell type secretes a specific hormone or hormones. In general, the anterior pituitary hormones are regulated by (1) secretion of hypothalamic releasing factors, (2) feedback effects of the hormones secreted by target glands, and (3) direct effects of other mediating neurotransmitters.

The anterior pituitary secretes tropic hormones that affect the physiologic function of specific target organs (see Fig. 21.7). These hormones can be grouped into three categories: corticotropin-related hormones, glycoproteins, and somatotropins (Table 21.4). Corticotropin-related hormones include melanocyte-stimulating hormone (MSH), which promotes the pituitary secretion of melanin to darken skin color, and adrenocorticotropic hormone (ACTH), which regulates the release of cortisol from the adrenal cortex. Also included in the corticotropic hormones are β-lipotropin, which plays a role in fat catabolism, and β-endorphins, which impact pain perception, body temperature, and food and water intake.

The glycoprotein hormones follicle-stimulating hormone (FSH) and luteinizing hormone (LH) influence reproductive function and are discussed in Chapter 24. Thyroid-stimulating hormone (TSH), also a glycoprotein hormone, regulates the activity of the thyroid gland. The roles of ACTH and TSH are discussed later in this chapter.

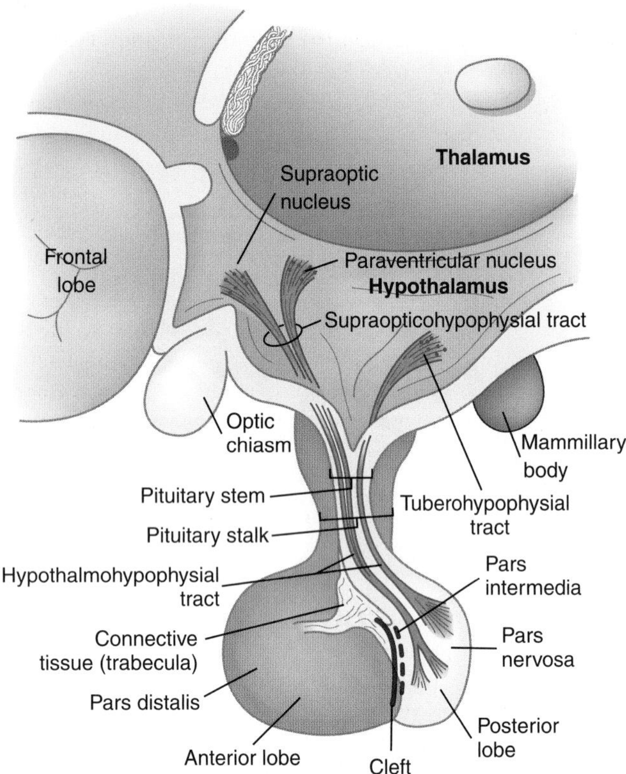

Fig. 21.10 Nerve Tracts from Hypothalamus to Posterior Lobe of Pituitary Gland.

TABLE 21.3 Hypothalamic Hormones

Hormone	Action
Target the Anterior Pituitary for Release	
Thyrotropin-releasing hormone (TRH)	Stimulates release of thyroid-stimulating hormone (TSH); modulates prolactin secretion
Gonadotropin-releasing hormone (GnRH)	Stimulates release of follicle-stimulating hormone (FSH) and luteinizing hormone (LH)
Somatostatin	Inhibits release of growth hormone (GH) and TSH
Growth hormone–releasing hormone (GHRH)	Stimulates release of GH
Corticotropin-releasing hormone (CRH)	Stimulates release of adrenocorticotropic hormone (ACTH) and β-endorphin
Substance P	Inhibits synthesis and release of adrenocorticotropic hormone (ACTH); stimulates secretion of GH, FSH, LH, and prolactin
Prolactin-inhibiting hormone (PIH, dopamine)	Inhibits synthesis and secretion of prolactin
Prolactin-releasing hormone (PRH)	Stimulates secretion of prolactin
Travel to Posterior Pituitary for Release	
Antidiuretic hormone (ADH)	Increases water reabsorption through the renal collecting ducts to reduce plasma osmolarity
Oxytocin	Stimulates contraction of the uterus and milk ejection in lactating women

TABLE 21.4 Tropic Hormones of the Anterior Pituitary and Their Functions

Hormone	Target Organs	Functions
Corticotropin-Related Hormones		
Adrenocorticotropic hormone (ACTH)	Adrenal gland (cortex)	Increased steroidogenesis (cortisol and androgenic hormones); synthesis of adrenal proteins contributing to maintenance of adrenal gland
Melanocyte-stimulating hormone (MSH)	Anterior pituitary	Promotes secretion of melanin and lipotropin by anterior pituitary; makes skin darker
Somatotropic Hormones		
Growth hormone (GH)	Muscle, bone, liver	Regulates metabolic processes related to growth and adaptation to physical and emotional stressors, muscle growth, increased protein synthesis, increased liver glycogenolysis, increased fat mobilization
	Liver	Induces formation of somatomedins, or insulin-like growth factors (IGFs) that have actions similar to insulin
Prolactin	Breast	Milk production
Glycoprotein Hormones		
Thyroid-stimulating hormone (TSH)	Thyroid gland	Increased production and secretion of thyroid hormoneIncreased iodide uptake; promotes hypertrophy and hyperplasia of thymocytes
Luteinizing hormone (LH)	*In women:* granulosa cells *In men:* Leydig cells	Ovulation, progesterone production Testicular growth, testosterone production
Follicle-stimulating hormone (FSH)	*In women:* granulosa cells *In men:* Sertoli cells	Follicle maturation, estrogen production Spermatogenesis
β-Lipotropin	Adipose cells	Fat breakdown and release of fatty acids
β-Endorphins	Adipose cells; brain opioid receptors	Analgesia; may regulate body temperature, food and water intake

The somatotropic hormones have diverse effects on body tissues and include GH and prolactin. Growth hormone secretion is controlled by two hormones from the hypothalamus: GHRH, which increases GH secretion; and somatostatin, which inhibits GH secretion. GH is essential to normal tissue growth and maturation and also impacts aging, sleep, nutritional status, stress, and reproductive hormones. In the bone, GH stimulates epiphyseal growth and increases osteoclast and osteoblast activity, resulting in increased bone mass. GH also increases amino acid transport in muscles. Other functions of GH include lipolysis and enhancement of hepatic protein synthesis.

Many of the anabolic functions of GH are mediated, at least in part, by the insulin-like growth factors (IGFs), also known as the *somatomedins*. There are two primary forms of IGF, IGF-1 and IGF-2, of which IGF-1 is the most biologically active. They both circulate bound to a group of IGF-binding proteins (IGFBPs) modulating their availability. IGF-1 binds to IGF-1 receptors, mediating the anabolic effects of GH. IGF-1 also binds to insulin receptors, providing an insulin-like effect on skeletal muscle. IGF-2 has important effects on fetal growth but suppresses GH in the adult. Because of the anabolic effects of GH and IGF-1, they can be used to treat growth disorders, increase muscle mass, and potentially slow the aging process; however, there are concerns about their safety, with potential links to increased rates of cancer.[9]

Prolactin primarily functions to induce milk production during pregnancy and lactation. It has immune stimulatory effects and modulates immune and inflammatory responses with both physiologic and pathologic reactions. Its synthesis and release are increased by stimulation of the nipples and mammary gland during nursing. Vasoactive intestinal polypeptide, serotonin, and growth factors also stimulate the synthesis of prolactin. Release of prolactin is inhibited by dopamine.

Posterior Pituitary

The embryonic posterior pituitary (neurohypophysis) is derived from the hypothalamus and is comprised of three parts: (1) the median eminence, located at the base of the hypothalamus; (2) the pituitary stalk; and (3) the infundibular process, also known as the *pars nervosa* or *neural lobe*. The median eminence is composed largely of the nerve endings of axons from the ventral hypothalamus. It often is designated as part of the posterior pituitary and contains at least 10 biologically active hypothalamic releasing hormones, as well as the neurotransmitters dopamine, norepinephrine, serotonin, acetylcholine, and histamine. The pituitary stalk contains the axons of neurons that originate in the supraoptic and paraventricular nuclei of the hypothalamus and connects the pituitary gland to the brain. Axons originating in the hypothalamus terminate in the pars nervosa, which secretes the hormones of the posterior pituitary (see Fig. 21.10).

The posterior pituitary secretes two polypeptide hormones: (1) ADH, also called *arginine vasopressin*; and (2) oxytocin. These hormones differ by only two amino acids. They are synthesized—along with their binding proteins, the neurophysins—in the supraoptic and paraventricular nuclei of the hypothalamus (see Fig. 21.10). They are packaged in secretory vesicles and are moved down the axons of the pituitary stalk to the pars nervosa for storage. The posterior pituitary thus can be seen as a site for both storing and releasing hormones synthesized in the hypothalamus. The release of ADH and oxytocin is mediated by cholinergic and adrenergic neurotransmitters. The major stimulus to both ADH and oxytocin release is glutamate, whereas the major inhibitory input is through gamma-aminobutyric acid (GABA). Before release into the circulatory system, ADH and oxytocin are split from the neurophysins and are secreted in unbound form.

Antidiuretic hormone. The major homeostatic function of the posterior pituitary is the control of plasma osmolality as regulated by antidiuretic hormone (ADH) (see Chapter 3). At physiologic levels, ADH increases the permeability of the distal renal tubules and collecting ducts (see Chapter 37). This increased permeability leads to increased water reabsorption into the blood, thus concentrating the urine and reducing serum osmolality. These effects may be inhibited by hypercalcemia, prostaglandin E, and hypokalemia.

The secretion of ADH is regulated primarily by the osmoreceptors of the hypothalamus, located near or in the supraoptic nuclei. As plasma osmolality increases, these osmoreceptors are stimulated, the rate of ADH secretion increases, thirst is stimulated (which increases water intake), and more water is reabsorbed by the kidney. This causes the plasma to become diluted back to its set-point osmolality. ADH has no direct effect on electrolyte levels, but by increasing water reabsorption, serum electrolyte concentrations may decrease because of a dilutional effect.[2]

ADH secretion also is stimulated by decreased intravascular volume, as monitored by baroreceptors in the left atrium, in the carotid arteries, and in the aortic arches. A volume loss of 7% to 25% acts through these receptors to stimulate ADH secretion. Stress, trauma, pain, exercise, nausea, nicotine, exposure to heat, and drugs, such as morphine, also increase ADH secretion. ADH secretion decreases with decreased plasma osmolality, increased intravascular volume, hypertension, alcohol ingestion, and an increase in estrogen, progesterone, or angiotensin II levels.

Physiologic levels of ADH do not significantly impact vessel tone. However, ADH was originally named *vasopressin* because, at extremely high levels, it causes vasoconstriction and a resulting increase in arterial blood pressure. For example, high doses of ADH (given as the drug vasopressin) may be administered to achieve hemostasis during hemorrhage and to raise blood pressure in shock states.

Oxytocin. Oxytocin is responsible for contraction of the uterus and milk ejection in lactating women and may affect sperm motility in men. In both genders, oxytocin has an antidiuretic effect similar to that of ADH. In women, oxytocin is secreted in response to suckling and mechanical distention of the female reproductive tract. Oxytocin binds to its receptors on myoepithelial cells in the mammary tissues and causes contraction of those cells, which increases intramammary pressure and milk expression ("let-down" reflex). Oxytocin acts on the uterus near the end of labor to enhance the effectiveness of contractions, promote delivery of the placenta, and stimulate postpartum uterine contractions, thereby preventing excessive bleeding. The function of this hormone is discussed in detail in Chapter 24.

Pineal Gland

The pineal gland is located near the center of the brain (see Fig. 21.1) and is composed of photoreceptive cells that secrete melatonin. It is innervated by noradrenergic sympathetic nerve terminals controlled by pathways within the hypothalamus. Melatonin release is stimulated by exposure to dark and inhibited by light exposure. It is synthesized from tryptophan, which is first converted to serotonin and then to melatonin. Melatonin regulates circadian rhythms and reproductive systems, including the secretion of the GnRHs and the onset of puberty. It also plays an important role in immune regulation and is postulated to impact the aging process. Further effects of melatonin include increasing nitric oxide release from blood vessels, removing toxic oxygen free radicals, and decreasing insulin secretion. Melatonin has been used therapeutically in humans to help with sleep disturbances, jet lag, and psychological and inflammatory disorders. Its utility for numerous other disorders is being explored.

Thyroid and Parathyroid Glands

The thyroid gland, located in the neck just below the larynx, produces hormones that control the rates of metabolic processes throughout the body. The four parathyroid glands are near the posterior side of the thyroid and function to control serum calcium levels (Fig. 21.11).

Thyroid Gland

Two lobes of the thyroid gland lie on either side of the trachea, inferior to the thyroid cartilage and joined by a small band of tissue termed the isthmus (see Fig. 21.11). The pyramidal lobe is superior to the isthmus. The normal thyroid gland is not visible on inspection, but it may be palpated on swallowing, which causes it to be displaced upward.

The thyroid gland consists of follicles that contain follicular cells surrounding a viscous substance called *colloid* (Fig. 21.12). The follicular cells synthesize and secrete the thyroid hormones. Neurons terminate on blood vessels within the thyroid gland and on the follicular cells themselves, so neurotransmitters (acetylcholine, catecholamines) may directly affect the secretory activity of follicular cells and thyroid blood flow. Approximately a 2-month supply of thyroid hormone is stored in the gland.

Also found in the thyroid are parafollicular cells, or C cells (see Fig. 21.12). C cells secrete various regulatory peptides, including calcitonin and, in much smaller quantities, the neuropeptides ghrelin, serotonin, and somatostatin. At high levels, calcitonin, also called *thyrocalcitonin*, lowers serum calcium levels by inhibiting bone-resorbing osteoclasts. However, in humans the metabolic consequences of calcitonin deficiency or excess do not appear to be significant. (Bone resorption is explained in Chapter 43). Calcitonin can be used therapeutically to treat a number of bone disorders, including osteogenesis imperfecta, osteoporosis, osteoarthritis, hypercalcemia, Paget bone disease, and metastatic cancer of the bone. The precursor molecule to calcitonin, called *procalcitonin*, is a stress hormone that is elevated in infectious and

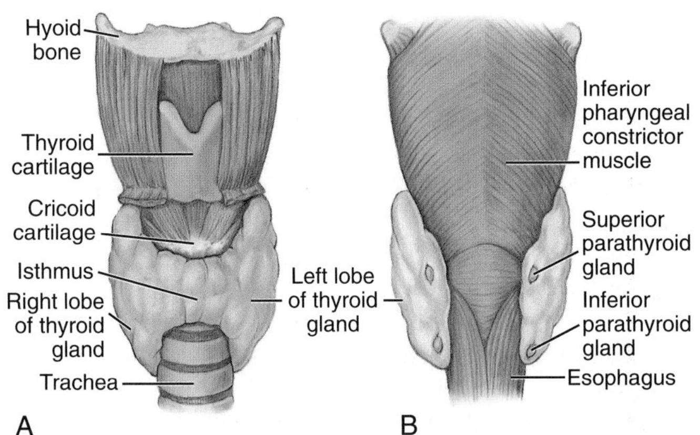

Fig. 21.11 Thyroid and Parathyroid Glands. **(A)** Anterior view. **(B)** Posterior view. (From Fehrenbach MJ, Herring SW. *Illustrated anatomy of the head and neck*, 4th edition. St. Louis: Saunders; 2012.)

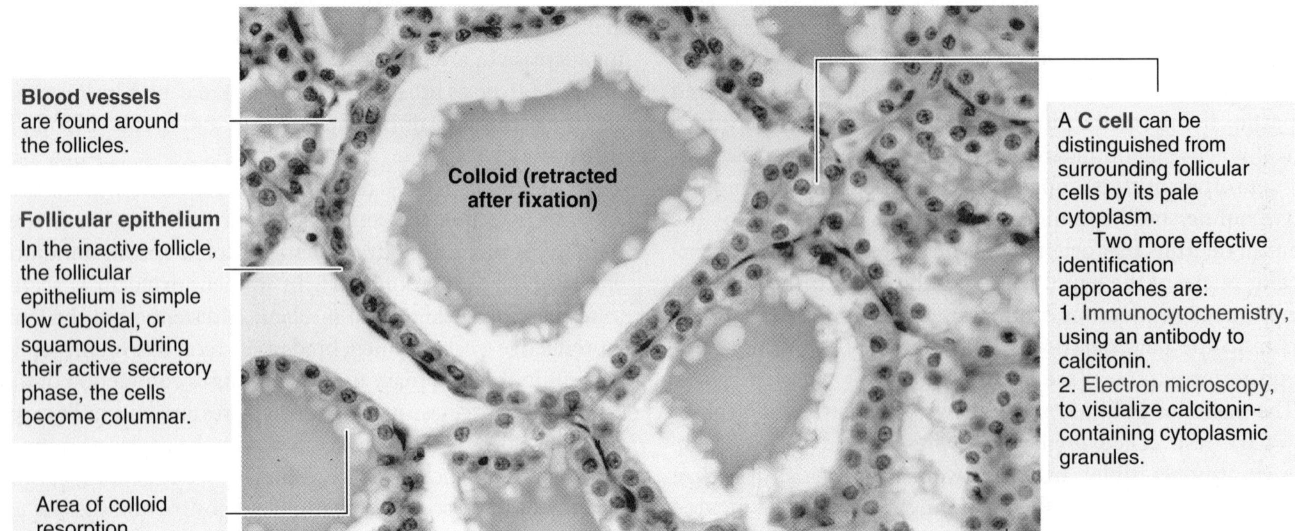

Fig. 21.12 Thyroid Follicle Cells.

inflammatory disorders, and its measurement can aid in the diagnosis of these serious diseases.[10,11]

Regulation of thyroid hormone secretion. Thyroid hormone (TH) is regulated through a negative-feedback loop involving the hypothalamus, the anterior pituitary, and the thyroid gland (see Fig. 21.2A). This loop is initiated by thyrotropin-releasing hormone (TRH), which is synthesized and stored within the hypothalamus. TRH is released into the hypothalamic-pituitary portal system and circulates to the anterior pituitary, where it stimulates the release of TSH. TRH levels increase with exposure to cold or stress and from decreased levels of T_4.

Thyroid-stimulating hormone (TSH) is a glycoprotein synthesized and stored within the anterior pituitary. When TSH is secreted by the anterior pituitary, it circulates to bind with TSH receptors on the plasma membrane of the thyroid follicular cells. The primary effects of TSH on the thyroid gland include (1) an immediate increase in the release of stored thyroid hormones, (2) an increase in iodide uptake and oxidation, (3) an increase in thyroid hormone synthesis, and (4) an increase in the synthesis and secretion of prostaglandins by the thyroid. TSH also increases growth of the thyroid gland by stimulating thymocyte hyperplasia and hypertrophy and decreasing apoptosis. As TH levels rise, there is a negative-feedback effect on the HPA to inhibit TRH and TSH release, which then results in decreased TH synthesis and secretion. TH synthesis is also controlled by serum iodide levels and by circulating selenium-dependent enzymes, called *deiodinases*, which inactivate the precursor molecule thyroxine. Thyroid gland hormones and their regulation and function are summarized in Table 21.5.

Synthesis of thyroid hormone. Thyroid hormone synthesis is summarized in these steps:

1. Uniodinated thyroglobulin (a large glycoprotein) is produced by the endoplasmic reticulum of the thyroid follicular cells.
2. Tyrosine (an amino acid) is incorporated into the thyroglobulin of follicular cells as it is synthesized.
3. Iodide (the inorganic form of iodine) is actively transferred from the blood into the colloid by carrier proteins located in the outer membrane of the follicular cells. This active transport system is called the *iodide trap* and is very efficient at accumulating the trace amounts of iodide from the blood.
4. Iodide is oxidized and quickly attaches to tyrosine within the thyroglobulin molecule.
5. Coupling of iodinated tyrosine forms thyroid hormones. Triiodothyronine (T_3) is formed from the coupling of monoiodotyrosine (one iodine atom and tyrosine) and diiodotyrosine (two iodine atoms and tyrosine). Tetraiodothyronine (T_4), commonly known as thyroxine, is formed from the coupling of two diiodotyrosines.
6. Thyroid hormones are stored attached to thyroglobulin within the colloid until they are released into the circulation.

The thyroid gland normally produces 90% T_4 and 10% T_3. Once released into the circulation, T_3 and T_4 are primarily transported bound to thyroxine-binding globulin (TBG), though some TH is transported by thyroxine-binding prealbumin (transthyretin), albumin, or lipoproteins. The bound form serves as a reservoir, whereas the unbound (free) form is active. In the body tissues, most of the T_4 is converted to T_3, which acts on the target cell.

TABLE 21.5 Thyroid Gland Hormones and Their Regulation and Functions

Hormone	Regulation	Functions
Thyroxine (T_4) and triiodothyronine (T_3)	Levels are controlled by TSH Released in response to metabolic demand Influences on amount secreted: Sex Pregnancy Gonadal and adrenocortical-increased steroids = ↑ levels Exposure to extreme cold = ↑ levels Nutritional state Chemicals GHIH = ↓ levels Dopamine = ↓ levels Catecholamines = ↑ levels	Regulates protein, fat, and carbohydrate catabolism in all cells Regulates metabolic rate of all cells Regulates body heat production Insulin antagonist Maintains growth hormone secretion, skeletal maturation Affects CNS development Necessary for muscle tone and vigor Maintains cardiac rate, force, and output Maintains secretion of GI tract Affects respiratory rate and oxygen utilization Maintains calcium mobilization Affects RBC production Stimulates lipid turnover, free fatty acid release, and cholesterol synthesis
Calcitonin	Elevated serum calcium—major stimulant for calcitonin Other stimulants Gastrin Calcium-rich foods (regardless of serum Ca^{++} levels) Pregnancy Lowered serum calcium—suppresses calcitonin release	Lowers serum calcium by opposing bone-resorbing effects of PTH, prostaglandins, and calciferols by inhibiting osteoclastic activity Lowers serum phosphate levels May also decrease calcium and phosphorus absorption in GI tract

CNS, Central nervous system; *GHIH*, growth hormone–inhibiting hormone; *GI*, gastrointestinal; *PTH*, parathyroid hormone; *RBC*, red blood cell; *TSH*, thyroid-stimulating hormone.

From Monahan FD, Sands JK, Neighbors M, et al. *Phipps' medical-surgical nursing: Health and illness perspectives*, 8th edition. St. Louis: Mosby; 2007.

Actions of thyroid hormone. TH has a significant effect on the growth, maturation, and function of cells and tissues throughout the body. TH binds to intracellular receptor complexes and then influences the genetic expression of specific proteins. TH is essential for normal growth and neurologic development in the fetus and infant and affects metabolic, neurologic, cardiovascular, and respiratory functioning across the life span. In addition, TH is required for the metabolism and function of blood cells, normal muscle functioning, the integrity of skin, nails, and hair, and for normal skeletal growth and maintenance of bone mass. Similar to some steroid hormones, TH also affects cell metabolism by altering protein, fat, and glucose metabolism and, as a result, increasing heat production and oxygen consumption.

TH has permissive effects throughout the body, optimizing the actions of other hormones and neurotransmitters. These effects can become very pronounced when there are either high or low levels of circulating thyroid hormones. For example, in the heart, T_3 stimulates the synthesis of specific contractile proteins, sarcolemmal ion pumps, and membrane receptors. Therefore, in hyperthyroidism, which is associated with elevated levels of thyroid hormones, cardiac effects include increased heart rate and cardiac output, as well as the development of cardiomyopathy. Thyroid hormones also affect the respiratory center, contributing to the normal hypoxic and hypercapnic drives. In severe hypothyroidism, ventilation can become very depressed. Thyroid hormone also plays a role in metabolic disorders and liver disease (see Emerging Science Box: Thyromimetics and Liver Disease). Hypothyroidism is also associated with impaired bone formation, and hyperthyroidism is associated with osteoporosis, hypercalcemia, and hypercalciuria.

Parathyroid Glands

Normally, two pairs of small parathyroid glands are present behind the upper and lower poles of the thyroid gland (see Fig. 21.11). However, their number may range from two to six. The parathyroid glands produce parathyroid hormone (PTH), which is the single most important factor in the regulation of the serum calcium concentration. The overall effect of PTH secretion is to increase serum calcium concentration and decrease the concentration of serum phosphate. A decrease in serum-ionized calcium level stimulates PTH secretion. On release, PTH enters the circulation in unbound form and attaches to plasma membrane receptors in target tissues. To achieve regulation of serum calcium concentration, PTH acts directly on bone with at least two effects. In acute hypocalcemia, PTH secretion stimulates osteoblasts to release factors that cause osteoclast proliferation, maturation, and release of acidic enzymes, such as cathepsin. These enzymes mobilize calcium release from bone (bone resorption), which increases the serum calcium level (Fig. 21.13). There is bone remodeling with chronic stimulation by PTH, a process in which bone is broken down and re-formed. Paradoxically, when PTH is administered intermittently and at a low dose, it stimulates bone formation. This observation led to the use of synthetic PTH for treatment of osteoporosis.[12]

PTH also acts on the kidney to increase calcium reabsorption in the distal tubules of the nephron while phosphate and bicarbonate reabsorption are decreased in the proximal tubules. The resultant increase in the serum calcium concentration inhibits PTH secretion. 1,25-Dihydroxy-vitamin D3 (the active form of vitamin D) is activated by the kidney and works as a cofactor with PTH to promote calcium and phosphate absorption in the gut and enhance bone mineralization. Vitamin D also plays an important role in metabolic processes and controlling inflammation. It has been found to be deficient in the majority of individuals in the United States (see Emerging Science Box: Vitamin D Deficiency).

EMERGING SCIENCE BOX

Thyromimetics and Liver Disease

An emerging field of research is focusing on thyromimetics due to the possible role thyroid hormones may play in the pathogenesis of non-alcoholic fatty liver disease (NAFLD) and non-alcoholic steatohepatitis (NASH) disease. These two liver diseases are closely linked to metabolic syndrome (diabetes mellitus type 2, dyslipidemia, and obesity), which also plays a role in endocrine disorders such as hypothyroidism. While the pathophysiologic processes continue to be explored through research, insulin resistance, both hepatic and peripheral, as well as metabolic syndrome are proposed as possible mechanisms. Currently, possible treatment options for NAFLD are in phase 3 clinical trials. These treatments focus on substitution therapy for hypothyroidism, specifically thyroid hormone receptor (THR) agonist and its metabolites, along with lifestyle modifications.

Data from Kizivat T, et al. Hypothyroidism and nonalcoholic fatty liver disease: Pathophysiological associations and therapeutic implications. *Journal of Clinical and Translational Hepatology*, 2020;8(3):347–353; Hazam R, et al. Hypothyroidism and non alcoholic fatty liver disease. *Journal of Endocrinology and Metabolism*, 2020;10(2):45–48.

EMERGING SCIENCE BOX

Vitamin D Deficiency

Vitamin D is essential for bone health and is widely used for the prevention and treatment of postmenopausal osteoporosis and renal osteodystrophy. Inadequate serum levels of vitamin D have been linked to numerous disorders, including infections, cancer, heart disease, dementia, diabetes, chronic pain syndromes, and autoimmune disorders, but cause and effect has never been established. However, recent reviews have found that there is still inadequate evidence that vitamin D supplementation reduces the risk for any of these nonskeletal conditions. Still, many health organizations recommend an increased intake of vitamin D–containing foods (seafood, vitamin D–fortified juices, and milk products), increased exposure to sunlight, and supplementation with vitamin D. The Institute of Medicine currently recommends 400 to 800 units of vitamin D per day for children and adults and 400 units for infants up to 12 months of age.

Vitamin D deficiency has been found to affect more than 75% of all Americans, and more than 90% of Americans with pigmented skin. Interestingly, in a "vitamin D paradox," Black Americans with markedly low levels of vitamin D are still found to have high bone density levels compared to white Americans. Further research in this area is needed to determine next steps and gather data on the actual benefits of treating Black Americans for vitamin D deficiency.

Data from Brown LL, et al. The vitamin D paradox in Black Americans: A systems-based approach to investigating clinical practice, research, and public health—Expert panel meeting report. *BMC Proceedings*, 2018;12(Suppl 6):6; LeFevre ML, et al. Vitamin D screening and supplementation in community-dwelling adults: Common questions and answers. *American Family Physician*, 2018;97(4):254–260; Mihos CG, et al. Vitamin D deficiency and supplementation in cardiovascular disorders. *Cardiology in Review*, 2017;25(4):189–196; Mondul AM, et al. Vitamin D and cancer risk and mortality: State of the science, gaps, and challenges. *Epidemiologic Reviews*, 2017;39(1):28–48; National Institutes of Health, Office of Dietary Supplements. *Vitamin D*. Updated March 24, 2020. https://ods.od.nih.gov/factsheets/VitaminD-HealthProfessional/; Pilz S, et al. Vitamin D: Current guidelines and future outlook. *Anticancer Research*, 2018;38(2):1145–1151.

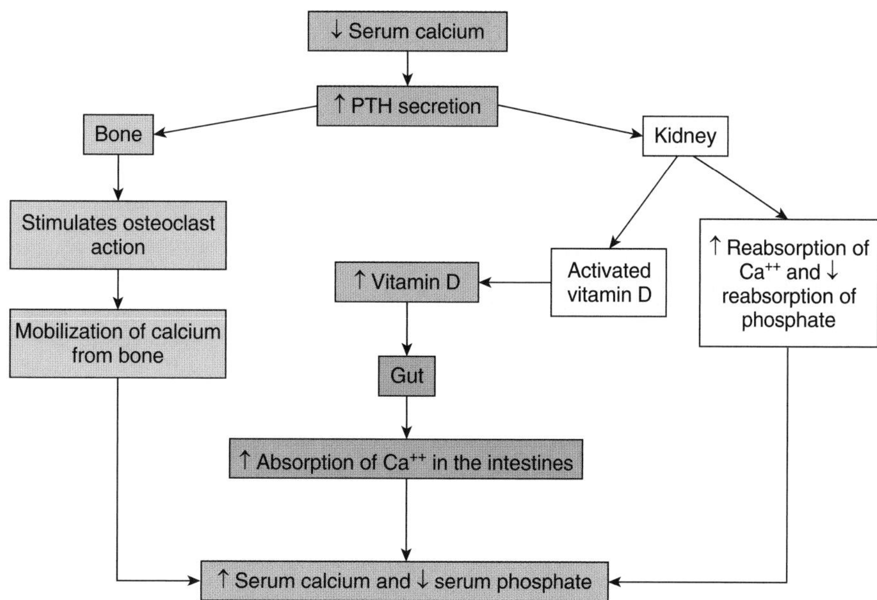

Fig. 21.13 The Role of Parathyroid Hormone *(PTH)* and Vitamin D in Calcium Metabolism.

Phosphate and magnesium concentrations also affect PTH secretion. An increase in the serum phosphate level decreases the serum calcium level by causing calcium-phosphate precipitation into soft tissue and bone, which indirectly stimulates PTH secretion. Hypomagnesemia in persons with normal calcium levels acts as a mild stimulant to PTH secretion; however, in persons with hypocalcemia, hypomagnesemia decreases PTH secretion.

Another hormone that plays an important role in calcium and bone physiology is parathyroid hormone–related protein (PTHrP). This hormone is synthesized in many adult and fetal tissues and affects tissues around it in a paracrine fashion with multiple metabolic effects. It has similar biologic properties to PTH and uses the same receptors but has other actions mediated by different regions within the molecule. It is important for endochondral bone formation and bone remodeling.[13]

Endocrine Pancreas

The pancreas is both an endocrine gland that produces hormones and an exocrine gland that produces digestive enzymes. (The exocrine function of the pancreas is discussed in Chapter 40.) The pancreas is located behind the stomach, between the spleen and the duodenum (Fig. 21.14). The pancreas houses pancreatic islets (islets of Langerhans), which are small islands of hormone-producing cells. The islets of Langerhans have four types of hormone-secreting cells: alpha cells, which secrete glucagon; beta cells, which secrete insulin and amylin; delta cells, which secrete gastrin and somatostatin; and F (or PP) cells, which secrete pancreatic polypeptide. These hormones regulate carbohydrate, fat, and protein metabolism. (The pancreas is illustrated in Fig. 21.14.) Nerves from both the sympathetic and the parasympathetic divisions of the autonomic nervous system innervate the pancreatic islets.

The perfusion of the anterior lobe of the pancreas, where alpha, beta, and delta cells are most numerous, comes from branches of the superior mesenteric artery. The posterior lobe is perfused by branches of the celiac artery. The pancreatic islets receive 10% of the pancreatic blood flow but represent only 1% of pancreatic mass. This is necessary for oxygenation and delivery of islet hormones to target cells.

Insulin

The beta cells of the pancreas synthesize insulin from the precursor proinsulin, which is formed from a larger precursor molecule, preproinsulin. Proinsulin is composed of A peptide and B peptide, which are connected by a C peptide and two disulfide bonds. C peptide is cleaved by proteolytic enzymes, leaving the bonded A and B peptides as the insulin molecule. Insulin circulates freely in the plasma and is not bound to a carrier. C peptide level can be measured in the blood and used as an indirect measurement of serum insulin synthesis.

Secretion of insulin is regulated by chemical, hormonal, and neural control. The primary stimulus for insulin secretion is an increase in blood levels of glucose. Insulin secretion also is stimulated by the parasympathetic nervous system, usually before eating a meal. Other factors stimulating insulin secretion include some amino acids (leucine, arginine, and lysine) and gastrointestinal hormones (glucagon, gastrin, cholecystokinin, secretin). Insulin secretion diminishes in response to low blood levels of glucose (hypoglycemia), high levels of insulin (through negative feedback to the beta cells), and sympathetic stimulation of the beta cells in the islets. Prostaglandins also inhibit insulin secretion.

Insulin is an anabolic hormone that promotes glucose uptake, primarily in liver, muscle, and adipose tissue. It also increases the synthesis of proteins, carbohydrates, lipids, and nucleic acids. The net effect of insulin in these tissues is to stimulate protein and fat synthesis and decrease blood glucose level. Insulin also facilitates the intracellular transport of potassium (K^+), phosphate, and magnesium. Table 21.6 summarizes the

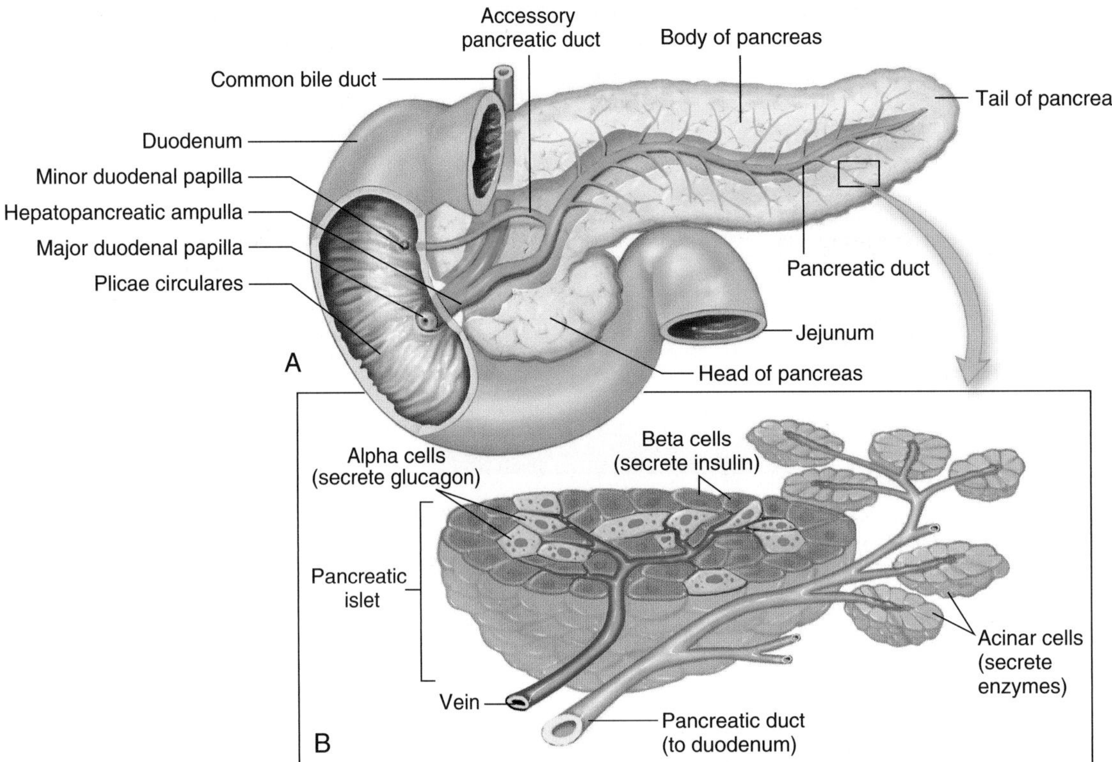

Fig. 21.14 **The Pancreas. (A)** Pancreas dissected to show main and accessory ducts. The main duct may join the common bile duct, as shown here, to enter the duodenum by a single opening at the major duodenal papilla, or the two ducts may have separate openings. The accessory pancreatic duct is usually present and has a separate opening into the duodenum. **(B)** Exocrine glandular cells (around small pancreatic ducts) and endocrine glandular cells of the pancreatic islets (adjacent to blood capillaries). Exocrine pancreatic cells secrete pancreatic juice, alpha endocrine cells secrete glucagon, and beta cells secrete insulin. (From Patton KT, Thibodeau GA. *Structure & function of the body*, 15th edition. St. Louis: Mosby; 2016.)

actions of insulin. Insulin is metabolized in the liver and kidney by enzymes that split disulfide bonds. Very little insulin is excreted unchanged in the urine.

At the target cell, insulin signaling is initiated when insulin binds and activates its cell surface receptor tyrosine kinase. These receptors are found on cells throughout the body.[4] Insulin receptor binding sends a cascade of signals to activate glucose transporters (GLUT) for entry of glucose into the cell. The primary GLUT is called GLUT4. It is stored in cellular vesicles until activated by the insulin receptor and is then translocated to the cell surface where it facilitates the diffusion of glucose into the cell. Translocation of GLUT4 to the cell surface is associated with a 10- to 21-fold increase in glucose diffusion into the cell, particularly in skeletal and cardiac muscle, liver, and adipose cells (Fig. 21.15). The brain, red blood cells, kidney, and lens of the eye do not require insulin for glucose transport.

The sensitivity of the insulin receptor is a key component in maintaining normal cellular function. Insulin sensitivity is affected by age, weight, abdominal fat, and physical activity. Insulin resistance has been implicated in numerous diseases, including hypertension, heart disease, and type 2 diabetes mellitus. Adipocytes release a number of hormones and cytokines that are altered in obesity and have an important impact on insulin sensitivity (see Chapter 23). The most effective measures shown to improve insulin sensitivity in humans are weight loss and exercise.

Amylin

Amylin (or islet amyloid polypeptide) is a peptide hormone co-secreted with insulin by beta cells in response to nutrient stimuli. It regulates blood glucose concentration by delaying gastric emptying and suppressing glucagon secretion after meals. Amylin also has a satiety effect, which reduces food intake. Through these mechanisms, amylin works with insulin to prevent hyperglycemia.

Glucagon

Glucagon is antagonistic to the effects of insulin, acting to increase blood glucose during fasting, exercise, and hypoglycemia. Glucagon release is stimulated by low glucose levels and sympathetic stimulation and is inhibited by high glucose levels. Amino acids, such as alanine, glycine, and asparagine, also stimulate glucagon secretion. A protein-rich meal has the same effect. Glucagon is produced by the alpha cells of the pancreas and by cells lining the gastrointestinal tract. Glucagon acts primarily in the liver and increases the blood glucose concentration by stimulating glycogenolysis and gluconeogenesis in muscle and lipolysis in adipose tissue. The lypolysis has a ketogenic effect caused by the metabolism of free fatty acids in the liver. These effects have led to the hypothesis that increased glucagon secretion is as important as insulin insufficiency in the pathogenesis of type 2 diabetes mellitus.[14]

TABLE 21.6 Insulin Actions

	Sites of Insulin-Promoted Synthesis		
Actions	**Liver Cells**	**Muscle Cells**	**Adipose Cells**
Glucose uptake	Increased	Increased	Increased
Glucose use	—	—	Increased glycerol phosphate
Glycogenesis	Increased	Increased	—
Glycogenolysis	Decreased	Decreased	—
Glycolysis	Increased	Increased	Increased
Gluconeogenesis	Increased	—	—
Other	Increased fatty acid synthesis	Increased amino acid uptake	Increased fat esterification
	Decreased ketogenesis	Increased protein synthesis	Decreased lipolysis
	Decreased urea cycle activity	Decreased proteolysis	Increased fat storage

Pancreatic Somatostatin

Pancreatic somatostatin is produced by delta cells of the pancreas in response to food intake and is essential in carbohydrate, fat, and protein metabolism. It is different from hypothalamic somatostatin, which inhibits the release of GH and TSH. Pancreatic somatostatin is involved in regulating alpha-cell and beta-cell function within the islets by inhibiting secretion of insulin, glucagon, and pancreatic polypeptide.

Incretins

The incretin hormones are secreted from endocrine cells in the gastrointestinal tract in the presence of carbohydrates, proteins, and fats. The incretin hormones control postprandial glucose levels by promoting glucose-dependent insulin secretion, inhibiting glucagon synthesis, promoting hepatic glucose secretion, and delaying gastric emptying. Incretins also enhance beta-cell mass and replenish intracellular stores of insulin. Gastric inhibitory polypeptide (GIP) and glucagon-like peptide-1 (GLP-1) are incretin hormones.

Gastrin, Ghrelin, and Pancreatic Polypeptide

Pancreatic gastrin stimulates the secretion of gastric acid. It is postulated that fetal pancreatic gastrin secretion is necessary for adequate islet cell development. Ghrelin stimulates

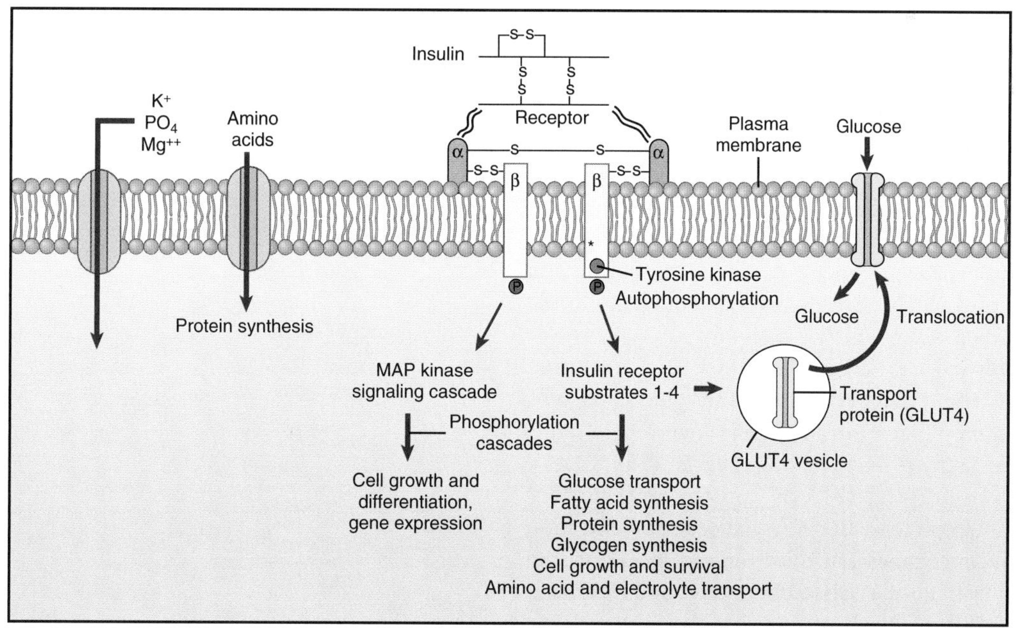

Fig. 21.15 Insulin Action on Cells. Binding of insulin to its receptor causes autophosphorylation of the receptor, which then itself acts as a tyrosine kinase that phosphorylates insulin receptor substrates 1-4 *(IRS-1-4)*. Numerous target enzymes, such as protein kinase B and mitogen-activated protein (MAP) kinase, are activated, and these enzymes have a multitude of effects on cell function. The glucose transporter *(GLUT4)* is recruited to the plasma membrane, where it facilitates glucose entry into the cell. The transport of amino acids, potassium, magnesium, and phosphate into the cell is also facilitated. The synthesis of various enzymes is induced or suppressed, and cell growth is regulated by signal molecules that modulate gene expression. (Redrawn from Levy MN, Koeppen BM, Stanton BA, eds. *Berne & Levy principles of physiology*, 4th edition. St. Louis: Mosby; 2006.)

GH secretion, controls appetite, and plays a role in obesity and the regulation of insulin sensitivity. Pancreatic polypeptide is released in response to hypoglycemia and protein-rich meals. It decreases pancreatic secretion of fluid and bicarbonate, promotes gastric secretion, antagonizes cholecystokinin, and is frequently increased in pancreatic tumors and in diabetes.[15]

Adrenal Glands

The adrenal glands are paired, pyramid-shaped organs behind the peritoneum and close to the upper pole of each kidney (see Fig. 21.1). Each gland is surrounded by a capsule, embedded in fat, and well supplied with blood from the aorta and phrenic and renal arteries. Venous return from the left adrenal gland is to the renal vein, and from the right adrenal gland is to the inferior vena cava.

Each adrenal gland consists of two separate portions—an outer cortex and an inner medulla. These two portions have different embryonic origins, structures, and hormonal functions. The adrenal cortex and medulla function like two separate but interrelated glands (Fig. 21.16).

Adrenal Cortex

The adrenal cortex accounts for 80% of the weight of the adult gland. The cortex is histologically subdivided into the following three zones:

1. The zona glomerulosa, the outer layer, constitutes about 15% of the cortex and primarily produces the mineralocorticoid aldosterone.
2. The zona fasciculata, the middle layer, constitutes 78% of the cortex and secretes the glucocorticoids cortisol, cortisone, and corticosterone.
3. The zona reticularis, the inner layer, constitutes 7% of the cortex and secretes mineralocorticoids (aldosterone), adrenal androgens and estrogens, and glucocorticoids.

The cells of the adrenal cortex are stimulated by ACTH from the pituitary gland. All hormones of the adrenal cortex are synthesized from low-density lipoprotein cholesterol. The best-known pathway of steroidogenesis involves the conversion of cholesterol to pregnenolone, which is then converted to the major corticosteroids.

Glucocorticoids

Functions of the glucocorticoids. The glucocorticoids are steroid hormones that have metabolic, neurologic, anti-inflammatory, and growth-suppressing effects (Fig. 21.17). These functions have direct effects on carbohydrate metabolism. These hormones increase the blood glucose concentration by promoting gluconeogenesis in the liver and by decreasing uptake of glucose into muscle cells, adipose cells, and lymphatic cells and by suppressing insulin secretion. They are released under stress conditions, which results in increased glucose for the brain.[34] In extrahepatic tissues, the glucocorticoids stimulate protein catabolism and inhibit amino acid uptake and protein synthesis. In extrahepatic tissues, the glucocorticoids stimulate protein catabolism and inhibit amino acid uptake and protein synthesis. The ultimate long-term effect of chronic stress on the body is protein catabolism and muscle wasting, increased lipolysis, insulin resistance, and hyperglycemia.[16]

The glucocorticoids act at several sites to suppress immune and inflammatory reactions. Adaptive immunity is affected by a glucocorticoid-mediated inhibitory effect on the proliferation of T lymphocytes, primarily T-helper lymphocytes. There is a greater adverse effect on T-helper 1 cell cytokine production (including antiviral interferons) than there is on T-helper 2 cell cytokine production, and therefore, greater depression of cellular immunity than humoral immunity (see Chapter 8). They affect innate immunity through several pathways, including inhibition of antigen presentation by dendritic cells and decreased activity of pattern recognition receptors on the surface of macrophages (see Chapter 7). Glucocorticoids also decrease immune and inflammatory responses by decreasing natural killer cell activity; by blocking phospholipase A and the synthesis of prostaglandins, thromboxanes, and leukotrienes; and by inhibiting inflammatory gene expression. In addition, glucocorticoids suppress the synthesis, secretion, and actions of chemical mediators involved in inflammatory and immune responses, including histamine, adhesion molecules, inducible cyclooxygenase, and inducible nitric oxide synthase.[17]

Glucocorticoids increase resistance to the severe inflammatory response to lipopolysaccharide (LPS, a bacterial endotoxin) through the inhibition of cytokines, chemokines, certain hormones, and neurotransmitters. In addition, glucocorticoids

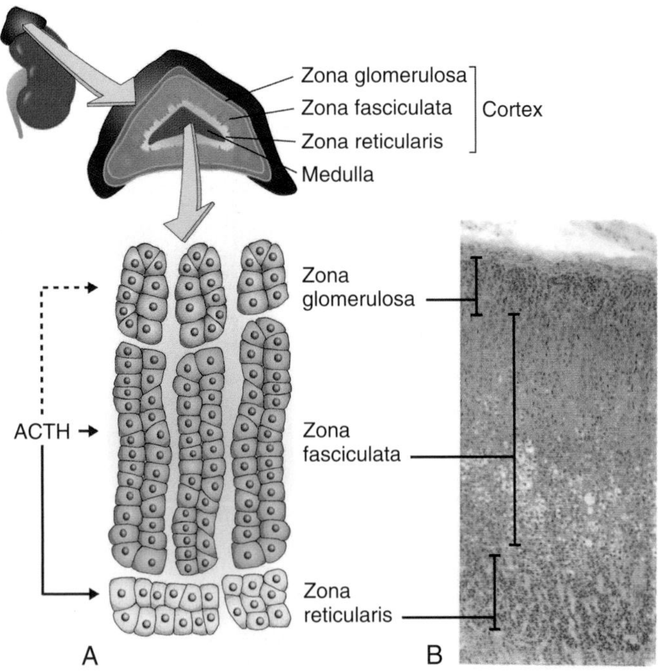

Fig. 21.16 Structure of the Adrenal Gland Showing Cell Layers (Zonae) of the Cortex. (A) Adrenal glands. Each gland consists of a cortex and a medulla. The cortex has three layers: zona glomerulosa, zona fasciculata, and zona reticularis. **(B)** A portion of the medulla is visible at the lower right in the photomicrograph (×35) and at the bottom of the drawing. *ACTH*, Adrenocorticotropic hormone. (A, From Damjanov I. *Pathophysiology*. Philadelphia: Saunders; 2008; B, From Kierszenbaum A. *Histology and cell biology*. St. Louis: Mosby; 2002.)

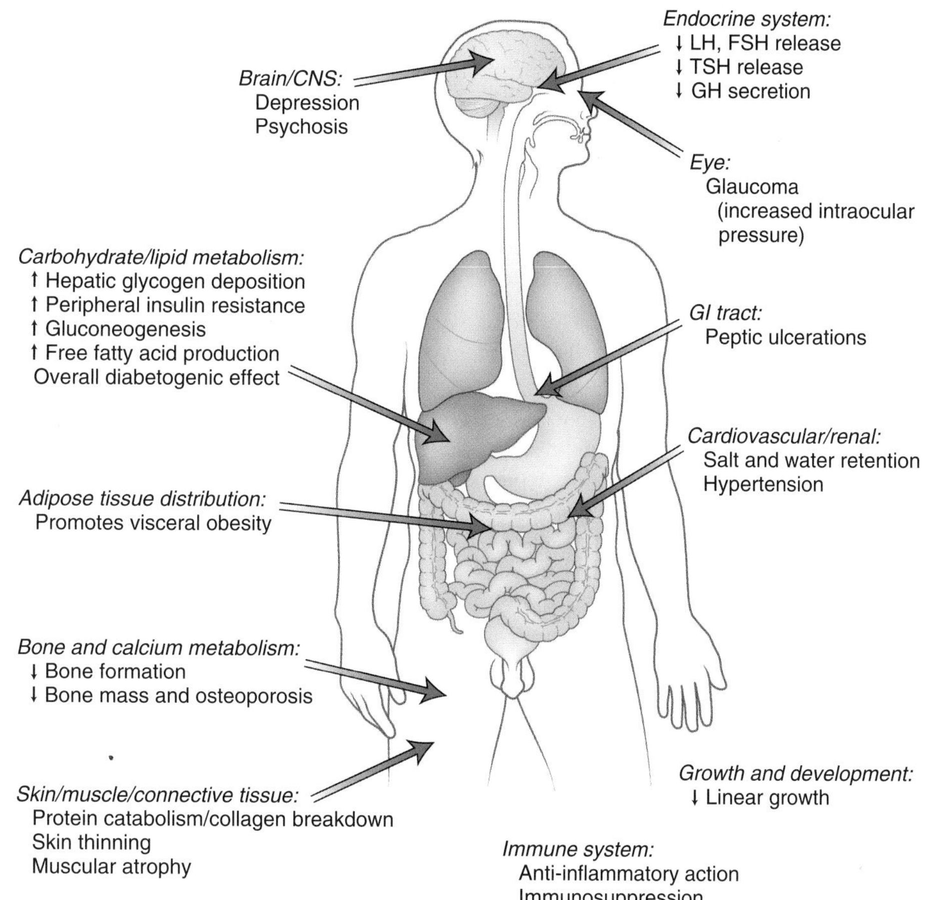

Fig. 21.17 Effects of Glucocorticoids on the Body. *CNS*, Central nervous system; *FSH*, follicle-stimulating hormone; *GH*, growth hormone; *GI*, gastrointestinal; *LH*, Luteinizing hormone; *TSH*, thyroid-stimulating hormone. (From Stewart PM, Krone NP. The adrenal cortex. In: Melmed S, Polonsky KS, Larsen PR, et al., eds. *Williams textbook of endocrinology*, 12th edition. Philadelphia: Saunders; 2011.)

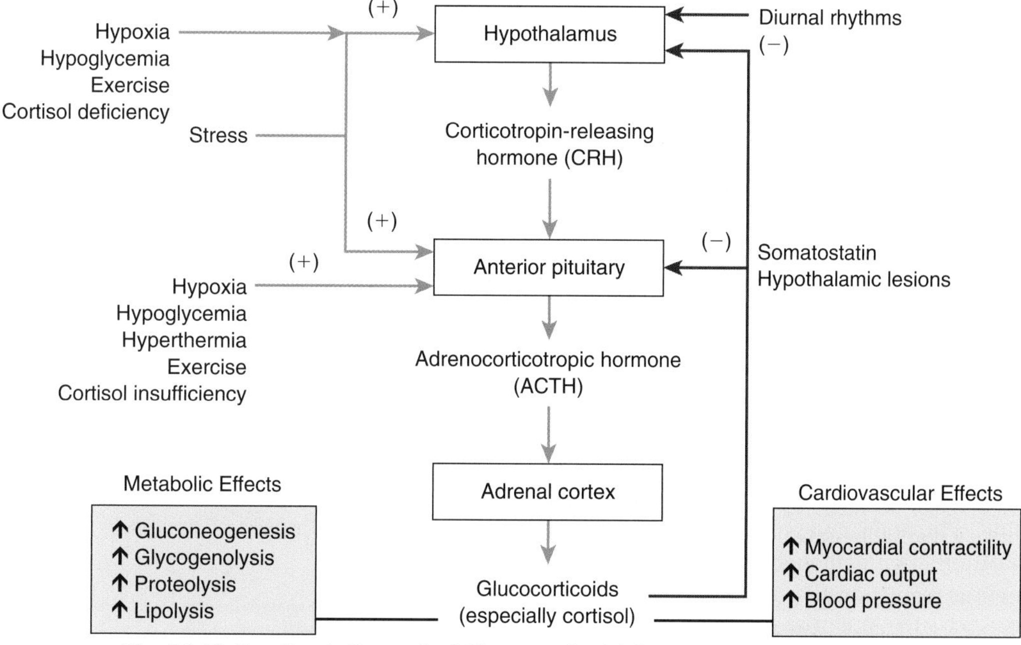

Fig. 21.18 Feedback Control of Glucocorticoid Synthesis and Secretion.

stimulate anti-inflammatory cytokines. Lysosomal membranes are also stabilized, decreasing the release of proteolytic enzymes. This suppression of innate and adaptive immunity by glucocorticoids means that infection and poor wound healing are some of the most problematic complications of the use of glucocorticoids in the treatment of disease. Similarly, psychologic and physiologic stress increases glucocorticoid production, which provides a pathway for the well-described decrease in immunity seen in both acute and chronic stress conditions (see Chapter 11).[18,19]

Glucocorticoids appear to potentiate the effects of catecholamines, including sensitizing the arterioles to the vasoconstrictive effects of norepinephrine, thus increasing the blood pressure. Thyroid hormone and GH effects on adipose tissue are also potentiated by glucocorticoids. Other effects of glucocorticoids include inhibition of bone formation, inhibition of ADH secretion, and stimulation of gastric acid secretion. A metabolite of cortisol may act like a barbiturate and depress nerve cell function in the brain, accounting for the noted effects on mood, such as anxiety and depression, associated with steroid level fluctuation in disease or stress. Pathologically high levels of glucocorticoids increase the number of circulating erythrocytes (leading to polycythemia), increase the appetite, promote fat deposition in the face and cervical areas, increase uric acid excretion, decrease serum calcium levels, suppress the secretion and synthesis of ACTH, and interfere with the action of GH so that somatic growth is inhibited.[20]

Cortisol. The most potent naturally occurring glucocorticoid is cortisol. It is the main secretory product of the adrenal cortex and is needed to maintain life and protect the body from stress (see Fig. 11.2). Cortisol circulates in bound form attached to albumin but is primarily bound to the plasma protein transcortin. A smaller amount circulates in free form and diffuses into cells with specific intracellular receptors for cortisol. Cortisol has a biologic half-life of approximately 90 minutes. It is primarily metabolized by the liver.

Cortisol secretion is regulated primarily by the hypothalamus and the anterior pituitary gland (Fig. 21.18). Corticotropin-releasing hormone (CRH) is produced by several nuclei in the hypothalamus and stored in the median eminence. Once released, CRH travels through the portal vessels to stimulate the production of ACTH, which is the main regulator of cortisol secretion.

Three factors appear to be primarily involved in regulating the secretion of ACTH: (1) negative-feedback effects of high circulating levels of cortisol; (2) diurnal rhythms, with peak levels during sleep; and (3) psychological and physiologic stress increases ACTH secretion, leading to increased cortisol levels. (Neurologic mechanisms regulating sleep are discussed in Chapter 16.)

There also is evidence that there is synthesis and secretion of glucocorticoids from extra-adrenal tissue including the thymus, lung, intestine, skin, brain, and possibly heart in response to immune stimulation. This is thought to provide autocrine and paracrine immune regulation and control of inflammation. Dysregulation of extra-adrenal glucocorticoid production can contribute to autoimmune and inflammatory diseases.[21]

Once ACTH is secreted, it binds to specific plasma membrane receptors on the cells of the adrenal cortex and on other extra-adrenal tissues. Because both adrenal and extra-adrenal tissues have ACTH receptors, a number of effects result from stimulation by ACTH (Box 21.1). ACTH stimulates the cells of the adrenal cortex to immediately synthesize and secrete cortisol. In healthy people, the secretory patterns of ACTH and cortisol are nearly identical. After secretion, 10% to 15% of cortisol circulates unbound, while the rest is bound to albumin or a plasma glycoprotein called *transcortin.* The levels of transcortin play a role in the HPA feedback system controlling cortisol secretion. Transcortin levels are significantly elevated by increased estrogen levels that occur with pregnancy and hormone therapy. The unbound portion is free to diffuse into cells, but only those cells with specific intracellular glucocorticoid receptors respond to cortisol stimulation. ACTH is rapidly inactivated in the circulation, and the liver and kidneys eliminate the deactivated hormone.

Mineralocorticoids: aldosterone. Mineralocorticoid steroids directly affect ion transport by epithelial cells, causing sodium retention and potassium and hydrogen loss. Aldosterone is the most potent naturally occurring mineralocorticoid and conserves sodium by increasing the activity of the sodium pump of epithelial cells in the nephron. (The sodium pump is described in Chapter 1.)

The initial stages of aldosterone synthesis occur in the adrenal zona fasciculata and zona reticularis. The final conversion of corticosterone to aldosterone occurs in the zona glomerulosa. Aldosterone synthesis and secretion is regulated primarily by the renin-angiotensin system (described in Chapter 37). The renin-angiotensin system is activated by sodium and water depletion, increased potassium levels, and a diminished effective blood volume (Fig. 21.19). Angiotensin II is the primary stimulant of aldosterone synthesis and secretion; however, sodium and potassium levels also may directly affect aldosterone secretion. ACTH acutely stimulates aldosterone secretion but is secondary to angiotensin II and potassium.

When sodium and potassium levels are within normal limits, approximately 50 to 250 mg of aldosterone is secreted daily. Of the secreted aldosterone, 50% to 75% binds to plasma proteins. The proportion of unbound aldosterone contributes to its rapid metabolic turnover in the liver, its low plasma concentration,

BOX 21.1 Effects of Adrenocorticotropic Hormone

Adrenal

Maintenance of gland size
Depletion of ascorbic acid
Activation of adenylyl cyclase
Conversion of cholesterol to pregnenolone
Accumulation of cholesterol for steroid hormone synthesis
Secretion of cortisol and adrenal androgens

Extra-Adrenal

Stimulation of melanocytes
Activation of tissue lipase

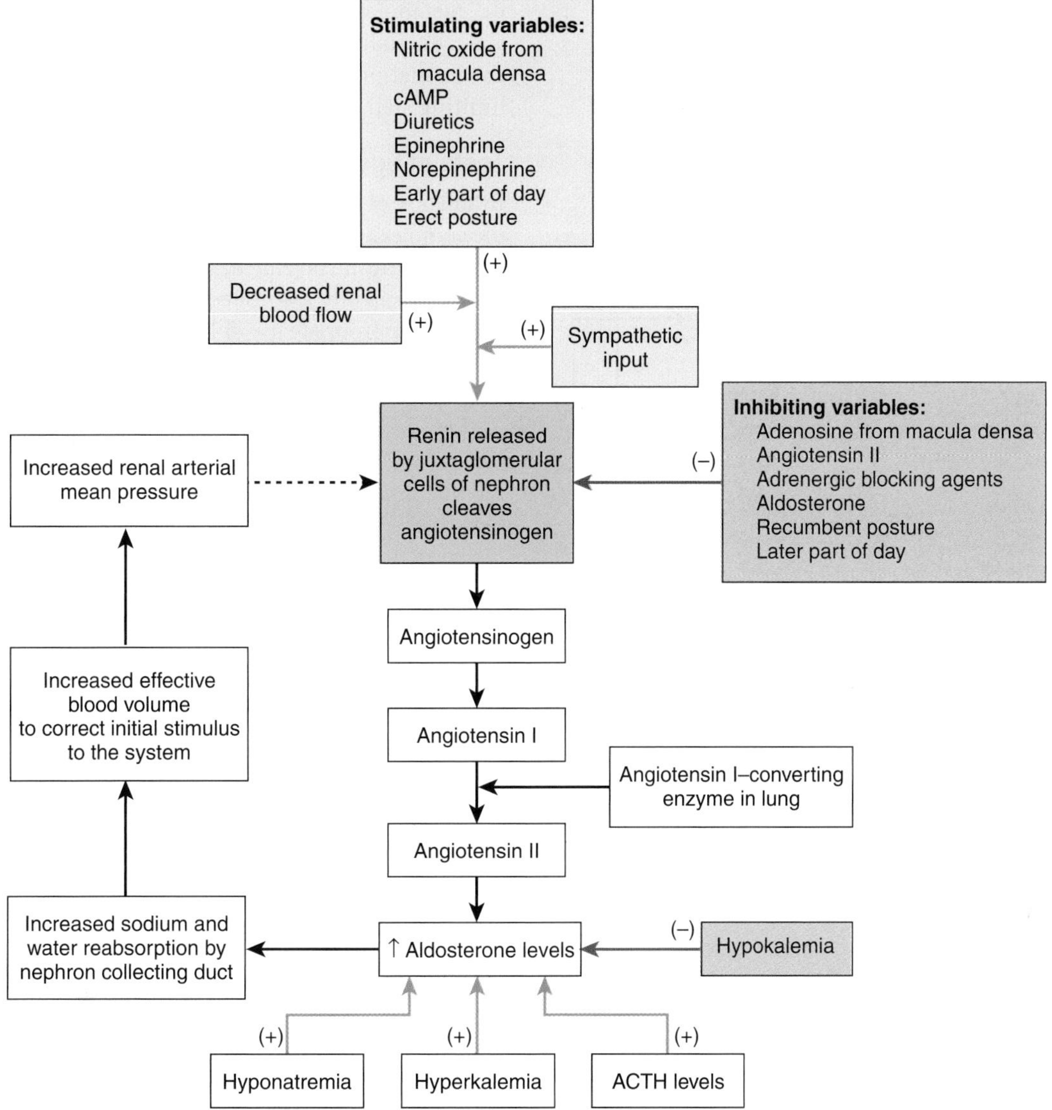

Fig. 21.19 Feedback Mechanisms Regulating Aldosterone Secretion. *ACTH,* Adrenocorticotropic hormone; *cAMP,* cyclic adenosine monophosphate.

and its short half-life (about 15 minutes). Aldosterone is metabolized in the liver and is excreted by the kidney.

Aldosterone maintains extracellular volume and blood pressure by acting on distal nephron epithelial cells to increase reabsorption of sodium and excretion of potassium and hydrogen. This renal effect takes 90 minutes to 6 hours. Fluid and electrolyte regulation is addressed in more detail in Chapter 3. Other effects of aldosterone include enhancement of cardiac muscle contraction, stimulation of ectopic ventricular activity through secondary cardiac pacemakers in the ventricles, stiffening of blood vessels with increased vascular resistance, and decrease in fibrinolysis. Pathologically elevated levels of aldosterone have been implicated in the myocardial changes associated with heart failure.[22]

Adrenal estrogens and androgens. The healthy adrenal cortex secretes minimal amounts of estrogen and androgens. ACTH appears to be the major regulator. Some of the weakly androgenic substances secreted by the cortex (dehydroepiandrosterone [DHEA], androstenedione) are converted by peripheral tissues to stronger androgens, such as testosterone, thus accounting for some androgenic effects initiated by the adrenal cortex. Peripheral conversion of adrenal androgens to estrogens is enhanced in aging or obese persons, as well as in those with liver disease or hyperthyroidism. The biologic effects and metabolism of the adrenal sex steroids do not vary from those produced by the gonads (see Chapter 24).

Adrenal Medulla

The adrenal medulla, together with the sympathetic division of the autonomic nervous system, is embryonically derived from neural crest cells. The chromaffin cells (pheochromocytes) of the adrenal medulla secrete and store the catecholamines epinephrine (adrenaline) and norepinephrine (noradrenaline). Both are synthesized from the amino acid phenylalanine (Fig. 21.20). Only 30% of circulating epinephrine comes from the adrenal medulla (the other 70% is released from nerve

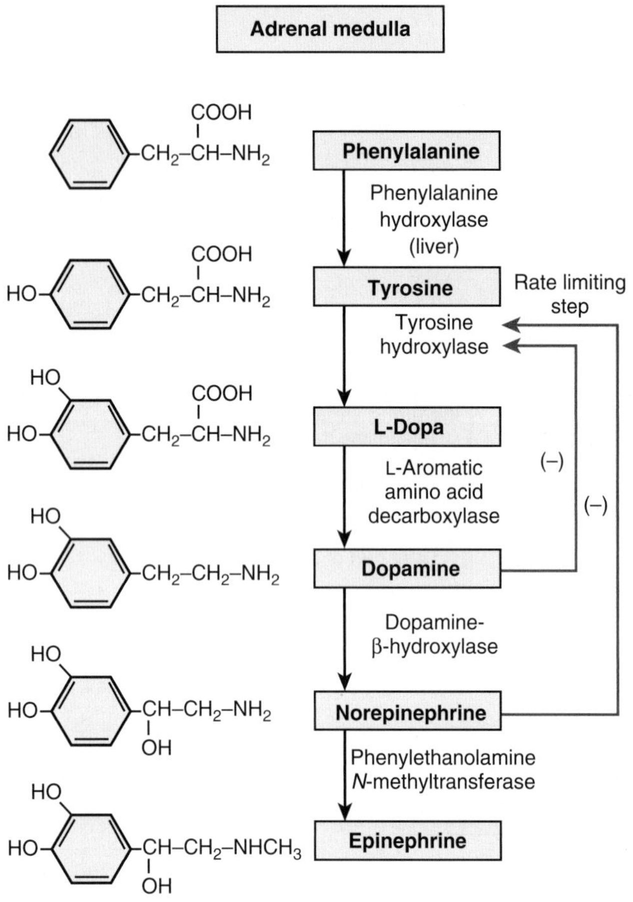

Fig. 21.20 Synthesis of Catecholamines.

terminals), and the medulla is only a minor source of norepinephrine. The adrenal medulla functions as a sympathetic ganglion without postganglionic processes. Sympathetic cholinergic preganglion fibers terminate on the chromaffin cells and secrete catecholamines directly into the bloodstream. The catecholamines acting in the blood are therefore hormones and not neurotransmitters.

Physiologic stress to the body (e.g., traumatic injury, hypoxia, hypoglycemia) triggers the exocytosis of the storage granules from chromaffin cells, with release of epinephrine and norepinephrine into the bloodstream. Secretion of adrenal catecholamines is also increased by ACTH and the glucocorticoids. Once released, the catecholamines remain in the plasma for only seconds to minutes. The catecholamines exert their biologic effects after binding to plasma membrane receptors (α_1, α_2, β_1, β_2, and β_3) in target cells. This binding activates the adenylyl cyclase system (an intracellular second messenger system). Catecholamines have diverse effects on the entire body. Their release and the body's response have been characterized as the "fight or flight" response (stress response) (see Figs. 11.2 and 11.4 and Tables 11.3 and 11.4). Metabolic effects of catecholamines promote hyperglycemia through a variety of mechanisms, including interference with the usual glucose regulatory feedback mechanisms. Catecholamines are rapidly removed from the plasma by neuron absorption for storage in new cytoplasmic granules, or metabolically inactivated and excreted in the urine. Catecholamines also directly inhibit secretion by decreasing the formation of the enzyme tyrosine hydroxylase (the rate-limiting step, see Fig. 21.20).

Tests of Endocrine Function

Evaluation of the endocrine system is challenging because of (1) the complexity of the clinical presentation as a result of multiple organ system involvement, (2) the nonspecific nature of complaints frequently associated with endocrine dysfunction, and (3) the inappropriate use of laboratory test interpretations.

Tests of the endocrine system involve several general types of clinical evaluation. Measurement of hormone level is accomplished by RIA, by ELISA, and, less commonly, by bioassay. Radioimmunoassay (RIA), a technique for measuring the minute quantities of hormones in the blood, uses antibodies and radiolabeled hormones to determine the quantity of hormone in the plasma. Enzyme-linked immunosorbent assay (ELISA) also is used to determine circulating hormone levels. This method is similar to that of RIA but is less expensive and easier to conduct. Instead of radiolabeled hormones, an enzyme-labeled hormone is used. A bioassay involves the use of graded doses of hormone in a reference preparation and then comparison of the results with an unknown sample. Bioassays are used more commonly in investigative endocrinology than in clinical laboratories. If the serum level is greater or less than the reference values, more definitive tests are required to determine the source of the problem.

Measurement of individual hormones does not always permit differentiation between normal and abnormal values when hormone levels are changing over time. For an accurate interpretation, the broad normal range of some hormones requires knowledge of previous hormonal levels and timed sampling. Stimulation and suppression tests that determine the response to exogenous stimulants or inhibitors can help to decipher some of these complexities.

Indirect assessment of hormonal function often includes measurement of concentrations of serum glucose and electrolytes that are affected by the endocrine process. Evaluation of hormonal function also may include radiographic imaging of specific glands.

AGING AND THE ENDOCRINE SYSTEM

The precise relationship between aging and the endocrine system is not clear. Perhaps most important, the question of whether changes in endocrine function are a consequence or a cause of aging has yet to be resolved. These relationships have been difficult to identify, in part because of a number of age-related variables that may coexist, such as acute and chronic nonendocrine disease; use of medications; alterations in diet, body composition, and weight; and changes in sleep-wake cycles. However, the endocrine system is so integral to health that changes in endocrine function have been used as "biomarkers" for unhealthy aging.

Investigation into the role of the endocrine glands and their interactions in the aging process has generated much data, although the evidence is contradictory. There are complex changes within the HPA; altered biologic activity of hormones, altered circulating levels of hormones, altered secretory response of the endocrine glands, altered metabolism of hormones, loss of circadian control of hormone secretion, and effects of oxidative stress and inflammation are among the findings. Changes in secretion of hypothalamic regulatory factors and hormones or changes in hypothalamic feedback sensitivity may contribute to alterations in control of an optimal internal environment.[23]

The dynamic equilibrium of the endocrine system also may be affected by altered secretion of neurotransmitters within certain areas of the brain, affecting hypothalamic and pituitary function. Such alterations may include an excess or deficit in secretion of pituitary hormones and loss of appropriate secretory pattern of those hormones. Loss of endocrine steady states may be associated with or contribute to aging.[24]

Thyroid Gland

Changes in thyroid structure and function occur with aging.[25] Structurally, some glandular atrophy and fibrosis occur with nodularity and increasing inflammatory infiltrates. These infiltrative changes may reflect age-related autoimmune damage. Clinical signs of thyroid disease are more difficult to detect in older adults. Overall, it is estimated that there is some evidence of thyroid dysfunction in 5% to 10% of older adult women. The presence of thyroid nodules increases after the age of 70 years. Changes relative to thyroid hormone and its function are more difficult to assess and much of the available data are contradictory. Overall, TSH secretion is thought to increase slightly, but there is controversy regarding whether this is normal aging or the presence of hypothyroidism with risk for adverse consequences.[26]

Treatment for thyroid deficiency is also affected by aging. The appropriate dose for TH replacement is often lower in older adults because the peripheral metabolism of TH decreases with age. In addition, TH must be replaced slowly in older adults with coronary artery disease to prevent angina and myocardial infarction.

Endocrine Pancreas

It is estimated that 40% to 50% of individuals older than age 65 have impaired glucose tolerance or diabetes, and there is an age-dependent decline in beta-cell function.[27] With aging, pancreatic cell regeneration declines, and there is fibrosis and shrinkage of the extracellular matrix and fat accumulation in the exocrine tissues.[28]

Dysfunction of the pancreas with decreased insulin secretion of beta cells and insulin receptors and increased insulin resistance have all been documented and may be related to changes in adipokine physiology.[29] These changes have significant implications for many target organs, particularly the cardiovascular system, which is increasingly at risk for both vascular (hypertension, atherosclerosis, glomerulosclerosis) and cardiac (infarction, failure) disorders.

Growth Hormone and Insulin-Like Growth Factors

The amounts of GH and IGF decline with aging, a process that has been called the *somatopause*. This decline in anabolic stimuli is linked to decreases in muscle size and function, decreased amounts of fat and bone mass, and changes in reproductive and cognitive function. Some studies have shown that GH resistance and declines in GH are associated with longevity in animals, but there is inconsistent data for humans.[30]

Parathyroid Glands

Age-related increases in PTH secretion, known as secondary hyperparathyroidism, occur in older adults. It is associated with low levels of calcitriol and calcium and related to a decline in renal conversion of vitamin D3 to calcitriol. Calcium malabsorption and hypocalcemia lead to increased bone remodeling and cortical bone thinning and porosity. Calcium intake, especially in women, also tends to decrease with aging and, combined with a decline in estrogen, contributes to osteoporosis (see Chapter 44).[31] The average daily intake of 450 to 500 mg/day causes a negative calcium balance greater than 40 mg/day and may be related to the absolute bone loss of approximately 1.5% per year. Older adults show decreased intestinal adaptation to variations in calcium intake. The elevated levels of parathyroid hormone have been linked to an increase in mortality in older adults, many of whom also have a mild, persistent hypercalciuria, which indicates a defective renal mechanism for responding to decreased calcium intake. Decreased circulating levels of vitamin D are common in older adults, especially those in long-term care institutions. Vitamin D deficiency has been linked to not only osteoporosis but also cancer, autoimmune diseases, diabetes, cardiovascular disease, and mental health disorders. The parathyroid gland, kidney, and choroid plexus secrete the Klotho protein, which, when overexpressed, has antiaging effects (see Emerging Science Box: Klotho Protein and Aging).

Adrenal Glands

The adrenal cortex loses some weight and has more fibrous tissue after the age of 50 years. Age diminishes negative feedback on the secretion of cortisol, due to impaired sensitivity of the hypothalamic-pituitary axis. There is an age-related decrease in the metabolic clearance rate of the glucocorticoids. The metabolic clearance of cortisol decreases with an age-related decline in liver and kidney function. Decreased clearance and reduced use of cortisol contribute to higher circulating cortisol levels, but diurnal variation is maintained. Because feedback mechanisms are intact, the higher cortisol levels cause a decrease in cortisol secretion. The chronic elevation in cortisol can impair recovery from stressful stimuli and contribute to loss of muscle mass, hypertension, osteopenia, visceral obesity, diabetes, suppressed immunity, and a decline in cognitive function.[32]

Plasma levels of the adrenal androgens, as well as urinary excretion of the metabolic end products, decrease gradually but

EMERGING SCIENCE BOX

Klotho Protein and Aging

Klotho is a protein known to have antiaging effects and is expressed primarily in the kidney distal tubules, parathyroid glands, and choroid plexus of the brain and in lesser amounts in many other organ tissues. The transmembrane form of Klotho protein functions as an obligatory co-receptor with endocrine fibroblast growth factor-23 (FGF23), which is important for the regulation of vitamin D metabolism and subsequently blood phosphate levels. In addition, the extracellular domain of the protein is secreted into the blood, cerebrospinal fluid, and urine. Decreased plasma, urinary, and renal Klotho levels are associated with normal aging, chronic kidney disease, salt-sensitive hypertension, cancers, osteoporosis, atherosclerosis, coronary artery disease, and increased mortality. Klotho also is known to have a tumor suppressor function. In contrast, overexpression of the Klotho gene results in reversal of the aging process, neuroprotection, and increased longevity in mammals. Klotho may derive much of its antiaging powers from its ability to regulate telomerase length and activity in stem cells. Finally, the Klotho protein is a powerful regulator of a wide variety of cellular transport systems, including ion channels, transport proteins, and the Na^+-K^+-ATPase pump. These functions can be stimulatory or inhibitory, and more research is needed to determine how these processes have antiaging effects and how their disruption contributes to disease. Recombinant human Klotho protein has been developed, and efforts are in progress to target its function in both health and disease.

Data from Cheikhi A, et al. An elephant in aging research. *Journals of Gerontology - Series A Biological Sciences and Medical Sciences,* 2019;74(7):1031–1042; Kuro-O M. The Klotho proteins in health and disease. Nature Reviews. *Nephrology,* 2019;15(1):27–44; Ullah M, et al. Klotho deficiency accelerates stem cells aging by impairing telomerase activity. *Journals of Gerontology - Series A Biological Sciences and Medical Sciences,* 2019;74:1396–1407.

dramatically with age, to as much as 50% to 70% of the young adult level. This change in adrenal function has been called the *adrenopause* and is correlated with decreased synthesis activity of DHEA.

This change appears to reflect a decline in the function of the zona reticularis. In postmenopausal women, this decline in adrenal androgen secretion is especially important because nearly all sex steroids after menopause come from adrenal and ovarian production of androgen precursors converted to estrogens in the periphery. In older adult men, adrenal androgen production accounts for more than half of circulating testosterone levels.

Antidiuretic Hormone and Aldosterone

Although hyponatremia is a common finding in older adults, it appears related to changes in renal function or sensitivity rather than to ADH-related mechanisms. Morphologic studies have not shown significant age-related degenerative changes in the neuroendocrine pathways that regulate the synthesis and secretion of ADH. However, it appears that ADH secretion is augmented when stimulated by changes in osmotic concentration, whereas baroreceptor-mediated ADH secretion is reduced, producing the syndrome of inappropriate ADH secretion (SIADH), common in older adults.[33] The secretion of aldosterone from the adrenal cortex declines with aging and is associated with decreased renin and an increased risk for hyperkalemia.[32]

SUMMARY REVIEW

Mechanisms of Hormonal Regulation

1. The endocrine system has five general functions: (1) differentiation of the reproductive and central nervous systems in the developing fetus; (2) stimulation of sequential growth and development during childhood and adolescence; (3) coordination of the male and female reproductive systems, which makes sexual reproduction possible; (4) maintenance of an optimal internal environment throughout life; and (5) initiation of corrective and adaptive responses when emergency demands occur.
2. Hormones are chemical messengers synthesized by endocrine glands and, when released, trigger intracellular responses.
3. Hormones have specific rates and rhythms of secretion: diurnal, pulsatile/cyclic, and patterns dependent on other circulating substances.
4. Hormones have specific negative- and positive-feedback mechanisms. Positive feedback occurs when a neural, chemical, or endocrine response increases the synthesis and secretion of a hormone. Negative feedback occurs when a changing chemical, neural, or endocrine response to a stimulus decreases the synthesis and secretion of a hormone.
5. Hormones affect only target cells with appropriate receptors and then act on these cells to initiate specific cell functions or activities.
6. Hormone receptors on target cells have two main functions: (1) to recognize and bind specifically and with high affinity to their particular hormones; and (2) to initiate a signal to appropriate intracellular effectors.
7. Receptors for hormones may be located on the plasma membrane or in the intracellular compartment of a target cell.
8. Water-soluble (peptide) hormones circulate throughout the body in unbound form. They bind with a receptor on a target cell's plasma membrane, acting as a first messenger. This binding signals the cell to generate a second messenger inside the cell. The second messenger communicates with the cell nucleus and mediates the action of the hormone on the target cell.
9. Lipid-soluble (steroid) hormones freely cross the plasma membrane by diffusion. These hormones diffuse directly into the cell nucleus and bind to nuclear receptors. Rapid responses of steroid hormones (non-genomic responses) may be mediated by plasma membrane receptors.

Structure and Function of the Endocrine Glands

1. The hypothalamic-pituitary axis (HPA) forms the structural and functional basis for the neuroendocrine system.
2. The hypothalamus is connected to the pituitary gland by the pituitary stalk. The hypothalamus regulates anterior pituitary function by secreting releasing or inhibiting hormones and factors into the portal circulation.
3. Hypothalamic hormones include prolactin-releasing hormone (PRH), which stimulates secretion of prolactin; prolactin-inhibiting hormone (PIH, dopamine), which inhibits prolactin secretion; thyrotropin-releasing hormone (TRH), which affects release of thyroid hormones; growth hormone-releasing hormone (GHRH), which stimulates the release of growth hormone (GH); somatostatin, which inhibits the release of GH and thyroid-stimulating hormone (TSH); gonadotropin-releasing hormone (GnRH), which facilitates the release of follicle-stimulating hormone (FSH) and luteinizing hormone (LH); corticotropin-releasing hormone (CRH), which facilitates the release of adrenocorticotropic hormone (ACTH) and endorphins; and substance P, which inhibits ACTH release and stimulates the release of a variety of other hormones.
4. The pituitary gland consists of anterior and posterior portions that have different functional relationships to the hypothalamus.
5. Hormones of the anterior pituitary are regulated by (1) secretion of hypothalamic-releasing factors, (2) feedback effects from hormones secreted by target organs, and (3) mediating effects of neurotransmitters.
6. Hormones of the anterior pituitary include corticotropin-related hormones (ACTH, melanocyte-stimulating hormone [MSH], β-lipotropin, β-endorphins), somatotropic hormones (GH, prolactin), and glycoprotein hormones (FSH, LH, TSH).
7. The posterior pituitary secretes antidiuretic hormone (ADH), which also is called vasopressin, and oxytocin.
8. ADH controls serum osmolality, increases permeability of the renal tubules to water, and causes vasoconstriction when administered pharmacologically in high doses.
9. Oxytocin causes uterine contraction and lactation in women and may have a role in sperm motility in men. In both men and women, oxytocin has an antidiuretic effect similar to that of ADH.
10. The pineal gland secretes melatonin, which regulates circadian rhythms and reproduction.
11. The two-lobed thyroid gland contains follicles, which secrete some of the thyroid hormones, and C cells, which secrete calcitonin.
12. Regulation of thyroid hormone (TH) involves a negative-feedback loop initiated by TRH and involving the hypothalamus, anterior pituitary, thyroid gland, and numerous biochemical variables.
13. TSH, which is synthesized and stored in the anterior pituitary, stimulates secretion of TH by activating intracellular processes, including uptake of iodine necessary for the synthesis of TH in the thyroid gland.
14. Synthesis of TH depends on the glycoprotein thyroglobulin, which contains a precursor of TH, tyrosine. Tyrosine then combines with iodine to form precursor molecules of the thyroid hormones thyroxine (T_4) and triiodothyronine (T_3). These hormones are then stored within thyroid colloid until released into the circulation.
15. When released into the circulation, T_3 and T_4 are bound by carrier proteins in the plasma, which store these hormones and provide a buffer for rapid changes in hormone levels. The free form is the active form.
16. Thyroid hormones alter protein synthesis and have a wide range of metabolic effects on proteins, carbohydrates, lipids, vitamins, and other hormones and neurotransmitters. TH also affects heat production and cardiac function.
17. The paired parathyroid glands are located behind the upper and lower poles of the thyroid. These glands secrete parathyroid hormone (PTH), an important regulator of serum calcium and phosphate levels.
18. PTH secretion increases levels of ionized calcium and decreases levels of phosphate in the plasma. In the kidney, PTH increases reabsorption of calcium and decreases reabsorption of phosphorus.
19. The endocrine pancreas contains the islets of Langerhans, which consist of alpha cells, beta cells, delta cells, and F cells. These cells secrete hormones that regulate carbohydrate, fat, and protein metabolism in the body.
20. Alpha cells produce glucagon, which is secreted inversely to blood glucose concentrations and helps increase blood glucose.
21. Beta cells synthesize insulin and secrete amylin. Insulin is a hormone that regulates blood glucose concentrations and overall body metabolism of fat, protein, and carbohydrates. Amylin suppresses glucagon secretion and has a satiety effect.
22. Delta cells secrete somatostatin, which inhibits glucagon and insulin secretion.
23. F cells secrete pancreatic polypeptide, which inhibits gallbladder contraction and exocrine pancreatic secretion.
24. The paired adrenal glands are situated above the kidneys. Each gland consists of an outer adrenal cortex, which secretes steroid hormones, and an inner adrenal medulla, which secretes catecholamines.
25. The steroid hormones secreted by the adrenal cortex are synthesized from cholesterol. These hormones include glucocorticoids, mineralocorticoids, and adrenal androgens and estrogens.
26. Glucocorticoids directly affect carbohydrate metabolism by increasing blood glucose concentration through gluconeogenesis in the liver and by decreasing uptake of glucose. Glucocorticoids also inhibit immune and inflammatory responses, suppress growth, and promote protein catabolism.
27. The most potent naturally occurring glucocorticoid is cortisol, which is necessary for the maintenance of life and for protection from stress. Secretion of cortisol is regulated by the hypothalamus and anterior pituitary.

28. Cortisol secretion is related to secretion of ACTH, which is stimulated by corticotropin-releasing hormone (CRH). ACTH binds with receptors of the adrenal cortex, which activates intracellular mechanisms and leads to cortisol release.
29. Mineralocorticoids are steroid hormones that directly affect ion transport epithelial cells, causing sodium retention and potassium and hydrogen loss.
30. Aldosterone is the most potent of the naturally occurring mineralocorticoids. Its primary role is conserving sodium by increasing the activity of the sodium pump of epithelial cells. The principal site of aldosterone action is the kidney, where it causes sodium reabsorption and potassium and hydrogen excretion. Aldosterone secretion is regulated primarily by the renin-angiotensin system and by sodium and potassium levels.
31. Androgens and estrogens secreted by the adrenal cortex act in the same way as those secreted by the gonads.
32. The adrenal medulla secretes the catecholamines epinephrine and norepinephrine. Physiologic stress to the body triggers their release.
33. Catecholamines bind with various target cells and are taken up by neurons or excreted in the urine. Catecholamines cause a range of metabolic effects (e.g., hyperglycemia) characterized as the "fight or flight" response.
34. Several assay methods are used to measure levels of hormones in the plasma. Radioimmunoassay (RIA) compares the proportion of radiolabeled and nonradiolabeled hormone against standard reference curves. Enzyme-linked immunosorbent assay (ELISA) is a method similar to RIA, but uses a radiolabeled enzyme rather than a radiolabeled hormone. Bioassays use graded doses of hormone in a reference preparation and then compare the results with an unknown sample to determine the hormone level.

Aging and the Endocrine System

1. Endocrine changes that may be associated with aging include altered biologic activity of hormones, altered circulating levels of hormones, altered secretory responses of endocrine glands, altered metabolism of hormones, loss of circadian control of hormone release, and changes in secretion of hypothalamic regulatory hormones.
2. Cellular damage associated with aging, genetically programmed cell change, and chronic wear and tear may contribute to endocrine gland dysfunction or alterations in the responsiveness of target organs.
3. Aging apparently causes atrophy of the thyroid gland and is associated with infiltrative glandular changes. Secretion of thyroid hormones may diminish with age.
4. Aging causes pancreatic fat deposition and is associated with a decrease both in insulin secretion and in insulin sensitivity. In addition, there is an age-dependent decline in beta-cell function.
5. Growth hormone levels decrease with aging, leading to decreased bone and muscle mass.
6. Aging is associated with alterations in calcium steady states, which may be related to alterations in PTH secretion from the parathyroid glands.
7. Age-related changes in adrenal function include synthesis of glucocorticoids and a decrease in levels of adrenal androgens. The effects of these changes, however, are offset by feedback mechanisms that maintain glucocorticoid levels and by gonadal secretion of androgens.
8. The kidney, choroid plexus, and parathyroid gland secrete the Klotho protein, which has antiaging effects.

REFERENCES

1. Narumi S, Hasegawa T. TSH resistance revisited. *Endocr J.* 2015;62(5):393–398.
2. Barabás K, et al. Rapid non-classical effects of steroids on the membrane receptor dynamics and downstream signaling in neurons. *Horm Behav.* 2018;104:183–191.
3. Ahmed WS, Geethakumari AM, Biswas KH. Phosphodiesterase 5 (PDE5): structure-function regulation and therapeutic applications of inhibitors. *Biomed Pharmacother.* 2020;134:111128.
4. Phillips JE. Inhaled phosphodiesterase 4 (PDE4) inhibitors for inflammatory respiratory diseases. *Front Pharmacol.* 2020;11:259.
5. Lv J, et al. Development of Bruton's tyrosine kinase inhibitors for rheumatoid arthritis. *Curr Med Chem.* 2018;25(42):5847–5859.
6. Burger JA. Bruton tyrosine kinase inhibitors: present and future. *Cancer J.* 2019;25(6):386–393.
7. Fontaine C, et al. The impact of estrogen receptor in arterial and lymphatic vascular diseases. *Int J Mol Sci.* 2020;21(9):3244.
8. Thomas P. Membrane androgen receptors unrelated to nuclear steroid receptors. *Endocrinology.* 2019;160(4):772–781.
9. Boguszewski CL. Boguszewski MCDS: Growth hormone's links to cancer. *Endocr Rev.* 2019;40(2):558–574.
10. Azzini AM, et al. A 2020 review on the role of procalcitonin in different clinical settings: an update conducted with the tools of the Evidence Based Laboratory Medicine. *Ann Transl Med.* 2020;8(9):610.
11. Gregoriano C, et al. Role of procalcitonin use in the management of sepsis. *J Thorac Dis.* 2020;12(Suppl 1):S5–S15.
12. Thompson JC, et al. Abaloparatide and the spine: a narrative review. *Clin Interv Aging.* 2020;15:1023–1033.
13. Lai NK, Martinez D. Physiological roles of parathyroid hormone-related protein. *Acta Biomed.* 2019;90(4):510–516.
14. Hædersdal S, et al. The role of glucagon in the pathophysiology and treatment of type 2 diabetes. *Mayo Clin Proc.* 2018;93(2): 217–239.
15. Maxwell JE, et al. Elevated pancreatic polypeptide levels in pancreatic neuroendocrine tumors and diabetes mellitus: causation or association? *Pancreas.* 2014;43(4):651–656.
16. Sharma VK, Singh TG. Chronic stress and diabetes mellitus: interwoven pathologies. *Curr Diabetes Rev.* 2020;16(6):546–556.
17. Ingawale DK, Mandlik SK, Patel SS. An emphasis on molecular mechanisms of anti-inflammatory effects and glucocorticoid resistance. *J Complement Integr Med.* 2015;12(1):1–13.
18. Barnes PJ. How corticosteroids control inflammation: Quintiles Prize Lecture 2005. *Br J Pharmacol.* 2006;148(3):245–254.
19. Mitre-Aguilar IB, Cabrera-Quintero AJ, Zentella-Dehesa A. Genomic and non-genomic effects of glucocorticoids: implications for breast cancer. *Int J Clin Exp Pathol.* 2015;8(1): 1–10.
20. Mazziotti G, Giustina A. Glucocorticoids and the regulation of growth hormone secretion. *Nat Rev Endocrinol.* 2013;9(5): 265–276.

21. Slominski RM, et al. Extra-adrenal glucocorticoid biosynthesis: implications for autoimmune and inflammatory disorders. *Genes Immun*. 2020;21(3):150–168.
22. Tsai CH, et al. Left ventricular remodeling and dysfunction in primary aldosteronism. *J Hum Hypertens*. 2021;35(2):131–147.
23. Diamanti-Kandarakis E, et al. Mechanisms in endocrinology: aging and anti-aging: a combo-endocrinology overview. *Eur J Endocrinol*. 2017;176(6):R283–R308.
24. Vitale G, Salvioli S, Franceschi C. Oxidative stress and the ageing endocrine system. *Nat Rev Endocrinol*. 2013;9(4):228–240.
25. Franceschi C, et al. The aging thyroid: a reappraisal within the geroscience integrated perspective. *Endocr Rev*. 2019;40(5):1250–1270.
26. Duntas LH. Thyroid function in aging: a discerning approach. *Rejuvenation Res*. 2018;21(1):22–28.
27. Gamage S, et al. Potential role of E4orf1 protein in aging-associated impairment in glycemic control. *J Diabetes Complications*. 2019;33(3):261–265.
28. Wang L, Zheng S. Pancreatic senescence and its clinical manifestations. *Aging Med (Milton)*. 2020;3(1):48–52.
29. Gulcelik NE, et al. Adipocytokines and aging: adiponectin and leptin. *Minerva Endocrinol*. 2013;38(2):203–210.
30. Bartke A. Growth hormone and aging. *Rev Endocr Metab Disord*. 2021;22(1):71–80.
31. Bhattarai HK, et al. Vitamin D, calcium, parathyroid hormone, and sex steroids in bone health and effects of aging. *J Osteoporos*. 2020;2020:9324505.
32. Yiallouris A, et al. Adrenal aging and its implications on stress responsiveness in humans. *Front Endocrinol (Lausanne)*. 2019;10:54.
33. Cowen LE, Hodak SP, Verbalis JG. Age-associated abnormalities of water homeostasis. *Endocrinol Metab Clin North Am*. 2013;42(2):349–370.
34. Kuo T, et al. Regulation of glucose homeostasis by glucocorticoids. *Adv Exp Med Biol*. 2015;872:99–126.

22

Alterations of Hormonal Regulation

Jodi A. Allen

http://evolve.elsevier.com/Rogers/pathophysiology/

CHAPTER OUTLINE

Functions of the endocrine system involve complex interactions between hormones and most body systems that maintain dynamic steady states and influence tissue growth and reproductive capabilities. Endocrine system dysfunction is usually caused by hypersecretion or hyposecretion of the various hormones, leading to abnormal hormone concentrations in the blood. Dysfunction also may result from abnormal cell receptor function or from altered intracellular response to the hormone–receptor complex.

MECHANISMS OF HORMONAL ALTERATIONS

Significantly elevated or significantly depressed hormone levels may result from two primary mechanisms: (1) inappropriate amounts of hormone delivered to the target cell, or (2) inappropriate responses by the target cell (Table 22.1). Inappropriate amounts of hormone can result from disorders of endocrine glands, causing them to synthesize too little or too much hormone, failure of feedback systems designed to control hormone release, dysfunctional or ectopically produced hormones (hormones produced from nonendocrine sources), or defects in delivery of the hormone in the bloodstream.

Target cells may not respond appropriately to hormonal stimulation for a number of reasons. Target cells may have too many or too few cell surface receptors. Those receptors may be abnormal and insensitive, or they may be blocked or stimulated by antibodies. There also may be intracellular disorders that cause a failure of the target cell to respond to receptor stimulation. For example, there may be inadequate synthesis of second messengers, such as cyclic adenosine monophosphate (cAMP), or the cell may respond abnormally to the second messenger if levels of intracellular enzymes or proteins are altered (second messengers for various hormones are listed in Table 21.2).

ALTERATIONS OF THE HYPOTHALAMIC–PITUITARY SYSTEM

The most common cause of apparent hypothalamic dysfunction is interruption of the pituitary stalk. Such interruptions prevent hypothalamic hormones from reaching the pituitary gland. Damage to the pituitary stalk can be caused by destructive lesions, rupture after head injury, surgical transection, or tumor. Without hypothalamic hormones, the pituitary releases inadequate amounts of follicle-stimulating hormone (FSH), luteinizing hormone (LH), adrenocorticotropic hormone (ACTH), thyroid-stimulating hormone (TSH), and growth hormone (GH) (Fig. 22.1). The control of prolactin is predominantly inhibitory by hypothalamic dopamine. It does not have endocrine target tissue and therefore lacks a regulatory feedback pathway. The effects of these changes in pituitary hormones are discussed later in this chapter.

Diseases of the Posterior Pituitary

Diseases of the posterior pituitary cause either increased or decreased secretion of antidiuretic hormone (ADH, arginine vasopressin [AVP]). An excess amount of this hormone

TABLE 22.1 Mechanisms of Hormone Alterations

Inappropriate Amounts of Hormone Delivered to Target Cell	Inappropriate Response by Target Cell
Inadequate Hormone Synthesis 1. Inadequate quantity of hormone precursors 2. Secretory cell unable to convert precursors to active hormone	***Cell Surface Receptor–Associated Disorders*** 1. Decrease in the number of receptors 2. Impaired receptor function 3. Presence of antibodies against specific receptors
Failure of Feedback Systems 1. Do not recognize positive feedback, leading to inadequate hormone synthesis 2. Do not recognize negative feedback, leading to excessive hormone synthesis	
Dysfunctional or Ectopic Hormones 1. Inadequate biologically free hormone 2. Hormone degraded at an altered rate 3. Circulating inhibitors 4. Ectopic production of hormones	**Intracellular Disorders** 1. Inadequate synthesis of a second messenger 2. Intracellular enzymes or proteins are altered
Dysfunctional Delivery System 1. Inadequate blood supply 2. Inadequate carrier proteins	

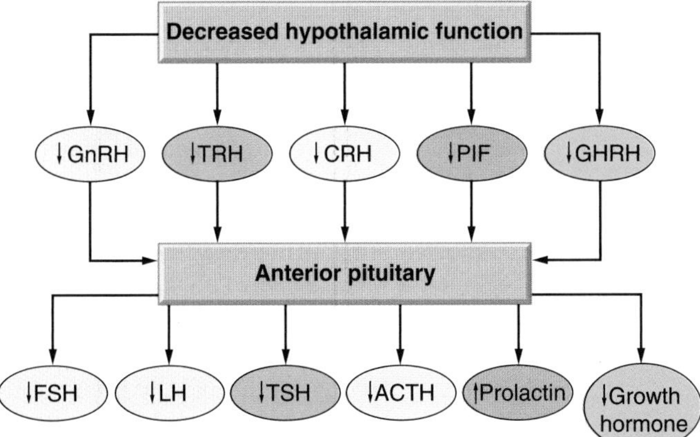

Fig. 22.1 Loss of Hypothalamic Hormones. *ACTH*, Adrenocorticotropic hormone; *CRH*, corticotropin-releasing hormone; *FSH*, follicle-stimulating hormone; *GHRH*, growth hormone–releasing hormone; *GnRH*, gonadotropin-releasing hormone; *LH*, luteinizing hormone; *PIF*, prolactin inhibitory factor (probably dopamine); *TRH*, thyrotropin-releasing hormone; *TSH*, thyroid-stimulating hormone.

TABLE 22.2 Signs and Symptoms of Diabetes Insipidus and Syndrome of Inappropriate Antidiuretic Hormone Secretion

Signs and Symptoms	DI	SIADH
Urine output	High	Low (no hypovolemia)
Urine osmolality	Low (<100–200 mOsm/L)	High (>800 mOsm/L)
Urine specific gravity	Low (<1.010)	High (>1.020)
Serum sodium	Hypernatremia (>145 mEq/L)	Hyponatremia (<135 mEq/L)
Serum osmolality	Hyperosmolar (>300 mOsm/L)	Hypoosmolar (<285 mOsm/L)
Symptoms	Polyuria, thirst, high urine output, signs of dehydration	Water retention, low urine output, nausea, vomiting, mental changes

DI, Diabetes insipidus; *SIADH*, syndrome of inappropriate antidiuretic hormone.

results in water retention, whereas deficiencies in the amount or response to ADH result in water loss. These complex pathophysiologic states not only have significant clinical effects on the modulation of body fluids and electrolytes, but also affect cognitive and emotional responses to stress.

Syndrome of Inappropriate Antidiuretic Hormone Secretion

The syndrome of inappropriate ADH secretion (SIADH) results from ADH release in the absence of normal physiologic stimuli from the pituitary gland, nonpituitary sources of ADH, or the continued action of ADH on vasopressin receptors.[1,2] SIADH is characterized by hypotonic and euvolemic hyponatremia along with urinary hyperosmolarity. SIADH can be idiopathic or due to multiple causes including neurological disease, pulmonary disease, malignant diseases, medications, or acute conditions such as stress, pain, and general anesthesia. Non-osmotic stimuli also mediate release of ADH via the afferent parasympathetic nervous system from high- and low-pressure receptors in the atria and carotid and artery during hemodynamic stress. Central nervous system disorders that may cause SIADH include encephalitis, meningitis, intracranial hemorrhage, tumors, and trauma. Pulmonary disorders associated with SIADH include pneumonia (e.g., tuberculosis), asthma, cystic fibrosis, and respiratory failure requiring mechanical ventilation. A common cause of SIADH is the ectopic production of ADH by tumors, such as cancers of the lung, stomach, pancreas, bladder, prostate, and endometrium; lymphomas; and sarcomas.

Iatrogenic causes of SIADH include surgery and medications. Any surgery can result in increased ADH secretion for as long as 5 to 7 days after surgery. The precise mechanism is uncertain, but likely related to fluid and volume changes after surgery, the amount and type of intravenous fluids given, and the use of narcotic analgesics. Medications are an important cause of SIADH, especially in the elderly. These include narcotics, general anesthetics, antidepressants, antipsychotics, chemotherapeutic agents, and nonsteroidal anti-inflammatory drugs.[2]

Pathophysiology. The cardinal features of SIADH are the result of enhanced renal free water retention. ADH induces the insertion of a water channel protein, called *aquaporin-2*, into the tubular luminal membrane, which increases water reabsorption by the kidneys (renal function is discussed in Chapter 37). This results in an expansion of extracellular fluid volume that leads to dilutional hyponatremia (low serum sodium concentration), high urinary osmolarity, high urinary sodium concentration, absence of edema, or clinical signs of volume depletion.[3] Urine is inappropriately concentrated with respect to serum osmolarity because water is reabsorbed that normally would be excreted.

Clinical Manifestations. The symptoms of SIADH result from hyponatremia (see Chapter 3) and are determined by its severity and rapidity of onset. Thirst, impaired taste, anorexia, dyspnea on exertion, fatigue, and dulled sensorium occur when the serum sodium level decreases rapidly. Gastrointestinal (GI) symptoms, including vomiting and abdominal cramps, occur with a drop in sodium concentration from 130 to 120 mEq/L. There is weight gain from water retention, but peripheral edema is absent. Serum sodium levels below 115 mEq/L cause confusion, lethargy, muscle twitching, and convulsions; severe and sometimes irreversible neurologic damage may occur. Symptoms usually resolve with correction of hyponatremia.

Evaluation and Treatment. A diagnosis of SIADH is based on these findings: (1) serum hypoosmolality and hyponatremia, (2) urine hyperosmolarity (i.e., urine osmolality is greater than expected for the concomitant serum osmolality), and (3) the absence of conditions that can alter volume status (e.g., adrenal or thyroid dysfunction, congestive heart failure, or renal insufficiency) (Table 22.2). It is important to remember that the diagnosis of SIADH requires normal renal, cardiac, hepatic, adrenal, and thyroid function. In particular, hypothyroidism and adrenal insufficiency must be excluded.[4]

The treatment of SIADH involves the correction of any underlying causal problems, as well as fluid restriction with careful monitoring of serum sodium and neurologic symptoms. In severe SIADH, emergency correction of severe hyponatremia by careful administration of hypertonic saline and administration of vasopressin receptor antagonists (vaptans) may be required. Resolution usually occurs within 3 days. If hyponatremia is corrected too rapidly, a severe neurologic syndrome called *central pontine myelinolysis* can ensue.

Diabetes Insipidus

Diabetes Insipidus (DI) is characterized by insufficient ADH activity, leading to polyuria (frequent urination) and polydipsia (frequent drinking). The three major forms of DI are:

1. *Neurogenic* or *central DI.* Caused by the insufficient secretion of ADH, it occurs when any organic lesion of the hypothalamus, pituitary stalk, or posterior pituitary interferes with ADH synthesis, transport, or release. Causative lesions include primary brain tumors, traumatic brain injury, hypophysectomy, aneurysms, thrombosis, infections, and immunologic disorders. It can also be caused by hereditary disorders that affect ADH genes or result in structural changes in the pituitary gland.
2. *Nephrogenic DI.* Caused by inadequate response of the renal tubules to ADH. Acquired nephrogenic DI is caused by disorders and drugs that damage the renal tubules. These disorders include pyelonephritis, amyloidosis, destructive uropathies, and polycystic kidney disease. Drugs that may induce a reversible form of nephrogenic DI include lithium carbonate, colchicine, amphotericin B, loop diuretics, general anesthetics, and demeclocycline. There are several genetic causes of nephrogenic DI, including a mutation in the gene that codes for aquaporin-2, which is one of the water transport channels in the renal tubule.[5]
3. *Primary polydipsia* or *Excessive thirst appreciation.* A rare form of DI, called *gestational DI*, is associated with pregnancy in which the level of the vasopressin-degrading enzyme vasopressinase is increased, resulting in ADH deficiency. Clinical manifestations are usually mild and do not require treatment.

Pathophysiology. Individuals with DI have a partial to total inability to concentrate urine. Insufficient ADH activity causes excretion of large volumes of dilute urine, leading to increased plasma osmolality. In conscious individuals, the thirst mechanism is stimulated and induces polydipsia. Dehydration develops rapidly without ongoing fluid replacement. If the individual with DI cannot conserve as much water as is lost in the urine, serum hypernatremia and hyperosmolality occur. Concentrations of other serum electrolytes generally are not affected. Neurogenic (central) DI is the clinical manifestation of destruction of the neurons of the hypothalamus/posterior pituitary axis, with consequent loss of AVP secretion. The syndrome is caused by a wide variety of acquired or congenital lesions.[6]

Clinical Manifestations. The clinical manifestations of DI include polyuria, nocturia, continuous thirst, and polydipsia. The urine output is varied but can increase from the normal output of 1 to 2 L/day to as much as 8 to 12 L/day. Individuals with long-standing DI develop a large bladder capacity and hydronephrosis (see Chapter 38). Neurogenic DI usually has an abrupt onset, whereas nephrogenic DI usually has a more gradual onset. Table 22.2 compares the signs and symptoms of DI and SIADH. A history of lithium therapy may raise the possibility of NDI, whereas previous brain injury or neurosurgical intervention may indicate neurogenic (central) DI.[6]

Evaluation and Treatment. The criteria for the diagnosis of DI include polyuria, polydipsia, low urine specific gravity (<1.010), low urine osmolality (<200 mOsm/kg), hypernatremia, high serum osmolality (300 mOsm or more depending on water intake), and continued diuresis despite a serum sodium level of 145 mEq/L or greater. The diagnosis of DI is generally confirmed through a two-step water deprivation testing in which urine output is maintained despite dehydration. Other measurements that are useful in diagnosis are serum and urine osmolality, serum electrolytes, ADH levels, and radioimmunoassay for AVP. DI must be distinguished from other polyuric states, including diabetes mellitus, osmotically induced diuresis, and psychogenic polydipsia. Therefore, an evaluation for underlying reversible central or renal causes should be undertaken.

Dipsogenic or *primary polydipsia* may be confused with DI, but it is particularly important not to misdiagnose primary polydipsia as neurogenic (central) DI, because inappropriate therapy with desmopressin can lead to dangerous hyponatremia in individuals who continue to drink excessively.[6] Primary polydipsia is usually the result of a psychiatric condition that causes the chronic ingestion of extremely large quantities of fluid, which washes out the renal concentration gradient, resulting in partial resistance to ADH.

Treatment of neurogenic (central) DI is based on the extent of the ADH deficiency. Fluid replacement using oral or intravenous routes is usually adequate. Some individuals require ADH replacement with the synthetic vasopressin analog desmopressin (DDAVP). Once a diagnosis of neurogenic (central) DI is made, magnetic resonance imaging (MRI) of the hypothalamic-pituitary region is required to establish whether there is a structural lesion that is responsible for AVP deficiency. Management of nephrogenic DI requires treatment of any reversible underlying disorders, discontinuation of etiologic medications, and correction of associated electrolyte disorders.[6] Drugs that potentiate the action of otherwise insufficient amounts of endogenous ADH, such as thiazide diuretics, chlorpropamide, carbamazepine, and clofibrate, may be used in individuals with incomplete ADH deficiency.

Diseases of the Anterior Pituitary

Hypopituitarism

Hypopituitarism is characterized by the absence of one or more anterior pituitary hormones or the complete failure of all anterior pituitary hormone functions.[7] The most common causes of hypopituitarism are pituitary infarction or space-occupying lesions. Pituitary infarction may occur when there is significant blood loss or hypovolemic shock. This also may occur in women during the postpartum period (Sheehan syndrome). Space-occupying lesions include pituitary adenomas or aneurysms, which can enlarge and compress the pituitary gland. Other causes of hypopituitarism include traumatic brain injury, removal or destruction of the gland, infections (e.g., meningitis, syphilis, tuberculosis), autoimmune hypophysitis, and certain drugs (e.g., bexarotene, carbamazepine, ipilimumab). A rare congenital form of hypopituitarism results from an early mutation of the prophet of pituitary transcription factor *(PROP-1)* gene, which affects embryonic pituitary development.

Pathophysiology. The pituitary gland is highly vascular and relies heavily on portal blood flow from the hypothalamus. It is therefore vulnerable to ischemia and infarction. Infarction results in tissue necrosis and edema with swelling of the gland. Over time, fibrosis of pituitary tissue occurs, and the symptoms of hypopituitarism develop. Adenomas and aneurysms may compress otherwise normal secreting pituitary cells and lead to compromised hormonal output. These lesions further impede blood supply because of enlargement of the pituitary within the fixed compartment of the sella turcica.

Clinical Manifestations. The signs and symptoms of hypofunction of the anterior pituitary are variable and depend on which hormones are affected. In panhypopituitarism, all hormones are deficient, and the individual suffers from multiple complications.

ACTH deficiency with associated loss of cortisol is a potentially life-threatening disorder. Symptoms of cortisol insufficiency include nausea, vomiting, anorexia, fatigue, and weakness. Hypoglycemia results from increased insulin sensitivity, decreased glycogen reserves, and decreased gluconeogenesis associated with hypocortisolism. ACTH deficiency also is associated with changes in aldosterone secretion, with resulting decreases in the glomerular filtration rate and urine output.

TSH deficiency causes cold intolerance, skin dryness, lethargy, and decreased metabolic rate. The symptoms usually are less severe than those of primary hypothyroidism.

The onset of FSH and LH deficiencies in women of reproductive age is associated with amenorrhea and atrophy of the vagina, uterus, and breasts. In postpubertal males, the testicles atrophy and facial hair growth is diminished. Both men and women experience decreased body hair and diminished libido.

GH deficiency in children is manifested by growth failure and a condition known as *hypopituitary dwarfism* (Fig. 22.2). Symptoms of chronic adult GH deficiency syndrome include increased body fat, decreased strength and lean body mass, osteoporosis, reduced sweating, dry skin, and psychological problems, including depression, social withdrawal, fatigue, loss of motivation, and a diminished feeling of well-being. Dyslipidemias and atherosclerotic cardiovascular disease may occur.

Evaluation and Treatment. The diagnostic evaluation of suspected pituitary disease includes simultaneous measurements of the levels of tropic hormones from the pituitary and target endocrine glands. Imaging of the pituitary (MRI or computed tomography [CT] scans) is critical to assess for anatomic lesions, such as tumors.

Management of hypopituitarism requires correction of the underlying disorder as quickly as possible. Replacement of target gland hormones that are deficient is essential (such as cortisol, thyroid hormone (TH), GH, and sex-specific steroid hormones). In cases of acute circulatory collapse, immediate therapy with glucocorticoids and intravenous fluids is critical.

Hyperpituitarism: Primary Pituitary Neuroendocrine Tumors

Pituitary neuroendocrine tumors (previously known as pituitary adenomas) usually are benign, slow-growing tumors that arise from cells of the anterior pituitary.[8] The cause of pituitary neuroendocrine tumors is not known, and most occur sporadically. Altered gene expression is commonly detected,

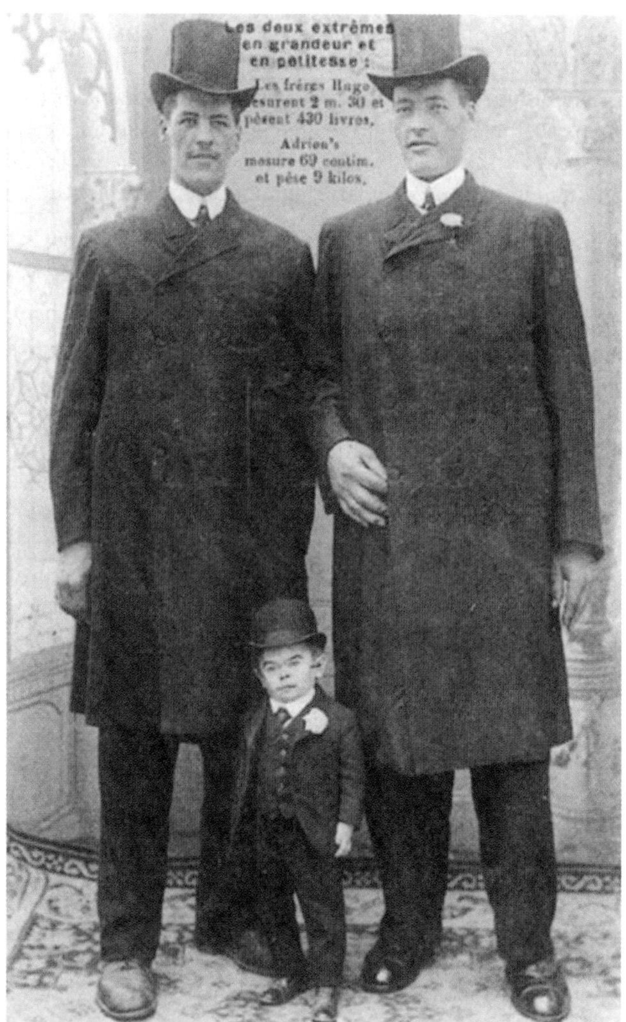
en grandeur et
en petitesse :
Les frères Hugo
pèsent 430 livres,
et pèse 9 kilos.

Fig. 22.2 Hypopituitary Dwarfism and Pituitary Giantism. A pituitary giant and dwarf contrasted with normal-size men. Excessive secretion of growth hormone by the anterior lobe of the pituitary gland during the early years of life produces giants of this type, whereas deficient secretion of this substance produces well-formed dwarfs. (From Enderle A. Dwarfism and gigantism in historical picture postcards. *Journal of the Royal Society of Medicine,* 1998;91(5):273–278. https://doi.org/10.1177/014107689809100511)

and familial pituitary neuroendocrine tumors occur as part of syndromes affecting other organs, such as multiple endocrine neoplasia type 1. About 50% are microscopic (microadenomas) found incidentally, are hormonally silent, and do not pose significant hazards to the individual. Larger tumors (macroadenomas) are associated with morbidity and mortality attributable to alterations in hormone secretion or to invasion or impingement of surrounding structures.[9,10]

Pathophysiology. Local expansion of the neuroendocrine tumor may impinge on the optic chiasma and cause various visual disturbances. If the tumor is locally aggressive, invasion of the cavernous sinuses may occur, resulting in compromise of cranial nerve function. Extension to the hypothalamus disturbs control of wakefulness, thirst, appetite, and temperature.

Hormonal effects of a neuroendocrine tumor include hypersecretion from the tumor itself and hyposecretion from surrounding pituitary cells. The adenomatous tissue secretes the hormone of the cell type from which it arose, without regard to regulatory feedback mechanisms (autonomous function). Because of the pressure exerted by the tumor in the unexpandable bony sella turcica, hyposecretion from those cells that are most sensitive to pressure is common (FSH-and LH-secreting cells).

Clinical Manifestations. The clinical manifestations of pituitary neuroendocrine tumors are related to tumor growth and hormone hypersecretion or hyposecretion. Increased tumor size causes headache, fatigue, neck pain or stiffness, and seizures. Visual changes include visual field impairments (often beginning in one eye and progressing to the other) and temporary blindness. If the tumor infiltrates other cranial nerves, neuromuscular function is affected.

Pituitary neuroendocrine tumors are most often associated with increased secretion of GH and prolactin. Gonadotropic hyposecretion results in menstrual irregularity in women, decreased libido, and receding secondary sex characteristics in both men and women. If the tumor exerts sufficient pressure, thyroid and adrenal hypofunction may occur because of a lack of TSH and ACTH, resulting in the symptoms of hypothyroidism and hypocortisolism, respectively.

Evaluation and Treatment. Diagnosis of pituitary neuroendocrine tumor involves physical and laboratory evaluations, including pertinent hormone assays and radiographic examination of the skull (MRI [preferred] or contrast-enhanced CT). The goal of treatment is to protect the individual from the effects of tumor growth and to control hormone hypersecretion while minimizing damage to appropriately secreting portions of the pituitary. Depending on tumor size and type, individuals may be treated by administration of specific medications to suppress tumor growth, transsphenoidal tumor resection, or radiation therapy, including stereotactic treatments.

Hypersecretion of Growth Hormone: Acromegaly

Acromegaly results from increased release of GH and insulin-like growth factor 1 (IGF-1). It almost always is caused by a GH-secreting pituitary neuroendocrine tumor.[11] Acromegaly is usually diagnosed in adults in the 40- to 59-year-old age group, although it is often present for years before diagnosis. It is a slow progressive disease and, if untreated, is associated with a decreased life expectancy. Deaths from acromegaly are caused by heart disease secondary to hypertension and coronary artery disease, stroke, diabetes mellitus, or malignancy (colon or lung cancers).

Pathophysiology. With a GH-secreting neuroendocrine tumor, only slight elevations of GH and IGF-1 can stimulate growth. In children and adolescents whose epiphyseal plates have not yet closed, the effect of increased GH levels is termed giantism (see Fig. 22.2). Skeletal growth is excessive, with some individuals becoming 8 or 9 feet tall. In the adult, epiphyseal closure has occurred, and increased amounts of GH and IGF-1 cause connective tissue proliferation and increased cytoplasmic matrix, as well as bony proliferation that results in the characteristic appearance of acromegaly (Fig. 22.3).

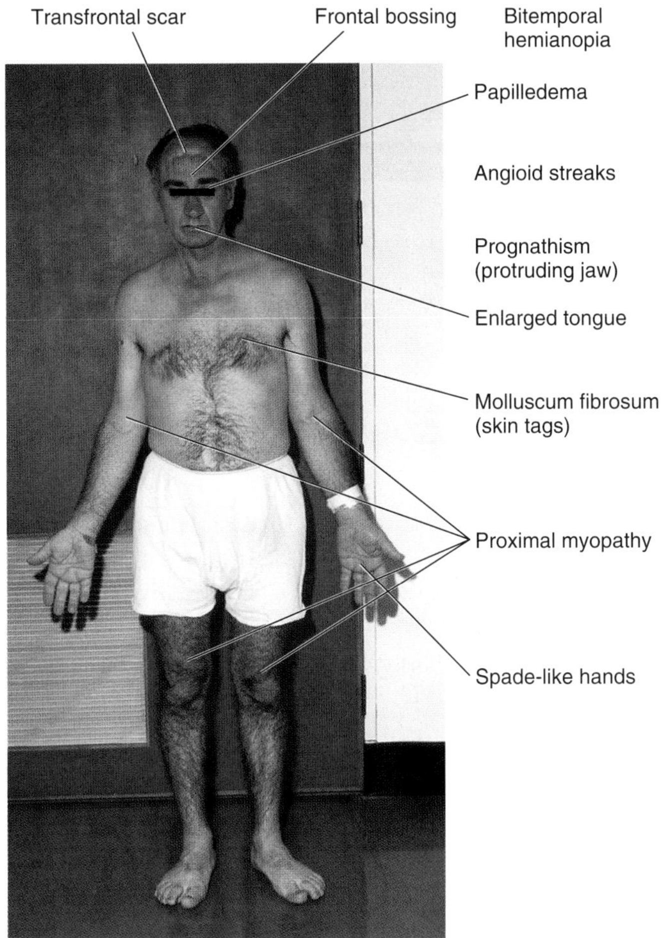

Fig. 22.3 Acromegaly. (From Talley NJ, O'Connor S. Clinical examination, 7th edition. Australia: Churchill Livingstone; 2014.)

GH also has significant effects on glucose, lipid, and protein metabolism. Hyperglycemia results from adipocyte inflammation and GH inhibition of peripheral glucose uptake and increased hepatic glucose production, followed by compensatory hyperinsulinism and, finally, insulin resistance. Diabetes mellitus occurs when the pancreas cannot secrete enough insulin to offset the effects of GH. Excessive levels of GH and IGF-1 also affect the cardiovascular system with calcium influx in cardiomyocytes, enhanced cardiac contractility, and cardiomyocyte growth. Hypertension, cardiomegaly, and left ventricular heart failure are seen in one-third to one-half of individuals with acromegaly. GH also acts on the renal tubules to increase phosphate reabsorption, leading to mild hyperphosphatemia. Approximately 20% of GH-secreting tumors also secrete prolactin. Because the adenoma becomes increasingly a space-occupying lesion, hypopituitarism may occur because of compression of surrounding hormone-secreting cells.

Clinical Manifestations. With connective tissue proliferation, individuals with acromegaly have an enlarged tongue, interstitial edema, enlarged and overactive sebaceous and sweat glands (leading to increased body odor), and coarse skin and body hair. Bony proliferation involves periosteal vertebral growth and enlargement of the bones of the face, hands, and feet (see Fig. 22.3). The lower jaw and forehead also protrude.

Increased IGF-1 levels cause ribs to elongate at the bone–cartilage junction, leading to a barrel-chested appearance, and increased proliferation of cartilage in joints, which causes backache and arthralgias. With bony and soft tissue overgrowth, nerve entrapment occurs, leading to peripheral nerve damage manifested by weakness, muscular atrophy, foot drop, and sensory changes in the hands.

Symptoms of diabetes mellitus, such as polyuria and polydipsia, may occur. Acromegaly-associated hypertension is usually asymptomatic until heart failure symptoms develop. Increased tumor size results in central nervous system symptoms of headache, seizure activity, visual disturbances, and papilledema. If compression hypopituitarism occurs, gonadotropin secretion may be affected, causing amenorrhea in women and sexual dysfunction in men. Increased prolactin results in hypogonadism.

Evaluation and Treatment. Diagnosis is confirmed by clinical features of the disease, MRI scans, and elevated levels of GH and IGF-1. The goals of treatment are to normalize or reduce GH secretion and relieve or prevent complications related to tumor expansion. The treatment of choice is transsphenoidal surgical removal of the GH-secreting neuroendocrine tumor. Radiation therapy may be effective when rapid control of GH levels is not essential, when the individual is not a good surgical candidate, or when hyperfunction persists after subtotal resection. Somatostatin analogs (e.g., octreotide or lanreotide) normalize IGF-1 and GH levels. Dopaminergic agonists may be helpful, especially if the tumor also secretes prolactin. Cardiovascular, metabolic, and symptoms of tumor compression often improve with treatment. Skeletal abnormalities are irreversible.

Prolactinoma

Pituitary tumors that secrete prolactin, prolactinomas, are the most common hormonally active pituitary tumors. Other conditions, such as renal failure, polycystic ovarian disease, primary hypothyroidism, breast stimulation, or even the stress of venipuncture, can increase prolactin levels. Prolactin is under tonic inhibitory hypothalamic control through the secretion of dopamine. Thus, medications that block the effects of dopamine can increase prolactin levels. These include some antipsychotics, metoclopramide, tricyclic antidepressants, and methyldopa. Estrogens can increase prolactin concentration by stimulating hyperplasia of prolactin-secreting cells. Any process that interferes with the delivery of dopamine from the hypothalamus to the lactotrophs (pituitary stalk tumor, pituitary stalk transection, or compressive pituitary tumor) also results in hyperprolactinemia. Because thyrotropin-releasing hormone (TRH) stimulates prolactin secretion, prolactin may be elevated in individuals with primary hypothyroidism.

Pathophysiology. The hallmark of a prolactinoma is sustained increases in the levels of serum prolactin, also known as hyperprolactinemia, which has multiple effects on female and male reproductive organs.[12] Pathologic elevations of prolactin suppress LH and FSH, resulting in estrogen and progesterone deficiency in women and low testosterone levels in men.

Hypopituitarism may occur because of the compression of surrounding hormone-secreting cells. Central nervous system symptoms may develop because of growth and pressure of the tumor within the sella turcica. These complications are especially common with what are called macro (>1 cm in diameter) or giant (>4 cm in diameter) prolactinomas.

Clinical Manifestations. Women with hyperprolactinemia generally present with galactorrhea (nonpuerperal milk production) and menstrual disturbances, including amenorrhea. Estrogen deficiency also may cause hirsutism, and fractures may occur because of osteopenia or osteoporosis. Hyperprolactinemia in men causes gynecomastia, hypogonadism, and erectile dysfunction, although they often are not diagnosed until they develop symptoms related to the increasing size of the tumor (i.e., headache or visual impairment).

Evaluation and Treatment. The diagnostic evaluation of hyperprolactinemia includes a careful history to exclude medications that may cause elevations in prolactin concentration. Screening for hypothyroidism is mandatory. MRI scanning of the pituitary is indicated to determine the size and location of an adenoma.

Dopaminergic agonists (bromocriptine and cabergoline) are the treatment of choice for prolactinomas. Decreases in tumor size and restoration of fertility in previously anovulatory women are common. In individuals resistant or intolerant to these medications, transsphenoidal surgery and radiotherapy are options. New chemotherapeutic and targeted molecular therapies are being explored in selected cases.

ALTERATIONS OF THYROID FUNCTION

Disorders of thyroid function develop as a result of primary dysfunction or disease of the thyroid gland or, secondarily, as a result of pituitary or hypothalamic alterations. Primary thyroid disorders result in either increased or decreased TH levels. These disorders also cause secondary feedback effects on pituitary TSH. For example, when there are primary elevations in the TH level, the TSH level will secondarily decrease because of negative feedback. When the TH level is decreased because of a condition affecting the thyroid gland, the TSH level will be elevated. Central (secondary) thyroid disorders are related to disorders of the anterior pituitary gland that affect thyroid function. When there is excessive TSH production, the thyroid follicular cells are stimulated and secrete excessive THs. The TH levels become elevated secondary to the primary elevation of the TSH concentration. The reverse is true with inadequate TSH production.

The majority of primary thyroid diseases are idiopathic and caused by autoimmune mechanisms that affect the gland. Although the exact genetic and environmental influences are not known, some individuals experience a predominantly cellular autoimmune response (some antithyroid autoantibodies also are involved) with resultant destruction of the thyroid gland, leading to hypothyroidism. Others experience a predominantly antibody-mediated autoimmune response that stimulates the gland, leading to hyperthyroidism. The most common autoimmune hypothyroid condition is called *chronic lymphocytic thyroiditis (also called Hashimoto thyroiditis)* with thyroid infiltration of T lymphocytes and follicular destruction.[13] The most common autoimmune hyperthyroid condition is called *Graves disease* (Fig. 22.4).[14,15]

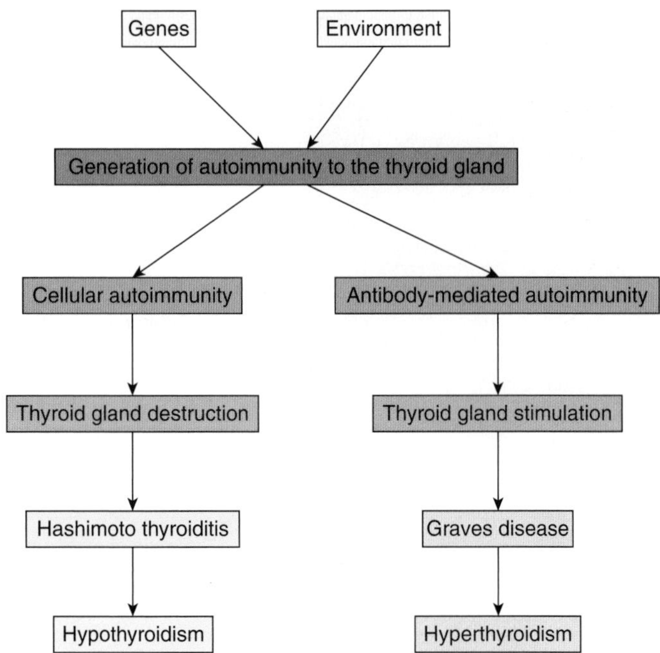

Fig. 22.4 Autoimmune Mechanisms in Primary Thyroid Disease.

Thyrotoxicosis/Hyperthyroidism

Pathophysiology. Thyrotoxicosis is a condition that results from any cause of increased TH levels and can result from dysfunction of the pituitary, the thyroid gland, ectopic thyroid tissue, or the ingestion of excessive amounts of TH medication. Hyperthyroidism is a form of thyrotoxicosis in which excess amounts of TH are secreted from the thyroid gland (Fig. 22.5).[16] *Primary hyperthyroidism* results from thyroid gland dysfunction and is most commonly caused by Graves disease, toxic multinodular goiter, and solitary toxic adenoma. *Central (secondary) hyperthyroidism* is less common and is caused by TSH-secreting pituitary adenomas. Each condition is associated with a specific pathophysiology and manifestations; however, all forms of thyrotoxicosis share some common characteristics.

Clinical Manifestations. The clinical features of thyrotoxicosis are attributable to the metabolic effects of increased circulating levels of THs. This results in an increased metabolic rate, with heat intolerance and increased tissue sensitivity to stimulation by the sympathetic nervous system. The major manifestations are summarized in Fig. 22.6 and Table 22.3.

Evaluation and Treatment. Elevated serum thyroxine (T_4) and triiodothyronine (T_3) levels and suppressed serum TSH levels are diagnostic for primary hyperthyroidism. By contrast, central (secondary) hyperthyroidism caused by TSH-secreting pituitary tumors is characterized by normal to increased TSH levels despite elevated TH concentrations. Treatment is directed at controlling excessive TH production, secretion, or action and involves antithyroid drug therapy, radioactive iodine therapy (absorbed only by thyroid tissue, causing death of cells), or surgical removal of nodules or part of the thyroid gland. A major complication of all forms of treatment for hyperthyroidism is excessive ablation of the gland, leading to hypothyroidism.

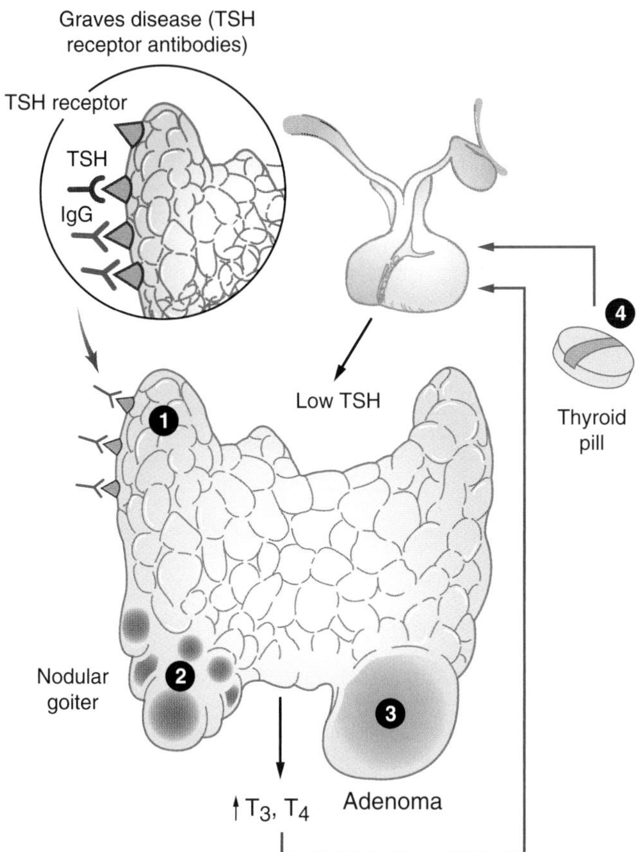

Fig. 22.5 Common Causes of Hyperthyroidism. Hyperthyroidism may have several causes, among them: *1,* Graves disease; *2,* toxic multinodular goiter; *3,* follicular adenoma; *4,* thyroid medication. *TSH,* thyroid stimulating hormone. (Adapted from Damjanov I. *Pathology for the health professions,* 4th edition. St Louis: Saunders; 2012.)

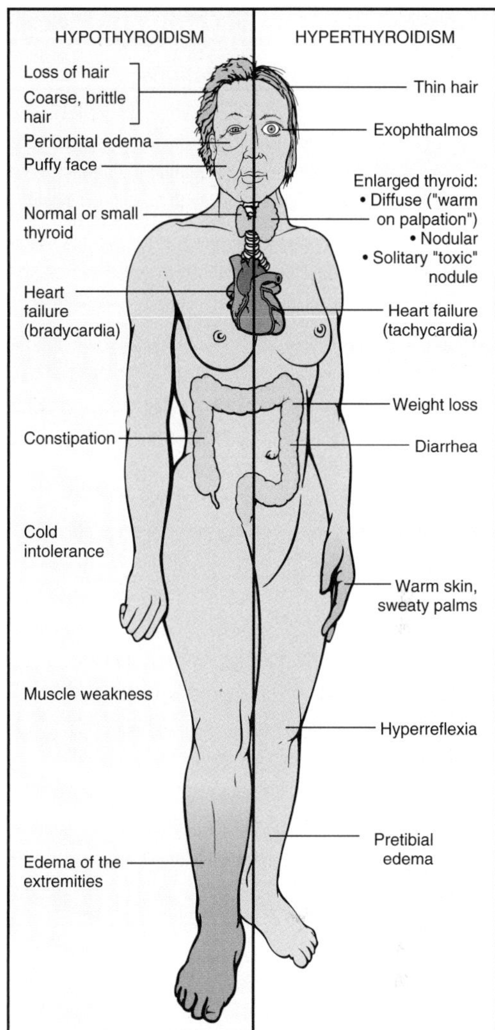

Fig. 22.6 Clinical Manifestations of Hyperthyroidism and Hypothyroidism. (From Damjanov I. *Pathology for the health professions,* 4th edition. St Louis: Saunders; 2012.)

Hyperthyroid Conditions

Graves disease. Graves disease is the underlying cause of 60% to 80% of cases of hyperthyroidism with a prevalence of approximately 3% of women and 0.5% of men in the United States.[17] Although the exact cause of Graves disease is not known, genetic factors interacting with environmental triggers play an important role in the pathogenesis. Graves disease is classified as an autoimmune disease and results from a form of type II hypersensitivity (see Chapter 9) in which there is stimulation of the thyroid by autoantibodies directed against the TSH receptor. These autoantibodies, called *thyroid-stimulating immunoglobulins* (TSIs; also called *thyroid-stimulating antibodies* [TSAbs] or *thyroid receptor antibodies* [TRAbs]), override the normal regulatory mechanisms. TSI stimulation of TSH receptors in the gland results in hyperplasia of the gland (goiter) and increased synthesis of TH, especially of T_3. Increased levels of TH result in the classic signs and symptoms of hyperthyroidism illustrated in Fig. 22.6. TSH production by the pituitary is inhibited through the usual negative feedback loop.

Autoimmunity also contributes to the two major distinguishing clinical manifestations of Graves disease (ophthalmopathy and dermopathy [pretibial myxedema]) (Fig. 22.7). Two categories of ophthalmopathy associated with Graves disease are (1) functional abnormalities resulting from hyperactivity of the sympathetic division of the autonomic nervous system (lag of the globe on upward gaze and of the upper lid on downward gaze) and (2) infiltrative changes involving the orbital contents with enlargement of the ocular muscles. These changes affect more than half of individuals with Graves disease. Orbital connective tissue accumulation, inflammation, and edema of the orbital contents result in exophthalmos (protrusion of the eyeball), periorbital edema, and extraocular muscle weakness leading to diplopia (double vision). The individual may experience irritation, pain, lacrimation, photophobia, blurred vision, decreased visual acuity, papilledema, visual field impairment, exposure keratosis, and corneal ulceration.

TABLE 22.3 Systemic Manifestations of Hyperthyroidism

System	Clinical Manifestations	Mechanisms Underlying Clinical Manifestations
Endocrine	Enlarged thyroid gland (goiter) (97%–99% of cases); systolic or continuous bruit over thyroid; increased cortisol degradation; hypercalcemia and decreased parathyroid hormone secretion; diminished sensitivity to exogenous insulin	Hyperactivity of the thyroid gland; excess bone resorption leading to hypercalcemia and a disruption of PTH-regulating mechanisms; increased insulin degradation
Reproductive	Oligomenorrhea or amenorrhea; erectile dysfunction and decreased libido; increased serum estradiol and estrone levels but lower than normal levels of free estradiol and estrone	Menstrual cycle alterations that may be related to hypothalamic or pituitary disturbances; increase in sex hormone–binding globulin
Gastrointestinal	Weight loss; increased peristalsis leading to less formed and more frequent stools; nausea, vomiting, anorexia, abdominal pain; increased use of hepatic glycogen stores and of adipose and protein stores; decrease in serum lipid levels (including triglycerides, phospholipids, and cholesterol); changes in vitamin metabolism leading to decrease in tissue stores of vitamins	Increased catabolism leading to the body's inability to meet its metabolic needs; increased glucose absorption; increase in cholesterol excretion in feces and cholesterol conversion to bile salts; impaired conversion of B vitamins to their coenzymes, causing increased need for water-soluble and fat-soluble vitamins
Integumentary	Excessive sweating, flushing, and warm skin; heat intolerance; hair fine, soft, and straight; temporary hair loss; nails that grow away from nail beds, palmar erythema	Hyperdynamic circulatory state
Sensory (eyes)	Ocular manifestations including elevated upper eyelid leading to decreased blinking and a staring quality; fine tremor of lid; infiltrative ocular changes associated with Graves disease	Overactivity of Müller muscle; inflammation of retroorbital contents
Cardiovascular	Increased cardiac output and decreased peripheral resistance; tachycardia at rest; loud heart sounds; supraventricular dysrhythmias, left ventricular dilation and hypertrophy	Hypermetabolism and need to dissipate heat
Nervous	Restlessness; short attention span; compulsive movement; fatigue; tremor; insomnia; increased appetite; emotional lability	Not clearly defined; alterations in cerebral metabolism resulting from excess thyroid hormone
Pulmonary	Dyspnea; reduced vital capacity	Weakness of respiratory muscles

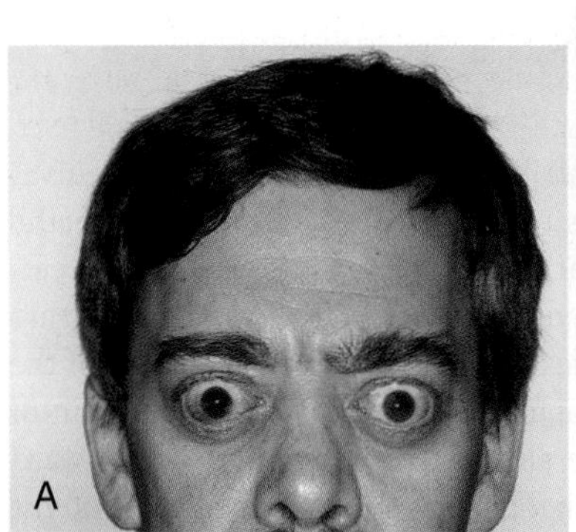

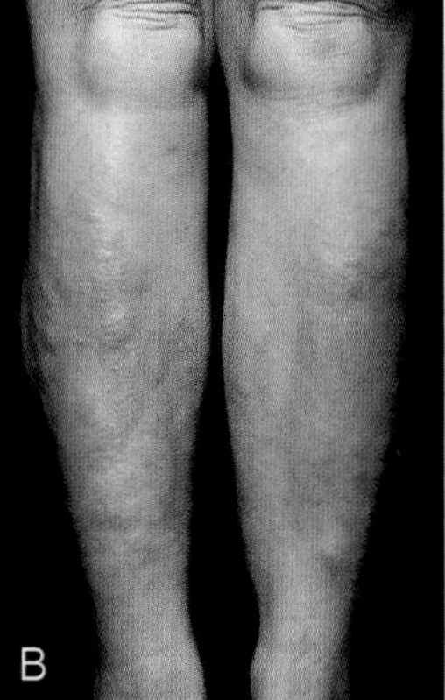

Fig. 22.7 Ophthalmopathy and Pretibial Edema in Graves Disease. (A) Exophthalmos (large and protruding eyeballs, often in association with a large goiter). **(B)** Pretibial myxedema associated with Graves disease; note lumpy and swollen appearance from accumulation of connective tissue and pinkish purple discoloration. (A, From Belchetz P, Hammond P. *Mosby's color atlas and text of diabetes and endocrinology*. Edinburgh: Mosby; 2003; B, From Habif T. *Clinical dermatology*, 5th edition. St Louis: Mosby; 2009.)

A small number of individuals with Graves disease who have very high levels of TSI experience pretibial myxedema (Graves dermopathy), characterized by subcutaneous swelling on the anterior portions of the legs and by indurated and erythematous skin. Graves dermopathy is associated with TSI stimulation of fibroblasts and T lymphocytes, causing excessive amounts of hyaluronic acid production in the dermis and subcutaneous tissue. These manifestations occasionally appear on the hands, giving the appearance of clubbing of the fingers (thyroid acropachy). Fig. 22.8 provides an overview of the pathophysiology of Graves disease.

Hyperthyroidism resulting from nodular thyroid disease. The thyroid gland normally enlarges in response to the increased demand for TH that occurs in puberty, pregnancy, and iodine-deficient states, as well as in individuals with immunologic, viral, or genetic disorders. When the condition resulting in increased TH resolves, TSH secretion normally subsides, and the thyroid gland returns to its original size.

Irreversible changes can occur in some follicular cells so that these cells form nodules that function autonomously and produce excessive amounts of TH. Toxic multinodular goiter occurs when there are several hyperfunctioning nodules leading

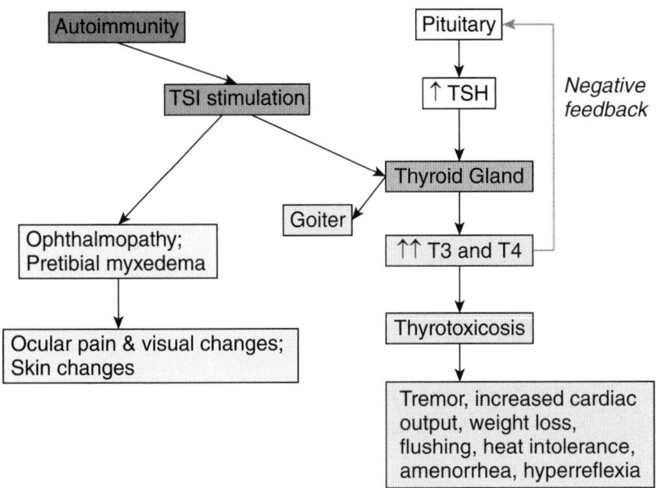

Fig. 22.8 Pathophysiology of Graves Disease. *TSI*, Thyroid-stimulating immunoglobulins (antibodies); *TSH*, thyroid-stimulating hormone; T_3, triiodothyronine; T_4, tetraiodothyronine.

to hyperthyroidism. Unlike Graves disease, there is absence of an autoimmune stimulus. If only one nodule is hyperfunctioning, it is termed toxic adenoma.

The classic clinical manifestations of hyperthyroidism (see Fig. 22.6) usually develop slowly, and exophthalmos and pretibial myxedema do not occur. Nodules may be palpable on physical examination, and there is increased uptake of radioactive iodine.

There is an increased incidence of malignancy in toxic nodular goiter, so most individuals should undergo a fine-needle aspiration biopsy of suspicious nodules before treatment. Treatment consists of a combination of radioactive iodine (may increase risk of solid cancer-related death, including breast cancer death),[18] surgery, and antithyroid medications.

Thyrotoxic crisis. Thyrotoxic crisis (thyroid storm) is a rare but dangerous worsening of the thyrotoxic state in which TH levels rise dramatically and death can occur within 48 hours without treatment. The condition may develop spontaneously but usually occurs in individuals who have undiagnosed or partially treated Graves disease and who are subjected to physiologic stress, such as infection, pulmonary or cardiovascular disorders, trauma, seizures, surgery (especially thyroid surgery), obstetric complications, or dialysis.

The systemic manifestations of thyrotoxic crisis include hyperthermia; tachycardia, especially atrial tachydysrhythmias; heart failure; agitation or delirium; and nausea, vomiting, or diarrhea contributing to fluid volume depletion. Treatment includes drugs that block TH synthesis (i.e., propylthiouracil or methimazole), β blockers, glucocorticoids, iodine, and supportive care.

Hypothyroidism

Hypothyroidism results from deficient production of TH by the thyroid gland. Primary hypothyroidism is the most common disorder of thyroid function, affecting 4% to 7% of the U.S. population, and occurs more commonly in women.[19] It may be primary, central, or subclinical. Primary hypothyroidism accounts for the majority of all cases. Central (secondary) hypothyroidism is much less common and is related to either pituitary or hypothalamic failure. Subclinical hypothyroidism is a mild thyroid failure estimated to occur in 13 million U.S. adults, most commonly in women and older adults.[20] It is characterized by elevated serum TSH levels with normal levels of circulating TH (T3, Free T4, Total T4). Progression to blatant hypothyroidism is common over time.[19]

Pathophysiology. In *primary hypothyroidism*, loss of thyroid function leads to decreased production of TH and increased secretion of TSH and TRH. The most common causes of primary hypothyroidism in adults include autoimmune thyroiditis (chronic lymphocytic thyroiditis), iatrogenic loss of thyroid tissue after surgical or radioactive treatment for hyperthyroidism or after head and neck radiation therapy, medications (e.g., lithium and amiodarone), and endemic iodine deficiency. Iodine, required for the production of TH, is not produced naturally by the body and is obtained through dietary intake. Iodine deficiency is relatively rare in the United States because of the use of iodized salt and fortified foods.[19] Infants and children may present with hypothyroidism because of congenital defects. *Central (secondary) hypothyroidism* is caused by the pituitary's failure to synthesize adequate amounts of TSH or a lack of TRH. Pituitary tumors that compress surrounding pituitary cells or the consequences of their treatment are the most common causes of central hypothyroidism. Other causes include traumatic brain injury, subarachnoid hemorrhage, pituitary infarction, or metabolic disorders including insulin resistance or hyperglycemia, dyslipidemia, obesity, and endothelial dysfunction.[21] Hypothalamic dysfunction results in low levels of TH, TSH, and TRH.

Clinical Manifestations. Hypothyroidism generally affects all body systems and occurs insidiously over months or years. Decreased TH levels lower energy metabolism and heat production. The individual develops a low basal metabolic rate, cold intolerance, lethargy, and slightly lowered basal body temperature (see Fig. 22.6). The decrease in the level of TH leads to excessive TSH production, which stimulates thyroid tissue and causes a goiter (Table 22.4).

The characteristic sign of severe or long-standing hypothyroidism is myxedema, which results from the altered composition of the dermis and other tissues. The connective tissue fibers are separated by large amounts of protein and mucopolysaccharide. This complex binds water, producing nonpitting, boggy edema, especially around the eyes, hands, and feet and in the supraclavicular fossae (Fig. 22.9). The tongue and laryngeal and pharyngeal mucous membranes thicken, producing thick, slurred speech and hoarseness. Myxedema coma, a medical emergency, is a diminished level of consciousness associated with severe hypothyroidism. Signs and symptoms include hypothermia without shivering, hypoventilation, hypotension, hypoglycemia, and lactic acidosis. Older individuals with comorbid conditions, such as pulmonary or urinary infections, congestive heart failure, or cerebrovascular accident, and with moderate or untreated hypothyroidism are

TABLE 22.4 **Systemic Manifestations of Hypothyroidism**

System	Clinical Manifestations	Mechanisms Underlying Clinical Manifestations
Neurologic	Confusion, syncope, slowed speech and thinking, memory loss; lethargy, headaches, hearing loss, night blindness; slow, clumsy movements; cerebellar ataxia; slow α-wave activity and loss of amplitude in EEG; reduced cAMP response to epinephrine, glucagons, and PTH stimulation; decreased appetite	Decreased cerebral blood flow leading to cerebral hypoxia; reduced intracellular processes caused by decreased β-adrenergic activity that may be related to a decrease in the number of β-adrenergic receptor sites
Endocrine	Increased TSH production in primary hypothyroidism; enlarged pituitary thyrotropes, increase in serum prolactin levels with galactorrhea; decreased rate of cortisol turnover but with normal serum cortisol levels	Impaired TH synthesis or defects in iodide trapping leading to compensatory TSH production; chronic overstimulation of thyrotropes of TRH and by TSH synthesis; stimulation of lactotropes by TRH related to increased prolactin levels; decreased deactivation of cortisol
Reproductive	Decreased androgen secretion in men, increased estriol formation in women; low total hormone values but with increased amounts of unbound hormone; anovulation, decreased libido, menorrhagia, and a high incidence of spontaneous abortion in women; erectile dysfunction, decreased libido, and oligospermia in men	Altered metabolism of estrogens and androgens; decreased levels of sex hormone–binding globulin
Hematologic	Decrease in red cell mass leading to normocytic, normochromic anemia; macrocytic anemia associated with vitamin B_{12} deficiency and inadequate folate or iron absorption in the GI tract	Decreased basal metabolic rate and reduced oxygen requirements; decreased production of erythropoietin; possible relationship between TH and optimal hematologic response to vitamin B_{12}
Cardiovascular	Reduction in stroke volume and heart rate causing lowered cardiac output; increased peripheral vascular resistance to maintain systolic blood pressure can cause hypertension; normal response to exercise but with alterations in circulatory system at rest (prolonged circulation time and decreased blood flow to tissues); cool skin and cold tolerance; enlarged heart; decreased intensity of heart sounds and variety of ECG changes (sinus bradycardia, prolonged PR interval, depressed P waves, flattened or inverted T waves, and low-amplitude QRS complexes); cardiac tamponade (although rare) (see Chapter 32)	Decreased metabolic demands and loss of regulatory and rate-setting effects of TH; protein-mucopolysaccharide–rich fluid in the pericardial sac associated with enlarged heart; pericardial effusions associated with heart sounds and ECG changes Increases in peripheral vascular resistance and increased blood volume can cause hypertension
Pulmonary	Dyspnea; myxedematous changes in respiratory muscles leading to hypoventilation and carbon dioxide retention, which contribute to myxedema coma	Pleural effusions associated with dyspnea, although effusions may be asymptomatic
Renal	Reduced renal blood flow and glomerular filtration rate leading to decreased renal excretion of water; increase in total body water and dilutional hyponatremia; reduced production of erythropoietin	Hemodynamic alterations associated with reduced blood flow and filtration; increased total body water related to decreased excretion and mucinous deposits in tissue
GI	Constipation, weight gain, and fluid retention; decreased absorption of most nutrients; decreased protein metabolism leading to retarded skeletal and soft tissue growth and slightly positive nitrogen balance; edema; decreased glucose absorption and delayed glucose uptake; elevated serum lipid values	Reduced intake and reduced peristaltic activity that may progress to fecal impaction; water absorption related to prolonged transit time; fluid retention associated with myxedematous changes; edema associated with high concentrations of exchangeable albumin in the extravascular space caused by increased capillary permeability to proteins; depressed insulin degradation; depressed lipid synthesis and degradation
Musculoskeletal	Muscle aching and stiffness; slow movement and slow tendon jerk reflexes; decreased bone formation and resorption, increased bone density; aching and stiffness in joints	Decreased rate of muscle contraction and relaxation contributing to slow movement and reflexes
Integumentary	Dry, flaky skin; dry, brittle head and body hair; reduced growth of nails and hair; slow wound healing	Reduced sweat and sebaceous gland secretion
	Myxedema	Accumulation of hyaluronic acid, which binds water and causes a puffy appearance
	Cool skin	Decreased circulation to skin

cAMP, Cyclic adenosine monophosphate; *ECG*, electrocardiogram; *EEG*, electroencephalogram; *GI*, gastrointestinal; *PTH*, parathyroid hormone; *TH*, thyroid hormone; *TRH*, thyrotropin-releasing hormone; *TSH*, thyroid-stimulating hormone.

particularly at risk for developing myxedema coma. It also may occur after overuse of narcotics or sedatives or after an acute illness in hypothyroid individuals. Symptoms of hypothyroidism in older adults should not be attributed to expected age-related changes.

Evaluation and Treatment. The diagnosis of primary hypothyroidism is made by documentation of the clinical symptoms of hypothyroidism and measurement of increased serum levels of TSH and decreased serum levels of TH (total T_3 and both total and free T_4). Central hypothyroidism is diagnosed

EMERGING SCIENCE BOX

Combination Therapy for the Treatment of Hypothyroidism

Combination therapy for hypothyroidism was the mainstay of treatment during the late 1800s–mid 1900s. The therapy could include thyroid transplant, thyroid extracts, thyroglobulin, and/or desiccated thyroid. A combination levothyroxine (LT4) and liothyronine (LT3) were noted to restore metabolic effects of thyroid hormone secretions. Due to thyrotoxic symptoms related to this combination therapy, monotherapy with levothyroxine was introduced in the 1970s. Now decades later, clinicians are noting trends in the ability of LT4 alone to normalize basal metabolic rate, cholesterol levels, and satisfaction due to persistent signs and symptoms of hypothyroidism. There is a growing body of evidence supporting physiologic thyroid replacement regimens with the goal of restoring thyroid hormone action within all tissues. This knowledge creates a shift back toward combination therapy as the standard of treatment. A slow-release form of oral LT3 has been developed and applied to rats with hypothyroidism, showing a stabilization of serum T3 levels. There have been no results from human trials as of this writing. Researchers are confident that the development of a long-acting formulation of LT3 in conjunction with LT4 will minimize risk of thyrotoxic symptoms and mimic endogenous thyroid signaling. We could see more individuals with euthyroidism, improvement in cholesterol levels, and overall well-being. What is old could be new again.

Data from McAninch EA, et al. The swinging pendulum in treatment for hypothyroidism: From (and toward?) combination therapy. *Frontiers in Endocrinology,* 2019;10:1–11; Chiovato L, et al. Hypothyroidism in context: Where we've been and where we're going. *Advances in Therapy,* 2019;36:S47–S58.

by finding low TH and low serum TSH levels. Alluded to earlier, subclinical hypothyroidism is diagnosed by an elevation in TSH level with normal levels of circulating TH. Hormone replacement therapy with the hormone levothyroxine is the treatment of choice for both primary and central thyroid disorders (Emerging Science Box: Combination Therapy for the Treatment of Hypothyroidism).

Hypothyroid Conditions

Chronic lymphocytic thyroiditis (Hashimoto disease). The most common cause of primary hypothyroidism in the United States is chronic lymphocytic thyroiditis (Hashimoto disease), which results in gradual, inflammatory destruction of thyroid tissue. This disorder is linked with several genetic risk factors and is often associated with other autoimmune conditions. Infiltration of the thyroid with autoreactive T lymphocytes, antithyroid antibodies (antithyroid peroxidase and antithyroglobulin antibodies), and natural killer cells induces inflammation, glandular apoptosis, and tissue destruction (Fig. 22.10).

Uncommon causes of hypothyroidism. Other, less common causes of hypothyroidism are subacute thyroiditis and postpartum thyroiditis. Subacute thyroiditis (de Quervain thyroiditis) is a rare nonbacterial inflammation of the thyroid gland often preceded by a viral infection. It is accompanied by fever, tenderness, an increase in erythrocyte sedimentation rate, enlargement of the thyroid gland, and transient hypothyroidism before the gland recovers normal activity. Symptoms may last for 2 to 4 months, and nonsteroidal anti-inflammatory drugs or corticosteroids usually resolve symptoms. Postpartum thyroiditis (PPT) is an autoimmune disease associated with antibodies to thyroid peroxidase. PPT has a prevalence of about 5% and generally occurs up to 6 months after birthing with a course similar to that seen in subacute thyroiditis. Individuals who develop PPT need to be monitored for permanent hypothyroidism. Iatrogenic hypothyroidism results from ablation of the thyroid gland during treatment for hyperthyroid conditions.

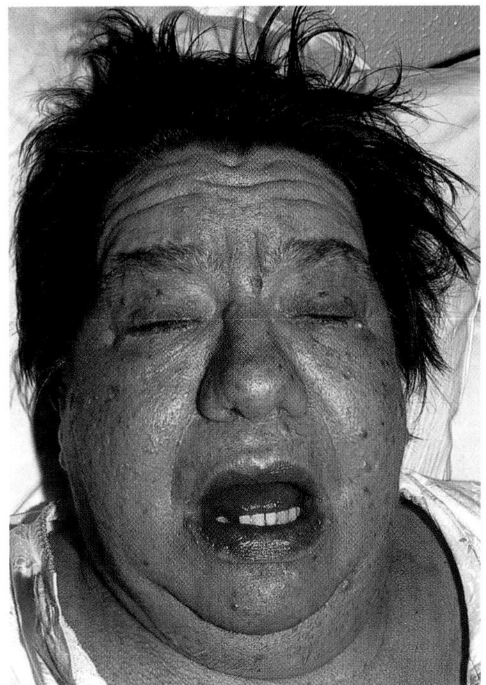

Fig. 22.9 Myxedema. Note edema around eyes and facial puffiness. The hair is dry. (From Bolognia JL, et al. *Dermatology,* 3rd edition. St. Louis: Mosby; 2012.)

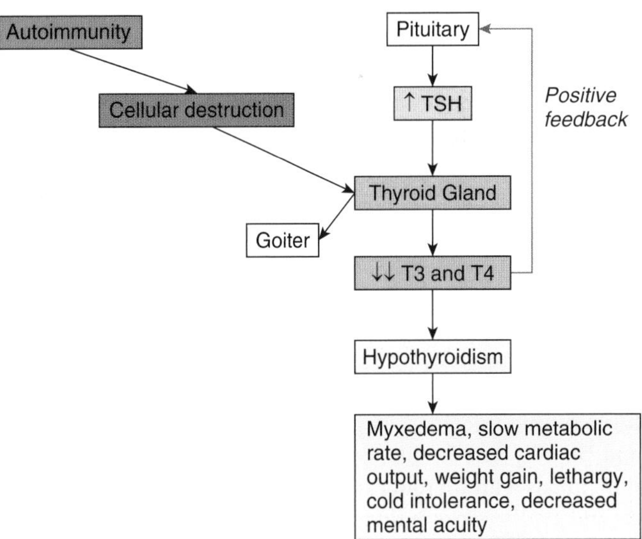

Fig. 22.10 Pathophysiology of Hashimoto Thyroiditis. *TSH,* Thyroid-stimulating hormone; T_3, triiodothyronine; T_4, tetraiodothyronine.

Congenital hypothyroidism. Hypothyroidism in infants occurs when thyroid tissue is absent (thyroid dysgenesis) or with hereditary defects in TH synthesis. Thyroid dysgenesis occurs more often in female infants, with permanent abnormalities in about 1 of every 4000 live births. The affected fetus is dependent on maternal thyroxine for the first 20 weeks of gestation, then becomes deficient in TH. TH is essential for fetal growth and for the development of brain tissue, so the infant will suffer developmental and cognitive disabilities if left untreated. Hypothyroidism may not be evident at birth. Symptoms may include high birth weight, hypothermia, delay in passing meconium, and neonatal jaundice. Cord blood can be examined in the first days of life for measurement of T_4 and TSH levels. The probability of normal growth and intellectual function is high if treatment with levothyroxine is started before the child is 3 or 4 months old. The earlier TH replacement is initiated, the better the child's outcome.

Without early screening, hypothyroidism may not be evident until after 4 months of age. Symptoms include difficulty eating, hoarse cry, and protruding tongue caused by myxedema of oral tissues and vocal cords; hypotonic muscles of the abdomen with constipation, abdominal protrusion, and umbilical hernia; subnormal temperature; lethargy; excessive sleeping; slow pulse rate; and cold, mottled skin. Skeletal growth is stunted because of impaired protein synthesis, poor absorption of nutrients, and lack of bone mineralization. The child will be dwarfed with short limbs, if not treated. Dentition is often delayed. Cognitive disability varies with the severity of hypothyroidism and the length of delay before treatment is initiated.

Thyroid carcinoma. Thyroid carcinoma is the most common endocrine malignancy and is the seventh most common cancer in the United States in women.[22] Exposure to ionizing radiation, especially during childhood, is the most consistent causal factor. Papillary and follicular thyroid carcinomas are the most frequent, and medullary and anaplastic thyroid carcinomas are less common.

The cancer is typically discovered as a small thyroid nodule or metastatic tumor in the lungs, brain, or bone. Changes in voice and swallowing and difficulty breathing are related to tumor growth impinging on the trachea or esophagus. The diagnosis of thyroid cancer is generally made by ultrasonography and then by fine-needle aspiration of a thyroid nodule. Most individuals with thyroid carcinoma have normal T_3 and T_4 levels and are therefore euthyroid.

Treatment may include partial or total thyroidectomy, TSH suppression therapy (levothyroxine), radioactive iodine therapy (in iodine-concentrating tumors), postoperative radiation therapy, and chemotherapy (especially in anaplastic carcinoma).[23] New insights into the molecular pathogenesis of thyroid carcinoma are leading to new therapies.

ALTERATIONS OF PARATHYROID FUNCTION

Hyperparathyroidism

Hyperparathyroidism is characterized by greater than normal secretion of parathyroid hormone (PTH) with associated hypercalcemia. Hyperparathyroidism is classified as primary, secondary, or tertiary.

Pathophysiology. Primary hyperparathyroidism is characterized by inappropriate excess secretion of PTH by one or more of the parathyroid glands.[24] It is one of the most common endocrine disorders. Approximately 80% to 85% of cases are caused by parathyroid adenomas, another 10% to 15% result from parathyroid hyperplasia, and approximately 1% of cases are caused by parathyroid carcinoma. In addition, primary hyperparathyroidism may be caused by a variety of genetic causes, especially the genes that cause multiple endocrine neoplasia.

In primary hyperparathyroidism, PTH secretion is increased and is not under the usual feedback control mechanisms. The calcium level in the blood rises because of increased bone resorption and GI absorption of calcium but fails to inhibit PTH secretion by the parathyroid gland. Some individuals with primary hyperparathyroidism maintain normal levels of calcium despite elevated levels of PTH and are diagnosed only when they develop osteoporosis.

Secondary hyperparathyroidism is a compensatory response of the parathyroid glands to chronic hypocalcemia, which is commonly associated with decreased activation of vitamin D in individuals with renal failure (see Chapter 38). Secretion of PTH is elevated, but not enough to achieve normal calcium levels because of insufficient levels of activated vitamin D. Other causes of secondary hyperparathyroidism include a dietary deficiency of vitamin D or calcium; decreased intestinal absorption of vitamin D or calcium; and ingestion of drugs, such as phenytoin, phenobarbital, and laxatives, which either accelerate the metabolism of vitamin D or decrease intestinal absorption of calcium.

Tertiary hyperparathyroidism can develop after any long-standing period of hypocalcemia, such as is seen with chronic dialysis, renal transplantation, or GI malabsorption. Parathyroid chief cell hyperplasia leads to excessive secretion of PTH and may cause hypercalcemia (cellular adaptation is discussed in Chapter 2).

Clinical Manifestations. Hypercalcemia and hypophosphatemia are the hallmarks of primary hyperparathyroidism. Hypercalcemia and hypophosphatemia may be asymptomatic or affected individuals may present with symptoms related to the muscular, nervous, and GI systems, including fatigue, headache, depression, anorexia, and nausea and vomiting. Excessive osteoclastic and osteocytic activity causes bone resorption, resulting in osteoporosis, pathologic fractures, kyphosis of the dorsal spine, and compression fractures of the vertebral bodies (bone resorption is discussed in Chapter 44).

Hypercalcemia means that the renal tubules must filter large amounts of calcium, leading to hypercalciuria and production of an abnormally alkaline urine. PTH hypersecretion enhances renal phosphate excretion and results in hypophosphatemia and hyperphosphaturia (see Chapter 3). The combination of these three variables—hypercalciuria, alkaline urine, and hyperphosphaturia—predisposes the individual to the formation of calcium stones, particularly in the renal pelvis or renal collecting ducts. These stones may be associated with infections and impaired renal function. Chronic hypercalcemia also is associated with mild insulin resistance, necessitating increased insulin secretion to maintain normal glucose levels (Table 22.5).

Secondary hyperparathyroidism, caused by renal disease, presents clinically not only with the complications of bone

TABLE 22.5 Manifestations of Primary Hyperparathyroidism

Symptoms	Responsible Derangements	Mechanisms
Renal colic, nephrolithiasis, recurrent urinary tract infections, renal failure	Hypercalciuria, hyperphosphaturia, proximal renal tubular bicarbonate leak, urine pH >6	Calcium phosphate salts precipitate in alkaline urine, renal pelvis, and collecting ducts; calcium oxalate stones also formed
Abdominal pain, peptic ulcer disease	Hypercalcemia-stimulated hypergastrinemia	Elevated hydrochloric acid secretion
Pancreatitis	Hypercalcemia	Etiology of relationship unknown
Bone disease, osteitis fibrosa and osteitis cystica, osteoporosis	PTH-stimulated bone resorption, metabolic acidosis	Osteoporosis now more commonly encountered, but other disorders are more specific for hyperparathyroidism
Muscle weakness, myalgia	PTH excess, possible direct effect on striated muscle and on nerves	Characteristic myopathic changes in muscle histology (neuropathy of type I and type II muscle fibers)
Neurologic and psychiatric problems (impaired memory, confusion, depression, anxiety, psychosis)	Hypercalcemia	Neuropathy; electroencephalographic changes present
Polyuria, polydipsia	Hypercalcemia	Direct effect on renal tubule to decrease responsiveness to antidiuretic hormone
Constipation	Hypercalcemia	Decreased peristalsis of gastrointestinal tract
Anorexia, nausea, and vomiting	Hypercalcemia	Central stimulation of vomiting center
Hypertension	Renal disease, direct effect of calcium on arterial smooth muscle, pheochromocytoma	Plasma renin activity elevated or normal
Arthralgia and arthritis	Gout, pseudogout, periarticular classification	Hyperuricemia, chronic renal failure with high calcium phosphate product

PTH, Parathyroid hormone.
Data from Flint PW, et al. *Cummings otolaryngology: Head & neck surgery,* 5th edition. St. Louis: Mosby.

resorption but also with the symptoms of hypocalcemia and hyperphosphatemia, such as muscle spasms and cardiovascular complications (see Chapter 3).

Evaluation and Treatment. The diagnosis of primary hyperparathyroidism is suggested by the concurrent findings of elevated PTH levels and an increased ionized calcium concentration. Imaging procedures are used to localize adenomas before surgery. Observation of asymptomatic individuals with mild hypercalcemia is recommended; these individuals are advised to avoid dehydration and limit dietary calcium intake. Definitive treatment of more severe primary hyperparathyroidism involves surgical removal of the solitary adenoma or, in the case of hyperplasia, complete removal of three and partial removal of the fourth hyperplastic parathyroid glands.

If the serum calcium concentration is low despite elevated levels of PTH, secondary hyperparathyroidism is likely. Evaluation for renal function may indicate chronic renal disease. Treatment for secondary hyperparathyroidism in chronic renal disease requires calcium replacement, dietary phosphate restriction and phosphate binders, and vitamin D replacement. Treatment also may include calcimimetics, which work to increase parathyroid calcium receptor sensitivity, thus lowering PTH levels.

Hypoparathyroidism

Hypoparathyroidism (abnormally low PTH levels) is most commonly caused by damage to the parathyroid glands during thyroid surgery. This occurs because of the anatomic proximity of the parathyroid glands to the thyroid (Fig. 21.11). Hypomagnesemia is another cause of low PTH levels. Hypoparathyroidism also is associated with genetic syndromes, including familial hypoparathyroidism and DiGeorge syndrome (see Chapter 9). There is an inherited condition called *pseudohypoparathyroidism* that causes a defect in tissue responsiveness to PTH. Pseudohypoparathyroidism is associated with hypocalcemia despite normal to elevated levels of PTH.

Pathophysiology. No matter the cause, the absence of PTH impairs resorption of calcium from bone and the renal tubules, leading to hypocalcemia. Deficient PTH also stimulates increased renal reabsorption of phosphate, leading to hyperphosphatemia. Hyperphosphatemia further lowers the calcium concentration by inhibiting the activation of vitamin D, thereby lowering the GI absorption of calcium.

Hypomagnesemia inhibits PTH secretion. Hypomagnesemia may be related to chronic alcoholism, malnutrition, malabsorption, increased renal clearance of magnesium caused by the use of aminoglycoside antibiotics or certain chemotherapeutic agents, or prolonged magnesium-deficient parenteral nutritional therapy. When serum magnesium levels return to normal, however, PTH secretion returns to normal.

Clinical Manifestations. Symptoms associated with hypopara thyroidism are primarily those of hypocalcemia (see Chapter 3). Hypocalcemia causes muscle spasms, which can progress to tetany, dry skin, and loss of body and scalp hair. Irreversible complications include hypoplasia of developing teeth, horizontal ridges

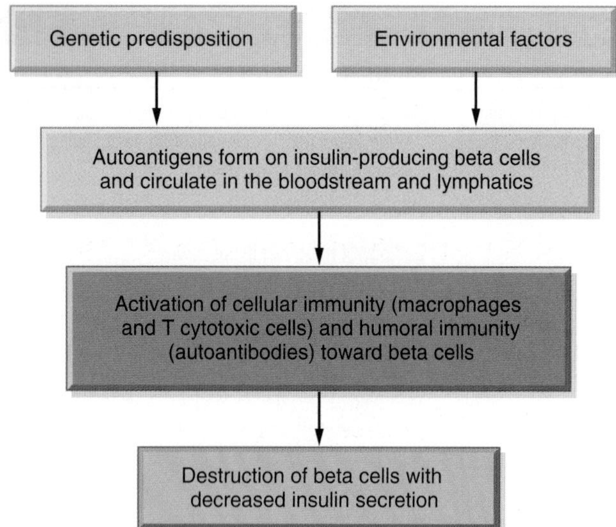

Fig. 22.11 Pathophysiology of Type 1 Diabetes Mellitus.

on the nails, cataracts, basal ganglia calcifications (which may be associated with a parkinsonian syndrome), and bone deformities, including brachydactyly and bowing of the long bones.

Evaluation and Treatment. A low PTH level, along with a low serum calcium concentration and a high phosphorus level in the absence of renal failure, intestinal disorders, or nutritional deficiencies, suggests hypoparathyroidism. Measurement of the serum magnesium level and urinary calcium excretion also can help in diagnosis. Treatment is directed toward alleviation of the hypocalcemia. In acute states, this involves parenteral administration of calcium, which corrects the serum calcium concentration within minutes. Chronic maintenance of the serum calcium level is achieved with pharmacologic doses of cholecalciferol (vitamin D_3) and oral calcium. PTH hormone replacement with recombinant human parathyroid hormone (rhPTH) is safe and effective.

DYSFUNCTION OF THE ENDOCRINE PANCREAS: DIABETES MELLITUS

Diabetes mellitus is a group of metabolic diseases characterized by hyperglycemia resulting from defects in insulin secretion, insulin action, or both. In 2018, an estimated 34.2 million individuals (10.5%) in the United States had diabetes, and another 7.3 million (21.4%) were estimated to be undiagnosed.[25] The American Diabetes Association (ADA)[26] classifies four categories of diabetes mellitus:

1. Type 1 diabetes (caused by autoimmune β-cell destruction, usually leading to absolute insulin deficiency)
2. Type 2 diabetes (caused by progressive loss of β-cell insulin secretion, frequently with a background of insulin resistance)[27]
3. Gestational diabetes mellitus (GDM) (diabetes diagnosed in the second or third trimester of pregnancy that was not clearly overt diabetes prior to gestation)
4. Specific types of diabetes mellitus due to other causes

Specific types of diabetes include monogenic diabetes syndromes (e.g., neonatal diabetes and maturity-onset diabetes of the young [MODY]), disease of the exocrine pancreas (e.g., cystic fibrosis and pancreatitis), and drug- or chemical-induced diabetes (e.g., glucocorticoid use in the treatment of human immunodeficiency virus [HIV] infection and/or acquired immunodeficiency syndrome [AIDS] or after organ transplantation) (Table 22.6).

The diagnosis of diabetes mellitus is based on glycated hemoglobin (HbA_{1C}) levels; fasting plasma glucose (FPG) levels; oral glucose tolerance testing (OGTT); or random glucose levels in an individual with symptoms (Box 22.1).[26] Glycated hemoglobin refers to the permanent attachment of glucose to hemoglobin molecules and reflects the average plasma glucose exposure over the life of a red blood cell (RBC) (approximately 120 days). It provides a more accurate measure for monitoring long-term control of blood glucose levels.

The ADA classification "categories at increased risk for diabetes" (or prediabetes) describes nondiabetic elevations of the HbA_{1C}, FPG, or 2-hour plasma glucose value during an OGTT (see Box 22.1).[26] The Centers for Disease Control and Prevention (CDC) estimates that 88 million U.S. adults (34.5%) aged 18 years or older have prediabetes.[24]

This classification includes impaired glucose tolerance (IGT), which results from diminished insulin secretion; and impaired fasting glucose (IFG), which is caused by enhanced hepatic glucose output. Individuals with IGT and IFG are at increased risk of cardiovascular disease and premature death and carry up to a 50% 5-year risk of developing diabetes, particularly type 2 diabetes. Thus, prevention of diabetes with lifestyle interventions is essential.

Types of Diabetes Mellitus

Diabetes Mellitus Type 1

Diabetes mellitus type 1 accounts for 5% to 10% of diabetes cases and is the most common pediatric chronic disease. It currently affects approximately 187,000 U.S. children younger than 20, and the incidence is increasing.[25] Between 10% and 13% of individuals with newly diagnosed type 1 diabetes have a first-degree relative (parent or sibling) with type 1 diabetes, and there is a 50% concordance rate in twins. Diagnosis is rare during the first 9 months of life and peaks at 12 years of age (Table 22.7).

Pathophysiology. Two distinct types of type 1 diabetes have been identified: idiopathic and autoimmune. *Idiopathic diabetes mellitus type 1* is far less common than autoimmune diabetes, has a strong genetic component, and occurs mostly in people of Asian or African descent. Affected individuals have no evidence of β-cell autoimmunity and have varying degrees of insulin deficiency.

Autoimmune diabetes mellitus type 1 is a slowly progressive disease that destroys β cells of the pancreas. There are strong genetic associations with histocompatibility leukocyte antigen (HLA) class II alleles *HLA-DQ* and *HLA-DR*. Environmental factors that have been implicated include exposure to certain drugs, foods, and viruses. These gene-environment interactions

TABLE 22.6 Classification and Characteristics of Diabetes Mellitus

Name	Characteristics
Type 1 β-cell destruction leading to absolute insulin deficiency; immune-mediated diabetes is most common form (≈90%)	Cellular-mediated autoimmune destruction of pancreatic β cells Individual prone to ketoacidosis Little or no insulin secretion Insulin dependent 75% of individuals develop before 30 years of age; can occur up to the tenth decade Usually not obese
Idiopathic (≈10%)	No defined etiologies; absolute requirement for insulin replacement therapy in affected individuals may be sporadic
Type 2 Progressive loss of b-cell insulin secretion frequency on the background of insulin resistance	Usually not insulin dependent but may be insulin requiring Individual not ketosis prone (but may form ketones under stress) Obesity common in the abdominal region Generally occurs in those older than 40 years, but the frequency is rapidly increasing in children Strong genetic predisposition Often associated with hypertension and dyslipidemia
Other Specific Types Genetic defects of β-cell function	**1.** Genetic abnormalities that decrease the ability of the β cell to secrete insulin: **2.** Maturity-onset diabetes of youth (MODY) includes six specific autosomal dominant mutations including genes for hepatocyte nuclear factor-1α (HNF-1α; *MODY 3*), glucokinase (*MODY 2*), HNF-4α (*MODY 1*), insulin-promoter factor-1(IPF-1; *MODY 4*), HNF-1β (*MODY 5*), and NeuroD1 (*MODY 6*) **3.** Defects in mitochondrial deoxyribonucleic acid (DNA) Other (including an inability to convert proinsulin to insulin)
Genetic defects in insulin action	Mutations in the insulin receptor with hyperinsulinism or hyperglycemia or severe diabetes
Diseases of the exocrine pancreas	Any process that diffusely injures the pancreas, including pancreatitis, neoplasia, and cystic fibrosis
Endocrinopathies	Endocrine disorders including acromegaly, Cushing syndrome, glucagonoma, pheochromocytoma, hyperthyroidism, somatostatinoma, and aldosteronoma
Drug- or chemical-induced β-cell dysfunction	Commonly associated drugs include glucocorticoids, treatment of HIV/AIDS, and after organ transplantation although many others may be implicated
Infections	β-cell destruction by viruses including cytomegalovirus, congenital rubella
Uncommon forms of immune-mediated diabetes mellitus	Anti–insulin receptor antibodies Reported with "stiff man syndrome" and individuals receiving interferon-α
Other genetic syndromes sometimes associated with diabetes mellitus	Down, Klinefelter, Turner, and Wolfram syndromes
Gestational Diabetes Mellitus (GDM) Any degree of glucose intolerance with onset or first recognition during pregnancy	Insulin resistance combined with inadequate insulin secretion in relation to hyperglycemia Women who are obese, older than 25 years of age, have a family history of diabetes, have a history of previous GDM, or are of certain ethnic groups (Hispanic, Native American, Asian, or black) are at increased risk of developing GDM The metabolic stress of pregnancy may uncover a genetic tendency for type 2 diabetes mellitus

GDM, Gestational diabetes mellitus; *MODY*, maturity-onset diabetes of youth.
Data from American Diabetes Association. *Diabetes Care.* 2017;40(Suppl. 1):S11–S24.

result in the formation of autoantigens that are expressed on the surface of pancreatic β cells and circulate in the bloodstream and lymphatics (see Fig. 22.11). Cellular immunity (T-cytotoxic cells and macrophages) and humoral immunity (autoantibodies against islet cells, insulin, glutamic acid decarboxylase [GAD], and other cytoplasmic proteins) are stimulated, resulting in β-cell destruction and apoptosis. Over time, 80% to 90% of the insulin-secreting β cells of the islet of Langerhans are destroyed, insulin synthesis declines, and hyperglycemia develops.

Insulin normally suppresses secretion of glucagon, and thus hypoinsulinemia leads to a marked increase in glucagon secretion. In addition to the decline in insulin secretion, there

BOX 22.1 Diagnostic Criteria for Diabetes Mellitus

1. HbA_{1C} (as measured in a DCCT-referenced assay) ≥6.5%
   OR
2. FPG ≥126 mg/dL; fasting is defined as no caloric intake for at least 8 h
   OR
3. 2-h plasma glucose ≥200 mg/dL during OGTT
   OR
4. In an individual with classic symptoms of hyperglycemia or hyperglycemic crisis, a random plasma glucose ≥200 mg/dL

In the absence of unequivocal hyperglycemia, criteria 1 through 3 diagnosis requires two abnormal test results from the same sample or in two separate test samples.

Categories of Increased Risk for Diabetes

1. FPG 100–125 mg/dL
2. 2-h PG 140–199 mg/dL during OGTT
3. HbA_{1C} 5.7%–6.4%

DCCT, Diabetes Control and Complications Trial; *FPG,* fasting plasma glucose; *HbA_{1C},* hemoglobin A_{1C} or glycated hemoglobin; *OGTT,* oral glucose tolerance testing; *PG,* plasma glucose.
Data from American Diabetes Association. Classification and diagnosis of diabetes: standards of medical care in diabetes—2020. Diabetes Care. 2020;43(Suppl. 1):S14–S31. Available from https://care.diabetesjournals.org/content/diacare/suppl/2019/12/20/43.Supplement_1.DC1/Standards_of_Care_2020.pdf.

is decreased secretion of amylin (another β-cell hormone), which also leads to an increase in glucagon. Glucagon, a hormone produced by the α cells of the islets, acts in the liver to increase the blood glucose level by stimulating glycogenolysis and gluconeogenesis. Thus, both a lack of insulin and a relative excess of glucagon contribute to hyperglycemia in type 1 diabetes.

The natural history of type 1 diabetes involves a long preclinical period before insulin deficiency and hyperglycemia develop. Glucose accumulates in the blood and appears in the urine as the renal threshold for glucose is exceeded, producing an osmotic diuresis and symptoms of polyuria and thirst (Table 22.8). Wide fluctuations in blood glucose levels occur. Insulin deficiency also causes protein and fat breakdown, resulting in weight loss. Excessive metabolism of fats and proteins leads to high levels of circulating ketones, causing a condition known as *diabetic ketoacidosis* (DKA) (see the Acute Complications of Diabetes section).

Although most individuals with type 1 diabetes are of normal or decreased weight, there are increasing numbers of individuals who have both type 1 diabetes and the clinical manifestations of metabolic syndrome, including obesity, dyslipidemia, and hypertension (Box 22.2). These individuals are at high risk for chronic complications of diabetes, including heart disease and stroke.

TABLE 22.7 Epidemiology and Etiology of Diabetes Mellitus in the United States

	Type 1 Diabetes: Primary β-Cell Defect or Failure	Type 2 Diabetes: Insulin Resistance With Inadequate Insulin Secretion
Incidence		
Frequency	5%–10% of all cases of diabetes mellitus Prevalence rate is 0.17%	Accounts for most cases (≈90%–95%) Prevalence rate for adults is 10.9%
Change in incidences	Incidence is increasing	Incidence in adults more than tripled in the past 3 decades
Characteristics		
Age at onset	Peak onset at age 11–13 years (slightly earlier for girls than for boys); rare in children younger than 9 months and adults older than 30 years	Risk of developing diabetes increases after age 40 years
Sex	Similar in males and females	Similar in males and females
Racial distribution	Rates for whites 1.5–2 times higher than for other ethnic groups	Risk is highest for African Americans and Native Americans
Weight	Generally normal or underweight	Obesity is common and is a frequent contributing factor to precipitate type 2 diabetes among those susceptible
Etiology		
Common theory	*Autoimmune:* genetic and environmental factors, resulting in gradual process of autoimmune destruction in genetically susceptible individuals *Nonautoimmune:* Unknown	Genetic susceptibility (polygenic) combined with environmental determinants; defects in β-cell function combined with insulin resistance Associated with long-duration obesity
Presence of antibody	Autoantibodies to insulin and to glutamic acid decarboxylase (GAD_{65})	Autoantibodies not present
Insulin resistance	Insulin resistance at diagnosis is unusual, but may occur as individual ages and gains weight	Insulin resistance is virtually universal and multifactorial in origin
Insulin secretion	Severe insulin deficiency or no insulin secretion at all	Typically increased at time of diagnosis, but progressively declines over course of illness

Data from American Diabetes Association. Standards of medical care in diabetes—2020. *Diabetes Care.* 2020;43(Suppl. 1):S1–S212. https://care.diabetesjournals.org/content/diacare/suppl/2019/12/20/43.Supplement_1.DC1/Standards_of_Care_2020.pdf.; Centers for Disease Control and Prevention (CDC). National diabetes statistics report. https://www.cdc.gov/diabetes/data/statistics/statistics-report.html.

TABLE 22.8 Clinical Manifestations and Mechanisms for Type 1 Diabetes Mellitus

Manifestation	Rationale
Polydipsia	Because of elevated blood glucose levels, water is osmotically attracted from body cells, resulting in intracellular dehydration and stimulation of thirst in hypothalamus
Polyuria	Hyperglycemia acts as an osmotic diuretic; amount of glucose filtered by glomeruli of kidney exceeds that which can be reabsorbed by renal tubules; glycosuria results, accompanied by large amounts of water lost in urine
Polyphagia	Depletion of cellular stores of carbohydrates, fats, and protein results in cellular starvation and a corresponding increase in hunger
Weight loss	Weight loss occurs because of fluid loss in osmotic diuresis and loss of body tissue as fats and proteins are used for energy
Fatigue	Metabolic changes result in poor use of food products, contributing to lethargy and fatigue
Recurrent infections (e.g., boils, carbuncles, and bladder infection)	Growth of microorganisms is stimulated by increased glucose levels; tissue ischemia and neuropathy contribute to the risk of infection; diabetes also is associated with systemic immunocompromise
Prolonged wound healing	Impaired blood supply hinders healing
Genital pruritus	Hyperglycemia and glycosuria favor fungal growth; candidal infections, resulting in pruritus, are a common presenting symptom in women
Visual changes	Blurred vision occurs as water balance in eye fluctuates because of elevated blood glucose levels; microvascular disease resulting in diabetic retinopathy may ensue
Paresthesias	Paresthesias are common manifestations of diabetic neuropathies
Cardiovascular symptoms (e.g., chest pain, extremity pain, and neurologic deficits)	Diabetes contributes to macrovascular disease with formation of atherosclerotic plaques that involve coronary, peripheral, and cerebral vessels

Clinical Manifestations. The common clinical manifestations of type 1 diabetes result from both insulin deficiency and hyperglycemia. These manifestations are described in Table 22.8. Acute complications also may include hypoglycemia and DKA, which are described later in this chapter. Chronic complications include renal, nervous system, cardiac, peripheral vascular, retinal, and bony tissue dysfunction.

Evaluation and Treatment. The criteria for diagnosis of type 1 diabetes are the same as those for type 2 diabetes (see Box 22.1). To estimate the severity of β-cell destruction, C-peptide, a component of proinsulin released during insulin production, can be measured in the serum as a surrogate for insulin levels. An individual with residual pancreatic β cell function will have detectable levels of C-peptide, but a negligible amount of C-peptide can point to the diagnosis of type 1 diabetes. Individuals with hyperglycemia and at risk for type 1 diabetes can be tested for a variety of autoantibodies, such as zinc transporter 8 (ZnT8Ab) or tyrosine phosphatases. If two or more of the autoantibodies are positive in conjunction with diagnostic hyperglycemia, then the diagnosis of type 1 diabetes is confirmed. It is important to note that antibody testing itself is not a diagnostic requirement for type 1 diabetes. Other important aspects of evaluation include looking for evidence of acute and chronic complications of type 1 diabetes.

There are no approved treatments for preventing destruction of the β cells. Currently, treatment regimens are designed to achieve optimal glucose level control (as measured by the HbA_{1C} value) without causing episodes of significant hypoglycemia. A comprehensive, person-centered collaborative management plan is essential.[26] Management requires individual planning according to type of disease, age, and activity level, but all individuals require some combination of insulin therapy, meal planning, an exercise regimen, and glucose monitoring. There are several different types of insulin preparations available, and there are new technologies for more physiologic insulin delivery systems. Many different kinds of therapies are being tested to prevent the autoimmune destruction of β cells, including immunosuppression with antirejection drugs and stem cell transplantation (Emerging Science Box: Pancreatic β Cell Regeneration as a Plausible Diabetic Therapy).

BOX 22.2 Criteria for the Diagnosis of Metabolic Syndrome

Three of these five traits must be present:

1. Increased waist circumference as determined by population- and country-specific definitions (>40 inches in men; >35 inches in women in the United States)
2. Plasma triglycerides ≥150 mg/dL
3. Plasma high-density lipoprotein cholesterol <40 mg/dL (men) or <50 mg/dL (women)
4. Blood pressure: systolic ≥130 and/or diastolic ≥85 mm Hg
5. Fasting plasma glucose ≥100 mg/dL and <126 mg/dL, or 2-h OGTT ≥140 mg/dL, or HbA_{1c} ≥5.7% to 6.4% or currently on oral drug treatment for elevated glucose without diagnosis of diabetes mellitus

Drug treatment for these conditions is an alternative indicator.

From Rosenzweig JL, Bakris GL, Berglund LF, et al. Primary prevention of ASCVD and T2DM in patients at metabolic risk: An endocrine society clinical practice guideline. *Journal of Clinical Endocrinology Metabolism,* 2019;9(104):3939–3985. https://academic.oup.com/jcem/article/104/9/3939/5540926.

Diabetes Mellitus Type 2

Diabetes mellitus type 2 (non–insulin-dependent diabetes mellitus) is a metabolic disorder that has reached pandemic dimensions all over the world, affecting 400 million people worldwide, and 10.9% of adults in the United States.[26,28] Prevalence is highest among American Indians and Alaska Natives (14.7%) and lowest among non-Hispanic whites (7.5%). There also is an increased prevalence of type 2 diabetes in children, especially in obese children (see Table 22.7).

Genetic abnormalities combined with environmental influences result in the basic pathophysiologic mechanisms of type 2 diabetes, which are insulin resistance and decreased insulin secretion by β cells (Fig. 22.12). The most well-recognized risk factors are family history, age, obesity, hypertension, poor diet, and physical inactivity. More than 60 genes have been identified that are associated with type 2 diabetes, including those that code for β-cell mass, β-cell function (ability to sense blood glucose levels, insulin synthesis, and insulin secretion), proinsulin and insulin molecular structures, insulin receptors, hepatic synthesis of glucose, glucagon synthesis, and cellular responsiveness to insulin stimulation.

There is increasing evidence that diet, including diet during pregnancy (both undernutrition and overnutrition), influences the long-term risk of type 2 diabetes in children and adults. Diets high in fruits, vegetables, fiber, and nuts reduce risk; diets high in simple carbohydrates, saturated fats, and red meat are associated with an increased risk. Weight gain and a lack of exercise also contribute to the risk for diabetes mellitus type 2.

Pathophysiology. Diabetes mellitus type 2 is a chronic and metabolic disease characterized by defects in pancreatic insulin secretion and (or) insulin effect on target tissues, generating a persistent state of hyperglycemia, inducing metabolic alteration, cell death, and inflammation.[28] Insulin resistance is defined as a suboptimal response of insulin-sensitive tissues (especially liver, muscle, and adipose tissue) to insulin. Several mechanisms are involved in abnormalities of the insulin signaling pathway and contribute to insulin resistance. These include an abnormality of the insulin molecule, high amounts of insulin antagonists, down-regulation of the insulin receptor, and alteration of glucose transporter (GLUT) proteins.

Obesity is one of the most important contributors to insulin resistance and diabetes and acts through several important mechanisms:

1. Adipokines (cytokines produced by adipose tissue): Increased serum levels of leptin (leptin resistance) and decreased levels of adiponectin result in inflammation and decreased insulin sensitivity.
2. Free fatty acids (FFAs): Increased FFAs, along with intracellular deposits of triglycerides and cholesterol, lead to decreased tissue responses to insulin.
3. Inflammation: Adipocyte-associated proinflammatory macrophages and inflammatory cytokines released from adipocytes induce insulin resistance and are cytotoxic to β cells.
4. Mitochondrial dysfunction: Decreased insulin-induced mitochondrial activity leads to insulin resistance.

EMERGING SCIENCE BOX

Pancreatic β Cell Regeneration as a Plausible Diabetic Therapy

The key pathophysiologic indicator for diabetes is an absolute deficiency (diabetes mellitus type 1) or inadequate supply (diabetes mellitus type 2) of functioning β-cells that produce insulin. Insulin resistance is a biproduct of the lack of functional β cells and is the primer for the cascade of negative health effects associated with a diabetes diagnosis. Replenishing β cells can alleviate the burden of disease and research has been underway to better understand regeneration of β cells via animal studies. Emerging science has shown that transdifferentiation of pancreatic cells such as ductal cells, acinar cells, and islet cells have produced functional β cells in mice and rats. There have been recent findings that propose the possibility of endogenous regeneration in humans. Understanding pathophysiology of diabetes brings many questions to the forefront: What is the ability to regenerate β cells in humans in vivo? How is the autoimmune characteristic of diabetes mellitus type 1 addressed so that regeneration is not merely immediate, but long lasting? How do β cells become re-sensitized after prolonged deactivation, secondary to hyperglycemia, as with diabetes mellitus type 2? Regardless, the research continues, and the foundation has been laid for identification of drugs already approved that have the potential to increase regenerative pathways for β cell functionality.

Data from Aguayo Mazzucato C, et al. Pancreatic β cell regeneration as a possible therapy for diabetes. *Cell Metabolism,* 2018;27(1):57–67; Balak JRA, et al. Highly efficient ex vivo lentiviral transduction of primary human pancreatic exocrine cells. *Scientific Reports,* 2019;9(1):15870.

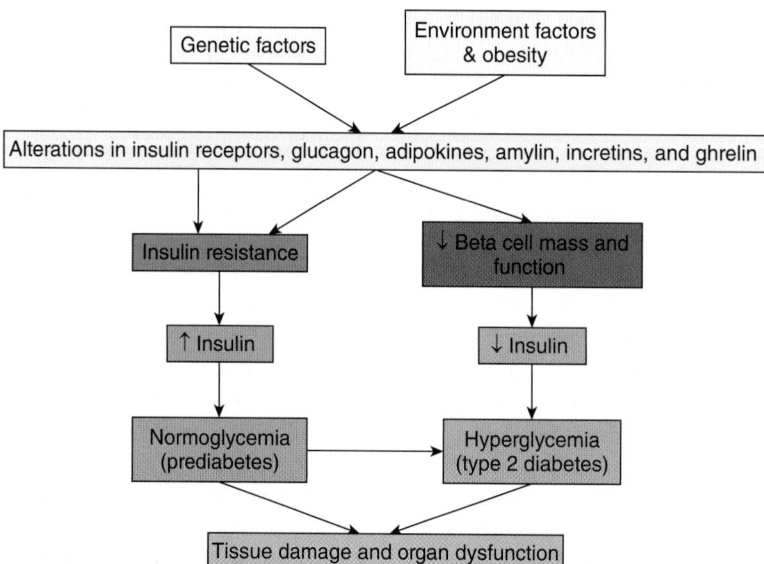

Fig. 22.12 Pathophysiology of Type 2 Diabetes Mellitus.

5. Hyperinsulinemia: Obesity is correlated with hyperinsulinemia and decreased insulin receptor density.

Compensatory hyperinsulinemia prevents the clinical appearance of diabetes for many years. Eventually, however, a decrease in β-cell mass and a reduction in normal β-cell function develops and leads to a relative deficiency of insulin activity.

The glucagon concentration is increased in type 2 diabetes because pancreatic α cells become less responsive to glucose inhibition, resulting in an increase in glucagon secretion. These abnormally high levels of glucagon increase the blood glucose level by stimulating glycogenolysis and gluconeogenesis. As was discussed under type 1 diabetes, type 2 diabetes also is associated with a deficiency in amylin, further increasing glucagon levels. Pramlintide, a synthetic analog of amylin, is used for treatment in type 2 diabetes.

Hormones released from the GI tract play a role in insulin resistance, β-cell function, and diabetes. Ghrelin is a peptide produced in the stomach and pancreatic islets that regulates food intake, energy balance, and hormonal secretion. Decreased levels of circulating ghrelin have been associated with insulin resistance and increased fasting insulin levels. The incretins are a class of peptides that are released from the GI tract in response to food intake and function to increase the secretion of insulin and have many other positive effects on metabolism. The most studied incretin is called *glucagon-like peptide 1* (GLP-1), and studies have demonstrated that β-cell responsiveness to GLP-1 is reduced both in prediabetes and in type 2 diabetes. Incretin therapies include GLP-1 receptor agonists (GLP-1 RAs) and dipeptidyl peptidase IV (DPP-IV) inhibitors, which can help control postprandial glucose levels by promoting glucose-dependent insulin secretion.

The kidneys also influence the pathophysiology of type 2 diabetes. Renal reabsorption of glucose through the sodium-glucose cotransporter 2 (SGLT2) is an important controller of serum glucose levels, and medications aimed at blocking it have resulted in decreased measurements for blood glucose level, weight, and blood pressure.

As you have learned, many organs contribute to insulin resistance, chronic hyperglycemia, and the consequences of type 2 diabetes. These causes and consequences are summarized in Fig. 22.13, and the complications of type 2 diabetes will be discussed later in this chapter.

Clinical Manifestations. The clinical manifestations of type 2 diabetes are nonspecific. The individual with type 2 diabetes may show some classic symptoms of diabetes, such as polyuria and polydipsia, but more often will have nonspecific symptoms, such as fatigue, pruritus, recurrent infections, visual changes, or symptoms of neuropathy (paresthesia or weakness). The affected individual is often overweight, dyslipidemic, and hypertensive. The increased morbidity and mortality rates related to diabetes mellitus type 2 are often associated with vascular complications, such as cardiovascular diseases, nephropathy, retinopathy, endothelial dysfunction, dyslipidemia, and an increase of oxidative stress, which is also due to inflammation (Emerging Science Box: Inflammation and Its Importance to the Pathophysiology of Insulin Resistance in Prediabetes and Diabetes Mellitus Type 2).[29,30]

Evaluation and Treatment. The diagnostic criteria for type 2 diabetes are the same as those for type 1 (see Box 22.1). Metabolic syndrome is a constellation of disorders (central obesity, dyslipidemia, prehypertension, and an elevated FPG) that confer a high risk of developing type 2 diabetes and associated cardiovascular complications (see Box 22.2).

As with type 1 diabetes, the goal of treatment for individuals with type 2 diabetes (and metabolic syndrome) is the restoration of near-euglycemia (normal blood glucose) levels and correction of related metabolic disorders. Prevention and treatment of type 2 diabetes, especially in those individuals with prediabetes, focuses on lifestyle modifications as the cornerstone modality.[31] Diet should match activity levels and include more complex carbohydrates (rather than simple sugars), foods low in fats, adequate protein, and fiber. Obesity management results in improved glucose tolerance. Bariatric surgery improves glycemic control, decreases the risk of cardiovascular disease, and promotes weight loss in those morbidly obese.[26]

EMERGING SCIENCE BOX

Inflammation and Its Importance to the Pathophysiology of Insulin Resistance in Prediabetes and Diabetes Mellitus Type 2

Insulin resistance is the hallmark of prediabetes and progression to diabetes mellitus type 2 with a myriad of pathophysiologic mechanisms that contribute to its occurrence. Systemic inflammation is an underlying current among these mechanisms, contributing to cardiometabolic conditions commonly identified with the diagnosis of diabetes mellitus type 2. A persistent state of hyperglycemia in prediabetes can trigger oxidative stress and inappropriate uptake of proinflammatory markers, which promote vascular dysfunction. Data from the Framingham Offspring study has shown a positive association between frequency of insulin resistance and the amount of urinary 8-epi-prostaglandin F2α (8-epi-PGF2α), an oxidative stress marker, present. This marker was specifically identified in groups with an elevated risk of diabetes such as those with IFG and obesity. Angiopoietin-like protein 2 (ANGPTL2), a proinflammatory cytokine, is predominantly secreted from adipose tissue and the macrophages that accumulate within it. These macrophages influence chronic low-grade inflammation which lead to systemic inflammation, insulin resistance, and increased lipid accumulation in the liver. High serum levels of ANGPTL2 have been identified in the development of renal diabetic disease due to the positive correlation with albumin-to-creatinine ratio and negative correlations with the glomerular filtration rate. Understanding the cascade of inflammation that occurs with insulin resistance can aid in identification of priority lifestyle modifications to combat it with the diagnosis of prediabetes and use of appropriate pharmacologic measure that contribute to the decrease of inflammation with the diagnosis of diabetes mellitus type 2.

Data from Luc K, et al. Oxidative stress and inflammatory markers in prediabetes and diabetes. *Journal of Physiology and Pharmacology,* 2019;70(6):10.26402/jpp.2019.6.01. doi:10.26402/ jpp.2019.6.01; Pivari F, et al. Curcumin and type 2 diabetes mellitus: Prevention and treatment. *Nutrients,* 2019;11(8):1837. Published August 8, 2019. doi:10.3390/ nu11081837; Sasaki Y, et al. Angiopoietin life protein 2 (ANGPTL2) promotes adipose tissue macrophage and T lymphocyte accumulation and leads to insulin resistance. *PLoS One,* 2015;10(7):e0131176. Published July 1, 2015. doi:10.1371/journal.pone.0131176.

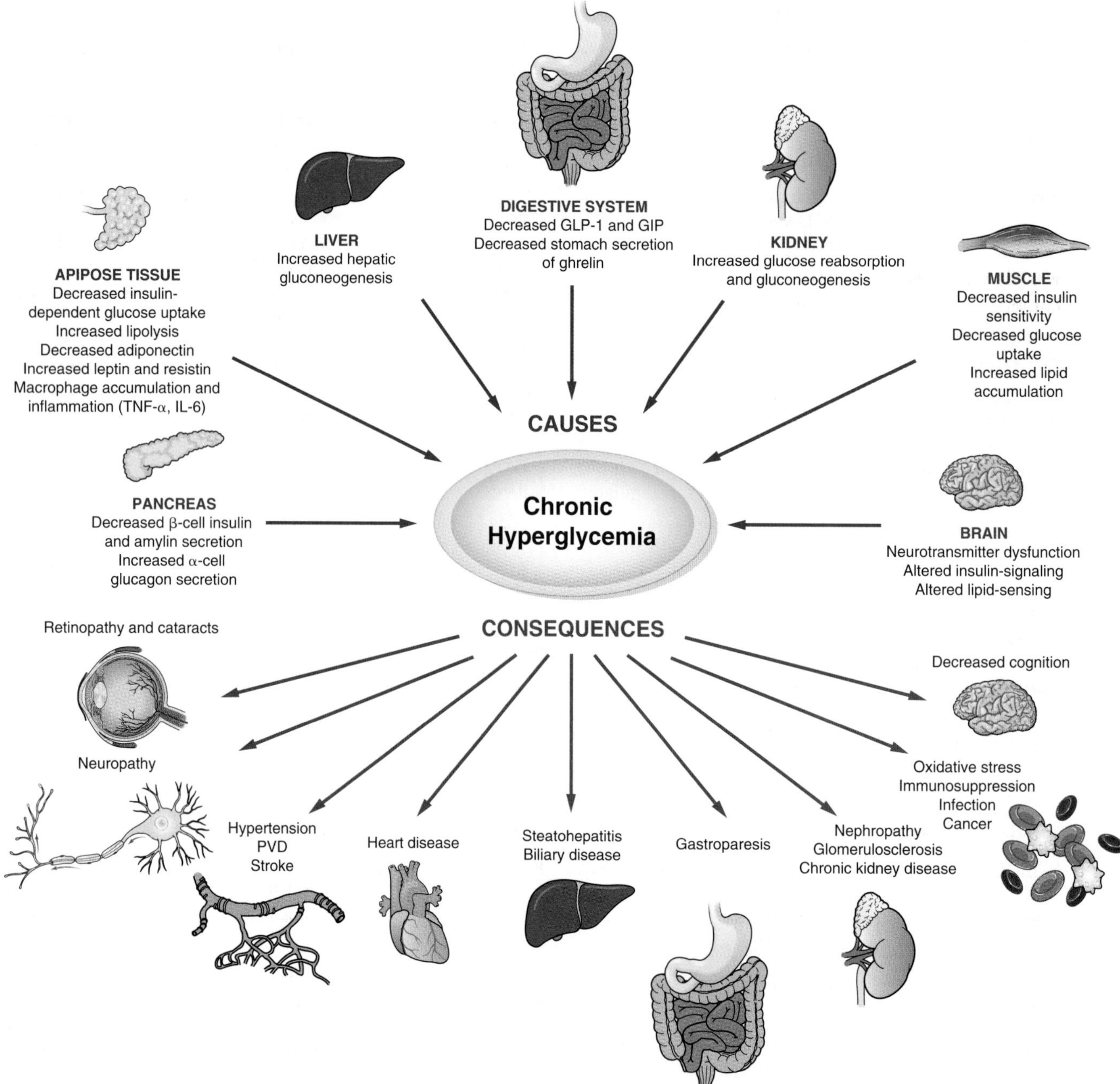

Fig. 22.13 Multiorgan Causes and Common Consequences of Chronic Hyperglycemia in Type 2 Diabetes. *GLP-1*, Glucagon-like peptide 1; *GIP*, gastric inhibitory polypeptide; *IL*, interleukin; *PVD*, peripheral vascular disease; *TNF*, tumor necrosis factor.

For individuals who require further intervention, oral and/or non-insulin antidiabetic agents are indicated (Table 22.9).[26] Currently, metformin is considered the primary pharmacologic choice for the treatment of type 2 diabetes. If the HbA_{1C} target is not maintained over 3 months, a GLP-1 receptor agonist (incretin) may be added.[26,31]

If treatment goals are still not met, a combination of drugs, including SGLT2 inhibitors, may be required. Insulin therapy may be needed in the later stage of type 2 diabetes because of loss of β-cell function, which is progressive over time (Emerging Science Box: Smart Pens for Improved Safety and Efficacy of Insulin Therapy).

Gestational Diabetes Mellitus and Specific Types of Diabetes Mellitus From Other Causes

As listed in Table 22.7 the ADA classification of diabetes mellitus not only includes the most common forms of diabetes (type

TABLE 22.9 Non-insulin Antidiabetic Medications

Drug Type	Mechanisms of Metabolic Control
α-Glycosidase inhibitor (miglitol and acarbose)	Delays carbohydrate absorption in gut by inhibiting disaccharidases
Biguanide (metformin)	Decreases hepatic glucose production and increases insulin sensitivity and peripheral glucose uptake
Meglitinides (glinides; repaglinide and nateglinide)	Stimulate insulin release from pancreatic β cells
Sulfonylureas (glyburide, glipizide, glimepiride)	Stimulate insulin release from pancreatic β cells
Peroxisome proliferator–activated receptor-γ agonists (thiazolidinediones, pioglitazone, and rosiglitazone)	Increase insulin sensitivity, particularly in adipose tissue
Bile acid sequestrant (colesevelam, cholestyramine, and colestipol)	Unknown; theories include decreased hepatic glucose production, increased insulin secretion, and increased incretin release
GLP-1 receptor agonists (exenatide, liraglutide, lixisenatide, exenatide extended-release, albiglutide, and dulaglutide)	Increase insulin secretion, decrease glucagon secretion, decrease rate of gastric emptying, decrease appetite, weight loss
DPP-IV inhibitors (sitagliptin, saxagliptin, alogliptin, and linagliptin)	Increase insulin secretion, decrease glucagon secretion, decrease rate of gastric emptying, decrease appetite
Amylin mimetics (pramlintide)	Decrease glucagon secretion, decrease rate of gastric emptying, and decrease appetite
SGLT2 inhibitor; In clinical trials: canagliflozin, dapagliflozin, empagliflozin	Inhibits proximal tubular renal transport of glucose, decreasing glucose reabsorption and increasing renal excretion of glucose independent of insulin
Bromocriptine mesylate	Increases CNS dopamine, reducing sympathetic nervous activity, hepatic glucose production, and lipolysis

CNS, Central nervous system; *DPP-IV*, dipeptidyl peptidase-IV; *GLP-1*, glucagon-like peptide-1; *SGLT2*, sodium-glucose cotransporter 2.
Data from Brietzke SA. Oral antihyperglycemic treatment options for type 2 diabetes mellitus. *Medical Clinics of North America*, 2015;99(1):87–106; Tran L, Zielinski A, Roach AH, et al. Pharmacologic treatment of type 2 diabetes: Oral medications. *Annals of Pharmacotherapy*, 2015;49(5):540–556.

1 and type 2) but also encompasses GDM and specific types of diabetes mellitus from other causes.

Gestational diabetes mellitus (GDM) complicates approximately 7% of pregnancies and is defined as diabetes diagnosed in the second or third trimester of pregnancy that was not clearly overt diabetes prior to gestation.[26] In most cases, this hyperglycemia is the result of IGT due to pancreatic β-cell dysfunction on a background of chronic insulin resistance. Risk factors for GDM include overweight and obesity, advanced maternal age, and a family history of any form of diabetes.[32] An OGTT is used to confirm the diagnosis. However, this definition means that many women with previously undiagnosed type 1 or type 2 diabetes are diagnosed with GDM, and many of them have progressive disease after delivery. Therefore, the ADA recommends that women with risk factors for diabetes be screened at their initial prenatal visit and that women diagnosed during pregnancy should continue to be monitored postpartum and at least every 3 years for persistent or recurrent diabetes.[26] Careful glucose control prenatally, during pregnancy, and after delivery is essential to the short- and long-term health of both mother and baby.

EMERGING SCIENCE BOX

Smart Pens for Improved Safety and Efficacy of Insulin Therapy

Insulin pens have improved convenience, accuracy of dosing, medication adherence, and decreased hypoglycemia risk since introduced as an option for insulin administration. Despite these benefits, there have been challenges for clinicians to optimize glycemic control due to limited information on insulin dose and timing of injection. FDA-approved smart insulin pens provide a record of the amount of insulin and timing of each dose which is transmitted wirelessly to a mobile application on a smartphone. The application, which is user-specific, can track current insulin-on-board, make dose recommendations, and will prepare a report to send to a preferred healthcare provider. The automaticity of the information going to the person and clinician supports treatment plan adherence, insulin dose accuracy and appropriateness, and continuity of care between person and provider. Emerging science boasts a new digital diabetes bionetwork where physiology, behavior, and environment can be evaluated in real time to prevent adverse drug effects, such as hypoglycemia, with insulin use. If cost can be controlled, smart pens could reduce the risk and burden of insulin use and improve overall diabetes care.

Data from Klonoff DC, et al. Smart pens will improve insulin therapy. *Journal of Diabetes Science and Technology*, 2018;12(3):551–553; Gildon BW. InPen Smart insulin pen system: Product review and user experience. *Diabetes Spectrum*, 2018;31(4):354–358.

Specific types of diabetes from other causes include monogenic diabetes syndromes (e.g., MODY), disease of the exocrine pancreas (e.g., cystic fibrosis), and drug- or chemical-induced diabetes (e.g., with glucocorticoid use, in the treatment of HIV/AIDS, or after organ transplantation). Maturity-onset diabetes of youth (MODY) usually presents before 25 years of age and includes at least 13 genetic mutations that affect critical enzymes involved in β-cell function but with little impact on insulin action.[26] The diagnosis of MODY should be considered in individuals who have atypical clinical presentations, who are diagnosed within the first 6 months of life (neonatal diabetes), and who have a strong family history of diabetes. Diagnosis includes genetic testing for the three most common forms of MODY. Management is similar to that used for type 2 diabetes. Diabetes also can result from pancreatic damage incurred through the effects of cystic fibrosis, medications, and immunosuppression after organ transplantation.

Acute Complications of Diabetes Mellitus

The major acute complications of diabetes mellitus are hypoglycemia, DKA, and hyperosmolar hyperglycemic nonketotic

TABLE 22.10 Common Acute Complications of Diabetes Mellitus

Hypoglycemia in Persons With Diabetes Mellitus	Diabetic Ketoacidosis	Hyperglycemic Nonketotic Syndromes
Synonyms		
Insulin shock, insulin reaction	Diabetic coma syndrome	Hyperosmolar hyperglycemia nonketotic coma
Persons at Risk		
Individuals taking insulin Individuals with rapidly fluctuating blood glucose levels Individuals with type 2 diabetes taking non-insulin antidiabetic medications	Individuals with type 1 diabetes Individuals with undiagnosed diabetes	Older adults with type 2 diabetes, nondiabetic persons with predisposing factors, such as pancreatitis; individuals with undiagnosed diabetes
Predisposing Factors		
Excessive insulin or non-insulin antidiabetic agents, lack of sufficient food intake, excessive physical exercise, abrupt decline in insulin needs (e.g., renal failure, immediately postpartum), simultaneous use of insulin-potentiating agents or β-blocking agents that mask symptoms	Stressful situation such as infection, accident, trauma, emotional stress; omission of insulin; medications that antagonize insulin	Infection, medications that antagonize insulin, comorbid condition
Typical Onset		
Rapid	Slow	Slowest
Presenting Symptoms		
Adrenergic reaction: pallor, sweating, tachycardia, palpitations, hunger, restlessness, anxiety, tremors Neurogenic reaction: fatigue, irritability, headache, loss of concentration, visual disturbances, dizziness, hunger, confusion, transient sensory or motor defects, convulsions, coma, death	Malaise, dry mouth, headache, polyuria, polydipsia, weight loss, nausea, vomiting, pruritus, abdominal pain, lethargy, shortness of breath, Kussmaul respirations, fruity or acetone odor to breath	Polyuria, polydipsia, hypovolemia, dehydration (parched lips, poor skin turgor), hypotension, tachycardia, hypoperfusion, weight loss, weakness, nausea, vomiting, abdominal pain, hypothermia, stupor, coma, seizures
Laboratory Analysis		
Serum glucose <30 mg/dL in newborn (first 2–3 days) and <55–60 mg/dL in adults	Glucose levels >250 mg/dL, reduction in bicarbonate concentration, increased anion gap, increased plasma levels of β-hydroxybutyrate, acetoacetate, and acetone	Glucose levels >600 mg/dL, lack of ketosis, serum osmolarity >320 mOsm/L, elevated blood urea nitrogen and creatinine levels

syndrome (HHNKS).[33] A comparison of these complications is summarized in Table 22.10.

Hypoglycemia in diabetes is sometimes called *insulin shock* or *insulin reaction*. Individuals with type 1 diabetes require insulin to manage their diabetes and are at more risk for hypoglycemia than those with type 2 diabetes because they have more severe deficits in their ability to control serum glucose levels. Significant drops in blood sugar most often occur when there is an unexpected change in caloric intake or exercise without appropriate modification of insulin dosing. Hypoglycemia sometimes occurs in type 2 diabetes during treatment with insulin or non-insulin antidiabetic medications. Symptoms include pallor, tremor, anxiety, tachycardia, palpitations, diaphoresis, headache, dizziness, irritability, fatigue, poor judgment, confusion, visual disturbances, hunger, seizures, and coma. Treatment requires immediate replacement of glucose either orally or intravenously. Glucagon for home use can be prescribed for individuals who are at high risk. Prevention is achieved with individualized management of medications and diet, monitoring of blood glucose levels, and education.

Diabetic ketoacidosis (DKA) is a serious complication related to a deficiency of insulin and an increase in the levels of insulin counterregulatory hormones (catecholamines, cortisol, glucagon, GH) (Fig. 22.14). DKA is much more common in type 1 diabetes because insulin is more deficient (see Table 22.10). It is characterized by hyperglycemia, acidosis, and ketonuria. Insulin normally stimulates lipogenesis and inhibits lipolysis, thus preventing fat catabolism. With insulin deficiency, lipolysis is enhanced and there is an increase in the amount of nonesterified fatty acids delivered to the liver. The consequence is increased glyconeogenesis, contributing to hyperglycemia and the production of ketone bodies (acetoacetate, hydroxybutyrate, and acetone) by the mitochondria of the liver at a rate that exceeds peripheral use. Accumulation of ketone bodies causes a drop in pH, resulting in metabolic acidosis and transient hyperkalemia. Symptoms of DKA include Kussmaul respirations

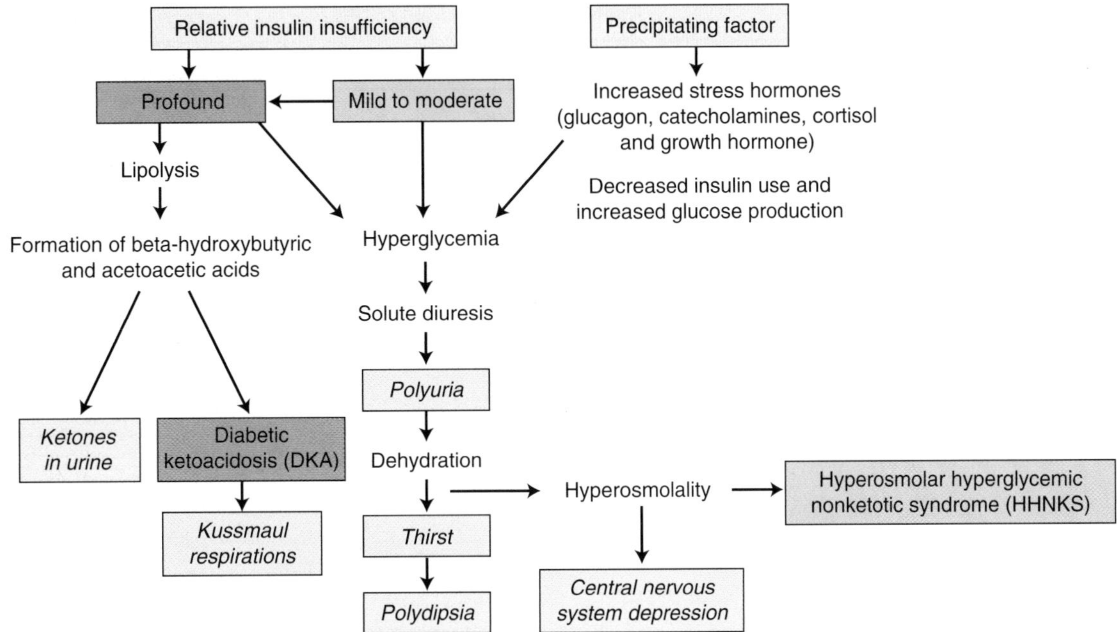

Fig. 22.14 Pathophysiology of Diabetic Ketoacidosis and Hyperosmolar Hyperglycemic Nonketotic Syndrome in Diabetes Mellitus.

(hyperventilation in an attempt to compensate for the acidosis), postural dizziness, central nervous system depression, ketonuria, anorexia, nausea, abdominal pain, thirst, and polyuria. DKA is managed with a combination of fluids, insulin, and electrolyte replacement.

Hyperosmolar hyperglycemic nonketotic syndrome (HHNKS) is an uncommon but significant complication of diabetes mellitus type 2 with a high overall mortality. It occurs more often in elderly individuals who have other comorbidities, including infections or cardiovascular or renal disease. HHNKS differs from DKA because type 2 diabetes is characterized by a lesser degree of insulin deficiency, which therefore prevents lipolysis and the production of ketones (see Fig. 22.14). However, hyperglycemia is usually more profound in HHNKS leading to more polyuria and fluid deficiency. Therefore, the clinical features of HHNKS include a very high serum glucose concentration and osmolarity without metabolic acidosis. Clinical manifestations include severe dehydration; loss of electrolytes (especially potassium); and neurologic changes, such as stupor. Management includes fluid, insulin, and electrolyte replacement.

Chronic Complications of Diabetes Mellitus

A number of serious complications are associated with any type of poorly controlled diabetes mellitus. Most complications are associated with insulin resistance or deficit and chronic hyperglycemia. Insulin resistance or deficit renders cells unable to process glucose normally, so they resort to a number of alternative pathways for glucose metabolism, particularly through activation of the polyol pathway. This pathway results in the accumulation of sorbitol and glutathione, both of which contribute to chronic tissue damage. Hyperglycemia leads to a number of deleterious effects, including abnormalities in intracellular communication (e.g., protein kinase C pathways) and the attachment of glucose to proteins, lipids, and nucleic acids (glycation). Therefore, glycation creates what are called *advanced glycation end products* (AGEs), which interfere with many crucial cellular processes. The cumulative effect of these abnormal processes leads to the microvascular (damage to capillaries; retinopathies, nephropathies, and neuropathies) and macrovascular (damage to larger vessels; coronary artery, peripheral vascular, and cerebral vascular disease) complications of chronic diabetes mellitus (Table 22.11).

Microvascular Disease

Diabetic microvascular complications are characterized by occlusion of capillaries, with associated ischemia of tissues.[34] It is a leading cause of blindness, diabetic nephropathy (including end-stage kidney failure), and various neuropathies. Approximately half of the individuals diagnosed with diabetes mellitus type 2 develop peripheral neuropathy. This progressive disorder is chronic, affecting the peripheral nervous system and characterized by allodynia, pain, and paresthesia symptoms. Neuropathies are caused by axonal degeneration and segmental demyelination. The frequency and severity of complications appear to be proportional to the duration of the disease (more or less than 10 years) and the status of glycemic control. Hypoxia and ischemia accompany microvascular disease, especially in the eye, kidney, and nerves. Many individuals with type 2 diabetes will present with microvascular complications because of the long duration of asymptomatic hyperglycemia that generally precedes diagnosis. This underscores the need to screen for diabetes.

Diabetic retinopathy. Diabetic retinopathy is a leading cause of blindness worldwide and is a common complication of type 2

TABLE 22.11 Chronic Complications of Diabetes Mellitus

Complications	Pathologic Mechanisms	Associated Symptoms
Microvascular		
Retinopathy	Microaneurysms, exudates, hemorrhages, formation of new blood vessels, scarring, retinal detachment. Macular edema may also occur.	Progresses from no visual changes to loss of visual acuity and blindness. Symptoms worsened by hyperosmolar lens edema and cataract formation.
Nephropathy	Glomerulosclerosis, glomerular perfusion and pressure changes, protein glycation	Microalbuminuria and hypertension slowly progressing to end-stage kidney failure
Neuropathy	Oxidative stress, poor perfusion and ischemia, loss of nerve growth factor	Sensorimotor polyneuropathy progressing to distal paresthesias in feet and hands, muscle wasting, Charcot joints, falls and injuries. Autonomic neuropathy progressing to postural hypotension, gastroparesis, urinary retention, and erectile dysfunction.
Skin and foot lesions	Loss of sensation, poor perfusion, suppressed immunity, and increased risk of infection	Pressure ulcers and delayed wound healing; abscess formation; necrosis and gangrene of toes and feet; infection and osteomyelitis
Macrovascular		
Cardiovascular	Accelerated atherosclerosis	Hypertension, coronary artery disease, cardiomyopathy, and heart failure
Cerebrovascular	Same as above	Increased risk for ischemic and thrombotic stroke
Peripheral vascular	Same as above	Claudication, nonhealing ulcers, gangrene
Infection		
	Impaired immunity, tissue ischemia, recurrent trauma, delayed wound healing, urinary retention	Skin and wound infections, urinary tract infections, increased risk for sepsis

diabetes because of the likelihood of long-standing hyperglycemia before diagnosis. Most individuals with diabetes will eventually develop retinopathy and also are more likely to develop cataracts and glaucoma (see Chapter 16).

Diabetic retinopathy results from relative hypoxemia, damage to retinal blood vessels, RBC aggregation, and hypertension (Fig. 22.15).[35] The three stages of retinopathy that lead to loss of vision are *nonproliferative* (stage I), characterized by an increase in retinal capillary permeability, vein dilation, microaneurysm formation, and superficial (flame-shaped) and deep (blot) hemorrhages; *preproliferative* (stage II), a progression of retinal ischemia, with areas of poor perfusion that culminate in infarcts; and *proliferative* (stage III), the result of neovascularization (angiogenesis) and fibrous tissue formation within the retina or optic disc. Traction of the new vessels on the vitreous humor may cause retinal detachment or hemorrhage into the vitreous humor, with severe blurring or loss of vision. Macular edema is the leading cause of blurred vision among persons with diabetes. Blurring of vision also can be a consequence of hyperglycemia and sorbitol accumulation in the lens. Dehydration of the lens, aqueous humor, and vitreous humor also reduces visual acuity.

Diabetic nephropathy. Diabetes is the most common cause of chronic kidney disease and end-stage renal disease in the world. Nearly half of individuals with diabetes mellitus develop diabetic nephropathy.[36] Renal glomerular changes occur early

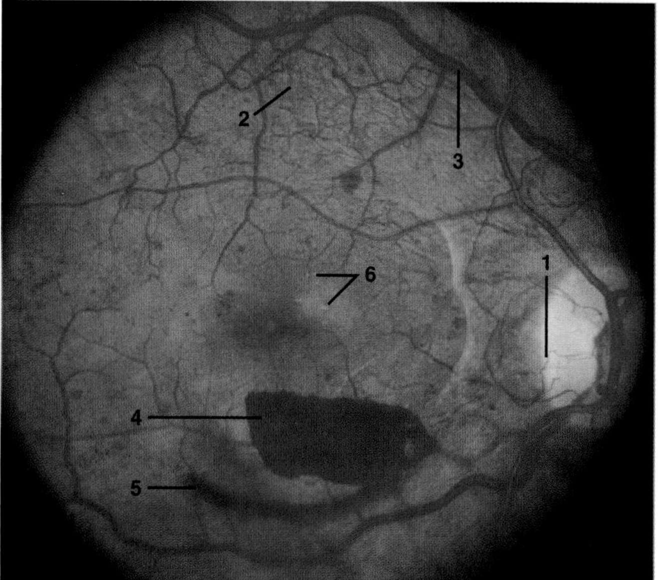

Fig. 22.15 Diabetic Retinopathy. Neovascularization is present at the optic nerve **(1)** and along vascular pathways **(2)**. Retinal veins are engorged **(3)** and a preretinal boat-shaped hemorrhage **(4)** is present below the fovea. A more diffuse mild vitreous hemorrhage **(5)** is present below the preretinal hemorrhage. A few small, hard exudates are visible in the fovea **(6)**. (From Palay DA, Krachmer JH. *Primary care ophthalmology,* 2nd edition. St. Louis: Mosby; 2006.)

in diabetes mellitus, occasionally preceding the overt manifestation of the disease. The glomeruli are injured by hyperglycemia with protein glycation (bonding of a glucose molecule to a protein), high renal blood flow (hyperfiltration), and intraglomerular hypertension exacerbated by systemic hypertension (Fig. 22.16). There is progressive glomerulosclerosis and decreased glomerular blood flow and glomerular filtration that can progress to renal failure. Tubulointerstitial fibrosis also develops in advanced stages of disease. Loss of autoregulation of renal blood flow and anemia contribute to hypoxia. Hyperglycemia and glomerular hyperfiltration increase tubular reabsorption of glucose promoting inflammation and activation of growth factors and fibroblasts. The consequence is tubulointerstitial fibrosis which contributes to renal failure.[37]

Microalbuminuria is the first manifestation of diabetic kidney dysfunction and signals the onset of systemic diabetic complications. Before proteinuria, no clinical signs or symptoms of progressive glomerulosclerosis are likely to be evident. Later, hypoproteinemia, reduction in plasma oncotic pressure, fluid overload, anasarca (generalized body edema), and hypertension may occur. As renal function continues to deteriorate, individuals with type 1 diabetes may experience hypoglycemia (because of loss of renal insulin metabolism), which necessitates a decrease in insulin therapy. As the glomerular filtration rate drops below 10 mL/min, uremic signs, such as nausea, lethargy, acidosis, anemia, and uncontrolled hypertension, occur (see Chapter 38 for a discussion of renal failure). Early diagnosis and control of hypertension and hyperglycemia decreases the severity of nephropathy and delays the onset of end-stage kidney disease.

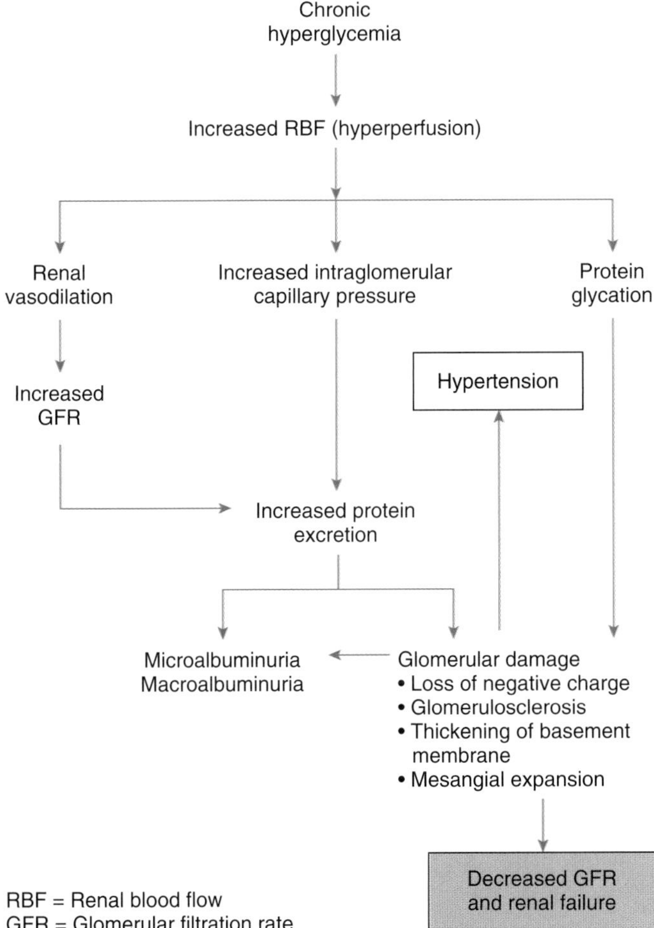

Fig. 22.16 Diabetic Nephropathy.

Diabetic neuropathies. Diabetic neuropathy is the most common complication of diabetes. The underlying pathologic mechanism includes metabolic and vascular factors related to chronic hyperglycemia with ischemia and demyelination contributing to neural changes and delayed conduction. Both somatic and peripheral nerve cells show diffuse or focal damage, resulting in polyneuropathy.[38,39] Loss of pain, temperature, and vibration sensation is more common than motor involvement and often involves the extremities first in the hands and feet. Motor neuropathies can affect muscle groups, particularly of the legs and feet, contributing to deformity and unstable balance. Peripheral neuropathy can cause Charcot arthropathy, a progressive deterioration of weight-bearing joints, typically in the foot and ankle. Distal neuropathies combined with vascular complications, infection, or injury can lead to amputation (Fig. 22.17).

Autonomic neuropathies include delayed gastric emptying, diabetic diarrhea, altered bladder function (e.g., decreased sensation of bladder fullness, urge or overflow incontinence), impotence, orthostatic hypotension, and heart rate variability, with both tachycardia and bradycardia. Neuropathy may occur during periods of "good" glucose control and may be the initial clinical manifestation of diabetes mellitus type 2. Chronic hyperglycemia also can cause cognitive dysfunction with alterations in learning and memory.

Macrovascular Disease

Macrovascular disease (lesions in large- and medium-sized arteries) increases morbidity and mortality and increases the risk for hypertension, accelerated atherosclerosis, cardiovascular disease, stroke, and peripheral vascular disease (PVD), particularly among individuals with diabetes mellitus type 2 (atherosclerosis is discussed in Chapter 32). Children with poorly controlled diabetes have higher risk for macrovascular complications within 1 to 2 decades. The process tends to be more severe and accelerated in the presence of other risk factors, including obesity, hyperlipidemia, and smoking.

Cardiovascular disease. Cardiovascular disease is the primary cause of death of people with diabetes, with higher risk for women. Hypertension often coexists with diabetes mellitus. Diabetes also is associated with deleterious changes in serum lipids, including high levels of low-density lipoproteins (LDLs), and low levels of high-density lipoproteins (HDLs). The combination of diabetes, hypertension dyslipidemia, and obesity (metabolic syndrome) greatly increases the risk for atherosclerotic cardiovascular disease, particularly CAD and stroke. CAD results from vessel injury related to insulin resistance and hyperglycemia, leading to accelerated atherosclerosis (see Chapter 32). In general, the prevalence of CAD increases with the duration but not the severity of diabetes, and the onset can be silent.

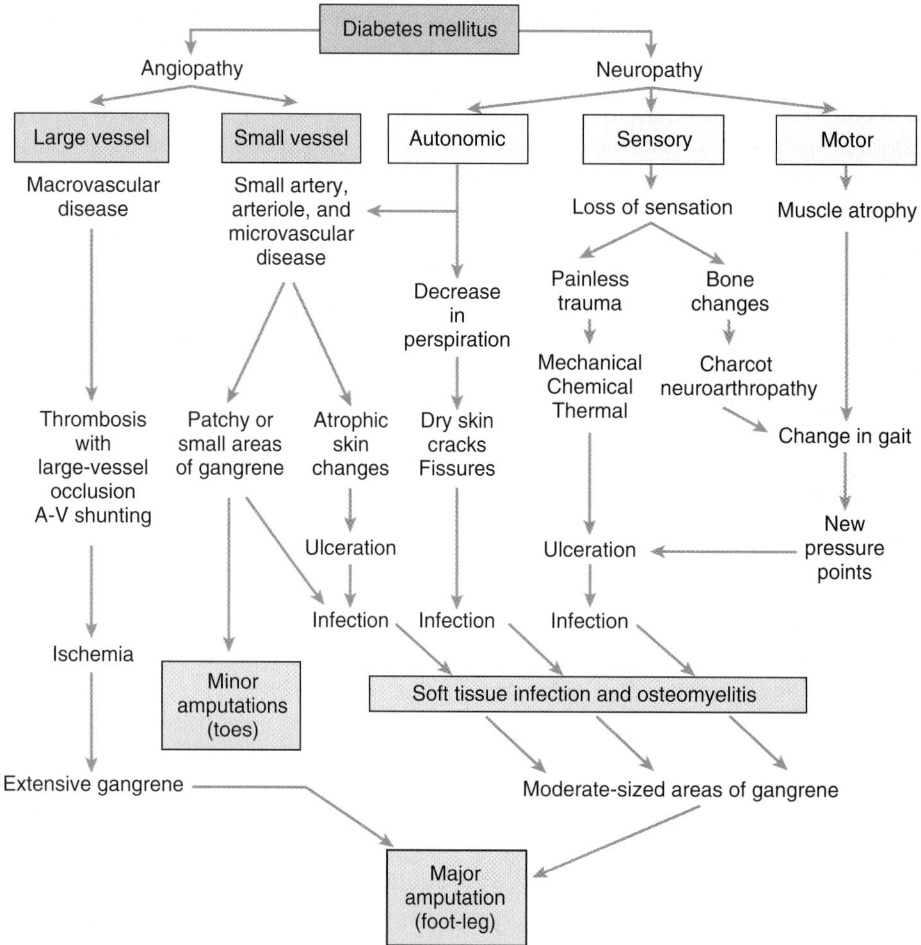

Fig. 22.17 How Foot Lesions of Diabetes Lead to Amputation. (From Levin ME, et al. *The diabetic foot,* 5th edition. St. Louis: Mosby; 1993.)

The incidence of *congestive heart failure* is higher in individuals with diabetes, even without myocardial infarction. This may be related to cardiomyopathy and the presence of increased amounts of collagen in the ventricular wall and ventricular hypertrophy. There is reduced mechanical compliance of the heart during filling with diastolic and, eventually, systolic failure (heart disease is described in Chapter 32).

Stroke. Stroke is twice as common in those with diabetes (particularly type 2 diabetes) as in the nondiabetic population. As in CAD, accelerated atherosclerosis of the cerebral vessels results from insulin resistance and hyperglycemia, especially when associated with hypertension and hyperlipidemia (see Chapter 18).

Peripheral vascular disease. Diabetes mellitus increases the incidence of PVD. Age, duration of diabetes, genetics, and additional risk factors (smoking, hyperlipidemia, hypertension) influence the development and management of PVD. PVD in those with diabetes is more diffuse and often involves arteries below the knee. Occlusions of the small arteries and arterioles can lead to claudication (pain from reduced blood flow during exercise), ulcers, gangrene, and amputation. The lesions begin as ulcers and progress to osteomyelitis or gangrene, requiring amputation (see Fig. 22.17). Peripheral neuropathies and an increased risk for infection advance the disease.

Infection

Diabetic individuals are more prone to develop common infections, like cystitis, enteric infections, skin and soft tissue infections, external otitis, pneumonia, appendicitis, and peritonitis as well as rare and severe infections, such as emphysematous pyelonephritis.[40]

The individual with diabetes is at an increased risk for infection throughout the body for several reasons:

1. *The senses.* Impaired vision caused by retinal changes and impaired touch caused by neuropathy lead to loss of protection, with injury and repeated trauma, open wounds, and soft tissue or osseous infection, particularly in the legs and feet.
2. *Hypoxia.* Once skin integrity is compromised, susceptibility to infection increases as a result of hypoxia. In addition, the glycated hemoglobin in the RBCs impedes the release of oxygen to tissues and contributes to delayed wound healing.
3. *Pathogens.* Some pathogens proliferate rapidly because of increased glucose in body fluids, which provides an excellent source of energy.

4. *Blood supply*. Decreased blood supply results from vascular changes and reduces the supply of white blood cells to the affected area.
5. *Suppressed immune response*. Chronic hyperglycemia impairs both innate and adaptive immune responses, including abnormal chemotaxis and vasoactive responses, and defective phagocytosis.

ALTERATIONS OF ADRENAL FUNCTION

Disorders of the Adrenal Cortex

Disorders of the adrenal cortex are related either to hyperfunction or to hypofunction. Hyperfunction that causes increased secretion of cortisol (hypercortisolism) leads to Cushing disease or Cushing syndrome. Hyperfunction that causes increased secretion of adrenal androgens or estrogens leads to virilization or feminization. Hyperfunction that causes increased levels of aldosterone leads to hyperaldosteronism, which may be primary or secondary. These syndromes often have overlapping features. Hypofunction of the adrenal cortex leads to Addison disease.

Hypercortical Function (Cushing Syndrome, Cushing Disease)

Cushing syndrome (chronic hypercortisolism) refers to the clinical manifestations resulting from chronic exposure to excess cortisol regardless of cause. Cushing disease refers to excess endogenous secretion of ACTH.[41,42] *ACTH-dependent hypercortisolism* (about 80% of cases) results from overproduction of pituitary ACTH by a primary pituitary corticotroph adenoma (most common and can occur at any age) or by an ectopic secreting nonpituitary tumor, such as a small cell carcinoma of the lung (more common in older adults). *ACTH-independent hypercortisolism* is caused by cortisol secretion from a rare benign or malignant tumor of one or both adrenal glands (more common in children). A Cushing-like syndrome may develop as a side effect of long-term pharmacologic administration of glucocorticoids.

Pathophysiology. With ACTH-dependent hypercortisolism, the excess ACTH stimulates excess production of cortisol and there is loss of feedback control of ACTH secretion. In individuals with ACTH-dependent hypercortisolism, secretion of both cortisol and adrenal androgens is increased, and cortisol-releasing hormone is inhibited. In contrast, ACTH-independent secreting tumors of the adrenal cortex generally secrete only cortisol. Elevated cortisol levels suppress CRH and ACTH levels. When the secretion of cortisol by the tumor exceeds normal cortisol levels, symptoms of hypercortisolism develop.

Clinical Manifestations. Weight gain is the most common feature and results from the accumulation of adipose tissue in the trunk, facial, and cervical areas. These characteristic patterns of fat deposition have been respectively described as “truncal obesity,” “moon face,” and “buffalo hump” (Figs. 22.18 and 22.19).

Glucose intolerance occurs because of cortisol-induced insulin resistance and increased gluconeogenesis and glycogen storage by the liver. Overt diabetes mellitus develops in approximately 20% of individuals with hypercortisolism. Polyuria is a manifestation of hyperglycemia and resultant glycosuria.

Protein wasting is caused by the catabolic effects of cortisol on peripheral tissues. Muscle wasting leads to muscle weakness. In bone, loss of the protein matrix leads to osteoporosis, with pathologic fractures, vertebral compression fractures, bone and back pain, kyphosis, and reduced height. Cortisol interferes with the action of GH in long bones; thus, children who present with short stature may be experiencing growth retardation related to Cushing syndrome rather than GH deficiency. Bone disease may contribute to hypercalciuria and resulting renal stones.

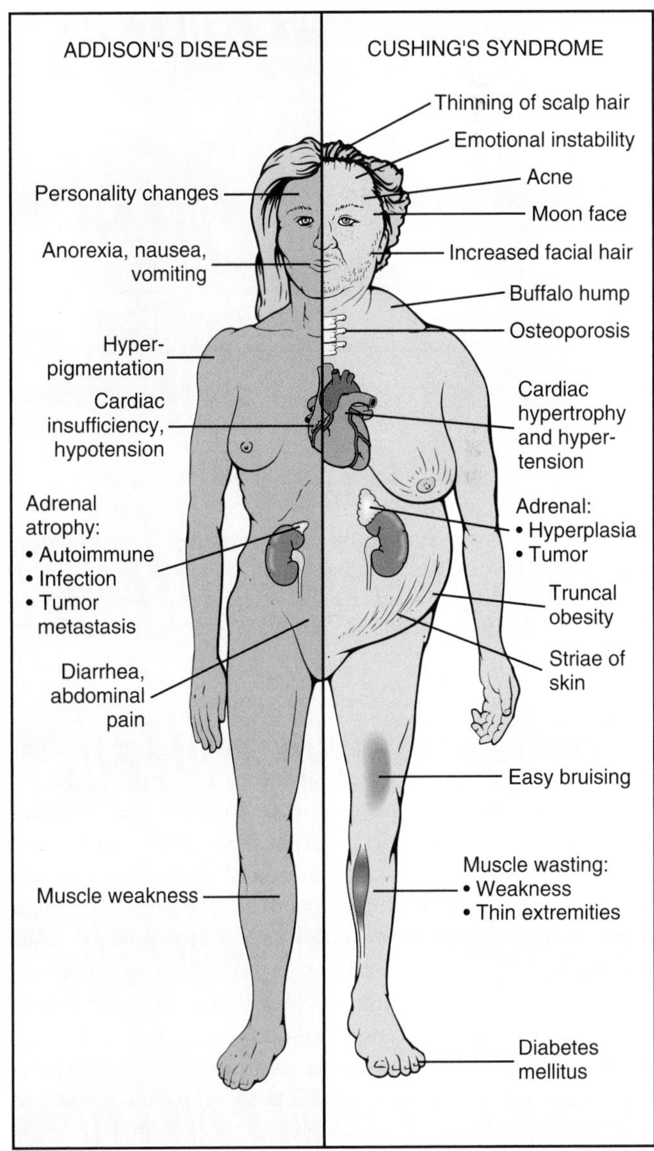

Fig. 22.18 Symptoms of Addison and Cushing Diseases. (From Goodman CC, Kelly Snyder TE. *Differential diagnosis for physical therapists*, 5th edition. Philadelphia: Saunders; 2013.)

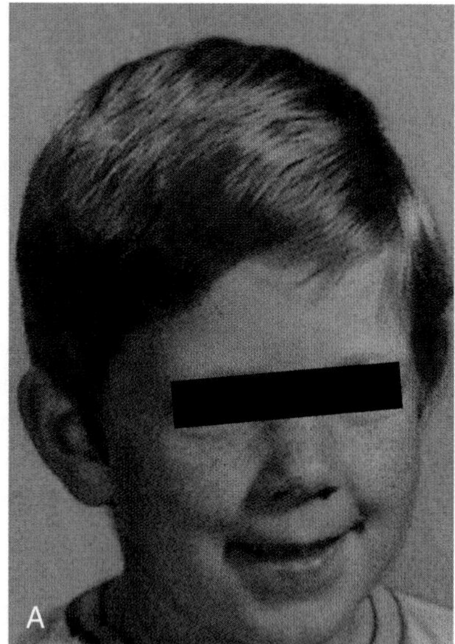

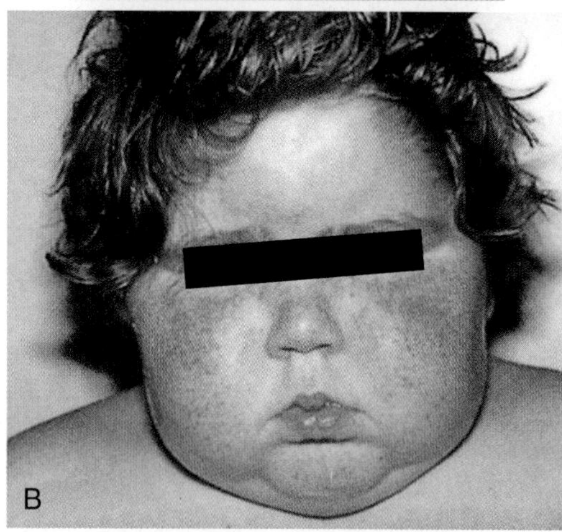

Fig. 22.19 Cushing Syndrome. (A) Individual before onset of Cushing syndrome. **(B)** Individual 4 months later. Moon facies is clearly demonstrated. (From Zitelli BJ, et al. *Zitelli and Davis' atlas of pediatric physical diagnosis,* 6th edition. London: Saunders; 2012.)

In the skin, loss of collagen leads to thin, weakened integumentary tissues through which capillaries are more visible and are easily stretched by adipose deposits. Together, these changes account for the characteristic purple striae seen in the trunk area. Loss of collagenous support around small vessels makes them susceptible to rupture, leading to easy bruising, even with minor trauma. Thin, atrophied skin is also easily damaged, leading to skin breaks and ulcerations. Bronze or brownish hyperpigmentation of the skin, mucous membranes, and hair occurs when there are very high levels of ACTH.

With elevated cortisol levels, vascular sensitivity to catecholamines increases significantly, leading to vasoconstriction and hypertension. Mineralocorticoid effects promote hypokalemia and sodium and water retention with transient weight gain. Suppression of the immune system and increased susceptibility to infections also occur. Approximately 50% of individuals with Cushing syndrome experience irritability and depression, disturbed sleep, difficulty concentrating, memory loss, and, rarely, schizophrenia-like psychosis. Females with ACTH-dependent hypercortisolism may experience symptoms of increased adrenal androgen levels (virilism), with increased hair growth (especially facial hair), acne, and oligomenorrhea. Rarely, unless an adrenal carcinoma is involved, do androgen levels become high enough to cause changes of the voice, recession of the hairline, and hypertrophy of the clitoris.

Evaluation and Treatment. Routine laboratory examinations may reveal hyperglycemia, glycosuria, hypokalemia, and metabolic alkalosis. A variety of laboratory tests are used to confirm the diagnosis of hypercortisolism and to determine the underlying disorder. These include serum and urinary cortisol levels, serum ACTH levels, and dexamethasone suppression testing. Late-evening salivary cortisol levels are used as a screening. Tumors are diagnosed using imaging procedures.

Treatment is specific for the cause of hypercorticoadrenalism and includes surgery, medication, and radiation. Differentiation between pituitary, ectopic, and adrenal causes is essential for effective treatment. Without treatment, individuals with Cushing syndrome have a high risk for developing overwhelming infection and significant complications from generalized arteriosclerosis and hypertensive disease.

Congenital Adrenal Hyperplasia

Congenital adrenal hyperplasia results from an inherited deficiency of an enzyme that is critical in cortisol biosynthesis in the adrenal gland. Because cortisol is not produced efficiently, the concentration of ACTH increases and causes adrenal hyperplasia, which results in the overproduction of mineralocorticoids or androgens, or both. The most common form is a 21-hydroxylase deficiency, which involves both mineralocorticoid and cortisol synthesis. Affected female children are virilized, and infants of both sexes exhibit salt wasting. Prenatal diagnosis is available, and treatment guidelines have been developed. Disease management requires treatment with glucocorticoids and mineralocorticoids and management of sex steroid excess.

Hyperaldosteronism

Hyperaldosteronism is characterized by excessive adrenal secretion of aldosterone. Both primary and secondary forms of hyperaldosteronism can occur.

Primary hyperaldosteronism (Conn syndrome, primary aldosteronism) is caused by excessive secretion of aldosterone from an abnormality of the adrenal cortex, usually a single benign aldosterone-producing adrenal adenoma.[43,44] Bilateral adrenal nodular hyperplasia and adrenal carcinomas account for the remainder of cases.

Secondary hyperaldosteronism results from an extra-adrenal stimulus of aldosterone secretion, most often through the secretion of excess angiotensin II in response to decreased circulating blood volume (e.g., in dehydration, shock, or hypoalbuminemia) and decreased delivery of blood to the kidneys (e.g., renal artery stenosis, heart failure, or hepatic cirrhosis).

Here, the activation of the renin-angiotensin system and subsequent aldosterone secretion may be seen as compensatory, although in some instances (e.g., congestive heart failure) the increased circulating volume further worsens the condition. Other causes of secondary hyperaldosteronism are Bartter syndrome, a renal tubular defect causing hypokalemia, and renin-secreting tumors of the kidney.

Pathophysiology. In *primary hyperaldosteronism*, pathophysiologic alterations are caused by excessive aldosterone secretion and the fluid and electrolyte imbalances that ensue. Hyperaldosteronism promotes (1) increased renal sodium and water reabsorption with corresponding hypervolemia (see Chapter 3) and hypertension and (2) renal excretion of hydrogen and potassium (see Chapter 3). The extracellular fluid volume overload, hypertension, and suppression of renin secretion are characteristic of primary disorders. Hypokalemic alkalosis, changes in myocardial conduction, and skeletal muscle weakness may be seen, particularly with severe potassium depletion.

In *secondary hyperaldosteronism*, renin secretion is stimulated by pressure-initiated cellular changes at the juxtaglomerular apparatus (see Chapter 37). This leads to an increase in angiotensin II and aldosterone with sodium and water retention and increased circulating blood volume.

Clinical Manifestations. Hypertension, hypokalemia, and hypervolemia are the hallmarks of primary hyperaldosteronism, and renin levels are suppressed. Hypertension is resistant to treatment and can lead to the development of left ventricular dilation and hypertrophy, vascular disease, and kidney disease. Edema is often absent.

Evaluation and Treatment. Various clinical and laboratory evaluations are useful in assessing hyperaldosteronism:

1. Measurement of blood pressure: hypertension is usually present.
2. Serum and urinary electrolyte levels: hypernatremia and metabolic alkalosis may be present.
3. Plasma aldosterone-to-renin ratio and aldosterone suppression testing: an increased aldosterone-to-renin ratio is present in primary hyperaldosteronism.
4. Imaging techniques may be used to localize an aldosterone-secreting adenoma.

Treatment includes management of hypertension, hypervolemia, and hypokalemia, most often with aldosterone receptor antagonists, such as spironolactone, eplerenone, or angiotensin-converting enzyme (ACE) inhibitors. If an aldosterone-secreting adenoma is present, it must be surgically removed.

Hypersecretion of Adrenal Androgens and Estrogens

Hypersecretion of adrenal androgens and estrogens may be caused by adrenal tumors (adenomas or carcinomas), Cushing syndrome, or defects in steroid synthesis. The clinical syndrome that is manifested depends on the hormone secreted, the sex of the individual, and the age at which the hypersecretion is initiated. Hypersecretion of estrogens causes feminization, the development of female secondary sex characteristics. Hypersecretion of androgens causes virilization, the development of male secondary sex characteristics (Fig. 22.20).

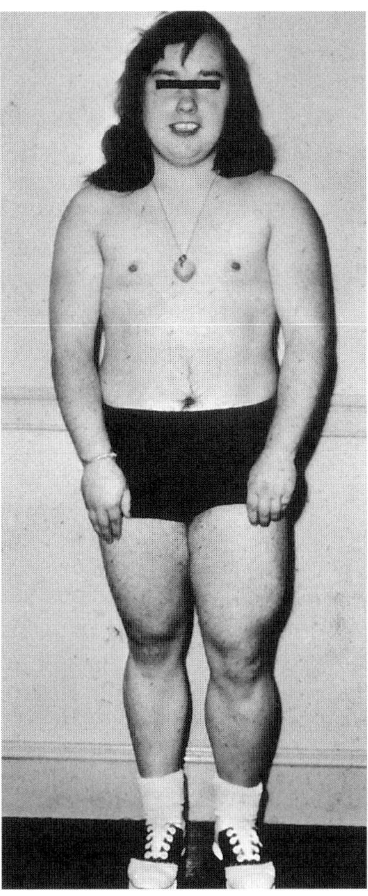

Fig. 22.20 Virilization. Virilization of a young girl by an androgen-secreting tumor of the adrenal cortex. Masculine features include lack of breast development, increased muscle bulk, and hirsutism (excessive hair). (From Thibodeau GA, Patton KT. *The human body in health & disease,* 4th edition. St. Louis: Mosby; 2010.)

The effects of an estrogen-secreting tumor are most evident in males and result in gynecomastia, testicular atrophy, and decreased libido. In female children, such tumors may lead to early development of secondary sex characteristics. The changes caused by an androgen-secreting tumor are more easily observed in females and include excessive face and body hair (hirsutism), clitoral enlargement, deepening of the voice, amenorrhea, acne, and breast atrophy. In children, virilizing tumors promote precocious sexual development and bone aging. Treatment of adrenal tumors usually involves surgical excision.

Adrenocortical Hypofunction

Hypocortisolism (low levels of cortisol secretion) develops either because of inadequate stimulation of the adrenal glands by ACTH or because of a primary inability of the adrenals to produce and secrete the adrenocortical hormones. Sometimes there is partial dysfunction of the adrenal cortex, so only synthesis of cortisol, aldosterone, or the adrenal androgens is affected.

Addison disease. Primary adrenal insufficiency is termed Addison disease. It is relatively rare, occurring most often in adults aged 30 to 60 years, although it may appear at any time.

In the United States, Addison disease is most commonly caused by autoimmune mechanisms that destroy adrenal cortical cells. Chronic infections that affect the adrenal gland, such as tuberculosis, account for the majority of cases of primary adrenal insufficiency in underdeveloped countries.

Pathophysiology. Addison disease is characterized by inadequate corticosteroid and mineralocorticoid synthesis and elevated levels of serum ACTH (loss of negative feedback). Idiopathic Addison disease (organ-specific autoimmune adrenalitis) causes adrenal atrophy and hypofunction and is an organ-specific autoimmune disease resulting from autoantibodies and autoreactive T cells that attach the adrenal cortical cells. It may occur in childhood (type 1) or adulthood (type 2) and is associated with other autoimmune diseases, especially Hashimoto thyroiditis, pernicious anemia, and idiopathic hypoparathyroidism. In some cases, Addison disease may be inherited as an autosomal recessive trait (Mechanisms of inheritance are described in Chapter 4). The adrenal glands in idiopathic Addison disease are smaller than normal and may be misshapen.

Clinical Manifestations. The symptoms of Addison disease are the result of hypocortisolism and hypoaldosteronism and are often nonspecific. With mild to moderate hypocortisolism, symptoms begin with weakness and easy fatigability. Skin changes, including hyperpigmentation and vitiligo, may occur. As the condition progresses, anorexia, nausea, vomiting, and diarrhea may develop. Of greatest concern is the development of hypotension that can progress to complete vascular collapse and shock. This is known as *adrenal crisis*, or Addisonian crisis, and most often develops in individuals who have undiagnosed disease and experience a physiologic stress.

Evaluation and Treatment. Serum and urine levels of cortisol are depressed with primary hypocortisolism, and ACTH levels are increased. Because of dehydration, blood urea nitrogen levels may increase. The serum glucose level is low. Eosinophil and lymphocyte counts often are elevated. Hyperkalemia is seen in Addison disease and may cause mild alkalosis (see Chapter 3). The ACTH stimulation test may be used to evaluate serum cortisol levels.

The treatment of Addison disease involves lifetime glucocorticoid and mineralocorticoid replacement therapy, together with dietary modifications and correction of any underlying disorders. The individual's diet should include at least 150 mEq of sodium per day; sodium intake should be increased if the individual experiences excessive sweating or diarrhea. With acute stressors (e.g., infection, surgery, or trauma), additional cortisol must be administered.

Secondary hypocortisolism. Secondary hypocortisolism commonly results from prolonged administration of exogenous glucocorticoids; they suppress ACTH secretion and cause adrenal atrophy, resulting in inadequate corticosteroidogenesis once the exogenous glucocorticoids are withdrawn. Decreased ACTH secretion also can result from pituitary infarction, pituitary tumors that compress ACTH-secreting cells, or hypophysectomy. In all instances of low ACTH levels, adrenal atrophy occurs, and endogenous adrenal steroidogenesis is depressed. Clinical manifestations of secondary hypocortisolism are similar to those of Addison disease, although hyperpigmentation usually does not occur. The renin-angiotensin system usually is normal, so aldosterone and potassium levels also tend to be normal.

Tumors of the Adrenal Medulla

Hyperfunction of the adrenal medulla is caused by pheochromocytomas (chromaffin cell tumors) or sympathetic paragangliomas of the adrenal medulla. These are rare tumors, but 10% to 20% are malignant and may metastasize. Occurrence is usually sporadic, although nearly half are associated with genetic markers that may be inherited.

Pathophysiology. Pheochromocytomas and sympathetic paragangliomas cause excessive production of norepinephrine, although large tumors secrete both epinephrine and norepinephrine. Approximately 5% of people with these tumors have no symptoms, apparently because the tumor is nonfunctioning. Such tumors can, however, release catecholamines, especially in response to a stressor, such as surgery.

Clinical Manifestations. The clinical manifestations of a pheochromocytoma and sympathetic paragangliomas are related to the chronic effects of catecholamine secretion and include persistent hypertension, headache, pallor, diaphoresis, tachycardia, and palpitations. Hypertension results from increased peripheral vascular resistance and may be sustained or paroxysmal. An acute episode of hypertension related to hypersecretion of catecholamines may follow specific events, such as exercise, excessive ingestion of tyrosine-containing foods (aged cheese, red wine, beer, yogurt), ingestion of caffeine-containing foods, external pressure on the tumor, and induction of anesthesia. Hypertension unresponsive to drug therapy is often the first indication of a pheochromocytoma. Headaches appear because of sudden changes in catecholamine levels in the blood, affecting cerebral blood flow. Hypermetabolism and sweating are related to chronic activation of sympathetic receptors in adipocytes, hepatocytes, and other tissues. Glucose intolerance may occur because of catecholamine-induced inhibition of insulin release by the pancreas. These tumors tend to be extremely vascular and can rupture, causing massive and potentially fatal hemorrhage.

Evaluation and Treatment. Symptoms of pheochromocytoma can be insidious or intermittent and difficult to diagnose. A diagnosis is made when increased catecholamine production is found in the blood or urine. The site of the tumor is then determined using abdominal imaging techniques. Because of the possibility of metastasis, whole-body scanning may be done. Genetic testing can guide therapy.

Management of catecholamine excess is essential to prevent hypertensive emergencies and requires the use of α- and β-adrenergic blockers. The usual treatment of pheochromocytoma is surgical excision of the tumor. Medical therapy is continued to stabilize blood pressure before, during, or after surgery. Malignant pheochromocytoma is rarely curable and is usually managed by a combination of surgical debulking of the tumor combined with chemotherapy.

SUMMARY REVIEW

Mechanisms of Hormonal Alterations

1. Abnormalities in endocrine function may be caused by elevated or depressed hormone levels that result from (1) disorders within glands that cause them to synthesize abnormal amounts of hormone, (2) faulty feedback systems, (3) dysfunctional or ectopically produced hormones, or (4) defects in carrying the hormone in the bloodstream.
2. Target cells may fail to respond to hormones because of (1) cell surface receptor–associated disorders, or (2) intracellular disorders.

Alterations of the Hypothalamic–Pituitary System

1. Dysfunction in the action of hypothalamic hormones is most commonly related to interruption of the connection between the hypothalamus and pituitary—the pituitary stalk.
2. Disorders of the posterior pituitary include syndrome of inappropriate antidiuretic hormone (ADH) secretion (SIADH) and diabetes insipidus. SIADH is characterized by abnormally high ADH secretion; diabetes insipidus is characterized by abnormally low ADH secretion.
3. In SIADH, high ADH levels cause retention of excess free water, leading to hyponatremia and hypoosmolality. SIADH is caused by ectopic production of ADH by tumors, surgical procedures, pulmonary disorders, and central nervous system disorders.
4. Diabetes insipidus may be neurogenic, also known as central (caused by insufficient amounts of ADH), or nephrogenic (caused by an inadequate response to ADH). Low ADH results in excess free water loss leading to hypernatremia and hyperosmolality. Its principal clinical features are polyuria and polydipsia.
5. Diseases of the anterior pituitary include hypopituitarism, hyperpituitarism, acromegaly, and prolactinoma.
6. Hypopituitarism is characterized by the absence of anterior pituitary hormones or the complete failure of all anterior pituitary hormone functions. The most common causes of hypopituitarism are pituitary infarction or space-occupying lesions.
7. Hypopituitarism can affect any or all of the pituitary hormones and symptoms may range from mild to life-threatening, depending on the hormone affected. Adrenocorticotropic hormone (ACTH) deficiency is a potentially life-threatening disorder. Growth hormone (GH) deficiency causes increased body fat, decreased muscle mass, and psychologic problems in adults, and hypopituitary dwarfism in children.
8. Hyperpituitarism is caused by pituitary neuroendocrine tumors. These are usually benign, slow-growing tumors that arise from cells of the anterior pituitary.
9. Expansion of a pituitary neuroendocrine tumor causes both neurologic and secretory effects. Pressure from the expanding tumor causes hyposecretion of surrounding cells, dysfunction of the optic chiasma (leading to visual disturbances), dysfunction of the hypothalamus, and some cranial nerves.
10. Hypersecretion of GH in adults causes acromegaly and is most commonly the result of a pituitary neuroendocrine tumor. Prolonged, abnormally high levels of GH lead to proliferation of body and connective tissue and slowly developing renal, thyroid, and reproductive dysfunction.
11. Excessive GH secretion in children with open epiphyseal plates causes giantism.
12. Prolactinomas, pituitary tumors that secrete prolactin, result in galactorrhea, hirsutism, amenorrhea, hypogonadism, and osteopenia.

Alterations of Thyroid Function

1. Alterations in thyroid function can be primary or secondary. Primary thyroid diseases are caused by dysfunction or disease of the thyroid gland, usually the result of autoimmunity, leading to either increased or decreased thyroid hormone (TH) levels. Secondary thyroid disorders are related to disorders of pituitary gland thyroid-stimulating hormone (TSH) function.
2. Thyrotoxicosis is a general condition resulting from elevated TH levels. Hyperthyroidism is defined as excessive secretion of TH from the thyroid gland. Common clinical manifestations include increased metabolic rate, heat intolerance, and weight loss.
3. Graves disease, the most common form of hyperthyroidism, is caused by an autoimmune mechanism that stimulates the TSH receptors on the thyroid gland. It is characterized by thyrotoxicosis and circulating thyroid-stimulating immunoglobulins. The two distinguishing clinical manifestations are ophthalmopathy and dermopathy (pretibial myxedema).
4. Toxic nodular goiter and toxic multinodular goiter occur when there are independently functioning follicular cells that form adenomas, which produce excessive TH.
5. Thyrotoxic crisis is a severe form of hyperthyroidism that is often associated with physiologic stress.
6. Hypothyroidism is caused by deficient production of TH by the thyroid gland. Primary hypothyroidism has increased levels of TSH and is caused by autoimmune thyroiditis, loss of thyroid tissue, medications, and iodine deficiency. Secondary hypothyroidism has decreased levels of TSH and is caused by hypothalamic or pituitary dysfunction.
7. Symptoms of hypothyroidism depend on the degree of TH deficiency. Common manifestations include decreased energy metabolism, cold intolerance, decreased heat production, lethargy, and myxedema.
8. Myxedema is a sign of hypothyroidism caused by alterations in connective tissue with water-binding proteins that lead to edema and thickened mucous membranes. Myxedema coma is a severe form of hypothyroidism that may be life-threatening without emergency medical treatment.
9. Autoimmune thyroiditis (Hashimoto disease) is the most common cause of primary hypothyroidism in the United States and involves autoimmune destruction of the thyroid gland and gradual loss of thyroid function.

10. Subacute thyroiditis is a nonbacterial inflammation of the thyroid gland that is often preceded by a viral infection.
11. Postpartum thyroiditis generally occurs up to 6 months after giving birth. Iatrogenic hypothyroidism results from ablation of the thyroid gland during treatment for hyperthyroid conditions.
12. Congenital hypothyroidism is the absence of thyroid tissue during fetal development or defects in hormone synthesis and, if untreated, can lead to severe physical and cognitive disorders.
13. Thyroid carcinoma is associated with exposure to ionizing radiation, especially in childhood.

Alterations of Parathyroid Function

1. Hyperparathyroidism, which may be primary, secondary, or tertiary, is characterized by greater than normal secretion of parathyroid hormone (PTH). Hyperparathyroidism leads to neuromuscular symptoms, bone damage, and renal stones.
2. Primary hyperparathyroidism is caused by an interruption of the normal mechanisms that regulate calcium and PTH levels. Hallmark manifestations include hypercalcemia and hypophosphatemia.
3. Secondary hyperparathyroidism is a compensatory response to hypocalcemia and often occurs with chronic renal failure and vitamin D deficiency.
4. Tertiary hyperparathyroidism develops after long-standing hypocalcemia, especially in individuals undergoing renal dialysis or transplantation.
5. Hypoparathyroidism, defined by abnormally low PTH levels, is caused by thyroid surgery, autoimmunity, or genetic mechanisms.
6. The lack of circulating PTH in hypoparathyroidism causes hypocalcemia, hyperphosphatemia, and decreased bone resorption.

Dysfunction of the Endocrine Pancreas: Diabetes Mellitus

1. Diabetes mellitus is a group of metabolic diseases characterized by hyperglycemia resulting from defects in insulin secretion, insulin action, or both.
2. A diagnosis of diabetes mellitus is based on elevated plasma glucose concentrations and measurement of glycated hemoglobin. Classic signs and symptoms are often present as well.
3. Diabetes mellitus is classified as type 1, type 2, or gestational.
4. Diabetes mellitus type 1 is caused by autoimmune β-cell destruction, usually leading to absolute insulin deficiency. It is characterized by loss of β cells, presence of islet cell antibodies, lack of insulin, excess of glucagon, and altered metabolism of fat, protein, and carbohydrates.
5. In diabetes mellitus type 1, hyperglycemia causes polyuria and polydipsia resulting from osmotic diuresis. Hypoglycemia and diabetic ketoacidosis may be seen.
6. Diabetes mellitus type 2 is caused by progressive loss of β-cell insulin secretion frequently on the background of insulin resistance. Genetic susceptibility is triggered by environmental factors. The most compelling environmental risk factor for type 2 diabetes is obesity.
7. In the obese, many factors, including metabolic syndrome, altered adipokines, increased fatty acids, inflammation, and hyperinsulinemia, contribute to the development of insulin resistance and hyperglycemia.
8. Early in the course of diabetes mellitus type 2, hyperinsulinemia occurs in order to overcome underlying insulin resistance. Over time, however, the weight and number of β cells decrease, and insulin levels decline. There also are decreased levels of amylin, ghrelin, and incretins and glucagon concentration is increased. All contribute to chronic hyperglycemia.
9. Gestational diabetes is glucose intolerance diagnosed during the second or third trimester of pregnancy.
10. The category other specific types of diabetes include monogenetic forms of diabetes called maturity-onset diabetes of youth (MODY).
11. Acute complications of diabetes mellitus include hypoglycemia, diabetic ketoacidosis, and hyperosmolar hyperglycemic nonketotic syndrome.
12. Hypoglycemia in diabetes is a complication related to insulin treatment.
13. Diabetic ketoacidosis (DKA) develops when there is an absolute or relative deficiency of insulin and an increase in the insulin counterregulatory hormones of catecholamines—cortisol, glucagon, and growth hormone. DKA presents with hyperglycemia, acidosis, and ketonuria.
14. Hyperosmolar hyperglycemic nonketotic syndrome is pathophysiologically similar to DKA, although a lack of ketosis resulting in acidosis indicates some level of insulin action. Severe dehydration and electrolyte imbalance are present.
15. Chronic complications of diabetes mellitus include microvascular disease (e.g., neuropathy, retinopathy, nephropathy), macrovascular disease (e.g., coronary artery disease, stroke, peripheral vascular disease), and infection.
16. Microvascular disease is characterized by obstruction of capillaries and decreased tissue perfusion.
17. Macrovascular disease associated with diabetes mellitus is most often related to the proliferation of atherosclerotic plaques in the arterial wall.
18. The incidence of coronary heart disease, peripheral vascular disease, and stroke is greater in those with diabetes than in nondiabetic individuals.
19. Individuals with diabetes are at risk for a variety of infections. Infection may be related to sensory impairment and resulting injury, hypoxia, increased proliferation of pathogens in elevated concentrations of glucose, decreased blood supply associated with vascular damage, and impaired immune protection.

Alterations of Adrenal Function

1. Disorders of the adrenal cortex are related to hyperfunction (secreting too much hormone) or hypofunction (secreting too little hormone).
2. Increased secretion of cortisol (hypercortisolism) is usually caused by Cushing disease (pituitary-dependent) and very rarely can be caused by ectopic production of ACTH. Complications include obesity, diabetes, protein wasting, immune suppression, and mental status changes.

3. Congenital adrenal hyperplasia is a genetic disorder with overproduction of mineralocorticoids or androgens, or both.
4. Excessive aldosterone secretion causes hyperaldosteronism, which may be primary or secondary. Primary hyperaldosteronism is caused by an abnormality of the adrenal cortex. Secondary hyperaldosteronism involves renin and angiotensin secretion in response to renal underperfusion.
5. Hyperaldosteronism promotes increased sodium reabsorption (with corresponding hypervolemia), increased extracellular volume (which is variable), hypokalemia related to renal reabsorption of sodium, and excretion of potassium.
6. Hypersecretion of adrenal androgens and estrogens can be a result of adrenal tumors, either adenomas or carcinomas; Cushing syndrome; or defects in steroid synthesis. Hypersecretion of estrogens causes feminization, the development of female secondary sexual characteristics. Hypersecretion of androgens causes virilization, the development of male secondary sexual characteristics.
7. Hypocortisolism, or low levels of cortisol, is caused secondarily by inadequate adrenal stimulation by ACTH or because of primary adrenal insufficiency, termed Addison disease.
8. Addison disease is characterized by elevated ACTH levels with inadequate corticosteroid and mineralocorticoid synthesis.
9. Manifestations of Addison disease are related to hypocortisolism and hypoaldosteronism. Symptoms include weakness, fatigability, hyperpigmentation, vitiligo, anorexia, vomiting, and diarrhea. The development of hypotension can progress to complete vascular collapse and shock, known as adrenal crisis, or Addisonian crisis.
10. Secondary hypocortisolism commonly results from prolonged administration of exogenous glucocorticoids that suppress ACTH secretion. Decreased ACTH secretion also can result from pituitary infarction, pituitary tumors, or hypophysectomy. In all instances of low ACTH levels, adrenal atrophy occurs, and endogenous adrenal steroidogenesis is depressed.
11. Hyperfunction of the adrenal medulla is usually caused by a pheochromocytoma, a catecholamine-producing tumor. Symptoms of catecholamine excess include hypertension, palpitations, tachycardia, glucose intolerance, excessive sweating, and constipation.

REFERENCES

1. Mentrasti G, et al. Syndrome of Inappropriate Antidiuretic Hormone Secretion (SIADH): Optimal Management. *Therapeutics and Clinical Risk Management* (2020)16:663–672.
2. Mentrasti G, et al. Syndrome of inappropriate antidiuretic hormone secretion (SIADH): optimal management. *Ther Clin Risk Manag*. 2020;16:663–672.
3. Pintaldi S, et al. SIADH versus adrenal insufficiency: a life-threatening misdiagnosis. *Ital J Pediatr*. 2019;45:23.
4. Jones DP. Syndrome of inappropriate secretion of antidiuretic hormone and hyponatremia. *Pediatr Rev*. 2018;39:27.
5. Kavanagh C, Uy NS. Nephrogenic diabetes insipidus. *Pediatr Clin North Am*. 2019;66(1):227–234.
6. Garrahy A, Moran C, Thompson CJ. Diagnosis and management of central diabetes insipidus in adults. *Clin Endocrinol (Oxf)*. 2019;90(1):23–30.
7. Chung TT, Koch CA, Monson JP. Hypopituitarism. In: Feingold KR, ed. *Endotext [Internet]*. South Dartmouth, MA: MDText.com; 2000. Updated July 25, 2018. Available at https://www.ncbi.nlm.nih.gov/books/NBK278989/. (Accessed September 7, 2021).
8. Lopes MBS. World Health Organization 2017 Classification of Pituitary Tumors. *Endocrinol Metab Clin North Am*. 2020;49(3):375–386.
9. Molitch ME. Diagnosis and treatment of pituitary adenomas: a review. *JAMA*. 2017;317(5):516–524.
10. Drummond J, et al. Clinical and pathological aspects of silent pituitary adenomas. *J Clin Endocrinol Metab*. 2019;104(7):2473–2489.
11. Colao A, et al. Acromegaly. *Nat Rev Dis Primers*. 2019;5(1):20 Published correction appears in *Nat Rev Dis Primers* 5(1):72, 2019.
12. Samperi I, Lithgow K, Karavitaki N. Hyperprolactinaemia. *J Clin Med*. 2019;8(12):2203.
13. Silvia de Morais N, et al. The impact of Hashimoto's thyroiditis on thyroid nodule cytology and risk of thyroid cancer. *J Endocr Soc*. 2019;3(4):791–800.
14. Bartalena L. Graves' disease: complications. In: De Groot LJ, ed. *Endotext [Internet]*. South Dartmouth, MA, 2000, MDText.com; 2000 –. Last update February 20, 2018. Available at http://www.ncbi.nlm.nih.gov/books/NBK285551/. (Accessed September 7, 2021).
15. Bobanga ID, McHenry CR. Treatment of patients with Graves' disease and the appropriate extent of thyroidectomy. *Best Pract Res Clin Endocrinol Metab*. 2019;33(4):101319.
16. LiVolsi VA, Baloch ZW. The pathology of hyperthyroidism. *Front Endocrinol (Lausanne)*. 2018;9:737.
17. Kahaly GJ, et al. 2018 European Thyroid Association Guideline for the Management of Graves' Hyperthyroidism. *Eur Thyroid J*. 2018;7(4):167–186.
18. Kitahara CM, et al. Association of radioactive iodine treatment with cancer mortality in patients with hyperthyroidism. *JAMA Intern Med*. 2019;179(8):1034–1042. Published correction appears in *JAMA Intern Med* 179(8):1152, 2019.
19. Rogers J. Understanding the most commonly billed diagnoses in primary care: hypothyroidism. *Nurse Prac J*. 2020;45(12):36–42.
20. Feller M, et al. Association of thyroid hormone therapy with quality of life and thyroid-related symptoms in patients with subclinical hypothyroidism: a systematic review and meta-analysis. *JAMA*. 2018;320(13):1349–1359.
21. Yang L, et al. Circulating Angplt3 and Angptl8 are increased in patients with hypothyroidism. *Biomed Res Int*. 2019;2019:3814687.
22. American Cancer Society (ACS): *Cancer Facts and Figures 2021*, Atlanta, GA: ACS; 2019. Available at https://www.cancer.org/content/dam/cancer-org/research/cancer-facts-and-statistics/annual-cancer-facts-and-figures/2021/cancer-facts-and-figures-2021.pdf. (Accessed September 7, 2021).
23. Choudhury PS, Gupta M. Differentiated thyroid cancer theranostics: radioiodine and beyond. *Br J Radiol*. 2018;91(1091):20180136.

24. Walker MD, Silverberg SJ. Primary hyperparathyroidism. *Nat Rev Endocrinol.* 2018;14(2):115–125.
25. Centers for Disease Control and Prevention (CDC): *National Diabetes Statistics Report, 2020.* Atlanta, GA: CDC; 2020. Page last reviewed August 28, 2020. Available at https://www.cdc.gov/diabetes/data/statistics/statistics-report.html. (Accessed September 7, 2021).
26. American Diabetes Association Standards of medical care in diabetes—2020. *Diabetes Care.* 2020;43(Suppl. 1):S1–S212. Available at https://care.diabetesjournals.org/content/diacare/suppl/2019/12/20/43.Supplement_1.DC1/Standards_of_Care_2020.pdf. (Accessed September 7, 2021).
27. Bellou V, et al. Risk factors for type 2 diabetes mellitus: an exposure-wide umbrella review of meta-analyses. *PLoS One.* 2018;13(3):e0194127.
28. Pivari F, et al. Curcumin and type 2 diabetes mellitus: prevention and treatment. *Nutrients.* 2019;11(8):1837.
29. Luc K, et al. Oxidative stress and inflammatory markers in prediabetes and diabetes. *J Physiol Pharmacol.* 2019;70(6):809–824.
30. Stehouwer CDA. Microvascular dysfunction and hyperglycemia: a vicious cycle with widespread consequences. *Diabetes.* 2018;67(9):1729–1741.
31. Rogers J, Allen J. Understanding the most commonly billed diagnoses in primary care: diabetes mellitus type 2. *Nurse Pract.* 2020;45(9):48–54.
32. Plows JF, et al. The pathophysiology of gestational diabetes mellitus. *Int J Mol Sci.* 2018;19(11):3342.
33. Baldrighi M, et al. Hyperglycemic hyperosmolar state: a pragmatic approach to properly manage sodium derangements. *Curr Diabetes Rev.* 2018;14(6):534–541.
34. Paul S, Ali A, Katare R. Molecular complexities underlying the vascular complications of diabetes mellitus – a comprehensive review. *J Diabetes Complications.* 2020;34(8):107613.
35. Gardner TW, Davila JR. The neurovascular unit and the pathophysiologic basis of diabetic retinopathy. *Graefes Arch Clin Exp Ophthalmol.* 2017;255(1):1–6.
36. Lin YC, et al. Update of pathophysiology and management of diabetic kidney disease. *J Formos Med Assoc.* 2018;117(8):662–675.
37. Yu SM, Bonventre JV. Acute kidney injury and progression of diabetic kidney disease. *Adv Chronic Kidney Dis.* 2018;25(2):166–180.
38. Juster-Switlyk K, Smith AG. Updates in diabetic peripheral neuropathy. *F1000Res.* 2016;5(F1000 Faculty Rev):738 Available at https://doi.org/10.12688/f1000research.7898.1. (Accessed September 7, 2021).
39. Azmi S, et al: An update on the diagnosis and treatment of diabetic somatic and autonomic neuropathy. *F1000Res* 8(F1000 Faculty Rev):186. Available at https://doi.org/10.12688/f1000research.17118.1. (Accessed September 7, 2021).
40. Akash MSH, et al. Diabetes-associated infections: development of antimicrobial resistance and possible treatment strategies. *Arch Microbiol.* 2020;202(5):953–965.
41. Castinetti F, et al. Cushing's disease. *Orphanet J Rare Dis.* 2012;7:41.
42. Nishioka H, Yamada S. Cushings disease. *J Clin Med.* 2019;8(11):1951.
43. Gyamlani G, et al. Primary aldosteronism: diagnosis and management. *Am J Med Sci.* 2016;352(4):391–398.
44. Vaidya A, et al. The expanding spectrum of primary aldosteronism: implications for diagnosis, pathogenesis, and treatment. *Endocr Rev.* 2018;39(6):1057–1088.

23

Obesity, Starvation, and Anorexia of Aging

Jodi A. Allen and Julia L. Rogers

http://evolve.elsevier.com/Rogers/pathophysiology/

CHAPTER OUTLINE

Obesity is one of the most common and costly chronic diseases in the world. The causes are complex, multifactorial, and associated with an increased risk of many comorbid diseases. Alternatively, starvation and anorexia of aging also are common conditions. This chapter presents an overview of the function of adipose tissue and the pathophysiology of obesity, starvation, and anorexia of aging.

ADIPOSE TISSUE

Adipose tissue provides insulation and mechanical support, secretes hormone like signaling molecules known as *adipokines*, and contributes to immune cell function. It is the body's major energy reserve to fuel other tissues. Adipocytes are fat-storing cells that store calories in the form of triglycerides (triglycerol), synthesize triglycerides from glucose, and mobilize energy in the form of free fatty acids (FFAs) and glycerol. Adipose tissue is classified according to color as white adipose tissue (WAT), brown adipose tissue (BAT), and beige adipose tissue (bAT). These tissue types are found in different locations within the body and have different functions.[1] Most adipose tissue in the body is WAT.

White adipocytes, which are derived from connective tissue, are located in visceral (central) and subcutaneous (peripheral) stores of WAT. WAT also is found in muscle, providing mechanical protection and sliding of muscle bundles, as well as in bone marrow. WAT contains various cells, including macrophages, mast cells, neutrophils, fibroblasts, endothelial cells, blood vessels, nerves, and precursor adipocytes. White adipocytes contain a single triglyceride fat droplet or vacuole. A low nutritional state, stimulation of the beta adrenergic sympathetic nervous system and release of catecholamines (epinephrine and norepinephrine), activates lipolysis in WAT to release FFAs and glycerol into the circulation. FFAs and glycerol can then be used for energy metabolism.

Subcutaneous or peripheral adipose tissue expands by increased adipocyte size (hypertrophy) and number (hyperplasia).[2] The alterations in precursor cell commitment and subcutaneous adipose tissue adipogenesis are associated with metabolic complications of obesity. Adipogenesis is the formation of new fat cells from preadipocytes. These adipocytes are smaller and have a greater fat storage capacity. Subcutaneous fat has higher leptin production, lower adiponectin production, lower production of inflammatory cytokines, and lower association with insulin resistance. Expansion of subcutaneous fat is a healthier expansion of fat tissue and is associated with fewer complications of obesity.

Visceral adipose tissue is located in the abdomen and surrounding intra-abdominal organs. Visceral WAT is more likely to store fat by adipocyte hypertrophy. Visceral adipocytes store fat as triglycerides, primarily in the form of very-low-density lipoprotein (VLDL), derived from hepatic and dietary sources. Visceral fat is more hormonally active than subcutaneous fat and releases leptin and inflammatory mediators. Excess visceral fat is associated with impaired lipid and glucose metabolism, insulin resistance, metabolic syndrome, and an increased risk of cardiovascular disease and cancer.[1] Thus, the complications of obesity are related to where fat is stored, not just the accumulation of fat stores.

Estrogen and estrogen receptors have a role in fat metabolism. They enhance the deposition of WAT in the subcutaneous tissue and inhibit it in visceral tissue. This may explain the higher incidence of peripheral obesity among premenopausal women and the increase in central obesity with menopause and in men.[3]

Bone marrow adipose tissue (MAT) is found in all bones, and it increases with obesity and age in long bones. With obesity, MAT releases adipokines that affect osteoblast and osteoclast function and alters hematopoiesis. In general, excessive MAT is associated with osteoporosis and fractures.[4]

Brown adipocytes form BAT and are derived from muscle tissue and have multiple lipid droplets. They are rich in mitochondria that contain iron, which gives them a brown color. Exposure to cold, activation of the sympathetic nervous system, catecholamines, and activation of triiodothyronine (T_3) stimulate BAT to generate heat rapidly through the oxidation of FFAs, acids, and glucose. This is known as *nonshivering thermogenesis;* it occurs at a rate 50-fold greater than in WAT and protects against obesity and metabolic syndrome.[5] Estrogen-related receptors also participate in nonshivering thermogenesis in BAT.[6] Neonates generate body heat from BAT primarily located in the interscapular and perirenal regions. It traditionally was thought that BAT did not persist into adult life. However, positron emission tomography (PET) scanning has shown that adults also have BAT. It is most common in lean individuals, usually located in the neck, supraclavicular, axillary, paravertebral, and mediastinal regions.[7]

There is an inverse relationship between the amount of BAT and both body mass index (BMI) and age. Interindividual differences in BAT-mediated thermogenesis may explain some of the variability in obesity susceptibility and the increased prevalence of obesity with aging. Variation in BAT and bAT also may be factors in the natural regulation of weight reduction.

Located within WAT, particularly in subcutaneous fat stores, are beige—or "brite" (from "brown in white")—adipocytes that form bAT. Beige adipocytes are a subpopulation of white adipocytes that also contain multiple mitochondria but not in the numbers associated with BAT. Beige adipocytes emerge within WAT with chronic exposure to cold and exercise, produce heat, and increase energy expenditure. This is known as the *beiging* or *browning* of WAT. The bAT disappear with elevated ambient temperatures and with warm adaptation revert to WAT.[8] Leptin and insulin together promote bAT, increasing energy expenditure and weight loss. bAT is diminished in obesity. Because the beiging (browning) of adipose tissue protects against obesity and metabolic syndrome, efforts are in progress to discover whether there is a therapeutic way to stimulate the synthesis and activity of BAT and bAT as an approach to preventing or treating obesity and diabetes mellitus.[9]

Adipose Tissue as an Endocrine Organ

Adipose tissue is an endocrine organ, and adipocytes secrete adipokines. Adipokines are cell-signaling proteins that function like hormones, having autocrine, paracrine, and endocrine actions. Adipokines include all the biologically active substances synthesized by WAT. They are necessary for numerous functions in body tissues.[10] These substances function in the regulation of appetite, food intake and energy expenditure, lipid storage, insulin secretion and sensitivity, immune and inflammatory responses, coagulation, fibrinolysis, angiogenesis, fertility, vascular homeostasis, blood pressure regulation, and bone metabolism. Excess WAT causes dysregulation of the secretion and function of adipokines, contributing to the many complications of obesity.

Adipokines are important to understand because they are targets of both experimental and currently available drugs and weight loss programs used to treat obesity and its complications. Examples of adipokines are provided as a reference in Box 23.1 (a summary of adipokines and their role in caloric intake, energy metabolism, and obesity is presented later in this chapter). The regulation of food intake and energy balance is summarized next.

Regulation of Food Intake and Energy Balance

Regulation of food intake and energy balance is a complex process controlled by central and peripheral physiological signals.[11] Centrally, the arcuate nucleus (ARC) in the hypothalamus regulates food intake and energy metabolism by balancing the opposing effects of two sets of neurons. One set of neurons promotes appetite, stimulates eating, and decreases metabolism (anabolic). These are known as *orexigenic neurons*, which are stimulated by molecules called *orexins*. Another set of neurons suppresses appetite, inhibits eating, and increases metabolism. These are known as *anorexigenic neurons*, which are stimulated by molecules called *anorexins*. The hypothalamic orexin and anorexin signaling pathways are transmitted through the autonomic nervous and endocrine systems to regulate and balance appetite, food intake, energy metabolism, and body temperature. The hypothalamus also communicates with higher brain centers related to reward, pleasure, memory, and addictive behavior. These higher centers can override hypothalamic control of food intake and satiety, which increases consumption of highly palatable foods and results in increased fat stores.[12] Peripherally, the gastrointestinal tract secretes a number of hormones (Box 23.2) that also control hunger and satiety. In addition, adipokines can function as orexins or anorexins and provide peripheral signals for the control of food intake and energy expenditure. They are described in the Adipokines and Obesity section later in the chapter.

OBESITY

Obesity is an increase in body adipose tissue and an endocrine and metabolic disorder that has become epidemic worldwide. Obesity is defined differently in adults and children. In adults, it is a BMI that exceeds 30 kg/m^2. In children, it is a BMI greater than or equal to the age- and sex-specific 95th percentile of the growth charts published in 2000 by the Centers for Disease Control and Prevention (CDC).[13]

Obesity develops when caloric intake exceeds caloric expenditure in genetically susceptible individuals. Between 2017 and 2018, the prevalence of obesity among U.S. adults was 42.4% and 19.3% among children and adolescents between ages 2 and 19 years.[14,15] Children tend to become obese adults. Ethnic differences also are seen in the rates of obesity: Hispanics (44.8%), non-Hispanic blacks (49.6%), non-Hispanic whites (42.2%), and non-Hispanic Asians (17.4%).[15]

BOX 23.1 Examples of Adipokines Secreted by Adipose Tissue

Adipokines

Increased in Obesity

Leptin (Leptin Resistance)

Inhibits appetite and stimulates energy expenditure

Satiety (hunger/appetite suppression) and regulation of eating behavior by hypothalamus

Sympathoactivation

Insulin sensitizing in liver and skeletal muscle

Modulating role in reproduction, angiogenesis, immune response, blood pressure control, and osteogenesis

Promotes inflammation (a harmful effect)

Angiopoietin-Related Protein 2 (a Vascular Endothelial Growth Factor)

Insulin resistance

Promotes inflammation

Angiotensinogen, Angiotensin Type 1 and Type 1 Receptors, Renin, and Angiotensin-Converting Enzyme

Vasoconstriction

Inflammation

Lipogenesis

Insulin resistance

Retinol-Binding Protein 4 (RBP4) (From Visceral White Adipose Tissue [WAT]; Role Not Clear)

Promotes insulin resistance in muscle

Promotes angiogenesis

Visfatin (From Visceral WAT)

Mimics insulin, binds to insulin receptors, and promotes insulin sensitivity

Promotes adhesion of monocytes to endothelial cells and promotes plaque instability (harmful in cardiac disease)

Decreased in Obesity

Adiponectin

Insulin sensitizing

Anti-inflammatory

Antiatherogenic

Apelin

Improves insulin sensitivity in muscle

Promotes vasodilation by blocking angiotensin

Promotes cardiac contractility

Proinflammatory Cytokines (Increased in Obesity)

Interleukin-6

Promotes insulin resistance

Inhibits adipogenesis

Decreases adiponectin secretion

Promotes inflammation

Monocyte Chemoattractant Protein 1

Attracts macrophages

Promotes insulin resistance

Promotes atherogenesis

Macrophage Products

Plasminogen activator inhibitor 1 (from visceral WAT)

Promotes clot formation (inhibits fibrinolysis) by inhibiting tissue plasminogen activator and urokinase (also released by endothelial cells)

Promotes insulin resistance

Prostaglandin E2 and leukotriene B4

Promotes inflammation

Tumor necrosis factor-alpha

Promotes insulin resistance

Promotes inflammation

Data from Giralt M, Cereijo R, Villarroya F. Adipokines and the endocrine role of adipose tissues. *Handbook of Experimental Pharmacology*, 2016;233:265–282; Luo L, Liu M. Adipose tissue in control of metabolism. *Journal of Endocrinology*, 2016;231(3):R77–R99.

BOX 23.2 Gastrointestinal Hormones and Obesity

Ghrelin: Stomach (decreased in obesity, but increased after eating; role in obesity not clear)
Stimulates hunger and controls gastric motility and acid secretion, stimulates growth hormone

Glucagon-like peptide 1 (GLP-1): Large intestine (decreased in obesity)
Stimulates insulin secretion; inhibits glucagon release; slows gastric emptying to reduce postprandial hyperglycemia, increases satiety

Peptide YY: Small intestine (decreased in obesity)
Reduces appetite, inhibits gastric motility, increases energy expenditure

Cholecystokinin: Small intestine (probably increased in obesity)
Increases satiation; reduces food intake; stimulates gallbladder contraction, release of pancreatic enzymes and insulin; slows gastric emptying

Obesity is the fifth leading cause of death globally and accounts for high health care costs worldwide.[16] Three leading causes of death in the United States are associated with obesity: cardiovascular disease, type 2 diabetes mellitus, and cancer (liver, advanced prostate, ovarian, gallbladder, kidney, colorectal, esophageal, postmenopausal breast, pancreatic, endometrial, and stomach).[17] Obesity is also a risk factor for hypertension, stroke, hyperlipidemia, gallstones, nonalcoholic steatohepatitis (NASH), gastroesophageal reflux, hiatal hernia, osteoarthritis, infectious disease, asthma, obstructive sleep apnea, and chronic kidney disease.[18] However, some studies have shown that mild obesity in older individuals is associated with lower mortality (the obesity paradox), particularly in individuals with hypertension and coronary heart disease, but the mechanisms are not clear.[19] The causes and consequences of obesity are multiple and complex, and rapidly advancing research is underway on the causal mechanisms, complications, and treatment.

Genotype and gene–environment interactions are important predisposing factors. Single-gene defects (monogenic defects)

are rare, and obesity is usually polygenic and associated with other phenotypes, such as endocrine disorders (e.g., diabetes mellitus and hypothyroidism) and intellectual disability (e.g., Down and Prader-Willi syndromes).[20] Metabolic abnormalities that contribute to obesity include Cushing syndrome, Cushing disease, polycystic ovary syndrome, growth hormone (GH) deficiency, hypothyroidism, and hypothalamic injury. Contributing environmental factors include food intake (low nutrient, energy-dense foods), physical inactivity, obesogens, and socioeconomic status (both high and low income). Obesity also is associated with adverse social and psychological consequences, including depression and mood disorders.[21]

Pathophysiology. The pathophysiology of obesity is complex and involves the interaction of peripheral and central neuroendocrine pathways, numerous adipokines, hormones, and neurotransmitters (Fig. 23.1).[22,23] The adipocyte is the cellular basis of obesity. Excess fat is stored in mature white adipocytes when energy balance is positive (excess caloric intake in relation to energy expenditure). These adipocytes undergo hypertrophy and adipogenesis (hyperplasia), store triglycerol, and secrete adipokines. Adipokines circulate in the blood at concentrations that increase or decrease in relation to body fat mass and provide signals to the central nervous system for regulation of hunger, satiety, and energy balance, as described previously. WAT accumulation causes dysfunction in the regulation and interaction of this signaling system and contributes to the complications and consequences of obesity.[24]

Adipokines and Obesity

Leptin is a product of the obesity gene (*Ob* gene) and is expressed primarily by adipocytes. Leptin levels increase after eating and act on the hypothalamus to inhibit orexigenic neurons and stimulate anorexigenic neurons to suppress appetite and increase energy expenditure. At low leptin levels (i.e., during fasting), leptin stimulates food intake and reduces energy expenditure. This balance regulates body weight and energy expenditure within a fairly narrow range. Leptin levels increase as the number of adipocytes increases. However, high leptin levels are ineffective at decreasing appetite and energy expenditure, a condition associated with obesity and known as central *leptin resistance* (Fig. 23.2).

Leptin resistance fails to inhibit orexigenic hypothalamic satiety signaling and promotes overeating and excessive weight gain. Leptin also regulates hepatic gluconeogenesis, insulin sensitivity, and glucose and lipid metabolism in liver, muscle, and adipose tissue. Peripheral leptin resistance (i.e., in muscle and adipose tissue) results in hyperglycemia, hyperinsulinemia, and hyperlipidemia and also stimulates macrophages and endothelial cells to produce proinflammatory mediators. The cause of leptin resistance is unknown. It may be related to a defect in leptin transport, an inability of leptin to cross the blood–brain barrier, an alteration in the permissive effect of leptin, or a defect in or suppression of the leptin receptor. The low-grade inflammation that accompanies obesity also is thought to contribute to leptin resistance. Chronic hyperleptinemia also stimulates the sympathetic nervous system, oxidative stress, chronic low-grade inflammation, and ventricular hypertrophy and contributes to the pathogenesis of hypertension, atherosclerosis, cardiovascular disease, type 2 diabetes, and cancer associated with obesity.[25,26]

Adiponectin, which is produced primarily by visceral adipose tissue but also by cardiomyocytes and skeletal muscle, increases energy expenditure. It also has insulin-sensitizing and anti-inflammatory properties. Plasma levels of adiponectin decrease with visceral obesity, and resistance to adiponectin action develops. Decreased adiponectin levels are associated with increased hepatic gluconeogenesis, insulin resistance, decreased skeletal muscle glucose uptake, and increased levels of inflammatory mediators, such as interleukin-6 (IL-6) and tumor necrosis factor-alpha (TNF-α). Adiponectin serves as an anti-inflammatory and antiatherogenic plasma protein; it also has an important role in vascular remodeling, and it is cardioprotective. Decreased levels of adiponectin are associated with type 2 diabetes mellitus and an increased risk for coronary artery disease resulting from hyperlipidemia, hypertension, and factors that promote thrombosis and inflammation.[27]

Decreased beta cell function and insulin resistance are associated with obesity. The mechanisms are not clear, but an association exists between hyperlipidemia and increased fat storage, macrophages and inflammation, and alterations in adipokines. Leptin resistance and decreased adiponectin also contribute to insulin resistance. Insulin resistance results in hyperinsulinemia, hyperglycemia, and a predisposition to type 2 diabetes mellitus. Retinol-binding protein 4 (binds vitamin A) is an adipokine produced both in the liver and by adipocytes. It is increased in visceral adiposity and contributes to inflammation and insulin resistance in the liver and muscles; it also is associated with cardiovascular disease and may contribute to hepatic steatosis (fatty liver).[28]

Endocannabinoids (i.e., anandamide) are arachidonic acid derivatives (unsaturated, essential fatty acids) expressed in both the brain and peripheral nerve tissues. They have effects on endocannabinoid (CB) receptors in orexigenic pathways. They increase appetite, enhance nutrient absorption, stimulate lipogenesis, and increase WAT accumulation by acting at both central (CB1 receptor) and peripheral sites (CB2 receptor). They also inhibit energy expenditure and thermogenesis. An increase in endocannabinoids is proposed to be associated with visceral obesity.[29] Angiotensinogen (AGT) is produced in the liver and by adipocytes and is increased in obesity. AGT is the precursor to angiotensin 1 (AGTI), which is then converted to angiotensin 2 (AGTII). The effects of AGTII include vasoconstriction, renal retention of sodium and water, and release of aldosterone. Increased AGTII from adipose tissue also promotes lipogenesis, oxidative stress, inflammation, and insulin resistance. All of these effects contribute to the complications associated with obesity.[30] Gastrointestinal hormones also play a role in the complex pathophysiology of obesity (see Box 23.2). The most significant ones are reviewed next.

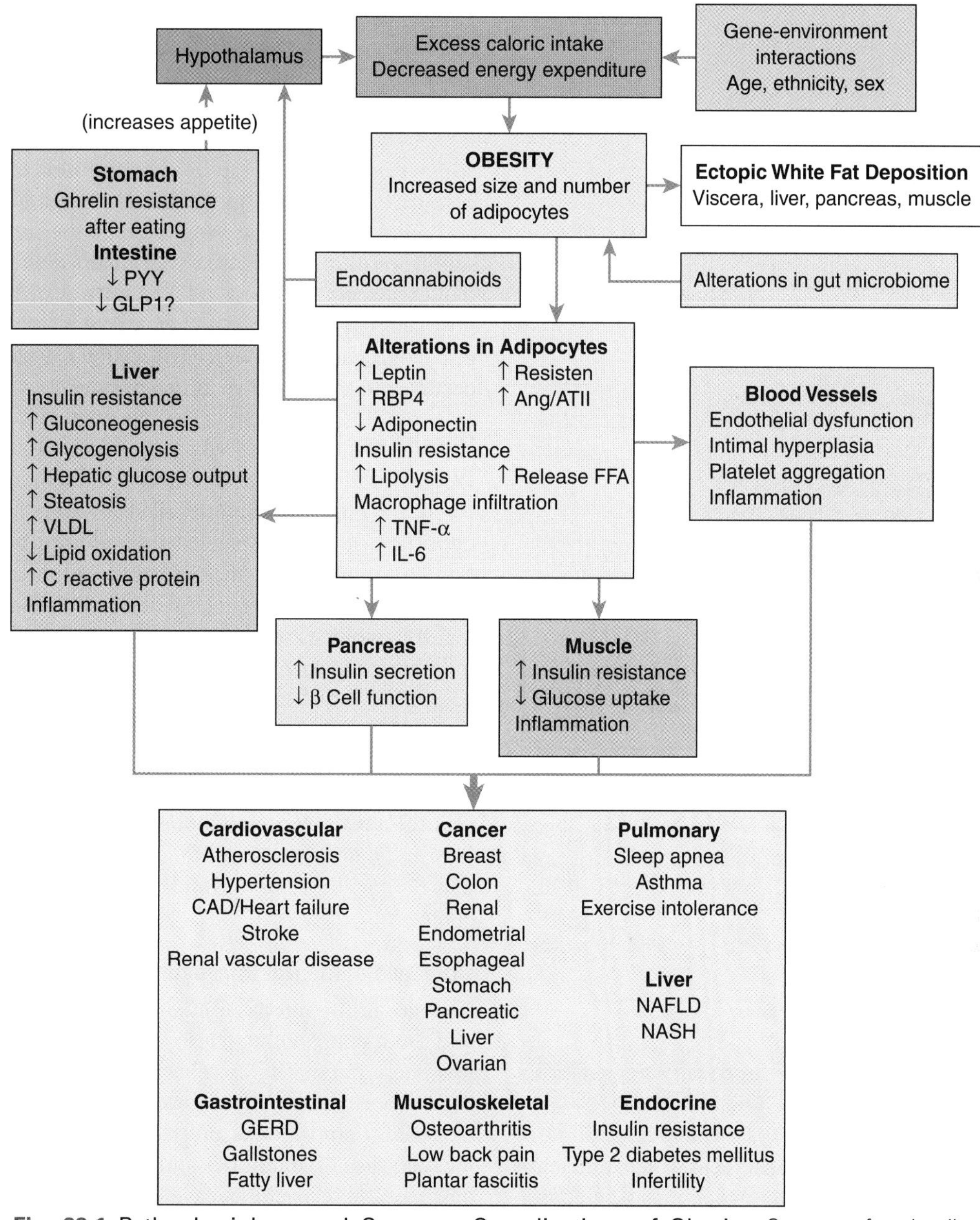

Fig. 23.1 Pathophysiology and Common Complications of Obesity. See text for details. *Ang/ATII*, Angiotensinogen/angiotensin 2; *CAD*, coronary artery disease; *FFA*, free fatty acids; *GERD*, gastroesophageal reflux disease; *GLP1*, glucagon-like peptide 1; *IL-6*, interleukin-6; *PYY*, intestinal peptide YY; *RBP4*, retinol-binding protein 4; *TNF-α*, tumor necrosis factor-alpha; *VLDL*, very-low-density lipoprotein. *NAFLD*, nonalcoholic fatty liver disease and *NASH*, nonalcoholic steatohepatitis.

Ghrelin is produced by the stomach gastric mucosa. Ghrelin stimulates food intake and fat storage and prevents life-threatening hypoglycemia by inhibiting insulin secretion and stimulating glucagon secretion. It increases in response to fasting and chronic caloric restriction and decreases after food intake. Ghrelin is thought to have antilipolytic effects and stimulates lipogenesis in visceral WAT, leading to an increase in body weight and body fat mass. Ghrelin also stimulates the release of GH from anterior pituitary cells, the release of gastric acid, gastrointestinal motility, and pancreatic secretion of insulin. It has satiety, vasodilatory, and cardioprotective effects. An elevation in FFAs and GH after eating normally decreases the release of ghrelin. However, obesity is associated with a decreased plasma level of ghrelin, and plasma ghrelin levels do not fall after eating. This is known as *ghrelin resistance*. The mechanisms for this response

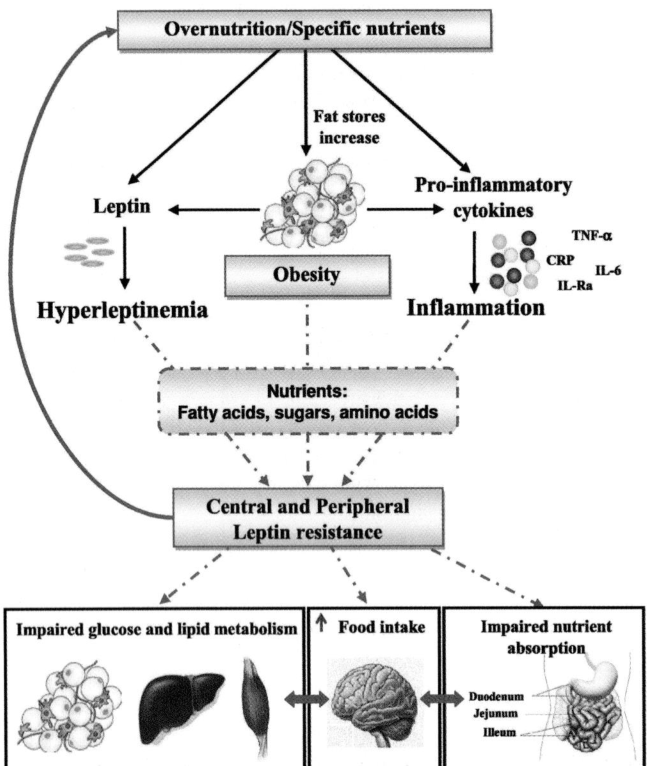

Fig. 23.2 Leptin Resistance and Obesity. *IL*, Interleukin; *TNF-α*, tumor necrosis factor-alpha; *CRP*, C-reactive protein. (From Sáinz N, Barrenetxe J, Moreno-Aliaga MJ, et al. Leptin resistance and diet-induced obesity: Central and peripheral actions of leptin. *Metabolism*, 2015;64(1):35–46. https://doi.org/10.1016/j.metabol.2014.10.015)

are not clear, and the role of ghrelin in obesity has yet to be clearly defined.[31]

Glucagon-like peptide 1 (GLP-1) is an anorexigenic hormone secreted by intestinal endocrine cells when nutrients enter the small intestine. GLP-1 stimulates pancreatic glucose-dependent insulin secretion, decreases blood glucose levels, delays gastric emptying, suppresses appetite, increases satiety, and increases energy expenditure. GLP-1 levels may be decreased in obese individuals, and a GLP-1 receptor analogue has been approved to treat both obesity and type 2 diabetes mellitus.[32]

Peptide YY (PYY) is released from intestinal endocrine cells in response to nutrients entering the intestine. PPY inhibits gastric motility and mucosal secretion and increases satiety and decreases appetite by acting on the medullary brain stem. PYY decreases with obesity.[33]

Cholecystokinin (CCK) is secreted by proximal small intestinal cells after food intake. Its actions include gallbladder contraction, release of pancreatic enzymes and insulin, satiation, and reduced food intake. Work is in progress to develop type 1 CCK receptor (CCK1R) agonists for the treatment of obesity.[34]

Lipotoxicity

Chronic positive energy balance and obesity can overwhelm fat storage by adipocytes, resulting in altered lipid metabolism and insulin resistance. Normally, insulin can inhibit lipolysis by activation of insulin receptors in adipocytes. With obesity, adipocytes are resistant to insulin inhibition of lipolysis. With a chronic increased energy intake, the increase in adipocyte size and number in visceral WAT exceeds the supporting vascular supply, resulting in hypoxia and inflamed and fibrotic adipose tissues. Excess lipolysis and FFAs are distributed to nonadipose cells (e.g., kidney, liver, heart, skeletal muscle). When their utilization capacity is exceeded, cellular dysfunction or death occurs, and this is known as *lipotoxicity*.[35]

Obesity and Inflammation

Obesity produces a state of chronic, low-grade inflammation in WAT. The enlarged adipose cell size results in apoptosis, local hypoxia, cell and mechanical stress, and promotes inflammation. Proinflammatory macrophages, lymphocytes, neutrophils, and mast cells infiltrate enlarged adipocytes and release inflammatory cytokines (e.g., TNF-α, and IL-6) (see Box 23.1).[36] The inflammatory state is supported by increased leptin, decreased adiponectin, and increased resistin (a hormone released by macrophages that promotes insulin resistance and inflammation). The inflammatory state, immune dysregulation, accelerated lipolysis, and lipotoxicity contribute to the development of insulin resistance, metabolic syndrome (see Chapter 22 and Box 22.2), and the complications of obesity, including type 2 diabetes mellitus, cardiovascular disease, kidney disease, NASH, and cancer.[2]

Obesity and the Gut Microbiome

Changes in the intestinal microbiome also are associated with and are a contributing cause of obesity, although the mechanisms are not clear. Microbes (mostly bacteria) are found in high concentration in the lower gastrointestinal tract, and the bacterial composition is affected by genetics, diet, geographical location, use of antibiotics and other medications, and energy balance. These bacteria have considerable variability among individuals and participate in the breakdown of complex carbohydrates, nutrient absorption, vitamin synthesis, inflammatory responses, gut permeability, and bile acid metabolism. Gut microbial fermentation of dietary fiber produces short chain fatty acids (acetate, butyrate, and propionate), which function as energy sources and signaling molecules that affect the host's energy metabolism and inflammation.

More studies are needed to determine how changes in microbiota contribute to body weight regulation, metabolism, low-grade inflammation, and increased adiposity and how manipulation of the gut microbiota can assist in preventing or treating obesity.[37]

Clinical Manifestations. Obesity usually presents with different forms or phenotypes of adipose tissue distribution and/or extent of metabolic abnormalities.[38] Visceral obesity (also known as intra-abdominal, central, or masculine obesity) occurs when the distribution of body fat is localized around the abdomen and upper body, resulting in an apple shape. Visceral obesity is associated with accelerated lipolysis and has an increased risk for chronic systemic inflammation, metabolic syndrome, obstructive sleep apnea syndrome, type 2 diabetes mellitus, cardiovascular complications, osteoarthritis, and cancer. Visceral venous blood drains into the portal vein, contributing to higher liver synthesis of plasma lipids and increasing the risk of nonalcoholic fatty liver disease (NAFLD) and NASH.[39]

Peripheral obesity (also known as subcutaneous, gluteal-femoral, or feminine obesity) occurs when the distribution of body fat is extraperitoneal and distributed around the thighs and buttocks and through the muscle, resulting in a pear shape. It is more common in premenopausal women. Peripheral and subcutaneous fat is less metabolically active and lipolytic and releases fewer adipokines (particularly adiponectin) than visceral fat. Risk factors are still present for the complications of obesity, but they are less severe than for visceral obesity.[40]

Obesity has been described in relation to the extent of metabolic abnormalities that are present. However, there is no universally accepted definition or guidelines to describe metabolic health for the phenotypes or the potentially transient nature of a metabolically healthy status. Depending on the phenotype, there are associated differences in adipose tissue distribution, metabolism, lipid profiles, and gut microbiota. There are modifiable lifestyle factors (diet, exercise, smoking, alcohol use, psychological stress, geographical location), and unmodifiable factors (age, sex, ethnicity, and genetics) that also play a role, all of which add to the complexity of a uniform definition. Continued development of clarity and consensus regarding criteria and parameter guidelines will facilitate research designs and personalized treatment decisions. Box 23.3 presents a summary of the proposed phenotype characteristics.

BOX 23.3 Obesity Metabolic Phenotypes

Metabolically unhealthy normal-weight obesity (MUHNW)

- Individuals with a normal body weight and BMI (18.5–25 kg/m^2) but a body fat percentage greater than 30%, ectopic fat distribution (fat in liver, skeletal muscle, heart, and pancreatic tissues) with increased subcutaneous abdominal fat.
- Increases in inflammatory adipokines, insulin resistance, and increased risk for metabolic syndrome, type 2 diabetes mellitus (T2DM), cardiovascular disease (CVD), and a higher mortality than a normal weight healthy population.
- Metabolically healthy obesity (MHO)—{benign or uncomplicated obesity}
  - Individuals with an elevated BMI (>30 kg/m^2) and less visceral adiposity without metabolic abnormalities (i.e., normal insulin sensitivity—fasting glucose concentrations), normal lipid values and C-reactive protein and absence of hypertension. Increased risk for insulin resistance, metabolic syndrome, T2DM and cardiovascular disease after many years of obesity.

Metabolically unhealthy obesity (MUO).

- BMI over 30 kg/m^2 and body fat percentage over 30% with excess visceral fat. Waist circumferences greater than 40 inches (102 cm) in men and 35 inches (88 cm) in women. Elevated fasting glucose, dyslipidemia, and hypertension. At high risk to develop metabolic syndrome progression, T2DM, and CVD and consequently, higher mortality.

Data from Brandão I, Martins MJ, Monteiro R. Metabolically healthy obesity-heterogeneity in definitions and unconventional factors. *Metabolites*, 2020;10(2):48; Duque AP, Rodrigues LF Jr., Mediano MFF, et al. Emerging concepts in metabolically healthy obesity. *American Journal of Preventive Cardiology*, 2020;10(2):48–61; Eckel N, Li Y, Kuxhaus O, et al. Transition from metabolic healthy to unhealthy phenotypes and association with cardiovascular disease risk across BMI categories in 90 257 women (the Nurses' Health Study): 30 year follow-up from a prospective cohort study. *Lancet Diabetes and Endocrinology*, 2018;6(9):714–724.

Evaluation and Treatment. All children and adults should be screened for obesity. Several methods are available for estimating or measuring the amount of adipose tissue: anthropometric measurements, including weight, height, and circumferences or various body diameters (i.e., waist-to-hip ratios and waist circumference); skinfold thickness (measured with skinfold calipers); ultrasound to measure peripheral body fat; and bioelectric impedance and underwater hydrostatic weighing to calculate total body fat. The only method for directly measuring total body fat is by dual-energy x-ray absorptiometry (DXA) scanning, an enhanced type of x-ray imaging.

In clinical practice, anthropometric and body diameter measures are most commonly used to calculate the BMI because they are the easiest to measure and most cost-effective. Body mass indices have been established based on height, weight, age, sex, and ethnicity. Overweight is defined as a BMI greater than 25 kg/m^2, and obesity is a BMI greater than 30 kg/m^2. BMI charts are available for children ages 2 to 20 years; these can be used for comparison during adulthood, because obese children generally become obese adults.

However, the BMI does not measure the amount and location of body fat. The waist circumference (more than 40 inches [102 cm] for men and more than 35 inches [88 cm] for women) adds information to assist with disease risk assessment in general practice. Obesity risk assessment is available from the American Association of Clinical Endocrinologists and the American College of Endocrinology.[41] No specific diagnostic criteria for obesity have been established.

Obesity is a chronic disease for which various treatment approaches have been used, including correction of metabolic abnormalities and individually tailored lifestyle interventions, such as weight reduction diets and exercise programs. Additional treatments include psychotherapy, behavioral modification, self-motivation, and support systems.[42,43] Several drugs have been approved for the pharmacologic management of obesity.[44]

Currently, bariatric surgical procedures (i.e., the Roux-en-Y gastric bypass, adjustable gastric banding, and sleeve gastrectomy) offer the most significant reduction in weight, reduction in comorbidities, and decrease in insulin resistance for the treatment of obesity.[45] Efforts are continuing to identify the molecular and neuroendocrine causes of obesity. This will lead to more specific and personalized prevention and treatment strategies (see Emerging Science Box: SGLT-2 Use for the Treatment of Obesity).

EMERGING SCIENCE BOX
SGLT-2 Use for the Treatment of Obesity

Efficacy and safety of sodium-glucose co-transporter 2 (SGLT-2) inhibitors have been well studied for the treatment of diabetes mellitus type 2. Beyond its ability to lower blood glucose, SGLT-2 inhibitors have also exhibited beneficial effects on body weight and systolic blood pressure and have shown to decrease risk for major cardiovascular and renal events. SGLT-2 inhibitors cause body weight loss by way of glucose excretion, or calorie loss, in the kidneys. Weight loss with use of SGLT-2 inhibitors has been consistent in multiple studies related to individuals with diabetes mellitus type 2, whether the SGLT-2 is prescribed as a mono or combination therapy. Exhibited weight loss appears to be dose dependent and often minimal on its own; however, in combination with glucagon-like peptide 1 receptor agonists (GLP1-RAs)—which naturally suppresses appetite—greater weight loss and maintenance of weight loss was observed versus SGLT-2 monotherapy alone. The majority of studies completed have only included individuals with the diagnoses of obesity *and* diabetes mellitus type 2, but there are ongoing trials studying the effects of SGLT-2 inhibitors in obesity *without* the diagnosis of diabetes. While lifestyle modification remains the mainstay for treatment of obesity, pharmacological modalities are an attractive and less invasive alternative to surgical intervention. Medication management options increase the ability to provide person-centered care to patients, especially if one medication can improve multiple conditions, overall health quality, and longevity.

Data from Pereira MJ, et al. Emerging role of SGLT-2 inhibitors for the treatment of obesity. *Drugs*, 2019;79(3):219–230; Williams DM, et al. Drug therapy in obesity: A review of current and emerging treatments. *Diabetes Therapy*, 2020;11(6):1199–1216.

EMERGING SCIENCE BOX
Weight Loss

Intermittent fasting has become a growing trend for weight loss with the increase in obesity. Intermittent fasting refers to regular periods with no or very limited caloric intake. For example, an individual may fast daily for 16 h or fast for 24 h on alternate days, or fast for 2 days per week on non-consecutive days. Caloric consumption during fasting can range from 0% to 25% of the individual's caloric needs. Current studies suggest that not only does intermittent fasting cause a reduction in weight (0.8% to 13.0% of baseline weight), but this type of diet could reduce the risk of cardiovascular disease. Recent evidence indicates that meal timing may influence circadian rhythm, and as a result, may directly or indirectly affect cardiometabolic risk. Researchers continue to study the effects of intermittent fasting on hypertension, dyslipidemia, and diabetes. Intermittent fasting may exert its effects through multiple pathways, including reducing oxidative stress, optimization of circadian rhythms, and ketogenesis. Currently, the evidence shows that intermittent fasting can trigger a metabolic switch from glucose-based to ketone-based energy. This switch can increase resistance to stress and overall improvement of longevity with an inverse relationship on the incidence of diseases, including cancer and obesity.

Data from Dong TA, et al. Intermittent fasting: A heart healthy dietary pattern? *American Journal of Medicine*, 2020;133(8):901–907. https://doi.org/10.1016/j.amjmed.2020.03.030. Epub 2020 Apr 21. PMID: 32330491; PMCID: PMC7415631; Effects of intermittent fasting on health, aging, and disease. *New England Journal of Medicine*, 2020;382(3):298 https://doi.org/10.1056/NEJMx190038. Erratum for: *New England Journal of Medicine*, 2019 Dec 26;381(26):2541–2551. PMID: 31940711; Welton S, et al. Intermittent fasting and weight loss: Systematic review. *Canadian Family Physician*, 2020;66(2):117–125. PMID: 32060194; PMCID: PMC7021351.

STARVATION

Malnutrition is lack of nourishment from inadequate amounts of calories, protein, vitamins, or minerals and is caused by an improper diet, alterations in digestion or absorption, chronic disease, or a combination of these factors. Starvation is a reduction in energy intake related to inadequate food sources that leads to weight loss. Short-term starvation and long-term starvation have different effects. Therapeutic short-term starvation is part of many weight reduction programs because it causes an initial rapid weight loss that reinforces the individual's motivation to diet (see Emerging Science Box: Weight Loss for more information). Therapeutic long-term starvation is used in medically controlled environments to facilitate rapid weight loss in morbidly obese individuals. Pathologic long-term starvation can be caused by poverty; food shortages; chronic diseases of the cardiovascular, pulmonary, hepatic, and digestive systems; malabsorption syndromes; human immunodeficiency virus (HIV) infection; cancer; and anorexia nervosa.[46]

Short-term starvation, or extended fasting, consists of several days of total dietary abstinence or deprivation. The body responds with mechanisms to protect protein mass. For 4 to 6 hours after the last meal, the body is in a well-fed state and its energy requirements are supplied by glucose from recently ingested carbohydrates. Once all available energy has been absorbed from the intestine, glycogen in the liver is converted to glucose through glycogenolysis—the splitting of glycogen into glucose. This process peaks within 4 to 8 hours, and gluconeogenesis begins. Gluconeogenesis is the formation of glucose from noncarbohydrate molecules: lactate, pyruvate, amino acids, and the glycerol portion of fats from lipolysis. Like glycogenolysis, gluconeogenesis takes place within the liver. Both of these processes deplete stored nutrients and, thus, cannot meet the body's energy needs indefinitely. Lipolysis and proteins continue to be catabolized to a minimal degree, providing carbon for the synthesis of glucose.[47]

Long-term starvation begins after several days of dietary abstinence and eventually causes death from proteolysis. Absolute deprivation of food (e.g., that associated with famine) causes marasmus, or protein-energy malnutrition (loss of muscle mass, body fat depletion, and absence of edema). Protein deprivation in the presence of carbohydrate intake is called kwashiorkor (loss of muscle mass with sustained body fat and peripheral edema). Marasmic kwashiorkor (edematous, severe childhood malnutrition) is a combination of chronic energy deficiency and chronic or acute protein deficiency and inadequate micronutrients.[48,49] These conditions are described in Chapter 42.

Anorexia is loss of appetite. Anorexia nervosa is a psychological cause of long-term starvation (Box 23.4). Cachexia (also known as cytokine-induced malnutrition) is skeletal muscle wasting, causing muscle atrophy with involuntary loss of weight leading to, fatigue, and weakness. Muscle atrophy

BOX 23.4 Diagnostic Criteria for Eating Disorders

Anorexia Nervosa

Persistent restriction of energy intake leading to significantly low body weight (in context of what is minimally expected for age, sex, developmental trajectory, and physical health).

Either an intense fear of gaining weight or of becoming fat, or persistent behavior that interferes with weight gain (even though significantly low weight).

Disturbance in the way one's body weight or shape is experienced, undue influence of body shape and weight on self-evaluation, or persistent lack of recognition of the seriousness of the current low body weight.

Subtypes:
- Restricting type
- Binge-eating/purging type

Bulimia Nervosa

Recurrent episodes of binge eating. An episode of binge eating is characterized by both of the following:
- Eating, in a discrete period of time (e.g., within any 2-h period), an amount of food that is definitely larger than most people would eat during a similar period of time and under similar circumstances.
- A sense of lack of control overeating during the episode (e.g., a feeling that one cannot stop eating or control what or how much one is eating).

Recurrent inappropriate compensatory behavior in order to prevent weight gain, such as self-induced vomiting; misuse of laxatives, diuretics, or other medications; fasting; or excessive exercise.

The binge eating and inappropriate compensatory behaviors both occur, on average, at least once a week for 3 months.

Self-evaluation is unduly influenced by body shape and weight.

The disturbance does not occur exclusively during episodes of anorexia nervosa.

Binge Eating Disorder[a]

Recurrent episodes of binge eating. An episode of binge eating is characterized by both of the following:
- Eating, in a discrete period of time (e.g., within any 2-h period), an amount of food that is definitely larger than most people would eat during a similar period of time and under similar circumstances.
- A sense of lack of control overeating during the episode (e.g., a feeling that one cannot stop eating or control what or how much one is eating).

The binge eating episodes are associated with three or more of the following:
- Eating much more rapidly than normal.
- Eating until feeling uncomfortably full.
- Eating large amounts of food when not feeling physically hungry.
- Eating alone because of feeling embarrassed by how much one is eating.
- Feeling disgusted with oneself, depressed, or very guilty afterward.
- Marked distress regarding binge eating is present.
- Binge eating occurs, on average, at least once a week for 3 months.
- Binge eating is not associated with the recurrent use of inappropriate compensatory behaviors as in bulimia nervosa and does not occur exclusively during the course of bulimia nervosa or anorexia nervosa methods to compensate for overeating, such as self-induced vomiting.

[a]NOTE: Binge eating disorder is less common but much more severe than overeating. Binge eating disorder is associated with more subjective distress regarding the eating behavior, and commonly other co-occurring psychologic problems

Data from American Psychiatric Association (APA). *DSM-5: Diagnostic and statistical manual of mental disorders*, 5th edition. Arlington, VA: Author; 2013:338–345.

is a result of negative protein and energy balance secondary to reduced food intake and abnormal metabolism.[50] Systemic inflammation caused by inflammatory mediators (e.g., TNF-α, interferon-γ, IL-1, IL-6, and IL-8), an increased catabolic response, and metabolic abnormalities are associated with the cachexia.[51] Cancer, congestive heart failure, chronic obstructive pulmonary disease, acquired immunodeficiency syndrome (AIDS), rheumatoid arthritis, tuberculosis, and other major chronic progressive proinflammatory diseases are contributable pathophysiological processes. While individuals may experience one or the other, anorexia and cachexia often occur together.[51] (Fig. 23.3).

The major metabolic characteristic of long-term starvation is a decreased dependence on gluconeogenesis and an increased use of ketone bodies (products of lipid and pyruvate metabolism) as a cellular energy source. During long-term starvation, depressed insulin levels and increased levels of glucagon, cortisone, epinephrine, and GHs promote lipolysis in adipose tissue. Lipolysis liberates fatty acids—which supply energy to cardiac and skeletal muscle cells—and ketone bodies—which sustain brain tissue. Fatty acid, or ketone body, oxidation meets most of the energy needs of the cells. (Some glucose is still needed as fuel for brain tissue and red blood cells.) Once the supply of adipose tissue is depleted, proteolysis begins. The breakdown of muscle and visceral protein is the last process the body engages in to supply energy for life. Death results from severe alterations in electrolyte balance and loss of renal, pulmonary, and cardiac function.[52]

Adequate ingestion of appropriate nutrients is the obvious treatment for starvation. In medically induced starvation, the body is maintained in a ketotic state until the desired amount of adipose tissue has been lysed. Starvation imposed by chronic disease, long-term illness, malabsorption syndromes, and chronic eating disorders is treated with enteral or parenteral nutrition (Box 23.5). Perioperative or critical care management of nutrition is necessary to prevent unnecessary starvation.[53] Care must be taken to prevent refeeding syndrome (Box 23.6) during the treatment of long-term starvation.

ANOREXIA OF AGING

Anorexia of aging describes a decrease in appetite or food intake in older adults. It can occur in illness-free individuals and with an adequate food supply. The resulting undernutrition leads to adverse outcomes and may affect up to 30% of independently living elders with higher incidence occurring in hospital and extended care nursing faciltities.[54] The anorexia of aging results from multiple age-related changes, including reduced energy needs, waning hunger, diminished senses of smell and taste, decreased production of saliva, altered gastrointestinal satiety control mechanisms, and the presence of comorbidities (Fig. 23.4). The neuroendocrine system physiologically

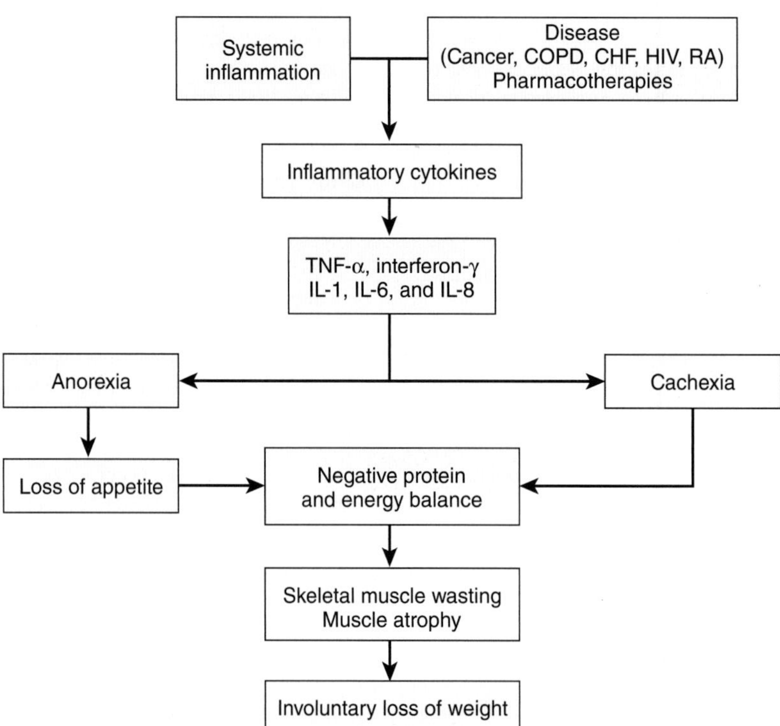

Fig. 23.3 Pathogenesis of Anorexia and Cachexia. *COPD,* Chronic obstructive pulmonary disease; *CHF,* congestive heart failure; *HIV,* human immunodeficiency virus; *RA,* rheumatoid arthritis.

BOX 23.5 Complications of Anorexia Nervosa and Bulimia

Anorexia Nervosa Complications

Cardiac

- Bradycardia
- Dysrhythmia
- Left ventricular atrophy
- Mitral valve prolapse
- Pericardial effusion
- Sudden cardiac death

Dermatological

- Acrocyanosis
- Hair thinning
- Xerosis

Endocrine

- Amenorrhea
- Estrogen decreased in females and testosterone decreased in males
- Euthyroid sick syndrome
- Hypoglycemia
- Hypogonadal related to reduced pulsed hypothalamic gonadotropin releasing hormone secretion
- Hypothyroidism: cold intolerance
- Low libido
- Preterm birth
- Thermoregulation impaired

Gastrointestinal

- Abdominal bloating

Anorexia Nervosa Complications

- Abdominal pain
- Constipation related to slowed peristalsis
- Dysphagia related to weakened oropharyngeal muscles
- Early Satiety
- Gastroparesis
- Liver function test abnormalities related to malnutrition; elevated transaminases
- Pelvic floor dysfunction
- Postprandial fullness

Hematological

- Anemia
- Leukopenia
- Thrombocytopenia

Metabolic

- Electrolyte Imbalances (hypokalemia; hypophosphatemia; hypomagnesemia; hyponatremia)

Musculoskeletal

- Osteoporosis: decreased bone mineral density
- Stress fracture risk from decreased bone formation and increased bone resorption

Neurological

- Brain atrophy
- Cognitive function impairment
- Taste and smell abnormalities

Continued

BOX 23.5 Complications of Anorexia Nervosa and Bulimia—cont'd

Anorexia Nervosa Complications

Bulimia Complications

Self-Induced Vomiting

- Dyspepsia
- Dysphagia
- Electrolyte and acid base disorders (hypokalemia; metabolic alkalosis)
- Gastric reflux
- Hoarse voice
- Parotid gland enlargement
- Tooth erosion
- Vocal cord inflammation

Laxative Abuse

- Diarrhea
- Electrolyte and acid base disorders (hypokalemia; hyperphosphatemia; metabolic alkalosis)
- Hemorrhoids
- Rectal Prolapse

Data from Donaldson AA, Gordon CM. Skeletal complications of eating disorders. *Metabolism*, 2015;64(9):943–951; Sangvai D. Eating disorders in the primary care setting. *Primary Care*, 2016;43(2):301–312; Sato Y, Fukudo S. Gastrointestinal symptoms and disorders in patients with eating disorders. *Clinical Journal of Gastroenterology*, 2015;8(5):255–263; Westmoreland P, Krantz MJ, Mehler PS. Medical complications of anorexia nervosa and bulimia. *American Journal of Medicine*, 2016;129(1):30–37; Cass K, McGuire C, Bjork I, et al. Medical complications of anorexia nervosa. *Psychosomatics*, 2020;61(6):625–631; Gibson D, Watters A, Cost J, et al. Extreme anorexia nervosa: Medical findings, outcomes, and inferences from a retrospective cohort. *Journal of Eating Disorders*, 2020;8(1):1–10.

BOX 23.6 Refeeding Syndrome

Refeeding syndrome is a life-threatening condition that occurs in severely malnourished individuals when parenteral or enteral nutritional therapy is initiated. During starvation, loss of body minerals causes the movement of phosphate, magnesium, and potassium ions out of the cells and into the plasma. When refeeding starts, an increase in insulin levels stimulates the movement of glucose and these ions back into the cells, and the plasma concentrations can decrease to dangerously low levels, causing hypophosphatemia, hypomagnesemia, hypokalemia, hyponatremia, hypocalcemia, and vitamin deficiency (particularly thiamin). Alterations usually occur within 72 h after the start of nutritional therapy.

Hypophosphatemia contributes to alterations in red blood cell shape and function, contributing to tissue hypoxia and increased respiratory drive. Rapid expansion of the extracellular fluid volume also can occur with carbohydrate refeeding and may cause fluid overload. The consequences of these alterations include life-threatening dysrhythmias, congestive heart failure, muscle weakness (including respiratory muscles), and death. Individuals at greatest risk are those with starvation from any cause, including anorexia nervosa, chronic diseases, aging, morbid obesity with massive weight loss, and prolonged fasting. Refeeding syndrome is prevented by identifying at-risk individuals; slowly reinstituting feeding (about 20 kcal/kg/day for the first few days); and monitoring plasma levels of phosphate, potassium, magnesium, and calcium during the change from catabolic to anabolic metabolism.

Data from Aubry E, Friedli N, Schuetz P, et al. Refeeding syndrome in the frail elderly population: Prevention, diagnosis and management. *Clinical and Experimental Gastroenterology*, 2018;11:255–264; Crook MA. Refeeding syndrome: Problems with definition and management. *Nutrition*, 2014;30(11–12):1448–1455; Friedli N, Baumann J, Hummel R. Refeeding syndrome is associated with increased mortality in malnourished medical inpatients: Secondary analysis of a randomized trial. *Medicine (Baltimore)*, 2020;99(1):e18506. https://doi.org/10.1097/MD.0000000000018506; Reber E, Friedli N, Vasiloglou MF, et al. Management of refeeding syndrome in medical inpatients. *Journal of Clinical Medicine*, 2019;8(12):2202. Published 2019 Dec 13. https://doi.org/10.3390/jcm8122202; Reintam Blaser A, Berger MM. Early or late feeding after ICU admission? *Nutrients*, 2017;9(12):E1278.

regulates appetite with multiple hormones implicated as mediators of hunger and satiety.[54]

Centrally, aging is associated with decreased orexigenic signals (e.g., levels of ghrelin or ghrelin resistance and reduced hypothalamic receptors, or both) and increased anorexigenic signals (e.g., decreased levels of leptin, insulin, PYY, and CCK), which lead to loss of appetite and diminished food intake (see Box 23.2). Chronic low-grade inflammation with elevated cytokines also can contribute to delayed gastric emptying and decreased motility of the small intestine. Risk factors for the anorexia of aging include functional impairments and deficiencies (e.g., loss of vision, poor dentition, dysphagia, inability to prepare foods); medical and psychiatric conditions (e.g., malabsorption syndromes, chronic disease, cancer, and depression); loneliness and grief; medications, including polypharmacy; social isolation; and abuse or neglect.[55] Progression of the underlying causes of anorexia (e.g., chronic obstructive pulmonary disease, congestive heart failure) increases the workload of breathing, which decreases energy reserves required to eat and digest food. The consequences of anorexia of aging include malnutrition, physical frailty, mitochondrial dysfunction, reduced regenerative capacity, increased oxidative stress, and imbalanced hormones. There are several tools available to screen for anorexia of aging in elderly individual. Early intervention improves the overall well-being of older individuals experiencing anorexia. Currently, no specific treatments exist for the anorexia of aging, although exercise, nutrition, and other supportive strategies are used. Exercise is a key strategy in treating elderly individuals with anorexia. Exercise improves appetite and oral intake, but has other beneficial effects, such as elevating mood and building muscle and strength. Nutrition also plays a vital role. It is recommended that older adults aged 65 years and above maintain a dietary protein intake of 0.9 to 1.2 g/kg/day and individuals with acute or chronic diseases

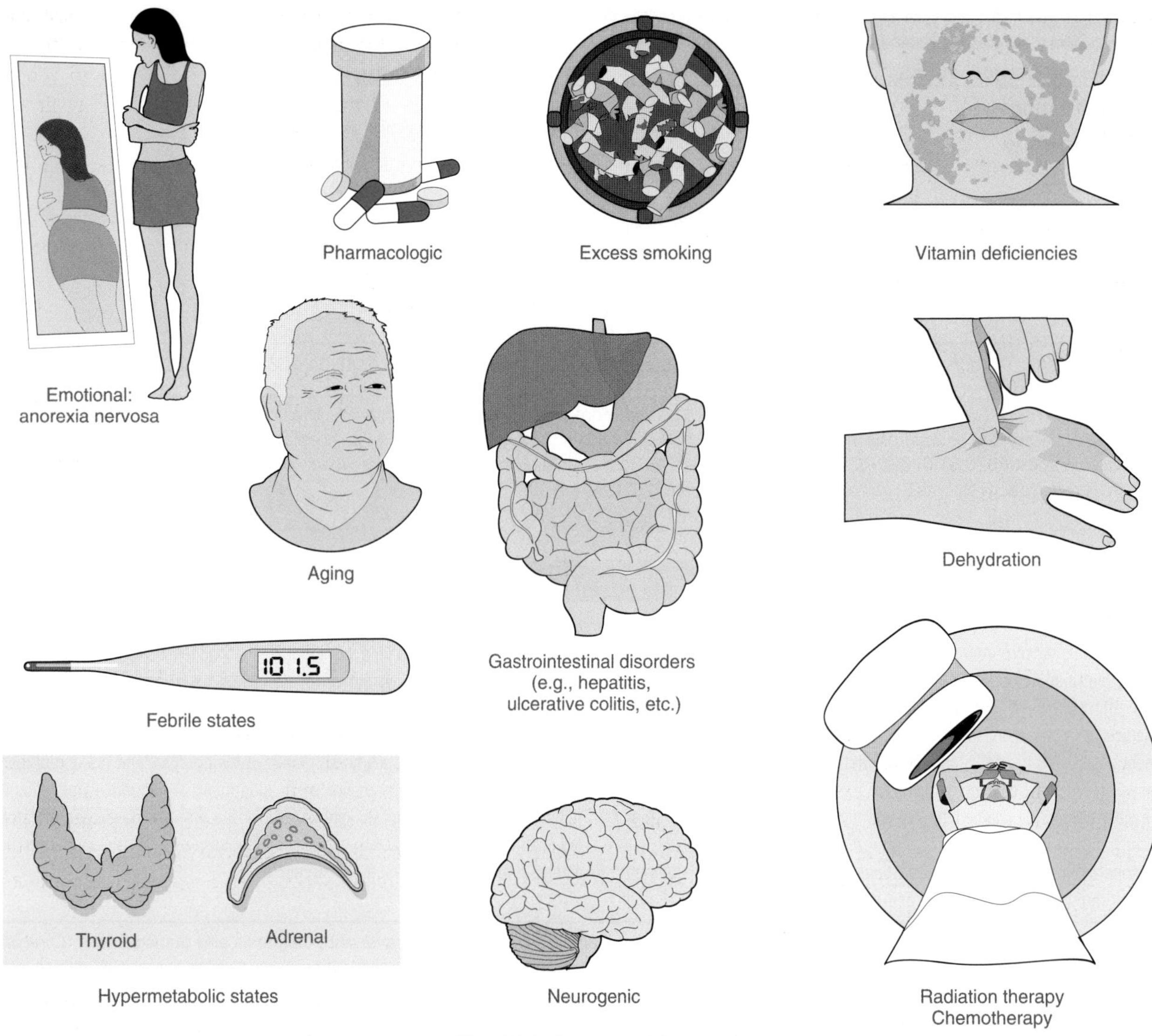

Fig. 23.4 Causes of Anorexia.

should intake 1.2 to 1.5 g/kg/day.[56] Other supportive interventions to help mitigate the effects of anorexia of the aging include improved food access and appearance, dental and eye care, and social stimulation. Pharmaceutical agents (e.g., megestrol acetate and dronabinol) are not recommended in elderly persons because the risk does not outweigh the benefit. Anorexia of aging is common; however, it should not be accepted as a normal consequence of aging. Mortality rates have been shown to be higher in those with anorexia of aging and unintentional weight loss.[57]

SUMMARY REVIEW

Adipose Tissue

1. Adipose tissue provides insulation and tissue support and is the body's major energy reserve, storing and releasing triglycerides and glycerol.
2. Adipose tissue is classified according to color: WAT, BAT, and bAT.
3. WAT contains macrophages, mast cells, neutrophils, fibroblasts, endothelial cells, blood vessels, nerves, and precursor adipocytes.
4. WAT is the largest fat depot and is located in visceral (central) and subcutaneous (peripheral) sites. It also is located in muscle and bone marrow.
5. White adipocytes store fat as a single lipid droplet or vacuole.
6. With a positive energy balance, WAT storage increases by adipocyte hypertrophy (more common in visceral fat) and adipogenesis (hyperplasia, more common in subcutaneous fat).

7. Estrogen enhances the deposition of subcutaneous fat compared to visceral fat.
8. BAT has multiple lipid droplets that are rich in mitochondria containing iron, which gives them a brown color. Exposure to cold, sympathetic activation and release of catecholamines, and activation of T_3 generates heat through free fatty acid oxidation (nonshivering thermogenesis).
9. Both neonates and adults have BAT, but not in the amounts of WAT.
10. bAT emerges within WAT with exposure to cold and exercise. This is known as the beiging of WAT.
11. BAT and bAT both protect against obesity and metabolic syndrome.
12. MAT is found in all bones. With obesity, MAT releases adipokines that affect osteoblast and osteoclast function. Excessive MAT is associated with osteoporosis and fractures.
13. Adipose tissue is an endocrine organ that secretes hormones, called *adipokines*, with autocrine, paracrine, and endocrine actions necessary for metabolic function and immune responses.
14. Regulation of food intake and energy balance are accomplished by balancing opposing sets of neurons in the arcuate nucleus: orexigenic neurons (promote appetite, stimulate eating, and decrease metabolism) and anorexigenic neurons (suppress appetite, inhibit eating, and increase metabolism). Peripherally, gastrointestinal hormones and adipokines also control food intake and energy expenditure.
15. Brain centers related to reward, pleasure, memory, and addictive behavior can override hypothalamic control of food intake and satiety, causing increased fat stores by increasing consumption of highly palatable foods.

Obesity

1. Obesity is an increase in body adipose tissue and an endocrine and metabolic disorder that develops when caloric intake exceeds energy expenditure. Obesity is defined as a BMI greater than 30 kg/m^2 in adults and a BMI greater than or equal to the age- and sex-specific 95th percentile of the 2000 CDC growth charts in children.
2. Obesity is an epidemic that has occurred worldwide in both adults and children. It is the fifth leading cause of death globally. Three leading causes of death in the United States are associated with obesity: cardiovascular disease, type 2 diabetes mellitus, and certain cancers. Obesity also increases the risk for numerous other systemic disorders.
3. Single-gene (rare) and polygenic disorders and metabolic disorders are associated with obesity, as are gene–environment interactions.
4. Adipokines and gastrointestinal hormones are altered with obesity and contribute to associated complications.
5. Leptin resistance occurs when leptin levels increase with obesity and promote overeating and excessive weight gain, hyperglycemia, hyperinsulinemia, and hyperlipidemia. It also stimulates macrophages and endothelial cells to produce proinflammatory mediators.
6. Adiponectin levels decrease with obesity, contributing to insulin resistance, inflammation, and hyperlipidemia.
7. Retinol-binding protein 4 levels are increased in visceral adiposity and promote insulin resistance and hepatic steatosis.
8. Endocannabinoids are increased in obesity and promote appetite, enhance nutrient absorption, stimulate lipogenesis, and inhibit energy expenditure.
9. Angiotensinogen and angiotensin 2 increase in obesity, promoting vasoconstriction, inflammation, lipogenesis, oxidative stress, and insulin resistance.
10. Gastrointestinal hormones (ghrelin, GLP-1, PYY, and CCK) also provide signals that control food intake and energy expenditure and are involved in the pathophysiology of obesity.
11. Ghrelin increases with obesity and stimulates food intake, promotes the release of growth hormone, and stimulates lipogenesis. It also has satiety, vasodilatory, cardioprotective, and antiproliferative effects; its role in obesity is not clear.
12. GLP-1 promotes insulin secretion, delays gastric emptying, suppresses appetite, increases satiety, increases energy expenditure, and is decreased with obesity.
13. PYY inhibits gastric motility, decreases appetite, and is decreased with obesity.
14. CCK is released after food intake and stimulates insulin secretion and satiation, decreases food intake, and is reduced in obesity.
15. Lipotoxicity occurs with excess adipocyte fat storage and lipolysis with distribution of free fatty acids to peripheral organs, resulting in cellular dysfunction and death.
16. Obesity is a state of chronic low-grade inflammation caused by expansion of adipocyte macrophages, neutrophils, lymphocytes, and mast cells, which release inflammatory mediators.
17. The chronic inflammation, alterations in adipokine action, and accelerated lipolysis related to excessive fat contribute to the complications of obesity, particularly insulin resistance, type 2 diabetes mellitus, cardiovascular disease, and cancer.
18. Changes in the intestinal microbiome also are associated with and are a contributing cause of obesity, although the mechanisms are not clear.
19. Obesity has two major phenotypes: visceral obesity (also known as intra-abdominal, central, or masculine obesity) and peripheral obesity (also known as subcutaneous, gluteal-femoral, or feminine obesity). Visceral obesity has the greatest risk for accelerated lipolysis, chronic inflammation, insulin resistance, and associated complications.
20. Normal-weight obesity describes individuals with a normal body weight and BMI but with greater than 30% body fat. These individuals are at risk for metabolic dysregulation, increases in inflammatory cytokines, insulin resistance, increased risk for cardiovascular disease, and higher mortality.
21. Treatment of obesity may include correction of metabolic abnormalities and individually tailored lifestyle interventions (diets, exercise, behavioral modifications, self-motivation) and psychotherapy. The current most effective treatment for extreme obesity is bariatric surgery.
22. New drugs are being developed that target specific molecules and will provide a personalized approach to treatment.

Starvation

1. The body responds to short-term starvation (several days of total dietary abstinence or deprivation) with mechanisms to protect protein mass, using the processes of glycogenolysis and gluconeogenesis. Neither of these processes can meet the body's energy needs indefinitely because they deplete stored nutrients.
2. Long-term starvation (begins after several days of dietary abstinence) results in an initial decreased dependence on gluconeogenesis and an increased use of ketone bodies as a cellular energy source, followed by lipolysis in adipose tissue. In the absence of adequate nutrition, long-term starvation results in proteolysis, with death resulting from severe alterations in electrolyte balance and loss of renal, pulmonary, and cardiac function.
3. Anorexia is a loss of appetite, whereas anorexia nervosa is a psychological cause of long-term starvation.
4. Cachexia is involuntary weight loss with associated muscle wasting and atrophy. The atrophy is due to negative protein and energy balance. Cachexia can be caused by chronic progressive proinflammatory disease processes.
5. The major metabolic characteristic of long-term starvation is a decreased dependence on gluconeogenesis and an increased use of ketone bodies (products of lipid and pyruvate metabolism) as a cellular energy source.
6. Treatment is management of nutrition through parenteral nutrition; however, it is important to prevent refeeding syndrome.

Anorexia of Aging

1. Anorexia of aging is a decrease in appetite or food intake in older adults that leads to undernutrition, resulting in a decline in function and an increased risk for morbidity and mortality.
2. Contributing factors related to aging include diminished sensory functions, poor dentition, decreased gastric emptying, decreased hunger and satiety, effects of medications, and social isolation and neglect.
3. Consequences of anorexia of aging include malnutrition, physical frailty, mitochondrial dysfunction, reduced regenerative capacity, increased oxidative stress, and imbalanced hormones.
4. No specific treatments exist for the anorexia of aging, although exercise, nutrition, and other supportive strategies are used.

REFERENCES

1. Schoetti T, Fischer IP, Ussar S. Heterogeneity of adipose tissue in development and metabolic function. *J Exp Biol*. 2018;221 (Pt Suppl 1). jeb162958.
2. Longo M, et al. Adipose tissue dysfunction as determinant of obesity-associated metabolic complications. *Int J Mol Sci*. 2019;20(9):2358.
3. Bracht JR, et al. The role of estrogens in the adipose tissue milieu. *Ann N Y Acad Sci*. 2020;1461(1):127–143.
4. Suchacki KJ, Cawthorn WP. Molecular interaction of bone marrow adipose tissue with energy metabolism. *Curr Mol Biol Rep*. 2018;4(2):41–49.
5. Jung SM, Sanchez-Gurmaches J, Guertin DA. Brown adipose tissue development and metabolism. *Handb Exp Pharmacol*. 2019;251:3–36.
6. Xu Y, López M. Central regulation of energy metabolism by estrogens. *Mol Metab*. 2018;15:104–115.
7. Leitner BP, et al. Mapping of human brown adipose tissue in lean and obese young men. *Proc Natl Acad Sci U S A*. 2017;114(32):8649–8654.
8. Paulo E, Wang B. Towards a better understanding of beige adipocyte plasticity. *Cells*. 2019;8(12):1552.
9. Maurer S, Harms M, Boucher J. The colorful versatility of adipocytes: white-to-brown transdifferentiation and its therapeutic potential in man. *FEBS J*. 2021;288:3628–3646.
10. Maximus PS, et al. Adipocytokines: are they the theory of everything? *Cytokine*. 2020;133:155144.
11. Abdalla MM. Central and peripheral control of food intake. *Endocr Regul*. 2017;51(1):52–70.
12. Gadde KM, et al. Obesity: pathophysiology and management. *J Am Coll Cardiol*. 2018;71(1):69–84.
13. Centers for Disease Control and Prevention (CDC) Last reviewed August 27, 2021. Available at https://www.cdc.gov/obesity. Accessed. *Overweight and obesity*. Atlanta, GA: CDC; September 14, 2020.
14. Centers for Disease Control and Prevention (CDC) Last reviewed April 5, 2021. Available at https://www.cdc.gov/obesity/data/childhood.html. Accessed. *Childhood obesity facts*. Atlanta, GA: CDC; September 14, 2020.
15. Centers for Disease Control and Prevention (CDC) Last reviewed June 7, 2021. Available at https://www.cdc.gov/obesity/data/adult.html. Accessed. *Adult obesity facts*. Atlanta, GA: CDC; September 14, 2020.
16. European Association for the Study of Obesity (EASO) Available at https://easo.org/media-portal/statistics/. Accessed. *Obesity statistics*. Middlesex, UK: EASO; September 14, 2020.
17. Lauby-Secretan B, et al. Body fatness and cancer— viewpoint of the IARC Working Group. *N Engl J Med*. 2016;375:794–798.
18. Ansari S, Haboubi H, Haboubi N. Adult obesity complications: challenges and clinical impact. *Ther Adv Endocrinol Metab*. 2020;11 2042018820934955.
19. Wang S, Ren J. Obesity paradox in aging: from prevalence to pathophysiology. *Prog Cardiovasc Dis*. 2018;61(2):182–189.
20. Endalifer ML, Diress G. Epidemiology, predisposing factors, biomarkers, and prevention mechanism of obesity: a systematic review. *J Obes*. 2020:6134362 2020.
21. Milano W, et al. Depression and obesity: analysis of common biomarkers. *Diseases*. 2020;8(2):23.
22. Heymsfield SB, Wadden TA. Mechanisms, pathophysiology, and management of obesity. *N Engl J Med*. 2017;376(3): 254–266.
23. Chait A, den Hartigh LJ. Adipose tissue distribution, inflammation and its metabolic consequences, including diabetes and cardiovascular disease. *Front Cardiovasc Med*. 2020;7:22.
24. Zorena K, et al. Adipokines and obesity. Potential link to metabolic disorders and chronic complications. *Int J Mol Sci*. 2020;21(10):3570.
25. Friedman J. The long road to leptin. *J Clin Invest*. 2016;126(12):4727–4734.
26. Poetsch MS, Strano A, Guan K. Role of leptin in cardiovascular diseases. *Front Endocrinol (Lausanne)*. 2020;11:354.
27. Choi HM, Doss HM, Kim KS. Multifaceted physiological roles of adiponectin in inflammation and diseases. *Int J Mol Sci*. 2020;21(4):1219.

28. Blaner WS. Vitamin A signaling and homeostasis in obesity, diabetes, and metabolic disorders. *Pharmacol Ther*. 2019;197: 153–178.
29. Murphy T, Le Foll B. Targeting the endocannabinoid CB1 receptor to treat body weight disorders: a preclinical and clinical review of the therapeutic potential of past and present CB1 drugs. *Biomolecules*. 2020;10(6):855.
30. Lefranc C, et al. Mitochondrial oxidative stress in obesity: role of the mineralocorticoid receptor. *J Endocrinol*. 2018;238(3):R143–R159.
31. Sovetkina A, et al. The physiological role of ghrelin in the regulation of energy and glucose homeostasis. *Cureus*. 2020;12(5):e7941.
32. Krieger JP. Intestinal glucagon-like peptide-1 effects on food intake: physiological relevance and emerging mechanisms. *Peptides*. 2020;131:170342.
33. Lafferty RA, Flatt PR, Irwin N. Emerging therapeutic potential for peptide YY for obesity-diabetes. *Peptides*. 2018;100:269–274.
34. Miller LJ, Desai AJ. Metabolic actions of the type 1 cholecystokinin receptor: its potential as a therapeutic target. *Trends Endocrinol Metab*. 2016;27(9):609–619.
35. Montgomery MK, De Nardo W, Watt MJ. Impact of lipotoxicity on tissue "cross talk" and metabolic regulation. *Physiology (Bethesda)*. 2019;34(2):134–149.
36. Zatterale F, et al. Chronic adipose tissue inflammation linking obesity to insulin resistance and type 2 diabetes. *Front Physiol*. 2020;10:1607.
37. Xiao H, Kang S. The role of the gut microbiome in energy balance with a focus on the gut-adipose tissue axis. *Front Genet*. 2020;11:297.
38. Goossens GH. The metabolic phenotype in obesity: fat mass, body fat distribution, and adipose tissue function. *Obes Facts*. 2017;10(3):207–215.
39. Nd AM. Non-alcoholic fatty liver disease, an overview. *Integr Med (Encinitas)*. 2019;18(2):42–49.
40. Kwok KH, Lam KS, Xu A. Heterogeneity of white adipose tissue: molecular basis and clinical implications. *Exp Mol Med*. 2016;48:e215.
41. Garvey WT, et al. American Association of Clinical Endocrinologists and American College of Endocrinology Comprehensive Clinical Practice Guidelines for Medical Care of Patients With Obesity. *Endocr Pract*. 2016;22(suppl 3):1–205.
42. Tsai AG, Bessesen DH. Obesity. *Ann Intern Med*. 2019;170(5):ITC33–ITC48.
43. Severin R, et al. Precision medicine in weight loss and healthy living. *Prog Cardiovasc Dis*. 2019;62(1):15–20.
44. Dragano NRV, et al. Recent updates on obesity treatments: available drugs and future directions. *Neuroscience*. 2020;437: 215–239.
45. Roth AE, Thornley CJ, Blackstone RP. Outcomes in bariatric and metabolic surgery: an updated 5-year review. *Curr Obes Rep*. 2020;9:380–389.
46. Jensen GL, Wheeler D. A new approach to defining and diagnosing malnutrition in adult critical illness. *Curr Opin Crit Care*. 2012;18(2):206–211.
47. Finn PF, Dice JF. Proteolytic and lipolytic responses to starvation. *Nutrition*. 2006;22(7–8):830–844.
48. Benjamin O, Lappin SL. *Kwashiorkor*. *StatPearls*. Treasure Island, FL: StatPearls Publishing; 2021. Last updated July 22, 2021. Available at. https://www.ncbi.nlm.nih.gov/books/NBK507876/. Accessed September 14, 2021.
49. Titi-Lartey OA, Gupta V. *Marasmus*. *StatPearls*. Treasure Island, FL: StatPearls Publishing; 2021. Last updated July 30, 2021. Available at. https://www.ncbi.nlm.nih.gov/books/NBK559224/. Accessed September 14, 2021.
50. Crawford J. What are the criteria for response to cachexia treatment? *Ann Palliat Med*. 2019;8(1):43–49.
51. Peixoto da Silva S, et al. Cancer cachexia and its pathophysiology: links with sarcopenia, anorexia and asthenia. *J Cachexia Sarcopenia Muscle*. 2020;11(3):619–635. 2020.
52. Berkley JA, et al. Prognostic indicators of early and late death in children admitted to district hospital in Kenya: cohort study. *BMJ*. 2003;326(7385):361.
53. Reintam Blaser A, Berger MM. Early or late feeding after ICU admission? *Nutrients*. 2017;9(12):E1278.
54. Johnson KO, et al. Differences in circulating appetite-related hormone concentrations between younger and older adults: a systematic review and meta-analysis. *Aging Clin Exp Res*. 2020;32(7):1233–1244.
55. Jadczak AD, Visvanathan R. Anorexia of aging - an updated short review. *J Nutr Health Aging*. 2019;23(3):306–309.
56. Courtney-Martin G, et al. Protein requirements during aging. *Nutrients*. 2016;8(8):492.
57. Wysokiński A, et al. Mechanisms of the anorexia of aging—a review. *Age (Dordr)*. 2015;37(4):9821.

24

Structure and Function of the Reproductive Systems

Karen C. Turner

http://evolve.elsevier.com/Rogers/pathophysiology/

CHAPTER OUTLINE

The male and female reproductive systems have several anatomic and physiologic features in common. Most obvious is their major function—reproduction—through which a 23-chromosome female gamete, the ovum (pl., ova), and a 23-chromosome male gamete, the spermatozoon (sperm cell), unite to form a 46-chromosome zygote that is capable of developing into a new individual. The male reproductive system produces sperm that can be transferred to the female reproductive tract. The female reproductive system produces the ovum; if the ovum is fertilized, it is then called the embryo and developing fetus. These functions are determined not only by anatomic structures but also by complex hormonal, neurologic, and psychogenic factors.

DEVELOPMENT OF THE REPRODUCTIVE SYSTEMS

The structure and function of both male and female reproductive systems depend on steroid hormones called sex hormones and their precursors. Cholesterol is the precursor for steroid hormones, including sex hormones (e.g., estrogen and testosterone). Other hormones that are not steroid hormones (e.g., gonadotropins) also support reproduction. The actions of both sex and reproductive hormones are summarized in Table 24.1. Sex and reproductive hormones act on target tissues by binding with cellular receptors (see Chapter 21 hormonal regulation). Hormonal effects on the reproductive systems begin during embryonic development and continue in varying degrees throughout life.

Sexual Differentiation and Hormone Production in Utero

Initially, in embryonic development, the reproductive structures of male and female embryos are homologous (the same) or undifferentiated. They consist of one pair of primary sex organs, or gonads, and two pairs of ducts—the wolffian ducts and the müllerian ducts (Fig. 24.1). The müllerian ducts are the precursor of the internal female sex organs (oviducts, uterus, cervix, and upper vagina). Müllerian ducts are initially formed regardless of genotypic sex and require no sex-determining region on the Y chromosome *(SRY)* signaling for development. *SRY* signaling is required in males to cause regression of the müllerian ducts, which in turn prevents the development of the female reproductive tract. The wolffian ducts are the precursor of male internal sex organs (secrete testosterone and promote the development of the male sex organs). Both pairs of ducts empty into an opening called the *urogenital sinus.*

The first sign of development of reproductive organs (male or female) occurs during the fifth week of gestation. Between

TABLE 24.1 Summary of Female and Male Sex and Reproductive Hormones

Hormone (Source)	Action in Females	Action in Males
Dehydroepiandrosterone (DHEA) (adrenal gland, ovary, other tissues)	Converted to androstenedione and then to estrogens, testosterone, or both	Converted to androstenedione and then to estrogens, testosterone, or both
Estrogens (estrone, estradiol, estriol) (ovary and placenta, small amounts in other tissues)	Stimulates development of female sexual characteristics: maturation of breast, uterus, and vagina; promotes proliferative development of endometrium during menstrual cycle; during pregnancy promotes mammary gland development, fetal adrenal gland function, and uteroplacental blood flow (see Box 24.1)	Growth at puberty, growth plate fusion in bone, prevention of apoptosis of germ cells
Testosterone (adrenal glands from DHEA, testes)	Libido, learning, sleep, protein anabolism, growth of muscle and bone; growth of pubic and axillary hair; activation of sebaceous glands, accounting for some cases of acne during puberty	Stimulates spermatogenesis, stimulates development of primary and secondary sexual characteristics, promotes growth of muscle and bone (anabolic effect); growth of pubic and axillary hair; activates sebaceous glands, accounting for some cases of acne during puberty; maintains libido
Gonadotropin-releasing hormone (GnRH) (hypothalamus-neuroendocrine cells)	Stimulates secretion of gonadotropins (FSH and LH) from anterior pituitary	Stimulates secretion of gonadotropins (FSH and LH) from anterior pituitary
Follicle-stimulating hormone (FSH) (anterior pituitary, gonadotroph cells)	Gonadotropin; promotes development of ovarian follicles; stimulates estrogen secretion	Gonadotropin; promotes development and growth of testes and stimulates spermatogenesis by Sertoli cells
Luteinizing hormone (LH) (anterior pituitary, gonadotroph cells)	Gonadotropin; triggers ovulation; promotes development of corpus luteum	Gonadotropin; stimulates testosterone production by Leydig cells of testis
Inhibin (ovary and testes)	Inhibits FSH production in anterior pituitary (perhaps by limiting GnRH)	Inhibits FSH production in anterior pituitary
Human chorionic gonadotropin (hCG) (placenta)	Supports corpus luteum, which secretes estrogen and progesterone during first 7 weeks of pregnancy	
Activin (ovary)	Stimulates secretion of FSH and pituitary response to GnRH and FSH binding in dominant granulosa cells	
Progesterone (ovary and placenta)	Promotes secretory changes in endometrium during luteal phase of menstrual cycle; quiets uterine myometrium (muscle) activity and prevents lactogenesis during pregnancy	
Relaxin (corpus luteum, myometrium, and placenta)	Inhibits uterine contractions during pregnancy and softens pelvic joints and cervix to facilitate childbirth	

6 and 7 weeks' gestation, the male embryo differentiates under the influence of testes-determining factor (TDF), a protein expressed by the *SRY* gene. When the *SRY* gene is expressed, male gonadal development prevails. TDF stimulates the male gonads to develop into the two testes, and by 8 weeks' gestation, testosterone secretion begins. Müllerian inhibitory hormone (MIH), secreted by Sertoli cells in the testes, promotes degeneration of the müllerian ducts. Without MIH, the müllerian ducts would develop, and the wolffian ducts would degenerate with loss of male sex organ development. The Leydig cells secrete testosterone and promote Wolffian duct development, which differentiates into the epididymis, vas deferens, seminal vesicles, and ejaculatory ducts. By 9 months' gestation, the male gonads (testes) have descended into the scrotum. The testes produce sperm after puberty.

Female gonadal development occurs in the absence of *SRY* expression and with the expression of other genes. The presence of *estrogen* and the absence of *testosterone* and MIH cause degeneration in the wolffian ducts and maintenance of the müllerian ducts. At 6 to 8 weeks' gestation, the two female gonads develop into ovaries, which will produce ova. By the tenth week, the wolffian ducts deteriorate, and the upper ends of the müllerian ducts become the fallopian tubules, whereas the lower ends join to become the uterus, cervix, and upper two-thirds of the vagina (see Fig. 24.1). The fallopian tubes will carry ova from the ovaries to the uterus during a female's reproductive years. Lack of testosterone and the presence of estrogen promote the development of external genitalia (lower end of vagina, labia, and clitoris).

Like the internal reproductive structures, the external structures develop from homologous embryonic tissues. During the first 7 to 8 weeks' gestation, both male and female embryos develop an elevated structure called the *genital tubercle* (Fig. 24.2). Testosterone is necessary for the genital tubercle to differentiate into external male genitalia; otherwise, female

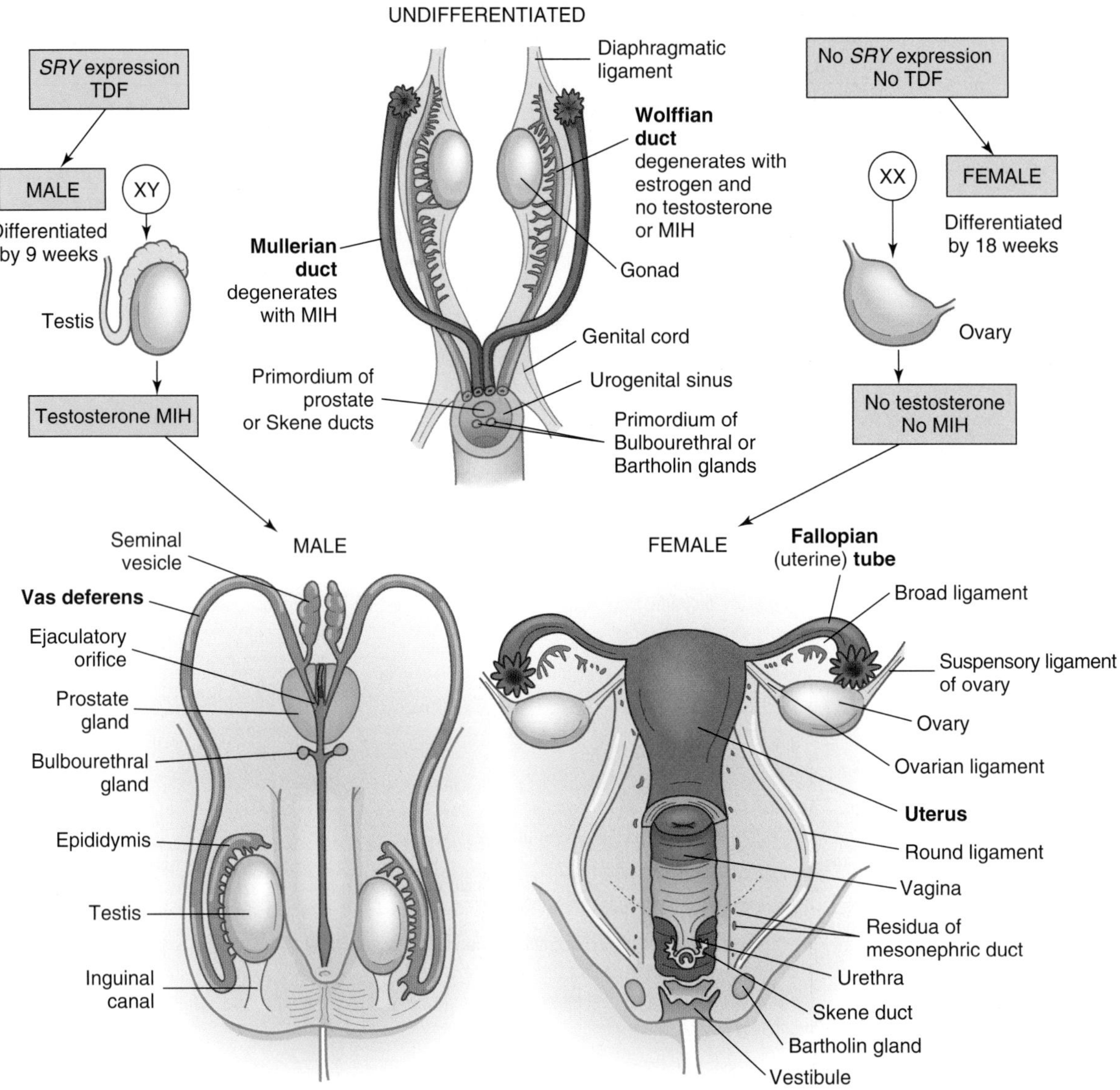

Fig. 24.1 Embryonic Sexual Differentiation. Embryonic and fetal development of the internal genitalia. *MIH,* Müllerian inhibitory hormone; *SRY,* gene that produces TDF; *TDF,* testosterone development factor; see text for additional details.

genitalia develop, which may occur even in the absence of ovaries, possibly because of the presence of placental estrogens.

Anterior pituitary development begins between the fourth and fifth weeks of fetal life, and the vascular connection between the hypothalamus and the pituitary is established by the 12th week. Gonadotropin-releasing hormone (GnRH) is produced in the hypothalamus by 10 weeks' gestation and controls the production of two gonadotropins, luteinizing hormone (LH) and follicle-stimulating hormone (FSH), by the anterior pituitary gland. In the female fetus, high levels of FSH and LH are excreted. FSH and LH stimulate the production of estrogen and progesterone by the ovary. The production of FSH and LH increases until about 28 weeks' gestation when the production of estrogen and progesterone by the ovaries and placenta is high enough to result in the decline of gonadotropin production. Production of primitive female gametes (ova) occurs solely during fetal life. From puberty to menopause, one female gamete matures per menstrual cycle. Production of the male gametes (sperm) begins at puberty; after that, millions are produced daily, usually for life.

By the end of pregnancy, a sensitive negative-feedback system, which includes the gonadostat, is operative in the human fetus. The gonadostat responds to high placental estrogen levels by releasing low levels of GnRH. Soon after birth, steroid hormones levels drop because of the withdrawal of maternal placental hormones. Hypothalamic pulsatile GnRH is secreted, and gonadotropins LH and FSH are released. Their levels peak at 3 to 6 months for boys and at 12 to 18 months for girls, and then fall steadily. The gonadotropins will be suppressed until the onset of puberty.

Puberty and Reproductive Maturation

Adolescence is the stage of human development between childhood and adulthood and includes social, psychological, and

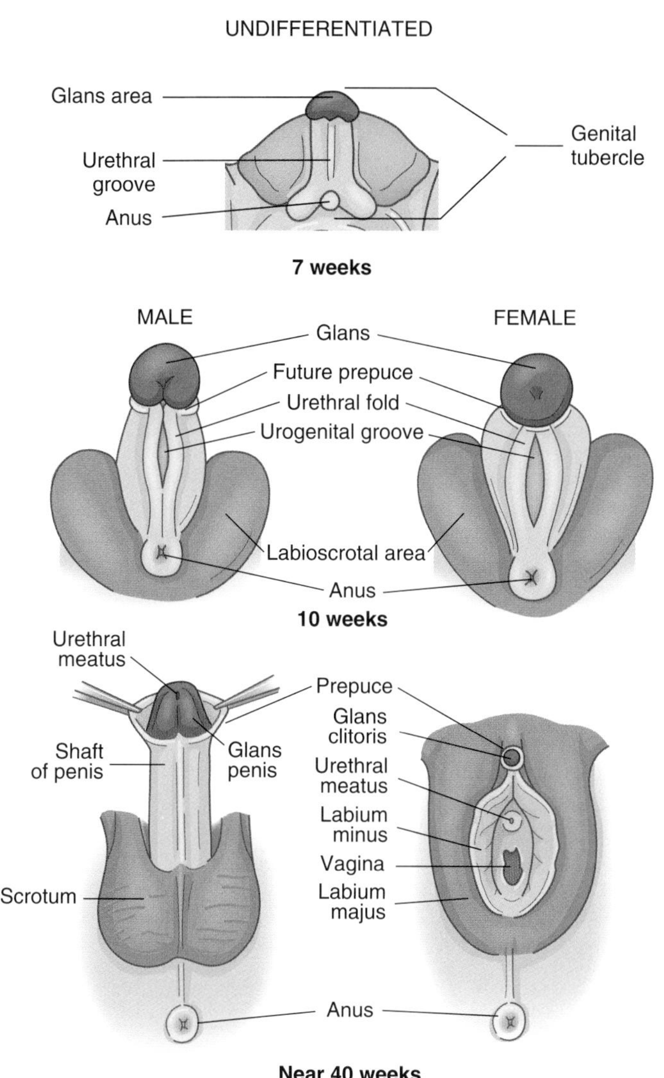

Fig. 24.2 External Genitalia Development. Embryonic and fetal development of the external genitalia.

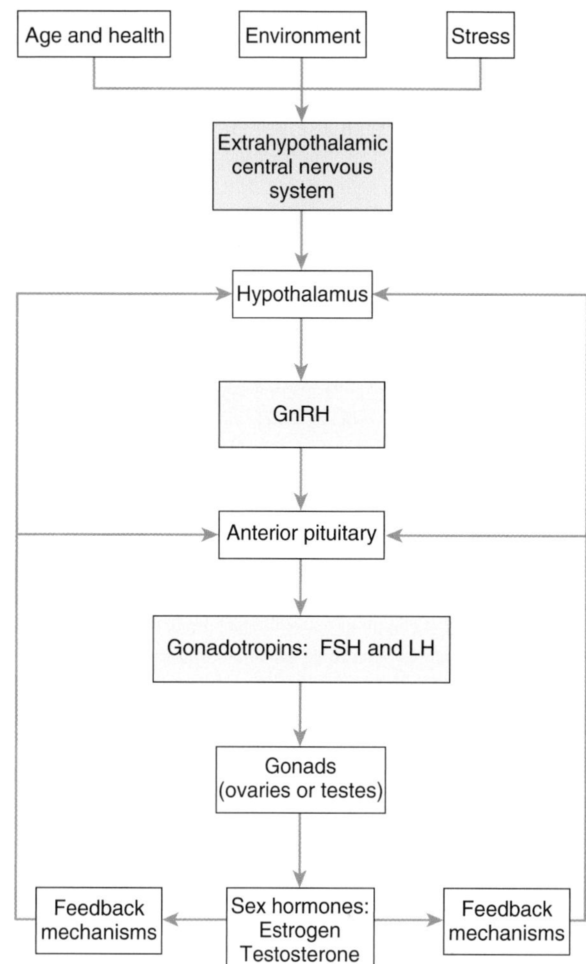

Fig. 24.3 Hormonal Stimulation of the Gonads. The hypothalamic-pituitary-gonadal axis. *FSH*, Follicle-stimulating hormone; *GnRH*, gonadotropin-releasing hormone; *LH*, luteinizing hormone.

biologic changes. Puberty is the onset of sexual maturation and differs from adolescence. Genetics, environment, ethnicity, general health, and nutrition can influence the timing of puberty. In females, puberty begins at about age 8 to 9 years with thelarche (breast development). In males, it begins later, at about age 11 years.

Reproductive maturation involves the hypothalamic-pituitary-gonadal axis, the central nervous system, and the endocrine system (Fig. 24.3). There is a sequential series of hormonal events that promote sexual maturation as puberty approaches. Nocturnal gonadotropin secretion (i.e., LH and FSH) and an increased response in the pituitary to GnRH occur about 1 year before puberty. This, in turn, stimulates gonadal maturation (gonadarche) with estradiol secretion in females and testosterone secretion in males. Estradiol causes thelarche, maturation of the reproductive organs (vagina, uterus, ovaries), and deposition of fat in the female's hips. Estrogen and increased production of growth factors cause rapid skeletal growth in both males and females. Testosterone causes the growth of the testes, scrotum, and penis. A positive feedback loop is created with gonadotropins stimulating the gonads to produce more sex hormones. The most important hormonal effects occur in the gonads. In males, the testes begin to produce mature sperm that are capable of fertilizing an ovum. Male puberty is complete with the first ejaculation that contains mature sperm. In females, the ovaries begin to release mature ova. Female puberty is complete at the time of the first ovulatory menstrual period. Before puberty, there also is an increase in adrenal androgen in both sexes, known as adrenarche. Adrenal androgens are converted to testosterone and estradiol and contribute to the growth of axillary and pubic hair and activation of sweat and sebaceous glands during puberty. Puberty is complete when an individual is capable of reproduction.

Puberty is a time during which some individuals begin to experience gender dysphoria. Gender dysphoria refers to the discomfort, distress, disharmony, and conflict caused by the discrepancy between a person's gender identity and their personal sense of self as a man or woman, their associated primary or secondary sexual characteristics, and their expected social

EMERGING SCIENCE BOX

Gender Reassignment and Gender Affirming Hormone Therapy

Transgender individuals are much more likely to experience anxiety, depression, and suicide attempts than cisgender individuals. Many transgender individuals choose gender-affirming hormone therapy (GAHT) to align with their gender identity and reduce gender dysphoria. Many transgender individuals also choose body modification with gender-affirming surgery, but that option is not the focus here.

Individuals choosing GAHT must demonstrate a consistent and persistent gender-variant identity that meets the criteria for gender dysphoria as categorized by the Diagnostic and Statistical Manual of Mental Disorders, Fifth Edition (2013 American Psychiatric Association, Washington, DC). Guidelines are available to assist clinicians with the hormonal management of individuals seeking GAHT (Hembree et al., 2017, details cited below). The goal of hormone therapy is to suppress endogenous sex hormone secretion determined by the person's genetic/gonadal sex and maintain sex hormone levels within the normal range for the person's affirmed gender. Hormone treatment is currently not recommended for prepubertal gender-dysphoric/gender-incongruent persons. Prior to beginning therapy, medical and mental health conditions that can be exacerbated by hormone depletion and treatment with sex hormones need to be evaluated and managed. Testosterone regimens are prescribed for transgender men (female to male) and estrogen (e.g., 17 beta-estradiol) augmented by antiandrogens (e.g., spironolactone) are prescribed for transgender women (male to female). Dosages are individually determined and monitored to maintain physiologic hormone levels and to achieve and maintain desired feminine and masculine characteristics. GAHT reduces fertility, and individuals desiring genetic offspring can consider oocyte/embryo or semen cryopreservation.

Hormone therapy requires ongoing preventive health care for the management of modifiable risk factors. Transgender women receiving estrogen and antiandrogens are at risk for thromboembolic disease (venous thrombosis and pulmonary embolism), cardiovascular and cerebrovascular disease, hypertriglyceridemia, osteoporosis, and breast cancer. Transgender men receiving testosterone are at risk for erythrocytosis, cardiovascular and cerebrovascular disease, dyslipidemia (low HDL, high LDL), hypertension, and breast, cervical and uterine cancer. Research is in progress to determine the long-term effects and safety profiles of hormone therapy and on cardiovascular health as cardiovascular disease is the leading cause of death in the transgender population undergoing GAHT.

GAHT has significant positive psychological effects on both adolescents and adults. Research tends to support that GAHT reduces symptoms of anxiety and depression, lowers perceived and social distress, and improves the quality of life and self-esteem for transgendered individuals.

Data from Connelly PJ, et al. Gender-affirming hormone therapy, vascular health and cardiovascular disease in transgender adults. *Hypertension.* 2019;74(6):1266–1274; Dutra E, et al. Cardiovascular implications of gender-affirming hormone treatment in the transgender population. *Maturitas.* 2019;129: 45–49; Fernandez JD, et al. Assessment of gender-affirming hormone therapy requirements. *LGBT Health.* 2019;6(3):101–106; Hembree WC, et al. Endocrine treatment of gender-dysphoric/gender-incongruent persons: an endocrine society clinical practice guideline. *J Clin Endocrinol Metab.* 2017;102(11):3869–3903. Erratum in: *J Clin Endocrinol Metab.* 103(2):699. Erratum in: *J Clin Endocrinol Metab.* 103(7):2758–2759. PMID: 28945902; Iwamoto SJ, et al. Health considerations for transgender women and remaining unknowns: a narrative review. *Ther Adv Endocrinol Metab.* 2019;30. doi:10:2042018819871166; Nguyen HB, et al. Gender-affirming hormone use in transgender individuals: impact on behavioral health and cognition. *Curr Psychiatry Rep.* 2018;20(12):1–9; Radix A. Hormone therapy for transgender adults. *Urol Clin North Am.* 2019;46(4), 467–473.

gender roles. Transgender is a term used to describe individuals whose gender identity or expression differs from their sex assigned at birth. Many transgender individuals choose hormonal or surgical interventions to reduce gender dysphoria (see Emerging Science Box: Gender Reassignment and Gender Affirming Hormone Therapy).

THE FEMALE REPRODUCTIVE SYSTEM

The function of the female reproductive system is to produce mature ova; then, if fertilization occurs, the female reproductive system provides protection and nourishment to the fetus until it is expelled at birth.

External Genitalia

The external genitalia protect body openings and play an important role in sexual functioning. Fig. 24.4 shows the external female genitalia, known collectively as the vulva or pudendum. The major structures are as follows:

Mons Pubis

The mons pubis is a fatty layer of tissue over the pubic symphysis (joint formed by the union of the pubic bones) that protects the joint during sexual intercourse. During puberty, it becomes covered with pubic hair, and sebaceous and sweat glands become more active. Estrogen causes the fat to be deposited under the skin giving it a mound-like shape.

Labia Majora and Minora

The labia majora (sing., labium majus) is composed of two folds of skin arising at the mons pubis and extending back to the fourchette, forming a cleft. During puberty, the amount of fatty tissue increases, pubic hair grows on lateral surfaces, and sebaceous glands on hairless medial surfaces secrete lubricants. This structure is highly sensitive to temperature, touch, pressure, and pain and protects the inner structures of the vulva. It is homologous to the male scrotum (see Fig. 24.2).

The labia minora (sing., labium minus) is composed of two smaller, thinner, asymmetric folds of skin within the labia majora that form the clitoral hood (prepuce) and frenulum, then split to enclose the vestibule, and converge near the anus to form the fourchette. The labia minora are hairless, pink, and moist; they are well supplied by nerves, blood vessels, and sebaceous glands that secrete bactericidal fluid with a distinctive odor that lubricates and waterproofs vulvar skin. The labia swell with blood during sexual arousal.

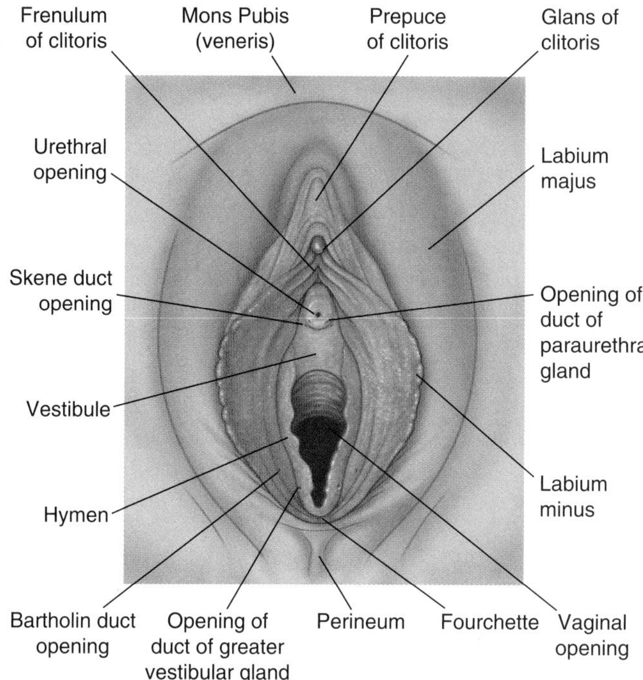

Fig. 24.4 External Female Genitalia. (Modified from Drake R, Vogl AW, Mitchell A, et al. *Gray's atlas of anatomy*, 3rd edition. Philadelphia: Churchill Livingstone; 2020.)

Clitoris

The clitoris is a richly innervated erectile organ between the labia minora. It is a small, cylindric structure having a visible glans and a shaft that lies beneath the skin; the clitoris is homologous to the penis. It secretes smegma, which has a unique odor that may be sexually arousing. Like the penis, the clitoris is a major site of sexual stimulation and orgasm. With sexual arousal, erectile tissue fills with blood, causing the clitoris to enlarge slightly.

Vestibule

The vestibule is an area protected by the labia minora that contains the external opening of the vagina, called the *introitus* or vaginal orifice. A thin, perforated membrane, the *hymen*, may cover the introitus. The vestibule also contains the opening of the urethra, or *urinary meatus* (orifice). These structures are lubricated by two pairs of glands: Skene glands and Bartholin glands. The ducts of the Skene glands (also called the *lesser vestibular* or *paraurethral glands*) open on both sides of the urinary meatus. The ducts of the Bartholin glands *(greater vestibular* or *vulvovaginal glands)* open on either side of the introitus. In response to sexual stimulation, Bartholin glands secrete mucus that lubricates the inner labial surfaces, as well as enhances the viability and motility of sperm. Skene glands help lubricate the urinary meatus and the vestibule. In response to sexual excitement, the highly vascular tissue just beneath the vestibule also fills with blood and becomes engorged.

Perineum

The perineum is an area with less hair, skin, and subcutaneous tissue lying between the vaginal orifice and anus. Unlike the rest of the vulva, this area has little subcutaneous fat, so the skin is close to the underlying muscles. The perineum covers the muscular *perineal body*, a fibrous structure that consists of elastic fibers and connective tissue and serves as the common attachment for the bulbocavernosus, external anal sphincter, and levator ani muscles. The perineum varies in length from 2 to 5 cm or more and has elastic properties. The length of the perineum and the elasticity of the perineal body influence tissue resistance and injury during childbirth.

Internal Genitalia

Vagina

The vagina is an elastic, fibromuscular canal that is 9 to 10 cm long in a reproductive-age female. It extends up and back from the introitus to the lower portion of the uterus. As Fig. 24.5 shows, the vagina lies between the urethra (and part of the bladder) and the rectum. Mucosal secretions from the upper genital organs, menstrual fluids, and products of conception leave the body through the vagina. During coitus, the penis enters the vagina. During sexual arousal, the vagina lengthens and widens, and the vaginal wall becomes engorged with blood, much like the labia minora and clitoris. Engorgement pushes some fluid to the surface of the mucosa, enhancing lubrication. The vaginal wall does not contain mucus-secreting glands; rather, secretions drain into the vagina from the endocervical glands or from the Bartholin and Skene glands of the vestibule. The vagina also functions as the birth canal during childbirth. Its elasticity and relatively sparse nerve supply enhance the vagina's function in this role. During childbirth, the pelvic floor muscles and rugae of the vagina stretch to facilitate the passage of the infant.

The vaginal wall is lined with a mucous membrane of squamous epithelial cells that thickens and thins in response to hormones, particularly estrogen. The squamous epithelial membrane is continuous with the membrane that covers the lower part of the uterus. In females of reproductive age, the mucosal layer is arranged in transverse wrinkles, or folds, called rugae (sing., ruga), that permit stretching during coitus and childbirth. Below the mucosal layer are three more layers: fibrous connective tissue containing numerous blood and lymphatic vessels, smooth muscle and connective tissue, and a rich network of blood vessels.

The upper part of the vagina surrounds the cervix, the lower end of the uterus (see Fig. 24.5). The recessed space around the cervix is called the fornix of the vagina. The posterior fornix is "deeper" than the anterior fornix because of the angle at which the cervix meets the vaginal canal. In most females, this angle is about 90 degrees. A pouch called the cul-de-sac separates the posterior fornix and the rectum.

Two factors help maintain the self-cleansing action of the vagina and defend it from infection, particularly during the reproductive years. They are (1) an acid-base balance that discourages the proliferation of most pathogenic bacteria and (2) the thickness of the vaginal epithelium. Before

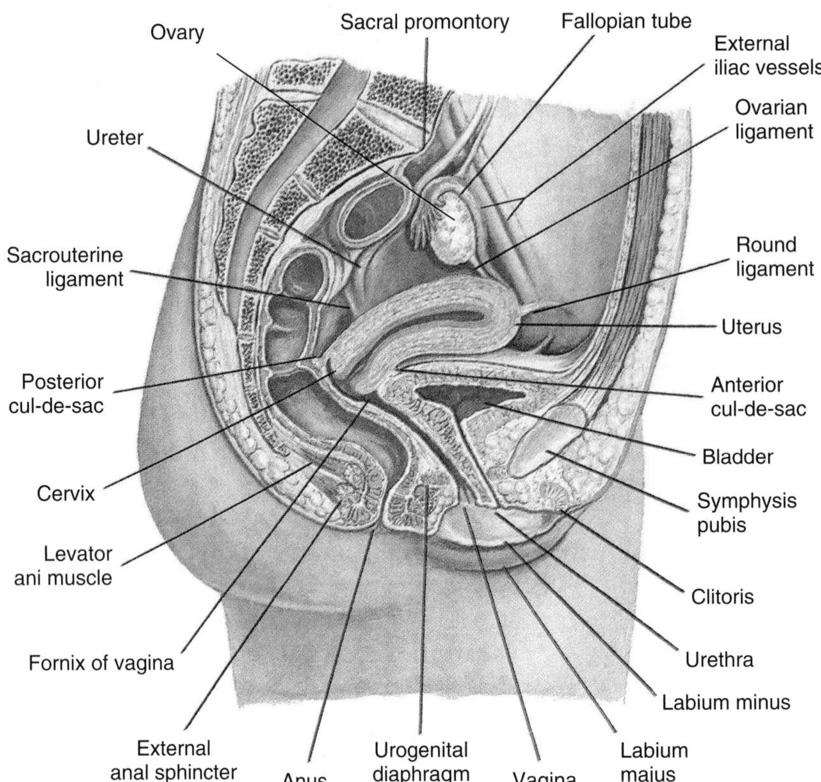

Fig. 24.5 Internal Female Genitalia and Other Pelvic Organs. (From Ball JW, et al. Seidel's *Guide to Physical Examination*. 8th ed. St Louis: Mosby; 2015.)

puberty, vaginal pH is about 7.0 (neutral), and the vaginal epithelium is thin. At puberty, the pH becomes more acidic (4.0 to 5.0), and the squamous epithelial lining thickens. These changes are maintained until menopause (cessation of menstruation) when the pH rises again to more alkaline levels and the epithelium thins. Therefore, protection from infection is greatest during the years when a female is most likely to be sexually active. Both defense factors are greatest when estrogen levels are high, and the vagina contains a normal population of *Lactobacillus acidophilus*, a harmless resident bacterium that helps maintain pH at acidic levels. Any condition that causes vaginal pH to rise—such as douching or use of vaginal sprays or deodorants, the presence of low estrogen levels, or destruction of *L. acidophilus* by antibiotics—lowers vaginal defenses against infection.

Uterus

The uterus is a hollow, pear-shaped organ whose lower end opens into the vagina. It anchors and protects a fertilized ovum, provides an optimal environment while the ovum develops, and pushes the fetus out at birth. In addition, the uterus plays an important role in sexual response and conception. During sexual excitement, the opening of the lower uterus (the cervix) dilates slightly. At the same time, the uterus increases in size and moves upward and backward, creating a tenting effect in the midvagina that results in the cervix "sitting" in a pool of semen. During orgasm, rhythmic contractions facilitate the movement of sperm through the cervical os while also enhancing physical pleasure.

At puberty, the uterus attains its adult size and proportions and descends from the abdomen to the lower pelvis, between the bladder and the rectum (see Fig. 24.5). The uterus of a mature, nonpregnant female is approximately 7 to 9 cm long and 6.5 cm wide, with muscular walls 3.5 cm thick, enlarging by about 1 cm in all dimensions after pregnancy.[1] It is loosely held in position by ligaments, peritoneal tissue folds, and the pressure of adjacent organs, especially the urinary bladder, sigmoid colon, and rectum. In most females, the uterus is tipped forward (anteverted) so that it rests on the urinary bladder. However, it may be tipped backward (retroverted), and various degrees of forward or backward flexion are normal (Fig. 24.6).

The uterus has two major parts: the corpus (body of the uterus) and the cervix (Fig. 24.7). The top of the corpus, above the insertion of the fallopian tubes, is called the fundus. The diameter of the uterine cavity is widest at the fundus and narrowest at the isthmus, just above the cervix (see Fig. 24.5). The cervix, or "neck of the uterus," extends from the isthmus to the vagina. The passageway between the upper opening (the internal os) and the lower opening (the external os) of the cervix is called the endocervical canal (see Fig. 24.7). The entire uterus, like the upper vagina, is innervated exclusively by motor and sensory fibers of the autonomic nervous system.

The uterine wall is composed of three layers (see Fig. 24.7). The perimetrium (parietal peritoneum) is the outer serous membrane that covers the uterus. The myometrium is the thick, muscular middle layer. It is thickest at the fundus, apparently to facilitate birth. The endometrium, or uterine lining, is

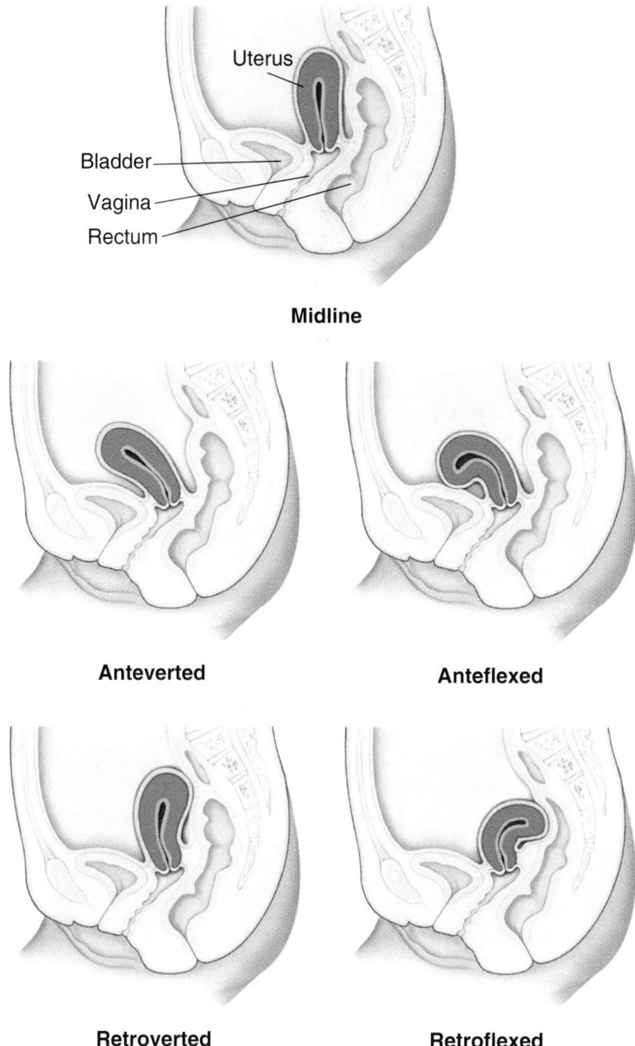

Fig. 24.6 Variations in Uterine Positions.

composed of a functional layer (superficial compact layer and spongy middle layer) and a basal layer. The functional layer of the endometrium responds to the sex hormones estrogen and progesterone. Between puberty and menopause, this layer proliferates and is shed monthly. The basal layer, which is attached to the myometrium, regenerates the functional layer after shedding (menstruation).

The endocervical canal does not have an endometrial layer but is lined with columnar epithelial cells. It is continuous with the lining of the outer cervix and vagina, which are lined with squamous epithelial cells. The point where the two types of cells meet is called the *transformation zone*, or squamous-columnar junction (see Fig. 25.20). The transformation zone is vulnerable to the human papillomavirus (HPV), especially HPV types 16 and 18, which can lead to cervical dysplasia or carcinoma in situ. Cells of the transformation zone are removed for examination during a Papanicolaou (Pap test) smear.

The cervix acts as a mechanical barrier, protecting the uterus from infectious microorganisms from the vagina. The external cervical os is a very small opening that contains thick, sticky mucus (the mucous "plug") during the luteal phase of the menstrual cycle and throughout pregnancy. During ovulation, the mucus changes under the influence of estrogen and forms watery strands, or spinnbarkeit mucus, to facilitate the transport of sperm into the uterus. In addition, the downward flow of cervical secretions moves microorganisms away from the cervix and uterus. In females of reproductive age, the pH of these secretions is inhospitable to many bacteria. Further, mucosal secretions contain enzymes and antibodies (mostly immunoglobulin A [IgA]) of the secretory immune system. Uterine pathophysiologic disorders include infection, displacement of the uterus within the pelvis, benign growths (fibroids) of the uterine wall, hyperplasia of the endometrium, endometriosis, and cancer (see Chapter 25).

Fallopian Tubes

The two fallopian tubes (oviducts, uterine tubes) enter the uterus bilaterally just beneath the fundus (see Fig. 24.7). They direct the ova from the spaces around the ovaries to the uterus. From the uterus, the fallopian tubes curve up and over the two ovaries. Each tube is 8 to 12 cm long and about 1 cm in diameter, except at its ovarian end, which resembles the bell of a trumpet and is fringed or fimbriated (infundibulum). The fimbriae (fringes) move, creating a current that draws the ovum into the infundibulum. Once the ovum enters the fallopian tube, cilia (hairlike structures) and peristalsis (muscle contractions) keep it moving toward the uterus.

The ampulla, or distal third, of the fallopian tube is the usual site of fertilization (see Fig. 24.7). Sperm released into the vagina travel upward through the endocervical canal and uterine cavity and enter the fallopian tubes. If an ovum is present in either tube, fertilization can occur. Whether or not the ovum encounters sperm, it continues to travel through the fallopian tube to the uterus. If fertilized, the ovum (then called a *blastocyst*) implants itself in the endometrial layer of the uterine wall. If not fertilized, the ovum fragments and leaves the uterus with menstrual fluids. Disorders that affect the fallopian tubes (e.g., congenital malformations, infection, and inflammation) can block the path of both sperm and the ovum and may cause infertility or ectopic (tubal) pregnancy.

Ovaries

The ovaries, the female gonads, are the primary female reproductive organs (Fig. 24.8). Their two main functions are secretion of female sex hormones and development and release of female gametes, or ova.

The almond-shaped ovaries are located on both sides of the uterus and are suspended and supported by a portion of the broad ligament (the mesovarium component), ovarian ligaments, and suspensory ligaments (see Fig. 24.7). The ovaries are smaller than their male homologs, the testes. In females of reproductive age, each ovary is about 3 to 5 cm long, 2.5 cm wide, and 2 cm thick, weighing 4 to 8 g. Size and weight vary slightly during each phase of the menstrual cycle (see the Menstrual (Ovarian) Cycle section).

The central part of the ovary, or medulla, is composed of connective tissue and contains many small arteries, veins, and

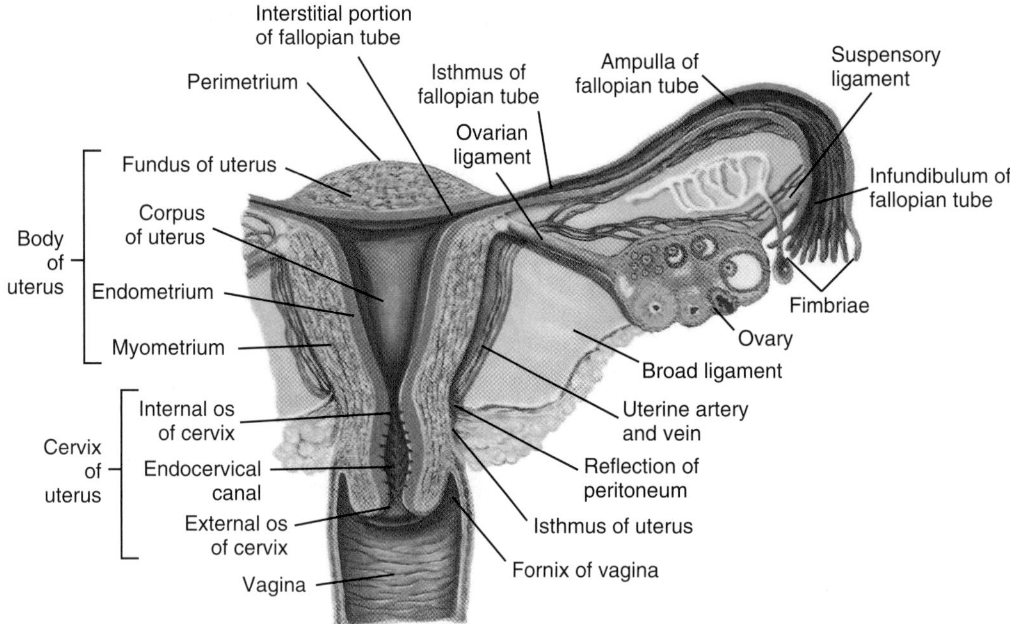

Fig. 24.7 Cross Section of Uterus, Fallopian Tube, and Ovary. (From Solomon B, et al. *Seidel's guide to physical examination*, 9th edition. Elsevier; 2019.)

lymphatics that enter at the hilum. Surrounding the medulla is the cortex. At birth, the cortex of each ovary contains approximately 1 to 2 million ova within primordial (immature) ovarian follicles. By puberty, the number ranges between 300,000 and 500,000, and some of the follicles and the ova within them begin to mature. Follicles grow and undergo atresia continuously and irrevocably throughout a woman's life. Between puberty and menopause, the ovarian cortex always contains follicles and ova in various stages of development (primary and secondary follicles). Once every menstrual cycle (about every 28 days), one of the follicles reaches maturation and discharges its ovum through the ovary's outer covering, the germinal epithelium. During the reproductive years, 400 to 500 ovarian follicles mature completely and release an ovum (ovulation). The remaining follicles either fail to develop at all or degenerate without maturing completely and are known as atretic follicles (see Fig. 24.8).

After the release of the mature ovum (ovulation), the follicle develops into another structure, the corpus luteum (see Fig. 24.8). If fertilization occurs, the corpus luteum enlarges and begins to secrete hormones that maintain and support pregnancy. If fertilization does not occur, the corpus luteum secretes these hormones for approximately 14 days and then degenerates, which triggers the maturation of another follicle. The ovarian cycle—the process of follicular maturation, ovulation, corpus luteum development, and corpus luteum degeneration—is continuous from puberty to menopause, except during pregnancy or hormonal contraceptive use. At menopause, this process ceases, and the ovaries atrophy to the point that they cannot be felt during a pelvic examination.

Sex hormones are secreted by cells present within the ovarian cortex, including two types of cells in the ovarian follicle—theca cells (produce androgens that migrate to granulosa cells) and granulosa cells (convert androgens to estradiol)—and cells of the corpus luteum (secrete primarily progesterone, estrogen, and inhibin) (see Fig. 24.8). These cells all contain receptors for gonadotropins (LH, FSH) or for sex hormones, which are discussed in the next section.

Female Sex Hormones

The sex hormones are all steroid hormones and are synthesized from cholesterol (see Chapter 21). The dominant female sex hormones, estrogen and progesterone, are produced primarily by the ovaries (see Table 24.1). During fetal development, infancy, and childhood, sex hormone production is low. At puberty, hormone production surges, triggering sexual maturation and the development of secondary sex characteristics. From puberty to menopause, the sex hormones are produced cyclically; production surges and diminishes monthly, creating the ovarian and uterine changes associated with the menstrual cycle. These hormones also are produced in higher levels during pregnancy by the placenta, inhibiting ovulation. Individual effects of sex hormones depend on the amount and concentration in the blood.

Both male and female sex hormones are present in all adults. However, the female body contains low levels of testosterone and other androgens, and the male body contains low levels of estrogen.

Estrogens and Androgens

Estrogen is a generic term for any of three similar hormones derived from cholesterol: estradiol, estrone, and estriol. Estradiol (E2) is the most potent and plentiful of the three and is principally produced (95%) by the ovaries (ovarian follicle and corpus luteum). Limited amounts are secreted by the cortices of the adrenal glands and the placenta during pregnancy. Androgens are converted to estrone in ovarian and adipose

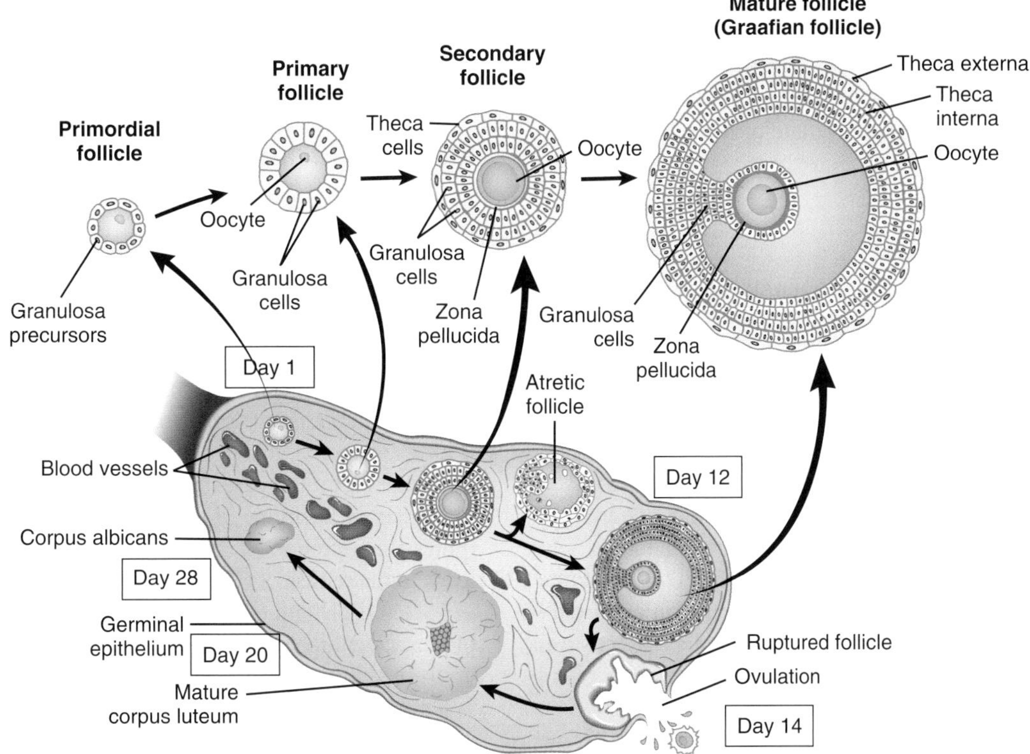

Fig. 24.8 Cross Section of Ovary and Development of an Ovarian Follicle. Schematic representation (not to scale) of the structure of the ovary, showing the various stages in the development of the follicle and its successor structure, the corpus luteum. (Adapted from Berne RM, Levy MN, eds. *Physiology*, 5th edition. St. Louis: Mosby; 2003.)

tissue; estriol is the peripheral metabolite of estrone and estradiol.

Estrogen has numerous biologic effects, many of which involve interactions with other hormones. It is needed for the maturation of reproductive organs, development of secondary sex characteristics, growth, and maintenance of pregnancy. It also is needed for many nonreproductive effects, including closure of long bones after the pubertal growth spurt (in both males and females), maintenance of bone and skin, and systemic organ function (see Table 24.1 and Box 24.1). After menopause, the ovaries dramatically reduce the production of estradiol, and secretion of estrone is markedly diminished (see the Aging and the Female Reproductive System section). At this time, the majority of estradiol is derived from intracellular synthesis in peripheral tissues. Estradiol acts locally to meet physiologic needs according to cell type and is then inactivated without systemic effects.[2]

Like other steroid hormones, estrogens are derived from cholesterol in a complex, enzyme-mediated series of reactions. The hypothalamus secretes GnRH in a pulsatile manner that stimulates gonadotropin (LH and FSH) release from the anterior pituitary. Gonadotropins trigger the ovarian production of estrogen. The primary function of LH is to stimulate theca cells of the ovarian follicle to produce androgens, mainly androstenedione. (Androgens are discussed further under the section titled Male Sex and Reproductive Hormones.) Some of these androgens are converted to estrogen by the theca cells themselves, and others diffuse into the granulosa cells. Within the granulosa layer, FSH induces conversion (aromatization) of androgens to estrogens. Estrogens are then released into the bloodstream.

BOX 24.1 Summary of Nonreproductive Effects of Estrogen

- Estrogens (including estrone, estradiol, estriol) function through estrogen receptors alpha and beta, have different roles in different cells and tissues and have paracrine or intracrine function.
- Maintains bone density by antagonizing effects of parathyroid hormone.
- Acts in the liver to decrease cholesterol level, increase high-density lipoprotein (HDL) level, and decrease low-density lipoprotein (LDL) level (antiatherosclerotic); promotes fat deposition.
- Maintains nervous system (neurotrophic and neuroprotective); facilitates memory and cognition.
- Increases collagen content, dermal thickness, elasticity, water content, and healing ability of the skin.
- Protects against chronic kidney disease in individuals without diabetes.
- Prevents vascular injury and early atheroma formation through endothelial mechanisms.
- Inhibits platelet adhesiveness.
- Can promote inflammation and have variable effects on immunity.
- Promotes clotting; increased risk of thromboembolism (only estrogen associated with pregnancy or use in contraceptive pills or hormone replacement therapy).

Although androgens are primarily male sex hormones produced in the testes, small amounts are produced in the adrenal cortex in both males and females and in the ovaries in females. Some androgens (dehydroepiandrosterone and its metabolite androstenedione) are precursors of estrogens (estrone, estradiol) (see Table 24.1). At puberty, androgens contribute to the skeletal growth spurt and cause the growth of pubic and axillary hair. Androgens also activate sebaceous glands, accounting for some cases of acne during puberty, and play a role in libido.

Progesterone

Luteinizing hormone from the anterior pituitary stimulates the corpus luteum to secrete progesterone, the second major female sex hormone. With estrogen, progesterone controls the ovarian menstrual cycle. LH surge occurs when there is a peak level of estrogen, about 24 to 36 hours before ovulation. LH promotes luteinization of the granulosa in the dominant follicle, resulting in progesterone production and the development of blood vessels and connective tissue. During the follicular phase, the ovary and adrenal glands each contribute approximately 50% of progesterone production. Conversely, large amounts are cyclically secreted from the ovary while the corpus luteum is active for about 9 to 13 days after ovulation. (The complementary and opposing effects of progesterone and estrogen are listed in Table 24.2.) Progesterone secreted by the corpus luteum stimulates the thickened endometrium to become more complex in preparation for implantation of a blastocyte. If conception and implantation do occur, the corpus luteum persists and secretes progesterone (and estrogen) until the placenta is well established at approximately 8 to 10 weeks' gestation and undertakes progesterone production.

Progesterone is sometimes called the *hormone of pregnancy*. Progesterone's effects in pregnancy include:

- maintaining the thickened endometrium;
- relaxing the smooth muscle in the myometrium, which prevents premature contractions and helps the uterus to expand;
- thickening (hypertrophy) the myometrium, which prepares it for the muscular work of labor;
- promoting the growth of lobules and alveoli in the breast in preparation for lactation, but preventing lactation until the fetus is born and then promoting lactation in collaboration with prolactin after birth;
- preventing additional maturation of ova by suppressing FSH and LH, thereby stopping the menstrual cycle;
- providing immune modulation, allowing tolerance against fetal antigens (the mother's immune system does not attack the fetus); and
- preventing preterm birth.

Menstrual (Ovarian) Cycle

In addition to pregnancy, the obvious manifestation of female reproductive functioning is menstrual bleeding (the menses), which starts with menarche (first menstruation) and ends with menopause (cessation of menstrual flow for 1 year). In the United States, the age of first menstruation is about 12 years.[3]

The onset of menarche appears to be related to body weight, especially a high percentage of body fat (a high ratio of fat to lean tissue), which many trigger a change in the metabolic rate and lead to hormonal changes associated with early menarche. The hormone leptin increases before the onset of menarche. Leptin (a regulatory hormone of appetite and energy metabolism) promotes the secretion of kisspeptin from the hypothalamus and leads to the release of GnRH, which in turn enhances the release of FSH and LH and estradiol, triggering ovulation and the onset of puberty. A high percentage of body fat is associated with higher levels of leptin. Childhood obesity is associated with an increase in leptin and with early menarche (age 11 years or younger).[4]

Cycles are not ovulatory at first and may vary in length from 10 to 60 days or more. As adolescence proceeds, regular patterns of menstruation and ovulation are established at intervals ranging between 21 and 45 days.[5] Menstruation continues to recur in a recognizable and characteristic pattern during adulthood, with the length of the menstrual cycle varying considerably among individuals. The commonly accepted cycle average is 28 (25 to 30) days, with rhythmic intervals of 21 to 35 days considered normal (Fig. 24.9). Approximately 4 to 10 years before menopause, cycles begin to lengthen again with variation related to changing hormone levels.[6]

Phases of the Menstrual Cycle

The menstrual (ovarian) cycle (see Fig. 24.9) is the process of menstruation (menses) in the uterine endometrium and ovulation in the ovary. The cycle consists of the follicular/proliferative phase (postmenstrual) followed by the luteal/secretory

TABLE 24.2 Complementary and Opposing Effects of Estrogen and Progesterone

Structure	Effect of Estrogen	Effect of Progesterone
Vaginal mucosa	Proliferation of squamous epithelium; increase in glycogen content of cells; layering (cornification) of cells	Thinning of squamous epithelium; decornification
Cervical mucosa	Production of abundant fluid secretions that favor survival and enhance motility of sperm	Production of thick, sticky secretions that tend to plug cervical os
Fallopian tube	Increase of motility and ciliary action	Decrease of motility and ciliary action
Uterine muscle	Increase of blood flow; increase of contractile proteins; increase of uterine muscle and myometrial excitability to action potential; increase of sensitization to oxytocin	Relaxation of myometrium; decrease of sensitization to oxytocin
Endometrium	Stimulation of growth; increase in number of progesterone receptors	Activation of glands and blood vessels; accumulation of glycogen and enzymes; decrease in number of estrogen receptors
Breasts	Growth of ducts; promotion of prolactin effects	Growth of lobules and alveoli; inhibition of prolactin effects

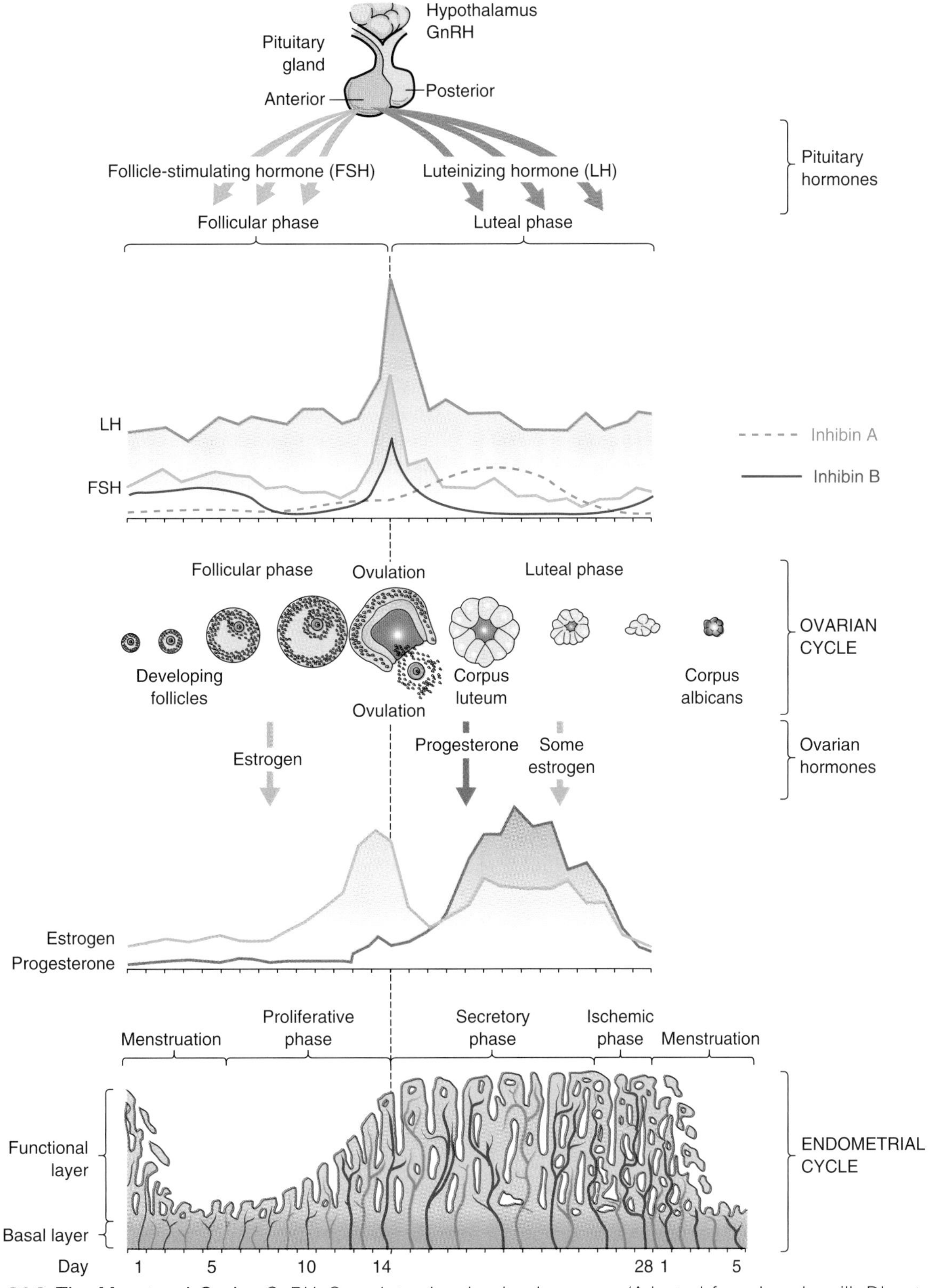

Fig. 24.9 The Menstrual Cycle. *GnRH*, Gonadotropin-releasing hormone. (Adapted from Lowdermilk DL, et al. *Maternity and women's health care*, 10th edition. St. Louis: Mosby; 2012.)

phase (premenstrual) and then the ischemic/menstrual phase if conception does not occur. These are named for processes that occur in the ovary (follicular and luteal phases) and the uterine endometrium (proliferative, secretory, and ischemic phases) during the menstrual cycle.

During menstruation (menses), the functional layer of the endometrium disintegrates and is discharged through the vagina. Menstruation is followed by the follicular/proliferative phase. This phase is named for two simultaneous processes: maturation of an ovarian follicle and proliferation of the uterine endometrium (see Fig. 24.9). During this phase, GnRH and a balance between activin and inhibin levels from the granulosa cells contribute to the increase of FSH level, which stimulates a number of follicles. The result is a rescue of a dominant ovarian follicle from normal dissolution by days 5 to 7 of the cycle. Together, estrogen and FSH make the granulosa cells of the primary follicle more sensitive to FSH and promote LH stimulation, which causes a more rapid secretion of follicular estrogen. A surge in the levels of both LH and FSH is then required for final follicular growth and ovulation. Estrogen levels increase, and inhibin B inhibits the secretion of FSH level by the granulosa cells in the dominant follicle. This drop in FSH concentration decreases the growth of less developed follicles (see Fig. 24.8). Estrogen causes cells of the endometrium to proliferate.

Ovulation is the release of an ovum from a mature follicle and marks the beginning of the luteal/secretory phase of the menstrual cycle. The ovarian follicle begins its transformation into a corpus luteum (see Fig. 24.8), hence the name *luteal phase*. Pulsatile secretion of LH from the anterior pituitary stimulates the corpus luteum to secrete progesterone, estrogen, and inhibin A (suppresses FSH secretion), which in turn initiates the secretory phase of endometrial development. Estrogen maintains the thickness of the endometrium, and progesterone stimulates the growth of glands and blood vessels in the endometrium. The glands begin to secrete a thin, glycogen-containing fluid, hence the name *secretory phase*. At this point, one of the following two paths occurs:

- If conception and implantation do not occur, the corpus luteum degenerates and ceases its production of progesterone and estrogen. Without progesterone or estrogen to maintain it, the endometrium enters the ischemic ("blood-starved") phase and disintegrates, hence the name ischemic/menstrual phase. Menstruation then occurs, marking the beginning of another cycle.
- If conception occurs, the nutrient-laden endometrium is ready for implantation. Human chorionic gonadotropin (hCG) is secreted 3 days after fertilization by the blastocytes and maintains the corpus luteum once implantation occurs at about day 6 or 7. Levels of hCG can be detected in maternal blood and urine 8 to 10 days after ovulation. The production of estrogen and progesterone will continue until the placenta can adequately maintain hormonal production.

Ovulatory cycles appear to have a minimum length of 24 to 26.5 days: the ovarian follicle requires 10 to 12.5 days to develop, and the luteal phase appears fixed at 14 days (±3 days). Menstrual blood flow usually lasts 3 to 7 days but may be between 2 and 8 days and still be considered within normal limits. Bleeding is consistently scant to heavy and varies from 30 to 80 ml, with most blood loss occurring during the first 3 days of menses. Menstrual discharge consists of blood, mucus, and desquamated endometrial tissue and does not clot under normal circumstances. It is usually dark and produces a characteristic musty odor on oxidation. Environmental factors such as severe emotional stress, illness, malnutrition, obesity, extreme exercise, and seasonal variation may affect the length of the menstrual cycle.[7,8]

Cervical mucus also undergoes cyclic changes during the menstrual cycle. During the proliferative phase, the cervical mucus is thin and watery. Peak estrogen levels occur just before ovulation and maximally stimulate the cervical glands to produce mucus. Cervical mucus becomes abundant and more elastic (spinnbarkeit). In the presence of estrogen, tiny channels develop in the mucus, which allows sperm access to the interior of the uterus. Changes in the consistency of cervical mucus can be used to identify fertile intervals. After ovulation, the ovary begins to secrete progesterone under the influence of the corpus luteum. The amount of cervical mucus is reduced, becomes thicker and stickier, and blocks sperm migration.

The vaginal epithelium also responds to the cyclic hormonal changes of the menstrual cycle. Under the influence of estrogen, cells of the vaginal epithelium become thicker during the follicular/proliferative phase. After ovulation, layers of keratinized cells overgrow the basal epithelium (cells become larger and flatter), a process known as cornification. Near the end of the luteal phase, leukocytes invade the vaginal epithelium, removing the outer layers in a process termed decornification with thinning of the epithelium.

Basal body temperature (BBT) undergoes characteristic biphasic changes during menstrual cycles in which ovulation occurs. During the follicular phase, the BBT fluctuates around 98°F (37°C). During the luteal phase, the average temperature increases by 0.4°F to 1.0°F (0.2°C to 0.5°C). At the end of the luteal phase, 1 to 3 days before the onset of menstruation, BBT declines to follicular-phase levels. The shift in temperature is related to ovulation, corpus luteum formation, and increased serum progesterone levels. Progesterone acts on the thermoregulatory center of the hypothalamus to increase body temperature. Changes in BBT are used to estimate ovulatory cycles but when used alone may not be the best method to support fertility awareness.[9]

Hormonal Control

Hormonal control of the menstrual cycle depends on complex interactions among the hypothalamus, the anterior pituitary, and the ovaries (or hypothalamic-pituitary-ovarian [HPO] axis) (Table 24.3). Hormonal control is dependent on negative and positive ovarian feedback mechanisms. In the hypothalamus, kisspeptin activates the release of GnRH to stimulate the gonadotropin production of FSH and LH. The constant and pulsatile release of GnRH is critical to the timing of the menstrual cycle. GnRH is secreted into the hypophyseal portal system and travels to the anterior pituitary, where it stimulates the secretion of LH and FSH. FSH and LH are released from the anterior pituitary in pulses that correspond to the pulsatile secretion of GnRH.

During the early follicular phase, estrogen levels rise steadily and, through negative feedback, suppress FSH and positively increase the production of LH. During the late follicular phase, the preovulatory rise in progesterone concentration facilitates the positive feedback of estrogen; estrogen levels begin to increase, stimulating a surge of LH secretion from the anterior pituitary. The midcycle surge of LH and FSH induces ovulation. A nonsteroidal ovarian factor, gonadotropin surge–attenuating factor (GnSAF), may antagonize the effect of estrogen on the pituitary and regulate the surge of LH at midcycle.[10] Rising estrogen and progesterone levels during the luteal phase may inhibit the anterior pituitary and

TABLE 24.3 **Hormonal Feedback Mechanism in the Menstrual Cycle**

Phase of Cycle and Ovarian Hormone Levels	Feedback to Hypothalamus and Anterior Pituitary	Resultant GnRH, FSH, and LH Levels	Ovarian and Menstrual Events
Early follicular phase: estrogen levels low; minute amount of progesterone secreted	Negative and inhibitory	All low	Ovarian follicle develops; endometrium proliferates
Late follicular (preovulatory) phase: estrogen levels high; progesterone increases with small surge before ovulation	Positive and stimulatory	All surge; LH dominates	Process of ovulation begins; endometrial proliferation complete
Ovulatory phase: estrogen levels dip; progesterone levels begin to rise	Negative and inhibitory	All fall sharply	Corpus luteum begins to develop; endometrium enters secretory phase
Early luteal phase: estrogen and progesterone levels high; progesterone dominates	Negative and inhibitory	All continue to decline, but gradually	Corpus luteum fully developed; endometrium ready for implantation
Late luteal phase: estrogen and progesterone levels fall sharply	Negative and inhibitory; feedback lessens slightly	All rise slightly	Corpus luteum regresses; endometrium breaks down; menstruation begins
Menstrual phase: estrogens levels low; minute amount of progesterone secreted	Negative and inhibitory	All low	More ovarian follicles begin to develop; functional layer of endometrium is shed

FSH, Follicle-stimulating hormone; *GnRH*, gonadotropin-releasing hormone; *LH*, luteinizing hormone.

thus reduce LH and FSH secretion. Just before the onset of menstruation, FSH and LH levels begin to increase slightly, probably because of declining estrogen and progesterone levels (see Fig. 24.9).

A variety of growth factors and autocrine/paracrine peptides influence hormonal control and follicular response. During the early follicular stage, FSH stimulates FSH receptors and LH receptors and the release of insulin-like growth factor one, as well as the production of inhibin and activin in the ovary. Activin from granulosa cells stimulates the secretion of FSH and increases the pituitary response to GnRH, and increases FSH binding in the granulosa cells in the dominant follicle. FSH stimulates inhibin secretion from granulosa cells, and it, in turn, suppresses FSH synthesis. Inhibin B is primarily secreted in the follicular phase of the cycle but sharply spikes when ovulation occurs. Inhibin A is secreted in the luteal phase and further suppresses FSH. Inhibin also restrains prolactin and growth hormone release, interferes with GnRH receptors, and promotes the breakdown of intracellular gonadotropins. In summary, the balance between activin and inhibin regulates FSH secretion. Follistatin inhibits activin and boosts inhibin activity. Inhibin and activin also regulate LH stimulation of androgen synthesis (required for ovarian estrogen biosynthesis) in theca cells.[11] Fig. 24.9 depicts fluctuating estrogen, progesterone, gonadotropin, and inhibin levels. Research continues to advance understanding of the function and structural complexity of these polypeptides and their interaction with GnRH, gonadotropins, and sex hormones.[12]

STRUCTURE AND FUNCTION OF THE BREAST

The breasts are modified sebaceous glands that lie on the ventral surface of the thorax, within the superficial fascia of the chest wall. They extend vertically from the second rib to the sixth or seventh intercostal space and laterally from the side of the sternum to the midaxillary line. Breast tissue also may extend into the axilla; this tissue is known as the *tail of Spence*.

Female Breast

The adult female breast is composed of 15 to 20 pyramid-shaped lobes that are separated and supported by suspensory (Cooper) ligaments (Fig. 24.10). Each lobe contains 20 to 40 lobules, which subdivide further into many functional units called acini (sing., acinus). Each acinus is lined with a layer of epithelial cells capable of secreting milk during lactation and a layer of subepithelial cells capable of contracting to squeeze milk from the acinus. The acini empty into a network of lobular collecting ducts, which empty into interlobular collecting and ejecting ducts. Ductal elongation and organized branching are achieved with collagen fiber alignment. The ducts reach the skin through openings (pores) in the nipple. The lobes and lobules are surrounded and separated by muscle strands and fatty connective tissue. The amount of fatty connective tissue varies among individuals depending on weight, genetic, and endocrine factors; this contributes to the diversity of breast size and shape and the function of the mammary epithelium. Fat increases in the breast after menopause and is a local source of estrogen and other steroid hormones.[13]

An extensive capillary network surrounds the acini and is supplied by branches of the internal mammary, thoracoacromial, internal and lateral thoracic, and intercostal arteries. Venous return follows arterial supply, with relatively rapid emptying into the superior vena cava. The breasts receive sensory innervation from branches of the second through sixth intercostal nerves and the cervical plexus. This accounts for the fact that breast pain may be referred to the chest, back, scapula, medial arm, and neck. Lymphatic drainage of the breast occurs largely through axillary nodes, but there may be a predominance of superficial mammary

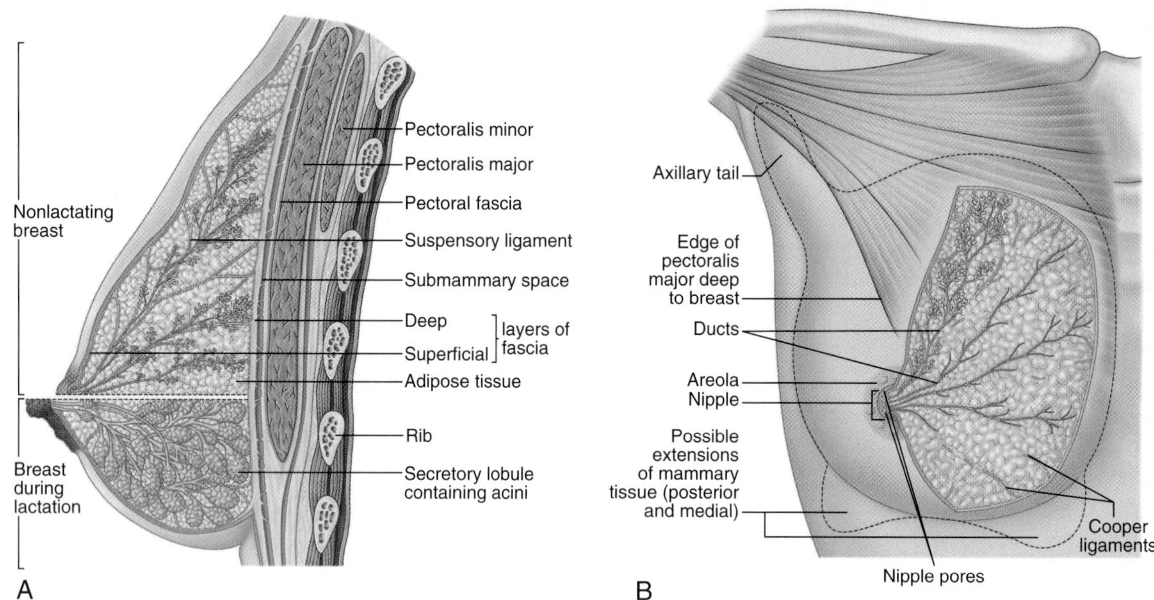

Fig. 24.10 Schematic Diagram of the Breast. (A) Lactating breast. **(B)** Structure of the breast. (From Standring S. *Gray's anatomy*, 42nd edition. London: Elsevier; 2021.)

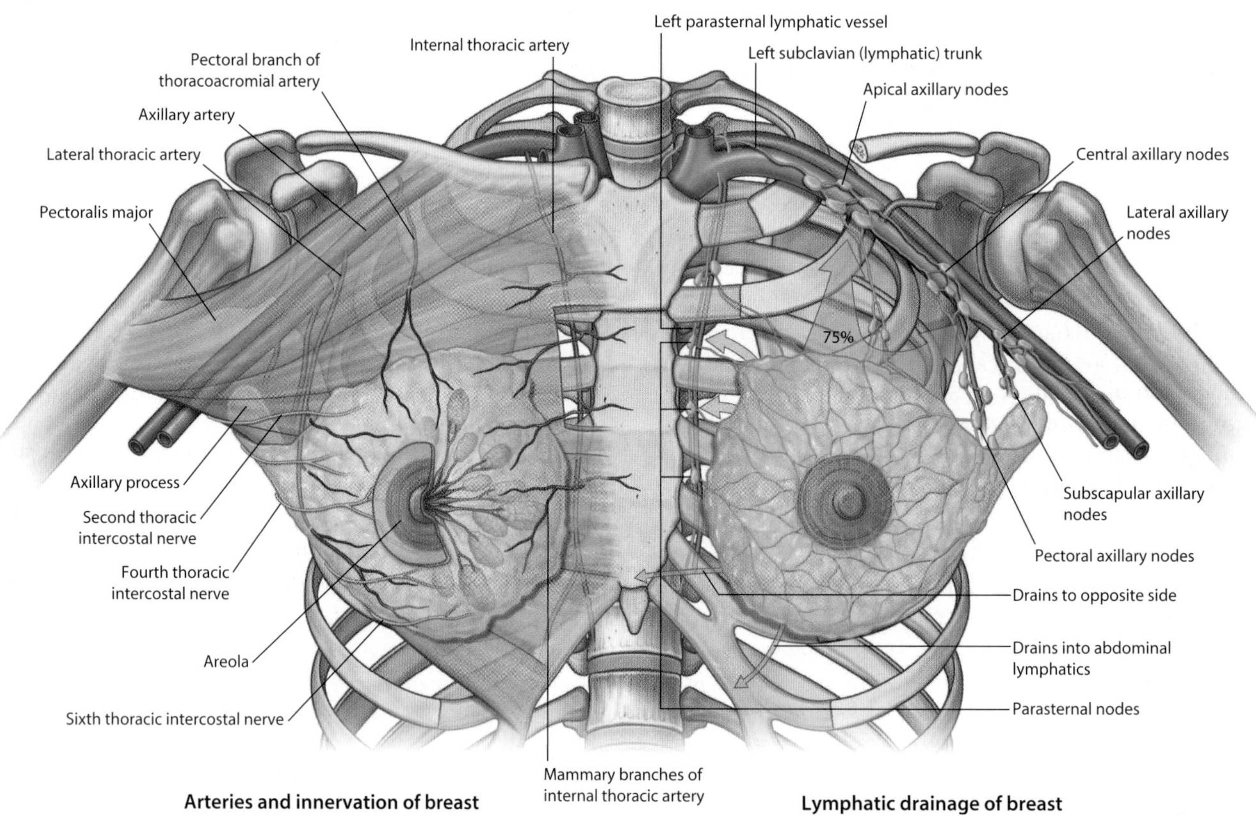

Fig. 24.11 Vasculature, Innervation, and Lymphatic Drainage of the Female Breast. (From Standring S. *Gray's atlas of anatomy*, 42nd edition. London: Elsevier; 2021.)

routes with resultant asymmetry between a person's breasts. Lymphatic drainage from one breast may drain to the opposite side and is a factor in cancer metastasis (Fig. 24.11).

The nipple is a pigmented cylindric structure usually located in the fourth or fifth intercostal space. It measures 0.5 to 1.3 cm in diameter and is approximately 10 to 12 mm in height when erect. On its surface lie multiple pores, one from each lobe. The areola is the pigmented circular area around the nipple. It may be 15 to 60 mm in diameter. A number of sebaceous glands, the glands of Montgomery, are located within the areola and aid in the lubrication of the nipple during lactation. The nipple and areola contain smooth muscles, which receive motor innervation from the sympathetic nervous system. Breast-feeding, sexual stimulation, and exposure to cold cause the nipple to become erect.

The fetal and early postnatal development of breast tissue does not depend on hormones, although fetal breast tissue does become progressively responsive to hormonal stimulation. The neonatal breasts are rudimentary, containing 10 to 12 branching ducts. During childhood, breast growth is latent, and growth of the nipple and areola keeps pace with body surface growth. (Male breast development normally does not progress any further.) At the onset of puberty in the female, growth hormone, insulin-like growth factor 1 (IGF1), and estrogen stimulate mammary growth. Thelarche is usually the first sign of puberty in the female. Full differentiation and development of breast tissue occur over approximately four years and are mediated by the levels of several hormones, including estrogen, progesterone, prolactin, growth hormone, thyroid and parathyroid hormones, insulin, and cortisol. Estrogen promotes the increase in the size of the breast by the formation of a mass of tissue under the areola, increases the size and pigmentation of the areola, and promotes the development of the lobular ducts. The breast cells of *parous* females (those who have given birth) are different than those of females who never become pregnant, as the expansion of acini only occurs with pregnancy when the mammary gland prepares for lactation. During menopause, the lobules of the parous breast involute to prepregnancy composition and become identical to the nulliparous breast.[14]

During the reproductive years, the breast undergoes cyclic changes in response to changes in the levels of estrogen and progesterone associated with the menstrual cycle. Estrogen promotes the development of the lobular ducts; progesterone stimulates the development of cells lining the acini. During the follicular/proliferative phase of the menstrual cycle, high estradiol levels increase the vascularity of breast tissue and stimulate the proliferation of ductal and acinar tissue. This effect is sustained into the luteal/secretory phase of the cycle. During this phase, progesterone levels increase and contribute to the breast changes induced by estradiol. Specific effects of progesterone include dilation of the ducts and conversion of the acinar cells into secretory cells. Most females experience some degree of premenstrual breast fullness, tenderness, and increased breast nodularity. Breast volume may increase as much as 10 to 30 ml. Because the length of the menstrual cycle does not allow for complete regression of new cell growth, breast growth continues at a slow rate until approximately 35 years of age. Because of the cyclic changes that occur in breast tissue, breast examination should be conducted at the conclusion of or a few days after the menstrual cycle, when hormonal effects are minimal and breasts are at their smallest and least tender.

The function of the female breast is primarily to provide a source of nourishment for the newborn. During pregnancy, the breast remodels into a milk-secreting organ and reaches its ultimate mature developmental stage. With increased levels of estrogen, the lobules further differentiate. Progesterone stimulates the development of cells lining the alveoli to produce milk. Lactation (milk production) occurs after childbirth in response to increased levels of prolactin. Prolactin secretion, in turn, increases by continued breastfeeding. Oxytocin, another hormone released during and after delivery, controls milk ejection from alveolar cells. Milk is continuously secreted into the alveolar lumen and is stored there until suckling by the infant stimulates oxytocin, which triggers the let-down reflex. The alveoli empty into a network of lactiferous ducts. These ducts reach the skin through 9 or 10 pores in the nipple.

Physiologically, breast milk is the most appropriate nourishment for newborns. Colostrum, produced in low quantities in the first few days postpartum, is rich in immunologic components, including secretory IgA, lactoferrin, leukocytes, and developmental factors, such as epidermal growth factor. The nutrient composition changes over time to meet the changing digestive capabilities and nutritional requirements of the infant. Secretory IgA and nonspecific antimicrobial factors, such as lysosomes and lactoferrin, protect the infant against infection. During lactation, high prolactin levels interfere with hypothalamic-pituitary hormones that stimulate ovulation. This mechanism suppresses the menstrual cycle and can prevent ovulation.

Male Breast

Until puberty, the development of the male breast is similar to that of the female breast. In the absence of sufficiently high levels of estrogen and progesterone, and with antagonistic effects of androgens, the male breast does not develop any further. The normal male breast consists mostly of fat with a small, underdeveloped nipple and a few ductlike structures in the subareolar area. The male breast may appear enlarged in obese males because of the accumulation of fatty tissue. During puberty, some males experience benign gynecomastia (benign proliferation of male breast glandular tissue), a condition in which the breasts enlarge temporarily as a result of hormonal fluctuations and which should be differentiated from any underlying systemic disorders.

THE MALE REPRODUCTIVE SYSTEM

The external genitalia in males perform the major functions of reproduction. Sperm are produced in the male gonads (testes) and delivered by the penis to the female vagina. The internal male genitalia consist of conducting tubes and fluid-producing glands, all of which aid in the transport of sperm from the testes to the urethral opening of the penis. The male reproductive and urinary structures are shown in Fig. 24.12.

External Genitalia

Testes

The testes (sing., testis) are the essential organs of male reproduction. Like the ovaries, the testes have two functions: (1) production of gametes (i.e., sperm) and (2) production of sex hormones (i.e., androgens and testosterone).

During embryonic and fetal life, the testes develop within the abdomen (see Fig. 24.1). About 3 months before birth, the testes start to descend toward the developing scrotum (Fig. 24.13). About 1 month before birth, they enter twin passageways called inguinal canals. Vaginal processes created by outpouchings of the peritoneum (lining of the abdominal cavity) also descend

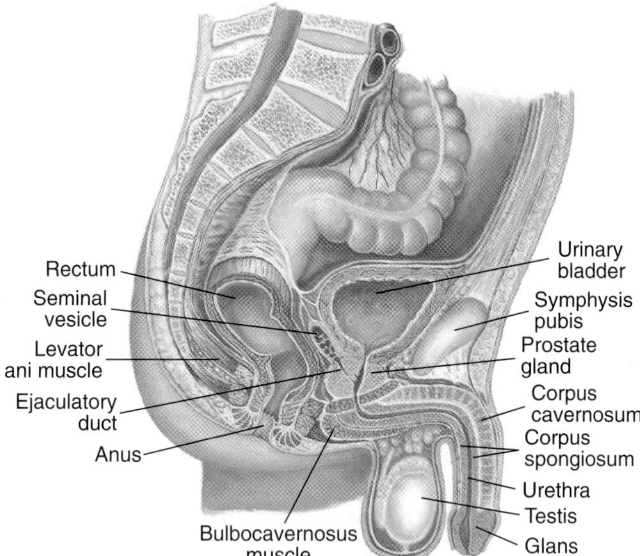

Fig. 24.12 Structure of the Male Reproductive Organs. (From Ball JW, et al. *Seidel's guide to physical examination*, 9th edition. St. Louis: Mosby; 2019.)

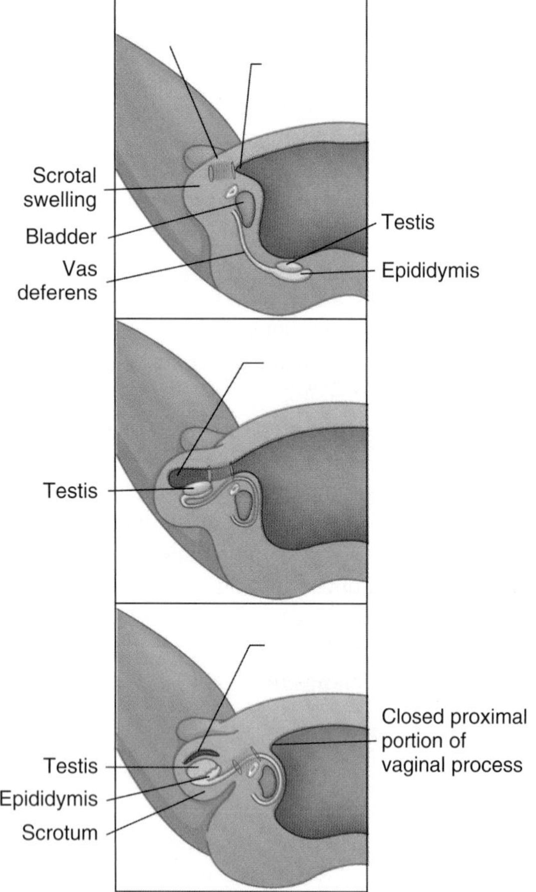

Fig. 24.13 Descent of a Testis. The testes descend from the abdominal cavity to the scrotum during the last 3 months of fetal development.

through the inguinal canals. When descent is complete, the abdominal end of each vaginal process closes, and the scrotal end of each process becomes the outer covering of the testis, the tunica vaginalis. (See Fig. 24.16, A for the inguinal canal in a mature adult.) Failure of the testes to descend through the inguinal canal is known as cryptorchidism.

Fig. 24.14 shows a sagittal section of a mature testis. The adult testis is oval and varies considerably in length (3 to 6 cm), width (2 to 3.5 cm), depth (3 to 4 cm), and weight (10 to 40 g). The testis is almost entirely surrounded by an outer covering called the tunica vaginalis, which separates the testis from the scrotal wall, and an inner covering called the tunica albuginea. Inward extensions of the tunica albuginea form septa that separate the testis into about 250 compartments, or lobules, each of which contains several tortuously coiled ducts called seminiferous tubules. The seminiferous tubules constitute the bulk (80%) of testicular volume and are the site of sperm production. (Sperm production is described in the Spermatogenesis section.) The tissue surrounding these ducts contains blood and lymphatic vessels, fibroblastic support cells, macrophages, mast cells, and Leydig cells, which occur in clusters and produce androgens, chiefly testosterone.

The two ends of each seminiferous tubule join and leave the lobule through the tubulus rectus, which leads to the central portion of the testis, the rete testis. The sperm then move through the efferent tubules, or vasa efferentia, to the epididymis, where they mature.

The testes are innervated by adrenergic fibers whose sole function is to regulate blood flow to the Leydig cells. Arterial blood from the internal spermatic and differential arteries flows over the surface of the testes before entering the parenchyma (functional tissues). Surface flow cools the blood to temperatures to approximately 35°C to 36°C, which promotes spermatogenesis.[15] Additionally, the testes are suspended outside the pelvic cavity to facilitate cooling.

Epididymis

The epididymis (pl., epididymides) is a comma-shaped structure that curves over the posterior portion of each testis (see Fig. 24.14). It consists of a single, densely packed, and markedly coiled duct measuring 5 to 7 cm in length (but about 6 meters in length when uncoiled). The epididymis has structural and physiologic functions. Its structural function is to conduct sperm from the efferent tubules to the vas deferens, whereas physiologic functions include sperm maturation, mobility, and fertility. When sperm enter the head of the epididymis, they are not fully mature or motile, nor can they fertilize an ovum. During the 12 or more days sperm take to travel the length of the epididymis, they receive nutrients and testosterone, and their capacity for fertilization is enhanced.[16] After traveling the length of the epididymis, sperm are stored in the epididymal tail and vas deferens. The vas deferens is a duct with muscular layers capable of powerful peristalsis that transports sperm toward the urethra (see Fig. 24.14). The vas deferens enters the pelvic cavity through the spermatic cord.

Scrotum

The testes, epididymides, and spermatic cord are enclosed and protected by the scrotum, a skin-covered, fibromuscular sac homologous to the female labia majora (see Fig. 24.2). The skin of the scrotum is thin and has rugae (wrinkles or folds), which enable it to enlarge or relax away from the body. At puberty, the scrotal skin darkens, develops active sebaceous glands, and becomes sparsely covered with hair. Just under the skin lies a layer of connective tissue (fascia) and smooth muscle, the tunica dartos (see Fig. 24.14). The tunica dartos also forms a septum that separates the two testes. Exposure to cold temperatures causes the tunica dartos to contract, pulling the testes close to the warm body. In warm temperatures, the tunica dartos relaxes, suspending the testes away from body heat. These mechanisms promote optimal temperatures for spermatogenesis. In addition, scrotal sensitivity to touch, pressure, temperature, and pain protects the testes from potential harm. During sexual excitement, the scrotal skin and tunica thicken, the scrotum tightens and lifts, and the spermatic cords shorten, partially elevating the testes toward the body. As excitement plateaus, the engorged testes increase 50% in size, rotate anteriorly, and flatten against the body, signaling impending ejaculation.

Penis

The penis has two main functions: delivery of sperm to the female vagina and elimination of urine. Embryonically, the penis is homologous to the female clitoris (see Fig. 24.2).

Fig. 24.12 shows a sagittal section of the adult penis and its anatomic relation to other urogenital structures, and Fig. 24.15 shows a cross section of the shaft of the penis. Internally, the penis consists of the urethra and three compartments or sinusoids: two corpora cavernosa (sing., corpus cavernosum) and the corpus spongiosum separated by Buck fascia. Like the testes, these compartments are enclosed by the fibrous tunica albuginea. The urethra passes through the corpus spongiosum and ends at a sagittal slit in the glans.

Externally, the penis consists of a shaft with a tip (the glans) that contains the opening of the urethra (see Fig. 24.14). The skin of the glans folds over the tip of the penis, forming the prepuce, or foreskin. At birth, the foreskin is adhered to the glans. Penile erections, which commonly occur, cause the adhesions

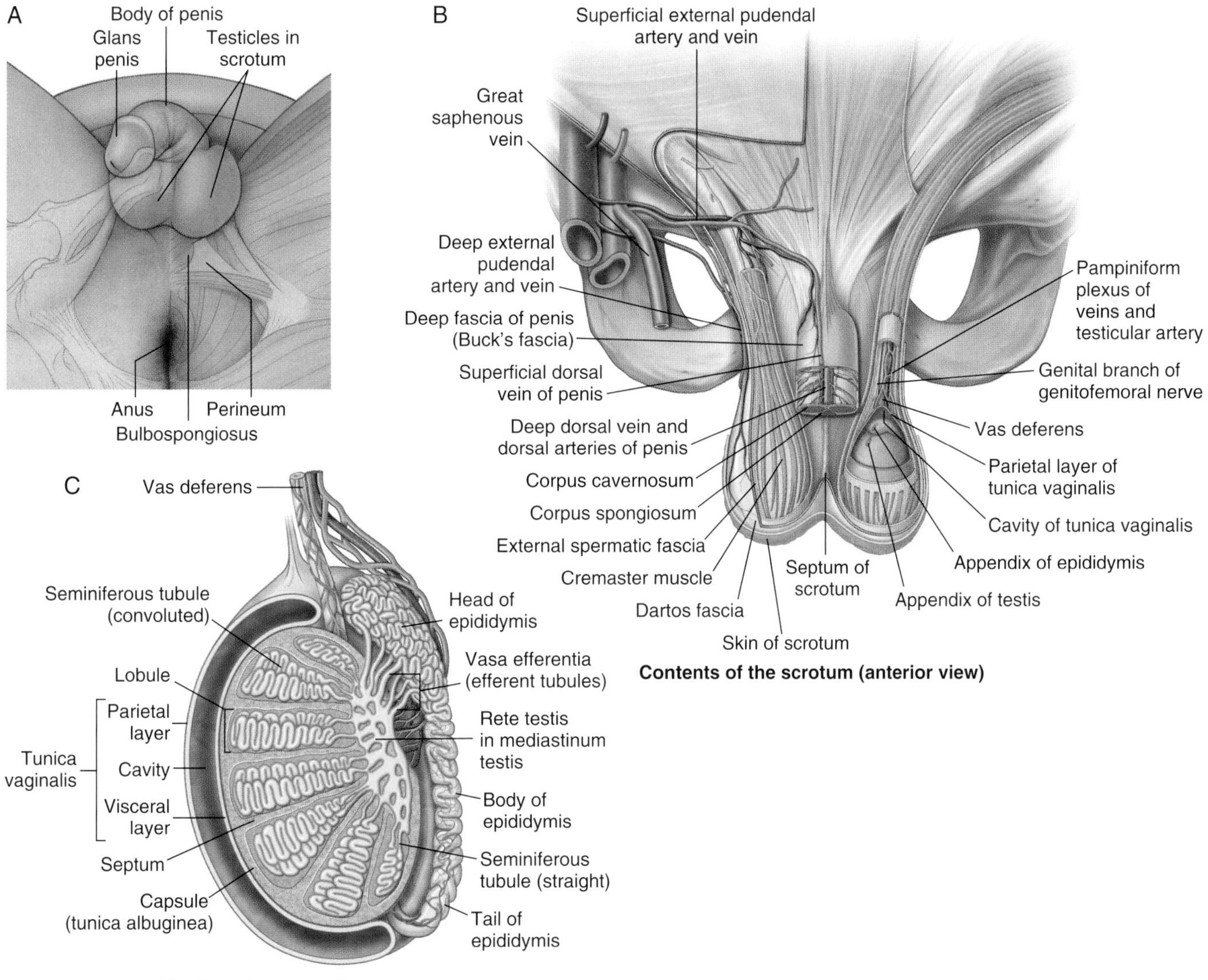

Fig. 24.14 Male Genitalia: **(A)** External, **(B)** Internal, and **(C)** Sagittal Views of the Scrotum and Testes. (Modified from Drake R, Vogl AW, Mitchell A, et al. *Gray's atlas of anatomy*, 3rd edition. Philadelphia: Churchill Livingstone; 2020.)

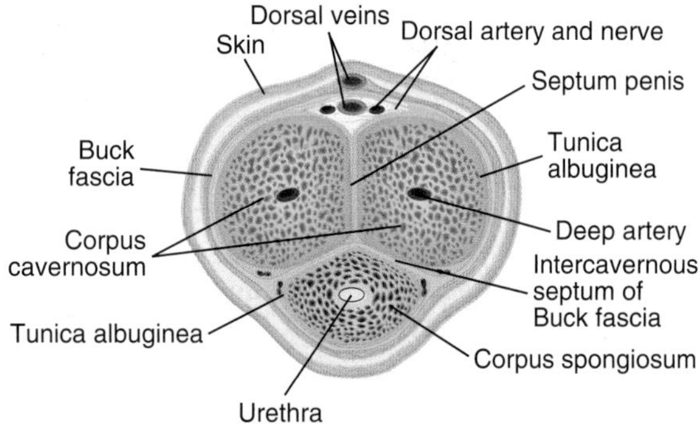

Fig. 24.15 Cross Section of the Penis. The Buck fascia is the blue layer separating the corpora cavernosa from the corpus spongiosum. (From Thompson JM, et al., eds. *Mosby's clinical nursing*, 5th edition. St. Louis: Mosby; 2002.)

to break so that by age 3 years, the foreskin becomes completely retractable. The skin of the penis is continuous with that of the groin, scrotum, and inner thighs. It is hairless, movable, and darker than the surrounding skin.

Penetration of the female vagina is made possible by the erectile reflex, a process in which erectile tissues within the corpora cavernosa and corpus spongiosum become engorged with blood, generally 20 to 50 mL. The erectile tissues consist of vascular spaces, or chambers, supplied with blood by arterioles (small arteries). Usually, the arterioles are constricted so that not much blood flows through the erectile tissues. Sexual stimulation, however, causes the arterioles to dilate and fill with blood, expanding the erectile tissues and causing an erection. The corpora cavernosa increases in length and width and becomes rigid. Erection apparently is maintained by compression or constriction of veins that drain the corpora cavernosa and corpus spongiosum. When sexual stimulation ceases, or orgasm and ejaculation occur, these veins open, blood flows out of the arterioles, and the penis becomes flaccid (soft and pendulous). Erection is under the control of the autonomic nervous system but can be stimulated or inhibited by CNS input.

Stimulation of the glans, which is endowed with copious sensitive nerve endings, provides maximum erotic sensation. With sexual arousal, skin color deepens, the glans doubles in size, and the urethral meatus dilates. Ejaculation occurs with frequent, strong contractions of the vas deferens, epididymis, seminal vesicles, prostate, urethra, and penis. Erection and ejaculation can occur independently of each other, but it is not common.[17]

Erections begin in utero and continue throughout life, but ejaculation does not occur until sperm production begins at puberty. Growth of the penis and scrotal contents continues well past puberty, however, and may not be complete until the late teens or early twenties. Penis size, when flaccid, varies considerably; with an erection, the difference in penis size diminishes.

Internal Genitalia

Fig. 24.12 shows the anatomy of the internal genitalia and their relation to other pelvic organs. The internal genitalia consist of ducts and glands.

- *Ducts* consist of two vasa deferentia, the ejaculatory duct and the urethra. They conduct sperm and glandular secretions from the testes to the urethral opening of the penis.
- *Glands* consist of the prostate gland, two seminal vesicles, and two Cowper (bulbourethral) glands. They secrete fluids that serve as a vehicle for sperm transport and create a nutritious alkaline medium that promotes sperm motility and survival. Together the sperm and the glandular fluids compose semen.

Sperm leaves the epididymides and travels rapidly through the internal ducts (emission). Emission occurs just seconds before ejaculation, at the moment when sexual arousal peaks. It always leads to ejaculation.

Emission occurs as smooth muscle in the walls of the epididymides and vasa deferentia begins to contract rhythmically, pushing sperm and epididymal secretions through the vasa deferentia. Each vas deferens is a firm, elastic, fibromuscular tube that begins at the tail of the epididymis, enters the pelvic cavity within the spermatic cord, loops up and over the bladder, and ends in the prostate gland (Fig. 24.16). Sperm are conducted by peristaltic contractions of smooth muscle in the walls of the vas deferens.

The seminal vesicles are glands about 4 to 6 cm long that lie behind the urinary bladder and in front of the rectum. As sperm leave the ampulla (wide portion) of the vas deferens, the seminal vesicles secrete a nutritive, glucose-rich fluid into the ejaculate (semen). The seminal vesicles provide fructose as a source of energy for ejaculated sperm and secrete prostaglandins that promote smooth muscle contraction, assisting with sperm transport. The ducts of the seminal vesicles join the ampulla of the vas deferens to become the ejaculatory duct, which contracts rhythmically during emission and ejaculation. As seen in Figs. 24.12 and 24.16B, the ejaculatory duct joins the urethra, where both pass through the prostate gland. During emission and ejaculation, a sphincter (muscle surrounding a duct) closes, preventing urine from entering the prostatic urethra.

The prostate gland is about the size of a walnut, surrounds the urethra, and is composed of glandular alveoli and ducts embedded in fibromuscular tissue. The prostate gland has three zones (see Fig. 24.16A), which are significant in the study of prostate cancers. Prostate growth, development, and function are regulated by androgens and the androgen receptor. Nerves required for penile erection travel along the posterolateral surface of the prostate.

Included in prostate epithelial secretions are prostate-specific antigen (PSA), cytokeratins, prostate-specific membrane antigen (PSMA), and prostate-specific acid phosphatase. Prostate secretions contribute to the ejaculate. While semen moves through the prostatic portion of the urethra, the prostate gland contracts rhythmically and secretes prostatic fluid (a thin, milky substance with an alkaline pH that helps sperm survive in the acidic environment of the female reproductive tract) into the mixture. In addition, clotting enzymes and fibrinolysin in prostatic fluids help to mobilize sperm after ejaculation.

Bulbourethral glands (Cowper glands) are the last pair of glands to add fluid to the ejaculate; their ducts secrete mucus into the urethra near the base of the penis. Ejaculation occurs

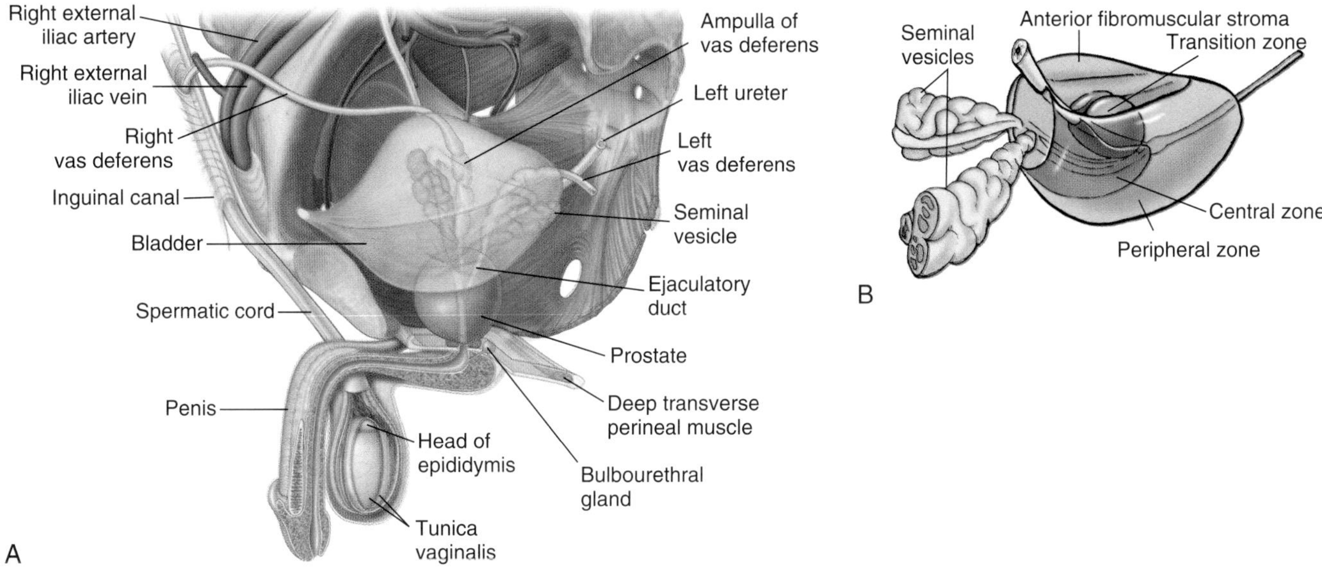

Fig. 24.16 Male Reproductive Ducts, Glands, and Seminal Vesicles. **(A)** Zones of the prostate. The peripheral zone, accounting for 70% of the prostate gland, is the site of origin of ≤70% of prostate cancers; the central zone, approximately 25% of the prostate gland, gives rise to only 1% to 5% of prostate cancers; and the transition zone, approximately 5% to 10% of the prostate gland, gives rise to 20% of prostate cancers and is the site of origin of benign prostatic hyperplasia (BPH) **(B)**, Glands and ducts within the male reproductive system. (A, From Drake R, et al. *Gray's atlas of anatomy*, 3rd edition. Philadelphia: Elsevier; 2020. B, Copyright Baylor College of Medicine, Houston, TX.)

as semen reaches the base of the penis, where muscles rhythmically contract and expel semen. Normally a male ejaculates between 2 and 6 ml of semen, containing 75 million to 400 million sperm. About 98% of the ejaculate consists of glandular fluids, 60% to 70% of the volume originates from the seminal vesicles, and 20% from the prostate. The ejaculate of a man who has undergone a vasectomy (a surgical procedure that prevents sperm from entering the vas deferens) is reduced by about 2%.

Spermatogenesis

Spermatogenesis (the production of sperm) begins at puberty and continues for life. In this respect, spermatogenesis differs markedly from oogenesis (production of primordial ova), which occurs during fetal life only. Spermatogenesis takes place within the seminiferous tubules of the testes (Fig. 24.17). The basement membrane of each seminiferous tubule is lined with diploid (46-chromosome) germ cells called spermatogonia (sing., spermatogonium). These cells undergo continuous mitotic division. Some spermatogonia move away from the basement membrane and mature, becoming **primary spermatocytes**. These undergo meiosis, cell division that results in two haploid (23-chromosome) cells called secondary spermatocytes. The secondary spermatocytes also undergo meiosis, resulting in four spermatids. Spermatids then differentiate into spermatozoa, or sperm, each of which contains 23 chromosomes (Fig. 24.18).

The development of spermatids into sperm depends on the presence of Sertoli cells (nondividing support cells) within the seminiferous tubules. Spermatids attach themselves to the Sertoli cells (see Fig. 24.17), where they receive nutrients and hormonal signals (e.g., testosterone) necessary to develop into sperm.

The process of spermatogenesis, from the mitotic division of a spermatogonium to the maturation of the spermatids, takes about 70 to 80 days. Mature sperm migrate from the seminiferous tubules to the epididymides, where their capacity for fertilization continues to develop. Although they are completely mature by the time they are ejaculated, the sperm do not become motile (capable of movement) until they are activated by biochemicals in the epididymis and in the female reproductive tract (known as sperm capacitation).

Male Sex and Reproductive Hormones

The male sex hormones are androgens. Testosterone, the primary male sex hormone, and other androgens are produced mainly by Leydig cells of the testes, but they are also produced by the adrenal glands in both males and females and by the ovary in females (see Table 24.1). In males, sex hormone production is relatively constant and does not occur in a cyclic pattern, as it does in females.

The physiologic actions of androgen are related to the growth and development of male tissues and organs. Androgens are responsible for the fetal differentiation and development of the male urogenital system and have some effects on the fetal brain. After birth, the Leydig cells become dormant until activated by the gonadotropins during puberty. Then androgens cause the sex organs to grow and secondary sex characteristics to develop.

Testosterone affects nervous and skeletal tissues, bone marrow, skin and hair, and sex organs. It has an anabolic effect on skeletal muscle tissue, thereby contributing to the difference in body weight and composition between males and females. Testosterone also stimulates the growth of the musculature and cartilage of the larynx, causing a permanent deepening

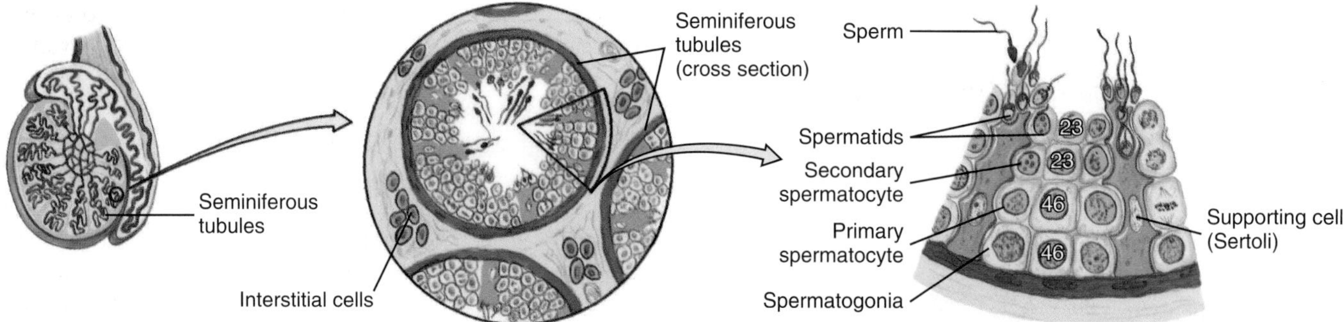

Fig. 24.17 Seminiferous Tubule and Spermatogenesis. Cross section of a seminiferous tubule showing the different cell types. Interstitial cells that produce testosterone are between the seminiferous tubules. Spermatids in the lumen become sperm by a process called spermiogenesis. The numbers in white represent the number of chromosomes. (From Applegate E. *The anatomy and physiology learning system*, 4th edition. St. Louis: Saunders; 2011.)

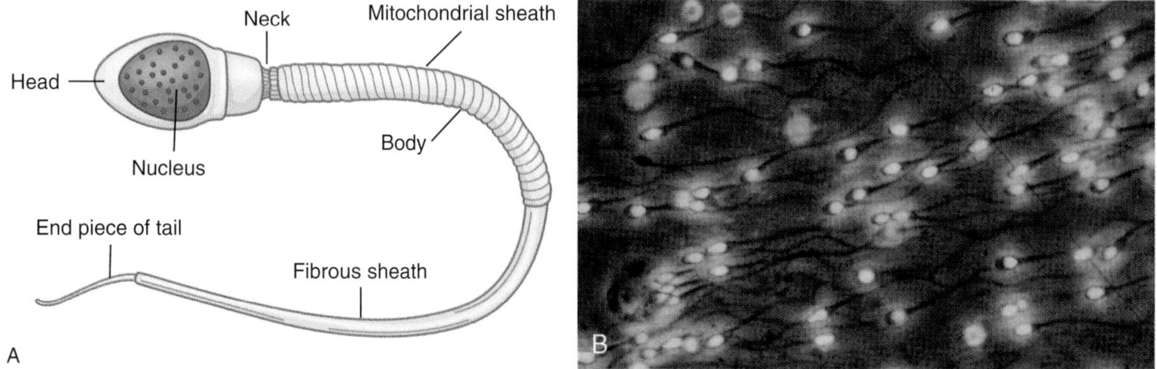

Fig. 24.18 Mature Sperm Cell (Spermatozoon). (A) Anatomy of mature sperm cell. **(B)** Human sperm with nuclear material glowing with a fluorescent dye. (B From Lennart Nilsson.)

of the voice. Testosterone directly stimulates the bone marrow and indirectly stimulates renal erythropoietin production to achieve increased hemoglobin and hematocrit levels. Because sebaceous gland activity is stimulated by testosterone, acne may develop. Hair becomes coarser in texture, and facial, axillary, and pubic hair grows in male patterns. Testosterone is required for spermatogenesis and for the secretion of fluid by the prostate gland, seminal vesicles, and bulbourethral glands. Testosterone is also associated with libido (sex drive). Other, less-understood effects of testosterone include regulatory proteins involved in glycolysis, glycogen synthesis, insulin action, and lipid and cholesterol metabolism.

The regulation of androgen production and spermatogenesis is achieved by a complex feedback system involving the extrahypothalamic CNS, the hypothalamus, the anterior pituitary, the testes, and the androgen-sensitive end organs. These make up the hypothalamic-pituitary-testicular (HPT) axis (Fig. 24.19). These relationships are essentially the same in females (see Fig. 24.3). Extrahypothalamic influences include such variables as physiologic and psychologic stress, which may inhibit or augment hypothalamic activity. In the hypothalamus, neurotransmitters regulate GnRH synthesis and pulsatile release (about every 3 hours) into the hypophyseal portal veins. Norepinephrine stimulates GnRH secretion, and serotonin and dopamine inhibit GnRH secretion. GnRH is transported by portal flow to the median eminence of the pituitary gland, where it binds to receptors and stimulates the synthesis and secretion of the gonadotropins LH and FSH. These gonadotropins are named for their effects in the female reproductive system but have important effects on the male system as well. LH acts on the Leydig cells to regulate testosterone secretion. FSH acts on the seminiferous tubule Sertoli cells to promote spermatogenesis. FSH secretion is inhibited by inhibin secreted by the Sertoli cells. Similar to their action in the female gonad, inhibin functions as an autocrine/paracrine regulator in the male gonad. Inhibin inhibits the proliferation of spermatogonia by regulating pituitary FSH levels. In addition, inhibin facilitates LH stimulation of androgen biosynthesis in Leydig cells.[18]

Ninety-eight percent of testosterone, the major steroid hormone produced by the testes, binds to either sex hormone-binding globulin (SHBG) (50%) or albumin (48%). The remaining 2% remains unbound in the plasma and is free to enter cells and wield its metabolic effects. Changes in the amount of available SHBG affect the amount of testosterone within tissues. The testes secrete only 25% of circulating estrogen (estradiol). The majority is produced by the peripheral conversion of testosterone and androstenedione. Estrogens help regulate GnRH and LH secretion. Peripheral conversion of testosterone also

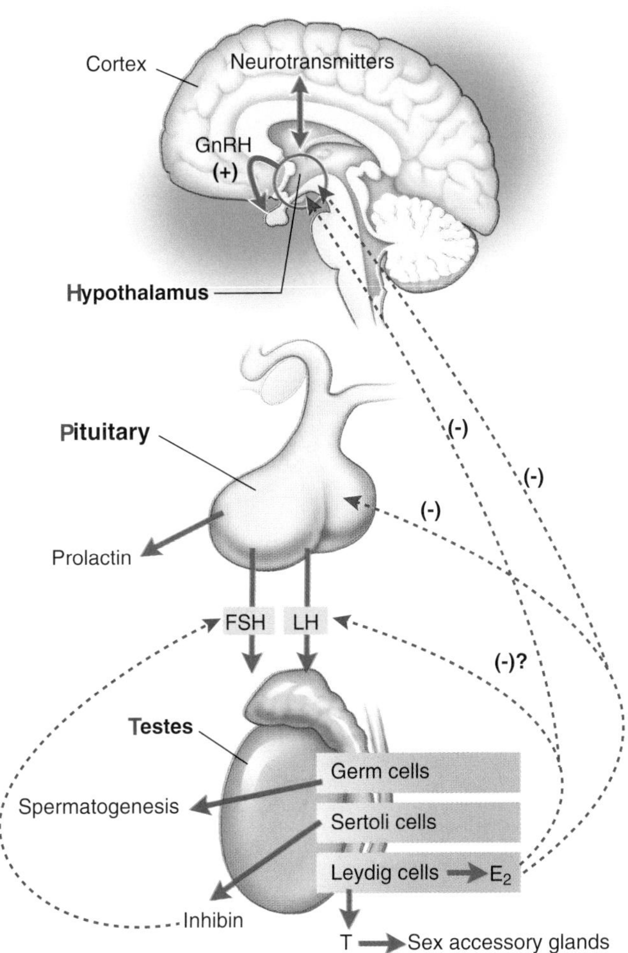

Fig. 24.19 Schematic Representation of Activity Along the Hypothalamus-Pituitary-Testicular *(HPT)* Axis. E_2, Estrogen; *FSH*, follicle-stimulating hormone; *GnRH*, gonadotropin-releasing hormone; *LH*, luteinizing hormone; *T*, testosterone.

produces dihydrotestosterone (DHT), another potent androgen. DHT is necessary for external virilization during embryogenesis and androgen activity beginning at puberty and continuing throughout adulthood. Prolactin, a polypeptide synthesized and secreted from the pituitary, helps maintain the biosynthesis of testosterone. However, elevated prolactin levels are associated with low levels of testosterone.[19]

In summary, hormones secreted at each level of the HPT axis control and coordinate testicular function (see Fig. 24.19). This control is exerted through positive and negative feedback signals by (1) sex steroids that inhibit hypothalamic GnRH secretion and pituitary LH responsiveness to GnRH; and (2) testicular inhibin that inhibits pituitary FSH and, possibly, circulating estrogens (E_2). Any disruption along the HPT axis may lead to hypogonadism or infertility.

TESTS OF REPRODUCTIVE FUNCTION

Diagnostic tests of the male and female reproductive systems may be performed to detect the presence of endometriosis or cancerous lesions or identify the presence of sexually transmitted infections. Most commonly, however, tests of reproductive function are performed when infertility exists. In cases of infertility, both partners are examined, and several diagnostic evaluations may be completed. The types of tests available to assess reproductive function and fertility are summarized in Table 24.4. A list of serum hormone tests and normal values is found in Table 24.5. The male is evaluated for number, amount, structure, and motility of sperm and obstruction along the reproductive tract. Tests for females determine whether (1) the reproductive tract (cervix, uterus, fallopian tubes) is adequately patent to allow for the passage of ovum and sperm, (2) ovulation occurs normally, (3) the endometrium is responding normally to hormones, and (4) reproductive tissues are free of tumors or infections. Hormonal assays evaluate the adequacy of pituitary function and target organ response. The position and size of organs or the presence of tumors can be detected by direct observation procedures using a laparoscope or by ultrasound, radiographic, and other imaging studies.[20]

AGING AND REPRODUCTIVE FUNCTION

Aging and the Female Reproductive System

Menopause is the cessation of ovulation and menses caused by ovarian failure. It is a normal developmental and transitional event that is universally experienced by the average age of 51 years with a range of 40 to 60 years. Premature menopause is the cessation of ovulation before 40 years of age. A number of factors are thought to influence the age of menopause, including genetics, socioeconomic status, race, parity, oral contraceptive use, early menarche, and lifestyles such as smoking or weight.[21] The term "climacteric" refers to gradual changes of ovarian function that start before menopause and result in the symptoms associated with loss of ovarian function.[22] For clarity, the term *menopause* will be used here. Reproductive changes are caused primarily by declining ovarian function and a resulting decrease in ovarian hormone secretion.

Perimenopause is the transitional period between reproductive and nonreproductive years and can last 1 to 8 years. About 5 to 10 years before menopause, approximately 90% of females note mild to extreme variability in frequency and quality of menstrual flow. Changes in hormones occur during this time, including erratically higher estradiol levels, decreased progesterone levels (in normal ovulatory, short luteal phase, or anovulatory cycles), and a disturbed ovarian-pituitary-hypothalamic feedback relationship with higher LH levels. A decrease in the sensitivity of the target tissue receptors and the development of perimenopausal symptoms are commonly experienced. Symptoms usually begin with a lengthening of the menstrual cycle, which correlates with anovulatory cycles. Unpredictable or irregular ovulation uniformly precedes menopause. The perimenopause experience varies among females and from cycle to cycle in the same person.

Menopause is defined by the point that marks 12 consecutive months of amenorrhea. This means that it is determined retrospectively after a female has not had a menstrual period for 1 year. It is characterized by loss of ovarian function, low

TABLE 24.4 Tests of Reproductive Function/Fertility

Test	Description
Basic Assessment	
Semen analysis (two samples at least 2 weeks apart)	Determines number, motility, and structure of sperm cells
Sperm DNA fragmentation	Determines the percentage of sperm DNA strand breaks and likelihood of infertility
White blood cells	Determines presence of bacteria/leukocytes
Immunologic tests	Detects antibody to sperm
Other Assessments	
Basal body temperature	Determines whether ovulation has occurred
FSH level	Day 2–3 of cycle to measure ovarian reserve
Estradiol	Day 2–3 of cycle to measure ovarian reserve
Progesterone	Midluteal phase—1 week before menses
Prolactin	Day 3 of cycle
TSH level	Day 3 of cycle
Urinary LH	Day 11 of cycle
Cervical mucus	Evaluates presence of ovulation from estrogenic effects at ovulation; mucus also may be examined for pH, glucose, or proteins or cultured for presence of infection
Postcoital cervical mucus (Sims-Huhner test)	Tests ability of sperm to penetrate and maintain motility in cervical mucus 2–4 hours after coitus approximately 1 day before ovulation
Zona binding test or hamster penetration test	Nonliving oocytes are surgically removed and bisected; sperm added to the hemi-oocyte to test fertilizing capability
Ultrasound vaginal scanning	Provides superior quality resolution of the uterine, fallopian, and ovarian structures; also can be used to study folliculogenesis, ovulation, and luteogenesis to detect abnormalities
More Specialized Tests	
Endometrial biopsy	Determines whether ovulation has occurred by obtaining endometrial tissue on day 26 of 28-day menstrual cycle (or postovulatory day 12)
Hysterosalpingogram	Assessment of uterus and fallopian tubes for obstructions using transuterine injection of contrast material and radiography; performed 1–2 days after cessation of menses
Laparoscopy (pelvic endoscopy)	Visualization of reproductive organs using a laparoscope inserted within the pelvic cavity through the abdomen to assess structure or determine presence of adhesions, endometriosis, tumors, or infection
Hysteroscopy	Visualization of uterine cavity using modified cystoscope inserted through cervical os; best done during first 14 days of cycle
Transvaginal ultrasound	Identifies endometrial development

FSH, Follicle-stimulating hormone; *TSH*, thyroid-stimulating hormone; *WBC*, white blood cell.

estrogen and progesterone levels, and high FSH and LH levels (Fig. 24.20). Early menopause is the 5 years after menopause onset. Late menopause follows and continues until death.

The primary changes of perimenopause and menopause are as follows:

- *Ovarian changes:* Beginning in utero, the number of follicles steadily decreases through activation, maturation, and atresia. Around 37 to 38 years of age, females experience accelerated follicular loss, which ends when the supply of follicles is depleted at menopause. This accelerated loss is correlated with increased FSH stimulation, declining inhibin production, slightly elevated estradiol levels, and decreasing amounts of anti-müllerian hormone (normally decreases FSH effects) (see Fig. 24.20). Attenuated LH surges are associated with impaired hypothalamic responses to estradiol positive feedback. The ovarian response to high FSH level recruits increasing numbers of follicles (Box 24.2); these follicles only partially develop, with a net effect of irregular ovulation, lower progesterone levels, depleted follicle reserve, and infertility. The ovaries begin to decrease in size around age 30; this decrease accelerates after age 60. Of the 500,000 follicles present at the onset of puberty, the number dwindles to between 100 and 1000 with menopause.[31] Table 24.6 summarizes endocrine events occurring during perimenopause. Table 24.7 provides a template to visualize the complex physiology of perimenopause and the dynamic changes that occur during this time.
- *Uterine changes:* The increase in anovulatory cycles allows for proliferative growth of the endometrium. With this longer exposure to unopposed estrogen and greater thickness

TABLE 24.5 Serum Hormone Values

Hormone	Value
Serum progesterone	Normal = >10 ng/dL, presumptive evidence of ovulation; draw level between days 20 and 25 of 28-day cycle or 6–10 days postovulation <10 ng/mL = inadequate luteal function <3 ng/mL suggests anovulation
Serum testosterone	Normal = 300–1200 ng/dL; must be interpreted with serum LH and FSH levels
Resulting from diurnal and pulsatile pattern, need serial blood draws	Low values in male hypogonadism
Serum FSH and LH	FSH = <22 international units/L
Resulting from diurnal and pulsatile pattern, need serial blood draws	LH = 4–24 international units/LHigh levels in males indicate primary testicular disease; low levels in males indicate hypogonadism caused by hypothalamic-pituitary dysfunction

FSH, Follicle-stimulating hormone; *LH*, luteinizing hormone.

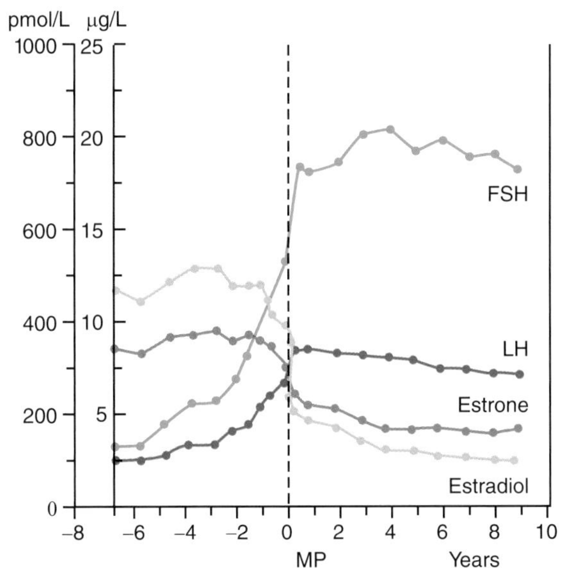

Fig. 24.20 Perimenopausal Hormone Transition. Mean circulating hormone levels. *FSH*, Follicle-stimulating hormone; *LH*, luteinizing hormone; *MP*, menopause.

BOX 24.2 Changes in Ovarian Follicle Maturation

Changes in ovarian folliculogenesis during perimenopause leads to endogenous overstimulation

- ↑ FSH → ovarian hyperstimulation → ↑ number of follicles recruited (net effect of follicular depletion) → ↑ estradiol
- ↓ Follicular reserve → ↓ inhibin and ↑ activin in FP and LP → ↑ FSH → ↑ number of follicles recruited, partial development, infrequent ovulation → ↑ estrogen (E_2) and ↓ progesterone

FP, Follicular phase; *FSH*, follicle-stimulating hormone; *LP*, luteal phase

TABLE 24.6 Endocrine Events Associated With Perimenopause

Hormone Changes	Effects
Estradiol (E_2) levels	Erratic and intermittent increase
Mean FP level 1 greater than mean FP level in younger women	First in FP (inverse relationship between length of FP and estradiol level)
FP level may be greater than midcycle peak level in fertile women	Later during premenstrual phase
Ovulatory cycles	Short or insufficient LP (decreased fertility)
Progesterone levels	Decreased in ovulatory cycle; minimal during anovulatory cycles
Anovulatory cycles	Increased to about 50%; perhaps more in later perimenopause
FSH levels	Variable, then increased
LH levels	Normal initially, then increased
Inhibin levels	Correlate with progesterone levels

FP, Follicular phase; *FSH*, follicle-stimulating hormone; *LH*, luteinizing hormone; *LP*, luteal phase.

of the endometrium, 50% of perimenopausal females will experience dysfunctional uterine bleeding that is heavy and unpredictable. Increased endometrial bleeding is correlated with a change from ovulatory to anovulatory cycles and is associated with unopposed high estrogen levels the week before menses. Estrogen causes endometrial tissue to thicken. However, without corresponding stromal support from progesterone, estrogen production leads to heavier periods, menometrorrhagia (excessive bleeding often caused by submucosal myomas and endometrial polyps), or metrorrhagia (midcycle bleeding) (Table 24.8). In the past, this has put females at high risk for hysterectomy or endometrial ablation. Medical and hormonal management is the first line of therapy if the uterus is normal.[23]

- *Breast tissue changes:* Breast tissue becomes involuted, fat deposits and connective tissue increase, and breasts are reduced in size and firmness. There can be an increase in white adipose tissue inflammation with elevated aromatase levels (increases circulating estrogen), particularly in obese women.[24]
- *Genitourinary tract changes:* The ovaries shrink; the uterus atrophies; and the vagina shortens, narrows, and loses some elasticity. Lubrication of the vagina diminishes, and vaginal pH increases, creating a higher incidence of vaginitis. The cervix atrophies; the cervical os shrinks; vaginal epithelium atrophies; labia majora and minora become less prominent; some pubic hair is lost; urethral tone declines along with muscle tone throughout the pelvic area; urinary frequency or urgency, urinary tract infections, and incontinence may occur. Regular sexual activity and orgasm may diminish some of these changes. Sexually active females have less vaginal atrophy.

TABLE 24.7 Postulated Perimenopausal Transition Time Line

Phase	Menstrual Physiology	Hormonal Changes	Symptomatology
A	Regular, ovulatory cycles Short cycles, short FP	Intermittent ↑ E_2 FSH usually normal Intermittent ↑ FP FSH Low inhibin	Increased breast tenderness, mood swings, fluid retention, premenstrual symptoms Early morning night sweats (vasomotor symptoms) Weight gain, migraine headaches, heavy flow
B	Regular cycles with disturbances in ovulation Short LP Insufficient LP Anovulatory cycles	Intermittent ↑ FP FSH E_2 often ↑ Inhibin inappropriately low	Heavy flow ↑ Premenstrual symptoms ↑ Dysmenorrhea Predictable or ↑ vasomotor symptoms before flow
C	Onset of perimenopause Alternating short, long, or skipped cycles	E_2 often quite ↑ E_2 normal or low ↑ FSH (slight) ↑ LH Low inhibin	Vasomotor symptoms during waking hours Vasomotor symptoms more persistent, remain cyclic before flow
D	Onset of oligomenorrhea 50% of cycles anovulatory Heavy flow may predict onset of oligomenorrhea	↑ Progesterone with ovulation Persistent ↓ FSH ↑ LH ↑ E_2 Low inhibin	↑ Vasomotor symptoms ↑ Signs/symptoms of high estrogen after long periods without flow Flow light but unpredictable
E	Final menstrual period plus 1 year	↑ FSH and LH ↓ or normal E_2 Consistent low inhibin ↓ Progesterone	↑ Intensity and frequency of vasomotor symptoms (although vasomotor symptoms may disappear) ↓ Cramps and premenstrual-type symptoms without subsequent flow ↓ Breast, mood, and fluid symptoms

E_2, Estradiol; *FP*, follicular phase; *FSH*, follicle-stimulating hormone; *LP*, luteal phase.

TABLE 24.8 Impact of High Estrogen Levels on Menstrual Cycle and Symptomatology

Associated Physiologic Change	Signs/Symptoms
Short follicular phase (FP)	Short cycles
Long FP	Long cycles
Thickened endometrium	Heavy, long, or unpredictable flow (including clotting and flooding)[a]
Increase in glandular cells without stromal support produced by progesterone → unstable endometrium	Midcycle spotting Menorrhagia
Possible increased production of prostaglandins within endometrial tissue	Metrorrhagia Dysmenorrhea Breast tenderness, modularity, enlargement Water retention Emotional stress; new or unpredictable mood swings Weight gain Vasomotor symptoms New onset of migraine headaches; exacerbation of headaches Increased premenstrual symptoms

[a]Symptoms aggravated by anovulatory cycles; leads to dysfunctional uterine bleeding.

- *Skeletal changes:* Bone mass is reduced, leading to increased brittleness and porosity, which increases the risk of osteoporosis and fracture, particularly in the lumbar spine and femoral neck.[25]
- *Cardiovascular changes:* The risk of cardiovascular disease increases significantly and is the leading cause of death in postmenopausal females. Blood pressure and total LDL cholesterol increase, and HDL cholesterol decreases. There is an increased risk for metabolic syndrome.[26]
- *Systemic changes:* Vasomotor flushes are characterized by a rise in skin temperature, dilation of peripheral blood vessels, increased blood flow in the hands, increased skin conductance, and a transient increase in heart rate followed by a temperature drop and profuse perspiration over the area of flush distribution. This usually occurs in the face and neck and may radiate into the chest and other parts of the body. Night sweats, dizziness, nausea, headaches, or palpitations may accompany the flush. These flushes can vary in frequency, intensity, and duration and are experienced by up to 85% of perimenopausal to postmenopausal females from 1 to 15 years. The physiology of vasomotor flushes is poorly understood. Interestingly, emerging evidence shows that the intensity of vasomotor flushes may be associated with an increased risk for cardiovascular disease.[27]
- *Other changes:* Emotional stress with unpredictable mood swings, weight gain, migraine headaches, insomnia, and depression often accompany the change in estrogen levels.

Lower estrogen levels decrease skin thickness and diminish skin elasticity, thereby causing increased skin dryness, wrinkling, and poor wound healing. Alopecia and unwanted facial hair are common.[28] Hormone replacement therapy can relieve the symptoms of menopause, but risks and benefits must be evaluated for each person.

Menopause increases the risk of ovarian, breast, and uterine cancers. The risk is greater in females who began menstruating before age 12 or experience menopause after age 55. Females who menstruate longer than normal during a lifetime are exposed to more estrogen and have more ovulations. A longer exposure to estrogen increases the risk of uterine and breast cancers and having more ovulations than normal increases the risk of ovarian cancer.

Aging and the Male Reproductive System

Males maintain reproductive capacity longer than females. There is no known discrete event comparable to menopause that characterizes aging of the male reproductive system, although the term andropause is sometimes used to describe the changes associated with male aging and lower levels of testosterone. Gradual changes do occur, and aging in the male reproductive system is characterized by hypogonadism, testosterone deficiency, erectile dysfunction, and proliferative disorders of the prostate gland (see Chapter 26). Aging changes are also influenced by chronic diseases and the use of medications.[29]

Components of male sexual behavior include both sexual drive and erectile and ejaculatory capacity. Libido, or sexual drive, is a complex phenomenon that is influenced significantly by health status and environmental, social, and psychological factors. In males older than 40 years, organic factors and chronic disease (e.g., vascular, endocrine, and neurologic disorders) are involved in more than half of the cases of male sexual dysfunction. Aging causes specific physical changes that may influence erectile and ejaculatory capabilities. Alterations in sexual response include the need for longer stimulation to achieve a full erection; slower and less forceful ejaculation, with less pelvic muscle involvement; decreased vasocongestive response; and longer refractory period (time during which erection and ejaculation are not possible), up to 24 hours in some men.

The testes undergo several age-related structural changes, including decreased weight, atrophy, and softening. Degenerative changes in the seminiferous tubules may include thickening of the basement membrane; increase in lumen size; germ cell (spermatogonium) arrest and a decrease in spermatogenic activity; and collapse of tubules, followed by complete obstruction caused by sclerosis and fibrosis. Areas of mild to severe degenerative change may be interspersed with areas having intact tubules. These morphologic changes may result from atherosclerosis (arterial clogging) in the testicular vascular bed. Alterations of the seminiferous tubules do not appear to diminish sperm counts (20 million sperm per milliliter of semen is estimated as the minimum concentration for fertility), but they do reduce fertility because a greater percentage of the sperm lack motility or have structural abnormalities.

About 20% of healthy males more than 60 years of age and 30% to 50% older than 80 years of age have testosterone levels below the reference range, and about 2% have hypogonadism. Aging can cause changes in the production of male sex hormones, levels of SHBG, and responsiveness of target tissue receptors. Hormone synthesis by the testes and testicular responsiveness to the gonadotropins (FSH and LH) are diminished, and pituitary secretion of these gonadotropins is elevated. The reduced levels of testosterone may be related to alterations in the Leydig cells, the testosterone producers of the testes. The number of Leydig cells and their function decrease as age increases, perhaps because of decreased arterial perfusion of the testes, and varicoceles and decreased LH or responsiveness to LH. Decreases in testosterone with advancing age and symptoms of libido loss, erectile dysfunction, loss of muscle mass, increased body fat, anemia, osteoporosis, depressed mood, decreased vitality, sweating, and hot flushes are described as late-onset hypogonadism.[30]

Even if testosterone levels are not decreased, older males may have less unbound testosterone in their blood, decreasing the amount of unbound hormone available to stimulate target tissues. Decreased testosterone levels have several effects, including functional deterioration of the accessory sex organs (the prostate gland, seminal vesicles, epididymis, and ductus deferens); loss of muscle mass, strength, and endurance; increased visceral fat, osteopenia, and cognitive decline; and, in many men, decrease in libido. This last effect also may be caused by alterations in other variables that affect libido. Modifiable risk factors for low testosterone levels and symptoms of androgen deficiency include health status and waist circumference.

SUMMARY REVIEW

Development of the Reproductive Systems

1. Differentiation of female and male genitalia begins around 7 to 8 weeks of embryonic development when the gonads of genetically male embryos begin to secrete male sex hormones, primarily testosterone, under the influence of *SRY* gene expression and testosterone-determining factor (TDF). Female gonadal development occurs in the absence of *SRY* gene expression. Until that time, the primitive reproductive organs of males and females are homologous (the same).
2. Production of primitive female gametes (ova) occurs solely during fetal life. From puberty to menopause, one female gamete matures per menstrual cycle. Production of male gametes (sperm) begins at puberty; after that, millions are produced daily, usually for life.
3. Puberty is the onset of sexual maturation. Adolescence is a stage of human development between childhood and adulthood and includes social, psychological, and biologic changes.
4. The structure and function of both male and female reproductive systems depend on interactions among the central nervous system (hypothalamus), the endocrine system (anterior pituitary), the gonads (ovaries, testes), and the

hypothalamic-pituitary-gonadal axis. A set of complex neurologic and hormonal interactions accelerate at puberty and lead to sexual maturation and reproductive capability.

5. One year before puberty, secretion of gonadotropin-releasing hormone (GnRH), follicle-stimulating hormone (FSH), and luteinizing hormone (LH) stimulate the gonads (ovaries and testes) to secrete female (estrogen and progesterone) or male sex hormones (testosterone). These stimulate the maturation of the gonads, reproductive organs, and breasts (in females). Puberty is complete in females with the first ovulatory menstrual period and is complete in males with the first ejaculation that contains mature sperm.

The Female Reproductive System

1. The function of the female reproductive system is to produce mature ova and, when they are fertilized, to protect and nourish them through embryonic and fetal life and expel them at birth.
2. The external female genitalia are the mons pubis, labia majora, labia minora, clitoris, vestibule (urinary and vaginal openings), Bartholin and Skene glands, and perineum. They protect body openings and may play a role in sexual functioning.
3. The internal female genitalia are the vagina, uterus, fallopian tubes, and ovaries. Although all these organs are needed for reproduction, the ovaries are the most essential because they produce the female gametes and female sex hormones.
4. The vagina is a fibromuscular canal that receives the penis during sexual intercourse and is the exit route for menstrual fluids and products of conception. The vagina leads from the introitus (its external opening) to the cervical portion of the uterus.
5. The uterus is the hollow, muscular organ in which a fertilized ovum develops until birth. The uterine walls have three layers: the endometrium (lining), myometrium (muscular layer), and perimetrium (outer covering, which is continuous with the pelvic peritoneum). The endometrium proliferates (thickens) and is shed in response to cyclic changes in levels of female sex hormones. The cervix is the narrow, lower portion of the uterus that opens into the vagina.
6. The two fallopian tubes extend from the uterus to the ovaries. Their function is to direct ova from the spaces around the ovaries to the uterus. Fertilization normally occurs in the distal third of the fallopian tubes.
7. From puberty to menopause, the ovaries are the site of (1) ovum maturation and release and (2) production of female sex hormones (estrogen, progesterone) and androgens. The female sex hormones are involved in sexual differentiation and development, the menstrual cycle, pregnancy, and lactation. Although they are primarily male sex hormones, androgens in females are precursors of female sex hormones and contribute to the prepubertal growth spurt, pubic and axillary hair growth, and activation of sebaceous glands.
8. Estrogen (primarily estradiol) is produced by cells in the developing ovarian follicle (the structure that encloses the ovum). Progesterone is produced by cells of the corpus luteum, the structure that develops from the ruptured ovarian follicle after ovulation (ovum release). Androgens are produced within the ovarian follicle, adrenal glands, and adipose tissue.
9. The average menstrual cycle lasts 25 to 30 days and consists of three phases, which are named for ovarian and endometrial changes: the follicular/proliferative phase, the luteal/secretory phase, and the ischemic menstrual phase.
10. The follicular/proliferative phase is the maturation of an ovarian follicle, the proliferation of the uterine endometrium, and the release of the ovum. FSH stimulates follicle and ovum maturation, then a surge of LH causes ovulation. Estrogen causes proliferation of the endometrium.
11. During the luteal/secretory phase, the ovum transforms into the corpus luteum. LH stimulates the corpus luteum to secrete progesterone and estrogen. Progesterone stimulates blood vessel and glandular growth, and estrogen maintains the thickened endometrium. Glands in the endometrium begin to secrete a thin, glycogen-containing fluid, hence the name *secretory phase.*
12. During the ischemic/menstrual phase, the corpus luteum degenerates, production of progesterone and estrogen drops sharply, and the "starved" endometrium degenerates and is shed, causing menstruation.
13. Cyclic changes in hormone levels also cause thinning and thickening of the vaginal epithelium, thinning and thickening of cervical secretions, and changes in basal body temperature.

Structure and Function of the Breast

1. The basic functional unit of the female breast is the lobe, a system of ducts that branches from the nipple to milk-producing units called *lobules*. Each breast contains 15 to 20 lobes, which are separated and supported by Cooper ligaments. The lobules contain *acini cells*, which are convoluted spaces lined with epithelial cells. Contraction of the subepithelial cells of each acinus moves milk into the system of ducts that leads to the nipple.
2. Until puberty, the female and male breasts are similar, consisting of a small, underdeveloped nipple and some fatty and fibrous tissue. At puberty, however, a variety of hormones (estrogen, progesterone, prolactin, growth hormone, insulin, cortisol) cause the female breast to develop into a system of glands and ducts that is capable of producing and ejecting milk.
3. During the reproductive years, breast tissue undergoes cyclic changes in response to hormonal changes of the menstrual cycle.
4. Milk production occurs in response to prolactin, a hormone that is secreted in larger amounts after childbirth. Milk ejection is under the control of oxytocin, another hormone of pregnancy and lactation.
5. The male breast does not develop because of the absence of sufficiently high levels of estrogen and progesterone and antagonistic effects of androgens.

The Male Reproductive System

1. The function of the male reproductive system is to produce male gametes (sperm) and deliver them to the female reproductive tract.

2. The external male genitalia are the testes, epididymides, scrotum, and penis. The internal genitalia are the vas deferens, ejaculatory duct, prostatic and membranous sections of the urethra, seminal vesicles, prostate gland, and bulbourethral glands.
3. The testes (male gonads) are paired glands suspended within the scrotum. The testes have two functions: spermatogenesis (sperm production) and the production of male sex hormones (androgens, chiefly testosterone).
4. The epididymis is a long, coiled tube arranged in a comma-shaped compartment that curves over the top and rear of the testis. The epididymis receives sperm from the testis and stores them while they develop further. Sperm travel the length of the epididymis and then are ejaculated into the vas deferens, which transports sperm to the urethra.
5. The scrotum is a skin-covered, fibromuscular sac that encloses the testes and epididymides, which are suspended within the scrotum by the spermatic cord. The scrotum keeps these organs at optimal temperatures for sperm survival (about 1°C to 2°C lower than body temperature) by contracting in cold environments and relaxing in warm environments.
6. The penis has two functions: delivery of sperm and elimination of urine.
7. The penis is a cylindric organ consisting of three longitudinal compartments (two corpora cavernosa and one corpus spongiosum) and the urethra. The urethra runs through the corpus spongiosum. The corpora cavernosa and corpus spongiosum consist of erectile tissue. Externally the penis consists of a shaft and a tip, which is called the *glans*.
8. Sexual intercourse is made possible by the erectile reflex, in which tactile or psychogenic stimulation of the parasympathetic nerves causes arterioles in the corpora cavernosa and corpus spongiosum to dilate and fill with blood, causing the penis to enlarge and become firm.
9. Emission, which occurs at the peak of sexual arousal, is the movement of semen from the epididymides to the penis. Ejaculation, which is a continuation of emission, is the pulsatile ejection of semen from the penis.
10. Spermatogenesis is a continuous process because spermatogonia, the primitive male gametes, undergo continuous mitosis within the seminiferous tubules of the testes. Some spermatogonia develop into primary spermatocytes, which divide meiotically into secondary spermatocytes and then spermatids. The spermatids develop into sperm with the help of nutrients and hormonal signals from Sertoli cells.
11. Production of the male sex hormones (androgens) is controlled by interactions among the hypothalamus, anterior pituitary, and gonads. The male hormones are produced steadily rather than cyclically, however.

Tests of Reproductive Function

1. Diagnostic tests are performed to evaluate fertility and detect disease.
2. Evaluation of fertility includes reproductive hormone assays and assessment of structural alteration or infections and the determination of normal ovulation or adequate sperm motility and count.

Aging and Reproductive Function

1. Perimenopause is the transitional period between reproductive and nonreproductive years in females. During this transition, the ovaries produce erratic and high levels of estrogen that contribute to such symptoms as hot flashes, breast tenderness and nodularity, and migraine headaches. Menstrual cycles shorten and then become irregular as anovulation occurs.
2. Menopause, the point that marks 12 consecutive months of amenorrhea, includes atrophic changes in the ovaries, vagina, and breast.
3. Males maintain reproductive capacity into their later years. In some males, there are gradual changes with testosterone deficiency, hypogonadism, proliferative disorders of the prostate, erectile dysfunction, and some loss of muscle mass and strength. Andropause is an androgen deficiency in the aging male.

REFERENCES

1. Lenz GM, ed. *Comprehensive gynecology*. ed 6 St Louis: Mosby; 2012.
2. Labrie F. All sex steroids are made intracellularly in peripheral tissues by the mechanisms of intracrinology after menopause. *J Steroid Biochem Mol Biol*. 2015;145C:133–138.
3. Hoyt LT, et al. Timing of puberty in boys and girls: implications for population health. *SSM Popul Health*. 2020;10:100549.
4. Huang A, Reinehr T, Roth CL. Connections between obesity and puberty: invited by Manuel Tena-Sempere, Cordoba. *Curr Opin Endocr Metab Res*. 2020;14:160–168.
5. Critchley HOD, et al. Physiology of the endometrium and regulation of menstruation. *Physiol Rev*. 2020;100(3):1149–1179.
6. Harlow SD. Menstrual cycle changes as women approach the final menses: what matters? *Obstet Gynecol Clin North Am*. 2018;45(4):599–611.
7. Matteson KA, Zaluski KM. Menstrual health as a part of preventive health care. *Obstet Gynecol Clin North Am*. 2019;46(3):441–453.
8. Huhmann K. Menses requires energy: a review of how disordered eating, excessive exercise, and high stress lead to menstrual irregularities. *Clin Ther*. 2020;42(3):401–407.
9. Simmons RG, Jennings V. Fertility awareness-based methods of family planning. *Best Pract Res Clin Obstet Gynaecol*. 2020;66:68–82.
10. Messinis IE, et al. Gonadotropin surge-attenuating factor: a nonsteroidal ovarian hormone controlling GnRH-induced LH secretion in the normal menstrual cycle. *Vitam Horm*. 2018;107:263–286.
11. Wijayarathna R, de Kretser DM. Activins in reproductive biology and beyond. *Hum Reprod Update*. 2016;22(3):342–357.
12. Appiah Adu-Gyamfi E, et al. Activin and inhibin signaling: from regulation of physiology to involvement in the pathology of the female reproductive system. *Cytokine*. 2020;133:155105.
13. Kothari C, Diorio C, Durocher F. The importance of breast adipose tissue in breast cancer. *Int J Mol Sci*. 2020;21(16):5760.
14. Macias H, Hinck L. Mammary gland development. *Wiley Interdiscip Rev Dev Biol*. 2012;1(4):533–557.

15. Hassanin AM, Ahmed HH, Kaddah AN. A global view of the pathophysiology of varicocele. *Andrology*. 2018;6(5):654–661.
16. James ER, et al. The role of the epididymis and the contribution of epididymosomes to mammalian reproduction. *Int J Mol Sci*. 2020;21(15):5377.
17. Abdel-Hamid IA, Ali OI. Spontaneous ejaculation: a focused review for the clinicians. *Sex Med Rev*. 2021;9(3):406–422.
18. Schlatt S, Ehmcke J. Regulation of spermatogenesis: an evolutionary biologist's perspective. *Semin Cell Dev Biol*. 2014;29:2–16.
19. Duskin-Bitan H, Shimon I. Prolactinomas in males: any differences? *Pituitary*. 2020;23(1):52–57.
20. Flyckt R, Falcone T. Infertility: a practical framework. *Cleve Clin J Med*. 2019;86(7):473–482.
21. Mishra GD, et al. EMAS position statement: predictors of premature and early natural menopause. *Maturitas*. 2019;123:82–88.
22. Blümel JE, et al. Menopause or climacteric, just a semantic discussion or has it clinical implications? *Climacteric*. 2014;17(3):235–241.
23. Goldstein SR, Lumsden MA. Abnormal uterine bleeding in perimenopause. *Climacteric*. 2017;20(5):414–420.
24. Brown KA, et al. Menopause is a determinant of breast aromatase expression and its associations with BMI, inflammation, and systemic markers. *J Clin Endocrinol Metab*. 2017;102(5): 1692–1701.
25. Karlamangla AS, Burnett-Bowie SM, Crandall CJ. Bone health during the menopause transition and beyond. *Obstet Gynecol Clin North Am*. 2018;45(4):695–708.
26. Mumusoglu S, Yildiz BO. Metabolic syndrome during menopause. *Curr Vasc Pharmacol*. 2019;17(6):595–603.
27. Thurston RC. Vasomotor symptoms: natural history, physiology, and links with cardiovascular health. *Climacteric*. 2018; 21(2):96–100.
28. Rzepecki AK, et al. Estrogen-deficient skin: the role of topical therapy. *Int J Women's Dermatol*. 2019;5(2):85–90.
29. Bhasin S, et al. Age-related changes in the male reproductive system. In: Feingold KR, ed. *Endotext [Internet]*. South Dartmouth, MA: MDText.com, Inc; 2000–2018. Updated 2018 December 14, 2018. Available at. https://www.ncbi.nlm.nih.gov/books/NBK278998/. Accessed August 14, 2021.
30. Nieschlag E. Late-onset hypogonadism: a concept comes of age. *Andrology*. 2020;8(6):1506–1511.
31. Hall JE. Endocrinology of the menopause. *Endocrinol Metab Clin North Am*. 2015;44(3):485–496.

25

Alterations of the Female Reproductive System

Corinne M. Djuric, Suzanne M. Ruiz, and Kathryn L. McCance

http://evolve.elsevier.com/Rogers/pathophysiology/

CHAPTER OUTLINE

Alterations of the female reproductive system span a wide range of clinical presentations, from delayed sexual development and suboptimal sexual performance to structural and functional abnormalities. Many common reproductive disorders carry potentially serious physiologic and psychological consequences. Sexual or reproductive dysfunction, such as impotence or infertility, can dramatically affect self-concept, relationships, and overall quality of life. Conversely, organic and psychosocial problems, such as alcoholism, depression, situational stressors, chronic illness, and medications can affect ovulation, menstruation, sexual performance, and fertility. These individuals may also be risk factors for the development of some types of reproductive tract cancers.[1,2]

ABNORMALITIES OF THE FEMALE REPRODUCTIVE TRACT

Normal development of the female reproductive tract requires the absence of testosterone during embryonic and fetal life (see Chapter 24). The resulting fusion of the two paramesonephric (müllerian) ducts produces the normal cervix and the uterus with an internal cavity. The distal portions of the paramesonephric ducts remain independent and form the two fallopian/uterine tubes. Alterations in the normal process include errors in cellular sensitivity to testosterone (androgen insensitivity) or failures of cell line migration, resulting in changes in the structure of the reproductive organs.

Androgen insensitivity occurs in its most extreme form and is discussed briefly in this chapter because of the often-resulting female phenotype, despite a male genotype. Androgen insensitivity syndrome (AIS) is caused by an X-linked (recessive pattern) genetic mutation in cellular androgen receptors that results in an end-organ insensitivity to testosterone, which normally acts as the catalyst for the development of the male reproductive system in embryonic development. Three types of AIS include complete androgen insensitivity syndrome (CAIS), partial androgen insensitivity syndrome (PAIS), and mild androgen insensitivity syndrome (MAIS).[3] AIS is characterized by a female phenotype or feminization (i.e., undermasculinization) of the external genitalia at birth, abnormal secondary sexual development in puberty, and infertility in individuals with a 46,XY karyotype.

Complete androgen insensitivity syndrome (CAIS) occurs when the body cannot use androgens at all.[3] Individuals with CAIS have external sex characteristics of females, but have a vagina with a short canal (sometimes called a blind-ending) with no uterus; therefore they do not menstruate and are infertile. They are typically raised as females with a female sex identity. Affected children have male internal organs or testes (which may be palpable within the labia majora, inguinal ring, or abdominal cavity) that produce testosterone (and estrogen). Breast development may be normal, but pubic and axillary hair is often sparse. CAIS and PAIS are associated with a rare but increased risk of gonadal germ cell cancer (GGCC). Issues in management include decisions on sex assignment, gonadectomy and timing, fertility, hormone replacement, psychological outcomes, and genetic counseling.[4–7] The risks of osteopenia and osteoporosis are higher in those with early gonadectomy.[8] Partial androgen insensitivity (PAIS) (also a common cause of male infertility) has a varied phenotype from the residual androgen receptor. Persons with PAIS (also called *Reifenstein syndrome*) can have genitalia that look typically female, genitalia that have both male and female characteristics, or genitalia that look typically male. These individuals are raised as males or as females and may have a male or female sex identity. Those with mild androgen insensitivity syndrome are born with male sex characteristics but are often infertile and may experience breast enlargement at puberty.

Other abnormalities of the uterus, cervix, and fallopian/uterine tubes have multifactorial origins, often the result of an interaction between genetic predisposition and environmental factors. Such interactions result in müllerian duct abnormalities. Some medications, chemicals, and toxins have been implicated as a direct cause of uterine abnormalities. An example, diethylstilbestrol (DES) was prescribed from 1938 until 1971 as a drug to prevent miscarriages. DES affected cell development, causing abnormal internal reproductive structural defects, infertility, and a predisposition to cancer (see Chapter 13). Most uterine abnormalities stem from abnormal cell migration in the müllerian ducts during key moments in fetal development (Fig. 25.1). Uterine abnormalities are rarely diagnosed until the woman has trouble becoming pregnant or carrying a baby to term, because the uterus is capable of menstruation but may have difficulty supporting a growing fetus. Uterine malformations are usually diagnosed by ultrasound during pregnancy or with magnetic resonance imaging (MRI). The prognosis depends on the severity of the malformation and the location and size of the placenta and fetus. Some abnormalities can be surgically corrected to improve the outcome of subsequent pregnancies. Abnormalities of the lower genital tract also can result in women having two vaginas or a vaginal septum (a thin membrane dividing the vaginal vault). For most women this does not create functional problems, but it can be surgically corrected if needed.[9,10]

ALTERATIONS OF SEXUAL MATURATION

The process of sexual maturation, or puberty, is marked by the development of secondary sex characteristics, rapid growth, and, ultimately, the ability to reproduce. A variety of congenital

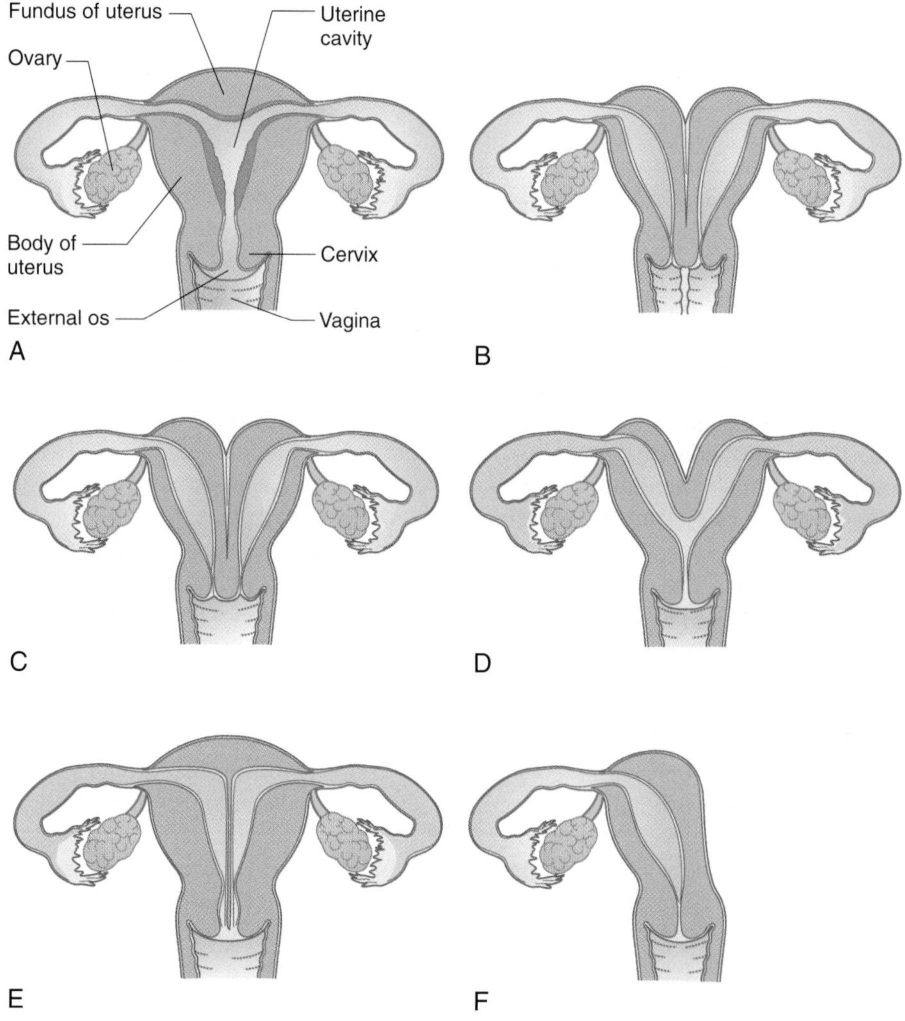

Fig. 25.1 Uterine Malformations. Congenital uterine abnormalities. **(A)** The normal configuration of the uterus and the ovaries. **(B)** Double uterus with a double vagina. **(C)** A single vagina. **(D)** Bicornuate uterus. **(E)** A uterus with a midline septum. **(F)** Unicornuate uterus. (From de Bruyn R. *Pediatric ultrasound,* 2nd edition. London: Churchill Livingstone; 2010.)

and endocrine disorders can disrupt the timing of puberty. These disorders may cause puberty to occur too late *(delayed puberty)* or too early *(precocious puberty)*. Both types involve an inappropriate onset of sex hormone production by the gonads and have potential implications for the child's social interactions and self-esteem.

The age of puberty is multifactorial, involving genetic and environmental components. The onset of puberty is 8 to 13 years of age and appears to be occurring earlier for girls. Females of African, Hispanic, and Latino descent begin puberty up to 1 year sooner than the average young female. The earlier onset appears primarily in breast development and not age of menarche. Puberty may also be accelerated by obesity.

Delayed or Absent Puberty

Delayed puberty is characterized by the absence of pubertal signs past the normal age range for the typical population. One of the first signs of puberty in girls is thelarche, or breast development, which typically begins by 13 years of age. In delayed puberty, these secondary sex characteristics develop later, but there are clear variations according to race and ethnicity that need consideration at the time of diagnosis. Delayed puberty is diagnosed if there is no breast development by age 13, which is 2 to 2.5 standard deviations greater than the mean age of pubertal onset. Pubic hair may be present because that is largely dependent on adrenal rather than gonadal function. Delayed puberty may have significant psychosocial implications and an increased risk for inadequate skeletal development and mineralization due to the rapid skeletal growth during that time. The majority of bone development and mineralization is achieved during adolescence. Estrogen plays a major role in this process, and a lack of circulating estrogen puts individuals at risk for inadequate bone density in adulthood.[11]

In most cases, delayed puberty is a physiologic (constitutional) delay. Hormonal levels are normal, the hypothalamic-pituitary-gonadal (HPG) axis is intact, and maturation is slowly occurring. Often, an underlying condition or illness unrelated to gonadal function is responsible for the delayed development (Table 25.1).

A delay in the production of gonadotropin-releasing hormone (GnRH) from the HPG axis further delays production of the gonadotropins: luteinizing hormone (LH) and follicle-stimulating hormone (FSH), which ultimately delays gametogenesis. The G protein–coupled receptor 54 (GPR54) has been identified as the gatekeeper gene for activation of the BnRH axis. GPR54 is required for the normal function of this axis, and data suggest that the ligand kisspeptin-1 may act as a neurohormonal regulator of the GnRH axis.[11–13]

Given the numerous etiologies contributing to the occurrence of delayed puberty, a thorough evaluation should be conducted that includes past medical history, birth history, family history, social history, and a physical examination. It is essential to review the child's growth curve based on appropriate age, sex, height, weight, and body mass index (BMI). If further work-up is warranted, a bone age can help to determine the child's growth status. Before ordering lab and imaging tests, the child's predicted target height should be plotted.[14] Laboratory and diagnostic work-up may consist of x-ray studies for bone age, measurement of thyroid function, determination of serum levels of prolactin, measurement of adrenal and gonadal steroids, radioimmunoassay of plasma gonadotropins, and screening for systemic disorders. Adolescents with high gonadotropin levels require a karyotype to rule out genetic causes, and those with low levels need skull imaging to rule out pituitary or central nervous system (CNS) pathology (infiltrate or tumor).[14,15]

Treatment of delayed puberty depends on the cause. The goals of treatment are the development of secondary sex characteristics and fertility (if possible) and the promotion of bone growth and mineralization.[12] The treatment for certain variations of delayed puberty requires lifelong hormone replacement therapy (HRT), synthetic GnRH, or sex hormone administration solely or in combinations.[13] This physiologic delay tends to be familial, is less common in girls than boys, and is diagnosed often retrospectively once pubertal progression is complete. Treatment is seldom needed unless the delayed puberty is causing psychosocial problems.

Precocious Puberty

Precocious puberty is the onset of sexual characteristics (breast or pubic hair development) 2 to 2.5 standard deviations below the mean age of onset of puberty in the racial and ethnic context of the individual. Precocious puberty is categorized into

TABLE 25.1 Frequency and Common Causes of Delayed Puberty Other Than Constitutional Delay of Growth and Puberty

Delayed Puberty	Hypergonadotropic Hypogonadism	Permanent Hypogonadotropic Hypogonadism	Functional Hypogonadotropic Hypogonadism
Male (assigned at birth)	5%–10%	10%	20%
Female (assigned at birth)	25%	20%	20%
Common causes	Turner syndrome, gonadal dysgenesis, chemotherapy, radiation therapy	Tumors or infiltrative diseases of the central nervous system, GnRH deficiency (isolated hypogonadotropic hypogonadism, Kallmann syndrome), combined pituitary-hormone deficiency, chemotherapy, or radiation therapy	Systemic illness (inflammatory bowel disease, celiac disease, anorexia nervosa, or bulimia), hypothyroidism, excessive exercise

GnRH, Gonadotropin-releasing hormone.
Data from Palmert MR, Dunkel L. Clinical practice. Delayed puberty. New *England Journal of Medicine*, 2012;366(5):443–453.

three groups: central precocious puberty (GnRH dependent), peripheral precocious puberty (GnRH independent), and benign pubertal variants.[16] Premature development of secondary sex characteristics causes premature closure of the epiphysis of long bones, which results in lifelong short stature and often carry profound psychosocial consequences.[17,18] Precocious puberty can be a sign of pathologic conditions; therefore all cases of precocious puberty require thorough evaluation.

Central precocious puberty, or true precocious puberty, is GnRH dependent and occurs when the HPG axis is working normally but prematurely.[17] Central precocious puberty results from failure of the central inhibition of the GnRH pulse generator because of a CNS abnormality. Causes can be idiopathic or can include CNS lesion, genetics, previous excess of sex steroid exposure, or pituitary gonadotropin-secreting tumors.[19,20] Most cases of precocious puberty in females are idiopathic, and in males there is usually an underlying pathology. Several conditions include CNS tumors, CNS injury, genetics, certain syndromes (e.g., neurofibromatosis type 1), and environmental or familial factors.[16] Recently, mutations in the imprinted gene MKRN3 were discovered as a cause of familial central precocious puberty.[19–22]

Peripheral precocious puberty, or gonadotropin-independent precocious puberty, is an excess of estrogens secreted from the gonads or adrenal glands from exogenous sources.[16] Some causes of peripheral precocious puberty include: Ovarian cysts, ovarian tumors, primary hypothyroidism (Van Wyk and Grumback syndrome), adrenal pathology, exogenous sex steroids, endocrine-disrupting chemicals, and McCune-Albright syndrome.[16,23] Benign pubertal variants include isolated premature thelarche, pubarche, self-limiting vaginal bleeding, and nonprogressive precocious puberty. The etiology of benign pubertal variants is characterized by not fitting into any other category of precocious puberty and is not followed by progressive development. However, close monitoring is still important to ensure that the variant is, in fact, benign and does not progress.

The diagnosis and cause of premature development are often straightforward. A thorough history and physical examination are done to determine the impetus of the process and to rule out life-threatening CNS, ovarian, or adrenal neoplasms. A family history and social history help to exclude or include certain genetic conditions as well as environmental, medication, and hormonal exposures. Children with precocious puberty may have a tendency toward obesity. Treatment for all forms of precocious puberty is aimed to identify and remove the underlying cause. Work-up typically starts with laboratory evaluation of LH, FSH, and estradiol.[24] Urinary gonadotropins are useful in the assessment and management of precocious puberty.[25,26] Management goals include arresting maturation until developmentally appropriate, maximizing eventual adult height, and reducing emotional problems. Because many of these children are obese and childhood obesity is predictive of morbidity in adolescence and adulthood, it is important for clinicians to include assessment and management of obesity in conjunction with the treatment of precocious puberty.[24–26]

DISORDERS OF THE FEMALE REPRODUCTIVE SYSTEM

Hormonal and Menstrual Alterations

Dysmenorrhea

Primary dysmenorrhea is recurrent, painful menstruation associated with the release of prostaglandins in ovulatory cycles but not with pelvic disease. Primary dysmenorrhea begins a few days before menstruation and persists for 48 to 72 hours.[27] Women are more likely to report primary dysmenorrhea if they are younger than 30 years old; have not given birth; have a history of sexual assault, premenstrual syndrome (PMS), or sterilization; are heavy tobacco or alcohol users; have a family history of dysmenorrhea; or have a BMI less than 20.[28] In contrast, secondary dysmenorrhea is painful menses in the presence of a pelvic pathologic condition. Secondary dysmenorrhea manifests later in the reproductive years and may occur any time in the menstrual cycle.[29]

Pathophysiology. Primary dysmenorrhea results from excessive prostaglandin synthesis of $F_2\alpha$ ($PGF_2\alpha$), a potent myometrial stimulant and vasoconstrictor, found in secretory endometrium. Elevated levels of prostaglandins, especially PGF2α and PGE2α, increase myometrial contractions, constrict endometrial blood vessels, and enhance nerve hypersensitivity, which results in pain.[30,31] These changes can lead to ischemia and endometrial shedding. Increased synthesis of prostaglandins may result from increased cyclooxygenase (COX) enzyme activity. Inflammatory mediators produced in leukocytes (leukotrienes) also contribute to increased levels of pain. The first 48 hours of menstruation correlate with higher prostaglandin levels, which may contribute to pain.[29] Women who experience severe primary dysmenorrhea appear to have a heightened pain sensitivity and possibly an alteration in their pain modulating system which puts them at higher risk for functional pain disorders (e.g., fibromyalgia) later in life.[32] Women who are anovulatory because they use oral contraceptives rarely have primary dysmenorrhea.[28]

Secondary dysmenorrhea results from disorders such as endometriosis (most common cause), endometritis (infection), adenomyosis, pelvic inflammatory disease (PID), obstructive uterine or vaginal anomalies, inflammation, uterine fibroids, polyps, tumors, cysts, ovarian cysts, pelvic congestion syndrome, or nonhormonal intrauterine devices (IUDs).[18]

Clinical Manifestations. The chief symptom of dysmenorrhea is pelvic pain associated with the onset of menses. The severity is directly related to the length and amount of menstrual flow. The pain often radiates into the groin and may be accompanied by fatigue, backache, anorexia, nausea, vomiting, diarrhea, syncope, insomnia, and headache. The latter symptoms are caused by the entry of prostaglandins and their metabolites into the systemic circulation. Secondary dysmenorrhea has very similar symptoms but in response to an underlying causative pathology.[29]

Evaluation and Treatment. A thorough medical history and pelvic examination can differentiate primary dysmenorrhea from secondary dysmenorrhea. Nonsteroidal antiinflammatory drugs (NSAIDs) (e.g., ibuprofen) are the treatment of choice because they reduce COX enzyme activity and thus prostaglandin production. NSAIDs are effective in the majority of women with primary dysmenorrhea and are most effective if started at the first sign of bleeding or cramping.[33] However, long-term use of NSAIDs has been associated with multiple side effects.[34] In women who desire contraception, dysmenorrhea may be relieved with hormonal contraceptives. Hormonal contraception inhibits ovulation and reduces endometrial proliferation, thereby decreasing prostaglandin synthesis and myometrial contractility. Regular exercise and stress reduction are thought to prevent or reduce symptoms. Complimentary approaches for treatment include local application of heat, herbs, yoga, relaxation, psychotherapy, massage, hypnosis, vitamins (E, B, C) and supplements (calcium and magnesium), acupressure, and acupuncture.[27]

Primary Amenorrhea

Amenorrhea is the lack of menstruation in females of reproductive age. Primary amenorrhea is the failure of menarche and the absence of menstruation by age 14 years without the development of secondary sex characteristics or by age 16 years regardless of the presence of secondary sex characteristics. In contrast, secondary amenorrhea is defined as the cessation of previous menses for more than 6 months.[35]

Pathophysiology. Normal menstruation depends on the structure and function of the genital outflow tract, including the uterus, ovaries, pituitary gland, and hypothalamus. If any of these components are nonfunctional, bleeding cannot occur.[36,37] The most common causes of amenorrhea (aside from pregnancy) include anatomic defects, elevated FSH levels, hyperprolactinemia, hypothalamic amenorrhea, or polycystic ovary syndrome (PCOS) (Table 25.2).[38] Anatomic defects, including absence of the vagina and uterus, are a disorder associated with amenorrhea. Genetically normal females without a uterus or vagina usually have normal ovarian function. Therefore skeletal growth occurs and secondary sex characteristics develop in the proper sequence, but menstruation does not occur because the uterus is too small or malformed to produce substantial endometrium. Other disorders related to amenorrhea involve the ovary, primarily genetic disorders (e.g., Turner syndrome), and AIS. Gonadal dysgenesis includes Turner syndrome, which accounts for approximately 43% of primary amenorrhea cases.[39] The target organs (e.g., ovaries) in AIS are completely resistant to the action of androgens, resulting in a lack of estrogen. Without primitive gametes and follicles, follicular development and estrogen secretion cannot occur. Lack of estrogen accounts for failure of secondary sex characteristic development and amenorrhea, although there are high levels of circulation FSH and LH.[40] Disorders of the anterior pituitary gland, including tumors, may result in failure of signaling to the ovaries through FSH and LH secretion. Examples of such defects include hydrocephalus, craniopharyngiomas, and other space-occupying lesions of the CNS. The target (the ovary) does not receive the necessary signals, and ovulation and menstruation do not occur. In some cases, these lesions develop between the onset and conclusion of puberty. Therefore skeletal growth may occur and secondary sex characteristics may develop, but sexual maturation is interrupted before menarche. Finally, CNS disorders that primarily involve hypothalamic defects, prevent secretion of GnRH; thus there is no signaling to the pituitary to release FSH and LH. The ovary does not receive the hormonal signals required to stimulate estrogen production, and ovulation and menstruation do not occur. Because the ovarian hormones are absent, estrogen-dependent sex characteristics do not develop. CNS tumors can cause these disruptions in the hypothalamic-pituitary-ovarian axis.[41]

TABLE 25.2 Common Causes of Primary Amenorrhea

Anatomic Defects Uterus and vagina are partially or completely lacking in the presence of otherwise normal female sexual characteristics.Other defects include imperforate hymen or transverse vaginal septum	The diagnosis is typically müllerian agenesis Accounts for ~10% of cases Create a partial or complete vaginal blockage
Elevated Follicle-Stimulating Hormone Indicate gonadal dysfunction	Individuals with XX chromosomes, gonadal failure refers to ovarian failure and isolated absence of the vagina or cervix
Hyperprolactinemia Prolactin	Involved in many reproductive functions; Prolactin secretion inhibits secretion of gonadotropin-releasing hormone (GnRH), which negatively modulates the secretion of pituitary hormones
Hypothalamic Amenorrhea Cessation or absence of menses	Functional disorder of the hypothalamus
Polycystic Ovary Syndrome (PCOS) Most common cause of amenorrhea in females with evidence of androgen excess; common reproductive and endocrinologic disorder	Three characteristics include: hyperandrogenism, polycystic ovaries, and ovulatory dysfunction.
Other Hypopituitarism, weight loss, anorexia nervosa, GnRH deficiencyConstitutional delay of puberty, chronic systemic disease, or acute illness	

Data from Gasner A, Rehman A. *Primary Amenorrhea.* StatPearls [Internet]. Treasure Island, FL: StatPearls Publishing; 2021.

Clinical Manifestations. The major clinical manifestation of primary amenorrhea is the absence of the first menstrual period. The cause of the amenorrhea determines whether secondary sex characteristics and height are affected.

Evaluation and Treatment. Diagnosis of primary amenorrhea is based on the history and physical examination. It is necessary to first rule out pregnancy. The Tanner scale should be used to stage pubertal development to determine whether secondary sexual characteristics are present. Absence of these sexual characteristics indicates that a female has never been exposed to estrogen. If ovarian steroid hormone levels are low, the individual has the appearance of an immature female. Pelvic ultrasound is used to confirm the presence or absence of a uterus.[39] Laboratory studies may be required to document abnormal levels of gonadotropins or ovarian hormones or the presence of genetic conditions. Diagnostic imaging, including ultrasonography and MRI, is used to document structural abnormalities.[42,43]

Treatment involves correction of any underlying disorders and implementation of HRT to induce the development of secondary sex characteristics. Although surgical alteration of the genitalia may be undertaken to correct structural abnormalities, it should be postponed until the individual can make a truly informed decision.[39] Hormonal manipulation or embryo transplantation may make pregnancy possible for women with primary amenorrhea who have a normal uterus.

Secondary Amenorrhea

Secondary amenorrhea is the absence of menstruation for a time equivalent to three or more cycles in women who previously had regular menstrual cycles or 6 months in females with irregular menstrual cycles. A wide variety of disorders and physiologic conditions is associated with secondary amenorrhea.[35] Secondary amenorrhea is common during early adolescence, pregnancy, lactation, and the perimenopausal period, primarily because of anovulation.[44] The most common causes (after pregnancy) are thyroid disorders (e.g., hypothyroidism); hyperprolactinemia; hypothalamic-pituitary-ovarian (HPO) interruption secondary to excessive exercise, stress, or weight loss; and PCOS. The factors leading to secondary amenorrhea also may cause primary amenorrhea in a young woman who has not begun to menstruate.

Pathophysiology. The pathophysiology is dependent on the causes of secondary amenorrhea (Fig. 25.2). Hormonal causes include pregnancy, lactation, thyroid dysfunction, hyperprolactinemia, hyperandrogenism (including PCOS), hypogonadotropic hypogonadism (hypothalamic-pituitary dysfunction), and suppression of the endometrium by hormonal birth control. Structural causes include damage to the endometrium (Asherman syndrome) and obstruction of the outflow tract (cervical stenosis). An excess of ovarian hormones disrupts feedback relationships within the HPO axis, preventing ovulation. Depressed ovarian hormone levels also cause amenorrhea by preventing ovulation. Lack of ovulation, termed *anovulation*, may result from increased levels of prolactin, decreased levels of gonadotropins, irregular secretion of gonadotropins, or abnormally low levels of CNS neurotransmitters. Any of these variables can alter the feedback mechanism that ovarian hormones have on the hypothalamus and pituitary.

High levels of prolactin are physiologic during lactation because it increases milk production and suppresses ovulation, preventing closely spaced pregnancies. However, high levels of prolactin not related to lactation are abnormal and will disrupt the menstrual cycle. Hyperprolactinemia (overproduction of prolactin by the pituitary) may have indirect effects that lead to decreased secretion of GnRH by the hypothalamus. The result is a reduction in FSH and LH secretion followed by anovulation and secondary amenorrhea. Hyperprolactinemia can have many causes, including medication side effects, hypothyroidism, excessive nipple stimulation, and pituitary tumors.[45]

Clinical Manifestations. The major manifestation of secondary amenorrhea is the absence of menses after previous menstrual periods, infertility, vasomotor flushes, vaginal atrophy, acne, and osteopenia. Hirsutism (abnormal hairiness) may also be present, depending on the underlying cause of the amenorrhea.

Evaluation and Treatment. Pregnancy is the most common cause of secondary amenorrhea and must be ruled out before any further evaluation. A thorough history and physical examination are important because the menstrual cycle may stop or become irregular in response to stress, exposure to severe emotional stress, extreme exercise, dietary changes, eating disorders,

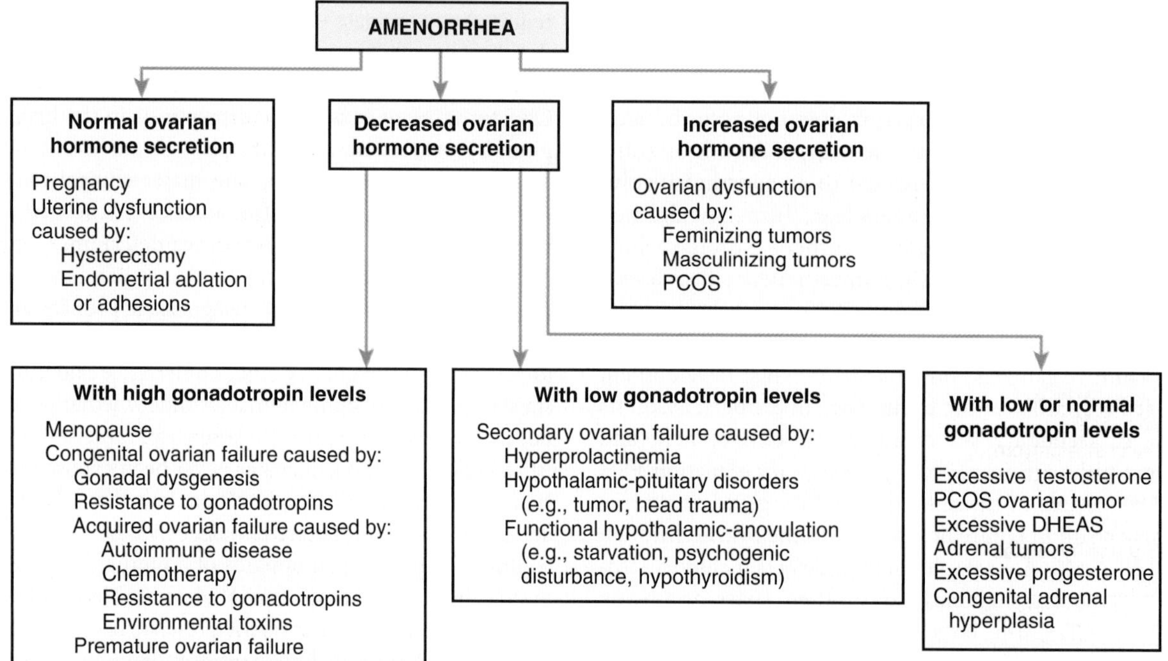

Fig. 25.2 Causes of Secondary Amenorrhea. Of note, hypothyroidism is a relatively common condition and should be ruled out as the cause of hyperprolactinemia before more extensive evaluation (i.e., computed tomography or magnetic resonance imaging) occurs. *DHEAS*, Dehydroepiandrosterone sulfate; *PCOS*, polycystic ovary syndrome.

or sleep abnormalities.[46] After ruling out pregnancy and PCOS, initial laboratory evaluation includes measurement of thyroid-stimulating hormone (TSH) and prolactin levels. Elevated prolactin levels warrant further investigation, which could include performing a progestin challenge; measurement of gonadotropins (FSH), estrogen, and testosterone; and ultrasonography of the outflow tract and/or ovaries, MRI, or both.[35]

Treatment of amenorrhea depends on the cause and on the woman's psychological need for cycle stability. Treatments may include replacing deficient hormones (e.g., estrogens, thyroid hormone, glucocorticoids, gonadotropins) or correcting underlying pathologic conditions.[41] A diagnosis of PCOS may be treated with an insulin-sensitizing agent, such as metformin, as well as ovulation-inducing drugs if fertility is desired. Asherman syndrome is treated with hysteroscopic lysis of lesions, and cervical stenosis is treated with cervical dilation. The goals of therapy include correcting the underlying pathology, achieving fertility, and preventing complications of treatment.

Abnormal Uterine Bleeding

Abnormal uterine bleeding (AUB) is bleeding that is abnormal in duration, volume, frequency, or regularity and has been present for the majority of 6 months, outside of pregnancy.[47] AUB may be acute or chronic and is classified by the cause of bleeding using an internationally recognized PALM-COEIN acronym (**P**olyp, **A**denomyosis, **L**eiomyoma, **M**alignancy [and hyperplasia]-**C**oagulopathy, **O**vulatory disorders, **E**ndometrial, **I**atrogenic, and **N**ot otherwise classified) (Fig. 25.3). Approximately one-third of females will experience AUB in their lifetime, with irregularities most commonly occurring at menarche and perimenopause.[47]

Acute AUB is excessive bleeding that requires immediate treatment. Acute AUB can occur on its own or as a part of chronic AUB. Chronic AUB is irregularities in menstrual bleeding for most of the previous 6 months.[48] Some structural changes, such as endocervical polyps, endometrial polyps, or leiomyomas, may be asymptomatic and not the primary cause of AUB.[47] In the 2018, AUB secondary to anticoagulants was moved from the coagulopathy category to the iatrogenic category by the International Federation of Gynecology and Obstetrics (FIGO) system. Conditions included in the "*not otherwise classified*" were PID, chronic liver disease, and cervicitis. The prevalence of AUB among reproductive-aged women internationally is estimated as 3% to 30%, with a higher incidence occurring around menarche and perimenopause. Because many women do not seek health care for their symptoms, the exact prevalence is uncertain. In premenstrual or menopausal women, any bleeding is considered abnormal. For reproductive-aged women, normal uterine bleeding is every 28 days with variation up to 7 days. Bleeding more frequently than every 21 days, or less frequently than every 35 days, is considered abnormal. Menstrual bleeding for longer than 7 days also is considered abnormal.[49] AUB is the leading cause for hysterectomy in the United States.

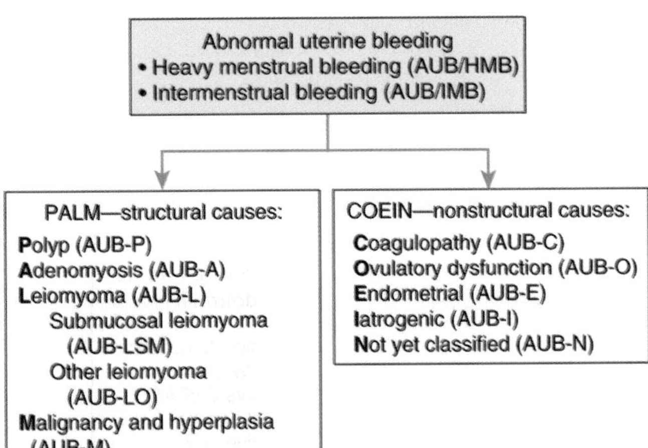

Fig. 25.3 PALM-COEIN System for Classification of Abnormal Uterine Bleeding. *AUB*, Abnormal uterine bleeding. (Modified from Critchley HOD, Fraser IS. The FIGO classification of causes of abnormal uterine bleeding: Malcolm G. Munro, Hilary O.D. Crithcley, Ian S. Fraser, for the FIGO Working Group on Menstrual Disorders. *International Journal of Gynecology & Obstetrics*, 2011;113:3–13.)

Pathophysiology. The majority of AUB is associated with lack of ovulation. Normal, regular periods are the result of a complex interplay between the hypothalamus, pituitary, ovary, and uterine endometrium. Disruptions in this system can affect the amount and structure of the uterine endometrium, causing it to shed irregularly or heavily. Although anovulatory AUB may occur at any time during the reproductive years and many conditions are associated with irregular ovulation, it tends to occur in adolescents and perimenopausal women more frequently because women at the edges of their productive years are more likely to ovulate irregularly. The formation of a follicle and its rupture to release an ovum are important components of the menstrual cycle. As the follicle forms, it produces estrogen, which causes proliferation of the endometrium. Following ovulation, the remaining portions of the follicle, known as the corpus luteum, release progesterone. The progesterone acts on the proliferating endometrium to limit growth and cause changes in the vasculature of the endometrium. This limits bleeding during endometrial shedding.

If a follicle forms but never releases the ovum, the follicle may continue to produce estrogen, encouraging endometrial proliferation beyond the normal 14-day time. In addition, the lack of progesterone causes the thickened endometrium to be unable to shed in a predictable fashion without excessive blood loss. Women who fail to ovulate experience irregularities in their menstrual bleeding because of a lack of progesterone and, in some cases, an excess of estrogen.

Without ovulation, menstrual flow may become irregular, excessive, or both, resulting from the large quantity of tissue available for bleeding and the random breakdown of tissue that results in exposure of vascular channels. Derangements to the clotting pathways (coagulopathies or iatrogenic) can lead to abnormal bleeding with prolonged and excessive flow. Stasis does not occur because the normal control mechanisms (i.e., vasoconstrictive rhythmicity, tight coiling of spiral vessels, and orderly collapse) are absent from the lack of progesterone. Unopposed estrogen induces a progression of endometrial responses beginning with proliferation, hyperplasia, and adenomatous hyperplasia. Over a course of many years, unopposed estrogen may end with atypia and carcinoma.

Abnormal menstrual bleeding also can result from defects of the corpus luteum, resulting in progesterone deficiencies, or from abnormalities of the uterus or cervix. Examples include endometrial polyps, uterine fibroids, or even uterine or cervical cancers. Coagulation defects also can cause heavy and AUB and should be suspected in younger women with a history of extensive bruising or bleeding during dental procedures. Iatrogenic AUB can be caused by IUDs or long-acting contraceptive implants or medications, such as anticoagulants, steroids, digitalis, phenytoin, or hypothalamic depressants.[50,51]

Clinical Manifestations. AUB is characterized by unpredictable and variable bleeding in terms of amount and duration. Especially during perimenopause, dysfunctional bleeding also may involve flooding and the passing of large clots, leading to excessive blood loss. Excessive bleeding can lead to iron deficiency anemia and its associated symptoms, including fatigue or shortness of breath. AUB also may cause pain, decreased productivity, and sexual dysfunction.

Evaluation and Treatment. The first step in the evaluation of AUB is to establish the cause of bleeding. Evaluation includes a thorough history, physical examination, and transvaginal ultrasound. Laboratory evaluation includes a pregnancy test, complete blood count (CBC), ferritin, thyroid function tests, coagulation studies, gonadotropins, and prolactin if indicated. If no cause is found, it is usually assumed that the bleeding is caused by lack of regular ovulation. Based on the PALM-COEIN acronym, specific treatment goals are indicated for each category (Box 25.1). Therapeutic goals include preventing or controlling abnormal bleeding, identifying underlying disease, and inducing regular menstrual cycles. Treatment varies greatly by the age of the woman and her desire for current and future fertility.[52,53]

BOX 25.1 Treatment Guidelines According to PALM-COEIN

Polyps are treated through surgical resection.

Adenomyosis is treated by hysterectomy. Less often, adenomyomectomy is performed.

Leiomyomas (fibroids) are treated according to the individual's desire, include both medical and surgical management for fertility, medical comorbidities, pressure symptoms, and distortion of the uterine cavity. Surgical options include uterine artery embolization, endometrial ablation, or hysterectomy. Medical management options include a levonorgestrel-releasing intrauterine device (IUD), GnRH agonists, systemic progestins, and tranexamic acid with nonsteroidal antiinflammatory drugs (NSAIDs).

Malignancy or hyperplasia can be treated through surgery, ± adjuvant treatment depending on the stage, progestins in high doses when surgery is not an option, or palliative therapy, such as radiotherapy.

Coagulopathies leading to abnormal uterine bleeding (AUB) can be treated with tranexamic acid or desmopressin (DDAVP).

Ovulatory dysfunction can be treated through lifestyle modification in women with obesity, polycystic ovary syndrome (PCOS), or other conditions where anovulatory cycles are suspected. Endocrine disorders, for example Cushing syndrome, are corrected using appropriate medications, such as cabergoline for hyperprolactinemia and levothyroxine for hypothyroidism.

Endometrial disorders have no specific treatment because mechanisms are not clearly understood.

Iatrogenic causes of AUB are based on offending drug(s). If a contraception method is suspected, alternative methods are considered, such as the levonorgestrel-releasing IUD, combined oral contraceptive pills (in monthly or extended cycles), or systemic progestins. If other medications are suspected but cannot be discontinued, the aforementioned methods can also help to control AUB.

Not otherwise classified causes of AUB include endometritis and arteriovenous malformations (AVMs). Endometritis can be treated with antibiotics and AVMs with embolization.

Data from American College of Obstetricians and Gynecologists (ACOG) committee opinion no. 557: Management of acute abnormal uterine bleeding in nonpregnant reproductive-aged women. *Obstetrics and Gynecology,* 2013;121(4):891–896; Whitaker L, Critchley HOD. Abnormal uterine bleeding. *Best Practice and Research in Clinical Obstetrics and Gynaecology,* 2016;34:54–65; Cheong Y, Cameron IT, Critchley HOD. Abnormal uterine bleeding. *British Medical Bulletin,* 2017;123(1):103–114; Davis, E Sparzak PB. Abnormal uterine bleeding. In: *StatPearls* [Internet]. Treasure Island: StatPearls Publishing; 2021.

Polycystic Ovary Syndrome

Polycystic ovary syndrome (PCOS) remains one of the most common endocrine disturbances affecting women. The National Institutes of Health (NIH) criteria for the diagnosis of PCOS require at least two of these three conditions: menstrual irregularity, hyperandrogenism, and appearance of polycystic ovaries on ultrasonography. International criteria (Androgen Excess-PCOS Society Criteria, Rotterdam Criteria) also include any two of the three conditions. The Rotterdam definition is the most widely used PCOS classification.[54] Polycystic ovaries do not have to be present to diagnose PCOS, and their presence alone does not establish the diagnosis. Signs and symptoms of PCOS can vary over time, with metabolic syndrome becoming more prominent with age.[55]

Pathophysiology. No single factor fully accounts for the abnormalities of PCOS. PCOS is a heterogeneous disorder with different manifestations and phenotypes.[54] Box 25.2 summarizes the phenotypes. The more criteria met by an individual with PCOS, the more severe a particular phenotype is considered.[54] Hyperandrogenic state is a cardinal feature in the pathogenesis of PCOS. Two-thirds of cases of PCOS are due to functional ovarian hyperandrogenism (FOH). It is characterized by dysregulation of androgen secretion with an increased response of 17-hydroxyprogesterone (17-OHP) to gonadotropin stimulation. Other PCOS cases have atypical FOH detectable by testosterone elevation after suppression of adrenal androgen production. Approximately 3% of cases of PCOS have

BOX 25.2 Phenotypes of Polycystic Ovary Syndrome

- Hyperandrogenism and ovulatory dysfunction.
- Hyperandrogenism and polycystic ovarian morphology.
- Oligo-ovulation and polycystic ovarian morphology.
- Hyperandrogenism, oligo-ovulation, and polycystic ovarian morphology.

From Steering Committee of the National Institutes of Health Evidence-Based Methodology Workshop on Polycystic Ovary Syndrome Evidence-based Methodology Workshop on Polycystic Ovary Syndrome Final Report https://prevention.nih.gov/docs/programs/pcos/FinalReport.pdf (National Institute of Health, Bethesda MD, USA 2012).

an isolated functional adrenal hyperandrogenism. The rest of the cases of PCOS are mild.[56,57]

Glucose intolerance/insulin resistance and hyperinsulinemia often occur concurrently and markedly aggravate the hyperandrogenic state, thus contributing to the severity of signs and symptoms of PCOS. A metabolic syndrome of obesity-related and/or intrinsic insulin resistance occurs in approximately half of PCOS individuals, and the compensatory hyperinsulinism has tissue specific effects that intensify hyperandrogenism.[56]

PCOS is proposed as resulting from a vicious circle of androgen excess favoring abdominal adipose tissue deposition and visceral adiposity by inducing insulin resistance and compensatory hyperinsulinism, which further allows androgen secretion by the ovaries and adrenal glands in women with PCOS (Fig. 25.4).[54] Weight gain tends to aggravate symptoms, whereas weight loss may ameliorate some of the metabolic and endocrine events. Avoidance of these epigenetic initiators and maintenance of healthy habits in women with PCOS, at least in theory, may be more protective for their fetuses and would to some extent prevent the nongenetic inheritance of PCOS and its metabolic comorbidities. Inappropriate gonadotropin secretion triggers the beginning of a vicious cycle that perpetuates anovulation. Typically, levels of FSH are low or below normal, and the LH level is elevated. Persistent LH level elevation causes an increase in the concentration of androgens (dehydroepiandrosterone sulfate [DHEAS] from the adrenal glands and testosterone, androstenedione, and dehydroepiandrosterone [DHEA] from the ovary). Androgens are converted to estrogen in peripheral tissues, and increased testosterone levels cause a significant reduction (approximately 50%) in the sex hormone–binding globulin (SHBG) level, which in turn causes increased levels of free estradiol. Elevated estrogen levels trigger a positive feedback response in LH and a negative feedback response in FSH. Because FSH levels are not totally depressed, new follicular growth is continuously stimulated but not to full maturation and ovulation. The accumulation of follicular tissue in various stages of development allows an increased and relatively constant production of steroids in response to gonadotropin stimulation. Thus PCOS is characterized by excessive production of both androgen and estrogen.

Increased androgens contribute to premature follicular failure (atresia) and persistent anovulation. Persistent anovulation causes enlarged polycystic ovaries, characterized by a smooth, pearly white capsule (Fig. 25.5). This characteristic appearance

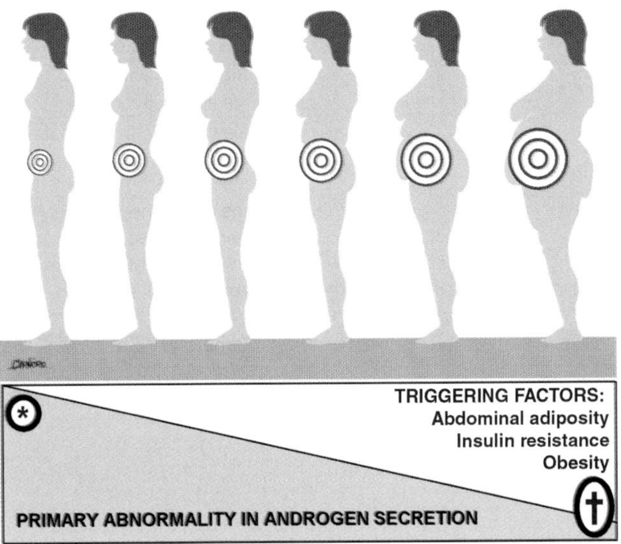

Fig. 25.4 Abdominal Adiposity and Polycystic Ovary Syndrome. An interplay between polycystic ovary syndrome (PCOS) and abdominal adiposity At one extreme *(*)*, for some individuals, the disorder is severe enough to result in PCOS even in the absence of triggering factors. At the other extreme *(†)*, a very mild defect in androgen secretion is amplified by the coexistence of abdominal adiposity, obesity and/or insulin resistance. All individuals share a primary defect in androgen secretion. (Modified and reproduced with permission from Escobar-Morreale HF, San Millan JL. Abdominal adiposity and the polycystic ovary syndrome. *Trends in Endocrinology and Metabolism,* 2007;18:266–272, copyright Elsevier, 2007 and Escobar-Morreale HF, Santacruz E, Luque-Ramirez M, Botella Carretero JI. Prevalence of "obesity-associated gonadal dysfunction" in severely obese men and women and its resolution after bariatric surgery: A systematic review and meta-analysis. *Human Reproduction Update,* 2017;23:390–408, Copyright Oxford University Press, 2017.)

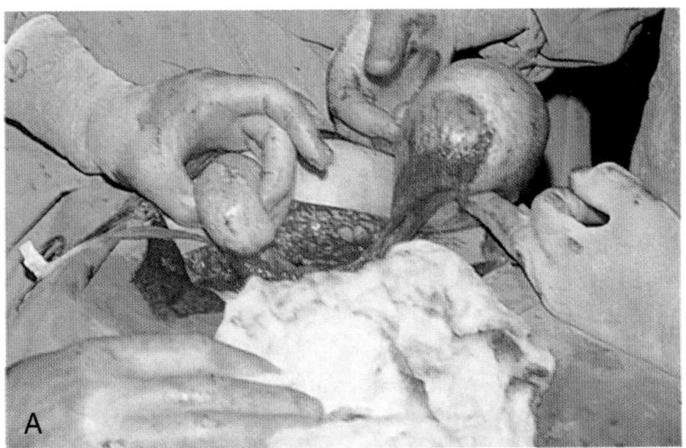

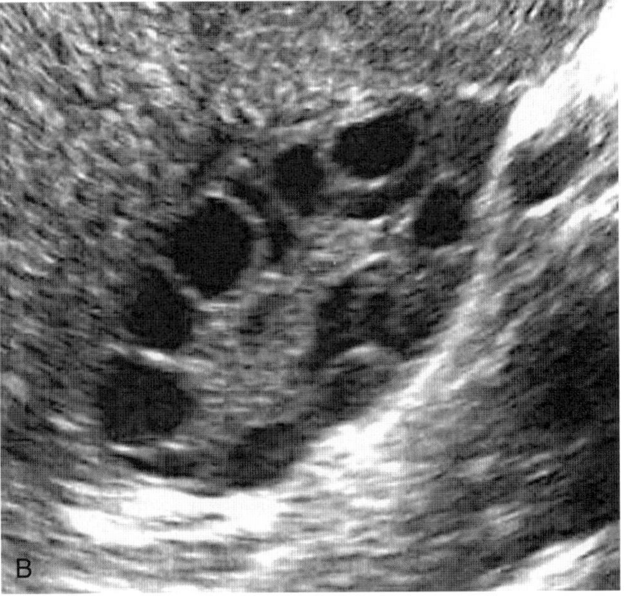

Fig. 25.5 Polycystic Ovary. (A) Surgical view of polycystic ovaries. **(B)** Ultrasound of polycystic ovary. (A, From Symonds EM, Macpherson MBA. *Diagnosis in color: Obstetrics and gynecology.* London: Mosby-Wolfe; 1997; B, From King J. Polycystic ovary syndrome. *Journal of Midwifery and Women's Health,* 2006;51(6):415–422. Reprinted with permission.)

is caused by an increase of surface area along with an increased volume, growing atretic follicles, thickening of the tunica, increasing cortical stromal thickening, and an increase in subcortical stroma. With advancing age, menstrual irregularities may improve, but the incidence of metabolic syndrome and type 2 diabetes mellitus (T2DM) increases. Women with PCOS have a three times greater incidence of uterine cancer later in life than normally cycling women because of an anovulatory lack of progesterone. Without treatment for anovulation, the risk for endometrial cancers increases because of the effects of unopposed estrogen.[56,58]

Clinical Manifestations. Clinical manifestations of PCOS usually appear within 2 years of puberty but may appear after a period of normal menstrual function and pregnancy. Signs and symptoms related to anovulation and hyperandrogenism are presented in Box 25.3, including a summary of hormonal disturbances and complications of PCOS. Multiple morbidities are associated with PCOS, including metabolic syndrome, infertility, impaired glucose tolerance, T2DM, cardiovascular risk, depression, obstructive sleep apnea (OSA), endometrial cancer, and nonalcoholic fatty liver disease/nonalcoholic steatohepatitis (NAFLD/NASH).[59–61]

Evaluation and Treatment. Diagnosis of PCOS is based on evidence of androgen excess, chronic anovulation, and sonographic evidence of polycystic ovaries, with at least two of the three criteria evident. As stated previously, polycystic ovaries do not have to be present and, conversely, their presence alone does not establish the diagnosis. Tests for impaired glucose tolerance are recommended. In female adolescents, evidence of hyperandrogenism in the setting of irregular menses must be present before PCOS is diagnosed. Principles of treatment for PCOS are outlined in Box 25.4. Goals of treatment include reversing signs and symptoms of androgen excess, instituting cyclic menstruation, restoring fertility, and ameliorating any associated metabolic and/or endocrine disturbances.[62]

Treatment of PCOS often includes use of combined oral contraceptives for the management of symptoms (e.g., hirsutism, acne) and to establish regular menses. Treatments for obese or overweight women with PCOS include lifestyle modifications, such as regular exercise and weight loss. Reductions in weight can dramatically improve insulin sensitivity and the return of ovulatory cycles. Women with insulin resistance or those who do not respond to contraceptive therapy may benefit from the insulin sensitizer metformin. Bariatric surgery is an alternative for women with severe obesity and PCOS.[63] Progesterone therapy is recommended to oppose estrogen's effects on the endometrium and as a means to initiate monthly withdrawal bleeding (at the expense of continued hirsutism) if combined oral contraceptives are not used and pregnancy is not desired.[58,62,64] Management of PCOS is a nearly lifelong process because the effects of the syndrome persist past childbearing years. Appropriate primary care is needed to control the systemic features of PCOS so that it has minimal impact on a woman's life and health outcomes.

BOX 25.3 Clinical Manifestations of Polycystic Ovary Syndrome

Obesity
Hirsutism
Menstrual disturbance
Oligomenorrhea
Amenorrhea
Regular menstruation
Hyperandrogenism
Infertility
Asymptomatic (20% of those with polycystic ovary syndrome [PCOS])

Hormonal Disturbances

Increased insulin
Decreased sex hormone–binding globulin (SHBG)
Increased androgens (testosterone, androstenedione)
Increased dehydroepiandrosterone (DHEA) (occurs in 50% of women)
Increased luteinizing hormone (LH) (genetic variant LH-β subunit)
Increased prolactin
Increased leptin, especially in obesity
Suggested decreased insulin-like growth factor 1 (IGF-1) receptors on theca cells
Possible decreased estrogen receptors (intraovarian and along hypothalamic-pituitary axis)

Possible Late Sequelae

Dyslipidemia—increased low-density lipoproteins (LDLs), decreased high-density lipoproteins (HDLs), increased triglycerides
Diabetes mellitus (30% of women with or without obesity will develop type 2 diabetes mellitus by age 30)
Cardiovascular disease; hypertension
Endometrial hyperplasia and carcinoma (anovulatory women are hyperestrogenic)

Other

Sleep apnea
Nonalcoholic fatty liver disease
Women with PCOS are at increased risk of gestational diabetes mellitus, pregnancy-induced hypertension, preterm birth, and perinatal mortality

Adapted from Azziz R, Carmina E, Dewailly D, et al. The Androgen Excess and PCOS Society criteria for the polycystic ovary syndrome: The complete task force report. *Fertility and Sterility*, 2009;91(2):456–488; Boomsma CM, Fauser BCJM, Macklon NS. Pregnancy complications in women with polycystic ovary syndrome. *Seminars in Reproductive Medicine*, 2008;26(1):72–84; Diamanti-Kandarakis E. Polycystic ovarian syndrome: pathophysiology, molecular aspects and clinical implications. *Expert Reviews in Molecular Medicine*, 2008;10(2):e3; Spritzer PM, Motta AB. Adolescence and polycystic ovary syndrome: Current concepts on diagnosis and treatment. *International Journal of Clinical Practice*, 2015;69:1236–1246; Escobar-Morreale HF. Polycystic ovary syndrome: definition, aetiology, diagnosis and treatment. *Nature Reviews Endocrinology*, 2018;142:271–284.

Premenstrual Disorders Syndrome

Premenstrual syndrome (PMS) and premenstrual dysphoric disorder (PMDD) are the cyclic recurrence (in the luteal phase of the menstrual cycle) of distressing physical, psychological, or behavioral changes that impair interpersonal relationships or interfere with usual activities. Symptoms for PMS and PMDD begin after ovulation during the luteal phase and persist up to 4 days into the menstrual cycle. The prevalence of PMS and PMDD is difficult to determine, possibly because of the wide-ranging nature of accepted symptoms. It is estimated that 12% of menstruating women are significantly affected by these disorders, with 2% to 5% meeting criteria for PMDD.[65]

BOX 25.4 Principles of the Treatment of Polycystic Ovary Syndrome

- No universal treatment for polycystic ovary syndrome (PCOS) exists.
- Treatment is symptom oriented.
- Other than lifestyle recommendations, individuals with mild symptoms might not require any intervention.
- No drugs are currently approved specifically for PCOS.
- Targets for pharmacologic treatment should consider androgen excess, oligo-ovulation, and insulin resistance.
- Treatment should be chronic and dynamic and adapted to the changing circumstances, personal needs, and expectations of the individual.

From Escobar-Morreale HF. Polycystic ovary syndrome: definition, aetiology, diagnosis and treatment. *Nature Reviews Endocrinology,* 2018;142:271–284.

Pathophysiology. The psychological and physiologic changes of PMS/PMDD occur in the luteal phase of ovulatory cycles and are linked with the complex hormonal changes of the menstrual cycle. Neurotransmitters, such as serotonin (SE), gamma-aminobutyric acid (GABA), and norepinephrine (NE), have demonstrated interactions with estrogen and progesterone and have established mood and behavior effects, including negative mood, irritability, aggression, and impulse control.[66] The differential behavioral response to estrogen and progesterone in PMDD is accompanied by ovarian steroid-related alterations in the neuronal circuit activity underlying reward, social cognition, and affective states.[67] There is evidence that supports a relationship between the severity and frequency of PMS/PMDD and reports of low well-being, major affective disorder, and personal characteristics, such as increased stress, poor nutrition, lack of exercise, low self-esteem, perfectionism, history of sexual abuse, and family conflict. In turn, when PMS/PMDD is distressing, the quality of interpersonal relationships and self-image are negatively affected.[68]

In addition, neurotransmitters may have mediating or moderating roles on symptom manifestation. Sex steroids also interact with the renin-angiotensin-aldosterone system (RAAS), which could explain some PMS/PMDD signs and symptoms (e.g., water retention, bloating, weight gain).[69] A predisposition to PMS occurs in families. Recently, expression of the ESC/E(Z) gene network was found to be systemically disturbed in PMDD.[65]

Clinical Manifestations. Nearly 300 physical, emotional, and behavioral symptoms have been attributed to PMS/PMDD. The pattern of symptom frequency and severity is more important than specific complaints. Emotional symptoms, particularly depression, anger, irritability, and fatigue, have been reported as the most prominent and the most distressing, whereas physical symptoms (abdominal bloating and fatigue) seem to be the least prevalent and problematic. PMS is characterized by the presence of both physical and behavior symptoms that negatively affect the woman's life. PMDD is a severe form of PMS in which symptoms such as anger, irritability, and internal tension are most prominent. The presence of underlying physical or psychological disease may be aggravated in the premenstrual phase and must be diagnosed and treated independently of PMS/PMDD.

Evaluation and Treatment. Diagnosis of PMS or PMDD is based on the health history, menstrual cycle history, symptoms, and the timing of symptoms (present *only* in the week or two prior to the period) using the Daily Record of Severity of Problems (DRSP) form. PMDD is diagnosed using the *Diagnostic and Statistical Manual of Mental Disorders*, 5th edition (DSM-5) criteria, which is presented in Box 25.5. Current management is treatment of symptoms. For many women, nonpharmacologic therapies, such as regular exercise, appropriate sleep, diet, stress reduction, acupuncture, and cognitive-behavioral therapy (CBT) with or without medication, may be effective in controlling symptoms.[70,71]

If nonpharmacologic methods fail or symptoms are severe, pharmacologic intervention is indicated. Two major forms of prescription treatment include hormonal cycle regulation and selective serotonin reuptake inhibitor (SSRI) antidepressants. SSRIs can be administered in three different dosing therapies: daily, luteal phase only (starting on cycle day 14), or symptom-onset only therapy. If a woman does not desire immediate fertility, the oral contraceptive pill containing estrogen and progesterone may regulate her menstrual cycle and decrease levels of circulating steroidal hormones.[72–74]

Infection and Inflammation

Infections of the genital tract may result from exogenous or endogenous microorganisms. Exogenous pathogens are most

BOX 25.5 Diagnostic Criteria for Premenstrual Dysphoric Disorder

A. Five or more of the symptoms listed in this box—occur in most cycles during the week before menses onset, improve within a few days after menses onset, and diminish in the week post menses
B. One (or more) of these symptoms must be present:
   a. Marked affective lability
   b. Marked irritability or anger or increased interpersonal conflicts
   c. Marked anxiety, tension
C. One (or more) of these symptoms must also be present:
   a. Decreased interest
   b. Difficulty concentrating
   c. Easy fatigability, low energy
   d. Increase or decrease in sleep
   e. Feelings of being overwhelmed
   f. Physical symptoms (e.g., breast tenderness, muscle or joint aches, "bloating" or weight gain)

Note: Criteria A through C must be present for most menstrual cycles in the preceding year.

D. Symptoms are associated with significant distress or interferences with work, school, and relationships.
E. The disturbance is *not* an exacerbation of another disorder, such as major depression, panic disorder, persistent depressive disorder, or a personality disorder.
F. Criterion A should be confirmed by prospective daily ratings in at least two symptomatic cycles.
G. The symptoms are not due to the physiologic effects of a substance or another medical condition.

Data from The American Psychiatric Association. *Diagnostic and statistical manual of mental disorders—DSM-5-TR* 5th ed. Washington: Author; 2022.

often sexually transmitted (see Chapter 27). Endogenous causes of infection include microorganisms that are normally resident in the vagina, bowel, or vulva. Infection occurs if these microorganisms migrate to a new location or overproliferate when the immune system and other defense mechanisms are impaired. Skin disorders that can affect the vulva include reactive dermatitis, contact dermatitis, psoriasis, and impetigo. (For a discussion of skin disorders, see Chapter 46.)

Pelvic Inflammatory Disease

Pelvic inflammatory disease (PID) is an acute inflammatory process caused by infection. It may involve any or all organs in the upper genital tract: the uterus, fallopian tubes, or ovaries. Typically, it is an ascending infection, spreading from the lower genital tract (Fig. 25.6).[75] In its most severe form, the entire peritoneal cavity can be affected. Inflammation of the fallopian tubes is termed salpingitis (Fig. 25.7), and inflammation of the ovaries is called oophoritis. Most cases of PID are caused by sexually transmitted microorganisms, such as *Chlamydia trachomatis* and *Neisseria gonorrhoeae*, that migrate from the vagina to the uterus, fallopian tubes, and ovaries. PID is very common in the United States and around the world and carries with it immediate and long-term health implications, including infertility and increased risk of ectopic pregnancy, for women and their sexual partners.[76] Risk factors include intercourse with multiple partners, age, previous history of PID, IUD implantation, and tubal ligation.

Pathophysiology. Infection of the upper female genital track leads to inflammatory damage, including scarring, adhesions, and partial or total obstruction of the fallopian tubes.[75] Loss of the ciliated epithelial cells along the fallopian tube lining results in impaired ovum transport and increases the risk for infertility, ectopic pregnancy, and adhesions that can lead to chronic pelvic pain.[77] Two sexually transmitted infectious causes of PID are gonorrhea and chlamydia. The microorganisms that cause these infections can infect the vagina and cervix, and if the normal vaginal microbial flora is disrupted, the pathogens can more easily ascend through the cervix (see Fig. 25.6).[78]

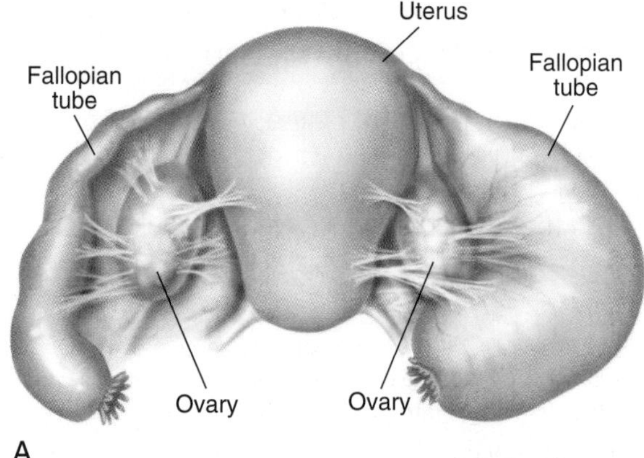

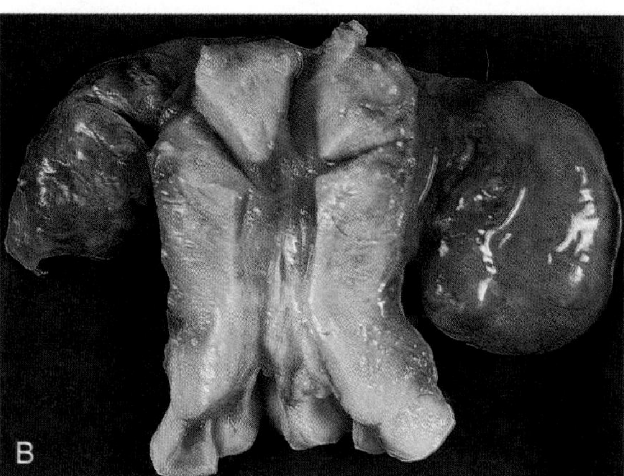

Fig. 25.7 Salpingitis. (A) Advanced pyosalpinx. Note the swollen fallopian tube. **(B)** Bilateral, retort-shaped, swollen, sealed tubes and adhesions of the ovaries are typical of salpingitis. (A, From Ball J, Dains JE, Flynn JA, Solomon BS, Stewart RW. *Seidel's guide to physical examination*, 8th edition. St. Louis: Mosby; 2015; B, From Damjanov I, Linder J, eds. *Anderson's pathology*, 10th edition. St. Louis: Mosby; 1996.)

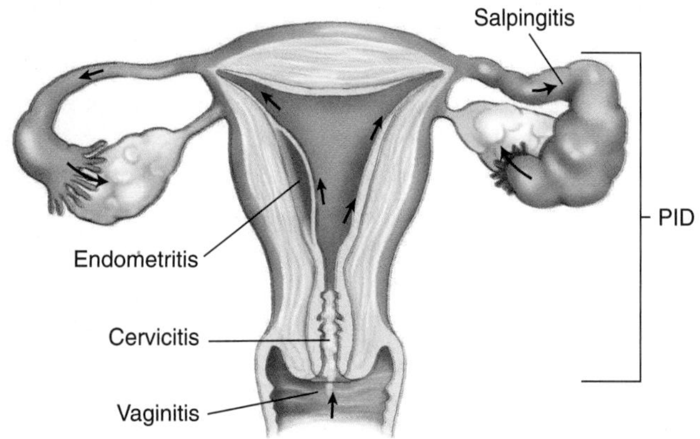

Fig. 25.6 Ascension of Pelvic Inflammatory Disease. Microorganisms from the lower genital track ascend into the endometrium, fallopian tubes, and peritoneum to cause endometriosis-salpingitis-peritonitis (pelvic inflammatory disease *[PID]*). The arrows indicate the "flow" of microorganisms from the lower genital tract to the upper genital tract. This is noted as an ascending infection in the text. (Adapted from Brooks M. *Exploring medical language*, 8th edition. St. Louis: Mosby; 2012.)

Many anaerobic bacteria have been implicated as increasing the risk of PID because they alter the pH of the vaginal environment and may decrease the integrity of the mucus blocking the cervical canal.[75] Bacterial vaginosis (BV) is present in up to 66% of women with PID. In addition, other pathogens are frequently isolated and include anaerobes (e.g., *Peptostreptococcus* species, *Bacteroides* species, *Gardnerella vaginalis*), respiratory pathogens *(Haemophilus influenzae, Streptococcus pneumonia, Staphylococcus aureus)*, genital tract mycoplasmas *(Mycoplasma hominis, Mycoplasma genitalis, Ureaplasma urealyticum)*, and enteric pathogens (*Escherichia coli, Bacteroides fragilis*, group B streptococci), which have been identified in acute PID and account for approximately 15% of cases.[75] Therefore, although *N. gonorrhoeae* and *C. trachomatis* are the main pathogens in PID, the disease is actually polymicrobial in origin and is treated with a broad spectrum of antibiotics to ensure that all the causative agents are eliminated.[78,79]

The infection may induce changes in the columnar epithelium lining of the upper reproductive tract, causing permanent damage. The subsequent inflammatory response causes localized edema and sometimes obstruction or necrosis of the area. Gonorrhea gonococci attach to the fallopian tubes and excrete a substance that is toxic to the tubal mucosa, increasing inflammation and damage. Chlamydia enter the tubal cells and replicate, bursting the cell membrane as they reproduce and causing permanent scarring. Scarring increases the risk of a later ectopic pregnancy because the mobility of an egg through the fallopian tubes is slowed by damaged cilia. Scarring and adhesions also can result in chronic pelvic pain and, potentially, an increased risk of uterine cancer.[80,81]

Clinical Manifestations. The clinical manifestations of PID vary from asymptomatic to sudden, severe abdominal pain with fever. It also may present with mild to moderate abdominal or pelvic pain, dysuria (difficult or painful urination), vaginal discharge, dyspareunia (pain with sexual intercourse), and/or abnormal vaginal bleeding.[75] An asymptomatic cervicitis may be present for some time before PID develops. The first sign of the ascending infection may be the onset of low bilateral abdominal pain, often characterized as dull and steady with a gradual onset. Symptoms are more likely to develop during or immediately after menstruation. The pain of PID may worsen with walking, jumping, intercourse, or other activities involving movement.

Evaluation and Treatment. PID often has limited or vague clinical symptoms, leading to undertreatment and long-term health effects. PID is a substantial health risk to a woman; therefore the Centers for Disease Control and Prevention (CDC) encourages clinicians to consider PID as a likely diagnosis when a sexually active woman has abdominal or pelvic tenderness and *one* of these conditions: cervical motion tenderness, uterine tenderness, or adnexal tenderness. Box 25.6 lists the diagnostic criteria for PID.

No laboratory tests or studies are needed to begin treatment; however, additional information can improve the specificity of the diagnosis. Abdominal pain in women can have many causes, and it is important to rule out other diagnoses (Fig. 25.8). This can be done while the person is being treated for PID.[61]. A pregnancy test may be done to exclude the possibility of an ectopic pregnancy as an alternate etiology of the pelvic pain.[75] If vaginal or cervical discharge is present, microscopy of the discharge is recommended along with obtaining nucleic acid amplification tests (NAATs) for *C. trachomatis* and *N. gonorrhoeae*. Testing for other sexually transmitted infections (STIs), such as human immunodeficiency virus (HIV) and *Treponema pallidum* (syphilis), is considered. Although laboratory testing may help to confirm the diagnosis, NAATs can typically take several hours to days to obtain a result. Negative results do not exclude the diagnosis. Therefore prompt and early treatment is advised.[78] Histopathologic examination from a biopsy is rarely done, but should be done if there is a doubt about the diagnosis.[75] Prompt antibiotic treatment can prevent severe damage to the reproductive organs and prevent infertility or a future ectopic pregnancy.[78]

BOX 25.6 Diagnostic Criteria for Pelvic Inflammatory Disease

Minimum Criteria (One or More Needed for Diagnosis)

Cervical motion tenderness, *or*
Uterine tenderness, *or*
Adnexal tenderness

Additional Criteria That Increase Specificity of Diagnosis

Fever >38.3°C (>101°F)
Mucopurulent cervical or vaginal discharge, or cervical friability
Numerous white blood cells on saline wet prep
Elevated C-reactive protein
Elevated erythrocyte sedimentation rate
Documented infection with *Chlamydia trachomatis* or *Neisseria gonorrhoeae*

Definitive Criteria (Not Needed for Treatment)

Transvaginal ultrasound, magnetic resonance imaging showing thickened and fluid-filled tubes, *or*
Doppler studies indicating pelvic infection, and
Laparoscopic visualization of PID-related abnormalities, or
Endometrial biopsy with evidence of endometritis

From Centers for Disease Control and Prevention (CDC). *Pelvic Inflammatory Disease (PID) Treatment and Care.* Atlanta: U.S. Department of Health and Human Services; 2022. https://www.cdc.gov/std/pid/treatment.htm

The complications of PID can be significant; therefore rapid treatment is recommended even before the causative pathogen can be identified. Because treatment is empiric, it needs to be effective against a broad range of pathogens, especially chlamydia, gonococci, and anaerobic bacteria. Treatment is usually done on an outpatient basis unless the female has symptoms of advanced infection, cannot take oral medications, is pregnant, or exhibits other pathologies that cannot be excluded. The outpatient regimen recommended by the CDC is shown in Box 25.7.[78] Although alternative treatment regimens are available, the growing antibiotic resistance of gonorrhea limits antibiotic choices.

To prevent recurrence, sexual partners of women with PID should also receive treatment, even if they are asymptomatic. Women receiving treatment should be reevaluated by their care provider in 3 days to ensure that the antibiotic treatment is effective. Because women with a history of PID are at increased risk for ectopic pregnancy, they should seek care as soon as they know they are pregnant, because ectopic pregnancy is a major cause of maternal mortality. All sexually active women younger than age 25 should receive, at minimum, annual screening for chlamydia and gonorrhea, as should women older than age 25 who have a new sexual partner, more than one sexual partner, a partner who has been diagnosed with an STI, or a partner with more than one sexual partner.[78]

Vaginitis

Vaginitis is irritation or inflammation of the vagina, typically caused by infection, irritants, pathologies, or disruption of the normal vaginal flora. Vaginitis is characterized by complaints of vaginal irritation, itching, burning, odor, or abnormal

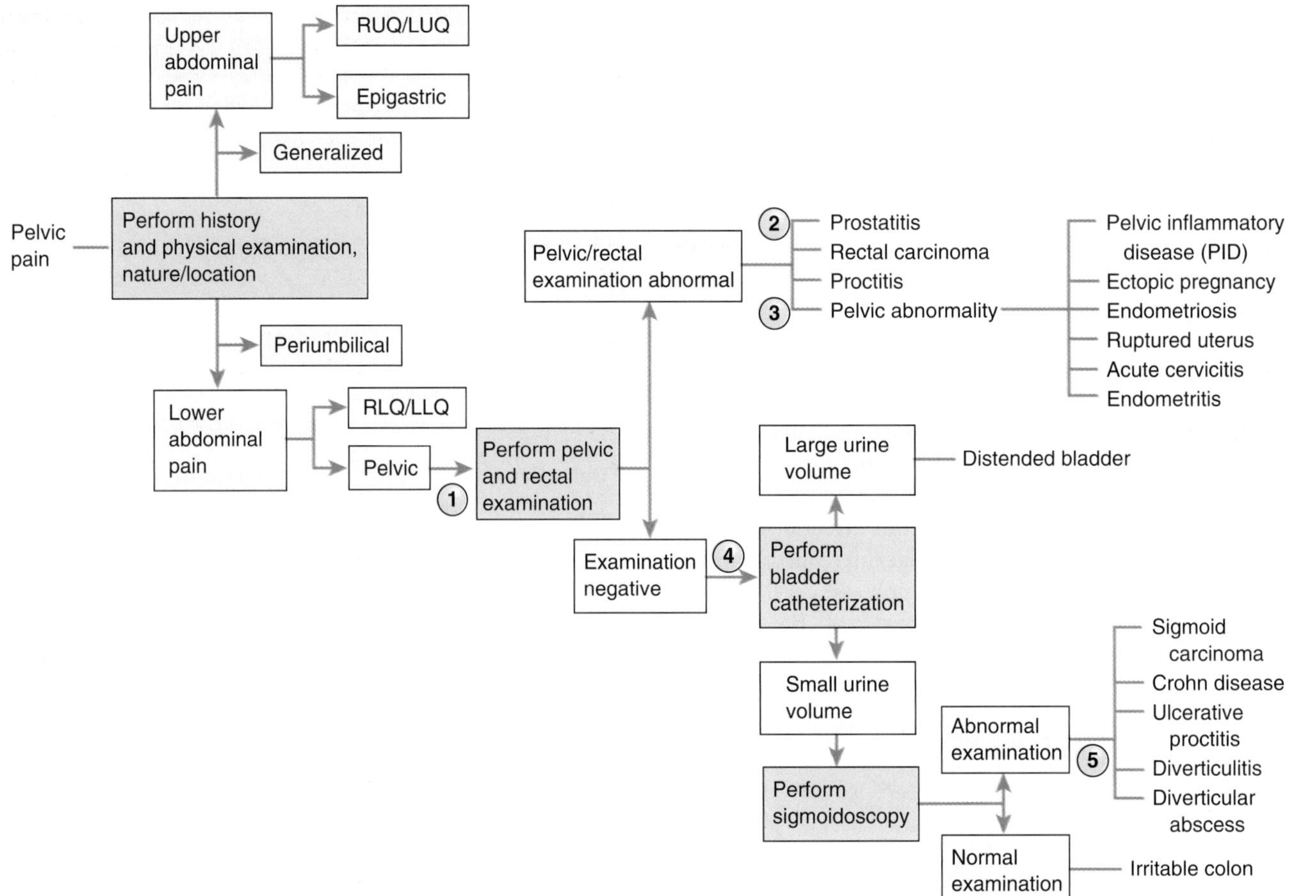

Fig. 25.8 Diagnostic Algorithm for Pelvic Pain. *LLQ*, Left lower quadrant; *LUQ*, left upper quadrant; *RLQ*, right lower quadrant; *RUQ*, right upper quadrant.

discharge. Clinically, it is characterized by an increase in white blood cells or abnormal cells, or both, observed on a saline wet prep examination. The major causes of vaginitis are overgrowth of normal flora, STIs, and vaginal irritation related to low estrogen levels during menopause (a condition known as *atrophic vaginitis*). The primary forms of vaginitis are vulvovaginal candidiasis, or yeast vaginitis, and BV, or trichomoniasis. Bacterial vaginosis (BV) is a noninflammatory condition resulting from an overgrowth of anaerobic bacteria. The overgrowth causes a shift in the composition of the vaginal flora and produces a malodorous vaginal discharge. Pain and itching are common manifestations.[82,83]

Pathophysiology. The development of vaginitis is related to alterations in the vaginal environment. This includes changes with complications in local defense mechanisms, such as skin integrity, immune reaction, and, particularly, vaginal pH. The pH of the vagina (normally 4 to 4.5) depends on cervical secretions and the presence of normal flora that help maintain an acidic environment. A neutral or alkaline pH normally occurs before puberty, after menopause, and during pregnancy. The acidic nature of vaginal secretions during the reproductive years provides protection against a variety of sexually transmitted pathogens and establishes a healthy microflora in the vagina. Changes in the vaginal pH may predispose a woman to infection. Variables that affect the vaginal pH and therefore the bactericidal nature of secretions and the predisposition to infection include semen and the use of douches, soaps, spermicides, feminine hygiene sprays, and deodorant menstrual pads or tampons. Another variable is having a condition associated with an increased glycogen content of vaginal secretions, such as pregnancy and diabetes. Antibiotics often destroy normal vaginal flora, facilitating the overgrowth of *Candida albicans* and causing a yeast infection. Increased vaginal alkalinity also may enhance susceptibility to trichomoniasis and BV.

Clinical Manifestations. Vaginal discharge is typically clear, milky, or cloudy with a slippery or clumpy texture. It is nonirritating, has a mild smell, and may yellow after drying. Throughout the menstrual cycle, the amount and texture of a woman's discharge change in response to hormonal fluctuation. Vaginal secretions increase at the time of ovulation, during pregnancy (because of increased estrogen levels), and with sexual arousal. Just before menstruation, vaginal discharge becomes thick and sticky. Unusual changes in the amount, color, or texture of the vaginal discharge may signal an infection, especially if the discharge is malodorous, irritating, or copious.

Evaluation and Treatment. Diagnosis is based on the history, physical examination, and examination of the discharge by wet mount. Infection is suggested by a marked change in color or

BOX 25.7 CDC-Recommended Treatment for Pelvic Inflammatory Disease: Intramuscular/Oral Regimens

Ceftriaxone 500mg IM in single dose
PLUS
Doxycycline 100mg PO twice a day for 14 days
WITH
Metronidazole 500mg PO twice a for 14 days
OR
Cefoxitin 2g IM in a single dose
AND
Probenecid 1g administered PO concurrently in a single dose
PLUS
Doxycycline 100mg PO twice a day for 14 days
WITH
Metronidazole 500mg PO twice a for 14 days
OR
Other parenteral third-generation
Cephalosporin (e.g., ceftizoxime or cefotaxime)
PLUS
Doxycycline 100mg PO twice a day for 14 days
WITH[a] or WITHOUT
Metronidazole 500mg PO twice a for 14 days

Data from Centers for Disease Control and Prevention (CDC). *Pelvic Inflammatory Disease (PID) Treatment and Care.* Atlanta: U.S. Department of Health and Human Services; 2021; Centers for Disease Control and Prevention (CDC). Page updated: November 9, 2021. https://www.cdc.gov/std/treatment-guidelines/pid.htm; Walker CK, Workowski KA, Washington AE, Soper D, Sweet RL. Anaerobes in pelvic inflammatory disease: Implications for the Centers for Disease Control and Prevention's guidelines for treatment of sexually transmitted diseases. *Clinical Infectious Diseases,* 1999;28(Supp 1):S29–S36.
CDC, Centers for Disease Control and Prevention; *IM,* intramuscularly; *PID,* pelvic inflammatory disease; *PO,* orally.

by a discharge that becomes copious, malodorous, or irritating. Treatment involves developing and maintaining an acidic environment, relieving symptoms (usually pruritus and irritation), and administering antimicrobial or antifungal medications to eradicate the infectious organism. If the infection can be sexually transmitted, the woman's partner will also need to be treated. Research suggests that probiotics, especially *Lactobacillus rhamnosus,* can encourage the proliferation of normal vaginal flora and reduce the incidence of vaginitis in women at risk for this disease.[84,85]

Cervicitis

Cervicitis is a nonspecific term used to describe inflammation of the cervix. The CDC defines cervicitis as having two major diagnostic signs: a purulent or mucopurulent (mucus and pus) discharge from the cervical os or endocervical bleeding (or both) induced by gently introducing a cotton swab into the cervix.[86] Cervicitis can have infectious or noninfectious causes; approximately half of all cases are caused by sexually transmitted pathogens. Chemicals and substances introduced into the vagina can cause cervicitis in addition to disruptions in the normal vaginal flora or microbiome. Age and risk factors are important in assessing a woman with cervicitis. Younger women are at risk for STIs and should be tested for chlamydia, gonorrhea, and trichomoniasis. More stubborn adolescent cases may involve group B streptococcus.[87] Older women with cervicitis may have STIs but are at risk for irritation from abnormal vaginal flora related to low vaginal estrogen levels. In cases where no infectious agent can be identified, pharmacologic therapy may still be effective. The CDC guidelines for the prevention and treatment include antimicrobial therapies, prevention counseling, vaccination, and contraceptive methods.[86] Surgery may be an option or necessary for unresponsive and chronic cases.[88]

Mucopurulent cervicitis (MPC) is usually caused by one or more sexually transmitted pathogens, such as *Trichomonas, Neisseria, Chlamydia, Mycoplasma,* or *Ureaplasma parvum.* Infection causes the cervix to become erythematous and edematous. A mucopurulent exudate drains from the external cervical os, and the individual may report vague pelvic pain, bleeding, or dysuria. The cervix often becomes friable, and bleeding can occur during sexual intercourse or with pelvic examinations (or both), as well as with Papanicolaou (Pap) smears. Because MPC is a symptom of PID, women at risk for STIs, especially those younger than age 26, should receive treatment for PID while awaiting the results of microbial testing. If the woman is not at risk for STIs, a thorough evaluation often reveals another cause for the inflammation.[86]

Vulvodynia

Vulvodynia (also referred to as *vulvitis, vestibulitis,* or *vulvovestibulitis* [VV]) is chronic pain of at least 3 months duration and inflammation of the vulva or vaginal vestibule (entrance of vagina), or both. The classification of vulvodynia is based on the location of the pain, whether it is localized or generalized, and whether the pain is provoked, unprovoked, or mixed. *Localized* is characterized by pain from a cause that usually does not cause pain (allodynia) to the vulvar vestibule area. *Generalized* is a diffuse pain pattern involving all of the pudendal nerve distribution and beyond. *Provoked* means any touch or stimulation that elicits pain, *unprovoked* is pain that occurs in the absence of touch or stimulation, and *mixed* is pain that varies with or without touch or stimulation. Individuals describe the pain as burning, stinging, soreness, irritation, dyspareunia, throbbing, itching, or rawness.[89]

Pathophysiology. The cause of vulvodynia is unknown. Theories suggest it is multifactorial in origin, including embryonic factors, chronic inflammation, genetic immune factors, nerve pathways, increased sensitivity to environmental factors (infection, trauma, irritants), hormonal changes, human papillomavirus (HPV), and oxalates. Although the inflammation of vulvodynia may be caused by contact dermatitis (e.g., exposure to soaps, detergents, lotions, sprays, shaving, menstrual pads/tampons, perfumed toilet paper, tight-fitting clothes), the condition may be more complex and represent abnormalities in three interdependent systems: the vestibular mucosa, pelvic floor musculature, and CNS pain regulatory pathways. The condition also may represent an autoimmune reaction or genetic and psychological links.

Clinical Manifestations. An important trigger is chronic inflammation caused by contact irritants, recurrent infections, hormonal changes, and chronic skin conditions. Overall, with normal sensations there is a heightened sensitivity. Vulvodynia can occur in the context of other pain conditions, such as irritable bowel syndrome, interstitial cystitis, recurrent yeast infections, and fibromyalgia.[90]

Evaluation and Treatment. Cotton swab testing is used to identify painful areas. For vulvar pain, treatment is focused on identifying and treating any infectious cause or comorbid contributor. However, laboratory tests and imaging are rarely required. Women are advised to avoid potential irritants; wear loose, cotton clothing; use mild soaps; and apply a vaginal emollient after bathing. Hot water may incite vulvar symptoms. Studies on treatments are limited but suggest that women may benefit from topical lidocaine (Xylocaine), estrogen cream, topical or systemic antidepressants, or anxiolytics; Botox injections into the affected nerve; dietary modifications; physical therapy; behavioral or sexual counseling (or both); acupuncture; or vestibulectomy. Biofeedback may help to relax the muscles of the pelvic floor and reduce pain.[91–93]

Bartholinitis

Bartholinitis, or Bartholin cyst, is an acute inflammation of one or both of the ducts that lead from the introitus (vaginal opening) to the Bartholin/greater vestibular glands (Fig. 25.9).

Pathophysiology. Most lesions of the Bartholin gland are cysts or abscesses. The usual causes are microorganisms that infect the lower female reproductive tract, such as streptococci, staphylococci, and sexually transmitted pathogens. Acute bartholinitis may be preceded by cervicitis, vaginitis, or urethritis.

Clinical Manifestations. Infection or trauma causes inflammatory changes that narrow the distal portion of the duct, leading to obstruction and stasis of glandular secretions. The obstruction, or cyst, varies from 1 to 8 cm in diameter and is located in the posterolateral portion of the vulva. The affected area is usually red and painful, and pus may be visible at the opening of the duct. The exudate should be cultured, specifically for gonorrhea and chlamydia. The individual may have fever and malaise.

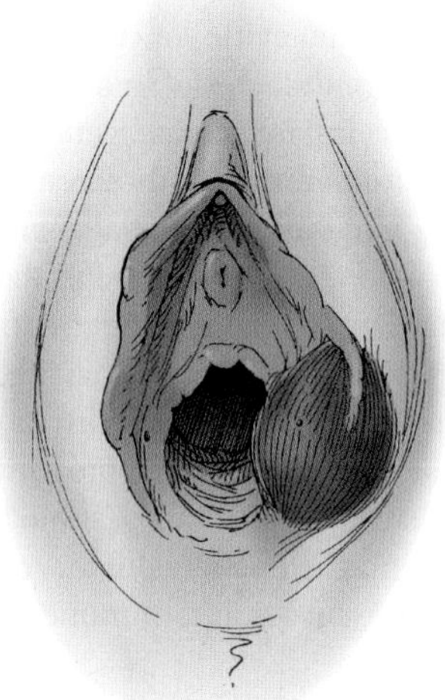

Fig. 25.9 Inflammation of Bartholin Gland. (Modified from Gershenson DM, DeCherney AH, Curry SL. *Operative gynecology,* 2nd edition. Philadelphia: Saunders; 2001. In Fuller JK. *Surgical technology,* 6th edition. Philadelphia: Saunders; 2013.)

Evaluation and Treatment. The diagnosis is based on the clinical manifestations reported and examined, and the identification of infectious microorganisms. Most cases of Bartholin cysts require no treatment. However, to prevent abscess formation, treatment is advised if the cysts are uncomfortable, large, or show signs of infection. Treatment has no consensus but may involve broad-spectrum antibiotics. Some clinicians attempt to drain the cyst using hot soaks, needle aspiration, insertion of a catheter, or marsupialization (cutting a slit and suturing the edges) of the infected gland.[94] No single treatment has proven superior for both relief and prevention of recurrence. Lesions in the form of carcinomas are a rare type of gynecologic tumor and are carefully monitored among postmenopausal women, who are more prone to Bartholin malignancy.[95]

Pelvic Organ Prolapse

The bladder, urethra, and rectum are supported by the endopelvic fascia and perineal muscles, particularly the levator ani group. This muscular and fascial tissue loses tone and strength with aging and may fail to maintain the pelvic organs in the proper position. Weak support of the bladder and rectum tends to cause movement toward the vagina and vaginal wall. The increased pressure causes the area becomes increasingly weaker. Progressive descent of the pelvic support structures may cause pelvic floor disorders, such as urinary and fecal incontinence, and pelvic organ prolapse.

Pelvic organ prolapse (POP) is the descent of one or more of these structures: the vaginal wall, uterus, or apex of the vagina (after a hysterectomy). Although more than 50% of women have some version of POP on physical examination, most women have no symptoms. When prolapse becomes severe, the function of the surrounding organs can be altered. POP is thought to be caused by direct trauma (e.g., childbirth), pelvic floor surgery, obesity, constipation, pelvic organ cancers, or damage to the pelvic innervation, particularly the pudendal nerve. However, risk factors in nulliparous women include occupational activities that require heavy lifting or chronic medical conditions, such as chronic lung disease or refractory constipation (chronically increased intra-abdominal pressure). The most frequently cited risk factors are aging, obesity, and hysterectomy. Other risk factors include a strong familial tendency (from family and twin studies) and possibly a multifactorial genetic component. Prolapse of the bladder, urethra, rectum, or uterus may occur many years after an initial injury to the supporting structure.[96] A list of symptoms and treatments of POP is contained in Box 25.8.

Uterine prolapse is descent of the cervix or entire uterus into the vaginal canal, and in severe cases the uterus falls completely through the vagina and protrudes from the introitus, creating ulceration and obvious discomfort. Fig. 25.10 illustrates the different degrees (grades) of uterine prolapse, showing descent of the cervix or the entire uterus into the vaginal canal. Grade 1 prolapse is not treated unless it causes discomfort. Grades 2 and 3 prolapse usually cause feelings of fullness, heaviness, and

BOX 25.8 Pelvic Organ Prolapse: Symptoms and Treatments

Symptoms	Treatment
Urinary Sensation of incomplete emptying of bladder Urinary incontinence Urinary frequency/urgency Bladder "splinting" to accomplish voiding	Depending on age of woman and cause and severity of condition: • Isometric exercises to strengthen pubococcygeal muscles (Kegel exercises) • Estrogen to improve tone and vascularity of fascial support (postmenopausal) • Pessary (a removable device) to hold pelvic organs in place
Bowel Constipation or feeling of rectal fullness or blockage Difficult defecation Stool or flatus incontinence Urgency Manual "splinting" of posterior vaginal wall to accomplish defecation	**Surgical** Reconstructive: autologous grafts; synthetic mesh/sling Obliterative (most extreme) Weight loss Avoidance of constipation Treatment of cough/lung conditions
Pain and Bulging Vaginal, bladder, rectum Pelvic pressure, bulging, pain Lower back pain	
Sexual Dyspareunia Decreased sensation, lubrication, arousal	

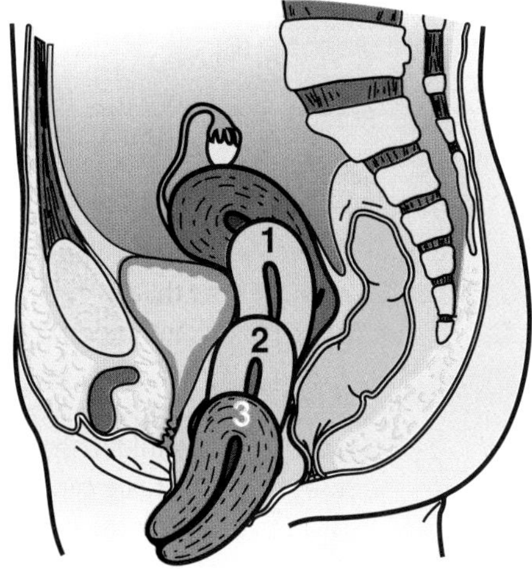

Fig. 25.10 Degrees of Uterine Prolapse. **Grade 1** prolapse is minimal and rarely requires correction. **Grade 2** prolapse has moderate symptoms. **Grade 3** prolapse is severe. The uterus is so low the cervix protrudes from the vagina. (From Phillips N. *Berry & Kohn's operating room technique,* 12th edition. Philadelphia: Mosby; 2013.)

collapse through the vagina. Symptoms of other pelvic floor disorders also may be present.[97]

Cystocele is descent of a portion of the posterior bladder wall and trigone into the vaginal canal and is usually caused by childbirth (Fig. 25.11). In severe cases, the bladder and anterior vaginal wall bulge outside the introitus. Symptoms are usually insignificant in mild to moderate cases. Increased bulging and descent of the anterior vaginal wall and urethra can be aggravated by vigorous activity, prolonged standing, sneezing, coughing, or straining and can be relieved by rest or by assumption of a recumbent or prone position. If the prolapse is large, women may complain of vaginal pressure.

A rectocele is the bulging of the rectum and posterior vaginal wall into the vaginal canal. Childbirth may increase damage, ultimately leading to a rectocele, but symptoms may not appear until after menopause. Genetic and familial predisposition and bowel habits contribute to rectocele development. Lifelong chronic constipation and straining may produce or aggravate a rectocele. A large rectocele may cause vaginal pressure, rectal fullness, and incomplete bowel evacuation. In severe cases, defecation may be difficult and can be facilitated by applying manual pressure to the posterior vaginal wall (see Fig. 25.11).

An enterocele is a herniation of the rectouterine pouch into the rectovaginal septum (between the rectum and the posterior vaginal wall). It can be congenital or acquired. Congenital enterocele rarely causes symptoms or progresses in size, but an acquired enterocele can result from muscular weakness caused by previous surgery, especially those through the vagina, or from pelvic relaxation disorders, such as uterine prolapse, cystocele, and rectocele. Most large enteroceles are found in grossly obese and older adults.

Treatment of POP depends on the severity of symptoms and the physical condition of the female. Treatment is often progressive with least invasive treatments tried first. Maintaining a healthy BMI, preventing constipation, and treating chronic cough or constipation will help. The pelvic floor muscles can be strengthened through Kegel exercises. Estrogen therapy may be necessary in postmenopausal women. A common first line treatment is a pessary, which is a removable device that, when placed into the vagina, holds the uterus in position. Surgical repair with or without hysterectomy is the treatment of last resort (see Box 25.8).[98] The US Food and Drug Administration (FDA) has advised the cessation of any sale of transvaginal synthetic mesh products for the repair of POP.[99]

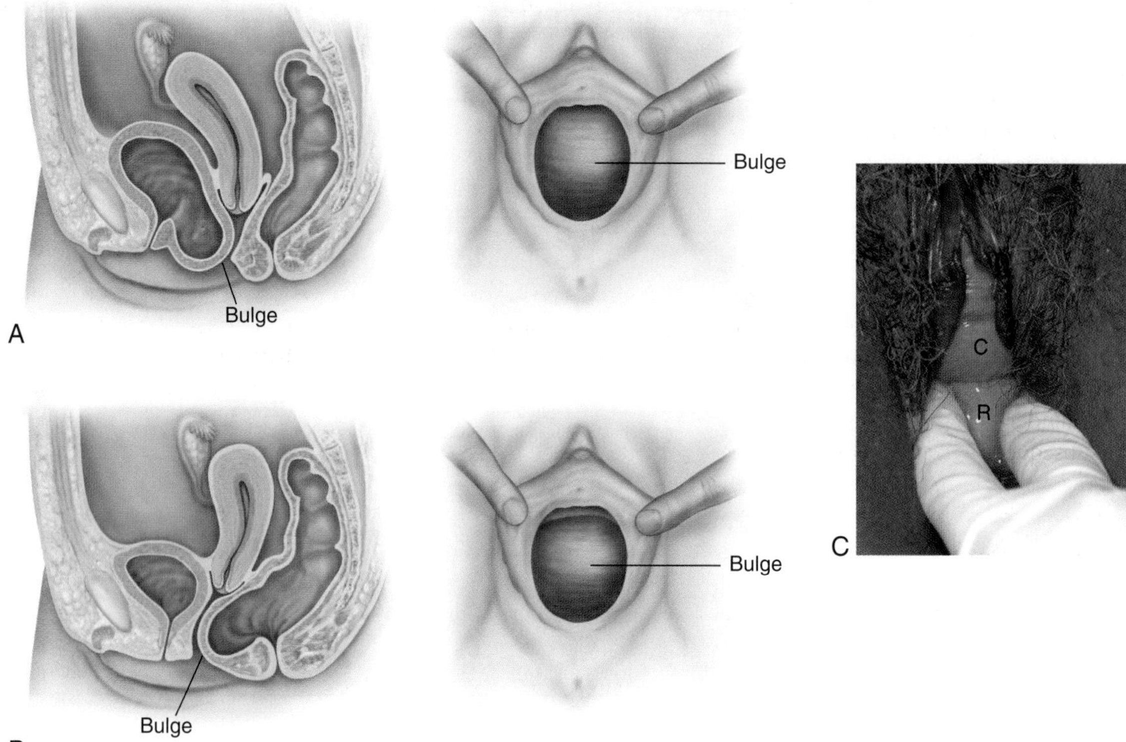

Fig. 25.11 Cystocele and Rectocele. **(A)** Grade 2: anterior vaginal wall prolapse. **(B)** Grade 2: posterior wall prolapse. **(C)** Photo slowing cystocele *(C)* and rectocele *(R)*. (A and B, From Seidel HM, et al. Mosby's guide to physical examination, 4th edition. St. Louis: Mosby; 1999; C, From Seidel HM, et al. *Mosby's guide to physical examination*, 7th edition. St. Louis: Mosby; 2011.)

Benign Growths and Proliferative Conditions

Benign Ovarian Cysts

Benign cysts of the ovary may occur at any time during the life span but are most common during the reproductive years and, in particular, at the extremes of those years (Fig. 25.12). An increase in benign ovarian cysts occurs when hormonal imbalances are more common (e.g., during puberty and menopause).[100] Benign ovarian cysts are quite common, comprising one-third of gynecologic hospital admissions. Two common causes of benign ovarian enlargement in ovulating women are follicular cysts and corpus luteum cysts. These cysts are called *functional cysts* because they are caused by variations of normal physiologic events. Follicular and corpus luteum cysts are unilateral. They are typically 5 to 6 cm in diameter but can grow as large as 8 to 10 cm. Most women are asymptomatic.

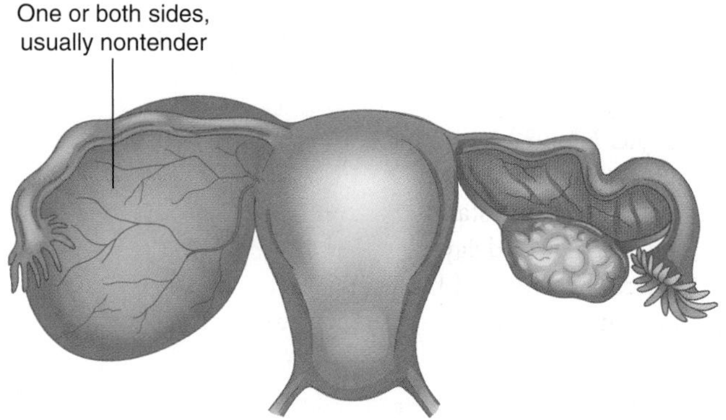

Fig. 25.12 Ovarian Cyst.

Benign cysts of the ovary are produced when a follicle or a number of follicles are stimulated but no dominant follicle develops and completes the maturation process. Every month approximately 120 follicles are stimulated, and in general, only 1 succeeds in ovulation of a mature ovum. Normally, in the early follicular phase of the menstrual cycle, follicles of the ovary respond to hormonal signals from the pituitary gland. The pituitary gland produces FSH to mature follicles in the ovary. As the follicles enlarge, granulosa cells in the follicle multiply and secrete estradiol. A dominant follicle will develop, and it secretes higher levels of estradiol, which stimulate the LH surge from the pituitary. A small cyst on the ovary during the follicular phase is normal. The LH surge stimulates the follicle to rupture, releasing the ovum and transforming the granulosa cells of the dominant follicle into the corpus luteum. If the dominant follicle develops properly before ovulation, the corpus luteum becomes vascularized and secretes progesterone. Progesterone arrests development of other follicles in both ovaries in that cycle. LH, proteolytic enzymes, and prostaglandins trigger follicular rupture and release of the ovum.

Follicular cysts are filled with fluid and can be caused by a transient condition in which the dominant follicle fails to rupture or one or more of the nondominant follicles fail to regress.

This disturbance is not well understood. It may be that the hypothalamus does not receive or send a message strong enough to increase FSH levels to the degree necessary to develop or mature a dominant follicle. The hypothalamus monitors blood levels of estradiol and progesterone; when the FSH level is low, the estradiol concentration does not increase enough to stimulate LH. Research indicates that when progesterone is not being produced, the hypothalamus releases GnRH to increase the FSH level.[101] FSH continues to stimulate follicles to mature; the granulosa cells grow, and, presumably, the estradiol level increases. This abnormal cycle continues to stimulate follicular size and causes follicular cysts to develop. Although individuals may experience no symptoms, some have pelvic pain, a sensation of feeling bloated, tender breasts, and heavy or irregular menses. After several subsequent cycles in which hormone levels once again follow a regular cycle and progesterone levels are restored, cysts usually are absorbed or regress. Follicular cysts can be random or recurrent events.

Follicular cysts can vary in size and symptoms from one episode to the next and often can recur. Most are fluid filled. The more solid an ovarian cyst, the greater the change of malignancy. Follicular cysts can be treated with combined estrogen-progestin oral contraceptives because they block the HPG axis, effectively quieting the ovary. However, progestin-only contraceptives increase the likelihood of developing follicular cysts because ovarian function is diminished but not suppressed, leading to an increased number of immature follicles.[100]

A *corpus luteum cyst* may normally form by the granulosa cells left behind after ovulation. This cyst is highly vascularized but usually limited in size, and with the normal menstrual cycle it spontaneously regresses. With an imbalance in hormones, low LH and progesterone levels may cause an abnormal or hemorrhagic cyst. In some cases, large cysts can rupture and cause hemorrhage.[102]

Corpus luteum cysts are less common than follicular cysts, but luteal cysts typically cause more symptoms, particularly if they rupture. Manifestations include dull, unilateral pelvic pain and amenorrhea or delayed menstruation, followed by irregular or heavier than normal bleeding. Rupture occasionally occurs and can cause massive bleeding, with excruciating pain; immediate surgery may be required. Corpus luteum cysts usually regress spontaneously in nonpregnant women. A persistent corpus luteum cyst is a normal finding within the first trimester of pregnancy because the corpus luteum produces progesterone to support the pregnancy until the placenta is established.[100] Following the development of a large, painful, or hemorrhagic cyst, oral contraceptives can be used to prevent cysts from forming in the future.

Dermoid cysts are ovarian teratomas that contain elements of all three germ layers; they are common ovarian neoplasms. These growths may contain mature tissue including skin, hair, sebaceous and sweat glands, muscle fibers, cartilage, and bone. Dermoid cysts are usually asymptomatic and are found incidentally on pelvic examination. Dermoid cysts have malignant potential and need careful evaluation for removal.[100]

Torsion of the ovary is a rare complication of ovarian cysts or tumors or enlargement of the ovary and can occur at any age in females. If a cyst is sufficiently large, it can cause the ovary to twist on its ligaments, pinching the blood supply to the ovary and causing extreme pain. *Ovarian torsion* is rare, but it is a gynecologic emergency. It usually presents with acute, severe, unilateral abdominal or pelvic pain and is treated surgically.[103]

Endometrial Polyps

An endometrial polyp is a benign mass of endometrial tissue that contains a variable number of glands, stroma, and blood vessels. Endometrial polyps are usually solitary and can occur anywhere within the uterus. Polyps are structurally diverse and are usually classified as hyperplastic, atrophic (or inactive), or functional. Hyperplastic polyps are often pedunculated (stalk- or mushroom-like) and may be mistaken for endometrial hyperplasia or, if large, for adenosarcoma (Fig. 25.13). Although polyps most often develop in women between the ages of 40 and 50 years, they can occur at all ages. Risk factors include advancing age, obesity, nulliparity, early menarche or late menopause (or both), diabetes, estrogenic states (i.e., anovulatory cycles and unopposed estrogen), treatment with tamoxifen, and hypertension. The coexistence of a separate endometrial atypical hyperplasia (AH) or adenocarcinoma is possible, but malignancy is extremely rare.

Endometrial polyps are a common cause of intermenstrual bleeding or even excessive menstrual bleeding and suboptimal fertility. Polyps resulting in abnormal bleeding have twice the rate of malignancy of asymptomatic polyps. The diagnosis is made by transvaginal sonography or hysteroscopy. The lesions can be removed with small, curved forceps, but there is a high rate of spontaneous resolution. Polypectomy can be performed through hysteroscopy for symptomatic women, for those at risk for malignancy, or for women who are struggling to conceive.[104]

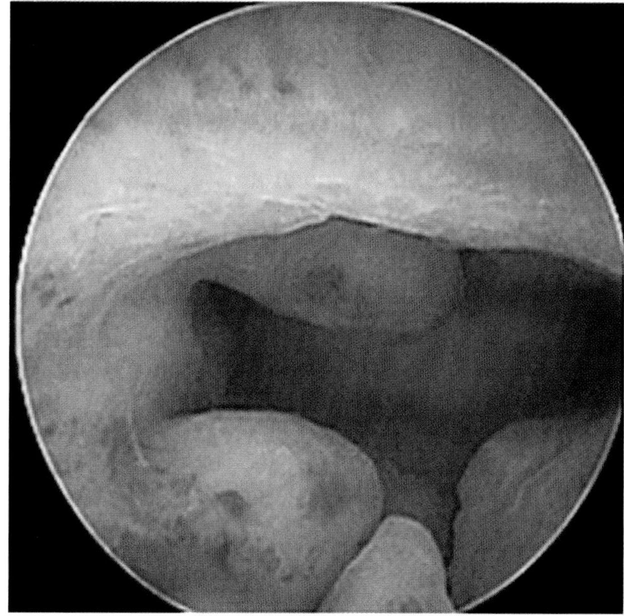

Fig. 25.13 Uterine Polyps Visible Through Hysteroscopy. (From Cheng C, Zhao T, Xue M, Wan Y, Xu D. Use of suction curettage in operative hysteroscopy. *Journal of Minimally Invasive Gynecology*, 2009;16(6):739–342.)

Leiomyomas

Leiomyomas, commonly called myomas or uterine fibroids, are benign tumors that develop from smooth muscle cells in the myometrium (Fig. 25.14). Leiomyomas are the most common benign tumors of the uterus, affecting 70% to 80% of all females, and most remain small and asymptomatic. The prevalence increases in females ages 30 to 50 years but decreases with menopause. The incidence of leiomyomas in Black and Asian females is two to five times higher than that in White females. On average, the age of onset for Black females is 10 years earlier than it is for White females.[105]

The cause of uterine leiomyomas is unknown, although their size appears to be related to estrogen and progesterone, growth factors, angiogenesis, and apoptosis. An increase in familial aggregation may indicate genetic factors as important, and leiomyomas exhibit nonrandom chromosomal abnormalities.[106] Because leiomyomas are estrogen and progesterone sensitive, uterine leiomyomas are not seen before menarche, are common during the reproductive years, and generally shrink after menopause. Tumors in pregnant females enlarge rapidly but often decrease in size after the end of the pregnancy. Risk factors include Black race, age, family history, nulliparity, time since last birth, obesity, postmenopausal hormone use, and hypertension. Lifestyle risk factors include diet, food additive consumption, soybean milk consumption, caffeine and alcohol consumption, smoking, lack of physical activity, and stress.[105,106] Conversely, the use of oral contraceptives or the injectable contraceptive depot medroxyprogesterone acetate, smoking, low BMI, and parity reduce fibroid risk.[105]

Pathophysiology. The formation and growth of uterine leiomyomas is not well understood; however, genetics, environmental factors, steroid hormones (estrogen and progesterone), and angiogenesis all play a role.[107] Fibroid development begins with a single uterine smooth muscle cell (myometrium). Leiomyomas are benign monoclonal neoplasms that occur as a single fibroid or multiples throughout the uterus. Leiomyomas are classified as subserous, submucous, or intramural, according to their location within the various layers of the uterine wall (see Fig. 25.14). Mutations in the mediator subcomplex 12 *(MED12)* gene have been identified in approximately 70% of uterine leiomyomas.[108] Degeneration and necrosis may occur when the leiomyoma outgrows its blood supply, which is more common in larger tumors and is frequently accompanied by pain.

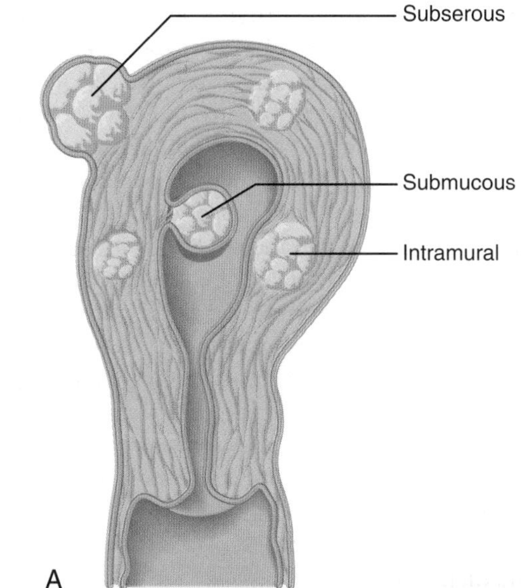

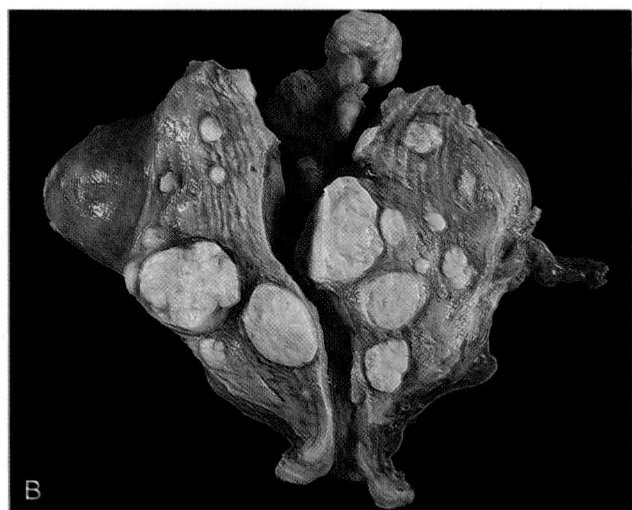

Fig. 25.14 Leiomyomas. **(A)** Uterine section showing the whorl-like appearance and locations of leiomyomas (also called *uterine fibroids*). **(B)** Sagittal section showing multiple leiomyomas. Typical, well-circumscribed, solid, light gray nodules distort the uterus. (B, From Damjanov I, Linder J. Pathology: *A color atlas*. St. Louis: Mosby; 2000.)

Clinical Manifestations. The major clinical manifestations of leiomyomas are abnormal vaginal bleeding, pain, and symptoms related to pressure on nearby structures. Fibroids also may contribute to infertility and subfertility, as well as obstruction during birth if the fibroids are large enough. The leiomyoma can make the uterine cavity larger, thereby increasing the endometrial surface area. This enlargement may account for the increased menstrual bleeding associated with leiomyomas. Although pain is not an early symptom, it occurs with the devascularization of larger leiomyomas and is associated with blood vessel compression that limits the blood supply to adjacent structures. Because the fibroid is relatively slow growing, enabling adjacent structures to adapt to pressure, symptoms of abdominal pressure develop slowly. Pressure on the bladder may contribute to urinary frequency, urgency, and dysuria. Pressure on the ureter may cause it to become distended "upstream" from the pressure point. Ectosigmoid pressure may lead to constipation. Larger fibroids may cause a sensation of abdominal or genital heaviness.

Evaluation and Treatment. Uterine leiomyomas are suspected when bimanual examination discloses irregular, nontender nodularity of the uterus. Transvaginal ultrasound is the gold standard for imaging and confirming the diagnosis, but current recommendations do not require serial imaging.[109] Treatment depends on the symptoms, tumor size, individual's age, reproductive status, preference, and overall health. Most leiomyomas are asymptomatic, with surveillance being the preferred management.

Hormonal contraceptives, GnRH agonist (Leuprolide), and NSAIDs are used in the medical management to decrease the severity of bleeding, relieve pain, and shrink the myoma. A progestin-only IUD may be helpful for women who wish to reduce their bleeding and decrease the size of the tumors if their uterine cavity is not completely blocked by large fibroids. GnRH agonists are usually a temporary management for those close to menopause or as a presurgical treatment. Side effects are similar to those of decreased levels of estrogen and include hot flashes and osteoporosis. Various selective estrogen receptor modulators have been studied alone and in conjunction with GnRh agonists and appear effective, although more research is needed, especially because these agents may decrease bone density.[110] Nonpharmalogic therapies include green tea extract, curcumin (the active ingredient in turmeric), vitamin D, and herbal preparations used in Chinese medicines.[111] Prevention of fibroids involves lifestyle factors and includes exercise, reducing obesity, and diet.[105]

Surgical treatments may include endometrial ablation, uterine artery embolization (UAE), myomectomy, MRI-guided focused ultrasound surgery, and hysterectomy. The most commonly performed procedure for fibroid-related bleeding and pain is a hysterectomy. Endometrial ablation is an alternative to surgery in those with heavy or abnormal bleeding. However, with submucosal fibroids, there is a larger risk of a failed procedure because the fibroids cause disruption of the uterine cavity, which can prevent proper cauterization.[109] UAE is a minimally invasive procedure for those who want to preserve fertility. The procedure is effective to control bleeding; however, there are limited studies to show preservation of fertility.[109,112] Myomectomy is an invasive option for those who want to preserve fertility and avoid hysterectomy. The outcome is highly dependent on the location and size of the fibroid, and there is no large randomized trial showing that it can improve fertility.[109] MRI-guided focused ultrasound surgery uses MRI and ultrasound to focus the fibroid and then cauterize. It is a new treatment that needs clinical evidence to support long-term effectiveness.[109] Benefits and risks of all treatments should be carefully considered, as should the desire for future pregnancy.

Adenomyosis

Adenomyosis is the presence of endometrial tissue within the uterine myometrium. Migration of endometrial cells into the myometrial layers occurs as a result of an unknown mechanism. Estrogen and progesterone likely play a role and, perhaps, metaplasia of müllerian tissue. Unlike endometriosis, the tissue does not respond to cyclic hormone changes.[113] Diagnosis of adenomyosis often is made during the late reproductive years; however, because it is commonly diagnosed after hysterectomy, the time of diagnosis may not be associated with the onset. Risk factors include conditions leading to increased estrogen exposure (increased parity, early menarche, short menstrual cycles, elevated BMI, oral contraceptive pill (OCP) use, tamoxifen use) and prior uterine surgery (e.g., dilation and curettage, cesarean section, myomectomy).[114,115]

Pathophysiology. Adenomyosis is the presence of endometrial stroma and glandular tissue within the smooth muscle of the myometrium. Endometrial proliferation, driven by estrogen, leads to the symptoms from different mechanisms. Adenomyosis leads to increased prostaglandins and results in dysmenorrhea. Heavy menstrual bleeding involves increased vascularization, abnormal uterine contractions, and increased cell-signaling molecules, such as prostaglandins, eicosanoids, and estrogen.[114,115]

Clinical Manifestations. Adenomyosis may be asymptomatic or may be associated with abnormal menstrual bleeding, anemia, dysmenorrhea, uterine enlargement, uterine tenderness during menstruation, chronic pelvic pain, dyspareunia, and infertility. Secondary dysmenorrhea becomes increasingly severe as the disease progresses.[114]

Evaluation and Treatment. On bimanual exam, the uterus is enlarged (two to three times the expected size), globular, and most tender just before or after menstruation. The enlarged uterus is often referred to as "boggy."[115] The diagnosis is confirmed by two-dimensional (2D) and three-dimensional (3D) ultrasonography as well as MRI.[116]

Treatment decisions are based on managing symptoms and preserving future fertility. Medical management includes NSAIDs for pain, hormonal contraceptives (e.g., levonorgestrel IUD) to reduce the estrogenic effects, androgenic hormones (e.g., danazol) to shrink the displaced tissue, and aromatase inhibitors (e.g., Arimidex).[115] Surgical options include endometrial ablation, hysteroscopic endometrial and adenomyoma resection, laparoscopic resection of adenoma, high-intensity focused ultrasonography (HIFU), and UAE.[117] Treatment decisions are based on managing symptoms and preserving future fertility.

Endometriosis

Endometriosis is the presence of functioning endometrial tissue or implants outside the uterus. The definition is limited because the disorder is complex and heterogenous involving pathobiologic, symptomatic, and multisystemic changes.[118] The ectopic (out of place) endometrium responds to the normal hormonal fluctuations of the menstrual cycle. Common sites of implantation of ectopic tissue include the ovaries, uterine ligaments (mostly broad and uterosacral), pouch of Douglas, and fallopian tubes.[119,120] Endometriotic implants are found outside of pelvic locations and include the gastrointestinal tract, lungs, diaphragm, abdomen, and pericardium.[121] Endometriosis primarily affects younger (premenopausal) women, with a peak incidence in the third decade. However, the incidence of endometriosis is difficult to determine, especially in asymptomatic adolescent and fertile women.[118,122,123] Endometriosis is the most common cause of chronic pelvic pain in women. It is the third most common reason for hysterectomy and is associated with a higher risk for infertility and cancers, especially ovarian cancer.[124]

The cause of endometriosis is multifaceted. In 1927, researchers found that endometriosis was linked to the implantation of endometrial cells during retrograde menstruation, in which menstrual fluids move through the fallopian tubes and into the pelvic cavity.[125] Women with obstructed menstrual flow do have a higher incidence of endometriosis. However, it is now known that retrograde menstruation occurs in almost all women but not all women develop endometriosis. Intracaitary endometriaum and extrauterine endometriotic tissue are composed of mesenchymal progenitor/stem cells with alternate programming. GATA-binding factor-6 overexpression transforms endometrial stromal cells, and steroidogenic factor-1 overexpression causes excessive production of estrogen. This excess estrogen drives the inflammation especially in the presence of pathologically high levels of estrogen receptor-B. Progesterone receptor (PR) deficiency causes progesterone resistance. A genetic predisposition to endometriosis has been documented, and genetic polymorphisms have been identified. These altered cells have been found to harbor multiple cancer-causing mutations, such as KRAS, which has been associated with ovarian cancer.[124]

Pathophysiology. Endometrial implants can occur throughout the body but generally occur in the pelvic and abdominal cavities. The most common sites of implantation are the ovaries, uterine ligaments, rectovaginal septum, and the pelvic peritoneum (Fig. 25.15). Other sites of implantation are the sigmoid colon, small intestine, rectum, appendix, bladder, uterus, vulva, vagina, cervix, lymph nodes, extremities, pleural cavity, lungs, laparotomy scars, and hernial sacs.

The growth of endometrial lesions depends on estrogen. Endometrial lesions are affected by various ovarian hormones. Endometrial remodeling is a cyclical process during which time the endometrium responds to estrogenic stimulation in a uniformed manner. Endometrial hyperplasia results from continuous estrogen stimulation that is unopposed by progesterone. The cyclic changes are influenced by blood supply and the presence of glandular and stromal cells. With an adequate blood supply, the ectopic endometrium proliferates, breaks down, and bleeds with the normal menstrual cycle. The proliferative response is regulated by progestogenic effects. The bleeding causes inflammation, triggering a cascade of cellular inflammatory mediators, including cytokines, chemokines, growth factors, and protective factors (leukocyte protease inhibitor and superoxide dismutase). Eventually, the inflammation leads to fibrosis, scarring, adhesions, and pain.

Infertility is common in women with endometriosis. The exact mechanism is unknown but may result from mechanical interference with ovulation or ovum transport through the fallopian tube because of adhesions and the effects of inflammation and cytokine activity. However, the infertility also could be a result of the underlying autoimmune disorder that caused the endometriosis in the first place. The overactive response to estrogen and the underactive response to progesterone seem to impair the endometrial receptivity to blastocyst implantation, which decreases the chance of successful pregnancy. Women with endometriosis who achieve pregnancy naturally or through in vitro fertilization (IVF) also seem to be at higher risk for poor obstetric outcomes, including preterm birth, small-for-gestational-age newborns, and placental complications.[126]

Clinical Manifestations. The clinical manifestations of endometriosis vary in frequency and severity and can mimic other pelvic diseases (e.g., PID, ovarian cysts, and irritable bowel syndrome). Heterogeneity of symptoms is high. Individuals may be asymptomatic or present with symptoms, which include infertility, pelvic pain, dyschezia (pain on defecation), dyspareunia, and, less commonly, constipation and abnormal vaginal bleeding. If implants are located within the pelvis, an asymptomatic pelvic mass having irregular, movable nodules and a fixed, retroverted uterus are found on examination. Most symptoms can be explained by the proliferation, breakdown, and bleeding of the ectopic endometrial tissue, with subsequent formation of adhesions. However, in most instances, the degree of endometriosis is not related to the frequency or severity of symptoms. For example, dysmenorrhea does not appear to be related to the degree of endometriosis. With involvement of the rectovaginal septum or the uterosacral ligaments, dyspareunia develops. Dyschezia, a hallmark symptom of endometriosis, occurs with bleeding of ectopic endometrium in the rectosigmoid musculature and subsequent fibrosis. Approximately 25% to 40% of women with infertility have endometriosis. The relationship between endometriosis and infertility is strong; however, the *degree* of disease is not as closely associated. More simply, women with untreated minimal to mild disease may have high pregnancy rates or may experience infertility.

Evaluation and Treatment. A presumptive diagnosis is based on the previously described symptoms, but pelvic laparoscopic visualization (ideally, with histologic verification) is the standard for diagnosis.[118] Less invasive testing includes imaging, genetic tests, biomarkers, or micro ribonucleic acid (miRNA), but further research is required before they can be recommended in routine clinical care. Ovarian endometrioma and deep nodular forms of disease can be detected through ultrasound and MRI.[127–129] Different classification systems have been introduced to categorize endometriosis. Some focus more on surgical findings and other with symptoms. It appears that the major drawback of all existing classification systems is that not one of them links the severity of the pain with the disease findings. As of now, no single global classification system exists.[130,131]

Treatment is based on preventing progression of the disease, alleviating pain, and restoring fertility. A multidisciplinary team approach using medical therapies that suppress systemic or local estrogen, decrease tissue proliferation, and reduce inflammation are the most common modalities. The combination of estrogen and progesterone or progestin-only oral birth control pills is a first line, widely used approach for dysmenorrhea or chronic pelvic pain, with or without presumed endometriosis.[132] GnRH agonists (i.e., leuprolide acetate, goserelin acetate, and nafarelin acetate) are a second line treatment to suppress systemic estrogen levels. Other treatment may include GnRH antagonists (e.g., Elagolix), which decrease hormones and reduce endometriosis-associated pelvic pain.[133] Aromatase inhibitors are used as off-label treatment for women resistant to hormone therapy (HT). However, long-term use is restricted because of bone-density loss, vasomotor side effects (flushing and hot flashes), and increased multiple-pregnancy rates.[118] Overall, hormonal treatments are contraindicated for women with endometriosis who wish to conceive.[118] Endometriosis-associated pain is treated with

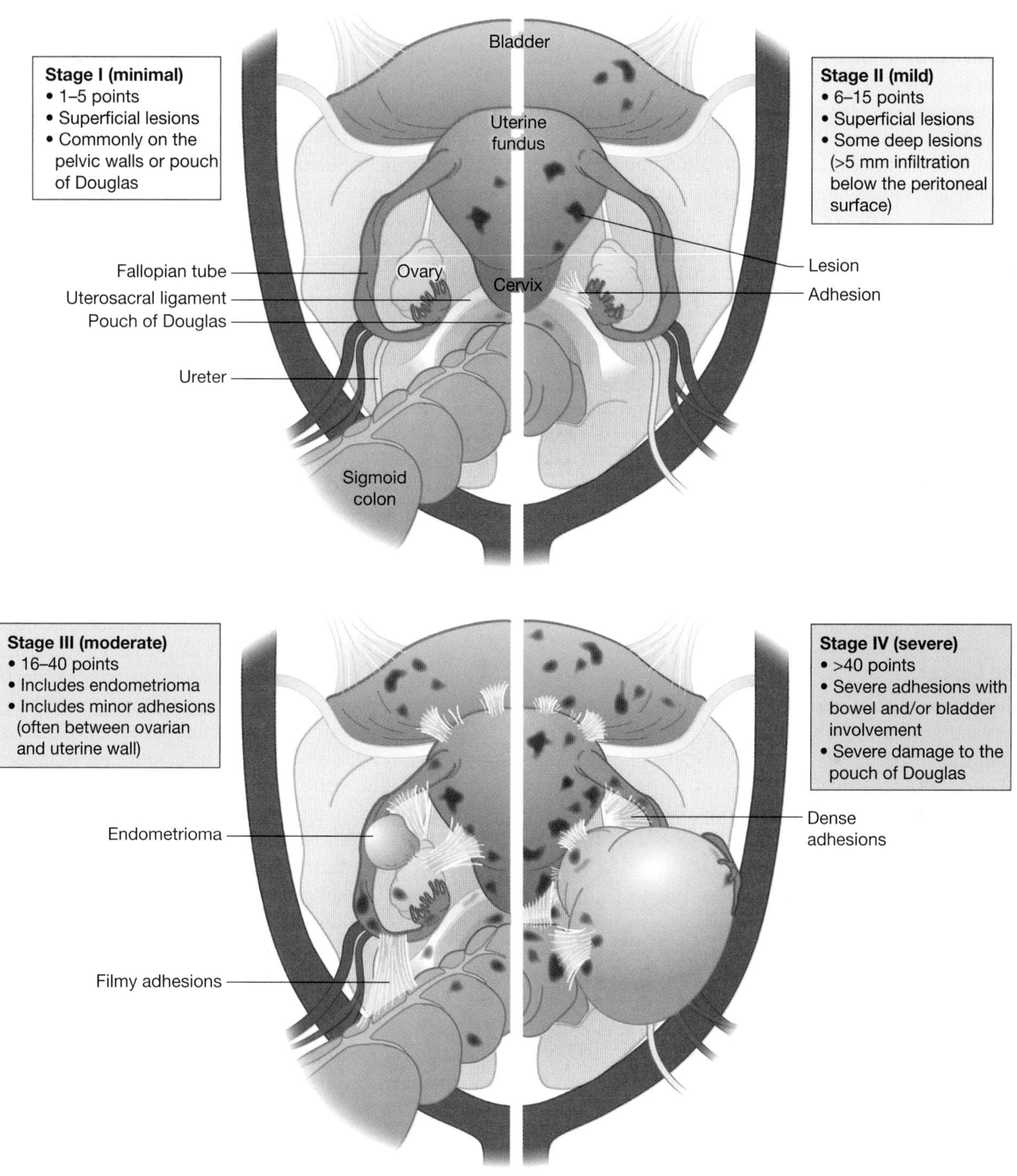

Fig. 25.15 Staging of Endometriosis. The revised American Fertility Society and American Society of Reproductive Medicine staging system of endometriosis is a points system based on location, extent, and depth of disease in relation to pelvic structures. The uterus, fallopian tubes, ovaries, ovarian fossae (the shallow depression on the lateral wall of the pelvis where the ovary lies), uterosacral ligaments, rectovaginal septum, and pouch of Douglas (portion of the peritoneal cavity between the rectum and the posterior wall of the peritoneum between the uterus and bladder) are often affected. The stages are shown as stage I, stage II, stage III, and stage IV. Critical is the severity of the disease according to this system and does not correlate with the severity and location of symptoms. For example, women with stage I (mild) disease may experience severe pain and/or infertility, whereas women with stage IV (severe) may be asymptomatic. (Adapted from Zondervan KT, Becker CM, Koga K, Missmer SA, Taylor RN, Viganò P. Endometriosis. *Nature Reviews Disease Primers*, 2018;4:9. Available at https://doi.org/10.1038/s41572-018-0008-5.)

analgesics, acetaminophen, and NSAIDs. Complementary therapies may include pelvic physical therapy and cognitive therapy. In women with hormone-resistant pain, surgical treatment is considered.[118] Conservative surgical treatment includes laparoscopic removal of endometrial implants with conventional or laser techniques. Endometriosis-associated pain is the leading indication for hysterectomy in females 30 to 34 years of age and accounts for 18% of all hysterectomies.[134] All treatments have risks or side effects, and recurrent symptoms develop in most females within a few years, even with surgical treatments. Females should be fully informed of all options and understand the risk-to-benefit ratio of treatments, especially nonreversible treatments.[135]

Cancer

Malignant tumors of the female reproductive system are common. Because the pelvis and abdomen are poorly innervated and designed to accommodate a growing fetus, cancers of the female reproductive tract can often grow large before causing pain. Reproductive cancers are likely to be diagnosed early if there are symptoms; for example, vaginal bleeding prompts the individual to seek treatment. Clear screening guidelines and techniques have proven beneficial in early detection and intervention, resulting in lower mortality.[1]

Cervical Cancer

Each year more than a half a million women are diagnosed with cervical cancer.[136] Globally, cervical cancer is the fourth most common cancer among women, causing more than 300,000 deaths worldwide.[137,138] Cervical cancer incidence rates declined by more than half between 1975 (14.8 per 100,000) and 2014 (6.9 per 100,000). The decline is attributed to the widespread use of screening, primarily with the Pap test, immunization efforts, and hand-held technology accessibility.[139] Estimated new cases for 2021 in the United States are 14,480, with 4290 deaths.[140] High-risk subtypes of HPV are the main cause of cervical cancer. HPV screening and vaccination programs are effective methods in disease prevention.[136] Box 25.9 summarizes the major risk factors for cervical cancer.

BOX 25.9 Risk Factors for Cervical Cancer

Chronic infection by high-risk oncogenic types of human papillomavirus (HPV).

Risk factors are those associated with acquiring HPV and impaired immune response to HPV, or both.

Risk Factors include:

Early age of sexual intercourse
Multiple sexual partners or a high-risk partner
Immunosuppression (e.g., organ transplantation, immunodeficiency disorders [HIV])
History of sexually transmitted infection
History of HPV-related vulvar or vaginal dysplasia
Lack of screening and underscreening
Tobacco smoke and cessation of smoking reduced risk by twofold

Data adapted from Cohen PA, Jhingran A, Oaknin A, Denny L. Cervical cancer. *The Lancet*, 2019;393:169–182.

Pathophysiology. Human papillomavirus (HPV) is a necessary condition in the development of almost all precancerous and cancerous cervical lesions. HPVs are DNA viruses grouped into high and low risk based on their genotypes. There are 15 high-risk HPVs currently identified. HPV-16 accounts for approximately 60% of cervical cancer cases, HPV-18 accounts for another 10%, and the other HPV types account for less than 5%.[141] Genital HPV infections are very common, and it is estimated that most sexually active women will contract HPV at some point in their lifetime. Most of these infections are asymptomatic, do not cause tissue changes detected on the Pap test, and resolve spontaneously. However, high-risk HPV may persist, increasing the risk of developing cervical precursor lesions (cervical intraepithelial neoplasia [CIN]) and eventual carcinoma (Fig. 25.16). It is unknown as to why some females are able to clear HPV infection and others cannot. Women with multiple sexual partners, a male partner with multiple previous or current sexual partners, young age at first sexual intercourse, high parity, immunosuppression, a long history of the use of oral contraceptives, certain human leukocytic antigen (HLA) subtypes, and use of nicotine are more likely to be infected.

The cervix is lined by two types of epithelial cells: squamous cells at the outer aspect and columnar glandular cells along the inner canal. The site of the cellular transformation zone, called the *squamocolumnar junction*, is illustrated in Fig. 25.17. The transformation zone is most susceptible to the oncogenic effects of HPV. Squamous cervical cancer accounts for most cervical precursor lesions and cancer and originates in the transformation zone or the glandular epithelium above the transformation zone.[141,142] In this zone, columnar epithelium is constantly being replaced by squamous epithelium in a process known as metaplasia (see Chapter 2). Metaplasia may be affected by hormonal levels. Because metaplastic cells are at increased risk of incorporating foreign or abnormal genetic material, neoplastic changes are most common in the transformation zone.

Young females are especially vulnerable to HPV because of their cervical anatomy. Squamous epithelial cells in older females cover the portions of the cervix that protrude into the vagina, and columnar epithelial cells line the inner portions of the cervical canal. The location of the transformation zone changes as females age and in response to estrogen and vaginal pH changes. In adolescent and mature females, a large portion of their cervix is covered with columnar epithelium, a condition known as squamous metaplasia. Hence the younger a female is when she contacts HPV, the more sensitive cervical cells are exposed. This is one reason vaccinations against HPV are aimed at individuals before the initiation of sexual activity.

Many chromosomes may contain genes that relate to HPV-linked cervical cancer. Like other cancers, cervical cancer requires the accumulation of genetic alterations for carcinogenesis to occur. Several genetic mutations have been identified, including some that have not been seen in other cancers. Several chromosome regions with recurrent loss of heterozygosity (LOH) have been identified. In addition, other genes may influence a female's receptivity to HPV. HPV may upregulate the

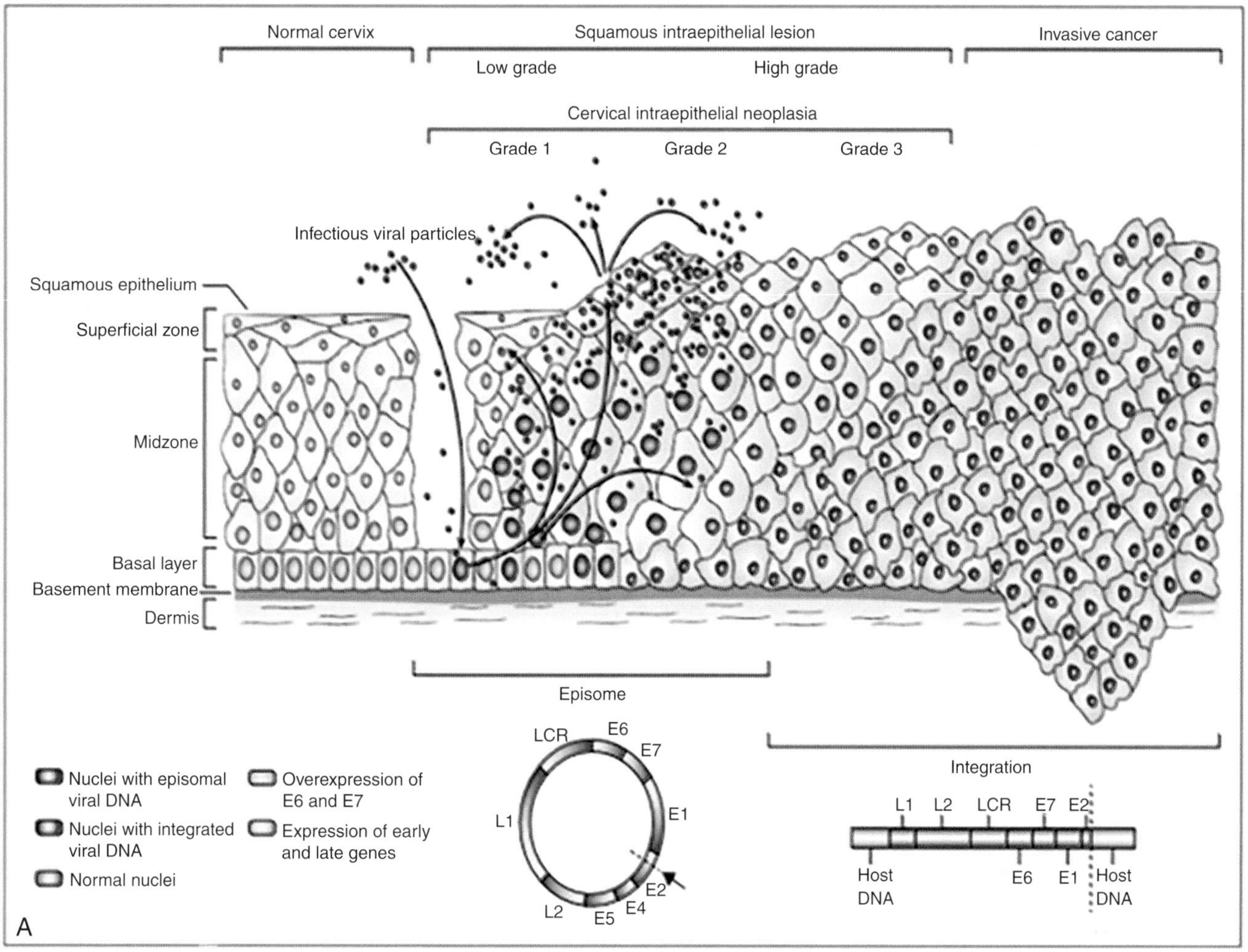

Normal cervix
Squamous intraepithelial lesion
Invasive cancer
Low grade
High grade
Cervical intraepithelial neoplasia
Grade 1
Grade 2
Grade 3
Infectious viral particles
Squamous epithelium
Superficial zone
Midzone
Basal layer
Basement membrane
Dermis
Episome
LCR
E6
E7
E1
L1
E2
E4
E5
L2
Integration
L1 L2 LCR E7 E2
Host DNA
E6 E1
Host DNA
Nuclei with episomal viral DNA
Nuclei with integrated viral DNA
Normal nuclei
Overexpression of E6 and E7
Expression of early and late genes
A

Mature squamous cells
Immature squamous cells
Squamocolumnar junction
Columnar glandular cells
B

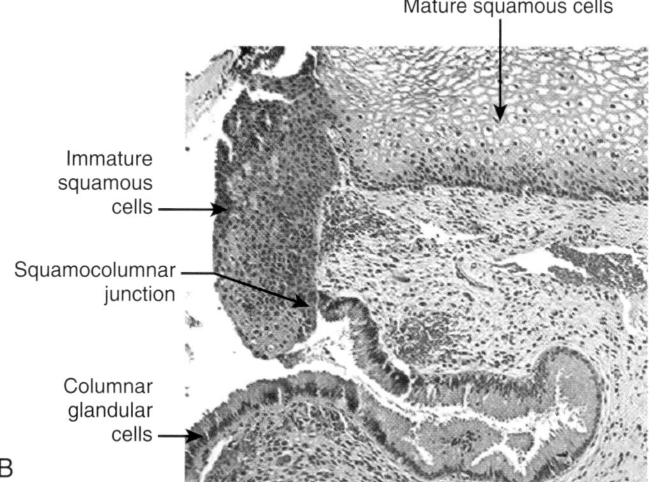

Fig. 25.16 Pathogenesis of Cervical Cancer. **(A)** Normal cervix and progression of cervical intraepithelial neoplasia (CIN) to invasive cervical cancer from persistent human papillomavirus (HPV) infection. The ability of HPV to act as a carcinogen depends on viral E6 and E7 proteins. These proteins interfere with the activity of key tumor suppressor proteins, p53 and RB, respectively. The overall effect of E6 and E7 proteins is increased proliferation of host cells now prone to acquire additional mutations and lead to carcinogenesis. **(B)** Normal epithelium, then HPV infection progressing to CIN stage I. With more time, persistent HPV infections progress to precancerous lesions CIN II and CIN III and eventually to cervical cancer. Most cervical lesions do not progress to cervical cancer. (A, Reprinted with permission from Elsevier. From Crosbie EJ, et al: *Lancet* 2013;382:889-899 with permission in Cohen PA, et al: *Lancet* 2019;393:169-82; B, From Symonds EM, Macpherson MBA. *Color atlas of obstetrics and gynecology*. London: Mosby; 1994.)

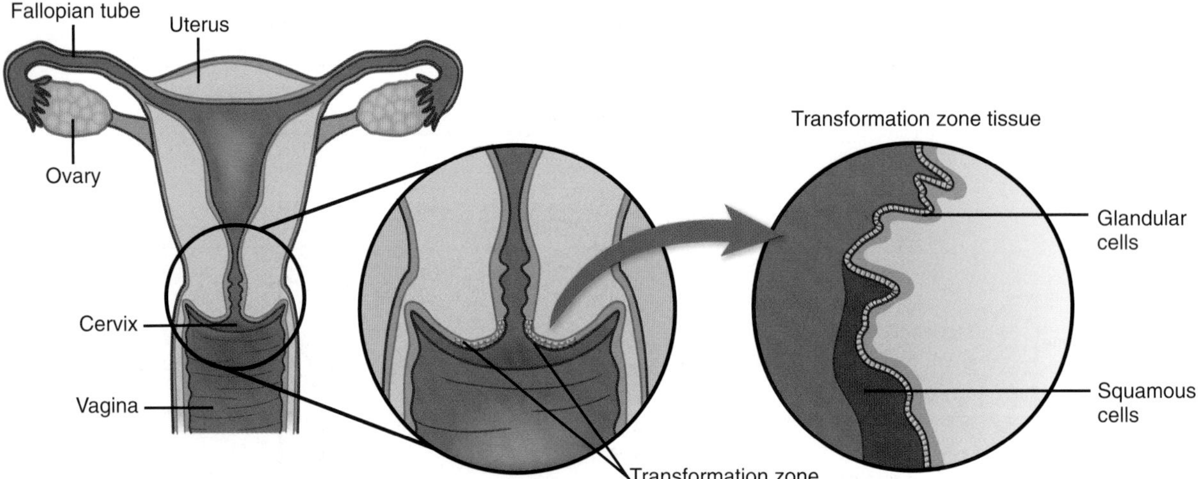

Fig. 25.17 Cervical Squamocolumnar Junction. Showing a transition from mature, glycogenized squamous epithelium, immature squamous metaplastic cells, and columnar endocervical glandular epithelium. The two types of epithelial cells lining the cervix: squamous cells and columnar glandular cells. (From Kumar V, Abbas AK, Aster JC, Cotran RS, Robbins SL. Robbins & Cotran pathologic basis of disease, 10th edition. Philadelphia: Elsevier; 2021.)

E6 and E7 oncoproteins in certain gene sequences, causing a greater production of vascular epidermal growth factor, which allows the tumor to promote blood vessel growth toward the proliferating cells, fueling growth (see Fig. 25.16A). These viral proteins impair the ability to repair DNA damage or to regulate telomerase, which leads to cellular immortalization. Overall, these alterations promote increased proliferation of cells prone to acquire more mutations that can lead to carcinogenesis.[143]

Clinical Manifestations. Cervical cancer in the early stages is often asymptomatic. Symptoms in advancing cervical cancer may include postcoital or abnormal vaginal bleeding or discharge.[144] Vaginal discharge is a less common presenting symptom and may be serosanguineous or yellowish in color with a foul odor. Bleeding and discharge are subtle and are likely to be disregarded by premenopausal females. Postmenopausal females are more likely to seek medical attention if these signs appear. Advanced disease may cause urinary (e.g., passage of urine through the vagina) or rectal (e.g., feces through the vagina) symptoms and pelvic or back pain along with anemia.

Evaluation and Treatment. Females should be screened for cervical cancer and their risk for future cervical cancer through Pap and HPV testing.

A Pap test involves the noninvasive collection of cellular samples from the surface of the cervix during a pelvic examination. Cervical cytologic examination is most accurate if cells are obtained from both the endocervix and the ectocervix (the transformation zone), which involves placing the collection device into the cervical os. Diagnosis is based on histopathologic assessment of a cervical biopsy. A colposcopy with biopsy is performed in symptomatic women with cytology suggestive of invasion without visible lesions.[136] A cone biopsy is necessary if cancer is suspected either clinically or on cervical cytology but is not confirmed on histopathologic review of cervical biopsies (Fig. 25.18).[136] If invasive carcinoma is found, lymphangiography, CT scan, MRI, ultrasonography, or radioimmunodetection methods are used for staging according to the FIGO guidelines, but it is not necessary to use all modalities on every individual.[136] The FIGO staging system was revised in 2018 and now includes lymph node status, similar to the system used by the American Joint Committee on Cancer (Table 25.3).[136,145]

Treatment depends on the degree of neoplastic change, stage of tumor, location of the lesion, and the extent of metastatic spread. Treatment includes surgery (hysterectomy), radiation therapy, chemotherapy, and targeted treatment. The prognosis is excellent with early detection and treatment.

The prevention of HPV infection through HPV vaccines is the key to substantially reducing the risk of cervical cancer. HPV also can cause anal cancer and mouth/throat (oropharyngeal) cancer, as well as cancer of the vulva, vagina, and penis. HPV vaccination is recommended for preteen individuals at age 11 or 12 through the age of 26. HPV vaccine recommendations are outlined in Table 25.4 and in Chapter 27, Box 27.5.[146]

Vaginal Cancer

Primary cancer of the vagina is the rarest of the female genital cancers, accounting for 1% to 2% of all female reproductive cancers.[147] It is rare because most of these lesions (80% to 90%) represent metastases from another primary site.[148] The metastases come from other reproductive organs such as the cervix, endometrium, or ovary but also can come from distant sites such as the colon, breast, and pancreas.[148]

Pathophysiology. Vaginal cancer is a heterogenous disease. Estimated new cases in the United States for 2021 are 8180 and estimated deaths 1530.[140] Vaginal and cervical cancers are thought to have a similar epidemiology. They both start as intraepithelial lesions, occur in females who have been sexually

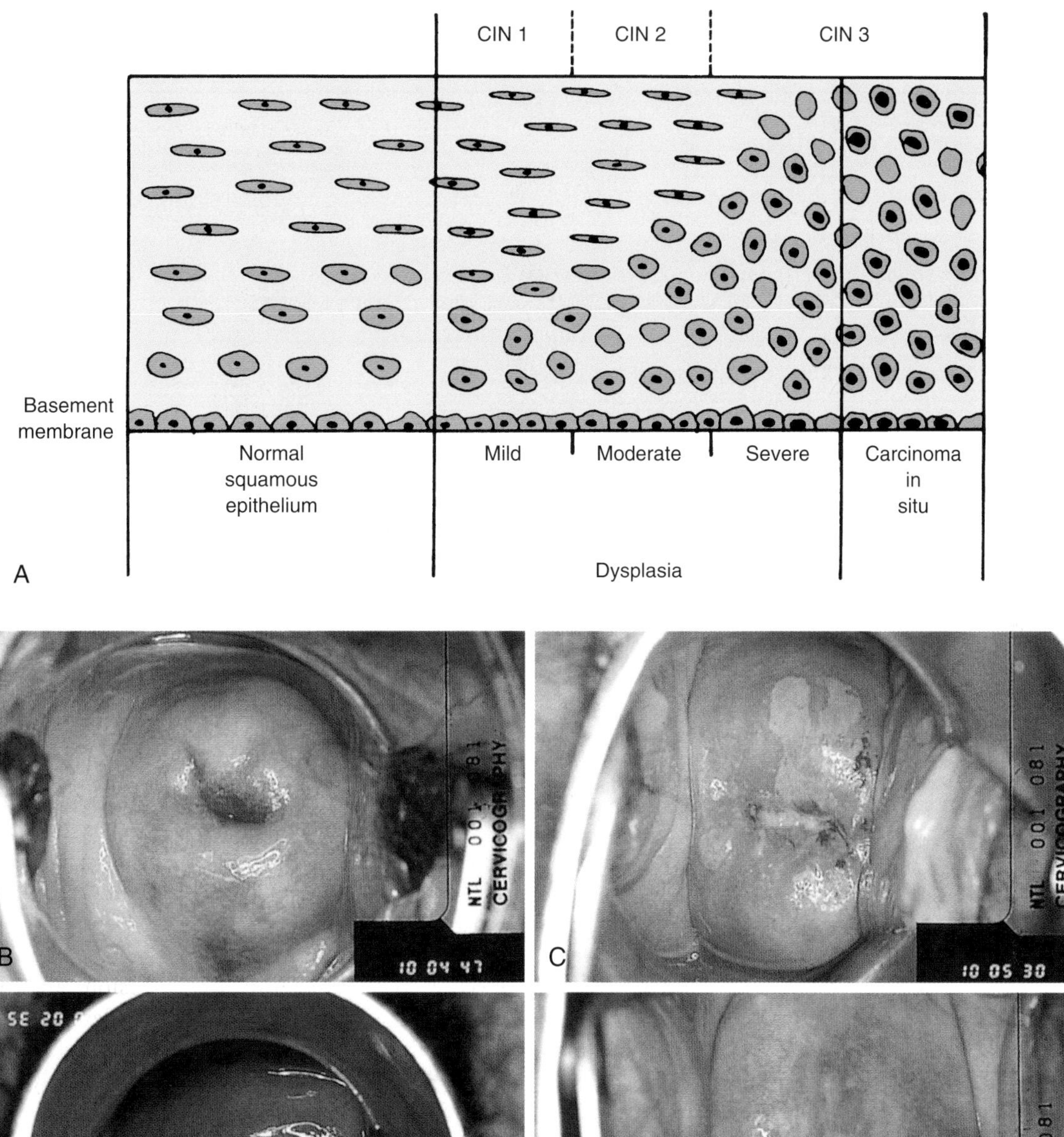

Fig. 25.18 Cervical Intraepithelial Neoplasia. **(A)** Diagram of cervical endothelium showing progressive degrees of cervical intraepithelial neoplasia *(CIN).* **(B)** Normal multiparous cervix. **(C)** CIN stage 1. Note the white appearance of part of the anterior lip of the cervix associated with neoplastic changes. **(D)** CIN stage 2. Lesions reflected in distant capillaries. **(E)** CIN stage 3. Lesion predominantly around the external os. (A, From Herbst AL, et al. *Comprehensive gynecology,* 2nd edition. St. Louis: Mosby; 1992. B–E, From Symonds EM, Macpherson MBA. *Color atlas of obstetrics and gynecology.* London: Mosby-Wolfe; 1994.)

active, and are associated with HPV infection. Although HPV is an established carcinogen for vaginal cancer, not all vaginal cancers are caused by HPV.[149] Like cervical cancer, the high-risk subtypes of HPV are responsible for cancers of the head and neck and vulva or vagina. As with cervical cancer, the HPV-16 subtype accounts for most of the HPV-positive females for both cancers.[150] Other risk factors include increasing age, smoking, previous cervical cancer, exposure to DES, history of radiotherapy, or hysterectomy.[147,151,152]

More than 90% of women with vaginal cancer have squamous cell carcinoma. The remaining 10% are adenocarcinomas, sarcomas (rare), and melanomas (rare). Nonsquamous types of cancer

TABLE 25.3 Staging of Cervical Tumors Staging of Cancer

	TNM	FIGO
Primary tumor cannot be assessed	TX	..
No evidence of primary tumor	T0	..
Carcinoma in situ (preinvasive)	Tis	..
Cervical carcinoma confined to the cervix (without extension to uterine corpus)	T1	I
Invasive carcinoma diagnosed only by microscopy, stromal invasion with a maximum depth of 5.0 mm measured from the base of the epithelium, and horizontal spread of 7.0 mm or less; vascular space involvement, venous or lymphatic, does not affect classification	T1a	IA
Measured stromal invasion no greater than 3.0 mm and lateral spread no greater than 7.0 mm	T1a1	IA1
Measured stromal invasion greater than 3.0 mm and no greater than 5.0 mm, and horizontal spread no greater than 7.0 mm	T1a2	IA2
Clinically visible lesion confined to the cervix or microscopic lesion greater than Tla or IA2	T1b	IB
Clinically visible lesion no greater than 4.0 cm in greatest dimension	T1b1	IB1
Clinically visible lesion greater than 4.0 cm in greatest dimension	T1b2	IB2
Cervical carcinoma invades beyond the uterus but not the pelvic wall or lower third of vagina	T2	II
Tumor without parametrial invasion	T2a	IIA
Clinically visible lesion no greater than 4.0 cm in greatest dimension	T2a1	IIA1
Clinically visible lesion greater than 4.0 cm in greatest dimension	T2a2	IIA2
Tumor with parametrial invasion	T2b	IIB
Tumor extends to pelvic wall, involves lower third of vagina, causes hydronephrosis, or a combination of all symptoms, or non-functioning kidney	T3	III
Tumor involves lower third of vagina, without extending to the pelvic wall	T3a	IIIA
Tumor extends to pelvic wall, causes hydronephrosis or non-functioning kidney, or both	T3b	IIIB
Tumor invades mucosa of bladder or rectum, extends beyond the true pelvis, or both (bullous oedema is not sufficient to classify a tumor as T4 or IV)	T4	IV
Tumor invades mucosa of bladder or rectum (bullous oedema is not sufficient to classify a tumor as T4 or IV)	T4a	IVA
Tumor extends beyond the true pelvis	T4b	IVB
TNM is a cancer staging system, where T is associated with the size of the primary tumor. N with the nodal involvement, and M with metastatic disease		

FIGO, International Federation of Gynecology and Obstetrics; *TNM*, **T** refers to the size and extent of the main tumor; **N** refers to the the number of nearby lymph nodes that have cancer; **M** refers to cancer metastasis.

TABLE 25.4 Human Papillomavirus Vaccine Recommendations

Eligible individual: Girls and boys ages 11–12 years old are eligible for the HPV vaccine series. However, the vaccination series can be started at age 9. Some adults age 27 through 45 who were not already vaccinated may wish to receive the vaccination after speaking with their health care provider. HPV vaccination in this age range provides less benefit because more people have already been exposed.

Age	Recommendation
9–14 years old	• 2-dose schedule is recommended for people who get the first dose before 15 years old. The second dose should be given 6–12 months after the first dose. • If the second dose is administered after a shorter interval, a third dose should be administered at a minimum of 12 weeks after the second dose.
15–26 years old	• 3-dose schedule • The second dose should be given 1–2 months after the first dose, and the third dose should be given 6 months after the first dose • The minimum intervals are 4 weeks between the first and second dose, 12 weeks between the second and third doses and 5 months between the first and third dose.
Immunocompromised, aged 9–26	• 3-dose schedule
27–45 years old	• Some adults may decide to get the HPV vaccine (just starting sexual encounters, not previously adequately vaccinated)

Data adapted from the Centers for Disease Control and Prevention. HPV vaccine information for clinicians. Available at https://www.cdc.gov/hpv/hcp/schedules-recommendations.html

are more common in younger women. Vaginal sarcomas can develop in children younger than 5 years, and adenocarcinomas are the most common in females younger than age 30 years.[152,153]

Clinical Manifestations. Vaginal cancer can be asymptomatic until late in the progression. The main clinical manifestations include abnormal vaginal bleeding or bloody discharge. Other manifestations include dyspareunia, pelvic pain, vaginal mass, vaginal discharge, vulvar pruritus, constipation, or dysuria.[148]

Evaluation and Treatment. Diagnosis of vaginal cancer includes history and physical examination, pelvic exam, cervical cytology (Pap smear), and HPV test. Other testing may include rectovaginal exam, a speculum exam, palpation of inguinal nodes, colposcopy, and biopsy. Biopsy is still the gold standard to diagnose vaginal cancer. Table 25.5 contains the stages of vaginal cancer. There are no specific laboratory tests in diagnosing vaginal cancer.[148] Once the diagnosis of cancer is known and the size and extent of the lesion are determined, FIGO encourages using CT, MRI, or positron emission tomography (PET) scan to guide therapy.[148] Treatment depends on these findings and on the age of the individual. Three main types of treatment are surgery, radiation therapy, and chemotherapy. New treatments being tested in clinical trials include immunotherapy and radiosensitizers. Vaginal cancer can recur after it has been treated.[154] Recurrence and survival rates vary greatly by stage, size of the tumor, grade of the tumor, whether the cancer is within the vagina, whether there are signs and symptoms at diagnosis, and whether the cancer has just been diagnosed or has recurred. Once the diagnosis of vaginal carcinoma is made, coordinated care needs to be prompt. The involvement of social workers, nurses, radiation oncologists, and gynecologic oncologists is critical.[148]

Vulvar Cancer

Cancer of the vulva most often affects the labia majora and less often the labia minora, clitoris, or vaginal glands. The incidence of vulvar cancer over the past 30 years has steadily increased. Age-adjusted rates for new vulvar cancer cases have been increasing 0.6% each year from 2008 through 2017.[155] Estimated number of new cases is 6330 and estimated deaths 1560 in 2022.[155]

Pathophysiology. The majority (90%) are squamous cell carcinomas. Melanoma subtypes are also common, whereas basal cell carcinoma and Paget disease of the vulva are rare. A history of HPV infection is related to 20% to 80% of vulvar cancers, depending on type; however, HPV-related lesions have a better prognosis than those that are not positive for HPV.[156] Previous squamous dysplasia of the vagina or cervix is a major risk factor, as are HPV infection, HPV-associated vulvar intraepithelial neoplasia, smoking, and HIV infections. Other risk factors include increased age, coexisting autoimmune conditions, organ transplant recipients, immunosuppressed individuals, many sexual partners, first sexual intercourse at a young age, and a history of abnormal Pap test results.[154,157]

Clinical Manifestations. Females in their 60s typically present with symptoms and are more likely to present with advanced disease as opposed to other malignant conditions. The most common symptoms are vulvar irritation, pruritis, and vulvar lesions, which may be a hard ulcerated area of the vulva, large cauliflower lesions, or lesions similar to those of chronic dermatitis. There also may be abnormal bleeding and pain. Early detection is critical.

Evaluation and Treatment. Biopsy confirms the diagnosis. Diagnosis and staging of vulvar cancer include physical examination and history, pelvic examination, Pap smear, HPV test, biopsy (may be examined under anesthesia), colposcopy, and imaging studies (MRI, CT, PET/CT).[154] The main treatment for vulvar cancer is ablative or excisional surgery. Radiation and chemotherapy may be used if the cancer cannot be removed with surgery. Prognosis depends on the lesion size and location, histology, and lymph node involvement. Risk of metastasis increases with tumor size. The 5-year survival rate depends on the extent of the lesion, treatment, and overall health of the woman. Cancer caught in the early stages has a greater 5-year survival rate, with progressively poorer prognosis with advancing stages.

Endometrial Cancer

Endometrial cancer begins in the cells lining the uterus or endometrium and is a prevalent gynecologic malignancy. Most cases occur in postmenopausal females, with a peak incidence in the late 50s to early 60s. It is the sixth most common cancer and the 14th leading cause of cancer death worldwide.[158] Incidence is highest in North America and Europe and lowest in middle-income countries, such as India and South Africa. Incidence rates have been increasing worldwide.[158] The rise in incidence is thought to be caused by factors that affect hormones, such as rising rates of obesity and shifting reproductive trends (e.g., having fewer children). The primary risk factor for endometrial cancer is prolonged exposure to unopposed estrogen (without progesterone). Exposure to unopposed estrogen includes estrogen-only HRT, tamoxifen use, early menarche, late menopause, nulliparous status (never having a child), and failure to ovulate

TABLE 25.5 FIGO Carcinoma of the Vagina

FIGO Nomenclature	
Stage I	The carcinoma is limited to the vaginal wall.
Stage II	The carcinoma has involved the subvaginal tissue but has not extended to the pelvic wall.
Stage III	The carcinoma has extended to the pelvic wall.
Stage IV	The carcinoma has extended beyond the true pelvis or has involved the mucosa of the bladder or rectum; bullous edemas as such does not permit a case to be allotted to stage IV. IVa—tumor invades bladder and/or rectal mucosa and/or direct extension beyond the true pelvis. IVb—spread to distant organs

FIGO, Fédération Internationale de Gynécologie et d'Obstétrique. Adapted from FIGO Committee on Gynecologic Oncology.

Data from PDQ® Adult Treatment Editorial Board. *PDQ Vaginal Cancer Treatment*. Bethesda, MD: National Cancer Institute. Updated February 22, 2021. Available at: https://www.cancer.gov/types/vaginal/hp/vaginal-treatment-pdq. Accessed June 11, 2021. [PMID: 26389242]

BOX 25.10 Epidemiologic and Genetic Risk Factors for Endometrial Cancer

Epidemiologic Risk Factors

Endometrioid endometrial cancer (EC) is an estrogen-dependent tumor type associated with obesity, diabetes, unopposed estrogen use, nulliparity, early menarche, and late menopause. Increasing age is a risk factor for serous and clear cell ECs. Tamoxifen use increases the risk of developing EC; histologic subtypes enhanced in users of tamoxifen are serous EC, high-grade endometrioid ECs, and carcinosarcoma.

Genetic Risk Factors

Increased genetic risk for development of EC is correlated with Lynch syndrome, polymerase proofreading-associated polyposis, and Cowden syndrome.

- Lynch syndrome autosomal dominant cancer syndrome, highly penetrant caused by germline mutation in a mismatch repair gene (*MLH1, MSH2, MSH6,* or *PMS2*), or by deletion in germline within *EPCAM* leading to epigenetic silencing of the adjacent *MSH2* gene. Mutation carriers have increased risk of EC and colorectal cancer, as well as cancers of the ovary, stomach, kidney, urinary tract, biliary tract, small intestine, and skin. Approximately 2%–6% of ECs are attributed to Lynch syndrome.
- Polymerase proofreading-associated polyposis is an autosomal dominant cancer susceptibility syndrome attributed to germline mutations of *POLD1* or *POLE. POLD1* mutation carriers are at increased risk of colorectal cancer. Predisposition to EC has not been established in *POLE* mutation carriers.
- Cowden syndrome is a condition with phosphatase and tensin homologue (PTEN) mutation carriers having an increased predisposition for developing multiple hamartomas and cancers of the breast, thyroid, endometrium, colorectum, kidney, and skin.

Data from Urick ME, Bell DW. Clinical actionability of molecular targets in endometrial cancer. *Nature Reviews Cancer*, 2019;19:510–521.

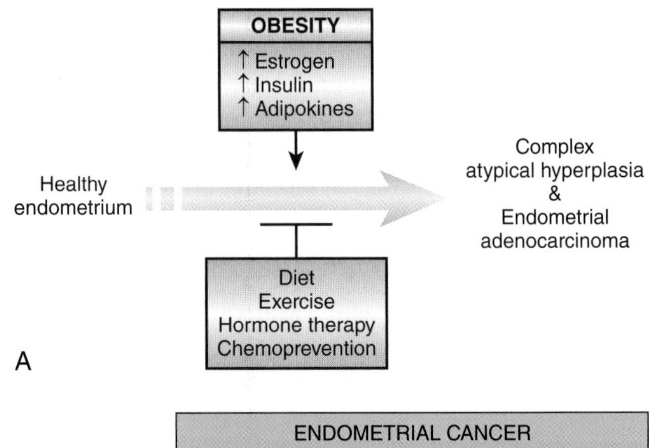

	ENDOMETRIAL CANCER	
	DECREASES RISK	INCREASES RISK
Convincing		Body fatness[1]
Probable	Physical activity[2] Coffee[3]	Glycemic load

1 The panel interpreted BMI (including BMI at age 18-25 years), measures of abdominal girth, and adult weight gain as interrelated aspects of body fatness as well as fat distribution
2 Physical activity of all types; occupational, household, transport and recreational
3 The effect is found in both caffeinated and decaffeinated coffee and cannot be attributed to caffeine

B

Fig. 25.19 Food, Nutrition, Physical Activity, and Endometrial Cancer. (A) Overview of obesity's contribution to the progression of endometrial cancer, and preventive strategies. The T-shaped bar indicates factors that reduce the risk of endometrial cancer. (See the text for a full discussion.) **(B)** Convincing and probable data on reducing and increasing the risk of endometrial cancer. (A, From Schmandt RE, Iglesias DA, Co NN, Lu KH. Understanding obesity and endometrial cancer risk: Opportunities for prevention. *American Journal of Obstetrics and Gynecology,* 2011;205(6):518–525; B, This material has been reproduced from the World Cancer Research Fund/American Institute for Cancer Research. Diet, Nutrition, Physical Activity and Cancer: a Global Perspective. Continuous Update Project Expert Report 2018. Available at dietandcancerreport.org.)

(i.e., PCOS and anovulatory cycles typical of the late reproductive years). Box 25.10 summarizes the epidemiologic and genetic risk factors for endometrial cancer. Another risk factor is obesity (elevated BMI as well as waist-to-hip ratio) because it is a known source of endogenous estrogen. Although related to obesity, other risk factors include diabetes, chronic inflammation, and lack of physical activity (Fig. 25.19).[159–161] Parity (having given birth to at least one child) reduced the risk of cancer.[162]

Pathophysiology. Endometrial hyperplasia is associated with prolonged estrogenic stimulation of the endometrium. Endometrial hyperplasia and carcinoma share acquired genetic alterations in genes linked to carcinogenesis (Fig. 25.20).[163–165] Progesterone inhibits estrogen-driven growth in the uterus. The antagonistic effects of progesterone on the estrogen-induced proliferation and growth occur mostly during the luteal phase and are dependent on the presence of functional PR expression. The interactions between the epithelial and stromal cells of the endometrium may determine the eventual role in the actions of progesterone. The delicate balance of the PR isoforms can tip the scales to foster endometrial hyperplasia and atypia and enhance expression of uterine growth factors. Dysregulation of isoform expression can lead to abnormal function and precancerous changes.

Clinical Manifestations and Evaluation and Treatment. AUB is the most common clinical manifestation of endometrial cancer. Females that are postmenopausal, obese, or with unopposed estrogenic conditions (i.e., anovulatory cycles) should be evaluated in the event of unscheduled or persistent, irregular vaginal bleeding.[166,167] Pain and weight loss are symptoms of more advanced disease. MRI is useful in diagnosis and locoregional spread of the tumor. Transvaginal ultrasound may be used to measure endometrial thickness, and with the rising incidence of endometrial cancer, earlier diagnosis is imperative. If the endometrium is abnormally thick (defined as >5 mm), then further testing, such as an endometrial biopsy, is done.[168] Treatment is based on the extent of the disease and may include progestin therapy for simple hyperplasia (orally or through LNG-IUD), curettage for carcinoma in situ (CIS), total abdominal hysterectomy, chemotherapy, and radiation. Metformin is being studied as a possible strategy for preventing and treating certain cancers, including endometrial cancer.[166,169]

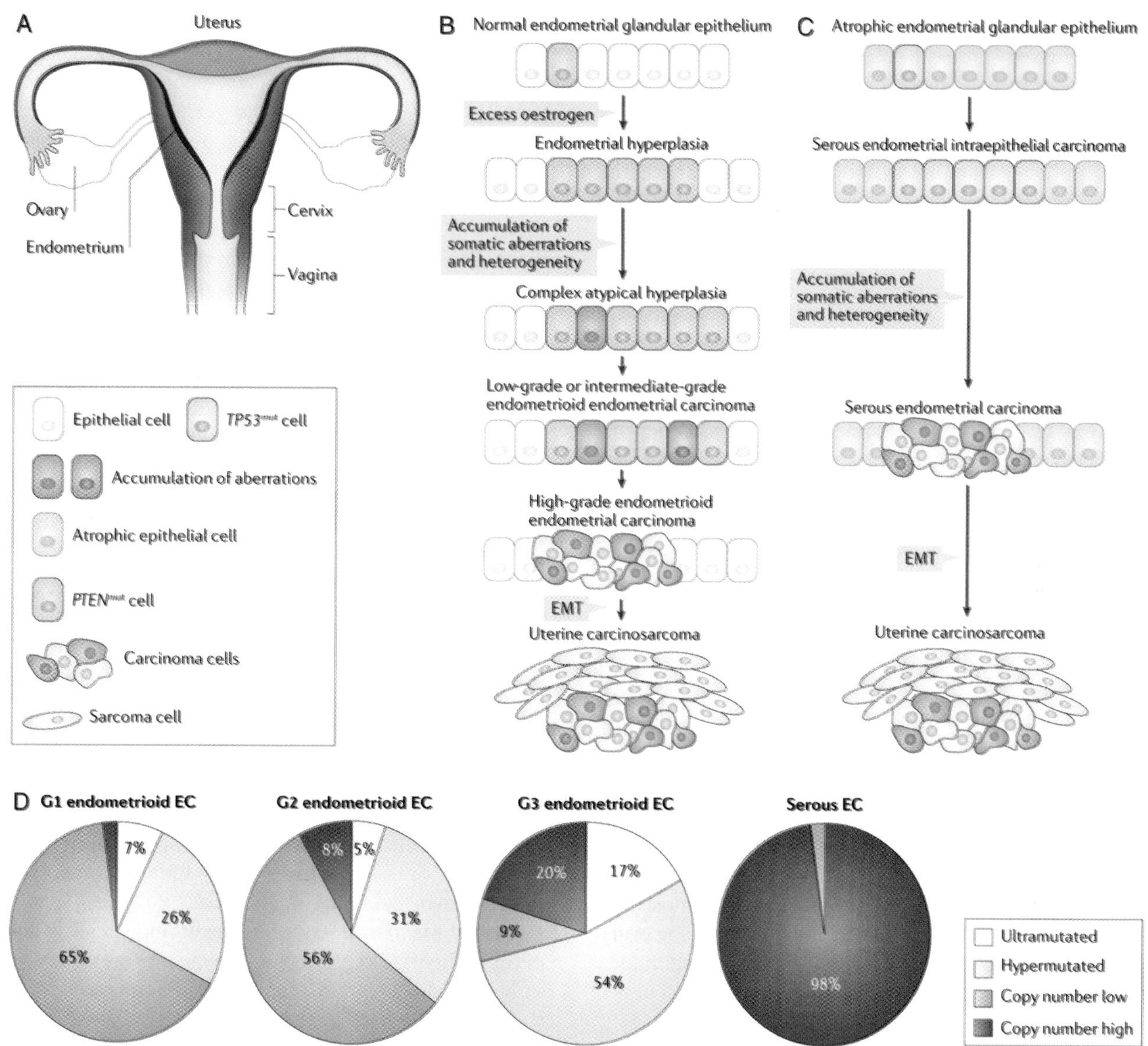

Fig. 25.20 Endometrial Hyperplasia, Complex Atypical Hyperplasia, Endometrial Carcinoma. (A) Female reproductive system showing the endometrium *(dark red).* (B) Depictions of the initiation and progression of endometrioid and (C) serous endometrial cancers (ECs) from the normal and atrophic endometrial glandular epithelium, via precursor lesions (complex atypical hyperplasia and serous endometrial intraepithelial carcinoma). Coloring shows the columnar epithelial that have acquired somatic mutations; intratumoral heterogeneity is shown by differentially colored epithelial cells. PTEN mutation and TP53 mutation, respectively, are early events in the etiology of many endometrioid and serous ECs. In some instances, carcinomas (especially, high-grade carcinomas, undergo epithelial-mesenchymal transition [EMT]; see Chapter 12). EMT gives rise to uterine carcinosarcomas, tumors that have epithelial carcinoma cells and sarcoma cells *(blue).* (D) Pie charts show the distribution (% of total tumors) of low-grade or intermediate-grade (G1 and G2, respectively) endometrioid EC, high-grade (G3) endometrioid EC, and serous EC among the four molecular subgroups described in The Cancer Genome Atlas. (From Urick ME, Bell DW. Clinical actionability of molecular targets in endometrial cancer. *Nature Reviews Cancer,* 2019;19:510–521. https://doi.org/10.1038/s41568-019-0177-x.)

Ovarian Cancer

Ovarian cancer is the seventh most common cancer in women and the eighth most common cause of cancer death. Estimates for 2021 in the United States for new ovarian cancer cases are 21,410 and cancer deaths 13,770, with a 5-year survival rate just less than 45%.[1,170] The understanding of incidence patterns both within and between populations is essential to revealing potential causes of and risk factors for ovarian cancer. The highest age-adjusted incidence rates are observed in developed parts of the world, including North America and Central and Eastern Europe; the lowest such rates are seen in Asia and Africa. In the Unitted States, racial differences in epidemiology mimic the observed international variation, with rates highest in non-Hispanic whites followed by American Indians and Alaska Natives, Hispanics, non-Hispanic Blacks, and Asian and Pacific Islanders.[171,172] Migration studies show that moving from countries with low rates to those with high rates results in greater risk, demonstrating the importance of nongenetic factors. The strongest risk factor for ovarian cancer is a positive family history of breast or ovarian cancer; a personal history of cancer also increases the risk.[173] There is increased incidence, advanced stage, and lower reported survival in postmenopausal females with ovarian cancer,[171] whereas parity poses a protective role.[171,174]

Pathophysiology. The pathogenesis of ovarian cancer is not fully understood. The majority of ovarian tumors are sporadic and are not caused by inherited genetic factors. These cancers are acquired as somatic mutations in the *TP53* gene and occur in almost half of all ovarian cancers.[175] However, in 10% to 15% of cases, a genetic predisposition is found. In cases that cluster in families, the genetic basis for the disease and the pattern of inheritance is unclear. However, there is association with the breast cancer susceptibility gene 1 *(BRCA1)* and a smaller number with mutations of *BRCA2* or mismatched repair genes (hereditary nonpolyposis colorectal cancer [HNPCC] syndrome). Females and families who are more susceptible to cancer may have errors in the ability to repair cellular DNA, related to abnormalities in several genes responsible for repair of damaged DNA.[176,177] Previously, the majority of ovarian cancers were thought to arise from just epithelial cells that cover the ovarian surface or line subserosal cysts. Newer evidence suggests that tumors arise from three ovarian components: (1) from the fimbriae of fallopian tubes and from deposits of endometriosis; (2) from germ cells, which are pluripotent and migrate to the ovary from the yolk sac; and (3) from stromal cells, including the sex cords, which precede endocrine changes of the postnatal ovary. Some ovarian tumors remain too difficult to classify.[170]

The normal ovary contains three major cell types: (1) germ cells, derived from the endoderm, which differentiate into oocytes; (2) hormone-producing cells (estrogen and progesterone) within the ovary; and (3) epithelial cells (derived from the müllerian duct) that cover the ovary and line inclusion cysts. Both benign and malignant tumors come from each of the three ovarian cell types.[178] The two major types of ovarian cancer are epithelial ovarian neoplasms and germ-cell neoplasms. Most ovarian malignancies are epithelial ovarian that develop from the surface epithelium of the ovary or the epithelium that lines cysts immediately beneath the ovarian surface or may be cells that have migrated from precursor lesions in the fallopian tubes (Fig. 25.21). Most epithelial cancers seem to arise from a single cell that is cloned. This occurs because of a loss of tumor-suppressor genes and activation of oncogenes. Ovarian cancer is heterogenous with four histologic types of epithelial ovarian cancers: serous, endometrioid, clear cell, and mucinous.[171] The histologic types also have different behaviors and characteristics.[179] Tumors are often classified as type I (low grade) and type II (high grade) based on their cellular type. Type I tumors grow more slowly and are genetically stable.[171] Type II tumors often grow rapidly and aggressively and often have genetic mutations along with a poorer prognosis.[171] Gross appearances of serous tumors are shown in Fig. 25.22.

Germ-cell tumors are derived from the primitive germ cells (gametes) of the embryonic gonad and may be malignant or benign. The benign cystic teratoma accounts for approximately 10% of all ovarian tumors. These tumors represent an error in meiosis that results in the formation of ectoderm, endoderm, and mesoderm cell lines. Hair, teeth, and skin can be visualized within cystic teratomas. If the germ-cell tumor is malignant, it tends to be highly aggressive and rapidly growing with a poor prognosis. Cystic hygromas and other germ-cell tumors can occur on the ovaries of females at any age. Germ-cell tumors in children can be particularly aggressive.

Clinical Manifestations. In general, individuals with ovarian cancer have no *early* symptoms. Symptoms are nonspecific and can be missed but tend to arise in the late stage (stage III or stage IV) when the tumors have grown to a very large size. Presenting symptoms include abdominal fullness, bloating, nausea, abdominal distension, early satiety, change in bowel habits, urinary symptoms, back pain, dyspareunia, and weight loss (Fig. 25.23).[171] The vague symptoms may occur months before the diagnosis.[180]

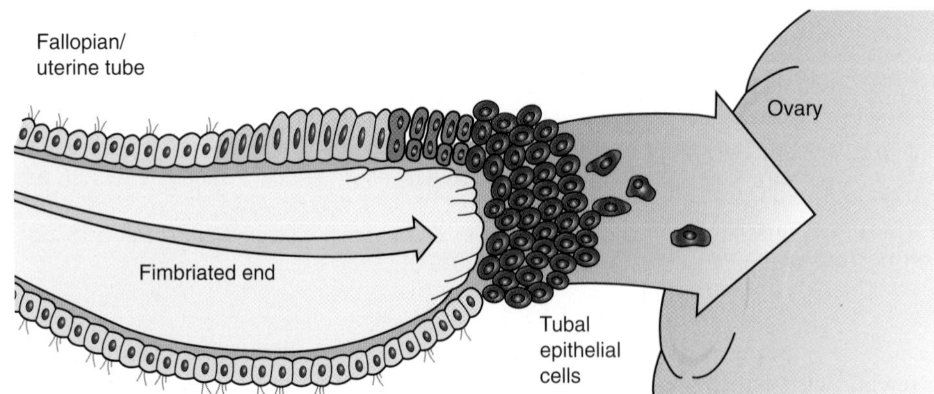

Fig. 25.21 Migration of Epithelial Cells from the Fallopian/Uterine Tubes to the Ovary. (Adapted from Kurman RJ, Shih I-M. The origin and pathogenesis of epithelial ovarian cancer: A proposed unifying theory. *American Journal of Surgical Pathology,* 2010; 34(3):433–443. https://doi.org/10.1097/pas.0b013e3181cf3d79)

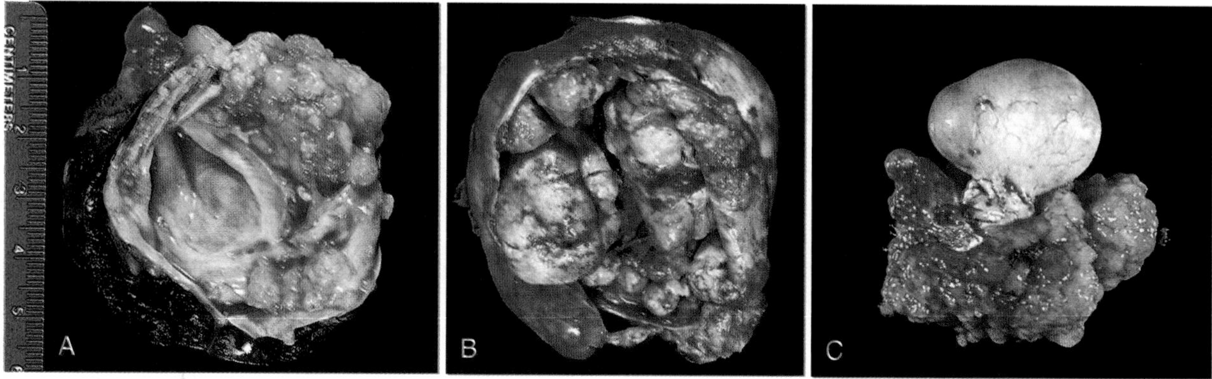

Fig. 25.22 Gross Appearances of Serous Tumors of the Ovary. **(A)** Serous borderline tumor opened to display a cyst cavity lined by papillary tumor growth. **(B)** Carcinoma. The cyst is opened to reveal a large, bulky tumor mass. **(C)** Another borderline tumor growing on the ovarian surface. (From Kumar V, Abbas AK, Fausto N, Robbins SL, Cotran RS. *Robbins and Cotran pathologic basis of disease*, 10th edition. Philadelphia: Elsevier; 2021.)

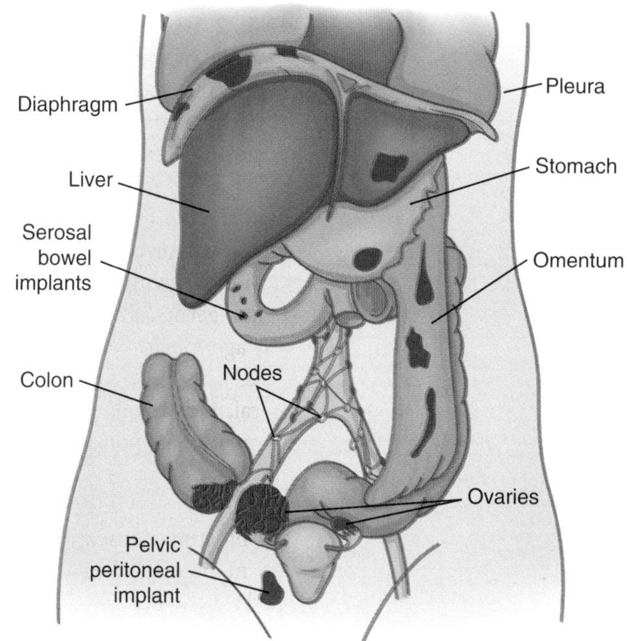

Fig. 25.23 Metastasis of Ovarian Cancer. Pattern of spread for epithelial cancer of the ovary.

Gastrointestinal manifestations may include dyspepsia, vomiting, and alterations in bowel habits caused by mechanical obstruction. Abnormal vaginal bleeding may occur if the postmenopausal endometrium is stimulated by hormone-secreting tumor. The tumor may cause ulcerations through the vaginal wall that result in bleeding. There can be a feeling of pressure in the pelvis or leg pain. Tumors that obstruct vascular channels can cause venous and, occasionally, arterial thrombosis. Alterations in coagulability also may occur, contributing to clot formation. Metastasis often causes pleural effusion with diminished breath sounds.

Evaluation and Treatment. A thorough physical exam, including rectovaginal examination on an empty bladder, should be performed.[171] In advanced cases, a palpable pelvic mass or ascites or diminished breath sounds may be found in the presence of pleural effusions. However, given the location of the ovaries, assessing abnormalities on routine gynecologic examination poses difficulty, especially in obese women. Minimally invasive testing should be considered in women with symptoms of disease. Initial work-up should include blood work and transvaginal ultrasound. The blood test, which measures the protein cancer antigen 125 (CA 125), is increased in approximately 80% of nonmucinous ovarian cancers. The CA 125 is an evaluative laboratory test that looks for specific cancer markers. However, CA 125 is also elevated in the presence of endometriosis, benign ovarian cysts, myomas, and pregnancy. Some types of germ cell and adenocarcinoma may be associated with increased levels of α-fetoprotein (AFP), hCG, and CA 125. A new marker, human epididymis protein 4 (HE4), is being further evaluated. HE4 has been found to be more sensitive to serous and endometrioid subtypes of ovarian cancer. A combination of higher CA 125 and HE4 levels are thought to be predictive of malignant ovarian cancer.[181]

If initial tests are suspicious for a cancerous mass, diagnosis is confirmed by biopsy and the extent of the disease is determined by ultrasound, CT, PET, MRI, or other imaging techniques. Staging of disease may include other studies such as upper gastrointestinal series, barium enema, intravenous pyelogram (IVP), mammography, and lymphography. The FIGO staging system is described in Table 25.6.

The initial approach to treatment is surgery to determine the stage of disease and to remove as much of the tumor as possible. Future treatment, which requires a skilled, multidisciplinary team, is then customized based on the stage of the cancer, the woman's desires, the cell type, and the sensitivity of the cancer cells. Advanced-stage ovarian cancer is treated with primary reductive surgery, followed by platinum-based chemotherapy.[182] Radiation and chemotherapy are common adjunct treatments.[183] Even after initially effective treatment, the majority of females will relapse.[171] Prophylactic removal of the ovaries and fallopian tubes is associated with increased survival rates among females who carry the BRCA mutation and is considered for those who do not desire fertility.

TABLE 25.6 FIGO Staging of Carcinoma of the Ovary

Stage	Characteristics
I	Growth limited to ovaries
II	Growth involves one or both ovaries and also other organs (i.e., uterus, bladder, colon)
III	Cancer involves one or both ovaries, and one or both of these are present: (1) cancer has spread beyond pelvis to lining of abdomen, (2) cancer has spread to lymph nodes
IV	Growth involves one or both ovaries, with distant metastases to lungs, liver, or other organs outside peritoneal cavity
Recurrent	Cancer recurs after completion of treatment

FIGO, The International Federation of Gynecologists and Obstetricians.

New therapies under investigation include monoclonal antibodies, epidermal growth factor receptor, gene therapy, small-molecular-weight inhibitors, and routine screening modalities. There is no sensitive and specific test for ovarian cancer for screening low-risk females. Routine screening of individuals without risk factors has not been shown to be beneficial and may cause harm because more females have unnecessary surgical procedures due to false-positives. Unfortunately, currently there are not sufficient data to support effective screening in the general population.[184,185]

However, research is ongoing for a cost-effective routine screening method.

Sexual Dysfunction

Sexual dysfunction is the lack of satisfaction with sexual function resulting from pain or a deficiency in sexual desire, arousal, or orgasm/climax. Sexual function and dysfunction result from a complex interplay of the individual, culture, and physiology.[186] Sexual issues are multifaceted and often very difficult to diagnose. Both organic and/or psychosocial disorders are implicated in sexual dysfunction. Studies show that up to 50% of adult women have some form of sexual dysfunction.[187]

The sexual response cycle is a complex process involving the brain, sympathetic and parasympathetic nervous systems, the systemic and local vascular, and local innervation. Any disruption in these systems can affect sexual response. Chronic medical conditions can greatly affect both sexual desire and sexual function (Table 25.7). Acute illness and infections also can affect the woman's desire and ability to engage in fulfilling sexual activity. Medications can disrupt the sexual response. Antihypertensives and antidepressants are commonly associated with sexual problems.[188] Surgeries near the genital area can disrupt nerve pathways, and hysterectomy may affect sexual function because the uterus, cervix, and vagina are involved in sexual response and orgasm. The mind is a large component of sexual response, and any stressor that affects the woman can affect her sexual response, including her feelings about her sexuality and relationship, as well as past sexual abuse.[189]

TABLE 25.7 Possible Effects of Chronic Disease on Sexual Functioning in Women

Disease	Sexual Function
Cerebral palsy	Intact genital sensations, decreased lubrication; difficulty with sexual activity/positioning because of muscle spasticity, rigidity, or weakness; pain with positioning caused by contracture of knees and hips or because of increased spasms with arousal
Cerebrovascular accident (CVA)	Difficulties in sexual positioning and sensitivity because of impaired motor strength, coordination, or paralysis; decreased libido with stroke on dominant side of brain
Diabetes	Diminished intensity of orgasm and gradual decline in ability to achieve orgasm; decreased lubrication or recurrent vaginal infections with resultant dyspareunia
Chronic renal failure	Decreased arousal; increasingly rare and less intense orgasms; decreased lubrication
Rheumatoid arthritis (RA)	Painful sexual activity/positions because of swollen, painful joints, muscular atrophy, and joint contracture; decreased libido because of pain, fatigue, or medication; genital sensations remain intact
Systemic lupus erythematosus (SLE)	Similar to RA; decreased lubrication and vaginal lesions result in painful penetration
Myocardial infarction (MI)	Most literature male oriented; problems related to medications
Multiple sclerosis (MS)	Diminished genital sensitivity; decreased lubrication; declining orgasmic ability; difficulty with sexual activity because of muscle weakness, pain, or incontinence
Spinal cord injury	Reflex sexual response with injury above sacral area; disrupted response with lesion at or below sacrum; loss of sensation, decreased lubrication; spasticity, incontinence, or pain with arousal; continued orgasmic sensations or sensations diffused in general or to specific body parts, such as breast or lips

A thorough history, including complete past medical, family, medication, and social history including any history of abuse, is needed to assess for sexual dysfunction. Testing can be appropriate to determine organic dysfunction and includes a CBC, comprehensive metabolic panel (CMP), glycated hemoglobin (HbA1c), as well as testing for STIs when indicated (Fig. 25.24). The American College of Obstetricians and Gynecologists divides sexual dysfunction into four categories: disorders of desire, arousal, orgasm, and sexual pain.[190]

Disorders of desire (hypoactive sexual desire, decreased libido) are the most common sexual dysfunction in women.[189] The prevalence of hypoactive sexual desire increases with age and may be a biologic manifestation of depression, dissatisfaction with partner relationships, a history of sexual or physical

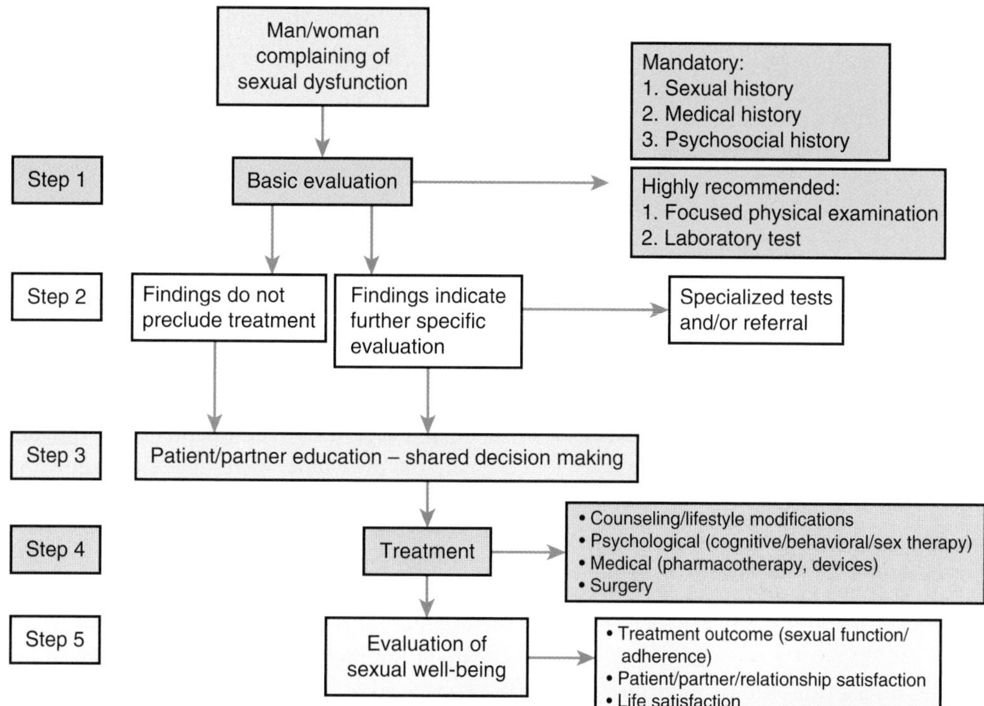

Fig. 25.24 Diagnostic and Treatment Algorithm for Sexual Dysfunction. The International Consultation in Sexual Medicine stepwise diagnostic and treatment algorithm for sexual dysfunction in men and women. (From Hatzichristou D, Rosen RC, Derogatis LR, et al. Recommendations for the clinical evaluation of men and women with sexual dysfunction. *Journal of Sexual Medicine,* 2010;7(1pt2):337–348.)

abuse, alcohol or other substance abuse, prolactin-secreting pituitary tumors, or testosterone deficiency. Medications, such as the β-adrenergic blockers used for heart disease, may inhibit sexual desire. The medication flibanserin has been shown to activate dopamine and norepinephrine in the brain which increases sexual desire. Treatment with exogenous testosterone, the antidepressant bupropion, and sexual and psychological therapy has shown to increase sexual desire in women.[189]

Anorgasmia (orgasmic dysfunction) is the inability of a woman to reach or achieve orgasm. It ranges from difficulty in arousal to lack of orgasm. Any chronic illness may affect arousal. Specific disorders that may block orgasm are diabetes, alcoholism, neurologic disturbances, hormonal deficiencies, and pelvic disorders (e.g., infections, trauma, and surgical scarring). Narcotics, tranquilizers, antidepressants (especially SSRIs), and antihypertensive medications also can inhibit orgasm.[186]

Dyspareunia (painful intercourse) is common. Women may experience pain at any time from the beginning of arousal to after intercourse. The pain may have a burning, sharp, searing, or cramping quality and may be described as external, vaginal, deep abdominal, or pelvic. A variety of psychosocial and organic causes have been identified. Inadequate lubrication may make penetration or intercourse difficult or painful. Low estrogen levels, common with menopause and lactation, can decrease vaginal lubrication. Drugs with a drying effect (e.g., antihistamines, certain tranquilizers, and marijuana) can decrease lubrication. Infections and skin problems of the vulva and the vagina are a frequent cause of acute onset dyspareunia. The use of products such as spermicides and fragrances on the sensitive vaginal mucosa may increase the risk of irritation. Disorders of the vaginal opening, such as scarring from female genital mutilation, episiotomy, or an intact hymen, also can cause discomfort. Deep pelvic disorders such as infection, tumors, and cervical or uterine pathologies also can cause pain with intercourse.

Vaginismus is an involuntary muscle spasm in response to attempted penetration. Vaginismus is often a response to previous painful penetration. Common psychological causes include prior sexual trauma and fear of sex. Organic causes are similar to those that cause dyspareunia, including vulvodynia. Even after the underlying organic problem is detected and successfully treated, vaginismus may persist.

Sexual dysfunction may develop as a coping mechanism. Women with a history of sexual trauma—rape, incest, or molestation—often have problems with desire, arousal, or orgasm or experience pain with sexual activity. In extreme cases, total sexual aversion may develop.[191] At other times, sexual dysfunction may be a symptom of marital or relationship problems. Because sexual dysfunction has many causes, assessment and treatment should be holistic, individualized, and culturally sensitive.[192,193]

Impaired Fertility

Infertility affects approximately 15% of all couples and is defined as the inability to conceive over 1 year of unprotected intercourse. Fertility can be impaired by factors in the male

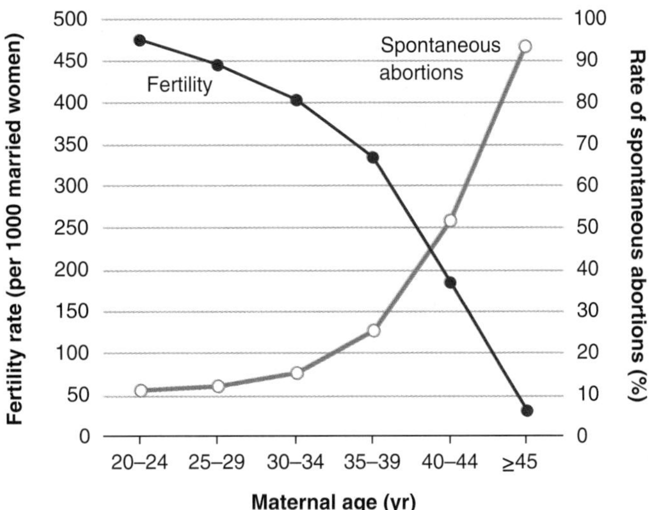

Fig. 25.25 Relationship of Fertility and Miscarriage with Maternal Age. (From Heffner LJ. Advanced maternal age—How old is too old? *New England Journal of Medicine,* 2004;351(19):1927–1929.)

or female, or in both partners. The rate of infertility may be increasing because of increased rates of STIs, environmental exposures, delayed childbearing, or lack of previous reporting. There is a greater utilization of medical services for infertility now than ever previously recorded.[194]

Pathophysiology. Causes of infertility include ovulatory disorder, abnormal semen, blockage of the fallopian tubes, endometriosis, and unexplained infertility. Most cases of infertility involve the female, caused in part by the complexity of the female reproductive cycle and tract. Ovulatory factors account for approximately 40% of female infertility. Regular ovulation occurs as a result of a functioning hypothalamic/pituitary axis. Ovulation can be disrupted by hormonal imbalances (e.g., TSH, estrogen, progesterone), chronic conditions, and stress. Age is a major factory in female fertility because the regularity of ovulation and the quality of ova decrease with age (Fig. 25.25). Approximately 20% of cases are because of abnormalities of the reproductive tract, such as tubal pathologies. Endometriosis, adhesions, and scarring from PID are major contributors to blockages within the female reproductive tract. The remaining 20% of female infertility cases are caused by rare conditions or unknown etiology.[195,196]

Fallopian tube dysfunction may result from acute pelvic infections such as chlamydia or gonorrhea. Adhesions from a pelvic infection, abdominal surgery, or endometriosis may cause blockage of one or both fallopian tubes, preventing access of the sperm to the ovum. The fertilized ovum must implant on a receptive endometrium. Receptivity may be greatly diminished by fibroids or inadequate molecular or cellular preparation of the implantation site. Male infertility contributes to approximately 40% of cases of infertility (see Chapter 26).

Evaluation and Treatment. Before the performance of basic fertility tests, a complete history is obtained that includes (1) coital (sex) timing and frequency in relation to menstrual cycle, (2) an in-depth assessment and charting of the menstrual cycle, (3) a reproductive history, including previous pregnancies from both partners and their outcome, (4) a medical history of systemic disease, (5) current medications, (6) previous surgeries, (7) a sexual history, including any previous STIs, and (8) exposure to toxins. Testing starts with the least invasive test or procedure and advances in complexity and, possibly, invasiveness. The most common test for male infertility is the semen analysis. Hormonal assays may be helpful. Pelvic examination, ultrasound, and hysterosalpingogram (HSG), and MRI can help determine anatomy and fallopian/uterine tube patency. Chromosomal analyses of the couple may reveal mutations that result in early embryo loss.[197]

Treatment of infertility aims at correcting underlying pathologies or overriding the deficient system. Male infertility is discussed separately (see Chapter 26). Anovulation in the female can be overcome with ovulation-inducing drugs. Blockages within the female reproductive tract can be bypassed with IVF.

Assisted reproductive technologies (ARTs) have enabled women and couples to conceive and bear children. However, there are questions about the health and long-term safety of infants conceived with assisted reproduction (e.g., concerns about the high rate of twins and preterm births in pregnancies conceived with ARTs). In addition, children born through ART have a higher rate of birth defects even when other variables are controlled.[198,199] Several explanations of the causes of these outcomes suggest that the birth defects may be the result of epigenetic changes that occur when the expression of the embryo's DNA is affected by the very early environment of the blastocysts, although it is not clear if damage done through the fertilization and implantation procedures themselves is caused by an underlying medical condition contributing to the infertility. Importantly, research in this area and in the field of epigenetics is ongoing.[199]

DISORDERS OF THE FEMALE BREAST

Galactorrhea

Galactorrhea (inappropriate lactation) is milk production from the breast not related to pregnancy or lactation. Milk production 1 year after cessation of breastfeeding is nonlactational and is considered galactorrhea.[200] The production of milk is affected by several hormones, including prolactin, estrogens, and thyrotropin-releasing hormone (TRH).[201] Box 25.11 includes hypothalamic-pituitary causes and non–hypothalamic-pituitary causes.

BOX 25.11 Etiology of Galactorrhea

Hypothalamic-Pituitary Causes

Prolactinomas

Non–prolactin-secreting pituitary tumor and infiltrative disorders of the pituitary stalk/hypothalamus

Non–hypothalamic-pituitary causes

Hypothyroidism

Medications (risperidone, clozapine, olanzapine, aripiprazole, metoclopramide, domperidone, tricyclic antidepressants, opioids, verapamil)

Renal failure

Chest wall lesions

Idiopathic hyperprolactinemia

Galactorrhea, which also can occur in men, may involve one or both breasts and is not usually associated with breast cancer.

The incidence of galactorrhea is difficult to estimate because of differences among definitions of the condition, examination techniques, and populations of women who have been studied. The prevalence ranges from 0.4% in an unselected adult population to as high as 9% to 17% in women with reproductive disorders.[200] Women with PCOS have a high reported prevalence of 17%.[202]

Pathophysiology. Galactorrhea is a manifestation of pathophysiologic processes elsewhere in the body rather than a primary breast disorder. These processes are chiefly hormone imbalances or exogenous, including drugs, estrogen, and stimulation of the nipples.[200]

Galactorrhea caused by hyperprolactinemia is manifested by the spontaneous appearance of a milky secretion from multiple duct openings, usually from both breasts. Estrogens cause hyperprolactinemia by inhibiting hypothalamic dopamine and by stimulating lactotrophs directly. High levels of estrogen in pregnancy cause lactotroph hyperplasia and can further increase the growth of a preexisting prolactinoma. Hyperprolactinemia also is associated with excess secretion of estrogen from ovaries.[200] Unilateral, spontaneous, serous, or serosanguineous discharge from a single duct usually is caused by an intraductal papilloma. Bloody discharge suggests cancer; bilateral, sticky, multicolored discharge from multiple ducts is often caused by ductal ectasia; and purulent discharge indicates a subareolar abscess.

Clinical Manifestations. Inappropriate lactation is manifested by milky white or green breast secretions from one or both breasts of nonpregnant, nonlactating females. Most females with galactorrhea experience menstrual abnormality and changes in libido. Most males experience erectile dysfunction.[200] If a pituitary process is involved, the female usually experiences hirsutism and infertility; if a hypothalamic lesion is present, CNS symptoms may be reported, such as intractable headache, visual field disturbances, sleep disturbances, and abnormal temperature, thirst, or appetite.

Evaluation and Treatment. Galactorrhea in nulliparous or parous females who have not breast-fed for 12 months must be thoroughly evaluated. After ruling out breast pathologies, therapy is directed toward the cause of hyperprolactinemia. Evaluation includes a variety of diagnostic tests. Serum prolactin levels are measured, and at least two positive results are needed to diagnose hyperprolactinemia. Prolactin levels higher than 25 to 30 ng/mL (measured by radioimmunoassay) are considered elevated. Those in the range of 75 to 100 ng/mL are possibly caused by a pituitary tumor until proven otherwise. Serum thyroxine (T_4) and TSH levels are measured to rule out hypothyroidism, and LH and FSH levels are obtained if the individual is amenorrheic. Treatment for galactorrhea consists of identifying and treating the cause. Medical therapy is typical, and surgical or radiation therapy is rarely required. The main treatments are bromocriptine or cabergoline.[200] Surgery or radiation therapy is rarely required.

Benign Breast Disease and Conditions

Benign breast disease (BBD) is a range of noncancerous changes in the breast. Numerous benign alterations in ducts and lobules occur in the breast, including lumps, cysts, sensitive nipples, and itching. The most common symptoms reported by women are pain, a palpable mass, or nipple discharge; the majority of these prove to have a benign cause. Major determinants of the risk of breast cancer after a diagnosis of BBD include histologic or biologic features, or both; previous biopsy; and degree of family history.[203,204] Benign epithelial lesions can be broadly classified as (1) nonproliferative breast lesions, (2) proliferative breast disease without atypia, and (3) atypical (atypia) hyperplasia. The majority of nonproliferative benign lesions are not precursors of cancer and generally are not associated with an increased risk of breast cancer.

Nonproliferative Breast Lesions

Nonproliferative epithelial breast lesions are usually not associated with an increased risk of breast cancer. The nonproliferative lesions include (1) simple breast cysts, (2) galactocele, (3) papillary apocrine change, and (4) mild hyperplasia of the usual type. Terms such as fibrocystic changes (FCCs) (or physiologic nodularity and cysts), fibrocystic disease, chronic cystic mastitis, and mammary dysplasia refer to nonproliferative lesions but are not clinically useful because they are a heterogeneous group of diagnoses.[204] Simple cysts (fluid-filled sacs) are the most common nonproliferative breast lesion and are a specific type of lump that commonly occurs in women in their 30 s, 40 s, and early 50 s. Cysts are categorized by imaging characteristics as simple, complex, or complicated. It is estimated that 50% to 80% of women normally experience some of these changes. The prevalence of fibrocystic lesions is probably related to hormonal changes, which in turn are affected by genetic background, age, parity, history of lactation, and use of caffeine and exogenous hormones. Cysts often rupture, with release of secretory material into the adjacent tissue. The resulting chronic inflammation and scarring fibrosis contribute to the palpable firmness of the breast. Fibrous tissue increases progressively until menopause and regresses thereafter.

Simple cysts do not require medical management unless they are large and painful. In this circumstance, aspiration can be completed under ultrasound guidance. If the aspirate is bloody, the fluid should be sent for cytology. *Complicated or complex cysts* can be aspirated to complete resolution with ultrasound guidance. If complete resolution is not obtained, percutaneous biopsy of the remaining cyst should be completed. Aspiration cytology has been related to tumor cell seeding; therefore a needle gauge of 22 or less should be used.[205]

Galactoceles are cystic collections of fluid often caused by an obstructed milk duct.[204] They present as soft cystic masses on physical examination and may appear as an indeterminate mass on mammography, unless the classic fat-fluid level is seen.[204] Ultrasound may show a complex mass. Clinical history and aspiration yield a milky substance. Once the diagnosis is made, excision is not necessary, and there is no increased risk of subsequent breast cancer.[204] Papillary apocrine change is an increase in ductal epithelial cells that has apocrine changes or an eosinophilic cytoplasm. Mild hyperplasia of the usual type is an increase in the number of epithelial cells within a duct that is more than two cells, but not more than four cells, in depth.

Proliferative Breast Lesions Without Atypia

Proliferative breast lesions without atypia are characterized by the proliferation of ductal epithelium or stroma, or both, without cellular signs of abnormality (atypia, or deviation from normal). Five structurally diverse lesions are discussed next.

Usual ductal hyperplasia (UDH) is additional or proliferating epithelial cells that fill and distend the ducts and lobules. They are usually an incidental finding on mammography. The cells can vary in size and shape, but they retain features of benign cells.[204] No additional treatment is needed, and chemoprevention is not recommended.[204]

Intraductal papillomas can occur as solitary or multiple lesions. *Solitary papillomas* are a monotonous (sameness) array of papillary cells that grow from the wall of the cyst into the lumen of the duct. Growth occurs within a dilated duct often near or beside the nipple, causing benign nipple discharge. These papillomas *can* harbor areas of atypia or ductal carcinoma in situ (DCIS). Newer data suggest that not all papillomas diagnosed by core needle biopsy (CNB) require surgical excision; however, surgical excision is warranted when a CNB demonstrates papilloma with atypical cells.[204]

Diffuse papillomatosis (multiple papillomas) may present as breast masses, nodules on ultrasound, or the cause of nipple discharge. Diffuse papillomatosis is defined as a minimum of five papillomas within a localized segment of breast tissue.[204] Although the breast cancer risk is small, these lesions require surgical excision.

Sclerosing adenosis is a lobular lesion with increased fibrous tissue and scattered glandular cells.[204] No treatment is needed, and chemoprevention is not indicated.

Radial scar (RS) (also called *complex sclerosing lesions*) refers to an irregular, radial proliferation of ductlike small tubules entrapped in a dense central fibrosis. RSs are usually discovered when a breast lesion or radiologic abnormality is biopsied or removed. Rarely are RSs discovered by mammography, which cannot reliably differentiate between these lesions and speculated carcinoma.[204] Although controversy exists about the need for surgical excision, there is some evidence that RSs may be premalignant lesions and can slowly progress from scar to hyperplasia to carcinoma.[204]

Simple fibroadenomas are benign solid tumors that contain glandular and fibrous lesions.[204] In approximately 20% of cases, multiple fibroadenomas can occur in the same breast or bilaterally.[204] The etiology for fibroadenomas is unknown but appears to be hormonal because they can persist during the reproductive years and can increase in size during pregnancy or with estrogen therapy. They usually regress after menopause.[204] They are more common among women between 15 and 35 years of age. Fibroadenomas are now considered proliferative lesions, and the histologic features influence the risk of breast cancer. There is no increased risk of breast cancer in the majority of women with a simple fibroadenoma. It is not necessary to excise all biopsy-proven fibroadenomas.[204] Disadvantages of excisional surgery include scarring at the incision site, dimpling of the breast from the removal of the tumor, damage to the breast's duct system, and mammographic changes (e.g., architectural distortion, skin thickening, increased focal density).[204] If a biopsy-proven fibroadenoma is asymptomatic, it can then be left in place.[204]

Proliferative Breast Lesions With Atypia

Atypical hyperplasia (AH) is an increase in the number of cells (or proliferation) with the cells having some variation in structure (*—atypia)*. AH is associated with a moderately increased risk of breast cancer and is characterized by two forms: ductal hyperplasia and atypical lobular hyperplasia. Atypical ductal hyperplasia (ADH) refers to abnormal proliferating cells in breast ducts. Atypical lobular hyperplasia (ALH) refers to proliferation of cells in the lumen of lobular units. Approximately 60% of the subsequent breast cancers in women with AH occur in the ipsilateral breast (same side) as the biopsy.[206–208]

It appears that menopausal status at the time of benign breast biopsy influences the magnitude of the subsequent breast cancer risk. For women who were premenopausal at the time of their breast biopsy, the risk of breast cancer was greater in those with ALH than among women with ADH.[208] Among women who were postmenopausal at the time of benign breast biopsy, the risk was similar for ALH and ADH.[208] Overall, ADH and ALH are viewed best as "markers" of a generalized, bilateral increase in breast cancer risk.[204,208] The younger a woman is when she receives a diagnosis of AH, the higher the risk that breast cancer will develop.[209]

Evaluation and Treatment. Breast problems are diagnosed from a multimodal approach that combines physical examination, mammography, ultrasonography, possibly MRI, and biopsy. The dense breast tissue often seen in young women can make mammographic interpretation extremely difficult (Box 25.12). Surgical excision was historically recommended after a CNB identified ADH or ALH; however, newer data suggest that routine excision of all atypical lesions may not be necessary.[204]

Treatment of cysts consists largely of relieving symptoms. Reduction in the consumption of caffeinated beverages (e.g., cola,) and chocolate, which can cause overstimulation for some women, may reduce pain and nodularity. Given time, the cysts may disappear without treatment.

Women with AH are advised to stop oral contraceptives and avoid HRT.[204] Certain selective estrogen modulators, such as tamoxifen and raloxifene, or an aromatase inhibitor may be considered for chemoprevention for women with AH after a thorough discussion of risks and benefits. A deficiency in iodine is hypothesized as contributing to the development of breast pathology and cancer. Therefore, although quite controversial, another preventive factor may be iodine.[210,211]

Breast Cancer

Except for skin cancer, breast cancer is the most common cancer in American females, regardless of race and ethnicity. In the United States, it is estimated that 284,200 females will be diagnosed with breast cancer, and 44,130 deaths will ensue in 2021.[1] Breast cancer is the most common cause of death from cancer among Hispanic females, and the second most common cause of death from cancer among White, Black, Asian/Pacific Islander, and American Indian/Alaska Native females.[212] The number of new cases worldwide of breast cancer in both sexes was estimated at 2.3 million and the number of deaths as 684,996 for all ages and both sexes.[213]

The causes of breast cancer have been difficult to define because each female has a different genetic profile, which is called genetic heterogeneity. Genetic heterogeneity is common

BOX 25.12 Breast Cancer Screening Mammography

Joann G. Elmore, MD, MPH

The idea behind screening healthy individuals for disease is the hope that we can diagnose disease early, when more treatment options are available and when we can positively affect the life of the individual. Screening programs for the entire population of a country are a large undertaking and usually require careful consideration and extensive resources. Therefore we need to make certain the test has a high level of accuracy, with reasonable costs and disadvantages, the disease is not too rare, and the treatment is effective for individuals who are diagnosed because of the screening.

Women have been encouraged to undergo breast cancer screening for many decades. Early screening programs encouraged women to perform self-breast exams and also to have their clinician perform a breast exam in the office—subsequent data have shown that these screening techniques lead to false-positive exams, and no studies have shown an association of these exams with a reduction in mortality. Most guideline groups no longer recommend breast self-exam or clinician breast exam for screening.

Breast cancer screening with mammography continues to be recommended by many groups, although the benefits are less than we had hoped and we are learning more about the harms. Mammography is an x-ray exam that takes views of each breast. The recommended age for the first mammogram and the frequency of screening vary among guidelines and countries. The US Preventive Services Task Force periodically reviews the evidence and issues guidelines to help aid discussions with women about screening.

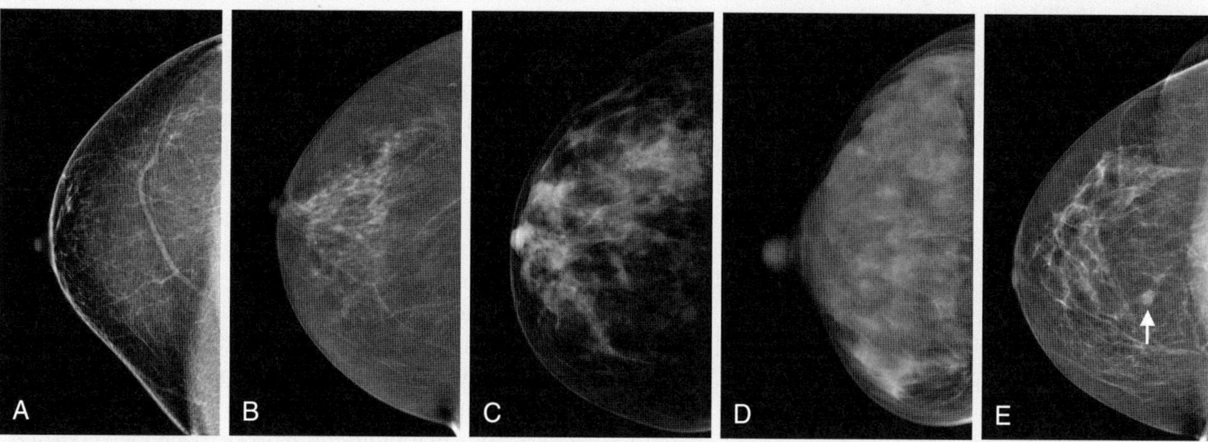

Mammographic Views of Various Breast Densities **A**, Almost entirely fat. **B**, Scattered fibroglandular densities. **C**, Heterogeneously dense. **D**, Extremely dense. **E**, Mammogram showing invasive cancer. (From Fuller MS, Lee CI, Elmore JG. Breast cancer screening: an evidence-based update. *Med Clin North Am.* 2015;99[3]:451–468; images provided by Christoph I. Lee, MD, MSHS.)

The benefits, risks, and accuracy of mammography screening depend on numerous factors, including a woman's age and breast density (see Figure), and the time interval between screening exams. Possible risks of screening are important to consider because screening at a population level involves testing healthy individuals; we are to "first, do no harm," and screening can have potential harms.

No medical test is perfect. Approximately 10% of screening mammograms in the United States are interpreted as "abnormal," requiring additional testing. The great majority of women with these "abnormal" exams do not have breast cancer; this is called a *false-positive result.* The false-positive results lead to additional diagnostic testing, which can result in anxiety and morbidity for women. It is estimated that at least 50% of women in the United States who are screened annually for a decade will have experienced at least one false-positive examination.

Another harm of screening mammography is overdiagnosis—a *diagnosis* of cancer that would never have harmed the woman during her lifetime; such diagnoses can be either of a preinvasive lesion (e.g., ductal carcinoma in situ [DCIS]) or of invasive breast cancer. With more women undergoing screening with mammography, we have seen a sharp increase in the number of women *diagnosed* with DCIS and early-stage breast cancer. By definition, DCIS is not an invasive carcinoma and not an immediate life-threatening cancer—it is confined to the duct—but DCIS is often treated as if it is an invasive early-stage breast cancer. Even though women with DCIS are at increased risk of a subsequent, invasive breast cancer *diagnosis,* most women with DCIS are never subsequently diagnosed with invasive cancer and treatment of DCIS does not alter mortality. Some discussion has centered on changing the name of DCIS lesions to better differentiate preinvasive DCIS from invasive cancer because the term *carcinoma* is similar to the term *cancer.* However, it is not likely that the name will be changed because of its current common use.

Unfortunately, we are not able to identify which women with a new diagnosis of DCIS or invasive breast cancer have the type of lesion that is so low risk that it will never harm them during their lifetime. Thus most women undergo treatment, which can include either lumpectomy and radiation therapy or mastectomy. This is overtreatment if the DCIS or invasive cancer was overdiagnosed. Estimates of the prevalence of overdiagnosis vary in the literature from 10%–50%, with many groups suggesting that approximately 1 in 5 women with a new diagnosis of breast cancer are overdiagnosed; more research is clearly needed.

Women with abnormalities noted on screening mammography are often asked to return for additional diagnostic imaging and sometimes even a breast biopsy. Some women think that a breast biopsy will provide an immediate and definitive diagnosis; however, this is not always the case. Pathologists have been noted to disagree on the diagnoses of atypia and DCIS.

Balancing the benefits and harms of breast cancer screening is not an easy task for women or their clinicians. Every woman should be encouraged to make an informed decision.

From Elmore JG. Solving the problem of overdiagnosis. *New England Journal of Medicine*, 2016;375(15):1483–1486; Elmore JG, Barton MB, Moceri VM, Polk S, Arena PJ, Fletcher SW. Ten-year risk of false positive screening mammograms and clinical breast examinations. *New England Journal of Medicine*, 1998;338(16):1089–1096; Elmore JG, Longton GM, Carney PA, et al. Diagnostic concordance among pathologists interpreting breast biopsy specimens. *Journal of the American Medical Association*, 2015;313(11):1122–1132; Fuller MS, Lee CI, Elmore JG. Breast cancer screening: An evidence-based update. *Medical Clinics of North America*, 2015;99(3):451–468; Elmore JG, Wild DMG, Nelson HD, Katz DL. *Jekel's epidemiology, biostatistics, preventive medicine, and public health*, 5th edition. Philadelphia: Elsevier; 2020; Pace LE, Keating NL. A systematic assessment of benefits and risks to guide breast cancer screening decisions. *Journal of the American Medical Association*, 2014;311(13):1327–1335; U.S. Preventive Services Task Force (USPSTF). Screening for breast cancer: U.S. Preventive Services Task Force recommendation statement. *Annals of Internal Medicine*, 2009;151(10):716–726; U.S. Preventive Services Task Force (USPSTF). *Final Recommendation Statement Breast Cancer: Screening.* Available at https://www.uspreventiveservicestaskforce.org/Page/Document/RecommendationStatementFinal/breast-cancer-screening1.

among individuals but also at the level of the tumor itself, involving both genetic and epigenetic processes. Phenotypic heterogeneity is the result of tumor cell plasticity and, combined with genetic factors of the tumor, determines whether cells resist environmental stress, such as from the surrounding microenvironment (e.g., hypoxia, entering dormancy) and metastasizing.[214] The most important of the dominant genes are the breast cancer susceptibility genes *(BRCA1, BRCA2)* (see Pathophysiology section).

Risk

Although breast cancer is a multifactorial disease involving a complex web of interacting factors, risk is related to timing, duration, and pattern of exposures. Risk factors and possible causes of breast cancer can be divided into the following categories: age, gender, personal and family history of breast cancer, histologic, genetic, and reproductive risk factors, exogenous hormone use, and environmental factors (Table 25.8).

TABLE 25.8 Factors That Increase the Relative Risk for Breast Cancer in Women

Relative Risk	Factor
>4.0	Age (65+ vs. <65 years, although risk increases across all ages until age 80) Atypical hyperplasia Lobular carcinoma in situ Pathogenic genetic variations (e.g., *BRCA1, BRCA2, PALB2, TP53*)
2.1–4.0	Ductal carcinoma in situ High endogenous hormone levels (postmenopausal) High-dose radiation to chest (e.g., Hodgkin lymphoma treatment) Mammographically dense breasts Two or more first-degree relatives with breast cancer
1.1–2.0	Alcohol consumption Early menarche (<11 years) Excess body weight High endogenous estrogen or testosterone levels (premenopausal) Late age at first full-term pregnancy (>30 years) Late menopause (>55 years) Never breastfed a child No full-term pregnancies One first-degree relative with breast cancer Obesity (postmenopausal) Personal history of ovarian or endometrial cancer Physical inactivity Proliferative breast disease without atypia (usual ductal hyperplasia, fibroadenoma) Recent and long-term use of menopausal hormone therapy containing estrogen and progestin Recent hormonal contraceptive use Weight gain in adulthood Tall height

Data from American Cancer Society (ACS). *Breast Cancer Facts & Figures 2019–2020*. Atlanta, GA: Author; 2020.

The Institute of Medicine reports that the two most strongly associated environmental factors are exposure to ionizing radiation and combined postmenopausal HT.[215] Ionizing radiation (e.g., x-rays, CT scans, and fluoroscopy) is a known mutagen and an established carcinogen for breast cancer. To date, only accidentally or medically induced radiation has been demonstrated to exert a carcinogenic effect on the breast.

The female reproductive hormones (estrogens, progesterone, and prolactin) have a major role and effect on mammary gland development and breast cancer (Fig. 25.26). Physiologic concentrations of estradiol increase the mitogenic activity of epithelial cells[216]; therefore increasing blood levels of estradiol increase the risk of breast cancer. Early menarche, late menopause, and short menstrual cycles all increase the risk, whereas menopause slows the *rate* of increase of breast cancer and oophorectomy reduces the risk. Environmental chemicals affect estrogen metabolism and contribute to breast cancer. Xenoestrogens are synthetic chemicals that mimic the actions of estrogens and are found in many pesticides, fuels, plastics, detergents, and drugs. The most significant chemicals may be polychlorinated biphenyls (PCBs), such as dichlorodiphenyltrichloroethane (DDT), pesticides (dieldrin, aldrin, heptachlor, and others), bisphenol A (pervasive in polycarbonate plastics), tobacco smoke (active and passive), dioxins (vehicle exhaust, incineration, contaminated food supply), alkylphenols (detergents and cleaning products), metals, phthalates (makes plastics flexible, some cosmetics), parabens (antimicrobials), food additives (recombinant bovine somatotropin [rBST] and zeranol to enhance growth in cattle and sheep), menopausal hormone treatment (MHT) (i.e., HRT), and others.

Other risks associated with breast cancer include increased alcohol consumption, the use of insulin therapy, sulfonylurea medications, obesity, and weight gain after menopause.[217–220] Ethanol increases estrogen concentrations through several mechanisms: (1) increase in aromatase activity; (2) inhibition in estrogen breakdown; (3) decrease of melatonin secretion, which inhibits estrogen production; and (4) increase in hepatic oxidative stress that interferes with estrogen metabolism.[221] Excess adiposity is positively associated with breast cancer recurrence and breast cancer–specific mortality among both premenopausal and postmenopausal women. Excess adipose tissue increases the risk from cellular pathways that involve hormonal regulation, cellular proliferation, and immunity. The increase in breast cancer risk with increasing BMI among postmenopausal females is most likely the result of increases in levels of estrogens by aromatase activity in adipose tissue. However, studies of hormones secreted by adipose tissue, *leptin* and *adiponectin*, may underlie the association between obesity and breast cancer risk. From molecular mechanism studies, leptin enhances breast cancer cell proliferation by inhibiting cell death (pro-apoptosis) signaling pathways and by increasing in vitro sensitivity to estrogens. A sedentary lifestyle may increase cancer risk through several mechanisms, including increased insulin resistance, increased inflammation, and decreased immune function. Epidemiologic studies demonstrate that physical activity lowered the risk of breast cancer in both premenopausal and postmenopausal women, and decreased the mortality in breast

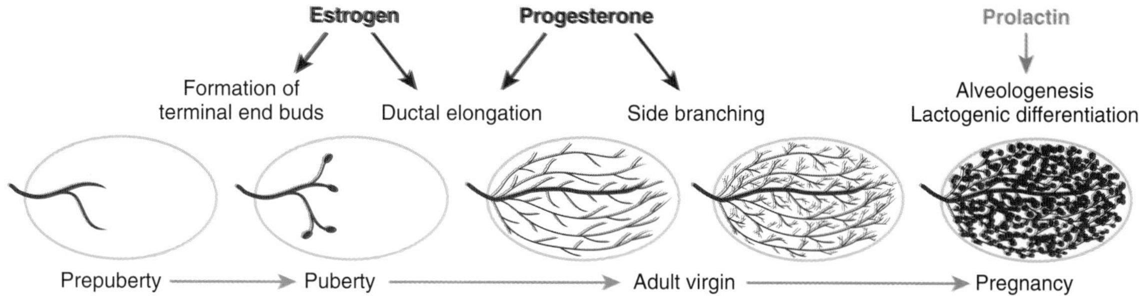

Fig. 25.26 Mammary Gland Development in the Mouse. Schematic representation of distinct stages of postnatal mammary gland development. (From Brisken C, Hess, K, Jeitziner R. Progesterone and overlooked endocrine pathways in breast cancer pathogenesis. *Endocrinology,* 2015;156(10):3442–3450.)

cancer survivors and improved their physiologic and immune functions.[222-224] Dietary factors also influence the risk of breast cancer.

Dietary factors also influence the risk of breast cancer. Dietary fiber may decrease the risk of breast cancer through modification of the estrogen concentration and stimulation of intestinal microflora. A recent meta-analysis revealed that every increment in dietary fiber of 10 g/day was associated with a significant reduction in breast cancer risk.[225,226]

Types

Most breast cancers are adenocarcinomas and first arise from the ductal/lobular epithelium as carcinoma in situ (CIS), which is a proliferation of epithelial cells that is confined to the ducts and lobules by the basement membrane (BM). Tumors of the infiltrating (invasive) ductal type do not grow to a large size, but they metastasize early (Fig. 25.27). This type accounts for 70% of breast cancers. Table 25.9 summarizes some types of breast cancer.

Ductal and Lobular Carcinoma in Situ

Ductal carcinoma in situ (DCIS) is a heterogeneous group of proliferative lesions limited to breast ducts and lobules without invasion of the BM. When DCIS breaches the BM and invades adjacent stroma, microinvasion (MI) is said to be present. Approximately 84% of all in situ disease is DCIS; the remainder is mostly lobular carcinoma in situ. DCIS occurs predominantly in females but can occur in males. Because DCIS is almost exclusively detected by mammography, the large increase in the incidence of DCIS over the past 20 years can be attributed to screening.[227] Approximately 49,290 cases of DCIS will be diagnosed in females in 2021.[1] Because DCIS looks like invasive cancer, the presumption was that these lesions were the precursors of cancer; therefore early removal and treatment would reduce cancer incidence and mortality.[228] However, long-term epidemiologic studies have demonstrated that the removal of 50,000 to 60,000 DCIS lesions annually has not been accompanied by a reduction in the incidence of invasive cancer; therefore low- to intermediate-grade DCIS does not need to be a target for screening or early detection.[229]

Lobular Carcinoma In Situ

Lobular carcinoma in situ (LCIS) originates from the terminal duct lobular unit. Unlike DCIS, LCIS has a uniform appearance—the cells expand but do not distort involved spaces; thus the lobular structure is preserved. The cells grow in noncohesive clusters, usually because of a loss of the tumor-suppressive adhesion protein E-cadherin. LCIS is found as an incidental lesion from a biopsy and not from mammography because it is not associated with calcifications or stromal reactions that produce mammographic densities (MDs). LCIS has an incidence of approximately 1% to 6% of all carcinomas and does not increase with mammographic screening. With biopsies in both breasts, LCIS is bilateral in 20% to 40% of cases, compared with 10% to 20% of cases of DCIS.

The cells of AH, LCIS, and invasive lobular carcinoma are structurally identical. Loss of cellular adhesion because of dysfunction of E-cadherin results in a rounded shape without attachment to adjacent cells, increasing the risk of invasion. E-cadherin functions as a tumor-suppressor protein and may be lost in neoplastic proliferations from various mechanisms, including mutation. LCIS is a risk factor for invasive carcinoma, which develops in 25% to 35% of women over a period of 20 to 30 years. Unlike DCIS, the risk is almost as high in the contralateral breast as in the ipsilateral breast.

Pathophysiology. Breast cancer is a heterogeneous disease with diverse molecular, biologic, phenotypic, and pathologic changes. Tumor heterogeneity results from the genetic, epigenetic, and microenvironmental influences that occur as tumors progress. Most breast cancers develop due to DNA damage and genetic mutations. Inheritance factors of procancerous genes *BRCA1* and *BRCA2* play a role in the development of breast cancer. Up to 25% of hereditary cases are because of a mutation in one of the highly penetrant genes (*BRCA1, BRCA2, PTEN, TP53, CDHI,* and *STKII*), which confer up to an 80% lifetime risk of breast cancer.[230] An additional 2% to 3% of cases are because of a mutation in a rare, moderate penetrant gene (e.g., *CHEK2, BRIP 1, ATM,* and *PALB2*).[230] BRCA1 (breast cancer 1 gene), located on chromosome 17, is a tumor-suppressor gene; therefore any mutation in the gene may inhibit or alter its suppressor function, leading to uncontrolled cell proliferation.[230] BRCA2 (breast cancer 2 gene) is located on chromosome 13.[230]

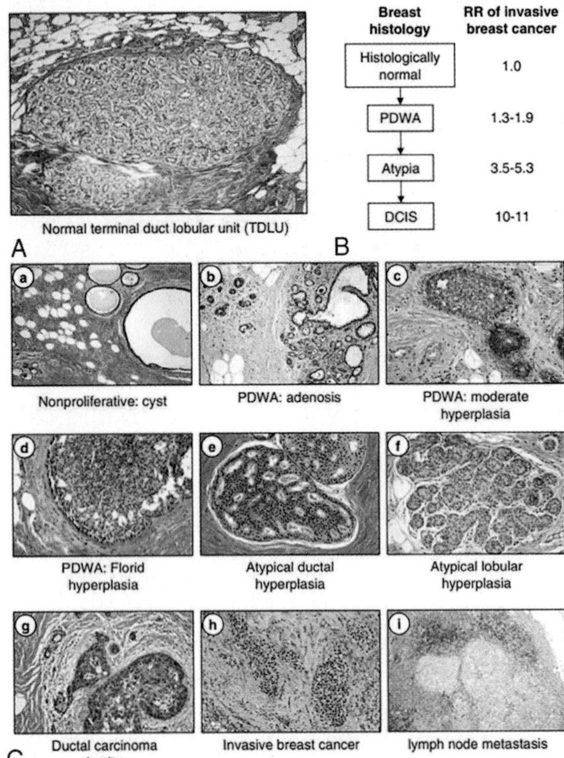

Fig. 25.27 Pathologic Characteristics Associated With Breast Cancer Progression. **(A)** Normal terminal duct lobular unit (TDLU), the anatomic structure where breast cancer originates, numerous acini surrounded by interlobular stroma. **(B)** Model of progression from normal epithelium through benign breast disease to invasive breast cancer. Women with proliferative disease without atypia (PDWA) have an increased lifetime risk for cancer development relative risk (RR) of 1.3 to 1.9; women with atypical hyperplasia (atypia) have RR of 3.5 to 5.3; women with ductal carcinoma in situ (DCIS) have RR of 10 to 11. **(C)** Stages of progression from benign breast disease to invasive, metastatic breast cancer. *a*, Nonproliferative disease showing mammary cysts from TDLU. *b*, Proliferative disease without atypia (PDWA): adenosis, a proliferative lesion characterized by increased number or size of glandular structures. *c*, PDWA: moderate hyperplasia, with an increased number of epithelial cells in breast ducts and lobules with 5 or more cells above the basement membrane. *d*, PDWA: florid hyperplasia with hyperplastic cells, in solid clusters distending the lumens. *e*, Atypical ductal hyperplasia, epithelial hyperplasia and monotonous cytologic features suggesting expansion of a cell population. *f*, Atypical lobular hyperplasia with enlarged lobules some involvement with acini expanded with monotonous dyshesive epithelial cells. *g*, DCIS, a malignant proliferation of epithelial cells remaining within the basement membrane; some surrounding inflammatory infiltrate. *h*, Invasive breast cancer, malignant cells have invaded the surrounding stromal tissues. *i*, Lymph node metastasis. (From Cichon MA, Degnim AC, Visscher DW, Radisky DC. Microenvironmental influences that drive progression from benign breast disease to invasive breast cancer. *Journal of Mammary Gland Biology and Neoplasia*, 2010;15(4):389–397.)

Males who develop breast cancer are more likely to have a *BRCA2* mutation than a *BRCA1* mutation (Chapter 26).

The immune system normally attacks cells with abnormal DNA or abnormal growth; however, this mechanism fails in those individuals with breast cancer, leading to tumor growth and metastatic spread. Cells communicate through paracrine or contact-dependent signaling from ligands, which is mediated from components of the microenvironment, such as blood vessels, immune cells, and fibroblasts (see Chapter 2). Cancer cells also communicate using the same system, and the cooperative behavior of these groups of cells can influence cancer progression. In advanced primary carcinomas, cancer cells recruit a variety of cell types into the surrounding stroma, including fibroblasts, myofibroblasts, granulocytes, macrophages, mesenchymal stem cells, and lymphocytes. Tissue involution involves massive epithelial cell death, recruitment and activation of fibroblasts, stromal remodeling, and immune cell infiltration, including macrophages with similarities to microenvironments present during wound healing and tumor progression.[231,232]

Once a founding tumor clone is established, genomic instability may assist through the establishment of other subclones and contribute both to tumor progression and to therapy resistance. Phenotypic plasticity is exemplified by a distinctive phenotype called epithelial-mesenchymal transition (EMT). EMT is involved in the generation of tissues and organs during embryogenesis, is essential for driving tissue plasticity during development, and is an unintentional process during cancer progression. Activation of an EMT program during cancer development often requires signaling between cancer cells and neighboring stromal cells (Fig. 25.28). The EMT-associated reprogramming is involved in many cancer cell characteristics, including suppression of cell death or apoptosis and senescence, is reactivated during wound healing, and is resistant to chemotherapy and radiation therapy. Overall, interactions of cancer cells with adjacent tumor-associated stromal cells may induce malignant cell phenotypes (Fig. 25.29).

Stromal fibroblasts adjacent to the breast tumor express aromatase, actively induce local estrogen production, and signal crosstalk between estrogen and growth factors, all of which affect the progression of breast carcinoma (Fig. 25.30).

Remodeling or reprogramming of the breast during postpregnancy involution is important because it involves inflammatory and "wound healing–like" tissue reactions known as reactive stroma or inflammatory stroma. These tissue reactions increase the risk for tumor invasion and may facilitate the transition of CIS to invasive carcinoma. Overall, for breast cancer, the long-term protective effects of pregnancy affect remodeling of the stromal microenvironment by causing apoptosis and involution. In postlactational involution, the mammary gland regresses and remodels to its prepregnant state, whereby fibroblasts secrete proteases that degrade the ECM proteins. Consequently, the increased release of bioactive matrix fragments can promote tumor growth, motility, and invasion.[233]

TABLE 25.9 Types of Breast Carcinoma and Major Distinguishing Features

	Distinguishing Features
Carcinoma of the Mammary Ducts	
Papillary	Well-delineated cystic masses in multiple areas; hemorrhage often present; majority appear in 40- to 60-year age group; often involves skin
Intraductal (comedo)	Often accompanied by evidence of inflammation; well-circumscribed tumors within duct; well-differentiated tumor cells; rarely ulcerates skin
Infiltrating Carcinoma	
Ductal (no specific type [NST])	Fibrous, firm, glistening, gray-tan mass with chalky streaks, mixture of patterns; may cause discharge from nipple; represents about 70%–80% of all breast cancers
Mucinous	Usually large (>3 cm in diameter), circumscribed, and encapsulated, glistening appearance, varies in color; two types: pure and mixed; pure tumor is surrounded by mucin; infrequent; found in lateral half of breast; tends to occur in women after age 70
Medullary	Encapsulated and grows very large (7–8 cm in diameter); commonly surrounded by lymphocytic inflammatory infiltrate; occurs after age 50
Tubular	Well-differentiated with orderly tubules in center (stroma) of mass; can be associated with noninfiltrating ductal carcinoma; occurs in women about age 50; nodal metastasis infrequent; occurrence is rare
Adenoid cystic	Very rare; well-circumscribed, painless mass arising from nipple and areola
Metaplastic	Involves cartilage or bone, mixed tumors or osteogenic sarcomas
Squamous cell	Frequent in black people; originates in ductal epithelium
Carcinoma of the Mammary Lobules	
Lobular carcinoma in situ	Found in individuals with fibrocystic disease; localized to upper breast quadrants; 15%–35% risk of becoming invasive; occurs frequently in mid-40s; infiltrating variety occurs in early 50 s
Infiltrating lobular	Infiltrates from duct; firm mass with chalky streaks
Paget disease	Eczema of nipple that extends to areola; cancer usually found underneath nipple; poorly circumscribed; large Paget cells arise from duct and directly invade nipple; history of scaly, red rash spreading from nipple; lesion palpable beneath nipple, often bilateral; occurs in middle age
Inflammatory carcinoma	Not a histologic type; fairly diffuse within breast tissue, diffuse edema of overlying skin; extremely undifferentiated, very rare; most metastasize to axilla
Sarcoma of the Breast	
Cystosarcoma phyllodes	Usually large (>17 cm in diameter); mostly localized but can rupture through skin; rarely metastasizes to lymph nodes; history of painless nodule present for years before it forms a large mass; ulceration and bleeding of skin often present; occurs in wide age range (13–77 years)
Fibrosarcoma	Well-circumscribed, firm, and usually does not involve skin or nipple; well-differentiated to extremely undifferentiated; arises from connective tissue; extremely rare (e.g., liposarcoma, angiosarcoma)

Hormones, commonly estrogen, may act as accelerators, as well as initiators, delay involution, and influence the susceptibility of the breast epithelium to environmental carcinogens. Hormones control the differentiation of the mammary gland epithelium, thereby regulating the rate of stem cell division. A vast majority of breast cancers are *initially* hormone dependent (estrogen positive [ER+] and/or progesterone positive [PR+]), with estrogens playing a crucial role in their development. Estrogens control processes critical for cellular functions by regulating activities and expression of key signaling molecules. These processes include regulation of receptor activity and receptor interaction with other intracellular proteins and DNA.

Endogenous estrogen may promote the progression of ER-negative breast cancer by stimulating cancer-associated fibroblasts to secrete factors from the microenvironment, which can recruit bone marrow–derived cells to the tumor microenvironment exerting tumor-promoting effects.[234] Estrogens can modulate immune function in the mammary gland. For example, estradiol can promote a proinflammatory phenotype in macrophages and estrogen can promote immunosuppression.

Progesterone also plays a complex role in breast physiology and carcinogenesis (Fig. 25.31).[216] In the breast, cell proliferation occurs during the luteal phase of the menstrual cycle and is accompanied by changes in the microenvironment.[235–237]

Dormant cells appear to perpetuate carcinogenesis and form the precursors of eventual metastatic relapse and, sometimes, rapid recurrence. These dormant cells are called minimal residual disease. Cancer metastases require that primary

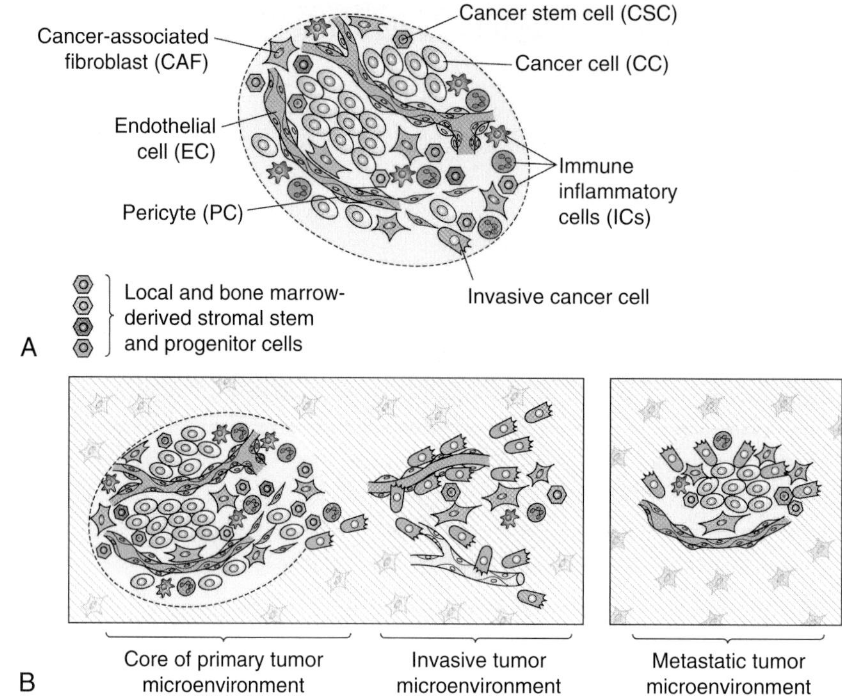

Fig. 25.28 Cells of the Tumor Microenvironment. **(A)** Distinct cell types constitute most solid tumors, including breast tumors. Both the main cellular tissue, called *parenchyma*, and the surrounding tissue, or stroma, of tumors contain cell types that enable tumor growth and progression. For example, the immune-inflammatory cells present in tumors can include both tumor-promoting and tumor-killing subclasses of cells. **(B)** The microenvironment of tumors. Multiple stromal cell types create a succession of tumor microenvironments that change as tumors invade normal tissue, eventually seeding and colonizing distant tissues. The organization, numbers, and phenotypic characteristics of the stromal cell types and the extracellular matrix *(hatched background)* evolve during progression and enable primary, invasive, and metastatic growth. (The premalignant stages are not shown.) (Data from Hanahan D, Weinberg R. Hallmarks of cancer: The next generation. *Cell*, 2011;144:646–674.)

tumor cells evolve the ability to intravasate into the lymphatic system or vasculature, and extravasate into and colonize secondary sites.

Clinical Manifestations. The majority of carcinomas of the breast occur in the upper outer quadrant, where most of the glandular tissue of the breast is located. The lymphatic spread of cancer to the opposite breast, to lymph nodes in the base of the neck, and to the abdominal cavity is caused by obstruction of the normal lymphatic pathways or destruction of lymphatic vessels by surgery or radiotherapy. The less common inner quadrant tumors may spread to mediastinal nodes or Rotter nodes, which are located between the pectoral muscles. Internal mammary chain nodes also are common sites of metastasis. Metastases from the vertebral veins can involve the vertebrae, pelvic bones, ribs, and skull. The lungs, kidneys, liver, adrenal glands, ovaries, and pituitary gland are also sites of metastasis.

The first sign of breast cancer is usually an irregularly shaped, firm, painless lump. Pain is rarely a sign of breast cancer. Other presenting signs include palpable nodes in the axilla, retraction of tissue (dimpling) (Fig. 25.32), or bone pain caused by metastasis to the vertebrae in rare cases. Table 25.10 summarizes the clinical manifestations of breast cancers. Manifestations vary according to the type of tumor and stage of disease.

Evaluation and Treatment. Clinical breast examination, mammography, ultrasound, MRI, biopsy, hormone receptor assays, and gene expression profiling are used in evaluating breast alterations and cancer. Conventional x-ray mammography is one of the most valuable diagnostic tools for imaging of the breast and is the common preventive screening method for breast cancer. Currently, full-field digital mammography (FFDM) is frequently used. The USPSTF periodically reviews the evidence and issues guidelines to aid women about screening mammography (see Box 25.12).

Continuous technical development has led to several new imaging techniques, including digital breast tomosynthesis (DBT), phase contrast x-ray imaging, thermography,[238] and CT of the breast, as well as ultrasound and MRI. Despite technical innovations, except for ultrasound and MRI, these modalities require exposure of breast tissue to ionizing radiation.

Percutaneous breast biopsy is the preferred method of diagnosis because risks are minimal compared with surgical excisional biopsy. Most of the United States enacted laws mandating that mammography facilities report breast density, but inconsistent

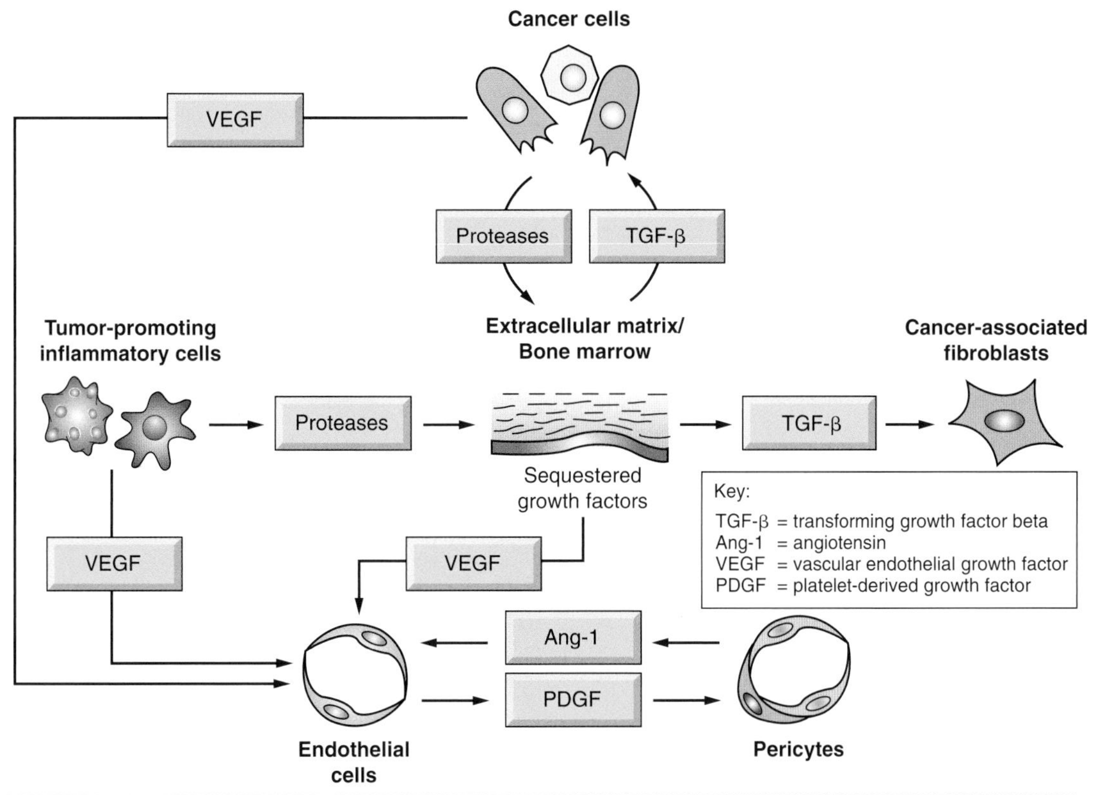

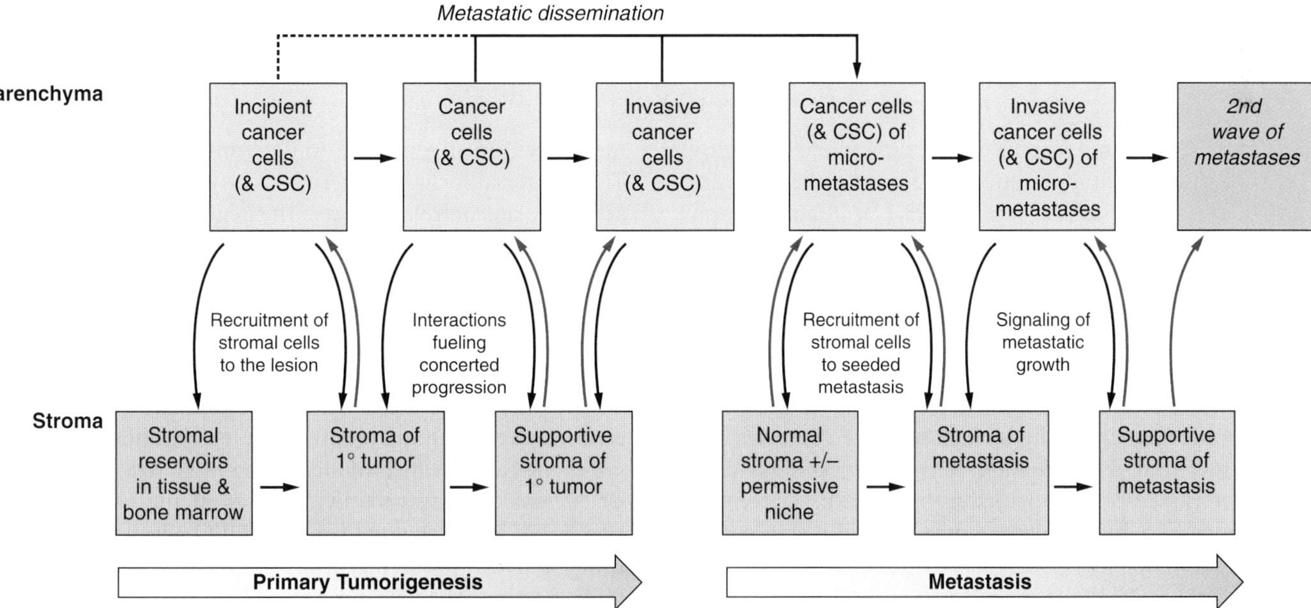

Fig. 25.29 Signaling Interactions in the Tumor Microenvironment During Malignant Progression. *Upper panel*, Numerous cell types constitute the tumor microenvironment and are orchestrated and maintained by reciprocal interactions. *Lower panel*, The reciprocal interactions between the breast main tissue (parenchyma) and the surrounding stroma are important for cancer progression and growth. Certain organ sites of "fertile soil" or "metastasis niches" facilitate metastatic seeding and colonization. Cancer stem cells are involved in some or all stages of tumor development and progression. (Adapted from Hanahan D, Weinberg R. Hallmarks of cancer: The next generation. *Cell*, 2011;144:646–674.)

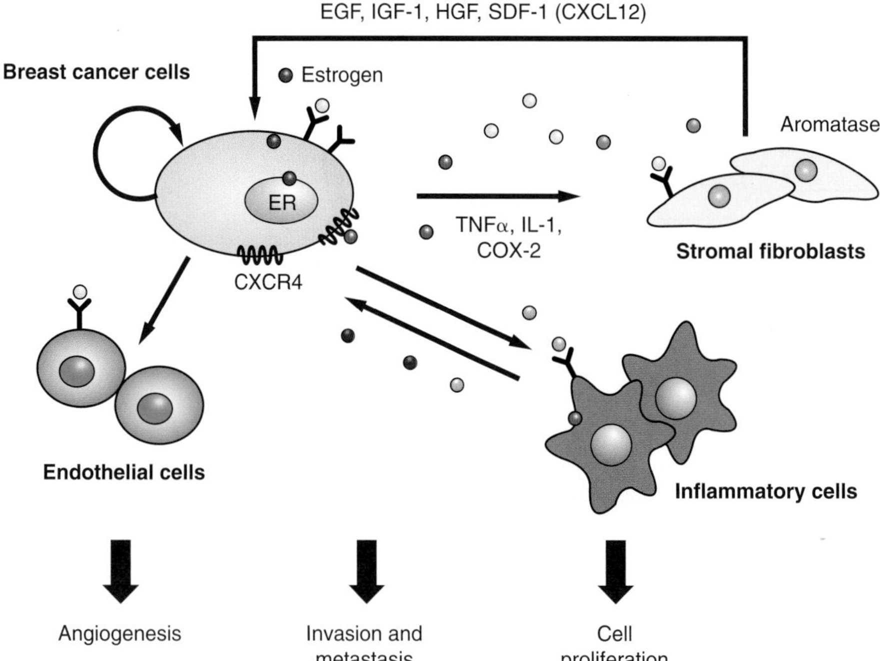

Fig. 25.30 Breast Cancer Cells and Stromal Fibroblasts Produce Estrogen. In the microenvironment of breast carcinoma, breast cancer cells interact with different stromal cells through the secretion of growth factors and cytokines. Fibroblasts adjacent to cancer cells produce estrogen through the expression of the enzyme aromatase, which is induced by several factors including tumor necrosis factor-alpha *(TNF-α)*, interleukin-1 *(IL-1)*, and cyclooxygenase-2 *(COX-2)*. *EGF*, Epidermal growth factor; *ER*, estrogen receptor; *HGF*, hepatocyte growth factor; *IGF*, insulin-like growth factor; *SDF-1*, stromal-derived factor 1 also known as *CXCL12* or chemokine 12. These interactions lead to cancer cell proliferation, angiogenesis, and metastasis. (Adapted from Yamaguchi Y, Hayashi S. Estrogen-related cancer microenvironment of breast carcinoma. *Endocrine Journal*, 2009;56(1):1–7.)

guidelines have caused confusion.[239] Mammographic density (MD) is the radiologic appearance of the breast, reflecting variations in breast composition (see Box 25.12). Mammographic breast density appears white or dense on a mammogram, is expressed as a percentage of the mammogram, and is a strong and consistent risk factor for breast cancer.[240–242]

A new hand-held breast-scanning device, called iBreastExam (iBE), can be used by community health workers to screen for breast abnormalities. With the increasing incidence of breast cancer worldwide, especially for low-resource countries, such a device is critical. iBE technology is free of radiation and uses a piezoelectric sensor array, which can measure tissue compression and stiffness by top-down touching of the skin surface. The device can enhance clinical breast examination sensitivity by 19% while maintaining high specificity (94%) and a negative predictive value of 98%. This is a promising tool for early detection of relevant lesions, and it is useful in younger females with dense breasts.[243–245] iBE received FDA approval as an aid in documenting palpable breast lesions from a clinical breast exam; it is to be used by qualified health care professionals and is not intended for home use. It currently is being used in low-resource countries.

Treatment is based on the extent or stage of the cancer. The extent of the tumor at the primary site, the presence and extent of lymph node metastases, and the presence of distant metastases are all evaluated to determine the stage of disease. Treatment can include surgery with or without radiotherapy to achieve local control of cancer. The benefit of surgery for treatment is that it eliminates cancer bulk and the diversity of cancer cells, including therapy-resistant cells.[246] Systemic therapy in the form of chemotherapy, hormonal therapy, targeted therapy, or combination therapy is indicated when there is a risk for metastatic relapse. Minimal residual disease may remain after initial chemotherapy, radiotherapy, and surgery. Current treatments preferentially kill proliferating cells, but dormant cells are not proliferating, which renders them more resistant to almost all current treatments.[246] Evidence from the US Agency for Healthcare Research and Quality (AHRQ) shows that estrogen combined with progestogen has both beneficial effects (fewer osteoporotic fractures) and harmful effects (increased risk of breast cancer, gallbladder disease, venous thromboembolic events, and stroke). The AHRQ published a systematic review from 283 trials comparing the effectiveness of treatments for menopausal symptoms.[247]

Options for those who have a positive test for the *BRCA1* or *BRCA2* mutation include surveillance to detect cancers early, prophylactic surgery (i.e., bilateral mastectomy and bilateral salpingo-oophorectomy), risk factor avoidance, and promotion of breast-feeding. There is emerging science that suggests vitamin D may play a pivotal role in cancer prevention in addition to its

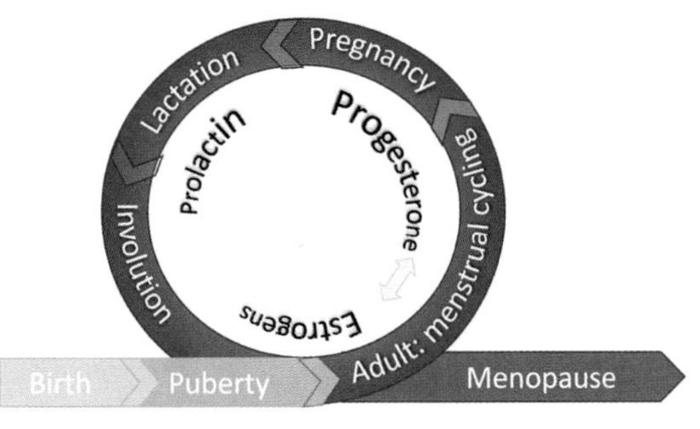

- Variation in levels across lifespan
- Dependence on other hormones

Progesterone plays a complex role in breast physiology and carcinogenesis:

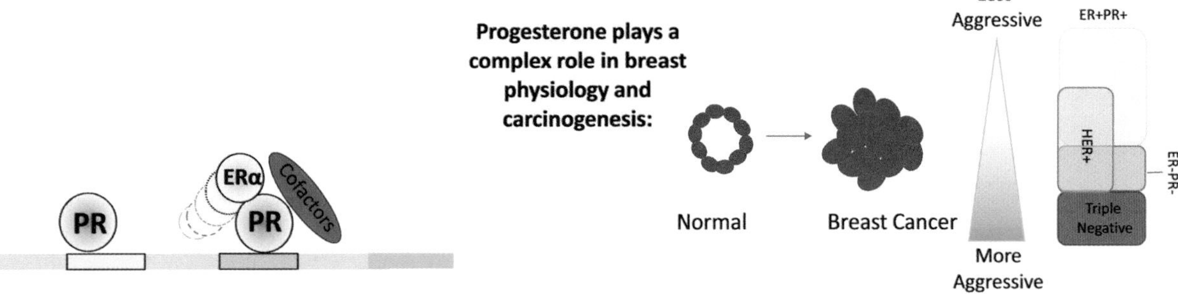

- Dependence of PR transcription on ERα-mediated transcriptional events
- Progesterone promotes differentiation and proliferation primarily via paracrine actions between PR+ and PR- breast cells

Fig. 25.31 A Graphical Presentation of Progesterone's Complex Role in Breast Physiology and Carcinogenesis. (From Trabert B, Sherman ME, Kannan N, Stanczyk FZ. Progesterone and breast cancer. *Endocrine Reviews,* 2020;41(2):320–344, https://doi.org/10.1210/endrev/bnz001.)

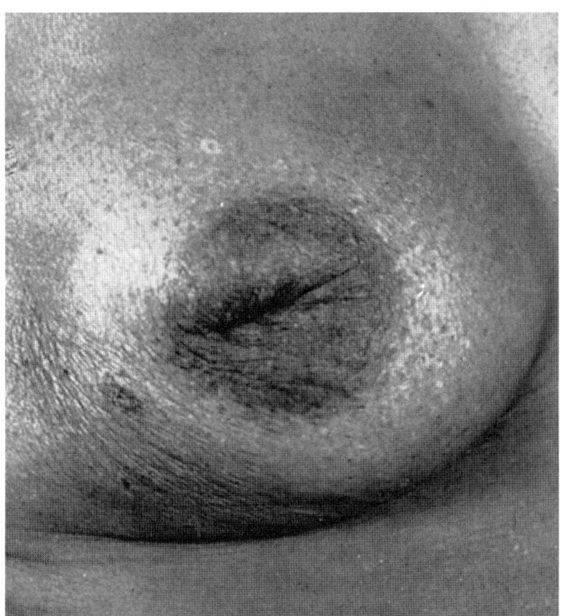

Fig. 25.32 Retraction of Nipple Caused by Carcinoma. (From del Regato JA, Spjut HJ. *Ackerman and del Regato's cancer: Diagnosis, treatment, and prognosis,* 6th edition. St. Louis: Mosby; 1985.)

TABLE 25.10 Clinical Manifestations of Breast Cancer

Clinical Manifestation	Pathophysiology
Local pain	Local obstruction caused by tumor
Dimpling of skin	Can occur with invasion of dermal lymphatics because of retraction of Cooper ligament or involvement of pectoralis fascia
Nipple retraction	Shortening of mammary ducts
Skin retraction	Involvement of suspensory ligament
Edema	Local inflammation or lymphatic obstruction
Nipple/areolar eczema	Paget disease
Pitting of skin (similar to surface of an orange *[peau dorange]*)	Obstruction of subcutaneous lymphatics, resulting in accumulation of fluid
Reddened skin, local tenderness, and warmth	Inflammation
Dilated blood vessels	Obstruction of venous return by a fast-growing tumor; obstruction dilates superficial veins
Nipple discharge in a nonlactating woman	Spontaneous and intermittent discharge caused by tumor obstruction
Ulceration	Tumor necrosis
Hemorrhage	Erosion of blood vessels
Edema of arm	Obstruction of lymphatic drainage in axilla
Chest pain	Metastasis to lung

EMERGING SCIENCE BOX
Vitamin D and Breast Cancer

Epidemiologic studies have identified that vitamin D may play a role in cancer prevention in addition to its role in bone metabolism. Vitamin D as a prohormone is metabolized in the liver and kidney, which produces calcitriol. Calcitriol then binds to the vitamin D receptor and regulates the expression of varied genes. Hormonally active calcitriol exerts antiproliferative, proapoptotic, and antiinflammatory effects. These properties have demonstrated anticancer effects in breast cancer cells. A study by Krishnan and colleagues found that dietary vitamin D_3 exhibits substantial tumor inhibitory effects in animal tissue of breast cancer equal to those of calcitriol. In a secondary analysis of the **VIT**amin D and Omeg**A**-3 Tria**L** (VITAL) randomized clinical trial, findings suggested dietary vitamin D_3 might reduce the risk of advanced cancer in individuals with normal body mass index. A study measuring the metabolite serum 25-hydroxyvitamin D also found that low levels were associated with poor prognosis in women with breast cancer. Studies continue to further evaluate appropriate vitamin D levels, recommended supplements, and further potential protective effects of vitamin D and cancers.

Data from Chandler PD, et al. Effect of vitamin D3 supplements on development of advanced cancer: A secondary analysis of the VITAL Randomized Clinical Trial. *JAMA Network Open,* 2020;3(11):e2025850, Erratum in *JAMA Network Open,* 2020;3(12):e2032460; Jeon SM, et al. Exploring vitamin D metabolism and function in cancer. *Experimental and Molecular Medicine,* 2018;50(4):20; Krishnan AV, et al. Equivalent anticancer activities of dietary vitamin D and calcitriol in an animal model of breast cancer: Importance of mammary CYP27B1 for treatment and prevention. *Journal of Steroid Biochemistry and Molecular Biology,* 2013;136:289–295; and Yao S, et al. Association of serum level of vitamin D at diagnosis with breast cancer survival: A case-cohort analysis in the pathways study. *JAMA Oncology,* 2017;3(3):351–357.

role in bone metabolism (see Emerging Science Box: Vitamin D and Breast Cancer.)

DCIS should be considered a "risk factor" for invasive cancer and should prompt targeting for preventive strategies. Radiation therapy should not be routinely offered after lumpectomy for DCIS lesions that are not high-risk, because the absolute risk reduction in mortality was minimal (relative risk reduction in mortality of 23%).[248] Treatments for LCIS include close clinical follow-up and mammographic screening, tamoxifen, and bilateral prophylactic mastectomy.

The prognosis of stage 0 and stage I breast cancer has a 100% 5-year survival rate. Stage II and stage III has a 5-year survival rate of approximately 93% and 72%, respectively. However, as breast cancer spreads and metastasizes, the prognosis worsens. The 5-year survival rate is 22% for stage IV breast cancer.

SUMMARY REVIEW

Abnormalities of the Female Reproductive Tract

1. Abnormalities of the female reproductive tract have multifactorial causes, including genetics and environmental factors. Common abnormalities include uterine agenesis or structural malformations of the vagina, uterus, and fallopian tubes.

Alterations of Sexual Maturation

1. Sexual maturation, or puberty, is marked by the development of secondary sex characteristics, rapid growth and ultimately, the ability to reproduce. The normal range for the onset of puberty is now 8 to 13 years of age and can vary geographically and ethnically.
2. Delayed puberty is the onset of sexual maturation after these ages.
3. Precocious puberty is the onset before these ages.
4. Treatment depends on the etiology of the alteration in sexual maturation.

Disorders of the Female Reproductive System

1. The female reproductive system can be altered by hormonal imbalances, infectious microorganisms, inflammation, structural abnormalities, and benign or malignant proliferative conditions.
2. Primary dysmenorrhea is painful menstruation not associated with pelvic disease. It results from excessive synthesis of $PGF_2\alpha$. It often results from excessive synthesis of prostaglandins, which cause the myometrium to contract and constrict blood vessels, resulting in ischemic pain.
3. Secondary dysmenorrhea results from endometriosis, pelvic adhesions, inflammatory disease, uterine fibroids, or adenomyosis.
4. Primary amenorrhea is the continued absence of menarche and menstrual function by 13 years of age without the development of secondary sex characteristics or by 15 years of age if these changes have occurred.
5. Secondary amenorrhea is the absence of menstruation for a time equivalent to three or more cycles in women who have previously menstruated. Secondary amenorrhea is associated with many disorders and physiologic conditions.
6. Abnormal uterine bleeding (AUB) is heavy or irregular bleeding in the absence of organic disease.
7. Polycystic ovary syndrome (PCOS) is a condition in which excessive androgen production is triggered by inappropriate secretion of gonadotropins. This hormonal imbalance prevents ovulation and causes enlargement and cyst formation in the ovaries, excessive endometrial proliferation, and often hirsutism. Insulin resistance and hyperinsulinemia play a key role in androgen excess.
8. Premenstrual syndrome (PMS) is the cyclic recurrence of physical, psychological, or behavioral changes distressing

enough to disrupt normal activities or interpersonal relationships. Emotional symptoms, particularly depression, anger, irritability, and fatigue, are reported as the most distressing symptoms; physical symptoms tend to be less problematic.

9. Premenstrual dysmorphic disorder (PMDD) is a severe form of PMS.
10. Infection and inflammation of the female genitalia can result from microorganisms that are present in the environment and often are sexually transmitted or from overproliferation of microorganisms that normally populate the genital tract.
11. Pelvic inflammatory disease (PID) is an acute inflammatory process caused by infection. Many infections are sexually transmitted, and microorganisms that comprise the vaginal flora are implicated. PID is a substantial health risk to women, and untreated PID can lead to infertility.
12. Vaginitis is irritation or inflammation of the vagina, typically caused by infection. It is usually caused by sexually transmitted pathogens or *Candida albicans*, which causes candidiasis.
13. Bacterial vaginosis (BV) is the most common microbiologic syndrome reported among women of childbearing age. It is characterized by a shift in the vaginal flora from the dominant *Lactobacillus* to a polymicrobial flora. It is correlated with a wide array of health issues, including preterm births, PID, and increased susceptibility to HIV infection. No one microorganism can identify all cases of BV.
14. Cervicitis, which is infection of the cervix, can be acute (mucopurulent cervicitis) or chronic. Its most common cause is a sexually transmitted pathogen.
15. Vulvovestibulitis (VV) is an inflammation of the skin of the vulva. It can be caused by chemical and mechanical irritants, allergens, skin disorders, nerve problems, or vaginal infection, such as candidiasis.
16. Bartholinitis, also called *Bartholin cyst*, is an infection of the ducts that lead from the Bartholin glands to the surface of the vulva. Infection blocks the glands, preventing the outflow of glandular secretions.
17. Pelvic organ prolapse—uterine prolapse, cystocele, rectocele, and urethrocele—is caused by the relaxation of muscles and fascial supports, usually as a result of advancing age or after childbirth or other trauma. They are more likely to occur in women with a familial or genetic predisposition.
18. Benign growths and proliferative conditions of the female reproductive tract tend to affect the ovaries or uterine tissues (endometrial polyps, leiomyomas, and endometriosis).
19. Benign ovarian cysts develop from mature ovarian follicles that do not release their ova (follicular cysts) or from a corpus luteum that persists abnormally instead of degenerating (corpus luteum cyst). Cysts usually regress spontaneously.
20. Endometrial polyps consist of benign overgrowths of endometrial tissue and often cause abnormal bleeding.
21. Leiomyomas, also called *myomas* or *uterine fibroids*, are benign tumors arising from the smooth muscle layer of the uterus, the myometrium. Prevalence increases in women between ages 30 and 50; most myomas remain small and asymptomatic.
22. Adenomyosis is the presence of endometrial glands and stroma within the uterine myometrium.
23. Endometriosis is the presence of functional endometrial tissue (i.e., tissue that responds to hormonal stimulation) at sites outside the uterus. Endometriosis causes an inflammatory reaction at the site of implantation and is a cause of infertility.
24. Most cancers of the female genitalia involve the uterus (particularly the cervix), cervix, and ovaries. Cancer of the vagina is rare.
25. Cervical cancer arises from the cervical epithelium and is triggered by HPV. The cellular transformational zone is called the *squamocolumnar junction*. The progressively serious neoplastic alterations are CIN (cervical intraepithelial neoplasia, also known as cervical dysplasia), cervical CIS (carcinoma in situ), and invasive cervical carcinoma. Cocarcinogens include immune responses, hormonal responses, and other environmental factors that determine regression or persistence of the HPV infection.
26. The HPV vaccination can substantially reduce the risk of cervical cancer as well as oropharyngeal and anal cancers. It is approved for girls and boys aged 11 through 26.
27. Primary cancer of the vagina is rare. Risk factors include age 60 or older, exposure to DES, infection with HPV-16, infection with HIV, and genital warts. The relationship of developing precancerous cell changes (called vaginal intraepithelial neoplasia) is controversial.
28. Risk factors for vulvar cancer include infection with HPV infection or squamous dysplasia of the vagina or cervix. Symptoms include chronic vulvar irritation, pruritus, bloody discharge, and a hard-ulcerated area of the vulva or cauliflower-like lesion. Peak incidence is in postmenopausal women, but younger women can be affected.
29. Endometrial cancer is the most common cancer of the pelvic region. Primary risk factors for endometrial cancer include exposure to unopposed estrogen (e.g., estrogen-only hormone replacement therapy, tamoxifen, early menarche, late menopause, nulliparity, failure to ovulate), chronic hyperinsulinemia, hyperglycemia, body fatness and adult weight gain, chronic inflammation, lack of physical exercise.
30. Risk factors for ovarian cancer include increased number of total lifetime ovulations (early menarche, late menopause), advancing age, genetic factors, family history, overweight and obesity, height, reproductive/hormonal factors, HRT, endometriosis, diabetes, previous cancer, smoking, asbestos, use of talc-based powder, and ionizing radiation.
31. BRCA1, BRCA2, and HNPCC gene abnormalities are linked with ovarian cancer. Ovarian cancer causes more deaths than any other genital cancer in women due to its presentation in advanced disease. New methods are being explored for routine screening.

Sexual Dysfunction

1. Sexual dysfunction is the lack of satisfaction with sexual function as a result of pain or a deficiency in sexual desire, arousal, or orgasm/climax.

2. Sexual function and dysfunction result from a complex set of personal and biologic factors that interact with the culture. Both organic and psychosocial disorders can be implicated in sexual dysfunction.

Impaired Fertility

1. Infertility, or the inability to conceive after 1 year of unprotected intercourse, affects approximately 15% of all couples. Fertility can be impaired by factors in the male, female, or both partners.
2. Female infertility decreases with age, and older women may opt for intervention sooner than younger women. It results from dysfunction of the normal reproductive process: menses and ovulation, fallopian tube function (transport of the egg to the uterus, and the tube as a site of fertilization), ovarian dysfunction, and implantation of the fertilized egg into a receptive endometrium.
3. Treatment depends on the cause of the infertility—ovulation disorders and tubal blockages are the most common pathologies.

Disorders of the Female Breast

1. Most disorders of the breast are disorders of the mammary gland (i.e., the female breast).
2. Galactorrhea, or inappropriate lactation, is the persistent secretion of a milky substance by the breasts of a woman who is not in the postpartum state or nursing an infant. Its most common cause is nonpuerperal hyperprolactinemia—a rise in serum prolactin levels.
3. Benign breast conditions are numerous and involve both ducts and lobules. Benign epithelial lesions can be broadly classified according to their future risk of developing breast cancer as (1) nonproliferative breast lesions, (2) proliferative breast disease, and (3) atypical (atypia) hyperplasia.
4. Nonproliferative lesions include simple breast cysts, papillary apocrine change, and mild hyperplasia of the usual type.
5. Proliferative breast lesions without atypia are diverse and include usual ductal hyperplasia, intraductal papillomas, sclerosing adenosis, radial scar, and simple fibroadenoma.
6. Proliferative breast lesions with atypia include ADH and ALH.
7. DCIS refers to a heterogeneous group of proliferations limited to breast ducts and lobules without invasion of the basement membrane. LCIS originates from the duct lobular unit.
8. Breast cancer is the most common form of cancer in women and second to lung cancer as the most common cause of cancer death. However, the inclusion of DCIS with invasive breast cancer statistics is controversial. Breast cancer is a heterogeneous disease with diverse molecular, phenotypic, and pathologic changes.
9. The major risk factors for breast cancer are reproductive factors, such as nulliparity; hormonal factors and growth factors (e.g., excessive estradiol and insulin-like growth factor [IGF]-1), familial factors (e.g., a family history of breast cancer), and environmental factors (e.g., ionizing radiation). Two factors that have emerged as important are delayed involution of the mammary gland and breast density. Physical activity and avoiding postmenopausal weight gain may be risk-reducing factors.
10. A dominating belief in the field of cancer research is that epithelial function depends on the *entire* tissue, including the stroma or microenvironment. Breast cancer is now known as a tissue-based disease with a possible abnormal, aberrant wound healing and inflammatory stromal (reactive stroma) component.
11. Models of breast carcinogenesis include three interrelated themes: gene addiction, phenotype plasticity, and cancer stem cells. The exact molecular events leading to breast cancer invasion are complex and not completely understood. These events involve genetic and epigenetic alterations and cancer cell and stromal interactions. New concepts for breast cancer metastases include tumor dormancy and vascular mimicry.
12. Most breast cancers arise from the ductal epithelium and then may metastasize to the lymphatics, opposite breast, abdominal cavity, lungs, bones, kidneys, liver, adrenal glands, ovaries, and pituitary glands.
13. The first clinical manifestation of breast cancer is usually a small, painless lump in the breast. Other manifestations include palpable lymph nodes in the axilla, dimpling of the skin, nipple and skin retraction, nipple discharge, ulcerations, reddened skin, and bone pain associated with bony metastases.

REFERENCES

1. American Cancer Society (ACS) *Cancer Facts & Figures 2021*. Atlanta, GA: ACS; 2019. https://www.cancer.org/content/dam/cancer-org/research/cancer-facts-and-statistics/annual-cancer-facts-and-figures/2021/cancer-facts-and-figures-2021.pdf. (Accessed May 11, 2022).
2. McCool-Myers Predictors of female sexual dysfunction: a systematic review and qualitative analysis through gender inequality paradigms. *BMC Womens Health*. 2018;18:108.
3. Gottlieb B, Trifiro MA. Androgen insensitivity syndrome. In: Adam MP, Ardinger HH, Pagon RA, eds. *GeneReviews®*. Seattle, WA: University of Washington, Seattle; 2017. Initial posting March 24, 1999. Last update May 11, 2017. Available at https://www.ncbi.nlm.nih.gov/books/NBK1429/. (Accessed May 11, 2022).
4. Tyutyusheva N, et al. Complete androgen insensitivity syndrome: from bench to bed. *Int J Mol Sci*. 2021;22(3):1264.
5. Batista RL, et al. Androgen insensitivity syndrome: a review. *Arch Endocrinol Metab*. 2018;62(2):227–235.
6. Chaudhry S, et al. Frequency of gonadal tumours in complete androgen insensitivity syndrome (CAIS): a retrospective case-series analysis. *J Pediatr Urol*. 2017;13(5):498.
7. Tack LJW, et al. Management of gonads in adults with androgen insensitivity: an international study. *Horm Res Paediatr*. 2018;90(4):236–246.
8. Kosti K, Athanasiadis L, Goulis DG. Long-term consequences of androgen insensitivity syndrome. *Maturitas*. 2019;127:51–54.
9. Acién P, Acién M. The presentation and management of complex female genital malformations. *Hum Reprod Update*. 2016;22(1):48–69.
10. Venetis CA, et al. Clinical implications of congenital uterine anomalies: a meta-analysis of comparative studies. *Reprod Biomed Online*. 2014;29(6):665–683.

11. Cattran AM, et al. Bone density and timing of puberty in a longitudinal study of girls. *J Pediatr Adolesc Gynecol.* 2015;28(3):170–172.
12. Abitbol L, Zborovski S, Palmert MR. Evaluation of delayed puberty: what diagnostic tests should be performed in the seemingly otherwise well adolescent? *Arch Dis Child.* 2015;101(8):767–771.
13. Trotman GE. Delayed puberty in the female patient. *Curr Opin Obstet Gynecol.* 2015;28(5):366–372.
14. Tang C, Gondal AZ, Damian M. *Delayed puberty. StatPearls.* Treasure Island, FL: StatPearls Publishing; 2021. Last update August 7, 2021. Available at https://www.ncbi.nlm.nih.gov/books/NBK544322/. (Accessed May 11, 2022).
15. Kaplowitz PB. Delayed puberty. *Pediatr Rev.* 2010;31(5): 189–195.
16. Kota AS, Ejaz S. *Precocious puberty. StatPearls.* Treasure Island, FL: StatPearls Publishing; 2021. Last update July 25, 2021. Available at https://www.ncbi.nlm.nih.gov/books/NBK544313/. (Accessed May 11, 2022).
17. Bertelloni S, et al. Central precocious puberty: adult height in girls treated with quarterly or monthly gonadotropin-releasing hormone analog triptorelin. *Horm Res Paediatr.* 2015;84(6):396–400.
18. Roberts C. Psychosocial dimensions of early-onset puberty and its treatment. *Lancet Diabetes Endocrinol.* 2016;4(3):195–197.
19. Chemaitilly W, et al. Central precocious puberty following the diagnosis and treatment of paediatric cancer and central nervous system tumours: presentation and long-term outcomes. *Clin Endocrinol (Oxf).* 2016;84:361.
20. van Iersel L, et al. Hypothalamic-pituitary disorders in childhood cancer survivors: prevalence, risk factors and long-term health outcomes. *J Clin Endocrinol Metab.* 2019;104:6101.
21. Simon D, et al. Mutations in the maternally imprinted gene MKRN3 are common in familial central precocious puberty. *Eur J Endocrinol.* 2016;174:1.
22. Valadares LP, et al. MKRN3 mutations in central precocious puberty: a systematic review and meta-analysis. *J Endocr Soc.* 2019;3:979.
23. Schoelwer M, Eugster EA. Treatment of peripheral precocious puberty. *Endocr Dev.* 2016;29:230–239.
24. Kaplowitz P, Bloch C. Section on Endocrinology, American Academy of Pediatrics: Evaluation and referral of children with signs of early puberty. *Pediatrics.* 2016;137(1):e20153732.
25. Lucaccioni L, et al. The measurement of urinary gonadotropins for assessment and management of pubertal disorder. *Hormones (Athens).* 2016;15:377.
26. Shim YS, et al. Random urinary gonadotropins as a useful initial test for girls with central precocious puberty. *Endocr J.* 2019;66:891.
27. Sharghi M, et al. An update and systematic review on the treatment of primary dysmenorrhea. *JBRA Assist Reprod.* 2019;23(1):51–57.
28. Iacovides S, Avidon I, Baker FC. What we know about primary dysmenorrhea today: a critical review. *Hum Reprod Update.* 2015;21(6):762–778.
29. Mendiratta V, Lentz GM. Primary and secondary dysmenorrhea, premenstrual syndrome, and premenstrual dysphoric disorder: etiology, diagnosis, management. In: Gershenson DM, ed. *Comprehensive gynecology.* ed 8 Philadelphia, PA: Elsevier; 2022:768–780. e4.
30. Ghafourian M, et al. The role of CD16+, CD56+, NK (CD16+/CD56+) and B CD20+ cells in the outcome of pregnancy in women with recurrent spontaneous abortion. *Int J Womens Health Reprod Sci.* 2015;3:61–66. Available at https://doi.org/10.15296/ijwhr.2015.10. (Accessed May 11, 2022).
31. Xu Y, et al. Effects of acupoint-stimulation for the treatment of primary dysmenorrhea caompared with NSAIDs: a systematic review and meta-analysis of 19 RCTs. *BMC Complement Altern Med.* 2017;17:436.
32. Wei SY, et al. Changes in functional connectivity of pain modulatory systems in women with primary dysmenorrhea. *Pain.* 2016;157(1):92–102.
33. Marjoribanks J, et al. Nonsteroidal anti-inflammatory drugs for dysmenorrhea. *Cochrane Database Syst Rev.* 2015;7:CD001751.
34. Navvabi Rigi S, et al. Comparing the analgesic effect of heat patch containing iron chip and ibuprofen for primary dysmenorrhea: a randomized controlled trial. *BMC Womens Health.* 2012;12:25.
35. Lord M, Sahni M: Secondary amenorrhea. : StatPearls. Treasure Island, FL, 2021, StatPearls Publishing. Last updated July 19, 2021. Available at https://www.ncbi.nlm.nih.gov/books/NBK431055/. (Accessed May 11, 2022).
36. Sarathi V, et al. A challenging case of primary amenorrhoea. *BMJ Case Rep 2018:bcr2018225447*, 2018.
37. Jacobson MH, et al. Thyroid hormones and menstrual cycle function in a longitudinal cohort of premenopausal women. *Paediatr Perinat Epidemiol.* 2018;32(3):225–234.
38. Klein DA, et al. A systematic approach to diagnosis and management. *Am Family Physician.* 2019;100(1):39–48.
39. Gasner A, Rehman A: Primary amenorrhea. StatPearls. Treasure Island, FL, 2021, StatPearls Publishing. Last update September 8, 2021. Available at https://www.ncbi.nlm.nih.gov/books/NBK554469/. (Accessed May 11, 2022).
40. Marsh CA, Grimstad FW. Primary amenorrhea: diagnosis and management. *Obstet Gynecol Surv.* 2014;69(10):603–612.
41. Lobo R. Primary and secondary amenorrhea and precocious puberty. In: Gershenson DM, ed. *Comprehensive gynecology.* ed 8 Philadelphia, PA: Elsevier; 2022:781–800. e4.
42. Eggermann T, et al. Search for altered imprinting marks in Mayer-Rokitansky-Küster-Hauser patients. *Mol Genet Genomic Med.* 2018;6(6):1225–1228.
43. Deligeoroglou E, et al. Evaluation and management of adolescent amenorrhea. *Ann N Y Acad Sci.* 2010;1205:23–32.
44. Chandeying P, Pantasri T. Prevalence of conditions causing chronic anoulation and the proposed algorithm for anovulation evaluation. *J Obstet Gynecol Res.* 2015;41(7):1074–1079.
45. Samperi I, Lithgow K, Karavitaki N. Hyperprolactinaemia. *J Clin Med.* 2019;8(12):2203.
46. Rebar R. Evaluation of amenorrhea, anovulation, and abnormal bleeding. In: Feingold KR, ed. *Endotext.* South Dartmouth, MA: MDText.com, Inc.; 2018. Last update January 15, 2018. Available at https://www.ncbi.nlm.nih.gov/books/NBK279144/. (Accessed May 11, 2022).
47. Munro MG, et al. FIGO Menstrual Disorders Committee: The two FIGO systems for normal and abnormal uterine bleeding symptoms and classification of causes of abnormal uterine bleeding in the reproductive years: 2018 revisions. *Int J Gynaecol Obstet.* 2018;143(3):393–408.
48. ACOG committee opinion no. 557: management of acute abnormal uterine bleeding in nonpregnant reproductive-aged women, *Obstet Gynecol* 121(4):891–896, 2013.
49. Ryntz T, Lobo RA. Abnormal uterine bleeding: etiology and management of acute and chronic excessive bleeding. In: Gershenson DM, ed. *Comprehensive gynecology.* ed 8 Philadelphia, PA: Elsevier; 2022:594–605. e4.
50. Benetti-Pinto CL, et al. Abnormal uterine bleeding. *Rev Bras Ginecol Obstet.* 2017;39(7):358–368.

51. Khafaga A, Goldstein SR. Abnormal uterine bleeding. *Obstet Gynecol Clin North Am.* 2019;46(4):595–605.
52. Oberman E, Rodriguez-Triana V. Abnormal uterine bleeding: treatment options. *Clin Obstet Gynecol.* 2018;61(1):72–75.
53. Marnach ML, Laughlin-Tommaso SK. Evaluation and management of abnormal uterine bleeding. *Mayo Clin Proc.* 2019;94(2):326–335.
54. Escobar-Morreale HF. Polycystic ovary syndrome: definition, aetiology, diagnosis and treatment. *Nat Rev Endocrinol.* 2018;142:271–284.
55. El Hayak S, et al. Poly cystic ovarian syndrome: an updated overview. *Front Physiol.* 2016;7:124.
56. Rosenfield RL, Ehrmann DA. The pathogenesis of polycystic ovary syndrome (PCOS): the hypothesis of PCOS as functional ovarian hyperandrogenism revisited. *Endocr Rev.* 2016;37(5):467–520.
57. Rasquin Leon LI, Anastasopoulou C, Mayrin JV. *Polycystic ovarian disease. StatPearls.* Treasure Island, FL: StatPearls Publishing; 2021. Last update July 21, 2021. Available at https://www.ncbi.nlm.nih.gov/books/NBK459251/. (Accessed May 11, 2022).
58. Ecklund LC, Usadi RS. Endocrine and reproductive effects of polycystic ovarian syndrome. *Obstet Gynecol Clin North Am.* 2015;42(1):55–65.
59. Ding DC, et al. Association between polycystic ovarian syndrome and endometrial, ovarian, and breast cancer: a population-based cohort study in Taiwan. *Medicine (Baltimore).* 2018;97(39):e12608.
60. Zang C, et al. Lysyl oxidase blockade ameliorates anovulation in polycystic ovary syndrome. *Hum Reprod.* 2018;33(11):2096–2106.
61. Norman RJ, Teede HJ. A new evidence-based guideline for assessment and management of polycystic ovary syndrome. *Med J Aust.* 2018;209(7):299–300.
62. Bednarska S, Siejka A. The pathogenesis and treatment of polycystic ovary syndrome: what's new? *Adv Clin Exp Med.* 2017;26(2):359–367.
63. Escobar-Morreale HF, et al. Prevalence of obesity-associated gonadal dysfunction in severely obese men and women and its resolution after bariatric surgery: a systematic review and meta-analysis. *Hum Reprod Update.* 2017;23:390–408.
64. Jin P, Xie Y. Treatment strategies for women with polycystic ovary syndrome. *Gynecol Endocrinol.* 2018;34(4):272–277.
65. Dubey N, et al. The ESC/E(Z) complex, an effector of response to ovarian steroids, manifests an intrinsic difference in cells from women with premenstrual dysphoric disorder. *Mol Psychiatry.* 2017;22(8):1172–1184.
66. Schiller CE, et al. Reproductive steroid regulation of mood and behavior. *Compr Physiol.* 2016;6(3):1135–1160.
67. Schmidt PJ, et al. Effects of estradiol withdrawal on mood in women with past perimenopausal depression: a randomized clinical trial. *JAMA Psychiatry.* 2015;72:714–726.
68. Schmalenberger KM, et al. Predictors of premenstrual impairment among women undergoing prospective assessment for premenstrual dysphoric disorder: a cycle-level analysis. *Psychol Med.* 2017;47:1585.
69. Hantsoo L, Epperson CN. Premenstrual dysphoric disorder: epidemiology and treatment. *Curr Psychiatry Rep.* 2015;17(11):87.
70. Mohebbi Dehnavi Z, Jafarnejad F, Sadeghi Goghary S. The effect of 8 weeks aerobic exercise on severity of physical symptoms of premenstrual syndrome: a clinical trial study. *BMC Womens Health.* 2018;18:80.
71. Yonkers KA, Simoni MK. Premenstrual disorders. *Am J Obstet Gynecol.* 2018;218:68.
72. Eisenlohr-Moul TA, et al. Treatment of premenstrual dysphoria with continuous versus intermittent dosing of oral contraceptives: results of a three-arm randomized controlled trial. *Depress Anxiety.* 2017;34:908.
73. Marjoribanks J, et al. Selective serotonin reuptake inhibitors for premenstrual syndrome. *Cochrane Database Syst Rev.* 2013;2013(6):CD001396.
74. Yonkers KA, et al. Symptom-onset dosing of sertraline for the treatment of premenstrual dysphoric disorder: a randomized clinical trial. *JAMA Psychiatry.* 2015;72:1037.
75. Jennings LK, Krywko DM. *Pelvic inflammatory disease. StatPearls.* Treasure Island, FL: StatPearls Publishing; 2021. Last update May 13, 2021. Available at https://www.ncbi.nlm.nih.gov/books/NBK499959/. (Accessed May 11, 2022).
76. Tabacco L, et al. Relationship status and sexual behaviors in post-pelvic inflammatory disease (PID) affected urban young women: a sub-study of a randomized trial. *Int Arch Nurs Health Care.* 2018;4(1):088.
77. Ross J, et al. 2017 European guideline for the management of pelvic inflammatory disease. *Int J STD AIDS.* 2018;29(2):108–114.
78. Centers for Disease Control and Prevention (CDC) *Pelvic inflammatory disease (PID) treatment and care.* Atlanta, GA: CDC; 2021. Page last reviewed July 22, 2021. Available at https://www.cdc.gov/std/pid/treatment.htm. (Accessed May 11, 2022).
79. Haggerty CL, et al. Identification of novel microbes associated with pelvic inflammatory disease and infertility. *Sex Transm Infect.* 2016;92(6):441–446.
80. Chayachinda C, Rekhawasin T. Reproductive outcomes of patients being hospitalised with pelvic inflammatory disease. *J Obstet Gynaecol.* 2017;37(2):228–232.
81. Brunham RC, Gottlieb SL, Paavonen J. Pelvic inflammatory disease. *N Engl J Med.* 2015;372(21):2039–2048.
82. Eckert LO, Lentz GM. Genital tract infections. In: Gershenson DM, ed. *Comprehensive gynecology.* ed 8 Philadelphia, PA: Elsevier; 2022:515–542.
83. McCord E, Rahn D. Gynecologic infection. In: Hoffman BL, ed. *Williams gynecology.* ed 3 New York: McGraw-Hill; 2016:50–85.
84. Palmeira-de-Oliveira R, Palmeira-de-Oliveira A, Martinez-de-Oliveira J. New strategies for local treatment of vaginal infections. *Adv Drug Deliv Rev.* 2015;92:105–122.
85. Recine N, et al. Restoring vaginal microbiota: biological control of bacterial vaginosis. A prospective case–control study using *Lactobacillus rhamnosus* BMX 54 as adjuvant treatment against bacterial vaginosis. *Arch Gynecol Obstet.* 2016;293(1):101–107.
86. Workowski KA, Bolan GA. Sexually transmitted diseases treatment guidelines 2015. *MMWR Recomm Rep 64(RR-.* 2015;3:1–137.
87. Hester EE, Middleman AB. A clinical conundrum: chronic cervicitis. *J Pediatr Adolesc Gynecol.* 2019;32(3):342–344.
88. Mattson SK, Polk JP, Nyirjesy P. Chronic cervicitis: presenting features and response to therapy. *J Low Genit Tract Dis.* 2016;20(3):e30–e33.
89. De Andres J, et al. Vulvodynia—an evidence -based literature review and proposed treatment algorithm. *Pain Pract.* 2016;16(2):204–236.
90. Bergeron S, et al. Vulvodynia. *Nat Rev Dis Primers.* 2020;6(1):36.
91. Hersh JE. Vulvodynia in adolescents: presentation, diagnosis and treatment options. *Curr Opin Obstet Gynecol.* 2018;30(5):293–299.
92. Vieira-Baptista P, et al. Diagnosis and management of vulvodynia in postmenopausal women. *Maturitas.* 2018;108:84–94.
93. Barnabei VM. Vulvodynia. *Clin Obstet Gynecol.* 2020;63(4):752–769.
94. Lee MY, et al. Clinical pathology of Bartholin's glands: a review of the literature. *Curr Urol.* 2015;8(1):22–25.

95. Illingworth B, et al. Evaluation of treatments for Bartholin's cyst or abscess: a systematic review. *BJOG*. 2020;127(6):671–678.
96. Barber MD. Pelvic organ prolapse. *BMJ*. 2016;354:i3853.
97. Chen CJ, Thompson H: Uterine prolapse. StatPearls. Treasure Island, FL, 2021, StatPearls Publishing. Last update November 5, 2021. Available at https://www.ncbi.nlm.nih.gov/books/NBK564429/. (Accessed May 11, 2022).
98. Tso C, et al. Nonsurgical treatment options for women with pelvic organ prolapse. *Nurs Womens Health*. 2018;22(3):228–239.
99. The American College of Obstetricians and Gynecologists and the American Urogynecologic Society INTERIM UPDATE: This Practice Bulletin is updated as highlighted to reflect the US Food and Drug Administration order to stop the sale of transvaginal synthetic mesh products for the repair of pelvic organ prolapse. Pelvic organ prolapse. *Female Pelvic Med Reconstr Surg*. 2019;25(6):397–408.
100. Hoffman BL. Pelvic mass. In: Hoffman BL, ed. *Williams Gynecology*. ed 3 New York: McGraw-Hill; 2016:202–229.
101. Bulun SE. Physiology and pathology of the female reproductive axis. In: Melmed S, ed. *Williams Textbook of Endocrinology*. ed 14, Philadelphia: Elsevier; 2020:574 +.
102. Dolan MS, Hill C, Valea FA. Benign gynecologic lesions: vulva, vagina, cervix, uterus, oviduct, ovary, ultrasound imaging of pelvic structures. In: Gershenson DM, ed. *Comprehensive gynecology*. ed 8 Philadelphia, PA: Elsevier; 2022:362–408.e6.
103. American College of Obstetricians and Gynecologists' Committee on Practice Bulletins—Gynecology Practice bulletin no. 174: evaluation and management of adnexal masses. *Obstet Gynecol*. 2016;128(5):e210–e226.
104. Bueloni-Dias FN, et al. Metabolic syndrome as a predictor of endometrial polyps in postmenopausal women. *Menopause*. 2016;23(7):759–764.
105. Stewart EA, et al. Epidemiology of uterine fibroids: a systematic review. *BJOG*. 2017;124(10):1501–1512.
106. Wise LA, Laughlin-Tommaso SK. Epidemiology of uterine fibroids: from menarche to menopause. *Clin Obstet Gynecol*. 2016;59(1):2–24.
107. Stewart EA. Uterine fibroids. *Lancet*. 2001;357(9252):293.
108. Wu X, et al. Subtype-specific tumor-associated fibroblasts contribute to the pathogenesis of uterine leiomyoma. *Cancer Res*. 2017;77(24):6891–6901.
109. Barjon K, Mikhail LN. *Uterine leiomyomata. StatPearls*. Treasure Island, FL: StatPearls Publishing; 2021. Last update August 11, 2021. Available at https://www.ncbi.nlm.nih.gov/books/NBK546680/. (Accessed May 11, 2022).
110. Donnez J, et al. Emerging treatment options for uterine fibroids. *Expert Opin Emerg Drugs*. 2018;23(1):17–23.
111. Bartels CB, et al. An evidence-based approach to the medical management of fibroids: a systematic review. *Clin Obstet Gynecol*. 2016;59(1):30–52.
112. De La Cruz MS, Buchanan EM. Uterine fibroids: diagnosis and treatment. *Am Fam Physician*. 2017;95(2):1100–1107.
113. Taran FA, et al. Epidemiology, risk factors, clinical phenotype and surgical and interventional alternatives to hysterectomy. *Geburtshilfe Frauenheilkd*. 2013;73(9):924–931.
114. Struble J, Reid S, Bedaiwy MA. Adenomyosis: a clinical view of a challenging gynecologic condition. *J Minim Invasive Gynecol*. 2016;23(2):164–185.
115. Gunther R, Walker C. *Adenomyosis. StatPearls*. Treasure Island, FL: StatPearls Publishing; 2021. Last update July 22, 2021. Available at https://www.ncbi.nlm.nih.gov/books/NBK539868/. (Accessed May 11, 2022).
116. Chapron C, et al. Diagnosing adenomyosis: an integrated clinical and imaging approach. *Hum Reprod Update*. 2020;26(3):392–411.
117. Dueholm M. Minimally invasive treatment of adenomyosis. *Best Pract Res Clin Obstet Gynaecol*. 2018;51:119–137.
118. Zondervan KT, Becker CM, Missmer SA. Endometriosis. *N Engl J Med*. 2020;382:1244–1256.
119. Klemmt PA, Starzinski-Powitz A. Molecular and cellular pathogenesis of endometriosis. *Curr Womens Health Rev*. 2018;14:106–116.
120. Vercellini P, et al. Endometriosis: pathogenesis and treatment. *Nat Rev Endocrinol*. 2013;10:261–275.
121. Alimi Y, et al. The clinical anatomy of endometriosis: a review. *Cureus*. 2018;10(9):e3361.
122. Shafrir AL, et al. Risk for and consequences of endometriosis: a critical epidemiologic review. *Best Pract Res Clin Obstet Gynaecol*. 2018;51:1–15.
123. The World Bank *Population Ages 15–64 (% of population). World Bank Staff Estimates Based on Age/Sex Distributions of United Nations Population Division's World Population Prospects: 2019 Revision*. Washington, DC: The World Bank; 2019. Available at https://data.worldbank.org/indicator/SP.POP.1564.TO.ZS. (Accessed May 11, 2022).
124. Bulun SE, et al. Endometriosis. *Endocr Rev*. 2019;40(4):1048–1079.
125. Sampson JA. Peritoneal endometriosis due to the menstrual dissemination of endometrial tissue into the peritoneal cavity. *Am J Obstet Gynecol*. 1927;14(4):422–469.
126. Vannuccini S, et al. Infertility and reproductive disorders: impact of hormonal and inflammatory mechanisms on pregnancy outcome. *Hum Reprod Update*. 2016;22(1):104–115.
127. Kiesel L, Sourouni M. Diagnosis of endometriosis in the 21st century. *Climacteric*. 2019;22(3):296–302.
128. Zondervan KT, et al. Endometriosis. *Nat Rev Dis Primers*. 2018;4(1):9.
129. Nisenblat V, et al. Imaging modalities for the non-invasive diagnosis for endometriosis. *Cochrane Database Syst Rev*. 2016;2(2):CD009591.
130. Andres MP, Borrelli GM, Abrão MS. Endometriosis classification according to pain symptoms: can the ASRM classification be improved? *Best Pract Res Clin Obstet Gynaecol*. 2018;51:111–118.
131. Rolla E. Endometriosis: advances and controversies in classification, pathogenesis, diagnosis, and treatment. *F1000Res*. 2019;8(F1000 Faculty Rev-529).
132. Agarwal SK, et al. Clinical diagnosis of endometriosis: a call to action. *Am J Obstet Gynecol*. 2019;220(4):354.e1–354.e12.
133. Taylor HS, et al. Treatment of endometriosis-associated pain with elagolix, an oral GnRH antagonist. *N Engl J Med*. 2017;377:28–40.
134. Whiteman MK, et al. Inpatient hysterectomy surveillance in the United States, 2000–2004. *Am J Obstet Gynecol*. 2008;198(1):34.e1–34.e7.
135. Dunselman GA, et al. ESHRE guideline: management of women with endometriosis. *Hum Reprod*. 2014;29:400–412.
136. Cohen PA, et al. Cervical cancer. *Lancet*. 2019;393:169–182.
137. Bray F, et al. Global cancer statistics 2018: GLOBOCAN estimates of cancer incidence and mortality for 36 cancers in 185 countries. *CA Cancer J Clin*. 2018;68:394–424.
138. Vu M, et al. Cervical cancer worldwide. *Curr Probl Cancer*. 2018;42(5):457–465.
139. Kessler TA. Cervical cancer: prevention and early detection. *Semin Oncol Nurs*. 2017;33(2):172–183.
140. American Cancer Society (ACS) *Estimated Number of New Cases and Deaths by Sex*. Atlanta, GA: ACS; 2022. Available at https://www.cancer.org/content/dam/cancer-org/research/cancer-facts-and-statistics/annual-cancer-facts-and-

figures/2022/estimated-number-of-new-cancer-cases-and-deaths-by-sex.pdf. (Accessed May 11, 2022).
141. Kumar V, Abbas AK, Aster JC. ,. *Robbins & Cotran Pathologic Basis of Disease*. ed 10 Philadelphia, PA: Elsevier; 2021.
142. Prendiville W, Sankaranarayanan R. *IARC Technical Report, no.45: Colposcopy and Treatment of Cervical Precancer*. Lyon, France: International Agency for Research on Cancer (IARC); 2017. Available at https://publications.iarc.fr/Book-And-Report-Series/Iarc-Technical-Publications/Colposcopy-And-Treatment-Of-Cervical-Precancer-2017. (Accessed May 11, 2022).
143. Pańczyszyn A, Boniewska-Bernacka E, Głąb G. Telomeres and telomerase during human paillomavirus-induced carcinogenesis. *Mol Diagn Ther*. 2018;22(4):421–430.
144. Centers for Disease Control and Prevention (CDC) *What are the Symptoms of Cervical Cancer?*. Atlanta, GA: CDC; 2021. Page last reviewed December 14, 2021. Available at https://www.cdc.gov/cancer/cervical/basic_info/symptoms.htm. (Accessed May 11, 2022).
145. Bhatla N, et al. Revised FIGO staging for carcinoma of the cervix uteri. *Int J Gynecol Obstet*. 2019;145:129–135.
146. Centers for Disease Control and Prevention (CDC) *Human Papillomavirus (HPV)*. Atlanta, GA: CDC; 2021. Page last reviewed July 23, 2021. Available at https://www.cdc.gov/hpv/index.html. (Accessed May 11, 2022).
147. Adams TS, Cuello MA. Cancer of the vagina. *Int J Gynaecol Obstet*. 2018;143(Suppl 2):14–21.
148. Kaltenecker B, Tikaria R. *Vaginal cancer. StatPearls*. Treasure Island, FL: StatPearls Publishing; 2021. Last update July 19, 2021. Available at https://www.ncbi.nlm.nih.gov/books/NBK559126/. (Accessed May 11, 2022).
149. Siegler E, et al. Vulvar and vaginal cancer, vulvar intraepithelial neoplasia 3 and vaginal intraepithelial neoplasia 3: experience of a referral institute. *Isr Med Assoc*. 2016;18(5):286–289.
150. Smith JS, et al. Human papillomavirus type-distribution in vulvar and vagina cancers and their associated precursors. *Obstet Gynecol*. 2009;113(4):917–924.
151. Cancer.Net *Vaginal Cancer: Risk Factors and Prevention*. Alexandria, VA: American Society of Clinical Oncology (ASCO); October 2021. Available at https://www.cancer.net/cancer-types/vaginal-cancer/risk-factors-and-prevention. (Accessed May 11, 2022).
152. PDQ Adult Treatment Editorial Board: Vaginal cancer treatment (PDQ®): health professional version. : PDQ Cancer Information Summaries. Bethesda, MD, 2021, National Cancer Institute. Published online February 24, 2021. Available at https://www.ncbi.nlm.nih.gov/books/NBK65801/. (Accessed May 11, 2022).
153. Cross NM, et al. Vaginal Ewing sarcoma: an uncommon clinical entity in pediatric patients. *J Clin Imaging Sci*. 2017;7:17.
154. PDQ® Adult Treatment Editorial Board *Vaginal cancer treatment (PDQ®)–health professional version*. Bethesda, MD: National Cancer Institute; 2021. Updated February 24, 2021. Available at https://www.cancer.gov/types/vaginal/hp/vaginal-treatment-pdq. (Accessed May 11, 2022).
155. National Cancer Institute (NCI) *SEER Cancer Stat Facts: Vulvar Cancer*. Bethesda, MD: NCI; 2022. Available at https://seer.cancer.gov/statfacts/html/vulva.html. (Accessed May 11, 2022).
156. Wakeham K, et al. HPV status and favorable outcome in vulvar squamous cancer. *Int J Cancer*. 2017;140(5):1134–1146.
157. Pepas L, et al. Medical intervention for high grade vulval intraepithelial neoplasia. *Cochrane Database Syst Rev*. 2011;4:CD007924.
158. Lortet-Tieulent J, et al. International patterns and trends in endometrial cancer incidence, 1978–2013. *J Natl Cancer Inst*. 2018;110(4):354–361.
159. Onstad MA, Schmandt RE, Lu KH. Addressing the role of obesity in endometrial cancer risk, prevention, and treatment. *J Clin Oncol*. 2016;34(35):4225–4230.
160. Staff S, et al. Endometrial cancer risk factors among Lynch syndrome women: a retrospective cohort study. *Br J Cancer*. 2016;115(3):375–381.
161. Dominick S, et al. Levonorgestrel intrauterine system for endometrial protection in women with breast cancer on adjuvant tamoxifen. *Cochrane Database Syst Rev*. 2015;12:CD007245.
162. Raglan O, et al. Risk factors for endometrial cancer: an umbrella review of the literature. *Int J Cancer*. 2019;145(7):1719–1730.
163. Cancer Genome Atlas Research Network Kandoth C, et al. Integrated genomic characterization of endometrial carcinoma. *Nature*. 2013;497(7447):67–73. Erratum in *Nature* 500(7461):242, 2013.
164. Liu Y, et al. Clinical significance of CTNNB1 mutation and Wnt pathway activation in endometrioid endometrial carcinoma. *J Natl Cancer Inst*. 2014;106(9). dju245.
165. Cherniack AD, et al. Integrated molecular characterization of uterine carcinosarcoma. *Cancer Cell*. 2017;31(3):411–423.
166. Mahdy H, Casey MJ, Crotzer D. *Endometrial cancer. StatPearls*. Treasure Island, FL: StatPearls Publishing; 2021. Last update August 25, 2021. Available at https://www.ncbi.nlm.nih.gov/books/NBK525981/. (Accessed May 11, 2022).
167. Clarke MA, et al. Association of endometrial cancer risk with postmenopausal bleeding in women: a systematic review and meta-analysis. *JAMA Intern Med*. 2018;178:1210–1222.
168. Suri V, Arora A. Management of endometrial cancer: a review. *Rev Recent Clin Trials*. 2015;10(4):309–316.
169. Lu KH, Broaddus RR. Endometrial cancer. *N Engl J Med*. 2020;383:2053–2064.
170. Kroeger Jr PT, Drapkin R. Pathogenesis and heterogeneity of ovarian cancer. *Curr Opin Obstet Gynecol*. 2017;29(1):26–34.
171. Arora T, Mullangi S, Lekkala MR. *Ovarian cancer. StatPearls*. Treasure Island, FL: StatPearls Publishing; 2022. Last updated January 4, 2022. Available at https://www.ncbi.nlm.nih.gov/books/NBK567760/. (Accessed May 11, 2022).
172. Chandra A, et al. Ovarian cancer: current status and strategies for improving therapeutic outcomes. *Cancer Med*. 2019;8(16):7018–7031.
173. Torre LA, et al. Ovarian cancer statistics. *CA Cancer J Clin*. 2018;68(4):284–296.
174. Momenimovahed Z, et al. Ovarian cancer in the world: epidemiology and risk factors. *Int J Womens Health*. 2019;11:287–299.
175. National Institutes of Health (NIH) *MedlinePlus: ovarian cancer*. Bethesda, MD: NIH; 2020. Page last updated on August 18, 2020. Page last reviewed February 1, 2019. Available at https://medlineplus.gov/genetics/condition/ovarian-cancer/. (Accessed May 11, 2022).
176. Neff RT, Senter L, Salani R. BRCA mutation in ovarian cancer: testing, implications and treatment considerations. *Ther Adv Med Oncol*. 2017;9(8):519–531.
177. Antoniou A, et al. Average risks of breast and ovarian cancer associated with BRCA1 or BRCA2 mutations detected in case series unselected for family history: a combined analysis of 22 studies. *Am J Hum Genet*. 2003;72:1117–1130.
178. Karnezis AN, et al. The disparate origins of ovarian cancers: pathogenesis and prevention strategies. *Nat Rev Cancer*. 2016;17(1):65–74.

179. Reid BM, Permuth JB, Sellers TA. Epidemiology of ovarian cancer: a review. *Cancer Biol Med.* 2017;14(1):9–32.
180. Lheureux S, et al. Epithelial ovarian cancer. *Lancet.* 2019;393(10177):1240–1253.
181. Dochex V, et al. Biomarkers and algorithms for diagnosis of ovarian cancer: CA125, HE4, RMI, and ROMA, a review. *J Ovarian Res.* 2019;12(1):28.
182. PDQ® Adult Treatment Editorial Board *Ovarian Epithelial, Fallopian Tube, and Primary Peritoneal Cancer Treatment (PDQ®)–Health Professional Version.* Bethesda, MD: National Cancer Institute; 2021. Updated April 1, 2022. Available at https://www.cancer.gov/types/ovarian/hp/ovarian-epithelial-treatment-pdq. (Accessed May 11, 2022).
183. Stewart C, Ralyea C, Lockwood S. Ovarian cancer: an integrated review. *Semin Oncol Nurs.* 2019;35(2):151–156.
184. Henderson JT, Webber EM, Sawaya GF. Screening for ovarian cancer: updated evidence report and systematic review for the US Preventive Services Task Force. *JAMA.* 2018;319(6):595–606.
185. Mathis J, et al. Ovarian cancer screening in the general population. *Horm Mol Biol Clin Investig.* 2019;41(3). 2019. Available at https://doi.org/10.1515/hmbci-2019-0038. (Accessed May 11, 2022).
186. Levin RJ, et al. The physiology of female sexual function and the pathophysiology of female sexual dysfunction (Committee 13A). *J Sex Med.* 2016;13(5):733–759.
187. Nappi PR, et al. Female sexual dysfunction (FSD): prevalence and impact on quality of life (QoL). *Maturitas.* 2016;94:87–91.
188. Dean J. Medication and sexual dysfunction. In: Wylie K, ed. *ABC of Sexual Health.* West Sussex, UK: John Wiley & Sons; 2015:51–54.
189. Parish SJ, Hahn SR. Hypoactive sexual desire disorder: a review of epidemiology, biopsychology, diagnosis, and treatment. *Sex Med Rev.* 2016;4(2):103–120.
190. American College of Obstetricians and Gynecologists' Committee on Practice Bulletins—Gynecology Female sexual dysfunction: ACOG practice bulletin clinical management guidelines for obstetrician-gynecologists, number 213. *Obstet Gynecol.* 2019;134(1):e1–e18. Available at https://doi.org/10.1097/aog.0000000000003324. (Accessed May 11, 2022).
191. Carreiro AV, et al. Sexual dysfunction risk and quality of life among women with a history of sexual abuse. *Int J Gynaecol Obstet.* 2016;134(3):260–263.
192. Wheeler LJ, Guntupalli SR. Female sexual dysfunction: pharmacologic and therapeutic interventions. *Obstet Gynecol.* 2020;136(1):174–186.
193. Clayton AH, Valladares Juarez EM. Female sexual dysfunction. *Med Clin North Am.* 2019;103(4):681–698.
194. Vander Borght M, Wyns C. Fertility and infertility: definition and epidemiology. *Clin Biochem.* 2018;62:2–10.
195. Marshburn PB. Counseling and diagnostic evaluation for the infertile couple. *Obstet Gynecol Clin North Am.* 2015;42(1):1–14.
196. Dickey RP. Evaluation of women with unexplained infertility. In: Schattman G, Perelman RO, Esteves SC, eds. *Unexplained Infertility.* New York: Springer; 2015:213–221.
197. Dishuck CF, et al. Advanced imaging in female infertility. *Curr Urol Rep.* 2019;20(11):77.
198. Stern JE, et al. Adverse pregnancy and birth outcomes associated with underlying diagnosis with and without assisted reproductive technology treatment. *Fertil Steril.* 2015;103(6):1438–1445.
199. Boulet SL, et al. Assisted reproductive technology and birth defects among liveborn infants in Florida, Massachusetts, and Michigan, 2000–2010. *JAMA Pediatr.* 2016;170(6):e154934.
200. Gosi SKY, Garla VV. *Galactorrhea. StatPearls.* Treasure Island, FL: StatPearls Publishing; 2021. Last update August 27, 2021. Available at https://www.ncbi.nlm.nih.gov/books/NBK537115/. (Accessed May 11, 2022).
201. Huang W, Molitch ME. Evaluation and treatment of galactorrhea. *Am Fam Physician.* 2012;85(11):11073–11080.
202. Vroonen L, Daly AF, Beckers A. Epidemiology and management challenges in prolactinomas. *Neuroendorinology.* 2019;109(1):20–27.
203. Ashbeck EL, et al. Benign breast biopsy diagnosis and subsequent risk of breast cancer. *Cancer Epidemiol Biomarkers Prev.* 2007;16(3):467–472.
204. Sabel MS. *Overview of Benign Breast Diseases.*: UpToDate, Inc.; 2022. Literature review current through January 2022. Last updated December 1, 2021. Available at https://www.uptodate.com/contents/overview-of-benign-breast-diseases. (Accessed February 20, 2022).
205. Shyamal K, Girish HC, Murgod S. Risk of tumor cell seeding through biopsy and aspiration cytology. *J Int Soc Prev Community Dent.* 2014;4(1):5–11.
206. Dupont WD, Page DI. Risk factors for breast cancer in women with proliferative breast disease. *N Engl J Med.* 1985;312: 146–151.
207. Page DL, et al. Atypical hyperplastic lesions of the female breast. A long-term follow -up study. *Cancer.* 1985;55:2698–2708.
208. Sanders M, et al. Continued observation of the natural history of low-grade ductal carcinoma in situ reaffirms proclivity for local recurrence even after more than 30 years of follow-up. *Mod Pathol.* 2015;28(5):662–669.
209. Hartmann LC, et al. Understanding the premalignant potential of atypical hyperplasia through its natural history: a longitudinal cohort study. *Cancer Prev Res (Phila).* 2014;7:211–217.
210. Iodine Monograph. *Altern Med Rev.* 2010;15(3):273–278.
211. Rappaport J. Changes in dietary iodine explains increasing incidence of breast cancer with distant involvement in young women. *J Cancer.* 2017;8(2):174–177.
212. Centers for Disease Control and Prevention (CDC) *Breast Cancer Statistics.* Atlanta, GA: CDC; 2021. Page last reviewed June 8, 2021. Available at https://www.cdc.gov/cancer/breast/statistics/index.htm. (Accessed May 11, 2022).
213. International Agency for Research on Cancer (IARC) *Breast Global Cancer Observatory (GLOBOCAN) 2020.* Lyon, France: IARC; 2020. Available at https://gco.iarc.fr/today/data/factsheets/cancers/20-Breast-fact-sheet.pdf. (Accessed May 11, 2022).
214. Senft D, Ronai ZE. Adaptive stress responses during tumor metastasis and dormancy. *Trends Cancer.* 2016;2(8):429–442.
215. Institute of Medicine *Breast Cancer and the Environment: A Life Course Approach.* Washington, DC: The National Academies Press; 2012. Available at https://doi.org/10.17226/13263. (Accessed May 11, 2022).
216. Trabert B, et al. Progesterone and breast cancer. *Endocr Rev.* 2020;41(2):320–3444.
217. Mourouti N, et al. Diet and breast cancer: a systematic review. *Int J Food Sci Nutr.* 2015;66:1–42.
218. Ferrini K, et al. Lifestyle, nutrition and breast cancer: facts and presumptions for consideration. *Ecancermedicalscience.* 2015;9:557.
219. Michels KB, et al. Diet and breast cancer: a review of the prospective observational studies. *Cancer.* 2007;109(Suppl 12):2712–2749.
220. Ahmadieh H, Azar ST. Type 2 diabetes mellitus, oral diabetic medications, insulin therapy, and overall breast cancer risk. *ISRN Endocrinol.* 2013;2013:181240.

221. De Cicco P, et al. Nutrition and breast cancer: a literature review on prevention, treatment and recurrence. *Nutrients.* 2019;11(7):1514.
222. Kim J, et al. The effects of physical activity on breast cancer survivors after diagnosis. *J Cancer Prev.* 2013;18(3):193–200.
223. Pizot C, et al. Physical activity, hormone replacement therapy and breast cancer risk: a meta-analysis of prospective studies. *Eur J Cancer.* 2016;52:138–154.
224. Hardefeldt PJ, et al. Physical activity and weight loss reduce the risk of breast cancer: a meta-analysis of 139 prospective and retrospective studies. *Clin Breast Cancer.* 2018;18(4):e601–e612.
225. Chen S, et al. Dietary fibre intake and risk of breast cancer: a systematic review and meta-analysis of epidemiological studies. *Oncotarget.* 2016;7(4):80980–80989.
226. Aune D, et al. Dietary fiber and breast cancer risk: a systematic review and meta-analysis of prospective studies. *Ann Oncol.* 2012;23(6):1394–1402.
227. Kerlikowske K. Epidemiology of ductal carcinoma in situ. *J Natl Cancer Inst Monogr.* 2010;41:139–141.
228. Esserman L, Yau C. Rethinking the standard for ductal carcinoma in situ treatment. *JAMA Oncol.* 2015;1(7):881–883.
229. Lin C, et al. I-SPY TRIAL Investigators: Locally advanced breast cancers are more likely to present as interval cancers: results from the I-SPY 1 TRIAL (CALGB 150007/150012, ACRIN 6657, InterSPORE Trial). *Breast Cancer Res Treat.* 2012;132(3):871–879.
230. Shiovitz S, Korde LA. Genetics of breast cancer: a topic in evolution. *Ann Oncol.* 2015;26(7):1291–1299.
231. Jindal S, et al. Postpartum breast involution reveals regression of secretory lobules mediated by tissue-remodeling. *Breast Cancer Res.* 2014;16(2):R31.
232. Radisky DC, Hartmann LC. Mammary involution and breast cancer risk: transgenic models and clinical studies. *J Mammary Gland Biol Neoplasia.* 2009;14(2):181–191.
233. Schedin P. Pregnancy-associated breast cancer and metastasis. *Nat Rev Cancer.* 2006;6:281–291.
234. Gupta PB, et al. Systemic stromal effects of estrogen promote the growth of estrogen receptor-negative cancers. *Cancer Res.* 2007;67:2062–2071.
235. Longacre TA, Bartow SA. A correlative morphologic study of human breast and endometrium in the menstrual cycle. *Am J Surg Pathol.* 1986;10:382–393.
236. Masters JR, Drife JO, Scarisbrick JJ. Cyclic variation of DNA synthesis in human breast epithelium. *J Natl Cancer Inst.* 1977;58:1263–1265.
237. Brisken C. Progesterone signalling in breast cancer: a neglected hormone coming into the limelight. *Nat Rev Cancer.* 2013;13(6):385–396.
238. PDQ® Screening and Prevention Editorial Board *Breast Cancer Screening (PDQ®)—Health Professional Version.* Bethesda, MD: National Cancer Institute; 2022. Updated February 10, 2022. Available at: https://www.cancer.gov/types/breast/hp/breast-screening-pdq. (Accessed May 11, 2022).
239. PDQ® Screening and Prevention Editorial Board *Cancer Screening Overview (PDQ®)—Health Professional Version.* Bethesda, MD: National Cancer Institute; 2019. Updated June 29, 2021. Available at https://www.cancer.gov/about-cancer/screening/hp-screening-overview-pdq. (Accessed May 11, 2022).
240. Rice MS, et al. Breast cancer research in the Nurses' Health Studies: exposures across the life course. *Am J Public Health.* 2016;106(9):1592–1598.
241. Boyd NF, et al. Mammographic density and breast cancer risk: current understanding and future prospects. *Breast Cancer Res.* 2011;13(6):223.
242. Krishnan K, et al. Longitudinal study of mammographic density measures that predict breast cancer risk. *Cancer Epidemiol Biomarkers Prev.* 2017;26(4):651–660.
243. Roach RB, et al. A cost-effective handheld breast scanner for use in low-resource environments: a validation study. *World J Surg Oncol.* 2016;14(1):277.
244. Somashekhar SP, et al. Noninvasive and low-cost technique for early detection of clinically relevant breast lesions using a handheld point-of-care medical device (iBreastExam); prospective three-arm-triple-blinded comparative study. *Indian J Gynecol Oncol.* 2016;14:26. Available at https://doi.org/10.1007/s40944-016-0057-1.
245. Xu X, et al. Breast tumor detection using piezoelectric fingers: first clinical report. *J Am Coll Surg.* 2013;216(6):1168–1173.
246. Lambert AW, Pattabiraman DR, Weinberg RA. Emerging biological principles of metastasis. *Cell.* 2017;168(4): 670–691.
247. Grant MD, et al: Menopausal Symptoms: Comparative Effectiveness of Therapies. Rockville, MD, 2015, Agency for Healthcare Research and Quality. Comparative Effectiveness Reviews, No. 147. Available at https://www.ncbi.nlm.nih.gov/books/NBK285463/. (Accessed May 11, 2022).
248. Giannakeas V, et al. Association of radiotherapy with survival in women treated for ductal carcinoma in situ with lumpectomy or mastectomy. *JAMA Netw Open.* 2018;1(4):e181100.

26

Alterations of the Male Reproductive System

George W. Rodway and Kathryn L. McCance

http://evolve.elsevier.com/Rogers/pathophysiology/

CHAPTER OUTLINE

Alterations of the male reproductive system span a wide range of concerns, from delayed sexual development and suboptimal sexual performance to structural and functional abnormalities. Many common male reproductive disorders carry potentially serious physiologic and psychological consequences.

ALTERATIONS OF SEXUAL MATURATION

The process of sexual maturation, or puberty, is marked by the development of secondary sex characteristics, rapid growth, and, ultimately, the ability to reproduce. A variety of congenital and endocrine disorders can disrupt the timing of puberty. Puberty that occurs too late (delayed puberty) or too early (precocious puberty) is caused by the inappropriate onset of sex hormone production. While the average age of pubertal onset appears to be decreasing for girls, the age of pubertal onset (9 to 14 years) has remained essentially unchanged for boys.[1] Generally, boys tend to mature later than girls, around 14 years of age. In males, the first sign of maturity is enlargement of the testes and thinning of the scrotal skin.

Puberty: Premature, Delayed, and Contrasexual Development

Premature puberty or precocious puberty is early development of secondary sexual characteristics and is defined as pubertal development of secondary sexual characteristics before age 9 in males and before age 8 in females. Delayed puberty is based on the absence of breast development by age 13 or absence of menarche by age 16 for females and lack of testicular enlargement by age 14 for males.[2–4] Contrasexual development occurs when male or female children develop features of the opposite gender (e.g., feminization in boys mainly gynecomastia; virilization in girls).[5] Although contrasexual development is less common in boys, it is typically related to estrogen secreting tumors.[6] About 3% of children living in North America experience delayed development of secondary sex characteristics.[7]

Precocious puberty for either gender is caused by premature adrenarche (an increase in the production of androgens by the adrenal cortex that usually occurs during the eighth or ninth year of life), central nervous system and pituitary lesions, constitutional and idiopathic precocious puberty, McCune–Albright syndrome, or exogenous sex hormones (also see Chapter 25). Causes unique to males include gonadotropin secreting tumors, benign gynecomastia of adolescence, and familial gynecomastia. Table 26.1 presents the causes and pathophysiology of precocious puberty. Excess adiposity during childhood influences growth patterns and pubertal development. Obesity increases the risk of developing early puberty in children (see Chapter 23).[8–10]

In about 95% of cases, a constitutional delay of puberty and growth (CDPG) is a normal physiologic event. Hormonal levels are normal, the hypothalamic-pituitary-gonadal axis is intact, and maturation is slowly occurring. Males with CDPG are generally healthy, but may appear short for age.[1] At birth, they are average size; however, the rate of growth slows down around 3 to 6 months of age and at 3 or 4 years of age, they will be growing below but parallel to the third percentile line.[1] As their male peers experience puberty and a growth spurt, affected males will continue to have a lower growth velocity

TABLE 26.1 Causes and Pathophysiology of Precocious Puberty

Causes of Precocious Puberty Shared by both genders	Premature adrenarche	Premature presence of pubic or axillary hair, possible sebaceous gland activity (before 6 years old). Plasma DHEAS is usually elevated to pubertal levels. FSH, LH, estradiol, testosterone are typical in children before puberty. GnRH shows prepubertal levels and ACTH test may exclude congenital adrenal hyperplasia.
	CNS and pituitary lesions typically present with normal stages of puberty but occurs prematurely.	Children may have bone age greater than chronological age. Visual defects may present. MRI may be necessary.
	Constitutional/idiopathic precocious puberty more often in girls than boys. It is considered idiopathic if no family links or no discovered causes.	Child responds to GnRH test with pubertal levels of sex hormones, including FSH and LH. Bone age higher than chronological age. Other causes must be ruled out such as CNS pathology and elevated levels of adrenal hormones.
	McCune-Albright syndrome	Associated with café-au-lait spots, polyostotic fibrous dysplasia and precocious puberty.
	Exogenous sex hormones (oral contraceptives, anabolic hormones.	Metabolites are found in the urine (urinalysis can rule out). Children will lack pubic hair. Boys will have small testicles, girls darkened areolae.
Causes of Precocious Puberty unique to males	Gonadotropin secreting tumors	Secrete hCG-like components similar function in signaling to LH, results in premature puberty in boys. Girls have the benefit of FSH in the ovaries so no premature development. Tumors that produce hCG include hepatomas, teratomas, and germinomas of the pineal gland. Benign gynecomastia of adolescence in mid to late puberty is common. The breast is tender and usually resolves on its own. Familial gynecomastia appears during puberty and has a genetic link, either x-linked recessive or sex-linked dominant.

From Breehl L, Caban O. *Physiology, puberty*. StatPearls Treasure Island, FL: StatPearls Publishing; 2021.

TABLE 26.2 Tanner Staging for Puberty Assessment for Males

Tanner Stage	Genitalia	Pubic Hair	Growth	Other
1	Testes <2.5 cm	Villus hair only	2.0–2.4 inches per year	Adrenarche
2	Testes 2.5–3.2 cm Thinning and reddening of the saotum	Sparse hair at penis base	2.0–2.4 inches per year	Decreases in body fat
3	Testes 3.3–4.0 cm Increase of penis length	Thicker curly hair spreads to the pubis	2.8–3.2 inches per year	Gynecomastia, voice break, increased muscle mass
4	Testes 4.1–4.5 cm, penis growth darkening: of scrotum	Adult hair does not spread to thighs	4.0 inches per year	Axillary hair, voice change, acne
5	Testes >4.5 cm, adult genitalia	Adult hair spreads to medial thigh	Deceleration, cessation	Facial hair, muscle mass increases

From Breehl L, Caban O. *Physiology, puberty*. StatPearls [Internet]. Treasure Island, FL: StatPearls Publishing; 2021.

(2 to 4 cm/year) and pubertal delay (Table 26.2). Their growth spurt occurs at a later age, generally between 15 to 17 years of age.[11] Sometimes, it is often difficult to differentiate between CDPG and hypogonadotropic hypogonadism.[1] Treatment is seldom needed unless the delayed puberty is causing psychosocial problems (e g., low self-esteem or poor academic performance).[1,12] The other 5% of cases are caused by the disruption of the hypothalamic-pituitary-gonadal axis or by the outcomes of a systemic disease (Box 26.1). The reproductive system, hypothalamus, pituitary gland, adrenal glands, ovaries, and testes are all involved in the changes of puberty. Human gonadal function is partially controlled by luteinizing hormone (LH) and follicle-stimulating hormone (FSH), the release of which is regulated by the pulsatile secretion of hypothalamic gonadotropin-releasing hormone (GnRH).[13] The zona reticularis of the adrenal cortex produces the hormones responsible for adrenarche and function separately from the hypothalamic-pituitary-gonadal axis.[5] With the onset of puberty adrenal androgens can lead to the development of acne, axillary hair, body odor, and pubic hair.

A thorough evaluation should be conducted that includes physical examination and medical and family history. The history should specifically target known contributors to delayed puberty.[13] Measurement of hormone levels may include testosterone, estradiol, FSH, and LH. A GnHR stimulation test is done to determine a central or peripheral cause. Treatment depends on the cause. The goal of treatment is the development of secondary sex characteristics and fertility. Hormone replacement

BOX 26.1 Causes of Delayed Puberty

Hypergonadotropic Hypogonadism: Low Testosterone, Increased Follicle-Stimulating Hormone and Luteinizing Hormone

1. Gonadal dysgenesis, most commonly Turner syndrome (45, X/46, XX; structural X or Y abnormalities, or mosaicism)
2. Klinefelter syndrome (47, XXY)
3. Bilateral gonadal failure
   a. Traumatic or infectious
   b. Postsurgical, postirradiation, or postchemotherapy
   c. Autoimmune
   d. Idiopathic empty scrotum or vanishing testes syndrome (congenital anorchia)

Hypogonadotropic Hypogonadism: Low Testosterone, Decreased Luteinizing Hormone, Depressed Follicle-Stimulating Hormone

1. Reversible
   a. Physiologic delay
   b. Weight loss/anorexia
   c. Strenuous exercise
   d. Severe obesity
   e. Illegal drug use; also use of marijuana in particular
   f. Primary hypothyroidism
   g. Congenital adrenal hyperplasia
   h. Cushing syndrome
   i. Prolactinomas
2. Irreversible
   a. Gonadotropin-releasing hormone (GnRH) deficiency (Kallmann syndrome) or idiopathic hypogonadotropic hypogonadism (IHH)
   b. Hypopituitarism
   c. Congenital central nervous system defects
   d. Other pituitary adenomas
   e. Craniopharyngioma
   f. Malignant pituitary tumors

Systemic Disease

1. Delayed puberty can occur in several illnesses
   a. Cystic fibrosis
   b. Sickle cell disease
   c. Celiac disease
   d. Diabetes mellitus
   e. Poor nutrition and long-term use of glucocorticoids

therapy can be used when there is insufficient sex hormone secretion, such as testosterone for males.[14,15]

DISORDERS OF THE MALE REPRODUCTIVE SYSTEM

Disorders of the Urethra

Urethritis and urethral strictures are common disorders of the male urethra. Urethral carcinoma, an extremely rare form of cancer, can occur in men older than 60 years.

Urethritis

Urethritis is an inflammatory process that is usually, but not always, caused by a sexually transmitted microorganism (see Chapter 27). Infectious urethritis caused by *Neisseria gonorrhoeae* is often called *gonococcal urethritis (GU);* urethritis caused by other microorganisms is called *nongonococcal urethritis (NGU).* Nonsexual origins of urethritis include inflammation or infection because of urologic procedures, insertion of foreign bodies into the urethra, anatomic abnormalities, or trauma. Noninfectious urethritis is rare and is associated with the ingestion of wood, ethyl alcohol, or turpentine. It is also seen with reactive arthritis.

Symptoms of urethritis include urethral tingling or itching or a burning sensation, and frequency and urgency with urination. The individual may note a purulent or clear mucus-like discharge from the urethra. Nucleic acid detection amplification tests allow early detection of *N. gonorrhoeae* and *Chlamydia trachomatis* in urine studies. Treatment consists of appropriate antibiotic therapy for infectious urethritis and avoidance of future exposure or mechanical irritation.

Urethral Strictures

A urethral stricture is a narrowing of the urethra, causing obstructive symptoms and affecting quality of life (Fig. 26.1).[16] Most urethral strictures result from injury to the urethral mucosa and surrounding tissues. Strictures can develop anywhere along the length of the male urethra and are due to several etiologies. The strictures are sometimes classified into anterior and posterior, where anterior comprises 92.2% of cases.[16] The World Health Organization (WHO) recommends a different nomenclature for classification into seven segments: urethral meatus, fossa navicularis, penile, bulbar, membranous, prostatic urethra, and bladder neck.[17] The etiology of strictures is divided into four main categories: idiopathic, iatrogenic, inflammatory, and traumatic. Idiopathic causes are the result of unrecognized repetitive minor perineal traumas.[16] Nearly 45% of all strictures

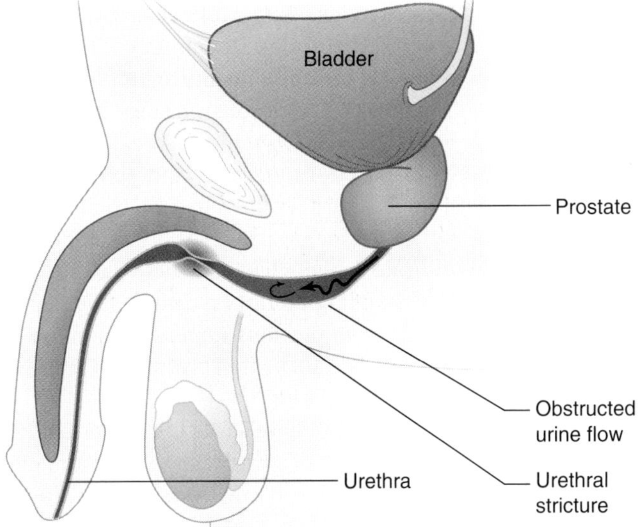

Fig. 26.1 Urethral Stricture. From damage and fibrosis, the diameter of the urethra duct is less than normal and is called a urethral stricture.

are iatrogenic and include those from trans-urethral resections (TUR) (41%), prolonged catheterization (36%), cystoscopy (12.7%), hypospadias repair (6.3%), radical prostatectomy (2% to 9%), and prostate cancer radiotherapy (3.4%) with the highest rate in high-dose-rate brachytherapy.[16,19,20] Children who have hypospadias repair have a 10% risk of developing urethral strictures later in life.[16] Inflammatory strictures are the result of post-infectious inflammation which leads to narrowing of the lumen and weakening of the epithelium. Post-infectious processes that cause inflammation include gonococcal urethritis, chlamydia, tuberculosis, and schistosomiasis.[16] Recurrent urinary tract infections (UTIs) and Lichen sclerosis (LS) are other causes of urethral strictures.[16,17]

Urethral strictures are common with a prevalence in the United States about 200 per 100,000 in younger men and more than 600 per 100,000 in men older than 65.[16,18] Estimated worldwide prevalence is 229 to 627 per 100,000.[21] Male urethral strictures account for 5000 hospital admissions yearly and 1.5 million clinic visits.[22]

Pathophysiology. An injury to the urethral epithelium or direct trauma to corpus spongiosum can cause urine to leak into the underlying area (corpus spongiosum).[16] The injury is then followed by inflammation and fibrous changes. Fibrous tissue causes contraction, which compresses the urethral lumen.[22] The urethral epithelium undergoes metaplasia to stratified squamous epithelium. These changes make the area more vulnerable to pressure changes and stretch causing tears in the mucosa, which leads to increased urine leakage into the corpus spongiosum. Eventually, the alterations lead to fibrous changes and stricture.[23]

Clinical Manifestations. Most individuals present with progressive obstructive voiding symptoms, such as a weak stream.[16] Severity of symptoms varies widely especially in those with a slow progression or a discrete stricture where they may have absence of such symptoms.[16] These individuals may compensate with adaptive detrusor hypertrophy. Other obstructive symptoms include urinary hesitancy, intermittency, and dribbling.[24] The symptom most notably associated with strictures is the feeling of incomplete emptying. With acute obstruction, individuals can present with hematuria and commonly with UTIs.[16] Symptoms are troublesome and affect quality of life.

Evaluation and Treatment. A thorough history is required to determine the underlying etiology. Included is a history of interventions, previous infections, trauma, comorbidities, and an appropriate past medical history.[24] A physical exam is done with palpation of the urethra for any palpable fibrous tissue. Pale skin patches may indicate lichen sclerosus. These patches may be confined to the surrounding urethral meatus.[16] It is important to identify any scars from previous surgery.[16] Examination of the prostate is done to ascertain benign prostatic hyperplasia (BPH), prostate cancer, or prostatitis.[23,24]

Laboratory blood tests do not have a role in diagnosing urethral strictures; however, an elevated white blood cell count may reveal an infectious process. Lower urinary tract flow studies provide a detailed assessment of the urethra; the preferred initial investigation is with uroflowmetry.[16] A triphasic uroflowmetry-based model can aid in distinguishing the voiding patterns of healthy individuals versus those with benign prostatic obstruction or those with urethral strictures. A maximum flow (Qmax) of less than 15 mL/s raises the suspicion of lower urinary tract stricture. The shape of the curve can help with the diagnosis as urethral strictures typically produce a plateau at the level of Qmax.[16] Reliable results from uroflowmetry studies are based on 150 mL in volume.[24–26]

Urethroscopy or cystoscopy can also be used to diagnose urethral stricture, and it can be done under local anesthesia (flexible cystoscopy).[16] Occasionally, the scope is unable to pass through the stricture in order to assess the length or the state of the urethra proximal to it, which causes the inability to provide information about the surrounding fibrosis. Hence, although it is of limited diagnostic value, it can provide a quick diagnosis in case of clinical doubt.[23,24,26] If clinical data are suggesting a stricture, urethrography is performed. If the individual is relaxed, a retrograde urethrography (RUG) can visualize the entire urethra up to the bladder.[16] However, RUG will not provide sufficient information if the stricture is significant and inadequate distention of the proximal urethra occurs.[16] With this situation, a voiding cystourethrography (VCUG) will provide useful additional information. This is done by either asking the individual to void after the bladder is filled with contrast from the RUG or by introducing the contrast through a suprapubic catheter.[16] The combination of RUG and VCUG can provide a sufficient image of the entire urethra providing information about the location, number, length, and severity of strictures. Thus, RUG and VCUG are definitive diagnostic tools.[16] These studies, however, have limitations when interpreting the images because of the position of the stricture and the state of the proximal urethra, as these techniques provide only a 2D image of a 3D structure.[23,24] The use of computed tomography (CT) voiding urethrography or sonoelastography also has utility and provides images of the stricture and its characteristics.[27,28] If cancer is suspected to be the cause of the stricture, MRI can provide quality images and show the location of the tumor.[24] Assessment of the bladder and upper urinary tract is mainly done with ultrasonography.[23]

If symptoms are not troublesome, treatment should not be offered.[16] Without bladder thickness or incomplete emptying, there is no need for any intervention.[16] Acute complications caused by the stricture must be addressed first before offering treatment for the stricture.[16] Individuals presenting with acute urinary retention are given a suprapubic bladder fistula, and any existing UTI is treated with antibiotics. Afterward, definitive treatment for the stricture should be undertaken.[26]

Urethral stricture treatment can be divided into transurethral (dilation, internal urethrotomy) and open surgical (stricture resection and anastomosis, urethroplasty and perineal urethrostomy). Importantly, with any of the treatment options, recurrence tends to happen especially with long strictures and previously treated ones.[16,26]

Disorders of the Penis

Phimosis and Paraphimosis

Phimosis and paraphimosis are both disorders in which the foreskin (prepuce) is “too tight” to move easily over the glans

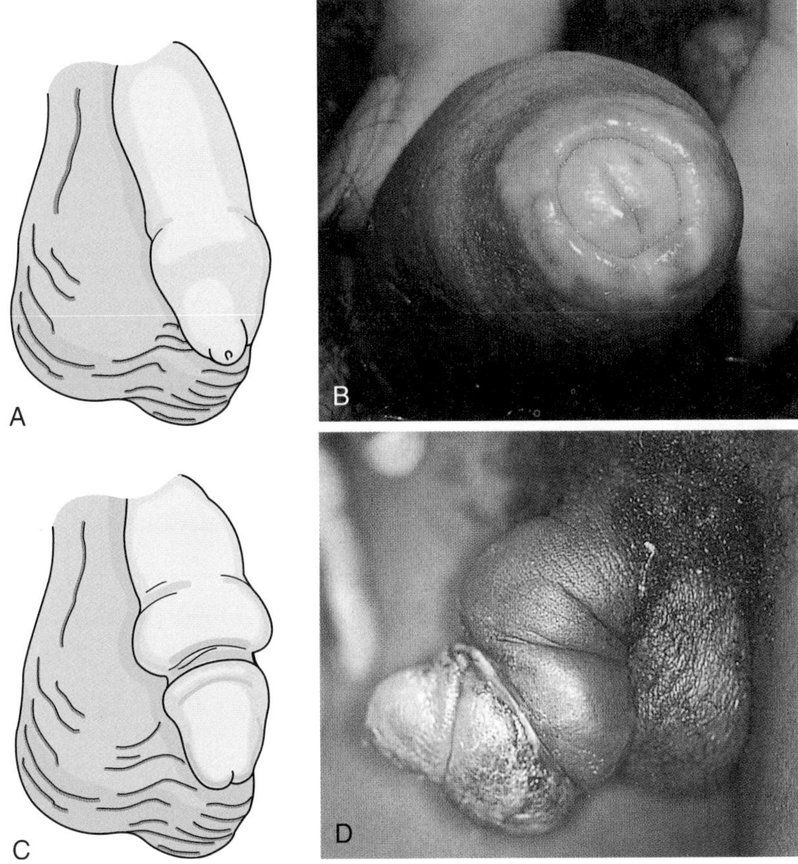

Fig. 26.2 Phimosis and Paraphimosis. (A) Phimosis: the foreskin has a narrow opening that is not large enough to permit retraction over the glans. **(B)** Lesions on the prepuce secondary to infection cause swelling, and retraction of the foreskin may be impossible. Circumcision is usually required. **(C)** Paraphimosis: the foreskin is retracted over the glans but cannot be reduced to its normal position. Here it has formed a constricting band around the penis. **(D)** Ulcer on the retracted prepuce with edema. (A and C, From Monahan FD, et al. *Phipps' medical-surgical nursing: Health and illness perspectives*, 8th edition. St. Louis: Mosby; 2007; B, From Taylor PK. *Diagnostic picture tests in sexually transmitted diseases*. St. Louis: Mosby; 1995; D, From Morse SA, et al. *Atlas of sexually transmitted diseases and AIDS*, 4th edition. London: Saunders; 2011.)

penis. Phimosis is a condition in which the foreskin cannot be retracted back over the glans (Fig. 26.2A), whereas paraphimosis is the opposite: the foreskin is retracted and cannot be moved forward (reduced) to cover the glans (see Fig. 26.2C). Both conditions can cause penile pathologic conditions.

Phimosis is normal in babies and toddlers; the foreskin will not retract because it is still attached to the glans. In older children it may be the result of a skin condition that has caused scarring. Phimosis can occur at any age and is commonly caused by poor hygiene and chronic infection (see Fig. 26.2B and D). It rarely occurs with normal foreskin. In adults, phimosis can sometimes be caused by sexually transmitted infections (STIs). It is associated with different skin conditions such as eczema, psoriasis, lichen planus, and lichen sclerosus.

Reasons for seeking treatment include edema, erythema, tenderness of the prepuce (foreskin), purulent discharge, dysuria, *balanitis* (inflammation of the head of the penis), and *balanoposthitis* (thick discharge underneath the foreskin). Circumcision, if desired, is performed after infection has been eradicated. Complications of phimosis include balanitis, posthitis (inflammation of foreskin), and paraphimosis.

Paraphimosis occurs in uncircumcised males when the foreskin becomes trapped behind the corona of the glans penis.[29] It can lead to strangulation of the glans, painful vascular changes, distal venous engorgement, edema, and necrosis.[29] Paraphimosis mostly occurs iatrogenically, when the foreskin is retracted for cleaning, preparation of a urinary catheter, penile examination, or procedures such as cystoscopy.[29,30] Caregivers who regularly change Foley catheters should replace the foreskin at the end of the procedure to prevent the development of paraphimosis.[29]

Evaluation of an individual with paraphimosis includes a history of any recent catheterizations, instrumentation, cleaning, or other procedures.[30] The person should be asked about cleaning techniques of the penis and if the foreskin is retracted for any reason.[29] The individual should also be asked if he is circumcised or uncircumcised.[29] In those with circumcision, it is still possible to develop paraphimosis.[29] If a Foley catheter is in place, it is recommended to review the reason why the catheter

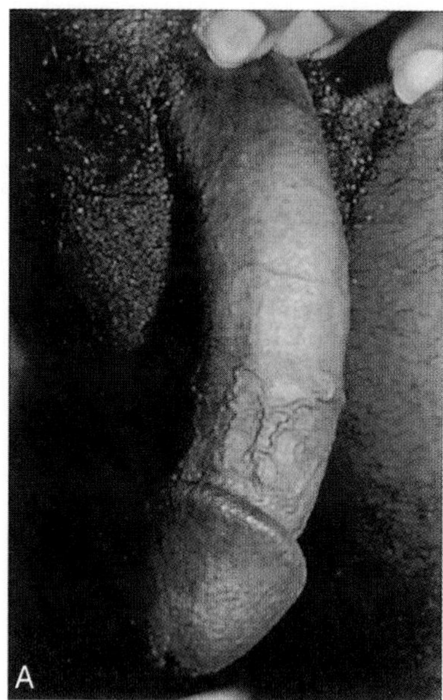

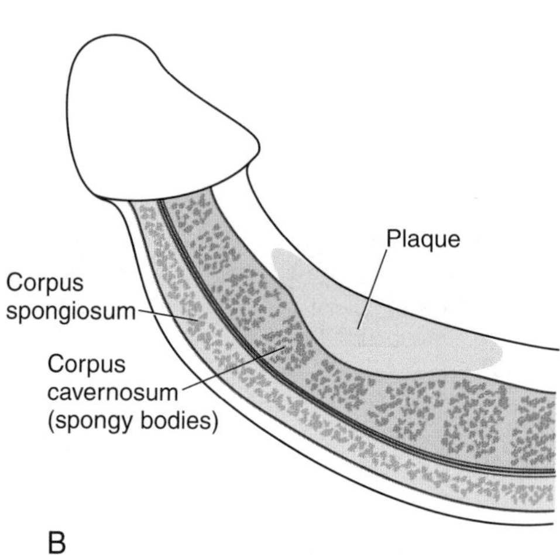

Fig. 26.3 Peyronie Disease (PD). (A) This person complained of pain and deviation of his penis to one side on erection. **(B)** Schematic of the corpus spongiosum, tunica albuginea, and fibrous plaque showing point of curvature. PD is a wound disorder that affects the tunica albuginea of the penis. Its occurrence appears to be after injury or trauma. Abnormal scar tissue develops into plaque under the skin of the penis, causing er-ectile curvature. (A, From Taylor PK. *Diagnostic picture tests in sexually transmitted diseases.* St. Louis: Mosby; 1995; B, From Koesterman JL. *Buck's Step-by-Step Medical Coding,* 2022 Edition, St. Louis: Elsevier; 2022)

was needed and if any difficulties were present in placing the catheter.[29] Most of the time, it is not necessary to remove the catheter to reduce the paraphimosis.[30] Paraphimosis is a urologic emergency. If the foreskin cannot be reduced by manual reduction methods, surgery must be performed to prevent necrosis of the glans caused by constricted blood vessels. An elective circumcision or dorsal slit procedure is strongly recommended in all individuals who have had a significant paraphimosis because of a great risk of recurrence.[29]

Peyronie Disease

Peyronie disease (PD) is a progressive non-malignant disorder of the penis that results in an abnormal curvature when erect (Fig. 26.3). The abnormal curvature is the result of scar tissue in the erectile tissue; the exact mechanism, however, for the formation of the scar tissue remains unknown.[31] PD is a disorder of wound healing of the tunica albuginea, resulting in fibrosis or scarring. In the United States, PD is reported to affect more than 1 in 10 men.[32] The prevalence of PD ranges from 0.3% to 20.3% depending on the variability of several factors, such as country or self-report versus physician report.[33] PD is common in many sexual disorders, such as erectile dysfunction (ED) and impaired sexual performance, causing significant distress to those affected and their partners.[31,34]

Each corpus cavernosum has a sheath of elastic fibers called the tunica albuginea, which has predominantly type 1 collagen fibers (see Fig. 26.3B).[31] The two corpora cavernosa are separated by a condensation of the tunica albuginea in the midline, which forms a septum that attaches to the top and bottom of the penis.[31] A fibrous plaque then forms in the tunica albuginea of the corpora cavernosa. The fibrous plaque is inelastic and changes the smooth upward curvature of the erect penis to a more crimped appearance. Why the plaque forms is uncertain, but the most accepted theory is trauma to the penis.[31] Other theories include microvascular injury, chromosomal instability of fibroblasts as part of plaque formation, changes in the inducible nitric oxide pathways, and human leukocyte antigen (HLA) subtype.[35–37] Better understanding of the risk factors will help to identify who will develop PD. Susceptible men may include those who engage in vigorous sexual activities or non-sexual activities, such as sport events that may be associated with micro-injuries to the penis.[31] Box 26.2 shows modifiable and non-modifiable risk factors for PD from different levels of evidence.

Pathophysiology. The hallmark of PD is the tunical fibrosis of the corpora cavernosa resulting in plaques (see Fig. 26.3B).[31] The main characteristics include deposition of abnormal clumps of collagen with disordered, fragmented, and scant elastic fibers.[38–40] Other findings include the presence of fibrin in 95% of PD plaques.[41] Deposition of fibrin is consistent with the hypothesis that microvascular injury results in fibrin deposition in the tissue space.[41] Abnormal inflammation and wound healing may be responsible for the increased cellularity around the tunica, which results in perivascular lymphocyte infiltrate surrounding or within the tunica itself.[39,42–46] It seems clear that the avoidance of injury or trauma to the penis reduces the risk of development of PD.

Clinical Manifestations. There are two phases in PD, acute and chronic. The first 6 to 18 months of PD is considered the acute phase and progresses with penile deformity and associated

BOX 26.2 Modifiable and Non-Modifiable Risk Factors for Peyronie Disease

- *Penile injury*—Previous injury is a strong predictor of developing Peyronie disease (PD)[1]. Genital or perineal trauma, iatrogenic injury, including catheterization, cystoscopy, and transurethral resection of the prostate, all increase the risk of PD.[1–3]
- *Connective tissue disorders*—PD is associated with certain fibroproliferative diseases such as Dupuytren disease (DD) or contracture and plantar fasciitis.[4] Suggests a significant pathophysiologic and genetic interaction between these two superficial fibrosing disorders. The prevalence of DD in 415 men with PD was 22.1%.[5] The prevalence of DD is reported to be between 1% and 7.3% adding evidence that these conditions may have overlapping mechanisms and predisposing genetic factors.[6] Many studies have linked PD to other systemic fibrotic diseases including idiopathic pulmonary fibrosis, Paget disease of the bone, retroperitoneal fibrosis, scleroderma, polyfibromatosis, and systemic sclerosis.[1]
- *Family history*—Genetic factors linked to PD are complex and reviewed by Gabrielsen.[7] Evidence of a genetic link exists and the interaction with penile trauma may increase the risk for genetically susceptible men.
- *Hypogonadism*—Both the risk of developing and the severity of PD is enhanced by hypogonadism. A prevalence of 74.4% of PD was reported in 121 individuals with hypogonadal testosterone levels less than 300.[8] Additionally, the degree of curvature was higher in the hypogonadal group compared with men with PD with normal testosterone levels. These data were corroborated by another study with 106 persons.[9] Serum testosterone levels influence wound healing and testosterone deficiency in those with PD increases the severity of PD by affecting penile deformity, plaque size, and erectile dysfunction.[9] Androgens have an essential role in wound healing by modulating matrix metalloproteinases[1] and in deficient states, the normal healing process is disrupted, thus increasing the risk of developing PD.[1]
- *Diabetes*-May enhance the fibrotic process involved in PD.[1] From a study of 206 diabetic patients 20.3% had PD, and penile curvature was present in 82.1%.[10] A higher prevalence of PD in those with diabetes has been reported in other studies.[11–14]
- *Smoking and alcohol*-There is limited data on the associations of smoking, as well as for alcohol.
- *Age*-Men in their 60 s are more commonly affected by PD[15] and the age at time of diagnosis varies from 52–57 years old.[16–19] PD can present at any age including as young as 21 years.[17]

REFERENCE

1. Sandean DP, Lotfollahzadeh S. *Peyronie Disease. [Updated 2021 Dec 3]. StatPearls [Internet]*. Treasure Island (FL): StatPearls Publishing; 2022. Available from: https://www.ncbi.nlm.nih.gov/books/NBK560628/.
2. Bjekic MD, lajinac HD, Sipetic SB, et al. Risk factors for Peyronie's disease: A case control study. *BJU Int.* 2006;97(3):570–574.
3. Carrieri MP, Serraino D, Palmiotto F, et al. A case-control study on risk factors for Peyronie's disease. *J Clin Epidemiol.* 1998;51(6):511–515.
4. Meyers AL, Marquart MJ. *Plantar fibromatosis. StatPearls [Internet]*. Treasure Island, FL: StatPearls Publishing; 2020.
5. Nugteren HM, Nijman JM, de Jong IJ, et al. The association between Peyronie's and Dupuytren's disease. *Int J Impot Res.* 2011;23(4):142–145.
6. Dibenedetti DB, Nguyen D, Zografos L, et al. Prevalence, incidence, and treatments of Dupuytren's disease in the United States: Results from a population based study. *Hand (N Y).* 2011;6(2):149–158.
7. Gabrielsen JS. Peyronie's disease: Is it genetic or not? *Transl Androl Urol.* 2020;9(Suppl 2):S262–S268.
8. Moreno SA, Morgentaler A. Testosterone deficiency and Peyronie's disease: Pilot data suggesting a significant relationship. *J Sex Med.* 2009;6(6):1729–1735.
9. Nam HJ, Park HJ, Park NC. Does testosterone deficiency exaggerate the clinical symptoms of Peyronie's disease? *Int J Urol.* 2011;18(11):796–800.
10. Arafa M, Eid H, El-Badry A, et al. The prevalence of Peyronie's disease in diabetic patients with erectile dysfunction. *Int J Impot Res.* 2007;19:213–217.
11. Stuntz M, Perlaky A. des Vignes F, et al. The prevalence of Peyronie's disease in the United States: A population-based study. *PLoS One.* 2016;11(2):e0150157.
12. Tefekli A, Kandirali E, Erol B, et al. Peyronie's disease: A silent consequence of diabetes mellitus. *Asian J Androl.* 2006;8(1): 75–79.
13. Kadioglu A, Tefekli A, Erol B, et al. A retrospective review of 307 men with Peyronie's disease. *J Urol.* 2002;168(3):1075–1079.
14. El-Sakka AI, Tayeb KA. Peyronie's disease in diabetic patients being screened for erectile dysfunction. *J Urol.* 2005;174(3):1026–1030.
15. Mulhall JP, Schiff J, Guhring P. An analysis of the natural history of Peyronie's disease. *J Urol.* 2006;175(6):2115–2118. [discussion 2118].
16. El-Sakka AI. Prevalence of Peyronie's disease among patients with erectile dysfunction. *Eur Urol.* 2006;49(3):564–569.
17. Kadioglu A, Sanli O, Akman T, et al. Factors affecting the degree of penile deformity in Peyronie disease: An analysis of 1001 patients. *J Androl.* 2011;32(5):502–508.
18. Lindsay MB, Schain DM, Grambsch P, et al. The incidence of Peyronie's disease in Rochester, Minnesota, 1950 through 1984. *J Urol.* 1991;146(4):1007–1009.
19. Schwarzer U, Sommer F, Klotz T, et al. The prevalence of Peyronie's disease: Results of a large survey. *BJU Int.* 2001;88(7):727–730.

pain in either the erect and/or flaccid states.[31] Treatment is not recommended in this phase. The chronic phase is a plateau of symptoms for about 3 to 6 months; the deformity remains stable with some or complete improvement in pain.[31] It is with this phase that treatment is initiated.[31]

Evaluation and Treatment. A thorough history and examination is key for the diagnosis of PD. The history should include a detailed presenting complaint, as well as past medical and surgical history. For PD, a sexual history is important. Box 26.3 indicates how to determine if the person is in the acute phase or chronic phase.[31]

An accurate physical exam of penile deformity is necessary for planning care.[47,48] American Urology Association (AUA) guidelines include examination of the penis in the flaccid and erect state. Examination in the erect state can be performed after intracavernosal injection of vasoactive agents.[49] Ultrasound after intracavernosal injection is superior to photographs or vacuum erectile device-assisted erection to accurately determine the type and degree of PD deformity. Duplex doppler penile ultrasound is best for assessing plaque size, location, and calcification, as well as etiology.[31] Laboratory blood tests have a limited role for diagnostic testing except when hypogonadal cause is suspected.[31] The individual should, however, be screened for comorbidities such as diabetes, cardiovascular disease, and other fibroproliferative conditions.

BOX 26.3 To Help Determine Acute Versus Chronic Phase of Peyronie Disease

- *Deformity*: Have the person describe the deformity. Include the direction and degree of deformity
- *Pain*: If pain is present is it associated with both flaccid and erect states or only the erect state.
- *Erection*: the degree of rigidity, ability to sustain it, presence of nocturnal erections
- *Trauma*: History of penile trauma/fracture, urologic procedures, or surgeries
- *Family history*: Any history of Peyronie disease or Dupuytren disease
- *Medical/surgical history*: Diabetes, hypertension, and cardiovascular disease
- *Social history*: Sexual history, smoking, alcohol use, recreational use
- *Psychosocial history*: How has PD affected the person, mood, relationships, self-esteem, and depression

A discussion of all available treatments is critical. The individual's distress over symptoms and the level of concern and willingness to undergo treatment is important to consider in the decision-making process.[31] Treatment consists of both non-surgical and surgical interventions. Non-surgical approaches include a variety of oral and injectable therapies. Very few of these strategies, however, have well-designed, double-blind, placebo-controlled, randomized trials.[31] The lack of quality research for these approaches is an obstacle for determining the best patient-centered interventions. Surgical indications include: (1) a deformity that impairs sexual relations, (2) stable deformity without pain for at least three months, (3) substantial plaque calcification, and (4) failed nonsurgical management.[31] Main criteria for a surgical approach include: (1) nature and location of the deformity, (2) immensity of penile deformity, (3) baseline erection function, (4) penile dimensions, (5) surgeon's experience, and (6) individual's preference.[50] Complications of surgery may include postoperative ED, infection, penile hematoma, penile pain, and recurrence of curvature.[31] Penile prosthesis placement is appropriate for men with ED, severe deformity refractory to medical treatment, or profound penile instability.[31] Prosthesis placement may be complicated because of the presence of plaque and corporal fibrosis, making the dilation of the

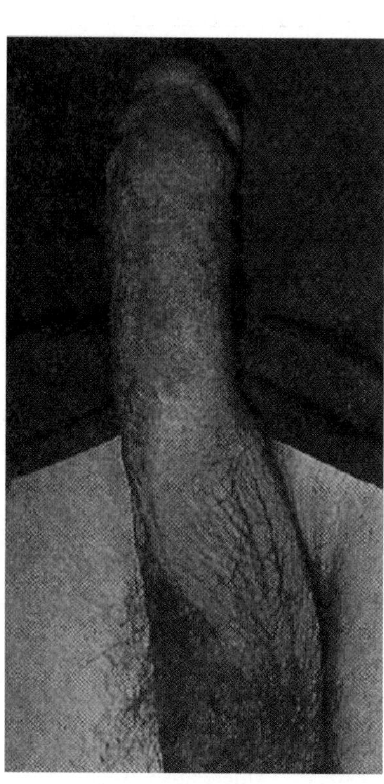
A

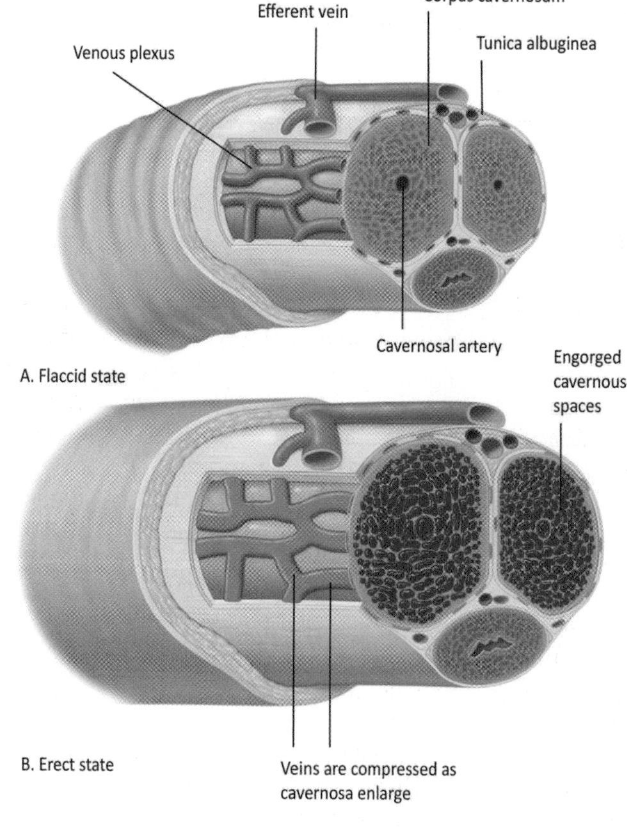

B

Fig. 26.4 Priapism. (A) Erect penis. (B). With priapism the corpus cavernosum is engorged with compressed veins. (A, From Lloyd-Davies RW. *Color atlas of urology*, 2nd edition. London: Wolfe Medical; 1994; B, From uroweb, 2017; B, From European Association of Urology © 2018 patients. uroweb. All rights reserved.)

corpora difficult and increasing the risk for corporal perforation.[31] There are associated psychosocial factors reported with PD, which include embarrassment, distress, self-image factors, mood, intimacy issues, and depression. Therefore, psychosocial support is an important aspect of treatment.

Priapism

Priapism is a disorder of prolonged, rigid penile erection in the absence of appropriate stimulation. Definitions of duration vary, but an erection lasting four hours or longer is considered priapism (Fig. 26.4).[51] Broad categories of priapism include ischemic, nonischemic, and recurrent ischemic. Ischemic causes are an emergency to prevent progression to complete and irreversible ED.[51] The etiology of priapism is determined by arterial flow with low flow (ischemic) and high flow (non-ischemic). The causes of ischemic priapism are numerous and include some hemoglobinopathies, such as sickle cell disease, thalassemia (see Chapter 30), and hypercoagulable state (see Chapter 29).[51] Other causes are vasoactive medications, including ED medications (phosphodiesterase 5 [PDE 5] inhibitors and intracavernous injections), antidepressants (e.g., Trazadone), and illicit drugs, such as cocaine.[51] Less common causes include neurologic disorders, infections, and neoplastic diseases. Recurrent ischemic causes of priapism have some of the same underlying etiologic factors as ischemic priapism except for dysregulated signaling of nitric oxide (NO) in intermittent ischemic episodes.[52] Nonischemic priapism is less common and results from trauma. Iatrogenic injury is a cause from surgical interventions, congenital malformations, or cancer.[51] In a small subset of individuals, no underlying cause or explanation is found.[53,54]

Priapism has a bimodal presentation and peaks at ages 7 to 10 and 20 to 50 years.[51] In two-thirds of individuals the cause is use of intracavernosal drugs used to treat ED. Sickle cell disease accounts for a high number of cases (between 40% and 80%).[51] Sickle cell cases of priapism are mostly seen in African Americans.[55]

Pathophysiology and Clinical Manifestations. Ischemic priapism is a disease of low arterial blood inflow into the corpora cavernosa resulting in a rigid and prolonged erection (see Fig. 26.3A). Venous blood becomes trapped in the corpora cavernosa with increasing pressure which results in tissue ischemia and associated penile pain (see Fig. 26.3B).[51] Priapism typically does not cause engorgement of the glans penis and corpus spongiosum.[51] Nonischemic priapism is caused by unregulated arterial blood flow into the corpora cavernosa without venous trapping. These individuals usually do not develop tissue ischemia; thus, the presentation is mostly painless.[56]

Evaluation and Treatment. A complete history is essential to understand the etiology and document the type of priapism. The history reveals an erection of an abnormally long time in the absence of stimulation with associated penile pain.[51] Critical questions include the duration of symptoms, previous treatments received, injection therapy utilized, erectile function before the priapism episode, current medications, and history of underlying disorders known to provoke priapism. If the etiology is not determined from the history, then laboratory evaluation is performed to determine penile hemodynamics, metabolism, and any underlying diseases that may be contributory.[51] If sickle cell disease is suspected, then hemoglobin S measurements are done.[51]

Ischemic priapism is an emergency. An erection lasting longer than 4 hours mandates early intervention to decrease the potential of irreversible damage and ED. Emergency department management is focused on achieving detumescence or diminution of erection. Several medications can be utilized while waiting for more advanced treatment; however, failure of oral therapies is common with about 75% failure rate.[51] In this situation, the need to perform corporal aspiration of blood is done with concurrent intracavernous injection of a sympathomimetic agent. Surgical intervention consists of shunt procedures with the underlying goal of reducing corporal pressures and, ultimately, penile pain.[53,57,58]

Non-ischemic priapism is typically managed conservatively because of the low probability of penile damage. The initial intervention should be an observation with treatment utilizing topical ice packs. Although aspiration can be completed for diagnostic purposes, it generally does not result in complete detumescence.[51] Many individuals elect to avoid surgery because of inherent risks of ED, and some are reported to maintain their capacity to obtain and maintain an erection despite years of non-ischemic priapism.[51] If a surgical procedure is desired, the general approach is selective embolization or direct ligation of the dysfunctional cavernous artery fistula.[51]

Balanitis

Balanitis is an inflammation of the glans penis (Fig. 26.5). Men present with penile pain and erythema. It affects about 3% to 11% of males during their lifetime. Posthitis is an inflammation of the foreskin or prepuce. Balanoposthitis involves both the glans and foreskin and occurs only in uncircumcised males.[59,60] Balanoposthitis occurs in approximately 6% of uncircumcised males.[61] Balanitis and balanoposthitis often occur together, and the terms are used interchangeably. Although balanitis is not a STI, infectious etiologies of balanitis include certain fungi like yeast, and bacteria or viruses (including those that cause STIs such as gonorrhea).[61] While the actual disease is not transferable from one person to another, the transfer of the infecting organisms that cause balanitis is possible.[61] Recurrent balanoposthitis is a warning for occult diabetes, and these individuals

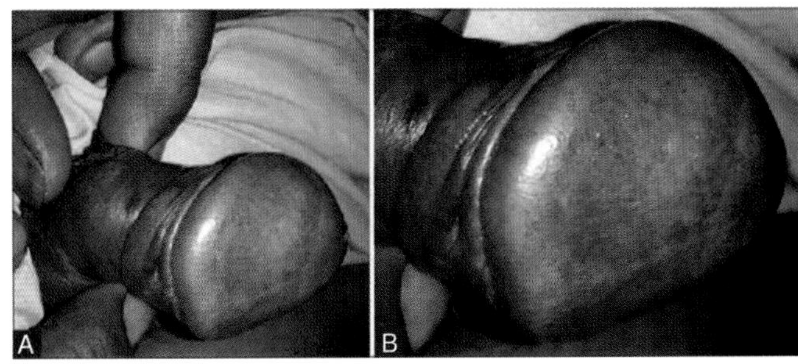

Fig. 26.5 Balanitis. Orange-red shiny plaque on the glans penis and undersurface of the prepuce with multiple pin point sized red spots. (From Dayal S, Sahu P. Zoon balanitis: A comprehensive review. *Indian J Sex Transm Dis AIDS.* 2016;37(2):129–138.)

BOX 26.4 Etiologies of Balanitis

Infectious Etiologies

- Candida species (most associated with diabetes)
- Group B and group A beta-hemolytic streptococci
- Neisseria gonorrhea
- Chlamydia species
- Anaerobic infection
- Human papillomavirus
- Gardnerella vaginalis
- Treponema pallidum (syphilis)
- Trichomonas species
- Borrelia vincentii and Borrelia burgdorferi

Noninfectious Etiologies

- Poor personal hygiene (most common)
- Chemical irritants (e.g., spermicides, detergents, perfumed soaps and shower gels, fabric conditioners)
- Edematous conditions, including congestive heart failure (right sided), cirrhosis, and nephrosis
- Drug allergies (e.g., tetracycline, sulfonamide)
- Morbid obesity
- Allergic reaction (condom latex, contraceptive jelly)
- Fixed-drug eruption (sulfa, tetracycline)
- Plasma cell infiltration (Zoon balanitis)
- Autodigestion by activated pancreatic transplant exocrine enzymes
- Trauma
- Neoplastic conditions

should have blood glucose screening and evaluation by a urologist.

Balanitis is associated with inadequate hygiene and phimosis in uncircumcised males leading to infection. The moist and warm environment under the uncircumcised penile foreskin encourages the growth of organisms such as fungi.[61] Fungal infections are the most identifiable, with most infections from *Candida albicans*.[62] *C. albicans* is normally present on the skin of the glans and considered normal flora. The yeast can cause infection particularly with poor hygiene, overgrowth, or changes in pH. Other etiologies exist and are listed in Box 26.4.[61]

Balanitis can occur at any age and affects about 1 in every 25 boys and 1 in 30 uncircumcised males over the lifetime. The highest risk group is boys under 4 years of age and uncircumcised males.[61] The risk of balanitis decreases when boys reach the age of 5 years, and the foreskin is easier to retract. Circumcised males have a 68% lower prevalence of balanitis than uncircumcised males, and those with balanitis have a 3.8-fold increase in risk of penile cancer.[63] Box 26.5 presents risk factors for balanitis.

Pathophysiology and Clinical Manifestations. Balanitis occurs from the accumulation of smegma beneath the foreskin. Smegma is a whitish sebaceous secretion of dead skin (epithelial cells) and sebum or oily secretions produced by the sebaceous glands. In normal circumstances, smegma helps in the lubrication of the foreskin, decreasing friction and irritation. Tight foreskin, poor hygiene, and smegma are key for bacterial and fungal overgrowth leading to irritation and inflammation. White curd-like exudate is suspicious of candida infection. The yeast *C. albicans* is the most common fungal infection but other etiologies exist (psoriasis or lichen planus, allergic reactions, and less likely premalignant

BOX 26.5 Risk Factors for Balanitis

- Presence of foreskin
- Morbid obesity
- Poor hygiene
- Diabetes (particularly males with uncontrolled diabetes), probably due to glucose on the skin, encouraging bacterial and fungal growth
- Nursing home environment
- Condom catheters
- Sensitivity to chemical irritants (i.e., soaps and lubricants)
- Edematous conditions: Congestive heart failure, nephrosis
- Reactive arthritis
- Sexually transmitted infections

From Wray A, Velasquez J. *Balanitis*. StatPearls [Internet]. Treasure Island, FL: StatPearls; 2020.

condition).[61] Without treatment, edema can occur promoting progression of balanitis. Inflammation and edema together can promote adherence of the foreskin to the glans.[61] Clinical manifestations include pain, tight shiny skin unable to retract on the glans, redness (see Fig. 26.5), soreness, itching, smegma, foul-smelling discharge from under the foreskin, painful urination, swollen glands near the penis, and sores on the glans. More severe symptoms may present in diabetic and immunosuppressed individuals.[63]

Evaluation and Treatment. The diagnosis of balanitis is visual, based on the clinical appearance and presence of lesions. Evaluation may include bacterial culture (in the presence of purulent exudate), herpes simplex virus (HSV) testing (with vesicular or ulcerative lesions), syphilis testing (presence of an ulcer), testing for scabies, trichomonas, and *Mycoplasma genitalium* (presence of urethritis). The mobility of the foreskin is assessed to exclude the complications of phimosis and paraphimosis. Hygienic care with frequent washing and drying of the prepuce is a preventive measure, but excessive genital washing with soap aggravates the disease. For balanoposthitis, topical antifungals usually for one to three weeks are the appropriate choice. First-line therapies are imidazoles such as clotrimazole 1% twice daily, and miconazole 1% twice daily.[61] In those with severe inflammation, the addition of fluconazole 150 mg stat orally or the combination of a topical imidazole with a low-potency topical steroid (e.g., hydrocortisone 0.5%) twice daily, often is successful.[61] With a concern for concomitant cellulitis, treatment with a first-generation cephalosporin is appropriate. Circumcision is recommended for recurrent and intractable episodes in immunosuppressed and diabetic persons. Female sexual partners of men with balanitis should be offered testing for candida. Treatment to both partners will reduce the infection for the couple.[64]

Tumors of the Penis

Tumors of the penis are not common. The most frequent are the benign epithelial tumor condyloma acuminatum and penile carcinomas.

Condyloma acuminatum is a benign tumor caused by HPV, a microorganism that causes a STI (see Chapter 27). HPV type 6 and, less often, type 11, are the most frequent types and can cause a common wart and moist surface of the external genitalia. Giant condyloma (Buschke-Löwenstein) affect older men and may be 5 to 10 cm in size. Atypia may be evident in long-standing giant condyloma, and assessment of other HPV subtypes may be indicated to distinguish the lesion from a noninvasive warty carcinoma.

Penile Cancer

Penile squamous cell carcinoma (PSCC) is a rare cancer with orphan disease designation and a prevalence of 0.1 to 1 per 100,000 men in high-income countries.[65] Globally, penile cancer is rare with 26,000 cases estimated per year.[65] It can affect men 40 to 70 years of age; two-thirds of men are diagnosed at 65 years of age or older. Observed trends of early onset (≤64 years of age) are thought to be associated with changes in sexual practice that increases exposure to STIs and HPV infection.[66] Although the exact cause is unknown, risk factors include HPV infection, smoking, chronic inflammatory conditions (i.e., lichen sclerosus),[67] and psoriasis treatments (psoralens and ultraviolet A; PUVA).[68] Penile cancer is more common in men with phimosis and when circumcision is performed in adulthood. However, circumcision at birth appears to decrease the risk.[69]

Pathophysiology. The standardized term for precursor lesions of penile cancer is penile intraepithelial neoplasia (PeIN).[65] PeIN is divided into two subtypes: a differentiated subtype, typically lichen sclerosus-associated, and an undifferentiated HPV-associated subtype.[70–72] PeIN are all squamous lesions confined to the epidermis by an intact basement membrane. Most PeIN lesions are HPV positive and have several HPV genotypes (HPV6, HPV11, or HPV 16).[65] HPV 16 is a concerning genotype because of its frequency and susceptibility to malignancy.[65] Estimated progression of HPV 16 infection to PeIN is up to 2% of cases within 2 years.[73]

Table 26.3 presents the WHO 2016 classification of PSCC of both HPV-related and non-HPV-related categories; each category has several different histologies. Best understood is the HPV-related biological pathway leading to penile carcinogenesis (Fig. 26.6) Persistent or recurrent exposure to HPV results in the integration of HPV deoxyribonucleic acid (DNA) into the host genome of penile tissue with eventual transformation into a malignant phenotype. Several chronic penile conditions, including balanoposthitis, phimosis, and lichen sclerosus, are risk factors for the development of penile cancer and share a common mechanism of inducing cyclooxygenase 2 (COX2) expression. COX2 has been associated with differentiated PeIN and primary and distant PSCC.[74] COX2 overexpression creates the overproduction of prostaglandins, notably prostaglandin E_2 and thromboxanes, leading to angiogenesis, proliferation, and invasion. Non-HPV-mediated penile carcinogenesis occurs through several gene alterations: amplifications, deletions, mutations, loss of heterozygosity, and/or epigenetic changes (see also Chapters 4, 6, and 12).[65]

Clinical Manifestations. Clinical appearance of penile cancer is presented in Fig. 26.7. Because of decreased public awareness and embarrassment or shame, the majority of penile cancers have a delayed presentation but are clinically apparent.[75] The anatomical location on the penis and the exophytic appearance are distinct features. Tumor location typically arises on the mucosal surfaces of the penis, and in a review of 2000 cases, the tumor was mainly on the glans (35% to 48%) or inner prepuce (13% to 21%), with a small percentage on the penile shaft (2%).[76,77] The lesions are mainly painless and if under a phimotic foreskin, can be associated with a purulent discharge.[78] Ulcerative lesions have a wider differential diagnosis than exophytic lesions and are not diagnosed until histologically proven on either an incisional or punch biopsy for larger and glandular lesions or excisional biopsy for foreskin lesions.[65]

TABLE 26.3 World Health Organization 2016 Pathologic Classification of Squamous Cell Carcinoma of the Penis

Non–HPV-Related Squamous Cell Carcinoma
Squamous cell carcinoma, usual type
Pseudohyperplastic carcinoma
Pseudoglandular carcinoma
Verrucous carcinoma
Carcinoma cuniculatum
Papillary squamous cell carcinoma
Adenosquamous carcinoma
Sarcomatoid (spindle cell) carcinoma
Mixed squamous cell carcinoma
HPV-Related Squamous Cell Carcinoma
Basaloid squamous cell carcinoma
Papillary-basaloid carcinoma
Warty carcinoma
Warty-basaloid carcinoma
Clear cell squamous carcinoma
Lymphoepithelioma-like carcinoma
Others

HPV, Human papillomavirus.
From Cubilla A, Velazquez EF, Amin MB, et al. The World Health Organisation 2016 classification of penile carcinomas: A review and update from the International Society of Urological Pathology expert-driven recommendations. *Histopathology*, 2018;72(6):893–904, In Kumar V, et al. *Robbins & Cotran Pathologic basis of disease*, 10th ed, 2021.

Evaluation and Treatment. Currently, there is no dedicated screening program for PSCC.[65] Clinical examination assesses the lesion size, location (glans, shaft, or foreskin), and morphology (papillary, nodular, ulcerating, fungating, or flat).[65] Clinically obvious are tumors of the penis with exophytic lesions. The majority of tumors are squamous cell carcinomas (SCCs 95%) which are predicted on appearance and location.[65] Diagnostic problems arise when the cancer is occluded under the foreskin or originates from the within the distal urethra. Even when it is very visible, small cancers or low-grade disease may be difficult to differentiate from benign genital dermatoses.[79]

Imaging is essential for cancer staging, surgical planning, and identification of skip lesions within the corpora cavernosa.[65]

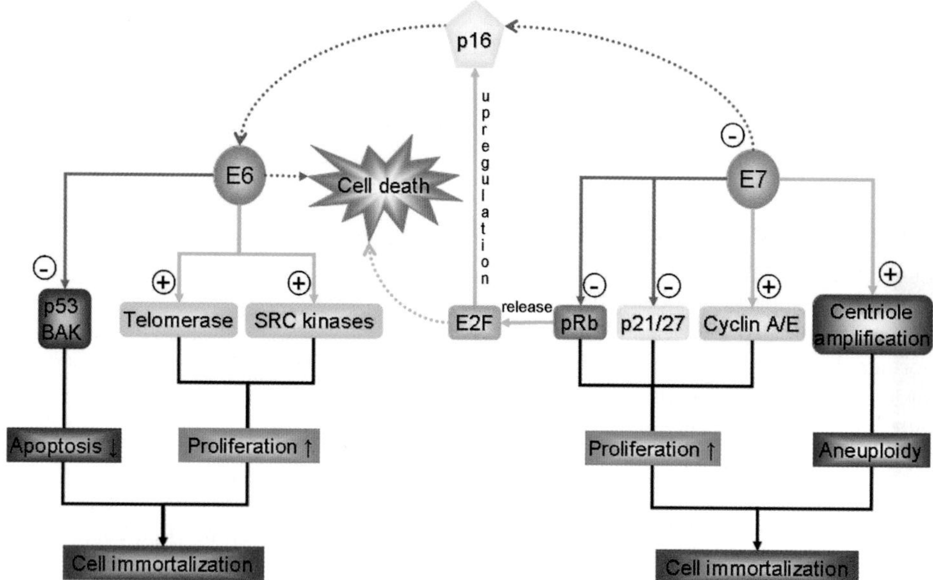

Fig. 26.6 Molecular Pathogenesis in HPV-Associated Penile Carcinogenesis. HPV E6 and E7 oncoproteins interact with cellular pathways and induce cell immortalization. E6 activates telomerase and proto-oncogene tyrosine-protein kinase (SRC kinases) and inhibits p53 and BAK. E7 inhibits the tumor suppressor protein pRb, which causes the release of the E2F transcription factor, allowing E2F to interact with the cellular transcription machinery and stimulate upregulation of the tumor suppressor gene *(CDKN2A)*, which encodes the protein p16 ^{INK4a} (p16). pRb inactivation releases p16 from its negative feedback control, causing a paradoxical increase in the levels of this protein. This attempts to inhibit uncontrolled cellular replication. More simply, p16 is overexpressed in HPV-related tumors in an unsuccessful attempt to stop cell proliferation. E7 stimulates cyclin A and cyclin E; inactivates cyclin-dependent kinase inhibitors p21 and p27, which help to regulate cell cycle control (see Chapter 1); and induces centriole amplification, leading to excessive cell proliferation and aneuploidy. BAK, BCL-2 homologous antagonist/killer; *CDKN2A*, cyclin-dependent kinase inhibitor 2A. (From Boulet G, Horvath C, Vanden Broeck D, et al. Human papillomavirus: E6 and E7 oncogenes. *Int J Biochem Cell Biol.* 2007;39(11):2006–2011.)

Penile ultrasound and MRI are the preferred types of imaging for the primary lesion.[65] Cross-sectional imaging such as CT allows disease staging at diagnosis and identification of abnormal inguinal or lymphadenopathy and distant metastatic disease.[65] The diagnostic pathway confirms the histological subtype, extent of invasion, and metastatic disease to regional or distant lymph nodes.[65] Palpation of the glans and penile shaft is associated with the extent of invasion into the corpus spongiosum or corpus cavernosum.[80] These data enable surgical planning, including the requirement for either a glansectomy or partial penectomy.[65] Generally, a diagnostic biopsy is mandatory in the management of solid tumors. With palpable inguinal lymph nodes, fine needle aspiration (FNA) confirming PSCC within the lymph nodes negates the need for a penile biopsy in the presence of a clinically obvious PSCC. The results would not change the treatment decision-making for an individual with metastatic disease.[65] Most invasive lesions located on the prepuce or glans can be excised using penis-preserving procedures.

In the United States, the 5-year survival rate for penile cancer that has not spread after initial diagnosis is 80%.[81] In the United Kingdom, about 40% of men are diagnosed with localized penile cancer, which has a 5-year overall survival rate of approximately 90%; however, with metastases the prognosis worsens considerably.[65,82] Importantly, the overall prognosis has not improved in Europe and in the US since 1990. This may be due to late-stage initial diagnosis and limited improvements in care and management.[65,83]

Disorders of the Scrotum, Testis, and Epididymis

Disorders of the Scrotum

Men may seek treatment for painful or painless scrotal masses. Masses may be serious (cancer or torsion) or benign (hydrocele or cyst) and may require immediate surgical intervention or allow for careful observation. Varicocele, hydrocele, and spermatocele are common intrascrotal disorders. Varicoceles are dilated tortuous veins of the pampiniform plexus, the venous sinuses that drain the testicles (Fig. 26.8). Although usually painless, varicoceles are clinically significant because they are the most identified cause of abnormal semen analysis, low sperm count, decreased sperm motility, and altered sperm morphology.[84] The right internal spermatic vein terminates directly into the low-pressure inferior vena cava. On the left side, it joins with the somewhat high-pressure left renal vein, thus explaining why most clinically detectable varicoceles are on the left side.[85]

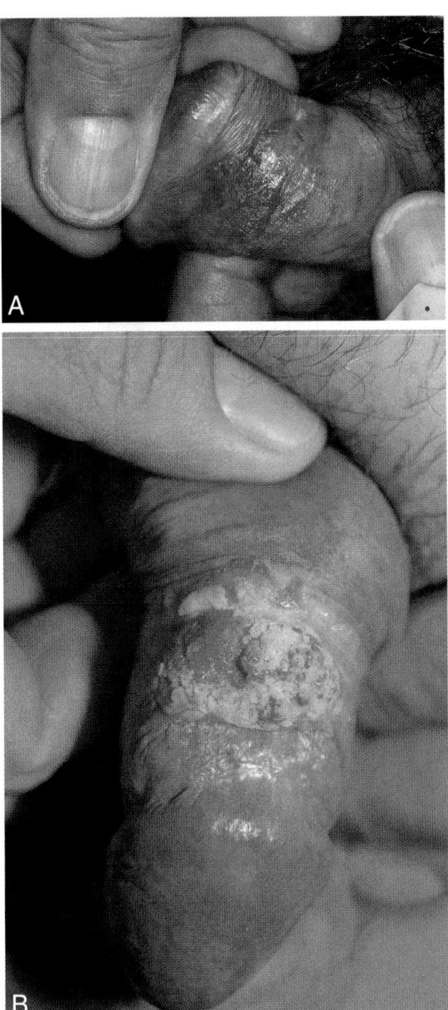

Fig. 26.7 Clinical Appearance in a Few Cases of Premalignant Lesions and Penile Cancer. (A) Non-HPV penile intraepithelial neoplasia (PeIN). **(B)** HPV-related invasive squamous cell carcinoma of the penis. (Courtesy Reinhard Kirnbauer, MD, and Petra Lenz, MD)

Varicocele occurs in 15% to 20% of males and in about 40% of infertile males.[85] It is unclear how a varicocele disrupts the production, structure, and function of sperm, but there are several theories since the association of varicocele with infertility is well known.[85] Varicoceles are classified as small, medium, and large.

The cause of varicocele is unknown. One hypothesis is that it develops from a backup of blood flow in the internal spermatic vein that causes venous engorgement and is detectable on scrotal examination.[86,87] Varicoceles are more common in the left testicle (80% to 90%), but if it is identified in the left testicle, there is a 30% to 40% probability that it is a bilateral condition.[85] Rare causes of varicocele include deep vein thrombosis, renal arteriovenous malformations, and thrombosis of the pampiniform plexus.[85] Risk factors that increase the risk of male infertility include tobacco smoking and mutations in the gene glutathione S-transferase Mu1, which also may increase the risk for a varicocele.[85]

Pathophysiology and Clinical Manifestations. The main concern with a varicocele is infertility. Many men with varicoceles are fertile; however, others may have sperm that is compromised in structure and function, numbers, or motility.[85] The most accepted theory for sperm impairment is that increased blood flow leads to higher intratesticular temperatures.[88]

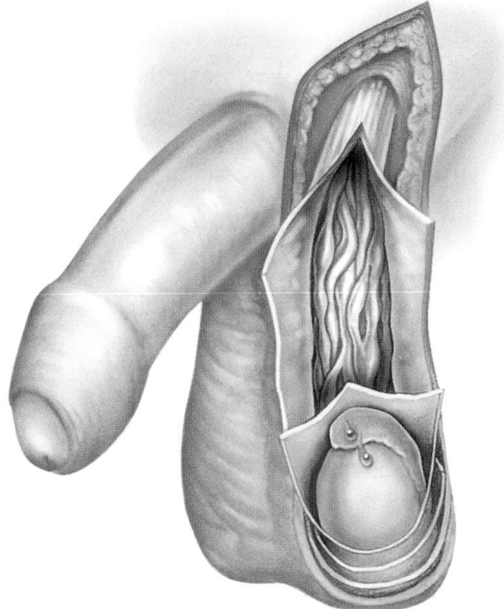

Fig. 26.8 Varicocele. Dilation of veins within the spermatic cord. (From Ball JW, et al. *Seidel's guide to physical examination*, 8th edition. St. Louis: Mosby; 2015.)

Progression from untreated varicoceles does not usually cause pain, although there are exceptions. Orchialgia or chronic testicular pain, when associated with varicoceles, is described as aching, dull, or throbbing and rarely can be acute, stabbing, or sharp.[89] Large varicoceles may cause testicular failure and result in lower hormonal production, oligospermia, and testicular atrophy.[83] Nuclear DNA integrity may be altered which links to sperm motility, viability, counts, and abnormal structure.[90] Varicoceles can cause a reduction in testosterone production in the testes by the Leydig cells.[85]

Evaluation and Treatment. After a complete history and physical examination, the varicocele is confirmed with high-resolution color-flow Doppler ultrasound.[85] Thermal imaging, another non-invasive and painless non-contact method, may also be used for evaluation.[91–93] A stress pattern is an abnormal semen analysis from a microscopic exam and includes a low sperm count, poor motility, and an increase in the percentage of abnormal sperm.[85] A possibility for a right-sided varicocele is renal cell carcinoma. A right-sided renal vein thrombus can expand into the vena cava forming venous obstruction causing spermatic vein obstruction and a right-sided varicocele. In this case, CT imaging is recommended.[94]

There are no effective medical treatments. Varicocelectomy improves the serum testosterone level in greater than 80% of individuals, with a mean increase between 100 and 140 ng/mL, and therefore may be a viable surgical option to permanently treat low testosterone levels in hypogonadal men with significant varicoceles.[85] Surgery is usually done as an outpatient procedure. Avoidance of the vas deferens and the testicular artery during surgery is mandatory.[95–98]

Percutaneous embolization from interventional radiology is usually reserved for open surgical failures or recurrences.[85] The process involves a catheter from the femoral vein, up the vena cava, laterally into the left renal vein and then inferiorly into the spermatic vein. An 89% success rate is reported with this approach.[85]

Identification of small anastomosing vessels is a strength of the microsurgical techniques.[85] This technique also permits better identification of the testicular artery, thus minimizing its unintentional injury.[85] Some pediatric urologists prefer a retroperitoneal, laparoscopic approach which allows for control of the spermatic vein near its insertion into a left renal vein; however, this technique has a fairly high recurrence rate of 15%.[85]

Complications include hematoma, hydrocele, infection, scrotal tissue injury, and arterial injury to the testis that may cause the loss of the testicle.[85] It is not clear which procedure improves male fertility more.[85] After surgery about 70% of individuals have improved semen factors and 40% to 60% have improved conception rates.[85] Surgery for infertility is not recommended for subclinical varicoceles by most experts because it typically does not affect fertility or sperm factors.[85,99] Recently, the use of intraoperative indocyanine green angiography has been used to help identify the testicular artery during dissection.[100]

A hydrocele is an abnormal collection of fluid between the layers of tunica vaginalis of testis (Fig. 26.9).[101] Accumulation of fluid can cause great enlargement of the scrotal sac. Hydroceles can be either congenital or acquired. Acquired hydrocele (secondary) occurs from an underlying condition including infection (filariasis, tuberculosis of the epididymis, syphilis), injury (trauma, post-herniorrhaphy hydrocele), or malignancy.[102] In children the main cause of hydrocele is patency of processus vaginalis (embryonic pouch of peritoneum carried into the scrotum by the descent of the testicle; in the scrotum forms the tunica vaginalis). At birth, approximately, 80% to 90% of term male infants possess a patent processus vaginalis, and this figure declines to about 25% to 40% at two years of age.[102]

Worldwide the cause in adults is filariasis (*Wuchereria* bancrofti), affecting 120 million people in more than 73 countries.[102,103] Iatrogenic causes are either trauma or post-herniorrhaphy complications.[102]

Hydroceles vary in size, and most are asymptomatic. The most important feature on physical examination is a tense, smooth scrotal mass that easily transilluminates. Transillumination, or holding a light behind the scrotum, can help distinguish a hydrocele from a hernia or a solid mass. Surgery is the treatment of choice and is warranted when the hydrocele becomes complicated or symptomatic.[102] A man presenting with a hydrocele in his third or fourth decade needs careful evaluation for testicular cancer.

Spermatoceles (epididymal cysts) are benign cystic collections of fluid of the epididymis located between the head of the epididymis and the testis. Spermatoceles are filled with a milky fluid containing sperm and are usually painless (Fig. 26.10). Spermatoceles that cause significant pain or discomfort are excised. Both spermatoceles and epididymal cysts present clinically as discrete, firm, freely mobile masses distinct from the testis that may be transilluminated.[104,105] Usually, however, spermatoceles are asymptomatic or produce mild discomfort that is relieved by scrotal support.

Fig. 26.9 Hydrocele. Accumulation of clear fluid between the visceral (inner) and parietal (outer) layers of the tunica vaginalis.

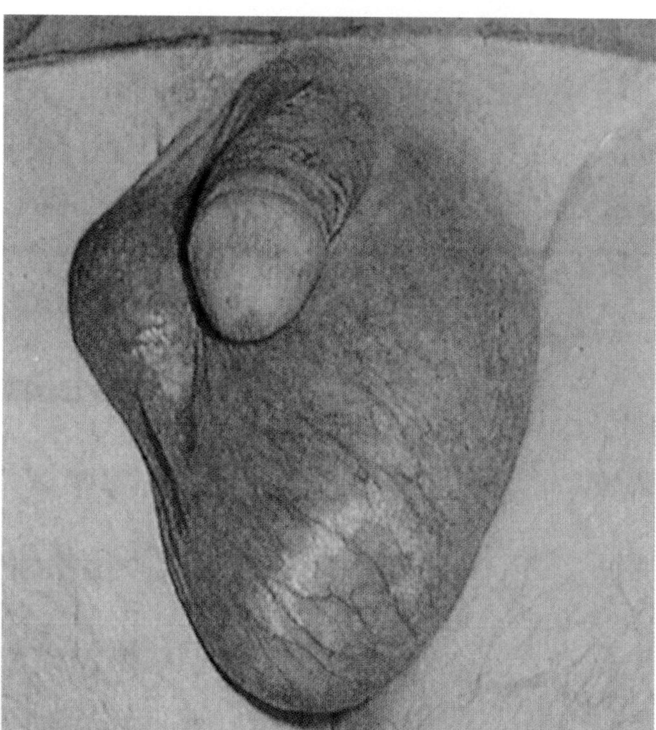

Fig. 26.10 Spermatocele. Retention cyst of the head of the epididymis or of an aberrant tubule or tubules of the rete testis. The spermatocele lies outside the tunica vaginalis; therefore, on palpation it can be readily distinguished and separated from the testis. (From Lloyd-Davies RW et al. *Color atlas of urology*, 2nd edition. London: Wolfe Medical; 1994.)

Cryptorchidism

Cryptorchidism is the absence of at least one testicle from the scrotum. It is the most common birth defect of the male genitalia.[106] The testicle may be in several locations along the "path of descent," such as high in the retroperitoneal abdomen to the inguinal ring, in the inguinal canal, ectopic from the path of descent, hypoplastic, dysgenetic, absent, or unilateral (two-thirds). About 80% of cryptorchid testes descend by the third month making the incidence approximately 1%. About 3% of full-term and 30% of premature male infants are born with one or both testicles undescended.[107] Cryptorchidism may occur on both sides but is more common with the right testicle.[106] Undescended testicles are associated with decreased fertility in bilateral cases, and in up to 10% in unilateral cases, increased germ cell tumors (risk <1%), testicular torsion, inguinal hernias, and certain psychological problems.[106] Without surgical correction, an undescended testicle often descends during the first three months of life.[106] Testicular dysgenesis syndrome (TDS) includes cryptorchidism, hypospadias, testicular cancer, and poor semen quality. TDS is thought to be due to harmful environmental factors that interfere with embryonal programming and gonadal development during fetal life (Fig. 26.11).[108]

Normal testicular descent depends on a normal hypothalamic-pituitary-gonadal axis. The main risk factor for undescended testes is birthweight followed by family history.[106] Typically, in full-term infants, the cause of cryptorchidism cannot be determined, making this a common, though sporadic, unknown birth defect.[106] Overall, genetics with maternal and environmental factors may disrupt hormones and physical changes that affect testicular development and descent. See Box 26.6 for other underlying risk factors.[106,107,109] Cryptorchidism occurs in about 1.5% to 4% of fathers and 6% of brothers of those affected. Heritability in first-degree male relatives is estimated at 0.5% to 1%.[106] For unknown reasons there is an association between cryptorchidism and autism. Cryptorchidism and neurodevelopmental disorders may have shared genetic or in utero/early postnatal risk factors, which need much more investigation.[110]

Pathophysiology and Clinical Manifestations. One mechanism for the reduced function of cryptorchid testes is temperature. Additionally, it is probable that hormone deficiencies may result in lack of testicular descent and impair the development of spermatogenic tissue.[111] Men with undescended testes may have reduced fertility even after orchiopexy (surgery to move an undescended testicle).[112] Risk of testicular cancer if orchiopexy is done before puberty is about 3 times that of the general population.[106] The risk is 5 to 6 times higher when orchiopexy is done after puberty.[106]

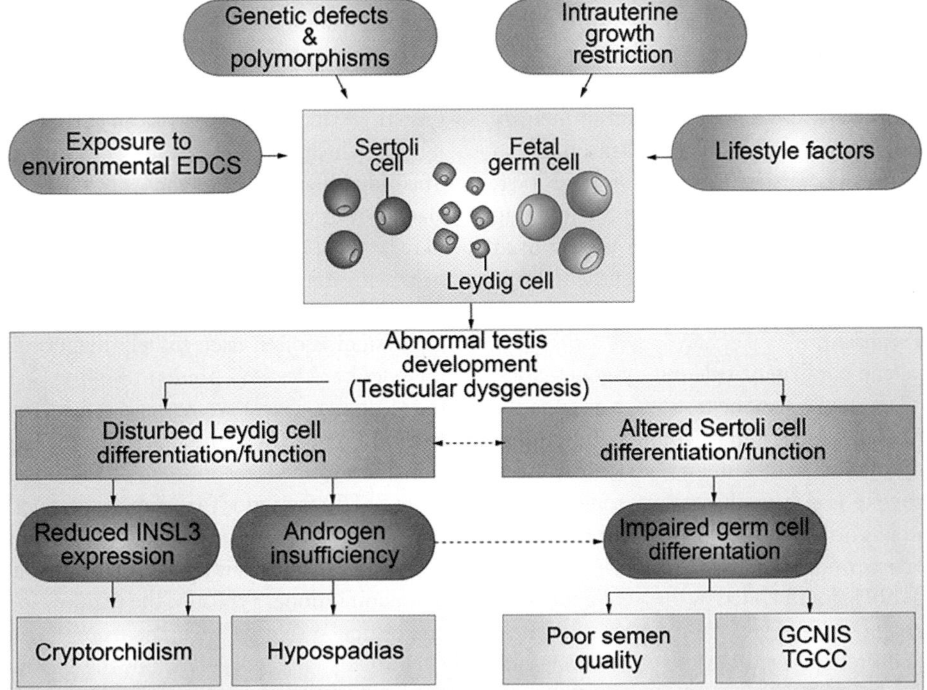

Fig. 26.11 Testicular Dysgenesis Syndrome. Working model of testicular dysgenesis syndrome (TDS) development may involve the following four key aspects: environmental exposure, genetic factors, intrauterine growth disorders, and lifestyle factors. These factors contribute to abnormal testis development which involve disturbed Leydig cell differentiation and altered Sertoli cell differentiation. Disturbed Leydig cell differentiation reduces insulin-like factor 3 (INSL3) and results in androgen insufficiency and altered Sertoli cell differentiation which leads to impaired germ cell function. *EDCS*, Endocrine-disrupting chemicals; *GCNIS*, germ cell neoplasia in situ; *TGCC*, testicular germ cell cancer. (From Xing J-S, Bai Z-M. Is testicular dysgenesis syndrome a genetic, endocrine, or environmental disease, or an unexplained reproductive disorder? *Life Sci.* 2018;194:120–129.)

BOX 26.6 Risk Factors for Cryptorchidism

- Premature infants born before the descent of the testicles
- Small for gestational age infants
- Smaller placental weight
- Chemical endocrine disruptors may interfere with normal fetal hormone balance
- Maternal obesity
- Maternal diabetes
- Maternal exposure to Diethylstilbestrol (DES)
- Pesticides
- Alcohol consumption during pregnancy (5 or more drinks per week, 3x increase)
- Cigarette smoking
- Family history
- Cosmetics use
- Exposure to phthalate (DEHP)
- Ibuprofen
- Preeclampsia (The more severe the preeclampsia, the greater the risk of cryptorchidism)
- Congenital malformation syndromes—Down syndrome, Prader–Willi syndrome, and Noonan syndrome
- Persistent Mullerian Duct Syndrome
- In vitro fertilization

Data from Wray A, Velasquez J. *Balanitis.* StatPearls [Internet]. Treasure Island, FL: StatPearls; 2020.

Evaluation and Treatment. AUA guidelines indicate that experienced providers can palpate more than 70% of cryptorchid testes by physical examination and need no imaging.[106] The challenge in the other 30% of cases, with a nonpalpable testis, is to "confirm absence or presence of the testis and to identify the location of the viable nonpalpable testis."[106] Ultrasound can be used but has a sensitivity and specificity at 45% and 78%, respectively.[106] CT is not recommended because of the ionizing radiation exposure and expense.[106] MRI is more widely used and has greater sensitivity and specificity.[106] Presently, there is no radiological test that can conclude, with 100% accuracy and reliability, that a testis is absent.[113]

A genetic karyotype can confirm or rule out dysgenetic primary hypogonadism.[106] Certain hormone tests, such as gonadotropins and anti-mullerian (AMH) may confirm functional testicles, as well as stimulation with human chorionic gonadotropin (HCG) to provoke a rise in the testosterone level.[106] Further testing may be important in some cases with the likelihood of detecting intersex conditions.[112]

Hormonal therapy is not recommended by the AUA guidelines to induce testicular descent.[112] However, the American Pediatric Association Guidelines do recommend the use of hormones for those with undescended testis associated with Prader-Willi syndrome.[112] The rationale is that a therapeutic trial of HCG is indicated for treatment of undescended testes before surgery, because infants with low muscle tone who are at high risk for underlying respiratory compromise should avoid general anesthesia.[112]

According to AUA guidelines, surgery is recommended for congenital undescended testes between the ages of 6 and 18 months.[106] Many experts recommend surgery, around 6 months to optimize testicular growth and fertility. For premature babies, corrected age is used to determine surgery timing. Germ loss increases and fertility decreases the longer the cryptorchid testis remains untreated. Thus, early orchidopexy is the usual, standard remedy.[114]

Individuals with bilateral undescended testes who receive orchidopexies as adults are usually infertile and azoospermic (complete absence of sperm from the fluid ejaculated during orgasm).[115] For both acquired (testis documented normal before diagnosis) and entrapped (after hernia repair) undescended testes, surgery is recommended shortly after diagnosis. With retractile testes, a yearly physical examination is recommended because of the 2% to 50% reported risk of a retractile testis becoming an acquired undescended testis.[106] In those with a history of cryptorchidism and treatment, testicular cancer risk and infertility remains somewhat increased compared to the general population.[116]

Testicular Torsion and Testicular Appendages

Testicular torsion occurs when a testicle rotates twisting the spermatic cord and interrupting its blood supply (Fig. 26.12). In most individuals the testicle rotates between 90 and 180 degrees; complete torsion is rare and can quickly decrease viability of the testicle. Torsion of the testis is one of several conditions that cause an acute scrotum, which is testicular pain and swelling. The testicle will become tender, swollen, and erythematous. It is a urologic emergency. Differentiation between testicular torsion and two other common causes of an acute scrotum is based on physical examination and history (Table 26.4).[117]

Testicular torsion can occur at any age, including pre- or perinatal, but is most common in adolescents (during periods of growth).[118] It often presents as an abrupt onset of unilateral scrotal pain which may be constant, intermittent, but not positional.[118] The individual may have nausea or vomiting. There may be associated lower abdominal and inguinal pain, and these symptoms may be the presenting complaint rather than scrotal pain.[118] To help with diagnosis, the cremasteric reflex and the Prehn sign are not as reliable as once thought.[118] However, the TWIST scoring system is often used to help diagnose testicular torsion and includes hard testis (2 points), swelling (2 points), nausea/vomiting (1 point), absent cremasteric reflex (1 point), and high riding testis (1 Point). The higher the score, the higher probability of torsion. Ultrasound is recommended for those individuals with a low score.[118] Ultrasound is the primary diagnostic method, and color flow Doppler is used to evaluate both venous and arterial flow.[118] If urological intervention is not immediately available manual detorsion is done. Typically, the window for surgical intervention and testicular salvage is 6 hours from the onset of pain.[118]

Testicular appendages include the appendix testis (a remnant of the müllerian duct) and the appendix epididymis (a remnant of the wolffian duct). Torsion of the appendages is more common than testicular torsion and not as critical. During early-onset, severe tenderness is noted with palpation near the head of the epididymis or testis, palpation of an isolated tender nodule, and/or visualizing a blue dot appearance on the testis. All of these characteristics aid in differentiating torsion of the appendages from testicular torsion. The blue dot is due to the cyanotic torsed appendage.[118] The testicular appendage tends to calcify and degenerate over two weeks, and usually surgical treatment is not required.[118]

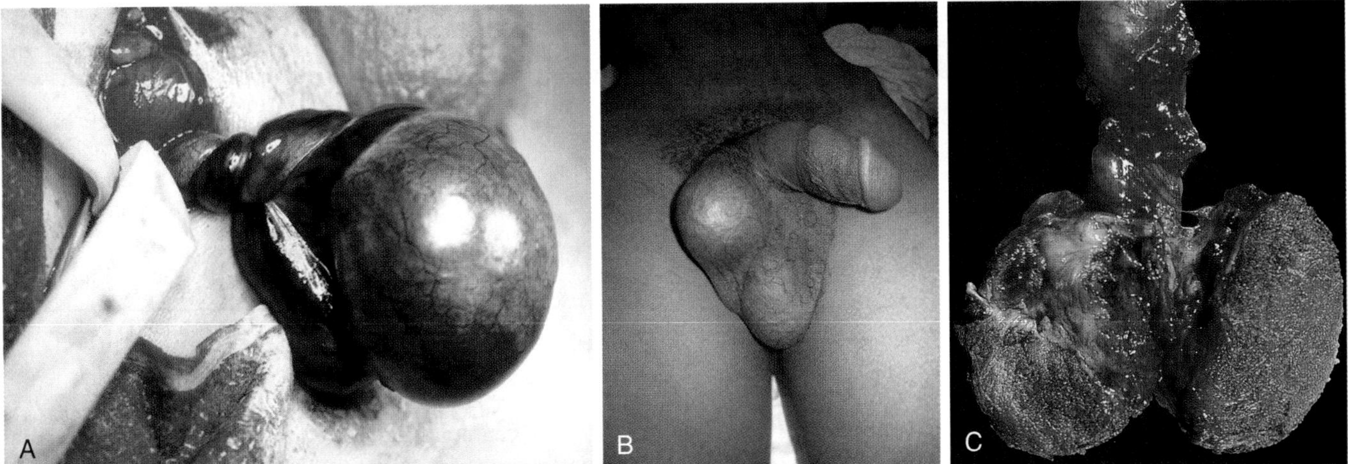

Fig. 26.12 **Torsion of the Testis.** **(A)** Left testicular torsion in an adolescent with acute scrotum; the testis is necrotic. **(B)** Late phase torsion in an adolescent with severe testicular pain 1 month previously. Note the absence of inflammation and the high position of the testis in the scrotum. **(C)** The testes appear dark red and partially necrotic owing to hemorrhagic infarction. (A and B, From Kliegman RM et al. *Nelson's textbook of pediatrics*, 19th edition. Philadelphia: Saunders; 2011. C, From Damjanov I, Linder J, eds. *Anderson's pathology*, 10th edition. St. Louis: Mosby; 1996.)

TABLE 26.4 Diagnosis of Selected Conditions Responsible for the Acute Scrotum

Condition	Onset of Symptoms	Age	Tenderness	Urinalysis	Cremasteric Reflex	Treatment
Testicular torsion	Acute	Early puberty	Diffuse	Negative	Negative	Surgical exploration
Appendiceal torsion	Subacute	Prepubertal	Localized to upper pole	Negative	Positive	Bed rest and scrotal elevation
Epididymitis	Insidious	Adolescence	Epididymal	Positive or negative	Positive	Antibiotics

Orchitis

Orchitis is an acute inflammation of the testis and is usually unilateral (Fig. 26.13). On presentation, it can be acute and symptomatic, or asymptomatic and chronic.[119] Isolated orchitis is rare and usually accompanied by an infection of the epididymis.[120] Box 26.7 presents the various bacteria and viruses that cause orchitis. It develops in 14% to 35% of post-pubertal individuals with mumps.[120]

Pathophysiology. There are two differences between orchitis and other infections of the male accessory sex organs: (1) the primary route of infection to the testis is blood-borne dissemination,[121] and (2) viruses are the significant infecting microorganisms.[120] Mumps virus is responsible for most of the cases of isolated orchitis. Common risk factors include a preexisting history of epididymitis, unprotected sexual contact, multiple sexual partners, long-term use of a urinary catheter, bladder outlet obstruction (BOO), and lack of immunization with measles, mumps, and rubella (MMR) vaccination (vaccination reduces the risk after mumps)[122]; however, cases of orchitis have been reported after receiving the MMR vaccine.[123]

Clinical Manifestations. The individual usually presents with acute onset of testicular pain, which initially involves one testis, and may spread to the entire scrotum. Other symptoms

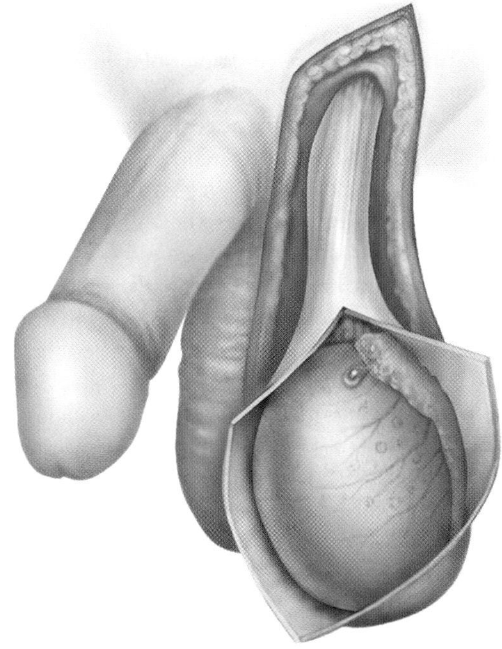

Fig. 26.13 **Orchitis.** (From Ball JW et al. *Seidel's guide to physical examination*, 8th edition. St. Louis: Mosby; 2015.)

BOX 26.7 Bacteria and Viruses That Cause Orchitis

- In young individuals orchitis is usually viral; mumps and rubella are most common
- Other viruses include coxsackievirus, varicella, echovirus, and cytomegalovirus
- Bacterial origins include *Escherichia coli, Klebsiella pneumoniae, Pseudomonas aeruginosa*, and *Staphylococcus* and *Streptococcus* species
- In sexually active males common bacteria are *Neisseria gonorrhoeae, Chlamydia trachomatis*, and *Treponema pallidum*
- In immunocompromised males causes of orchitis are *Mycobacterium avium* complex, *Cryptococcus neoformans, Toxoplasma gondii, Haemophilus parainfluenzae*, and *Candida albican.*

may include fever, malaise, fatigue, and chills.[120] Physical examination findings may include testicular enlargement, scrotal edema, tenderness, induration, and possibly erythema.[120] If orchitis is accompanied by epididymitis, the epididymis may be enlarged. Cremasteric reflex is normal in affected individuals. Mumps orchitis may also present with parotid enlargement, which is usually present 4 to 8 days after onset of parotitis.[120]

Evaluation and Treatment. Laboratory blood tests are generally not helpful but urethral swabs and urine samples are routinely obtained, as are cultures to rule out UTI and diagnose any STIs.[120] Healthcare providers must distinguish between torsion and inflammation of the testis when individuals present in the emergency department.[120] Antibiotics are not used for viral causes. Supportive therapies include bed rest, antipyretics, analgesics, scrotal support, and hot or cold packs for analgesics.[120] Bacterial infections are treated with antibiotics. STIs are treated according to CDC guidelines (see Chapter 27). Sexual partners of those with an STI should receive treatment.

Cancer of the Testis

Testicular cancer is the most common solid malignancy in young adult men, and its incidence in the last two decades has risen worldwide.[116,124,125] Testicular cancer accounts for approximately 1% of newly diagnosed cancer in men worldwide; it is the most common malignancy among men ages 14 and 44 years.[116] Germ cell neoplasia in situ (GNIS) is known as the precursor lesion to malignant testicular germ cell tumors (TGCTs).[116,126] In western countries, the incidence of testicular cancer continues to increase with an estimated 9470 cases and 440 deaths in the United States in 2021.[124] Globally, the estimated incidence is 74,458 and 9334 estimated deaths.[127] In the United States, it is more common in white men (6.9 per 100,000 males) than in African Americans (1.2 per 100,000 males).[116] Despite the high incidences of testicular cancer in Europe, North America, Australia, and New Zealand, these areas account for only one-fifth of mortalities.[116] The highest mortality rates are reported in western Asia.[128] The most consistent risk factor for testicular cancer is cryptorchidism, which increases the risk almost fivefold.[116]

An important and causal pathway to cryptorchidism, hypospadias, low sperm count, and testicular cancer is disrupted signaling to endogenous hormones by prenatal xenobiotic exposure.[129,130] Emerging evidence suggests that postnatal environmental or lifestyle factors such as diet or environmental exposures to endocrine-disrupting chemicals influence testicular cancer development.[131] During the 20th century, populations of industrialized countries worldwide have experienced a decline in total fertility rates (TFR, average number of live births/woman). Simultaneously, a rise in testicular germ cell cancer (TGCC) has occurred globally.[132] Additionally, other male reproductive problems, several of which are linked to testicular cancer, including disorders of spermatogenesis, are widespread.[132] Therefore, investigators have proposed possible etiological roles of environmental, epigenetic, and genetic factors to account for these trends. The most common epidemiological risk factors, however, are summarized in Box 26.8.[133]

BOX 26.8 Most Common Epidemiological Risk Factors Testicular Cancer

- Cryptorchidism
- Infections-HPV, EBV, CMV, Parvovirus B-19, and HIV
- Testicular trauma
- High maternal estrogen level
- Carcinoma in situ (intratubular germ cell neoplasia
- Prior history of testis cancer or extragonadal germ cell tumor
- Family history

HPV, Human papilloma virus; *EBV*, Epstein-Barr virus; *CMV*, cytomegalovirus; *HIV*, human immunodeficiency virus.

Germ cell tumors were traditionally classified by histological composition. Another way for classification has also been the germ cell lineage and the age of onset of testicular cancer: pediatric, adolescent, or adult.[116] In 2016, the WHO published a classification system combining categories and defining the two major entities of TGCTs as GCNIS-related TGCTs and non-GNIS-related TGCTs (Box 26.9).[134,135]

Pathophysiology. GCNIS is regarded as the precursor lesion to malignant testicular germ cell tumors (TGCTs).[116] Germ-cell tumors are observed secondary to a carcinogenic event in utero that results in an intratubular germ-cell neoplasia.[136] Intratubular germ-cell neoplasia is derived from gonocytes (cell that produces gametes) that have failed to differentiate into spermatogonia.[133,137] During puberty these cells attain invasive potential because of hormonal changes.[133] Seminomas are comprised of transformed germ cells that are blocked in their differentiation.[133] Embryonal carcinoma cells resemble undifferentiated stem cells, and their gene expression is like those of stem cells and intratubular germ-cell neoplasms.[138,139] Choriocarcinomas and yolk-sac tumors have extraembryonic (situated outside the embryo) differentiation, and teratomas have somatic differentiation.[133]

The origin of TGCT likely initiates in early embryogenesis and appears to be part of the TDS, where some early gonocytes are blocked in their differentiation. They are tightly regulated by epigenetic modifications (specific transcription factors discussed earlier) in terms of microRNA expression and DNA methylation retaining their early primordial germ cells (PGCs),

BOX 26.9 WHO Classification for Testicular Cancer

1. **Germ Cell Tumors**
   - Germ cell neoplasia in situ (GCNIS)
2. **Derived from Germ Cell Neoplasia in Situ (GCNIS)**
   - Seminoma
   - Embryonal carcinoma
   - Yolk sac tumor, post-pubertal type
   - Trophoblastic tumor
   - Teratoma, post-pubertal type
   - Teratoma with somatic-type malignancies
   - Mixed germ cell tumors
3. **Germ Cell Tumors Unrelated to GCNIS**
   - Spermatocytic tumor
   - Yolk sac tumor, pre-pubertal type
   - Mixed germ cell tumor, pre-pubertal type
4. **Sex Cord/Stromal Cell Tumors**
   - Leydig cell tumor
   - Malignant Leydig cell tumor
   - Sertoli cell tumor

Malignant Sertoli cell tumor
Large cell calcifying Sertoli cell tumor
Intratubular large cell hyalinizing Sertoli cell neoplasia

- Granulosa cell tumor

Adult type
Juvenile type

- Thecoma/fibroma group of tumors
- Other sex cord/gonadal stromal tumors

Mixed
Unclassified

- Tumors containing both germ cell and sex cord/gonadal stromal

Gonadoblastoma

5. **Miscellaneous Non-specific Stromal Cell Tumors**
   - Ovarian epithelial tumors
   - Tumors of collecting ducts and rete testes

Adenoma
Carcinoma

- Tumors of paratesticular structures

Adenomatoid tumor
Mesothelioma (epithelioid, biphasic)
Epididymal tumors

- Cystadenoma of the epididymis
- Papillary cystadenoma
- Adenocarcinoma of the epididymis
- Mesenchymal tumors of the spermatic cord and the testicular adnexa

Data From Gaddam SJ, Chesnut GT. *Testicle cancer*. StatPearls [Internet]. Treasure Island, FL: StatPearls; 2021.

or gonocyte changes progressing to testicular cancer.[140,141] Formation of different histologic subtypes may be associated with distinct gene expression through epigenetic regulation, including DNA methylation.[133,142]

Clinical Manifestations. Most men with testicular tumors present with a palpable lump that may or may not be painful (Fig. 26.14).[116] Rarely do they present with signs of metastatic disease such as cachexia, breathlessness, or hemoptysis.[116] Occurring gradually, it may be accompanied by a sensation of testicular heaviness or a dull ache in the lower abdomen. Sometimes, the testis is unable to be completely palpated because

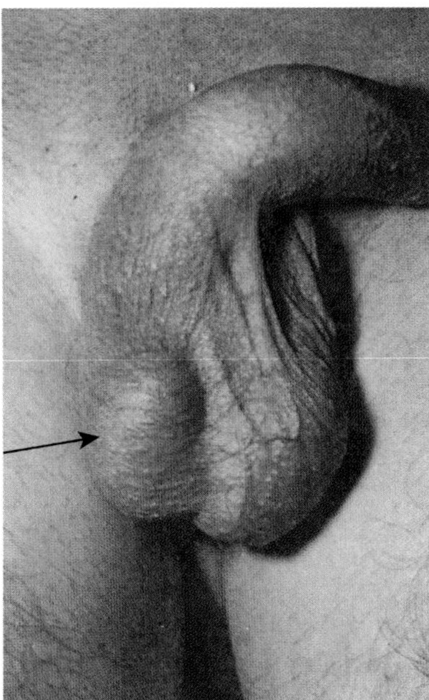

Fig. 26.14 Testicular Tumor. (From Wolfe J. 400 *Self-assessment picture tests in clinical medicine*. London: Wolfe Medical; 1984.)

BOX 26.10 Manifestations of Metastatic Disease Testicular Cancer

- Systemic symptoms: weight loss, anorexia, malaise,
- Pulmonary metastasis: shortness of breath or cough
- Lymphatic metastasis: cervical or supraclavicular lymphadenopathy
- Retroperitoneal disease: bulky retroperitoneal disease can present as back pain or compression on the gonadal veins leading to findings of varicocele
- Vascular obstruction or thrombosis resulting in lower extremity edema
- Retroduodenal metastasis: nausea, vomiting, or gastrointestinal hemorrhage
- Central or peripheral nervous system metastasis: symptoms from the cerebral, spinal cord, or peripheral nerve root involvement.

of the presence of a hydrocele. Uncommonly, individuals present with manifestations of metastatic disease (Box 26.10).[133]

Evaluation and Treatment. Evaluation begins with a thorough history, and careful physical examination, which generally will reveal a firm intratesticular lesion. Included are questions about the history of cryptorchidism, orchiopexy, or inguinal repair as an infant.[133] Questions include a family history of testicular cancer in father or brother. Unless proven otherwise, findings of any solid mass should be considered testicular cancer. The contralateral testis is examined because 0.6% of individuals have a synchronous contralateral testis tumor.[133] The primary imaging is with trans-scrotal ultrasound.[143–145] Ultrasound imaging, combined with physical examination for the diagnosis of testicular cancer, provides almost 100% sensitivity.[146] All individuals with TGCTs have further imaging with abdominopelvic CT scans. Additional scans are done in those with elevated serum tumor markers (AFP, α-fetoprotein; β-hCG, β-subunit of HCG; LDH, lactate dehydrogenase).[133] Further evaluation includes serum tumor markers (AFP, HCG, and LDH), which should be done before any intervention, including orchiectomy.[133] Many new immunohistochemical markers have been studied for diagnostic purposes. Counseling includes the possibility of infertility, testicular prosthesis if desired, and sperm banking with bilateral testicular pathology.[143,144] Persons should be referred to an oncology specialist for staging and treatment of cancer.

Epididymitis

Epididymitis is an inflammation of the epididymis testis, the tubular structure located on the posterior and superior part of the testis where sperm mature prior to ejaculation.[147] Testis proximity to the epididymis can cause the infection or inflammatory process to spread to the testis itself, which is known as epididymo-orchitis.[148] Epididymitis is the most common cause of acute scrotal pain in adults with more than 600,000 men in the Unites States affected yearly.[147] Most cases of epididymitis result from retrograde flow of urine, which commonly occurs in elderly males, and from STIs in males 20 to 40 years old (Fig. 26.15).[147] Approximately 50% of cases of sexually transmitted microorganisms in males less than 39 years old include *N. gonorrhoeae* or *C. trachomatis*. After 39 years of age, the most common etiologic agents are *Escherichia coli* and other coliform bacteria located in the gastrointestinal tract.[147]

Pathophysiology. The main etiology of epididymitis is bacterial infection. Pathogens from STIs can be introduced during sexual intercourse and move through the genitourinary (GU) tract to the epididymis.[147] Whereas, pathogens from UTIs cause epididymitis due to retrograde flow of urine or from stagnation of urine along the GU tract. Although rare, epididymitis may result from a chemical inflammation caused by the reflux of sterile urine into the ejaculatory ducts. Repetitive movement creating mobility of the scrotum can create inflammation of the testes or epididymis.[147] Young males prior to sexual maturity can develop epididymis as an inflammatory process from repetitive sports (e.g., jumping, running). Viral infection (e.g., mumps virus) can infect the testis resulting in epididymitis or epididymo-orchitis.[147] Chemical epididymitis can result from exercising or having sexual intercourse with a full bladder. Certain medications also can cause epididymitis, such as amiodarone used in the treatment of cardiac dysrhythmia.

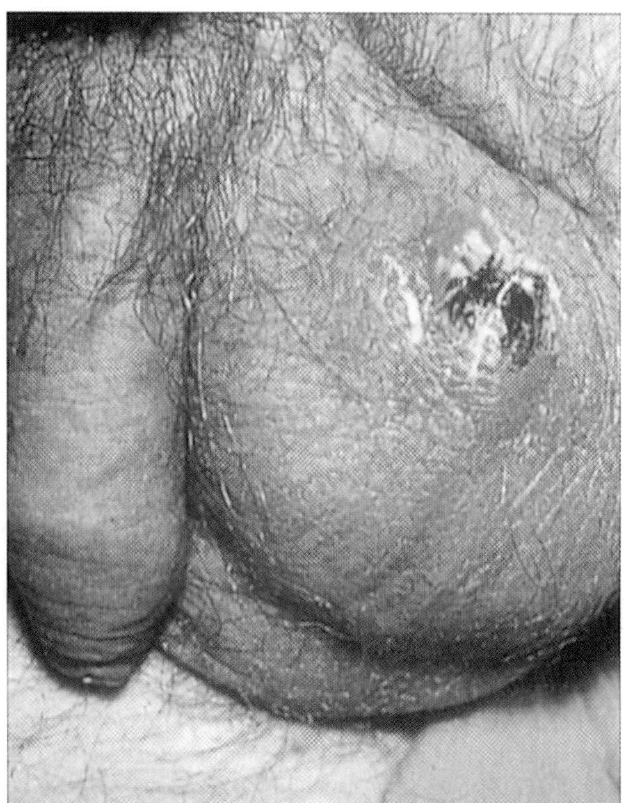

Fig. 26.15 Epididymitis Secondary to Gonorrhea or Nongonococcal Urethritis. (This infection has spread to the testes, and rupture through the scrotal wall is threatened. (From Taylor PK. *Diagnostic picture tests in sexually transmitted disease.* London: Mosby; 1995.)

Clinical Manifestations. The main symptom of epididymitis is scrotal or inguinal pain caused by inflammation of the epididymis and surrounding tissues. Onset of pain is gradual rather than acute.[147] Flank pain may occur if, as the urethra passes over the spermatic cord, edematous swelling of the cord then obstructs the urethra. The individual may have pyuria, bacteriuria, urinary frequency, urgency, or incontinence, and a history of urethral discharge. The scrotum on the involved side is erythematous and edematous. The tail of the epididymis, near the lower pole of the testis, usually swells first; swelling then ascends to the head of the epididymis. The spermatic cord also may be swollen and tender. Tender inguinal adenopathy may also be present.

Evaluation and Treatment. A careful history should focus on repetitive activities such as sports, complete sexual history including exposure to STIs, possibility of traumatic injury, and problems associated with GU tract, such as previous UTIs, prostatitis, or surgical procedures.[147] A physical exam will likely show swelling of the scrotum and palpation of the scrotum will reveal scrotal tenderness, usually unilaterally. The hallmark of epididymitis is tenderness upon palpation of the testis along the posterior and superior area.[147] Additionally, the tenderness may indicate epididymo-orchitis or orchitis. A urethral discharge may be demonstrated from physical exam of the penis.

Evaluation begins with a urinalysis; the presence of red blood cells and white blood cells, though nonspecific, may indicate an acute infectious or inflammatory condition. The definitive diagnosis is based on culture or Gram stain. A urethral swab is done where STI is considered after obtainment of the sexual history. Ultrasound can assess anatomy and vascular flow to the testis. It can demonstrate inflammation of the epididymis and testis in cases of epididymitis and epididymo-orchitis. It is critical to rule out the possibility of testicular torsion as a cause of scrotal pain. Pain from epididymitis is usually gradual; the pain of testicular torsion typically is very abrupt.[147]

Treatment includes antibiotic therapy for the infection itself. Improvement in pain and swelling occurs in many cases by using ice.[149–151] If the individual does not steadily improve, reevaluation is necessary within a few days for possible complications. The individual's sexual partner should be treated with antibiotics if the causative microorganism is a sexually transmitted pathogen.

Disorders of the Prostate Gland

Benign Prostatic Hyperplasia

Benign prostatic hyperplasia (BPH) is nonmalignant growth or hyperplasia of prostate tissue (Fig. 26.16). It is not a premalignant lesion. BPH is a common cause of lower urinary tract symptoms (LUTS) and is the most common benign prostatic disease in men older than 50 years. Several definitions exist when describing BPH such as BOO, LUTS, and benign prostatic enlargement (BPE). BPH, the preferred term, is a histologic description (hyperplasia); BPE describes the increased size of the gland (typically secondary to BPH); and BOO describes the obstruction of flow.[152] Another term, benign prostatic obstruction, refers to those with BPE who present with BOO.[153] With population aging, the incidence and prevalence of BPH and LUTS have increased rapidly.[154] Age is a significant predictor of both development of BPH and later LUTS, with 50% of men over the age of 50 having evidence of BPH and then development of LUTS, with a linear increase with age.[152] BPH prevalence in the United States is as high as 70% in those between 60 and 69 years of age and more than 80% in men over 70 years.[152]

Risk factors for BPH include increasing age, metabolic syndrome, diabetes, obesity, hypertension, diet, sex hormone levels, and genetic factors.[152,154] Metabolic syndrome includes hypertension, glucose intolerance/insulin resistance, and dyslipidemia. Meta-analysis has shown those with metabolic syndrome and obesity have significantly higher prostate volume.[155] LUTS is associated with increased levels of glycated hemoglobin (HbA1c).[156] Observational studies have shown an associated risk of BPH with obesity.[157,158] Proposed mechanisms of these associations include increased levels of systemic inflammation and increased levels of estrogens.[159,160]

Pathophysiology. The cause of BPH is unknown.[161] Current causative theories for BPH focus on aging, the levels and ratios of endocrine factors (e.g., androgens and estrogens [androgen/estrogen ratio]), the role of chronic inflammation, and the effects of autocrine/paracrine growth-stimulating and growth-inhibiting factors (see Emerging Science Box: Benign Prostatic Hyperplasia). These factors may include insulin-like growth factors (IGFs), epidermal growth factor, nerve growth factor, fibroblast factors, IGF binding proteins, and transforming growth factor-beta (TGF-β).[162] Inflammation in men with BPH can be related to underlying metabolic syndrome and/or obesity (see Chapter 23).[152,154] Human prostate stromal cells can actively contribute to the inflammatory process from the induction of inflammatory cytokines and chemokines.

Although androgens, such as dihydrotestosterone (DHT), are necessary for normal growth, their role in BPH remains

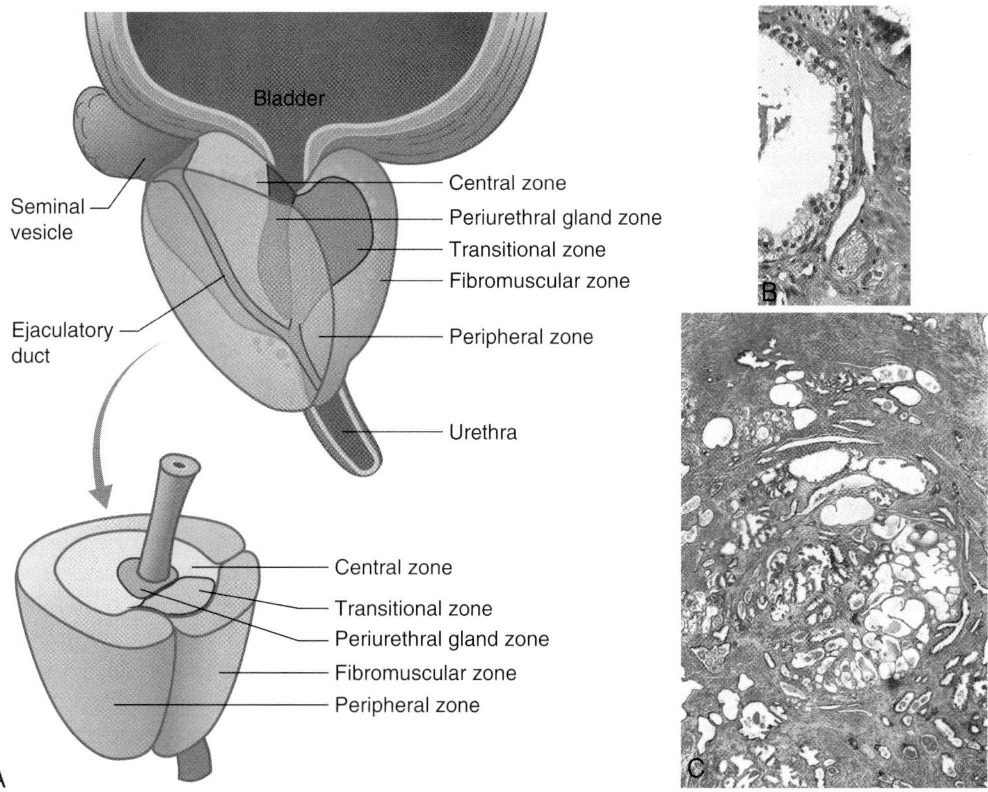

Fig. 26.16 Benign Prostatic Hypertrophy. (A) The transitional zone is the principal site of benign prostatic hypertrophy (BPH). Size of the prostate gland remains stable until approximately 40 years of age, then hyperplasia of the gland develops. **(B)** Histological slides are presented of both a normal prostate and BPH tissue. **(C)** The BPH slide shows pleomorphism (stromal/epithelial ratio) and proliferation of the glandular epithelial cells. (From Chughtai B, Forde JC, Thomas DDM, et al. Benign prostatic hyperplasia. *Nat Rev Dis Primers*. 2016;2:16031. https://doi.org/10.1038/nrdp.2016.31)

EMERGING SCIENCE BOX

Benign Prostatic Hyperplasia

Similar to prostate cancer, benign prostatic hyperplasia (BPH) occurs more often in Westernized countries (e.g., United States, United Kingdom, and Canada). BPH is the most common benign neoplasm of aging men and is present in approximately 8% of men in the fourth decade of life but up to 90% of men in the ninth decade. Overall, no clear patterns have emerged with risk of BPH and race. Being overweight or obese with central fat distribution (i.e., around the abdomen) increases the risk of developing BPH. Surgical procedures, including less invasive modalities, are generally indicated for failure of medical therapy, refractory urinary retention, recurrent urinary tract infection, persistent hematuria, bladder stones, or renal insufficiency.

Data from Langan RC. Benign prostatic hyperplasia. *Primary Care*, 2019;46:223–232.

unclear. With aging, circulating androgens are associated with BPH and prostate enlargement. Androgens are proposed as factors disrupting the *balance* of growth factor signaling pathways and stromal/epithelial interactions, creating a growth-promoting and tissue-remodeling microenvironment. However, BPH is a multifactorial disease, including lifestyle factors, and not all men respond well to currently available treatments, which suggests that factors other than androgens are involved.[163] For example, other effects related to estrogens include apoptosis, aromatase expression, and paracrine regulation that may be important for stimulating inflammation. The prostate is an estrogen target tissue, and estrogens directly and indirectly affect growth and differentiation of the prostate. Estrogens and selective estrogen receptor (ER) modulators have been shown to promote or inhibit prostate proliferation, signifying potential roles in BPH.[164] Testosterone, the primary circulating androgen in men, also can be metabolized through CYP19/aromatase into the potent estrogen, estradiol-17β. The precise role of endogenous and exogenous estrogens in directly affecting prostate growth and differentiation is an understudied area.

Increased levels of specific inflammatory mediators include IL-2, IL-4, IL-7, IL-17, IFN γ, and their appropriate receptors.[165–167] Chronic inflammation in BPH is associated with upregulation of COX2 in the glandular epithelium, generating pro-inflammatory prostaglandins which also cause prostate cell proliferation.[168,169] The remodeled stroma promotes local inflammation with altered cytokine, reactive oxygen/nitrogen species, and chemoattractants. The resultant increased oxygen demands of proliferating cells cause a local hypoxia that induces angiogenesis and changes to fibroblasts.

BPH begins in the periurethral glands, which are the inner glands or layers of the prostate. The prostate enlarges as nodules form and grow (nodular hyperplasia), and glandular cells enlarge. The development of BPH occurs over a prolonged period, and changes within the urinary tract are slow and insidious.

Clinical Manifestations. As nodular hyperplasia and cellular enlargement progress, tissues that surround the prostatic urethra compress it, usually, but not always, causing bladder outflow obstruction. These symptoms are called the *lower urinary tract symptoms* (LUTS). LUTS can be divided into storage (frequency, nocturia, urgency) and voiding (stream, straining, hesitancy, prolonged micturition) symptoms.[152] These symptoms help to differentiate other causes of urinary symptoms such as UTI/overactive bladder, and identify the site affected (bladder versus prostate).[152] Men with BPH typically identify the most prominent symptoms of nocturia, poor stream, hesitancy, or prolonged micturition.[152] As the obstruction progresses, often over several years, the bladder cannot empty all the urine, and the increasing volume leads to long-term urine retention. The volume of urine retained may be great enough to produce uncontrolled "overflow incontinence" with any increase in intra-abdominal pressure. At this stage, the force of the urinary stream is significantly reduced, and more time is required to initiate and complete voiding. Hematuria, bladder or kidney infection, bladder calculi, acute urinary retention (hydroureter), hydronephrosis, and renal insufficiency are common complications.[170] The impact of LUTS on quality of life can be assessed using the American Urological Association Symptom Score (AUASS) as well as the International Prostate Symptom Score (IPSS).[171]

Evaluation and Treatment. The diagnosis is made from a medical history, physical examination, and laboratory tests, including urinalysis. Prostate-specific antigen (PSA) testing is used with caution and should not be done to investigate BPH routinely.[152] PSA levels may be increased in several conditions (large prostate, infection, catheterization, prostate cancer) and can cause unnecessary anxiety and trigger more investigations.[152] Careful review of symptoms is necessary. Ultrasound scans are used for evidence of hydronephrosis and indicated for men with high residual volumes or renal impairment.[152] Urine flow studies are done to assess volume of urine passed over time.[152] Flexible cystoscopy is only used to investigate "red flag" symptoms, such as hematuria/suspected bladder cancer and urethral strictures.[152]

In those men with LUTS, treatment options range from watchful waiting to medical and surgical intervention and depend on the degree of "discomfort or bother" or disease burden.[152] α_1-Adrenergic blockers (Tamsulosin and Alfuzosin) result in stromal smooth muscle relaxation and thus improve urinary flow. Alpha-reductase inhibitors (finasteride and dutasteride) block conversion of testosterone to DHT, causing shrinkage of the prostate. It takes several weeks to show noticeable improvement and six months to show maximal effectiveness.[154]

Antiandrogen agents lower the PSA level by 50% after 6 months of therapy with prostate volume decreasing up to 25%.[152] Worsening BOO can cause bladder detrusor instability, increasing urgency, or overactive bladder and frequency. These symptoms can be relieved with muscarinic receptor antagonists by blocking muscarinic receptors on detrusor muscle and reducing smooth muscle tone.[152] The combination of an alpha-blocker and alpha-reductase inhibitor are used to achieve improvements in voiding symptoms.[172,173]

The guidelines for surgery in BPH are outlined by the European Association of Urology (EAU) and include[174]: (1)

refractory urinary retention, (2) recurrent UTIs, (3) hematuria refractory to medical treatment (other causes excluded), (4) renal insufficiency, (5) bladder stones, (6) increased post-void residual, and (7) high-pressure chronic retention (absolute indication). Over the years, surgical innovations have increased with minimally invasive procedures. Recommended procedures include transurethral incision of the prostate, transurethral resection for the prostate, and newer techniques of laser vaporization and holmium laser enucleation, which have largely replaced open prostatectomy.[152] Bipolar diathermy has mostly replaced monopolar diathermy techniques for transurethral resection of the prostate (TURP).[152] Meta-analysis for HoLEP (Holmium laser enucleation of the prostate) has shown improved Qmax (flow rate), reduction in post-void residual, and lowered IPSS score as compared to TURP.[152]

Prostatitis

Prostatitis is an infection or inflammation of the prostate gland that presents as several syndromes with varying clinical features (Fig. 26.17). The term *prostatitis* is defined as microscopic inflammation of the tissue of the prostate gland. Prostatitis syndromes have been classified by the National Institutes of Health as (1) acute bacterial prostatitis (ABP), (2) chronic bacterial prostatitis (CBP), (3) chronic pelvic pain syndrome (CPPS), and (4) asymptomatic inflammatory prostatitis (Box 26.11). ABP and CBP are mostly caused by gram-negative Enterobacteriaceae and *Enterococci* species that originate in the gastrointestinal flora. Nonbacterial prostatitis (CP/CPPS) syndromes are caused by a cascade of inflammatory, immunologic, neuroendocrine, and neuropathic mechanisms, such that the initiating cause is unknown.

BOX 26.11 National Institutes of Health Classification of Prostatitis Syndrome

This system, developed for clinical research purposes, can be simplified for use in primary care practice (see text).

Category I, or acute bacterial prostatitis (ABP), is an acute infection of the prostate and is manifested by systemic signs of infection and a positive urine culture result.

Category II, or chronic bacterial prostatitis (CBP), is a chronic bacterial infection in which bacteria are received in significant numbers from a purulent prostatic fluid. These bacteria are thought to be the most common cause of recurrent urinary tract infection in men.

Category III, or chronic pelvic pain syndrome (CPPS), is diagnosed when no pathologic bacteria can be localized to the prostate (culture of expressed prostatic fluid or postprostatic massage urine specimen) and is further divided into IIIa and IIIb. Category IIIa is inflammatory CPPS, in which a significant number of white blood cells (WBCs) are localized to the prostate; category IIIb is noninflammatory.

Category IV is asymptomatic inflammatory prostatitis in which bacteria or WBCs are localized to the prostate, but individuals are asymptomatic.

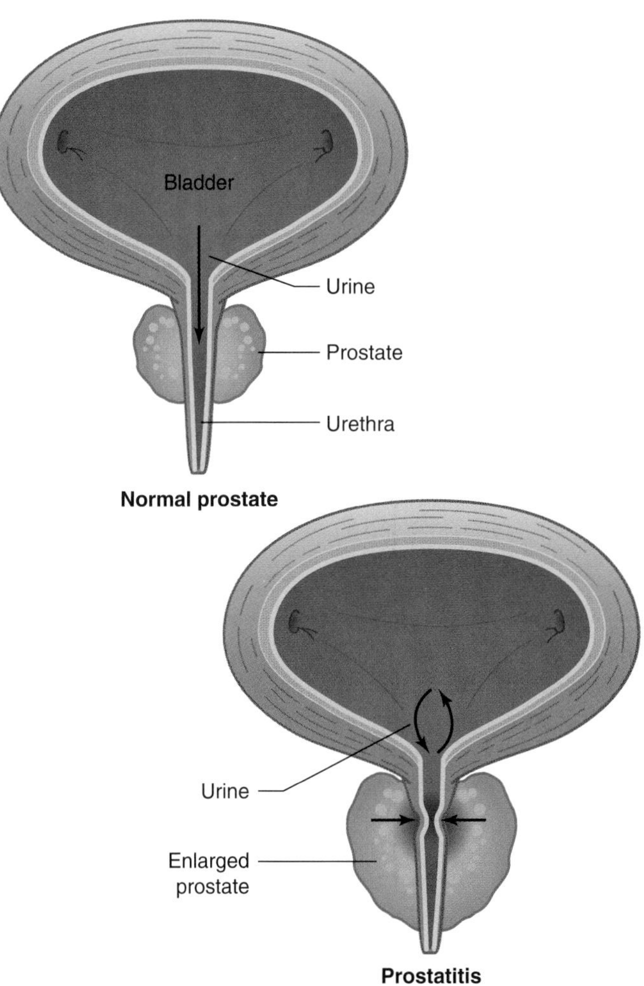

Fig. 26.17 Prostatitis. Simple schematic of a normal prostate gland and an enlarged prostate gland secondary to prostatitis.

Acute bacterial prostatitis (ABP, category I) is an ascending infection of the urinary tract that tends to occur in men between the ages of 30 and 50 years, but it is also associated with BPH in older men. In general, ABP is rare and often associated with BOO or an immunocompromised state. Infection stimulates an inflammatory response in which the prostate becomes enlarged, tender, firm, or boggy. The most common organism is *E. coli*, which is identified in approximately 50% to 90% of infections. *Klebsiella* species, *Proteus*, *Pseudomonas aeruginosa*, and *Serratia* species also are common gram-negative cultured microorganisms. Sometimes implicated are gram positive organisms such as *Enterococcus* species and *Staphylococcus* species as well as organisms from STIs, including *N. gonorrhoeae, C. trachomatis*, and *Ureaplasma urealyticum*.[175] Immunocompromised individuals are at an increased risk for BP from atypical organisms such as *Salmonella* species, *Mycobacterium* species, *Staphylococcus* species, and others.[175] Fungal and viral etiologies need consideration, especially with immunosuppressed states. Although Enterobacteriaceae are the most common causative microorganisms in both ABP and CBP, gram-positive and atypical microorganisms are more likely in CBP than in ABP. The role of gram-positive microorganisms in CBP is debated, but they sometimes are isolated in culture.[176,177]

The onset of prostatitis may be acute and unrelated to previous illnesses. It may follow prostate manipulation from procedures such as transrectal prostate biopsy, transurethral prostate biopsy, cystoscopy, and catheterization.[175,178,179] Box 26.12 provides a summary of risk factors.[173] In young men, common

BOX 26.12 Summary of Risk Factors for Bacterial Prostatitis

- Phimosis
- Intraprostatic ductal reflux
- Unprotected vaginal/anal intercourse
- Sexually transmitted infections
- Sexual abuse
- Development of a urinary tract infection
- Indwelling catheter
- Transurethral biopsy/surgery
- Prostate manipulation
- Urethral stricture
- Benign prostatic hyperplasia
- Diabetes
- Urethritis
- Congenital abnormality of the ureter

causes include an ascending infection following anal or vaginal intercourse. In older males, two common causes are prolonged catheterization and instrumentation.[175]

ABP usually presents with abrupt symptoms of infection. A sudden onset of malaise, low back, rectal, and perineal pain, fever, and chills. Other common symptoms include dysuria, inability to empty the bladder, nocturia, urinary retention, and painful ejaculation. The individual also may have symptoms of lower urinary tract obstruction, such as a slow, small, "narrowed" urinary stream, which may be a medical emergency. Acute inflammatory prostatic edema can compress the urethra, causing urinary obstruction. Systemic signs of infection include sudden onset of a high fever (up to 40° C [104° F]), fatigue, arthralgia, and myalgia. Prostatic pain may occur, especially when the individual is in an upright position, because the pelvic floor muscles tighten with standing, and compression of the prostate gland occurs. Palpation discloses an enlarged, extremely tender, and swollen prostate that is firm, indurated, and warm to the touch.

Once ABP is suspected, based on history and physical examination, a midstream urinalysis and urine culture is recommended. If a person meets sepsis criteria or has significant medical comorbidities, blood cultures, lactic acid, metabolic panel, and complete blood count are obtained. Although imaging is not required in all cases, a CT or transrectal ultrasound (TRUS) may be done to evaluate a prostatic abscess in individuals who are immunocompromised, at risk of bacteremia, or are not responding to treatment.[175] With ABP and individuals presenting with acute urinary retention, urology is consulted for possible suprapubic catherization.[175] Prostatic massage may express enough secretions from the urethra for direct bacterial examination. The four-glass test is a test of four different samples: voided urine, mid-stream urine, expressed prostatic secretions, and post-prostate massage urine. The 2-glass test is performed by obtaining pre-massage and post-massage urine samples. The 4-glass is not performed often, as it is difficult for the individual and the supporting evidence is poor.[180,181]

To resolve the infection and control its spread, individuals may require antibiotics. In severe cases (individuals meet sepsis criteria, have urinary retention, treatment failure/resistant organisms), the individual is hospitalized and treated with intravenous antibiotics, followed by oral antibiotics. Complications include urinary retention, progression to chronic prostatitis, epididymitis, or pyelonephritis. At least 10% of individuals develop chronic pain.[175]

Chronic bacterial prostatitis (CBP (category II) is characterized by recurrent urinary tract symptoms. The pathophysiology of CBP is less well known and may involve the development of bacterial biofilms.[182]

CBP presents more subtly than ABP. The symptoms of CBP are chronic and recurring and less severe than ABP.[175] Although men with CBP do not usually appear acutely ill, their quality of life can be significantly impacted.[175] These men have chronic asymptomatic bacteriuria. The prostate may be tender but typically not inflamed, and men may present with sexual dysfunction (SD).[175]

CBP evaluation is appropriately performed by a urologist or in consultation with one. Diagnosis of CBP is best done by a urologist using either the Meares and Stamey four-glass test or the simpler two-glass pre-massage and post-massage test, and possibly semen sample with urodynamic studies.[175]

Treatment for CBP is guided by culture results, and initiating treatment emergently is not warranted because treatment can wait for culture results.[175] Typically, duration of treatment is two to six weeks.[175] Those who fail to respond to medical therapy may have a surgical procedure for an abscess.[175] Decreased fertility has been associated with massive bacterial infection of the prostate. A prostatic abscess is rare but may occur in those with indwelling catheters. Healthcare providers need to be aware that unnecessary urethral catheterization should be avoided. Education should be provided to individuals on barrier protection if participating in anal sex. Also, education is needed on adequate hydration and the use of antipyretics. Close communication between team members and the urologist is critical to lower morbidity and improve outcomes.[183,184]

Chronic prostatitis/chronic pelvic pain syndrome (CP/CPPS, category III) has no real consensus on its definition, etiology, and pathophysiology. The heterogeneity of the disorder has created major difficulties in defining CP/CPPS. One proposal is that CP/CPPS is logically defined as a set of associated symptoms rather than a single entity of disease.[185] Four elements are necessary to diagnose CP/CPPS and include: (1) symptoms occurring in perineal and/or low abdominal area, (2) infection and or inflammatory changes of the prostate with laboratory evidence of abnormal findings, (3) clinical presentations, mainly pain and discomfort derived from or associated with the prostate and lower urinary tract, and (4) symptoms appearing after an inducible cause with varied incubation times.[185] Shoskes divided CP/CPPS into six subtypes by clinical presentation, subjective presentation, and psychosocial background: urinary (U), psychosocial (P), organ specific (O), infection (I), neurologic/systemic (N), and tenderness (T), altogether UPOINT.[186]

A working group of the International Continence Society (ICS) published nine clinical domains: lower urinary tract, female genital, male genital, gastrointestinal, musculoskeletal, neurological, psychological, sexual, and comorbidities.[187] These publications provide further support for symptom-oriented diagnosis and treatment.

Recommendations for diagnosis include the phenotype-based diagnosis of CP/CPPS[186] and UPOINT.[188,189] Associated symptoms are linked to varicocele, irritable bowel syndrome, and melena.[190–193]

The terminology of CPPS by ICS is used for measuring scales and locations of pain.[187] The NIH-Chronic Prostatitis Symptom Index (NIH-CPSI) and the consensus guideline by the Prostatitis Expert Reference Group are useful instruments for initial review of symptom severity and follow-up of treatment results.[185] Other taxonomies exist, including the International Association for the Study of Pain (IASP) and the EAU.

Definitive diagnosis and selection of an effective treatment are frustrations encountered by individuals and their urology care providers.[185] A multimodal approach to treatment for CP/CPP includes both pharmacologic and nonpharmacologic therapies. Pharmacologic treatment includes antimicrobials, α-blockers, anti-inflammatory and immunomodulatory agents, phytotherapy, phosphodiesterase inhibitors, antidepressants, neuromodulatory agents, and hormonal agents. The nonpharmacologic therapies include pelvic floor physical therapy, myofascial trigger point release, acupuncture, extracorporeal shock wave therapy (ESWT), and psychological support.[194]

Cancer of the Prostate

Prostate cancer affects millions of men worldwide.[195] It is the second most common cancer in men after lung cancer, accounting for 7% of newly diagnosed cancers in men globally and 15% of men in developed regions.[196] Globally, prostate cancer accounts for 1,148,515 estimated new cases and 375,304 estimated deaths (see Emerging Science Box: Prostate Cancer).[195] The regions of highest incidence are Australia, New Zealand, Oceania, North America, Europe, and Brazil. The lowest incidence of prostate cancer is found in low-income nations, including South Asia, Central Asia, and Sub-Saharan Africa, but these regions have the highest rates of annual increase in incidence.[197,198] In the United States estimated new cases of prostate cancer for 2021 is 248,530 and estimated deaths is 34,130.[199] Studies in Europe with long-term follow-up data have shown that repeated screening increases detection of all prostate cancers (including those that are indolent)[200,201] and reduces prostate cancer-specific mortality.[200,201] Overall, the majority of prostate cancers tend to grow slowly and are low-grade and low-risk with limited aggressiveness.[202]

EMERGING SCIENCE BOX

Prostate Cancer

Prostate cancer is the second most frequent cancer diagnosis made in males and the fifth leading cause of death worldwide. Prostate cancer incidence rates during the most recent 5 years have declined (five countries) or stabilized (35 countries), after increasing for many years. In contrast, rates continued to increase for four countries in Eastern Europe and Asia. During the most recent 5 data years, mortality rates among 76 countries examined increased (three countries), remained stable (59 countries), or decreased (14 countries). There is no evidence yet on how to prevent prostate cancer; however, it is possible to lower the risk by limiting high-fat foods, increasing intake of fruits and vegetables, and increasing activity with exercise.

Data from Culp MB, et al. Recent global patterns in prostate cancer incidence and mortality rates. *European Urology*, 2020;77:38–52; Rawla P. Epidemiology of prostate cancer. *World Journal of Oncology*, 2019;10(2):63–89. doi:10.14740/wjon1191.

The known major risk factors for prostate cancer are age, ethnicity, obesity, and family history.[202,203] Across age ranges, black men and men with a family history of prostate cancer have an increased risk of developing and dying of prostate cancer. Black men are approximately twice as likely to succumb to prostate cancer compared with men of other races in the United States, and the reason for this disparity is unknown. Other risk factors include increased height, hypertension, lack of exercise, Agent Orange exposure, and the typical Western diet.[202,204–206] Androgens and androgen receptor (AR) function have major roles in the development and progression of prostate cancer.[207] Although the cause of prostate cancer is unknown, genetics play a role. Men with a first-degree relative (father or brother) with prostate cancer have twice the general population risk, and risk increases more with an affected brother than an affected father.[208] Prostate cancer-associated genetic changes are copy number alterations (CNAs) or gene structural rearrangements (see Pathophysiology discussion).[209,210] Acquired genetic and epigenetic alterations are involved in the development of prostate cancer.[161]

Diet, obesity, and microbiota. Although evidence exists for a dietary role in prostate cancer, the epidemiologic evidence is inconsistent. The nutrients in the epidemiology of prostate cancer that have received the most attention include carotenoids, fat, vitamin E, vitamin D/calcium, and selenium. Less studied are isoflavones, curcumin, lycopene, green tea, omega-3 polyunsaturated fats, and sulforaphane. Associations between obesity and prostate cancer are not clear because of inconsistencies, but obesity seems to be negatively associated with more indolent prostate cancer and positively associated with more aggressive disease and a worse outcome.[211–216] Several biological mechanisms have been proposed to understand how obesity may be related to prostate cancer. First, obesity may be associated with a low physical activity level, suspected to increase the risk of prostate cancer.[217] Second, obese men have higher levels of insulin and IGF[218,219] reported to promote carcinogenesis and inhibit apoptosis.[220–222] Last, experimental and epidemiological studies also suggested that chronic inflammation may be associated either with initiation or progression of several cancers, including prostate cancer.[223–228] Importantly, it has been suggested that obesity promotes a low-grade inflammation state that may contribute to cancer development (see Chapter 23).[211]

Hormones. Prostate cancer develops in an androgen-dependent epithelium and is usually androgen sensitive. The significance of androgens for maintaining the growth and survival of prostate cancer cells is noted from the therapeutic effect of castration or treatment with antiandrogens, which mostly induce disease regression.[161] Over time, most tumors become resistant to androgen blockage (see section Evaluation and Treatment). Androgens are synthesized not only in the testis, accounting for 50% to 60% of the total testosterone in the prostate, but also in the prostate gland itself. In a process called intraprostatic conversion, the hormone dehydroepiandrosterone (DHEA) produced by the adrenal glands is converted to testosterone and then into DHT in the prostate (Fig. 26.18). Additionally, prostate cancer cells have been reported to make androgens from cholesterol (i.e., de novo).

Estrogens also may have a role in prostate cancer development. Normal human prostate stem progenitor cells express ER-α and ER-β. Their roles in prostate cancer are discussed in the pathophysiology section.

Chronic inflammation. Chronic inflammation may be an important risk factor for prostatic adenocarcinoma. Possible causes of prostate inflammation are shown in Fig. 26.19. Chronic inflammation involves autocrine/paracrine growth-stimulating and growth-inhibiting factors. These factors include IGFs, epidermal growth factors, fibroblast factors, and TGF-β, as well as several others. Recent data show that human prostate stromal cells can actively contribute to the inflammatory process from the induction of inflammatory cytokines and chemokines. Importantly, continuous input from TGF-β and IGF in the tumor microenvironment or stroma results in cancer progression.

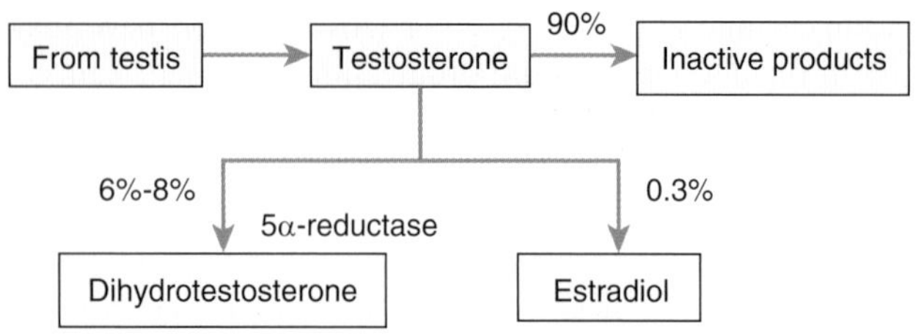

Fig. 26.18 Testosterone and Conversion to Dihydrotestosterone.

Pathophysiology. More than 95% of prostatic neoplasms are adenocarcinomas, and most occur in the periphery of the prostate (Figs. 26.20 and 26.21). Prostatic adenocarcinoma is a heterogeneous group of tumors with a diverse spectrum of molecular and pathologic characteristics and, therefore, diverse clinical behaviors and challenges. The cells of origin of a prostatic adenocarcinoma are thought to originate from the basal or luminal prostate epithelial cells, and genetic mutation is thought to be the primary driver of prostate carcinogenesis.[198] Interactions of environmental factors and genetic factors contribute to the notable differences in incidence of prostate cancer worldwide. Migration studies have shown the importance of environmental factors; for example, men of Asian descent living in Asia are at lower risk of prostate cancer than white men living in the United States, but the risk within Asian men reaches

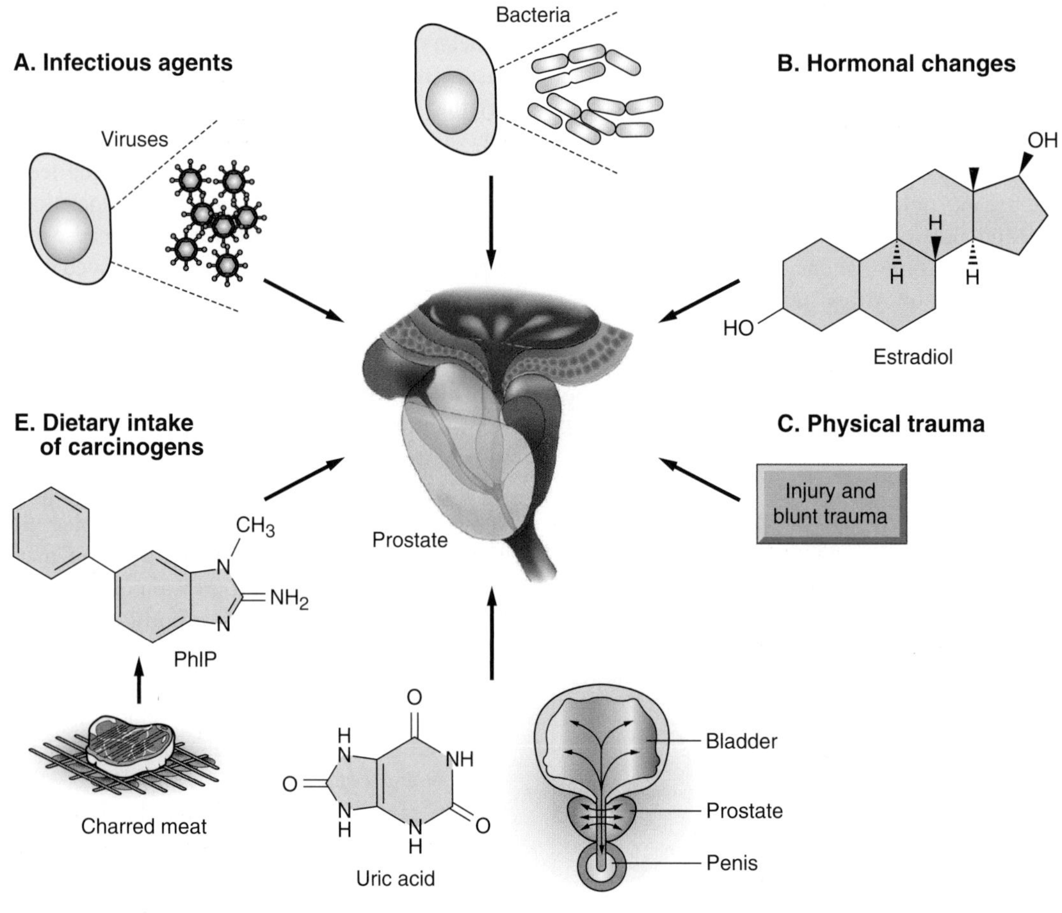

Fig. 26.19 Possible Causes of Prostate Inflammation. (A) Infection, including viruses, bacteria, fungi, and parasites. (B) Hormones, for example, estrogen at key times during development. (C) Physical trauma, any type of blunt physical injury. (D) Urine reflex. (E) Certain dietary factors (see text).

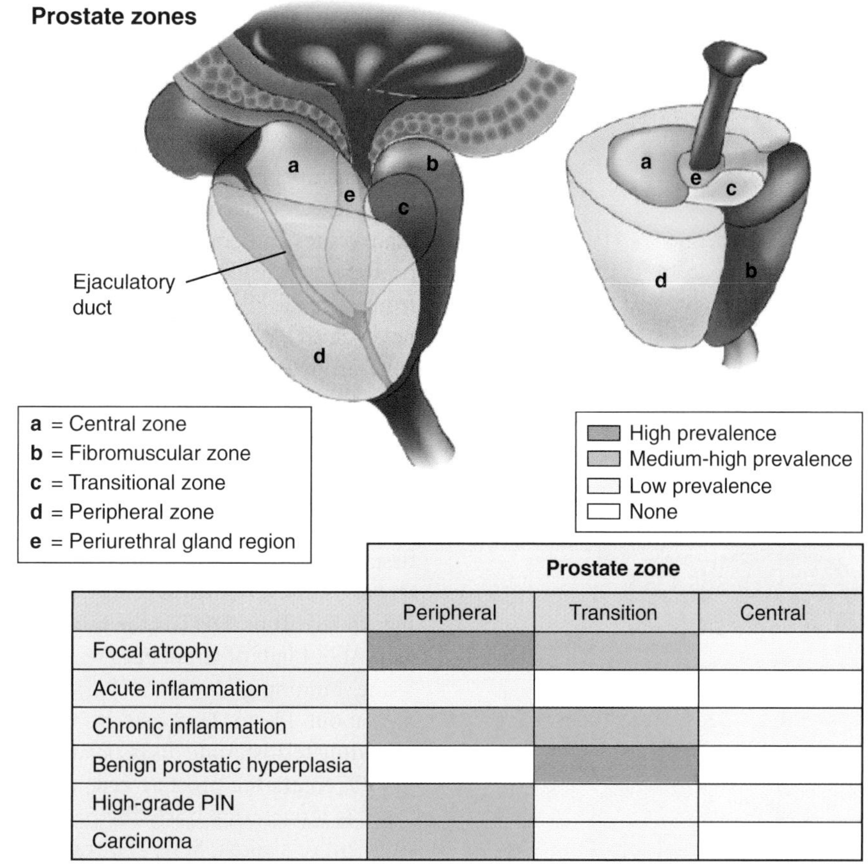

	Prostate zone		
	Peripheral	Transition	Central
Focal atrophy			
Acute inflammation			
Chronic inflammation			
Benign prostatic hyperplasia			
High-grade PIN			
Carcinoma			

Fig. 26.20 Prostate Zones, Benign Prostatic Hyperplasia, and Prostate Cancer Locations.

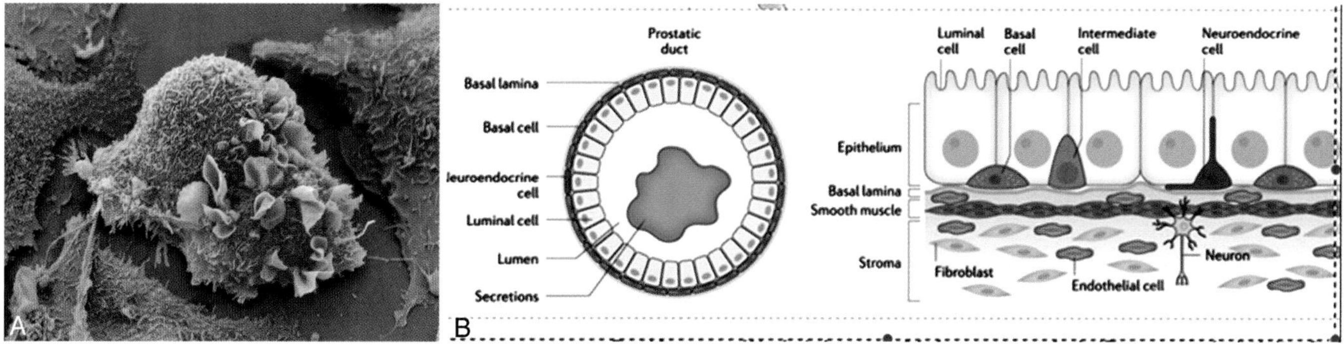

Fig. 26.21 **Photomicrograph of Prostate Cancer Cells. (A)** Pink ruffled cells are prostate cancer cells. **(B)** The cells of origin of prostate adenocarcinoma are thought to be from the basal or luminal prostate epithelial cells. (A, From Cancer Research UK, London Research Institute, Electron Microscopy Unit. B, From Rebello RJ, Oing C, Knudsen KE, et al. Prostate cancer. *Nat Rev Dis Primers.* 2021;7:9)

levels like white men when living in the United States.[229] Studies of twins and families show genetic predisposing factors. Many inherited germline variants have been identified and associated with prostate cancer risk, for example, variants that influence an important oncogene, *MYC*. Other rare variants have been identified and linked to high risk of early onset, aggressive disease including loss of function mutations in *BRCA2* and in DNA mismatch repair genes.[230] The rare mutations with the highest risk are those in *BRCA2* (sevenfold to eightfold) and *HOX13* mutations (threefold increased relative risk).[231] Acquired genetic and epigenetic alterations can alter the expression of tumor suppressor genes and oncogenes. The most common (~50%) genetic alteration in the prostate is a chromosomal rearrangement that juxtaposes (puts close together) the coding sequence of an ETS family transcription factor gene (e.g., *ERG* or *ETV1*) next to the androgen regulated *TMPRSS2* promotor. TMPRSS2 is an androgen-regulated cell surface serine protease[232] and plays an important role in prostate cancer invasion, extracellular matrix degradation, invasion, tumor growth, and metastasis (Fig. 26.22).[233]

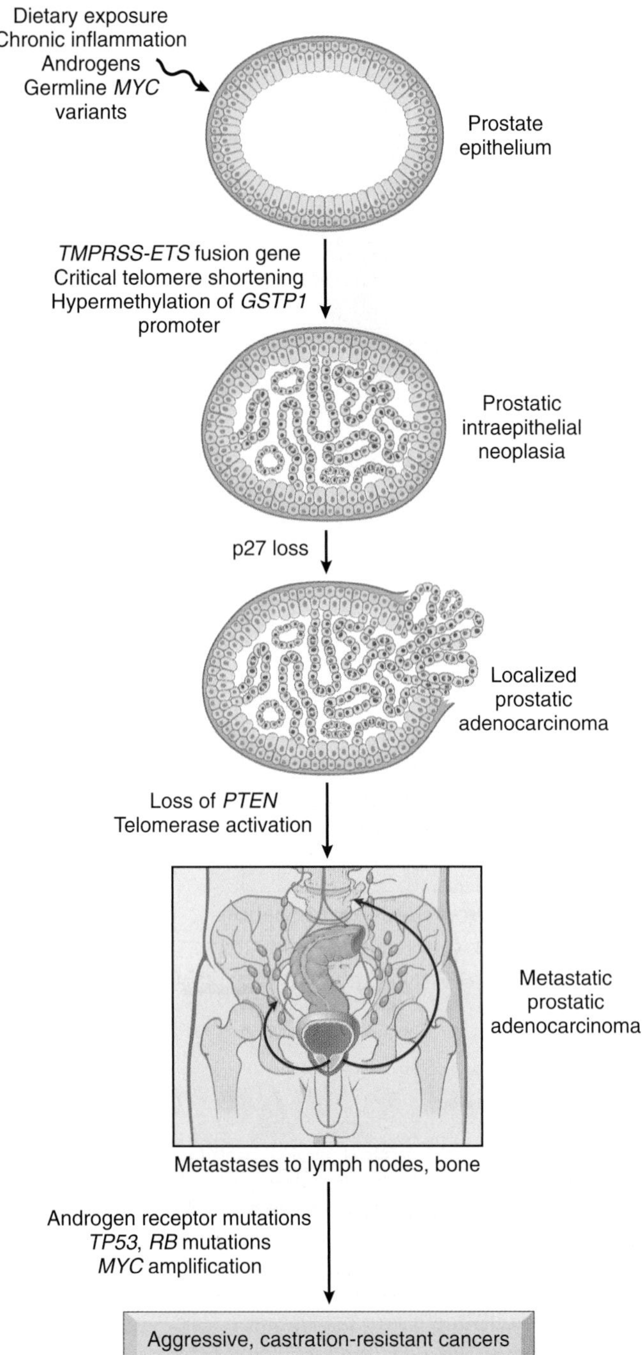

Fig. 26.22 Interaction of Environmental and Genetic Risk Factors and Acquired Genetic and Epigenetic Alterations Leading to Prostate Cancer Development and Progression. Prostate cancer is thought to be strongly associated with the accumulation of acquired somatic mutations over a man's lifetime. Risk factors include many environmental factors interacting with genes and epigenetic factors. Prostate cancer is highly heterogenous and individuals have a combination of one or more of these genetic changes. For example, *TMPRSS2-ETS* fusion, *PTEN* and *RB1* deletion, *TP53* mutation, and amplification of *MYC* are common genetic changes in all stages of prostate cancer. Although still debated, a putative precursor lesion, prostatic intraepithelial neoplasia (PIN), occurs in some cases of prostate cancer. (From Kumar V, Abbas AK, Aster JC. *Robbins & Cotran pathologic basis of disease*, 10th edition. Elsevier; 2021.)

Hormonal factors. Just as the testicles are the male equivalent of the female ovaries, the prostate is the male equivalent of the female uterus; in both situations they originate from the same embryonic cells. This may be important in understanding the role of the associated hormones testosterone (T), DHT, and estrogens in prostate cancer development (Fig. 26.23). The relationship between hormones and the pathophysiology of prostate carcinogenesis is incomplete and controversial. The main issues and controversies include (1) sources of androgen production outside of the testes, or extratesticular sources (e.g., from adrenal DHEA and from prostate tissue cholesterol [de novo] itself); (2) the role of prostatic AR; (3) the role of estrogens, aromatase enzyme, and the ERs ERα and ERβ; and (4) the role of the surrounding microenvironment or stroma.

Testicular testosterone provides the main source of androgens in the prostate and is the major circulating androgen. The adrenal cortex contributes the far less potent DHEA that promotes synthesis of androgens in the prostate. In the target tissues, and to a lesser extent in the testes themselves, testosterone is converted to DHT by the enzyme 5α-reductase (see Fig. 26.18). Thus, DHT is the most potent intraprostatic androgen. About half of circulating testosterone is bound to sex hormone–binding globulin (SHBG), about half binds to albumin, and about 1% to 2% exists in a free state. Free testosterone, including testosterone disassociated from albumin and possibly SHBG, enters the prostate cell, where it is converted to DHT. DHT is a paracrine hormone because it affects the local environment or stroma. Several intraprostatic enzymes encoded by genes HSD3A and HDS3B are activated by DHT and are important components of intraprostatic androgen regulation. The growth, differentiation, and maintenance of the prostate gland depend mainly on androgens and are the basis of the antiandrogenic therapies for the treatment of primary prostate cancer. Development and physiology of the prostate is also directly regulated by somatotrophic hormones, such as insulin, prolactin, and growth hormone, retinoic acid, and estrogen.[234]

Prostate cancer growth and progression relies on the activation of the AR by testosterone (T), or its more potent metabolite, DHT. AR is associated with the origins of prostate tumors and with the recurrence of androgen independent cancer.[235] Estrogens are mediated by the ER. The two subtypes, ERα and ERβ, are the products of different genes and have different physiological roles (see below discussion).[234] Both ERα and ERβ are expressed in the prostate and in adults ERα and ERβ are preferentially found in the stroma and the epithelium, respectively.[234] ER expression, like the AR, might be suppressed by methylation of its promoters; this epigenetic alteration is suggested to be involved in both BPH and prostate cancer development.[236,237] It is well known that circulating androgens are converted into estrogens in various peripheral tissues by the enzyme aromatase.[238] Aromatase was also identified in the human prostate, suggesting that the human prostate is able to perform the aromatization reaction and is a logical local source of estrogen production (see Fig. 26.18).[239]

Estrogen effects are determined by the two receptors ER-α and ER-β. It is ER-α activation that is thought to contribute to prostate carcinogenesis and has been implicated with tumor

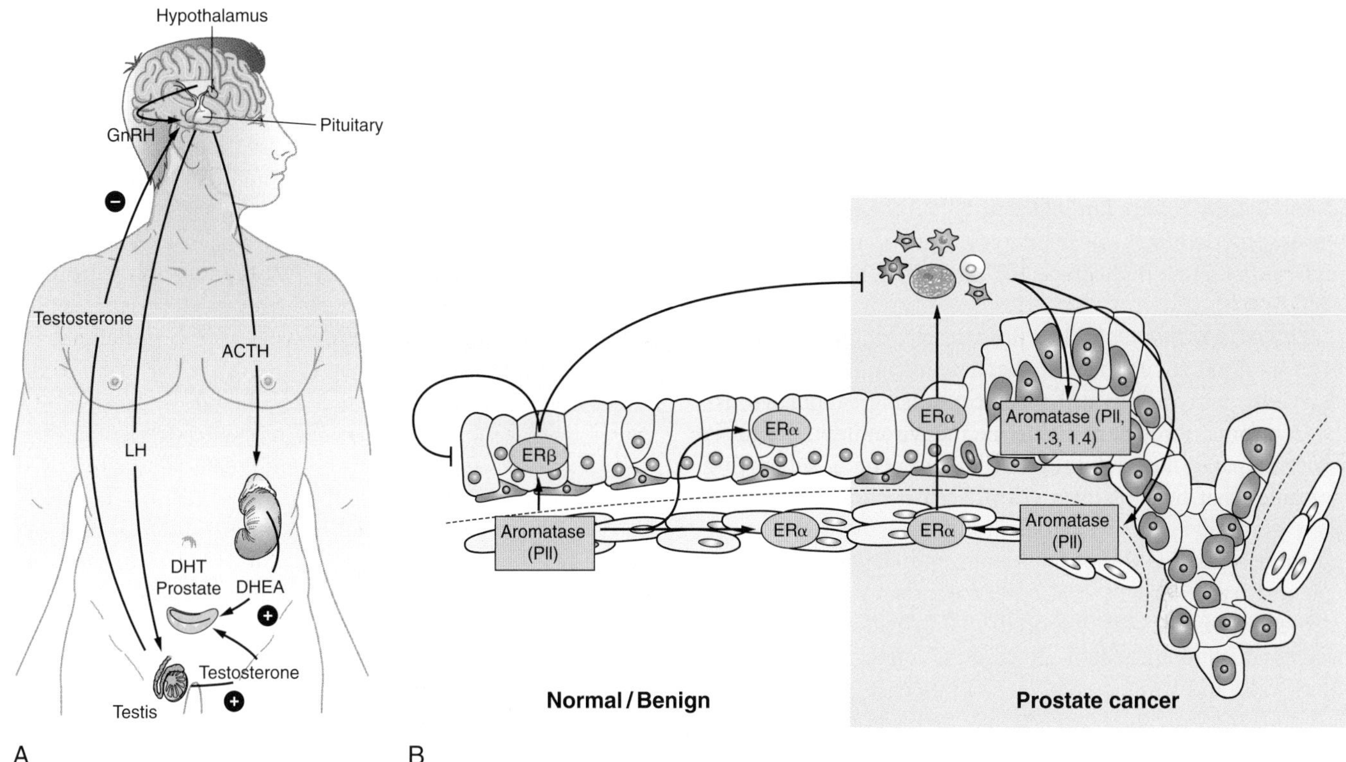

Fig. 26.23 Sources of Androgens and Aromatase and Estrogen Signaling in the Prostate. (A) Body sources of androgens in the prostate gland. Hypothalamic gonadotropin-releasing hormone *(GnRH)* causes the release of luteinizing hormone *(LH)* from the anterior pituitary gland. LH stimulates the testes to produce testosterone, which accumulates in the blood. Pituitary adrenocorticotropic hormone *(ACTH)* release stimulates the adrenal glands, which secrete the androgen precursor dehydroepiandrosterone *(DHEA)* into the blood. DHEA is converted into testosterone and then into dihydrotestosterone *(DHT)* in the prostate. (B) Aromatase, and estrogen signaling in the prostate. In normal and benign tissue, aromatase is expressed within the stroma and regulated by promoter PII. Estrogen then exerts its effects in an autocrine fashion through the stromal ER-α receptor and in a paracrine fashion through both ER-α and ER-β receptors. With prostate cancer, aromatase is now expressed within the tumor cells and in stromal cells and is regulated by aromatase promoters 1.3, 1.4, and PII. Thus, estrogen exerts its effects in an autocrine way through stromal and epithelial ER-α and ER-β. Consequently, the increased levels of estrogen and abnormal ER-α signaling promote inflammation, which increases aromatase expression and the development of a positive feedback cycle. Inflammation drives aromatase expression, thus increasing estrogen, which in turn promotes further inflammation. *ER*, Estrogen receptor. (A, Adapted from Labrie F. Blockade of testicular and adrenal androgens in prostate cancer treatment. *Nat Rev Urol.* 20 1;8:73–80. B, From Ellem SJ, Risbridger GP. Aromatase and regulating the estrogen: Androgen ratio in the prostate gland. *J Steroid Biochem Mol Biol.* 2010;118(4–5):246–251.)

progression.[240,241] In contrast, ER-β has been shown to be reduced in localized malignant lesions of the prostate as compared to benign lesions, thus supporting an anti-proliferative role in prostate tissue.[242] In addition to the ER-α and ER-β, the G protein—coupled estrogen receptor (GPER), a member of the G-protein family found in the endoplasmic reticulum, has been found to have differential expression between BTH and prostate cancer.[243] High estrogen and low T levels have been shown to lead to inflammation with aging and to the emergence of precancerous lesions.[244] The mechanism is not clearly understood and may involve estrogen-generated oxidative stress and DNA toxicity, and it requires androgen-mediated and ER–mediated processes, such as changes in sex steroid metabolism and receptor status.[245] In addition, there are changes in the balance between autocrine/paracrine growth-stimulatory and growth-inhibitory factors, such as the IGFs.

Prostate epithelial neoplasia. A precursor lesion, prostatic epithelial neoplasia (PIN) may be more concentrated in prostates containing cancer and is noted in proximity to cancer. However, the final fate of PIN is unknown, including the possibilities of latency, invasion, and even regression. The current working model of prostate carcinogenesis suggests that repeated cycles of injury and cell death occur to the prostate epithelium because of damage (i.e., from oxidative stress) from inflammatory responses.[226,246] The direct injury is hypothesized as a response to infections; autoimmune disease;

circulating carcinogens or toxins, or both, from the diet; or urine that has refluxed into the prostate (see Fig. 26.19). The resultant manifestation of this injury is focal atrophy or prostate intraepithelial atrophy (PIA). Biologic responses cause an increase in proliferation and a massive increase in epithelial cells that have a phenotype intermediate between basal cells and mature luminal cells.[226,246,247] Molecular genetic and epigenetic changes can increase genetic instability that might progress to high-grade PIN and early prostate cancer formation.[248].

Stromal environment. The prostate gland is composed of secretory luminal epithelium, basal epithelium, neuroendocrine cells, and various cell types comprising supportive tissue or stroma. Stroma, or tissue microenvironment, produces autocrine/paracrine factors as well as structural supporting molecules that help regulate normal cell behavior and organ homeostasis.[249] Stromal microenvironment in prostate cancer is altered compared to normal stroma and exhibits features of a wound repair stroma.[250] Stromal components in the tumor microenvironment are important contributions to tumor progression and metastasis. Reciprocal interactions between tumor cells and stromal components influence the metastatic, dormancy-related, and stem cell–like potential of tumor cells. The stromal compartment of the tumor is complex and includes inflammatory/immune cells, vascular endothelial cells, fibroblasts, myofibroblasts, adipocytes, and components of the extracellular matrix.[251]

Epithelial-mesenchymal transition (EMT) was first described in embryonic development and is observed in several solid tumors (see Chapter 12).[252] Cells that undergo EMT become more migratory and invasive and gain access to vascular vessels. Numerous studies have shown that these transition states (EMT and mesenchymal-epithelial transition [MET]) are a consequence of tumor-stromal interactions.[253]

Clinical Manifestations. Prostatic cancer often causes no symptoms until it is far advanced. The first manifestations of disease are those of BOO: slow urinary stream, hesitancy, incomplete emptying, frequency, nocturia, and dysuria. Unlike the symptoms of obstruction caused by BPH, the symptoms of obstruction caused by prostatic cancer are progressive and do not remit. Local extension is usually posterior, although late in the disease the tumor may invade the rectum or encroach on the prostatic urethra and cause BOO (obstructing the upper urinary tract ureters) (Fig. 26.24). Rectal obstruction also may occur, causing the individual to experience large bowel obstruction or difficulty in defecation. Prostatic cancer and its treatment also can affect sexual functioning. Symptoms of late disease include bone pain at sites of bone metastasis, edema of the lower extremities, enlargement of lymph nodes, liver enlargement, pathologic bone fractures, and mental confusion associated with brain metastases. The spread of cancer through blood vessels is illustrated in Fig. 26.25. The most common sites of distant metastasis are the lymph nodes, bones, lungs, liver, and adrenals. The pelvis, lumbar spine, femur, thoracic spine, and ribs are the most common sites of bone metastasis.

Evaluation and Treatment. Screening for prostatic cancer includes PSA blood test and DRE. The issue of prostate cancer screening is controversial. Evidence is lacking on whether PSA screening or DRE reduces the mortality from prostate cancer or that the benefits outweigh the harms of screening.[254] Nonetheless, the PSA test is commonly used in the diagnosis and management of prostate cancer. For men aged 55 to 69 years, the decision to undergo periodic PSA-based screening for prostate cancer should be an individual one and should include discussion with their health care providers of the potential benefits and harms of screening. Screening for prostate cancer in any man 70 years or older is not recommended. Screening offers a small potential benefit to reduce the chance of death from prostate cancer in some men.[255] PSA screening may reduce the prostate cancer mortality risk but is associated with false positive

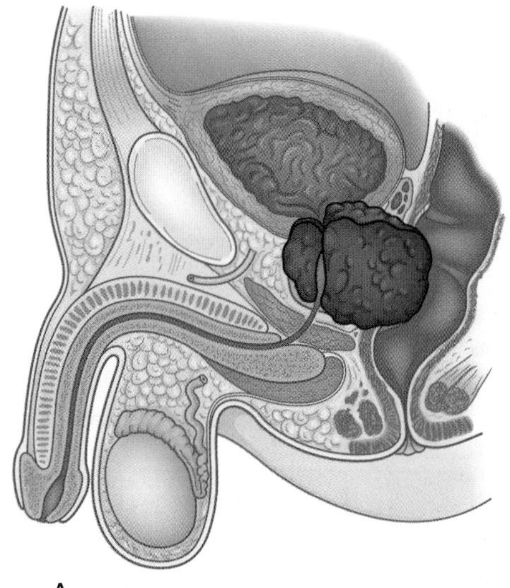

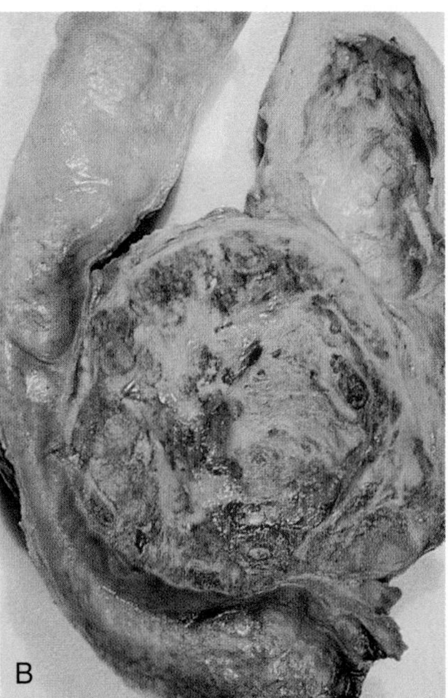

Fig. 26.24 Carcinoma of the Prostate. (A) Schematic of carcinoma of the prostate. **(B)** Carcinoma of the prostate extending into the rectum and urinary bladder. (B, From Damjanov I, Linder J, eds. *Pathology*: A color atlas. St. Louis: Mosby; 2000.)

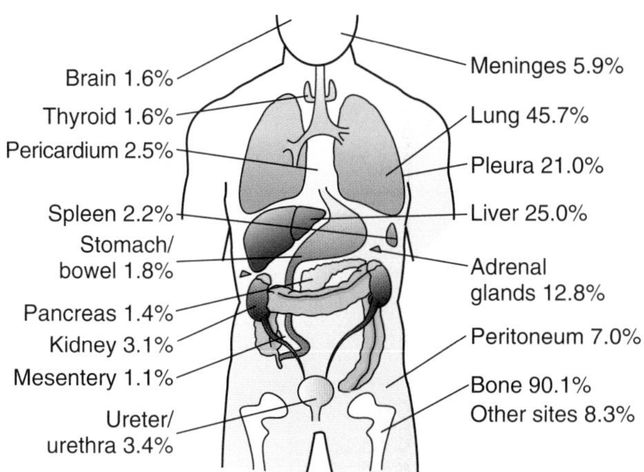

Fig. 26.25 Distribution of Hematogenous Metastases in Prostate Cancer. The results are from a study of 556 men with metastatic prostate cancer. (Adapted from Budendorf L, Schöpfer A, Wagner U, et al. Metastatic patterns of prostate cancer: An autopsy study of 1,589 patients. *Hum Pathol.* 2000;31:578.)

BOX 26.13 AJCC Stage Groupings Prostate Cancer

Grade Group	Gleason Score	Gleason Pattern
1	≤6	≤3+3
2	7	3+4
3	7	4+3
4	8	4+4, 3+5, or 5+3
5	9 or 10	4+5, 5+4, or 5+5

Adapted from AJCC: Prostate. In: Amin MB, Edge SB, Greene FL, et al., eds. *AJCC cancer staging manual*, 8th edition. New York: Springer, 2017, pp. 715–26.
AJCC, American Joint Committee on Cancer.
From PDQ® Adult Treatment Editorial Board. PDQ prostate cancer treatment. Bethesda, MD: National Cancer Institute. Updated February 12, 2021. Available at: https://www.cancer.gov/types/prostate/hp/prostate-treatment-pdq (accessed May 8, 2022).

results, biopsy complications, and overdiagnosis. DRE may detect early prostatic carcinomas, but it has low sensitivity and specificity. Cancer diagnosis is confirmed through tissue biopsy and microscopic examination of tissue. Lymphography, bone scans, MRI, and CT scans also may be used to determine metastasis to lymph, bone, or other adjacent tissue. Important for treatment is to accurately measure the size of the index (longest) tumor and its percentage Gleason grade of differentiation.[256]

Treatment of prostatic cancer depends on the stage of the neoplasm, the anticipated effects of treatment, and the age, general health, and life expectancy of the individual. Options include no treatment; surgical treatments, such as total prostatectomy, TURP, or cryotherapy; nonsurgical treatments, such as radiation therapy, hormone therapy, or chemotherapy; watchful waiting; and any combination of these treatment modalities. In addition, new approaches are using immunotherapy. Palliative treatment is aimed at relieving urinary, bladder outlet, or colon obstruction; spinal cord compression; and pain. Box 26.13 shows the stage groupings for prostate cancer. Prognosis and survival rates have improved steadily over the past 50 years. The 5-year relative survival rate for the vast majority (89%) of men diagnosed with local (74.3% of cancers) cancer approaches 100% but drops to 30% for those diagnosed with distant-stage disease.[257]

Treatment for prostate cancer may lead to stress incontinence or loss of urinary control, which may or may not return to normal after several weeks or months, and SD. Sensation of orgasm is not usually affected, but smaller amounts of ejaculate will be produced, or men may experience a "dry" ejaculate because of retrograde ejaculation.

Sexual Dysfunction: Erectile Dysfunction

Male SD is not a single disease.[258] It involves the whole process of sexual activity including sexual arousal, penis erection, insertion, and ejaculation. Sexual dysfunction is the impairment of any or all these processes and can be caused by various physiologic, psychological, and emotional factors. Until the late 1970s, most cases of male SD were considered psychogenic. Now there is evidence that up to 90% of cases involve organic factors (Fig. 26.26). Most of these disorders cause erectile dysfunction (ED).[259] ED is the most prevalent among diseases in SD and the most challenging to treat successfully.[258] Reportedly, 52% of 40- to 70-year-old men suffer from ED; it is closely associated to age and other comorbidities.[260,261] Epidemiological evidence suggests that impotence has affected 10 million American men.[262] Various implicated risk factors for SD are presented in Box 26.14.

Pathophysiology. SD is complex and involves both risk and pathogenic factors. Pathogenic factors include endothelial dysfunction,[263] neurogenic factors,[264] hormonal pathways, and hemodynamic factors.[263] Men with ED have more endothelial damage than men without ED, and ED may be the first symptom of endothelial injury.[258] Penile erection requires a series of coordinated and complex events involving neuronal pathways, vascular response, and psychosomatic stimulation.[258] All of these actions are mediated by activation of the NO-cGMP dilator pathway.[265] NO released by the cavernous nerve terminals initiates erection, and NO from endothelial cells maintains the erection.[261]

Cyclic guanosine monophosphate (cyclic GMP) is stimulated by NO, and GMP enters the smooth muscle. Protein kinase G is activated by cyclic GMP which opens potassium channels while closing calcium channels.[261] Low intracellular calcium causes the intracavernosal smooth tissue to relax which allows arterial flow and veno-occlusive activity. The erection is then maintained with minimal blood flow moving into or out of the corpora. The process reverses when the corporal smooth muscle contracts again with the degraded GMP by the penile enzyme, phosphodiesterase. ED arises when any of these processes are disrupted by pathological changes.[261]

Endocrine regulation is critical for successful sexual development and for normal sexual function. Failure of the pituitary gland to maintain relative ratio of endogenous levels likely disrupts processes in sexual function.[258] Testosterone is the most important androgen for libido and spermatogenesis. Androgen deficiency can lead to SD, ED, loss of libido, and a decline in reproductive capacity.[258]

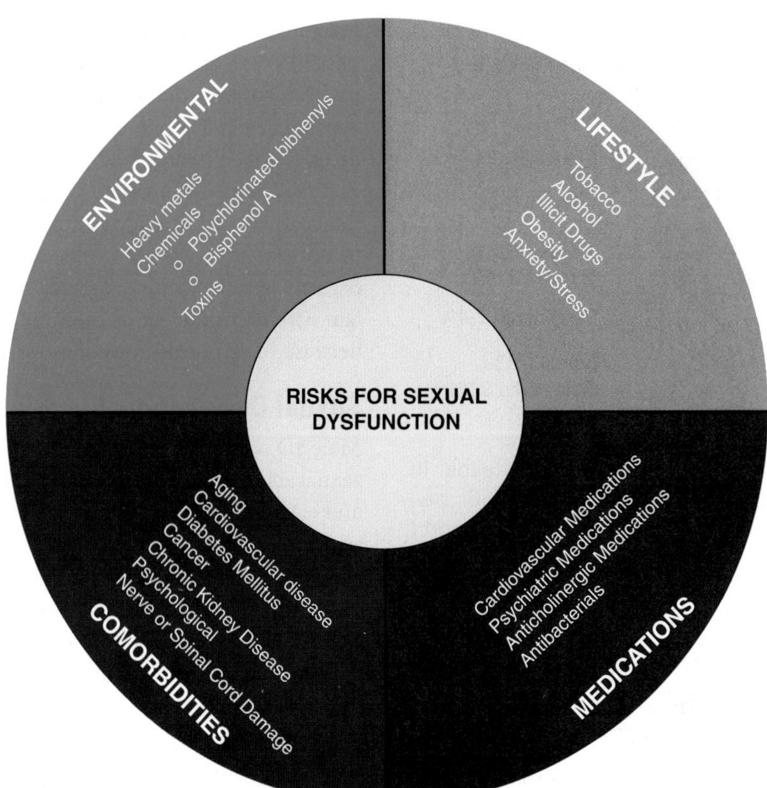
ENVIRONMENTAL
Heavy metals
Chemicals
o Polychlorinated bibhenyls
o Bisphenol A
Toxins
LIFESTYLE
Tobacco
Alcohol
Illicit Drugs
Obesity
Anxiety/Stress
RISKS FOR SEXUAL DYSFUNCTION
Aging
Cardiovascular disease
Diabetes Mellitus
Cancer
Chronic Kidney Disease
Psychological
Nerve or Spinal Cord Damage
COMORBIDITIES
Cardiovascular Medications
Psychiatric Medications
Anticholinergic Medications
Antibacterials
MEDICATIONS

Fig. 26.26 Risk Factors of Sexual Dysfunction.

BOX 26.14 Implicated Risk Factors for Sexual Dysfunction in Males

- Altered lifestyle
- Stressful living conditions
- Chronic diseases: cardiovascular, hypertension, hyperlipidemia, diabetes, chronic kidney disease, reproductive cancers, stroke, neurodegenerative, disorders, epilepsy, spinal cord injury, sleep apnea, chronic obstructive pulmonary disease (COPD), sequela of priapism, benign prostatic hyperplasia, lower urinary tract symptoms
- Diverse environmental pollutants: endocrine disruptors, heavy metals, radiation, estrogenic and destructive chemicals (bisphenol A, phthalates, organochlorine), lead exposure
- Drug side effects examples: anti-hypertensives, clofibrate, cimetidine, digoxin, anti-neoplastic, and various hormonal agents, recreational, others
- Psychological disturbances: depression, performance anxiety
- Dose-dependent alcohol intake
- Traumatic: pelvic fractures, spinal cord injuries
- Iatrogenic: post transurethral resection of the prostate
- Smoking
- Obesity
- Increased age
- Testosterone deficiency syndrome
- Hypogonadism

Emotional and psychologic response (e.g., anxiety, depression, and loss of self-esteem) to chronic illness can affect sexual functioning. In other chronic conditions, SD is associated with low energy levels and loss of libido. The pathophysiologic mechanisms responsible for such changes are not known.

Evaluation and Treatment. A complete medical history, detailed sexual history, and physical examination are required. A complete list of all medications and supplements is necessary. Use of a scoring system is easier for individuals, with 100% being the best and hardest erection they ever had, 0% being completely flaccid, and 50% being firm enough for penetration.[261] A valid questionnaire called the International Index of Erectile Function (IIEF) is also available for individuals to complete in private.[266] Having the sexual partner present for the history greatly improves the outcome of the treatment process.[261] Obvious cases of psychogenic ED are referred to an appropriate mental health professional.

There are no specific tests required for the initial evaluation of ED. Routine blood testing includes a CBC, electrolytes, baseline renal and liver function tests, HgbA1c to screen for diabetes, and a lipid profile.[261] A morning testosterone level is recommended by the 2018 AUA Guidelines for Erectile Dysfunction, but it is not necessary unless there are symptoms of hypogonadism, such as loss of sexual desire or testicular atrophy.[261] Other tests may include LH prolactin (with hypogonadism), sickle cell in the African/Caribbean patient, and thyroid function. Because there is no effective cure for ED, identification of the underlying cause is useful only for detecting other potential health issues and comorbidities.[261] Thus, the focus changes from expensive diagnostic testing that will not significantly affect the outcome, to facilitating treatment selection after a candid and detailed discussion of reasonable therapeutic options.

Lifestyle modifications are the initial treatment recommendations. This approach improves erectile function and reduces cardiovascular risk. Lifestyle recommendations include increased physical activity, switching to a Mediterranean diet and/or nutritional counseling, drug, alcohol, and smoking cessation, and optimal control of diabetes, lipids, and cholesterol. If possible, these recommendations are given to both the patient and his partner. The drug history is carefully reviewed to remove or alter problem medications. Studies have shown some efficacy in treating mild to moderate ED with L-arginine supplementation.[267] Oral phosphodiesterase-5 inhibitors (PDE-5 inhibitors) are the first-line treatment of ED.[261] Importantly, PDE-5 inhibitors do not *initiate* the erectile response. Sexual stimulation is required to release NO from the vascular endothelium and penile nerve endings to begin the erectile process. PDE-5 inhibitors are effective and have an overall success rate of up to 76%.[268] The most common side effects (sildenafil) are headache, flushing, upset stomach, abnormal vision, nasal congestion, muscle pain, and dizziness. Known interactions of sildenafil and heart medications prompted the FDA to urge caution in those men who have experienced heart attack, stroke, or other serious cardiovascular events within six months of starting therapy. They should not be used at all with nitrates due to possible dangerous and significant hypotension.[261] Different PDE-5 inhibitors have varying half-lives which can influence the individual's final decision. Testosterone supplementation appears to be more effective for low libido than ED.[269,270] External vacuum device therapy is safe, effective, and the most inexpensive long-term therapy for ED.[261] Intracavernosal injection therapy has been reported as effective in up to 94% of individuals.[271] Prostaglandin E1 is relatively expensive and somewhat painful when injected into the corpora.[261] Combination therapy, such as Trimix or QuadMix, and is prepared by a compounding pharmacy. Side effects from intracavernosal injection include pain, priapism, bleeding, bruising, and scarring.[261] It is critical to warn individuals not to increase the injected dosage without the approval of their healthcare provider, not to mix it with other ED agents such as PDE-5 inhibitors, and to go to the nearest Emergency Department for reversal therapy if their erection lasts longer than 4 hours to prevent permanent damage to the corpora.[261] Penile revascularization surgery is done in a very small subgroup of individuals (typically young men), about 5% of all persons with ED.[272]

DISORDERS OF THE MALE BREAST

Gynecomastia

Gynecomastia is the overdevelopment of breast tissue in a male. It appears more during certain ages of hormonal change such as birth, adolescence, and old age.[273] The incidence is greatest among adolescents and men older than 65 years. Gynecomastia results from hormonal alterations, which may be idiopathic or caused by systemic disorders, drugs including thiazides, digoxin, estrogens, phenothiazines, and theophylline, hypogonadism, or liver and kidney failure.[273] Marijuana is also associated with gynecomastia. Chemotherapeutic drugs known to cause gynecomastia include methotrexate, alkylating agents, imatinib, and vinca alkaloids. The most common drugs are those with estrogen-like actions, including cimetidine, spironolactone, ketoconazole, and finasteride. Contributing disorders associated with gynecomastia are breast cancer, adrenal disease, thyroid disease, cirrhosis, renal failure, hypogonadism, and malnutrition.[273] Most cases of gynecomastia are idiopathic; however, it is known to involve an imbalance of the estrogen/testosterone (estrogen/T) ratio.[274,275]

The normal estrogen/T ratio can be altered in one of two ways. First, estrogen levels may be excessively high, although T levels are normal. This is the case in drug-induced and tumor-induced hyperestrogenism. Second, T levels may be extremely low, although estrogen levels are normal, as is the case in hypergonadism. Gynecomastia also can be caused by alterations in breast tissue responsiveness to hormonal stimulation. Breast tissue may have increased responsiveness to estrogen or decreased responsiveness to androgen. Alterations of responsiveness may cause many cases of idiopathic gynecomastia.

Hormone-induced gynecomastia is usually bilateral. Pubertal gynecomastia is a self-limiting phenomenon that usually disappears within 4 to 6 months. Senescent gynecomastia usually regresses spontaneously within 6 to 12 months. Gynecomastia also is often seen in males receiving estrogen therapy such as in preparation for sex reasignment surgery or gender affirming surgery.

Pathophysiology. Gynecomastia is the result of enlargement of breast glandular tissue and adipose tissue. Estrogen is responsible for the growth of glandular tissue, as well as the suppression of testosterone. Estrogen suppresses LH, which is responsible for testicular secretion of testosterone. The hormonal imbalance leads to gynecomastia. Three types of gynecomastia related to the length of the condition are florid, fibrous, and intermediate. Florid gynecomastia is seen in early stages of the condition, four months or less, with an increase in ductal tissue and vascularity.[273] Fibrous gynecomastia is noted after a year duration with more stromal fibrosis and few ducts. Intermediate gynecomastia, seen after one year, is thought to be a progression from florid to fibrous.

Evaluation and Treatment. The diagnosis of gynecomastia is based on a complete history and physical examination. A careful review of all medications and recreational drug use is obtained. During the physical exam, the head and neck are examined for any abnormal masses or thyroid changes. The breasts and axilla regions are examined for masses, skin changes, nipple discharge, asymmetry, and tenderness. The testes are examined for asymmetry, enlargement, masses, or atrophy.[273] Males with feminizing characteristics have endocrine and genetic testing.[273] Identification and treatment of the cause are likely to be followed by resolution of the gynecomastia. The man should be taught to perform breast self-examination and is examined at 6- and 12-month intervals if the gynecomastia persists. All unilateral breast enlargement in men warrants an evaluation for malignancy; workup includes fine-needle aspiration, cytology, mammography, ultrasound, and biopsy. If the underlying condition is treated, yet persists for longer than a year, surgical treatment is suggested.[276–278]

Male Breast Cancer

Male breast cancer (MBC) accounts for 0.26% of all male cancers and 1.1% of all breast cancers. In 2021, estimated new cases of MBC were 2650 and deaths 530.[199] Global incidence rates were generally less than 1 per 100,000 man-years, in contrast to much higher rates in females.[279] It is seen most after the age of 60 years, with the peak incidence between 60 and 69 years (men tend to be diagnosed at an older age than women). However, it has been reported in males as young as 6 years old and in adolescents. Klinefelter syndrome is the strongest risk factor for developing male breast carcinoma. Other risk factors include germline mutation in *BRCA1* or *BRCA2*, but familial cases usually have *BRCA2* rather than *BRCA1* mutations.[280]

Obesity increases the risk of MBC. Testicular disorders, including cryptorchidism, mumps, orchitis, and orchiectomy, are related to risk. The relationship between these factors and the risk of disease is not clearly defined.

Recent data on the most frequent molecular subtypes of MBC appears to be different from those for female breast cancers. Luminal A and luminal B are most common, and basal-like, unclassifiable triple-negative, and *HER2*-driven MBCs are rare.[280]

Male breast tumors often resemble carcinoma of the breast in women (see Breast Cancer in Chapter 25). The majority of MBCs express estrogen and progesterone receptors. The malignant male breast lesion is usually a unilateral solid mass located near the nipple. Because the nipple is commonly involved, crusting and nipple discharge are typical clinical manifestations. Other findings include skin retraction, ulceration of the skin over the tumor, and axillary node involvement. Patterns of metastasis are similar to those in females.

The diagnosis of cancer is confirmed by biopsy. Because of delays in seeking treatment, MBC tends to be advanced at the time of diagnosis and therefore is likely to have a poor prognosis. Treatment protocols are like those for female breast cancer, and endocrine therapy is used for MBC as male tumors are hormone dependent. The mainstay of treatment is modified mastectomy with axillary node dissection to assess the stage and prognosis. Because 90% of tumors are hormonal receptor positive, tamoxifen is standard adjuvant therapy. For metastatic disease, hormonal therapy is the main treatment, but chemotherapy also can provide palliation. An orchiectomy may need to be performed to treat metastatic disease to the testes.

SUMMARY REVIEW

Alterations of Sexual Maturation

1. Sexual maturation, or puberty, is marked by the development of secondary sex characteristics, rapid growth, and ultimately, the ability to reproduce. Puberty begins later in boys than in girls; the onset of 9 to 14 years has remained unchanged in boys.
2. Precocious puberty is early development of secondary characteristics in boys before age 9. Contrasexual development occurs when male or female children develop features of the opposite gender. Delayed puberty in boys is when their growth spurt occurs later (15 to 17 years) and seldom requires treatment.

Disorders of the Male Reproductive System

1. Disorders of the urethra include urethritis (infection of the urethra) and urethral strictures (narrowing or obstruction of the urethral lumen caused by scarring).
2. Most cases of urethritis result from sexually transmitted pathogens. Urologic instrumentation, foreign body insertion, trauma, or an anatomic abnormality can cause urethral inflammation with or without infection.
3. Urethritis causes urinary symptoms, including a burning sensation during urination (dysuria), frequency, urgency, urethral tingling or itching, and a clear or purulent discharge.
4. Strictures mostly result from injury to the urethral mucosa and surrounding tissues. Etiologies include idiopathic, iatrogenic, inflammatory, and traumatic. Urethral strictures are common in the United States.
5. Pathophysiology of stricture is injury to the urethral epithelium from any of the specific etiologies causing a leak of urine to the corpus spongiosum or by direct trauma to the corpus spongiosum.
6. Manifestations of urethral stricture include those of bladder outlet obstruction: urinary frequency and hesitancy, mild dysuria, double urinary stream or spraying, and dribbling after voiding.
7. Phimosis and paraphimosis are penile disorders involving the foreskin (prepuce). In phimosis, the foreskin cannot be retracted over the glans. In paraphimosis, the foreskin is retracted and cannot be reduced (returned to its normal anatomic position over the glans). Phimosis is caused by poor hygiene and chronic infection. In adults it can be caused by sexually transmitted infections. Paraphimosis can constrict the penile blood vessels, preventing circulation to the glans.
8. The hallmark of Peyronie disease is the tunical fibrosis of the corpora cavernosa resulting in plaques. Fibrosis prevents engorgement on the affected side, causing a lateral curvature during erection. Peyronie disease can cause painful erection, painful intercourse for both partners, and poor erection distal to the involved area. It is a disorder of wound healing of the tunica albuginea.
9. Priapism is a disorder of prolonged, painful erection in the absence of appropriate stimulation. The causes of priapism are numerous and include hemoglobinopathies, sickle cell disease, thalassemia, vasoactive medications, intracavernous injections, antidepressants, and less commonly neurologic infections, and neoplastic diseases. Pathophysiology of priapism includes ischemic and nonischemic changes.
10. Balanitis is an inflammation of the glans penis. Posthitis is inflammation of the foreskin or prepuce. It is associated with phimosis, inadequate cleansing under the foreskin, skin disorders, and pathogens (e.g., *Candida albicans*).

Balanoposthitis involves both the glans and foreskin and occurs only in uncircumcised males.

11. Balanitis is associated with inadequate hygiene and phimosis in uncircumcised males leading to infection. Other etiologies include chemical irritants, edematous conditions, drug allergies, morbid obesity, allergic reaction, trauma, neoplastic disorders, and others.
12. Condyloma acuminatum is a benign tumor caused by HPV.
13. Cancer of the penis is rare. It can affect men 40 to 70 years of age, Risk factors include HPV, smoking, chronic inflammatory conditions, certain treatments for psoriasis, obesity, and poor penile hygiene. The precursor lesion of penile cancer is penile intraepithelial neoplasia (PeIN).
14. Varicocele, hydrocele, and spermatocele are common disorders of the scrotum.
15. A varicocele is an abnormal dilation of the veins within the spermatic cord and is classically described as a "bag of worms." Varicoceles are one of the most identified scrotal abnormalities and abnormal findings among infertile men.
16. A hydrocele is an abnormal collection of fluid between the layers of the tunica vaginalis of testis.
17. A spermatocele is a cyst located between the testis and epididymis that is filled with fluid and sperm.
18. Cryptorchidism is the absence of at least one testicle from the scrotum and is the most common birth defect of the male genitalia. About 80% of cryptorchid testes descend by the third month making the incidence about 1%. The main risk factor for undescended testes is birthweight followed by family history.
19. Testicular torsion occurs when a testicle rotates twisting the spermatic cord and interrupting its blood supply. Torsion of the testis is a surgical emergency and must be corrected within 6 hours from the onset of pain to preserve normal testicular function.
20. Orchitis is an acute inflammation of the testes and is usually unilateral. Common risk factors include a preexisting history of epididymitis, unprotected sexual contact, multiple sexual partners, long-term use of a urinary catheter, bladder outlet obstruction, and lack of immunization with MMR vaccination.
21. Testicular cancer is very uncommon and usually affects men between 14 and 44 years of age. It is, however, increasing worldwide and the etiology is not well documented. The most consistent risk factor is cryptorchidism, which increases risk of testicular cancer fivefold. Germ cell neoplasia (GNIS) is known as the precursor lesion to malignant testicular germ cell tumors (TGCTs). Germ-cell tumors are observed secondary to a carcinogenic event in utero. During puberty hormonal changes increase the invasive potential of these neoplasms.
22. Epididymitis, an inflammation of the epididymis testis, is commonly caused by a sexually transmitted pathogen (mostly bacteria) in younger men and from retrograde flow of urine in elderly males.
23. Benign prostatic hyperplasia is nonmalignant growth or hyperplasia of prostate tissue. This condition becomes symptomatic as the enlarging prostate compresses the urethra, causing symptoms of bladder outlet obstruction and urine retention.
24. Prostatitis is an infection or inflammation of the prostate gland. Prostatitis syndromes have been classified by the National Institutes of Health as (1) acute bacterial prostatitis (ABP), (2) chronic bacterial prostatitis (CBP), (3) chronic pelvic pain syndrome (CPPS), and (4) asymptomatic inflammatory prostatitis.
25. Prostate cancer is the most diagnosed, non–skin cancer in American males, and the incidence varies greatly worldwide. Risk factors include age, ethnicity, obesity, family history, height, hypertension, lack of exercise, Agent Orange exposure, and Western diet. Although the cause is unknown, genetics plays a role. Androgens and androgen receptor (AR) function have major roles in the development and progression of prostate cancer. Chronic inflammation may be an important risk factor for prostate adenocarcinoma.
26. Most cancers of the prostate are adenocarcinomas that develop at the periphery of the gland.
27. Sexual dysfunction in males can be caused by any physical or psychological factor that impairs erection, emission, or ejaculation. Erectile dysfunction is the most prevalent.
28. Spermatogenesis (sperm production by the testes) can be impaired by disruptions that reduce testosterone secretion and by testicular trauma, infection, atrophy from any cause, systemic illness involving high fever, ingestion of various drugs, exposure to environmental toxins, and cryptorchidism.

Disorders of the Male Breast

1. Gynecomastia is the overdevelopment of breast tissue in a male. The incidence is greatest among adolescents and men older than 65 years of age.
2. Gynecomastia can result from systemic disorders, drugs, neoplasms, or idiopathic causes. Most cases are idiopathic and involve an imbalance of the estrogen/testosterone ratio.
3. Breast cancer is relatively uncommon in males, but it has a poor prognosis because men tend to delay seeking treatment until the disease is advanced. The incidence is greatest in men in their sixties.

REFERENCES

1. Tang C, Gondal AZ, Damian M. *Delayed puberty*. In: *StatPearls*. Treasure Island, FL: StatPearls Publishing; 2021. Last update August 7, 2021. Available at https://www.ncbi.nlm.nih.gov/books/NBK544322/. (Accessed February 22, 2022).
2. Sultan C, et al. Disorders of puberty. *Best Pract Res Clin Obstet Gynaecol*. 2018;48:62–89.
3. Palmert MR, Dunkel L. Clinical practice. Delayed puberty. *N Engl J Med*. 2012;366(5):443–453.
4. Bozzola M, et al. Delayed puberty versus hypogonadism: a challenge for the pediatrician. *Ann Pediatr Endocrinol Metab*. 2018;23(2):57–61.
5. Breehl L, Caban O. Physiology, puberty. In: *StatPearls*. Treasure Island, FL: StatPearls Publishing; 2021. Last update April 21, 2021. Available at https://www.ncbi.nlm.nih.gov/books/NBK534827/. (Accessed February 22, 2022).

6. Blondell RD, Foster MB, Dave KC. Disorders of puberty. *Am Fam Physician*. 1999;60(1):209–218, 223–224.
7. Jospe N. Disorders of pubertal development. In: Osborn LM, ed. *Pediatrics*. Philadelphia: Mosby; 2005.
8. De Leonibus C, Marcovecchio ML, Chiarelli F. Update on statural growth and pubertal development in obese children. *Pediatr Rep*. 2012;4:e35.
9. Marcovecchio ML, Chiarelli F. Obesity and growth during childhood and puberty. *World Rev Nutr Diet*. 2013;106:135–141.
10. Kansra AR, Lakkunarajah S, Jay MS. Childhood and adolescent obesity: a review. *Front Pediatr*. 2020;8:581461.
11. Stanhope R, Preece MA. Management of constitutional delay of growth and puberty. *Arch Dis Child*. 1988;63(9):1104–1110.
12. Whittemore BJ, et al. Endocrine and metabolic disorders. In: Burns CE, ed. *Pediatric Primary Care*. St. Louis: Saunders; 2012.
13. Smaldone A, et al. Endocrine and metabolic diseases. In: Burns CE, ed. *Pediatric Primary Care*. St. Louis: Saunders; 2016.
14. Fenichel P. Delayed puberty. *Endocr Dev*. 2012;22:138–159.
15. Raivio T, Miettinen PJ. Constitutional delay of puberty versus congenital hypogonadotropic hypogonadism: genetics, management and updates. *Best Pract Res Clin Endocrinol Metab*. 2019;33:1–14.
16. Abdeen BM, Badreldrin MD. Urethral strictures. In: *StatPearls*. Treasure Island, FL: StatPearls Publishing; 2021. Last update October 21, 2021. Available at https://www.ncbi.nlm.nih.gov/books/NBK564297/. (Accessed February 22, 2022).
17. Latini JM, et al. SIU/ICUD Consultation On Urethral Strictures: epidemiology, etiology, anatomy, and nomenclature of urethral stenoses, strictures, and pelvic fracture urethral disruption injuries. *Urology*. 2014;83(3 Suppl):S1–S7.
18. Smith TG. Current management of urethral stricture disease. *Indian J Urol*. 2016;32(1):27–33.
19. Kranz J, et al. [Urethral stricture rate after prostate cancer radiotherapy: five -year data of a certified prostate cancer center]. *Urologe A*. 2017;56(3):336–341. German.
20. Chi AC, Han J, Gonzalez CM. Urethral strictures and the cancer survivor. *Curr Opin Urol*. 2014;24(4):415–420.
21. Liaw A, Rickborn L, McClung C. Incidence of urethral stricture in patients with adult acquired buried penis. *Adv Urol*. 2017 7056173, 2017.
22. Hampson LA, McAninch JW, Breyer BN. Male urethral strictures and their management. *Nat Rev Urol*. 2014;11(1):43–50.
23. Mundy AR, Andrich DE. Urethral strictures. *BJU Int*. 2011;107(1):6–26.
24. Verla W, et al. Comprehensive review emphasizing anatomy, etiology, diagnosis, and treatment of male urethral stricture disease. *Biomed Res Int*. 2019 9046430, 2019.
25. Lambert E, et al. Validated uroflowmetry-based predictive model for the primary diagnosis of urethral stricture disease in men. *Int J Urol*. 2018;25(9):792–798.
26. Tritschler S, et al. Urethral stricture: etiology, investigation, and treatments. *Dtsch Arztebl Int*. 2013;110(13):220–226.
27. Lv XG, et al. The application of CT voiding urethrography in the evaluation of urethral stricture associated with fistula: a preliminary report. *Int Urol Nephrol*. 2016;48(8):1267–1273.
28. Talreja SM, et al. Comparison of sonoelastography with sonourethrography and retrograde urethrography in the evaluation of male anterior urethral strictures. *Turk J Urol*. 2016;42(2):84–91.
29. Bragg BN, Kong EL, Leslie SW. Paraphimosis. In: *StatPearls*. Treasure Island, FL: StatPearls Publishing; 2021. Last update August 12, 2021. Available at https://www.ncbi.nlm.nih.gov/books/NBK459233/. (Accessed February 22, 2022).
30. Choe JM. Paraphimosis: current treatment options. *Am Fam Physician*. 2000;62(12):2623–2626, 2628.
31. Sandean DP, Lotfollahzadeh S. Peyronie disease. In: *StatPearls*. Treasure Island, FL: StatPearls Publishing; 2021. Last update December 3, 2021. Available at https://www.ncbi.nlm.nih.gov/books/NBK560628/. (Accessed February 22, 2022).
32. Dibenedetti DB, et al. Population-based study of Peyronie's disease: prevalence and treatment patterns in the United States. *Adv Urol*. 2011:282503, 2011.
33. Arafa M, et al. The prevalence of Peyronie's disease in diabetic patients with erectile dysfunction. *Int J Impot Res*. 2007;19(2):213–217.
34. Davis SN, et al. Female partners of men with Peyronie's disease have impaired sexual function, satisfaction, and mood, while degree of sexual interference is associated with worse outcomes. *J Sex Med*. 2016;13(7):1095–1103.
35. Gonzalez-Cadavid NF, Rajfer J. Mechanisms of disease: new insights into the cellular and molecular pathology of Peyronie's disease. *Nat Clin Pract Urol*. 2005;2(6):291–297.
36. Nyberg LM, et al. Identification of an inherited form of Peyronie's disease with autosomal dominant inheritance and association with Dupuytren's contracture and histocompatibility B7 cross-reacting antigens. *J Urol*. 1982;128(1):48–51.
37. Willscher MK, Cwazka WF, Novicki DE. The association of histocompatibility antigens of the B7 cross-reacting group with Peyronie's disease. *J Urol*. 1979;122(1):34–35.
38. Brock G, et al. The anatomy of the tunica albuginea in the normal penis and Peyronie's disease. *J Urol*. 1997;157(1):276–281.
39. Davis CJ. The microscopic pathology of Peyronie's disease. *J Urol*. 1997;157(1):282–284.
40. El-Sakka AI, et al. Histological and ultrastructural alterations in an animal model of Peyronie's disease. *Br J Urol*. 1998;81(3):445–452.
41. Somers KD, Dawson DM. Fibrin deposition in Peyronie's disease plaque. *J Urol*. 1997;157(1):311–315.
42. Devine CJ, et al. Proposal: trauma as the cause of the Peyronie's lesion. *J Urol*. 1997;157(1):285–290.
43. Diegelmann RF. Cellular and biochemical aspects of normal and abnormal wound healing: an overview. *J Urol*. 1997;157(1):298–302.
44. Gholami SS, et al. Peyronie's disease: a review. *J Urol*. 2003;169(4):1234–1241.
45. Jalkut M, Gonzalez-Cadavid N, Rajfer J. New discoveries in the basic science understanding of Peyronie's disease. *Curr Urol Rep*. 2004;5(6):478–484.
46. Mulhall JP, et al. Basic fibroblast growth factor expression in Peyronie's disease. *J Urol*. 2001;165(2):419–423.
47. Bacal V, et al. Correlation of degree of penile curvature between patient estimates and objective measures among men with Peyronie's disease. *J Sex Med*. 2009;6(3):862–865.
48. Ralph D, et al. The management of Peyronie's disease: evidence-based 2010 guidelines. *J Sex Med*. 2010;7(7):2359–2374.
49. Ohebshalom M, et al. Measurement of penile curvature in Peyronie's disease patients: comparison of three methods. *J Sex Med*. 2007;4(1):199–203.
50. Levine LA, Lenting EL. A surgical algorithm for the treatment of Peyronie's disease. *J Urol*. 1997;158(6):2149–2152.

51. Siberman M, Stormont G, Hu EW. Priapism. In: *StatPearls*. Treasure Island, FL: StatPearls Publishing; 2021. Last update June 16, 2021. Available at https://www.ncbi.nlm.nih.gov/books/NBK459178/. (Accessed February 22, 2022).
52. Lagoda G, et al. Sustained nitric oxide (NO)-releasing compound reverses dysregulated NO signal transduction in priapism. *FASEB J*. 2014;28(1):76–84.
53. Carnicelli D, Akakpo W. [Priapism: diagnosis and management]. *Prog Urol*. 2018;28(14):772–776.
54. Bai WJ, Hu HB. [Considerations on priapism]. *Zhonghua Nan Ke Xue*. 2018;24(8):675–680.
55. Quint R, et al. Priapism in sickle cell disease: beware of neuroleptics. *Am J Hematol*. 2018;93:E211–E213.
56. La Favor JD, et al. Molecular profile of priapism associated with low nitric oxide bioavailability. *J Proteome Res*. 2018;17(3):1031–1040.
57. Vreugdenhil S, de Jong IJ, van Driel MF. [Priapism is an emergency]. *Ned Tijdschr Geneeskd*. 2018;162:D2895 Dutch.
58. Gandhi J, et al. Clinical utility of hyperbaric oxygen therapy in genitourinary medicine. *Med Gas Res*. 2018;8(1):29–33.
59. Edwards S. Balanitis and balanoposthitis: a review. *Genitourin Med*. 1996;72(3):155–159.
60. Vohra S, Badlani G. Balanitis and balanoposthitis. *Urol Clin North Am*. 1992;19(1):143–147.
61. Wray AA, Velasquez J, Khetarpal S. Balanitis. In: *StatPearls*. Treasure Island, FL: StatPearls Publishing; 2021. Last update August 9, 2021. Available at https://www.ncbi.nlm.nih.gov/books/NBK537143/. (Accessed February 22, 2022).
62. Lisboa C, et al. Infectious balanoposthitis: management, clinical and laboratory features. *Int J Dermatol*. 2009;48(2):121–124.
63. Morris BJ, Krieger JN. Penile inflammatory skin disorders and the preventive role of circumcision. *Int J Prev Med*. 2017;8:32.
64. Edwards SK, et al. 2013 European guideline for the management of balanoposthitis. *Int J STD AIDS*. 2014;25(9):615–626.
65. Thomas A, et al. Penile cancer. *Nat Rev Dis Primers*. 2021;7:11.
66. Hansen BT, et al. Trends in incidence, mortality and survival of penile squamous cell carcinoma in Norway 1956-2015. *Int J Cancer*. 2018;142(8):1586–1593.
67. Clouston D, Hall A, Lawrentschuk N. Penile lichen sclerosis (balanitis xerotica obliterans). *BJU Int*. 2011;108(Suppl 2):14–19.
68. Clark PE, et al. National Comprehensive Cancer Network: Penile cancer: clinical practice guidelines in oncology. *J Natl Compr Canc Netw*. 2013;11(5):594–615.
69. Larke NL, et al. Male circumcision and penile cancer: a systematic review and meta-analysis. *Cancer Causes Control*. 2011;22(8):1097–1110.
70. Ingles DJ, et al. Human papillomavirus (HPV) genotype- and age-specific analyses of external genital lesions among men in the HPV Infection in Men (HIM) study. *J Infect Dis*. 2015;211(7):1060–1067.
71. Sudenga SL, et al. Genital humanpapillomavirus infection progression to external genital lesions: the HIM study. *Eur Urol*. 2016;69(1):166–173.
72. Oertell J, et al. Differentiated precursor lesions and low-grade variants of squamous cell carcinomas are frequent findings in foreskins of patients from a region of high penile cancer incidence. *Histopathology*. 2011;58(6):925–933.
73. Spiess PE, et al. Pathophysiological basis of human papillomavirus in penile cancer: key to prevention and delivery of more effective therapies. *CA Cancer J Clin*. 2016;66(6):481–495.
74. De Paula AAP, et al. The impact of cyclooxygenase-2 and vascular endothelial growth factor C immunoexpression on the prognosis of penile carcinoma. *J Urol*. 2012;187(1):134–140.
75. Lucky MA, Rogers B, Parr NJ. Referrals into a dedicated British penile centre and sources of possible delay. *BMJ*. 2009;85(7):527–530.
76. Hernandez BY, et al. Burden of invasive squamous cell carcinoma of the penis in the United States, 1998-2003. *Cancer*. 2008;113(10 Suppl):2883–2891.
77. Barnholtz-Sloan JS, et al. Incidence trends in primary malignant penile cancer. *Urol Oncol*. 2007;25(5):361–367.
78. Favorito LA, et al. Epidemiologic study on penile cancer in Brazil. *Int Braz J Urol*. 2008;34(5):587–591. discussion 591–593.
79. Shim TN, et al. Benign male genital dermatoses. *BMJ*. 2016;354:i4337.
80. Lont AP, et al. A comparison of physical examination and imaging in determining the extent of primary penile carcinoma. *BJU Int*. 2003;91(6):493–495.
81. American Cancer Society (ACS) *Survival Rates for Penile Cancer*. Atlanta, GA: ACS; 2021. Last revised January 26, 2021. Available at https://www.cancer.org/cancer/penile-cancer/detection-diagnosis-staging/survival-rates.html. (Accessed February 22, 2022).
82. Djajadiningrat RS, et al. Contemporary management of regional nodes in penile cancer-improvement of survival. *J Urol*. 2014;191(1):68–73.
83. Verhoeven RHA, et al. Population-based survival of penile cancer patients in Europe and the United States of America: no improvement since 1990. *Eur J Cancer*. 2013;49(6):1414–1421.
84. Yetkin E, Ozturk S. Dilating vascular diseases: pathophysiology and clinical aspects. *Int J Vasc Med*. 2018 9024278, 2018.
85. Leslie SW, Sajjad H, Siref LE. Varicocele. In: *StatPearls*. Treasure Island, FL: StatPearls Publishing; 2021. Last update December 26, 2021. Available at https://www.ncbi.nlm.nih.gov/books/NBK448113/. (Accessed February 22, 2022).
86. Arafa M, et al. Correlation of oxidation-reduction potential with hormones, semen parameters and testicular volume. *Andrologia*. 2019;51(5):e13258.
87. Reesink DJ, et al. Sneeze and pop: a ruptured varicocele; analysis of literature, guided by a well-documented case report. *BMC Urol*. 2019;19(1):14.
88. Vaganée D, et al. Testicular asymmetry in healthy adolescent boys. *BJU Int*. 2018;122(4):654–666.
89. Cho CL, Esteves SC, Agarwal A. Indications and outcomes of varicocele repair. *Panminerva Med*. 2019;61(2):152–163.
90. Kohn TP, et al. The effect of subclinical varicocele on pregnancy rates and semen parameters: a systematic review and meta-analysis. *Curr Urol Rep*. 2018;19(7):53.
91. Hannick JH, et al. Prevalence, Doppler ultrasound findings, and clinical implications of the nutcracker phenomenon in pediatric varicoceles. *Urology*. 2019;128:78–83.
92. Shakeri S, et al. Inter-observer agreement on varicoceles diagnosis among patients referred to Shiraz Namazi Hospital. *Int J Reprod Biomed*. 2018;16(10):649–652.
93. Rocher L, et al. Ultrasensitive Doppler as a tool for the diagnosis of testicular ischemia during the Valsalva maneuver: a new way to explore varicoceles? *Acta Radiol*. 2019;60(8):1048–1056.
94. Hadad Z, Norup K, Petersen C. [Right-sided varicocele testis as the only sign of right-sided renal tumour]. *Ugeskr Laeger*. 2016;178(5):V05140307 Danish.
95. Yan S, et al. Should the current guidelines for the treatment of varicoceles in infertile men be re-evaluated? *Hum Fertil (Camb)*. 2021;24(2):78–92.

96. Jensen CFS, et al. CopMich Collaborative: Male infertility problems of patients with strict sperm morphology between 5-14% may be missed with the current WHO guidelines. *Scand J Urol.* 2018;52(5–6):427–431.
97. Silay MS, et al. Treatment of varicocele in children and adolescents: a systematic review and meta-analysis from the European Association of Urology/European Society for Paediatric Urology Guidelines Panel. *Eur Urol.* 2019;75(3):448–461.
98. Colpi GM, et al. European Academy of Andrology guideline Management of oligo-astheno-teratozoospermia. *Andrology.* 2018;6(4):513–524.
99. Rodriguez Peña M, et al. Predictors of improved seminal parameters and fertility after varicocele repair in young adults. *Andrologia.* 2009;41(5):277–281.
100. Cho CL, et al. Use of indocyanine green angiography in microsurgical subinguinal varicocelectomy - lessons learned from our initial experience. *Int Braz J Urol.* 2017;43(5):974–979.
101. Dagur G, et al. Classifying hydroceles of the pelvis and groin: an overview of etiology, secondary complications, evaluation, and management. *Curr Urol.* 2017;10(1):1–14.
102. Huzaifa M, Moreno MA. Hydrocele. In: *StatPearls.* Treasure Island, FL: StatPearls Publishing; 2021. Last update July 12, 2021. Available at https://www.ncbi.nlm.nih.gov/books/NBK559125/. (Accessed February 22, 2022).
103. Sherchand JB, et al. Mapping of lymphatic filariasis in Nepal. *Filaria J.* 2003;2(1):7.
104. Rioja J, et al. Adult hydrocele and spermatocele. *BJU Int.* 2011;107(11):1852–1864.
105. Lundström KJ, et al. Epidemiology of hydrocele and spermatocele; incidence, treatment and complications. *Scand J Urol.* 2019;53:134–138.
106. Leslie SW, Sajjad H, Villanueva CA. Cryptorchidism. In: *StatPearls.* Treasure Island, FL: StatPearls Publishing; 2021. Last update September 17, 2021. Available at https://www.ncbi.nlm.nih.gov/books/NBK470270/. (Accessed February 22, 2022).
107. Khatwa UA, Menon PS. Management of undescended testis. *Indian J Pediatr.* 2000;67(6):449–454.
108. Xing J-S, Bai Z-M. Is testicular dysgenesis syndrome a genetic, endocrine, or environmental disease, or an unexplained reproductive disorder? *Life Sci.* 2018;194:120–129.
109. Shin J, Jeon GW. Comparison of diagnostic and treatment guidelines for undescended testis. *Clin Exp Pediatr.* 2020;63(11):415–421.
110. Chen J, et al. Cryptorchidism and increased risk of neurodevelopmental disorders. *J Psychiatr Res.* 2018;96:153–161.
111. Hadziselimovic F. On the descent of the epididymo-testicular unit, cryptorchidism, and prevention of infertility. *Basic Clin Androl.* 2017;27:2.
112. Braga LH, Lorenzo AJ, Romao RLP. Canadian Urological Association-Pediatric Urologists of Canada (CUA-PUC) guideline for the diagnosis, management, and followup of cryptorchidism. *Can Urol Assoc J.* 2017;11(7):E251–E260.
113. Berger C, et al. Nonpalpable testes: ultrasound and contralateral testicular hypertrophy predict the surgical access, avoiding unnecessary laparoscopy. *J Pediatr Urol.* 2018;14(2):163.e1–163.e7.
114. Rodprasert W, et al. Hypogonadism and cryptorchidism. *Front Endocrinol (Lausanne).* 2019;10:906.
115. Thorup J, Cortes D. Surgical management of undescended testis - timetable and outcome: a debate. *Sex Dev.* 2019;13(1):11–19.
116. Cheng L, et al. Testicular cancer. *Nat Rev Dis Primers.* 2018;4(1):29.
117. Ludvigson AE, Beaule LT. Urologic emergencies. *Surg Clin North Am.* 2016;96(3):407–424.
118. Schick MA, Sternard BT. Testicular torsion. In: *StatPearls.* Treasure Island, FL: StatPearls Publishing; 2021. Last update August 2, 2021. Available at https://www.ncbi.nlm.nih.gov/books/NBK448199/. (Accessed February 22, 2022).
119. Pilatz A, et al. [Orchitis]. *Urologe A.* 2019;58(6):697–710. German.
120. Azmat CE, Vaitla P. Orchitis. In: *StatPearls.* Treasure Island, FL: StatPearls Publishing; 2021. Last update November 11, 2021. Available at https://www.ncbi.nlm.nih.gov/books/NBK553165/. (Accessed February 22, 2022).
121. Krieger JN. Epididymitis, orchitis, and related conditions. *Sex Transm Dis.* 1984;11(3):173–181.
122. Hahné S. Mumps vaccine effectiveness against orchitis. *Emerg Infect Dis.* 2012;18(1):191–193.
123. Kanda T, et al. Case of mumps orchitis after vaccination. *Int J Urol.* 2014;21(4):426–428.
124. Howlader N, et al, eds. *SEER Cancer Statistics Review (CSR) 1975-2018.* Bethesda, MD: National Cancer Institute; 2021. Released April 15, 2021. Available at https://seer.cancer.gov/csr/1975_2018/. (Accessed February 22, 2022).
125. Ghazarian AA, et al. Future of testicular germ cell tumor incidence in the United States: forecast through 2026. *Cancer.* 2017;123(12):2320–2328.
126. Berney DM, et al. Germ cell neoplasia in situ (GCNIS): evolution of the current nomenclature for testicular pre-invasive germ cell malignancy. *Histopathology.* 2016;69(1):7–10.
127. Sung H, et al. Global cancer statistics 2020: GLOBOCAN estimates of incidence and mortality worldwide for 36 cancers in 185 countries. *CA Cancer J Clin.* 2021;71(3):209–249.
128. Park JS, et al. Recent global trends in testicular cancer incidence and mortality. *Medicine (Baltimore).* 2018;97(37):e12390.
129. Skakkebaek NE, Meyts ER, Main KM. Testicular dysgenesis syndrome: an increasingly common developmental disorder with environmental aspects. *Hum Reprod.* 2001;16(5):972–978.
130. Hemminki K, Li X. Cancer risks in Nordic immigrants and their offspring in Sweden. *Eur J Cancer.* 2002;38(18):2428–2434.
131. Giannandrea F, Fargnoli S. Environmental factors affecting growth and occurrence of testicular cancer in childhood: an overview of the current epidemiological evidence. *Children (Basel).* 2017;4(1):1.
132. Skakkebaek NE, et al. Male reproductive disorders and fertility trends: influences of environment and genetic susceptibility. *Physiol Rev.* 2016;96:55–97.
133. Gaddam SJ, Chesnut GT. *Testicle cancer.* In: StatPearls. Treasure Island, FL: StatPearls Publishing; 2021. Last update November 7, 2021. Available at https://www.ncbi.nlm.nih.gov/books/NBK563159/. (Accessed February 22, 2022).
134. Moch H, et al. The 2016 WHO classification of tumours of the urinary system and male genital organs-part a: renal, penile, and testicular tumours. *Eur Urol.* 2016;70(1):93–105.
135. Humphrey PA, et al. The 2016 WHO classification of tumours of the urinary system and male genital organs-part b: prostate and bladder tumours. *Eur Urol.* 2016;70(1):106–119.
136. Chieffi P, Chieffi S. Molecular biomarkers as potential targets for therapeutic strategies in human testicular germ cell tumors: an overview. *J Cell Physiol.* 2013;228(8):1641–1646.
137. Rajpert-De Meyts E. Developmental model for the pathogenesis of testicular carcinoma in situ: genetic and environmental aspects. *Hum Reprod Update.* 2006;12(3):303–323.

138. Sperger JM, et al. Gene expression patterns in human embryonic stem cells and human pluripotent germ cell tumors. *Proc Natl Acad Sci U S A*. 2003;100(23):13350–13355.
139. Almstrup K, et al. Genome-wide gene expression profiling of testicular carcinoma in situ progression into overt tumours. *Br J Cancer*. 2005;92(10):1934–1941.
140. Baroni T, et al. On the origin of testicular germ cell tumors: from gonocytes to testicular cancer. *Front Endocrinol (Lausanne)*. 2019;10:343.
141. Garolla A, De Giorgi U, Milardi D. Editorial: Testicular cancer: new insights on the origin, genetics, treatment, fertility, general health, quality of life and sexual function. *Front Endocrinol (Lausanne)*. 2020;11:41.
142. Koul S, et al. Characteristic promoter hypermethylation signatures in male germ cell tumors. *Mol Cancer*. 2002;1:8.
143. Stephenson A, et al. Diagnosis and treatment of early stage testicular cancer: AUA Guideline. *J Urol*. 2019;202(2):272–281.
144. Gilligan T, et al. Testicular cancer, version 2.2020, NCCN Clinical Practice Guidelines in Oncology. *J Natl Compr Canc Netw*. 2019;17(12):1529–1554.
145. Wood L, et al. Canadian consensus guidelines for the management of testicular germ cell cancer. *Can Urol Assoc J*. 2010;4(2):e19–e38.
146. Kreydin EI, et al. Testicular cancer: what the radiologist needs to know. *AJR Am J Roentgenol*. 2013;200(6):1215–1225.
147. Rupp TJ, Leslie SW. Epididymitis. In: *StatPearls*. Treasure Island, FL: StatPearls Publishing; 2021. Last update August 12, 2021. Available at https://www.ncbi.nlm.nih.gov/books/NBK430814/. (Accessed February 22, 2022).
148. Liu W, Li YY, Shang XJ. [Mycoplasma genitalium and male urogenital diseases: an update]. *Zhonghua Nan Ke Xue*. 2018;24(7):645–650. Chinese.
149. Bodie M, et al. Addressing the rising rates of gonorrhea and drug-resistant gonorrhea: there is no time like the present. *Can Commun Dis Rep*. 2019;45(2–3):54–62.
150. Yamamichi F, et al. What are the differences between older and younger patients with epididymitis? *Investig Clin Urol*. 2017;58(3):205–209.
151. Janier M, et al. la section MST de la SFD: [Epididymo-orchitis]. *Ann Dermatol Venereol*. 2016;143(11):765–766.
152. Ng M, Baradhi M. Benign prostatic hyperplasia. In: *StatPearls*. Treasure Island, FL: StatPearls Publishing; 2021. Last update August 11, 2021. Available at https://www.ncbi.nlm.nih.gov/books/NBK558920/. (Accessed February 22, 2022).
153. Abrams P. New words for old: lower urinary tract symptoms for "prostatism". *BMJ*. 1994;308(6934):929–930.
154. Chughtai B, et al. Benign prostatic hyperplasia. *Nat Rev Dis Primers*. 2016;2:16031.
155. Gacci M, et al. Metabolic syndrome and benign prostatic enlargement: a systematic review and meta-analysis. *BJU Int*. 2015;115(1):24–31.
156. Rohrmann S, et al. Association between markers of the metabolic syndrome and lower urinary tract symptoms in the Third National Health and Nutrition Examination Survey (NHANES III). *Int J Obes (Lond)*. 2005;29(3):310–316.
157. Kristal AR, et al. Race/ethnicity, obesity, health related behaviors and the risk of symptomatic benign prostatic hyperplasia: results from the prostate cancer prevention trial. *J Urol*. 2007;177(4):1395–1400. quiz 1591.
158. Parsons JK, et al. Metabolic factors associated with benign prostatic hyperplasia. *J Clin Endocrinol Metab*. 2006;91(7):2562–2568.
159. Furukawa S, et al. Increased oxidative stress in obesity and its impact on metabolic syndrome. *J Clin Invest*. 2004;114(12):1752–1761.
160. De Nunzio C, et al. The correlation between metabolic syndrome and prostatic diseases. *Eur Urol*. 2012;61(3):560–570.
161. Kumar V, Abbas A, Aster J. *Robbins & Cotran Pathologic Basis of Disease*. ed 10 : Elsevier; 2021.
162. Gandaglia G, et al. The role of prostatic inflammation in the development and progression of benign and malignant diseases. *Curr Opin Urol*. 2016;27(2):99–106.
163. Nicholson TTM, Ricke WA. Androgens and estrogens in benign prostatic hyperplasia: past, present and future. *Differentiation*. 2011;82(4–5):184–199.
164. Wynder JL, et al. Estrogens and male lower urinary tract dysfunction. *Curr Urol Rep*. 2015;16(9):61.
165. Kramer G, Mitteregger D, Marberger M. Is benign prostatic hyperplasia (BPH) an immune inflammatory disease? *Eur Urol*. 2007;51(5):1202–1216.
166. Kramer G. Increased expression of lymphocyte-derived cytokines in benign hyperplastic prostate tissue, identification of the producing cell types, and effect of differentially expressed cytokines on stromal cell proliferation. *Prostate*. 2002;52(1):43–58.
167. Steiner GE, et al. cytokine expression pattern in benign prostatic hyperplasia infiltrating T cells and impact of lymphocytic infiltration on cytokine mRNA profile in prostatic tissue. *Lab Invest*. 2003;83:1131–1146.
168. Chughtai B, et al. Inflammation and benign prostatic hyperplasia: clinical implications. *Curr Urol Rep*. 2011;12:274–277.
169. Wang W, Bergh A, Damber J-E. Chronic Inflammation in benign prostate hyperplasia is associated with focal upregulation of cyclooxygenase-2, Bcl-2, and cell proliferation in the glandular epithelium. *Prostate*. 2004;61(1):60–72.
170. Bachmann A, de la Rosette J, eds. *Benign Prostatic Hyperplasia and Lower Urinary Tract Symptoms in Men*. New York: Oxford University Press; 2012. Available at https://oxfordmedicine.com/view/10.1093/med/9780199572779.001.0001/med-9780199572779. (Accessed February 22, 2022).
171. Barry MJ, et al. Measurement Committee of the American Urological Association. The American Urological Association symptom index for benign prostatic hyperplasia. *J Urol*. 2017;197(2S):S189–S197.
172. Roehrborn CG, et al. The effects of combination therapy with dutasteride and tamsulosin on clinical outcomes in men with symptomatic benign prostatic hyperplasia: 4-year results from the CombAT study. *Eur Urol*. 2010;57(1):123–131.
173. Regadas RP, et al. Urodynamic effects of the combination of tamsulosin and daily tadalafil in men with lower urinary tract symptoms secondary to benign prostatic hyperplasia: a randomized, placebo-controlled clinical trial. *Int Urol Nephrol*. 2013;45(1):39–43.
174. de la Rosette JJ, et al. European Association of Urology. EAU Guidelines on benign prostatic hyperplasia (BPH). *Eur Urol*. 2001;40(3):256–263. discussion 264.
175. Davis NG, Silberman M. *Bacterial acute prostatitis. StatPearls*. Treasure Island, FL: StatPearls Publishing; 2021. Last update October 7, 2021. Available at https://www.ncbi.nlm.nih.gov/books/NBK459257/. (Accessed February 22, 2022).
176. Carroll DE, et al. *Staphylococcus aureus* prostatic abscess: a clinical case report and a review of the literature. *BMC Infect Dis*. 2017;17(1):509.
177. Lee DS, et al. Acute bacterial prostatitis and abscess formation. *BMC Urol*. 2016;16(1):38.

178. Kim SJ, et al. Risk factors for acute prostatitis after transrectal biopsy of the prostate. *Korean J Urol.* 2010;51(6):426–430.
179. Campeggi A, et al. Acute bacterial prostatitis after transrectal ultrasound-guided prostate biopsy: epidemiological, bacteria and treatment patterns from a 4-year prospective study. *Int J Urol.* 2014;21(2):152–155.
180. Mouraviev V, McDonald M. An implementation of next generation sequencing for prevention and diagnosis of urinary tract infection in urology. *Can J Urol.* 2018;25(3):9349–9356.
181. Lee Y, et al. Risk factor analysis of ciprofloxacin-resistant and extended spectrum beta-lactamases pathogen-induced acute bacterial prostatitis in Korea. *J Korean Med Sci.* 2016;31(11):1808–1813.
182. Khan FU, et al. Comprehensive overview of prostatitis. *Biomed Pharmacother.* 2017;94:1064–1076.
183. Gill BC, Shoskes DA. Bacterial prostatitis. *Curr Opin Infect Dis.* 2016;29(1):86–91.
184. Yoon BI, et al. Acute bacterial prostatitis: how to prevent and manage chronic infection? *J Infect Chemother.* 2012;18(4):444–450.
185. Zhang J, et al. Chronic prostatitis/chronic pelvic pain syndrome: a disease or symptom? Current perspectives on diagnosis, treatment, and prognosis. *Am J Mens Health.* 2020;14(1). 1557988320903200, Available at https://doi.org/10.1177/1557988320903200. (Accessed February 22, 2022).
186. Shoskes DA, Nickel JC, Kattan MW. Phenotypically directed multimodal therapy for chronic prostatitis/chronic pelvic pain syndrome: a prospective study using UPOINT. *Urology.* 2010;75(6):1249–1253.
187. Doggweiler R, et al. A standard for terminology in chronic pelvic pain syndromes: a report from the chronic pelvic pain working group of the International Continence Society. *Neurourol Urodyn.* 2017;36(4):984–1008.
188. Hao ZY, et al. The prevalence of erectile dysfunction and its relation to chronic prostatitis in Chinese men. *J Androl.* 2011;32(5):496–501.
189. Li HJ, Kang DY. Prevalence of sexual dysfunction in men with chronic prostatitis/chronic pelvic pain syndrome: a meta-analysis. *World J Urol.* 2016;34(7):1009–1017.
190. Li HJ, et al. [Investigation of chronic prostatitis and altered bowel habits]. *Zhonghua Nan Ke Xue.* 2002;8(5):338–340. Chinese.
191. Lotti F, et al. The association between varicocele, premature ejaculation and prostatitis symptoms: possible mechanisms. *J Sex Med.* 2009;6(10):2878–2887.
192. Pavone C, et al. Correlation between chronic prostatitis syndrome and pelvic venous disease: a survey of 2,554 urologic outpatients. *Eur Urol.* 2000;37(4):400–403.
193. Vicari E, et al. High frequency of chronic bacterial and non-inflammatory prostatitis in infertile patients with prostatitis syndrome plus irritable bowel syndrome. *PLoS One.* 2011;6(4):e18647.
194. Pena VN, et al. Diagnostic and management strategies for patients with chronic prostatitis and chronic pelvic pain syndrome. *Drugs Aging.* 2021;38:845–886.
195. Global Cancer Observatory (GLOBOCAN) *International Agency for Research on Cancer.* : World Health Organization; 2021. Available at https://gco.iarc.fr/today/data/factsheets/populations/900-world-fact-sheets.pdf. (Accessed February 22, 2022).
196. Bray F, et al. Global cancer statistics 2018: GLOBOCAN estimates of incidence and mortality worldwide for 36 cancers in 185 countries. *CA Cancer J Clin.* 2018;68(6):394–424.
197. Wong MCS, et al. Global incidence and mortality for prostate cancer: analysis of temporal patterns and trends in 36 countries. *Eur Urol.* 2016;70(5):862–874.
198. Rebello RJ, et al. Prostate cancer. *Nat Rev Dis Primers.* 2021;7:9.
199. American Cancer Society (ACS): *Cancer facts & figures 2021*, Atlanta, GA, 2019, ACS. Available at https://www.cancer.org/content/dam/cancer-org/research/cancer-facts-and-statistics/annual-cancer-facts-and-figures/2021/cancer-facts-and-figures-2021.pdf. (Accessed February 22, 2022).
200. Schröder FH, et al. Screening and prostate cancer mortality: results of the European randomized study of screening for prostate cancer (ERSPC) at 13 years of follow-up. *Lancet.* 2014;384(9959):2027–2035.
201. Hugosson J, et al. A 16-yr follow-up of the European randomized study of screening for prostate cancer. *Eur Urol.* 2019;76(1):43–51.
202. Leslie SW, et al. Prostate cancer. In: *StatPearls.* Treasure Island, FL: StatPearls Publishing; 2021. Last update September 17, 2021. Available at https://www.ncbi.nlm.nih.gov/books/NBK470550/. (Accessed February 22, 2022).
203. Gann PH. Risk factors for prostate cancer. *Rev Urol.* 2002;4(Suppl 5):S3–S10.
204. Kaiser A, et al. The evolving role of diet in prostate cancer risk and progression. *Curr Opin Oncol.* 2019;31(3):222–229.
205. Lin PH, Aronson W, Freedland SJ. Nutrition, dietary interventions and prostate cancer: the latest evidence. *BMC Med.* 2015;13:3.
206. Mullins JK, Loeb S. Environmental exposures and prostate cancer. *Urol Oncol.* 2012;30(2):216–219.
207. Klap J, Schmid M, Loughlin KR. The relationship between total testosterone levels and prostate cancer: a review of the continuing controversy. *J Urol.* 2015;193(2):403–413.
208. Bruner DW, et al. Relative risk of prostate cancer for men with affected relatives: systematic review and meta-analysis. *Int J Cancer.* 2003;107(5):797–803.
209. Baca SC, et al. Punctuated evolution of prostate cancer genomes. *Cell.* 2013;153:666–677.
210. Hieronymus H, et al. Copy number alteration burden predicts prostate cancer relapse. *Proc Natl Acad Sci U S A.* 2014;111(30):11139–11144.
211. Lavalette C, et al. Abdominal obesity and prostate cancer risk: epidemiological evidence from the EPICAP study. *Oncotarget.* 2018;9(77):34485–34494.
212. Renehan AG, et al. Body-mass index and incidence of cancer: a systematic review and meta-analysis of prospective observational studies. *Lancet.* 2008;371:569–578.
213. Bergström A, et al. Overweight as an avoidable cause of cancer in Europe. *Int J Cancer.* 2001;91:421–430.
214. Discacciati A, Orsini N, Wolk A. Body mass index and incidence of localized and advanced prostate cancer—a dose-response meta-analysis of prospective studies. *Ann Oncol.* 2012;23:1665–1671.
215. MacInnis RJ, English DR. Body size and composition and prostate cancer risk: systematic review and meta-regression analysis. *Cancer Causes Control.* 2006;17:989–1003.
216. Harding JL, et al. Comparison of anthropometric measures as predictors of cancer incidence: a pooled collaborative analysis of 11 Australian cohorts. *Int J Cancer.* 2015;137:1699–1708.
217. Kruk J, Czerniak U. Physical activity and its relation to cancer risk: updating the evidence. *Asian Pac J Cancer Prev.* 2013;14:3993–4003.
218. Giovannucci E, Michaud D. The role of obesity and related metabolic disturbances in cancers of the colon, prostate, and pancreas. *Gastroenterology.* 2007;132:2208–2225.

219. World Cancer Research Fund, American Institute for Cancer Research: Continuous update project expert report; 2018. Available at https://www.wcrf.org/wp-content/uploads/2021/02/prostate-cancer-report.pdf. (Accessed February 22, 2022).
220. Cao Y, et al. Prediagnostic plasma IGFBP-1, IGF-1 and risk of prostate cancer. *Int J Cancer*. 2015;136:2418–2426.
221. Roddam AW, et al. Insulin-like growth factors, their binding proteins, and prostate cancer risk: analysis of individual patient data from 12 prospective studies. *Ann Intern Med*. 2008;149:461–471. W83–W88.
222. Nandeesha H. Insulin: a novel agent in the pathogenesis of prostate cancer. *Int Urol Nephrol*. 2009;41:267–272.
223. Balkwill F, Mantovani A. Inflammation and cancer: back to Virchow? *Lancet*. 2001;357(9255):539–545.
224. Coussens LM, Werb Z. Inflammation and cancer. *Nature*. 2002;420:860–867.
225. De Marzo AM, et al. Proliferative inflammatory atrophy of the prostate: implications for prostatic carcinogenesis. *Am J Pathol*. 1999;155(6):1985–1992.
226. De Marzo AM, et al. Inflammation in prostate carcinogenesis. *Nat Rev Cancer*. 2007;7:256–269.
227. Mantovani A, et al. Cancer-related inflammation. *Nature*. 2008;454:436–444.
228. Thapa D, Ghosh R. Chronic inflammatory mediators enhance prostate cancer development and progression. *Biochem Pharmacol*. 2015;94:53–62.
229. Kimura T, et al. Epidemiology of prostate cancer in Asian countries. *Int J Urol*. 2018;25(6):524–531.
230. Kirchhoff T, et al. BRCA mutations and risk of prostate cancer in Ashkenazi Jews. *Clin Cancer Res*. 2004;10(9):2918–2921.
231. Karlsson R, et al. A population-based assessment of germline *HOXB13* G84E mutation and prostate cancer risk. *Eur Urol*. 2014;65(1):169–176.
232. Lin CY, et al. Purification and characterization of a complex containing matriptase and a Kunitz-type serine protease inhibitor from human milk. *J Biol Chem*. 1999;274:18237–18242.
233. Ko CJ, et al. Androgen-induced TMPRSS2 activates matriptase and promotes extracellular matrix degradation, prostate cancer cell invasion, tumor growth, and metastasis. *Cancer Res*. 2015;75:2949–2960.
234. Simoes GF, et al. An overview on prostate pathophysiology: new insights into prostate cancer clinical diagnosis. In: Gaze D, ed. *Pathophysiology - Altered Physiological States*. London: IntechOpen; 2018. Available at https://www.intechopen.com/chapters/59625. (Accessed February 22, 2022).
235. Feldman BJ, Feldman D. The development of androgen-independent prostate cancer. *Nat Rev Cancer*. 2001;1(1):34–45.
236. Li SC, et al. Altered expression of extracellular matrix and proteinases in Noble rat prostate gland after long-term treatment with sex steroids. *Prostate*. 2001;49:58–71.
237. Li LC. Frequent methylation of estrogen receptor in prostate cancer: correlation with tumor progression. *Cancer Res*. 2000;3:702–706.
238. Simpson E, et al. Local estrogen biosynthesis in males and females. *Endocr Relat Cancer*. 1999;6(2):131–137.
239. Tsugaya M, et al. Aromatase mRNA levels in benign prostatic hyperplasia and prostate cancer. *Int J Urol*. 1996;3(4):292–296.
240. Mishra S, et al. Estrogen and estrogen receptor alpha promotes malignancy and osteoblastic tumorigenesis in prostate cancer. *Oncotarget*. 2015;6(42):44388–44402.
241. Dobbs RW, et al. Estrogens and prostate cancer. *Prostate Cancer Prostatic Dis*. 2019;22:185–194.
242. Levakov AF, et al. The expression and localization of estrogen receptor beta in hyperplastic and neoplastic prostate lesions. *Vojnosanit Pregl*. 2015;72(10):906–913.
243. Rago V, et al. Identification of the G-protein-coupled estrogen receptor (GPER) in human prostate: expression site of the estrogen receptor in the benign and neoplastic gland. *Andrology*. 2016;4(1):121–127.
244. Ellem SJ, Risberger GP. Aromatase and regulating the estrogen: androgen ratio in the prostate gland. *J Steroid Biochem Mol Biol*. 2010;118(4–5):246–251.
245. Bosland MC. Sex steroids and prostate carcinogenesis: integrated, multifactorial working hypothesis. *Ann N Y Acad Sci*. 2006;1089:168–176.
246. Tewari AK, et al. Inflammation and prostate cancer. *Adv Exp Med Biol*. 2018;1095:41–65.
247. Taverna G, et al. Inflammation and prostate cancer: friends or foe? *Inflamm Res*. 2015;64(5):275–286.
248. Zhou M. High-grade prostatic intraepithelial neoplasia, PIN-like carcinoma, and intraductal carcinoma of the prostate. *Mod Pathol*. 2018;31:71–79.
249. Montico F, et al. Reactive stroma in the prostate during late life: the role of microvasculature and antiangiogenic therapy influences. *Prostate*. 2015;75(14):1643–1661.
250. Tuxhorn JA, et al. Reactive stroma in human prostate cancer: induction of myofibroblast phenotype and extracelluar matrix remodelling. *ClinCancer Res*. 2002;8(9):2912–2923.
251. Krušlin B, Ulamec M, Tomas D. Prostate cancer stroma: an important factor in cancer growth and progression. *Bosn J Basic Med Sci*. 2015;15(2):1–8.
252. Yadavalli S, et al. Data-driven discovery of extravasation pathway in circulating tumor cells. *Sci Rep*. 2017;7:43710.
253. Friedlander TW, Premasekharan G, Paris PL. Looking back, to the future of circulating tumor cells. *Pharmacol Ther*. 2014;142(3):271–280.
254. PDQ Screening and Prevention Editorial Board. *PDQ® Prostate Cancer Screening—Health Professional Version*. Bethesda, MD: National Cancer Institute; 2021. Available at https://www.cancer.gov/types/prostate/hp/prostate-screening-pdq. (Accessed February 22, 2022).
255. U.S. Preventive Services Task Force (US PSTF). Screening for prostate cancer: U. S. Preventive Services Task Force recommendation statement. *JAMA*. 2018;319:1901–1913.
256. Fitzpatrick JM, Banu E, Oudard S. Prostate-specific antigen kinetics in localized and advanced prostate cancer. *BJU Int*. 2009;103(5):578–587.
257. National Cancer Institute (NCI), Surveillance Research Program (SRP) *Cancer Stat Facts: Prostate Cancer*. Bethesda, MD: Division of Cancer Control and Population Sciences, Surveillance, Epidemiology, and End Results Program (SEER); 2021. Available at https://seer.cancer.gov/statfacts/html/prost.html. (Accessed February 22, 2022).
258. Chen L, et al. Male sexual dysfunction: a review of literature on its pathological mechanisms, potential risk factors, and herbal drug intervention. *Biomed Pharmacother*. 2019;112:108585.
259. Aversa A, et al. Phosphodiesterase 5 inhibitors in the treatment of erectile dysfunction. *Curr Pharm Des*. 2006;12(27):3467–3484.
260. Feldman HA, et al. Impotence and its medical and psychosocial correlates: results of the Massachusetts Male Aging Study. *J Urol*. 1994;151(1):54–61.
261. Sooriyamoorthy T, Leslie SW. Erectile dysfunction. In: *StatPearls*. Treasure Island, FL: StatPearls Publishing; 2021. Last update August 12, 2021. Available at https://www.ncbi.nlm.nih.gov/books/NBK562253/. (Accessed February 22, 2022).

262. Tan HM, Tong SF, Ho CC. Men's health: sexual dysfunction, physical, and psychological health—is there a link? *J Sex Med.* 2012;9(3):663–671.
263. Karabakan M, et al. Significance of serum endothelial cell specific molecule-1 (Endocan) level in patients with erectile dysfunction: a pilot study. *Int J Impot Res.* 2017;29(4):175–178.
264. Aversa A, et al. Endothelial dysfunction and erectile dysfunction in the aging man. *Int J Urol.* 2010;17(1):38.
265. Ryan JG, Gajraj J. Erectile dysfunction and its association with metabolic syndrome and endothelial function among patients with type 2 diabetes mellitus. *J Diabetes Complicat.* 2012;26(2):141.
266. Neijenhuijs KI, et al. The International Index of Erectile Function (IIEF)—a systematic review of measurement properties. *J Sex Med.* 2019;16(7):1078–1091.
267. Rhim HC, et al. The potential role of arginine supplements on erectile dysfunction: a systemic review and meta-analysis. *J Sex Med.* 2019;16(2):223–234.
268. Goldstein I, Tseng LJ. Efficacy and safety of sildenafil by age in men with erectile dysfunction. *J Sex Med.* 2016;13(5):852–859.
269. Snyder PJ, et al. Testosterone Trials Investigators: Effects of testosterone treatment in older men. *N Engl J Med.* 2016;374(7):611–624.
270. Brock G, et al. Effect of testosterone solution 2% on testosterone concentration, sex drive and energy in hypogonadal men: results of a placebo controlled study. *J Urol.* 2016;195(3):699–705.
271. Linet OI, Ogrinc FG. Efficacy and safety of intracavernosal alprostadil in men with erectile dysfunction. The Alprostadil Study Group. *N Engl J Med.* 1996;334(14):873.
272. Molodysky E, et al. Penile vascular surgery for treating erectile dysfunction: current role and future direction. *Arab J Urol.* 2013;11(3):254–266.
273. Vandeven HA, Pensler JM. Gynecomastia. In: *StatPearls.* Treasure Island, FL: StatPearls Publishing; 2021. Last update August 13, 2021. Available at https://www.ncbi.nlm.nih.gov/books/NBK430812/. (Accessed February 22, 2022).
274. Jin Y, Fan M. Treatment of gynecomastia with prednisone: case report and literature review. *J Int Med Res.* 2019;47(5): 2288–2295.
275. Guilmette J, Nosé V. Paraneoplastic syndromes and other systemic disorders associated with neuroendocrine neoplasms. *Semin Diagn Pathol.* 2019;36(4):229–239.
276. Reisenbichler E, Hanley KZ. Developmental disorders and malformations of the breast. *Semin Diagn Pathol.* 2019;36(1): 11–15.
277. Sollie M. Management of gynecomastia-changes in psychological aspects after surgery-a systematic review. *Gland Surg.* 2018;7(Suppl 1):S70–S76.
278. Chesebro AL, Rives AF, Shaffer K. Male breast disease: what the radiologist needs to know. *Curr Probl Diagn Radiol.* 2019;48(5):482–493.
279. Ferzoco RM, Ruddy KJL. The epidemiology of male breast cancer. *Curr Oncol Rep.* 2016;18(1):1.
280. Deb S, et al. The cancer genetics and pathology of male breast cancer. *Histopathology.* 2016;68(1):110–118.

27

Sexually Transmitted Infections

William E. Somerall, Jr.

http://evolve.elsevier.com/Rogers/pathophysiology/

CHAPTER OUTLINE

Newly acquired sexually contracted infections affect more than 26 million Americans per year, and half of those individuals are younger than 25 years of age (Box 27.1).[1–4] **Sexually transmitted infections (STIs)** are called the hidden epidemic by the Centers for Disease Control and Prevention (CDC).[1] They account for nearly $16 billion in healthcare costs in the United States.[5] STIs are so prevalent yet rarely discussed. Complications of STIs include short- and long-term morbidity, which can affect physical, emotional, and financial well-being, and even mortality.[5]

In the past, an infection transmitted through sexual intercourse was called a *venereal disease*. However, the term venereal disease has been replaced with STI. STIs are contracted by genital contact or through contact with infected blood or body fluids. Infections can be transmitted directly through touch, or the infectious agent can be transmitted by an object, known as a **fomite**. STIs such as **syphilis, gonorrhea, chlamydia**, hepatitis, and human immunodeficiency virus (HIV) also can be transmitted from mother to child during pregnancy and birth, a process known as **vertical transmission**.

Many infected individuals are not screened for STIs because symptoms are absent, minor, or transient, or because health services are inaccessible, unaffordable, or culturally insensitive. When individuals do not know they have an STI, they often fail to prevent transmission to others. With adequate screening and early treatment and education, the prevalence and sequelae of STIs can be greatly reduced.

Behaviors are the greatest risk factor for STI acquisition. Individuals who have unprotected intercourse or genital/oral contact, especially with non-monogamous or multiple partners, are at the greatest risk. Certain populations as defined by age, behaviors, geographic location, traits, or race/ethnicity have a higher incidence of STIs. This increase is usually a result of increased risky behaviors by individuals in this group, but it can also be due to physical or cultural characteristics that contribute to transmission. For example, rates of gonorrhea, chlamydia, vaginitis, cervical condyloma, genital warts, and pelvic inflammatory disease (PID) are highest in adolescents and decline exponentially with increasing age (Fig. 27.1). Adolescents more often engage in risky behaviors and have a greater number of sexual partners than older adults. Individuals entering correctional facilities, such as jails, also have higher rates of STI prevalence related to their risky behaviors before incarceration.[1]

Some populations are at greater risk because of the pathophysiology of STI transmission. Transmission of many STIs is enhanced when the infectious agent contacts mucous membranes, such as the mouth, oropharynx, vagina, rectum, and the inner foreskin, which provide a more favorable environment for transmission than skin. Therefore women, uncircumcised men, and men who are the receptive partner in oral or anal sex are at increased risk.[1] In addition, prolonged contact with infectious body fluids also increases transmission, which occurs when semen is deposited in the vagina or rectum. Young women also are at greater risk for STI acquisition when compared with older women, which is related to the position of susceptible cells on the surface of their cervix.

STI transmission is enhanced when the infectious agent has contact with broken skin or blood vessels. Sexual contact that is damaging to the genitals increases STI acquisition. This is the case with penile-rectal penetration, as well as forced genital contact. Broken or friable skin caused by genital infections or trauma also can increase the risk of STI transmission. As a result, if an individual has one STI, susceptibility increases when exposed to other STIs.

Race and ethnicity are not direct factors in STI acquisition. STIs are prevalent in all socioeconomic and racial/ethnic groups. Publicly available data suggest a greater prevalence in minority groups or among people with low socioeconomic status, which may reflect greater STI reporting from public clinics that serve marginalized groups when compared with private providers who are not required to report all infections to authorities. Race and ethnicity alone do not alter STI risk but rather act as risk markers that correlate with other more fundamental determinants of health status, such as (1) poverty, (2) access to quality care, and (3) health-seeking behavior. In some geographic areas, racial, ethnic, or socioeconomic groups may be more or less likely to engage in at-risk behaviors such as intravenous (IV) drug use and

BOX 27.1 Sexually Transmitted Infection Statistical Summary from 2019 Centers for Disease Control and Prevention Report

Each year in the United States:

- 20 million individuals contract a sexually transmitted infection.
- $16 billion is spent on sexually transmitted infection (STIs), not including long-term healthcare costs.
- Only half of people who need STI screening receive needed services.

Chlamydia cases:

- 1.8 million cases were reported a 19% increase since 2015.

Gonorrhea cases:

- 616,392 cases were reported in 2019, a 56% increase since 2015.
- Increasing antibiotic resistance means that gonorrhea may soon become resistant to all known treatments.

Syphilis cases:

- There was a 74% overall increase in cases reported since 2015.
- The syphilis rate is highest among men who have sex with men.

Viral STIs affect more than 70 million people in the United States:

- The use of the human papillomavirus (HPV) vaccine has demonstrated positive effects on the rates of HPV acquisition in the United States.
- 26 billion STIs in 2018 with almost half of new STIs among youth aged 15-24 in the United States.
- There are 18.6 million individuals living with herpes simplex-2.

Data from Centers for Disease Control and Prevention (CDC). *Sexually Transmitted Disease 2022.* Washington, DC: U.S. Department of Health and Human Services; 2022. https://www.cdc.gov/std/default.htm.

unprotected sex. Healthcare providers should provide risk-appropriate screening based on behaviors and physiologic risk factors without racial profiling. To assist clinicians, the CDC regularly publishes a comprehensive guideline detailing STI screening, evaluation, and treatment that specifies current at-risk groups. This guide and its corresponding smartphone app are the best sources of current information on STI screening and treatment because this area of clinical care changes rapidly.

An STI can be caused by bacteria, viruses, protozoa, parasites, or fungi (Table 27.1). Transmission rates and prevalence depend on the characteristics of the pathogen and complex factors associated with behavioral and societal factors. Bacterial, protozoan, parasitic, and fungal STIs can be successfully treated once diagnosed, but viral STIs cannot be cured by pharmacologic means alone and, depending on the virus, affected individuals have the potential to carry or transmit the virus throughout their life.

Treatment or symptom management of STIs depends on the causative pathogen. Treatments change frequently based on drug resistance and availability of medications. The treatment is personalized based on the individual's medical needs and personal preferences. Treatment of the individual and his or her sexual partner(s) is often complicated by inadequate access to medical care, drug cost, and privacy concerns.[1] Many states have enacted legislation to allow sexual partners to be treated without having to go to a clinic for an examination and prescription.[6,7] This practice is recommended and supported by many health organizations.[8,9]

Prevention of STIs involves a multifaceted approach. This includes encouraging behavioral changes such as decreasing the number of sexual partners or using condoms to decrease transmission. Preexposure prophylaxis (PrEP), including vaccines for hepatitis and **human papillomavirus (HPV)**, has been used to protect populations against viral STIs before exposure.[10] Medications also may be used to prevent acquisition of STIs as PrEP (e.g., emtricitabine/tenofovir) and postexposure prophylaxis (PEP), especially in the prevention of HIV.[10] Early treatment of STIs prevents transmission to new hosts and decreases the risk of additional STIs. Testing and treatment are especially helpful in preventing vertical transmission.

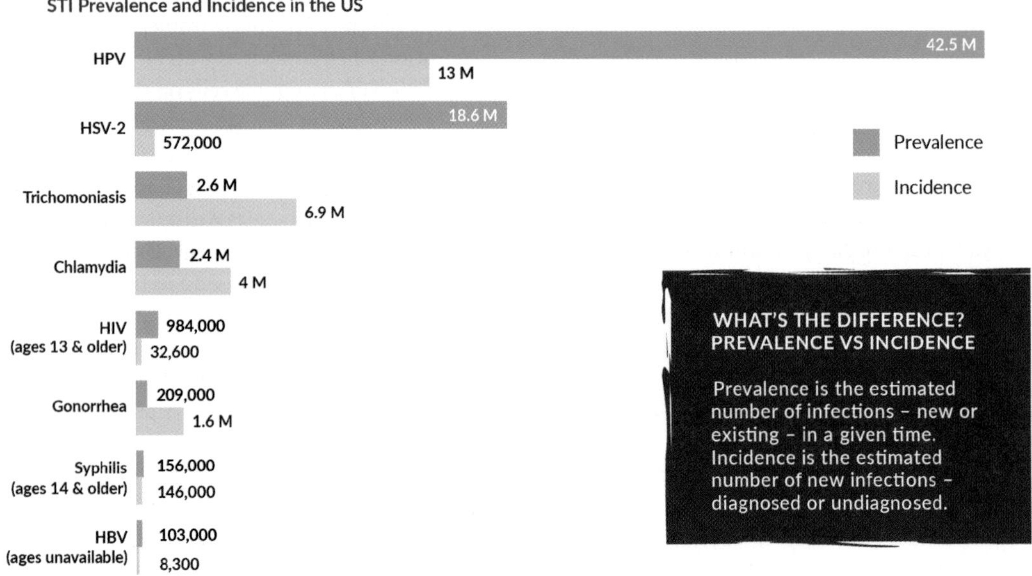

Fig. 27.1 Prevalence and Incidence of Sexually Transmitted Infections. (From Centers for Disease Control and Prevention [CDC]. *CDC Prevention Infographics; Division of STD Prevention, National Center for HIV, Viral Hepatitis, STD, and TB Prevention, Centers for Disease Control and Prevention, page last reviewed;* 2022. http://www.cdc.gov/std/products/infographics.htm.)

TABLE 27.1 Currently Recognized Sexually Transmitted Infections

Causal Microorganism	Infection
Bacteria	
Campylobacter	Campylobacter enteritis
Calymmatobacterium granulomatis	Granuloma inguinale
Chlamydia trachomatis	Urogenital infections; lymphogranuloma venereum
Polymicrobial	
Gardnerella vaginalis interaction with anaerobes *(Bacteroides and Mobiluncus* spp.) and genital mycoplasmas	Bacterial vaginosis
Haemophilus ducreyi	Chancroid
Mycoplasma	Mycoplasmosis
Neisseria gonorrhoeae	Gonorrhea
Shigella	Shigellosis
Treponema pallidum	Syphilis
Viruses	
Cytomegalovirus	Cytomegalic inclusion disease
Hepatitis B virus (HBV)	Hepatitis
Hepatitis C virus (HCV)	Hepatitis
Herpes simplex virus (HSV)	Genital herpes
Human immunodeficiency virus (HIV)	Acquired immunodeficiency syndrome (AIDS)
Human papillomavirus (HPV)	Condylomata acuminata, cervical dysplasia, and cervical cancer
Molluscum contagiosum virus	Molluscum contagiosum
Zika virus	Zika virus disease
Protozoa	
Entamoeba histolytica	Amebiasis; amebic dysentery
Giardia lamblia	Giardiasis
Trichomonas vaginalis	Trichomoniasis
Ectoparasites	
Pthirus pubis	Pediculosis pubis
Sarcoptes scabiei	Scabies
Fungus	
Candida albicans	Candidiasis

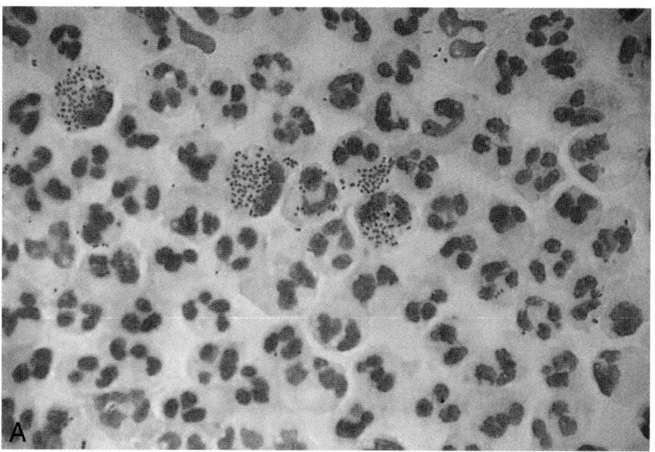

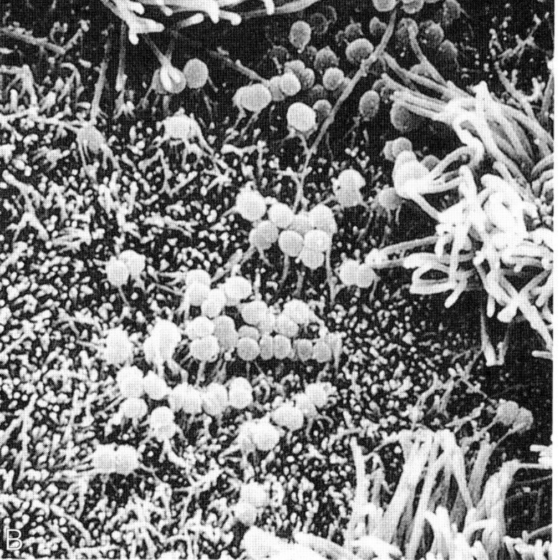

Fig. 27.2 **(A)** A Gram stain picture of *Neisseria gonorrhoeae.* (From Goldman L, Schafer AI. *Goldman-Cecil medicine,* 26th edition. Philadelphia: Elsevier; 2020.) **(B)** Gonococci. Scanning electron microscopy showing gonococci attaching to the nonciliated cells of human uterine/fallopian tube mucosa. (From Morse SA, et al., eds. *Atlas of sexually transmitted diseases and AIDS,* 3rd edition. London: Mosby; 2003.)

SEXUALLY TRANSMITTED UROGENITAL INFECTIONS

Bacterial Infections

Gonorrhea

Gonorrhea is caused by Neisseria gonorrhoeae, aerobic, non-spore-forming, oxidase-positive, gram-negative diplococci, organisms that usually appear in pairs with adjacent, slightly flattened sides (Fig. 27.2A). The rates for gonorrhea have increased in part because of widespread testing using more accurate nucleic acid amplification tests (NAATs).[11] In 2019, the CDC reported a total of 616,392 new cases, with as many as 1,000,000 cases undiagnosed.[5] This represents a 92% increase from the record low in 2009, including a 5.9% increase from 2018 to 2019. The rate of increase has occurred in all ethnic/racial groups and in all regions of the United States. The increase is consistently higher in men as compared with women.[10]

The risk of developing gonorrhea from intercourse with an infected male partner is 50% to 80% for women, and with an infected female partner, it is 20% to 30% for men. The risk increases threefold to fourfold for men after four exposures to an infected partner. Men who have sex with infected men have a greater risk of contracting gonorrhea if they are the receptive partner.[12]

Transmission of gonococcal infection generally requires direct contact of epithelial (mucosal) surfaces, such as occurs during vaginal, oral, or anal intercourse. Infection in adults can be maintained in the vagina, rectum, oropharynx, or urethra.[13] A pregnant woman can transmit gonorrhea to her fetus through infected cervical and vaginal secretions that contact the baby's mucosal surfaces during birth. Following vertical transmission, the newborn eyes can be infected and can result in blindness if untreated.

Treatment for gonorrhea is becoming more difficult because of rapidly developing resistance to available antibiotics. In 2019, the CDC reported that more than half of infections were resistant to at least one antibiotic.[10]

Prior to 2021, both the CDC and the World Health Organization (WHO) advised dual drug treatment for gonorrhea to effectively treat infection and prevent increasing resistance.[10] In 2021, the CDC STI Treatment Guidelines indicated that dual therapy may increase harm to the microbiome and currently recommend using only ceftriaxone for treating gonorrhea in the United States.[10,14] Antimicrobial resistance is increased in populations that frequently have oral or anal receptive intercourse, such men who have sex with men (MSM). The CDC states it is reasonable to expect that gonorrhea may become resistant to all known antibiotics soon.[10,14]

Pathophysiology. Humans are the only natural hosts for *N. gonorrhoeae*. Hair-like filaments on the gonococci, called *pili*, appear to help the microorganisms attach themselves to host cells: the epithelial cells of mucous membranes (Fig. 27.2B). Columnar, transitional, and stratified squamous epithelial cells are most often infected. First, the gonococci attach to the plasma membranes (cell walls) of these cells, and then they invade the cells and begin to damage the mucosa. In general, a quick leukocytic (inflammatory) response and exudate occurs at the site of infection.

In women, the endocervical canal (inner portion of the cervix) is a common site of initial gonococcal infection, although urethral colonization and infection of glands (paraurethral [Skene] glands and greater vestibular [Bartholin] glands) near the urethra and vagina also are common. Several factors facilitate ascent of gonococci into the uterus and the fallopian tubes, where they can cause PID. Among these factors are (1) disintegration of the cervical mucous plug and an increase in vaginal pH to greater than 4.5 during menstruation, (2) uterine contractions that may cause retrograde menstruation into the fallopian/uterine tubes, and (3) various microbes that possess virulent potentiating factors for chlamydia or gonococcal PID. Bacteria (*N. gonorrhoeae, Chlamydia trachomatis*) may adhere to sperm and be transported to the fallopian/uterine tubes. Once gonococci are in the fallopian/uterine tubes, progressive mucosal and submucosal invasion of the tissues causes sloughing of normal, ciliated tubal epithelium and a marked inflammatory response causing the tubes to fill with exudate (see Chapter 25 for more discussion on PID).

In men, the gonococci typically infect the urethra or rectum. In men, untreated urethral infection can cause epididymitis and potentially lead to urethral stricture, fistula formation, and sterility. However, a few men maintain asymptomatic infections for long periods of time.[8]

Concurrent or isolated oropharyngeal and anorectal infection can be found in infected men and women and may be difficult to detect with common testing mechanisms.[12] These sites are associated with greater antibiotic resistance than urethral or vaginal infection and may need additional treatment and monitoring.[12] One hypothesis for the increase in resistant strains in populations with a high prevalence of oral and anal intercourse is that the oral and rectal mucosae normally contain many nonpathogenic forms of *Neisseria* bacteria. These bacteria are often exposed to antibiotics used for other non-STI conditions; however, instead of being eliminated, they develop antibiotic resistance. Gonococci frequently share plasmids and DNA across species, a process known as *conjugation*, facilitating the transfer of antibiotic resistance.[11] When the oropharynx and the rectum are infected by *N. gonorrhoeae*, the pathogens meet antibiotic-resistant bacteria that share plasmids and DNA. As the *N. gonorrhea* proliferate, they can acquire antibiotic resistance before being spread to new individuals through oral sexual contact.[11]

Clinical Manifestations. The clinical manifestations of gonorrhea can be categorized as local or systemic and uncomplicated or complicated. Uncomplicated local infections include urethral infections in men and urogenital infections in women. Although infection can initially be asymptomatic, most infected men will develop painful urination or purulent penile discharge, or both, within a week of infection.[10] These severe symptoms encourage most men in developed countries to seek treatment.[10] However, some men may have only a slight discharge or urethral itching (pruritus). As many as 5% to 10% of infected men never have signs or symptoms of gonorrhea. Most cases of untreated gonococcal urethritis resolve spontaneously after several weeks. More than 95% of men are asymptomatic by 6 months after infection (although they may still be infectious).

In women, the incubation period varies, but those who develop symptoms usually manifest within 10 days of exposure or 1 to 2 days after the next menstrual period. More than half of gonorrhea infections in women are initially asymptomatic. Symptoms often do not appear until the infection has spread to the upper reproductive tract (uterus, fallopian/uterine tubes, and ovaries). Symptoms may include dysuria, increased vaginal discharge, abnormal menses (increased flow or dysmenorrhea), dyspareunia, lower abdominal/pelvic pain, and fever. Pelvic examination may identify cervical friability and erythema (redness) with mucopurulent discharge from the cervical os (Fig. 27.3). There may be discharge from the paraurethral (Skene) or greater vestibular (Bartholin) glands if these sites are involved.

Anorectal gonorrhea occurs more commonly in MSM but is also found in women both as an isolated finding and with coexisting urogenital gonorrhea.[1] Symptoms of anorectal gonorrhea range from mild anal pruritus (itching), mucopurulent rectal discharge, and slight rectal bleeding to severe rectal pain, tenesmus (painful and ineffectual straining at stool), and constipation. Findings on physical exam may include anal erythema and discharge and evidence of mucosal damage to the anus and rectum, such as friability, edema, and purulent exudate.

Gonococcal pharyngitis occurs after oral sexual contact with an infected partner. Symptomatic pharyngitis is indistinguishable from any other bacterial pharyngitis and can

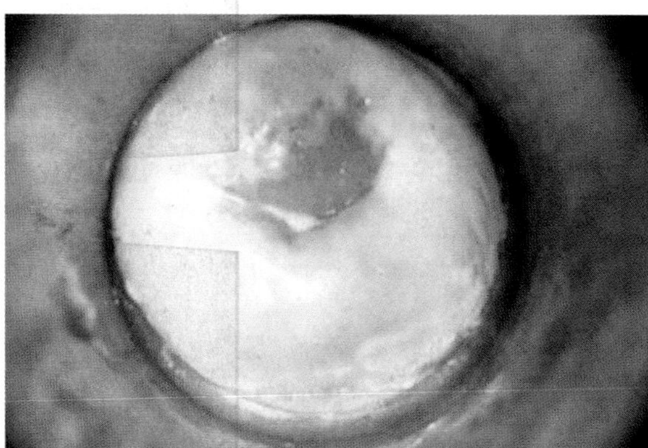

Fig. 27.3 Gonococcal Cervicitis. The cervix is involved in 85% to 90% of cases in women, but discharge is profuse enough to be recognized in only 10%. (From Centers for Disease Control and Prevention [CDC]. *STD Clinical* Slides *[website]*. www.cdc.gov/std/training/clinicalslides/slides-dl.htm. Accessed December 6, 2020.)

include fever, lymphadenopathy, and tonsillitis. However, 60% of people with oropharyngeal infections are asymptomatic.[8] In addition, many clinicians neglect to test for oropharyngeal gonorrhea because they do not screen for unprotected oral sex. Cure rates for this type of gonorrhea are much lower because of inadequate antibiotic concentrations in oral tissue.[11] Other sites of uncomplicated local infections include the eyes, leading to conjunctivitis; this condition occurs almost exclusively in newborns born vaginally to infected mothers. Primary cutaneous infections have also been reported and usually manifest as a localized ulcer of the genitalia, perineum, proximal lower extremities, or fingers.

Complicated gonococcal infections in men include prostatitis, epididymitis, lymphangitis, and urethral stricture. Complicated gonococcal infections in women include bartholinitis and endometritis (infection of the uterine lining). Further spread into the fallopian tubes and peritoneum is known as *PID* and can result in severe inflammation and scarring. The onset of PID symptoms may be rapid and usually occurs during menses.[15] Women may experience chills, fever, nausea, vomiting, and lower abdominal/pelvic pain that worsens with movement, such as walking, coughing, sneezing, or intercourse. Abdominal palpation often discloses bilateral lower quadrant tenderness and rebound tenderness from peritoneal irritation.[8] Marked motion tenderness of the cervix and internal genitalia is often noted during pelvic examination (Chandelier sign).

PID resulting from any pathogen contributes to infertility through a variety of mechanisms. During infection, the delicate ciliated epithelium of the uterine tubes is permanently damaged. The lack of regular cilia movement can impair the transit of sperm and fertilized ova.[15] Scarring and adhesions of the tubes may further impair fertility. Up to 18% of women who have been diagnosed with PID experience later infertility. Because fertilization occurs in the midportion of the fallopian tube, ectopic pregnancy rates in this population are as high as 9% partially due to slowed motility of the cilia and scarring in the fallopian tubes.[15]

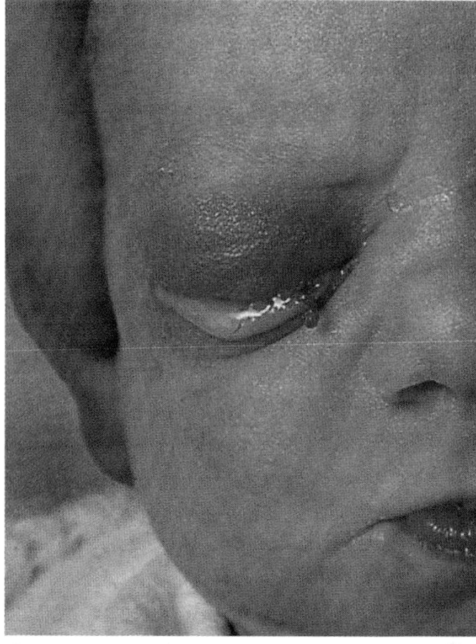

Fig. 27.4 Gonococcal Ophthalmia Neonatorum. Examiner should be gloved. (From McMillan A, Scott GR. *Sexually transmitted infections*, 2nd edition. London: Churchill Livingstone; 2000.)

Disseminated gonococcal infection (DGI) is a rare systemic complication caused by the spread of infection through the bloodstream. Symptoms of this life-threatening condition include a generalized rash, severe joint pain, meningitis, and endocarditis.[8] Gonococcal strains that can cause DGI may cause genital inflammation before systemic dissemination.[8]

If during pregnancy a mother has gonorrhea at the time of delivery, she can transmit the infection to her child. Most states require that all infants receive prophylactic ophthalmic antibiotics to prevent gonococcal eye infection (**ophthalmia neonatorum**) (Fig. 27.4). Topical antibiotics may not be effective in eliminating neonatal infection, and systemic treatment is indicated for all newborns with known exposure.[8] Untreated infection causes bilateral corneal ulceration, with a profuse yellow or gray purulent exudate, and is followed by necrosis, scarring, and blindness. Newborns born to infected mothers also may develop gonorrheal rhinitis, anorectal infection, or an abscess at the site of electrode placement for fetal monitoring. Onset of symptoms generally occurs 1 to 12 days after birth.[8]

Evaluation and Treatment. Because of the large percentage of infected women without symptoms, routine genital tract screening for at-risk women (i.e., those younger than age 25, pregnant, or with a new sexual partner) is recommended.[16] Men should be screened according to risk factors and symptoms.[16,17] Clinical signs and symptoms are not sufficient for the differential diagnosis. The test that is used should be selected based on the suspected site of infection. Nucleic acid hybridization tests can be used on samples collected from the vagina and urethra (of adult males and females; female children but not male children), as well as urine (except in boys).[16,17] Culture should be used to diagnose infections of the rectum, oropharynx, and conjunctiva of both sexes and all ages, as well as any site on boys.[14,15] Microscopic evaluation of Gram-stained slides of specimens from symptomatic men also can be used for diagnosis and is deemed positive for *N. gonorrhoeae* if gram-negative diplococci with typical "kidney bean" morphology are seen inside polymorphonuclear leukocytes.

N. gonorrhoeae has developed resistance to many antibiotics and has the real potential to become resistant to all current treatments.[16,17] There is currently only one CDC-recommended drug (ceftriaxone) to treat gonorrhea, although less-effective alternatives are available.[16,17] To prevent further drug resistance, the CDC and WHO recommend a multidrug treatment for gonorrhea that also is effective against chlamydia.[16,17] The CDC is closely observing the drug resistance of gonorrhea through monitoring of samples obtained at clinics around the country. In 2019, the CDC reported increased resistance to azithromycin particularly in MSM (8.8%) compared with men having sex with women (3.3%).[16]Treatment guidelines are updated regularly, and the most recent edition, found on the CDC website or app, should be used. Current CDC treatment guidelines for uncomplicated gonorrheal infections are listed in Box 27.2.[16] Complicated infections require IV antibiotic therapy and possibly hospitalization.[16]Sexual partners also are assessed and treated according to these protocols, and sexual contact is avoided until treatment is completed. Condoms for all genital contact, including oral sex, are strongly recommended to prevent future infection.

BOX 27.2 Centers for Disease Control and Prevention Recommended Regimens for Uncomplicated Gonococcal Infections, 2020

Regimen for uncomplicated gonococcal infections of the cervix, urethra, or rectum:

Ceftriaxone 500 mg IM as a single dose for persons weighing <150 kg (300 lb)

- For persons weighing ≥150 kg (300 lb), 1 g of IM ceftriaxone should be administered.
- If chlamydial infection has not been excluded, providers should treat for chlamydia with doxycycline 100 mg orally twice daily for 7 days. During pregnancy, azithromycin 1 g as a single dose is recommended to treat chlamydia.

Alternative regimens for uncomplicated gonococcal infections of the cervix, urethra, or rectum if ceftriaxone is not available:

Gentamicin 240 mg IM as a single dose plus azithromycin 2 g orally as a single dose OR cefixime 800 mg orally as a single dose. If treating with cefixime, and chlamydial infection has not been excluded, providers should treat for chlamydia with doxycycline 100 mg orally twice daily for 7 days. During pregnancy, azithromycin 1 g as a single dose is recommended to treat chlamydia.

Recommended regimen for uncomplicated gonococcal infections of the pharynx:

Ceftriaxone 500 mg IM as a single dose for persons weighing <150 kg (300 lb)

- For persons weighing ≥150 kg (300 lb), 1 g of IM ceftriaxone should be administered.
- If chlamydia coinfection is identified when pharyngeal gonorrhea testing is performed, providers should treat for chlamydia with doxycycline 100 mg orally twice a day for 7 days. During pregnancy, azithromycin 1 g as a single dose is recommended to treat chlamydia.
- No reliable alternative treatments are available for pharyngeal gonorrhea. For persons with a history of a beta-lactam allergy, a thorough assessment of the reaction is recommended.[a]
- For persons with an anaphylactic or other severe reaction (e.g., Stevens Johnson syndrome) to ceftriaxone, consult an infectious disease specialist for an alternative treatment recommendation.

IM, Intramuscular.

[a]CDC. Sexually transmitted diseases treatment guidelines. *MMWR Recomm Rep.* 2015;64(No. RR-3). https://www.cdc.gov/mmwr/preview/mmwrhtml/rr6403a1.htm.

Syphilis

Syphilis, caused by the spirochete *Treponema pallidum*, is a disease with local and systemic manifestations that stretch over years and has been well-known throughout history. With the advent of antibiotics and intensive public health efforts during and after World War II, the prevalence of syphilis declined sharply (Fig. 27.5).[18]

Rates of syphilis reached a record low of 2.1 cases per 100,000 in 2000.[19] However, since this all-time low, in 2019, 129,813 cases of syphilis in all stages were reported, an increase of 11.2% during 2018 to 2019.[16] Men account for nearly 82% to 91% of all new cases of syphilis, whereas rates between sexes were equivalent two decades ago.[18] While rates of syphilis have decreased among MSM, MSM accounts for more than 56.7% of all cases of primary and **secondary syphilis**.[2,19,20] **Congenital syphilis (CS)**, caused by vertical transmission of the spirochete from mother to fetus, also has experienced resurgence in the United States. After years of decline, the rate of CS has increased each year since 2013. In 2019, CS was reported in 1870 cases, or 48.5 cases per 100,000 live births. This represents an increase of 41.4% from 2018 to 2019. Reported stillbirths also increased from 79 to 94 from 2018 to 2019.[21] This increase reflects the increase in primary and secondary syphilis.

Pathophysiology. *T. pallidum*, the cause of syphilis, is an anaerobic spirochete bacterium that can grow in any human organ or tissue but cannot be cultured in vitro. When viewed through dark-field microscopy, the *Treponema* (individual microorganism) resembles a corkscrew, with regular, tight spirals and a rotary motion.

Because the bacterium is present in exudate from moist mucosal or cutaneous lesions, the spirochete is usually transmitted to others during the first few years of infection.[8] Transmission generally occurs through minor abrasions during sexual intercourse but can occur extragenitally as well. Although condoms can decrease the likelihood of infection, if lesions are present on areas not covered during intercourse, transmission can occur even with safer sex practices.

The course of untreated syphilis consists of four stages based on clinical findings: primary, secondary, latent, and tertiary (Box 27.3); the division between stages is not always apparent, and the drug of choice is the same for all stages.[8]

Primary syphilis begins at the site of bacterial invasion (Fig. 27.6), where *T. pallidum* multiplies in the epithelium and produces a granulomatous tissue reaction called a **chancre**. Some microorganisms drain with lymph into adjacent lymph nodes. Within the nodes and at the site of the chancre, the cell-mediated and humoral immune responses are stimulated.

Secondary syphilis is systemic. During this stage, blood-borne bacteria spread to all major organ systems. The secondary

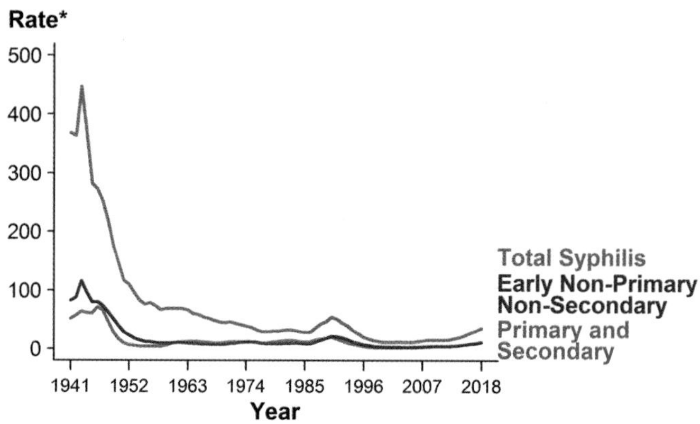

* Per 100,000.

Fig. 27.5 **Syphilis Cases Reported in 2018.** In 2018, a total of 35,063 cases of P&S syphilis were reported in the United States, yielding a rate of 10.8 cases per 100,000 population. This rate represents a 14.9% increase compared with 2017 (9.4 cases per 100,000 population) and a 71.4% increase compared with 2014 (6.3 cases per 100,000 population). (From Centers for Disease Control and Prevention. https://www.cdc.gov/std/stats18/figures/35.htm.)

BOX 27.3 Progression of Untreated Syphilis

Stage I, primary syphilis—local invasion: *Treponema pallidum* multiplies in epithelium, producing granulomatous tissue reaction (chancre); lymph-containing microorganisms drain into adjacent lymph nodes and stimulate immune responses

Stage II, secondary syphilis—systemic disease: blood-borne bacteria spread to all major organ systems; immune system suppresses infection and symptoms regress spontaneously

Stage III, latent syphilis—silent infection: transmission of infection possible even though there are no clinical signs of infection

Stage IV, tertiary syphilis—noninfectious disease: significant morbidity and mortality occur; destructive skin, bone, and soft tissue lesions, or gummas, result from severe hypersensitivity; cardiovascular complications (aneurysms, heart valve insufficiency, heart failure) and neurosyphilis develop

Antibiotic resistance is rapidly increasing for this pathogen; please check current guidelines at the Centers for Disease Control and Prevention website at www.cdc.gov and search "gonorrhea."

stage is followed by a period during which the immune system can suppress the infection. Even without treatment, spontaneous resolution of the skin lesions occurs, and the individual enters the latent stage of infection.

Latent syphilis may be subdivided into early and late stages; however, no specific criteria delineate one from the other.[8] Medical history and serologic studies can show that syphilis is present, but the individual has no clinical manifestations. Transmission remains possible during this phase.

Tertiary syphilis is the most severe stage, involving significant morbidity and mortality. The pathogenesis of syphilitic manifestations at this stage remains unclear. The destructive skin, bone, and soft tissue lesions (called gummas) of tertiary syphilis probably are caused by a severe hypersensitivity reaction to the microorganism. Within the cardiovascular system, infection with *T. pallidum* may cause aneurysms, heart valve insufficiencies, and heart failure.

CS is caused by vertical transmission and is estimated to cause 500,000 fetal and neonatal deaths every year worldwide.[22] Syphilis becomes a systemic disease shortly after maternal infection and can be transmitted to the fetus as early as the ninth week of gestation because the spirochete can pass through the placental membrane to infect the fetus. Intrauterine infection causes fetal or perinatal death in 40% of affected infants and may lead to perinatal complications in more than 70% of cases. Many live-born infants have permanent, lifelong morbidity, including congenital abnormalities.[22] The risk of CS is estimated at up to 80% in primary syphilis and declines with advancing stages of the disease.[22] However, simple treatment with penicillin is 98% effective at preventing vertical transmission, thereby decreasing morbidity and mortality if the disease can be diagnosed early in fetal development.[23]

Primary Stage

Clinical Manifestations. In adults, the incubation period of syphilis ranges from 12 days to 12 weeks after exposure and averages 3 weeks. A sore, or *hard chancre*, develops at the site of treponemal entry. Typically, the chancre is an eroded, painless, firm, and indurated (hard) ulcer up to 2 cm in diameter. Firm, enlarged, and nontender regional lymph nodes accompany chancres. Typical chancres of the penis and vulva are shown in Fig. 27.6. Syphilitic chancres are not always typical, and syphilis should be considered in the presence of any open lesion. With secondary infection, chancres can become necrotic and painful. Lesions on the fingers may be dry, scaly, and papular or moist and vegetative. If left untreated, the chancre of primary syphilis heals in 2 to 8 weeks and then spontaneously disappears, usually without leaving a scar.

Secondary Stage

Clinical manifestations of secondary syphilis usually develop 6 weeks after the first appearance of the chancre but may overlap with those of the primary stage. Systemic symptoms are variable and can include low-grade fever, malaise, sore throat, hoarseness, anorexia, generalized adenopathy, headache, joint pain, and skin or mucous membrane lesions or rashes. Cutaneous (skin) rashes are generally papulosquamous (raised and scaly), but any variation or combination of macular (flat), papular (raised), and pustular (pus-filled) lesions may be seen. Lesions are often widespread and bilateral, appearing on the palms and soles (Fig. 27.7). Some lesions become hypertrophied, flat, moist, and wart-like or vegetative (e.g., cauliflower-like). These lesions, called condylomata lata, are highly contagious and develop on the perineum, vulva, and groin of women (Fig. 27.8) and around the inner thigh and anal area in men and women. Besides skin sores, oral mucous membrane lesions (known as *mucous patches*), lymphadenopathy, pruritus, and alopecia are common. Some individuals develop anemia, leukocytosis, increased erythrocyte sedimentation rate (ESR), hepatitis, transitory proteinuria, arthritis, electrocardiographic abnormalities, and central nervous system (CNS) symptoms. Regardless of

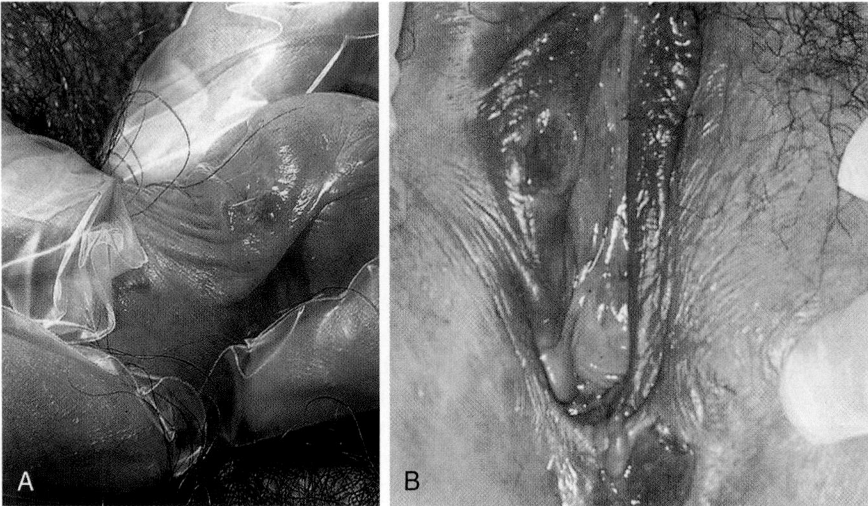

Fig. 27.6 Primary Syphilis. (**A**) Penile chancre. (**B**) Vulval chancres; the labia and perineum show induration and edema of chancres. (A, From McMillan A, Scott GR. *Sexually transmitted infections*, 2nd edition. London: Churchill Livingstone; 2000; B, Courtesy Barbara Romanowski, MD, from Morse SA, et al., eds. *Atlas of sexually transmitted diseases and AIDS*, 4th edition. London: Saunders; 2013.)

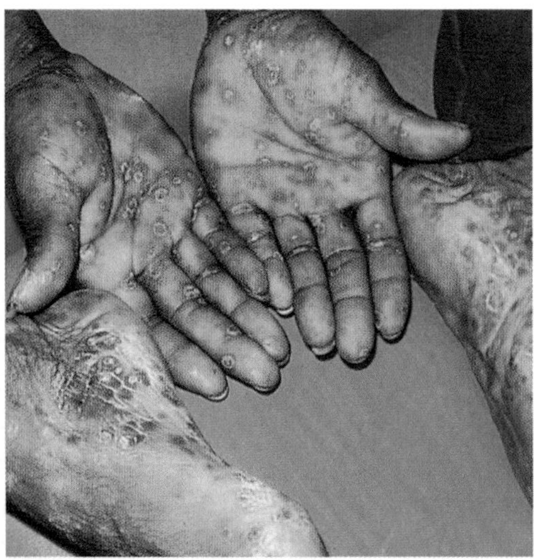

Fig. 27.7 Secondary Syphilis. Secondary syphilis to the palms and plantar surfaces. (From Morse S, et al., eds. *Atlas of Sexually Transmitted Diseases and AIDS*. 4th ed. London: Saunders; 2013.)

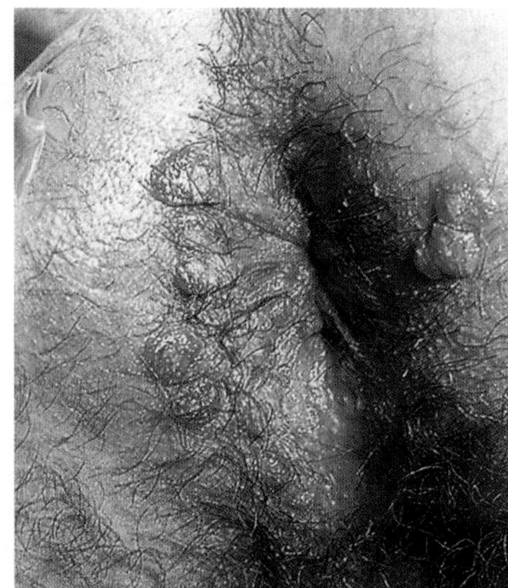

Fig. 27.8 Condylomata Lata. Broad-based, moist, dark-field–positive condylomata lata of the perineum. (From McMillan A, Scott GR. *Sexually transmitted infections*, 2nd edition. London: Churchill Livingstone; 2000.)

treatment, cutaneous lesions generally heal in 2 to 10 weeks. Within the CNS, the presence of *T. pallidum* in cerebrospinal fluid may cause the manifestations of neurosyphilis, including altered mental status and meningitis, which can occur within any stage of syphilis infection but are more common in early stages of infection.[8]

Latent and Tertiary Stages

The asymptomatic, latent stage of syphilis may be as short as 1 year or as long as a lifetime. After the latent stage, tertiary syphilis may present with gummas, cardiovascular lesions, and neurosyphilis manifestations, including *tabes dorsalis* and general paresis caused by demyelination of the spinal cord.[8] Tertiary syphilis is rare because of the widespread availability of antibiotics.

Congenital Syphilis

Although considered rare, CS was relatively stable from 2008 until 2013, when a significant increase in incidence occurred. Since 2013, the rate of CS has increased from 9.2 cases/100,000 births to 48.5 cases/100,000 births in 2019. When compared with the CS rates in 2015 with rates in 2019, the relative increase was 291.1%. Cases were reported in 43 states and the District of Columbia.[21]

CS can cause fetal death (79 in 2018 and 94 in 2019)[21] or growth abnormalities, including changes in the fetal bones, teeth, and neurologic system. Affected newborns can have a variety of manifestations of the disease, including growth abnormalities, rashes, hepatosplenomegaly, jaundice, and CNS involvement, including blindness and deafness. A classically reported late manifestation of CS is notched incisors (Hutchinson teeth) (Fig. 27.9).

Evaluation and Treatment. Numerous dermatologic disorders can mimic the skin lesions of secondary syphilis, making differential diagnosis difficult. Laboratory confirmation is important. Two categories of serologic testing exist: nontreponemal antigen tests and treponemal antibody tests.[8] Nontreponemal antigen tests, such as the Venereal Disease Research Laboratory (VDRL) antigen and the rapid plasma reagin (RPR) tests, demonstrate the presence of *reagin* (a group of antibodies present in syphilis) in serum and provide indirect evidence of infection (Box 27.4). These tests yield a positive result (presence of reagin) in more than 50% of individuals with primary syphilis and in 100% of individuals in the secondary phase of disease and can be useful in screening and assessing response to treatment.[8]

Because the VDRL and RPR tests have high rates of false-positives, a treponemal test is performed if the screening test is positive. Treponemal tests are serologic-specific tests that are used to assess antibody response to *T. pallidum* and include enzyme immunoassays (EIAs), chemiluminescence immunoassays, the fluorescent treponemal antibody absorption (FTA-ABS) test, and the passive *T. pallidum* particle agglutination (TP-PA) assay.[8] Studies indicate that because of increased sensitivity and specificity (98% and 97.5%) of enzyme-linked immunosorbent assays (ELISAs) for *T. pallidum*, the ELISA test has the potential to replace VDRL and RPR for screening.[24]

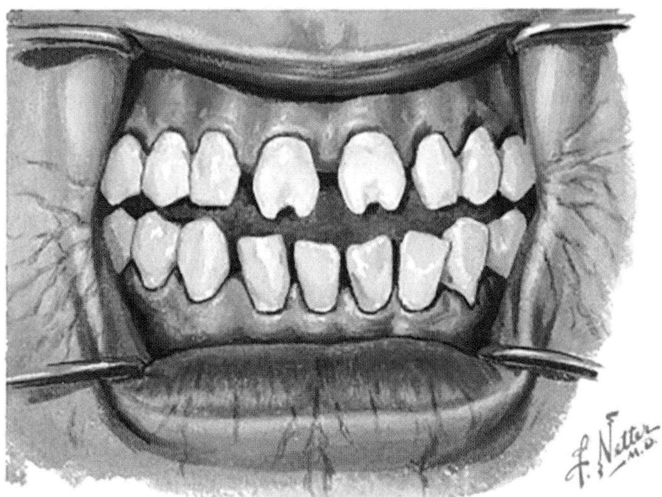

Hutchinson's teeth, scars of healed rhagades (congenital syphilis)

Fig. 27.9 Hutchinson Teeth. (From Jong EC, Stevens DL. *Netter's Infectious Diseases*. Philadelphia: Saunders; 2012.)

BOX 27.4 False-Positive Serologic Tests for Syphilis

Reasons for False-Positive, Nontreponemal Reactions (VDRL, RPR)

Transient Reactions (<6 Months)

Technical error (low titer)
Mycoplasma pneumonia
Enterovirus infections
Infectious mononucleosis
Pregnancy
Narcotic abuse
Advanced tuberculosis
Scarlet fever
Viral and atypical pneumonia
Brucellosis
Rat-bite fever
Leptospirosis
Measles
Mumps
Lymphogranuloma venereum
Malaria
Trypanosomiasis
Varicella

Chronic Reactions (>6 Months)

Malaria
Leprosy
Systemic lupus erythematosus
Narcotic abuse
Other connective tissue diseases
Elderly population
Hashimoto thyroiditis
Rheumatoid arthritis
Reticuloendothelial malignancy
Familial false-positive reaction
Idiopathic

Reasons for False-Positive, Treponemal-Specific Reactions (FTA-ABS)

Technical error
Inefficient sorbents
Healthy individuals without syphilis
Genital herpes simplex
Pregnancy
Lupus erythematosus (skin only or systemic)
Alcoholic cirrhosis
Scleroderma
Mixed connective tissue disease

RPR, rapid plasma reagin; *VDRL*, Venereal Disease Research Laboratory.

Preferred treatment for all stages of syphilis is parenteral injection of benzathine penicillin G. Other types of penicillin are not as effective. If the individual has manifested signs of the disease for less than 1 year, a single intramuscular dose is appropriate. If signs have been present for more than 1 year or they are asymptomatic and assumed to be in late latent syphilis, the treatment is three weekly injections. The CDC is the best source for current information on treatment regimens.[25]

Penicillin therapy also is appropriate for pregnant women to prevent vertical transmission.[25] There is no evidence to date that *T. pallidum* has developed resistance to penicillin. In fact, it is highly sensitive; however, because of the slow replication time, serum levels must be maintained for 7 to 14 days. Men and nonpregnantwomen who are allergic to penicillin may receive oral doxycycline, 100 mg twice daily for 14 days, or tetracycline, 500 mg four times per day for 14 days. Pregnant women with a penicillin allergy should be desensitized and then treated with benzathine penicillin G as recommended by the CDC because the other available antibiotics cause lifelong discoloration of the forming teeth of the fetus.[26]

Repeated assessment of VDRL or RPR titers is used to determine effectiveness of treatment. Because the results of the VDRL and RPR testing are not interchangeable, the same test should be used for repeat testing. Titers should decrease fourfold if treatment was successful. Sexual partners also are tested and treated, and the use of condoms is recommended until effective treatment is verified.

Newborns of mothers with documented syphilis need careful evaluation after birth. Definitive diagnosis of CS is complicated by the presence of maternal antibodies in the newborn's blood. Treatment decisions are made based on maternal status, clinical symptoms of CS, and comparison of maternal and neonatal titers.[23] If the infant requires treatment, penicillin is the drug of choice with carefully titrated dosing depending on fetal weight and the day of treatment, and the CDC is the best source of current information.[23]

Chancroid

Chancroid, or soft chancre, is an acute infectious disease that is caused by *Haemophilus ducreyi*, a gram-negative bacillus. The incidence of chancroid is decreasing worldwide, and is infrequently seen in the United States.[1] Sporadic outbreaks occur throughout the world and tend to be associated with sex workers and illicit drug use, when individuals continue to engage in intercourse despite a painful genital lesion.[27] Chancroid is a risk factor for HIV acquisition, and existing HIV infection is a risk factor for chancroid infection with exposure.[8]

Pathophysiology. *H. ducreyi* is a gram-negative bacillus with rounded ends. It is commonly observed in small chains or clusters along mucous strands under a microscope. Transmission can occur through sexual contact and autoinoculation, but there is no evidence for vertical transmission.[8] Chancroid lesions are found throughout the genital area. Initially, the papule enlarges; then erodes into a soft, circumscribed ulcer containing a superficial exudate of varying size and presentation.[27] Beneath the ulcer is a lesion characterized by edema, endothelial proliferation, and a base of granulation tissue. Adjacent lymph nodes are acutely inflamed and full of polymorphonuclear leukocytes and necrotic cells.

Clinical Manifestations. Chancroid has an incubation period of 3 to 10 days.[27] Women are generally asymptomatic but, depending on the site of infection, can present with less obvious symptoms (dysuria, dyspareunia, vaginal discharge, pain on defecation, or rectal bleeding). Constitutional symptoms are unusual. An initial vesicopustular lesion forms at the site of inoculation and erodes to form a soft ulcer with a necrotic base, surrounding erythema, and a ragged, serpiginous (spreading) border (Fig. 27.10). Unilateral, painful, local lymphadenopathy presents in approximately half of infected individuals. Inguinal buboes (unilocular abscess of the inguinal lymph nodes) develop 7 to 10 days after the initial chancre and fill with exudate. In 25% to 60% of cases, the buboes spontaneously rupture out onto the skin, spreading the infection through autoinoculation.

Ulcers on the foreskin may lead to phimosis or paraphimosis see Chapter 26. Other complications of chancroid include balanitis, secondary infections, necrosis, and fistula formation. Lesions may take months or years to heal and cause scarring.[8]

Evaluation and Treatment. Chancroid is easily confused with other types of genital ulcers, particularly those of syphilis, genital herpes, and granuloma inguinale (see Fig. 27.10). Unlike the syphilitic ulcer, the chancroid ulcer is painful, tender, and nonindurated and inguinal lymphadenopathy is pronounced. Microscopic analysis of a Gram-stained smear from the chancroid helps to identify the microorganism. Definitive diagnosis depends on recovery of *H. ducreyi* from cultured specimens; however, the culture medium is not commercially available.[28] Diagnosis depends on the clinical presentation of a painful genital ulcer with inguinal lymphadenopathy and with negative testing for syphilis and herpes simplex virus (HSV).[28] In addition, HIV testing is recommended because chancroid is a cofactor for transmission of HIV.

Resistance to recommended antibiotics has emerged in isolated instances worldwide. Treatment recommendations include a single intramuscular injection of ceftriaxone (250 mg) or a single dose of oral azithromycin (1 g). Effective oral multiple-dose regimens include ciprofloxacin, 500 mg orally twice daily for 3 days, or erythromycin, 500 mg three times daily for 7 days. Persons infected with HIV and uncircumcised men have higher rates of treatment failure and may require a longer treatment regimen. Treatment failure requires more intensive assessment for coinfection with other diseases.[28] Simultaneous treatment of sexual partners and use of condoms are recommended to prevent reinfection (see Emerging Science Box: New Therapeutics for Human Immunodeficiency Virus Prevention and Treatment).

Granuloma Inguinale

Granuloma inguinale (donovanosis) is a chronic, progressively destructive bacterial infection caused by *Klebsiella granulomatis*, a gram-negative intracellular bacterium. Although sexually transmitted, granuloma inguinale has a low transmission rate between sexual partners.[27] Infection through fecal contamination and autoinoculation also is possible.[27] As with all genital ulcerative diseases, granuloma inguinale plays a role in HIV transmission.[27] Granuloma inguinale very rarely occurs in the United States[27]; it is more prevalent in some tropical and

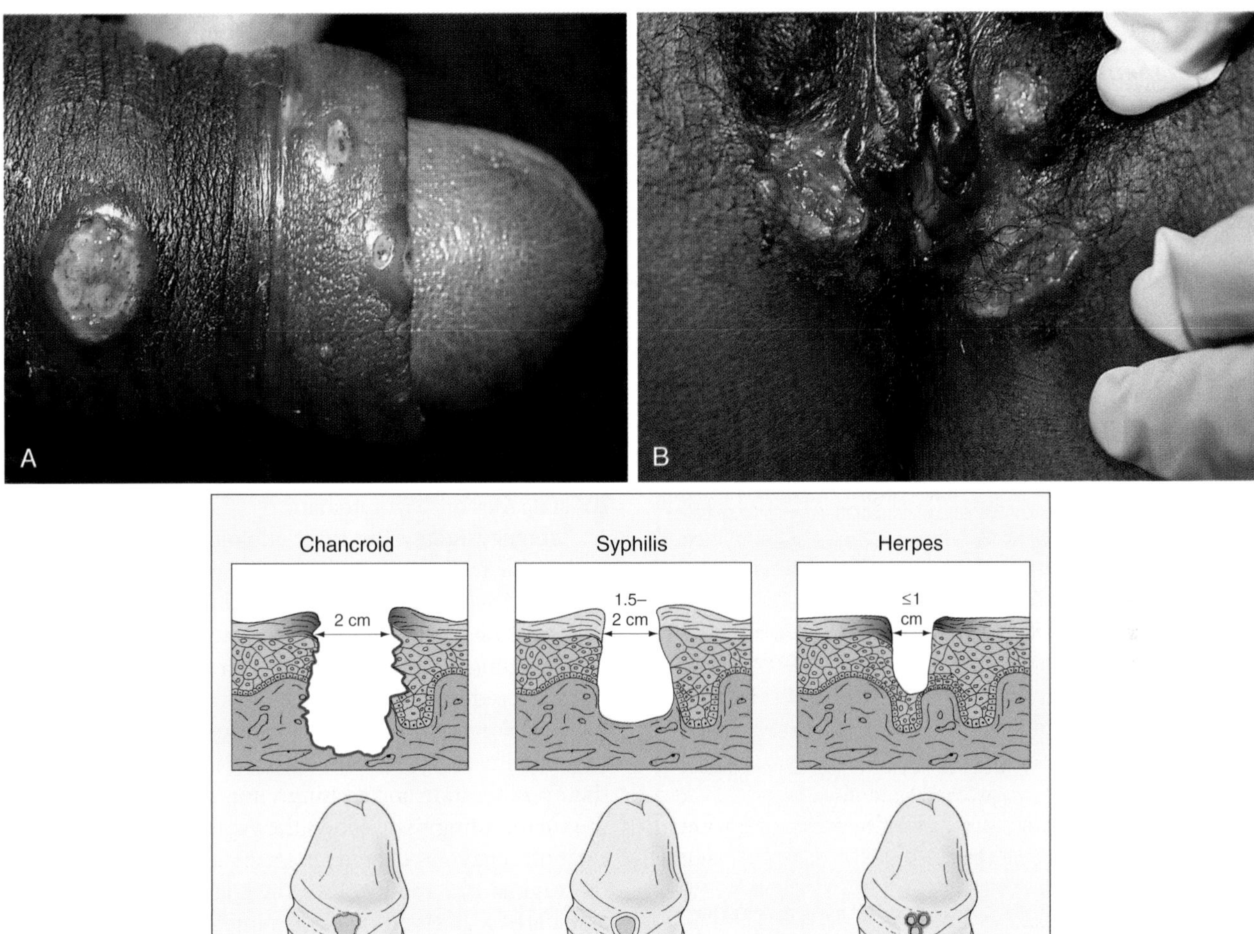

Fig. 27.10 Chancroid. (A) Ulcers on the penile shaft. (B) Multiple vulvar lesions. (C) Differences in clinical appearance among chancroid, syphilis, and genital herpes. (From Morse SA, et al., eds. *Atlas of sexually transmitted diseases and AIDS*, 4th edition. London: Saunders; 2013.)

subtropical parts of the world (India, New Guinea, Africa, central Australia, and to less extent the Caribbean and Brazil). With increased ease of travel, this may become more common in other parts of the world.

Pathophysiology. *K. granulomatis* is a gram-negative, nonsporing, nonmotile, encapsulated rod not easily cultured in the laboratory. After an individual is infected, bacteria survive and multiply within vacuoles of large histiocytic cells or polymorphonuclear leukocytes. The bacteria reproduce within these cells, and a vacuole may contain 20 to 30 microorganisms. These bacteria-filled vacuoles, identified by Charles Donovan in 1905, are termed Donovan bodies. Donovan bodies, when present, in tissue smears of material from the lesions are considered pathognomonic for diagnosis, but this test is difficult even in well-equipped laboratories.[29]

The incubation period of granuloma inguinale is 8 to 80 days. As lesions begin to form, single lesions often coalesce with nearby lesions or form new lesions by autoinoculation of nearby skin surfaces. Progression from the initial nodule to a large, granuloma-heaped ulcer occurs slowly. These lesions are vascularized and bleed easily.[29] Secondary infection may occur, increasing tissue damage and residual scarring. The disease may spread to the bones, joints, and liver.

Clinical Manifestations. The primary site for development of the lesions in men is the distal penis and in women the vaginal introitus. The initial lesion is an indurated, sharply defined, painless, subcutaneous nodule that is often preceded and accompanied by itching. Nodules bleed easily and contain abundant red, beefy-looking granulation tissue. These lesions spread as the disease progresses. Secondary infection may occur, increasing tissue damage and residual scarring. Although systemic symptoms are rare, the disease may spread to the bones, joints, and liver. In some cases, infection spreads to the inguinal area and produces pseudobuboes. In these instances, the affected lymph nodes are not directly affected, but the surrounding area may be infected and abscessed.

EMERGING SCIENCE BOX

New Therapeutics for Human Immunodeficiency Virus Prevention and Treatment

Although most sexually transmitted infections (STIs) can be cured with early diagnosis and therapeutic intervention, infection with the human immunodeficiency virus (HIV) still poses great risk to those persons who acquire the infection. Although there is still no cure for HIV, with proper treatment, those with HIV are now living longer and with less morbidity.

In recent years, significant work has been done to decrease the transmission and the acquisition of HIV through sexual contact. Preexposure prophylaxis (PrEP), first approved in 2012 using either the combination of emtricitabine with tenofovir disoproxil fumarate (Truvada) or emtricitabine with tenofovir alafenamide (Descovy) can reduce the risk of HIV acquired through sexual contact and by injected drug use by 99% and 74%, respectively, when taken appropriately and when used in conjunction with safe sexual practices using condoms. Early studies of women using a monthly vaginal ring containing dapivirine have shown that the risk of acquiring HIV is reduced by approximately 27%–34%. Since January 2021, the World Health Organization recommends the use of the dapivirine vaginal ring for women at risk of HIV infection.

In 2019, a long-acting, monthly injectable combination of cabotegravir and rilpivirine was approved for use in Canada and in 2021 was approved in the United States in 2021 for individuals who are already virologically suppressed. Rates of suppression were as high as 93.6%.

Data from https://www.hiv.gov/hiv-basics/hiv-prevention/using-hiv-medication-to-reduce-risk/pre-exposure-prophylaxis; https://www.cdc.gov/hiv/risk/prep/index.html Powell VE, et al. Update on HIV preexposure prophylaxis: Effectiveness, drug resistance, and risk compensation. *Current Infectious Disease Reports*, 2019;21(28); https://doi.org/10.1007/s11908-019-0685-6; Baeten JM, et al. MTN-020–ASPIRE Study Team. Use of a vaginal ring containing dapivirine for HIV-1 prevention in women. New England Journal of Medicine, 2016;375(22):2121–2132. https://doi.org/10.1056/NEJMoa1506110; https://www.who.int/news/item/26-01-2021-who-recommends-the-dapivirine-vaginal-ring-as-a-new-choice-for-hiv-prevention-for-women-at-substantial-risk-of-hiv-infection; https://www.fda.gov/news-events/press-announcements/fda-approves-first-extended-release-injectable-drug-regimen-adults-living-hiv.

Evaluation and Treatment. Although the clinical manifestations of this disease are important for diagnosis, confirmation involves microscopic examination for Donovan bodies in a smear or biopsy specimen. Currently, there is not a US Food and Drug Administration (FDA)-approved laboratory test for detection of *K. granulomatis*.[29]

Many antibiotics successfully treat *K. granulomatis*. With effective antibiotic treatment, lesions begin to heal in 7 days, but treatment is continued for at least 3 weeks and until all lesions are healed. The recommended oral therapy is azithromycin, 1 g orally once weekly or 500 mg daily for 3 weeks or more or until lesions have completely healed. Alternative regimens include doxycycline, 100 mg twice a day for at least 3 weeks; erythromycin base, 500 mg four times a day for at least 3 weeks; or trimethoprim-sulfamethoxazole, 160 mg/800 mg, double-strength oral tablet twice a day for at least 3 weeks.[29] Despite effective initial therapy, relapses can occur 6 to 18 months later. Prolonged follow-up is necessary as is treatment of sexual partners. Because other STIs frequently coexist, individuals should be tested for chlamydia, gonorrhea, syphilis, hepatitis B, and HIV.

Bacterial Vaginosis

Bacterial vaginosis (BV) (previously called nonspecific vaginitis, nonspecific vaginosis, or *Haemophilus, Corynebacterium*, or *Gardnerella* vaginitis) is a sexually associated condition but is not necessarily considered an STI. The condition is associated with sexual contact, including genital touching and digital penetration, oral sex, and penile penetration. Although BV occurs mostly in sexually active women of reproductive age, it can affect women, especially menopausal women, who are not sexually active. Prevalence rates vary from 17% among women in family planning clinics to 37% among some groups of pregnant women. A majority of women clinically diagnosed with BV state they are asymptomatic.[30]

Pathophysiology. The exact etiology of BV is unknown but is thought to be a disruption of normal vaginal flora that is associated with sexual contact. *Gardnerella vaginalis* and various anaerobes, including *Mycoplasma hominis, Bacteroides*, and *Mobiluncus*, interact and proliferate when lactobacilli (the normal predominant vaginal flora) are decreased or absent. Bacteria adhere to vaginal epithelium and form a scaffolding-like biofilm to which other bacteria can adhere, facilitating their proliferation and causing a noninflammatory response in the surrounding tissues.[31] As the vaginal microbiome changes, catabolic enzymes degrade proteins into amines which elevate the vaginal pH and produce the characteristic fish-like odor associated with BV. BV has been implicated in PID, chorioamnionitis, preterm labor, and postpartum endometritis. In addition, BV increases a woman's risk of contracting other STIs, such as HIV.[30]

Clinical Manifestations. BV is characterized by a thin, gray, homogeneous, and malodorous discharge that adheres to the vaginal walls but is often copious enough to drain from the vagina. Occasionally, the discharge is bubbly or frothy. The normal vaginal pH is usually 5 to 5.5. Because odor is intensified by contact with alkaline secretions, including semen (pH 5.2 to 8.2) and menstrual discharge (pH 6.3 to 6.9), women often complain of a strong, foul, fish-like vaginal odor particularly after intercourse and during menses. Male and female partners of infected women may harbor the microorganisms responsible for BV but have no signs or symptoms.

Evaluation and Treatment. Diagnosis of BV can be made on the basis of the presence of three of four of the following criteria, known as *Amsel criteria:* (1) the presence of homogeneous, adherent gray or white vaginal discharge; (2) a vaginal pH greater than 4.5; (3) a positive amine odor in the presence of an alkali, such as potassium hydroxide, known as the *whiff test;* and (4) the presence of clue cells on wet mount.[30] *Clue cells* are considered pathognomonic for BV. They are vaginal epithelial cells that are covered with bacteria, causing them to look as if they were sprinkled with pepper. The saline wet mount also may show the absence of lactobacilli and few or no leukocytes. There also is a commercially available test, Affirm VPIII, that uses DNA hybridization to detect *G. vaginalis*. Cultures for BV are not recommended; however, high-risk individuals should be screened for gonorrhea and chlamydia.[30]

The most commonly used treatment for BV is a course of oral metronidazole (Flagyl), 500 mg twice daily for 7 days; 0.75% metronidazole vaginal gel, once daily for 5 days; or clindamycin cream 2% applied vaginally for 7 days.[30] Alternative regimens include tinidazole, 2 g orally once daily for 2 days or 1 g orally for 5 days; oral clindamycin, 300 mg twice daily for 7 days; or clindamycin ovules, 100 mg intravaginally for 3 days.[30] Treatment for BV should be personalized based on the woman's needs and behaviors. For example, metronidazole and tinidazole strongly react with alcohol and should not be used by women who cannot or will not eliminate alcohol ingestion for the full duration of treatment plus an additional 24 hours. In addition, the ovules can weaken latex condoms and diaphragms. Women who are asymptomatic for BV do not need treatment.[30]

BV treatment in women infected with HIV is the same as that in individuals who are HIV negative. The CDC currently recommends treatment of symptomatic BV in pregnancy to reduce the risk of poor perinatal outcomes, including preterm birth.[30]

Chlamydia

Chlamydia is the common name for infections caused by *C. trachomatis*. *C. trachomatis* is responsible for a variety of syndromes, including acute urethral syndrome, nongonococcal urethritis (NGU), mucopurulent cervicitis, and PID. Chlamydia is a leading cause of preventable infertility and ectopic pregnancy. In 2019, with more than 1.8 million new cases of infections reported, chlamydia was the most common reportable STI in the United States.[32] Because chlamydia is often asymptomatic, it is estimated that just over a million unreported infections occur annually. This represents a 19% increase since 2014.[1] Rates of chlamydia infections are increasing in all age groups, areas of the country, and racial/ethnic groups. This increase probably reflects the continued expansion of screening efforts and the increased use of more sensitive diagnostic tests, as well as an actual increase in incidence.[33] The majority of reported cases of chlamydia are in people younger than 26 years old, but the incidence in older adults is increasing.[1] Up to 90% of women with *C. trachomatis* infection are asymptomatic, which can delay diagnosis and increase the risk of long-term health sequelae.[33] Without timely treatment, 10% to 20% of women will have the infection spread to the uterus and uterine tubes.[33] Although the rate of chlamydia in men is lower than women, with increased use of urine screening testing, there was an increase of 32.1% in men from 2015 to 2019. This increased number of men include MSM, bisexual, and men who have sex with both men and women.[32]

Risk groups for chlamydia include age younger than 26, recent new sexual partner, and drug use or other risky behaviors.[1] Like gonorrhea, *Chlamydia* infection can be transmitted from mother to infant during birth and can cause eye infections and pneumonia in affected newborns.[33]

Pathophysiology. *C. trachomatis* is a gram-negative obligate intracellular bacterium that lacks the ability to reproduce without a host cell. It is differentiated from other bacteria by its unique two-part growth cycle. The first part consists of an elementary body that is small and resilient and is able to survive extracellularly.[34] Once this elementary body attaches itself to a receptor host cell, it is able to enter by endocytosis. Once inside the cell, the second part of the cycle begins and the microorganism becomes a metabolically active parasite, reproducing within the cell until the cell is destroyed and ruptures, disseminating up to 1000 new elementary bodies. Infection with *C. trachomatis* produces an inflammatory reaction that results in permanent scarring of tissues.[34]

Because they are not part of the normal urogenital tract flora, *Chlamydia* microorganisms are always pathogens even though infection is often asymptomatic. Numerous serotypes, or strains, of *C. trachomatis* have been identified. Some cause urogenital infection; some, blindness; and others, lymphogranuloma venereum (LGV), which is discussed in the next section.[34] The strains of *C. trachomatis* that cause urogenital infection require squamous-columnar and columnar-epithelial cells as hosts. *C. trachomatis* infects and disrupts superficial tissues, causing damage and scarring, but does not seem to invade or destroy deeper tissues.[35]

In newborns, several sites may be inoculated with *Chlamydia* when passing through the infected maternal cervix. These include the eye, nasopharynx, rectum, and vagina. The infant may also aspirate infected secretions with its first breaths, resulting in chlamydial pneumonitis and substantial newborn morbidity.[32]

Clinical Manifestations. Chlamydial infections are asymptomatic in up to 90% of adults.[32] Urogenital infections caused by *Chlamydia* closely parallel those caused by gonorrhea. Both microorganisms infect superficial genital tract tissues, such as mucosa of the urethra and cervix, and both can invade the epididymis, the fallopian/uterine tubes, and (rarely) the hepatic capsule. Table 27.2 lists the pathophysiologic similarities of chlamydial and gonococcal infections. Men and women have different responses to the infection.

The rate of chlamydial infection in men appears to be rising, with a 32.1% increase in diagnoses from 2015 to 2019. The rate of infection among adolescent males (15 to 19 years old) who have sex with women increased by 32.8% in the same time.[32] This increase may be an expression of increased testing as a result of easier screening methods.

Although most men do not have symptoms even while contagious, chlamydial infection can cause NGU. Clinically, urethritis caused by gonorrhea and chlamydia cannot be differentiated: both have a 7- to 21-day incubation period and cause dysuria. Although urethral discharge in men may be similar in the two infections, chlamydial discharge tends to be more clear and gonococcal discharge more purulent. Men might note a clear, mucous discharge or mild burning with urination.

Chlamydial epididymitis can accompany urethritis in men and is characterized by fever and a unilaterally painful, swollen scrotum. Chlamydial infection also causes proctitis (rectal inflammation) in men and women who have receptive anal intercourse. Chlamydial proctitis is generally mild, although it may, like gonorrheal proctitis, cause rectal bleeding, mucous discharge, and diarrhea. Reiter syndrome (urethritis, conjunctivitis,

TABLE 27.2 Similarity of Clinical Syndromes Caused by *Neisseria gonorrhoeae* and *Chlamydia trachomatis*

Site of Infection	CLINICAL SYNDROME	
	N. gonorrhoeae	*C. trachomatis*
Men		
Urethra	Urethritis	Urethritis
Epididymis	Epididymitis	Epididymitis
Rectum	Proctitis	Proctitis
Conjunctiva	Conjunctivitis	Conjunctivitis
Systemic	Disseminated gonococcal infection	Reiter syndrome
Women		
Urethra	Acute urethral syndrome	Acute urethral syndrome
Bartholin gland	Bartholinitis	Bartholinitis
Cervix	Cervicitis	Cervicitis; cervical atypia
Fallopian tube	Salpingitis	Salpingitis
Conjunctiva	Conjunctivitis	Conjunctivitis
Liver capsule	Perihepatitis	Perihepatitis
Systemic	Disseminated gonococcal infection	Arthritis-dermatitis syndrome

Data from Stamm WE, Holmes KK. *Chlamydia trachomatis* infections in the adult. In: Holmes KK, et al., eds. *Sexually transmitted diseases*. 2nd edition. New York: McGraw-Hill; 1990.

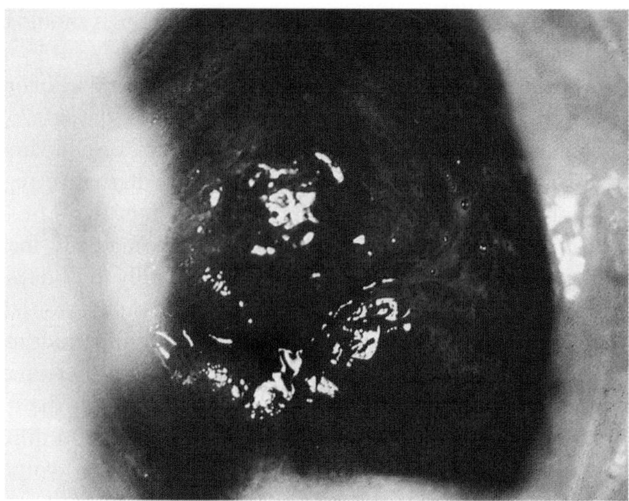

Fig. 27.11 Chlamydial Cervicitis. Beefy red mucosa of columnar epithelium of cervix. (Courtesy Paul Weisner. From Morse SA, et al., eds. *Atlas of sexually transmitted diseases and AIDS*, 4th edition. London: Saunders; 2013.)

arthritis, and characteristic mucocutaneous lesions) is also associated with untreated urogenital tract infections.

C. trachomatis can cause asymptomatic urethral infection or acute urethral syndrome (dysuria, urinary frequency, and presence of sterile pus in the urine) in infected women. Chlamydial infection of Bartholin/greater vestibular glands can cause purulent discharge leading to a Bartholin cyst. Women with chlamydial cervicitis may be asymptomatic or may have a yellow mucopurulent discharge from the cervical os and a hypertrophic, edematous, and friable area of cervical ectopy. The woman also may report intermenstrual or postcoital spotting. Although ectopy alone does not indicate a pathologic condition, an erythematous, raw, and friable cervix is suggestive of chlamydial cervicitis (Fig. 27.11).

Chlamydia infection is the leading cause of tubal infertility in women because of infectious damage to the fallopian tubes like that which may occur with gonorrhea. Risk factors for infertility include the duration and severity of infection and the lifetime number of chlamydial infections. Even women with asymptomatic salpingitis have a risk of subsequent infertility.[32]

The most common manifestations of chlamydial infections in the newborn are conjunctivitis and pneumonia. Prophylactic treatment with antibiotic eye ointment at birth does not provide complete protection against neonatal conjunctivitis and does not protect against neonatal pneumonia. IV antibiotics are needed for any child at risk of acquisition. Chlamydial conjunctivitis begins between 5 and 14 days after delivery, when the infant's eyes begin to water. This discharge may become purulent, and both eyes may become red and swollen.

Scarring of the conjunctivae may result, but this infection does not cause blindness. Infants with chlamydial pneumonia develop staccato coughing spells, nasal congestion, and fever at 3 to 11 weeks of age.

Evaluation and Treatment. Since most infections are asymptomatic, the CDC recommends widespread screening of at-risk groups. A complete detailing of groups needing annual screening can be found in their treatment guideline, on their website, or through their smartphone app.[32] All sexually active women who are 25 years old or younger should be screened annually. In addition, the CDC recommends that all women, regardless of age, be screened if they have a new sexual partner or their partner is not monogamous. Pregnant women should be routinely screened for *Chlamydia* at least once during pregnancy.[32]

Methods for diagnosing chlamydial infections include tissue culture, direct chlamydial EIA, fluorescein-labeled monoclonal antibody tests, and NAAT. Currently, tests using chlamydia-specific NAAT are the most sensitive and cost-effective tests available. In addition, NAAT is easy to use with a variety of specimen types.[32] Concurrent testing for gonorrhea can be done using the same swab. NAAT can be performed on samples taken from the vagina, endocervix, or urethra, or urine specimens can be used. The person should be tested from all locations of genital contact. The ease of NAAT testing means that screening can be performed without a clinician, if needed, because the individual can collect the specimen following basic instructions.[32]

C. trachomatis is susceptible to inexpensive, readily accessible antibiotics, and treatment should begin as soon as possible to prevent complications. Treatment includes antibiotic therapy for infected individuals and all sexual contacts. Abstinence or use of condoms during treatment and for 7 days after treatment is recommended. The CDC recommends observed, on-site treatment for both partners when feasible.[32]

Oral doxycycline, 100 mg twice daily for 7 days is the preferred treatment for chlamydial infection among adolescents and adults. Alternate regimens include azithromycin , 1 g given orally, as a single dose, or a 7-day course of oral levofloxacin 500 mg once daily for 7 days. Single-dose azithromycin is preferred if adherence to a multiple-dose, multiple-day regimen is not feasible for the individual. In pregnancy, oral azithromycin 1 g in a single dose is the drug of choice. A test of cure is needed only if there is concern that treatment of both partners was not successful. However, treatment failures are common, especially with multidose regimens and when the partner is not immediately provided with a prescription.[32]

Lymphogranuloma Venereum

C. trachomatis (invasive serovars of strains L1, L2, or L3) can cause a chronic STI known as lymphogranuloma venereum, which may be confused with syphilis, herpes, or chancroid. LGV was previously rare in the developed world but now is increasingly found in MSM and may spread to other populations.[36] The infection is acquired during sexual intercourse or through contact with contaminated exudate from active lesions. HIV infection increases the likelihood of acquisition and the severity of symptoms.[37] Because there is an increasing incidence of LGV in HIV-negative men, universal screening of MSM is recommended.[38]

Pathophysiology. The strain of *C. trachomatis* that causes LGV probably penetrates skin and mucous membranes through tiny abrasions. LGV spreads to genital and rectal lymphatic tissue, where it causes marked inflammation, necrosis, buboes, abscesses of inguinal lymph nodes, and infection of surrounding tissues. Healing occurs by fibrosis after several weeks or months and results in scarring, damaging the lymph nodes and disrupting their function. LGV can cause permanent lymphatic disruption and genital disfigurement. Affected nodes become chronically swollen, hardened, and enlarged. *C. trachomatis* also spreads systemically through the bloodstream and can enter the CNS.[8]

Clinical Manifestations. The primary lesion of LGV appears after an incubation period of 5 to 21 days. The lesion is most commonly a herpetiform (multivesicular) ulcer, but it can assume various forms. The ulcer generally is asymptomatic and inconspicuous and heals rapidly, leaving no scar. However, when contracted through receptive anal intercourse (a common current mode of transmission), the ulcer is never visible. When rectal infection occurs, LGV can cause an inflammatory response that mimics inflammatory bowel disease or proctocolitis.[8] Other signs of primary LGV include a large, tender lymphatic nodule (especially unilateral) or bubo, urethritis, and cervicitis. Although historically this infection resulted in three clinical stages, anorectal infection has become the most common location of infection and results in symptoms that mimic other primary care conditions.[27]

Clinical symptoms of anorectal infection mimic other inflammatory bowel conditions and include irregular bowel movements, multiple ulcerations of the rectal mucosa, mucopurulent rectal discharge, and rectovaginal fistulae in women. Individuals may have fever, rectal pain, and tenesmus. Rectal strictures, perirectal abscesses, and anal fissures may develop with untreated infection.[8]

Evaluation and Treatment. Clinical manifestations, history of sexual intercourse, and laboratory tests are used for LGV diagnosis. LGV is diagnosed with NAAT testing at the suspected site of infection. If clinical symptoms match LGV presentation, pharmacologic treatment should begin while waiting definitive diagnosis with test results.[36] The recommended treatment for LGV is oral doxycycline, 100 mg twice daily for 21 days. An alternative 21-day course of erythromycin base 500 mg four times daily or azithromycin 1 g orally once a week for 3 weeks also is effective. Sexual partners within the past 60 days should be treated.[36] Pregnant/lactating women should be treated with erythromycin or azithromycin. Persons with HIV are treated using the same but possibly prolonged treatment protocols as if they were HIV negative.

Viral Infections

Genital Herpes

Genital herpes, which causes painful blisters (cold sores), is a chronic, lifelong viral infection and is the most common infectious cause of genital ulcerations in the United States. Although HSV is not a reportable disease, the CDC reports that approximately 572,000 new individuals are infected each year.[39]

Recurrent infections are mostly asymptomatic (50% to 70%) and affect an estimated 50 million Americans annually.[1] Eighty percent of infected individuals do not know they have herpes. Genital herpes can be caused by either of the two serotypes of HSV: HSV-1 or HSV-2. Historically, HSV-1 lesions were more common around the mouth, whereas HSV-2 lesions were more frequently found in the genital area. However, both HSV-1 and HSV-2 are increasingly found in both the oral and the anogenital area.[1] HSV-2 outbreaks are more frequent and more severe, so serologic testing to determine the HSV subtype is warranted at diagnosis to guide suppression efforts.[8]

HSV infection is transmitted through contact with HSV-infected fluids or skin as occurs with genital skin or mucosal contact with a person shedding the virus. There is even the possibility that saliva alone can transmit the virus when placed on mucous membranes or genitals for lubrication.[40] Persons without symptoms probably transmit most infections. Asymptomatic viral shedding occurs on approximately 10% of days compared with 20% of days for those who are symptomatic. Transmission rates are not well identified. However, women and men who are the receptive partner for men are more susceptible to contracting herpes related to prolonged semen contact with the vaginal or rectal mucosa. Any type of rough intercourse that causes breaks in the skin surface increases transmission as well. It is estimated that a woman has an 80% to 90% risk of developing genital herpes after being exposed to an infected man.

Condoms reduce the risk of transmission, especially from males to females.[41] However, if lesions or shedding occur outside the area covered by the condom, transmission can still occur.[41] Female condoms offer a bit more protection from HSV because they cover and protect the vulva, but they do not eliminate risk. HSV infection greatly increases the risk of HIV acquisition. People with HSV are two to four times more likely to contract HIV if exposed, potentially because of skin splits that occur as a result of HSV infection.[39]

Neonatal infections can begin in utero or, more commonly, during the intrapartum or postpartum period. The risk of transmission of HSV to the neonate varies from less than 1% among women with recurrence of known herpes at term to up to 30% to 50% in women who acquire HSV near term.[39] Perinatal transmission can cause extensive morbidity and mortality. Intrauterine transmission is rare (only 5% of neonatal infections) but can occur through transplacental or ascending infection and can cause fetal malformations.[42]

Eighty-five percent of infections are transmitted during the intrapartum period.[42] Infants are at greatest risk if the mother has a primary infection acquired near the time of delivery rather than a recurrent infection or an infection acquired during the first half of pregnancy.[1] Ruptured membranes have a role in the development of HSV. Rupture of membranes for more than 4 hours increases the risk of the fetus contracting HSV. Internal fetal monitoring devices also increase the risk of vertical transmission because they break the fetal skin. Infants also may be exposed after birth through mouth-to-mouth kissing by family members; there have been several cases of infants exposed during ritual circumcision involving direct orogenital suction.[43]

Pathophysiology. After initial exposure and entry of the virus at mucocutaneous sites or abraded skin, the virus undergoes replication locally in the dermis and epidermis. This leads to cell destruction, transudation, and vesicle formation. The virus spreads to contiguous cells and eventually into sensory nerves. This process often causes a systemic, inflammatory immune response, especially with HSV-2 infection, that includes fever and malaise. In rare cases, the herpes can cause CNS manifestations. Painful lesions can last from days to weeks. Eventually, the virus is transported through the axon to the dorsal root, where it remains in a latent stage until it becomes reactivated. After oral infection, the latent virus resides in the trigeminal ganglion; after genital infection, the virus resides in the dorsal sacral nerve roots. During the latent period, the viral genome is maintained in the host cell nucleus without causing cell death.

Reactivation of latent infections often occurs during times of physical or emotional stress causing a recurrent infection. Compared with HSV-1 infections, reactivation of the HSV-2 infection is twice as common, and the likelihood of HSV-2 recurrent infections is 8 to 10 times that of HSV-1. Reactivation of HSV is not well understood but may be attributable to physical, hormonal, and immunologic stimuli. During reactivation, the viral genomes are transported through the peripheral sensory nerves back to the dermal surface.

Shedding of the virus occurs during outbreaks and also may occur when the person is asymptomatic, increasing the likelihood of transmission. Antiviral medications decrease asymptomatic viral shedding and should be considered as an adjunct to safe sex practices.

Clinical Manifestations. Three distinct syndromes associated with HSV infection are first-episode primary genital infection, first-episode non–primary HSV, and recurrent infections. The manifestations of each one depend on the individual's immune state. First-episode primary genital infection occurs when an individual has no antibodies to HSV-1 or HSV-2. Many primary infections with HSV are asymptomatic or the symptoms are not severe enough to warrant medical attention. If symptoms occur, the individual may have small (1 to 2 mm), multiple, vesicular lesions at the site of infection, usually on the labia minora, fourchette, penis, or mouth (Fig. 27.12). They also may appear on the cervix, buttocks, and thighs and are often painful and pruritic. These lesions usually last about 10 to 20 days. The lesions of HSV-1 and HSV-2 can be very small and almost indistinguishable to the naked eye or large and clustered into raw areas. These wet lesions actively shed virus for approximately 10 to 14 days, after which they heal by reepithelialization. Small lesions may coalesce into larger ulcers and become secondarily infected.

Systemic manifestations such as fever, malaise, myalgia, lymphadenopathy, and urinary retention often accompany primary HSV infection. Pharyngitis, aseptic meningitis,

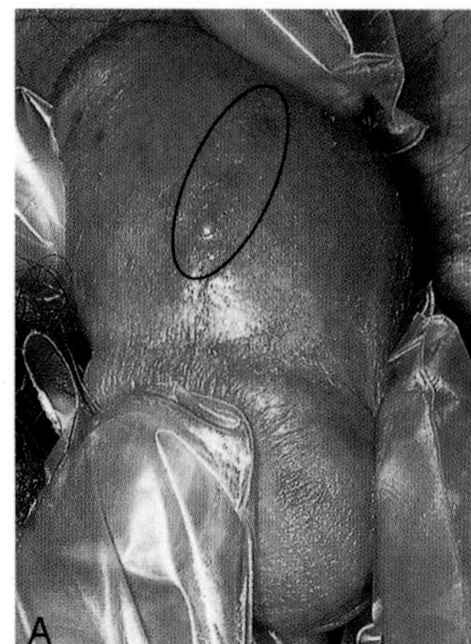

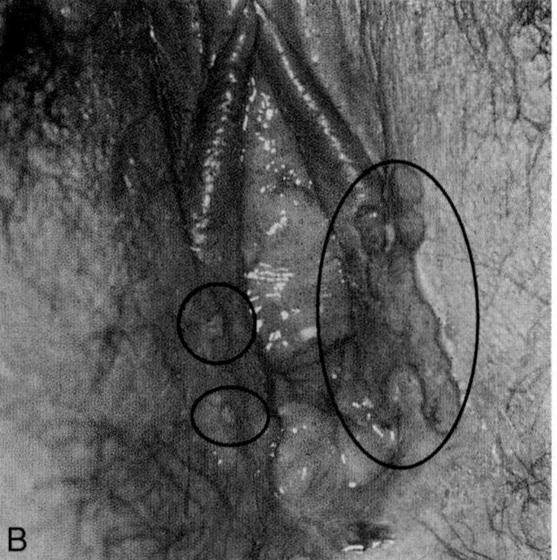

Fig. 27.12 Herpes Lesions. (A) Herpetic vesicles on the penis. **(B)** Herpetic ulceration of the vulva. (A, From McMillan A, Scott GR. *Sexually transmitted infections*, 2nd edition. London: Churchill Livingstone; 2000. B, From Morse SA, et al., eds. *Atlas of sexually transmitted diseases and AIDS*, 4th edition. London: Saunders; 2013.)

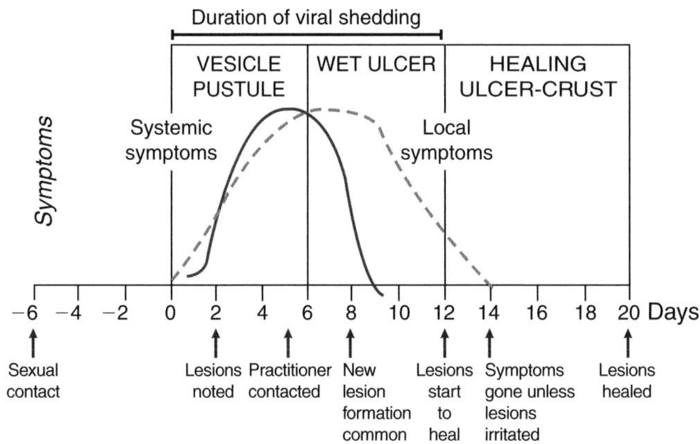

Fig. 27.13 Clinical Course of Primary Genital Herpes. (From Corey L. Genital herpes. In: Holmes KK, et al., eds. *Sexually transmitted diseases*, 2nd edition. New York: McGraw-Hill; 1990.)

and hepatitis also may accompany primary HSV infection. Fig. 27.13 illustrates the clinical course of primary genital HSV.

First-episode non–primary genital HSV occurs in individuals who have preexisting antibodies. In some individuals, the primary infection may not have had any clinical manifestations, but the HSV virus has become latent in the nerve root and can reactivate later in life. Compared with primary infection, the first episode of non–primary HSV is often milder with fewer lesions that are less painful and heal faster. Fewer systemic manifestations occur, and viral shedding is of shorter duration. However, the symptoms may be severe if the second infection occurs during a period of immunocompromised health status.

Recurrent infections usually produce mild local symptoms. The number of lesions is greatly reduced, and the lesions are less painful. Lesions are often unilateral, with crusting within 4 to 5 days. Recovery and healing are usually complete within 10 days. Asymptomatic viral shedding can occur with both HSV-1 and HSV-2 but is more common with HSV-2.[39]

Individuals infected with HSV-2 are more likely to experience recurrent infections. Recurrent infections occur on an average of five to eight times per year but may be more frequent in the first few years of infection. Individuals may experience prodromal symptoms (e.g., pruritus, tingling, dysesthesias) a few hours to 2 days before the eruption of lesions. Women may experience a vaginal discharge and dysuria, and 44% of men have dysuria.

Symptomatic HSV infection of the newborn may occur any time in the first month of life. Manifestations range from a local infection of the eyes, skin, or mucous membranes to a severe disseminated infection with CNS involvement. Approximately 70% of affected infants present with skin lesions. CNS involvement includes seizures and is associated with a mortality of more than 50% and extensive neurologic sequelae in survivors.[42]

Evaluation and Treatment. Genital HSV infection is suggested if typical genital lesions are present; painful genital lesions alone are enough to begin treatment. The CDC recommends serologic testing for diagnosis and to determine the virus subtype because the prognosis and the risk of transmission differ. Diagnosis of HSV-1 and HSV-2 with polymerase chain reaction (PCR) is much more rapid (6 to 14 hours) and more cost effective compared with previous viral cultures (7 to 14 days).

There is no cure for HSV, only symptom management and viral suppression treatments. All primary outbreaks should be treated with antiviral medications to prevent complications and speed healing.[44] Oral acyclovir, valacyclovir, penciclovir, and famciclovir are used for primary and periodic outbreaks and to prevent recurrences. Acyclovir has a better safety profile for pregnant and nursing women, but there is ongoing research supporting the safety of valacyclovir as well. IV acyclovir is reserved for very ill or severely immunocompromised individuals.[44]

Suppressive treatment is recommended for individuals with frequent or severe outbreaks and pregnant women at term with a history of herpes.[45] Suppressive treatment also may reduce asymptomatic viral shedding, decreasing transmission to sexual partners and infants born vaginally. Although there are few side effects with suppression drugs, the decision to take daily medication is complex for many individuals. Although male and female condoms offer some protection, individuals with HSV should refrain from all genital or oral contact when prodromal or symptomatic and understand that an undetermined risk of transmission exists even during asymptomatic periods.

Human Papillomavirus Infection

HPV infection is the most common symptomatic viral STI in the United States. Although more than 5.5 million cases are diagnosed yearly, the prevalence of 24 million cases is considered underestimated because HPV infection is often subclinical. More sensitive measures of HPV indicate that 50% of all sexually active people are infected with the virus at some point in their lives, although these numbers are expected to decrease sharply in response to widespread vaccination. The virus is easily transmissible through direct contact with lesions or infected secretions. Vertical transmission in utero and during vaginal birth also is possible.[46,47]

Approximately 150 different types of HPV have been identified.[48] More than 40 serotypes are unique to the stratified squamous epithelia of the anogenital area, although research is finding these same subtypes also may infect the oropharynx.[49] These are divided into high-risk serotypes (high risk of causing cancer) and low-risk serotypes (associated with benign genital lesions or warts: condylomata acuminata of the vulva, vagina, penis, and perianal areas).

Serotypes 6 and 11 are associated with 90% of genital warts. These low-risk, or nononcogenic, subtypes can coexist with the high-risk types but do not cause cancer independently. Genital warts are very contagious, with transmission rates among individuals estimated to be between 38% and 95%. Such a wide range is attributable to the subclinical nature of some infections and various influencing factors that include number of exposures, HPV type, location of lesions, and cellular immunity response.

High-risk, or oncogenic, types 16 and 18 are the most common, causing up to 70% of anogenital cancers (cervical, penile, vulvar, vaginal, anal), and are highly associated with oropharyngeal cancers (see Chapters 12, 13, and 25).[1] HPV-related cancers of the anogenital and oropharynx areas are more common than ovarian cancer in women and more common than brain cancer in men. In future generations, most of these cancers can be prevented through vaccination before HPV exposure.[49]

HPV infection is closely associated with multiple sexual partners and early onset of sexual activity and is most common in teens and young adults 16 to 25 years of age. Fortunately, most cases of HPV are transient, and 70% of healthy individuals will spontaneously eliminate the virus.[50] The persistence of the virus and the immune response play a role in the development of cancer following HPV exposure. Behaviors and conditions that affect overall health status affect the body's ability to clear HPV infection. Alcohol use, smoking, and HIV infection are strongly correlated with persistent HPV infection.[50]

Although three approved vaccines are available to protect against HPV (2-, 4-, and 9-valent), only the 9-valent vaccine is currently available in the United States.[48] Approved vaccines use noninfectious virus-like particles to induce an immune response. The CDC advises using the 9-valent vaccine because of greater prevention capability and cost-effectiveness.[48]

Routine HPV vaccination is recommended for all adolescents at age 11 or 12 but can start as early as age 11, with catch-up vaccination through age 26 if not previously vaccinated. If vaccination is begun before age 15, a two-dose schedule is recommended. For unvaccinated persons 27 to 45 years, the decision for vaccination is based on risk factors and shared decision making between provider and patent. For immunocompromised persons regardless of age, a three-dose vaccine schedule is recommended.[48] Prevention of HPV acquisition in young adults is important because they are more likely than older adults to contract STIs and because the cervix of younger women is more vulnerable to HPV. Public health officials are hopeful that vaccination of boys and girls before they become sexually active will decrease the burden of HPV infection in the future. Preliminary data suggest the effects of widespread vaccination that began in 2006 are already becoming apparent (Box 27.5).[51,52] There are even some reports that vaccination of pregnant women can decrease vertical transmission during vaginal birth because maternal antibodies to HPV cross the placenta.[53]

The immune system is prepared to eliminate the virus through the immune response when previously vaccinated. When an individual has not been vaccinated, he or she may or may not be able to clear this viral infection. Although most HPV subtypes are not associated with abnormal cellular growth, high-risk HPV subtypes cause cellular changes that can lead to cell proliferation, causing warts or cancer.

Pathophysiology. HPV is a nonenveloped, circular, double-stranded DNA virus.[50] Transmission of the virus occurs through close physical contact with infected skin, mucosa, or fluids; however, the exact transmissibility of the virus into the cell is unknown. The initial infection follows trauma to the epithelium that allows the virus to reach and infect the basal cells of the epithelium, which appear to be supportive of viral propagation. Such minor trauma may occur during sexual intercourse. HPV may enter the nuclear DNA and change the expression of cell proteins, leading either to increased but noncancerous cell growth (e.g., warts) or to unchecked cell growth (e.g., cancer). It is not known exactly why some HPV serotypes are cleared from cells whereas other serotypes cause cellular transformations, but immune response and other cofactors play a role.[50] HPV infection may occur months to years before symptoms appear, such as warts or precancerous lesions.

Clinical Manifestations. Genital warts, condylomata acuminata, are soft, skin-colored, white-pink to red-brown discrete growths. They may occur singly or in clusters, may be broad at the base or pedunculated, and may be feathery or smooth. Sometimes the warts enlarge to form cauliflower-like masses on the male frenulum, glans, foreskin, urinary meatus, shaft, scrotum, or anus and on the female labia, clitoris, perineum, vagina, or anus (Fig. 27.14). Although the lesions are usually not painful, they may cause dyspareunia (painful intercourse) and may be friable and bleed easily. Some individuals complain of pruritus. Common locations for condylomata are the on the

BOX 27.5 Human Papillomavirus Vaccine

Every year in the United States:

- Nearly 1 in 4 adults have at least one strain of human papillomavirus (HPV).
- About 12,000 women are diagnosed with HPV-related cervical cancer.
- Almost 4000 women die from HPV-related cervical cancer.
- About 1900 men are diagnosed with HPV-related penile or anal cancer.

Vaccines are available in the United States to vaccinate 2, 4, or 9 strains of high-risk HPV:

- Vaccines are recommended for females and males beginning at age 11 years and up to age 26 depending on gender and risk factors.
- The Centers for Disease Control and Prevention (CDC) currently recommends children ages 11–12 years receive two doses of HPV vaccine rather than the previously recommended three doses; the second dose should be given 6–12 months after the first dose.
- Vaccines are highly effective in preventing high-risk HPV types associated with cervical cancer; they have been proven safe and effective by the CDC, with ongoing safety monitoring.
- Vaccines are not recommended for pregnant women because their safety is not yet established, but preliminary reports suggest that HPV vaccination in pregnancy may decrease vertical transmission during vaginal birth.
- Vaccinated women still need cervical cancer screening at regular intervals.
- The three-injection vaccine series is covered by most insurance plans, Medicaid, and the Vaccines for Children (VFC) program if individuals meet eligibility requirements, including age and financial need.

For more information, visit the Centers for Disease Control and Prevention (CDC). STD website at www.cdc.gov/std/default.htm.
Data from Centers for Disease Control and Prevention (CDC). *Human Papillomavirus (HPV)*. Atlanta, GA: U.S. Department of Health and Human Services; 2022. https://www.cdc.gov/hpv/hcp/schedules-recommendations.html#:~:text=HPV%20vaccination%20provides%20the%20most,vaccinated%20when%20they%20were%20younger. Accessed February 21, 2022; Centers for Disease Control and Prevention (CDC). *Multi-, Routine-, & Non-Routine-Vaccine VISs*. Atlanta, GA: U.S. Department of Health and Human Services; 2022. www.cdc.gov/vaccines/hcp/vis/index.html.

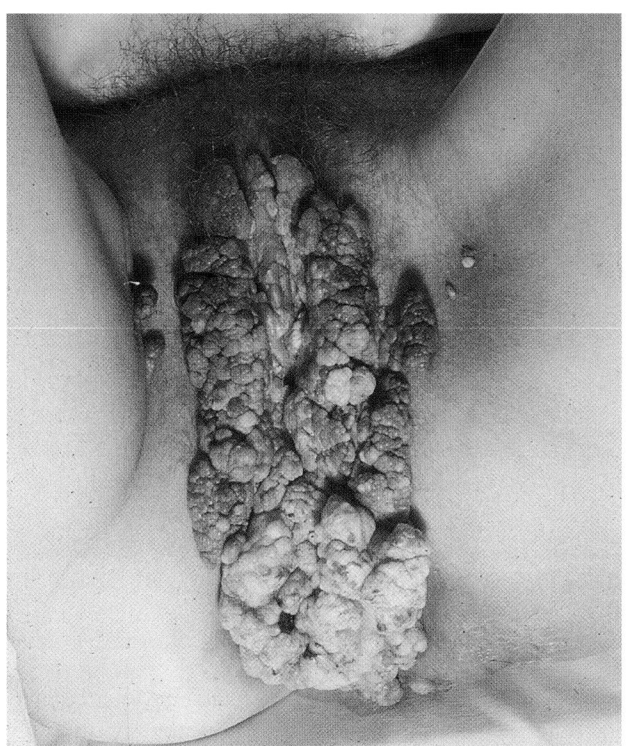

Fig. 27.14 Condylomata Acuminata—Vulva and Perineum. The clinical diagnosis was giant condylomata. Such large and confluent lesions should be carefully examined and multiple biopsies obtained to rule out underlying malignancy. (From Morse SA, et al., eds. *Atlas of sexually transmitted diseases and AIDS*, 4th edition. London: Saunders; 2013.)

vaginal introitus, the shaft of the penis, and under the foreskin. However, warts can be in any location infected by HPV along the reproductive tract, anus, and oropharynx.[8,31] Laryngeal papillomas can occur in infants and children whose mothers had genital warts at the time of delivery. Clinical manifestations of laryngeal warts include stridor, hoarseness, abnormal cry, cough, and respiratory distress.[53]

Precancerous changes related to HPV often do not have any visible manifestations. Because the lesions are not painful early detection is often hampered. In addition, cervical and anal cancers may not cause symptoms until late into the disease process. Routine screening for cervical cancer (see later) was begun to increase early detection since clinical symptoms are minimal.

Evaluation and Treatment. In general, the diagnosis of condylomata acuminata is made based on clinical manifestations. Verrucous, fleshy-pink lesions caused by HPV must be differentiated from condylomata lata (the whitish gray, flat lesions) of secondary syphilis. Because HPV infection often accompanies other STIs, testing for gonorrhea, chlamydia, and syphilis and wet prep for other vaginal organisms should be performed.

Treatments for external genital warts are considered cosmetic—not curative—and include individual-applied therapies (podofilox, imiquimod, and sinecatechins) and provider-administered therapies (cryotherapy, podophyllin resin, trichloroacetic acid [TCA], bichloroacetic acid [BCA], and surgery). Vaginal, urethral, or anal warts can be treated in the clinic using topical medications, cryotherapy, or surgical excision; the CDC provides specific guidance on therapies based on wart location and pregnancy status. Cervical and anal warts require additional screening to exclude more extensive lesions.[48] Success of treatment depends on response of the immune system. Surgical excision is the treatment for laryngeal warts in infants.

With currently available cytologic technology for cervical cell evaluation, the identification of both nononcogenic and oncogenic strains of HPV is readily available. In women who are unscreened, the identification of cervical cancer may be delayed because of poor innervation of the upper pelvis, allowing cancerous masses to grow large before causing symptoms. The development of the Papanicolaou, or "Pap," smear helped to reduce deaths related to cervical cancer by 80% since the 1950s.[54] Ideally, persistent HPV infections can be identified to encourage greater screening for abnormal cellular changes. The appropriate screening for nongenital HPV infection is controversial because there are no guidelines delineating who should be screened for anal and oropharyngeal infection.

Following the development of the Pap smear, women were advised to have yearly Pap tests to detect cancer. However, over time, it became apparent that, although younger women often had abnormal Pap tests, they were often able to clear HPV infection and resolve cellular changes without treatment. Treatment of women younger than 20 years of age provides little to no benefit in reducing later rates of cervical cancer but results in pain, anxiety, and increased healthcare costs. Therefore the US Preventive Services Health Task Force, the American College of Obstetricians and Gynecologists, and many other national cancer agencies recommended that Pap smear testing begin only after 21 years of age.[55,56]

Women ages 21 to 29 should receive just Pap testing every 3 years, whereas women 30 to 65 years of age may receive Pap testing with HPV screening every 5 years (preferred) or Pap testing alone every 3 years. After 65 years of age, Pap testing and HPV screening are no longer recommended for women with previous normal testing results, because the risk of new malignancy is low. Women who have had a hysterectomy with removal of the uterine cervix for a noncancerous condition do not need Pap smears or HPV testing for the rest of their lives. Although the HPV vaccine does reduce the risk for cervical cancer, it does not change the frequency or need for Pap and HPV testing at this time.[56]

If the results of a Pap test are abnormal, the woman's cervix will be further evaluated using colposcopy, which involves applying 3% acetic acid (vinegar) and using magnification to examine the cervix for changes indicative of cancer or precancerous lesions. HPV-infected cells will appear white when exposed to acetic acid. In some developing countries with limited laboratory facilities, this test alone is used to screen for cervical cancer. Following visual investigation of the cervix during colposcopy, the clinician biopsies suspicious areas for further evaluation. Treatment of precancerous and cancerous lesions varies and involves removal or destruction of the affected cells through excision or ablation.

Although infection with high-risk HPV strains is a risk factor for development of anogenital cancers, as well as cervical cancer, there is no consensus on screening for rectal and anal cancers.[49] Anyone who engages in receptive anal intercourse is at risk for rectal HPV and subsequent development of anal cancer. Women are approximately twice as likely as men to develop anal cancer, but MSM remain at risk.[49] It is hoped that the need for treatment of HPV-related genital conditions will decrease as more children and young adults are vaccinated for HPV before becoming sexually active.[46]

Molluscum Contagiosum

Molluscum contagiosum is a benign viral infection of the skin in children and adults. For detailed information, see Chapter 47. In adults, the disease is more commonly sexually transmitted and affects the lower abdomen, genitalia, and perianal area.[27] Molluscum contagiosum in adults is most common in men 20 to 29 years of age and in those with multiple sexual partners. Treatment for sexually transmitted molluscum contagiosum is the same as that for the nonsexually transmitted form of the disease; the CDC also includes information in their regularly updated guidelines.[8]

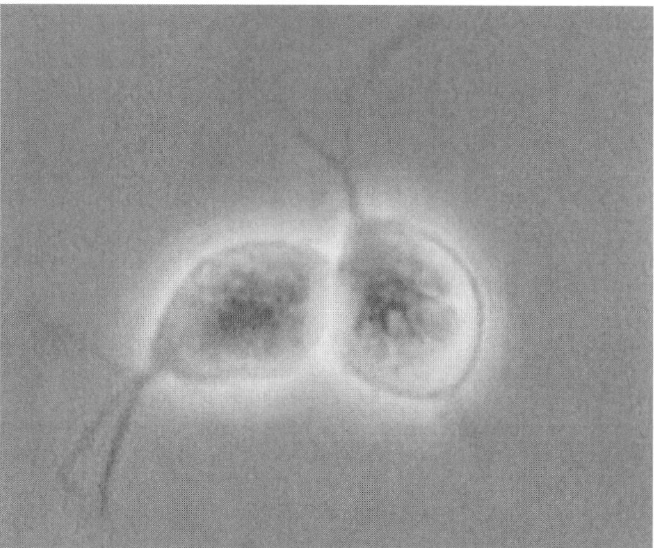

Fig. 27.15 Trichomonas vaginalis. (From CDC Public Health Information Library [PHIL].)

Parasitic Infections

Trichomoniasis

Trichomonas vaginalis, commonly known as "*trich*," is estimated to be the most prevalent nonviral STI worldwide. Trichomonas affects more than 3.7 million people in the United States. Trichomoniasis affects greater than 11% of women older than 40 and is the most common nonviral STI in this age range.[1] The high rate of asymptomatic infection aids the spread of this pathogen. Male-female vaginal intercourse is the most common route of transmission.[1] Although sexual transmission is clearly the most common means of disease spread, transmission through fomites is theoretically possible.

Pathophysiology. *T. vaginalis* is an anaerobic, unicellular, flagellated, parasitic protozoan that adheres to and damages squamous epithelial cells (Fig. 27.15). It is primarily spread through penile-vaginal sex, although anal sex and oral sex could be potential routes of infection.[38] Because this protozoan selectively affects squamous epithelia, the vaginal and urethral tissues in women are often infected, as are periurethral (Skene) and greater vestibular (Bartholin) glands. The endocervical canal is not affected because it is lined with columnar epithelium. In men, the urethra is the most common site of infection, although the protozoans, called trichomonads, can infect the epididymis and (rarely) the prostate. Uncircumcised men are more likely to become infected after exposure than circumcised men.[8] There are no conclusive data that the rectum or the oropharynx is a reservoir for infection.[8]

Clinical Manifestations. Manifestations of vaginal trichomoniasis range from none to severe. Up to 85% of those infected have minimal or no symptoms.[57] Vaginal discharge and internal pruritus are the most common manifestations of infection. Dyspareunia and dysuria also are fairly common. Some women report an increase in symptoms immediately after menses. Vaginal secretions can be copious, frothy, malodorous, and yellow-green to gray-green. On examination, the vaginal walls may appear erythematous and sore. Small, punctate red marks, sometimes called *strawberry spots*, are sometimes visible on the vaginal walls and cervix. Most men with trichomoniasis are asymptomatic but may have scant intermittent discharge, slight pruritus, and mild dysuria.[57]

Evaluation and Treatment. All women reporting abnormal vaginal discharge should be tested for trichomoniasis.[57] NAAT is the most sensitive and specific method for detection of *T. vaginalis* infection. Samples for testing can be obtained from the woman's endocervix, vagina, or urine. Samples for men ideally come from the penile meatus, but urine is acceptable as well. Self-collection of samples is acceptable; some tests have even been shown to be accurately used in self-testing,[57] which can aid diagnosis, especially in cases of recurrence. A microscopic examination of vaginal fluid mixed with saline (wet prep) was previously widely used to detect the presence of this protozoan, but, with a sensitivity of just greater than 50%, the wet prep is much less accurate than NAAT testing.[57] However, this method can be used when other tests are unavailable or cost prohibitive.

On microscopic examination, the ovoid microorganism is slightly larger than a polymorphonuclear leukocyte and has one rounded, flagellated end and one slightly pointed, flagellated end. The flagella give the trichomonads their characteristic twisting motility.

The recommended treatment of choice for trichomoniasis in women is metronidazole 500 mg orally two times daily for 7 days. For men, a single oral 2 g dose of metronidazole (Flagyl) is recommended. An alternative and more expensive regimen for women and men is tinidazole 2 g orally in a single dose. Metronidazole vaginal gel is not recommended.[57] These drugs have intense disulfiram-like reaction which causes severe nausea and vomiting when taken with alcohol; thus individuals must be able to abstain from all alcohol products for 3 days after treatment. Sexual partners, even if asymptomatic, also should be treated. There are high rates of reinfection and the CDC advises a 3-month follow-up after treatment for a test of cure.[8]

T. vaginalis infection in pregnant women is associated with an increased risk of preterm birth through unknown mechanisms that may be linked with inflammation.[58] The 2-g single dose of metronidazole can be used to treat pregnant women. However, it is not clear if treatment improves outcomes and metronidazole therapy may actually increase the rate of preterm delivery.[59,60] An alternative dosing regimen is available for lactating women, or the woman can abstain from breast-feeding for 12 to 24 hours after taking the drug.

Scabies

Scabies, a common parasitic infection caused by *Sarcoptes scabiei*, is spread by close skin-to-skin and sexual contact.[61] Although scabies is more common in children and the elderly than in adults,[61] sexual transmission is the most frequent cause of infection in adults.[8] (Detailed information on scabies is contained in Chapter 47.)

Pathophysiology. The discussion of scabies is presented in Chapter 47.

Clinical Manifestations. The classic symptom of scabies is intense pruritus, which increases at night. Pruritus is a result of a reaction to the presence of the *S. scabiei* mite. This reaction may take weeks with initial infection but only 24 hours if the person has been previously infected. The groin and buttocks are common locations for sexually transmitted scabies. Fig. 27.16 shows the typical sites of scabies burrows. The typical burrow of *S. scabiei* is a short, linear, curved, or S-shaped line (Fig. 27.17). There may be small, erythematous, excoriated larval papules near the burrows. Secondary infections are common and are caused by scratching. Even after successful treatment, some individuals will continue to experience pruritus for several weeks.[61]

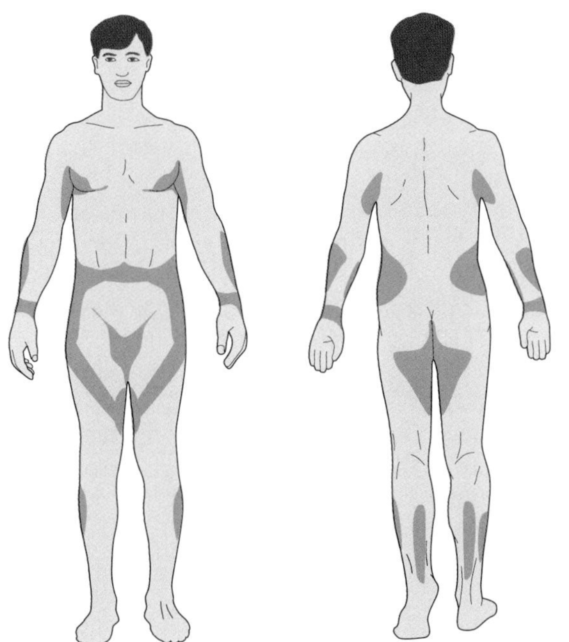

Fig. 27.16 Distribution of Skin Lesions of Sarcoptes scabiei Infestation. Unshaded areas are rarely affected in healthy adults. (From Morse SA, et al., eds. *Atlas of sexually transmitted diseases and AIDS*, 3rd edition. London: Mosby; 2003.)

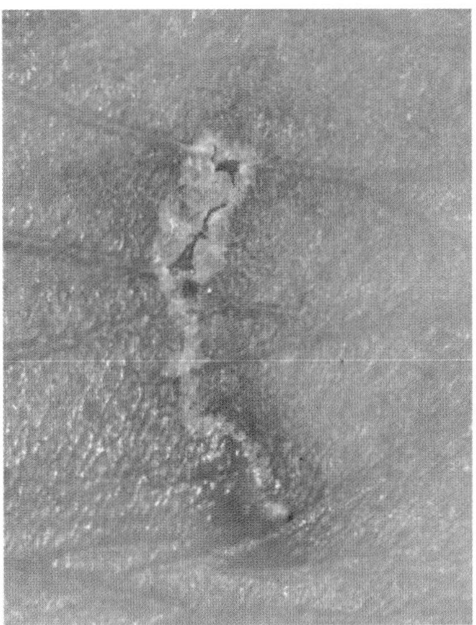

Fig. 27.17 Scabies Burrow. An **S**-shaped burrow with a tiny vesicle at one end. (From Marks JG, Miller JJ. *Lookingbill and Marks' principles of dermatology*, 4th edition. St. Louis: Saunders; 2006.)

Evaluation and Treatment. The diagnosis of scabies is often made clinically when risk factors are present. Microscopic identification of the mite, eggs, larvae, or feces is ideal because the symptoms of scabies can imitate many dermatologic conditions. Superficial scrapings from an intact papule or burrow can be observed under the microscope. An application of 10% potassium hydroxide (KOH) to the skin scrapings facilitates mite visualization.

Preferred treatment is topical application of 5% permethrin massaged into the skin and left for 8 to 14 hours or ivermectin dosed at 200 μg/kg/dose orally and repeat the same dose again in 1 weeks. Ivermectin is an oral antiparasitic agent approved for the treatment of worm infestations. Evidence suggests that oral ivermectin may be a safe and effective treatment for scabies; however, ivermectin is not FDA-approved for this use.[61] Lindane (1%) lotion or cream also is effective if applied thinly to all areas of the body below the neck and washed thoroughly 8 hours after application. Because of its toxicity, lindane should be reserved for those who cannot tolerate any other therapy. Lindane should not be used during pregnancy or on children younger than 10 years old.[61] Pregnant women should be treated with permethrin.[61] Close household and sexual contacts should be examined and treated if infected.[61] To prevent reinfestation, clothing and bed linens should be washed and dried in a machine at high temperatures or kept away from body contact for 72 hours.[61]

Pediculosis Pubis

Pthirus pubis, or crab louse, is one of three species of lice that infest humans. *P. pubis* is commonly transmitted by intimate sexual contact or by contact with infected linens and causes pediculosis pubis, or "crabs." It is highly contagious; there is a 95% chance of contracting lice during a single sexual encounter. Fomites are a common method of infection because crabs can live away from the body for several days. The transfer of lice from pubic hair is probably mechanical, assisted by scratching, fingernails, and towels rather than by self-propulsion. Pubic lice usually infect the perineal and axillary hair and occasionally the hair of the trunk, beard, scalp, and eyelashes.

Pathophysiology. The crab louse has a 25- to 30-day life cycle that consists of five stages, all of which occur on the host: the egg (or nit) stage, three nymphal stages, and an adult stage. The white-gray nits of crab lice, found "glued" to hairs, are oval, 0.8 by 0.3 mm in length and hatch in 5 to 10 days (Fig. 27.18). In the adult stage, pubic lice are gray, are approximately 1 mm in length, and have a segmented body and claws to cling to hairs. They bite into the host's skin to feed on blood, causing itching and pain.

Clinical Manifestations. The mites are visible, facilitating self-identification of infestation. Symptoms range from mild pruritus to severe, intolerable itching, depending on the individual's sensitivity to louse bites. Allergic sensitization occurs in approximately 5 days, when itching, erythema, and inflammation may worsen. Excessive scratching may lead to secondary infection.

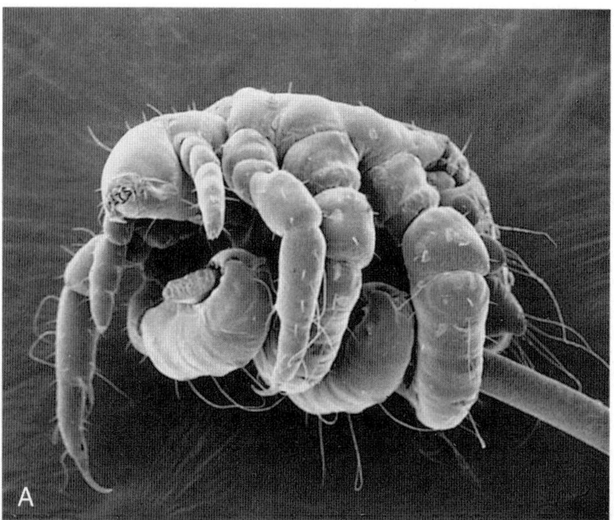

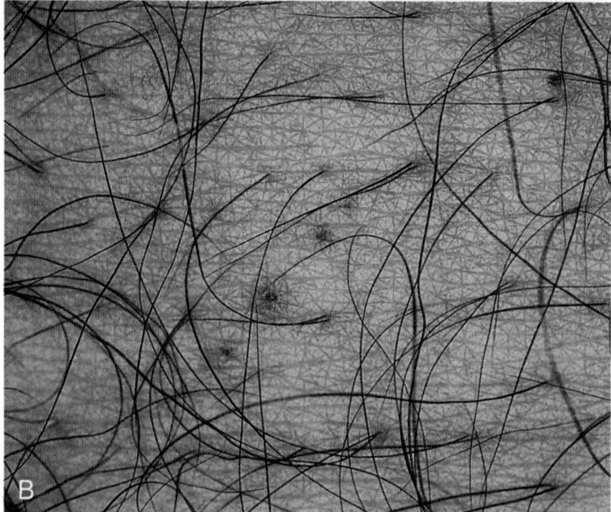

Fig. 27.18 Pubic Louse and Crab Louse. (A) Pubic louse *(Pthirus pubis)* encircling a pubic hair; the claw-like legs produce a firm grip. **(B)** Crab louse bites *(P. pubis)*. (From Morse SA, et al., eds. *Atlas of sexually transmitted diseases and AIDS*, 4th edition. London: Saunders; 2013.)

Evaluation and Treatment. The individual usually presents with a history of itching in the infected area. Because the lice and nits are visible to the naked eye, a thorough clinical examination permits definitive diagnosis. Pediculosis pubis is treated with 1% permethrin cream rinse to the affected areas and washed off after 10 minutes or with piperonyl butoxide, an over-the-counter pyrethrin. For nonocular infections, the pediculicide is applied to infested and adjacent hairy areas and washed off after a specified time. Remaining nits can be removed with a fine-toothed comb. Permethrin is the first line treatment. However, drug resistance is widespread and increasing. Malathion and ivermectin are alternative regimens, although ivermectin does not adequately kill the eggs and requires redosing at 2 weeks. Malathion is undesirable because of its long duration of application and odor. Lindane is a higher-level treatment that should be reserved for when other treatments have failed. Because of the risk of toxicity, lindane cannot be used by pregnant women.[8] Sexual contacts from the past month should be treated regardless of symptoms, and household contacts should be examined and treated if needed. Clothing and bed linens should be machine washed and dried at high temperatures or kept away from body contact for 72 hours.[8]

SEXUALLY TRANSMITTED INFECTIONS OF OTHER BODY SYSTEMS

The effects of some STIs extend beyond the urogenital tract. Many disorders have varied methods of transmission that may include nonsexual means. Although the major mode of transmission may be by oral ingestion or by direct contact with blood or body fluids (e.g., sharing of needles among drug users, blood transfusions, vertical transmission from mother to baby, health worker exposures), infection can be transmitted through intimate sexual contact as well. Anal contact and physically damaging sex can increase the transmission of many of these infections.

Among the most serious of these infections are acquired immunodeficiency syndrome (AIDS) caused by the HIV and hepatitis (all types). Worldwide, the main mode of transmission of HIV and hepatitis B is through sexual intercourse (primarily male female), but nonsexual exposure to infected blood and body fluids, especially through needle sharing, contributes to infection rates. The epidemiology, modes of transmission, pathophysiology, clinical manifestations, and evaluation and treatment of AIDS and hepatitis are discussed in detail in Chapters 10 and 42,respectively.

Sexual transmission of less serious but often debilitating infections, such as shigellosis and giardiasis, and systemic diseases, such as Epstein-Barr virus and cytomegalovirus infections, also can occur, although nonsexual transmission is more common. Table 27.3 provides a list of several gastrointestinal and systemic infections that are known to be transmitted by intimate sexual contact but in which the mode of transmission is primarily through other routes.

TABLE 27.3 Infections With Known Sexual Transmissibility: Main Mode of Transmission by Other Means

Infection/Disease	Main Route of Transmission
Gastrointestinal Infections	
Shigellosis caused by *Shigella* bacteria	Contact with infected feces Hand-to-mouth
Campylobacter enteritis caused by *Campylobacter jejuni* bacteria	Primarily an animal pathogen Hand-to-mouth
Giardiasis caused by *Giardia lamblia* protozoa	Contaminated drinking water Hand-to-mouth
Amebiasis caused by *Entamoeba histolytica* protozoa	Contaminated drinking water Hand-to-mouth
Hepatitides A and C (liver infection and inflammation)	Hepatitis A: contact with infected feces; hand-to-mouth Hepatitis C: blood-borne pathogen; direct exposure to contaminated blood; sexual transmission very uncommon
Systemic Diseases	
Epstein-Barr virus	Mucous membrane (oral) exposure
Cytomegalovirus	Body fluids; exposure via close interpersonal contact or direct transfer
Zika virus	Primary spread through bites from infected mosquitos but may be transmitted sexually and across the placental membrane

EMERGING SCIENCE BOX

Treatment Effectiveness for Hepatitis C

In 2018, it was estimated there were 50,300 cases of acute hepatitis C virus (HCV) in the United States, with an estimated 2.4 million people living with chronic HCV. HCV is primarily transmitted through exposure to infected blood or blood containing body fluids. Although not truly classified as a sexually transmitted infection (STI), the transmission of HCV is spread through sex with an individual when blood is present. This is particularly seen in men who have sex with men, particularly with HIV-positive partners, or with an infected woman during her menstrual cycle. Transmission can also occur from an infected mother to her infant during pregnancy. In 2018, it was estimated there were 50,300 cases of acute HCV in the United States, with an estimated 2.4 million people living with chronic HCV. Of those infected, 5%–25% will develop cirrhosis within 10–20 years, with an additional 1%–4% acquiring hepatocellular carcinoma. Liver failure develops in approximately 5% HCV-infected individuals, of whom 15%–20% will die in the following year.

Currently, HCV is treatable with oral antiviral therapy resulting in cure for more than 90%. Recommended treatment regimens include direct-acting antiviral (DAA) combinations glecaprevir/pibrentasvir (Mavyret) for 8 weeks, sofosbuvir/velpatasvir (Epclusa) for 12 weeks, or ledipasvir/sofosbuvir (Harvoni). In addition, the oral treatment is better tolerated than previously used interferons.

Although these drugs are expensive, the cost savings of treatment is difficult to assess. However, early studies indicate that treatment with DAAs can improve quality of life at a reduced cost for longer periods of time when compared without treatment.

Data from https://www.cdc.gov/hepatitis/hcv/hcvfaq.htm#:~:text=In%202018%2C%20a%20total%20of,C%20cases%20occurred%20in%202018; https://www.cdc.gov/hepatitis/hcv/hcvfaq.htm#d8; https://www.fda.gov/consumers/consumer-updates/hepatitis-c-treatments-give-patients-more-options; Breskin A, Westreich D, Hurt CB, et al. The effects of hepatitis C treatment eligibility criteria on all-cause mortality among people with human immunodeficiency virus. Clinical Infectious Diseases, 2019;69(9):1613–1620. https://doi.org/10.1093/cid/ciz008.

AIDS, Acquired immunodeficiency syndrome; *CNS*, Central nervous system; *HIV*, human immunodeficiency virus.

Hepatitis

Hepatitis is a liver infection that can be caused by six types of viruses: hepatitis A, B, C, D, E, and G. Each virus causes a syndrome of acute, icteric (jaundice-producing) liver inflammation. Additional information about hepatitis is found in Chapter 42. Of the three most common types, A, B, and C, the hepatitis B virus (HBV) is most sexually transmitted. Hepatitis A, like most other predominantly enteric infections, may be considered an STI because of anal-oral transmission, and vaccination is advised for MSM.[62]

Although hepatitis C virus (HCV) is not recognized as an STI, sexual exposure, particularly for individuals with multiple partners, MSM, and individuals with HIV, increases risk of transmission (Fig. 27.19) (see Emerging Science Box: Treatment Effectiveness for Hepatitis C).[63,64]

Hepatitis B prevalence varies dramatically worldwide, with some geographic areas having more than 10% of the population infected with the virus.[65] There are an estimated 21,600 new cases of HBV infection in the United States each year, and more than 2.2 million people are chronically infected.[66]

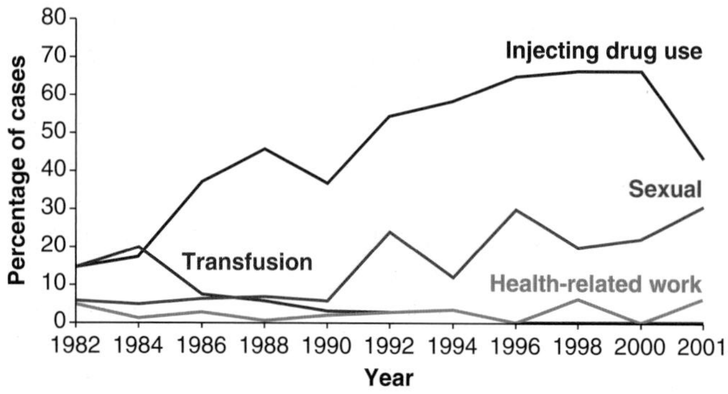

Fig 27.19 Risk for Hepatitis C Exposure. Comparison of injecting drug use *(blue)*, transfusions *(purple)*, health-related work *(green)*, and sexual exposure *(red)*. Note the rise in sexually transmitted incidences. (From Centers for Disease Control and Prevention [CDC]. *Hepatitis C: What Clinicians and Other Health Professionals Need to Know*, 2000. www.cdc.giv/ncid/diseases/hepatitis/c_training/edu/intro.)

Those at risk for HBV infection in the United States are infants born to hepatitis-infected mothers, healthcare workers, individuals who have sex with HBV-infected persons, people with diabetes, and immigrants from areas of high HBV prevalence.[66] Widespread screening of pregnant women and vaccination of all infants since 1991 have decreased the rate of infection in the United States by more than 80% and are expected to have lasting effects into future decades.[67] Vaccination of healthcare workers also has decreased infection rates.[68]

Transmission of HBV can occur through needle puncture, blood transfusion, cuts or abrasions in the skin, and absorption by mucosal surfaces. Direct contact with infected body fluids, such as semen and vaginal fluid, may transmit the infection. HBV can survive dry and outside the body for up to 1 week, making it easily infectious on fomites.

In the United States, seropositivity generally increases with age.[66] This is a function of more time for exposure as well as the lack of routine vaccination before the 1990s. However, the younger a person is when he or she contracts the virus, the greater likelihood of chronic infection.[62] Perinatal transmission of HBV is relatively common, especially in developed countries without routine screening of pregnant women. Neonates whose mothers are infectious have a 90% chance of becoming chronically infected with HBV during labor or delivery if they do not receive treatment but a 1% risk if they receive adequate treatment.[68] Infants of infected mothers should receive HBV vaccine and immunoglobulin against hepatitis within 12 hours of birth to reduce risk. The vaccine and immunoglobulin combination successfully prevents chronic carrier status in 99% of infants.[68] Although HBV is in many maternal body fluids, it is not found in breast milk, and breast-feeding is still encouraged for mothers with HBV.[69] More information about the pathology, diagnosis, and treatment of hepatitis is covered in Chapter 42.

Acquired Immunodeficiency Syndrome

Epidemiology, modes of transmission, pathophysiology, clinical manifestations, and evaluation and treatment of AIDS are discussed in detail in Chapter 10.

SUMMARY REVIEW

Sexually Transmitted Urogenital Infections

1. Sexually transmitted diseases many be more common in certain populations related to increased physiologic risk for acquisition (e.g., with younger women or with men who have sex with men) or insufficient access to quality healthcare (e.g., with lower socioeconomic groups, racial/ethnic minorities, and marginalized groups).
2. Gonorrhea is a sexually transmitted communicable disease that can be local or systemic. Complications include pelvic inflammatory disease (PID), sterility, and disseminated infection.
3. Gonorrhea can be passed to the fetus from the mother and typically manifests as an eye infection 1 to 12 days after birth. Ophthalmic antibiotic prophylaxis alone is not sufficient to prevent vertical transmission.
4. Although gonorrhea may become resistant to available antibiotics, the CDC no longer recommends multiple drug therapy in the United States.
5. Syphilis is an sexually transmitted infections (STIs) that becomes systemic shortly after infection. The four stages of the disease are (a) primary syphilis with chancre formation at the site of infection; (b) secondary syphilis with systemic spread to all body systems; (c) latent syphilis with minimal symptoms or the development of skin lesions; and (d) tertiary syphilis, the most severe stage, with destruction of bone, skin, soft tissue, and neurologic tissues.
6. Congenital syphilis contributes to prematurity of the newborn with bone marrow depression, central nervous system involvement, renal failure, and intrauterine growth retardation.
7. Syphilis is diagnosed with serologic testing and is treated with injectable penicillin.
8. With chancroid infection *(Haemophilus ducreyi)*, women are generally asymptomatic. Men may develop inflamed, painful genital ulcers and inguinal buboes. The incubation period is 1 to 14 days. Single-dose therapy with injectable ceftriaxone or oral azithromycin for both partners is recommended. Persons with HIV may require a longer treatment regimen.
9. Granuloma inguinale (donovanosis) is rare in the United States. The bacteria are gram-negative and survive within macrophages. Localized nodules coalesce to form granulomas and ulcers on the penis in men and on the labia in women. Antibiotics provide effective treatment.

10. Although not a true STI, bacterial vaginosis (BV) is a sexually associated condition caused by an overgrowth of anaerobic bacteria that produce aromatic amines and raise the pH of the vagina, promoting further bacterial growth (without an inflammatory response) and a fishy odor. "Clue cells" are found on the wet mount. Metronidazole (Flagyl) provides effective treatment. BV has been associated with PID, chorioamnionitis, preterm labor, and postpartum endometritis. Treatment of male sexual partners is not recommended.
11. Chlamydia *(Chlamydia trachomatiti)*, the most common bacterial STI in the United States, is a leading preventable cause of infertility and ectopic pregnancy. *C. trachomatis* localizes to epithelial tissue and can spread throughout the urogenital tract or pass from the infected mother to the eyes and respiratory tract of newborn infants during birth. *C. trachomatis* is susceptible to inexpensive, readily accessible antibiotics. Single-dose azithromycin is the drug of choice for infected individuals and all sexual contacts. Because of the asymptomatic nature of chlamydia and the potential sequelae of infection, widespread screening is recommended by the CDC.
12. Lymphogranuloma venereum *(invasive strains of C. trachomatis)* is a chronic STI uncommon in the United States. The lesion begins as a skin infection and spreads to the lymph tissue, causing inflammation, necrosis, buboes, and abscesses of the inguinal lymph nodes. Primary lesions appear on the penis and scrotum in men and on the cervix, vaginal wall, and labia in women. Secondary lesions involve inflammation and swelling of the lymph nodes with formation of large buboes that rupture and drain. A 21-day or longer course of oral doxycycline or erythromycin is needed for treatment. Treatment of sexual partners is recommended.
13. Genital herpes simplex virus (HSV) is the most common genital ulceration in the United States and is caused by either HSV-1 or HSV-2. Lesions initially appear as groups of vesicles that progress to ulceration with pain, lymphadenopathy, and fever. HSV can pass from mother to fetus. Women with active lesions should be delivered by cesarean section to avoid vertical transmission.
14. HSV infection is lifelong and can result in an initial outbreak and subsequent outbreaks. Individuals are contagious during outbreaks and episodes of asymptomatic viral shedding. Acyclovir reduces symptoms but does not cure the disease. Recurrent infections are most often attributable to HSV-2 and are generally milder and of shorter duration.
15. HPV is associated with the development of cervical dysplasia and cancer as well as condylomata acuminata. The high-risk strains of HPV (HR-HPV) that are precursors to the development of cervical cancer do not cause genital warts. Testing is available to detect HR-HPV and a vaccine is now available for the HPV types with highest risk for cervical cancer.
16. Condylomata acuminata (genital warts) are sexually transmitted and highly contagious. The velvety cauliflower-like lesions occur in the genital and anal areas, vagina, and cervix and are painless. Condylomata can be transmitted to the infant at birth.
17. Molluscum contagiosum is a benign viral infection of the skin. It is transmitted by skin-to-skin contact in children and adults. In adults, it tends to occur on the genitalia and is transmitted by sexual contact.
18. Trichomoniasis *(Trichomonas vaginalis)* causes vaginitis in women and urethritis in men. Both partners usually are infected. Women usually have a copious, malodorous, gray-green discharge with pruritus. Men usually are asymptomatic. Metronidazole is the treatment for both sexes.
19. Scabies *(Sarcoptes scabiei)* is a parasitic infection that spreads by skin-to-skin and sexual contact. The scabies mite burrows through the skin, depositing eggs, causing intense pruritus, especially at night. Treatment consists of topical application of a pediculicide.
20. Pediculosis pubis (crabs) *(Pthris pubis)* is commonly transmitted sexually. The lice bite into the skin for nutrition. Symptoms include mild and severe pruritus. Topical application of prescription or over the counter pediculicides is effective treatment.

Sexually Transmitted Infections of Other Body Systems

1. Systemic diseases known to be sexually transmitted include AIDS (see Chapter 10), cytomegalovirus infection, and Epstein-Barr virus.
2. Transmission of hepatitis B virus (HBV) can occur through needle puncture, blood transfusion, cuts in the skin, and contact with infected body fluids.
3. Hepatitis B infection poses significant health risks including chronic liver disease and hepatocellular cancer. Immunization against hepatitis B is the most effective means of preventing transmission. Universal vaccination of infants and children is recommended, as well as vaccination of high-risk adults.
4. The risk of perinatal transmission of HBV is high for infants of HBV-infected mothers unless they receive immunoglobulin and are vaccinated.
5. Hepatitis C is generally transmitted percutaneously but sexual transmission appears possible.

REFERENCES

1. Centers for Disease Control and Prevention (CDC) *Sexually transmitted disease surveillance 2019*. Atlanta, GA: CDC; 2021. Page last reviewed July 29, 2021. Available at https://www.cdc.gov/std/statistics/2019/default.htm. (Accessed August 24, 2021).
2. Kreisel KM, et al. Sexually transmitted infections among US women and men: prevalence and incidence estimates, 2018. *Sex Transm Dis*. 2021;48(4):208–214.
3. Weinstock HS, et al. STI prevalence, incidence, and costs in the United States: new estimates, new approach. *Sex Transm Dis*. 2021;48(4):207.
4. Workowski KA, et al. Sexually transmitted infections treatment guidelines, 2021. *MMWR Recomm Rep*. 2021;70(4):1–187. Available at https://doi.org/10.15585/mmwr.rr7004a1. (Accessed August 24, 2021).
5. Centers for Disease Control and Prevention (CDC): Sexually transmitted infections prevalence, incidence, and cost estimates in the United States. STIs at a glance, Atlanta, GA, CDC. Page last reviewed

January 25, 2021. Available at https://www.cdc.gov/std/statistics/prevalence-2020-at-a-glance.htm. (Accessed August 24, 2021).
6. Cramer R, et al. The legal aspects of expedited partner therapy practice: do state laws and policies really matter? *Sex Transm Dis.* 2013;40(8):657–662.
7. Centers for Disease Control and Prevention (CDC) *Legal status of expedited partner therapy (EPT).* Atlanta, GA: CDC; 2021. Page last reviewed April 19, 2021. Available at https://www.cdc.gov/std/ept/legal/default.htm. (Accessed August 24, 2021).
8. Centers for Disease Control and Prevention (CDC): *Sexually transmitted infections treatment guidelines, 2021.* Atlanta, GA: CDC; 2021. Page last reviewed July 22, 2021. Available at https://www.cdc.gov/std/treatment-guidelines/default.htm. (Accessed August 24, 2021).
9. Cuffe KM, et al. Assessing partner services provided by state and local health departments, 2018. *Sex Transm Dis.* 2021;48(6):429–435.
10. Centers for Disease Control and Prevention (CDC): *Sexually transmitted infections treatment guidelines, 2021.* Atlanta, GA: CDC; 2021. Page last reviewed July 22, 2021. Available at https://www.cdc.gov/std/treatment-guidelines/default.htm. (Accessed February 21, 2022).
11. Centers for Disease Control and Prevention (CDC): *National overview of STDs, 2019. Gonorrhea.* Atlanta, GA: CDC; 2021. Page last reviewed April 13, 2021. Available at https://www.cdc.gov/std/statistics/2019/overview.htm#Gonorrhea. (Accessed August 24, 2021).
12. Patton ME, et al. Extragenital gonorrhea and chlamydia testing and infection among men who have sex with men—STD surveillance network, United States, 2010–2012. *Clin Infect Dis.* 2014;58(11):1564–1570.
13. Lewis D. Will targeting oropharyngeal gonorrhoea delay the further emergence of drug-resistant *Neisseria gonorrhoeae* strains? *Sex Transm Infect.* 2015;91(4):234–237.
14. Centers for Disease Control and Prevention (CDC): *Gonococcal infections among adolescents and adults.* Atlanta, GA: CDC; 2021. Page last reviewed July 29, 2021. Available at https://www.cdc.gov/std/treatment-guidelines/gonorrhea-adults.htm. (Accessed August 24, 2021).
15. Brunham RC, Gottlieb SL, Paavonen J. Pelvic inflammatory disease. *N Engl J Med.* 2015;372(21):2039–2048.
16. Centers for Disease Control and Prevention (CDC): *Gonococcal infections.* Atlanta, GA: CDC; 2021. Page last reviewed July 22, 2021. Available at https://www.cdc.gov/std/treatment-guidelines/gonorrhea.htm. (Accessed August 24, 2021).
17. Centers for Disease Control and Prevention (CDC): *Screening recommendations and considerations referenced in treatment guidelines and original sources.* Atlanta, GA: CDC; 2021. Page last reviewed August 12, 2021. https://www.cdc.gov/std/treatment-guidelines/screening-recommendations.htm. (Accessed August 24, 2021).
18. Centers for Disease Control and Prevention (CDC): *National overview of STDs, 2019. Syphilis.* Atlanta, GA: CDC; 2021. Page last reviewed April 13, 2021. Available at https://www.cdc.gov/std/statistics/2019/overview.htm#Syphilis. (Accessed August 24, 2021).
19. Centers for Disease Control and Prevention (CDC): Sexually transmitted infections treatment guidelines, 2021. Syphilis, Atlanta, GA, 2021, CDC. Page last reviewed July 22, 2021. Available at https://www.cdc.gov/std/treatment-guidelines/syphilis.htm. (Accessed August 24, 2021).
20. Centers for Disease Control and Prevention (CDC): *Syphilis & MSM (men who have sex with men)—CDC fact sheet.* Atlanta, GA: CDC; 2021. Page last reviewed July 22, 2021. Available at https://www.cdc.gov/std/syphilis/stdfact-msm-syphilis.htm. (Accessed August 24, 2021).
21. Centers for Disease Control and Prevention (CDC): *National overview—sexually transmitted disease surveillance, 2019.* Atlanta, GA: CDC; 2021. Page last reviewed July 22, 2021. Available at https://www.cdc.gov/std/statistics/2019/overview.htm#CongenitalSyphilis. (Accessed August 24, 2021).
22. Gomez GB, et al. Untreated maternal syphilis and adverse outcomes of pregnancy: a systematic review and meta-analysis. *Bull World Health Organ.* 2013;91(3):217–226.
23. Centers for Disease Control and Prevention (CDC) *Sexually transmitted infections treatment guidelines, 2021. Congenital syphilis.* Atlanta, GA: CDC; 2021. Page last reviewed July 22, 2021. Available at https://www.cdc.gov/std/treatment-guidelines/congenital-syphilis.htm. (Accessed August 24, 2021).
24. Solaimalai D, et al. Enzyme-linked immunosorbent assay (ELISA) versus venereal disease research laboratory test (VDRL) and rapid plasma reagin test (RPR) for screening of syphilis in pregnant women. *Int J Gynecol Obstet.* 2020;150:103–107.
25. Centers for Disease Control and Prevention (CDC): *Sexually transmitted infections treatment guidelines, 2021.* Atlanta, GA: CDC; 2021. Available at https://www.cdc.gov/std/treatment-guidelines/STI-Guidelines-2021.pdf. (Accessed August 24, 2021).
26. Centers for Disease Control and Prevention (CDC): *Sexually transmitted infections treatment guidelines, 2021. Managing persons who have a history of penicillin allergy.* Atlanta, GA: CDC; 2021. Page last reviewed July 22, 2021. Available at https://www.cdc.gov/std/treatment-guidelines/penicillin-allergy.htm. (Accessed August 24, 2021).
27. Basta-Juzbašić A, Čeović R. Chancroid, lymphogranuloma venereum, granuloma inguinale, genital herpes simplex infection, and molluscum contagiosum. *Clin Dermatol.* 2014;32(2):290–298.
28. Centers for Disease Control and Prevention (CDC): *Sexually transmitted infections treatment guidelines, 2021. Chancroid.* Atlanta, GA: CDC; 2021. Page last reviewed July 22, 2021. Available at https://www.cdc.gov/std/treatment-guidelines/chancroid.htm. (Accessed August 24, 2021).
29. Centers for Disease Control and Prevention (CDC): *Sexually transmitted infections treatment guidelines, 2021. Granuloma inguinale (donovanosis).* Atlanta, GA: CDC; 2021. Page last reviewed July 22, 2021. Available at https://www.cdc.gov/std/treatment-guidelines/donovanosis.htm. (Accessed August 24, 2021).
30. Centers for Disease Control and Prevention (CDC): *Sexually transmitted infections treatment guidelines, 2021. Bacterial vaginosis.* Atlanta, GA: CDC; 2021. Page last reviewed July 22, 2021. Available at https://www.cdc.gov/std/treatment-guidelines/bv.htm. (Accessed August 24, 2021).
31. Verstraelen H, Swidsinski A. The biofilm in bacterial vaginosis: implications for epidemiology, diagnosis and treatment. *Curr Opin Infect Dis.* 2013;26(1):86–89.
32. Centers for Disease Control and Prevention (CDC): *Sexually transmitted infections treatment guidelines, 2021. Chlamydial infection.* Atlanta, GA: CDC; 2021. Page last reviewed July 22, 2021. Available at https://www.cdc.gov/std/treatment-guidelines/chlamydia.htm. (Accessed August 24, 2021).
33. Centers for Disease Control and Prevention (CDC): *National Overview—Sexually Transmitted Disease Surveillance, 2019. Chlamydia.* Atlanta, GA: CDC; 2021. Page last reviewed April 13, 2021. Available at https://www.cdc.gov/std/statistics/2019/overview.htm#Chlamydia. (Accessed August 24, 2021).
34. Elwell C, Mirrashidi K, Engel J. Chlamydia cell biology and pathogenesis. *Nat Rev Microbiol.* 2016;14(6):385–400.

35. Quayle A. The innate and early immune response to pathogen challenge in the female genital tract and the pivotal role of epithelial cells. *J Reprod Immunol.* 2002;57(1):61–79.
36. Centers for Disease Control and Prevention (CDC): *Sexually transmitted infections treatment guidelines, 2021. Lymphogranuloma venereum (LGV).* Atlanta, GA: CDC; 2021. Page last reviewed July 22, 2021. Available at https://www.cdc.gov/std/treatment-guidelines/lgv.htm. (Accessed August 24, 2021).
37. Van der Bij AK, et al. Diagnostic and clinical implications of anorectal lymphogranuloma venereum in men who have sex with men: a retrospective case-control study. *Clin Infect Dis.* 2006;42(2):186–194.
38. van Aar F, et al. Increasing trends of lymphogranuloma venereum among HIV-negative and asymptomatic men who have sex with men, the Netherlands, 2011 to 2017. *Euro Surveill.* 2020;25(14):1900377.
39. Centers for Disease Control and Prevention (CDC): *Genital herpes—CDC fact sheet (detailed).* Atlanta, GA: CDC; 2021. Page last reviewed July 22, 2021. Available at https://www.cdc.gov/std/herpes/stdfact-herpes-detailed.htm. (Accessed August 24, 2021).
40. Kaufman HE, et al. HSV-1 DNA in tears and saliva of normal adults. *Invest Ophthalmol Vis Sci.* 2005;46(1):241–247.
41. Magaret AS, et al. Effect of condom use on per-act HSV-2 transmission risk in HIV-1, HSV-2-discordant couples. *Clin Infect Dis.* 2016;62(4):456–461.
42. James SH, Kimberlin DW. Neonatal herpes simplex virus infection: epidemiology and treatment. *Clin Perinatol.* 2015;42(1):47–59.
43. Madan RP, et al. Neonatal herpes infection associated with direct orogenital suction during ritual Jewish circumcision. *J Pediatric Infect Dis Soc.* 2015;4(3):283–284.
44. Centers for Disease Control and Prevention (CDC): *Sexually transmitted infections treatment guidelines, 2021. Genital herpes.* Atlanta, GA: CDC; 2021. Page last reviewed July 22, 2021. Available at https://www.cdc.gov/std/treatment-guidelines/herpes.htm. (Accessed August 24, 2021).
45. American College of Obstetricians and Gynecologists (ACOG): Management of genital herpes in pregnancy. ACOG practice bulletin, number 220. *Obstet Gynecol.* 2020;135(5):e193–e202.
46. Trottier H, et al. Human papillomavirus (HPV) perinatal transmission and risk of HPV persistence among children: design, methods and preliminary results of the HERITAGE study. *Papillomavirus Res.* 2016;2:145–152.
47. Viens LJ, et al. Human papillomavirus–associated cancers—United States, 2008–2012. *MMWR Morb Mortal Wkly Rep.* 2016;65:661–666.
48. Centers for Disease Control and Prevention (CDC): *Sexually transmitted infections treatment guidelines, 2021. Human papillomavirus (HPV) infection.* Atlanta, GA: CDC; 2021. Page last reviewed July 22, 2021. Available at https://www.cdc.gov/std/treatment-guidelines/hpv.htm. (Accessed August 24, 2021).
49. Pytynia KB, Dahlstrom KR, Sturgis EM. Epidemiology of HPV-associated oropharyngeal cancer. *Oral Oncol.* 2014;50(5):380–386.
50. Moreira ED, et al. Incidence, clearance, and disease progression of genital human papillomavirus infection in heterosexual men. *J Infect Dis.* 2014;210(2):192–199.
51. Hariri S, et al. Monitoring effect of human papillomavirus vaccines in US population, emerging infections program, 2008–2012. *Emerg Infect Dis.* 2015;21(9):1557–1561.
52. Centers for Disease Control and Prevention (CDC): *Vaccines and preventable diseases. HPV vaccine recommendations.* Atlanta, GA: CDC; 2020. Page last reviewed March 17, 2020. Available at https://www.cdc.gov/vaccines/vpd/hpv/hcp/recommendations.html. (Accessed August 24, 2021).
53. Shah KV. A case for immunization of human papillomavirus (HPV) 6/11–infected pregnant women with the quadrivalent HPV vaccine to prevent juvenile-onset laryngeal papilloma. *J Infect Dis.* 2013;209(9):1307–1309.
54. Siegel RL, Miller KD, Jemal A. Cancer statistics, 2015. *CA Cancer J Clin.* 2015;65(1):5–29.
55. Massad LS, et al. 2012 ASCCP Consensus Guidelines Conference. 2012 updated consensus guidelines for the management of abnormal cervical cancer screening tests and cancer precursors. *Obstet Gynecol.* 2013;121(4):829–846.
56. Preventive Services Task Force US, et al. Screening for cervical cancer: US Preventive Services Task Force Recommendation Statement. *JAMA.* 2018;320(7):674–686.
57. Centers for Disease Control and Prevention (CDC): *Sexually transmitted infections treatment guidelines, 2021. Trichomoniasis.* Atlanta, GA: CDC; 2021. Page last reviewed July 22, 2021. Available at https://www.cdc.gov/std/treatment-guidelines/trichomoniasis.htm. (Accessed August 24, 2021).
58. Silver BJ, et al. *Trichomonas vaginalis* as a cause of perinatal morbidity: a systematic review and meta-analysis. *Sex Transm Dis.* 2014;41(6):369–376.
59. Gülmezoglu AM, Azhar M. Interventions for trichomoniasis in pregnancy. *Cochrane Database Syst Rev.* 2011;2011(5):CD000220.
60. Kim TG, et al. *Trichomonas vaginalis* in pregnancy: patterns and predictors of testing, infection, and treatment. *Obstet Gynecol.* 2020;135(5):1136–1144.
61. Romani L, et al. Prevalence of scabies and impetigo worldwide: a systematic review. *Lancet Infect Dis.* 2015;15(8):960–967.
62. Centers for Disease Control and Prevention (CDC) *Sexually transmitted infections treatment guidelines, 2021. Hepatitis A virus (HAV) infection.* Atlanta, GA: CDC; 2021. Page last reviewed July 22, 2021. Available at https://www.cdc.gov/std/treatment-guidelines/hav.htm. (Accessed August 24, 2021).
63. Tohme RA, Holmberg SD. Is sexual contact a major mode of hepatitis C virus transmission? *Hepatology.* 2010;52(4):1497–1505.
64. Centers for Disease Control and Prevention (CDC): *Sexually transmitted infections treatment guidelines, 2021. Hepatitis C virus (HAV) infection.* Atlanta, GA: CDC; 2021. Page last reviewed July 22, 2021. Available at https://www.cdc.gov/std/treatment-guidelines/hcv.htm. (Accessed August 24, 2021).
65. Ott J, et al. Global epidemiology of hepatitis B virus infection: new estimates of age-specific HBsAg seroprevalence and endemicity. *Vaccine.* 2012;30(12):2212–2219.
66. Centers for Disease Control and Prevention (CDC): *2019 Viral hepatitis surveillance report.* Atlanta, GA: CDC; 2021. Page last reviewed May 19, 2021. Available at https://www.cdc.gov/hepatitis/statistics/2019surveillance/index.htm. (Accessed October 11, 2021).
67. Schillie S, et al. Update: shortened interval for postvaccination serologic testing of infants born to hepatitis B-infected mothers. *MMWR Morb Mortal Wkly Rep.* 2015;64(39):1118–1120.
68. Schillie S, et al. CDC guidance for evaluating health-care personnel for hepatitis B virus protection and for administering postexposure management. *MMWR Recomm Rep.* 2013;62(10):1–19.
69. Chen X, et al. Breastfeeding is not a risk factor for mother-to-child transmission of hepatitis B virus. *PLoS One.* 2013;8(1):e55303.

28

Structure and Function of the Hematologic System

Karen C. Turner

http://evolve.elsevier.com/Rogers/pathophysiology/

CHAPTER OUTLINE

All the body's tissues and organs require oxygen and nutrients to survive. These essential needs are provided by the blood that circulates through miles of vessels found throughout the human body. The red blood cells provide the oxygen and the fluid portion of the blood carries the nutrients. The blood cleans discarded waste from the tissues; transports hormones; moves white blood cells (WBCs), platelets, and other components necessary to protect the body from injury and infection and initiate healing; and provides thermal regulation to maintain organs and tissues within an acceptable range of temperatures.

COMPONENTS OF THE HEMATOLOGIC SYSTEM

Composition of Blood

Blood consists of various cells that circulate suspended in a solution of protein and inorganic materials (plasma), which is approximately 91% water and 9% dissolved substances (solutes) (Fig. 28.1). The blood volume amounts to about 6 quarts (5.5 L) in adults. The continuous movement of blood guarantees that critical components are available to all parts of the body to carry out their chief functions: (1) delivery of substances needed for cellular metabolism in the tissues, (2) removal of the wastes of cellular metabolism, (3) defense against invading microorganisms and injury, and (4) maintenance of acid–base balance.

Plasma and Plasma Proteins

In adults, plasma accounts for 50% to 55% of blood volume (see Fig. 28.1). Plasma is a complex aqueous liquid containing a variety of organic and inorganic elements (Table 28.1). The concentration of these elements varies, depending on diet, metabolic demand, hormones, and vitamins. Plasma differs from serum in that serum is free of clotting proteins (e.g., fibrinogen). The clotting proteins may interfere with some diagnostic tests.

Plasma contains a large number of proteins (plasma proteins) that make up about 7% of the total plasma weight. These vary in structure and function and can be classified primarily into two major groups, albumin and globulins, plus a small amount of clotting proteins. Most plasma proteins are produced by the liver. The major exception is antibody, which is produced by plasma cells (B cells) in the lymph nodes and other lymphoid tissues (see Chapter 8).

Albumin (about 57% of total plasma protein) serves as a carrier molecule for the normal components of blood and for drugs that have low solubility in water (e.g., free fatty acids, lipid-soluble hormones, thyroid hormones, bile salts). Its most essential role is regulation of the passage of water and solutes through the capillaries. Albumin molecules are large and do not diffuse freely through the vascular endothelium, and thus they maintain the critical colloidal osmotic pressure (or oncotic pressure) that regulates the passage of fluids and electrolytes into the surrounding tissues (see Chapters 1 and 3). Water and solute particles tend to diffuse out of the arterial portions of

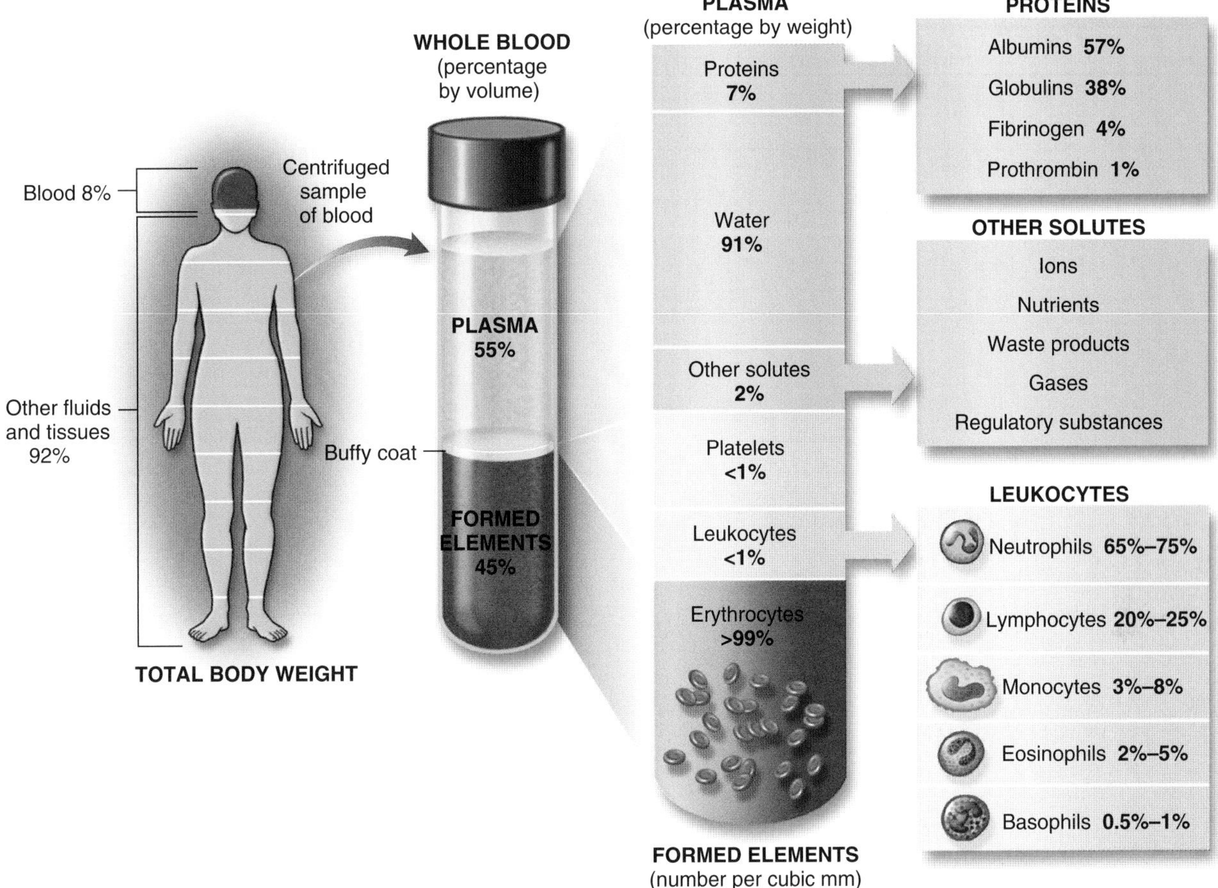

Fig. 28.1 Composition of Whole Blood. Approximate values for the components of blood in a normal adult. (From Patton KT, Thibodeau GA. *The human body in health & disease*, 7th edition. St. Louis: Mosby; 2018.)

the capillaries because blood pressure (hydrostatic pressure) is greater in arterial than in venous blood vessels. Water and solutes move from tissues into the venous portions of the capillaries, where the pressures are reversed, oncotic pressure being greater than intravascular pressure or hydrostatic pressure (see Fig. 3.1). In the case of decreased production of albumin (e.g., cirrhosis, other diffuse liver diseases, protein malnutrition) or excessive loss of albumin (e.g., certain kidney diseases, extensive burns), the reduced plasma oncotic pressure leads to excessive movement of water and solutes into the tissue and decreased blood volume.

Most of the remaining plasma proteins are globulins (about 38% of total plasma protein), which are often classified by their properties in an electric field (serum electrophoresis). Under the normal conditions used to perform serum electrophoresis, albumin is the most rapidly moving protein. The globulins are classified into alpha, beta, and gamma groups by their movement relative to albumin. Alpha (α) globulins (those moving most closely to albumin) include high-density lipoproteins [HDLs], prothrombin, and proteins that transport hormones. Beta (β) globulins include low-density lipoproteins (LDLs). Gamma (γ) globulins (those with the least movement) consist primarily of immunoglobulin G (IgG) (see Chapter 8).

Plasma proteins also can be classified by function: clotting, defense, transport, or regulation. The clotting factors or **proteins** promote coagulation and stop bleeding from damaged blood vessels. Fibrinogen is the most plentiful of the clotting factors and is the precursor of the fibrin clot (see Fig. 28.19). Proteins involved in defense, or protection, against infection include antibodies (immunoglobulins) and complement proteins (see Chapters 8 and 9). Transport proteins specifically bind and carry a variety of inorganic and organic molecules, including iron (transferrin), copper (ceruloplasmin), lipids and steroid hormones (lipoproteins) (see Chapter 1), and vitamins (e.g., retinol-binding protein for vitamin A transport). The plasma lipids, triglycerides, phospholipids, cholesterol, and fatty acids are transported through the blood as complexes with plasma proteins; they are known as *lipoproteins* (see Chapters 1 and 32). Regulatory proteins include a variety of enzymatic inhibitors (e.g., α_1-antitrypsin) that protect the tissues from damage; precursor molecules (e.g., kininogen) that are converted into active biologic molecules when needed; and protein hormones (e.g., cytokines) that communicate between cells.

TABLE 28.1 **Organic and Inorganic Components of Arterial Plasma**

Constituent	Major Functions
Water	Medium for carrying all other constituents
Electrolytes Na^+ K^+ Ca^{2+} Mg^{2+} Cl^- HCO_3^- Phosphate (mostly HPO_4^-)	Maintain H_2O in extracellular compartment; act as buffers; function in membrane excitability
Proteins Albumins Globulins Fibrinogen Transferrin Ferritin	Provide colloid osmotic pressure of plasma; act as buffers; bind other plasma constituents (e.g., lipids, hormones, vitamins, minerals); clotting factors; enzymes; enzyme precursors; antibodies (immunoglobulins); hormones; transporters
Gases CO_2 content	By-product of oxygenation, most CO_2 content is from HCO_3^- and acts as buffer
O_2	Oxygenation
N_2	By-product of protein catabolism
Nutrients Glucose and other carbohydrates Total amino acids Total lipids Cholesterol Individual vitamins Individual trace elements Iron	Provide nutrition and substances for tissue repair
Waste products Urea	End product of protein catabolism
Creatinine (from creatine)	End product from energy metabolism
Uric acid (from nucleic acids)	End product from protein metabolism
Bilirubin (from heme)	End product of red blood cell destruction
Individual hormones	Functions specific to target tissue

BUN, Blood urea nitrogen; *Ca^{2+}*, calcium; *Cl^-*, chloride; *CO_2*, carbon dioxide; *H_2O*, water; HCO_3^-, bicarbonate; HPO_4^-, phosphorus; *K^+*, potassium; *Mg^{2+}*, magnesium; *N_2*, nitrogen; *Na^+*, sodium.

Data from Vander AJ, et al. *Human physiology: The mechanisms of body function.* New York: McGraw-Hill; 2001.

Plasma also contains several charged inorganic ions that regulate cell function, osmotic pressure, and blood pH. These include the electrolytes sodium, potassium, calcium, chloride, and phosphate (Electrolytes are described in Chapters 1 and 3).

Cellular Components of the Blood

The cellular elements of the blood are broadly classified as red blood cells (erythrocytes), WBCs (leukocytes), and platelets (thrombocytes) (Fig. 28.2). The components of the blood are listed in Table 28.2.

Erythrocytes. Erythrocytes (red blood cells [RBCs]) are the most abundant cells of the blood, occupying approximately 48% of the blood volume in men and about 42% in women. Erythrocytes are formed in the bone marrow, and there are 4.2 to 6.2 million erythrocytes/mm^3 circulating in normal blood. Erythrocytes are primarily responsible for tissue oxygenation. The erythrocyte contains hemoglobin (Hb), which carries the gases, and electrolytes, which regulate gas diffusion through the cell's plasma membrane. The mature erythrocyte lacks a nucleus and cytoplasmic organelles (e.g., mitochondria), so it cannot synthesize protein or carry out oxidative reactions. Because it cannot undergo mitotic division, the erythrocyte has a limited life span (approximately 100 to 120 days), ages, and is removed from the circulation, primarily in the spleen, to be replaced by new erythrocytes.

The erythrocyte's size and shape is ideally suited to its function as a gas carrier. It is a small disk with two unique properties: (1) a *biconcave* shape and (2) the capacity to be *reversibly*

TABLE 28.2 Cellular Components of the Blood

Cell	Structural Characteristics	Function	Life Span
Erythrocyte (red blood cell)	Nonnucleated cytoplasmic disk containing hemoglobin	Gas transport to and from tissue cells and lungs	80–120 days
Leukocyte (white blood cell)	Nucleated cell	Body defense mechanisms	See specific cells below
Neutrophil	Segmented polymorphonuclear granulocyte	Phagocytosis, particularly during early phase of inflammation	4 days
Eosinophil	Segmented polymorphonuclear granulocyte	Control of inflammation, phagocytosis, defense against parasites, allergic reactions	8–12 days
Basophil	Segmented polymorphonuclear granulocyte	Mast cell–like functions, associated with allergic reactions	Few hours to days
Monocyte and macrophage	Large mononuclear phagocyte	Phagocytosis; mononuclear phagocyte system	Months or years
Lymphocyte	Mononuclear immunocyte	Humoral and cell-mediated immunity	Days or years, depending on type
Natural killer cell	Large granular lymphocyte	Defense against some tumors and viruses	Unknown
Platelet	Irregularly shaped cytoplasmic fragment (not a cell)	Hemostasis after vascular injury; normal coagulation and clot formation/retraction; release of growth factors	8–11 days

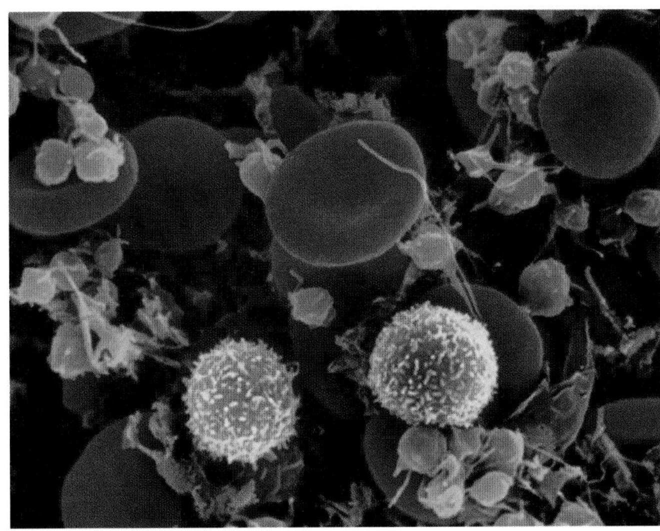

Fig. 28.2 Blood Cells and Platelets. Leukocytes are spherical and have irregular surfaces with numerous extending pili. Leukocytes are the cotton candy–like cells *(yellow)*. Erythrocytes are flattened spheres with a depressed center *(red)*. Platelets are the smaller *(green)* cell fragments. (Copyright Dennis Kunkel Microscopy, Inc.)

deformed. The flattened, biconcave shape (see Fig. 28.2) provides a surface area/volume ratio that is optimal for gas diffusion into and out of the cell and for deformity. During its life span, the erythrocyte, which is 6 to 8 μm in diameter, repeatedly circulates through splenic sinusoids and capillaries that are only 2 μm in diameter. Reversible deformity enables the erythrocyte to assume a more compact torpedo-like shape, squeeze through the microcirculation (diapedesis), and return to normal (Fig. 28.3).

Erythrocytes are also part of the innate immune system. Erythrocytes catch bacteria in the blood stream by electric charge attraction and kill them by oxycytosis, the release of oxygen from oxyhemoglobin (oxygen-dependent killing). The decomposed bacteria are then cleared in the liver and spleen. Oxycytosis is complimentary to leukocytosis (phagocytosis) as leukocytes cannot recognize and attach bacteria in the blood because of the velocity of blood flow.[1]

Leukocytes. Leukocytes (WBCs) (see Fig. 28.2) defend the body against organisms that cause infection and also remove debris, including dead or injured host cells of all kinds. The leukocytes act primarily in the tissues but are transported in the circulation. The average adult has approximately 5000 to 10,000 leukocytes/mm^3 of blood.

Leukocytes are classified according to structure as either granulocytes or agranulocytes and according to function as either phagocytes or immunocytes (cells that create immunity; see Chapter 8). The granulocytes, which include neutrophils, basophils, eosinophils, and mast cells, are all phagocytes. (Phagocytic action is described in Chapter 7.) Of the agranulocytes, the monocytes and macrophages are phagocytes, whereas the lymphocytes are immunocytes. Fig. 28.4 shows a microscopic image of the various types of leukocytes.

Granulocytes. The granulocytes are formed in the red bone marrow and have a nucleus with several lobes (polymorphonuclear) and many membrane-bound granules in their cytoplasm. These granules contain enzymes capable of killing microorganisms and catabolizing debris ingested during phagocytosis. The granules also contain powerful biochemical mediators with inflammatory and immune functions. These mediators, along with the digestive enzymes, are released from granulocytes in response to specific stimuli and affect other cells in the

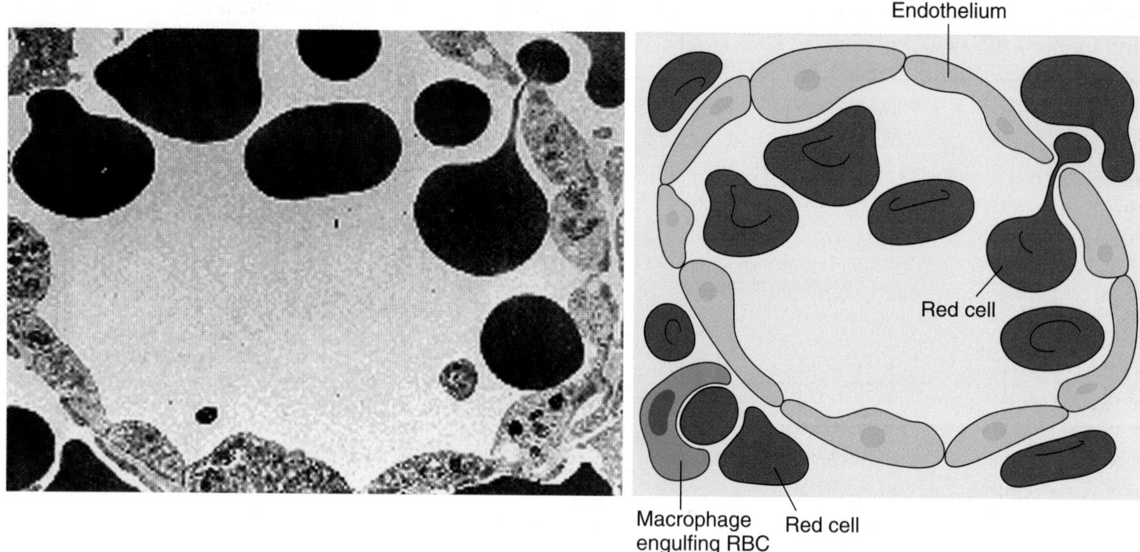

Fig. 28.3 Red Cells Moving in the Spleen. Transmission electron micrograph and schematic drawing of erythrocytes in the process of moving by diapedesis from the red pulp cords into the sinus lumen. They resume their normal shape after squeezing through. Note the degree of deformability required for red cells to pass through the wall of the sinus. *RBC*, Red blood cell. (From Damjanov I, Linder J, eds. *Anderson's pathology*, 10th edition. St. Louis: Mosby; 1996. Schematic from Kumar V, Fausto N, Abbas A. *Robbins & Cotran pathologic basis of disease*, 7th edition. St. Louis: Saunders; 2005.)

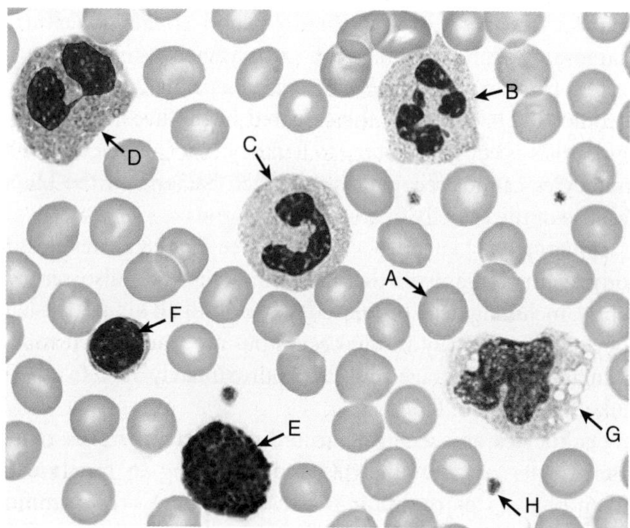

Fig. 28.4 Leukocytes. Normal cells in peripheral blood. *A*, Erythrocyte (red blood cell); *B*, neutrophil (segmented); *C*, neutrophil (banded); *D*, eosinophil; *E*, basophil; *F*, lymphocyte; *G*, monocyte; *H*, platelet. (From Keohane E, Smith L, Walenga J. *Rodak's hemotology*, 5th edition. St. Louis: Saunders; 2016.)

circulation. The biochemical mediators have vascular and intercellular effects, and the enzymes participate in the breakdown of debris from sites of infection or injury. Granulocytes are capable of amoeboid movement, by which they migrate through vessel walls (diapedesis) and then to sites where their action is needed. They have a life span of only a few hours or days.

The neutrophil (polymorphonuclear neutrophil [PMN]) is the most numerous and best understood of the granulocytes.

EMERGING SCIENCE BOX

Tumor Associated Neutrophils

The role of tumor-associated neutrophils (TANs) in cancer is complex and can include both the killing of cancer cells (N1 neutrophils) or the promotion of tumor growth and metastasis (N2 neutrophils). The variance in function is related to significant genetic variation among populations of neutrophils. Tumors can induce myelopoiesis and recruit immature neutrophils to the tumor microenvironment (TME) where these cells undergo reprogramming and transitioning to myeloid-derived suppressor cells with a pro-tumorigenic phenotype (N2 neutrophils). These N2 neutrophils produce a broad range of mediators and growth factors to promote DNA instability resulting in tumor growth, angiogenesis, and metastasis. Tumor cells are also captured by neutrophil extracellular traps which facilitate their migration to distant sites. N2 neutrophils also suppress the anti-tumor activity of tumor-infiltrating cytotoxic T lymphocytes and exclude these cells from the TME. An elevated neutrophil-to-lymphocyte ratio (NLR) has been correlated with poor responses to cancer therapy. Realization of the pro-tumorigenic activities of N2 TANs has resulted in the evaluation of a range of adjunctive strategies targeting the recruitment of these cells and/or the harmful activities of their mediators of immunosuppression.

Data from Rapoport BL, et al. Role of the neutrophil in the pathogenesis of advanced cancer and impaired responsiveness to therapy. *Molecules*, 2020;25(7):1618; Sagiv JY, et al. Phenotypic diversity and plasticity in circulating neutrophil subpopulations in cancer. *Cell Reports*, 2015;10(4):562–573; Zhang Y, et al. Targeting and exploitation of tumor-associated neutrophils to enhance immunotherapy and drug delivery for cancer treatment. *Cancer Biology and Medicine*, 2020;17(1):32–43. doi:10.20892/j.issn.2095-3941.2019.0372.

Neutrophils constitute about 65% to 75% of the total leukocyte count in adults. The results vary by laboratory and populations studied.

The cytoplasm of neutrophils contains small lysosomal granules and a central nucleus with two to five distinct lobes. Immature neutrophils are called *bands* or *stabs*. Mature neutrophils are called *segmented neutrophils* because of the characteristic appearance of their nucleus (see Fig. 28.4). Neutrophils reach a fully mature state in the bone marrow, where these mature neutrophils are called the *marrow neutrophil reserve*. Normally it takes about 14 days for neutrophils to develop from early precursors, but this process is accelerated by infection and treatment with colony-stimulating factors.

Neutrophils are the chief phagocytes of early inflammation. Soon after bacterial invasion or tissue injury, neutrophils migrate out of the capillaries and into the damaged tissue, where they phagocytize and destroy contaminating microorganisms and debris. Neutrophils also release nuclear DNA onto extracellular pathogens to control their growth and proliferation and aid the killing of bacteria. These extracellular DNA deposits are termed *neutrophil extracellular traps (NETs)*, and are a phagocytosis-independent anti-microbial pathway. In addition to their crucial role in fighting infection, neutrophils play a complex role in tumors. (see Emerging Science Box: Tumor Associated Neutrophils). Neutrophils are sensitive to the environment in damaged tissue (e.g., low pH, enzymes released from damaged cells) and die in 1 or 2 days. The breakdown of dead neutrophils releases digestive enzymes from their cytoplasmic granules. These enzymes dissolve cellular debris and prepare the site for healing. (This final function, called *débridement*, is described in Chapter 7.)

Eosinophils, which have large, coarse granules, constitute only about 2% to 5% of the normal leukocyte count in adults. Using a spectrum of pattern-recognition receptors, eosinophils are capable of amoeboid movement and phagocytosis. Unlike neutrophils, eosinophils ingest antigen-antibody complexes and are induced by immunoglobulin E (IgE)–mediated hypersensitivity reactions to attack parasites by release of toxic molecules. Eosinophils also mediate immunity against bacterial, viral, and fungal infections by presenting bacterial, viral, and parasitic antigen to cytotoxic T cells. IL-5 promotes the maturation and migration of eosinophils during the inflammatory response. Eosinophilic inflammation mediated by IL-5, particularly from T helper cells, and other cytokines, contributes to the type 2 hypersensitivity response associated with asthma and other chronic eosinophilic inflammatory diseases (see Chapter 9). During inflammation, eosinophil death and cytolysis is known as *extracellular trap cell death (ETosis)*, which differs from the processes of accidental necrosis or apoptosis. Eosinophil extracellular trap products consist of damage-associated molecular patterns (DAMPs) that are able to activate both the innate and adaptive immune systems (see Chapters 7 and 8).[2] Eosinophils also release IL-4 important for tissue repair and regeneration in muscle and liver.[3]

Eosinophil secondary granules contain toxic chemicals (e.g., major basic protein, eosinophil cationic protein, eosinophil peroxidase, eosinophil-derived neurotoxin) that are highly destructive to parasites and viruses. Eosinophil granules also contain a variety of enzymes (e.g., histaminase) that help control inflammatory processes. Eosinophils also release proinflammatory molecules, including leukotrienes, prostaglandins, platelet-activating factor (PAF), and a variety of cytokines (e.g., IL-1, IL-4, IL-6, tumor necrosis factor-alpha [TNF-α], and granulocyte-macrophage colony-stimulating factor [GM-CSF]). Type I and type II hypersensitivity allergic reactions and asthma are characterized by high circulating eosinophil counts (see Chapters 9 and 36). The eosinophils may be involved in a dual role: regulation of inflammation and contribution to the destructive inflammatory processes observed in allergic reactions (e.g., the lungs of persons with asthma and eosinophilic esophagitis).

Basophils, which make up less than 1% of leukocytes, are structurally similar to the mast cells (see Fig. 28.4). Basophils contain cytoplasmic granules that have an abundant mixture of biochemical mediators, including histamine, chemotactic factors, proteolytic enzymes (e.g., elastase, lysophospholipase), and an anticoagulant (heparin). Stimulation of basophils also induces synthesis of vasoactive lipid molecules (e.g., leukotrienes) and cytokines, including IL-6, which affects differentiation of type 1 T-helper cells (Th1 cells) (focus on intracellular parasites) and type 2 T-helper cell (Th2 cells) (focus on extracellular parasites). Basophils are a particularly rich source of the cytokine IL-4, which preferentially guides B-cell differentiation toward plasma cells that secrete IgE (see Chapter 8).

The number of basophils is often increased at sites of allergic inflammatory reactions and parasitic infection, particularly ectoparasites (e.g., ticks). IgE receptors on the basophil induce degranulation at sites of IgE-mediated hypersensitivity reactions and contribute to the local inflammatory response.

Mast cells are highly similar to basophils but are generated from a different set of precursor cells in the bone marrow, from which they migrate in an immature form into tissues. Mast cells reside in vascularized connective tissues just beneath body epithelial surfaces, including the submucosal tissues of the respiratory and gastrointestinal tracts, as well as in the dermal layer that lies just below the surface of the skin. Mast cells play a central role in inflammation. Activation and degranulation of the mast cells affect a great number of other cells, including those involved in inflammation (e.g., vascular endothelial cells, smooth muscle cells, circulating platelets and leukocytes, nerves) and healing (e.g., fibroblasts), as well as glandular cells and cells of the immune system. Their activation contributes greatly to increased permeability of blood vessels and synthesis of mediators producing smooth muscle contraction (see Fig 7.4).

Agranulocytes. The agranulocytes—monocytes, macrophages, and lymphocytes—contain relatively fewer granules than granulocytes. Monocytes and macrophages make up the mononuclear phagocyte system (MPS) (see Chapter 7). Both monocytes and macrophages participate in the immune and inflammatory response, being powerful phagocytes. They also ingest dead or defective host cells, particularly blood cells.

The mononuclear phagocyte system (MPS), also known as the *reticuloendothelial system* or *macrophage system*, consists of specialized endothelial cells: promonocytes and their precursors in the bone marrow; monocytes in the peripheral blood; and a portion of macrophages that reside in the tissues, remaining there for months or perhaps years. Cells of the MPS ingest and destroy (by phagocytosis) unwanted materials, such as foreign protein particles, circulating immune complexes, microorganisms, debris from dead or injured cells, defective or injured erythrocytes, and dead neutrophils.

Monocytes are immature macrophages. They are the largest normal blood cell and have a horseshoe-shaped nucleus (see Fig. 28.4). Monocytes are formed and released by the bone marrow into the bloodstream. As they mature, monocytes migrate into a variety of tissues (e.g., liver [Kupffer cells], spleen, lymph nodes, peritoneum, gastrointestinal tract, brain [microglia], and bone) and differentiate into tissue macrophages with tissue-specific functions (Table 28.3). Monocytes also differentiate into myeloid linage dendritic cells and disseminate to lymphoid organs and body surfaces such as the skin and mucous membranes. Both macrophages and dendritic cells are part of the MPS. Other monocytes may migrate out of blood vessels and differentiate into macrophages in response to infection or inflammation. Macrophages are generally larger and are more active as phagocytes than monocytes. Dendritic cells frequently extend projections *(dendrites)* into the tissue and assume a "neuron-like" appearance. The origin and turnover of many of the tissue macrophages are not precisely known. It seems clear that once monocytes leave the circulation, they do not return. They can survive many months or even years.

The normal role of macrophages is to remove old and damaged cells and large molecular substances from the blood. Cellular targets of macrophage phagocytosis include circulating senescent or damaged erythrocytes and platelets (removed primarily in spleen), dead neutrophils (in the circulation and at sites of inflammation), and cells undergoing apoptosis. Noncellular targets include antigen-antibody complexes, cellular debris, products of coagulation, and macromolecules (such as lipids and carbohydrates synthesized by the body as the result of faulty metabolism, as in storage diseases). Macrophages remove and kill contaminating microorganisms in the blood (mostly in the liver and spleen) and at sites of infection. Macrophages and, particularly, dendritic cells are the major "antigen-processing" and "antigen-presenting" cells that initiate immune responses (see Chapter 8). Macrophages initiate wound healing and tissue remodeling and, if activated by cytokines from T cells, secrete a large array of biologically active chemicals that if uncontrolled result in chronic inflammation and tissue injury (see Chapter 7).

TABLE 28.3 Mononuclear Phagocyte System

Name of Cell	Location
Committed Stem Cells	Bone marrow
Monoblasts	Bone marrow
Promonoblasts	Bone marrow
Monocytes	Bone marrow and peripheral blood
Macrophages	Tissue
Kupffer cells	Liver macrophages
Alveolar macrophages	Lung
Histiocytes	Connective tissue
Macrophages	Bone marrow
Fixed and free macrophages	Spleen and lymph nodes
Pleural and peritoneal macrophages Adipose macrophages	Serous cavities Adipose (fat) tissue
Microglial cells	Nervous system
Mesangial cells	Kidney
Osteoclasts	Bone
Langerhans cells	Skin
Dendritic cells	Lymphoid tissue, lining of respiratory and gastrointestinal tracts

Modified from Kumar V, et al. *Robbins & Cotran pathologic basis of disease*, 9th edition. Philadelphia: Saunders; 2015.

Lymphocytes constitute about 20% to 25% of the total leukocyte count and are the primary cells of the immune response (see Fig. 28.4 and Chapter 8). Lymphocytes arise from lymphoid stem cells in the bone marrow and subsequently develop and reproduce in the lymphatic tissues as mature T cells, B cells, or plasma cells. The lymphocytes do not contain any enzyme-filled digestive vacuoles. The life span of the lymphocyte can be days, months, or years, depending on its type and subtype.

Natural killer (NK) cells, which resemble large granular lymphocytes, recognize cells that do not express "self" proteins (self-antigens) on their plasma membrane or that contain foreign or abnormal antigens such as cancer cells or some virus-infected cells without prior exposure to these antigens (see Chapters 7 and 8). Hence, they are named *natural killer cells* as they do not require exposure to antigen for activation to differentiate them from T-cytotoxic cells which are induced by antigen. NK cells also have the capacity to activate T cells and phagocytes and produce a variety of cytokines that can regulate immune responses. The predominant form of NK cells develops in the bone marrow and circulates in the blood, and is found mainly in the peripheral blood and spleen where it accounts for 5% to 10% of the circulating lymphoid pool. NK cells develop independent of the thymus, although some NK precursors are found in the thymus and may develop into NK T cells, which will then have markers of both NK cells and T cells.[4]

Platelets. Platelets (thrombocytes) are not true cells, but rather irregularly discoid-shaped cytoplasmic fragments that lack a nucleus and deoxyribonucleic acid (DNA) and are incapable of mitotic division. Platelets are essential for blood coagulation and control of bleeding. They are formed in the bone marrow by fragmentation of very large cells (40 to 100 μm in diameter) known as megakaryocytes. They contain cytoplasmic granules (e.g., dense granules, alpha granules, and lysosomes) and can release adhesive proteins and coagulation and growth factors when stimulated by injury to a blood vessel. Platelets can assume different shapes and form adhesive pseudopodia (long surface extensions) that increase their surface area and promote interconnectedness and adherence to collagen fibers in damaged vascular walls, plugging vascular openings to control bleeding (Fig. 28.5).

The normal platelet concentration is about 150,000 to 400,000 platelets/mm^3 of circulating blood, although the normal ranges may vary slightly from laboratory to laboratory. An additional one-third of the body's available platelets are in a reserve pool in

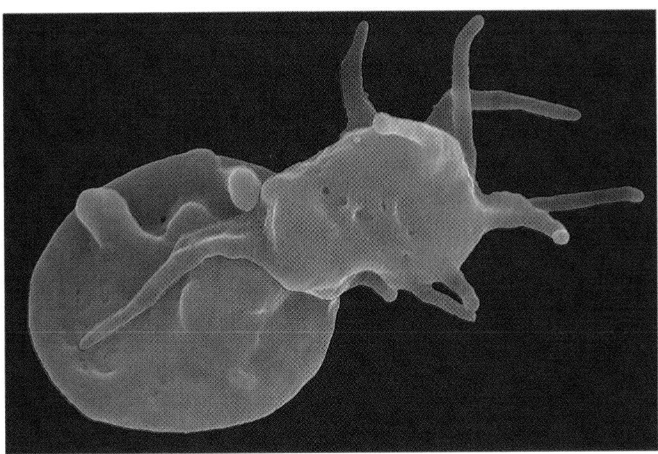

Fig. 28.5 Colored Micrograph of Platelets. The platelet on the left is moderately activated, with a generally round shape and the beginning of formation of pseudopodia (foot-like extensions from the membrane). The platelet on the right is fully activated, with extensive pseudopodia. (Copyright Dennis Kunkel Microscopy, Inc.)

the spleen. A platelet circulates for approximately 8 to 11 days, and is then removed by macrophages, mostly in the spleen.

Lymphoid Organs

The lymphoid system is closely integrated with the circulatory system. The lymphoid organs, some of which are merely aggregations of lymphoid tissue, are classified as primary or secondary. The primary lymphoid organs are the thymus and the bone marrow. The secondary lymphoid organs consist of the spleen, lymph nodes, tonsils, and Peyer patches in the ileum of the small intestine. All of the lymphoid organs link the hematologic and immune systems in that they are sites of residence, proliferation, differentiation, or function of lymphocytes and mononuclear phagocytes (monocytes and macrophages) (see Chapter 8). The liver, which is primarily a digestive organ and is described in Chapter 40, synthesizes both coagulant and anticoagulant proteins.

Spleen

The spleen is the largest of the lymphoid organs. It serves as a site of fetal hematopoiesis, filters blood-borne antigens, cleanses the blood through the action of mononuclear phagocytes, initiates an immune response to blood-borne microorganisms, destroys aged erythrocytes, and serves as a reservoir for blood.

The spleen is a concave, encapsulated organ that weighs about 150 g and is about the size of a fist. It is located in the left upper abdominal cavity, curved around a portion of the stomach. Strands of connective tissue (trabeculae) extend throughout the spleen from the splenic capsule, dividing it into compartments that contain masses of lymphoid tissue called *splenic pulp* (white and red) (Fig. 28.6). The spleen is interlaced with many blood vessels, some of which can distend to store blood. Blood that circulates through the spleen comes from the splenic artery, which branches from the descending aorta and reenters the circulatory system through the splenic vein and into the portal vein.

Arterial blood that enters the spleen first encounters the white splenic pulp, which consists of masses of lymphoid tissue containing macrophages and lymphocytes, primarily T lymphocytes in proximity to the arterioles (the periarterial lymphoid sheath) (see Fig. 28.6). Cellular clumps (lymphoid follicles) are formed in the white pulp around the splenic arterioles. The lymphoid follicles consist primarily of B lymphocytes and are the chief sites of immune function within the spleen. Here blood-borne antigens encounter lymphocytes, initiating the immune response and the conversion of lymphoid follicles into germinal centers in the middle of the follicle where B cells proliferate and differentiate during the humoral immune response (see Chapter 8).

Some of the blood that enters the terminal capillaries continues through the microcirculation and enters highly distensible storage areas, called *venous sinuses*, in the red pulp of the spleen. The venous sinuses (and the red pulp) can store more than 300 mL of blood. Passive dilation of the venous sinuses enables the spleen to increase its storage capacity as needed by the body. Sudden reductions in blood pressure cause the sympathetic nervous system to stimulate constriction of the sinuses and expel as much as 200 mL of blood into the venous circulation, helping restore blood volume or pressure in the circulation and increasing the hematocrit by as much as 4%.

The endothelial lining of the venous sinuses is discontinuous (having gaps between endothelial cells) and therefore extremely permeable, allowing blood cells to exit the circulation. The red pulp contains a system of loosely interconnected resident macrophages that provide the principal site of splenic filtration. Because of the slow circulation in the sinuses, the macrophages easily phagocytose old, damaged, or dead blood cells of all kinds (but chiefly erythrocytes), microorganisms, macromolecules, and particles of debris. Hemoglobin from phagocytosed erythrocytes is catabolized, and heme (iron) is stored in the cytoplasm of the macrophages or released back into the blood (see Fig. 28.15). The macrophages also can remove particulate inclusions containing denatured hemoglobin (Heinz bodies) from erythrocytes without harming the cells themselves. Blood that filters through the red pulp then moves through the venous sinuses and into the portal circulation (blood flowing to the liver).

The spleen is not absolutely necessary for life or for adequate hematologic function. However, splenic absence as a result of any cause (atrophy, traumatic injury, or removal because of disease) has several secondary effects on the body. For example, leukocytosis (high levels of circulating leukocytes) often occurs after splenectomy, suggesting that the spleen exerts some control over the rate of proliferation of leukocyte stem cells in the bone marrow or their release into the bloodstream. Circulating levels of iron also may decrease, reflecting the spleen's role in the iron cycle (see the Iron Cycle section). The immune response to encapsulated bacteria (e.g., *Streptococcus pneumoniae* [pneumococcus], *Neisseria meningitidis* [meningococcus], and *Haemophilus influenzae*), which is primarily an IgM response, may be severely diminished, resulting in increased susceptibility to disseminated infections and sepsis. An increase in morphologically defective blood cells within the circulation after the loss of the spleen helps confirm the spleen's role in removing old or damaged cells. Thrombocytosis and thrombosis are complications of splenectomy and requires anticoagulation therapy.[5]

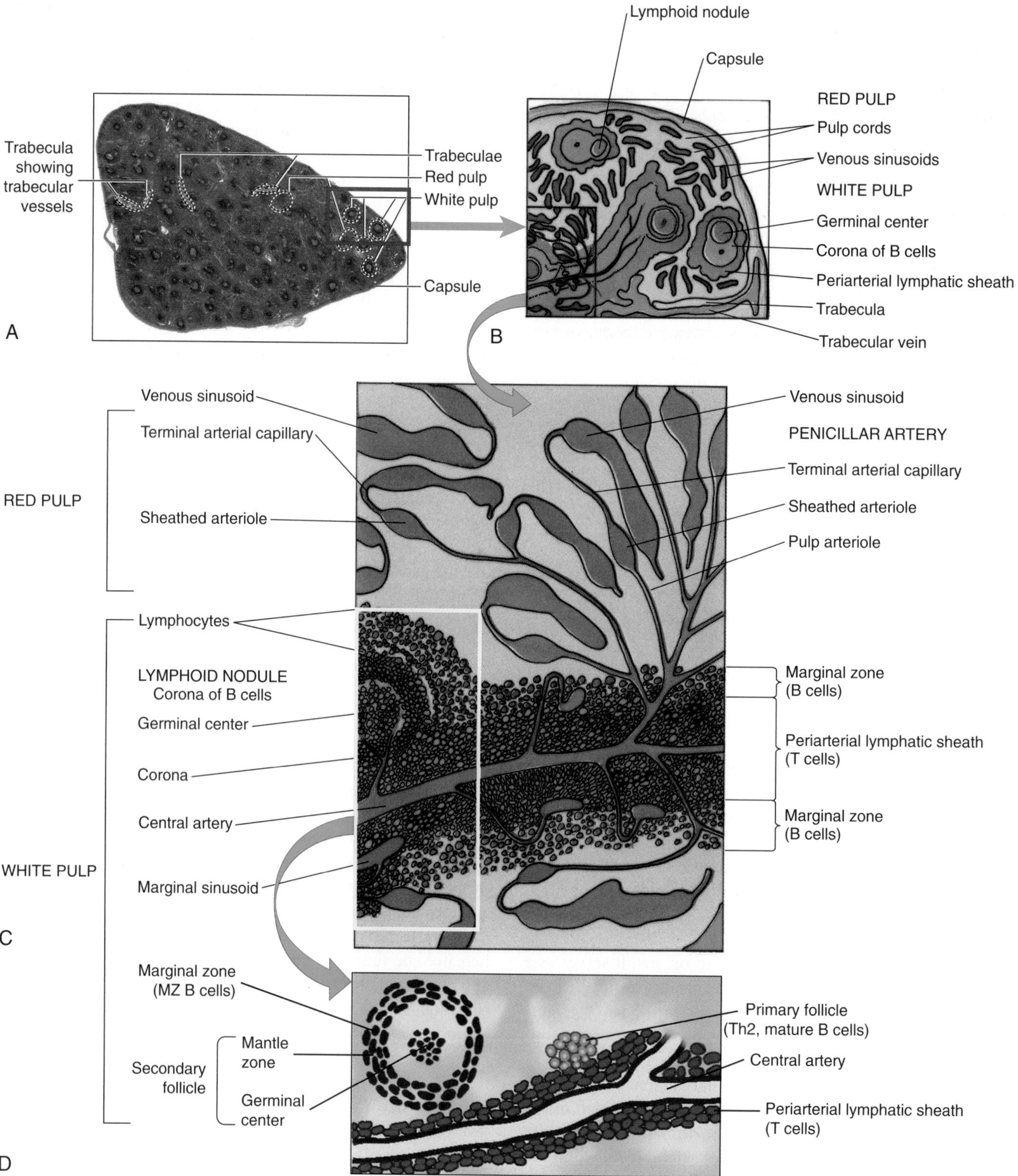

Fig. 28.6 Splenic Architecture. (A) Cross-section of the spleen. The spleen is enclosed in a capsule with the interior pulp divided into compartments by strands of connective tissue. The splenic pulp contains regions that are rich in lymphocytes *(white pulp)* and those containing erythrocytes *(red pulp)*. **(B)** Subcapsular splenic structures. **(C)** Magnified view of red and white pulp structures. **(D)** The splenic artery branches into trabecular arteries and then to central arteries frequently surrounded by a periarterial lymphoid sheath, primarily containing T cells. The secondary lymphoid follicles contain B cells that are proliferating in response to antigen. *Th2*, T-helper 2 cells. (A, From Telser AG, Young JK, Baldwin KM. *Elsevier's integrated histology*. St. Louis: Mosby; 2007; B and C, From Gartner LP, Hiatt JL. *Color textbook of histology*, 3rd edition. Philadelphia: Elsevier; 2007; D, From Hoffman R, et al. *Hematology: Basic principles and practice*, 6th edition. Philadelphia: Churchill Livingstone; 2013.)

Lymph Nodes

Structurally lymph nodes are part of the lymphatic system. Lymphatic vessels collect interstitial fluid from the tissues and transport it, as lymph, through vessels of increasing size to the thoracic duct, which drains into the superior vena cava and returns the lymph to the circulation. Lymph nodes are distributed throughout the body and provide filtration of the lymph during its journey through the lymphatics. Each lymph node is enclosed in a fibrous capsule, branches of which (trabeculae) extend inward to partition the node into several compartments. Reticular fibers of connective tissue divide the compartments into a meshwork throughout the lymph node. The node consists of outer (cortex) and inner (paracortex) cortical areas and an inner medulla. Lymph enters through multiple small afferent lymphatic vessels into the subcapsular sinus, just beneath the capsule, and drains into the cortical sinuses to the medullary sinuses, from which the lymph is collected and leaves the node by way of the efferent lymphatic vessel. Blood flows into the lymph nodes through the lymphatic artery, which ends in groups of postcapillary venules distributed throughout the outer cortex. The blood is drained through the lymphatic vein.

Functionally, lymph nodes are part of the hematologic and immune systems and are the primary site for the first encounter between antigen and lymphocytes. Lymphocytes enter the lymph node from the blood through specialized postcapillary venules called high endothelial venules (HEVs) by means of diapedesis across the endothelial lining (Fig. 28.7). Within the secondary lymph nodes, naïve T and B lymphocytes are segregated into different regions. B lymphocytes tend to migrate preferentially to nodes in the cortex and medulla, whereas T lymphocytes

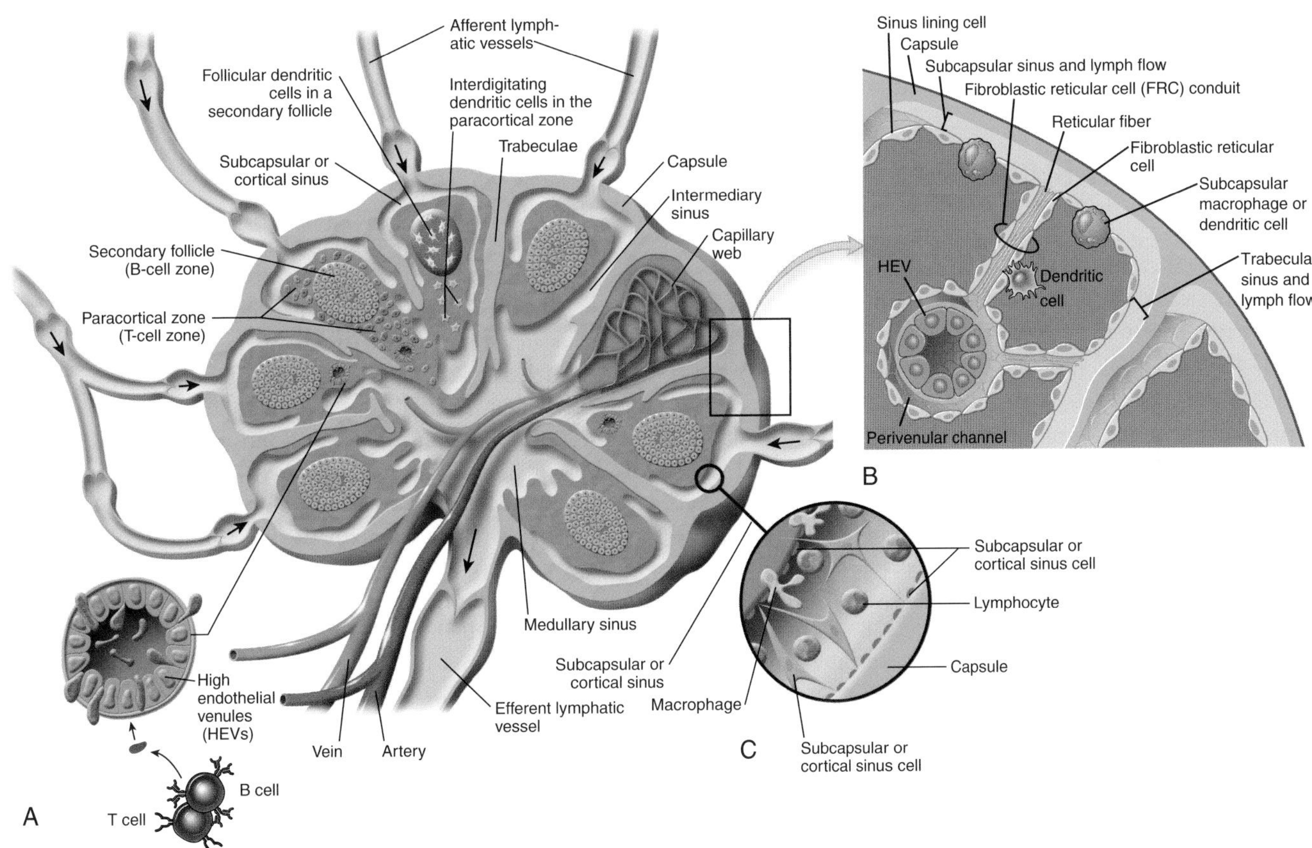

Fig. 28.7 Lymph Node Architecture. (A) Cross section showing ingoing and outgoing lymph vessels (afferent and efferent), blood supply, compartmentalization of the B-cell region (secondary follicle), T-cell region (paracortical zone) with precapillary or high endothelium venules, follicular interdigitating dendritic cells, medullary sinus, intermediate sinus, and subcapsular or cortical sinus. Naive B and T lymphocytes enter through the high endothelial venule (HEV), shown in cross section, and are drawn to different areas of the node by chemokines that are produced in these areas and bind selectively to either cell type. **(B)** Cellular composition of the lymph node cortex depicting the route of lymph drainage from the subcapsular sinus, through fibroreticular cell conduits, to the perivenular channel around the high endothelial venule (HEV). Dendritic cells pick up antigen from peripheral sites of antigen entry and enter the lymph node through the afferent lymph vessels and migrate to the T-cell region of the node. **(C)** Cellular composition of subcapsular sinus. (A and C, From Paulsen F. *Sobottta atlas of human anatomy*. Vol. 1, 15th edition. Philadelphia: Elsevier; 2013; B, From Abbas AK, Pillai S. *Cellular and molecular immunology*, 9th edition. Philadelphia: Saunders; 2015.)

predominantly migrate to the paracortex. Macrophages reside in the lymph node; help filter the lymph of debris, foreign substances, and microorganisms; and provide antigen-processing functions. The dendritic cells encounter and process antigens (see Chapter 8) and microorganisms in other tissues, then enter the lymph node through the afferent lymph vessels, and migrate throughout the nodes. The reticular network provides adhesive surfaces for trapping large numbers of phagocytes and lymphocytes and facilitates their organization into follicles or primary nodules. The presence of antigen, either removed from the lymph by macrophages or presented on the surface of dendritic cells, results in the production of secondary nodules containing germinal centers. In the germinal centers lymphocytes, particularly B cells, respond to antigenic stimulation by undergoing proliferation and further differentiation into memory cells and plasma cells (see Chapter 8). Plasma cells migrate to the medullary cords. The B-lymphocyte proliferation in response to a great deal of antigen (e.g., during infection) may result in lymph node enlargement and tenderness (reactive lymph node), which can be palpable during a physical examination.

DEVELOPMENT OF BLOOD CELLS

Bone Marrow

Bone marrow is confined to the cavities of bone and is the primary site of residence of hematopoietic stem cells (HSCs). The bone marrow environment provides HSC self-renewal, proliferation, differentiation, and apoptosis, and supports the developing progenitor cells.

Adults have two kinds of bone marrow: red marrow (active or hematopoietic marrow; also called myeloid tissue) and yellow marrow (inactive marrow). Bone cavities contain only red marrow at birth. The large quantity of fat in adult marrow is responsible for its yellow appearance. Not all bones contain active marrow. In adults, active marrow is found primarily in the flat bones of the pelvis (34%), vertebrae (28%), cranium and mandible (13%), sternum and ribs (10%), and in the extreme proximal portions of the humerus and femur (4% to 8%). Stem cells for transplant are commonly harvested from the flat bones of the pelvis. Inactive marrow predominates in cavities of other bones. (Bones are discussed further in Chapter 43.)

The hematologic compartment of the bone marrow consists of a variety of cellular and specialized molecular microenvironments, called bone marrow niches (Fig. 28.8). The niches provide essential autocrine, endocrine, and paracrine signals as well as direct cell-to-cell interactions necessary for the ability of HSCs to self-renew and to differentiate into all blood-cell lineages.

At least two populations of stem cells are found in bone marrow niches. Hematopoietic stem cells (HSCs) are progenitors of all the cell types of myeloid and lymphoid lineages (see Fig. 28.10). Mesenchymal stem cells (MSCs) are stromal cells (connective tissue cells) that can differentiate into a variety of cells, including osteoblasts (produce bone), adipocytes (store fat), chondrocytes (produce cartilage), sinusoidal endothelial cells, fibroblasts, and other stromal cells (connective tissue cells). The stromal cells secrete substances that form an extracellular matrix critical for cell growth and for anchoring developing blood cell progenitors in the bone marrow. Both populations of stem cells undergo continuous proliferation and self-renewal in the niches of the microenvironment of the bone marrow so that additional HSCs and MSCs are produced to replace those undergoing differentiation.

Hematopoietic niches are specialized microenvironments within the bone marrow that promote the maintenance of stem cells and regulate their function. The two main niches are the endosteal niche located close to endosteal bone, and the perivascular niche located more centrally near blood vessels and venous sinusoids. Different cell types reside in each niche. The primary cells of the *endosteal niche* are osteocytes, osteoblasts, osteoclasts, megakaryocytes, and macrophages. Osteoblasts are derived from MSCs and are responsible for construction of bone and support myelopoiesis through the release of soluble factors. Osteocytes are terminally differentiated osteoblasts and are the mature cell of the bone matrix. They are indirectly involved in the maintenance of the HSC pool through their interaction with osteoblasts. Osteoclasts are cells which originate from mononuclear cells of the HSC lineage and remodel bone by resorption. Additionally, osteoblasts can promote differentiation of B cells and osteoclasts can present antigen to T cells and are phagocytic, providing a link to immune function.[6]

Megakaryocytes and macrophages promote HSC migration and proliferation in the perivascular niches of the bone marrow. Megakaryocytes lie close to vascular sinuses where they produce platelets releasing them into the blood stream. Macrophages are also important for erythroid proliferation, differentiation, and maturation and supplying iron. Bone marrow adipocytes are a subpopulation of stromal adipocytes located throughout the bone marrow and support HSC maintenance.

Perivascular niches contain two specialized MSCs: chemokine ligand 12 (CXCL12)-abundant sinusoidal reticular (CAR) cells and periarteriolar and sinusoidal nestin-expressing cells. These cells closely interact with HSCs and provide intercellular signaling and cross-talk through several HSC regulatory molecules important for retention, expansion, maintenance, and quiescence or dormancy (prevents cell exhaustion and maintain their numbers throughout life) of HSCs. These regulatory molecules include CXCL12 (promotes retention and expansion of HSCs), stem cell factor (SCF, stimulates hematopoiesis), vascular cell adhesion molecule 1 (VCAM-1, promotes HSC retention), secreted protein angiopoietin 1 (ANG1, promotes quiescence or HSC stemness or ability to self-replicate), and transforming growth factor-beta (TGF-β, regulates quiescence and self-renewal).[7] The sympathetic nervous system acts with SCF to promote HSC maintenance and retention and regulates HSC mobilization.[8] The perivascular niche is also essential for gas exchange and delivery of nutrients and waste removal in the bone marrow.[9]

Hematopoietic marrow is vascularized by the primary arteries of the bones. Arterial vessels enter the bone, branch near the endosteum into smaller arterioles and capillaries, and drain into venous sinusoids. These sinuses coalesce into a large central sinus in the central cavity. Hematopoietic marrow and yellow

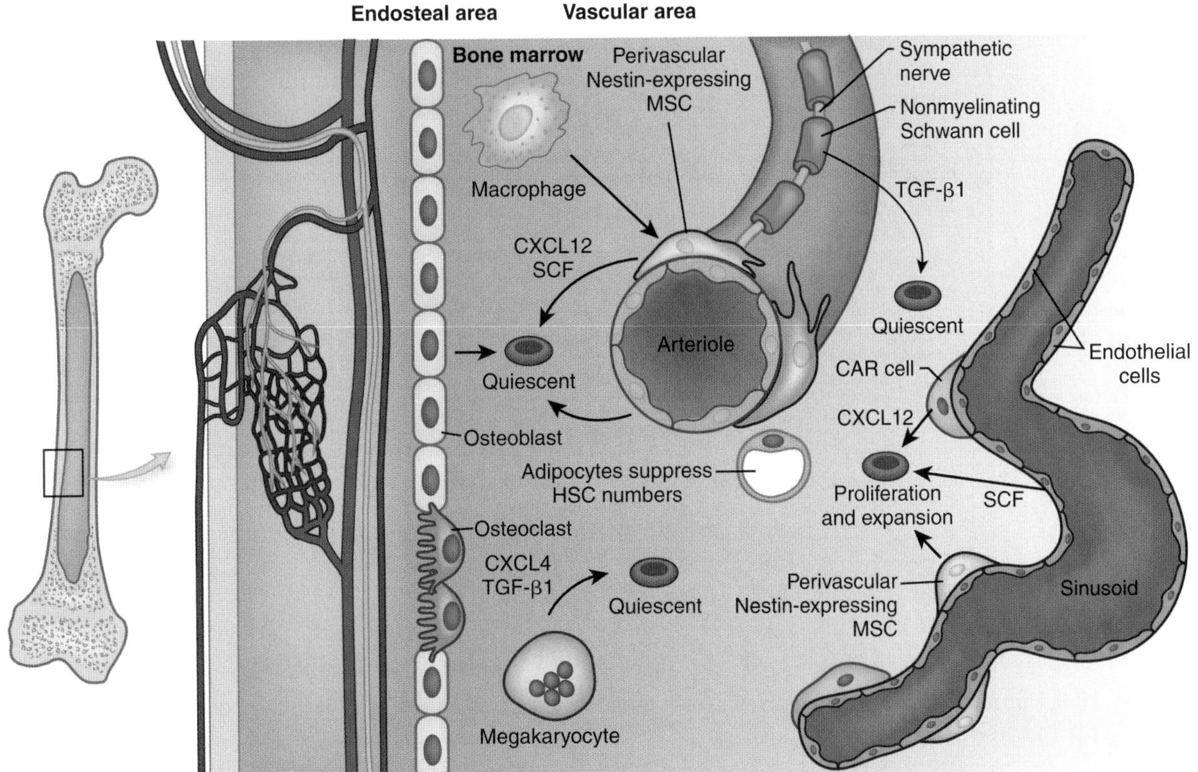

Fig. 28.8 Bone Marrow Stem Cell Niches. Stem cell niches are microenvironments where stem cells undergo hematopoiesis into all forms of blood cells. Stem cell niches retain and maintain adult quiescent hematopoietic stem cells (HSCs) and are activated to promote cell self-renewal, proliferation, and differentiation to form new cells. The fate of individual HSCs is determined by interactions with specialized cells within the niches. *CAR*, CXCL12-abundant reticular cells; *CXCL4*, chemokine ligand 4 (also known as *platelet factor 4*); *CXLC12*, chemokine ligand 12; *MSC*, mesenchymal stem cells; *SCF*, stem cell factor; *TGF-β1*, transforming growth factor-beta 1. (Adapted from Boulais PE, Frenette PS. Making sense of hematopoietic stem cell niches. *Blood*, 2015;125(17):2621–2629; Schepers K, Campbell TB, Passegué E. Normal and leukemic stem cell niches: insights and therapeutic opportunities. *Cell Stem Cell*, 2015;16(3):254–267.)

marrow fill the spaces surrounding the network of venous sinuses. Newly produced blood cells traverse narrow openings between endothelial cells (diapedesis) in the venous sinus walls and thus enter the circulation. The low blood flow of the arteriole/sinusoid network limits gas exchange, creates a relatively hypoxic microenvironment, and maintains HSC dormancy.

Cellular Differentiation

All humans originate from a single cell (the fertilized egg) that has the capacity to proliferate and eventually differentiate into the huge diversity of cells of the human body. After fertilization, the egg divides over a 5-day period to form a hollow ball (blastocyst) that implants on the uterus. Until about 3 days after fertilization, each cell (blastomere) is undifferentiated and retains the capacity to differentiate into any cell type. During this period, the outer layer of cells of the blastocyte has undergone differentiation and commitment to become the placenta. Cells of the inner cell mass, however, continue to have unlimited differentiation potential (currently referred to as being *embryonic pluripotent stem cells*) and can grow into different kinds of tissue—blood, nerves, heart, bone, and so forth. After implantation, cells of the inner cell mass begin differentiation into other cell types. *Differentiation* is a multistep process and results in intermediate groups of stem cells with more limited, but still impressive, abilities to differentiate into many different types of cells. These are known as *multipotent stem cells* and include the HSCs (Fig. 28.9).

Within the bone marrow niches, each type of blood cell originates from HSCs that proliferate and differentiate under control of a variety of cytokines and growth factors (Table 28.4). As with all stem cells, the HSCs are self-renewing (they have the ability to proliferate without further differentiation) so that a relatively constant population of stem cells is available. Some HSCs will continue differentiation into hematopoietic progenitor cells. Progenitor cells retain proliferative capacity but are *committed* to possible further differentiation into particular (unipotent) lineages of hematologic cells. The cell lineages include lymphoid lineages (T and B lymphocytes, NK cells) and myeloid lineages (monocytes, macrophages, neutrophils, basophils, eosinophils, megakaryocyte/platelets, and erythrocytes) (Fig. 28.10).

Several cytokines participate in hematopoiesis, particularly colony-stimulating factors (CSFs or hematopoietic growth factors),

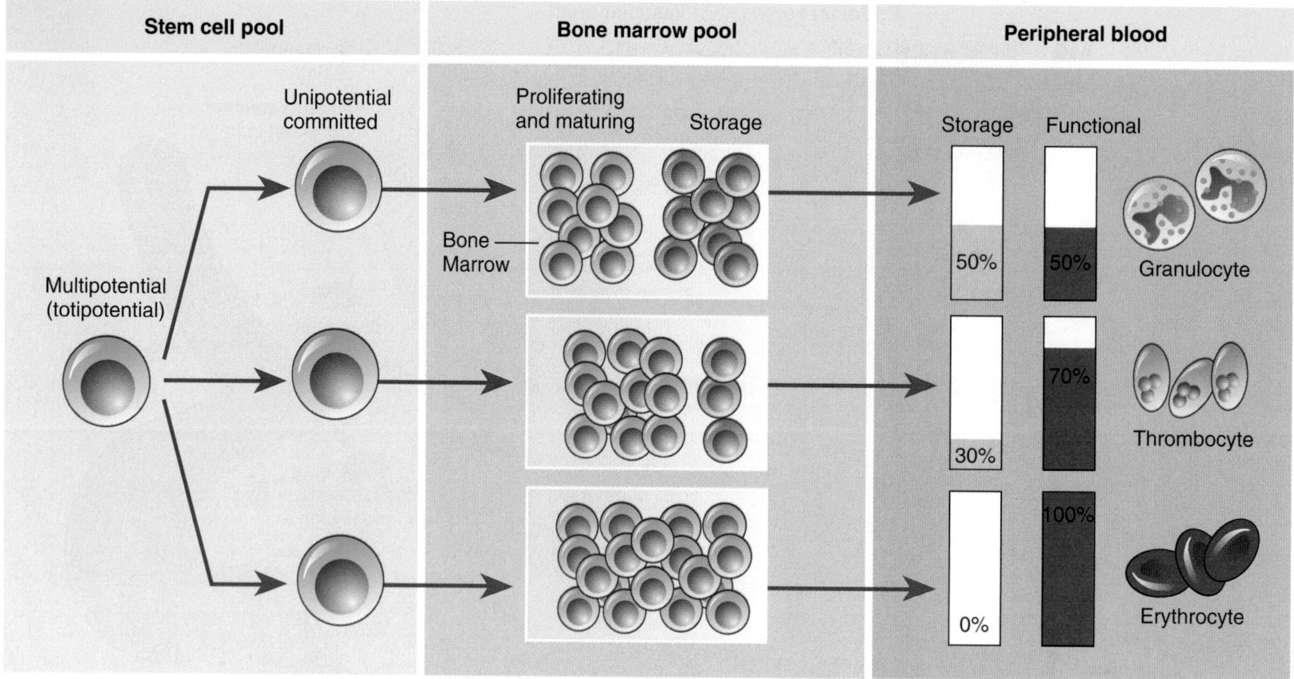

Fig. 28.9 Hematopoiesis. Hematopoiesis from the stem cell pool; activity mainly in the bone marrow and in the peripheral blood.

TABLE 28.4 Human Hematopoietic Growth Factors (Cytokines, Colony-Stimulating Factors)

Factor	Cell Origin	Primary Cell Stimulated
M-CSF	Macrophage, lymphocyte, fibroblast, endothelial cell, osteoblast	Monocyte progenitor to monocyte
GM-CSF	Macrophage, T cell, endothelial cell, fibroblast, mast cell	Common myeloid progenitor to granulocyte progenitor and monocyte progenitor
G-CSF	Macrophage, fibroblast, endothelial cell	Granulocyte progenitor to neutrophil
IL-2	Th cell	T-cell progenitor to T cell
IL-3	T cell, monocyte/macrophage, stromal cell	Common myeloid progenitor to progenitors for megakaryocyte, erythroid, granulocyte, and monocyte series
IL-4	Th cell	B-cell progenitor to B cell
IL-5	Th cell, mast cell	Common myeloid progenitor to eosinophilz
IL-7	Stromal cell, intestinal epithelium	Hematopoietic stem cell to common lymphoid progenitor Common lymphoid progenitor to progenitor B cell, pro NK cell, and progenitor T cell Progenitor T cell to T cell and progenitor B cell to B cell
IL-11	Stromal cell	Megakaryocyte progenitor to megakaryocyte
IL-15	Monocyte/macrophage	NK progenitor to NK cell
Erythropoietin	Peritubular kidney cell and Kupffer cell	Common myeloid progenitor to erythrocyte progenitor Erythrocyte progenitor to erythrocyte
Thrombopoietin	Liver, kidney, skeletal muscle	All cells in megakaryocyte lineage from common myeloid progenitor to platelet
Stem cell factor	Stromal cell in bone marrow and many other cells	Hematopoietic progenitor to common myeloid progenitor Common myeloid progenitor to progenitors for megakaryocyte, erythroid, granulocyte, and monocyte series

G-CSF, Granulocyte colony-stimulating factor; *GM-CSF*, granulocyte-macrophage colony–stimulating factor; *IL*, interleukin; *M-CSF*, macrophage colony-stimulating factor; *NK*, natural killer; *pro*, progenitor; *Th*, T helper.

which stimulate the proliferation of progenitor cells and their progeny and initiate the maturation events necessary to produce fully mature cells (see Table 28.4 and Fig. 28.10). Multiple cell types in hematopoietic organs, including endothelial cells, fibroblasts, granulocytes, monocytes, and lymphocytes, produce the necessary CSFs

Hematopoiesis in the bone marrow occurs in two separate pools: the stem cell pool and the bone marrow pool (see Fig. 28.9). The stem cell pool is the product of self-renewal that maintains the number of pluripotent stem cells and partially committed progenitor cells. The bone marrow pool, the largest

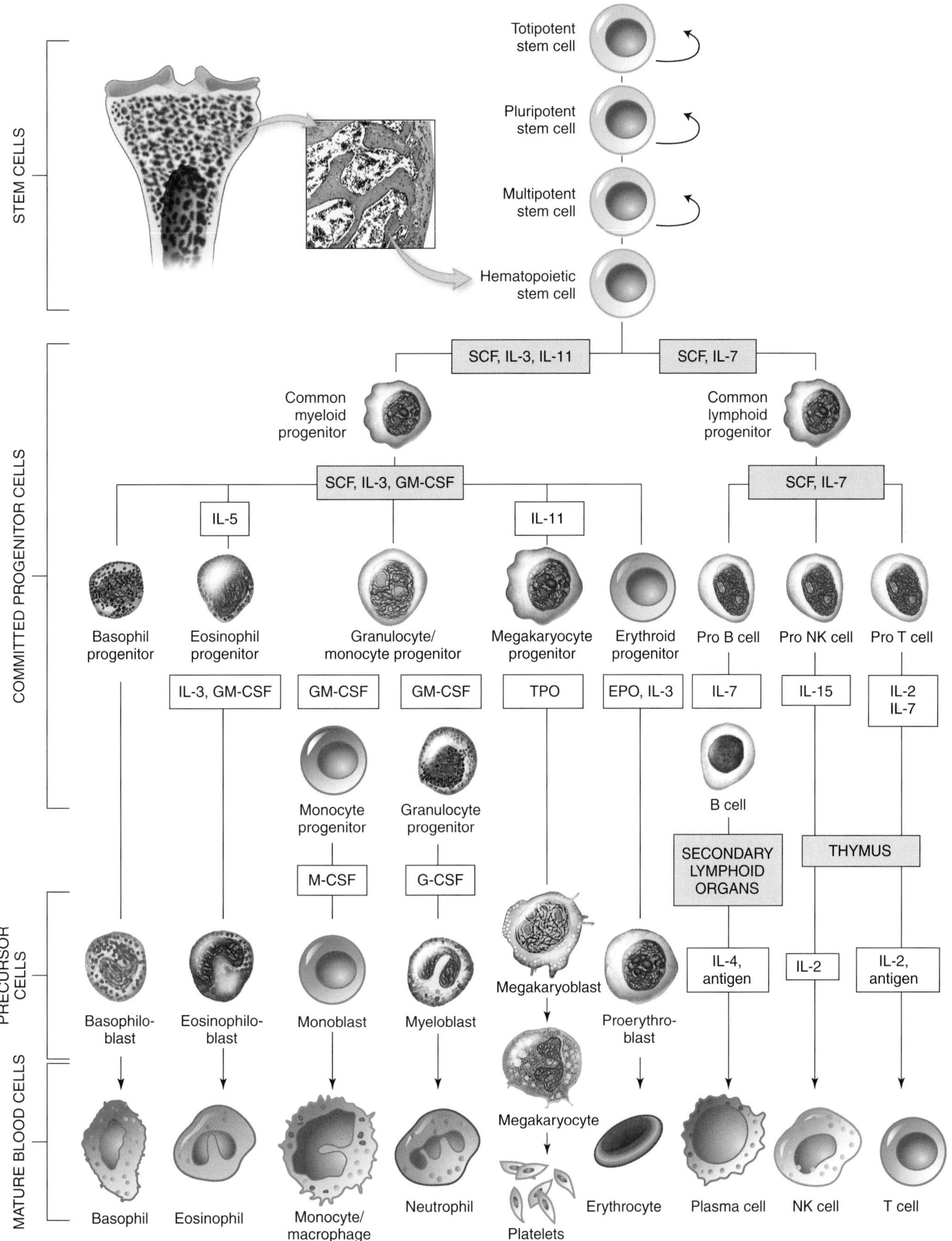

Fig. 28.10 Differentiation of Hematopoietic Cells. Curved arrows indicate proliferation and expansion of prehematopoietic stem cell populations. Yellow boxes are the hematopoietic growth factors needed for proliferation and differentiation (see Table 28.4) *EPO*, Erythropoietin; *G-CSF*, granulocyte colony-stimulating factor; *GM-CSF*, granulocyte-macrophage colony–stimulating factor; *IL*, interleukin; *M-CSF*, macrophage colony-stimulating factor; *NK*, natural killer; *SCF*, stem cell factor; *TPO*, thrombopoietin. (Modified from Patton K. *Anatomy and Physiology*. 10th ed. Elsevier; 2019.)

pool, contains cells that are proliferating and maturing in preparation for release into the circulation and mature cells that are stored for later release into the peripheral blood. The peripheral blood also contains two pools of cells: those in the circulation and those stored around the walls of the blood vessels (often called the marginating storage pool). The marginating storage pool primarily consists of neutrophils that adhere to the endothelium in vessels where the blood flow is relatively slow. These cells can rapidly move into tissues and mucous membranes when needed (e.g., during an inflammatory response).

Under certain conditions, the levels of circulating hematologic cells need to be rapidly replenished. Medullary hematopoiesis can be accelerated by any or all of three mechanisms: (1) conversion of yellow bone marrow, which does not produce blood cells, to red marrow, by the actions of erythropoietin (a hormone produced primarily by the kidney that stimulates erythrocyte production); (2) faster proliferation of stem cells into progenitor cells; and (3) faster differentiation of progenitor cells.

Hematopoiesis

The typical human requires about 100 billion new blood cells per day. Hematopoiesis is the production of blood cells. Blood cell production is constantly ongoing, occurring in the liver and spleen of the fetus, but only within the bone marrow (medullary hematopoiesis) after birth. This process involves the biochemical stimulation of populations of relatively undifferentiated cells to undergo mitotic division (i.e., proliferation) and maturation (i.e., differentiation) into mature hematologic cells (Fig. 28.10). Although proliferation and differentiation are usually sequential, certain blood cells proliferate and differentiate simultaneously. Erythrocytes and neutrophils generally differentiate fully before entering the blood, but monocytes and lymphocytes continue to mature in the blood and in secondary lymphatic organs.

Hematopoiesis continues throughout life, increasing in response to a need to replenish aged or destroyed circulating cells or in response to infection. In general, long-term stimuli, such as chronic diseases, cause a greater increase in hematopoiesis than do acute conditions, such as hemorrhage. Various abnormalities in medullary hematopoiesis have been identified and are discussed in Chapter 29.

Extramedullary hematopoiesis is blood cell production in tissues other than bone marrow, primarily the liver and spleen, but less frequently in the lymph nodes, adrenal glands, cartilage, adipose tissue, intrathoracic areas, and kidneys. Extramedullary hematopoiesis is usually a sign of disease and can occur in pernicious anemia, sickle cell anemia, thalassemia, hemolytic disease of the newborn (erythroblastosis fetalis), hereditary spherocytosis (abnormal sphere-shaped RBCs), and certain leukemias.

Development of Erythrocytes

Erythropoiesis is the development of RBCs. In the confines of the bone marrow, progenitor cells proliferate and differentiate into large, nucleated proerythroblasts, which are committed to producing erythroid cells (Fig. 28.11). The proerythroblast, which has ribosomes and can produce protein, differentiates through several intermediate forms of erythroblast (sometimes called **normoblast**) while progressively eliminating most intracellular structures (including the nucleus), synthesizing hemoglobin, and becoming more compact, eventually assuming the shape and characteristics of an erythrocyte.

The last immature form is the reticulocyte, which is anucleate and contains a mesh-like (reticular) network of ribosomal ribonucleic acid (rRNA). The reticulocyte contains polyribosomes (for globin synthesis) and mitochondria (for oxidative metabolism and heme synthesis). The reticulocyte matures into an erythrocyte within 24 to 48 hours. During this period, mitochondria and ribosomes disappear and the cell becomes smaller and more disc-like. With these final changes, the erythrocyte loses its capacity for hemoglobin synthesis and oxidative metabolism. Reticulocytes remain in the marrow approximately 1 day and are released into the venous sinuses. They continue to mature in the bloodstream and may travel to the spleen for several days of additional maturation. The normal reticulocyte count is 1% of the total RBC count. Approximately 1% of the body's circulating erythrocyte mass normally is generated every 24 hours. Therefore, the reticulocyte count is a useful clinical index of erythropoietic activity and indicates whether new red cells are being produced.

Regulation of erythropoiesis. In healthy humans, the total volume of circulating erythrocytes remains surprisingly constant. Most steps of erythropoiesis are primarily under the control of a feedback loop involving erythropoietin (EPO) and other cytokines (see Table 28.4). In conditions of tissue hypoxia, EPO is secreted primarily by the peritubular cells of the kidney (Fig. 28.12). Rising circulating levels of EPO cause a compensatory increase in erythrocyte production. The normal steady-state rate of production of 2.5 million erythrocytes per second

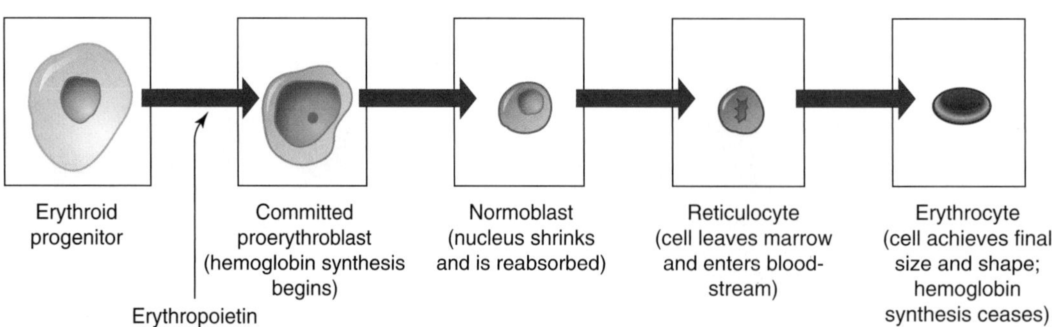

Fig. 28.11 Erythrocyte Differentiation. Erythrocyte differentiation from large, nucleated progenitor cells to small nonnucleated erythrocytes.

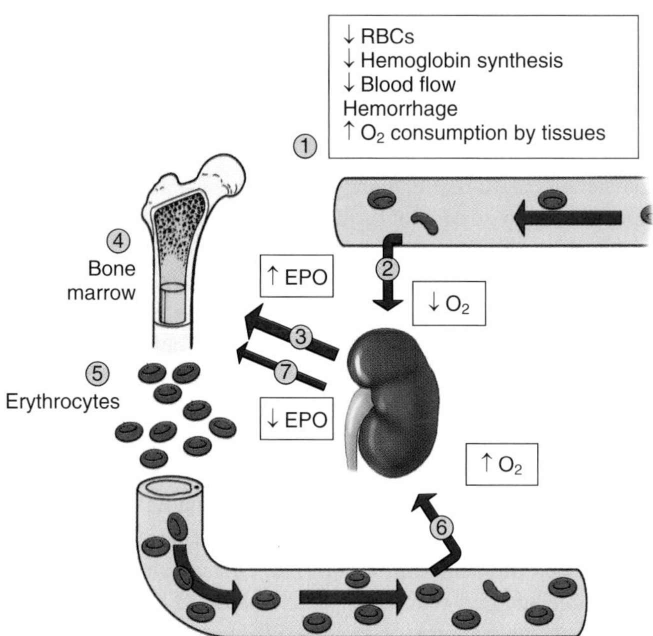

Fig. 28.12 Role of Erythropoietin in Regulation of Erythropoiesis. *(1)* Decreased arterial oxygen levels result in decreased tissue oxygen (hypoxia) that *(2)* stimulates the kidney to increase production *(3)* of erythropoietin. Erythropoietin is carried to the bone marrow *(4)* and binds to erythropoietin receptors on proerythroblasts, resulting in increased red cell production *(5)*. The increased release of red cells into the circulation frequently corrects the hypoxia in the tissues. Perception of normal oxygen levels by the kidney *(6)* causes diminished production *(7)* of erythropoietin (negative feedback) and a return to normal levels of erythrocyte production. *EPO*, Erythropoietin; O_2, oxygen in the blood and tissue; *RBCs*, red blood cells.

can increase to 17 million per second under anemic or low-oxygen states, such as high-altitude environments or pulmonary disease. Thus the body responds to reduced oxygenation of blood in two ways: (1) by increasing the intake of oxygen through increased respiration and (2) by increasing the oxygen-carrying capacity of the blood through increased erythropoiesis.

Recombinant human erythropoietin (r-HuEPO) is used in individuals with anemia secondary to decreased EPO from chronic renal failure. An immediate effect of EPO administration is an increase in the blood reticulocyte count, followed by increasing levels of erythrocytes. The most significant side effect is increased blood pressure.

Hemoglobin synthesis. Erythrocytes form hemoglobin in the bone marrow. Hemoglobin (Hb), the oxygen-carrying protein of the erythrocyte, constitutes approximately 90% of the cell's dry weight. Hb-packed blood cells take up oxygen in the lungs and exchange it for carbon dioxide in the tissues. A single erythrocyte can contain as many as 300 hemoglobin molecules. Hb increases the oxygen-carrying capacity of blood by 100-fold. Each Hb molecule is composed of two pairs of polypeptide chains (the globins) and four colorful complexes of iron plus protoporphyrin (the hemes), which are responsible for the blood's ruby-red color and oxygen-carrying capacity (Fig. 28.13).

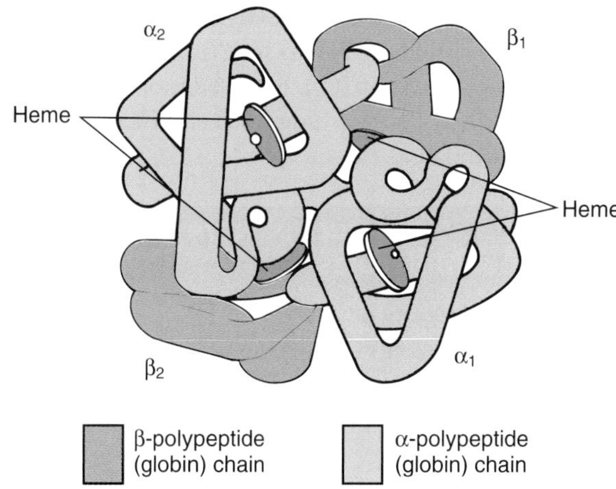

Fig. 28.13 Molecular Structure of Hemoglobin. Molecule is spherical and contains a pair of α-polypeptide chains, a pair of β-polypeptide chains, and four heme groups.

Each polypeptide chain contains approximately 150 amino acids and is arranged in a knotted-sausage configuration. The chains assemble to form a tetrahedron containing two pairs of identical chains. Several variants of Hb exist (Table 28.5), and they differ only slightly in primary structure based on the use of different polypeptide chains: alpha, beta, gamma, delta, epsilon, or zeta (α, β, γ, δ, ε, or ζ, respectively). Hb A, the most common type in adults, is composed of two α- and two β-polypeptide chains ($\alpha_2\beta_2$) (see Fig. 28.13). A normal variant, fetal Hb (Hb F), is a complex of two α- and two γ-polypeptide chains ($\alpha_2\gamma_2$) that binds oxygen with a much greater affinity than adult Hb. Other variants are genetic mutations associated with various diseases (see Chapter 29).[10]

Heme is a large, flat, iron-protoporphyrin disc that is synthesized in the mitochondria and can carry one molecule of oxygen (O_2). Thus, an individual Hb molecule with its four hemes can carry four oxygen molecules. If all four oxygen-binding sites are occupied by oxygen, the molecule is said to be saturated. Through a series of biochemical reactions, protoporphyrin, a complex four-ringed molecule, is produced and bound with ferrous iron. It is crucial that the iron be correctly charged; reduced ferrous iron (Fe^{2+}) can bind oxygen in the lungs and release it in the tissues, whereas ferric iron (Fe^{3+}) cannot. Binding of O_2 to ferrous iron temporarily oxidizes Fe^{2+} to Fe^{3+} (oxyhemoglobin), but after the release of O_2 the body reduces the iron to Fe^{2+} and reactivates the Hb (deoxyhemoglobin [reduced hemoglobin]). Without reactivation, the Fe^{3+}-containing Hb (methemoglobin) cannot bind O_2. An excess of ferric iron occurs with certain drugs and chemicals, such as nitrates and sulfonamides, and reduces oxygen-carrying capacity.

Hb undergoes a conformational change when binding O_2. When one of the iron molecules binds O_2, the porphyrin ring changes shape, increasing the exposure of the three remaining iron atoms to O_2. This greatly increases the affinity for the oxygen-carrying capacity of Hb, as occurs in the lungs. When oxygen is unloaded from Hb, the oxygen-carrying capacity of hemoglobin is low, facilitating the transport of carbon dioxide back to the lungs.

Several other molecules can competitively bind to deoxyhemoglobin. Carbon monoxide (CO) directly competes with O_2 for binding to Fe^{2+} with an affinity that is about 200-fold greater than that of O_2. Thus even a small amount of CO can dramatically decrease the ability of Hb to bind and transport O_2. Hb also binds carbon dioxide (CO_2), but at a binding site separate from where O_2 binds. In the lungs, CO_2 is released, allowing hemoglobin to bind O_2.

TABLE 28.5 Structure of Normal Hemoglobin Molecules

Type of Hemoglobin (Hb)	Identity of Polypeptide Chain	Significance
HbA	$\alpha_2\beta_2$	92% of adult Hb
HbA_{1c}	α_2 (β-*NH*-glucose)	5% of adult Hb; increased in diabetes (see Chapter 22)
HbA_2	$\alpha_2\delta_2$	2% of adult Hb; increased in β-thalassemia (see Chapter 29)
HbF	$\alpha_2\gamma_2$	Major fetal Hb from the third through ninth month of gestation; promotes oxygen transfer across platelets; increased in β-thalassemia
Hb Gower I	ε_4 or $\zeta_2\beta_2$	Present in early embryo; function unknown
Hb Gower II	$\alpha_2\varepsilon_2$	Present in early embryo; function unknown
Hb Portland	$\zeta_2\gamma_2$	Present in early embryo; function unknown

NH, Amine.

Erythrocytes may also play a role in the maintenance of vascular relaxation and blood flow. Nitric oxide (NO) produced by blood vessels is a major mediator of relaxation and dilation of the vessel walls. In the lungs, Hb can concurrently bind O_2 to the Fe^{2+} and NO to cysteine residues in the globins. As Hb transfers its O_2 to tissue, it may also shed small amounts of NO, contributing to dilation of the blood vessels and helping transfer of the O_2 into tissues.

Nutritional requirements for erythropoiesis. Normal development of erythrocytes and synthesis of hemoglobin depend on an optimal biochemical state and adequate supplies of the necessary building blocks, including protein, vitamins, and minerals (Table 28.6). If these components are lacking for a prolonged time, erythrocyte production slows and anemia (insufficient numbers of functional erythrocytes) may result (see Chapter 29).

Erythropoiesis cannot proceed in the absence of vitamins, especially B_{12}, folate (folic acid), B_6, riboflavin, pantothenic acid, niacin, ascorbic acid, and vitamin E. Dietary vitamin B_{12} is a large molecule that requires a protein secreted by parietal cells into the stomach (intrinsic factor [IF]) for transport across the ileum. Once absorbed, vitamin B_{12} is stored in the liver and used as needed in erythropoiesis. Defects in IF production lead to decreased B_{12} absorption, which may lead to pernicious (megaloblastic) anemia.

Folate is the second most important vitamin for erythrocyte production and maturation. Folate is necessary for DNA and ribonucleic acid (RNA) synthesis in precursor RBCs. Lack of folate results in an increase in abnormally large, nucleated

TABLE 28.6 Nutritional Requirements for Erythropoiesis

Nutrient	Role in Erythropoiesis	Consequence of Deficiency[a]
Protein (amino acids)	Structural component of plasma membrane	Decreased strength, elasticity, and flexibility of membrane; hemolytic anemia
Synthesis of hemoglobin		Decreased erythropoiesis and life span of erythrocytes
Cobalamin (vitamin B_{12})	Synthesis of DNA, maturation of erythrocytes, facilitator of folate metabolism	Macrocytic (megaloblastic) anemia
Folate (folic acid)	Synthesis of DNA and RNA, maturation of erythrocytes	Macrocytic (megaloblastic) anemia
Vitamin B_6 (pyridoxine)	Heme synthesis	Microcytic-hypochromic anemia
Vitamin B_2 (riboflavin)	Oxidative reactions	Normocytic-normochromic anemia
Vitamin C (ascorbic acid)	Iron metabolism, acts as reducing agent to maintain iron in its ferrous (Fe^{2+}) form	Normocytic-normochromic anemia
Pantothenic acid	Heme synthesis	Unknown in humans[b]
Niacin	None, but needed for respiration in mature erythrocytes	Unknown in humans
Vitamin E	Heme synthesis (?); protection against oxidative damage in mature erythrocytes	Hemolytic anemia with increased cell membrane fragility; shortens life span of erythrocytes in individual with cystic fibrosis
Iron	Hemoglobin synthesis	Iron deficiency anemia
Copper	Optimal mobilization of iron from tissues to plasma	Microcytic-hypochromic anemia

[a]See Chapter 29.
[b]Although pantothenic acid is important for optimal synthesis of heme, experimentally induced deficiency failed to produce anemia or other hematopoietic disturbances.
DNA, Deoxyribonucleic acid; *RNA*, ribonucleic acid.
Data from Lee GR, et al. *Wintrobe's Clinical Hematology*, 9th edition. Philadelphia: Lea & Febiger; 1993; Harmening DM. *Clinical hematology and fundamentals of hemostasis*, 3rd edition. Philadelphia: FA Davis; 1997.

precursor RBCs (megaloblasts) with a reduced capacity to carry O_2. Folate is absorbed principally in the upper small intestine and is stored in the liver. Folate deficiency is more common than vitamin B_{12} deficiency and occurs more rapidly. Folate stores can be depleted within a few months, whereas vitamin B_{12} depletion can take years. Folate supplements are prescribed for pregnant women because pregnancy increases the demand for folate. Supplements may prevent anemia and can protect against neural tube defects because folate is also required for embryonic neural tube closure (see Chapter 20).

Normal destruction of senescent erythrocytes. After about 120 days in the circulation, old erythrocytes are removed by tissue macrophages, primarily in the spleen.[11] Although mature erythrocytes lack nuclei, mitochondria, and the endoplasmic reticulum, they do have cytoplasmic enzymes capable of glycolysis (anaerobic glucose metabolism) and production of small quantities of adenosine triphosphate (ATP). ATP provides the energy needed to maintain cell function and keep its plasma membrane pliable. Metabolic processes diminish as the erythrocyte ages, so less ATP is available to maintain plasma membrane function. The aged or senescent red cell becomes increasingly fragile and loses its reversible deformability due to disruption of the anchorage between the cytoskeleton and the plasma membrane, thus becoming susceptible to rupture while passing through narrowed regions of the microcirculation.

Additionally, the plasma membrane of senescent red cells undergoes phospholipid rearrangement, signaling macrophages (primarily in the spleen) to selectively remove and sequester the senescent red cells. If the spleen is dysfunctional or absent, macrophages in the liver (Kupffer cells) assume control of this process. The erythrocytes are digested by proteolytic and lipolytic enzymes in the phagolysosomes (digestive vacuoles) of the macrophage. The heme and globin dissociate easily, and the globin is broken down into its component amino acids. The iron in hemoglobin is oxidized, forming Fe^{3+} (methemoglobin), and recycled.

During digestion of Hb in the macrophage, porphyrin reduces to unconjugated bilirubin, which is conjugated (made water soluble) and excreted from the liver into the intestine or into bile (Fig. 28.14). Bacteria in the intestinal lumen transform conjugated bilirubin into urobilinogen. Although a small portion is reabsorbed and excreted by the kidneys, most urobilinogen is excreted in feces. Conditions causing accelerated erythrocyte destruction increase the load of serum unconjugated bilirubin, increased liver conjugation of bilirubin, and increased urinary excretion of urobilinogen. Gallstones (cholelithiasis) can result from a chronically elevated rate of bilirubin excretion.

Iron cycle. Approximately 67% of total body iron is bound to heme in erythrocytes (Hb), and about 5% to 10% is bound to heme-containing myoglobin in muscle cells. Approximately 30% is stored in mononuclear phagocytes (i.e., macrophages) and hepatic parenchymal cells as either ferritin (iron bound to protein) or hemosiderin (intracellular bound iron). The remaining 3% (less than 1 mg) is lost daily in urine, sweat, bile, sloughing of epithelial cells from the skin and intestinal mucosa, and minor bleeding, as occurs with menstruation in women. There is no excretory mechanism for iron. Unbound, or free, iron is toxic to human cells. Approximately 25 mg of iron is required daily for erythropoiesis; only 1 to 2 mg of iron is dietary, and the remainder is obtained from continual recycling of iron from erythrocytes through a process known as the iron cycle.[12] Pregnant women require more iron to meet the needs of the placenta and growing fetus.

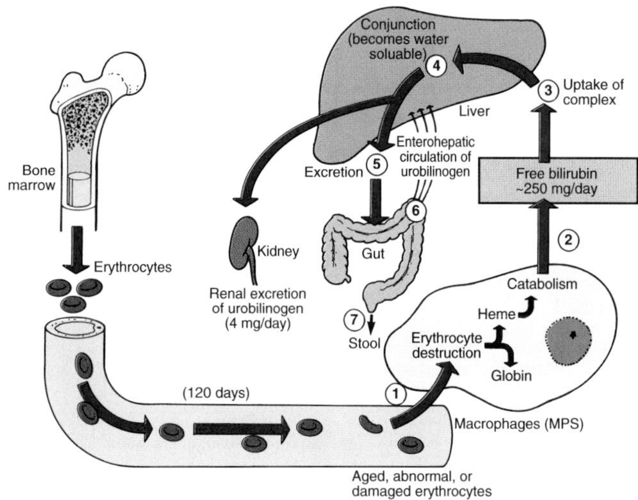

Fig. 28.14 Metabolism of Bilirubin Released by Heme Breakdown. *(1)* Senescent red blood cells (RBCs) are consumed by macrophages. During digestion, *(2)* the porphyrin in the RBC reduces to bilirubin. *(3)* Bilirubin is taken up by the liver, where it is *(4)* conjugated by glucuronyl transferase and then is *(5)* excreted as bile. *(6)* Bacteria in the intestine transform conjugated bilirubin into urobilinogen, *(7)* most of which is excreted in feces. *MPS*, Mononuclear phagocyte system.

The methemoglobin released from the breakdown of senescent or damaged erythrocytes is dissociated by the enzyme heme oxygenase, and the iron is released into the bloodstream, where it binds again to transferrin or is stored in the macrophage's cytoplasm as ferritin or hemosiderin (Fig. 28.15). A minute amount of iron is stored in muscle cells by the heme-containing protein myoglobin. Unavailable stores of iron are present in cytochromes, catalases, and peroxidase enzymes.

Ferritin is the major intracellular iron storage protein. Apoferritin is ferritin without attached iron and can store thousands of atoms of iron. Apoferritin binds to free Fe^{2+} and stores it as Fe^{3+}, becoming ferritin. Excess accumulations of iron produce large intracellular iron storage complexes, known as hemosiderin. Hemosiderin is visible as an iron-based pigment under a light microscope as cell inclusions. The iron within deposits of hemosiderin is poorly available because it is not water-soluble, but it is available when iron requirements increase. The most common cause of hemosiderin deposition is simple bruising. Hemosiderin in small amounts within iron-rich tissues (i.e., spleen, liver, bone marrow) is considered normal. Large aggregates or its presence in tissue, such as the lungs or subcutaneous tissue, suggests a pathologic condition known as hemosiderosis.

Iron from either dietary sources, release of iron stores, or erythrocyte catabolism is transported in the blood bound to apotransferrin, thus becoming transferrin. Under normal conditions, only one-third of the iron-binding sites on transferrin molecules are occupied. Apotransferrin is a glycoprotein

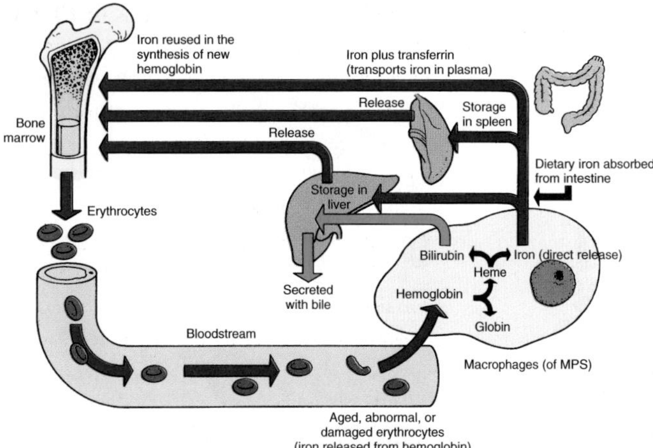

Fig. 28.15 Iron Cycle. Iron released from gastrointestinal epithelial cells circulates in the bloodstream associated with its plasma carrier, transferrin. It is delivered to erythroblasts in bone marrow, where most of it is incorporated into hemoglobin. Mature erythrocytes circulate for approximately 120 days, after which they become senescent and are removed by the mononuclear phagocyte system *(MPS).* Macrophages of the MPS (mostly in the spleen) break down ingested erythrocytes and return iron to the bloodstream directly or after storing it as ferritin or hemosiderin.

synthesized primarily by hepatocytes in the liver but also produced in small quantities by tissue macrophages, submaxillary and mammary glands, and ovaries or testes. Iron for hemoglobin production is carried by transferrin to the bone marrow, where it binds to transferrin receptors on erythroblasts. Transferrin receptors are on the plasma membrane of all nucleated cells, but at particularly high levels on erythroid precursors and rapidly proliferating cells (e.g., lymphocytes), and are thought to be the only route of cellular entry for transferrin-attached iron. Transferrin is recycled (transferrin cycle) by intracellular dissociation of iron from transferrin and secretion of the resultant apotransferrin to the bloodstream. The iron is transported to the erythroblast's mitochondria (the site of Hb production), where the enzyme heme synthetase inserts Fe^{2+} into protoporphyrin to form heme. Heme then is bound to globin to form Hb. Iron not used in erythropoiesis is stored temporarily as ferritin or hemosiderin and later excreted or recycled.

Splenic red pulp macrophages are specialized for iron recycling with increased expression of proteins for the uptake of hemoglobin, the breakdown of heme, and the export of iron.[13] The body's iron homeostasis is primarily controlled by the hormone hepcidin. Hepcidin is the regulator of the systemic transportation of iron.[14] It is a protein synthesized in the liver and released into the plasma, where it is bound with high affinity to α_2-macroglobulin and with less affinity to albumin. Hepatocellular hepcidin production is regulated physiologically by the levels of iron in the body, rate of erythropoiesis, and percentage of oxygen saturation. Hepatocytes (liver cells) sense levels of circulating iron by means of receptors for transferrin. Excess iron is stored in hepatocytes and macrophages, and hepatocytes sense these levels by means of receptors for bone morphogenetic protein (BMP), most likely BMP-6, which is a growth factor produced to a large extent by bone marrow sinusoid endothelial cells. Hepcidin production also can be induced by inflammation through IL-6 and other inflammatory cytokines, produced in response to infection or chronic conditions such as cancer.

Hepcidin regulates iron levels through its binding capacity to ferroportin, which is a transmembrane iron exporter found in the plasma membrane of cells that transport or store iron, including macrophages, hepatocytes, enterocytes (intestinal cells), and erythrocytes. The body's total iron balance is maintained through controlled absorption rather than excretion. Dietary iron (primarily as Fe^{2+}) is transported directly across the membranes of enterocytes in the duodenum and proximal jejunum and is carried in the plasma by transferrin. (Transport mechanisms are described in Chapter 1.) Hepcidin induces internalization and degradation of ferroportin, thus leading to increased intracellular iron stores, decreased dietary iron absorption, and decreased levels of circulating iron. Decreased production of hepcidin leads to release of stored iron and increased dietary absorption. Thus, if the body's iron stores are low or the demand for erythropoiesis increases, dietary iron is transported rapidly through the epithelial cell and into the plasma. If body stores are high and erythropoiesis is not increased, iron transport is stopped. Hepcidin production also can be induced by inflammation. During inflammation, increased levels of hepcidin lead to sequestering of iron as a result of down-regulation of ferroportin expression on macrophages and enterocytes and thus can cause anemia.

Development of Leukocytes

Leukocytes consist of lymphocytes, granulocytes, and monocytes (their pathways of differentiation are shown in Fig. 28.10). Most of the leukocytes arise from stem cells in the bone marrow. HSCs differentiate into two populations of progenitor cells: common lymphoid progenitors and common myeloid progenitors. Lymphopoiesis (lymphocytopoiesis) is the generation of lymphocytes from lymphoid progenitor cells released into the bloodstream to undergo further maturation in the primary and secondary lymphoid organs (see Chapter 8).

Myelopoiesis is the development of granulocytes (neutrophils, eosinophils, and basophils) and monocytes from the differentiation of myeloid progenitor cells in the bone marrow. The common myeloid progenitors differentiate into progenitors for basophils, mast cells, eosinophils, and megakaryocytes, and into granulocyte/monocyte progenitors. The granulocyte/monocyte progenitors further differentiate into monocyte progenitors and granulocyte progenitors, which develop into monocytes/macrophages and neutrophils, respectively. Development from HSCs to common granulocyte-monocyte progenitors primarily is under the control of SCF, IL-3, and GM-CSF, whereas further differentiation into granulocytic and monocytic progenitors is controlled by granulocyte colony stimulating factor (G-CSF) and macrophage stimulating factor (M-CSF), respectively (see Table 28.4 and Fig. 28.10).

Monocytic progenitors undergo development into monocytes within 24 hours and are released into the circulation. Monocytes mature into various forms of macrophages, a process that is usually completed within 1 or 2 days after their release.

Progenitor cells for granulocytes normally fully mature in the bone marrow into neutrophils, eosinophils, and basophils. The ultimate phenotype is determined by relative local bone marrow concentrations of early- and late-acting cytokines, including GM-CSF, G-CSF, IL-3, IL-5, SCF, and others (see Table 28.4). Granulocytes are released into the blood within 10 to 14 days of development. The bone marrow selectively retains immature granulocytes as a reserve pool that can be rapidly mobilized in response to the body's needs.

Most leukocytes exist in the body from days to years, depending on type (e.g., mature neutrophils live for hours and some macrophages live for years). Maintenance of optimal levels of granulocytes and monocytes in the blood depends on the availability of pluripotent stem cells in the marrow, induction of these into committed stem cells, timely release of new cells from the marrow, and mobilization of the granulocyte reserve pool. Leukocyte production increases in response to infection, to the presence of steroids, and to reduction or depletion of reserves in the marrow. It is also associated with strenuous exercise, convulsive seizures, heat, intense radiation, paroxysmal tachycardias, pain, nausea and vomiting, and anxiety.

Development of Platelets

Thrombopoiesis is the development of platelets. Platelets (thrombocytes) are derived from stem cells and progenitor cells that differentiate into megakaryocytes (see Fig. 28.10). During thrombopoiesis, the megakaryocyte nucleus enlarges and becomes extremely polyploidy (up to 100-fold or more of the normal amount of DNA) without cellular division. Concurrently, the numbers of cytoplasmic organelles (e.g., internal membranes, granules) increase and the cell develops cellular surface elongations and branches that progressively fragment into platelets. A single large (up to 100 μm) megakaryocyte may produce thousands of smaller platelets (2 to 3 μm). Like erythrocytes, platelets released from the bone marrow lack nuclei but contain granules that promote their stickiness. About two-thirds of platelets enter the circulation, and the remainder resides in the splenic pool.

Thrombopoietin (TPO), a hormone growth factor, stimulates the production and differentiation of megakaryocytes and is the main regulator of the circulating platelet numbers.[15] TPO is primarily produced by the liver and induces platelet production in the bone marrow. Platelets express receptors for TPO and, when circulating platelet levels are normal, TPO is adsorbed onto the platelet surface and prevented from accessing the bone marrow and initiating further platelet production. When platelet levels are low, however, the amount of TPO exceeds the number of available platelet TPO receptors, and free TPO can enter the bone marrow. During inflammation IL-6 induces increased production of TPO, which increases production of newly formed platelets, which are more thrombogenic.

Platelets circulate in the bloodstream for about 8 to 10 days before beginning to lose their ability to perform thrombogenic activity and biochemical reactions. Senescent platelets are sequestered and destroyed in the spleen by macrophage phagocytosis.

MECHANISMS OF HEMOSTASIS

Hemostasis is the arrest of bleeding by formation of blood clots at sites of vascular injury (Fig. 28.16). As a result of hemostasis, damaged blood vessels may maintain a relatively steady state of blood volume, pressure, and flow. Three equally important interactive components of hemostasis are the vasculature (endothelial cells and subendothelial matrix), platelets, and clotting factors. The general sequence of events in hemostasis is as follows:

1. Vascular injury leads to a transient arteriolar vasoconstriction to limit blood flow to the affected site.
2. Damage to the endothelial cell lining of the vessel exposes prothrombogenic subendothelial connective tissue matrix, leading to platelet adherence and activation and formation of a *hemostatic plug* to prevent further bleeding (primary hemostasis).
3. Tissue factor, produced by the endothelium, collaborates with secreted platelet factors and activated platelets to activate the clotting (coagulation) system to form fibrin clots and further prevent bleeding (secondary hemostasis).
4. The fibrin/platelet clot contracts to form a more permanent plug, and regulatory pathways are activated (fibrinolysis) to limit the size of the plug and begin the healing process.

The relative importance of the hemostatic mechanisms clearly varies with vessel size. Damage to large vessels cannot easily be controlled by hemostasis but requires vascular contraction and dramatically decreased blood flow into the damaged vessels (Table 28.7).

Function of Blood Vessel Endothelium

The vessel walls consist of a layer of endothelial cells that adhere to an underlying subendothelial matrix of connective tissue.

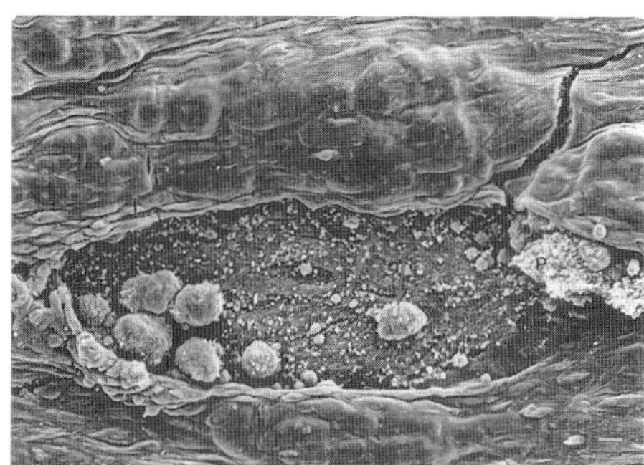

Fig. 28.16 Platelet Adhesion. After endothelial denudation, platelets and leukocytes *(blue arrows)* adhere to the subendothelium in a monolayer fashion. (From Zipes DP, et al. *Braunwald's heart disease: A textbook of cardiovascular medicine*, 8th edition. Philadelphia: Saunders; 2019, as reproduced from Faggiotto A, Ross R. Studies of hypercholesterolemia in the nonhuman primate. II. Fatty streak conversion to fibrous plaque. *Arteriosclerosis*. 1984;4:341–356.)

TABLE 28.7 Types of Bleeding: Sources, Vessel Size, and Sealing Requirements

Types and Sources of Bleeding	Involved Vessel	Size	Sealing Requirements
Pinpoint petechial hemorrhage (blood leakage from small vessels)	Capillary	Smallest	Generally direct sealing
	Venule	↓	Mostly fused platelets
	Arteriole		Mostly fused platelets
Ecchymosis (large, soft tissue bleeding)	Vein		Vascular contraction, fused platelets, perivascular and intravascular hemostatic factor activation
Rapidly expanding "blowout" hemorrhage	Artery	Largest	Greater vascular contraction, more fused platelets, greater perivascular and intravascular hemostatic factor activation

Modified from Harmening DM, ed. *Clinical hematology and fundamentals of hemostasis*, 3rd edition. Philadelphia: FA Davis; 1997.

The matrix contains a variety of proteins, including collagen, fibronectin, and laminins. Endothelial cells adhere to the matrix and to each other through receptors that are expressed only on the intercellular and basal surfaces.

Under normal conditions the endothelium actively regulates blood flow and prevents spontaneous activation of platelets and the clotting system. Endothelial cells produce nitric oxide (NO), also known as endothelium-derived vasorelaxant factor (EDRF),[16] and synthesize prostacyclin (prostaglandin I2 [PGI2]), both of which are vasodilators that modulate blood flow and pressure and maintain platelets in an inactive state. Synergism between PGI_2 and NO is significant. PGI_2 production varies a great deal in response to stimuli, whereas NO is released continually to regulate vascular tone. Endothelium also produces adenosine diphosphatase, which degrades adenosine diphosphate (ADP), a potent activator of platelets.

The endothelial cell surface contains antithrombotic molecules, such as glycosaminoglycans (e.g., heparan sulfate), thrombomodulin, and plasminogen activators. These limit platelet activation and fibrin deposition. Although thrombomodulin and plasminogen activators help control hemostasis in normal vessels, their effects are magnified during vascular damage and clot formation.

As a result of damage to the vessels, the endothelial cell barrier is frequently compromised, the remaining endothelial cells are activated by products of tissue damage, and the underlying subendothelial matrix is exposed. Endothelial cells contain intracellular structures that contain von Willebrand factor (vWF, clotting factor VIII), which is released during vascular injury and activates platelets for hemostasis.

Function of Platelets

Platelets normally circulate freely, suspended in plasma, in an unactivated state. The roles of platelets are to (1) contribute to regulation of blood flow into a damaged site by induction of vasoconstriction (vasospasm); (2) initiate platelet–platelet interactions (adhesion and aggregation) and attachment to injured endothelium, resulting in formation of a platelet plug to stop further bleeding; (3) release granules that activate the coagulation (or clotting) cascade to stabilize the platelet plug; and (4) initiate repair processes, including clot retraction and clot dissolution (fibrinolysis) and release of growth factors.[17]

The normal platelet count ranges from 150,000 to 400,000/mm^3. Thrombocytopenia (abnormally low numbers of platelets) develops if the platelet count drops below 100,000/mm^3, and an individual may experience longer than normal clotting times. Spontaneous major bleeding episodes do not generally occur unless the platelet count falls below 20,000/mm^3. If platelet numbers are elevated (thrombocytosis), the risk for spontaneous blood clots (thrombosis), stroke, or heart attack is increased.

Damage to the vessel initiates a process of platelet activation: (1) increased platelet *adhesion* to the damaged vascular wall; (2) *activation* leading to platelet degranulation, which stimulates changes in platelet shape and biochemistry; (3) *aggregation* as platelet–vascular wall and platelet-platelet adherence increases; and (4) activation of the clotting system and development of an immobilizing meshwork of platelets and fibrin.

Adhesion

Normally platelets are generally observed "rolling" along the margins of vessels. At sites of vessel injury, however, platelets become adherent to the site of endothelial damage, where the subendothelial matrix is exposed and endothelial cells have released vWF and decreased their antithrombotic activities (Fig. 28.17). Platelet adhesion is mostly mediated by the binding of platelet surface receptor glycoprotein Ib (GPIb) to vWF. The vWF protein is found in the subendothelial matrix and is released by endothelial cells and platelets. Platelet adhesion narrows the diameter of the blood vessel, resulting in increasing shear forces that could strip platelets off the vessel surface. However, those same forces induce conformational changes in the vWF molecule that result in increased affinity with the adhesive GPIb, thus stabilizing the adherent platelet.

Platelet adhesion is also facilitated by other interactions between platelet receptors and exposed molecules of the subendothelial matrix. For instance, adhesion is increased through binding of the platelet collagen receptors GPVI and integrin $\alpha_2\beta_1$ to exposed collagen in the matrix.

Activation

As a result of interactions with the endothelium or the subendothelial matrix, as well as exposure to inflammatory mediators produced by the endothelium and other cells, the platelets are activated. Activation results in reorganization of the platelet cytoskeleton, leading to dynamic changes in platelet shape from smooth spheres to those with spiny projections (increases surface area) (see Fig. 28.5) and degranulation (also called the platelet-release reaction) and resulting in the release of various potent biochemicals.

Platelets contain three types of granules: dense bodies, alpha granules, and lysosomes. The contents of the dense bodies and alpha granules are particularly important in hemostasis. The dense bodies contain ADP, serotonin, and calcium. ADP recruits and activates other platelets through specific receptors. During activation the platelet plasma membrane experiences several important changes, including becoming ruffled and sticky; undergoing cellular spreading to make tight contacts between neighboring platelets, causing the platelet plug to seal the injured endothelium; and externalizing the phospholipid phosphatidylserine, which provides a matrix for activation of clotting factors. Serotonin is a vasoactive amine that functions like histamine and increases vasodilation and vascular

I. Subendothelial exposure

- Occurs after endothelial sloughing
- Platelets begin to fill endothelial gaps
- Promoted by thromboxane A_2 (TXA_2)
- Inhibited by prostacyclin I_2 (PGI_2)
- Platelet function depends on many factors, especially calcium

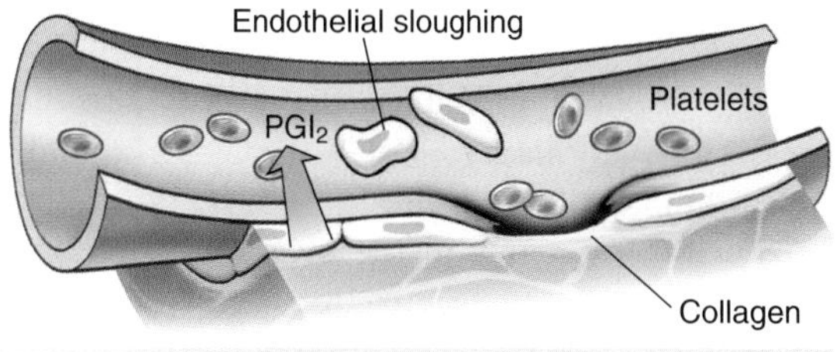

II. Adhesion

- Adhesion is initiated by loss of endothelial cells (or rupture or erosion of atherosclerotic plaque), which exposes adhesive glycoproteins such as collagen and von Willebrand factor (vWF) in the subendothelium. vWF and, perhaps, other adhesive glycoproteins in the plasma deposit on the damaged area. Platelets adhere to the subendothelium through receptors that bind to the adhesive glycoproteins (GPIb, GPIa/IIa, GPIIb/IIIa).

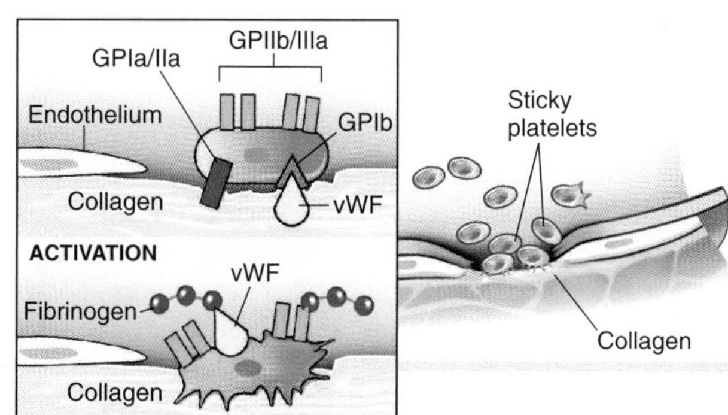

III. Activation

- After platelets adhere they undergo an activation process that leads to a conformational change in GPIIb/IIIa receptors, resulting in their ability to bind adhesive proteins, including fibrinogen and vWF
- Changes in platelet shape
- Formation of pseudopods
- Activation of arachidonic pathway

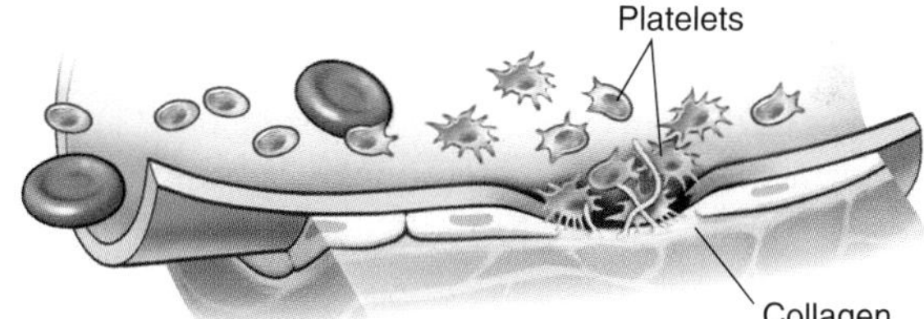

IV. Aggregation

- Induced by release of TXA_2
- Adhesive glycoproteins bind simultaneously to GPIIb/IIIa on two different platelets
- Stabilization of the platelet plug (blood clot) occurs by activation of coagulation factors, thrombin, and fibrin
- Heparin neutralizing factor enhances clot formation

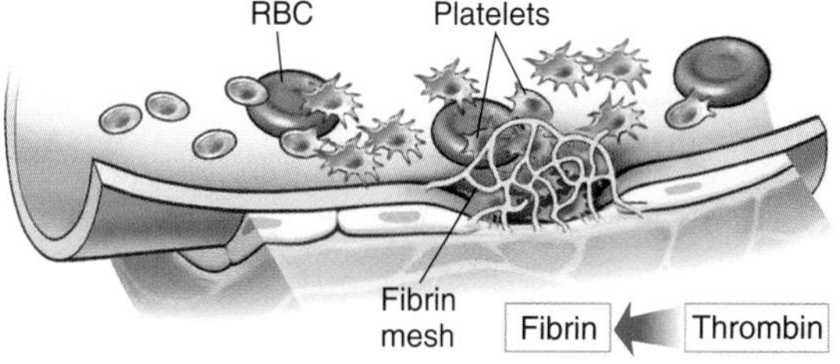

V. Platelet plug formation

- RBCs and platelets enmeshed in fibrin

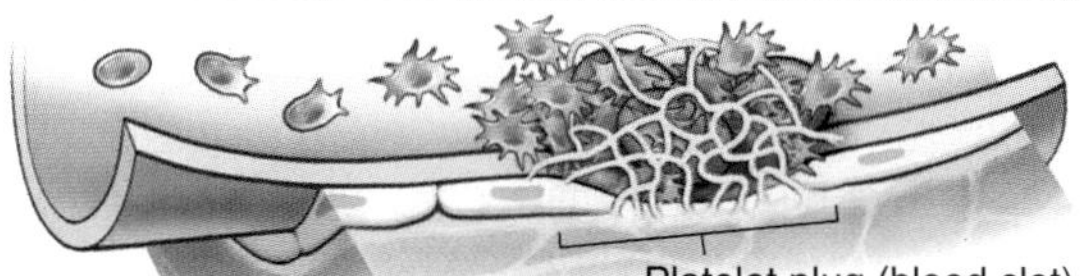

VI. Clot retraction and clot dissolution

- Clot retraction, using large number of platelets, joins the edges of the injured vessel
- Clot dissolution is regulated by thrombin and plasminogen activators

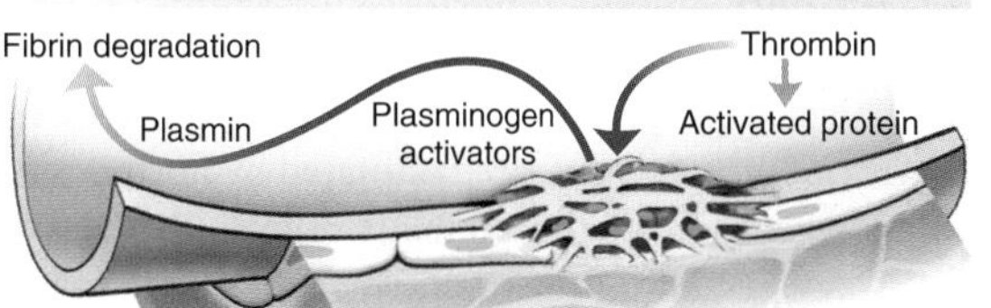

Fig. 28.17 Blood Vessel Damage, Platelet Activation, Blood Clot, and Clot Dissolution.

permeability. Calcium is necessary for many of the adhesive interactions as well as for intracellular signaling mechanisms that control platelet activation.

Alpha granules contain a mixture of clotting factors (e.g., fibrinogen), growth and angiogenic factors (e.g., platelet-derived growth factor [PDGF], vascular endothelial growth factor [VEGF], basic fibroblast growth factor), and angiogenesis inhibitors (e.g., platelet factor 4, thrombospondin, inhibitors of metalloproteinases). Platelet factor 4 also is a heparin-binding protein and enhances clot formation at the site of injury. Depending on the particular stimulus, platelets may selectively release promoters or inhibitors of angiogenesis. Many of these mediators either promote or inhibit platelet activity and the eventual process of clot formation. PDGF stimulates smooth muscle cells and promotes tissue repair.

Platelet lysosomes have a role in the digestion of phagocytic and cytosolic components, similar to that in nucleated cells. Lysosomal contents also may have important extracellular functions, such as supporting receptor cleavage, fibrinolysis and degradation of extracellular matrix components, and remodeling of the vasculature.[18]

Platelets also initiate production of the prostaglandin derivative thromboxane A2 (TXA2), which counters the effects of PGI_2 produced by endothelial cells. TXA_2 causes vasoconstriction and promotes the degranulation of platelets, increases expression of platelet fibrinogen receptors, and stimulates platelet aggregation, whereas PGI_2 promotes vasodilation and inhibits platelet degranulation. Arachidonic acid metabolism by cyclooxygenase (COX) is a major pathway for blood platelet activation. An isoform of cyclooxygenase (COX-1) converts arachidonic acid to TXA_2 in platelets. Aspirin at low doses specifically and irreversibly inactivates COX-1, decreasing production of TXA_2 and decreasing platelet activation and aggregation.[19] Daily intake of low doses of aspirin leads to more than 95% inhibition of TXA_2 in just a few days.

Other stimuli of platelet activation include epinephrine, thrombin, and collagen. Thrombin and collagen are particularly strong stimuli. Thrombin cleaves the extracellular domain of G-protein–coupled protease-activated receptors (PARs), thereby initiating transmembrane signaling.

Aggregation

Platelet aggregation is stimulated primarily by TXA_2 and ADP, which induce functional fibrinogen receptors on the platelet. The glycoprotein IIb/IIIa (GPIIb/IIIa) complex (also called *integrin* $\alpha IIb\beta_3$) undergoes a conformational change during activation to become a calcium-dependent receptor for fibrinogen, allowing it to bind other matrix proteins (e.g., fibronectin, fibrinogen, thrombospondin). Although the GPIIb/IIIa complex is the most abundant fibrinogen receptor on the platelet, receptors for vWF and collagen also contribute to the process. Interplatelet aggregation and clot retraction, which forms the *primary hemostatic plug*, are facilitated by fibrinogen bridges between receptors on the platelets. The GPIIb/IIIa–fibrinogen pathway is essential for the formation of a thrombus and as such is an important therapeutic target for blockage by antiplatelet drugs. In addition, fibrin strands within the clot shorten and become denser and stronger, helping the clot to approximate the edges of the injured vessel wall and sealing the site of injury. Contraction of myosin and actin filaments in the platelet cytoskeleton mediates *platelet contraction* and fusion of the platelet mass into a *secondary hemostatic plug*. Contraction expels serum from the fibrin meshwork, resulting in greater packing and increased strength.

If blood vessel injury is minor, hemostasis is achieved temporarily by formation of the platelet plug within 3 to 5 minutes of injury. Platelet plugs adhere to damaged vessel walls and seal the many minute ruptures that occur daily in the microcirculation, particularly in capillaries. With too few platelets, numerous small hemorrhagic areas called *purpuras* develop under the skin and throughout the tissues (see Chapter 29). If primary hemostasis is inadequate to prevent further bleeding, the process proceeds through secondary hemostasis to create a larger complex of more tightly interactive platelets within a matrix created by activation of the clotting system.

Function of Clotting Factors

A blood clot is a meshwork of protein strands that stabilizes the platelet plug and traps other cells, such as erythrocytes, phagocytes, and microorganisms (see Fig. 28.16). The strands are made of fibrin, which is produced by the clotting (coagulation) system. The clotting system was described in Chapter 7 and consists of a family of proteins that circulate in the blood in inactive forms (proenzymes). The proteins of the clotting system are all produced in liver hepatocytes. Initiation of the system results in sequential activation (cascade) of proteolytic enzymes which activate downstream enzymes in the system until a fibrin clot is created (Table 28.8).

The clotting system is commonly presented as two pathways of initiation: the extrinsic pathway (also known as the *tissue factor pathway*) and the intrinsic pathway (also known as the *contact activation pathway*). These two pathways join to form a common pathway, with activation of factor X, which proceeds to thrombin, fibrin, and clot formation. These pathways are controlled by anticoagulant proteins. The extrinsic pathway is activated when there is vascular injury and blood escapes into the tissue, with activation of tissue factor. The process is a normal mechanism of hemostasis. Tissue factor (TF) (also called tissue thromboplastin) is abundant in vascular subendothelium, in the surrounding larger blood vessels, and body organs, particularly the skin, brain, lungs, kidney, and placenta. There also are receptors for TF on activated monocytes. With vessel trauma and bleeding, TF binds with high affinity to circulating activated factor VII (TF/VIIa), initiating the clotting pathway. TF mediates a number of changes in disease-related activities, including inflammation, tumor angiogenesis metastasis, cell migration, and clotting associated with atherosclerosis (Fig. 28.18). The extrinsic pathway is evaluated in vitro by adding TF to a sample of plasma and measuring the prothrombin time (time to form a fibrin clot).

Factor XIIa (Hageman factor), prekallikrein (PK), and high-molecular-weight kininogen (HK; activates factor XII) initiate the intrinsic coagulation pathway through activation of the downstream substrate factor XI. The terms *intrinsic* or *contact* mean that the pathway is activated within the blood

TABLE 28.8 Coagulation Factors and Synonyms

Factor	Synonym	Primary Function
I	Fibrinogen	Source of fibrin to form clot
II	Prothrombin	Source of thrombin that activates fibrinogen, V, VII, VIII, XI, XIII, protein C, platelets
Tissue factor (thromboplastin)	Previously called *factor III*	Cofactor for factor VIIa
Calcium	Previously called *factor IV*	Cofactor for clotting factor binding to phosphatidylserine
V	Labile factor	Va is cofactor in prothrombinase complex
VII	Stable factor, proconvertin	VIIa forms complex with tissue factor and activates factors IX and X
VIII	Antihemophilic factor	VIIIa is component of tenase complex
IX	Christmas factor	IXa is component of tenase complex, activates factor X
X	Stuart-Prower factor	Xa is component of prothrombinase complex, activates prothrombin
XI	Plasma thromboplastin antecedent	XIa activates factor IX
XII	Hageman (contact) factor	XIIa activates factor XI
XIII	Fibrin-stabilizing factor	XIIIa cross-links fibrin

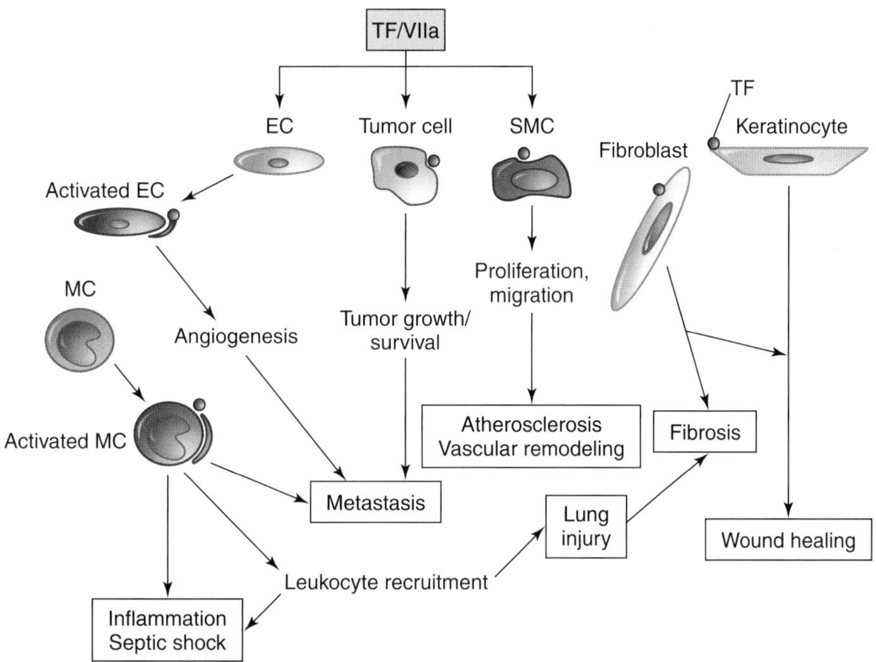

Fig. 28.18 Tissue Factor (TF) and Disease. Factor VIIa signaling through TF expressed on the surface of cells mediates changes in disease-related cellular activities. EC, Endothelial cell; MC, monocyte/macrophage; SMC, smooth muscle cell. (Modified from Rao LV, Pendurthi UR. Tissue factor-factor VIIa signaling. *Arteriosclerosis, Thrombosis, and Vascular Biologyl*, 2005;25(1):47–56.)

vessel by contact with anionic (negatively charged) surfaces (e.g., exposure of subendothelial collagen from vessel damage) or other substances without the action of TF. The intrinsic pathway is not a significant pathway for normal hemostasis but is a pathophysiologic surface defense mechanism against foreign proteins, microbial pathogens, and artificial materials. Individuals with deficiencies in intrinsic pathway components (e.g., factor XI, factor XII) do not have disruption of hemostasis or prolonged bleeding with the exception of hemophilia C (deficiency of factor XI that usually causes mild bleeding).

In the activation of the intrinsic pathway, factor XIIa recruits HK that is complexed with PK. Factor XIIa activates PK to kallikrein, which in turn generates more factor XIIa and amplifies the pathway. Factor XIIa also activates HK to release bradykinin (a proinflammatory mediator). Other exogenous artificial surfaces also can activate factor XII (e.g., use of tubing for blood flow during hemodialysis, cardiopulmonary bypass, or extracorporeal membrane oxygenation) and require anticoagulation therapy. More recently it has been discovered that naturally occurring polyphosphates (e.g., RNA and DNA from injury in arterioles), activated platelets, neutrophil extracellular traps, and cell membranes from bacteria can activate the intrinsic pathway and promote thrombin formation and thrombosis. The intrinsic pathway also may be essential for stabilization of thrombi and prevention of embolism.[20]

It is important to recognize that factor XIa and factor IXa can be generated by routes independent of factor XIIa (e.g., thrombin also can activate factor XI, as well as factors V and VIII). Thrombin activation of XI and IX is a feedback mechanism that amplifies the coagulation pathway and maintains the clot over time.

Activated platelets are important participants in clotting as previously described. The phosphatidylserine-rich surface produced during platelet activation provides a matrix on which several important complexes of clotting factors are formed. These include the intrinsic pathway's *tenase complex* (factor X and activated factors VIII and IX) that activates factor X and the *prothrombinase complex* (prothrombin and activated factors X and V) that activates prothrombin into thrombin. Thrombin then converts fibrinogen into fibrin, which polymerizes into a fibrin clot (see Fig. 28.16). Thrombin has broad activity in the inflammatory response. In addition to producing fibrin, thrombin is an activator of other coagulation proteins (e.g., factors V, VIII, XI, XIII), platelets (e.g., aggregation, degranulation), endothelial cells (e.g., up-regulation of adhesion molecules for leukocytes, increased NO, PGI_2, PDGF), and monocytes (e.g., cytokine secretion and increased receptors for endothelial cells). In addition to these pathways, RBCs can also promote clotting, particularly when there are diseases that affect the vasculature or there is an increase in the concentration of RBCs (see Emerging Science Box: Red Bloods Cells and Hemostasis).

Control of Hemostatic Mechanisms

Blood normally remains fluid despite the continual presence of clotting factors and platelets in the circulation. This is because under normal conditions, spontaneous activation of hemostasis is prevented by factors residing on the endothelial cell surface. These include thrombin inhibitors (e.g., antithrombin III), tissue factor inhibitors (e.g., tissue factor pathway inhibitor), and mechanisms for degrading activated clotting factors (e.g., protein C). When the endothelium is damaged, it transitions to the hemostatic action (vasoconstriction, platelet and clotting factor activation) described previously.

Antithrombin III (AT-III) is a circulating inhibitor of plasma serine proteases. AT-III is produced by the liver and binds to heparin sulfate found naturally on the surface of endothelial cells, or with heparin administered clinically to prevent thrombosis. Heparin induces a change in AT-III that greatly enhances its capacity to inhibit thrombin and other activated clotting factors. Under normal conditions the presence of endothelial cell heparan sulfate and the available AT-III in the circulation cooperate to protect the vessels from the effects of spontaneously activated thrombin. Acquired AT-III deficiencies can result from infection with bacteria that produce AT-III inhibitors, sepsis, liver disease, and nephrotic syndrome and lead to venous thrombosis and pulmonary embolism (PE).

Tissue factor pathway inhibitor (TFPI) is produced by endothelial cells and platelets and is the primary inhibitor of the initiation of blood clotting. TFPI forms complexes with and reversibly inhibits factor Xa. The resultant TFPI/Xa complex inhibits the extrinsic coagulation initiation complex TF/VIIa and prothrombinase (converts prothrombin to thrombin) and thus inhibits clotting.[21]

Thrombomodulin is a transmembrane thrombin-binding protein on the surface of endothelial cells and a receptor for thrombin. When thrombin binds to thrombomodulin, it no longer serves as a procoagulant and cannot activate platelets, convert fibrinogen to fibrin, or amplify fibrin generation. Protein C in the circulation binds to thrombomodulin-thrombin complex and is rapidly converted to activated protein C. Activated protein C, in association with a cofactor (protein S), degrades factors Va and VIIIa, inhibits fibrin formation, and inhibits coagulation. Deficiencies of AT-III, protein C, or protein S are important inherited causes of hypercoagulation

EMERGING SCIENCE BOX

Red Bloods Cells and Hemostasis

Red blood cells (RBCs) contribute to clotting and hemostasis by the expression of adhesive proteins, aggregation, hemolysis, and release of extracellular microvesicles and interaction with platelets and fibrin. Exposure of phosphatidylserine from the RBC wall promotes clotting via thrombin formation through a factor XII-dependent pathway without tissue factor activity. RBC interaction with the endothelial wall of vessels is normally minimal, but with pathological conditions such as retinal venous occlusion, hypertension, diabetic mellitus, and stroke there is increased adhesion of RBCs and increased thrombosis. Erythrocyte volume (hematocrit) affects blood viscosity and flow velocity, particularly in veins. High hematocrit slows blood flow velocity and is associated with thrombus formation. There is an increase in platelet margination, adhesion, and activation and prothrombotic activity. Slower flow velocity also promotes rouleaux formation (linear arrays of stacked red blood cells) and promotes thrombus formation particularly in veins. On the other hand, low hematocrit is associated with bleeding. RBCs are incorporated into blood clots and can play a role in the contraction of clots by platelets, adherence to fibrin, and the lysis of clots by fibrinolysis. RBC modulation of clot structure affects clot stability, embolization, and the efficacy of anticoagulation and therapeutic thrombolysis. Changes in RBC membrane deformability with increased stiffness or rigidity of RBC walls makes movement through the microvasculature difficult, increases thrombotic potential, and enhances platelet aggregation. These changes are associated with diseases such as autoimmune hemolytic anemia, sickle cell disease, thalassemia, hereditary spherocytosis, and xerocytosis. The multifactorial mechanisms of the role of RBCs is complex and not fully understood, emphasizing the need for further investigation.

Data from Alamin AA. The role of red blood cells in hemostasis. *Seminars in Thrombosis and Hemostasis*, 2020;47(1):26–31; Pretini V, et al. Red blood cells: Chasing interactions. *Frontiers in Physiology*, 2019;10:945; Weisel JW, et al. Red blood cells: The forgotten player in hemostasis and thrombosis. *Journal of Thrombosis and Haemostasis*, 2019;17(2):271–282.

(increased clotting). Expression of thrombomodulin and the endothelial cell protein C receptor is down-regulated by cytokines and other products of inflammation (e.g., IL-1α, TNF-α, endotoxin), thereby enhancing clot formation. Activated protein C inhibits the adhesion of neutrophils to the endothelium, but during inflammation neutrophil elastase enzymatically removes thrombomodulin from the endothelial cell surface and regulates clot formation.[22]

Retraction and Lysis of Blood Clots

After a clot is formed, it retracts, or "solidifies." Fibrin strands shorten, becoming denser and stronger, which approximates the edges of the injured vessel wall and seals the site of injury. Retraction is facilitated by the large numbers of platelets trapped within the fibrin meshwork. The platelets contract and "pull" the fibrin threads closer together while releasing a factor that stabilizes the fibrin. Contraction expels serum from the fibrin meshwork. This process usually begins within a few minutes after a clot has formed, and most of the serum is expelled within 20 to 60 minutes.[23]

Lysis (breakdown) of blood clots is carried out by the fibrinolytic system (Fig. 28.19). Another plasma protein, plasminogen, is converted to plasmin by several products of coagulation and inflammation, especially by the enzymatic action of tissue plasminogen activator (t-PA). Endothelial cells express t-PA, which is activated maximally after binding to fibrin. Another activator of plasminogen is urokinase-like plasminogen activator (u-PA). The u-PA binds to a specific cellular u-PA receptor (u-PAR), causing activation of plasminogen. This urokinase is the major activator of fibrinolysis in the *extravascular*, or tissue, compartment, whereas t-PA is largely involved in *intravascular* fibrinolysis. Several cancers appear to use membrane-bound u-PA to digest intercellular matrix and greatly facilitate tumor invasion and metastasis. Both t-PA and u-PA have been used

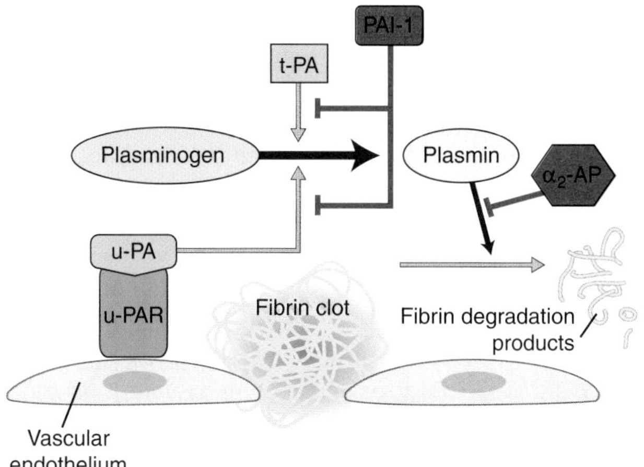

Fig. 28.19 The Fibrinolytic System. Fibrinolysis is initiated by the binding of plasminogen to fibrin. Although tissue plasminogen activator *(t-PA)* initiates intravascular fibrinolysis, urokinase plasminogen activator *(u-PA)* is the major activator of fibrinolysis in tissue (extravascular). Plasmin digests the fibrin into smaller soluble pieces (fibrin degradation products). *u-PAR,* Urokinase-like plasminogen activator receptor.

clinically to treat diseases associated with a blood clot (e.g., PE, myocardial infarction, stroke).

As with most components of inflammation, plasmin interacts greatly with other factors. In addition to activation by t-PA and u-PA, plasminogen is activated to plasmin by thrombin, fibrin, factor XIIa, factor XIa, and kallikrein. Plasmin is proteolytic to several substrates, and cleaves fibronectin, fibrin, thrombospondin, laminin, and vWF. Cross-linked fibrin is deposited in tissues around wounds, inflammatory sites, and tumors. Fibrin removal is an important biologic process, for intravascular and extravascular spaces, with various controlling mechanisms that can lead to abnormalities of fibrin accumulation and thrombotic events and can be a structural barrier to tumor invasion.

Plasmin is an enzyme that dissolves clots (fibrinolysis) by degrading fibrin and fibrinogen into fibrin degradation products (FDPs). A major FDP is D-dimer. Measurement of levels of circulating d-dimer (a small protein fragment of fibrin degradation) has been used for diagnosis because D-dimer can be elevated in cases of deep venous thrombosis (DVT) or PE.

CLINICAL EVALUATION OF THE HEMATOLOGIC SYSTEM

Tests of Bone Marrow Function

Several abnormal conditions in the numbers or morphology of circulating blood cells or suspected infection of the marrow may justify further investigation of the bone marrow. Usually bone marrow is aspirated from the sternum or pelvis using a needle. In children a bone marrow aspirate can be obtained from the vertebrae or the femur. The aspirate is examined microscopically and may be cultured if infection (e.g., fungi, mycobacteria, brucellosis, typhoid fever) is suspected. Microscopic evaluation may also include flow cytometry, chromosome analysis, or polymerase chain reaction (PCR) related to the presence of atypical cells, the presence of atypical numbers of normal cells, and the absence of particular cell types. A normal bone marrow aspirate contains stromal cells (fibroblasts, macrophages, osteoblasts, adipocytes), stem cells (hematopoietic, mesenchymal, and endothelial), and immature and mature forms of blood cells (erythrocytes, leukocytes, platelets) (Fig. 28.20A). The differential cell count of a bone marrow aspirate involves examining approximately 400 nucleated cells under oil-immersion magnification and counting populations of cells differentiated on the basis of morphology. The relative number of each type of stem cell is expressed as a fraction of 400 (Table 28.9).

Bone marrow iron stores, primarily in macrophages, can be examined using special stains (e.g., Prussian blue) for iron-containing granules. A direct measure of iron stores also can be obtained only from liver biopsy specimens, although bone marrow is preferred because it is a safer procedure and because bone marrow is the immediate source of iron destined for erythrocyte production.

Bone marrow aspiration is an important diagnostic test for severe central defects in hematopoiesis (e.g., aplastic anemia, metabolic anemias arising from insufficient iron or inadequate

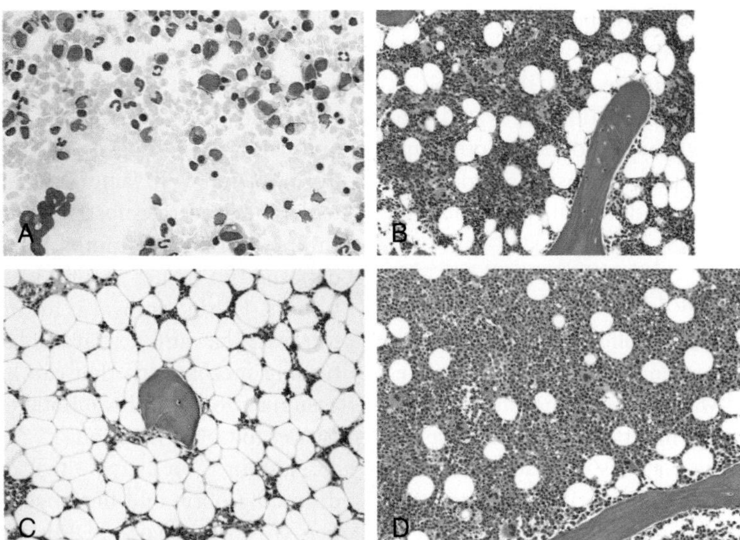

Fig. 28.20 Bone Marrow Samples. (A) Normal bone marrow aspirate stained by the May-Grünwald/Giemsa technique. **(B–D)** Bone marrow biopsies representing conditions of normal cellularity **(B)**, hypocellularity **(C)** as would be seen in conditions of bone marrow depletion such as aplastic anemia, and hypercellularity **(D)** as seen in malignant conditions. (A and C, From Hoffbrand V, et al. *Color atlas of clinical hematology*, 4th edition. Philadelphia: Mosby; 2013; B–D, From Jaffe E. *Hematology*. Philadelphia: Saunders; 2010.)

TABLE 28.9 Differential Cell Counts in Bone Marrow with Age

Developing Cells in Marrow	Birth	1 Month–1 Year	1–4 Years	4–12 Years	Adult
Erythrocytic series	14	8	19	21	20
Lymphocytic series	14	47	22	18	17
Eosinophilic series	3	3	6	3	3
Neutrophilic series	60	33	50	52	57
Myeloid/erythroid ratio	4:3	4:0	1:3	2:5	1:3

NOTE: Values are percentages of cell types counted during examination of a marrow specimen containing approximately 400 nucleated cells.

EPO, thrombocytopenia, and neutropenia). Examination of the bone marrow is also useful to diagnose B-lymphocyte immune deficiencies, nonmalignant myeloproliferative disorders (e.g., polycythemia vera), and lymphoid/monocytic malignancies (e.g., leukemias, myelomas, lymphomas). This test can also be used to monitor the effects of chemotherapy on malignancies that have invaded the bone marrow. A marrow aspirate that is richly cellular implies normal or increased hematopoiesis but does not indicate whether marrow activity is effective.

Results from bone marrow aspiration are sometimes limited because this technique disturbs the architecture of the marrow and only provides an analysis of the general cellularity (numbers of constituent cells) of the marrow. On occasion, analysis of an aspirate may only suggest the presence of a malignancy or a central defect in hematopoiesis without being clearly confirmatory, or the sample may be inadequate for diagnosis of bone marrow fibrosis. In these cases the need for a bone marrow biopsy may be indicated.

During a biopsy, a special needle is used to obtain a "core" or cylindrical sample of bone and marrow in which the three-dimensional structure of the marrow is preserved. The biopsy specimens provide the most reliable and complete information about marrow cellularity (see Fig. 28.20B–D). Obtaining a bone marrow biopsy is, however, usually more painful and expensive than aspiration. Therefore biopsy is not performed unless insufficient information is obtained from aspiration.

Blood Tests

Blood tests provide information about the absolute and relative numbers of blood cells in a specimen of blood, as well as various structural and functional characteristics of the cells, and usually provide the initial justification for performing a bone marrow aspiration. Deviations from the normal differential distribution and the presence of abnormal or immature cells can reflect disease, physiologic states (e.g., pregnancy, infancy, old age), injury, or dysfunction in almost any part of the body. Blood tests that reflect chiefly hematologic disorders are listed in Table 28.10.

PEDIATRICS AND THE HEMATOLOGIC SYSTEM

Blood cell counts tend to rise above adult levels at birth and then decline gradually throughout childhood. Table 28.11 lists normal ranges during infancy and childhood. The immediate rise in values is the result of accelerated hematopoiesis during

TABLE 28.10 **Blood Tests for Hematologic Disorders**

Cell Type and Test	Property Evaluated by Test	Possible Hematologic Cause of Abnormal Findings
Erythrocytes		
Red cell count	Number (in millions) of erythrocytes/μL of blood	Altered erythropoiesis, anemias, hemorrhage, Hodgkin disease, leukemia
Mean corpuscular volume	Size of erythrocytes	Anemias, thalassemias
Mean corpuscular hemoglobin (MCH)	Amount of hemoglobin in each erythrocyte (by weight)	Anemias, hemoglobinopathy
Mean corpuscular hemoglobin concentration (MCHC)	Concentration of hemoglobin in each erythrocyte (percentage of erythrocyte occupied by hemoglobin)	Anemias, hereditary spherocytosis
Hemoglobin determination	Amount of hemoglobin (by weight)/dL of blood	Anemias
Hematocrit determination	Percentage of a given volume of blood that is occupied by erythrocytes	Hemorrhage, polycythemia, erythrocytosis, anemias, leukemia
Reticulocyte count	Number of reticulocytes/μL of blood (also expressed as percentage of reticulocytes in total red cell count)	Hyperactive or hypoactive bone marrow function
Erythrocyte osmotic fragility test	Cellular shape (biconcavity), structure of plasma membrane	Anemias, hemolytic disease caused by ABO or Rh blood group incompatibility, Hodgkin disease, polycythemia vera, thalassemia major
Hemoglobin electrophoresis	Relative percentage of different types of hemoglobin in erythrocytes	Sickle cell disease, sickle cell trait, hemoglobin C disease, hemoglobin C trait, thalassemias
Sickle cell test	Presence of hemoglobin S in erythrocytes	Sickle cell trait, sickle cell anemia
Glucose-6-phosphate dehydrogenase (G6PD) deficiency test	Deficiency of G6PD in erythrocytes	Hemolytic anemia
Hemoglobin Metabolism		
Serum ferritin determination	Depletion of body iron (potential deficiency of heme synthesis)	Iron deficiency anemias
Total iron-binding capacity (TIBC)	Amount of iron in serum plus amount of transferrin available in serum (mcg/dL)	Hemorrhage, iron deficiency anemia, hemochromatosis, hemosiderosis, iron overload, anemias, thalassemias
Transferrin saturation	Percentage of transferrin that is saturated with iron	Acute hemorrhage, hemochromatosis, hemosiderosis, sideroblastic anemia, iron deficiency anemia, iron overload, thalassemias
Porphyrin analysis (protoporphyrin analysis)	Concentration of protoporphyrin in erythrocytes (mcg/dL); an indicator of iron-deficient erythropoiesis	Megaloblastic anemia, congenital erythropoietic porphyria
Direct antiglobulin test (DAT)	Antibody binding to erythrocytes	Hemolytic disease of the newborn, autoimmune hemolytic anemia, drug-induced hemolytic anemia, transfusion reaction
Antibody screen (indirect Coombs test)	Detection of antibodies to erythrocyte antigens (other than the ABO antigens)	Same as for DAT
Leukocytes		
Differential white cell count (absolute number of a type of leukocyte/μL of blood)	See below	See below
Neutrophil count	Neutrophils/μL	Myeloproliferative disorders, hematopoietic disorders, hemolysis, infection, immune deficiency
Lymphocyte count	Lymphocytes/μL	Infectious lymphocytosis, infectious mononucleosis, hematopoietic disorders, anemias, leukemia, lymphosarcoma, Hodgkin disease, primary immune deficiency
Plasma cell count	Plasma cells/μL	Infectious mononucleosis, lymphocytosis, plasma cell leukemia, primary immune deficiency
Monocyte count	Monocytes/μL	Hodgkin disease, infectious mononucleosis, monocytic leukemia, non-Hodgkin lymphoma, polycythemia vera, primary immune deficiency

(Continued)

TABLE 28.10 Blood Tests for Hematologic Disorders—cont'd

Cell Type and Test	Property Evaluated by Test	Possible Hematologic Cause of Abnormal Findings
Eosinophil count	Eosinophils/μL	Hematopoietic disorders
Basophil count	Basophils/μL	Chronic myelogenous leukemia, hemolytic anemias, Hodgkin disease, polycythemia vera
Platelets and Clotting Factors		
Platelet count	Number of circulating platelets (in thousands)/μL of blood	Anemias, multiple myeloma, myelofibrosis, polycythemia vera, leukemia, disseminated intravascular coagulation (DIC), hemolytic disease of the newborn, idiopathic thrombocytopenic purpura, transfusion reaction, lymphoproliferative disorders
Bleeding time	Duration of bleeding following a standardized superficial puncture wound of the skin, integrity of the platelet plug; measured in minutes following puncture	Leukemia, anemias, DIC, fibrinolytic activity, purpuras, hemorrhagic disease of the newborn, infectious mononucleosis, multiple myeloma, clotting factor deficiencies, thrombasthenia, thrombocytopenia, von Willebrand disease
Clot retraction test	Platelet number and function, fibrinogen quantity and use; measured in hours, which is required for expression of serum from a clot incubated in a test tube	Acute leukemia, aplastic anemia, factor XIII deficiency, increased fibrinolytic activity, Hodgkin disease, hyperfibrinogenemia or hypofibrinogenemia, idiopathic thrombocytopenic purpura, multiple myeloma, polycythemia vera, secondary thrombocytopenia, thrombasthenia
Platelet adhesion studies	Ability of platelets to adhere to foreign surfaces	Anemia, macroglobulinemia, Bernard-Soulier syndrome, multiple myeloma, myeloid metaplasia, plasma cell dyscrasias, thrombasthenia, thrombocytopathy, von Willebrand disease
Platelet aggregation tests	Ability of platelets to adhere to one another	Afibrinogenemia, Bernard-Soulier syndrome, thrombasthenia, hemorrhagic thrombocythemia, myeloid metaplasia, plasma cell dyscrasias, platelet-release defects, polycythemia vera, preleukemia, sideroblastic anemia, von Willebrand disease, Waldenström macroglobulinemia, hypercoagulability
Whole blood clotting time (Lee-White coagulation time)	Overall ability of blood to clot; measured in minutes in a test tube	Afibrinogenemia, clotting factor deficiencies, excessive fibrinolysis, hemorrhagic disease of the newborn, hypofibrinogenemia, hypoprothrombinemia, leukemia
Circulating anticoagulants (immunoglobulin G [IgG] or M [IgM] antibodies that inhibit coagulation)	Presence of antibodies that neutralize clotting factors and inhibit coagulation, as indicated by prolonged clotting time, prothrombin time, or partial thromboplastin time	Afibrinogenemia, presence of fibrin-fibrinogen degradation products, macroglobulinemia, multiple myeloma, DIC, plasma cell dyscrasias
Partial thromboplastin time (PTT)	Effectiveness of clotting factors (except factors VII and VIII), effectiveness of intrinsic pathway of coagulation cascade; measured in seconds in a test tube	Presence of circulating anticoagulants, DIC, clotting factor deficiencies, excessive fibrinolysis, hemorrhagic disease of the newborn, hypofibrinogenemia and afibrinogenemia, prothrombin deficiency, von Willebrand disease, acute hemorrhage
Prothrombin time (PT)	Effectiveness of activity of prothrombin, fibrinogen, and factors V, VII, and X; effectiveness of vitamin K–dependent coagulation factors of the extrinsic and common pathways of the coagulation cascade; measured in seconds in a test tube	Hypofibrinogenemia, dysfibrinogenemia, and afibrinogenemia; presence of circulating anticoagulants; DIC; deficiency of factors V, VII, or X; presence of fibrin degradation products, increased fibrinolytic activity, hemolytic jaundice, hemorrhagic disease of the newborn; acute leukemia, polycythemia vera, prothrombin deficiency, multiple myeloma
Thrombin time	Quantity and activity of fibrinogen; measured in seconds in a test tube	Hypofibrinogenemia, dysfibrinogenemia, and afibrinogenemia; presence of circulating anticoagulants; hemorrhagic disease of the newborn, polycythemia vera; increase in fibrin-fibrinogen degradation products; increased fibrinolytic activity
Fibrinogen assay	Amount of fibrinogen available for fibrin formation	Acute leukemia, congenital hypofibrinogenemia or afibrinogenemia, DIC, increased fibrinolytic activity, severe hemorrhage
Fibrin-fibrinogen degradation products (fibrin-fibrinogen split products)	Fibrinogenic activity as measured by levels of fibrin-fibrinogen degradation products (in mcg/mL of blood)	Transfusion reactions, DIC, internal hemorrhage in the newborn, deep vein thrombosis, pulmonary embolism

DAT, Direct antiglobulin test; *DIC*, disseminated intravascular coagulation.

Data from Garrels M, Oatis CS. *Laboratory and diagnostic testing in ambulatory care: A guide for health care professionals*, 3rd edition. St. Louis: Saunders; 2015; Hudnall D. *Hematology: A pathophysiologic approach*. St. Louis: Mosby; 2012.

TABLE 28.11 **Mean Hematologic Differential Counts from Birth to Adulthood**

Hematologic Differential	Newborn (Cord Blood)	2 Weeks of Age	3 Months of Age	6 Months to 6 Years of Age	7–12 Years of Age	Adult
Hemoglobin (g/dl)	16.8	16.5	12	12	13	13
Hematocrit (%)	55	50	36	37	38	40
Reticulocytes (%)	5	1	1	1	1	1
Leukocytes (WBCs/mm^3)	18,000	12,000	12,000	10,000	8000	8000
Neutrophils (%)	61	40	30	45	55	55
Lymphocytes (%)	31	48	63	48	38	35
Eosinophils (%)	2	3	2	2	2	2
Monocytes (%)	6	9	5	5	5	5
Platelets (10^3/mm^3)	290	252	150–400	150–400	150–400	150–400

WBCs, White blood cells.

fetal life and the increased numbers of cells that result from the trauma of birth and cutting of the umbilical cord.

Average blood volume in the full-term neonate is about 85 mL/kg of body weight. The premature infant has a slightly larger blood volume of 90 mL/kg of body weight. In both full-term and premature infants, blood volume decreases during the first few months. Thereafter the average blood volume is about 75 to 80 mL/kg, which is similar to that of older children and adults.

The hypoxic intrauterine environment stimulates EPO production in the fetus and accelerates fetal erythropoiesis, producing polycythemia (excessive proliferation of erythrocyte precursors) in the newborn. After birth, the oxygen from the lungs saturates arterial blood, and more oxygen is delivered to the tissues. In response to the change from a placental to a pulmonary oxygen supply during the first few days of life, levels of EPO and the rate of blood cell formation decrease. The active rate of fetal erythropoiesis is reflected by the large numbers of immature erythrocytes (reticulocytes) in the peripheral blood of full-term neonates. After birth, the number of reticulocytes decreases by 50% every 12 hours, so it is rare to find an elevated reticulocyte count after the first week of life. During this period of rapid growth, the rate of erythrocyte destruction is greater than that in later childhood and adulthood. In full-term infants, the normal erythrocyte life span is 60 to 80 days; in premature infants, it may be as short as 20 to 30 days; and in children and adolescents, it is the same as that in adults—100 to 120 days.

The postnatal fall in hemoglobin and hematocrit values is more marked in premature infants than it is in full-term infants. Fetal hemoglobin has higher affinity for oxygen compared to adult globins, which presumably allows for efficient maternal–embryonic gas exchange in the placental environment. In preschool and school-aged children, hemoglobin, hematocrit, and RBC counts gradually rise. Metabolic processes within the erythrocytes of neonates differ significantly from those found in erythrocytes of normal adults. The relatively young population of erythrocytes in newborns consumes greater quantities of glucose than do erythrocytes in adults. Platelet counts in full-term neonates are comparable with those in adults and remain so throughout infancy and childhood.

Most coagulation factors (both procoagulants and anticoagulants) in children reach adult levels by 6 months of age, and some not until adolescence. Children have quantitative and qualitative differences in clotting factors that result in decreased risk for thrombosis without increased risk for bleeding (developmental hemostasis) because the reduction of procoagulant and anticoagulant proteins is balanced. Laboratory values for hemostasis (e.g., prothrombin time and activated partial thromboplastin time) are referenced by age.[24]

WBCs develop and mature during fetal life, including neutrophils, monocyte-macrophages, eosinophils, and lymphocytes, but the function of the cells at birth is weak because the cells are immature. At birth the lymphocyte count is high, and it continues to rise during the first year of life. Then it steadily declines until the lower value seen in adults is reached. The lymphocytes of children also tend to have more cytoplasm and less compact nuclear chromatin than do the lymphocytes of adults. A possible explanation is that children tend to have more frequent viral infections, some of which are subclinical, and are receiving vaccinations, both of which are associated with atypical lymphocytes.

The neutrophil count, like the lymphocyte count, is high at birth and rises during the first days of life. After 2 weeks, the neutrophil count falls to within or below the normal adult range. Although the exact age can vary, by approximately 7 years of age, the neutrophil count is the same as that of an adult. The eosinophil count is higher in the first year of life and higher in children than in teenagers or adults. Monocyte counts also are high in the first year of life but then decrease to adult levels.

Newborn infants are at risk for impaired phagocytosis, bacterial infections, and delayed wound healing. Immature lymphocytes also increase the risk for viral infection, and there is a weak response to the production of antibodies and a poor response to foreign antigens. Protection against infectious disease is provided by passive IgG antibody transfer from the mother transplacentally and in breast milk. By 2 months of age the WBCs have matured enough for the infant to begin receiving protection from infectious disease by vaccination. As the child ages, immunity is further enhanced by intercurrent infection and vaccinations, with the formation of antibodies and memory T cells that provide lifelong protection.

AGING AND THE HEMATOLOGIC SYSTEM

Blood composition changes little with age, although some components may be altered by iron deficiency. Values of total serum iron level, total iron-binding capacity, and intestinal iron absorption are all decreased somewhat in elderly persons. The erythrocyte life span is normal, although the erythrocytes are replenished more slowly after bleeding and their deformability decreases with advanced age.[25] Hemoglobin levels may be low, and the plasma membranes of erythrocytes become increasingly fragile, with portions being lost, presumably because of physical trauma inflicted during circulation. Chronic inflammation and the presence of chronic disease, including diabetes mellitus, chronic heart disease, chronic renal insufficiency, and Parkinson disease, are associated with suppressed erythropoiesis and anemia occurring in older adults.[26] Lymphocyte function decreases with age, causing changes in cellular immunity and some decline in T-cell function. The humoral immune system is less able to respond to antigenic challenge and to vaccination.

Platelet count remains relatively stable during middle age (25 to 60 years old) but falls in older people (greater than 60 years),[27] yet platelet adhesiveness increases, which may be related to oxidative stress. Fibrinogen levels and levels of factors V, VII, and IX and also vWF tend to be increased. In addition, thrombin generation and platelet activation are enhanced in older adults. Consequently, there is an increased incidence of venous thromboembolism.[28]

SUMMARY REVIEW

Components of the Hematologic System

1. Blood consists of a variety of components—about 91% water and 9% solutes. In adults, the total blood volume is approximately 5.5 L.
2. Plasma, a complex aqueous liquid, contains two major groups of plasma proteins: albumins and globulins.
3. The cellular elements of blood are the red blood cells (erythrocytes), white blood cells (leukocytes), and platelets.
4. Erythrocytes are the most abundant cells of the blood, occupying approximately 48% of the blood volume in men and approximately 42% in women. Erythrocytes are responsible for tissue oxygenation.
5. Leukocytes are fewer in number than erythrocytes and constitute approximately 5000 to 10,000 cells/mm^3 of blood. Leukocytes defend the body against infection and remove dead or injured host cells.
6. Leukocytes are classified as either granulocytes (neutrophils, eosinophils, basophils) or agranulocytes (monocytes/macrophages, lymphocytes, natural killer cells).
7. The mononuclear phagocyte system (MPS) is composed of monocytes in bone marrow and peripheral blood and macrophages in tissue. Cells of the MPS ingest and destroy unwanted materials, such as foreign protein particles, circulating immune complexes, microorganisms, debris from dead or injured cells, defective or injured erythrocytes, and dead neutrophils.
8. Platelets are irregularly shaped anuclear cytoplasmic fragments. Platelets are essential for blood coagulation and control of bleeding.
9. The lymphoid organs are sites of residence, proliferation, differentiation, or function of lymphocytes and mononuclear phagocytes.
10. 10 The spleen is the largest lymphoid organ and functions as the site of fetal hematopoiesis, filters and cleanses the blood, and acts as a reservoir for lymphocytes and other blood cells.
11. The lymph nodes are the site of development or activity of large numbers of lymphocytes, monocytes, and macrophages.

Development of Blood Cells

1. Bone marrow consists of red (active or hematopoietic) marrow and yellow (inactive) marrow.
2. The hematopoietic marrow consists of a variety of cellular and molecular microenvironments called niches. Niches support the hematopoietic stem cells by direct cell-to-cell signaling and production of growth factors and cytokines important for retention, expansion, maintenance, and quiescence.
3. The bone marrow contains multiple populations of stem cells. Hematopoietic stem cells develop into blood cells. Mesenchymal stem cells develop into osteoblasts, adipocytes, chondrocytes, sinusoidal endothelial cells, fibroblasts, and other stromal cells.
4. Osteoblasts (responsible for construction of bone) and osteoclasts (remodel bone by resorption) produce cytokines that affect proliferation and maintenance of hematopoietic cells.
5. Specific hematopoietic growth factors (e.g., colony-stimulating factors) are necessary for the adequate production of myeloid, erythroid, lymphoid, and megakaryocytic lineages.
6. Hematopoiesis, or blood cell production, occurs in the liver and spleen of the fetus and in the bone marrow after birth.
7. Hematopoiesis involves two stages: mitotic division (i.e., proliferation) and maturation (i.e., differentiation). Each type of blood cell has parent cells called stem cells.
8. Hematopoiesis continues throughout life to replace blood cells that grow old and die, are killed by disease, or are lost through bleeding.
9. Regulation of erythropoiesis (development of red blood cells) is mediated by erythropoietin, which is secreted by the kidneys in response to tissue hypoxia. Erythropoietin causes a compensatory increase in erythrocyte production if the oxygen content of the blood decreases because of anemia, high altitude, or pulmonary disease.
10. Hemoglobin, the oxygen-carrying protein of the erythrocyte, enables the blood to transport 100 times more oxygen than could be transported dissolved in plasma alone.

11. Erythropoiesis depends on the presence of vitamins (especially vitamin B_{12}, folate, vitamin B_6, riboflavin, pantothenic acid, niacin, ascorbic acid, and vitamin E).
12. The iron cycle reutilizes iron released from old or damaged erythrocytes. Iron binds to transferrin in the blood, is transported to macrophages, and is stored in the cytoplasm as ferritin.
13. Iron homeostasis is controlled by hepcidin, a small hormone produced by hepatocytes, which regulates ferroportin, the principal transporter of iron from stores in hepatocytes and macrophages and from intestinal cells that absorb dietary iron.
14. Myelopoiesis is the development of granulocytes (neutrophils, eosinophils, and basophils) and monocytes from the differentiation of myeloid progenitor cells in the bone marrow. Granulocytes are released into the blood and are either functioning cells that circulate in the blood or stored cells that are stored around the walls of blood vessels (marginating storage pool). Monocytes are released into the blood and travel to various tissues to become tissue macrophages and dendritic cells.
15. Lymphocytes, which are generated from lymphoid progenitor cells in a process called lymphopoiesis, are released into the bloodstream to undergo further maturation in the primary and secondary lymphoid organs.
16. Platelets develop from megakaryocytes by a process called thrombopoiesis, which is controlled by thrombopoietin. During thrombopoiesis, megakaryocytes undergo mitosis but not cell division and the cytoplasm and plasma membrane fragment into platelets.

Mechanisms of Hemostasis

1. Hemostasis, or arrest of bleeding, involves (1) vasoconstriction (vasospasm), (2) formation of a platelet plug, (3) activation of the clotting cascade, (4) formation of a blood clot, and (5) clot retraction and clot dissolution.
2. The normal vascular endothelium prevents spontaneous clotting by producing factors such as nitric oxide (NO) and prostacyclin I_2 (PGI_2) that relax the vessels and prevent platelet activation.
3. Platelet activation involves three linked processes: (1) adhesion, (2) activation, and (3) aggregation.
4. A blood clot is a meshwork of protein strands that stabilizes the platelet plug. The strands are made of fibrin. Fibrin is the end product of the coagulation cascade.
5. Lysis of blood clots is the function of the fibrinolytic system. Plasmin, a proteolytic enzyme, splits fibrin and fibrinogen into fibrin degradation products that dissolve the clot.

Clinical Evaluation of the Hematologic System

1. Tests of bone marrow function include bone marrow aspiration and bone marrow biopsy.
2. Cells contained in the marrow specimen are assessed with respect to (a) relative numbers of stem cells and their developing daughter cells, and (b) morphologic structure.

Pediatrics and the Hematologic System

1. Blood cell counts tend to rise above adult levels at birth and then decline gradually throughout childhood. Platelet counts in full-term neonates are comparable with those in adults and remain so throughout infancy and childhood.
2. White blood cells develop during fetal life but the function of the cells at birth is weak as the cells are immature.
3. Newborn infants are at risk for impaired phagocytosis, bacterial infections, and delayed wound healing. Immature lymphocytes also increase risk for viral infection and there is a weak response to the production of antibodies and a poor response to foreign antigens.

Aging and the Hematologic System

1. Blood composition changes little with age. Erythrocyte replenishment may be delayed after bleeding, presumably because of iron deficiency.
2. Lymphocyte function appears to decrease with age. Particularly affected is a decrease in cellular immunity.
3. Platelet numbers decrease with age, but adhesiveness increases.

REFERENCES

1. Minasyan H. Phagocytosis and oxycytosis: two arms of human innate immunity. *Immunol Res*. 2018;66(2):271–280.
2. Aoki A, et al. Eosinophils: cells known for over 140 years with broad and new functions. *Allergol Int*. 2021;70(1):3–8.
3. Weller PF, Spencer LA. Functions of tissue-resident eosinophils. *Nat Rev Immunol*. 2017;17(12):746–760.
4. Yang Y, et al. Natural killer cells in inflammatory autoimmune diseases. *Clin Transl Immunology*. 2021;10(2):e1250.
5. Gong C, et al. The best anticoagulation strategy for cirrhotic patients who underwent splenectomy: a network meta-analysis. *Gastroenterol Res Pract*. 2017;2017:9216172.
6. Madel MB, et al. Immune function and diversity of osteoclasts in normal and pathological conditions. *Front Immunol*. 2019;10:1408.
7. Boulais PE, Frenette PS. Making sense of hematopoietic stem cell niches. *Blood*. 2015;125(17):2621–2629.
8. Aerts-Kaya F, et al. Neurological regulation of the bone marrow niche. *Adv Exp Med Biol*. 2020;1212:127–153.
9. Galán-Díez M, Cuesta-Domínguez Á, Kousteni S. The bone marrow microenvironment in health and myeloid malignancy. *Cold Spring Harb Perspect Med*. 2018;8(7):a031328.
10. Ahmed MH, Ghatge MS, Safo MK. Hemoglobin: structure, function and allostery. *Subcell Biochem*. 2020;94:345–382.
11. Lew VL, Tiffert T. On the mechanism of human red blood cell longevity: roles of calcium, the sodium pump, PIEZO1, and Gardos channels. *Front Physiol*. 2017;8:977.
12. Wallace DF. The regulation of iron absorption and homeostasis. *Clin Biochem Rev*. 2016;37(2):51–62.
13. Sukhbaatar N, Weichhart T. Iron regulation: macrophages in control. *Pharmaceuticals (Basel)*. 2018;11(4):137.
14. Xu Y, Alfaro-Magallanes VM, Babitt JL. Physiological and pathophysiological mechanisms of hepcidin regulation: clinical implications for iron disorders. *Br J Haematol*. 2021;193(5): 882–893.

15. Noetzli LJ, French SL, Machlus KR. New insights into the differentiation of megakaryocytes from hematopoietic progenitors. *Arterioscler Thromb Vasc Biol.* 2019;39(7):1288–1300.
16. Krüger-Genge A, et al. Vascular endothelial cell biology: an update. *Int J Mol Sci.* 2019;20(18):4411.
17. Gianazza E, et al. Platelets in healthy and disease states: from biomarkers discovery to drug targets identification by proteomics. *Int J Mol Sci.* 2020;21(12):4541.
18. Sang Y, et al. Interplay between platelets and coagulation. *Blood Rev.* 2021;46:100733.
19. Yan AR, et al. Effectiveness of platelet function analysis-guided aspirin and/or clopidogrel therapy in preventing secondary stroke: a systematic review and meta-analysis. *J Clin Med.* 2020;9(12):3907.
20. Winter WE, et al. Clotting factors: clinical biochemistry and their roles as plasma enzymes. *Adv Clin Chem.* 2020;94:31–84.
21. Subramaniam S, et al. Post-transcriptional, post-translational and pharmacological regulation of tissue factor pathway inhibitor. *Blood Coagul Fibrinolysis.* 2018;29(8):668–682.
22. Amiral J, Seghatchian J. Revisiting the activated protein C-protein S-thrombomodulin ternary pathway: impact of new understanding on its laboratory investigation. *Transfus Apher Sci.* 2019;58(4):538–544.
23. de Witt SM, et al. Insights into platelet-based control of coagulation. *Thromb Res.* 2014;133(Suppl 2):S139–S148.
24. Nair AB, Parker RI. Hemostatic testing in critically ill infants and children. *Front Pediatr.* 2021;8:606643.
25. Lazari D, et al. The relationship between aggregation and deformability of red blood cells in health and disease. *Front Physiol.* 2020;11:288.
26. de Las Cuevas Allende R, Díaz de Entresotos L, Conde Díez S. Anaemia of chronic diseases: pathophysiology, diagnosis and treatment. *Med Clin (Barc).* 2021;156(5):235–242.
27. Jones CI. Platelet function and ageing. *Mamm Genome.* 2016;27(7–8):358–366.
28. Wang Q, Zennadi R. Oxidative stress and thrombosis during aging: the roles of oxidative stress in RBCs in venous thrombosis. *Int J Mol Sci.* 2020;21(12):4259.

29

Alterations of Hematologic Function

Sean McConnell and Valentina L. Brashers

http://evolve.elsevier.com/Rogers/pathophysiology/

CHAPTER OUTLINE

Alterations of erythrocyte function involve either insufficient or excessive numbers of erythrocytes in the circulation or normal numbers of cells with abnormal components. Anemias are conditions in which there are too few erythrocytes or an insufficient volume of erythrocytes in the blood. Polycythemias are conditions in which erythrocyte number or volume is excessive. Each of these conditions has many causes and shares pathophysiologic manifestations with other disease states.

Disorders involving white blood cells (leukocytes) can range from increased numbers of leukocytes (leukocytosis) in response to infections, or proliferative disorders (e.g., leukemia), to decreased numbers of leukocytes (e.g., leukopenia). Many hematologic and nonhematologic malignancies metastasize to the bone marrow and affect leukocyte production. Thus, a large portion of this chapter is devoted to malignant disease.

The primary role of clotting (hemostasis) is to stop bleeding through an interaction of endothelium lining the vessels, platelets, and clotting factors. Several disease states increase or decrease clotting in at least one of the three main components of the clotting process.

ANEMIA

Classification and General Characteristics

Anemia is a reduction in the total number of erythrocytes in the circulating blood or a decrease in the quality or quantity of hemoglobin. The term anemia refers to a true decrease in erythrocyte number, rather than a relative decrease due to increases in plasma volume (hemodilution). The overall prevalence of anemia is approximately 10% to 15% of individuals in the United States affecting approximately 40% of men and 22% of women over the age of 85.[1]

Anemias commonly result from (1) blood loss (acute or chronic), (2) impaired erythrocyte production, (3) increased erythrocyte destruction, or (4) a combination of these three factors (Fig. 29.1). Anemias are classified based on etiology (e.g., acute blood loss or anemia of inflammation [AI]) or by the changes that affect the size, shape, or substance of the erythrocyte. The most common classification of anemias is based on the changes that affect the cell's size and hemoglobin content (Table 29.1). Terms used to identify anemias reflect these characteristics. Terms that end with *-cytic* refer to cell size, and those that end with *-chromic* refer to hemoglobin content. Additional terms describing erythrocytes found in some anemias are anisocytosis (assuming various sizes) and poikilocytosis (assuming various shapes).

Clinical Manifestations. The main clinical effect of anemia is a reduced oxygen-carrying capacity of the blood resulting in tissue hypoxia. Symptoms of anemia vary, depending on the body's ability to compensate for the reduced oxygen-carrying capacity. Anemia that is mild and starts gradually is usually easier to compensate and may cause problems for the individual only during physical exertion. As red cell reduction continues, symptoms become more pronounced and alterations in specific organs and compensation effects are more apparent. Compensation generally involves the cardiovascular, respiratory, and hematologic systems (Fig. 29.2).

A reduction in the number of blood cells causes a reduction in the consistency and volume of blood. Initial compensation

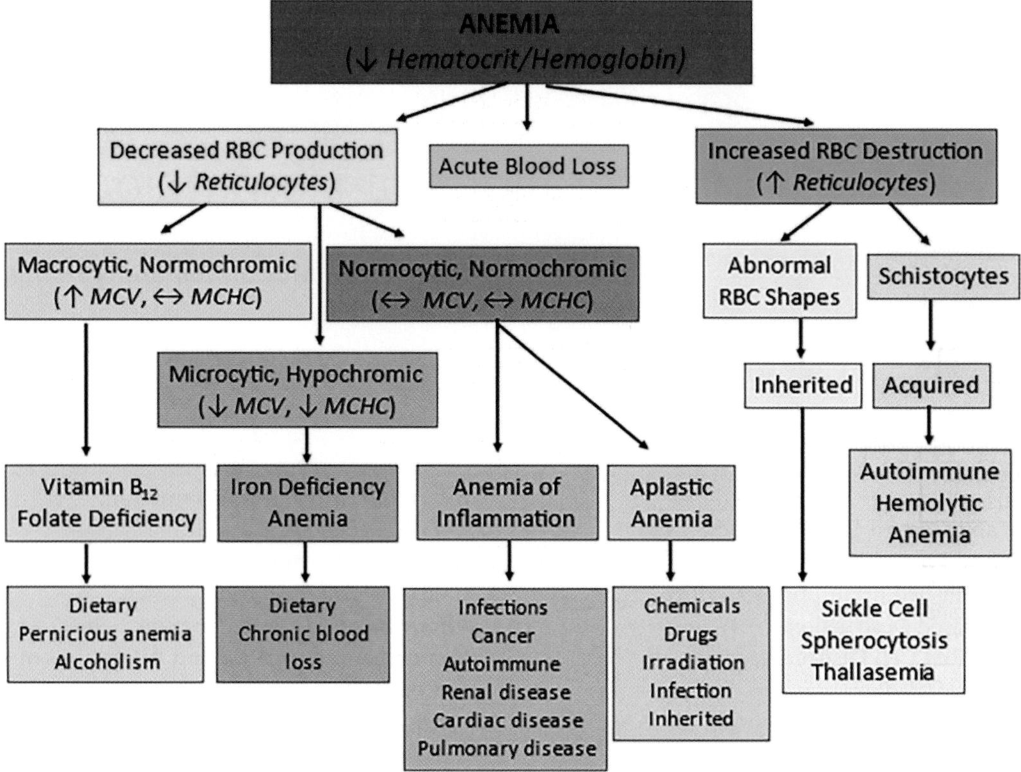

Fig. 29.1 Classification of Anemia. Anemias can be classified into three major categories: acute blood loss, decreased RBC production in which reticulocytes are decreased, and increased RBC destruction in which reticulocyte counts are increased. Further classification relies on the size (*-cytic*), color (*-chromic*), and shape of the cells. Based on these factors, the most common types and causes of anemia can be identified. *MCHC*, Mean corpuscular hemoglobin concentration; *MCV*, mean corpuscular volume.

TABLE 29.1 Morphologic Classification of Anemias

Structure of Erythrocytes	Name and Mechanism of Anemia	Primary Cause
Macrocytic-normochromic anemia: large, abnormally shaped erythrocytes, normal hemoglobin concentrations	Pernicious anemia: lack of vitamin B_{12}; abnormal DNA and RNA synthesis in erythroblast; premature cell death	Congenital or acquired deficiency of intrinsic factor (IF); genetic disorder of DNA synthesis
	Folate deficiency anemia: lack of folate; premature cell death	Dietary folate deficiency
Microcytic-hypochromic anemia: small, abnormally shaped erythrocytes and reduced hemoglobin concentration	Iron deficiency anemia: lack of iron for hemoglobin; insufficient hemoglobin	Chronic blood loss, dietary iron deficiency, disruption of iron metabolism or iron cycle
	Sideroblastic anemia: dysfunctional iron uptake by erythroblasts and defective porphyrin and heme synthesis	Congenital dysfunction of iron metabolism in erythroblasts, acquired dysfunction of iron metabolism as result of myelodysplastic syndromes, dietary deficiencies, drugs or toxins
Normocytic-normochromic anemia: normal size, normal hemoglobin concentration	Posthemorrhagic anemia: blood loss	Increased erythropoiesis; iron depletion
	Aplastic anemia: insufficient erythropoiesis	Depressed stem cell proliferation
	Anemia of Inflammation; diminished erythropoiesis	Defects in iron metabolism
Anemia with abnormal cell shapes or the presence of schistocytes	Hemolytic anemia: premature destruction (lysis) of mature erythrocytes in circulation	Autoimmune targeting of erythrocyte antigens
	Sickle cell anemia: abnormal hemoglobin synthesis, abnormal cell shape with susceptibility to damage, lysis, and phagocytosis	Congenital dysfunction of hemoglobin synthesis
	Hereditary spherocytosis: destruction of mature erythrocytes that have abnormal cell membranes and spherical shapes	Genetic mutations leading to changes in erythrocyte membrane structure
	Thalassemia: impaired synthesis of α- or β-chain of hemoglobin A; phagocytosis	Genetic defect of globin synthesis

DNA, Deoxyribonucleic acid; *RNA*, ribonucleic acid.

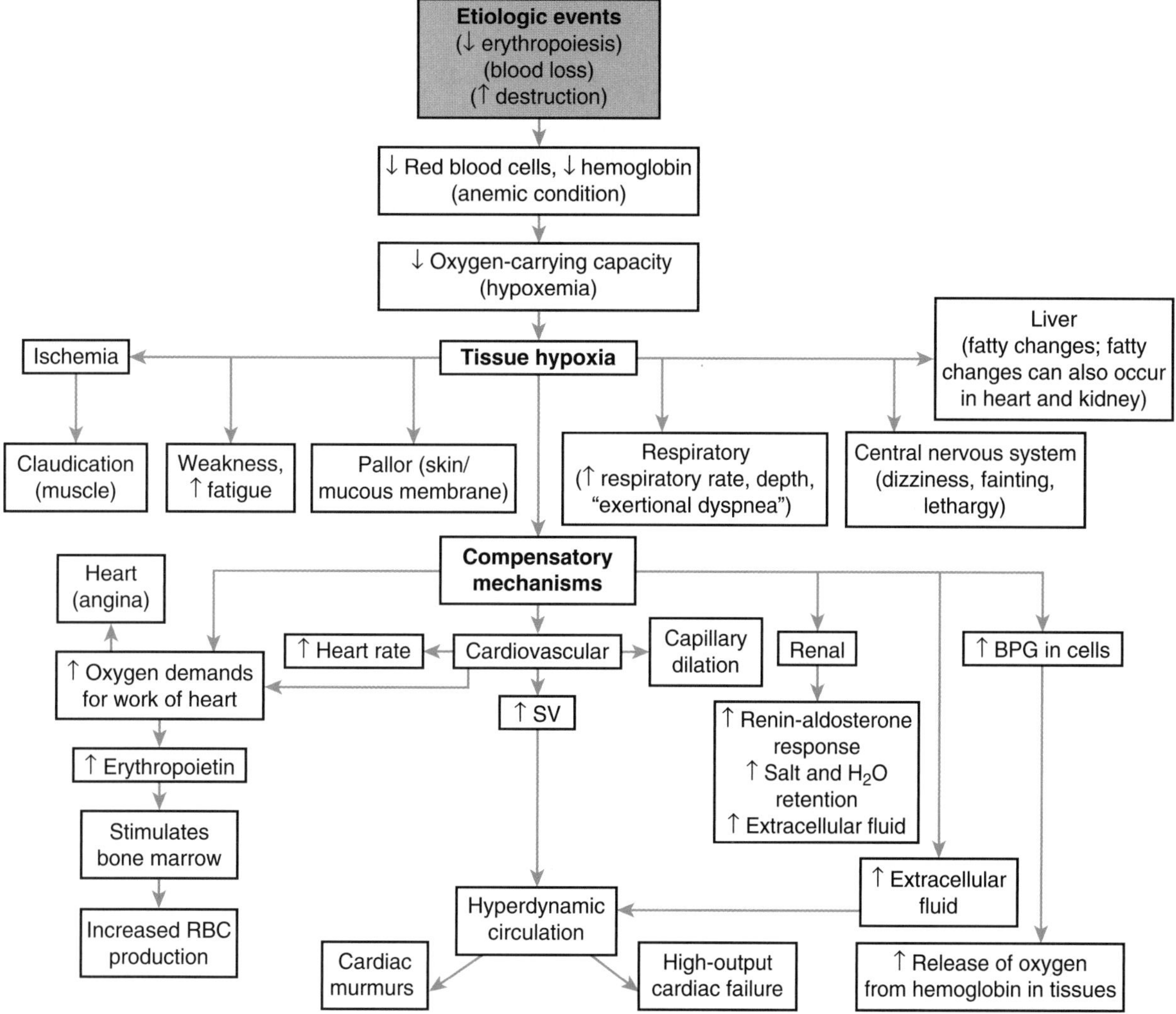

Fig. 29.2 Progression and Manifestations of Anemia. *BPG*, Bisphosphoglycerate; *SV*, stroke volume.

for cellular loss is movement of interstitial fluid into the blood, causing an increase in plasma volume. This movement maintains an adequate blood volume, but the viscosity (thickness) of the blood decreases. The "thinner" blood flows faster and more turbulently than normal blood, causing a hyperdynamic circulatory state. This hyperdynamic state creates cardiovascular changes—increased stroke volume and heart rate. These changes may lead to cardiac dilation and heart valve insufficiency if the underlying anemic condition is not corrected.

Hypoxemia, reduced oxygen level in the blood, further contributes to cardiovascular dysfunction by causing dilation of arterioles, capillaries, and venules in the systemic circulation, thus increasing flow through them. Increased peripheral blood flow and venous return further contributes to an increase in heart rate and stroke volume in a continuing effort to meet normal oxygen demand and prevent cardiopulmonary congestion. These compensatory mechanisms may lead to heart failure.

Tissue hypoxia creates additional demands and effects on the pulmonary and hematologic systems. The rate and depth of breathing increase, in an effort to increase oxygen availability, accompanied by an increase in the release of oxygen from hemoglobin (see Chapter 34). All these compensatory mechanisms may cause individuals to experience shortness of breath (dyspnea), a rapid and pounding heartbeat, dizziness, and fatigue. In mild chronic cases, these symptoms may be present only when there is an increased demand for oxygen (e.g., during physical exertion), but in severe cases, symptoms may be experienced even at rest.

Manifestations of anemia may be seen in other parts of the body. The skin, mucous membranes, lips, nail beds, and conjunctivae become either pale because of reduced hemoglobin concentration or yellowish (jaundiced) because of accumulation of end products of red cell destruction (hemolysis) if that is the cause of the anemia. Tissue hypoxia of the skin results in impaired healing and loss of elasticity, as well as thinning and early graying of the hair. Nervous system manifestations may occur in which the cause of anemia is a deficiency of vitamin B_{12}. Myelin degeneration may occur, causing a loss of nerve fibers in the spinal cord, resulting in paresthesia (numbness), gait disturbances, extreme weakness, spasticity, and reflex abnormalities. Decreased oxygen supply to the gastrointestinal (GI) tract often produces abdominal pain, nausea, vomiting, and anorexia. Low-grade fever (<101°F [38.3°C]) occurs in some anemic individuals and may result from the release of inflammatory pyrogens from ischemic tissues.

EMERGING SCIENCE BOX

Traumatic Coagulopathy

Emerging is the understanding that persons with bleeding trauma are already developing complications of coagulopathy upon hospital admission. Onequarter to one-third of hemorrhaging trauma patients suffer from traumatic coagulopathy. The presence of coagulopathy is related to an increased risk of multiple organ failure and death (see Chapter 48). Terms for coagulopathy that accompanies trauma include acute traumatic coagulopathy, early coagulation of trauma, acute coagulopathy of trauma-shock, trauma-induced coagulopathy, and trauma-associated coagulopathy. Acute coagulopathy associated with traumatic injury is now recognized as a multifactorial condition caused by preexisting factors such as age, genetic background, comorbidities and medications (e.g., oral anticoagulants), and trauma-related factors such as bleeding-induced shock, tissue-related thrombin-thrombomodulin-complex generation, coagulation factor consumption, and activation of the anticoagulant and fibrinolytic pathways. One of the primary mechanisms of the coagulopathy is activation of protein C system.

In addition to its contribution to uncontrolled bleeding, traumatic coagulopathy and trauma-associated inflammation combine to exacerbate organ dysfunction and thromboembolic complications. The early phase of the process is characterized by hemorrhage, and the late phase (6–24 h after injury) by a hypercoagulability. Adding to this complexity, structural damage and metabolic changes in erythrocytes cause them to contribute to coagulopathy by their adherence to the endothelium, activation of platelets, exposure of prothrombotic factors, release of prothrombotic microparticles, and resistance to thrombolysis (see Chapter 28). Recent guidelines recommend that individuals be transferred directly to trauma centers to improve outcomes. Treatments for traumatic coagulopathy include tranexamic acid, fresh frozen plasma, and coagulation factor concentrates.

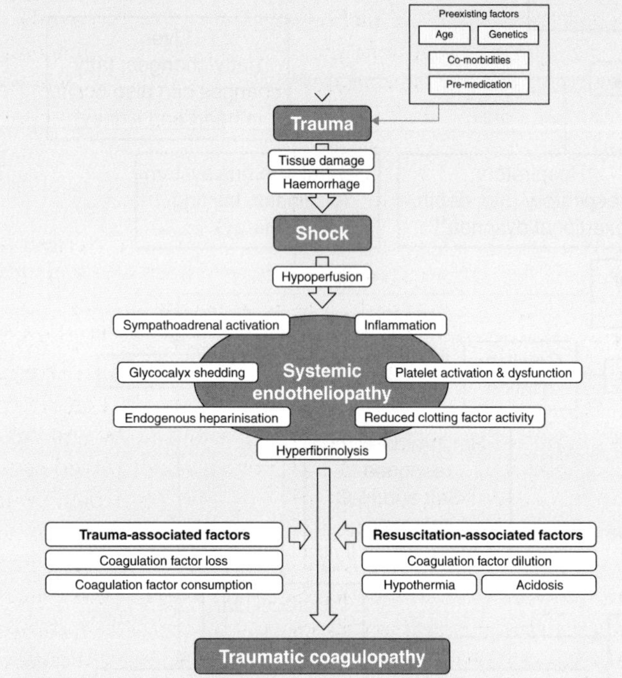

Figure adapted from Spahn DR, et al: the European guideline on the management of major bleeding and coagulopathy following trauma: Fifth edition, Crit Care 23:98,2019. https://ccforum.biomedcentral.com/articles/10.1186/s13054-019-2347-3/figures/1.

Data from Alamin AA. The role of red blood cells in hemostasis. *Seminars in Thrombosis and Hemostasis*, 2021;47(1):26–31; Gangloff C, et al. New considerations on pathways involved in acute traumatic coagulopathy: The thrombin generation paradox. *World Journal of Emergency Surgery*, 2019;14:57; Gratz J, et al. Trauma-induced coagulopathy and massive bleeding: Current hemostatic concepts and treatment strategies. *Hamostaseologie*, Sep 7, 32894876, 2020Epub ahead of print; Kornblith LZ, et al. Trauma-induced coagulopathy: The past, present, and future. *Journal of Thrombosis and Haemostasis*, 2019;17(6):852–862; Maegele M. The European perspective on the management of acute major hemorrhage and coagulopathy after trauma: summary of the 2019 updated european guideline. *Journal of Clinical Medicine*, 2021;10(2):362; Wang IJ, et al. FIBTEM improves the sensitivity of hyperfibrinolysis detection in severe trauma patients: A retrospective study using thromboelastometry. *Scientific Reports*, 2020;10:6980.

When the onset of anemia is severe or acute (e.g., hemorrhage), the initial compensatory mechanism is peripheral blood vessel constriction, which diverts blood flow to essential vital organs. Decreased blood flow detected by the kidneys activates the renin-angiotensin response, causing salt and water retention in an attempt to increase blood volume (see Chapters 31 and 37). These situations are emergencies and require immediate intervention to correct the underlying problem that caused the acute blood loss; therefore, long-term compensatory mechanisms do not develop.

Therapeutic interventions for slowly developing anemic conditions should focus on treatment of the underlying condition with improvement of associated symptoms. Therapies include dietary correction, administration of supplemental vitamins or iron, removal of toxic agents (e.g., drugs), and interventions that are directed at treating hemolytic conditions (e.g., sickle cell disease). Transfusion therapy is used when anemia is severe and cannot be reversed quickly.

Anemias of Blood Loss

Acute Blood Loss

Posthemorrhagic anemia is a normocytic-normochromic anemia (see Table 29.1) caused by acute blood loss. Acute blood loss is mainly a loss of intravascular volume, and its effects depend on the rate of hemorrhage. If the blood loss is rapid, it can lead to cardiovascular collapse, shock, and death. A major cause of acute blood loss is trauma. Severe trauma is a rising global problem, resulting in an annual worldwide death rate of more than 5 million or 9% of mortalities.[2,3] Uncontrolled posttraumatic bleeding is the leading cause of potentially preventable death among injured individuals. Table 29.2 presents classification of estimated blood loss for a 70 kg male based on initial presentation. The pathophysiologic mechanism of traumatic injury is an evolving field of study. Emerging is the understanding that persons with bleeding trauma are already developing complications of coagulopathy upon hospital admission. The presence of coagulopathy is related to an increased risk of multiple organ failure and death (see Emerging Science Box: Traumatic Coagulopathy).

Within 24 hours of acute blood loss, lost plasma is replaced from the movement of water and electrolytes from tissues and interstitial spaces into the intravascular system. The hematocrit becomes lowered because of resulting hemodilution. Red blood cells are normocytic and normochromic (i.e., mean corpuscular volume [MCV] and mean corpuscular hemoglobin concentration [MCHC] are within normal range). A rapid elevation

TABLE 29.2 Classification of Estimated Blood Loss[a]

	Class I	Class II	Class III	Class IV
Blood loss (mL)	Up to 750	750–1500	1500–2000	>2000
Blood loss (% blood volume)	Up to 15	15–30	30–40	>40
Pulse rate (beats/min)	<100	100–120	120–140	>140
Systolic blood pressure	Normal	Normal	Decreased	Decreased
Pulse pressure	Normal or increased	Decreased	Decreased	Decreased
Respiratory rate (breaths/min)	14–20	20–30	30–40	>35
Urine output (mL/h)	>30	20–30	5–15	Negligible
Central nervous system/mental state	Slightly anxious	Mildly anxious	Anxious, confused	Confused, lethargic
Initial fluid replacement	Crystalloid	Crystalloid	Crystalloid and blood	Crystalloid and blood

[a]For a 70-kg man.
Data from Rossaint R, Bouillon B, Cerny V, et al. The European guideline on management of major bleeding and coagulopathy following trauma: Fourth edition. *Critical Care*, 2016;20:100.

of circulating neutrophils occurs within a few hours due to a release of leukocytes from the bone marrow into the circulation. The platelet count can rise significantly during the early recovery from acute blood loss. Erythropoietin is stimulated from the reduction in tissue oxygenation and increases bone marrow production of erythrocytes. However, iron stores may be depleted due to loss of red blood cells from the body, and erythropoiesis may be impeded. To restore blood volume, saline, dextran, albumin, or plasma is typically used, and with large blood losses it may be necessary to transfuse fresh whole blood.

Red blood cell transfusion is an option for both acute and chronic blood loss. However, transfusion of critically ill individuals may worsen the outcome and increase morbidity and mortality. Stored red blood cells undergo structural and metabolic impairments including formation of toxic products, phosphatidylserine exposure, and shedding of microparticles. These changes promote thrombotic complications such as deep venous thrombosis (DVT) after infusion.[4] In an effort to improve patient outcomes, patient blood management is a patient-centered and multidisciplinary approach to effectively manage anemia, reduce iatrogenic blood loss, and improve outcomes for those with anemia.[5]

Chronic Blood Loss

Anemia from chronic blood loss occurs if the loss is greater than the replacement capacity of the bone marrow. Hemorrhage that is slow and chronic produces less prominent adaptations, but an iron deficiency anemia (IDA) may develop. In adults, an otherwise unexplained IDA should be evaluated for an occult source of blood loss such as a bleeding ulcer or a malignancy.

Anemias of Diminished Erythropoiesis

There are many varied anemias of diminished red cell production that can be classified according to the underlying mechanism (Table 29.3). IDA is the most common type of anemia in the world. Other common anemias of diminished red cell production are the result of ineffective erythrocyte DNA synthesis caused by nutritional deficiencies of vitamin B_{12} (cobalamin) or folate (folic acid). IDA causes a microcytic anemia, whereas deficiencies of vitamin B_{12} and folate cause macrocytic (megaloblastic) anemias (Fig. 29.3).

Macrocytic (Megaloblastic)—Normochromic Anemias

The macrocytic (megaloblastic) anemias are characterized by large stem cells (megaloblasts) in the marrow (Fig. 29.4) that mature into erythrocytes that are unusually large in size (macrocytic; elevated MCV) thickness, and volume (see Fig. 29.3C). The most common etiology for macrocytic anemias is vitamin B12 or folate deficiencies. Vitamin B12 is dependent on dietary B12 intake. Plants and vegetables contain little cobalamin and strictly vegetarian and macrobiotic diets do not provide adequate amounts. Folate is found in green leafy vegetables, fruits, nuts, eggs, and meats. Both vitamin B12 and folate levels can be affected by disorders that decrease absorption of these vitamins from the gut, and by increased demand for these nutrients in conditions such as pregnancy, hyperthyroidism, chronic infection, and disseminated cancer. Another important cause of megaloblastic anemia is medications that interfere with DNA synthesis such as chemotherapeutic drugs.

The defective erythrocytes in megaloblastic anemias die prematurely, which decreases their numbers in the circulation, causing anemia. Premature death of damaged erythrocytes, eryptosis, is a common mechanism of cellular loss in individuals with anemia secondary to nutritional deficiencies, infections (e.g., malaria, mycoplasma), chronic diseases (e.g., diabetes, renal disease), genetic diseases (e.g., beta-thalassemia, glucose-6-phosphate dehydrogenase [G6PD] deficiency, sickle cell anemia), and myelodysplastic syndrome.[6]

Deoxyribonucleic acid (DNA) synthesis and cell division are blocked or delayed in megaloblastic anemias. Defective DNA synthesis causes red cell growth and development to proceed at unequal rates. However, ribonucleic acid (RNA) replication and protein (hemoglobin) synthesis proceed normally. Asynchronous development leads to an overproduction of hemoglobin during prolonged cellular division, creating a larger than normal erythrocyte with a disproportionately small nucleus. With each cell division, the disproportion between increased RNA and cell size and decreased DNA becomes more apparent.

Pernicious anemia. Pernicious anemia (PA) is a type of megaloblastic anemia and is caused by vitamin B_{12} (cobalamin) deficiency due to intestinal malabsorption. The main disorder in PA is the absence of intrinsic factor (IF) which is essential for the absorption of vitamin B12 in the ileum (see Chapter 28). *Pernicious* means highly injurious or destructive and reflects the fact that this condition was once fatal. It most commonly affects

TABLE 29.3 Classification of Anemia According to Underlying Mechanism

Mechanism	Specific Examples
Blood Loss	
Acute blood loss	Trauma
Chronic blood loss	Gastrointestinal tract lesions, gynecologic disturbances[a]
Anemias of Diminished Erythropoiesis	
Inherited Defects	
Defects leading to stem cell depletion	Fanconi anemia, telomerase defects
Defects affecting erythroblast maturation	Thalassemia syndromes
Acquired Defects	
Deficiencies affecting DNA synthesis	B_{12} and folate deficiencies
Deficiencies affecting hemoglobin synthesis	Iron deficiency anemia
Erythropoietin deficiency	Renal failure, anemia of chronic disease
Immune-mediated injury of progenitors	Aplastic anemia, pure red cell aplasia
Inflammation-mediated iron sequestration	Anemia of inflammation
Primary hematopoietic neoplasms	Acute leukemia, myelodysplasia, myeloproliferative disorders
Space-occupying marrow lesions	Metastatic neoplasms, granulomatous disease
Infections of red cell progenitors	Parvovirus B19 infection
Unknown mechanisms	Endocrine disorders, hepatocellular liver disease
Anemias of Increased Destruction (Hemolysis)	
Inherited Defects	
Red cell membrane disorders	Hereditary spherocytosis, hereditary elliptocytosis
Enzyme deficiencies	
Hexose monophosphate shunt enzyme deficiencies	G6PD deficiency, glutathione synthetase deficiency
Glycolytic enzyme deficiencies	Pyruvate kinase deficiency, hexokinase deficiency
Hemoglobin abnormalities	
Deficient globin synthesis	Thalassemia syndromes
Structurally abnormal globins (hemoglobinopathies)	Sickle cell disease, unstable hemoglobins
Acquired Defects	
Deficiency of phosphatidylinositol-linked glycoproteins	Paroxysmal nocturnal hemoglobinuria
Antibody-mediated destruction	Hemolytic disease of the newborn (Rh disease), transfusion reactions, drug-induced, autoimmune disorders
Mechanical trauma	
Microangiopathic hemolytic anemias	Hemolytic uremic syndrome, disseminated intravascular coagulation, thrombotic thrombocytopenia purpura
Cardiac traumatic hemolysis	Defective cardiac valves
Repetitive physical trauma	Bongo drumming, marathon running, karate chopping
Infections of red cells	Malaria, babesiosis
Toxic or chemical injury	Clostridial sepsis, snake venom, lead poisoning
Membrane lipid abnormalities	Abetalipoproteinemia, severe hepatocellular liver disease
Sequestration	Hypersplenism

[a]Most often cause of anemia is iron deficiency, not bleeding.
G6PD, Glucose-6-phosphate dehydrogenase.
Data from Kumar V, Abbas A, Aster JC. *Robbins & Cotran pathologic basis of disease*, 10th edition. Philadelphia: Elsevier; 2021.

individuals older than age 30 who are of Northern European descent; however, it is now recognized in all populations and ethnic groups.

Deficiency of IF may be congenital. It is more often acquired as the result of an autoimmune process or conditions that damage the gastric mucosa. Congenital IF deficiency is a genetic disorder with an autosomal recessive inheritance pattern. Approximately 20% of individuals with PA have a family member with PA, although the pattern of transmission has not been identified.[7] PA most commonly is caused by autoimmune

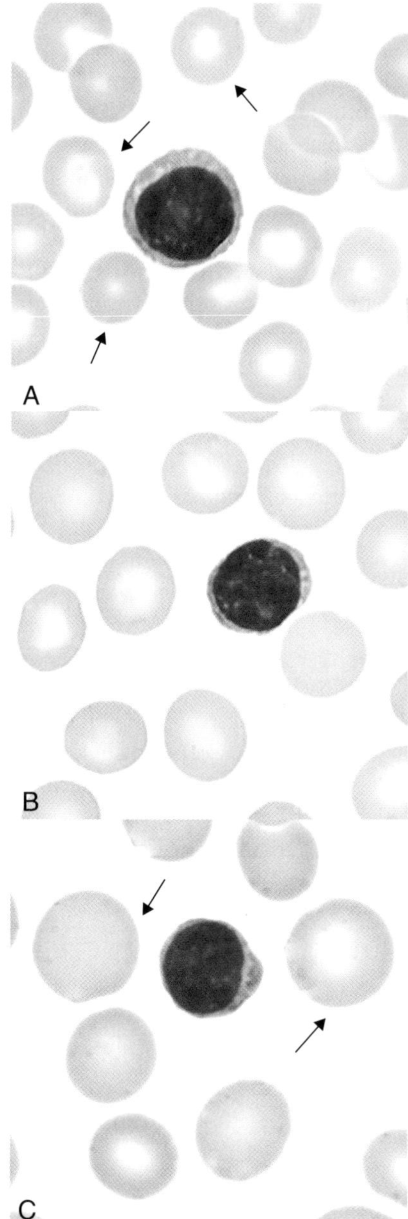

Fig. 29.3 Variations in Size of Erythrocytes (A) Microcytes (mean cell volume [MCV] <80 fL) associated with iron deficiency anemia, thalassemia minor, chronic inflammation (some cases), lead poisoning, hemoglobinopathies (some), and sideroblastic anemia. (B) Normocytes (mean cell volume [MCV] 80–100 fL). Normal erythrocytes are approximately the same size as the nucleus of a small lymphocyte. (C) Macrocytes (mean cell volume [MCV] >100 fL). Associated with vitamin B12 deficiency, folate deficiency, liver disease, neonates, and reticulocytosis. (From Rodak BF, Carr JH. *Clinical hematology atlas*. 5th edition. St. Louis: Elsevier; 2017)

processes directed against gastric parietal cells or IF itself. It may be a component of a cluster of autoimmune diseases affecting endocrine organs such as autoimmune thyroiditis and type 1 diabetes mellitus.[8] Chronic infection with *Helicobacter pylori* is also implicated. Other causes include surgical removal of the stomach, resection of the ileum, and tapeworms. Environmental conditions that may contribute to the development of PA include excessive alcohol intake and smoking.

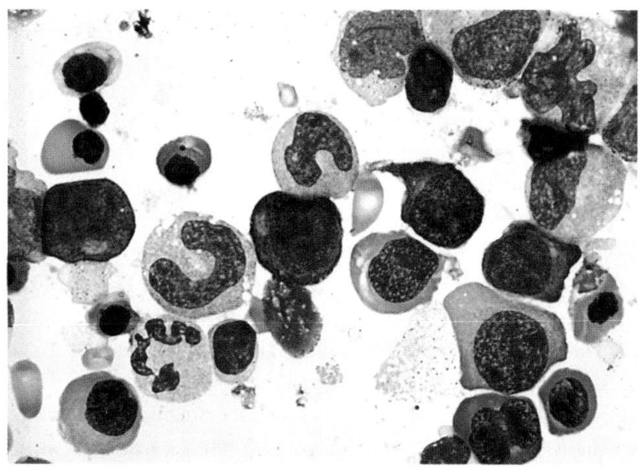

Fig. 29.4 Bone Marrow Aspirate from Individual With Pernicious Anemia. Bone marrow aspirate smear from an individual with megaloblastic red blood cell precursors and giant metamyelocytes. The chromatin in the red blood cell nuclei is more dispersed than that in normal red blood cell precursors at comparable stages of maturation; the giant metamyelocytes have dispersed nuclear chromatin in contrast to a normal metamyelocyte, which has condensed chromatin (Wright-Giemsa stain). (From Damjanov I, Linder J, eds. *Anderson's pathology*, 10th edition. St. Louis: Mosby; 1996.)

Pathophysiology. Individuals with autoimmune PA commonly have two types of antibodies: one to parietal cells and the other to IF or its binding site in the small bowel.[7] IF deficiency in PA is most often associated with type A chronic atrophic (autoimmune) gastritis, whereby autoantibodies destroy parietal and zymogenic (relating to an enzyme) cells leading to gastric atrophy (see Chapter 41). *H. pylori* infection may cause an increase in antibody production. These autoantibodies often target gastric H+-K+ adenosine triphosphate (ATP)ase, which is the major protein constituent of parietal cell membranes. Early in progression of disease, the gastric submucosa becomes infiltrated with inflammatory cells. These cells include autoreactive T cells, which initiate gastric mucosal injury and trigger the formation of autoantibodies. Gastric mucosal injury and atrophy result in a deficiency of all secretions of the stomach—hydrochloric acid (achlorhydria), pepsin, and IF. Without adequate IF, vitamin B12 malabsorption develops. Vitamin B_{12} is essential for nuclear maturation and DNA synthesis in red blood cells. Deficiencies lead to an anemia characterized by abnormal RBC precursor cells in the bone marrow (megaloblasts) and enlarged mature RBCs in the circulation (macrocytes). In addition, there is an increased risk for gastric cancer in individuals with chronic gastritis and PA.

Approximately 40% to 60% of individuals with PA have autoantibodies to intrinsic factor antibodies (IFA) directly leading to vitamin B_{12} malabsorption in the ileum. Many of these individuals have a history of IDA and gastric achlorhydria. Individuals with unexplained IDA should be screened for autoimmune gastritis and PA.[7]

Clinical Manifestations. PA develops slowly (over 20 to 30 years), so by the time an individual seeks treatment, it is usually severe. Early symptoms are often ignored because they are nonspecific and vague and include infections, mood swings, and GI, cardiac, or kidney ailments.[9] When the hemoglobin level has decreased to 7 to 8 g/dL, the individual experiences classic symptoms of PA: weakness, fatigue, paresthesia of feet and fingers, difficulty walking, loss of appetite, abdominal pain, weight loss, and a sore tongue that is smooth and beefy red (glossitis). The skin may become "lemon yellow" (sallow), caused by a combination of pallor and jaundice. Hepatomegaly and splenomegaly, indicating right-sided heart failure, may be present in the elderly.

Neurologic manifestations result from nerve demyelination that may produce neuronal death. The most frequently recognized deficit is a sensory neuropathy resulting in a loss of position and vibration sense that is especially prominent in the feet leading to ataxia.[10] The spinal cord is affected, causing weakness and spasticity. Vision may also be impaired. Early diagnosis and treatment improve chances of recovery, and while only a small percentage experience a complete neurological recovery, most individuals experience some improvement in symptoms after treatment.[11] The cerebrum also may be involved with manifestations of affective disorders, most commonly depression. Low levels of vitamin B_{12} have been associated with neurocognitive disorders and Alzheimer disease.

Evaluation and Treatment. Diagnosis of PA is based on clinical manifestations and test results demonstrating a macrocytic (high MCV) normochromic (normal MCHC) anemia (see Table 29.1) and low serum levels of vitamin B_{12}. Reticulocyte counts are decreased. Confirmatory studies include bone marrow aspiration, detection of circulating antibodies against parietal cells and IF, and gastric biopsy.[9]

Replacement of vitamin B_{12} (cobalamin) is the treatment of choice. Initial injections of vitamin B_{12} are administered weekly until the deficiency is corrected, followed by monthly injections for the remainder of the individual's life. Conventional practice assumed that oral preparations were ineffective because the lack of IF meant there would be continued malabsorption of vitamin B_{12}. However, high doses of orally administered vitamin B_{12} can be absorbed across the small bowel in many individuals and can be considered as an alternative treatment for PA.[7] The effectiveness of B_{12} replacement therapy is determined by a rising reticulocyte count. Blood counts return to normal within 5 to 6 weeks. PA cannot be cured, so maintenance therapy is lifelong. Treated individuals should be monitored for the development of gastric cancer and IDA.

Folate deficiency anemia. A deficiency of folic acid results in a megaloblastic anemia having the same pathologic consequences as those caused by vitamin B_{12} deficiency. Folate (folic acid) is an essential vitamin required for RNA and DNA synthesis within the maturing erythrocyte. Humans are totally dependent on dietary intake of folate to meet the daily requirement of 50 to 200 mg/day. It is estimated that at least 10% of North Americans are folate deficient, but the incidence has been decreasing in the United States since the fortification of foods with folate and the increased use of folate supplements. Increased amounts are required for lactating and pregnant females, and deficiencies of folate can cause neural tube defects in the developing fetus. Folate deficiency occurs more often than B_{12} deficiency, particularly in alcoholics and individuals with chronic malnourishment. Inflammatory bowel disease (ulcerative colitis) may be the underlying cause of folate malabsorption in some individuals, and treatment with sulfasalazine decreases folate absorption from the gut.

Folate is absorbed from the upper small intestine and does not require any other element (e.g., IF) to facilitate absorption. After absorption, folate circulates through the liver, where it is stored. Folates are coenzymes required for the synthesis of thymine and purines (adenine and guanine) and the conversion of homocysteine to methionine.[12] Deficient production of thymine affects cells undergoing rapid division (e.g., bone marrow cells undergoing erythropoiesis) resulting in megaloblastic precursor cells and a macrocytic anemia.

Clinical manifestations are similar to those apparent in individuals with PA. Specific manifestations include cheilosis (scales and fissures of the mouth), stomatitis (inflammation of the mouth), and painful ulcerations of the buccal mucosa and tongue characteristic of burning mouth syndrome. *Burning mouth syndrome* also may be secondary to other disorders (e.g., extremely dry mouth, infection, autoimmune disease, nutritional deficiencies, and other conditions) and is not diagnostic for folate deficiency. Dysphagia, flatulence, and watery diarrhea may be present, as well as histologic changes in the GI tract similar to those seen in celiac disease (see Chapter 42). Neurologic manifestations, if present, may be caused by thiamine deficiency, which often accompanies folate deficiency in malnourished individuals.

Evaluation of folate deficiency is based on clinical manifestations, the appearance of macrocytic RBCs (high MCV) in the blood, and the measurement of serum folate levels. Treatment requires administration of oral folate preparations until adequate blood levels are obtained and manifestations are reduced or eliminated. Long-term therapy is not necessary if the appropriate dietary adjustments are made to maintain adequate intake. Manifestations of anemia disappear within 1 to 2 weeks after administration of folate.

Megaloblastic anemia caused by medications. Many drugs can directly affect DNA synthesis and thereby interfere with RBC maturation leading to megaloblastic anemia.[12] These drugs include immunomodulatory drugs (e.g., azathioprine and leflunomide), chemotherapeutics (e.g., fluorouracil and methotrexate), allopurinol, and trimethoprim (sulfa drug).[12] Other medications reduce vitamin B_{12} or folate absorption. Management includes discontinuation of the drug if possible, or if not, vitamin supplementation is indicated.

Microcytic-Hypochromic Anemias

The microcytic-hypochromic anemias are characterized by abnormally small erythrocytes (low MCV) (see Figs. 29.1 and 29.3A) that contain reduced amounts of hemoglobin (low MCHC). Sideroblastic anemia can cause erythrocytes to be microcytic and hypochromic, (see Table 29.1), but IDA is far more common.

Iron deficiency anemia. IDA is the most common nutritional disorder worldwide, affecting 10% to 20% of the world's population, occurring in both developed and developing countries.[13] The causes of IDA include (1) dietary deficiency, (2) impaired absorption (e.g., celiac disease, disorders of fat absorption), (3) increased requirement, (4) chronic blood loss, and (5) chronic diarrhea.

IDA is common in the United States, particularly in toddlers, adolescent girls, and women of childbearing age. Other populations at risk for IDA include those living in poverty, infants consuming cow's milk (decreased bioavailability of iron), older individuals ingesting restricted diets, and teenagers with poor diets (junk food). An increased prevalence of iron deficiency has been observed in those with eating disorders, as well as in overweight children, adolescents, and women.[13] Premenopausal women have an increased iron requirement, especially during pregnancy and with excessive menstrual bleeding. Increased requirement also is a major cause of iron deficiency in growing infants, children, and adolescents. Other causes of IDA include bariatric surgery and surgical procedures that decrease stomach acidity.

Both sexes may have IDA secondary to bleeding as a result of gastric or duodenal ulcers, hiatal hernia, esophageal varices, cirrhosis, hemorrhoids, inflammatory bowel disease, or cancer. In fact, unexplained IDA in a male or a postmenopausal woman may be the first indication of GI disease.

Children in developing countries often are affected by chronic parasite infestations that result in blood and iron loss that is greater than dietary intake, thus causing IDA. Treatment of helminth infections improves the anemia as well as appetite and growth. *H. pylori* infection impairs iron uptake and is a cause of iron-refractory or iron-dependent anemia of previously unknown origin in adults. Children in resource-poor conditions often are exposed to unsafe levels of toxins such as lead (see Chapter 2). Chronic lead poisoning can produce a mild microcytic anemia, and the absorption of lead can prevent the normal addition of iron to heme molecules resulting in IDA.[14] Furthermore, IDA is associated with pica, which can lead to ingestion of lead-containing paint and soil. IDA and lead poisoning can act synergistically to cause anemia more severe than would either condition alone. Treatment for iron deficiency is associated with a decrease in lead levels.

Pathophysiology. IDA is a hypochromic-microcytic anemia (see Fig. 29.3A) and occurs when iron stores are depleted. Inadequate dietary intake and excessive blood loss deplete iron stores and reduce hemoglobin synthesis. When total body stores of iron are low, iron deprivation for erythroblasts and other tissues occurs. In some cases, iron stores may be sufficient, but delivery is inadequate to maintain heme synthesis, thus producing a functional or relative iron deficiency. For example, inflammation can cause withholding of iron from the plasma, particularly through the action of the peptide hepcidin, the main regulator of systemic iron balance (see Chapter 28).[15] Hepcidin inhibits iron transfer to the plasma by binding to ferroportin, causing it to be endocytosed and degraded.[16]

Iron in the form of hemoglobin is in constant demand by the body. Iron is recyclable; therefore, the body maintains a balance between iron that is contained in hemoglobin and iron that is in storage and available for future hemoglobin synthesis (see Chapter 28). Blood loss disrupts this balance by creating a need for more iron, thus depleting the iron stores more rapidly to replace the iron that is lost from the body due to bleeding.

Iron contributes to immune function by regulating several immune mechanisms. Acquired *hypoferremia* (deficiency of iron in the blood) due to a decrease in hepcidin may be part of the body's response to infection.[17] Many pathogens require iron for survival; thus, hypoferremia would hamper their growth. In contrast, neutrophils and macrophages require adequate iron to function appropriately in the innate immune response to infection. The precise benefits or detriments of iron deficiency and immunity remain under investigation.

IDA occurs when the demand for iron exceeds the supply and develops slowly through three overlapping stages. Stage I is characterized by decreased bone marrow iron stores; hemoglobin and serum iron remain normal. In stage II, iron transportation to bone marrow is diminished, resulting in iron-deficient erythropoiesis. Stage III begins when the small hemoglobin-deficient cells enter the circulation to replace the normal aged erythrocytes that have been removed from the circulation. The manifestations of IDA appear in stage III, when there is depletion of iron stores and diminished hemoglobin production.

Clinical Manifestations. Symptoms of IDA begin gradually, and individuals may not seek medical attention until hemoglobin levels have decreased to about 7 to 8 g/dL. Nonspecific early symptoms include fatigue, weakness, shortness of breath, and pale earlobes, palms, and conjunctivae (Fig. 29.5A). As the condition progresses and becomes more severe, structural and functional changes occur in epithelial tissue. Koilonychia or *spoon-shaped* fingernails become brittle, thin, and coarsely ridged as a result of impaired capillary circulation (see Fig. 29.5B). Other

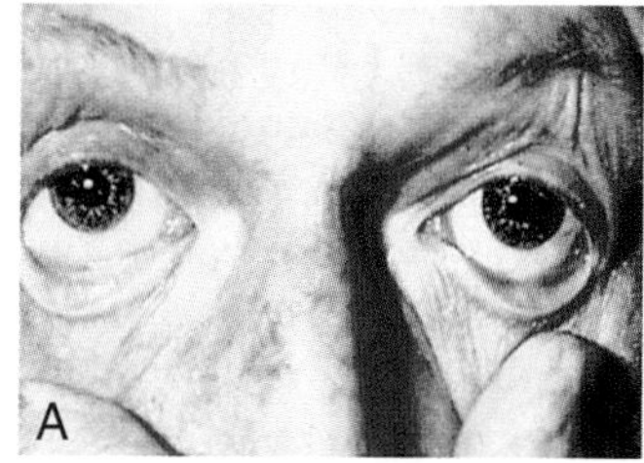

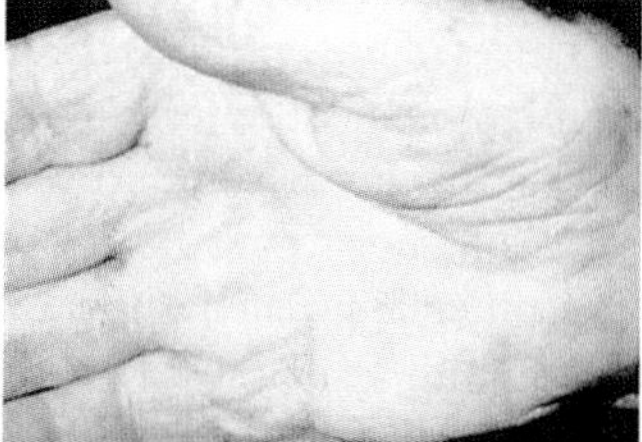
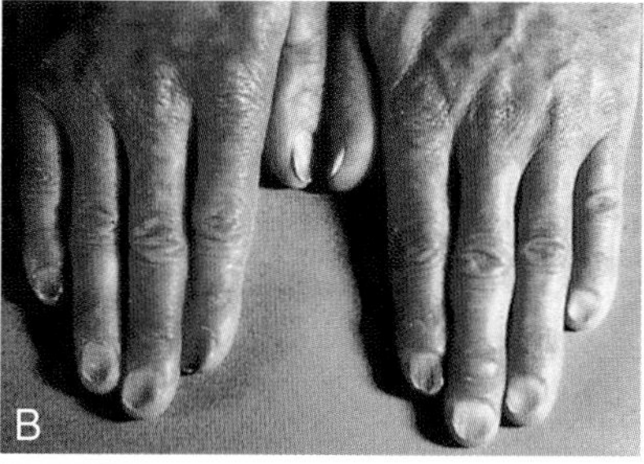

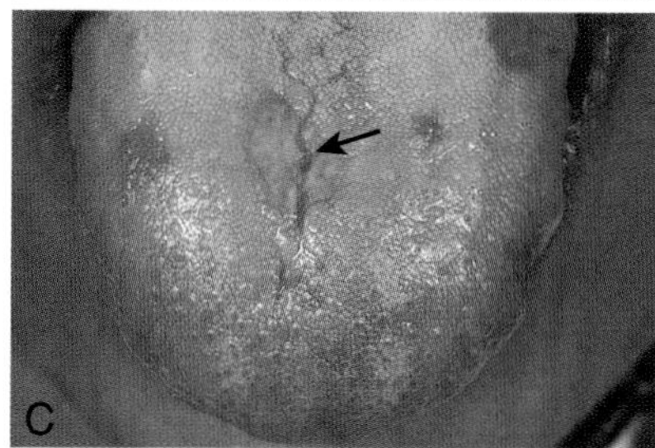

Fig. 29.5 Manifestations of Iron Deficiency Anemia. (A) Pallor and iron deficiency. Pallor of the skin, mucous membranes, and palmar creases in an individual with a hemoglobin level of 9 g/dL. Palmar creases become as pale as the surrounding skin when the hemoglobin level approaches 7 g/dL. **(B)** Koilonychia. The nails are concave, ridged, and brittle. **(C)** Glossitis. Tongue of individual with iron deficiency anemia has bald, fissured appearance caused by loss of papillae and flattening. (From Hoffbrand AV, Pettit JE, Vyas P. *Color atlas of clinical hematology*, 4th edition. London: Mosby; 2009; B, Courtesy Dr. S.M. Knowles.)

manifestations include cheilosis (scales and fissures of the mouth), stomatitis (inflammation of the mouth), and painful ulcerations of the buccal mucosa and tongue characteristic of burning (glossitis) (see Fig. 29.5C). Difficulty in swallowing (dysphagia) is associated with an esophageal *web*, a thin, concentric extension of normal esophageal tissue consisting of mucosa and submucosa at the juncture between the hypopharynx and esophagus. Dysphagia is worsened by hyposalivation. Individuals with IDA also exhibit gastritis, neuromuscular changes, headache, irritability, tingling, numbness, and vasomotor disturbances. Alterations in gait are rare. Iron deficiency in children is associated with numerous adverse manifestations, especially cognitive impairment. Cognitive impairment may be long-lasting and irreversible (see Chapter 30).

Evaluation and Treatment. Initial evaluation is based on symptoms and decreased levels of hemoglobin and hematocrit and the finding of microcytic (low MCV) and hypochromic (low MCHC) erythrocytes in the blood. Decreased serum iron, ferritin, and transferrin saturation levels are also found. A sensitive indicator of heme synthesis is the amount of free erythrocyte protoporphyrin (FEP) within erythrocytes.

An initial step in treatment of IDA is to identify and eliminate sources of blood loss. Oral iron replacement therapy is indicated, and hematocrit levels should improve within 1 to 2 months of therapy. Parenteral iron replacement is used in instances of uncontrolled chronic blood loss, intolerance to oral iron replacement, intestinal malabsorption, or poor adherence to oral therapy. Serum ferritin level is a more precise measurement of improvement. A rapid decrease in fatigue, lethargy, and other associated symptoms is generally seen within the first month of therapy. Replacement therapy may continue for many months. Menstruating females may need daily oral iron replacement therapy until menopause.

Normocytic-Normochromic Anemia

Some causes of anemia do not change the size, color, or shape of erythrocytes (see Figs. 29.1 and 29.3B). Two important causes of normocytic-normochromic anemia are AI and aplastic anemia (AA).

Anemia of inflammation. Anemia of inflammation (AI) (also called anemia of chronic inflammation and anemia of chronic disease [ACD]), is a mild to moderate anemia resulting from decreased erythropoiesis and impaired iron utilization in individuals with chronic diseases that produce systemic inflammation (e.g., infections, cancer, and chronic inflammatory or autoimmune diseases). It is one of the most common conditions encountered in medicine. Table 29.4 lists some of these causes of AI. AI is a common type of anemia in hospitalized individuals where it is observed in individuals with chronic obstructive pulmonary disease (COPD) and congestive heart failure (CHF); in persons with critical illnesses after acute events such as major surgery, severe trauma, myocardial infarction, and sepsis; and in the elderly. The elderly may be predisposed to AI related to age-associated hematopoietic changes with increased concentrations of inflammatory cytokines. More than 50% of elderly individuals who reside in nursing homes have anemia, with two-thirds of cases being AI or unexplained. The elderly with characteristics of AI without an underlying malignancy or inflammatory condition are described as having primary defective iron utilization syndrome.

TABLE 29.4 Underlying Causes of Anemia of Inflammation

Associated Diseases	Estimated Prevalence (%)
Infections: Acute and chronic; viral infections including HIV infection, bacterial, parasitic, fungal	18–95
Cancer: Hematologic, solid tumor	30–63
Systemic Inflammatory Disorders: Rheumatoid arthritis, systemic lupus erythematosus, inflammatory bowel disease, vasculitis, or systemic sclerosis, sepsis	33–60
Aging: Due to the presence of inflammatory conditions or chronic kidney disease in older aging individuals	33
Chronic Disorders: Chronic obstructive pulmonary disease, congestive heart failure, chronic kidney disease, immune-mediated diseases	Unknown
Other: Critical illnesses after acute events, major surgery, severe trauma, myocardial infarction, obesity, anemia of the elderly	Unknown

CKD, Chronic kidney disease.
Data from Weiss G, Schett G. Anaemia in inflammatory rhematic diseases. *Nature Reviews Rheumatology*, 2013;9(4):205–215; Weiss G, Ganz T, Goodnough LT. Anemia of inflammation. *Blood*, 2016;133(1):40–50; Nemeth E, Ganz T. Anemia of inflammation. *Hematology/Oncology Clinics of North America*. 2014;28(4):671–681. Fraenkel PG. Anemia of inflammation: a review. *The Medical Clinics of North America*. 2017;101(2):285–296; Weiss G, Ganz T, Goodnough LT. Anemia of inflammation. Blood. 2019 Jan 3;133(1):40-50. doi: 10.1182/blood-2018-06-856500. Epub 2018 Nov 6. PMID: 30401705; PMCID: PMC6536698.

Pathophysiology. AI usually develops after 1 to 2 months of disease activity. The initial severity is related to the underlying disorder, but, although persistent, it usually does not progress. AI results from a combination of (1) decreased erythrocyte life span, (2) suppressed production of erythropoietin, (3) ineffective bone marrow response to erythropoietin, and (4) altered iron metabolism and iron dynamics in macrophages. During chronic inflammation, a large variety of cytokines are released by lymphocytes, macrophages, and the affected tissue. Inflammatory cytokines increase hepcidin levels, which reduces iron absorption, sequesters iron in macrophages, and suppresses erythropoietin production (Fig. 29.6).[16] Impaired iron metabolism is partially the result of iron sequestration (Emerging Science Box: Regulation of Iron Metabolism). Normal iron transport by transferrin also may be decreased as a result of inflammation-related increases in the levels of circulating lactoferrin and apoferritin.

The erythropoietic defect in AI is failure to increase erythropoiesis in response to decreased numbers of erythrocytes. In part, decreased erythropoiesis results from diminished production of erythropoietin by the kidneys. In addition, the failure in erythropoiesis may reflect decreased responsiveness of erythroid progenitors to erythropoietin. Decreased availability of iron would diminish the rate of erythropoiesis. Proliferation of erythroid cells also is inhibited by proinflammatory cytokines. Loss of integrins may prevent adequate interaction with stromal cells and matrix proteins and inhibit erythropoiesis.

Erythrocyte destruction is the result of eryptosis (described earlier in this chapter). Most of the diseases responsible for AI cause damage to erythrocytes resulting in macrophage activity. Platelet function also may be defective in these individuals, which results in chronic bleeding and loss of erythrocytes.

Clinical Manifestations. AI is usually in the mild to moderate range. Individuals may be asymptomatic, or the anemia may be a chance clinical finding. If there is a significant drop in hemoglobin levels, clinical manifestations of anemia appear.

Evaluation and Treatment. Initially, AI is normocytic-normochromic, but with persistence it becomes hypochromic and microcytic (see Table 29.1). AI is characterized by low levels of circulating iron and reduced levels of transferrin. The most significant finding of AI is very high total body iron storage, although inadequate iron is released from the bone marrow for erythropoiesis. A first indication of AI is often a failure to respond to conventional iron replacement therapy. Levels of erythropoietin are generally lower than expected for the degree of anemia. Individuals frequently present with low or normal total iron-binding capacity (TIBC), normal or high serum ferritin levels, and low concentrations of soluble transferrin receptor. It occasionally may be difficult to differentiate AI from IDA.

Use of erythropoietin in treatment of AI associated with arthritis, malignancies, and acquired immunodeficiency syndrome (AIDS) has met with limited success. Individuals with severe anemia secondary to chronic kidney disease (CKD) can be treated successfully with erythropoietin and treatments to increase iron stores. However, the optimal degree of restoration of hemoglobin levels has not been determined; a return to normal levels increases the risk of hypertension, stroke, and death.[18] The principal treatment is easement of the underlying disorder. Individuals with AI, but without evidence of inflammatory or infectious conditions, should be screened for malignancies.

Aplastic anemia. Aplastic anemia (AA) is a hematopoietic failure of the bone marrow leading to a reduction in the effective production of mature blood cells and resulting in peripheral pancytopenia (anemia, neutropenia, and thrombocytopenia), which is a reduction or absence of all three blood cell types. (Fig. 29.7) The incidence of AA in the United States is low; however, the incidence in developing countries is higher related to greater exposure to certain chemicals known to cause AA. The incidence is bimodal, with one peak occurring between 15 and 25 years of age and a second peak occurring in individuals older than age 60. AA is equally distributed between genders.

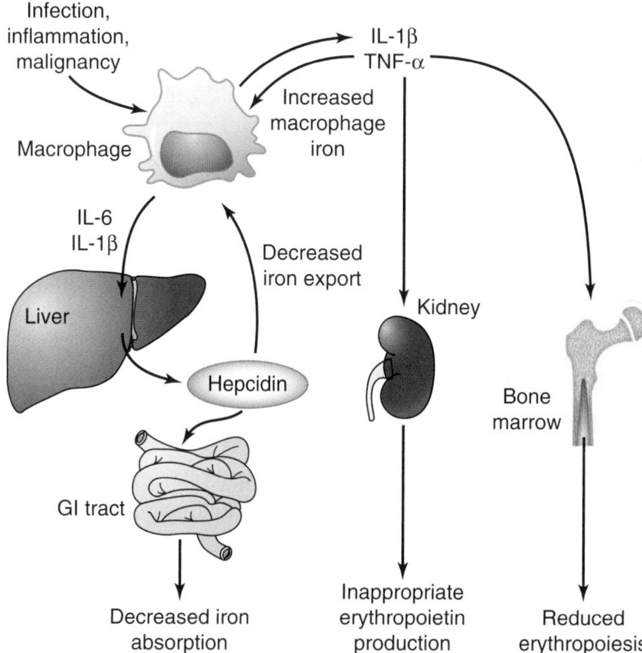

Fig. 29.6 Mechanism for the Anemia of Inflammation. *GI,* Gastrointestinal; *IL-6,* interleukin-6; *IL-1β,* interleukin-1β; *TNF-α,* tumor necrosis factor-α.

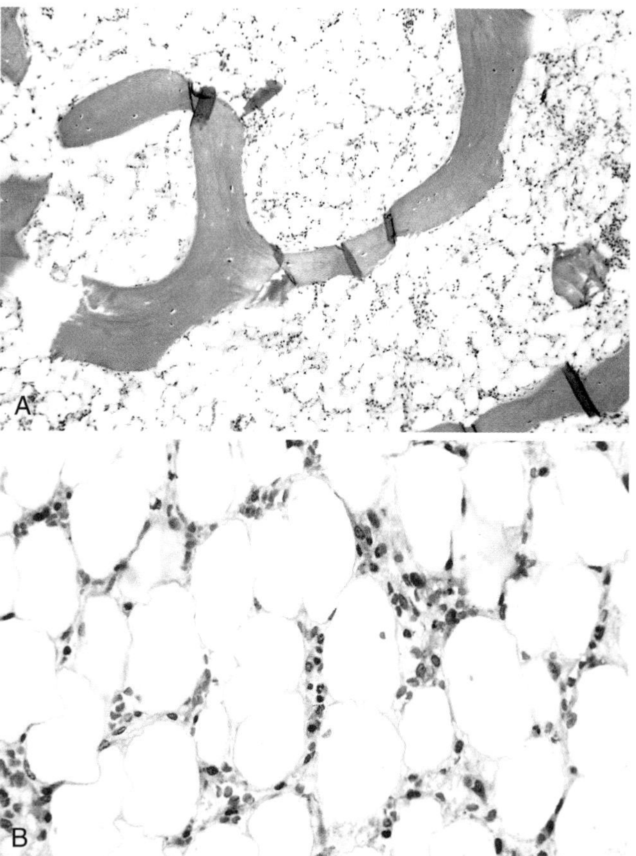

Fig. 29.7 Aplastic Anemia. The common pathology of the bone marrow replaced by fat can result from chemical or physical damage (iatrogenic; benzene); immune destruction (mainly T cells); and as a constitutional defect in genes important in maintenance of cell integrity and immune regulation. (A) Low power. (B) High power. (From Kumar V, Abbas A, Aster J. *Robbins & Cotran pathologic basis of disease*, 10th edition. Philadelphia: Elsevier; 2021.)

BOX 29.1 Major Causes of Aplastic Anemia

Acquired
- Idiopathic
- Acquired stem cell defects
- Immune mediated

Chemical Agents
- Dose related
  - Alkylating agents
  - Antimetabolites
  - Benzene
  - Chloramphenicol
  - Inorganic arsenicals
- Idiosyncratic
  - Chloramphenicol
  - Phenylbutazone
  - Organic arsenicals
  - Methylphenylethylhydantoin
  - Carbamazepine
  - Penicillamine
  - Gold salts

Physical Agents
- Whole-body irradiation
- Viral infections
- Hepatitis (unknown virus)
- Cytomegalovirus infections
- Epstein-Barr virus infections
- Herpes zoster (varicella zoster)

Inherited
- Fanconi anemia
- Telomerase defects

From Kumar V, Abbas A, Aster J. *Robbins & Cotran pathologic basis of disease*, 10th edition. Philadelphia: Elsevier; 2021.

Idiopathic AA (primary acquired; autoimmune) accounts for approximately 75% of all confirmed cases. *Secondary* AA, which accounts for approximately 15% of cases, is caused by a variety of known chemical agents and ionizing radiation (Box 29.1). Total body irradiation is a well-described cause of AA and in certain instances may be used therapeutically for this effect in the treatment of certain cancers or for organ and bone marrow transplantation (BMT). Infections also are known to cause AA, with viruses being the most common agent, including the human immunodeficiency virus (HIV), Epstein-Barr virus (EBV), and hepatitis (non-A, non-B, non-C, and non-G forms of the virus). Persistent parvovirus B19 infection also has been identified as producing bone marrow failure resulting in AA.

Another condition associated with AA is pure red cell aplasia (PRCA), in which only the erythrocytes are affected. PRCA is a rare disorder and has been associated with autoimmune, viral, and neoplastic (leukemias) disorders; infiltrative disorders of the bone marrow (myelofibrosis); renal failure; hepatitis; mononucleosis; and systemic lupus erythematosus (SLE). It also is a well-recognized but infrequent complication of allogeneic BMT, particularly when there is donor-recipient ABO mismatch. A thymoma often is found in association with PRCA and is also present in Diamond-Blackfan syndrome, a congenital disorder.

AA is associated with one or more somatic mutations. A subset of these is found to have defective telomerase RNA, resulting in shortened telomere.[19] A very small percentage of AA cases are linked to inherited genetic alterations. Fanconi anemia is a rare genetic anemia characterized by pancytopenia resulting from defects in DNA repair. This anemia develops early in life and is accompanied by multiple congenital anomalies.

Pathophysiology. The characteristic lesion of AA is a hypocellular bone marrow that has been replaced with fat. Although the pathogenesis is not fully defined, AA results from loss of hematopoietic stem cells (HSCs) or their progenitors at various stages of differentiation. Two etiologies and mechanisms are observed: an immune-mediated destruction of bone marrow progenitor cells (idiopathic AA) and an intrinsic abnormality of stem cells (secondary AA).

Several immune abnormalities are found in individuals with idiopathic AA including dysregulated CD4 +, CD8 +, natural killer, and Th-17 T-cell responses and reduced numbers of regulatory T cells.[20] Elevations of circulating levels of inflammatory or myelosuppressive cytokines, such as interferon-gamma (IFN-γ), tumor necrosis factor-alpha (TNF-α), and transforming growth factor-beta (TGF-β) are seen. The initial immune response may be triggered by pathogens, drugs, or chemicals, or by neoantigens through epigenetic mechanisms. It also is interesting that transient and persistent bone marrow hypoplasia has been linked to many microorganisms, and the interaction between the gut microbiota and immune system is hypothesized as an initial insult in the development of bone marrow failure syndromes such as AA.[21]

In secondary AA, stem cells and the bone marrow microenvironment may be altered from exposure to drugs, infectious agents, or other environmental factors.[20] Somatic changes in stem cell chromosomes may trigger these autoimmune processes and may contribute to the development of myelodysplastic syndrome and leukemia in individuals with AA.[19,20]

Clinical Manifestations. The onset of symptoms in AA is related to the rapidity with which the bone marrow is destroyed and replaced. Approximately 50% of AA cases progress rapidly, with a high risk of death from overwhelming infection or bleeding. In some cases, the rate of decline is slow, and the individual may adapt progressively to a new level of hematologic function. This condition is referred to as hypoplastic anemia rather than AA.

Initial symptoms depend on which cell line is affected. Rapidly progressing disease is usually associated with hypoxemia, pallor, and weakness. Other symptoms include fever and dyspnea and rapidly developing signs of hemorrhaging if platelets are affected (e.g., unexplained bruising, nosebleeds, bleeding gums, bleeding in the GI tract, prolonged bleeding at sites of minor injury). A more insidious onset over weeks or months is characterized by progressive weakness and fatigue with gradually developing signs of hemorrhaging. Major hemorrhage may occur from any organ at any time; however, it is generally observed in the late stages and is often secondary to other events. In both rapid onset and slow onset AA, diminished leukocyte production may result in a progressive frequency and prolongation of infections. Ulcerations of the mouth and pharynx or a low-grade cellulitis in the neck may be seen. Neurologic changes may become evident when hemorrhages have occurred within the system.

Evaluation and Treatment. AA is suspected if levels of circulating erythrocytes, leukocytes, and platelets are diminished. The diagnosis is confirmed by bone marrow biopsy. The bone marrow usually has reduced cellularity (e.g., less than 25% normal cellularity). The morphology of the few remaining hematopoietic cells is usually normal. Occasionally the erythrocytes are macrocytic, with anisocytosis and poikilocytosis, and may appear immature.

Bone marrow and, most recently, peripheral blood stem cell transplantation (SCT) from a histocompatible sibling often cures the underlying bone marrow failure. Before transplantation, the recipient usually receives radiation or chemotherapy to deplete the bone marrow of disease-causing precursor cells. Infection and graft-versus-host (GVH) disease are major contributors to premature death after transplantation.[22]

For those individuals unable to undergo BMT or who lack a suitable sibling donor, immunosuppression remains the treatment of choice. Drugs like antithymocyte globulin (ATG) and cyclosporine suppress the activity of autoimmune cells. Corticosteroids are often used concurrently with ATG and cyclosporine. The addition of recombinant hematopoietic growth factors (e.g., granulocyte-macrophage colony–stimulating factor [GM-CSF], IL-6, and epoetin) to immunosuppressive therapy can produce significant additional benefit in both children and adults. A promising new treatment for AA is the oral thrombopoietin (TPO) receptor agonist eltrombopag which improves HSC maintenance and expansion.[23]

Anemias of Increased Destruction

Hemolytic anemia is premature accelerated destruction of erythrocytes, either episodically or continuously. They can be inherited or acquired (see Fig. 29.1). Hemolytic anemias may develop due to destruction outside of blood vessels or intravascularly. *Extravascular hemolysis* is the destruction of erythrocytes by macrophages which are abundant in the spleen, bone marrow, and liver. Macrophages will phagocytose erythrocytes that have been opsonized by antibodies, erythrocytes with structural alterations of the membrane surface, or erythrocytes that have become more rigid due to intracellular defects. *Intravascular hemolysis* most often is caused by antibody-mediated complement fixation. It can also be caused by mechanical injury, intracellular parasites, or exogenous toxic factors (e.g., clostridial sepsis, snake venom, lead poisoning). Although compensatory erythropoiesis provides new erythrocytes to replace those that are lost, if destruction outpaces production, then anemia develops. Hemolytic anemias may be either congenital or acquired.

Congenital hemolytic anemias result from intrinsic defects in erythrocytes, including the red cell membrane (e.g., hereditary spherocytosis, paroxysmal nocturnal hemoglobinuria), enzymatic pathways (e.g., glucose6-phosphate dehydrogenase deficiency), and hemoglobin synthesis (e.g., the thalassemia syndromes, sickle cell anemia) (see Chapter 30).

Acquired hemolytic anemias are usually immunologic, such as erythrocyte destruction caused by autoantibodies against erythrocyte antigens (e.g., autoimmune hemolytic anemia), isohemagglutinins (e.g., mismatched erythrocyte transfusions), or allergic reactions against drug antigens adsorbed onto the erythrocyte surface (drug-induced hemolytic anemia). Isohemagglutinins, erythrocyte antigens, autoantibodies, and allergic reactions are discussed in Chapter 9.

Pathophysiology. Autoimmune hemolytic anemias (AIHAs) are acquired disorders caused by autoantibodies, complement, or both, directed against antigens on the surface of erythrocytes. Aging, genetic background, autoimmune disorders, infections, medications, cancers (especially lymphomas), and organ transplants are risk factors for AIHA development. Recent studies implicate T- and B-cell dysregulation, reduced T regulatory cell function, and impaired lymphocyte apoptosis.[24] Five types of AIHAs have been described: (1) warm reactive antibody type, (2) cold agglutinin type, (3) cold hemolysin type (paroxysmal cold hemoglobinuria), (4) alloimmune hemolytic anemia, and (5) drug-induced hemolytic anemia. This classification is based on the optimal temperature at which the antibody binds to erythrocytes and the mechanism of erythrocyte destruction.

Warm autoimmune hemolytic anemia is the most common form of AIHA accounting for about 1/3 of cases.[24] Approximately half of the cases are associated with other diseases, especially lymphomas but also chronic lymphocytic leukemia, other neoplastic disorders, or SLE. The anemia is caused by immunoglobulin G (IgG) antibodies that bind to erythrocytes at normal body temperature. The most common targets of these antibodies are Rh antigens on the erythrocyte surface.[25] The IgG-coated erythrocytes bind to the Fc receptors on monocytes and splenic macrophages and are removed by phagocytosis (see Chapter 9).

Cold agglutinin autoimmune hemolytic anemia is mediated by immunoglobulin M (IgM) antibodies and occurs less often than warm antibody hemolysis. These antibodies optimally bind to erythrocytes at colder temperatures (lower than 31°C [87.8°F]). Cold agglutinin autoantibodies may appear acutely during recovery from certain infectious disorders, particularly infectious mononucleosis (IM), *Mycoplasma pneumoniae*, and disseminated tuberculosis (TB). Chronic cold agglutinin AIHAs also can occur in association with lymphoid neoplasm and other unknown or idiopathic conditions. IgM autoantibodies are directed against erythrocyte carbohydrate antigens on the surface of erythrocytes.[25] In the colder areas of the body (e.g., fingers, toes, nose, ears, exposed skin), particularly during cold weather, the IgM autoantibodies bind to circulating erythrocytes where they activate complement leading to phagocytosis by mononuclear phagocytes in the liver and spleen (see Chapter 9). The IgM is rapidly released when the blood recirculates and warms. The severity of hemolysis is variable and may result in a progressive chronic anemia. Prolonged exposure to the cold may lead to gangrene.

Cold hemolysin autoimmune hemolytic anemia (paroxysmal cold hemoglobinuria) is a disorder in which exposure to cold initiates acute intravascular hemolysis that, unlike cold agglutinin anemia, is severe enough to cause hemoglobinuria. The acute form occurs primarily in children younger than the age of

10 years and is usually preceded by an upper respiratory tract infection or flulike symptoms. Viral infections with measles, mumps, or varicella, as well as *M. pneumoniae* infections, have also been linked to an onset of paroxysmal cold hemoglobinuria. The anemia may be rapidly progressing and associated with fever, reddish brown urine, hemoglobinuria, jaundice, abdominal pains, and pallor, with about 25% of individuals presenting with hepatomegaly and splenomegaly.

A transfusion reaction is an example of alloimmune hemolytic anemia (see Chapter 9). Transfused blood that is mismatched for ABO antigens is destroyed by preexisting isohemagglutinins in the recipient. Isohemagglutinins, which are generally IgM antibodies, activate complement, resulting in a rapid intravascular hemolysis. The individual may immediately experience fever, chills, dyspnea, and hypotension and may progress to shock.

Drug-induced hemolytic anemia is a form of immune hemolytic anemia usually resulting from an allergic reaction against foreign antigens (e.g., antibiotics) (see Chapter 9). A low molecular weight drug may function as a hapten and bind to proteins on the surface of erythrocytes. IgG antibody is directed against the drug or against the unique antigen formed by the binding of the drug and erythrocyte protein (Fig. 29.8A). This leads to opsonization of the erythrocyte and phagocytosis by macrophages in the liver. Autoimmunity also can occur due to the formation of immune complexes which attach to erythrocytes and activate complement (see Fig. 29.8B). This mechanism also may explain some of the anemia observed in other immune complex conditions, such as SLE. Rarely, a drug (e.g., methyldopa) initiates the formation of cross-reactive antibodies that bind with erythrocyte antigens leading to phagocytosis by macrophages (see Fig. 29.8C).

Clinical Manifestations. The presence and severity of signs and symptoms of hemolytic anemia depend on the degree of anemia and hemolysis and the success of compensatory erythropoiesis.[24] Bone marrow is capable of increasing red cell production up to eight times its normal rate. When accelerated erythrocyte production is incapable of keeping up with destruction, anemia develops. The severity of anemia varies widely among individuals, even in those who have the same underlying illness. Severe disease may be diagnosed shortly after birth or within the first year of life. Mild to moderate anemia is more common because the shortened erythrocyte survival time is offset by increased erythropoiesis. Some individuals have no symptoms of anemia, and the underlying hemolytic process remains undetected unless some other complications develop during the course of the disease. Acute conditions that disrupt the delicate equilibrium of accelerated erythropoiesis and erythrocyte destruction may precipitate a crisis. The most common type of crisis is aplastic and results from failure of bone marrow erythrocyte production.

Jaundice (icterus) is present when heme release from destroyed erythrocytes exceeds the liver's ability to conjugate and excrete bilirubin (see Chapter 41). Adults with mild or moderate hemolytic anemia may not have icterus, or it may be visible only in the sclera, and thus remains unnoticed. Cardiovascular and respiratory manifestations vary with the degree of anemia. Thromboembolism may occur, and pulmonary embolism is a common finding during autopsies of individuals with immune hemolytic anemia.[25] Individuals with congenital hemolytic disorders demonstrate splenomegaly, and in some cases, the spleen

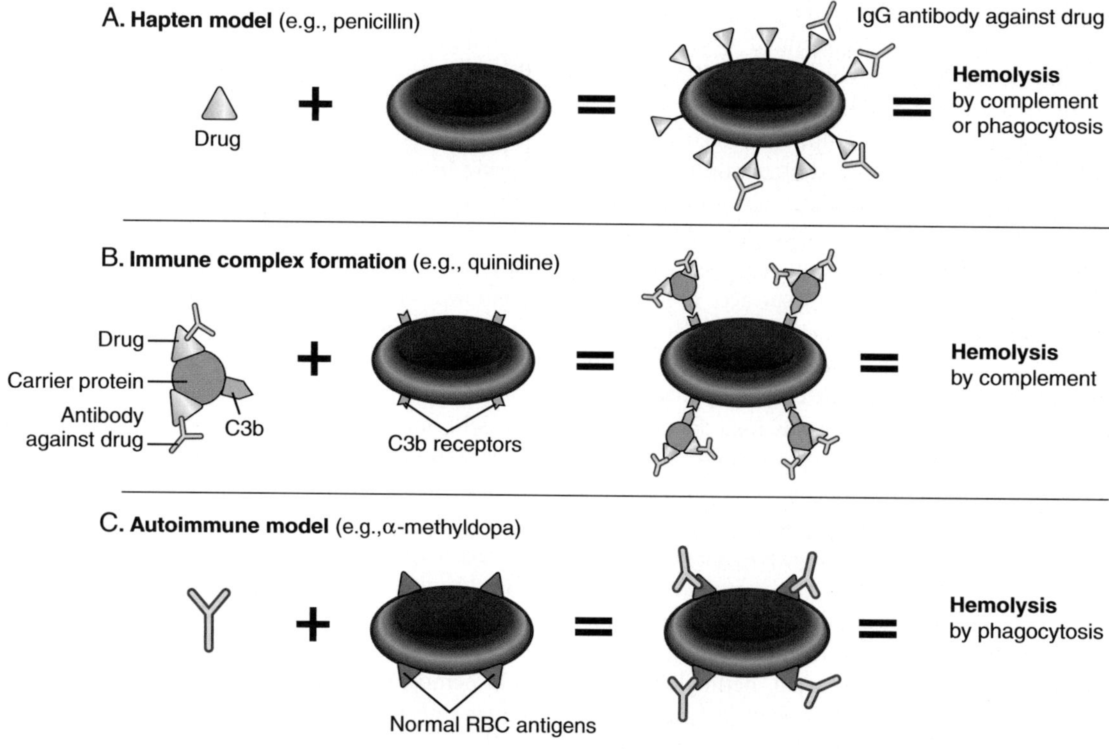

Fig. 29.8 Models of Drug-Induced Hemolytic Anemia.

may become quite enlarged. Children who have hemolytic anemia may develop skeletal abnormalities caused by expansion of erythroid bone marrow during the active phase of growth and development.

Evaluation and Treatment. Diagnosis of AIHA is based on clinical manifestations and blood tests. A normocytic- normochromic anemia, in which the erythrocytes are damaged or have abnormal shapes (schistocytes), combined with increased numbers of reticulocytes are indicative of hemolysis. Studies to detect the presence of autoantibodies (Direct Antiglobulin Test [DAT]) are performed and have 90% to 95% sensitivity in diagnosing AIHA.[25] Bone marrow biopsy may be indicated in certain individuals. Evaluation for the underlying cause of the hemolysis is conducted.

Acquired hemolytic anemias are treated by removing the cause or treating the underlying disorder when possible. Folate is given to prevent megaloblastic anemia because long-term erythrocyte turnover increases folate requirements. Corticosteroids are used for initial treatment in most cases, with a response rate of over 80%.[25] However some individuals relapse unless the underlying cause can be removed. The most commonly used second-line treatment is administration of rituximab (monoclonal antibody that reduces the number of B lymphocytes and thus antibody production), although it may be used as initial therapy for cold agglutinin AIHA. Third-line treatments may include splenectomy and the use of more potent immune-suppressive medications.[25] Most treatments for AIHA confer an increased risk for infection, and individuals should be monitored carefully. Acute fulminating hemolytic anemia (hemolytic crisis) is treated with fluid and electrolyte replacement to prevent shock and renal damage, which may be caused by erythrocyte debris clogging the kidney tubules. Transfusions of blood products is reserved for severe life-threatening acute anemia. If repeated transfusion is required, an erythropoiesis-stimulating agent may be used.[24]

MYELOPROLIFERATIVE RED CELL DISORDERS

Hematologic dysfunction results from an overproduction of cells, as well as a deficiency. One or more hematopoietic lines may be overproduced in the marrow in response to exogenous (e.g., exposure to radiation, drugs) or endogenous (e.g., physiologic compensatory response, immune disorder) signals. Excessive red cell production is classified as polycythemia. Polycythemia exists in two forms: relative and absolute. Relative polycythemia results from hemoconcentration of the blood associated with dehydration that may be caused by decreased water intake, diarrhea, excessive vomiting, or increased use of diuretics. Its development is usually of minor consequence and resolves with fluid administration or treatment of underlying conditions.

Absolute polycythemia consists of two types: primary and secondary (Table 29.5). *Primary polycythemia* comes in two forms. The more common form (but still rare) is polycythemia vera which occurs in older adults and is a type of malignancy of erythrocyte precursor cells in the bone marrow. Familial (congenital) polycythemia is most often caused by an autosomal dominant mutation of the erythropoietin receptor of erythroid progenitors causing hypersensitivity to erythropoietin and leading to increased rate of erythropoiesis.[26] Familial polycythemia also can be caused by inherited defects in hemoglobin (e.g., Chesapeake Hb, San Diego Hb) which have a greater affinity for oxygen, causing isolated erythrocytosis in asymptomatic individuals. *Secondary polycythemia* is the most common type of polycythemia and is most often a physiologic response to hypoxia leading to increases in erythropoietin secretion. Chronic hypoxia is found in individuals living at higher altitudes (>10,000 ft), smokers with increased blood levels of carbon dioxide (CO), and individuals with COPD or heart failure, or both. Secondary polycythemia caused by nonphysiologic responses results from the production of erythropoietin by certain tumors (see Table 29.5).

TABLE 29.5 Disorders Classified as Polycythemia

Type of Polycythemia	Mechanism of Increased Erythropoiesis	Cause of Associated Disorder
Primary polycythemia 1. Polycythemia vera	Excessive proliferation of erythroid precursors in marrow	Mutation in the Janus kinase 2 gene (JAK2 gene) resulting in increased intracellular stimulation of cell division
2. Familial (congenital) polycythemia	Increased sensitivity of stem cell to erythropoietin; or production of abnormal hemoglobin (Chesapeake Hb, San Diego Hb)	Inherited mutation of the erythropoietin receptor of erythroid progenitors causing hypersensitivity to erythropoietin; or the production of abnormal hemoglobin which has a greater affinity for oxygen
Secondary polycythemia	Physiologic increase in erythropoietin secretion by kidneys in response to underlying systemic disorder	Tissue hypoxia caused by cardiopulmonary disorders (chronic obstructive pulmonary disease, congestive heart failure), decreased barometric pressure, cardiovascular malformations causing mixing of arterial and venous blood, methemoglobinemia, carboxyhemoglobinemia, smoking, obesity
	"Nonphysiologic"[a] increase in erythropoietin secretion	Renal disorders, cerebellar hemangioblastomas, hepatoma (liver tumor), ovarian carcinoma, uterine leiomyoma, pheochromocytoma, adrenocortical hypersecretion

[a] *Nonphysiologic* means that there is no obvious physiologic explanation for hypersecretion of erythropoietin.

Polycythemia Vera

Polycythemia vera (PV) is a slowly growing blood cancer in which the bone marrow makes too many red blood cells. PV is quite rare, with a peak incidence between the ages of 60 and 80 years. However, PV has been observed in individuals younger than the age of 40. Males are twice as likely as females to develop PV. It is more common in whites of Eastern European Jewish ancestry. PV is rarely seen in children or in multiple members of a single family; however, an autosomal dominant form exists that causes increased secretion of erythropoietin. Median survival for PV is 15 years; however, the survival rate for individuals 40 and younger is 37 years.[27]

PV is one of several disorders collectively known as *myeloid malignancies* (Box 29.2). These disorders all result from abnormal regulation of the HSCs. Specifically, the common pathogenic feature is the presence of a mutation in the Janus kinase 2 gene (***JAK2*** gene). Normally, the *JAK2* gene makes a protein that helps the body produce blood cells. When JAK2 is mutated, there is an increased intracellular stimulation of cell division and an overproduction of blood cells.[27] Because of numerous characteristics (e.g., overproduction of different blood cells, marrow hypercellularity, or fibrosis) shared by these disorders and a lack of specific molecular markers, the diagnosis can be quite challenging. The major characteristics shared by these disorders include (1) involvement of a hematopoietic progenitor cell, (2) overproduction of one or more of the formed elements in blood in the absence of a defined stimulus, (3) dominance by a transformed progenitor cell, (4) hypercellular bone marrow or fibrosis, (5) chromosomal (cytogenetic) abnormalities, (6) predisposition to thrombus formation and hemorrhage, and (7) spontaneous transformation to leukemia.

Pathophysiology. PV is a stem cell disorder with hyperplastic and neoplastic bone marrow alterations. It is characterized by an abnormal uncontrolled proliferation of red blood cells (frequently with increased levels of white blood cells [leukocytosis] and platelets [thrombocytosis]). The polycythemia is responsible for most of the clinical symptoms, including an increase in blood volume and viscosity. Proliferation of erythroid progenitors occurs in the bone marrow independent of the hormone erythropoietin. More than 95% of individuals with PV have an acquired mutation in the tyrosine kinase *JAK2* gene.[27] Normal JAK2 protein increases the activity of the erythropoietin receptor and is self-regulatory so that JAK2 activity diminishes over time. The mutation associated with PV negates the self-regulatory activity of JAK2 so that the erythropoietin receptor is constantly active regardless of the level of erythropoietin. Overall, the mutated tyrosine kinases bypass normal controls, causing growth factor–independent proliferation and survival of marrow progenitors or precursor cells. The cause of the mutation is unknown.

Increased numbers of erythrocytes and other blood cells increase the blood viscosity. This alters blood flow and creates a hypercoagulable state that results in thrombotic occlusion of blood vessels. Tissue injury (ischemia) and death (infarction) are the outcomes of blood vessel blockage. These outcomes are directly correlated with hematocrit levels. Increases in numbers

BOX 29.2 2016 World Health Organization Classification of Myeloid Malignancies

Acute Myeloid Leukemia (AML) and Related Neoplasms	Chronic Myeloid Neoplasms
AML with recurrent genetic abnormalities	Myeloproliferative neoplasms (MPN)
AML with myelodysplasia-related changes	1. Chronic myeloid leukemia, BCR-ABL1+
Therapy-related myeloid neoplasms	2. Chronic neutrophilic leukemia, often CSF3R mutated
AML, not otherwise specified	3. Chronic eosinophilic leukemia, not otherwise specified
Myeloid sarcoma	4. MPN, unclassifiable (MPN-U)
Down associated myeloid proliferations	5. Polycythemia vera (PV)
	6. Essential thrombocythemia (ET)
	7. Primary myelofibrosis (PMF)
	Mastocytosis
	Myeloid/lymphoid neoplasms with eosinophilia and PDGFRA, PDGFRB, FGFR1, or PCM1⊠JAK2 mutations
	Myelodysplastic/myeloproliferative neoplasms (MDS/MPN)
	Myelodysplastic syndromes (MDS)
	Myeloid neoplasms with germ line predisposition

Definition of Smoldering Multiple Myeloma

Both criteria must be met:

Serum monoclonal protein (IgG or IgA) $\geq$ 30 g/L or urinary monoclonal protein $\geq$ 500/24 h and/or clonal bone marrow plasma cells 10%–60%

Absence of myeloma-defining events or amyloidosis

PET-CT, 18F-Labeled fluorodeoxyglucose PET with CT.

Adapted from Tefferi A, Barbui T. Polycythemia vera and essential thrombocythemia: 2021 update on diagnosis, risk-stratification and management. *American Journal of Hematology*, 2020;95(12):1599–1613; Rajkumar SV, Dimopoulos MA, Palumbo A, et al. International Myeloma Working Group updated criteria for the diagnosis of multiple myeloma. *Lancet Oncology*, 2014;15(12):e538–e548.

of thrombocytes, as well as production of dysfunctional platelets, also contribute to this hypercoagulable condition. Leukemia develops in approximately 3% of individuals with PA, and fibrotic transformation of the bone marrow limits survival in 15%.[28]

Clinical Manifestations. Clinical manifestations of PV are a result of the increased red cell mass and hematocrit leading to increased blood volume and viscosity. This combined with thrombosis leads to symptoms of ischemia in vital organs (pain, hypoxia, decreased peripheral circulation). Circulatory alterations caused by the thick, sticky blood give rise to other manifestations, such as plethora (ruddy, red color of the face, hands, feet, ears, and mucous membranes) and engorgement of retinal and cerebral veins. Other symptoms may include headache, drowsiness, delirium, mania, psychotic depression, chorea, and visual disturbances. Individuals frequently have an enlarged spleen with abdominal pain and discomfort. Death from cerebral thrombosis is approximately five times greater in individuals with PV.

Cardiovascular function, despite the vascular alterations, remains relatively normal. Cardiac workload and output remain constant; however, increased blood volume does increase blood pressure. Coronary blood flow may be affected, precipitating angina, although cardiovascular infarctions are uncommon. Other cardiovascular manifestations include Raynaud phenomenon and thromboangiitis obliterans.

A unique feature of PV, and helpful in diagnosis, is the development of intense, painful itching that appears to be intensified by heat or exposure to water *(aquagenic pruritus)* so that individuals avoid exposure to water, particularly warm water when bathing or showering. The intensity of itching is related to the concentration of mast cells in the skin and is generally not responsive to antihistamines or topical lotions.

Evaluation and Treatment. PV may be suspected because of clinical features, such as a thrombotic event, splenomegaly, or aquagenic pruritus. Blood and laboratory findings confirm the diagnosis. Diagnostic criteria include a hemoglobin greater than 16.5 g/dL or a hematocrit greater than 49% in men and greater than 48% in women.[27] Erythrocytes appear normal, but anisocytosis may be present. There also may be moderate increases in white blood cells and platelets. A bone marrow examination demonstrates proliferation of precursor cells and the presence of a *JAK2* mutation which confirms the diagnosis. Serum erythropoietin levels are decreased.

Treatment of PV consists of reducing red cell proliferation and blood volume, controlling symptoms, and preventing clogging and clotting of the blood vessels. In low-risk individuals (e.g., those younger than age 60 or with no history of thrombosis and without risk factors for cardiovascular disease), the recommended therapy is phlebotomy (300 to 500 mL at a time to reduce erythrocytosis and blood volume) and low-dose aspirin. Frequent phlebotomies also reduce iron levels, a condition that impedes erythropoiesis.[28]

In high-risk PV, systemic anticoagulation is indicated. Hydroxyurea, a nonalkylating myelosuppressive, is the drug of choice for myelosuppression because of a reduced incidence to cause leukemia and thrombosis. IFN-α or busulfan are used when other forms of treatment have failed. Ruxolitinib inhibits the JAK2 pathway and is showing positive results in multiple studies.[28]

Iron Overload

Iron overload can be primary, as in hereditary hemochromatosis (HH), or secondary. The secondary causes of iron overload include anemias with inefficient erythropoiesis (e.g., AA), dietary iron overload, or conditions that require repeated blood transfusions or iron dextran injections.

Hereditary Hemochromatosis

Hemochromatosis is caused by excessive iron absorption. Hereditary hemochromatosis (HH) is a common inherited iron overload disorder characterized by excessive absorption of iron. It is due to a deficiency of hepcidin or to decreased binding of hepcidin to ferroportin, the transmembrane protein that exports iron outside the cell (Fig. 29.9).[29] HH is characterized by increased iron absorption from the GI tract, with subsequent tissue iron deposition. Excess iron is deposited first in the liver and pancreas, followed by the heart, joints, and endocrine glands. Excess iron causes tissue damage that can lead to diseases such as cirrhosis, diabetes, heart failure, arthropathies, and impotence.

Pathophysiology. Different forms of HH result from mutations in various genes that play important roles in regulating absorption, transport, and storage of iron. HH is classified by type (1, 2, 3, and 4) based on which proteins involved in iron homeostasis are affected. Type 1 HH is the most frequent form and is characterized by one of two mutations of the human homeostatic iron regulator (HFE) gene. These mutations result in decreased synthesis of hepcidin. Hepcidin is a hormone secreted by the liver in response to increased serum iron, and it inhibits iron absorption from the intestine by degrading ferroportin-1. (see Chapter 28). Most affected individuals have a homozygous C282Y mutations in the HFE gene (type 1a).[30] Less common is H63D mutation, which by itself does not cause significant iron overload, but may become clinically significant when associated with excessive alcohol intake or hepatitis C infection or may act as a cofactor in combination with C282Y. This combined C282Y/H63D genotype is classified as HH type 1b.[29] The other HH genotypes have a much lower prevalence. Type 2 HH, also called juvenile hemochromatosis, is associated with mutations in either the HJV gene or the hepatic antimicrobial protein (HAMP) gene leading to hepcidin deficiency. Type 2 is the most severe form of primary iron overload and develops in younger individuals. Type 3 HH is associated with mutations in the transferrin receptor 2 (TFR2) gene, also leading to hepcidin deficiency. Type 4 A HH results from autosomal dominant mutations in the ferroportin gene (SLC40A1) These mutations disrupt the export function of ferroportin despite normal levels of hepcidin. Intracellular iron rises in association with low levels of plasma iron and normal levels of transferrin saturation but elevated levels of serum transferrin. Type 4B HH results from resistance of ferroportin to hepcidin.[29]

In all types of HH, iron accumulates in tissues and organs disrupting their normal function.[30] In the liver, this accumulation of iron may lead to the development of cirrhosis and

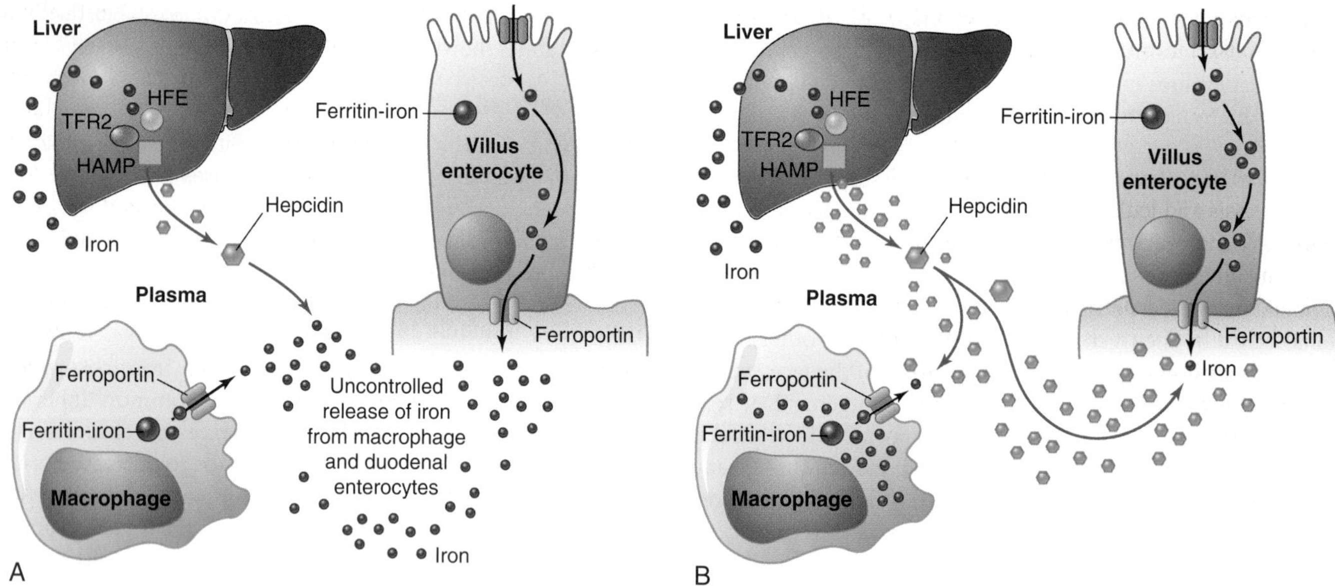

Fig. 29.9 Hemochromatosis. **(A)** Mutations in genes affecting HFE, TFR2, or HAMP lead to decreased levels of hepcidin causing excessive absorption of iron. **(B)** Mutations to ferroportin cause decreased binding of hepcidin and iron accumulation within cells. *HAMP*, Hepatic antimicrobial protein; *HFE*, human homeostatic iron regulator protein; *TFR2*, transferrin receptor 2. (Adapted from Pietrangelo A. Hereditary hemochromatosis. Biochimica et Biophysica Acta (BBA). *Molecular Cell Research*, 2006;1763(7):700–710.)

hepatocellular carcinoma.[31] Cardiac complications are the second-leading cause of death in HH and include cardiomyopathy, arrhythmias, and heart failure. HH injures the pancreatic β-islet cells and contributes to the development of hepatic insulin resistance leading to diabetes in 13% to 23% of affected individuals.[29] Iron deposits in the skin lead to increased melanin deposition, causing bronzing. Arthropathy most commonly involves the second and third metacarpophalangeal joints.

Clinical Manifestations. Clinical HH, more common in men than women, is characterized by excessive storage of iron in the liver, skin, pancreas, heart, joints, and testes. Fatigue and arthralgias are the most common symptoms encountered early in the disease. Other early symptoms may include weakness and weight loss. The risk of cirrhosis is significantly increased when the serum ferritin level is higher than 1000 ng/mL.[29] Upper right quadrant abdominal pain, ascites, and edema indicate liver dysfunction and cirrhosis. Symptoms of heart failure (dyspnea, orthopnea, edema) may develop. Other findings include progressive increase in skin pigmentation, diabetes mellitus, arthritis, and hypogonadism. Most individuals are diagnosed as a result of elevated liver function tests found during routine health screening.

Evaluation and Treatment. The American College of Gastroenterology (ACG) published guidelines for diagnosis and management of hemochromatosis in 2019.[29] Serum transferrin saturation and serum ferritin are the first-line diagnostic tests for HH. Individuals with abnormal results should undergo genetic testing. Magnetic resonance imaging is used to estimate hepatic iron concentration. However, if another source of liver disease is suspected, liver biopsy is indicated. First-degree relatives of individuals diagnosed with HH should be screened for mutations.

Phlebotomy is first-line treatment, with a goal of reducing serum ferritin to 50 to 100 ng/mL.[29] Therapeutic phlebotomy to remove excess iron is indicated in the presence of iron overload or evidence of end-organ damage (e.g., advanced cirrhosis, cardiac failure, skin pigment changes, or diabetes). Initially, phlebotomy may be needed weekly, but once therapeutic ferritin levels are reached, phlebotomy may be needed only every 2 to 3 months. Iron chelation therapy can be used in selected individuals who cannot tolerate phlebotomy and may decrease the risk for development of cirrhosis and hepatocellular cancer but is associated with numerous side effects. Individuals should be instructed to refrain from drinking alcohol, taking iron supplements, and consuming raw fish or shellfish. Vaccination against hepatitis A and B is advised. Regular screening for the development of hepatocellular carcinoma should be performed every 6 months.[31]

ALTERATIONS OF LEUKOCYTE FUNCTION

Leukocyte function (infection fighting) is affected if too many or too few white cells are present in the blood or if the cells that are present are structurally or functionally defective. Quantitative leukocyte disorders result from decreased production in the bone marrow or accelerated destruction of cells in the circulation. In addition, quantitative alterations occur in response to infections.

Qualitative leukocyte disorders consist of disruptions of leukocyte function. Phagocytic cells (granulocytes, monocytes, macrophages) may lose their ability to act as effective phagocytes, and the lymphocytes may lose their ability to respond to antigens. (Disruptions of inflammatory and immune processes caused by leukocyte disorders are described in Chapter 7.)

Other leukocyte alterations include IM and cancers of the blood—leukemia and multiple myeloma (MM).

Quantitative Alterations of Leukocytes

Leukocytosis is present when the count is higher than normal; leukopenia is present when the count is lower than normal. Leukocytosis and leukopenia may affect a specific type of white blood cell and may result from a variety of physiologic conditions and alterations.

Leukocytosis occurs as a normal protective response to physiologic stressors, such as invading microorganisms, strenuous exercise, emotional changes, temperature changes, anesthesia, surgery, pregnancy, and some drugs, hormones, and toxins. It also is caused by pathologic conditions, such as malignancies and hematologic disorders. Unlike leukocytosis, leukopenia is never normal and is defined as an absolute blood cell count less than 4000 cells/μL. Leukopenia is associated with a decrease in neutrophils, which increases risk for infection. The absolute neutrophil count (ANC) is calculated by multiplying the white blood cell count by the percent of band and segmented neutrophils. The ANC is classified as mild (1000 to 1500 cells/μL), moderate (500 to 1000 cells/μL), or severe (<500 cells/μL). When the ANC is less than 500/μL, the possibility for life-threatening infections is high. Leukopenia may be caused by radiation, anaphylactic shock, autoimmune disease (e.g., SLE), immune deficiencies (see Chapter 9), and certain drugs, such as glucocorticoids and chemotherapeutic agents.

Granulocytes and Monocytes

Increased numbers of circulating granulocytes (neutrophils, eosinophils, basophils) and monocytes are chiefly a physiologic response to infection. Increased numbers also occur as a result of myeloproliferative disorders that increase stem cell proliferation in the bone marrow.

Decreased numbers occur when infectious processes deplete the supply of circulating granulocytes and monocytes, drawing them out of the circulation and into infected tissues faster than they can be replaced. Decreases also can be caused by disorders that suppress marrow function, such as severe congenital neutropenia or immune-related neutropenia.

Granulocytosis—an increase in granulocytes (neutrophils, eosinophils, or basophils)—begins when stored blood cells are released. Neutrophilia is another term that may be used to describe *granulocytosis* because neutrophils are the most numerous of the granulocytes (Table 29.6). Neutrophilia occurs in the early stages of infection or inflammation and is established when the absolute count exceeds 7500/μL. Release and depletion of stored neutrophils stimulates granulopoiesis to replenish neutrophil reserves.

When the demand for circulating mature neutrophils exceeds the supply, immature neutrophils (and other leukocytes) are released from the bone marrow. Premature release of the immature cells is responsible for the phenomenon known as a shift-to-the-left, or leukemoid reaction. This refers to the microscopic detection of disproportionate numbers of immature leukocytes in peripheral blood smears. Many diagrams present cellular differentiation and maturation progressing from left to right within the drawing, instead of vertically as shown in Fig. 28.10. The early release of immature white cells prevents the completion of the sequence and shifts the distribution of leukocytes in the blood toward those on the left side of the diagram. This phenomenon is also seen in the blood smear of individuals with leukemia, hence the term *leukemoid reaction*. As infection or inflammation diminishes, and granulopoiesis replenishes circulating granulocytes, a shift-to-the-right, or return to normal, occurs.

Neutropenia is a condition associated with a reduction in circulating neutrophils and exists clinically when the neutrophil count is less than 2000/μL. Reduction in neutrophils occurs in severe prolonged infections when production of granulocytes cannot keep up with demand. Severe neutropenia, granulocytopenia (less than 500/μL), or agranulocytosis (complete absence of granulocytes in blood) is usually secondary to arrested hematopoiesis in the bone marrow or massive cell destruction in the circulation. Chemotherapeutic agents used to treat hematologic and other malignancies cause bone marrow suppression. Several other drugs cause agranulocytosis, which occurs rarely but carries a high mortality of 10% to 50%. Clinical manifestations of agranulocytosis include severe infection (particularly of the respiratory system) leading to septicemia, general malaise, fever, tachycardia, and ulcers in the mouth and colon. If this condition remains untreated, sepsis caused by agranulocytosis results in death within 3 to 6 days.

Other causes of neutropenia, in the absence of infection, may be (1) decreased neutrophil production or ineffective granulopoiesis, (2) reduced neutrophil survival, and (3) abnormal neutrophil distribution and sequestration. Neutropenia also is classified as primary or secondary, and primary disorders are further identified as congenital or acquired. Primary acquired neutropenia is associated with multiple conditions. The megaloblastic anemias (vitamin B_{12} and folate deficiency), as well as starvation and anorexia nervosa, cause neutropenia because of an inadequate supply of vitamins and nutrients for protein production.

Congenital defects in neutrophil production include cyclic neutropenia, neutropenia with congenital immunodeficiencies, and multiple syndromes. Reduced neutrophil survival and abnormal distribution and sequestration are usually secondary to other disorders. Neutropenia occurs in a variety of immunologic disorders, particularly SLE, rheumatoid arthritis, Felty and Sjögren syndromes, splenomegaly, and drug-related causes.

Eosinophilia is an absolute increase (>450/μL) in the total number of circulating eosinophils. Allergic disorders (type 1) associated with asthma, hay fever, parasitic infections, and drug reactions often cause eosinophilia. Hypersensitivity reactions trigger the release of eosinophilic chemotaxic factor of anaphylaxis (ECF-A), and histamine from mast cells attracts eosinophils to the area. Mast cells release interleukin-5 (IL-5), which stimulates the bone marrow to produce more eosinophils into the blood. Areas with abundant mast cells, such as the respiratory and GI tracts, are commonly affected. Eosinophilia also may occur in dermatologic disorders, eosinophilia-myalgia syndrome, and parasitic invasion.

Eosinopenia, a decrease in the number of circulating eosinophils, generally is caused by migration of eosinophils into inflammatory sites. It also may be seen in Cushing syndrome

TABLE 29.6 Other Conditions Associated With Neutrophils, Eosinophils, Basophils, Monocytes, and Lymphocytes

Condition	Cause	Example
Neutrophil		
Neutrophilia (granulocytosis)	Inflammation or tissue necrosis	Surgery, burns, MI, pneumonitis, rheumatic fever, rheumatoid arthritis
	Infection	Bacterial: gram-positive (staphylococci, streptococci, pneumococci), gram-negative (*Escherichia coli, Pseudomonas* species)
	Physiologic	Exercise, extreme heat or cold, third-trimester pregnancy, emotional distress
	Hematologic	Acute hemorrhage, hemolysis, myeloproliferative disorder, chronic granulocytic leukemia
	Drugs or chemicals	Epinephrine, steroids, heparin, histamine, endotoxin
	Metabolic	Diabetes (acidosis), eclampsia, gout, thyroid storm
	Neoplasm	Liver, GI tract, bone marrow
Neutropenia	Primary neutropenia	Cyclic neutropenia, neutropenia with congenital immunodeficiencies, and multiple syndromes
	Congenital	
	Acquired	Megaloblastic anemias (vitamin B_{12} and folate deficiency), leukemia, aplastic anemia starvation, anorexia nervosa, radiation, chemotherapy,
	Decreased marrow production, ineffective granulopoiesis	
	Secondary neutropenia Increased destruction, reduced survival, abnormal distribution	Splenomegaly, hemodialysis, autoimmune disease (rheumatoid arthritis, systemic lupus erythematous, Felty syndrome, Sjögren syndrome)
	Prolonged infection	Gram-negative (typhoid), viral (influenza, hepatitis B, measles, mumps, rubella), severe infections, protozoal infections (malaria)
Eosinophil		
Eosinophilia	Allergy	Asthma, hay fever, drug sensitivity
	Infection	Parasites (trichinosis, hookworm), chronic (fungal, leprosy, TB)
	Malignancy	CML, lung, stomach, ovary, Hodgkin disease
	Dermatosis	Pemphigus, exfoliative dermatitis (drug-induced)
	Drugs	Digitalis, heparin, streptomycin, tryptophan (eosinophilia-myalgia syndrome), penicillins, propranolol
Eosinopenia	Stress response	Trauma, shock, burns, surgery, mental distress
	Drugs	Steroids (Cushing syndrome)
Basophil		
Basophilia	Inflammation	Infection (measles, chickenpox), hypersensitivity reaction (immediate)
	Hematologic	Myeloproliferative disorders (CML, polycythemia vera, Hodgkin lymphoma, hemolytic anemia)
	Endocrine	Myxedema, antithyroid therapy
Basopenia	Physiologic	Pregnancy, ovulation, stress
	Endocrine	Graves disease
Monocyte		
Monocytosis	Infection	Bacterial (subacute bacterial endocarditis, TB), recovery phase of infection
	Hematologic	Myeloproliferative disorders, Hodgkin disease, agranulocytosis
	Physiologic	Normal newborn
Monocytopenia	Rare	
Lymphocyte		
Lymphocytosis	Physiologic	4 months to 4 years
	Acute infection	Infectious mononucleosis, CMV infection, pertussis, hepatitis, mycoplasma pneumonia, typhoid
	Chronic infection	Congenital syphilis, tertiary syphilis
	Endocrine	Thyrotoxicosis, adrenal insufficiency
	Malignancy	ALL, CLL, lymphosarcoma cell leukemia
Lymphocytopenia	Immunodeficiency syndrome	AIDS, agammaglobulinemia
	Lymphocyte destruction	Steroids (Cushing syndrome), radiation, chemotherapy
		Hodgkin lymphoma
		CHF, renal failure, TB, SLE, aplastic anemia

AIDS, Acquired immunodeficiency syndrome; *ALL*, acute lymphocytic leukemia; *CHF*, congestive (left) heart failure; *CLL*, chronic lymphocytic leukemia; *CML*, chronic myelogenous leukemia; *CMV*, cytomegalovirus; *GI*, gastrointestinal; *MI*, myocardial infarction; *SLE*, systemic lupus erythematosus; *TB*, tuberculosis.

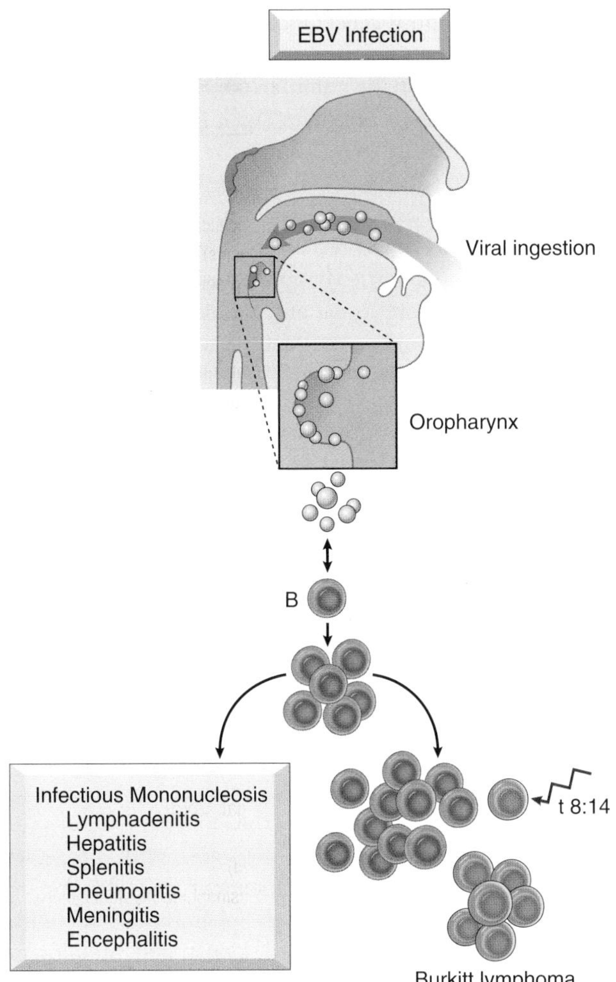

Fig. 29.10 Outcomes of Epstein-Barr Virus (EBV). In individuals with normal immune function, infection is typically asymptomatic or leads to mononucleosis. With immunodeficiency, proliferation of B cells may be uncontrolled and progress to the development of B-cell neoplasms. Individuals without evidence of immunodeficiency can also develop EBV-positive neoplasms. In Burkitt lymphoma, the individual's susceptibility to EBV causes B cells to undergo genetic alterations (usually an 8;14 chromosomal translocation). EBV also is implicated in Hodgkin lymphoma, nasopharyngeal carcinoma, and other rare non-Hodgkin lymphomas. (From Kumar V, Abbas A, Aster JC. *Robbins & Cotran pathologic basis of disease*, 9th edition. Philadelphia: Saunders; 2015.)

and as a result of stress caused by surgery, shock, trauma, burns, or mental distress.

Basophilia, an increase in the number of circulating basophils, is rare and generally is a response to inflammation and immediate hypersensitivity reactions. Basophils contain histamine that is released during an allergic reaction. Increased numbers of basophils are seen in myeloproliferative disorders, such as chronic myeloid leukemia and myeloid metaplasia.

Basopenia (also known as *basophilic leukopenia*) is a decrease in circulating numbers of basophils. It is seen in hyperthyroidism, acute infection, ovulation and pregnancy, and long-term therapy with steroids.

Monocytosis is an increase in numbers of circulating monocytes (generally >800/μL). It is often transient and not related to a dysfunction of monocyte production. If present, it is usually associated with neutropenia during bacterial infections, particularly in the late stages or recovery stage, when monocytes are needed to phagocytize surviving microorganisms and debris. Increased monocytes also may indicate marrow recovery from agranulocytosis. Monocytosis is often seen in chronic infections such as TB, brucellosis, listeriosis, and subacute bacterial endocarditis (SBE). Monocytosis has been found to correlate with the extent of myocardial damage after myocardial infarctions. Monocytopenia, a decrease in the number of circulating monocytes, is rare but has been identified with hairy cell leukemia and prednisone therapy.

Lymphocytes

Quantitative alterations of lymphocytes occur when lymphocytes are activated by antigenic stimuli, usually microorganisms (see Chapters 7 and 8). Lymphocytosis (absolute lymphocytosis) is an increase in the number or proportion of lymphocytes in the blood. It is rare in acute bacterial infections and is seen most in acute viral infections, particularly those caused by the EBV, a causative agent in IM.

Lymphocytopenia is a decrease in the number of circulating lymphocytes in the blood. It may be attributed to (1) abnormalities of lymphocyte production associated with neoplasias and immune deficiencies and (2) destruction by drugs, viruses, or radiation. It is also known to occur without any detectable cause. The lymphocytopenia associated with heart failure and other acute illnesses may be caused by elevated cortisol levels. Lymphocytopenia is a major problem in AIDS. AIDS-related lymphocytopenia is caused by HIV, which destroys T-helper lymphocytes. (For a detailed discussion of AIDS, see Chapter 9.) Other conditions associated with increases or decreases in these specific types of white blood cells are listed in Table 29.6.

Infectious Mononucleosis

Infectious mononucleosis (IM) is a benign, acute, self-limiting, lymphoproliferative clinical syndrome characterized by acute viral infection of B lymphocytes (B cells). It is associated with several human tumors, such as B-cell and T-cell lymphomas, Hodgkin lymphoma (HL), and nasopharyngeal carcinoma.[32] The virus has been linked to posttransplant lymphoproliferative diseases (PTLDs), and gastric carcinoma.[33] The most common cause is EBV. EBV is a ubiquitous herpesvirus and accounts for most IM cases. Other viruses that cause symptoms resembling IM include cytomegalovirus (CMV), adenovirus, HIV, hepatitis A, influenza A and B, and rubella, as well as the bacteria *Toxoplasma gondii*, *Corynebacterium diphtheriae*, and *Coxiella burnetii*. The classic symptoms of IM are pharyngitis, lymphadenopathy, and fever. In individuals with immunodeficiency, the proliferation of infected B cells may be uncontrolled and can lead to the development of B-cell lymphomas.[34] Individuals who are coinfected with malaria or HIV are at increased risk of developing EBV-associated lymphomas, including Burkitt lymphoma (BL). EBV also is etiologically linked to subgroups of HL.

EBV has not been documented from environmental sources, thus humans are considered the major reservoir. More than 90% of individuals worldwide have antibodies to EBV.[33,35] Approximately 50% to 85% of children are infected with EBV by age 4. These early infections are usually asymptomatic and provide immunity to EBV; thus, early EBV infections rarely develop into IM. IM may arise when the initial infection occurs during adolescence or later, but still only results in IM in 35% to 50% of these individuals. Symptomatic IM usually affects young adults between ages 15 and 35 years, with the peak incidences occurring between ages 15 and 24 years; males have a later peak (18 to 24 years) than females. The overall incidence rate for this age group is 6 to 8 cases per 1000 persons per year. Children from low socioeconomic environments are particularly susceptible to infections with EBV. IM is uncommon in individuals older than age 40; however, if it does occur, IM is more commonly caused by CMV.

Transmission of EBV involves (1) person-to-person, (2) breastfeeding, and (3) sexual transmission.[35] From *person-to-person transmission* the virus is shed in salivary secretions at high levels for a prolonged time.[35] After the onset of illness, viral oral shedding persists for a median duration of about six months.[36] Once a person is infected with EBV, the virus may be intermittently shed in the oropharynx for decades.[36,37]

EBV has been isolated from healthy *breastfeeding* mothers, however, it is still not considered an important route of transmission.[35] Transmission may occur *sexually* because it has been isolated in cervical and male seminal fluid. In a study of university students in Scotland, sexual activity before college admission was significantly associated with EBV seropositivity and the seropositive status increased with the number of sexual partners.[38] A longitudinal study also found that EBV was associated with sexual activity in young women.[39] The virus also may be secreted in other mucosal secretions of the genital, rectal, and respiratory tracts, as well as blood. The infection begins with widespread invasion of the B lymphocytes, which have receptors for EBV. The virus initially infects the oropharynx, nasopharynx, and salivary epithelial cells with later spread into lymphoid tissues and B cells. Once the virus enters the bloodstream, the infection spreads systemically.

Pathophysiology. In the immunocompetent individual, unaffected B cells produce antibodies (IgG, IgA, IgM) against the virus. At the same time, there is a massive activation and proliferation of cytotoxic T cells (CD8) that are directed against EBV-infected cells (see Chapter 8). The immune response against EBV-infected cells is largely responsible for the cellular proliferation in the lymphoid tissue (lymph nodes, spleen, tonsils, and, occasionally, liver). Sore throat and fever are caused by inflammation at the site of initial viral entry and initial infection (the mouth and throat). Outcomes of EBV are presented in Fig. 29.10.

Clinical Manifestations. The incubation period for IM is approximately 30 to 50 days. Early flulike symptoms, such as headache, malaise, joint pain, and fatigue, may appear during the first 3 to 5 days, although some individuals are without symptoms. At the time of diagnosis, the individual commonly presents with the *classic group of symptoms*: fever, sore throat (pharyngitis), cervical lymph node enlargement, and fatigue. The pharyngitis is usually diffuse with a whitish or grayish green thick exudate. It can be painful, causing the individual to seek treatment. Characteristics with progression may include a generalized lymphadenopathy, enlarged spleen, and atypical activated T lymphocytes (mononucleosis cells) in the blood (Fig. 29.11). IM is usually self-limiting, and recovery occurs in a few weeks. Fatigue, however, may last for 1 to 2 months after resolution of the infection.

Severe clinical complications are rare. With progression of IM, general lymph node enlargement may develop with enlargement of the spleen and liver. Splenomegaly is clinically evident 50% of the time and is demonstrated radiologically 100% of the time. Difficulty in detecting splenomegaly with physical examination contributes to the underestimation of actual enlargement. Splenic rupture is rare (only 0.1% to 0.5% of all cases) and can occur spontaneously as a result of mild trauma, arising primarily in men younger than 25 years of age and between days 4 and 21 after the onset of symptoms. It is the most common cause of death related to IM. Other causes of fatalities are hepatic failure, extensive bacterial infection, and

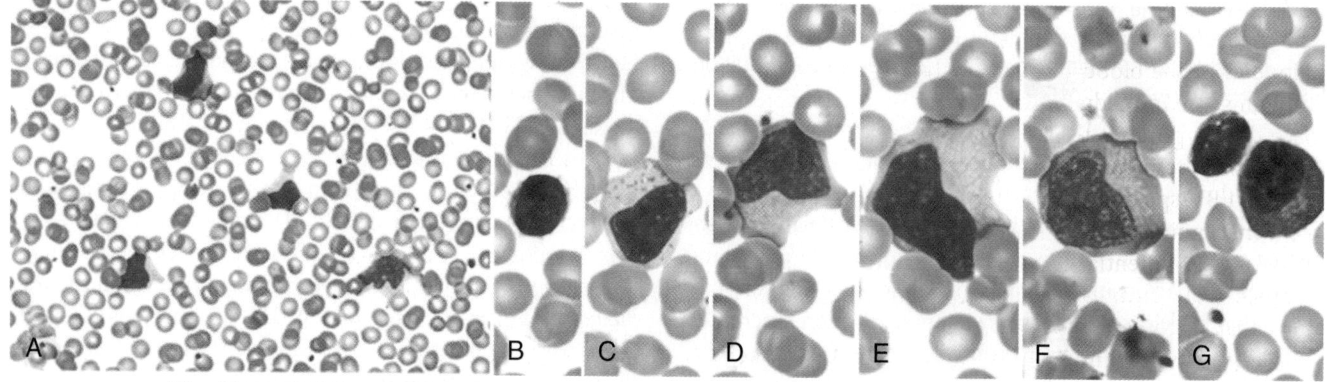

Fig. 29.11 Peripheral Blood Smear in Infectious Mononucleosis. Low power **(A)** shows moderately high white blood cell count and a high number of reactive, or "atypical," lymphocytes. Higher power **(B–G)** illustrates the spectrum of lymphoid morphology, including small resting lymphocytes **(B)** for comparison, large granular lymphocytes **(C)**, atypical forms **(D–F)** (also referred to as reactive lymphs), and circulating plasma cells **(G)**. (From Hoffman R, et al. *Hematology*, 6th edition. Philadelphia: Churchill Livingstone; 2013.)

viral myocarditis. Other organ systems are rarely involved, but such involvement may be present with characteristic manifestations, such as fulminant hepatitis with jaundice and anemia, encephalitis, meningitis, Guillain-Barré syndrome, and Bell palsy. Eye manifestations may include eyelid and periorbital edema, dry eyes, keratitis, uveitis, and conjunctivitis. Reye syndrome has been known to develop in children with EBV infection. Pulmonary and respiratory failure has been documented but is more likely to occur in immunocompromised individuals. A generalized maculopapular, urticarial, or petechial rash may emerge; however, the mechanisms for the rash are not clear.[35] Approximately 3% to 10% of adults older than 40 years of age have never been infected with EBV and are susceptible to IM later in life. In these individuals, the classic symptoms are not generally present, making diagnosis more difficult.

Evaluation and Treatment. Children commonly present with fever, pharyngitis, lymphadenitis, and manifestations discussed earlier. Young adults present with malaise, fatigue, and lymphadenopathy and often a fever of unknown origin. Palatal petechiae, splenomegaly, and posterior cervical adenopathy are very suggestive of IM, and the absence of cervical lymphadenopathy and fatigue make the diagnosis less likely.[35] The blood of affected individuals contains an increased number of white blood cells or lymphocytosis (absolute count $>4500/\mu L$, or on peripheral count $>50\%$ with many atypical lymphocytes ($\geq 10\%$).[35] The diagnosis of IM depends on the following specific findings: (1) an increase in the number of lymphocytes, commonly based on Hoagland criteria of at least 50% lymphocytes and at least 10% atypical lymphocytes in the blood, and (2) a positive heterophile antibody (heterogeneous group of IgM antibodies that are agglutinins against nonhuman red blood cells [e.g., sheep, horse]) reaction (Monospot test). Although a rising titer of specific antibodies for EBV antigens can be used to make the diagnosis, the results of the heterophile test type return more quickly; and it may not be necessary for individuals with a reactive heterophile antibody.[35] Use of the Monospot test is, however, limited because other infections (e.g., CMV, adenovirus) and toxoplasmosis also produce heterophilic antibodies. Thus, 5% to 15% of Monospot tests yield false-positive results. False-negative rates are highest during the beginning of clinical symptoms.[35] Heterophilic antibodies in the blood increase as the condition progresses, although some individuals and children younger than 4 years of age do not produce them. Diagnosis of EBV infection specifically may be increased with newer viral-specific tests that identify EBV-specific antibodies. Not all individuals with fever, pharyngitis, and lymphadenopathy have infection due to EBV. Other potential causative organisms include group A streptococcus, *Arcanobacterium haemolyticum*, CMV, acute HIV, or rarely *Toxoplasma gondi*.[35]

IM is usually self-limiting and medical intervention is rarely required. Treatment is supportive and consists of rest and alleviation of symptoms with analgesics and antipyretics. Aspirin is avoided with children because of its association with Reye syndrome. Streptococcal pharyngitis, which occurs in 20% to 30% of cases, is treated with penicillin or erythromycin, not ampicillin—ampicillin is known to cause a rash. Bed rest with avoidance of strenuous activity and contact sports is indicated. Steroids are not recommended for routine cases of IM; however, they may be used in cases with *severe* complications such as impending airway obstruction or other organ involvement (central nervous system [CNS] manifestations, thrombocytopenic purpura, myocarditis, pericarditis).[40] Severe complications require emergent consultation with an otolaryngologist. Acyclovir has been used in immunocompromised individuals, but significant clinical benefit has not been shown and is not considered standard therapy. In the rare event of splenic rupture, the treatment has been removal of the spleen and continues to be the choice in hemodynamically unstable individuals.

Lymphoid Neoplasm: Leukemias

Leukemia is a clonal malignant disorder of the bone marrow and usually, but not always, of the blood. The common pathologic feature of all forms of leukemia is an uncontrolled proliferation of malignant leukocytes, causing an overcrowding of bone marrow and decreased production and function of normal hematopoietic cells. Chromosomal abnormalities and translocations are common in the majority of leukemias. When genes become mutated, they create genomic aberrations that block cell maturation and activate pro–growth signaling pathways that prevent apoptotic cell death.

With time, the overall classification of leukemia has become increasingly complex with notable changes. These changes have created a blurring between the once discrete categories *lymphoma* and *leukemia*. Some cancers known as *lymphoma* have *leukemic* presentations, and evolution to leukemia is not unusual during the progression of incurable lymphoma. The World Health Organization (WHO) currently groups the lymphoid neoplasms into five broad categories, which are defined by the cell of origin:

1. Precursor B-cell neoplasms (immature B cells)
2. Peripheral B-cell neoplasms (mature B cells)
3. Precursor T-cell neoplasms (immature T cells)
4. Peripheral T-cell and NK (natural killer)-cell neoplasms (mature T cells and NK cells)
5. Hodgkin lymphoma (Reed-Sternberg [RS] cell and variants)

The 2016 revision of the WHO classification of lymphoid neoplasms clarifies the diagnosis and management of lymphoid neoplasms, details expanding genetic/molecular criteria for some neoplasms and their clinical correlates, and refers to investigations for targeted treatment strategies.[41] Most lymphoid neoplasm classifications relate to stages of cell differentiation of B-cell or T-cell differentiation (Fig. 29.12A). Fig. 29.12B provides a simple schematic overview of the main types of leukemia.

Acute leukemia is characterized by undifferentiated or immature cells, usually a blast cell. The onset of disease is abrupt and rapid. Without treatment, disease progression results in a short survival time. In chronic leukemia, the predominant cell is more differentiated but does not function normally, with a relatively slow progression. There are four general types of leukemia: acute lymphocytic (ALL), acute myelogenous (AML), chronic lymphocytic (CLL), and chronic myelogenous (CML).

Leukemia occurs with varying frequencies at different ages and is more common in adults than in children. More than

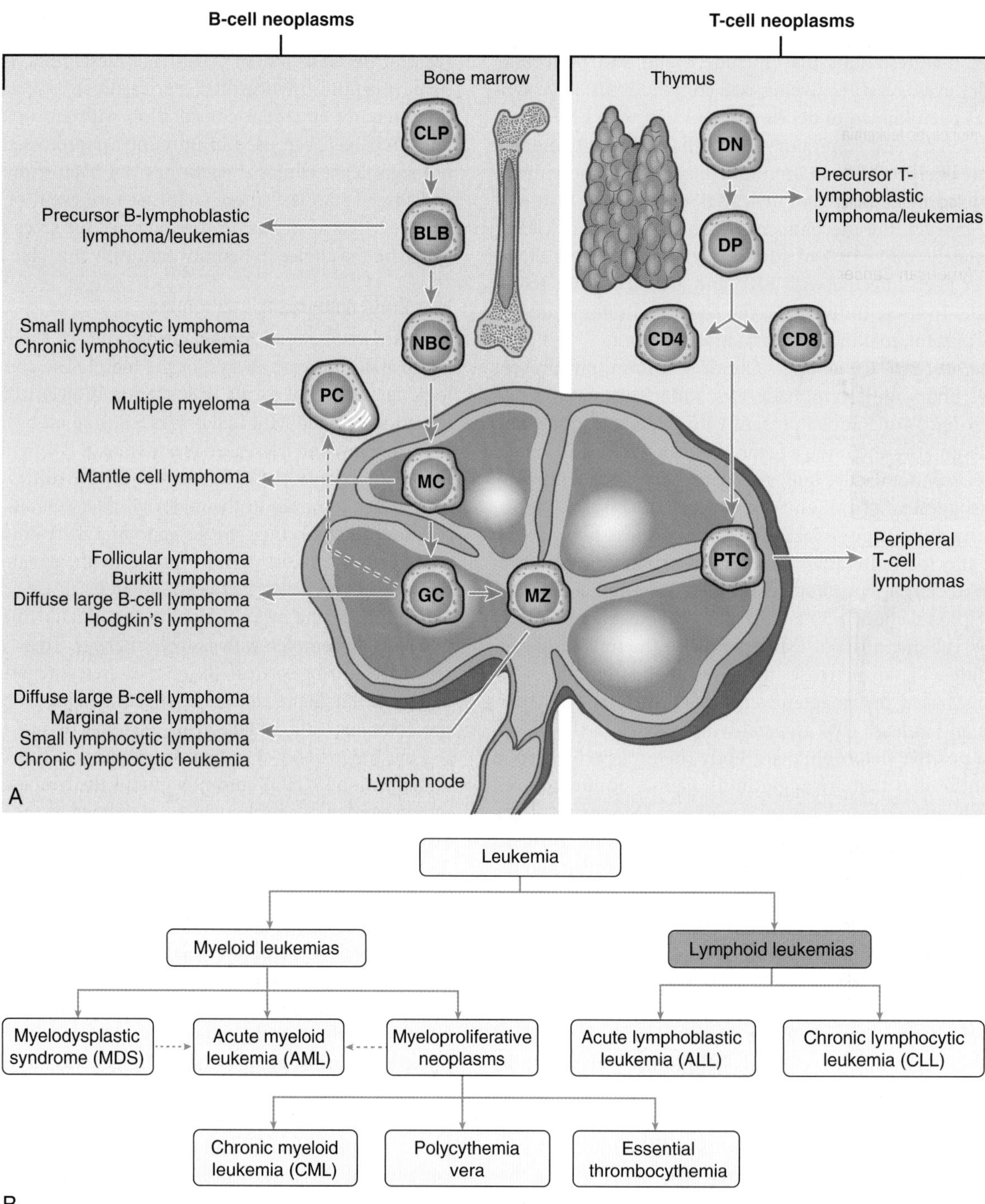

Fig. 29.12 Origin of Lymphoid Neoplasms. (A) Specific lymphoid tumors emerge from stages of B- and T-cell differentiation. **(B)** Overview of main types of leukemia. Acute myeloid leukemia *(AML)* may arise de novo or be preceded by myelodysplastic phase. Not all cases of myelodysplastic syndrome (MDS) evolve to AML *(dashed line)*. Some myelodysplastic neoplasms can transform into AML, although very rarely *(dotted line)*. *BLB*, Pre-B lymphoblast; *CLP*, common lymphoid precursor; *DN*, CD4/CD8 double-negative pro-T cell; *DP*, CD4/CD8 double-positive pre-T cell; *GC*, germinal-center B cell; *MC*, mantle B cell; *MZ*, marginal zone B cell; *NBC*, naïve B cell; *PTC*, peripheral T cell. (A, From Kumar V, Abbas A, Aster JC. *Robbins & Cotran pathologic basis of disease*, 9th edition. Philadelphia: Saunders; 2015. B, From Khwaja A, et al. Acute myeloid leukaemia. *Nature Reviews Disease Primers*, 2016;2:16010.)

TABLE 29.7 Estimated New Cases and Deaths from Leukemia in the United States—2021

Types of Leukemia	TOTAL NEW CASES (Proportion of New Cases) (%)	NEW CASES BY SEX Male	NEW CASES BY SEX Female	DEATHS BY SEX Male	DEATHS BY SEX Female
All types	61,090 (100)	35,530	25,560	13,900	9,760
Acute lymphocytic leukemia	5,690 (12)	3,000	2,690	900	680
Chronic lymphocytic leukemia	21,250 (30)	13,040	8,210,	2,620	1,700
Acute myelogenous leukemia	20,240 (36)	11,230	9,010	6,620	4,780
Chronic myelogenous leukemia	9,110 (11)	5,150	3,960	680	540
Other	4,800 (11)	3,110	1,690	3,080	2,060

Data from American Cancer Society. *Cancer Facts and* Figures—2021. Atlanta: The Society; 2021.

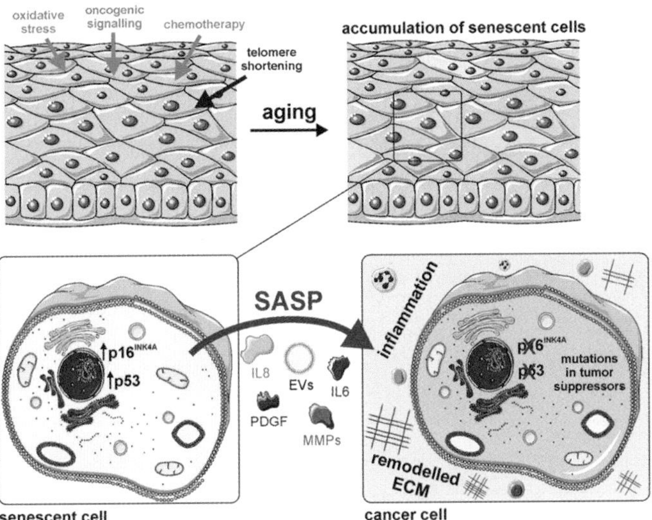

Fig. 29.13 Cellular Senescence Produces a Pro-tumorigenic Microenvironment. Various stimuli lead to cellular senescence and their accumulation in aged tissues. The senescent state is characterized by activation of the potent tumor suppressors p16INK4a and /or p53, as well as by secretion of cytokines *(IL-6, IL-8)*, growth factors *(PDGF)*, matrix metalloproteinases *(MMPs)*, and extracellular vesicles *(EVs)*. This senescence-associated secretory phenotype *(SASP)* produces a pro-tumorigenic microenvironment by causing extracellular matrix remodeling and inflammation. (From Schosserer M, Grillari J, Brietenbach M. The dual role of cellular senescence in developing tumors and their response to cancer therapy front. *Oncology*, 2017;23. https://doi.org/10.3389/fonc.2017.00278.)

61,090 cases of leukemia were estimated for 2021, with males having a higher incidence than females (Table 29.7). Estimated deaths for 2021 was 23,660 individuals.[42] CLL and AML are the most common types in adults, but CML is also a common leukemia in adults (see Chapter 30 for leukemia in children).

Over the past 2 decades, the rates of induced remission and survival in most forms of leukemia have increased. Current 5-year relative survival rates range from 29% for AML to 86% for CLL, and as high as 91% for children and adolescents younger than 15 years of age with ALL.[43] Risk factors for the onset of leukemia include environmental factors, genetic factors, and other diseases (see Acute Leukemias and Chronic Leukemias sections for further discussion on risk factors).

Pathophysiology. All leukemias have certain pathophysiologic features in common. Most lymphoid neoplasms arise from B-cell and T-cell differentiation pathways (see Fig. 29.12A). The hypothesis of origin for leukemias is "clonal disorders driven by genetically abnormal progenitor cells or stem-like cancer cells (SLCCs)." The majority (85% to 90%) of lymphoid neoplasms are of B-cell origin, followed by T-cell tumors and, rarely, NK-cell tumors. Abnormal immature white blood cells, called leukemic blasts, fill the bone marrow and can spill into the blood. Leukemic blasts literally "crowd out" the bone marrow, compete for growth factors, and cause cellular proliferation of the other cell lines to decrease or cease. For example, AML is an age -related disease that is very dependent on the bone marrow microenvironment (see section on acute myeloid leukemia).[44] Tissues accumulate senescent cells with increasing age, characterized by an irreversible arrest of cell proliferation and the secretion of proinflammatory cytokines, chemokines, and growth factors, broadly called the senescence-associated secretory phenotype (SASP) (Fig. 29.13). Leukemic blasts induce a *senescent phenotype* in the stromal cells within the bone marrow microenvironment driven by the protein (cell cycle regulator) p16INK4a expression. Deletion of these senescent p16INK4a-expressing bone marrow stromal cells (BMSCs) slows tumor progression and extends survival.[44] The senescent response may have evolved to *suppress* the development of cancer, but also to assist tissue repair and regeneration. Because senescent cells gradually increase with age as does cancer, the senescent response may become *maladaptive* with age, and emerging evidence reveals that they contribute to several age-related phenotypes and pathologies.[45–47] Additionally, blast cell longevity is promoted by adipocytes. Emerging studies are revealing that bone marrow adipocytes support the survival and proliferation of AML blasts (see AML section for further discussion).[48]

Normal granulocytic-monocytic, lymphocytic, erythrocytic, and megakaryocytic progenitor cells can cease to function, leading to pancytopenia (a reduction in all cellular components of the blood). Genetic translocations (mitotic errors) are observed in leukemic cells. The most common genetic abnormality is the reciprocal translocation between chromosomes 9 and 22—t(9;22) (q34;q11), the Philadelphia chromosome. The Philadelphia chromosome was first observed in persons with CML and is present in 95% of those with CML,

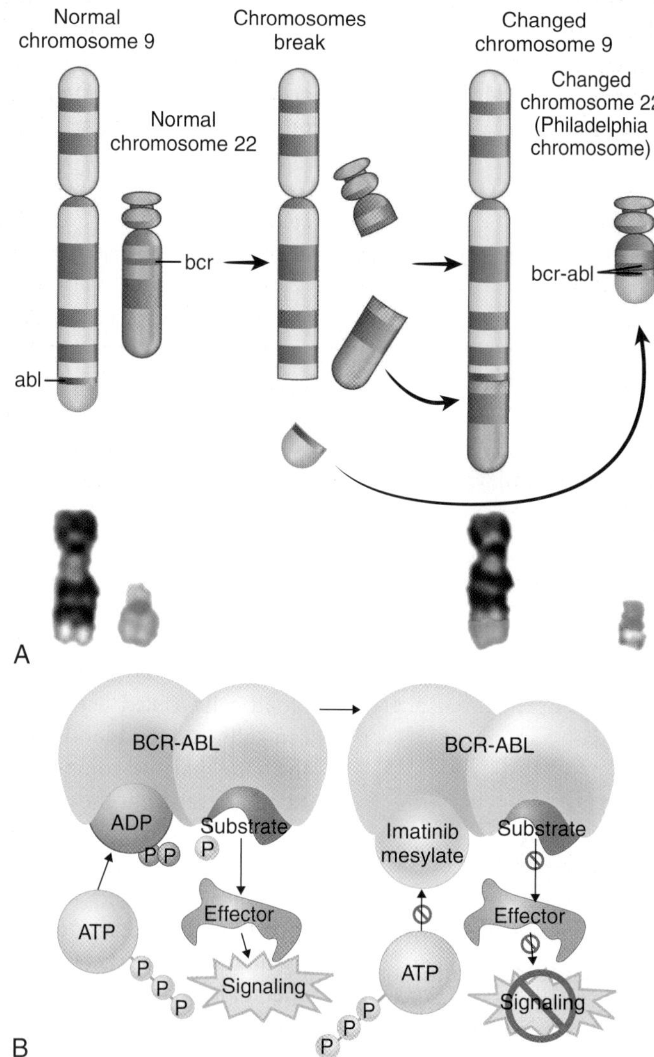

Fig. 29.14 Philadelphia Chromosome. The Philadelphia chromosome is an example of a reciprocal chromosomal translocation that results in an abnormal gene product responsible for a clinical disorder. **(A)** An exchange occurs between the long arm of chromosome 9 (black chromosome) and the long arm of chromosome 22 (blue chromosome); t(9;22)(q34;q11). **(B)** Mechanism of action of imatinib. By occupying the ATP-binding pocket of the ABL kinase domain, imatinib prevents substrate phosphorylation and downstream activation of signals, thus inhibiting the leukemogenic effects of BCR-ABL1 on cells in chronic myelogenous leukemia. *ADP,* Adenosine diphosphate; *ATP,* adenosine triphosphate; *BCR-ABL,* Breakpoint cluster region-Abelson; *P,* phosphate group. (A, Top portion from Rakel R, Bope E. *Conn's current therapy.* Philadelphia: Saunders; 2008; lower portion from Yanoff M, Duker J. *Ophthalmology,* 3rd edition. Edinburgh: Mosby; 2009; B From Goldman L, Schafer AI. *Goldman's Cecil medicine,* 24th edition. Philadelphia: Saunders; 2012.)

up to 3% of individuals with AML, about 25% of adults with ALL, and 10% of children with ALL.[49,50] This translocation results in the novel fusion of the *BCR1* gene region from chromosome 22 and the proto-oncogene *ABL1* from chromosome 9 (Fig. 29.14). The BCR-ABL1 joining results in the expression of a unique fused oncoprotein, BCR-ABL1. The ABL1 protein excessively activates intracellular pathways that promote cell proliferation, decrease sensitivity to apoptosis, and cause premature release of immature cells into the circulation. The BCR-ABL1 variant proves to be essential for transformation into leukemic cells. In most leukemias and lymphomas a single major genetic abnormality, such as the t(9;22) translocation, does not lead to an aggressive malignancy. The initial event is usually followed by a series of secondary genetic changes. Therefore, the original tumor becomes genetically unstable and diverse. In most cases leukemic cells are ejected into the blood where they accumulate. These cells also may infiltrate and accumulate in the liver, spleen, lymph nodes, and other organs throughout the body. The presentation of large numbers of leukemic cells in the blood may be one of the most dramatic indicators of leukemia; however, leukemia is still a primary disruption of the bone marrow.

Acute leukemias. Acute leukemias include two types: acute lymphocytic leukemia (ALL) and acute myelogenous leukemia (AML). ALL is a disease of the bone marrow, an aggressive, fast-growing leukemia with too many *lymphoblasts* (immature lymphocyte with altered morphology) or lymphocytes in the bone marrow and peripheral blood. It also is called *acute lymphoblastic leukemia.*

AML is a disease of the bone marrow, an aggressive fast-growing leukemia, and highly heterogenous disease. AML is a malignancy of the stem cell precursors of the myeloid lineage [red blood cells, platelets, and white blood cells (except B and T cells)].[51] It is characterized by overproduction of neoplastic clonal myeloid stem cells or *myeloblasts* (i.e., immature white blood cells that are not lymphoblasts).[51,52] It is also called *acute myeloblastic leukemia, acute myeloid leukemia*, or *acute nonlymphocytic leukemia* (*ANLL*). The WHO updated guidelines distinguish six groups of AML: (1) AML with recurrent genetic abnormalities, (2) AML with myelodysplasia-related changes, (3) Therapy-related myeloid neoplasms, (4) AML not Otherwise Specified, (5) Myeloid sarcoma, and (6) Myeloid proliferations related to Down syndrome.[53]

Acute leukemias are seen in both sexes and in all ages. AML is the more common acute leukemia in adults, with the median age at diagnosis around 70 years. There is a rise in the age-related incidence around 40 to 50 years of age, and a steep increase from 60 to 64 years of age. Mortality for all acute leukemias in the United States is about 7 per 100,000. In children younger than 15 years, leukemia accounts for one-third of all deaths from cancer (see chapter 30). North America and Scandinavian countries have the highest mortality; Eastern European countries, Asia (except Japan), and Central America have the lowest mortality. The higher mortality in Japan is the result of the atomic bombs dropped in World War II.[54] Black and Hispanic people have increased mortality compared with whites.[55]

More than 5690 new cases of ALL and 20,240 cases of AML were estimated for 2021, with more than 2480 deaths from ALL and 18,020 deaths from AML.[42]

Increased risk for ALL has been linked to exposure to x-rays before birth, being exposed to ionizing radiation (postnatally), past treatment with chemotherapy, certain chemical exposures (e.g., benzene, glues, detergents, art supplies, paint strippers), certain viral infections (see below), age (children and adults over age 50), race/ethnicity (more common in whites), gender (more common in males), and certain genetic conditions.[56] Leukemia has a statistically significant tendency to reappear in families. Controversial and unproven, increased risk in adults also has been linked to exposure to cigarette smoke. Large doses of ionizing radiation in particular result in an increased incidence of myelogenous leukemia. There is growing concern about the effect of low-dose radiation on subsequent risk of leukemia.[57] Infections with HIV or hepatitis C virus increase the risk for lymphoid neoplasms. It is now widely accepted that some types of leukemia are caused by infection with the human T-cell leukemia/lymphoma virus-1 (HTLV-1).

Acute leukemia also may develop secondary to certain acquired disorders, such as CML, CLL, HL, and others. Unlike other forms of leukemia, ALL develops at different rates in different geographic locations and the reason is unclear. People from developed countries and those of higher socioeconomic categories have an increased incidence of ALL. AML can arise in people *de novo*, those with an underlying hematological disorder, or as a consequence of prior treatment.[52] It is the most frequently reported secondary cancer after high doses of chemotherapy for HL, non-Hodgkin lymphoma (NHL), MM, ovarian cancer, and breast cancer.

Pathophysiology. ALL presumably progresses from malignant transformation of immature B- or T-cell progenitor cells (like a stem cell) (Fig. 29.15).[16] Most cases of ALL occur in children and often in the first decade (see Chapter 30). Although adults account for about 20% of all cases, their mortality rate is significantly higher. The significant difference between the incidence of ALL in adults and children may be because of differences in the biology of the disease (see Chapter 30).

Chromosomal aberrations in ALL disrupt normal B- and T-cell development by causing the dysregulation of expression and function of transcription factors. Most T-ALLs have mutations in *NOTCH1*, a gene necessary for normal T-cell development. Many B-ALLs have mutations affecting genes required for differentiation of early precursor cells, such as *PAX5, TCF3, ETV6*, and *RUNX1*.[16] By altering these "prime" regulatory factors, the mutations promote maturation arrest and increased self-renewal, creating a stem-cell like phenotype.[16] The identification of mutations found in ALL is ongoing and includes mutations that drive cell growth and mutations that increase tyrosine kinase activity and RAS signaling.

AML is the most common adult leukemia. Driver mutations in AML include four categories:

1. *Transcription factor mutations that disrupt normal myeloid differentiation.* For example, the two most common chromosomal rearrangements, t(8;21) and inv(16), alter the genes RUNX1 and CBFB, respectively.[16]
2. *Mutation of signaling proteins that promote pro-growth/survival pathways.* An example for AMLs is the t(15;17) which often have activating mutations in FLT3, a receptor tyrosine kinase that mimics normal growth factor signaling and promotes cellular proliferation and survival.
3. *Mutations of genes that regulate or maintain the epigenome.* Some of these mutations may lead to abnormal DNA methylation (see Chapter 6).
4. *Mutation of TP53 or genes that regulate p53.* AMLs with these alterations have complex karyotypes, significant dysplasia, and a poor prognosis due to resistance to standard therapies.[16]

More simply, genetic alterations in AML alter genes that encode transcription factors needed for normal myeloid differentiation; consequently, differentiation becomes arrested. These mutations affect the epigenome, suggesting that epigenetic alterations are key in AML. Mutations may lead to proliferation by activating

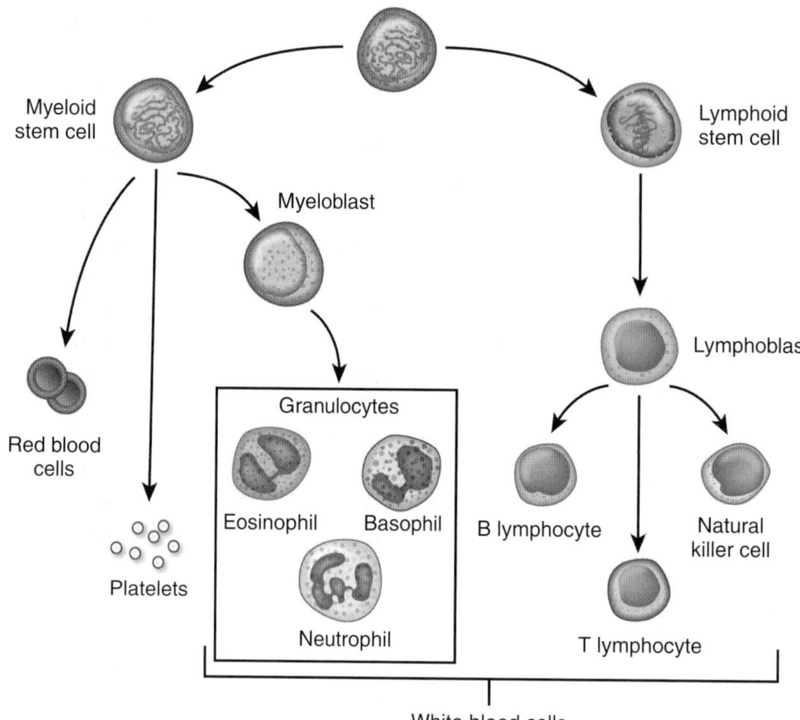

Fig. 29.15 Leukemia Arises From Stem-Like Cells. A blood stem cell undergoes multiple steps to finally become a red blood cell, platelet, or white blood cell. (© 2007 Terese Winslow LLC, U.S. Govt. has certain rights.)

growth factor signaling, as well as a decreased rate of apoptosis. Thus, the bone marrow and peripheral blood are characterized by leukocytosis and a predominance of blast cells. With an increase in immature blasts, they displace normal myelocytic blood cells, megakaryocytes, and erythrocytes. This displacement can lead to complications of bleeding, anemia, and infection. Several hereditary conditions are known to increase the risk for AML (e.g., Down syndrome, Fanconi aplastic anemia, Bloom syndrome, and others).

Numerous interactions between the bone marrow microenvironment and HSCs determine the balance between the proliferation, differentiation, and homeostasis of the stem cell compartment. Changes in this tightly regulated network promote malignant transformation.[58] Leukemic blast cells interact with the perivascular niche (Fig. 29.16). Secreted factors and cell-cell interactions regulate the survival, proliferation, and resistance of AML cells in the perivascular niche. Understanding these interactions will help to define targeted therapies.

Clinical Manifestations. Within days to a few weeks of the first symptoms is an abrupt stormy onset, which is more prevalent in ALL. The clinical manifestations of all varieties of acute leukemia are generally similar. Mechanisms associated with common manifestations are summarized in Table 29.8. Signs and symptoms related to bone marrow depression include fatigue caused by anemia, bleeding resulting from thrombocytopenia, and fever caused by infection. Bleeding may occur in the skin, gums, mucous membranes, and GI tract. Visible signs include petechiae and ecchymosis, as well as discoloration of the skin, gingival bleeding, hematuria, and midcycle or heavy menstrual bleeding.

Infection sites include the mouth, throat, respiratory tract, lower colon, urinary tract, and skin and may be caused by gram-negative bacilli *(Escherichia coli), Pseudomonas aeruginosa*, and *Klebsiella pneumoniae*. Fever is an early sign and is often accompanied by chills.

Anorexia is accompanied by weight loss, diminished sensitivity to sour and sweet tastes, wasting of muscle, and difficulty swallowing. Liver, spleen, and lymph node enlargement occurs more commonly in ALL than in AML. Liver and spleen enlargement commonly occur together. The leukemic individual often experiences abdominal pain and tenderness. Pain in the bones and joints is thought to result from leukemia infiltration with secondary stretching of the periosteum.

Neurologic manifestations are common and may be caused by either leukemic infiltration or cerebral bleeding. Headache, vomiting, papilledema, facial palsy, blurred vision, auditory disturbances, and meningeal irritation can occur if leukemic cells infiltrate the cerebral or spinal meninges.

Evaluation and Treatment. Diagnosis is made through examination of blood cells and bone marrow. For ALL, diagnostic confusion with AML, hairy cell leukemia, and malignant lymphoma is not uncommon. It is critical to obtain an accurate diagnosis because of the differences in treatment and prognosis of ALL and AML. Also critical is that bone marrow aspirates should be done

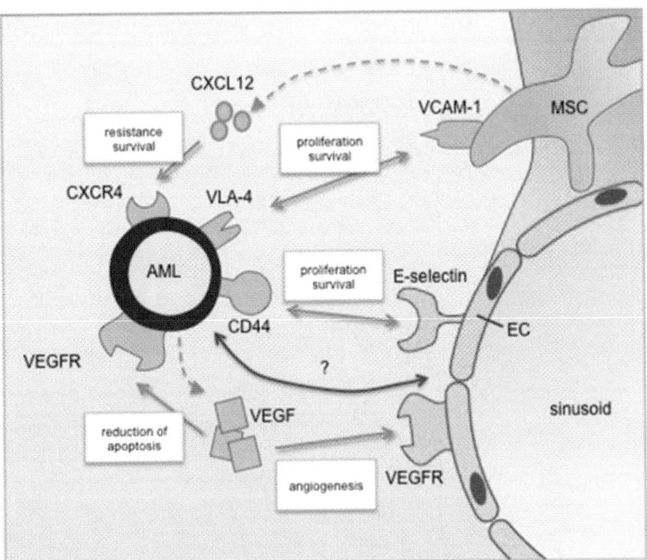

Fig. 29.16 Leukemic Blast Cells Interact With the Perivascular Niche. A tight relationship between leukemic cells and endothelial cells supports AML development and progression. Understanding these pathways (autocrine and paracrine) is critical for targeted therapy development. *AML*, Acute myeloid leukemia; *CXCL12*, C-X-C motif chemokine12; *CXCR4*, C-X-C chemokine receptor 4; *EC*, endothelial cell; *MSC*, mesenchymal stromal cell; *VEGF*, vascular endothelial growth factor; *VEGFR*, vascular endothelial growth factor receptor; *VCAM-1*, vascular cell adhesion molecule1; *VLA-4*, very late antigen 4. (From Behrmann L, Wellbrock J, Fiedler W. Acute myeloid leukemia and the bone marrow niche—Take a closer look. *Frontiers in Oncology*, 2018;8. https://doi.org/10.3389/fonc.2018.00444.)

by an experienced oncologist, hematologist, hematopathologist, or general pathologist experienced in interpreting conventional and specially stained specimens. The morphologic aspects of leukemia cells are seen in Fig. 29.17.

Chemotherapy, used in various combinations, is the treatment of choice for leukemia.[59] Successful treatment of ALL is control of bone marrow and systemic disease and the treatment (or prevention) of sanctuary-site disease, especially the CNS.[59] Treatment is divided into three phases: remission induction, CNS prophylaxis, and post remission.[59] CNS prophylaxis is achieved with chemotherapy (intrathecal and /or high-dose systemic therapy) and, in some cases, cranial radiation therapy.[60] Other types of treatment include chemotherapy with stem cell transplant and other drug therapy. Supportive measures include antibiotics, antifungals, antivirals, and blood transfusions.[60] It is critical that stem cell transplants be done in hospitals with very experienced staff for both the procedure and the recovery phase.

There are an increasing number of targeted treatment strategies to treat AML, yet patient outcomes remain poor. Relapses after chemotherapy continues to be a major obstacle, driving demand for new treatment approaches.[61] Attainment of complete remission requires aggressive treatment. However, particularly problematic in persons greater than 60 years is a diminished tolerance for intensive chemotherapy and increased treatment-related toxicity, leading to an estimated treatment-related mortality from 10% to 30%.[62] Determining who is fit or unfit for standard treatments among older adults remains a challenge.[63]

Historically, maintenance therapy for AML was administered for several years but it has not been shown to benefit persons with AML in several studies. However, two strategies have shown a benefit: (1) midostaurin in individuals with *FLT3*-mutated AML and (2) oral azacytidine.[64]

Post remission therapy appears to be more effective when given immediately after remission is achieved. Factors influencing increased survival rate include the use of combined and multimodality treatment methods; improved supportive services, such as nutritional support; and antimicrobial treatment. The presence of the Philadelphia chromosome (observed in about 5% of children with ALL, in 30% of adults with ALL, and occasionally in AML) is a poor prognostic indicator. Dramatic responses, however, have been achieved in B-ALL with chimeric antigen receptor T cells against the B-cell antigen CD19, but with associated toxicities that are sometimes fatal and with high economic costs.[16]

Myelosuppression is both a consequence of leukemia and a treatment for the disease. Hematologic support with blood products and granulocyte colony-stimulating factor (G-CSF) or GM-CSF has effectively shortened the time of neutropenia and improved survival by reducing the risk for infection.

Chronic leukemias. The two main types of chronic leukemia are (1) chronic lymphocytic leukemia (CLL) and (2) chronic myelogenous leukemia (CML). CLL is a disorder of structurally mature but immunologically immature lymphocytes. It is manifested by progressive accumulation of these cells in the blood, bone marrow, and lymphatic tissues.[65] In adults, CLL is the most common leukemia in the Western world. It is a slow-growing cancer. CLL and small lymphocytic lymphoma (SLL) differ only in the amount of proliferation of peripheral blood lymphocytes.

CML is also called *chronic granulocytic leukemia* and *chronic myeloid leukemia*. It is classified as a myeloproliferative neoplasm (MPN). CML is a slowly progressing disease with increased numbers of maturing granulocytic precursors in the bone marrow, which usually includes elevated proportions of eosinophils and basophils.[16] The peripheral blood reveals a leukocytosis, often exceeding 100,000 cells/mm^3.[16] CML is mostly a disease of adults but can occur in children or adolescents (see Chapter 30). The peak incidence is the fifth to sixth decades. Individuals with chronic leukemia have a longer life expectancy, usually extending several years from the time of diagnosis.

It is estimated 21,250 new cases of CLL and 4320 deaths, and 9110 new cases of CML and 1220 deaths in 2021.[42] CML is one of a group of diseases called myeloproliferative disorders—acquired abnormalities in signaling pathways that lead to growth factor–independent proliferation. The only known cause of CML is exposure to ionizing radiation.

Exposure to pesticides, deltamethrin,[66] and herbicides[67] has been associated with the development of CLL.[68] The most convincing association is Agent Orange used during the Vietnam War.[69,70] Radon has shown a similar relationship.[71] The link with ionizing radiation is controversial. An underlying immune defect may be involved because respiratory tract infections,

TABLE 29.8 Clinical Manifestations and Related Pathophysiology in Leukemia

Clinical Manifestations	Laboratory Abnormalities	Cause	Comments
Anemia	Relative *proportion* of erythroblasts to total count (decreased in anemia) is key	Decreased stem cell input or ineffective erythropoiesis, or both	In acute leukemia, anemia is usually present from beginning, often first symptom noticed, and severe; mild form without symptoms is common in CML and CLL; hemorrhage common in acute forms, occasional in CML, but rare in CLL
Bleeding (purpura, petechiae, ecchymosis, hemorrhage)	Decreased and possibly abnormal platelets	Reduction in megakaryocytes leading to thrombocytopenia	Bleeding more common in acute than in chronic leukemia
Infection	Increased multisegmented neutrophils	Opportunistic organisms; decreased protection resulting from granulocytopenia or immune deficiency secondary to chemotherapy, corticosteroids, and disease process	Major sites of infection: oral cavity, throat, lower colon, urinary tract, lungs, and skin; prevention of infection focuses on restoring host defenses, decreasing invasive procedures, and reducing colonization of microorganisms
Weight loss	Decreased 24-h urinary creatinine excretion; hypoalbuminemia	Condition can be attributed to pain, depression, chemotherapy, radiation therapy, loss of appetite, and alterations in taste	Severe weight loss may be related to excess production of TNF-α
Bone pain	Often no radiographic evidence of bone problems	Result of bone infiltration by leukemic cells or intramedullary infection	If combination drug regimens are ineffective, radiation therapy is used
Liver, spleen, and lymph node enlargement	Biopsy abnormal for liver and spleen	Leukemic cell infiltration	Lymph nodes also undergo leukemia proliferation in CLL
Elevated uric acid level	Normal excretion of uric acid is 300–500 mg/day; leukemic individual can excrete 50 times more	Increased catabolism of protein and nucleic acid; urate precipitation increased from dehydration caused by anorexia or fever and drug therapy	Hyperuricemia is present in both acute leukemia and CML; treatment focuses on increasing urine pH or decreasing acid production with drug allopurinol

CLL, Chronic lymphocytic leukemia; *CMA*, chronic myelocytic leukemia; *RBC*, red blood cell; *TNF-α*, tumor necrosis factor-α.

cellulitis, and herpes zoster can portend the diagnosis of CLL.[72–74] Additionally, hypogammaglobulinemia is common in CLL and can precede the diagnosis.[68,75,76]

Among leukemias, CLL has the highest incidence of familial association, with first-degree relatives having more than an eightfold higher likelihood of developing the disease.[68,77] Contrarily, the low CLL incidence among Asians/Pacific Islanders, particularly Japanese, does not increase when living in the United States.[68,78] These observations strongly imply involvement of inheritable susceptibility alleles that promote or prevent disease.[68,79] Consistent with these findings is recent work with persons with CLL and myeloma revealing the shared risk loci affecting genes involved in B-cell development.[80] Susceptible genes can influence many points along the B-cell differentiation pathways.[68]

Pathophysiology. CML is defined by the fusion oncoprotein *BCR-ABL1*.[81] The Philadelphia chromosome with a shortened chromosome 22 and reciprocal translocation t(9;220 (q34;q11.2) occurs in 90% to 95% of patients (see Fig. 29.14).[81] The presence of the BCR-ABL1 protein is responsible for initiation of CML (Fig. 29.18).

CLL involves malignant transformation and accumulation of B lymphocytes co-expressing low levels of surface immunoglobulin (IG) of a single IG light (L) chain type. Unlike most other lymphoid malignancies, CLL rarely involves chromosomal translocations. The most common genetic disturbances are deletions of 13q14.3, 11q, and 17p and trisomy 12q.[16] Studies of chromosome 13 reveal two incriminating microRNAs miR-15a and miR-16-1 tumor suppressor genes.[16] Loss of these miRs is thought to result in overexpression of the anti-apoptotic protein BCL2.[16,68] Overexpression of BCL2 is observed in CLL and *small lymphocytic lymphoma* (SLL; therefore, both neoplasms are often discussed together (*CLL/SLL*). B lymphocytes with a CLL phenotype can be found in the blood of normal individuals, sometimes years before the diagnosis, and is called *monoclonal B-cell lymphocytosis (MBL)*.[68] Annually, only 1% of subjects with MBL progress to CLL requiring treatment.[68] MBL and CLL have similar mutation burdens with less found in MBL, consistent with the stepwise unfolding from one to the other.[68] Individuals with MBL, as in CLL, may have a more global immune defect. Such individuals have a higher incidence of severe infections and non-hematologic cancers and may have an increased incidence of hypogammaglobulinemia.[68]

Clinical Manifestations. Chronic leukemia advances slowly and insidiously. Approximately 70% of individuals with CLL are asymptomatic at the time of diagnosis. When symptoms do appear, the most common finding is lymphadenopathy. The most significant effect of CLL is suppression of humoral

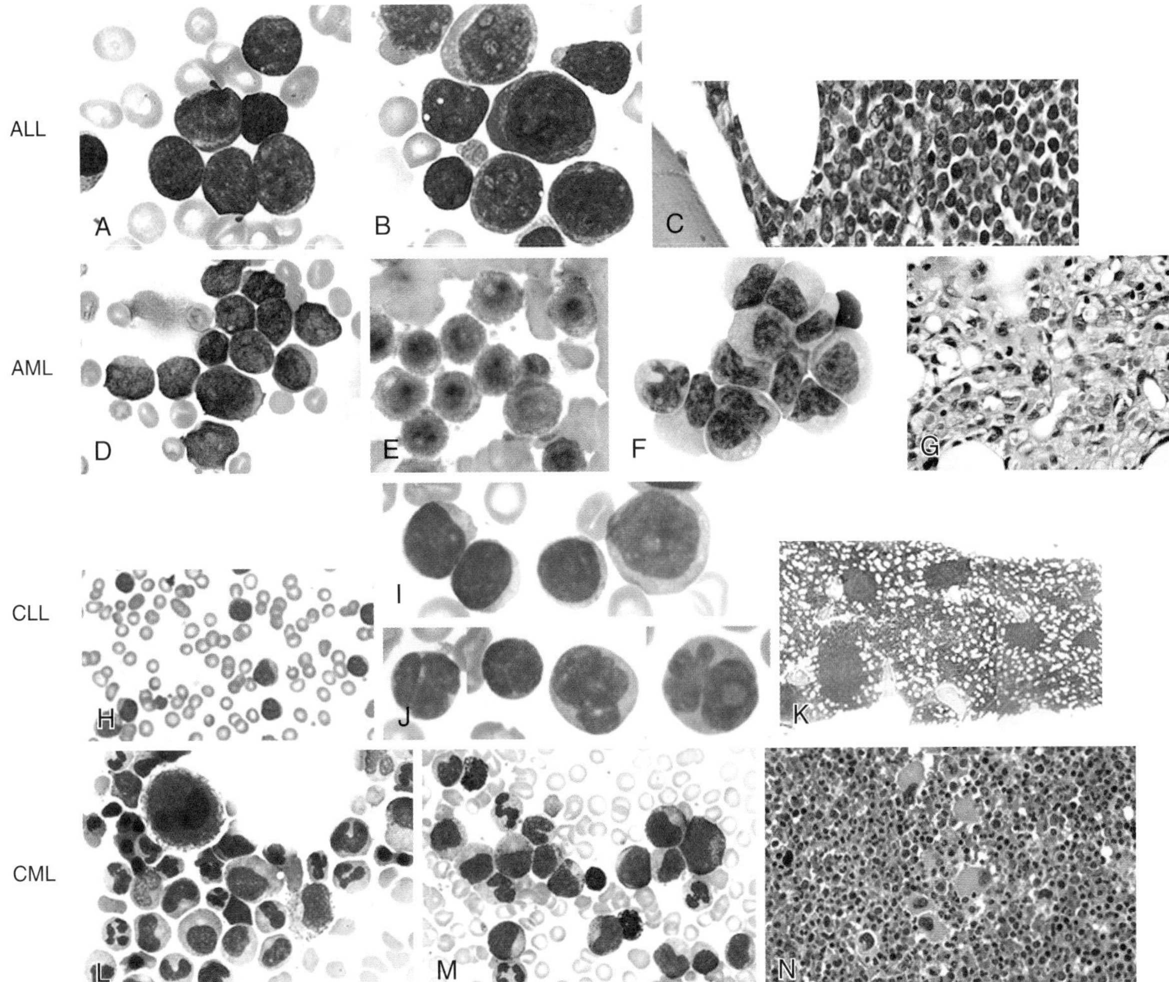

Fig. 29.17 Morphologic Aspects of Leukemia Cells. Acute lymphoblastic leukemia *(ALL)* (A–C). **(A)** Typical uniform lymphoblasts with intermediate-sized nuclei, fine but "smudgy" chromatin, absence of nucleoli, and scant cytoplasm. **(B)** Lymphoblasts with more cytologic variation, including variability in size, number of nucleoli, and amount of cytoplasm. **(C)** Histologic features of ALL in bone core biopsy. Acute myeloid leukemia *(AML)* (D–G). **(D)** Acute myeloblastic leukemia with minimal or no maturation. The cells are myeloblasts with dispersed chromatin and variable amounts of agranular cytoplasm. Some display medium-sized, poorly defined nucleoli. **(E)** Acute monoblastic leukemia; characteristic monoblasts with round nuclei and delicate chromatin and prominent nucleoli. Cytoplasm is abundant. **(F)** Acute monocytic leukemia with most of the cells in this field being promonocytes. Monoblasts and an abnormal monocyte also are present. **(G)** Marrow biopsy of acute megakaryoblastic leukemia containing large and small blasts and atypical megakaryocytes. Chronic lymphocytic leukemia *(CLL)* (H–K). **(H)** Peripheral blood smear typically shows lymphocytosis. Cytologic features of CLL cells differ. **(I)** Classic cells have a small nucleus with a "soccer ball" chromatin pattern. **(J)** Some cases have increased large cells, or prolymphocytes, with more open chromatin and prominent "punched-out" nucleoli (prolymphocyte, right side). **(K)** The bone marrow can show nodular infiltrates of CLL cells. Chronic myelogenous leukemia *(CML)* (L–N). **(L)** Peripheral smear shows marked leukocytosis attributable to a granulocytic proliferation of all stages with particularly increased myelocytes and absolute basophilia. **(M)** Bone core biopsy illustrates markedly hypercellular marrow attributable to granulocytic proliferation and increased small hypolobated megakaryocytes. **(N)** Bone marrow aspirate shows granulocytic proliferation and small, "dwarf" megakaryocyte. (A–C and H–N, From Hoffman R, et al. *Hematology: Basic principles and practice*, 6th edition. Philadelphia: Churchill Livingstone; 2013. D–G, From Abeloff M, et al. *Abeloff's clinical oncology*, 4th ed. Philadelphia: Churchill Livingstone; 2008.)

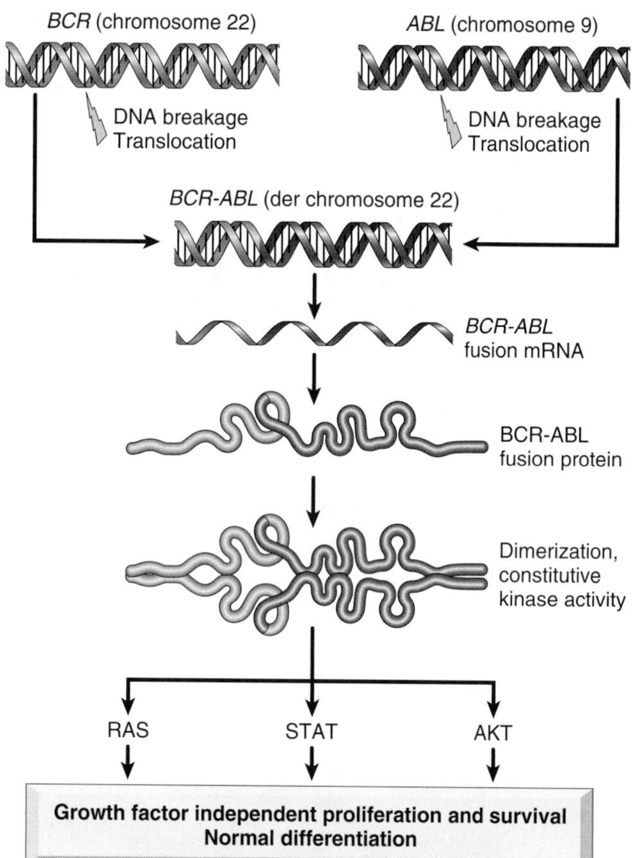

Fig. 29.18 Pathogenesis of Chronic Myeloid Leukemia. The breakage and joining of *BCR* and *ABL* creates the chimeric fusion gene *BCR-ABL*. *BCR-ABL* genetically encodes an active BCR-ABL intracellular tyrosine kinase (an enzyme that controls intracellular "on-off" switches). The ABL kinase in turn induces signaling through the same pro-growth and pro-survival pathways that are activated by normal hematologic growth factors. Altogether the activation of many downstream pathways drives growth factor–independent proliferation and survival of bone marrow progenitors. *der chromosome* is a structurally rearranged chromosome. *AKT*, Serine/threonine kinases; *BCR-ABL*, breakpoint cluster region-Abelson; *RAS*, rat sarcoma; *STAT*, signal transducer and activator of transcription. (From Kumar V, et al. *Robbins & Cotran pathologic basis of disease*, 9th edition. St. Louis: Elsevier; 2015.)

immunity and increased infection with encapsulated bacteria. Frequently, the level of neutrophils is depressed, which adds to the risk of infection. Invasion of most organ cells is uncommon, but infiltration does occur in lymph nodes, liver, spleen, and salivary glands. CNS involvement is rare. Approximately 10% of individuals develop a more aggressive malignancy, usually a diffuse large B-cell lymphoma. In these individuals, extreme fatigue, weight loss, night sweats, low-grade fever, elevated levels of the enzyme lactic dehydrogenase, hypercalcemia, anemia, and thrombocytopenia are common.

Individuals with CML may progress through three phases of the disease: a chronic phase, during which symptoms may not be apparent, often never requiring treatment; an accelerated phase, during which the primary symptoms develop and require treatment; and a terminal blast phase ("blast crisis") necessitating treatment. The accelerated phase is characterized by excessive proliferation and accumulation of malignant cells. Splenomegaly is prominent and becomes painful, but lymphadenopathy generally is not present. Liver enlargement also occurs, but liver function is rarely altered. Hyperuricemia is common and produces gouty arthritis. Infections, fever, and weight loss also are seen often. The terminal blast phase is characterized by rapid and progressive leukocytosis with an increase in basophils. In the later stages of the terminal phase, which then resembles AML, blast cells or promyelocytes predominate and the individual experiences a "blast crisis."

The acute effects of CML resemble those of acute leukemia but with more prominent and painful splenomegaly. Lymphadenopathy generally is found only in the acute phase of the disease. Hyperuricemia is usually present and produces gouty arthritis. Infections, fever, and weight loss are common findings with CML.

Evaluation and Treatment. Diagnosis of chronic leukemia depends on laboratory analyses of peripheral blood and bone marrow. Diagnosis of CLL is based on detection of a monoclonal B-cell lymphocytosis in the blood. The cells must have the characteristic immunophenotype (CD5+, CD19+, CD20 [weak], CD23+) at levels more than 5000 cells/μL over a sustained period (usually 4 weeks). Confusion with other diseases may be avoided by determination of cell surface markers.

Treatment of CLL ranges from periodic observation with treatment of infection, hemorrhage, or immunologic complications. Because the disease mostly occurs in the elderly and the rate of progression is slow, it is often simply observed until the disease progresses. Randomized trials show no survival advantage for immediate versus delayed treatment of those individuals with early-stage disease. For individuals with progressing CLL, treatment with conventional doses of chemotherapy is not curative; selected individuals treated with allogeneic SCT have achieved prolonged disease-free survival. Antileukemic therapy is frequently unnecessary in uncomplicated early disease. From older clinical trials (1970s through the 1990s), the median survival for all individuals ranges from 8 to 12 years. However, a large variation in survival exists, ranging from several months to a normal life expectancy. Treatment must be individualized based on the clinical behavior of the disease. The complexity and variability in clinical course and in leukemia biology warrants the use of algorithms that have been devised to better predict outcomes and response to therapy.[68] For example, individual's age, disease stage (Rai or Binet systems), TP53 disruption, immunoglobulin heavy chain variable region gene (IgHV) mutation status, and serum β2-microglobulin levels are included in the Chronic Lymphocytic Leukemia International Prognostic Index (CLL-IPI).[82]

Complications of pancytopenia, including hemorrhage and infection, are a major cause of death. Typically, individuals with CLL survive 10 years or more. Those with certain risk factors, however, have a more aggressive disease, shortening survival to less than 3 years.

Diagnosis of CML involves fluorescent *in situ* studies of the *BCR/ABL* translocation on the bone marrow aspirate or on the peripheral blood of individuals. A small subset of patients has *BCR/ABL* detectable only by reverse transcriptase-polymerase chain reaction (RT-PCR).[83] Treatment of individuals with CML is usually initiated when the diagnosis is established. Establishment is done by the presence of an elevated white blood cell count, splenomegaly, thrombocytosis, and identification of the *BCR/ABL* translocation.[83]

Current treatment modalities for CML do not cure the disease or prevent blastic transformation. Standard treatment consists of combined chemotherapy, biologic response modifiers, and allogenic BMT or SCT. BMT or SCT use is limited by donor availability and high toxicity in older adults (older than 65 years). Imatinib mesylate (Gleevec), a tyrosine kinase inhibitor, led to changes in the management of CML. Other tyrosine kinase inhibitors have been developed; however, concerns about disease persistence and resistance still exist.[84] Gleevec produces a complete cytogenic response in more than 80% of newly diagnosed persons; however, it does not cure CML because it does not kill leukemia stem cells both in the laboratory and in vivo.

ALTERATIONS OF LYMPHOID FUNCTION

Lymphadenopathy

Lymphadenopathy is characterized by enlarged lymph nodes (Fig. 29.19). Lymph node enlargement occurs because of an increase in the size and number of its germinal centers caused by proliferation of lymphocytes and monocytes (immature phagocytes) or invasion by malignant cells. Normally, lymph nodes are not palpable or are barely palpable. Enlarged lymph nodes are palpable and often also may be tender or painful to touch, although not in all situations.

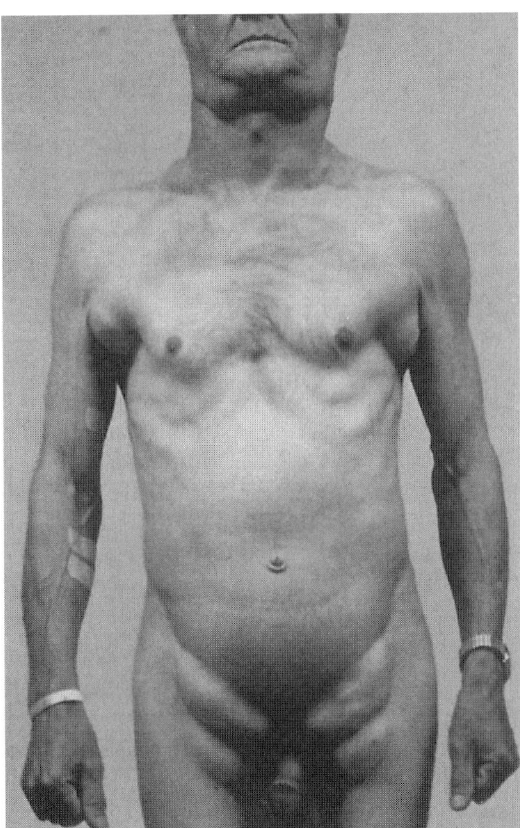

Fig. 29.19 Lymphadenopathy. Individual with lymphocyte leukemia with extreme but symmetric lymphadenopathy. (Courtesy Dr. A.R. Kagan, Los Angeles. From del Regato JA, et al. *Cancer: Diagnosis, treatment, and prognosis*, 6th edition. St. Louis: Mosby; 1985.)

Localized lymphadenopathy usually indicates drainage of an area associated with an inflammatory process or infection (reactive lymph node). *Generalized lymphadenopathy* occurs less often and is usually seen in the presence of infections, autoimmune diseases, or disseminated malignancy. Palpable nodes, however, do not always indicate serious disease and may indicate a minor trauma or infection. The location and size of the enlarged nodes are important factors in diagnosing the cause of the lymphadenopathy, as are the individual's age, sex, and geographic location. Generalized lymphadenopathy occurs with NHLs, CLL, histiocytosis, and disorders that produce lymphocytosis. In general, lymphadenopathy results from four types of conditions: (1) neoplastic disease, (2) immunologic or inflammatory conditions, (3) endocrine disorders, or (4) lipid storage diseases. Diseases of unknown cause, including autoimmune diseases and reactions to drugs, also may lead to generalized lymphadenopathy.

Malignant Lymphomas

Lymphomas consist of a diverse group of neoplasms that develop from the proliferation of malignant lymphocytes in the lymphoid system. The WHO publishes the Revised European American Lymphoma (REAL) classification based on the cell type from which the lymphoma probably originated. The basic groups include *HL* and *NHL*. Three major groups of lymphoid malignancies based on morphology and cell lineage include (1) B-cell neoplasms, (2) T-cell neoplasms, and (3) NK-cell neoplasms. MM, which was previously classified independently, is included as a B-cell lymphoma. NHL can be further divided into cancers that have an *indolent*, slow-growing course, and those with an *aggressive*, fast-growing, course. Both HL and NHL occur in children and adults, and the overall treatment and prognosis depend on the stage and type of lymphoma.

Lymphoma is the most common blood cancer in the United States. Incidence rates of lymphoma differ with respect to age, sex, geographic location, and socioeconomic class. The estimated new cases of lymphoma include 8830 cases of HL and 81,560 cases of NHL.[42] It was estimated in 2021 that 20,720 will die from NHL and 960 from HL. Since the early 1970s, the incidence of NHL has nearly doubled. The exact reason for this increase remains a mystery; however, a modest portion of the increase had been attributed to lymphomas developing in association with immune deficiencies, including AIDS and organ transplants. Conversely, the incidence of HL has declined over the same time period, especially among older adults.

In general, lymphomas are the result of genetic mutations or viral infection. Globally, however, the incidence of lymphoma is increased in more developed countries (except for BL); therefore, investigators are studying the following potential risk factors: diet, obesity, metabolic syndrome, sedentary lifestyle, stress, advances in medical care and access, increases in longevity, and exposure to compounds from industrialization. Malignant transformation produces a cell with uncontrolled and excessive growth

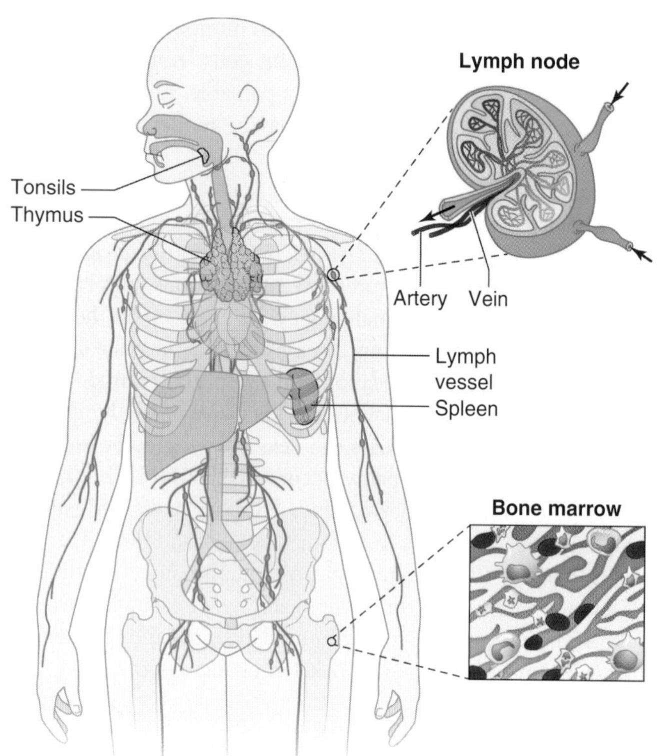

Fig. 29.20 Lymphomas Start in Lymph Nodes or Lymphoid Tissue.

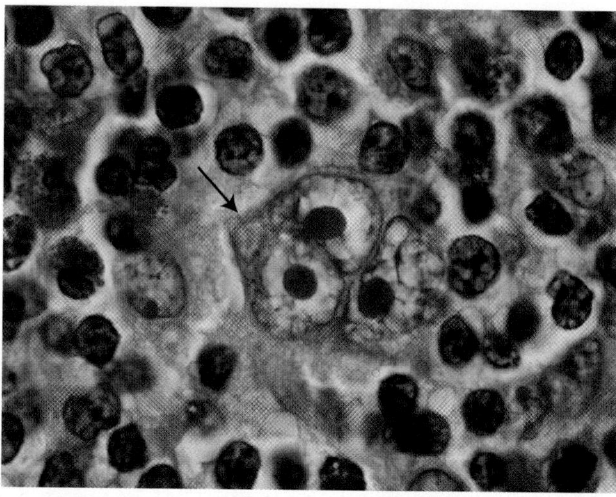

Fig. 29.21 Lymph Nodes. Diagnostic Reed-Sternberg cell *(arrow)*. A large multinucleated or multilobed cell with inclusion body–like nucleoli surrounded by a halo of clear nucleoplasm. (From Damjanov I, Linder J, eds. *Anderson's pathology*, 10th edition. St. Louis: Mosby; 1996.)

that accumulates in the lymph nodes and other sites, producing tumor masses. Lymphomas usually start in the lymph nodes or lymphoid tissues of the stomach or intestines (Fig. 29.20).

Hodgkin Lymphoma

Hodgkin lymphoma (HL) is a malignant lymphoma that progresses from one group of lymph nodes to another and includes the development of systemic symptoms and the presence of multinucleated cells derived from B lymphocytes called Hodgkin and Reed-Sternberg (HRS) cells (see the Pathophysiology section). Estimates of new cases of HL include 8480 cases in 2020 and 970 deaths.[42] The incidence of HL is slightly higher in females and occurs mostly in young adults and less frequently in elderly individuals.[85] The overall incidence of HL is low, about 2 to 3/100,000 individuals of European ancestry[86]; however, HL is one of the most common cancers diagnosed in young adults (see Chapter 30). HL peaks at two different ages: early in life in the second and third decades and later in life during the sixth and seventh decades. Incidence is greater in whites than blacks and lower in Hispanic Americans, Asians/Pacific Islanders, American Indians, and Alaskan natives.[87]

HL has unique characteristics among human cancers, including young age of onset; rarity of malignant cells or HRS cells and are usually present within a microenvironment with lots of immune effector cells; a high cure rate, even when the individual presents with metastatic spread; and a particular sensitivity to radiation therapy.[85]

EBV has been linked to the pathogenesis of HL, but the virus is detected in only a small subset of cases, and absolute risk for HL after EBV infections is very small.[88] Individuals with HIV infection or AIDS are at increased risk of HL *since* the introduction of highly active retroviral therapy (HAART).[89]

Pathophysiology. The HRS cell represents the malignant transformed lymphocyte (Fig. 29.21). HRS cells are often large and binucleate with occasional mononuclear variants. HRS cells are necessary for the diagnosis of HL. In rare instances, cells resembling HRS cells can be found in benign illnesses, as well as in other forms of cancer, including NHLs and solid tissue cancers and in IM.

The neoplastic HRS cells originate from a germinal center or post-germinal center B cell.[16] The triggering mechanism for the malignant transformation of cells remains unknown. Classic HL appears to be derived from a B cell in the germinal center that has not undergone successful immunoglobulin gene rearrangement (see Chapter 8) and would normally be induced to undergo apoptosis. Survival of this cell may be linked to infection with EBV. Laboratory and epidemiologic studies have linked HL with EBV infections. The HRS cells secrete and release cytokines (e.g., IL-10, TGF-β) that result in the accumulation of inflammatory cells in the tumor microenvironment, which produces the local and systemic effects (Fig. 29.22). The inflammatory cell infiltrate produces molecules that bind to proteins expressed on the cell membrane of the HRS cell.[85] These cellular interactions lead to activation of pathways that support the growth and survival of the HRS cells. Tumor-associated macrophages have been reported to be the prominent cells that support HRS cell growth and participate in forming an immune-prosperous niche.[85]

Clinical Manifestations. Many clinical features of HL can be explained by the complex action of cytokines and other growth factors that are secreted and released by the malignant cells. These substances induce infiltration and proliferation of inflammatory cells, resulting in an enlarged, painless lymph node in the neck (often the first sign of HL) (Fig. 29.23A and B).

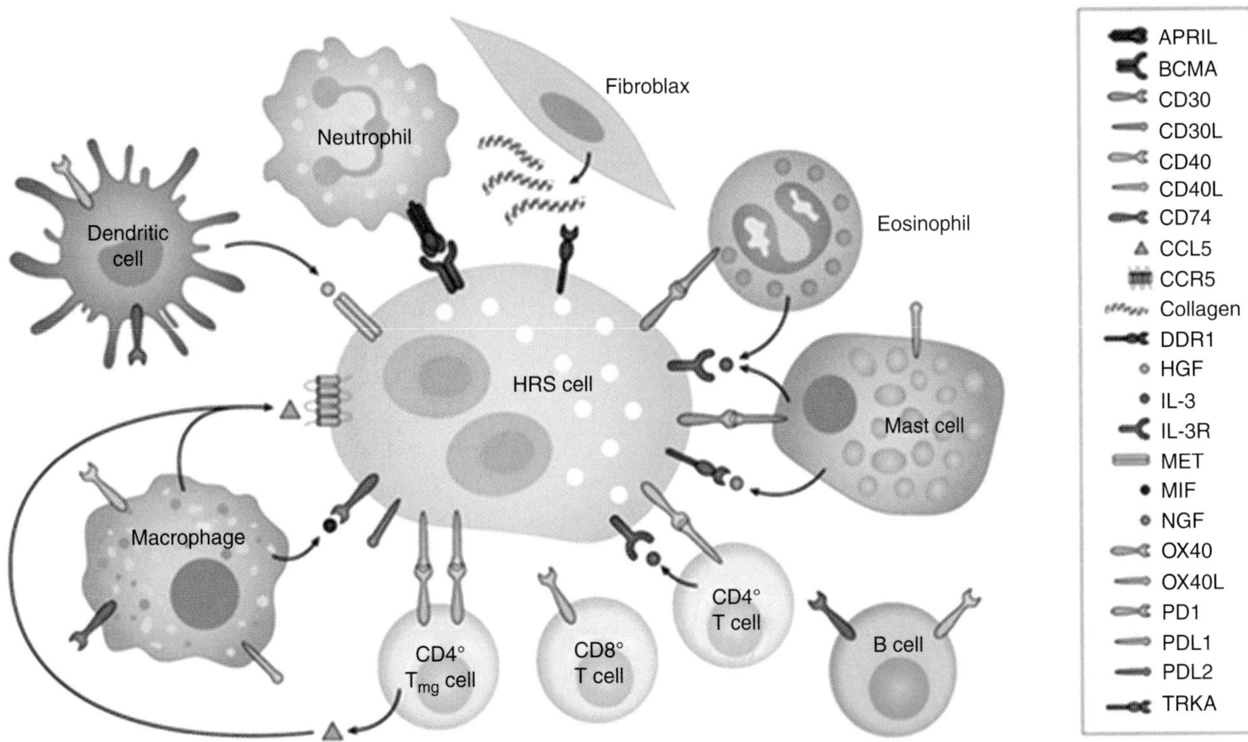

Fig. 29.22 Hodgkin Disease and the Tumor Microenvironment. A diagnostic Hodgkin and Reed-Sternberg (HRS) cell surrounded by the inflammatory tumor microenvironment. The range of microenvironment changes are associated with all four types of classic Hodgkin lymphoma (cHL). The inflammatory cell infiltrate produces molecules that bind to the cell membrane of the HRS cell. These interactions lead to pathways that support the growth and survival of the HRS cells. APRIL, A proliferation-inducing ligand; BCMA, B cell maturation antigen; CD30L, CD30 ligand; CD40, CD40 ligand; CCR5, CC-chemokine receptor 5; DDR1, discoidin domain receptor 1: HGF, hepatocyte growth factor; IL3R, IL-3 receptor; Met, protooncogene Met; MIF, migration inhibitory factor: NGF, nerve growth factor; OX40, OXO40L receptor; OX40L, OX40 ligand; TRKA, tyrosine kinase receptor. (From Connors J, Cozen W, Steidl C, et al. Hodgkin lymphoma. *Nature Reviews Disease Primers*, 2020;6(1). https://doi.org/10.1038/s41572-020-0189-6.)

The discovery of an asymptomatic mediastinal mass on routine chest x-ray is not uncommon. The cervical, axillary, inguinal, and retroperitoneal lymph nodes are commonly affected in HL (Fig. 29.24). Local symptoms caused by pressure and obstruction of lymph nodes are the result of the lymphadenopathy.

About one-third of individuals will have some common systemic symptoms, such as intermittent fever, without other symptoms of infection, drenching night sweats, itchy skin (pruritus), and fatigue. These constitutional symptoms accompanied by weight loss are associated with a poor prognosis.

Although HL rarely arises in the lung, mediastinal and hilar node adenopathy can cause secondary involvement of the trachea, bronchi, pleura, or lungs. Retroperitoneal nodes can involve vertebral bodies and nerves and can cause displacement of ureters. Spinal cord involvement is more common in the thoracic and lumbar regions than in the cervical region. Skin lesions, although uncommon, include psoriasis and eczematoid lesions, causing itching and scratching.

As a result of direct invasion from mediastinal lymph nodes, pericardial involvement can cause pericardial friction rub, pericardial effusion, and engorgement of neck veins. The GI tract and urinary tract are rarely involved. Anemia is often found in individuals with HL accompanied by a low serum iron level and reduced iron-binding capacity. Other laboratory findings include elevated sedimentation rate, leukocytosis, and eosinophilia. Leukopenia occurs in advanced stages of HL.

Splenic involvement in HL depends on histologic type. In mixed cellularity and lymphocytic deletion types of HL, the spleen is involved in 60% of cases. With lymphocyte and nodular sclerosis types, 34% of cases involve the spleen.

Evaluation and Treatment. Treatment depends on the stage of HL. Because of the variability in symptoms, early definitive detection may be challenging. Asymptomatic lymphadenopathy can progress undetected for several years. Diagnosis is made from physical examination and history; complete blood count (CBC); and blood chemistry studies, including sedimentation

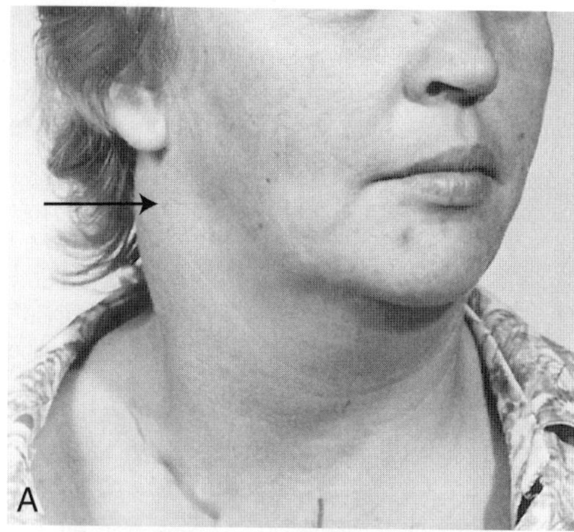

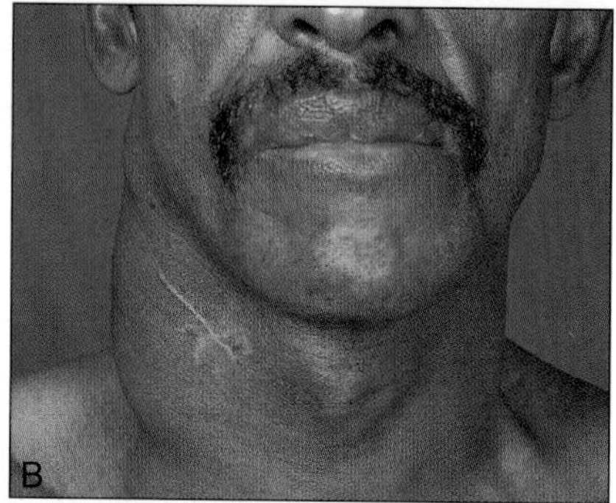

Fig. 29.23 Hodgkin Lymphoma and Enlarged Cervical Lymph Node. Typical enlarged cervical lymph node in the neck **(A)** *(arrow)* of a 35-year-old woman with Hodgkin lymphoma and **(B)** *(arrow)* of a man with Hodgkin lymphoma. The scar of a previous biopsy incision is well healed. (A, From del Regato JA, et al. *Cancer: Diagnosis, treatment, and prognosis*, 6th edition. St. Louis: Mosby; 1985. B, From Hoffbrand AV, Petit JE, Vyas P. *Color atlas of clinical hematology*, 4th edition. Philadelphia: Mosby, Elsevier; 2009.)

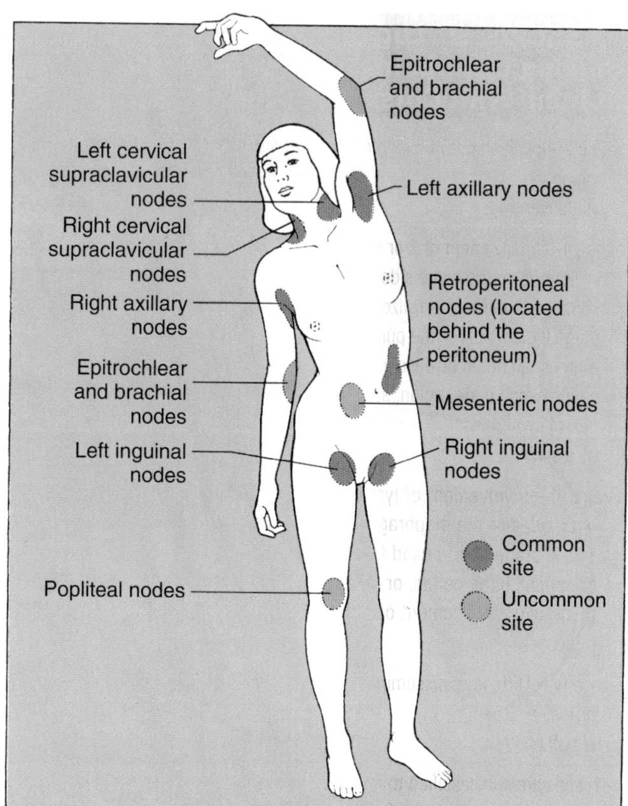

Fig. 29.24 Common and Uncommon Involved Lymph Node Sites for Hodgkin Lymphoma.

rate, and imaging. Radiologic examination may include CT scans of the neck, chest, abdomen, and pelvis; or metabolic imaging with positron emission tomography–computed tomography (PET-CT).[90] Occasionally, biopsy of suspicious nodes is needed if imaging studies are indeterminate and treatment decisions are affected by confirmation of involvement.[88] The current staging system for HL is the Lugano classification derived from Ann Arbor staging with Cotswolds modifications (Table 29.9).[88]

Pretreatment evaluation includes history and physical exam, laboratory studies, imaging (PET/CT), and specialized studies to determine the individual's fitness for treatment and to determine the disease stage.[88] MRI can be used for anatomical imaging of PET-positive lesions to characterize involvement of certain organs (e.g., brain, liver). CNS involvement with HL is rare; if involved, it should be evaluated by MRI. Persons with neurologic findings should also undergo lumbar puncture with cytology.[88] Exploratory laparotomy, with or without splenectomy, was used frequently in the past, but is not used now because of associated morbidity and improved imaging.[88] Prognostic indicators include clinical stage, histologic type, tumor cell concentration and tumor burden, constitutional symptoms, and age of the individual.

The effectiveness of treatment is related to the age, sex, and general health of the individual; signs and symptoms; stage of the disease; blood test results; type of HL; and classification of the disease as recurrent or progressive. HL in adults usually can be cured with early diagnosis and treatment. Treatment approaches include chemotherapy and radiation options. Radiation therapy alone is almost never used to treat individuals newly diagnosed with early favorable disease.[90] When mediastinal radiation will encompass the left side of the heart or will increase breast cancer risk in young female patients, proton therapy may be considered to reduce the radiation dose to organs at risk. When used as a single modality, radiation therapy is delivered to the neck, chest, and axilla (mantle field) and then to an abdominal field to treat para-aortic nodes and the spleen (splenic pedicle). In some individuals, pelvic nodes are treated with a third field. The three fields constitute *total nodal radiation therapy*.[90] Treatment for pregnant women includes watchful waiting and steroid therapy. Treatment with chemotherapy or radiation therapy, or both, may increase the risk of second cancers, cardiovascular disease, and other health problems for many months or years after treatment. The National Cancer Institute has developed tables to assist with understanding the treatment options. Persons with HL who are older than 60 years may have more treatment-related morbidity and mortality.

Non-Hodgkin Lymphomas

Non-Hodgkin lymphomas (NHLs) are a heterogeneous group of lymphoid tissue neoplasms with differing biologic and clinical

TABLE 29.9 Lugano Classification for Staging Lymphomas (Derived from Ann Arbor Staging With Cotswolds Modifications)

Stage I—Involvement of a single lymph node region (e.g., cervical, axillary, inguinal, mediastinal) or lymphoid structure such as the spleen, thymus, or Waldeyer ring.
Stage II—Involvement of 2 or more lymph node regions or lymph node structures on the same side of the diaphragm. Hilar nodes should be considered to be "lateralized" and when involved on both sides, constitute stage II disease. For the purpose of defining the number of anatomic regions, all nodal disease within the mediastinum is considered to be a single lymph node region, and hilar involvement constitutes an additional site of involvement. The number of anatomic regions should be indicated by a subscript (e.g., II-3).
Stage III—Involvement of lymph node regions or lymphoid structures on both sides of the diaphragm. This may be subdivided to stage III.1 or 111.2: stage III.1 is used for persons with involvement of the spleen or splenic hilar, celiac, or portal nodes; and stage III.2 is used for those with involvement of the paraaortic, iliac, inguinal, or mesenteric nodes.
Stage IV—Diffuse or disseminated involvement of 1 or more extranodal organs or tissue beyond that designated "E," with or without associated lymph node involvement.
All cases are subclassified to indicate the absence (A) or presence (B) of the systemic symptoms of significant unexplained fever, night sweats, or unexplained weight loss exceeding 10% of body weight during the 6 months prior to diagnosis.
The designation "E" refers to extranodal contiguous extension (i.e., proximal or contiguous extranodal disease) that can be encompassed within an irradiation field appropriate for nodal disease of the same anatomic extent. More extensive extranodal disease is designated stage IV.
Bulky disease: A single nodal mass, in contrast to multiple smaller nodes, of 10 cm or ≥ {1/3} of the transthoracic diameter at any level of thoracic vertebrae as determined by CT; record the longest measurement by CT scan. The term T (used in the Ann Arbor staging system) is no longer necessary.
The subscript "RS" is used to designate the stage at the time of relapse.

CT, Computed tomography.
From National Comprehensive Cancer Network: Hodgkin lymphoma. In NCCN practice guidelines, Version 2.2014: Hodgkin lymphoma (originally adapted from Carbono PP et al: Cancer Res 31[11]:1860–1861, 1971.

patterns of activity and responses to treatment. For unknown reasons, NHL incidence rates increased worldwide from 1950 to 2000, tripling in adults older than 65 years of age.[91,92] The previously used generic classification of NHL has been reclassified in the WHO/REAL scheme into (1) B-cell neoplasms, which include a variety of lymphomas and myelomas that originate from B cells at various stages of differentiation; and (2) T-cell and NK-cell neoplasms, which include lymphomas that originate from either T or NK cells. These cancers are differentiated from HL by lack of HRS cells and other cellular changes not characteristic of HL.

More than 81,560 new cases of NHL and 20,720 deaths are estimated for 2021.[42] The median age of diagnosis is 67 years, with a higher occurrence in men than women. Gene changes related to NHL are usually acquired during life and not inherited. However, having a family history of lymphoma (HL, NHL, CLL) does seem to increase the risk of lymphoma.[42] The highest incidences are in North America, Europe, Oceania, and several African countries. Part of the increased incidence has been attributed to diagnostic improvements as well as AIDS-related cancers after the HIV epidemic. Conversely, the mortality has risen at a slower rate. It is thought that newer treatment modalities are improving survival rates.

Risk factors for adult NHL include being older, male, or white and having one of the following: immunosuppression (e.g., HIV/AIDS, organ transplantation), viruses and other pathogens (EBV, HTLV, HHV8, Hepatitis C, SV40, and *H. pylori*), autoimmune and chronic inflammatory disorders (rheumatoid arthritis, Sjogren syndrome, celiac, and SLE), occupational exposure (pesticides like phenoxy acids, organophosphates, and organochlorines).[93]

Pathophysiology. NHL is a progressive clonal expansion of B cells, T cells, or NK cells. B cells account for 85% to 90% of NHLs, with most of the remainder being T cells and rarely NK cells. A very small percentage originates from macrophages. The key pathogenic mechanisms include immunosuppression, especially in relation to T-cell function and loss of control of latent EBV infection, and chronic antigen stimulation[93] as above. Chronic antigenic stimulation increases B-cell proliferation, which can lead to random genetic mistakes, particularly immunoglobulin gene rearrangements. Immunosuppression in a variety of medical conditions increases the risk of NHL. For example, dysregulation or suppression of T-cell function occurs with HIV/AIDS and organ transplantation, which promotes EBV driven B-cell proliferation and transformation.[93] Oncogenes may be activated by chromosomal translocations or the tumor-suppressor loci may be inactivated by deletion or mutation of chromosomes. Certain subtypes may have altered genomes by oncogenic viruses. Infections are characterized by their pathogenic effects and include those that directly transform lymphocytes (e.g., HTLV1, HIV, EBV [particularly in parts of Africa for BL], HHV8), infections that weaken the immune system (e.g., HIV), and infections that cause chronic immune stimulation (e.g., *H. pylori*, *Chlamydophilia psittaci*, *Campylobacter jejuni*, hepatitis C).[94] Various subtypes of NHL are identified by specific diagnostic markers related to various cytogenetic lesions. The most common type of chromosomal alteration in NHL is translocation, which disrupts the genes encoded at the breakpoints. Unlike HL, NHL spreads in a less predictable way and spreads widely early.

Clinical Manifestations. Clinical manifestations of NHL usually begin as localized or generalized lymphadenopathy, similar to HL. Differences in clinical features are noted in Table 29.10. The cervical, axillary, inguinal, and femoral lymph node chains are the most affected sites. Generally, the swelling is painless, and the nodes have enlarged and transformed over a period of months or years. Other sites of involvement are the nasopharynx, GI tract, bone, thyroid, testes, and soft tissue.

TABLE 29.10 Clinical Differences Between Non-Hodgkin Lymphoma and Hodgkin Lymphoma

Characteristics	Non-Hodgkin Lymphoma	Hodgkin Lymphoma
Nodal involvement	Multiple peripheral nodes	Localized to single axial group of nodes (i.e., cervical, mediastinal, paraaortic)
	Mesenteric nodes and Waldeyer ring commonly involved	Mesenteric nodes and Waldeyer ring rarely involved
Spread	Noncontiguous	Orderly spread by contiguity
B symptoms[a]	Uncommon	Common
Extranodal involvement	Common	Rare
Extent of disease	Rarely localized	Often localized

[a]Fever, weight loss, night sweats.

EMERGING SCIENCE BOX

Immunotherapy

Immunotherapy can stimulate or direct an individual's own immune system to target cancer cells. Several types of drugs, biologic, and cellular therapies can activate or suppress specific immune responses. Examples include immune checkpoint inhibitors ([ICIs], e.g., CTLA-4, PD-1, or PD-L1 antibodies), cytokines, immunomodulating agents (e.g., lenalidomide), monoclonal antibodies to tumor antigens (e.g., CD26), cancer vaccines based on tumor-mutated antigens (neo-antigens), oncolytic viruses (OVs), adoptive cell transfer (ACT), and chimeric antigen receptor (CAR) T-cell therapies. Immunotherapies have the potential to induce durable responses and even in some cases cure persons with certain forms of cancer that previously had extremely poor prognosis such as metastatic melanoma. Some of these approaches have therapeutic potential across many forms of cancer, while others are highly specific to a molecular subtype. Genomic sequencing or other precision oncology approaches are used to identify alterations in a person's cancer amenable to targeted or personalized therapies. Other approaches include harvesting a person's immune cells and engineering them to recognize the person's cancer cells via gene therapy and genome editing. Key opportunities include identifying predictive biomarkers of response, while challenges for immunotherapies include navigating unique toxicities (e.g., immune-related adverse events) and ensuring equitable access, given the unprecedented financial burden associated with many of these treatments.

Data from Albertini MR. The age of enlightenment in melanoma immunotherapy. *Journal for ImmunoTherapy of Cancer*, 2018;6(1):80. Published 2018 Aug 22. doi:10.1186/s40425-018-0397-8; Riley RS, et al. Delivery technologies for cancer immunotherapy. *Nature Reviews Drug Discovery*, 2019;18(3):175–196. doi:10.1038/s41573-018-0006-z; Sanmamed MF, et al. A paradigm shift in cancer immunotherapy: from enhancement to normalization. *Cell*, 2018;175(2):313–326. doi:10.1016/j.cell.2018.09.035; Velcheti V, et al. Basic overview of current immunotherapy approaches in cancer. *American Society of Clinical Oncology Educational Book*, 2016;35:298–308. doi:10.1200/EDBK_156572; Yang Y. Cancer immunotherapy: Harnessing the immune system to battle cancer. *Journal of Clinical Investigation*, 2015;125(9):3335–3337. doi:10.1172/JCI83871.

Some individuals have retroperitoneal and abdominal masses with symptoms of abdominal fullness, back pain, ascites (fluid in the peritoneal cavity), skin rash or itchy skin, fatigue, fever of unknown origin, drenching night sweats, and leg swelling.

Lymphomas are classified as low, intermediate, or high grade. A low-grade lymphoma, which also may be termed *indolent*, has a slow progression. Individuals with low-grade lymphoma commonly present with a painless, peripheral adenopathy. Spontaneous regression of these nodes may occur, mimicking the presence of an infection. Night sweats with an elevated temperature (more than 38°C [100.4°F]) and weight loss, as well as extra nodular involvement, are not commonly present in the early stages but are common in advanced or end-stage disease. *Cytopenia*, or reduction in the number of blood cells, reflective of bone marrow involvement is often observed. Hepatomegaly is common; splenomegaly is present in approximately 40% of individuals. Fatigue and weakness are more prevalent with advanced stages.

Intermediate and high-grade lymphomas, which are more aggressive, have a more varied clinical presentation. A high-grade lymphoma also may be termed *aggressive*.

Evaluation and Treatment. The primary means for diagnosis of NHL is biopsy. A common finding in NHL is noncontiguous lymph node involvement, which is not common in HL. Staging is determined from physical exam, blood tests, radiologic studies (PET and CT), biopsy, and examination of bone marrow aspirate (often, but not always done).

Treatment for NHL is quite diverse and depends on type (B cell or T cell), tumor stage, histologic status (low, intermediate, or high grade), symptoms, age, and presence of comorbidities. Depending on the type (B cell or T cell) of the tumor, stage of disease, and aggressiveness of the tumor, treatment is usually initiated at the time of diagnosis. However, because treatment is not curative for some low-grade indolent lymphomas that are widely disseminated, observation without treatment may be the most appropriate choice. These indolent tumors are often not symptomatic for the individual, and this approach improves quality of life. In some individuals the disease may be so slow growing that treatment is not needed for an extended period.

Treatment with chemotherapy alone may be adequate for many individuals, although radiation therapy is often included. Low-dose chemotherapy has been followed by autologous SCT in some NHLs or for recurrent disease. Immunotherapies are emerging (see Emerging Science Box: Immunotherapy). Treatment using monoclonal antibody alone or in combination with radiation therapy (radioimmunotherapy) also is being used. Rituximab-based chemoimmunotherapy has improved the response and survival of people with follicular lymphoma.[95]

Individuals with NHL can survive for extended periods. A partial remission may be achieved in some cases in which evidence of the disease remains, but the disease does not progress. Survival with nodular lymphoma ranges up to 15 years, but those with diffuse disease generally do not survive as long. Overall, the survival rates of NHL are less than those for HL. Survival rates for NHL with modern treatment are over 60% at 5 years.

Burkitt leukemia/lymphoma adult. Burkitt lymphoma is a B-cell NHL with unique clinical and epidemiologic features. It is highly aggressive and is the fastest growing human tumor.

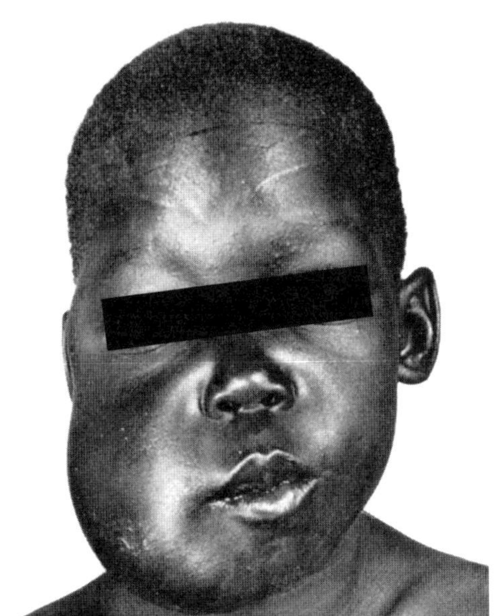

Fig. 29.25 **Burkitt Lymphoma.** Burkitt lymphoma involving the jaw in a young African boy. (Courtesy I. Magrath MD, Bethesda MD. From Zitelli BJ, et al. *Zitelli and Davis' atlas of pediatric physical diagnosis*, 6th edition. Philadelphia: Saunders; 2012.)

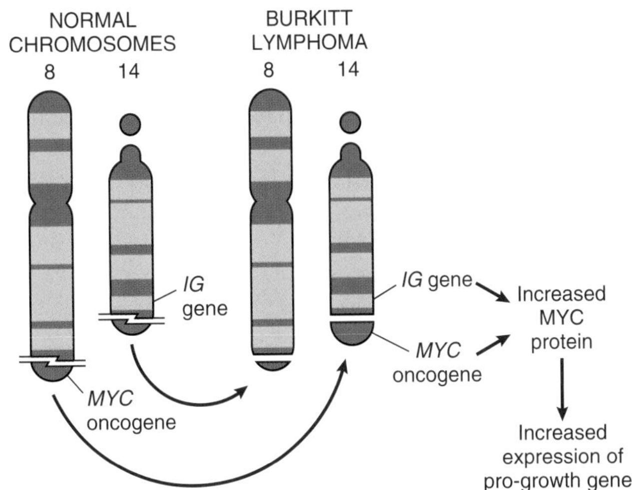

Fig. 29.26 **Burkitt Lymphoma Cells.** The 8,14 chromosomal translocation and associated oncogenes in Burkitt lymphoma.

It is derived from germinal or post-germinal center B cells.[96] There are three main types of BL: endemic, nonendemic, and immunodeficiency related. *Endemic* BL commonly occurs in Africa and is linked to the EBV, and *nonendemic* BL occurs worldwide. *Immunodeficiency-related* BL is most often seen in individuals with AIDS. BL occurs most often in children and young adults (see Chapter 30). Endemic cases, usually from Africa, involve a rapidly growing tumor of the jaw and facial bones (Fig. 29.25). In the United States, BL is rare, usually involves the abdomen, and is characterized by extensive bone marrow invasion and replacement. BL and Burkitt leukemia are classified as different manifestations of the same disease.[97] With advances in diagnostic criteria, many older studies included a heterogenous patient population that contained those who today would not be diagnosed with BL by current criteria.[96,97]

Pathophysiology. The different clinical subtypes of BL (e.g., endemic, nonendemic, and immunodeficiency related) probably arise from B cells at different stages of development.[96,97] Virtually all cases of BL are associated with chronic EBV infection. Perhaps suppression of the immune system by other illnesses (e.g., HIV infection, chronic malaria) increases the individual's susceptibility to EBV. B cells are particularly sensitive because of specific surface receptors for EBV. As a result, the B cell undergoes chromosomal translocations that result in overexpression of the myelocytomatosis (*c*-MYC) proto-oncogene and loss of control of cell growth (Fig. 29.26). The most common translocation (75% of individuals) is between chromosomes 8 (containing the *c-MYC* gene) and 14 (containing the immunoglobulin heavy chain genes). Other translocations have been reported between chromosome 8 and chromosomes 2 or 22, which contain genes for immunoglobulin light chains.

Clinical Manifestations. In non-African BL the most common presentation is abdominal swelling. Manifestations of most tumors occur at extra nodal sites. More advanced disease may involve the eye, ovaries, kidneys, or glandular tissue (breast, thyroid, tonsils) and presents with type B symptoms (night sweats, fever, weight loss). Common manifestations may include nausea and vomiting; loss of appetite or change in bowel habits, or both; GI bleeding; symptoms of an acute abdominal condition; intestinal perforation; and renal failure.

Evaluation and Treatment. Usually indicative of BL is the presence of tumors in the jaw and facial bones, enlarged lymph nodes, and bone marrow containing malignant B cells. Laboratory studies include CBC, electrolytes, liver and renal function tests, lactate dehydrogenase (LDH), hepatitis B, HIV, and uric acid.[96,97] Treatment is aggressive multidrug regimens, such as combination chemotherapy. There is no role for radiation therapy in treatment of people with BL.[96,97]

Plasma Cell Malignancy

Multiple Myeloma

Multiple myeloma (MM) is a clonal plasma cell cancer characterized by the neoplastic proliferation of plasma cells producing a monoclonal immunoglobulin.[98] The plasma cells proliferate in the bone marrow (Fig. 29.27). These masses are associated with *lytic bone lesions* (round, punched-out regions of bone) (Fig. 29.28A and B). Uncommon variants include *solitary myeloma (plasmacytoma)* with a single mass in bone or soft tissue and *smoldering myeloma*, which is defined by a lack of symptoms and a high plasma abnormal antibody called the M protein.

Myeloma cells reside in the bone marrow and are usually not found in the peripheral blood. As the number of myeloma cells increases, fewer red blood cells, white blood cells, and platelets are produced. It may occasionally spread to other tissues, especially in very advanced stages of the disease. For unknown reasons, the reported incidence of MM has doubled in the past 2 decades. About 34,920 new cases and 12,410 deaths are estimated for 2021.[42] MM occurs in all races, but the incidence in blacks is about twice that of whites. It rarely occurs before the age of 40 years—the median age of diagnosis is between 65 and 74 years. It is slightly more common in men (7.7 estimated new cases per 100,000 persons) than in women (4.9 new cases per 100,000 persons). Other risk factors include overweight or obesity, Agent Orange, and a history of monoclonal gammopathy of undetermined significance (MGUS; see Clinical Manifestations) or plasmacytoma.[98] MM has been observed in some irradiated populations including Hiroshima and Nagasaki, where the relative risk increased with dose in males and females aged 20 to 59 at the time of bombing and was not apparent until 20 years later. No excess risk of MM was evident in 150,000 women who were followed for more than 15 years after radiation therapy for carcinoma of the uterine cervix.[99]

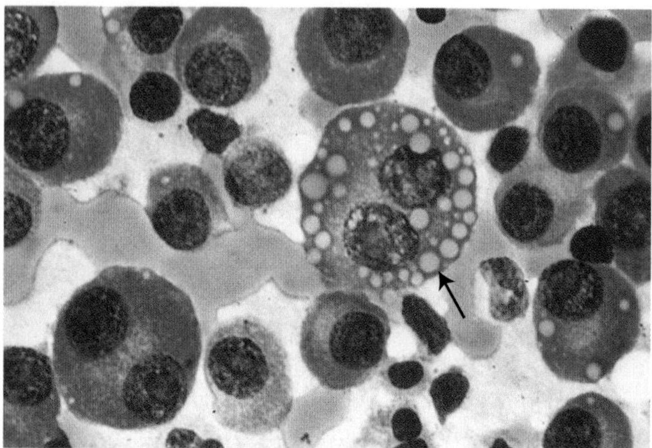

Fig. 29.27 Multiple Myeloma, Bone Marrow Aspirate. Normal marrow cells are largely replaced by plasma cells, including atypical forms with multiple nuclei *(arrow)*, and cytoplasmic droplets *containing* immunoglobulin. (From Kumar V, et al. *Robbins and Cotran pathologic basis of disease*, 9th edition. Philadelphia: Saunders; 2015.)

Pathophysiology. MM is a plasma cell neoplasia that causes lytic bone lesions (bony disease; radiologically appears as punched-out defects), hypercalcemia, renal failure, anemia, and immune abnormalities. It is a biologically complex disease with significant heterogeneity (wide range of genetic abnormalities, differences in clinical response, and survival in those with the same treatment). Multiple mutations in different pathways alter the intrinsic biology of the plasma cell, generating the features of myeloma. Although some steps in these pathways are identified, many are unknown.[98] Defining the main, or driver, mutations and heterogeneity is essential for treatment decisions. Many myelomas are aneuploid and, in most individuals with myeloma, chromosomal translocations are the most common. Development of further secondary genetic alterations increases progression to an aggressive MM. Investigators are studying various epigenetic alterations and interactions with extracellular matrix proteins. For example, myeloma cells interact and secrete peptides that adhere to stromal cells, inducing cytokines that promote inflammation. Myeloma cells are prone to the accumulation of misfolded protein, such as unpaired immunoglobulin chains. Misfolded proteins activate apoptosis.

Malignant plasma cells arise from one clone of B cells that produce abnormally large amounts of one class of immunoglobulin (usually IgG, occasionally IgA, and rarely IgM, IgD, or IgE). The malignant transformation may begin early in B-cell development, possibly before encountering antigen in the secondary lymphoid organs. The myeloma cells return either to the bone marrow or to other soft tissue sites. Cytokines, particularly IL-6, have been identified as essential factors that promote the growth and survival of MM cells (lymphocytes and cytokines are described in Chapters 7 and 8). IL-6 in particular acts as an osteoclast-activating factor and stimulates osteoclasts to reabsorb bone. This process results

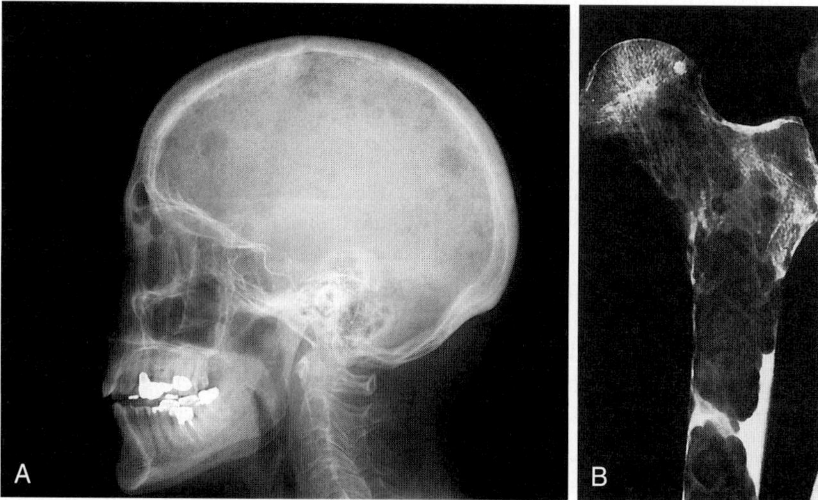

Fig. 29.28 Osteolytic Lesions in Individuals With Multiple Myeloma. (A) Radiograph showing skull lesions in a client with myeloma. **(B)** Radiograph of femur showing extensive bone destruction caused by tumor. Note absence of reactive bone formation. (A, From *Abeloff M, et al. Abeloff's clinical oncology*, 4th edition. Philadelphia: Churchill Livingstone; 2008. B, From Kissane JM, ed. *Anderson's pathology*, 9th edition. St. Louis: Mosby; 1990.)

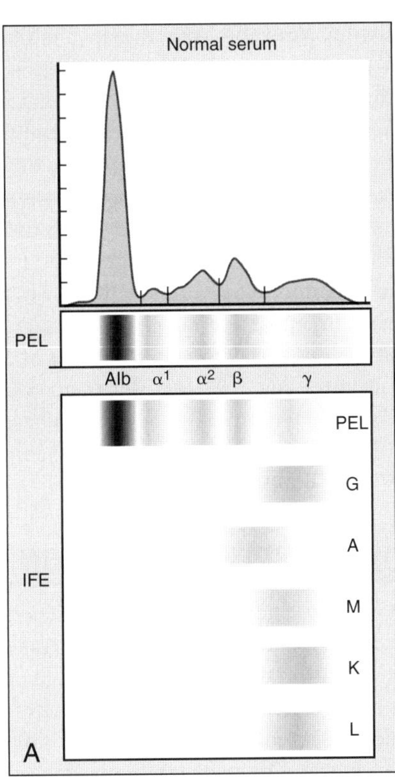

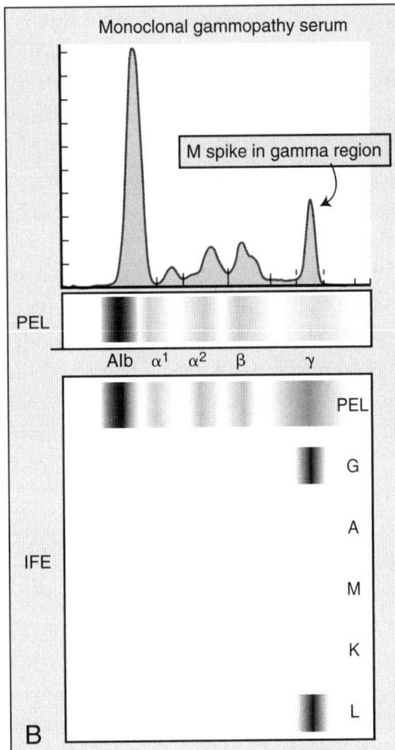

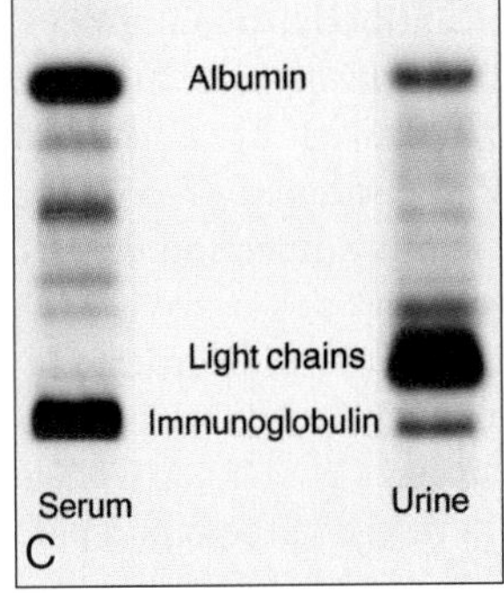

Fig. 29.29 M Protein. Serum protein electrophoresis *(PEL)* is used to screen for M proteins in multiple myeloma (MM). **(A)** In normal serum the proteins separate into several regions between albumin *(Alb)* and a broad band in the gamma *(γ)* region, where most antibodies (gamma globulins) are found. Immunofixation *(IFE)* can identify the location of IgG *(G)*, IgA *(A)*, IgM *(M)*, and kappa *(κ)*, and lambda *(λ)* light chains. **(B)** Serum from an individual with MM contains a sharp M protein *(M spike)*. The M protein is monoclonal and contains only one heavy chain and one light chain. In this instance the IFE identifies the M protein as an IgG containing a lambda light chain. **(C)** Serum and urine protein electrophoretic patterns in an individual with MM. Serum demonstrates an M protein *(Immunoglobulin)* in the gamma region, and the urine has a large amount of the smaller sized light chains with only a small amount of the intact immunoglobulin. (A and B, From Abeloff M, et al. *Abeloff's clinical oncology*, 4th edition. Philadelphia: Churchill Livingstone; 2008. C, From McPherson R, Pincus M. *Henry's clinical diagnosis and management by laboratory methods*, 22nd edition. Edinburgh: Saunders; 2012.)

in bone lesions and hypercalcemia (high calcium levels in the blood) attributable to the release of calcium from the breakdown of bone.

The antibody produced by the transformed plasma cell is frequently defective, containing truncations, deletions, and other abnormalities, and is often referred to as a *paraprotein* (abnormal protein in the blood). Because of the large number of malignant plasma cells, the abnormal antibody, or M protein, becomes the most prominent protein in the blood (Fig. 29.29). Suppression of normal plasma cells by the myeloma results in diminished or absent normal antibodies. The excessive amount of M protein also may contribute to many of the clinical manifestations of the disease. Frequently, the myeloma produces free immunoglobulin light chain (Bence Jones protein) that is present in the blood and urine and contributes to damage of renal tubular cells.

Clinical Manifestations. MM is characterized by elevated levels of calcium in the blood (hypercalcemia), renal failure, anemia, and bone lesions. The hypercalcemia and bone lesions result from infiltration of the bone by malignant plasma cells and stimulation of osteoclasts to reabsorb bone. This process results in the release of calcium (hypercalcemia) and the development of lytic lesions of bone (see Fig. 29.28A and B). Destruction of bone tissue causes pain, the most common presenting symptom, and pathologic fractures. The bones most involved, in decreasing order of frequency, are the vertebrae, ribs, skull, pelvis, femur, clavicle, and scapula. Spinal cord compression, because of the weakened vertebrae, occurs in about 10% of individuals.

A condition called amyloidosis may occur, in which antibody proteins increase and stick together in peripheral nerves and organs, such as the kidney and heart. Signs and symptoms of amyloidosis include fatigue, purple spots on the skin, enlarged tongue, diarrhea, edema, and numbness or tingling in the legs and feet.

Proteinuria is observed in 90% of individuals. Renal failure may be either acute or chronic and is usually secondary to the hypercalcemia. Bence Jones protein may lead to damage of the proximal tubules. Anemia is usually normocytic and normochromic and results from inhibited erythropoiesis caused by tumor cell infiltration of the bone marrow.

The high concentration of paraprotein in the blood may lead to hyperviscosity syndrome. The increased viscosity interferes with blood circulation to various sites (brain, kidneys, extremities). Hyperviscosity syndrome is observed in up to 20% of persons. Additional neurologic symptoms (e.g., confusion, headaches, blurred vision) may occur secondary to hypercalcemia or hyperviscosity.

Suppression of the humoral (antibody-mediated) immune response results in repeated infections, primarily pneumonias, and pyelonephritis. The most involved microorganisms are encapsulated bacteria that are particularly sensitive to the effects of antibody; pneumonia caused by *Streptococcus pneumoniae, Staphylococcus aureus*, or *K. pneumoniae;* or pyelonephritis caused by *E. coli* or other gram-negative organisms. Cell-mediated (T-cell) function is relatively normal. Overwhelming infection is the leading cause of death from MM.

MM is a progressive disorder and is often preceded by a condition known as monoclonal gammopathy of undetermined significance (MGUS). MGUS is diagnosed by the presence of an M protein in the blood or urine without additional evidence of MM.[100] MGUS is present in approximately 1% of the general population and in 3% of individuals older than 70 years. Although MGUS is considered a benign condition and requires no treatment, *about 1% of individuals with MGUS progress to malignant plasma cell disorders.*[16] Progression of MM after MGUS advances to asymptomatic MM and finally symptomatic MM. Asymptomatic MM also may be referred to as smoldering myeloma. Smoldering myeloma is usually characterized by the presence of an M protein and clonal bone marrow plasma cells, but with no indication of end-organ damage.

Evaluation and Treatment. Diagnosis of MM is made by symptoms and radiographic and laboratory studies; a definitive diagnosis requires a bone marrow biopsy. The International Myeloma Working Group's new criteria for the diagnosis of MM and smoldering MM are presented in Box 29.2. Several types of radiologic studies document the presence of bone lesions and areas of destruction. Optimal use of imaging methods is provided by the International Myeloma Working Group for imaging at different stages.[101] Quantitative measurements of immunoglobulins (IgG, IgM, IgA) are usually done, and serum electrophoretic analysis reveals increased levels of M protein. Bence Jones protein may be observed in the urine or serum by immunoelectrophoresis, or in the serum using available enzyme-linked immunosorbent assays (ELISAs). However, variants of MM include individuals in which only free light chain is produced and a rare variant that produces only free heavy chain; about 1% of cases are non-secretory so that neither M protein nor Bence Jones protein is produced. Measurement of another protein, free β2-microglobulin, is used as an indicator of prognosis or effectiveness of therapy.

Treatment options include combinations of chemotherapy; other drug therapy; targeted therapy; high-dose chemotherapy with stem cell transplant; biologic therapy; radiation therapy (bone lesions of the spine); and, sometimes, surgery. New therapies, called *proteasome inhibitors*, are emerging. Dose intensification improves outcomes in younger persons; however, long-term remissions occur in a minority of people. Gene expression profiling (GEP) helps improve the treatment of MM because it identifies prognostic subgroups and defines the molecular pathways associated with these subgroups. Newer agents (e.g., bortezomib, lenalidomide) have expanded therapeutic regimens for end-stage myeloma. Preliminary results show lenalidomide may delay the development of MM in those with smoldering myeloma.[102,103] The 5-year survival rate for all stages of MM is 54%.[43] Approval of new drugs has changed the management of MM, and research for survival improvement is ongoing.

ALTERATIONS OF SPLENIC FUNCTION

The complexities of splenic function are not totally understood, and its mysteries are still being studied. The normal functions of the spleen that may affect disease states include (1) phagocytosis of blood cells and particulate matter (e.g., bacteria), (2) antibody production, (3) hematopoiesis, and (4) sequestration of formed blood elements. The spleen is known as a *secondary lymphoid organ* and is the site for maturation and storage of T and B lymphocytes playing a role in the synthesis of IgG.[104] The spleen is part of the mononuclear phagocyte system and is involved in all systemic inflammations, hematopoietic disorders, and many metabolic disorders.

In the past, splenomegaly (enlargement of the spleen) has been associated with various disease states. It is now recognized that splenomegaly is not necessarily pathologic; an enlarged spleen may be present in certain individuals without any evidence of disease. Splenomegaly may be, however, one of the first physical signs of underlying conditions, and its presence should not be ignored. In conditions in which splenomegaly is present, the normal functions of the spleen may become overactive, producing a syndrome known as hypersplenism.

Current criteria indicating the presence of hypersplenism include (1) cytopenias (anemia, leukopenia, thrombocytopenia, or combinations of these), (2) cellular bone marrow, (3) splenomegaly, and (4) improvement after splenectomy. Some individuals may seek treatment for problems even though they have not met all these clinical criteria; thus, the relevance and significance of hypersplenism are still uncertain. Primary hypersplenism is recognized when no etiologic factor has been identified; secondary hypersplenism occurs in the presence of another condition.

Pathophysiology. Specific conditions causing splenomegaly and resulting hypersplenism are many (Box 29.3). Different pathologic processes that produce splenomegaly are described briefly.

Acute inflammatory or infectious processes cause splenomegaly because of an increased demand for defensive activities. An acutely enlarged spleen secondary to infection may become so filled with erythrocytes that their natural rubbery resilience is lost, and they become fragile and vulnerable to blunt trauma.

BOX 29.3 Disorders Associated With Splenomegaly Infections

Nonspecific splenitis of various blood-borne infections (particularly infectious endocarditis)
- Infectious mononucleosis
- Tuberculosis
- Typhoid fever
- Brucellosis
- Cytomegalovirus
- Syphilis
- Malaria
- Histoplasmosis
- Toxoplasmosis
- Kala-azar
- Trypanosomiasis
- Schistosomiasis
- Leishmaniasis
- Echinococcosis

Congestive states related to portal hypertension
- Cirrhosis of the liver
- Portal or splenic vein thrombosis
- Cardiac failure

From Kumar V, Abbas A, Aster J. *Robbins & Cotran pathologic basis of disease*, 10th edition. Philadelphia: Elsevier; 2021.

Splenic rupture is a complication associated with IM; rupture occurs mostly in males between days 4 and 21 of acute illness.

Congestive splenomegaly is accompanied by ascites, portal hypertension, and esophageal varices and is most seen in those with hepatic cirrhosis. Splenic hyperplasia develops in disorders that increase splenic workload and is associated most with various types of anemia (hemolytic) and chronic myeloproliferative disorders (i.e., polycythemia vera).

Infiltrative splenomegaly is caused by engorgement by the macrophages with indigestible materials associated with various "storage diseases." Tumors and cysts cause actual growth of the spleen. Neoplastic involvement of the spleen is rare except in myeloid and lymphoid tumors.[16]

Clinical Manifestations. The most common physical symptom is vague abdominal discomfort.[104] Abdominal bloating, distended abdomen, anorexia, and/or early satiety may occur.[104] Those individuals with acute infection may present with fever, rigors, malaise, and focal infectious symptoms. Cirrhosis is the main cause of congestive splenomegaly; other causes include, for example, hepatitis. Other symptoms include those from anemia (lightheadedness and dyspnea), easy bruising, bleeding, or petechiae.[104] Overactivity of the spleen results in hematologic alterations that affect all blood components. Sequestering of red blood cells, granulocytes, and platelets results in a reduction of all circulating blood cells. The spleen may sequester up to 50% of the red blood cell population, thereby upsetting the normal physiologic concentration of red blood cells in the circulation. The rate of splenic pooling is directly related to spleen size and the degree of increased blood flow through it. Sequestering exposes the red blood cells to splenic conditions that accelerate destruction, further contributing to the decreased red blood cell concentration. Anemia is the result of these combined activities. Anemia may be further potentiated by an increase in blood volume, which produces a *dilutional effect* on the already reduced concentration of red blood cells. The dilutional effect, as well as the removal and destruction of red blood cells, depends primarily on the degree of splenomegaly.

White blood cells and platelets also are affected by sequestering, although not to the same degree as the red blood cell. Again, the size of the spleen is the determining factor in the number of cells sequestered.

Evaluation and Treatment. Treatment of splenomegaly is targeted at treating the underlying disease and protecting individuals from complications of splenomegaly itself. Splenic rupture is a serious and feared complication of splenomegaly.[104] Treatment includes splenectomy; however, it may not always be indicated. A splenectomy is considered necessary to alleviate the destructive effects on red blood cells. Clinical indicators should determine the need for splenectomy, not necessarily specific conditions. Splenectomy for splenic rupture is no longer considered mandatory because of the possibility of overwhelming sepsis after removal. Repair and preservation are now considered before the decision to remove the spleen. Splenectomy also may be performed as treatment for hairy cell leukemia, Felty syndrome, agnogenic myeloid metaplasia, thalassemia major, Gaucher disease, hemodialysis, splenomegaly, splenic venous thrombosis, and thrombotic thrombocytopenia purpura (TTP).

Individuals are able to lead normal lives after splenectomy, but blood cell abnormalities often exist after removal of the spleen (i.e., red blood cells become thinner, broader, and wrinkled; white blood cell counts initially increase and then plateau; platelet counts rise after surgery and then stabilize). A major postoperative complication after splenectomy is *overwhelming post-splenectomy infection (OPSI)*. It is a rare but rapidly fatal infection. Unless treated in time, OPSI may rapidly progress to septic shock and possibly disseminated intravascular coagulation (DIC). OPSI can be prevented by educating patients, vaccination, and antibiotic prophylaxis.[105]

HEMORRHAGIC DISORDERS AND ALTERATIONS OF PLATELETS AND COAGULATION

The arrest of bleeding, or hemostasis, depends on adequate numbers of platelets, normal levels of coagulation factors, and absence of defects in vessels walls. The spectrum of abnormal bleeding varies widely from massive bleeds, such as rupture of large vessels like the aorta, to small bleeds in skin or mucosal membranes. Diminished or excessive levels of coagulation factors can lead to defective hemostasis or spontaneous and unnecessary clotting. (Hemostasis is discussed in Chapter 28.) Diminished hemostasis results in either internal or external hemorrhage, defined as copious or heavy discharge of blood from blood vessels. A classification of hemorrhagic disorders is included in Table 29.11.

Purpuric disorders, red or purple discolored spots on skin, occur when there is a deficiency of normal platelets necessary to plug damaged vessels or prevent leakage from the tiny tears

TABLE 29.11 Classification of Hemorrhagic Disorders

Type of Defect	Example	Manifestation
Defects of primary hemostasis	Platelet defects or von Willebrand disease	Usually present with small bleeds in skin or mucosal membrane; bleeds are usually petechiae (<3-mm min hemorrhages) or purpuras (>3-mm red-purple discolorations); common in capillaries; also includes epistaxis (nose bleeds), GI bleeds, or excessive menstruation
Defects of secondary hemostasis	Coagulation factor defects	Bleeds into soft tissue, muscle, or joints; intracranial bleeds may occur
Generalized defects of small vessels	Palpable purpura and ecchymoses	Extravasated blood creates a palpable mass (or palpable purpura), ecchymoses (simply called a *bruise*), or a larger palpable lesion (or hematoma); systemic disorders disrupt small blood vessels, called vasculitis

that occur daily in capillaries. More serious internal bleeding occurs from events that simply overwhelm hemostatic mechanisms, such as rupture of large blood vessels, trauma, and diseases associated with massive hemorrhage including abdominal aneurysm (also see the Anemias of Blood Loss section). Between these smaller bleeds and massive bleeds are deficiencies of coagulation factors found with the hemophilias (see Chapter 30). Disorders that result in spontaneous clotting can develop from genetic disorders of the clotting system components or from acquired diseases that activate clotting. These disorders are known collectively as thromboembolic disease. Additionally, any disorder of the blood that predisposes to clotting of blood or thrombosis is called hypercoagulability (thrombophilia).

Disorders of Platelets

Quantitative or qualitative abnormalities of platelets can interrupt normal blood coagulation and prevent hemostasis. The quantitative abnormalities are *thrombocytopenia*, a decrease in the number of circulating platelets, and *thrombocythemia*, an increase in the number of platelets. Qualitative disorders affect the structure or function of individual platelets and can coexist with the quantitative disorders. Qualitative disorders usually prevent platelet adherence and aggregation, preventing formation of a platelet plug.

Thrombocytopenia

Thrombocytopenia is defined as a platelet count less than 150,000 platelets/μL of blood.[106] Hemorrhage associated with minor trauma does not appreciably increase until the count falls below 50,000 platelets/μL. Spontaneous bleeding without trauma can occur with counts ranging from less than 10,000 platelets /μL to less than 20,000/μL and surgical bleeding with counts below 50,000/μL.[107] Counts less than 10,000 platelets/μL can result in skin manifestations (e.g., petechiae, ecchymoses, and larger purpuric spots) or frank bleeding from mucous membranes. Severe

BOX 29.4 Common Causes of Thrombocytopenia

Primary immune thrombocytopenia (primary ITP)

- Drug-induced immune thrombocytopenia:
  - Heparin-induced thrombocytopenia (HIT)
  - Quinine
  - Sulfonamides, ampicillin, vancomycin, piperacillin
  - Acetaminophen, ibuprofen, naproxen
  - Cimetidine
  - Glycoprotein IIb/IIIa inhibitors
  - Other over the counter remedies, supplements, foods like African bean, sesame seeds, walnuts, and beverages (herbal teas and cranberry juice)
- Drug-induced non-immune thrombocytopenia. Valproic acid, daptomycin, linezolid cause thrombocytopenia by dose-dependent suppression of platelet production.
- Infections:
  - Viral: HIV, hepatitis C, Epstein-Barr virus, parvovirus, mumps, varicella, rubella, Zika viral infections
  - Sepsis causes bone marrow suppression.
  - Helicobacter pylori
  - Leptospirosis, brucellosis, anaplasmosis, and other tick-borne infections are associated with thrombocytopenia.
  - Malaria, babesiosis intracellular parasite infections are associated with both thrombocytopenia and hemolytic anemia
- Hypersplenism due to chronic liver disease
- Chronic alcohol abuse
- Nutrient deficiencies (folate, vitamin B12, copper)
- Autoimmune disorders: systemic lupus erythematosus, rheumatoid arthritis
- Pregnancy. Mild thrombocytopenia presents in gestational thrombocytopenia; moderate-severe thrombocytopenia can occur in preeclampsia and HELLP (hemolysis, elevated liver enzymes, low platelet count) syndrome

Other Causes Include

- Myelodysplasia
- Malignancy: cancer with chronic DIC, cancer with marrow suppression (leukemia, lymphoma, solid tumors)
- Paroxysmal nocturnal hemoglobinuria (PNH)
- Thrombotic microangiopathy (TMA)
  - Thrombotic thrombocytopenic purpura (TTP)
  - A hemolytic uremic syndrome (HUS) caused by Shiga toxin-producing organism (E. coli and Shigella), seen in children.
  - Drug-induced TMA: quinine, specific chemotherapy agents
  - Antiphospholipid antibody syndrome
- Aplastic anemia
- Inherited thrombocytopenia. Often seen in children, rare in adults
  - Von Willebrand disease type 2
  - Alport syndrome
  - Wiskott-Aldrich syndrome
  - Fanconi syndrome.
  - Thrombocytopenia-absent radius syndrome
  - Bernard–Soulier syndrome
  - May-Hegglin anomaly

Data from Jinna S, Khandhar PB. *Thrombocytopenia.* Treasure Island, FL: StatPearls Publishing; 2020.

spontaneous bleeding may result if the count is less than 10,000 platelets/μL and can be fatal if it occurs in the GI tract, respiratory tract, or CNS. Thrombocytopenia is associated with risk of thrombosis in conditions like heparin-induced thrombocytopenia (HIT), antiphospholipid antibody syndrome (APS), DIC, thrombotic microangiopathy (TMA), and paroxysmal nocturnal hemoglobinuria (PNH).[107] Common causes of thrombocytopenia are included in Box 29.4. Normal platelet counts vary by age, sex, and ethnicity. Women, young people, and non-Hispanic blacks have slightly higher platelet counts.[108]

Before the diagnosis of thrombocytopenia is made, pseudothrombocytopenia must be ruled out. This phenomenon occurs in approximately 1 in 1000 to 1 in 10,000 laboratory samples and results from an error in platelet counting when a blood sample is analyzed by an automated cell counter. Platelets in the blood sample may become nonspecifically agglutinated by immunoglobulins in the presence of ethylenediaminetetraacetic acid (EDTA), a preservative in banked blood. The agglutinated platelets are not counted, thus giving an apparent, but false, thrombocytopenia. Thrombocytopenia also may be falsely diagnosed because of a dilutional effect observed after massive transfusion of platelet-poor packed cells to treat a hemorrhage. This occurs when more than 10 units of blood have been transfused within a 24-hour period. The hemorrhage that necessitated the transfusion also accelerates the loss of platelets, contributing to the pseudothrombocytopenic state. Splenic sequestering of platelets in hypersplenism (congestive) also induces an apparent thrombocytopenia, as does hypothermia (less than 25°C [77°F]), which is reversed when temperatures return to normal, suggesting an increased platelet sequestration in response to chilling.

Pathophysiology. Thrombocytopenia results from decreased platelet production, increased destruction, or both. The condition may be either congenital or acquired and may be either primary or secondary to other acquired or congenital conditions. Thrombocytopenia secondary to congenital conditions occurs in many different diseases, although each is relatively rare.

Acquired thrombocytopenia is more common and may occur as a result of decreased platelet production secondary to viral infections (e.g., EBV, rubella, CMV, HIV), drugs (e.g., valproic acid, daptomycin, certain chemotherapeutic agents, chronic ethanol abuse), nutritional deficiencies (vitamin B_{12} or folic acid in particular), chronic renal failure, bone marrow suppression (e.g., AA), radiation therapy, or bone marrow infiltration by cancer. Most common forms of thrombocytopenia are the result of increased platelet destruction. Examples include HIT idiopathic (immune) TTP, TTP, and DIC (discussed in the Disorders of Coagulation section). The spleen can also hold on to too many platelets; it normally stores about one-third of the body's platelets.[106] Dilutional thrombocytopenia presents after massive fluid resuscitation and massive blood transfusion.[107]

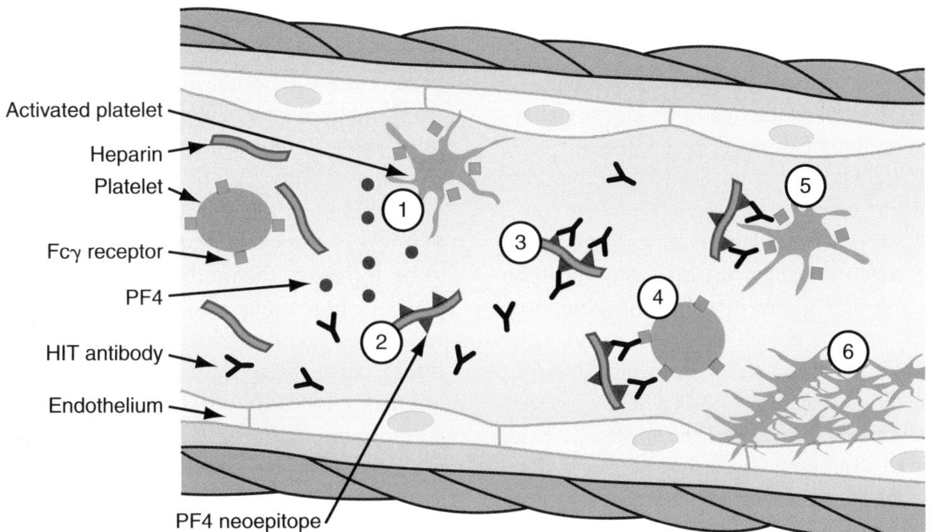

Fig. 29.30 Pathogenesis of Heparin Induced Thrombocytopenia (HIT). *(1)* Activated platelets release procoagulant proteins from α-granules, including platelet factor 4 (PF4). Administered heparin binds PF4 *(2)*, which undergoes a conformational change and expresses a new antigen (neoepitope). Individuals with HIT produce an immunoglobulin G (IgG) antibody that specifically reacts *(3)* with multiple identical neoepitopes on the heparin-PF4 complex. The reaction forms heparin-PF4-IgG immune complexes. Platelets express FcγRIIa receptors (Fcγ receptor) that react *(4)* with the Fc portion of IgG in immune complexes. Cross-linking of Fc receptors *(5)* results in FcγRIIa-dependent platelet activation. The activated platelets mediate a series of events that lead to further activation of the coagulation cascade, resulting in thrombin generation. Further release of PF4 from newly activated platelets leads to a cycle of continuing platelet activation and *(6)* formation of a primary clot. The reaction can be enhanced by the release of platelet-derived microparticles that are rich in surface phosphatidylserine and increase activation of coagulation and by the binding of heparin-PF4 complexes and HIT-IgG to the vascular endothelium (not shown).

Heparin-induced thrombocytopenia. Heparin is a common cause of drug-induced thrombocytopenia. Approximately 4% of individuals treated with unfractionated heparin develop HIT. The incidence is lower (about 0.1%) with the use of low-molecular-weight heparin. HIT is an immune-mediated, adverse drug reaction caused by IgG antibodies against the heparin–platelet factor 4 complex leading to platelet activation through platelet Fc γIIa receptors (Fig. 29.30) (see Chapter 9). The release of additional platelet factor 4 from activated platelets and activation of thrombin lead to increased platelet consumption and a decrease in platelet counts beginning 5 to 10 days after administration of heparin.

Clinical Manifestations. The hallmark of HIT is thrombocytopenia. A decrease of approximately 50% in the platelet count is observed in more than 95% of individuals. However, 30% or more of those with thrombocytopenia are also at risk for venous or arterial thrombosis because a *prothrombotic state* is caused by antibody binding to platelets, inducing activation, aggregation, and consumption (thus the term *thrombocytopenia* in the syndrome name) of platelets. Venous thrombosis is more common and results in DVT and pulmonary emboli. Arterial thrombosis affects the lower extremities, causing limb ischemia. Arterial thrombosis may lead to cerebrovascular accidents and myocardial infarctions. Other major arteries also may be affected (e.g., renal, mesenteric, upper limb). Although platelet counts are low, bleeding is uncommon.

Evaluation and Treatment. Diagnosis is primarily based on clinical observations. Evaluation of persons with isolated thrombocytopenia includes a CBC, a peripheral blood smear, and HIV and HCV tests. Liver enzymes and coagulation tests are done in those with liver disease. A bone marrow biopsy is indicated in conditions when the cause of thrombocytopenia is unclear, and when a hematologic disorder is suspected.[107]

The individual presents with dropping platelet counts after 5 days or longer of heparin treatment. On average, platelet counts may fall to 60,000/μL. Because most individuals have undergone surgery and the onset of symptoms, including thrombosis, may be delayed until after release from the hospital, other possible causes of thrombocytopenia (e.g., infection, other drug reactions) must be considered. Tests are available to measure anti-heparin–platelet factor 4 antibodies. The sensitivity of this test is extremely high (>90%), but the specificity is less because of false-positive reactions (e.g., those receiving dialysis). Treatment is the withdrawal of heparin and use of alternative anticoagulants.

Repeat and routine monitoring is done in asymptomatic, mild thrombocytopenic individuals. Thrombocytopenic emergency conditions that require immediate action include suspected HIT, TTP, HUS, drug-induced ITP, pregnancy with severe thrombocytopenia, bleeding with severe thrombocytopenia, urgently needed invasive procedure in the presence of severe thrombocytopenia, leukopenia, and AA.[107]

Immune thrombocytopenia purpura. The most common cause of thrombocytopenia secondary to increased platelet destruction is immune thrombocytopenic purpura (ITP). ITP may be acute or chronic. The acute form presents in childhood and typically lasts 1 to 2 months with a complete remission. In some children, however it may last for up to 6 months and may progress to the chronic condition in 7% to 28% of children (see Chapter 30). Acute ITP is usually secondary to infections (particularly viral) or other conditions that lead to large amounts of antigen in the blood, such as drug allergies or SLE. HIV-associated disease is now the most common cause of ITP, especially in males between 20 and 50 years of age.[109] Sometimes an identical form of autoimmune thrombocytopenia is associated with CLL, lymphomas, IM, and other infections.[109] The antigen usually forms immune complexes with circulating antibody (anti-platelet IgG antibodies); it is thought that the immune complexes bind to Fc receptors on platelets, leading to their destruction in the spleen. The acute form of ITP usually resolves as the source of antigen is resolved (infection) or removed (drugs).

Chronic ITP is caused by autoantibodies against platelet-specific antigens. This form is more commonly observed in adults, being most prevalent in women between 20 and 40 years of age, although it can be found in all ages. The chronic form tends to get progressively worse. It can occur from a variety of predisposing conditions or exposures (secondary) or have no known risk factors (primary). The autoantibodies are generally of the IgG class and are against one or more of several platelet glycoproteins (e.g., GPIIb/IIIa, GPIIb/IX, GPIa/IIa). The antibodies bind directly to the platelet antigens, after which the antibody-coated platelets are recognized and removed from the circulation by macrophages in the spleen.

Clinical Manifestations. Initial manifestations range from minor bleeding problems (development of petechiae and purpura) over the course of several days to major hemorrhage from mucosal sites (epistaxis, hematuria, menorrhagia, bleeding gums). Rarely will an individual present with intracranial bleeding or other sites of internal bleeding.

During pregnancy, a woman with ITP may have a newborn that is also thrombocytopenic. If the fetal platelets express the same antigen as the mother, the maternal antibody will coat the platelets, potentially resulting in thrombocytopenia in utero. A variant of neonatal thrombocytopenia *(neonatal alloimmune thrombocytopenia)* occurs when the mother does not have ITP but makes IgG antibodies against an antigen inherited from the father found on fetal platelets but not on maternal platelets.

Evaluation and Treatment. Diagnosis of ITP is based on a history of bleeding and associated symptoms (weight loss, fever, headache). Physical examination includes notations on the type, location, and severity of bleeding. In addition, evidence of infections (bacterial, HIV and other viral), medication history, family history, and evidence of thrombosis are assessed. Other diagnostic tests include CBC and peripheral blood smear. Unlike some other forms of thrombocytopenia, there is usually no evidence of splenectomy. Testing for antiplatelet antibodies is usually not helpful. Although most cases of ITP are associated with elevated levels of IgG on platelets, other forms of thrombocytopenia also have a high incidence of platelet-associated antibodies; thus, the specificity is low (49% to 66%).[110] In addition, some cases of ITP will not present with elevated platelet-associated antibodies. The sensitivity is 78% to 92%; therefore, a negative test does not rule out ITP.

The acute form of ITP usually resolves without major clinical consequences, but the chronic form, like many autoimmune diseases, is variable with multiple remissions and exacerbations. Treatment is palliative, not curative, and focuses on prevention of platelet destruction. Initial therapy for ITP is glucocorticoids (e.g., prednisone), which suppress the immune response and prevent sequestering and further destruction of platelets. If steroid therapy is ineffective, other reagents have been used. Treatment with intravenous immunoglobulin (IVIG) is used to prevent major bleeding. The response rate is 80%, but the effects are transient, lasting only days to a few weeks. Anti-Rh_0(D) immune globulin (anti-D) has been used with limited success to treat individuals who are Rh-positive. Newer drug therapies are now available.

If other therapies are ineffective, splenectomy is considered to remove the site of platelet destruction. However, splenectomy is not without risks and approximately 10% to 20% of individuals who undergo a splenectomy suffer a relapse and require further treatment. In that situation, it is thought that the liver has become the site for platelet destruction. If splenectomy is unsuccessful and life-threatening thrombocytopenia persists, more aggressive immunosuppressive medications are usually recommended. Because of potential complications, these medications are reserved for individuals who are severely thrombocytopenic and refractive to other therapies. Zidovudine is effective in raising platelet counts in those with HIV-associated ITP.[109]

Thrombotic thrombocytopenia purpura. Thrombotic thrombocytopenia purpura (TTP; also known as Moschcowitz disease) is a multisystem disorder characterized by TMA (small or microvessel disease) in which platelets aggregate and cause occlusion of arterioles and capillaries within the microcirculation. Aggregation may lead to increased platelet consumption and organ ischemia. TTP is relatively uncommon, occurring in about 5 per 1 million individuals per year. The incidence is increasing and does appear to be an actual increase and not just the result of improved recognition. One suspected etiologic factor for TMA, thrombotic thrombocytopenic purpura, and hemolytic-uremic syndrome is drug-induced, and a recent report found definite evidence from three drugs: quinine, cyclosporine, and tacrolimus.

There are two types of TTP: familial and acquired idiopathic. The familial type is the rarer type and is usually chronic, relapsing, and typically seen in children. When the disease is recognized and treated early, the child experiences predictable recurring episodes at approximately 3-week intervals that are responsive to treatment. Acquired TTP is more common and more acute and severe. It occurs mostly in females in their thirties and is rarely observed in infants or older adults.

Platelet aggregation and microthrombi formation is found throughout the entire vascular system, causing damage to multiple organs. The most susceptible organs for damage include the kidney, brain, and heart. Also affected are the pancreas, spleen, and adrenal glands. The thrombi are composed of platelets with minimal fibrin and red cells, differentiating them from thrombi secondary to intravascular coagulation. Most cases of TTP are related to a dysfunction of the plasma metalloprotease ADAMTS13 (Fig. 29.31A and B). This enzyme is responsible for digesting large precursor molecules of von Willebrand factor (vWF) produced by endothelial cells into smaller molecules. Defects in ADAMTS13 result in expression of large-molecular-weight vWF on the endothelial cell surface and the formation of large aggregates of platelets, which can break off and

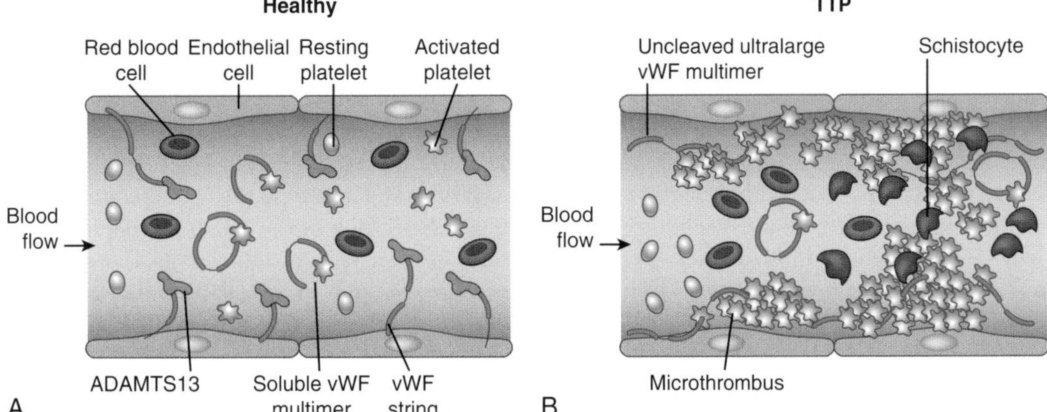

Fig. 29.31 Thrombotic Thrombocytopenic Purpura. (A) A microvessel (arteriole or capillary) in a healthy individual. Normal proteolysis by ADAMTS13 of ultra-large von Willebrand factor *(vWF)* strings anchored to or secreted from stimulated microvascular endothelial cells. (B) A microvessel in thrombotic thrombocytopenic purpura *(TTP)*. Cleavage of secreted or anchored ultralarge vWF is severely reduced when ADAMTS13 activity is less than 10% of normal level. The results include excessive microthrombi formation, shear stress injury to red blood cells (schistocytes) flowing through microvessels that are partially occluded by platelet clumps (producing hemolysis), and perhaps damage from activation of the alternative complement pathway on the uncleaved ultralarge vWF strings. (From Hovinga JAK, Coppo P, Lämmle B, et al. Thrombotic thrombocytopenic purpura. *Nature Reviews Disease Primers*, 2017;3:17020.)

form occlusions in smaller vessels.[111] People with TTP (about 80%) have less than 5% of normal plasma ADAMTS13 levels. Although deficiency of ADAMS-13 is necessary to cause TTP, it is not sufficient to induce the clinical syndrome.[111] The hypothesis of a "second trigger" helps to explain that such conditions as infections, pregnancy, and inflammation increase plasmatic vWF level moving to overt TTP.[111,112] Most individuals with familial TTP are homozygous for mutations in ADAMTS13. Acquired TTP of unexplained origin is associated in individuals with an IgG autoantibody against ADAMTS13.

Clinical Manifestations. Chronic relapsing TTP is a rare familial form of TTP observed in children and usually recognized and successfully treated (see Chapter 30). The acquired acute idiopathic TTP is much more common and more severe. Early diagnosis and treatment are essential because TTP may prove fatal within 90 days of onset. TTP is clinically related to and must be distinguished from other thrombotic microangiopathic conditions, including hemolytic uremic syndrome (HUS), malignant hypertension, preeclampsia, and pregnancy induced HELLP (*h*emolysis, *el*evated *l*iver enzymes, *l*ow *p*latelet count) syndrome.

Acute idiopathic TTP is characterized by a *pathognomonic pentad* (characteristic for a particular disease; group of five). However, only 20% to 30% of those with acute idiopathic TTP present with the classic pentad. These include (1) extreme thrombocytopenia (less than 20,000 platelets/μL), (2) intravascular hemolytic anemia, (3) ischemic signs and symptoms most often involving the CNS (about 65% present with memory disturbances, behavioral irregularities, headaches, or coma), (4) kidney failure (affecting about 65% of individuals), and (5) fever (present in about 33% of individuals with TTP). It is not mandatory that all five be present to begin treatment.

Evaluation and Treatment. The initial findings may be very nonspecific and include weakness, headache, confusion, nausea, vomiting, and diarrhea.[111] The more prevalent findings are a significant thrombocytopenia (usually <30,000/μL of blood) and microangiopathic hemolytic anemia.[110] Both findings are associated with their relative signs of cutaneous and mucosal bleeding, weakness, and dyspnea.[111] A routine blood smear usually shows fragmented red cells *(schistocytes)* produced by shear forces when red cells are in contact with the fibrin mesh in clots that form in the vessels. As a result of tissue injury, serum levels of LDH may be very high, and low-density lipoprotein (LDL) levels may be elevated. The presence of an LDH level 1 times the upper normal value, a cardiac troponin level greater than 0.25 ng/mL on diagnosis, and older age are associated with treatment refractoriness and death.[111,113,114] Tests for antibody on red cells are negative, excluding immune hemolytic anemia.

Importantly, prompt treatment can significantly reduce the death rate. Therapeutic plasma exchange (TPE) with fresh frozen plasma, which replenishes functional ADAMTS13, is the treatment of choice, achieving a 70% to 85% response rate. Additionally, steroids (glucocorticoids) are administered. In the absence of major organ damage, this approach may lead to complete recovery with no long-term complications. The anti-CD20 monoclonal antibody rituximab has shown some success in people who are refractory to plasma exchange. In other individuals rituximab is started immediately. Relapse does occur, generally within the first year of treatment, although recurrences have been reported as late as 20 years after treatment.[115] The transfusion of platelets is debated, and studies suggest this may be harmful. The studies lack rigor; they should not be used to make a liberal policy for transfusion. The use of platelets should be limited to individuals with overt bleeding or before invasive procedures.[111] Individuals who do not respond to conventional treatment may be candidates for splenectomy; however, postoperative hemorrhage remains a dangerous complication. Immunosuppression therapy has been successful in some individuals.

Thrombocythemia

Thrombocythemia (also called thrombocytosis) is defined as a platelet count greater than 450,000/μL of blood. Thrombocythemia may be primary or secondary (reactive) and is usually asymptomatic until the count exceeds 1 million/μ. Then intravascular clot formation (thrombosis), hemorrhage, or other abnormalities can occur.

Pathophysiology. Essential (primary) thrombocythemia (ET) is a chronic, MPN characterized by excessive platelet production resulting from a defect in the bone marrow megakaryocyte progenitor cells. Abnormal blood clotting commonly occurs in individuals with essential thrombocythemia causing many clinical manifestations. Other disease features include leukocytosis, splenomegaly, thrombosis, bleeding, microcirculatory symptoms, itching (or pruritus), and risk of leukemic or bone marrow fibrotic transformation. The most mutated genes in ET are the *JAK2* (in 60%), calreticulin *CALR* (in 20%), or *MPL* (in 3%).[116] The *JAK2* mutation induces overactivity in cell signaling from JAK2 protein. JAK2, a tyrosine kinase, is an essential player downstream of cytokine receptors, such as the TPO (affects platelet proliferation) and erythropoietin (EPO, affects erythrocyte proliferation) receptors. More simply, both EPO and TPO convey their signals and consequent proliferation through JAK2. Along with increased platelets, there may be a concomitant increase in the number of red cells, indicating a myeloproliferative disorder; however, the increase in red cells is not to the extent seen in PV. Red blood cells in ET tend to aggregate and adhere to the endothelium and contribute to the blockage of flow in the microvasculature and altered interactions between platelets and the vascular endothelium. The *JAK2* is more common in middle-aged individuals, with most cases occurring between ages 50 and 60 years.[116] There is no known sex preference, however, a Mayo clinic retrospective study (n = 1076) showed a higher incidence in women (67%).[116] There also is a rare hereditary type of ET called *familial essential thrombocythemia (FET)* that is inherited in an autosomal dominant pattern.

Secondary thrombocythemia may occur after splenectomy because platelets that normally would be stored in the spleen remain in circulating blood. The increase in platelets may be gradual, with thrombocythemia not occurring for up to 3 weeks after splenectomy. Reactive thrombocythemia may occur during some inflammatory conditions, such as rheumatoid arthritis and cancers. In these conditions, excessive production of some cytokines (e.g., IL-6, IL-11) may induce increased production of TPO in the liver, resulting in increased megakaryocyte proliferation. Reactive thrombocythemia also may occur during a variety of physiologic conditions, such as after exercise.

Clinical Manifestations. Clinical manifestations vary among individuals. Those with ET are at risk for large-vessel arterial or venous thrombosis, although the most common complication is microvasculature thrombosis leading to ischemia in the fingers, toes, or cerebrovascular regions. The primary presenting symptoms of microvasculature thrombosis are erythromelalgia, headache, and paresthesia. Other constitutional symptoms include night sweats, weight loss, and splenomegaly.[116] Erythromelalgia is unilateral or bilateral warm, congested, red hands and feet with painful burning sensations, particularly in the forefoot sole and one or more toes. The lower extremities are affected more often, and only one side may be involved. The pain is initiated by standing, exercise, or warmth and relieved by elevation and cooling. In extreme situations, acrocyanosis (bluish or purple coloring of hands or feet) and gangrene may result.

Arterial thrombosis is more common than venous thrombosis and may involve the coronary and renal arteries. DVT of the lower extremities and pulmonary embolism are the major sites for venous involvement. Other common venous sites include intra-abdominal venous thrombosis (portal and hepatic). People with prior history of thrombotic events have a much higher chance of developing a cerebral, cardiac, or peripheral arterial thrombus and, less often, developing a pulmonary embolism or DVT. The IPSET-revised score also considers the *JAK2*V617F mutation as well as classical risk variables.[117] Conversion to acute leukemia is found in less than 10% of persons with ET.[118] Symptoms related to microvascular thrombosis in the CNS include headache, dizziness with paresthesia, transient ischemic attacks (TIAs), strokes, visual disturbances, and seizures. Major thrombotic events, not directly related to the platelet count, occur in about 20% to 30% of individuals with ET. Prior history of thrombotic events, advanced age, and duration of thrombocytosis are predictors of future thrombotic complications. Individuals older than age 60 are at greatest risk.

Although thrombosis is the more common symptom, hemorrhage can also occur. Sites for bleeding include the GI tract, skin, mucous membranes, urinary tract, gums, teeth sockets after extraction, joints, eyes, and brain. GI bleeding may be mistaken for a duodenal ulcer. Hemorrhage is not severe and generally occurs in the presence of very high platelet counts; transfusions are required only occasionally. Bleeding and clotting may occur simultaneously, and individuals will not necessarily be "bleeders" or "clotters."

Evaluation and Treatment. Initial diagnosis is not difficult, and as many as two-thirds of cases are diagnosed from a routine CBC. Secondary thrombocytosis also may occur as a moderate rise in the platelet count that resolves with treatment or resolution of the underlying condition. The WHO criteria for the diagnosis of ET require the following four criteria be met: (1) sustained platelet count of at least 450×10^9/L; (2) bone marrow biopsy showing proliferation of enlarged mature megakaryocytes and no increase of granulocyte or erythrocyte precursors; (3) failure to meet the criteria of PV, myelofibrosis, CML, or other myelodysplastic syndrome; and (4) presence of *JAK2*V617F,*CALR*, or *MPL* mutation.[119] Because ET can be mistaken for CML, careful differentiation is necessary because treatment varies significantly.

Treatment of ET is directed toward preventing thrombosis or hemorrhage. Reducing the platelet count remains a significant treatment issue. Hydroxyurea, a nonalkylating myelosuppressive agent, has been the drug of choice to suppress platelet production. However, there are persistent concerns that long-term use may cause progression to other myelodysplastic disorders, particularly AML or myelofibrosis, although this has not been proven.[120] Another drug used to treat ET is IFN. IFN has a response rate of 80% but may not be effective for everyone because of side effects. Anagrelide interferes with platelet maturation rather than production, thus not interfering with red and white cell growth and development. Low-dose aspirin may be effective to alleviate erythromelalgia and transient neurologic manifestations. ET is not necessarily considered life-threatening but, in those older than age 60 and who have had previous incidences of thrombosis, complications are more common and have a higher risk of mortality. The most important determinant of survival among individuals with ET is age, with a median survival ranging from 8.1 years among those older than 70 years of age to 34.7 years among those younger than 40 years of age.[116]

Alterations of Platelet Function

Qualitative alterations in platelet function are characterized by an increased bleeding time in the presence of a normal platelet count. Associated clinical manifestations include spontaneous petechiae and purpura, and bleeding from the GI tract, genitourinary tract, pulmonary mucosa, and gums. Congenital alterations in platelet function *(thrombocytopathies)* are quite rare and may be categorized into several types of disorders (also see Chapter 30).

Acquired disorders of platelet function are more common than the congenital disorders and may be categorized into three principal causes: (1) drugs, (2) systemic inflammatory conditions, and (3) hematologic alterations.

Multiple drugs are known to interfere with platelet function in several ways: inhibition of platelet membrane receptors, inhibition of prostaglandin pathways, and inhibition of phosphodiesterase activity. Aspirin is the most used drug that affects platelets. It irreversibly inhibits cyclooxygenase function for several days after administration. Nonsteroidal anti-inflammatory drugs also affect cyclooxygenase, although in a reversible fashion.

Systemic disorders that affect platelet function are chronic renal disease, liver disease, cardiopulmonary bypass surgery, and severe deficiencies of iron or folate and antiplatelet antibodies associated with autoimmune disorders. Hematologic disorders associated with platelet dysfunction include CMPDs, MM, leukemias, myelodysplastic syndromes, and dysproteinemias.

Disorders of Coagulation

Disorders of coagulation are usually caused by defects or deficiencies of one or more of the clotting factors. (Normal function of the clotting factors is described in Chapter 28) Qualitative or quantitative abnormalities interfere with or prevent the enzymatic reactions that transform clotting factors, circulating as plasma proteins, into a stable fibrin clot (see Fig. 28.17). Some clotting factor defects are inherited and involve a single factor, such as the hemophilias and von Willebrand disease, caused by deficiencies of specific clotting factors. Other coagulation defects are acquired and tend to result from deficient synthesis of clotting factors by the liver. Causes include liver disease and dietary deficiency of vitamin K.

Other coagulation disorders are attributed to pathologic conditions that trigger coagulation inappropriately, engaging the clotting factors and causing detrimental clotting within blood vessels. For example, any cardiovascular abnormality that alters normal blood flow by acceleration or deceleration or obstruction can create conditions in which coagulation proceeds within the vessels. An example of this is thromboembolic disease, in which blood clots obstruct blood vessels. Coagulation is also stimulated by the presence of *tissue factor* that is released by damaged or dead tissues. Vasculitis, or inflammation of the blood vessels, along with vessel damage activates platelets, which in turn activates the coagulation cascade. In extensive or prolonged vasculitis, blood clot formation can suppress mechanisms that normally control clot formation and dissolution, leading to clogging of the vessels. In each of these acquired conditions, normal hemostatic function proves detrimental to the body by consuming coagulation factors excessively or by overwhelming normal control of clot formation and breakdown (fibrinolysis) (see Fig. 28.19).

Impaired Hemostasis

Impaired hemostasis, or the inability to promote coagulation and the development of a stable fibrin clot, is commonly associated with liver dysfunction, which may be caused by either specific liver disorders or lack of vitamin K.

Vitamin K deficiency. Vitamin K, a fat-soluble vitamin, is required for the synthesis and regulation of prothrombin, the procoagulant factors (VII, IX, X), and the anticoagulant factors within the liver (proteins C and S). Unknown is the contribution of vitamin K to the overall supply by the intestinal flora. The primary source of vitamin K is found in green leafy vegetables. The most common cause of vitamin deficiency is parenteral nutrition in combination with antibiotics that destroy normal gut flora. Rarely is the deficiency caused by a lack of dietary intake; however, bulimia can suppress vitamin K–dependent activity. Parenteral administration of vitamin K is the treatment of choice and usually results in correction of the deficiency within 8 to 12 hours. Fresh frozen plasma also may be administered but is usually reserved for individuals with life-threatening hemorrhages or those who require emergency surgery.

Liver disease. Liver disease (e.g., acute or chronic hepatocellular diseases, cirrhosis), vitamin K deficiency, or liver surgery includes hemostatic derangements with defects in the clotting or fibrinolytic systems and platelet function. The hepatic (parenchyma) cells produce most of the factors involved in hemostasis; therefore, damage to the liver frequently results in diminished production of factors involved in clotting. Factor VII level is the first to decline after liver damage because of its rapid turnover. Factor IX levels are less affected and do not decline until the liver destruction is well advanced. The liver also is a major site for production of plasminogen and α_2-antiplasmin of the fibrinolytic system, as well as TPO and the metalloprotease ADAMTS13. Diminished TPO may lead to thrombocytopenia from decreased platelet production. Decreased production of ADAMTS13 results in increased levels of large precursor molecules of vWF, which leads to the formation of large aggregates of platelets.

With severe liver disease, such as cirrhosis, most clotting factors are significantly depressed. Levels of clotting system regulators, such as antithrombin, protein C, protein S, and fibrinogen, also are diminished. The fibrinolytic system is commonly active because of plasmin inhibitor and other activators that are unaffected. Thrombocytopenia occurs in affected individuals because of diminished TPO and ADAMTS13, as well as increased sequestration (pooling) of platelets in the spleen, which is frequently enlarged in cirrhosis and is associated with portal hypertension. Thus, these individuals may appear to have a condition similar to DIC (see the Consumptive Thrombohemorrhagic Disorders section).

Treatment of hemostasis alterations in liver disease must be comprehensive to cover all aspects of dysfunctions. Fresh frozen plasma administration is the treatment of choice; however, not all individuals tolerate the volume needed to adequately replace all deficient factors. Alternative modalities include the addition of exchange transfusions and platelet concentration to plasma administration.

Consumptive Thrombohemorrhagic Disorders

Consumptive thrombohemorrhagic disorders are a heterogeneous group of conditions that demonstrate the entire spectrum of hemorrhagic and thrombotic pathologic findings. Symptoms range from the subtle to the devastating and generally are intermediary disease processes that complicate a vast number of primary disease states. These disorders are also characterized by confusion and controversy related to their diagnosis, treatment, and management. No one definition can cover all possible varieties of these disorders; however, DIC is most used in the clinical setting to describe a pathologic condition associated with hemorrhage and thrombosis.

Disseminated intravascular coagulation. Disseminated intravascular coagulation (DIC) is an acquired clinical syndrome characterized by widespread activation of coagulation resulting in formation of fibrin clots in medium and small vessels or microvasculature throughout the body. DIC can be acute, subacute, or chronic. DIC is secondary to a wide variety of well-defined clinical conditions, specifically those capable of activating the clotting cascade (see Pathophysiology and Box 29.5).[121] Widespread clotting may lead to blockage of blood flow to organs, resulting in multiple organ failure. The excess clotting may result in consumption of platelets and clotting factors, leading to tendency to bleed despite widespread clots.

The clinical course of DIC is largely determined by the stimulus intensity, host response, and comorbidities and ranges from an acute, severe, life-threatening process that is characterized by massive hemorrhage and thrombosis to a

BOX 29.5 Clinical Conditions Associated With Disseminated Intravascular Coagulation

Sepsis or Severe Infection
Potentially from any microorganism, including malaria

Trauma
Serious head injury
Head injury
Fat metabolism
Burns

Liver Diseases
Fulminant hepatitis
Severe liver cirrhosis

Heat Stroke
Organ Destruction
Severe pancreatitis

Malignancy
Solid tumors
Hematologic cancers

Obstetrical Calamities
Preeclampsia or eclampsia
Placental abruption
Amniotic fluid embolism
HELLP (hemolysis, elevated liver enzymes, and low platelet count) syndrome
Acute fatty liver
Sepsis during pregnancy

Vascular Abnormalities
Hemangioma
Leaking or ruptured aneurysm (such as in the aorta)
Aortic aneurysm
Kasabach-Merritt syndrome
Other vascular malformations

Severe Toxic or Immunologic Reactions
Snake bite
Recreational drug use
Severe transfusion reaction
Transplant rejection

Data from Gando S, Levi M, Toh C-H. Disseminated intravascular coagulation. *Nature Reviews Disease Primers*, 2016;2:16037.

chronic, low-grade condition. The chronic condition includes subacute hemorrhage and diffuse microcirculatory thrombosis. DIC may be localized to one specific organ or generalized, involving multiple organs.

The diagnosis of DIC has been challenging because of the complexity and wide variations in clinical manifestations. Diagnostic criteria have been established and include a systemic thrombohemorrhagic disorder with laboratory evidence of (1) clotting activation, (2) fibrinolytic activation, (3) coagulation inhibitor consumption, and (4) biochemical evidence of end-organ damage or failure.

Sepsis is the most common condition associated with DIC. Gram-negative microorganisms, as well as some gram-positive microorganisms, fungi, protozoa (malaria), and viruses (influenza, herpes), are capable of precipitating DIC by causing damage to the vascular endothelium. Gram-negative endotoxins are the primary cause of endothelial damage. The adenocarcinomas most frequently associated with DIC include the lung, pancreas, colon, and stomach. Direct tissue damage (e.g., massive trauma, extensive surgery, severe burns) also results in release of tissue factor (TF), an initiator of DIC, by the endothelium. Severe trauma, especially to the brain, can induce DIC. DIC occurs in about two-thirds of individuals with a systemic inflammatory response (SIRS) to trauma. Some complications of pregnancy also are associated with DIC; incidences range from 50% for women with placental abruptions to less than 10% for severe preeclampsia. Other causes of DIC have been identified, most notably blood transfusion. Transfused blood dilutes the clotting factors, as well as circulating naturally occurring antithrombins. In hemolytic transfusion reactions, the endothelium is damaged by complement-mediated reactions.

Pathophysiology. The pathophysiology of DIC is complex. DIC results from abnormally widespread and ongoing activation of clotting—*coagulopathy*—in small and midsize vessels that alters the microcirculation, leading to ischemic necrosis in various organs, particularly the kidney and lung. Concomitantly, DIC can be caused by the imbalance between the coagulant system and the fibrinolytic system (which generates plasmin) to maintain normal circulation (Fig. 29.32). DIC can cause widespread deposition of fibrin in the microcirculation that leads to ischemia, microvascular thrombotic obstruction, and organ failure (Fig. 29.33).

Seemingly paradoxical, DIC involves both widespread clotting and bleeding because of simultaneous procoagulant activation, fibrinolytic activation, and consumption of platelets and coagulation factors, which results directly in serious bleeding (see Fig. 29.33).

DIC is not a disease but is secondary to a variety of conditions (see Box 29.5) because of activation of the clotting cascade. The common pathway for DIC appears to be excessive and widespread exposure to TF. This may occur by several mechanisms:

1. Damage to the vascular endothelium results in exposure to TF.
2. When stimulated by inflammatory cytokines, endothelial cells and monocytes express surface TF.
3. Endotoxin triggers the release of many cytokines that can both promote and cause progression of DIC.
4. Sepsis is associated with many cytokines, interleukins, and platelet activating factor (PAF) that promote DIC as well as activate endothelial cells that stimulate thrombi development.
5. TF may be released directly into the bloodstream from circulating white blood cells.

TF binds clotting factor VII, which leads to conversion of prothrombin to thrombin and formation of fibrin clots (see Fig. 28.18). This pathway appears to be the primary route by which DIC is initiated.

Not only is the clotting system extensively activated in DIC, but also the activities of the predominant natural anticoagulants (TF pathway inhibitor, antithrombin III, protein C) are greatly diminished. During DIC, the activation of clotting is prolonged

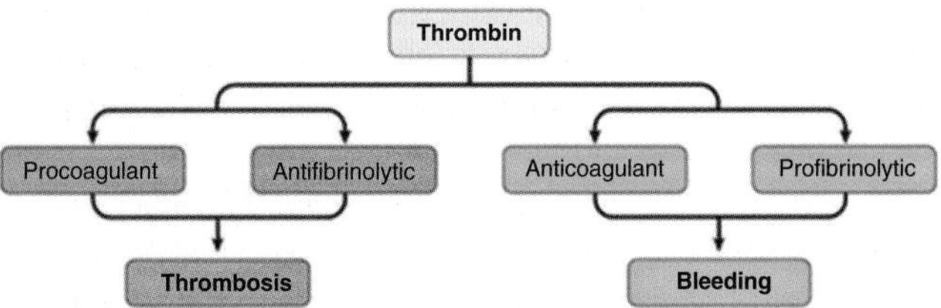

Fig. 29.32 Imbalance Between the Coagulant System and the Fibrinolytic System. Increased thrombin generation in disseminated intravascular coagulation leads to bleeding and/or thrombosis depending on the presiding change of the dynamic balance in both coagulant and fibrinolytic outcomes. (From Gando S, Levi M, Toh CH. Disseminated intravascular coagulation. *Nature Reviews Disease Primers*, 2016;2(1). https://doi.org/10.1038/nrdp.2016.37.)

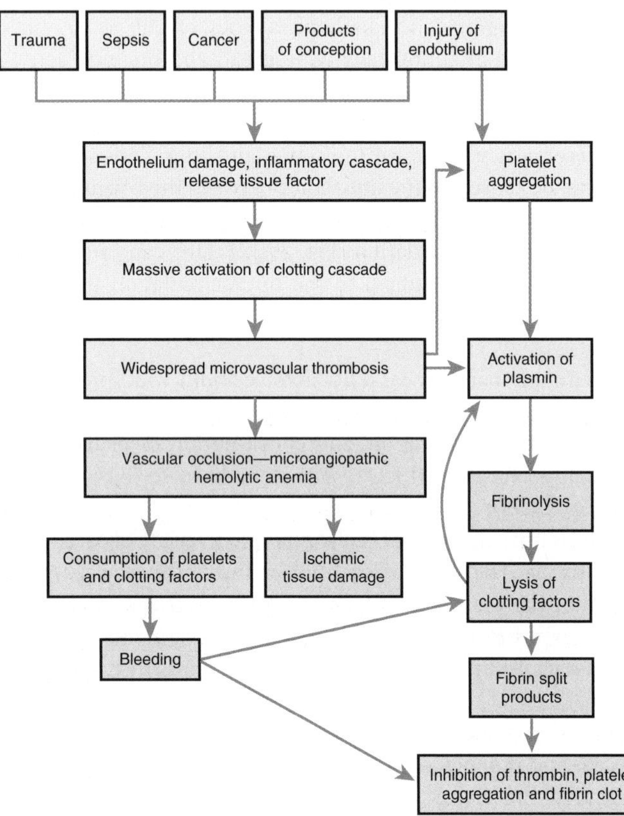

Fig. 29.33 Pathophysiology of Disseminated Intravascular Coagulation. See text.

and is a result of certain conditions (e.g., bacteremia or endotoxemia); thrombin generation is increased and is insufficiently balanced by impaired anticoagulant systems, such as antithrombin and protein C. The overall result is fibrin generation and deposition in the vascular system. In early DIC, plasmin (naturally occurring clot busting or fibrinolytic agent) produced from endothelial cells causes fibrinolysis to maintain circulation. Bleeding can occur with excess fibrinolytic activity. However, fibrinolysis becomes blunted by high levels of plasminogen activator inhibitor-1 (PAI-1), a fibrinolytic inhibitor. Over time the activity of plasmin is diminished by PAI-1. Although some fibrinolytic activity remains, the level is inadequate to control the systemic deposition of fibrin. The slow breakdown of fibrin by plasmin produces fibrin split products (FSPs) (also known as fibrin degradation products [FDPs]). These products are powerful anticoagulants that are normally removed from blood by fibronectin and macrophages. FSPs, along with thrombin, induce further cytokine release from monocytes, contributing to endothelial damage and TF release. During DIC, the presence of FSPs is prolonged. Low levels of fibronectin suggest a poor prognosis.

Although thrombosis is generalized and widespread, individuals with DIC are paradoxically at risk for hemorrhage. Hemorrhage is secondary to the abnormally high consumption of clotting factors and platelets, as well as the anticoagulant properties of FSPs, which interfere with fibrin mesh formation or polymerization. Both thrombin and FSPs have a high affinity for platelets and cause platelet activation and aggregation—an event that occurs early in the development of DIC—which facilitates microcirculatory coagulation and obstruction in the initial phase. However, platelet consumption exceeds production, resulting in a thrombocytopenia that increases bleeding.

Activation of clotting also leads to activation of other inflammatory pathways, including the kallikrein-kinin and complement systems (see Chapter 7). With sepsis, TNF first reaches a peak, followed by an increase in IL-6 and IL-1.[121] Other cytokines are released and produce cytokine release syndrome (CRS), which is a life-threatening complication induced by hyperinflammatory responses.[122] Activation of these systems contributes to increased vascular permeability, hypotension, and shock. Activated complement components also induce platelet destruction, which initially contributes to the thrombosis and later to the thrombocytopenia.

The deposition of fibrin clots in the circulation interferes with blood flow, causing widespread organ hypoperfusion. This condition may lead to ischemia, infarction, and necrosis, further potentiating and complicating the existing DIC process by causing further release of TF and eventually organ failure. Manifestations of multisystem organ dysfunction and failure ultimately result.

In addition to initiation of clotting by TF, DIC may be precipitated by direct proteolytic activation of factor X. This has been described as "thrombin mimicry" and is the result of proteases directly converting fibrinogen to fibrin. These proteases may come from snake venom, some tumor cells, or the pancreas and liver, where they are respectively released during episodes of pancreatitis and various stages of liver disease. Direct proteolytic activity appears to be independent of any type of damage to the endothelium or tissue.

Whatever initiates the process of DIC, the cycle of thrombosis and hemorrhage persists until the underlying cause of the DIC is removed or appropriate therapeutic interventions are used.

Clinical Manifestations. Clinical signs and symptoms of DIC present a wide spectrum of possibilities, depending on the underlying disease process that initiates DIC and whether the DIC is acute or chronic (see Box 29.5). Most symptoms are the result of either bleeding or thrombosis. Acute DIC presents with rapid development of hemorrhaging (oozing) from venipuncture sites, arterial lines, or surgical wounds or development of ecchymotic lesions (purpura, petechiae) and hematomas. Other sites of bleeding include the eyes (sclera, conjunctiva), the nose, and the gums. Most individuals with DIC demonstrate bleeding at three or more unrelated sites, and any combination may be observed. Shock of variable intensity, out of proportion to the amount of blood loss, also may be observed. Hemorrhaging into closed compartments of the body can occur and may precede the development of shock.

Manifestations of thrombosis are not always as evident, even though it is often the first pathologic alteration to occur. The initial observations may be bleeding and sometimes very extensive hemorrhage. Several organ systems are susceptible to microvascular thrombosis associated with dysfunction: cardiovascular, pulmonary, central nervous, renal, and hepatic systems. Acute and accurate clinical interpretations are critical to preventing progression of DIC that may lead to multisystem organ dysfunction and failure. (Multiple organ dysfunction and failure are discussed further in Chapter 48.) Indicators of multisystem dysfunction include changes in level of consciousness or behavior, confusion, seizure activity, oliguria, hematuria, hypoxia, hypotension, hemoptysis, chest pain, and tachycardia. Symmetric cyanosis of fingers and toes (blue finger/toe syndrome), nose, and breast may be observed and indicates macrovascular thrombosis. This may lead to infarction and gangrene that may require amputation. Jaundice also is observed and most likely results from red cell destruction rather than liver dysfunction.

Individuals with chronic or low-grade DIC do not present with the overt manifestations of hemorrhaging and thrombosis but instead have subacute bleeding and diffuse thrombosis; these individuals are described as having *compensated DIC*, or *non-overt DIC*. The major characteristic of this state is an increased turnover and decreased survival time of the components of hemostasis: platelets and clotting factors. Occasionally, diffuse or localized thrombosis develops, but this is infrequent.

Evaluation and Treatment. Persons with DIC should be treated at hospitals with appropriate critical care and subspecialty expertise, such as hematology, blood bank, or surgery.[123] Individuals who present without those capabilities and who are able to be transferred should be referred immediately to a hospital that has those resources.[123] No single laboratory test can be used to effectively diagnose DIC. Diagnosis is based primarily on clinical symptoms and confirmed by a combination of laboratory tests. The person must present with a clinical condition that is known to be associated with DIC. The most used combination of laboratory tests usually confirms thrombocytopenia or a rapidly decreasing platelet count on repeated testing, prolongation of clotting times, the presence of FSPs, and decreased levels of coagulation inhibitors. Platelet counts below 100,000/μL or a progressive decrease in platelet counts is very sensitive for DIC, although not greatly specific. These changes usually indicate consumption of platelets.

The standard coagulation tests (e.g., prothrombin time [PT], activated partial thromboplastin time [aPTT]) also have a high degree of sensitivity, but they are not highly specific for DIC. As a result of consumption of circulating clotting factors, these tests are usually abnormal, ranging from shortened to prolonged times. However, conditions other than DIC may prolong clotting times.

Detection of FSPs is more specific for DIC. Detection of D-dimers is a widely used test for DIC. A D-dimer is a molecule produced by plasmin degradation of cross-linked fibrin in clots. D-Dimers in the blood can be quantified using ELISA tests that include commercially available and highly specific monoclonal antibody against the D-dimer. Agglutination tests for other FSPs are available. Levels of FSPs are elevated in the plasma in 95% to 100% of cases; however, they are less specific and only document the presence of plasmin and its action on fibrin. ELISAs for markers of thrombin activity are sometimes used.

Levels of coagulation inhibitors (e.g., antithrombin III [AT-III], protein C) can be measured by assays that rely on function or by ELISAs that quantify the amount of the specific inhibitor. AT-III levels can provide key information for diagnosing and monitoring therapy of DIC. Initial levels of functional AT-III are low in DIC because thrombin is irreversibly complexed with activated clotting factors and AT-III.

Treatment of DIC is directed toward (1) eliminating the underlying pathologic condition, (2) controlling ongoing thrombosis, and (3) maintaining organ function. Elimination of the underlying pathologic condition is the initial intervention in the treatment phase in order to remove the trigger for activation of clotting. Once the stimulus is gone, production of coagulation factors in the liver leads to restoration of normal plasma levels within 24 to 48 hours.

Control of thrombosis is more difficult to attain. Heparin has been used for this; however, its use is controversial because its mechanism of action is binding to and activating AT-III, which is deficient in many types of DIC. Currently, heparin is indicated only in certain types of situations related to DIC.[123] For instance, heparin seems to be effective in DIC caused by a retained dead fetus or associated with acute promyelocytic leukemia. Organ function is compromised by microthrombi, and there is a risk of losing an extremity because of vascular occlusion; therefore, heparin is also indicated in these conditions. Heparin's usefulness, however, for DIC that is precipitated by septic shock has not been established and so is contraindicated in that instance; heparin is also contraindicated when there is evidence of postoperative bleeding, peptic ulcer, or CNS bleeding.

Replacement of deficient coagulation factors, platelets, and other coagulation elements is gaining recognition as an effective treatment modality. Their use is not without controversy, however, because a major concern with replacement therapy is the possible risk of adding components that will increase the rate of thrombosis. Clinical judgment is the key factor in determining whether replacement is to be used as a treatment modality. Several clinical trials are evaluating replacement of anticoagulants (i.e., AT-III, protein C). Antifibrinolytic drugs also are used in treatment but are limited to instances of life-threatening bleeding that have not been controlled by blood component replacement therapy.

Maintenance of organ function is achieved by fluid replacement to sustain adequate circulating blood volume and maintain

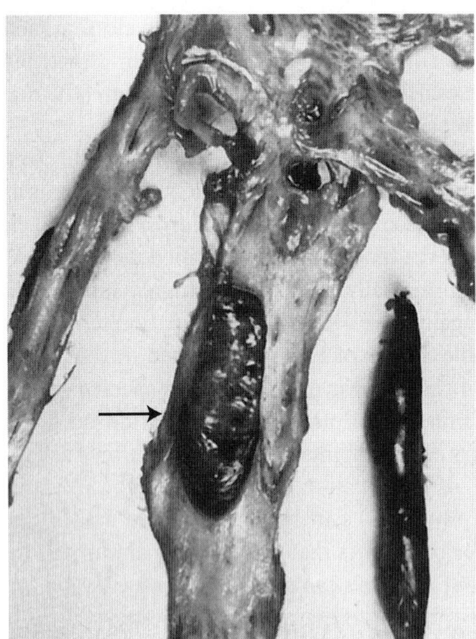

Fig. 29.34 Thrombus. Thrombus arising in valve pocket at upper end of superficial femoral vein *(arrow)*. Postmortem clot on the right is shown for comparison. (From McLachlin J, Paterson JC. Some basic observations on venous thrombosis and pulmonary embolism. *Surgery, Gynecology and Obstetrics*, 1951;93(1):1–8.)

optimal tissue and organ perfusion. Fluids may be required to restore blood pressure, cardiac output, and urine output to normal parameters.

Thromboembolic Disorders

Certain conditions within the blood vessels predispose an individual to develop clots spontaneously. Close to 100,000 people die each year of blood clots, and 1 in 4 people who have the clot in their lungs—*a pulmonary embolism*—die without warning (see Chapter 35). *Venous thromboembolism* (VTE) affects about 900,000 Americans each year, and 3 in 10 people who have a clot will have another episode within 10 years. Blood clots can happen to anyone, and they are often preventable. Early diagnosis is critical to prevent death.[124] A stationary clot attached to the vessel wall is called a thrombus (Fig. 29.34). A thrombus is composed of fibrin and blood cells and can develop in either the arterial or the venous system. Arterial thrombi form under conditions of high blood flow and are composed mostly of platelet aggregates held together by fibrin strands. Venous thrombi form under conditions of low flow and are composed mostly of red cells with larger amounts of fibrin and few platelets.

A thrombus eventually reduces or obstructs blood flow to tissues or organs, such as the heart, brain, or lungs, depriving them of essential nutrients critical to survival. A thrombus also has the potential to detach from the vessel wall and circulate within the bloodstream (referred to as an embolus). The embolus may become lodged in smaller blood vessels, blocking blood flow into the local tissue or organ and leading to ischemia. A pulmonary embolism (PE) is life-threatening and can cause sudden death.[124] Episodes of thromboembolism are life-threatening depending on the *site* of vessel occlusion. Risk factors for venous thromboembolism (VTE), include older age, malignancy, inflammatory disorders (e.g., 4.7% risk in those with rheumatoid arthritis), and inherited thrombophilia.[125] Deep vein thrombosis (DVT) for lower extremity ranges from 88 to 112/100,000 person-years and increases with age.[125] Postthrombotic syndrome is persistent symptoms, signs of chronic venous insufficiency, or both and occurs in 25% to 50% of patients 3 to 6 months after DVT diagnosis.[125] Catheter-directed fibrinolysis with or without mechanical thrombectomy is appropriate in those with iliofemoral obstruction, severe symptoms, and a low risk of bleeding.[125] Newer direct oral anticoagulants including rivaroxaban, apixaban, dabigatran, and edoxaban are considered noninferior to warfarin (absolute rate of recurrent VTE or VTE-related death, 2.0% vs. 2.2%).[125] Major bleeding occurs in 1.1% of individuals treated with direct oral anticoagulants versus 1.8% treated with warfarin.[125]

More aggressive therapy may be indicated for such conditions as pulmonary embolism, coronary thrombosis, or thrombophlebitis. Streptokinase, tissue plasminogen activator (t-PA), and urokinase activate the fibrinolytic system and are administered to accelerate the lysis of known thrombi. These drugs are known as fibrinolytic or thrombolytic therapy and are prescribed with a high degree of caution because they can cause hemorrhagic complications.

The risk for developing spontaneous thrombi is related to several factors, referred to as the Virchow triad: (1) injury to the blood vessel endothelium, (2) abnormalities of blood flow (turbulence or stasis), and (3) hypercoagulability of the blood (see Chapter 32).

Endothelial injury to blood vessels can result from atherosclerosis (plaque deposits on arterial walls) (see Chapter 32). Atherosclerosis initiates platelet adhesion and aggregation, promoting the development of atherosclerotic plaques that enlarge, causing further damage and occlusion. Other causes of vessel endothelial injury may be related to hemodynamic alterations associated with hypertension and turbulent blood flow. Injury is also caused by radiation injury, exogenous chemical agents (e.g., toxins from cigarette smoke), endogenous agents (e.g., cholesterol), bacterial toxins or endotoxins, or immunologic mechanisms.

Sites of turbulent blood flow in the arteries and stasis of blood flow in the veins increase the risk for thrombus formation. In areas of turbulence, platelets and endothelial cells may be activated, leading to thrombosis. In sites of stasis, platelets may remain in contact with the endothelium for prolonged lengths of time, and clotting factors that would normally be diluted with fresh flowing blood are not diluted and may become activated. The most common clinical conditions that predispose to venous stasis and subsequent thromboembolic phenomena are major surgery (e.g., orthopedic surgery), acute myocardial infarction, CHF, limb paralysis, travel, spinal injury, malignancy, advanced age, the postpartum period, and bed rest longer than 1 week. Turbulence and stasis occur with ulcerated atherosclerotic plaques, hyperviscosity (polycythemia), and conditions with deformed red cells (e.g., sickle cell anemia).

Hypercoagulability, *or thrombophilia*, increases the risk for venous thrombosis. Hypercoagulability is differentiated according to whether it results from primary (hereditary) or secondary (acquired) causes (see Chapter 32).

Hereditary thrombophilias. Thrombophilias can result from both inherited conditions and, more commonly, acquired conditions. Several inherited conditions increase the risk of developing thrombosis, and most are autosomal dominant. Thus, individuals who are homozygous for the mutation are at greatest risk for thrombosis. These include mutations in platelet receptors, coagulation proteins, fibrinolytic proteins, and other factors. The mutations that have been most strongly linked as risk factors for venous thrombosis or for arterial thrombosis involving coronary artery disease or stroke include those that affect fibrinogen, prothrombin (G20210A variant), and factor V (factor V Leiden) of the coagulation system. Other inherited thrombophilias are risk factors mostly for venous thrombosis and in some cases arterial ischemic stroke, including deficiencies in protein C and protein S.[126,127] Other hereditary thrombophilias are less common.

Tests to diagnose inherited thrombophilias include PT; partial thromboplastin time; and levels of protein C, protein S, and AT-III. More elaborate tests to detect precise mutations in factor V, prothrombin, or MTHFR may be indicated. Management is based on the underlying defect and may include long-term anticoagulation.[128]

Acquired hypercoagulability. Deficiencies in proteins S and C and AT-III may be acquired and contribute to a hypercoagulable state. Conditions associated with an acquired protein deficiency include DIC, liver disease, infection, DVT, acute respiratory distress syndrome, L-asparaginase therapy, HUS, and TTP. The postoperative state also predisposes an individual to protein C or S deficiency; however, its role in contributing to DVT remains unclear.

Acquired hypercoagulable states include *antiphospholipid syndrome (APS)*. APS is an autoimmune syndrome characterized by autoantibodies against plasma membrane phospholipids and phospholipid-binding proteins. As with most autoimmune diseases, the predominantly affected individual is female and of reproductive age. Those with APS are at risk for both arterial and venous thrombosis (Fig. 29.35) and a variety of obstetric complications, including pregnancy loss and preeclampsia/eclampsia. In severe cases the individual may die from recurrent major thrombus formation. The pathophysiology is related to autoantibodies directly reacting with platelets or endothelial cells (increasing the risk for thrombosis) or the placental surface (resulting in damage to the placenta). The predominant diagnostic tests measure prolongation of laboratory blood coagulation tests related to an antibody inhibitor (lupus anticoagulant) and specific ELISAs for antibodies against phospholipids (e.g., anticardiolipin antibody) or proteins that bind to phospholipids (e.g., β_2-glycoprotein I). Highly effective therapy (i.e., unfractionated or low-molecular-weight heparin with low-dose aspirin) is available to prevent the obstetric complications.

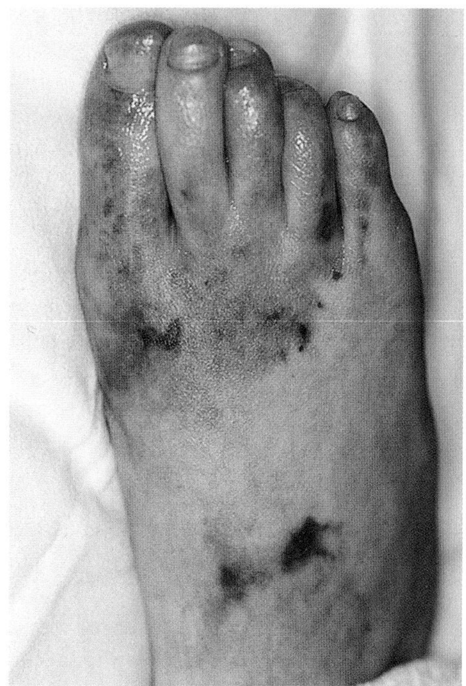

Fig. 29.35 Arterial Thrombosis Associated Antiphospholipid Antibodies. A 12-year-old girl with systemic lupus erythematosus and antiphospholipid antibodies with painful cutaneous vasculitis of the right foot. Arterial thrombosis documented by angiography resulted in cyanosis of the large toe. Symptoms resolved with treatment with heparin and corticosteroids. (From Kliegman R, et al. *Nelson textbook of pediatrics*, 18th edition. Philadelphia: Saunders; 2007.)

SUMMARY REVIEW

Anemia

1. Anemia is defined as a reduction in the number or volume of circulating red cells or a decrease in the quality or quantity of hemoglobin.
2. The most common classification of anemias is based on changes in the cell size—represented by the cell suffix *-cytic*—and changes in the cell's hemoglobin content—represented by the suffix *-chromic.*
3. Clinical manifestations of anemia can be found in all organs and tissues throughout the body. Decreased oxygen delivery to tissues causes fatigue, dyspnea, dizziness, compensatory tachycardia, and organ dysfunction.
4. Posthemorrhagic anemia is caused by acute blood loss, often caused by trauma. Complete recovery is possible if acute blood loss is not severe.
5. Macrocytic (megaloblastic) anemias are characterized by unusually large stem cells (megaloblasts) in the marrow that mature into very large erythrocytes (macrocytic). Macrocytic anemias are caused most by deficiency of vitamin B_{12} or folate. Pernicious anemia can be fatal, usually because of heart failure, unless vitamin B_{12} replacement is given (lifelong replacement is required). Folate deficiency anemia is treated with folate supplements, but long-term therapy is not necessary if dietary adjustments are made to increase folate intake.

6. Microcytic-hypochromic anemias are characterized by abnormally small red cells with unusually reduced hemoglobin content. The most common cause is iron deficiency.
7. Iron deficiency anemia (IDA) is the most common nutritional disorder worldwide. The causes of IDA include (1) dietary deficiency, (2) impaired absorption, (3) increased requirement, (4) chronic blood loss, (5) impaired absorption, and (6) chronic diarrhea.
8. IDA usually develops slowly, with a gradual, insidious onset of nonspecific symptoms, including fatigue, weakness, shortness of breath, and pale earlobes, palms, and conjunctivae. Once the source of blood loss is identified and corrected, iron replacement therapy can be initiated.
9. Normocytic-normochromic anemias are characterized by insufficient numbers of normal erythrocytes.
10. Anemia of inflammation is caused by inflammatory cytokines which increase hepcidin levels. The increased levels reduce iron absorption, sequester iron in macrophages, and suppress erythropoietin production. Altogether these changes cause decreased production of red blood cells and impaired iron utilization in people with chronic systemic diseases or chronic inflammation. It is a common anemia found in hospitalized individuals and is usually in the mild to moderate range of anemias.
11. Aplastic anemia is caused by a reduction in the effective production of mature cells by the bone marrow, causing a reduction or absence of all three blood cell types (pancytopenia). Hemolytic anemia is the premature accelerated destruction of erythrocytes.

Myeloproliferative Red Cell Disorders

1. Myeloproliferative disorders involve an overproduction of cells resulting from abnormal regulation of hematopoietic stem cells. Polycythemia is an excessive red cell production.
2. Polycythemia vera is a slow-growing blood cancer in which the bone marrow makes too many red blood cells. It is a stem cell disorder with hyperplastic and neoplastic bone marrow alterations characterized by abnormal uncontrolled proliferation of erythrocytes, frequently with increased white blood cells and platelets. Polycythemia is responsible for most of the clinical symptoms, including increased blood volume and viscosity.
3. Treatment of polycythemia vera includes frequent phlebotomies and aspirin in low-risk individuals. Hydroxyurea is the drug of choice for myelosuppression. Polycythemia vera may spontaneously convert to acute myelogenous leukemia.
4. Hereditary hemochromatosis is a common inherited disorder of iron metabolism characterized by increased gastrointestinal iron absorption with subsequent iron deposition in the liver, pancreas, heart, joints, and endocrine glands. Periodic phlebotomy is effective at removing excess iron.

Alterations of Leukocyte Function

1. Quantitative alterations of leukocytes (too many or too few) can be caused by bone marrow dysfunction or premature destruction of cells in the circulation. Many quantitative changes in leukocytes occur in response to invasion by microorganisms.
2. Leukocytosis is a condition in which the leukocyte count is higher than normal and is usually a response to physiologic stressors and pathologic conditions, such as malignancies and hematologic disorders.
3. Leukopenia is present when the leukocyte count is lower than normal and is caused by radiation, anaphylactic shock, autoimmune disease, immune deficiencies, and certain drugs. A decrease in neutrophils increases the risk for infection.
4. Granulocytosis (or neutrophilia) is an increase in circulating granulocytes—neutrophils, eosinophils, or basophils—that occurs in response to infection and inflammation. Granulocytopenia (or neutropenia), a significant decrease in the number of neutrophils, is often caused by chemotherapeutic agents, severe infection, and radiation. Agranulocytosis is a complete absence of granulocytes in the blood.
5. Eosinophilia (increase in circulating eosinophils) results most commonly from allergic disorders and parasitic invasion. Eosinopenia (decrease in circulating eosinophils) is generally caused by the migration of eosinophils into inflammatory sites.
6. Basophilia (increase in circulating basophils) is rare and generally is a response to inflammation and immediate hypersensitivity reactions. Basopenia (decrease in circulating basophils) is seen in hyperthyroidism, acute infection, ovulation and pregnancy, and long-term steroid therapy.
7. Monocytosis (increase in circulating monocytes) is often transient and occurs during the late or recuperative phase of infection. Monocytopenia (decrease in circulating monocytes) is rare but may occur with hairy cell leukemia and prednisone therapy.
8. Lymphocytosis is an increase in the number or proportion of lymphocytes in the blood and is most caused by viral infections. Lymphocytopenia is a decrease in the number of circulating lymphocytes and is associated with neoplasias, immune deficiencies, and destruction by drugs, viruses, or radiation.
9. Infectious mononucleosis (IM) is an acute, self-limiting infection of B lymphocytes most associated with the Epstein-Barr virus (EBV), which is transmitted from person-to-person (salivary secretions), breastfeeding, and sexual contact (cervical and seminal fluid). The classic symptoms of IM are pharyngitis, lymphadenopathy, and fever. The proliferation of infected B cells may be uncontrolled and lead to B-cell and T-cell lymphomas. Treatment of IM consists of rest and symptomatic treatment.
10. The common pathologic feature of all forms of leukemia is an uncontrolled proliferation of malignant leukocytes, overcrowding the bone marrow and resulting in decreased production and function of the other blood cell lines.
11. The classification of leukemias is complex, because the once discrete categories of lymphoma and leukemia have been blurred.

12. The World Health Organization (WHO) groups lymphoid neoplasms into five categories defined by cell of origin: (1) precursor B-cell neoplasms (immature B cells), (2) peripheral B-cell neoplasms (mature B cells), (3) precursor T-cell neoplasms (immature T cells), (4) peripheral T-cell and NK (natural killer)-cell neoplasms (mature T cells and NK cells), and (5) Hodgkin lymphoma (Reed-Sternberg cell and variants).
13. Acute leukemia is characterized by undifferentiated or immature cells. The onset of disease is abrupt and rapid, and, without treatment, disease progression results in a short survival time. In chronic leukemia, the predominant cell is more differentiated but does not function normally, with a relatively slow progression.
14. All leukemias have certain pathophysiologic features in common. Abnormal immature white blood cells, called leukemic blasts, fill the bone marrow and spill into the blood. The blasts overcrowd the marrow and cause cellular proliferation of the other cell lines to cease. Leukemic blasts induce a *senescent phenotype* in stromal cells within the bone marrow microenvironment. Blast cell longevity is promoted by adipocytes.
15. Acute leukemias include acute lymphocytic leukemia (ALL) and acute myelogenous leukemia (AML).
16. Increased risk for ALL has been linked to prenatal exposure to x-rays, postnatal exposure to ionizing radiation, past treatment with chemotherapy, certain chemical exposures, certain viral infections, age, race/ethnicity, gender, and certain genetic conditions. AML can arise in people de novo, those with an underlying hematological disorder, or as a consequence of prior treatment. It is the most frequently reported secondary cancer after high doses of chemotherapy for HL, NHL, MM, ovarian cancer, and breast cancer.
17. The major clinical manifestations of acute leukemia include fatigue caused by anemia, bleeding caused by thrombocytopenia, fever secondary to infection, anorexia, and weight loss.
18. Treatment varies depending on the type of leukemia and includes chemotherapy, radiation therapy, stem cell transplant, and other drug therapy.
19. Chronic leukemias include chronic lymphocytic leukemia (CLL) and chronic myelogenous leukemia (CML).
20. CLL is a disorder of structurally mature but immunologically immature lymphocytes. In adults, CLL is the most common leukemia in the Western world.
21. Exposures associated with CLL include pesticides, deltamethrin and herbicides, Agent Orange, and radon. The role of ionizing radiation is controversial. Hypogammaglobulinemia is common in CLL and can precede the diagnosis. Genetic studies strongly imply involvement of inheritable susceptibility alleles that promote or prevent disease. CLL has the highest incidence of familial association.
22. CML is classified as a myeloproliferative neoplasm, is a slowly progressing disease with increased numbers of granulocytic precursors in the bone marrow, which usually includes elevated proportions of eosinophils and basophils. Megakaryocytes are also increased in the bone marrow and some with dysphasia.
23. The only known cause of CML is exposure to ionizing radiation.
24. CLL involves malignant transformation and accumulation of B lymphocytes and rarely involves chromosomal translocations.
25. The Philadelphia chromosome is present in more than 90% to 95% of persons diagnosed with CML.
26. Most individuals with chronic leukemia are asymptomatic at the time of diagnosis, but the most common finding is lymphadenopathy.
27. Treatments for progressing CLL include chemotherapy and in selected individuals stem cell transplantation. In early disease antileukemic therapy is frequently unnecessary. Treatments for CML do not cure the disease, but include chemotherapy, biologic response modifiers, and stem cell transplant.

Alterations of Lymphoid Function

1. Lymphadenopathy is enlarged lymph nodes. Lymphadenopathy results from four types of conditions: (1) neoplastic disease, (2) immunologic or inflammatory conditions, (3) endocrine disorders, or (4) lipid storage diseases.
2. Lymphomas consist of a diverse group of neoplasms that develop from the proliferation of malignant lymphocytes in the lymphoid system. The WHO classification of lymphomas based on the cell type it originated from include Hodgkin lymphoma (HL) and non-Hodgkin lymphoma (NHL). Classification based on morphology and cell lineage include B-cell neoplasms, T-cell neoplasms, and natural killer (NK) cell neoplasms. Two *basic* categories of lymphomas are HL and NHL.
3. In general, lymphomas are the result of genetic mutations or viral infection. Globally, however, the incidence of lymphoma is increased in more developed countries. Malignant transformation produces a cell with uncontrolled and excessive growth that accumulates in the lymph nodes and other sites, producing tumor masses.
4. HL is a malignant lymphoma that progresses from one group of lymph nodes to another and is characterized by abnormal cells called Hodgkin and Reed-Sternberg cells (HRS). EBV has been linked to the pathogenesis of HL. Only a few people that have been infected with EBV develop HL. Genome-wide studies have identified genetic risk variants mostly in immune-related genes.
5. The neoplastic HRS cells originate from a germinal center or post-germinal center B cell. The HRS cells secrete and release cytokines that result in accumulation of inflammatory cells in the tumor microenvironment, which produces the local and systemic effects.
6. An enlarged, painless lymph node, most commonly in the neck, is an initial sign of HL; however, asymptomatic lymphadenopathy can progress undetected for years.
7. Treatment of HL includes chemotherapy and radiation options. Treatment with chemotherapy or radiation

therapy, or both, may increase the risk of second cancers, cardiovascular disease, and other health problems months or years after treatment.

8. The NHLs are a heterogeneous group of lymphoid tissue neoplasms. NHL is a progressive clonal expansion of B cells, T cells, or NK cells, with B cells accounting for the majority of NHLs. Oncogenes may be activated by chromosomal translocation or by deletion of tumor-suppressor genes. Certain subtypes may have altered genomes by oncogenic viruses.
9. Risk factors for NHL include being older, male, or white with immunosuppression, certain viruses, *Helicobacter pylori*, autoimmune and chronic inflammatory disorders, occupational exposures, for example certain pesticides, and radiation exposure. Previous treatment of both radiation and chemotherapy increases risk of NHL.
10. The key pathogenic mechanisms include immunosuppression and chronic antigen stimulation, which increases B-cell proliferation leading to random genetic mistakes notably immunoglobulin rearrangement.
11. Generally, with NHL, the swelling of lymph nodes is painless, and the nodes enlarge and transform over a period of months or years. The cervical, axillary, inguinal, and femoral lymph node chains are the most affected sites.
12. Treatment for NHL may include chemotherapy, radiation therapy, monoclonal antibody therapy, and watchful waiting.
13. Burkitt leukemia/lymphoma (BL) is a B-cell NHL. It is highly aggressive and is the fastest growing human tumor. There are three main types of BL: endemic (common in Africa and linked to EBV), nonendemic (occurs worldwide), and immunodeficiency-related (found in individuals with AIDS). The rapidly growing tumor involves the jaw and facial bones and sometimes the abdomen.
14. Virtually all cases of BL are associated with chronic EBV infection.
15. Treatment for BL is aggressive multidrug regimens, such as combination chemotherapy.
16. Multiple myeloma (MM) is a clonal plasma cell cancer characterized by the neoplastic proliferation of plasma cells producing a monoclonal immunoglobulin. The plasma cells proliferate in the bone marrow. The multiple malignant tumor masses of plasma cells are scattered throughout the skeletal system (lytic bone lesions) and sometimes found in soft tissue. The common presentation of MM is characterized by elevated levels of calcium in the blood, renal failure, anemia, and lytic bone lesions.
17. Multiple mutations in different pathways alter the intrinsic biology of the plasma cell, generating the features of myeloma. The exact cause of MM is unknown, but risk factors include overweight or obesity, Agent Orange, possibly other certain chemicals, and a history of monoclonal gammopathy of undetermined significance (MGUS). MM has been observed in some irradiated populations.
18. Treatment options for MM include combinations of chemotherapy; other drug therapy; targeted therapy; high-dose chemotherapy with stem cell transplant; biologic therapy; radiation therapy; and, sometimes, surgery.

9.5 Alterations of Splenic Function

1. Splenomegaly (enlargement of the spleen) may be considered normal in certain individuals, but its presence is associated with various diseases.
2. Splenomegaly results from (1) acute inflammatory or infectious processes, (2) congestive disorders, (3) infiltrative processes, and (4) tumors or cysts.
3. Hypersplenism (overactivity of the spleen) results from splenomegaly. Hypersplenism results in sequestering of the blood cells, causing increased destruction of red blood cells, leukopenia, and thrombocytopenia.

Hemorrhagic Disorders and Alterations of Platelets and Coagulation

1. The arrest of bleeding is called hemostasis. Copious or heavy discharge of blood from blood vessels is called hemorrhage.
2. Quantitative or qualitative abnormalities of platelets can interrupt normal blood coagulation and prevent hemostasis.
3. Thrombocytopenia is characterized by a platelet count below 150,000/μL of blood; a count less than 50,000/μL increases the potential for hemorrhage associated with minor trauma. A count less than 10,000 platelets/μL can cause spontaneous bleeding without trauma.
4. Thrombocytopenia exists in primary or secondary forms and can be congenital or acquired. Acquired thrombocytopenia is associated with viral infections, drugs, nutritional deficiencies, chronic renal failure, cancer, radiation therapy, and bone marrow hypoplasia.
5. Common forms of thrombocytopenia include heparin-induced thrombocytopenia, idiopathic (immune) thrombocytopenia purpura, thrombotic thrombocytopenia purpura, and disseminated intravascular coagulation.
6. Thrombocythemia is characterized by a platelet count more than 450,000 platelets/μL of blood and is symptomatic when the count exceeds 1 million/μL, at which time the risk for intravascular clotting (thrombosis) is high.
7. Thrombocythemia is a myeloproliferative neoplasm characterized by excessive platelet production resulting from a defect in the bone marrow megakaryocyte progenitor cells. It also can include an increase in red blood cell production.
8. Qualitative alterations in normal platelet function prevent platelet plug formation and may result in prolonged bleeding times. Acquired disorders of platelet function are more common than congenital disorders.
9. Disorders of coagulation are usually caused by defects or deficiencies of one or more clotting factors. Coagulation is stimulated by the presence of tissue factor that is released by damaged or dead tissues.
10. Coagulation is impaired when there is a deficiency of vitamin K because of insufficient production of prothrombin and synthesis of clotting factors VII, IX, and X, often associated with liver diseases.
11. Disseminated intravascular coagulation (DIC) is an acquired clinical syndrome characterized by widespread activation of coagulation, resulting in formation of fibrin clots in medium and small vessels or microvasculature throughout the body. Widespread clotting may lead to blockage of blood flow to

organs, resulting in multiple organ failure. The excessive clotting may result in consumption of platelets and clotting factors, leading to a tendency to bleed despite widespread clots.

12. DIC is secondary to a wide variety of clinical conditions, with sepsis being the most common. Massive cytokine release can produce cytokine release syndrome (CRS) which is life-threatening induced by a hyperinflammatory process.
13. For a diagnosis of DIC, the person must present with a clinical condition that is known to be associated with DIC. The most used combination of laboratory tests usually confirms thrombocytopenia, or a rapidly decreasing platelet count on repeated testing, prolongation of clotting times, the presence of fibrin split products, and decreased levels of coagulation inhibitors.
14. Treatment of DIC is directed toward (1) eliminating the underlying pathologic condition, (2) controlling ongoing thrombosis, and (3) maintaining organ function.
15. Thromboembolic disease results from a fixed (thrombus) or moving (embolus) clot that blocks flow within a vessel, denying nutrients to tissues distal to the occlusion; death can result when clots obstruct blood flow to the heart, brain, or lungs.
16. The Virchow triad refers to three factors that influence the risk of developing spontaneous thrombi: (1) injury to the blood vessel endothelium, (2) abnormalities of blood flow, and (3) hypercoagulability of the blood.

REFERENCES

1. [No authors listed]: QuickStats: prevalence of anemia among adults aged ≥65 years, by sex and age group—National Health and Nutrition Examination Survey, 2013–2016, *MMWR Morb Mortal Wkly Rep* 67:1198, 2018. Available at https://doi.org/10.15585/mmwr.mm6742a8. (Accessed November 18, 2021).
2. Rossaint R, et al. The European guideline on management of major bleeding and coagulopathy following trauma: fourth edition. *Crit Care*. 2016;20:100.
3. World Health Organization (WHO) *Injuries and violence: the facts, 2014*. Geneva, Switzerland: WHO; 2014. Available at https://apps.who.int/iris/bitstream/handle/10665/149798/9789241508018_eng.pdf. (Accessed November 18, 2021).
4. Weisel JW, Litvinov RI. Red blood cells: the forgotten player in hemostasis and thrombosis. *J Thromb Haemost*. 2019;17:271–282.
5. Meybohm P, et al. Simplified international recommendations for the implementation of patient blood management (SIR4PBM). *Perioper Med (Lond)*. 2017;6:5.
6. Repsold L, Joubert AM. Eryptosis: an erythrocyte's suicidal type of cell death. *Biomed Res Int*. 2018;2018:9405617.
7. Ammouri W, et al. Pernicious anemia: mechanisms, diagnosis and management. *European Medical Journal Hematology*. 2020;1(1):71–80. Available at https://www.emjreviews.com/hematology/article/pernicious-anaemia-mechanisms-diagnosis-and-management/. (Accessed November 18, 2021).
8. Zulfiqar AA, Andres E. Association pernicious anemia and autoimmune polyendocrinopathy: a retrospective study. *J Med Life*. 2017;10(4):250–253.
9. Oo TH. Diagnostic difficulties in pernicious anemia. *Discov Med*. 2019;28(155):247–253.
10. Gwathmey KG, Grogan J. Nutritional neuropathies. *Muscle Nerve*. 2020;62(1):13–29.
11. Mohamed M, et al. Pernicious anaemia. *BMJ*. 2020;369:m1319.
12. Socha DS, et al. Severe megaloblastic anemia: vitamin deficiency and other causes. *Cleve Clin J Med*. 2020;87(3):153–164.
13. Lopez A, et al. Iron deficiency anaemia. *Lancet*. 2016;387:907–916.
14. Goldman RH, Weissmann L. A diagnosis to chew on. *N Engl J Med*. 2019;381(5):466–473.
15. Pasricha S, et al. Iron deficiency. *Lancet*. 2020;397(10270):233–248.
16. Kumar V, Abbas A, Aster J, eds. *Robbins & Cotran pathologic Basis of Disease*. 10 ed: Elsevier; 2020.
17. Cronin SJF, et al. The role of iron regulation in immunometabolism and immune-related disease. *Front Mol Biosci*. 2019;6:116.
18. Fishbane S, Spinowitz B. Update on anemia in ESRD and earlier stages of CKD: core curriculum 2018. *Am J Kidney Dis*. 2018;71(3):423–435.
19. Brzeźniakiewicz-Janus K, Rupa-Matysek J, Gil L. Acquired aplastic anemia as a clonal disorder of hematopoietic stem cells. *Stem Cell Rev Rep*. 2020;16(3):472–481.
20. Wang L, Liu H. Pathogenesis of aplastic anemia. *Hematology*. 2019;24(1):559–566.
21. Zhao XC, et al. Excellent response of severe aplastic anemia to treatment of gut inflammation: a case report and review of the literature. *World J Clin Cases*. 2020;8(2):425–435.
22. Andrea B, Giammarco S. Stem cell transplantation in aplastic anemia: Impact on choices for first line therapy. *Hemasphere*. 2019;3(52):15–17.
23. Fan X, et al. Eltrombopag for patients with moderate aplastic anemia or uni-lineage cytopenias. *Blood Adv*. 2020;4(8):1700–1710.
24. Michalak SS, et al. Autoimmune hemolytic anemia: current knowledge and perspectives. *Immun Ageing*. 2020;17:38.
25. Jäger U, et al. Diagnosis and treatment of autoimmune hemolytic anemia in adults: Recommendations from the First International Consensus Meeting. *Blood Rev*. 2020;41:100648.
26. Aljabry MS. Primary familial and congenital polycythemia: the forgotten entity. *Journal of Applied Hematology*. 2018;9(2):39–44. Available at http://www.doi.org/10.4103/joah.joah_30_18. (Accessed November 18, 2021).
27. Tefferi A, Barbui T. Polycythemia vera and essential thrombocythemia: 2021 update on diagnosis, risk-stratification and management. *Am J Hematol*. 2020;95(12):1599–1613.
28. Guglielmelli P, Vannucchi AM. Current management strategies for polycythemia vera and essential thrombocythemia. *Blood Rev*. 2020;42:100714.
29. Kowdley KV, et al. ACG clinical guideline: hereditary hemochromatosis. *Am J Gastroenterol*. 2019;114:1202–1218.
30. Brissot P, et al. Haemochromatosis. *Nat Rev Dis Primers*. 2018;4:18016.
31. Jayachandran A, et al. Association between hereditary hemochromatosis and hepatocellular carcinoma: a comprehensive review. *Hepatoma Res*. 2020;6:8.
32. Sullivan JL. *Clinical Manifestations and Treatment of Epstein-Barr Virus Infection*. Waltham, MA: UpToDate Inc; 2021. Literature review current through October 2021. Last updated May 26, 2021. Available at https://www.uptodate.com/contents/clinical-manifestations-and-treatment-of-epstein-barr-virus-infection. (Accessed November 18, 2021).
33. Smatti MK, et al. Epstein-Barr virus epidemiology, serology, and genetic variability of LMP-1 oncogene among healthy population: an update. *Front Oncol*. 2018;8:211.

34. Crombie JL, LaCasce AS. Epstein Barr virus associated B-cell lymphomas and iatrogenic lymphoproliferative disorders. *Front Oncol.* 2019;9:109.
35. Aronson MD, Auwaerter PG. *Infectious Mononucleosis.* Waltham, MA: UpToDate Inc; 2021. Literature review current through October 2021. Last updated March 19, 2021. Available at https://www.uptodate.com/contents/infectious-mononucleosis. (Accessed November 18, 2021).
36. Balfour HH, et al. Behavioral, virologic, and immunologic factors associated with acquisition and severity of primary Epstein-Barr virus infection in university students. *J Infect Dis.* 2013;207(1):80.
37. Vetsika EK, Callan M. Infectious mononucleosis and Epstein-Barr virus. *Expert Rev Mol Med.* 2004;6(23):1.
38. Higgens CD, et al. A study of risk factors for acquisition of Epstein-Barr virus and its subtypes. *J Infect Dis.* 2007;195(4):474.
39. Woodman CBJ, et al. Role of sexual behavior in the acquisition of asymptomatic Epstein-Barr virus infection: a longitudinal study. *Pediatr Infect Dis J.* 2005;24(6):498–502.
40. Rezk E, et al. Steroids for symptom control in infectious mononucleosis. *Cochrane Database Syst Rev.* 2015;2015(11):CD004402.
41. Swerdlow SH, et al. The 2016 revision of the World Health Organization classification of lymphoid neoplasms. *Blood.* 2016;127(20):2375–2390.
42. American Cancer Society (ACS) *Cancer Facts & Figures 2021.* Atlanta, GA: ACS; 2021. Available at https://www.cancer.org/research/cancer-facts-statistics/all-cancer-facts-figures/cancer-facts-figures-2021.html. (Accessed November 18, 2021).
43. National Cancer Institute (NCI) *SEER*Explorer: an Interactive Website for SEER Cancer Statistics.* Bethesda, MD: NCI; 2020. Available at https://seer.cancer.gov/explorer/. (Accessed November 18, 2021).
44. Abdul-Aziz AM, et al. Acute myeloid leukemia induces protumoral p16INK4a-driven senescence in the bone marrow microenvironment. *Blood.* 2019;133(5):446–456.
45. Campisi J. Aging, cellular senescence, and cancer. *Annu Rev Physiol.* 2013;75:685–705.
46. deKeizer PL. The fountain of youth by targeting senescent cells? *Trends Mol Med.* 2017;23(1):6–17.
47. Munoz-Espin Serrano M. Cellular senescence: from physiology to pathology. *Nat Rev Mol Cell Biol.* 2014;15(7):482–496.
48. Shafat MS, et al. Leukemic blasts program bone marrow adipocytes to generate a protumoral microenvironment. *Blood.* 2017;129(10):1310–1332.
49. Pui CH, et al. Philadelphia chromosome-like acute lymphoblastic leukemia. *Clin Lymphoma Myeloma Leuk.* 2017;17(8):464–470.
50. Reboursiere E, et al. Rare but authentic Philadelphia-positive acute myeloblastic leukemia: two case reports and a literature review of characteristics, treatment and outcome. *Hematol Oncol Stem Cell Ther.* 2015;8(1):28–33.
51. Pelcovits A, Niroula R. Acute myeloid leukemia: a review. *R I Med J (2013).* 2020;103(3):38–40.
52. Kouchkovsky De, Abdul-Hay M. Acute myeloid leukemia: a comprehensive review and 2016 update. *Blood Cancer J.* 2016;6:e441.
53. Arber DA, et al. The 2016 revision to the World Health Organization classification of myeloid neoplasms and acute leukemia. *Blood.* 2016;127(20):2391–2405.
54. Hsu WL, et al. The incidence of leukemia, lymphoma and multiple myeloma among atomic bomb survivors: 1950-2001. *Radiat Res.* 2013;179(3):361–382.
55. Kirtane K, Lee SJ. Racial and ethnic disparities in hematologic malignancies. *Blood.* 2017;130(15):1699–1705.
56. American Cancer Society (ACS) *Risk Factors for Acute Lymphocytic Leukemia (ALL).* Atlanta, GA: ACS; 2018. Last revised October 17, 2018. Available at https://www.cancer.org/cancer/acute-lymphocytic-leukemia/causes-risks-prevention/risk-factors.html. (Accessed November 18, 2021).
57. Nikkilä A, et al. Radiation exposure from computerized tomography and risk of childhood leukemia: Finnish register-based case-control study of childhood leukemia (FRECCLE). *Haematologica.* 2018;103(11):1873–1880.
58. Ribeiro-Filho AC, et al. Traditional and advanced cell cultures in hematopoietic stem cell studies. *Cells.* 2019;8(12):1628.
59. PDQ® Adult Treatment Editorial Board *Adult Acute Lymphoblastic Leukemia Treatment (PDQ®)—Health Professional Version.* Bethesda, MD: National Cancer Institute; 2002. Available at https://www.cancer.gov/types/leukemia/hp/adult-all-treatment-pdq. (Accessed November 18, 2021).
60. Nelson R. *Blood Transfusions in Leukemia a Deterrent to Hospice Care.* New York: Medscape Medical News, WebMD LLC; 2017. Available at https://www.medscape.com/viewarticle/889858. (Accessed November 18, 2021).
61. Behrmann L, Wellbrook J, Fiedler W. Acute myeloid leukemia and the bone marrow niche—take a closer look. *Front Oncol.* 2018;8:444.
62. Klepin HD. Elderly acute myeloid leukemia: assessing risk. *Curr Hematol Malig Rep.* 2015;10:118–125.
63. Klepin HD. Definition of unfit for standard acute myeloid leukemia therapy. *Curr Hematol Malig Rep.* 2016;11:537–544.
64. PDQ® Adult Treatment Editorial Board *Adult Acute Myeloid Leukemia Treatment (PDQ®)—Health Professional Version.* Bethesda, MD: National Cancer Institute; 2021. Updated January 13, 2021. Available at https://www.cancer.gov/types/leukemia/hp/adult-aml-treatment-pdq. (Accessed November 18, 2021).
65. Hallek M, Shanafelt TD, Eichhorst B. Chronic lymphocytic leukaemia. *Lancet.* 2018;391(10129):1524–1537.
66. Leon ME, et al. Pesticide use and risk of non-Hodgkin lymphoid malignancies in agricultural cohorts from France, Norway, and the USA: a pooled analysis from the AGRICOH Consortium. *Int J Epidemiol.* 2019;48:1519–1535.
67. Alavanja MC, et al. Non-Hodgkin lymphoma risk and insecticide, fungicide and fumigant use in the agricultural health study. *PLoS One.* 2014;9(10):e109332.
68. Chiorazzi N, Chen SS, Rai KR. Chronic lymphocytic leukemia. *Cold Spring Harb Perspect Med.* 2021;11:a0355220.
69. Baumann Kreuziger LM, Tarchand G, Morrison VA. The impact of Agent Orange exposure on presentation and prognosis of patients with chronic lymphocytic leukemia. *Leuk Lymphoma.* 2014;55:63–66.
70. Mescher C, et al. The impact of Agent Orange on prognosis and management in patients with chronic lymphocytic leukemia: a National Veteran Affairs Tumor Registry study. *Leuk Lymphoma.* 2018;59:1348–1355.
71. Schwartz GG, Klug MG. Incidence rates of chronic lymphocytic leukemia in US states are associated with residential radon levels. *Future Oncol.* 2016;12:165–174.
72. Landgren O, et al. Acquired immune-related and inflammatory conditions and subsequent chronic lymphocytic leukaemia. *Br J Haematol.* 2007;139:791–798.

73. Landgren O, et al. Respiratory tract infections and subsequent risk of chronic lymphocyctic leukemia. *Blood*. 2007;109:2198–2201.
74. Lesley AA, Ola L, Eric AE. Common community acquired infections and subsequent risk of chronic lymphocytic leukaemia. *Br J Haematol*. 2009;147:444–449.
75. Lenders JW, et al. Combined immunodeficiency preceding chronic lymphocytic leukemia. *Blut*. 1984;48:171–175.
76. Tsai H-T, et al. Evidence of serum immunoglobulin abnormalities up to 9.8 years before diagnosis of chronic lymphocytic leukemia: a prospective study. *Blood*. 2009;114:4928–4932.
77. Goldin LR, et al. Familial risk of lymphoproliferative tumors in families of patients with chronic lymphocytic leukemia: results from the Swedish Family-Cancer Database. *Blood*. 2004;104(6):1850–1854.
78. Gale RP, et al. Decreased chronic lymphocytic leukemia incidence in Asians in Los Angeles County. *Leuk Res*. 2000;24:665–669.
79. Law PJ, et al. Genome-wide association analysis implicates dysregulation of immunity genes in chronic lymphocytic leukaemia. *Nat Commun*. 2017;8:14175.
80. Went M, et al. Genetic correlation between multiple myeloma and chronic lymphocytic leukaemia provides evidence for shared aetiology. *Blood Cancer J*. 2018;9(1):1.
81. Eden RE, Coviello JM. *Chronic myelogenous leukemia. StatPearls*. Treasure Island, FL: StatPearls Publishing; 2021. Last update July 26, 2021. Available at https://www.ncbi.nlm.nih.gov/books/NBK531459/. (Accessed November 18, 2021).
82. International CLL-IPI Working Group An International prognostic index for patients with chronic lymphocytic leukemia (CLL-IPI): a meta-analysis of individual patient data. *Lancet Oncol*. 2016;17(6):779–790.
83. PDQ® Adult Treatment Editorial Board *Chronic Myelogenous Leukemia Treatment (PDQ®)—Health Professional Version*. Bethesda, MD: National Cancer Institute; 2021. Updated March 5, 2021. Available at https://www.cancer.gov/types/leukemia/hp/cml-treatment-pdq. (Accessed November 18, 2021).
84. Arrigoni E, et al. Concise review: chronic myeloid leukemia: stem cell niche and response to pharmacologic treatment. *Stem Cells Transl Med*. 2018;7(3):305–314.
85. Connors JM, et al. Hodgkin lymphoma. *Nat Rev*. 2020;6:61.
86. National Cancer Institute (NCI) Surveillance Epidemiology and End Results (SEER) Program *Cancer Stat Facts: Hodgkin Lymphoma*. Bethesda, MD: NCI; 2019. Available at https://seer.cancer.gov/statfacts/hmtl/hodg.html. (Accessed November 18, 2021).
87. National Cancer Institute (NCI) Surveillance Epidemiology and End Results (SEER) Program: SEER Cancer Statistics Review 1975-2014: *Hodgkin lymphoma*, Bethesda, MD, 2019, NCI. Available at https://seer.cancer.gov/archive/csr/1975_2014/results_merged/sect_09_hodgkins.pdf. (Accessed November 18, 2021).
88. LaCasce AS, Ng AK. *Hodgkin Lymphoma: Epidemiology and Risk Factors*. Waltham, MA: UpToDate Inc; 2021. Literature review current through October 2021. Topic last updated January 22, 2020. Available at https://www.uptodate.com/contents/hodgkin-lymphoma-epidemiology-and-risk-factors. (Accessed November 18, 2021).
89. International Agency for Research on Cancer (IARC) *A Review of Human Carcinogens. Part B: Biological Agents. IARC Monographs on the Evaluation of Carcinogenic Risks to Humans*. Volume 100B. Lyon, France: IARC; 2012. (IARC Working Group on the Evaluation of Carcinogenic Risks to Humans, Lyon, France, 24 February 24, 2009, to March 3, 2009). Available at https://publications.iarc.fr/119. (Accessed November 18, 2021).
90. PDQ® Adult Treatment Editorial Board *Adult Hodgkin lymphoma treatment (PDQ®)—health professional version*. Bethesda, MD: National Cancer Institute; 2021. Updated October 29, 2021. Available at https://www.cancer.gov/types/lymphoma/hp/adult-hodgkin-treatment-pdq. (Accessed November 18, 2021).
91. Fisher SG, Fisher RI. The epidemiology of non-Hodgkin's lymphoma. *Oncogene*. 2004;23:6524–6534.
92. Han YY, Dinse GE, Davis DL. Temporal and demographic patterns of non-Hodgkin's lymphoma incidence in Pennsylvania. *Int J Occup Environ Health*. 2010;16(1):75–84.
93. Singh R, et al. Non-Hodgkin's lymphoma: a review. *J Family Med Prim Care*. 2020;9:1834–1840.
94. American Cancer Society (ACS) *Non-Hodgkin Lymphoma Causes, Risk Factors, and Prevention*. Atlanta, GA: ACS; 2020. Available at https//www.cancer.org/content/dam/CRC/PDF/Public/8718.00.pdf. (Accessed November 18, 2021).
95. Feugier P, Filliatre-Clement L. Recent advances in the first-line treatment of follicular non-Hodgkin lymphoma. *F1000Research*. 2019;8(F1000 Faculty Rev):294.
96. Brown JR, Freedman AS, Aster JC. *Pathobiology of Burkitt Lymphoma in Adults*. Waltham, MA: UpToDate Inc; 2021. Literature review current through October 2021. Last updated October 29, 2021. Available at https://www.uptodate.com/contents/pathobiology-of-burkitt-lymphoma. (Accessed November 18, 2021).
97. Freedman AS, Friedberg JW. *Treatment of Burkitt Leukemia/Lymphoma in Adults*. Waltham, MA: UpToDate Inc; 2021. Literature review current through October 2021. Last updated May 14, 2021. Available at https://www.uptodate.com/contents/treatment-of-burkitt-leukemia-lymphoma-in-adults. (Accessed November 18, 2021).
98. Laubach JP. *Multiple myeloma: clinical features, laboratory manifestations, and diagnosis*. Waltham, MA: UpToDate Inc; 2021. Literature review current through October 2021. Last updated May 14, 2021. Available at https://www.uptodate.com/contents/multiple-myeloma-clinical-features-laboratory-manifestations-and-diagnosis. (Accessed November 18, 2021).
99. National Research Council (US) Committee on the Biological Effects of Ionizing Radiation (BEIR V) *Health Effects of Exposure to Low Levels of Ionizing Radiation: Beir V*. Washington, DC: National Academies Press; 1990. Available at https://www.ncbi.nlm.nih.gov/books/NBK218708/. (Accessed November 18, 2021).
100. Kim EB, Yee AJ, Raje N. Treatment of smoldering multiple myeloma: ready for prime time? *Cancers (Basel)*. 2020;12(5):1223.
101. Hillengass J, et al. International Myeloma Working Group consensus recommendations on imaging in monoclonal plasma cell disorders. *Lancet Oncol*. 2019;20(6):e302.
102. Lonial S, et al. Randomized trial of lenalidomide versus observation in smoldering multiple myeloma. *J Clin Oncol*. 2020;38(11):1126–1137.
103. National Cancer Institute (NCI) *Drug shows Promise in Slowing Progression of Smoldering Myeloma to Cancer*. Bethesda, MD: NCI; 2019. Available at https://www.cancer.gov/news-events/cancer-currents-blog/2019/lenalidomide-slows-progression-smoldering-myeloma. (Accessed November 18, 2021).
104. Chapman J, et al. *Splenomegaly. StatPearls*. Treasure Island, FL: StatPearls Publishing; 2021. Last update August 11, 2021. Available at https://www.ncbi.nlm.nih.gov/books/NBK430907/. (Accessed November 18, 2021).
105. Tahir F, Ahmed J, Malik F. Post-splenectomy sepsis: a review of the literature. *Cureus*. 2020;12(2):e6898.

106. National Heart Lung Blood Institute (NHLBI) *Thrombocytopenia*. Bethesda, MD: NHLBI; 2021. Available at https://www.nhlbi.nih.gov/health-topics/thrombocytopenia. (Accessed November 18, 2021).
107. Jinna S, Khandhar PB. *Thrombocytopenia. StatPearls*. Treasure Island, FL: StatPearls Publishing; 2021. Last update July 25, 2021. Available at https://www.ncbi.nlm.nih.gov/books/NBK542208/. (Accessed November 18, 2021).
108. Segal JB, Moliterno AR. Platelet counts differ by sex, ethnicity, and age in the United States. *Ann Epidemiol*. 2006;16(2):123–130.
109. Vaillant AAJ, Gupta N. *ITP-immune thrombocytopenic purpura. StatPearls*. Treasure Island, FL: StatPearls Publishing; 2020. Last update December 30, 2020. Available at https://www.ncbi.nlm.nih.gov/books/NBK537240/. (Accessed November 18, 2021).
110. Kistangari G, McCrae KR. Immune thrombocytopenia. *Hematol Oncol Clin North Am*. 2013;27(3):495–520.
111. Nuñez Zuno JA, Khaddour K. *Thrombotic thrombocytopenic purpura evaluation and management. StatPearls*. Treasure Island, FL: StatPearls Publishing; 2021. Last update July 31, 2021. Available at https://www.ncbi.nlm.nih.gov/books/NBK470585/. (Accessed November 18, 2021).
112. Mead TJ, Apte SS. ADAMTS proteins in human disorders. *Matrix Biol*. 2018;71-72:225–239. Available at https://doi.org/10.1016/j.matbio.2018.06.002. (Accessed November 18, 2021).
113. Fox LC, et al. Consensus opinion on diagnosis and management of thrombotic microangiopathy in Australia and New Zealand. *Intern Med J*. 2018;48(6):624–636.
114. Nagalla S, Sarode R. Recent advances in understanding and management of acquired thrombocytopenia. *F1000Res*. 2018;7:68.
115. Sadler JE. Pathophysiology of thrombotic thrombocytopenic purpura. *Blood*. 2017;130(10):1181–1188.
116. Tefferi A, Pardanani A. Essential thrombocytopenia. *N Engl J Med*. 2019;381:2135–2144.
117. Guglielmelli P, et al. Validation of the IPSET score for thrombosis in patients with prefibrotic myelofibrosis. *Blood Cancer J*. 2020;10(2):21.
118. Ayres-Silva JP, et al. Genetic alterations in essential thrombocythemia progression to acute myeloid leukemia: a case series and review of the literature. *Front Oncol*. 2018;8:32.
119. Barbui T, et al. The 2016 WHO classification and diagnostic criteria for myeloproliferative neoplasms: document summary and in-depth discussion. *Blood Cancer J*. 2018;8(2):15.
120. Tefferi A, Barbui T. Polycythemia vera and essential thrombocythemia: 2017 update on diagnosis, risk-stratification, and management. *Am J Hematol*. 2017;92(1):94–108.
121. Gando S, Levi M, Toh CH. Disseminated intravascular coagulation. *Nat Rev Dis Primers*. 2016;2:16037.
122. Kang S, et al. Il-6 trans -signaling induces plasminogen activator inhibitor-1 from vascular endothelial cells in cytokine release syndrome. *Proc Natl Acad Sci U S A*. 2020;117(36):22351–22356.
123. Levi MM, et al. *Disseminated Intravascular Coagulation (DIC) Treatment and Management*. New York: Medscape Medical News, WebMD LLC; 2020. Updated December 6, 2020. Available at https://emedicine.medscape.com/article/199627-treatment. (Accessed November 18, 2021).
124. Centers for Disease Control and Prevention (CDC) *Impact of Blood Clots on the United States*. Atlanta, GA: CDC; 2020. Page last reviewed February 7, 2020. Available at https://www.cdc.gov/ncbddd/dvt/infographic-impact.html. (Accessed November 18, 2021).
125. Chopard R, Albertsen IE, Piazza G. Diagnosis and treatment of lower extremity venous thromboembolism: a review. *JAMA*. 2020;324(17):1765–1776.
126. Nakashima MO, Rogers HJ. Hypercoagulable states: an algorithmic approach to laboratory testing and update on monitoring of direct oral anticoagulants. *Blood Res*. 2014;49(2):85–94.
127. Chiasakul T, et al. Inherited thrombophilia and the risk of arterial ischemic stroke: a systematic review and meta-analysis. *J Am Heart Assoc*. 2019;8(19):e012877.
128. Moran J, Bauer KA. Managing thromboembolic risk in patients with hereditary and acquired thrombophilias. *Blood*. 2020;135(5):344–350.

30

Alterations of Hematologic Function in Children

Lauri A. Linder and Anne Harvey

http://evolve.elsevier.com/Rogers/pathophysiology/

CHAPTER OUTLINE

This chapter briefly explains fetal and neonatal hematopoiesis and postnatal changes in the blood as a foundation for understanding the pathophysiology of specific blood disorders in childhood. Among the diseases that affect erythrocytes are acquired disorders, such as iron deficiency anemia (IDA), hemolytic disease of the newborn, and anemia of infectious disease; and inherited disorders, such as glucose-6-phosphate dehydrogenase (G6PD) deficiency, hereditary spherocytosis, sickle cell disease, and the thalassemias. Disorders of coagulation and platelets include inherited hemorrhagic diseases, such as the hemophilias, and antibody-mediated hemorrhagic diseases, which include immune thrombocytopenia, autoimmune neonatal thrombocytopenias, and autoimmune vascular purpuras. Finally, leukocyte disorders, such as leukemia and the lymphomas (non-Hodgkin lymphoma as well as Hodgkin lymphoma), are discussed.

FETAL AND NEONATAL HEMATOPOIESIS

As the developing embryo becomes too large for oxygenation of tissues by simple diffusion, the production of erythrocytes begins within the vessels of the yolk sac. Shortly after 2 weeks of gestation, circulating erythrocytes play a significant role in delivering oxygen to the tissues. At approximately the eighth week of gestation, the site of erythrocyte production shifts from the vessels to the liver sinusoids, and the production of leukocytes and platelets begins in the liver and spleen. Erythropoiesis in the liver and, to a lesser extent, in the spleen and lymph nodes, peaks at approximately 4 months. Hepatic blood formation declines steadily thereafter but does not disappear entirely during the remainder of gestation. By the fifth month of gestation, hematopoiesis begins to occur in the bone marrow and increases rapidly until hematopoietic (red) marrow fills the entire bone marrow space. By the time of delivery, the marrow is the only significant site of hematopoiesis.

In neonates and young infants, hematopoietic marrow progressively fills the bony cavities of the entire axial skeleton (skull, vertebrae, ribs, and sternum), the long bones of the limbs, and many intramembranous bones. (These structures are described in Chapter 43). Fatty (yellow) marrow gradually replaces hematopoietic marrow in some bones. During childhood, hematopoietic tissue retreats centrally to the vertebrae, ribs, sternum, pelvis, scapulae, skull, and proximal ends of the femur and humerus.

In diseases characterized by hemolysis, erythrocyte production can increase as much as 12 times the normal level because erythropoietin causes hematopoietic marrow to increase in volume. Initially, hematopoietic marrow expands from the ends of the long bones toward the middle of the shafts, replacing fatty marrow. Next, blood cell production begins to occur outside the marrow cavities, especially in the liver and spleen. Extramedullary hematopoiesis is more likely to occur in children than in adults because the bony cavities of children already are filled with red marrow (Fig. 30.1), which is the reason hemolytic disease causes especially pronounced enlargement of the spleen and liver in children.

The erythrocytes undergo striking changes during gestation, particularly during the first two trimesters, at which time they nearly double in numbers and in hemoglobin content. A proportionate increase in hematocrit level also occurs. By the end of gestation, the erythrocyte count has more than tripled, but the size of each erythrocyte has decreased.

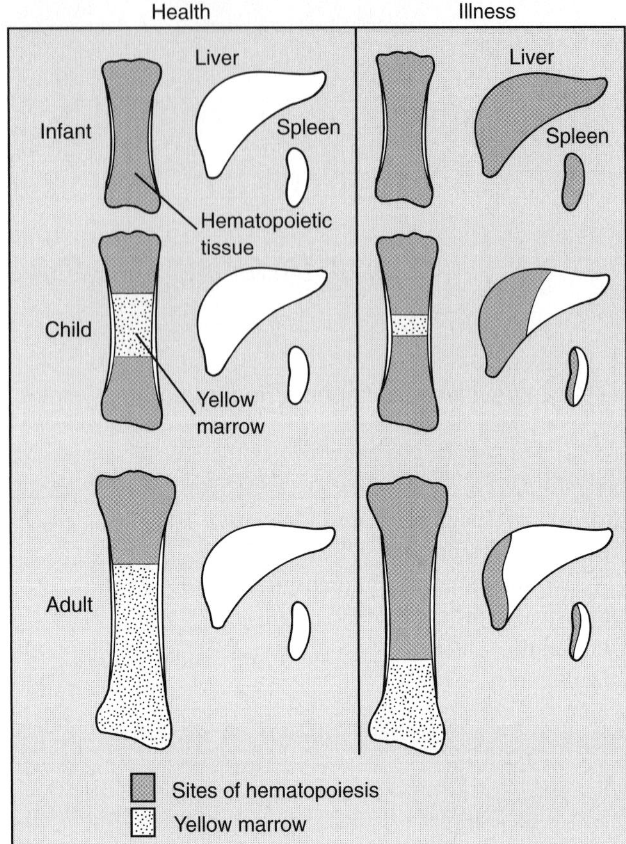

Fig. 30.1 Sites of Hematopoiesis in Health and Illness. With normal maturation, red marrow is partly replaced by yellow marrow in the shafts of the long bones. In adults, red marrow is largely restricted to the proximal ends of the femur and humerus. In response to hemolysis, red marrow replaces yellow marrow in the long bones. In infants, whose long bones already are filled with red marrow, additional hematopoiesis takes place in the liver and spleen. In children and adults, red marrow can replace yellow marrow in response to hemolysis, necessitating less hematopoiesis in the liver and spleen.

A biochemically distinct type of hemoglobin is synthesized during fetal life. The three embryonic hemoglobin molecules (Gower 1, Gower 2, and Portland) have different combinations of alpha, epsilon, zeta, and gamma chains, and fetal hemoglobin (HbF) molecules are composed of two α and two γ chains of polypeptides. Adult hemoglobin HbA_1 molecules are composed of two α chains and two β chains, and adult hemoglobin HbA_2 molecules are composed of 2 α chains and two δ chains. (The structure of an adult hemoglobin molecule is illustrated in Fig. 28.13 and types of hemoglobin are defined in Table 28.5). A transcriptional regulation mechanism promotes γ-chain synthesis and inhibits β- and δ-chain synthesis in utero. This results in production of embryonic or fetal hemoglobin. After birth, γ-chain synthesis is inhibited, whereas β- and δ-chain synthesis is facilitated, resulting in production of adult hemoglobin types.

Fetal hemoglobin has greater affinity for oxygen than does adult hemoglobin because it interacts less readily with an enzyme (2,3-diphosphoglycerate [2,3-DPG]) that inhibits hemoglobin-oxygen binding. The decreased inhibitory effects of 2,3-DPG enable fetal blood to transport oxygen despite the relative lack of oxygen in the intrauterine environment. The increased affinity for oxygen enables HbF to bind with maternal oxygen in the placental circulation.

During the first trimester, nearly all of the hemoglobin in the fetus is embryonic, but some HbA can be detected. Therefore, some disorders of adult hemoglobin, such as sickle cell anemia and thalassemia major, can be identified as early as 16 to 20 weeks of gestation. In the 6-month fetus, HbF constitutes 90% of the total hemoglobin. This percentage then declines. At birth, neonatal hemoglobin consists of 70% HbF, 29% HbA, and 1% HbA_2. Between 6 and 12 months of age, normal adult hemoglobin percentages are established (see Chapter 28).

POSTNATAL CHANGES IN THE BLOOD

Blood cell counts tend to rise to higher than adult levels at birth and then decline gradually throughout childhood. Table 30.1 lists normal ranges during infancy and childhood. The immediate rise in values is the result of the accelerated hematopoiesis during fetal life, the increased numbers of cells that result from the trauma of birth, and the cutting of the umbilical cord. These events surrounding the birth also are accompanied by the presence of large numbers of immature erythrocytes and leukocytes (particularly granulocytes) in peripheral blood (see Chapter 28). As the infant develops over the first 2 to 3 months of life, the numbers of these immature blood cells decrease.

Average blood volume in the full-term neonate is 85 mL/kg of body weight. The premature infant has a proportionately larger blood volume of 90 to 100 mL/kg of body weight. In both full-term and premature infants, blood volume relative to body weight decreases during the first few months. By 3 years of age, a child's average blood volume is 75 to 77 mL/kg, which is similar to that of older children and adults.

Erythrocytes

The hypoxic intrauterine environment stimulates erythropoietin production in the fetus. This accelerates fetal erythropoiesis, producing polycythemia (excessive proliferation of erythrocyte precursors) of the newborn. After birth, the oxygen from the lungs saturates arterial blood, and the amount of oxygen delivered to the tissues increases. In response to the change from a placental to a pulmonary oxygen supply during the first few days of life, levels of erythropoietin and the rate of blood cell formation decrease. The very active rate of fetal erythropoiesis is reflected by the large numbers of immature erythrocytes (reticulocytes) in the peripheral blood of full-term neonates. The number of reticulocytes decreases abruptly during the first few days after birth, which is associated with decreased erythropoietin production.[1] Finding an elevated reticulocyte count after the first week of life is rare. A decrease in extramedullary hematopoiesis also occurs at this time. In the peripheral blood, the erythrocyte count drops for 6 to 8 weeks after birth. During this period of rapid growth, the rate of erythrocyte destruction is greater than that in later childhood and adulthood. In full-term infants, the normal erythrocyte

TABLE 30.1 Hematologic Values During Infancy and Childhood (US-Based Reference Values)

Age	Hemoglobin (g/dL) Range	Hematocrit (%) Range	Reticulocytes (%) Range	MCV (fl) Range	Leukocytes (WBC/mm³) Range	Neutrophils (%) Range	Lymphocytes (%) Range	Eosinophils (%) Range	Monocytes (%) Range
0–30 days	15.0–24.0	44–70	0.4–1.2	99–115	9.1–34.0	57–67	25–33	1–3	3–7
1–23 months	10.5–14.0	32–42	0.1–2.9 (1–3 months) 0.5–1.5 (≥3 months)	72–88	6.0–14.0	57–67	25–33	1–3	3–7
2–9 years	11.5–14.5	33 - 43	0.5–1.5	76–90	4.0–12.0	57–67	25–33	1–3	3–7
10–17 years M	12.5–16.1	36–47	0.5–1.5 (≥3	78–95	4.0–10.5	57–67	25–33	1–3	3–7
10–17 years F	12.0–15.0	35–45	0.5–1.5	78–95	4.0–10.5	57–67	25–33	1–3	3–7
Adult									
18+ years M	13.5–18.0	42–52	0.5–1.5	78–100	4.0–10.5	57–67	25–33	1–3	3–7
18+ years F	12.5–16.0	37–47	0.5–1.5	78–100	4.0–10.5	57–67	25–33	1–3	3–7

fl, Femtoliters; *MCV*, mean corpuscular volume; *WBC*, white blood cells.
From Kliegman RM, et al., eds. *Nelson textbook of pediatrics*, 21st edition. Philadelphia: Saunders; 2020.

life span is 60 to 80 days; in premature infants it may be as short as 20 to 30 days; and in children and adolescents, it is the same as that in adults—120 days (see Mechanisms of hemolysis are described in Chapter 28).

In the premature infant, the postnatal decrease in hemoglobin and hematocrit values is more marked than in the full-term infant. In the preschool and school-age child, hemoglobin, hematocrit, and red blood cell (RBC) count values rise gradually. In males and females, these values first begin to diverge in adolescence. In the female, the gradual hemoglobin level increase continues into early puberty, at which time it stabilizes. In the male, the hemoglobin level increase keeps pace with growth and maturation and eventually surpasses that of the female. This higher value of hemoglobin level in the mature male is related to androgen secretion.

Metabolic processes within the erythrocytes of neonates differ significantly from those of erythrocytes in the normal adult. The relatively young population of erythrocytes in the newborn consumes more glucose than do erythrocytes in adults. Several enzymes that regulate glucose consumption are increased in the erythrocytes of neonates, with a subsequent increase in the rate of glycolysis.

Leukocytes and Platelets

The lymphocytes of children tend to have more cytoplasm and less compact nuclear chromatin than do the lymphocytes of adults. The significance of these differences is unknown. One possible explanation is that children tend to have more frequent viral infections, which are associated with atypical lymphocytes. Even minor infections, in which the child fails to exhibit clinical manifestations of illness, or administration of immunizations may result in lymphocyte changes.[2]

The lymphocyte count is high at birth and continues to rise in some healthy infants during the first year of life. A steady decline occurs throughout childhood and adolescence until lower adult values are reached. Whether these developmental variations are physiologic or are a pathologic response to frequent viral infections and immunizations in children is not known.

In healthy neonates, the neutrophil count peaks 6 to 12 hours after birth and then declines over the next few days of life.[3] Neutrophil counts also are slightly higher in female neonates compared with males. After 2 weeks of life, neutrophil counts fall to within or below normal adult ranges. By approximately 4 years of age, the neutrophil count is similar to that of an adult. White children have slightly higher counts than black children.[4]

The eosinophil count is elevated in the first year of life relative to children, teenagers, or adults.[5,6] Monocyte counts are elevated through the preschool years and then decrease to adult levels. No relationship between age and basophil count has been found. Platelet counts in full-term neonates are comparable to platelet counts in adults and remain so throughout infancy and childhood.[5]

DISORDERS OF ERYTHROCYTES

Anemia is the most common blood disorder in children. Although anemia is not a disease state in and of itself, its presence may be associated with an underlying pathophysiologic process. Like anemia in adults, anemias occurring in children result from inadequate erythropoiesis or early destruction of erythrocytes. Iron deficiency is the most common cause of inadequate erythropoiesis. Iron deficiency can result from insufficient dietary intake or chronic loss of iron caused by bleeding. The hemolytic anemias of childhood are either inherited, acquired, or both. They may be divided into disorders that result from destruction caused by (1) intrinsic abnormalities of the erythrocytes and (2) damaging factors external to the erythrocytes.

The most dramatic form of acquired congenital hemolytic anemia is hemolytic disease of the fetus and newborn (HDFN), also termed *erythroblastosis fetalis*. HDFN is an alloimmune disorder in which the maternal blood and fetal blood are antigenically incompatible, causing the mother's immune system to produce antibodies against fetal erythrocytes. Fetal erythrocytes that have been bound to maternal antibodies are recognized as foreign or defective by the fetal mononuclear phagocyte system and are removed from the circulation by phagocytosis, usually in the fetal spleen. (For a complete discussion of HDFN, see Hemolytic Disease of the Fetus and Newborn.) Other acquired hemolytic anemias—some of which begin in utero—include those caused by infections or the presence of toxins.

The inherited forms of hemolytic anemia result from intrinsic defects of the child's erythrocytes, any of which can lead to erythrocyte destruction by the mononuclear phagocyte system. Structural defects include abnormal RBC size and abnormalities of plasma membrane structure (spherocytosis). Intracellular defects include enzyme deficiencies, the most common of which is glucose-6-phosphate dehydrogenase (G6PD) deficiency; and defects of hemoglobin synthesis, which manifest as sickle cell disease or thalassemia, depending on which component of hemoglobin is defective. These and other causes of childhood anemia, some more common than others, are listed in Table 30.2.

Acquired Disorders

Iron Deficiency Anemia

IDA is the most common nutritional disorder worldwide, with the highest incidence occurring between 6 months and 2 years of age. Its prevalence in the United States is greatest among toddlers, adolescent girls, and women of childbearing age. Iron is *critical* to the developing child, especially for normal brain development. Without it, the damage from the periods of IDA is irreversible. The clinical manifestations of IDA are mostly related to inadequate hemoglobin synthesis. The incidence of IDA is not related to gender or race; however, socioeconomic factors are important because they affect nutrition.

IDA can result from (1) dietary lack of iron, (2) problems with iron absorption, (3) blood loss, and (4) increased requirement for iron. During the first few years of life, IDA most often results from inadequate iron intake. During childhood and adolescence, blood loss is the most common cause of IDA. Chronic IDA from occult (hidden) blood loss may be caused by a gastrointestinal lesion, parasitic infestation, or hemorrhagic disease. A reasonable hypothesis for infants and young children who develop IDA is that they have chronic intestinal blood loss induced by exposure to a heat-labile protein in cow's milk. Such exposure causes an inflammatory gastrointestinal reaction that

TABLE 30.2 **Anemias of Childhood**

Cause	Examples of Anemic Condition
Blood Loss	
Trauma	Iron deficiency anemia
Gastrointestinal lesion	
Parasitic infestation	
Hemorrhagic disease	
Decreased Red Cell Production or Hemoglobin Synthesis	
Decreased stem cell population in marrow (congenital or acquired pure red cell aplasia)	Normocytic-normochromic anemia
Decreased erythropoiesis despite normal stem cell population in marrow (infection, inflammation, cancer, chronic renal disease, congenital dyserythropoiesis)	Normocytic-normochromic anemia
Deficiency of a Factor or Nutrient Needed for Erythropoiesis	
Cobalamin (vitamin B_{12}), folate	Megaloblastic anemia
Iron	Microcytic-hypochromic anemia
Increased or Premature Hemolysis	
Alloimmune disease (maternal-fetal Rh, ABO, or minor blood group incompatibility)	Autoimmune hemolytic anemia
Autoimmune disease (idiopathic autoimmune hemolytic anemia, symptomatic systemic lupus erythematosus, lymphoma, drug-induced autoimmune processes)	Autoimmune hemolytic anemia
Inherited defects of plasma membrane structure (spherocytosis, elliptocytosis, stomatocytosis) or cellular size or both (pyknocytosis)	Hemolytic anemia
Infection (bacterial sepsis, congenital syphilis, malaria, cytomegalovirus infection, rubella, toxoplasmosis, disseminated herpes)	Hemolytic anemia
Intrinsic and inherited enzymatic defects (deficiencies) of G6PD, pyruvate kinase, 5′-nucleotidase, glucose phosphate isomerase	Hemolytic anemia
Inherited Defects of Hemoglobin Synthesis	
Structurally abnormal globins	Sickle cell anemia
Deficient globin synthesis	Thalassemia
Other Anemias	
Disseminated intravascular coagulation (see Chapter 29)	Hemolytic anemia
Galactosemia	Hemolytic anemia
Prolonged or recurrent respiratory or metabolic acidosis	Hemolytic anemia
Blood vessel disorders (cavernous hemangiomas, large vessel thrombus, renal artery stenosis, severe coarctation of aorta)	Hemolytic anemia

ABO; Type A, type B, type O blood; *G6PD*; glucose-6-phosphate dehydrogenase.

damages the mucosa and results in diffuse microhemorrhage. Growing evidence indicates that cellular components of both innate and adaptive immunity play significant roles during the pathogenesis of cow's milk allergy.[7,8]

Dietary lack of iron is less common in developed countries, where iron is readily absorbed from heme found in meat. In developing countries, food may be less available. Although iron is found in plants, it is a more poorly absorbed form.[9] In the United States, rates of IDA have remained relatively unchanged over the past 10 years.[10] Infants are at increased risk for IDA because milk has only very small amounts of iron. The bioavailability of iron from breast milk, however, is higher than that from cow's milk. In developed countries, including the United States, excessive consumption of cow's milk remains an important predisposing factor for severe IDA.[11] Presently, only low-quality evidence for use of micronutrient powders in pregnant women and in the general population is available.[12,13] Impaired absorption is found in the context of chronic diarrhea, fat malabsorption, and celiac disease. Evidence also is emerging from international studies regarding genetic polymorphisms that may contribute to altered iron absorption in cases of refractory IDA with a familial component.[14,15]

Children in developing countries are often affected by chronic parasite infestations that result in blood and iron loss greater than dietary intake. However, a recent systematic review addressing outcomes of anti-helminthic treatments in adolescent girls and women failed to show an effect on anemia and iron deficiency.[16] Newer evidence is emerging related to a potential protective benefit of iron deficiency against malaria in parts of the world where malaria is endemic.[17] Additional research is needed to establish causality and to determine interventions to minimize adverse health consequences of IDA while maintaining the protective benefit. The association of IDA with lead (Pb) poisoning remains controversial. The role of *Helicobacter pylori* infection in relation to IDA is an area of ongoing investigation. While gastric colonization with *H. pylori* containing the sabA gene is associated with IDA, an understanding of its underlying pathophysiology is limited.[18]

Pathophysiology. No matter the cause, a deficiency of iron produces a hypochromic-microcytic anemia. In the early stages, however, the body may respond by increasing RBC activity in the bone marrow, which may temporarily prevent the development of anemia. As the body's iron stores are depleted, anemia develops (also see Chapter 29). Alterations in hepcidin have an essential role in diseases involving disturbances of iron metabolism (see Chapters 28 and 29). Low serum levels of ferritin and transferrin saturation lead to lowered hemoglobin and hematocrit levels (see Mechanisms of iron depletion are described in Chapter 29).

Clinical Manifestations. The symptoms of mild anemia—listlessness and fatigue—may go unnoticed in infants and young children, who are unable to describe these symptoms. Clinical indicators of anemia also are nonspecific, such as general irritability, decreased activity tolerance, weakness, and lack of interest in play, and may be attributed to other causes. As a result, parents may not note persistent changes in the child's behavior until moderate anemia has developed. In mild to moderate IDA (hemoglobin level of 6 to 10 g/dL), compensatory mechanisms of tissue oxygenation, such as increased amounts of 2,3-DPG within erythrocytes and a shift of the oxyhemoglobin dissociation curve, may be so effective that few clinical manifestations are apparent. Other clinical manifestations, such as pallor, anorexia, tachycardia, and systolic murmurs, are often not present until hemoglobin levels fall below 5 g/dl.

Other symptoms and signs of chronic IDA include splenomegaly, widened skull sutures, decreased physical growth, developmental delays, *pica* (a behavior in which nonfood substances, such as clay or ice, are eaten). Weight is not necessarily an indicator of IDA because children may be obese, underweight, or normal weight. Consequences of IDA are significant and may include altered neurologic and intellectual function, especially involving attention span, alertness, and learning ability.

Evaluation and Treatment. The evaluation and treatment of IDA are similar in children and adults (see Chapter 29). The diagnosis of IDA is confirmed by laboratory tests. These tests include hemoglobin, hematocrit, serum iron, ferritin levels and the total iron binding capacity. Obtaining a thorough history of the child's present illness and dietary history and performing a complete physical examination also are essential to the evaluation and subsequent clinical management of IDA. Oral administration of a simple ferrous salt is usually sufficient. Taking iron supplements with a vitamin C source helps promote absorption.[19] If liquid iron supplements are used, they should be given with a straw or a dropper placed back on the tongue to prevent staining the teeth. Iron therapy is continued for at least 2 months after erythrocyte indexes have returned to normal to replenish iron stores.[20]

Dietary modification is required to prevent recurrences of IDA. Intake of iron-rich foods is increased, and the intake of cow's milk may be restricted, with the exact amount restricted to 16 to 32 ounces per day depending on the child's age. Limiting milk intake makes the child hungrier for other iron-rich foods and prevents gastrointestinal blood loss in children whose anemia is aggravated or caused by inflammatory reactions to proteins in cow's milk.

Hemolytic Disease of the Fetus and Newborn

The most common cause of hemolytic anemia in newborns is alloimmune disease. Hemolytic disease of the fetus and newborn (HDFN) (erythroblastosis fetalis) can occur only if antigens on fetal erythrocytes differ from antigens on maternal erythrocytes. The antigens present on erythrocytes are determined genetically. They may be type A, B, or O, and they may or may not include Rh antigen D. Erythrocytes that express Rh antigen D are called Rh-positive; those that do not are called Rh-negative. The frequency of Rh negativity is higher in whites (15%) than in blacks (5%), and it is rare in Asians. Maternal-fetal incompatibility exists if mother and fetus differ in ABO blood type or if the fetus is Rh-positive and the mother is Rh-negative. (The antigenic properties of erythrocytes are described in Chapter 9).

Most cases of HDFN are caused by ABO incompatibility, which occurs if the mother and fetus have different ABO blood types. Although ABO incompatibility occurs in about 20% to 25% of all pregnancies, only 1 in 10 cases of ABO incompatibility results in HDFN. About 1 in 3 cases of HDFN is caused by Rh incompatibility, which occurs when the fetus is Rh-positive and the mother is Rh-negative. Rh incompatibility occurs in less than 10% of pregnancies and rarely causes HDFN in the first incompatible fetus. Typically, erythrocytes from the first incompatible fetus cause the mother's immune system to produce antibodies. These antibodies then can affect the fetuses of subsequent incompatible pregnancies. Even after five or more pregnancies, however, only 5% of women have babies with hemolytic disease. Some minor blood antigens also may be involved.

Pathophysiology. Three conditions must be present for HDFN to occur:

1. the mother's blood contains preformed antibodies against fetal erythrocytes or produces them when exposed to fetal erythrocytes,
2. sufficient amounts of antibody (usually immunoglobulin G [IgG] class) cross the placenta and enter fetal blood, and
3. IgG binds with sufficient numbers of fetal erythrocytes to cause widespread antibody-mediated hemolysis or splenic removal (antibody-mediated cellular destruction is described in Chapter 9).

In most cases of HDFN, the mother has blood type O, and the fetus has blood type A or B. Maternal antibodies may be formed against type B fetal erythrocytes if the mother has blood type A or against type A fetal erythrocytes if the mother has blood type B.

ABO incompatibility can cause HDFN even if fetal erythrocytes do not escape into the maternal circulation during pregnancy because the blood of most adults already contains anti-A or anti-B antibodies. These antibodies are produced on exposure to certain foods or infection by gram-negative bacteria. As a result, IgG against type A or B erythrocytes is usually already present in maternal blood and can enter the fetal circulation during the first incompatible pregnancy. Anti-O antibodies do not exist because type O erythrocytes are not antigenic.

Anti-Rh antibodies, on the other hand, form only in response to the presence of Rh-positive erythrocytes from the fetus in the blood of an Rh-negative mother. This exposure typically occurs when fetal blood is mixed with the mother's blood at the time of delivery. Exposure may also occur through transfused blood, and, rarely, previous sensitization of the mother by her own mother's incompatible blood.

The first Rh-incompatible pregnancy generally presents no difficulties for the fetus because few fetal erythrocytes cross the placental barrier during the pregnancy. When the placenta detaches at birth, many fetal erythrocytes often enter the mother's bloodstream. If the mother is Rh-negative and the fetus is Rh-positive, the mother produces anti-Rh antibodies. The capacity of the mother's immune system to produce anti-Rh antibodies depends on many factors, including her genetic capacity to make antibodies against the Rh antigen D, the amount of fetal-to-maternal bleeding, and the occurrence of any bleeding earlier in the pregnancy. These anti-Rh antibodies persist in the mother's bloodstream for a long time. If the next offspring is Rh-positive, the mother's anti-Rh antibodies can enter the bloodstream of the fetus and destroy the erythrocytes. Antibodies against Rh antigen D are of the IgG class and easily cross the placenta.

Antibody-coated fetal erythrocytes are usually destroyed through extravascular hemolysis, primarily by phagocytic cells in the spleen. As hemolysis proceeds, the fetus becomes anemic. Erythropoiesis accelerates, particularly in the liver and spleen. Immature nucleated cells (erythroblasts) are released into the bloodstream, hence the name ***erythroblastosis fetalis***. The degree of anemia depends on several factors: (1) the length of time the antibody has been in the fetal circulation, (2) the concentration of the antibody, and (3) the ability of the fetus to compensate for increased hemolysis. During the pregnancy, unconjugated (indirect) bilirubin, which forms during the breakdown of hemoglobin, is transported across the placental barrier into the maternal circulation and is excreted by the mother. Hyperbilirubinemia, an increase in bilirubin concentration in the blood occurs in the neonate shortly after birth because lipid-soluble unconjugated bilirubin is no longer excreted through the placenta.

HDFN is typically more severe in Rh incompatibility than in ABO incompatibility. ABO incompatibility may resolve after birth without life-threatening complications. Maternal-fetal incompatibility in which a mother with type O blood has a child with type A or B blood usually is so mild that it does not require treatment.

Rh incompatibility is more likely to result in severe or even life-threatening anemia, death in utero, or damage to the central nervous system (CNS). Severe anemia alone can cause death because of cardiovascular complications. Extensive hemolysis can result in increased levels of unconjugated bilirubin in the neonate's circulation. If bilirubin levels exceed the liver's ability to conjugate and excrete bilirubin, it can be deposited in the brain, a condition known as kernicterus, causing cellular damage and, eventually, death if the neonate does not receive exchange transfusions.

Fetuses that do not survive anemia in utero are usually stillborn with gross edema in the entire body, a condition called hydrops fetalis. Death can occur as early as 17 weeks' gestation and results in spontaneous abortion.

Clinical Manifestations. Neonates with mild HDFN may appear healthy or slightly pale, with slight enlargement of the liver or spleen. Pronounced pallor, splenomegaly, and hepatomegaly indicate severe anemia, which predisposes the neonate to cardiovascular failure and shock. Life-threatening symptoms as a consequence of Rh incompatibility, however, are rare, largely because of the routine use of Rh immunoglobulin.

Because the maternal antibodies remain in the neonate's circulatory system after birth, erythrocyte destruction can continue causing hyperbilirubinemia and icterus neonatorum (neonatal jaundice) that occurs shortly after birth. Without replacement transfusions, in which the child receives Rh-negative erythrocytes, the bilirubin can be deposited in the brain, causing a condition termed kernicterus. If kernicterus develops, it can cause cerebral damage, including intellectual disabilities, cerebral palsy, high-frequency deafness, and even death (icterus gravis neonatorum).[21]

Evaluation and Treatment. Fetuses and neonates with ABO incompatibility typically do not require additional monitoring or treatment. Fetuses and infants at risk for HDFN because of Rh incompatibility may require additional monitoring and treatment. Routine evaluation of fetuses at risk for HDFN includes the Coombs test. The indirect Coombs test measures antibody in the mother's circulation and indicates whether the fetus is at risk for HDFN. The direct Coombs test measures antibody already bound to the surfaces of fetal erythrocytes. It is used primarily to confirm the diagnosis of antibody-mediated HDFN. If a prior history of fetal hemolytic disease is present, additional diagnostic tests are done to determine risk with the current pregnancy. These include maternal antibody titers, fetal blood sampling, amniotic fluid spectrophotometry, and ultrasound fetal assessment.[22]

Prevention is the key to managing HDFN that results from Rh incompatibility. Immunoprophylaxis through the use of Rh immune globulin (RhoGAM), a preparation of antibody against Rh antigen D (anti-D Ig), prevents an Rh-negative woman from producing antibodies. If an Rh-negative woman is given Rh immune globulin within 72 hours of exposure to Rh-positive erythrocytes, she will not produce antibody against the D antigen. As a result, the next Rh-positive baby she conceives will be protected. Updated United States and United Kingdom guidelines also state that if anti-D Ig is not given within 72 hours, every effort should be made to administer it within 10 days.[23,24]

The injected (anti-D Ig) antibodies remain in the mother's bloodstream long enough to prevent her immune system from producing its own anti-Rh antibodies but not long enough to affect subsequent offspring. The mother must be given Rh immune globulin injections after the birth of each Rh-positive baby and after a miscarriage. The mother also must be especially careful not to receive a transfusion containing Rh-positive blood because this would stimulate production of anti-Rh antibodies.

If antigenic incompatibility of the mother's erythrocytes is not discovered in time to administer Rh immune globulin and a child is born with HDFN, treatment consists of exchange transfusions in which the neonate's blood is replaced with new Rh-positive blood that is not contaminated with anti-Rh antibodies. This treatment is instituted during the first 24 hours of extrauterine life to prevent kernicterus. Phototherapy also is used to reduce the toxic effects of unconjugated bilirubin.

Jaundice and indirect hyperbilirubinemia are reduced when the infant is exposed to high-intensity light in the visible spectrum from 460 to 490 nm.[25] Bilirubin in the skin absorbs light energy, which converts the toxic unconjugated bilirubin into its conjugated water-soluble form that is excreted in the bile. Phototherapy also causes autosensitization that results in oxidation reactions. Breakdown products from the oxidation reactions are excreted by the liver and kidney without need for conjugation. The therapeutic effect of phototherapy depends on the light energy emitted in the effective wavelengths, the distance between the infant and the light source, and the amount of skin exposed. The rate of hemolysis and the infant's ability to excrete bilirubin also are factors in determining the effectiveness of phototherapy in lowering serum bilirubin levels.

Anemia of Infectious Disease

Infections of the newborn, often initially acquired by the mother and transmitted to the fetus, may result in a hemolytic anemia with clinical manifestations similar to those of HDFN. Congenital syphilis, toxoplasmosis, cytomegalic inclusion disease, rubella, coxsackievirus B infection, herpesvirus infection, and bacterial sepsis can cause hemolytic anemia in the neonate.

The exact mechanism of anemia caused by congenital infections is unclear. In some instances, it is related to direct injury of erythrocyte membranes or erythrocyte precursors by the infectious microorganism. In other instances, it results from traumatic destruction of erythrocytes during their passage through inflamed capillaries.

Anemia in Critically Ill Children

Anemia is a common occurrence in critically ill children (see Chapter 49). The causes are numerous and include decreased erythropoietin activity, poor iron use by the body, and blood loss from diverse conditions and consequences of treatment. A topic of ongoing discussion is whether transfusion of blood products, particularly packed RBCs, improves outcomes in critically ill children because of problems related to blood storage. New research is ongoing and needed to understand these problems, the development of new blood transfusion strategies, and blood substitutes.[26]

Inherited Disorders

A number of inherited and intrinsic erythrocyte conditions are known to cause hemolytic disease or increased hemolysis (see Table 30.2). These conditions may result from enzymatic abnormalities that disrupt metabolic processes and prevent normal biochemical balance within the cell, alterations of hemoglobin structure or synthesis, or plasma membrane defects accompanied by changes in erythrocyte size or shape.

Glucose-6-Phosphate Dehydrogenase Deficiency

Glucose-6-phosphate dehydrogenase (G6PD) deficiency is an inherited disorder caused by a genetic defect in the RBC enzyme G6PD, which is involved in the normal processing of carbohydrates. It is the most common disorder of RBCs, estimated to affect 200 to 400 million people worldwide. The deficiency occurs most often in tropical and subtropical regions of the Eastern Hemisphere including the Mediterranean region, Africa, the Middle East, and Asia. G6PD deficiency is an X-linked recessive disorder, most fully expressed in homozygous males, although partial expression is possible in heterozygous females because of mosaicism resulting from X-inactivation. (X-linked inheritance is discussed in Chapter 4). More than 200 mutations have been identified in the G6PD gene, almost all of which result in changes in single amino acids. The consequences of these mutations are decreased quantities of the G6PD enzyme or an enzyme with abnormal structure and function. The type of mutation that is present will determine the degree of deficiency and the associated clinical manifestations.[27]

G6PD is responsible for the first step in a pathway that converts glucose to ribose-5-phosphate. These initial chemical reactions usually produce another enzyme, nicotinamide adenine dinucleotide phosphate (NADPH), which helps protect cells from oxidative stress from reactive oxygen species. The deficiency of G6PD leads to damaged RBCs that can hemolyze, or rupture and break down prematurely.

Pathophysiology. G6PD enables erythrocytes to maintain normal metabolic processes despite injury from oxidative stressors. As a result, G6PD deficiency is usually asymptomatic unless exposure to a source of oxidative stress occurs. Deficient or abnormal enzyme function can cause abnormalities in the hexose monophosphate shunt or glutathione metabolism that impairs the ability of RBCs to protect themselves against oxidative stress injuries. Such injury can cause both an intravascular and an extravascular hemolysis. Sources of oxidative stress include exposure to certain classes of drugs (sulfonamides, nitrofurantoins, antimalarial agents, salicylates, or naphthaquinolones), ingestion of fava beans (a dietary staple in some Mediterranean areas and parts of Africa), hypoxemia, fever, acidosis, or infection. Infections associated with initiation of hemolysis include viral hepatitis, pneumonia, and typhoid fever. Erythrocyte damage in affected children begins after intense or prolonged exposure to one or more sources of oxidative stress and ceases when the stressors are removed. In black males, the G6PD defect becomes more pronounced as the erythrocyte ages. In other population groups the defect is profound even in young erythrocytes. A fetus with G6PD deficiency may experience an episode of hemolysis if the mother ingests a substance with oxidant properties, such as a salicylate (aspirin).

In the absence of G6PD, oxidative stressors damage hemoglobin and the plasma membranes of erythrocytes and possibly interfere with the activities of other enzymes within the cell. Hemoglobin is oxidized progressively to methemoglobin, sulfmethemoglobin, and denatured globin-glutathione complexes. Exposure to oxidizing substances results in the precipitation of insoluble hemoglobin inclusions, called *Heinz bodies*, within the cell. Plasma membrane damage and the presence of Heinz bodies cause hemolysis, primarily in the spleen.

Clinical Manifestations. In infants, G6PD deficiency may present as icterus neonatorum. The most common clinical manifestation of G6PD deficiency is acute hemolytic anemia, usually after infections or the ingestion of certain oxidative drugs or foods. Ingestion of fava beans can produce a severe hemolytic reaction in children with G6PD deficiency.

Hemolytic episodes are characterized by pallor, icterus, dark urine, back pain, and, in severe cases, shock, cardiovascular collapse, and death. When the child is not exposed to sources of oxidative stress, the child does not have anemia, and erythrocyte survival is normal.

Evaluation and Treatment. Reduced G6PD activity in erythrocytes is required for diagnosis. Immediately after a hemolytic episode, reticulocytes and young erythrocytes are evident. Because young erythrocytes have significantly higher enzyme activity than do older cells, laboratory evaluation should not be performed after a crisis. Doing so can result in a low to normal range, a false-negative result. Testing for suspected G6PD deficiency should be done when hemoglobin and reticulocytes are normal. G6PD deficiency also can be detected by electrophoretic analysis.

Prevention of hemolysis is the most important therapeutic measure. Prevention includes avoiding medications and dietary substances associated with hemolysis. Because of the high frequency of G6PD deficiency in areas of the world that are endemic for malaria, the World Health Organization (WHO) currently recommends testing for G6PD deficiency before administration of antimalarial medications in these regions.[28] When hemolysis occurs, supportive treatment may include blood transfusions and oral iron therapy. Spontaneous recovery generally follows treatment.

Hereditary Spherocytosis

Hereditary spherocytosis (HS) is an inherited disorder caused by defects in the membrane skeleton of RBCs. The changes cause RBCs to become spherical, less deformable, and vulnerable to destruction. Mutations in at least five genes that produce proteins necessary for the RBC membrane (*ANK1, EPB42, SLC4A1, SPTA1,* and *SPTB*) result in the HS phenotype. Proteins produced by these genes act as transporters for molecules in and out of the cells, attach to other proteins, and maintain the RBC's biconcave disc shape. Thus, these proteins help the cells to be flexible for RBC mobility from large blood vessels to capillaries. Altered RBC cell membranes result in a more rigid and spherical cell shape. These misshapen cells, or spherocytes, are vulnerable to destruction or hemolysis particularly in the splenic vessels. Ultimately, these damaged cells are removed from circulation in the spleen.

Pathophysiology. HS is transmitted as an autosomal dominant trait in about 75% of cases. The defect results from properties of its specialized membrane skeleton, which lies close to the internal surface of the plasma membrane. The affected proteins include spectrins and ankyrin, and their intrinsic defects in the membrane cause less deformability and increased vulnerability to splenic sequestration and destruction.

The spleen is intimately involved in the hemolytic process. The spherocyte is relatively rigid and passes with difficulty through the small openings between the splenic cords and sinuses initiating macrophage response. Circulation of blood to the spleen creates repeated circulation through a metabolic environment that results in sequestration and destruction of spherocytes.

Clinical Manifestations. The presenting signs of HS are ane mia, jaundice, and splenomegaly, which can be mild to severe depending on the individual's physiologic compensation. In these cases, the reticulocyte count will be elevated. In infancy, hemolytic anemia and hyperbilirubinemia may be severe.[29] Infants and children may have life-threatening anemia with clinical symptoms ranging from difficulty feeding, circumoral pallor, tachycardia, nasal flaring, and diaphoresis to lethargy. They also are at increased risk for gallstones because of the presence of extra bile pigment from hemolysis. Infection (specifically parvovirus),[30] fever, and stress stimulate the spleen to destroy more RBCs than usual, leading to a worsening anemia in a child with baseline anemia. The parvovirus also infects erythroid progenitor cells in the bone marrow resulting in an aplastic crisis.[31]

Evaluation and Treatment. Ascertaining a family history of spherocytosis is important. Laboratory findings include spherocytes in the peripheral blood smear *(spherocytosis)*, elevated reticulocyte count (with or without anemia), indirect hyperbilirubinemia, and a positive osmotic fragility test. An osmotic fragility test is performed by placing RBCs in a saline solution for 24 hours. Spherocytes do not tolerate saline solutions; as a result, they burst more readily than normal RBCs. In addition, flow cytometry can detect reductions in RBC transmembrane proteins. Band 3 Protein Reduction testing can confirm the diagnosis of HS. Treatment of HS is based on disease severity and some children or adolescents may require RBC transfusions; however, this is somewhat rare. Management includes regular monitoring for anemia and splenomegaly. Daily folic acid supplementation supports the increased production of healthy RBCs. In the past, splenectomy was the first line of treatment. Currently, however, splenectomy is only recommended for those children more than 5 years of age with severe anemia or splenomegaly. Some children who develop gallstones may undergo splenectomy and cholecystectomy. Partial splenectomy, in which only a portion of the spleen is removed, is being performed on children with HS to decrease the risk of postsplenectomy complications.[31]

Sickle Cell Disease

Sickle cell disease is a group of autosomal recessive disorders characterized by the production of an atypical type of hemoglobin, hemoglobin S (HbS; sickle hemoglobin) within the erythrocytes. The hemoglobin molecule consists of four protein subunits called α-globin and two subunits called β-globin. The hemoglobin B *(HbB)* gene provides instructions for making protein β-globin. HbS is formed as a result of a genetic point mutation (missense mutation) in β-globin in which one amino acid (valine) replaces another (glutamic acid) (Fig. 30.2). Abnormal versions of β-globin can cause erythrocytes to distort into a sickle shape. Other mutations in the *HbB* gene lead to other versions of β-globin, such as hemoglobin C (HbC) and hemoglobin E (HbE). *HbB* gene mutations also can affect the quantity of β-globin, such as low levels of β-globin found in β-thalassemia.

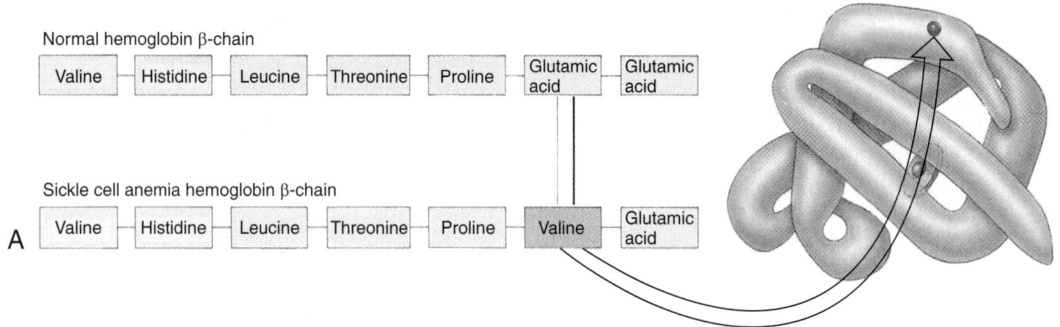

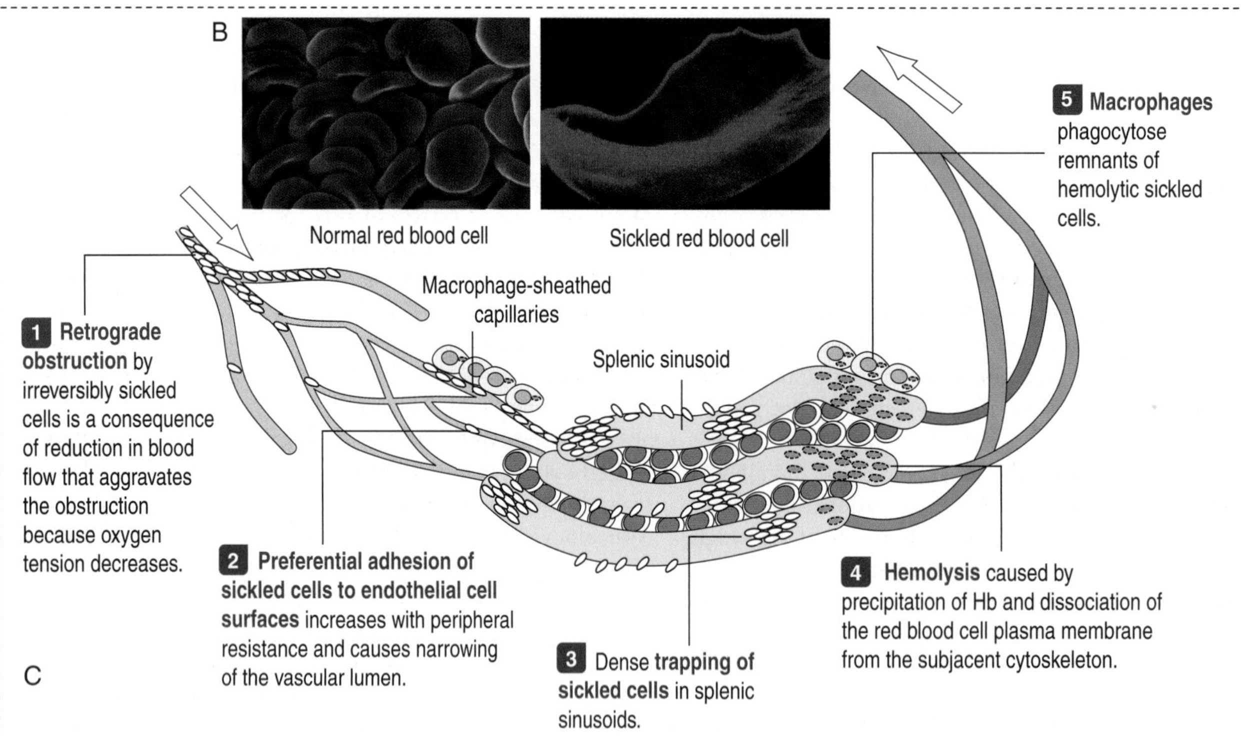

A. Sickle cell anemia is determined by the substitution of normal hemoglobin (Hb A) by hemoglobin S (Hb S) caused by a point mutation (replacement of the nucleotide triplet CTC coding glutamic acid at the mRNA level [GAG] by the CAC triplet [GUG] coding for valine) that modifies the physicochemical properties of the β-globin chain of hemoglobin. B. Color enhanced electron micrographs of normal red bloods and sickled red blood cells. C. All hemoglobin is abnormal in homozygous individuals for the mutant gene, and red blood cells show a sickling deformity and hemolytic anemia in the presence or absence of normal oxygen tension. Heterozygous individuals contain a mixture of Hb A and Hb S, and sickling and anemia are observed when the tension of oxygen decreases.

Irreversibly sickled red blood cells are trapped within the splenic sinusoids and are destroyed by adjacent macrophages. Hemolysis may also occur in the macrophage-sheathed capillaries of the red pulp.

Fig. 30.2 Brief Summary of Sickle Cell. (From Kierzenbaum AL, Tres LL. *Histology and cell biology: An introduction to pathology*, 4th edition. Philadelphia: Saunders; 2015.)

TABLE 30.3 Inheritance of Sickle Cell Disease

Hemoglobin Inherited From First Parent	Hemoglobin Inherited From Second Parent	Form of Sickle Cell Disease in Child
HbS (an abnormal hemoglobin)	HbS	Sickle cell anemia: homozygous inheritance in which child's hemoglobin is mostly HbS, with remainder HbF (fetal hemoglobin)
HbS	Defective or insufficient α- or β-chains of HbA (alpha- or beta-thalassemia)	Sickle cell–thalassemia disease (heterozygous inheritance of HbS and alpha- or beta-thalassemia)
HbS	HbC or D (both abnormal hemoglobins)	Sickle cell–hemoglobin C (or D) disease (heterozygous inheritance of hemoglobin S and either C or D)
HbS	Normal hemoglobins (mostly HbA)	Sickle cell trait, carrier state (heterozygous inheritance of HbS and normal hemoglobin)

The most prevalent types of sickle cell disease are sickle cell anemia, sickle cell–thalassemia disease, and sickle cell–HbC disease (Table 30.3). (See Chapter 4 for a discussion of genetic inheritance of disease.) SCD is inherited in an autosomal recessive pattern in which each parent carries one copy of the mutated gene. Sickle cell anemia (SCA; HbSS), a homozygous form, is the most severe.[32] The most prevalent SCD genotypes include homozygous hemoglobin SS (HbSS, or sickle cell anemia) and the compound heterozygous conditions hemoglobin Sβ^0-thalassemia (Hbβ^0-thalassemia), hemoglobin Sβ-thalassemia (HbSβ^+-thalassemia), and hemoglobin SC disease (HbSC).[33] HbSS and HbSβ^0-thalassemia are clinically similar and are, therefore, commonly referred to as *sickle cell anemia (SCA);* these genotypes are associated with the most severe clinical manifestations. Sickle cell trait (HbAS), in which the child inherits HbS from one parent and normal hemoglobin (HbA) from the other. This heterozygous carrier state rarely has clinical manifestations and is not regarded as a form of SCD. All forms of SCD are lifelong conditions.[34]

Sickle cell disease affects millions of people worldwide and is most common among persons with ancestry from sub-Saharan Africa. Although less common, it also is present among individuals with ancestry from Mediterranean countries, the Arabian Peninsula, parts of India, and Spanish-speaking areas of South America. Approximately 100,000 individuals living in the United States have SCD,[33] and most infants with SCD born in the United States are now identified by routine neonatal screening. In the United States, sickle cell anemia is most common in black people, with a reported incidence of around 1 in 365 live births.[33] In the general population, the risk of two black parents having a child with sickle cell anemia is 0.7%. Sickle cell–HbC disease occurs in 1 in 800 births, and sickle cell–thalassemia is even less common (1 in 1700 births).

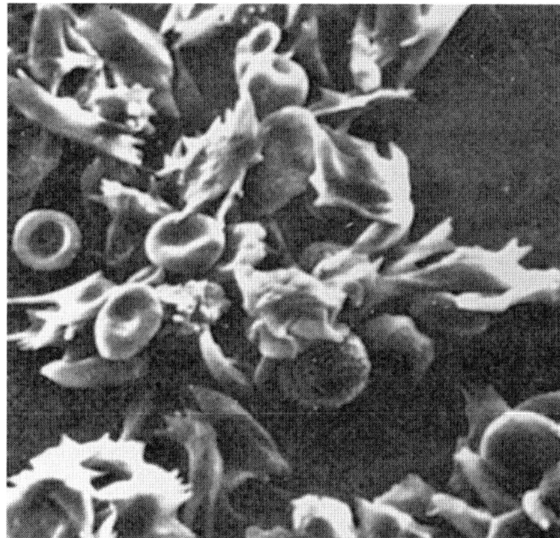

Fig. 30.3 Scanning Electron Micrograph of Normal and Sickle-Shaped Red Blood Cells Together. The irregularly shaped cells are the sickle cells; the circular cells are the normal blood cells. (From Raven PH, Johnson GB. *Biology*, 3rd edition. St. Louis: Mosby; 1992.)

Between 1 and 3 million Americans and more than 100 million individuals worldwide are estimated to be heterozygous carriers for the sickle cell trait (HbAS).[34] Sickle cell trait is present in 7% to 13% of African Americans. Its prevalence in African countries, such as Nigeria and the Democratic Republic of Congo, may be as high as 30%.[35] The sickle cell trait may provide protection against lethal forms of malaria. This results in a genetic advantage for carriers who reside in regions of the world that are endemic for malaria, such as sub-Saharan Africa and some Mediterranean countries.

Under conditions of decreased oxygen tension and dehydration, HbS stretches and elongates. Repeated cycles of deoxygenation and oxygenation cause the HbS molecule to polymerize and stiffen. These polymers can damage the RBC structure, leading to sickle-shaped RBCs. This change causes several pathologic consequences: the sickle-shaped RBCs die prematurely leading to hemolytic anemia, microvascular obstruction, and ischemic tissue damage (Fig. 30.3).

Two effective disease therapies for SCD are hydroxyurea and chronic transfusion.[32] The role of curative treatments including hematopoietic stem cell transplantation (HSCT) and gene therapy (GT) for SCD are increasing. See Emerging Science Box: Gene Therapy for Sickle Cell. Although data are encouraging, additional studies are needed to assess efficacy and long-term outcomes.[36]

Pathophysiology. The sickling process is an occasional, intermittent phenomenon that can be triggered or sustained by one or more of the following stressors: decreased oxygen tension (Po_2) of the blood (e.g., hypoxemia), acidosis (decreased pH), increased plasma osmolality, decreased plasma volume, and low temperature (Fig. 30.4). Low temperatures can precipitate sickle crisis, presumably because of vasoconstriction.[37]

EMERGING SCIENCE BOX

Gene Therapy for Sickle Cell

Historically, the clinical management of sickle cell disease has been largely supportive. With the advancement of technology and supportive care strategies, curative treatments, including hematopoietic stem cell transplant and gene therapy are emerging. Gene therapy for sickle cell disease involves editing one of two genes of interest in the individual's hematopoietic stem cells using CRISPR/Cas9 technology. Editing a gene of interest allows its function and expression to be changed. Currently available clinical trials that include gene therapy for sickle cell disease are targeting two genes of interest: HBB and BCL11A, each of which has a different role in the phenotypic expression of sickle cell disease.

HBB provides the code for the beta-globin protein. A point mutation in HBB results in the production of hemoglobin S, which is associated with the sickling process. Gene editing replaces the incorrect base, thymine, with the correct base adenine. When this sequence is introduced into the individual's hematopoietic stem cells, they will then produce the correct beta-globin protein.

BCL11A is a transcription factor. Under normal conditions, expression of the BCL11A gene is responsible for the transition to the production of adult hemoglobin rather than fetal hemoglobin. Current gene editing techniques modify the expression of BCL11A so that it reverts back to producing fetal hemoglobin rather than adult hemoglobin. By producing fetal hemoglobin, the sickling process is prevented.

The gene therapy process involves the removal of some of the individual's hematopoietic stem cells to allow for gene editing. After the gene sequence of interest, HBB or BCL11A, is edited, a virus is used as a vector to introduce it into the harvested stem cells. The individual receives chemotherapy to create space for the newly modified stem cells. The stem cells are then infused back into the individual with the goal that the cells will express the newly edited version of the gene of interest.

Data from Bourzac K. Gene therapy: Erasing sickle-cell disease. *Nature*, 2017; 549:S28–S30; Cai L, et al. A universal approach to correct various HBB gene mutations in human stem cells for gene therapy of beta-thalassemia and sickle cell disease. *Stem Cells Translational Medicine*, 2018;7(1):87–97; Kalkan BM, et al. Development of gene editing strategies for human B-globin (HBB) gene mutations. *Gene*, 2020;734:144398; Orkin SH, et al. Emerging genetic therapy for sickle cell disease. *Annual Review of Medicine*, 2019;70:257–271.

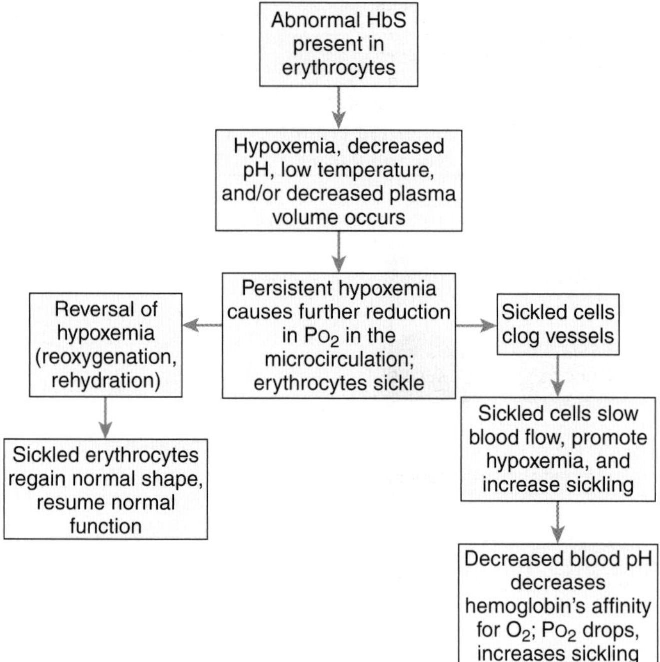

Fig. 30.4 Sickling of Erythrocytes.

The pathophysiology of the sickling process includes erythrocyte derangement, chronic hemolysis (hemolytic anemia), microvascular occlusions, and tissue damage. HbS is soluble and usually causes no problem when it is properly oxygenated; therefore, deoxygenation is probably the most important variable in determining the occurrence of sickling. Other significant variables that affect sickling include interaction of HbS with other types of hemoglobin in the cell, mean cell hemoglobin concentration (MCHC), intracellular pH, and transit times of erythrocytes through the microcirculation. Among individuals who are heterozygous for sickle cell trait, the presence of other types of Hb prevents sickling except under conditions of severe hypoxia.

As the sickling process begins, intracellular dehydration increases the MCHC, which increases sickling. A decrease in pH reduces the oxygen affinity of hemoglobin, resulting in a further increase in the quantity of deoxygenated HbS regardless of the oxygen tension. These changes, in turn, increase the sickling process. Inflammation in the microcirculation will slow erythrocyte transit times because blood flow is sluggish with adhesion of leukocytes to activated endothelial cells. Increased osmolality of the plasma draws water out of the erythrocytes. The result is sickling by raising the relative HbS content in erythrocytes. Investigators are studying the optimal intravenous fluid to increase erythrocyte deformability and biomechanical properties.[38]

Sickling causes damage to erythrocytes through several mechanisms, including (1) *membrane derangements* occur because as HbS units (polymers) grow they protrude through the membrane skeleton by only the lipid layer, causing changes in membrane structure: (2) membrane derangement leads to *changes in ionic flow* with an influx in Ca^{++} ions, which induces cross-linking of membrane proteins and activation of an ion channel that induces the efflux of K^+ and H_2O; and (3) with time the damaged *cells are converted to end-stage*, nondeformable or stiff and irreversibly sickled cells (Fig. 30.5). Recent studies have shown that elevated red cell levels of the enzyme *sphingosine kinase 1 (SPH1)* underlie sickling and disease progression by increasing *sphingosine 1-phosphate (S1P)* production in the blood.[39,40] S1P level, a bioactive lipid enriched in red cells, is elevated in red cells and plasma of mice and humans with SCD.[40] S1P also is a signaling molecule that regulates diverse biologic functions including inflammation.[41] Additionally, investigators demonstrated that the compound 5C can inhibit *SPHK1* and, thus, has antisickling properties.[42] These data are important for identifying the structure of the sickling process to assess potential new therapeutics.

Some cells remain sickled even with full oxygenation and are vulnerable to hemolysis. Polymerization of sickled hemoglobin is central to the disorder. Polymerization stiffens the

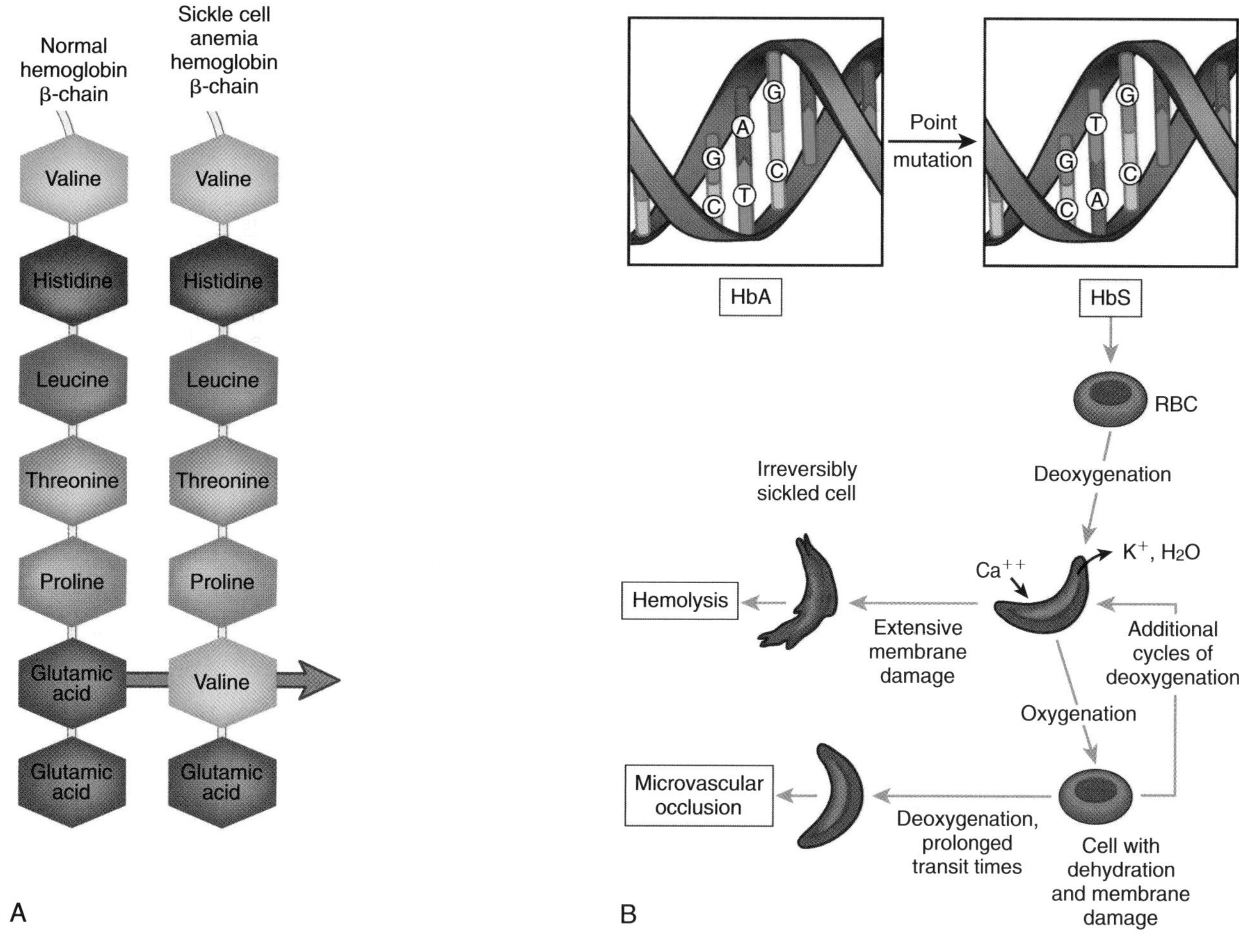

Fig. 30.5 Sickle Cell Disease Pathogenesis. See text for discussion. (A and B, Adapted from Kumar V, Abbas AK, Aster JC. *Robbins and Cotran pathologic basis of disease*, 9th edition. Philadelphia: Elsevier Saunders; 2015.)

sickled erythrocyte, changing it from a flexible, beneficial cell to an inflexible one where HbS molecules stack into polymers that starve and damage tissues. The pathogenesis of SCD derives from the tendency of HbS molecules to stack into polymers even when deoxygenated and assemble into needle-like fibers within cells, producing the distorted crescent-like sickle or holly-leaf shape (see Figs. 30.2 and 30.3). Sickled cells undergo hemolysis in the spleen or become sequestered there, causing blood pooling and infarction of splenic vessels. The anemia that follows triggers erythropoiesis in the marrow and, in extreme cases, in the liver.[43,44]

The pathogenesis of microvascular occlusions, a main feature of SCD is not fully understood. This process is responsible for the most serious and urgent manifestations of SCD. Microvascular occlusions are not related to the quantity of irreversibly sickled cells in the blood. Rather, they are dependent on understated RBC membrane damages and other local factors, such as inflammation or vasoconstriction, that tend to decrease blood flow or arrest red cells through the microcirculation.[45] Sickled RBCs express higher than normal amounts of adhesion molecules and are sticky. During inflammatory reactions, leukocyte release of meditators increases the expression of adhesion molecules on endothelial cells. These reactions further promote sickled erythrocytes to become arrested during movement through the microvasculature.[45] The sluggish and stagnant red cells within the inflamed vascular vessels result in extended exposure to low oxygen tension, sickling, and vascular obstruction. Lysed sickle erythrocytes release hemoglobin. This free hemoglobin can bind and inactivate nitric oxide (NO), which is a powerful vasodilator and inhibitor of platelet aggregation. A decrease in blood pH reduces hemoglobin's affinity for oxygen leading to an increasing fraction of deoxygenated HbS at any oxygen tension and predisposition to sickling. As less oxygen is taken up by hemoglobin in the lungs, the Po_2 drops, promoting additional sickling.

Sickling usually is not permanent. Most sickled erythrocytes regain a normal shape after reoxygenation, a return of the Po_2 to normal, and rehydration. Irreversible sickling is caused by permanent plasma membrane damage, which in turn is caused by sickling. In persons with sickle cell anemia, in which the erythrocytes contain a high percentage of HbS (75% to 95%), up to 30% of the erythrocytes can become irreversibly sickled.

The extent, severity, and clinical manifestations of sickling depend to a great extent on the percentage of hemoglobin that is HbS. That is why homozygous inheritance of HbS produces the severest form of SCD—sickle cell anemia. The presence of sickle

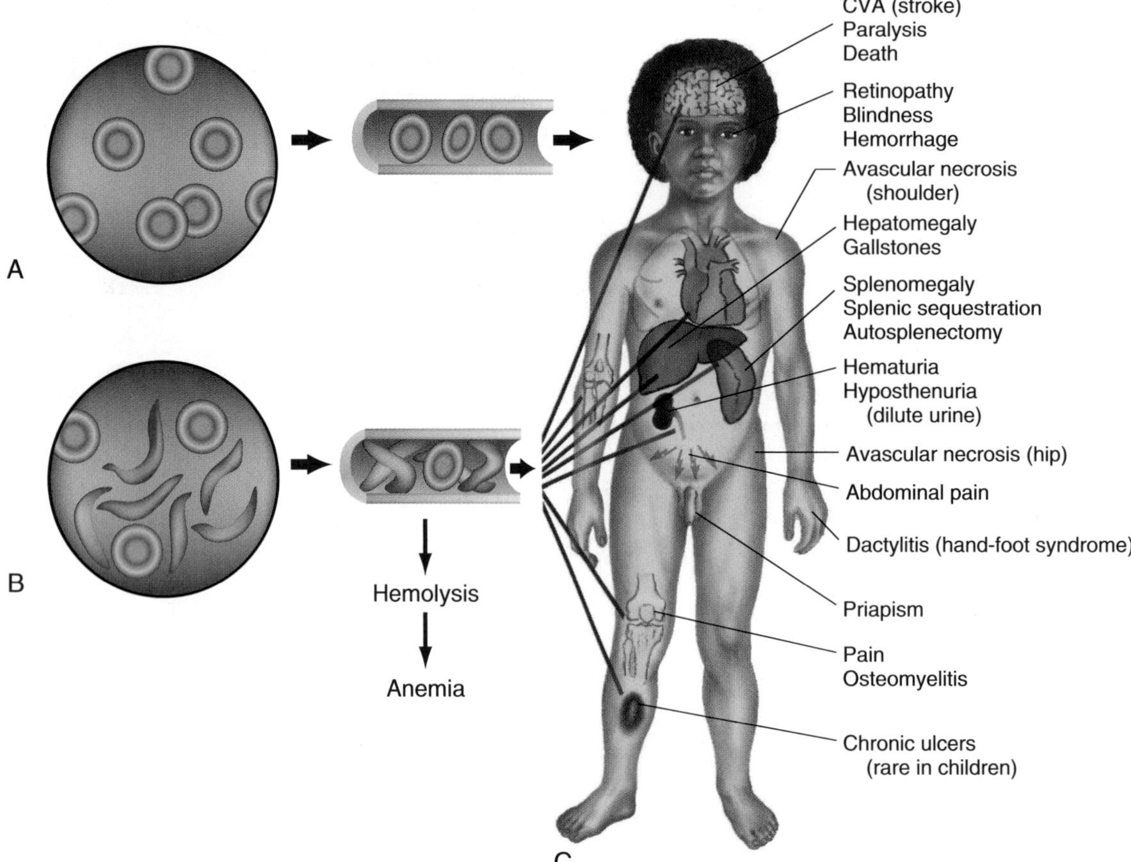

Fig. 30.6 Differences between effects of normal **(A)** and sickled **(B)** red blood cells on blood circulation and selected consequences in a child. **(C)** Tissue effects of sickle cell anemia. *CVA*, Cerebrovascular accident. (A and B, Adapted from Hockenberry MJ, et al., eds. *Wong's nursing care of infants and children*, 10th edition. St. Louis: Mosby; 2015.)

cell trait rarely results in sickling because these individuals also produce normal HbF and HbA which do not contribute to sickling at all. Anemia persists because HbF does not live 120 days.

Clinical Manifestations. The clinical manifestations of sickle cell disease can vary. Some individuals have mild symptoms; others suffer from repeated vasoocclusive crises. The clinical manifestations of sickle cell disease usually do not appear until the infant is at least 6 months old. At this time, postnatal concentrations of HbF decrease, causing concentrations of HbS to rise (Fig. 30.6). Two key attributes of SCD contribute to its presentation: the first is its nature to be a chronic disease with acute exacerbations; the second is that it is a condition affecting RBCs that supply oxygen to all cells of the body. As a consequence, SCD can affect any part of the body. Sites of specific dysfunction are shown in Fig. 30.7.

The general manifestations of hemolytic anemia from the sickling process include pallor, fatigue, jaundice, and irritability. Extensive sickling can precipitate four types of acute manifestations, often referred to as *crises*: (1) vaso-occlusive crisis, (2) aplastic crisis, (3) sequestration crisis, or rarely (4) hyperhemolytic crisis.

Vasoocclusive crisis (pain crisis). This type of crisis involves hypoxic injury and infarction that can cause severe pain in the microcirculation. The frequency of this type of crisis is variable and unpredictable because it may develop spontaneously or be precipitated by infection, exposure to cold, dehydration, low Po_2, acidosis (low pH), or localized hypoxemia. Vaso-occlusive crises are extremely painful, and the specific cause of this sensory pain is not well characterized.[46,47]

As blood flow is obstructed by sickled cells, vasospasm occurs, and a logjam effect blocks all blood flow through the vessel. Unless the process is reversed, thrombosis and infarction of local tissue occur. Vasoocclusive crisis may last for days or even weeks, with an average duration of 4 to 6 days. The most common sites include bones, lungs, spleen, liver, brain, and penis. Painful bone crises are common in young children and are difficult to distinguish from acute osteomyelitis. These bone alterations can manifest as painful swelling of the hands and feet (*hand-foot syndrome* or *dactylitis*).

A high-risk type of vaso-occlusive crisis involving the lungs is known as acute chest syndrome. It typically presents with fever, cough, chest pain, and accumulations of lung infiltrates. The complications in the lungs create a worsening cycle of hypoxemia, sickling, and vaso-occlusion. Acute chest syndrome remains a leading cause of death among people with SCD.[48,49] *Priapism*, or prolonged erection of the penis, can lead to hypoxic

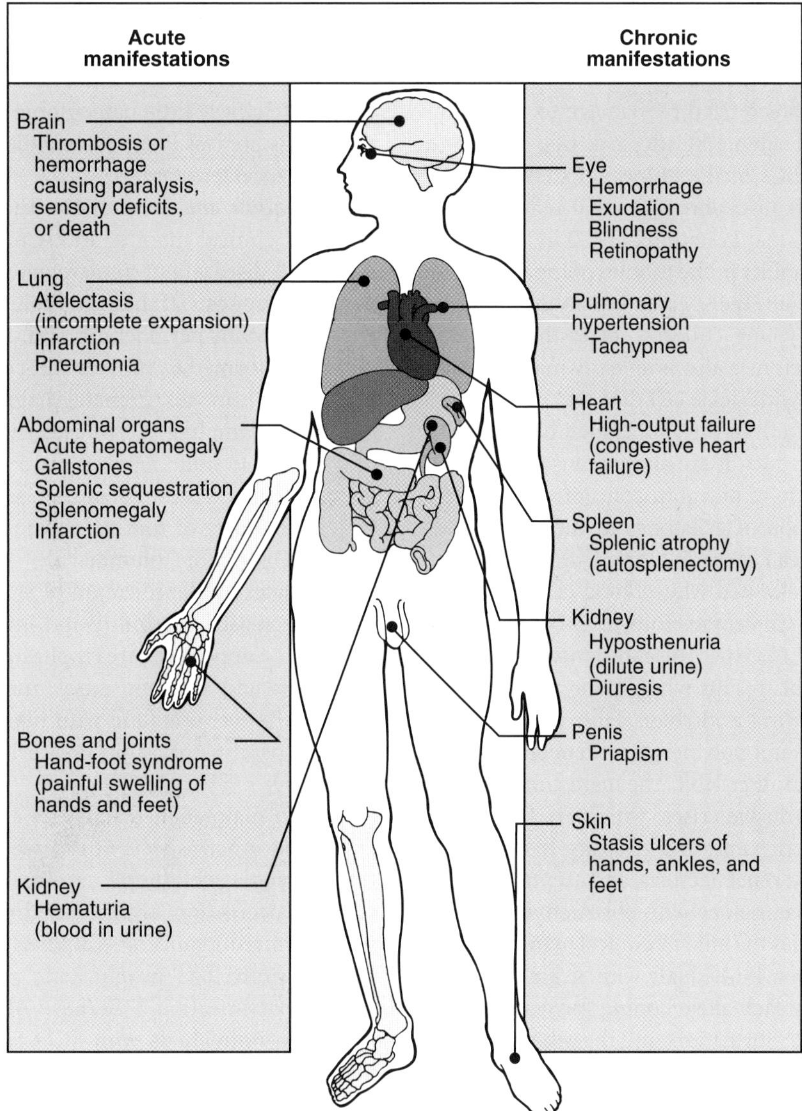

Fig. 30.7 Clinical Manifestations of Sickle Cell Disease.

damage and erectile dysfunction. Vaso-occlusion in vessels to the brain can result in stroke. Chronic vaso-occlusion in vessels to the kidneys results in end-stage renal disease.

Aplastic crisis. This type of crisis involves profound anemia caused by a transient cessation in RBC production despite a need for new RBCs. In sickle cell anemia, erythrocyte survival is only 10 to 20 days; however, the bone marrow is typically able to compensate to replace RBCs that are lost through hemolysis. Aplastic crisis is often precipitated by a viral infection, such as parvovirus B1. The virus causes temporary shutdown of RBC production with an accompanying sudden drop in hemoglobin level with an extremely low reticulocyte count. This type of crisis typically lasts 7 to 10 days.

Sequestration crisis. This type of crisis is typically seen only in children less than 5 years of age. It occurs when large amounts of sickled RBCs become acutely pooled in the liver and spleen. Because the spleen can hold as much as one-fifth of the body's blood supply, hypovolemia and, sometimes shock, can occur (see Chapter 49). The risk of mortality is high if the condition is not recognized and managed appropriately. Clinical management may include exchange transfusions.[32] Approximately half of children who experience sequestration crises will have recurrent episodes.

Hyperhemolytic crisis. This type of crisis, associated with an accelerated rate of RBC destruction, is unusual, but it may occur in association with certain drugs or infections. It is characterized by anemia, jaundice, and reticulocytosis. The concomitant presence of G6PD deficiency (see Glucose-6-Phosphate Dehydrogenase Deficiency) contributes to hyperhemolytic episodes, especially when combined with infections. It has also been reported as an acute or chronic reaction following a blood transfusion.

Infection is the most common cause of death related to sickle cell disease. Infection is also an important cause of disease-related morbidity, particularly for children with impaired splenic function. Sepsis and meningitis develop in as many as 10% of children with sickle cell anemia during the first 5 years of life. Splenic congestion and poor blood flow compromise splenic function and lead to splenic infarction. As a consequence, the risk of infection from *Pneumococcus pneumoniae* and *Haemophilus influenzae* is increased.

Glomerular disease, characterized by damage to the glomeruli allowing protein and often RBCs to leak into the urine, is caused by sickling of RBCs in the kidneys. Extensive damage to the glomeruli results in nephropathy that may progress to renal failure. The earliest manifestation of SCD in the kidney is hyposthenuria, or the inability of the tubules of the kidneys to concentrate urine. As a result, the specific gravity of the urine tends to be very low. In young children, hyposthenuria can result in bed-wetting. Proteinuria also is an early manifestation of nephropathy associated with sickle cell disease.

Cholecystitis, inflammation of the gallbladder, occurs when a gallstone blocks the cystic duct. It can also be caused by hemolysis resulting in an increase of bilirubin concentration, which in turn causes the formation of gallstones in the gallbladder. The presence of gallstones can cause right upper quadrant pain, nausea, vomiting, and an elevated white blood cell count and alkaline phosphatase level. Cholecystectomy may be required.

Sickle cell–hemoglobin C (HbC) disease is usually milder than sickle cell anemia. HbC results when lysine is substituted for glutamic acid in the amino acid chain. HbC is less soluble than HbA; however, it does not polymerize under conditions of decreased oxygen tension as does HbS. The main clinical problems are related to vasoocclusive crises, which are thought to result from higher hematocrit values and viscosity. In older children, sickle cell retinopathy, renal necrosis, and aseptic necrosis of the femoral heads can occur along with obstructive crises.

Sickle cell–thalassemia has the mildest clinical manifestations of all the sickle cell diseases. Individuals with sickle cell–thalassemia have mutations in each allele coding for hemoglobin. One mutation results in HbS formation, and the other is associated with β-thalassemia, which results in decreased production of hemoglobin. Even though most of the child's hemoglobin is HbS (60% to 90%), normal hemoglobins (HbA and HbF) also are present. The normal hemoglobins, particularly HbF, inhibit sickling. The erythrocytes tend to be small (microcytic) and to contain relatively little hemoglobin (hypochromic). As a result, these cells are less likely to occlude the microcirculation, even when in a sickled state.

Evaluation and Treatment. The parents' hematologic history and clinical manifestations may suggest that a child has sickle cell disease, but hematologic tests are necessary to confirm the diagnosis. If the sickle solubility test confirms the presence of HbS in peripheral blood, hemoglobin electrophoresis will be performed to provide information about the amount of HbS in erythrocytes. Prenatal diagnosis can be made by chorionic villus sampling (CVS) as early as 8 to 10 weeks' gestation or by amniotic fluid analysis at 15 weeks' gestation (Fig. 30.8). Hemoglobinopathies, including sickle cell disease, are now included as part of routine newborn screening in all 50 states and the District of Columbia.

Advances in identification of SCD and supportive care have led to decreased morbidity and improved survival of children with SCD. Supportive care emphasizes preventing consequences of anemia and avoiding crises, including adequate hydration, infection prevention, and pain management. Genetic counseling and psychologic support are important for the child and family.

Health maintenance activities are key to reduce the risk of crises and other aspects of disease-related morbidity. In addition to regular childhood vaccines, children with SCD should receive vaccination against pneumococcus and other encapsulated microorganisms. Children under 5 years of age may also be prescribed prophylactic penicillin to further reduce the risk of infection.[32] Because of the high infection-related mortality, individuals with SCD and their families should be instructed to seek immediate medical attention in the event of fever. Evidence-based guidance for screening for nephropathy,

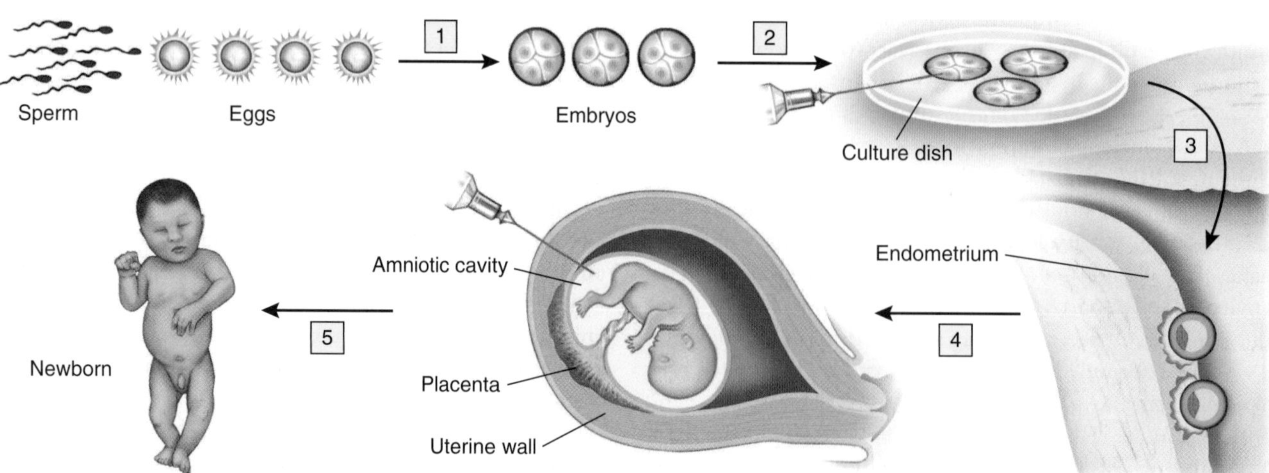

Fig. 30.8 Prepregnancy Sickle Cell Test. This technique has potential for detection of other inherited diseases. *(1)* Fertilization produces several embryos. *(2)* The embryos are tested for the presence of the gene. *(3)* The embryos without the gene are implanted. *(4)* Amniocentesis confirms whether the fetus (or fetuses) has the sickle cell gene. *(5)* Woman has a normal child.

hypertension, retinopathy, pulmonary disease, and the risk of stroke have been published by the National Heart, Lung, and Blood Institute.[32]

Sickle cell trait typically does not affect life expectancy or interfere with daily activities. On rare occasions, however, severe hypoxia caused by shock, vigorous exercising at high altitudes, flying at high altitudes in unpressurized aircraft, or undergoing anesthesia may precipitate vasoocclusive episodes in persons with sickle cell trait. Persons with sickle cell trait are at risk for hyphema with traumatic injury to the eye. Untreated hyphema may result in glaucoma and potential vision loss. In 2010, the National Collegiate Athletic Association implemented testing for sickle cell trait for all incoming student athletes. While having sickle cell trait does not disqualify the individual from participation in athletics, the goal of this testing is to ensure the safety of student athletes.[50]

Treatment advances since the late 1980s have significantly decreased morbidity and mortality in children with SCD. Aggressive management of fever, early diagnosis of *acute chest syndrome* (hypoxia, anemia, progressive multilobar pneumonia, fat emboli), and proper pain management can improve quality of life and prognosis for these children. Treatment of SCD consists of supportive care aimed at preventing consequences of anemia and avoiding crises. Crises can be prevented by avoiding fever, infection, acidosis, dehydration, constricting clothes, and exposure to cold. Immediate correction of acidosis and dehydration with appropriate intravenous fluids is imperative. Infections require aggressive antibiotic therapy, and infections can be reduced by vaccination. Oxygen is not needed unless the child becomes hypoxic. Pain associated with SCD is very complex, requiring accurate assessment and multimodal management.[51,52]

A common treatment for sickle cell disease is hydroxyurea. Hydroxyurea inhibits deoxyribonucleic acid (DNA) synthesis, which causes an increase in HbF concentration. HbF will not sickle. It also provides an anti-inflammatory effect by decreasing leukocyte production. These outcomes are thought to decrease mechanisms that lead to crises.

Two new medications were approved by the US Food and Drug Administration for use in individuals with sickle cell disease in 2019.[32] Voxelotor is an oral medication approved for individuals 12 years of age and older. It is proposed to inhibit HbS polymerization and the sickling process by modifying the affinity between hemoglobin and oxygen.[53] Crizanlizumab is a monoclonal antibody against the adhesion molecule P-selectin. P-selectin is involved in the underlying process by which blood cells adhere to blood vessel walls, thereby contributing to vasoocclusion.[54] Crizanlizumab is administered as an IV infusion.

Transfusion therapy can decrease morbidity and mortality associated with sickle cell disease, particularly in those at increased risk for stroke.[32] Despite these benefits, it can result in iron overload in the liver, heart, and endocrine glands causing disruption of normal function, including delayed physical and sexual development and heart disease. Chelation therapy to remove excess iron is often required for individuals with SCD who require chronic transfusion of RBCs

HSCT offers the only cure for sickle cell disease; however, it is not without important risks. Observational studies to date have demonstrated improved survival and prevention of long-term complications. Additional studies are needed to evaluate benefits and risks by comparing individuals based on disease severity.[55] Current research is seeking to reduce the toxicities associated with transplantation while optimizing long-term outcomes. Clinical trials evaluating the feasibility of GT using an RNA viral vector are presently underway. One type of trial seeks to inhibit the BCL11a gene with the goal of increasing hemoglobin F production, thereby creating a sickle cell trait phenotype.[56]

Thalassemias

The alpha- and beta-thalassemias are autosomal recessive disorders that result in impaired synthesis of one of the two chains—α or β—of adult hemoglobin (HbA). The disorder was named thalassemia, which is derived from the Greek word for *sea*, because it was initially described in people with origins near the Mediterranean Sea. Beta-thalassemia, in which synthesis of the β-globin chain is slowed or defective, is most prevalent among Greek, Italian, some Arab, and Sephardic Jewish people. Alpha-thalassemia, in which the α chain is affected, is most common among Chinese, Vietnamese, Cambodian, and Laotian people. Both alpha- and beta-thalassemias are common among black people.

Beta-thalassemias are more common than alpha-thalassemias. The classification is based on the genes that control α- or β-chain synthesis. It also is based on the combination of mutations within these genes and whether they are homozygous or heterozygous. The anemia associated with both alpha- and beta-thalassemia is a microcytic-hypochromic hemolytic anemia.

Pathophysiology. The β-thalassemias are caused by mutations in the *HBB* gene that decrease the synthesis of β-globin chains and lead to anemia, tissue hypoxia, and RBC hemolysis. The β-thalassemias are classified into three types depending on the severity of symptoms: thalassemia major, intermedia, or minor. Both beta-thalassemia major (Cooley anemia) and beta-thalassemia intermedia are inherited in an autosomal recessive pattern in which both copies of the *HBB* gene in each cell have mutations; however, beta thalassemia major is more severe. β-globin chain production is moderately depressed in the heterozygous form, beta-thalassemia minor, and is known as beta-thalassemia trait. In a small percentage of families, the *HBB* gene mutation, associated with beta-thalassemia major, is inherited in an autosomal dominant manner.[57]

The mutations associated with beta-thalassemia are classified as (1) β^0 mutations or absent β-globin synthesis and (2) β^+ mutations with reduced amounts of β-globin synthesis. More than 200 different causative mutations have been identified, and most are point (missense) mutations. The clinical classification of β-thalassemias is based on the severity of the anemia, which is dependent on the type of mutation (β^0 or β^+ allele) and whether the individual is homozygous or heterozygous for mutations.[57] Individuals who have β-thalassemia major, a β^0/β^0 genotype, will lack HbA and have severe anemia. Those with β^+/β^+ or β^0/β^+ genotypes, β-thalassemia intermedia, may produce small amounts of HbA. β-Chain production is depressed

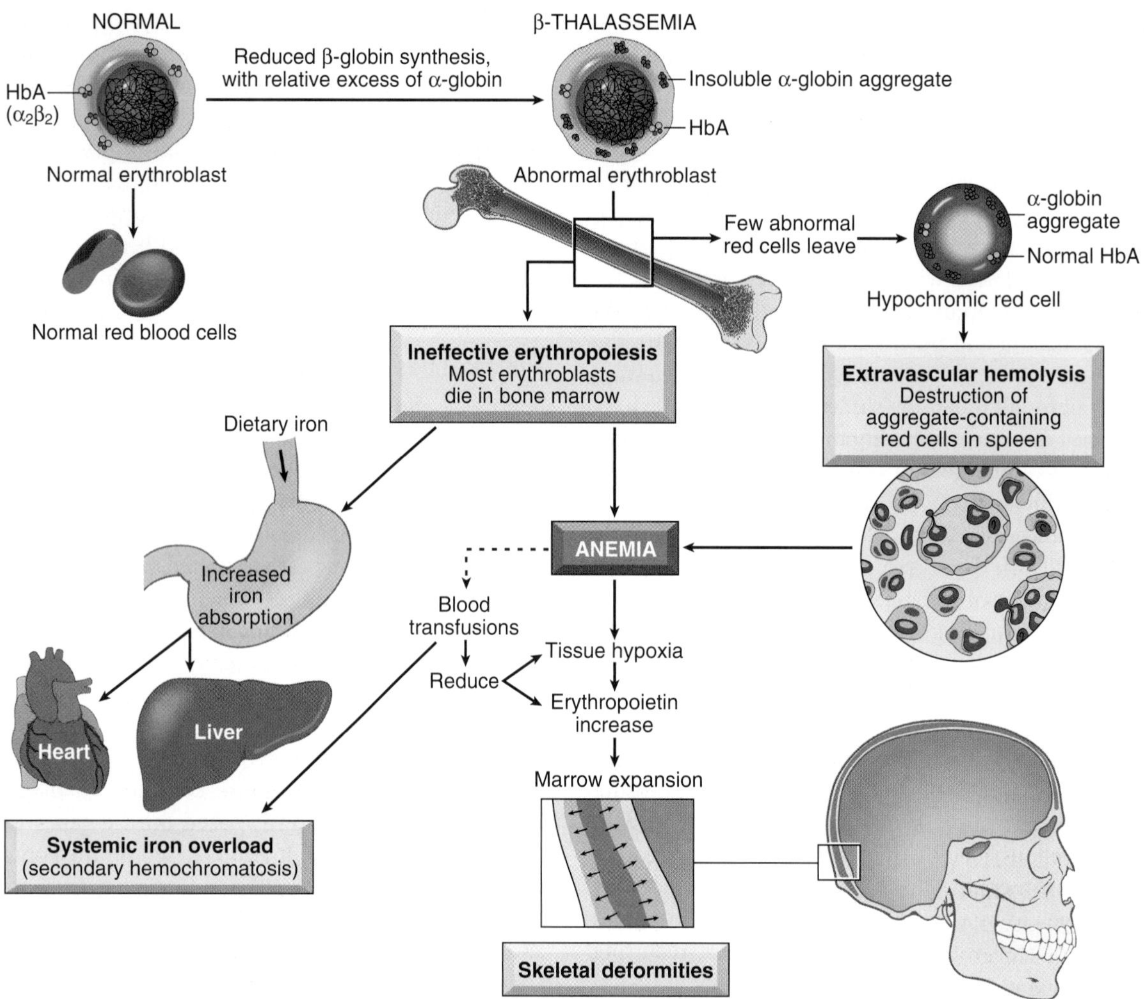

Fig. 30.9 **Pathogenesis of β-Thalassemia Major.** The aggregates of unpaired α-globin chains are a hallmark of the disease. Blood transfusions can diminish the anemia, but they add to the systemic iron overload. (From Kumar V, Abbas AK, Aster JC. *Robbins and Cotran pathologic basis of disease*, 9th edition. Philadelphia: Elsevier Saunders; 2015.)

in the heterozygous form, thalassemia minor (β^0 or β^+ allele); and anemia, if present, is mild. The predominant type of hemoglobin is HbF and typically comprises more than 90% of the total hemoglobin among individuals who are homozygous for mutations. HbA_2 levels are variable among individuals who are homozygous but may be increased among individuals with beta thalassemia minor.[58]

The depression of β-chain synthesis that occurs in beta-thalassemia results in erythrocytes having a reduced amount of hemoglobin and accumulations of free α chains (Fig. 30.9). Free α-chains are unstable and easily precipitate in the cell. Most erythroblasts that contain precipitates are destroyed by mononuclear phagocytes in the marrow. Destruction results in ineffective erythropoiesis and anemia. Some of the precipitate-carrying cells mature and enter the bloodstream. These cells are destroyed prematurely in the spleen, resulting in mild hemolytic anemia.

The alpha (α)thalassemias result from deletions involving the *HBA1* and *HBA2* genes. These genes provide instructions for making a protein called α-globin, a subunit of hemoglobin. The different types of α-thalassemia result from mutations in one or more of the four alleles involved in producing α-globin. These alleles include the two copies of the *HBA1* gene and the two copies of the *HBA2* gene that are present in each cell. The characteristic features of α-thalassemia are anemia, weakness, fatigue, and other more severe complications. The four types of α-thalassemia include

1. ***Hb Bart syndrome*** is the most severe form of α-thalassemia and is caused by loss-of-function mutations in all four α-globin alleles. In an attempt to compensate, Hb Barts, which contains γ-globin chains, is produced. These γ-globin chains have a high affinity for oxygen; however, they do not deliver oxygen to the tissues of the developing fetus. As a result, hydrops fetalis develops, and signs of fetal distress may become evident in the third trimester of pregnancy. Although most cases are fatal, intrauterine transfusions may save the baby.[59]
2. HbH disease results from a loss-of-function in three of the four α-globin alleles. These individuals have an excess of beta-globin chains within the RBCs that form beta-4

tetramers, known as *hemoglobin H* (HbH). HbH also does not carry oxygen effectively, which leads to anemia and other related consequences.[59,60]

3. Alpha thalassemia minor or alpha thalassemia trait occurs when mutations are present in two alleles. Although the amount of α-globin will be reduced, some normal hemoglobin will still be produced and therefore cause fewer health problems. Affected individuals may have microcytic RBCs and slight anemia.[59]
4. Silent α-thalassemia carrier results from a mutation in one of the four α-globin alleles. These individuals typically have no related clinical manifestations but can pass the mutated allele on to their children.[59]

Clinical Manifestations. Beta-thalassemia minor causes mild to moderate microcytic-hypochromic anemia. The degree of reticulocytosis depends on the severity of the anemia. Hemolysis of immature, and therefore fragile, erythrocytes may cause a slight elevation in serum iron and indirect bilirubin levels. Persons with beta-thalassemia minor may be asymptomatic; however, they may experience mild splenomegaly, bronze coloring of the skin, and hyperplasia of the bone marrow. These individuals are less likely to experience life-threatening complications.

If untreated, persons with beta-thalassemia major may become quite ill and have impaired physical growth and development. Skeletal changes begin in infancy and include spinal impairment that impedes linear growth and causes subsequent upper and lower limb-length discrepancy. Deformity of the facial bones in response to hyperplastic marrow results in a characteristic chipmunk-like facial appearance, as the nasal bridge, mandible, and maxilla widen. Osteopenia, osteochondrosis, or both also may develop. The severe anemia resulting from this condition can cause a significant cardiovascular burden with high-output congestive heart failure. For persons with thalassemia that require regular transfusions, progressive hemosiderosis will occur. If not managed carefully from infancy into adulthood, death may occur. Today, careful management with regular blood transfusions and compliance with chelation therapy can increase the life span significantly.

Persons who inherit the mildest form of α-thalassemia (silent α-thalassemia trait) usually are symptom free or have mild microcytosis. Alpha-thalassemia minor has clinical manifestations similar to those of beta-thalassemia minor: mild microcytic-hypochromic anemia, reticulocytosis, bone marrow hyperplasia, increased serum iron concentrations, and mild to moderate splenomegaly.

The clinical manifestations of HbH disease are variable based on the specific characteristics of the mutations that are present in the three affected alleles.

Alpha-thalassemia major (Hb Barts) causes hydrops fetalis, whereby the developing fetus suffers from severe tissue anoxia and may develop fulminant intrauterine congestive heart failure. Signs of fetal distress became evident by the third trimester of pregnancy. In the past, severe tissue anoxia led to death in utero; now many such infants are saved by intrauterine transfusions.

Evaluation and Treatment. Evaluation of thalassemia is based on the familial disease history, clinical manifestations, and blood tests. Diagnostic tests include peripheral blood smears that show a microcytic, hypochromic anemia and target cells. Hemoglobin electrophoresis typically indicates decreased amounts of HbA and increased amounts of HbF after age 12 months and may be useful in diagnosing beta thalassemia. However, to diagnose α-thalassemia, targeted deletion analysis is recommended.

Prenatal diagnosis may be performed, and families with an affected fetus will be referred for genetic counseling. Identification of thalassemia is now included as part of routine newborn screening for hemoglobinopathies in all 50 states and the District of Columbia. Molecular genetic testing of at-risk siblings should be offered to allow for early diagnosis and appropriate treatment. Women with thalassemia intermedia who have never received a blood transfusion or who received a minimal quantity of blood are at risk for severe alloimmune anemia if blood transfusions are required during pregnancy.[61] Treatment for thalassemia is largely supportive. Typical treatment involves a regular transfusion program and chelation therapy to reduce transfusion iron overload. Individuals with milder forms of thalassemia rarely require transfusion. These individuals are at risk for iron overload secondary to increased intestinal absorption of iron from ineffective erythropoiesis.[61] Optimal clinical management may decrease the need for splenectomy. Treatment of thalassemia intermedia is based on the individual's symptoms, and splenectomy may be performed for those who are more symptomatic. These individuals may also require sporadic red cell transfusions, folic acid supplementation, and iron chelation.[61] The only available definitive cure for thalassemia major is allogeneic HSCT from a matched family or unrelated donor or cord blood transplantation from a related donor.[61] In addition, ongoing clinical trials are investigating the use of GT strategies for thalassemia.[62,63]

DISORDERS OF COAGULATION AND PLATELETS

Inherited Hemorrhagic Disease

Table 30.4 provides a summary of the coagulation factors and deficiencies associated with clinical bleeding. Not all the disorders are discussed in this chapter because some are extremely rare (congenital dysfibrinogenemias), and others have no clinical significance. For example, Hageman factor deficiency is a condition with profound laboratory deficiency of factor XII yet is associated with no clinical defects in humans.

Hemophilias

Awareness of a serious bleeding disorder in males was documented nearly 2000 years ago in the Babylonian Talmud, which exempted those boys having male relatives prone to excessive bleeding from the rite of circumcision. In 1803, the first description of this disorder appeared in the medical literature, where it was noted to be X-linked and associated with joint bleeding and crippling.

TABLE 30.4 The Coagulation Factors

Clotting factors	Synonym	Disorder
I	Fibrinogen	Congenital deficiency (afibrinogenemia) and dysfunction (dysfibrinogenemia)
II	Prothrombin	Congenital deficiency or dysfunction
V	Labile factor, proaccelerin	Congenital deficiency (parahemophilia)
VII	Stable factor or proconvertin	Congenital deficiency
VIII	Antihemophilic factor (AHF)	Congenital deficiency is hemophilia A (classic hemophilia)
IX	Christmas factor	Congenital deficiency is hemophilia B
X	Stuart-Power factor	Congenital deficiency
XI	Plasma thromboplastin antecedent	Congenital deficiency, sometimes referred to as hemophilia C
XII	Hageman factor	Congenital deficiency is *not* associated with clinical symptoms
XIII	Fibrin-stabilizing factor	Congenital deficiency

The hemophilias are a group of inherited bleeding disorders resulting from mutations in the genes responsible for coagulation factors. Until 1952 the term *hemophilia* was reserved for deficiency of factor VIII (antihemophilic factor). Since then, two additional coagulation proteins, factor IX (plasma thromboplastin component) and factor XI (plasma thromboplastin antecedent), have been identified. Deficiencies in these two clotting factors are associated with similar clinical manifestations and are regarded as hemophilia B and hemophilia C, respectively. Collectively, inherited deficiencies of these three plasma clotting factors—VIII, IX, XI—account for 90% to 95% of the hemorrhagic bleeding disorders.

Types of hemophilia. Hemophilia has a wide range of clinical severity. The most prevalent types of hemophilia are hemophilia A (classic hemophilia or factor VIII deficiency) and hemophilia B (Christmas disease or factor IX deficiency). Hemophilia A results from mutations in the *F8* gene, which codes for factor VIII, an essential cofactor for factor IX in the coagulation cascade. It is the most common hereditary disease associated with life-threatening bleeding. Hemophilia B results from a mutation in the *F9* gene, which codes for factor IX. Because both factors VIII and IX function together to activate factor X, hemophilias A and B are clinically indistinguishable. The alterations or deficiencies of these coagulation factors decrease the ability to form blood clots in response to injury. The decreased or ineffective blood clotting leads to continuous bleeding.

Hemophilias A and B occur with varying degrees of clinical severity, depending on concentrations of clotting factor VIII or IX in the blood. Severe hemophilia (concentration of clotting factors less than 1% of normal) is associated with spontaneous bleeding. This manifestation of hemophilia is associated with mutations that eliminate the activity of factors VIII or XI. In moderate hemophilia (1% to 5% of normal), bleeding may occur with injury, trauma, or surgery; in the mild form (6% to 50% of normal), bleeding typically occurs only after severe trauma or surgery. Moderate and mild hemophilia are associated with mutations that reduce but do not eliminate the activity of these coagulation factors.[63]

Hemophilia is equally prevalent across racial groups. The incidence of hemophilia A is approximately 1 in 5000 male births. Hemophilia B is five times less common, with an incidence of approximately 1 in 20,000 male births.[64] Hemophilia C, which results from a deficiency of Factor XI is inherited as an autosomal recessive condition and is extremely rare. It affects approximately 1 in 1,000,000 individuals.[65] The worldwide prevalence of severe hemophilia is estimated to be around 400,000 people. A recent meta-analysis of worldwide registry data, however, suggests that approximately 1,125,000 males are living with hemophilia, with manifestations ranging from mild to severe disease.[66]

Pathophysiology. As X-linked recessive conditions, hemophilias A and B are most frequently inherited from a mother who is heterozygous, that is, a carrier, for a mutation in either the *F8* or *F9* gene. Approximately 30% of cases, however, result from a new mutation. This new mutation can occur in either a carrier female or in an affected male. Multiple types of genetic mutations are associated with hemophilias A and B. More than 2000 unique mutations have been identified for hemophilia A,[67] and more than 1000 mutations have been described for hemophilia B.[68] The type of mutation also affects the phenotype, or severity, of the disease. Mutations tend to be identical among affected members of a given family; however, mutations often differ across families.[69]

The *F8* and *F9* genes are located on the long arm of the X chromosome. A mutation in either of these genes typically results in either deficient or abnormal function of the corresponding clotting factor. Because males have only one copy of the X chromosome, the mutation results in the clinical manifestations of hemophilia. Females who are heterozygous carriers typically do not experience excessive bleeding. However, 50% of female carriers have lower than normal clotting factor levels. Those females without a sufficient quantity of normal functioning clotting factor may have bleeding similar to a male with mild hemophilia. Because X-inactivation, or lyonization (see Chapter 4), is a random process, phenotypes of females who are heterozygous carriers can vary. Although very uncommon, it is plausible for a female to be homozygous for mutations in the *F8* or *F9* gene and therefore have hemophilia.

Inversions in introns 1 and 22 of the factor VIII gene are the most frequently observed mutations and account for the most severe cases of hemophilia A.[68] Point mutations, in which a single base in the DNA is inserted in the place of another base, are another type of mutation that causes hemophilia. This type of mutation comprises the majority of unique mutations associated with hemophilia.[67] When a point mutation gives rise to a de novo stop codon (nonsense mutation), translation of the protein ceases, and a shortened version of the protein is synthesized. Usually, the protein is destroyed intracellularly and never reaches the plasma. A point mutation defect also is associated with severe hemophilia, that is, with coagulant activity levels below 1%. Point mutations resulting in the substitution of one amino acid for another can cause phenotypes of varying severity. The altered amino acid chain can destroy protein function, activation, or folding; inhibit intracellular processing; or cause protein clearance.[69]

Clinical Manifestations. The clinical manifestations and severity of hemophilia depend largely on the level of factor VIII and IX activity. Children with severe hemophilia also manifest prolonged bleeding times at different ages. Many boys with hemophilia are circumcised without excessive bleeding. Normal hemostasis is achieved in these infants because clotting is activated through the extrinsic coagulation cascade, which does not involve factors VIII, IX, or XI.

During the first year of life, spontaneous bleeding often is minimal, but hematoma formation may result from immunizations and from firm holding (e.g., under the arms), and joint bleeding may occur. Most children with severe hemophilia initiate prophylactic factor administration around the time they become mobile (e.g., crawling, pulling to stand).

Joint bleeding, or hemarthrosis, is the most characteristic type of bleeding in hemophilia. The joints most often affected are the knees, ankles, and elbows.[70] Hemarthrosis causes pain, limits joint mobility, and predisposes the child to degenerative joint changes. Bleeding into muscles, usually from trauma, also can occur. Oral bleeding is common in the setting of traumatic injury to the mouth or dental surgery. Spontaneous painless hematuria is relatively common in hemophilia; it does not result in significant blood loss but requires evaluation. Hematuria accompanied by pain requires prompt evaluation and treatment. Spontaneous epistaxis may also occur. Although troublesome, it tends to be a minor complication.

Recurrent bleeding—spontaneous and after minor trauma—is a lifelong problem. Intracranial bleeding, bleeding of internal organs, and bleeding into the tissues of the neck, chest, or abdomen are all life-threatening. Delayed or suboptimal treatment of these bleeding episodes may lead to permanent brain injury, loss of organ function, or death.

Evaluation and Treatment. Because hemophilia most often manifests as an inherited disease, a positive family history may expedite a diagnosis of hemophilia. When a mother who is a known or suspected carrier is pregnant, prenatal genetic testing through CVS or amniocentesis may reveal a diagnosis of hemophilia. In the absence of a positive family history, a personal bleed history, laboratory testing, family history, and physical assessment contribute to a thorough evaluation and accurate diagnosis. In general, those with hemophilia A or B will have a prolonged partial thromboplastin time (PTT) and the prothrombin time (PT) will be normal. Measuring factor VIII and factor IX levels also is necessary for diagnosis.

Most children with hemophilia A can be treated with recombinant factor VIII, and most children with hemophilia B can be treated with recombinant factor IX. Recombinant factor is reconstituted in a small volume of diluent, administered by slow intravenous push, and raises the factor level almost immediately.

Primary prophylaxis consists of regular infusions of factor VIII or IX with the goal of preventing joint bleeding. It is usually given to children with severe hemophilia. A 5-year, multicenter trial, which has now become the standard of care,[71,72] found prophylaxis initiated in children between 6 and 30 months of age to be effective in the prevention of joint bleeding, structural joint damage, and frequency of bleeding in boys with factor VIII deficiency. Recent multisite trials have demonstrated the safety and efficacy of pegylated, recombinant factors VIII and IX. These pegylated products have extended half-lives and require less frequent dosing.[73,74] Newer generation products are fully produced in human cell lines and help reduce the risk of the development of inhibitors that limit the efficacy of the infused product.[75] Recently approved substitution therapies using monoclonal antibodies have shown great promise in the management of bleeding in hemophilia. Ongoing investigation of rebalancing therapies and GT may transform disease severity and management.

von Willebrand Disease

von Willebrand disease is an inherited condition with variable clinical manifestations and hematologic findings resulting from a deficiency or dysfunction in von Willebrand factor. von Willebrand factor binds factor VIII and platelets to the blood vessel wall as part of the clotting process. As a result, factor VIII activity may be decreased in individuals with von Willebrand disease. Over 80% of cases of von Willebrand disease demonstrate an autosomal dominant pattern of inheritance; however, some cases demonstrate an autosomal recessive or compound heterozygous pattern. The pattern of inheritance depends on the type of mutation that is present.[67] The clinical management of von Willebrand disease will depend on the underlying subtype that is present.

Congenital Hypercoagulability and Thrombosis

Hereditary bleeding disorders, such as hemophilia, have been recognized and treated for centuries; however, the counterpart of these disorders, thrombophilia, has not been recognized until the past 50 years. The inherited thrombophilic conditions generally are caused by defects in the clotting factors that inhibit clot formation; thus, the balance between bleeding and clotting is directed toward the clotting aspects of hemostasis. In general, thromboses in children in the absence of some type of triggering event such as a vascular access catheter, infection, or heart disease are rare and comprise less than 5% of thrombotic events in children. For these spontaneous events, approximately 60% have some type of hereditary basis.[76] A recent study investigating genetic mutations in 115 adolescents and young adults presenting with thrombotic events identified single-gene mutations in two-thirds of this sample, and some individuals had more than one mutation.[77] Ongoing studies are needed to further investigate the specific roles of these mutations as well as the clinical management of children and adolescents who present with a thrombotic event. Current guidance supports testing for inherited thrombophilia if (1) identification of a thrombophilic mutation or defect might explain the basis for the event, (2) a positive test would have implications for the child or adolescent's clinical management, or (3) testing might help identify asymptomatic family members and provide guidance in avoiding risk factors for future thrombotic events.[78]

Defects in specific proteins (C and S) and antithrombin (AT) and resistance to activated protein C (APC) and hyperhomocysteinemia are the main recognized causes of inherited thrombophilia. Both proteins C and S inhibit coagulation and depend on vitamin K for synthesis in the hepatocytes of the liver. Decreased levels of either of these proteins interfere with the normal homeostatic balance of procoagulant and anticoagulant activity at the endothelial level. Protein C and S deficiency states predispose affected individuals to thrombosis, especially venous thrombosis of the lower extremities.

Protein C deficiency is inherited in an autosomal dominant manner and results from mutations in the *PROC* gene. Its prevalence is approximately 0.2% to 0.4% in the general population. Genetic mutations may result in quantitative (type I) or qualitative (type II) deficiencies of protein C. *Type I deficiencies* involve a reduction in both biologic and immunologic activity of protein C. Type I is caused by deletion of the entire gene. *Type II deficiencies* are less common and result in decreased functional levels of protein C activity despite the presence of a normal level of protein C.[79]

Individuals who are heterozygous for protein C mutations have levels that are 50% to 60% of normal. They may develop superficial thrombophlebitis, deep venous thrombosis, or pulmonary embolism in their late teens and early 20 s. Individuals with homozygous mutations have less than 1% of normal levels of protein C and tend to develop thrombosis of the cutaneous vessels with large areas of skin necrosis. Arterial thrombosis is rare among individuals with protein C deficiency.

Neonatal purpura fulminans is a fatal syndrome found in neonates who are homozygous or compound heterozygous for types I and II protein deficiency. Ecchymosis becomes apparent on the first day of life and develops around the head, trunk, and extremities and often is accompanied by cerebral thrombosis and infarction. The ecchymotic areas often coalesce, and ulceration and necrosis develop. Treatment is largely supportive and includes administration of fresh frozen plasma (FFP) and heparinization; however, the condition is often fatal.

Treatment for protein C deficiency depends on the clinical manifestations. Individuals who are asymptomatic may not require therapy unless a strong family history of thrombosis is present. Heparin is the treatment for acute episodes of thrombosis caused by protein C deficiency. The need for long-term therapy is varied and will be individualized to the person with attention to prior family history. Supplemental protein C concentrates (human) also are available and have been approved for use in children.[80]

Protein S deficiency results from mutations in the *PROS1* gene and is similar to protein C deficiency. Its autosomal dominant pattern of inheritance is also similar. The severity of the clinical manifestations varies. Approximately 60% to 80% of affected individuals will develop a venous thrombosis at some point during their lives.[81]

Protein S deficiency exists in three forms: type I, type II, and type III.[82] *Type I* deficiency is identified as a quantitative deficiency and manifests as low levels of total protein S antigen and free protein S antigen. *Type II* deficiency is identified as a qualitative deficiency with normal levels of free and total protein S antigen but reduced protein S activity. *Type III deficiency* results in low free protein S levels; however, the total plasma concentration of protein S is normal. Type III deficiency has not been established as a risk factor for venous or arterial thromboembolism.

The clinical manifestations of Protein S deficiency vary across individuals. Approximately half of individuals who are heterozygous for mutations will experience a thrombotic event before age 55. Other manifestations include superficial thrombophlebitis and pulmonary emboli. Although clots may occur spontaneously in individuals with protein S deficiency, risk factors, such as increasing age and immobility, can raise the risk of thrombus formation.

Homozygotes demonstrate severe manifestations of the condition and may develop a form of purpura fulminans in the neonatal period. The homozygous state also may lead to intrauterine death. Treatment with heparin, warfarin (Coumadin), and protein C concentrate is similar to that for protein C deficiency.

Antithrombin III (AT III) deficiency is inherited as an autosomal dominant condition. Most individuals are heterozygous for a mutation. AT III deficiency results from mutations in the *SERPINC1* gene and exists in forms type I and type II. Type I is a quantitative deficiency of the AT III antigen resulting from decreased production. Type II is characterized by decreased functional activity. Normal levels of AT III are present; however, their activity is reduced.[83]

Individuals with AT III deficiency are at risk for early development of venous thrombosis and pulmonary embolism. These events often occur in the middle to late teens, but they can occur as early as 10 years of age. The deep veins of the lower extremities are usually involved, most commonly the iliofemoral vein. Other sites include the mesenteric veins, vena cava, renal veins, and retinal veins. Cerebral thromboses also have been described, and arterial thrombotic events are rare. In some cases, thrombosis is precipitated by surgery, trauma, pregnancy, oral contraceptives, and infection.

The treatment of choice for AT III deficiency is heparin. Antiplatelet agents (e.g., aspirin, dipyridamole) may be used, as well as AT III concentrates.

Antibody-Mediated Hemorrhagic Disease

Antibody-mediated hemorrhagic diseases are caused by the immune response. Antibody-mediated destruction of platelets or antibody-mediated inflammatory reactions to allergens damage blood vessels and cause seepage into tissues. The thrombocytopenic purpuras may be intrinsic or idiopathic. They also may be transient phenomena transmitted from mother to fetus. The inflammatory, or "allergic," purpuras, although rare, occur in response to allergens in the blood. All of these disorders first appear during infancy or childhood.

Primary Immune Thrombocytopenia

Primary immune thrombocytopenia (ITP) (previously referred to as idiopathic thrombocytopenic purpura) is the most common of the thrombocytopenic purpuras of childhood. It is a disorder of platelet consumption in which autoantibodies bind to the plasma membranes of platelets. Antibody binding causes platelet sequestration and destruction by mononuclear phagocytes in the spleen and other lymphoid tissues at a rate that exceeds the ability of the bone marrow to produce them. The destruction of platelets is triggered by drugs, infections, lymphomas, or an unknown cause.

ITP is defined further based on the phases of the illness and established criteria for evaluating the response to therapy.[84] Specific phases include *newly diagnosed ITP*, within 3 months of diagnosis; *persistent ITP*, describing individuals with 3 to 12 months of diagnosis who have not achieved remission or complete response off therapy; *chronic ITP*, symptoms lasting longer than 12 months; and *severe ITP*, the presence of bleeding that requires treatment either at diagnosis or following initiation of treatment.

Pathophysiology. The autoantibodies that produce the destruction are often of the IgG class and are usually against the platelet membrane glycoproteins (IIb-IIIa or Ib-IX). Approximately 70% of cases of ITP are preceded by a viral illness (e.g., cytomegalovirus [CMV], Epstein-Barr virus [EBV], parvovirus, or respiratory tract infection), suggesting that viral sensitization has occurred. The typical interval between infection and onset of purpura is 1 to 3 weeks.

Clinical Manifestations. Bruising and a generalized petechial rash often develop acutely about 1 to 3 weeks after a viral illness. Petechiae can develop into ecchymoses. Asymmetric bruising is typical and is found most often on the legs and trunk. Hemorrhagic bullae of the gums, lips, and other mucous membranes may be prominent. Epistaxis (nose bleeding) may be severe and difficult to control. Except for signs of bleeding, the child appears well. The principal changes are found in the spleen, bone marrow, and blood. The acute phase of the disease associated with spontaneous hemorrhages lasts 1 to 2 weeks, but thrombocytopenia often persists. Intracranial hemorrhage is the most serious complication of ITP; however, the incidence is less than 1%. In some cases, the onset of ITP is more gradual, and clinical manifestations consist of moderate bruising and a few petechiae.

Evaluation and Treatment. Laboratory examination reveals an isolated low platelet count. The few platelets observed on a peripheral smear are large, reflecting increased bone marrow production. The Ivy bleeding time is prolonged. Bone marrow aspiration is not recommended for children with typical features of ITP. The primary management for children newly diagnosed with ITP, with no or mild bleeding (skin manifestations), is only observation regardless of the platelet count. When non-life-threatening mucosal bleeding or diminished quality of life is present, a short burst of corticosteroids is recommended.[84]

Even without treatment, the prognosis for children with ITP is excellent: 75% recover completely within 3 months. After the initial acute phase, spontaneous clinical manifestations subside. By 6 months after onset, 80% to 90% of affected children have regained normal platelet counts. ITP that persists longer than 12 months in children is considered chronic. Thrombopoietin receptor agonists (TPO-RA) are recommended for the management of children with ITP who are unresponsive to first-line therapies.[84]

Autoimmune Neonatal Thrombocytopenias

Antibody-mediated thrombocytopenic purpura occurs in neonates in either autoimmune or alloimmune form. Both forms are characterized by the immunologic destruction of platelets by autoantibodies (IgG) against tissue-specific antigens expressed by the platelets (i.e., platelet-specific antigens).

Autoimmune neonatal thrombocytopenia was first noted in the early 1950s when it was observed that mothers with ITP often delivered infants who were transiently thrombocytopenic. Neonatal thrombocytopenia was observed in approximately 50% of infants at risk and lasted an average of 1 month. As platelet counts returned to normal, a concomitant drop in the level of maternal antiplatelet antibody on the child's platelets occurred. The antibody is directed against antigens common to maternal and neonatal platelets. The prognosis generally is favorable, and the frequency of intracranial hemorrhage is rare (1% to 3% of cases). Medical management of affected infants is to prevent the severe thrombocytopenia that can cause significant morbidity by administering intravenous immunoglobulins.

Neonatal alloimmune thrombocytopenia purpura (NAIT) is less common and is estimated to occur in 1 to 2 per 1000 live births. NAIT is caused by maternal immunization against fetal paternally derived platelet-specific antigens (similar to rhesus [Rh] disease). The mother has a normal platelet count, whereas the fetus can be severely thrombocytopenic.

The diagnosis of NAIT is confirmed by detection in the maternal serum of antibody that reacts with platelets from the infant and father but not with platelets from the mother. In approximately 75% to 85% of cases, NAIT recurs in subsequent pregnancies. Purpura usually develops in the affected infant shortly after delivery, and intracranial, renal, and gastrointestinal hemorrhages are possible. The mortality rate from intracranial hemorrhage has been estimated at 10% to 15%. Management of the newborn with NAIT includes an immediate cranial ultrasound because of the significant risk of intracranial hemorrhage. Severely thrombocytopenic newborns (<10,000/μl) or newborns with intracranial or visceral hemorrhages should receive a matched platelet transfusion (maternal or homozygous human platelet antigen 1b [HPA-1b] donor) as soon as possible. If maternal platelets are used, they must be processed to remove platelet alloantibodies. Newborn thrombocytopenia is difficult to predict because newborn platelet counts do not correlate with maternal platelet counts or antiplatelet antibody titers.[85]

Most of the life-threatening clinical manifestations of transient neonatal thrombocytopenia and NAIT can be avoided through cesarean delivery. If the mother has antiplatelet disease, however, surgery can result in hemorrhage and serious maternal morbidity. Maternal morbidity resulting from NAIT during pregnancy is low (less than 5%): the principal maternal risk is bleeding from surgical incisions during cesarean delivery. The incidence of transient thrombocytopenia in infants born to mothers with NAIT is about 50%. If all deliveries were cesarean, half the mothers would undergo cesarean delivery unnecessarily. Conversely, if all deliveries were vaginal, half the infants—those with thrombocytopenia—would be at risk for intracranial bleeding. Therefore, in the absence of any clear benefit to the neonate (given the low rate of intracranial hemorrhage in infants born to mothers with ITP), cesarean delivery should be reserved for the usual obstetric indications.

Autoimmune Vascular Purpura

Autoimmune vascular purpura (allergic purpura) is caused by antibody-mediated injury of blood vessel walls, typically arterioles and capillaries. The exact cause of the inflammatory reaction is unknown but is believed to result from exposure to foreign proteins or chemicals in the blood such as microorganisms, drugs, or other chemicals.

Autoimmune vascular purpura usually is seen in young children. Its incidence decreases among adolescents and adults and occurs only rarely in older adults. The average age at onset is 5 years, with a slightly higher proportion of males affected. Purpura occurs as vessel integrity is disrupted by inflammatory processes, causing effusion of serosanguineous exudate to perivascular tissues.

Clinical manifestations include headache, anorexia, fever, abdominal pain, constipation, arthralgias and urticaria, and erythema that are located symmetrically on the proximal portions of the extremities, particularly on the legs and buttocks, and may be accompanied by itching or paresthesias. Abdominal pain results from hemorrhage into the bowel, which may lead to colic, nausea, and vomiting. These symptoms may precede the appearance of skin lesions. The pain usually is midabdominal but may radiate to other parts of the abdomen. Joint pain and tenderness may be present, but hemarthrosis does not occur. Periarticular swelling and edema of the hands and feet are common and may precede the onset of abdominal pain and purpura. Subacute glomerulonephritis occurs in some cases but usually is reversible.

The characteristic skin lesions (purpura and cutaneous manifestations of allergy), accompanied by a history of joint and abdominal pain, are suspicious for diagnosis. Laboratory test results often reveal no major abnormalities. Attacks may last several weeks and may recur at odd intervals and with changing manifestations with each episode. Treatment, if necessary, consists of symptom management, often with analgesics and nonsteroidal anti-inflammatory medications.

NEOPLASTIC DISORDERS

Leukemia

Leukemia is cancer of the blood-forming tissues, such as the bone marrow, that most often produces abnormal white blood cells called leukemic cells. Once in the blood, leukemic cells can spread to other organs, such as the lymph nodes, spleen, and brain. Leukemia is the most common malignancy in children and adolescents. Of the types of acute childhood leukemia, 75% to 80% of leukemias in children are derived from the lymphoid line and are classified as *acute lymphoblastic leukemia (ALL)*. The remaining 20% to 25% are derived from the myeloid line and are classified as *acute myeloid leukemia (AML)* and *related neoplasms*. The related neoplasms include acute promyelocytic, myelomonocytic, and myelomonoblastic leukemias, as well as the very rare erythroid leukemia.[86] A very small percentage of acute leukemias have characteristics of both the lymphoid and myeloid line and are classified as acute leukemia of ambiguous lineage. Chronic leukemias are rare in children and account for fewer than 5% of cases. Leukemia accounts for 25% of cases of cancer in black children and 34% of cases of cancer in white children.

In the United States, over 50% of all cases of ALL are diagnosed in individuals less than 20 years of age with new cases most prevalent among children between 2 and 6 years of age.[86] The incidence of ALL is greatest among children aged 2 to 3 years (>90 cases per 1 million per year) with rates decreasing to fewer than 30 cases per million by age 8. Since 1975, the incidence of ALL has gradually increased.[87] New cases of leukemia have been rising on average 0.3% a year in the last 10 years. ALL affects more white and Hispanic than black children and more males than females. The incidence of ALL is also higher in Western and industrialized nations.[88] ALL is more common in boys than girls and among Hispanic and white children than among black and Asian American children. AML is slightly more common during the first 2 years of life and during the teenage years. It occurs about equally among boys and girls of all races; however, recent studies suggest increasing rates among Asian children and those of Hispanic ethnicity.[89,90]

Types of Leukemia

A number of different classifications are used for the leukemias. First, acute leukemia is differentiated from chronic leukemia. Second, the cell line determines whether lymphoid cells or myeloid cells are involved. In acute leukemia, this difference separates ALL from AML and vice versa. Categories of ALL are further identified based on their presumed origin from bursa-equivalent cells (B cells) of cases of ALL and thymic cells (T cells) of normal lymphocytes. B-cell ALL comprises 80% to 85% of cases of ALL, and approximately 15% to 20% of cases are T-cell ALL. (See Chapter 29 for a discussion of leukemias in adults.)

Cytogenic studies of leukemic cells are performed routinely at most major treatment centers during the diagnostic process. Abnormal morphologic characteristics, as well as abnormalities in the number of copies of chromosomes, are often found in leukemic cells. Hyperdiploidy (the presence of greater than the diploid [46] number of chromosomes) is associated with a good prognosis. Common translocations associated with ALL are TEL-AML1, MLL rearrangements, and BCR-ABL. TEL-AML1 is the most common abnormality (in 20% to 30% of cases) and occurs when the *TEL* gene on chromosome 12p13 fuses with the *AML1* gene on chromosome 21q22. TEL-AML1 is associated with a favorable outcome. MLL rearrangements are translocations between the *MLL* gene on chromosome 11q23 and other partner chromosomes. One of the most noted MLL rearrangements involves chromosome 4 as the partner chromosome t(4;11). This specific MLL rearrangement occurs most frequently among leukemia in infants less than 1 year of age and is associated with a poor prognosis despite intensive therapy.[91] A translocation involving the long arms of chromosomes 9 and 22, t(9;22)(q34;q11), also described as the Philadelphia chromosome, occurs in more than 95% of cases of chronic myeloid leukemia (CML) yet is also present in about 2% to 3% of cases of ALL.[86] The specific breakpoint, however, varies in CML and ALL. The translocation results in the generation of the *BCR-ABL* fusion gene. The bcr-abl protein that is produced by this fusion gene results in unregulated tyrosine kinase activity.

Classification of childhood leukemia has become a complex but essential process to determine treatment. The WHO has developed a classification scheme based on a comprehensive system that uses morphology, immunophenotyping, cytogenetic, and clinical features.[86] Immunophenotyping using flow cytometry is used to distinguish between lymphoblastic and nonlymphoblastic leukemia. Molecular cytogenetic techniques, such as fluorescence in situ hybridization (FISH), allow for further detection of specific genetic abnormalities associated with leukemia subtypes. Next-generation sequencing (NGS) techniques, including whole genome and whole exome sequencing, are supporting further investigation of the molecular basis of childhood leukemia as well as planning treatment.[92] (See Emerging Science Box: Molecular Characterization of Childhood Leukemia and Treatment Considerations.)

EMERGING SCIENCE BOX

Molecular Characterization of Childhood Leukemia and Treatment Considerations

The presence of the Philadelphia chromosome, which involves a translocation between chromosomes 9 and 22 has been well-described in a subset of children with acute lymphoblastic leukemia. This translocation results in the formation of the *BCR-ABL* fusion gene. The protein produced by this gene results in unregulated tyrosine kinase activity within the cell. Historically, cure rates for children with Philadelphia positive (Ph+) acute lymphoblastic leukemia (ALL) have been poor. The use of tyrosine kinase inhibitors, in combination with chemotherapy, have resulted in improved cure rates.

In recent years, another molecular subtype of ALL that involves altered tyrosine kinase activity has been discovered. This subtype has been designated Philadelphia chromosome-like ALL or Ph-like ALL. It is present in approximately 12% of children and 21% of adolescents with ALL. It is also more prevalent among children and adolescents of Hispanic ethnicity and those with Down syndrome. As with Ph+ ALL, Ph-like ALL has been associated with poorer outcomes. Although the pattern of gene expression in Ph-like ALL is similar to that of Ph+ ALL, the bcr-abl protein is not produced. Ph-like ALL is genetically heterogeneous and is further defined by its gene expression profile and underlying tyrosine kinase alteration. Determining the tyrosine kinase alteration that is present can then guide the selection of a tyrosine kinase inhibitor to be used as part of the child's treatment.

Tyrosine kinase inhibitors differ from traditional chemotherapy in that they block intracellular signals rather than interfere with DNA synthesis. Tyrosine kinase inhibitors are also administered orally. Although this group of medications is associated with improved survival, treatment outcomes can depend on the individual's adherence to the prescribed treatment. Optimizing outcomes for individuals affected with this subtype of leukemia involves early identification of its molecular characteristics and then supporting affected children, adolescents, and their families in adhering to the prescribed treatment.

Data from Harvey RC, et al. Clinical diagnostics and treatment strategies for Philadelphia chromosome-like acute lymphoblastic leukemia. *Blood Advances*, 2020;4(1):218–228; Pui C-H, et al. Philadelphia chromosome-like acute lymphoblastic leukemia. *Clinical Lymphoma, Myeloma & Leukemia*, 2017;17(8):464–470.

Etiology. The exact cause of most childhood cancer, including leukemia, is unknown. The occurrence of leukemia in monozygotic twins is estimated as being as high as 25%. About 5% of all childhood cancers are caused by inherited mutations. Genetic mutations that predispose the child to cancer development can occur during fetal development. Genetic conditions associated with leukemia include Down syndrome, neurofibromatosis, Li-Fraumeni syndrome, Shwachman-Diamond syndrome, Bloom syndrome, Fanconi anemia, and ataxia-telangiectasia.[93] AML in children is sometimes associated with loss or deletion of chromosome 7 in the leukemia cells. AML can develop from preexisting myeloproliferative disorders that also are preleukemia syndromes, such as myelodysplastic syndrome. Epigenetic modifications, including DNA methylation, have been proposed as mediating events between environmental exposures and subsequent disease development.[94,95]

Multiple types of exposures have been investigated in relation to the development of leukemia. Many studies have shown that exposure to ionizing radiation (prenatal exposure to x-rays and postnatal exposure to high doses) can lead to the development of childhood leukemia and possibly other cancers.[96] There is recent concern for performing computed tomography (CT) scans in children. The increased use of these scans combined with wide variability in radiation doses has resulted in many children receiving a high dose of radiation.[97] Studies of other possible environmental risk factors, including parental exposure to cancer-causing chemicals, prenatal exposure to pesticides, childhood exposure to common infectious agents, and living near a nuclear power plant, have so far produced inconsistent results. Higher risks of cancer have not been seen in children of individuals treated for sporadic cancer (cancer not caused by an inherited mutation).[98,99]

Exposure to prenatal and postnatal smoking has also been investigated in relation to the development of leukemia and other childhood cancers. A recent meta-analysis identified an association between the development of ALL and paternal smoking in both the preconception and prenatal periods.[100] Paternal smoking before, during, and after a pregnancy was identified as contributing to an increased risk of both ALL and AML in another recent meta-analysis; however, maternal smoking was not.[101]

Prenatal exposure to pesticides is hypothesized to increase the risk of childhood leukemia by resulting in oxidative stress leading to the generation of free radicals that induce breaks in the DNA of early hematopoietic stem cells. Results of recent meta-analyses support associations between parental exposure to pesticides and other potential environmental toxins before or during pregnancy and subsequent development of childhood leukemia.[102,103]

Chemicals such as benzene have been associated with the development of AML in adults. Recent meta-analyses provide evidence of a possible association between benzene exposure, occurring in the context of traffic-related air pollution and childhood leukemia.[104,105] Previous treatment with chemotherapy for other cancer types is also a risk factor for developing ALL and AML.[91]

Studies investigating other types of exposures have had inconclusive results. Leukemic "clusters" that represent a greater number of leukemia cases occurring in a particular geographic location have raised speculation about environmental factors or infectious patterns of transmission. Follow-up studies, however, have not provided evidence of increased risk in the context of these exposures.[106,107]

Pathophysiology. ALL involves immature B (pre-B) or T (pre-T) cells called lymphoblasts. As leukemia develops, the bone marrow becomes dense with lymphoblasts that replace the normal marrow and disrupt normal function. Many of the chromosomal abnormalities documented in ALL cause dysregulation of the expression and function of transcription factors required for normal B-cell and T-cell development.[108,109] The mutations can include both gain of function and loss of function that are required for normal development.

AML is caused by acquired oncogenic mutations that impair differentiation, resulting in the accumulation of immature myeloid blasts in the marrow and other organs. Epigenetic alterations are frequent in AML and have a central role. The bone marrow crowding by blast cells produces marrow failure and complications, including anemia, thrombocytopenia, and neutropenia. AML is very heterogeneous because myeloid cell differentiation is very complex. Leukemia, whether ALL or AML, is typically distinguished from lymphoma by the presence of greater than 20% leukemic blasts in the bone marrow.

Clinical Manifestations. The onset of leukemia may be abrupt or insidious. Children with leukemia may present with symptoms only a few weeks before diagnosis. Regardless of how leukemia develops, the most common symptoms reflect consequences of bone marrow failure. These include decreased levels of RBCs and platelets, as well as changes in white blood cells. Pallor, fatigue, petechiae, purpura, bleeding, and fever generally are present. Approximately 45% of children present with a hemoglobin level below 7 g/dL. Three-quarters of children with ALL have platelet counts less than 100,000/mm^3 at diagnosis, and 28% have platelet counts less than 20,000/mm^3. Epistaxis, excessive bruising, and hematuria may occur in children with severe thrombocytopenia. Half of all children newly diagnosed with AML have platelet counts less than 50,000/mm^3. Disseminated intravascular coagulation occurs more commonly with AML, particularly with promyelocytic leukemia. The granules in the leukemic promyelocytes likely possess thromboplastin activity.

Fever can be present as a result of (1) infection associated with the decrease in functional neutrophils and (2) hypermetabolism associated with the ongoing rapid growth and destruction of leukemic cells. In most children with ALL, the total white blood count at diagnosis is less than 10,000/mm^3, and with AML, most present with white cell counts less than 50,000/mm^3. In a few children, however, the peripheral white blood count at presentation may be greater than 100,000/mm^3. White blood cell counts greater than 200,000/mm^3 can cause leukostasis, an intravascular clumping of cells resulting in infarction and hemorrhage, usually in the brain and lung. The three most important favorable prognostic factors are age at diagnosis (2 to 10 years), initial leukocyte count ($<$50,000/mm^3), and initial response to treatment.

Renal failure as a result of hyperuricemia (high uric acid levels) can be associated with ALL, particularly at diagnosis or during the initial phase of treatment. Uric acid levels rise as an end product of purine metabolism from cellular destruction. Because the major excretory pathway is through the kidney, urates can precipitate in renal tubules or ureters and can lead to oliguria and acute renal failure. Renal failure is typically preventable if uric acid levels are monitored, and initial management is aimed at optimal hydration and blockage of further uric acid formation by administration of the drug allopurinol. Rasburicase, a medication that directly inhibits existing uric acid, may be administered to children with elevated uric acid levels and deemed at increased risk for renal failure.[110]

Extramedullary invasion with leukemic cells can occur in nearly all body tissue. Most children with ALL have some extramedullary involvement at diagnosis. Leukemic invasion of tissue other than bone marrow is believed to represent metastatic infiltration. Hepatosplenomegaly and lymphadenopathy, resulting from extramedullary hematopoiesis, occur in nearly half of children with ALL, but they are less common in children with AML.

The CNS is a common site of infiltration of extramedullary leukemia. Less than 10% of children with ALL, however, will have CNS involvement at diagnosis. The most common symptoms of CNS involvement relate to increased intracranial pressure, causing early morning headaches, nausea, vomiting, irritability, and lethargy. Gonadal involvement with testicular infiltration also may occur.

Leukemic infiltration into bones and joints is common. Reports of bone or joint pain actually lead to the diagnosis of leukemia in some children. In most children, bone pain is characterized as migratory, vague, and without areas of swelling or inflammation. In some cases, however, joint pain is the primary symptom, and some swelling is associated with the pain. Occasionally, these children are initially misdiagnosed as having rheumatoid arthritis. Other organs reported to be sites of leukemic invasion include the kidneys, heart, lungs, thymus, eyes, skin, and gastrointestinal tract. Skin involvement is more common in AML than in ALL.

Evaluation and Treatment. Leukemia is diagnosed through blood tests and examination of peripheral blood smears. A bone marrow aspiration is usually performed to further characterize the leukemia. The blast cell is the hallmark of acute leukemia (Fig. 30.10A). The blast cell is a relatively undifferentiated cell characterized by diffusely distributed nuclear chromatin, with one or more nucleoli and basophilic cytoplasm (Fig. 30.10B).

Healthy children have less than 5% blast cells in the bone marrow and none in the peripheral blood. In ALL, the bone marrow often is replaced by 80% to 100% blast cells. The bone marrow, at the time of diagnosis, is typically considered hypercellular and is composed of a homogeneous population of cells. Counts of normally developing RBCs, granulocytes, and platelets are typically reduced. Occasionally, the marrow appears hypocellular, making the diagnosis difficult to differentiate from aplastic anemia. When this occurs, bone marrow biopsy or biopsy of extramedullary sites is necessary to confirm the diagnosis.

Approximately 85% of children with ALL will become 5-year survivors of their illness. Chemotherapy, using a combination

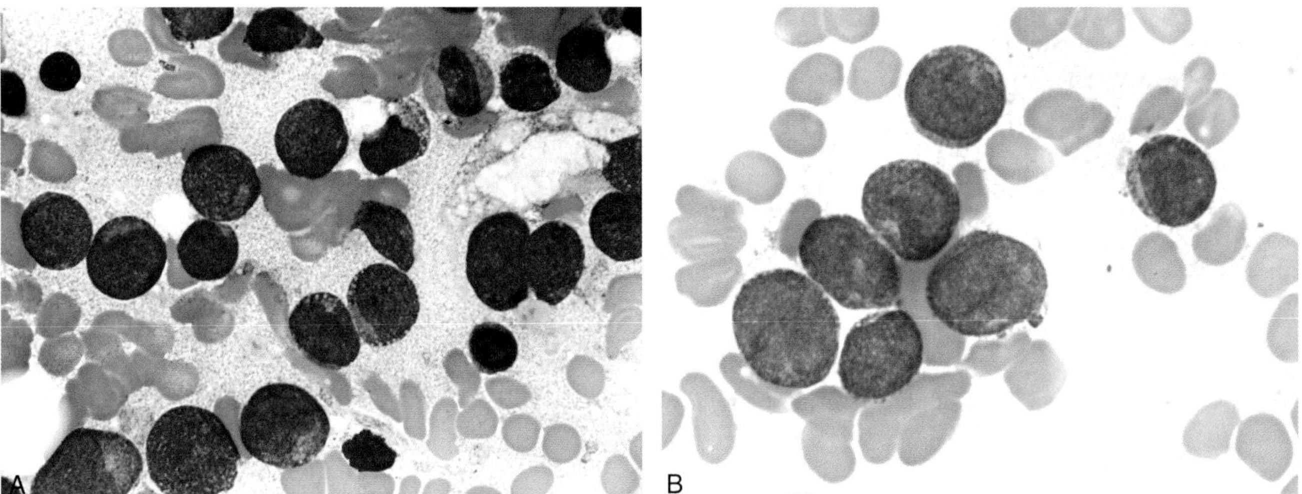

Fig. 30.10 Blast Cells Acute Myeloid Leukemia Without Maturation. (A) Bone marrow smear with numerous blast cells and **(B)** blast cells (shown in purple) with basophilic cytoplasm. (From Naeim F, Nagesh Rao P, Song SX, et al. Acute myeloid leukemia, not otherwise specified. *Atlas of Hematopathology*, 2018; 345–374. https://doi.org/10.1016/b978-0-12–809843-1.00022-x.)

of medications, is the treatment of choice for acute leukemia. Radiation of the CNS is used only in selected cases. Identification of various risk groups among children with ALL has led to the development of different intensities of drug protocols. As a result, treatment can be targeted specifically for a particular risk group. For example, enhanced technologies to detect minimal residual disease have improved the ability to identify children who are at increased risk of relapse. These children are then able to receive intensified treatment with emerging therapeutic approaches, including bi-specific antibodies earlier in their course of treatment.[111] Children who experience relapses of ALL may receive hematopoietic stem cell transplants. Treatment with chimeric antigen receptor T cells (CAR-T cells) is also showing promise.[93]

AML is more difficult to treat than ALL. Combination chemotherapy is the most common approach to treatment. Those children with unfavorable cytogenetic markers and those who experience a relapse of their disease will often undergo HSCT.[112]

CML accounts for less than 5% of childhood leukemias. Biologically targeted therapies, specifically tyrosine kinase inhibitors (TKIs), are becoming the mainstay of treatment, specifically for individuals whose disease has the *BCR/ABL* translocation.[112] TKIs are administered orally, and several are now approved for use in children. Treatment requires continued adherence to the medication regimen, and the health impact of long-term TKI therapy is not yet known.

Lymphomas

Lymphoma (Hodgkin lymphoma [HL] and non-Hodgkin lymphoma [NHL]) develops from the proliferation of malignant lymphocytes in the lymphoid system (see Chapters 14 and 29). Lymphomas arise from discrete tissue masses and involve some recognizable stage of lymphocyte B- or T-cell differentiation. The WHO provides a classification scheme for lymphoma that was updated in 2016 (also see Chapter 29).[113]

Lymphomas are the third most common type of childhood cancer, behind leukemia and CNS tumors, and represent about 11% of all cases of childhood cancer. Around 1800 children younger than 20 years of age are diagnosed with lymphoma in the United States each year.[114] NHL (including Burkitt lymphoma) occurs more often than Hodgkin lymphoma. Either group of diseases is rare before the age of 5 years, and the relative incidence increases throughout childhood. Boys are more likely to be diagnosed with lymphoma than are girls. Children with inherited or acquired immunodeficiency syndromes, such as Wiskott-Aldrich syndrome, ataxia-telangiectasia, and Bloom syndrome, are at particular risk for developing NHL.

Non-Hodgkin Lymphoma

Non-Hodgkin lymphomas (NHLs) are cancers of immune cells. NHLs are a large and diverse group of tumors. NHL typically arises at extranodal sites and spreads in a noncontiguous or unpredictable manner. Some tumors develop more slowly, whereas others develop more quickly and aggressively. Some mature B-cell lymphomas present more like leukemia. Childhood NHL typically becomes evident as a diffuse disease and can be further subdivided into four major types: (1) mature B-cell non-Hodgkin lymphoma (Burkitt and Burkitt-like lymphoma and Burkitt leukemia); (2) lymphoblastic lymphoma; and (3) anaplastic large cell lymphoma.[115] The common types of NHL in children are different from those in adults. The most common types of NHL in children are Burkitt lymphoma (40%), lymphoblastic lymphoma (25% to 30%), and large cell lymphoma (10%).

Pathophysiology. Burkitt lymphoma will be discussed as an example of the pathogenesis of NHL in children. Burkitt lymphoma includes three clinical variants: sporadic, endemic, and immunodeficiency associated. Each of these variants is associated with translocations of the *MYC* gene on chromosome 8 that lead to increased MYC protein levels.[115] MYC is a transcription factor, meaning that it influences the rate of transcription of DNA into messenger RNA. Overexpression of MYC further increases the expression of genes required for aerobic glycolysis, called the *Warburg effect* (see Chapter 12). Many Burkitt lymphomas are associated with latent infection of the EBV.[116] EBV is present in nearly all cases of endemic Burkitt lymphoma, which occur mostly among individuals living in areas of the world where malaria is highly prevalent. Malaria is believed to reduce resistance to EBV, thereby increasing susceptibility to lymphoma. EBV is also present in 15% to 20% of sporadic cases of Burkitt lymphoma and about 25% of tumors associated with human immunodeficiency virus (HIV) infection.[116,117] Other immunodeficiency conditions that increase the risk for Burkitt and other NHLs include receipt of a solid organ transplant, Wiskott-Aldrich syndrome, ataxia-telangiectasia, and Bloom syndrome.

Clinical Manifestations. NHL can arise from any lymphoid tissue. Signs and symptoms therefore are specific for the involved site. Some children have such widespread involvement that no original site can be determined. Because some childhood NHL is rapidly progressive, symptoms are often present only a few weeks before diagnosis is made. Rapidly enlarging lymphoid tissue and painless lymphadenopathy are common in about one-third of children with abdominal sites of involvement, usually representing a gastrointestinal origin for the disease. Symptoms often include abdominal pain and vomiting, but a palpable mass is not always present. The other common site of childhood NHL is the chest region. Associated signs of NHL include swelling of the lymph nodes in the neck, underarm, stomach, or groin; trouble swallowing; a painless lump or swelling in a testicle; weight loss for unknown reason; night sweats; and possibly trouble breathing. Involvement of facial bones, particularly the jaw, is common in endemic Burkitt lymphoma.

Evaluation and Treatment. Diagnosis is made by physical exam and health history, followed by a needle biopsy of disease sites, usually the involved lymph nodes, tonsils, spleen, liver, bowel, or skin. Burkitt lymphoma is very aggressive and responds well to treatment. With intensive chemotherapy, most children and young adults can be cured.

Hodgkin Lymphoma

Hodgkin lymphoma (HL) is a group of lymphoid neoplasms that, unlike NHL, arises in a single chain of lymph nodes and spreads first in a contiguous way to lymphoid tissue. HL is characterized by the presence of Hodgkin and Reed-Sternberg cells (HRS), which are large cells that come from the germinal center of B cells (Fig. 30.11). HL is a common type of cancer in young adults and adolescents but rare in childhood. The WHO has identified five types of HL: (1) nodular sclerosis, (2) mixed cellularity, (3) lymphocyte rich, (4) lymphocyte depletion, and (5) lymphocyte predominance (also see Chapter 29). Similar expression of HRS cells occurs in the first four types; therefore, they are considered the *classic* types. In the lymphocyte predominance type, the HRS cell is distinctive but different than the others. Risk factors for HL include having EBV, being infected with HIV or other immunologic disorders (immunodeficiencies, autoimmune lymphoproliferative syndrome), having a personal history of mononucleosis, and having a parent or sibling with a personal history of HL.[118] Relatively few cases of HL are diagnosed in children before age 5 years, and HL is much more prevalent among males than females (M:F = 5.3) in this age group. Among adolescents 15 to 19 years of age, however, the incidence of HL is slightly greater in females (M:F = 0.8). The incidence of HL gradually increases through age 11 years, with a marked increase through adolescence that continues into the 30 s.

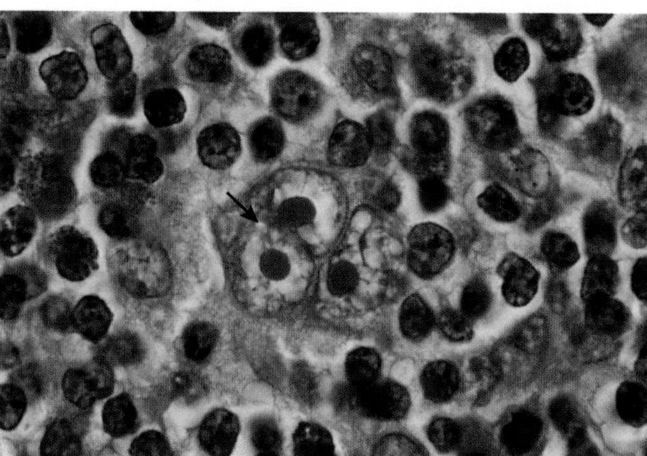

Fig. 30.11 Diagnostic Reed-Sternberg Cell. A large multinucleated or multilobated cell with inclusion body–like nucleoli *(arrow)* surrounded by a halo of clear nucleoplasm. (From Damjanov I, Linder J. *Pathology: A color atlas*. St. Louis: Mosby; 2000.)

Pathophysiology. The HRS cells fail to express most of the normal B-cell markers, as well as those of T-cells. The causes of the genetic rearrangements or reprogramming are not fully known but are thought to be the result of widespread epigenetic changes.

The abnormal pattern of gene expression in HRS cells suggests that the activity of many transcription factors is also altered.[119] NGS studies have identified mutations in signaling pathways, including transcription factor nuclear factor-kappa B (NF-κB) and other epigenetic regulators. Abnormalities in the activation of NF-κB may be influenced by EBV infection. NF-κB is involved in many biologic processes, including inflammation, immunity, cell growth, differentiation, and apoptosis. EBV-infected B cells, resembling Reed-Sternberg cells, are found in lymph nodes in individuals with infectious mononucleosis, suggesting that the EBV proteins may have a role in changes of the B cells into HRS cells.[120] Altered expression of major histocompatibility class antigens may allow HRS cells to avoid the normal host immune response.[121]

Clinical Manifestations. Painless lymphadenopathy in the lower cervical chain, with or without fever, is the most common symptom in children. These nodes are firm and rubbery and may be sensitive to palpation if they have grown rapidly. Other lymph nodes and organs also may be involved (Fig. 30.12). At least two-thirds of individuals have mediastinal involvement that may cause symptoms ranging from

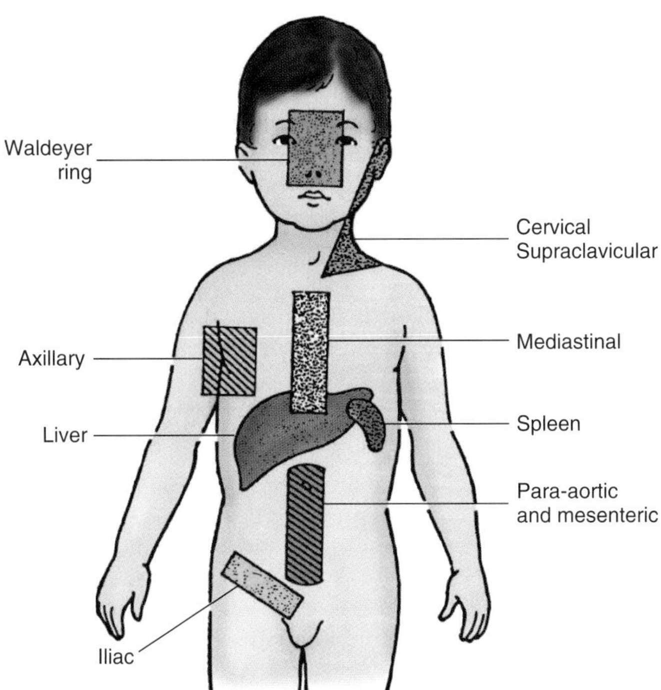

Fig. 30.12 Main Areas of Lymphadenopathy and Organ Involvement in Hodgkin Lymphoma. (From Hockenberry MJ, et al., eds. *Wong's nursing care of infants and children*, 10th edition. St. Louis: Mosby; 2015.)

a nonproductive cough to tracheal or bronchial compression leading to airway obstruction. Extranodal primary sites in Hodgkin lymphoma are rare. Systemic symptoms at the time of diagnosis may include fatigue, anorexia, weight loss, malaise, drenching night sweats, and pruritus. Intermittent fever is present in 30% of children, and weight loss may be present.

Evaluation and Treatment. The Ann Arbor staging system considers extent and location of disease, as well as substage classifications that consider systemic symptoms (presence of fever of 38°C [100.4°F] for 3 consecutive days, drenching night sweats, or unexplained loss of 10% or more of body weight in the 6 months preceding diagnosis), extranodal manifestations, or bulky disease. Combination chemotherapy used with or without low-dose radiation has been an effective treatment, with long-term cure rates reported from 90% to 95%.[118]

Historically, survivors had a much greater risk of developing a secondary cancer, such as lung cancer, melanoma, and breast cancer. Treatment protocols have been modified to minimize the use of radiotherapy and use less toxic chemotherapy. Targeted therapies, including monoclonal antibodies such as brentuximab vedotin and immune checkpoint inhibitors, may have a greater role in treating Hodgkin lymphoma.

SUMMARY REVIEW

Disorders of Erythrocytes

1. Anemia is the most common blood disorder in children. Like the anemias of adulthood, the anemias of childhood are caused by ineffective erythropoiesis or premature destruction of erythrocytes.
2. Iron deficiency anemia (IDA) is the most common nutritional disorder worldwide. Its incidence is greatest among children between 6 months and 2 years of age. Iron is critical for the developing child and without it, damage from the periods of IDA is irreversible.
3. Regardless of its cause, IDA produces a hypochromic-microcytic anemia. Symptoms of mild anemia are often nonspecific, so parents may not notice changes until moderate anemia has developed.
4. Hemolytic disease of the fetus and newborn (HDFN) results from incompatibility between the maternal and the fetal Rh factors or blood type (ABO). Maternal antibodies (anti-Rh antibodies) form in response to the presence of fetal incompatible (Rh-positive) erythrocytes in the blood of an Rh-negative mother. The maternal antibodies then enter the fetal circulation and cause hemolysis of fetal erythrocytes. ABO incompatibility can cause HDFN even if fetal erythrocytes do not escape into the maternal circulation during pregnancy.
5. The key to treatment of HDFN resulting from Rh incompatibilities lies in prevention or immunoprophylaxis.
6. Sickle cell disease is a group of disorders characterized by the production of abnormal hemoglobin S (HbS) within the erythrocytes. It is most common among people with ancestry from sub-Saharan Africa.
7. Sickle cell disease is an inherited, autosomal recessive disorder expressed as sickle cell anemia, sickle cell–thalassemia disease, or sickle cell–HbC disease, depending on mode of inheritance. Sickle cell anemia, in which the individual is homozygous for HbS, is the most severe. Sickle cell–thalassemia and sickle cell–HbC disease are compound heterozygous forms in which the child inherits HbS from one parent or another type of abnormal hemoglobin from the other parent. All forms of sickle cell disease are lifelong conditions.
8. Sickle cell trait, in which the child inherits HbS from one parent and normal hemoglobin (HbA) from the other, is a heterozygous carrier state that rarely has clinical manifestations.
9. Sickle cell disease causes a change in the shape of red blood cells into the sickle shape. Sickling is triggered by decreased oxygen or dehydration. Most sickled erythrocytes regain a normal shape after reoxygenation and rehydration.
10. The alpha- and beta-thalassemias are inherited autosomal recessive disorders. These conditions result in an impaired rate of synthesis of one of the two chains—α or β—of adult hemoglobin (HbA).

Disorders of Coagulation and Platelets

1. Hemorrhagic diseases can be either inherited (hemophilias) or antibody-mediated (primary immune thrombocytopenia [ITP]).

2. The hemophilias are a group of inherited bleeding disorders resulting from mutations in the genes responsible for coagulation factors.
3. Hemophilia A (factor VIII deficiency) and hemophilia B (factor IX deficiency) are caused by mutations in the genes coding for factors VIII and IX, factors essential in the coagulation cascade. Because factors VIII and IX function together, hemophilia A and B are clinically indistinguishable. Hemophilia A is the most common hereditary disease associated with life-threatening bleeding.
4. Hemophilias A and B are inherited as X-linked recessive conditions. Approximately one-third of cases, however, are the result of a spontaneous mutation in the involved gene.
5. The antibody-mediated hemorrhagic diseases are a group of disorders caused by the immune response. Antibody-mediated destruction of platelets or antibody-mediated inflammatory reactions to allergens damage blood vessels and cause seepage into tissues.
6. ITP is the most common disorder of platelet consumption in which antiplatelet antibodies bind to the plasma membranes of platelets. ITP results in platelet sequestration and destruction by mononuclear phagocytes at a rate that exceeds the ability of the bone marrow to produce them.

Neoplastic Disorders

1. Leukemia is cancer of the blood-forming tissues, such as the bone marrow, that most often produces abnormal white blood cells called leukemic cells.
2. About 75% of childhood leukemias are acute lymphoblastic leukemia (ALL). The remaining cases are classified as acute myeloid leukemia (AML) and related neoplasms. Chronic leukemias are rare in children.
3. The cause of most childhood cancer, including leukemia, is unknown. About 5% of all childhood cancers are caused by inherited mutations. Genetic mutations that predispose the child to cancer development can occur during fetal development.
4. Exposure to ionizing radiation can lead to the development of childhood leukemia and possibly other cancers.
5. ALL causes dysregulation of the expression and function of transcription factors required for normal B- and T-cell development.
6. Epigenetic alterations are frequent in AML and have a central role in its development.
7. The onset of leukemia may be abrupt or insidious. The most common symptoms reflect consequences of bone marrow failure and can include decreased levels of red blood cells and platelets, as well as changes in white blood cells.
8. The lymphomas of childhood are Hodgkin lymphoma (HL) and non-Hodgkin lymphoma (NHL).
9. Lymphomas are proliferations of malignant lymphocytes that arise from discrete tissue masses. Lymphoid neoplasms involve some recognizable stage of lymphocyte B- or T-cell differentiation.
10. Some lymphomas occasionally have leukemic presentations, and evolution to leukemia is not unusual during the progression of incurable lymphoma.
11. The lymphomas of childhood are Hodgkin lymphoma (HL) and non-Hodgkin lymphoma (NHL).
12. NHLs are cancers of immune cells. Children with inherited or acquired immunodeficiency syndromes have an increased risk of developing NHL.
13. The most common types of NHL in children are Burkitt lymphoma, lymphoblastic lymphoma, and large cell lymphoma. Most Burkitt lymphomas are latently infected with the Epstein-Barr virus (EBV).
14. HL is a group of lymphoid cancers. HL arises in a single chain of lymph nodes and spreads first in a contiguous way to lymphoid tissue.
15. HL is characterized by the presence of Reed-Sternberg cells, which are large cells derived from the germinal center of B cells.

REFERENCES

1. Christensen RD, et al. Reference intervals for reticulocyte parameters of infants during their first 90 days after birth. *J Perinatol.* 2016;36:61–66.
2. Nagaoka H. Immunization and infection change the number of recombination activating gene1 (Rag) expressing B cells in the periphery by altering immature lymphocyte production. *J Exp Med.* 2000;191:2113–2120.
3. Schmutz N, et al. Expected ranges for blood neutrophil concentrations of neonates: the Manroe and Mouzinho charts revisited. *J Perinatol.* 2008;28:275–281.
4. Lim EM, et al. Race-specific WBC and neutrophil count reference intervals. *Int J Lab Hematol.* 2010;32(6 Pt 2):590–597.
5. Aldrimer M, et al. Population-based pediatric reference intervals for hematology, iron and transferrin. *Scand J Clin Lab Invest.* 2013;73:253–261.
6. Christensen RD, et al. Reference ranges for blood concentrations of eosinophils and monocytes during the neonatal period defined from over 63,000 records in a multihospital health-care system. *J Perinatol.* 2010;30:540–545.
7. Jo J, et al. Review article: role of cellular immunity in cow's milk allergy: pathogenesis, tolerance induction, and beyond. *Mediators Inflamm.* 2014;2014:249784.
8. Caubet JC, et al. Humoral and cellular responses to casein in patients with food protein-induced enterocolitis to cow's milk. *J Allergy Clin Immunol.* 2017;139:572–583.
9. Cerami C. Iron nutriture of the fetus, neonate, infant, and child. *Ann Nutr Metab.* 2017;71(Suppl 3):8–14.
10. Gupta PM, et al. Iron, anemia, and iron deficiency among young children in the United States. *Nutrients.* 2016;8:330.
11. Parkin PC, et al. Severe iron-deficiency anaemia and feeding practices in young children. *Public Health Nutr.* 2016;19: 716–722.
12. Suchdev PS, Pena-Rosas JP, De-Regil LM. Multiple micronutrient powders for home (point-of-use) fortification in pregnant women. *Cochrane Database Syst Rev.* 2015(6):CD011158.
13. Das JK, et al. Food fortification with multiple micronutrients: Impact on health outcomes in general population. *Cochrane Database Syst Rev.* 2019;12(12):CD011400.
14. Al-Jamea LH, et al. Genetic analysis of TMPRSS6 gene in Saudi female patients with iron deficiency anemia. *Hematol Oncol Stem Cell Ther.* 2021;14(1):41–50.

15. Shinta D, et al. The association of *TMPRSS6* gene polymorphism and iron intake with iron status among under-two-year-old children in Lombok, Indonesia. *Nutrients*. 2019;11:878.
16. Ghogomu ET, et al. Deworming in non-pregnant adolescent girls and adult women: A systematic review and meta-analysis. *BMC Syst Rev*. 2018;7:239.
17. Muriuki JM, et al. Iron status and associated malaria risk among African children. *Clin Infect Dis*. 2019;68:180701814.
18. Kato S, et al. *Helicobacter pylori sabA* gene is associated with iron deficiency anemia in childhood and adolescence. *PLoS One*. 2017;12:e0184046.
19. Sourabh S, et al. Favourable improvement in haematological parameters in response to oral iron and vitamin C combination in children with Iron Refractory Iron Deficiency Anemia (IRIDA) phenotype. *Blood Cells Mol Dis*. 2019;75:26–29.
20. Lopez A, et al. Iron deficiency anaemia. *Lancet*. 2016;387(10021):907–916.
21. Rennie JM, et al. Learning from claims: hyperbilirubinaemia and kernicterus. *Arch Dis Child Fetal Neonatal Ed*. 2019;104:F202–F204.
22. Zwiers C, et al. The near disappearance of fetal hydrops in relation to current state-of-the-art management of red cell alloimmunization. *Prenat Diagn*. 2018;38:943–950.
23. American College of Obstetricians and Gynecologists (ACOG) Committee on Practice Bulletins Obstetrics, practice bulletin no 181: prevention of RhD alloimmunization *Obstet Gynecol*. 1302017e57–e70.
24. McBain RD, et al. Anti-D administration in pregnancy for preventing Rhesus alloimmunization. *Cochrane Database Syst Rev*. 2015(9):CD000020.
25. Hansen TWR, et al. Sixty years of phototherapy for neonatal jaundice - from serendipitous observation to standardized treatment and rescue for millions. *J Perinatol*. 2020;40:180–193.
26. Doctor A, et al. Recommendations on RBC transfusion in general critically ill children based on hemoglobin and/ or physiologic thresholds from the Pediatric Critical Care Transfusion and Anemia Expertise Initiative. *Pediatr Crit Care Med*. 2018;19(9S Suppl 1):S98–S113.
27. Gomez-Manzo S, et al. Glucose-6-phosphate dehydrogenase: update and analysis of new mutations around the world. *Int J Mol Sci*. 2016;17:2069.
28. World Health Organization: Testing for G6PD deficiency for safe use of primaquine in radical cure of *P. vivax* and *P. ovale* malaria. Policy brief. 2016. Available at https://apps.who.int/iris/bitstream/handle/10665/250297/WHO-HTM-GMP-2016.9-eng.pdf;jsessionid=B98209FFADE7540C209F2F76FCAB90B2?sequence=1. (Accessed November 8, 2021).
29. Christensen RD, Yaish HM, Gallagher PG. A pediatrician's practical guide to diagnosing and treating hereditary spherocytosis in neonates. *Pediatrics*. 2015;135(6):1107–1114.
30. Cilla N, et al. Transient aplastic crisis triggered by parvovirus B19 in a family with hereditary spherocytosis. *IDCases*. 2020;21:e00802.
31. Manciu S, et al. Long-term evaluation of the outcomes of subtotal laparoscopic and robotic splenectomy in hereditary spherocytosis. *World J Surg*. 2020;44:2220–2228.
32. National Institutes of Health (NIH) *Evidence report evidence-based management of sickle cell disease: expert panel report, 2014*. Bethesda, MD: U.S. Department of Health and Human Services, National Institutes of Health, National Heart, Lung and Blood Institute; 2014. Available at https://www.nhlbi.nih.gov/sites/default/files/media/docs/sickle-cell-disease-report%20020816_0.pdf. (Accessed November 8, 2021).
33. National Heart, Lung, & Blood Institute (NHLBI) *Sickle cell disease*. Bethesda, MD: NHLBI; 2020. Last updated September 1, 2020. Available at https://www.nhlbi.nih.gov/health-topics/sickle-cell-disease. (Accessed November 8, 2021).
34. American Society of Hematology (ASH) *Sickle cell trait*. Washington, DC: ASH; 2021. Available at https://www.hematology.org/education/patients/anemia/sickle-cell-trait. (Accessed November 8, 2021).
35. DeBaun MR, Galadanci NA: Sickle cell disease in sub-Saharan Africa. *UpToDate*; 2020. Literature review current through October, 2021. Topic last updated September 3, 2021. Available at https://www.uptodate.com/contents/sickle-cell-disease-in-sub-saharan-africa. (Accessed November 8, 2021).
36. Rotin LE, et al. Allogeneic hematopoietic stem cell transplant versus gene therapy in sickle cell disease: a systematic review. *Blood*. 2019;134(Suppl 1):4714.
37. Piel FB, et al. Associations between environmental factors and hospital admissions for sickle cell disease. *Haematologica*. 2017;104:666–675.
38. Carden MA, et al. Normal saline is associated with increased sickle red cell stiffness and prolonged transit times in a microfluidic model of the capillary system. *Microcirculation*. 2017;24:e12353.
39. Sun K, et al. Structural and functional insight of sphingosine 1-phosphate-mediated pathogenic metabolic reprogramming in sickle cell disease. *Sci Rep*. 2017;7:15281.
40. Weigert A, et al. Sphignosine-1-phosphate and macrophage biology—how the sphinx tames the big eater. *Front Immunol*. 2019;10:1706.
41. Darrow MC, et al. Visualizing red blood cell sickling and the effects of inhibition of sphingosine kinase 1 using soft X-ray tomography. *J Cell Sci*. 2016;129(18):3511–3517.
42. Voskou S, et al. Oxidative stress in β-thalassemia and sickle cell disease. *Redox Biol*. 2015;6:226–239.
43. Zhang D, et al. Neutrophils, platelets, and inflammatory pathways at the nexus of sickle cell disease. *Blood*. 2016;127(7):801–809.
44. Nader E, et al. The red blood cell-inflammation vicious circle in sickle cell disease. *Front Immunol*. 2020;11:454.
45. Lu X, et al. A microfluidic platform to study the effects of vascular architecture and oxygen gradients on sickle blood flow. *Microcirculation*. 2017;24(5):e12357.
46. Brandow AW, et al. Children and adolescents with sickle cell disease have worse cold and mechanical hypersensitivity during acute painful events. *Pain*. 2019;160:407–416.
47. Field JJ, DeBaun MR: Acute chest syndrome in adults with sickle cell disease, *UpToDate*. Literature review current through October, 2021. This topic last updated June 8, 2020. Available at https://www.uptodate.com/contents/acute-chest-syndrome-in-adults-with-sickle-cell-disease. (Accessed November 8, 2021).
48. Jain S, Bakshi N, Krishnamurti L. Acute chest syndrome in children with sickle cell disease. *Pediatr Allergy Immunol Pulmonol*. 2017;30:191–201.
49. Farooq S, Abu Omar M, Salzman GA. Acute chest syndrome in sickle cell disease. *Hosp Pract*. 2018;46(3):144–151.
50. National Collegiate Athletics Association (NCAA) *Sickle cell trait*. Indianapolis, IN: NCAA; 2021. Available at http://www.ncaa.org/sport-science-institute/sickle-cell-trait. (Accessed November 8, 2021).
51. Balsamo L, et al. Improving care for sickle cell pain crisis using a multidisciplinary approach. *Pediatrics*. 2019;143:e20182218.

52. Shah N, et al. Evaluation of vaso-occlusive crises in United States sickle cell patients: a retrospective claims-based study. *J Health Econ Outcomes Res*. 2019;6:106–117.
53. AlDallal SM. Voxelotor: a ray of hope for sickle cell disease. *Cureus*. 2020;12(2):e7105.
54. Ataga KI, et al. Crizanlizumab for the prevention of pain crises in sickle cell disease. *N Engl J Med*. 2017;376:429–439.
55. Oringanje C, Nemecek E, Oniyangi O. Hematopoietic stem cell transplant for people with sickle cell disease. *Cochrane Database Syst Rev*. 2020;7:CD007001.
56. National Library of Medicine (NLM) *Gene transfer for sickle cell disease*. Bethesda, MD: NLM; 2021. Available at https://clinicaltrials.gov/ct2/show/NCT03282656. (Accessed November 8, 2021).
57. National Library of Medicine (NLM) *Medline Plus: Beta thalassemia, from Genetics Home Reference*. Bethesda, MD: NLM; 2020. Page last updated August 18, 2020. Page last reviewed September 1, 2015. Available at https://medlineplus.gov/genetics/condition/beta-thalassemia/. (Accessed November 8, 2021).
58. Thein SL. The molecular basis of β-thalassemia. *Cold Spring Harb Perspect Med*. 2013;3:a011700.
59. National Library of Medicine (NLM) *Medline Plus: Alpha thalassemia, from Genetics Home Reference*. Bethesda, MD: NLM; 2020. Page last updated August 18, 2020. Page last reviewed June 1, 2017. Available at https://medlineplus.gov/genetics/condition/alpha-thalassemia/. (Accessed November 8, 2021).
60. Genetic Testing Registry (GTR) *Hemoglobin H disease*. Bethesda, MD: GTR; 2020. Available at https://www.ncbi.nlm.nih.gov/gtr/conditions/C3161174/. (Accessed November 8, 2021).
61. Origa R. β-thalassemia. *Genet Med*. 2017;19:609–619.
62. Origa R: Beta-thalassemia. In Adam MP, et al, editors. *GeneReviews®* [Internet]. Seattle, WA, 2021, University of Washington, Seattle. Initial posting September 28, 2020. Updated February 4, 2021. Available at https://www.ncbi.nlm.nih.gov/books/NBK1426/. (Accessed November 8, 2021).
63. Karponi G, Zogas N. Gene therapy for beta-thalassemia: updated perspectives. *Appl Clin Genet*. 2019;12:167–180. Available at https://doi.org/10.2147/TACG.S178546. (Accessed November 8, 2021).
64. National Library of Medicine (NLM) *Medline Plus: hemophilia*. Bethesda, MD: NLM; 2021. Page last updated on September 20, 2021. Topic last reviewed April 18, 2016. Available at https://medlineplus.gov/hemophilia.html. (Accessed November 8, 2021).
65. Jayakrishnan T. Hemophilia C: a case report with updates on diagnosis and management of a rare bleeding disorder. *J Hematol*. 2019;8:144–147.
66. Iorio A, et al. Establishing the prevalence and prevalence at birth of hemophilia in males: a meta-analytic approach using national registries. *Ann Intern Med*. 2019;171:540–546.
67. McVey JH, et al. The European Association for Haemophilia and Allied Disorders (EHAD) coagulation factor variant databases: important resources for haemostasis clinicians and researchers. *Haemophilia*. 2020;26:306–313.
68. Rallapalli PM, et al. An interactive mutation database for human coagulation factor IX provides novel insights into the phenotypes and genetics of haemophilia B. *J Thromb Haemost*. 2013;11:1329–1340.
69. Konkle BA, Huston H, Nakaya Fletcher S: Hemophilia A. In: Adam MP, et al, editors. *GeneReviews®* [Internet]. Seattle, WA, 2021, University of Washington, Seattle. Initial posting September 21, 2000. Updated June 22, 2017. Available at https://www.ncbi.nlm.nih.gov/books/NBK1404/. (Accessed November 8, 2021).
70. van Vulpen LFD, et al. Synovitis and synovectomy in haemophilia. *Haemophilia*. 2021;27(suppl 3):96–102.
71. Manco-Johnson MJ, et al. Prophylaxis versus episodic treatment to prevent joint disease in boys with severe hemophilia. *N Engl J Med*. 2007;357:535–544.
72. Ljung R. Aspects of prophylactic treatment of hemophilia. *Thromb J*. 2016;14(Suppl 1):30.
73. Konkle BA, et al. Pegylated, full-length, recombinant factor VIII for prophylactic and on-demand treatment of severe hemophilia A. *Blood*. 2015;126(9):1078–1085.
74. Santagostino E, et al. Long-acting recombinant coagulation factor IX albumin fusion protein (rIX-FP) in hemophilia B: results of a phase 3 trial. *Blood*. 2016;127(14):1761–1769.
75. Lissitchkov T, et al. Efficacy and safety of simoctocog alfa (Nuwiq®) in patients with severe hemophilia A: a review of clinical trial data from the GENA program. *Ther Adv Hematol*. 2019;10 2040620719858471.
76. Revel-Vilk CA, et al. Prothrombotic conditions in an unselected cohort of children with venous thromboembolic disease. *J Thromb Haemost*. 2003;1:915–921.
77. Yokus O, et al. Risk factors for thrombophilia in young adults presenting with thrombosis. *Int J Hematol*. 2009;90(5):583–590.
78. van Ommen CH, Nowak-Göttl U. Inherited thrombophilia in pediatric venous thromboembolic disease: why and who to test. *Front Pediatr*. 2017;5:50.
79. National Library of Medicine (NLM) *Genetics home reference: protein C deficiency*. Bethesda, MD: NLM; 2020. Page last updated August 18, 2020. Page last reviewed May 1, 2013. Available at https://medlineplus.gov/genetics/condition/protein-c-deficiency/. (Accessed November 8, 2021).
80. National Library of Medicine (NLM) *Drug Information Portal: Ceprotin*. Bethesda, MD: NLM; 2021. Last updated: November 2021. Available at https://druginfo.nlm.nih.gov/drugportal/name/ceprotin. (Accessed November 8, 2021).
81. National Library of Medicine (NLM) *Genetics home reference: protein S deficiency*. Bethesda, MD: NLM; 2020. Page last updated August 18, 2020. Page last reviewed October 1, 2009. Available at: https://medlineplus.gov/genetics/condition/protein-s-deficiency/. (Accessed November 8, 2021).
82. Genetics and Rare Diseases Information Center (GARD). *Protein S deficiency*, Gaithersburg, MD, no date, GARD. Available at https://rarediseases.info.nih.gov/diseases/4524/protein-s-deficiency. (Accessed November 8, 2021).
83. National Library of Medicine (NLM) *Genetics home reference: SERPINC1 gene*. Bethesda, MD: NLM; 2020. Page last updated August 18, 2020. Page last reviewed: August 1, 2009. Available at https://medlineplus.gov/genetics/gene/serpinc1/#conditions. (Accessed November 8, 2021).
84. Neunert CE, et al. American Society of Hematology 2019 guidelines for immune thrombocytopenia. *Blood Adv*. 2019;3(23):3829–3866.
85. Peterson JA, et al. Neonatal alloimmune thrombocytopenia: pathogenesis, diagnosis and management. *Br J Haematol*. 2013;161:3–14.
86. Arber DA, et al. The 2016 revision to the World Health Organization Classification of Myeloid Neoplasms and Acute Leukemia. *Blood*. 2016;127(20):2391–2405.
87. Howlader N, ed. *SEER Cancer Statistics Review, 1975-2018*. Bethesda, MD: National Cancer Institute; 2021. Based on November 2020 SEER data submission. Posted to the SEER web site April 2021. Available at https://seer.cancer.gov/csr/1975_2018/. (Accessed November 8, 2021).

88. Bonaventure A, et al. Worldwide comparison of survival from childhood leukaemia for 1995-2009 by subtype, age, and sex (CONCORD-2): a population-based study of individual data for 89,828 children from 198 registries in 53 countries. *Lancet Haematol.* 2017;4:e202–e217.
89. Giddings BM, et al. Childhood leukemia incidence in California: high and rising in the Hispanic population. *CA J Clin.* 2016;122:2867–2875.
90. Oksuzyan S, et al. Race/ethnicity and the risk childhood leukemia: a case-control study in California. *J Epidemiol Community Health.* 2015;69:795–802.
91. Guest EM, Stam RW. Updates in the biology and therapy for infant acute lymphoblastic leukemia. *Curr Opin Pediatr.* 2016;29(1):20–26.
92. Coccaro N, et al. Next-generation sequencing in acute lymphoblastic leukemia. *Int J Mol Sci.* 2019;20:2929.
93. PDQ® Pediatric Treatment Editorial Board: PDQ Childhood Acute Lymphoblastic Leukemia Treatment, Bethesda, MD: National Cancer Institute. Updated October 7, 2021. Available at https://www.cancer.gov/types/leukemia/hp/child-all-treatment-pdq. (Accessed November 8, 2021).
94. Cao L-L, et al. The clinical values of dysregulated DNA methylation and demethylation intermediates in acute lymphoblastic leukemia. *Hematology.* 2019;24:567–576.
95. Langie SA, et al. DNA methylation and the hygiene hypothesis: connecting respiratory allergy and childhood acute lymphoblastic leukemia. *Epigenomics.* 2019;11:1519–1537.
96. Berrington de Gonzalez A, et al. Relationship between paediatric CT scans and subsequent risk of leukaemia and brain tumours: assessment of the impact of underlying conditions. *Br J Cancer.* 2016;114:388–394.
97. Baysson H, et al. Exposure to CT scans in childhood and long-term cancer risk: a review of epidemiological studies. *Bull Cancer.* 2016;103:190–198.
98. Kenney LB, et al. Improving male reproductive health after childhood, adolescent, and young adult cancer: progress and future directions for survivorship research. *J Clin Oncol.* 2018;36:2160–2168.
99. van Dorp W, et al. Reproductive function and outcomes in female survivors of childhood, adolescent, and young adult cancer: a review. *J Clin Oncol.* 2018;36:2169–2180.
100. Cao Y, et al. Paternal smoking before conception and during pregnancy is associated with an increased risk of childhood acute lymphoblastic leukemia: a systematic review and meta-analysis of 17 case-control studies. *J Pediatr Heamtol Oncol.* 2020;42:32–40.
101. Chunxia D, et al. Tobacco smoke exposure and the risk of childhood acute lymphoblastic leukemia and acute myeloid leukemia: a meta-analysis. *Medicine (Baltimore).* 2019;98:e16454.
102. Van Maele-Fabry G, et al. Household exposure to pesticides and risk of leukemia in children and adolescents: updated systematic review and meta-analysis. *Int J Hyg Environ Health.* 2019;222: 49–67.
103. Chen M, et al. Residential exposures to pesticide during childhood and childhood cancers: a meta-analysis. *Pediatrics.* 2015;136:719–729.
104. Gong Z-H, et al. A meta-analysis of traffic-related air pollution and risk of childhood leukemia. *J Pediatr Hematol Oncol.* 2019;41:267–274.
105. Fillipini T, et al. Association between outdoor air pollution and childhood leukemia: a systematic review and dose-response meta-analysis. *Environ Health Perspect.* 2019;127:46002.
106. Chen J, et al. An ecological study of cancer incidence in Port Hope, Ontario from 1992 to 2007. *J Radiol Prot.* 2013;33:227–242.
107. Laurier D, et al. Epidemiological studies of leukaemia in children and young adults around nuclear facilities: a critical review. *Radiat Prot Dosimetry.* 2008;132:182–190.
108. Weimels JL, et al. GWAS in childhood acute lymphoblastic leukemia reveals novel genetic associations at chromosomes 17q12 and 8q24.21. *Nat Commun.* 2018;9(1):286.
109. Pi W-C, et al. E2A-PBX1 functions as a coactivator for RUNX1 in acute lymphoblastic leukemia. *Blood.* 2020;136:11–23.
110. Russell TB, Kram DE. Tumor lysis syndrome. *Pediatr Rev.* 2020;41(1):20–26.
111. National Library of Medicine (NLM) *Phase 3 trial of blinatumomab vs standard chemotherapy in pediatric subjects with high-risk (HR) first relapse B-precursor acute lymphoblastic leukemia (ALL).* Bethesda, MD: NLM; 2020. Available at https://clinicaltrials.gov/ct2/show/NCT02393859. (Accessed November 8, 2021).
112. PDQ® Pediatric Treatment Editorial Board: *PDQ childhood acute myeloid leukemia/other myeloid malignancies treatment.* Bethesda, MD: National Cancer Institute; 2021. Updated September 21, 2021. Available at https://www.cancer.gov/types/leukemia/hp/child-aml-treatment-pdq. (Accessed November 8, 2021).
113. Swerdlow SH, et al. The 2016 revision of the World Health Organization Classification of Lymphoid Neoplasms. *Blood.* 2016;127:2375–2390.
114. American Cancer Society (ACS) *Cancer Facts & Figures 2020.* Atlanta, GA: ACS; 2020. Available at https://www.cancer.org/content/dam/cancer-org/research/cancer-facts-and-statistics/annual-cancer-facts-and-figures/2020/cancer-facts-and-figures-2020.pdf. (Accessed November 8, 2021).
115. PDQ® Pediatric Treatment Editorial Board *PDQ childhood non-Hodgkin lymphoma treatment.* Bethesda, MD: National Cancer Institute; 2021. Updated October 8, 2021. Available at https://www.cancer.gov/types/lymphoma/hp/child-nhl-treatment-pdq. (Accessed November 8, 2021).
116. Khan G, et al. Global and regional incidence, mortality and disability-adjusted life-years for Epstein-Barr virus-attributable malignancies, 1990-2017. *BMJ Open.* 2020;10:e037505.
117. Navan M, et al. The presence of Epstein Barr virus significantly impacts the transcriptional profile in immunodeficiency-associated Burkitt lymphoma. *Front Microbiol.* 2015;6:556.
118. PDQ® Pediatric Treatment Editorial Board *PDQ childhood Hodgkin lymphoma treatment.* Bethesda, MD: National Cancer Institute; 2021. Updated September 30, 2021. Available at https://www.cancer.gov/types/lymphoma/hp/child-hodgkin-treatment-pdq. (Accessed November 8, 2021).
119. Mata E, et al. Analysis of the mutational landscape of classic Hodgkin lymphoma identifies disease heterogeneity and potential therapeutic targets. *Oncotarget.* 2017;8:111386–111395.
120. Carbone A, et al. The impact of EBV and HIV infection on the microenvironmental niche underlying Hodgkin lymphoma pathogenesis. *Int J Cancer.* 2017;140:1233–1245.
121. Reichel J, et al. Flow sorting and exome sequencing reveal the oncogenome of primary Hodgkin and Reed-Sternberg cells. *Blood.* 2015;125:1061–1072.

31

Structure and Function of the Cardiovascular and Lymphatic Systems

Karen C. Turner and Valentina L. Brashers

http://evolve.elsevier.com/Rogers/pathophysiology/

CHAPTER OUTLINE

The functions of the circulatory system include delivery of oxygen, nutrients, hormones, immune system components, and other substances to body tissues and removal of the waste products of metabolism. Delivery and removal are achieved by an extensive array of tubes—the blood and lymphatic vessels—connected to a pump—the heart. The heart continuously pumps blood through the blood vessels in collaboration with other systems, particularly the nervous and endocrine systems, which are intrinsic regulators of the heart and blood vessels. Immune system components, nutrients, and oxygen are supplied by the immune, digestive, and respiratory systems; gaseous wastes of metabolism are expired through the lungs; and other wastes are removed by the kidneys and digestive tract.

The vascular endothelium also is a key component of the circulatory system and is sometimes considered a separate endocrine organ. This endothelium is a multifunctional tissue whose health is essential to normal vascular, immune, and hemostatic system function. Endothelial dysfunction is a critical factor in the development of vascular and other diseases (see Chapter 32).

CIRCULATORY SYSTEM

The heart is composed of two conjoined pumps moving blood through two separate circulatory systems in sequence: one pump supplies blood to the lungs, whereas the second pump delivers blood to the rest of the body. Structures on the right side, or right heart, pump blood through the lungs. This system is termed the pulmonary circulation and is described in Chapter 34. The left side, or left heart, sends blood throughout the systemic circulation, which supplies all of the body except the lungs (Fig. 31.1). These two systems are serially connected; thus the output of one becomes the input of the other.

Arteries carry blood from the heart to all parts of the body, where they branch into arterioles and even smaller vessels, ultimately becoming a fine meshwork of capillaries. Capillaries allow the closest contact and exchange between the blood and the interstitial space, or interstitium—the environment in which cells live. Venules and then veins next carry blood from the capillaries back to the heart. Some of the plasma or liquid part of the blood passes through the walls of the capillaries into the interstitial space. This fluid, called ***lymph***, is returned to the cardiovascular system by vessels of the lymphatic system. The lymphatic system is a critical component of the immune system as described in Chapters 7 and 8.

HEART

The adult heart is about the size of a fist and weighs between 250 and 350 g. The heart lies obliquely (diagonally) in the

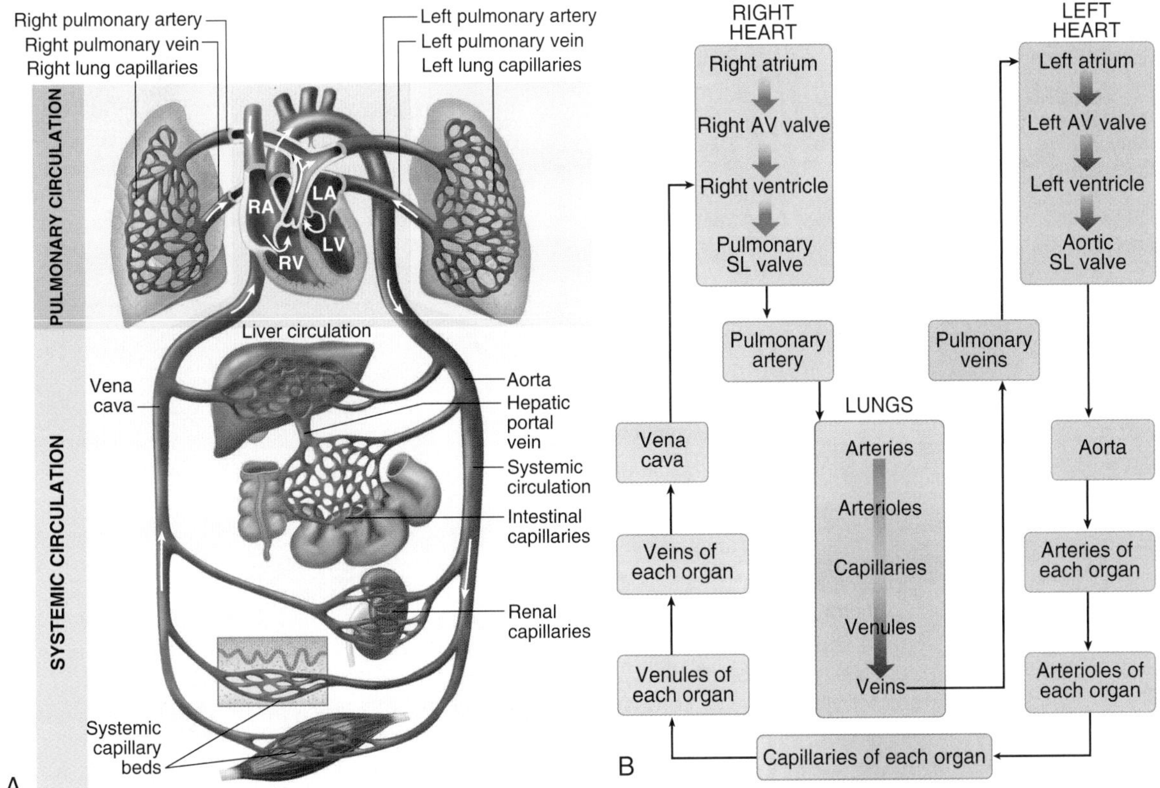

Fig. 31.1 Diagram of the Pulmonary and Systemic Circulatory Systems and Flow Chart of the Direction of Blood Flow. **(A)** The right heart pumps unoxygenated blood *(blue)* through the pulmonary circulation, where oxygen enters the blood and carbon dioxide is exhaled, and the left heart pumps oxygenated *(red)* blood to and from all the other organ systems in the body. **(B)** Blood flow begins at the left ventricle of the heart; the blood flows to the arteries, arterioles, capillaries of each body organ, venules, veins, right atrium, right ventricle, pulmonary artery, lung capillaries, pulmonary veins, and left atrium and then returns to the left ventricle. (B, Adapted from Patton KT, Thibodeau GA. *The human body in health & disease*, 7th edition. St. Louis: Mosby; 2018.)

mediastinum, the area above the diaphragm and between the lungs. Heart structures can be categorized by function:

1. *Structural support of heart tissues and circulation of pulmonary and systemic blood through the heart.* This category includes the heart wall and fibrous skeleton enclosing and supporting the heart and dividing it into four chambers; the valves directing flow through the chambers; and the great vessels conducting blood to and from the heart.
2. *Maintenance of cardiac metabolism.* This category includes all the vessels of the coronary circulation—the arteries and veins that serve the metabolic needs of all the heart cells—and the heart's lymphatic vessels.
3. *Stimulation and control of heart action.* Among these structures are the nerves and specialized muscle cells that direct the rhythmic contraction and relaxation of the heart muscles, propelling blood throughout the pulmonary and systemic circulatory systems.

Structures that Direct Circulation Through the Heart

The complex anatomy and physiology of the heart serve to accept blood from the venous system and propel it unidirectionally through the right heart into the lungs, then through the left heart and out into the systemic arterial circulation (Fig. 31.2A). This process ensures the delivery of oxygenated blood into the systemic circulation and maintains tissue perfusion.

Heart Wall

The three layers of the heart wall—the epicardium, myocardium, and endocardium—are enclosed in a double-walled membranous sac, the pericardium (see Fig. 31.2B). The pericardial sac has several functions: provides stability of the heart within the thorax, reduces friction between the heart and the mediastinal structures, limits the size of the heart chambers, provides a barrier to the spread of infection, and it contains pain receptors and mechanoreceptors that can cause reflex changes in blood pressure and heart rate.[1] The fibrous pericardium is composed of tough connective tissue that surrounds but does not attach to the heart. Within this outer layer are the parietal pericardium which adheres to the internal surface of the fibrous pericardium, and the visceral pericardium which adheres to the heart (see Fig. 31.2B). These two layers are separated by a fluid-containing space called the pericardial cavity. The pericardial fluid (about 20 mL) is secreted by cells of the mesothelial layer

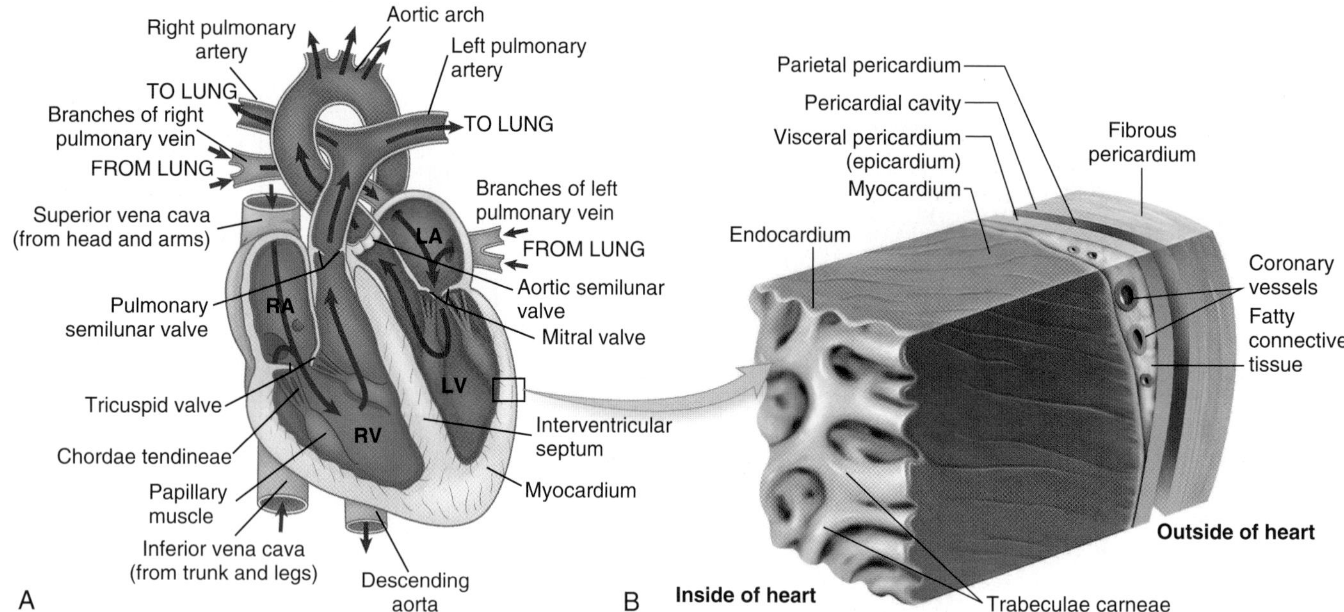

Fig. 31.2 Structures that Direct Blood Flow Through the Heart and Wall of the Heart. (A) The *arrows* indicate the path of blood through the chambers, valves, and major vessels. **(B)** This section of the heart wall shows the fibrous pericardium, the parietal and visceral layers of the serous pericardium (with the pericardial space between them), the myocardium, and the endocardium. Note the fatty connective tissue between the visceral layer of the serous pericardium (epicardium) and the myocardium. Note also that the endocardium covers tubular projections of myocardial muscle tissue called trabeculae. (Revised from Applegate E. *The anatomy and physiology learning system*, 4th edition. St. Louis: Saunders; 2011.)

of the pericardium and lubricates the membranes that line the pericardial cavity, enabling them to slide smoothly over one another with minimal friction as the heart beats. The amount and character of the pericardial fluid are altered if the pericardium is inflamed (see Chapter 32).

The smoothness of the outer layer of the heart, the epicardium, also minimizes the friction between the heart wall and the pericardial sac. The thickest layer of the heart wall, the myocardium, is composed of cardiac muscle and is anchored to the heart's fibrous skeleton. The thickness of the myocardium varies tremendously from one heart chamber to another. Thickness is related to the amount of resistance the muscle must overcome to pump blood from the different chambers. The heart muscle cells, cardiomyocytes, provide the contractile force needed for blood to flow through the heart and into the pulmonary and systemic circulations. About 0.5% to 1% of the cardiomyocytes are replaced annually; thus over a lifetime only about half of these muscle cells are replaced.[2] There is great interest in finding therapies that will increase the rate of cardiomyocyte replacement for persons who have suffered a myocardial infarction or have heart failure from another cause because the limited myocyte turnover is insufficient to restore contractile function (see Emerging Science Box: Myocardial Regeneration).[3]

The internal lining of the myocardium, the endocardium, is composed of connective tissue and squamous cells (see Fig. 31.2B). This lining is continuous with the endothelium that lines all the arteries, veins, and capillaries of the body, creating a continuous, closed circulatory system.

Great Vessels

Blood moves into and out of the heart through several large veins and arteries (see Fig. 31.2A). The right heart receives venous deoxygenated blood from the systemic circulation through the superior and inferior venae cavae, which join and then enter the right atrium. Blood leaving the right ventricle enters the pulmonary circulation through the pulmonary artery, which divides into right and left branches to transport deoxygenated blood from the right heart to the lungs. The pulmonary arteries branch further into the pulmonary capillary beds, where oxygen and carbon dioxide exchange occurs (see Fig. 31.1B).

Four pulmonary veins, two from the right lung and two from the left lung, carry oxygenated blood from the lungs to the left side of the heart. The oxygenated blood moves through the left atrium and ventricle, out into the aorta that subsequently branches into the systemic arteries that supply the body.

Chambers of the Heart

The heart has four chambers: the left atrium, the right atrium, the right ventricle, and the left ventricle. These chambers form two pumps in series: the right heart is a low-pressure system pumping blood through the lungs, and the left heart is a high-pressure system pumping blood to the rest of the body (see Fig. 31.2A). The atria are smaller than the ventricles and have thinner walls. The ventricles have a thicker myocardial layer and constitute much of the bulk of the heart. The wall of the right ventricle is about 4 to 5 mm thick, and that of the more muscular left ventricle is 8 to 12 mm thick.[1] The ventricles are formed

EMERGING SCIENCE BOX

Myocardial Regeneration

Myocardial infarction causes the loss of some of the muscle cells needed to maintain cardiac output, thus increasing the risk of heart failure in survivors. Given that heart failure is a growing problem with a poor prognosis in both the United States and internationally, finding an effective therapy is a critical need.

To replace the approximately 1 billion cardiomyocytes that are estimated to be lost with a myocardial infarction, researchers have identified four possible approaches: (1) accelerating the rate of heart cell division, (2) inserting new cells into the heart, (3) stimulating the heart muscle precursor cells already in the heart, and (4) reprogramming other cells so that they will become cardiomyocyte precursor cells. To stimulate adult heart cells to enter the cell cycle and thus accelerate cell division, various signaling molecules, such as neuregulin and fibroblast growth factor 1, have been used with some success. Currently the most promising cell types that have been injected into the heart include cells from the bone marrow, cardiac-derived cells taken from myocardial biopsies, and human pluripotent stem cells. Although there are cardiac progenitor or precursor cells in the heart, their rate of division is not adequate to replace lost tissue after an infarction. Some of the methods being investigated to stimulate these cardiomyocytes or other progenitor cells in the heart include treatment with peptides that act as growth factors, and some types of modified ribonucleic acids (RNAs) that produce vascular endothelial growth factor (VEGF). Reprogramming from one cell type into a pluripotent stem cell has been attempted with fibroblasts with some success. Each of these four approaches to replacing cardiomyocytes after injury comes with its own set of risks and challenges. Associated risks include increasing the chances for tumor development, damage to other organs, and myocardial scarring.

A barrier to using embryonic cells to replace adult heart tissue is that energy metabolism of the embryonic and adult heart is quite distinct. During embryonic development the relatively hypoxic embryonic heart utilizes anaerobic glycolysis as a main source of energy, whereas adult cardiomyocytes utilize the oxygen-dependent mitochondrial oxidative phosphorylation as an energy source. Therefore, to further advance this field, it is necessary to study changes in oxygenation of cardiomyocytes.

Data from Cho HM, et al. Cardiomyocyte death and genome-edited stem cell therapy for ischemic heart disease. *Stem Cell Reviews and Reports*. 2021;17:1264–1279; Gong R, et al. Regulation of cardiomyocyte fate plasticity: a key strategy for cardiac regeneration. *Nature Signal Transduction Targeted Therapy*, 2021;6:31; He L, et al. Heart regeneration by endogenous stem cells and cardiomyocyte proliferation: Controversy, fallacy, and progress. *Circulation*, 2020;142:275–291; Braga L, et al. Non-coding RNA therapeutics for cardiac regeneration. *Cardiovascular Research*, 2021;117(3):674–6931; Mancuso A, et al. Cardiac stem cell-loaded delivery systems. A new challenge for myocardial tissue regeneration. *International Journal of Molecular Sciences*, 2020;21(2):7701; Murry CE, et al. Stem cells and the heart—The road ahead. *Science*, 2020;67:854–855; Riching AS, et al. Cardiac regeneration: new insights into the frontier of ischemic heart failure therapy. *Frontiers in Bioengineering and Biotechnology*, 2021;8:1585; Vadivel S, et al. Inflammation in myocardial injury: Stem cells as potential immunomodulators for myocardial regeneration and restoration. *Life Sciences*. 2020;250:117582.

by a continuum of muscle fibers originating from the fibrous skeleton at the base of the heart.

The wall thickness of each cardiac chamber depends on the amount of pressure or resistance it must overcome to eject blood. The two atria have the thinnest walls because they are low-pressure chambers that serve as storage units and channels for blood that is emptied into the ventricles. Normally, there is little resistance to flow from the atria to the ventricles. The ventricles, on the other hand, must propel the blood all the way through the pulmonary or systemic vessels. The ventricular myocardium must be strong enough to pump against pressures within the pulmonary or systemic vessels. The mean pulmonary artery pressure, the force the right ventricle must overcome, is only 15 mm Hg, whereas the mean arterial pressure the left ventricle must pump against is about 92 mm Hg. Because the pressure is markedly higher in the systemic circulation, the wall of the left ventricle is about three times thicker than that of the right ventricle.

The right ventricle is shaped like a crescent or triangle, enabling a bellows-like action that efficiently ejects large volumes of blood through the pulmonary semilunar valve into the low-pressure pulmonary system. The larger left ventricle is bullet shaped, which allows it to generate enough pressure to eject blood through a relatively larger aortic semilunar valve into the high-pressure systemic circulation.

The ventricles are structurally more complex than the atria. Each ventricle contains muscle fibers that divide it roughly into an inflow tract, which receives blood from the atrium, and an outflow tract, which sends blood to the circulation (see Fig. 31.2A).

Blood normally does not flow between the chambers of the right and left sides of the heart. The atria are separated by the interatrial septum, and the ventricles by the interventricular septum. However, because the fetus does not depend on the lungs for oxygenation, there is an opening before birth between the right and left atria, called the foramen ovale, that facilitates circulation. This opening closes functionally at the time of birth as the higher pressure in the left atrium pushes a flap, the septum primum, over the hole. In 75% to 80% of infants these septa are permanently fused within the first year of life (see Chapter 33).

Valves of the Heart

Four valves in the heart direct blood flow in one direction through the heart chambers (Fig. 31.3). The atrioventricular (AV) valves are termed such because they fall between the atria and ventricles. The AV valve openings are composed of tissue flaps called *leaflets* or *cusps*, which are attached at the upper margin to a ring in the heart's fibrous skeleton and by the chordae tendineae at the lower end to the papillary muscles (see Fig. 31.2A). The papillary muscles, extensions of the myocardium, help hold the cusps together and downward at the onset of ventricular contraction, thus preventing their backward expulsion or prolapse into the atria. The AV valve in the right heart is called the tricuspid valve because it has three cusps. The tricuspid opening (orifice) has the largest diameter of all the heart valves.[1] The left atrioventricular valve is a bicuspid (two-cusp) valve called the mitral valve. The tricuspid and mitral valves function as a unit because the atria, fibrous rings, valvular tissue, chordae tendineae, papillary muscles, and ventricular

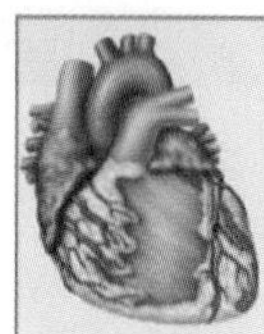

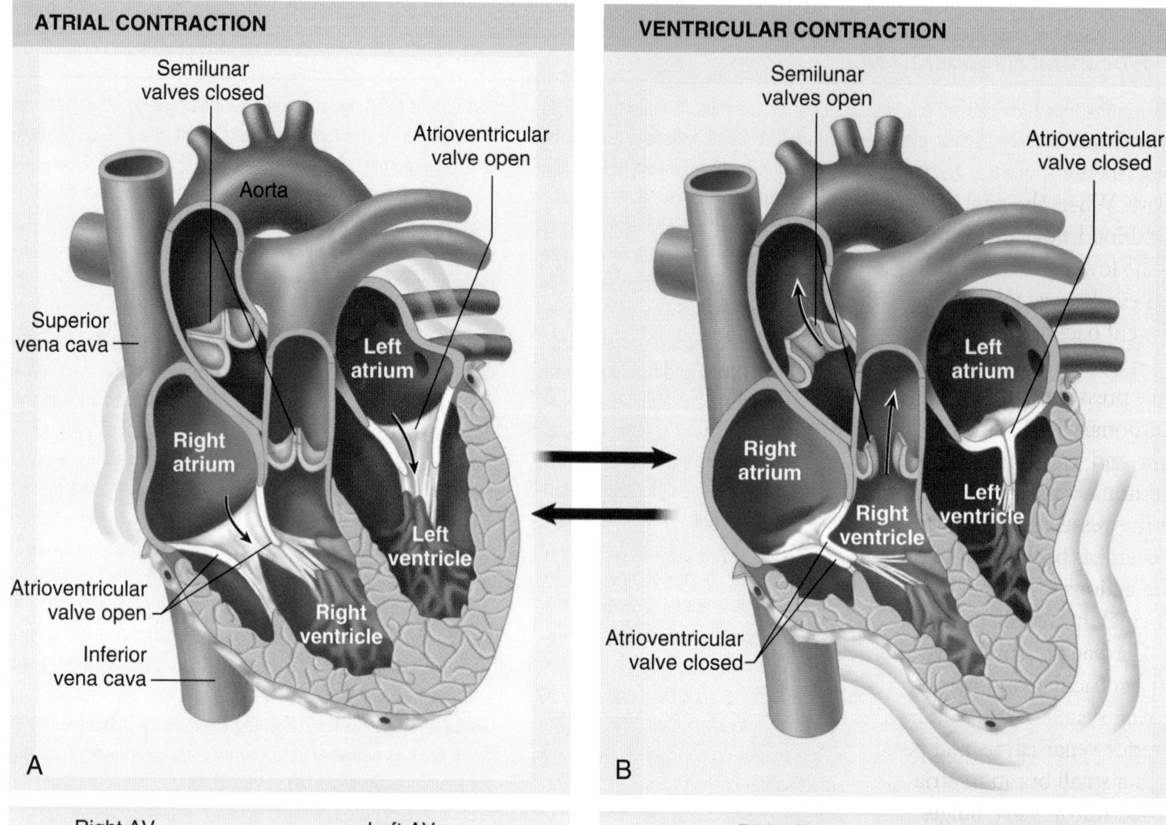

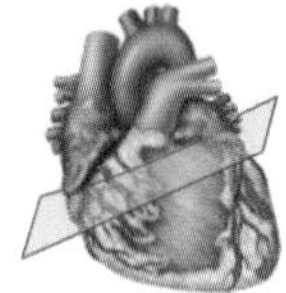

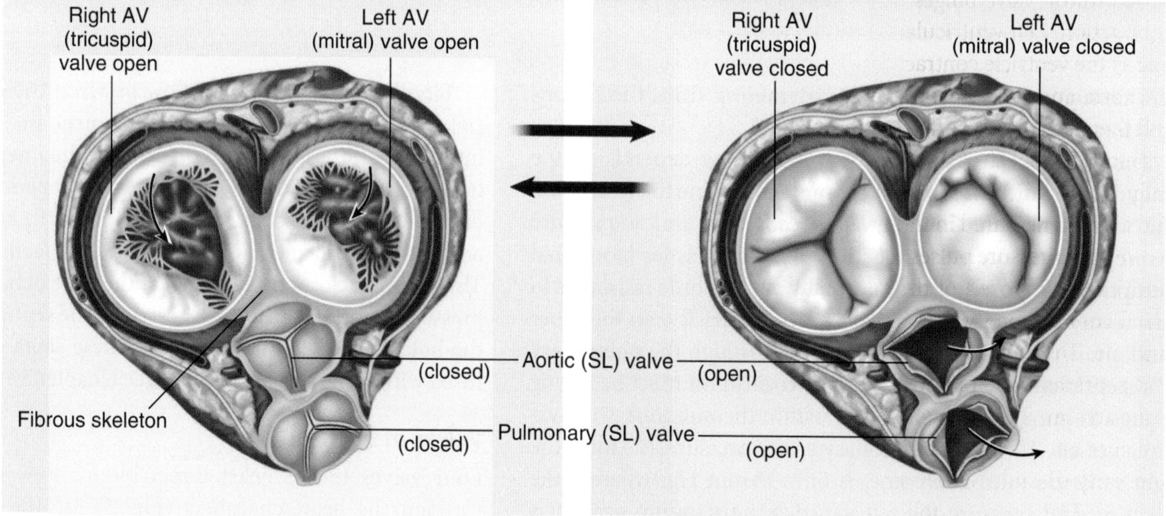

Fig. 31.3 Blood Flow Through the Heart During a Single Cardiac Cycle. **(A)** During diastole, blood flows into atria, the atrioventricular valves are pushed open, and blood begins to fill the ventricles. Atrial systole squeezes the blood remaining in the atria into the ventricles. **(B)** During ventricular systole, the ventricles contract, pushing the blood out through the semilunar valves into the pulmonary artery (right ventricle) and the aorta (left ventricle). (From Patton KT, Thibodeau GA. *Structure & function of the body*, 15th edition. St. Louis: Elsevier; 2016.)

walls are connected. Collectively, these six structures are known as the mitral and tricuspid complex. Damage to any one of the six components of this complex can alter function significantly and contribute to heart failure.

The other two valves in the heart are called the semilunar valves. These valves have three cup-shaped cusps that arise from the fibrous skeleton. Blood leaves the right ventricle through the pulmonary semilunar valve, and it leaves the left ventricle through the aortic semilunar valve (see Figs. 31.2 and 31.3).

Fibrous Skeleton of the Heart

Four rings of dense fibrous connective tissue provide a firm anchorage for the attachments of the atrial and ventricular musculature, as well as the valvular tissue (see Fig. 31.3). The fibrous rings are adjacent and form a central, fibrous supporting structure collectively termed the *annuli fibrosi cordis*.

Intracardiac Pressures

Four heart valves, four chambers, and the pressure gradients they maintain ensure that blood only flows one way through the heart. When the ventricles are relaxed, the two AV valves open and blood flows from the relatively higher pressure in the atria to the lower pressure in the ventricles. As the ventricles contract, ventricular pressure increases and causes these valves to close and prevent backflow into the atria. The semilunar valves of the heart open when intraventricular pressure exceeds aortic and pulmonary pressures, and blood flows out of the ventricles and into the pulmonary and systemic circulations. After ventricular contraction and ejection, intraventricular pressure decreases and the pulmonary and aortic semilunar valves close when the pressure in the vessels is greater than the pressure in the ventricles, thus preventing backflow into the right and left ventricles, respectively. The actions of the heart valves are shown in Figs. 31.2 and 31.3. Normal intracardiac pressures are shown in Table 31.1.

Cardiac pressure curves depicted in Fig. 31.4 include left atrial, left ventricular, and aortic pressures. Left atrial pressures increase during systole as the atrium receives blood from the superior and inferior venae cavae, and peaks during atrial contraction. In addition, a small bump in atrial pressure occurs early in systole as the closed mitral valve bulges into the left atrium during ventricular contraction. Left ventricular pressure increases rapidly during systole as the ventricle contracts, then falls rapidly as blood flows into the aorta and ventricular volume decreases. Aortic pressure rises and then falls after blood from the left ventricle is distributed to the systemic arterial circulation during diastole. This is reflected clinically in the difference between systolic and diastolic blood pressures when measured in the arm with a blood pressure cuff.

Venous pressure pulses (like that seen in the jugular vein of the neck) are composed of three waves. The a wave is generated by atrial contraction, which actively fills the right ventricle in end-diastole. The c wave occurs after the a wave during early systole and represents the bulging of the closed tricuspid valve into the right atrium. The v wave corresponds to the passive increase in pressure and volume of the right atrium as it fills in late systole and early diastole. Other aspects of falling venous pressure are defined. The x descent follows the c wave and reflects movement of the lower portion of the right atrium toward the right ventricle during the final phases of ventricular systole The y descent corresponds to the abrupt termination of the downstroke of the v wave during early diastole after the tricuspid valve opens and the right ventricle starts to fill passively.

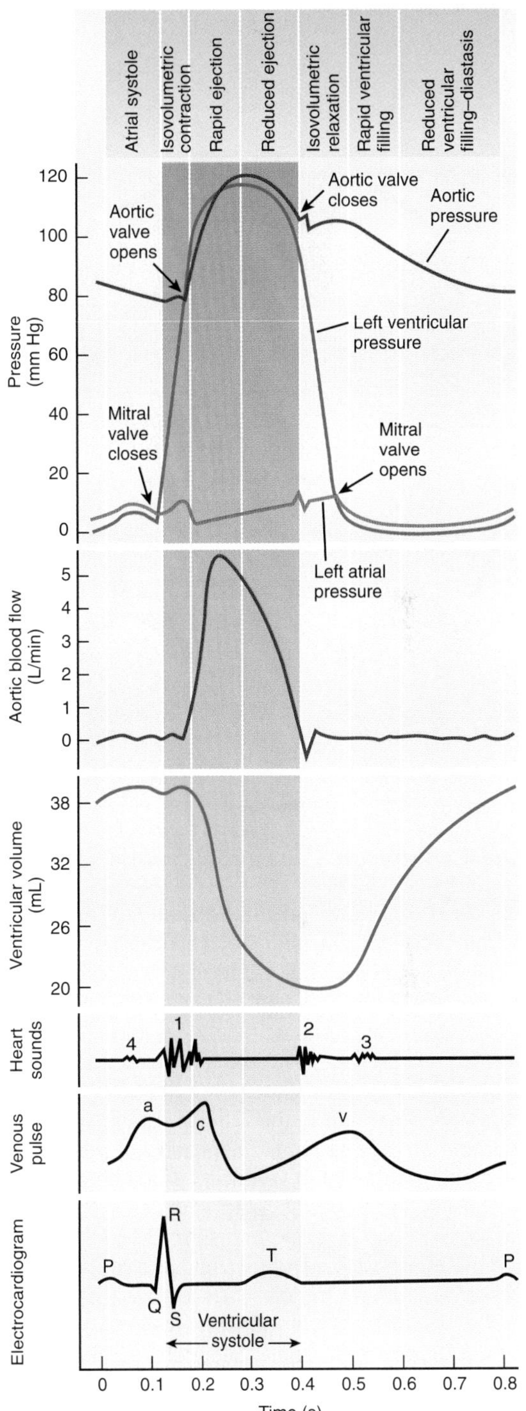

Fig. 31.4 Composite Chart of Heart Function. This chart is a composite of several diagrams of heart function (cardiac pumping cycle, blood pressure, blood flow, volume, heart sounds, venous pulse, and an electrocardiogram [ECG]), all on the same time scale.

TABLE 31.1 Normal Intracardiac Pressures

	Mean (mm Hg)	Range (mm Hg)
Right atrium	4	0–8
Right ventricle		
Systolic	24	15–28
End-diastolic	4	0–8
Left atrium	7	4–12
Left ventricle		
Systolic	130	90–140
End-diastolic	7	4–12

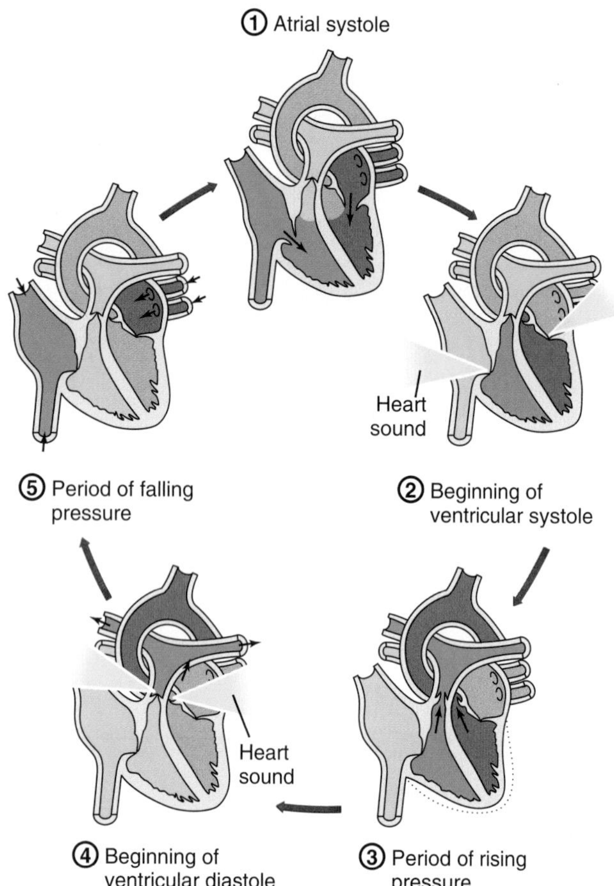

Fig. 31.5 The Five Phases of the Cardiac Cycle. *1,* Atrial systole. The atria contract, pushing blood through the open tricuspid and mitral valves into the ventricles. The semilunar valves are closed. *2,* Beginning of ventricular systole. The ventricles contract, increasing pressure within the ventricles. The tricuspid and mitral valves close, causing the first heart sound. *3,* Period of rising pressure. The semilunar valves open when pressure in the ventricle exceeds that in the arteries. Blood spurts into the aorta and pulmonary arteries. *4,* Beginning of ventricular diastole. Pressure in the relaxing ventricles drops below that in the arteries. The semilunar valves snap shut, causing the second heart sound. *5,* Period of falling pressure. Blood flows from the veins into the relaxed atria. The tricuspid and mitral valves open when pressure in the ventricles falls below that in the atria. (Adapted from Solomon E. *Introduction to human anatomy and physiology,* 4th edition. St. Louis: Saunders; 2016.)

Blood Flow during the Cardiac Cycle

The pumping action of the heart consists of contraction and relaxation of the heart muscle, or myocardium. Each ventricular contraction and the relaxation that follows it constitute one cardiac cycle (Fig. 31.5). During the period of relaxation, termed diastole, blood fills the ventricles. The ventricular contraction that follows, termed systole, propels the blood out of the ventricles and into the pulmonary and systemic circulations. Contraction of the left ventricle occurs slightly earlier than contraction of the right ventricle.

During ventricular systole, blood from the veins of the systemic circulation enters the thin-walled right atrium from the superior and inferior venae cavae (see Figs. 31.2 and 31.3). Venous blood from the coronary circulation enters the right atrium through the coronary sinus. The right atrium fills, which, along with the falling right ventricular pressures, allows the right AV (tricuspid) valve to open and fill the right ventricle during ventricular diastole (occasionally called *atrial systole*). The same sequence of events occurs a split second earlier in the left heart. The four pulmonary veins, two from the right lung and two from the left lung, carry blood from the pulmonary circulation to the left atrium. As the left atrium fills and left ventricular pressure falls, the mitral valve opens and blood flows into the left ventricle. Left atrial contraction, termed *atrial kick*, provides significant increases in the volume of blood entering the left ventricle at the end of diastole. Filling of the right and left ventricles occurs during one period of diastole. Five phases of the cardiac cycle can be identified (see Figs. 31.4 and 31.5). The cardiac cycle is said to *begin* with the opening of the mitral and tricuspid valves and atrial contraction, and to *end* with the closing of the mitral and tricuspid valves and passive ventricular filling. As blood is pushed through the inflow and outflow tracts of the ventricles, it flows around the crista supraventricularis—the muscle that separates the inflow from the outflow tracts—and is mixed by passing through the strands of the trabeculae carneae.

Structures that Support Cardiac Metabolism: Coronary Circulation

The myocardium and other heart structures are supplied with oxygen and nutrients by the coronary circulation, which is the part of the systemic circulation that occurs within the blood vessels of the heart muscles. The coronary arteries originate at the upper edge of the aortic semilunar valve cusps (Fig. 31.6A and B) and receive blood through openings in the aorta called the coronary ostia. The cardiac veins empty into the right atrium through another ostium, the opening of a large vein called the coronary sinus (see Fig. 31.6C). (The Regulation of the Coronary Circulation section describes the regulation of this mechanism, which is similar to regulation of flow through systemic and pulmonary vessels.)

Coronary Arteries

The major coronary arteries, the right coronary artery (RCA) and the left coronary artery (LCA) (see Fig. 31.6A), traverse the epicardium, myocardium, and endocardium and branch to become arterioles and then capillaries. The LCA arises from a single ostium behind the left cusp of the aortic semilunar valve. It generally divides into the left anterior descending (LAD) artery (supplies blood to portions of the left and right ventricles and much of the interventricular septum), and the circumflex artery (supplies blood to the left atrium and the lateral wall of the left ventricle). The RCA originates from an ostium behind the right aortic cusp. It branches into the conus (supplies blood to the upper right ventricle), right marginal branch (supplies the right ventricle to the apex), and posterior descending branch (supplies smaller branches to both ventricles). Because women's hearts weigh proportionally less than men's hearts, the coronary arteries are smaller in women.

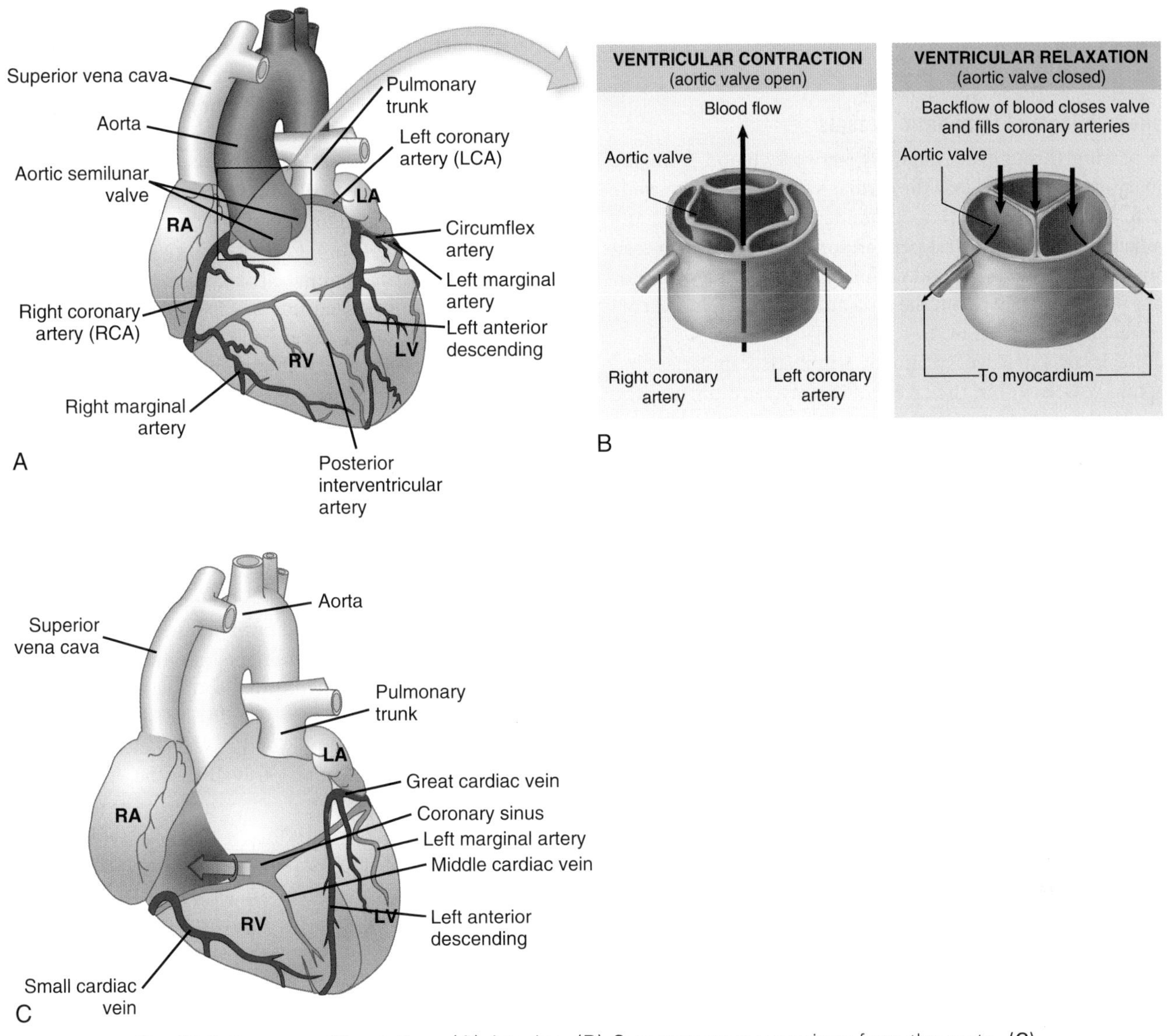

Fig. 31.6 Coronary Circulation. **(A)** Arteries. **(B)** Coronary artery openings from the aorta. **(C)** Veins. Both A and C are anterior views of the heart. Vessels near the anterior surface are more darkly colored than vessels of the posterior surface seen through the heart. (A and C, From Patton KT, Thibodeau GA. *Anatomy & physiology*, 7th edition. St. Louis: Mosby; 2010. B, Patton KT, Thibodeau GA. *The human body in health & disease,* 6th edition. St. Louis: Mosby; 2014.)

Collateral Arteries

Collateral arteries are connections, or *anastomoses*, between branches of the same coronary artery or connections of branches of the right coronary artery with branches of the left. The epicardium contains more collateral vessels than the endocardium. New collateral vessels are formed through two processes: arteriogenesis (new artery growth branching from preexisting arteries) and angiogenesis (growth of new capillaries within a tissue). This collateral growth is stimulated by shear stress, an increased blood flow speed within and just beyond areas of stenosis, or narrowing, as well as the production of growth factors and cytokines. The collateral circulation assists in supplying blood and oxygen to myocardium that has become ischemic following gradual stenosis of one or more major coronary arteries (coronary artery disease). Unfortunately, diabetes, which predisposes to coronary artery disease, also impedes collateral formation because of increased production of antiangiogenic factors, such as endostatin and angiostatin. Current research is focused on identifying whether some factors that stimulate collateral growth might be useful treatments for myocardial ischemia.[4]

Coronary Capillaries

The heart requires an extensive capillary network to function. Blood travels from the arteries to the arterioles and then into the capillaries, where oxygen and other nutrients enter the myocardium while waste products enter the blood. At rest, the heart extracts 70% to 80% of the oxygen delivered to it, and coronary blood flow is directly correlated with myocardial oxygen consumption. Any alteration of the cardiac muscles dramatically affects blood flow in the capillaries. For example, in ventricular hypertrophy (enlargement of the ventricular myocardium), the capillary network does not expand along with muscle fiber size. Therefore, the same number of capillaries must now perfuse a larger area. This results in decreased exchange of oxygen and nutrients.

Coronary Veins and Lymphatic Vessels

After passing through the capillary network, blood from the coronary arteries drains into the cardiac veins located alongside the arteries. Most of the venous drainage of the heart occurs through veins in the visceral pericardium. The veins then feed into the great cardiac vein and coronary sinus on the posterior surface of the heart, between the atria and ventricles, in the coronary sulcus (see Fig. 31.6C).

There is an extensive system of lymphatic capillaries and collecting vessels within the layers of the myocardium and the valves. With cardiac contraction, the lymphatic vessels drain fluid to lymph nodes in the anterior mediastinum that empty into the superior vena cava. The cardiac lymphatics maintain tissue fluid homeostasis, allow immune cells to move in and out of the heart tissue, aid in nutritional lipid transport, and participate in reverse cholesterol transport (see Emerging Science Box: Coronary Lymphatics in Health and Disease).[5]

Structures that Control Heart Action

Life depends on continuous repetition of the cardiac cycle (systole and diastole), which requires the transmission of electrical impulses, termed cardiac action potentials, through the myocardium.[6] (Action potentials are described in Chapters 1 and 3.) As an electrical impulse passes from cell to cell (fiber to fiber) in the myocardium, it stimulates an intracellular process that results in fiber shortening—that is, muscular contraction or systole. Between action potentials, the fibers relax and return to their resting length, causing diastole. The muscle fibers of the myocardium are electrically coupled so that action potentials pass from cell to cell very rapidly and efficiently. The myocardial structures that allow the action potentials to move so rapidly through the heart are the gap junctions in the intercalated discs. In the intercalated discs, the channel-forming proteins, called connexins, form pores in the gap junctions.[7] As a result of these structures plus the heart's conduction system, an action potential generated in one part of the myocardium passes very quickly throughout the heart, causing rapid, organized, sequential contraction of the atria and then the ventricles.

The myocardium contains its own conduction system—a collection of specialized cells that enable the myocardium to generate and transmit action potentials without input from the nervous system (Fig. 31.7). Cells that initiate signals are called pacemakers. The pacemaker cells are concentrated at two sites in the myocardium, called *nodes:* the sinoatrial node and the atrioventricular node. The cardiac cycle is stimulated by these nodes of specialized cells. Although the heart is innervated by the autonomic nervous system (both sympathetic and parasympathetic fibers), neural impulses are not needed to maintain the cardiac cycle. Thus the heart will beat in the absence of any innervation, one of the many factors that allow heart transplantation to be successful. The cardiac cycle is adjusted to the physical needs of the body by the autonomic fibers.

Heart action is also influenced by substances delivered to the myocardium in coronary blood. Nutrients and oxygen are needed for cellular survival and normal function. Hormones and biochemical substances, including medications, can affect the strength and duration of myocardial contraction and the degree and duration of myocardial relaxation. Normal or appropriate function depends on the supply of these substances, which is why coronary artery disease can seriously disrupt heart function.

Conduction System

Normally, electrical impulses arise in the sinoatrial (SA) node (sinus node), the usual pacemaker of the heart. The SA node is located at the junction of the right atrium and superior vena cava, just superior to the tricuspid valve (see Fig. 31.7). It sits only 1 mm beneath the visceral pericardium, making it vulnerable to injury and disease, especially pericardial inflammation. The SA node is nourished by the sinus node artery, which passes through the center of the node. The SA node is heavily

EMERGING SCIENCE BOX

Coronary Lymphatics in Health and Disease

The primary function of the cardiac lymphatic vasculature is to maintain tissue fluid homeostasis and prevent edema formation. Cardiac lymphatics also have several other essential functions. For example, the heart and coronary vessels rely on the lymphatics for transport of lipids and lipoproteins (cholesterol) in and out of cardiac and coronary tissues. Also crucial is the role of the lymphatics in modulating the inflammatory response to injury and pathogens. Cardiac lymphatics regulate innate and adaptive immune responses, and macrophages in the lymphatic system contribute to the regeneration of cardiac tissue after myocardial infarction. Without adequate lymphatic function, edema and chronic immune responses contribute to fibrotic remodeling of the myocardium. In atherosclerotic cardiovascular disease, myocardial infarction, and heart failure, lymphatics are disrupted and the generation of new lymphatic vessels is decreased. Recently, pharmacologic stimulation of lymphangiogenesis has been shown to improve cardiac function and reduce myocardial fibrosis during heart failure development after myocardial infarction. Methods under investigation for stimulating cardiac lymphangiogenesis include injection of vascular endothelial growth factor-C (VGEF-C), adenovirus vector-mediated VEGF-C gene therapy, and intravenous epicardium-specific peptide adrenomedullin administration. Early results are promising.

Data from Brakenhielm E, et al. Role of cardiac lymphatics in myocardial edema and fibrosis: JACC review topic of the week. *Journal of the American College of Cardiology*, 2020;76:735–744; Lim GB. Reduced lymphatic drainage promotes HFpEF and atherosclerosis. *Nature Reviews Cardiology*, 2021;18:149; Klaourakis K, et al. The evolving cardiac lymphatic vasculature in development, repair and regeneration. *Nature Reviews Cardiology*, 2021. https://doi.org/10.1038/s41569-020-00489-x; Liu X, et al. New insights about the lymphatic vasculature in cardiovascular diseases. *F1000Res.* 2019;8:*F1000 Faculty Rev-1811*; Trincot CE, et al. Adrenomedullin induces cardiac lymphangiogenesis after myocardial infarction and regulates cardiac edema via connexin 43. *Circulation Res.* 2019;124:101–113; Vuorio T, et al. Cardiac lymphatics—A new avenue for therapeutics? *Trends in Endocrinology and Metabolism*, 2017;28:285–296; Zhang Y, et al. Functions and regeneration of mature cardiac lymphatic vessels in atherosclerosis, myocardial infarction, and heart failure. *Lymphatic Research and Biology*, 2018;16:507–515.

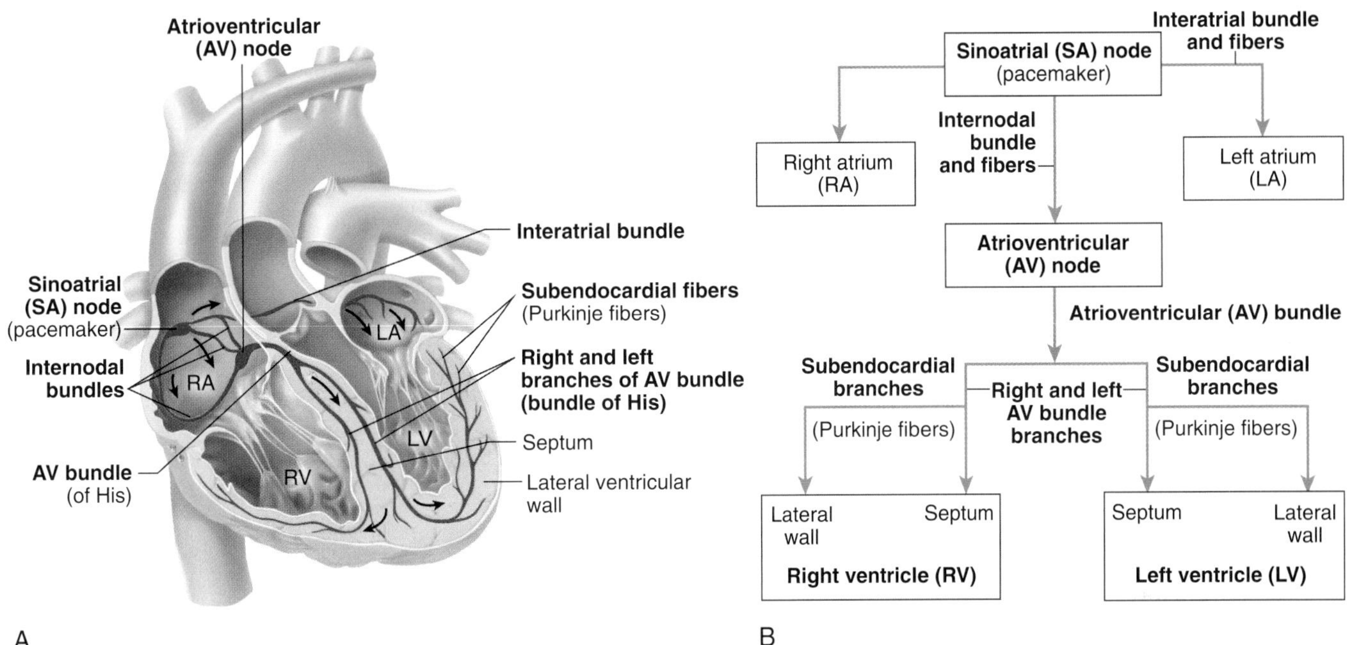

Fig. 31.7 Conduction System of the Heart. Specialized cardiac muscle cells *(boldface type)* in the wall of the heart rapidly initiate or conduct an electrical impulse throughout the myocardium. Both the sketch of the conduction system (A) and the flowchart (B) show the origin and path of conduction. The signal is initiated by the SA node (pacemaker) and spreads to the rest of the right atrial myocardium directly, to the left atrial myocardium by way of a bundle of interatrial conducting fibers, and to the AV node by way of three internodal bundles. The AV node then initiates a signal that is conducted through the ventricular myocardium by way of the AV bundle (of His) and subendocardial branches (Purkinje fibers). (From Patton KT, Thibodeau GA. *The human body in health & disease*, 7th edition. St. Louis: Mosby; 2018.)

innervated by both sympathetic and parasympathetic nerve fibers. In the resting adult the SA node generates about 60 to 100 action potentials per minute, depending on the age and physical condition of the person. Each action potential travels rapidly from cell to cell and through the atrial myocardium as well as through interatrial and internodal fibers, carrying the action potential onward to the atrioventricular (AV) node, as well as causing both atria to contract, beginning systole (see Fig. 31.7).

The AV node, located in the right atrial wall superior to the tricuspid valve and anterior to the ostium of the coronary sinus, conducts the action potentials onward to the ventricles. It is innervated by nerves from the autonomic parasympathetic ganglia that serve as receptors for the vagus nerve and cause slowing of impulse conduction through the AV node.

Conducting fibers from the AV node converge to form the bundle of His (atrioventricular bundle), within the posterior border of the interventricular septum. The bundle of His then gives rise to the right and left bundle branches. The right bundle branch (RBB) is thin and travels without much branching to the right ventricular apex. Because of its thinness and relative lack of branches, the RBB is susceptible to interruption of impulse conduction by damage to the endocardium. The left bundle branch (LBB) divides into two branches, or fascicles. The left anterior bundle branch (LABB) passes the left anterior papillary muscle and the base of the left ventricle and crosses the aortic outflow tract. Damage to the aortic valve or the left ventricle can interrupt this branch. The left posterior bundle branch (LPBB) travels posteriorly, crossing the left ventricular inflow tract to the base of the left posterior papillary muscle. This branch spreads diffusely through the posterior inferior left ventricular wall. Blood flow through this portion of the left ventricle is relatively nonturbulent, so the LBB is somewhat protected from injury caused by wear and tear.

The Purkinje fibers are the terminal branches of the RBB and LBB (see Fig. 31.7). They extend from the ventricular apexes to the fibrous rings and penetrate the heart wall to the outer myocardium. The first areas of the ventricles to be excited are portions of the interventricular septum. The septum is activated from both the RBB and the LBB. The extensive network of Purkinje fibers promotes the rapid spread of the impulse to the ventricular apexes. The basal and posterior portions of the ventricles are the last to be activated.

Cardiac excitation. From the SA node, the impulse that begins systole spreads throughout the right atrium at a conduction velocity of about 35 cm/s.[8] The action potential is delayed in the region of the AV node, possibly because of electrophysiologic differences in the cells that comprise the AV region. Conduction velocity within the node is about 10 cm/s, markedly slower than conduction through the atria. The delay between atrial and ventricular excitation permits an additional boost to ventricular filling by atrial contraction (atrial kick). From the AV node the impulse travels from the AV bundle and through the bundle branches to the Purkinje fibers. Conduction velocities in the AV and Purkinje fibers are the most rapid in the heart.

Ventricular activation occurs sequentially in three phases: (1) septal activation, (2) apical activation, and (3) basal (upper) and posterior activation. The first areas of the ventricles to be excited are portions of the interventricular septum. The septum is activated from both the RBB and the LBB, although the impulse travels from left to right. The extensive network of Purkinje fibers promotes the rapid spread of the impulse to the ventricular apexes. *Activation* traverses the heart wall from the inside outward (from the endocardium to the epicardium). The basal and posterior portions of the ventricles are the last to be activated. *Deactivation*, which begins in diastole, occurs in the opposite direction, spreading from the outside inward (epicardium to endocardium). All areas of the ventricle recover at about the same time.

Propagation of cardiac action potentials. Electrical activation of the muscle cells, termed depolarization, is caused by the movement of ions, including sodium, potassium, calcium, and chloride, across cardiac cell membranes. Deactivation, called repolarization, occurs the same way. (Movement of ions across cell membranes is described in Chapter 1; electrical activation of muscle cells is described in Chapter 43.)

Movement of ions into and out of the cell creates an electrical (voltage) difference across the cell membrane, called the *membrane potential.* The resting membrane potential of myocardial cells is between −80 and −90 mV, whereas that of the SA node is between −50 and −60 millivolts and that of the AV node is between −60 and −70 mV.[8] During depolarization, the inside of the cell becomes less negatively charged as positive ions move inside. In cardiac cells, as in other excitable cells, when the resting membrane potential (in millivolts) becomes less negative with depolarization and reaches the threshold potential for cardiac cells, a cardiac action potential is fired. The various phases of the cardiac action potential are related to changes in the permeability of the cell membrane to sodium, potassium, chloride, and calcium. *Threshold* is the point at which the cell membrane's selective permeability to these ions is temporarily disrupted, leading to an "all or nothing" depolarization. Drugs that alter the movement of these ions (e.g., calcium) have profound effects on the action potential and can alter heart rate. If the resting membrane potential becomes more negative because of a decrease in the extracellular potassium concentration (hypokalemia), it is termed *hyperpolarization.*

Normal myocardial cell depolarization and repolarization occur in five phases numbered 0 through 4 (Fig. 31.8). Phase 0 consists of depolarization. This phase lasts 1 to 2 ms and represents rapid sodium entry into the cell. Phase 1 is early repolarization, in which calcium slowly enters the cell. Phase 2, also called the *plateau*, is a continuation of repolarization, with slow entry of calcium and sodium into the cell. Potassium is moved out of the cell during phase 3, with a return to resting membrane potential in phase 4.[8] The time between action potentials corresponds to diastole.

The phases of depolarization and repolarization occur somewhat differently in the SA and AV node cells, a difference that enables these cells to generate cardiac action potentials independently. The cells of the Purkinje fibers, atria, and ventricles begin with a negative

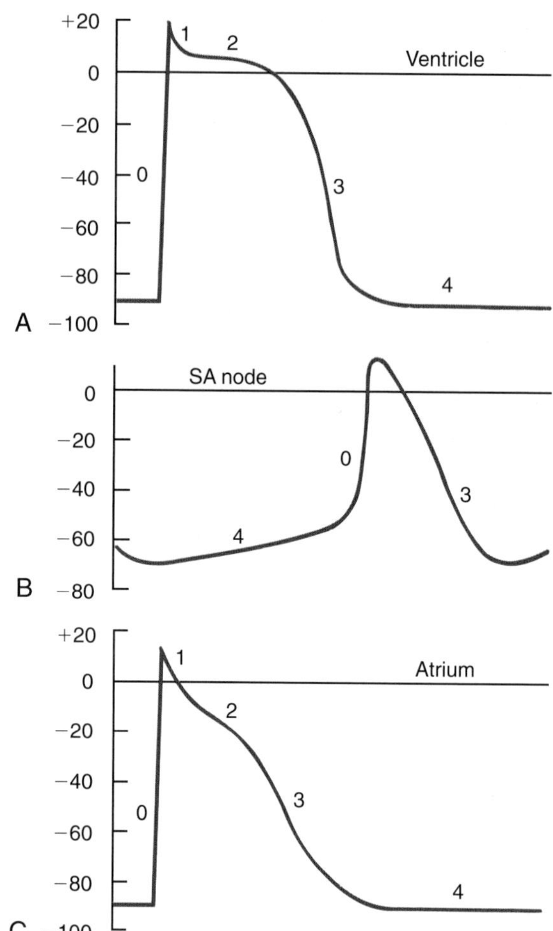

Fig. 31.8 Cardiac Action Potentials. **(A)** Ventricle. **(B)** Sinoatrial *(SA)* node. **(C)** Atrium. Sweep velocity in (B) is half that in (A) or (C). (Modified from Koeppen BM, Stanton BA. *Berne and Levy Physiology*, 6th edition. Philadelphia: Mosby; 2010.)

resting membrane potential and proceed to a rapid upstroke, or depolarization (phase 0), a rapid early repolarization (phase 1), a plateau (phase 2), and a rapid later repolarization (phase 3) (see Fig. 31.8 A and C). The fast inward current of phase 0 is mediated by sodium ions flowing through "fast channels" in the cell membrane and causes the rapid upstroke of the action potential in Purkinje fibers, atria, and ventricles. In contrast, the cells of the SA and AV nodes begin with a less negative resting membrane potential, proceed to a slow upstroke (phase 0), and usually lack a plateau (phase 2) (see Fig. 31.8B). The slow inward current, mediated by calcium through transient and long-lasting channels and sodium ions flowing through "slow channels" of the cell membrane, is responsible for the action potential of the SA node and the AV node. Hence, drugs that block calcium have profound effects on the slow inward current and can alter heart rate. Slow channel-blocking drugs, such as verapamil, are used to treat a variety of cardiovascular disorders.

The absolute refractory period, during which no new cardiac action potential can be initiated by a stimulus, no matter the strength, follows depolarization. The absolute refractory period corresponds to the time needed for the reopening of channels that permit sodium and calcium influx (phase 0 through half of phase 3). A relative refractory period occurs near the end of repolarization. During this time, the membrane can be depolarized again but only by a greater than normal stimulus. Abnormal refractory periods as a result of disease can cause abnormal heart rhythms or dysrhythmias, including ventricular fibrillation and cardiac arrest (see Chapter 32).

The electrocardiogram. An electrocardiogram originates from myocardial cell electrical activity as recorded by skin electrodes and is the summation of all the cardiac action potentials (Fig. 31.9). The P wave represents atrial depolarization. The PR interval is a measure of time from the onset of atrial activation to the onset of ventricular activation. The PR interval represents the time necessary for electrical activity to travel from the sinus node through the atrium, AV node, and His-Purkinje system to activate ventricular myocardial cells. The QRS complex represents the sum of all ventricular muscle cell depolarization. The configuration and amplitude of the QRS complex may vary considerably among individuals. During the ST interval, the entire ventricular myocardium is depolarized. The QT interval is sometimes called the *electrical systole* of the ventricles but the time it takes varies inversely with the heart rate. The T wave represents ventricular repolarization.

Automaticity. Automaticity, or the property of generating spontaneous depolarization to threshold, enables the SA and AV nodes to generate cardiac action potentials without any external stimulus. Cells capable of spontaneous depolarization are called automatic cells. The automatic cells of the cardiac conduction system can stimulate the heart to beat even when it is transplanted and thus has no innervation. Spontaneous depolarization is possible in automatic cells because the membrane potential of these special cells does not actually "rest" during the phase 4 return to the resting membrane potential. Instead, it slowly depolarizes toward threshold during the diastolic phase of the cardiac cycle. Because threshold is approached during diastole, return to the resting membrane potential in automatic cells is called diastolic depolarization. The electrical impulse normally begins in the SA node because its cells depolarize more rapidly than other automatic cells.

Rhythmicity. Rhythmicity is the regular generation of an action potential by the heart's conduction system. The SA node sets the pace because normally it has the fastest rate of depolarization. The SA node depolarizes spontaneously 60 to 100 times per minute. If the SA node is damaged, the AV node can become the heart's pacemaker at a rate of about 40 to 60 spontaneous depolarizations per minute. Eventually, however, conduction cells in the atria usually take over from the AV node. Purkinje fibers are capable of spontaneous depolarization but at an even slower rate than the AV node. Therefore the Purkinje fibers only function as pacemakers when the SA and AV nodes are diseased or there is interruption to movement of electrical current through the heart.

Cardiac Innervation

Sympathetic and parasympathetic nerves. Although the heart's nodes and conduction system are able to generate action potentials independently, the autonomic nervous system influences both the *rate* of impulse generation (firing), depolarization, and repolarization of the myocardium, and the *strength* of

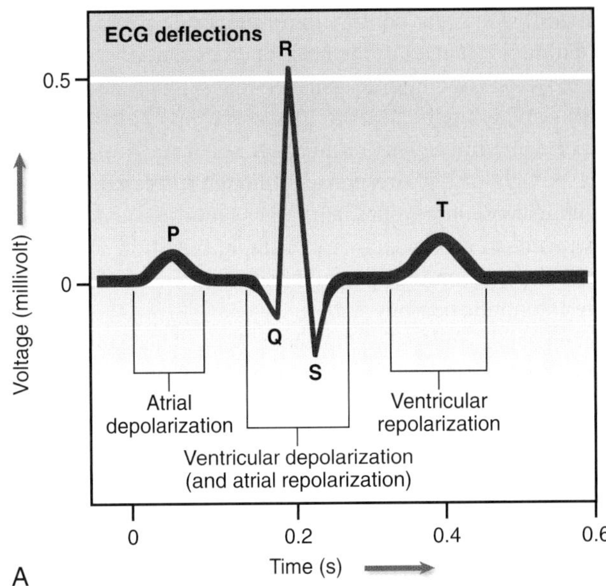

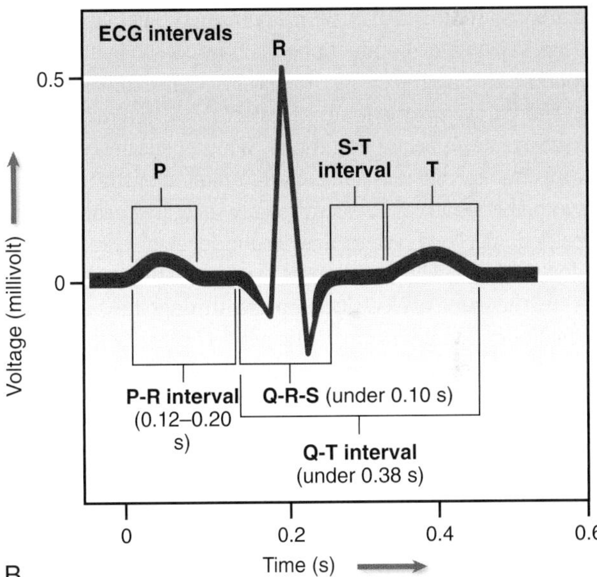

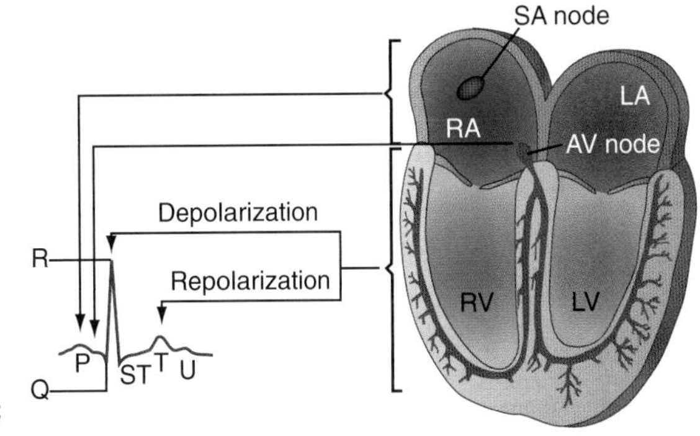

Fig. 31.9 Electrocardiogram (ECG) and Cardiac Electrical Activity. (A) Normal ECG. Depolarization and repolarization. (B) ECG intervals among P, QRS, and T waves. (C) Schematic representation of ECG and its relationship to cardiac electrical activity. *AV*, Atrioventricular; *LA*, left atrium; *LBB*, left bundle branch; *LV*, left ventricle; *RA*, right atrium; *RBB*, right bundle branch; *RV*, right ventricle.

atrial and ventricular contraction. Autonomic neural transmission produces changes in the heart and circulatory system faster than metabolic or humoral agents. Speed is important, for example, in stimulating the heart to increase its pumping action with increased physical activity or during times of stress and fear—the so-called fight or flight response. Although increased delivery of oxygen, glucose, hormones, and other blood-borne factors sustains increased cardiac activity, the rapid initiation of increased activity depends on the sympathetic and parasympathetic fibers of the autonomic nervous system.

Sympathetic and parasympathetic nerve fibers innervate all parts of the atria and ventricles and the SA and AV nodes. Efferent sympathetic and parasympathetic fibers join at the cardiac plexus, a neural junction located at the root of the aorta in front of the trachea. The cardiovascular center in the brainstem responds to input from higher brain centers and from sensory receptors in the periphery and modulates sympathetic and parasympathetic nerve activation (Fig. 31.10) In general, sympathetic stimulation increases electrical conductivity and the strength of myocardial contraction, and vagal parasympathetic nerve activity does the opposite, slowing the conduction of action potentials through the heart and reducing the strength of contraction. Thus the sympathetic and parasympathetic nerves affect the speed of the cardiac cycle (heart rate, or beats per minute). Sympathetic nervous activity enhances myocardial performance. Stimulation of the SA node by the sympathetic nervous system rapidly increases heart rate. The sympathetic nervous system may also induce an increased influx of calcium (Ca^{2+}), which increases the contractile strength of the heart and the speed of electrical impulses through the heart muscle and the nodes. Finally, sympathetic nerves influence the diameter of the coronary vessels. Increased sympathetic discharge dilates the coronary vessels by causing the release of vasodilating metabolites resulting from increased myocardial contraction.

The parasympathetic nervous system affects the heart through the vagus nerve, which releases acetylcholine. Receptors for acetylcholine are found in the myocardium and coronary vessels of the heart. Acetylcholine causes a decreased heart rate, slows conduction through the AV node, and reduces myocardial contraction strength.

Adrenergic receptor function. Sympathetic neural stimulation of the myocardium and coronary vessels depends on the presence of G-protein–coupled adrenergic receptors, which bind specifically with neurotransmitters of the sympathetic nervous system. The effects of sympathetic stimulation depend on whether the α- or β-adrenergic receptors are most plentiful on cells of the effector tissue and whether the neurotransmitter is norepinephrine or epinephrine. Individual variations in receptor structure also influence receptor responsiveness.[9] There are five types of adrenergic receptors: β_1, β_2, β_3, α_1, and α_2. (Each of the α-adrenergic receptors also has three subtypes, so some sources indicate that there are nine types of adrenergic receptors.) Overall, cardiovascular structures have more β- than α-receptors; therefore, effects mediated by the β-receptors predominate. Norepinephrine is released by postsynaptic sympathetic nerve endings in the heart, whereas epinephrine is mainly released by the adrenal medulla and reaches the heart through the bloodstream.

The β_1-receptors are found mostly in the heart, specifically the conduction system (AV and SA nodes, Purkinje fibers) and the atrial and ventricular myocardium. The β_2-receptors are found in the heart and also on vascular smooth muscle. Stimulation of both the β_1- and β_2-receptors results in an increase in heart rate (chronotropy) and force of myocardial contraction (inotropy).[6] In addition, stimulation of the β_2-receptors results in vasodilation because of the location of the receptors on vascular smooth muscle. Overall β_1 and β_2 stimulation enables the heart to pump more blood, and β_2 stimulation also increases coronary blood flow. In the heart, stimulation of β_3-receptors found in the myocardium and coronary vessels opposes the effects of β_1- and β_2-receptor stimulation and decreases myocardial contractility (negative inotropic effect).[9] Thus, β_3-receptors may provide a "safety mechanism" to prevent overstimulation of the heart by the sympathetic nervous system.

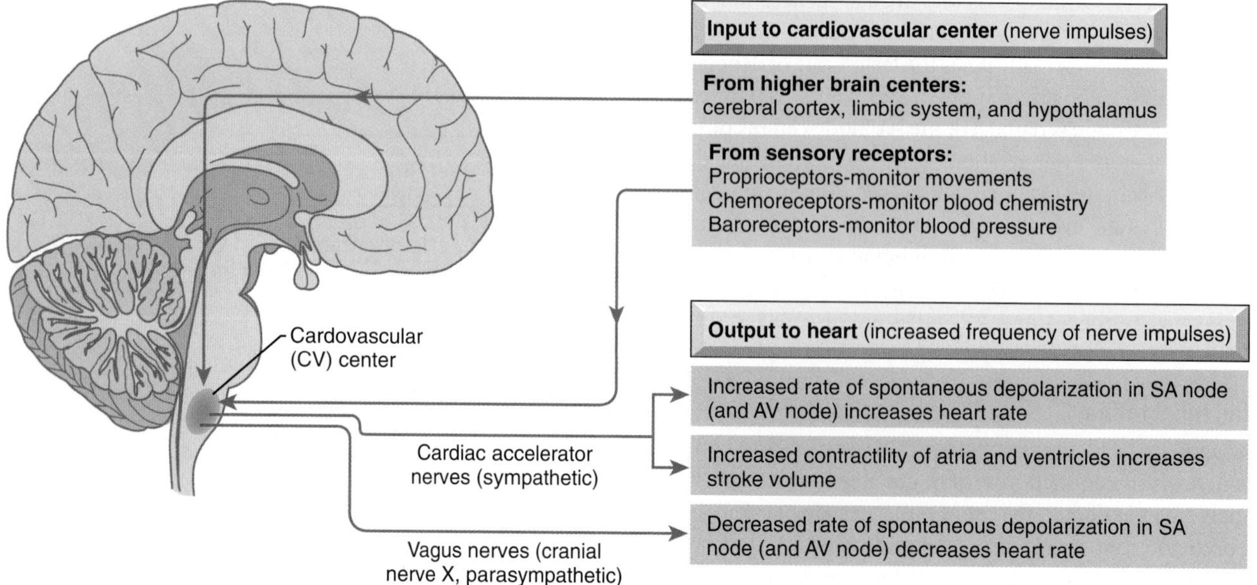

Fig. 31.10 Autonomic Innervation of the Cardiovascular System. Input to the cardiovascular center and output to the heart.

Norepinephrine binding with α_1-receptors, all of which are postsynaptic in the systemic and coronary arteries, causes smooth muscle contraction and thus vasoconstriction. One of the subtypes of α_2-receptors is located on the sympathetic ganglia and nerve terminals. The effect of norepinephrine on these receptors is to inhibit release of more norepinephrine, which promotes vasodilation, thus providing another safety mechanism to prevent excess blood pressure elevation. Dysfunction of α- and β-adrenergic receptors can occur in many conditions (e.g., diabetes, hypertension) and has been implicated in the pathogenesis of many cardiac diseases, including heart failure, myocardial ischemia, and dysrhythmias (see Chapter 32).

Myocardial Cells

Cardiomyocytes are composed of long, narrow fibers that contain bundles of longitudinally arranged myofibrils; a nucleus; mitochondria; an internal membrane system (the sarcoplasmic reticulum); cytoplasm (sarcoplasm); and a plasma membrane (the sarcolemma), which encloses the cell (Fig. 31.11).[6] Cardiac and skeletal muscle cells also have an "external" membrane system made up of transverse tubules (T tubules) formed by inward pouching of the sarcolemma. The sarcoplasmic reticulum forms a network of channels that surrounds the muscle fiber.

Because the myofibrils in both cardiac and skeletal fibers consist of alternating light and dark bands of protein, the fibers appear striped, or striated. The dark and light bands of the myofibrils create repeating longitudinal units, called *sarcomeres*, which are between 1.6 and 2.2 μm long (Fig. 31.12). The length of these sarcomeres determines the limits of myocardial stretch

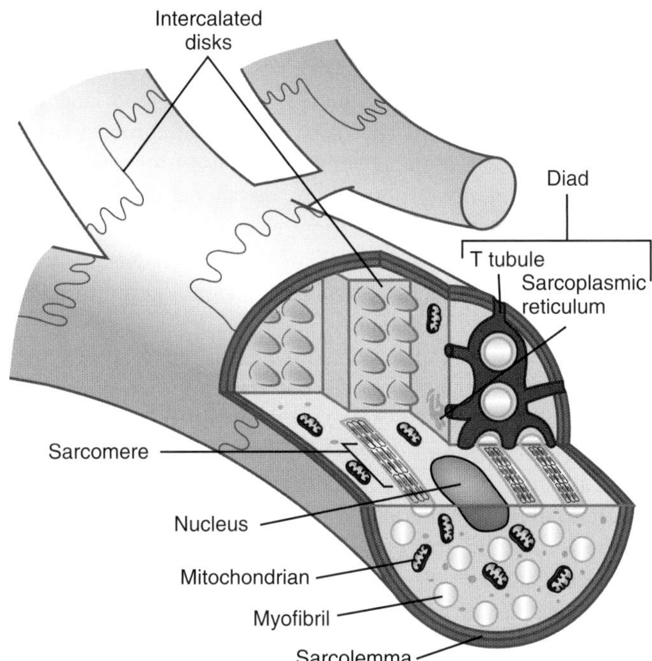

Fig. 31.11 Cardiac Muscle Fiber. Unlike other types of muscle fibers, cardiac muscle fibers are typically branched with junctions, called intercalated discs, between adjacent myocytes. Like skeletal muscle cells, cardiac muscle cells contain sarcoplasmic reticula and T tubules, although these structures are not as highly organized as in skeletal muscle fibers.

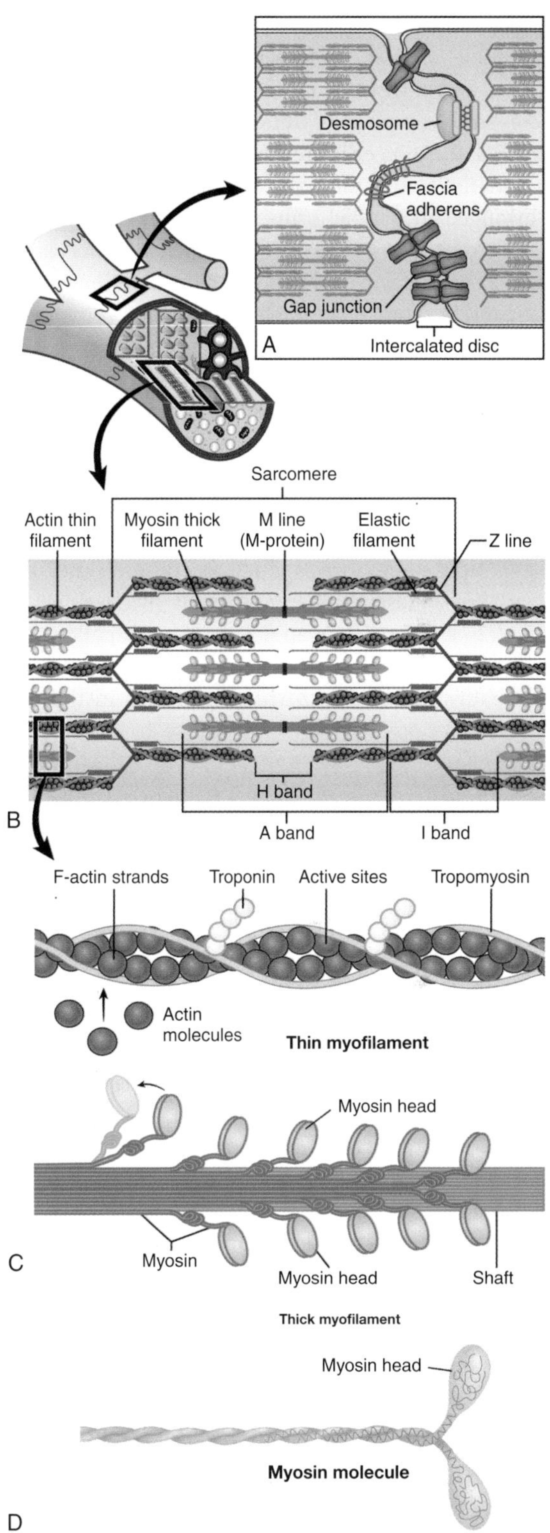

Fig. 31.12 Structure of a Sarcomere, Myofilaments, and Myosin. (A) Structure of the intercalated disc with three types of junctions. (B) The sarcomere is the basic contractile unit of a muscle cell. The Z line is the anchor for the contractile elements actin and myosin. Actin attaches directly to the Z line, whereas myosin is attached to it by elastic titin filaments. The myosin filaments are connected to each other by M-protein at the M line. The A, H, and I bands refer to parts of the sarcomere as they were originally seen by light microscopy. (C) Thin myofilament and thick myofilament. (D) Myosin molecule.

at the end of diastole and subsequently the force of contraction during systole. Alterations in sarcomere size are seen in both physiologic and pathologic myocardial hypertrophy.

There are a number of differences between cardiac and muscle cells. Cardiac cells are arranged in branching networks throughout the myocardium, whereas skeletal muscle cells tend to be arranged in parallel units throughout the length of the muscle. Cardiac fibers have only one nucleus, whereas skeletal muscle cells have many nuclei. Differences between cardiac and skeletal muscle often relate to heart function. Some of these functions include:

1. *Transmit action potentials quickly from cell to cell.* Myocardial cells are all electrically and mechanically connected within the wall of a particular heart chamber. Electrical impulses are transmitted rapidly from cardiac fiber to cardiac fiber because the network of fibers connects at intercalated discs, which are thickened portions of the sarcolemma. The intercalated discs contain three junctions: desmosomes, or macula adherens; fascia adherens, which mechanically attach one cell to another; and gap junctions, which allow the electrical impulse to spread from cell to cell through a low-resistance pathway (see Fig. 31.12A). Changes in the function of these junctional elements may cause an increased risk of arrhythmias.[10]
2. *Maintain high levels of energy synthesis.* Unlike skeletal muscle, the heart cannot rest and is in constant need of energy, which is supplied by molecules such as adenosine triphosphate (ATP). Therefore, the cytoplasm surrounding the bundles of myofibrils in each cardiomyocyte contains a large number of mitochondria (25% to 35% of cell volume, versus 3% to 8% of cell volume in skeletal muscle). Cardiac muscle cells have more mitochondria than skeletal muscle cells to provide the necessary respiratory enzymes for aerobic metabolism and supply quantities of ATP sufficient for the constant action of the myocardium.
3. *Gain access to more ions, particularly sodium and potassium, in the extracellular environment.* Cardiac fibers contain more T tubules than do skeletal muscle fibers (see Fig. 31.11). This increased closeness to the T tubules gives each myofibril in the myocardium faster access to molecules needed for the transmission of action potentials, a process that involves transport of sodium and potassium through the walls of the T tubules. Because the T tubule system is continuous with the extracellular space and the interstitial fluid, it facilitates the rapid transmission of the electrical impulses from the surface of the sarcolemma to the myofibrils inside the fiber. This rapid transmission activates all the myofibrils of one fiber simultaneously. The sarcoplasmic reticulum is located around the myofibrils. As an action potential is transmitted through the T tubules, it induces the sarcoplasmic reticulum to release its stored calcium, thus activating the contractile proteins actin and myosin.

The sarcomere. Within each myocardial sarcomere are myosin and actin molecules that are grouped together to form filaments. Myosin molecules resemble golf clubs with two large, ovoid heads at one end of the shaft (see Fig. 31.12D). The bilobed heads contain an actin-binding site and a site of ATPase activity. About 200 myosin molecules are bundled together with their heads facing outward, forming a single thick filament. Actin molecules resemble beads, and they are strung into two chains that wind around each other, forming a thin filament (see Fig. 31.12C).

Several proteins are also present in the sarcomere. A tropomyosin molecule (a relaxing protein) lies alongside actin molecules. Troponin, another relaxing protein, associates with the tropomyosin molecule. The troponin complex itself has three components. *Troponin T* aids in binding of the troponin complex to actin and tropomyosin; *troponin I* inhibits the ATPase of actomyosin; and *troponin C* contains binding sites for the calcium ions involved in contraction. *Troponin T* and *I* molecules are released into the bloodstream during myocardial injury. They can be measured to evaluate if a myocardial infarction or other damage has occurred. The sarcomere also contains a giant elastic protein, titin, which attaches myosin to the Z line, acts as a spring, and influences myocardial stiffness. The titin structure affects myocardial diastolic filling and has been found to play a role in heart failure.[11]

Where thick filaments overlap with thin filaments, a central dark band is formed, called the anisotropic band, or A band (see Fig. 31.12B). The light bands of the sarcomere, called isotropic bands or I bands, contain only actin molecules and no myosin. The center of the sarcomere is a less dense region called the H band, which contains only myosin molecules and no actin. Thick filaments are held together by M-protein molecules that form a central thin, dark M line.[7] Thin filaments of actin extend from each side of the Z line, a dense fibrous structure at the center of each I band. The area from one Z line to the next Z line defines one sarcomere.

Myocardial metabolism. Cardiomyocytes depend on the constant production of ATP, which is synthesized within the mitochondria mainly from glucose, fatty acids, and lactate. If the myocardium is underperfused because of coronary artery disease, anaerobic metabolism must be used for energy (see Chapter 1). Energy produced by metabolic processes fuels muscle contraction and relaxation, electrical excitation, membrane transport, and synthesis of large molecules. Normally, the amount of ATP produced supplies sufficient energy to pump blood throughout the system.

Cardiac work is expressed as myocardial oxygen consumption ($M\dot{V}O2$), which is closely correlated with total cardiac energy requirements. The $M\dot{V}O2$ is determined by three major factors: (1) the amount of wall stress during systole, estimated by measuring the systolic blood pressure; (2) the duration of systolic wall tension, measured indirectly by the heart rate; and (3) the contractile state of the myocardium, which is not measured clinically.

The coronary arteries deliver oxygen (O_2) to the myocardium. Approximately 70% to 75% of this O_2 is used immediately by cardiac muscle, leaving little O_2 in reserve. Because the O_2 content of the blood and the amount of O_2 extracted from the blood cannot be increased under normal circumstances, any increased energy needs can be met only by increasing coronary blood flow. The $M\dot{V}O2$ increases with exercise and decreases with hypotension and hypothermia. As myocardial metabolism and consumption of O_2 increase, the concentration of local vasoactive metabolic factors increases. Some of these (e.g., adenosine, nitric oxide, and prostaglandins) dilate coronary arterioles, thus increasing coronary blood flow. Aging reduces the efficiency of myocardial metabolism and may contribute to the development of heart failure.[12]

Myocardial Contraction and Relaxation

Myocardial contractility is a change in developed tension at a given resting fiber length, which basically is the ability of the heart muscle to shorten. Each sarcomere serves as the basic contractile unit of a muscle cell. The outward-facing heads of myosin molecules are called *cross-bridges* because they can form force-generating bridges by binding with exposed actin molecules. Once bound, the myosin molecules effectively pull the thin filaments toward the center of the sarcomere, shortening the sarcomere and resulting in contraction. This process is known as the cross-bridge theory of muscle contraction (Fig. 31.13). Anatomically, contraction occurs when the sarcomere shortens, causing adjacent Z lines to move closer together. The width of the A band, which contains the thick myosin filaments, is unchanged whereas the I band becomes narrower as the overlap between the thick and thin filaments increases. The degree of shortening depends on the amount of overlap between the thick and thin filaments.

Cross-bridge cycling. The ovoid head-end of the myosin contains a binding site for actin and a separate enzymatic site that catalyzes the breakdown of ATP to adenosine diphosphate (ADP) and inorganic phosphate (P_i) (see Fig. 31.13). This reaction releases the chemical energy stored in ATP. The splitting of ATP occurs on the myosin molecule before it attaches to actin, but the ADP and inorganic phosphate released remain bound to the active site on myosin.

The binding of this high-energy myosin-actin to form a cross-bridge releases the energy stored in myosin (i.e., ADP and P_i), producing the force necessary for movement of the cross-bridge. With the attachment of actin to myosin at the cross-bridge, the myosin head molecule undergoes a position change, exerting traction on the rest of the myosin bridge, causing the thin filaments to slide past the thick filaments (see Fig. 31.13D). During contraction each cross-bridge undergoes several cycles of attachment, movement, and dissociation from the thin filaments. The rate of cross-bridge cycling is linked to systolic function and cardiac output.[13]

Calcium and excitation-contraction coupling. Excitation-contraction coupling is the process by which an action potential arriving at the muscle fiber plasma membrane triggers the cycle, leading to cross-bridge formation and contraction. Cycle activation depends on calcium availability, and the amount of force developed is regulated by how much the concentration of calcium ions increases within the cardiomyocytes. Calcium enters the myocardial cell from the interstitial fluid after electrical excitation that increases membrane calcium permeability. Two types of calcium channels are identified in cardiac tissues. The *L-type*, or long-lasting, channels are the predominant type of calcium channels and are the channels blocked by calcium channel–blocking drugs (verapamil, nifedipine, diltiazem). The major effect of these medications is to decrease the strength of cardiac contraction. The *T-type*, or transient, channels are much less abundant in the heart and are not blocked by currently available calcium channel–blocking drugs and are being investigated.

Calcium entering the cell triggers the release of additional calcium from the two storage sites within the sarcomere. Calcium ions then diffuse toward the myofibrils, where they bind with troponin. The calcium-troponin complex interaction facilitates the contraction process (see Fig. 31.13). In the resting state, troponin is bound to actin and the tropomyosin molecule covers the sites where the myosin heads bind to actin, thereby preventing interaction between actin and myosin. Calcium binds to troponin, which ultimately results in tropomyosin moving troponin, thus

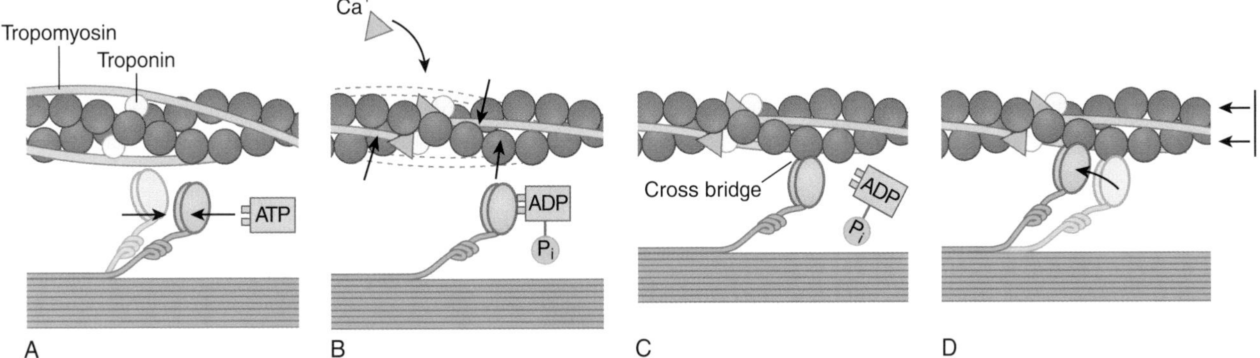

Fig. 31.13 Cross-Bridge Theory of Muscle Contraction. **(A)** Each myosin cross-bridge in the thick filament moves into a resting position after an adenosine triphosphate *(ATP)* molecule binds and transfers its energy. **(B)** Calcium ions released from the sarcoplasmic reticulum bind to troponin in the thin filament, allowing tropomyosin to shift from its position blocking the active sites of actin molecules. **(C)** Each myosin cross-bridge then binds to an active site on a thin filament, displacing the remnants of ATP hydrolysis—adenosine diphosphate *(ADP)* and inorganic phosphate *(P_i)*. **(D)** The release of stored energy from step A provides the force needed for each cross-bridge to move back to its original position, pulling actin along with it. Each cross-bridge will remain bound to actin until another ATP molecule binds to it and pulls it back into its resting position (A). (Adapted from *Thibodeau GA, Patton KT. Anatomy & physiology*, 4th edition. St. Louis: Mosby; 1999.)

uncovering the binding sites. Myosin and actin can now form cross-bridges, and ATP can be dephosphorylated to adenosine diphosphate (ADP). Under these circumstances, sliding of the thick and thin filaments can occur, and the muscle contracts.

Myocardial relaxation. Relaxation is as vital to optimal cardiac function as contraction, and calcium, troponin, and tropomyosin also facilitate relaxation. After contraction, free calcium ions are actively pumped out of the cell back into the interstitial fluid or taken back into storage by the sarcoplasmic reticulum and tubule system. As the concentration of calcium within the sarcomere decreases, troponin releases its bound calcium. The tropomyosin complex moves and blocks the active sites on the actin molecule, preventing cross-bridge formation with the myosin heads. If the ability of the myocardium to relax is impaired, it can lead to increased diastolic filling pressures and eventually heart failure (see Chapter 32).

Factors Affecting Cardiac Output

Cardiac performance can be evaluated by measuring the cardiac output. Cardiac output is calculated by multiplying the heart rate in beats per minute by the stroke volume (volume of blood ejected during systole) in liters per beat. Normal adult cardiac output is about 5 L/min at rest, given a heart rate of about 70 beats/min and a normal stroke volume of about 70 mL.

With each heartbeat, the ventricles eject much of their blood volume, and the percentage of total end-diastolic ventricular volume ejected per beat is called the ejection fraction. The ejection fraction is calculated by dividing the stroke volume by the end-diastolic volume. The end-diastolic volume of the normal ventricle is about 70 to 80 mL/m^2, and the normal ejection fraction of the resting heart, measured with gated myocardial perfusion imaging, was 66% ± 8% for women and 58% ± 8% for men. The ejection fraction is increased by factors that increase contractility, such as increased sympathetic nervous system activity. A decrease in the ejection fraction may indicate ventricular failure. The effects of aging on cardiovascular function are summarized in Table 31.2.

The factors that determine cardiac output are (1) preload, (2) afterload, (3) myocardial contractility, and (4) heart rate. Preload, afterload, and contractility all affect stroke volume (Fig. 31.14).

TABLE 31.2 Cardiovascular Function in Elderly Adults

Determinant	Resting Cardiac Performance	Exercise Cardiac Performance[a]
Cardiac output	Unchanged	Decreases because of a decrease in maximum heart rate
Heart rate	Slight decrease	Increases less than in younger people
Stroke volume	Slight increase	No change
Ejection fraction	Unchanged	Decreased
Afterload	Increased	Increased
End-diastolic volume	Unchanged	Increased
End-systolic volume	Unchanged	Increased
Contraction	Decreased velocity	Decreased
Myocardial wall stiffness	Increased	Increased
Maximum oxygen consumption	Not applicable	Decreased
Plasma catecholamines	—	Increased

[a]Changes in healthy men and women up to age 80 years as compared to those 20 years of age.
Data from Lakatta EG, et al. Aging and cardiovascular disease in the elderly. In: Fuster V, et al., eds. *Hurst's the heart,* 13th edition. Philadelphia: McGraw-Hill; 2011.

Preload

Preload is the volume and pressure inside the ventricle at the end of diastole (ventricular end-diastolic volume [VEDV] and pressure [VEDP]). Preload is determined by two primary factors: (1) the amount of blood left in the ventricle after systole (end-systolic volume) and (2) the amount of venous blood returning to the ventricle during diastole. *End-systolic volume* is dependent on the strength of ventricular contraction and the resistance to ventricular emptying. *Venous return* is dependent on blood volume and flow through the venous system and the atrioventricular valves. Clinically, preload is estimated by measuring the central venous pressure (CVP) for the right side of the heart and the pulmonary artery wedge pressure (cross-sectional pressure) for the left side. Normal values for these two estimates are 1 to 5 mm Hg and 4 to 12 mm Hg, respectively. Heart failure can occur because of an increase in preload (VEDV), which causes a decline in stroke volume and also increases VEDP (see Chapter 32). Increased VEDP causes pressures to increase or "back up" into the pulmonary or systemic venous circulation, increasing plasma outflow through the vessel walls, causing fluid to accumulate in lung tissues (pulmonary edema) or in peripheral tissues (peripheral edema).

Frank-starling law of the heart. Cardiac muscle, like other muscle, increases its strength of contraction when it is stretched up to a certain point. The Frank-Starling law of the heart, or the length-tension relationship of cardiac muscle, relates resting sarcomere length, expressed as the volume of blood in the heart at the end of diastole (end-diastolic volume), to tension generation, described as development of left ventricular pressure. Thus, the volume of blood in the heart at the end of diastole (the length of its muscle fibers) is directly related to the force of contraction during the next systole. Although the change in pressure is related to the volume of the ventricle and, consequently, to the length of the ventricular muscle fibers, preload (i.e., filling pressure) is commonly used as an index of ventricular volume. The length-tension mechanism is the main mechanism by which the normal right and left ventricles maintain equal minute outputs even though their stroke outputs may vary considerably during normal respiration. For example, changes in volume occur when an individual assumes a reclining position after being in a standing position; the volume of blood returning to the heart temporarily increases. The right ventricle stretches to accommodate this

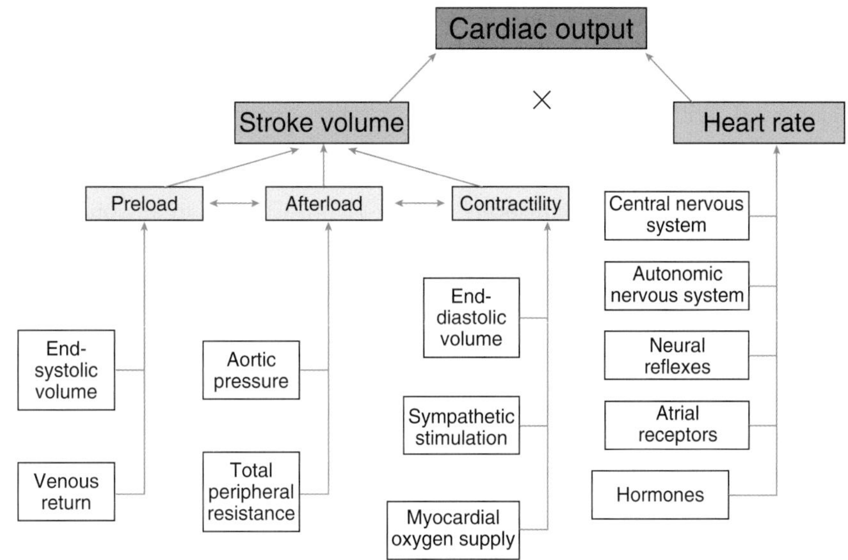

Fig. 31.14 Factors Affecting Cardiac Performance. Cardiac output, the amount of blood (in liters) ejected by the heart per minute, depends on the heart rate (beats per minute) and stroke volume (milliliters of blood ejected during ventricular systole).

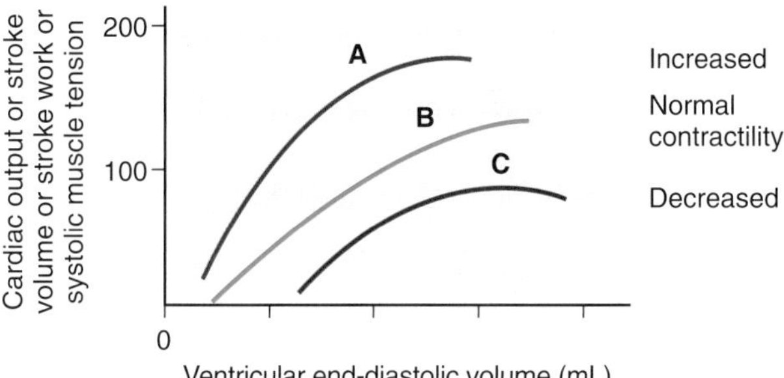

Fig. 31.15 Frank-Starling Law of the Heart. The relationship between length and tension in the heart. The end-diastolic volume determines the end-diastolic length of ventricular muscle fibers and is proportional to tension generated during systole, as well as to cardiac output, stroke volume, and stroke work. A change in myocardial contractility causes the heart to perform on a different length-tension curve. **(A)** Increased contractility; **(B)** normal contractility; **(C)** heart failure or decreased contractility. (See text for further explanation.)

increase in volume and thereby increases its force of contraction. A larger stroke volume (i.e., the amount of blood ejected per beat) is pumped to the lungs, generating higher pressures. Pulmonary vascular pressure increases, causing a rise in the left ventricular filling pressure or preload. Left ventricular volume and pressure increase. The left ventricle pumps a larger stroke volume, and arterial vascular pressure rises.

The mechanical function of the heart is characterized by a number of length-tension curves (Fig. 31.15). Factors that increase contractility, such as sympathetic nerve stimulation, cause the heart to operate on a higher length-tension curve (curve *A* in Fig. 31.15). A higher tension or increase in ventricular stroke volume is generated without a necessary change in left ventricular end-diastolic volume (LVEDV) or fiber length. Heart failure (curve *C* in Fig. 31.15) is characterized by a lower length-tension curve. The Frank-Starling law of the heart may not apply to dilated or failing hearts because their fibers are already stretched beyond their optimal length. The failing heart responds to increased filling or stretch with a progressive decline in the force of contraction. Thus at the same left ventricular end-diastolic volume (LVEDV) as curves *A* and *B* (see Fig. 31.15), the force of contraction of stroke volume is decreased (Fig. 31.15C).

The cross-bridge arrangement with the sarcomere partially accounts for the length-tension mechanism of cardiac muscle. According to the Frank-Starling law, the longer the initial resting length of the cardiac muscle fiber (optimal length is between 2.2 and 2.4 mm), the greater the strength of contraction. At 2.2 mm an optimal number of active cross-bridges exist between actin and myosin. However, if the fibers are stretched beyond 2.2 to 2.4 mm, the force of contraction decreases because actin and myosin become partially disengaged, disrupting many of the cross-bridges. Excessive stretching, to about 3.65 mm, causes actin and myosin to become completely disengaged so that tension (force of contraction) drops to zero. The relationship between stretch and contraction can be compared with that of a rubber band. Up to a certain point, the more the rubber band is stretched the farther it will fly when one end is released; beyond that point, however, the rubber band will break but, of course, the myocardium does not actually break.

Laplace law. Laplace law states that wall tension is related directly to the product of intraventricular pressure and internal radius, and inversely related to the wall thickness as shown in the Laplace equation:

$$T(p \times r)/\mu m$$

where T = wall tension, p = intraventricular pressure, r = internal radius of the sphere, and μm = wall thickness. In other words, the amount of tension generated in the ventricular wall (or any chamber or vessel) to produce a given intraventricular pressure depends on the size (radius and wall thickness) of the ventricle.

Laplace law is useful for understanding aneurysm formation, distensibility in blood vessels, and the effects of ventricular dilation on myocardial contraction. Dilation is an important factor in heart failure (see Chapter 32). With a dilated ventricle, myocardial fibers in the wall must develop greater tension to produce a given pressure within the ventricle. The disadvantage of dilation is that the increased force, or tension, in the myocardial fibers required to develop a given pressure inside a dilated ventricle decreases the rate of fiber shortening, thereby decreasing the ability of the ventricle to eject blood.

Afterload

Ventricular afterload is the resistance to ejection of blood from the ventricle. It is the load the muscle must move during contraction. The aortic systolic pressure is an index of afterload. Pressure in the ventricle must exceed the aortic pressure before blood can be pumped out during systole. Low aortic pressures (decreased afterload) enable the heart to contract more rapidly and efficiently, whereas high aortic pressures (increased afterload) slow contraction and cause higher workloads against which the heart must function to eject blood. Increased aortic pressure is usually the result of increased systemic vascular resistance (SVR), sometimes referred to as total peripheral resistance (TPR). In individuals with hypertension, increased SVR means that afterload is chronically elevated, resulting in increased ventricular workload and hypertrophy of the myocardium. SVR is calculated by dividing the mean arterial pressure by the cardiac output; the normal range is 700 dyne/s/cm^{-5}. The most sensitive measure of afterload is SVR. In some individuals, changes in afterload are the result of aortic valvular disease.

Myocardial Contractility

Stroke volume, or the volume of blood ejected per beat during systole, also depends on the *force* of contraction, myocardial contractility, or the degree of myocardial fiber shortening. Three major factors determine the force of contraction (see Fig. 31.14):

1. *Changes in the stretching of the ventricular myocardium caused by changes in VEDV (preload).* As discussed previously, increased venous return to the heart distends the ventricle, thus increasing preload, which increases the stroke volume and, subsequently, cardiac output, up to a certain point. However, an excessive increase in preload leads to decreased stroke volume.
2. *Alterations in the inotropic stimuli of the ventricles.* Hormones, neurotransmitters, or medications that affect contractility are called inotropic agents. The most important endogenous positive inotropic agents are epinephrine and norepinephrine released from the sympathetic nervous system. The most important negative inotropic agent is acetylcholine released from the vagus nerve. Many medications have positive or negative inotropic properties that can have significant effects on cardiac function. In sepsis, a variety of cytokines, including tumor necrosis factor-alpha (TNF-α), and interleukin-1β, have been shown to impair myocardial contractility.[14]
3. *Adequacy of myocardial oxygen supply.* O_2 and carbon dioxide levels (tensions) in the coronary blood also influence contractility. With severe hypoxemia (arterial O_2 saturation less than 50%), contractility is decreased. Moderate degrees of hypoxemia may increase contractility by enhancing the myocardial response to circulating catecholamines.

Preload, afterload, and contractility all interact with one another to determine stroke volume and cardiac output (see Fig. 31.14). Changes in any one of these factors can result in deleterious effects on the others, resulting in heart failure (see Chapter 32).

Heart Rate

As described previously, SA node activity is the primary determinant of the heart rate. The average heart rate in healthy adults is about 70 beats/min; in children it is typically greater. This rate diminishes by 10 to 20 beats/min during sleep and can accelerate to more than 100 beats/min during muscular activity or emotional excitement. In well-conditioned athletes, the resting heart rate is normally about 50 to 60 beats/min. In highly trained or elite athletes, the resting heart rate can be below 50 beats/min; these athletes also have a greater stroke volume and lower peripheral resistance in active muscles than they had before training. The control of heart rate includes activity of the central nervous system, autonomic nervous system, neural reflexes, atrial receptors, and hormones (see Fig. 31.14).

Heart rate variability. Heart rate varies naturally with many factors such as exercise, anxiety, temperature, and hormones (e.g., estrogen). This ability of the heart to change rate is called heart rate variability (HRV) and is a measure of cardiac autonomic function. For example, heart rate varies with respiration, the rate increasing with inspiration and decreasing with expiration. This normal alteration in rhythm pattern, called sinus arrhythmia, is caused by changes that occur within the chest cavity because of respiration. Inspiration results in stretch and an associated increase in firing of the SA node that increases heart rate. The stretch is reduced with expiration and the SA node firing rate slows, resulting in a decrease in heart rate. Adequate amounts of HRV in response to physiologic conditions is believed to be an important indicator of health.

Many pathophysiologic factors are linked to decreased HRV, including neurologic disease (e.g., parkinsonian syndrome, multiple sclerosis), cardiovascular disease (e.g., coronary artery disease, heart failure), inflammation, alcohol and drug consumption, occupational exposures, exposure to electromagnetic fields, air pollution, and others.[15] Recent studies have documented the relationship between psychological stress, lack of effective coping mechanisms, and mental health disorders with decreased heart rate variability.[16] A decrease in HRV may indicate that the individual is vulnerable to complications from their underlying conditions. For example, a decrease in HRV is associated with a higher risk of cardiovascular events and mortality in individuals with cardiovascular disease.[17]

Cardiovascular control centers in the brain. The cardiovascular vasomotor control center is in the medulla and pons areas of the brainstem, with additional areas in the hypothalamus, cerebral cortex, and thalamus. The hypothalamic centers regulate cardiovascular responses to changes in temperature, the cerebral cortex centers adjust cardiac reaction to a variety of emotional states, and the brainstem control center regulates heart rate and blood pressure.

The nerve fibers from the cardiovascular control center synapse with autonomic neurons that influence the rate of firing of the SA node. As previously discussed, an increased heart rate occurs with sympathetic (adrenergic) stimulation. When the parasympathetic nerves to the heart are stimulated (primarily via the vagus nerve), the heart rate slows and the sympathetic nerves to the heart, arterioles, and veins are inhibited. At rest, the heart rate in healthy individuals is primarily under the control of parasympathetic stimulation. Administration of drugs that block parasympathetic function (anticholinergic) or physical interruption of the vagus nerve causes significant tachycardia (abnormally fast heart rate) because this inhibitory parasympathetic influence is lost.

Neural reflexes. Output from the baroreceptor reflexes influences short-term regulation of the vascular smooth muscle of resistance arteries, myocardial contractility, and heart rate, all components of blood pressure control. The baroreceptors or pressoreceptors are located in the aortic arch and carotid arteries. If blood pressure decreases, the baroreceptor reflex accelerates the heart rate, increases myocardial contractility, and increases vascular smooth muscle contraction in the arterioles, thus raising blood pressure. This reflex is critical to maintaining adequate tissue perfusion. When the blood pressure increases, the baroreceptors increase their rate of discharge, sending neural impulses over a branch of the glossopharyngeal nerve (cranial nerve IX) and through the vagus nerve to the cardiovascular control centers in the medulla. These reflexes increase parasympathetic activity and decrease sympathetic activity, causing the resistance arteries to dilate, decreasing myocardial contractility and the heart rate. The role of baroreceptors in influencing blood pressure is discussed in more detail later in this chapter.

Atrial receptors. Mechanoreceptors that influence the heart rate exist in both atria. They are located where the veins, venae cavae, and pulmonary veins enter their respective atria. The Bainbridge reflex is the name for the changes in the heart rate that may occur after intravenous infusions of blood or other fluid. The change in heart rate is thought to be caused by a reflex mediated by these atrial volume receptors that are innervated by the vagus nerve (volume receptors are thought to respond to increased plasma volume). Although this reflex can be elicited in humans, its relevance is uncertain at this time. Stimulation of these atrial receptors also increases urine volume, presumably because of a neurally mediated reduction in antidiuretic hormone. In addition, peptides of the atrial natriuretic family are released from atrial tissue in response to the increases in blood volume. These peptides have diuretic and natriuretic (salt excretion) properties, resulting in decreased blood volume and pressure. The atrial natriuretic peptides also have been shown to relax vascular smooth muscle and oppose myocardial hypertrophy, leading to measurement of blood levels to evaluate clinical status and raising interest in their use as therapeutic agents (see Chapter 32).

Hormones and biochemicals. Hormones and other biochemically active substances affect the arteries, arterioles, venules, capillaries, and contractility of the myocardium. Norepinephrine, mainly released as a neurotransmitter from the adrenal medulla, dilates vessels of the liver and skeletal muscle and also causes an increase in myocardial contractility. Epinephrine dilates vessels of the liver and skeletal muscle and causes an increase in myocardial contractility. Some adrenocortical hormones, such as hydrocortisone, increase the effects of the catecholamines—norepinephrine and epinephrine.

Thyroid hormone, specifically triiodothyronine, causes increases in both heart rate and contractility, resulting in an increase in cardiac output; it also decreases systemic vascular resistance. Triiodothyronine acts directly on the cardiac myocytes to cause gene transcription and cellular changes that result in more calcium release from the sarcoplasmic reticulum.[18] Awareness of these changes helps to understand the cardiovascular changes that occur with thyroid diseases. Growth hormone, working together with insulin-like growth factor-1 (IGF-1), also has been shown to increase myocardial contractility.[19] Decreases in levels of growth hormone or thyroid hormone may result in bradycardia (heart rate below 60 beats/min), reduced cardiac output, and low blood pressure. (Other hormones are discussed in the Regulation of Blood Pressure section.)

SYSTEMIC CIRCULATION

The arteries and veins of the systemic circulation are illustrated in Fig. 31.16. Oxygenated blood leaves the left side of the heart through the aorta and flows into the systemic arteries. These arteries branch into small arterioles, which branch into the smallest vessels, the capillaries, where nutrient and waste product exchange between the blood and tissues occurs. Blood from the capillaries then enters tiny venules that join to form the larger veins, which return venous blood to the right heart (see Fig. 31.1B). Peripheral vascular system is the term used to describe the part of the systemic circulation that is outside of the chest or abdomen, consisting primarily of the vessels that supply blood to the extremities. Cerebrovascular system is the term used to describe the vessels that supply blood to the neck, head, and brain.

Structure of Blood Vessels

Blood vessel walls are composed of three layers: (1) the tunica intima (innermost, or intimal, layer), (2) the tunica media (middle, or medial, layer), and (3) the tunica externa or adventitia (outermost, or external, layer), which also contains nerves and lymphatic vessels. These layers are illustrated in Fig. 31.17. Blood vessel walls vary in thickness, depending on the thickness or absence of one or more of these three layers. Cells of the larger vessel walls are nourished by the vasa vasorum, small vessels located in the tunica externa, and innervated by perivascular nerves. The vasa vasorum arises from the blood vessel itself or from other vessels nearby.

Adults are capable of growing new blood vessels through three processes, all of which are important in wound healing but also contribute to tumor growth. The three processes are angiogenesis, arteriogenesis, and vasculogenesis. Both angiogenesis and arteriogenesis occur by growth of new vessels that branch from existing vessels. Angiogenesis is branching of small vessels, such as capillaries, whereas arteriogenesis occurs by branching

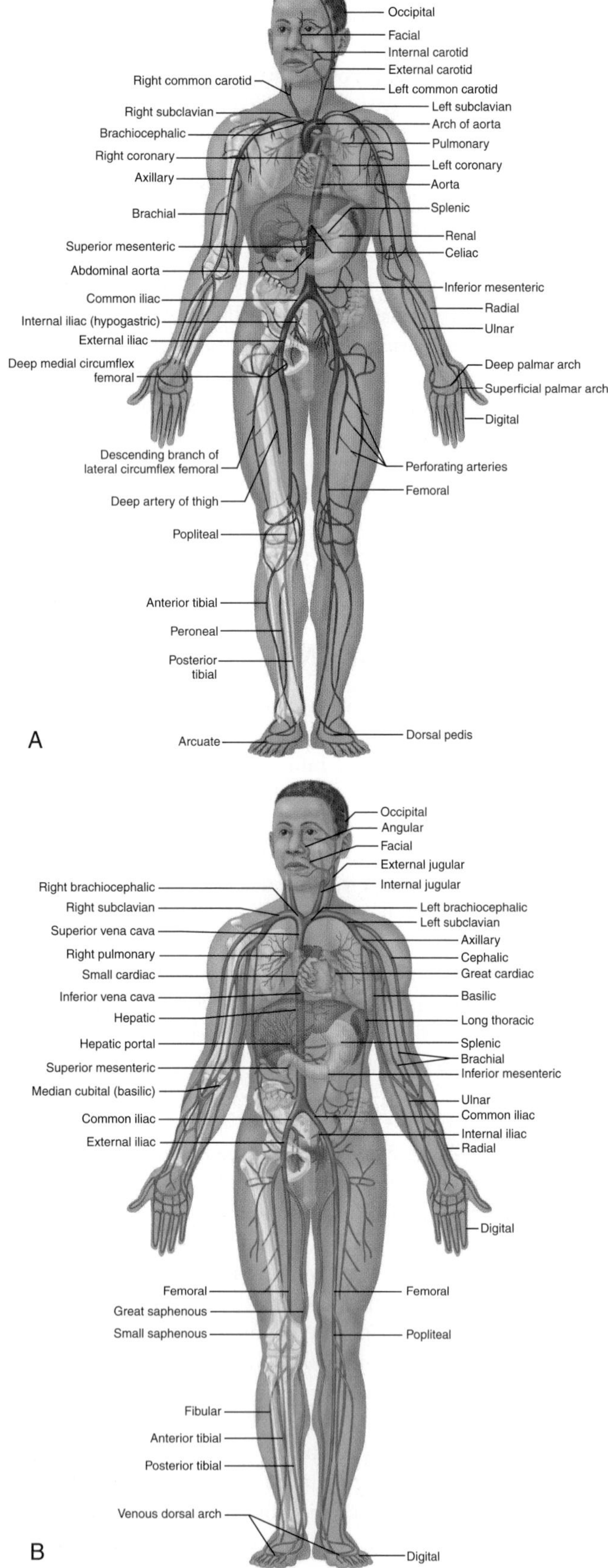

Fig. 31.16 Circulatory System. (A) Principal arteries of the body. **(B)** Principal veins of the body. (From Patton KT, Thibodeau GA. *The human body in health & disease*, St. Louis: Elsevier; 2018.)

from larger vessels, such as arterioles. Vasculogenesis is a term that refers to the growth of vessels from progenitor or stem-like cells that originate in the bone marrow and other body tissues.

Arterial Vessels

An artery is a thick-walled, pulsating blood vessel transporting blood away from the heart. In the systemic circulation, arteries carry oxygenated blood. When the iron in hemoglobin is oxygenated, it turns bright red, which is why arterial vessels are often color-coded red in illustrations (see Fig. 31.17). Arterial walls are composed of elastic connective tissue, fibrous connective tissue, and smooth muscle. There are two types of arteries: elastic and muscular. Elastic arteries have a thick tunica media with more elastic fibers than smooth muscle fibers. Elastic arteries are located close to the heart and include the aorta and its major branches and the pulmonary trunk. Elasticity allows the vessel to absorb energy and stretch as blood is ejected from the heart during systole. During diastole, elasticity promotes recoil of the arteries, maintaining blood pressure within the vessels.

Muscular arteries, consisting of the medium and small size arteries, are farther from the heart than the elastic arteries. They contain more muscle fibers and fewer elastic fibers than the elastic arteries and they function to distribute blood to arterioles throughout the body (see Fig. 31.17). Because their smooth muscle can contract or relax, they play a role in blood flow control and in directing flow to body parts with the highest need at any point in time. For example, during exercise more blood is sent to the skeletal muscles, while after a meal more blood is directed to the gut and liver. Contraction narrows the vessel lumen (the internal cavity of the vessel), which diminishes flow through the vessel (vasoconstriction). When the smooth muscle layer relaxes, more blood flows through the vessel lumen (vasodilation).

An artery becomes an arteriole where the diameter of its lumen narrows to less than 0.5 mm. Arterioles are mainly composed of smooth muscle and regulate the flow of blood into the capillaries by constricting or dilating to either slow or increase the flow of blood into the capillaries (Fig. 31.18). The thick smooth muscle layer of the arterioles is a major determinant of the resistance blood encounters as it flows through the systemic circulation.

The capillary network is composed of connective channels called metarterioles and "true" capillaries (see Fig. 31.18). Metarterioles have discontinuous smooth muscle cells in their tunica media, whereas capillaries have no smooth muscle cells. There is a ring of smooth muscle called the precapillary sphincter at the point where capillaries branch from metarterioles. As the sphincters contract and relax, they regulate blood flow through the capillary beds. The precapillary sphincters help to maintain arterial pressure and regulate selective flow to vascular beds.

Capillaries are composed solely of a layer of endothelial cells surrounded by a basement membrane (see Fig. 31.17). Their thin walls and unique structure make possible the rapid exchange of water; small soluble molecules; some larger molecules, such as albumin; and cells of the innate and adaptive components of the immune system between the blood and the interstitial fluid. Based on their structure, three types of capillaries have been described: *continuous*, *sinusoid*, and *fenestrated*. In the renal glomerulus,

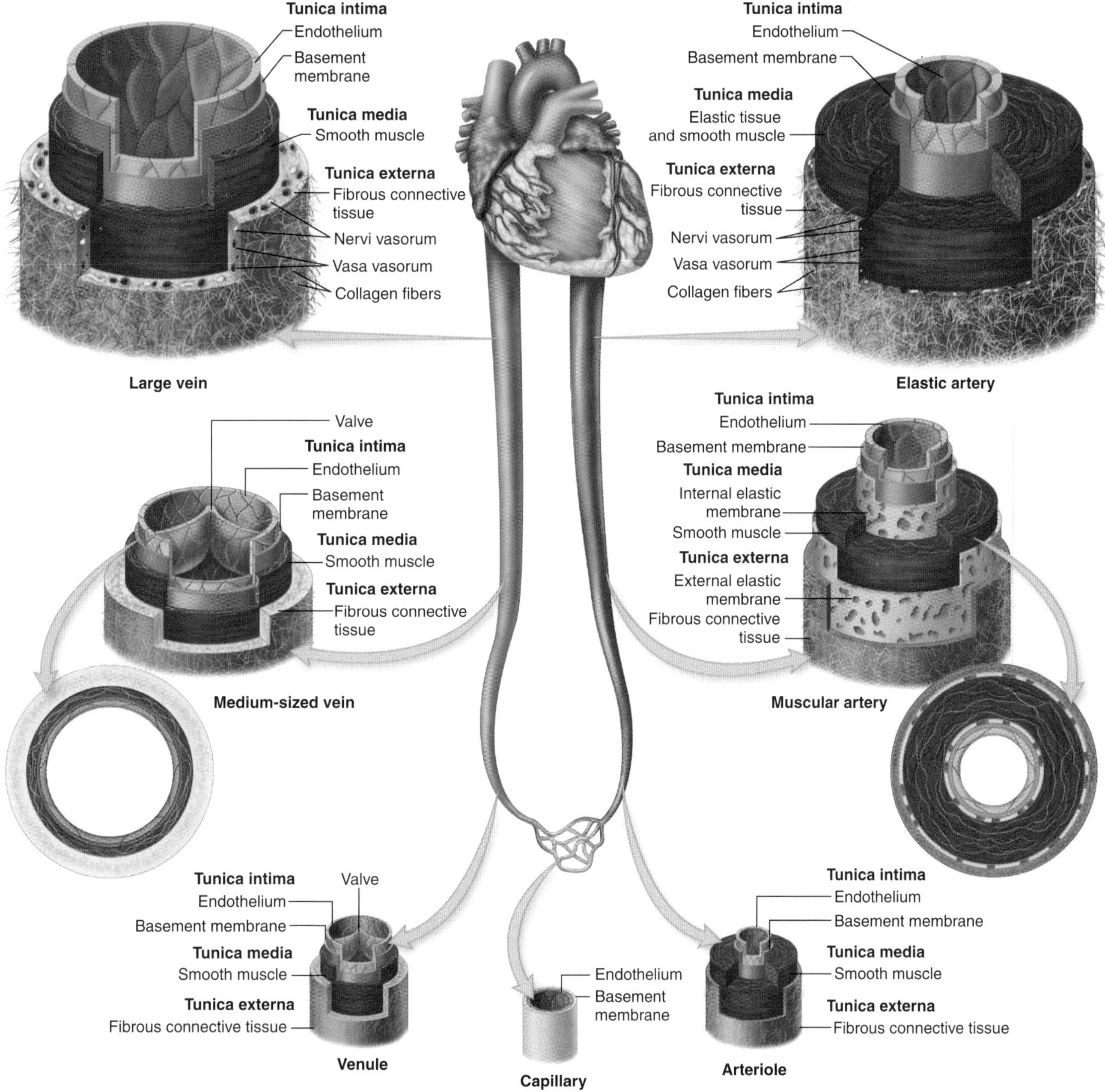

Fig. 31.17 Structure of Blood Vessels, and an Artery and Vein. Structure of blood vessels. The tunica externa of the veins are color-coded *blue* and the arteries *red.* (From Patton KT. *Anatomy & physiology*, 10th edition. St. Louis: Elsevier; 2019.)

for example, the endothelial cells contain oval windows or pores termed fenestrations, which are covered by a thin diaphragm. Sinusoid capillaries are found in the liver and bone marrow.

Substances pass between the capillary lumen and the interstitial fluid (1) through junctions between endothelial cells, (2) through fenestrations in endothelial cells, (3) in vesicles moved by active transport across the endothelial cell membrane, or (4) by diffusion through the endothelial cell membrane (Fig. 31.19B). A single capillary may be only 0.5 to 1 mm in length and 0.01 mm in diameter, but the capillaries are so numerous their total surface area may be more than 600 m^2 (about 100 football fields).

Endothelium

The vascular endothelium, or blood vessel lining, is important to several body functions and is sometimes considered a separate endocrine organ. All tissues depend on a blood supply, and the blood supply depends on endothelial cells, which form the lining, or endothelium, of the blood vessel (see Fig. 31.19). In addition to substance transport, the vascular endothelium has important roles in coagulation, antithrombogenesis, and fibrinolysis; immune system function; tissue and vessel growth and wound healing; and vasomotion, the contraction and relaxation of vessels. Table 31.3 summarizes some of the more important endothelial functions. Because of its varying roles, the actual structure of the endothelium

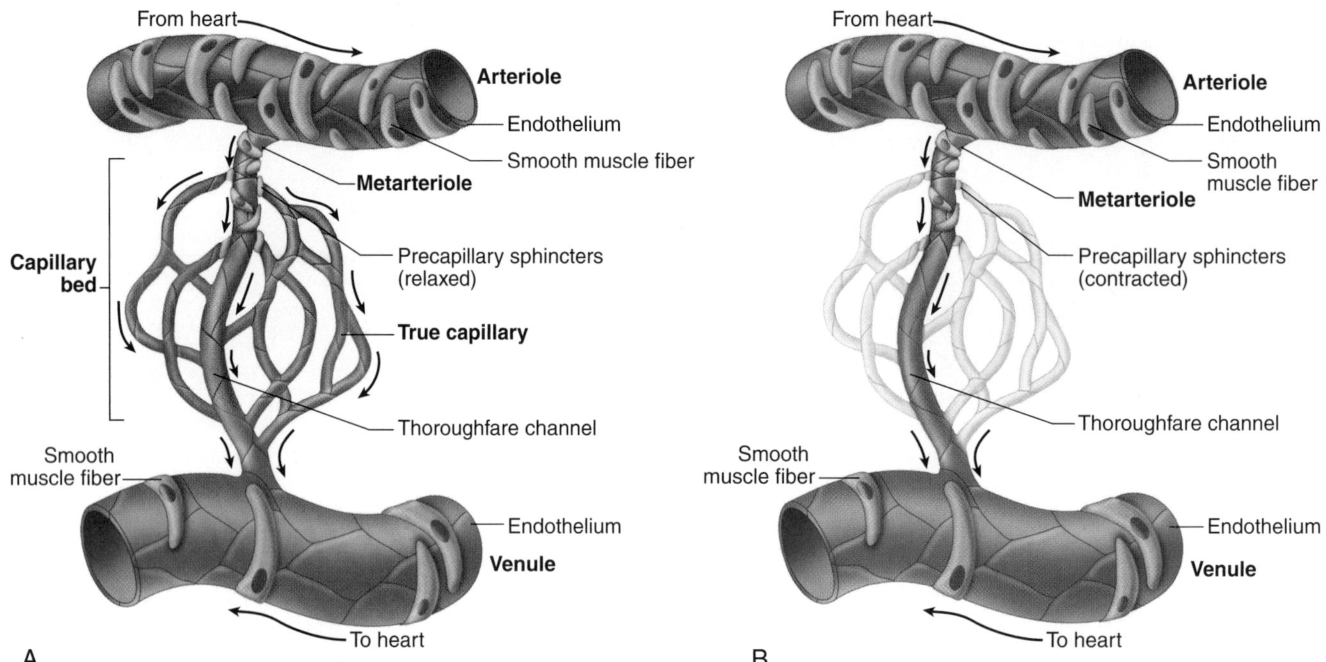

Fig. 31.18 Microcirculation. Control of local blood flow through a capillary network is regulated by altering the tone of precapillary sphincters surrounding arterioles and metarterioles. **(A)** Sphincters are relaxed, permitting blood flow to enter the capillary bed. **(B)** With sphincters contracted, blood flows from the metarteriole directly into the thoroughfare channel, bypassing the capillary bed. (From Patton KT. *Anatomy & physiology*, 10th edition. St. Louis: Mosby; 2019.)

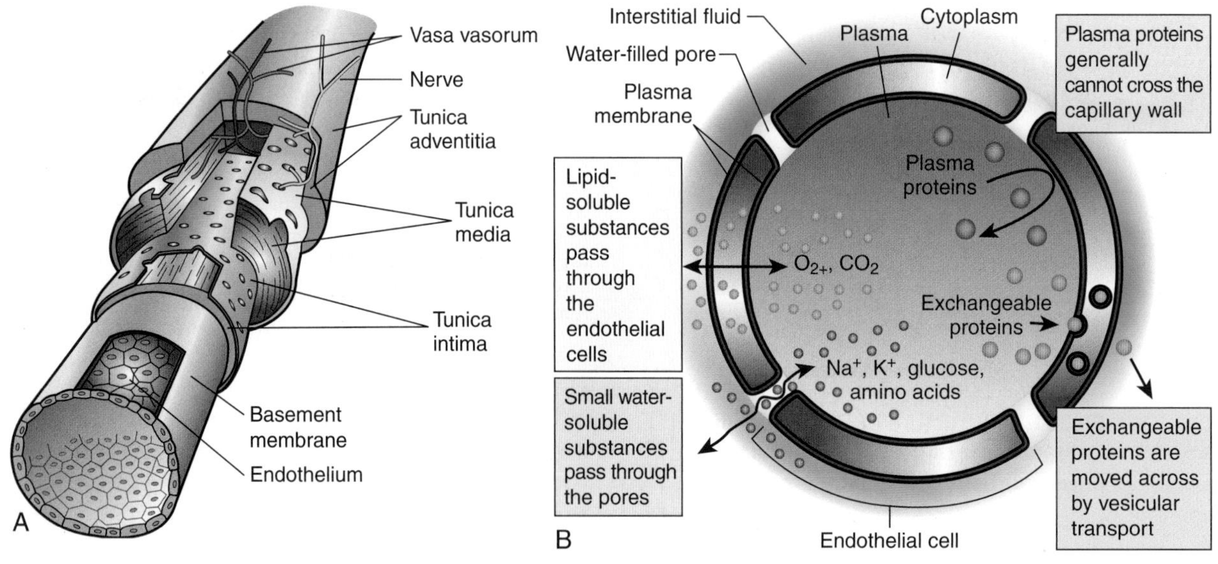

Fig. 31.19 Vascular Endothelium. **(A)** This shows the endothelial cells in context with the entire blood vessel. The endothelial cells arrange themselves as a single-layer lining that has numerous critical functions (see Table 31.3). **(B)** The endothelium supports numerous functions through synesis and release of vasoactive fibers.

may vary in different vascular beds. For example, within lymph nodes the endothelial cells of specialized venules, called *high endothelial venules*, are uniquely structured to support the movement of lymphocytes from the blood into the lymph node.[20] Endothelial injury and dysfunction are central processes in many of the most common and serious cardiovascular disorders, including hypertension and atherosclerosis (see Chapter 32).

Veins

Compared with arteries, veins are thin walled with more fibrous connective tissue and have a larger diameter (see Fig. 31.17). A given vein is larger than the artery that lies within the same sheath. Veins also are more numerous than arteries. The smallest venules downstream from the capillaries have an endothelial lining and are surrounded by connective tissue.

TABLE 31.3 Functions of the Endothelium

Function	Actions Involved
Filtration and permeability	Facilitates transport of large molecules via vesicular transport movement through intercellular junctions Facilitates transport of small molecules via movement of vesicles, through opening of tight junctions, and across cytoplasm
Vasomotion	Stimulates vascular relaxation through production of nitric oxide, prostacyclin, and other vasodilators Stimulates vascular constriction through production of endothelin-1 and of angiotensin II by the action of endothelial angiotensin-converting enzyme on angiotensin I
Hemostatic balance	Endothelial surface is normally antithrombotic and maintains a balance between procoagulant and anticoagulant factors, as well as profibrinolytic and antifibrinolytic factors Anticoagulant factors include prostacyclin, nitric oxide, antithrombin, thrombomodulin, tissue factor pathway inhibitor, and heparins Procoagulant factors include tissue factor (factor VII), factor VIII, factor V, and plasminogen activator inhibitor-1 (PAI-1) Profibrinolytic factors are tissue- and urokinase-type plasminogen activating factor and PAI-1 Antifibrinolytic factor is tissue plasminogen activator
Inflammation/ immunity	Expresses chemotactic agents and adhesion molecules that support white blood cells (including monocytes, neutrophils, and lymphocytes) moving into tissues Expresses receptors for oxidized lipoproteins, allowing them to enter vascular intima
Angiogenesis/ vessel growth	Releases growth factors, such as endothelin-1, and heparins for vascular smooth muscle cells
Lipid metabolism	Expresses receptors for lipoprotein lipase and low-density lipoproteins (LDLs)

From Griendling KK., Harrison DG, Alexander RW. Biology of the vessel wall. In: Fuster V, Walsh RA, Harrington RA, eds. *Hurst's the heart*, 13th edition. Philadelphia: McGraw-Hill; 2011; Rajendran P, Rengarajan T, Thangavel J, et al. The vascular endothelium and human diseases. *International Journal of Biological Sciences*, 2013;9(10):1057–1069.

The largest venules have some smooth muscle fibers in their thin tunica media. The venous tunica externa has less elastic tissue than that in arteries, so veins do not recoil as much or as rapidly after distention. Like arteries, veins receive nourishment from tiny vasa vasorum.

Some veins, typically in the legs, contain valves to facilitate the one-way flow of blood toward the heart (Fig. 31.20). These valves are folds of the tunica intima and resemble the semilunar valves of the heart. Backflow in veins of the legs is stopped as the flaps of the valves fill with blood and block the vessel. The position of the valves also facilitates blood flow in the proper direction during venous compression. When a person stands up, contraction of the skeletal muscles of the legs compresses the deep veins of the legs and assists the flow of blood toward the heart and against the force of gravity. This important mechanism of venous return is called the muscle pump (see Fig. 31.20B).

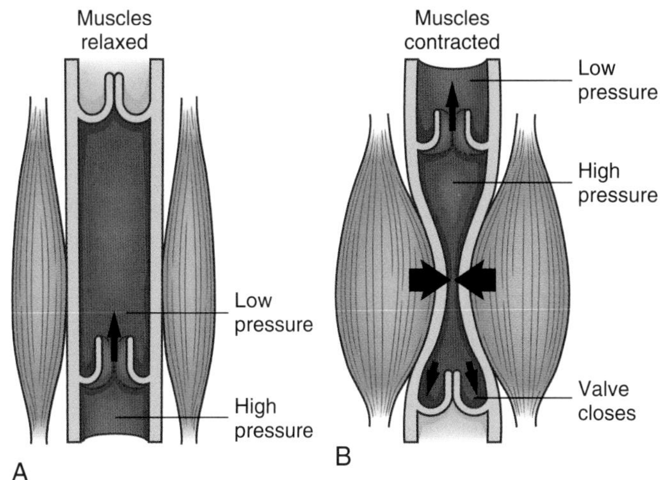

Fig. 31.20 Venous Valves and the Muscle Pump. In veins, one-way valves aid circulation by preventing backflow of venous blood when pressure in a local area is low. **(A)** Blood is moved toward the heart as valves in the veins are forced open by pressure from volume of blood downstream and the neighboring muscles are relaxed. **(B)** When pressure below the valve drops, blood begins to flow backward but fills the "pockets" formed by the valve flaps, pushing the flaps together and thus blocking further backward flow. Contraction in the adjacent muscles and the valves of the systemic veins assist in the return of unoxygenated blood to the right heart.

Factors Affecting Blood Flow

Blood flow, the amount of fluid moved per unit of time, is usually expressed as liters or milliliters per minute (L/min or mL/min). Factors that influence blood flow include pressure, resistance, velocity, laminar versus turbulent flow, and compliance, with the most important of these being pressure and resistance.

Pressure and Resistance

Pressure in a liquid system is the force exerted on the liquid per unit area and is expressed clinically as millimeters of mercury (mm Hg), or torr (1 torr = 1 mm Hg). Blood flow to an organ depends partly on the pressure difference between the arterial and venous vessels supplying that organ. Fluid moves from the arterial "side" of the capillaries where the pressure is higher to the venous side where the pressure is lower.

Resistance is the opposition to blood flow. Most opposition to blood flow results from the diameter and length of the vessels. Changes in blood flow through an organ result from changes in the vascular resistance within the organ because of increases or decreases in vessel diameter and the opening or closing of vascular channels. Resistance in a vessel is inversely related to blood flow—that is, increased resistance leads to decreased blood flow. The Poiseuille law indicates that resistance is directly related to tube length and blood viscosity and inversely related to the radius of the tube to the fourth power (r^4). Resistance to flow cannot be measured directly, but it can be calculated if the pressure difference and flow volumes are known. Resistance to blood flow in a single vessel is determined by the radius and length of the blood vessel and by the blood viscosity.

The most important factor determining resistance *in a single vessel* is the radius or diameter of the vessel's lumen. Small changes in the lumen's radius or diameter lead to large changes in vascular resistance. Because vessel length is relatively constant but lumen size is quite variable, length is not as important as lumen size in determining flow through a single vessel. Clinically, vasoconstriction of arterioles will decrease blood flow to organs perfused by those vessels, whereas vasodilation will increase perfusion. Vasoconstriction or vasodilation of multiple arterioles leads to changes in TPR that may cause a rise of fall in systemic blood pressure.

Blood vessel radius is usually the key factor in determining the TPR because viscosity, the consistency of the fluid, is relatively constant. Thick fluids move more slowly and cause greater resistance to flow than thin fluids—just think of honey as compared to water. The viscosity of blood depends on the red cell content. The greater the percentage of red cells in the blood, the more viscous the blood. This relationship is expressed as the hematocrit. A high hematocrit value reduces flow through the blood vessels, particularly the microcirculation (arterioles, capillaries, venules). An elevated hematocrit level is relatively rare. Conditions with elevated hematocrits include a lack of body water, cyanotic congenital heart disease (see Chapter 33), or polycythemia (see Chapter 29), and can lead to increased cardiac work as a result of increased vascular resistance.

Resistance to flow through a *system of vessels*, or total resistance, depends not only on characteristics of individual vessels, but also on whether the vessels are arranged in *series* (end to end) or in *parallel* (side to side) and on the total cross-sectional area of the system. Vessels arranged in parallel provide less resistance than vessels arranged in series. Blood flowing through the distributing arteries, beginning with branches off the aorta and ending at arterioles in the capillary bed, encounters more resistance than blood flowing through the capillary bed itself, where flow is distributed among many short, tiny branches arranged in parallel (Fig. 31.21). The total cross-sectional area of the arteriolar system is greater than that of the arterial system, yet the greater number of arterioles arranged in series leads to great resistance to flow in the arteriolar system. In contrast, the capillary system has a larger number of vessels arranged in parallel than the arteriolar system, and the total cross-sectional area is much greater; thus there is lower resistance overall through the capillary system. The resulting slow velocity of flow in each capillary is optimal for capillary-tissue exchange.

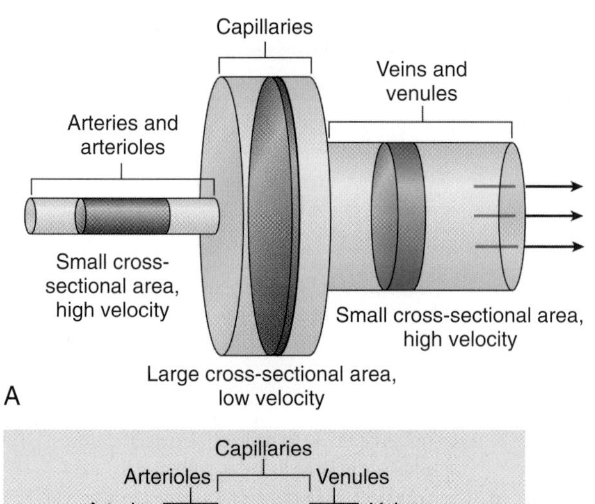

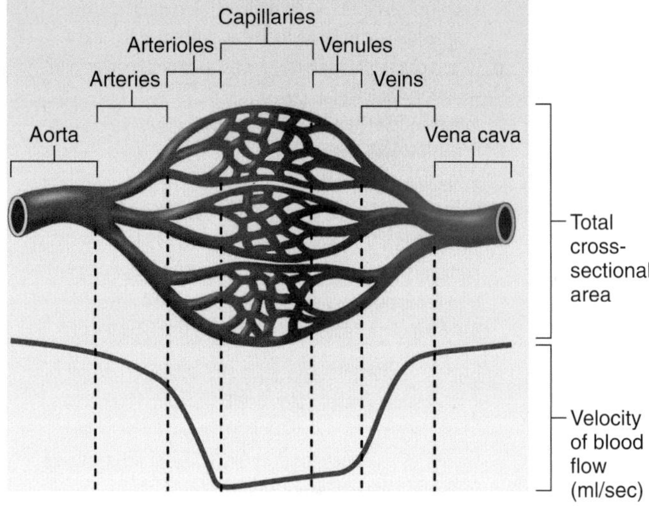

Fig. 31.21 Relationship Between Cross-Sectional Area and Velocity of Blood Flow. (A) Small and large cross-sectional areas and their relationship to velocity changes. **(B)** Total cross-sectional area of different kinds of blood vessels with velocity of blood flow (mL/s). Blood flows with great speed in the large arteries. However, branching of arterial vessels increases the total cross-sectional area of the arterioles and capillaries, reducing the flow rate. When capillaries merge into venules and venules merge into veins, the total cross-sectional area decreases, causing the flow rate to increase. (From Patton KT. *Anatomy & physiology*, 10th edition. St. Louis: Elsevier; 2019.)

Velocity

Blood velocity, or speed, is the *distance* blood travels in a unit of time, usually centimeters per second (cm/s). It is directly related to blood flow (the *amount* of blood moved per unit of time) and inversely related to the cross-sectional area of the vessel in which the blood is flowing (see Fig. 31.21). As blood moves from the aorta to the capillaries, the total cross-sectional area of the vessels increases and the velocity decreases.

Laminar Versus Turbulent Flow

Flow through a tubular system can be either laminar or turbulent. Blood flow through the vessels, except where vessels split or branch, is usually laminar. In laminar flow, concentric layers of molecules move "straight ahead," with each layer flowing at a slightly different velocity (Fig. 31.22A). The cohesive attraction between the fluid and the vessel wall prevents the molecules of blood that are in contact with the wall from moving at all. The next thin layer of blood is able to slide slowly past the stationary layer and so on until, at the center, the blood velocity is greatest. Large vessels have room for a large center layer; therefore they have less resistance to flow and greater flow and velocity than smaller vessels.

Where flow is obstructed, the vessel turns or branches, or blood flows over rough surfaces, the flow becomes turbulent with whorls or eddy currents that produce noise, causing a bruit (vascular murmur) to be heard on auscultation (see Fig. 31.22B). Resistance increases with turbulence, which

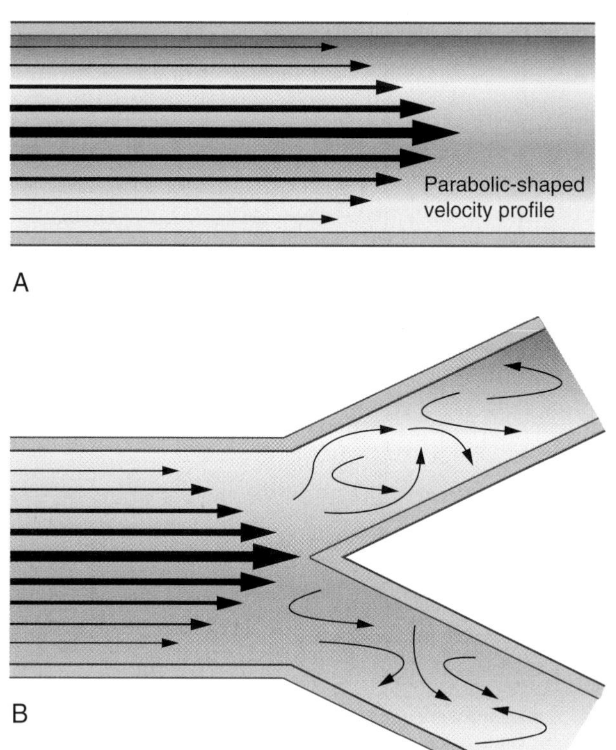

Fig. 31.22 Laminar and Turbulent Blood Flow. (A) Laminar flow. Fluid flows in long, smooth-walled tubes as if it is composed of a large number of concentric layers. (B) Turbulent flow. Turbulent flow is caused by numerous small currents flowing crosswise or oblique to the long axis of the vessel, resulting in flowing whorls and eddy currents.

frequently occurs in areas with atherosclerotic plaque (e). Wall shear stress (WSS) is the complex interaction between the vessel wall's endothelial layer and blood hemodynamics. Much investigation is on the consequences of lower WSS and the promotion of atherosclerotic plaque development distal to an induced stenosis.[21] Clarifying WSS and the perivascular changes with inflammation, macrophage activation, medial thinning, and plaque disruption is critical to understanding the pathogenesis of atherosclerosis.

Vascular Compliance

Vascular compliance is the increase in volume a vessel can accommodate with a given increase in pressure. Compliance depends on factors related to the nature of a vessel wall, such as the ratio of elastic fibers to muscle fibers in the wall. Elastic arteries are more compliant than muscular arteries. The veins are more compliant than either type of artery because they have less smooth muscle, and they can serve as storage areas for the circulatory system.

Compliance determines a vessel's response to pressure changes. For example, a large volume of blood can be accommodated by the venous system with only a small increase in pressure. In the less compliant arterial system, where smaller volumes and higher pressures are normal, even small changes in blood volume can cause significant changes in arterial pressure.

Stiffness is the opposite of compliance. Several conditions and disorders can cause stiffness, with the most common being aging and atherosclerosis (see Chapter 32). Increases in stiffness of arterial walls increases peak arterial pressure at a given volume of blood.

Regulation of Blood Pressure

Arterial Pressure

The arterial blood pressure is determined by the cardiac output multiplied by the peripheral resistance (Fig. 31.23). The systolic blood pressure is the highest arterial blood pressure after ventricular contraction or systole. The diastolic blood pressure is the lowest arterial blood pressure that occurs during ventricular filling or diastole. The mean arterial pressure (MAP), which is the average pressure in the arteries throughout the cardiac cycle, depends on the elastic properties of the arterial walls and the mean volume of blood in the arterial system. MAP can be approximated from the measured values of the systolic (P_s) and diastolic (P_d) pressures as follows:

$$\text{MAP} = P_d + \frac{1}{3}(P_s - P_d)$$

The normal range for MAP is 70 to 110 mm Hg. The difference between the systolic pressure and the diastolic pressure ($P_s - P_d$) is called the pulse pressure and typically is between 40 and 50 mm Hg. The pulse pressure is directly related to arterial wall stiffness and stroke volume.

During a wide range of physiologic conditions, including changes in body position, muscular activity, and circulating blood volume, arterial pressure is regulated within a fairly narrow range to maintain tissue perfusion, or blood supply to the capillary beds. The major factors and relationships that regulate arterial blood pressure are summarized in Fig. 31.23.

Effects of Cardiac Output

The cardiac output (minute volume) of the heart can be changed by alterations in the heart rate, stroke volume (volume of blood ejected during each ventricular contraction), or both. An increase in cardiac output without a decrease in peripheral resistance will cause the MAP and flow rate to increase. The higher arterial pressure increases blood flow through the arterioles. On the other hand, a decrease in the cardiac output causes a drop in the MAP and arteriolar flow if peripheral resistance stays constant (Table 31.4).

Effects of Total Peripheral Resistance

Total resistance in the systemic circulation, known as either SVR or TPR, is primarily a function of arteriolar diameter. If cardiac output remains constant, arteriolar constriction raises the MAP by reducing the flow of blood into the capillaries, whereas arteriolar dilation has the opposite effect. Reflex control of total cardiac output and peripheral resistance includes (1) sympathetic stimulation of the heart, arterioles, and veins; and (2) parasympathetic stimulation of the heart (Fig. 31.24). The cardiovascular center in the medulla receives input from arterial baroreceptors and chemoreceptors throughout the vascular system and then modifies vagal and sympathetic output

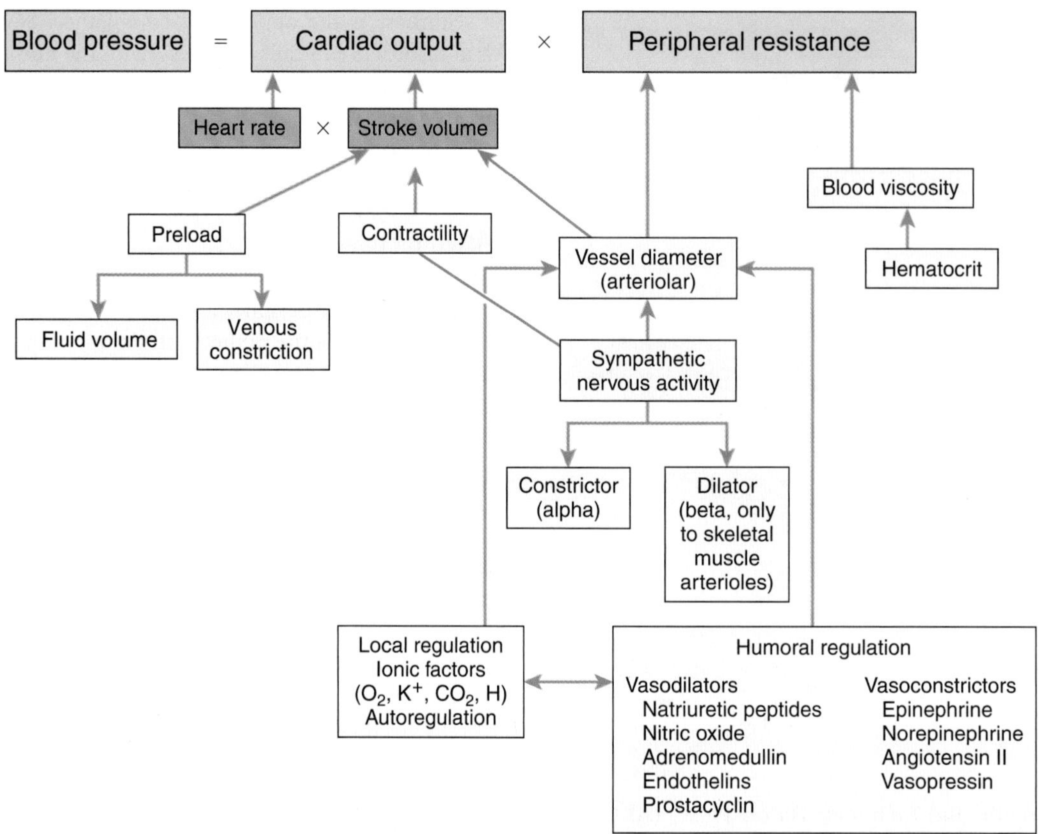

Fig. 31.23 Factors Regulating Blood Pressure. *O_2*, Oxygen; *K^+*, potassium; *CO_2*, carbon dioxide; *H*, hydrogen.

TABLE 31.4 Factors that Affect Mean Arterial Pressure and Capillary Flow

	Mean Arterial Pressure	Capillary Flow
Peripheral Resistance[a]		
Increased	Increased	Decreased
Decreased	Decreased	Increased
Heart Rate[b]		
Increased	Increased	Increased
Decreased	Decreased	Decreased
Stroke Volume[c]		
Increased	Increased	Increased
Decreased	Decreased	Decreased

[a]Cardiac output maintained constant.
[b]Peripheral resistance and stroke volume constant.
[c]Peripheral resistance and heart rate constant.
From Little RC. *Physiology of the Heart and Circulation*. 3rd ed. St Louis: Mosby; 1985.

to control heart rate and contractility, plus vascular diameter. Vasoconstriction is regulated by an area of the brainstem that maintains a constant (tonic) output of norepinephrine from sympathetic fibers in the peripheral arterioles. This tonic activity is essential for maintenance of blood pressure.

Baroreceptors. As discussed previously, baroreceptors are stretch receptors located predominantly in the aorta and in the carotid sinus (see Fig. 31.24A). They respond to pressure-related changes in smooth muscle fiber length by altering their rate of discharge and supply sensory information to the cardiovascular center in the brainstem. When activated (stretched), the baroreceptors decrease cardiac output by lowering the heart rate, stroke volume, and peripheral resistance, and thus lower blood pressure.

Arterial chemoreceptors. Specialized areas within the medulla oblongata, aortic arch, and carotid arteries are sensitive to concentrations of O_2, carbon dioxide (CO_2), and hydrogen ions (pH) in the blood (see Fig. 31.24B). Although these chemoreceptors are most important for respiratory control, they also transmit impulses to the medullary cardiovascular centers that regulate blood pressure. A decrease in arterial oxygen concentration (hypoxemia), an increase in arterial $PaCO_2$ concentration, or to a lesser extent a decrease in arterial blood pH causes a reflexive increase in heart rate, stroke volume, and blood pressure.

Effects of hormones. Hormones influence blood pressure regulation through their effects on vascular smooth muscle and blood volume. By constricting or dilating the arterioles in organs, hormones can (1) increase or decrease the blood flow in response to the body's needs, (2) redistribute blood volume during hemorrhage or shock, and (3) regulate heat loss. The key vasoconstrictor hormones include angiotensin II,

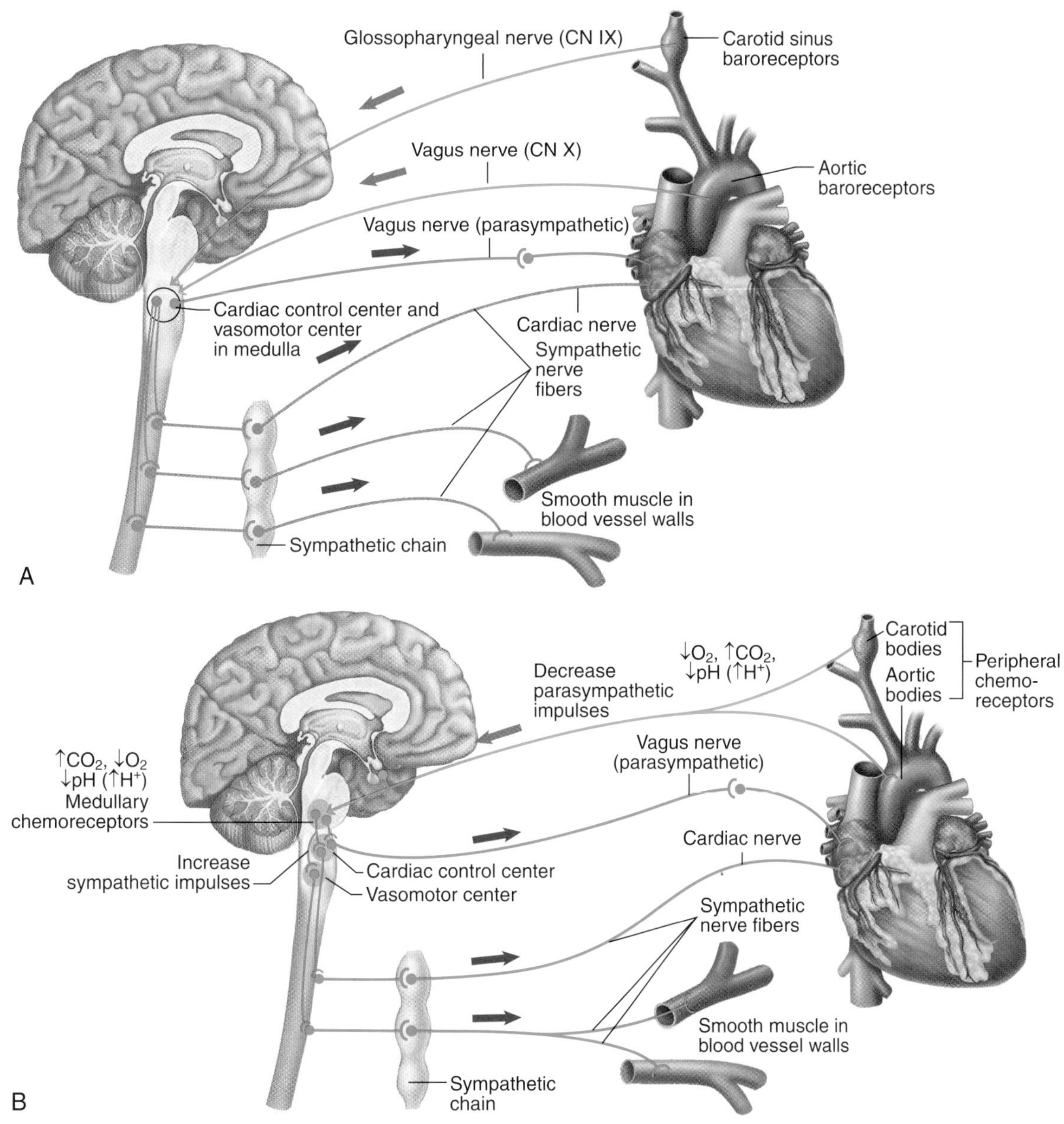

Fig. 31.24 Baroreceptors and Chemoreceptor Reflex Control of Blood Pressure. **(A)** Baroreceptor reflexes. **(B)** Vasomotor chemoreflexes. *CN*, Cranial nerve; O_2, oxygen; CO_2, carbon dioxide; H^+, hydrogen. (Modified from Patton KT. *Anatomy & physiology*, 10th edition. St. Louis: Elsevier; 2019.)

antidiuretic hormone (ADH; vasopressin), epinephrine, and norepinephrine. The main vasodilator hormones are the atrial natriuretic hormones, nitric oxide, adrenomedullin, and endothelins. By causing fluid retention or loss, aldosterone, ADH, and the natriuretic hormones can influence stroke volume and thus blood pressure. A variety of other hormones, including adipokines and insulin, may be related to the hypertension that occurs with chronic conditions, such as adiposity and diabetes mellitus. However, these factors have not been clearly demonstrated to play a role in blood pressure regulation in healthy individuals.

Vasoconstrictor hormones. The vasoconstrictor hormones include epinephrine; norepinephrine; angiotensin II, which is part of the renin-angiotensin-aldosterone system (RAAS) (see Chapters 5 and 32); and ADH. Epinephrine, the catecholamine hormone released from the adrenal medulla, causes vasoconstriction in most vascular beds except the coronary, liver, and skeletal muscle circulations. Norepinephrine mainly acts as a neurotransmitter; however, some also is released from the adrenal medulla. When the RAAS is activated, angiotensin II (ANG II) binds to the AT_1 receptor and serves as a potent vasoconstrictor. Other RAAS pathways oppose this action (see Fig. 32.2). High levels of aldosterone also can increase vascular tone.

ADH and aldosterone also affect blood pressure by increasing blood volume through their influence on fluid reabsorption in the kidney and by stimulating thirst. ADH causes the reabsorption of water from tubular fluid in the distal tubule and collecting duct of the nephron. Aldosterone, the end product of

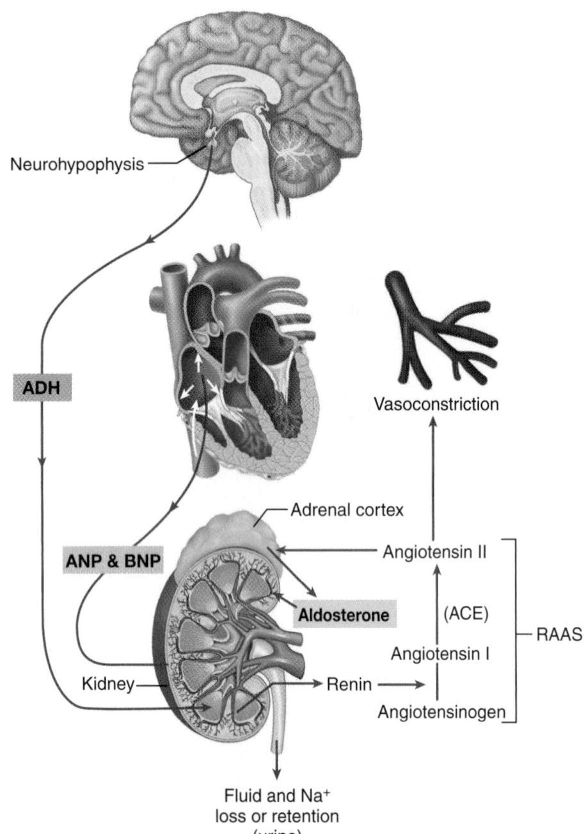

Fig. 31.25 Three Mechanisms That Influence Total Plasma Volume. Antidiuretic hormone *(ADH)* mechanism and renin-angiotensin-aldosterone system *(RAAS)* to increase water and sodium retention by the kidney and thus increase total plasma volume. Atrial natriuretic peptide *(ANP)* and B-type natriuretic peptide *(BNP)* antagonize these mechanisms by promoting water and sodium loss, thus promoting a decrease in total plasma volume. *ACE,* Angiotensin-converting enzyme; *Na⁺,* sodium. (Modified from Patton, K. T. [2019]. *Anatomy & physiology* [10th ed.]. St Louis: Elsevier.) ACE, Angiotensin-converting enzyme; *Na⁺*, sodium. (Modified from Patton KT. *Anatomy & physiology*, 10th edition. St. Louis: Elsevier; 2019.)

the RAAS, stimulates the reabsorption of sodium, chloride, and water from the same locations in the kidney (Fig. 31.25; also see Chapters 3 and 22).

Vasodilator hormones. There are numerous vasodilator hormones, most of which have other important effects on blood volume and vascular function. The natriuretic peptides (NPs) include atrial natriuretic peptide (ANP), B-type natriuretic peptide (BNP), C-type natriuretic peptide (CNP), and urodilatin. These hormones function as both vasodilators and regulators of sodium and water excretion (natriuresis and diuresis) (see Chapter 3). ANP and BNP are released from myocytes in heart. Increased pressure or diastolic volume in the heart stimulates the release of these peptide hormones which then stimulate secretion of sodium and water from the kidney (see Fig. 31.25). Serum levels of BNP are increased in many types of cardiac disease including heart failure, hypertension, pulmonary embolism, valvular heart disease, and chronic coronary artery disease, and can be used to predict prognosis. Neprilysin is a drug that prevents the degradation of the natriuretic peptides and can be used in combination with other medications for the treatment of severe acute heart failure (see Chapter 32).[22] Many studies are underway to develop other medications that can mimic the positive effects of the natriuretic peptides.[23]

Other vasodilating mediators include nitric oxide (NO), adrenomedullin (ADM), the endothelins, and prostacyclin. These mediators are being investigated to determine if they or their inhibitors might be useful drugs for the treatment of cardiovascular diseases or if their levels might be useful in determining the prognosis of persons with known disease. Nitric oxide (NO) is a soluble gas continuously synthesized in endothelial cells by the enzyme nitric oxide synthase (NOS). NO has a wide range of biologic properties that maintain vascular homeostasis, including modulation of vascular dilator tone, regulation of local cell growth, and protection of the vessel from injurious consequences of platelets and cells circulating in blood. NO plays a crucial role in the normal endothelial function. An emerging list of conditions, including those commonly associated as risk factors for atherosclerosis such as hypertension, hypercholesterolemia, smoking, diabetes mellitus, and heart failure, is associated with diminished release of nitric oxide into the arterial wall because of impaired synthesis or excessive oxidative degradation (Fig. 31.26).[24,25] Adrenomedullin (ADM), a peptide with powerful vasodilatory activity, is present in numerous tissues. It has been found to have numerous cardiovascular effects, including a role in fetal cardiovascular system development and vasodilation. ADM is released by endothelial cells in conditions of vascular wall stress and plays a role in controlling vascular tone and blood pressure.[26] The endothelins are a family of three structurally similar peptides (ET-1, ET-2, and ET-3) and four receptors produced in cells in the vascular smooth muscle, the endothelium, the kidneys, and other organs. Understanding the physiologic and pathologic roles of these peptides has been complicated by the fact that endothelin binding to some receptors causes vasodilation and natriuresis, whereas binding to other receptors causes the opposite response—vasoconstriction plus sodium and water retention. Inhibitors to ET-1 have been approved for the treatment of pulmonary hypertension (see Chapter 35).

Prostacyclin is a vasodilator that is produced by the actions of cyclooxygenases (COX-1 and COX-2) on arachidonic acid. It has the additional properties of opposing clot formation (antithrombotic), decreasing platelet activity, and inhibiting the release of growth factors from macrophages and the endothelial cells. Nonsteroidal antiinflammatory drugs (NSAIDs) that inhibit these cyclooxygenases have been associated with cardiovascular disease risk in healthy people and in those with a known cardiovascular disease.[27]

Venous Pressure

The main determinants of venous blood pressure are (1) the volume of fluid within the veins and (2) the compliance (distensibility) of the vessel walls. The venous system typically accommodates about 66% of the total blood volume at any time, with venous pressure averaging less than 10 mm Hg. The systemic arteries accommodate about 11% of the total blood volume, with an average arterial pressure (blood pressure) of about

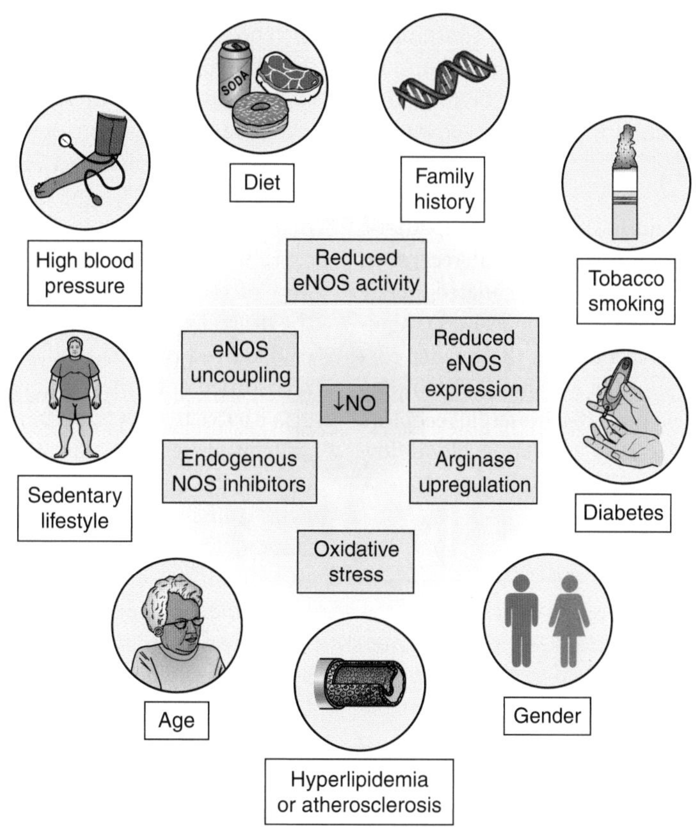

Fig. 31.26 Lifestyle Factors Associated With Reduced Bioavailability of Nitric Oxide (NO). *eNOS*, Endothelial nitric oxide synthase. (Adapted from Lundberg JO, Gladwin MT, Weitzberg E. Strategies to increase nitric oxide signalling in cardiovascular disease. *Nature Review Drug Discovery*, 2015;14:623–641.)

100 mm Hg; the remainder of the blood volume is within the heart, capillaries, and pulmonary circulation.

The sympathetic nervous system controls venous compliance. The walls of the veins are highly innervated by sympathetic fibers that control venous smooth muscle. Rather than constriction that would occur in the arteries, smooth muscle contraction in the veins results in stiffening of the vessel walls. This stiffening reduces venous distensibility and increases venous blood pressure, thus forcing more blood through the veins and into the right heart.

Two other mechanisms that increase venous pressure and venous return to the heart are (1) the skeletal muscle pump and (2) the respiratory pump. During skeletal muscle contraction, the veins within the muscles are partially compressed, causing decreased venous capacity and increased return to the heart (see Fig. 31.20B). The respiratory pump acts during inspiration, when the veins of the abdomen are partially compressed by the downward movement of the diaphragm. Increased abdominal pressure moves blood toward the heart.

Regulation of the Coronary Circulation

Coronary blood flow is directly proportional to the perfusion pressure and inversely proportional to the vascular resistance of the coronary bed. Coronary perfusion pressure is the difference between pressure in the aorta and pressure in the coronary vessels. Thus, aortic pressure is the driving pressure for the arteries and arterioles that perfuse the myocardium. Vasodilation and vasoconstriction maintain coronary blood flow despite stresses imposed by the constant contraction and relaxation of the heart muscle and despite shifts (within a physiologic range) of coronary perfusion pressure.

Several unique anatomic factors influence coronary blood flow. Because of their anatomic location, the aortic valve cusps can obstruct coronary blood flow by occluding the openings of the coronary arteries during systole. Also during systole, the coronary arteries are compressed by ventricular contraction. The resulting systolic compressive effect is particularly evident in the subendocardial layers of the left ventricular wall and can greatly increase resistance to coronary blood flow, with the result that most left ventricular coronary blood flow occurs during diastole. During the period of systolic compression, when flow is slowed or stopped, myoglobin, a protein in heart muscle that binds O_2, provides the supply of O_2 to the myocardium. Myoglobin's O_2 levels are replenished during diastole.

Autoregulation

Autoregulation (automatic self-regulation) enables organs to regulate blood flow by altering the resistance (diameter) in their arterioles. Autoregulation in the coronary circulation maintains the blood flow at a nearly constant rate at perfusion pressures (MAP) between 60 and 140 mm Hg when other influencing factors are held constant. Thus autoregulation helps to ensure constant coronary blood flow despite shifts in the perfusion pressure within the stated range.

Given that blood flow is directly related to pressure and inversely related to resistance, for flow to stay constant as pressure decreases, resistance also has to decrease; therefore the mechanisms underlying autoregulation must be related to control of smooth muscle contraction in the arteriolar walls.

Autonomic Regulation

Although the coronary vessels themselves contain sympathetic (α- and β-adrenergic) and parasympathetic neural receptors, coronary blood flow during regular activity is regulated locally by the factors that cause autoregulation. During exercise, however, the vasodilating effects of β_2-receptors on the smaller coronary resistance arteries are responsible for about 25% of any increase in blood flow. At the same time, α-adrenergic receptors in larger arteries cause vasoconstriction to direct the blood flow to the inner layers of the myocardium.

LYMPHATIC SYSTEM

The lymphatic system is a one-way network of lymphatic vessels and the lymph nodes (Figs. 31.27 and 31.28) that is important for immune function, fluid balance, and transport of lipids, hormones, and cytokines and is considered to be part of the circulatory system. Every day about 3 liters of fluid filters out of venous capillaries in body tissues and is not reabsorbed (Fig. 31.29). This fluid becomes the lymph that is carried by the lymphatic vessels to the chest, where it enters the venous circulation. The lymphatic vessels run in the same sheaths with the arteries and veins. (Lymph nodes and lymphoid tissues are described in Chapters 8 and 28.) The lymphatic capillaries are closed at the distal ends, as shown in Fig. 31.29.

In this pumpless system, a series of valves ensures one-way flow of the excess interstitial fluid (now called *lymph*) toward the heart. Lymph consists primarily of water and small amounts of dissolved proteins, mostly albumin, that are too large to be reabsorbed into the less permeable blood capillaries. Lymph also carries two types of immune system cells: lymphocytes and antigen-presenting cells. The antigen-presenting cells are carried to the next lymph node in the system, whereas lymphocytes traffic between lymph nodes. Once within the lymphatic system, lymph travels through lymphatic venules and veins that drain into one of two large ducts in the thorax: the right lymphatic duct and the thoracic duct. The right lymphatic duct drains lymph from the right arm and the right side of the head and thorax, whereas the larger thoracic duct receives lymph from the rest of the body (see Fig. 31.28). The right lymphatic duct and the thoracic duct drain lymph into the right and left subclavian veins, respectively.

Lymphatic veins are thin walled like the veins of the cardiovascular system. In larger lymphatic veins, endothelial flaps form valves similar to those in blood-carrying veins. The valves allow lymph to flow in only one direction, because lymphatic vessels are compressed intermittently by skeletal muscle contraction, pulsating expansion of the artery in the same

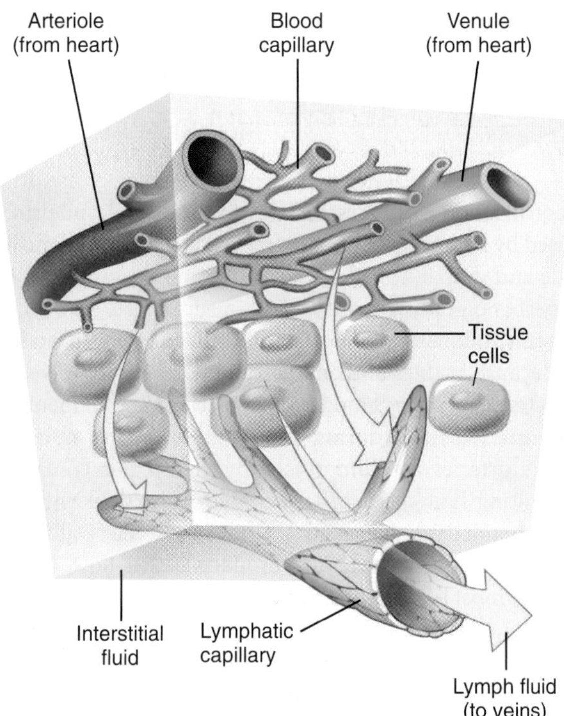

Fig. 31.27 Role of the Lymphatic System in Fluid Balance. Fluid from plasma flowing through the capillaries moves into interstitial spaces. Although most of this interstitial fluid is either absorbed by tissue cells or reabsorbed by blood capillaries, some of the fluid tends to accumulate in the interstitial spaces. This lymph then diffuses into the lymphatic vessels that carry it to the lymph nodes and then into the systemic venous blood. Green is used to diagram the lymphatic vessels although the lymphatic vessels, particularly the smaller ones, are almost transparent. (Modified from Thibodeau GA, Patton KT. *Structure & function of the body,* 13th edition. St. Louis: Elsevier; 2008.)

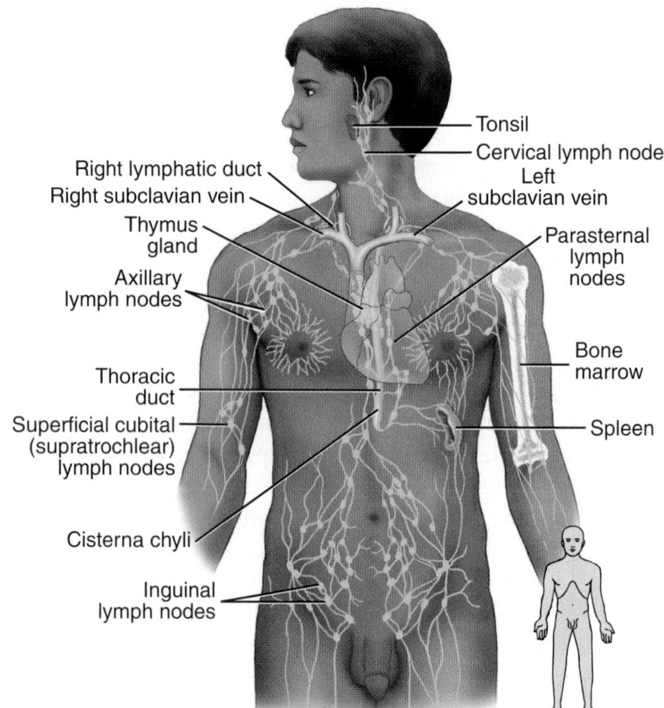

Fig. 31.28 Principal Organs of the Lymphatic System. (From VanMeter KC, Hubert RJ. *Microbiology for the healthcare professional.* St. Louis: Mosby; 2010.)

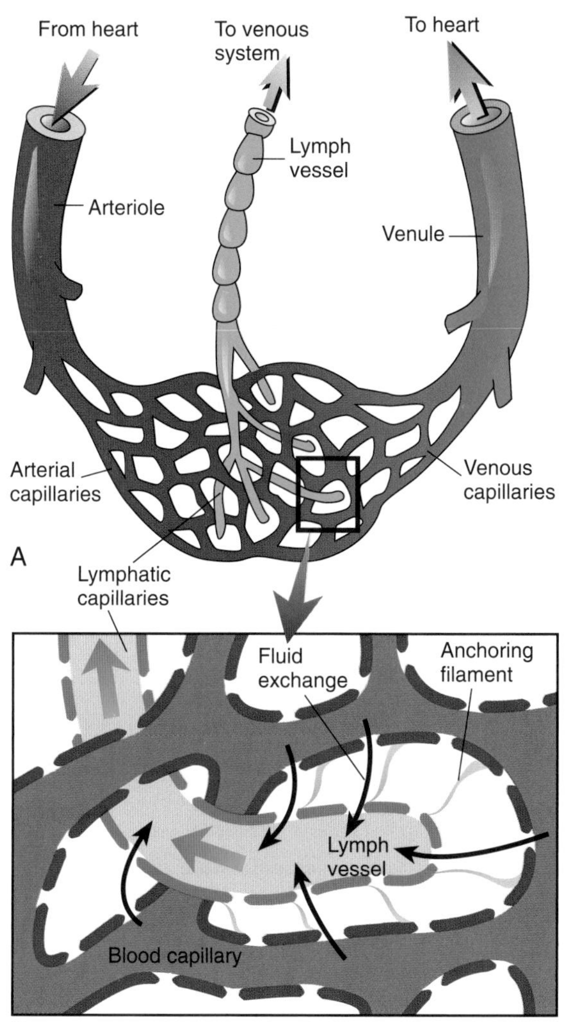

Fig. 31.29 Lymphatic Capillaries. **(A)** Schematic representation of lymphatic capillaries. **(B)** Anatomic components of microcirculation.

sheath, and contraction of the smooth muscles in the walls of the lymphatic vessels.

As lymph is transported toward the heart, it is filtered through thousands of bean-shaped lymph nodes clustered along the lymphatic vessels (see Fig. 31.28). Lymph enters the nodes through afferent lymphatic vessels, filters through the sinuses in the node, and leaves by way of efferent lymphatic vessels. Lymph flows slowly through a node, allowing phagocytosis of foreign substances within the node and delivery of lymphocytes. (Phagocytosis is described in Chapter 7.)

TESTS OF CARDIOVASCULAR FUNCTION

Assessment of the individual with suspected cardiovascular disorders begins with a thorough history for determination of risk factors and symptoms. A careful physical examination looking for evidence of tissue ischemia, pulmonary congestion, and cardiac dysfunction is next. Blood samples are taken and sent for a variety of tests. For many individuals, these basic steps will be complemented with methods that measure heart and vascular function with greater specificity. Cardiac function can be evaluated using indicators calculated from pressures and flow rates in the heart and vessels. Table 31.5 defines the indicators most often used in the clinical setting. The normal values for several testing methods are different for men and women.

Cardiac and Coronary Artery Evaluation

Many sophisticated tests are used to evaluate and diagnose cardiac or coronary artery diseases, and new ones are being developed each year. Some of the more commonly used modalities include chest x-ray, electrocardiography, echocardiography, stress testing, single-photon emission computed tomography (SPECT), computed tomography (CT), magnetic resonance imaging (MRI), electrophysiology studies, and catheterization with angiography.

Chest Radiograph Examination

Chest x-rays allow for the examination of the size and contour of the heart and related structures. Evidence of chamber enlargement, pericardial disease, pulmonary edema, valvular calcification, ventricular hypertrophy, and pathology of the great vessels may be visualized. Chest x-ray also is useful to assess for appropriate placement of invasive cardiac conduction devices and for any complications caused by these devices (e.g., pneumothorax or hemothorax; see Chapter 35). A chest x-ray examination is a routine part of a cardiac examination.

Electrocardiography

Electrocardiography, typically a 12-lead electrocardiogram (ECG), gives information about heart rate and rhythm; the effects of activities of daily life, exercise, electrolytes, drugs, and disease on electrical activity in the heart; and the electrical orientation of the cardiac muscle (see Fig. 31.9). An ECG provides no direct information about the contractile state or mechanical performance of the heart.

Serial 12-lead ECGs are of primary importance in establishing the presence of myocardial ischemia and infarction or conduction defects and dysrhythmias. This examination has become part of the routine hospital preadmission/admission assessment, even when the admitting diagnosis is not cardiac in nature, because it establishes baseline information about the electrical function of the heart. Also, recent ECGs can be compared with ECGs obtained from the same individual in the past. Changes in the ECG over time assist in determining the cause, amount, or nature of changes in cardiac anatomy and physiology. Ambulatory electrocardiographic or Holter monitoring is used to evaluate rhythm changes that may occur in persons during activities of daily living. Cell phone technology also is rapidly advancing to enable ECG recording and relaying to healthcare providers.

Echocardiography

Echocardiography is the most widely used noninvasive modality for evaluating the structures of the heart. Ultrasound beams reflected by cardiovascular structures produce shapes that can be visualized and can allow for recognition of altered cardiac anatomy. It is used to evaluate for suspected coronary artery disease, heart failure, valvular disease, infective endocarditis, cardiomyopathies, pericardial disease, prosthetic valve function, congenital heart disease, and

TABLE 31.5 Indicators of Cardiac Function

Indicator	Definition[a]	Common Cause of Abnormality
Heart rate (HR)	Number of heartbeats (cardiac cycles) per minute Normal adult value: 70 beats/min	Ischemia, electrolyte disturbances, drug toxicity
Cardiac output (CO)	Amount of blood (in L) moved by the heart in 1 min Normal range: 4–8 L/min	Decrease indicates heart failure Increase indicates decreased systemic vascular resistance, common in sepsis
Cardiac index (CI)	Relationship between cardiac output and body surface area (BSA, in m^2) Normal range: 2.8–4.2 L/min/m^2	Decrease indicates heart failure Increase indicates decreased systemic vascular resistance, common in sepsis
Stroke volume (SV)	Amount of blood (in mL) ejected by the left ventricle during systole (i.e., per beat) Normal range: 60–100 mL/beat	Decrease indicates heart failure Increase indicates decreased systemic vascular resistance, common in sepsis
Stroke volume index (SVI)	Relationship between stroke volume and body surface area Normal range: 33–47 mL/beat/m^2	Decrease indicates heart failure Increase indicates decreased systemic vascular resistance, common in sepsis
Ejection Fraction (EF)	Percentage of total ventricular end-diastolic volume ejected with each beat Normal range 50%–75%	Decrease indicates heart failure
Oxygen consumption index ($\dot{V}_2$)	Amount of oxygen (in mL) consumed per minute in relation to BSA	Decrease: sedation, anesthesia, hypothermia Increase: elevated temperature, sepsis, seizures
Stroke work index (SWI)	Amount of work (expressed as done) by the left or right ventricle per systole per square meter of BSA Normal value: 35 g/m^2	Decreases within specific ranges indicate cardiogenic or hypovolemic shock (see Chapter 48) Increase: elevated systemic vascular resistance
Systemic mean arterial pressure (MAP)	Mean blood pressure (in mm Hg) in the systemic arteries Normal range: 70–100 mm Hg	Elevated: epinephrine release, diseases of arteries, primary hypertension Decreased: cardiac failure, decreased vascular resistance of sepsis
Pulmonary vascular resistance (PVR)	Relationship among cardiac output, preload, and afterload, expressed as units of force of resistance per second per centimeter of water Normal value: <250 dynes/s/cm^{-5}	Increased: acute respiratory distress syndrome (ARDS), pneumonia, primary pulmonary hypertension, congestive heart failure Decreased: late shock
Systemic vascular resistance (SVR)	Same definition as for PVR Normal range: 770–1500 dynes/s/cm^{-5}	Increased: epinephrine release Decreased: inflammatory response

[a]Values given are for adults at rest.

aortic diseases. Through the use of one-dimensional (M-mode), two-dimensional, and three-dimensional echocardiographic techniques and combining them with Doppler and color flow imaging, accurate assessments of cardiac output, ejection fraction, and valvular function can be obtained.[28] Advances in technology now allow both intracardiac and transesophageal echocardiography for evaluation of the heart anatomy and physiology.

Exercise or Stress Testing

Cardiac activity during exercise is examined during a stress test when an intervention is used to increase myocardial work. Stress testing elicits signs and symptoms of heart disease and coronary artery disease that may not appear at rest. Echocardiography or continuous 12-lead ECG and blood pressure measurements are obtained before, during, and after the study. Cardiac stress from exercise is usually induced by having the individual walk on a treadmill. Other, less frequently used forms of exercise include static exercise (hand ergometry or chemical stress), stair climbing (the Stairmaster's double two-step), arm ergometry, and bicycle ergometry. The individual exercises until the maximal heart rate for gender and age is reached or until other subjective or objective indicators of cardiac dysfunction or distress appear. Subjective indicators include chest pain, extreme fatigue, extreme dyspnea, leg pain, or the individual's request to stop the test. Objective criteria include ST-segment elevation or depression, SA node or atrial dysrhythmias, AV node dysrhythmias, ventricular dysrhythmias, elevated or decreased blood pressure, signs of cerebral hypoxia, and signs of circulatory insufficiency.[29] One limitation of this test is that it cannot be used in persons whose capacity for exercise is limited.

Stress testing also may be used to evaluate either fitness for noncardiac surgery or progress in recovery after myocardial infarction or cardiac surgery. Graded exercise in individuals with low- to moderate-risk chest pain evaluated in an emergency department can be used as a prognostic indicator of adverse cardiac events. When a differential diagnosis for chest pain has been difficult to determine, stress testing may help distinguish coronary artery insufficiency from other causes of pain. The risks associated with stress testing include dysrhythmias, myocardial infarction, and death. The risk is greater when the test is performed soon after an acute ischemic event.

Stress testing with ECG monitoring may not be sensitive enough to detect and localize areas of the myocardium at risk for ischemia and infarction. Currently, most stress testing includes the injection of a radiotracer that is absorbed by active heart cells. When the heart is scanned, during and after stress testing, areas where the radiotracer is not taken up by ischemic cells can be seen and those locations indicate areas of myocardial damage.

Single-Photon Emission Computed Tomography

Single-photon emission computed tomography (SPECT) is typically used to evaluate individuals for coronary artery disease and myocardial ischemia during stress testing. A radiotracer (usually thalium-201 or technetium) is injected intravenously and is absorbed and retained for a while by healthy myocytes.[30] Photons are emitted from the radiotracer in the myocardium in proportion to perfusion of the tissue. A gamma camera visualizes the photons, and views are taken from 360 degrees by CT, which digitizes the information and provides a three-dimensional view of myocardial perfusion. Data about where the myocardium absorbs the tracer normally, slowly, or not at all can be correlated with existing myocardial disease and can help quantify ischemic risk. A new development, high-speed SPECT, has the advantage of taking less time and, thereby, requiring less radiotracer, which decreases radiation exposure for the person being examined Positron emission tomography (PET) scanning also can be used to assess myocardial perfusion and metabolism.[30]

Computed Tomography and Magnetic Resonance Imaging

Computed tomography (CT) and magnetic resonance imaging (MRI) are used to evaluate cardiac anatomy and physiology. Techniques such as ECG gating (timing of data gathering to the cardiac cycle), electron beam CT, and spiral CT have improved the ability of tomography to visualize cardiac structures.[31] The high resolution of CT can provide information about calcification of coronary vessels and cardiac valves. Information about coronary artery calcification is being used to improve risk classification for coronary artery disease. It also is a tool for evaluating large-vessel disease. Concerns and debate continue, however, about the radiation risks and use of variable protocols.

MRI is based on the principle that the frequency of energy (resonant frequency) given up by a nucleus is exactly proportional to the surrounding magnetic field. The anatomy and physiology of the great blood vessels and myocardium are depicted in three dimensions with excellent resolution. Ventricular function can be evaluated using indexes of ventricular function, such as ejection fraction. Rapidly moving sequences (MRI) can determine regional wall motion and myocardial deformation. Flow direction and velocity also can be quantitatively determined. Stress testing also can be done with MRI using the drug dobutamine to increase the cardiac workload instead of exercise.[32]

Electrophysiology Studies

In-depth evaluation of electrical conduction within the heart can provide important information about the nature and causes of dysrhythmias, such as atrial and ventricular tachycardias and heart block. This evaluation is often referred to as *electrophysiologic mapping* of the myocardium. There are many types of electrophysiology studies that are specific to certain conduction disorders but they have the common goal of documenting abnormal conduction pathways.[33] Furthermore, the techniques used may also allow for ablation of unwanted pathways or the appropriate placement of pacemakers and implantable defibrillators. Mapping can include the use of echocardiography and CT scanning.

One example of an electrophysiology study is AV bundle electrocardiography. Two electrode-tipped catheters are inserted percutaneously into the femoral vein, floated up the inferior vena cava, and positioned in or near the right atrium during AV bundle (His bundle) electrocardiography. AV bundle electrocardiography can detect secondary sites of impulse generation (ectopic foci), as well as accessory pathways of conduction. Other conduction defects and the effects of drugs on conduction also can be illuminated. Risks related to this procedure can be grave and include dysrhythmias, death, vessel or heart perforation, clot or plaque embolization, and kidney failure.

Cardiac Catheterization and Angiography

One or both sides of the heart can be examined using cardiac catheterization. This invasive procedure requires the use of fluoroscopy and strict sterile techniques and takes place in a specially equipped catheterization laboratory. Local anesthetic is administered, and a catheter is introduced percutaneously into the vasculature and passed caudally into the atrium and ventricle. For a right-heart catheterization, the catheter is placed in either the jugular, subclavian, brachial, or femoral veins. The femoral artery is commonly used for a left-heart study. Once the catheter has been guided into the heart chambers, pressures are recorded, blood samples are obtained to examine oxygen content, and a contrast medium is injected to visualize chamber function and valve patency.

Cardiac catheterization provides a means to visualize the chambers of the heart continuously, although for a short time. A great deal of information can be obtained about heart structure and function.[34] Pressures in each chamber and across heart valves can be precisely measured, along with timing of events in the cardiac cycle. Of particular value is the ability to compare the oxygen content of blood in each heart chamber. Risks for this procedure that have decreased over time include the development of dysrhythmias. Death can occur secondary to cardiac arrest after ventricular fibrillation.

Fluoroscopic visualization of the coronary arteries and left-heart structures using contrast dye is called coronary angiography or arteriography. Like cardiac catheterization, this study takes place in a catheterization laboratory using local anesthesia and a sterile field. A catheter is threaded into the left ventricle through the femoral artery. A ventriculogram generally is performed first. Contrast dye is injected into the apex of the ventricle, and the next few cardiac cycles are visualized and filmed.

Like cardiac catheterization, coronary angiography is used to gain information about the structure and function of the ventricles and related valves. After the ventriculogram, catheters are introduced individually into the ostia of the coronary arteries. When the catheter is in position, a small volume of contrast dye is mechanically and rapidly injected into the artery and the results are visualized and filmed. Dye injection is repeated with the individual tilted at various angles to afford views of the artery other than the anteroposterior view.

The risks of coronary angiography are similar to those of cardiac catheterization, with exceptions. As the blood supply to the cardiac muscle is briefly interrupted when dye is introduced into the coronary arteries, angina (chest pain) caused by ischemia (lack of oxygen) is much more common. Coronary artery spasms also can occur. Interrupted flow also causes decreased heart rate (bradycardia), as well as some tachydysrhythmias, hypotension, and ST-segment depression.

Systemic Vascular Evaluation

The systemic vascular system can be studied by a variety of techniques in order to evaluate for adequate flow rates, vascular obstruction, and structural defects. These techniques include Doppler ultrasonography, CT and MRI, venography, and arteriography.

Arterial Pressure Pulse Waveform Analysis

Pulsation, described by the flow of blood through an artery during the cardiac cycle, can be drawn as a waveform plotting pressure against time (Fig. 31.30). The waveform can be obtained noninvasively by placing a transducer on the skin over the carotid artery while the individual's head is turned slightly away from the transducer. The amplitude and shape of arterial waveforms can provide information about the elasticity of the arterial wall, or its inverse—the stiffness of the wall.

Doppler Ultrasonography Studies

A Doppler study is done using a microphone that amplifies and records the sounds made by blood flowing in peripheral vessels. The Doppler microphone is placed over the vessel to be studied, and sounds related to obstructions to flow, vessel wall mobility, and heart murmurs are transmitted through a lubricating gel to the microphone. The audio findings can be digitized into visual findings that can be analyzed for flow velocity and volume. These studies are useful in the evaluation for abnormalities of venous flow (e.g., deep venous thrombosis) and arterial flow (e.g., embolism). Ultrasound also is used to calculate the thickness of arterial walls, yielding a reading called *intimal-medial thickness*. Carotid intimal-medial thickness is used to assess for atherosclerosis.[28]

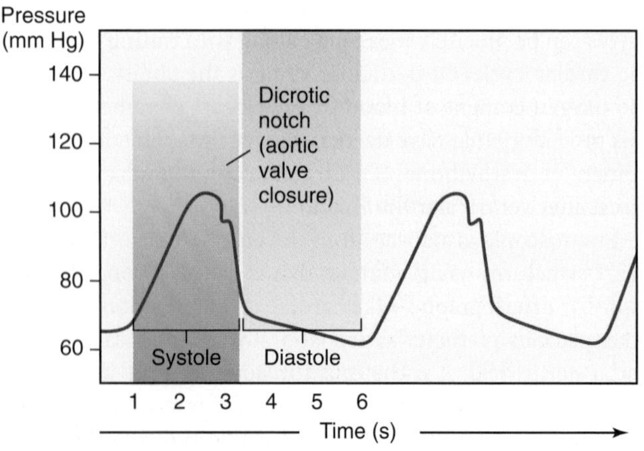

Fig. 31.30 Arterial Pressure Pulse Waveforms.

Computed Tomography and Magnetic Resonance Imaging

CT and MRI are used to evaluate the systemic circulation, providing information about the structure of the great vessels. Either can be used to evaluate for aneurysms and dissections of the thoracic or abdominal aorta. CT also is used to assess for vessel calcification and provide some insights into the risk for stroke and myocardial infarction through evaluation of the carotid and coronary vessels.

Venography and Arteriography

Radiopaque dye can be injected through intravenous or intra-arterial catheters to allow for visualization of the internal structure, diameter, and patency of veins and arteries. Venography is performed primarily in the lower extremity to assess for the presence of thrombi in the large veins of the leg. Arteriography (angiography) can be used in almost any vascular system, including the great vessels and the pulmonary, coronary (see previously in this chapter), cerebral, mesenteric, renal, hepatic, and peripheral arteries. Risks include rupture, dissection, thrombosis, embolization, or organ infarction involving the arterial system being studied.

AGING AND THE CARDIOVASCULAR SYSTEM

Cardiovascular disease is the most common cause of morbidity and mortality in older adults in Western society and in much of the rest of the world (see Chapter 32). Age is a key driver of cardiovascular risk, in large measure due to the increased prevalence of risk factors such as hypertension, hyperlipidemia, and sedentary lifestyle in older individuals. For example, lipoprotein removal from tissues is decreased with aging, contributing to the risk of cardiovascular disease.[35] The most relevant age-associated physiologic changes in cardiovascular performance include myocardial and blood vessel stiffening, changes in neurogenic control over vascular tone, increased occurrence of atrial fibrillation, and loss of exercise capacity plus left ventricular hypertrophy and fibrosis. These changes pose considerable consequences with increased demand for flow, with changes in posture, or with disease. Cardiovascular aging occurs at the cellular level and includes genomic instability, epigenetic changes, inflammation and mitochondrial oxidative stress, and endothelial senescence.[36]

Arterial stiffening occurs with aging even in the absence of clinical hypertension. It can, however, be an important contributor to systolic hypertension and its associated risks for cardiovascular events, dementia, and death. These changes result from alterations within the vascular media, including age-associated changes in cross-linking of collagen, an increase in the amount of collagen, deposition of calcium, and changes in the nature of elastin, the extracellular matrix, inflammatory molecules, endothelial cell function, and reactive oxygen species. The increased arterial stiffness may not be related strictly to an age-associated change in vascular structure but may be caused by changes in baroreceptor activity. Baroreceptor activity may decrease with age, slowing physiologic adjustment to changes in blood pressure and posture. In persons older than age 60, pulse pressure, which is directly influenced by arterial stiffness, is a better predictor of cardiovascular disease than either diastolic or systolic blood pressure (see Chapter 32).

Left ventricular hypertrophy and fibrosis also are more common in the aging population, even in the absence of high blood pressure. As the arterial system becomes stiffer the ventricles must work harder to pump blood throughout the body, thus contributing to hypertrophy. Fibrosis, calcification, and increase in stiffness also impact valvular function, particularly the function of the atrioventricular valves. These changes make valvular disease a greater risk for the elderly, along with an increased risk of heart failure related to the left ventricular hypertrophy and stiffness.

Stress testing is used to uncover functional capacity losses that are not apparent at rest. In contrast to the subtle age effects on resting cardiac tests, more dramatic changes occur during exercise. Table 31.2 summarizes age-associated changes at rest and during exercise. Overall, long-term exercise conditioning in older individuals increases aerobic capacity, improves left ventricular function, and decreases arterial stiffness so that cardiovascular diseases may be prevented or delayed in older adults. Although the risks and benefits of pharmacologic and invasive strategies must always be assessed carefully, lack of cardiovascular health is a strong predictor of disability in the elderly,[37] and many older adults can live longer and healthier lives if appropriate preventive and treatment regimens are offered, even quite late in life.

The advent of genomic medicine and a deeper exploration of molecular changes with aging continue to enhance understanding of the myriad changes in people's bodies as they age.[36] The ongoing hope is that as understanding of the causative factors related to cardiovascular decline with aging improves, therapeutics that arrest or slow these changes may be developed.

SUMMARY REVIEW

Circulatory System

1. The circulatory system is part of the body's transport and communication systems. It delivers O_2, nutrients, metabolites, hormones, neurochemicals, proteins, and blood cells, including lymphocytes and leukocytes, throughout the body and carries metabolic wastes to the kidneys, lungs, and liver for excretion.
2. The circulatory system consists of the heart and the blood and lymphatic vessels and is made up of two separate but conjoined, serially connected pump systems: the pulmonary circulation and the systemic circulation. The lymphatic system is a one-way network consisting of lymphatic vessels and lymph nodes.
3. The low-pressure pulmonary circulation is driven by the right side of the heart; its function is to deliver blood to the lungs for oxygenation.
4. The higher-pressure systemic circulation is driven by the left side of the heart and functions to provide oxygenated blood, nutrients, and other key substances to body tissues and transport waste products to the lungs, kidneys, and liver for excretion.
5. The lymphatic vessels collect fluids from the interstitium and return the fluids to the circulatory system; lymphatic vessels also deliver antigens, microorganisms, and cells to the lymph nodes.

Heart

1. The heart consists of four chambers (two atria and two ventricles), four valves (two atrioventricular valves and two semilunar valves), a muscular wall, a fibrous skeleton, a conduction system, nerve fibers, systemic vessels (the coronary circulation), and openings where the great vessels enter the atria and ventricles.
2. The heart wall, which encloses the heart and divides it into chambers, is made up of three layers: the epicardium (outer layer), the myocardium (muscular layer), and the endocardium (inner lining). The heart lies within the pericardium, a double-walled sac.
3. The myocardial layer of the two atria, which receive blood entering the heart, is thinner than the myocardial layer of the ventricles, which have to be stronger to squeeze blood out of the heart.
4. The right and left sides of the heart are separated by portions of the heart wall called the *interatrial septum* and the *interventricular septum.*
5. Deoxygenated (venous) blood from the systemic circulation enters the right atrium through the superior and inferior venae cavae. From the right atrium, the blood passes through the right atrioventricular (tricuspid) valve into the right ventricle. In the ventricle, the blood flows from the inflow tract to the outflow tract and then through the pulmonary semilunar valve (pulmonary valve) into the pulmonary artery, which delivers it to the lungs for oxygenation.
6. Oxygenated blood from the lungs enters the left atrium through the four pulmonary veins (two from the left lung and two from the right lung). From the left atrium, the blood passes through the left atrioventricular valve (mitral valve) into the left ventricle. In the ventricle, the blood flows from the inflow tract to the outflow tract and then through the aortic semilunar valve (aortic valve) into the aorta, which delivers it to systemic arteries of the entire body.
7. There are four heart valves. The atrioventricular valves ensure one-way flow of blood from the atria to the ventricles. The semilunar valves ensure one-way blood flow from the right ventricle to the pulmonary artery and from the left

ventricle to the aorta. The valves are supported by a fibrous skeleton.

8. The pumping action of the heart consists of two phases: diastole, during which the myocardium relaxes and the ventricles fill with blood; and systole, during which the myocardium contracts, forcing blood out of the ventricles. A cardiac cycle consists of one systolic contraction and the diastolic relaxation that follows it. Each cardiac cycle represents one heartbeat.
9. Coronary circulation provides O_2 and nutrients to the myocardium and other heart structures. Oxygenated blood enters the coronary arteries through openings from the aorta, and deoxygenated blood from the coronary veins enters the right atrium through the coronary sinus.
10. The conduction system of the heart generates and transmits electrical impulses (cardiac action potentials) that stimulate systolic contractions. The autonomic nerves (sympathetic and parasympathetic fibers) can adjust heart rate and force of contraction, but they do not originate the heartbeat.
11. The normal electrocardiogram is the sum of all cardiac action potentials. The P wave represents atrial depolarization; the QRS complex is the sum of all ventricular cell depolarizations. The ST interval occurs when the entire ventricular myocardium is depolarized.
12. Cardiac action potentials are generated by the sinoatrial node at a rate of 60 to 100 impulses per minute. The impulses can travel through the conduction system of the heart, stimulating myocardial contraction as they go.
13. Each cardiac action potential travels from the SA node to the AV node to the bundle of His (atrioventricular bundle), through the bundle branches, and finally to the Purkinje fibers and ventricular myocardium, where the impulse stops. It is prevented from reversing its path by the refractory period of cells that have just been polarized. The refractory period ensures that diastole (relaxation) will occur, thereby completing the cardiac cycle.
14. Cells of the cardiac conduction system have the properties of automaticity and rhythmicity. Automatic cells return to threshold and depolarize rhythmically without an outside stimulus. The cells of the sinoatrial node depolarize faster than other automatic cells, making it the natural pacemaker of the heart. If the SA node is disabled, the next fastest pacemaker, the AV node, takes over.
15. Adrenergic receptor number, type, and function govern autonomic (sympathetic) regulation of heart rate, contractile force, and the dilation or constriction of coronary arteries. The presence of specific receptors on the myocardium and coronary vessels determines the effects of the neurotransmitters norepinephrine and epinephrine.
16. Unique features that distinguish myocardial cells from skeletal cells enable myocardial cells to transmit action potentials faster (through intercalated discs), synthesize more ATP (because of a large number of mitochondria), and have readier access to ions in the interstitium (because of an abundance of transverse tubules). These combined differences enable the myocardium to work constantly, which is not required by skeletal muscle.
17. Cross-bridges between actin and myosin enable contraction. Calcium ions interacting with the troponin complex help initiate the contraction process. Subsequently, myocardial relaxation begins as troponin releases calcium ions.
18. Cardiac performance is affected by preload, afterload, myocardial contractility, and heart rate.
19. Preload, or pressure generated in the ventricles at the end of diastole, depends on the amount of blood in the ventricle. Afterload is the resistance to ejection of the blood from the ventricle. Afterload depends on pressure in the aorta.
20. Myocardial stretch determines the force of myocardial contraction; thus the greater the stretch, the stronger the contraction up to a certain point. This relationship is known as the Frank-Starling law of the heart.
21. Contractility is the potential for myocardial fiber shortening during systole. It is determined by the amount of stretch during diastole (i.e., preload) and by sympathetic stimulation of the ventricles.
22. The heart rate is determined by the sinoatrial node and by components of the autonomic nervous system, including cardiovascular control centers in the brain, receptors in the aorta and carotid arteries, and hormones, including catecholamines (epinephrine, norepinephrine).

Systemic Circulation

1. Blood flows from the left ventricle into the aorta and from the aorta into arteries that eventually branch into arterioles and capillaries, the smallest of the arterial vessels. O_2, nutrients, and other substances needed for cellular metabolism pass from the capillaries into the tissues, where they are taken up by the cells. Capillaries also absorb metabolic waste products from the tissues.
2. Venules, the smallest veins, receive capillary blood. From the venules, the venous blood flows into larger and larger veins until it reaches the venae cavae, through which it enters the right atrium.
3. Vessel walls have three layers: the tunica intima (inner layer), the tunica media (middle layer), and the tunica externa (the outer layer).
4. Layers of the vessel wall differ in thickness and composition from vessel to vessel, depending on the vessel's size and location within the circulatory system. In general, the tunica media of arteries close to the heart has more elastic fibers (elastic arteries) because these arteries must be able to distend during systole and recoil during diastole. Arteries farther from the heart contain more smooth muscle fibers (muscular arteries) because they constrict and dilate to control blood pressure and volume within specific capillary beds.
5. Blood flow into the capillary beds is controlled by the contraction and relaxation of smooth muscle bands (precapillary sphincters) at junctions between metarterioles and capillaries.
6. Endothelial cells line the blood vessels. The endothelium is a life-support tissue; it functions as a filter (altering permeability), changes in vasomotion (constriction and dilation), and is involved in clotting and inflammation.

7. Blood flow through the veins is assisted by the contraction of skeletal muscles (the muscle pump), and backward flow is prevented by one-way valves, which are particularly important in the deep veins of the legs.
8. Blood flow is affected by blood pressure, resistance to flow within the vessels, velocity of the blood, anatomic features that may cause turbulent or laminar flow, and compliance (distensibility) of the vessels.
9. The Poiseuille law states that resistance is directly related to tube length and blood viscosity, and inversely related to the radius of the tube.
10. Total resistance, or the resistance to flow within the entire systemic circulatory system, depends on the combined lengths and radii of all the vessels within the system and on whether the vessels are arranged in series (greater resistance) or in parallel (lesser resistance).
11. Blood flow is also influenced by neural stimulation (vasoconstriction or vasodilation) and by autonomic features that cause turbulence within the vascular lumen (e.g., protrusions from the vessel wall, twists and turns, vessel branching).
12. Arterial blood pressure is influenced and regulated by factors that affect cardiac output (heart rate, stroke volume), total resistance within the system, and blood volume.
13. ADH, the RAAS system, and NPs can all alter blood volume and thus blood pressure.
14. Venous blood pressure is influenced by blood volume within the venous system and compliance of the venous walls.
15. Blood flow through the coronary circulation is governed by the same principles as flow through other vascular beds plus two adaptations dictated by cardiac dynamics. First, blood flows into the coronary arteries during diastole rather than systole, because during systole the cusps of the aortic semilunar valve block the openings of the coronary arteries. Second, systolic contraction inhibits coronary artery flow by compressing the coronary arteries.
16. Autoregulation enables the coronary vessels to maintain optimal perfusion pressure despite systolic compression.
17. Myoglobin in heart muscle stores O_2 for use during the systolic phase of the cardiac cycle.

The Lymphatic System

1. The vessels of the lymphatic system run in the same sheaths as the arteries and veins.
2. Lymph (interstitial fluid) is absorbed by lymphatic venules in the capillary beds and travels through ever larger lymphatic veins until it empties through the right lymphatic duct or thoracic duct into the right or left subclavian veins, respectively.
3. As lymph travels toward the thoracic ducts, it passes through thousands of lymph nodes clustered around the lymphatic veins. The lymph nodes are sites of immune function and are ideally placed to sample antigens and cells carried by the lymph from the periphery of the body into the central circulation.

Tests of Cardiovascular Function

1. The evaluation of an individual with known or suspected cardiovascular disease must include a careful history and physical examination including assessment of risk factors, symptoms, vital signs, level of consciousness, mucous membrane color, and cardiopulmonary functioning.
2. Important tests for cardiac disorders are ECG and Holter monitoring, which detect disturbances of impulse generation or conduction.
3. Stress tests elicit clinical manifestations of cardiovascular disease that might not be present at rest.
4. The sensitivity of stress testing is improved by the use of radiotracer imaging techniques such as SPECT.
5. Echocardiography detects structural and functional cardiac abnormalities over time.
6. Cardiac catheterization is used to measure the oxygen content and pressure of blood in the heart's chambers and to inject contrast media for x-ray examination of the size and shape of the chambers and valves. Injection of contrast medium into the coronary arteries (coronary angiography), on the other hand, permits visualization of the coronary circulation and every tissue perfused by the coronary arteries.
7. Evaluation of the systemic vascular system can include arterial pressure pulse waveform analysis, Doppler ultrasonography, venography, and arteriography.

Aging and the Cardiovascular System

1. Cardiovascular disease is the most common cause of morbidity and mortality in older adults in Western society and in much of the rest of the world. In addition, age is a key driver of cardiovascular risk, which explains why it is the primary cause of death in persons older than age 65.
2. The most common cardiovascular disease condition is hypertension followed by coronary atherosclerosis, for which hypertension is a risk factor.
3. It is challenging to determine the normal physiologic changes in cardiac function with aging because many pathologic changes are usually present and physical fitness is variable in older people as well.
4. The most relevant age-associated physiologic changes in cardiovascular performance include myocardial and blood vessel stiffening, changes in neurogenic control over vascular tone, increased occurrence of atrial fibrillation, and loss of exercise capacity plus left ventricular hypertrophy and fibrosis.
5. With active risk reduction, physical activity, and disease management, older adults can have markedly improved cardiovascular health.

REFERENCES

1. Susan Standring S. *Gray's anatomy: the anatomical basis of clinical practice*. ed 42 : Elsevier; 2021.
2. Elhelaly WM, et al. Redox regulation of heart regeneration: an evolutionary tradeoff. *Front Cell Dev Biol*. 2016;4:137.
3. He L, et al. Heart regeneration by endogenous stem cells and cardiomyocyte proliferation: controversy, fallacy, and progress. *Circulation*. 2020;142:275–291.

4. Jamaiyar A, et al. Cardioprotection during ischemia by coronary collateral growth. *Am J Physiol Heart Circ Physiol.* 2019;316:H1–H9.
5. Brakenhielm E, Alitalo K. Cardiac lymphatics in health and disease. *Nat Rev Cardiol.* 2019;16(1):56–68.
6. Pappano AJ, Wier WG. The cardiac pump. In: Pappano AJ, Wier WG, eds. *Cardiovascular physiology*. ed 11 Philadelphia: Elsevier; 2019.
7. Rodríguez-Sinovas A, et al. Connexins in the heart: Regulation, function and involvement in cardiac disease. *Int J Mol Sci.* 2021;22(9):4413.
8. Tomaselli GF, Rubart M, Zipes DP. Mechanisms of cardiac arrhythmias. In: Bonow R, Mann D, Tomaselli G, eds. *Braunwald's heart disease: a textbook of cardiovascular medicine*. ed 11 : Elsevier; 2019:619–647.
9. de Lucia C, Eguchi A, Koch WJ. New insights in cardiac β-adrenergic signaling during heart failure and aging. *Front Pharmacol.* 2018;9:904.
10. Zhao G, et al. Intercalated discs: cellular adhesion and signaling in heart health and diseases. *Heart Fail Rev.* 2019;24(1):115–132.
11. Koser F, Loescher C, Linke WA. Posttranslational modifications of titin from cardiac muscle: how, where, and what for? *FEBS J.* 2019;286:2240–2260.
12. Sithara T, Drosatos K, Metabolic Complications in Cardiac Aging. *Front Physiol.* 2021:12:66497.
13. Chung JH, et al. Impact of heart rate on cross-bridge cycling kinetics in failing and nonfailing human myocardium. *Am J Physiol Heart Circ Physiol.* 2019;317:H640–H647.
14. L'Heureux M, et al. Sepsis-induced cardiomyopathy: a comprehensive review. *Curr Cardiol Rep.* 2020;22(5):35.
15. Fatisson J, Oswald V, Lalonde F. Influence diagram of physiological and environmental factors affecting heart rate variability: an extended literature overview. *Heart Int.* 2016;11(1):e32–e40.
16. Perna G, et al. Heart rate variability: Can it serve as a marker of mental health resilience?: Special Section on "Translational and Neuroscience Studies in Affective Disorders" Section Editor, Maria Nobile MD, PhD *J Affect Disord.* 2632020754–761.
17. Fang SC, Wu YL, Tsai PS. Heart rate variability and risk of all-cause death and cardiovascular events in patients with cardiovascular disease: a meta-analysis of cohort studies. *Biol Res Nurs.* 2020;22:45–56.
18. Zeng B, et al. Thyroid hormone diminishes Ca2+ overload induced by hypoxia/reoxygenation in cardiomyocytes by inhibiting late sodium current and reverse-Na+/Ca2+ exchange current. *Pharmacology.* 2020;105:63–72.
19. Isgaard J, et al. GH and the cardiovascular system: an update on a topic at heart. *Endocrine.* 2015;48(1):25–35.
20. Ager A. High endothelial venules and other blood vessels: critical regulators of lymphoid organ development and function. *Front Immunol.* 2017;8:45.
21. Genkel VV, Kuznetcova AS, Shaposhnik II. Biomechanical forces and atherosclerosis: from mechanism to diagnosis and treatment. *Curr Cardiol Rev.* 2020;16(3):187–197.
22. Ambrosy AP, et al. Angiotensin receptor-neprilysin inhibition based on history of heart failure and use of renin-angiotensin system antagonists. *J Am Coll Cardiol.* 2020;76:1034–1048.
23. Goetze Cardiac natriuretic peptides. *Nat Rev Cardiol.* 2020;17:698–717.
24. Oikonomou E, et al. Coronary artery disease and endothelial dysfunction: novel diagnostic and therapeutic approaches. *Curr Med Chem.* 2020;27:1052–1080.
25. Zuchi C, et al. Role of endothelial dysfunction in heart failure. *Heart Fail Rev.* 2020;25(1):21–30.
26. Iring A, et al. Shear stress–induced endothelial adrenomedullin signaling regulates vascular tone and blood pressure. *J Clin Invest.* 2019;129(7):2775–2791.
27. Rane MA, et al. Risks of cardiovascular disease and beyond in prescription of nonsteroidal anti-inflammatory drugs. *J Cardiovasc Pharmacol Ther.* 2020;25(1):3–6.
28. Solomon SD, et al. Echocardiography. In: Bonow R, Mann D, Tomaselli G, eds. *Braunwald's heart disease: a textbook of cardiovascular medicine.* ed 11 : Elsevier; 2019:174–251.
29. Balady GJ, Morise AP. Exercise electrocardiographic testing. In: Bonow R, Mann D, Tomaselli G, eds. *Braunwald's heart disease: a textbook of cardiovascular medicine.* ed 11 : Elsevier; 2019:154–173.
30. Udelson JE, Dilsizian V, Bonow RO. Nuclear cardiology. In: Bonow R, Mann D, Tomaselli G, eds. *Braunwald's heart disease: a textbook of cardiovascular medicine.* ed 11 : Elsevier; 2019:261–300.
31. Min JK. Cardiac computed tomography. In: Bonow R, Mann D, Tomaselli G, eds. *Braunwald's heart disease: a textbook of cardiovascular medicine.* ed 11 : Elsevier; 2019:321–347.
32. Kwong RY. Cardiovascular magnetic resonance imaging. In: Bonow R, Mann D, Tomaselli G, eds. *Braunwald's heart disease: a textbook of cardiovascular medicine.* ed 11 : Elsevier; 2019:301–320.
33. Tomaselli GF, Zipes DP. Approach to the patient with cardiac arrhythmias. In: Bonow R, Mann D, Tomaselli G, eds. *Braunwald's heart disease: a textbook of cardiovascular medicine.* ed 11 : Elsevier; 2019:597–603.
34. Herrmann J. Cardiac catheterization. In: Bonow R, Mann D, Tomaselli G, eds. *Braunwald's heart disease: a textbook of cardiovascular medicine.* ed 11 : Elsevier; 2019:348–373.
35. Maranhao RC, Pala D, Freitas FR. Lipoprotein removal mechanisms and aging: implications for the cardiovascular health of the elderly. *Curr Opin Endocrinol Diabetes Obes.* 2020;27(2):104–109.
36. Paneni F, et al. The aging cardiovascular system. *J Am Coll Cardiol.* 2017;69:1952–1967.
37. Jin Y, et al. Cardiovascular health is associated with disability among older community dwelling men and women. *J Aging Health.* 2019;31(8):1339–1352.

32

Alterations of Cardiovascular Function

Valentina L. Brashers

http://evolve.elsevier.com/Rogers/pathophysiology/

CHAPTER OUTLINE

Cardiovascular disease is the leading cause of death, both in the United States and worldwide. Disorders of the veins, arteries, and heart comprise the scope of cardiovascular disease. Current understanding of the pathophysiology of cardiovascular disease is focused on genetic, neurohumoral, inflammatory, and metabolic mechanisms that underlie tissue and cellular alterations.

DISEASES OF THE VEINS

Varicose Veins and Chronic Venous Insufficiency

A varicose vein is a vein in which blood has pooled, producing distended, tortuous, and palpable vessels (Fig. 32.1). Risk factors include age, female sex, family history of varicose veins, obesity, pregnancy, deep venous thrombosis (DVT), and previous leg injury. Varicose veins typically involve the saphenous veins of the leg and are caused by (1) injury or disease involving the saphenous vein valves or (2) gradual venous distention caused by the action of gravity on blood in the legs.

If a valve is damaged, volume and pressure increase within the vessel. The vein swells as it becomes engorged and surrounding tissue becomes edematous because increased hydrostatic pressure pushes plasma through the stretched vessel wall. Venous distention develops over time, especially in individuals who habitually stand for long periods, wear constricting garments, or cross the legs at the knees, which diminishes the action of the muscle pump (see Fig. 31.20). Genetic factors, female sex, and pregnancy are contributing factors. Eventually the pressure in the vein damages venous valves, rendering them incompetent and unable to maintain normal venous pressure.

Varicose veins and valvular incompetence can progress to chronic venous insufficiency, especially in sedentary obese individuals and those who smoke. Chronic venous insufficiency (CVI) is inadequate venous return over a long period of time. Venous hypertension, circulatory stasis, and tissue hypoxia cause an inflammatory reaction and changes in the extracellular matrix in vessels. Endothelial cells express adhesion molecules bringing leukocytes and fibroblasts to the area. Collagen synthesis increases vascular wall thickening and fibrosclerotic remodeling of the veins. The microcirculation is impaired contributing to more inflammation and tissue hypoxia. Approximately one-third of those with varicose veins develop significant skin changes.[1] Symptoms include edema of the lower extremities and hyperpigmentation of the skin of the feet and ankles. Poor circulation makes tissues vulnerable to trauma and infection resulting in the formation of venous stasis ulcers (Fig. 32.2) and cellulitis.

Evaluation of CVI includes careful physical examination of pulses and skin, followed by Doppler ultrasound and measurement of ankle brachial pressure index. Identification of the underlying cause is crucial to effective management.[2] Treatment of varicose veins and CVI begins conservatively with elevating the legs, wearing compression bandages or stockings, and performing physical exercise. In those with venous ulcers, the choice of compression materials and their proper use is essential to obtaining improvement in symptoms and ulcer healing.[1] Advanced wound care techniques including skin grafting,

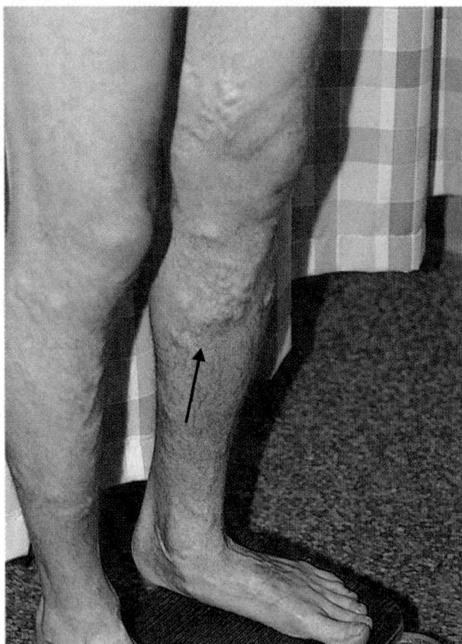

Fig. 32.1 Varicose Veins of the Leg (Arrow). (From Robbins SL, Cotran RS, Kumar V, et al. *Robbins and Cotran pathologic basis of disease*, 8th edition. Philadelphia: Saunders; 2010. Courtesy Dr. Magruder C. Donaldson, Brigham and Women's Hospital, Boston, MA.)

mesenchymal stem cells, and autologous platelet rich plasma may be indicated for large non-healing ulcers.[2] Invasive management for venous obstruction and dilation includes endovenous ablation, sclerotherapy or surgical ligation, conservative vein resection (phlebectomy), and vein bypass.

Thrombus Formation in Veins

A thrombus is a blood clot that remains attached to a vessel wall. A detached thrombus is a thromboembolus. The Centers for Disease Control and Prevention estimates that venous thrombi and associated thromboembolism affect about 900,000 people and cause nearly 100,000 deaths in the United States per year.[3] Deep venous thrombosis (DVT) occurs primarily in the lower extremity. Venous thrombi are more common than arterial thrombi because flow and pressure are lower in the veins than in the arteries. Three factors (triad of Virchow) promote venous thrombosis: (1) venous stasis, (2) venous endothelial damage, and (3) hypercoagulable states (see Chapter 29).

Venous stasis occurs in conditions that limit flow through the local or systemic venous circulation. For example, immobility (e.g., stroke, spinal cord injury, casting) prevents the muscular pump (see Fig. 31.20) from increasing blood flow from the lower extremity to the inferior vena cava and right atrium. Similarly, heart failure results in increased diastolic filling pressures causing reduced venous return. Accumulation of clotting factors and platelets leads to thrombus formation in the vein, often near a venous valve. Further platelet aggregation leads to the thrombus propagating (growing) proximally.

Damage to endothelial cells can occur due to trauma (e.g., orthopedic injury or surgery), the use of caustic intravenous medications, or the use of invasive venous procedures (e.g., peripherally inserted central catheters). The healthy vascular endothelium serves as a barrier between the blood and the prothrombotic subendothelium. It also expresses several anticoagulant factors including protein C receptors and tissue factor pathway inhibitor. In the presence of endothelial damage, endothelial cells lose their anticoagulant properties and instead express adhesion molecules that promote inflammatory cell and platelet activation.[4] Polymorphonucleocytes infiltrate the vessel wall and produce neutrophil extracellular traps (NETs) (see Chapter 7) that cause additional inflammatory damage to the endothelium and promote clotting.

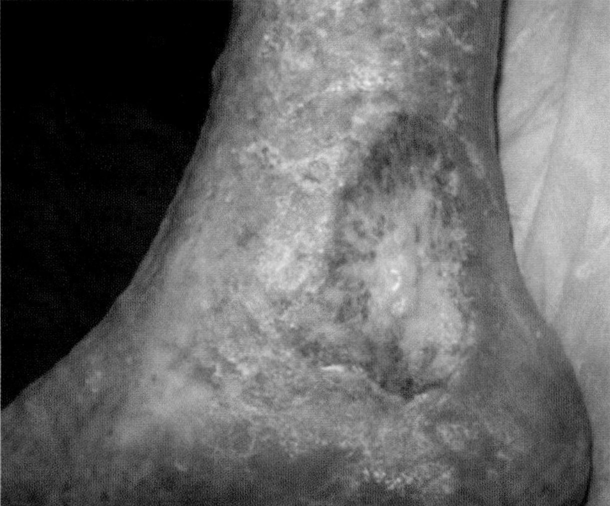

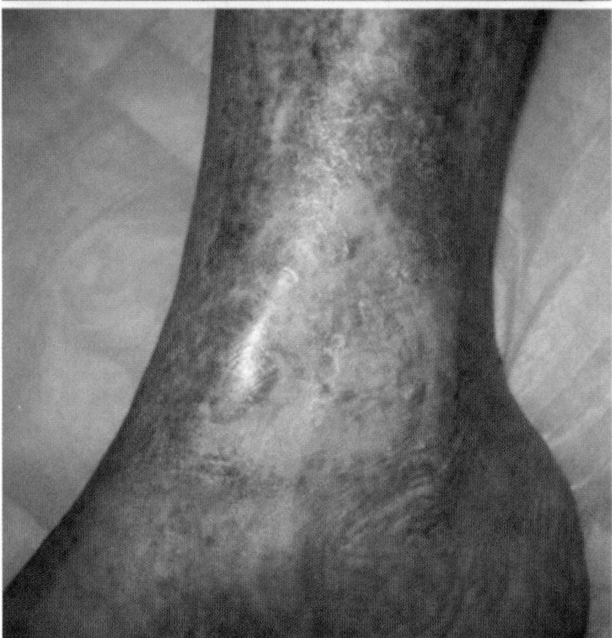

Fig. 32.2 Venous Stasis Ulcer. Typical venous ulcer, healed after 11 weeks of compression therapy using high pressure Unna boot bandages. (From Caprini JA, Partsch H, Simman R. Venous ulcers. *Journal of the American College of Clinical Wound Specialists*, 2013;4(3):54–60. doi:10.1016/j.jccw.2013.11.001.)

Many individuals develop DVT because of transient or prolonged hypercoagulability states. Pregnancy is associated with both hypercoagulability and venous stasis in the lower extremities. Active cancer is estimated to be the cause of approximately

20% of all cases of venous thromboembolism, especially hematologic malignancies and those involving the pancreas, stomach, lung, brain, ovaries, and kidneys.[5] In malignancy-related DVT, a hypercoagulable state is created by the cancer cells themselves. Tissue factor produced by cancer cells activates coagulation, fibrin synthesis, and platelet activation. Many cancer cells also produce plasminogen activator inhibitor-1 which inhibits the fibrinolytic system.[6] Some infections also are associated with hypercoagulability and venous thromboembolism. For example, systemic inflammation that results from infections such as bacterial sepsis or SARS-CoV-2 induced Coronavirus Disease 2019 (COVID-19) are associated with a high risk for the development of DVT.[7,8] Inherited hypercoagulability states increase the risk for DVT, especially in association with other risk factors, such as immobility or pregnancy. The most common inherited hypercoagulability state is factor V Leiden mutation, which affects 3% to 8% of the population and is estimated to be the cause of 20% to 25% of venous thromboembolism cases. Factor V Leiden results from a single point mutation in the Factor V gene which causes an inadequate anticoagulant response to activated protein C.[9] Individuals may develop DVT without apparent cause or after a relatively minor risk event such as airplane travel. This mutation also increases the risk of DVT recurrence after treatment. Other inherited hypercoagulability states are caused by prothrombin mutations and deficiencies of protein C, protein S, and antithrombin.

Venous thrombosis is often asymptomatic and affected individuals may be unaware that they are at risk for serious complications until they develop symptoms of thromboembolism to the lungs (pulmonary embolism, see Chapter 35). In some cases, venous inflammation causes pain and redness of the overlying tissues and skin. If the thrombus creates significant obstruction to venous blood flow, increased pressure in the vein behind the clot may lead to edema of the extremity. Most thrombi will eventually dissolve without treatment; however, untreated DVT is associated with a high risk of thromboembolization. Persistent venous obstruction may lead to CVI and postthrombotic syndrome with associated pain, edema, and ulceration of the affected limb.[4]

Because DVT is usually asymptomatic and difficult to detect clinically, prevention is important in at-risk individuals. Risk stratification algorithms are used to identify and manage at-risk individuals. Common approaches to prevention include early ambulation, pneumatic compression devices, and prophylactic anticoagulation. If thrombosis is suspected, a serum D dimer is measured. If it is negative, the diagnosis of DVT is unlikely. If the D-dimer is elevated, diagnosis of DVT is confirmed by a Doppler ultrasonography. Current guidelines recommend that uncomplicated DVT should be managed at home rather than in the hospital unless there is limb-threatening venous obstruction, high risk of bleeding, or severe pain.[10] Direct oral anticoagulants (e.g., dabigatran, apixaban, edoxaban, rivaroxaban) have been shown to have a favorable benefit-to-risk ratio and are rapidly becoming the treatments of choice.[10] Thrombolytic therapy (intravenous or catheter directed) or placement of an inferior vena cava filter may be indicated in selected individuals. Treatment is continued for 3 to 6 months at which time anticoagulation may be discontinued, or continued indefinitely for those with irreversible underlying risk factors.[10]

Superior Vena Cava Syndrome

Superior vena cava syndrome (SVCS) is a progressive occlusion of the superior vena cava (SVC) that leads to venous distention in the upper extremities and head. The most common cause is bronchogenic cancer followed by lymphomas and metastasis of other cancers. The incidence of device-related thromboses as a cause of SVCS is increasing.[11] Other less common causes include tuberculosis, mediastinal fibrosis, and cystic fibrosis. The SVC is a relatively low-pressure vessel that lies in the closed thoracic compartment; therefore space-occupying lesions can easily compress the SVC. The SVC is surrounded by lymph nodes and abuts the right mainstem bronchus, which commonly becomes involved in thoracic cancers which may compress the SVC during tumor growth. The SVC also can be occluded by the presence of large thrombi. Invasive therapies (pacemaker wires, central venous catheters, and pulmonary artery catheters) with associated thrombosis now account for nearly half of cases of SVCS.

Clinical manifestations of SVCS are edema and venous distention in the upper extremities and face, including the ocular beds. Affected persons complain of a feeling of fullness in the head or tightness of shirt collars, necklaces, and rings. Cerebral edema may cause headache, visual disturbance, and impaired consciousness. The skin of the face and arms may become purple and taut, and capillary refill time is prolonged. Respiratory distress may be present because of bronchial compression. In infants, SVCS can lead to hydrocephalus.

Diagnosis is made by chest x-ray, Doppler studies, computed tomography (CT), magnetic resonance imaging (MRI), and ultrasound. SVCS is an oncologic emergency. Treatment for malignant disorders can include radiation therapy, surgery, chemotherapy, and the administration of diuretics, steroids, and anticoagulants, as necessary. Treatment for moderate to severe nonmalignant causes may include endovascular therapy such as balloon angioplasty or bypass surgery using various grafts. Severe symptoms require thrombolysis, balloon angioplasty, placement of intravascular stents, and/or surgery.[11]

DISEASES OF THE ARTERIES

Hypertension

Hypertension is consistent elevation of systemic arterial blood pressure. It results from a sustained increase in peripheral vascular resistance (PVR), an increase in circulating blood volume and cardiac output, or both. Hypertension is defined as a sustained systolic blood pressure (SBP) of 130 mm Hg or a diastolic blood pressure (DBP) of 80 mm Hg or greater (Table 32.1). According to the American Heart Association, 51.7% of men and 42.8% of women over the age of 20 in the United States have hypertension, and the lifetime risk for developing hypertension is between 70% and 86%, with white females having the lowest risk and black males the highest risk.[12] Most affected individuals do not have their hypertension under control. Between 2007 and 2017, hypertension-related deaths in the United States increased from 18.3 per 100,000 to 23.0 per 100,000, probably related to increasing rates of obesity and diabetes.[13] The chance of developing primary hypertension increases with age, although children are being diagnosed with increasing frequency (see Chapter 33). The prevalence of hypertension is higher in Blacks and in those with diabetes. Those who fall into the category called elevated blood pressure (SBP 120 to 129 mm Hg and DBP < 80 mm Hg) are at risk for developing hypertension unless lifestyle modification is instituted. All stages of hypertension are associated with increased risk for target organ disease events, such as myocardial infarction (MI), kidney disease, and stroke.

TABLE 32.1 Classification of Blood Pressure for Adults Age 18 Years and Older

Category	Systolic (mm Hg)		Diastolic (mm Hg)
Normal	<120	AND	<80
Elevated	120–129	AND	<80
Stage 1 hypertension	130–139	OR	80–89
Stage 2 hypertension	≥140	OR	≥90
Hypertensive crisis	≥180	AND/OR	>120

Data from Whelton PK, Carey RM, Aronow WS, et al. 2017 ACC/AHA/AAPA/ABC/ACPM/AGS/APhA/ASH/ASPC/NMA/PCNA Guideline for the prevention, detection, evaluation, and management of high blood pressure in adults: a report of the American College of Cardiology/American Heart Association Task Force on Clinical Practice Guidelines. *Hypertension.* 2018;71(6):e13–e115.

Most cases (90% to 95%) of hypertension are diagnosed as primary hypertension (also called essential or idiopathic hypertension). Secondary hypertension is caused by an underlying disease process or medication that raises PVR or cardiac output. This form of hypertension accounts for only 5% to 10% of cases.[14] Examples include renal vascular or parenchymal disease, adrenocortical tumors, adrenomedullary tumors (pheochromocytoma), and drugs (oral contraceptives, corticosteroids, antihistamines). If the cause is identified and removed before permanent structural changes occur, blood pressure returns to normal.

Primary Hypertension

A specific cause for primary hypertension has not been identified. Primary hypertension is the result of a complicated interaction of genetics and the environment mediated by a host of neurohumoral effects that influence intravascular volume and PVR (Algorithm 32.1). Genetic predisposition to hypertension

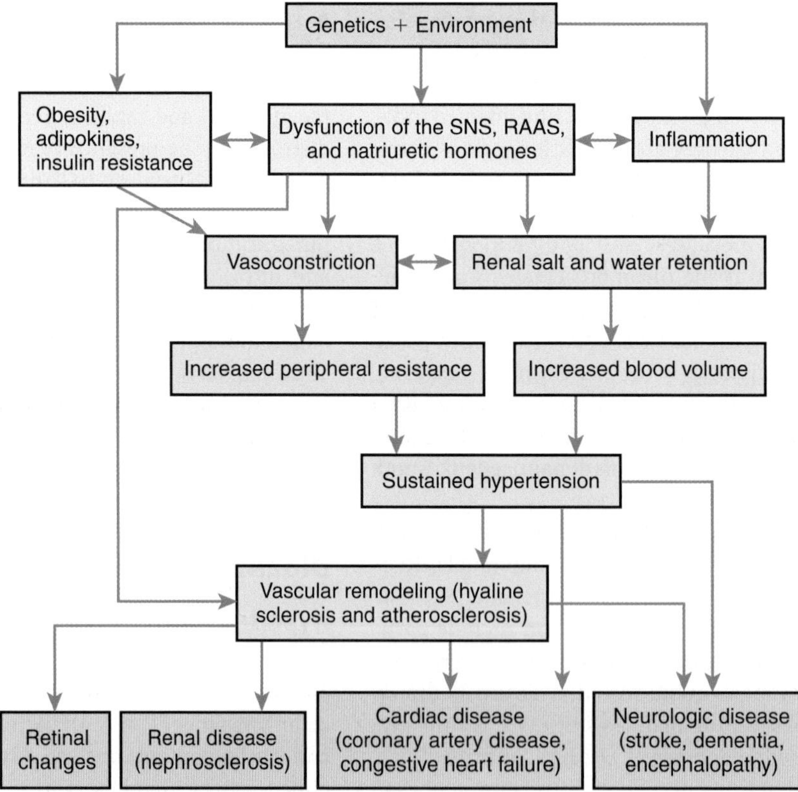

Algorithm 32.1 Pathophysiology of Hypertension. Numerous genetic vulnerabilities have been linked to hypertension and these, in combination with environmental risks, cause neurohumoral dysfunction (sympathetic nervous system *[SNS]*, renin-angiotensin-aldosterone *[RAA]* system, natriuretic hormones) and promote inflammation and insulin resistance. Insulin resistance, obesity-related adipokine alterations, and neurohumoral dysfunction contribute to sustained systemic vasoconstriction and increased peripheral vascular resistance. Inflammation contributes to renal dysfunction, which, in combination with the neurohumoral alterations, results in renal salt and water retention and increased blood volume. Increased peripheral vascular resistance and increased blood volume are two primary causes of sustained hypertension. Sustained hypertension leads to blood vessel sclerosis and associated damage to the retina, kidney, heart, and brain.

is thought to be polygenic and associated with epigenetic changes influenced by diet and lifestyle. Genetic risks include defects in renal sodium excretion, insulin sensitivity, activity of the sympathetic nervous system (SNS) and the renin-angiotensin-aldosterone system (RAAS), and cell membrane sodium or calcium transport. Risk factors for primary hypertension relate to age, sex, race, and dietary factors (see *Risk Factors:* Primary Hypertension). Many of these factors are also risk factors for other cardiovascular disorders. In fact, obesity, hypertension, dyslipidemia, and glucose intolerance often are found together in a condition called the metabolic syndrome (see Chapter 22).

RISK FACTORS
Primary Hypertension

Family history
Advancing age
Cigarette smoking
Obesity
Heavy alcohol consumption
Sex (men > women before age 55, women > men after 55)
Black race
High dietary sodium intake
Low dietary intake of potassium, calcium, magnesium
Glucose intolerance and diabetes

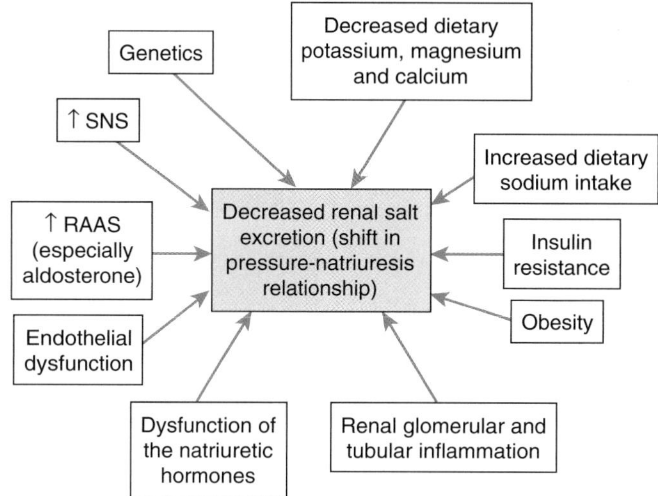

Fig. 32.3 Factors that Cause a Shift in the Pressure-Natriuresis Relationship. Numerous factors have been implicated in the pathogenesis of sodium retention in individuals with hypertension. These factors cause less renal excretion of salt than would normally occur with increased blood pressure. This is called a shift in the pressure-natriuresis relationship and is thought to be a central process in the pathogenesis of primary hypertension. *RAAS,* Renin-angiotensin-aldosterone system; *SNS,* sympathetic nervous system.

Pathophysiology. Multiple mechanisms contribute to the pathophysiology of hypertension including changes in the SNS, the RAAS, and natriuretic peptides. Inflammation, endothelial dysfunction, obesity-related hormones, and insulin resistance also contribute. Increased vascular volume is related to a decrease in renal excretion of salt, often referred to as a shift in the pressure-natriuresis relationship (Fig. 32.3). This means that for a given blood pressure, individuals with hypertension tend to secrete less salt in their urine.

As described in Algorithm 32.1, genetic and environmental risks lead to changes in neurohormones, insulin resistance, and inflammation. Obesity contributes to these changes through changes in adipokines and increased inflammation. The combination of all of these factors cause sodium and water retention and peripheral vasoconstriction leading to sustained hypertension and organ damage.

Increased SNS activity causes accelerated heart rate and systemic vasoconstriction. These changes increase both cardiac output and peripheral vascular resistance, thus raising the blood pressure. Additional mechanisms of SNS-induced hypertension include structural changes in blood vessels (vascular remodeling), renal sodium retention (shift in pressure-natriuresis curve), insulin resistance, increased renin and angiotensin levels, and procoagulant effects.

In hypertensive individuals, overactivity of the classical pathway of the RAAS directly causes salt and water retention and increased vascular resistance (Algorithm 32.2). This RAAS pathway begins when angiotensinogen is synthesized in the liver and is released into the blood. There it is cleaved to angiotensin I (Ang I) by renin which is secreted from the juxtaglomerular apparatus (JGA) in the kidney. Angiotensin-converting enzyme 1 (ACE1) in the lung and in tissues catalyzes the formation of angiotensin II (Ang II). Ang II binds with several receptors, the most important of which are AT1 and AT2. AT1 receptor binding results in vasoconstriction (increases vascular resistance) and aldosterone secretion by the adrenal cortex (increases salt and water retention) leading to hypertension and edema. AT1 receptor binding by Ang II also activates the SNS and acts as a growth factor contributing to vascular and myocardial remodeling, inflammation, insulin resistance, and platelet activation. Vascular remodeling is structural change in vessel walls that results in permanent increases in PVR and contributes to atherogenesis. Taken together, these effects contribute to atherosclerosis, ischemic heart disease, myocardial hypertrophy, and heart failure. Medications such as ACE inhibitors, angiotensin receptor blockers (ARBs), and aldosterone blockers oppose the activity of the RAAS and are effective in reducing blood pressure and protecting against target organ damage.

In contrast, when Ang II binds to the AT2 receptor, it functions to oppose the effects of AT1 stimulation. Ang II binding to the AT2 receptor causes vasodilation and decreased remodeling and has anti-inflammatory and antioxidant effects. An imbalance between these two receptor pathways is linked to primary hypertension (see Algorithm 32.2). A second RAAS pathway uses angiotensin converting enzyme 2 (ACE2) to create Ang (1–7) which binds to MAS receptors in vascular, cardiac, and pulmonary tissues. It serves to downregulate AT1 receptors, promotes antihypertensive vasodilation, and reduces cardiovascular remodeling.[15] MAS receptor binding by Ang (1–7) also provides cerebrovascular and metabolic protective effects. In addition, the ACE2 pathway is highly expressed in lungs with the ability to mitigate cardiopulmonary diseases

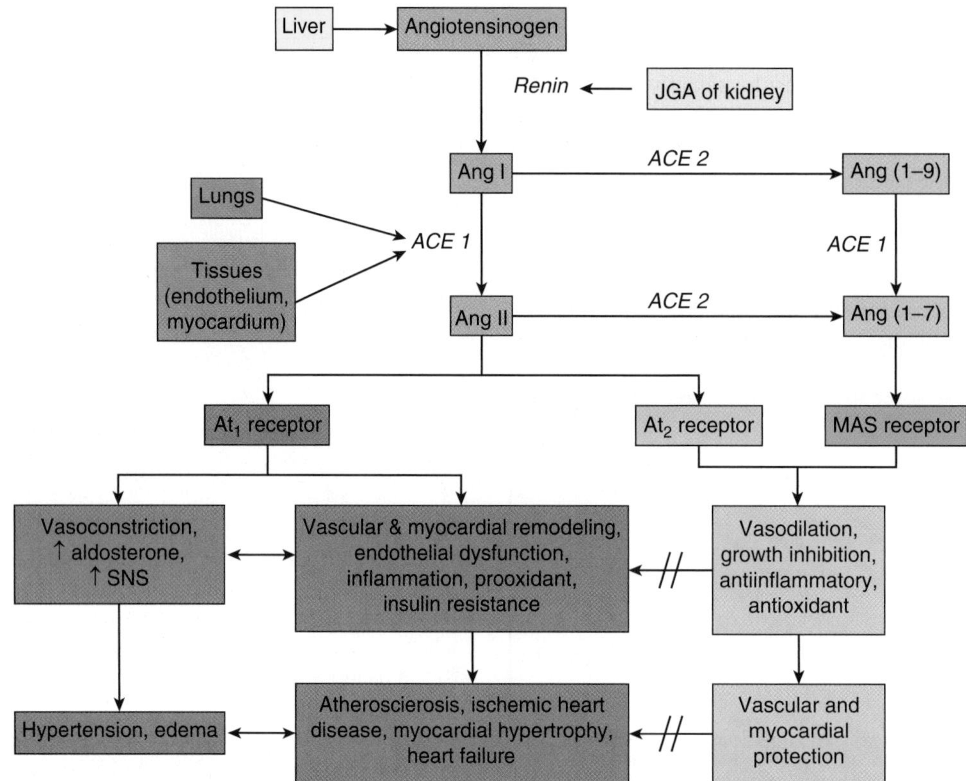

Algorithm 32.2 The Renin-Angiotensin-Aldosterone System and Its Effects on Tissues The classical pathway of the renin-angiotensin-aldosterone system (RAAS) begins when angiotensinogen is synthesized in the liver and is released into the blood. There it is cleaved to angiotensin I *(Ang I)* by renin which is secreted from the juxtaglomerular apparatus *(JGA)* in the kidney. Angiotensin-converting enzyme 1 *(ACE1)* in the lung and in tissues catalyzes the formation of angiotensin II *(Ang II)*. Ang II binds with several receptors, the most important of which are AT1 and AT2. AT1 receptor binding results in vasoconstriction (increases vascular resistance) and aldosterone secretion by the adrenal cortex (increases salt and water retention) leading to hypertension and edema. AT1 receptor binding by Ang II also acts as a growth factor leading to vascular and myocardial remodeling as well as inflammation and insulin resistance. Taken together, these effects contribute to atherosclerosis, ischemic heart disease, myocardial hypertrophy and heart failure. In contrast, Ang II binding to the AT2 receptor causes vasodilation, decreased remodeling and has anti-inflammatory and antioxidant effects. Another pathway of the RAAS uses the enzyme ACE2 to form Angiotensin (1–7) from Angiotensin (1–9). Ang (1–7) binds to the MAS receptor and provides additional protection against the negative vascular and myocardial effects of Ang II. *SNS*, Sympathetic nervous system.

such as inflammatory lung disease associated with COVID-19.[16] New therapies aimed at potentiating the ACE2 pathway are in development.[17]

Dysfunction of the natriuretic hormones plays an important role in the pathogenesis of hypertension. These hormones include atrial natriuretic peptide (ANP), B-type natriuretic peptide (BNP), C-type natriuretic peptide (CNP), and urodilatin. Together they modulate renal sodium (Na^+) excretion and require adequate potassium, calcium, and magnesium intake to function properly. ANP and BNP are released when there is mechanical stretch of the myocardium. After binding to the natriuretic receptor, they stimulate salt and water loss by the kidney (natriuresis), contribute to arteriolar vasodilation, and reduce RAAS activation.[18] Dysfunction of these hormones, along with alterations in the RAA system and the SNS, causes a shift in the pressure-natriuresis relationship leading to increased blood volume and blood pressure. Decreased activity of the natriuretic peptides also is linked to vascular and cardiac remodeling. With inadequate natriuretic function, there is a compensatory increase in natriuretic peptide serum levels. High levels of these peptides therefore indicate dysfunction and are linked to an increased risk for ventricular hypertrophy, atherosclerosis, and heart failure in individuals with hypertension. Salt restriction combined with adequate intake of dietary potassium, magnesium, and calcium improves natriuretic peptide function. Diuretics promote renal salt and water excretion and are a mainstay of hypertensive treatment. Drugs that block the degradation of the natriuretic peptides by blocking the enzyme neprilysin are currently used in combination with angiotensin receptor blockers (ARNi) (e.g., sacubitril/valsartan) for the treatment of heart failure, and are being evaluated for the treatment of hypertension, but may be associated with decreased cognitive function.[19,20]

Innate and adaptive immunity with associated inflammation play a role in the pathogenesis of hypertension. Activation of immunity results in chronic inflammation with damage to endothelial cells, decreased production of vasodilators (such as nitric oxide), vascular remodeling, and smooth muscle contraction. The contributions of diet, obesity, insulin resistance, and activation of the RAAS to the development of hypertension are likely to be mediated in part by increased systemic inflammation.[21] Neuroinflammation is linked to increased SNS activity.[22] Inflammation also contributes to insulin resistance, decreased natriuresis, and autonomic dysfunction.

Obesity accounts for 65% to 75% of primary hypertension.[23] Obesity and increased caloric intake contribute to adipocyte dysfunction and ectopic fat deposition throughout the cardiovascular system. Adipocytes secrete adipokines, including leptin and adiponectin. The primary function of leptin is to interact with the hypothalamus to control body weight through appetite inhibition and increased metabolic rate (see Chapter 23). Adiponectin is a protein produced by adipose tissue but is reduced in obesity. With obesity, increased leptin and decreased adiponectin have been found to increase sympathetic nervous system and renin-angiotensin-aldosterone system activity, contribute to insulin resistance, decrease renal sodium excretion, promote inflammation, and stimulate myocyte hypertrophy. Other adipokines that are altered in obesity-related cardiovascular diseases include resistin, omentin, visfatin, and perivascular adipose tissue–derived relaxing factor. Obesity also is linked with endothelial dysfunction which contributes to vasoconstriction and arterial remodeling. Taken together, these obesity-related changes result in vasoconstriction, salt and water retention, and renal dysfunction that contribute to the development of hypertension. Weight loss is an essential treatment for obesity-related hypertension. In severe obesity, bariatric surgery has been shown to cause long-standing remission of hypertension in many individuals, although those with severe hypertension requiring multiple medications are less likely to benefit.[24,25]

Insulin resistance is common in hypertension, even in individuals without clinical diabetes. Insulin resistance is associated with decreased endothelial release of nitric oxide and other vasodilators. It also affects renal function and causes renal salt and water retention. Insulin resistance promotes overactivity of the SNS and RAAS. The interactions among obesity, hypertension, insulin resistance, and lipid disorders in metabolic syndrome result in a high risk of cardiovascular disease.[26]

Given the complexity of all the factors that contribute to its pathophysiology, primary hypertension is now being considered a metabolic disease that results from the interaction of genes, diet, neurohormones, adipokines, immune cytokines, and gut microbiota (see Emerging Science Box: Hypertension as a Metabolic Disease). These discoveries are leading to new approaches to hypertension

Complicated hypertension. As hypertension becomes more severe and chronic, tissue damage can occur in the blood vessels and tissues leading to target organ damage in the heart, kidney, brain, and eyes. Cardiovascular complications of sustained hypertension include left ventricular hypertrophy, angina pectoris, heart failure, coronary artery disease, myocardial infarction, and sudden death.[14] Myocardial hypertrophy is mediated by the SNS and RAAS. Hypertrophy is characterized by a myocardium that is thickened, scarred, and less able to relax during diastole, leading to heart failure with preserved ejection fraction. Over time, the increased size of the heart muscle increases demand for oxygen delivery, the contractility of the heart is impaired, and the individual is at risk for myocardial infarction and heart failure with reduced ejection fraction. Vascular complications include hyaline sclerosis and accelerated atherosclerosis that can affect perfusion to any vascular bed. Hypertension also can contribute to the formation, dissection, and rupture of aneurysms (outpouchings in vessel walls). Renal manifestations of complicated hypertension include

EMERGING SCIENCE BOX

Hypertension as a Metabolic Disease

As the complex mechanisms that link obesity with hypertension are being elucidated, there is increasing appreciation for the concept of hypertension as a metabolic disorder. This concept derives from an increased understanding of the many ways that diet, gut function and microbiota, neurohormones, and adipose tissue composition and function work together to influence cardiovascular health and disease. For example, it is now believed that high salt intake not only causes hypertension in genetically predisposed individuals, it also may directly contribute to the development of obesity and diabetes. Furthermore, a high-salt diet causes gut microbiota dysbiosis, alters nutrient uptake from the intestines, and negatively impacts gastrin-induced natriuresis. There are interactions between the gut, the brain, adipose tissue, and the kidney that affect vascular tone. Obesity is not only linked to changes in adipokines such as leptin and adiponectin, but there are other hormones released from adipose tissue that are linked to changes in fat deposition and vascular function including apelin, omentin, and visfatin. Further complicating these relationships is the discovery that visceral and perivascular adipose tissue are independently associated with insulin resistance, dyslipidemia, and hypertension even in individuals with a healthy body mass index (BMI). Changes in glucocorticoid function are linked to obesity-related hypertension, and may be associated with stress even in perinatal development. Inflammatory and immune cells are also impacted by obesity-related metabolic changes resulting in chronic inflammation and immune-mediated damage to blood vessels and to renal tissue. These complex interactions reinforce the benefits of lifestyle interventions (diet, exercise, weight loss) and provide multiple potential opportunities for future hypertension therapies aimed at specific mechanisms of metabolic dysfunction.

Data from Dalmasso C, et al. Sensory signals mediating high blood pressure via sympathetic activation: Role of adipose afferent reflex. *American Journal of Physiology - Regulatory Integrative and Comparative Physiology*, 2020;318(2):R379–R389; Facchi JC, et al. Perinatal programming of metabolic diseases: the role of glucocorticoids. *Metabolism*, 2020;104:154047; Manor O, et al. Health and disease markers correlate with gut microbiome composition across thousands of people. *Nature Communications*, 2020;11:206; Palmu J, et al. Association between the gut microbiota and blood pressure in a population cohort of 6953 individuals. *Journal of the American Heart Association*, 2020;9(15):e016641; Saxton SN, et al. Mechanistic links between obesity, diabetes, and blood pressure: Role of perivascular adipose tissue. *Physiological Reviews*, 2019;99(4):1701–1763; Smiljanec K, et al. Sodium, hypertension, and the gut: Does the gut microbiota go salty? *American Journal of Physiology - Heart and Circulatory Physiology*, 2019;317(6):H1173–H1182; Tanaka M, et al. Hypertension as a metabolic disorder and the novel role of the gut. *Current Hypertension Reports*, 2019;21:63; Witkowski M, et al. Gut microbiota and cardiovascular disease. *Circulation Research*, 2020;127(4):553–370.

nephrosclerosis, renal arteriosclerosis, and renal insufficiency or failure. Microalbuminuria (small amounts of protein in the urine) occurs in many individuals with HTN and is now recognized as an early sign of impending renal dysfunction and increased risk for cardiovascular events. Complications specific to the retina include retinal vascular sclerosis, exudation, and hemorrhage. Cerebrovascular complications include transient ischemia, stroke, cerebral thrombosis, aneurysm, hemorrhage, and dementia. The pathologic effects of complicated hypertension are summarized in Table 32.2.

Clinical Manifestations. The early stages of hypertension have no clinical manifestations other than elevated blood pressure; for this reason, hypertension is called a silent disease. Some hypertensive individuals never develop signs, symptoms, or complications, whereas others become very ill, and hypertension can be a cause of death. If elevated blood pressure is not detected and treated, it becomes established, setting the stage for the complications of hypertension that begin to appear during the fourth, fifth, and sixth decades of life.

Most clinical manifestations of hypertensive disease are caused by complications that damage organs and tissues outside the vascular system. Besides elevated blood pressure, the signs and symptoms therefore tend to be specific for the organs or tissues affected. Evidence of heart disease, renal insufficiency, central nervous system dysfunction, impaired vision, impaired mobility, vascular occlusion, or edema can all be caused by sustained hypertension.

Evaluation and Treatment. Diagnosis of hypertension requires the measurement of blood pressure on at least two separate occasions, averaging two readings at least 2 minutes apart, with the following conditions: the person is seated, the arm is supported at heart level, the person must be at rest for at least 5 minutes, and the person should not have smoked or ingested any caffeine in the previous 30 minutes. Diagnostic tests for further evaluation of hypertension may include ambulatory 24-hour blood pressure monitoring to detect night-time blood pressure variations and the presence of white-coat or masked hypertension (blood pressures that are elevated or normal only during office blood pressure measurement) in selected individuals.[27] Other evaluative studies should include measurement of electrolytes, glucose, and lipids, and an electrocardiogram (ECG). Individuals who have elevated blood pressure are assumed to have primary hypertension unless their history, physical examination, or initial diagnostic screening indicates secondary hypertension. Once the diagnosis is made, a careful evaluation for other cardiovascular risk factors and for end-organ damage should be done (e.g., echocardiography, carotid ultrasound, renal evaluation).

Treatment of primary hypertension depends on its severity. Management begins with lifestyle modification including exercise, and dietary modifications including reducing salt intake, smoking cessation, and weight loss. In 2021 the American College of Cardiology recommended that individuals with Stage 1 hypertension who are at low risk for cardiovascular disease but who do not respond to lifestyle modification should consider beginning pharmacologic therapy.[28] Pharmacologic treatment is recommended for individuals with Stage 1 hypertension who have existing or are at high risk for atherosclerotic cardiovascular disease, and for those who have Stage 2 hypertension. The 2017 American College of Cardiology/American Heart Association guidelines recommend medications including diuretics, ACE inhibitors or ARBs, and calcium channel blockers.[27] These guidelines were largely affirmed by the International Society of Hypertension in 2020.[29] The choice of medications depends upon several factors including race and ethnicity, gender, age, and comorbidities such as heart disease, diabetes, and renal disease. Combinations of different types of antihypertensive medications may be indicated. Careful follow-up to support continued adherence, determine the response, and monitor for potential side effects of these medications is important. Other therapies for selected individuals include mineralocorticoid receptor antagonists and renal denervation.

Treatment goals include returning blood pressure to normotensive levels in most individuals, which can reduce the risk for stroke, dementia, and cardiovascular complications.[27,30] Older adults with hypertension also benefit from blood pressure reduction treatments but should be managed carefully with treatment goals adjusted by age and underlying comorbidities.[27]

Hypertensive crisis. Hypertensive crisis (malignant hypertension) is rapidly progressive hypertension in which systolic pressure is ≥180 mm Hg and/or diastolic pressure is ≥120 mm

TABLE 32.2 Pathologic Effects of Sustained, Complicated Primary Hypertension

Site of Injury	Mechanism of Injury	Pathologic Effect
Heart		
Myocardium	Increased workload combined with diminished blood flow through coronary arteries	Left ventricular hypertrophy, myocardial ischemia, heart failure
Coronary arteries	Accelerated atherosclerosis (coronary artery disease)	Myocardial ischemia, myocardial infarction, sudden death
Kidneys	Reduced blood flow, increased arteriolar pressure, RAAS and SNS stimulation, and inflammation	Glomerulosclerosis and decreased glomerular filtration, end-stage renal disease
Brain	Reduced blood flow and oxygen supply; weakened vessel walls, accelerated atherosclerosis	Transient ischemic attacks, cerebral thrombosis, aneurysm, hemorrhage, acute brain infarction
Eyes (retinas)	Retinal vascular sclerosis, increased retinal artery pressures	Hypertensive retinopathy, retinal exudates and hemorrhages
Aorta	Weakened vessel wall	Dissecting aneurysm
Arteries of lower extremities	Reduced blood flow and high pressures in arterioles, accelerated atherosclerosis	Intermittent claudication, gangrene

RAAS, Renin-angiotensin-aldosterone system; *SNS*, sympathetic nervous system.

Hg and is associated with advanced bilateral retinopathy, encephalopathy, or microangiopathy.[27] It can occur in those with primary hypertension, but the reason some people develop this complication and others do not is unknown. Other causes include complications of pregnancy, cocaine or amphetamine use, reaction to certain medications, adrenal tumors, and alcohol withdrawal. High arterial pressure renders the cerebral arterioles incapable of regulating blood flow to the cerebral capillary beds. High hydrostatic pressures in the capillaries cause vascular fluid to exude into the interstitial space. Retina exhibit hemorrhages, cotton wool spots, and papilledema. If blood pressure is not reduced, cerebral edema and cerebral dysfunction (encephalopathy) increase until death occurs. Besides encephalopathy, hypertensive crisis can cause hemolysis and thrombocytopenia, angiopathy, myocardial infarction, cardiac failure with pulmonary edema, aortic dissection, uremia, and cerebrovascular accident (stroke) and is considered a medical emergency. A rapid evaluation for underlying cause and cardiovascular and neurologic complications is indicated, with rapid institution of medications such as beta- or alpha-blockers, calcium channel blockers, and nitrates.[27] It is likely that in many cases, individuals who present with hypertensive crisis have poorly controlled underlying chronic hypertension, and careful follow-up and management is crucial.

Orthostatic (Postural) Hypotension

The term orthostatic (postural) hypotension (OH) refers to a decrease in SBP of at least 20 mm Hg or a decrease in DBP of at least 10 mm Hg within 3 minutes of moving to a standing position. It is a common condition in individuals accessing community and primary care clinics (prevalence 17% to 19%) and affects nearly one third of individuals in residential care or nursing homes, especially those with dementia and Parkinson disease.[31] OH affects men more often than women, and usually occurs between the ages of 40 and 70 years. It is a significant risk factor for falls and associated injury and for increased mortality.

OH is often associated with disorders that affect autonomic nervous function. Normally when an individual stands, the gravitational changes on the circulation are compensated by a baroreceptor-mediated reflex that stimulates the SNS. This causes arteriolar and venous constriction and increased heart rate upon standing. Other compensatory mechanisms include mechanical factors, such as the closure of valves in the venous system, contraction of the leg muscles, and a decrease in intrathoracic pressure. These mechanisms are dysfunctional or inadequate in individuals with orthostatic hypotension; consequently, upon standing, blood pools in the lower extremities and normal arterial pressure cannot be maintained.

Orthostatic hypotension may be acute or chronic. Acute orthostatic hypotension is common in older adults and occurs when the normal regulatory mechanisms are inadequate as a result of (1) altered body chemistry, (2) drug action (e.g., antihypertensives, antidepressants), (3) prolonged immobility, (4) starvation, (5) physical exhaustion, (6) volume depletion (e.g., dehydration, diuresis, potassium or sodium depletion), or (7) any condition that results in venous pooling (e.g., pregnancy, extensive varicosities of the lower extremities).

Chronic orthostatic hypotension may be (1) secondary to a specific disease or (2) primary (idiopathic). Secondary causes include neurogenic OH which results from diseases of the central or peripheral nervous systems that affect autonomic function (e.g., spinal cord injury, Parkinson disease, multiple system atrophy, intracranial tumors, cerebral infarcts, Wernicke encephalopathy, and peripheral neuropathies). Other causes of secondary OH are adrenal insufficiency and metabolic disorders (e.g., diabetes, porphyria). Cardiovascular autonomic neuropathy is a common cause of OH in persons with diabetes affecting up to 20% of diabetic individuals and is often overlooked.[32] Chronic OH also can occur in those taking antihypertensive medications. It is interesting to note that although OH is common in older individuals being treated for hypertension, those who undergo intensive treatment and achieve good control of their systolic blood pressure are less likely to develop OH than those who are treated less intensively, likely due to favorable effects of improved blood pressure on autonomic function.[33] Many other medications also can cause OH including nitrates, antidepressants, phosphodiesterase inhibitors, and dopamine agonists.[32]

OH can be asymptomatic. In those with symptoms, it often is characterized by dizziness, blurring or loss of vision, and syncope. In neurogenic OH, symptoms often worsen during exercise and after meals. When possible, acute OH and secondary chronic OH are managed by correction of the underlying condition. Chronic primary OH and irreversible secondary OH are managed with a combination of nondrug and drug therapies.[34] Nonpharmacologic interventions include avoidance of caffeine and alcohol, increased fluid and salt intake, frequent small low-glycemic meals, sleeping with the head of the bed raised, and waist-high stockings or abdominal binders. Pharmacologic management includes mineralocorticoids (e.g., fludrocortisone) and vasoconstrictors (e.g., midodrine, droxidopa). Norepinephrine reuptake inhibitors are being studied.[32]

Aneurysm

An aneurysm is a localized dilation or outpouching of a vessel wall or cardiac chamber. True aneurysms involve weakening in all three layers of the arterial wall (Fig. 32.4A). Most are fusiform and circumferential, whereas *saccular aneurysms* are basically spherical in shape. False aneurysms are an extravascular hematoma that communicates with the intravascular space. A common cause of this type of lesion is a leak between a vascular graft and a natural artery.

Vascular aneurysms most commonly occur in the thoracic or abdominal aorta, and in the cerebrovascular system. Major risk factors for aneurysm formation include hypertension and atherosclerosis. Chronic hypertension results in mechanical and shear forces that contribute to inflammation and remodeling resulting in weakening of the vessel wall. Atherosclerotic plaque formation also causes inflammatory changes that erode the vessel wall. Additional risk factors include gene polymorphisms that are linked to the production of growth factors, myosin, and proteases.[35] Infections, such as syphilis, collagen disorders (such as Marfan syndrome), and traumatic injury to the chest or abdomen, also can cause aortic aneurysms. There are rare inherited syndromes that are characterized by aneurysm formation at an early age.

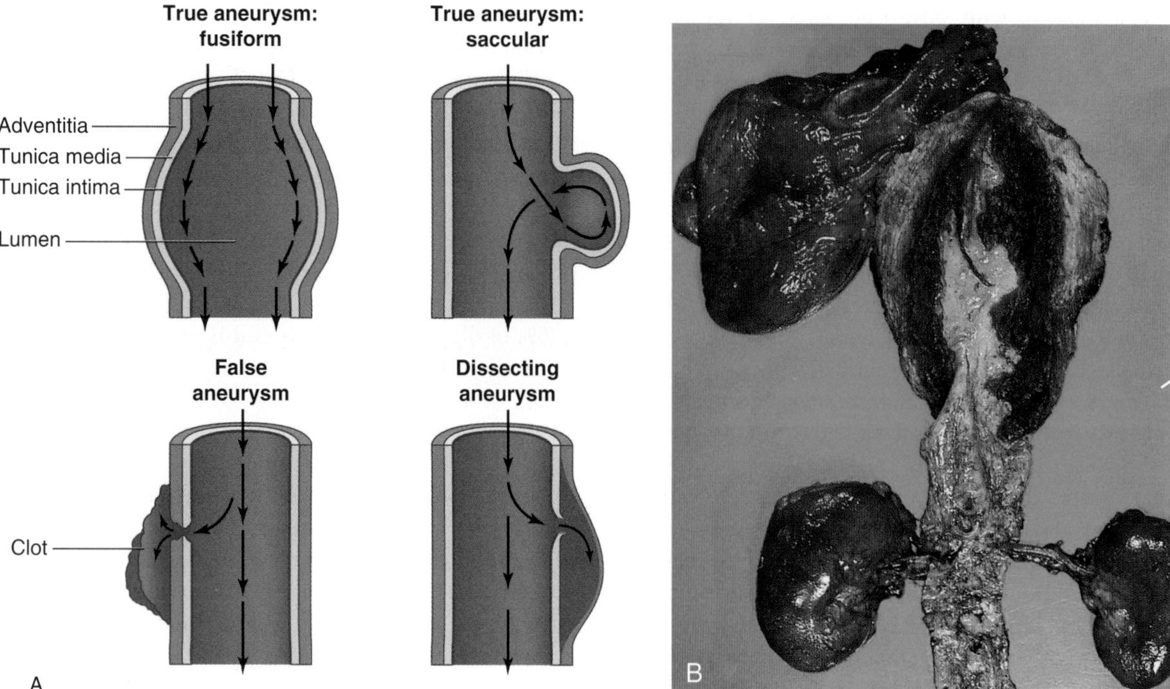

Fig. 32.4 Longitudinal Sections Showing Types of Aneurysms. (A) True aneurysms are caused by bulging of all three layers of the vessel wall and can be circumferential (fusiform) or can form a bulge on one side of the vessel (saccular). False aneurysms are a collection of clotted blood just outside of the vessel due to a break all the way through the vessel wall, usually caused by trauma. Dissecting aneurysms result from a partial break in the vessel wall such that blood is pushed between the tunica media and the adventitia. **(B)** Dissecting aneurysm of thoracic aorta *(arrow)*. (B, From Damjanov I, Linder J, eds. *Anderson's pathology*, 10th edition. St. Louis: Mosby; 1996.)

The aorta is particularly susceptible to aneurysm formation because of constant stress on the vessel wall and the absence of penetrating vasa vasorum in the media layer. Chronic inflammation of the wall of the aorta is considered the primary cause of aortic aneurysms leading to weakening of the intima and medial layers. Neutrophils, macrophages, and T and B lymphocytes enter the aortic wall, and cytokines produced by these cells cause an inflammatory response. Proteases are released that destroy tissues and contribute to extracellular matrix remodeling, apoptosis and calcification of vascular smooth muscle cells, and decreased wall elasticity.[36] These chronic inflammatory changes are potentiated in individuals with atherosclerosis and hypertension, which are found in more than half of all individuals with aneurysms.

Formation of a cardiac ventricular wall aneurysm most often occurs when intraventricular tension stretches noncontracting infarcted muscle. Acutely infarcted myocardium is characterized by a weak and thin layer of necrotic tissue that bulges with each contraction. With time the aneurysm becomes more fibrotic, but continues to bulge with each systole, thus acting as a "reservoir" and reducing stroke volume.

Clinical manifestations of aneurysms depend on where the aneurysm is located. Aortic aneurysms often are asymptomatic until they rupture and then cause severe pain and hypotension. Thoracic aortic aneurysms can cause dysphagia (difficulty swallowing) and dyspnea (breathlessness). An aneurysm that impairs flow to an extremity causes symptoms of ischemia. Cerebral aneurysms, which often occur in the circle of Willis, are associated with signs and symptoms of increased intracranial pressure and stroke. (Cerebral aneurysms are described in Chapter 18.) Aneurysms in the heart present with dysrhythmias, heart failure, and embolism of clots to the brain or other vital organs.

The diagnosis of an aneurysm is usually confirmed by ultrasonography, CT, MRI, or angiography. Medical treatment for small asymptomatic aortic aneurysms includes cessation of smoking, reduction of blood pressure, and initiation of cholesterol lowering medications (statins) and antiplatelet drugs. None of these treatments can fully prevent the progression of these aneurysms, and their growth must be monitored closely. Potential new medical therapies being explored include the diabetes drug metformin, blockers of specific inflammatory pathways, and stem cells.[36] For aneurysms that are dilating rapidly or have become large, either open or endovascular surgical repair is indicated and usually includes replacement with a prosthetic graft.[37]

Aortic aneurysms can be complicated by the acute aortic syndromes, which include aortic dissection, hemorrhage into the vessel wall, or vessel rupture. Dissection of the layers of the arterial wall occurs when there is a tear in the intima and blood is pushed between the tunica media and the adventitia of the wall of the artery (see Fig. 32.4B). Dissections can involve any part of the aorta (ascending, arch, or descending) and can disrupt flow through arterial branches. Symptoms include severe pain in the neck, jaw, chest, back, or abdomen. Emergent evaluation and surgical intervention are critical. Chest CT angiography is the diagnostic technique of choice.[38] Surgical intervention is often emergent.

Thrombus Formation in Arteries

As in venous thrombosis, arterial thrombi develops when intravascular conditions promote activation of coagulation or when there is stasis of blood flow. These conditions include those in which there is intimal irritation or roughening (such as in percutaneous or surgical procedures and trauma), inflammation, infection, low intravascular volume and pressures, or obstructions that cause blood stasis and pooling within the vessels. Damage to the endothelium leads to activation of the clotting cascade and platelet adherence. An anatomic change in an artery (such as an aneurysm) can contribute to thrombus formation, particularly if the change results in a pooling of arterial blood. Valvular thrombi are most commonly associated with inflammation of the endocardium (endocarditis) and rheumatic heart disease. Widespread arterial thrombus formation can occur in shock when systemic inflammation activates the intrinsic and extrinsic pathways of coagulation, resulting in microvascular thrombosis throughout the systemic arterial circulation (see Chapter 48).

Arterial thrombi pose two potential threats to the circulation. First, the thrombus may grow large enough to occlude the artery, causing ischemia in tissue supplied by the artery. Second, the thrombus may dislodge, becoming a thromboembolus that travels through the vascular system until it occludes flow into a distal systemic vascular bed.

Diagnosis of arterial thrombi is usually accomplished through the use of Doppler ultrasonography and angiography. Pharmacologic treatment involves the administration of anticoagulants or thrombolytics. A balloon-tipped catheter can be used to remove or compress an arterial thrombus.

Embolism

Embolism is the obstruction of a vessel by an embolus—a bolus of matter circulating in the bloodstream. The embolus may consist of a dislodged thrombus; an air bubble; an aggregate of amniotic fluid; an aggregate of fat, bacteria, or cancer cells; or a foreign substance. The types of emboli are summarized in Table 32.3. Most emboli arise from venous or arterial thrombi and travel in the bloodstream until they reach a vessel through which they cannot pass. Pulmonary emboli originate on the venous system (mostly from the deep veins of the legs) or in the right heart; arterial emboli most commonly originate in the left heart and are associated with thrombus formation associated with MI, valvular disease, left heart failure, endocarditis, and dysrhythmias.

Embolism causes ischemia or infarction in tissues distal to the obstruction, producing organ dysfunction and pain. Infarction and subsequent necrosis of a central organ are life-threatening. For example, occlusion of a coronary artery will cause an MI whereas occlusion of a cerebral artery causes a stroke (see Chapter 18).

TABLE 32.3 Types of Emboli

Type	Characteristics
Arteries	
Arterial thromboembolism	Dislodged thrombus; source is usually from heart; most common sites of obstruction are lower extremities (femoral and popliteal arteries), coronary arteries, and cerebral vasculature
Veins	
Venous thromboembolism	Dislodged thrombus; source is usually from lower extremities; obstructs branches of pulmonary artery
Air embolism	Bolus of air displaces blood in vasculature; source usually room air entering circulation through IV lines; trauma to chest also may allow air from lungs to enter vascular space
Amniotic fluid embolism	Bolus of amniotic fluid; extensive intra-abdominal pressure attending labor and delivery can force amniotic fluid into bloodstream of mother; introduces antigens, cells, and protein aggregates that trigger inflammation, coagulation, and immune responses
Bacterial embolism	Aggregates of bacteria in bloodstream; source is subacute bacterial endocarditis or abscess
Fat embolism	Globules of fat floating in bloodstream associated with trauma to long bones; lungs in particular are affected
Foreign matter	Small particles or fibers introduced during trauma or through an IV or intra-arterial line; coagulation cascade is initiated and thromboemboli form around particles

Peripheral Vascular Diseases

Thromboangiitis Obliterans (Buerger Disease)

Thromboangiitis obliterans (Buerger disease) is a highly inflammatory autoimmune disease of the peripheral arteries. It is strongly associated with smoking. Thromboangiitis obliterans is characterized by the formation of thrombi filled with inflammatory and immune cells. Inflammatory cytokines and toxic oxygen free radicals contribute to accompanying vasospasm. Over time, these thrombi become organized and fibrotic and result in permanent occlusion of small- and medium-sized arteries in the feet and sometimes in the hands.

The chief symptom of thromboangiitis obliterans is pain and tenderness of the affected part, usually affecting more than one extremity. Clinical manifestations include rubor (redness of the skin), which is caused by dilated capillaries under the skin, and cyanosis, which is caused by tissue ischemia. Chronic ischemia causes the skin to become thin and shiny and serious ulcers may occur. In advanced disease, profound ischemia of the extremities can cause gangrene necessitating amputation. Thromboangiitis obliterans also has been associated with cerebrovascular disease (stroke), mesenteric disease, and rheumatic symptoms (joint pain).

Diagnosis of thromboangiitis obliterans is made by identification of the following common features—age <45 years, smoking history, evidence of peripheral ischemia—and by exclusion of other causes of arterial insufficiency. The most important part of treatment is cessation of cigarette smoking. Other measures include vasodilators and exercises aimed at improving circulation to the foot or hand. Endovascular procedures can improve outcomes in selected individuals. Stem cell therapy for skin ulcers have been shown to improve healing and symptoms.[39,40]

Raynaud Phenomenon

Raynaud phenomenon (RP) is characterized by attacks of vasospasm in the small arteries and arterioles of the fingers and, less commonly, the toes. Approximately 90% of individuals with RP have primary Raynaud phenomenon, which is a common vasospastic disorder of unknown origin affecting up to 5% of adults.[41] Genetic factors have been implicated. Secondary Raynaud phenomenon is associated with systemic diseases, particularly collagen vascular disease (progressive systemic sclerosis [scleroderma]), vasculitis, malignancy, pulmonary hypertension, chemotherapy, cocaine use, hypothyroidism, thoracic outlet syndrome, trauma, serum sickness, or long-term exposure to environmental conditions such as cold temperatures or vibrating machinery in the workplace. Blood vessels in affected individuals demonstrate dysfunctional autonomic vascular thermoregulation.[41] In addition, endothelial dysfunction with an imbalance in endothelium-derived vasodilators (e.g., nitric oxide) and vasoconstrictors (e.g., endothelin-1) is seen. Platelet activation also may play a role. It tends to affect young women and is characterized by vasospastic attacks triggered by brief exposure to cold, vibration, or emotional stress. Genetic predisposition may play a role in its development.

The clinical manifestations of the vasospastic attacks of either disorder are changes in skin color and sensation caused by ischemia. Attacks tend to be bilateral, and manifestations usually begin at the tips of the digits and progress to the proximal phalanges. Vasospasm causes pallor, numbness, and the sensation of coldness in the digits. Sluggish blood flow resulting from ischemia may cause the skin to appear cyanotic. Rubor, throbbing pain, and paresthesias follow as blood flow returns. Skin color returns to normal after the attack, but frequent, prolonged attacks interfere with cellular metabolism, causing the skin of the fingertips to thicken and the nails to become brittle. In severe, chronic Raynaud phenomenon, ischemia can eventually cause ulceration and gangrene.

The diagnosis of RP is based on clinical presentation and nailfold capillaroscopy or infrared thermography. A search for underlying secondary causes should be conducted. Treatment of RP begins with avoidance of stimuli that trigger attacks (e.g., cold temperatures, emotional stress) and cessation of cigarette smoking to eliminate the vasoconstricting effects of nicotine. If attacks of vasospasm become frequent or prolonged, vasodilators (e.g., calcium channel blockers, alpha blockers, ACE inhibitors) are administered.[41] Sympathectomy or botulinum injection may be indicated in severe cases.

Atherosclerosis

Arteriosclerosis is a condition characterized by thickening and hardening of the vessel wall. Atherosclerosis is a form of arteriosclerosis that is caused by the accumulation of lipid-laden macrophages within the arterial wall, which leads to the formation of a lesion called a plaque. Atherosclerosis is a pathologic process that can affect vascular systems throughout the body and is the leading cause of peripheral artery disease, CAD, and cerebrovascular disease. (Atherosclerosis of the coronary arteries is described later in this chapter, and atherosclerosis of the cerebral arteries is described in Chapter 18.)

Pathophysiology. Atherosclerosis is an inflammatory disease that begins with injury to the endothelial cells that line artery walls.[42] Pathologically, the lesions progress from endothelial injury and dysfunction to fatty streak to fibrotic plaque to complicated lesion (Fig. 32.5). Possible causes of endothelial injury include the common risk factors for atherosclerosis, such as smoking, hypertension, diabetes, increased levels of low-density lipoprotein (LDL), decreased levels of high-density lipoprotein (HDL), and autoimmunity. Other "nontraditional" risk factors include increased serum markers for inflammation and thrombosis (e.g., high-sensitivity C-reactive protein [hs-CRP]), troponin I, adipokines, infection, and air pollution. These risk factors are discussed in more detail in the following section on CAD (see the section on Coronary Artery Disease, Myocardial Ischemia, and Acute Coronary Syndromes).

Injured endothelial cells become inflamed. Inflamed endothelial cells cannot make normal amounts of antithrombic and vasodilating cytokines and express adhesion molecules that bind macrophages and other inflammatory and immune cells (Fig. 32.6). Macrophages release numerous inflammatory cytokines (e.g., tumor necrosis factor-alpha [TNF-α], interferons, interleukins, C-reactive protein) and enzymes that further injure the vessel wall.[43] Toxic oxygen free radicals generated by the inflammatory process cause oxidation (i.e., addition of oxygen) of LDL that has accumulated in the vessel intima. Oxidized LDL causes additional adhesion molecule expression with the recruitment of monocytes that differentiate into macrophages. These macrophages penetrate into the intima, where they engulf oxidized LDL, and are then called foam cells. When they accumulate in significant amounts, they form a lesion called a fatty streak (see Figs. 32.6 and 32.7). Once formed, fatty streaks produce more toxic oxygen free radicals, and secrete additional inflammatory mediators resulting in progressive damage to the vessel wall. In addition, oxidized LDL and foam cells serve as damage-associated molecular patterns (DAMPs; see Chapter 7) and activate macrophage release of inflammatory cytokines and recruit autoreactive T cells leading to autoimmune vascular injury.[44–46] Selected lipid lowering and antihypertensive medications may improve atherosclerotic disease progression through their antiinflammatory effects (see Emerging Science Box: Lipid-Lowering and Antihypertensive Medication Effects on Atherosclerosis-Associated Inflammation). Increasing understanding of the pivotal role of inflammation and autoimmunity in the pathogenesis of atherosclerosis has led to significant research into potential antiinflammatory treatments.[42,47]

Macrophages also release growth factors that stimulate smooth muscle cell proliferation. Smooth muscle cells in the region of endothelial injury proliferate, produce collagen, and migrate over the fatty streak, forming an atherosclerotic plaque (see Fig. 32.7).[48] The plaque may calcify, protrude into the vessel lumen, and obstruct blood flow to distal tissues (especially during exercise), which may cause symptoms (e.g., angina or intermittent claudication).

Many plaques are "unstable," meaning they are prone to rupture. These plaques are clinically silent and do not affect luminal blood flow significantly until they erode and rupture (see

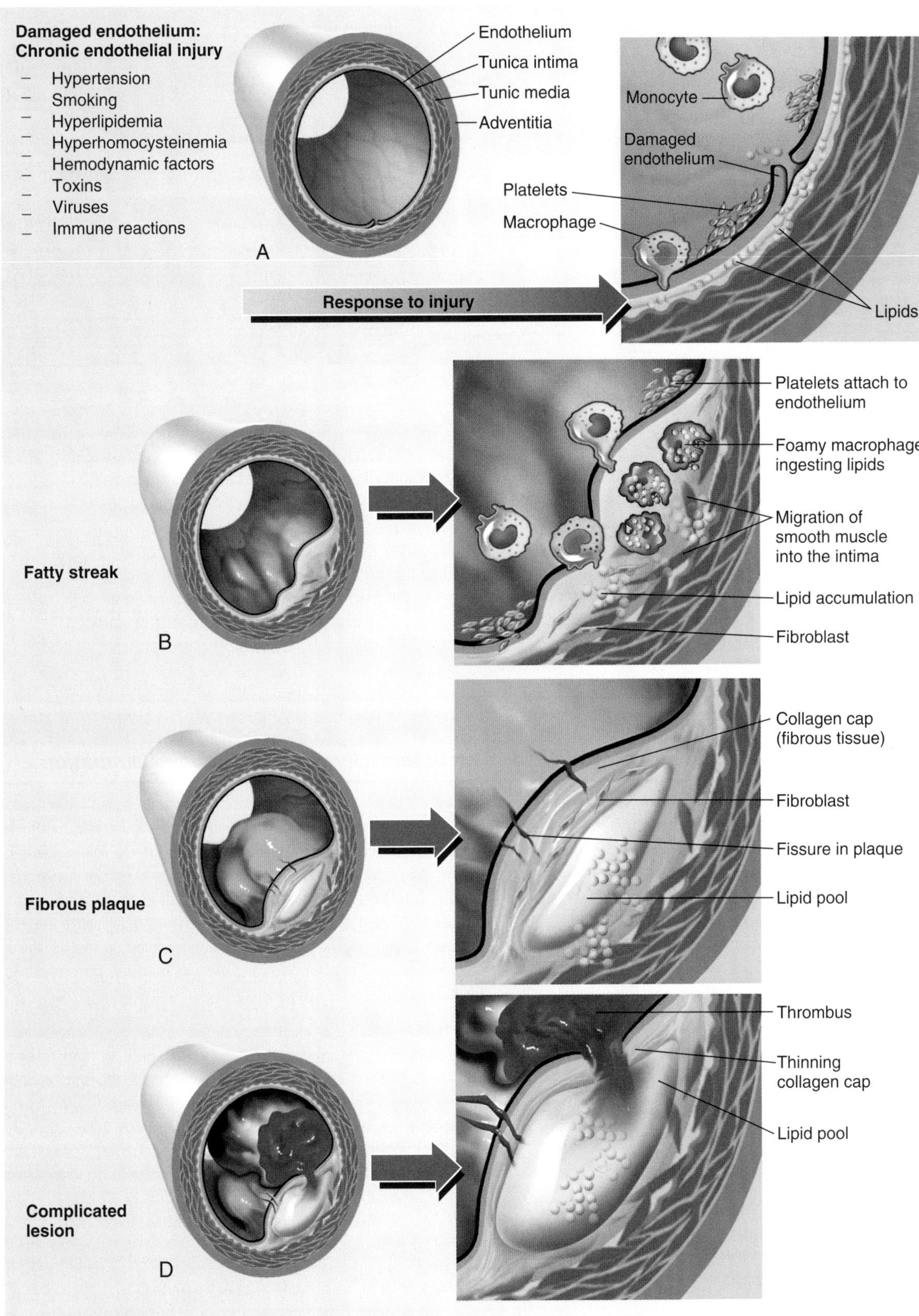

Fig. 32.5 Progression of Atherosclerosis. **(A)** Damaged endothelium. **(B)** Diagram of fatty streak and lipid core formation (see Fig. 32.6 for a diagram of oxidized low-density lipoprotein [LDL]). **(C)** Diagram of fibrous plaque. Raised plaques are visible: some are yellow; others are white. **(D)** Diagram of complicated lesion; thrombus is red; collagen is blue. Plaque is complicated by red thrombus deposition.

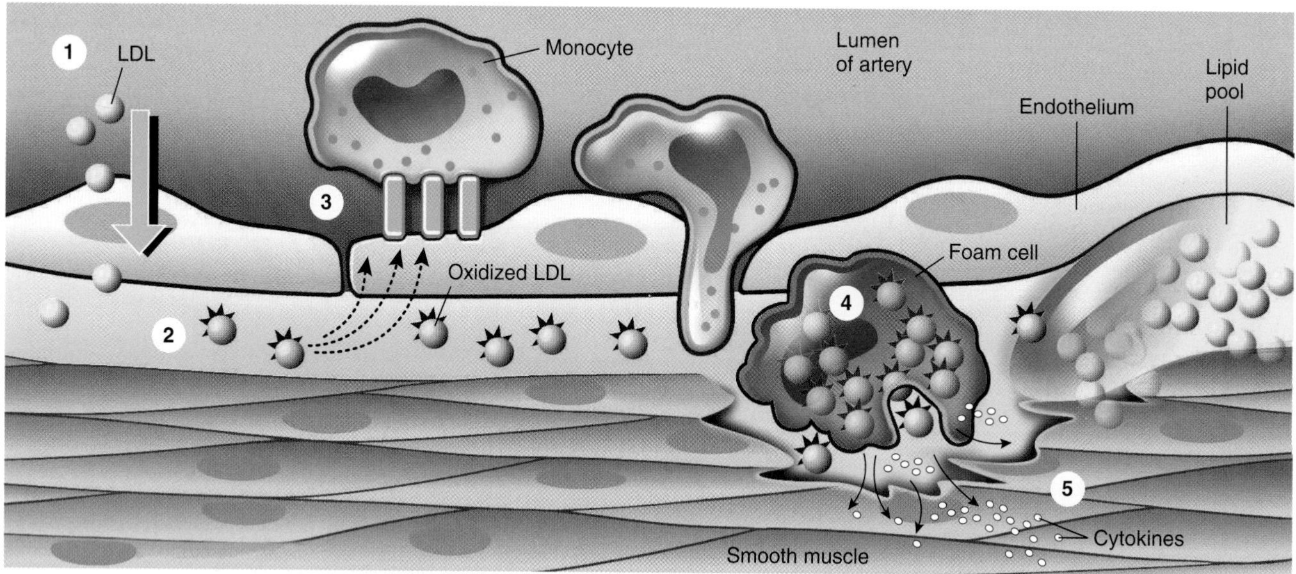

Fig. 32.6 Low-Density Lipoprotein Oxidation. *(1)* Low-density lipoprotein *(LDL)* enters the arterial intima through an intact endothelium. *(2)* In hypercholesterolemia, the influx of LDL exceeds the eliminating capacity and an extracellular pool of LDL is formed. *(3)* Intimal LDL oxidized through the action of free oxygen radicals generates proinflammatory cytokines that induce endothelial expression of the adhesion molecules. Monocytes bind to the adhesion molecules and differentiate into macrophages, which then *(4)* internalize oxidized LDL and become foam cells. *(5)* Foam cells accumulate forming a fatty streak and release many inflammatory cytokines that damage the vessel wall. (Modified from Crawford MH, Dim Arco JP, Paulus WJ. *Cardiology*, 3rd edition. London: Mosby; 2010.)

EMERGING SCIENCE BOX

Lipid-Lowering and Antihypertensive Medication Effects on Atherosclerosis-Associated Inflammation

Atherosclerosis and coronary artery disease are the result of chronic inflammatory and immune processes involving the vessel wall. The use of several types of lipid-lowering and antihypertensive drugs is associated with a decreased risk for coronary artery disease and associated ischemic events. There is increasing evidence that the positive effects of these medications are related not only to their lowering of serum lipid levels or blood pressure, but also to their antiinflammatory effects within the vasculature. The most widely used lipid lowering medications are the HMG-CoA reductase inhibitors, which are collectively referred to as statins. Statins not only decrease LDL synthesis, but also have multiple other effects including improved nitric oxide production by the vascular endothelium, inhibition of smooth muscle cell proliferation, decreased T cell activation, decreased vascular inflammation, and decreased C-reactive protein levels in the serum. Statins also have been shown to contribute to fibrotic and calcific stabilization of plaques, thus reducing their likelihood for rupture. Treatment with the proprotein convertase subtilisin/Kexin Type 9 (PCSK9) antibodies inhibits degradation of the LDL receptor and thus lowers serum LDL. In addition, this drug inhibits macrophage uptake of oxidized LDL thus reducing foam cell formation, and inhibits activation of the inflammatory nuclear factor kappa B (NF-κB). The antihypertensive medications angiotensin converting enzyme (ACE) inhibitors suppress autoreactive T lymphocytes and lower levels of interleukin 6. Beta blockers decrease production of toxic oxygen radicals by neutrophils and decrease the number of activated macrophages. Successful treatment specifically targeting inflammation in atherosclerotic coronary artery disease has been achieved with blockade of interleukin 1 beta (IL-1β) by canakinumab, a human monoclonal IL-1β antibody. Canakinumab reduces cardiovascular events and mortality in individuals who have a history of myocardial infarction and an elevated C-reactive protein. However, individuals treated with canakinumab have an increased risk for serious infection. Agonists of CD (cluster of differentiation) 31—a molecule expressed by inflammatory cells—has been found to promote the healing of injured arteries in animals. Attempts to advance vaccination strategies to modulate the adaptive immune component of atherogenesis are underway. Modulation of the gut microbiome to reduce systemic inflammation provides another approach to the prevention and treatment of atherosclerosis. Many other antiinflammatory treatments for atherosclerosis and coronary artery disease are being researched.

Data From Almeida SO, et al. Effect of statins on atherosclerotic plaque. *Trends in Cardiovascular Medicine*, 2019;29(8):451–455; Bäck M, et al. Inflammation and its resolution in atherosclerosis: mediators and therapeutic opportunities. *Nature Reviews Cardiology*, 2019;16(7):389–406; Caligiuri G. CD31 as a therapeutic target in atherosclerosis. *Circulation Research*, 2020;126:1178–1189; Libby P. Inflammation in atherosclerosis—No longer a theory. *Clinical Chemistry*, 2021;67(1):131–142; Nilsson J, et al. Vaccination strategies and immune modulation of atherosclerosis. *Circulation Research*, 2020;126:1281–1296; Peng R, et al. Vascular macrophages as a target for modulation in vascular diseases. *Journal of Immunology Research*, 2020:8131754; Witkowski M, et al. Gut microbiota and cardiovascular disease. *Circulation Research*, 2020;127(4):553–570; Wolf D, et al. Immunity and inflammation in atherosclerosis. *Circulation Research*, 2019;124(2):315–327; Zhao TX, et al. Targeting the immune system in atherosclerosis: JACC state-of-the-art review. *Journal of the American College of Cardiology*, 2019;73(13):1691–1706.

the section on Coronary Artery Disease, Myocardial Ischemia, and Acute Coronary Syndromes). Rupture of unstable plaques occurs due to the degradative effects of inflammatory cytokines and enzymes, wall stress, and neurohumoral changes.[49] Plaques that have ruptured are called complicated plaques. Once rupture occurs, exposure of underlying tissue results in platelet

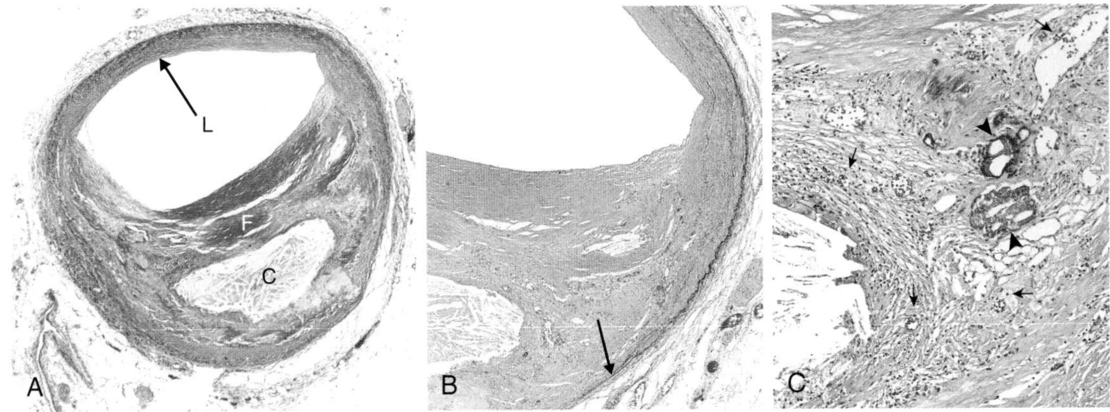

Fig. 32.7 Histologic Features of Atheromatous Plaque in the Coronary Artery. **(A)** Overall architecture demonstrating fibrous cap *(F)* and a central necrotic (largely lipid) core *(C)*. The lumen (*L*) has been moderately narrowed. Note that a segment of the wall is plaque free *(arrow)*, so that there is an eccentric lesion. In this section, collagen has been stained blue (Masson trichrome stain). **(B)** Higher power photograph of a section of the plaque shown in **(A)** stained for elastin *(black)*, demonstrating that the internal and external elastic membranes are destroyed and the media of the artery is thinned under the most advanced plaque *(arrow)*. **(C)** Higher magnification photomicrograph at the junction of the fibrous cap and core, showing scattered inflammatory cells, calcification *(arrowhead)*, and neovascularization *(small arrows)*. (From Kumar V, Abbas A, Aster J. *Robbins basic pathology*, 9th edition. St. Louis: Saunders; 2007.)

adhesion, initiation of the clotting cascade, and rapid thrombus formation. The thrombus may suddenly occlude the affected vessel, resulting in ischemia and infarction. Aspirin or other antithrombotic agents are used to prevent this complication of atherosclerotic disease.

Clinical Manifestations. Atherosclerosis presents with symptoms and signs that result from inadequate perfusion of tissues because of obstruction of the vessels that supply them. Partial vessel obstruction may lead to transient ischemic events, often associated with exercise or stress. As the lesion becomes complicated, increasing obstruction with superimposed thrombosis may result in tissue infarction. Obstruction of peripheral arteries can cause significant pain and disability. CAD caused by atherosclerosis is the major cause of myocardial ischemia. Atherosclerotic obstruction of the vessels supplying the brain is the major cause of stroke. Often, more than one vessel will become involved with this disease process such that an individual may present with symptoms from several ischemic tissues at the same time, and disease in one area may indicate that the individual is at risk for ischemic complications elsewhere.

Evaluation and Treatment. In evaluating individuals for the presence of atherosclerosis, obtaining a complete health history (including risk factors and symptoms of ischemia) is essential. Physical examination may reveal arterial bruits and evidence of decreased blood flow to tissues. Laboratory data that include measurements of levels of lipids, blood glucose, and hs-CRP are also indicated. Judicious use of x-ray films, electrocardiography, ultrasonography, nuclear scanning, CT, MRI, and angiography may be necessary to identify affected vessels, particularly coronary vessels.

Current management of atherosclerosis is focused on detection and treatment of preclinical lesions with drugs aimed at stabilizing and reversing plaques before they rupture. Once a lesion obstructs blood flow, the primary goal in the management of atherosclerosis is to restore adequate blood flow to the affected tissues. If an individual has presented with acute ischemia (e.g., MI, stroke), interventions are specific to the diseased area (discussed further under those topics). In situations in which the disease process does not require immediate intervention, management focuses on reduction of risk factors and prevention of plaque progression. This includes implementation of an exercise program, cessation of smoking, and control of contributing factors such as hypertension, diabetes, and dyslipidemia. Management of atherosclerotic risk factors is discussed further in the Coronary Artery Disease, Myocardial Ischemia, and Acute Coronary Syndromes section.

Peripheral Artery Disease

Peripheral artery disease (PAD) refers to atherosclerotic disease of arteries that perfuse the limbs, especially the lower extremities. PAD affects an estimated 6.5 million Americans aged > 40 years.[12] The risk factors for PAD are the same as those previously described for atherosclerosis. It is especially prevalent in smokers and older adults with diabetes.

Lower extremity ischemia resulting from arterial obstruction in PAD can be gradual or acute. In most individuals, gradually increasing atherosclerotic changes in arterial walls is associated with endothelial cell dysfunction, decreases in endogenous vasodilators such as endothelin -1, and the tendency for thrombosis.[50] This leads to obstruction to arterial blood flow and exercise-related ischemia. In the iliofemoral vessels, this may result in leg pain with ambulation called intermittent claudication. If a thrombus forms over the atherosclerotic lesion, complete obstruction of blood flow can occur acutely, causing severe pain, loss of pulses, and skin color changes in the affected extremity. Critical limb ischemia may lead to gangrene.

Evaluation for PAD requires a careful history and physical examination that focuses on finding evidence of atherosclerotic disease (e.g., bruits), determining a difference in blood pressure measured at the ankle versus the arm (ankle-brachial index), and measuring blood flow using duplex ultrasound, CT angiography, or magnetic resonance angiography. Treatment begins with risk factor reduction including smoking cessation, exercise, diabetes and hypertension management, and treatment for dyslipidemia.[50] Symptomatic PAD should be managed with vasodilators in combination with antiplatelet medications. Newer vasodilators such as cilostazol and anticoagulants such as rivaroxaban may be indicated.[51,52] If acute or refractory symptoms occur, emergent invasive catheterization followed by percutaneous or surgical revascularization may be needed.

Coronary Artery Disease, Myocardial Ischemia, and Acute Coronary Syndromes

Coronary artery disease (CAD) caused by atherosclerosis is the primary cause of heart disease in the United States. CAD can diminish the myocardial blood supply until deprivation impairs myocardial metabolism enough to cause myocardial ischemia, a local state in which the cells are temporarily deprived of blood supply. The cells remain alive but cannot function normally. Persistent ischemia or the complete occlusion of a coronary artery causes the acute coronary syndromes, including MI *(heart attack)*.

Development of Coronary Artery Disease

An estimated 20.1 million Americans have coronary heart disease, which constitutes a prevalence of 7.2% in adults over 20 years of age and 22% to 34% in those over 80. In 2018, coronary heart disease was the leading cause of death attributable to cardiovascular disease in the United States, with mortality reaching over 365,000 deaths.[12] Risk factors for CAD are the same as those for atherosclerosis and can be categorized as conventional (major) versus nontraditional (novel) and as modifiable versus nonmodifiable. Conventional or major risk factors for CAD that are nonmodifiable include (1) advanced age, (2) male sex or women after menopause, and (3) family history. Aging and menopause are associated with increased exposure to risk factors and poor endothelial healing. Family history may contribute to CAD through genetics and shared environmental exposures. Modifiable major risks include (1) dyslipidemia, (2) hypertension, (3) cigarette smoking, (4) diabetes and insulin resistance, (5) obesity, (6) sedentary lifestyle, and (7) atherogenic diet. Fortunately, modification of these factors can dramatically reduce the risk for CAD.

Genes. An individual's risk of developing CAD and MI is impacted by both genetic and lifestyle factors. Recent studies have identified 37 genes that are likely causal for CAD.[53] Inheritance of genetic risks for dyslipidemia, diabetes, hypertension, and other risk factors is common. Epigenetic patterns are affected by the environment and can modulate gene expression. For example, dietary changes can alter the expression of genes related to dyslipidemia and the development of atherosclerotic lesions.[54]

Dyslipidemia. Using data from 2015-2018, it is estimated that over 90 million, or 38 %, of American adults have dyslipidemia.[12] The link between CAD and abnormal levels of lipoproteins is well documented. The term lipoprotein refers to lipids, phospholipids, cholesterol, and triglycerides bound to carrier proteins. The cycle of lipoprotein synthesis is complex. Dietary fat is packaged into particles known as chylomicrons in the small intestine. Chylomicrons primarily contain triglycerides. Some of the triglycerides may be removed and either stored by adipose tissue or used by muscle as an energy source. The chylomicron remnants, composed mainly of cholesterol, are taken up by the liver. A series of chemical reactions in the liver results in the production of several lipoproteins that vary in density and function. These include very-low-density lipoproteins (VLDLs) composed primarily of triglycerides and protein; LDLs, composed mostly of cholesterol and protein; and HDLs, composed mainly of phospholipids and protein. Although lipoproteins are necessary for many physiologic functions, they can accumulate in abnormal amounts in the serum.

Dyslipidemia (or dyslipoproteinemia) refers to abnormal concentrations of serum lipoproteins as defined by the Third Report of the National Cholesterol Education Program.[55] (Table 32.4). These abnormalities are the result of a combination of genetic and dietary factors. Primary or familial dyslipoproteinemias result from genetic defects that cause abnormalities in lipid-metabolizing enzymes and abnormal cellular lipid receptors.[56] Secondary causes of dyslipidemia include the existence of several common systemic disorders, such as diabetes, hypothyroidism, pancreatitis, and renal nephrosis, as well as the use

TABLE 32.4 Criteria for Dyslipidemia[a]

	Optimal	Near-Optimal	Desirable	Low	Borderline	High	Very High
Total cholesterol			<200		200–239	≥240	
Low-density lipoprotein	<100	100–129			130–159	160-189	≥190
Triglycerides			<150		150–199	200-499	≥500
High-density lipoprotein				<40		≥60	

[a]All units are milligrams per deciliter.

Data from Expert Panel on Detection, Evaluation, and Treatment of High Blood Cholesterol in Adults. Executive summary of the third report of the National Cholesterol Education Program (NCEP) expert panel on detection, evaluation, and treatment of high blood cholesterol in adults (Adult Treatment Panel III). *JAMA.* 2001;285:2486–2497.

of certain medications, such as some diuretics, glucocorticoids, interferons, and antiretrovirals.

LDL is responsible for the delivery of cholesterol to the tissues, and an increased serum concentration of LDL is a strong indicator of coronary risk. Serum levels of LDL are normally controlled by hepatic receptors that bind LDL and limit liver synthesis of this lipoprotein. Genetic predisposition to dyslipidemias, in combination with a high dietary intake of saturated fats, result in excess amounts of LDL in the bloodstream. Excess LDL migration into the vessel wall, oxidation, and phagocytosis by macrophages are key steps in the pathogenesis of atherosclerosis (see Fig. 32.6). LDL also plays a role in endothelial injury, inflammation, and immune responses that have been identified as being important in atherogenesis. The term *LDL* actually describes several types of LDL molecules. Measurement of LDL subfractions allows for a better prediction of coronary risk. For example, LDL-C and apolipoprotein B (structural protein found in both LDL and VLDL) measurements allow for the detection of the small, dense LDL particles that are the most atherogenic. Guidelines from the American Heart Association and the American College of Cardiology focus on treating dyslipidemia in the context of other risk factors.[57] Diet and medication are the mainstays of treatment for elevated LDL. The most commonly used medications are the 3-hydroxy-3-methyl-glutaryl-CoA reductase medications (statins); however, side effects limit their use in some individuals. New medications, such as the proprotein convertase subtilisin/kexin 9 (PCKS9) inhibitors, also effectively lower LDL. Lipid-lowering medications may have other beneficial effects on the vasculature (see Emerging Science Box: Lipid-Lowering and Antihypertensive Medication Effects on Atherosclerosis-Associated Inflammation).

Low levels of HDL cholesterol are an indicator of increased coronary risk, whereas high levels of HDL are associated with a significant reduction in coronary risk independent of age, smoking history, LDL levels, blood pressure, or weight.[58] HDL is responsible for "reverse cholesterol transport," which returns excess cholesterol from the tissues to the liver for processing or elimination in the bile. HDL also participates in endothelial repair and decreases thrombosis. It can be fractionated into several particle densities (HDL-2 and HDL-3) that have different effects on vascular function. Exercise, weight loss, fish oil consumption, and moderate alcohol use result in modest increases in HDL level. Pharmacologic interventions to increase HDL levels have largely been ineffective in reducing CAD risk.[59] Recent studies suggest that it is not only the serum levels of HDL that are key to determining CAD risk, but rather HDL functionality, which is harder to measure.[60] One approach is measurement of the cholesterol efflux capacity (an indirect measure of reverse cholesterol transport) which has been found to be inversely associated with atherosclerotic risk.[61]

Other lipoproteins associated with increased cardiovascular risk include elevated levels of serum VLDLs (triglycerides) and increased lipoprotein(a) levels. Triglycerides are associated with an increased risk for CAD, especially in combination with other risk factors such as diabetes. Lipoprotein(a) (Lp[a]) is a genetically determined molecular complex between LDL and a serum glycoprotein called apolipoprotein A and has been shown to be an important risk factor for atherosclerosis, especially in women. Lipoprotein(a) potentially contributes to cardiovascular disease through proatherogenic, proinflammatory, and prothrombotic effects.[62] Emerging therapies targeting elevated levels of Lp(a) may improve the management of individuals with CAD.[63]

Hypertension. Hypertension is responsible for a two- to threefold increased risk of atherosclerotic cardiovascular disease. It contributes to endothelial injury, a key step in atherogenesis. It also can cause myocardial hypertrophy, which increases myocardial demand for coronary flow (see Algorithm 32.2). Overactivity of the RAAS commonly found in hypertension also contributes to the genesis of atherosclerosis, and treatment of hypertension with medications that block the RAAS reduces CAD risk.

Cigarette smoking. Both direct and passive (environmental) smoking increase the risk of CAD. Smoking has a direct effect on endothelial cells and the generation of oxygen free radicals that contribute to atherogenesis. Nicotine stimulates the release of catecholamines (epinephrine and norepinephrine), which increase heart rate and peripheral vascular constriction. As a result, blood pressure increases, as do cardiac workload and oxygen demand. Cigarette smoking is associated with an increase in LDL levels and a decrease in HDL levels. The risk of CAD increases with heavy smoking and decreases when smoking is stopped.

Diabetes mellitus. Insulin resistance and diabetes mellitus are extremely important risk factors for CAD (see Chapter 22). Type 2 diabetes is associated with chronic vascular inflammation resulting from hyperglycemia, insulin resistance, and elevated levels of circulating insulin. Insulin resistance and diabetes have multiple effects on the cardiovascular system, including damage to the endothelium, thickening of the vessel wall, increased thrombosis, glycation of vascular proteins, and decreased production of endothelial-derived vasodilators, such as nitric oxide. Diabetes also is associated with dyslipidemia. Good diabetic control is linked to reduced risk for CAD.[64]

Obesity/adipokines/sedentary lifestyle. A sedentary lifestyle not only increases the risk of obesity but also has an independent effect on increasing CAD risk. Abdominal obesity has a strong link with increased CAD risk and is related to inflammation, insulin resistance, decreased HDL level, and increased blood pressure. Adipokines are a group of hormones released from adipose cells. Obesity causes increased levels of leptin and decreased levels of adiponectin that are associated with inflammation, endothelial injury, and thrombosis. Obesity-related changes in adipokines have been linked to hypertension, diabetes, and heart failure, as well as CAD. Excessive accumulation of perivascular adipose tissue leads to the paracrine release of vasoconstrictors and growth factors which have deleterious effects on vascular smooth muscle endothelial cells.[65] Perivascular fat tissue also affects local adipokine levels (especially leptin), as well as releases proinflammatory signals and promotes atherosclerotic plaque formation.[66,67] Weight loss, exercise, and healthy diet improve adipokine levels. Bariatric surgery procedures, such as gastric bypass, can provide sustained improvement in risk factors for cardiovascular disease, such as hypertension, dyslipidemia, and diabetes in selected individuals.[68,69]

Atherogenic diet. Diet plays a complex role in atherogenic risk. Diets high in salt, fats, trans-fats, and carbohydrates all have been implicated. There are many recommendations regarding diet modification to reduce coronary risk; one of the most effective is called the Mediterranean diet.

The traditional Mediterranean diet is characterized by a high intake of olive oil, fruits, nuts, vegetables, and cereals; moderate intake of fish and poultry; low intake of dairy products, red meat, processed meats, and sweets; and moderate intake of wine consumed with meals. The beneficial effects of the Mediterranean diet are hypothesized to include modulation of many different biologic components of cardiovascular health such as epigenetic control of genes associated with cardiovascular risk, modification of the gut microbiome, antiinflammatory and immune effects, and improvement in metabolic factors such as glucose tolerance and lipid metabolism. Dietary guidance to improve cardiovascular health had been published by the American Heart Association.[70]

Nontraditional risk factors. Nontraditional risk factors for CAD have been identified that can help with clinical decision-making about how best to manage individuals who also have established CAD or significant traditional risk factors.

Markers of inflammation and ischemia. Of the numerous markers of inflammation that have been linked to an increase in CAD risk, high-sensitivity C-reactive protein (hs-CRP) is the most important clinically. hs-CRP is a protein synthesized in the liver and is used as an indirect measure of atherosclerotic plaque–related inflammation. The primary use of hs-CRP is as an aid to decision-making about pharmacologic interventions for individuals with other risk factors for coronary disease.

Troponin I (TnI) is a serum protein whose measurement is used as a sensitive and specific diagnostic test to help identify myocardial injury during acute coronary syndromes. Highly sensitive TnI assays are used in individuals without a history of CAD to assess risk for future CHD events, mortality, and heart failure.

Chronic kidney disease. In individuals with chronic kidney disease (CKD), a decline in glomerular filtration rate is associated with an increasing risk for CAD. CKD is associated with dyslipidemia, endothelial injury, and vascular calcification, which contribute to atherogenesis.

Air pollution and ionizing radiation. Exposure to air pollution, especially roadway exposures, is strongly correlated with coronary risk. Fine particulate matter is the major cardiovascular risk component of air pollution and is considered the most important risk factor contributing to global cardiovascular mortality.[71] It is postulated that toxins in pollution contribute to macrophage activation, oxidation of LDL, thrombosis, and inflammation of vessel walls. Exposure to even low levels of ionizing radiation also has been linked to increased risk for CAD. Reducing exposure to air pollutants can reduce cardiovascular risk.[72]

Medications. Medications may contribute to CAD through their effect on lipid metabolism (e.g., protease inhibitors, diuretics, antirejection medications), clotting (e.g., estrogens and progesterones), or other effects on vascular function and tone. Nonsteroidal antiinflammatory drugs (NSAIDs) are linked to an increase in CAD-related ischemic events that can occur within weeks of beginning their use.[73] Likely mechanisms include increases in toxic oxygen radicals, vasoconstrictors, and thrombosis.

The microbiome. The microbiome is increasingly being recognized for its influence on cardiovascular disease risk. The impact of the microbiome on atherogenesis is likely related to its effects on underlying risk factors, as well as its role in modulating innate and adaptive immunity. Differences in the composition of the microbiome between those with CAD and healthy individuals have been documented. Changes in the microbiome have been found to have significant effects on the development of traditional risk factors for cardiovascular disease, such as diabetes and obesity. The identification of microbiota-controlled metabolites, such as trimethylamine N-oxide (TMAO), is shedding light on the link between diet and these risk factors.[74,75]

Transient Myocardial Ischemia

As described previously, CAD can diminish the myocardial blood supply causing ischemia. The process of atherosclerotic plaque progression can be gradual, which usually results in transient myocardial ischemic syndromes when demand for blood supply exceeds supply, but perfusion is restored before there is permanent damage to the heart muscle. Ischemia also can occur with coronary vasospasm even in the absence of atherosclerosis.

Pathophysiology. Myocardial ischemia develops if the flow or oxygen content of coronary blood is insufficient to meet the metabolic demands of myocardial cells (Algorithm. 32.3). Imbalances between coronary blood supply and myocardial demand can result from a number of conditions. The most common cause of decreased coronary blood flow and resultant myocardial ischemia is the formation of atherosclerotic plaques in the coronary circulation (CAD). As the plaque increases in size, it may partially occlude the vessel lumen, thus limiting coronary flow and causing ischemia especially during exercise. While these large plaques are often considered "stable," individuals with chronic atherosclerotic changes are still at risk for adverse events. Myocardial ischemia also can result from other causes of decreased blood and oxygen delivery to the myocardium, such as coronary spasm, hypotension, dysrhythmias, and decreased oxygen-carrying capacity of the blood (e.g., anemia, hypoxemia). Common causes of increased myocardial demand for blood include tachycardia, exercise, hypertension (hypertrophy), and valvular disease.

Factors that decrease coronary artery blood flow (e.g., atherosclerosis) or increase demand for myocardial blood supply (e.g., exercise) cause myocardial ischemia. Both transient and prolonged ischemia can cause abnormal or absent myocyte responses to electrical impulses through the myocardium leading to dysrhythmias or decreased contractility. Decreased ability of the heart to pump blood results in heart failure and contributes to decreased coronary perfusion, further compromising the supply of blood to the heart. Dysrhythmias also may lead to sudden death.

Myocardial cells become ischemic within 10 seconds of coronary occlusion, thus hampering pump function and

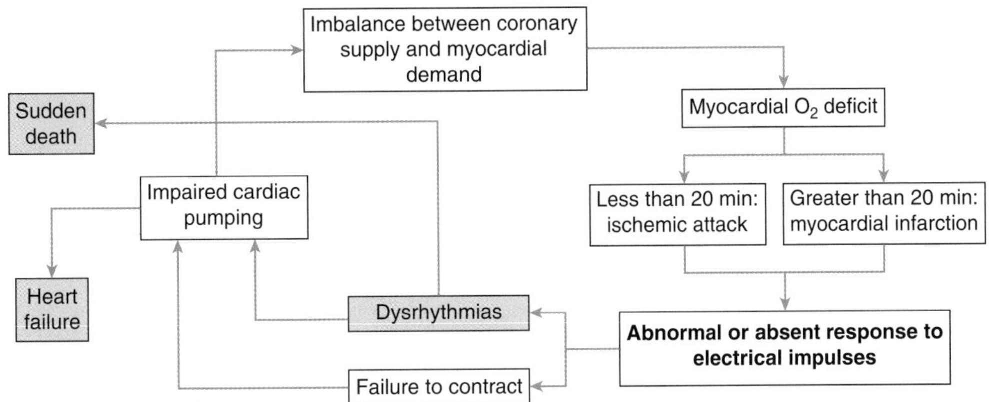

Algorithm 32.3 Cycle of Myocardial Ischemic Events. Factors that decrease coronary artery blood flow (e.g., atherosclerosis) or increase demand for myocardial blood supply (e.g., exercise) cause myocardial ischemia. Both transient and prolonged ischemia can cause abnormal or absent myocyte responses to electrical impulses through the myocardium leading to dysrhythmias or decreased contractility. Decreased ability of the heart to pump blood results in heart failure and decreased coronary perfusion, further compromising the supply of blood to the heart. Dysrhythmias may also lead to sudden death.

depriving the myocardium of a glucose source necessary for aerobic metabolism. Anaerobic processes take over, and lactic acid accumulates. After several minutes, the heart cells lose the ability to contract and cardiac output decreases. Cardiac cells remain viable for approximately 20 minutes under ischemic conditions. If blood flow is restored, aerobic metabolism resumes, contractility is restored, and cellular repair begins. If perfusion is not restored, myocardial infarction occurs.

Individuals with transient myocardial ischemia present clinically in several ways. Chronic coronary obstruction results in recurrent predictable chest pain called *stable angina*. Abnormal vasospasm of coronary vessels results in unpredictable chest pain called *vasospastic (Prinzmetal) angina*. Myocardial ischemia that does not cause detectable symptoms is called *silent ischemia*.

Stable angina pectoris. Angina is chest pain caused by myocardial ischemia. Atherosclerotic plaques partially obstruct coronary vessels, and affected vessels cannot dilate in response to increased myocardial demand associated with physical exertion or emotional stress. In stable angina pectoris, blood flow is restored with rest and the administration of nitrates, and necrosis of myocardial cells does not occur. The pain of stable angina is caused by the buildup of lactic acid or abnormal stretching of the ischemic myocardium that irritates myocardial nerve fibers. These afferent sympathetic fibers enter the spinal cord from levels C3 to T4, accounting for a variety of locations and radiation patterns of anginal pain. Discomfort may radiate to the neck, lower jaw, left arm, and left shoulder, or occasionally to the back or down the right arm.

Stable angina is typically experienced as transient substernal chest discomfort, ranging from a sensation of heaviness or pressure to moderately severe pain. Individuals often describe the sensation by clenching a fist over the left sternal border. The discomfort may be mistaken for indigestion. Pallor, diaphoresis, and dyspnea may be associated with the pain. Guidelines for the acute evaluation of chest pain recommend a careful symptom history and physical examination followed by diagnostic testing to include ECG, chest radiography, and measurement of serum biomarkers such as troponins.[76]

Many individuals with reversible myocardial ischemia will have a normal physical examination between events. Physical examination of those experiencing myocardial ischemia may disclose rapid pulse rate or extra heart sounds (gallops or murmurs), and pulmonary congestion indicating impaired left ventricular function. The presence of xanthelasmas (small fat deposits) around the eyelids or arcus senilis of the eyes (a yellow lipid ring around the cornea) suggests severe dyslipidemia and possible atherosclerosis. The presence of peripheral or carotid artery bruits suggests probable atherosclerotic disease and increases the likelihood that CAD is present. Electrocardiography detects distortion of electrical impulses across ischemic myocardium, and can be conducted during exercise stress testing to detect ischemic changes associated with stable angina. Transient ST segment depression and T wave inversion are characteristic signs of stable angina involving the endocardium, although ST elevation indicative of ischemia involving the full myocardial wall (transmural ischemia) may occur (Fig. 32.8). Serum troponin levels remain within normal limits. Stress radionucleotide imaging with single-photon emission computerized tomography (SPECT) is effective at identifying ischemia and estimating coronary risk. Other noninvasive tests for evaluating coronary atherosclerotic lesions include stress echocardiography and coronary CT angiography.[77]

The primary aims of therapy for myocardial ischemia and stable angina are to increase coronary blood flow, reduce myocardial oxygen consumption, and to reduce the risk for adverse cardiovascular events such as myocardial infarction. Coronary blood flow is improved by reversing vasoconstriction, reducing plaque growth and rupture, and preventing clotting. Myocardial oxygen demand is reduced by manipulation of blood pressure, heart rate, contractility, and left ventricular volume. Several classes of drugs are useful for increasing coronary flow and decreasing myocardial demand, especially nitrates, β-blockers, calcium channel blockers, and sodium ion channel inhibitors

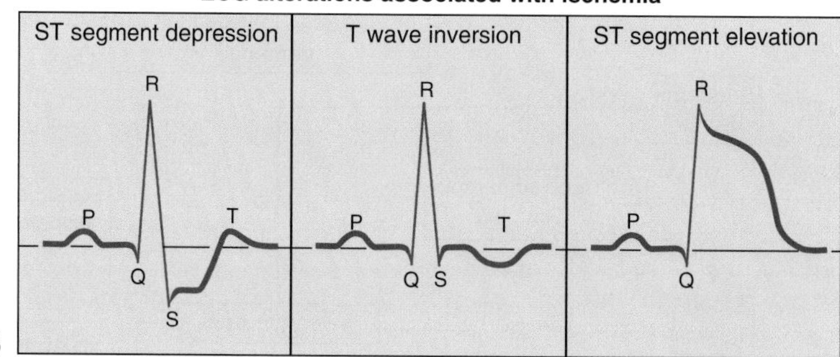

Fig. 32.8 Electrocardiogram *(ECG)* and Ischemia. **(A)** Normal ECG. **(B)** Electrocardiographic alterations associated with ischemia.

(e.g., nicorandil).[77] Antiplatelet medications are used to prevent thrombus formation. Percutaneous coronary intervention (PCI) is a procedure in which stenotic (narrowed) coronary vessels are dilated with a catheter. The use of PCI for stable angina may be associated with improvements in symptoms but does not reduce the risk for future MI or death.[78] Severe CAD also can be surgically treated by a coronary artery bypass graft (CABG), usually using the saphenous vein from the lower leg.[77,79]

Primary prevention of CAD is key to improving morbidity and mortality in those with stable angina. Primary prevention refers to reduction in CAD risk factors before the occurrence of a major ischemic event such as myocardial infarction, whereas secondary prevention refers to risk reduction after such an event. Primary prevention rests on the calculation of 10-year atherosclerotic cardiovascular disease risk, followed by the development of a comprehensive plan for lifestyle change to include exercise and dietary modifications.[80] Antihypertensive and lipid lowering medications should be prescribed as indicated by current guidelines.[27,28,57] In those individuals with diabetes, metformin, sodium-glucose cotransporter 2 (SGLT2) inhibitors, or a glucagon-like peptide-1 receptor agonist are recommended along with diet and exercise.[80]

It is estimated that half of women with stable angina do not have obstructive CAD, but rather have "microvascular angina," which results from vasoconstriction of small coronary arterioles deep in the myocardium. This form of myocardial ischemia may present with atypical chest pain, palpitations, sense of unease, and severe fatigue rather than typical angina; thus many women with this disorder are misdiagnosed. Small intramyocardial arterioles constrict in MVA due to endothelial dysfunction, decreased endogenous vasodilators, inflammation, changes in adipokines, and platelet activation. Evaluation for microvascular angina relies upon transthoracic Doppler echocardiography and positron emission tomography. The combination of calcium channel blockers or sodium ion channel inhibitors with statins has been shown to be effective in many women.[81]

Vasospastic (Prinzmetal) angina. Vasospastic angina is chest pain attributable to transient ischemia of the myocardium that occurs unpredictably and often at rest. Pain is caused by vasospasm of one or more major coronary arteries and can occur in those with or without coronary artery disease. The spasm may involve the large epicardial coronary arteries, or may occur in the microvasculature. Vasospasm may result from coronary smooth muscle hypercontractility, decreased vagal activity, endothelial dysfunction, magnesium deficiency, inflammation, oxidative stress, and hyperactivity of the SNS.[82] It can be triggered by hyperventilation, mental stress, smoking, alcohol, use of stimulants, or rapid eye movement sleep. Hypokalemia worsens symptoms and outcomes.[83] Vasospastic angina is diagnosed by matching clinical manifestations with documented transient ischemic changes on ECG. In some individuals, confirmation with coronary angiography combined with administration of a provocative agent (e.g., ergonovine) is needed. Management includes avoidance of triggers and the use of calcium channel blockers or nitrates. Although vasospastic angina is usually a benign condition, it can cause dysrhythmias and infarction, especially in those who also have atherosclerotic coronary lesions.[84]

Another form of vasospastic myocardial ischemia without coronary artery disease is called Takotsubo syndrome (TTS). TTS occurs primarily in postmenopausal women during mental or physical stress and is associated with acute transient heart failure. It is believed to be the result of increased catecholamine levels coupled with increased adrenergic receptor density and sensitivity in the myocardium.[85] It is usually reversible but can cause significant morbidity and mortality (see Emerging Science Box: Takotsubo Syndrome).

Silent ischemia. Silent ischemia is myocardial ischemia that does not cause detectable symptoms such as angina. Ischemia can be totally asymptomatic, or individuals may complain of fatigue, dyspnea, or a feeling of unease. It is believed to be more common than symptomatic angina.[86] The primary cause of silent ischemia is abnormalities in autonomic innervation, most commonly associated with diabetes mellitus. Other causes include surgical denervation during CABG or cardiac transplantation. Also of interest is silent ischemia occurring in some individuals during mental stress. Chronic stress has been linked to an increase in inflammatory cytokines and a hypercoagulable state that may contribute to acute ischemic events (see Chapter 11). Detection and management of silent ischemia is important because it may be an indicator of future serious cardiovascular events. Treatment is based on the degree of ischemia and the extent of underlying coronary disease.[86]

EMERGING SCIENCE BOX

Takotsubo Syndrome

Takotsubo syndrome (TTS) is an acute reversible heart failure syndrome associated with acute myocardial ischemia but without obstruction of coronary arteries. TTS usually is preceded by emotional or physical stress and occurs most commonly in postmenopausal women. It occurs in up to 2% of those presenting with suspected acute coronary syndrome. The pathophysiology of TTS includes increased density and sensitivity of adrenergic receptors coupled with a stress-induced catecholamine surge. Direct myocardial toxicity to high levels of adrenergic stimulation plus increased myocardial workload and coronary microvascular vasospasm cause acute ischemia. Inflammation with increased levels of interleukins has also been documented. The diagnosis rests on acute transient myocardial hypokinesis without evidence of epicardial coronary artery disease. There are transient ischemic changes seen on ECG along with modest increases in troponins. Echocardiography typically demonstrates ventricular apical ballooning that extends beyond the distribution of a single coronary artery. MRI may show ventricular dysfunction and edema in a noncoronary regional distribution pattern. Management includes beta blockers such as levosimendan and mechanical circulatory support. TTS carries substantial mortality due to arrhythmias, acute heart failure, cardiogenic shock, cardiac arrest, and thromboembolic events.

Data From Borodzicz S, et al. Autonomic nervous system in Takotsubo syndrome. *Heart Failure Reviews*, 2019;24(1):101–108; Boyd B, et al. Takotsubo cardiomyopathy: Review of broken heart syndrome. *Journal of the American Academy of Physician Assistants*, 2020;33:24–29; Dias A, et al. Takotsubo syndrome: State-of-the-art review by an expert panel—Parts 1 & 2. *Cardiovascular Revascularization Medicine*, 2019;20:70–79, and 153–166; Jha S, et al. Clinical management in the takotsubo syndrome. *Expert Review of Cardiovascular Therapy*, 2019;17(2):83–93; Lyon AR, et al. Pathophysiology of Takotsubo syndrome: JACC State-of-the-Art Review. *Journal of the American College of Cardiology*, 2021;77(7):902–911; Moscatelli S, et al. An emerging cardiovascular disease: Takotsubo syndrome. *BioMed Research International*, 2019:6571045; Rodriguez M, et al. Misconceptions and facts about Takotsubo syndrome. *American Journal of Medicine*. 2019;132(1):25–31; Zhang L, et al. Stress-induced cardiomyopathy. *Heart Failure Clinics*, 2019;15(1):41–53.

Acute Coronary Syndromes

The process of atherosclerotic plaque progression can be gradual. However, when there is sudden coronary obstruction caused by thrombus formation over a ruptured atherosclerotic plaque, the acute coronary syndromes result (Algorithm 32.4). Unstable angina is a form of acute coronary syndrome that is a harbinger of impending infarction. Myocardial infarction (MI) results when there is prolonged ischemia causing irreversible damage to the heart muscle. MI can be further subdivided into non-ST elevation MI (non-STEMI) and ST elevation MI (STEMI). Sudden cardiac death can occur as a result of any of the acute coronary syndromes.

An unstable atherosclerotic plaque has a core that is especially rich in deposited oxidized LDL, has a thin fibrous cap, and is prone to rupture (Fig. 32.9). Calcification of these plaques further destabilizes them.[87] These unstable plaques may not extend into the lumen of the vessel and may be clinically silent until they rupture. New methods are emerging for detecting unstable plaques before they rupture, thus identifying those individuals at highest risk for acute coronary syndromes.[88] Plaque rupture occurs because of the effects of shear forces, inflammation with release of multiple inflammatory mediators,

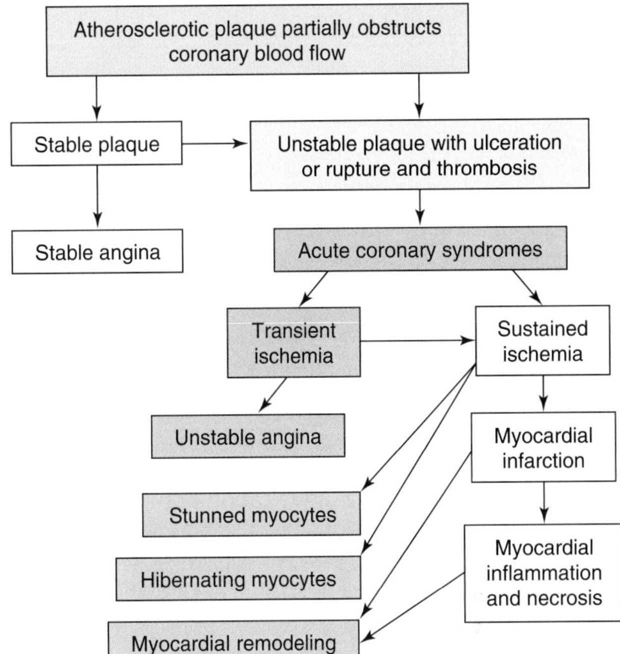

Algorithm 32.4 Pathophysiology of Acute Coronary Syndromes. The atherosclerotic process can lead to stable plaque formation and stable angina or can result in unstable plaques that are prone to rupture and thrombus. Thrombus formation on a ruptured plaque that disperses in less than 20 minutes leads to transient ischemia and unstable angina. If the vessel obstruction is sustained, myocardial infarction (MI) with inflammation and necrosis of the myocardium results. In addition, MI is associated with other structural and functional changes, including myocyte stunning and hibernation and myocardial remodeling.

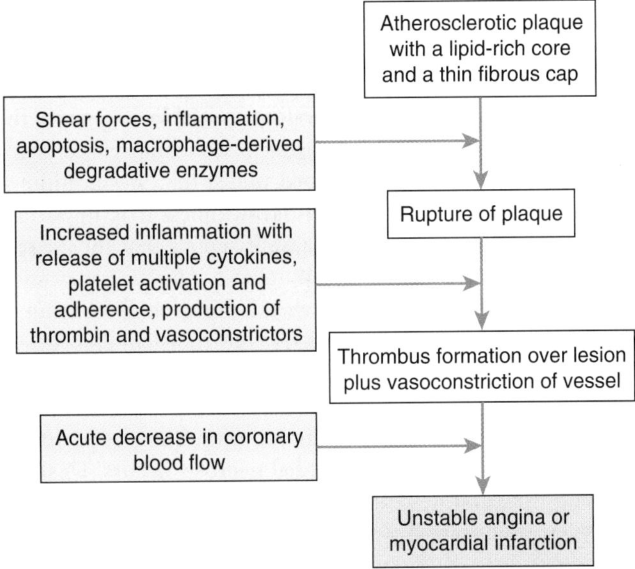

Fig. 32.9 Pathogenesis of Unstable Plaques and Thrombus Formation.

secretion of neutrophil- and macrophage-derived degradative enzymes, and apoptosis of cells at the edges of the lesions.[44] Exposure of the plaque substrate activates the clotting cascade. The resulting thrombus can form very quickly (Fig. 32.10A).

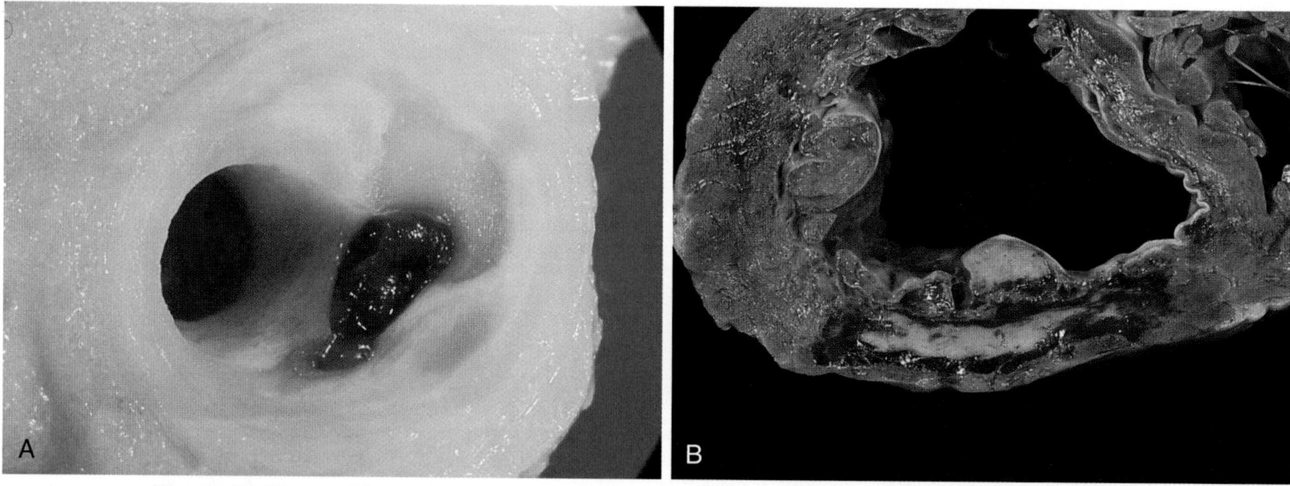

Fig. 32.10 Plaque Disruption and Myocardial Infarction. (A) Plaque disruption. The cap of the lipid-rich plaque has become torn, with the formation of a thrombus, mostly inside the plaque. **(B)** Myocardial infarction. This infarct is 6 days old. The center is yellow and necrotic with a hemorrhagic red rim. The responsible arterial occlusion is probably in the right coronary artery. The infarct is on the posterior wall. (From Damjanov I, Linder J, eds. *Anderson's pathology*, 10th edition. St. Louis: Mosby; 1996.)

Vessel obstruction is further exacerbated by the release of vasoconstrictors, such as thromboxane A_2 and endothelin. The thrombus may dissolve when only minimal myocyte damage has occurred (unstable angina), or it may persist causing prolonged ischemia with infarction of the heart muscle (MI) (see Fig. 32.10B).

Unstable angina. Unstable angina was once considered a separate type of acute coronary syndrome characterized by reversible myocardial ischemia and the absence of myocardial cell injury. However, the use of highly sensitive measurements of myocardial damage (hs-troponin I) has resulted in the recognition that most individuals with unstable angina do have some myocardial damage. Therefore, unstable angina is the first step in a progressive spectrum of ischemia-related myocardial injury and now is grouped under the classification of non-ST elevation acute coronary syndromes. It is important to recognize this syndrome because it signals that the atherosclerotic plaque has begun to rupture and infarction may soon follow. Unstable angina occurs when a fairly small fissuring or superficial erosion of the plaque leads to transient episodes of thrombotic vessel occlusion and vasoconstriction at the site of plaque damage. This thrombus is labile and occludes the vessel for no more than 10 to 20 minutes, with return of perfusion before large amounts of myocardial necrosis occurs. Unstable angina presents as new-onset angina, angina that is occurring at rest, or angina that is increasing in severity or frequency. Individuals may experience increased dyspnea, diaphoresis, and anxiety as the angina worsens. Physical examination may reveal evidence of ischemic myocardial dysfunction such as pulmonary congestion. The ECG most commonly shows ST segment depression and T wave inversion during pain that resolve as the pain is relieved. Serum levels of hs-troponin I are often slightly increased. Management of unstable angina requires immediate hospitalization with administration of nitrates and antithrombotics (e.g., aspirin, clopidogrel, abciximab, eptifibatide). Anticoagulants, such as low-molecular-weight heparin (enoxaparin), bivalirudin, or fondaparinux, are also given.[89,90] Beta-blockers, calcium channel blockers, and ACE inhibitors also may be used. Choices are based on symptoms, underlying conditions, and planned interventions. Lipid lowering medications such as statins should be administered. Rapid intervention with PCI also may be indicated if the individual's condition is refractory to medical treatment.[89,90]

Myocardial infarction. When coronary blood flow is interrupted for an extended period, infarction with myocyte necrosis occurs. This results in MI. Plaque progression, disruption, and subsequent clot formation are the same for MI as they are for unstable angina (see Algorithm 32.4 and Figs. 32.9 and 32.10). In this case, however, the thrombus is less labile and occludes the vessel for a prolonged period, such that myocardial ischemia progresses to myocyte necrosis and death. Pathologically, there are two major types of MI: subendocardial infarction and transmural infarction. Clinically, however, MI is categorized as non-ST segment elevation MI (non-STEMI) or ST segment elevation MI (STEMI).

If the thrombus disintegrates before complete distal tissue necrosis has occurred, the infarction will involve only the myocardium directly beneath the endocardium (subendocardial MI) (Fig. 32.11). This type of infarction usually will present with ST segment depression and T wave inversion without ST elevation; therefore, it is termed non-STEMI. It is important to recognize this form of acute coronary syndrome because recurrent clot formation on the disrupted atherosclerotic plaque is likely. If the thrombus lodges permanently in the vessel, the infarction will extend through the myocardium all the way from endocardium to epicardium (transmural MI), resulting in severe cardiac dysfunction (see Fig. 32.11). Transmural myocardial infarction usually will result in ST segment elevation on ECG, so it is

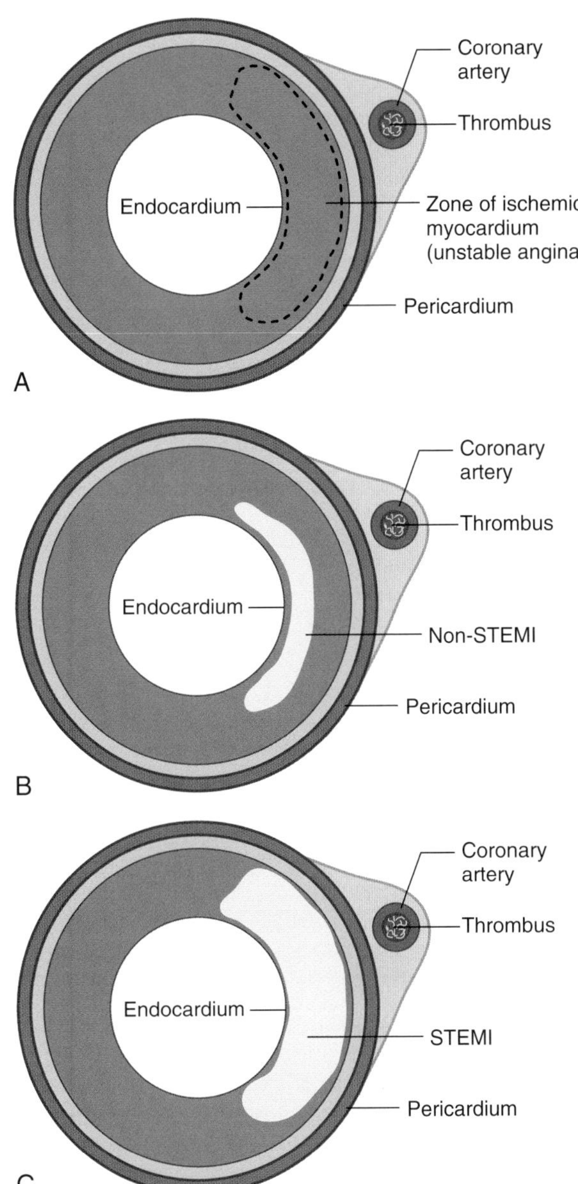

Fig. 32.11 Unstable Angina, non-ST elevation myocardial infarction *(STEMI)*, and STEMI. (A) Unstable angina. Coronary thrombosis leads to myocardial ischemia. **(B)** Non-STEMI. Persistent coronary occlusion leads to infarction of the myocardium closest to the endocardium. **(C)** STEMI. Continued coronary occlusion leads to transmural infarction extending from endocardium to pericardium.

called STEMI. Clinically, it is important to identify individuals with STEMI because they are at highest risk for serious complications and should receive definitive intervention without delay.

Pathophysiology. After 8 to 10 seconds of decreased blood flow, myocardial oxygen reserves are used quickly. Glycogen stores decrease as anaerobic metabolism begins. Unfortunately, glycolysis can supply only 65% to 70% of the total myocardial energy requirement and produces much less adenosine triphosphate (ATP) than aerobic processes. Hydrogen ions and lactic acid accumulate, making the myocardium more vulnerable to the damaging effects of lysosomal enzymes and may suppress impulse conduction and contractile function, thereby leading to heart failure.

Oxygen deprivation also is accompanied by electrolyte disturbances, specifically the loss of potassium, calcium, and magnesium from cells. Myocardial cells deprived of necessary oxygen and nutrients lose contractility, thereby diminishing the pumping ability of the heart. Ischemia causes the myocardial cells to release catecholamines, predisposing the individual to serious imbalances of sympathetic and parasympathetic function, irregular heartbeats (dysrhythmia), and heart failure. Catecholamines cause an increase in plasma concentrations of free fatty acids and glycerol, which can have a harmful detergent effect on cell membranes. Norepinephrine elevates blood glucose levels, which also contributes to myocardial dysfunction. Ang II is released during myocardial ischemia and causes peripheral vasoconstriction, coronary spasm, and fluid retention. It also is a growth factor for vascular smooth muscle cells, myocytes, and cardiac fibroblasts, resulting in structural changes in the myocardium called remodeling. Infiltration of inflammatory cells further contributes to tissue injury.

MI results in both structural and functional changes of cardiac tissues (Fig. 32.12). Cardiac cells can withstand ischemic conditions for about 20 minutes before irreversible hypoxic injury causes cellular death (apoptosis) and myocardial infarction. Gross tissue changes at the area of infarction may not become apparent for several hours, despite almost immediate onset (within 30 to 60 seconds) of electrocardiographic changes. Myocyte injury and necrosis result in the release of intracellular enzymes, such as creatine phosphokinase-myocardial bound (CPK-MB), and myocyte proteins, such as the troponins, through the damaged cell membranes into the interstitial spaces. The lymphatics absorb the enzymes and transport them into the bloodstream, where they can be detected by serologic tests.

Although restoration of blood flow is crucial to reducing infarct size, reperfusion of the ischemic myocardium triggers a process called reperfusion injury which can contribute as much as 50% to the overall infarct size (see Fig. 32.12).[91] Reperfusion injury involves the release of toxic oxygen free radicals, calcium flux, and pH changes that cause a sustained opening of mitochondrial permeability transition pores (mPTPs) and contribute to resultant cellular death. Ischemia and reperfusion also cause damage to the coronary circulation through endothelial injury, platelet activation, inflammation, and vasoconstriction.[92] Many studies are exploring ways to reduce the extent of injury in ischemia and reperfusion injury during myocardial infarction (see Emerging Science Box: Cardioprotection Therapies for Myocardial Infarction and Reperfusion Injury).

Cardiac tissue surrounding the area of necrosed tissue in myocardial infarction also undergoes changes. Myocardial stunning is a temporary loss of contractile function that persists for hours to days after perfusion has been restored (see Fig. 32.12). This pathophysiologic state can occur both after MI and in individuals who suffer ischemia during cardiovascular procedures or during CNS trauma. Stunning is caused by the alterations in electrolyte pumps and calcium homeostasis and by the release of toxic oxygen free radicals and contributes to heart failure, shock, and dysrhythmias.[93] Numerous interventions to limit the

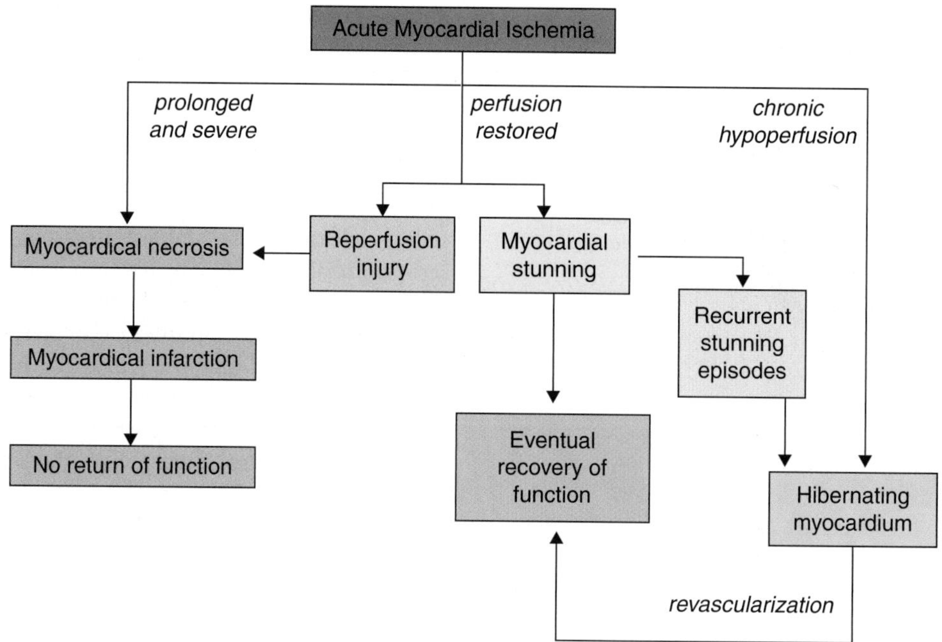

Fig. 32.12 Structural and Functional Changes Associated With Acute Myocardial Ischemia. Acute myocardial ischemia can result in prolonged and severe hypoperfusion, reperfusion, or chronic hypoperfusion. As a result, an acute coronary syndrome may be characterized by infarction, reperfusion injury, stunning, or hibernating myocardium. Recovery of function is not possible once myocardial tissue is necrosed, however stunned and hibernating myocardium may regain function after days, weeks, or even months, especially after appropriate revascularization procedures. (Adapted from Kloner RA. Stunned and hibernating myocardium: Where are we nearly 4 decades later? *Journal of the American Heart Association*, 2020;9:e015502.)

EMERGING SCIENCE BOX

Cardioprotection Therapies for Myocardial Infarction and Reperfusion Injury

Outcomes for individuals with myocardial ischemia and infarction have greatly improved through advances in the speed and efficacy of reperfusion strategies such as emergent percutaneous coronary interventions and thrombolytic medications. However, these reperfusion efforts cannot fully reverse established myocardial damage, and may contribute to infarct size through reperfusion injury. Numerous studies are exploring emerging therapies that may provide cardioprotection and reduce the extent of myocardial injury during and after ischemic events. For example, therapeutic angiogenesis using growth factors and progenitor cells has been shown to revascularize ischemic heart tissue. Techniques such as ischemic preconditioning promote neural pathways that have beneficial effects on myocyte resilience and function. Antiinflammatory and anti-immune therapeutics are also being explored. Stem cell approaches are of particular interest to researchers. These approaches include the intracoronary, intravenous, or intramuscular infusion of bone marrow, embryonic, mesenchymal, or cardiac stem cells. More recently, stem cell sheets are being created that are monolayers of stem cells that preserve cell-cell contact and their extracellular matrix resulting in enhanced effectiveness. To date, early animal and a few human clinical trials have shown that stem cell therapy is safe and has the potential to significantly improve cardiac function after myocardial infarction. Many further studies are underway.

Data from Attar A, et al. Mesenchymal stem cell transplantation after acute myocardial infarction: a meta-analysis of clinical trials. *Stem Cell Res Ther*, 2021;12:600; Cruz-Samperio R, et al. Cell augmentation strategies for cardiac stem cell therapies. *Stem Cells Transl Med*, 2021;10(6):855–866; Epstein JA, et al. Teasing the immune system to repair the heart. *New England Journal of Medicine*, 2020;382:1660–1662; Guo R, et al. Stem cell-derived cell sheet transplantation for heart tissue repair in myocardial infarction. *Stem Cell Research Therapy*, 2020;11:19; Gong R, et al. Regulation of cardiomyocyte fate plasticity: A key strategy for cardiac regeneration. *Signal Transduction Target Therapy*, 2021;6:31; Huynh K. Stem cell therapy improves heart function by triggering an acute immune response. *Nature Reviews Cardiology*, 2020;17:69; Johnson T, et al. Approaches to therapeutic angiogenesis for ischemic heart disease. *Journal of Molecular Medicine*, 2019;97(2):141–151; He L, et al. Heart regeneration by endogenous stem cells and cardiomyocyte proliferation: Controversy, fallacy, and progress. *Circulation*, 2020;142:275–291; Parviz Y, et al. Cellular and molecular approaches to enhance myocardial recovery after myocardial infarction. *Cardiovascular Revascularization Medicine*, 2019;20(4):351–364; Zuurbier CJ, et al. Innate immunity as a target for acute cardioprotection. *Cardiovascular Research*, 2019;115(7):1131–1142.

amount of stunning are being explored. Hibernating myocardium describes tissue that is persistently ischemic and undergoes metabolic adaptation to prolong myocyte survival until perfusion can be restored. Cardiomyocytes undergo downregulation of calcium-handling and mitochondrial proteins and upregulation of survival and stress proteins.[93] PCI or surgery aimed at reperfusion of hibernating myocardium can restore significant cardiac function (see Fig. 32.12).

Myocardial remodeling is a process that causes myocyte hypertrophy and loss of contractile function in the areas of the heart distant from the site of infarction. It can occur over days, weeks, and months after an acute ischemic event.[94] It is mediated by Ang II, aldosterone, catecholamines, adenosine, and inflammatory cytokines. It contributes to long-term myocardial dysfunction and heart failure. Remodeling can be limited through rapid restoration of coronary flow and the use of renin-angiotensin-aldosterone blockers and β-blockers after MI.

The severity of functional impairment depends on the size of the lesion and the site of infarction. Functional changes can include (1) decreased cardiac contractility with abnormal wall motion, (2) altered left ventricular compliance, (3) decreased stroke volume and ejection fraction, (4) increased left ventricular end-diastolic pressure (LVEDP), and (5) sinoatrial (SA) node malfunction. Life-threatening dysrhythmias and heart failure often follow MI.

With infarction, ventricular function is abnormal and the EF falls, resulting in increases in ventricular end-diastolic volume (VEDV). If the coronary obstruction involves the perfusion to the left ventricle, pulmonary venous congestion ensues; if the right ventricle is ischemic, increases in systemic venous pressures occur.

MI causes a severe inflammatory response that ends with wound repair (see Chapter 6).[95] Damaged cells undergo degradation, fibroblasts proliferate, and scar tissue is synthesized. Within 24 hours, leukocytes infiltrate the necrotic area, and proteolytic enzymes released from scavenger neutrophils degrade the necrotic tissue. Macrophages remove dead cells and secrete growth factors which help repair myocardial injury.[96] The collagen matrix that is deposited is initially weak, mushy, and vulnerable to reinjury. Unfortunately, it is at this time in the recovery period (10 to 14 days after infarction) that individuals feel more like increasing activities and may stress the newly formed scar tissue. After 6 weeks, the necrotic area is completely replaced by scar tissue, which is strong but cannot contract and relax like healthy myocardial tissue. These cellular and extracellular matrix changes contribute to sustained functional impairment of the heart often resulting in heart failure. Recent studies have shown that cardiac stem cells have regenerative capacity, and stem cell therapy may be a novel approach for cardiac muscle repair and regeneration (see Emerging Science Box: Cardioprotection Therapies for Myocardial Infarction and Reperfusion Injury).[97]

Clinical Manifestations. The first symptom of acute MI is usually sudden, severe chest pain. The pain is similar to that of angina pectoris but more severe and prolonged. It may be described as heavy and crushing, such as a "truck sitting on my chest." Radiation to the neck, jaw, back, shoulder, or left arm is common. Some individuals, especially those who are older or have diabetes, experience no pain, thus having a "silent" infarction. Infarction often simulates a sensation of unrelenting indigestion. Nausea and vomiting may occur because of reflex stimulation of vomiting centers by pain fibers. Vasovagal reflexes from the area of the infarcted myocardium also may affect the gastrointestinal tract.

Various cardiovascular changes are found on physical examination:

1. The SNS is reflexively activated to compensate, resulting in a temporary increase in heart rate and blood pressure.
2. Abnormal extra heart sounds reflect left ventricular dysfunction.
3. Pulmonary findings of congestion, including dullness to percussion and inspiratory crackles at the lung bases, can occur if the individual develops heart failure.
4. Peripheral vasoconstriction may cause the skin to become cool and clammy.

The number and severity of postinfarction complications depend on the location and extent of necrosis, the individual's physiologic condition before the infarction, and the availability of swift therapeutic intervention. Table 32.5 lists the most common complications of MI. Sudden cardiac death can occur in individuals with myocardial ischemia even if infarction is absent or minimal. Risk factors for sudden death are related to

TABLE 32.5 Complications of Myocardial Infarction

Type	Characteristics
Dysrhythmias	Caused by alterations of impulse conduction because of ischemia and electrolyte disturbances; sudden onset of tachycardia or bradycardia, palpitations, syncope, shock, or sudden death
Left ventricular failure	Characterized by pulmonary congestion, reduced myocardial contractility, and abnormal heart wall motion; cardiogenic shock may develop
Pericarditis	Inflammation of the pericardium associated with anterior chest pain that worsens with respiratory effort and pericardial friction rub; occurs 2–3 days after infarction
Dressler postinfarction syndrome	Delayed form of pericarditis that occurs 1 week to several months after acute myocardial infarction and thought to be immunologic response to necrotic myocardium; marked by pain, fever, friction rub, pleural effusion, and arthralgias
Organic brain syndrome	Occurs if blood flow to brain is impaired
Rupture of chordae tendinea	Caused by necrosis of tissue in or around papillary muscles; acute onset of severe valvular regurgitation
Aneurysm and rupture of wall or septae of infarcted ventricle	Aneurysm formation resulting from high chamber pressures and volume pushing against weakened ventricular wall; rupture of ventricular wall or septae between chambers when pressure becomes too great; rapid onset of shock
Systemic arterial thromboembolism	May disseminate from debris and clots that collect inside dilated aneurysmal sacs or from infarcted endocardium; can affect any system but especially targets cerebrovascular system with transient ischemic attacks and stroke
Pulmonary thromboembolism	Usually from deep venous thrombi of legs; acute onset of dyspnea and hypoxemia
Sudden death	Dysrhythmias frequently causative, particularly ventricular fibrillation

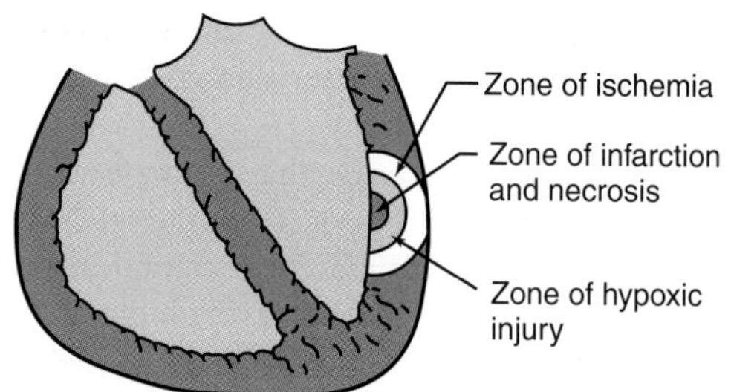

Fig. 32.13 Electrocardiographic Alterations Associated With the Three Zones of Myocardial Infarction.

an interaction among three factors: ischemia, left ventricular dysfunction, and electrical instability.

Evaluation and Treatment. There are several defined categories of myocardial infarction, each with their own criteria for diagnosis.[98] In general, the diagnosis of acute MI is made on the basis of history, physical examination, ECG results, and serial cardiac troponin elevations.

MI can occur in various regions of the heart wall and may be described as anterior, inferior, posterior, lateral, subendocardial, or transmural, depending on the anatomic location and extent of tissue damage from infarction. Twelve-lead ECGs help localize the affected area through identification of changes in ST segments and T waves. The infarcted myocardium is surrounded by a zone of hypoxic injury, which may progress to necrosis or return to normal, and adjacent to this zone of hypoxic injury is a zone of reversible ischemia (Fig. 32.13). A characteristic Q wave often develops on ECG some hours later in STEMI.

Cardiac troponin I (cTnI) is the most specific indicator of MI, and measurement of its level should be performed on admission to the emergency department. cTnI level elevation is detectable 2 to 4 hours after onset of symptoms. Additional measurements within 6 to 9 hours and again at 12 to 24 hours are recommended if clinical suspicion is high and previous samples were negative. Troponin levels also can be used to estimate infarct size and therefore the likelihood of complications. Additional laboratory data may reveal leukocytosis and elevated C-reactive protein (CRP), both of which indicate inflammation. The individual's blood glucose level is usually elevated and the glucose tolerance level may remain abnormal for several weeks.

Acute MI requires admission to the hospital, often directly into a coronary care unit. The individual should be given an aspirin immediately (ticlopidine if allergic to aspirin) along with nitrates and morphine for pain. Continuous monitoring of cardiac rhythms and enzymatic changes is essential, because the first 24 hours after onset of symptoms is the time of highest risk for sudden death. Non-STEMI is treated in the same way as unstable angina including antithrombotics, anticoagulation or PCI, or both.[89] STEMI is best managed with emergent PCI and antithrombotics.[99,100] Hyperglycemia is treated with insulin, and hyperlipidemia with statins. Recent studies suggest that intravenous statins given as a bolus during acute MI management may reduce infarct size, improve systolic contraction, and reduce remodeling.[101] ACE inhibitors should be prescribed as secondary prevention.[79] Individuals who are in shock require aggressive fluid resuscitation, ionotropic drugs, and possible emergent invasive procedures.

Bed rest, followed by gradual return to activities of daily living, reduces the myocardial oxygen demands of the compromised heart. Individuals not receiving thrombolytic or heparin infusion must receive DVT prophylaxis as long as their activity is significantly limited. Stool softeners are given to eliminate the need for straining. Education regarding appropriate diet and caffeine intake, smoking cessation, exercise, and other aspects of risk factor reduction is crucial for secondary prevention of recurrent myocardial ischemia.

DISORDERS OF THE HEART WALL

Disorders of the Pericardium

Pericardial disease is a localized manifestation of another disorder, such as infection (bacterial, viral, fungal, rickettsial, or parasitic); trauma or surgery; neoplasm; or a metabolic, immunologic, or vascular disorder (uremia, rheumatoid arthritis, systemic lupus erythematosus, periarteritis nodosa). The pericardial response to injury from these diverse causes may consist of pericarditis, pericardial effusion, or constrictive pericarditis.

Pericarditis

Pericarditis can be categorized as acute, recurrent, or chronic. Acute pericarditis is acute inflammation of the pericardium. The etiology of acute pericarditis is most often idiopathic or caused by viral infection by coxsackie, influenza, hepatitis, measles, mumps, varicella viruses, or human immunodeficiency virus (HIV). Other causes include MI, trauma, neoplasm, bacterial infection (especially tuberculosis), connective tissue disease (especially systemic lupus erythematosus and rheumatoid arthritis), or hypothyroidism. Iatrogenic causes include radiation therapy, cardiac surgery, pacemaker insertion, radiofrequency ablation, transcatheter aortic valve implantation, and PCI.[102] The pericardial membranes become inflamed with the release of inflammatory cytokines such as IL-1, and a pericardial effusion may develop that can be serous, purulent, or fibrinous (Fig. 32.14).

Symptoms may follow several days of fever and usually begin with the sudden onset of severe retrosternal chest pain that worsens with respiratory movements and when assuming a recumbent position. The pain may radiate to the back as a result of irritation of the phrenic nerve (innervates the trapezius muscles) as it traverses the pericardium. Individuals with acute pericarditis also report dysphagia, restlessness, irritability, anxiety, weakness, and malaise.

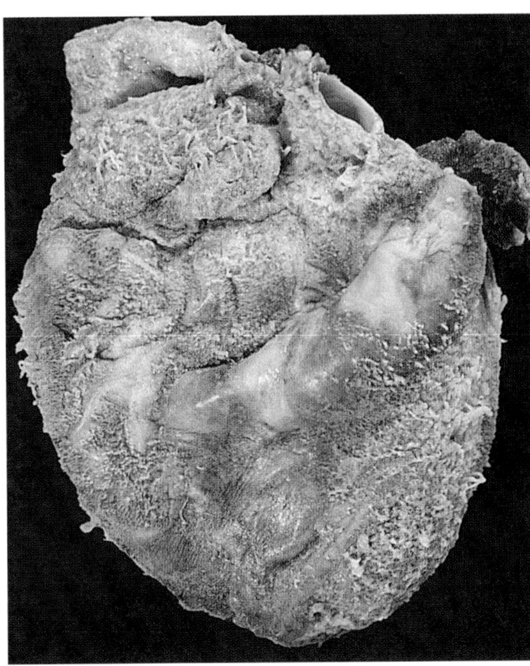

Fig. 32.14 Acute Pericarditis. Note shaggy coat of fibers covering the surface of heart. (From Damjanov I, Linder J. *Pathology: A color atlas*. St. Louis: Mosby; 2000.)

Physical examination often reveals low-grade fever and sinus tachycardia. An intermittent friction rub—a scratchy, grating sound—may be heard at the cardiac apex and left sternal border and is highly suggestive of pericarditis. The rub is caused by the roughened pericardial membranes rubbing against each other. Evidence of underlying infection or disease may also be evident. ECG findings may reflect inflammatory processes through PR segment depression and diffuse ST segment elevation (sometimes described as "saddle shaped") without Q waves, and they may remain abnormal for days or even weeks. Cardiac troponins may be slightly elevated in some individuals. Echocardiography is the primary imaging modality for diagnosis. Some individuals will require CT or cardiac magnetic resonance (CMR) evaluation. Acute pericarditis requires at least two of the following four criteria for diagnosis: (1) chest pain characteristics of pericarditis, (2) pericardial rub, (3) characteristic electrocardiographic changes, and (4) new or worsening pericardial effusion.[103]

Treatment for uncomplicated acute pericarditis consists of administration of antiinflammatory agents, such as salicylates and NSAIDs, and colchicine.[102] Exploration of the underlying cause is important. Approximately one-third of cases will be complicated by the development of recurrent pericarditis (symptoms return after 4 to 6 weeks without symptoms) and may require the administration of more aggressive antiinflammatory and immunosuppressive medications such as corticosteroids.[103] Other possible sequelae of pericarditis include chronic pericarditis (symptoms persist beyond 3 months), cardiac tamponade, or constrictive pericarditis.

Pericardial Effusion

Pericardial effusion is the accumulation of fluid in the pericardial cavity and can occur in all forms of pericarditis. Many are idiopathic (20%), but other causes, such as neoplasm, infection, renal failure, or hypothyroidism must be considered.[104] Analysis of the fluid obtained through pericardiocentesis allows for identification of the likely source of the fluid. The fluid may be a transudate, such as the serous effusion that develops with left heart failure, overhydration, or hypoproteinemia. More often, however, the fluid is an exudate, which reflects pericardial inflammation like that seen with acute pericarditis, MI, heart surgery, some chemotherapeutic agents, infections, and autoimmune disorders such as systemic lupus erythematosus. (Types of exudate are described in Chapter 7.) If the fluid is serosanguineous, the underlying cause is likely to be tuberculosis, neoplasm, uremia, or radiation, although some remain idiopathic. Effusions of frank blood are generally related to aneurysms, trauma, or coagulation defects. If chyle leaks from the thoracic duct, it may enter the pericardium and lead to cholesterol pericarditis.

If a pericardial effusion develops gradually, the pericardium can stretch to accommodate large quantities of fluid without compressing the heart. If the fluid accumulates rapidly, however, even a small amount (50 to 100 mL) may create sufficient pressure to cause cardiac compression, a serious condition known as tamponade. In tamponade, the pressure exerted by the pericardial fluid eventually equals or even exceeds diastolic pressure within the heart chambers, which interferes with right atrial filling. This causes increased venous pressure, systemic venous congestion, and signs and symptoms of right heart failure (distention of the jugular veins, edema, hepatomegaly). Decreased atrial filling also leads to decreased ventricular filling, decreased stroke volume, and reduced cardiac output. Life-threatening circulatory collapse may occur.

An important clinical finding is pulsus paradoxus, in which arterial blood pressure during expiration exceeds arterial pressure during inspiration by more than 10 mm Hg. Pulsus paradoxus in the setting of a pericardial effusion indicates tamponade and reflects impairment of diastolic filling of the left ventricle plus reduction of blood volume within all four cardiac chambers.

Other clinical manifestations of pericardial effusion are distant or muffled heart sounds, poorly palpable apical pulse, dyspnea on exertion, and dull chest pain. A chest x-ray film may disclose a "water-bottle configuration" of the cardiac silhouette. An echocardiogram (which often may be done at the bedside) can detect an effusion as small as 20 ml and is a reliable and accurate diagnostic test, although CT scans also may be done.

Treatment of pericardial effusion or tamponade consists of pericardiocentesis (aspiration of excessive pericardial fluid) and treatment of the underlying condition.[104] Persistent pain may be treated with analgesics, antiinflammatory medications, or steroids. Surgery may be required if the underlying cause of tamponade is trauma or aneurysm. A pericardial "window" may be surgically created to prevent tamponade.[105,106]

Constrictive Pericarditis

Constrictive pericarditis, or restrictive pericarditis (chronic pericarditis), is most commonly idiopathic or associated with viral infection, tuberculosis, radiation exposure, collagen vascular disorders, sarcoidosis, neoplasm, uremia, or cardiac surgery. In constrictive pericarditis, fibrous scarring with occasional

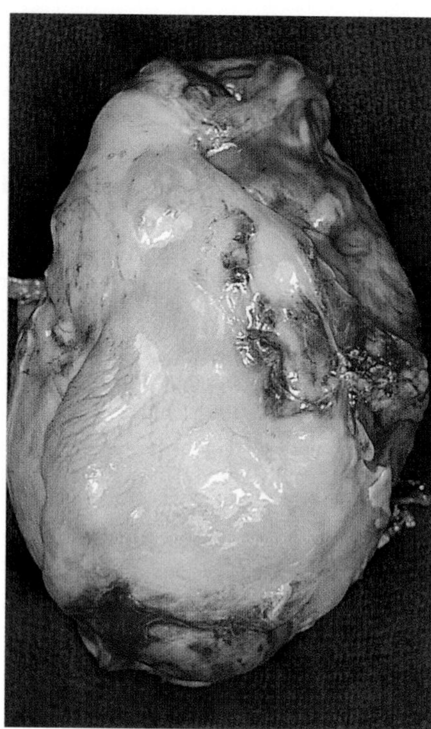

Fig. 32.15 Constrictive Pericarditis. The fibrotic pericardium encases the heart in a rigid shell. (From Damjanov I, Linder J. *Pathology: A color atlas*. St. Louis: Mosby; 2000.)

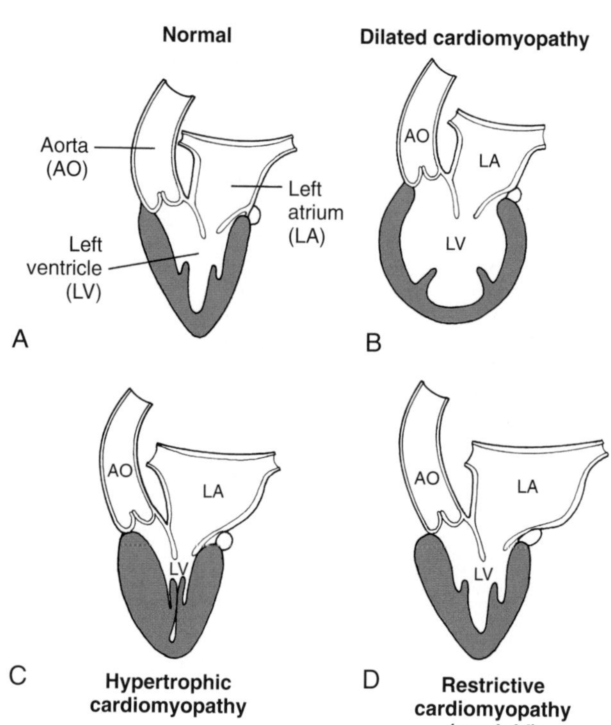

Fig. 32.16 Diagram Showing Major Distinguishing Pathophysiologic Features of the Three Types of Cardiomyopathy. **(A)** The normal heart. **(B)** In the dilated type of cardiomyopathy, the heart has a globular shape and the largest circumference of the left ventricle is not at its base but midway between apex and base. **(C)** In the hypertrophic type, the wall of the left ventricle is greatly thickened; the left ventricular cavity is small, but the left atrium may be dilated because of poor diastolic relaxation of the ventricle. **(D)** In the restrictive (constrictive) type, the left ventricular cavity is normal size, but, again, the left atrium is dilated because of the reduced diastolic compliance of the ventricle. (From Kissane JM, ed. *Anderson's pathology*, 9th edition. St. Louis: Mosby; 1990.)

calcification of the pericardium causes the visceral and parietal pericardial layers to adhere, obliterating the pericardial cavity. The fibrotic lesions encase the heart in a rigid shell (Fig. 32.15). Like tamponade, constrictive pericarditis compresses the heart and eventually reduces cardiac output. Unlike tamponade, however, constrictive pericarditis always develops gradually.

Symptoms are exercise intolerance, dyspnea on exertion, fatigue, and anorexia. Clinical assessment shows edema, distention of the jugular vein, hepatic congestion, and systemic hypotension. Restricted ventricular filling may cause a pericardial knock (early diastolic sound).

ECG findings include nonspecific ST and T wave abnormalities and atrial fibrillation (AF). Chest x-ray films often disclose prominent pulmonary vessels and calcification of the pericardium. CT, MRI, and transesophageal echocardiography are used to detect pericardial thickening and constriction and to distinguish constrictive pericarditis from restrictive cardiomyopathy. Pericardial biopsy may be needed to determine the etiology.

Initial treatment for constrictive pericarditis consists of restriction of dietary sodium intake and administration of diuretics to improve cardiac output. Management also may include use of antiinflammatory drugs and treatment of any underlying disorder such as tuberculosis. If these modalities are unsuccessful, surgical excision of the restrictive pericardium is indicated (pericardiectomy).[105]

Disorders of the Myocardium: Cardiomyopathies

The cardiomyopathies are a diverse group of diseases that affect the myocardium. Primary cardiomyopathies are disorders confined to the myocardium. Many primary cardiomyopathies are idiopathic; others are caused by ischemia, hypertension, inherited disorders, infections, toxins, myocarditis, or autoimmunity. Secondary cardiomyopathies occur in the context of disorders that affect other organs as well as the heart, such as infectious disease, toxin exposure, systemic connective tissue disease, infiltrative and proliferative disorders, or nutritional deficiencies. The cardiomyopathies are further categorized as dilated, hypertrophic, or restrictive, depending on their physiologic effects on the heart (Fig. 32.16).

Dilated Cardiomyopathy

Dilated cardiomyopathy most commonly results from ischemic heart disease or valvular disease. Non-ischemic non-valvular causes include diabetes, renal failure, alcohol or drug toxicity, peripartum complications, or infection. It also can be associated with inherited disorders such as muscular dystrophy, and genetic polymorphisms that affect cytoskeletal and sarcomere proteins (including truncated titin proteins) can be identified in up to 35% of individuals.[107] Four different phenotypic groups of dilated cardiomyopathies have been described: (1) mild systolic dysfunction, (2) autoimmune cardiomyopathy, (3) genetic with arrhythmias (atrial fibrillation or non-sustained ventricular

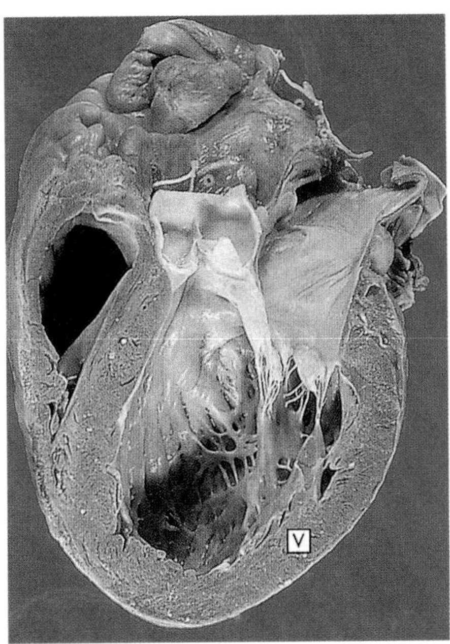

Fig. 32.17 Dilated Cardiomyopathy. The dilated left ventricle has a thin wall *(V)*. (From Stevens A, Lowe JS, Scott I. *Core pathology*, 3rd edition. London: Mosby; 2009.)

tachycardia), and (4) severe systolic dysfunction. Each of these types is characterized by different pathophysiologic mechanisms of metabolism, inflammation, and fibrosis.[108] Dilated cardiomyopathy results in impaired systolic function leading to increases in intracardiac volume, ventricular dilation, and heart failure with reduced EF (Fig. 32.17). Individuals complain of dyspnea, fatigue, and pedal edema. Findings on examination include a displaced apical pulse, S_3 gallop, peripheral edema, jugular venous distention, and pulmonary congestion. Diagnosis is confirmed by chest x-ray and echocardiogram, and management includes standard treatment of heart failure plus prevention of dysrhythmias.[109] Further management is determined by the specific cause of the cardiomyopathy. Ventricular assist devices and heart transplant are required in severe cases.

Hypertrophic Cardiomyopathy

Hypertrophic cardiomyopathy refers to two major categories of thickening of the myocardium: (1) hypertrophic cardiomyopathy (hypertrophic obstructive cardiomyopathy, asymmetric septal hypertrophic cardiomyopathy, or subaortic stenosis) and (2) hypertensive or valvular hypertrophic cardiomyopathy.

Hypertrophic cardiomyopathy. Hypertrophic cardiomyopathy (HCM) is the most common inherited cardiac disorder. The prevalence in young adults in the United States is estimated to be 1:200 to 1:500, while diagnosed symptomatic cases occur in about 1:3000 adults.[110] It results from autosomal dominant inheritance of mutations affecting genes encoding for cardiac sarcomere proteins and hypercontractility.[111] HCM is characterized by left ventricular hypertrophy with thickening of the septal wall (Fig. 32.18), which may cause outflow obstruction to the left ventricle outflow tract. Obstruction of left ventricular outflow can occur when the heart rate is increased, and the intravascular volume is decreased such as occurs with exercise. Other abnormalities include myocardial

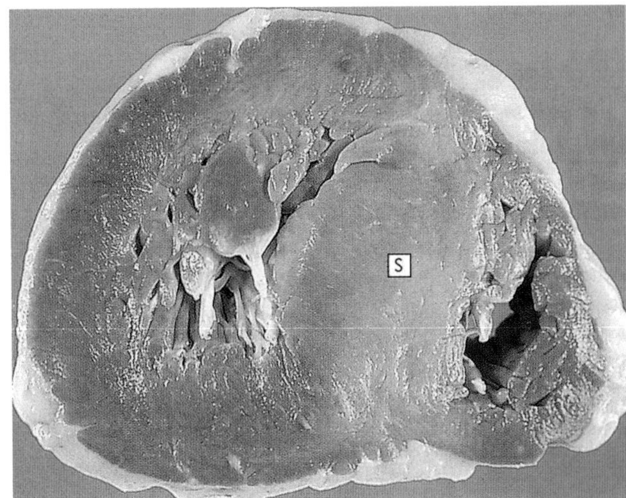

Fig. 32.18 Hypertrophic Cardiomyopathy. There is marked left ventricular hypertrophy. This often affects the septum *(S)*. (From Stevens A, Lowe JS, Scott I. *Core pathology*, 3rd edition. London: Mosby; 2009.)

fibrosis with diastolic dysfunction, abnormal mitral valve leaflets with mitral regurgitation, remodeled coronary vessels with myocardial ischemia, and the development of heart failure. Sudden death may occur, although increased awareness and management of HCM have reduced mortality rates to less than 1.0% per year.[110]

Recognition of HCM usually occurs after the development of symptoms such as palpitations, exercise intolerance, syncope, detection of a heart murmur, or abnormal ECG in a young person. Diagnosis is confirmed by echocardiography or MRI. Genetic testing and counseling are recommended for affected individuals and their families. Risk assessment for sudden death based on family history, extent of hypertrophy, development of syncope or heart failure, and presence of arrhythmias should be conducted.

Management begins with extensive discussions and shared decision-making with affected individuals and families about risks for HCM complications, lifestyle changes, and appropriate interventions. Moderate exercise is safe in most cases; however participation in high-intensity sports requires extensive evaluation and in-depth counseling about risks.[110] Management of symptoms may include beta blockers and calcium channel blockers. Implantable cardioverter defibrillator implantation significantly reduces mortality in high-risk individuals. Heart failure is managed in accordance with general heart failure guidelines.[110] Antiarrhythmic medications may be needed. Transaortic septal myectomy or septal ablation may be indicated in selected individuals. Mavacamten, a cardiac myosin inhibitor, was found to improve cardiac structure and function, symptoms, and quality of life in phase 3 trials for individuals with HCM.[112]

Hypertensive hypertrophic cardiomyopathy and valvular hypertrophic cardiomyopathy. Hypertensive hypertrophic cardiomyopathy and valvular hypertrophic cardiomyopathy occur because of increased resistance to ventricular ejection, which is commonly seen in individuals with hypertension or valvular stenosis (usually aortic). In this case, hypertrophy of the myocytes is an attempt to compensate for increased myocardial workload. Long-term dysfunction of the myocytes develops over time, with diastolic dysfunction appearing first and leading eventually to systolic dysfunction of the ventricle (see the Heart Failure section). Individuals with hypertensive hypertrophic cardiomyopathy may be asymptomatic or may complain of angina, syncope, dyspnea on exertion, and palpitations. Examination may reveal extra heart sounds (especially an S4) and murmurs. Echocardiography and cardiac catheterization can confirm the diagnosis. Management rests on appropriate treatment for the underlying condition.

Restrictive Cardiomyopathy

Restrictive cardiomyopathy is characterized by resistance to filling and increased diastolic pressure of either or both ventricles. Systolic function and wall thickness are normal. It may occur idiopathically or as a cardiac manifestation of systemic diseases, such as amyloidosis, scleroderma, sarcoidosis, lymphoma, and hemochromatosis, or a number of inherited storage diseases. Cardiac amyloidosis is caused by the deposition of excess light chain immunoglobulins leading to ventricular wall thickening and fibrosis.[113] The myocardium becomes rigid and noncompliant, impeding ventricular filling and raising filling pressures during diastole. The most common clinical manifestation of restrictive cardiomyopathy is right heart failure with systemic venous congestion. Cardiomegaly and dysrhythmias are common. A thorough evaluation for the underlying cause should be initiated (and may include myocardial biopsy). Treatment is aimed at managing heart failure and reversing the underlying cause when possible. Death occurs as a result of heart failure or dysrhythmias.

Disorders of the Endocardium

Disorders that involve the endocardium (the innermost lining of the heart wall) damage the cardiac valves. These disorders include valvular heart disease, acute rheumatic fever and rheumatic heart disease, and infective endocarditis.

Valvular Heart Disease

Valvular heart disease can be either congenital or acquired. The acquired forms are more common in adults and result from inflammatory, ischemic, traumatic, degenerative, or infectious alterations of valvular structure and function. Worldwide, the most common cause of acquired valvular dysfunction is degeneration or inflammation of the endocardium secondary to rheumatic heart disease (Table 32.6). In the United States degenerative-calcific disease is the most common cause, and a link between mitral annular calcification and atherosclerotic vascular disease has been established.[114] Structural alterations of the heart valves are caused by remodeling changes in the valvular

TABLE 32.6 Clinical Manifestations of Valvular Stenosis and Regurgitation

Manifestation	Aortic Stenosis	Mitral Stenosis	Aortic Regurgitation	Mitral Regurgitation	Tricuspid Regurgitation
Most common cause	Congenital bicuspid valve, degenerative (calcific) changes with aging, rheumatic heart disease	Rheumatic heart disease, mitral annular calcification (MAC)	Infective endocarditis; aortic root disease (connective tissue diseases, Marfan syndrome); dilation of aortic root from hypertension and aging	Myxomatous degeneration (mitral valve prolapse)	Congenital; secondary to pulmonary hypertension with cor pulmonale
Cardiovascular outcome (untreated)	Left ventricular hypertrophy followed by left heart failure; decreased coronary blood flow with myocardial ischemia	Left atrial hypertrophy and dilation with fibrillation, followed by right ventricular failure	Left ventricular hypertrophy and dilation, followed by left heart failure	Left atrial hypertrophy and dilation, followed by left heart failure	Right heart failure
Pulmonary effects	Pulmonary edema with dyspnea on exertion	Pulmonary edema with dyspnea on exertion	Pulmonary edema with dyspnea on exertion	Pulmonary edema with dyspnea on exertion	Dyspnea (may be caused by underlying lung disease)
Central nervous system effects	Syncope, especially on exertion	Stroke resulting from emboli (e.g., hemiparesis)	Syncope	None	None
Pain	Angina pectoris	Atypical chest pain	Angina pectoris	Atypical chest pain	Palpitations
Heart sounds	Systolic murmur heard best at right parasternal second intercostal space and radiating to neck	Low, rumbling diastolic murmur heard best at apex and radiating to axilla; accentuated first heart sound, opening snap	Diastolic murmur heard best at right parasternal second intercostal space and radiating to neck	Murmur throughout systole heard best at apex and radiating to axilla	Murmur throughout systole heard best at left lower sternal border

With data from Mann DL, Zipes DP, Libby P, et al., eds. *Braunwald's heart disease: A textbook of cardiovascular medicine*, 10th edition. St. Louis: Elsevier; 2014.

extracellular matrix and lead to stenosis, incompetence, or both. Previously undiagnosed, mild valvular heart disease is present in approximately half of individuals ≥65 years of age, and the prevalence of undiagnosed moderate or severe valvular heart disease may be as high as 6.4%.[12]

In valvular stenosis, the valve orifice is constricted and narrowed, so blood cannot flow forward and the workload of the cardiac chamber proximal to the diseased valve increases. Pressure (intraventricular or atrial) rises in the proximal chamber to overcome resistance to flow through the valve, necessitating greater exertion by the myocardium and producing myocardial hypertrophy. Although all four heart valves may be affected, those of the left heart (mitral and aortic valves) in adults are far more commonly affected than those of the right heart (tricuspid and pulmonic valves).

In valvular regurgitation (also called insufficiency or incompetence), the valve leaflets, or cusps, fail to shut completely, permitting blood flow to continue even when the valve is presumably closed. During systole or diastole, some blood leaks back into the chamber proximal to the diseased valve, which increases the volume of blood the heart must pump and increases the workload of both the atrium and the ventricle. Increased volume leads to chamber dilation, and increased workload leads to hypertrophy; both lead to cardiac dysfunction over time. For both valvular stenosis and regurgitation, over time. myocardial contractility diminishes, EF drops, diastolic pressure increases, and the ventricles fail from being overworked. Depending on the severity of the valvular dysfunction and the capacity of the heart to compensate, valvular alterations cause a range of symptoms and some degree of incapacitation (see Table 32.6).

In general, valvular disease is suspected when a heart murmur is detected, when symptoms develop, or when incidental findings of valvular abnormalities are detected on noninvasive testing.[115] Diagnosis rests on transthoracic echocardiography (TTE), which can be used to assess the severity of valvular obstruction or regurgitation before the onset of symptoms. CT or MRI may be indicated in certain settings. BNP measurements are obtained to assess cardiac chamber stress. ECG, chest x-ray, and exercise stress testing are often obtained. Cardiac catheterization may be needed if surgical intervention is planned. Valvular lesions are staged and appropriate management is determined by using four general categories: (1) at risk, (2) progressive, (3) asymptomatic severe, and (4) symptomatic severe.[115]

Management of valvular heart disease includes cardiovascular risk reduction and careful medical management. Regular exercise and diet modification to reduce overall cardiovascular risk are crucial. The maintenance of oral health is important to the prevention of infective endocarditis. Medical management most often is focused on reducing cardiac workload and improving systolic function, as well as treating established heart failure.[115] Valvular repair or replacement is indicated for progressive disease. The purpose of valvular repair or replacement is to improve symptoms and prolong survival, as well as to minimize complications such as asymptomatic irreversible heart failure, pulmonary hypertension, stroke, and AF. Anticoagulation either with a non-vitamin K oral anticoagulant or with warfarin is indicated in most individuals with valvular heart disease with or without atrial fibrillation, although warfarin is the antithrombotic of choice for those having undergone valve replacement.[115] Infectious endocarditis prophylaxis is recommended for those with prosthetic valves who are undergoing dental procedures that involve manipulation of gingival tissue or the periapical region of the teeth, or perforation of the oral mucosa.[115]

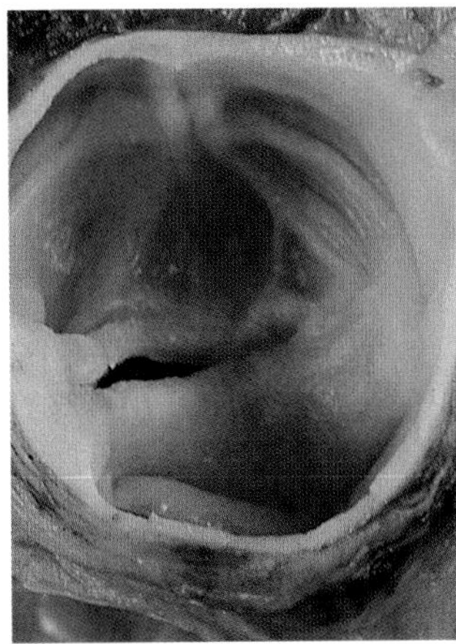

Fig. 32.19 Aortic Stenosis. Mild stenosis in valve leaflets of a young adult. (From Damjanov I, Linder J. *Pathophysiology: A color atlas.* St. Louis: Mosby; 2000.)

Aortic stenosis. Aortic stenosis is the most commonly diagnosed form of valvular heart disease, affecting nearly 2% of adults older than 65 years of age and nearly 10% of those over the age of 80.[116] It has three common causes: (1) congenital bicuspid valve, (2) degeneration with aging, and (3) inflammatory damage caused by rheumatic heart disease (Fig. 32.19). Congenital bicuspid aortic valve is found in 1% to 2% of the population. The valve functions normally at birth, but degenerates with fibrosis and calcification of the valve, causing stenosis as early as age 50. Degenerative aortic valve disease results from progressive deposition of calcium phosphate into all three cusps causing the valves to adhere to one another.[116] In addition, the aortic valve contains numerous inflammatory and immune cells such as macrophages, T lymphocyte, and B lymphocytes that play a causative role in aortic valve degeneration and calcification.[117] Rheumatic (post-inflammatory) aortic stenosis results from chronic inflammation of the valve leading to fibrosis, calcific degeneration, and fusion of the valve cusps. Aortic stenosis is associated with many risk factors for CAD, including hypertension, smoking, and dyslipidemia. Of interest, recent studies have identified a significant reduction in serum levels of zinc in individuals with calcific AS, which suggests a role of zinc metabolism in early valve degeneration.[114]

In aortic stenosis, the orifice of the valve narrows, causing resistance to blood flow from the left ventricle into the aorta (Algorithm 32.5). Outflow obstruction increases pressure within the left ventricle as it tries to eject blood through the narrowed opening. Left ventricular hypertrophy develops to compensate for the increased workload. Remodeling of the LV myocardium with fibrosis leads to a gradual decline in LV function with decreased cardiac output. Untreated aortic stenosis can lead to hypertrophic cardiomyopathy, myocardial ischemia or infarction, oliguria, stroke, heart failure, and pulmonary edema.

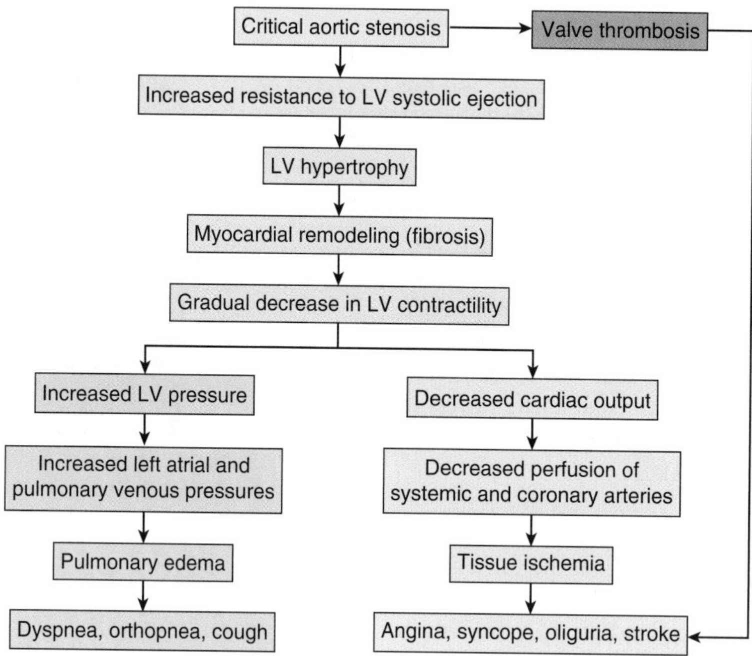

Algorithm 32.5 Pathophysiology of Aortic Stenosis. *LV*, Left ventricle.

Aortic stenosis usually develops gradually. Classic symptoms include angina, syncope, and dyspnea. Clinical manifestations include decreased stroke volume and narrowed pulse pressure (the difference between systolic and diastolic pressures). Heart rate is often slow, and pulses are delayed. Resistance to flow leads to a crescendo-decrescendo systolic heart murmur heard best at the right parasternal second intercostal space and may radiate to the neck. Echocardiography can be used to assess the severity of valvular obstruction before the onset of symptoms. Medical management includes vasodilator therapy to reduce resistance to ventricular ejection. Statins are prescribed for associated CAD, but have not been shown to prevent progression of AS.[114] Percutaneous placement of a prosthetic valve (transcatheter aortic valve implantation [TAVI]) is indicated for symptomatic and most asymptomatic individuals with severe stenosis. In a meta-analysis of four randomized controlled trials (RCTs) comparing TAVI and surgical valve replacement in low-risk individuals, TAVI was associated with a lower all-cause and cardiovascular mortality along with lower rates of new-onset atrial fibrillation, life-threatening bleeding, and acute kidney injury, but higher rates of paravalvular regurgitation and pacemaker implantation.[118] Surgical valve replacement may be indicated in selected individuals. Untreated aortic stenosis may result in irreversible fibrotic damage to the left ventricle.

Mitral stenosis. Mitral stenosis impairs the flow of blood from the left atrium to the left ventricle. Mitral stenosis is the most common form of rheumatic heart disease. Autoimmunity in response to group A β-hemolytic streptococcal M protein antigens leads to inflammation and scarring of the valvular leaflets. Scarring causes the leaflets to become fibrous and fused, and the chordae tendineae cordis become shortened (Fig. 32.20).

Another cause of narrowing of the mitral orifice is mitral annular calcification (MAC), which is a calcific degeneration of the mitral valve seen in 10% of the U.S. population and affecting up to 40% of those over the age of 70.[119] It is most common in those with risk factors for atherosclerotic coronary artery disease and chronic kidney disease. MAC only occasionally causes significant mitral stenosis by itself but can complicate the care of those with rheumatic mitral valve disease.

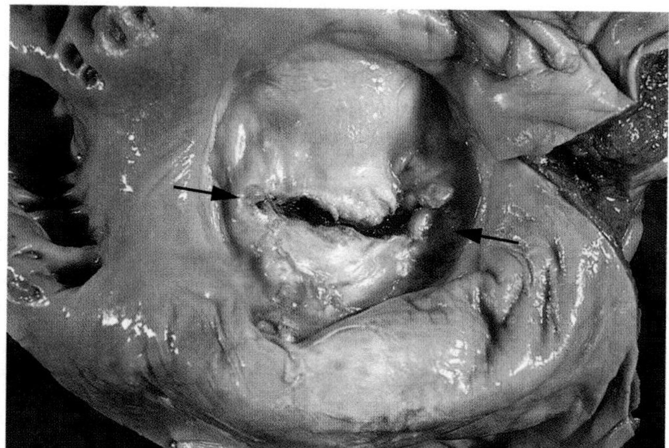

Fig. 32.20 Mitral Stenosis With Classic "Fish Mouth" Orifice (Arrows).

Impedance to blood flow results in incomplete emptying of the left atrium and elevated atrial pressure as the chamber tries to force blood through the stenotic valve. Continued increases in left atrial volume and pressure cause atrial dilation and hypertrophy (Algorithm 32.6). The risk of developing AF and dysrhythmia-induced thrombi is high. As mitral stenosis progresses, symptoms of decreased cardiac output occur, especially during exertion. Continued elevation of left atrial pressure and volume causes pressure to rise in the pulmonary circulation leading to pulmonary hypertension, pulmonary edema, and right ventricular failure.

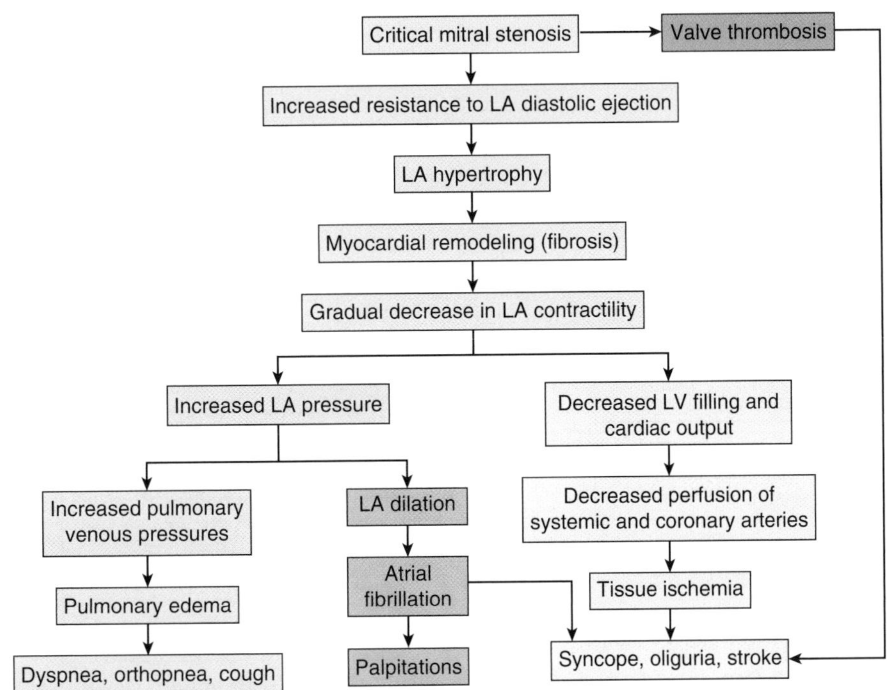

Algorithm 32.6 Pathophysiology of Mitral Stenosis. *LA*, Left atrium; *LV*, Left ventricle.

Blood flow through the stenotic valve results in a rumbling decrescendo diastolic murmur heard best over the cardiac apex and radiating to the left axilla. If the mitral valve is forced open during diastole, it may make a sharp noise called an opening snap. The first heart sound (S_1) is often accentuated and somewhat delayed because of increased left atrial pressure. Other signs and symptoms are generally those of pulmonary congestion and right heart failure. Atrial enlargement and valvular obstruction are demonstrated by chest x-ray films, electrocardiography, and echocardiography. Management includes use of anticoagulation therapy and control of heart rate. Mitral stenosis can often be repaired with clipping leaflets and opening the valve orifice (commissurotomy), or percutaneous balloon commissurotomy, but may require surgical valve replacement in advanced cases.[115,120] While untreated severe calcific mitral stenosis is associated with significant mortality in older adults, surgical or percutaneous interventions are associated with a high risk for procedural complications.[115,121]

Aortic regurgitation. Aortic regurgitation results from an inability of the aortic valve leaflets to close properly during diastole because of abnormalities of the leaflets, the aortic root and annulus, or both. It can be primary, caused by congenital bicuspid valve or degeneration in older adults; or secondary, resulting from chronic hypertension, rheumatic heart disease, bacterial endocarditis, syphilis, connective tissue disorders (e.g., Marfan syndrome and ankylosing spondylitis), appetite-suppressing medications, trauma, valvular surgery, or atherosclerosis. Myxomatous degeneration of the valve causing distortion of the valve leaflets occurs most often in those with hypertension.[122]

During systole, blood is ejected from the left ventricle into the aorta. During diastole, some of the ejected blood flows back into the left ventricle through the leaking valve (Algorithm 32.7). Volume overload occurs in the ventricle because it receives blood from the left atrium and from the aorta during diastole. As the end-diastolic volume of the left ventricle increases, myocardial fibers stretch to accommodate the extra fluid. Compensatory dilation permits the left ventricle to increase its stroke volume and maintain cardiac output. Ventricular hypertrophy also occurs as an adaptation to the increased volume and because of increased afterload created by the high stroke volume and resultant systolic hypertension. Over time, ventricular dilation and hypertrophy eventually cannot compensate for aortic incompetence, and heart failure develops.[122]

Clinical manifestations include widened pulse pressure resulting from increased stroke volume and diastolic backflow. Turbulence across the aortic valve during diastole produces a decrescendo murmur in the second, third, or fourth intercostal spaces parasternally and may radiate to the neck. Large stroke volume and rapid runoff of blood from the aorta cause prominent carotid pulsations and bounding peripheral pulses (Corrigan pulse). Other symptoms are usually associated with heart failure that occurs when the ventricle can no longer pump adequately. Dysrhythmias are a common complication of aortic regurgitation. The severity of regurgitation can be estimated by echocardiography, and valve replacement surgery may be delayed for many years through careful use of vasodilators such as ACE inhibitors and beta blockers.[115,122]

Mitral regurgitation. Mitral regurgitation can be primary (degenerative) because of mitral valve prolapse (MVP), rheumatic heart disease, infective endocarditis, MI, connective tissue diseases (Marfan syndrome), and dilated cardiomyopathy. It also can be secondary (functional) because of ischemic or nonischemic myocardial disease, which damages the chordae tendineae or the mitral annulus. Mitral regurgitation permits

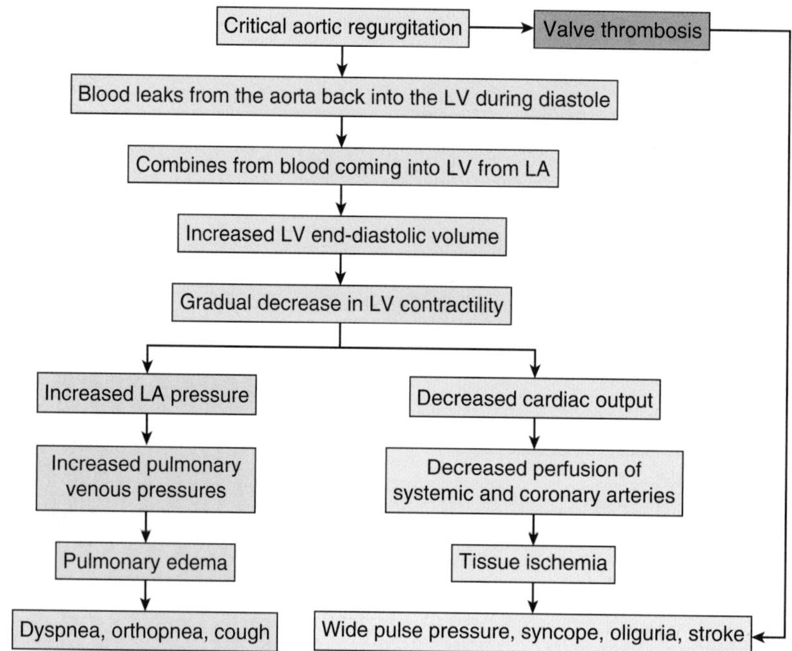

Algorithm 32.7 Pathophysiology of Aortic Regurgitation. *LA*, Left atrium; *LV*, Left ventricle.

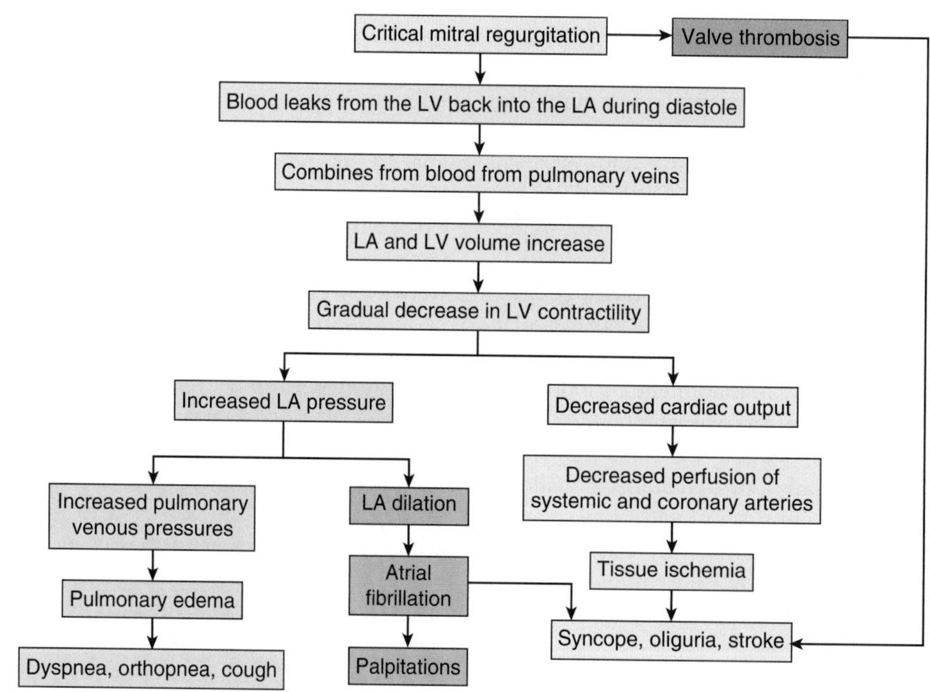

Algorithm 32.8 Pathophysiology of Mitral Regurgitation. *A*, Left atrium; *LV*, Left ventricle.

backflow of blood from the left ventricle into the left atrium during ventricular systole (Algorithm 32.8). The left atrium and ventricle become dilated and hypertrophied to maintain adequate cardiac output. As the left atrium enlarges, stretching of the atrial myocardium often leads to AF. As mitral valve regurgitation progresses, left ventricular function may become impaired to the point of failure. Eventually, increased atrial pressure leads to pulmonary hypertension and failure of the right ventricle. Most clinical manifestations are caused by heart failure. A characteristic holosystolic (throughout systole) murmur, heard best at the apex and that radiates into the back and axilla, suggests the underlying valvular abnormality, which is then confirmed by echocardiography. Mitral incompetence is usually well tolerated—often for years—until heart failure occurs, at which time transcatheter or surgical repair becomes necessary. Mitral valve replacement for chronic mitral regurgitation should not be performed unless mitral valve repair has been attempted and was unsuccessful.[115] In acute mitral regurgitation caused by MI, surgical repair must be done emergently.

Tricuspid regurgitation. Tricuspid regurgitation is a prevalent valvular disorder and is more common than tricuspid stenosis. Primary tricuspid regurgitation can be caused by congenital defects, rheumatic heart disease, endocarditis, or trauma. However, most cases of tricuspid regurgitation in adults are the result of annular dilatation related to chronic heart failure with pulmonary hypertension and dilation of the right ventricle, which pulls the valve leaflets apart.[123] Tricuspid valve incompetence leads to volume overload in the right atrium and ventricle, increased systemic venous blood pressure, and right heart failure. Management includes guideline-directed medical treatment for heart failure.[115] Some individuals require surgery, but operative mortality can be high, and new transcatheter approaches are emerging.[114,123] Pulmonic valve dysfunction can have the same consequences as tricuspid valve dysfunction.

Mitral Valve Prolapse Syndrome. In mitral valve prolapse syndrome (MVPS), one or both of the cusps of the mitral valve billow upward (prolapse) into the left atrium during systole (Fig. 32.21). MVP is the most common valve disorder in the United States, with a prevalence of nearly 3% of adults. MVP can be associated with inherited connective tissue disorders (Marfan syndrome, Ehlers-Danlos syndrome, osteogenesis imperfecta), suggesting that it results from a genetic or environmental disruption of valvular development during the fifth or sixth week of gestation. There also may be a relationship between symptomatic MVP and hyperthyroidism.

The most common cause of MVP is myxomatous degeneration of the leaflets. Valve leaflets undergoing abnormal biomechanics undergo degeneration of valve structure and tissue proliferation on the atrial side of the mitral leaflets contributing to prolapse.[114] Cusps become redundant, thickened, and scalloped because of changes in tissue proteoglycans, increased levels of proteinases, and infiltration by myofibroblasts.[124] MVP is the most common cause of mitral regurgitation which occurs if the ballooning valve permits blood to leak into the atrium.

Many cases of MVP are completely asymptomatic. Cardiac auscultation on routine physical examination may disclose a regurgitant murmur or midsystolic click, or echocardiography may demonstrate the condition in the absence of auscultatory findings. Symptomatic MVPs can cause palpitations, tachycardia, atypical chest pain, lightheadedness, syncope, fatigue, weakness, dyspnea, chest tightness, anxiety, depression, and panic attacks. Many symptoms are vague and puzzling and are unrelated to the degree of prolapse. Most individuals with MVP have an excellent prognosis, do not develop symptoms, and do not require any restriction in activity or medical management. Occasionally, β-blockers are needed to alleviate syncope, severe chest pain, or palpitations. If MVP is complicated by mitral regurgitation, it has a 10-year mortality of 19% and mitral valve prolapse-related events (stroke, heart failure, endocarditis, and mitral valve surgery) occur in 20% of individuals by 10 years.[125]

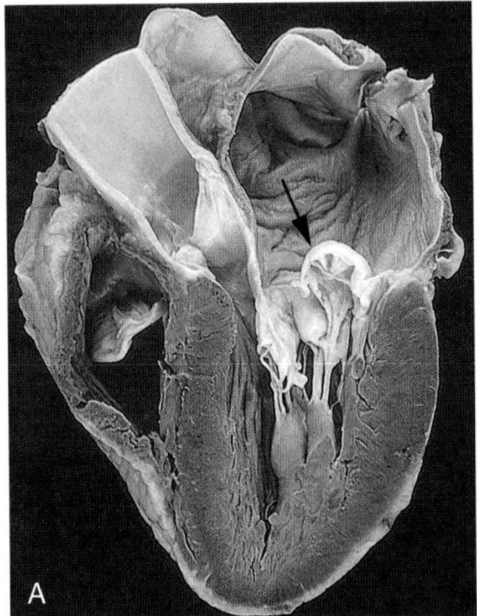

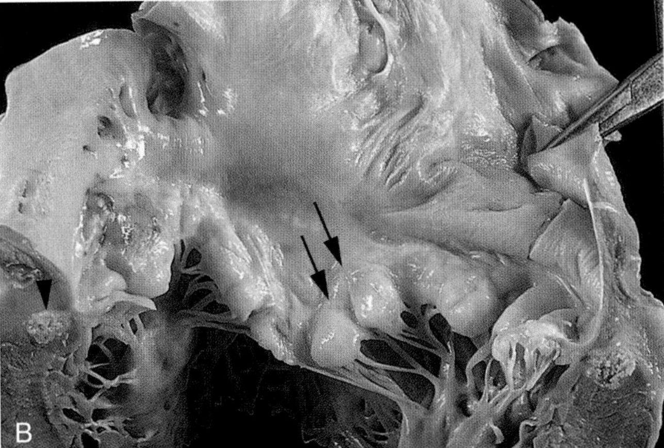

Fig. 32.21 Mitral Valve Prolapse (MVP). (A) Prolapsed mitral valve. Prolapse permits the valve leaflets to billow back *(arrow)* into the atrium during left ventricular systole. The billowing causes the leaflets to part slightly, permitting regurgitation into the atrium. **(B)** Looking down into the mitral valve, the ballooning *(arrows)* of the leaflets is seen. (Used with permission of Mayo Foundation for Medical Education and Research. All rights reserved.)

Acute Rheumatic Fever and Rheumatic Heart Disease

Acute rheumatic fever (ARF) is a systemic inflammatory disease caused by a delayed exaggerated immune response to infection by the group A β-hemolytic streptococcus. In its acute form, rheumatic fever is a febrile illness characterized by inflammation of the joints, skin, nervous system, and heart. Although decreasing in incidence in the United States, ARF is the cause of rheumatic heart disease (RHD) later in life, which affects 40 million people worldwide.[126] Acute rheumatic fever occurs most often in children between the ages of 5 and 15 years, whereas RHD is usually diagnosed in adults.

Pathophysiology. ARF can develop only as a complication of pharyngeal infection by group A β-hemolytic streptococcus. Streptococcal skin infections do not progress to acute rheumatic fever because the strains of the microorganism that affect the skin do not have the same antigenic molecules in their cell membranes and do not elicit the same kind of immune response. Acute rheumatic fever is the result of an abnormal humoral and cell-mediated immune response to group A streptococcal cell membrane antigens called M proteins (Fig. 32.22). This immune response cross-reacts with molecularly similar

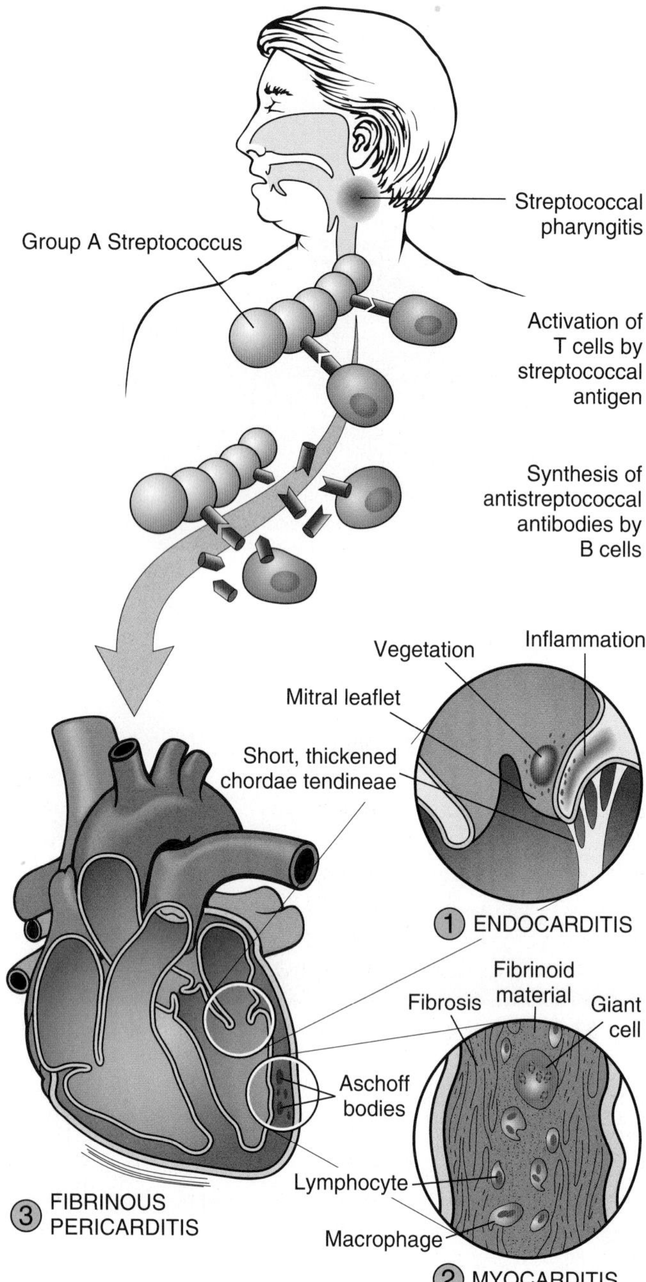

Fig. 32.22 Pathogenesis and Structural Alterations of Acute Rheumatic Heart Disease. Beginning usually with a sore throat, rheumatic fever can develop only as a sequel to pharyngeal infection by group A β-hemolytic streptococcus. Suspected as a hypersensitivity reaction, it is proposed that antibodies directed against the M proteins of certain strains of streptococci cross-react with tissue glycoproteins in the heart, joints, and other tissues. The exact nature of cross-reacting antigens has been difficult to define, but it appears that the streptococcal infection causes an autoimmune response against self-antigens. Inflammatory lesions are found in various sites; the most distinctive within the heart are called Aschoff bodies. The chronic sequelae result from progressive fibrosis because of healing of the inflammatory lesions and the changes induced by valvular deformities. (From Damjanov I. *Pathology for the health professions*, 4th edition. Philadelphia: Saunders; 2012.)

self-antigens in the heart, muscle, brain, and joints (molecular mimicry), causing an autoimmune response that results in diffuse, proliferative, and exudative inflammatory lesions in these tissues.[127] The inflammation may subside before treatment, leaving behind damage to the heart valves. Repeated attacks of acute rheumatic fever cause chronic proliferative changes with resultant tissue scarring, granuloma formation, and thrombosis.

Approximately 10% of individuals with rheumatic fever develop RHD, usually between the ages of 25 and 34. Valvulitis during clinical or subclinical ARF transitions to chronic valvular lesions that evolve over years.[128] The primary lesion in RHD involves the endocardium. Endocardial inflammation causes swelling of the valve leaflets, with secondary erosion along the lines of leaflet contact. Small, bead-like clumps of vegetation containing platelets and fibrin are deposited on eroded valvular tissue and on the chordae tendineae cordis. These lesions can become progressively adherent, and the leaflets may adhere to each other. Scarring and shortening of the involved structures occur over time.

If inflammation penetrates the myocardium (myocarditis), localized fibrin deposits develop that are surrounded by areas of necrosis. These fibrinoid necrotic deposits are called Aschoff bodies. Pericarditis also can occur, characterized by serofibrinous effusion within the pericardial cavity. Cardiomegaly and left heart failure may occur during episodes of untreated acute or recurrent rheumatic fever. Conduction defects and AF often are associated with rheumatic heart disease.

Clinical Manifestations. The common symptoms of acute rheumatic fever are fever, lymphadenopathy, arthralgia, nausea, vomiting, epistaxis (nosebleed), abdominal pain, and tachycardia. The major clinical manifestations of acute rheumatic fever usually occur singly or in combination 1 to 5 weeks after streptococcal infection of the pharynx. They are (1) carditis: murmur, chest pain, pericardial friction rub, ECG changes, valvular dysfunction; (2) polyarthritis: heat, redness, swelling, and pain that migrate among the large joints of the extremities; (3) chorea: sudden, aimless, irregular, involuntary movements; (4) erythema marginatum: nonpruritic, erythematous macules on the trunk that may fade in the center; and (5) subcutaneous nodules: palpable nodules over bony prominences and extensor tendons.

Evaluation and Treatment. Diagnosis of ARF is based on the Jones Criteria which combine symptoms and signs with laboratory evidence of systemic inflammation (elevated C-reactive protein or erythrocyte sedimentation rate). Echocardiography should be performed on anyone suspected of ARF to determine if subclinical carditis is present.[129] Supportive evidence for the diagnosis of rheumatic fever includes positive throat cultures and measurement of serum antibodies against the hemolytic factor streptolysin O. Several other antibody tests also are available.

Appropriate antibiotic therapy given within the first 9 days of group A β-hemolytic streptococcus infection usually prevents rheumatic fever.[128] Therapy for acute rheumatic fever is aimed at eradicating the streptococcal infection and involves a 10-day regimen of antibiotics. NSAIDs are used as antiinflammatory agents for both carditis and arthritis. Serious carditis may require corticosteroids and diuretics. Because recurrent rheumatic fever occurs in more than half of affected children, continuous prophylactic antibiotic therapy may be necessary for as long as 5 years. RHD may require surgical repair of damaged valves.

Infective Endocarditis

Infective endocarditis is a general term used to describe infection and inflammation of the endocardium—especially the cardiac valves. Over 80% of cases are caused by bacteria, especially streptococci, staphylococci, and enterococci. Other causes include viruses, fungi, rickettsia, and parasites (see *Risk Factors:* Infective Endocarditis).

RISK FACTORS

Infective Endocarditis

- Acquired valvular heart disease
- Implantation of prosthetic heart valves
- Congenital lesions associated with highly turbulent flow (e.g., ventricular septal defect)
- Previous attack of infective endocarditis
- Intravenous drug use
- Long-term indwelling intravenous catheterization (e.g., for pressure monitoring, feeding, hemodialysis)
- Implantable cardiac pacemakers
- Heart transplant with defective valve

Pathophysiology. The pathogenesis of infective endocarditis requires at least three critical elements:

1. *Endocardial damage.* Trauma, congenital heart disease, valvular heart disease, and the presence of prosthetic valves are the most common risk factors for endocardial damage that leads to infective endocarditis. Turbulent blood flow caused by these abnormalities usually affects the atrial surface of atrioventricular valves or the ventricular surface of semilunar valves. Endocardial damage exposes the endothelial basement membrane, which contains a type of collagen that attracts platelets and thereby stimulates sterile thrombus formation on the membrane. This causes an inflammatory reaction (nonbacterial thrombotic endocarditis).
2. *Adherence of blood-borne microorganisms to the damaged endocardial surface.* Bacteria may enter the bloodstream during injection drug use, trauma, dental procedures that involve manipulation of the gingiva, cardiac surgery, genitourinary procedures and indwelling catheters in the presence of infection, or gastrointestinal instrumentation, or they may spread from uncomplicated upper respiratory tract or skin infections. Bacteria adhere to the damaged endocardium using adhesins.
3. *Formation of infective endocardial vegetations* (Fig. 32.23). Bacteria infiltrate the sterile thrombi and accelerate fibrin formation by activating the clotting cascade. These vegetative lesions can form anywhere on the endocardium but usually occur on heart valves and surrounding structures. Although endocardial tissue is constantly bathed in antibody-containing blood and is surrounded by scavenging monocytes and polymorphonuclear leukocytes, bacterial colonies are inaccessible to host defenses because they are embedded in the protective fibrin clots and biofilms. This also makes them difficult to treat with antibiotics. Embolization from these vegetations can lead to abscesses and characteristic skin changes, such as petechiae, splinter hemorrhages, Osler nodes, and Janeway lesions.

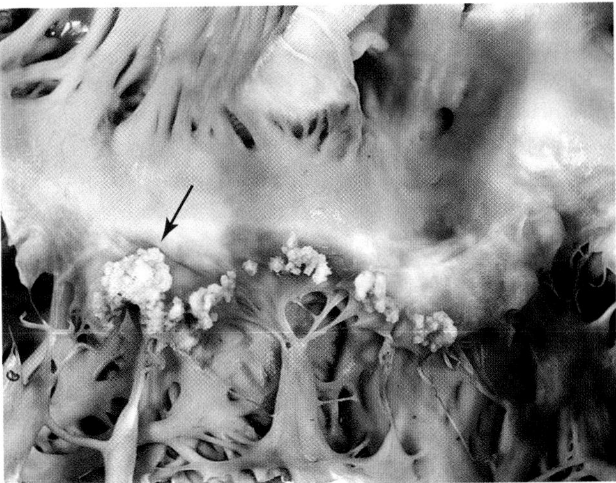

Fig. 32.23 Bacterial Endocarditis of Mitral Valve. The valve is covered with large, irregular vegetations *(arrow).* (From Damjanov I, Linder J. *Pathology: A color atlas.* St. Louis: Mosby; 2000.)

Clinical Manifestations. Infective endocarditis causes varying degrees of valvular dysfunction and may be associated with manifestations involving several organ systems, making diagnosis difficult. Signs and symptoms of infective endocarditis are caused by infection and inflammation, systemic spread of microemboli, and immune complex deposition. Microemboli can spread to splenic, renal, pulmonary, peripheral arterial, coronary, bone, CNS, and ocular circulations. The classic findings are fever; new or changed cardiac murmur; and petechial lesions of the skin, conjunctiva, and oral mucosa. Characteristic physical findings include Osler nodes (painful erythematous nodules on the pads of the fingers and toes) and Janeway lesions (nonpainful hemorrhagic lesions on the palms and soles). CNS complications are the most severe extracardiac complications and include stroke, abscess, and meningitis. Other manifestations include weight loss, back pain, night sweats, and heart failure.

Evaluation and Treatment. The Modified Duke criteria for the diagnosis of infective endocarditis include blood cultures positive for bacteria, evidence for endocardial involvement (by echocardiogram or by recognition of a new valvular regurgitation murmur), recognized risk factors, fever, vascular complications, and immunologic phenomena (e.g., Osler nodes).[115] Positron emission tomography (PET) may be required.[130] Serum C-reactive protein is elevated. Antimicrobial therapy is generally given for several weeks, beginning with intravenous and ending with oral administration.[115] Other drugs may be necessary to treat left heart failure secondary to valvular dysfunction. Surgery that involves excision of infected tissue with or without valve replacement may be needed for refractory infections, especially in those individuals who develop acute heart failure, highly resistant infections, or abscesses and emboli.[115,131] Persistent or relapsing infection requires the removal of implanted cardiac devices such as pacemakers, defibrillator systems, and prosthetic valves.[115]

Guidelines for the use of antibiotic prophylaxis before dental procedures to prevent infective endocarditis were updated in 2017.[132] Indications include prosthetic valves (including transcatheter-implanted grafts), prosthetic material used for cardiac valve repair, a history of infective endocarditis, unrepaired cyanotic congenital heart disease, and heart transplant with valvular defect.

MANIFESTATIONS OF HEART DISEASE

Heart Failure

In 2021, the first universal definition and classification of heart failure was published: "Heart failure is a clinical syndrome with symptoms and/or signs caused by a structural and/or functional cardiac abnormality and corroborated by elevated natriuretic peptide levels and/or objective evidence of pulmonary or systemic congestion."[133] Heart failure occurs when the heart is unable to generate an adequate cardiac output, causing inadequate perfusion of tissues, or when there is increased diastolic filling pressure of the left ventricle, or both, so that pulmonary capillary pressures are increased.

An estimated 6 million Americans over the age of 20 have heart failure, and the prevalence of heart failure has been predicted to increase by 46% by 2030. Heart failure results in 800,000 hospital admissions and 83,000 deaths per year in the United States.[12] Ischemic heart disease and hypertension are the most important predisposing risk factors. Another important risk factor is diabetes which has multiple effects on the myocardium (see Emerging Science Box: Diabetes and Heart Failure). Other risk factors include age, obesity, renal failure, valvular heart disease, cardiomyopathies, myocarditis, congenital heart disease, and excessive alcohol use. Numerous genetic polymorphisms have been linked to an increased risk for heart failure, including genes for cardiomyopathies, myocyte contractility, and neurohumoral receptors. Most heart failure results from dysfunction of the left ventricle (heart failure with reduced EF and heart failure with preserved EF). The right ventricle also may be dysfunctional, especially in pulmonary disease (right ventricular failure). Finally, some conditions cause inadequate perfusion despite normal or elevated cardiac output (high-output failure).

Left Heart Failure (Congestive Heart Failure)

Left heart failure is categorized as heart failure with reduced EF (systolic heart failure) or heart failure with preserved EF (diastolic heart failure). It is possible for these two types of heart failure to occur simultaneously in one individual.

Heart failure with reduced ejection fraction. Heart failure with reduced ejection fraction (HFrEF), or systolic heart failure, is defined as heart failure with an ejection fraction of ≤40% and an inability of the heart to generate an adequate cardiac output to perfuse vital tissues. An ejection fraction (EF) of ≤40% means that 40% or less of the total amount of blood in the left ventricle at the end of diastole is pushed out with each systolic contraction (normal EF is 55% to 70%). This definition of HFrEF was affirmed in 2021, and two additional categories of HFrEF were proposed: (1) heart failure with mildly reduced EF (HFmrEF), which is defined as HF with an EF of 41% to 49%, and (2) heart failure with improved EF (HFimpEF) defined as a baseline EF of ≤40%, a ≥10-point increase from baseline EF, and a second measurement of EF > 40%.[133]

Cardiac output depends on the heart rate and stroke volume. Stroke volume is estimated by measuring the EF and is influenced by three major determinants: (1) contractility, (2) preload, and (3) afterload (see Chapter 31). Contractility is reduced by diseases that disrupt myocyte activity. MI is the most common primary cause of decreased contractility. Other primary

EMERGING SCIENCE BOX

Diabetes and Heart Failure

The prevalence of diabetes in individuals with heart failure ranges from 25% to 40%, and two thirds of those with metabolic syndrome will eventually develop HFrEF. In addition to being a risk factor for dyslipidemia, coronary artery disease, and hypertension, diabetes has direct toxicity to the myocardium (diabetic cardiomyopathy). Myocytes are impacted by insulin resistance resulting in decreased efficacy of intracellular calcium efflux and decreased contractility. The deposition of damaging by-products of insulin resistance (advanced glycation end products [AGEs]) contributes to hypertrophic and fibrotic remodeling of the myocardium. In addition to structural changes, insulin resistance in type 2 diabetes leads to impairment of ATP production, which shifts myocyte metabolism toward fatty acid oxidation. In the failing heart, increased demand for oxygen and energy is coupled with a decreased ability to use fatty acids as an energy source and lipids are deposited into the myocardium causing lipotoxicity. Diabetes also contributes to autonomic dysfunction and inflammation in the heart, further compromising myocyte function. In addition to blocking renal reabsorption of glucose, the sodium-glucose cotransporter 2 (SLGT2) inhibitors increase renal sodium excretion and target many of the inflammatory, fibrotic, and neurohumoral mechanisms implicated in diabetes and heart failure. Clinical studies demonstrate improved cardiovascular outcomes for individuals with diabetes who are treated with these medications, and they are likely to become first-line medications for the treatment of diabetes and heart failure.

Data from Braunwald E. Diabetes, heart failure, and renal dysfunction: the vicious circles. *Progress in Cardiovascular Diseases*, 2019;62(4):298–302; Chen S, et al. Impact of glycemic control on the association of endothelial dysfunction and coronary artery disease in patients with type 2 diabetes mellitus. *Cardiovascular Diabetology*, 2021;20:64; Ding X, et al. Triglyceride–glucose index and the incidence of atherosclerotic cardiovascular diseases: a meta-analysis of cohort studies. *Cardiovascular Diabetology*, 2021;20:76; Dunlay SM, et al. Type 2 diabetes mellitus and heart failure: A scientific statement from the American Heart Association and the Heart Failure Society of America: This statement does not represent an update of the 2017 ACC/AHA/HFSA heart failure guideline update. *Circulation*, 2019;140(7):e294–e324; Ghosh RK, et al. Sodium glucose co-transporter 2 inhibitors and heart failure. *American Journal of Cardiology*, 2019;124(11):1790–1796; Murtaza G, et al. Diabetic cardiomyopathy—A comprehensive updated review. *Progress in Cardiovascular Disease*, 2019;62(4):315–326; Sposito AC, et al. Dapagliflozin effect on endothelial dysfunction in diabetic patients with atherosclerotic disease: A randomized active-controlled trial. *Cardiovascular Diabetology*, 2021;20:74; Vardeny O. The sweet spot: Heart failure prevention with SGLT2 inhibitors. *American Journal of Medicine*, 2020;133(2):182–185; Wilkinson MJ, et al. Heart failure and diabetes mellitus: Defining the problem and exploring the interrelationship. *American Journal of Cardiology*, 2019;124(Suppl. 1):S3–S11.

causes include myocarditis and cardiomyopathies, especially dilated cardiomyopathy and hypertensive hypertrophic cardiomyopathy. Myocardial ischemia and increased myocardial workload contribute to inflammatory, immune, and neurohumoral changes (activation of the SNS and RAAS) that mediate a process called ventricular remodeling. Ventricular remodeling results in disruption of the normal myocardial extracellular structure and causes progressive myocyte contractile dysfunction over time (Fig. 32.24). When contractility is decreased, stroke volume falls and left ventricular end-diastolic volume (LVEDV) increases. This causes dilation of the heart and an increase in preload.

Preload, or LVEDV, increases with decreased contractility or an excess of plasma volume (intravenous fluid administration, renal failure, mitral valvular disease). Increases in LVEDV stretch the heart and can actually improve cardiac output up to a certain point, but as preload continues to rise, dilation of the myocardium eventually leads to dysfunction of the sarcomeres and decreased contractility. This relationship is described by the Frank-Starling law of the heart (see Fig. 31.15). Dilation of the heart also stretches the coronary arteries causing them to narrow, diminishing blood flow to the myocardium and further compromising contractility. Decreased contractility means less blood is ejected from the heart and therefore leads to further increases in preload.

Increased afterload is most commonly a result of increased PVR seen with hypertension. Although much less common, it also can be the result of aortic valvular disease. With increased afterload, there is resistance to ventricular emptying and more workload for the ventricle (Algorithm 32.9). Sustained afterload is associated with high levels of Ang II and catecholamines leading to remodeling and eventual hypertensive hypertrophic cardiomyopathy. This results in an increase in oxygen demand by the thickened myocardium. A state of relative ischemia develops

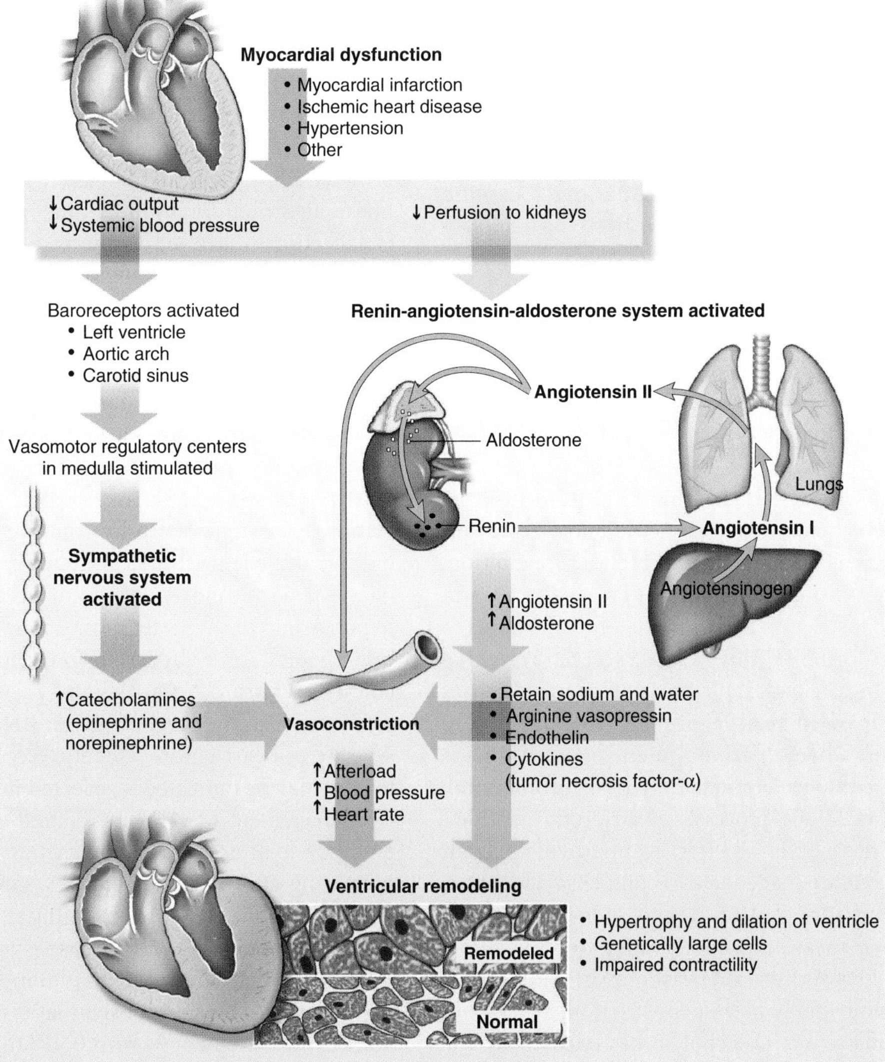

Fig. 32.24 Pathophysiology of Ventricular Remodeling. Myocardial dysfunction activates the renin-angiotensin-aldosterone and sympathetic nervous systems, releasing neurohormones (angiotensin II, aldosterone, catecholamines, and cytokines). These neurohormones contribute to ventricular remodeling. (Redrawn from Carelock J, Clark AP. Heart failure: Pathophysiologic mechanisms. *American Journal of Nursing*, 2001;101(12):27.)

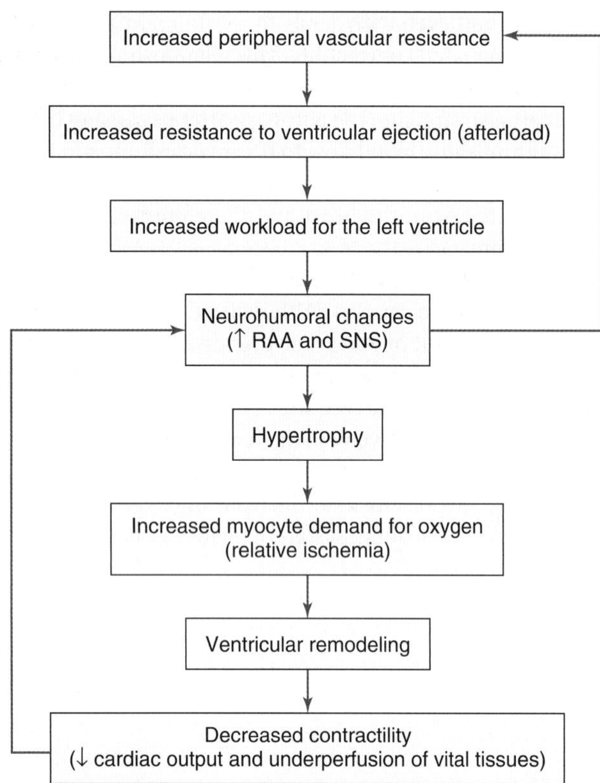

Algorithm 32.9 Role of Increased Afterload in the Pathogenesis of Heart Failure. *RAA*, Renin-angiotensin-aldosterone; *SNS*, sympathetic nervous system.

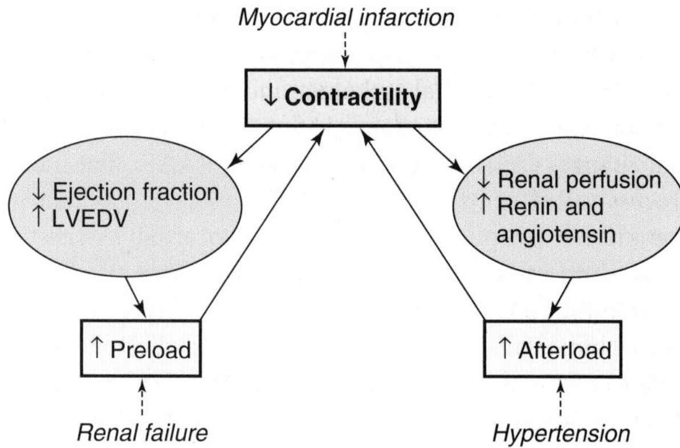

Fig. 32.25 Vicious Cycle of Heart Failure With Reduced Ejection Fraction. Although the initial insult may be one of primary decreased contractility (e.g., myocardial infarction), increased preload (e.g., renal failure), or increased afterload (e.g., hypertension), all three factors play a role in the progression of left heart failure. *LVEDV,* Left ventricular end-diastolic volume.

that contributes to alteration of the cardiac extracellular matrix which can disrupt the integrity of the muscle, decrease contractility, and increase the likelihood that the ventricle will dilate and fail.[134]

As cardiac output falls, renal perfusion diminishes and the RAAS is activated, which acts to increase PVR and plasma volume, thus further increasing afterload and preload. In addition, baroreceptors in the central circulation stimulate the SNS to cause yet more vasoconstriction and cause the hypothalamus to produce antidiuretic hormone. This vicious cycle of decreasing contractility, increasing preload, and increasing afterload causes progressive worsening of left heart failure (Fig. 32.25).

In addition to these hemodynamic interactions, HFrEF is characterized by a complex constellation of neurohumoral, inflammatory, and metabolic processes. Natriuretic peptides, especially BNP, are released in an effort to improve renal salt and water excretion but are inadequate to compensate for these neurohumoral perturbations. Ang II and aldosterone have direct toxicity to the myocardium, contributing to remodeling, myocyte death, and fibrosis. Arginine vasopressin (antidiuretic hormone [ADH]) contributes to vasoconstriction, renal fluid retention, and hyponatremia. Catecholamines released by the SNS are toxic to the myocardium and contribute to remodeling. Insulin resistance and diabetes not only contribute to heart failure but also are a complication of heart failure with changes in myocyte metabolism. Inflammatory cytokines, such as TNF-α, are released in heart failure, contributing to myocardial damage as well as systemic weight loss (cardiac cachexia). Finally, changes in the metabolic processes within the myocardium also are affected, with a decreased ability of the heart to produce energy and an increase in release of toxic metabolites. These neurohumoral, inflammatory, and metabolic aspects of left HFrEF have led to the routine use of combinations of medications that inhibit angiotensin, aldosterone, and catecholamines, and increase salt excretion in an effort to prevent long-term damage to the myocardium, as well as the exploration of new treatment modalities focused on reducing inflammation and improving myocardial metabolic function.

The clinical manifestations of left heart failure are the result of pulmonary vascular congestion and inadequate perfusion of the systemic circulation. Individuals experience dyspnea, orthopnea, cough of frothy sputum, fatigue, decreased urine output, and edema. Physical examination often reveals pulmonary edema (cyanosis, inspiratory crackles, pleural effusions), hypotension or hypertension, an S_3 gallop, and evidence of underlying CAD or hypertension. The diagnosis can be further confirmed with echocardiography showing decreased EF and cardiomegaly. The level of serum BNP is used to estimate the severity of heart failure. Genetic screening for underlying risk factors may be indicated in selected individuals.

Management of HFrEF is aimed at interrupting the worsening cycle of decreasing contractility, increasing preload, and increasing afterload. Current U.S. guidelines for management are based on the ACC/AHA staging system which uses risk, evidence of structural heart disease, symptoms, and response to treatment to guide therapeutic interventions.[135,136] A new staging system has been proposed that is very similar but adds biomarker measurement (serum BNP) to its criteria.[133]

The acute onset of left heart failure is most often the result of acute myocardial ischemia and must be managed in conjunction with management of the underlying coronary disease. Oxygen, nitrate, and morphine administration improves myocardial oxygenation and helps relieve coronary spasm while lowering preload through systemic venodilation. Inotropic drugs, such as dopamine, dobutamine, and milrinone, increase contractility and can help raise the blood pressure in hypotensive individuals. Diuretics reduce preload. ACE inhibitors, ARBs, and aldosterone blockers reduce both preload and afterload by decreasing aldosterone levels and reducing PVR. Finally, individuals with severe HFrEF failure may benefit from acute coronary bypass or PCI. These people often are supported with the intra-aortic balloon pump (IABP) or left ventricular assist devices (LVADs) until surgery can be performed.[135]

Management of chronic left heart failure is based on current guidelines and clinical severity.[135,136] The overall goals are to reduce preload and afterload. Loop diuretics are effective in reducing preload. A combination of ACE inhibitors and aldosterone blockers are indicated, along with β-blockers.[135–137] In 2021, interim heart failure guidance issued by the American College of Cardiology added angiotensin receptor-neprilysin inhibitors (sacubitril/valsartan) and sodium-glucose cotransporter-2 (SGLT2) inhibitors (dapagliflozin, empagliflozin) to treatment algorithms for new-onset and chronic heart failure.[138] SGLT2 inhibitors have been shown to offer a significant reduction in mortality and heart failure hospitalizations, and improvement of quality of life when added to current standard drugs.[139] Inotropic drugs are used for those with refractory symptoms or to control atrial dysrhythmias. Recently, the selective myosin activator omecamtiv mecarbil was shown to improve cardiac function in individuals with HRrEF.[140] Additional interventions, such as implantable cardioverter-defibrillators, cardiac resynchronization, and LVADs, may be indicated in selected individuals.[135,136] For those individuals with CAD, coronary bypass surgery or PCI may improve perfusion to ischemic myocardium (hibernating myocardium) and improve cardiac output. Surgical interventions that improve ventricular geometry or heart transplantation may need to be considered.[141] Experimental therapies, including gene and stem cell therapies, are being explored.[142,143] Those with severe heart failure unresponsive to treatment and ineligible for transplantation should receive palliative care.

Heart failure with preserved ejection function. Heart failure with preserved ejection function (HFpEF) is a clinical syndrome in which individuals have symptoms and signs of HF with a left ventricular ejection fraction ≥50%.[135,136] It is associated with decreased compliance of the left ventricle. This results in the inability of the heart to achieve a normal cardiac output without the requirement for elevated cardiac filling pressures due to decreased diastolic relaxation. It is the cause of over half of all cases of left heart failure, affecting >70% of individuals with HF over the age of 65.[144,145] The major risk factors for HFpEF include hypertension, aging, obesity, diabetes, myocardial ischemia, valvular heart disease, atrial fibrillation, pericardial disease, and cardiomyopathies.

In the aging individual with risk factors for HFpEF, numerous pathological changes occur within the endothelium and myocardium of the left ventricle (Algorithm 32.10). In many individuals, a persistent increase in afterload due to hypertension or valvular disease results in hypertrophic remodeling of the left ventricle and deleterious changes to the extracellular matrix.[146] HFpEF is now considered to be a multisystem syndrome involving the heart, lungs, kidneys, skeletal muscle, adipose tissue, blood vessels, and inflammatory/immune activation.[144] Systemic chronic inflammation associated with aging, diabetes, obesity, ischemia, and primary disease of the pericardium and myocardium contributes to cellular damage and collagen deposition with scarring.[144,145,147] Endothelial microvascular and mitochondrial dysfunction compound these effects.[148] As a result, there is decreased compliance

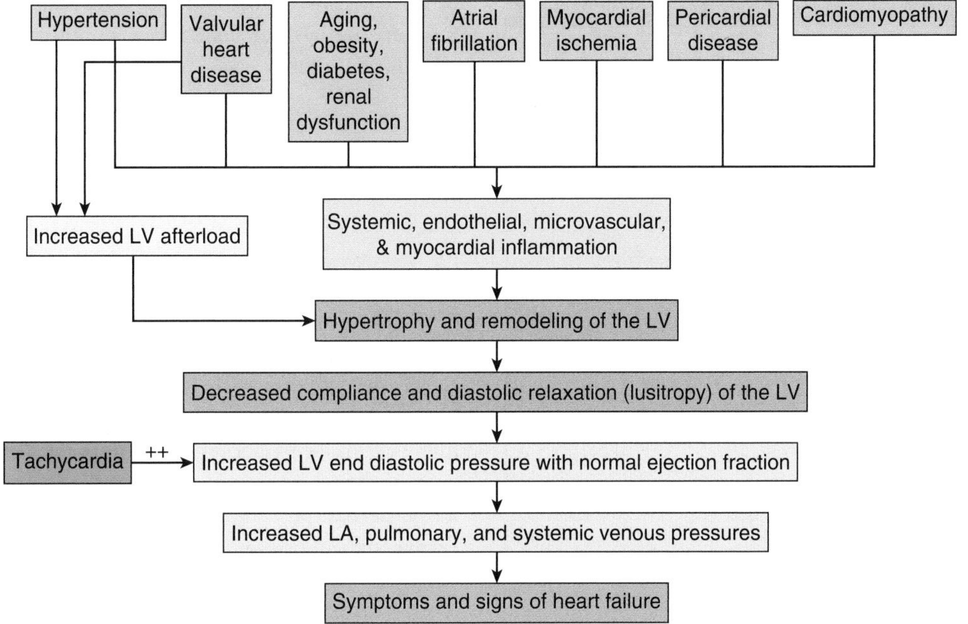

Algorithm 32.10 Pathophysiology of Heart Failure with Preserved Ejection Fraction *LA,* Left atrium; *LV,* Left ventricle.

of the left ventricle and abnormal diastolic relaxation. With decreased compliance and inadequate relaxation, the ventricle lumen is smaller than normal during diastole and cannot accept filling with blood without causing an increase in wall tension. Thus a normal LVEDV results in an increased LVEDP. This pressure is reflected back into the left atrium, pulmonary vessels, and systemic venous circulation. Left atrial hypertrophy, pulmonary hypertension, and right ventricular hypertrophy may develop. If pulmonary pressures are high enough, pulmonary edema occurs. The increase in pressure is made worse by rapid ventricular filling, so symptoms are worse with tachycardia (e.g., with exercise).

Individuals with early HFpEF present with dyspnea on exertion and fatigue. Evidence of pulmonary edema (inspiratory crackles on auscultation, pleural effusions) is usually not present in resting individuals without tachycardia but may develop over time. Late in diastole, atrial contraction with rapid ejection of blood into the noncompliant ventricle may give rise to an S_4 gallop. Other symptoms and signs in advanced disease include paroxysmal nocturnal dyspnea, jugular venous distension, and hepatomegaly. Electrocardiography often reveals evidence of left ventricular hypertrophy, and chest x-ray may show pulmonary congestion without cardiomegaly (Table 32.7). There also may be evidence of underlying coronary disease, hypertension, or valvular disease. Diagnosis is based on three factors: (1) signs and symptoms of heart failure, (2) normal left ventricular EF, and (3) evidence of diastolic dysfunction. The diagnosis is confirmed by clinical Doppler echocardiography, which demonstrates poor ventricular filling with normal EFs. In some individuals, invasive hemodynamic exercise testing may be needed.[149] BNP levels are usually elevated in more severe cases.

TABLE 32.7 Comparison of Heart Failure With Reduced Ejection Fraction (HFrEF) and Heart Failure With Preserved Ejection Fraction (HFpEF)

Characteristic	HFrEF	HFpEF
Sex	Male > female	Female > male
Left ventricular ejection fraction	Decreased	Normal
Left ventricular morphology	Remodeling with dominance of dilation	Remodeling with dominance of hypertrophy
Left ventricular chamber size	Increased	Decreased
Left ventricular end diastolic volume (LVEDV)	Increased	Normal
Left ventricular end diastolic pressure (LVEDP)	Increased	Increased
Chest radiography	Pulmonary congestion with cardiomegaly	Pulmonary congestion without cardiomegaly
Gallop	S_3	S_4

Management approaches for HFpEF are directed toward control of hypervolemia with thiazide or loop diuretics, the use of spironolactone and dual angiotensin-neprilysin inhibitors in selected individuals, exercise training, and management of associated comorbidities.[149] New therapies that target metabolic and immune signaling cascades are being developed.[144] Studies to evaluate the effectiveness of transcatheter interatrial shunts are underway.[150] Outcomes for individuals with HFpEF are as poor as those with HFrEF, and there has been little improvement in prognosis despite numerous new treatment trials.

Right Heart Failure

Right heart failure is defined as the inability of the right ventricle to provide adequate blood flow into the pulmonary circulation at a normal central venous pressure. It can result from left heart failure when an increase in left ventricular filling pressure is reflected back into the pulmonary circulation. As pressure in the pulmonary circulation rises, the resistance to right ventricular emptying increases. The right ventricle is poorly prepared to compensate for this increased afterload and will dilate and fail. When this happens, pressure will rise in the systemic venous circulation, resulting in peripheral edema and hepatosplenomegaly. Treatment relies on management of the left ventricular dysfunction as just outlined.

When right heart failure occurs in the absence of left heart failure, it is typically attributable to diffuse hypoxic pulmonary disease such as chronic obstructive pulmonary disease (COPD), cystic fibrosis, and acute respiratory distress syndrome (ARDS). These disorders result in pulmonary vasoconstriction, pulmonary hypertension, and an increase in right ventricular afterload (Algorithm 32.11). The mechanisms for this type of right ventricular failure (cor pulmonale) are discussed in Chapter 35. Finally, MI, cardiomyopathies, and pulmonic valvular disease interfere with right ventricular contractility and can lead to right heart failure.

High-Output Failure

High-output failure is the inability of the heart to adequately supply the body with blood-borne nutrients, despite adequate blood volume and normal or elevated myocardial contractility. In high-output failure, the heart increases its output, but the body's metabolic needs are still not met. Common causes of high-output failure are anemia, septicemia, hyperthyroidism, and beriberi (Algorithm 32.12).

Anemia decreases the oxygen-carrying capacity of the blood. Metabolic acidosis occurs as the body's cells switch to anaerobic metabolism (see Chapter 3). In response to metabolic acidosis, heart rate and stroke volume increase in an attempt to improve tissue perfusion. If anemia is severe, however, even maximum cardiac output does not supply the cells with enough oxygen for metabolism.

In septicemia, disturbed metabolism, bacterial toxins, and the inflammatory process cause systemic vasodilation and fever. Faced with a lowered systemic vascular resistance (SVR) and an elevated metabolic rate, cardiac output increases to maintain blood pressure and prevent metabolic acidosis. In overwhelming septicemia, however, the heart may not be able to raise its output enough to compensate for vasodilation. Body tissues show signs of inadequate blood supply despite a high cardiac output.

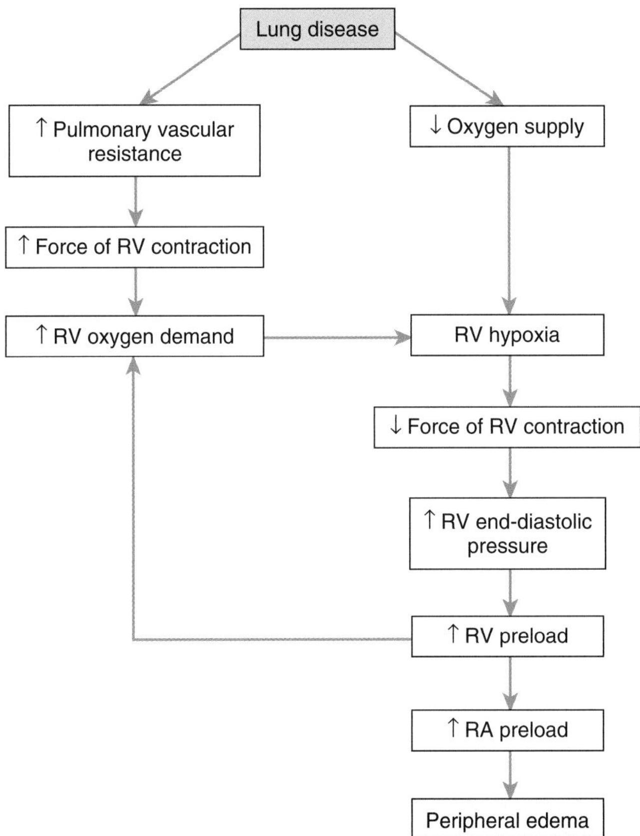

Algorithm 32.11 Right Heart Failure Due to Lung Disease. *RA*, Right atrial; *RV*, right ventricular.

Hyperthyroidism accelerates cellular metabolism through the actions of elevated levels of thyroxine from the thyroid gland. This may occur chronically (thyrotoxicosis) or acutely (thyroid storm). Because the body's increased demand for oxygen threatens to cause metabolic acidosis, cardiac output increases. If blood levels of thyroxine are high and the metabolic response to thyroxine is vigorous, even an abnormally elevated cardiac output may be inadequate.

In the United States, beriberi (thiamine deficiency) usually is caused by malnutrition secondary to chronic alcoholism. Beriberi actually causes a mixed type of heart failure. Thiamine deficiency impairs cellular metabolism in all tissues, including the myocardium. In the heart, impaired cardiac metabolism leads to insufficient contractile strength. In blood vessels, thiamine deficiency leads to peripheral vasodilation, which decreases SVR. Heart failure ensues as decreased SVR triggers increased cardiac output, which the impaired myocardium is unable to deliver. The strain of demands for increased output in the face of impaired metabolism may deplete cardiac reserves until low-output failure begins.

Dysrhythmias

A dysrhythmia, or arrhythmia, is a disturbance of heart rhythm. Normal heart rhythms are generated by the SA node and travel through the heart's conduction system, causing the atrial and ventricular myocardium to contract and relax at a regular rate that is appropriate to maintain circulation at various levels of physical activity (see Chapter 31). There are many types of dysrhythmias that arise from disorders of impulse formation. These include those that are the result from dysfunction of the SA node, or from the development of abnormal electrical activity arising elsewhere in the conduction system or myocardium. Many other dysrhythmias arise from disorders of impulse conduction through the cardiac conducting system or heart tissue. There are multiple causes

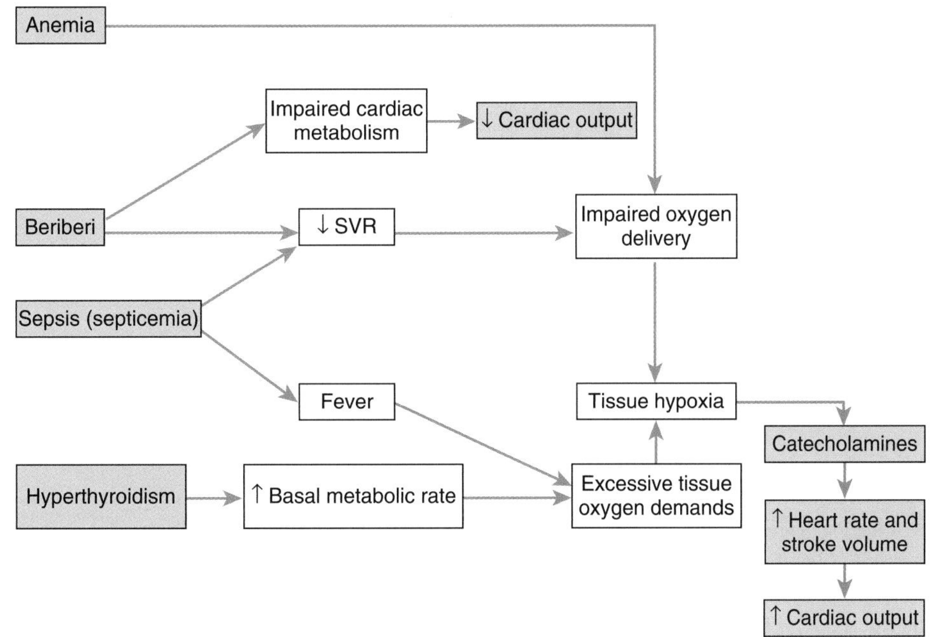

Algorithm 32.12 High-Output Failure. *SVR*, Systemic vascular resistance.

TABLE 32.8 Examples of Common Atrial and Ventricular Dysrhythmias and Cardiac Conduction Disorders

Pathophysiologic Type	Risk Factors	Clinical Manifestations	Acute Management
Atrial Dysrhythmias			
• Premature atrial contractions (PACs), • Atrial tachycardia, • Atrial flutter, • Atrial fibrillation, • Wolf-Parkinson White syndrome	Hypertension, ischemia, cardiomyopathy (e.g., hypertrophy), valvular heart disease, hyperthyroidism, alcohol/drugs, medications, inherited conduction abnormalities	Palpitations, lightheadedness, anxiety, dyspnea, chest pain, syncope, rapid or irregular pulse, hypotension, emboli (e.g., stroke)	Pharmacologic or electrical cardioversion, digoxin, calcium channel blockers, antiarrhythmics, pacemaker, catheter ablation, antithrombotics
Ventricular Dysrhythmias			
• Premature ventricular contractions (PVCs), • Ventricular flutter, • Ventricular tachycardia, • Torsades de pointes, • Ventricular fibrillation	Myocardial infarction, heart failure, electrolyte disorders, hypoxia, medications, hyperthyroidism, cardiomyopathy/myocarditis neuromuscular disorders, congenital heart disease, alcohol/drugs, underlying critical illness	Palpitations, lightheadedness, anxiety, dyspnea, chest pain, syncope, rapid, or irregular or absent pulse, hypotension	Cardioversion, antiarrhythmics, beta blockers, catheter ablation, pacing modalities
Sinus Node Dysfunction and Cardiac Conduction Disorders			
• Sinus node disease, • Atrioventricular block (first, second and third degree), • Atrioventricular disjunction, • Bundle branch block	Medications (e.g., beta blockers, calcium channel blockers, digoxin), myocardial infarction, infection (e.g., Lyme carditis), infiltrative disease (e.g., cardiomyopathy), sleep apnea, hypothyroidism, iatrogenic (e.g., surgery)	Fatigue, lightheadedness, syncope, coma, slow or irregular heart rate, hypotension	Vagolytics, sympathomimetics, theophylline, treatments specific for medication effects (e.g., intravenous calcium for calcium channel blocker toxicity), pacemaker, cardiac resynchronization,

Data from Al-Khatib SM, Stevenson WG, Ackerman MJ, et al. 2017 AHA/ACC/HRS guideline for management of patients with ventricular arrhythmias and the prevention of sudden cardiac death: A report of the American College of Cardiology/American Heart Association Task Force on Clinical Practice Guidelines and the Heart Rhythm Society. *Circulation*, 2018;138:e272–e391; January CT, Wann LS, Alpert JS, et al. 2014 AHA/ACC/HRS guideline for the management of patients with atrial fibrillation: A report of the American College of Cardiology/American Heart Association Task Force on Clinical Practice Guidelines and the Heart Rhythm Society in Collaboration with the Society of Thoracic Surgeons. *Circulation*, 2014;130:e199–e267; January CT, Wann LS, Calkins H, et al. 2019 AHA/ACC/HRS focused update of the 2014 AHA/ACC/HRS guideline for the management of patients with atrial fibrillation: A report of the American College of Cardiology/American Heart Association Task Force on Clinical Practice Guidelines and the Heart Rhythm Society in Collaboration with the Society of Thoracic Surgeons. *Circulation*, 2019;140:e125–e151; Kusumoto FM, Schoenfeld MH, Barrett C, et al. 2018 ACC/AHA/HRS guideline on the evaluation and management of patients with bradycardia and cardiac conduction delay: A report of the American College of Cardiology/American Heart Association Task Force on Clinical Practice Guidelines and the Heart Rhythm Society. *Circulation*, 2019;140:e382–e482.

for disorders affecting conduction through the heart including inherited abnormalities, ischemia, infection, underlying diseases, medications, and iatrogenic injury from surgery or percutaneous interventions. For all arrhythmias, the primary clinical manifestations are the result of changes in the delivery of blood to the vital tissues due to changes in pulse rate, cardiac output, and blood pressure. These changes can range from asymptomatic to life-threatening. Diagnosis begins with documenting characteristic changes in the ECG along with evaluation for underlying causes. Management is aimed at supporting adequate cardiac output with medications or electrical stimulation (cardioversion, pacemaker insertion, cardiac resynchronization techniques) while attempting to reverse the underlying etiology.

While there are many ways to categorize dysrhythmias, national management guidelines focus on three primary areas: atrial dysrhythmias, ventricular dysrhythmias, and sinus node dysfunction and conduction disorders.[151–154] Table 32.8 provides an overview of some of the most common examples of these three types of dysrhythmias.

SUMMARY REVIEW

Diseases of the Veins

1. Varicose veins are veins in which blood has pooled, usually in the saphenous veins of the leg. Varicose veins may be caused by damaged valves as a result of trauma to the valve or by chronic venous distention involving gravity and venous constriction.
2. Chronic venous insufficiency is inadequate venous return over a long period of time that causes pathologic ischemic changes in the vasculature, skin, and supporting tissues. Poor circulation makes tissues vulnerable to trauma and infection resulting in the formation of venous stasis ulcers.
3. A thrombus is a blood clot that remains attached to a vessel wall. Deep venous thrombosis results from stasis of blood flow, endothelial damage, or hypercoagulability. The most serious complication of deep venous thrombosis is pulmonary embolism.

4. Superior vena cava syndrome is a progressive occlusion of the superior vena cava that leads to venous distention in the upper extremities and head. Because this syndrome is usually caused by bronchogenic cancer, it is generally considered an oncologic emergency rather than a vascular emergency.

Diseases of Arteries

1. Hypertension is the elevation of systemic arterial blood pressure resulting from increases in cardiac output (blood volume), total peripheral vascular resistance, or both.
2. Hypertension can be primary, without a known cause, or secondary, caused by an underlying disease.
3. The risk factors for primary hypertension include a positive family history; male sex; advancing age; black race; obesity; high sodium intake; low magnesium, potassium, or calcium intake; diabetes mellitus; cigarette smoking; and heavy alcohol consumption.
4. Primary hypertension is the result of a complicated interaction of genetics and the environment mediated by neurohumoral effects that influence intravascular volume and peripheral vascular resistance. Pathophysiologic mechanisms include overactivity of the sympathetic nervous system; overactivity of the renin-angiotensin-aldosterone system; sodium and water retention by the kidneys; hormonal inhibition of sodium-potassium transport across cell walls; and complex interactions involving insulin resistance, inflammation, and endothelial function.
5. Secondary hypertension is caused by a disease process or medication that raises peripheral vascular resistance or cardiac output.
6. As hypertension becomes more severe and chronic, tissue damage can occur in the blood vessels and tissues leading to target organ damage in the heart, kidney, brain, and eyes. Hypertensive crisis is an extremely high blood pressure that can lead to cardiac failure, stroke, or death, and is considered a medical emergency.
7. Clinical manifestations of hypertension result from damage of organs and tissues outside the vascular system. These include heart disease, renal insufficiency, central nervous system dysfunction, impaired vision, impaired mobility, vascular occlusion, and edema.
8. Hypertension is managed with both pharmacologic and nonpharmacologic methods that lower the blood volume and the total peripheral vascular resistance.
9. Orthostatic hypotension is a drop in blood pressure that occurs upon standing. The compensatory vasoconstriction response to standing is replaced by a marked vasodilation and blood pooling in the muscle vasculature.
10. The clinical manifestations of orthostatic hypotension include dizziness, blurring or loss of vision, and syncope or fainting.
11. An aneurysm is a localized dilation of a vessel wall; the aorta is particularly susceptible.
12. Arterial thrombi develop similarly to venous thrombi. They may grow large enough to occlude the artery, or they can dislodge and become a thromboembolus that may occlude flow into a distal systemic vascular bed.
13. An embolus is a mobile aggregate of a variety of substances that occludes the vasculature. Sources of emboli include clots, air, amniotic fluid, bacteria, fat, and foreign matter. These emboli cause ischemia and necrosis when a vessel is totally blocked.
14. The most common source of arterial thrombotic emboli is the left heart and they are associated with thrombus formation associated with myocardial infarction, valvular disease, left heart failure, endocarditis, and dysrhythmias.
15. Peripheral vascular diseases include thromboangiitis obliterans and Raynaud phenomenon.
16. Thromboangiitis obliterans is an autoimmune disease of the peripheral arteries characterized by the formation of thrombi filled with inflammatory and immune cells. It is strongly associated with smoking.
17. Raynaud phenomenon is characterized by vasospastic attacks in the small arteries and arterioles of the fingers and the toes triggered by brief exposure to cold, vibration, or emotional stress.
18. Atherosclerosis is a form of arteriosclerosis that is characterized by thickening and hardening of the vessel wall. It is the leading cause of peripheral artery disease, coronary artery disease, and cerebrovascular disease.
19. Atherosclerosis is an inflammatory disease that begins with endothelial injury.
20. Following injury, important steps in atherogenesis include inflammation, adherence of macrophages, release of inflammatory mediators, oxidation of LDL, formation of foam cells and fatty streaks, and development of fibrous plaque.
21. Once a plaque has formed, it can rupture, resulting in clot formation and instability and vasoconstriction, which lead to obstruction of the lumen and inadequate oxygen delivery to tissues.
22. Peripheral artery disease is the result of atherosclerotic plaque formation in the arteries that supply the extremities, and it causes pain, loss of pulse, and skin color changes in the affected limb.
23. Coronary artery disease (CAD) caused by atherosclerosis can diminish the myocardial blood supply until deprivation impairs myocardial metabolism enough to cause myocardial ischemia, a local state in which the cells are temporarily deprived of blood supply.
24. Many risk factors contribute to the onset and escalation of CAD. Conventional (major) risk factors that are modifiable include dyslipidemia, smoking, hypertension, diabetes and insulin resistance, and obesity, sedentary lifestyle, and atherogenic diet. Conventional nonmodifiable risk factors include advanced age, male sex or women after menopause, and family history.
25. Nontraditional (novel) risk factors for CAD include markers of inflammation and ischemia, adipokines, chronic kidney disease, air pollution and ionizing radiation, medications, and the microbiome.
26. Myocardial ischemia develops if the flow or oxygen content of coronary blood is insufficient to meet the metabolic demands of myocardial cells. It is most commonly the result of coronary artery disease and the ensuing decrease in myocardial blood supply.
27. Atherosclerotic plaque progression can be gradual and cause stable angina pectoris, which is predictable chest pain caused by myocardial ischemia in response to increased demand (e.g., exercise) without infarction.

28. Prinzmetal angina, which results from coronary artery vasospasm, is chest pain attributable to transient ischemia of the myocardium that occurs unpredictably and often at rest.
29. Silent ischemia, myocardial ischemia that is asymptomatic, is an indicator of future serious cardiovascular events.
30. Sudden coronary obstruction because of thrombus formation on ruptured unstable atherosclerotic plaques causes the acute coronary syndromes. These include unstable angina and myocardial infarction.
31. Unstable angina results from rupture of an unstable plaque and subsequent thrombus formation with reversible myocardial ischemia.
32. Myocardial infarction is caused by rupture of an unstable plaque and thrombus formation leading to prolonged, unrelieved ischemia that interrupts blood supply to the myocardium. After about 20 minutes of myocardial ischemia, irreversible hypoxic injury causes cellular death and tissue necrosis.
33. Myocardial infarction is clinically classified as non-ST elevation myocardial infarction (non-STEMI) or ST elevation myocardial infarction (STEMI) based on electrocardiographic findings that suggest the extent of myocardial damage (subendocardial versus transmural).
34. An increase in plasma enzyme levels is used to diagnose the occurrence of myocardial infarction as well as indicate its severity. Elevations of the troponins are most predictive of a myocardial infarction.
35. Treatment of a myocardial infarction includes revascularization (thrombolytics or PCI) and administration of antithrombotics, ACE inhibitors, and beta-blockers. Pain relief and fluid management also are key components of care.

Disorders of the Heart Wall

1. Pericardial disease is a localized manifestation of another disorder, such as infection; trauma or surgery; neoplasm; or a metabolic, immunologic, or vascular disorder.
2. Acute pericarditis is acute inflammation of the pericardium. The pericardial membranes become inflamed and roughened, and a pericardial effusion may develop. Symptoms begin with sudden onset of severe chest pain that is worse with respirations or when lying down.
3. Pericardial effusion is the accumulation of fluid in the pericardial cavity. If the accumulation of fluid occurs rapidly, cardiac compression (tamponade) can occur.
4. In constrictive pericarditis, fibrous scarring with occasional calcification of the pericardium causes the pericardial layers to adhere. The fibrotic lesions encase the heart in a rigid shell which compresses the heart, reducing cardiac output.
5. Cardiomyopathies are a diverse group of diseases that affect the myocardium. The cardiomyopathies are categorized as dilated, hypertrophic, and restrictive. The size of the cardiac muscle walls and chambers may increase or decrease depending on the type of cardiomyopathy, thereby altering contractile activity.
6. Disorders of the endocardium damage the heart valves. Congenital or acquired disorders that result in stenosis (constricted or narrow valve), regurgitation (failure of valve to shut completely), or both can structurally alter the valves.
7. Characteristic heart sounds, cardiac murmurs, and systemic complaints assist in identification of an abnormal valve. If severely compromised function exists, a prosthetic heart valve may be surgically implanted to replace the faulty one.
8. Mitral valve prolapse (MVP) describes the condition in which the mitral valve leaflets do not position themselves properly during systole. MVP may be a completely asymptomatic condition or can result in unpredictable symptoms.
9. Rheumatic fever is an inflammatory disease that results from a delayed immune response to a streptococcal infection. Severe or untreated cases of rheumatic fever may progress to rheumatic heart disease, a potentially disabling cardiovascular disorder.
10. Infective endocarditis is a general term for infection and inflammation of the endocardium, especially the cardiac valves. Pathogenesis requires (1) endocardial damage, (2) adherence of blood-borne microorganisms to the damaged endocardial surface, and (3) formation of infective endocardial vegetations.

Manifestations of Heart Disease

1. Heart failure is when the heart is unable to generate an adequate cardiac output. Most causes of heart failure result from dysfunction of the left ventricle.
2. Left heart failure can be divided into heart failure with reduced ejection fraction (systolic) and heart failure with preserved ejection fraction (diastolic).
3. Heart failure with reduced ejection fraction (systolic heart failure) is caused by increased preload, decreased contractility, or increased afterload. These processes result in increased left ventricular end-diastolic volume and pressure that cause increased pulmonary venous pressures and pulmonary edema.
4. In addition to the hemodynamic changes of left ventricular failure, there is a neuroendocrine response that tends to exacerbate and perpetuate the condition.
5. The neuroendocrine mediators of heart failure include the sympathetic nervous system and the renin-angiotensin-aldosterone system; thus diuretics, beta-blockers, and angiotensin-converting enzyme (ACE) inhibitors are important components of the pharmacologic therapy.
6. Heart failure with preserved ejection fraction (diastolic heart failure) is a clinical syndrome characterized by the symptoms and signs of heart failure, a preserved ejection fraction, and abnormal diastolic function.
7. Heart failure with preserved ejection fraction means that the left ventricular end-diastolic pressure is increased, even if volume and cardiac output are normal.
8. Right heart failure is the inability of the right ventricle to provide adequate blood flow into the pulmonary circulation and can result from left heart failure or pulmonary disease.
9. High-output failure is the inability of the heart to adequately supply the body with blood-borne nutrients, despite adequate blood volume and normal or elevated myocardial contractility
10. A dysrhythmia (arrhythmia) is a disturbance of heart rhythm. Dysrhythmias range in severity from occasional

missed beats or rapid beats to disturbances that impair myocardial contractility and are life-threatening.

11. Dysrhythmias can be categorized into atrial arrhythmias, ventricular arrhythmias, and sinus node dysfunction and conduction disorders.

REFERENCES

1. Labropoulos N. How does chronic venous disease progress from the first symptoms to the advanced stages? A review. *Adv Ther.* 2019;36:13–19.
2. Ren SY, et al. Strategies and challenges in the treatment of chronic venous leg ulcers. *World J Clin Cases.* 2020;8(21):5070–5085.
3. Centers for Disease Control and Prevention. *Data and statistics on venous thromboembolism.* Last reviewed 02/07/2020. Available at https://www.cdc.gov/ncbddd/dvt/data.html. Accessed 16/01/22
4. Borgel D, et al. Inflammation in deep vein thrombosis: a therapeutic target? *Hematology.* 2019;24(1):742–750.
5. Mahajan A, et al. The epidemiology of cancer-associated venous thromboembolism: an update. *Semin Thromb Hemost.* 2019;45(4):321–325.
6. Caio J, et al. Cancer-associated thrombosis: the when, how and why. *Eur Respir Rev.* 2019;28(151):180119.
7. Bouck EG, et al. COVID-19 and sepsis are associated with different abnormalities in plasma procoagulant and fibrinolytic activity. *Arterioscler Thromb Vasc Biol.* 2020;41(1):401–414.
8. Longchamp G, et al. Proximal deep vein thrombosis and pulmonary embolism in COVID-19 patients: a systematic review and meta-analysis. *Thrombosis J.* 2021;19:15.
9. Mukesh Shrestha, Wei Li. Factor V Leiden and the risk of pulmonary embolism. *Cardiol Cardiovasc Med.* 2019;3:001–008.
10. Ortel TL, et al. American Society of Hematology 2020 guidelines for management of venous thromboembolism: treatment of deep vein thrombosis and pulmonary embolism. *Blood Adv.* 2020;4(19):4693–4738.
11. Azizi AH, et al. Superior vena cava syndrome. *JACC Cardiovasc Interv.* 2020;13(24):2896–2910.
12. Virani SS, et al. Heart disease and stroke statistics—2021 update: A report from the American Heart Association. *Circulation.* 2021;143:e254–e743.
13. Nambiar L, et al. Decade long temporal trends in U.S. hypertension related cardiovascular mortality. *J Am Coll Cardiol.* 2020;75(20):2644–2646.
14. Al Ghorani H, et al. Hypertension trials update. *J Hum Hypertens.* 2021;35(5):398–409.
15. Zhu H, et al. The role of SARS-CoV-2 target ACE2 in cardiovascular diseases. *J Cell Mol Med.* 2021;25(3):1342–1349.
16. Sharma RK, et al. ACE2 (angiotensin-converting enzyme 2) in cardiopulmonary diseases. *Hypertension.* 2020;76(3):651–661.
17. Povlsen AL, et al. The vasoactive Mas receptor in essential hypertension. *J Clin Med.* 2020;9(1):267.
18. Januzzi JL, Ibrahim NE. "Rebranding" natriuretic peptides. *Clin Chem.* 2021;67(1):4–5.
19. Salazar J, et al. Neprilysin: a potential therapeutic target of arterial hypertension? *Curr Cardiol Rev.* 2020;16(1):25–35.
20. Poorgolizadeh E, et al. Do neprilysin inhibitors walk the line? Heart ameliorative but brain threatening! *Eur J Pharmacol.* 2021;894:173851.
21. Angeli F, Reboldi G, Verdecchia P: The link between inflammation and hypertension: unmasking mediators, *Am J Hypertens.* 2021;34(7):683–685.
22. Haspula D, Clark MA. Neuroinflammation and sympathetic overactivity: mechanisms and implications in hypertension. *Auton Neurosci.* 2018;210:10–17.
23. Hall JE, et al. Obesity, kidney dysfunction and hypertension: mechanistic links. *Nat Rev Nephrol.* 2019;15(6):367–385.
24. Pareek M, Bhatt DL, Schiavon CA, Schauer PR. Metabolic surgery for hypertension in patients with obesity. *Circ Res.* 2019;124(7):1009–1024.
25. Gandotra C, et al. Characteristics and resolution of hypertension in obese African American bariatric cohort. *Sci Rep.* 2021;11:1683.
26. da Silva AA, et al. Role of hyperinsulinemia and insulin resistance in hypertension: metabolic syndrome revisited. *Can J Cardiol.* 2020;36(5):671–682.
27. Whelton PK, et al. 2017 ACC/AHA/AAPA/ABC/ACPM/AGS/APhA/ASH/ASPC/NMA/PCNA guideline for the prevention, detection, evaluation and management of high blood pressure in adults: a report of the American College of Cardiology/American Heart Association Task Force on Clinical Practice Guidelines. *Hypertension.* 2018;71(6):e13–e115.
28. Jones DW, et al. Management of stage 1 hypertension in adults with a low 10-year risk for cardiovascular disease: filling a guidance gap: a scientific statement from the American Heart Association. *Hypertension* 2021;77:e58–e67.
29. Unger T, et al. 2020 International Society of Hypertension Global Hypertension Practice Guidelines. *Hypertension.* 2020;75(6):1334–1357.
30. Zuo Y, et al: Antihypertensive treatment decrease stroke occurrence a prospective cohort study. *J Hypertension.* 2021;39(8):1652–1661.
31. McDonagh STJ, Mejzner N, Clark CE. Prevalence of postural hypotension in primary, community and institutional care: a systematic review and meta-analysis. *BMC Fam Pract.* 2021;22:1.
32. Palma JA, Kaufmann H. Management of orthostatic hypotension. *Continuum (Minneap Minn).* 2020;26(1):154–177.
33. Vargas F, Goyal P, Rich MW. *Effects of Intensive Blood Pressure Treatment on Orthostatic Hypotension: Expert Analysis.* Washington, DC: American College of Cardiology; 2021. Available at: https://www.acc.org/latest-in-cardiology/articles/2021/01/13/12/55/effects-of-intensive-blood-pressure-treatment-on-orthostatic-hypotension. Accessed 15.01.22.
34. Cheshire WP. Chemical pharmacotherapy for the treatment of orthostatic hypotension. *Exp Opin Pharmacother.* 2019;20(2):187–199.
35. Pinard A, Jones GT, Milewicz DM. Genetics of thoracic and abdominal aortic diseases. *Circ Res.* 2019;124:588–606.
36. Golledge J. Abdominal aortic aneurysm: update on pathogenesis and medical treatments. *Nat Rev Cardiol.* 2019;16:225–242.
37. Dulak A. Endovascular aneurysm repair. *J Vasc Endovasc Ther.* 2021;6(2):e101.
38. Ko JP, et al. Chest CT angiography for acute aortic pathologic conditions: pearls and pitfalls. *Radiographics.* 2021;41(2):399–424.
39. Cacione DG, et al. Stem cell therapy for treatment of thromboangiitis obliterans (Buerger's disease). *Cochrane Database Syst Rev.* 2018;10(10):CD012794.
40. Jeong ST, Ra JC. Treatment of Buerger's disease (thromboangiitis obliterans) with autologous adipose tissue-derived mesenchymal stem cell: report of three cases. *F1000Res.* 2019;8:2016.
41. Haque A, Hughes M. Raynaud's phenomenon. *Clin Med J.* 2020;20(6):580–587.
42. Libby P. Inflammation in atherosclerosis—no longer a theory. *Clin Chem.* 2021;67(1):131–142.
43. Barrett TJ. Macrophages in atherosclerosis regression. *Arterioscleros Thrombos Vasc Biol.* 2020;40(1):20–33.

44. Sterpetti AV. Inflammatory cytokines and atherosclerotic plaque progression: therapeutic implications. *Curr Atheroscleros Rep.* 2020;22:75.
45. Wang J, et al. HDAC3 protects against atherosclerosis through inhibition of inflammation via the microRNA-19b/PPARγ/NF-κB axis. *Atherosclerosis.* 2021;323:1–12.
46. Wolf D, Ley K. Immunity and inflammation in atherosclerosis. *Circ Res.* 2019;124(2):315–327.
47. Zhao TX, Mallat Z. Targeting the immune system in atherosclerosis: JACC State-of-the-Art Review. *J Am Coll Cardiol.* 2019;73(13):1691–1706.
48. Misra A, Fisher EA. Tipping the cap away from danger. *Nat Metab.* 2021;3:128–130.
49. Tomaniak M, et al. Vulnerable plaques and patients: state-of-the-art. *Eur Heart J.* 2020;41(31):2997–3004.
50. Campia U, et al. Peripheral artery disease: past, present, and future. *Am J Med.* 2019;132(10):1133–1141.
51. Bevan GH, Solaru KTW. Evidence-based medical management of peripheral artery disease. *Arterioscleros Thrombos Vasc Biol.* 2020;40:541–553.
52. Bonaca MP, et al. Rivaroxaban in peripheral artery disease after revascularization. *N Engl J Med.* 2020;382:1994–2004.
53. Shadrina AS, et al. Prioritization of causal genes for coronary artery disease based on cumulative evidence from experimental and in silico studies. *Sci Rep.* 2020;10:10486.
54. Rizzacasa B, et al. Epigenetic modification in coronary atherosclerosis: JACC Review Topic of the Week. *J Am Coll Cardiol.* 2019;74(10):1352–1365.
55. Expert Panel on Detection, Evaluation and Treatment of High Blood Cholesterol in Adults: Executive summary of the third report of the National Cholesterol Education Program (NCEP) Expert Panel on Detection, Evaluation, and Treatment of High Blood Cholesterol in Adults (Adult Treatment Panel III). *JAMA.* 2001;285(19):2486–2497.
56. Shah NP, Ahmed HM, Tang WHW. Familial hypercholesterolemia: detect, treat, and ask about family. *Cleve Clin J Med.* 2020;87:109–115.
57. Grundy SM, et al. 2018 AHA/ACC/AACVPR/AAPA/ABC/ACPM/ADA/AGS/APhA/ASPC/NLA/PCNA guideline on the management of blood cholesterol: a report of the American College of Cardiology/American Heart Association Task Force on Clinical Practice Guidelines. *Circulation.* 2019;139:e1082–e1143.
58. Tall AR. HDL in morbidity and mortality: a 40+ year perspective. *Clin Chem.* 2021;67(1):19–23.
59. Gulec S, Erol C. High-density lipoprotein cholesterol and risk of cardiovascular disease. *e-Journal of Cardiology Practice.* 2020;19(3). European Society of Cardiology. Available at: https://www.escardio.org/Journals/E-Journal-of-Cardiology-Practice/Volume-19/high-density-lipoprotein-cholesterol-and-risk-of-cardiovascular-disease. Accessed 15.01.22.
60. Barter P, Genest J. HDL cholesterol and ASCVD risk stratification: a debate. *Atherosclerosis.* 2019;283:7–12.
61. Hunjadi M, et al. HDL cholesterol efflux capacity is inversely associated with subclinical cardiovascular risk markers in young adults: THE Cardiovascular Risk in Young Finns Study. *Sci Rep.* 2020;10:19223.
62. Tsimikas S, et al. for the AKCEA-APO(a)-LRx Study Investigators: Lipoprotein(a) reduction in persons with cardiovascular disease. *N Engl J Med.* 2020;382:244–255.
63. Berman AN, Blankstein R. Current and future role of lipoprotein(a) in preventive cardiology. *Curr Opin Cardiol.* 2019;34(5):514–518.
64. Joseph JJ, et al. Comprehensive management of cardiovascular risk factors for adults with type 2 diabetes: A scientific statement from the American Heart Association. *Circulation* 2022; Published online ahead of print January 2022. Available at https://www.ahajournals.org/doi/10.1161/CIR.0000000000001040. Accessed 15.01.22
65. Chang L, Garcia-Barrio MT, Chen YE. Perivascular adipose tissue regulates vascular function by targeting vascular smooth muscle cells. *Arterioscleros Thrombos Vasc Biol.* 2020;40(5):1094–1109.
66. Antoniades C, Kotanidis CP, Berman DS. State-of-the-art review article. Atherosclerosis affecting fat: What can we learn by imaging perivascular adipose tissue? *J Cardiovasc Comput Tomogr.* 2019;13(5):288–296.
67. Kim HW, et al. Perivascular adipose tissue and vascular perturbation/atherosclerosis. *Arterioscleros Thrombos Vasc Biol.* 2020;40(11):2569–2576.
68. Adams TD, et al. Weight and metabolic outcomes 12 years after gastric bypass. *N Engl J Med.* 2017;377:1143–1155.
69. Singh P, et al. Impact of bariatric surgery on cardiovascular outcomes and mortality: a population-based cohort study. *Br J Surg.* 2020;107(4):432–442.
70. Lichtenstein AH, et al. 2021 Dietary guidance to improve cardiovascular health: A scientific statement from the American Heart Association. *Circulation.* 2021;144:e472–487.
71. Rajagopalan S, Al-Kindi SG, Brook RD. Air pollution and cardiovascular disease: JACC State-of-the-Art Review. *J Am Coll Cardiol.* 2018;72(17):2054–2070.
72. Mahlof EN, Bisognano JD. Reducing cardiovascular risk caused by air pollution: individuals can make a difference. *J Hum Hypertens.* 2020;34:805–806.
73. Schjerning AM, McGettigan P, Gislason G. Cardiovascular effects and safety of (non-aspirin) NSAIDs. *Nat Rev Cardiol.* 2020;17:574–584.
74. Kazemian N, et al. Gut microbiota and cardiovascular disease: opportunities and challenges. *Microbiome.* 2020;8:36.
75. Troseid M, et al. The gut microbiome in coronary artery disease and heart failure: current knowledge and future directions. *EBioMedicine.* 2020;52:102649.
76. Gulati M, et al. 2021 AHA/ACC/ASE/CHEST/SAEM/SCCT/SCMR Guideline for the evaluation and diagnosis of chest pain: Executive Summary: A report of the American College of Cardiology/American Heart Association Joint Committee on Clinical Practice Guidelines. *Circulation* 2021;144:e368–e454.
77. Fihn SD, et al. 2014 ACCF/AHA/ACP/AATS/PCNA/SCAI/STS Focused update of the guideline for the diagnosis and management of patients with stable ischemic heart disease: a report of the American College of Cardiology Foundation/American Heart Association Task Force on Practice Guidelines, and the American College of Physicians, American Association for Thoracic Surgery, Preventive Cardiovascular Nurses Association, Society for Cardiovascular Angiography and Interventions, and Society of Thoracic Surgeons. *J Am Coll Cardiol.* 2014;64(18):1929–1949.
78. Maron DJ, et al. Initial invasive or conservative strategy for stable coronary disease. *N Engl J Med.* 2020;382:1395.
79. Lawton JS, et al. 2021 ACC/AHA/SCAI guideline for coronary artery revascularization: Executive Summary: A report of the American College of Cardiology/American Heart Association Joint Committee on Clinical Practice Guidelines. Circulation Published online ahead of print December 2021. Available at https://www.ahajournals.org/doi/10.1161/CIR.0000000000001039. Accessed 15.01.22.

80. Arnett DK, et al. 2019 ACC/AHA Guideline on the Primary Prevention of Cardiovascular Disease: A Report of the American College of Cardiology/American Heart Association Task Force on Clinical Practice Guidelines. *Circulation*. 2019;140:e595–e646.
81. Merz CNB, et al. Treatment of coronary microvascular dysfunction. *Cardiovasc Res*. 2020;116(4):856–870.
82. Picard F, et al. Vasospastic angina: a literature review of current evidence. *Arch Cardiovasc Dis*. 2019;112(1):44–55.
83. Seo WW, et al. Admission serum potassium levels and prognosis of vasospastic angina. *Sci Rep*. 2021;11:5707.
84. Hao K, et al. Prognostic impacts of comorbid significant coronary stenosis and coronary artery spasm in patients with stable coronary artery disease. *J Am Heart Assoc*. 2021;10:e017831.
85. Lyon AR, et al. Pathophysiology of Takotsubo syndrome: JACC State-of-the-Art Review. *J Am Coll Cardiol*. 2021;77(7):902–911.
86. Indolfi C, et al. Old unsolved problems: when and how to treat silent ischaemia. *Eur Heart J Suppl*. 2020;22(Suppl_L):L82–L85.
87. Canet-Soulas E, et al. The elusive origin of atherosclerotic plaque calcification. *Front Cell and Dev Biol*. 2021;9:622736.
88. Liu W, et al. Relationship between coronary hyper-intensive plaques identified by cardiovascular magnetic resonance and clinical severity of acute coronary syndrome. *J Cardiovasc Magn Reson*. 2021;23:12.
89. Amsterdam EA, et al. AHA/ACC guideline for the management of patients with non-ST-elevation acute coronary syndromes: a report of the American College of Cardiology/American Heart Association Task Force on practice guidelines. *Circulation*. 2014;130(25):2354–2394.
90. Collet JP, et al. 2020 ESC Guidelines for the management of acute coronary syndromes in patients presenting without persistent ST-segment elevation: the Task Force for the management of acute coronary syndromes in patients presenting without persistent ST-segment elevation of the European Society of Cardiology (ESC). *Eur Heart J*. 2021;42(14):1289–1367.
91. Rossello X, Lobo-Gonzalez M, Ibanez B: Editor's Choice: Pathophysiology and therapy of myocardial ischaemia/reperfusion syndrome. *Eur Heart J Acute Cardiovasc Care*. 2019;8(5):443–456.
92. Hausenloy DJ, et al. The coronary circulation in acute myocardial ischaemia/reperfusion injury: a target for cardioprotection. *Cardiovasc Res*. 2019;115(7):1143–1155.
93. Heusch, G. Myocardial stunning and hibernation revisited. *Nat Rev Cardiol* 2021;18:522–536.
94. van der Bijl P, et al. Left ventricular post-infarct remodeling: implications for systolic function improvement and outcomes in the modern era. *JACC Heart Fail*. 2020;8(2):131–140.
95. Zuurbier CJ, et al. Innate immunity as a target for acute cardioprotection. *Cardiovasc Res*. 2019;115(7):1131–1142.
96. Nasser MI, et al. Macrophages: first guards in the prevention of cardiovascular diseases. *Life Sci*. 2020;250:117559.
97. Gong R, et al. Regulation of cardiomyocyte fate plasticity: a key strategy for cardiac regeneration. *Signal Transduct Target Ther*. 2021;6:31.
98. Thygesen K, et al. Fourth universal definition of myocardial infarction (2018). *J Am Coll Cardiol*. 2018;72(18):2231–2264.
99. O'Gara PT, et al. 2013 ACCF/AHA guideline for the management of ST-elevation myocardial infarction: a report of the American College of Cardiology Foundation/American Heart Association Task Force on practice guidelines. *Circulation*. 2013;127:e362–e425.
100. Ibanez B, et al. 2017 ESC Guidelines for the management of acute myocardial infarction in patients presenting with ST-segment elevation: the Task Force for the management of acute myocardial infarction in patients presenting with ST-segment elevation of the European Society of Cardiology (ESC). *Eur Heart J*. 2018;39(2):119–177.
101. Mendieta G, et al. Intravenous statin administration during myocardial infarction compared with oral post-infarct administration. *J Am Coll Cardiol*. 2020;75:1386–1405.
102. Chiabrando JG, et al. Management of acute and recurrent pericarditis. *J Am Coll Cardiol*. 2020;75(1):76–92.
103. Ismail TF. Acute pericarditis: update on diagnosis and management. *Clin Med (Lond)*. 2020;20(1):48–51.
104. Rosario J, et al. Pericardial effusion with tamponade: bedside ultrasonography saves another life. *Int J Emerg Med*. 2020;13:3.
105. Tuck BC, Townsley MM. Clinical update in pericardial diseases. *J Cardiothorac Vasc Anesth*. 2019;33:184–199.
106. Lazaros G, et al: Contemporary management of pericardial effusion, *Panminerva Med*. 2021;63(3):288–300.
107. Reichart D, et al. Dilated cardiomyopathy: from epidemiologic to genetic phenotypes: a translational review of current literature. *J Intern Med*. 2019;286(4):362–372.
108. Verdonschot JAJ, et al. Phenotypic clustering of dilated cardiomyopathy patients highlights important pathophysiological differences. *Eur Heart J*. 2021;42(2):162–174.
109. Schultheiss HP, et al. Dilated cardiomyopathy. *Nat Rev Dis Primers*. 2019;5(1):32.
110. Ommen SR, et al. 2020 AHA/ACC guideline for the diagnosis and treatment of patients with hypertrophic cardiomyopathy: a report of the American College of Cardiology/American Heart Association Joint Committee on Clinical Practice Guidelines. *Circulation*. 2020;142(25):e558–e631.
111. Makavos G, et al. Hypertrophic cardiomyopathy: an updated review on diagnosis, prognosis, and treatment. *Heart Fail Rev*. 2019;24:439–459.
112. Spertus JA, et al. Mavacamten for treatment of symptomatic obstructive hypertrophic cardiomyopathy (EXPLORER-HCM): health status analysis of a randomised, double-blind, placebo-controlled, phase 3 trial. *Lancet* 2021;397(10293):2467–2475.
113. McVeigh T, Tennyson C. Understanding and recognizing cardiac amyloidosis. *Journal of the American Association of Physician Assistants*. 2020;33:16–20.
114. Bermego J, Postigo A, Baumgartner H. The year in cardiovascular medicine 2020: valvular heart disease. *Eur Heart J*. 2021;42(6):647–656.
115. Otto CM, et al. 2020 ACC/AHA guideline for the management of patients with valvular heart disease: a report of the American College of Cardiology/American Heart Association Joint Committee on Clinical Practice Guidelines. *J Am Coll Cardiol*. 2021;77:e25–e197.
116. Fishbein GA, Fishbein MC. Pathology of the aortic valve: aortic valve stenosis/aortic regurgitation. *Curr Cardiol Rep*. 2019;21(8):81.
117. Raddatz MA, Madhur MS, Merryman WD. Adaptive immune cells in calcific aortic valve disease. *Am J Physiol Heart Circ Physiol*. 2019;317(1):H141–H155.
118. Zhang X, et al. Meta-Analysis comparing results of transcatheter versus surgical aortic-valve replacement in patients with severe aortic stenosis. *Am J Cardiol*. 2020;125(3):449–458.
119. Bedeir K, Kaneko T, Aranki S. Current and evolving strategies in the management of severe mitral annular calcification. *J Thorac Cardiovasc Surg*. 2019;157(2):555–566.
120. Fishbein GA, Fishbein MC. Mitral valve pathology. *Curr Cardiol Rep*. 2019;21(7):61.

121. Kato N, et al. The natural history of severe calcific mitral stenosis. *J Am Coll Cardiol.* 2020;75(24):3048–3057.
122. Flint N, et al. Aortic regurgitation. *Curr Cardiol Rep.* 2019;21(7):65.
123. Asmarats L, et al. Tricuspid valve disease: diagnosis, prognosis and management of a rapidly evolving field. *Nat Rev Cardiol.* 2019;16(9):538–554.
124. Althunayyan A, et al. Mitral valve prolapse. *Expert Rev Cardiovasc Ther.* 2019;17(1):43–51.
125. Wunderlich NC, et al. Degenerative mitral regurgitation: assessment, physical examination and imaging. *Curr Cardiol Rep.* 2019;21(8):85–98.
126. Nascimento BR, Beaton AZ. Rheumatic heart disease and socioeconomic development. *Lancet Glob Health.* 2019;7(10):E1297–E1299.
127. Cunningham MW. Molecular mimicry, autoimmunity, and infection: the cross-reactive antigens of group A Streptococci and their sequelae. *Microbiol Spectr.* 2019;7(4). Available at: https://doi.org/10.1128/microbiolspec.GPP3-0045-2018. Accessed 15.01.22.
128. Kumar RK, et al. Contemporary diagnosis and management of rheumatic heart disease: Implications for closing the gap: a scientific statement from the American Heart Association. *Circulation.* 2020;142(20):e337–e357.
129. Gerwitz MH, et al. Revision of the Jones Criteria for the diagnosis of acute rheumatic fever in the era of Doppler echocardiography. A Scientific Statement From the American Heart Association. *Circulation.* 2015;131(20):1806–1818.
130. El-Dalati S, et al. Clinical practice update on infectious endocarditis. *Am J Med.* 2020;133(1):44–49.
131. Baddour L, et al. Infective endocarditis in adults: diagnosis, antimicrobial therapy, and management of complications a scientific statement for healthcare professionals from the American Heart Association. *Circulation.* 2015;132:1–53.
132. Nishimura RA, et al. 2017 AHA/ACC focused update of the 2014 AHA/ACC guideline for the management of patients with valvular heart disease: a report of the American College of Cardiology/American Heart Association Task Force on Clinical Practice Guidelines. *Circulation.* 2017;135:e1159–e1195.
133. Bozkurt B, et al. Universal definition and classification of heart failure: a report of the Heart Failure Society of America, Heart Failure Association of the European Society of Cardiology, Japanese Heart Failure Society and Writing Committee of the Universal Definition of Heart Failure. *J Cardiac Fail.* 2021;27(4):387–413.
134. Sorrentino MJ. The evolution from hypertension to heart failure. *Heart Fail Clin.* 2019;15(4):447–453.
135. Yancy CW, et al. 2013 ACCF/AHA guideline for the management of heart failure: A report of the American College of Cardiology Foundation/American Heart Association Task Force on Practice Guidelines. *Circulation.* 2013;128:e240–e327.
136. Yancy CW, et al. 2017 ACC/AHA/HFSA focused update of the 2013 ACCF/AHA guideline for the management of heart failure: a report of the American College of Cardiology/American Heart Association Task Force on Clinical Practice Guidelines and the Heart Failure Society of America. *Circulation.* 2017;136:e137–e161.
137. Rossignol P, et al. Heart failure drug treatment. *Lancet.* 2019; 393(10175):1034–1044.
138. Writing Committee 2021 Update to the 2017 ACC Expert Consensus Decision Pathway for Optimization of Heart Failure Treatment: Answers to 10 pivotal issues about heart failure with reduced ejection fraction: A report of the American College of Cardiology Solution Set Oversight Committee. *J Am Coll Cardiol.* 2021;77(6):772–810.
139. Bauersachs J. Heart failure drug treatment: the fantastic four. *Eur Heart J.* 2021;42(6):681–683.
140. Teerlink JR, et al. for the GALACTIC-HF Investigators: Cardiac myosin activation with omecamtiv mecarbil in systolic heart failure. *N Engl J Med.* 2021;384:105–116.
141. Bhagra SK, Pettit S, Parameshwar J. Cardiac transplantation: indications, eligibility and current outcomes. *Heart.* 2019;105(3):252–260.
142. Cannata A, et al. Gene therapy for the heart: lessons learned and future perspectives. *Circ Res.* 2020;126(10):1394–1414.
143. Tehzeeb J, Manzoor A, Ahmed MM. Is stem cell therapy an answer to heart failure: a literature search. *Cureus.* 2019;11(10):e5959.
144. Mishra S, Kass DA. Cellular and molecular pathobiology of heart failure with preserved ejection fraction. *Nat Rev Cardiol.* 2021;18(6):400–423.
145. Pfeffer MA, Shah AM, Borlaug BA. Heart failure with preserved ejection fraction in perspective. *Circ Res.* 2019;124:1598–1617.
146. Slivnick J, Lampert BC. Hypertension and heart failure. *Heart Fail Clin.* 2019;15(4):531–541.
147. Upadhya B, Kitzman DW. Heart failure with preserved ejection fraction: new approaches to diagnosis and management. *Clin Cardiol.* 2020;43(2):145–155.
148. Elgendy IY, Pepine CJ. Heart failure with preserved ejection fraction: Is ischemia due to coronary microvascular dysfunction a mechanistic factor? *Am J Med.* 2019;132(6):692–697.
149. Borlaug BA. Evaluation and management of heart failure with preserved ejection fraction. *Nat Rev Cardiol.* 2020;17(9):559–573.
150. Normand C, et al. Beyond pharmacological treatment: an insight into therapies that target specific aspects of heart failure pathophysiology. *Lancet.* 2019;393(10175):1045–1055.
151. Al-Khatib SM, et al. 2017 AHA/ACC/HRS Guideline for management of patients with ventricular arrhythmias and the prevention of sudden cardiac death: a report of the American College of Cardiology/American Heart Association Task Force on Clinical Practice Guidelines and the Heart Rhythm Society. *Circulation.* 2018;138:e272–e391.
152. January CT, et al. 2014 AHA/ACC/HRS Guideline for the management of patients with atrial fibrillation: a report of the American College of Cardiology/American Heart Association Task Force on Clinical Practice Guidelines and the Heart Rhythm Society in Collaboration with the Society of Thoracic Surgeons. *Circulation.* 2014;130:e199–e267.
153. January CT, et al. 2019 AHA/ACC/HRS focused update of the 2014 AHA/ACC/HRS Guideline for the management of patients with atrial fibrillation: a report of the American College of Cardiology/American Heart Association Task Force on Clinical Practice Guidelines and the Heart Rhythm Society in Collaboration with the Society of Thoracic Surgeons. *Circulation.* 2019;140:e125–e151.
154. Kusumoto FM, et al. 2018 ACC/AHA/HRS Guideline on the evaluation and management of patients with bradycardia and cardiac conduction delay: a report of the American College of Cardiology/American Heart Association Task Force on Clinical Practice Guidelines and the Heart Rhythm Society. *Circulation.* 2019;140:e382–e482.

33

Alterations of Cardiovascular Function in Children

Melanie L. Scala and Casey Bor

http://evolve.elsevier.com/Rogers/pathophysiology/

CHAPTER OUTLINE

Cardiovascular disorders in children are classified as congenital or acquired. Congenital heart disease (CHD) is the most common. Early screening and improved surgical and perioperative care have resulted in improved outcomes. Acquired heart diseases such as Kawasaki disease and hypertension in children continue to present challenges to the practitioner. Although guidelines for diagnosing acquired diseases are available, work is still needed in developing standards of treatment and long-term follow-up protocols.

CONGENITAL HEART DISEASE

Congenital heart disease (CHD) is a structural abnormality of the heart and (or) great vessels that is present at birth. Incidence varies from 0.8% to 1.2% of live births worldwide. While several environmental and genetic risk factors have been linked to CHD, only 15% of cases can be attributed to a specific cause.[1] The relative lack of identifiable and modifiable environmental risks for most cases has limited the effectiveness of prevention measures for CHD. The environmental factors that have been linked to CHD are typically maternal and are listed with the associated congenital heart defect in Table 33.1.[2,3]

Several specific chromosomal aberrations are associated with CHD, although the mechanism of causation is often unknown (Table 33.2). The incidence of CHD is three to four times higher in siblings of affected children, and chromosomal defects account for about 6% of all cases of CHD. Down syndrome (trisomy 21), trisomies 13 and 18, Turner syndrome, 22q11.2 deletion syndrome (DiGeorge/Velofacialcardio syndromes),[4] and cri du chat syndrome (chromosome 5p deletion syndrome) have been associated with a relatively high incidence of heart defects.

The diagnosis and management of CHD continues to improve with the use of fetal echocardiography for early detection, early interventional catheterization, neonatal pulse oximetry pre discharge screening,[5] and refined surgical repair. However, children who survive corrective surgery for their CHD continue to be at risk for long-term morbidity, including heart failure, obstructive pulmonary disease, neurologic diseases, and psychiatric illness.[6] For many types of CHD, endocarditis prophylaxis is recommended, especially after transcatheter or surgical intervention.

Classification of Congenital Heart Disease

Congenital heart diseases can be broadly categorized into those that are most commonly associated with normal oxygen delivery to tissues (acyanotic) and those that are most often associated with a decrease in oxygen delivery to tissues (cyanotic). This categorization is not absolute however, because severe cases of any type of cardiac defect may eventually lead to heart failure and cyanosis. There are four major subcategories based on whether they increase or decrease pulmonary blood flow, obstruct blood flow, or mix desaturated and saturated blood within the chambers or great arteries (Fig. 33.1). By classifying lesions into these categories, one can predict the clinical and physiological sequelae of the type of congenital heart defect based on its category.

In normal cardiac physiology, the movement of blood through the right side of the heart and into the pulmonary system is separate from the blood flow through the left side of the heart into the systemic circulation (Fig. 33.2A). Abnormal movement from one side of the heart to the other is termed a shunt. A shunt typically occurs through a defect or hole between two chambers or blood vessels or through a patent ductus arteriosus (PDA). The direction of this shunt depends on multiple anatomic and physiologic factors, including pressure differences or the presence of any obstructions in the chambers or blood vessels distal to the defect.

Shunting of blood flow from the left heart into the right heart is called a left-to-right shunt and occurs in conditions

TABLE 33.1 **Environmental Factors Associated With Congenital Heart Defects**

Cause	Type of Congenital Heart Defect
Infection	
Intrauterine	PDA, PS, COA
Systemic viral	PDA, PS, COA
Rubella	PDA, PS, COA
Coxsackie B5	Endocardial fibroelastosis
Herpesvirus, cytomegalovirus	Can infect endothelial cells and vascular endothelium
Radiation	Studies of cancer survivors reveal radiation can cause atherosclerosis; myocardial, endocardial, and pericardial disease; conduction disturbances; and endothelial vessel disease
Metabolic Disorders	
Diabetes	VSD, cardiomegaly, transposition of the great vessels
Phenylketonuria	COA, PDA
Hypercalcemia	Supravalvular AS, PS; aortic hyperplasia
Drugs	
Alcohol	TOF, ASD, VSD
Lithium	Exact effect not known
Phenytoin	Embryonic dysrhythmia and valvular heart disease
Warfarin	ASD, PDA
Peripheral Conditions	
Increased maternal age	VSD, TOF (relationship unclear)
Antepartal bleeding	Various defects (relationship unclear)
Prematurity	PDA, VSD
High altitude	PDA, ASD (increased incidence)

AS, Aortic stenosis; *ASD*, atrial septal defect; *COA*, coarctation of the aorta; *PDA*, patent ductus arteriosus; *PS*, pulmonary stenosis; *TOF*, tetralogy of Fallot; *VSD*, ventricular septal defect.

TABLE 33.2 **Congenital Heart Disease in Selected Fetal Chromosomal Aberrations**

Conditions	Incidence of CHD (%)	Common Defects (in Decreasing Order of Frequency)
5p (cri du chat syndrome)	25	VSD, PDA, ASD
Trisomy 13 syndrome	90	VSD, PDA, dextrocardia
Trisomy 18 syndrome	99	VSD, PDA, PS
Trisomy 21 (Down syndrome)	50	AVSD, VSD
Turner syndrome (XO)	35	COA, AS, ASD
Klinefelter variant (XXXXY)	15	PDA, ASD
22q11.2 deletion syndrome	75–80	TOF, PA + VSD, IAA, truncus arteriosus, VSD, Aortic arch anomalies

AS, Aortic stenosis; *ASD*, atrial septal defect; *AVSD*, atrioventricular septal defect; *COA*, coarctation of the aorta; *PDA*, patent ductus arteriosus; *PS*, pulmonary stenosis; *VSD*, ventricular septal defect; *TOF*, Tetralogy of Fallot; *PA*, pulmonary atresia; *IAA*, interrupted aortic arch. From Park MK. *Pediatric cardiology for practitioners*, 6th edition. St. Louis: Mosby; 2014.

such as atrial septal defect (ASD) and ventricular septal defect (VSD) (see Fig. 33.2B). This type of shunt occurs because the pressure is higher on the left side of the heart than it is in the right side of the heart. A left-to-right shunt increases the volume in the right side of the heart and results in increased blood flow into the pulmonary circulation. Depending on the degree of shunting, this increase in pulmonary blood flow may cause affected children to develop symptoms of heart failure. Because blood continues to flow through the lungs before passing into the systemic circulation, there is no decrease in tissue oxygenation or cyanosis. Thus, defects that cause left-to-right shunt are termed acyanotic heart defects. There are other types of acyanotic heart defects where blood flow is obstructed as it leaves the ventricles, but there is no hole or defect to cause shunting. These lesions can result from partial or complete obstructions in either the right side of the heart, the left side of the heart, or both.

Cyanotic heart defects frequently cause shunting of blood from the right side of the heart directly into the left side of the heart (right-to-left shunt). A right-to-left shunt decreases blood flow through the pulmonary system, causing less-than-normal oxygen delivery to the tissues and resulting in a bluish discoloration of the skin called cyanosis (see Chapter 35). Tetralogy of Fallot is the most common cyanotic heart defect.[3] In this condition, narrowing of the pulmonary outflow tract increases right heart pressures, thus forcing blood through a defect in the ventricular septum into the left heart (see Fig. 33.2C). Other types of heart defects result in cyanosis due to the mixing of venous and arterial blood that enters the systemic circulation.

Most congenital heart defects are named to describe the underlying defect (e.g., valvular abnormalities, abnormal openings in the septa, and malformation or abnormal placement of the great vessels). Descriptions of the most common defects follow.

Defects With Increased Pulmonary Blood Flow

Patent Ductus Arteriosus

Patent ductus arteriosus (PDA) is failure of the fetal ductus arteriosus (DA) to close within hours after birth (Fig. 33.3). The most important risk factor for PDA is premature birth. Other risk factors include congenital rubella, perinatal asphyxia, and birth in high altitude places. Genetic risks are associated with inherited syndromes such as 22q11.2 deletion syndrome.[7]

Pathophysiology. The DA connects the aorta and pulmonary artery (PA) during fetal development and functions to bypass the lungs, which are still a fluid filled organ in utero. Between 10 and 15 hours after birth, higher oxygen concentrations in the

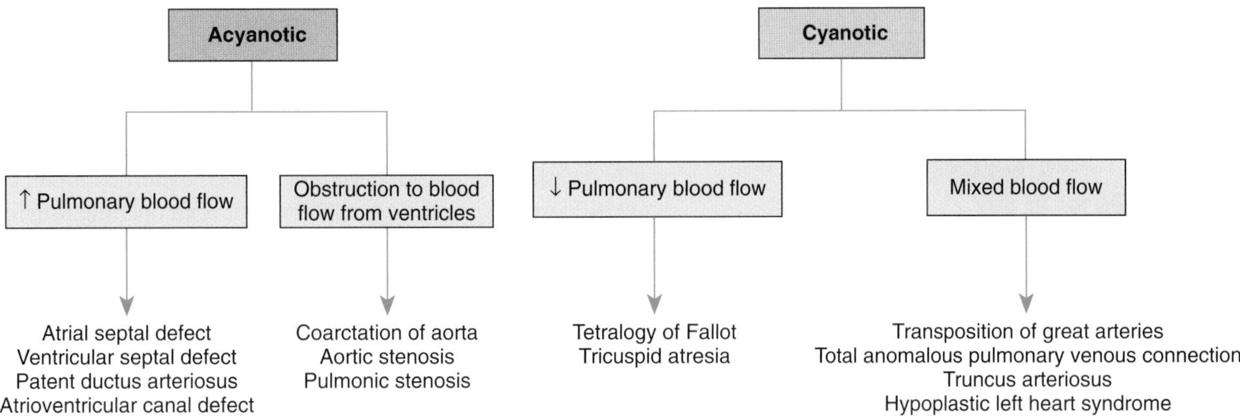

Fig. 33.1 Classification Systems for Congenital Heart Disease. Individual diseases are discussed later in this chapter. (From Hockenberry MJ, Wilson D. *Wong's nursing care of infants and children*, 10th edition. St. Louis: Mosby; 2016.)

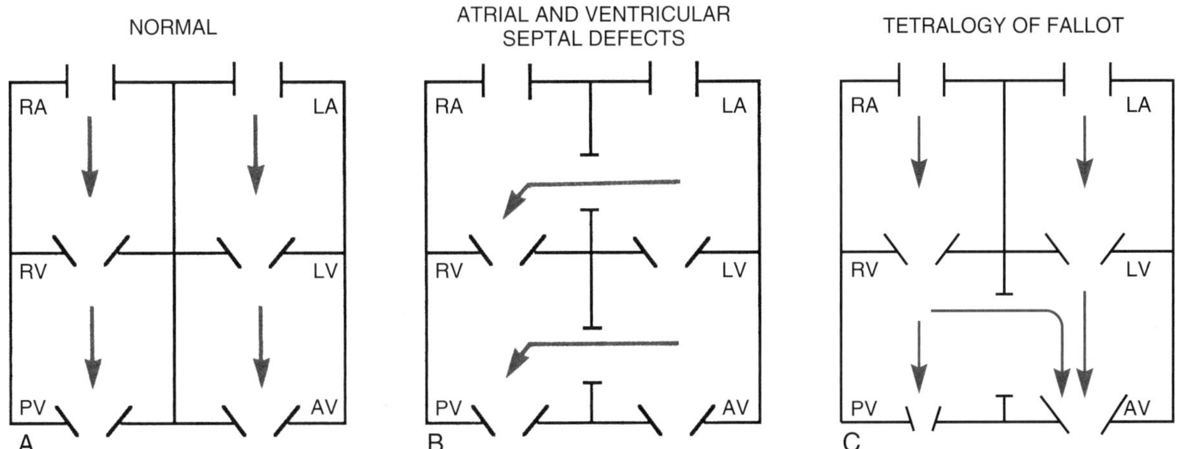

Fig. 33.2 Shunting of Blood in Congenital Heart Disease. (A) Normal. **(B)** Acyanotic defect. **(C)** Cyanotic defect. *AV*, Aortic valve; *LA*, left atrium; *LV*, left ventricle; *PV*, pulmonic valve; *RA*, right atrium; *RV*, right ventricle. (From Hockenberry MJ, Wilson D. *Wong's nursing care of infants and children*, 10th edition. St. Louis: Mosby; 2016.)

blood cause the DA to undergo muscle contraction and functionally close. Normally by the third week after birth, fibrous proliferation of the intimal layer causes permanent closure of the DA. Premature infants, neonates who suffer asphyxia, and infants born at higher altitudes have lower blood oxygen concentrations and therefore are more susceptible to PDA.

In PDA, the persistent patency of the DA allows blood to flow from the higher pressure aorta to the lower pressure PA, causing the blood to flood the lungs (left-to-right shunt). The amount of shunting determines the clinical manifestations. PDA can be classified into five different types (A-E), dependent on anatomical characteristics of the defect and the associated degree of obstruction. This is important in determining the urgency and type of management.[7]

Clinical Manifestations. Infants may be asymptomatic or show signs of pulmonary distress, such as dyspnea and tachypnea, fatigue, poor feeding or diaphoresis with feeding, and failure to thrive (FTT). There is a characteristic continuous, machinery-like murmur in both systole and diastole, heard best at the left upper sternal border. There can be a thrill to palpation. Aortic flow (run-off) into the lower pressure pulmonary circulation produces low diastolic blood pressure, widened pulse pressure, and bounding pulses. In preterm infants, PDA is associated with an increased risk for bronchopulmonary dysplasia, especially if they require prolonged intubation and mechanical ventilation (see Chapter 36).[8] Children are at risk for bacterial endocarditis and may develop chronic lung disease and pulmonary hypertension in later life from chronic excessive pulmonary blood flow.

Evaluation and Treatment. The diagnosis of PDA is confirmed by echocardiography. Administration of intravenous indomethacin or ibuprofen (nonsteroidal anti-inflammatory drugs [NSAIDs]) has proved successful in closing a PDA in premature infants and some newborns. Surgical closure of the PDA is indicated only when pharmacologic therapy has failed. There is evidence that successful surgical closure

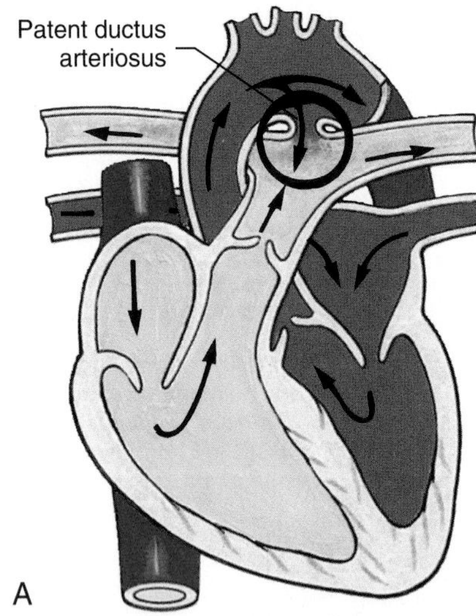

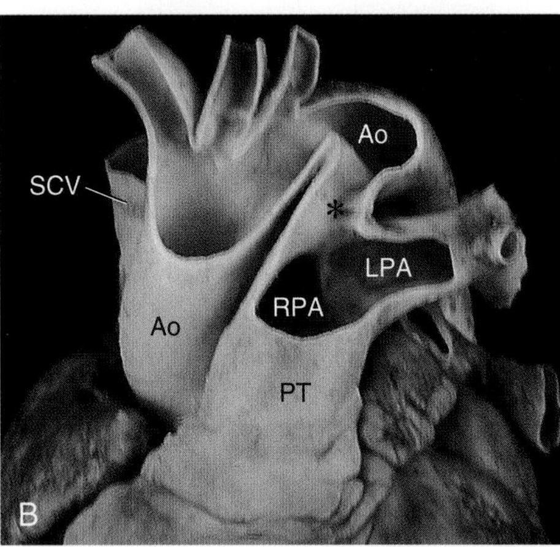

Fig. 33.3 Patent Ductus Arteriosus (PDA). (A) PDA with left-to-right shunt. **(B)** PDA *(asterisk)* in an adult with pulmonary hypertension. *Ao*, Aorta; *LPA*, left pulmonary artery; *RPA*, right pulmonary artery; *SCV*, subclavian vein. (A, From Hockenberry MJ, Wilson D. *Wong's nursing care of infants and children*, 10th edition. St. Louis: Mosby; 2016. B, From Damjanov I, Linder J, eds. *Anderson's pathology*, 10th edition. St. Louis: Mosby; 1996.)

in children at about 6 months of age is associated with a decreased risk for the development of chronic lung disease.[9] Closure of the PDA with an occlusion device during cardiac catheterization is performed in select children older than 6 months of age.[7] Both surgical and transcatheter procedures are considered low risk.[3] Transcatheter closure has also been performed successfully in premature infants, although more studies are needed.[10]

Atrial Septal Defect

Anatrial septal defect (ASD) is an opening in the septal wall between the two atria. This opening allows blood to shunt from the left atrium (LA) to the right atrium (RA) (Fig. 33.4). It is a common form of CHD and carries significant mortality and morbidity if not treated early.

Pathophysiology. There are three types of ASDs:

- Ostium primum atrial septal defect is an opening low in the atrial septum and may be associated with abnormalities of the mitral valve or atrioventricular canal (AVC).
- Ostium secundum atrial septal defect is an opening in the middle of the atrial septum and is the most common type.
- Sinus venosus atrial septal defect is an opening usually high in the atrial wall near the junction of the superior vena cava. In rare cases, the sinus venosus ASD opening may be located in the atrial wall near the junction of the inferior vena cava.

Another type of abnormal opening in the atrial septal wall is called a patent foramen ovale (PFO). Like the DA, the foramen ovale is part of normal fetal circulation and serves to bypass the pulmonary circulation in utero, usually closing after birth. When the lungs become functional, the pulmonary pressure decreases and the LA pressure exceeds that of the RA. This pressure change forces the septum to functionally close the foramen ovale. If it does not close, PFO results, and shunting from the LA to RA persists. In many types of CHD, the foramen ovale remains open as a component of more complex cardiac defects.[3]

Clinical Manifestations. Infants and children with an ASD are usually asymptomatic. If the ASD is not too large, nearly half will close spontaneously.[11] Infants with a large ASD may develop pulmonary overcirculation. In these infants, excessive pulmonary blood flow from left-to-right shunting causes dyspnea and tachypnea symptoms, commonly referred to as heart failure (HF). A systolic ejection murmur and a widely split-second heart sound (reflecting RV volume overload) are the expected findings on physical examination. Some older children and adults will experience shortness of breath with activity as the RV becomes less compliant with age. About 24% of adults have an asymptomatic PFO that does not require treatment, although clot formation and embolization to the brain may occur (cryptogenic stroke).

Evaluation and Treatment. The diagnosis of ASD is confirmed by echocardiography. Surgical closure requires open heart surgery and involves a pericardial patch or suture closure of the defect. Transcatheter device closure offers a less invasive alternative for children with an ASD that meets anatomic and size criteria.[12] Perioperative complications are common but are usually minor. Arrhythmias or complete heart block may occur.

Ventricular Septal Defect

A ventricular septal defect (VSD) is an opening of the septal wall between the ventricles (Fig. 33.5). VSDs are one of the most common types of congenital heart defects and account for 10% to 40% of all CHDs.[13]

Pathophysiology. VSDs are classified by location. Perimembranous ventricular septal defects are located high in the ventricular septal wall underneath the atrioventricular (AV) valves. Muscular ventricular septal defects are located low in the septal wall. VSDs also can be located in the inlet (AV canal type) or the outlet (also called subpulmonary or supracristal) portion of the ventricle. VSDs are similar to ASDs in that blood will shunt from left to right. The amount of shunting depends on the size of the defect. Depending on the size and

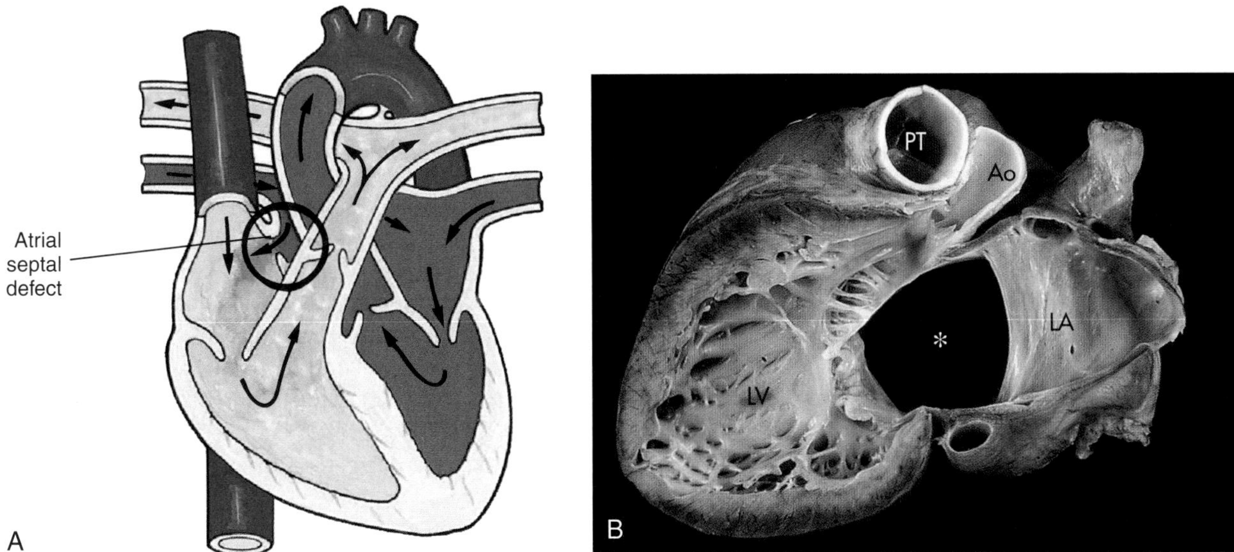

Fig. 33.4 Atrial Septal Defect. (A) Abnormal opening between the atria causing blood from the higher-pressure left atrium to flow into the lower-pressure right atrium. **(B)** Complete ASD *(asterisk)* form in children. *Ao,* Aorta; *LA,* left atrium; *LV,* left ventricle; *PT,* pulmonary artery trunk. (A, From Hockenberry MJ, Wilson D. *Wong's nursing care of infants and children,* 9th edition. St. Louis: Mosby; 2011. B, From Damjanov I, Linder J, eds. *Anderson's pathology,* 10th edition. St. Louis: Mosby; 1996.)

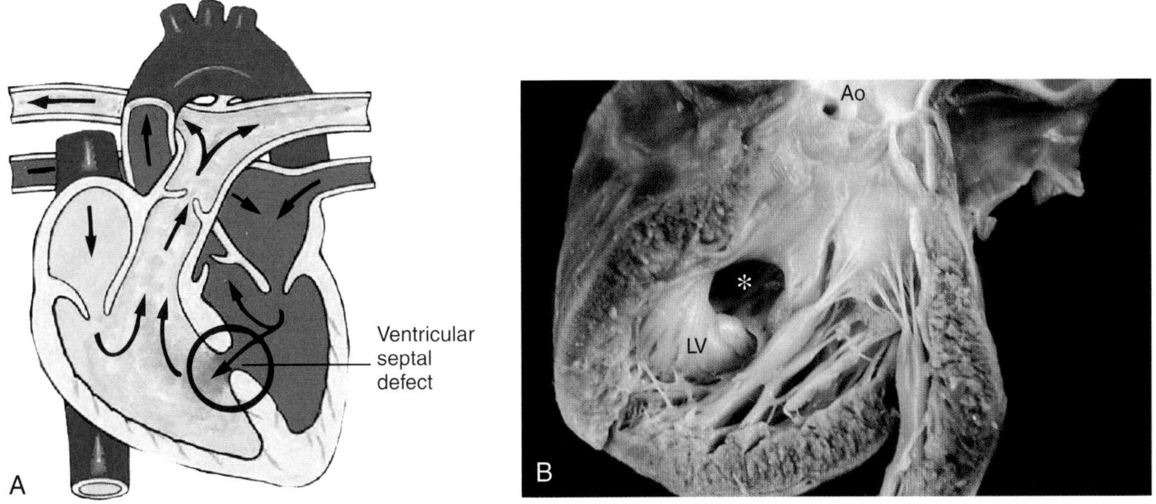

Fig. 33.5 Ventricular Septal Defect (VSD). (A) VSD with left-to-right shunt. **(B)** Muscular *(asterisk)* defect (opened left ventricle). *Ao,* Aorta; *LV,* left ventricle. (A, From Hockenberry MJ, Wilson D. *Wong's nursing care of infants and children,* 9th edition. St. Louis: Mosby; 2011. B, From Damjanov I, Linder J, eds. *Anderson's pathology,* 10th edition. St. Louis: Mosby; 1996.)

location, many VSDs close spontaneously, most often within the first 2 years of life.[3]

Clinical Manifestations. Depending on the size, location, and degree of shunting and pulmonary vascular resistance (PVR), children may have no symptoms, or they may have clinical evidence of excessive pulmonary blood flow. In the infant, excessive pulmonary blood flow from left-to-right shunting causes heart failure (HF), even though the heart muscle functions well with a VSD. In addition to dyspnea and tachypnea, these infants can have poor feeding, diaphoresis with feeding, and FTT. A loud, harsh, holosystolic (pansystolic) murmur and systolic thrill (a palpable tremor) is a classic finding on physical examination.

If the degree of shunting is significant and not corrected, the child is at risk for developing pulmonary hypertension. This condition develops over decades of life in response to the excessive pulmonary blood flow. Irreversible pulmonary hypertension can result in Eisenmenger syndrome, in which shunting of blood is reversed because of high pulmonary pressure and resistance; it results in a right-to-left shunt with cyanosis.

Evaluation and Treatment. The diagnosis of VSD is confirmed by echocardiogram and auscultatory findings. Cardiac catheterization may be needed to determine the hemodynamics and, in some instances, the location of other defects. Smaller VSDs require minimal treatment and may close completely or become small enough that surgical closure is not required. If the infant has severe HF or FTT that is unmanageable with medical therapy, early surgical repair is performed. Surgical repair involves open-heart surgery with cardiopulmonary bypass. The opening is either sutured closed or covered with a patch of pericardium or artificial material. Minimally invasive surgical closure techniques are proving effective and with a low incidence of adverse events.[14] Nonsurgical device closure in the catheterization laboratory is available, but only under restricted conditions, depending on the size and location of the defect.[15]

Atrioventricular Canal Defect

Atrioventricular canal (AVC) defect (atrioventricular septal defect, endocardial cushion defect) is the result of incomplete fusion of endocardial cushions (Fig. 33.6). Endocardial cushions fuse to form the septa that divide the four heart chambers and the mitral and tricuspid valves. When they do not develop properly, several types of AVC defects may occur. AVC is associated with extracardiac defects in about 75% of cases and is a common cardiac defect in children with trisomy 21 (Down syndrome).[16]

Pathophysiology. Complete AVC (CAVC) defect consists of an ostium primum ASD, an inlet VSD, and a single common five leaflet mitral and tricuspid valve. Partial AVC (PAVC) defect consists of an ostium primum ASD and a cleft in the mitral valve. The direction and pathways of flow are determined by pulmonary and systemic resistance, LV and RV pressures, the type of AVC defect, and the compliance of each chamber. Shunting is generally from left to right.

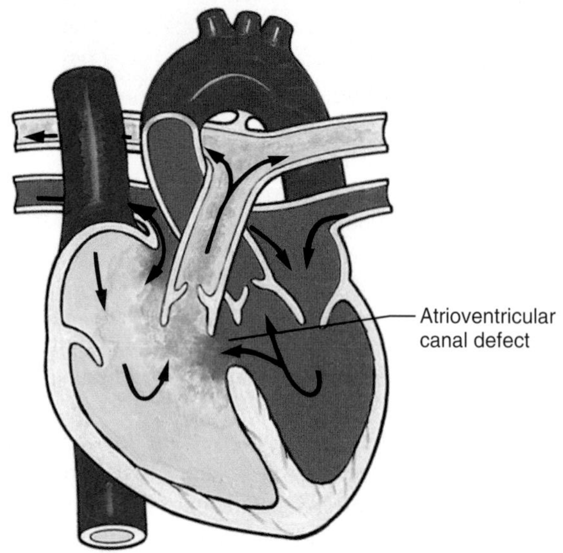

Fig. 33.6 Atrioventricular Canal (AVC) Defect. (From Hockenberry MJ, Wilson, D. *Wong's essentials of pediatric nursing*, 10th edition. St. Louis: Mosby; 2016.)

Clinical Manifestations. Infants and children with PAVC may have minimal symptoms. Infants with CAVC often display moderate to severe HF symptoms attributable to left-to-right shunting and pulmonary overcirculation. These include tachypnea and tachycardia, poor feeding, diaphoresis with feeding, and FTT. Those with a large left-to-right shunt will have a holosystolic murmur. Children with CAVC are at risk for developing irreversible pulmonary hypertension if the condition is left untreated.[3] Children with Down syndrome and CAVC are at a higher risk for developing pulmonary hypertension at a younger age.[17] Therefore, surgical correction of CAVC in these children is recommended by 4 months.[18]

Evaluation and Treatment. AVC is diagnosed with fetal echocardiography. Cardiac catheterization is rarely indicated but may be performed to evaluate the reversibility of pulmonary vascular disease. Initial treatment goals include aggressive medical management of HF and nutritional supplementation. Infants are followed closely for signs or symptoms of FTT. Complete surgical repair is indicated in most cases and typically is performed between 3 and 6 months of age to prevent irreversible pulmonary hypertension. This procedure consists of patch closure of the septal defects and reconstruction of the AV valve tissue (either repair of the mitral valve cleft or fashioning of two AV valves). Postoperative complications include heart block, dysrhythmias, mitral regurgitation and/or stenosis, or left ventricular outflow tract obstruction (LVOTO) requiring further surgical intervention or valve replacement.

Obstructive Defects

Coarctation of the Aorta

Coarctation of the aorta (COA) is an abnormal localized narrowing of the aorta just proximal to the insertion of the ductus arteriosus (Fig. 33.7). It is one of the most common types of CHD and commonly occurs along with other congenital valvular or septal defects.[19]

Pathophysiology. Before birth, the ductus arteriosus bypasses the obstruction caused by COA and allows for blood to flow from the PA into the distal aorta. However, once the ductus functionally closes within hours after birth, blood flow is restricted by the coarctation, preventing adequate perfusion of the systemic circulation including the lower extremities and organs. The left ventricle experiences increased resistance to systolic ejection (afterload) and undergoes hypertrophy that may lead to eventual heart failure. Clinically, there is increased blood pressure proximal to the defect (head and upper extremities, right greater than left) and decreased blood pressure distal to the obstruction (torso and lower extremities). If the COA goes undiagnosed, the child will develop collateral circulation in order to bypass the obstruction. These are small vessels arising from the subclavian arteries that join the intercostal arteries and flow into the descending aorta. Because of this, some cases of coarctation are not diagnosed until school age, adolescence, or adulthood and result in hypertension.

Clinical Manifestations. The location and severity of the COA determine whether an infant will become symptomatic

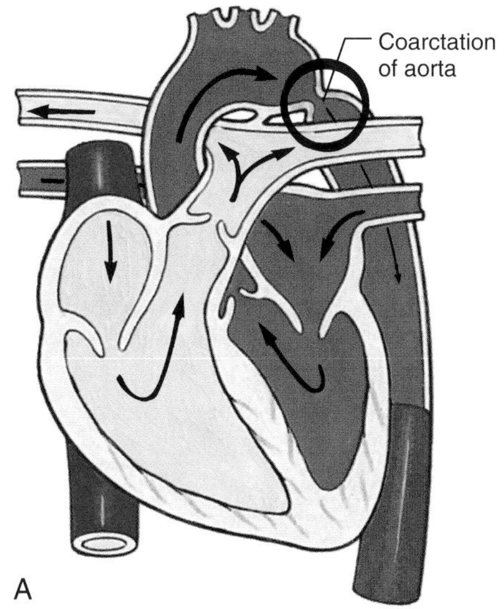

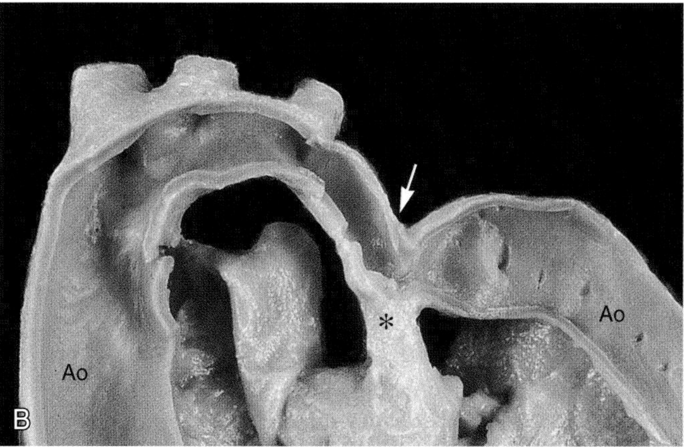

Fig. 33.7 **Postductal and Preductal Coarctation of the Aorta (COA).** **(A)** Postductal coarctation occurs distal to ("after") the insertion of the closed ductus arteriosus into the aortic arch. Preductal coarctation occurs proximal to ("before") the insertion of the patent ductus arteriosus. The coarctation consists of a flap of tissue that protrudes from the tunica media of the aortic wall. **(B)** Coarctation of the aorta with typical indentation of the aortic wall *(arrow)* opposite the ductal arterial ligament *(asterisk). Ao,* Aorta. (A, From Hockenberry MJ, Wilson, D. *Wong's essentials of pediatric nursing,* 10th edition. St. Louis: Mosby; 2016. B, From Damjanov I, Linder J, eds. *Anderson's pathology,* 10th edition. St. Louis: Mosby; 1996.)

after the ductus arteriosus closes. If the COA is severe, infants will present with low cardiac output, poor tissue perfusion, acidosis, and hypotension. Physical examination of the infant will reveal weak or absent femoral pulses. Some infants with COA will remain asymptomatic after the closure of the ductus arteriosus and will present later in childhood with unexplained upper extremity hypertension. Although rare, they also may experience dizziness, headaches, fainting, or epistaxis from hypertension. Children may complain of leg pain or cramping with exercise. Physical examination and measurement of upper and lower extremity blood pressures will often suggest the diagnosis. Children with COA have decreased or absent pulses in the lower extremities and a delay between the brachial and femoral pulses. In addition, they may have a systolic ejection murmur at the left interscapular area caused by turbulent blood flow through the narrowed portion of the aorta.

Evaluation and Treatment. Echocardiography is used to confirm the diagnosis. Magnetic resonance imaging (MRI) and computed tomography (CT) are used for surgical planning. In children with severe COA and shock, immediate initiation of continuous intravenous infusion of prostaglandin E_1 is imperative to maintain patency of the ductus arteriosus. These infants may require mechanical ventilation and vasoactive support pre-operatively. Once the symptomatic newborn is stabilized, emergent surgical correction is indicated. In an older child who has developed collateral circulation, symptoms of cardiogenic shock or end-organ dysfunction are absent and prostaglandin is not indicated. Surgical timing is urgent but not emergent.

Surgical correction consists of either resection of the narrowed portion of the aorta with an end-to-end anastomosis (a surgical connection between vessels), aortic arch augmentation, or enlargement of the constricted section using a portion of the left subclavian artery (commonly named the "subclavian flap"). Because this defect is outside the heart and pericardium, cardiopulmonary bypass is usually not required, and the operation is performed via a thoracotomy incision. However, COA repair may be part of a more complex operation, which would require a sternotomy incision and cardiopulmonary bypass. Postoperative hypertension is treated with an intravenous, short-acting β-blocker, followed by oral medications, such as an angiotensin-converting enzyme (ACE) inhibitor. Residual hypertension after the repair of COA seems to be related to increased age prior to repair; therefore, surgical intervention is recommended at the time of diagnosis.

Percutaneous balloon angioplasty to dilate the aorta, with or without stent implantation, may be a less invasive option for treating COA in selected individuals (infants older than 6 months of age) or for reducing residual postoperative COA. However, aortic aneurysm formation and blood vessel injury from arterial access can be complications of the procedure and may require surgical correction.[19]

Aortic Stenosis

Aortic stenosis (AS) is a narrowing or stricture of the outlet of the LV, causing resistance of blood flow from the LV into the aorta (Fig. 33.8). It commonly is the result of a bicuspid aortic valve. AS is a common form of congenital heart disease found in approximately 0.5% to 0.8% of the population.[20]

Pathophysiology. The pathophysiologic consequence of severe AS is hypertrophy of the LV wall, which eventually leads to increased LV end-diastolic pressure. Pressure backs up from the LV into the LA, causing pulmonary hypertension and pulmonary edema. If severe, there may be decreased cardiac output and poor perfusion of the systemic arterial circulation. Left ventricular hypertrophy impedes coronary artery perfusion and may result in myocardial ischemia and associated papillary muscle dysfunction leading to mitral insufficiency.

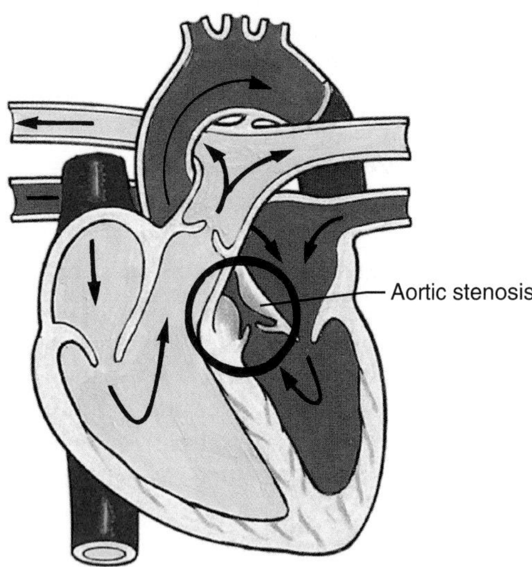

Fig. 33.8 Aortic Stenosis (AS). Narrowing of the aortic valve causes resistance to blood flow in the left ventricle, decreased cardiac output, left ventricular hypertrophy, and pulmonary congestion. (From Hockenberry MJ, Wilson, D. *Wong's essentials of pediatric nursing*, 10th edition. St. Louis: Mosby; 2016.)

There are three types of AS:

- Valvular aortic stenosis occurs because of malformed or fused cusps, resulting in a unicuspid or bicuspid valve. Valvular AS is a serious defect because the obstruction tends to be progressive. There may be sudden episodes of myocardial ischemia or low cardiac output that result in sudden death in late childhood or adolescence.
- Subvalvular aortic stenosis is a stricture caused by a fibrous ring below a normal valve or by a narrowed LV outflow tract in combination with a small aortic valve annulus (diameter at the base of the aortic root).
- Supravalvular aortic stenosis, a narrowing of the aorta just above the valve, occurs infrequently. It can occur as a single defect or as a part of Williams-Beuren syndrome, which also is characterized by an unusual elfin facial appearance and intellectual disability.[21]

Clinical Manifestations. Infants with severe AS demonstrate signs of decreased cardiac output, with faint pulses, hypotension, tachycardia, and poor feeding. These infants may progress to cardiogenic shock and evidence of end-organ hypoperfusion. A loud, harsh systolic ejection murmur is expected. In valvular AS, there may be an audible click during LV ejection as the stenosed valve partially opens. Many children with mild or moderate AS do not have symptoms. Older children may have complaints of epigastric pain and exercise intolerance. In rare cases, exertional chest pain, syncope, or sudden death may occur.

Evaluation and Treatment. A diagnosis of AS is confirmed by echocardiography. Treatment for subvalvular AS and supravalvular AS usually involves surgical excision of the area causing the constriction. Management of valvular AS depends on its severity. Mild to moderate valvular AS does not usually require intervention or restriction of activity, whereas more severe AS requires restriction of strenuous physical activity until correction of the stenosis is accomplished. The treatment of severe valvular AS varies. Dilation of the stenotic valve with balloon valvuloplasty is performed in the cardiac catheterization laboratory. This procedure avoids initial surgical intervention, but more than one-third of cases will require surgery for valve replacement within the next 6 years.[22] Surgical treatment for valvular AS depends on the severity of the stenosis, previous interventions, and the age of the child. Aortic valve commissurotomy (incision at the edges of the commissure, or joining point) or valvotomy may be used as an early intervention.[23] Both balloon valvuloplasty and valvotomy may result in significant aortic regurgitation (insufficiency) requiring valve replacement.[24] Aortic valve replacement may be done using a Ross procedure. This procedure involves replacing the aortic valve with the child's own pulmonary valve, then replacing the pulmonary valve with a cadaver allograft.[25] Mechanical valve replacement may be required if the valve is severely abnormal. If possible, mechanical valve replacement is usually deferred to minimize the number of valve replacements over a child's life related to growth. Aortic stenosis requires lifelong evaluation and treatment. Multiple surgical or catheterization interventions are expected.[3]

Pulmonic Stenosis

Pulmonic stenosis (PS) is a narrowing or stricture of the pulmonary valve that causes resistance to blood flow from the RV into the PA (Fig. 33.9). It is commonly associated with other congenital cardiac defects.

Pathophysiology. Similar to AS, the PS can be valvular, subvalvular, or supravalvular. In PS, the narrowed valve orifice increases the RV afterload and the RV myocardium hypertrophies. If the obstruction is severe, pressure may back up into the RA, causing atrial dilation. If there is a PFO or ASD, a right-to-left shunt may develop (cyanotic heart defect). Pulmonary atresia is an extreme form of PS, with total fusion of the valve leaflets (blood cannot flow to the lungs). Pulmonary atresia is usually associated with a hypoplastic RV and, sometimes, a VSD. In infants with severe pulmonary stenosis or pulmonary atresia without PFO or VSD, pulmonary blood flow and therefore oxygenation is dependent upon a PDA.[26]

Clinical Manifestations. Most infants are asymptomatic if the PS is mild to moderate. Newborns with severe PS or pulmonary atresia will be cyanotic (from a right-to-left shunt through an ASD) and may have signs of decreased cardiac output. A harsh systolic murmur, ejection click, and a thrill at the upper left sternal border is expected with PS.

Evaluation and Treatment. Echocardiography confirms the diagnosis and determines the severity of the PS. Mild PS is usually not progressive and often does not require intervention. Critical PS must be addressed immediately. Infants with severe PS or pulmonary atresia require continuous intravenous infusion of prostaglandin E_1 to keep the DA open and to maintain pulmonary blood flow and oxygenation. The treatment of choice for infants with moderate to severe PS is balloon angioplasty (see Fig. 33.9B).[27] This procedure is considered highly effective in reducing the pressure gradient across the pulmonic valve. In rare cases, surgical valvotomy may be required. Both valvotomy and balloon angioplasty may result in pulmonary valve incompetence, and long-term follow-up may reveal the

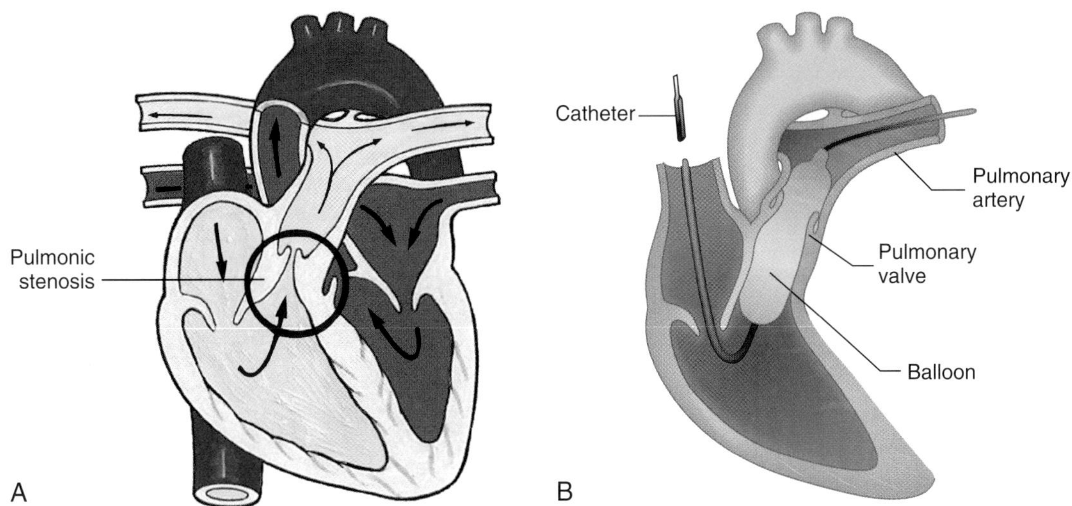

Fig. 33.9 Pulmonic Stenosis (PS). **(A)** The pulmonary valve narrows at the entrance of the pulmonary artery. **(B)** Balloon angioplasty is used to dilate the valve. A catheter is inserted across the stenotic pulmonic valve into the pulmonary artery, and a balloon at the end of the catheter is inflated while it is positioned across the narrowed valve opening. (A, From Hockenberry MJ, Wilson, D. *Wong's essentials of pediatric nursing*, 10th edition. St. Louis: Mosby; 2016.)

need for pulmonary valve replacement. Treatment for pulmonary atresia depends on the size of the pulmonary arteries, the size of the right ventricle, and whether there are associated cardiac defects. Initial treatment may consist of an aortopulmonary shunt to supply stable blood flow to the lungs and, later, a second procedure to connect the RV to the PA.

Defects With Decreased Pulmonary Blood Flow

Tetralogy of Fallot

Tetralogy of Fallot (TOF) occurs in 5% to 10% of all CHD and is the most common cyanotic heart defect. The classic form of TOF consists of four defects: (1) a large VSD, (2) PS, (3) an overriding aorta that straddles the VSD, and (4) RV hypertrophy (Fig. 33.10).

Pathophysiology. The pathophysiology associated with TOF varies widely, depending primarily on the degree of PS, the size of the VSD, and the pulmonary and systemic resistance to flow. In cases with a large VSD, pressures are equal in the RV and LV. Therefore, the major determinant of shunt direction through the VSD is the difference between pulmonary vascular resistance and systemic vascular resistance. If systemic resistance is more than pulmonary resistance, the shunt is from left to right (acyanotic; known as "pink tets"). If resistance to pulmonary flow is greater than systemic resistance, the shunt is from right to left, causing decreased pulmonary blood flow, decreased oxygen in the blood, and cyanosis. Physiologic compensation for low oxygen saturation (hypoxemia) in the systemic circulation is the production of more red blood cells (polycythemia), the development of collateral bronchial vessels, and enlargement of the nail beds (clubbing).

Clinical Manifestations. Some infants may be acutely cyanotic at birth. In others, the progression of hypoxia and cyanosis may be more gradual over the first year of life as the pulmonary stenosis worsens. The typical heart murmur of TOF is a pulmonary systolic ejection murmur caused by the obstruction in the outflow tract of the RV, which creates turbulence during systole. The enlarged RV may cause the left side of the chest to be more prominent, and a "heave" also may be palpated. Acute episodes of cyanosis and hypoxia can occur, called *hypercyanotic spells* or *"tet" spells*. Hypercyanotic spells (increased right-to-left shunt) may occur during crying, exertion, or after feeding.

Evaluation and Treatment. The diagnosis is confirmed with echocardiography. Additionally, chest radiograph shows the heart to be shaped like a boot (upturned apex because of small PA). Diagnostic cardiac catheterization is rarely indicated, except to define unusual coronary artery anatomy crossing the RV outflow tract that may complicate surgical palliation.

Management of hypercyanotic spells is aimed at decreasing the pulmonary vascular resistance and increasing the systemic vascular resistance to help promote left-to-right shunting. Therefore, placing the infant in a knee-chest position and administering oxygen and morphine sulfate are most commonly used to treat hypercyanotic spells. Older children with unrepaired TOF will use squatting to help with cyanosis because it increases peripheral vascular resistance (e.g., the knee-chest position). If prolonged or frequent, these spells are an indication for prompt evaluation and surgical treatment.

Elective pulmonary balloon valvuloplasty performed before 6 months of age in those with acyanotic TOF can delay surgical repair.[28] Indications for earlier surgical repair include increasing cyanosis or the development of hypercyanotic spells. Complete repair involves closure of the VSD, resection of the infundibular stenosis, and application of a pericardial patch to enlarge the RV outflow tract that can extend across the PV annulus (transannular patch). This repair may be done by full primary repair, which is associated with fewer reinterventions, or by staged repair, which is associated with less early mortality and morbidity.[29] Despite the greater risk for surgical mortality, early complete

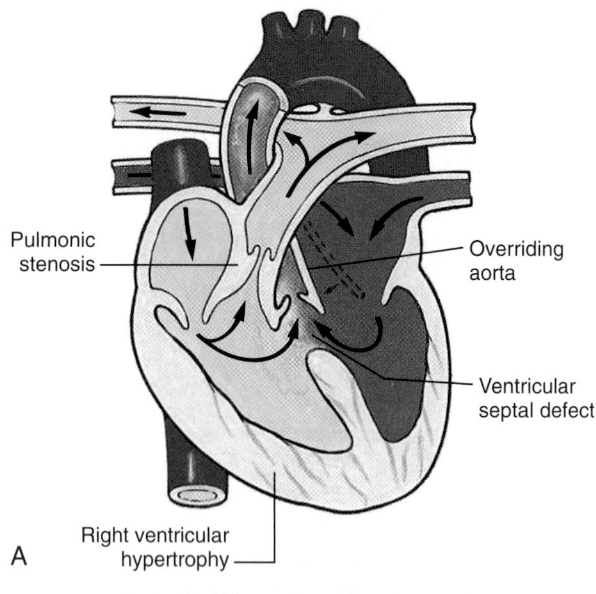

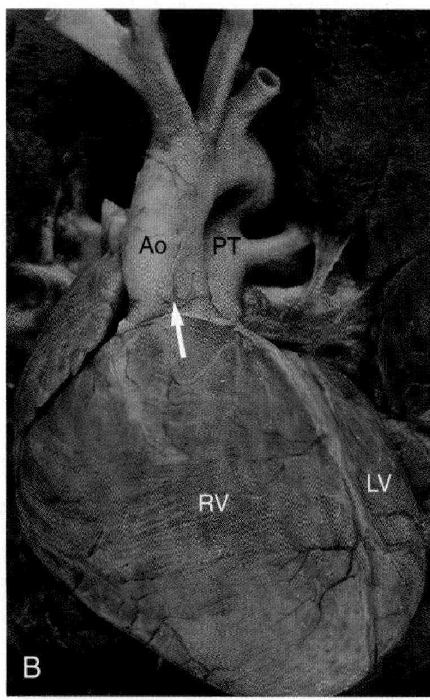

Fig. 33.10 Tetralogy of Fallot (TOF). (A) TOF hemodynamics. **(B)** Right ventricular *(RV)* hypertrophy and overriding aorta *(Ao, arrow). LV,* Left ventricle; *PT,* pulmonary artery trunk. (A, From Hockenberry MJ, Wilson, D. *Wong's essentials of pediatric nursing,* 10th edition. St. Louis: Mosby; 2016. B, From Damjanov I, Linder J, eds. *Anderson's pathology,* 10th edition. St. Louis: Mosby; 1996.)

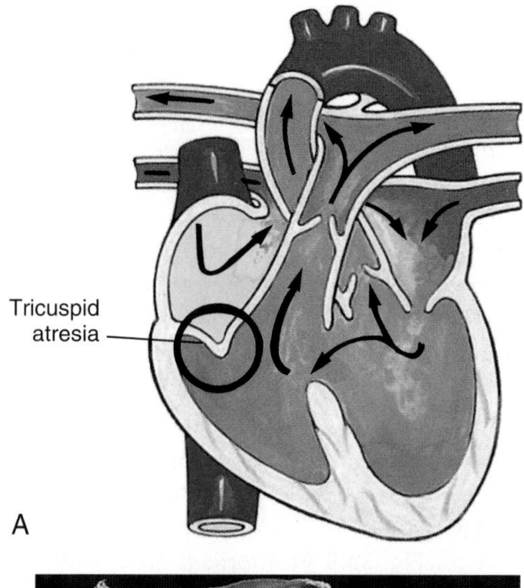

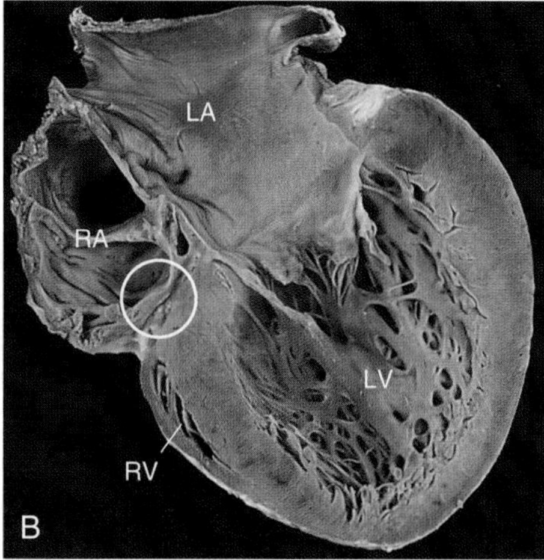

Fig. 33.11 Tricuspid Atresia. (A) Tricuspid atresia hemodynamics. **(B)** Small right ventricle *(RV)* slit of ventricular septal defect; left ventricle *(LV)* is enlarged. *LA,* Left atrium; *RA,* right atrium. (A, From Hockenberry MJ, *Wilson D. Wong's essentials of pediatric nursing,* 10th edition. St. Louis: Mosby; 2016. B, From Damjanov I, Linder J, eds. *Anderson's pathology,* 10th edition. St. Louis: Mosby; 1996.)

surgical repair is associated with survival rates to age 5 as high as 92%.[30] In a staged approach, the first stage is the placement of a palliative shunt from the subclavian or innominate artery to the PA, known as the *modified Blalock-Taussig* (using a prosthetic graft) or *classic Blalock-Taussig* (using the native subclavian artery) in order to increase pulmonary blood flow. This is done within the first few days of life and is followed at 2 to 6 months of age by the next surgical phase to achieve complete repair. Depending on the size of the pulmonary outflow tract, transcatheter pulmonary valve replacement can be a less invasive treatment for severe pulmonary insufficiency in selected individuals, and transcatheter techniques for total repair are being studied.[31] Children with tetralogy of Fallot remain at risk for lethal cardiac arrhythmias and right ventricular dysfunction even decades after the initial repair; therefore, continued monitoring of these individuals is indicated.[32]

Tricuspid Atresia

Tricuspid atresia is failure of the tricuspid valve to develop; consequently, there is no communication from the RA to the RV (Fig. 33.11). It accounts for approximately 1% of all new cases of CHD, and incidence is similar in both males and females. Risk factors for tricuspid atresia include trisomy 21, poorly controlled diabetes and excess alcohol consumption during pregnancy, and a family history of CHD.[33] Tricuspid atresia is associated with other defects including septal defects, hypoplastic or absent RV, enlarged MV and LV, and/or varying degrees of pulmonic stenosis.

Pathophysiology. In tricuspid atresia, deoxygenated blood returning to the RA flows through an ASD or a PFO to the LA. From there, the blood enters the LV and either goes into the systemic circulation through the aorta or through a VSD into the hypoplastic RV and into the lungs.[33] There is mixing of deoxygenated and oxygenated blood in the left side of the heart, resulting in systemic hypoxemia and mild cyanosis. Depending on the degree of PS and the size of the RV, a PDA is necessary to ensure blood flow into the pulmonary circulation. A PFO is required to maintain cardiac output due to lack of communication between the RA and RV.

Clinical Manifestations. Approximately half of affected children with tricuspid atresia will present with symptoms within the first day of life, and 80% by 1 month of age.[33] A murmur and cyanosis often are present in the newborn period. Tachycardia, dyspnea, fatigue, and poor feeding may be noted with excessive pulmonary blood flow and the development of HF. Older children may have signs of chronic hypoxemia with polycythemia and clubbing. Depending on the other defects associated with tricuspid atresia, the abnormal heart sounds heard on auscultation will have several components. The VSD causes a systolic regurgitant murmur which will be softer and shorter as the VSD enlarges. The second heart sound may be narrowly split due to decreased pulmonary blood, or only a single heart sound heard if PS or pulmonary atresia is present.

Evaluation and Treatment. Echocardiogram confirms the diagnosis of tricuspid atresia and may reveal the presence of associated defects. Pulse oximetry reveals hypoxemia. The neonate with PDA is treated with a continuous infusion of prostaglandin E_1 to maintain adequate pulmonary blood flow.[33] If the ASD is restrictive, a balloon atrial septostomy (creation of a hole between the atria) is performed during cardiac catheterization or under echocardiographic guidance at the bedside. Treatment is accomplished in staged procedures. First, the newborn gets a modified Blalock-Taussig shunt (subclavian or innominate artery to the PA) to supply blood flow to the lungs. Conversely, if the child is experiencing increased pulmonary blood flow, a PA band may be required.[33] Further surgery occurs between 4 to 8 months of age using the bidirectional Glenn shunt, in which the superior vena cava is anastomosed to the PA, the PA is tied off, and the shunt or PA band from the first procedure is removed. Finally, at 2 to 4 years of age, the pulmonary circulation is fully separated from the systemic circulation via a Fontan procedure, which is the routing of the inferior vena cava blood flow to the PA through a grafted or artificial tube called a conduit. Postoperative complications that prolong a hospital stay include pleural effusions, elevated pulmonary vascular resistance, and ventricular dysfunction. Exercise tolerance is limited in many children, and careful monitoring is needed throughout childhood.[34]

Mixing Defects

Transposition of the Great Arteries

In dextro-transposition of the great arteries (dTGA), the great vessels arise from the incorrect ventricles: the PA leaves the LV and the aorta exits the RV (Fig. 33.12). This is called ventriculoarterial discordance. dTGA is a cyanotic heart defect that accounts for 5% to 7% of all CHD.[35]

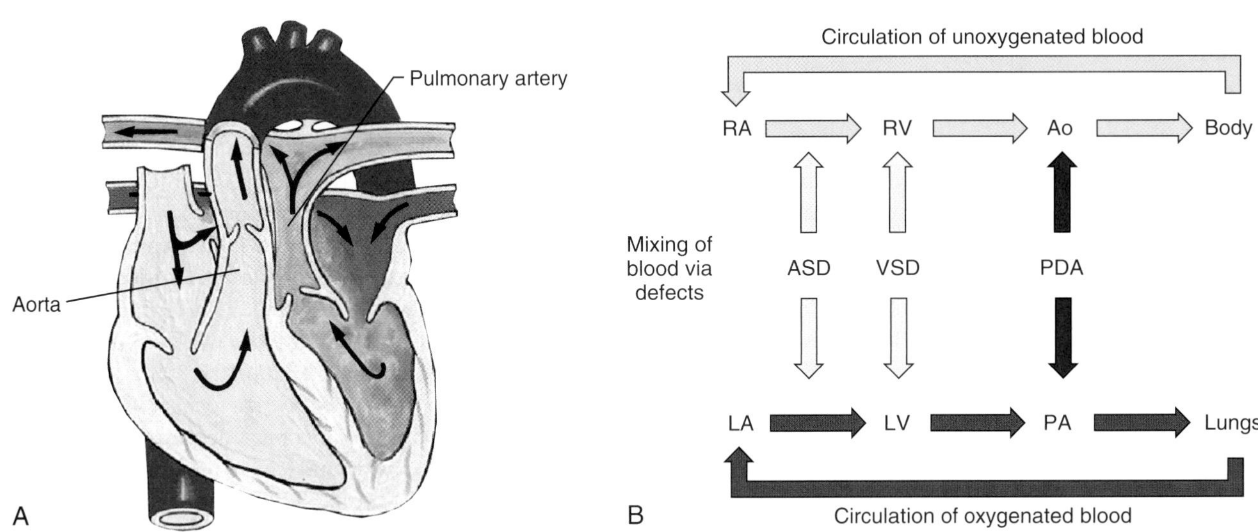

Fig. 33.12 Hemodynamics in Dextro-Transposition of the Great Arteries (dTGA). **(A)** Complete transposition of the great arteries with an intact interventricular septum. The aorta arises from the right ventricle and the pulmonary artery from the left ventricle. **(B)** Oxygen saturation in the separate, parallel circuits with transposition of the great vessels (TGV). Mixing of blood occurs only with the defects associated with TGV. *Ao*, Aorta; *ASD*, atrial septal defect; *LA*, left atrium; *LV*, left ventricle; *PA*, pulmonary artery; *PDA*, patent ductus arteriosus; *RA*, right atrium; *RV*, right ventricle; *VSD*, ventricular septal defect. (A, From Hockenberry MJ, Wilson D. *Wong's essentials of pediatric nursing*, 10th edition. St. Louis: Mosby; 2016.)

Pathophysiology. Because of the transposition of the PA onto the LV and the aorta onto the RV, there are two separate, parallel circuits in which deoxygenated blood circulates continuously through the systemic circulation and oxygenated blood circulates repeatedly through the pulmonary circulation. Associated defects, such as ASD, VSD, or PDA, permit mixing of saturated and desaturated blood, which is necessary to survive after birth and helps maintain adequate tissue oxygenation for a limited time.[36]

Clinical Manifestations. The degree of mixing permitted by the associated defects determines the type and severity of clinical manifestations. Children with limited communication between cardiac chambers are severely cyanotic, acidotic, and critically ill at birth. Those with large septal defects or a PDA may be less cyanotic but will develop heart failure if left untreated. Classically, no murmur is heard unless there is an associated VSD.[3]

Evaluation and Treatment. On chest radiograph, the heart has a characteristic shape, like an "egg on a string," with increased pulmonary vascular markings. Typically, the diagnosis is suspected from the physical examination and chest radiograph findings before confirming with echocardiography. Administration of intravenous prostaglandin E_1 to maintain the patency of the PDA is needed to increase oxygen delivery until the presence and size of associated defects can be determined. Enlargement of the PFO by balloon atrial septostomy may be performed during cardiac catheterization or under echocardiographic guidance at the bedside to increase mixing at the atrial level if a VSD is not present.

The preferred type of surgical repair for dTGA performed in the first days of life is the *arterial switch operation*, which involves

- transecting the great arteries and anastomosing the main PA to the native proximal aorta (just above the aortic valve) and anastomosing the ascending aorta to the native proximal PA, and,
- moving and reimplanting the coronary arteries with a *button* of tissue onto the new aortic outflow.

Reimplantation of the coronary arteries is critical to survival. The arterial switch procedure reestablishes normal circulation in series, with the LV acting as the systemic pump. Potential complications of the arterial switch include narrowing at the great artery surgical anastomosis sites, aortic valve regurgitation, or coronary artery insufficiency resulting in myocardial ischemia. Long-term results for the arterial switch operation are usually good, with overall long-term survival as high as 80%.[37] However, persistent LV myocardial stiffening and fibrosis can be detected in adolescents and adults.[38] Depending on the anatomy and severity of dTGA, other procedures, such as atrial switch surgery, may be chosen with similar positive outcomes.[39]

Total Anomalous Pulmonary Venous Connection

Total anomalous pulmonary venous connection (TAPVC), or *total anomalous pulmonary venous return (TAPVR)*, is characterized by failure of the pulmonary veins to join the LA during cardiac development (Fig. 33.13). It is a rare form of CHD.

Pathophysiology. In TAPVC, the pulmonary venous return is connected to the right side of the circulation rather than to the LA. The type of TAPVC is classified according to the location of pulmonary venous return connection:

- *Supracardiac:* Attachment above the diaphragm, usually to the superior vena cava via vertical or innominate vein (most common form)
- *Cardiac:* Direct attachment to the heart, usually to the RA or coronary sinus
- *Infracardiac:* Attachment below the diaphragm, such as to the inferior vena cava or portal or hepatic vein (most severe and least common form)
- *Mixed:* A combination of the various types[40]

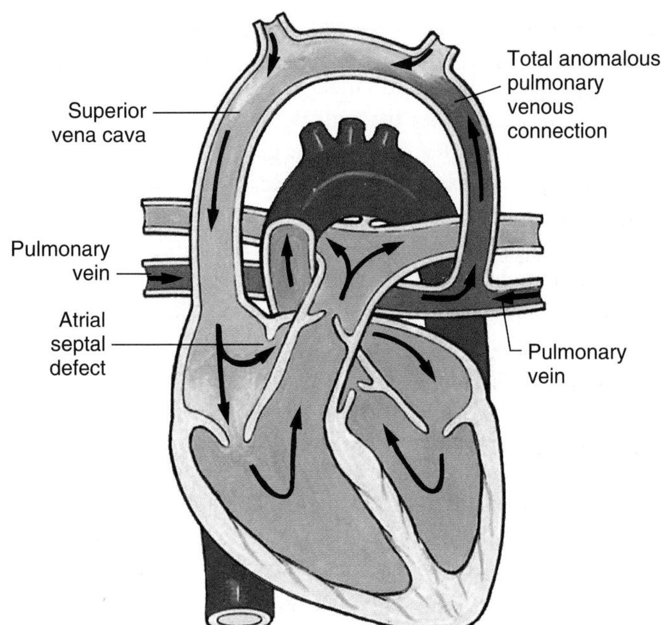

Fig. 33.13 Total Anomalous Pulmonary Venous Connection (TAPVC).

Physiologically, TAPVC can be differentiated into two groups: nonobstructive and obstructive, depending on the absence or presence of obstruction to the pulmonary venous drainage. In nonobstructive TAPVC, the RA receives all the blood that normally would flow into the LA. The presence and size of an associated ASD or PFO will determine the amount of blood that will shunt from the RA to the left side of the heart. If there is little communication between the atria, more blood will go to the RV than the LA, and there will be increased pulmonary blood flow, resulting in pulmonary edema as well as right heart enlargement. In the obstructive form of TAPVC, obstruction to pulmonary venous drainage decreases blood flow into the pulmonary circulation and leads to severe cyanosis and low cardiac output. Infracardiac TAPVC often is associated with obstruction of pulmonary venous drainage and has a higher mortality than the unobstructed types.

Clinical Manifestations. Cyanosis is the predominant clinical manifestation. The degree of cyanosis is inversely related to the amount of pulmonary blood flow. Children with unobstructed TAPVC may be asymptomatic until pulmonary vascular resistance decreases during infancy, causing increased pulmonary blood flow and signs and symptoms of pulmonary overcirculation. In obstructed TAPVC, cyanosis is severe and the infant's condition deteriorates rapidly, necessitating immediate surgical intervention, or death will occur. Murmur is not a common feature of TAPVC.

Evaluation and Treatment. Chest radiograph will reveal cardiomegaly and increased pulmonary vascular markings. In supracardiac TAPVC, the heart may have a snowman appearance. The diagnosis is typically confirmed with echocardiography but may require confirmative angiography. Timing of corrective repair depends on whether there is obstruction to pulmonary venous return. In nonobstructive types of TAPVC, repair can be delayed until early infancy. If there is obstruction, surgical repair is emergent. In general, the surgical approach consists of anastomoses of the common pulmonary vein to the LA, the ASD is partially closed, and the vertical vein (if present) may be ligated.[40] Potential complications include re-obstruction at the anastomosis site, atrial dysrhythmias, PA hypertension, and LV dysfunction. Long term survival is generally above 90% for those without significant postoperative pulmonary venous obstruction.[41]

Truncus Arteriosus

Truncus arteriosus (TA) is failure of normal septation and division of the embryonic outflow tract into a PA and an aorta, resulting in a single vessel that exits the heart, providing both pulmonary and systemic blood flow (Fig. 33.14). It is a rare form of cyanotic CHD and often is associated with 22q11.2 deletion syndrome.[42]

Pathophysiology. In TA, the common vascular trunk created by the lack of division between the PA and aorta has a single valve with either three or four leaflets. This valve may exhibit regurgitation, stenosis, or both. A VSD is always present and allows for mixing of the systemic and arterial circulations causing some degree of cyanosis. Once ejected from the heart, blood flows preferentially to the lower pressure PAs, causing increased pulmonary blood flow, although this can be altered due to the presence of other defects such as PS. The four types of TA are:

- *Type I:* A single pulmonary trunk arises near the base of the truncus and divides into the left and right PAs
- *Type II:* The left and right PAs arise separately from the posterior aspect of the truncus
- *Type III:* The PAs arise independently and from the lateral aspect of the truncus
- *Type IV:* The bronchial arteries arise from the descending aorta, also known as pseudotruncus

Types I and II constitute 85% of cases, with types III and IV comprising the remainder of cases.

Clinical Manifestations. Physical findings depend on the amount of pulmonary blood flow and the presence of other cardiac anomalies. If PS is present, a newborn will present with cyanosis. Conversely, if PS is not present, the newborn initially will have mild cyanosis and moderate HF. A harsh systolic regurgitant murmur is usually present along the left sternal border as a result of the VSD, and a systolic click at the apex and left upper sternal border indicating opening of the truncal valve.

Evaluation and Treatment. Chest radiograph will reveal cardiomegaly with biventricular and LA enlargement as well as increased pulmonary vascular markings. Conversely, if PS is present, heart size will be normal with decreased pulmonary vascular markings. The diagnosis is made by echocardiography. Corrective repair is performed in the first few days or weeks of life. It involves closing the VSD so that the blood flow from the LV outflow tract goes into the truncus, and excising the PAs from the aorta and attaching them to the RV through a tissue homograft (cadaver conduit).[42] Initial postoperative complications include dysrhythmias, truncal valve stenosis or insufficiency, and pulmonary hypertension.[43] Despite these potential complications, the overall uncomplicated 20-year survival after successful repair is over 75%.[44]

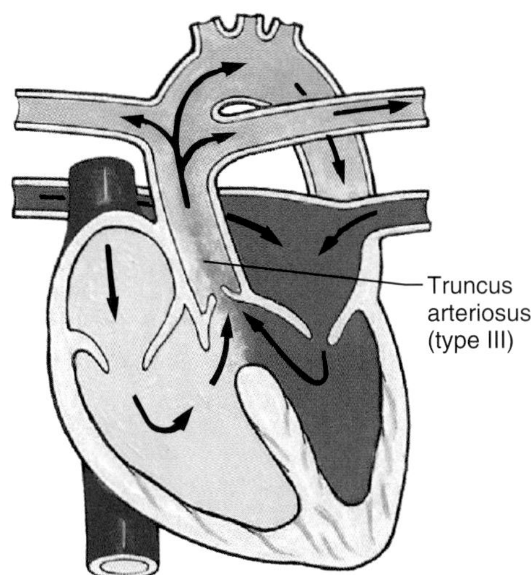

Fig. 33.14 Truncus Arteriosus (TA). The TA fails to divide into the pulmonary artery and aorta, and the interventricular septum fails to close at the top. Blood from both ventricles mixes in the TA and then enters the pulmonary and systemic circuits. (From Hockenberry MJ, Wilson D. *Wong's Essentials of Pediatric Nursing.* 10th ed. St Louis: Mosby; 2016.)

Hypoplastic Left Heart Syndrome

Hypoplastic left heart syndrome (HLHS) is abnormal development of the left side of the heart resulting in anatomic and functional inadequacy of the left ventricle to perform systemic perfusion.[45] Features include underdevelopment of the LV, aorta, and aortic arch, as well as small or absent mitral and aortic valves (Fig. 33.15).

Pathophysiology. In HLHS, most blood from the LA flows across the PFO to the RA, to the RV, and out the PA. A PDA then allows for blood to go to the descending aorta. The amount of blood that travels to the pulmonary and systemic circulation depends on the vascular resistance in each circuit. Retrograde blood flow from the PDA into the hypoplastic ascending aorta provides coronary and cerebral blood flow. Based on this, the presence of both an ASD or PFO and a PDA is critical for survival after birth.

Clinical Manifestations. HLHS may be detected by fetal echocardiogram. It presents in the early newborn period as mild cyanosis, tachypnea, and low cardiac output. Support of the systemic circulation is accomplished with prostaglandin E_1

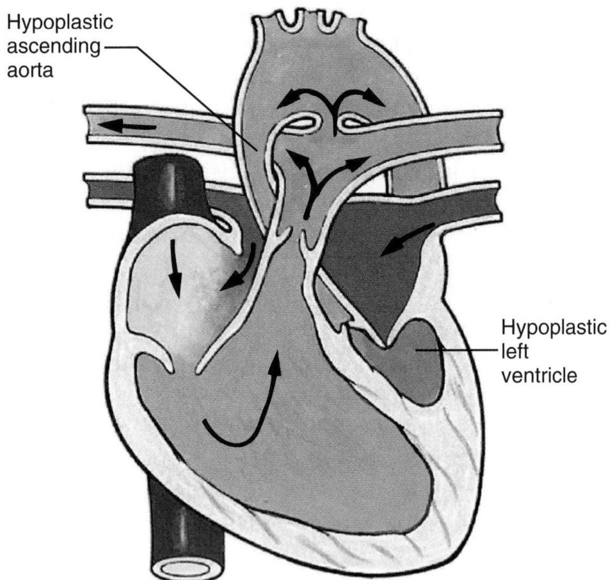

Fig. 33.15 Hypoplastic Left Heart Syndrome (HLHS). (From Hockenberry MJ, Wilson D. *Wong's essentials of pediatric nursing,* 10th edition. St. Louis: Mosby; 2016.)

infusion to maintain flow through the DA. If there is not an adequate ASD or PFO, immediate interventional cardiac catheterization or echocardiography-guided balloon atrial septostomy is needed. If HLHS is not suspected and the DA closes, there is progressive deterioration with cyanosis and decreased cardiac output, leading to cardiovascular collapse. If left untreated, HLHS is usually fatal in the first days of life due to shock and organ failure secondary to inadequate cardiac output and oxygen delivery.

Evaluation and Treatment. Echocardiography shows all the features of HLHS. Chest radiography shows cardiomegaly and increased pulmonary vascular congestion. Surgical intervention is a staged approach to provide pulmonary blood flow and relieve the work of the RV.[45] This includes:

- *Norwood procedure:* Anastomosis of the main PA to the aorta to create a new aorta (or neo-aorta), construction of shunt to provide pulmonary blood flow (either *modified Blalock-Taussig* shunt or RV-PA conduit), and creation of a large ASD. This is performed in the first few days of life.
- *Bidirectional Glenn procedure:* Anastomosis of the superior vena cava to the PA and ligation of previously placed shunt. This is completed around 4 months of life.
- *Fontan procedure:* Routing of the inferior vena cava blood flow to the PA with a grafted or artificial tube. This occurs at approximately 3 years of age.

Another option for high-risk infants with HLHS and other comorbidities, such as prematurity, is the Hybrid Stage I palliation. This involves placement of bilateral PA bands to restrict pulmonary blood flow and stenting of the PDA to provide stable systemic blood flow. The individual then undergoes the second and third stage of surgical interventions listed previously. Postoperative complications are different for each surgical intervention, although the development of heart failure is a risk at any point. Infants who are not candidates for staged procedures are offered palliative care. Heart transplantation may be possible for some individuals. While there are improved survival rates because of advances in surgical and medical technology, many infants and children with this complex CHD have long-term liver fibrosis, osteoporosis, and neurodevelopmental disabilities.[45] Research into stem-cell and gene therapies are showing promise (see Emerging Science Box: Stem Cell Therapies for Congenital Heart Disease).[46]

ACQUIRED CARDIOVASCULAR DISORDERS

Acquired heart diseases refer to disease processes or abnormalities that occur after birth. They result from various causes, such as congenital heart disease, infection, genetic disorders, autoimmune processes in response to infection, environmental factors, or autoimmune diseases. Examples of acquired heart diseases include heart failure, Kawasaki disease, systemic hypertension, myocarditis, rheumatic heart disease, and cardiomyopathy. This chapter discusses heart failure, Kawasaki disease, and systemic hypertension in children. Myocarditis, rheumatic heart disease, and cardiomyopathy are discussed in Chapter 32.

EMERGING SCIENCE BOX

Stem Cell Therapies for Congenital Heart Disease

Complex congenital heart defects such as COA, TGA, TOF, and HLHS are often termed "Critical Congenital Heart Defects." In the United States, approximately 25% of congenital heart defects fall into this category annually. These conditions have a shorter life expectancy than many other forms of CHD and/or have more long-term complications in survivors. In an effort to improve outcomes for these disorders, stem cell therapies are being studied. Most clinical trials have used mesenchymal stem cells (MSCs), autologous umbilical cord blood cells, or tissue-engineered stem cell grafts. MSCs have the ability to transform into functional cardiomyocytes and can contribute to myocardial repair and the growth of new blood vessels. Autologous umbilical cord blood cells have been used less often, but results from recent research trials look promising. Stem cells are introduced via intracoronary perfusion, or more commonly, by direct injection or implantation into the myocardium. Most successful studies have involved the use of stem cells for treatment of HLHS. For example, a recent study injected autologous umbilical cord blood-derived mononuclear cells directly into the right ventricular myocardium during the second stage of surgery for HLHS. Results show the procedure is safe, and continuing research into efficacy is ongoing. The current goal of cell-based therapies is to serve as an adjunct to surgery by maintaining right ventricular function and contributing to improved morbidity and mortality.

Data from Brown MA, et al. Update on stem cell technologies in congenital heart disease. *Journal of Cardiac Surgery,* 2020;35(1):174–179; Burkhart HM, et al. Autologous stem cell therapy for hypoplastic left heart syndrome: Safety and feasibility of intraoperative intramyocardial injections. *Journal of Thoracic and Cardiovascular Surgery,* 2019;158:1614–1623; Martinez J, et al. Safety and efficacy of cell therapies in pediatric heart disease: a systematic review and meta-analysis. *Stem Cell Research Therapy,* 2020;11(1):272; Friedman KG, et al. Fetal cardiac interventions: Where do we stand? *Archives of Cardiovascular Disease,* 2020;113:121–128; Saraf A, et al. Hypoplastic left heart syndrome: From bedside to bench and back. *Journal of Molecular Cell Cardiology,* 2019;135:109–118.

Heart Failure

Heart failure (HF) occurs when the heart is unable to maintain sufficient cardiac output to meet the metabolic demands of the body. It is a common complication of many congenital heart defects.[47] The likely etiology of new-onset HF is determined by the age of diagnosis. For example, HF that results from CHD with pulmonary overcirculation from a large left-to-right shunt is common in newborns and infants (Table 33.3), whereas HF in older children is most often due to acquired disorders such as viral myocarditis, rheumatic heart disease, autoimmune disorders, anemia, Kawasaki disease, and hypothyroidism.[48]

Pathophysiology. HF in children is most often a result of pulmonary venous hypertension and pulmonary venous congestion either from pulmonary overcirculation or LV dysfunction. RV failure is rare in childhood. The pathophysiology of HF due to pulmonary overcirculation that results from CHD is discussed earlier in this chapter. In LV dysfunction, the pathophysiologic mechanisms of HF in infants and children are similar to those in adults (see Chapter 32). Compensatory mechanisms, including the sympathetic nervous system and the renin-angiotensin-aldosterone system, are activated in the face of inadequate cardiac output. These hormones result in myocardial remodeling, LV hypertrophy, interstitial fibrosis, and changes in calcium handling in the sarcoplasmic reticulum and contractile proteins, resulting in direct cardiotoxicity.[47]

TABLE 33.3 Congenital Heart Defects Causing Heart Failure

Age	Congenital Heart Defect
Time of birth	HLHS Volume overload caused by tricuspid regurgitation (rare) AV fistula
Birth to 1 week	HLHS Aortic atresia TGA with VSD COA TAPVC with obstruction PDA in small premature infants
First 4 weeks	COA TAPVC Large left-to-right shunt caused by VSD, PDA in premature infants Tricuspid atresia Persistent TA with large left-to-right shunt All previously mentioned defects
4–6 weeks	TGA with VSD Large left-to-right shunt caused by endocardial cushion defect
6 weeks to 6 months	VSD
6 months	Endocardial fibroelastosis

AV, Arteriovenous; *COA*, coarctation of the aorta; *HLHS*, hypoplastic left heart syndrome; *PDA*, patent ductus arteriosus; *TA*, truncus arteriosus; *TAPVC*, total anomalous pulmonary venous connection; *TGA*, transposition of the great arteries; *VSD*, ventricular septal defect.

Modified from Park MK. *Pediatric cardiology for practitioners*, 6th edition. St. Louis: Mosby; 2014.

Clinical Manifestations. HF in infants is manifested as poor feeding and growth, often leading to FTT. Dyspnea, tachypnea, and diaphoresis may be accompanied by retractions, grunting, and nasal flaring. On physical exam, crackles and wheezing can be auscultated within the lungs, and a gallop is present when assessing heart sounds. Common skin changes, such as pallor or mottling, are often present (Box 33.1). Signs of systemic venous congestion, such as hepatomegaly, weight gain without caloric intake increase, and ascites, can be present but could be suggestive of other medical conditions such as renal or nutritional deficiencies.

Evaluation and Treatment. A thorough physical examination with emphasis on cardiac and pulmonary findings will often reveal the degree of HF. Plotting a child's growth (height, weight, head circumference) is an important method of assessing a child's health. Echocardiography is the gold standard for definitive diagnosis of structural and functional cardiac disease. A chest radiograph is useful in assessing the presence of cardiomegaly and signs of increased pulmonary circulation or pulmonary edema. An electrocardiogram (ECG) also should be performed to determine the presence of dysrhythmia or hypertrophy.

BOX 33.1 Clinical Manifestations of Heart Failure

Impaired Myocardial Function

Tachycardia
Sweating (inappropriate)
Decreased urinary output
Fatigue
Weakness
Restlessness
Anorexia
Pale, cool extremities
Weak peripheral pulses
Decreased blood pressure
Gallop
Cardiomegaly

Pulmonary Congestion

Tachypnea
Dyspnea
Retractions (infants)
Flaring nares
Exercise intolerance
Orthopnea
Cough, hoarseness
Cyanosis
Wheezing (rare)
Grunting

Systemic Venous Congestion

Weight gain
Hepatomegaly
Ascites
Neck vein distention (rare in children)
Peripheral edema (rare)

From Hockenberry MJ, Wilson D. *Wong's nursing care of infants and children*, 10th edition. St. Louis: Mosby; 2015.

HF in infants and children is classified on the basis of cardiac function and structure, which helps to determine treatment choices.[47] Management in pediatrics is extrapolated from adult guidelines as described by a pediatric cardiology taskforce in 2014.[49] Treatment is aimed at decreasing cardiac workload and increasing the efficiency of heart function. ACE inhibitors are the first-line treatment of HF. Aldosterone receptor antagonists improve mortality in children with HF. Digoxin may be used for selected children with left-to-right shunting lesions. In young children with acute HF, there is evidence that epinephrine is more effective than dobutamine in improving cardiac output, and milrinone provides improved contractility while reducing vascular resistance.[50] Diuretics are recommended in those with fluid overload. In severe cases of HF, angiotensin receptor neprilysin inhibitors and ivabradine may be considered.[47] End-stage HF requires anticoagulation, and mechanical circulatory support may be indicated to support the failing myocardium while awaiting cardiac transplantation.[51]

Kawasaki Disease

Kawasaki disease (KD), formerly known as mucocutaneous lymph node syndrome, is an acute systemic vasculitis that may result in myocarditis and coronary artery aneurysms. KD is a leading cause of acquired heart disease among children in the United States, although it remains far more prevalent in Asian countries such as Japan and Korea.[52] KD is primarily a condition of young children, with 80% of cases seen in children younger than 5 years of age, peaking in the toddler age group. Approximately 5% of cases are diagnosed in children 10 years or older whose disease often goes unrecognized until cardiac complications develop. Males are affected slightly more than females. In the United States, black individuals are affected twice as often as white individuals.

Pathophysiology. The etiology of KD remains unknown.[52] Current etiologic theories center on a normal immunologic response to an infectious, toxic, or antigenic substance, or an abnormal immune response to a common stimulus. The predominant theory is a genetic predisposition to the development of autoimmune response to inhaled viruses such as retroviruses, coronaviruses, or Epstein-Barr virus.[53] Dysbiosis of the intestinal microbiome and intestinal permeability may also play a role.

The innate and adaptive immune system responses in KD include the release of multiple inflammatory cytokines, increased serum levels of antibodies, and infiltration of vessel walls by neutrophils, macrophages, and lymphocytes. Additional immune changes include elevated activity of T helper 17 cells (Th17), a decrease in T regulatory cells, and a proliferation of T cytotoxic and B cells (see Chapter 8).[54] A necrotizing arteritis develops with the risk of aneurysm development, especially affecting the coronary arteries. An acute myocarditis also occurs in many individuals. Kawasaki disease progresses pathologically and clinically in these stages:

Stage I (days 1 through 12): Small capillaries, arterioles, and venules become inflamed, as does the heart itself (acute myocarditis).

Stage II (days 13 through 25): Inflammation spreads to larger vessels and aneurysms of the coronary arteries may develop (acute necrotizing vasculitis).

Stage III (days 26 through 40): Medium-sized arteries begin the granulation process which contributes to coronary artery thickening with increased risk for thrombosis.

Stage IV (day 41 and beyond): Myofibroblasts are activated, and vessels develop scarring, intimal thickening, calcification, and stenosis.

The acute myocarditis of KD may progress to left ventricular dysfunction. Fortunately, these pathophysiologic changes

EMERGING SCIENCE BOX

COVID-19 Post-Infective Myocarditis in Children

SARS-CoV-2 infection and resulting COVID-19 is associated with the development of Multisystem Inflammatory Syndrome in Children (MIS-C) (see Chapter 36). In addition to the pulmonary complications associated with MIS-C, injury to the cardiovascular system is common. Post-infective myocarditis can occur in the wake of many viral infections, including those caused by Coxsackievirus B virus, enteroviruses, influenza, rubella, and adenoviruses. However, children with COVID 19 post-infective myocarditis have a clinical picture that generally is more severe. Similar to Kawasaki disease, COVID-19 related MIS-C is recognized as a systemic vasculitis affecting not only the lung but all organs, including the myocardium. While some investigators have postulated that SARS-CoV-2 initiates Kawasaki disease itself, others consider COVID-19 post-infective myocarditis to be a separate entity and point to characteristics that differentiate the two. For example, while the two diseases share fever, rash, cheilitis, and adenopathy, children with COVID 19 are older (mean age 7 years vs. 3 years), have more digestive symptoms, and are more likely to develop shock and severe myocarditis. Similar to Kawasaki disease, children with COVID-19 post-infective myocarditis may develop coronary artery aneurysms. Management of COVID-19 post-infective myocarditis includes supportive therapy with oxygen and diuretics plus ionotropic medications and mechanical hemodynamic support if needed. Intravenous immunoglobulin (IVIG) and antiviral administration is associated with improved outcomes in affected children. The majority of children recover with few if any long term sequelae, including the resolution of coronary aneurysms. However, there is still the possibility of persistent or progressive cardiovascular complications, some of which may go undiagnosed and may result in serious morbidity and mortality later in life (e.g., coronary aneurysms). This has led to emerging recommendations that children who recover from COVID-19 MIS-C should undergo a cardiac evaluation before participating in sports and should be followed for potential cardiac complications into adulthood.

Data from Barach P, et al. Rethinking COVID-19 in children: Lessons learned from pediatric viral and inflammatory cardiovascular diseases. *Progress in Pediatric Cardiology,* 2020;22:101233. Advance online publication; Bordet J, Perrier S, Olexa C, et al. Paediatric multisystem inflammatory syndrome associated with COVID-19: Filling the gap between myocarditis and Kawasaki? *European Journal of Pediatrics,* 2020;21:1–8; Grimaud M, et al. Acute myocarditis and multisystem inflammatory emerging disease following SARS-CoV-2 infection in critically ill children. *Annals of Intensive Care,* 2020;10:69; Matsubara D, et al. Longitudinal assessment of cardiac outcomes of multisystem inflammatory syndrome in children associate with COVID-19 in fections. *J. Am Heart Assoc,* 2022;0:e23251; Riphagen S, et al. Hyperinflammatory shock in children during COVID-19 pandemic. *Lancet,* 2020;395:1607–1608; Tissières P, et al. SARS-CoV-2 post-infective myocarditis: The tip of COVID-19 immune complications? *Ann Intensive Care,* 2020;10:98.

are usually self-limiting and respond well to anti-inflammatory treatment.[53] However, some children present with Kawasaki shock syndrome, which is characterized by hypotension, poor perfusion, hyponatremia, coagulopathy, and anemia.[52] KD myocarditis is similar to that being seen in association with pediatric coronavirus disease 2019 (COVID-19) infection (see Emerging Science Box: COVID-19 Post-Infective Myocarditis in Children). Coronary artery aneurysms resulting from the necrotizing vasculitis occur in up to 25% to 30% of untreated children with Kawasaki disease, and early treatment is crucial to preventing this complication.[52] These aneurysms occur most frequently in males and those who either receive treatment late (after 10 days) or who are resistant to treatment.[55]

Clinical Manifestations. KD progresses in three stages (acute, subacute, and convalescent):

- *Acute phase*: The child with classic or typical KD has fever, conjunctivitis, oral changes ("strawberry" tongue), rash, erythema of the palms and soles, and lymphadenopathy, and is often irritable. During this phase, myocarditis in addition to vasculitis may develop.
- *Subacute phase*: Begins when the fever ends and continues until the clinical signs have resolved. It is at this time that the child is most at risk for coronary artery aneurysm development. Desquamation (skin peeling) of the palms and soles occurs at this time, as well as marked thrombocytosis.
- *Convalescent phase*: This phase is marked by the elevation of the erythrocyte sedimentation rate and C-reactive protein level, as well as by an increased platelet count. Arthritis or arthralgia of the joints may be present. This phase continues until all laboratory values return to normal—usually about 6 to 8 weeks after onset.

Evaluation and Treatment. The diagnosis and management of KD is based on guidelines published by the American Heart Association in 2017.[56] Initial diagnosis is made on the basis of clinical features, and the child must exhibit 5 days of fever along with four of five criteria presented in Box 33.2. Other supportive diagnostic findings include leukocytosis, anemia, hypoalbuminemia, increased c-reactive protein, thrombocytosis, and elevated liver enzymes. An echocardiogram is obtained at the time of diagnosis as a baseline measurement to assess for coronary aneurysms or inflammation. Serial echocardiograms are obtained after treatment to assess for the development of coronary aneurysms or regression of those present early in the course of the disease.

Treatment with aspirin and intravenous immunoglobulin during the acute phase significantly decreases the incidence of coronary aneurysms.[52] In severe cases, children may also receive corticosteroids or other anti-inflammatory agents such as infliximab, etanercept, or cyclosporin.[52] Refractory KD is the recurrence or persistence of fever after immunoglobulin infusion and requires retreatment and the use of high-dose anti-inflammatory agents.[52] Aspirin is continued until the manifestations of inflammation are resolved, but it may be used indefinitely in children with residual coronary artery abnormalities. Most children recover completely from KD, including regression of aneurysms. The most common cardiovascular complication is coronary thrombosis with myocardial infarction due to persistent coronary artery aneurysms.

BOX 33.2 Diagnostic Criteria for Kawasaki Disease

Classic KD is diagnosed in the presence of fever for at least 5 days together with at least 4 of the 5 following principal clinical features:

1. Bilateral conjunctival infection without exudation
2. Inflammation of the oral mucous membranes, such as erythema, dryness, and fissuring of the lips; oropharyngeal reddening; or "strawberry tongue"
3. Changes in the extremities, such as peripheral edema, peripheral erythema, and desquamation of the palms and soles, particularly periungual peeling
4. Polymorphous rash, often accentuated in the perineal area
5. Cervical lymphadenopathy (one lymph node >1.5 cm)

Modified from McCrindle BW, Rowley AH, Newburger JW, et al. Diagnosis, treatment, and long-term management of Kawasaki disease: A scientific statement for health professionals from the American Heart Association. *Circulation*, 2017;135:e927–e999.

Pediatric Hypertension

Pediatric hypertension (HTN) affects millions of children worldwide, and the prevalence is increasing, especially in developing countries.[57] Updated criteria for the diagnosis of HTN in children and adolescents was published in 2017 by the American Academy of Pediatrics.[58] Like in adults, blood pressure in children is categorized into Normal, Elevated, Stage 1, HTN, and Stage 2 HTN. For young children, these categories are determined by where the individual's blood pressure falls as a percentile of average readings for healthy children. For adolescents, the criteria for each of these categories is the same as those for adults (see Chapter 32). A summary of normative blood pressure levels for neonates and young children can be found in Table 33.4. Epidemiologic studies estimate that in the United States, up to

TABLE 33.4 Normative Blood Pressure Levels (Systolic/Diastolic Pressure [Mean]) by Dinamap Monitor in Children 5 Years Old or Younger

Age	Mean BP Levels (mm Hg)	90th Percentile	95th Percentile
1–3 days	64/41 (50)	75/49 (50)	78/52 (62)
1 months to 2 years	95/58 (72)	106/68 (83)	110/71 (86)
2–5 years	101/57 (74)	112/66 (82)	115/68 (85)

BP, Blood pressure.
Data from Park MK. *Pediatric cardiology for practitioners*, 6th edition. St. Louis: Mosby; 1989; modified from Park MK, Menard SM. Normative oscillometric blood pressure values in the first 5 years in an office setting. *American Journal of Diseases of Children*, 1989;143:860.

16% of children between the ages of 10 to 17 years have elevated blood pressure, and 2% to 4% have hypertension.[59]

Hypertension is classified into two categories:

- *primary (or essential) hypertension*, in which a specific cause cannot be identified
- *secondary hypertension*, in which a cause can be identified (Box 33.3)

BOX 33.3 Conditions Associated With Secondary Hypertension in Children

Renal Disorders

Congenital defects
- Polycystic kidney, ectopic kidney, horseshoe kidney, etc.
- Obstructive anomalies
- Hydronephrosis

Renal tumor
- Wilms tumor
- Retrovascular tumor

Abnormalities of renal arteries

Renal vein thrombosis

Acquired disorders
- Glomerulonephritis, acute or chronic
- Pyelonephritis
- Nephritis associated with collagen disease

Cardiovascular Disease

Coarctation of the aorta

Arteriovenous fistulae

Patent ductus arteriosus

Aortic or mitral insufficiency

Metabolic and Endocrine Diseases

Adrenal tumors
- Adenoma
- Pheochromocytoma
- Neuroblastoma
- Cushing syndrome
- Adrenogenital syndrome
- Hyperthyroidism
- Aldosteronism
- Hypercalcemia
- Diabetes mellitus

Neurologic Disorders

Space-occupying lesions of cranium (increased intracranial pressure)
- Tumors, cysts, hematoma
- Cerebral edema
- Encephalitis (including Guillain-Barré and Reye syndromes)

Miscellaneous Causes

Drugs (corticosteroids, oral contraceptives, pressor agents, amphetamines)

Burns

Genitourinary surgery

Trauma (e.g., stretching of femoral nerve with leg traction)

Insect bites (e.g., scorpion)

Intravascular overload (blood, fluid)

Hypernatremia

Toxemia of pregnancy

Heavy metal poisoning

From Hockenberry MJ, Wilson D. *Wong's essentials of pediatric nursing*, 10th edition. St. Louis: Mosby; 2015.

HTN in children differs from adult HTN in etiology and presentation. Low birth weight and an adverse intrauterine environment are linked to epigenetic modifications and alterations in renal, vascular, and autonomic functions.[60] Young children, when diagnosed with HTN, are often found to have secondary HTN caused by some underlying disease, such as renal disease or COA (see Box 33.3). An increased prevalence of primary HTN has been linked to the increasing prevalence of obesity and diabetes in children and adolescents. Primary HTN in children has been shown to cause subclinical organ damage, such as increased ventricular mass, carotid artery disease, and microalbuminuria.[61] Emerging data suggests that pediatric hypertension may also result in impaired cognition later in life.[62]

Pathophysiology. Primary hypertension is now the most common form of hypertension in children and adolescents. The pathophysiology of pediatric primary HTN has not been fully elucidated but is believed to result from a combination of modifiable and nonmodifiable risk factors (Algorithm 33.1). Similar to primary HTN in adults, the pathophysiology of pediatric HTN consists of a complex interaction between inflammatory processes, activation of the sympathetic nervous systems, upregulation of the renin-angiotensin-aldosterone system, increased sodium absorption, and increased vascular reactivity with the end result leading to hypertension. Additionally, obesity-linked increases in serum leptin, a hormone produced by adipose tissue, is associated with HTN in obese children.

Clinical Manifestations. Most children with systemic HTN are asymptomatic. Although the United States Preventive Task Force does not recommend routine screening for high blood pressure in children and adolescents, those with high body mass index, family history, or history of potential secondary causes of hypertension are at increased risk.[63] If hypertension is suspected, it is necessary that a thorough history, including family history of HTN and heart disease, as well as physical examination be obtained. The examination should include an accurate blood pressure measurement obtained in the right arm

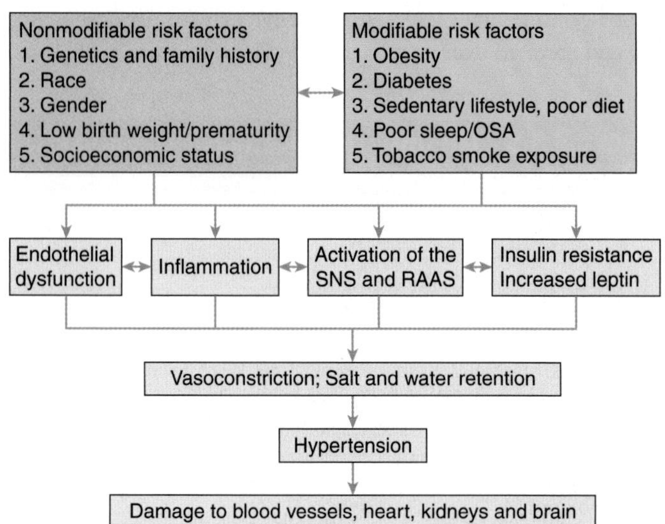

Algorithm 33.1 Proposed Mechanisms of Primary Hypertension in Children. *OSA*, Obstructive sleep apnea; *SNS*, sympathetic nervous system; *RAAS*, renin-angiotensin-aldosterone system.

with the arm supported at the level of the heart; three separate measurements using an appropriate-size cuff also are needed for an accurate blood pressure reading. In neonates, an oscillometric device (e.g., dynamap) should be used, and measurements should be obtained at least 90 minutes after feeding with the infant lying prone or supine.[57]

Evaluation and Treatment. The diagnosis and management of hypertension in children and adolescents is based on guidelines published by the American Academy of Pediatrics in 2017.[58] The history and physical examination should be directed at determining the etiology of HTN, such as COA or renal disease (Table 33.5). For example, blood pressure differences between upper and lower extremities and echocardiogram can be used to identify COA. Table 33.6 includes routine and special laboratory tests for HTN. If HTN is determined to be essential, or primary, in nature, nonpharmacologic therapy is used initially. Moderate weight loss and exercise can decrease systolic and diastolic pressures in many children. Appropriate diet, regular physical activity, and avoidance of smoking have been shown to be effective in reducing blood pressure. Ambulatory blood pressure monitoring has been shown to be more precise in the assessment of blood pressure in children and is more predictive of end-organ damage.[64] Medication therapy is controversial in children with primary HTN; however, when nonpharmacologic therapy fails, the approach is similar to the treatment of HTN in adults with the use of ACE inhibitors, angiotensin receptor blockers, and calcium channel blockers.[58] The current emphasis on preventive cardiology, especially for children, is significant because many investigators believe signs of atherosclerosis are present during childhood.

TABLE 33.5 Most Common Causes of Chronic Sustained Hypertension in Children

Age Group	Causes
Newborn	Renal artery thrombosis, renal artery stenosis, congenital renal malformation, coarctation of the aorta (COA), bronchopulmonary dysplasia
<6 years	Renal parenchymal disease, COA, renal artery stenosis
6–10 years	Renal artery stenosis, renal parenchymal disease, primary hypertension
>10 years	Primary hypertension, renal parenchymal disease

From Park MK. *Pediatric cardiology for practitioners*, 6th edition. St. Louis: Mosby; 2014.

TABLE 33.6 Routine and Special Laboratory Tests for Hypertension

Laboratory Tests	Significance of Abnormal Results
Urinalysis, urine culture, blood urea nitrogen, and creatinine levels	Renal parenchymal disease
Serum electrolyte levels (hypokalemia)	Hyperaldosteronism, primary or secondary Adrenogenital syndrome Renin-producing tumors
ECG, chest x-ray studies	Cardiac cause of hypertension, also baseline function
Intravenous pyelography (or ultrasonography, radionuclide studies, computed tomography of kidneys)	Renal parenchymal diseases Renovascular hypertension Tumors (neuroblastoma, Wilms tumor)
Plasma renin activity, peripheral	High-renin hypertension Renovascular hypertension Renin-producing tumors Some caused by Cushing syndrome Some caused by essential hypertension Low-renin hypertension Adrenogenital syndrome Primary hyperaldosteronism
24-hour urine collection for 17-ketosteroids and 17-hydroxycorticosteroids	Cushing syndrome Adrenogenital syndrome
24-hour urine collection for catecholamine levels and vanillylmandelic acid	Pheochromocytoma Neuroblastoma
Aldosterone	Hyperaldosteronism, primary or secondary Renovascular hypertension Renin-producing tumors
Renal vein plasma renin activity	Unilateral renal parenchymal disease Renovascular hypertension
Abdominal aortogram	Renovascular hypertension Abdominal COA Unilateral renal parenchymal diseases Pheochromocytoma
Intra-arterial digit subtraction angiography	Renovascular hypertension

COA, Coarctation of the aorta; *ECG*, electrocardiogram.
From Park MK. *Pediatric cardiology for practitioners*, 6th edition. St. Louis: Mosby; 2014.

SUMMARY REVIEW

Congenital Heart Disease

1. Congenital heart defects are heart defects present since birth, and some have associated causes, both environmental and genetic.
2. Environmental risk factors associated with the incidence of CHDs typically are maternal conditions and include infections, radiation, metabolic disorders, alcohol or drug intake, and perinatal conditions.
3. Genetic factors associated with congenital heart defects include, but are not limited to, Down syndrome, trisomy 13, trisomy 18, cri du chat syndrome, 22q11 deletion syndrome, and Turner syndrome.
4. Classification of congenital heart defects is based on whether they cause (1) increased pulmonary blood flow, (2) obstruction to flow, (3) decreased pulmonary blood flow, or (4) mixed desaturated and saturated blood within the chambers or great arteries of the heart.
5. Cyanosis, a bluish discoloration of the skin, indicates that the tissues are not receiving normal amounts of oxygenated blood. Cyanosis can be caused by defects that (1) restrict

blood flow into the pulmonary circulation, (2) overload the pulmonary circulation, causing pulmonary overcirculation, pulmonary edema, and respiratory difficulty, or (3) cause large amounts of unoxygenated blood to shunt from the pulmonary to the systemic circulation.

6. Congenital defects that maintain or create direct communication between the pulmonary and systemic circulatory systems cause blood to shunt from one system to another, mixing oxygenated and unoxygenated blood and increasing blood volume and, occasionally, pressure on the receiving side of the shunt.
7. The direction of shunting through an abnormal communication depends on differences in pressure and resistance between the two systems. Direction of shunt blood flow is always from an area of high pressure to an area of low pressure.
8. If the abnormal communication between the left and right circuits is large, volume and pressure overload in the pulmonary circulation can lead to left-sided HF.
9. Acyanotic congenital defects that increase pulmonary blood flow consist of abnormal openings (ASD, VSD, PDA, or AVC) that permit blood to shunt from left (systemic circulation) to right (pulmonary circulation). Cyanosis does not occur because the left-to-right shunt does not interfere with the flow of oxygenated blood through the systemic circulation.
10. An acyanotic defect caused by obstruction of ventricular outflow is commonly caused by PS or AS. In less severe obstruction, ventricular outflow remains normal because of compensatory ventricular hypertrophy stimulated by increased afterload and, in postductal COA, development of collateral circulation around the coarctation.
11. Cyanotic congenital defects in which saturated and desaturated blood mix within the heart or great arteries include TGA, TAPVC, TA, and HLHS.
12. In cyanotic heart defects that decrease pulmonary blood flow (TOF and tricuspid atresia), myocardial hypertrophy cannot compensate for restricted RV outflow. Flow to the lungs decreases, and cyanosis is caused by an insufficient volume of oxygenated blood and right-to-left shunt.
13. The initial treatment for CHD, depending on the defect, is aimed at controlling the level of HF symptoms or cyanosis. Interventional procedures in the cardiac catheterization laboratory and surgical palliation or repair are performed to establish a source of pulmonary blood flow or restore normal circulation.

Acquired Cardiovascular Disorders

1. Heart failure occurs when the heart is unable to maintain sufficient cardiac output to meet the metabolic demands of the body. HF in infants and young children is usually the result of congenital heart defects that increase blood volume in the pulmonary circulation. HF in older children is more often due to LV dysfunction that results from viral myocarditis, rheumatic heart disease, autoimmune disorders, anemia, Kawasaki disease, and hypothyroidism. A clinical manifestation of HF unique to children is FTT.
2. Acquired heart diseases are those that develop after birth. They may result from infection, genetic disorders, autoimmune processes or diseases, or environmental factors.
3. Kawasaki disease (KD) is an acute systemic vasculitis, or inflammation of the blood vessels, that also may result in the development of coronary artery aneurysms and thrombosis if untreated.
4. Systemic hypertension in children differs from HTN in adults in etiology and presentation. When significant HTN is found in young children, they should be evaluated for the presence of secondary HTN, most commonly renal disease or COA.

REFERENCES

1. Wu W, et al. Incidence and mortality trend of congenital heart disease at the global, regional, and national level, 1990–2017. *Medicine (Baltimore)*. 2020;99:e20593.
2. Allen HD, ed. *Moss and Adams' heart disease in infants, children, and adolescents including the fetus and young adults*. ed 9 Philadelphia: Lippincott Williams & Wilkins; 2016.
3. Park MK, Salamat M. *Pediatric cardiology for practitioners*. ed 7: Elsevier; 2021.
4. Unolt M, et al. Congenital heart diseases and cardiovascular abnormalities in 22q11.2 deletion syndrome: from well-established knowledge to new frontiers. *Am J Med Genet A*. 2018;176(10):2087–2098.
5. Martin GR, et al. Updated strategies for pulse oximetry screening for critical congenital heart disease. *Pediatrics*. 2020;146(1):e20191650.
6. Rainsadat A, et al. Chronic disease burden after congenital heart surgery: a 47 year population-based study with 99% follow-up. *JAMA*. 2020;9:9.
7. Brandão LdES, et al. Patent ductus arteriosus: update review. *Cardiol Angiol*. 2020;9(4):5–14. Available at: https://doi.org/10.9734/ca/2020/v9i430140. Accessed January 29. 2022.
8. Clyman RI, et al. Patent ductus arteriosus, tracheal ventilation, and the risk of bronchopulmonary dysplasia. *Pediatr Res*. Published online March 31, 2021. Available at: https://doi.org/10.1038/s41390-021-01475-w. Accessed January 29. 2022.
9. Bussmann N, et al. Patent ductus arteriosus shunt elimination results in a reduction in adverse outcomes: a post hoc analysis of the PDA RCT cohort. *J Perinatol*. 2021;41(5):1134–1141.
10. Garg R, et al. Transcatheter patent ductus arteriosus closure in extremely premature infants. *Progress in Pediatric Cardiology*. 2021;61:101366 Published online February 12, 2021. Available at: https://doi.org/10.1016/j.ppedcard.2021.101366. Accessed January 29. 2022.
11. Sawamura K, et al. Can the atrial septal defect size in newborn patient predict spontaneous closure? *Eur Heart J Cardiovasc Imaging*. 2021;22(Suppl 1):jeaa356.001. Available at: https://doi.org/10.1093/ehjci/jeaa356.001. Accessed January 29, 2022.
12. Han Y, Zhang X, Zhang F. Transcatheter and intraoperative device closure of atrial septal defect in infants under three years of age. *J Cardiothorac Surg*. 2020;15:9.
13. Cox K, et al. The natural and unnatural history of ventricular septal defects presenting in infancy: an echocardiography-based review. *J Am Soc Echocardiogr*. 2020;33:763–770.
14. Ren C, et al. Minimally invasive closure of transthoracic ventricular septal defect: postoperative complications and risk factors. *J Cardiothorac Surg*. 2021;16:30.

15. Mijangos-Vázquez R, et al. Transcatheter closure of perimembranous ventricular septal defects using different generations of amplatzer devices: multicenter experience. *J Intervent Cardiol.* 2020;2020:8948249. Available at: https://doi.org/10.1155/2020/8948249. Accessed January 29, 2022.
16. Pugnaloni F, et al. Genetics of atrioventricular canal defects. *Ital J Pediatr.* 2020;46:61.
17. Alhuzaimi AN, et al. Congenital heart defect and pulmonary hypertension in children with Down syndrome: clinical profile over two decades. *Cureus.* 2021;13(2):e13212.
18. Saji T. Clinical characteristics of pulmonary arterial hypertension associated with Down syndrome. *Pediatr Int.* 2014;56(3):297–303.
19. Cribbs MG. Coarctation: a review. *US Cardiol.* 2019;13:99–104.
20. Ancona R, Pinto SC. Epidemiology of aortic valve stenosis (AS) and of aortic valve incompetence (AI): Is the prevalence of AS/AI similar in different parts of the world? *e-Journal of Cardiology Practice.* 2020;18(10). European Society of Cardiology. Available at: https://www.escardio.org/Journals/E-Journal-of-Cardiology-Practice/Volume-18/epidemiology-of-aortic-valve-stenosis-as-and-of-aortic-valve-incompetence-ai. Accessed January 29, 2022.
21. Kumar P, et al. Williams-Beuren syndrome: the role of cardiac CT in diagnosis. *Methodist Debakey Cardiovasc J.* 2020;16:61–64.
22. Vergnat M, et al. Aortic stenosis of the neonate: a single-center experience. *J Thorac Cardiovasc Surg.* 2019;157:318–326. e1.
23. Buratto E, Konstantinov IE. Aortic valve surgery in children. *J Thorac Cardiovasc Surg.* 2021;161(1):244–250.
24. Saung MT, et al. Outcomes following balloon aortic valvuloplasty versus surgical valvotomy in congenital aortic valve stenosis: a meta-analysis. *J Invasive Cardiol.* 2019;31:E133–E142.
25. Buratto E, et al. Ross procedures in children with previous aortic valve surgery. *J Am Coll Cardiol.* 2020;76:1564–1573.
26. Gottschalk I, et al. Severe pulmonary stenosis or atresia with intact ventricular septum in the fetus: the natural history. *Fetal Diagn Ther.* 2020;47:420–428.
27. Camell MV, et al. Percutaneous management of pulmonary atresia with intact ventricular septum and critical pulmonary stenosis. *An Pediatr (Barc).* 2019;91:336–343.
28. Muneuchi J, et al. Early palliative balloon pulmonary valvuloplasty in neonates and young infants with tetralogy of Fallot. *Heart Vessels.* 2020;35(2):252–258.
29. Goldstein BH, et al. Comparison of management strategies for neonates with symptomatic tetralogy of Fallot. *J Am Coll Cardiol.* 2021;77:1093–1106.
30. Menaissy Y, et al. Total correction of tetralogy of Fallot in the first 60 days of life in symptomatic infants: Is it the gold standard? *Thorac Cardiovasc Surg.* 2020;68(1):45–50.
31. Rahmath MRK, Boudjemline Y. Tetralogy of Fallot will be treated interventionally within two decades. *Pediatr Cardiol.* 2020;41(3):539–545.
32. Cohen MI, et al. Preventing arrhythmic death in patients with tetralogy of Fallot: JACC Review Topic of the Week. *J Am Coll Cardiol.* 2021;77(6):761–771.
33. Sumal AS, Kyriacou H. Mostafa AMHAM: Tricuspid atresia: Where are we now? *J Card Surg.* 2020;35:1609–1617.
34. Huang L, et al. Long-term out-of-hospital health care use for Fontan survivors across childhood. *Ann Thorac Surg.* 2020;110:1372–1379.
35. Bravo-Valenzuela NJ, Peixoto AB, Araujo Júnior E. Prenatal diagnosis of transposition of the great arteries: an updated review. *Ultrasonography.* 2020;39(4):331–339.
36. Villafane J, et al. D-transposition of the great arteries: hot topics in the current era of the arterial switch operation. *J Am Coll Cardiol.* 2014;64:498–511.
37. Barrios PA, et al. Outcomes of treatment pathways in 240 patients with congenitally corrected transposition of great arteries. *J Thorac Cardiovasc Surg.* 2021;161(3):1080–1093.
38. Wang C, et al. Left ventricular stiffness in adolescents and young adults after arterial switch operation for complete transposition of the great arteries. *Pediatr Cardiol.* 2020;41:747–754.
39. Kari FA, et al. Repair of complex transposition of great arteries: up to 30 years of follow-up. *Ann Thorac Surg.* 2020;109:555–565.
40. Xiang M, et al. Mixed type of total anomalous pulmonary venous connection: diagnosis, surgical approach and outcomes. *J Cardiothorac Surg.* 2020;15:293.
41. Harada T, et al. Surgical results of total anomalous pulmonary venous connection repair in 256 patients. *Interact Cardiovasc Thorac Surg.* 2019;28(3):421–426.
42. Chikkabyrappa S, et al. Common arterial trunk: physiology, imaging, and management. *Semin Cardiothorac Vasc Anesth.* 2019;23(2):225–236.
43. Mastropietro CW, et al. Characteristics and operative outcomes for children undergoing repair of truncus arteriosus: a contemporary multicenter analysis. *J Thorac Cardiovasc Surg.* 2019;157(6):2386–2398. e4.
44. Naimo PS, et al. Truncus arteriosus repair: a 40-year multicentre perspective. *J Thorac Cardiovasc Surg.* 2021;161:230–240.
45. Metcalf MK, Rychik J. Outcomes in hypoplastic left heart syndrome. *Pediatr Clin North Am.* 2020;67:945–962.
46. Saraf A, et al. Hypoplastic left heart syndrome: from bedside to bench and back. *J Mol Cell Cardiol.* 2019;135:109–118.
47. Watanabe K, Shih R. Update of pediatric heart failure. *Pediatr Clin North Am.* 2020;67:889–901.
48. Price JF. Congestive heart failure in children. *Pediatr Rev.* 2019;40(2):60–70.
49. Kirk R, Dipchand AI, Rosenthal DN, eds. *ISHLT guidelines for the management of pediatric heart failure.* Birmingham, UK: University of Alabama at Birmingham; 2014.
50. Del Castillo S, Shaddy RE, Kantor PF. Update on pediatric heart failure. *Curr Opin Pediatr.* 2019;31:598–603.
51. Navaratnam M, Maeda K, Hollander SA. Pediatric ventricular assist devices: bridge to a new era of perioperative care. *Paediatr Anaesth.* 2019;29:506–518.
52. Zhu F, Ang JY. 2021 Update on the clinical management and diagnosis of Kawasaki disease. *Curr Infect Dis Rep.* 2021;23(3):3.
53. Noval Rivas M, Arditi M. Kawasaki disease: pathophysiology and insights from mouse models. *Nature Reviews Rheumatology.* 2020;16:391–405.
54. Hicar MD. Antibodies and immunity during Kawasaki disease. *Front Cardiovasc Med.* 2020;7:94.
55. Yan F, et al. Risk factors of coronary artery abnormality in children with Kawasaki disease: a systematic review and meta-analysis. *Front Pediatr.* 2019;7:374.
56. McCrindle BW, et al. Diagnosis, treatment, and long-term management of Kawasaki disease: a scientific statement for health professionals from the American Heart Association. *Circulation.* 2017;135:e927–e999.
57. Ashraf M, Irshad M, Parry NA. Pediatric hypertension: an updated review. *Clin Hypertens.* 2020;26:22.
58. Flynn JT, et al. Subcommittee on Screening and Management of High Blood Pressure in Children: Clinical Practice Guideline for Screening and Management of High Blood Pressure in Children and Adolescents. *Pediatrics.* 2017;140(3):e20171904.

59. Bell CS, Samuel JP, Samuels JA. Prevalence of hypertension in children: applying the new American Academy of Pediatrics clinical practice guideline. *Hypertension*. 2019;73:148–152.
60. Dissanayake HU, Skilton MR, Polson JW. Autonomic dysfunction in programmed hypertension. *J Hum Hypertens*. 2019;3:267–276.
61. Marcon D, Tagetti A, Fava C. Subclinical organ damage in children and adolescents with hypertension: current guidelines and beyond. *High Blood Press Cardiovasc Prev*. 2019;26(5):361–373.
62. Lande MB, Kupferman JC. Blood pressure and cognitive function in children and adolescents. *Hypertension*. 2019;73:532–540.
63. US Preventive Services Task Force Screening for high blood pressure in children and adolescents: US Preventive Services Task Force Recommendation Statement. *JAMA*. 2020;324(18):1878–1883.
64. Patel SS, Daniels SR. Ambulatory blood pressure monitoring in pediatrics. *Curr Hypertens Rep*. 2019;21(9):71.

34

Structure and Function of the Pulmonary System

Karen C. Turner and Valentina L. Brashers

http://evolve.elsevier.com/Rogers/pathophysiology/

CHAPTER OUTLINE

The primary function of the pulmonary system is the exchange of gases between the environmental air and the blood. The three steps in this process are (1) ventilation, the movement of air into and out of the lungs; (2) diffusion, the movement of gases between air spaces in the lungs and the bloodstream; and (3) perfusion, the movement of blood into the capillary beds of the lungs and out to body organs and tissues. The first two functions are carried out by the pulmonary system, and the third by the cardiovascular system (see Chapter 31). Normally the pulmonary system functions efficiently under a variety of conditions and with little energy expenditure.

STRUCTURES OF THE PULMONARY SYSTEM

The pulmonary system includes two lungs, the upper and lower airways, the blood vessels that serve these structures (Fig. 34.1), the diaphragm, and the chest wall (thoracic cage). The lungs are divided into lobes: three in the right lung (upper, middle, lower) and two in the left lung (upper, lower). Each lobe is further divided into segments and lobules. The mediastinum is the space between the lungs and contains the heart, great vessels, and esophagus. A set of conducting airways, or bronchi, delivers air to each section of the lung. The lung tissue that surrounds the airways supports them, preventing distortion or collapse of the airways as gas moves in and out during ventilation. The diaphragm is a dome-shaped muscle that separates the thoracic and abdominal cavities and is involved in ventilation.

The lungs are protected from a variety of exogenous contaminants in inspired air by a series of mechanical and cellular defenses (Table 34.1). These defense mechanisms are so effective that, in the healthy individual, contamination of the lung tissue itself, particularly by infectious agents, is relatively uncommon.

Conducting Airways

The conducting airways allow air into and out of the gas-exchange structures of the lung. The nasopharynx, oropharynx, and related structures are often called the *upper airway* (Fig. 34.2). These structures are lined with a ciliated mucosa with a rich vascular supply that warms and humidifies inspired air and removes foreign particles from it before it passes into the lungs. The mouth and oropharynx are used for ventilation when the nose is obstructed or when increased flow is required (e.g., during exercise). Filtering and humidifying are not as efficient with mouth breathing.

The larynx connects the upper and lower airways and consists of the endolarynx and its surrounding triangular-shaped bony and cartilaginous structures. The endolarynx is formed by two pairs of folds: the false vocal cords (supraglottis) and the true vocal cords. The slit-shaped space between the true cords forms the glottis (see Fig. 34.2). The vestibule is the space above the false vocal cords. The laryngeal box is formed of three large cartilages (epiglottis, thyroid, cricoid) and three smaller cartilages (arytenoid, corniculate, cuneiform) connected by ligaments. The supporting cartilages prevent the collapse of the larynx during inspiration and swallowing. The internal laryngeal muscles control vocal cord length and tension, and the external laryngeal muscles move the larynx as a whole. Both sets of muscles are important to swallowing, ventilation, and vocalization. The internal muscles contract during swallowing

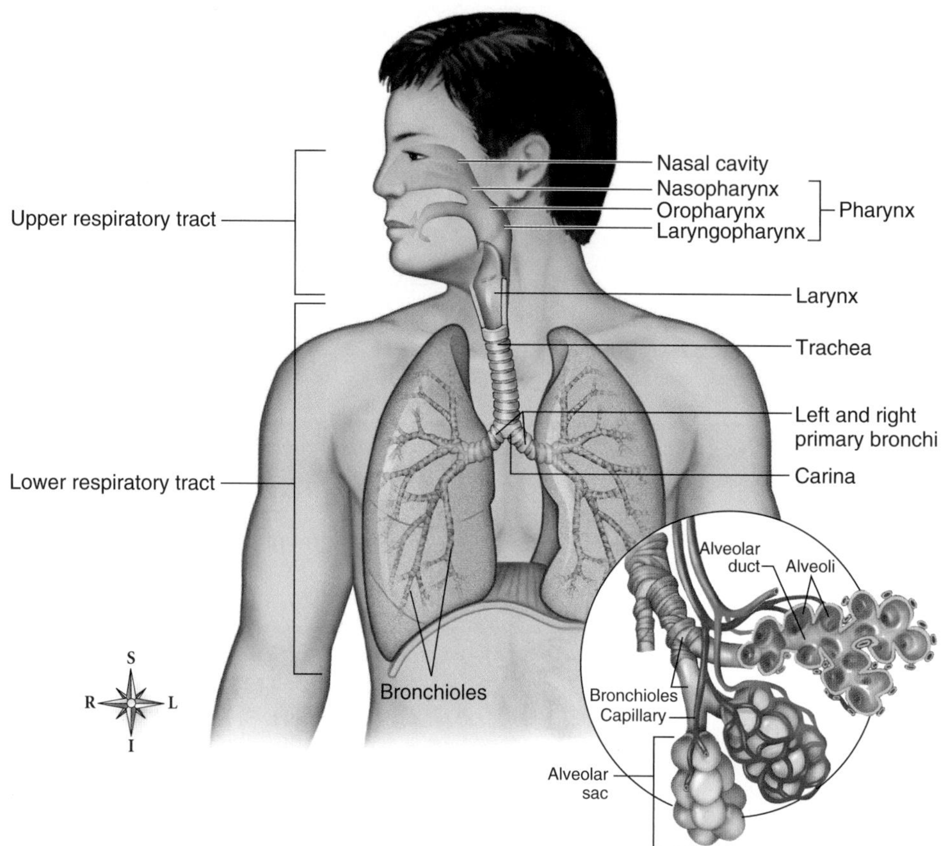

Fig. 34.1 Structure of the Pulmonary System. The upper and lower respiratory tracts (airways) are illustrated. The enlargement in the circle depicts the acinus, where oxygen and carbon dioxide are exchanged. (From Patton KT, Thibodeau GA. *Structure & function of the body*, 15th edition. St. Louis: Mosby; 2016.)

TABLE 34.1 Pulmonary Defense Mechanisms

Structure or Substance	Mechanism of Defense
Upper respiratory tract mucosa	Maintains constant temperature and humidification of gas entering the lungs; traps and removes foreign particles, some bacteria, and noxious gases from inspired air
Nasal hairs and turbinates	Trap and remove foreign particles, some bacteria, and noxious gases from inspired air
Branching airways	Disrupt laminar flow and enhance deposition of particles and pathogens on ciliated mucosa
Mucous blanket	Protects trachea and bronchi from injury; traps most foreign particles and bacteria that reach the lower airways
Innate immune proteins	Lysozyme, lactoferrin, defensins, surfactant protein (A [SP-A] and surfactant protein D [SP-D]), and immunoglobulin A (IgA); recognize and promote killing of pathogens
Cilia	Propel mucous blanket and entrapped particles toward the oropharynx, where they can be swallowed or expectorated
Alveolar macrophages	Ingest and remove bacteria and other foreign material from alveoli by phagocytosis (see Chapter 7)
Surfactant	Enhances phagocytosis of pathogens and allergens in alveoli; down-regulates inflammatory responses
Irritant receptors in nares (nostrils)	Stimulation by chemical or mechanical irritants triggers sneeze reflex, which results in rapid removal of irritants from nasal passages
Irritant receptors in trachea and large airways	Stimulation by chemical or mechanical irritants triggers cough reflex, which results in removal of irritants from the trachea and large airways

to prevent aspiration into the trachea. These muscles also contribute to voice pitch.

The trachea, which is supported by U-shaped cartilage, connects the larynx to the bronchi (sing., bronchus), the conducting airways of the lungs. The trachea branches into two bronchi at the carina (see Fig. 34.1). The carina is very sensitive and, when stimulated, can cause coughing and airway narrowing.[1] The left mainstem bronchus branches from the trachea at about a 45-degree angle. The right mainstem bronchus is slightly larger and more vertical than the left. Aspirated fluids or foreign

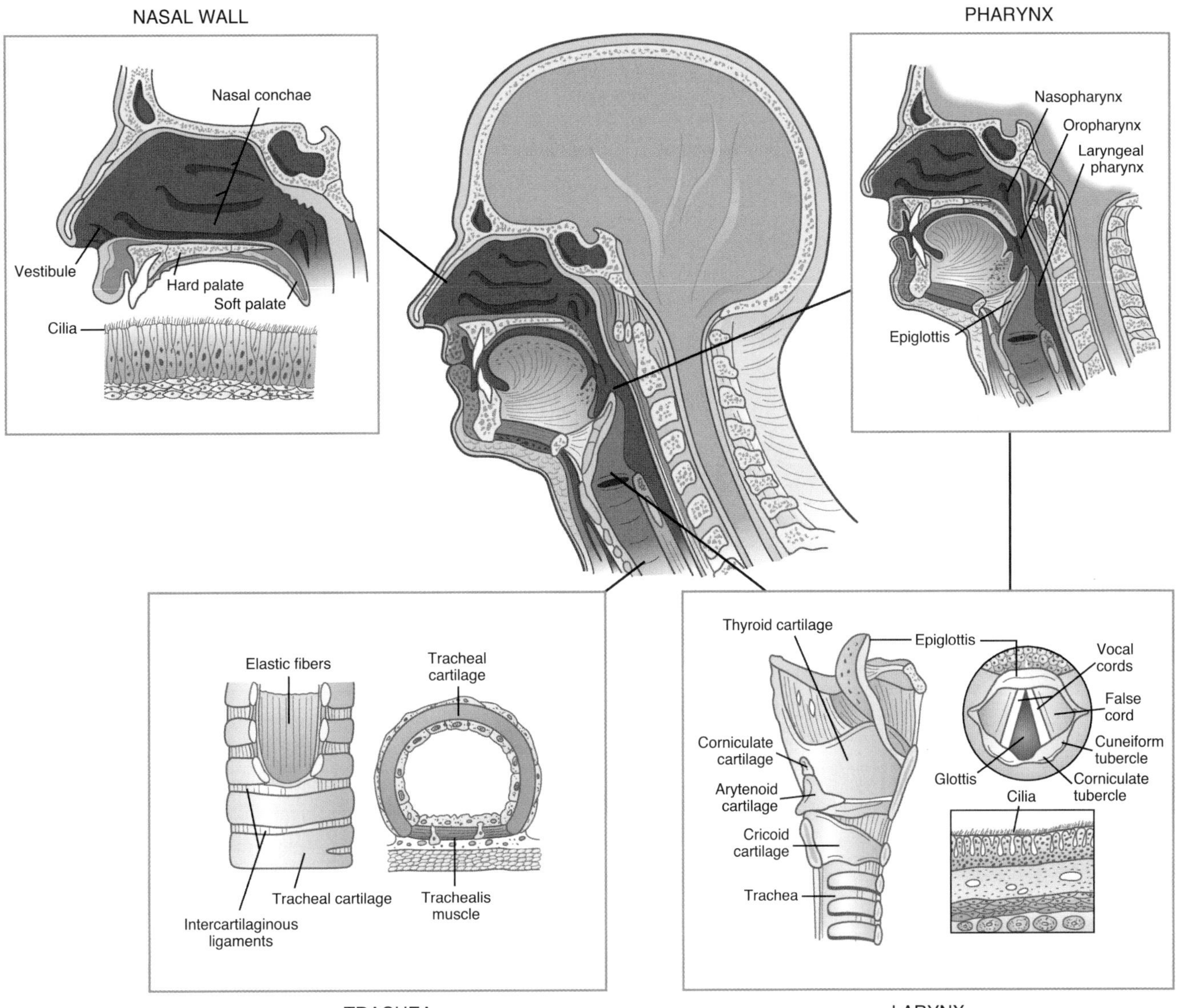

Fig. 34.2 Structures of the Upper Airway. (Redrawn from Thompson JM, McFarland GK, Hirsch JE, et al. *Mosby's clinical nursing*, 5th edition. St. Louis: Mosby; 2002.)

particles thus tend to enter the right lung rather than the left. The right and left main bronchi enter the lungs at the hila (sing., hilum), or "roots" of the lungs, along with the pulmonary blood and lymphatic vessels. From the hila, the main bronchi branch into lobar bronchi and then to segmental and subsegmental bronchi, and finally end in the smallest of the conducting airways, the terminal bronchioles (Fig. 34.3). With these multiple divisions, the cross-sectional area of the airways increases to 20 times that of the trachea. This results in a decreased velocity of airflow into the gas-exchange portion of the lung and allows for optimal gas diffusion.

The bronchial walls have three layers: an epithelial lining, a smooth muscle layer, and a connective tissue layer. In the large bronchi, the connective tissue layer contains cartilage. High columnar pseudostratified epithelium lines the larger airways and becomes progressively thinner, changing to columnar cuboidal epithelium in the bronchioles and squamous epithelium in the alveoli. The epithelial lining of the bronchi contains single-celled mucous-secreting goblet cells and ciliated cells. The goblet cells produce a mucous blanket that protects the airway epithelium. The mucus blanket is composed of periciliary fluid and airway liquid surface layers. When goblet cells detect microbes invading the bronchial tree, they secrete enzymes that improve the ability of the mucus they produce to trap the microbes in the mucous blanket.[2] Ciliated epithelial cells rhythmically beat this mucous blanket toward the trachea and pharynx, where it can be swallowed or expectorated by coughing. Toward the terminal bronchioles, ciliated cells and goblet cells become sparser, and smooth muscle and connective tissue layers thin (see Fig. 34.3).

Gas-Exchange Airways

The conducting airways terminate in the gas-exchange airways, including the respiratory bronchioles, alveolar ducts, and alveoli (sing., alveolus). A cluster of these three structures distal to a single terminal bronchiole is called an acinus (see Figs. 34.1

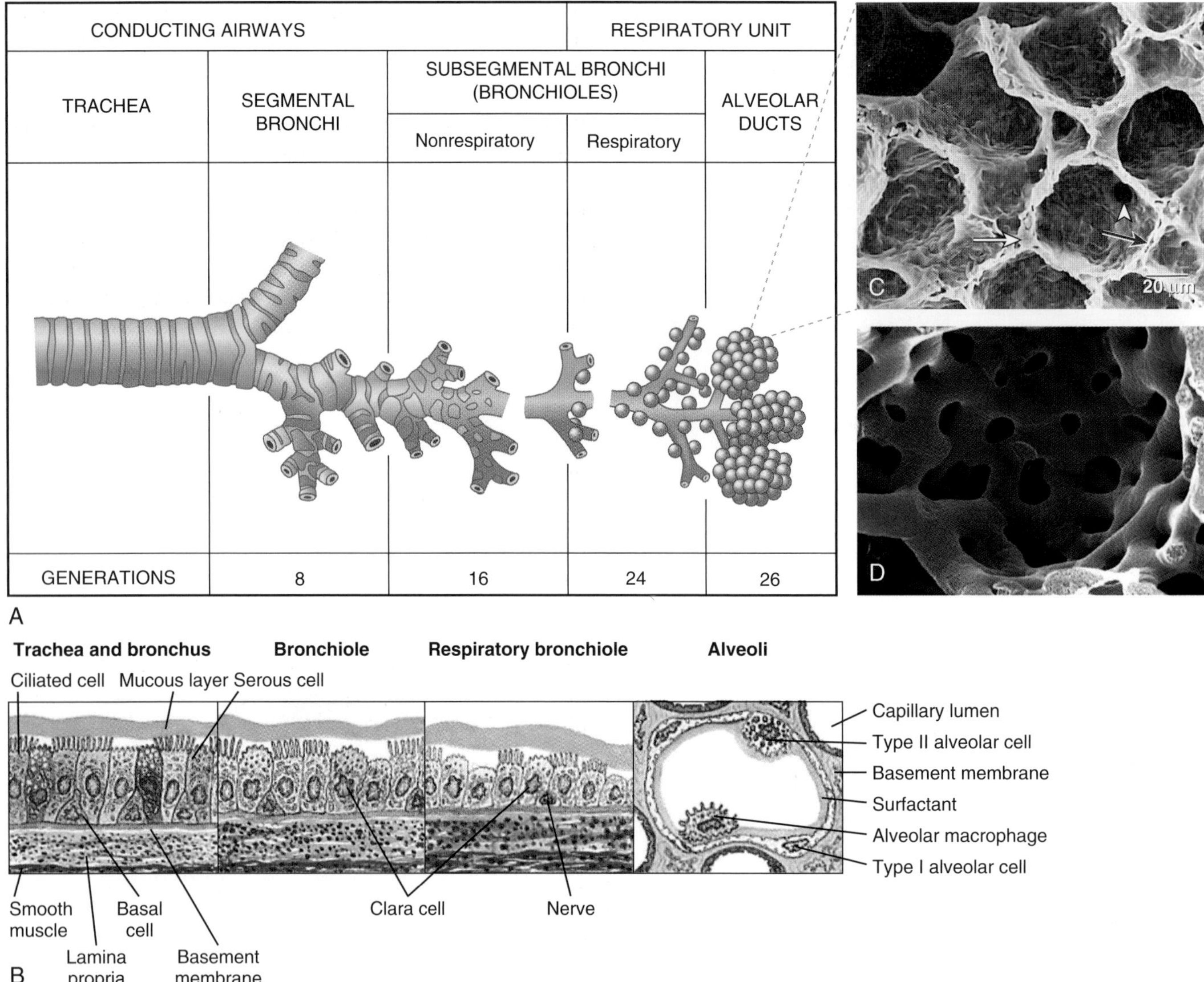

Fig. 34.3 Structures of the Lower Airway. **(A)** Structures of the lower respiratory airway. **(B)** Changes in the bronchial wall with progressive branching. Clara (club) cells secrete protective surfactant-type proteins. **(C)** Electron micrograph of alveoli: long white arrow identifies type II pneumocyte (secretes surfactant); white arrowhead identifies pores of Kohn; red arrow identifies alveolar capillary. **(D)** Plastic cast of pulmonary capillaries at high magnification. (A, Redrawn from Thompson JM, McFarland GK, Hirsch JE, et al. *Mosby's clinical nursing*, 5th edition. St. Louis: Mosby; 2002; B, From Wilson SF, Thompson JM. *Respiratory disorders*, St. Louis: Mosby; 1990; C, From Mason RJ, et al. *Murray and Nadel's textbook of respiratory medicine*, 5th edition. Philadelphia: Saunders; 2010; D, Courtesy A. Churg, MD, and J. Wright, MD, Vancouver, Canada. From Leslie, K. O., & Wick, M. R. *Practical pulmonary pathology: A diagnostic approach*, 2nd ed. Philadelphia: Saunders; 2011.)

and 34.3). The alveoli are the primary gas-exchange units of the lung, where oxygen (O_2) enters the blood and carbon dioxide (CO_2) is removed (Fig. 34.4). Tiny passages called *pores of Kohn* permit some air to pass through the septa from alveolus to alveolus, promoting collateral ventilation and even distribution of air among the alveoli. The lungs contain approximately 50 million alveoli at birth and 480 million by adulthood.

Alveolar cells provide a protective interface with the environment and are essential for adequate gas exchange, preventing entry of foreign agents, regulating ion and water transport, and maintaining the mechanical stability of the alveoli. The alveolar septa consist of an epithelial layer and a thin, elastic basement membrane but no muscle layer. Two major types of epithelial cells appear in the alveolus. Type I alveolar cells provide structure and are large, thin cells that comprise 95% of the surface across which gas exchange occurs.[3] Type II alveolar cells secrete surfactant, a lipoprotein that coats the inner surface of the alveolus and facilitates its expansion during inspiration, which lowers alveolar surface tension at end-expiration, thereby preventing lung collapse (atelectasis). Surfactant also plays a role in defending against infection.

Macrophages are the most numerous immune cells present in the lung environment and provide defense of the airway from the bronchi to the alveoli. Humans breathe over 10,000 L of non-sterile air per day, and potentially pathogenic microorganisms must be removed in order to prevent infection. In the alveoli, *alveolar macrophages* move through the pores of Kohn and patrol the alveoli, where they detect and ingest inhaled microorganisms without activating neutrophils and other elements of innate immunity.[4] They also provide protection by clearing surfactant from the lung and ingesting foreign materials that reach the alveolus, preparing these substances for removal through the lymphatics.[5] Phagocytosis and the mononuclear phagocyte system are described in Chapters 7 and 8. Surfactant and alveolar macrophages work together with the normal pulmonary microbiota to prevent lower lung infection. Pathogens must overcome these defense mechanisms in order to cause lower respiratory tract infection. Changes in the pulmonary microbiome are associated with many pulmonary diseases (see Emerging Science Box: The Pulmonary Microbiome).

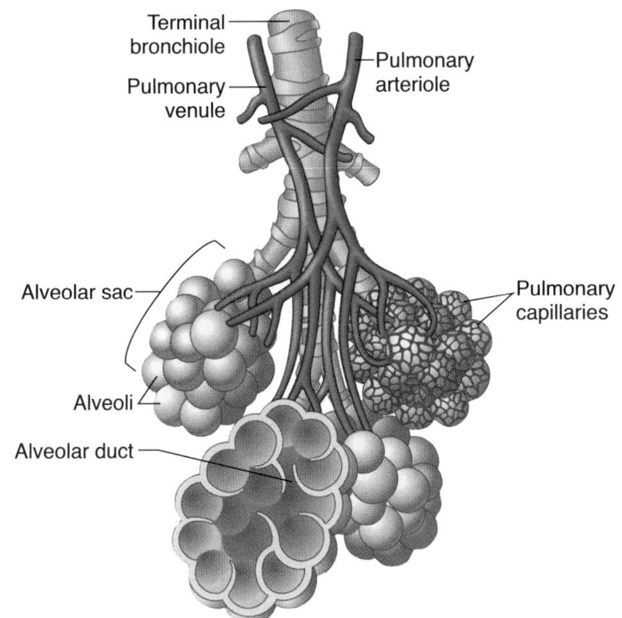

Fig. 34.4 Alveoli. Bronchioles subdivide to form tiny tubes called alveolar ducts, which end in clusters of alveoli called alveolar sacs. (Modified from Patton KT, Thibodeau GA. *The human body in health & disease*, 6th edition. St. Louis: Mosby; 2014.)

Pulmonary and Bronchial Circulation

The pulmonary circulation facilitates gas exchange, delivers nutrients to lung tissues, acts as a blood reservoir for the left ventricle, and serves as a filtering system that removes clots, air, and other debris from the circulation. The pulmonary vasculature is composed of three compartments connected in series: arteries, capillaries, and veins (Fig. 34.5).

Although the entire cardiac output from the right ventricle goes into the lungs, the pulmonary circulation has a lower pressure and resistance than the systemic circulation. Pulmonary arteries are exposed to about one-fifth the pressure of the systemic circulation and have a much thinner muscle layer. Pulmonary artery pressure is about 18 mm Hg, compared to 90 mm Hg in the aorta. Usually, about one-third of

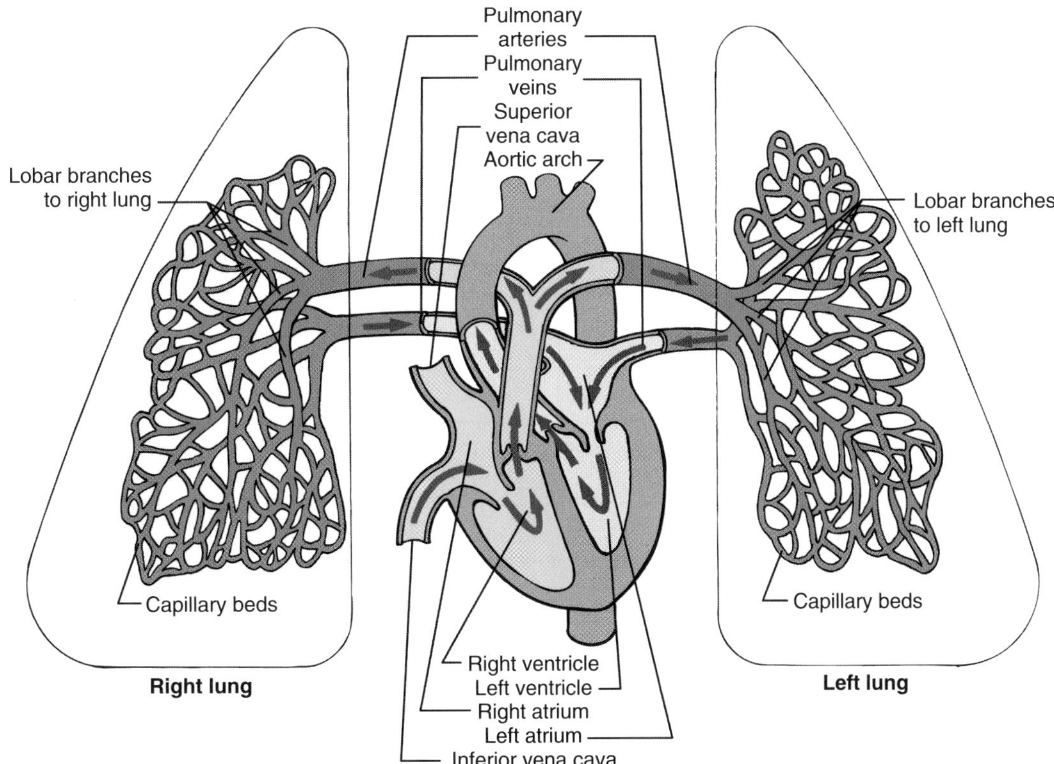

Fig. 34.5 The Pulmonary Circulation. The right and left pulmonary veins and arteries and the branching capillaries are illustrated. Note the pulmonary artery carries venous blood, and the pulmonary vein carries arterial blood.

EMERGING SCIENCE BOX

The Pulmonary Microbiome

Until recently, it was believed that the lower lungs were sterile. The first report of a healthy lung microbiome was published in 2010, and many more confirmatory articles have been published since then. The pulmonary microbiome is dynamic and is constantly influenced by the movement of air, mucus, and microbes in and out of the lung. The lung's natural defense mechanisms, such as the presence of bacteriostatic surfactant and active bronchial and alveolar macrophages, limit bacterial density along the mucosal surfaces, but those microorganisms that do survive provide important immunologic roles in preventing disease. There is an interaction between the oral and gut mucosa and the pulmonary microbiome (gut-lung axis), and these relationships are just beginning to be understood in terms of causing and treating lung disease.

A healthy pulmonary microbiome confers protection against many infectious and inflammatory conditions. Changes in lung microbiota (dysbiosis) have been associated with environmental impacts such as tobacco smoking, air pollution, and the use of corticosteroids and antibiotics. There is also increasing evidence that pulmonary dysbiosis is a contributing factor for a number of pulmonary disorders. For example, studies have found that Proteobacteria such as *Moraxella*, *Pseudomonas*, and *Enterobacteriaceae* are more prevalent in the airways of those with asthma. These microorganisms are postulated to accentuate the inflammatory processes that underlie asthma pathophysiology and may provide a link between diet, obesity, and asthma onset and severity. Similar links have been found between pulmonary and gut microbiota and the pathogenesis and clinical course of COPD, cystic fibrosis, idiopathic pulmonary fibrosis, and bronchiectasis. Recent studies suggest that pulmonary dysbiosis can have an adverse effect on the pathogenesis and clinical severity of coronavirus disease 2019 (COVID-19). Therapeutic interventions aimed at modifying the microbiome are undergoing intensive research, and early outcomes appear positive for several common pulmonary disorders.

Data from de Oliveira GLV, et al. Microbiota modulation of the gut-lung axis in COVID-19. *Frontiers in Immunology*, 2021;12:214; Dima E, et al. The lung microbiome dynamics between stability and exacerbation in chronic obstructive pulmonary disease (COPD): Current perspectives. *Respiratory Medicine*, 2019;157:1–6; Fromentin M, et al. Respiratory microbiome in mechanically ventilated patients: A narrative review. *Intensive Care Medicine*, 2021;47:292–306; Haiminen N, et al. Functional profiling of COVID-19 respiratory tract microbiomes. *Nature - Scientific Reports*, 2021;11:6433; Lipinski JH, et al. The evolving role of the lung microbiome in pulmonary fibrosis. *American Journal of Physiology - Lung Cellular and Molecular Physiology*, 2020;319(4):L675–682; Loverdos K, et al. Lung microbiome in asthma: Current perspectives. *Journal of Clinical Medicine*, 2019;8(11):1967; Peroni DG, et al. Microbiome composition and its impact on the development of allergic diseases. *Frontiers in Immunology*, 2020;11:700; Shukla SD, et al. Microbiome-focused asthma management strategies. *Current Opinion in Pharmacology*, 2019;46:143–149; Spagnolo P, et al. The role of the lung's microbiome in the pathogenesis and progression of idiopathic pulmonary fibrosis. *International Journal of Molecular Sciences*, 2019;20:5618.

the pulmonary vessels are filled with blood (perfused) at any given time. More vessels become perfused when right ventricular cardiac output increases. Therefore, increased delivery of blood to the lungs does not normally increase the mean pulmonary artery pressure significantly. During intense exercise, pulmonary arterial pressure may increase as much as 30 to 50 mm Hg, although the threshold above which the diagnosis of exercise pulmonary hypertension has not been fully established.[6] The pulmonary artery divides and enters the lung at the hila, branching with each main bronchus and with all bronchi at every division. Thus, every bronchus and bronchiole has an accompanying artery or arteriole. The arterioles divide at the terminal bronchioles to form a network of pulmonary capillaries around the acinus (see Fig. 34.4). Capillary walls consist of an endothelial layer and a thin basement membrane. The capillary endothelium is composed of two cell types. One type is composed of aerocytes specialized for gas exchange and allows leukocytes to enter the alveolus during inflammation. The other type is termed gCap and is specialized to regulate vasomotor tone and as progenitor cells for capillary repair.[3] The shared alveolar and capillary walls compose the alveolocapillary membrane, a very thin membrane made up of the alveolar epithelium, the alveolar basement membrane, an interstitial space, the capillary basement membrane, and the capillary endothelium (Fig. 34.6). Gas exchange occurs across this membrane. The extremely thin alveolar walls are easily damaged and can leak plasma and blood into the alveolar space. Any disorder that thickens the membrane impairs gas exchange.

Each pulmonary vein drains several pulmonary capillaries. Unlike the pulmonary arteries, which follow the branching bronchi, pulmonary veins are dispersed randomly throughout the lung and then leave the lung at the hila and enter the left atrium. They are similar to veins in the systemic circulation, but they have no valves.

The bronchial circulation is part of the systemic circulation, and it both moistens inspired air and supplies nutrients to the conducting airways, large pulmonary vessels, lymph nodes, and membranes (pleurae) that surround the lungs. The bronchial arteries supply blood to the trachea, bronchi and its branches, esophagus, visceral pleura, the vasa vasorum of the thoracic

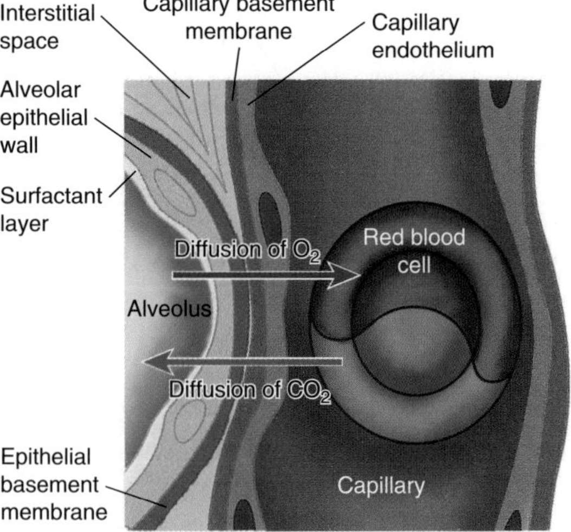

Fig. 34.6 Cross-Section Through an Alveolus Showing Histology of the Alveolar-Capillary Membrane (Respiratory Membrane). The dense network of capillaries forms an almost continuous sheet of blood in the alveolar walls, providing a very efficient arrangement for gas exchange. CO_2, Carbon dioxide; O_2, oxygen. (Adapted from Montague SE, Watson R, Herbert R. *Physiology for nursing practice*, 3rd edition. London: Elsevier; 2005.)

aorta, and the pulmonary arteries and to the nerves, pulmonary veins, and lymph nodes. The bronchial circulation does not participate in gas exchange.

The lung vasculature also includes deep and superficial pulmonary lymphatic capillaries through which fluid and alveolar macrophages can leave the alveoli to the terminal bronchioles, where they enter the lymphatic system. The superficial lymphatic capillaries drain the membrane that surrounds the lungs. Both deep and superficial lymphatic vessels leave the lung at the hilum through a series of mediastinal lymph nodes; thus many infectious or malignant processes in the lung also affect these nodes.[7] The lymphatic system plays an important role in both providing immune defense and keeping the lung free of fluid. (The lymphatic system is described in Chapter 31.)

Control of the Pulmonary Circulation

The caliber of pulmonary artery lumina decreases as smooth muscle in the arterial walls contracts. Contraction increases pulmonary artery pressure. Caliber increases as these muscles relax, decreasing blood pressure. Contraction (vasoconstriction) and relaxation (vasodilation) primarily occur in response to both local humoral conditions and the autonomic nervous system (ANS), as is the systemic circulation.

The most important cause of pulmonary artery constriction is a low alveolar partial pressure of oxygen (PAO_2), often termed hypoxic pulmonary vasoconstriction. This results from an increase in intracellular calcium levels in vascular smooth muscle cells in response to a low O_2 concentration and the presence of charged O_2 molecules, called *oxygen radicals*.[8] It can affect only one segment of the lung (i.e., one lobe that is obstructed, decreasing its PAO_2) or the entire lung. If only one segment of the lung is involved, the arterioles to that segment constrict, shunting blood to other, well-ventilated portions of the lung. This reflex improves the lung's efficiency by better matching ventilation and perfusion. If all segments of the lung are affected, however, vasoconstriction occurs throughout the pulmonary vasculature, and pulmonary hypertension (elevated pulmonary artery pressure) can result. The pulmonary vasoconstriction caused by a low PAO_2 values is reversible if the PAO_2 level is corrected. Chronic alveolar hypoxia can result in inflammation and structural changes in pulmonary arterioles, causing permanent pulmonary artery hypertension, which eventually leads to right heart failure (cor pulmonale) (see Chapter 35).

Acidemia also causes pulmonary artery constriction. If the acidemia is corrected, the vasoconstriction is reversed. (Respiratory acidosis and metabolic acidosis are described in Chapter 3.) An elevated partial pressure of carbon dioxide ($PaCO_2$) in the arterial blood value without a drop in pH does not cause pulmonary artery constriction. Other biochemical factors that affect the caliber of vessels in the pulmonary circulation are histamine, prostaglandins, endothelin, serotonin, nitric oxide, and bradykinin.

Chest Wall and Pleura

The chest wall (skin, ribs, intercostal muscles) protects the lungs from injury. The intercostal muscles of the chest wall, along with the diaphragm, accessory muscles, and abdominal muscles, perform the muscular work of breathing. The thoracic cavity is contained by the chest wall and encases the lungs (Fig. 34.7). A serous membrane called the pleura adheres firmly to the lungs and then folds over itself and attaches firmly to the chest wall. The membrane covering the lungs is the *visceral pleura;* that lining the thoracic cavity is the *parietal pleura*. The area between the two pleurae is called the pleural space, or pleural cavity. Normally, only a thin layer of fluid secreted by the pleura (pleural fluid) fills the pleural space, lubricating the pleural surfaces and allowing the two layers to slide over each other without separating. Pressure in the pleural space is usually negative or subatmospheric (−4 to −10 mm Hg).

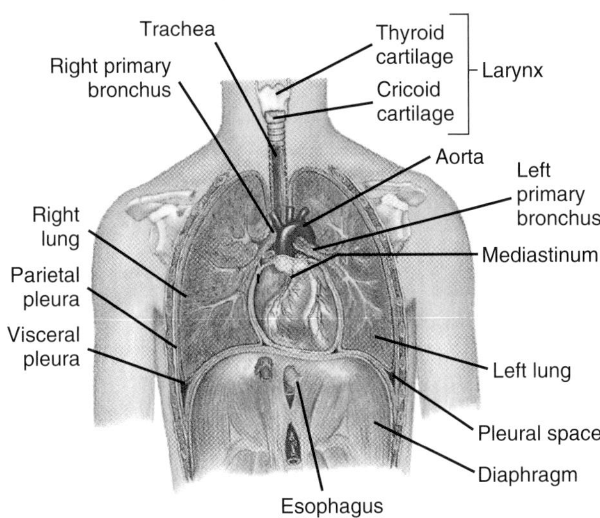

Fig. 34.7 Thoracic (Chest) Cavity and Related Structures. The thoracic (chest) cavity is divided into three subdivisions (left and right pleural divisions and mediastinum) by a partition formed by a serous membrane called the pleura. (From Thibodeau GA, Patton KT. *Anatomy & physiology*, 3rd edition. St. Louis: Mosby; 1996.)

FUNCTION OF THE PULMONARY SYSTEM

The pulmonary system (1) ventilates the alveoli, (2) diffuses gases into and out of the blood, and (3) perfuses the lungs so that the organs and tissues of the body receive blood that is rich in O_2 and deficient in CO_2. Each component of the pulmonary system contributes to one or more of these functions (Fig. 34.8).

Ventilation

Ventilation is the mechanical movement of gas or air into and out of the lungs. It is often misnamed *respiration*, which is actually the exchange of O_2 and CO_2 during cellular metabolism. The "respiratory rate" is actually the ventilatory rate, or the number of times gas is inspired and expired per minute. The volume of ventilation is calculated by multiplying the ventilatory rate (breaths per minute) by the volume or amount of air per breath (liters per breath, or tidal volume). This is called the minute volume (or minute ventilation [$\dot{V}$]) and is expressed in liters per minute. The effective ventilation is calculated by

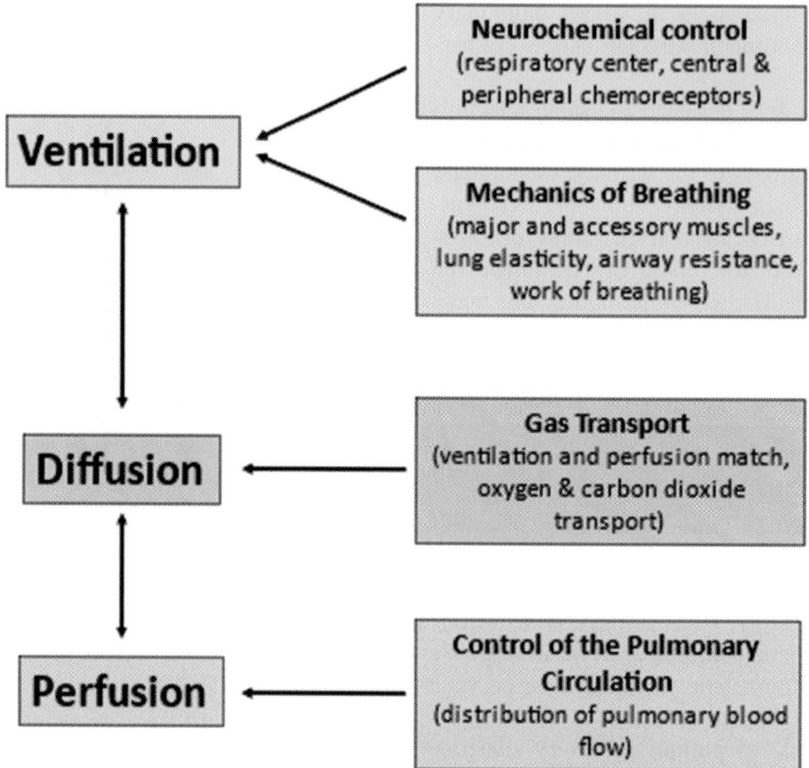

Fig. 34.8 Functional Components of the Respiratory System. The central nervous system responds to neurochemical stimulation of ventilation and sends signals to the chest wall musculature. The response of the respiratory system to these impulses is influenced by several factors that affect the mechanisms of breathing and, therefore, the adequacy of ventilation. Gas transport between the alveoli and pulmonary capillary blood depends on a variety of physical and chemical activities. Finally, the control of the pulmonary circulation plays a role in the appropriate distribution of blood flow.

multiplying the ventilatory rate by the tidal volume minus the dead space. Dead-space ventilation (V_D) is the volume of air per breath that does not participate in gas exchange. It is ventilation without perfusion. *Anatomic dead-space* is the volume of air in the conducting airways. *Alveolar dead-space* is the volume of air in unperfused alveoli.

CO_2, the gaseous form of carbonic acid (H_2CO_3), is produced by cellular metabolism. The lung eliminates about 10,000 milliequivalents (mEq) of H_2CO_3 per day in the form of CO_2, which is produced at the rate of approximately 200 mL/min. CO_2 is eliminated to maintain a normal partial pressure of arterial CO_2 ($PaCO_2$) of 40 mm Hg and normal acid-base balance (see Chapter 3 for a discussion of acid-base regulation). Adequate ventilation is necessary to maintain normal $PaCO_2$ levels. Diseases that limit the ventilatory rate or tidal volume, or both, decrease ventilation and result in CO_2 retention. The adequacy of alveolar ventilation *cannot* be accurately determined by observation of the ventilatory rate, pattern, or effort. If a healthcare professional needs to determine the adequacy of ventilation, an arterial blood gas analysis or capnography must be performed to determine if there is CO_2 retention.

Neurochemical Control of Ventilation

Breathing is usually involuntary because homeostatic changes in the ventilatory rate and volume are adjusted automatically by the nervous system to maintain normal gas exchange. Voluntary breathing is necessary for talking, singing, laughing, and deliberately holding one's breath. The mechanisms that control respiration are complex (Fig. 34.9).

The respiratory center in the brainstem controls respiration by transmitting impulses to the respiratory muscles, causing them to contract and relax. The respiratory center is composed of several groups of neurons located bilaterally in the brainstem: the pontine respiratory group (pneumotaxic and apneustic centers), the dorsal respiratory group (DRG), the ventral respiratory group (VRG), the pontine respiratory center, and the apneustic center.

The basic automatic rhythm of respiration is set by the VRG, a cluster of inspiratory nerve cells located in the medulla that sends efferent impulses to the diaphragm and inspiratory intercostal muscles. The DRG receives afferent input from peripheral chemoreceptors in the carotid and aortic bodies; from mechanical, neural, and chemical stimuli; and from receptors in the lungs, and it alters breathing patterns to restore normal blood gases. This is usually accompanied by a sensation of dyspnea (breathing discomfort) (see Emerging Science Box: Silent Hypoxemia in COVID-19). The pontine respiratory group does not generate primary rhythm but, rather, acts as a modifier of the rhythm established by the VRG. Breathing can be modified by input from

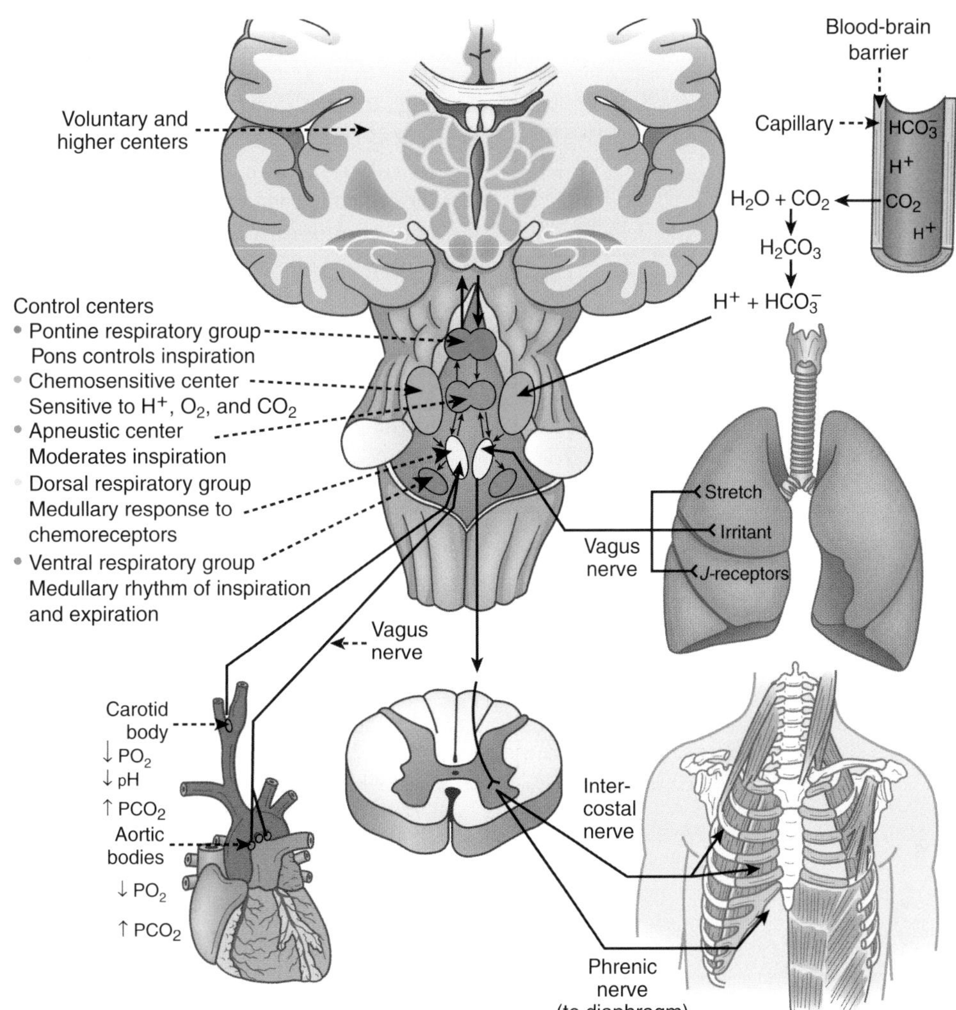

Fig. 34.9 Neurochemical Respiratory Control System. *CO_2,* Carbon dioxide; *H^+,* hydrogen; *H_2CO_3,* carbonic acid; HCO_3^-, bicarbonate; *PO_2,* partial pressure of oxygen.

the cortex, the limbic system, and the hypothalamus, and the pattern of breathing can be influenced by emotion, pain, and disease.

Chemoreceptors. Chemoreceptors monitor the pH, $PaCO_2$, and PaO_2 of arterial blood. Central chemoreceptors are located near the respiratory center and monitor arterial blood indirectly by sensing changes in the pH of cerebrospinal fluid (CSF) (see Fig. 34.9). As CO_2 accumulates in the blood because of decreased ventilation, it diffuses across the blood-brain barrier (the capillary wall separating the blood from the cells of the central nervous system) into the CSF until the partial pressure of CO_2 (PCO_2) is equal on both sides. CO_2 that has entered the CSF combines with water (H_2O) to form H_2CO_3, which subsequently dissociates into hydrogen ions (H^+) that are capable of stimulating acid-activated central chemoreceptors (the retrotrapezoid nucleus).[9]

As the central chemoreceptors sense the decrease in pH, they stimulate the respiratory center to increase the depth and rate of ventilation. Increased ventilation causes the partial pressure of carbon dioxide ($PaCO_2$) in the arterial blood to decrease below that of the CSF, and CO_2 diffuses out of the CSF, returning its pH to normal. In this way, $PaCO_2$ regulates ventilation through its effect on the pH (hydrogen ion content) of the CSF.

The central chemoreceptors are sensitive to very small changes in the pH of the CSF (equivalent to a 1 to 2 mm Hg change in PCO_2) and can maintain a normal $PaCO_2$ under many different conditions, including strenuous exercise. If inadequate ventilation, or hypoventilation, is long term (e.g., in chronic obstructive pulmonary disease [COPD]), these receptors become insensitive to small changes in $PaCO_2$ ("reset") and regulate ventilation poorly. In addition, prolonged increases

EMERGING SCIENCE BOX
Silent Hypoxemia in COVID-19

Silent (apathetic) hypoxemia is defined as a lack of dyspnea despite significant decreases in oxygen saturation of the blood. In healthy individuals, changes in lung mechanics, arterial oxygen and carbon dioxide levels, and inflammatory cytokines stimulate afferent impulses from pulmonary mechano-chemoreceptors (irritant, stretch, pulmonary C-fiber receptors) and peripheral and central chemoreceptors to the respiratory center in the brainstem. In response, the respiratory center sends efferent signals to the respiratory system that appropriately alter the respiratory rate and tidal volume. These compensatory mechanisms are usually accompanied by the sensation of dyspnea (a subjective experience of breathing discomfort). It has been noted, however, that considerable variation exists between individuals with respect to the amount of dyspnea experienced with various levels of hypoxemia. Some individuals experience severe dyspnea and panic, whereas others will experience very little dyspnea even when oxygen saturations fall below 70%. These latter individuals are considered to have silent hypoxemia. Silent hypoxemia can be seen in diseases such as atelectasis and cardiac shunts; however, it appears to be quite common in coronavirus infection 2019 (COVID-19). Hypotheses for silent hypoxemia in COVID-19 include a relative lack of early changes in pulmonary mechanics, viral interactions with hemoglobin, inhibition of carotid body responsiveness, and neuronal damage to the central nervous system. This is of particular concern because of the propensity of COVID-19 pneumonia to progress rapidly to severe respiratory failure despite a lack of dyspnea early in the course of infection. Careful monitoring of oxygen saturation and carbon dioxide levels is critical to identifying seriously ill individuals.

Data from Bickler PE, et al. "Silent" presentation of hypoxemia and cardiorespiratory compensation in COVID-19. *Anesthesiology*, 2021;134(2):262–269; Chandra A, et al. Silent hypoxia: A frequently overlooked clinical entity in patients with COVID-19. *BMJ Case Reports*, 2020;13(9):e237207; Dhont S, et al. The pathophysiology of "happy" hypoxemia in COVID-19. *Respiratory Research*, 2020;21:198; Nouri-Vaskeh M, et al. Dyspneic and non-dyspneic (silent) hypoxemia in COVID-19: Possible neurological mechanism. *Clinical Neurology and Neurosurgery*, 2020;198106217; Villadiego J, et al. Is carotid body infection responsible for silent hypoxemia in COVID-19 patients? *Function*, 2021:2(1)zqaa032; Wilkerson RG, et al. Silent hypoxia: A harbinger of clinical deterioration in patients with COVID-19. *American Journal of Emergency Medicine*, 2020;38(10):2243.e5–2243.e6.

in $PaCO_2$ result in renal compensation through bicarbonate (HCO_3^-) retention. This HCO_3^- gradually diffuses into the CSF, where it normalizes the pH and limits the effect on the ventilatory drive.

The peripheral chemoreceptors are located in aortic bodies, the aortic arch, and carotid bodies at the bifurcation of the carotids, near the baroreceptors. They are only somewhat sensitive to changes in pH and instead are sensitive primarily to PaO_2 levels. As the PaO_2 and pH decrease, peripheral chemoreceptors, particularly in the carotid bodies, send signals to the respiratory center to increase ventilation. However, the PaO_2 must drop well below normal (to approximately 60 mm Hg) before the peripheral chemoreceptors have much influence on ventilation. If the pH is decreased as well, ventilation increases much more than it would in response to either abnormality alone. The peripheral chemoreceptors become the major stimulus to ventilation when the central chemoreceptors are reset by chronic hypoventilation.

Lung receptors. Three types of lung sensory receptors send impulses from the lungs to the DRG:

1. Irritant receptors (rapidly adapting receptors) are found in the epithelium of all conducting airways. They are sensitive to noxious aerosols (vapors), gases, and particulate matter (e.g., inhaled dust), which cause them to initiate the cough reflex. Transient receptor potential (TRP) channels respond to irritant receptor activation and inflammatory stimuli and induce cough via the vagus nerve.[10] When stimulated, irritant receptors also cause bronchoconstriction and increased ventilatory rate. These receptors are located primarily in the proximal larger airways and are nearly absent in the distal airways; thus, it is possible for secretions to accumulate in the distal respiratory tree without initiating cough.
2. Stretch receptors (slowly adapting receptors) are located in the smooth muscles of the airways and are sensitive to increases in the size or volume of the lungs. They decrease the ventilatory rate and volume when stimulated, an occurrence sometimes referred to as the *Hering-Breuer expiratory reflex*. This reflex is active in newborns and assists with ventilation. In adults, this reflex is active only at high tidal volumes (e.g., with exercise and mechanical ventilation) and may protect against excess lung inflation.
3. Pulmonary C-fiber receptors (also known as *J-receptors* [juxtapulmonary capillary receptors]) are located near the capillaries in the alveolar septa and in other airway locations as nociceptors. They are sensitive to increased pulmonary capillary pressure, which stimulates them to initiate rapid, shallow breathing; laryngeal constriction on expiration; and mucus secretion; hypotension; and bradycardia. They may be associated with the sensation of dyspnea.[11]

Autonomic nervous system. The lung is innervated by the ANS (The structures and function of the ANS are discussed in detail in Chapter 15). Fibers of the sympathetic division of the ANS in the lung branch out from the upper thoracic and cervical ganglia (stellate ganglia) of the spinal cord. The primary sympathetic neurotransmitter in the lung is norepinephrine. Fibers of the parasympathetic division of the ANS travel in the vagus nerve to the lung, where they release acetylcholine. The parasympathetic and sympathetic divisions of the ANS control airway caliber (interior diameter of the airway lumen) by stimulating the bronchial smooth muscle to contract or relax. Bronchial smooth muscle tone depends on equilibrium, that is, equal stimulation of contraction and relaxation. The sympathetic nervous system's release of norepinephrine stimulates airway β-adrenergic receptors causing airway smooth muscle to relax (bronchodilation). The parasympathetic nervous system's release of acetylcholine stimulates two types of muscarinic receptors in the lung, M_2 and M_3. Stimulation of M_2 receptors limits the further release of acetylcholine, whereas stimulation of M_3 receptors causes airway smooth muscle to contract (bronchoconstriction) and increases mucous secretion. M_3 activation and associated bronchoconstriction occur if receptors in the airway epithelium are stimulated by irritants in inspired air, by inflammatory mediators (e.g., histamine, serotonin, prostaglandins, leukotrienes), by many drugs, and by humoral substances.[12] Muscarinic receptor antagonists are used to promote bronchodilation and reduce mucous secretion in conditions such as asthma and COPD (see Chapter 35).[13]

Mechanics of Breathing

The mechanical aspects of inspiration and expiration are known collectively as the *mechanics of breathing* and involve (1) major and accessory muscles of inspiration and expiration, (2) elastic properties of the lungs and chest wall, and (3) resistance to airflow through the conducting airways. Alterations in any of these properties increase the work of breathing or the metabolic energy needed to achieve adequate ventilation and oxygenation of the blood.

Major and accessory muscles. The major muscles of inspiration are the diaphragm and the external intercostal muscles (muscles between the ribs) (Fig. 34.10). The diaphragm is the primary muscle of ventilation and provides the anatomic separation between the thorax and the abdomen. It is a dome-shaped muscle that separates the abdominal and thoracic cavities. It has multiple intrathoracic attachments and is innervated by the paired phrenic nerves. When it contracts and flattens downward, it increases the volume of the thoracic cavity, creating a negative pressure that draws gas into the lungs through the upper airways and trachea. The phrenic nerves have both sensory and motor functions. They originate from the C3 to C5 spinal nerves and descend through the thorax to innervate the right and left hemidiaphragms. They provide sensory input from the pleura and upper peritoneum. They provide the only motor innervation of the diaphragm and are essential for stimulating adequate ventilation. Trauma to the cervical spine above C4, central nervous system disorders, neuropathies, and neuromuscular diseases (see Chapter 18) may lead to diaphragmatic paralysis and respiratory failure.[14] The right and left phrenic nerves pass close to the right hilum and left hila of the lung, respectively, and may be impacted by diseases such as tumors or trauma that damage the hilar regions causing hemiparalysis of the diaphragm. Prolonged mechanical ventilation can inhibit the function of the phrenic nerve making it more difficult to return to normal ventilation.[15] Contraction of the external intercostal muscles elevates the anterior portion of the ribs and increases the volume of the thoracic cavity by increasing its front-to-back (anterior-posterior [AP]) diameter. Although the external intercostal muscles may contract during quiet breathing, inspiration at rest is usually assisted by the diaphragm only.

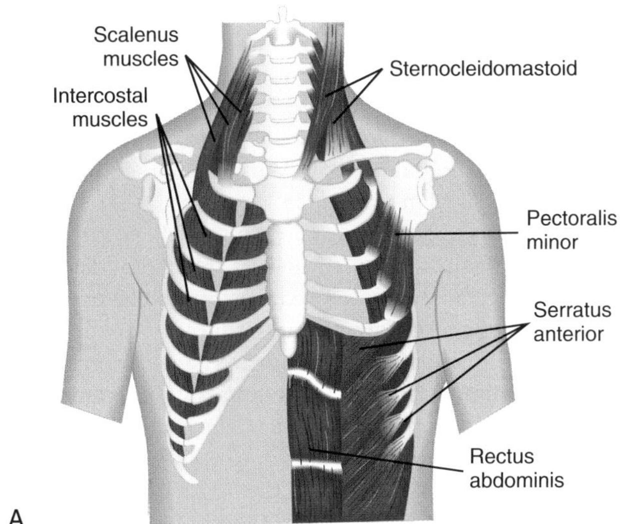

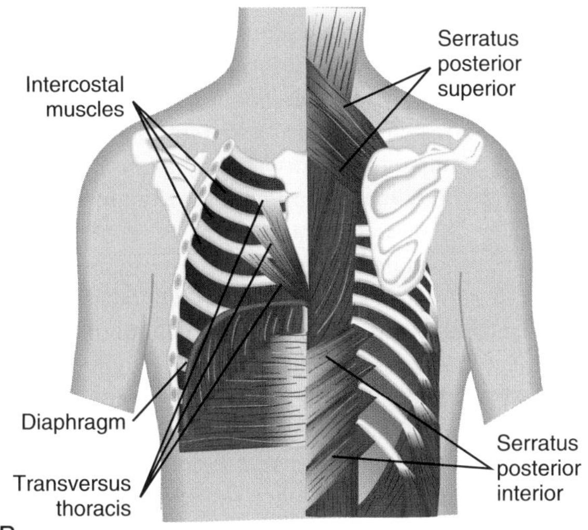

Fig. 34.10 Muscles of Ventilation. **(A)** Anterior view. **(B)** Posterior view. (Modified from Thompson JM, McFarland GK, Hirsch JE, et al. *Mosby's clinical nursing*, 5th edition. St. Louis: Mosby; 2002.)

The accessory muscles of inspiration are the sternocleidomastoid and scalene muscles. Like the external intercostal muscles, these muscles enlarge the thorax by increasing its AP diameter. The accessory muscles assist inspiration when the minute volume (volume of air inspired and expired per minute) is very high, such as during strenuous exercise or when the work of breathing is increased because of disease. The accessory muscles do not increase the volume of the thorax as efficiently as the diaphragm does.

There are no major muscles of expiration because normal, relaxed expiration is passive and requires no muscular effort. The accessory muscles of expiration, the abdominal and internal intercostal muscles, assist expiration when the minute volume is high, during coughing, or when airway obstruction is present. When the abdominal muscles contract, intra-abdominal pressure increases, pushing up the diaphragm and decreasing the volume of the thorax. The internal intercostal muscles pull down the anterior ribs, decreasing the AP diameter of the thorax.

Alveolar surface tension. Surface tension occurs at any gas-liquid interface and refers to the tendency for liquid molecules that are exposed to air to adhere to one another. This phenomenon can be seen in the way liquids "bead" when splashed on a waterproof surface.

Within a sphere, such as an alveolus, surface tension tends to make expansion difficult. According to the law of Laplace, the pressure *(P)* required to inflate a sphere is equal to two times the surface tension (2*T*) divided by the radius *(r)* of the sphere, or $P = 2T/r$. As the radius of the sphere (or alveolus) becomes smaller, more and more pressure is required to inflate it. If the alveoli were lined with a water-like fluid, taking breaths would be extremely difficult.

Alveolar ventilation, or distention, is made possible by surfactant, which lowers the surface tension by coating the air-liquid interface in the alveoli. Surfactant, a lipoprotein (90% lipids and 10% protein) produced by type II alveolar cells, includes two groups of surfactant proteins. One group consists of small hydrophobic molecules called surfactant B and C that have a detergent-like effect that separates the liquid molecules, thereby decreasing alveolar surface tension. These surfactant proteins line the alveolar side of the alveolocapillary membrane and, in effect, reverse the law of Laplace. As the radius of a surfactant-lined sphere (alveolus) becomes smaller, the surface tension *decreases*, and as the radius grows larger, the surface tension *increases*. This occurs because the surfactant molecules have much weaker intermolecular attraction than do liquid molecules. The surfactant molecules occupy most of the air-fluid interface and disrupt the intermolecular forces that tend to collapse the alveoli. Therefore, the alveoli are much easier to inflate at low lung volumes (i.e., after expiration) than at high volumes (i.e., after inspiration). The decrease in surface tension caused by surfactant also is responsible for keeping the alveoli free of fluid. If surfactant is not produced in adequate quantities, alveolar surface tension increases, causing alveolar collapse, decreased lung expansion, increased work of breathing, and severe gas-exchange abnormalities. Surfactant replacement therapy is used for a number of pulmonary diseases in which alveolar collapse (atelectasis) occurs.[16]

The other group of surfactant proteins is crucial in lung defense. Surfactant proteins A and D contribute to the control of lung inflammation by decreasing the release of proinflammatory mediators, preventing oxidative injury, and regulating the role of fibroblasts in airway remodeling.[17] These surfactant proteins have important antimicrobial effects, and defects in these proteins are linked to several lung disorders, including pneumonia, asthma, and COPD.[18]

Elastic properties of the lung and chest wall. The lung and chest walls have elastic properties that permit expansion during inspiration and return to resting volume during expiration. The elasticity of the lungs is caused both by elastin fibers in the alveolar walls surrounding the small airways and pulmonary capillaries and by surface tension at the alveolar air-liquid interface. The elasticity of the chest wall is the result of the configuration of its bones and musculature.

Elastic recoil is the tendency of the lungs to return to the resting state after inspiration. Normal elastic recoil permits passive expiration, eliminating the need for major muscles of expiration. Passive elastic recoil may be insufficient during labored breathing (high minute volume) when the accessory muscles of expiration may be needed. The accessory muscles are also used if disease compromises elastic recoil (e.g., in emphysema) or blocks the conducting airways.

Normal elastic recoil depends on an equilibrium between opposing forces of recoil in the lungs and chest wall. Under normal conditions, the chest wall tends to recoil by expanding outward. When the sternum is split to open the thoracic cavity, the chest wall moves outward laterally. The tendency of the chest wall to recoil by expanding is balanced by the tendency of the lungs to recoil or inward collapse around the hila. This reaction is caused by elastic recoil and surface tension in the alveoli. The opposing forces of the chest wall and lungs create the small negative intrapleural pressure.

A balance between the outward recoil of the chest wall and the inward recoil of the lungs occurs at the resting level, at the end of expiration. During inspiration, the diaphragm and intercostal muscles contract, air flows into the lungs, and the chest wall expands. Muscular effort is needed to overcome the resistance of the lungs to expansion. During expiration, the muscles relax, and the elastic recoil of the lungs causes the thorax to decrease in volume until a balance between the chest wall and lung recoil forces is reached (Fig. 34.11).

Compliance is the measure of lung and chest wall distensibility and is defined as volume change per unit of pressure change. It represents the relative ease with which these structures can be stretched and is, therefore, the opposite of elasticity. Compliance is determined by the alveolar surface tension and the elastic recoil of the lung and chest wall.

Increased compliance indicates that the lungs or chest wall is abnormally easy to inflate and has lost some elastic recoil. A decrease in compliance indicates that the lungs or chest wall is abnormally stiff or difficult to inflate. Compliance increases with normal aging and with disorders such as emphysema; it decreases in individuals with acute respiratory distress syndrome, pneumonia, pulmonary edema, and fibrosis. (These disorders are described in Chapter 35.)

Airway resistance. Airway resistance, which is similar to resistance to blood flow (described in Chapter 31), is determined by the length, radius, and cross-sectional area of the airways and by the density, viscosity, and velocity of the gas (Poiseuille's law). Resistance is computed by dividing the change in pressure (P) by the rate of flow (F), or $R = P/F$ (Ohm's law), and can easily be measured in the pulmonary function laboratory. Airway resistance is normally very low. One-half to two-thirds of total airway resistance occurs in the nose. The next highest resistance is in the oropharynx and larynx. Airway resistance also is affected by the diameter of the airways, and there is very little resistance in the conducting airways of the lungs because of their large cross-sectional area. Bronchodilation, which decreases resistance to airflow, is caused by β_2-adrenergic receptor stimulation. Bronchoconstriction, which increases airway resistance, can be caused by the stimulation of parasympathetic receptors in the bronchial smooth muscle and by numerous irritants and inflammatory mediators. Airway resistance can also be increased by edema of the bronchial mucosa and by airway obstructions, such as mucus, tumors, or foreign bodies. Pulmonary function tests (PFTs) measure lung volumes and flow rates and can be used to measure airway resistance and help diagnose certain lung diseases (see Tests of Pulmonary Function section).

Work of breathing. The work of breathing is determined by the muscular effort (and therefore oxygen and energy) required for ventilation. Normally very low, the work of breathing may increase considerably in diseases that disrupt the equilibrium between forces exerted by the lung and chest wall. More muscular effort is required when lung compliance decreases (e.g., in pulmonary edema), chest wall compliance decreases (e.g., in spinal deformity or obesity), or airways are obstructed by

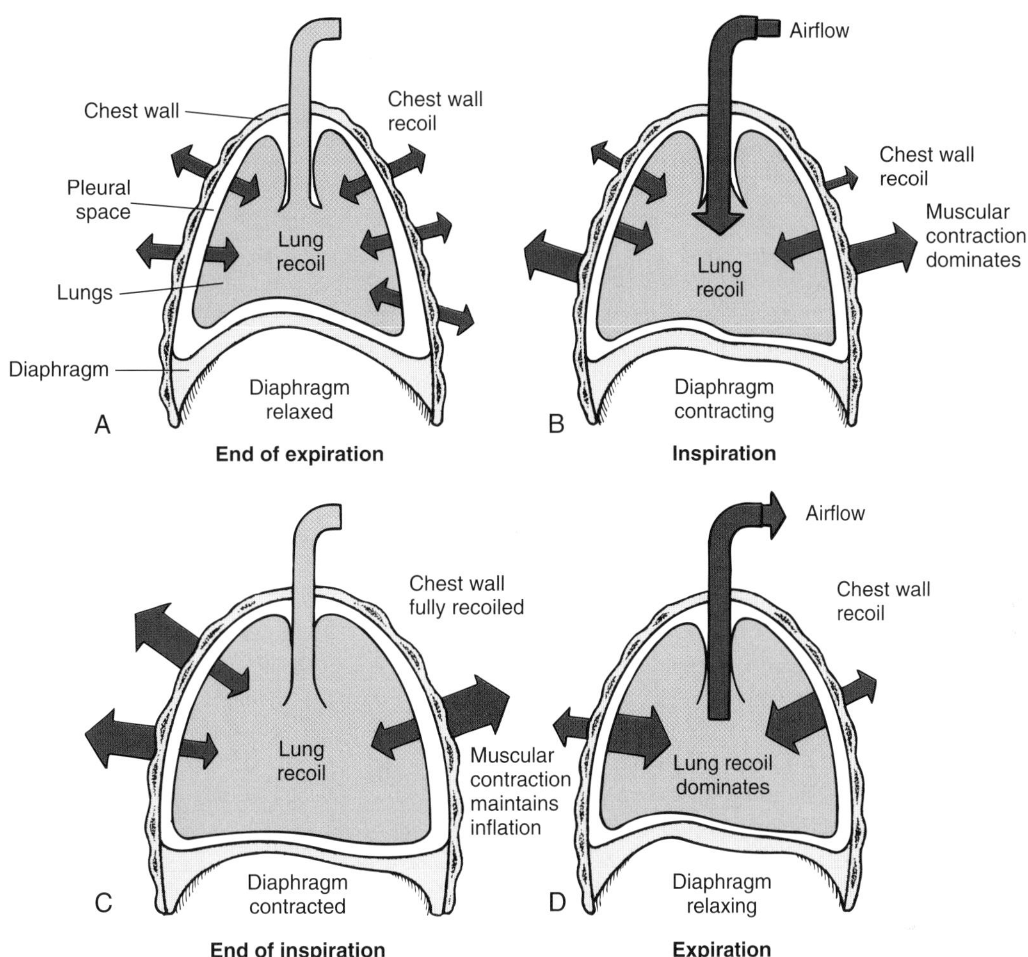

Fig. 34.11 Interaction of Forces During Inspiration and Expiration. **(A)** Outward recoil of the chest wall equals inward recoil of the lungs at the end of expiration. **(B)** During inspiration, contraction of respiratory muscles, assisted by chest wall recoil, overcomes the tendency of lungs to recoil. **(C)** At the end of inspiration, respiratory muscle contraction maintains lung expansion. **(D)** During expiration, respiratory muscles relax, allowing elastic recoil of the lungs to deflate the lungs.

bronchospasm or mucous plugging (e.g., in asthma or bronchitis). An increase in the work of breathing can result in a marked increase in O_2 consumption and an inability to maintain adequate ventilation.

Gas Transport

Gas transport is the delivery of O_2 to the cells of the body and the removal of CO_2. Delivery of O_2 has four steps: (1) ventilation of the lungs, (2) diffusion of O_2 from the alveoli into the capillary blood, (3) perfusion of systemic capillaries with oxygenated blood, and (4) diffusion of O_2 from systemic capillaries into the cells. Steps in the transport of CO_2 occur in reverse order: (1) diffusion of CO_2 from the cells into the systemic capillaries, (2) perfusion of the pulmonary capillary bed by venous blood, (3) diffusion of CO_2 into the alveoli, and (4) removal of CO_2 from the lung by ventilation. If any step in gas transport is impaired by a respiratory or cardiovascular disorder, gas exchange at the cellular level is compromised.

Measurement of Gas Pressure

The properties of air, once it enters the body, are determined by interactions among gas molecules at a given temperature. The millions of gas molecules are moving randomly, colliding with each other and with the wall of the space in which they are contained. These collisions exert pressure. If the same number of gas molecules is contained in a small and a large container, the pressure is greater in the small container because more collisions occur in the smaller space (Fig. 34.12). Heat increases the speed of the molecules, which increases the number of collisions and, therefore, the pressure.

Barometric pressure (P_B) (atmospheric pressure) is the pressure exerted by gas molecules in air at specific altitudes. At sea level, barometric pressure is 760 mm Hg, which is the sum of the pressures exerted by each gas in the air at sea level. The portion of the total pressure exerted by any individual gas is its partial pressure. At sea level, the air consists of O_2 (20.9%), nitrogen (78.1%), and a few other trace gases. The partial pressure of oxygen (PO_2) is equal to the percentage of O_2 in the air (20.9%) times the total P_B (760 mm Hg at sea level), or 159 mm Hg. At higher elevations, the P_B falls, and the amount of gases in the air decreases.

The amount of water vapor contained in a gas mixture is determined by the temperature of the gas and is unrelated to the barometric pressure. Gas that enters the lungs becomes saturated with

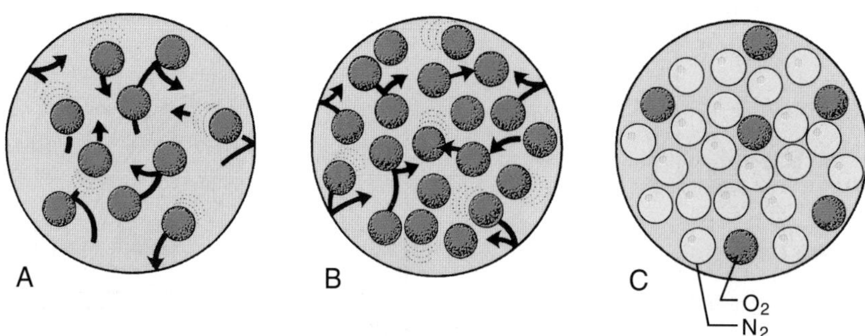

Fig. 34.12 Relationship Between Number of Gas Molecules and Pressure Exerted by the Gas in an Enclosed Space. **(A)** Theoretically, 10 molecules of the same gas exert a total pressure of 10 mm Hg within the space. **(B)** If the number of molecules is increased to 20, the total pressure is 20 mm Hg. **(C)** If there are different gases in the space, each gas exerts a partial pressure: here, the partial pressure of nitrogen *(yellow)* is 18, the partial pressure of oxygen *(blue)* is 6, and the total pressure is 24 mm Hg.

water vapor (humidified) as it passes through the upper airway. At body temperature (37°C [98.6°F]), water vapor exerts a pressure of 47 mm Hg regardless of the total P_B. The partial pressure of water vapor (PH_2O) must be subtracted from the P_B before the partial pressure of other gases in the mixture can be determined. In air saturated with water at sea level, the partial pressure of oxygen is $(760 - 47) \times 0.209 = 149$ mm Hg. All pressure and volume measurements made in pulmonary function laboratories specify the temperature and humidity of a gas at the time of measurement.

The percentage of O_2 in the inspired air is equal to the PO_2 (20.9%) and is called the fraction of inspired oxygen (FiO_2) in room air. The adequacy of ventilation to deliver O_2 to the alveoli cannot be measured directly but can be estimated by measuring the removal of CO_2 from the blood, as calculated by dividing the $PaCO_2$ by the respiratory quotient. The respiratory quotient describes the relationship between ventilation and perfusion of the lung and is considered to be 0.8.

The amount of oxygen in the alveoli (PAO_2) depends on the barometric pressure, the water vapor pressure, the amount of oxygen in the inspired air, the adequacy of ventilation as measured by the $PaCO_2$, and the respiratory quotient. The calculation of PAO2 using these parameters is called the alveolar gas equation:

$PAO_2 = (PB - PH_2O) \times FiO_2 - (PaCO_2/\text{respiratory quotient})$. For example, at sea level in an individual with normal ventilation, the amount of oxygen in the alveoli available for gas diffusion into the blood is calculated as $PAO_2 = (760 - 47) \times 0.209 - (40/0.8) = 99$ mm Hg (Fig. 34.13). Different values for PAO2 can be calculated if there are changes in the inspired oxygen content or the $PaCO_2$, which are common occurrences in clinical settings. All pressure and volume measurements made in pulmonary function laboratories specify the temperature and humidity of a gas at the time of measurement. Symbols used in the measurement of gas pressures and pulmonary ventilation are defined in Table 34.2.

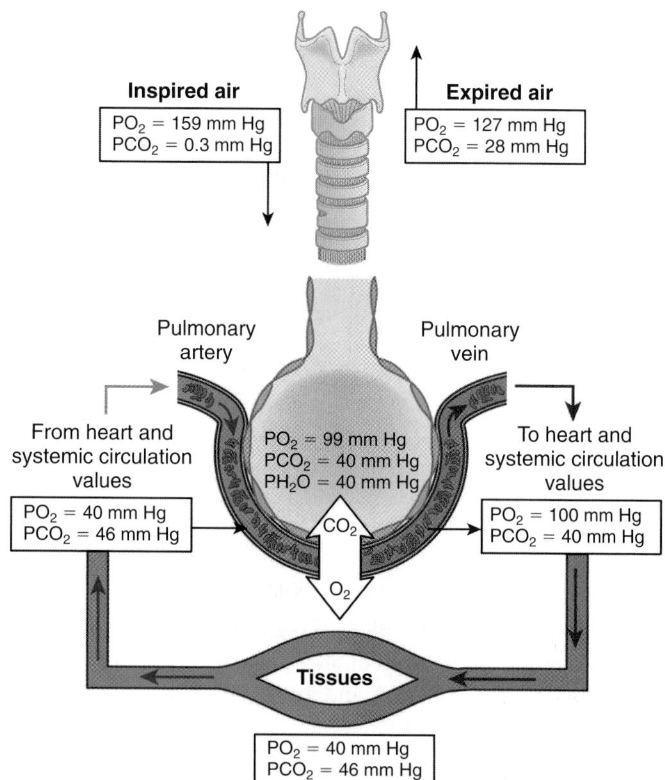

Fig. 34.13 Partial Pressure of Respiratory Gases in Normal Respiration. The numbers shown are average values near sea level. (Modified from Thompson JM, McFarland GK, Hirsch JE, et al. *Mosby's clinical nursing*, 5th edition. St. Louis: Mosby; 2002.)

Distribution of Ventilation and Perfusion

Effective gas exchange depends on an approximately even distribution of gas (ventilation) and blood (perfusion) in all portions of the lungs. The lungs are suspended from the hila in the thoracic cavity. When an individual is in an upright position (sitting or standing), gravity pulls the lungs down toward the diaphragm and compresses their lower portions, or bases. The alveoli in the upper portions, or apices, of the lungs contain a greater residual volume of gas and are larger and less numerous than those in the lower portions. Because surface tension increases as the alveoli become larger, the larger alveoli in the upper portions of the lung are more difficult to inflate (less compliant or less distensible) than the smaller alveoli in the lower portions of the lung. Therefore, during ventilation, most of the tidal volume is distributed to the bases of the lungs, where compliance is greater.

The heart pumps against gravity to perfuse the pulmonary circulation. As blood is pumped into the lung apices of a sitting or standing individual, some blood pressure is dissipated in overcoming gravity.

TABLE 34.2 Common Pulmonary Abbreviations

Symbol[a]	Definition
V	Volume or amount of gas
Q	Perfusion or blood flow
P	Pressure (usually partial pressure) of a gas
PiO_2	Partial pressure of inspired oxygen (varies with altitude)
PaO_2	Partial pressure of oxygen in arterial blood
PAO_2	Partial pressure of oxygen in alveolar blood
$PaCO_2$	Partial pressure of carbon dioxide in arterial blood
PH_2O	Partial pressure of water vapor
PN_2	Partial pressure of nitrogen
$P\bar{v}O_2$	Partial pressure of oxygen in mixed venous or pulmonary artery blood
$P(A-a)O_2$	Difference between alveolar and arterial partial pressure of oxygen (A–a gradient)
P_B	Barometric or atmospheric pressure
SaO_2	Saturation of hemoglobin (in arterial blood) with oxygen
$S\bar{v}O_2$	Saturation of hemoglobin (in mixed venous blood)
V_A	Alveolar ventilation—effective total lung capacity
V_D	Dead-space ventilation
V_E	Minute capacity
V_T	Tidal volume or average breath
$\dot{V}/\dot{Q}$	Ratio of ventilation to perfusion
FiO_2	Fraction (percent) of inspired oxygen (0.21)
FRC	Functional residual capacity
FVC	Forced vital capacity
FEV_1	Forced expiratory volume in 1 second
ERV	Expiratory reserve volume
IRV	Inspiratory reserve volume
IC	Inspiratory capacity

[a]Subscripts identify the particular gas, volume, or pressure being discussed. An overhead dot, such as in $\dot{V}/\dot{Q}$, means measurement over time, usually 1 minute.

From Kacmarek RM, Stoller JK, Heuer AJ. *Egan's fundamentals of respiratory care*, 11th edition. St. Louis: Mosby; 2017.

As a result, blood pressure at the apices is lower than that at the bases. Because greater pressure causes greater perfusion, the bases of the lungs are better perfused than the apices (Fig. 34.14). Thus, ventilation and perfusion are greatest in the same lung portions—the lower lobesin the upright position. If a standing individual assumes a supine or side-lying position, the areas of the lungs that are then most dependent become the best ventilated and perfused.

The distribution of perfusion in the pulmonary circulation also is affected by the alveolar pressure (gas pressure in the alveoli). The pulmonary capillary bed differs from the systemic capillary bed in that it is surrounded by gas-containing alveoli. If the gas pressure in the alveoli exceeds the blood pressure in the capillary, the capillary collapses, and flow ceases. This is most likely to occur in portions of the lung where blood pressure is lowest and alveolar gas pressure is greatest—that is, at the apex of the lung.

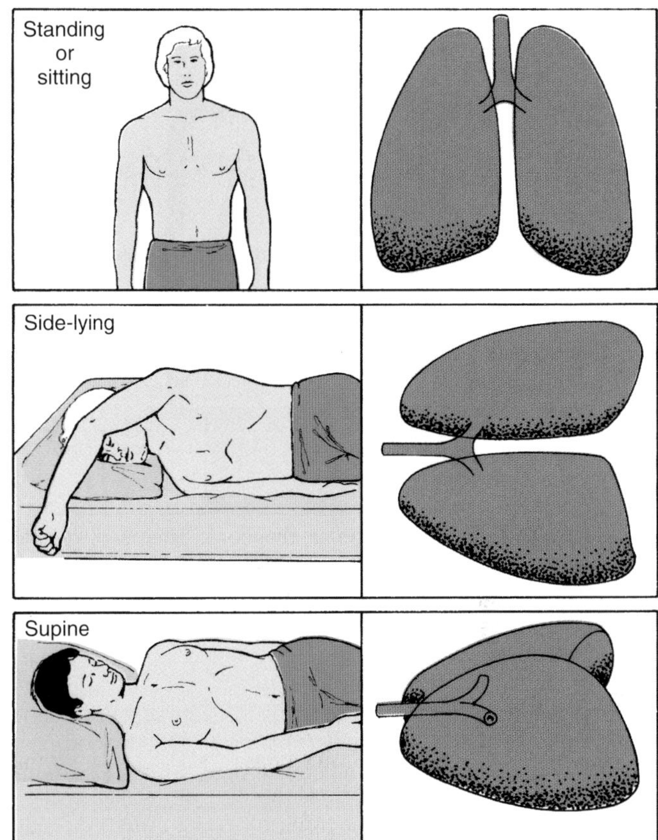

Fig. 34.14 Pulmonary Blood Flow and Gravity. The greatest volume of pulmonary blood flow normally will occur in the gravity-dependent areas of the lung. Body position has a significant effect on the distribution of pulmonary blood flow. The shaded areas represent gravity-dependent pulmonary blood flow.

The lungs are divided into three zones on the basis of relationships among all the factors affecting pulmonary blood flow. Alveolar pressure and the forces of gravity, arterial blood pressure, and venous blood pressure affect the distribution of perfusion, as shown in Fig. 34.15.

In zone I, the alveolar pressure exceeds the pulmonary arterial and venous pressures. The capillary bed collapses, and normal blood flow ceases. Normally zone I is a very small part of the lung at the apex. In zone II, the alveolar pressure is greater than the venous pressure but not the arterial pressure. Blood flows through zone II, but it is impeded to a certain extent by the alveolar pressure. Zone II is normally above the level of the left atrium. In zone III, both the arterial and venous pressures are greater than the alveolar pressure, and blood flow is not affected by the alveolar pressure. Zone III is in the base of the lung. Blood flow through the pulmonary capillary bed increases in regular increments from the apex to the base.

Although both blood flow and ventilation are greater at the base of the lungs than at the apices, they are not perfectly matched in any zone. Perfusion exceeds ventilation in the bases, and ventilation exceeds perfusion in the apices of the lung. The relationship between ventilation and perfusion is expressed as a ratio called the ventilation-perfusion ratio ($\dot{V}/\dot{Q}$). The normal

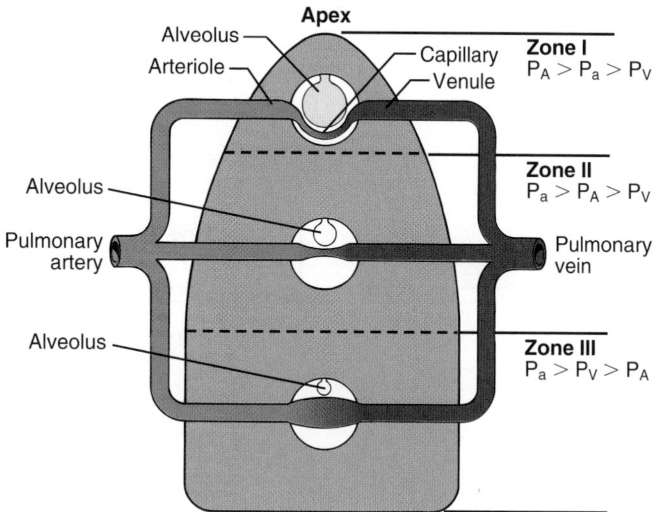

Fig. 34.15 Gravity and Alveolar Pressure. Effects of gravity and alveolar pressure on pulmonary blood flow in the three lung zones. In zone I, the alveolar pressure (P_A) is greater than the arterial pressure (P_a) and the venous pressure (P_V), and no blood flow occurs. In zone II, the P_a exceeds the P_A, but the P_A exceeds the P_V. Blood flow occurs in this zone, but the P_A compresses the venules (venous ends of the capillaries). In zone III, both the P_a and P_V are greater than the P_A, and blood flow fluctuates, depending on the difference between the P_A arterial pressure and the P_V.

$\dot{V}/\dot{Q}$ is called the respiratory quotient and is 0.8. This is the amount by which perfusion exceeds ventilation under normal conditions.

As described previously in this chapter, a low alveolar partial pressure of oxygen causes a reflex called hypoxic pulmonary vasoconstriction. Increases in carbon dioxide also contribute to pulmonary vasoconstriction.[19] If a segment of the lung experiences decreased alveolar oxygen and increased carbon dioxide, arterioles to that segment constrict, so that appropriate matching of ventilation and perfusion is restored.

Oxygen Transport

Approximately 1000 mL (1 L) of O_2 is transported to the cells of the body each minute. O_2 is transported in the blood in two forms: a small amount dissolves in plasma, and the remainder binds to hemoglobin molecules. Without hemoglobin, O_2 would not reach the cells in amounts sufficient to maintain normal metabolic function. (Hemoglobin is discussed in detail in Chapter 28, and cellular metabolism is explored in Chapter 1.)

Diffusion across the alveolocapillary membrane. The alveolocapillary membrane is ideal for O_2 diffusion because it has a large total surface area (70 to 100 m^2) and is very thin (0.5 μm). In addition, the PAO_2 (approximately 99 mm Hg at sea level) is much greater than that in capillary blood (approximately 40 mm Hg), a condition that promotes rapid diffusion down the concentration gradient from the alveolus into the capillary. Therefore, a pressure gradient of nearly 60 mm Hg facilitates the diffusion of O_2 from the alveolus into the capillary (see Fig. 34.13).

Blood remains in the pulmonary capillary for about 0.75 seconds, but only 0.25 seconds is required for the O_2 concentration to equilibrate (equalize) across the alveolocapillary membrane. Therefore, O_2 has ample time to diffuse into the blood, even during increased cardiac output, which speeds blood flow and shortens the time the blood remains in the capillary.

Determinants of arterial oxygenation. As O_2 diffuses across the alveolocapillary membrane, it dissolves in the plasma, where it exerts pressure (PaO_2). As the PaO_2 increases, O_2 moves from the plasma into the red blood cells (erythrocytes) and binds with hemoglobin molecules. O_2 continues to bind with hemoglobin until the hemoglobin-binding sites are filled, or *saturated.* O_2 then continues to diffuse across the alveolocapillary membrane until the PaO_2 (oxygen dissolved in plasma) and PAO_2 (oxygen in the alveolus) equilibrate, eliminating the pressure gradient across the alveolocapillary membrane. At this point, diffusion ceases (see Fig. 34.13).

The majority (97%) of the O_2 that enters the blood is bound to hemoglobin. The remaining 3% stays in the plasma and creates the PaO_2. The PaO_2 can be measured in the blood by obtaining an arterial blood gas measurement. The oxygen saturation (SaO_2) is the percentage of the available hemoglobin that is bound to O_2 and can be measured using a device called an *oximeter.* The total amount of oxygen carried in the blood is the oxygen content and is measured in milliliters per deciliter (1 dL = 100 mL) of blood. It is the combined value of the O_2 in oxygen-saturated hemoglobin and the O_2 dissolved in the blood.

To calculate the total arterial O_2 content, one must know (1) the hemoglobin concentration, or the amount of hemoglobin that is available to bind with oxygen (hemoglobin [Hb] in grams per deciliter); (2) the oxygen saturation, or the percentage of available hemoglobin that is bound to oxygen (SaO_2); and (3) the partial pressure of oxygen (PaO_2). The maximum amount of oxygen that can be transported by hemoglobin is 1.34 mL/g. The amount of oxygen that can be physically dissolved in blood is 0.003 mL/dL per mm Hg. With the specific values known, the oxygen content of arterial blood can be calculated. To calculate the oxygen content of venous blood, the partial pressure of mixed venous blood (PvO_2) and venous oxygen saturation (SvO_2) are substituted for the arterial values in the basic formula. Normal venous oxygen content is 15 to 16 mL/dL.

Because hemoglobin transports all but a small fraction of the O_2 carried in arterial blood, changes in the hemoglobin concentration affect the O_2 content of the blood. Decreases in the hemoglobin concentration below the normal value of approximately 15 g/dL of blood reduce the O_2 content, and increases in the hemoglobin concentration may increase O_2 content. An increased hemoglobin concentration is a major compensatory mechanism in pulmonary diseases that impair gas exchange. For this reason, measurement of the hemoglobin concentration is important in assessing individuals with pulmonary disease. If cardiovascular function is normal, the body's initial response to low O_2 content is to accelerate cardiac output. In individuals who also have cardiovascular disease, this compensatory mechanism is ineffective. An elevated hemoglobin level can compensate for an inability to accelerate cardiac output, making an increased hemoglobin concentration an even more important compensatory mechanism.

Oxyhemoglobin association and dissociation. When hemoglobin molecules bind with O_2, oxyhemoglobin (HbO_2) forms. Binding occurs in the lungs and is called *oxyhemoglobin association* or *hemoglobin saturation with oxygen* (SaO_2). The reverse process, in which O_2 is released from hemoglobin, occurs in the body tissues at the cellular level and is called *hemoglobin desaturation*. When hemoglobin saturation and desaturation are plotted on a graph, the result is a distinctive S-shaped curve known as the oxyhemoglobin dissociation curve (Fig. 34.16). For PaO_2 values less than 60 mm Hg, oxygen is readily unloaded to peripheral tissues, and hemoglobin's affinity for oxygen diminishes, reflecting the steep part of the curve. For PaO_2 values greater than 60 mm Hg, the curve becomes relatively flat, reflecting the maximum saturation of hemoglobin with oxygen in the lungs.

Several factors can change the relationship between the PaO_2 and the SaO_2, causing the oxyhemoglobin dissociation curve to shift to the right or left (see Fig. 34.16). At a PaO_2 of 26.6 mm Hg, hemoglobin is 50% saturated, known as P_{50}. An increase in the P_{50} value shifts the curve to the right, indicating hemoglobin's decreased affinity for O_2 or an increase in the ease with which oxyhemoglobin dissociates and O_2 moves into the cells. A larger partial pressure is necessary to maintain 50% oxygen saturation. A shift to the left depicts hemoglobin's increased affinity for O_2, which promotes association in the lungs and inhibits dissociation in the tissues. Lower partial pressure is necessary to maintain 50% oxygen saturation.

The oxyhemoglobin dissociation curve is shifted to the right by acidosis (low pH) and hypercapnia (increased $PaCO_2$). In the tissues, the increased levels of CO_2 and H^+ produced by metabolic activity decrease the affinity of hemoglobin for O_2, and O_2 is released into the tissues. The curve is shifted to the left by alkalosis (high pH) and hypocapnia (decreased $PaCO_2$). In the lungs, as CO_2 diffuses from the blood into the alveoli, the blood CO_2 level is reduced, and the affinity of hemoglobin for O_2 is increased so that more O_2 can be transported from the lungs into the tissues. The shift in the oxyhemoglobin dissociation curve caused by changes in the CO_2 and hydrogen ion concentrations in the blood is called the Bohr effect.

The oxyhemoglobin curve is also shifted by changes in body temperature and increased or decreased levels of 2,3-diphosphoglycerate (2,3-DPG), a substance normally present in erythrocytes. Hyperthermia and increased 2,3-DPG levels shift the curve to the right so that more O_2 is released into the tissues. Hypothermia and decreased 2,3-DPG levels shift the curve to the left.

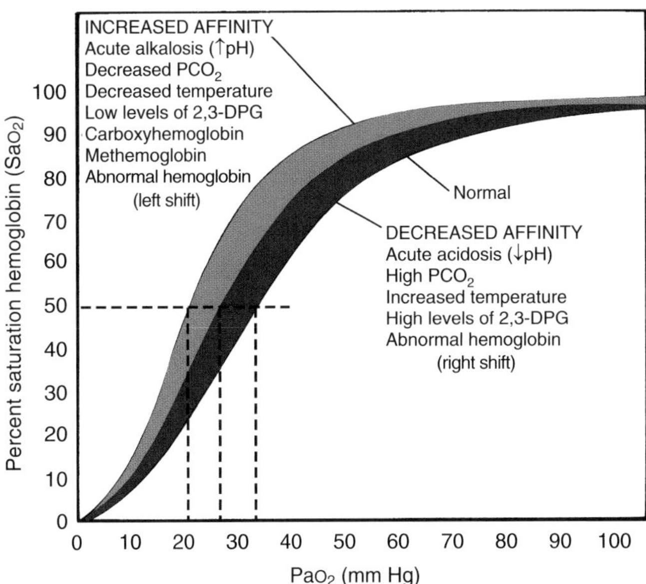

Fig. 34.16 Oxyhemoglobin Dissociation Curve. The horizontal or flat segment of the curve at the top of the graph is the arterial or association portion, or that part of the curve where oxygen (O_2) is bound to hemoglobin and occurs in the lungs. This portion of the curve is flat because partial pressure changes of O_2 between 60 and 100 mm Hg do not significantly alter the percentage saturation of hemoglobin with O_2 and allow adequate hemoglobin saturation at a variety of altitudes. If the relationship between the oxygen saturation of hemoglobin in arterial blood (SaO_2) and the partial pressure of oxygen in the arterial blood (PaO_2) were linear (in a downward sloping straight line) instead of flat between 60 and 100 mm Hg, there would be inadequate saturation of hemoglobin with O_2. The steep part of the oxyhemoglobin dissociation curve represents the rapid dissociation of O_2 from hemoglobin that occurs in the tissues. During this phase, there is rapid diffusion of O_2 from the blood into tissue cells. The P50 is the PaO_2 at which hemoglobin is 50% saturated, normally 26.6 mm Hg. A lower than normal P50 represents increased affinity of hemoglobin for O_2; a high P50 is seen with decreased affinity. Note that variation from the normal is associated with decreased (low P50) or increased (high P50) availability of O_2 to tissues (dashed lines). The shaded area shows the entire oxyhemoglobin dissociation curve under the same circumstances. 2,3-DPG, 2,3-Diphosphoglycerate; PaO_2, arterial pressure of oxygen; PCO_2, partial pressure of carbon dioxide. (From Lane EE, Walker JF. *Clinical arterial blood gas analysis*. St. Louis: Mosby; 1987.)

Carbon Dioxide Transport

Approximately 200 mL of CO_2 is produced by the tissues per minute at rest as a byproduct of cellular metabolism. This CO_2 equilibrates with carbonic acid (H_2CO_3) and must be eliminated continuously to prevent acidosis. The elimination of CO_2 by the lungs plays an important role in the regulation of acid-base balance (see Chapter 3).

CO_2 is carried in the blood in three ways: (1) dissolved in plasma, (2) transported as bicarbonate, and (3) combined with blood proteins to form carbamino compounds. As CO_2 diffuses out of the cells into the blood, it dissolves in the plasma. Approximately 10% of the total CO_2 in venous blood and 5% of the CO_2 in arterial blood are carried dissolved in the plasma. As CO_2 moves into the blood, it diffuses into the red blood cells. Within the red blood cells, CO_2, with the help of the enzyme carbonic anhydrase, combines with water to form carbonic acid and then quickly dissociates into H^+ and HCO_3^-. As carbonic acid dissociates, the H^+ binds to hemoglobin, where it is buffered, and the HCO_3^- moves out of the red blood cell into the plasma. Approximately 60% of the CO_2 in venous blood and

90% of the CO_2 in arterial blood are carried in the form of bicarbonate. The remainder combines with blood proteins, hemoglobin, in particular, to form carbamino compounds.

CO_2 is 20 times more soluble than O_2 and diffuses quickly from the tissue cells into the blood. The amount of CO_2 able to enter the blood is enhanced by the diffusion of O_2 out of the blood and into the cells. Reduced hemoglobin (hemoglobin that is dissociated from O_2) can carry more CO_2 than can hemoglobin saturated with O_2. Therefore, the drop in O_2 saturation at the tissue level increases the ability of hemoglobin to carry CO_2 back to the lung.

The diffusion gradient for CO_2 in the lung is only approximately 6 mm Hg ($PvCO_2$ = 46 mm Hg; $PACO_2$ = 40 mm Hg) (see Fig. 34.13). Yet CO_2 is so soluble in the alveolocapillary membrane that the CO_2 in the blood quickly diffuses into the alveoli, where it is removed from the lung with each expiration. Diffusion of CO_2 in the lung is so efficient that diffusion defects that cause hypoxemia (low O_2 content of the blood) do not as readily cause hypercapnia (excessive CO_2 in the blood).

The diffusion of CO_2 out of the blood and into the lungs also is enhanced by O_2 binding with hemoglobin. As hemoglobin binds with O_2, the amount of CO_2 carried by the blood decreases, and it is released into the alveoli. Thus, in the tissue capillaries, O_2 dissociation from hemoglobin facilitates the pickup of CO_2, and the binding of O_2 to hemoglobin in the lungs facilitates the release of CO_2 from the blood. This effect of O_2 on CO_2 transport is called the Haldane effect.

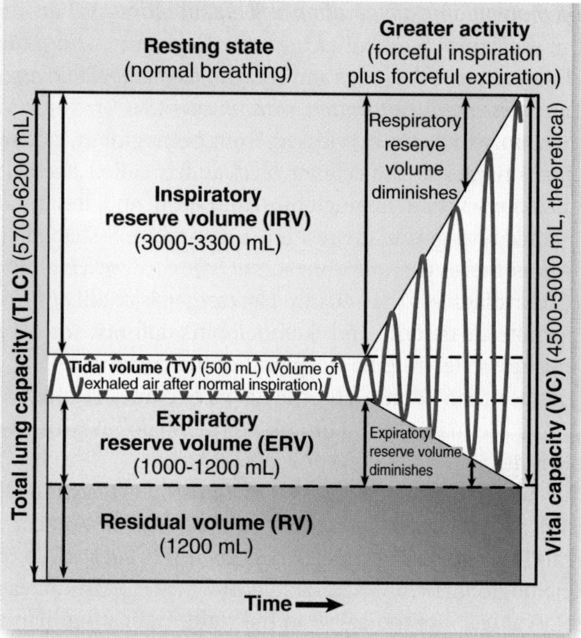

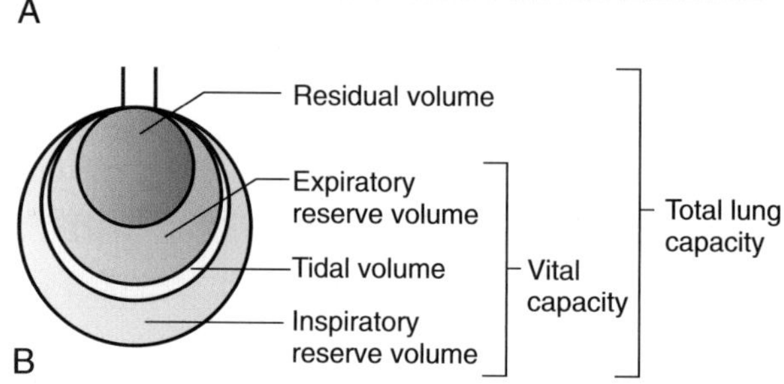

Fig. 34.17 Pulmonary Ventilation and Lung Capacities. **(A)** Spirogram. During normal, quiet respiration, the atmosphere and lungs exchange about 500 mL of air (VT). With a forcible inspiration, about 3300 mL more air can be inhaled (*IRV*). After a normal inspiration and normal expiration, approximately 1000 mL more air can be forcibly expired (*ERV*). Vital capacity is the amount of air that can be forcibly expired after a maximal inspiration and indicates, therefore, the largest amount of air that can enter and leave the lungs during respiration. Residual volume (*RV*) is the air that remains trapped in the alveoli. **(B)** Lung capacities. (From Patton KT, Thibodeau GA. *The human body in health & disease*, 7th edition. St. Louis: Mosby; 2018.)

TESTS OF PULMONARY FUNCTION

Several laboratory tests aid in the diagnosis and evaluation of pulmonary system abnormalities. Most of them are easy to perform at hospitals and clinics. They provide valuable information about the possible cause of a respiratory abnormality and evaluate the progression or resolution of disease.[20]

Pulmonary function testing includes spirometry, which measures the volume and flow of air inhaled and exhaled and is plotted against time (flow rate) during different breathing maneuvers. Several different types of spirometers are available. It is essential that these devices meet current standards and that they are used properly in order to achieve accurate results.[21] The procedure produces a spirogram, which is a record of the individual's ventilation in relation to time (Fig. 34.17). Clinically the most important spirometric tests are the forced vital capacity (FVC) and the forced expiratory volume in 1 second (FEV_1). (These tests and other important measurements are described in Table 34.3.) Spirometry enables clinicians to detect restrictive or obstructive deficits early in the course of disease. *Restrictive lung diseases* restrict the lungs' volume; the lungs are unable to expand normally, diminishing the amount of gas that can be inspired and reducing the FVC. *Obstructive lung diseases* affect gas flow; airflow into and out of the lungs is obstructed, reducing the FEV_1 (see Chapter 35).

Lung capacities, such as vital capacity (sum of inspiratory reserve volume, tidal volume, and expiratory reserve volume) and total lung capacity (sum of the vital capacity and the residual capacity), are always the sum of two or more volumes. Norms for volumes and capacities are based on age, sex, and height and are referred to as *predicted values*. Differences from predicted or changes from baseline values are taken into account in diagnosing and assessing respiratory disorders.

Pulmonary diffusing capacity (transfer factor) is a measure of the rate of gas diffusion across the alveolocapillary membrane. O_2, or more commonly carbon monoxide (CO), is used to measure diffusing capacity. CO has a high affinity for hemoglobin and is not limited by pulmonary blood flow and therefore is an excellent measure of diffusion. The measurement is made by determining how much CO is taken up by the blood and dividing this amount by the pressure gradient across the alveolocapillary membrane. Helium (an inert gas poorly soluble in alveolar blood and lung tissue) often is added to the gas mixture to obtain a simultaneous measurement of residual volume (RV), functional residual capacity (FRC), and total lung capacity (TLC). Individuals are asked to perform ventilatory maneuvers similar to those used in spirometry testing. A decreased diffusing capacity can be the result of an abnormal ventilation-perfusion ratio or an actual diffusion defect. For example, diffusing capacity is decreased in individuals with emphysema, where there is a decrease in the surface area of pulmonary capillaries available for gas exchange.

Oximetry is commonly performed for individuals with suggested or diagnosed pulmonary disease. It indirectly measures hemoglobin oxygen saturation and can suggest that the PaO_2 is low. However, it is prone to inaccurate measurements, particularly in individuals with poor peripheral circulation, and does not measure the $PaCO_2$ or pH of the blood. Capnography measures the amount of CO_2 in expired air and thus estimates $PaCO_2$, but this test is also prone to inaccuracy. Arterial blood gas analysis is the direct measurement of the pH and gas concentrations in arterial blood and provides more accurate and complete information about an individual's gas exchange and acid-base status. Acidosis (low pH), alkalosis (high pH), ventilatory alterations, and decreased PaO_2 can be diagnosed accurately only by arterial blood gas analysis. A blood gas report may be divided into an acid-base/ventilation portion and an oxygenation portion. (Normal values for arterial blood gases are given in Table 34.4; acid-base alterations are described in Chapter 3.)

Signs and symptoms of most respiratory abnormalities first appear when the system is stressed during exercise. Therefore, if pulmonary disease is suspected, the individual is evaluated at rest and during exercise. Evaluation during exercise usually entails spirometry and oximetry to monitor hemoglobin saturation. The exercise usually consists of riding a stationary bicycle or walking on a treadmill. Exercise testing enables clinicians to detect early changes in respiratory function and thus begin treatment. Exercise tests also are used in planning and evaluating exercise and rehabilitation programs.

Thoracic imaging techniques are among the most common examinations for diagnosis and detection of pulmonary disease and tumors and for evaluation of disease progression. Numerous techniques are available and include chest radiography, computed tomography (CT), magnetic resonance imaging (MRI), positron emission tomography, and ultrasonography. Pulmonary angiography is used for the detection of pulmonary embolism and pulmonary arteriovenous malformations. Techniques may be combined for the best evaluation of pulmonary structure and function.

TABLE 34.3 Values Measured by Spirometry

Symbol	Ventilatory Property Measured
FVC	Forced vital capacity; maximum amount of gas that can be displaced from the lung during a forced expiration
FEV_1	Forced expiratory volume in 1 second; maximum amount of air that can be expired from the lung in 1 second
FEV_1/FVC	Percentage of maximum inspiration that is expired in 1 second; usually 80% of FVC
FEV_3	Forced expiratory volume in 3 seconds; maximum amount of gas that can be expired in 3 seconds
FEV_3/FVC	Percentage of FVC that is expired in 3 seconds; usually 95% of FVC
$FEF_{25-75\%}$	Forced expiratory flow rate during the middle 50% of expiration; sometimes reported as maximum mid expiratory flow rate (MMFR)
MVV	Maximum voluntary ventilation
PEF	Peak expiratory flow

TABLE 34.4 Normal Ranges for Arterial and Mixed Venous Blood Gases

Measurement	Arterial Blood	Mixed Venous Blood[a]	Clinical Notes
Acid-base status (pH)	7.35–7.45	7.33–7.43	Most important acid-base value; detects acidosis or alkalosis
Partial pressure of carbon dioxide (PCO_2)	35–45 mm Hg	41–57 mm Hg	Measures adequacy of ventilation and respiratory contribution of acid-base abnormality (respiratory acidosis)
Bicarbonate concentration (HCO_3^-)	22–26 mEq/L	24–28 mEq/L	Measures metabolic contribution to acid-base abnormality (metabolic acidosis); calculated from pH and PCO_2
Base excess (BE)	−2 to +2	0 to +4	Reflects deviation of bicarbonate concentration from normal
Partial pressure of oxygen (PO_2) (sea level)	80–100 mm Hg	35–40 mm Hg	Indicates driving pressure that causes oxyhemoglobin binding; varies with age and barometric pressure
Saturation of hemoglobin with oxygen (SO_2)	96%–98%	70%–75%	Indicates abnormalities of oxyhemoglobin association and dissociation; may be measured directly or calculated from PCO_2, pH, and body temperature
Concentration of hemoglobin in the blood	15 g/dL	15 g/dL	Detects alterations of gas transport caused by anemia

[a]Mixed venous (pulmonary artery) blood is analyzed for critically ill individuals and those undergoing cardiac catheterization (it is not practical to withdraw samples except from a pulmonary artery catheter). Mixed venous blood gas analysis, in conjunction with arterial analysis, provides important information about the adequacy of cardiac output and tissue oxygenation.

GERIATRIC CONSIDERATIONS

Aging and the Pulmonary System

Most knowledge about pulmonary structure and function is based on norms for the middle-age years. Less is known about structure and function in the very young (see Chapter 36) and in older adults, but a few normal physiologic (developmental and degenerative) changes are known to occur from birth to old age. An understanding of these changes is needed to provide appropriate care and to differentiate between age-associated alterations and disease. Normal alterations in the pulmonary system that occur with aging include (1) loss of elastic recoil, (2) stiffening of the chest wall, (3) changes in gas exchange, and (4) increases in flow resistance. These changes, which affect lung volumes, are gradual and usually without adverse consequences in healthy individuals (Fig. 34.18). They are influenced by genetics, sociocultural factors, nutritional status, exercise, decreased immune function, respiratory disease, body size, sex, and race. Exposure to environmental toxins, such as some respiratory tract infections, tobacco smoke, air pollution, and occupational dusts, also contributes to decreased lung function with aging. These changes contribute to increased lung disease morbidity and mortality in older adults, including chronic obstructive lung disease, lung cancer, pulmonary fibrosis, and infection.

During adulthood and as age advances, the alveoli tend to lose alveoli wall tissue and capillaries. This process increases alveolar size, diminishes the alveolar surface area available for gas diffusion, and decreases airway support provided by normal lung tissues. These changes are similar to those seen in emphysema and diminish the elasticity of the lungs. Chest wall compliance decreases with age because the ribs become ossified (less flexible), and the joints become stiffer. As a result, the chest wall loses some of its ability to expand. In addition, respiratory muscle strength and endurance decrease by up to 20% by age 70. These mechanical changes in the lung and chest wall, along with structural changes in the alveoli, reduce the ventilatory capacity in older adults. Vital capacity decreases and residual volume increases; however, total lung capacity remains unchanged. These changes decrease ventilatory reserves and lead to decreased ventilation-perfusion ratios. With advancing age, there is also increased immune dysregulation, asymptomatic low-grade inflammation ("inflamm-aging"), and increased risk of infection.

Alterations in gas exchange are reflected by blood gas analysis. With advancing age, pH and $PaCO_2$ levels do not change much, even though it has been documented that the chemoreceptors become less sensitive to gas partial pressures with age. Older adults have a decreased compensatory response to hypercapnia and hypoxemia; however, the perception of dyspnea remains intact and is even enhanced. PaO_2 declines with age as a result of structural and mechanical changes, such as loss of alveolar surface area, thickening of plural septa, loss of lung elasticity, and increase in ventilation-perfusion mismatch. The maximum PaO_2 value in an older adult at sea level can be estimated by multiplying the person's age by 0.3 and subtracting the product from 100. For example, an 80-year-old individual would have an estimated maximum PaO_2 of 76 mm Hg ($0.3 \times 80 = 24$; $100 - 24 = 76$).

The decrease in PaO_2 and the diminished ventilatory reserve in an older adult lead to a decrease in exercise tolerance. Respiratory muscle strength and endurance decrease with age. Furthermore, older adults are at greater risk for respiratory depression caused by medications. Changes in respiratory structure and function can vary considerably from person to person, however. Changes also are affected by activity and fitness earlier in life.

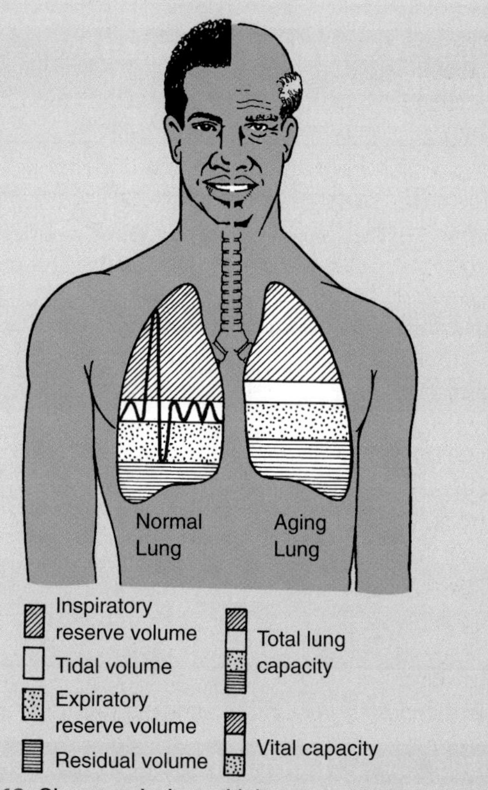

Figure 34.18 Changes in Lung Volumes with Aging. In aging, vital capacity decreases, and residual volume increases.

Data from Bowdish DME. The aging lung: Is lung health good health for older adults? *Chest.* 2019;155(2):391–400; Brandenberger C, Muhfield C. Mechanics of lung aging. *Cell Tissue Res.* 2017;367:469–480; Hardie JA, et al. Reference values for arterial blood gases in the elderly. *Chest.* 2004;125:2053–2060; Kim J, Im JS, Choi YH. Objectively measured sedentary behavior and moderate-to-vigorous physical activity on the health-related quality of life in US adults: the National Health and Nutrition Examination Survey 2003–2006. *Qual Life Res.* 2017;25:1315– 1326.

SUMMARY REVIEW

Structures of the Pulmonary System

1. The pulmonary system consists of the lungs, upper and lower airways, chest wall, and pulmonary and bronchial circulation.
2. Air is inspired and expired through the conducting airways: nasopharynx, oropharynx, trachea, bronchi, and bronchioles.
3. Gas exchange occurs in structures beyond the respiratory bronchioles: in the alveolar ducts and the alveoli. Together these structures compose the acinus.
4. The chief gas exchange units of the lungs are the alveoli. The membrane that surrounds each alveolus and contains the pulmonary capillaries is called the alveolocapillary membrane.
5. The gas-exchange airways are perfused by the pulmonary circulation, a separate division of the circulatory system. The bronchi and other lung structures are perfused by a branch of the systemic circulation called the bronchial circulation.

6. The pulmonary circulation is innervated by the autonomic nervous system (ANS), but vasodilation and vasoconstriction are controlled mainly by local and humoral factors, particularly arterial oxygenation and acid-base status.
7. The chest wall, which contains and protects the contents of the thoracic cavity, consists of the skin, ribs, and intercostal muscles, which lie between the ribs.
8. The chest wall is lined by a serous membrane called the parietal pleura; the lungs are encased in a separate membrane called the visceral pleura. The pleural space is the area where these two pleurae contact and slide over one another.

Function of the Pulmonary System

1. The pulmonary system (1) ventilates the alveoli, (2) diffuses gases into and out of the blood, and (3) perfuses the lungs so that the organs and tissues of the body receive blood that is rich in oxygen and deficient in carbon dioxide.
2. Ventilation is the process by which air flows into and out of the gas-exchange airways.
3. Most of the time, ventilation is involuntary. It is controlled by the sympathetic and parasympathetic divisions of the autonomic nervous system, which adjust airway caliber (by causing the bronchial smooth muscle to contract or relax) and control the rate and depth of ventilation.
4. Neuroreceptors in the lungs (lung receptors) monitor the mechanical aspects of ventilation. Irritant receptors sense the need to expel unwanted substances, stretch receptors sense lung volume (lung expansion), and J-receptors sense pulmonary capillary pressure.
5. Chemoreceptors in the circulatory system and brainstem sense the effectiveness of ventilation by monitoring the pH status of cerebrospinal fluid and the oxygen content (Po_2) of arterial blood.
6. Successful ventilation involves the mechanics of breathing: the interaction of forces and counterforces involving the muscles of inspiration and expiration, alveolar surface tension, elastic properties of the lungs and chest wall, and resistance to airflow.
7. The major muscle of inspiration is the diaphragm. When the diaphragm contracts, it moves downward in the thoracic cavity, creating a vacuum that causes air to flow into the lungs.
8. The type II alveolar cells produce surfactant, a lipoprotein that lines the alveoli. Surfactant reduces alveolar surface tension and permits the alveoli to expand as air enters.
9. Elastic recoil is the tendency of the lungs and chest wall to return to their resting state after inspiration. The elastic recoil forces of the lungs and chest wall are in opposition and pull on each other, creating the normally negative pressure of the pleural space.
10. Compliance is the ease with which the lungs and chest wall expand during inspiration. Lung compliance is ensured by an adequate production of surfactant, whereas chest wall expansion depends on elasticity.
11. The work of breathing is determined by the muscular effort required for ventilation and is normally very low. Work increases when lung or chest wall compliance decreases or airways are obstructed.
12. Gas transport depends on ventilation of the lungs, diffusion of oxygen across the alveolocapillary membrane, perfusion of systemic capillaries with oxygenated blood, and diffusion between systemic capillaries and tissue cells.
13. Efficient gas exchange depends on an even distribution of ventilation (gas) and perfusion (blood) within the lungs. Both ventilation and perfusion are greatest in the bases of the lungs because the alveoli in the bases are more compliant (their resting volume is low), and perfusion is greater in the bases as a result of gravity.
14. Almost all the oxygen that diffuses into pulmonary capillary blood is transported by hemoglobin, a protein contained within red blood cells. The remainder of the oxygen is transported dissolved in plasma.
15. Oxygen enters the body by diffusing down the concentration gradient, from high concentrations in the alveoli to lower concentrations in the capillaries. Diffusion ceases when alveolar and capillary oxygen pressures equilibrate.
16. Oxygen is loaded onto hemoglobin by the driving pressure exerted by PaO_2 in the plasma. As pressure decreases at the tissue level, oxygen dissociates from hemoglobin and enters tissue cells by diffusion, again down the concentration gradient.
17. Compared with oxygen, carbon dioxide is more soluble in plasma. Therefore carbon dioxide diffuses readily from tissue cells into plasma and from plasma into the alveoli. Carbon dioxide returns to the lungs dissolved in plasma, as bicarbonate, or in carbamino compounds (e.g., bound to hemoglobin).

Tests of Pulmonary Function

1. Spirometry measures the volume and flow rate of air during forced expiration.
2. The alveolar-arterial oxygen gradient is used to evaluate the cause of hypoxia.
3. Diffusing capacity is a measure of the gas diffusion rate at the alveolocapillary membrane.
4. Arterial blood gas analysis can be used to determine pH, oxygen, and CO_2 concentrations.
5. Thoracic imaging techniques are used to detect pulmonary disease and tumors and to evaluate disease progression.

Aging and the Pulmonary System

1. Aging affects the mechanical aspects of ventilation by decreasing chest wall compliance and elastic recoil of the lungs. Changes in these elastic properties reduce ventilatory reserve.
2. Aging causes loss of alveolar wall tissue and alveolar enlargement, thus diminishing the surface area available for gas diffusion.
3. Aging can cause the PaO_2 level to decrease but does not affect the $PaCO_2$ level.
4. Vital capacity decreases, and residual volume increases with age; however, total lung capacity remains unchanged.

REFERENCES

1. Kaplan AG. Chronic cough in adults: make the diagnosis and make a difference. *Pulm Ther*. 2019;5:11–21.
2. Cortez V, Schultz-Cherry S. The role of goblet cells in viral pathogenesis. *FEBS J*. 2021;288(24):7060–7072.
3. Gillich A, et al. Capillary cell-type specialization in the alveolus. *Nature*. 2020;586:785–789.
4. Neupane AS, et al. Patrolling alveolar macrophages conceal bacteria from the immune system to maintain homeostasis. *Cell*. 2020;183(1):110–125.e11.
5. Hume PS, et al. Localization of macrophages in the human lung via design-based stereology. *Am J Respir Crit Care Med*. 2020;201(10):1209–1217.
6. Simonneau G, et al. Haemodynamic definitions and updated clinical classification of pulmonary hypertension. *Eur Respir*. 2019;53:1801913.
7. Lee GM, et al. Lymphatic pathways of the thorax: predictable patterns of spread. *AJR Am J Roentgenol*. 2021;216(3):649–658.
8. Smith KA, Schumacker PT. Sensors and signals: the role of reactive oxygen species in hypoxic pulmonary vasoconstriction. *J Physiol*. 2019;597(4):1033–1043.
9. Guyenet PG, et al. The retrotrapezoid nucleus: central chemoreceptor and regulator of breathing automaticity. *Trends Neurosci*. 2019;42(11):807–824.
10. Xia Y, et al. Transient receptor potential channels and chronic airway inflammatory diseases: a comprehensive review. *Lung*. 2018;196:505–516.
11. Anand A, et al. dyspnea in Esenmenger syndrome and its amelioration by sildenafil: role of J receptors. *Int J Cardiol*. 2014;174:574–578.
12. De Virgiliis F, Di Giovann S. Lung innervation in the eye of a cytokine storm: neuroimmune interactions and COVID-19. *Nat Rev Neurol*. 2020;16:645–652.
13. Calzetta L, et al. The impact of muscarinic receptor antagonists on airway inflammation: a systematic review. *Int J Chron Obstruct Pulmon Dis*. 2021;16:257–279.
14. Ricoy J, et al. Diaphragmatic dysfunction. *Pulmonology*. 2019;25(4):223–235.
15. Laghi F, et al. Inhibition of central activation of the diaphragm: a mechanism of weaning failure. *J Appl Physiol*. 2020;129:366–376.
16. Hentschel R, et al. Surfactant replacement therapy: from biological basis to current clinical practice. *Pediatr Res*. 2020;88: 176–183.
17. Smole U, Kratzer B, Pickl WF. Soluble pattern recognition molecules: guardians and regulators of homeostasis at airway mucosal surfaces. *Eur J Immunol*. 2020;50(5):624–642.
18. Casals C, Garcia-Fojeda B, Minutti CM. Soluble defense collagens: sweeping up immune threats. *Mol Immunol*. 2019;112: 291–304.
19. Swenson ER. The unappreciated role of carbon dioxide in ventilation/perfusion matching. *Anesthesiology*. 2019;131(2): 226–228.
20. Gold WM, Doth LL. Pulmonary function testing. In: Mason RJ, et al. *Murray & Nadel's textbook of respiratory medicine*. ed 6 Philadelphia: Saunders; 2016:407–435.
21. Graham BL, et al. Standardization of spirometry 2019 update: an official American Thoracic Society and European Respiratory Society technical statement. *Am J Respir Crit Care Med*. 2019;200(8):e70–e88.

35

Alterations of Pulmonary Function

Mary Beth Winton and Valentina L. Brashers

http://evolve.elsevier.com/Rogers/pathophysiology/

CHAPTER OUTLINE

Pulmonary disease is often classified as acute or chronic, obstructive or restrictive, infectious or noninfectious, and malignant or benign. Signs and symptoms of lung disease are common and associated not only with primary lung disorders, but also with diseases of other organ systems, particularly the heart.

CLINICAL MANIFESTATIONS OF PULMONARY ALTERATIONS

Signs and Symptoms of Pulmonary Disease

Pulmonary disease is associated with many signs and symptoms such as dyspnea and cough, and their specific characteristics often help identify underlying pulmonary disorder. Other signs and symptoms include abnormal sputum, hemoptysis, altered breathing patterns, cyanosis, nail clubbing, and chest pain.

Dyspnea

Dyspnea, a subjective experience of breathing discomfort, is one of the most common symptoms of pulmonary disease. It is often described as breathlessness, air hunger, shortness of breath, or labored breathing. Often a person becomes preoccupied with breathing. Even though dyspnea is a common pulmonary complaint, it can be due to other conditions, such as acute pain, heart disease, trauma, and anxiety.

Dyspnea originates from interactions among multiple physiological, psychological, social, and environmental factors. Stimulation of many receptors can contribute to the sensation of dyspnea, including afferent receptors in the brain and brainstem, mechanoreceptors in the chest wall and upper airway, and central and peripheral chemoreceptors that sense the effectiveness of gas exchange. These receptors communicate with the central nervous system respiratory control center, which then sends signals to the cerebral cortex and to the mechanical portions of the respiratory system to modulate breathing (see Chapter 34). In many individuals with dyspnea, neuro-mechanical dissociation exists between the inspiratory neural drive to breathe and the ability of the respiratory system to respond mechanically.[1] Damage to the lung parenchyma, diffuse or focal disturbances of ventilation (e.g., pleural effusion, pneumothorax, asthma or muscle weakness), increased ventilatory demand (e.g., hypoxia, anemia, febrile states), alterations in gas exchange (e.g., pneumonia or pulmonary embolism [PE]), or decreases in compliance and ventilatory capacity (e.g., interstitial fibrosis or pulmonary edema) (see Chapter 34) can cause dyspnea.

Dyspnea may occur transiently or can become chronic. The magnitude of the experience of dyspnea may not directly correlate with the severity of the underlying disease. In fact, some individuals may not experience dyspnea even when they have very low blood oxygen levels (silent hypoxemia; see Chapter 34).[2] Dyspnea often first presents during exercise and is called dyspnea on exertion (DOE). DOE is common in individuals with underlying pulmonary disorders such as chronic obstructive pulmonary disease and asthma, and in those with heart failure. Orthopnea is dyspnea that occurs when an individual lies supine, which increases intrathoracic and intraabdominal pressure. This puts pressure on the diaphragm and the respiratory muscles and is usually relieved by standing. Paroxysmal nocturnal dyspnea (PND) occurs when individuals with pulmonary or cardiac disease awake at night with air hunger requiring the person to sit or stand to relieve the dyspnea.

More severe signs of dyspnea include nasal flaring and use of accessory muscles of respiration. Retractions (pulling inward of the intercostal or abdominal muscles during inspiration) can be seen in both children and in individuals with poorly developed thoracic musculature. Subjective complaints of dyspnea can be quantified by asking the individual to rate the level of dyspnea using an ordinal or visual analog scale. Dyspnea may be unrecognized in mechanically ventilated individuals and is often accompanied by pain and anxiety.

Cough

Cough is a protective reflex that helps clear the airways by an explosive expiration. Inhaled particles, accumulated mucus, inflammation, or the presence of a foreign body initiates the cough reflex by stimulating the irritant receptors in the epithelium of the airway. There are few such receptors in the most distal bronchi and the alveoli; thus, it is possible for significant amounts of secretions to accumulate in the distal respiratory tree without initiating the cough reflex. The cough reflex consists of inspiration, closure of the glottis and vocal cords, contraction of the expiratory muscles, and reopening of the glottis. These physiological changes cause a sudden, forceful movement of air through expiration that removes the offending substance. The effectiveness of the cough depends on the strength of the respiratory muscles and the depth of the inspiration. Those with an inability to cough effectively are at greater risk for pneumonia.

Acute cough is cough that resolves within 2 to 3 weeks of the onset of illness or resolves with treatment of the underlying condition. It can be caused by any upper or lower respiratory disease; but commonly is related to upper respiratory tract infections, allergic rhinitis, acute bronchitis, pneumonia, congestive heart failure, pulmonary embolus, or aspiration. *Chronic cough* is defined as cough that is persistent beyond 8 weeks.[3] In individuals who do not routinely inhale irritants such as tobacco smoke, the most common causes of chronic cough are postnasal drainage, asthma, bronchitis or bronchiectasis, and gastroesophageal reflux disease (GERD). Medications, such as angiotensin-converting enzyme (ACE) inhibitors, can also cause chronic cough. ACE inhibitor-related cough is believed to result from decreased breakdown in bradykinin and substance P, causing them to accumulate in the respiratory tract where they stimulate the cough reflex.[4] In persons who smoke or inhale toxins such as dust, sand, or chemicals, chronic bronchitis is the most common cause of chronic cough, although lung cancer must always be considered. Many cases may have no identifiable underlying cause.

Abnormal Sputum

Changes in the amount, color, and consistency of sputum provide information about the cause and progression of disease and the effectiveness of therapy. Expectorated sputum may look clear, foamy, purulent, or bloody. Purulent sputum can be yellow, green, or creamy in color. The gross and microscopic appearances of sputum enable the clinician to identify cellular debris or microorganisms, which aids in diagnosis and choice of therapy.

Hemoptysis is the coughing up of bloody sputum originating from the tracheobronchial branches of the pulmonary system.[5] Hemoptysis is sometimes confused with hematemesis, which is the vomiting of blood. Bloody sputum is often frothy and is usually bright red with an alkaline pH. Hematemesis is usually dark with a coffee-ground appearance, has an acidic pH, and is often mixed with food particles. Hemoptysis usually indicates lung cancer, bronchiectasis, or infection (pneumonia, tuberculosis, lung abscess).[6] Other causes include cancer or PE. The amount and duration of bleeding provide important clues about its source. Chest imaging, often combined with bronchoscopy, is used to confirm the site of bleeding.

Abnormal Breathing Patterns

Normal breathing (eupnea) is involuntary, rhythmic, and effortless. The average adult has a resting ventilatory rate of 8 to 16 breaths/min and tidal volume of 400 to 800 mL with occasional deeper breaths or sighs. Sighs are voluntary deep breathing, help to maintain normal lung function, are usually 1.5 to 2 times the normal tidal volume, and occur approximately 10 to 12 times per hour. Anxiety can cause sighing respirations, which consist of irregular breathing characterized by frequent, deep sighing inspirations.

The rate, depth, regularity, and effort of breathing undergo characteristic alterations in response to physiologic and pathophysiologic conditions. Patterns of breathing automatically adjust to minimize the work of respiratory muscles. Strenuous exercise or metabolic acidosis induces Kussmaul respiration (hyperpnea), which is characterized by a slightly increased ventilatory rate and very large tidal volumes.

Labored breathing occurs whenever there is an increased work of breathing, especially if the airways are obstructed. In large airway obstruction, a slow ventilatory rate (bradypnea), large tidal volume, increased effort, prolonged inspiration and expiration, and stridor or audible wheezing are typical. In small airway obstruction, a rapid ventilatory rate, small tidal volume, increased effort, prolonged expiration, and wheezing are often present. *Restricted breathing* is commonly caused by disorders, such as pulmonary fibrosis, that stiffen the lungs or chest wall and decrease compliance. Restricted breathing often results in small tidal volumes and tachypnea.

Shock and severe cerebral hypoxia contribute to gasping respirations that consist of irregular, quick inspirations with an expiratory pause. Cheyne-Stokes respirations are characterized by alternating periods of deep, shallow breathing and apnea. Apnea lasting 15 seconds or more is often followed by ventilations that increase in volume until a peak is reached; then ventilation (tidal volume) decreases again to apnea. Cheyne-Stokes respirations result from any condition that reduces blood flow to the brainstem, which in turn slows impulses sending information to the respiratory centers of the brainstem. Neurologic impairment above the brainstem can also be a contributing factor (see Chapter 17).

Hypoventilation and Hyperventilation

Hypoventilation is inadequate alveolar ventilation in relation to metabolic demands. Hypoventilation occurs when minute ventilation (respiratory rate × tidal volume) is reduced. It is caused by alterations in the drive to breathe (neurologic control) or the ability to respond to that drive (pulmonary mechanics). When alveolar ventilation is normal, carbon dioxide (CO_2) is removed from the lungs at the same rate as it is produced by cellular metabolism, and the arterial CO_2 pressure ($PaCO_2$) and alveolar CO_2 pressure ($PACO_2$) remain at normal levels. With hypoventilation, CO_2 removal lags behind CO_2 production, and the $PaCO_2$ increases, causing hypercapnia ($PaCO_2$ greater than 44 mm Hg) (see Table 34.2 for a definition of gas partial pressures and other common pulmonary abbreviations). Hypercapnia results in an increase in hydrogen ion concentration (i.e., an increase in carbonic acid) in the blood leading to a pH of less than 7.35 (respiratory acidosis) that can affect the function of many tissues throughout the body.

Hypoventilation is often overlooked until it is severe because the breathing pattern and ventilatory rate may appear to be normal, and changes in the tidal volume can be difficult to detect clinically. Measurement of the $PaCO_2$ (i.e., blood gas analysis) or the amount of CO_2 in the inspired and expired air (capnography) reveals the hypoventilation. Severe hypoventilation can cause secondary hypoxemia, somnolence, and disorientation.

Hyperventilation is alveolar ventilation exceeding metabolic demands. The lungs remove CO_2 faster than it is produced by cellular metabolism, resulting in a decreased $PaCO_2$, or hypocapnia ($PaCO_2$ <36 mm Hg). Hypocapnia results in a decrease in the concentration of hydrogen ions in the blood (i.e., a decrease in carbonic acid), leading to a pH of greater than 7.45 (respiratory alkalosis) that can interfere with tissue function. Hyperventilation commonly occurs with severe anxiety, acute head injury, pain, and in response to conditions that affect the lung and chest wall, especially those that cause hypoxemia. Like hypoventilation, hyperventilation can be determined by arterial blood gas analysis.

Cyanosis

Cyanosis is a bluish discoloration of the skin and mucous membranes caused by increasing amounts of desaturated or reduced hemoglobin (which is bluish) in the blood. *Peripheral cyanosis* results from poor blood circulation in the fingers and toes. It is most often caused by heart disease, intense peripheral vasoconstriction (such as that observed in persons who have Raynaud disease), or cold environments. Peripheral cyanosis is best seen in the nail beds. *Central cyanosis* is caused by decreased arterial oxygenation (low PaO_2) from decreased inspired oxygen (e.g., at high altitudes), central nervous system disorders that affect respiration, pulmonary diseases, or cardiac diseases. Central cyanosis is best assessed in the buccal mucous membranes and lips.

Lack of cyanosis does not necessarily indicate that oxygenation is normal. In adults, cyanosis is not evident until severe hypoxemia is present and, therefore, is an insensitive indicator of respiratory failure. Severe anemia (inadequate hemoglobin concentration) and carbon monoxide poisoning (in which hemoglobin binds to carbon monoxide instead of to oxygen) can cause inadequate oxygenation of tissues without causing cyanosis. Individuals with polycythemia (an abnormal increase in the number of red blood cells), however, may have cyanosis when oxygenation is adequate. Therefore, cyanosis must be interpreted in relation to the underlying pathophysiologic condition. If cyanosis is suspected, blood gas analysis should be done.

Clubbing

Clubbing is the selective bulbous enlargement of the end of a digit (finger or toe) (Fig. 35.1). It is recognized by measuring the nail-fold angle and phalangeal depth.[7] Its severity can be graded from 1 to 5 based on the extent of nail bed hypertrophy and the number of changes in the nails themselves. Clubbing of the nails is usually painless and develops gradually over weeks or months. The most common cause of clubbing in the United States is lung cancer.[7] Clubbing also is commonly associated with diseases that cause chronic hypoxemia, such as bronchiectasis, cystic fibrosis, pulmonary fibrosis, lung abscess, and congenital heart disease. Clubbing without underlying cancer or lung disease can occur in association with a variety of conditions including gastrointestinal disorders, hepatobiliary diseases, and endocrine disorders. Clubbing may be congenital.

The exact cause of clubbing is unknown. In lung cancer, some propose that platelet clumps escape filtration by the pulmonary bed and enter the systemic circulation. These platelets then release platelet-derived growth factor (PDGF), causing periosteal changes near the nail bed. In individuals with chronic hypoxemia, some suggest that decreased oxygen causes the release of vascular endothelial growth factor, which promotes proliferation of the connective tissue between the nail matrix and the distal phalanx.[8] Clubbing is rarely reversible.

Pain

Pain caused by pulmonary disorders originates in the pleurae, airways, or chest wall. Infection and inflammation of the pleura (pleurisy or pleuritis) cause sharp or stabbing pain (pleurodynia) when

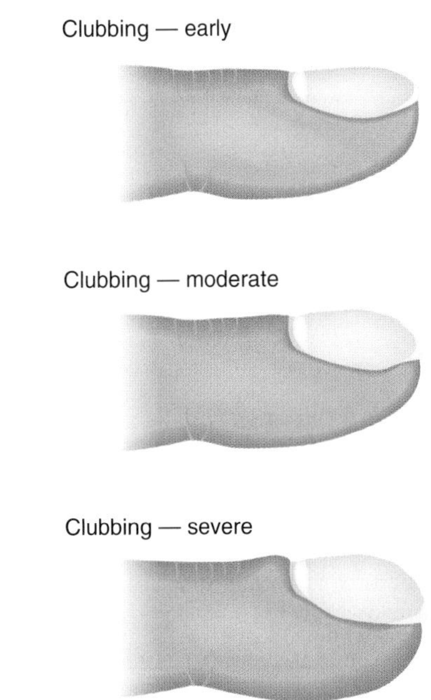

Fig. 35.1 **Clubbing of Fingers Caused by Chronic Hypoxemia.** (Modified from Seidel HM, et al. *Mosby's guide to physical examination*, 7th edition. St. Louis: Mosby; 2011.)

the pleura stretches during inspiration. The pain is usually localized to a portion of the chest wall, where a unique breath sound called a *pleural friction rub* may be heard over the painful area during inspiration. Laughing or coughing makes pleural pain worse.

Infection and inflammation of the trachea or bronchi (tracheitis or tracheobronchitis, respectively) can cause central chest pain that is pronounced after coughing. High blood pressure in the pulmonary circulation (pulmonary hypertension [PH]) can cause pain during exercise that is often mistaken for angina-like cardiac pain.

Pain in the chest wall is muscle pain or rib pain. Excessive coughing (which makes the muscles sore) and rib fractures or thoracic surgery produce such pain. Inflammation of the costochondral junction (costochondritis) also can cause chest wall pain. Chest wall pain can often be reproduced by pressing on the sternum or ribs.

Conditions Caused by Pulmonary Disease or Injury

Hypercapnia

Hypercapnia, increased $PaCO_2$, is caused by hypoventilation of the alveoli (Algorithm 35.1). CO_2 is easily diffused from the blood into the alveolar space, but it must be removed from the alveoli by ventilation to maintain a normal $PaCO_2$. Thus, minute ventilation (respiratory rate × tidal volume) determines not only the alveolar ventilation, but also the $PaCO_2$. Although respiratory rate is measured routinely, tidal volume is difficult to assess at the bedside, and hypoventilation can be overlooked. Therefore, if hypoventilation is suspected, it is important to obtain blood gas analysis or capnography to determine the severity of the hypercapnia and resultant respiratory acidosis (acid-base balance is described in Chapter 3).

Hypercapnia has many causes. Most are a result of a decreased drive to breathe or an inadequate ability to respond to ventilatory stimulation. Some of these causes include (1) depression of the respiratory center by drugs; (2) diseases of the medulla, including infections of the central nervous system or trauma; (3) abnormalities of the spinal conducting pathways, as in spinal cord disruption or poliomyelitis; (4) diseases of the neuromuscular junction or of the respiratory muscles themselves, as in myasthenia gravis or muscular dystrophy; (5) thoracic cage abnormalities, as in chest injury or congenital deformity; (6) large airway obstruction, as in tumors or sleep apnea; and (7) increased work of breathing or physiologic dead space, as in emphysema.

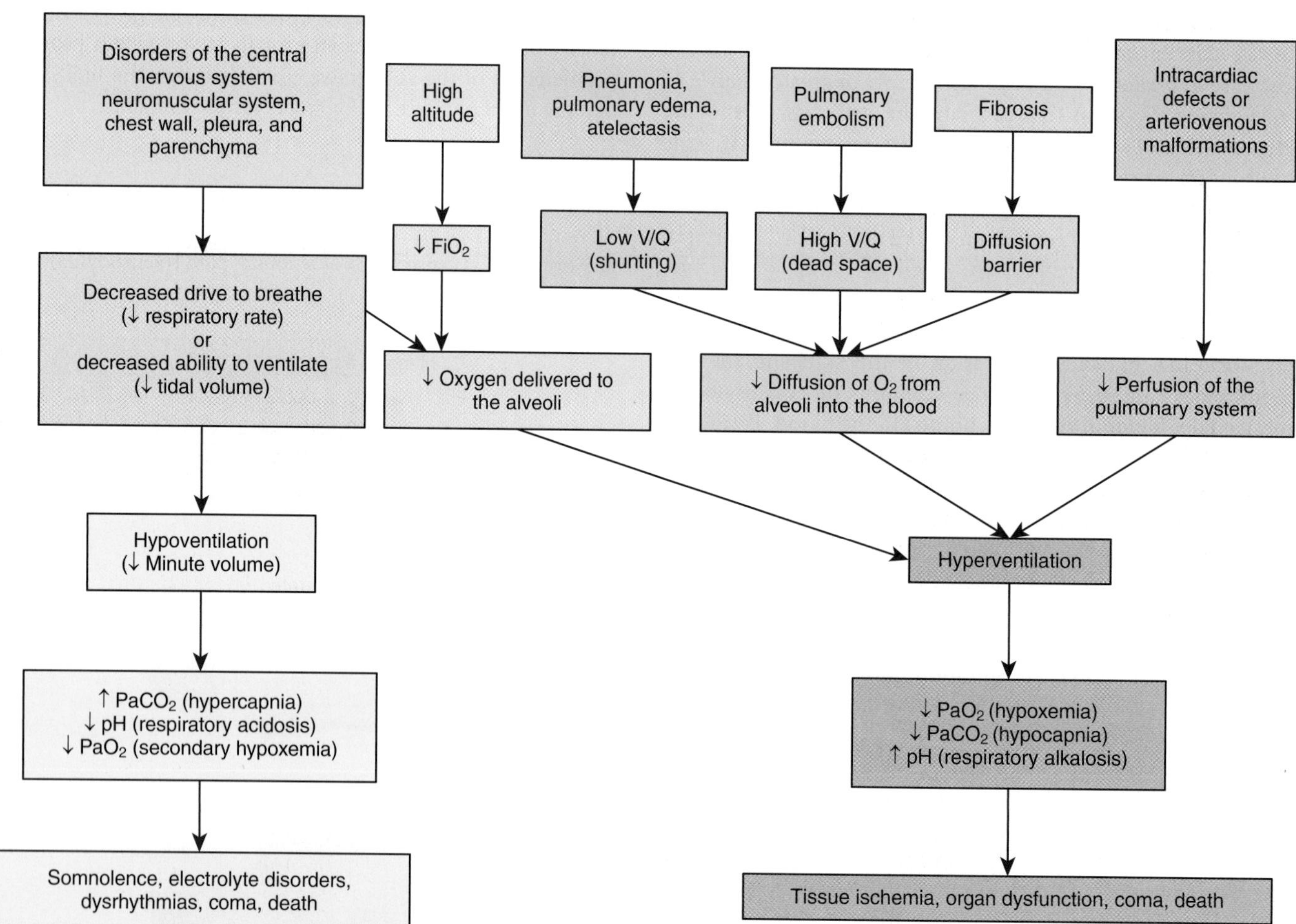

Algorithm 35.1 Hypercapnia and Hypoxemia. Disorders that diminish the respiratory rate or tidal volume lead to hypoventilation, hypercapnia, and respiratory acidosis. Disorders that decrease the amount of oxygen delivered to the alveoli, the diffusion of oxygen from the alveoli into the blood, or perfusion of the pulmonary system are associated with hyperventilation, hypoxemia, and a respiratory alkalosis.

Hypercapnia and the associated respiratory acidosis can cause dysrhythmias due to electrolyte abnormalities. High levels of arterial CO_2 cause cerebral vasodilation, resulting in somnolence and even coma. Alveolar hypoventilation with an increased alveolar CO_2 concentration limits the amount of oxygen available for diffusion into the blood, thereby leading to secondary hypoxemia.

Hypoxemia

Hypoxemia, or reduced oxygenation of arterial blood (reduced PaO_2), is caused by respiratory alterations, whereas hypoxia (or ischemia) is reduced oxygenation of cells in tissues. Hypoxemia results from problems with one or more of the major mechanisms of oxygenation Table 35.1 lists some of the common clinical causes of hypoxemia. Although hypoxemia can lead to tissue hypoxia, tissue hypoxia also can result from other abnormalities unrelated to alterations of pulmonary function, such as low cardiac output, anemia, or cyanide poisoning.

Hypoxemia results from problems with one or more of the major mechanisms of oxygenation (see Algorithm 35.1):

1. Oxygen delivery to the alveoli
   a. Minute ventilation (secondary hypoxemia)
   b. Oxygen content of the inspired air (FiO_2)
2. Diffusion of oxygen from the alveoli into the blood
   a. Balance between alveolar ventilation and perfusion ($\dot{V}/\dot{Q}$ match)
   b. Diffusion of oxygen across the alveolar capillary barrier
3. Perfusion of the pulmonary system

The amount of oxygen in the alveoli is the PAO_2 and is dependent on two factors. The first factor is the amount of alveolar minute ventilation (tidal volume × respiratory rate), as discussed previously in the Hypoventilation section. Hypoventilation results in an increase in the $PACO_2$ and a decrease in the amount of oxygen available in the alveoli for diffusion into the blood. This type of secondary hypoxemia is associated with hypercapnia and respiratory acidosis and can be corrected if alveolar ventilation is improved by increases in the rate and depth of breathing. The second factor is the presence of inadequate oxygen content of the inspired air. The amount of oxygen in inspired air is expressed as the percentage or fraction of air that is composed of oxygen, the FiO_2. The FiO_2 of air at sea level is 20.9%. Anything that decreases the FiO_2 (e.g., high altitude) decreases the PAO_2.

Diffusion of oxygen from the alveoli into the blood also is dependent on two factors. The first is the balance between the amount of air that enters alveoli ($\dot{V}$) and the amount of blood perfusing the capillaries around the alveoli ($\dot{Q}$). An abnormal ventilation-perfusion ratio ($\dot{V}/\dot{Q}$) is the most common cause of hypoxemia (Fig. 35.2). The normal $\dot{V}/\dot{Q}$ is 0.8 (also called the respiratory quotient) because some blood is normally shunted to the bronchial circulation so that ventilation is somewhat greater than perfusion. $\dot{V}/\dot{Q}$ mismatch refers to an abnormal distribution of ventilation and perfusion. Hypoxemia can be caused by inadequate ventilation of well-perfused areas of the lung (low $\dot{V}/\dot{Q}$), resulting in wasted perfusion. Mismatching of this type, called shunting, occurs in atelectasis, in asthma because of bronchoconstriction, and in pulmonary edema and pneumonia when alveoli are filled with fluid. A compensatory mechanism called hypoxic pulmonary

TABLE 35.1 Causes of Hypoxemia

MECHANISM	COMMON CLINICAL CAUSES
Decrease in inspired oxygen (decreased FiO_2)	High altitude Low oxygen content of gas mixture Enclosed breathing spaces (suffocation)
Hypoventilation of the alveoli (secondary hypoxemia)	Lack of neurologic stimulation of the respiratory center (oversedation, drug overdose, neurologic damage) Defects in chest wall mechanics (neuromuscular disease, trauma, chest deformity, air trapping) Large airway obstruction (laryngospasm, foreign body aspiration, neoplasm) Increased work of breathing (emphysema, severe asthma)
Ventilation-perfusion mismatch	Asthma Chronic bronchitis Pneumonia Acute respiratory distress syndrome Atelectasis Pulmonary embolism
Alveolocapillary diffusion abnormality	Edema Fibrosis Emphysema
Decreased pulmonary capillary perfusion	Intracardiac defects Intrapulmonary arteriovenous malformations

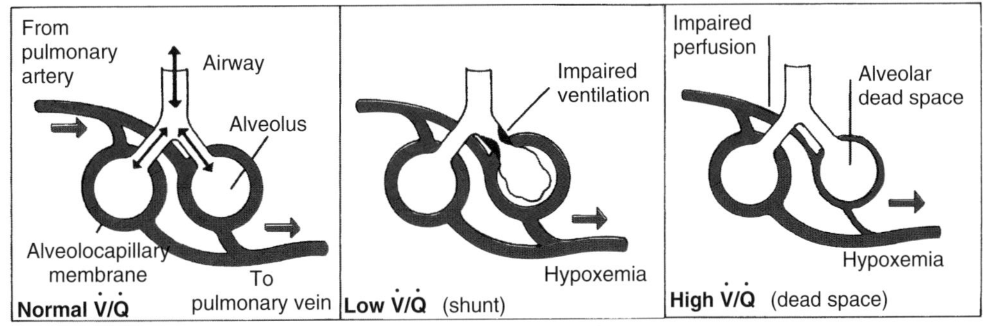

Fig. 35.2 Ventilation-Perfusion ($\dot{V}/\dot{Q}$) Abnormalities.

vasoconstriction causes arterioles that perfuse localized areas of shunting to constrict and reduce blood flow to the damaged lung tissue (see Chapter 34). This prevents wasted perfusion and sends the shunted blood to better functioning parts of the lung. This improves overall $\dot{V}/\dot{Q}$ matching and raises the PaO_2. However, in lung diseases that affect large portions of the lung, diffuse hypoxic pulmonary vasoconstriction can lead to elevated pulmonary artery pressures (PH) and lead to right heart failure, or *cor pulmonale* (see Cor Pulmonale under Pulmonary Vascular Disease section).

Hypoxemia also can be caused by poor perfusion of well-ventilated portions of the lung (high $\dot{V}/\dot{Q}$), resulting in wasted ventilation. The most common cause of high $\dot{V}/\dot{Q}$ is a pulmonary embolus that impairs blood flow to a segment of the lung. An area where alveoli are ventilated but not perfused is termed alveolar dead space. Increases in alveolar dead space also occur in diseases, such as emphysema, that destroy lung tissue.

The second factor affecting diffusion of oxygen from the alveoli into the blood is the alveolocapillary membrane. Diffusion of oxygen through the alveolocapillary membrane is impaired if the membrane is thickened, or the surface area available for diffusion is decreased. Thickened alveolocapillary membranes, as occur with edema and fibrosis, increase the time required for oxygen to diffuse from the alveoli into the capillaries. If diffusion is slowed enough, the oxygenation levels (PO_2) of alveolar gas and capillary blood do not have time to equilibrate during the fraction of a second that blood remains in the capillary. Hypercapnia is seldom produced by impaired diffusion because CO_2 diffuses so easily from capillary to alveolus.

Hypoxemia can also result when blood flow bypasses the lungs, allowing deoxygenated venous blood to return to the systemic circulation. This can occur when there are intracardiac defects that cause right-to-left shunting (see Chapter 33) or because of intrapulmonary arteriovenous malformations.

Hypoxemia is most often associated with a compensatory hyperventilation and the resultant respiratory alkalosis (i.e., decreased $PaCO_2$ and increased pH). However, in individuals with associated ventilatory difficulties, hypoxemia may be complicated by hypercapnia and respiratory acidosis. Hypoxemia results in widespread tissue dysfunction and, when severe, can lead to organ infarction. Clinical manifestations of acute hypoxemia may include cyanosis, confusion, tachycardia, edema, and decreased renal output.

Acute Respiratory Failure

Respiratory failure is defined as inadequate gas exchange, which is characterized as $PaO_2 \leq 60$ mm Hg (hypoxemic respiratory failure) and/or $PaCO_2 \geq 50$ mm Hg, pH ≤ 7.25 (hypercapnic respiratory failure). Respiratory failure can result from direct injury to the lungs, airways, or chest wall or indirectly because of disease or injury involving another body system, such as the brain, spinal cord, or heart. If the respiratory failure is primarily hypercapnic, it is the result of inadequate alveolar minute ventilation and the individual requires ventilatory support, such as with a bag-valve mask, noninvasive positive pressure ventilation, or intubation and the use of mechanical ventilation. If the respiratory failure is primarily hypoxemic, it is the result of inadequate exchange of oxygen between the alveoli and the capillaries and the individual must receive supplemental oxygen. Many people will have combined hypercapnic and hypoxemic respiratory failure and will require both kinds of support.

Of the many possible causes of respiratory failure, it is especially important to recognize that it is a potential complication of any major surgical procedure, especially those that involve the central nervous system, thorax, or upper abdomen. The most common postoperative pulmonary problems are atelectasis, pneumonia, pulmonary edema, and pulmonary emboli, each of which may cause respiratory failure. People who smoke or are obese are at particular risk, especially if they have preexisting lung disease. Limited cardiac reserve, neurologic disease, chronic renal failure, chronic hepatic disease, and infection also increase the tendency to develop postoperative respiratory failure.

Prevention of respiratory failure includes the recognition of at-risk individuals and the initiation of deep-breathing exercises and early ambulation to prevent atelectasis and the accumulation of secretions. Incentive spirometry provides individuals immediate feedback about tidal volumes, which encourages them to breathe more deeply. Humidification of inspired air can help loosen secretions. Antibiotics may be prescribed to treat infection. If severe respiratory failure develops, the individual may require mechanical ventilation or extracorporeal membrane oxygenation.

DISORDERS OF THE CHEST WALL AND PLEURA

Many conditions can affect the chest wall, pleura, or both, and compromise the function of the respiratory system. Chest wall disorders primarily affect tidal volume, resulting in hypoventilation and hypercapnia. Pleural diseases impact both ventilation and oxygenation.

Chest Wall Restriction

If the chest wall is deformed, traumatized, immobilized, or heavy from the accumulation of fat, the work of breathing increases, and ventilation may be compromised because of a decrease in tidal volume. The degree of ventilatory impairment depends on the severity of the chest wall restriction. Grossly obese individuals are often dyspneic on exertion or when recumbent. Individuals with severe kyphoscoliosis (bending and rotation of the spinal column, with distortion of the thoracic cage) often present with dyspnea on exertion that can progress to respiratory failure. Other musculoskeletal abnormalities that can impair ventilation are ankylosing spondylitis (see Chapter 44) and pectus excavatum (a deformity characterized by depression of the sternum).

Impairment of respiratory muscle function caused by neuromuscular diseases, such as poliomyelitis, muscular dystrophy, myasthenia gravis, and Guillain-Barré syndrome (see Chapters 18 and 45), also can restrict the chest wall and impair pulmonary function. Muscle weakness can result in hypoventilation, hypercapnia, inability to remove secretions, and hypoxemia.

Pain from chest wall injury, surgery, or disease can restrict the movement of the chest wall, causing significant hypoventilation.

Trauma to the thorax not only can restrict chest expansion because of pain but also can cause structural and mechanical changes that impair the ability of the chest to expand normally. Flail chest complicates up to 15% of chest trauma cases.[9] It results from the fracture of several consecutive ribs with or without fracture of the sternum. These multiple fractures result in instability of a portion of the chest wall, causing paradoxical movement of the chest with breathing. During inspiration, the negative intrathoracic pressure causes the unstable portion of the chest wall to move inward and during expiration it moves outward, impairing movement of gas.

In chest wall restriction, an increase in the respiratory rate can compensate for small decreases in tidal volume. However, as tidal volume decreases further, hypercapnic respiratory failure develops. Although alveolar function is usually preserved, hypoxemia occurs secondary to the hypoventilation. A diagnosis of chest wall restriction is made by pulmonary function testing (reduction in forced vital capacity [FVC]), arterial blood gas measurement and capnography (hypercapnia), and radiographs. Treatment is aimed at any reversible underlying cause, and supportive measures such as physiotherapy, pain management, and incentive spirometry are indicated. In severe cases, noninvasive or invasive mechanical ventilation may be indicated. Flail chest is managed with positive-pressure ventilation and surgical stabilization.[9]

Pleural Abnormalities

Pneumothorax

Pneumothorax is the presence of air or gas in the pleural space. It is caused by a rupture in either the visceral pleura (surrounds the lungs) or the parietal pleura (lines the inner surface of the chest wall) or both. As air separates the visceral and parietal pleurae, it destroys the negative pressure of the pleural space and disrupts the equilibrium between the elastic recoil forces of the lung and chest wall. This disequilibrium causes the affected part of the lung to collapse toward the hilum (Fig. 35.3), resulting in impaired oxygenation and ventilation.

Pneumothorax can be categorized as spontaneous or traumatic, and spontaneous pneumothorax can be categorized as primary or secondary.[10] *Primary spontaneous pneumothorax* occurs unexpectedly in healthy individuals (usually men) between 20 and 40 years of age and is caused by the spontaneous rupture of blebs (blister-like formations) on the visceral pleura. Bleb rupture, usually in the apices of the lungs, can occur during sleep, rest, or exercise. The cause of bleb formation is not known, but there appears to be a genetic component, and more than 80% of these individuals have been found to have emphysema-like changes in their lungs despite no history of smoking. *Secondary spontaneous pneumothorax* occurs in individuals with underlying respiratory disorders such as emphysema, cystic fibrosis, tuberculosis, lung cancer, and pneumonia in which the integrity of the visceral pleura is compromised. *Traumatic pneumothorax* may be due to punctures by a fractured rib or knife and bullet wounds. It also may result from complications of medical interventions *(iatrogenic pneumothorax)*, such as transthoracic needle aspiration or mechanical ventilation (barotrauma). Traumatic pneumothorax frequently involves both the visceral and parietal pleura.

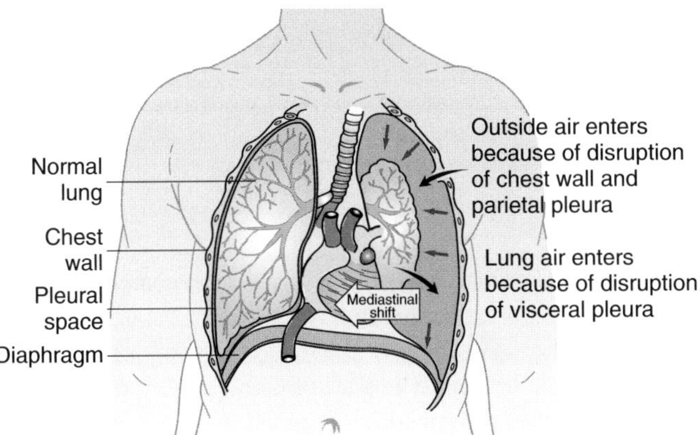

Fig. 35.3 Pneumothorax. Air in the pleural space causes the lung to collapse around the hilus and may push the mediastinal contents (heart and great vessels) toward the other lung.

Spontaneous or traumatic pneumothorax can present as either open or tension. In open (communicating) pneumothorax, air that is drawn into the pleural space during inspiration through the injured area is forced back out during expiration. Open pneumothorax usually results in partial lung collapse. In tension pneumothorax, the site of pleural rupture acts as a one-way valve, permitting air to enter the pleural space on inspiration but preventing its escape during expiration. As more air enters the pleural space, air pressure in the pleural space increases. Air pressure in the pleural space pushes against the lung, causing compression atelectasis. Both oxygenation and ventilation are severely impacted. As the pleural pressure continues to increase, it may press on the mediastinum, compressing and displacing the heart, great vessels, and trachea *(mediastinal shift)* (see Fig. 35.3). The pathophysiologic effects of tension pneumothorax are life-threatening.

Clinical manifestations of pneumothorax begin with sudden pleural pain, tachypnea, and dyspnea. Depending on the size of the pneumothorax, physical examination may reveal absent or decreased breath sounds and hyperresonance to percussion on the affected side. Tension pneumothorax may be complicated by severe hypoxemia, tracheal deviation away from the affected lung, and hypotension. The diagnosis of pneumothorax is confirmed with chest radiographs, ultrasound, and computed tomography (CT). Management of primary spontaneous pneumothorax is often possible in an ambulatory setting with placement of a small catheter into the pleural space equipped with one-way valve, although some individuals may require follow-up thoracic surgery to prevent recurrences.[11] In contrast, individuals with tension pneumothorax deteriorate rapidly, and immediate hospitalization and treatment are required. Pneumothorax is treated by aspiration, usually with insertion of a thoracostomy (chest) tube that is attached to a water-seal drainage system with suction. After the pneumothorax is evacuated and the pleural rupture has healed, the chest tube is removed. For individuals with persistent air leaks, other interventions may be needed, including pleurodesis (the instillation of substances such as talc into the pleural space) or surgery.[12]

Pleural Effusion

Pleural effusion is the presence of fluid in the pleural space. The source of the fluid is usually blood vessels or lymphatic vessels lying beneath the pleural space. Pleural effusions can be divided into five categories based on their mechanisms: transudative, exudative, empyema, hemothorax, and chylothorax (Table 35.2).

Transudative pleural effusions are often clear or slightly discolored and contain few cells and little protein. Transudation of fluid into the pleural space occurs because of changes in hemodynamic or oncotic pressures within the pulmonary vessels (see Chapter 3). Common examples include congestive heart failure, in which venous and left atrial pressures are increased pushing fluid into the pleural space, and hypoproteinemia (such as is seen with liver and kidney disorders), which decreases capillary oncotic pressure and promotes diffusion of water out of the capillaries. Exudative effusion occurs in response to inflammation, infection, or malignancy and involves inflammatory processes that increase capillary permeability. When stimulated by biochemical mediators of inflammation, tight junctions between capillary endothelial cells open, enabling leukocytes and plasma proteins to migrate out into affected tissues (see Chapter 7). Exudative effusions that occur in association with pneumonia are called *parapneumonic effusions*.[13] These often resolve with treatment of the underlying infection but can progress to empyema. Empyema is pleural effusion containing infectious microorganisms. It develops when the pulmonary lymphatics become blocked, leading to an outpouring of contaminated lymphatic fluid into the pleural space.[13] Empyema occurs most commonly in older adults and children as a complication of pneumonia, surgery, trauma, or bronchial obstruction from a tumor. Commonly documented infectious organisms include *Staphylococcus aureus, Escherichia coli, Klebsiella pneumoniae*, and anaerobic bacteria. Hemothorax is the presence of blood in the pleural space usually due to trauma, surgery, cancer, PE, or tuberculosis. Chylothorax results from a tear in the thoracic duct leading to the leakage of chyle into the pleural space. It is a rare complication of surgery and some malignancies. Most malignant pleural effusions are related to lung cancer, breast cancer, and lymphoma, occurring in an estimated one-third of individuals with lung cancer.[13]

Small collections of fluid may not affect lung function and remain undetected. Most will be removed by the lymphatic system once the underlying condition is resolved. Dyspnea, compression of the lung with impaired ventilation, and pleural pain are common in larger effusions. Mediastinal shift and cardiovascular complications occur in a large, rapidly developing effusions. Physical examination shows decreased breath sounds and dullness to percussion on the affected side. A pleural friction rub may be heard over areas of inflamed pleura.

The diagnosis is confirmed by chest imaging and thoracentesis. Chest radiographs may show large amounts of pleural fluid (Fig. 35.4). Thoracic ultrasound, CT, or MRI may be needed for smaller or more localized fluid collections. Thoracentesis can provide symptomatic relief, and examination of the fluid can assist in determining the type of effusion. The number and type of cells, the pH, and the presence or absence of microorganisms in the pleural fluid are determined.[13,14] In some cases, medical pleuroscopy and pleural biopsies may be needed to evaluate unexplained effusions.

Management depends on the type and cause of the pleural effusion.[15] Transudative effusions are managed by treating the underlying condition. Exudative effusions are also managed by treating the underlying condition; however, if the effusion is large, drainage is achieved through the placement of a chest tube. Management of empyema includes the administration of appropriate antimicrobials and drainage of the pleural space with a chest tube, often combined with the use of intrapleural enzyme therapy, such as deoxyribonuclease (stimulates pleural

TABLE 35.2 Mechanism of Pleural Effusion

Type of Fluid/Effusion	Source of Accumulation	Primary or Associated Disorder
Transudate (hydrothorax)	Watery fluid that diffuses out of capillaries beneath pleura (i.e., capillaries in lung or chest wall)	Cardiovascular disease that causes high pulmonary capillary pressures; liver or kidney disease that disrupts plasma protein production, causing hypoproteinemia (decreased oncotic pressure in blood vessels)
Exudate	Fluid rich in cells and proteins (leukocytes, plasma proteins of all kinds; see Chapter 5) that migrates out of capillaries	Infection, inflammation, or malignancy of pleura that stimulates mast cells to release biochemical mediators that increase capillary permeability
Pus (empyema)	Microorganisms and debris of infection (leukocytes, cellular debris) accumulate in pleural space	Pulmonary infections, such as pneumonia; lung abscesses; infected wounds
Blood (hemothorax)	Hemorrhage into pleural space	Traumatic injury, surgery, rupture, or malignancy that damages blood vessels
Chyle (chylothorax)	Chyle (milky fluid containing lymph and fat droplets) that moves from lymphatic vessels into pleural space instead of passing from gastrointestinal tract to thoracic duct	Traumatic injury, surgical procedure, infection, or disorder that disrupts lymphatic transport

The principles of diffusion are described in Chapter 1; mechanisms that increase capillary permeability and cause exudation of cells, proteins, and fluid are discussed in Chapter 5.

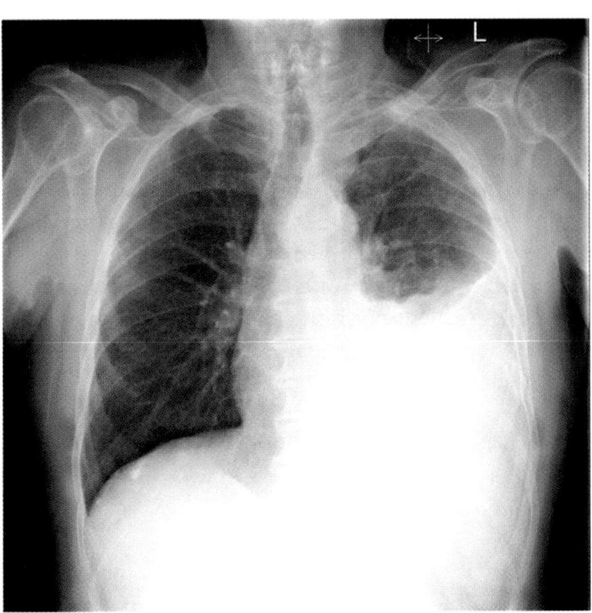

Fig. 35.4 Pleural Effusion. (From Tsitsias T, Santhirakumaran G, Jenkins M. Management of pleural effusions. *Surgery (Oxford),* 2020;38(5), 244–248. https://doi.org/10.1016/j.mpsur.2020.03.004.)

fluid formation, reduces pleural fluid viscosity, and promotes resolution of systemic inflammation) to achieve adequate drainage. Malignant exudative effusions may require placement of an indwelling pleural catheter and pleurodesis.[13] Hemothorax is managed surgically. Chylothorax may improve spontaneously or may require radiation (in the case of malignancy) or surgical management.

PULMONARY DISORDERS

Restrictive Lung Diseases

Restrictive lung diseases are characterized by decreased compliance (stiffness) of the lung tissue. This means that more effort is needed to expand the lungs during inspiration, which increases the work of breathing. Individuals with lung restriction have dyspnea, an increased respiratory rate, and a decreased tidal volume. Pulmonary function testing reveals a decrease in the FVC. Restrictive lung diseases also can cause $\dot{V}/\dot{Q}$ mismatch and affect the alveolocapillary membrane, which reduces the diffusion of oxygen from the alveoli into the blood and results in hypoxemia. Some of the most common restrictive lung diseases in adults are aspiration, atelectasis, bronchiectasis, bronchiolitis, pulmonary fibrosis, inhalation disorders, pneumoconiosis, allergic alveolitis, pulmonary edema, and acute respiratory distress syndrome.

Aspiration

Aspiration is the passage of fluid and solid particles into the lung. It accounts for 5% to 15% of community-acquired pneumonia cases, especially in older individuals.[16] An estimated 45% of the population aspirates while sleeping without causing disease.[17] Predisposing factors for clinically significant aspiration and aspiration pneumonia include dysphagia; absent cough reflex; altered level of consciousness caused by substance use, sedation, or anesthesia; endotracheal intubation; being bedridden; neurologic disorders such as dementia, stroke, and seizure disorders; home oxygen therapy; use of proton pump inhibitor medications; and feeding through a nasogastric tube.[17] In the upright individual, the right lung, particularly the right lower lobe, is more susceptible to aspiration than the left lung because the branching angle of the right mainstem bronchus is straighter than the branching angle of the left mainstem bronchus. In recumbent individuals, the superior segments of the lower lobes and the posterior segments of the upper lobes are most commonly affected.[18]

The characteristics of the aspirated material interact with host defenses leading to several possible pulmonary complications, including aspiration pneumonia, pneumonitis, pulmonary abscess, and airway obstruction. Aspiration of oral or pharyngeal secretions, including acidic gastric fluid, results in bronchial and alveolar inflammation and aspiration pneumonitis. Bronchial damage includes loss of ciliary function and bronchospasm. In the alveoli, acidic fluid damages the alveolocapillary membrane and diminishes surfactant production. Consequently, plasma and blood cells move from capillaries into the alveoli, and the lung becomes stiff and noncompliant. Aspiration of oral contents may lead to infection of the lung parenchyma resulting in aspiration pneumonia.[18] The type and number of microorganisms present in the oropharynx (oral microbiome) along with host defense mechanisms interact to determine the likelihood and severity of aspiration pneumonia. In recent years, the most common causative microorganisms have changed such that gram-negative aerobic bacteria are now more common than anaerobes.[16,17] Aspiration of large food particles has serious consequences. Solid food particles can obstruct a bronchus, resulting in bronchial inflammation and collapse of airways distal to the obstruction. If the aspirated solid is not identified and removed by bronchoscopy, a chronic, local inflammation develops that may lead to recurrent infection, abscess formation, and bronchiectasis.

Clinical manifestations of acute aspiration include the sudden onset of choking or intractable cough with or without vomiting. The development of aspiration pneumonitis is characterized by dyspnea, tachypnea, and tachycardia. Auscultation reveals both crackles and wheezes. Hypoxemia develops rapidly. Fever and purulent sputum production are common if aspiration pneumonia develops. Chronic aspiration is characterized by recurrent lung infections, chronic cough, or persistent wheezing over months and even years. Diagnosis is made by assessing risk factors, symptoms, and chest radiographs. In some individuals, bronchoscopy with bronchoalveolar lavage is indicated.

Preventive measures for individuals at risk include use of a semirecumbent position, surveillance of enteral feeding, use of promotility drugs, and avoidance of excessive sedation. Fasting for a minimum of 8 hours before surgery reduces the incidence of aspiration associated with general anesthesia. The use of nasogastric tubes to reduce stomach contents is controversial and has not been shown to reduce the incidence of aspiration.[16]

Oral hygiene may reduce the incidence of aspiration pneumonia. Speech-language pathologists employ a variety of feeding and swallowing techniques that can significantly reduce the risk of aspiration in selected individuals.

Treatment of aspiration pneumonitis includes use of supplemental oxygen and suctioning. Mechanical ventilation may be needed in severe cases. Routine administration of corticosteroids or antibiotics is not recommended for mild to moderate aspiration pneumonitis.[16] If aspiration pneumonia develops, the administration of antibiotics is indicated.[17]

Atelectasis

Atelectasis is the collapse of lung tissue. Atelectasis causes $\dot{V}/\dot{Q}$ mismatch, leading to hypoxemia. There are three types of atelectasis:

1. Obstructive (absorption) atelectasis results from obstructed or hypoventilated alveoli as the air is gradually absorbed out of the alveoli and into the blood. Mucous plugging or bronchogenic lung carcinoma are common causes of airway obstruction causing atelectasis.[19] Aspiration of a foreign body may also result in airway obstruction and atelectasis. A subset of obstructive atelectasis occurs due to hypoventilation of alveoli, especially in individuals who have undergone surgery or who have severe chest or abdominal pain. After surgery, individuals are often in pain, breathe shallowly, are reluctant to change position, and produce viscous secretions that tend to pool in dependent portions of the lung, causing obstruction of small airways. This type of atelectasis occurs in subsegmental portions of the lung forming 'platelike' lesions.
2. Compression atelectasis is caused by external pressure exerted by tumor, fluid, or air in the pleural space or by abdominal distention pressing on a portion of lung, causing alveoli to collapse.
3. Surfactant impairment (adhesive) atelectasis results from decreased production or inactivation of surfactant. Surfactant is necessary to reduce surface tension in the alveoli and thus prevent lung collapse during expiration. Surfactant impairment can occur because of premature birth and from any serious lung injury, such as aspiration, acute respiratory distress syndrome, anesthesia induction, or mechanical ventilation.

Clinical manifestations of atelectasis include dyspnea, cough, fever, and leukocytosis and therefore may be mistaken for infection. Prevention and treatment of atelectasis usually include deep-breathing exercises (often with the aid of an incentive spirometer), frequent position changes, and early ambulation. Deep breathing promotes ciliary clearance of secretions, stabilizes the alveoli by redistributing surfactant, and promotes collateral ventilation through the *pores of Kohn*, promoting expansion of collapsed alveoli (Fig. 35.5). Bronchoscopy may be needed to remove foreign bodies, or when complete or near-complete lung atelectasis has occurred.

Bronchiectasis

Bronchiectasis is persistent abnormal dilation of the bronchi. It usually occurs in conjunction with other respiratory conditions that are associated with chronic bronchial inflammation, such as cystic fibrosis. It also can occur due to prolonged atelectasis, aspiration of a foreign body, recurrent pulmonary infections (e.g., mycoplasma, viruses), tuberculosis, or congenital weakness of the bronchial wall. Bronchiectasis also is associated with a number of systemic disorders, such as rheumatologic disease, inflammatory bowel disease, and immunodeficiency syndromes (e.g., acquired immunodeficiency syndrome [AIDS]). There may be no known cause (idiopathic). Several classification schemes for bronchiectasis have been proposed based on underlying cause, pathologic features (e.g., cylindrical, saccular, varicose), microbiologic phenotypes, or clinical presentation. However, the heterogeneity of the disease process and associated clinical features has limited the clinical utility of these classification groupings.[20]

In most cases, the bronchiectasis results from recurrent inflammatory and infectious insults to the bronchial epithelium

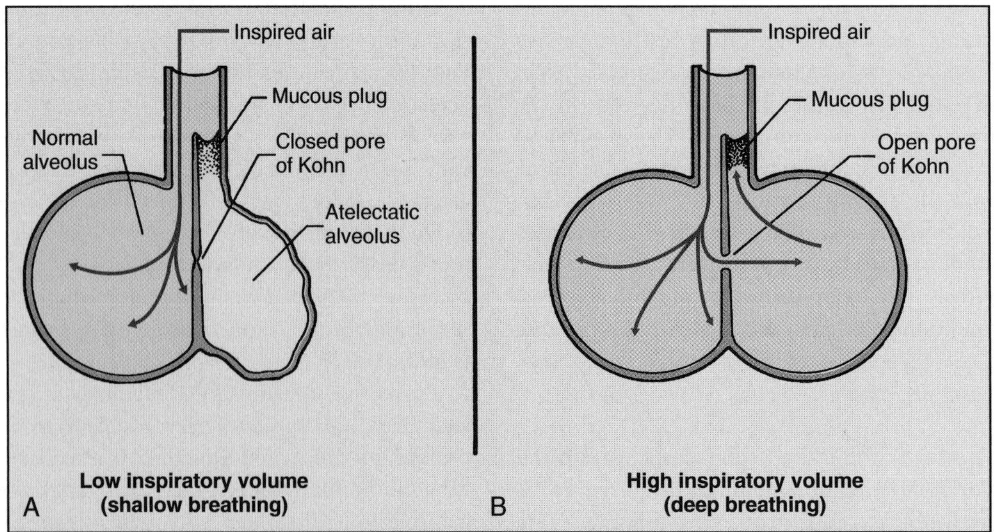

Fig. 35.5 Pores of Kohn. (A) Absorption atelectasis caused by a lack of collateral ventilation through the pores of Kohn. **(B)** Restoration of collateral ventilation during deep breathing.

leading to the infiltration of neutrophils and the release of neutrophil-derived proteases that destroy the elastic and muscular components of the bronchial walls.[21] This is followed by obstruction of the bronchial lumen, fibrosis, and permanent dilation. Chronic infection by *Pseudomonas aeruginosa* is common and is associated with more rapid lung function decline, more sputum production, and increased mortality.[22]

The primary symptom of bronchiectasis is a chronic productive cough. Dyspnea and fatigue are common. Recurrent lower respiratory tract infections lead to expectoration of copious amounts of foul-smelling, purulent sputum. Common signs include clubbing of the fingers (from chronic hypoxemia) and hemoptysis. Hypoxemia occurs due to $\dot{V}/\dot{Q}$ mismatch. Pulmonary function studies show decreases in the FVC and expiratory flow rates. The diagnosis is usually confirmed using high-resolution CT. Bronchiectasis is treated with antibiotics (inhaled or systemic), anti-inflammatory drugs, bronchodilators, mucolytic agents, chest physiotherapy, and supplemental oxygen.[21] Removal of the affected portion of the lung may be necessary. A lung transplant may be needed in advanced disease that is unresponsive to conventional treatment.[23]

Bronchiolitis

Bronchiolitis is a diffuse injury of the bronchioles (small airways with a diameter of 2 mm or less) resulting in inflammation and fibrosis. Primary bronchiolitis occurs most commonly in children due to viral infection. In adults, it most often results from smoking and chronic bronchitis but can occur in otherwise healthy individuals in association with an upper or lower respiratory tract infection. Bronchiolitis also occurs in association with interstitial lung diseases such as inhalational lung injury, hypersensitivity pneumonia, and pulmonary fibrosis. This type of bronchiolitis includes a fibrotic process that causes scarring of the lungs and is referred to as organizing pneumonia.[24] In severe lung injury, like that which may occur as a complication of lung or hematopoietic stem cell transplantation, the development of scarring and occlusion of the airways causes severe respiratory compromise and is referred to as bronchiolitis obliterans.[25]

Clinical manifestations of bronchiolitis include a rapid ventilatory rate, use of accessory muscles, low-grade fever, and a nonproductive cough. Wheezing may be heard. A $\dot{V}/\dot{Q}$ mismatch results in hypoxemia. The diagnosis of bronchiolitis is made by bronchoscopy with biopsy. Bronchiolitis is treated with chest physical therapy that includes humidified air administration, deep-breathing exercises, and postural drainage. Pharmacologic management includes antibiotics, corticosteroids, and immunosuppressive drugs. Careful handling of the lung tissue prior to surgery, tailored management of antirejection drugs, and the use of other medications (e.g., azithromycin and montelukast) can improve bronchiolitis obliterans outcomes after lung transplantation.[26]

Pulmonary Fibrosis

Pulmonary fibrosis is an excessive amount of fibrous or connective tissue in the lung. Pulmonary fibrosis can be idiopathic or caused by formation of scar tissue after active pulmonary disease (e.g., acute respiratory distress syndrome, pneumonia, inhalational injury). It may also be associated with autoimmune disorders (e.g., rheumatoid arthritis, progressive systemic sclerosis, sarcoidosis), inhalation of harmful substances (e.g., coal dust, asbestos), or chest irradiation. Fibrosis of the interstitial lung tissue around the alveoli causes decreased oxygen diffusion across the alveolocapillary membrane and hypoxemia. As the disease progresses, decreased lung compliance leads to an increased work of breathing, a decreased tidal volume, and resultant hypoventilation with hypercapnia. Diffuse pulmonary fibrosis has a poor prognosis.

Idiopathic pulmonary fibrosis (IPF) is a chronic progressive disease of unknown etiology. IPF is the most common of the fibrosing interstitial lung diseases, although its true prevalence is difficult to determine because of inconsistent diagnostic criteria.[27] It typically affects older individuals, and men are affected more often than women. Environmental factors such as smoking, viral infections, gastroesophageal reflux, inhalational injuries, and associated aberrant DNA methylation patterns are felt to be a critical component of the risk for IPF.[28] Many gene polymorphisms for inflammatory, immune, and fibrotic responses have been linked to the development of IPF. Mutations in the MUC5b gene are linked to airway mucociliary dysfunction and microbiome dysbiosis. Desmoplakin (DSP) variants contribute to changes in tissue architecture. Polymorphisms near the *AKAP13, ITGB6*, and *ELK1*genes have been identified that increase the risk of developing idiopathic pulmonary fibrosis (IPF) through increased growth factor and profibrotic cytokine production.[29]

The pathogenesis of IPF is felt to be multifactorial. Epithelial damage along with innate and adaptive immune responses involving neutrophils, macrophages, fibrocytes, and T lymphocytes result in the release of inflammatory cytokines and growth factors (e.g., transforming growth factor-β [TGF-β] and connective tissue growth factor [CTGF]).[30] Oxidative stress associated with activation of inflammatory and epithelial cells contributes to DNA damage, alveolar epithelial cell apoptosis, and the release of pro-fibrotic cytokines.[31] This initiates a fibrotic process that leads to interstitial and alveolar fibrin deposition, scarring, and "honeycombing" of the lung parenchyma. Dysfunctional surfactant production and alveolar collapse also occur.[32] Disease progression is highly variable, with some individuals demonstrating a slow decline, while others progress to death within a few years. Acute exacerbations may occur without clear provocation and accelerate decline.

IPF presents with dyspnea on exertion and dry cough. Auscultation reveals fine crackles. Many individuals also may present with symptoms and signs of comorbid conditions such as coronary artery disease, emphysema, and lung cancer. The diagnosis of IPF rests on the use of high-resolution CT scans and biopsies. Histological hallmarks include dense fibrosis and micro-honeycombing in the sub-pleural areas. Treatment includes pulmonary rehabilitation and symptom management along with psychosocial support, management of comorbidities, and palliative care. Two pharmacologic therapies aimed at decreasing the fibrotic process, nintedanib and pirfenidone, have been shown to slow disease progression in IPF.[33]

Lung transplant is indicated in selected individuals. New approaches to therapy are in development (Emerging Science Box: Future Treatments for Idiopathic Pulmonary Fibrosis).[29]

Inhalation Disorders

Exposure to toxic gases. Inhalation of gaseous irritants can cause significant respiratory dysfunction. Commonly encountered toxic gases include smoke, ammonia, hydrogen chloride, sulfur dioxide, chlorine, phosgene, and nitrogen dioxide. Inhalation injuries in burns can include heat, smoke particles, and toxic gases from household or industrial combustants. Inhaled toxins cause damage to the airway epithelium and promote mucus secretion, inflammation, mucosal edema, ciliary damage, pulmonary edema, and surfactant inactivation. The cellular effects of exposure to toxic gases are described in Chapter 2. Acute toxic inhalation frequently is complicated by acute respiratory distress syndrome and pneumonia. Initial symptoms include burning of the eyes, nose, and throat; coughing; chest tightness; and dyspnea. Hypoxemia is common. Treatment includes supplemental oxygen, mechanical ventilation, bronchodilators, corticosteroids, and support of the cardiovascular system. Most individuals respond quickly to therapy. Some, however, may improve initially and then deteriorate as a result of bronchiectasis or bronchiolitis.

Prolonged exposure to high concentrations of supplemental oxygen can result in a relatively rare condition in adults known as oxygen toxicity. The basic underlying mechanism of injury is a severe inflammatory response mediated by oxygen free radicals and lipid peroxidation of cell membranes. Damage to alveolocapillary membranes results in disruption of surfactant production, production of interstitial and alveolar edema, fibrosis, and a reduction in lung compliance. In infants, this can lead to a condition known as *bronchopulmonary dysplasia*, in which there is severe scarring of the lung. Treatment involves a reduction of the inspired oxygen concentration as soon as tolerated.

Pneumoconiosis. Pneumoconiosis represents any change in the lung caused by inhalation of inorganic dust particles. Pneumoconiosis often occurs after years of exposure to the offending particles, with progressive fibrosis of lung tissue. The dusts of silica and coal inhaled in the workplace are the most common causes of pneumoconiosis. These exposures result in disorders called silicosis and coal workers' lung. Asbestosis is another form of pneumoconiosis. Other causes include talc, fiberglass, clays, mica, slate, cement, and metals (cadmium, beryllium, tungsten, cobalt, aluminum, iron, indium, and titanium).

Deposition of these materials in the lungs causes chronic inflammation with scarring of the alveolocapillary membrane, resulting in pulmonary fibrosis and progressive pulmonary deterioration. Silica and coal particles create pulmonary nodules as well as fibrotic interstitial infiltrates. Smoking-related emphysema and tuberculosis infection are serious comorbidities in many individuals with silicosis and coal workers' lung. Asbestos is composed of long thin particles which cause not only interstitial fibrotic changes but also pleural disease and cancer (bronchogenic cancer and malignant mesothelioma).[34]

Clinical manifestations of pneumoconiosis include cough, chronic sputum production, dyspnea, decreased lung volumes (restriction), and hypoxemia. Bronchospasm with wheezing is often present. In most cases, diagnosis is made by obtaining a complete exposure and occupational history along with chest radiography. Lung biopsy is sometimes required to confirm the diagnosis. Treatment is usually palliative and focuses on preventing further exposure, management of associated hypoxemia and bronchospasm, and pulmonary rehabilitation.

EMERGING SCIENCE BOX

Future Treatments for Idiopathic Pulmonary Fibrosis

While the use of nintedanib and pirfenidone has been shown to slow the fibrotic process in idiopathic pulmonary fibrosis (IPF), long-term outcomes remain poor, and new therapies are needed. The pathophysiologic processes that contribute to the onset and progression of idiopathic pulmonary fibrosis are complex. Environmental factors interact with genetic and epigenetic factors to activate innate and adaptive immune responses culminating in interstitial fibrin deposition and alveolar collapse. Many new discoveries about these processes have been made. For example, the interaction between changes in the microorganisms that colonize the pulmonary system (microbiome) and genetic mutations is being elucidated. Pulmonary microbiome dysbiosis with the presence of bacteria such as *Escherichia* is felt to contribute to epithelial cell dysfunction and initiation of fibrosis. The gene Mucin-5B is important to innate immune responses to microorganisms. It is believed that polymorphisms of the Mucin-5B gene and associated alterations of MUC5B protein gene are linked to the risk of developing IPF through their impact on immune responses to pulmonary dysbiosis. Another exciting area of research focuses on the role of autotaxins, which are a group of enzymes involved in fibroblast recruitment and epithelial damage. Discoveries such as these have led to numerous studies toward new approaches to the treatment of IPF, such as modulation of the lung microbiome and autotaxin inhibitors. Pamrevlumab, which is an anti- connective tissue growth factor antibody, has shown promising efficacy in IPF in phase III trials. Other treatments being researched include pentraxin-2 analogues, which inhibit fibroblast maturation; leukotriene antagonists, which reduce inflammation; monoclonal antibodies to interleukins and growth factors; and medications that block the adaptive immune system.

Data from Hadjicharalambous MR, et al. Idiopathic pulmonary fibrosis: Pathogenesis and the emerging role of long non-coding RNAs. *International Journal of Molecular Science*, 2020;21(2):524; Podolanczuk AJ, et al. Idiopathic pulmonary fibrosis: Prime time for a precision-based approach to treatment with N-acetylcysteine. *European Medical Journal - Respiratory*, 2021;57:2003551; Richeldi L, et al. Current and Future Idiopathic Pulmonary Fibrosis Therapy. *American Journal of the Medical Sciences*, 2019;357(5):370–373; Sgalla G, et al. Phase three clinical trials in idiopathic pulmonary fibrosis. *Expert Opinion on Orphan Drugs*, 2021;9(1):1–11; Torrisi SE, et al. Evolution and treatment of idiopathic pulmonary fibrosis. *La Presse Médicale*, 2020;49(2):104025; Valenzuela C, et al. Ongoing challenges in pulmonary fibrosis and insights from the nintedanib clinical programme. *Respiratory Research*, 2020;21:7; Varone F, et al. Evaluation of the lung microbiome as a therapeutic target in the management of idiopathic pulmonary fibrosis: Role of antioxidant/antibiotic combination therapy. *European Review for Medical and Pharmacological Sciences*, 2019;23(14):6379–6386; Yoon HY, et al. Lung tissue microbiome Is associated with clinical outcomes of idiopathic pulmonary fibrosis. *Front Med*, 2021;8:744523.

Hypersensitivity pneumonitis. Hypersensitivity pneumonitis (extrinsic allergic alveolitis) is an inflammatory disease of the lungs caused by inhalation of organic particles. Many organic substances can cause this disorder, including grains, silage, bird droppings or feathers, wood and cork dust, animal pelts, coffee beans, fish meal, mushroom compost, and molds that grow on sugarcane, barley, and straw. Although it is often described as an allergic disease, it is not immunoglobulin E (IgE)-mediated. Rather the pathophysiology is of type III and type IV hypersensitivity with infiltration of T cytotoxic lymphocytes, inflammatory cells, autoantibodies, and resultant tissue damage (see Chapter 9).[35]

Hypersensitivity pneumonitis can be classified into acute, chronic non-fibrotic, or chronic fibrotic forms.[36] The acute form results from high-level exposure, causes fever, cough, and chills a few hours after exposure. Tachypnea and inspiratory crackles over the lower lung lobes are found on physical examination. Chronic hypersensitivity pneumonitis results from long-term, low-level exposure and may occur within weeks, months, or even years of exposure.[36] With continued exposure, pulmonary fibrosis develops with progressive dyspnea, fatigue, and weight loss. The diagnosis is made by obtaining a history of exposure and by performing serum antibody testing, chest radiography, high resolution CT, bronchoscopy with lavage, and, in some cases, lung biopsy.[37] Treatment consists of removal of the offending agent and administration of corticosteroids. New antifibrotic medications are being explored.[36]

Pulmonary Edema

Pulmonary edema is excess fluid in the lung. The normal lung maintains minimal fluid in interstitial tissues by lymphatic drainage and a balance among capillary hydrostatic pressure, capillary oncotic pressure, and capillary permeability. Chapter 3 provides further discussion on osmotic forces (hydrostatic and oncotic pressures). In addition, surfactant lining the alveoli repels water, keeping fluid from entering the alveoli. Pulmonary edema develops when these protective mechanisms are disrupted. Predisposing factors for pulmonary edema include heart disease, lung capillary injury, and processes that block the lymphatic vessels. The pathogenesis of pulmonary edema is shown in Algorithm 35.2.

The most common cause of pulmonary edema is left-sided heart disease. When the left ventricle fails, filling pressures on the left side of the heart increase and cause a concomitant increase in the pulmonary capillary hydrostatic pressure (see Chapter 32). When the hydrostatic pressure exceeds the oncotic pressure, fluid moves from the capillary into the interstitial space and alveoli. When the flow of fluid out of the capillaries exceeds the lymphatic system's ability to remove it, pulmonary edema develops.

Another cause of pulmonary edema is pulmonary or systemic injury that increases capillary permeability, as in cases of acute respiratory distress syndrome or inhalation of toxic gases. Damage to the alveolocapillary membrane and inflammation allow water, cells, and plasma proteins to leak out of the capillary and move into the interstitial space and alveoli. Pulmonary edema also can result from obstruction of the lymphatic system.

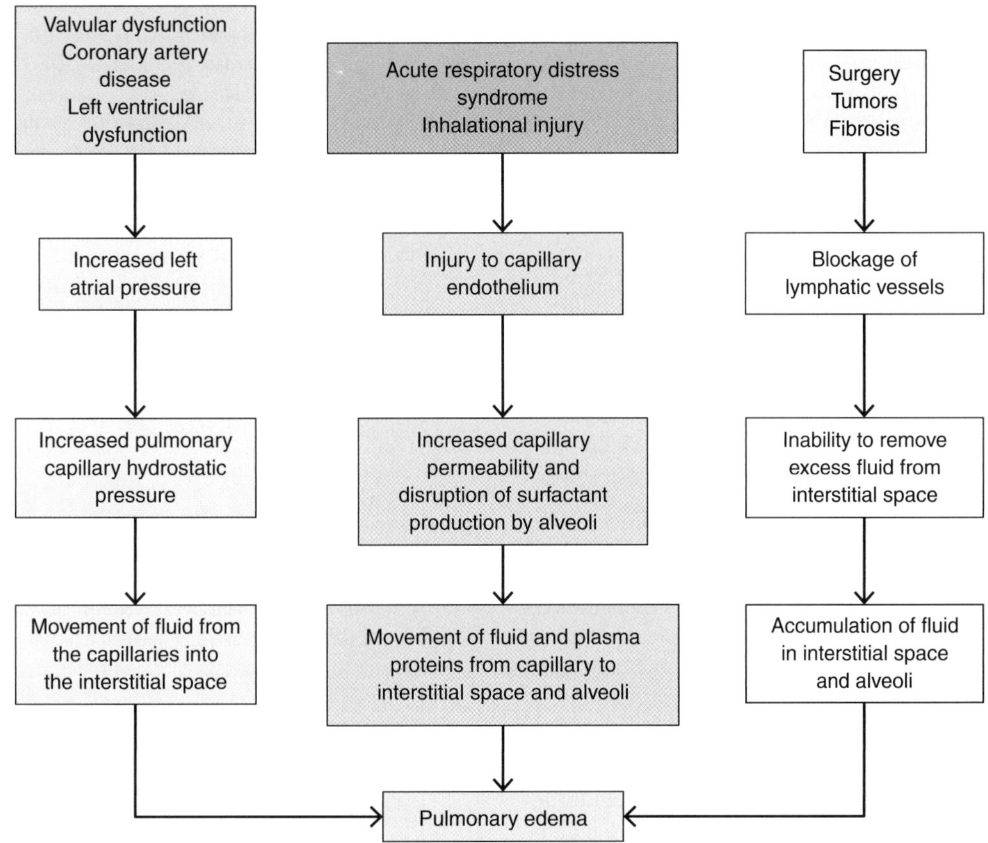

Algorithm 35.2 Pathogenesis of Pulmonary Edema.

This may occur during surgical procedures or because of the presence of tumors and fibrotic tissue. Fluid in the alveoli results in low a V· /Q· ratio and hypoxemia.

Clinical manifestations of pulmonary edema include dyspnea, tissue hypoxia, and increased work of breathing. Physical examination may reveal inspiratory crackles (rales) and dullness to percussion over the lung bases. In severe cases, pink, frothy sputum is expectorated, hypoxemia worsens, and hypoventilation with hypercapnia may develop.

The treatment of pulmonary edema depends on its cause. If the edema is caused by increased hydrostatic pressure resulting from heart failure, therapy is directed toward improving cardiac output with diuretics, vasodilators, and drugs that improve the contraction of the heart muscle (see Chapter 32). If the edema is the result of increased capillary permeability resulting from injury, the treatment is focused on removing the offending agent and implementing supportive therapy to maintain adequate ventilation and circulation. Individuals with either type of pulmonary edema require supplemental oxygen. Lymphatic blockage is managed by treating the underlying condition but may not be reversible. Mechanical ventilation may be needed if edema significantly impairs ventilation and oxygenation.

Acute Respiratory Distress Syndrome

Acute respiratory distress syndrome (ARDS) is a form of acute lung inflammation and diffuse alveolocapillary injury that results from direct pulmonary injury or from severe systemic inflammation. Although rare in the general population, it is estimated that 10% of individuals admitted to the ICU and 23% of all individuals requiring mechanical ventilation carry the diagnosis of ARDS.[38] Individuals with ARDS have an acute onset of bilateral infiltrates on a chest radiograph (i.e., pulmonary edema) and a persistent hypoxemia despite supplemental oxygen (low ration of PaO_2 to FiO_2). The most common predisposing factors are sepsis and multiple trauma. There are many other causes, including pneumonia, burns, aspiration, cardiopulmonary bypass surgery, pancreatitis, blood transfusions, drug overdose, inhalation of smoke or noxious gases, fat emboli, radiation therapy, and disseminated intravascular coagulation. The emergence of Coronavirus Disease-2019 (COVID-19) has resulted in a dramatic increase in the number of ARDS cases worldwide (Emerging Science Box: The Pathogenesis of the Acute Respiratory Distress Syndrome (ARDS) in COVID-19).[39] Several genetic and epigenetic factors have been identified that confer susceptibility to developing ARDS.[40] Several subphenotypes and endotypes of ARDS have been proposed (e.g., uninflamed versus hyperinflammatory forms), but to date, there is no clear clinical application of these classifications.[41] Despite advances in diagnosis and therapy, mortality remains at approximately 30% to 40%.[39]

Pathophysiology. All disorders causing ARDS result in an acute inflammatory lung injury characterized by diffuse alveolar damage and triggered by direct injury to the lung epithelium and/or by indirect biochemical injury to the endothelium.[38] Within 72 hours, damage to both pulmonary capillary endothelial cells and alveolar epithelial cells develops. Endothelial damage activates neutrophils, macrophages, and platelets with the

EMERGING SCIENCE BOX

The Pathogenesis of the Acute Respiratory Distress Syndrome in COVID-19 Infection

As described in Chapter 10, the pathogenesis of COVID-19 infection begins when SARS-CoV-2 binds its viral S spike protein with angiotensin-converting enzyme (ACE)-2 receptors on host respiratory epithelial cells. SARS-CoV-2 infection in the respiratory system can be divided into three clinical stages: viral infection, pulmonary involvement with inflammation, and fibrosis. The virus first enters and replicates in the epithelial cells of the upper respiratory tract, making it transmissible from person to person through speech-related aerosolization of viral particles. The virus is then tropic for ciliated lower airway epithelial cells and alveolar type II pneumocytes, both of which express the ACE-2 receptor. There follows an inflammatory response involving infiltration of large numbers of macrophages and neutrophils and the release of cytokines including interleukins, tumor necrosis factor alpha, and interferons, along with the activation of complement and clotting systems. This has been called a "cytokine storm" and results in diffuse alveolar and microvascular damage and thrombosis. Fluid leaks into the pulmonary interstitium resulting in $\dot{V}/\dot{Q}$ mismatch and hypoxemia. As the disease progresses, interstitial fibrosis and formation of hyaline membranes develop. In many individuals with COVID-19, these pathologic changes cause hypoxic pulmonary vasoconstriction, right-to-left shunting, and decreased pulmonary compliance like that seen in other forms of acute respiratory distress syndrome (ARDS). These individuals are severely dyspneic due to the increased work of breathing and frequently require mechanical ventilation with high levels of positive end-expiratory pressure (PEEP). However, in a significant proportion of those with ARDS associated with the COVID-19, there is little hypoxic pulmonary vasoconstriction and little reduction in lung compliance. These individuals are less likely to be severely dyspneic and may appear to be in much less overall respiratory distress. Mechanical ventilation with PEEP in these individuals may actually increase lung damage. Instead, a gradual escalation of oxygen therapy is indicated, including continuous positive airway pressure by means of noninvasive ventilation. Intubation with mechanical ventilation or extracorporeal membrane oxygenation (ECMO) are used only if these methods prove insufficient to maintain adequate gas exchange. Pharmacologic interventions that can be considered for COVID-19 associated ARDS include antivirals, monoclonal antibodies, corticosteroids, anticoagulants, inhaled vasodilators, bronchodilators, surfactant, and anti-immune therapies (see Chapter 10).

Data from Acosta MAT, et al. Pathogenesis of COVID-19- induced ARDS: Implications for an ageing population. *European Respiratory Journal*, 2020;56(3):2002049; Aslan et al. Acute respiratory distress syndrome in COVID-19: possible mechanisms and therapeutic management. *Pneumonia*, 2021;13:14; Bahari Z, et al. Pharmacological mechanism of immunomodulatory agents for the treatment of severe cases of COVID-19 infection. *Inflammation Research*, 2021;70:389–405; Kavianpour M, et al. The role of mesenchymal stromal cells in immune modulation of COVID-19: Focus on cytokine storm. *Stem Cell Research Therapy*, 2020;11(1):404; Matera MG, et al. Pharmacological management of COVID-19 patients with ARDS (CARDS): A narrative review. *Respiratory Medicine*, 2020;171:106114; Morris G, et al. The pathophysiology of S RS-CoV-2: a suggested model and therapeutic approach. *Life Sciences*, 2020;258:118166; Perchiazzi G, et al. The use of positive end expiratory pressure in patients affected by COVID-19: Time to reconsider the relation between morphology and physiology. *Best Practice and Research in Clinical Anaesthesiology*, 2020;34(3):561–567; Ratre YK, et al. Molecular mechanism, diagnosis, and potential treatment for novel coronavirus (COVID-19): A current literature review and perspective. *3 Biotech*, 2021;11(2):94; Sette A, et al. Adaptive immunity to SARS-CoV-2 and COVID-19. *Cell*, 2021;184(4):861–880; Schultze JL, et al. COVID-19 and the human innate immune system. *Cell*, 2021. https://doi.org/10.1016/j.cell.2021.02.029

release of inflammatory cytokines, resulting in greatly increased capillary membrane permeability, hypercoagulability, and pulmonary arteriolar vasoconstriction. Fluids, proteins, and blood cells leak from the capillary bed into the pulmonary interstitium and flood the alveoli (exudative phase). Alveolar ventilation is severely reduced, resulting in $\dot{V}/\dot{Q}$ mismatch and severe hypoxemia. Increasing respiratory rate results in an initial hypocapnia and respiratory alkalosis. Epithelial cell damage causes a reduction in surfactant production, resulting in atelectasis. Lung compliance declines, with associated decreases in tidal volume and the development of hypercapnia. The result of this overwhelming inflammatory response by the lungs is acute hypoxemic and hypercapnic respiratory failure. Within 4 to 14 days, there is resolution of the pulmonary edema, and the proliferative phase of ARDS begins. The intra-alveolar exudate becomes cellular granulation tissue, appearing as hyaline membranes that form a diffusion barrier for oxygen exchange and resulting in continued hypoxemia. The final stage (fibrotic stage) occurs within 14 to 21 days and consists of remodeling and fibrosis of the lung tissue. In severe cases, the fibrosis progressively obliterates the alveoli, respiratory bronchioles, and interstitium, leading to long-term respiratory compromise. Algorithm 35.3 summarizes the pathogenesis of ARDS.

Clinical Manifestations. The clinical manifestations of ARDS are progressive and include

1. Dyspnea and hypoxemia with poor response to oxygen supplementation
2. Initial hyperventilation and respiratory alkalosis
3. Decreased tissue perfusion, metabolic acidosis, and organ dysfunction
4. Increased work of breathing, decreased tidal volume, and hypoventilation
5. Hypercapnia, respiratory acidosis, and worsening hypoxemia
6. Respiratory failure, decreased cardiac output, hypotension, multiple organ dysfunction syndrome (MODS) and death

Evaluation and Treatment. The diagnosis is based on a history of the lung injury, physical examination, blood gas analysis, and chest radiographs. In 2012, a consensus definition described three major criteria for the diagnosis of ARDS: (1) onset within 1 week of known clinical insult or new or worsening respiratory symptoms; (2) bilateral opacities not fully explained by effusions, lobar/lung collapse, or nodules on chest x-ray or CT; and (3) respiratory failure not fully explained by cardiac failure or fluid to exclude hydrostatic edema if no ARDS risk factor is present.[42] Measurement of serum biomarkers (i.e., surfactant proteins, B-type natriuretic peptide [BNP], C-reactive protein [CRP], and interleukins) may aid in the diagnosis and prognosis of ARDS. Treatment is based on early detection, supportive therapy, and prevention of complications. Supportive therapy is focused on maintaining adequate oxygenation and ventilation while preventing further lung injury and infection. This often requires high flow nasal oxygen and various modes of mechanical ventilation, prone positioning, or extracorporeal oxygenation.[43] The risk of barotrauma increases as lung compliance decreases, making lung-protective strategies of ventilation (e.g., lowering tidal volume and driving pressure) essential in severe disease.[44] To date, no pharmacologic interventions have been consistently shown to improve morbidity or mortality, although corticosteroids continue to be recommended for moderate to severe ARDS.[39] New treatment strategies such as mesenchymal stem cell and exosome-based therapies are showing early promise.[45] COVID-19 related ARDS is treated with antivirals, monoclonal antibodies, corticosteroids, anticoagulants, inhaled vasodilators, bronchodilators, surfactant, and anti-immune therapies (see Emerging Science Box: The Pathogenesis of the Acute Respiratory Distress Syndrome (ARDS) in COVID-19).[39]

Obstructive Lung Diseases

Obstructive lung disease is characterized by narrowing of the airways, resulting in airway obstruction that is worse with expiration. More force is required to expire a given volume of air; thus, individuals have an increased work of breathing and must use their accessory muscles of expiration. Emptying of the lungs is slowed, as measured by a decreased forced expiratory volume in 1 second (FEV_1). Air is trapped in the lungs resulting in decreased tidal volume eventually leading to hypoventilation and hypercapnia. Changes in alveolar ventilation result in $\dot{V}/\dot{Q}$ mismatching and hypoxemia. The unifying symptom of obstructive lung diseases is dyspnea, and the unifying sign is wheezing. The most common obstructive diseases are asthma, chronic bronchitis, and emphysema. Because many individuals have chronic bronchitis with emphysema, these diseases together are often called *chronic obstructive pulmonary disease (COPD).*

Asthma

Asthma, as defined by the Global Initiative for Asthma (GINA) 2021 report, is a "...heterogenous disease, usually characterized by chronic airway inflammation. It is defined by the history of respiratory symptoms, such as wheeze, shortness of breath, chest tightness, and cough that vary over time and in intensity, together with variable expiratory airflow limitation."[46] The chronic inflammation causes bronchial hyperresponsiveness, constriction of the airways, and variable airflow obstruction that is reversible, although airflow limitation may become persistent with disease progression. Asthma occurs at all ages, affecting 7% of children (see Chapter 36) and 8% (approx. 20 million) adults in the United States.[47] It is more prevalent in women and in individuals who live below the poverty level.

Asthma is a familial disorder, and more than 120 genes have been identified that play a role in the susceptibility, pathogenesis, and treatment response of asthma.[48] Specific gene expressions may impart associated *phenotypes*, the most common of which are allergic asthma, non-allergic asthma, adult-onset asthma, asthma with persistent airflow limitation, and asthma with obesity. Classifying individuals with asthma into these phenotypes can guide therapies that target specific pathophysiologic pathways.[49] Allergic asthma (type I hypersensitivity; see Chapter 9) is the most common phenotype and is the primary focus of the information in this chapter, although overlap with other phenotypes is common. Asthma also can be classified into various *endotypes*, such as clinical characteristics, biomarkers, lung physiology, histopathology, epidemiology, and treatment response.

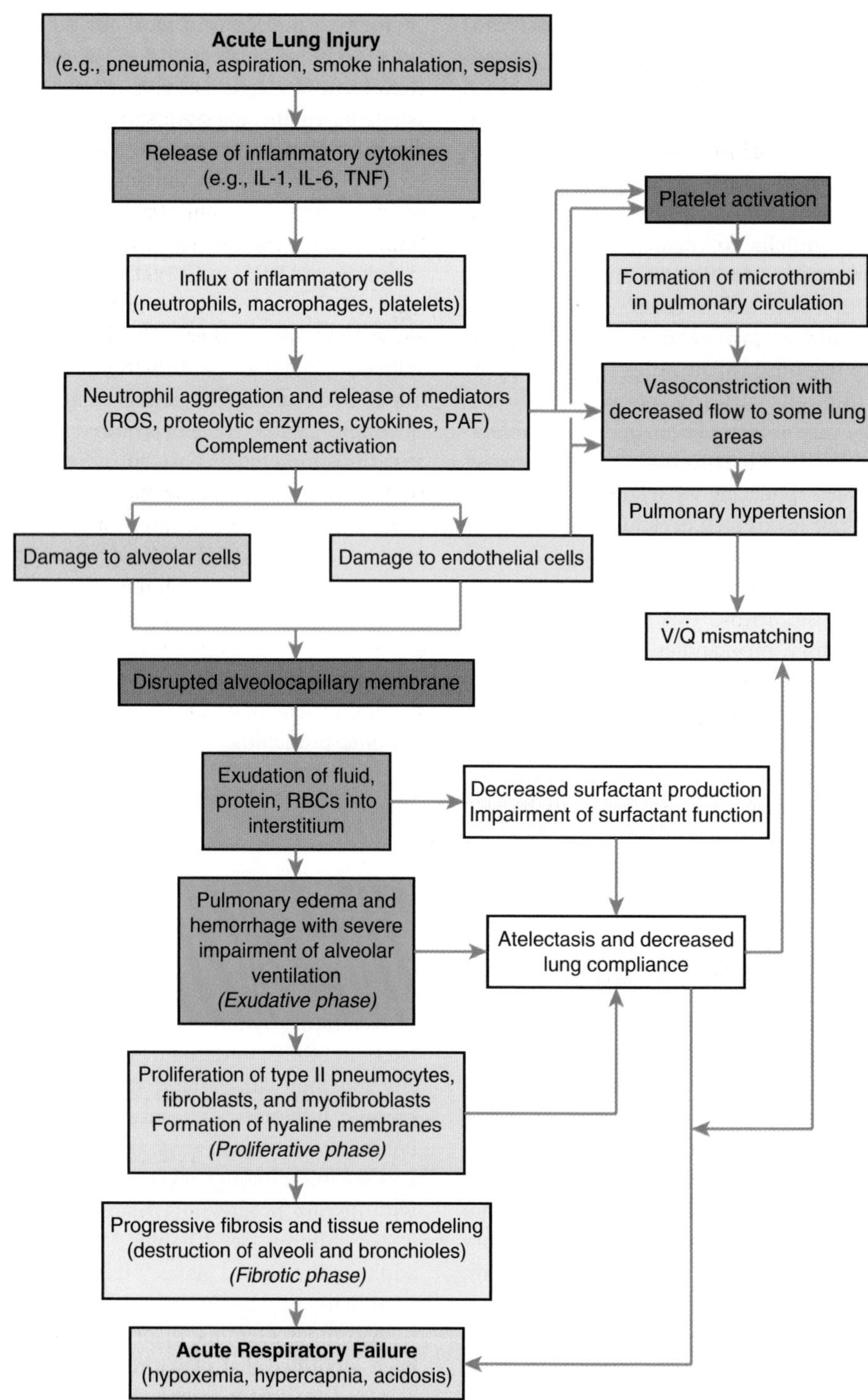

Algorithm 35.3 Pathogenesis of Acute Respiratory Distress Syndrome (ARDS). *IL-1,* Interleukin-1; *IL-6,* interleukin-6; *PAF,* platelet-activating factor; *RBCs,* red blood cells; *ROS,* reactive oxygen species; *TNF,* tumor necrosis factor.

Allergen exposure, urban residence, exposure to indoor and outdoor air pollution, tobacco smoke, recurrent respiratory tract viral infections, obesity, use of acetaminophen-containing medications, and GERD impact gene expression (epigenetics) and therefore the risk of developing asthma.[50] Exposure to high levels of certain allergens increases the risk for allergic asthma in sensitized individuals by promoting more type 1 hypersensitivity (see Chapter 9). The effect of infections is more complicated. Decreased exposure to certain infectious microorganisms appears to create an immunologic imbalance that favors the development of allergy and asthma (hygiene hypothesis). In contrast, exposure to several common respiratory viruses (e.g., respiratory syncytial virus) increases the risk of asthma. Furthermore, diet, immunization and antibiotic use, and indoor/outdoor activity patterns have been linked to asthma development.[51] The relationship between the microbiome and asthma risk is shedding light on these complex interactions. There is accumulating evidence of a cross-talk between gut and lung. Upper gastrointestinal microorganisms influence the airway microbiota primarily through aspiration. Dysbiosis of the gut can lead to dysbiosis in the lung via microorganisms traveling through the bloodstream. Airway dysbiosis is linked to allergen sensitization and the development of asthma.[52,53] Exposure to inhaled irritants can cause neutrophil activation, inflammation, and damage to airways independent of allergen sensitivity and may contribute to the onset of symptoms in both allergic and non-allergic asthma phenotypes. Obesity is associated with a chronic inflammatory state that sensitizes the bronchial mucosa to allergen and irritant exposure. Acetaminophen depletes glutathione levels in the respiratory tract, leading to oxidative stress, airway inflammation, and bronchoconstriction. GERD causes stimulation of the vagus nerve with the release of acetylcholine (ACh), which causes bronchoconstriction.

Pathophysiology. In allergic asthma, airway epithelial exposure to antigen initiates both an innate and an adaptive immune response in sensitized individuals (type I hypersensitivity; see Chapter 9). A concise overview of the pathophysiology of asthma is depicted in Algorithm 35.4. The immune response to epithelial antigen exposures includes many cells and cellular elements contributing to persistent inflammation of the bronchial mucosa and hyperresponsiveness of the airways.[54] These cells include dendritic cells (antigen-presenting macrophages), T-helper 2 (Th2) lymphocytes, B lymphocytes, mast cells, neutrophils, eosinophils, and basophils (see Chapter 8). There is both an early (immediate) asthmatic response and a late (delayed) response.

During the *early asthmatic response*, antigen exposure to the bronchial epithelium activates dendritic cells, which present antigen to T-helper cells. T-helper cells differentiate into Th2 cells, which release numerous cytokines. Of these, the most important in the pathogenesis of asthma include IL-4, which activates B lymphocytes (plasma cells), IL-5, which activates eosinophils, IL-13, which contributes to airway injury, and IL-33, which promotes the maturation of Th2 cells and the activation of mast cells, basophils, and eosinophils.[55] Plasma cells produce antigen-specific IgE, which binds to the surface of mast cells. Subsequent cross-linking of IgE molecules with the antigen causes mast cell degranulation and the release of inflammatory mediators, including histamine, bradykinins, leukotrienes, prostaglandins, platelet-activating factor, and interleukins. Together these inflammatory mediators cause vasodilation,

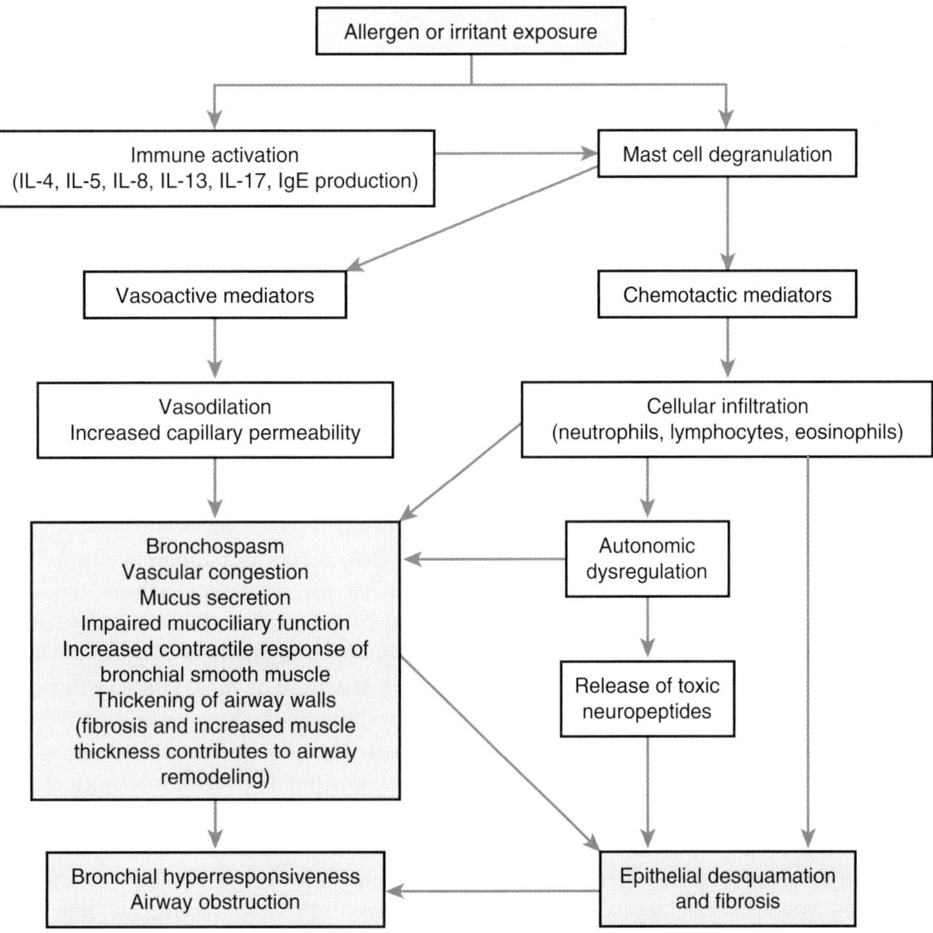

Algorithm 35.4 Overview of the Pathophysiology of Asthma. Allergen or irritant exposure results in a cascade of inflammatory events, leading to acute and chronic airway dysfunction. *IgE*, Immunoglobulin E; *IL*, interleukin.

increased capillary permeability, mucosal edema, bronchial smooth muscle contraction (bronchospasm), and mucus secretion with narrowing of the airways and obstruction to airflow. Inflammation also leads to increased ACh release by the pulmonary parasympathetic nervous system. ACh binds to the muscarinic 3 (M_3) receptor, further contributing to bronchospasm and mucus secretion.[56] Eosinophils release toxic neuropeptides that contribute to increased bronchial hyperresponsiveness (Figs. 35.6 and 35.7).

The *late asthmatic response* begins 4 to 8 hours after the early response. Chemotactic recruitment of eosinophils, neutrophils, and lymphocytes during the acute response causes a release of inflammatory mediators, again inciting bronchospasm, edema, and mucus secretion with obstruction to airflow. Synthesis of leukotrienes contributes to prolonged smooth muscle contraction. Eosinophils cause direct tissue injury with fibroblast proliferation and airway scarring. Damage to ciliated epithelial cells contributes to the accumulation of mucus and cellular debris, forming plugs in the airways. Untreated inflammation can lead to long-term airway damage resulting in subepithelial fibrosis and smooth muscle hypertrophy (airway remodeling) and may become irreversible.[57]

Airway obstruction increases resistance to airflow and expiratory flow rates. Decreased expiratory flow causes air trapping, hyperinflation of the lungs, and an increased work of breathing. Changes in resistance to airflow are not uniform throughout the lungs, and the distribution of inspired air is uneven, resulting in $\dot{V}/\dot{Q}$ mismatch and hypoxemia. Hyperventilation is triggered by lung receptors responding to airway obstruction and increased lung volume. The result is early hypoxemia with decreased $PaCO_2$ and increased pH (respiratory alkalosis). With progressive obstruction of expiratory airflow, air trapping becomes more severe, and the lungs and thorax become hyperexpanded, positioning the respiratory muscles at a mechanical disadvantage. This leads to a decrease in tidal volume, hypoventilation, increased $PaCO_2$, and respiratory acidosis. Respiratory acidosis signals respiratory failure.

Clinical Manifestations. Individuals are usually asymptomatic between attacks, and pulmonary function tests are normal. At the beginning of an asthmatic attack, the individual experiences chest constriction, expiratory wheezing, dyspnea, nonproductive cough, prolonged expiration, use of accessory muscles of respiration, tachycardia, and tachypnea. A pulsus paradoxus (decrease in systolic blood pressure during inspiration of more than 10 mm Hg) may be noted. Peak flow measurements should be obtained. Because the severity of blood–gas alterations is difficult to evaluate by clinical signs alone, arterial blood gas tensions should be measured if oxygen saturation falls below 90%.

If bronchospasm is not reversed by usual treatment measures, the individual is considered to have status asthmaticus (acute severe bronchospasm), and the situation becomes life-threatening. If status asthmaticus continues, hypoxemia worsens, expiratory flows and volumes decrease further, and effective ventilation decreases. Acidosis develops as the $PaCO_2$ level begins to rise. Ventilation may cease altogether, and a silent chest (no audible air movement) and a $PaCO_2$ greater than 70 mm Hg are ominous signs of impending death.

Evaluation and Treatment. The diagnosis of asthma is based on the history of symptom patterns and evidence of variable and reversible airflow limitation.[46] It is supported by a history of allergies and recurrent episodes of wheezing, dyspnea, and cough or exercise intolerance. These symptoms often are worse at night, vary over time and in intensity, and are triggered by exposure to allergens, irritants, changes in weather, and viral infections, Physical examination findings are often normal between episodes. Spirometry is used to document reversible decreases in FEV_1 during an induced attack. Careful assessment is critical to making the correct diagnosis since many other conditions may be mistaken for asthma, including heart disease, cystic fibrosis, vocal cord dysfunction, and medication-related cough. Allergy testing may be performed. Once the diagnosis is established, asthma is classified by severity.[46]

The evaluation of an acute asthma attack requires the rapid assessment of arterial blood gases and expiratory flow rates (using a peak flow meter) and a search for underlying triggers, such as infection. Hypoxemia and respiratory alkalosis are expected early during an acute attack. The development of hypercapnia with respiratory acidosis signals the need for mechanical ventilation. Management of the acute asthma attack is based on severity as determined by peak flow measurements. In those with severe exacerbation, immediate administration of oxygen, inhaled short-acting β-agonist bronchodilators, and systemic corticosteroids are indicated.[58] Careful monitoring of gas exchange and airway patency in response to therapy provides information necessary to determine whether hospitalization and noninvasive ventilation are necessary. Exhaled nitric oxide (FeNO) levels increasingly are used to follow response to therapy and can be used when other diagnostic modalities are inconclusive.[59] Antibiotics are not indicated for acute asthma unless there is a documented bacterial infection.

The goals of asthma management are to control symptoms and prevent exacerbation. Management decisions are guided by the GINA working group.[46] In addition, a 2020 Focused Updates to the Asthma Management Guidelines from the National Asthma Education and Prevention Program Coordinating Committee is available.[59] Management of chronic asthma begins with avoidance of allergens and irritants. Individuals with asthma tend to underestimate the severity of their asthma, and extensive education is important, including the use of a peak flow meter and adherence to an action plan. A stepwise approach for persistent asthma treatment is recommended. The use of continuous low-dose inhaled corticosteroids with or without long-acting beta-agonist (LABA) for even the mildest forms of asthma is most effective in managing symptoms. The use of short-acting beta-agonists (SABAs) is associated with an increased risk for severe exacerbations and should be reserved for those individuals with intermittent asthma symptoms[59] and those with persistent asthma who are well controlled and do not want to alter their current regimen or are unlikely to be adherent to low-dose inhaled corticosteroids alone.[46] Because of these adherence concerns, new recommendations also include the use of as-needed low dose inhaled corticosteroids combined with formoterol as an option for adults and adolescents with mild asthma.[46,60] For all categories of more severe

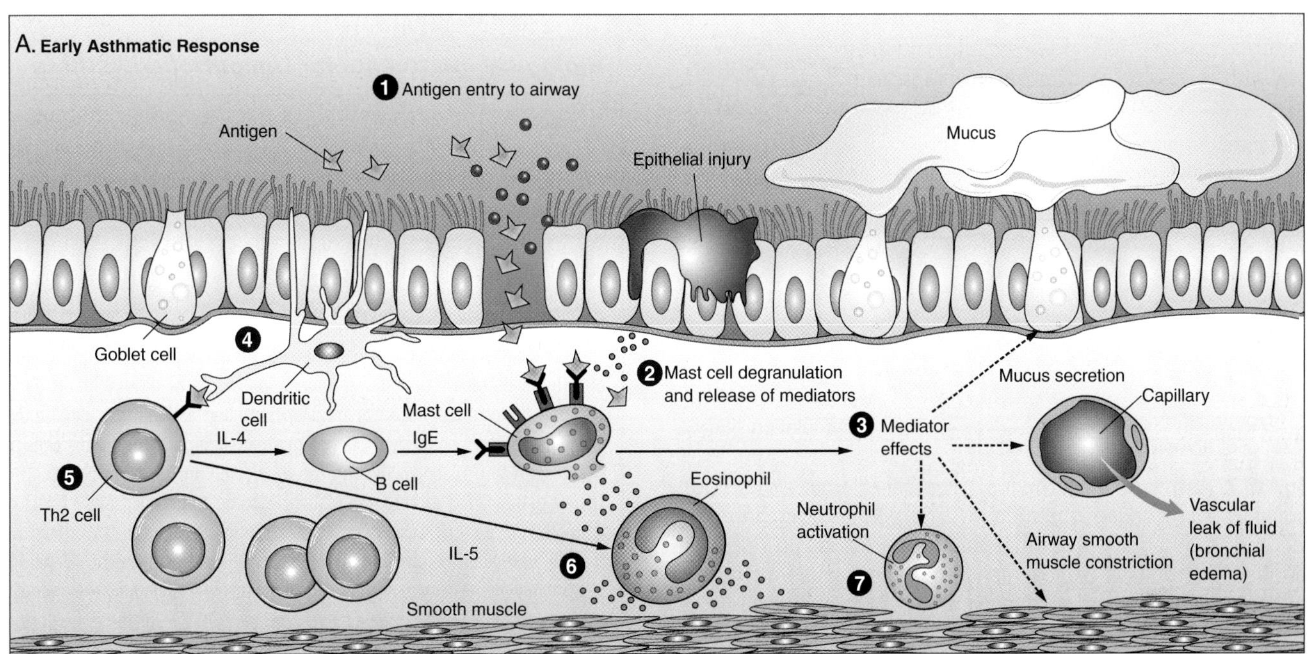

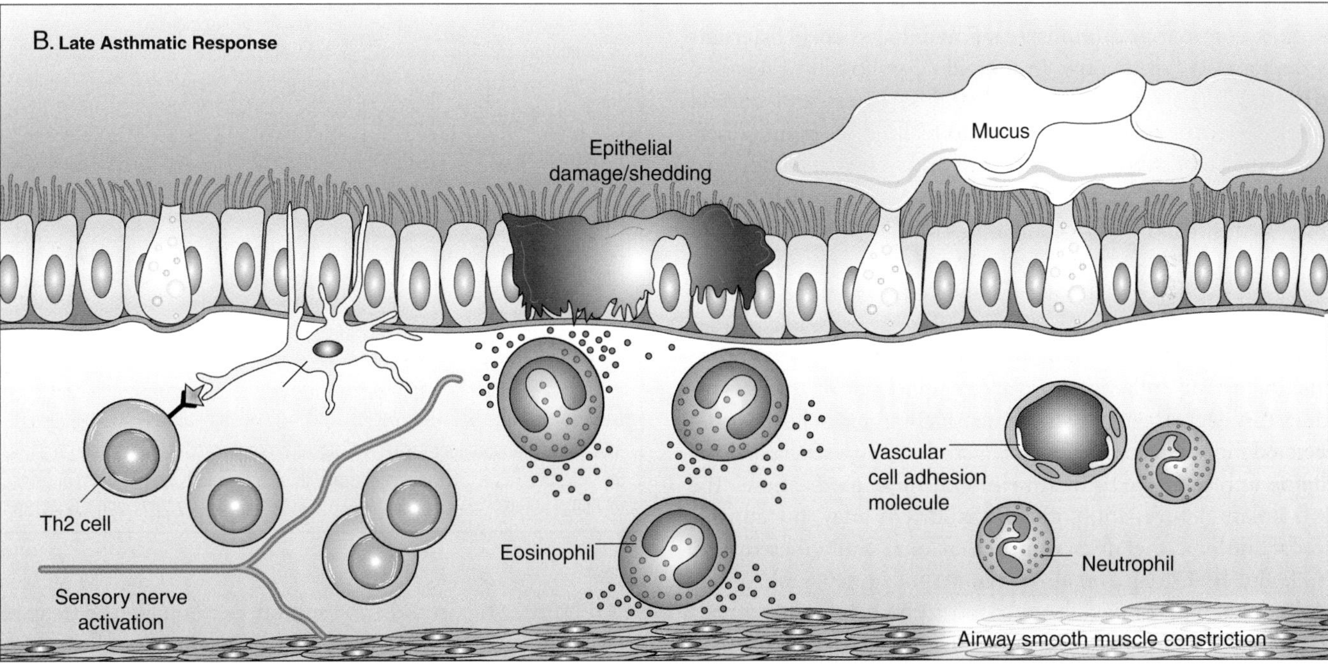

Fig. 35.6 Early and Late Asthmatic Response. (A) *Early response:* Inhaled antigen *(1)* binds to mast cells covered with preformed immunoglobulin E (IgE). Mast cells degranulate *(2)* and release inflammatory mediators, such as histamine, bradykinins, leukotrienes, prostaglandins, platelet-activating factor, and interleukins. Secreted mediators *(3)* induce active bronchospasm (airway smooth muscle constriction), edema from increased capillary permeability, and airway mucus secretion from goblet cells. At the same time, antigen is detected by *(4)* dendritic cells that process and present it to T-helper 2 *(Th2)* cells *(5)*, which produce interleukin-4 *(IL-4)* and many other interleukins (see text). IL-4 promotes switching of B cells to favor IgE production. Th2 cells also produce IL-5 *(6)*, which activates eosinophils. Many inflammatory cells, including neutrophils *(7)*, also contribute to the inflammatory process. **(B)** *Late response:* Areas of epithelial damage and shedding caused, at least in part, by toxicity of eosinophil products (major basic protein, eosinophilic cationic protein, eosinophil-derived neurotoxin, and eosinophil peroxidase). Many inflammatory cells are recruited by chemokines and upregulation of vascular cell adhesion molecules. Local T lymphocytes display a predominant Th2 cytokine profile. They produce IL-4 and IL-13, which promote switching of B cells to favor IgE production; and IL-3, IL-5, and granulocyte-macrophage colony–stimulating factor, which encourage eosinophil differentiation and survival. Inflammatory mediators also activate sensory nerves, further stimulating bronchoconstriction.

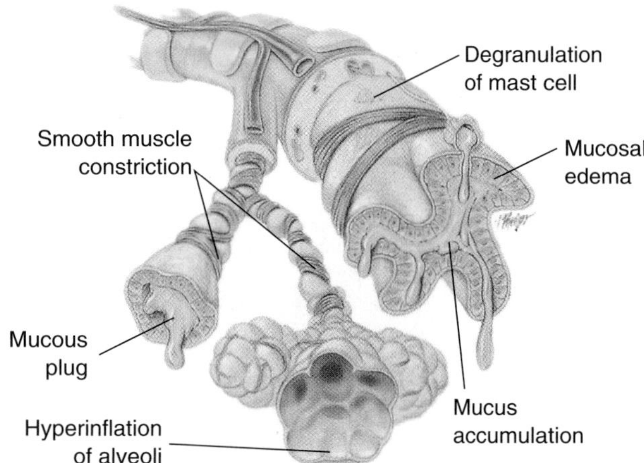

Fig. 35.7 Asthma. Thick mucus, mucosal edema, and smooth muscle spasm cause obstruction of small airways; breathing becomes labored and expiration is difficult. (Modified from Des Jardins T, Burton GG. *Clinical manifestations and assessment of respiratory disease*, 3rd edition. St. Louis: Mosby; 1955.)

asthma, continuous administration of inhaled corticosteroids is the mainstay of therapy. In individuals who fail to respond to initial management, it is essential to assess and correct problems such as incorrect inhaler technique, poor adherence, persistent exposure to allergens and irritants, comorbidities, and incorrect diagnosis before stepping up treatment. If these problems are addressed, and the individual is still not adequately controlled, LABAs, long-acting muscarinic antagonists (LAMAs), or leukotriene antagonists can be added.[46] Leukotrienes are products of arachidonate metabolism (see Chapter 7) which contribute to airway hypersensitivity, bronchospasm, and inflammatory injury. Blockage of these cytokines can decrease airway inflammation and bronchospasm in selected individuals with asthma.[61] In adults with severe asthma that is unresponsive to treatment with these medications, the anti-inflammatory antibiotic azithromycin may be considered.[46] Biologic therapies with monoclonal antibodies to IgE, IL-5, and IL-13 (e.g., omalizumab, mepolizumab, reslizumab, and benralizumab) have been found to be helpful as adjunctive therapy to inhaled steroids, and many new biologics are being developed (Emerging Science Box: Biological Treatments for Uncontrolled Asthma). Immunotherapy (allergy shots) has been shown to be an important tool in reducing asthma exacerbations, reducing the need for both long and short-acting asthma medications, and improving quality of life and FEV_1. Immunotherapy also can be given sublingually, although current recommendations state that sublingual immunotherapy should not be substituted for subcutaneous immunotherapy in those individuals with persistent asthma despite treatment.[59] In individuals in whom long-term control of symptoms has been achieved, careful step down in medications may be attempted.

EMERGING SCIENCE BOX

Biological Treatments for Uncontrolled Asthma

Approximately 10% of individuals with asthma suffer from severe disease that remains poorly controlled despite appropriate use of bronchodilators and high-dose inhaled corticosteroids. Many of these individuals have large numbers of activated lymphocytes and eosinophils that release high levels of inflammatory cytokines resulting in persistent disease, resistance to treatment, and progressive remodeling of airways. Among the most important of these cytokines are interleukin (IL)-4, IL-5, and IL-13. Other injurious cytokines include IL-17, IL-25, IL-33, and thymic stromal lymphopoietin. The recognition of these pathophysiologic changes in uncontrolled severe asthma has led to the development of tailored therapies that target specific pathways of airway inflammation. The first biologic developed to treat uncontrolled asthma was omalizumab. It is a monoclonal antibody that prevents the binding of IgE to mast cells and basophils. More recently, the role of eosinophils in the pathophysiology of severe asthma and airway remodeling is being targeted using monoclonal antibodies that block IL-5. Three drugs targeting IL-5 currently are approved for use and include mepolizumab, reslizumab, and benralizumab. Dopilumab is a monoclonal antibody that blocks both the IL-4 and the IL-13 receptors and has recently been approved for home use. All five of these monoclonal antibody drugs have been shown to improve symptoms, decrease the number and severity of exacerbations, and reduce the use of systemic corticosteroids in selected individuals with severe asthma. Emerging therapies aimed at other inflammatory and immune cytokines are being explored. Examples include the potential use of monoclonal antibodies that block receptors for thymic stromal lymphopoietin (tezpelumab), leukotrienes, IL-25, and IL-33.

Data from Assaf SM, et al. Biological treatments for severe asthma. *Current Opinion in Allergy and Clinical Immunology,* 2019;19(4):379–386; Corren J. New targeted therapies for uncontrolled asthma. *Journal of Allergy and Clinical Immunology: In Practice,* 2019;7(5):1394–1403; Krings JG, et al. Biologics for severe asthma: treatment-specific effects are important in choosing a specific agent. *Journal of Allergy and Clinical Immunology: In Practice,* 2019;7(5):1379–1392; Jappe U, et al. Biologics for atopic diseases: Indication, side effect management, and new developments. *Allergol Select,* 2021;5:1–25; Peters MC, et al. Intersection of biology and therapeutics: Type 2 targeted therapeutics for adult asthma. *Lancet,* 2020;395(10221):371– 383; Struß N, et al. Biologics in asthma management—Are we out of breath yet? *Allergol Select,* 2021;5: 96–102; Wu AC, et al. Biologic therapy in allergy practice: A new era in treatment has begun. *Journal of Allergy and Clinical Immunology,* 2021;9(3):118–1120.

Chronic Obstructive Pulmonary Disease

Chronic obstructive pulmonary disease (COPD) is defined by the Global Initiative for Chronic Obstructive Lung Disease (GOLD) 2022 report as "…a common, preventable and treatable disease characterized by persistent respiratory symptoms and airflow limitation that is due to airway and/or alveolar abnormalities usually caused by significant exposure to noxious particles or gases and influenced by host factors including abnormal lung development.[62] COPD is the most common chronic lung disease in the world, and the sixth leading cause of death in the United States, affecting as many as 10% of individuals in states where cigarette smoking is prevalent.[63] Risk factors for COPD include tobacco smoke (cigarette, pipe, cigar, and environmental tobacco smoke), occupational dusts and chemicals (vapors, irritants, and fumes), indoor air pollution from biomass fuel used for cooking and heating (in poorly vented dwellings), outdoor air pollution, factors that affect lung growth during gestation, certain infections such as tuberculosis, low socioeconomic status, and genetic abnormalities.[62] Evidence is emerging that the use of e-cigarettes (vaping) leads to an increased risk for COPD

(Emerging Science Box: E-Cigarettes and Respiratory Disease).[64] Changes in the lung microbiome also have been linked to the development of COPD.[65] At least 22 gene polymorphisms, as well as epigenetic susceptibilities, have been identified in association with COPD.[66] An inherited homozygous mutation in the gene responsible for α_1-antitrypsin synthesis occurs in 1 in 2000 persons of European descent and results in the development of COPD at an early age, even in individuals who never smoked.[67]

The two most common phenotypes of COPD are chronic bronchitis and emphysema. Chronic bronchitis is defined as hypersecretion of mucus and chronic productive cough that continues for at least 3 months of the year (usually the winter months) for at least 2 consecutive years. Emphysema is abnormal permanent enlargement of gas-exchange airways (acini) accompanied by destruction of alveolar walls without obvious fibrosis. Both phenotypes are associated with an enhanced chronic inflammatory response in the airways to noxious particles or gases. Exacerbations and comorbidities contribute to the overall severity of disease. The asthma-COPD overlap (ACO) is a phenotype of chronic respiratory disease where there is an overlap of the clinical symptoms of asthma and COPD.[68]

Pathophysiology. The pathologic changes of COPD occur in large central airways, small peripheral airways, and the lung parenchyma. In both chronic bronchitis and emphysema, chronic irritant exposure recruits neutrophils, macrophages, and lymphocytes to the lung, resulting in progressive damage from inflammation, oxidative stress, extracellular matrix proteolysis, and apoptotic and autophagic cell death.[62,66] Frequent infectious exacerbations and lung senescence with aging contribute to the progression of disease.

In chronic bronchitis, inspired irritants result in airway inflammation with infiltration of neutrophils, macrophages, and lymphocytes into the bronchial wall. Continual bronchial inflammation causes bronchial edema, an increase in the size and number of mucous glands and goblet cells in the airway epithelium, smooth muscle hypertrophy with fibrosis, and narrowing of airways. Thick, tenacious mucus is produced and cannot be cleared because of impaired ciliary function (Fig. 35.8), compromising the lung's defense mechanisms. These pathophysiological changes increase susceptibility to pulmonary infection, which contributes to injury and ineffective repair. Frequent infectious exacerbations from bacterial colonization of damaged airways are complicated by bronchospasm with dyspnea and productive cough. Exacerbations contribute to the overall severity and progression of disease. This process initially affects only the larger bronchi, but eventually, all airways are involved. The thick mucus and hypertrophied bronchial smooth muscle constrict the airways and lead to obstruction, particularly during expiration when the airways are narrowed. This expiratory obstruction traps air in the distal portions of the lung (hyperinflation), which expands the thorax and positions the respiratory muscles at a mechanical disadvantage. This leads to decreased tidal volume, hypoventilation, and hypercapnia. Airway obstruction also leads to $\dot{V}/\dot{Q}$ mismatch with hypoxemia.

In emphysema, there is destruction of alveolar walls resulting in abnormal permanent enlargement of gas-exchange airways. Obstruction results from inflammatory and destructive changes in lung tissues rather than mucus production as in chronic bronchitis. It most often is the result of inhalation of toxic gases such as cigarette smoke. Emphysema is characterized by inflammation and an imbalance between proteases and antiproteases, oxidative stress, and apoptosis of lung structural cells. An autoimmune response is triggered by infiltration of lymphocytes and the release of toxic immune cytokines.[62] These processes lead to the destruction of alveoli through the breakdown of elastin within the septa (Algorithm. 35.5). Alveolar destruction produces large air spaces within the lung parenchyma (bullae) and air spaces adjacent to pleurae (blebs) (Fig. 35.9).

EMERGING SCIENCE BOX

E-Cigarettes and Respiratory Disease

Electronic cigarette (e-cigarette) use has increased in the 10 years since they were introduced, especially among adolescents and young adults for which e-cigarette use has increased by over 1500% to an estimated 10.5% of middle school students and 27.5% of high school students. E-cigarettes include any nicotine delivery products, commonly known as "vapes." Although some previous studies suggests that e-cigarettes are more effective than nicotine replacement therapy with respect to 1-year smoking abstinence rates, more recent data are less conclusive and they are not benign in their effects on lung tissue. The use of e-cigarettes, especially those with multiple ingredients, exposes users to high levels of inhaled cytotoxic toxins including propylene glycol and vegetable glycerin. E-cigarettes also emit aldehydes (such as formaldehyde), as well as aerosolized particles, diacetyl, and volatile organic compounds. Exposure to these toxins results in airway inflammation (macrophage and neutrophil activation and cytokine release), capillary dysfunction, and alveolar injury along with increased susceptibility to respiratory infections. E-cigarette use is linked to both acute and chronic respiratory disease. In December 2019, an outbreak of e-cigarette product use-associated lung injury (EVALI) resulted in over 2500 hospitalizations and 54 deaths. In addition, emerging data demonstrates up to a 75% increase in risk for COPD in individuals who use e-cigarettes, especially those who use them daily. Many e-cigarette users also use combustible tobacco products, especially among the adolescents and young adults. Combined use of both e-cigarettes and combustible tobacco products confers up to a 3-fold increase in risk for COPD and asthma. Continued research on the impact of e-cigarette use on the prevalence of lung disorders, such as COPD and cancer is needed.

Data from American Lung Association. Overall tobacco trends. Retrieved from lung.org on February 4, 2022; American Lung Association. The impact of e-cigarettes on the lung. Retrieved from lung.org on February 4, 2022; Bhatta DN, et al. Association of e-cigarettte use with respiratory disease among adults: A longitudinal analysis. *American Journal of Preventative Medicine*, 2020;58(3):182–190; Colesar MT, et al. E-Cigarette or vaping product use-associated lung injury (EVALI) in an active duty service member. *Military Medicine*, 2021;186(1–2):e250–e253; Gotts JE, et al. What are the respiratory effects of e-cigarettes? *British Medical Journal*, 2019;366:l5275; Hajek P, et al. A randomized trial of e-cigarettes versus nicotine-replacement therapy. *New England Journal of Medicine*, 2019;380:629–637; Layden JE, et al. Pulmonary illness related to e-cigarette use in Illinois and Wisconsin—Final Report. *New England Journal of Medicine*, 2020;382:903–916; Osei AD, et al. Association between e-cagerette use and chronic obstructive pulmonary disease by smoking status: Behavioral risk factor surveillance system 2016 and 2017. *American Journal of Preventative Medicine*, 2020;58(3):336–342; Werner AK, et al. Hospitalizations and deaths associated with EVALI. *New England Journal of Medicine*, 2020;382:1589–1598.

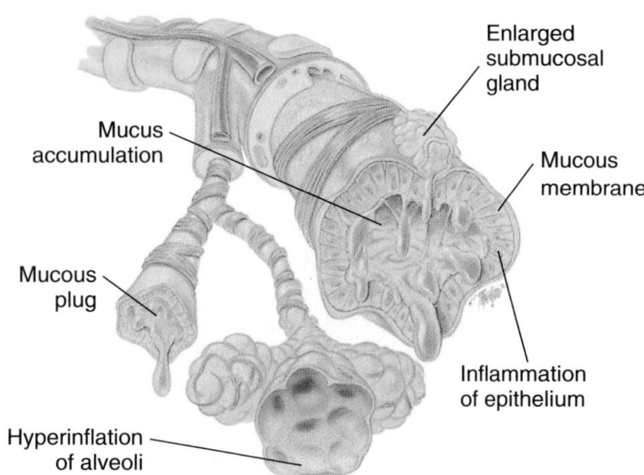

Fig. 35.8 Chronic Bronchitis. Inflammation and thickening of the mucous membrane, with accumulation of mucus and pus, leading to obstruction characterized by a productive cough. (Modified from Des Jardins T, Burton GG. *Clinical manifestations and assessment of respiratory disease*, 3rd edition. St. Louis: Mosby; 1995.)

Bullae and blebs are not effective in gas exchange and contribute to $\dot{V}/\dot{Q}$ mismatching and hypoxemia. The main mechanism of airflow limitation is loss of elastic recoil with collapse of the airways during expiration (Fig. 35.10). Air trapping causes hyperexpansion of the chest, placing the muscles of respiration at a mechanical disadvantage and increasing workload of breathing. This gradually progresses, leading to reduced tidal volumes so that many individuals will develop hypoventilation and hypercapnia. Persistent inflammation results in hyperreactivity of the bronchi causing bronchoconstriction. Acute bronchoconstriction may be partially reversible with bronchodilators. Continued destruction of alveolar walls and pulmonary capillaries causes pulmonary hypertension (PH) and *cor pulmonale* (see the Pulmonary Hypertension section). Approximately one-third of individuals with emphysema have significant eosinophilic inflammation, which contributes to airway injury and may predict lack of responsiveness to treatment.[66] Chronic inflammation also can have significant systemic effects. including weight loss, muscle weakness, and increased susceptibility to comorbidities.

Inherited α1-antitrypsin deficiency (primary emphysema) accounts for 1% to 3% of all cases of emphysema. Normally, α1-antitrypsin inhibits the action of proteolytic enzymes (e.g., elastases released by neutrophils) that serve to break down lung tissue. Without this inhibitory activity, neutrophils are recruited into the lung, protease activity is unopposed, and structural damage develops.[67] Deficiency of α1-antitrypsin is suggested in individuals who develop emphysema before 40 years of age and in individuals who never smoked but still develop the disease. Nonsmoking individuals with α1-antitrypsin deficiency develop COPD at an older age than those with the deficiency who also smoke. Hepatic fibrosis also may occur. Because there are emerging effective treatments, some experts now recommend that all individuals with diagnosed COPD be screened for alpha-1 antitrypsin deficiency. Family screening is indicated for those who test positive.[69] Supportive treatment for the lung disease associated with α1-antitrypsin deficiency is the same as treatment for COPD. Specific treatment with intravenous augmentation therapy using plasma-purified α1-antitrypsin slows disease progression.[69] New treatments, including gene therapy and stem cell technologies, are being explored.[70]

Clinical Manifestations. Dyspnea on exertion that progresses to marked dyspnea, even at rest, is the most common symptom of COPD.[71] In chronic bronchitis, individuals have a persistent productive cough, whereas in emphysema, cough is usually productive only during acute exacerbations. Table 35.3 provides a comparative list of the common clinical manifestations between chronic bronchitis and emphysema. The individual with COPD is often thin, has tachypnea with prolonged expiration, and must use accessory muscles for ventilation. The anteroposterior diameter of the chest is increased (barrel chest), and the chest has a hyperresonant sound with percussion. The individual often leans forward with arms extended and braced on knees when sitting and exhales through pursed lips (helps prevent expiratory airway collapse). As the disease progresses. marked hypoxemia leads to polycythemia (overproduction of erythrocytes) and cyanosis. If not reversed, respiratory failure leads to PH and eventually results in *cor pulmonale* with right heart failure and peripheral edema.

Evaluation and Treatment. Diagnosis of COPD is based on history of exposures, family history, respiratory symptoms, physical examination, chest imaging, and pulmonary function tests. Pulmonary function testing reveals airway obstruction (decreased FEV_1) that is progressive and unresponsive to bronchodilators. Chest x-ray may reveal changes in thoracic diameter, distended lung fields, and flattening of the diaphragm. High-resolution CT scanning provides detailed information about the underlying COPD phenotype which may help to guide management.[72] Oximetry should be obtained, and arterial blood gas analysis should be performed in those with significant hypoxemia. Hypoxemia may first occur with exercise but gradually progresses to hypoxemia at rest. Hypercapnia develops as air trapping worsens and the work of breathing increases. Serum eosinophil counts should also be obtained.

Prevention of COPD is the best treatment because pathologic changes are not reversible. By the time an individual seeks medical care for symptoms, considerable airway damage is present. If the individual stops smoking and receives optimal pharmacotherapy, disease progression can be slowed. Influenza, COVID-19, and pneumococcal vaccination should be kept up to date. Pharmacologic management is based on clinical severity as described by the GOLD classification for COPD (mild, moderate, severe, or very severe).[62] Initial treatment most often begins with a LAMA (e.g., tiotropium or revefenacin).[72] Additional medications that can be considered include LABA and inhaled glucocorticoids, and combinations of these may be beneficial for severe COPD (triple combination).[62] Inhaled corticosteroids are associated with an increased risk of pneumonia and should not be used alone. The addition of a phosphodiesterase E4 (PDE4) inhibitor (e.g., roflumilast) and a macrolide antibiotic (azithromycin) can be considered for those with moderate to severe COPD.[62]

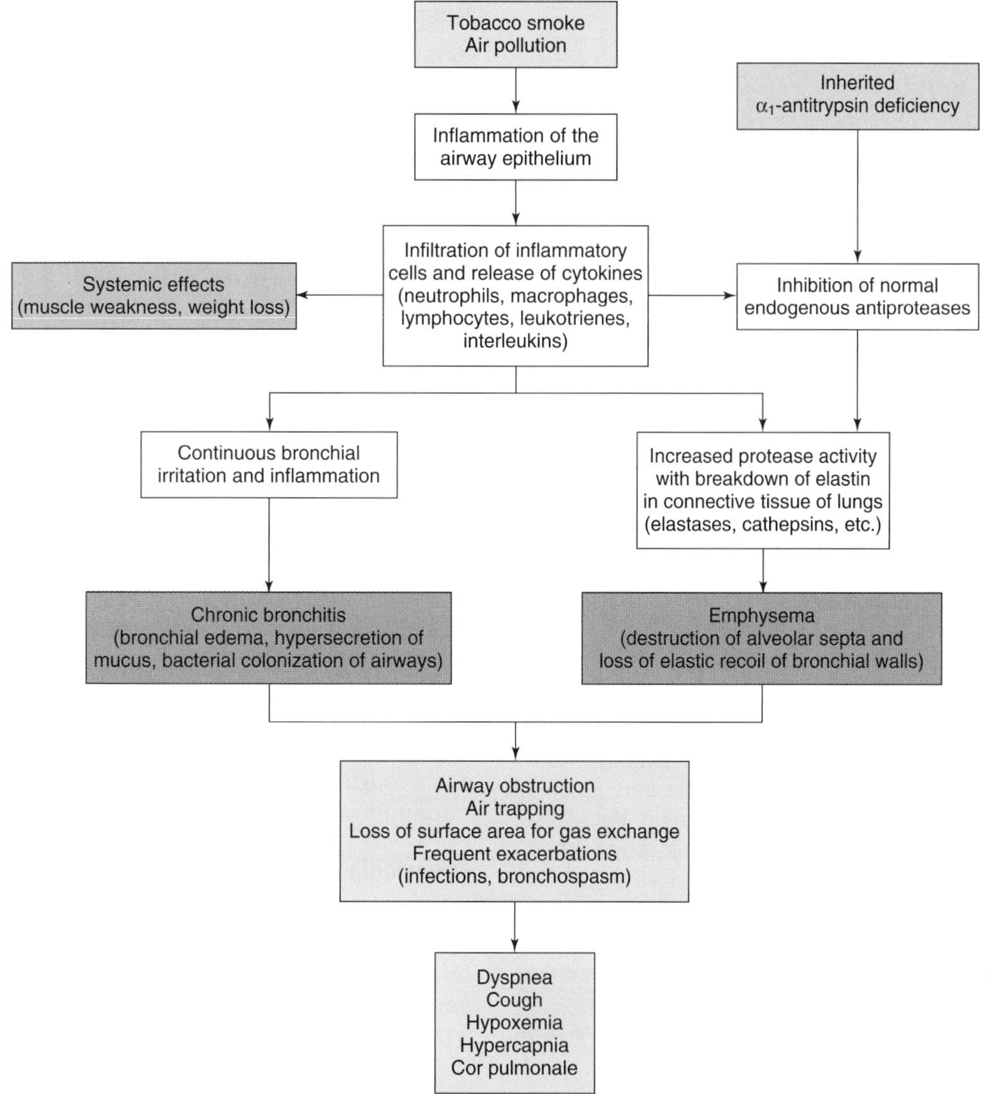

Algorithm 35.5 Pathogenesis of Chronic Bronchitis and Emphysema (Chronic Obstructive Pulmonary Disease).

Acute exacerbations of COPD are characterized by an increased dyspnea, cough, or sputum purulence. They most often are caused by bacterial or viral infection but may also occur due to changes in air quality or medication use. These exacerbations may be life-threatening and contribute to overall disease progression. Therapy includes bronchodilators (often given via nebulizer), systemic corticosteroids, and antibiotics.[72] If respiratory failure develops, high-flow nasal cannula or noninvasive ventilation are indicated.[73]

Pulmonary rehabilitation improves symptoms and quality of life in individuals with moderate to severe COPD, and efforts at creating effective programs using telehealth modalities are being developed.[62,74] Progressive pulmonary dysfunction with hypoxemia and hypercapnia may require long-term oxygen therapy and ventilation. Oxygen is titrated with care to individuals with severe hypoxemia and CO2 retention. Lung volume reduction surgery improves symptoms in selected individuals with severe COPD but is associated with significant postoperative

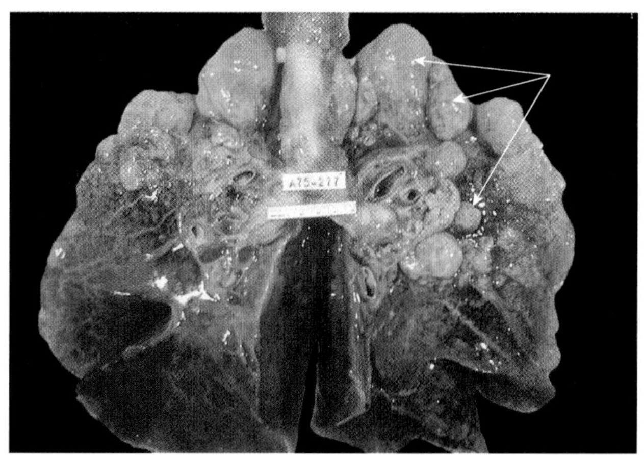

Fig. 35.9 Bullous emphysema with large apical and subpleural bullae (arrows). (From Kumar V, et al., eds. *Robbins basic pathology*, 8th edition. Philadelphia: Saunders/Elsevier; 2007.)

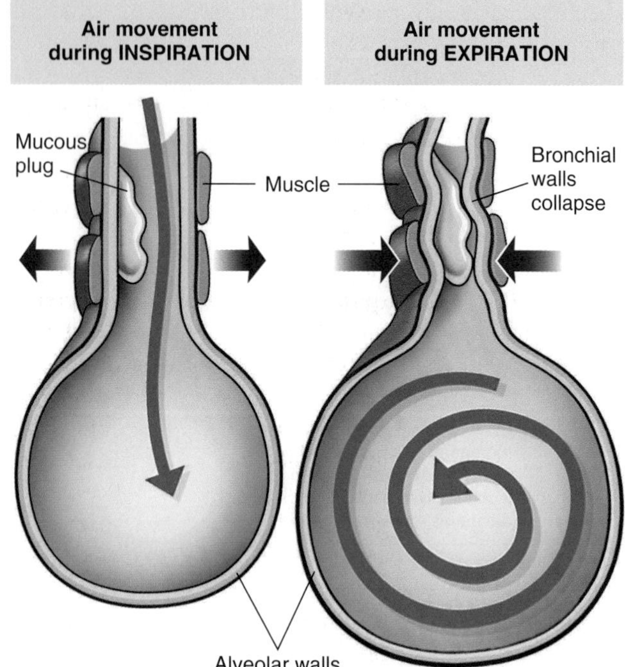

Fig. 35.10 Mechanisms of Air Trapping in Chronic Obstructive Pulmonary Disease. Mucous plugs and narrowed airways cause air trapping and hyperinflation of alveoli on expiration. During inspiration, the airways are pulled open, allowing gas to flow past the obstruction. During expiration, decreased elastic recoil of the bronchial walls results in collapse of the airways and prevents normal expiratory airflow.

TABLE 35.3 Clinical Manifestations of Chronic Obstructive Lung Disease

Clinical Manifestations	Bronchitis	Emphysema
Productive cough	Classic sign	With infection
Dyspnea	Late in course	Common
Wheezing	Intermittent	Common
History of smoking	Common	Common
Barrel chest	Occasionally	Classic
Prolonged expiration	Always present	Always present
Cyanosis	Common	Uncommon
Chronic hypoventilation	Common	Late in course
Polycythemia	Common	Late in course
Cor pulmonale	Common	Late in course

complications and new safer bronchoscopic techniques are emerging.[75] Lung transplantation can be considered, especially in younger individuals with inherited α1-antitrypsin deficiency. In addition, many comorbidities, such as bronchiectasis, cardiovascular disorders, metabolic diseases, bone disease, stroke, lung cancer, cachexia and muscle weakness, anemia, depression, and cognitive decline accompany COPD and require monitoring and therapy.

Respiratory Tract Infections

Respiratory tract infections are the most common cause of short-term disability in the United States. Most of these infections—the common cold, pharyngitis, and laryngitis—involve only the upper airways and are not discussed in this chapter. Infections of the lower respiratory tract occur most often in the very young and very old, smokers, or those with impaired immunity. However, viral pneumonias can occur in healthy individuals of any age.

Acute Bronchitis

Acute bronchitis is an acute infection or inflammation of the airways or bronchi and is usually self-limiting. Most cases of acute bronchitis are caused by viruses. Many of the clinical manifestations are similar to those of pneumonia (i.e., fever, cough, chills, malaise), but the physical examination does not reveal signs of pulmonary consolidation (i.e., dullness to percussion, crackles, egophony), and chest radiographs do not show infiltrates. Individuals with viral bronchitis usually have a nonproductive cough that occurs in paroxysms and is aggravated by cold, dry, or dusty air. Purulent sputum may be produced in bacterial bronchitis. Chest pain often develops from the effort of coughing. Treatment consists of rest, hydration, humidity, analgesics, and a cough suppressant, such as codeine. Antibiotics are indicated for bacterial bronchitis.

Pneumonia

Pneumonia is an infection of the lower respiratory tract caused by bacteria, viruses, fungi, protozoa, or parasites. It is estimated that lower respiratory tract infections affected nearly 500 million people and resulted in 1.23 million deaths globally in 2019.[76] Pneumonia accounts for over 45,000 deaths per year in the United States.[77]

Pneumonia can be categorized as community-acquired (CAP) or hospital-acquired (HAP).[76] CAP is defined as pneumonia that is acquired outside of the hospital setting. It is one of the most common reasons for hospitalization in the United States. Risk factors for pneumonia include age below 5 or above 70 years, compromised immunity, underlying lung disease, alcoholism, altered consciousness, impaired swallowing, smoking, malnutrition, immobilization, underlying cardiac or liver disease, and residence in a nursing home or other extended care facility. Other risk factors include the use of gastric acid suppressive agents or benzodiazepines.[78]

HAP denotes an episode of pneumonia that develops during hospitalization. It is the second most common nosocomial infection (urinary tract infection [UTI] is the most common) and has the greatest mortality. Ventilator-associated pneumonia (VAP) is a subset of HAP and is a nosocomial infection that occurs in many individuals who require intubation and mechanical ventilation. VAP affects nearly a third of all individuals in ICUs and has a higher mortality than HAP in nonventilated individuals. Risk factors for HAP include oropharyngeal colonization with resistant pathogens, presence of an endotracheal tube (intubation), impaired swallowing and cough reflex, and decreased level of consciousness.[76]

The causative microorganisms for pneumonia influence the clinical presentation of the individual, the treatment plan, and the prognosis. The mechanisms of viral and bacterial infection are reviewed in Chapter 10. The microorganisms that commonly cause CAP have changed in the past decade due to increasing numbers of individuals in the community who are immunocompromised, live in chronic care institutions, or have chronic underlying conditions. Viruses are now believed to be the most common cause of CAP. The most common cause of viral CAP is influenza, which occurs most often during the winter season. While usually a mild and self-limiting infection, influenza causes over 50,000 deaths annually in the United States.[79] Respiratory syncytial virus is another common cause of CAP. Pneumonias caused by Epstein Barr virus, herpes simplex virus, and cytomegalovirus primarily occur in immunocompromised individuals such as those with human immunodeficiency virus (HIV) infection (see Chapter 10). Viral pneumonia also can be a complication of another viral illness, such as chickenpox or measles (spread to the lungs from the blood). New or atypical forms of viral infection such as COVID-19 have affected previously healthy populations and pose a considerable threat for pandemics (see Chapter 10, Emerging Science Box: Severe Acute Respiratory Syndrome Coronavirus -2 and Coronavirus Disease 2019). The most common cause of bacterial CAP is *Streptococcus pneumoniae*, also known as the pneumococcus. Other common etiologic bacteria include *Legionella pneumophila, Moraxella catarrhalis*, and *Hemophilus influenzae*.[76] Atypical microorganisms such as *Chlamydophila pneumoniae* and *Mycoplasma pneumoniae* also cause CAP. Fungi are a less common cause of CAP except in the case of severe immunocompromise like that seen in individuals with HIV infection when *Pneumocystis jirovecii, Aspergillus*, and *Cryptococcus* infections may occur.[80] Unfortunately, there is increasing incidences of CAP caused by antibiotic-resistant organisms such as methicillin-resistant *S. aureus* (MRSA), *P. aeruginosa*, and *Enterobacteriaceae*.[81] The most common etiologic microorganisms in HAP are *S. aureus* and MRSA, *Enterobacteriaceae, P. aeruginosa, Acinetobacter* species, *K. pneumoniae*, and *Enterococcus coli*.[76,82] These microorganisms also cause pneumonia in individuals who recently have been discharged from the hospital or who live in long-term care facilities.

Pathophysiology. Viruses can enter the lower respiratory tract through direct inoculation or inhalation, spread from viral infections near the upper respiratory tract, or hematogenously. They target the airway and alveolar epithelial cells, especially pneumocytes. For example, in influenza, viral hemagglutinin (HA) binds to sialic acid residues expressed on epithelial cells, leading to viral entry into these cells.[83] Viral replication ensues, along with activation of both innate and adaptive immune responses. In severe viral pneumonias that can occur with influenza and COVID-19, a cytokine storm ensues which causes epithelial and endothelial damage, hypercoagulability, and increased vascular permeability leading to alveolar edema and ARDS (see Emerging Science Box: The Pathogenesis of the Acute Respiratory Distress Syndrome (ARDS) in COVID-19). Influenza and other respiratory viruses can set the stage for a secondary bacterial infection by damaging ciliated epithelial cells, which normally prevent pathogens from reaching the lower airways. Sloughing of destroyed bronchial ciliated epithelium occurs throughout the respiratory tract, preventing mucociliary clearance. Viral pneumonia is usually self-limiting and alveolar regeneration results in complete resolution of lung injury. However, bronchiectasis, irreversible atelectasis, long-term morbidity, and mortality occur in some individuals, especially the very young and very old.

In bacterial pneumonia, colonization of the upper respiratory tract followed by aspiration of oropharyngeal secretions is the most common route of lower respiratory tract infection.[76] Another route of infection is through the inhalation of certain microorganisms (e.g., *M. pneumoniae, C. pneumoniae, Legionella pneumoniae*) that have been released into the air when an infected individual coughs, sneezes, or talks, or from aerosolized water, such as that from contaminated respiratory therapy equipment. The pathogens then adhere to the upper airway epithelium where they escape from mucociliary clearance and evade host clearance through expression of host-mimicking or antigenically varying molecules.[76] They then enter the lower airways through inhalation. In VAP, bacteria form biofilms on the endotracheal tube, allowing bacteria to bypass protective mechanisms and directly invade the lung. Bacterial pneumonia also can occur when pathogens are spread to the lung hematogenously from infection elsewhere in the body or from intravenous (IV) drug use.

The most important guardian cell of the lower respiratory tract is the alveolar macrophage, which recognizes pathogens through its pattern-recognition receptors (e.g., Toll-like receptors) and phagocytoses them (see Chapters 7 and 8). Some bacteria (e.g., pneumococci) have capsules that make phagocytosis by alveolar macrophages more difficult, and opsonization with complement and antibodies is required (see Chapter 7). Macrophages present infectious antigens to the adaptive immune system, activating T cells and B cells with the induction of both cellular and humoral immunity (see Chapters 8). The release of TNF-α and interleukin-1 (IL-1) from macrophages, along with chemokines and chemotactic factors from mast cells and fibroblasts contributes to widespread inflammation and the recruitment of neutrophils from the capillaries into the alveoli. Neutrophils release neutrophil extracellular traps (NETs), which are essential to removing the invading microorganism but cause bystander damage to host lung tissue.[84] Adaptive immune activation leads to the production of antibodies and immune cytokines that activate lymphocytes. IL-17 and IL-22 activate epithelial cells to secrete antimicrobial proteins and stimulate epithelial repair mechanisms.[76] Inflammatory mediators, immune complexes, and toxins damage bronchial mucous membranes and alveolocapillary membranes, causing the alveoli and terminal bronchioles to fill with infectious debris and exudate causing $\dot{V}/\dot{Q}$ mismatching and hypoxemia. Some microorganisms cause further damage to lung tissue through the release of toxins. For example, pneumococci release pneumolysin, which is a pore-forming toxin that damages airway and alveolar cells and induces inflammatory cytokine release.[76] *Staphylococcus aeruginosa* organisms release alpha-hemolysin which damages epithelial cells.[85] The pathogenesis of bacterial pneumonia is outlined in Algorithm 35.6.

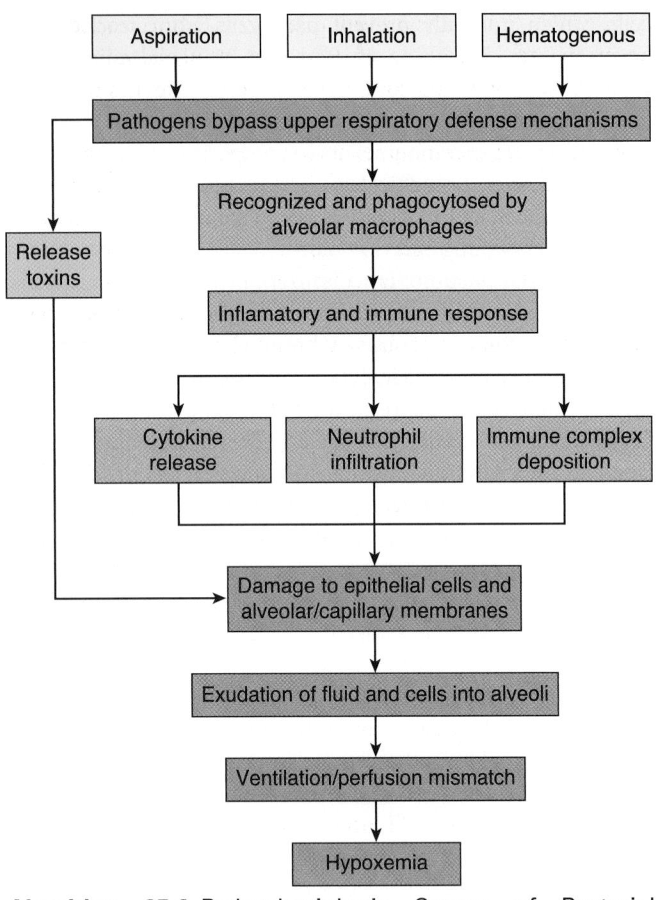

Algorithm 35.6 Pathophysiologic Course of Bacterial Pneumonia.

Clinical Manifestations. Most cases of pneumonia are preceded by a viral upper respiratory tract infection. Individuals then develop fever, chills, a cough (productive or dry), malaise, pleural pain, and sometimes dyspnea and hemoptysis. The physical examination may show signs of pulmonary consolidation, such as dullness to percussion, inspiratory crackles, increased tactile fremitus (palpable chest vibrations when a person speaks), and egophony ("E" to "A" change). A pleural effusion may develop. Individuals also may demonstrate symptoms and signs of underlying systemic disease or sepsis. Pneumonia may contribute to decreased left ventricular function, arrhythmias, ischemia, and infarction (see Chapter 32). Individuals hospitalized for pneumonia have an increased risk for cardiovascular disease whose symptoms may be erroneously attributed to pneumonia persistence or recurrence.

Evaluation and Treatment. The initial diagnosis of pneumonia is made based on the history of exposures and symptoms, followed by a careful physical examination (tachypnea, tachycardia, crackles, bronchial breath sounds, findings of pleural effusion). The white blood cell count is usually elevated, although it may be low if the individual is immunocompromised or has significant comorbidities. Chest radiographs show infiltrates that may involve a single lobe of the lung or may be more diffuse. No further evaluation is indicated for outpatients with mild to moderate CAP.[76] In the case of severe CAP requiring hospitalization, in those suspected of having MRSA or *P. aeruginosa*, or in HAP, the pathogen is identified by means of sputum characteristics (Gram stain and culture).[86] If sputum studies fail to identify the pathogen, further diagnostic studies may include blood cultures, thoracentesis, bronchoscopy, or lung biopsy. Serum procalcitonin can be used to assess severity of disease but should not be used to guide initial antibiotic therapy.[86] Urine and serum antigen rapid testing for pneumococcus or *Legionella* may be obtained for selected individuals.

Prevention of pneumonia includes avoidance of aspiration, respiratory isolation of infected individuals, and vaccination. Measures to prevent VAP include head of bed elevation, oral hygiene, hand hygiene, and the use of specialized endotracheal tubes.[87]

The first step in the management of pneumonia is establishing adequate ventilation and oxygenation. Hydration and good pulmonary hygiene (e.g., deep breathing, coughing, chest physical therapy) also are important. Viral pneumonia is treated with supportive therapy. Antivirals are indicated for hospitalized individuals.[86] Antibiotics should be given promptly for bacterial pneumonia. Empiric treatment with macrolide antibiotics is recommended for outpatients with CAP who are not suspected of having resistant infections. In severe CAP, HAP, and VAP, broad-spectrum antibiotics that cover resistant organisms are recommended.[86] New antibiotics with improved outcomes in resistant infections are being developed.[88] Opportunistic infections in immunocompromised individuals may be the result of several different microorganisms and often require multiple drugs, including antifungals.

Tuberculosis

Tuberculosis (TB) is an infection caused by *Mycobacterium tuberculosis*, a bacillus that usually affects the lungs but may invade other body systems. TB affects an estimated 10 million people worldwide, resulting in 1.6 million deaths and is the leading cause of death in the world from a curable infectious disease.[89] TB cases increased greatly during the mid-1990s because of AIDS, but both have decreased since 2000. Unfortunately, emerging multidrug-resistant strains are becoming more common. Emigration of infected individuals from high-prevalence countries, transmission in crowded institutional settings, homelessness, substance abuse, and lack of access to screening and medical care have contributed to the spread of TB.

Pathophysiology. TB is highly contagious and is transmitted from person to person in airborne droplets. In immunocompetent individuals, the *M. tuberculosis* is usually contained by the person's inflammatory and immune response systems. This results in latent TB infection (LTBI) and is associated with no clinical evidence of disease. Once the bacilli are inspired, they lodge in the lung, usually in the upper lobe, and cause localized nonspecific inflammation to the lung tissue. Some bacilli migrate through the lymphatics and become lodged in the lymph nodes, initiating an immune response. Alveolar macrophages and neutrophils engulf and isolate the bacilli, preventing them from spreading.[90] However, the bacterium can evade the person's defense mechanism within macrophages and resist lysosomal killing, forming a granulomatous lesion called a *tubercle* (see Chapter 7). Infected tissues within the tubercle die, forming cheeselike material called *caseation necrosis*. Collagenous scar tissue then grows around the tubercle, completing the isolation of bacilli. The immune response is complete after about 10 days, preventing further multiplication of bacilli.

Once bacilli are isolated in tubercles, tuberculosis may remain latent (LTBI) for life. If the immune system is impaired, reactivation with progressive disease can occur and may spread throughout the lung and through the blood and lymphatics to other organs, causing active pneumonia and extrapulmonary disease. Cancer, immunosuppressive medications (e.g., corticosteroids), poor nutritional status, renal failure, and HIV can reactivate the disease.

Clinical Manifestations. LTBI is asymptomatic. Symptoms of active disease often develop gradually and are not diagnosed until the disease has advanced. Common clinical manifestations include night sweats, fatigue, weight loss, lethargy, anorexia (loss of appetite), and a low-grade fever that usually occurs in the afternoon. A cough that produces purulent sputum develops slowly and becomes more frequent over several weeks or months. Dyspnea, chest pain, and hemoptysis may occur as the disease progresses. Extrapulmonary TB disease is common in HIV-infected individuals and may cause neurologic deficits, meningitis symptoms, bone pain, and urinary symptoms.

Evaluation and Treatment. Screening for tuberculosis is usually conducted using the tuberculin skin test (TST; purified protein derivative [PPD]). A positive PPD is not sensitive nor specific for TB infection. For example, a person who previously received a bacilli Calmette-Guérin (BCG) vaccine can have a false positive TB skin test, while immunocompromised individuals may be unable to react to the protein and therefore have a false negative test. High-risk individuals instead should be screened with the interferon-gamma release assay (IGRA). The diagnosis is confirmed through sputum stain and culture and chest radiographs. However, a positive result from a sputum culture can take up to 6 weeks.

Currently, the only tuberculosis vaccine licensed for use globally is BCG, although new advances in TB vaccine development are encouraging.[91] Prevention of reactivation of LTBI through the use of antituberculous medications is recommended for at-risk individuals, such as those with HIV and those initiating immunosuppressive therapy for other conditions.[92] Individuals with active TB must be kept in respiratory isolation until their sputum is negative for bacilli. In drug-susceptible TB, four antibiotics are given together for the first two months of treatment, followed by an additional four months of a two-drug combination.[93] Monitoring for adherence is important to prevent the development of resistant strains. Assessing individuals for toxicities and drug-to-drugs interactions is essential. Multidrug-resistant TB requires genotypic and phenotypic drug susceptibility testing, and new drugs are emerging that can improve treatment outcomes.[94,95]

Abscess Formation and Cavitation

An abscess (liquefactive necrosis) is a circumscribed area of suppuration and destruction of lung parenchyma. Abscesses often occur because of aspiration associated with alcohol abuse, seizure disorders, general anesthesia, and swallowing disorders. Abscess formation follows consolidation of lung tissue, in which inflammation causes alveoli to fill with fluid, pus, and microorganisms. Necrosis of consolidated tissue may lead to cavitation in which the abscess empties into a bronchus, forming a cavity. Abscess communication with a bronchus causes production of copious amounts of malodorous sputum and occasionally hemoptysis. Other clinical manifestations include fever, cough, chills, and pleural pain. The diagnosis is made by chest radiography and sputum analysis. Treatment includes appropriate antibiotics and chest physical therapy. Bronchoscopy may be needed to drain the abscess.

Pulmonary Vascular Disease

Blood flow through the lungs can be disrupted by disorders that occlude the vessels, increase pulmonary vascular resistance, or destroy the vascular bed. The consequences of altered pulmonary blood flow can result in severe and life-threatening changes in $\dot{V}/\dot{Q}$. Significant disorders include PE, PH, and cor pulmonale.

Pulmonary Embolism

Pulmonary embolism (PE) is occlusion of a portion of the pulmonary vasculature by an embolus. An estimated 900,000 people in the United States develop deep venous thrombosis (DVT)/PE, and sudden death is the first symptom in 25% of people who have a PE.[96] PE most commonly results from embolization of a clot from DVT involving the lower leg (see Chapter 32); this form of PE is often called venous thromboembolism (VTE). Other, less common types of emboli include tissue fragments, lipids, a foreign body, an air bubble, or amniotic fluid.

Risk factors for VTE include conditions and disorders that promote blood clotting because of venous stasis (immobilization, heart failure), injuries to the endothelial cells that line the vessels (trauma, infection, caustic IV infusions), and hypercoagulability (inherited coagulation disorders, malignancy, hormone replacement therapy, pregnancy, oral contraceptives). Increased risk for thrombosis associated with hemodynamic stasis, hypercoagulability, and endothelial injury is known as *triad of Virchow* (see Chapter 32). Individuals with cancer are at particular risk for VTE due to stasis of blood flow due to pressure of tumor on vessels, thrombogenic medications, chronic inflammation, and procoagulant molecules secreted by some cancer cells.[97] COVID-19 also is associated with a significantly increased risk for VTE.[98] Approximately 5% to 8% of the U.S. population has an inherited thrombophilia.[96] Inherited coagulation disorders include factor V Leiden mutation, prothrombin gene mutations, and deficiencies of antithrombin II, protein S, and protein C. It is now well recognized that systemic or localized bacterial and viral infections markedly increase the risk of both arterial thromboemboli and VTE in both inpatients and outpatients. For example, the incidence of VTE in individuals hospitalized for COVID-19 is estimated at 15% to 18% and arterial thromboemboli (acute coronary syndrome, stroke and other arterial emboli) at 4%.[99]

Pathophysiology. The effect of the embolus depends on the extent of pulmonary blood flow obstruction, the size of the affected vessels, and the nature of the embolus. As a result of the thrombus lodging in the pulmonary circulation, there is a release both of neurohumoral substances, such as serotonin, histamine, catecholamines, and angiotensin II, and of inflammatory mediators, such as endothelin, leukotrienes, thromboxanes, and toxic oxygen-free radicals. This causes widespread vasoconstriction that further impedes blood flow to the lung. Small pulmonary emboli typically cause $\dot{V}/\dot{Q}$ mismatch and associated hypoxemia without damaging the lung itself. More significant obstruction of the pulmonary vasculature leads to pulmonary artery vasoconstriction, PH, and an increased workload for the right ventricle (RV). Large emboli can cause pulmonary infarction, dysrhythmias, decreased cardiac output, shock, and death. If the embolus does not cause infarction, the clot is dissolved by the fibrinolytic system, and pulmonary function returns to normal. If pulmonary infarction occurs, shrinking and scarring develop in the affected area of the lung. The pathogenesis of PE caused by DVT is summarized in Algorithm 35.7.

Clinical Manifestations. In most cases, the clinical manifestations of PE are nonspecific and may be confused with many other pulmonary or cardiac conditions. Although most emboli originate from clots in the lower extremities, DVT is often asymptomatic, and clinical examination may not indicate the presence of clot. Therefore, evaluation of risk factors and predisposing factors is an important aspect of diagnosis.

The classic clinical presentation of PE is the sudden onset of pleuritic chest pain, dyspnea, tachypnea, tachycardia, and unexplained anxiety. Occasionally syncope or hemoptysis occurs. With large emboli, a pleural friction rub, pleural effusion, fever, and leukocytosis may be noted. Recurrent small emboli may not be detected until progressive incapacitation, precordial pain, anxiety, dyspnea, and right ventricular enlargement are exhibited. Massive occlusion causes severe PH and shock.

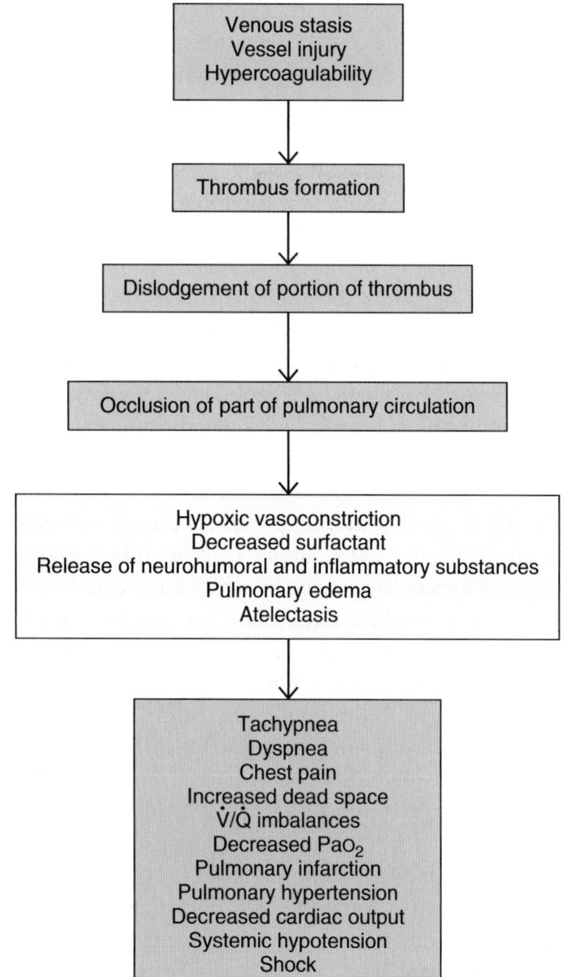

Algorithm 35.7 Pathogenesis of Pulmonary Embolism Caused by a Thrombus (Venous Thromboembolism). *PaO_2*, Arterial oxygen pressure; $\dot{V}/\dot{Q}$, ventilation-perfusion.

Evaluation and Treatment. The diagnosis of PE is made by assessing the clinical probability followed by measuring D-dimer levels in the blood (a product of thrombus degradation). Although these clinical predictive models are not completely accurate, in general if clinical probability is low and D-dimer levels are normal, the diagnosis of PE is excluded. If clinical probability is high or D-dimer is elevated, CT arteriography or magnetic resonance arteriography (MRA) is used to confirm the diagnosis.[100,101] Arterial blood gas analysis usually demonstrates hypoxemia and respiratory alkalosis. Measurement of the levels of BNP and troponin is useful in evaluating PE associated with right ventricular dysfunction. Testing for inherited hypercoagulability is recommended in those with unprovoked or recurrent DVT.

Prevention of PE includes elimination of predisposing factors for individuals at risk. Venous stasis in hospitalized persons is minimized by leg elevation, bed exercises, position changes, early postoperative ambulation, and pneumatic calf compression. Clot formation is also prevented by prophylactic anticoagulant therapy, most often with direct oral anticoagulant medications (DOACs; e.g., apixaban, dabigatran, rivaroxaban).[102]

Anticoagulant therapy is the primary treatment for PE. DOACs are now the treatment of choice for most individuals with stable oxygenation and hemodynamics who can be treated as outpatients.[100,103,104] Acute PE with significant symptoms and hypoxemia requires hospitalization and supportive care. Initial anticoagulant therapy usually includes factor Xa inhibitors (e.g., fondaparinux) or low-molecular-weight heparins (e.g., enoxaparin). The risk of recurrent VTE is high, especially in individuals with persistent risk factors. Therefore, long-term treatment with DOACs usually is indicated after discharge from the hospital. If the PE is associated with hemodynamic instability, an intravenous fibrinolytic agent, such as streptokinase, is indicated, and some individuals will require catheter-directed therapies or surgical thrombectomy.[103,105] In individuals who have contraindications to anticoagulation therapy, the placement of a filter in the inferior vena cava can prevent emboli from reaching the lungs. In some cases, these filters can be used during high-risk situations such as acute trauma, with retrieval after recovery.[106]

Pulmonary Hypertension

Pulmonary hypertension (PH) is defined as a mean pulmonary artery pressure greater than 25 mm Hg at rest (normal is 15 to 18 mm Hg). PH is classified by the WHO into five groups and multiple subgroups based on the cause. One major category of PH is termed pulmonary artery hypertension (PAH) and includes subcategories of idiopathic, heritable, drug and toxin-induced, and disorders associated with PAH (e.g., connective tissue disease). The other major categories of PH include PH caused by left-sided heart disease, PH caused by lung diseases and/or hypoxia, chronic thromboembolic PH, and PH with unclear multifactorial mechanisms (e.g., tumors, metabolic disorders, chronic renal failure). Left heart disease is the most common cause of PH, and COPD and interstitial fibrosis are the most common lung diseases associated with PH.

Pathophysiology. PAH is characterized by endothelial dysfunction with overproduction of vasoconstrictors, such as thromboxane and endothelin, and decreased production of vasodilators, such as prostacyclin and nitric oxide. Inflammation with infiltration of macrophages, neutrophils and lymphocytes, and the release of enzymes and vascular growth factors lead to fibrosis and vascular *remodeling* with permanent arteriolar narrowing and superimposed abnormal vasoconstriction.[107] Vasoconstriction causes resistance to pulmonary artery blood flow, thus increasing the pressure in the pulmonary arteries and RV. As resistance and pressure increase, the workload of the RV increases with subsequent right ventricular hypertrophy. Right heart failure may occur. PH from left heart disease is caused by increased filling pressures into the left heart (see Chapter 32). In PH caused by lung disease, damage to the lung parenchyma combined with hypoxic pulmonary vasoconstriction leads to increased pressures in the right heart and *cor pulmonale.* The pathogenesis of PH resulting from disease of the respiratory system is shown in Algorithm 35.8.

Clinical Manifestations. Symptoms of PH may not develop until late in the disease process. Manifestations of fatigue, chest discomfort, tachypnea, and dyspnea (particularly with exercise) are common. The physical examination may reveal peripheral edema, jugular venous distention, a precordial heave, and accentuation of the pulmonary component of the second heart sound.

Evaluation and Treatment. The first indication of PH may be an abnormality seen on a chest radiograph (enlarged right heart) or an electrocardiogram that shows right ventricular hypertrophy. Identification of underlying cardiac or pulmonary conditions is essential. Common diagnostic modalities used to determine the cause include a chest x-ray, echocardiography, and CT.

General therapies for PAH include administration of oxygen, diuretics, and anticoagulants; and avoidance of contributing factors, such as air travel, decongestants, nonsteroidal anti-inflammatories, pregnancy, and tobacco use. Pharmacologic interventions for PAH may include vasodilators such as calcium channel blockers, prostacyclin and its analogs, inhaled nitric oxide, endothelin receptor antagonists, phosphodiesterase-5 inhibitors, and soluble guanylate cyclase activators.[108] Selexipag, an oral, long-acting agonist of the prostacyclin receptor (IP receptor), recently has been shown to reduce morbidity and mortality in adults with PAH.[109] None of these drugs are curative, but they may improve morbidity and mortality. Individuals who do not achieve adequate clinical remission may require lung transplantation. Stem cell therapies are being explored.[110]

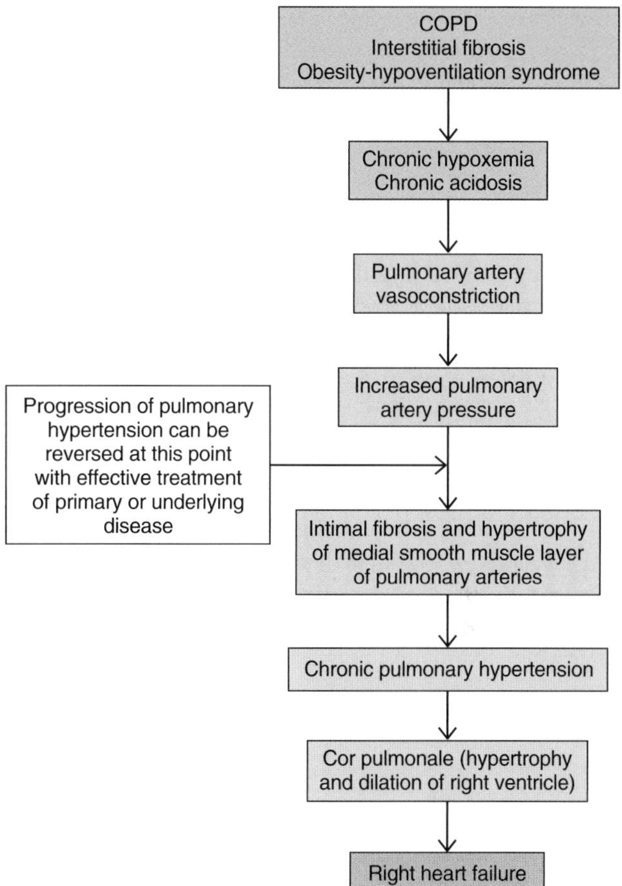

Algorithm 35.8 Pathogenesis of Pulmonary Hypertension and *Cor Pulmonale* Resulting from Respiratory Disease. *COPD,* Chronic obstructive pulmonary disease.

The most effective treatments for PH associated with cardiac and pulmonary disorders are supplemental oxygen and treatment of the underlying disease.

Cor Pulmonale

Cor pulmonale is right ventricular enlargement (hypertrophy, dilation, or both) due to pulmonary disorders that cause PH.

Pathophysiology. Chronic pulmonary disease associated with hypoxemia and hypercapnia cause pulmonary vasoconstriction and increased pressures in the pulmonary system. Cor pulmonale develops as PH exerts chronic pressure overload in the RV (see Algorithm 35.8). Pressure overload increases the work of the RV, resulting in hypertrophy of the normally thin-walled heart muscle. RV compliance decreases causing increasing pressures in the LV that are reflected to the RA and systemic venous circulation. This eventually progresses to dilation and failure of the ventricle.

Clinical Manifestations. The clinical manifestations of cor pulmonale may be obscured by underlying respiratory or cardiac disease and may appear only during exercise testing. The heart may appear normal at rest, but with exercise, cardiac output decreases due to decreased diastolic filling time for the RV. The electrocardiogram may show right ventricular hypertrophy. The pulmonary component of the second heart sound (i.e., closure of the pulmonic valve) may be accentuated, and a pulmonic valve murmur may be present. A tricuspid valve murmur may accompany the development of RV failure. Increased pressures in the systemic venous circulation cause jugular venous distention, hepatosplenomegaly, and peripheral edema.

Evaluation and Treatment. The diagnosis is based on the physical examination, thoracic imaging, and electrocardiography or echocardiography, or both. The treatment goal for cor pulmonale is to decrease the workload of the RV by lowering the pulmonary artery pressure. Treatment is the same as that for PH, and its success depends on reversal of the underlying lung disease.

Malignancies of the Respiratory Tract

Laryngeal Cancer

Cancer of the larynx (laryngeal cancer) represents less than 1% of all cancers in the United States. In 2021 it is estimated that there were 12,620 new cases and 3770 deaths due to laryngeal cancer, with a 5-year survival rate of 60.7%.[111] Laryngeal cancer is much more common in men than women, and the primary risk factor is tobacco smoking. The risk is heightened by the combination of smoking and alcohol consumption. The human papillomavirus (HPV types 6 and 11) also has been linked to both benign and malignant tumors of the larynx. There is evidence that GERD may also increase the risk for laryngeal cancer.[112]

Pathophysiology. Carcinoma of the true vocal cords (glottis) is more common than that of the supraglottic structures (structures above the glottis) (Fig. 35.11). Tumors of the subglottic area are rare. Squamous cell carcinoma is the most common cell type, although neuroendocrine carcinomas also occur. Metastasis develops by cells spreading into the draining lymph nodes, but distant metastasis is rare.

Clinical Manifestations. The presenting symptoms of laryngeal cancer include dysphagia, hoarseness (dysphonia), dyspnea, and cough. Progressive hoarseness can result in voice loss. Dyspnea is rare with supraglottic tumors but can be severe in subglottic tumors. Swallowing may initiate a cough reflex. Laryngeal pain is likely with supraglottic lesions.

Evaluation and Treatment. Early evaluation for dysphonia improves subsequent survival after the diagnosis and treatment of laryngeal cancer, while delay in evaluation is associated with greater mortality.[113] This makes education of at-risk individuals important. Evaluation for laryngeal cancer includes external inspection and palpation of the larynx and the lymph nodes of the neck. Indirect or direct laryngoscopy with biopsy provides a definitive diagnosis. Imaging procedures facilitate the identification of tumor boundaries and the degree of extension to surrounding tissue.

Combined treatment with surgery (transoral laser microsurgery and partial or total laryngectomy), chemotherapy, immunotherapy, and irradiation can result in cure in selected cases.[114] Larynx-preservation strategies are being used to preserve swallowing and speech whenever possible. Swallowing and speech therapy after treatment can significantly improve recovery. Voice restoration after total laryngectomy includes using esophageal speech, electrolarynx, or voice prosthesis, among others.

Lung Cancer

Lung cancer is the second most common cancer in the United States and the leading cause of cancer death. In 2021, it is estimated that there were 235,760 new cases (12.4% of all new cancer cases) and 131,880 deaths (21.7% of all cancer deaths).[115] Despite emerging new therapies, the overall 5-year survival remains low, at about 22%.

Cigarette smoking accounts for 80% to 90% of primary lung cancers, however only 15% of smokers develop lung cancer, suggesting a genetic susceptibility.[116] The reduction in smoking prevalence over the past 3 decades has led to a gradual decline in incidence, but many new cases of lung cancer occur in individuals who have already quit smoking. Smokers with COPD are at even greater risk. Other risk factors for lung cancer include aging, secondhand (environmental) smoke, radon gas exposure, occupational exposures to certain workplace toxins

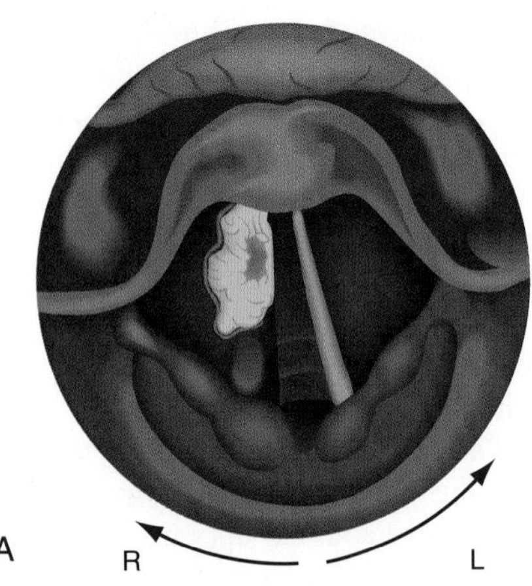

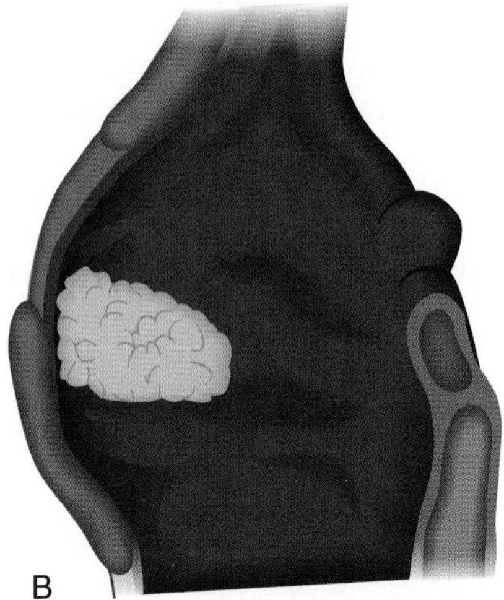

Fig. 35.11 Laryngeal Cancer. (A) Mirror view of carcinoma of the right false cord partially hiding the true cord. **(B)** Lateral view. (Redrawn from del Regato JA, et al. *Ackerman and del Regato's cancer*, 2nd edition. St. Louis: Mosby; 1985.)

(e.g., asbestos), radiation, and both indoor and outdoor air pollution. Environmental risk factors for cancer are discussed in Chapter 12. Genetic risks include polymorphisms of the genes responsible for growth factor receptors, angiogenesis, apoptosis, deoxyribonucleic acid (DNA) repair, and detoxification of inhaled smoke.

Types of lung cancer. Most primary lung cancers arise from cells that line the bronchi within the lungs and are therefore called *bronchogenic carcinomas*. Lung cancers are classified by cell type and molecular profiling. Although there are many types of lung cancer, they can be divided into two main categories: non–small cell lung carcinoma (NSCLC) and neuroendocrine tumors of the lung. The category of NSCLC accounts for 80% to 85% of all lung cancers and can be subdivided into three types of lung cancer: squamous cell carcinoma, adenocarcinoma, and large cell undifferentiated carcinoma. Neuroendocrine tumors of the lung also arise from the bronchial mucosa and include small cell carcinoma, large cell neuroendocrine carcinoma, and typical and atypical carcinoid tumors. Small cell carcinoma is the most common of these neuroendocrine tumors, accounting for approximately 15% to 20% of all lung cancers.

Other pulmonary tumors, such as mesotheliomas (associated with asbestos exposure), occur less commonly. Many cancers that arise in other organs of the body metastasize to the lungs; however, these are not considered primary lung cancers and are categorized by their site of origin. Characteristics of primary lung tumors, including clinical manifestations, are listed in Table 35.4.

Non-small cell lung cancer. Squamous cell carcinoma accounts for about 30% of bronchogenic carcinomas. These tumors are typically located near the hila and project into bronchi (Fig. 35.12A). Because of this central location, symptoms of a nonproductive cough or hemoptysis are common. Pneumonia and atelectasis are often associated with squamous cell carcinoma. Chest pain is a late symptom associated with large tumors. These tumors are often well localized and tend not to metastasize until late in the course of the disease.

Adenocarcinoma (tumor arising from glands) of the lung constitutes 35% to 40% of all bronchogenic carcinomas (Fig. 35.12B). Environmental tobacco smoke, occupational carcinogens, viruses, hormones, and positive family history are associated with this tumor type. Epidermal growth factor receptor (EGFR) mutations and anaplastic lymphoma kinase (ALK) gene rearrangements, as well as other tyrosine kinase inhibitors, are common in this type of lung cancer and are targets for therapy.[117,118] Pulmonary adenocarcinoma develops in a stepwise fashion through atypical adenomatous hyperplasia, adenocarcinoma in situ, and minimally invasive adenocarcinoma to invasive carcinoma. These tumors, which are usually smaller than 4 cm, more commonly arise in the peripheral regions of the pulmonary parenchyma. Individuals may be asymptomatic, and the tumors may be discovered by routine chest imaging in the early stages, or the individual may present with pleuritic chest pain and shortness of breath from pleural involvement by the tumor.

Included in the category of adenocarcinoma is bronchioloalveolar cell carcinoma. These tumors arise from terminal bronchioles and alveoli and are now being referred to as *adenocarcinoma in situ* or *minimally invasive adenocarcinoma*. They are slow-growing tumors with an unpredictable pattern of metastasis through the pulmonary arterial system and mediastinal lymph nodes.

TABLE 35.4 Characteristics of Lung Cancers

Tumor Type	Growth Rate	Metastasis	Means of Diagnosis	Clinical Manifestations and Treatment
Non–Small Cell Carcinoma				
Squamous cell carcinoma	Slow	Late, mostly to hilar lymph nodes	Biopsy, sputum analysis, bronchoscopy, electron microscopy, immunohistochemistry	Cough, hemoptysis, sputum production, airway obstruction, hypercalcemia; treated surgically, chemotherapy, radiation, and immunotherapy as adjunctive therapy
Adenocarcinoma	Moderate	Early, to lymph nodes, pleura, bone, adrenal glands, and brain	Radiography, fiberoptic bronchoscopy, electron microscopy	Pleural effusion; treated surgically, chemotherapy, and immunotherapy as adjunctive therapy
Large cell carcinoma	Rapid	Early and widespread	Sputum analysis, bronchoscopy, electron microscopy (by exclusion of other cell types)	Chest wall pain, pleural effusion, cough, sputum production, hemoptysis, airway obstruction resulting in pneumonia; treated surgically
Neuroendocrine Tumors of the Lung				
Small cell carcinoma	Very rapid	Very early; to mediastinum, lymph nodes, brain, bone marrow	Radiography, sputum analysis, bronchoscopy, electron microscopy, immunohistochemistry	Cough, chest pain, dyspnea, hemoptysis, localized wheezing, airway obstruction, signs and symptoms of excessive hormone secretion; treated by chemotherapy and ionizing radiation to thorax and central nervous system
Other Pulmonary Tumors				
Malignant pleural mesothelioma (MPM)	Rapid	Early, to lymph nodes, lungs, heart, bone	Radiography, thoracentesis	Chest pain, chronic cough, signs of pleural effusion; treated by surgery, chemotherapy, radiation, and immunotherapy

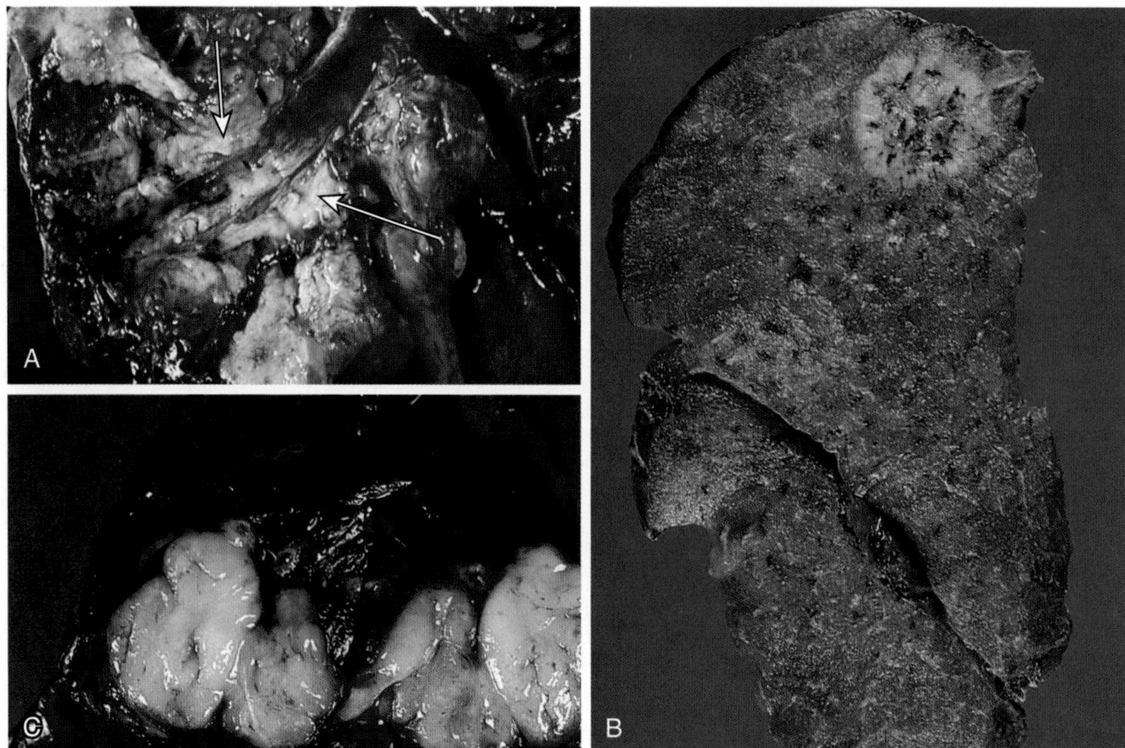

Fig. 35.12 Lung Cancer. **(A)** Squamous cell carcinoma. This hilar tumor originates from the main bronchus. **(B)** Peripheral adenocarcinoma. The tumor shows prominent black pigmentation, suggestive of having evolved in an anthracotic scar. **(C)** Small cell carcinoma. The tumor forms confluent nodules. On cross section, the nodules have an encephaloid appearance. (From Damjanov I, Linder J, eds. *Anderson's pathology*, 10th edition. St. Louis: Mosby; 1996.)

Large cell carcinomas constitute approximately 10% of bronchogenic carcinomas. These transformed epithelial cells have lost clear evidence of maturation and are considered an undifferentiated non–small cell carcinoma. These tumors arise from squamous, glandular, or neuroendocrine precursor cells, commonly arise centrally, and can grow to distort the trachea and cause widening of the carina.

Neuroendocrine tumors. Neuroendocrine tumors include small cell carcinoma, large cell neuroendocrine carcinoma, and bronchial carcinoids. Large cell neuroendocrine and bronchial carcinoids are rare.[119]

Small cell lung carcinoma (SCLC) is the most common type of neuroendocrine lung tumor and causes 25% of lung cancer deaths with an overall 5-year survival of less than 10%. Small cell carcinoma arises from neuroendocrine cells that contain neurosecretory granules. Most of these tumors are central in origin (hilar and mediastinal) (see Fig. 35.12C), have a rapid rate of growth, and tend to metastasize early and widely. Because these cells arise from neuroendocrine cells, they are often associated with ectopic hormone production. Ectopic hormone production is important to the clinician because resulting signs and symptoms, called *paraneoplastic syndromes* (see Chapter 12), may be the first manifestation of the underlying cancer. Examples include hyponatremia (antidiuretic hormone), Cushing syndrome (adrenocorticotropic hormone), hypocalcemia (calcitonin), gynecomastia (gonadotropins), carcinoid syndrome (serotonin), and Lambert-Eaton myasthenic syndrome (paneoplastic cerebellar degeneration).

Bronchial carcinoid tumors represent about 1% of all lung tumors. They are not related to smoking, may begin in childhood, and grow very slowly. Carcinoid tumors contain neuroendocrine-like hormones, but rarely produce hormone related symptoms. The tumors are usually discovered by chest imaging undertaken for an unrelated condition and can be cured by local surgical or bronchoscopic resection.

Other lung cancers. Malignant mesotheliomas arise from the mesothelial cells that line the pleura. Nearly 80% have been linked to asbestos exposure, although it may take up to 40 years after exposure for the tumor to be diagnosed. They are classified as epithelioid, sarcomatoid, and biphasic, although new classification categories are being proposed.[120] Clinical manifestations include dyspnea and chest pain. Chest imaging may reveal a pleural effusion, with the diagnosis confirmed by CT scanning, thoracentesis, thoracoscopy, and cytology. Management includes surgery, chemotherapy, radiation, and immunotherapy, although toxicities are high and outcomes poor in those with advanced disease.[121,122]

Pathophysiology. Tobacco smoke contains more than 7000 chemicals, 69 of which are classified as carcinogens.[123] Air pollution and other inhaled toxins also contain numerous carcinogens. These chemicals, along with an inherited genetic predisposition to cancers, result in tumor development. Once lung cancer is initiated by these carcinogen-induced mutations, tumor development is promoted by additional mutations that alter the production and response to growth factors that alter cell growth and differentiation and by the production of inflammatory mediators. The bronchial mucosa suffers multiple carcinogenic "hits" because of repetitive exposure to tobacco smoke, and, eventually, epithelial cell changes begin progressing from metaplasia to carcinoma in situ and finally to invasive carcinoma. Further tumor progression includes invasion of surrounding tissues and finally metastasis to distant sites, including the brain, bone marrow, and liver (see Chapter 12 for the details of cancer biology).

Clinical Manifestations. Table 35.4 summarizes the characteristic clinical manifestations according to tumor type. Approximately half of individuals eventually diagnosed with lung cancer develop a new cough, a third develop dyspnea, and a quarter develop hemoptysis.[116] Recurrent infections are also common. These symptoms are nonspecific and often attributed to smoking;, and when they are severe enough to motivate the individual to seek medical advice, the disease is often advanced. Symptoms of advanced disease such as dysphagia, weight loss, fatigue, bone pain, and paraneoplastic syndromes may be the first indication of underlying lung cancer.

Evaluation and Treatment. Annual screening for lung cancer with low-dose CT (LDCT) scans is recommended for adults age 50 to 80 who have 20 pack years or more of smoking history and either continue to smoke or have quit within the past 15 years or develops a health problem that substantially limits life expectancy or the ability or willingness to have curative lung surgery.[124] Most studies suggest that concerns about the high false-positive rate and considerable radiation exposure are outweighed by the estimated 20% reduction in lung cancer mortality as compared to plain radiographs.[116] Diagnostic tests for the evaluation of lung cancer include sputum cytologic studies, chest CT, bronchoscopy, PET scanning, and endobronchial ultrasound (EBUS)-guided bronchoscopic biopsy. Biopsy determines the cell type. The evaluation of lymph nodes and other organ systems, usually by FDG-PET scanning, is used to determine the stage of the cancer. The currently accepted system for the staging of non–small cell cancer is the TNM classification (*T* denotes the extent of the primary tumor, *N* indicates the nodal involvement, *M* describes the extent of metastasis) (see Chapter 12). This system,as applied to primary lung cancers, was updated in 2016 and includes a detailed description of each category with the aim of improving both clinical and research approaches toward management.[125] Long delays between diagnosis and staging may occur and can lead to progression of disease and poorer outcomes in individuals with NSCLC.[126] In contrast to NCSLC, small cell lung cancers are only staged as either limited (confined to the area of origin in the lung) or extensive.

The histologic cell type, the genotype, and the stage of the disease are major factors that influence the choice of therapy. For all types of early-stage NSLC, the preferred treatment is surgical resection.[127] Once metastasis has occurred, total surgical resection is more difficult, and survival rates dramatically decrease. Other treatment modalities include chemotherapy, dose-intensified irradiation, radiofrequency ablation, microwave ablation, cryotherapy, and brachytherapy. Molecular and immunotherapies have been approved that can increase the survival time for selected individuals (Emerging Science Box: Molecular and Immune Therapies for Lung Cancer).[117,128,129] Only 5% of individuals with SCLC can be treated surgically. Systemic chemotherapy and radiation are indicated in most cases.

EMERGING SCIENCE BOX

Molecular and Immune Therapies for Lung Cancer

A better understanding of the genetic and immunologic features of lung cancer cells has led to new treatment options. Molecular therapies are now available for both non–small cell carcinoma (NSCLC) and, to a lesser degree, for small cell carcinoma (SCLC). These therapies target specific cancer cell mutations and require molecular analysis of tumor cells to determine if an individual is likely to benefit from their use. Among the most effective molecular therapies for NSCLC are drugs that block the action of epidermoid growth factor receptor (EGFR) and include erlotinib, gefitinib, afatinib, osimertinib, dacomitinib, and necitumumab. These drugs have increased overall response rates to treatment and survival time in individuals whose cancer cells are positive for EGFR mutations. Other targets either approved or awaiting approval include drugs that block the effects of ALK and tyrosine-protein kinase ROS-1 mutations (crizotinib, ceritinib, entrectinib, lorlatinib). Drugs that block angiogenesis (bevacizumab and ramucirumab) are also used in selected individuals. Cancer cells have the capacity to prevent effective adaptive immune responses by activating molecules called immune checkpoint inhibitors, such as PDL-1 and CTLA-4, on the surface of T cells, thus shutting these cells off. Monoclonal antibodies can be used to block these immune checkpoint inhibitors and thus restore the immune response to the cancer. Immunotherapies currently approved by the U.S. Food and Drug Administration (FDA) for NSCLC that block PDL-1 or CTLA-4 include nivolumab, pembrolizumab, atezolizumab, durvalumab, avelumab, ipilimumab, and tremelimumab. Nivolumab can be considered for treatment of SCLC. These therapies can shrink tumors and prolong life but are rarely curative, and many have considerable side effects. New combinations of immunotherapy drugs used as first-line treatment for advanced lung cancer are being explored.

Data from Broderick SR. Adjuvant and neoadjuvant immunotherapy in non-small cell lung cancer. *Thoracic Surgery Clinics*, 2020;30(2):215–220; Cantelmo AR, et al. Angiogenesis inhibition in non-small cell lung cancer: a critical appraisal, basic concepts and updates from American Society for Clinical Oncology 2019. *Current Opinion in Oncology*, 2020;32(1):44–53; de Alencar VTL, et al. Immunotherapy as single treatment for non-small-cell lung cancer patients with brain metastases: A systematic review and meta-analysis— the META-L-BRAIN study. *Journal of Thoracic Oncology*. Published online: May 05, 2021; Hsu ML, et al. Principles of immunotherapy in non-small cell lung cancer. *Thoracic Surgery Clinics*, 2020;30(2):187–198; Liu L, et al. Efficacy and safety of first-line immunotherapy combinations for advanced non-small-cell lung cancer: A systematic review and network meta-analysis. *Journal of Thoracic Oncology*. Published online: April 08, 2021; Makuku R, et al. Current and future perspectives of PD-1/PDL-1 blockade in cancer immunotherapy. *Journal of Immunology Research*, 2021:Article 6661406; Makuku R, et al. Current and future perspectives of PD-1/PDL-1 blockade in cancer immunotherapy. *Journal of Immunology Research*, 2021:Article 6661406; Qiao M, et al. Immune checkpoint inhibitors in EGFR-mutated non-small cell lung cancer: Dusk or Dawn? *Journal of Thoracic Oncology*. 2021;16(8):1267-1288; Reckamp KL. Molecular targets beyond the big 3. *Thoracic Surgery Clinics*, 2020;30(2):157–164; Sanka K, et al. Immunotherapy for ALK-Rearranged non-small cell lung cancer: Challenges inform promising approaches. *Cancers*, 2021;13(6):476; Urwyler P, et al. Mechanisms of checkpoint inhibition-induced adverse events. *Clinical and Experimental Immunology*, 2020;200(2):141–154.

SUMMARY REVIEW

Clinical Manifestations of Pulmonary Alterations

1. Dyspnea is the feeling of breathlessness or shortness of breath, requiring the individual to become preoccupied with breathing.
2. Orthopnea is dyspnea that occurs when an individual lies flat, which causes the abdominal contents to exert pressure on the diaphragm.
3. Paroxysmal nocturnal dyspnea is dyspnea that occurs with pulmonary or cardiac disease, waking the individual while sleeping, gasping for air.
4. Coughing is a protective reflex that expels secretions and irritants from the airways. It can be acute or chronic.
5. Changes in the volume, consistency, or color of sputum may indicate underlying pulmonary disease.
6. Hemoptysis is expectoration of bloody mucus, usually due to infection or inflammation that damages the bronchi or lung parenchyma.
7. Abnormal breathing patterns are adjustments made by the body to minimize the work of respiratory muscles. They include Kussmaul, labored, restricted, gasping, Cheyne-Stokes respirations, and sighing.
8. Hypoventilation is decreased alveolar ventilation caused by altered pulmonary mechanics or neurologic control of breathing and results in increased $PaCO_2$ (hypercapnia).
9. Hyperventilation is increased alveolar ventilation produced by anxiety, head injury, pain, or severe hypoxemia and causes decreased $PaCO_2$ (hypocapnia).
10. Cyanosis is a bluish discoloration of the skin caused by desaturation of hemoglobin, polycythemia, or peripheral vasoconstriction.
11. Clubbing of the fingertips is associated with diseases that cause chronic hypoxemia, and it is rarely reversible.
12. Pain to the chest wall can result from infection and inflammation of the pleurae, trachea, bronchi, ribs, or respiratory muscles.
13. Hypercapnia is an increased $PaCO_2$ due to hypoventilation of the alveoli and is associated with respiratory acidosis. There are many causes of hypoventilation
14. Hypoxemia is a reduced PaO_2 caused by respiratory alterations, resulting in $\dot{V}/\dot{Q}$ mismatch.
15. Hypoxia is reduced oxygenation of cells, usually due to hypoxemia.
16. $\dot{V}/\dot{Q}$ match is the balance between the amount of air that enters the alveoli and amount of blood that is perfusing. An alteration in this balance can cause a $\dot{V}/\dot{Q}$ mismatch resulting in hypoxemia.
17. Respiratory failure is inadequate gas exchange that can result from direct injury to the lungs, airways, or chest wall or indirectly because of disease or injury involving another body system. It is classified as either hypoxemic or hypercapnic.

Disorders of the Chest Wall and Pleura

1. Restricted movement of the chest wall can occur by obesity and kyphoscoliosis, which compress the lungs, and by neuromuscular diseases that impair chest wall muscle function.
2. Flail chest results from rib or sternal fractures that disrupt the mechanics of breathing.
3. Pneumothorax is the accumulation of air in the pleural space caused by rupture of weakened areas of the pleura.
4. Tension pneumothorax is a life-threatening condition caused by trapping of air in the pleural space, producing displacement of the trachea, great vessels, and heart.
5. Pleural effusion is the accumulation of fluid in the pleural space resulting from disorders from capillaries underlying the pleura or from blockage or injury to lymphatic vessels that drain into the pleural space.
6. Empyema is the presence of pus in the pleural space (infected pleural effusion); it usually occurs because of lymphatic drainage from sites of bacterial pneumonia.

Pulmonary Disorders

1. Pulmonary disorders can be restrictive (limiting lung volumes) or obstructive (limiting airflow) or both.
2. Restrictive lung diseases are characterized by decreased lung compliance, requiring more effort to expand the lungs during inspiration, which increases the work of breathing. Individuals with lung restriction have dyspnea, an increased respiratory rate, and a decreased tidal volume.
3. Aspiration of food particles or pharyngeal or gastric secretions into the airways can cause obstruction, inflammation, or pneumonia.
4. Atelectasis is the collapse of alveoli resulting from compression of lung tissue, absorption of gas from obstructed alveoli, or decreased production of surfactant.
5. Bronchiectasis is abnormal dilation of the bronchi secondary to another pulmonary disorder, usually infection or inflammation.
6. Bronchiolitis is the inflammatory obstruction of small airways. It is most common in children.
7. Pulmonary fibrosis is excessive connective tissue in the lung that diminishes lung compliance; it may be idiopathic or caused by disease and is associated with chronic inflammation.
8. Inhalation of noxious gases or prolonged exposure to high concentrations of oxygen can damage the bronchial mucosa or alveolocapillary membrane and cause inflammation or acute respiratory failure.
9. Pneumoconiosis, which is caused by inhalation of dust particles in the workplace, can cause pulmonary fibrosis and progressive pulmonary deterioration.
10. Hypersensitivity pneumonitis (extrinsic allergic alveolitis) is an allergic or hypersensitivity reaction to many allergens causing lung inflammation.
11. Pulmonary edema is excess fluid in the lung caused by increased capillary hydrostatic pressure, decreased capillary oncotic pressure, or increased capillary permeability. Causes include left heart failure that increases capillary

hydrostatic pressure in the pulmonary circulation, inflammation of alveoli, or lymphatic obstruction.
12. Acute respiratory distress syndrome (ARDS) is a form of acute lung inflammation and diffuse alveolocapillary injury that results from direct pulmonary injury or from severe systemic inflammation. Endothelial damage results in increased capillary membrane permeability causing hypoxemia and remodeling of the tissue causes fibrosis.
13. Obstructive lung disease is characterized by airway obstruction that causes difficult expiration. Accessory muscles of expiration must be used, which increases the work of breathing. The unifying symptom of obstructive lung diseases is dyspnea, and the unifying sign is wheezing.
14. Asthma is a chronic inflammation that causes bronchial hyperresponsiveness, constriction of the airways, mucosal edema, increased mucus production, and variable airflow obstruction that can be reversible.
15. Chronic obstructive pulmonary disease (COPD) is a group of lung disorders with persistent airflow limitation due to chronic inflammatory response in the airways. COPD is usually progressive and includes asthma, bronchitis, and emphysema.
16. Chronic bronchitis causes airway obstruction resulting from inflammation, bronchial smooth muscle hypertrophy, and production of thick, tenacious mucus.
17. In emphysema, destruction of the alveolar septa and loss of passive elastic recoil lead to alveolar enlargement, airway collapse, obstruction of gas flow, and air trapping during expiration.
18. Respiratory tract infections are common and usually involve only the upper airways.
19. Acute bronchitis is usually a self-limiting inflammation or viral infection of the airways.
20. Pneumonia is infection of the lower respiratory tract caused by bacteria, viruses, fungi, protozoa, or parasites.
21. Pneumococcal *(Streptococcus pneumoniae)* is the most common cause of community acquired pneumonia.
22. Viral pneumonia can be severe, but is more often an acute, self-limiting lung infection usually caused by the influenza virus.
23. Tuberculosis (TB) is a lung infection caused by *Mycobacterium tuberculosis* (tubercle bacillus). In tuberculosis, the inflammatory response proceeds to isolate colonies of bacilli by enclosing them in tubercles and surrounding the tubercles with scar tissue. TB bacilli escape immune defenses by surviving within macrophages.
24. An abscess is a circumscribed area of suppuration and destruction of lung parenchyma, often caused by aspiration. Necrosis of consolidated tissue may lead to cavitation in which the abscess empties into a bronchus and cavity formation.
25. Pulmonary vascular diseases are caused by embolism, hypertension, or cor pulmonale in the pulmonary circulation.
26. Pulmonary embolism is a clot most often originating from deep venous thrombosis and causes vascular obstruction, $\dot{V}/\dot{Q}$ mismatch, hypoxemia, and pulmonary hypertension; it may or may not cause infarction.
27. Pulmonary artery hypertension (pulmonary artery pressure >25 mm Hg) can be caused by heritable defects, drugs, veno-occlusive disease, lung or heart disease, systemic disorders, and chronic pulmonary embolism.
28. Cor pulmonale is secondary to pulmonary artery hypertension and results in right ventricular enlargement or failure.
29. Laryngeal cancer occurs primarily in men, represents less than 1% of all cancers, and presents with a clinical symptom of progressive hoarseness.
30. Lung cancer, the most common cause of cancer death in the United States, is usually caused by tobacco smoking.
31. Lung cancer (bronchogenic carcinomas) cell types include non–small cell carcinoma (squamous cell, adenocarcinoma, and large cell) and neuroendocrine tumors (small cell lung carcinoma and bronchial carcinoid tumors). Each type arises in a characteristic site or type of tissue, causes distinctive clinical manifestations, and differs in likelihood of metastasis and prognosis.

REFERENCES

1. O'Donnell DE, et al. Dyspnea in COPD: new mechanistic insights and management implications. *Adv Ther*. 2020;37:41–60.
2. Bickler PE, Feiner JR, Lipnick MS, McKleroy W. "Silent" presentation of hypoxemia and cardiorespiratory compensation in COVID-19. *Anesthesiology*. 2021;134(2):262–269.
3. Davis JA, Gudi K. Approach to the patient with cough. *Med Clin North Am*. 2021;105:31–38.
4. Pinto B, et al. ACEI-induced cough: a review of current evidence and its practical implications for optimal CV risk reduction. *Indian Heart J*. 2020;72(5):345–350.
5. Cordovilla R, et al. Diagnosis and treatment of hemoptysis. *Arch Bronconeumol*. 2016;52(7):368–377.
6. Quigley N, Gagnon S, Fortin M. Aetiology, diagnosis and treatment of moderate-to-severe haemoptysis in a North American academic centre. *ERJ Open Res*. 2020;6(4):00204–02020.
7. Matsuura N. Schamroth sign. *CMAJ*. 2019;191(45):E1251.
8. Diebold M, Kuster S, Osthoff M. Reversible Hippocratic fingers in a patient with pneumonia. *Am J Med*. 2020;133:e9–e10.
9. Brascia D, et al. Surgical stabilization of flail chest after trauma: when, why and how to do it? *Current Challenges in Thoracic Surgery*. 2020;2(28).
10. Kelly C, Carlberg M, Madsen T. Spontaneous pneumothorax resulting in tension physiology. *Am J Emerg Med*. 2019;37(173):E1–173. E2.
11. Hallifax RJ, et al. Ambulatory management of primary spontaneous pneumothorax: an open-label, randomised controlled trial. *Lancet*. 2020;396(10243):39–49.
12. Hallifax R, Janssen JP. Pneumothorax—time for new guidelines? *Semin Respir Crit Care Med*. 2019;40(3):314–322.
13. Bedawi EO, et al. Advances in pleural infection and malignancy. *Eur Respir Rev*. 2021;30:200002.
14. Mercer RM. Interpreting pleural fluid results. *Clin Med*. 2019;19:213–217.
15. Aboudara M, Maldonado F. Update in the management of pleural effusions. *Med Clin North Am*. 2019;103:475–485.

16. Mandell LA, Niederman MS. Aspiration pneumonia. *N Engl J Med.* 2019;380:651–663.
17. Marin-Corral J, et al. GLIMP investigators: Aspiration risk factors, microbiology, and empiric antibiotics for patients hospitalized with community-acquired pneumonia. *Chest.* 2021;159(1):58–72.
18. Neill S, Dean N. Aspiration pneumonia and pneumonitis: a spectrum of infectious/noninfectious diseases affecting the lung. *Curr Opin Infect Dis.* 2019;32:152–157.
19. Patel TP, Karle EM, Krvavac A. Resorptive (obstructive) atelectasis. *BMJ Case Rep.* 2019;12(11):e232405.
20. Chang-Macchiu P, Traversi L, Polverino E. Bronchiectasis phenotypes. *Curr Opin Pulm Med.* 2019;25(3):281–288.
21. Imam JS, Duarte AG. Non-CF bronchiectasis: orphan disease no longer. *Respir Med.* 2020;166:105940.
22. Sibila O. Reducing Pseudomonas sputum density in bronchiectasis. *Eur Respir J.* 2021;57:2003390.
23. National Institute of Health, National Heart, Lung, & Blood Institute: Bronchiectasis. Available at: https://www.nhlbi.nih.gov/health-topics/bronchiectasis. Accessed February 2, 2022.
24. Ryu JH, et al. Recent advances in the understanding of bronchiolitis in adults. *F1000Res 9:F1000 Faculty Rev.* 2020;568
25. Chambers DC. Bronchiolitis obliterans syndrome 'endotypes' in haematopoietic stem cell transplantation. *Respirology.* 2019;24(5):408–409.
26. Arjuna A, et al. An update on current treatment strategies for managing bronchiolitis obliterans syndrome after lung transplantation. *Expert Rev Respir Med.* 2021;15(3):339–350.
27. Wakwaya Y, Brown KK. Idiopathic pulmonary fibrosis: epidemiology, diagnosis and outcomes. *Am J Med Sci.* 2019;357(5):359–369.
28. Luo QK, Zhang H, Li L. Research advances on DNA methylation in idiopathic pulmonary fibrosis. *Adv Exp Med Biol.* 2020;1255:73–81.
29. Jenkins G. Demystifying pulmonary fibrosis. *Am J Physiol Lung Cell Mol Physiol.* 2020;319:L554–L559.
30. Heukels P, et al. Inflammation and immunity in IPF pathogenesis and treatment. *Respir Med.* 2019;147:79–91.
31. Podolanczuk AJ, Noth I, Raghu G. Idiopathic pulmonary fibrosis: prime time for a precision-based approach to treatment with N-acetylcysteine. *Eur Respir J.* 2021;57:2003551.
32. Snijder J, et al. Pulmonary fibrosis: a disease of alveolar collapse and collagen deposition. *Expert Rev Respir Med.* 2019;13(7):615–619.
33. Kang J, Han M, Song JW. Antifibrotic treatment improves clinical outcomes in patients with idiopathic pulmonary fibrosis: a propensity score matching analysis. *Sci Rep.* 2020;10:15620.
34. Perlman DM, Maier LA. Occupational lung disease. *Med Clin North Am.* 2019;103:535–548.
35. Greenberger PA. Hypersensitivity pneumonitis: a fibrosing alveolitis produced by inhalation of diverse antigens. *J Allergy Clin Immunol.* 2019;143(4):1295–1301.
36. Costabel U, et al. Hypersensitivity pneumonitis. *Nat Rev Dis Primers.* 2020;6(1):65.
37. Raghu G, et al. Diagnosis of hypersensitivity pneumonitis in adults. An official ATS/JRS/ALAT Clinical Practice Guideline. *Am J Respir Crit Care Med.* 2020;202(3):e36–e69.
38. Kang M, Kempker JA. Definitions, epidemiology, clinical risk factors, and health disparities in acute respiratory distress syndrome. *Semin Respir Crit Care Med.* 2019;40(1):3–11.
39. Welker C, et al. 2021 acute respiratory distress syndrome update, with coronavirus disease 2019 focus. *J Cardiothorac Vasc Anesth.* 2021; Feb 27:S1053-0770(21)00188-9.
40. Lynn H, et al. Genomic and genetic approaches to deciphering acute respiratory distress syndrome risk and mortality. *Antioxid Redox Signal.* 2019;31(14):1027–1052.
41. Wildi K, et al. The discovery of biological subphenotypes in ARDS: a novel approach to targeted medicine? *J Intensive Care.* 2021;9(1):14.
42. ARDS Definition Task Force Ranieri VM, et al. Acute respiratory distress syndrome: the Berlin Definition. *JAMA.* 2012;307(23):2526–2533.
43. Ohshimo S. Oxygen administration for patients with ARDS. *J Intensive Care.* 2021;9:17.
44. Goligher EC, et al. Effect of lowering tidal volume on mortality in ARDS varies with respiratory system elastance. *Am J Respir Crit Care Med.* 2021;203(11):1378–1385.
45. Xu B, et al. Stem cell derived exosomes-based therapy for acute lung injury and acute respiratory distress syndrome: a novel therapeutic strategy. *Life Sci.* 2020;254:117766.
46. Global Initiative for Asthma (GINA): 2021 GINA Report, Global Strategy for Asthma Management and Prevention. https://ginasthma.org/gina-reports/. Accessed February 2, 2022.
47. Centers for Disease Control and Prevention (CDC) National Center for Health Statistics. *Most Recent National Asthma Data.* 2021 Available at: https://www.cdc.gov/asthma/most_recent_national_asthma_data.htm. Accessed February 2, 2022.
48. El-Husseini ZW, et al. The genetics of asthma and the promise of genomics-guided drug target discovery. *Lancet Respir Med.* 2020;8(10):1045–1056.
49. Schoettler N, Strek ME. Recent advances in severe asthma: from phenotypes to personalized medicine. *Chest.* 2020;157(3):516–528.
50. Long A, et al. Epigenetics and the environment in airway disease: asthma and allergic rhinitis. *Adv Exp Med Biol.* 2020;1253:153–181.
51. Renz H, Skevaki C. Early life microbial exposures and allergy risks: opportunities for prevention. *Nat Rev Immunol.* 2021;21:177–191.
52. Barcik W, et al. The role of lung and gut microbiota in the pathology of asthma. *Immunity.* 2020;52(2):241–255.
53. Chiu CY, et al. Cross-talk between airway and gut microbiome links to IgE responses to house dust mites in childhood airway allergies. *Sci Rep.* 2020;10:13449.
54. Peebles Jr RS, Aronica MA. Proinflammatory pathways in the pathogenesis of asthma. *Clin Chest Med.* 2019;40(1):29–50.
55. Lambrecht BN, Hammad H, Fahy JV. The cytokines of asthma. *Immunity.* 2019;50(4):975–991.
56. Calzetta L, et al. The impact of muscarinic receptor antagonists on airway inflammation: a systematic review. *Int J Chron Obstruct Pulmon Dis.* 2021;16:257–279.
57. Banno A, et al. Bidirectional interaction of airway epithelial remodeling and inflammation in asthma. *Clin Sci.* 2020;134(9):1063–1079.
58. Zaidan MF, Ameredes BT, Calhoun WJ. Management of acute asthma in adults in 2020. *JAMA.* 2020;323(6):563–564.
59. National Institute of Health, National Heart, Lung, & Blood Institute: *2020 Focused Updates to the Asthma Management Guidelines: A Report from the National Asthma Education and Prevention Program Coordinating Committee Expert Panel Working Group.* Available at: https://www.nhlbi.nih.gov/health-topics/all-publications-and-resources/2020-focused-updates-asthma-management-guidelines. Accessed February 2, 2022.
60. Tripple JW, Ameredes BT, Calhoun WJ. Outpatient management of chronic asthma in 2020. *JAMA.* 2020;323(6):561–562.

61. Yamamoto T, et al. Current state and future prospect of the therapeutic strategy targeting cysteinyl leukotriene metabolism in asthma. *Respir Investig*. 2019;57(6):534–543.
62. Global Initiative for Chronic Obstructive Lung Disease: *Global Strategy for the Diagnosis, Management, and Prevention of Chronic Obstructive Pulmonary Disease (GOLD) 2022 Report*. Available at: https://goldcopd.org/2022-gold-reports-2/. Accessed February 2, 2022.
63. Centers for Disease Control and Prevention (CDC): *Chronic obstructive pulmonary disease: data and statistics*. Available at https://www.cdc.gov/copd/data.html. Accessed February 2, 2022.
64. Osei AD, et al. Association between e-cigarette use and chronic obstructive pulmonary disease by smoking status: behavioral risk factor surveillance system 2016 and 2017. *Am J Prevent Med*. 2020;58:336–342.
65. Ramsheh MY, et al. Lung microbiome composition and bronchial epithelial gene expression in patients with COPD versus healthy individuals: a bacterial 16S rRNA gene sequencing and host transcriptomic analysis. *Lancet Microbe*. 2021;2(7):E300-310.
66. Agusti A, Hogg JC. Update on the pathogenesis of chronic obstructive pulmonary disease. *N Engl J Med*. 2019;381:1248–1256.
67. Strnad P, McElvaney NG, Lomas DA. Alpha1-antitripsin deficiency. *N Engl J Med*. 2020;382:1443–1455.
68. Tu X, et al. Asthma-COPD overlap: current understanding and the utility of experimental models. *Eur Respir Rev*. 2021;30:190185.
69. Strange C. Alpha-1 antitrypsin deficiency associated COPD. *Clin Chest Med*. 2020;41(3):339–345.
70. Lorincz R, Curiel DT. Advances in alpha-1 antitrypsin gene therapy. *Am J Respir Cell Mol Biol*. 2020;63(5):560–570.
71. Duffy SP, Criner GJ. Chronic obstructive pulmonary disease. *Med Clin North Am*. 2019;103 453–451.
72. Celli BR, Wedzicha JA. Update on the clinical aspects of chronic obstructive pulmonary disease. *N Engl J Med*. 2019;381:1257–1266.
73. Hill NS, et al. Noninvasive ventilatory support for acute hypercapnic respiratory failure. *Respir Care*. 2019;64(6):647–657.
74. Tsutsui M, Gerayeli F, Sin DD. Pulmonary rehabilitation in a post-COVID-19 world: telerehabilitation as a new standard in patients with COPD. *Int J Chron Obstruct Pulmon Dis*. 2021;16:379–391.
75. Abia-Trujillo D, et al. Bronchoscopic lung volume reduction: a new hope for patients with severe emphysema and air trapping. *Mayo Clin Proc*. 2021;96:464–472.
76. Torres A, et al. Pneumonia. *Nat Rev Dis Primers*. 2021;7:25.
77. Centers for Disease Control and Prevention (CDC) National Center for Health Statistics. *Pneumonia*. 2021 Reviewed January 25, 2021. Available at: https://www.cdc.gov/nchs/fastats/pneumonia.htm. Accessed February 2, 2022.
78. Feldman C, Shaddock E. Epidemiology of lower respiratory tract infections in adults. *Expert Rev Respir Med*. 2019;13(1):63–77.
79. Centers for Disease Control and Prevention (CDC). National Center for Health Statistics. *Influenza*. 2021 Reviewed April 9, 2021. Available at: https://www.cdc.gov/nchs/fastats/flu.htm. Accessed February 2, 2022.
80. José RJ, Periselneris JN, Brown JS. Opportunistic bacterial, viral and fungal infections of the lung. *Medicine (Abingdon)*. 2020;48(6):366–372.
81. Ho J, Ip M. Antibiotic-resistant community-acquired bacterial pneumonia. *Infect Dis Clin North Am*. 2019;33(4):1087–1103.
82. Lanks CW, Musani AI, Hsia DW. Community-acquired pneumonia and hospital-acquired pneumonia. *Med Clin North Am*. 2019;103(3):487–501.
83. Herold S, et al. Influenza virus-induced lung injury: pathogenesis and implications for treatment. *Eur Respir J*. 2015;45:1463–1478.
84. Grudzinska FS, et al. Neutrophils in community-acquired pneumonia: parallels in dysfunction at the extremes of age. *Thorax*. 2020;75(2):164–171.
85. Grousd JA, Rich HE, Alcorn JF. Host-pathogen interactions in gram-positive bacterial pneumonia. *Clin Microbiol Rev*. 2019;32(3):e00107–e00118.
86. Metlay JP, et al. Diagnosis and treatment of adults with community acquired pneumonia: an official clinical practice guideline of the American Thoracic Society and Infectious Diseases Society of America. *Am J Respir Crit Care Med*. 2019;200(7):e45–e67.
87. Coppadoro A, Bellani G, Foti G. Non-pharmacological interventions to prevent ventilator-associated pneumonia: a literature review. *Respir Care*. 2019;64(12):1586–1595.
88. Liapikou A, et al. Emerging antibiotics for community-acquired pneumonia. *Expert Opin Emerg Drugs*. 2019;24(4):221–231.
89. MacNeil A, et al. Global epidemiology of tuberculosis and progress toward achieving global targets—2017. *MMWR Morb Mortal Wkly Rep*. 2019;68(11):263–266.
90. Chai Q, Lu Z, Liu CH. Host defense mechanisms against Mycobacterium tuberculosis. *Cell Mol Life Sci*. 2020;77(10):1859–1878.
91. Schrager LK, et al. The status of tuberculosis vaccine development. *Lancet Infect Dis*. 2020;20(3):e28–e37.
92. World Health Organization (WHO). *Latent tuberculosis infection: updated and consolidated guidelines for programmatic management*. Geneva: World Health Organization; 2018. Available from: https://www.ncbi.nlm.nih.gov/books/NBK531235/. Accessed February 2, 2022.
93. World Health Organization (WHO). 2017 update. *Guidelines for treatment of drug-susceptible tuberculosis and patient care*. Geneva: World Health Organization; 2018. Available at: https://apps.who.int/iris/bitstream/handle/10665/255052/9789241550000-eng.pdf. Accessed February 2, 2022.
94. Lange C, et al. Management of patients with multidrug-resistant tuberculosis. *Int J Tuberc Lung Dis*. 2019;23(6):645–662.
95. Muthukrishnan L. Multidrug resistant tuberculosis—diagnostic challenges and its conquering by nanotechnology approach—an overview. *Chem Biol Interact*. 2021;337:109397.
96. Centers for Disease Control and Prevention (CDC): *Venous Thromboembolism (Blood Clots). Data and Statistics on Venous Thromboembolism*. Available at: https://www.cdc.gov/ncbddd/dvt/data.html. Accessed February 2, 2022.
97. Nasser NJ, Fox J, Agbarya A. Potential mechanisms of cancer-related hypercoagulability. *Cancers*. 2020;12(3):566.
98. Longchamp G, et al. Proximal deep vein thrombosis and pulmonary embolism in COVID-19 patients: a systematic review and meta-analysis. *Thromb J*. 2021;19:15.
99. Tan BK, et al. Arterial and venous thromboembolism in COVID-19: a study-level meta-analysis. *Thorax*. 2021;76:970-979.
100. Duffett L, Castellucci LA, Forgie MA. Pulmonary embolism: update on management and controversies. *BMJ*. 2020;370:m2177.
101. Simon M. Effectiveness of clinical decision tools in predicting pulmonary embolism. *Pulm Med*. 2021;2021:8880893.

102. MacDougall K, Spyropoulos AC. Prevention of venous thromboembolism in acutely ill medical patients: a new era. *Semin Respir Crit Care Med.* 2021;42:308–315.
103. Ortel TL, et al. American Society of Hematology 2020 guidelines for management of venous thromboembolism: treatment of deep vein thrombosis and pulmonary embolism. *Blood Adv.* 2020;4(19):4693–4738.
104. Nair S, et al. Treatment of acute venous thromboembolism. *Med Clin North Am.* 2020;104(4):631–646.
105. Tan CW, et al. Contemporary management of acute pulmonary embolism. *Semin Thorac Cardiovasc Surg.* 2020;32(3):396–403.
106. Kesselman A, et al. Current controversies in inferior vena cava filter placement: AJR expert panel narrative review. *AJR Am J Roentgenol.* 2021;216:563–569.
107. Klouda T, Yuan K. Inflammation in pulmonary arterial hypertension. *Adv Exp Med Biol.* 2021;1303:351–372.
108. Woodcock CSC, Chan SY. The search for disease-modifying therapies in pulmonary hypertension. *J Cardiovasc Pharmacol Ther.* 2019;24:334–354.
109. Panagiotidou E, Boutou A, Pitsiou G. An evaluation of selexipag for the treatment of pulmonary hypertension. *Expert Opin Pharmacother.* 2021;22:29–36.
110. Pu X, et al. Stem/progenitor cells and pulmonary arterial hypertension. *Arterioscler Thromb Vasc Biol.* 2021;41:167–178.
111. National Cancer Institute: Surveillance, Epidemiology and End Results Program: *Cancer Stat Facts: Laryngeal cancer.* Available at: https://seer.cancer.gov/statfacts/html/laryn.html. Accessed February 2, 2022.
112. Wang SM, et al. Gastroesophageal reflux disease: a risk factor for laryngeal squamous cell carcinoma and esophageal squamous cell carcinoma in the NIH-AARP Diet and Health Study cohort. *Cancer.* 2021;127(11):1871–1879.
113. Lu YA, et al. Seeking medical assistance for dysphonia is associated with an improved survival rate in laryngeal cancer: real-world evidence. *Diagnostics.* 2021;11:255.
114. Obid R, Redlich M, Tomeh C. The treatment of laryngeal cancer. *Oral Maxillofac Surg Clin North Am.* 2019;31(1):1–11.
115. National Cancer Institute. Surveillance, Epidemiology and End Results Program: *Cancer Stat Facts: Lung and Bronchus Cancer.* Available at: https://seer.cancer.gov/statfacts/html/lungb.html. Accessed February 2, 2022.
116. Nasim F, Sabath BF, Eapen GA. Lung cancer. *Med Clin North Am.* 2019;103(3):463–473.
117. Konig D, Prince SS, Rothschild SI. Targeted therapy in advanced and metastatic non-small cell lung cancer. An update on treatment of the most important actionable oncogenic driver alterations. *Cancers.* 2021;13:804.
118. Mustachio LM, Roszik J. Current targeted therapies for the fight against non-small cell lung cancer. *Pharmaceuticals.* 2020;13:374.
119. Metovic J, et al. Morphologic and molecular classification of lung neuroendocrine neoplasms. *Virchows Archiv.* 2021;478:5–19.
120. Beasley MB, Galateau-Salle F, Dacic S. Pleural mesothelioma classification update. *Virchows Archiv.* 2021;478(1):59–72.
121. Nasser A, et al. Three decades of malignant pleural mesothelioma: an Academic Centre experience. *Clin Lung Cancer.* 2021;22(5)441-448.
122. Uprety D. CheckMate 743: a glimmer of hope for malignant pleural mesothelioma. *Clin Lung Cancer.* 2021;22(2):71–73.
123. American Lung Association: *Health effects of smoking.* Last updated July 13, 2020. Available at: https://www.lung.org/quit-smoking/smoking-facts/health-effects/smoking. Accessed February 2, 2022.
124. US Preventive Task Force Screening for lung cancer: US Preventive Services Task Force Recommendation Statement. *JAMA.* 2021;325(10):962–970. 2021.
125. Detterbeck FC, et al. The IASLC lung cancer staging project: methodology and validation used in the development of proposals for revision of the stage classification of NSCLC in the forthcoming (eighth) edition of the TNM classification of lung cancer. *J Thorac Oncol.* 2016;11:1433–1446.
126. Bissonnette JP, et al. Non-small cell lung cancer stage migration as a function of wait times from diagnostic imaging: a pooled analysis from five international centres. *Lung Cancer.* 2021;155:136–143.
127. Handa Y, et al. Surgical procedure selection for stage I lung cancer: complex segmentectomy versus resection. *Clin Lung Cancer.* 2021;22(2):e224–e233.
128. Chen R, et al. Emerging therapeutic agents for advanced non-small cell lung cancer. *J Hematol Oncol.* 2020;13:58.
129. Montenegro GB, Farid S, Liu SV. Immunotherapy in lung cancer. *J Surg Oncol.* 2021;123:718–729.

36

Alterations of Pulmonary Function in Children

Valentina L. Brashers

http://evolve.elsevier.com/Rogers/pathophysiology/

CHAPTER OUTLINE

Alterations of respiratory function in children are influenced by physiologic development, which is determined by age, genetics, and environmental conditions. Infants, especially premature infants, are particularly vulnerable to a variety of respiratory disorders because of incomplete development of the airways, circulation, chest wall, and immune system. A variety of upper and lower airway infections can cause respiratory compromise or play a role in the pathogenesis of more chronic pulmonary disease. Pulmonary dysfunction can be categorized into disorders of either the upper or the lower airways.

DISORDERS OF THE UPPER AIRWAYS

Disorders of the upper airways can cause significant obstruction to airflow. Common causes of upper airway obstruction (UAO) in children are infections, foreign body aspiration, and obstructive sleep apnea. Congenital malformations, such as laryngomalacia and subglottic stenosis, may occur but are a less common cause of UAO.

Infections of the Upper Airways

Table 36.1 compares some of the more common upper airway infections.

Croup

Croup illnesses are all characterized by obstruction of the upper airways. The two most common croup illnesses are viral croup and recurrent croup (spasmodic croup). Diphtheria can be considered a croup illness but is now rare because of vaccinations.

Viral croup is an acute *laryngotracheobronchitis* and almost always occurs in children between 6 months and 3 years of age with a peak incidence at 2 years of age.[1] It most commonly is caused by parainfluenza. Other causes include respiratory syncytial virus (RSV), rhinovirus, adenovirus, rubella virus, or atypical bacteria. SARS-CoV-2 infection has been diagnosed in several children with croup.[2] The incidence of croup is higher in males, with higher incidence during the winter months. Recurrent (spasmodic) croup is two or more episodes of symptoms similar to viral croup, except without symptoms of respiratory tract infection. It usually occurs in older children. The etiology is unknown, but it can be associated with underlying congenital obstruction or airway narrowing, gastroesophageal reflux, and allergies.

Pathophysiology. The pathophysiology of viral croup is the result of subglottic (the area containing the vocal cords) inflammation and edema from the infection. The mucous membranes of the larynx are tightly adherent to the underlying cartilage, whereas those of the subglottic space are looser and thus allow accumulation of mucosal and submucosal edema (Fig. 36.1). The cricoid cartilage is structurally the narrowest point of the airway, making edema in this area critical to the development of airway obstruction. Recurrent croup also causes obstruction but with less inflammation and edema. As illustrated in Algorithm 36.1, increased resistance to airflow leads to increased work of breathing, which generates more negative intrathoracic pressure that, in turn, may exacerbate dynamic collapse of the upper airway.

Clinical Manifestations. Typically, a child with viral croup experiences rhinorrhea (runny nose), sore throat, and low-grade fever for a few days and then develops a harsh (seal-like), barking

TABLE 36.1 Comparison of Upper Airway Infections

Condition	Age	Onset	Etiology	Pathophysiology	Symptoms
Viral Croup (acute laryngotracheobronchitis)	6 months to 3 years	Usually gradual following a viral prodrome	Viral (e.g., parainfluenza, respiratory syncytial virus)	Inflammation from larynx to bronchi	Harsh cough; stridor; low-grade fever; may have nasal discharge, conjunctivitis; symptoms last 2–7 days
Spasmodic Croup	6 months to 5 years	Abrupt with absence of prodrome	Airway narrowing, gastroesophageal reflux, allergies	Noninflammatory edema of the larynx	Abrupt onset of cough and stridor without fever or viral symptoms; symptoms last 2–4 h then recur.
Bacterial tracheitis	1–12 years	Abrupt or after viral illness	*Staphylococcus aureus*/ methicillin resistant *S. aureus* (MRSA) *Haemophilus influenzae* type B Group A streptococci	Inflammation and edema of upper trachea, pseudomembrane formation	High fever; tachypnea, toxic appearance; harsh cough; purulent secretions
Acute epiglottitis	2–6 years; also in adults with a mean age of 45 years	Abrupt	*Streptococcus pneumoniae, Staphylococcus aureus, Moraxella*	Inflammation of supraglottic structures	Severe sore throat; high fever; stridor, toxic appearance; muffled voice; may drool; sits erect or leans forward
Peritonsillar abscess	>9 years	May be abrupt	S. pyogenes S. aureus/MRSA	Abscess within or around tonsil	Fever, malaise trismus (locked jaw), drooling, muffled voice

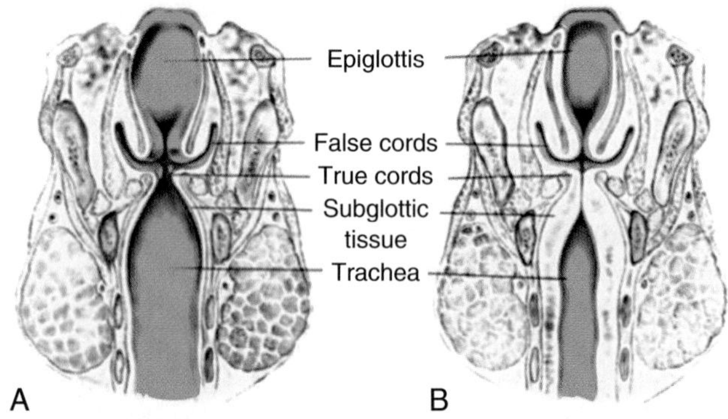

Fig. 36.1 The Larynx and Subglottic Trachea. (A) Normal epiglottis, laryngeal vocal cords, and trachea. **(B)** Narrowing and obstruction of laryngeal tissue around false and true vocal cords from edema caused by croup. (From Hockenberry MJ, Wilson D. *Wong's nursing care of infants and children.* 10th edition, St. Louis: Mosby; 2015.)

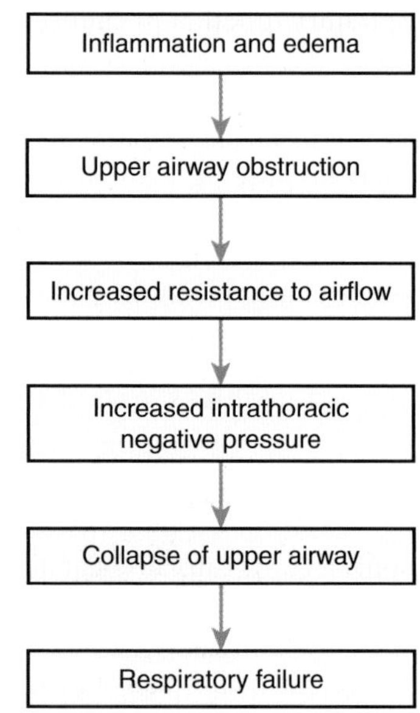

Algorithm 36.1 Upper Airway Obstruction With Croup.

cough, a hoarse voice, and inspiratory stridor (a harsh, vibratory sound). The quality of the voice, cough, and stridor may suggest the location of the obstruction (Fig. 36.2). Most cases resolve spontaneously within 24 to 48 hours. A young child with severe croup usually displays deep retractions (Fig. 36.3), agitation, tachycardia, and sometimes pallor or cyanosis.

Recurrent croup is characterized by a similar hoarseness, barking cough, and stridor. It is of sudden onset and usually occurs at night and without prodromal symptoms. It usually resolves quickly.

Evaluation and Treatment. The degree of symptoms determines the level of treatment. The most common tool for estimating croup severity is the Westley Croup Score.[3] Few cases require hospitalization, and most children with croup receive outpatient evaluation and management. These children usually have only mild stridor and appear alert, playful, and able to eat.

The mainstay of treatment for croup is oral or inhaled glucocorticoids which have been shown to reduce symptoms and shorten hospital stays.[4] The presence of stridor at rest, moderate or severe retractions of the chest, or agitation suggests severe disease and requires inpatient observation and treatment. For acute respiratory distress, nebulized epinephrine stimulates α- and β-adrenergic receptors promoting vasoconstriction, bronchodilation, and decreasing mucosal edema

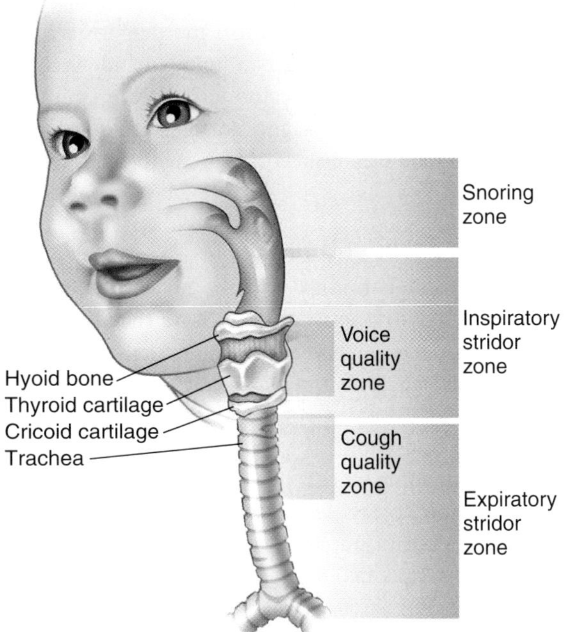

Fig. 36.2 Listening Can Help Locate the Site of Airway Obstruction. A loud, gasping snore suggests enlarged tonsils or adenoids. In inspiratory stridor, the airway is compromised at the level of the supraglottic larynx, subglottic region and vocal cords which are behind the thyroid cartilage, or upper trachea. Expiratory stridor results from a narrowing or collapse in the trachea or bronchi. Airway noise during both inspiration and expiration often represents a fixed obstruction of the vocal cords or subglottic space. Hoarseness or a weak cry is a by-product of obstruction at the vocal cords. If a cough is croupy, suspect constriction below the vocal cords. (Redrawn from Eavey RD. *Contemporary pediatrics*, 1986;3(6):79; original illustration by Paul Singh-Roy.)

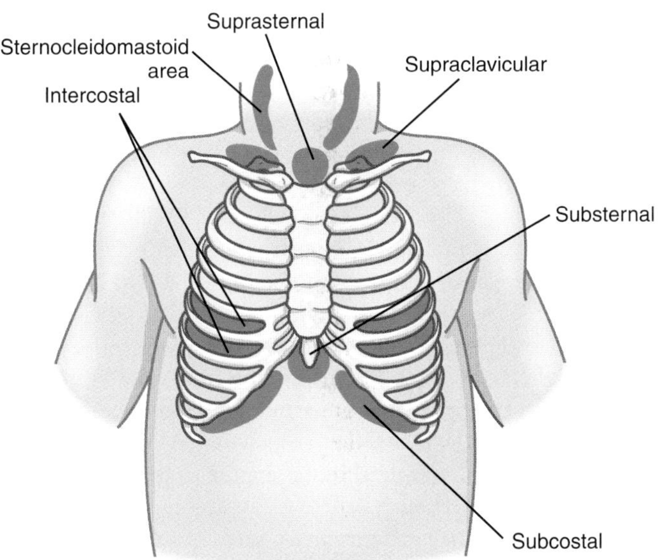

Fig. 36.3 Areas of Chest Muscle Retraction.

and airway secretions. Heliox (a helium-oxygen mixture) can be used in severe cases. This works by minimizing air flow resistance in the narrowed airway and decreases the work of breathing. In rare cases, croup may require placement of an endotracheal tube.

Bacterial Tracheitis

Bacterial tracheitis (pseudomembranous croup) is a relatively rare but potentially life-threatening condition with an estimated incidence of 0.1 cases per 100,000 children.[5] Most cases occur in children 6 years old or younger and follow a viral respiratory illness (influenza or parainfluenza). Bacterial tracheitis is caused most often by *Staphylococcus aureus* (including methicillin-resistant *S. aureus* [MRSA] strains), *Streptococcus pyogenes, Moraxella catarrhalis, Haemophilus influenzae*, or group A beta-hemolytic *Streptococcus* (GABHS).[5] Bacterial infection causes airway edema and copious purulent secretions which lead to airway obstruction that can be worsened by the formation of a tracheal pseudomembrane and mucosal sloughing. The acute clinical presentation usually includes tachypnea, stridor, hoarse voice, fever, cough, and/or increased secretions from the nose or mouth. Bacterial tracheitis is treated with immediate administration of antibiotics and may require emergent endotracheal intubation to prevent total UAO.

Acute Epiglottitis

Historically, acute epiglottitis was a disease mostly affecting children between the ages of 2 and 6 years of age and caused by *H. influenzae* type B (HiB). Since the advent of the *H. influenzae* vaccine, the overall incidence of acute epiglottitis has decreased significantly and it is increasingly an infectious disease of adults. Most cases are now caused by *Streptococcus pneumoniae, S. aureus*, and *Moraxella lacunata*.[6]

Pathophysiology. The epiglottis arises from the posterior tongue base and covers the laryngeal inlet during swallowing (see Fig. 36.1). Bacterial invasion of the mucosa with associated inflammation leads to the rapid development of edema, causing severe, life-threatening obstruction of the upper airway.

Clinical Manifestations. In the classic form of the disease, there is the sudden development of high fever, irritability, sore throat, inspiratory stridor, and severe respiratory distress. The affected individual appears anxious and has a voice that sounds muffled ("hot potato voice"). Drooling, absence of cough, a preference to sit, and dysphagia (inability to swallow) are common. In addition to appearing ill, the individual may adopt a position of leaning forward (tripoding) to try to improve breathing. Death can occur in a few hours. Pneumonia, cervical lymph node inflammation, otitis, and, rarely, meningitis or septic arthritis may occur during the course of epiglottitis.

Evaluation and Treatment. Acute epiglottitis is a life-threatening emergency. Efforts should be made to keep the individual calm and undisturbed. Physical examination of the throat should not be attempted because it may trigger laryngospasm and cause respiratory collapse. Soft tissue x-rays of the neck may reveal a widening of the epiglottis, although direct laryngoscopy is the gold standard for diagnosis.[6] With severe airway obstruction, the airway may be secured with intubation or emergency tracheotomy. The prompt administration of broad-spectrum antibiotics is indicated, and corticosteroids may be considered, although this remains controversial. Resolution with treatment is usually rapid.

Tonsillar Infections

Tonsillar infections (tonsillitis) are occasionally severe enough to cause UAO. Viral infections, such as infectious mononucleosis, are the most common cause of tonsillitis, although there continue to be significant numbers of cases of tonsillitis secondary to group A beta-hemolytic streptococcal and MRSA infection. Inflammation of the tonsils is associated with the release of numerous inflammatory cytokines, T lymphocyte activation, and tonsillar hypertrophy.[7] Significant swelling of the tonsils and pharynx occurs, and a tenacious membrane may cover the mucosa. The development of significant airway obstruction in tonsillar infections may require the use of corticosteroids, especially in the case of mononucleosis. The management of severe bacterial tonsillitis requires the use of antibiotics. Some children with recurrent tonsillitis benefit from tonsillectomy or adenotonsillectomy. Guidelines published in 2019 provide detailed information about indications for surgery and appropriate pre, intra, and postoperative care.[8] Recurrent and chronic tonsillitis along with persistent tonsillar hypertrophy may occur and may be related to changes in the tonsillar microbiome.[9]

Peritonsillar abscess is a collection of pus between the tonsillar capsule and the pharyngeal constrictor muscle (Fig. 36.4). It is usually unilateral and is most often a complication of acute tonsillitis that occurs when bacteria spread to the peritonsillar space via the salivary duct system.[10] These infections are often polymicrobial.[6] The mean age of onset is 12 years of age.[11] Abscesses can contribute to UAO, and descending mediastinitis, necrotizing fasciitis, and jugular vein obstruction may occur (see Table 36.1).[10] Symptoms in children include fever, sore throat, dysphagia, trismus, pooling of saliva, and muffled voice. Peritonsillar bulging and cervical adenopathy on the same side are usually visible. Intraoral ultrasound or computed tomography (CT) is used to confirm the diagnosis.[12] Surgical management is usually indicated and may include incision and drainage of the abscess, tonsillectomy, or needle aspiration followed by empiric antibiotics and corticosteroids.[6] Death can occur from spontaneous abscess rupture with aspiration or airway obstruction.

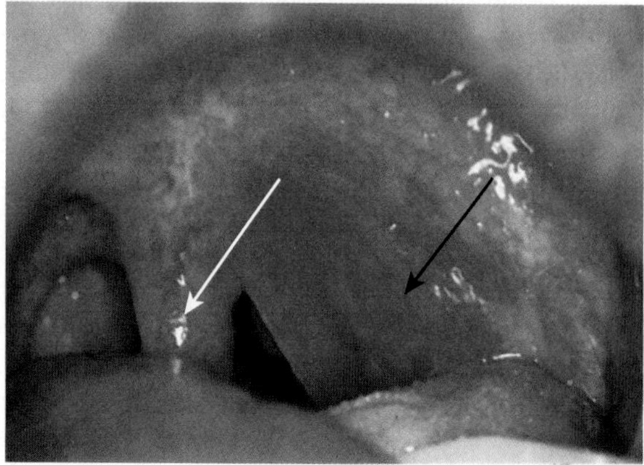

Fig. 36.4 Peritonsillar Abscess. If the tonsils are inflamed and appear asymmetrical with unilateral palatal swelling *(black arrow)* and uvular deviation *(white arrow)*, a peritonsillar abscess should be suspected. (From Goldman L, Schafer AI. *Goldman's Cecil medicine*, 24th edition. Philadelphia: Saunders; 2012.)

Aspiration of Foreign Bodies

Aspiration of foreign bodies into the airways is most common in children 1 to 4 years of age. More than 100,000 cases and 100 deaths occur each year.[13] Risk factors include age, sex, tracheobronchial anatomy, and external setting (e.g., age and type of guardian, urban vs rural residence, presence of other children in the household).[14] Most objects are expelled by the cough reflex, but some objects may lodge in the larynx, trachea, or bronchi. Large objects (e.g., hard candy, a bite of hot dog, nuts, seeds, popcorn, grapes, beans, toy pieces, fragments of popped balloons, or coins) may occlude the airway and become life-threatening (Fig. 36.5). Foreign bodies lodged in the larynx or upper trachea cause cough, stridor, hoarseness or inability to speak, respiratory distress, and agitation or panic.[15] With smaller objects, the aspiration event often is not witnessed or is not recognized when it happens because the coughing, choking, or gagging symptoms may resolve quickly.

If the child is acutely hypoxic and unable to move air, immediate action, such as sweeping the oral airway or performing abdominal thrusts (formerly called the *Heimlich maneuver*), may be required to prevent death. Otherwise, bronchoscopic removal should be performed urgently. If an aspirated foreign body is small enough, it will be transferred to a bronchus before becoming lodged. If the foreign body is lodged in the airway for a longer period of time, local irritation, granulation, obstruction, and infection will ensue. Thus, children may present with cough or wheezing, atelectasis, pneumonia, lung abscess, or blood-streaked sputum. Occult foreign body aspiration should be considered in children with chronic or recurrent respiratory diseases that are poorly explained, even in the absence of a previous history of aspiration.[16] These children are treated by prompt bronchoscopic removal of the object and administration of antibiotics as necessary.

Obstructive Sleep Apnea

Pediatric obstructive sleep apnea syndrome (OSAS) (also called obstructive sleep apnea or sleep-disordered breathing) results from partial or complete UAO obstruction that occurs during sleep with associated snoring, labored or obstructed breathing, and disrupted sleep patterns. Pediatric OSAS has an estimated prevalence of 1% to 5% and can occur at any age.[17] The prevalence is higher in obese children, as well as in vulnerable populations (Blacks, Hispanics, and preterm infants), and there may be a family history of OSAS. Other risk factors include adenotonsillar hypertrophy, allergic rhinitis, craniofacial abnormalities, and genetic disorders such as Down Syndrome. Possible influences early in life may include environmental smoke inhalation and socioeconomic status, together with genetic modifiers that promote airway inflammation.

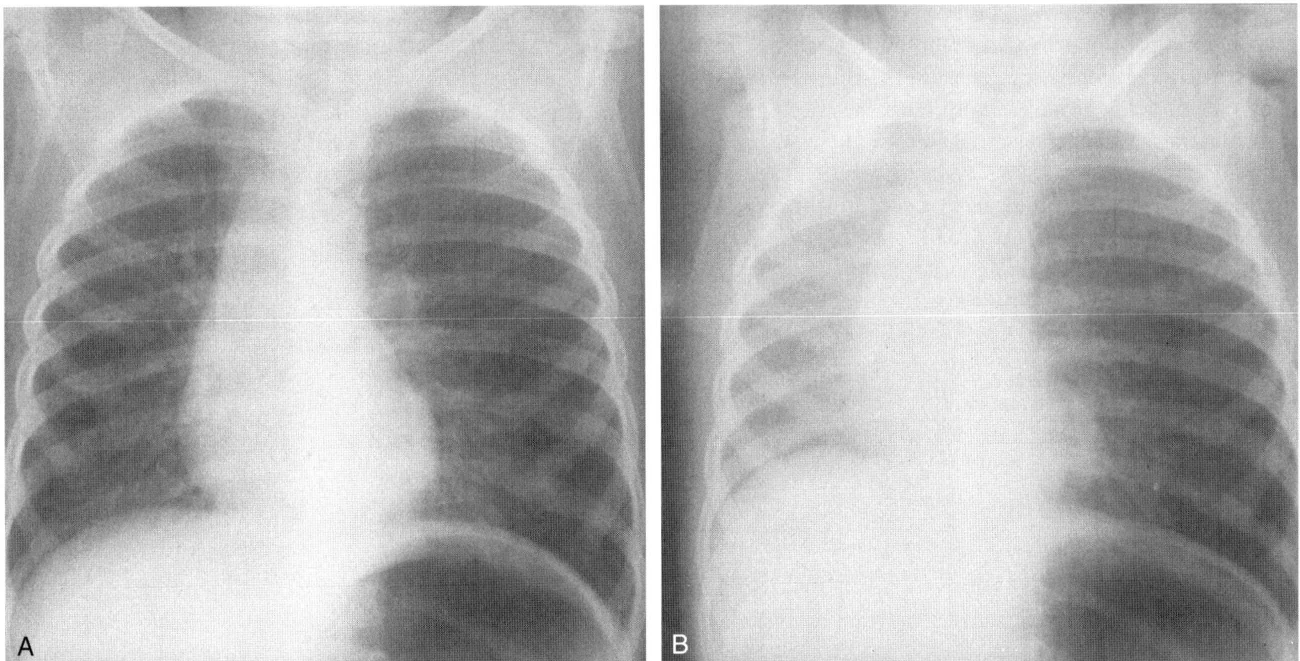

Fig. 36.5 Foreign Body Aspiration. Anteroposterior inspiratory (A) and expiratory (B) chest radiographs. Air trapping in the left lung is caused by a peanut in the left mainstem bronchus. (From Taussig LM, Landau LI. *Pediatric respiratory medicine*, 2nd edition. St. Louis: Mosby; 2008.)

Pathophysiology. Airway narrowing (adenotonsillar hypertrophy, craniofacial anomalies), increased upper airway collapsibility (obesity, neurologic disorders, Down syndrome), and airway inflammation (gastroesophageal reflux, asthma, allergy) are the common causes of OSAS. Airway obstruction can be partial or complete and is associated with atypical sleep patterns.[18] Obstruction of the upper airway during sleep results in cyclic episodes of increasing respiratory effort and changes in intrathoracic pressures with oxygen desaturation, hypercapnia, and arousal. The child goes back to sleep, and the cycle repeats. Infants are at risk because they have both anatomic and physiologic predispositions toward airway obstruction and gas exchange abnormalities.

Clinical Manifestations. Common manifestations of OSAS include snoring and labored breathing, sweating, and restlessness during sleep, which may be continuous or intermittent. There may be episodes of increased respiratory effort but no audible airflow, often terminated by snorting, gasping, repositioning, or arousal. Daytime sleepiness/napping is occasionally reported, as well as nocturnal enuresis. Cognitive and neurobehavioral impairment, excessive daytime sleepiness, impaired school performance, and poor quality of life are consequences of OSAS.

Evaluation and Treatment. The American Academy of Pediatrics guidelines for the diagnosis and treatment of OSAS recommend that all children should be screened for snoring.[19] Definitive evaluation is conducted using a polysomnographic sleep study. Imaging of the upper airway, including neck x-ray, CT, and magnetic resonance imaging (MRI), may be used to rule out tonsillar enlargement or upper airway narrowing.[20] If obstructive sleep apnea is caused by tonsillar enlargement, children most often are referred for tonsillectomy and adenoidectomy (T&A). For severely affected children who do not respond to T&A or who have different problems (e.g., obesity), the use of positive airway pressure (PAP) can improve symptoms and help prevent complications.[21] Anti-inflammatories, dental treatments, and weight loss can be considered.[19] Treatment is important to minimize associated morbidities such as hypertension, cardiovascular disease, learning difficulties, and behavioral issues.[18,22]

DISORDERS OF THE LOWER AIRWAYS

Lower airway disease is one of the leading causes of morbidity in the first year of life and continues to be an important component of other illnesses progressing into childhood. Pulmonary disorders commonly observed include disorders of prematurity, infections, aspiration pneumonitis, asthma, acute respiratory distress syndrome (ARDS), and cystic fibrosis.

Disorders of Prematurity

Surfactant Deficiency Disorder (Respiratory Distress Syndrome of the Newborn)

Surfactant deficiency disorder (SDD), also known as respiratory distress syndrome (RDS) of the newborn, is a significant cause of neonatal morbidity and mortality. It occurs almost exclusively in premature infants because the immature lung has not yet developed adequate surfactant production. SDD (RDS) occurs in most infants born before 28 weeks of pregnancy, and 50% to 60% of infants born at 29 weeks' gestation. Risk factors include prematurity, low birth weight, male sex, a sibling with SDD, cesarean delivery without labor, multiple pregnancy, diabetic mother, and perinatal asphyxia. The incidence has increased in the United States over the past two decades; however, death rates have declined since the introduction of antenatal steroid therapy and postnatal surfactant therapy.[23] In rare cases, SSD occurs in full-term neonates as the result of mutations in genes that control surfactant synthesis (*SFTPA1, SFTPA2, SFTPB, SFTPC, ABCA3, NKX2-1*).[24]

Pathophysiology. SDD (RDS) is caused by surfactant deficiency. Surfactant is a lipoprotein with a detergent-like effect that separates the liquid molecules inside the alveoli, thereby decreasing alveolar surface tension. Without surfactant, alveoli collapse at the end of each exhalation, decreasing the alveolar surface area available for gas exchange. Surfactant normally is not secreted by the alveolar cells until approximately 20 to 24 weeks' gestation (Fig. 36.6). Premature infants also are born

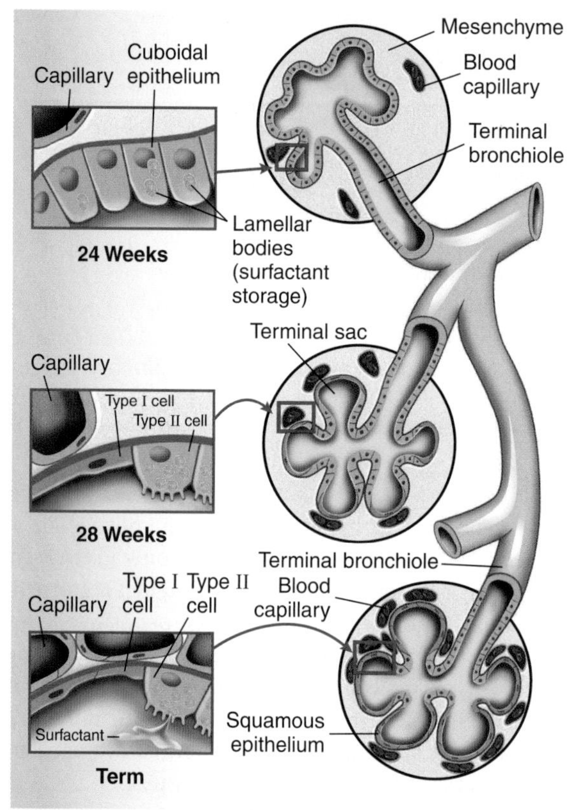

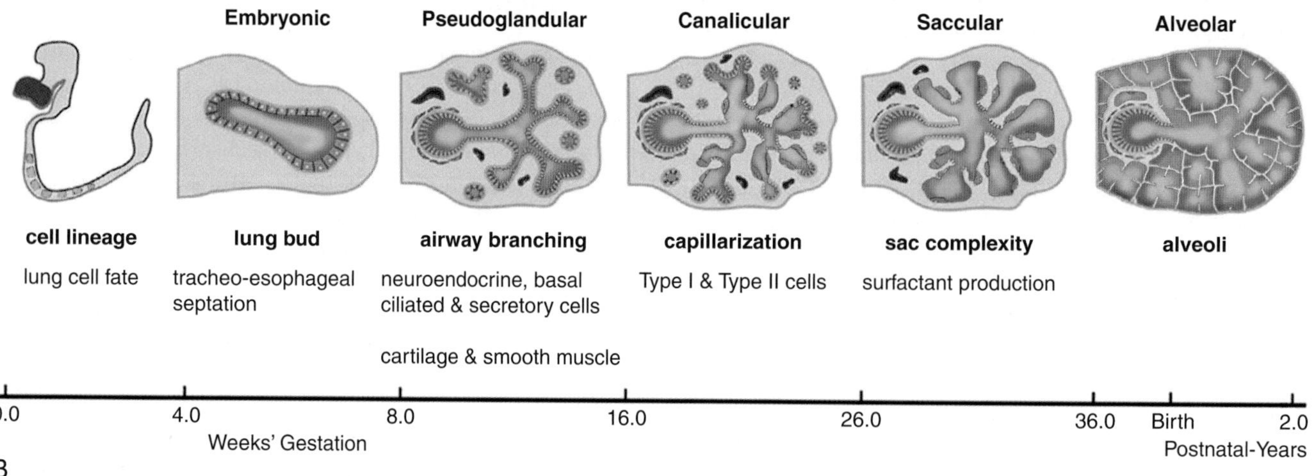

Fig. 36.6 Prenatal Development of the Alveolar Unit. **(A)** Epithelial cells differentiate into type II and type I cells. Mature type II cells (type II pneumocytes) store and secrete surfactant. Type I cells are derived from type II cells and consist of flattened epithelium overlying capillaries, thus forming part of the thin air-blood gas exchange membrane of the alveoli. **(B)** Time line for gestational development of alveoli.

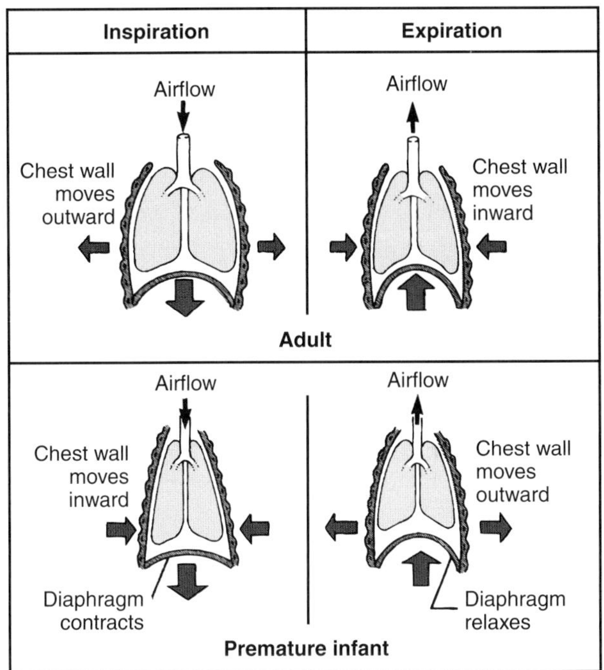

Fig. 36.7 Developmental Differences in the Chest Wall and Lung Mechanics. Differences in lung mechanics caused by differences in chest wall compliance (degree of rigidity) in premature infants and adults. (*Arrows* indicate direction of airflow, chest wall movement, and diaphragm movement.)

with underdeveloped and small alveoli that are difficult to inflate and have thick walls and inadequate capillary blood supply such that gas exchange is significantly impaired. The net effect is *atelectasis* (collapsed alveoli), resulting in hypoxemia. Atelectasis is difficult for the neonate to overcome because it requires a significant amount of work to open the alveoli with each breath. The infant's chest wall is weak and highly compliant and, thus, the rib cage tends to collapse inward with increased respiratory effort (Fig. 36.7). Increased work of breathing may result in hypercapnia. Hypoxia and hypercapnia cause pulmonary vasoconstriction, which increases intrapulmonary resistance and pulmonary hypoperfusion. Increased pulmonary vascular resistance may cause a partial return to fetal circulation, with right-to-left shunting of blood through the ductus arteriosus and foramen ovale (see Chapter 33). Inadequate perfusion of tissues and hypoxemia contribute to metabolic acidosis.

Many premature infants with SDD (RDS) will require mechanical ventilation, which is lifesaving, but damages the alveolar epithelium, leading to leakage of plasma proteins into the alveoli. These proteins result in fibrin deposits in the air spaces, which create the appearance of *hyaline membranes* (transparent or glassy appearance on microscopic examination) and contribute to the inactivation of any surfactant that may be present. The pathogenesis of SDD (RDS) is summarized in Algorithm 36.2.

Clinical Manifestations. Signs of SDD (RDS) appear within minutes of birth and include tachypnea (respiratory rate greater than 60 breaths/min), expiratory grunting, intercostal and subcostal, nasal flaring, and cyanosis. A characteristic chest x-ray appearance and hypoxemia that is refractory to the administration of supplemental oxygen are hallmarks of the condition. The severity tends to increase over the first hours of life. Apnea and irregular respirations occur as the infant tires. Clinical manifestations reach a peak within 3 days.

Evaluation and Treatment. The diagnosis is made on the basis of premature birth or other risk factors, chest radiographs, pulse oximetry measurements, and, if needed, analysis of amniotic fluid or tracheal aspirates to estimate lung maturity. For women at risk of preterm birth, antenatal treatment with glucocorticoids induces a significant and rapid acceleration of lung maturation and stimulation of surfactant production in the fetus and significantly reduces the incidence of SDD (RDS) and death.[23] The ultimate prevention for SDD (RDS) would be the prevention of premature birth.

Administration of exogenous surfactant (either synthetic or natural) within 15 to 30 minutes of birth is recommended as a prophylactic or preventive treatment for infants weighing between 500 g (1 lbs 1.65 oz) and 2000 g (4 lbs 6.5 oz). A thin catheter, nebulizer, or continuous positive airway pressure (CPAP) ventilation is used for administration. There is usually a dramatic improvement in oxygenation, as well as a decreased incidence of death, pneumothorax, and pulmonary interstitial emphysema from SDD (RDS).[25,26]

Supportive care includes oxygen administration and often such measures as mechanical ventilation. Mechanical ventilation can result in a proinflammatory state that may contribute to the development of chronic lung disease, such as bronchopulmonary dysplasia. Strategies that are lung protective include greater reliance on nasal CPAP, permissive hypercapnia, lower oxygen saturation targets, modulation of tidal volume (V_t) settings, and use of high-frequency oscillation.[27] Most infants survive SDD (RDS), and, in many cases, recovery may be complete within 10 to 14 days. However, the incidence of subsequent bronchopulmonary dysplasia is significant among very low birth weight infants.

Bronchopulmonary Dysplasia

Bronchopulmonary dysplasia (BPD), also known as *chronic lung disease of prematurity*, is a chronic, inflammatory lung disease associated with arrested pulmonary development and a need for supplemental oxygen. A National Institutes of Health (NIH) consensus definition published in 2001 described BPD as occurring in infants born at less than 32 weeks with the requirement of supplemental oxygen for at least 28 days and at 36 weeks postmenstrual age (PMA).[28] The definition also includes a graded severity determination that is dependent on required respiratory support at term (mild, moderate, and severe, based on oxygen requirements and ventilatory needs). A new consensus definition is being developed that includes the following criteria: (1) less than 32 weeks' gestational age, (2) persistent parenchymal lung disease, (3) radiographic confirmation of parenchymal lung disease, and (4) at 36 weeks PMA requires supplemental oxygen for at least 3 consecutive days to maintain arterial oxygen saturation in the 90% to 95% range.[29]

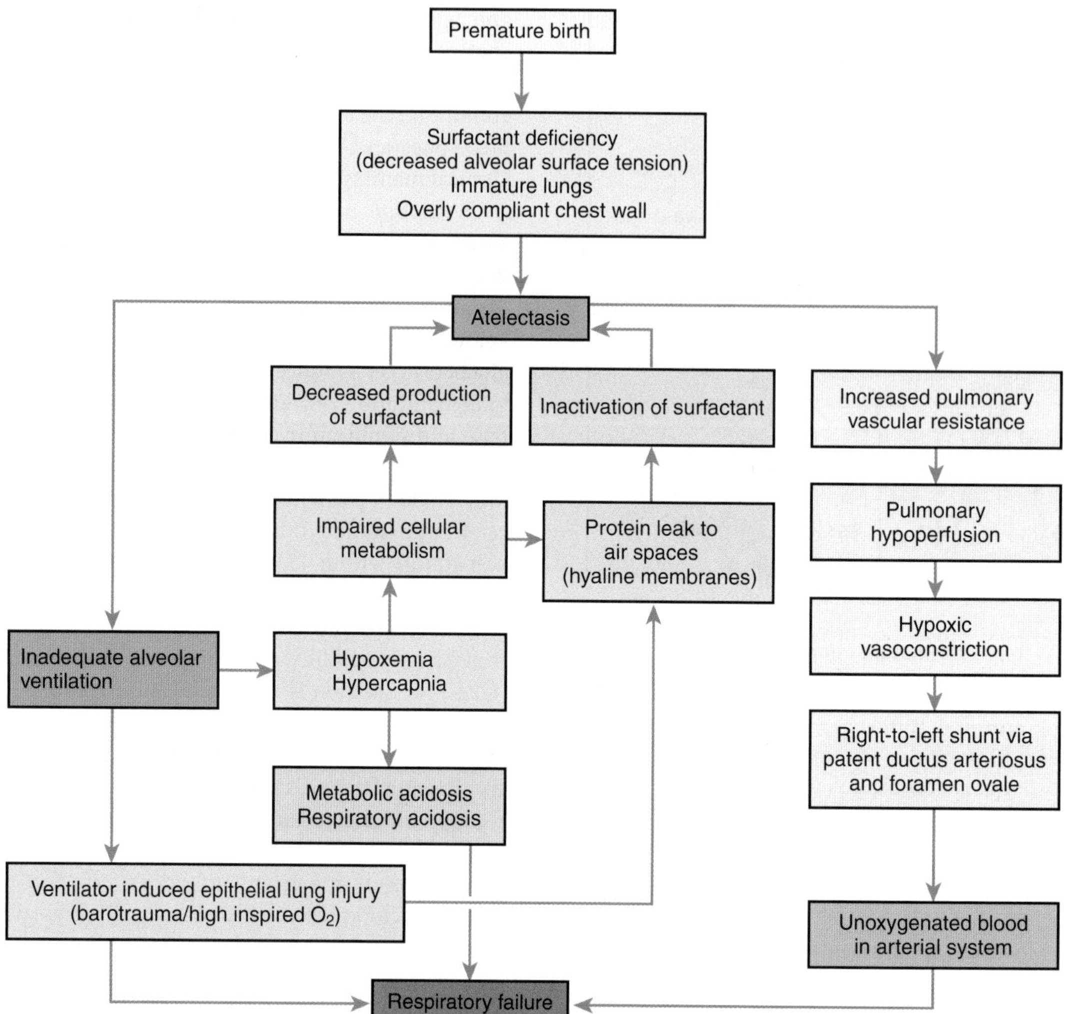

Algorithm 36.2 Pathogenesis of Surfactant Deficiency Disorder (Respiratory Distress Syndrome of the Newborn). *O_2*, Oxygen.

BPD is the major cause of chronic pulmonary disease associated with premature birth.[30] It occurs most commonly in infants with severe SDD (RDS) who require prolonged perinatal supplemental oxygen (at least 28 days) and positive pressure ventilation. Each year in the United States, BPD affects about 45% of infants born extremely preterm.[31]

The widespread use of antenatal glucocorticoids and postnatal surfactant has lessened the incidence and severity of SDD (RDS) and BPD. BPD now is occurring primarily in the smallest premature infants (23 to 28 weeks' gestation) who have received mechanical ventilation or those with other complicating risks. Maternal factors such as preeclampsia, placental dysfunction, and smoking are associated with a higher incidence of BPD.[32] Risk factors for BPD are summarized in *Risk Factors:* Bronchopulmonary Dysplasia.

Pathophysiology. Lung immaturity and inflammation contribute to the development of BPD. *Classic BPD* is characterized by airway injury, inflammation, and parenchymal fibrosis. With the initiation of surfactant therapy, what is called the *new BPD* is a form of arrested lung development that results from an aberrant repair response to antenatal and postnatal lung injury.[31] There is poor formation of the airway epithelium, alveolar structure, and

RISK FACTORS

Bronchopulmonary Dysplasia

- Maternal Factors
  - Placental insufficiency
  - Lack of antenatal steroids
  - Infection
  - Smoking
- Infant Predisposition
  - Premature birth (especially ≤28 weeks)
  - Genetic susceptibility
  - Male sex
  - Race
  - Altered microbiome
  - Sepsis
- Mechanical Ventilation
  - Volutrauma
  - Barotrauma
  - Atelectotrauma
- Supplemental oxygen administration
  - DNA damage
  - Lipid peroxidation
  - Protein oxidation

Data fromSahni and Bhandari.[33]

a decreased surface area for gas exchange. Abnormal bronchoalveolar attachments, imbalances in neural pathways, changes in smooth muscle mass, and airway hyperreactivity contribute to the pathogenesis of BPD.[34] Levels of proinflammatory cytokines, such as tumor necrosis factor-alpha (TNF-α), interleukin-1β (IL-1β), interleukin 6 (IL-6), and interleukin 8 (IL-8), are all elevated in the amniotic fluid or tracheal aspirates, or both, of preterm infants who later develop BPD. Inflammation invites neutrophils and macrophages to release reactive oxygen species and proteolytic enzymes, initiating oxidative and immune injury.[30] Other important mediators include growth factors such as insulin-like growth factor-1 and vascular endothelial growth factor, along with other profibrotic and angiogenic cytokines which contribute to lung damage and pulmonary hypertension.[30] Algorithm 36.3 illustrates the pathophysiology of BPD. Persistent inflammation contributes to airway epithelial injury, pulmonary capillary fibrosis, perfusion mismatch, pulmonary hypertension, and decreased exercise capacity.[35]

Clinical Manifestations. Clinically, the infant exhibits hypoxemia and hypercapnia caused by ventilation-perfusion mismatch and diffusion defects. The work of breathing increases, and the ability to feed may be impaired. Intermittent bronchospasm, mucus plugging, and pulmonary hypertension characterize the clinical course. In the most severely affected infants, dusky spells may occur with agitation, feeding, or gastroesophageal reflux. Infants with mild BPD may demonstrate only mild tachypnea and difficulty handling respiratory tract infections.

Evaluation and Treatment. An online risk estimator for BPD development has been created to help with early identification and management.[36] Chest x-ray and echocardiography are used to rule out other causes of respiratory distress. Infants with severe BPD require prolonged assisted ventilation with nasal CPAP or nasal intermittent positive pressure ventilation (IPPV). Diuretics are used to control pulmonary edema. Bronchodilators reduce airway resistance. Low dose systemic or inhaled corticosteroids improve respiratory function and reduce mortality, but dexamethasone is associated with an increased risk for neurologic and infectious complications.[37] Caffeine citrate administration to premature neonates within 2 days of birth reduces the risk for BPD as well as some cardiac and neurodevelopmental disorders. Vitamin A supplementation (necessary for normal lung development), and careful fluid and nutritional support are routinely used and have resulted in improved outcomes. Stem cell-based therapies and administration of growth factors are in clinical trials.[33] Children with BPD should be monitored into adulthood for the development of chronic lung disease.

Respiratory Tract Infections

Respiratory tract infections are common in children and are a frequent cause for emergency department visits and

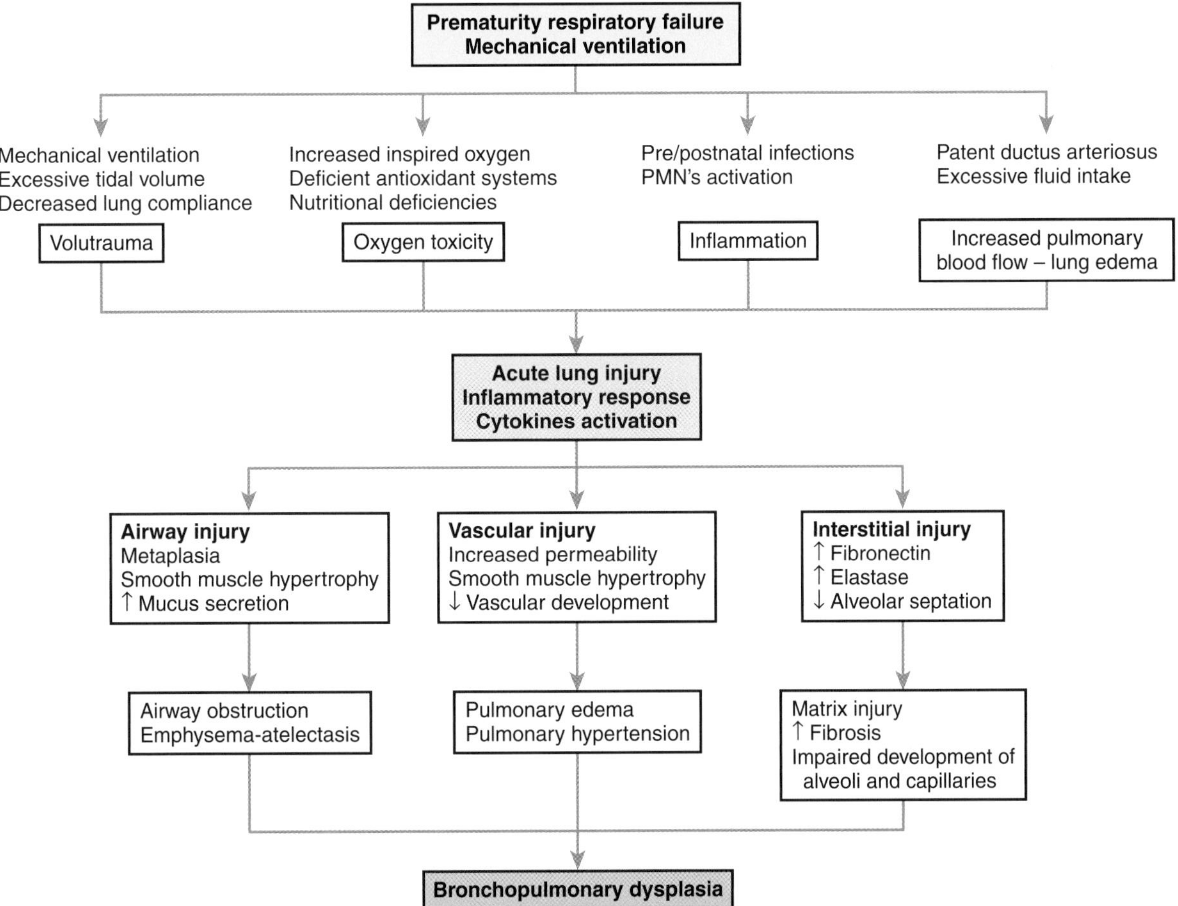

Algorithm 36.3 Pathophysiology of Bronchopulmonary Dysplasia. *PMN,* Polymorphonuclear neutrophil.

hospitalizations. The clinical presentation, child's age, season of the year, and environmental exposures can often provide clues to the etiologic agent, even when the agent cannot be proved.

Bronchiolitis

Bronchiolitis is the most common viral respiratory tract infection of the small airways that occurs almost exclusively in children younger than 2 years. It is the leading cause of hospitalization for infants during the winter season. The most common pathogen is respiratory syncytial virus (RSV), but bronchiolitis also may be caused by rhinovirus, adenovirus, influenza, parainfluenza virus, human metapneumovirus, and human bocavirus. Air pollution and cigarette smoke are linked to an increased risk for bronchiolitis. Healthy infants usually make a full recovery from RSV bronchiolitis, but infants who were premature (birth weight less than 2500 g) or who have underlying BPD, heart disease, or immune deficiency have a higher risk for a more severe or even deadly course.[38] Bronchiolitis has been linked to an increased risk for asthma later in childhood, particularly in those with a family history of asthma. Children who develop severe bronchiolitis and are found to have persistent RSV infection weeks after hospitalization are at greatest risk for recurrent wheezing and asthma by age 3 years.[39]

Pathophysiology. Viral infection causes necrosis of the bronchial epithelium and destruction of ciliated epithelial cells. There is infiltration with lymphocytes around the bronchioles and a cell-mediated hypersensitivity to viral antigens with the release of lymphokines causing inflammation, as well as activation of eosinophils, neutrophils, and monocytes.[40] The submucosa becomes edematous, and cellular debris and fibrin form plugs within the bronchioles. Edema of the bronchiolar wall, accumulation of mucus and cellular debris, and bronchospasm narrow many peripheral airways. Atelectasis occurs in some areas of the lung and hyperinflation in others. Airways become partially or completely occluded. The mechanics of breathing are disrupted by bronchiolitis. Airway narrowing causes obstruction of airflow that is worse on expiration. This leads to air trapping, hyperinflation, and increased functional residual capacity. Airway resistance and hyperinflation result in increased work of breathing and the development of hypercapnia in severe cases.

In rare cases, airway occlusion becomes severe and irreversible. This condition is known as bronchiolitis obliterans. This complication can occur after viral bronchiolitis, or it may occur after lung or bone marrow transplantation.[41]

Clinical Manifestations. Symptoms usually begin with rhinorrhea and cough. Over the next several days, systemic signs of decreased appetite, lethargy, and fever may develop. Increasing respiratory distress is evidenced by tachypnea, wheezing, and chest retractions. Very young infants may present with severe apnea before lower respiratory tract symptoms appear, and these apneas frequently require mechanical ventilation. Many children also may present with conjunctivitis or otitis media.

Evaluation and Treatment. Guidelines published in 2014 and reaffirmed in 2019 by the American Academy of Pediatrics are available for the evaluation, treatment, and prevention of bronchiolitis.[40,42] The diagnosis of bronchiolitis is made by reviewing the history, signs, and symptoms (e.g., rhinitis, cough, wheezing, chest retractions, tachypnea). Laboratory and radiologic examinations are not routinely performed.

Treatment for bronchiolitis is determined by the severity of the disease and the age of the child. Most cases are mild and require no specific treatment, and the child may be monitored as an outpatient. When treatment is indicated, it is primarily supportive in nature and may include high-flow nasal oxygen or noninvasive ventilation.[43] Bronchodilators, corticosteroids, and antibiotics are not recommended. Preventive treatment with RSV-specific monoclonal antibody (palivizumab) can reduce morbidity in infants with RSV bronchiolitis.[38,42] The American Academy of Pediatrics guidelines recommend the use of palivizumab prophylaxis for all infants born on or before 32 weeks gestation.[42] The National Perinatal Association also recommends the use of palivizumab in older preterm infants (born at 32 to 35 weeks gestation) who have additional risk factors.[44] Other preventive measures include the use of hand washing and alcohol-based decontamination, prevention of exposure to tobacco smoke, and promotion of infant breast feeding until at least 6 months of age.

Pneumonia

Pneumonia is infection and inflammation in the terminal airways and alveoli. Community-acquired pneumonia (CAP) is a major cause of morbidity and mortality in children, particularly in developing countries, although pneumonia related deaths among children globally have declined as a result of vaccines against *S. pneumoniae* and *H. influenzae*, antibiotic therapy, and improvements in education, nutrition, water, sanitation, and hygiene.[45] In the United States, CAP is the cause for over 100,000 pediatric hospitalizations annually.[46] The most common agents are viruses, and then bacteria and atypical microorganisms (e.g., mycoplasma) (Table 36.2). Risk factors for developing CAP are age younger than 2 years, overcrowded living conditions, winter season, recent antibiotic treatment, daycare attendance, and passive smoke exposure. Nutritional status, age, and underlying disease process influence morbidity and mortality rates related to CAP. Hospital-acquired pneumonia (HAP) is a nosocomial infection that occurs most commonly in those who are immunocompromised or who experience prolonged hospitalization for treatment of malignancy, trauma, surgery, or underlying chronic illness (see Chapter 35).

Pathophysiology. Viral pneumonia accounts for approximately 66% of childhood CAP requiring hospitalization.[47] RSV is the most common viral pneumonia in young children. A number of other viruses are important, including parainfluenza, influenza, human rhinovirus, human metapneumovirus, and adenoviruses. SARS-CoV-2 infection is most often asymptomatic or mild in children; however, a significant number of affected children do suffer serious complications such as multisystem inflammatory syndrome and require hospitalization (see Emerging Science Box: COVID-19 Infection in Children).[48] Acquisition of these viruses is by direct inoculation of the upper respiratory tract through inhalation of infectious secretions (droplet transmission), aerosol exposure, or from fomites in the child's environment (see Chapter 10). There is initial destruction of the ciliated epithelium of the distal airway with sloughing of cellular material and initiation of an inflammatory response. Alveolar injury results in loss of surfactant formation, hyaline

TABLE 36.2 Common Types of Pneumonia in Children

Type	Causal Agent	Age	Onset	Signs/Symptoms
Viral pneumonia	Respiratory syncytial virus (RSV), rhinovirus, influenza, adenovirus, parainfluenza, coronavirus	Neonates to 5 years	Acute or gradual, winter and early spring	Mild to high fever, cough, rhinorrhea, malaise, rales, rhonchi, wheezing, or apnea; variable radiographic pattern, may be severe requiring hospitalization
Pneumococcal pneumonia	*Streptococcus pneumoniae*	Usually 1 month to 4 years	Acute, occurs after an upper respiratory tract infection, winter and early spring	High fever, productive cough, pleuritic pain, increased respiration rate, decreased breath sounds in area of consolidation; lobar infiltrate on radiograph
Staphylococcal pneumonia	*Staphylococcus aureus* (including methicillin-resistant strains)	1 week to 2 years	Acute, winter	High fever, cough, respiratory distress, toxic appearance, sepsis; empyema or pneumatoceles common
Streptococcal pneumonia	Group B *Streptococcus*	Neonates	Acute, any season	Fussy, listless, tachypnea and retractions, pain in extremities, fever, meningitis, sepsis
Listeria pneumonia	*Listeria monocytogenes*	Neonates	May develop within hours of birth (early onset) or after several weeks (late onset)	Listlessness, poor feeding, respiratory distress, meningitis, sepsis
Atypical pneumonia	*Mycoplasma pneumoniae, Chlamydophila pneumoniae*	3 months to adolescents	Gradual	Low-grade fever, cough

Data adapted from Popovsky EY, Florin TA. Community-acquired pneumonia in childhood. *Reference Module in Biomedical Sciences,* 2020;B978-0-08–102723-3.00013–5.

EMERGING SCIENCE BOX

COVID-19 Infection in Children

Overall, children make up only 2%–8% of diagnosed Coronavirus Disease 19 (COVID-19) cases worldwide, although the number of asymptomatic infections is likely to be much higher. While most children have no or very mild symptoms during acute SARS-CoV-2 infection, a significant number develop a serious illness that occurs days to a few weeks after the initial infection. This condition is called multisystem inflammatory syndrome in children (MIS-C). As of late January 2022, 6,851 children with MIS-C were reported to state public health departments in the United States. The median age of patients with MIS-C was 9 years and 60% were male. The case definition for MIS-C according to the U.S. Centers for Disease Control and Prevention (CDC) includes the following:

- Age <21 years
- Temperature ≥38.0°C for ≥24 hours or subjective fever for ≥24 hours
- Severe illness (hospitalized) and ≥2 organ systems involved
- Laboratory evidence of inflammation
- Current or recent findings of positive by PCR; positive by serology; positive by antigen test; or COVID-19 exposure within prior 4 weeks
- No alternative diagnosis

While the pathogenesis of MIS-C continues to be delineated, both humoral and cellular autoimmune responses are implicated. It is postulated that SARS-CoV-2 serves as a superantigen eliciting an overwhelming immune response. Autoantibodies and T cell recognition of antigens expressed on infected cells, as well as the formation of antigen/antibody complexes, result in cellular damage and the release of numerous inflammatory cytokines such as interleukins 1 and 6, tumor necrosis factor alpha, and monocyte chemotactic factors. Neutrophils are activated and contribute to tissue damage. A hyperinflammatory condition results causing mucocutaneous, cardiac, pulmonary, renal, gastrointestinal, neurological injury as well as thrombotic complications and shock. Acute severe COVID-19 infection in children is considered distinct from MIS-C in that it occurs when viral titers are high, whereas the onset of MIS-C can be delayed for days or even weeks after the initial infection. Symptoms involving multiple organ systems including the gastrointestinal (abdominal pain and vomiting), mucocutaneous (rash), cardiac (chest pain), and neurocognitive (confusion, lethargy, somnolence) systems are common in those with MIS-C, whereas respiratory symptoms are not a prominent feature. Coronary artery aneurysms or arrhythmias affect approximately 10% of those with MIS-C, so once the diagnosis is made, additional testing should include echocardiogram, electrocardiogram, cardiac enzyme or troponin testing, and B-type natriuretic peptide. The CDC-recommended management includes fluid resuscitation, cardiac and respiratory support, corticosteroids, aspirin, and anticoagulants. Intravenous immunoglobulin and interleukin-1 or interleukin-6 antagonists may be used in severe cases. Approximately 60% of individuals require admission to intensive care, 40% require inotropic support, and 15% require mechanical ventilation. The overall mortality rate is around 2%. Close follow-up including cardiac reevaluation is indicated.

Data from Belay ED, et al. Trends in geographic and temporal distribution of US children with Multisystem Inflammatory Syndrome During the COVID-19 pandemic. *JAMA Pediatr.* 2021; 175(8):837–845; Centers for Disease Control and Prevention. Multisystem inflammatory syndrome. Available at https://www.cdc.gov/mis-c/hcp/. Accessed February 5, 2022; Centers for Disease Control and Prevention. Health department-reported cases of multisystem inflammatory syndrome in children (MIS-C) in the United States. Available at https://covid.cdc.gov/covid-data-tracker/#mis-national-surveillance. Accessed February 5, 2022; Dione A, et al. An update on multisystem inflammatory syndrome in children related to SARS-CoV-2. *Pediatr Infect Dis J.* 2022; 41(1):e6–e9; Feldstein LR, et al. Characteristics and outcomes of US children and adolescents with multisystem inflammatory syndrome in children (MIS-C) compared with severe acute COVID-19. *JAMA.* 2021;325(11):1074–1087; Giacalone M, et al. Multisystem inflammatory syndrome in children (MIS-C): a mini-review. *Int J Emerg Med.* 2021;14:50; McArdle AJ, et al. Treatment of multisystem inflammatory syndrome in children. *N Engl J Med.* 2021;385:11–22; Sharma C, et al. Multisystem inflammatory syndrome in children and Kawasaki disease: a critical comparison. *Nat Rev Rheumatol.* 2021;17:731–748; Son MBF, et al. Multisystem inflammatory syndrome in children- Initial therapy and outcomes. *N Engl J Med.* 2021;385:23–34; Sancho-Shimizu V, et al. SARS-CoV-2–related MIS-C: a key to the viral and genetic causes of Kawasaki disease? *J Exp Med.* 2021;218(6):e20210446.

membrane formation, and edema of the alveolar-capillary membrane.[46] Bacterial coinfections are common.

Bacterial pneumonia beyond the neonatal period most commonly is the result of infection with *S. pneumoniae*.[47] Other causative bacteria include *S. aureus* and atypical bacteria (see Table 36.2). Childhood immunization with the pneumococcal and *H. influenzae* vaccines has decreased the incidence of these two types of bacterial pneumonia in children younger than 2 years of age. Bacterial pneumonia usually begins with aspiration of bacteria that have colonized the nasopharynx.[45] A preceding viral infection sometimes sets the stage for bacterial infection by causing epithelial damage, reduced mucociliary clearance in the trachea and major bronchi, and a reduced immune response. Once in the alveolar region, bacteria encounter local host defenses, such as antibodies, complement, and cytokines, which prepare bacteria for ingestion by alveolar macrophages. Alveolar macrophages recognize bacteria with their surface receptors and phagocytose them. Macrophages release numerous inflammatory cytokines, and neutrophils are recruited into the lung. An intense, cytokine-mediated inflammation will ensue. Vascular engorgement, edema, and a fibrinopurulent exudate occur. Alveolar filling interferes with gas exchange and, if extensive, can lead to respiratory failure. If sepsis occurs at the same time, shock and end-organ hypoperfusion will cause metabolic acidosis. Staphylococcal pneumonia and group A streptococcal pneumonia can be particularly fulminant with a high incidence of accompanying empyema, pneumatocele (a lung lesion filled with air), and sepsis.

Pneumonia in neonates during the first 7 days of life (congenital or early onset pneumonia) is most often due to exposure to maternal pathogens during birth such as *Toxoplasma gondii, cytomegalovirus*, and *herpes simplex virus*.[46] Bacterial pathogens include group B *streptococcus* and *Listeria monocytogenes*. Risk factors include prematurity, low birth weight, and prolonged rupture of membranes. Late-onset neonatal pneumonia (greater than 7 days) may be caused by *S. aureus, S. pneumoniae*, or lower respiratory tract viruses.

Atypical pneumonia caused by Mycoplasma pneumoniae is a common cause of CAP for school-age children and young adults. It colonizes the respiratory tract in an estimated 21% of asymptomatic children and can cause symptomatic infections at any time of the year.[49] *Mycoplasma* can cause a wide spectrum of disease including rash, mucositis, upper airway infections, pneumonia, and autoimmune hemolytic anemia. Transmission occurs person to person, and there is a 2- to 3-week incubation period. *Mycoplasma* microorganisms lack cell walls but have a limiting membrane and a specialized receptor for attaching to ciliated respiratory epithelial cells. Local sloughing of cells occurs. Lymphocytic infiltration develops around the bronchi, along with neutrophil recruitment to the airway lumen. Complications, when they do occur, can include bronchopneumonia, parapneumonic pleural effusions, and necrotizing pneumonitis. Chlamydophila pneumoniae is clinically indistinguishable from *Mycoplasma* infection and is typically grouped with it as "atypical pneumonia."

Clinical Manifestations. Pneumonia in children has many overlapping features with other lower respiratory tract conditions such as asthma and bronchiolitis. Common clinical manifestations include dyspnea, fever, cough, crackles, wheezing, tachypnea, and tachycardia. Chest retractions, nasal flaring, emesis, and evidence of dehydration may develop. Bacterial pneumonia often is preceded by a viral illness followed by fever and increasingly productive cough. Occasionally, there is blood streaking of the sputum. In atypical pneumonia, the onset is usually gradual, resembling an upper respiratory tract infection but with low-grade fever, cough, and chest pain

Evaluation and Treatment. Guidelines have been developed to improve and aid assessment and management of pediatric pneumonia.[50] The diagnosis of pneumonia is based on clinical and laboratory findings. Identifying etiologic pathogens can be very difficult in children, especially because there is often overlap between bacterial and viral pathogens. The etiologic agent can sometimes be inferred from the age of the child and the clinical scenario. Chest x-rays and oximetry can assist in determining the extent of pulmonary involvement. The use of serum procalcitonin measurement as a biomarker for bacterial pediatric pneumonia is controversial. Measurement of serum surfactant protein D is an emerging clinical biomarker that may help predict pneumonia severity in children.[51] Several more specific microbiologic tests, such as sputum and blood cultures, and antigen detection assays (e.g., influenza, pneumococcus, *Mycoplasma, Chlamydophila*) are available.[46]

Many pneumonias may be treated on an outpatient basis; however, more severely ill children require oxygen supplementation and, occasionally, assisted ventilation. This is particularly true with infants who have a severe viral pneumonia that involves large portions of the lung, such as that seen with RSV. In addition, adequate hydration, proper nutrition, and supportive pulmonary therapy are required to reduce the duration and severity of illness. Many infected infants are markedly tachypneic and unable to coordinate their breathing with swallowing; they may require enteral feeding. Aspiration is always a risk with infants in respiratory distress.

Empiric antibiotic administration for bacterial pneumonias is dependent on age and severity assessment.[46] Local patterns of resistance must be considered when choosing appropriate antibiotics. Current guidelines recommend 10 days of antibiotic treatment; however, evidence is emerging that shorter courses (5 days) of antibiotics may be equally effective.[52] Pneumococcal pneumonias may require immune adjuvant therapies in addition to antibiotics. Prevention with vaccines against influenza and pneumococcal pneumonias is important in infants and young children.

Aspiration Pneumonitis

Aspiration pneumonitis is caused by a foreign substance, such as meconium, food, secretions (saliva or gastric), or environmental compounds, entering the lung and resulting in inflammation of the lung tissue. The aspiration of meconium from amniotic fluid can occur at birth. Children undergoing sedation or anesthesia may aspirate oral secretions contaminated with anaerobic bacteria or acidic stomach contents. Neurologically compromised children or children with chronic lung disease may have chronic pulmonary aspiration (CPA), which can cause progressive lung disease, bronchiectasis (chronically enlarged and scarred bronchi), and respiratory failure. CPA is the leading cause of death in children who are neurologically compromised because of failure of protective reflexes and difficulty swallowing (dysphagia).

The severity of lung injury after an aspiration incident is determined by the volume and pH of the material aspirated and the presence of pathogenic bacteria. A very low or an extremely high pH will cause a significant inflammatory response leading to damage to the bronchial epithelium followed by atelectasis and pneumonia.[53] Fibrosis and bronchiectasis may occur. With hydrocarbon fluid ingestions, lung injury is determined by the volatility and viscosity of the aspirated substance. A low-viscosity substance, such as gasoline or lighter fluid, is the most toxic; high-viscosity hydrocarbons, such as petroleum jelly or mineral oil, are much less likely to cause a pneumonitis.

Acute aspiration may present with the sudden onset of cough, dyspnea, and respiratory distress. CPA is characterized by cough, wheezing, and recurrent pneumonias. Evaluation includes chest radiography and arterial blood gases. Individuals suspected of CPA should be evaluated for dysphagia. Treatment for aspiration pneumonitis depends on the material aspirated. In children who aspirate significant amounts of toxic chemicals or acidic gastric contents, hospitalization and management for respiratory failure may be needed. Secondary bacterial pneumonia requires the use of broad-spectrum antibiotics. Children with CPA benefit from feeding and swallowing therapy. For selected children with neurologic disorders who have a large amount of upper respiratory tract secretions, anticholinergic medications, salivary gland injection with botulinum toxin A, or tracheotomy may be indicated.[53]

Asthma

Asthma is a chronic inflammatory disease characterized by bronchial hyperreactivity and reversible airflow obstruction, usually in response to an allergen (see Chapter 35). It is the most prevalent chronic disease in childhood, affecting approximately 7% of US children between birth and 17 years of age. Populations most affected include black and Puerto Rican children and those of low socioeconomic status.[54] Although 50% to 75% of children and adolescents with asthma are classified as having mild asthma, approximately one-third of severe exacerbations occur in this group.[55]

Childhood asthma results from a complex interaction between *genetic* susceptibility and *environmental* factors. Over 120 gene polymorphisms have been linked to the development of asthma, including genes for leukocyte function, cell surface receptors, susceptibility to certain infections, and autonomic function.[56] Important environmental risk factors for asthma include early exposure to allergens (e.g., dust mites, molds, cockroaches, cats), tobacco smoke, and air pollution. Gastroesophageal reflux and preterm birth are also risk factors. Exposure to respiratory pathogens such as fungi, some bacteria, and viruses (e.g., RSV) is associated with an increased risk for asthma in genetically predisposed individuals. Dysbiosis of the lung and gut microbiome also plays a major role in influencing the development of asthma in children.[57] Childhood obesity is strongly linked to asthma risk and severity (see Emerging Science Box: Obesity and Childhood Asthma).

EMERGING SCIENCE BOX

Obesity and Childhood Asthma

The association between childhood obesity and asthma risk and severity is well described. Obesity is linked to both allergic and nonallergic asthma phenotypes, including early-onset obese-asthma and late-onset obese-asthma. The pathophysiology that underlies this association is complex. There are genetic factors that are common to both obesity and asthma, as well as numerous epigenetic factors that are influenced by diet, sedentary lifestyle, and childhood exposures to environmental toxins. For example, low dietary fiber intake is linked with gut microbiome dysbiosis, systemic inflammation, and increased asthma risk. Obesity is a metabolically active state in which there are increased levels of inflammatory cytokines such as interleukin-1, interleukin-6, interferon gamma, and tumor necrosis factor alpha. The allergic immune cytokines interleukin-4, interleukin-5, and interleukin-13 are also increased. Furthermore, obesity results in an increased level of leptin which can increase levels of IgE and airway hyperreactivity. Insulin resistance and metabolic perturbations in obesity are linked with airway dysfunction. In addition to an increased risk for the development of asthma, obese individuals also are more likely to experience severe symptoms of dyspnea and chest tightness. Obese children with asthma are at increased risk for hospitalization for asthma-related respiratory distress and have a worse quality of life. Response to asthma medications is also decreased as compared to non-obese individuals with asthma. Management of obesity-related asthma is the same as for other types of asthma, with the addition of aggressive attempts at weight reduction. In children who accomplish significant weight loss, significantly improved asthma control and quality of life can be achieved.

Data from Dixon AE, et al. Diet and metabolism in the evolution of asthma and obesity. *Clinics in Chest Medicine,* 2019;40(1):97–106; Lang JE. Obesity and childhood asthma. *Current Opinion in Pulmonary Medicine,* 2019;25(1):34–43; Mohan A, et al. The effects of obesity in asthma. *Current Allergy Asthma Reports,* 2019;19(10):49; Palmo E, et al. Childhood obesity and respiratory diseases: Which link? *Children,* 2021;8:177; Papamichael MM, et al. Weight status and respiratory health in asthmatic children. *Lung,* 2019;197(6):777–782; Rastogi D. Pediatric obesity-related asthma: A prototype of pediatric severe non-T2 asthma. *Pediatric Pulmonology,* 2020;55(3):809–817; Santos LM, et al. The impact of weight loss beyond lung function: Benefit with respect to asthma outcomes. *Pulmonology,* 2019;25(6):313–319; van der Plaat DA. Mendelian randomisation supports causal link between obesity and asthma. *Thorax,* 2020;75(3):194–195.

Pathophysiology. The pathophysiology of asthma in children is similar to that for adults and is described in Chapter 35 (see Algorithm 35.4 and Figs. 35.6 and 35.7). Allergic asthma is initiated by a type I hypersensitivity reaction primarily mediated by T-helper 2 (Th2) lymphocytes, whose cytokines activate mast cells, eosinophilia, leukocytosis, and enhanced B-cell IgE production (see Chapter 9). As in adults, inflammation, bronchospasm, and mucus production in the airways lead to ventilation and perfusion mismatch with hypoxemia and to expiratory airway obstruction with air trapping and increased work of breathing. In young children, airway obstruction can be more severe because of the smaller diameter of their airways.

Most acute wheezing episodes in children with asthma are associated with viral respiratory tract infection (e.g., RSV, human rhinoviruses, and parainfluenza viruses).[58] In infants and toddlers younger than 2 years old, RSV is the most common. In older children and adults, rhinovirus (the "common cold" virus) is the major viral trigger. Bacterial respiratory tract infections also can trigger an acute asthma attack.

Clinical Manifestations. Clinical manifestations of an acute asthma attack include coughing, expiratory wheezing, and shortness of breath. Breath sounds may become faint when air movement is poor. The child may speak in clipped sentences or not at all because of dyspnea. The respiratory rate and heart rate are elevated. Nasal flaring and the use of accessory muscles with retractions in the substernal, subcostal, intercostal, suprasternal, or sternocleidomastoid areas are evident (see Fig. 36.3). Infants may appear to be "head bobbing" because of sternocleidomastoid muscle use. Pulsus paradoxus (a decrease in the systolic blood pressure of more than 10 mm Hg during inspiration) may be present. The child may appear anxious or may be sweating heavily, important signs of respiratory compromise.

Findings in chronic asthma may include persistent cough (often at night), wheezing when exposed to cold air or other irritants, exercise intolerance, and hyperinflation of the thorax (barrel chest). Clubbing should not be seen with asthma and, if present, should trigger evaluation for other conditions, such as cystic fibrosis. Exercise intolerance may indicate underlying asthma.

Evaluation and Treatment. Asthma is often underdiagnosed and undertreated, especially in preschool-age children, because asthma symptoms overlap with other respiratory illnesses, such as bronchitis or upper respiratory tract infections. The diagnosis of asthma is based on recurrent episodes of wheezing as well as a variety of risk factors, including a parental history of asthma, atopic dermatitis, sensitization to aeroallergens or foods, blood eosinophilia, or wheezing not associated with upper respiratory tract illnesses. The modified Asthma Predictive Index (mAPI) can be used to help with asthma diagnosis and is recommended by the NIH guidelines.[59] Confirmation of the diagnosis of asthma relies on pulmonary function testing using spirometry, which can be accomplished only after the child is 5 to 6 years of age. For younger children, an empirical trial of asthma medications is commonly initiated.

The goal of asthma therapy is to achieve long-term control by reduction in impairment and risk. Child and family education and appropriate allergen avoidance techniques should begin immediately. Care providers need to periodically assess asthma control in children. Key features for assessment include nighttime awakenings, interference with normal activities, use of short-acting β_2-agonists, pulmonary function testing, and exacerbations requiring steroids. Peak flow meters are often used to help guide treatment.

The pharmacologic treatment of asthma in children is essentially the same as that for adults and is initiated in a stepwise sequence based on asthma severity and the response to treatment (see Chapter 35). The Global Initiative for Asthma (GINA) provides recommendations for the use of inhaled corticosteroids and leukotriene receptor antagonists in children.[60] Management of asthma medications in children is often difficult because fluctuation in the severity of the symptoms is common. A Single Maintenance and Reliever (SMART) approach with an inhaled corticosteroid and a long-acting beta agonist is effective in reducing exacerbations and improving symptoms in most children 4 years and older.[55] Before therapy is augmented, care providers need to assess medication administration techniques, environmental controls, and comorbidities. For a reduction in therapy, the asthma needs to be under good control for a minimum of 3 months. Many children with less severe asthma outgrow the disease by adulthood.

Pediatric Acute Respiratory Distress Syndrome

Pediatric acute respiratory distress syndrome (PARDS) is a clinical syndrome in which there is pulmonary edema that is not the result of cardiac disease (noncardiogenic pulmonary edema). It is characterized by an acute onset of hypoxemia and pulmonary infiltrates. PARDS accounts for 1% to 10% of total admissions to pediatric intensive care units.[61] The risk for development of PARDS varies depending on age and the underlying cause. For example, children with underlying malignancies are at much higher risk for PARDS associated with infection with or without septic shock.[62] Mortality from PARDS in children remains high at about 24% and is higher in those who are immunocompromised, require vasopressors, or have multiple organ dysfunction.[63,64] Mortality in children with malignancy admitted to the ICU with PARDS may be as high as 80%.

Pathophysiology. PARDS results from a direct lung injury, such as pneumonia, aspiration, near-drowning, or smoke inhalation; or from a systemic insult, such as sepsis, pancreatitis, or multiple traumas. Some cases of adolescent PARDS have been linked to vaping.[65] Although less common than in adults, COVID-19 may cause of PARDS (see Emerging Science Box: COVID-19 Infection in Children). PARDS is characterized by an inflammatory response that causes alveolocapillary injury followed by leakage of fluid into the alveoli, coagulation, surfactant degradation, and fibrosis.[61] The steps in the pathophysiology of PARDS is the same as that described for ARDS in adults in Chapter 35 (see Algorithm 35.3).

Clinical Manifestations. Children with PARDS most commonly have suffered a known clinical insult, followed by increasing dyspnea, hypoxemia, and pulmonary infiltrates on chest x-ray. Initially, hyperventilation occurs, but carbon dioxide (CO_2) retention may ultimately develop because of inadequate functional air space and respiratory muscle fatigue. The severity of the overall picture is modified by comorbid factors, such as the presence of sepsis or multiorgan failure, and by the presence or absence of complications, such as nosocomial pneumonia.

Evaluation and Treatment. The evaluation of children with PARDS includes a physical examination, evaluation of blood gases, and imaging. The Pediatric Acute Lung Injury Consensus Conference has developed diagnostic criteria for PARDS which describe an onset within 7 days of clinical insult, new infiltrates on chest x-ray, edema not explained by fluid overload, or cardiac failure and hypoxemia. Perinatal causes of acute hypoxemia are excluded (i.e., lung disease related to prematurity, perinatal lung injury, congenital abnormalities, left ventricular failure, or fluid overload).[66] The degree of hypoxemia used to define the severity of PARDS uses the oxygenation index (OI), which is determined by the mean airway pressure and the ratio of supplemental oxygen to the PaO_2.

Treatment for PARDS remains supportive in nature, and the goals are to maintain adequate tissue oxygenation, minimize acute lung injury, and avoid iatrogenic pulmonary complications. Most children with PARDS require mechanical ventilation to promote alveolar ventilation and stabilization, and redistribution of alveolar edema fluid into the interstitium. Infants are at greater risk for ventilator-induced lung injury, and non-invasive ventilation, lung protective ventilation strategies, or extracorporeal membrane oxygenation (ECMO) should be considered. Prone positioning for severe PARDS improves oxygenation and reduces mortality.[61] Use of corticosteroids in PARDS is controversial but has been associated with improvements in lung function and survival in some studies.[67] Surfactant therapies appear promising in preclinical and clinical studies.[68] More research is needed regarding the long-term outcomes of PARDS.

Cystic Fibrosis

Cystic fibrosis (CF) is an autosomal recessive disease caused by inherited mutations in the *cystic fibrosis transmembrane conductance regulator* (CFTR) gene located on chromosome 7. These mutations result in defective epithelial chloride ion transport. There are over 2000 different variants of the CFTR gene. These mutations are divided into five classes with varying severity of disease expression: protein production mutations, protein processing mutations, gating mutations, conduction mutations, and insufficient protein mutations.[69]

In 2020 the Cystic Fibrosis Foundation Patient Registry reported 708 newly diagnosed individuals with CF in the U.S., and the median age at diagnosis was 3 months.[70] CF primarily affects Caucasians (approximately 95%). Due to improvement in treatment, median survival is 46.2 years and over half of people living with CF are 18 years or older.[71] The overall estimated carrier frequency for people in the United States is 1 in 35, while the frequency in US Caucasians is 1 in 20. Carriers are not affected by the mutation.

Pathophysiology. CF is a multiorgan disease that affects the lungs, digestive tract (see Chapter 42), and reproductive organs. *CFTR* gene mutations result in the abnormal expression of cystic fibrosis transmembrane conductance regulator (CFTR) protein, which is an activated chloride channel present on the surface of many types of epithelial cells lining airways, bile ducts, the pancreas, sweat ducts, paranasal sinuses, and vas deferens.[72] Without adequate CFTR function, chloride and water are not transported appropriately across epithelial membranes, resulting in thick, dehydrated mucus secretions. The most important effects are on the lungs, and respiratory failure is almost always the cause of death.

The typical features of CF lung disease are mucous plugging, chronic inflammation, and chronic infection of the small airways (Algorithm 36.4).[73] The mucous plugging results from increased production of mucus from more numerous and larger goblet cells, altered physicochemical properties of the mucus, and impaired mucociliary clearance. The depleted fluid in the mucus and impaired mobility of the cilia allow mucus to adhere to the airway epithelium, along with bacteria and injurious by-products from neutrophils. Neutrophils are present in great excess in the airways and release oxidants and proteases (i.e., elastase) that cause direct damage to lung structural proteins.[74] Microorganisms also induce airway cells to produce inflammatory mediators that destroy immunoglobulin G (IgG) and complement components important for opsonization and phagocytosis of pathogens, thus contributing to chronic infection (see Algorithm 36.4).

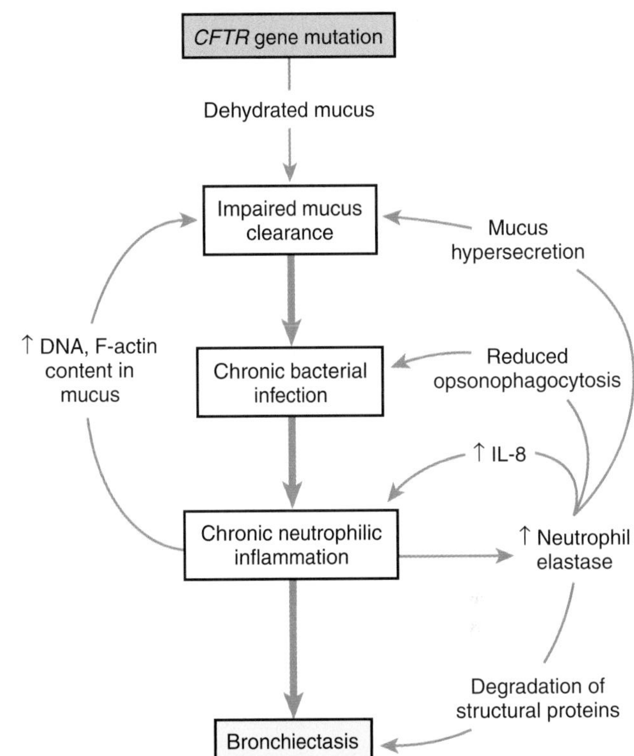

Algorithm 36.4 Pathogenesis of Cystic Fibrosis Lung Disease. *CFTR,* Cystic fibrosis transmembrane conductance regulator; *IL-8,* interleukin-8.

The CF airway microenvironment favors bacterial colonization, which leads to a bacterial biofilm that promotes chronic endobronchial infection. The biofilm resists beta-lactam antibiotics, and rapid mutation of the biofilm makes these children antibiotic resistant. Persistence of these microorganisms incites chronic local inflammation and airway damage, with microabscess formation, bronchiectasis, patchy consolidation and pneumonia, peribronchial fibrosis, and cyst formation (Fig. 36.8).[71] Peripheral bullae may develop, and pneumothorax may occur. Hemoptysis (coughing up blood) is sometimes life-threatening and may occur because of the erosion into enlarged bronchial arteries. Over time, pulmonary vascular remodeling occurs because of localized hypoxia and arteriolar vasoconstriction. Pulmonary hypertension and cor pulmonale may develop in the late stages of the disease (see Chapter 35).

Clinical Manifestations. Clinical manifestations of CF can vary from mild to severe, depending on the degree of gene

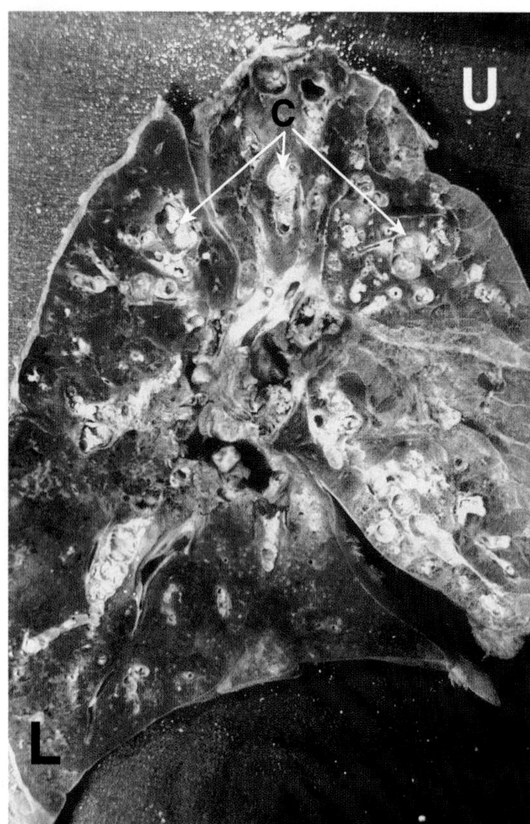

Fig. 36.8 Pathology of the Lung in End-Stage Cystic Fibrosis. Key features are widespread mucus impaction of the airways and bronchiectasis, especially from the upper lobe *(U; white arrows)*, with hemorrhagic pneumonia in the lower lobe *(L)*. Small cysts are present at the apex of the lung *(C)*. (From Kleinerman J, Vauthy P. *Pathology of the lung in cystic fibrosis*. Atlanta: Cystic Fibrosis Foundation; 1976.)

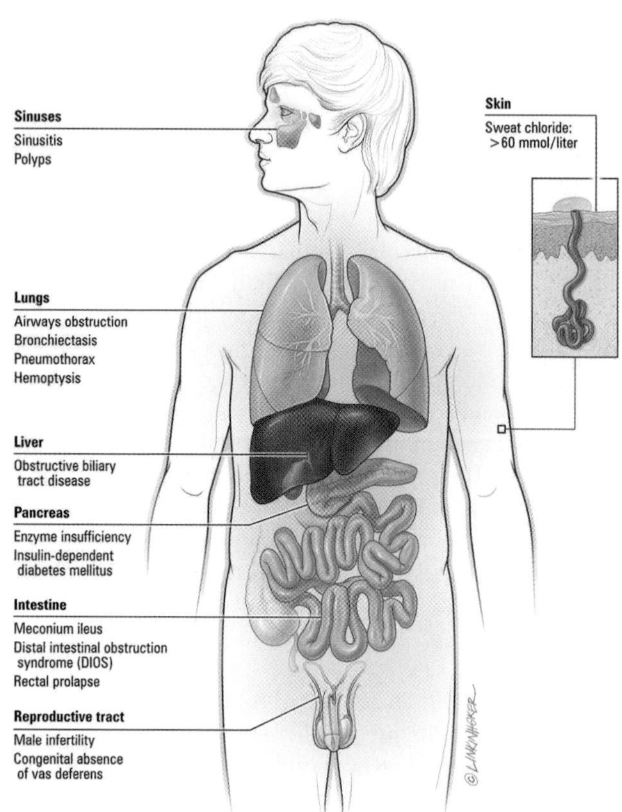

Fig. 36.9 Clinical Manifestations of Cystic Fibrosis. Cystic fibrosis affects many organs in the body. (From Dickinson KM, Collaco JM. Cystic fibrosis. *Pediatrics in Review*, 2021;42(2): 55–67. https://doi.org/10.1542/pir.2019-0212.)

mutation. The most common presenting symptoms of CF involve the respiratory or gastrointestinal/digestive systems (Fig. 36.9). Respiratory symptoms include persistent cough or wheeze, excessive sputum production, and recurrent or severe pneumonia. Physical signs that develop over time include barrel chest and digital clubbing. More subtle presentations include chronic sinusitis and nasal polyps. Gastrointestinal affects include malnutrition and intestinal obstruction (see Chapter 42).

Evaluation and Treatment. According to the Cystic Fibrosis Foundation, guidelines for the diagnosis of CF include one or more clinical features, a history of CF in a sibling, or a positive newborn screen plus laboratory evidence of an abnormality in the *CFTR* gene or the CFTR protein. Newborn screening for CF is universal throughout the United States and is essential to providing early, pre-symptomatic diagnosis and treatment, including nutritional counseling, early digestive enzyme replacement, and provision of psychosocial support to families. The standard method of screening newborns in most states is the IRT, a blood test which measures immunoreactive trypsinogen (a chemical made by the pancreas) and identifies DNA changes.[75] If the IRT test is positive, then a sweat test is performed before 4 weeks of age. Carrier testing to detect adult heterozygotes is available and enables informed reproductive choices before the birth of the first child with CF (25% chance if both parents are carriers).[76]

Treatment is primarily focused on pulmonary health and nutrition and prevention of persistent cycles of lung infection and inflammation.[77] Pancreatic enzyme therapy is initiated when pancreatic insufficiency and malabsorption are documented, along with fat soluble vitamin replacement.[71] Common pulmonary therapies include airway clearance therapy (chest physical therapy and related mechanical devices), use of bronchodilators, and the administration of solutions which liquefy mucus (e.g., aerosolized dornase alfa [an enzyme] and hypertonic saline). Different classes of oral, inhaled, or intravenous antibiotics are used to treat different pathogens and to overcome antibiotic resistance. High-dose ibuprofen is indicated for children older than 6 years.[77] CFTR modulators can restore the function of the *CFTR* gene in 90% of individuals with CF (see Emerging Science Box: CFTR Modulators).[78] Cell based therapies are under investigation.[79] Individuals with end-stage lung disease may consider lung transplantation.

EMERGING SCIENCE BOX

CFTR Modulators

An improved understanding of the cystic fibrosis transmembrane conductance regulator (CFTR) protein gene mutations led to the development CFTR modulating drugs. These modulator drugs have the ability to enhance the function of the CFTR gene and have been classified into five main groups depending on their effects: potentiators, correctors, stabilizers, read-through agents, and amplifiers. To date, four CFTR modulators have reached the market: ivacaftor(Kalydeco), lumacaftor/ivacaftor(Orkambi), tezacaftor/ivacaftor(Symdeko), and elexacaftor/tezacaftor/ivacaftor(Trikafta). These drug combinations have been found to be effective in achieving short- and long-term improvements in clinical outcomes for up to 90% of individuals with CF, transforming the disease into a treatable chronic condition. There is emerging evidence that starting these medications early in life before severe lung injury develops may halt disease progression. Unfortunately, it is as yet unclear if these treatments will prove safe and effective over decades of use, adherence issues need to be addressed, and these medications are very expensive. Furthermore, there remain rare CFTR mutations that are unresponsive to these treatments and will require additional innovative approaches such as gene and stem cell therapies.

Data from Burgel PR, et al. Real-life safety and effectiveness of lumacaftor-ivacaftor in patients with cystic fibrosis. *American Journal of Respiratory and Critical Care Medicine*, 2020;15:188–197; Gillan JL, et al. Targeting cystic fibrosis inflammation in the age of CFTR modulators: Focus on macrophages. *European Respiratory Journal*, 2021;57(6):2003502; epub ahead of print, 2020; Heijerman HGM, et al. Efficacy and safety of the elexacaftor plus tezacaftor plus ivacaftor combination regimen in people with cystic fibrosis homozygous for the F508del mutation: a double-blind, randomised, phase 3 trial. *Lancet*, 2019;394:1940–1948; Lopes-Pacheco M. CFTR Modulators: The changing face of cystic fibrosis in the era of precision medicine. *Frontiers in Pharmacology*, 2020;10:1662; Metha Z, et al. Adherence to cystic fibrosis transmembrane conductance regulator (CFTR) modulators: Analysis of a national specialty pharmacy database. *Journal of Drug Assessment*, 2021;10(1):62–67; Middleton PG, et al. Elexacaftor-Tezacaftor-Ivacaftor for cystic fibrosis with a single Phe508del allele. *New England Journal of Medicine*, 2019;381:1809–1819; Morrison CB, et al. Treatment of cystic fibrosis airway cells with CFTR modulators reverses aberrant mucus properties via hydration. *Eur Respir J.* 2022;59:2100185; Page A, et al. Lived experiences of individuals with cystic fibrosis on CFTR-modulators. *BMC Pulm Med* 2022;22:42; Pranke I, et al. Emerging therapeutic approaches for cystic fibrosis. From gene editing to personalized medicine. *Frontiers in Pharmacology*, 2019;10:121; Rusnati M, et al. Recent strategic advances in CFTR drug discovery: An overview. *International Journal of Molecular Sciences*, 2020;21:2407.

SUDDEN INFANT DEATH SYNDROME

Sudden Infant Death Syndrome (SIDS) is the most common cause of sudden unexpected infant death. It remains a disease of unknown cause. It is defined as sudden death of an infant under 12 months of age which remains unexplained after a thorough case investigation, including performance of a complete autopsy, examination of the death scene, and review of the clinical history.[80]

The incidence of SIDS is low during the first month of life, with the peak incidence at 2 to 4 months of age. It is unusual after 6 months of age. In 2019, there were approximately 1250 deaths due to SIDS.[81] SIDS almost always occurs during nighttime sleep, when infants are least likely to be observed. Clinical risk groups are summarized in *Risk Factors:* Sudden Infant Death Syndrome (SIDS). About 75% of all SIDS victims have no known predisposing clinical risk factor.

RISK FACTORS

Sudden Infant Death Syndrome

- Prone and side-lying sleeping positions
- Sleeping on soft bedding
- Overheated sleeping environment
- Lower socioeconomic status
- Mothers younger than 20
- Black or African American, Native Americans, Alaska Natives
- Low birth weight or growth-restricted infants
- Male infants
- Preterm delivery
- Multiple gestations
- Sibling who died of SIDS
- Smoking during pregnancy
- Exposure to tobacco smoke
- Lack of prenatal care
- Illicit drug use or binge-drinking
- Larger family size

Data from Moon RY; Task Force on Sudden Infant Death Syndrome. SIDS and other sleep-related infant deaths: Evidence base for 2016 updated recommendations for a safe infant sleeping environment. *Pediatrics*, 2016;138(5):e20162940.

The etiology of SIDS remains unknown but probably involves a combination of predisposing factors, including physiologic vulnerabilities and environmental stressors. A specific genetic cause for SIDS has not been identified; however, important risk factor genes include those involved in the regulation of the immune system and inflammation, cardiac abnormalities or arrhythmias, and brainstem function.[82] There is evidence for impaired autonomic regulation and failure of cardiovascular, ventilatory, and arousal responses. A prominent theory is that a subset of SIDS infants suffers from serotonergic abnormalities due to a lesion in the medullary reticular formation that leads to a failure of protective brainstem responses during sleep.[83] Other theories involve immune dysregulation, airway inflammation, and responses to bacterial pathogens from the nasopharynx or viral respiratory tract infections. Findings on autopsy in over 90% of SIDS cases reveal intrathoracic petechiae, unclotted heart chamber blood, congested lungs, and enlarged brain and thymus, suggesting a heterogeneous pathogenesis.[84]

Currently, the best strategy for reducing SIDS and sudden unexpected infant death during sleep seems to be avoidance of risk factors such as placing the infant supine, use of a firm mattress with no soft or loose bedding, and avoidance of parental smoking before and after birth. Other recommendations include breast feeding, recommended immunizations, and use of a pacifier at sleep time.[85] Parents of infants with clinical risk should be taught cardiopulmonary resuscitation (CPR) as a precaution. Some infants at risk for episodes of apnea and bradycardia may warrant cardiorespiratory monitoring after careful consideration of the individual situation.

SUMMARY REVIEW

Disorders of the Upper Airways

1. Viral croup is an acute laryngotracheobronchitis, usually caused by the parainfluenza virus. This infection causes swelling of the upper trachea. The typical sign is a seal-like barking cough, which appears after a few days of rhinorrhea, sore throat, and low-grade fever.
2. Recurrent (spasmodic) croup is characterized by a similar barking cough but occurs in older children and has a sudden onset at night, without fever. The etiology is unknown.
3. Acute epiglottitis is a potentially life-threatening airway infection; its incidence in children has decreased dramatically since the advent of the Hib vaccine. Now other pathogens, such as GABHS, *Candida* species, *S. aureus*, MRSA, and viral pathogens are usually the causative agents.
4. Tonsillar infections are usually caused by viral infections, such as infectious mononucleosis, and can be complicated by tonsillar and peritonsillar abscesses.
5. Aspiration of foreign bodies that lodge in the airways may cause cough, hoarseness, stridor or wheezing, and dyspnea. The severity depends on the location of the foreign body within the airway and the degree of obstruction. Blockage of the larynx or trachea can be fatal, whereas bronchial obstruction may not be diagnosed immediately.
6. OSAS results from partial or complete upper airway obstruction during sleep with associated snoring, labored or obstructed breathing, and disrupted sleep patterns.

Disorders of the Lower Airways

1. SDD (RDS of the newborn) usually occurs in premature infants who are born before surfactant production and alveolocapillary development are complete. Atelectasis and hypoventilation cause shunting, hypoxemia, and hypercapnia. Prenatal steroids and postnatal surfactant are beneficial preventive therapies.
2. BPD is the result of tissue injury and repair and disrupted alveolar development in the lungs of infants who required ventilatory support during a time when their lungs were underdeveloped because of their prematurity. Surfactant therapy has improved outcomes. Infants with BPD may require oxygen and additional therapies for many months.
3. Bronchiolitis is a viral lower respiratory tract infection that presents with a runny nose, wheezing, cough, and tachypnea in infants and is usually caused by infection with RSV. Infants with risk factors of prematurity or underlying lung or heart disease are at high risk and may receive RSV-specific monoclonal antibody to prevent RSV disease.
4. Pneumonia is infection and inflammation in the terminal airways and alveoli. Viral, bacterial, and atypical pneumonia cause varying degrees of illness in children. Bacterial CAP is one of the leading causes of hospitalization and is prevented with a polyvariant pneumococcal conjugate vaccine.
5. Aspiration pneumonitis is caused by inhalation of a foreign substance, such as food, milk, secretions, or environmental compounds into the lung, resulting in inflammation.
6. Asthma is a chronic inflammatory disease characterized by bronchial hyperreactivity and reversible airflow obstruction, usually in response to an allergen. Its origins are multifactorial and include genetic, allergic, and viral-triggered mechanisms.
7. ARDS is a clinical syndrome in which there is pulmonary edema that is not the result of cardiac disease; it is often a life-threatening condition. ARDS results from direct lung injury. There is progressive respiratory distress with severe hypoxemia and respiratory failure.
8. Cystic fibrosis is an autosomal recessive genetic disease that affects the epithelial lining of many organ systems, especially the respiratory and gastrointestinal systems. Airway secretions are particularly thick and tenacious, and the airways develop a chronic bacterial infection. Chronic infection, plugged airways, and severe inflammation cause long-term lung damage and ultimately death. New CFTR modulators are improving outcomes.

Sudden Infant Death Syndrome

1. SIDS is the leading cause of postnatal death for infants outside of the hospital setting. It is associated with a low birth weight, a prone sleeping position, and other environmental factors. There has been a significant reduction in SIDS cases since the widespread adoption of recommendations for safe sleep techniques for infants.

REFERENCES

1. Eskander A, de Almeida JR, Irish JC. Acute upper airway obstruction. *N Engl J Med*. 2019;381(20):1940–1949.
2. Aghdam MK, Mirzaee HS, Eftekhari K. Croup is one of the clinical manifestations of novel coronavirus in children. *Case Rep Pulmonol 2021*. 2021:8877182.
3. Li SF. The Westley croup score. *Acad Emerg Med*. 2003;10:289.
4. Gates A, Johnson DW, Klassen TP. Glucocorticoids for croup in children. *JAMA Pediatr*. 2019;173(6):595–596.
5. DeBlasio D, Real J. Tracheitis. *Pediatr Rev*. 2020;41(9):495–497.
6. Klein MR. Infections of the oropharynx. *Emerg Med Clin North Am*. 2019;37(1):69–80.
7. Geißler K, et al. Cytokine production in patients with recurrent acute tonsillitis: analysis of tonsil samples and blood. *Sci Rep*. 2020;10:13006.
8. Mitchell RB, et al. Clinical practice guideline: tonsillectomy in children (update)-executive summary. *Otolaryngol Head Neck Surg*. 2019;160(2):187–205.
9. Wu S, et al. Tonsillar microbiota: a cross sectional study of patients with chronic tonsillitis or tonsillar hypertrophy. *mSystems*. 2021;6(2):e01302–e01320.
10. Klug TE, Greve T, Hentze M. Complications of peritonsillar abscess. *Ann Clin Microbiol Antimicrob*. 2020;19:32.
11. Olsen BBC, Zonfrillo MR, Allister LM. Peritonsillar abscess in an infant. *J Pediatr*. 2020;227:320–321.
12. Gibbons RC, Costantino TG. Evidence-based medicine improves the emergent management of peritonsillar abscesses using point-of-care ultrasound. *J Emerg Med*. 2020;59(5):693–698.

13. Kim IA, et al. The national cost burden of bronchial foreign body aspiration in children. *Laryngoscope*. 2015;125(5):1221–1224.
14. Gan W, et al. Clinical analysis of tracheobronchial foreign body aspiration in children: a focus on external and intrinsic factors. *BMC Surg*. 2021;21:108.
15. Crane MD. Foreign body aspiration. *JAAPA*. 2019;32(7):48–49.
16. Liu B, et al. Occult foreign body aspirations in pediatric patients: 20-years of experience. *BMC Pulm Med*. 2020;20:320.
17. Tsukada E, et al. Prevalence of childhood obstructive sleep apnea syndrome and its role in daytime sleepiness. *PLoS One*. 2018;13(10):e0204409.
18. Giuca MR, et al. Pediatric obstructive sleep apnea syndrome: emerging evidence and treatment approach. *ScientificWorldJournal 2021*. 2021:5591251.
19. Marcus CL, et al. Clinical practice guideline: diagnosis and management of childhood obstructive sleep apnea syndrome. *Pediatrics*. 2012;130(3):576–584.
20. Quinlan CM, Otero H, Tapia IE. Upper airway visualization in pediatric obstructive sleep apnea. *Paediatr Respir Rev*. 2019;32:48–54.
21. Parmar A, Baker A, Narang I. Positive airway pressure in pediatric obstructive sleep apnea. *Paediatr Respir Rev*. 2019;31:43–51.
22. Gallucci M, et al. Cardiovascular issues in obstructive sleep apnoea in children: a brief review. *Paediatr Respir Rev*. 2021;38:45–50.
23. Kemp MW, Schmidt AF, Jobe AH. Optimizing antenatal corticosteroid therapy. *Semin Fetal Neonatal Med*. 2019;24(3):176–181.
24. van Moorsel CHM, van der Vis JJ, Grutters JC. Genetic disorders of the surfactant system: focus on adult disease. *Eur Respir Rev*. 2021;30:200085.
25. Hentschel R, et al. Surfactant replacement therapy: from biological basis to current clinical practice. *Nat Pediatr Res*. 2020;88:176–183.
26. Challis P, et al. Association of adherence to surfactant best practice uses with clinical outcomes among neonates in Sweden. *JAMA Netw Open*. 2021;4(5):e217269.
27. Jain D, Bancalari E. New developments in respiratory support for preterm infants. *Am J Perinatol*. 2019;36(S 02):S13–S17.
28. Jobe AH, Bancalari E. Bronchopulmonary dysplasia. *Am J Respir Crit Care Med*. 2001;163:1723–1729.
29. Higgins RD, et al. Bronchopulmonary dysplasia: executive summary of a workshop. *J Pediatr*. 2018;197:300–308.
30. Bonadies L, et al. Present and future of bronchopulmonary dysplasia. *J Clin Med*. 2020;9(5):1539.
31. Stoecklin B, Simpson SJ, Pillow JJ. Bronchopulmonary dysplasia: rationale for a pathophysiological rather than treatment based approach to diagnosis. *Paediatr Respir Rev*. 2019;32:91–97.
32. Mandell EW, et al. Drugs for the prevention and treatment of bronchopulmonary dysplasia. *Clin Perinatol*. 2019;46(2):291–310.
33. Sahni M, Bhandari V. Recent advances in understanding and management of bronchopulmonary dysplasia. *F1000Res*. 2020;9(F1000 Faculty Rev-703).
34. Ganguly A, Martin RJ. Vulnerability of the developing airway. *Respir Physiol Neurobiol*. 2019;270:103263.
35. Papagianis PC, Pillow JJ, Moss TJ. Bronchopulmonary dysplasia: pathophysiology and potential anti-inflammatory therapies. *Paediatr Respir Rev*. 2019;30:34–41.
36. Cuna A, et al. Usefulness of an online risk estimator for bronchopulmonary dysplasia in predicting corticosteroid treatment in infants born preterm. *J Pediatr*. 2018;197:23–28.
37. Filippone M, et al. Update on postnatal corticosteroids to prevent or treat bronchopulmonary dysplasia. *Am J Perinatol*. 2019;36(S 02):S58–S62.
38. Krilov LR, Anderson EJ. Respiratory syncytial virus hospitalizations in US preterm infants after the 2014 change in immunoprophylaxis guidance by the American Academy of Pediatrics. *J Perinatol*. 2020;40:1135–1144.
39. Mansbach JM, et al. Detection of respiratory syncytial virus or rhinovirus weeks after hospitalization for bronchiolitis and the risk of recurrent wheezing. *J Infect Dis*. 2021;223(2):268–277.
40. Silver AH, Naziff JM. Bronchiolitis. *Pediatr Rev*. 2019;40:568–576.
41. Burrows J, Thursfield R. Bronchiolitis obliterans - a review of this rare paediatric respiratory disorder. *Eur Respir J*. 2019;54(Suppl 63):PA1013.
42. Ralston SL, et al. Clinical practice guideline: the diagnosis, management, and prevention of bronchiolitis. *Pediatrics*. 2014;134(5):e1474–e1502.
43. Franklin D, Fraser JF, Schibler A. Respiratory support for infants with bronchiolitis, a narrative review of the literature. *Paediatr Respir Revews*. 2019;30:16–24.
44. National Perinatal Association: 2018 Respiratory syncytial virus (RSV) prevention clinical practice guideline: an evidence-based interdisciplinary collaboration. Lonedell, MO, 2018, National Perinatal Association. Available at: http://www.neonatologytoday.net/newsletters/nt-oct17.pdf. Accessed February 5, 2022.
45. Torres A, et al. Pneumonia. *Nat Rev Dis Primers*. 2021;7:25.
46. Popovsky EY, Florin TA. *Community-acquired pneumonia in childhood. Reference Module in Biomedical Sciences.* : Elsevier; 2020:00013–00015 B978-0-08-102723-3.
47. Yun KW, et al. Community-acquired pneumonia in children: myths and facts. *Am J Perinatol*. 2019;36(Suppl 52):554–557.
48. Jiang L, et al. COVID-19 and multisystem inflammatory syndrome in children and adolescents. *Lancet Infect Dis*. 2020;20:e276–e288.
49. Krafft C, Christy C. *Mycoplasma* pneumonia in children and adolescents. *Pediatr Rev*. 2020;41:12–19.
50. Bradley JS, et al. The management of community-acquired pneumonia in infants and children older than 3 months of age: clinical practice guidelines by the Pediatric Infectious Diseases Society and the Infectious Diseases Society of America. *Clin Infect Dis*. 2011;53:e25–e76.
51. Saleh NY, et al: Surfactant protein D: a predictor for severity of community-acquired pneumonia in children, *Pediatr Res*. Online ahead of print: 31 March 2021. Available at: https://doi.org/10.1038/s41390-021-01492-9. Accessed February 5, 2022
52. Same RG, et al. The association of antibiotic duration with successful treatment of community-acquired pneumonia in children. *J Pediatric Infect Dis Soc*. 2021;10(3):267–273.
53. Tutor JD. Dysphagia and chronic pulmonary aspiration in children. *Pediatr Rev*. 2020;41:236–244.
54. Centers for Disease Control and Prevention (CDC) National Center for Health Statistics. *Most Recent National Data*. 2021 Available at: https://www.cdc.gov/asthma/most_recent_national_asthma_data.htm. Accessed February 6, 2022.
55. Abrams EM, et al. Treatment of mild-to-moderate asthma in childhood and adolescence in 2021. *Lancet Respir Med*. 2021;9(5):443–445.

56. El-Husseini ZW, et al. The genetics of asthma and the promise of genomics-guided drug target discovery. *Lancet Respir Med.* 2020;8:1045–1056.
57. Barcik W, et al. The role of lung and gut microbiota in the pathology of asthma. *Immunity.* 2020;52(2):241–255.
58. Patel SJ, Teach SJ. Asthma. *Pediatr Rev.* 2019;40:549–567.
59. National Heart, Lung, and Blood Institute (NHLBI) *Asthma management guidelines: focused updates 2020.* Bethesda, MD: NHLBI; 2020. Last updated 14 July 2021. Available at: https://www.nhlbi.nih.gov/health-topics/asthma-management-guidelines-2020-updates. Accessed February 5, 2022.
60. Global Initiative for Asthma (GINA): *2021 GINA main report; 2021 GINA report, global strategy for asthma management and prevention.* Fontana, WI, 2021, GINA. Available at: https://ginasthma.org/gina-reports/. Accessed February 5, 2022.
61. Orloff KE, Turner DA, Rehder KJ. The current state of pediatric acute respiratory distress syndrome. *Pediatr Allergy Immunol Pulmonol.* 2019;32:35–44.
62. Zeng J, Qian S. Pediatric acute respiratory distress syndrome in children with malignancies. *Pediatr Crit Care Med.* 2021;22:204–205.
63. Yehya N, et al. Predicting mortality in children with pediatric acute respiratory distress syndrome: a pediatric acute respiratory distress syndrome incidence and epidemiology study. *Crit Care Med.* 2021;48(6):e514–e522.
64. Wong JJ, et al. Mortality in pediatric acute respiratory distress syndrome: a systematic review and meta-analysis. *J Intensive Care Med.* 2019;34(7):563–571.
65. Carroll BJ, et al. Impaired lung function following e-cigarette or vaping product use associated lung injury in the first cohort of hospitalized adolescents. *Pediatr Pulmonol.* 2020;55(7):1712–1718.
66. The Pediatric Acute Lung Injury Consensus Conference Group Pediatric acute respiratory distress syndrome: consensus recommendations from the Pediatric Acute Lung Injury Consensus Conference. *Pediatr Crit Care Med.* 2015;16(5):428–439.
67. Mitting RB, et al. Improved oxygenation following methylprednisolone therapy and survival in paediatric acute respiratory distress syndrome. *PLoS One.* 2019;14(11):e0225737.
68. De Luca D, et al. Surfactant therapies for pediatric and neonatal ARDS: ESPNIC expert consensus opinion for future research steps. *Crit Care.* 2021;25:75.
69. Cystic Fibrosis Foundation: *Types of CFTR mutations.* Bethesda, MD, undated, Cystic Fibrosis Foundation. Available at: https://www.cff.org/What-is-CF/Genetics/Types-of-CFTR-Mutations/. Accessed February 5, 2022.
70. Cystic Fibrosis Foundation *Patient registry 2020 annual data report.* Bethesda, MD: Cystic Fibrosis Foundation; 2020. Available at: https://www.cff.org/medical-professionals/patient-registry. Accessed February 5, 2022.
71. Dickinson KM, Collaco JM. Cystic fibrosis. *Pediatr Rev.* 2021;42(2):55–67.
72. Lopes-Pacheco M. CFTR modulators: the changing face of cystic fibrosis in the era of precision medicine. *Front Pharmacol.* 2019;10:1662.
73. Balazs A, Mall MA. Mucus obstruction and inflammation in early cystic fibrosis lung disease: emerging role of the IL-1 signaling pathway. *Pediatr Pulmonol.* 2019;54(Suppl 3):S5–S12.
74. Khan MA, et al. Progression of cystic fibrosis lung disease from childhood to adulthood: neutrophils, neutrophil extracellular trap (NET) formation, and NET degradation. *Genes (Basel).* 2019;10(3):183.
75. Cystic Fibrosis Foundation: *Testing for CF.* Bethesda, MD, no date, Cystic Fibrosis Foundation. Available at: https://www.cff.org/What-is-CF/Testing. Accessed February 5, 2022.
76. Cystic Fibrosis Foundation: *Carrier testing for cystic fibrosis.* Bethesda, MD, no date, Cystic Fibrosis Foundation. Available at: https://www.cff.org/What-is-CF/Testing/Carrier-Testing-for-Cystic-Fibrosis/. Accessed February 5, 2022.
77. Lahiri T, et al. Clinical practice guidelines from the cystic fibrosis foundation for preschoolers with cystic fibrosis. *Pediatrics.* 2016;137:e20151784.
78. Cystic Fibrosis Foundation: *CFTR modulator therapies.* Bethesda, MD, no date, Cystic Fibrosis Foundation. Available at: https://www.cff.org/Life-With-CF/Treatments-and-Therapies/Medications/CFTR-Modulator-Therapies/. Accessed February 5, 2022.
79. Allan KM, et al. Treatment of cystic fibrosis: from gene- to cell-based therapies. *Front Pharmacol.* 2021;12:241.
80. Behman-Temeus M, Clementine M. SIDS, BRUE and safe sleep guidelines. *Pediatr Rev.* 2019;40:443455.
81. Centers for Disease Control and Prevention (CDC): *Sudden unexpected infant death and sudden infant death syndrome: data and statistics.* Bethesda, MD, 2021, CDC. Page last reviewed: 28 April 2021. Available at: https://www.cdc.gov/sids/data.htm. Accessed February 5, 2022.
82. Johannsen EB, et al. The genetics of sudden infant death syndrome—towards a gene reference resource. *Genes (Basel).* 2021;12(2):216.
83. Kinney HC, Haynes RL. The serotonin brainstem hypothesis for the sudden infant death syndrome. *J Neuropathol Exp Neurol.* 2019;78(9):765–779.
84. Goldwater PN. SIDS, prone sleep position and infection: an overlooked epidemiological link in current SIDS research? Key evidence for the "infection hypothesis". *Med Hypotheses.* 2020;144:110114.
85. Horne RSC. Sudden infant death syndrome: current perspectives. *Intern Med J.* 2019;49:433–438.

37

Structure and Function of the Renal and Urologic Systems

Karen C. Turner

http://evolve.elsevier.com/Rogers/pathophysiology/

CHAPTER OUTLINE

The renal system consists of the kidneys. The primary function of the kidney is to maintain a stable internal environment for optimal cell and tissue metabolism. The kidneys accomplish these life-sustaining tasks by balancing solute and water transport, excreting metabolic waste products, conserving nutrients, and regulating acids and bases. The kidney also has an endocrine function and secretes the hormones renin for regulation of blood pressure, erythropoietin (Epo) for red blood cell production, and vitamin D_3 for calcium metabolism. The kidney also synthesizes glucose in a process called gluconeogenesis and releases it into the circulation when needed (Box 37.1). The formation of urine is achieved through the processes of glomerular filtration, tubular reabsorption, and secretion within the kidney. The bladder stores the urine received from the kidney by way of the ureters. Urine is then released from the bladder through the urethra.

STRUCTURES OF THE RENAL SYSTEM

Structures of the Kidney

The kidneys are paired organs located in the posterior region of the abdominal cavity behind the peritoneum. They lie on either side of the vertebral column with their upper and lower poles extending from the twelfth thoracic vertebra to the third lumbar vertebra (Fig. 37.1). The right kidney is slightly lower than the left and is displaced downward by the overlying liver. Each kidney is approximately 11 cm long, 5 to 6 cm wide, and 3 to 4 cm thick. A tightly adhering renal capsule surrounds each kidney, which is embedded in a mass of perirenal fat. The capsule and fatty layer are covered with a double layer of renal fascia, which is composed of fibrous tissue and attaches the kidney to the posterior abdominal wall. A cushion of adipose tissue and the position of the kidney between the abdominal organs and muscles of the back protect it from trauma.

The internal structures of the kidney are summarized in Fig. 37.2. The hilum is a medial indentation in the kidney and is the location of the entry and exit for the renal blood vessels, nerves, lymphatic vessels, and ureter. The outer layer of the kidney is called the cortex. The medulla forms the inner part of the kidney and consists of regions called pyramids. Renal columns are an extension of the cortex and extend between the pyramids to the renal pelvis. The apexes of the pyramids project into minor calyces (cup-shaped cavities) that unite to form major calyces. The minor and major calyces are chambers receiving urine from the collecting ducts and form the entry into the renal pelvis. The renal pelvis is an extension of the upper ureter. The walls of the calyces, pelvis, and ureter are lined with epithelial cells and contain smooth muscle cells that contract to move urine to the

BOX 37.1 The Kidney and Glucose Regulation

The human kidney contributes to the regulation of glucose concentration by making glucose through gluconeogenesis, by taking up glucose from the circulation, and by reabsorbing glucose from the glomerular filtrate. The human liver and kidneys release approximately equal amounts of glucose through gluconeogenesis in the postabsorptive state (4–12 h after meal ingestion). Other tissues lack the enzyme necessary for gluconeogenesis (glucose-6-phosphatase) and cannot participate in gluconeogenesis. In the postprandial state (up to 4 h after meal ingestion), although overall endogenous glucose release decreases substantially, renal gluconeogenesis accounts for 40% of glucose formed by gluconeogenesis.

About 180 g of glucose are normally filtered each day by the kidneys. Almost all of this is actively reabsorbed by means of sodium-glucose cotransporter 2 (SGLT2), a transmembrane protein expressed in the luminal border of the proximal tubule. This ensures sufficient energy is available during fasting periods. When plasma glucose concentrations exceed a threshold, the SGLT2 becomes saturated, and glucose appears in the urine. Individuals with diabetes mellitus have an increased transport maximum (T_m) for glucose from enhanced expression of SGLT2 and this contributes to hyperglycemia when there is poor glucose control. SGLT2 inhibitors are used for reducing hyperglycemia associated with diabetes mellitus, and they also have beneficial effects by stabilizing cellular metabolic stress and reducing glucose-mediated toxicity and inflammation in the kidneys and the heart.

Renal glucose release is stimulated by epinephrine and is inhibited by insulin. Insulin suppresses glucose release in both the liver and the kidney. The kidneys do not synthesize glycogen and, therefore, do not release glucose through glycogenolysis. In the postabsorptive state, the kidneys utilize about 10% of all glucose used by the body. When there is hypoglycemia, the liver initially releases glucose through glycogenolysis and then increases gluconeogenesis. The kidney also counter-regulates hypoglycemia through gluconeogenesis, which may explain in part why individuals with renal failure tend to develop hypoglycemia.

Data from Fernandes R. The controversial role of glucose in the diabetic kidney. *Porto Biomedical Journal,* 2021;6(1):e113; Vasquez-Rios G, Nadkarni GN. SGLT2 inhibitors: Emerging roles in the protection against cardiovascular and kidney disease among diabetic patients. *International Journal of Nephrology and Renovascular Disease,* 2020;13:281–296; Solini A. Role of SGLT2 inhibitors in the treatment of type 2 diabetes mellitus *Acta Diabetologica,* 2016;53(6):863–870.

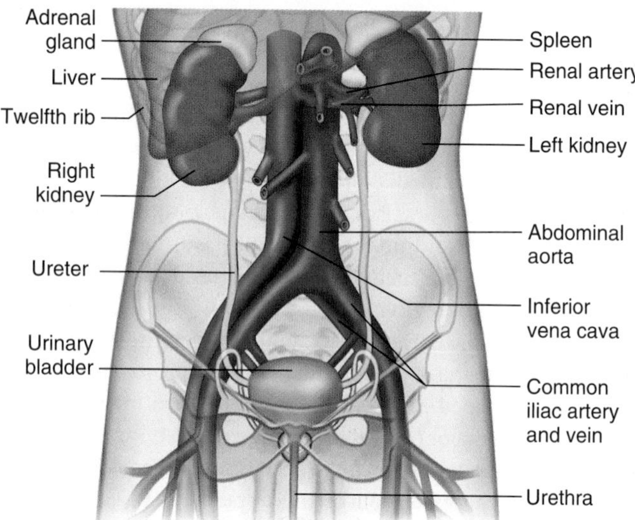

Fig. 37.1 Organs of the Urinary System. (From Patton KT, Thibodeau GA. *The human body in health & disease*, 7th edition. St. Louis: Mosby; 2018.)

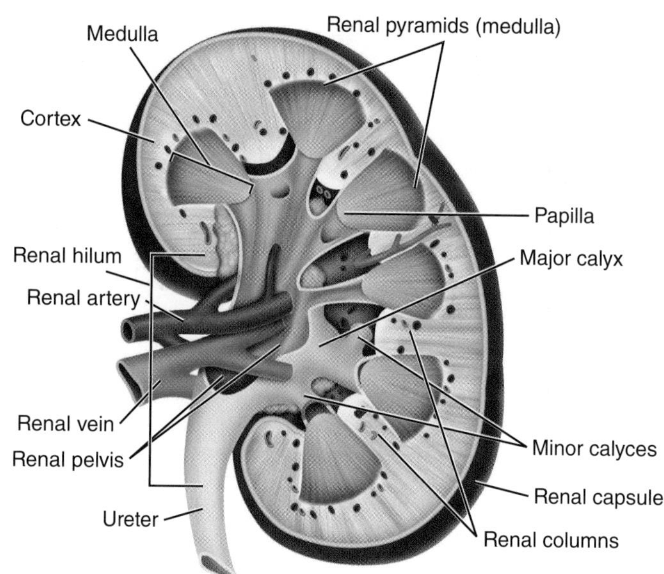

Fig. 37.2 Internal Structure of the Kidney. (From Solomon E. *Introduction to human anatomy and physiology*. 4th edition. St. Louis: Saunders; 2016.)

bladder. The lobe is the structural unit of the kidney. Each lobe is composed of a pyramid and the overlying cortex. There are about 14 to 18 lobes in each kidney.

Nephron

The nephron is the functional unit of the kidney. Each kidney contains approximately 1.2 million nephrons. The nephron is a tubular structure with subunits that include the renal corpuscle, proximal tubule (PT), loop of Henle, distal tubule, and collecting duct, all of which contribute to the formation of final urine (Fig. 37.3). The different structures of the epithelial cells lining various segments of the tubule facilitate the special functions of secretion and reabsorption (Fig. 37.4). The cortex contains the renal corpuscle, most of the PTs, and some segments of the distal tubule. The renal pyramids in the medulla contain the loops of Henle and collecting ducts. The kidney has three kinds of nephrons: (1) superficial cortical nephrons (85% of all nephrons), which originate close to the surface of the cortex or in the midcortex and extend partially into the medulla; (2) midcortical nephrons with short or long loops; and (3) juxtamedullary nephrons (about 12% of nephrons), which lie near and have long loops that extend deep into the medulla (about 40 mm) and are important for the concentration of urine (Fig. 37.5).

The renal corpuscle is composed of the glomerulus, Bowman (glomerular) capsule, and Bowman space. The glomerulus is a tuft of capillaries that loop into the Bowman space, like a fist pushed into bread dough. The Bowman space is continuous with the lumen of the renal tubules. Mesangial cells (shaped like smooth muscle cells) secrete the mesangial matrix (a type of connective tissue) and lie between and support the glomerular capillaries. Different mesangial cells contract like smooth muscle cells to regulate glomerular capillary blood

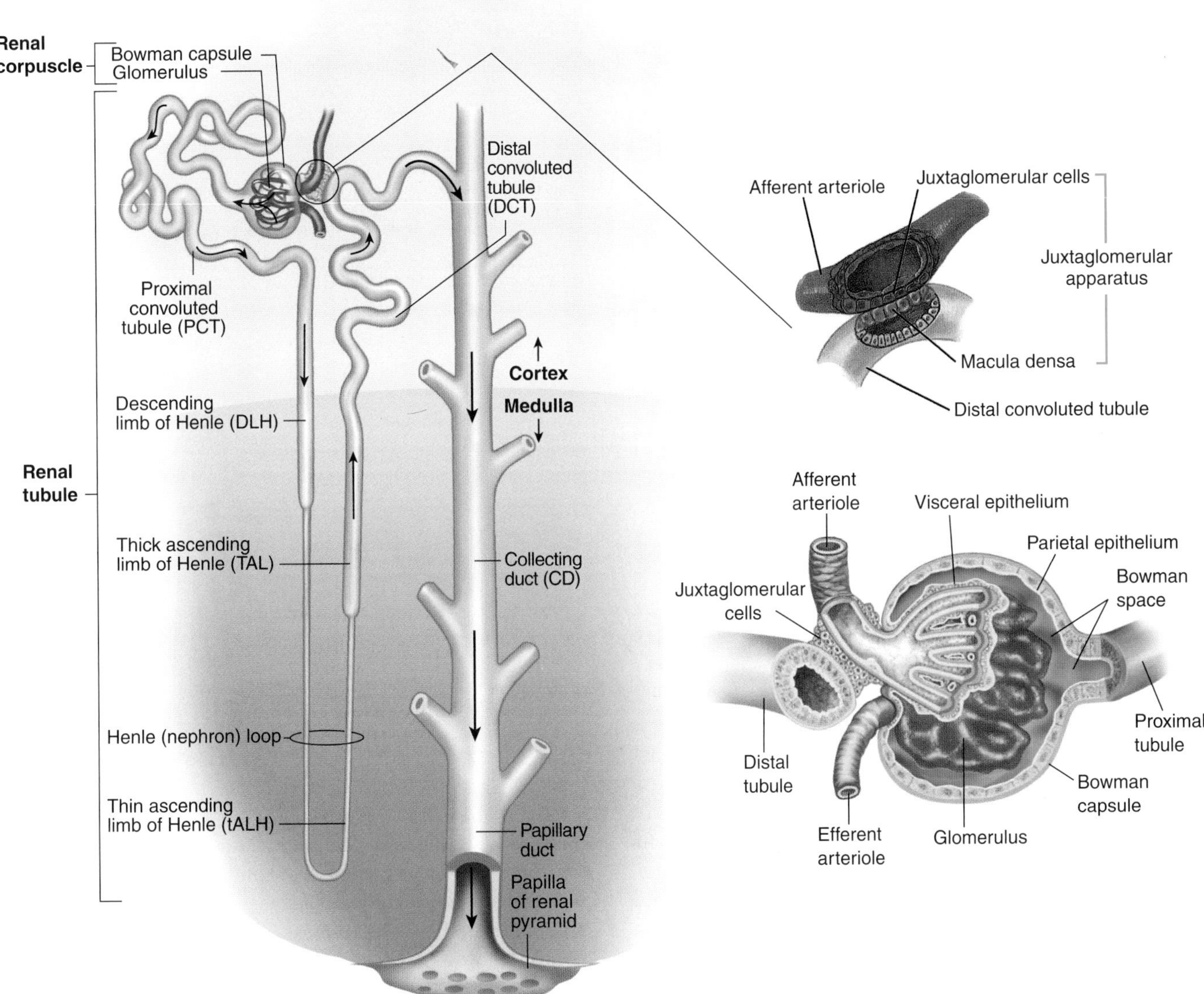

Fig. 37.3 Components of the Nephron. (From Patton, KT. *Anatomy and physiology,* 10th edition. St. Louis: Elsevier; 2019; Applegate EJ. *The anatomy and physiology learning system,* 4th edition. St. Louis: Saunders; 2011.)

flow. Mesangial cells also have phagocytic abilities similar to monocytes and release inflammatory cytokines and growth factors.

The glomerular filtration membrane filters blood components through three layers: (1) an inner capillary endothelium, (2) a middle basement membrane, and (3) an outer layer of capillary or visceral epithelium. The capillary endothelium is composed of cells in continuous contact with the basement membrane and contains pores. The pores are maintained by vascular epithelial growth factor (VEGF) produced by the visceral epithelium. The endothelial cells synthesize nitric oxide (a vasodilator) and endothelin-1 (a vasoconstrictor) that help regulate glomerular blood flow. The middle basement membrane is a selectively permeable membrane made up of a network of proteoglycans (type IV collagen) secreted and maintained by the epithelial cells. The epithelium has specialized cells called podocytes from which pedicles or projections radiate and adhere to the basement membrane. Pedicles from adjacent podocytes interlock, forming an elaborate network of intercellular clefts called filtration slits, or slit membranes (Fig. 37.6) that modulate filtration. Transcellular protein molecules ensure proper function of the filtration slits and, when altered, cause glomerular disease.[1]

The endothelium, basement membrane, and podocytes are covered with protein molecules bearing negative (anionic) charges that retard the filtration of anionic proteins, preventing proteinuria. The glomerular filtration membrane separates

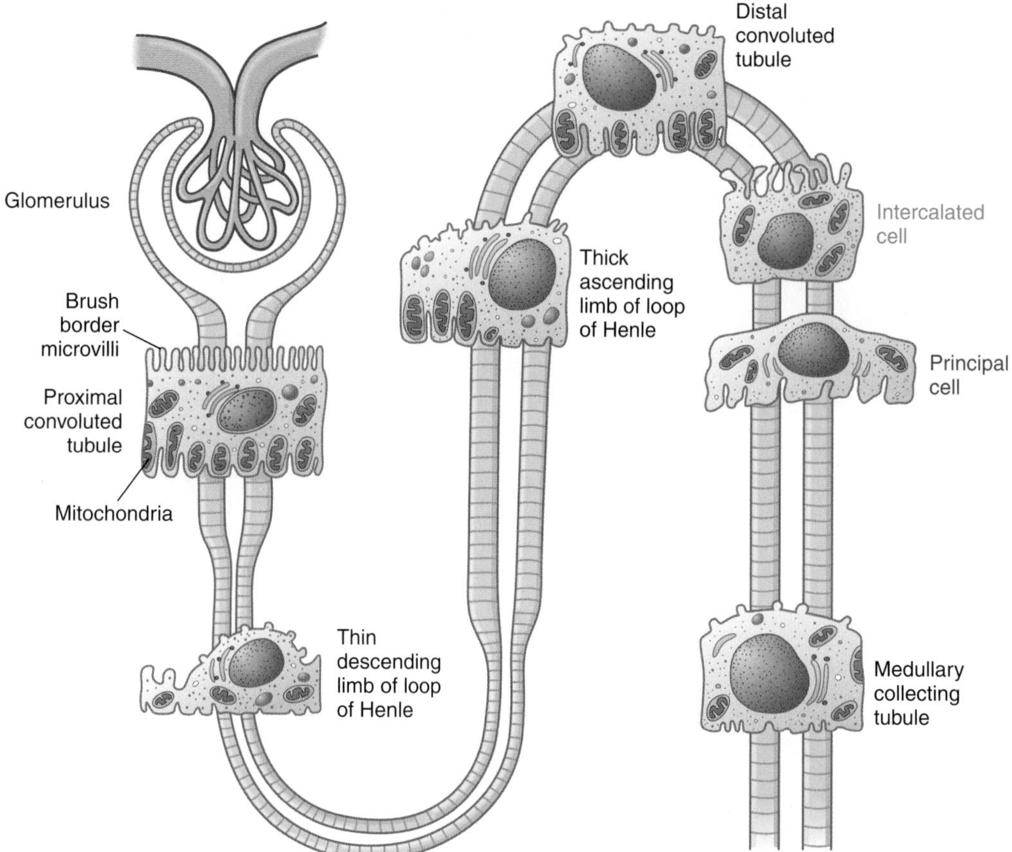

Fig. 37.4 Epithelial Cells of the Various Segments of Nephron Tubules. The proximal tubule is the only segment of the nephron that has a brush border, and the increased surface area promotes reabsorption of 50% of the glomerular filtrate.

the blood within the glomerular capillaries from the fluid (filtrate) in the Bowman space. The membrane allows all components of the blood to be filtered with the exception of blood cells and plasma proteins with a high molecular weight (most of the plasma proteins). The glomerular filtrate passes through the three layers of the glomerular membrane and forms the primary urine.

The glomerulus is supplied by the afferent arteriole and drained by the efferent arteriole. A group of specialized cells known as juxtaglomerular cells (renin-releasing cells) are located around the afferent arteriole where it enters the glomerulus. Between the afferent and efferent arterioles is the macula densa (sodium-sensing cells) of the distal tubule. Together the juxtaglomerular cells, macula densa cells, and mesangial cells form the juxtaglomerular apparatus (JGA). Control of renal blood flow (RBF), glomerular filtration, and renin secretion occurs at this site.

The proximal tubule, the first segment of the renal tubule, extends from the Bowman space. The PT has an initial convoluted segment that leads into a straight segment that descends toward the medulla (see Fig. 37.3). The wall of the proximal tubule consists of one layer of cuboidal epithelial cells with a surface layer of microvilli (a brush border) that increases the reabsorptive surface area. This is the only surface inside the nephron where the cells are covered with a brush border of microvilli (see Fig. 37.4). Sodium-coupled bicarbonate absorption from renal PTs provides a significant role in the maintenance of systemic acid/base balance (see Chapter 3). The early section of the PT also expresses a sodium glucose transporter (SGLT) known as SGLT2. SGLT2 belongs to a family of molecular carriers for transport of sugars, vitamins, amino acids, or smaller organic ions such as choline. SGLT2 reabsorbs approximately 90% of filtered glucose, and SGL2 inhibitors (gliflozins) have been developed as an oral medication for the treatment of type 2 diabetes mellitus (see Chapter 22).[2]

The PT joins the loop of Henle, which extends into the medulla. The loop is composed of a thin descending segment, a thin ascending segment, and a thick ascending segment. The thin descending segment is composed of squamous cells, has no active transport functions, and is highly permeable to water. The thin ascending segment is permeable to ions but not to water. The cells of the thick ascending segment are cuboidal and actively transport ions, particularly sodium, potassium, calcium, and magnesium into the interstitium, and pass urine into the distal convoluted tubule (see Fig. 37.14).

The distal tubule is shorter than the PT but also has straight and convoluted segments. It extends from the ascending loop of Henle to connecting tubules. An array of distal tubules joins into a connecting tubule and thus drains several nephrons. The connecting tubule then drains into a collecting duct. The

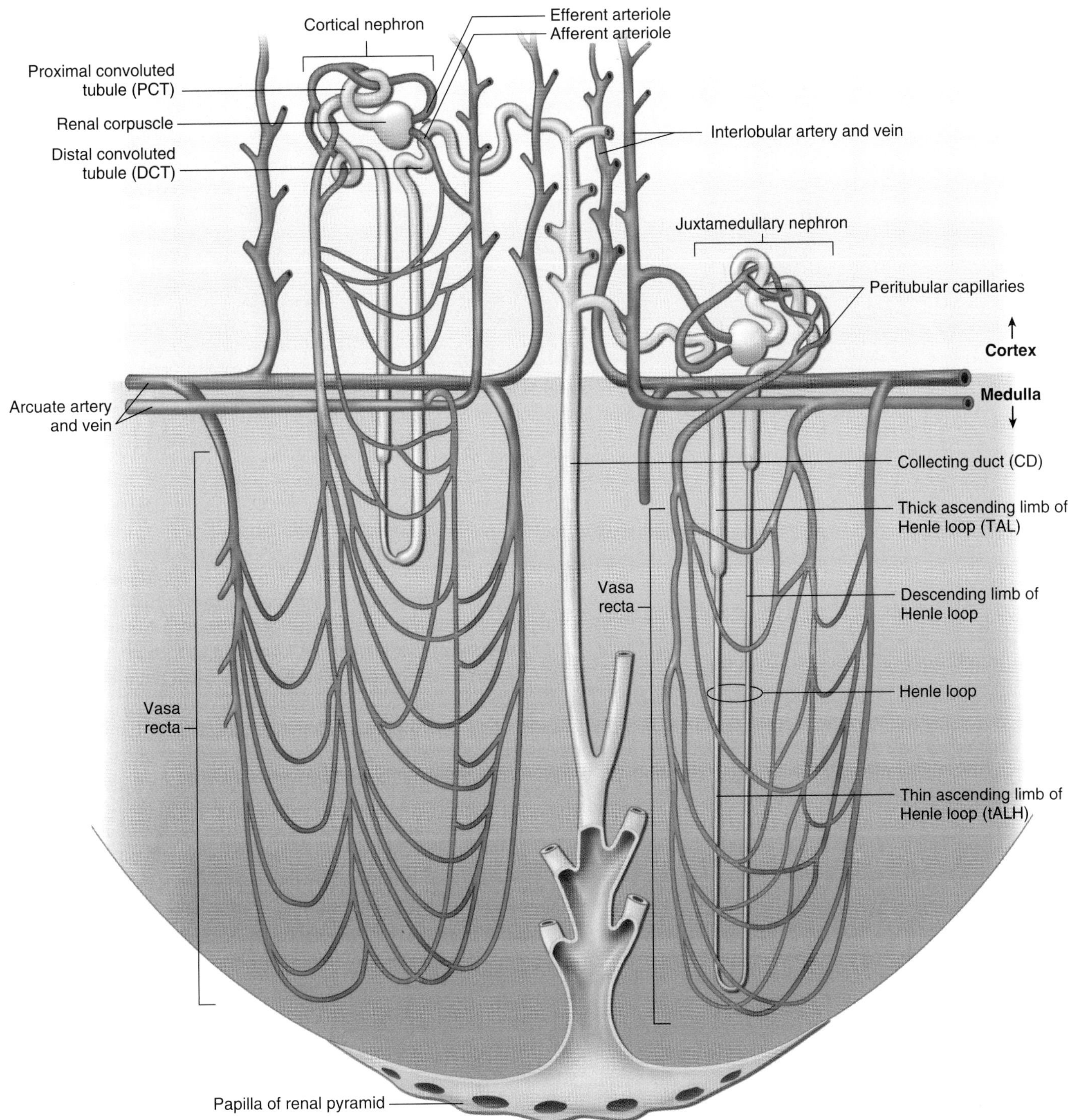

Fig. 37.5 Nephron Unit With Its Blood Vessels. Blood flows through nephron vessels as follows: interlobular artery, afferent arteriole, glomerulus, efferent arteriole, peritubular capillaries (around the tubules), venules, interlobular vein. (From Patton, KT. *Anatomy and physiology*, 10th edition. St. Louis: Elsevier; 2019:974.)

collecting duct is a large tubule that descends down the cortex and through the renal pyramids of the inner and outer medullae, draining urine into the minor calyx. In the distal tubule, principal cells reabsorb sodium and secrete potassium, and intercalated cells secrete hydrogen and reabsorb potassium and bicarbonate (see Fig. 37.4). These cells are important for maintaining fluid and electrolyte and acid-base balance.

Blood Vessels of the Kidney

The blood vessels of the kidney closely parallel the nephron's structure (see Fig. 37.5). The major vessels are as follows:

1. Renal arteries (see Fig. 37.2) arise as the fifth branches of the abdominal aorta, divide into anterior and posterior branches at the renal hilum, and then subdivide into lobar arteries supplying blood to the lower, middle, and upper thirds of the kidney.

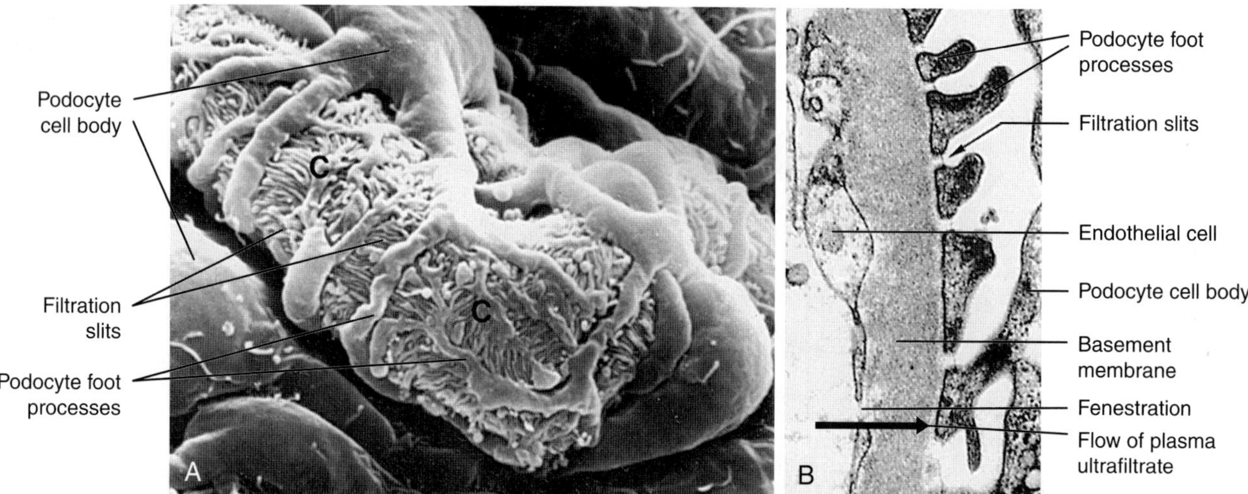

Fig. 37.6 Glomerular Capillary. (A) Scanning electron micrograph of normal glomerular capillary *(C)*. **(B)** Glomerular capillary wall (filtration membrane) (×40,000). Black arrow indicates direction of urine flow. (From Kissane JM, ed. *Anderson's pathology*, 9th edition. St. Louis: Mosby; 1990.)

2. Interlobar arteries are lobar subdivisions that travel down renal columns and between pyramids to form afferent glomerular arteries.
3. Arcuate arteries consist of branches of interlobar arteries at the cortical-medullary junction; they arch over the base of the pyramids and run parallel to the surface.
4. Glomerular capillaries consist of four to eight vessels and are arranged in a fistlike structure; they arise from the afferent arteriole and empty into the efferent arteriole, which carries blood to the peritubular capillaries. They are the major resistance vessels for regulating intrarenal blood flow (see Autoregulation of Intrarenal Blood Flow in the Renal Blood Flow section).
5. Peritubular capillaries surround convoluted portions of the proximal and distal tubules and the loop of Henle; they are adapted for cortical and juxtamedullary nephrons.
6. Vasa recta is a network of capillaries that forms loops and closely follows the loops of Henle; it is the only blood supply to the medulla (important for formation of concentrated urine).
7. Renal veins follow the arterial path in reverse direction and have the same names as the corresponding arteries; they eventually empty into the inferior vena cava. The lymphatic vessels also tend to follow the distribution of the blood vessels.

Urinary Structures

Ureters

The urine formed by the nephrons flows from the distal tubules and collecting ducts through the papillary ducts to the renal papillae (projections of the ducts) into the calyces, where it is collected in the renal pelvis (see Fig. 37.2). The urine is then funneled into the ureters (see Figs. 37.1 and 37.7). Each adult ureter is approximately 30 cm long and is composed of long, intertwining smooth muscle bundles. The lower ends pass through the posterior aspect of the bladder wall. The close approximation of smooth muscle cells in the ureter permits the direct transmission of electrical stimulation from one cell to another, resulting in downward peristaltic contraction, which propels urine into the bladder. Contraction of the bladder during micturition (urination) compresses the lower end of the ureter, preventing reflux. Peristalsis is maintained even when the ureter is denervated, so ureters can be transplanted.

Sensory innervation for the upper part of the ureter arises from sympathetic inputs from the tenth thoracic nerve. The innervation of lower segments arises from parasympathetic sacral nerves. Ureteral pain (e.g., pain from a kidney stone in the ureter) can be referred pain to the flank, umbilicus, vulva, or penis. The ureters have a rich blood supply. The upper part of the ureter is supplied by the renal arteries; the middle part is supplied by the common iliac arteries and branches from the abdominal aorta and gonadal arteries; and the lower part of the ureter is supplied mainly by branches from the internal iliac and vesical arteries.

Bladder and Urethra

The bladder is a bag made of smooth muscle fibers that forms the detrusor muscle with its smooth lining of uroepithelium. As the bladder fills with urine, it distends and the layers of uroepithelium within the lining slide past each other and become thinner as bladder volume increases. The uroepithelium (transitional epithelium) forms the interface between the urinary space and the underlying vasculature and connective, nervous, and muscle tissue. Uroepithelium also lines the urinary tract from the renal pelvis to the urethra. The uroepithelium maintains an important barrier function to prevent movement of water and solutes between the urine and the blood. It communicates information about urine pressure and composition to surrounding nerve and muscle cells. The trigone is a triangular area of smooth muscle between the openings of the two ureters and the urethra (see Fig. 37.7). The position of the bladder varies with sex and age. In infants and young children, the bladder

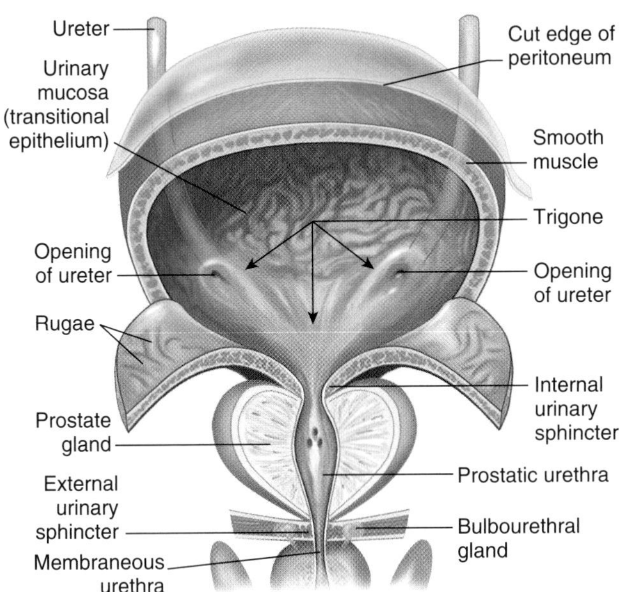

Fig. 37.7 Structure of the Urinary Bladder. Frontal view of a dissected urinary bladder (male) in a fully distended position. No prostate is present in females. (From Patton KT, Thibodeau GA. *The human body in health & disease*, 7th edition. St. Louis: Mosby, 2018.)

rises above the symphysis pubis, providing easy access for percutaneous aspiration. In adult females, the bladder is anterior to the vagina and inferior to the uterus. In adult males, the bladder lies between the pubic symphysis and rectum. The bladder has a profuse blood supply, accounting for the bleeding that readily occurs with trauma, surgery, or inflammation.

The urethra extends from the inferior side of the bladder to the outside of the body. A ring of smooth muscle forms the internal urethral sphincter at the junction of the urethra and bladder and is under involuntary muscle control. The external urethral sphincter is composed of striated skeletal muscle and is under voluntary motor control. The entire urethra is lined with mucus-secreting glands. The female urethra is short (3 to 4 cm). The male urethra is long (18 to 20 cm) and has three main segments: prostatic, membranous, and penile. The prostatic urethra is closest to the bladder. It passes through the prostate gland and contains the openings of the ejaculatory ducts. Prostatic enlargement can obstruct the flow of urine in this segment. The membranous urethra passes through the floor of the pelvis. The penile segment forms the remainder of the tube. It is surrounded by the corpus spongiosum erectile tissue and contains the openings of the bulbourethral glands (see Figs. 24.11 and 24.15).

The innervation of the bladder and internal urethral sphincter is supplied by parasympathetic fibers of the autonomic nervous system that arise from the sacral levels of the spinal cord (S2 to S4) and contribute to bladder contraction and urine emptying. Sympathetic fibers originate from T11-L2 and inhibit the bladder body and excite the lower bladder and proximal urethral sphincter to retain urine. Sensory fibers from the bladder and urethra may extend as high as the T6 portion of the spinal cord. Somatic motor neurons in the pudendal nerve innervate the striated external urethral sphincter. The detrusor muscle is innervated by sympathetic nervous system fibers from the lumbar spinal cord and parasympathetic fibers from the sacral spinal cord. The reflex arc required for micturition is stimulated by mechanoreceptors that respond to stretching of tissue, sensing bladder fullness, and sending impulses to the sacral level of the cord. When the bladder accumulates 250 to 300 mL of urine, the bladder contracts and the internal urethral sphincter relaxes through activation of the spinal reflex arc (known as the *micturition reflex*). At this time, a person feels the urge to void. The reflex can be inhibited or facilitated by impulses coming from the brain, resulting in voluntary control of micturition by the relaxation or contraction of the external sphincter.

RENAL BLOOD FLOW AND GLOMERULAR FILTRATION

The kidneys are highly vascular organs and usually receive 1000 to 1200 mL of blood per minute, or about 20% to 25% of the cardiac output. With a normal hematocrit of 45%, about 600 to 700 mL of blood flowing through the kidney per minute is plasma. Of the renal plasma flow (RPF), 20% (approximately 120 to 140 mL/min) is filtered at the glomerulus and passes into the Bowman capsule. (The remaining 80% of plasma flows through the efferent arterioles to the peritubular capillaries.) The filtration of the plasma per unit of time is known as the glomerular filtration rate (GFR) (e.g., 120 to 140 mL/min), which is directly related to the perfusion pressure of the glomerular capillaries. The ratio of glomerular filtrate to RPF per minute (e.g., 120/600 = 0.20) is called the *filtration fraction*. Normally, all but 1 to 2 mL/min of the glomerular filtrate is reabsorbed from nephron tubules and returned to the circulation by the peritubular capillaries.

The GFR is directly related to the RBF, which is regulated by intrinsic autoregulatory mechanisms, by neural regulation, and by hormonal regulation. In general, blood flow to any organ is determined by the arteriovenous pressure differences across the vascular bed. If the mean arterial pressure decreases or the vascular resistance increases, the RBF declines and urinary output decreases. Normal urinary output is about 30 mL/h minimum in adults or 0.5 to 1.0 mL/kg/h.

Autoregulation of Intrarenal Blood Flow

In the kidney, the autoregulation of the glomerular blood flow helps keep the GFR fairly constant over a range of systemic arterial pressures between 80 and 180 mm Hg (Fig. 37.8). This is necessary to maintain the clearance of metabolic wastes and the reabsorption of filtered electrolytes and nutrients by the renal tubules with the normal variations in systemic blood pressure. For example, systemic blood pressure increases during exercise and decreases during rest, but nephron blood flow and GFR remain fairly constant. This mechanism is known as the autoregulation of intrarenal blood flow.[3] It is maintained by two mechanisms working together to control the tone of the glomerular afferent arteriole. One mechanism responds to changes in afferent arterial pressure and another responds to changes in the sodium chloride concentration of the distal tubular fluid.

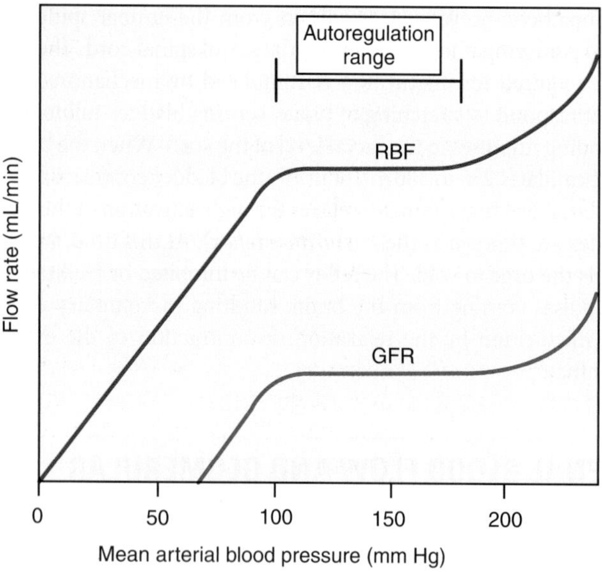

Fig. 37.8 Renal Autoregulation. Renal blood flow *(RBF)* and glomerular filtration rate *(GFR)* are stabilized in the face of changes in perfusion pressure.

1. When the systemic blood pressure (perfusion pressure) in the afferent arteriole of each nephron increases causing stretch of the vessel, an intrinsic autoregulatory myogenic mechanism of afferent arteriolar contraction increases resistance, thus maintaining constant flow and GFR and also protecting the glomerulus from high filtration pressure. The opposite occurs with a decrease in the systemic blood pressure.
2. The tubuloglomerular feedback mechanism (Fig. 37.9) involves the macula densa cells in the distal tubule, the renin secreting juxtaglomerular cells of the afferent arteriole and mesangial cells. The macula densa cells are adjacent to the extraglomerular mesangial cells, which fill the angle formed by the afferent and efferent arterioles of the glomerulus. This anatomic arrangement of macula densa cells, extraglomerular mesangial cells, afferent arteriolar smooth muscle cells, and renin-secreting cells of the afferent arterioles is known as the *juxtaglomerular apparatus.* As the blood pressure increases or decreases, the macula densa epithelial cells sense the resulting increase or decrease in the filtered amounts of sodium in the distal tubule. When the GFR and sodium concentration increase, the macula densa cells "feedback to" or stimulate afferent arteriolar vasoconstriction and decrease glomerular pressure and GFR, returning it to a normal range and preventing sodium loss. The decreased sodium load then entering the tubule inhibits tubuloglomerular feedback, shutting down the feedback system. When the blood pressure decreases, the juxtaglomerular cells secrete renin, resulting in an increase in blood pressure and an increase in GFR (See Section on Hormones and Other Factors Regulating RBF). Mesangial cells are also thought to contribute to afferent arteriolar vasoconstriction by contracting and secreting renin.[4]

Neural Regulation of Renal Blood Flow

The blood vessels of the kidney are innervated by sympathetic nerve fibers located primarily on afferent arterioles. When the systemic arterial pressure decreases, increased renal sympathetic nerve activity is mediated reflexively through the carotid sinus and the baroreceptors of the aortic arch. The renal sympathetic nerves release catecholamines. This stimulates afferent renal arteriolar vasoconstriction and decreases the RBF and GFR, increases renal tubular sodium and water reabsorption, and increases the systemic blood pressure. Decreased afferent renal sympathetic nerve activity produces the opposite effects. The integrated response regulates water and sodium balance. Renalase is a hormone released by the kidney, heart, and other organs. It is a growth factor that maintains renal tubular function and, as a monoamine oxidase, promotes the metabolism of catecholamines and, in this way, participates in lowering the blood pressure and GFR. Renalase also has a protective role in cardiovascular and chronic kidney diseases. (See Emerging Science Box: Renalase). The sympathetic nervous system also participates in hormonal regulation of the RBF (i.e., stimulates the renin-angiotensin-aldosterone system [RAAS]). There is no significant parasympathetic innervation. The innervation of the kidney arises primarily from the celiac ganglion and greater splanchnic nerve.

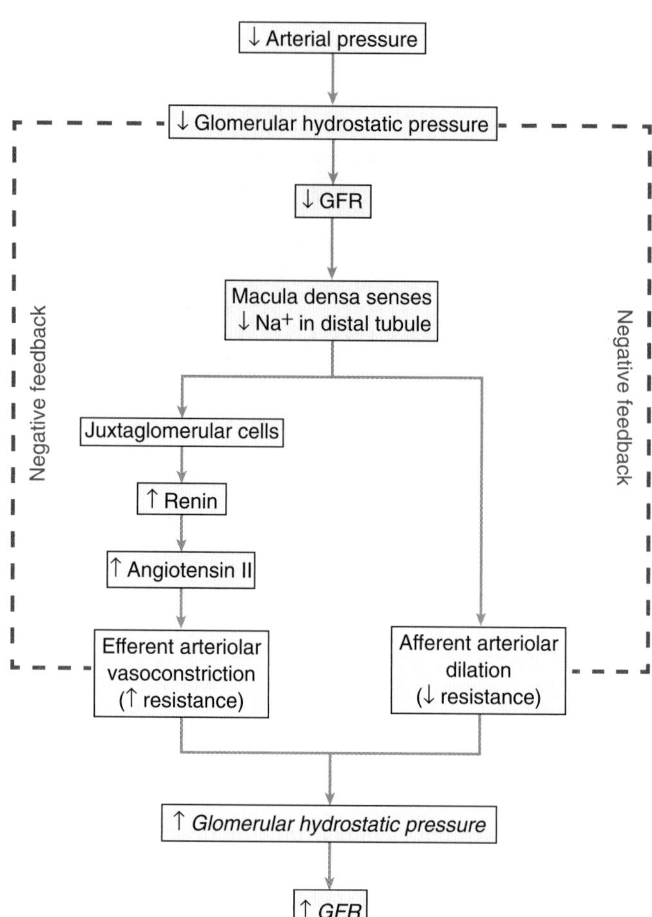

Fig. 37.9 Tubuloglomerular Feedback. Negative feedback increases glomerular hydrostatic pressure and GFR. See text for details. *GFR,* Glomerular filtration rate.

Hormones and Other Factors Regulating Renal Blood Flow

Hormones and other mediators can alter the resistance of the renal vasculature by stimulating vasodilation or

EMERGING SCIENCE BOX

Renalase

Renalase is highly expressed in the proximal tubule, but also in the heart, skeletal muscle and small intestine. Elevated plasma catecholamines activate renalase enzymatic activity and lead to a threefold to fourfold stimulation of renalase secretion, causing a significant fall in blood pressure. Renalase single nucleotide polymorphisms (a variation at a single position in a DNA sequence) are found to be associated with essential hypertension, higher left ventricular mass index, lower left ventricular ejection fraction, lower exercise capacity and ischemic stroke. Increases in renalase signaling, independent of its enzymatic activity in breaking down catecholamines, are known to improve cardiac and renal function by activating cytoprotective intracellular signals to lower blood pressure, protect ischemic tissue via anti-apoptotic and anti-inflammatory mechanisms, and promote atherosclerotic plaque stability in cardiovascular disease. Renal function also affects renalase levels, and serum renalase levels are higher in individuals with chronic kidney disease. Renalse may have a pathologic role in the survival and growth of cancer cells, particularly malignant melanoma. Anti-renalase therapy in mouse models decreased melanoma cell survival, and blocked tumor growth. Mechanisms of renalase regulation are not well understood, and elevations may be associated with increased production and secretion, limited filtration or increased reabsorption under conditions of increased demand in different disease states. Efforts are in progress to develop more standardized and validated methods to evaluate the activity and levels of renalase in tissue and body fluids, including blood and urine. These measures will help to distinguish the pathophysiological relevance and diagnostic/therapeutic utility of renalase as a biomarker of disease and guide the development of both replacement therapy and/or inhibition.

Data from Desir GV, et al. Renalase in hypertension and kidney disease. *Nephrology Dialysis Transplantation*, 2014;29(1):22–28; Hollander L, et al. Renalase expression by melanoma and tumor-associated macrophages promotes tumor growth through a STAT3- mediated mechanism. *Cancer Research*, 2016;76(13):3884–3894; Li Y, et al. Roles and mechanisms of renalase in cardiovascular disease: A promising therapeutic target. *Biomedicine and Pharmacotherapy*, 2020;131:110712; Serwin NM, et al. Serum-to-urine renalase ratio and renalase fractional excretion in healthy adults and chronic kidney disease patients. *BMC Nephrology*, 2020;21(1):77; Skrzypczyk P, et al. Renalase in children with chronic kidney disease. *Biomarkers*, 2019;24(7):638–644; Wiśniewska M, et al. Chronic kidney disease is associated with increased levels of renalase in serum and decreased in erythrocytes. *Polish Archives of Internal Medicine*, 2019;129(11):790–797.

vasoconstriction. A major hormonal regulator of RBF is the RAAS, which can increase systemic arterial pressure, reabsorption of sodium and water, and RBF. Renin is an enzyme formed and stored in the granular cells of the afferent arterioles of the JGA. Renin release is triggered by a decreased blood pressure in the afferent arterioles, a decreased sodium chloride concentration in the distal convoluted tubule, sympathetic nerve stimulation of β-adrenergic receptors on the juxtaglomerular cells, and the release of prostaglandins.

When renin is released, it cleaves an α-globulin (angiotensinogen produced by liver hepatocytes) in the plasma to form angiotensin I, which is physiologically inactive. In the presence of angiotensin-converting enzyme (ACE) produced from the pulmonary and renal endothelium, angiotensin I is converted to angiotensin II. Angiotensin II stimulates secretion of aldosterone by the adrenal cortex, is a potent vasoconstrictor, and stimulates antidiuretic hormone (ADH) secretion and thirst.

Numerous physiologic effects of the RAAS stabilize the systemic blood pressure and preserve the extracellular fluid volume during hypotension or hypovolemia. Actions include sodium reabsorption, systemic vasoconstriction, sympathetic nerve stimulation, and thirst stimulation, with an increased fluid intake. The effects of aldosterone combine with those of ADH in regulating blood volume (Fig. 37.10).

Natriuretic peptides are synthesized and released from the heart and are natural antagonists to the RAAS (see Fig. 3.5). Natriuretic peptides cause vasodilation, increase sodium and water excretion, and decrease the blood pressure. Thus, they assist in protecting the heart from volume overload. Urodilatin is a renal natriuretic peptide produced by cells in the distal tubule and collecting duct. It increases RBF, causing diuresis. Other hormones and mediators that influence RBF are summarized in Table 37.1.

KIDNEY FUNCTION

Nephron Function

The major function of the nephron is urine formation, which it does by performing many functions simultaneously (Fig. 37.11):

1. Filtering plasma at the glomerulus
2. Reabsorbing and secreting different substances along the tubular structures
3. Forming a filtrate of protein-free fluid (ultrafiltration)
4. Regulating the filtrate to maintain the body fluid volume, electrolyte composition, and pH within narrow limits

Glomerular filtration is the movement of fluid and solutes across the glomerular capillary membrane into the Bowman space. Tubular reabsorption is the movement of fluids and solutes from the tubular lumen into the peritubular capillary plasma. Tubular secretion is the transfer of substances from the plasma of the peritubular capillary to the tubular lumen (Fig. 37.12). The transport mechanisms are both active and passive (processes defined in Chapter 1). Excretion is the elimination of a substance in the final urine.

Glomerular Filtration

The fluid filtered across the glomerular capillary filtration membrane and released into the proximal convoluted tubule is protein free but contains electrolytes (e.g., sodium, chloride, and potassium) and organic molecules (e.g., creatinine, urea, and glucose) in the same concentrations as those found in plasma. As are other capillary membranes, the glomerulus is freely permeable to water and relatively impermeable to large colloids, such as plasma proteins. The molecule's size and the small size of the filtration slits in the glomerular epithelium affect the permeability of substances crossing the glomerulus and entering the PT. The negative charge along the filtration membrane further impedes the passage of negatively charged macromolecules, particularly proteins (because like forces repel each other). Positively charged macromolecules therefore permeate the membrane more readily than neutrally charged particles.

In addition to permeability, capillary pressures also affect glomerular filtration. The hydrostatic pressure within

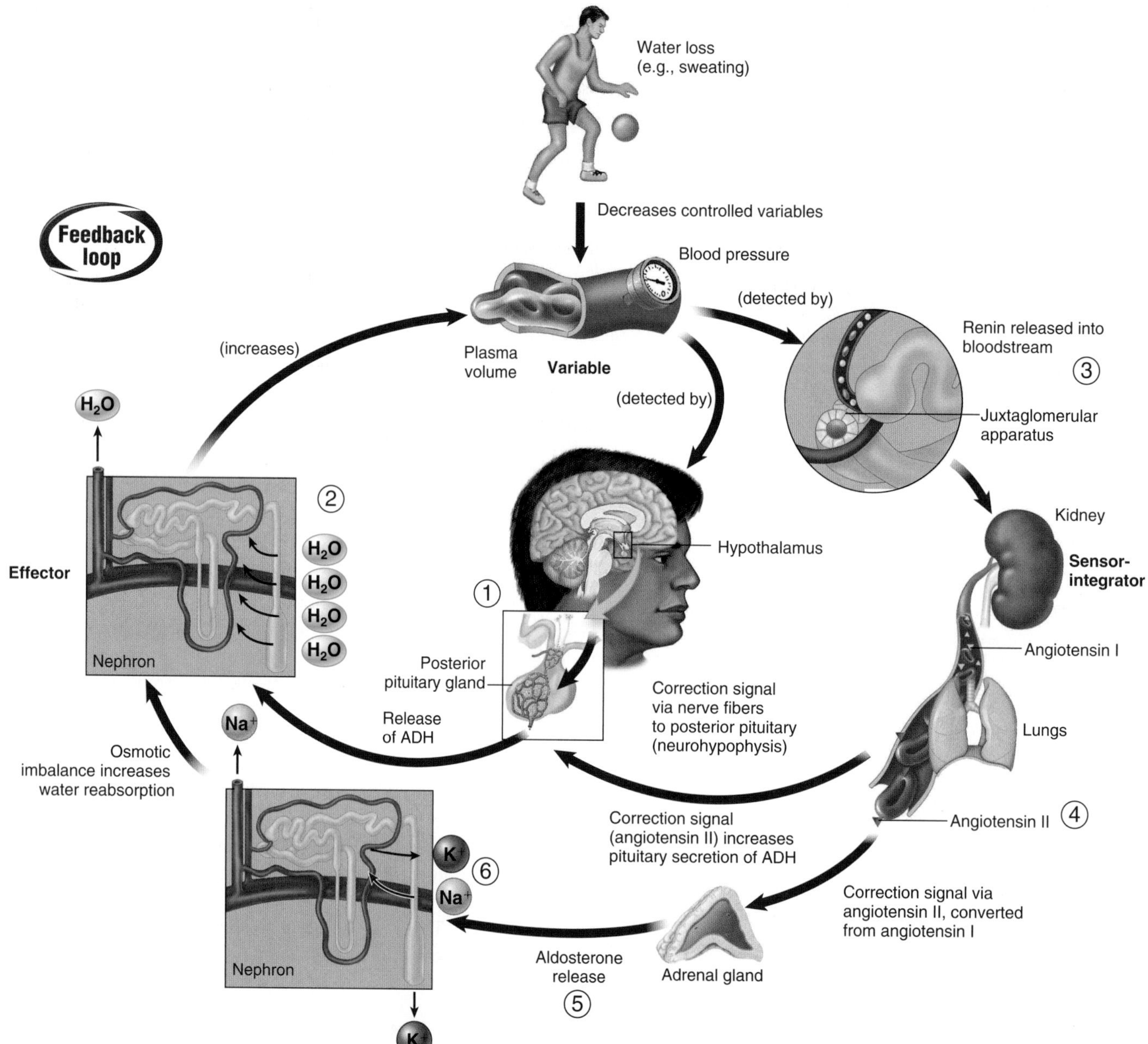

Fig. 37.10 Cooperative Roles of Antidiuretic Hormone (ADH) and Aldosterone in Regulating Urine and Plasma Volume. The drop in blood pressure that accompanies loss of fluid from the internal environment triggers the hypothalamus to rapidly release ADH from the posterior pituitary gland **(1)**. ADH increases water reabsorption by the kidney by increasing water permeability of the distal tubules and collecting ducts **(2)**. The drop in blood pressure also is detected by each nephron's juxtaglomerular apparatus, which responds by secreting renin **(3)**. Renin triggers the formation of angiotensin II **(4)**, which stimulates release of aldosterone from the adrenal cortex **(5)**. Aldosterone then slowly boosts water reabsorption by the kidneys by increasing reabsorption of Na^+**(6)**. Because angiotensin II also stimulates secretion of ADH, it serves as an additional link between the ADH and aldosterone mechanisms. (From Patton KT. *Anatomy & physiology*, 10th edition. St. Louis: Mosby; 2019)

the capillary is the major force for pushing water and solutes across the filtration membrane and into the Bowman capsule. This pressure is determined by the systemic arterial pressure and the resistances to blood flow in the afferent and efferent arterioles. Two forces oppose the filtration effects of the glomerular capillary hydrostatic pressure: (1) the hydrostatic pressure in the Bowman space, and (2) the effective oncotic pressure of the glomerular capillary blood. Remember, hydrostatic pressure is a pushing pressure, and oncotic pressure is a pulling pressure in relation to water. Because the fluid in the Bowman space normally contains only very small amounts of protein, it does not usually have an oncotic influence on the plasma of the glomerular capillary (Fig. 37.13).

TABLE 37.1 Hormones, Mediators, and Renal Blood Flow

Hormone or Mediator	Effect on Renal Blood Flow
Adenosine	Produced within kidney; causes vasoconstriction of afferent arteriole; decreases RBF and GFR
Angiotensin II	Produced systemically and within kidneys; constricts afferent and efferent arterioles; decreases RBF and GFR
Atrial and brain natriuretic peptides	Produced by atria and ventricles of the heart with hypertension and increased blood volume; cause vasodilation of afferent arteriole and vasoconstriction of efferent arteriole; modest increase in GFR with little change in RBF
Bradykinin	Produced in kidney from kininogen and causes vasodilation by release of nitric oxide and prostaglandins; increases RBF and GFR
Dopamine	Produced by the proximal tubule; increases RBF; inhibits renin secretion
Endothelin	Produced by renal vessel endothelial cells, mesangial cells, and distal tubule cells in response to bradykinin, angiotensin II, epinephrine, and stretch; most active with renal disease; profound vasoconstriction of afferent and efferent arterioles; decreases RBF and GFR
Histamine	Produced locally within the kidney; modulates RBF in basal state and during inflammation; increases RBF by decreasing afferent and efferent arteriolar resistance and does not decrease GFR
Nitric oxide	Produced by renal vessel endothelial cells with increased stretch and by stimulation of acetylcholine, histamine, bradykinin, ATP; increases vasodilation of afferent and efferent arterioles
Prostaglandins, PGI_2, PGE_2	Produced locally within kidney with decreased RBF; dampen vasoconstriction caused by sympathetic nerves and angiotensin II; prevent harmful vasoconstriction and renal ischemia
Urodilatin (a natriuretic peptide)	Produced by distal tubule and collecting duct when there is increased circulating volume and increased blood pressure; inhibits sodium and water reabsorption from medullary part of collecting duct, thereby producing diuresis

ATP, Adenosine triphosphate; *GFR*, glomerular filtration rate; *PGE2*, prostaglandin E2; *PGI2*, prostaglandin I2; *RBF*, renal blood flow.

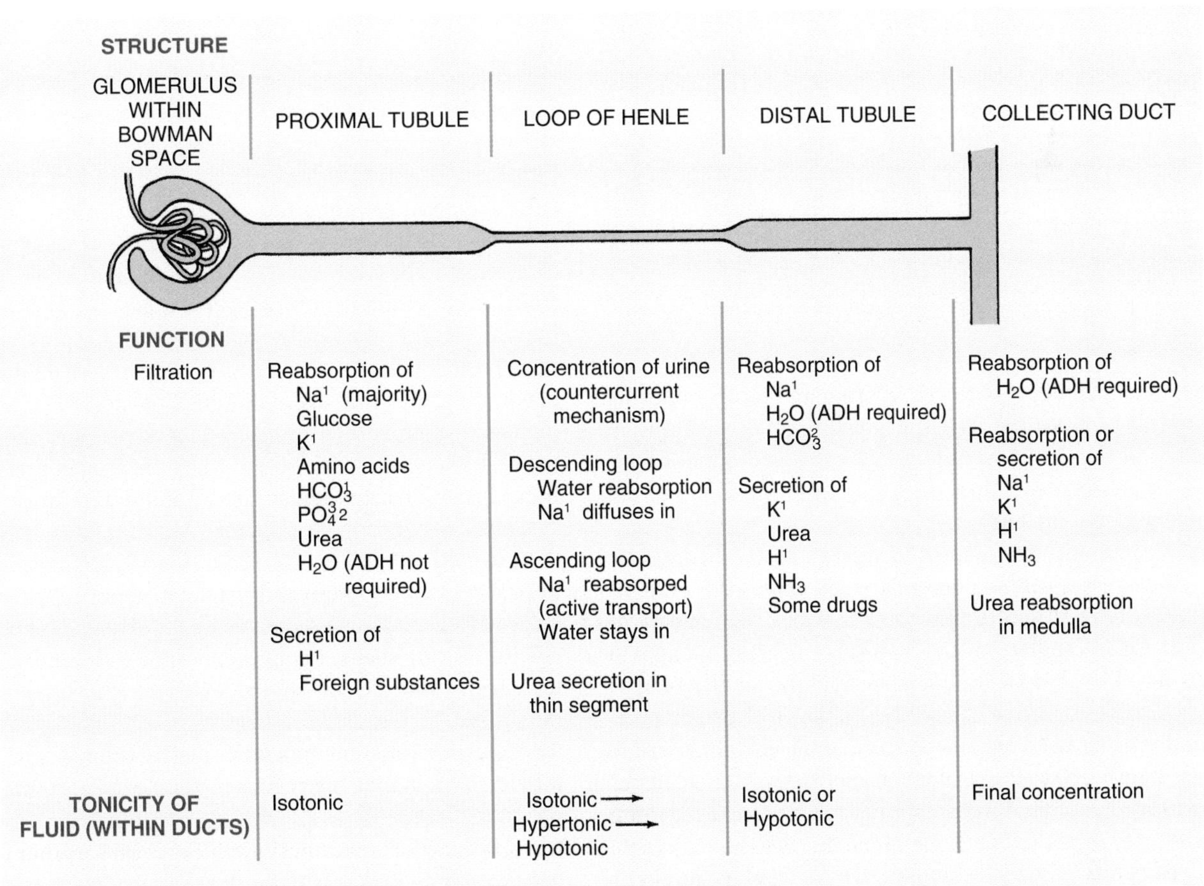

Fig. 37.11 Major Functions of Nephron Segments. *ADH*, Antidiuretic hormone. (Modified from Hockenberry MJ et al. *Wong's nursing care of infants and children*, 8th edition. St. Louis: Mosby; 2007.)

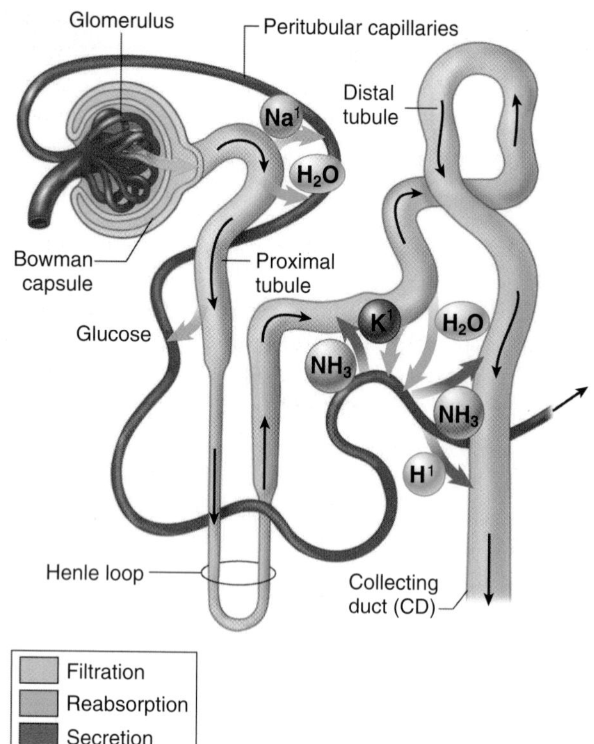

Fig. 37.12 Urine Formation: Glomerular Filtration, Tubular Reabsorption, and Tubular Secretion. These are the three processes by which the kidneys excrete urine. Water, electrolytes, glucose, and organic molecules are filtered at the glomerulus. Sodium and glucose are reabsorbed into peritubular capillaries by active transport from the proximal convoluted tubules, and water reabsorption follows by osmosis. Sodium is reabsorbed by active transport from distal convoluted tubules; more sodium is conserved when aldosterone is secreted. Osmotic reabsorption of water from the distal tubules occurs when antidiuretic hormone is present. Secretion of ammonia (NH_3), hydrogen, and potassium occurs from peritubular capillaries into distal tubules by active transport. (From Patton KT, Thibodeau GA. *The human body in health & disease*, 7th edition. St. Louis: Mosby; 2018.)

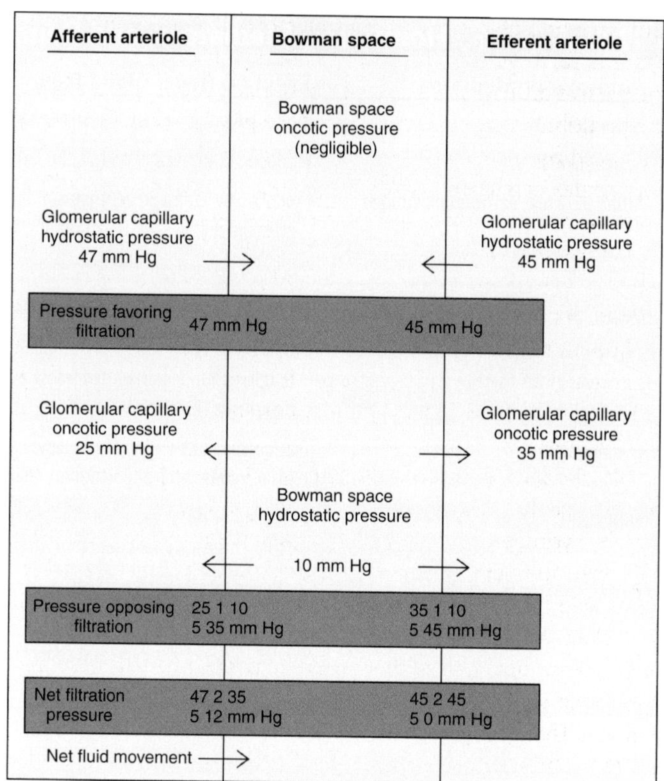

Fig. 37.13 Glomerular Filtration Pressures.

The combined effect of forces favoring and forces opposing filtration determines the filtration pressure. The net filtration pressure (NFP) is the sum of forces favoring and opposing filtration. The estimated values contributing to the forces of net filtration are presented in Fig. 37.13.

The plasma oncotic pressure increases and the hydrostatic pressure decreases in the glomerular capillary, as the protein-free fluid is filtered into the Bowman capsule. The increase in the glomerular capillary oncotic pressure is great enough to reduce the NFP to zero at the efferent end of the capillary and to stop the filtration process effectively. The low hydrostatic pressure and the increased oncotic pressure in the efferent arteriole then are transferred to the peritubular capillaries. This facilitates the reabsorption of fluid from the PTs back into the circulating blood.

Filtration rate. The total volume of fluid filtered by the glomeruli averages 180 L/day, or approximately 120 mL/min, a phenomenal amount considering the size of the kidneys. Because only 1 to 2 L of urine is excreted per day, 99% of the filtrate is reabsorbed into the peritubular capillaries and returned to the blood. The factors determining the GFR are directly related to the pressures that favor or oppose filtration (see Fig. 37.13). Obstruction of the outflow of urine (e.g., caused by strictures, stones, or tumors along the urinary tract) can cause a retrograde increase in hydrostatic pressure at the Bowman space and a decrease in the GFR. Low levels of plasma protein in the blood from severe malnutrition or liver disease can also result in a decrease in the glomerular capillary oncotic pressure, which increases the GFR. Excessive loss of protein-free fluid as a result of vomiting, diarrhea, use of diuretics, or excessive sweating can increase the glomerular capillary oncotic pressure and decrease the GFR. Renal disease also can cause changes in pressure relationships by altering capillary permeability and the surface area available for filtration (see Chapter 38).

Proximal tubule. By the end of the PT, approximately 60% to 70% of filtered sodium and water and about 50% of urea have been actively reabsorbed, along with 90% or more of potassium, glucose, bicarbonate, calcium, phosphate, amino acids, and uric acid. Chloride, water, and urea are reabsorbed passively but linked to the active transport of sodium (a cotransport mechanism). For some molecules, active transport in the renal tubules is limited as the carrier molecules become saturated, a phenomenon known as transport maximum (T_m). For example, when the carrier molecules for glucose reabsorption in the PT become saturated (i.e., with the development of hyperglycemia), the excess will be excreted in the urine, causing glucosuria.

Active reabsorption of sodium is the primary function of the convoluted segment of the PT. Water, most other electrolytes, and organic substances are cotransported with sodium. The osmotic force generated by active sodium transport promotes the passive diffusion of water out of the tubular lumen and into the peritubular capillaries. Passive transport of water is further enhanced by the elevated oncotic pressure of the blood in the peritubular capillaries, which is created by the previous filtration of water at the glomerulus. The reabsorption of water leaves an increased concentration of urea within the tubular lumen, creating a gradient for its passive diffusion to the peritubular plasma. As the positively charged sodium ions leave the tubular lumen, negatively charged chloride ions passively follow to maintain electroneutrality. Because the inner membrane of the proximal tubular cell has a limited permeability to chloride, chloride reabsorption lags behind that of sodium.

Bicarbonate is completely filtered at the glomerulus, and approximately 90% is reabsorbed in the PT. In the tubular lumen, hydrogen ions are actively exchanged for sodium. The hydrogen ions combine with bicarbonate ions and form carbonic acid (H_2CO_3), which rapidly breaks down, or dissociates, to carbon dioxide (CO_2) and water (H_2O). The CO_2 and H_2O then diffuse into the tubular cell, where the enzyme carbonic anhydrase again catalyzes the CO_2 and H_2O to form HCO_3^- and H^+. The H^+ is secreted into the tubular lumen again, and HCO_3^- combines with sodium and is transported to the peritubular capillary blood as $NaHCO_3$ (a sodium bicarbonate buffer). Bicarbonate is thus conserved. The hydrogen combines with hydroxide ion (OH^-) and is reabsorbed as water. Therefore, in the PT, these ions normally do not contribute to the urinary excretion of acid or the addition of acid to the blood.

In the PT, secretory transport mechanisms exist for creatinine, other organic bases, and endogenous and exogenous organic acids, including para-aminohippurate (PAH) and penicillin (Box 37.2). These secretory mechanisms eliminate drugs and other exogenous chemical products from the body, often after first conjugating (combining) them with sulfate and glucuronic acid in the liver. Many drugs and their metabolites are eliminated from the body in this way. When the renal tubules are damaged, metabolic by-products and drugs may accumulate, causing toxic levels in the body.

Normally, 99% of the glomerular filtrate is reabsorbed. When the GFR spontaneously decreases or increases, the renal tubules, primarily the PTs, automatically adjust their rate of reabsorption of sodium and water to balance the change in the GFR. Thus, a constant fraction of filtered sodium and water is reabsorbed from the PT. This prevents wide fluctuations in the excretion of sodium and water into the urine and is known as glomerulotubular balance (GTB). GTB and tubuloglomerular feedback together regulate sodium and water balance.

BOX 37.2 Substances Transported by Renal Tubules

Reabsorption	Secretion
Albumin	Choline
Ascorbate	Creatinine
Fructose	Histamine
Galactose	Methylguanidine
Glutamae	*para*-Aminohippurate
Glucose	Penicillin and many other drugs
Phosphate	Steroid glucuronides
Sulfate	Thiamine
Xylose	

Loop of Henle and distal tubule. Urine can be hypotonic, isotonic, or hypertonic, depending on the concentration or dilution of the urine. Urine concentration or dilution occurs principally in the loop of Henle, distal tubules, and collecting ducts. The structural features of the medullary hairpin loops allow the kidney to concentrate urine and conserve water for the body. The transition of the filtrate into the final urine reflects the concentrating ability of the loops. Final adjustments in urine composition are made by the distal tubule and collecting duct according to the body's needs.

Production of concentrated urine involves a countercurrent exchange system, in which fluid flows in opposite directions through the parallel tubes of the loop of Henle. A concentration gradient in the medulla causes fluid to be exchanged across the parallel pathways. The longer the loop the greater the concentration gradient. The concentration gradient increases from the cortex to the tip of the medulla. The *loops of Henle multiply the concentration gradient*, and the vasa recta blood vessels (located parallel to the loops of Henle) act as a *countercurrent exchanger* for maintaining the gradient. The process is initiated in the thick ascending limb of the loop of Henle with the active transport of chloride and sodium out of the tubular lumen and into the medullary interstitium (Fig. 37.14). Because the lumen of the ascending limb is impermeable to water, water cannot follow the sodium-chloride transport. This causes the ascending tubular fluid to become hypoosmotic and the medullary interstitium to become hyperosmotic.

The descending limb of the loop, which receives fluid from the PT, is highly permeable to water, but it is the only place in the nephron that does not actively transport either sodium or chloride. Sodium and chloride may, however, diffuse into the descending tubule from the interstitium. The hyperosmotic medullary interstitium causes water to move out of the descending limb, and the remaining fluid in the descending tubule becomes increasingly concentrated as it flows toward the tip of the medulla. When the tubular fluid rounds the loop and enters the ascending limb, sodium and chloride are removed, and water is retained as described previously. The fluid then becomes more and more dilute as it encounters the distal tubule.

The slow rate of blood flow and the hairpin structure of the vasa recta blood vessels allow blood to flow slowly through the medullary tissue without disturbing the osmotic gradient. When blood flows into the descending limb of the vasa recta, it encounters the increasing osmotic concentration gradient of the medullary interstitium. Water moves out, and sodium and chloride diffuse into the descending vasa recta. The plasma becomes increasingly concentrated as it flows toward the tip of the medulla.

As blood flows away from the tip of the medulla and toward the cortex, the surrounding interstitial fluid becomes comparatively more dilute. Water then moves back into the vasa

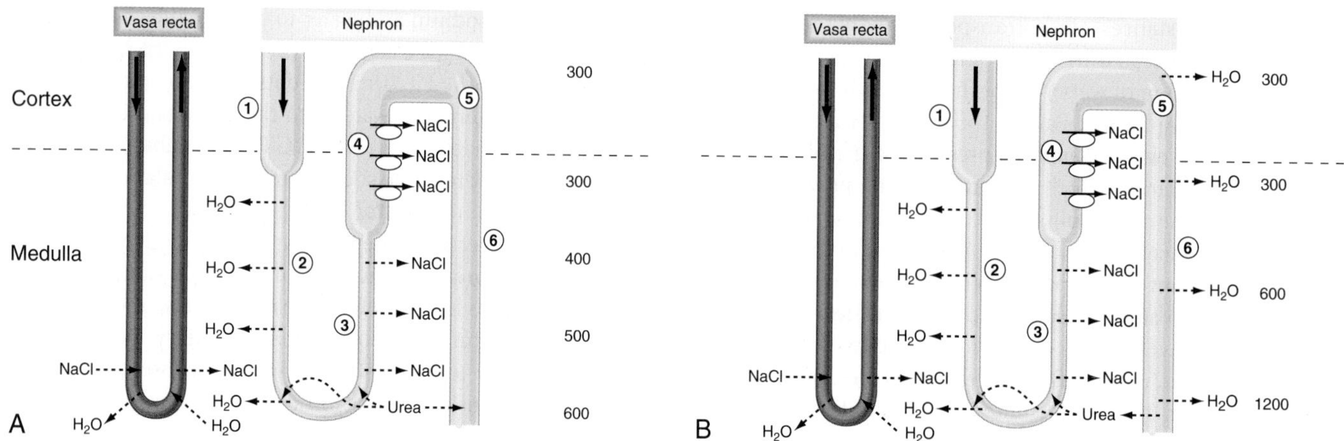

Fig. 37.14 Countercurrent Mechanism for Concentrating and Diluting Urine. (A) Urine dilution; **(B)** urine concentration. *1,* Filtrate isotonic to plasma. *2,* Descending thin limb permeable to water. *3,* Ascending thin limb impermeable to water; permeable to ions. *4,* Ascending thick limb actively transports NaCl; impermeable to water and urea. *5,* Distal tubule actively resorbs NaCl; resorbs water in presence of antidiuretic hormone. *6,* Medullary collecting duct actively resorbs NaCl, and slightly permeable to water and urea. (Note: Numbers on illustration represent milliosmoles [mOsm]). *H_2O,* water; *NaCl,* sodium chloride. See text for details. (From Koeppen BM, Stanton BA. *Berne and Levy physiology [updated],* 6th edition. St. Louis: Mosby; 2010.)

recta, and sodium and chloride diffuse out and the plasma again becomes more dilute. The net result is a preservation of the medullary osmotic gradient. If blood were to flow rapidly through the vasa recta, as occurs in some renal diseases, the medullary concentration gradient would be washed away and the ability to concentrate urine and conserve water would be lost. The efficiency of water conservation is related to the length of the loops of Henle: the longer the loops, the greater the ability to concentrate the urine, and the slower the flow of blood through the vasa recta.

Urea is the major constituent of urine, along with water. The glomerulus freely filters urea, and tubular reabsorption depends on the urine flow rate, with less reabsorption at higher flow rates. Approximately 50% of urea is excreted in the urine, and 50% is recycled within the kidney. This recycling contributes to the osmotic gradient within the medulla and is necessary for the concentration and dilution of urine (see Fig. 37.14). Because urea is an end product of protein metabolism, individuals with protein deprivation cannot maximally concentrate their urine.

Another function of the ascending loop of Henle is the production of uromodulin (also known as Tamm-Horsfall protein [THP]), the most abundant protein in human urine. This protein prevents the attachment of *Escherichia coli* to uroepithelial cell receptors by binding to the type 1 fimbria adhesin (FimH) and removing other uropathogens. It also modulates renal ion channel activity, salt/water balance, renal and systemic inflammatory responses, intertubular communication, mineral crystallization, and bacterial adhesion. Consequently, uromodulin participates in the countercurrent gradient formation for urine concentration, protects the uroepithelium from injury and kidney stone formation, regulates blood pressure, and functions as an immune regulatory molecule against infections in the urinary system.[5] Uromodulin is also a biomarker for the progression of kidney disease and genetic mutations that are associated with congenital urolithiasis, hereditary hyperuricemia/gout, and medullary cystic kidney diseases.[6]

The convoluted portion of the distal tubule is poorly permeable to water but readily reabsorbs ions and contributes to the dilution of the tubular fluid. The later, straight segment of the distal tubule and the collecting duct are permeable to water as controlled by ADH released from the posterior pituitary gland. Sodium is readily reabsorbed by the later segment of the distal tubule and collecting duct under the regulation of the hormone aldosterone (see Chapter 21). Potassium is actively secreted by principal cells and is reabsorbed in lesser amounts by intercalated cells in these segments. Potassium secretion is controlled by aldosterone and other factors related to the concentration of potassium in body fluids.

Hydrogen is secreted by the distal tubule and combines with nonbicarbonate buffers (i.e., ammonium and phosphate) for the elimination of acids in the urine. The distal tubule thus contributes to the regulation of acid-base balance by excreting hydrogen ions into the urine and by adding new bicarbonate to the plasma (see Fig. 3.13). The mechanism is similar to the conservation of bicarbonate by the PT, except that the hydrogen ion is excreted in the urine and influences the acid-base balance. The specific mechanisms of acid-base balance and acid excretion are described in Chapter 3.

Urine Composition

Urine is normally clear yellow or amber in color. Cloudiness may indicate the presence of bacteria, cells, or a high solute concentration. The pH ranges from 4.6 to 8.0, but it is normally acidic, providing protection against bacteria. The specific gravity ranges from 1.001 to 1.035. Normal urine does not contain glucose or blood cells and only occasionally contains traces of protein, usually in association with rigorous exercise.

Hormones and Nephron Function

Antidiuretic Hormone

The distal tubule in the cortex receives the hypoosmotic urine from the ascending limb of the loop of Henle. The specific gravity, or concentration, of the final urine is controlled by antidiuretic hormone (ADH), which is secreted from the posterior pituitary or neurohypophysis. ADH increases water permeability and reabsorption in the last segment of the distal tubule and along the entire length of the collecting ducts, which pass through the inner and outer zones of the medulla. The water diffuses into the ascending limb of the vasa recta and returns to the systemic circulation to maintain fluid balance. The excreted urine can have a high osmotic concentration, up to 1400 mOsm. The volume is normally reduced to about 1% of the amount filtered at the glomerulus.

Excess ADH secretion is therefore one cause of oliguria, or diminished excretion of urine, clinically defined as less than 400 mL/day or 30 mL/h. The syndrome of inappropriate secretion of ADH occurs when the posterior pituitary hypersecretes ADH, resulting in excess water reabsorption and water excess in the plasma (see Chapters 3 and 22). Inadequate secretion of ADH results in diabetes insipidus and causes the distal tubules and collecting ducts to become impermeable to water. Water remains in the tubular lumen and is excreted as a dilute and large volume of urine. (The mechanism for the regulation of ADH and plasma osmolality is described in Chapters 3 and 21.)

Aldosterone

Aldosterone is synthesized and secreted by the adrenal cortex under the regulation of the RAAS (see Chapter 21 and the previous discussion of the RAAS in this chapter). Aldosterone stimulates the epithelial cells of the distal tubule and collecting duct to reabsorb sodium (promoting water reabsorption) and increases the excretion of potassium and hydrogen ion.

Natriuretic Peptides

Natriuretic peptides are a group of vasoactive hormones that promote sodium and water excretion, including atrial natriuretic peptide (ANP or A-type natriuretic peptide), secreted from myocardial cells in the atria, brain natriuretic peptide (BNP or B-type natriuretic peptide), secreted from myocardial cells in the cardiac ventricles, and several other variants.[7] When the heart dilates during volume expansion or heart failure, ANP and BNP inhibit sodium and water absorption by the kidney tubules, inhibit secretion of renin and aldosterone, vasodilate the afferent arterioles, and constrict the efferent arterioles. The result is increased urine formation (diuresis), leading to a decrease in blood volume and blood pressure. *C-type natriuretic peptide* is secreted from the vascular endothelium; it causes vasodilation in the nephron and complements the action of ANP and BNP. *Urodilatin*, an extended form of ANP, is secreted by the distal convoluted tubules and collecting ducts that causes vasodilation and natriuretic and diuretic effects.

Diuretics as a Factor in Urine Flow

A diuretic is any agent enhancing the flow of urine. Clinically, diuretics interfere with renal sodium reabsorption and reduce the extracellular fluid volume. Diuretics are commonly used to treat hypertension and edema caused by heart failure, cirrhosis, and nephrotic syndrome. However, side effects may include dehydration, hypokalemia, systemic acidosis, metabolic alkalosis, nausea, and headache.

Diuretics are divided into five general categories: (1) osmotic diuretics, (2) carbonic anhydrase inhibitors (inhibitors of urinary acidification), (3) inhibitors of loop sodium or chloride transport, (4) potassium sparing (i.e., aldosterone receptor antagonists), and (5) aquaretics. (The physiologic mechanism related to each category is summarized in Table 37.2.)

Renal Hormones

Certain hormones are either activated or synthesized by the kidney. These hormones have significant systemic effects and include urodilatin (see earlier text), the active form of vitamin D, Epo, renin-angiotensin-aldosterone, and natriuretic hormones.

Vitamin D

Vitamin D is a hormone that is necessary for the absorption of calcium and phosphate by the small intestine. The normal serum concentration is 50 nmol/L (i.e., 20 ng/mL). It can be obtained in the diet or synthesized by the action of ultraviolet radiation (sun exposure) on cholesterol in the skin. These forms of vitamin D_3 (cholecalciferol) are inactive and require two hydroxylations (which adds an OH^- group to a compound) to establish a metabolically active form. The first hydroxylation occurs in the liver and the second in the kidneys. The renal hydroxylation step is stimulated by parathyroid hormone (see Chapter 21). The end product is 1,25-dihydroxy-vitamin D_3 (1,25-OH_2D_3), or calcitriol, the active form of vitamin D. Calcitriol is necessary for the absorption of calcium and phosphate by the small intestine. A decreased plasma calcium level (less than 10 mg/dL) stimulates the secretion of parathyroid hormone. Parathyroid hormone then stimulates a sequence of events to help return the plasma calcium concentration toward normal levels (9 to 10.5 mg/dL):

1. Calcium mobilization from bone
2. Synthesis of 1,25-dihydroxy-vitamin D_3
3. Absorption of calcium from the intestine
4. Increased renal calcium reabsorption
5. Decreased renal phosphate reabsorption

Fluctuations in the serum phosphate concentration also influence the renal hydroxylation of vitamin D. Decreased levels stimulate active 1,25-dihydroxy-vitamin D_3 formation, and increased levels inhibit formation. This results in compensatory changes in phosphate absorption from the bones and intestine. Individuals with renal disease have a deficiency of 1,25-OH_2D_3 and manifest symptoms of disturbed calcium and phosphate balance (see Chapters 3, 21, and 38).

Erythropoietin

Erythropoietin (Epo) is produced by the fetal liver and the adult kidney and is essential for normal erythropoiesis. Epo stimulates the bone marrow to produce red blood cells in response to tissue hypoxia and may have tissue protective effects. Erythrocyte production is discussed in Chapter 28. The stimulus for Epo

TABLE 37.2 Action of Diuretics

Diuretic	Site of Action	Action	Side Effects
Osmotic Diuretic			
Mannitol Glycerol Urea	Proximal tubule	Freely filtered but not reabsorbed; osmotically attracts water and diminishes sodium reabsorption	Hypokalemia, dehydration
Carbonic Anhydrase Inhibitors			
Acetazolamide	Proximal tubule	Inhibits carbonic anhydrase; blocks hydrogen ion secretion and reabsorption of sodium and bicarbonate	Hypokalemia, systemic acidosis, alkaline urine
Inhibitors of Sodium/Chloride Reabsorption (Loop Diuretics)			
Thiazides	Between end of ascending loop and beginning of distal tubule	Blocks sodium and chloride reabsorption; mildly suppresses carbonic anhydrase	Hypokalemia, metabolic alkalosis
Furosemide Ethacrynic acid Torsemide	Thick ascending limb of Henle loop	Blocks active transport of chloride, sodium, and potassium	Hypokalemia, uric acid retention
Bumetanide	Cortical vasodilation	Increased rate of urine formation	Hypokalemia, uric acid retention
Potassium Sparing			
Spironolactone Eplerenone	Distal tubule	Inhibits aldosterone, blocks sodium reabsorption, and results in potassium retention	Hyperkalemia, nausea, confusion, gynecomastia
Triamterene Amiloride	Distal tubule	Blocks sodium reabsorption and inhibits potassium excretion	Nausea, vomiting, headache, and amiloride granulocytopenia, skin rash
Aquaretics			
Vasopressin (V2 receptor) blockers (e.g., conivaptan)	Distal tubule and collecting ducts	Blocks action of antidiuretic hormone	Dehydration

release is decreased oxygen delivery in the kidneys. Oxygen-sensing Epo-producing cells are peritubular fibroblast-like cells located in the juxtamedullary cortex. The anemia of chronic renal failure, in which kidney cells have become nonfunctional, can be related to the lack of this hormone (see Chapter 38.)

TESTS OF RENAL FUNCTION

Renal Clearance

A number of specific renal functions can be measured by renal clearance. Renal clearance techniques or formulas determine how much of a substance can be cleared from the blood by the kidneys per given unit of time. The application of this principle permits an indirect measure of the GFR, tubular secretion, tubular reabsorption, and the RBF.

Clearance and Glomerular Filtration Rate

The GFR provides the best estimate of functioning renal tissue and is important for assessing or monitoring kidney damage and drug dosing. Damage to the glomerular membrane or loss of nephrons leads to a corresponding decrease in the GFR. Measurement of the GFR requires the use of a substance that does not influence GFR; has a stable plasma concentration; is not protein bound; is freely filtered at the glomerulus; is not secreted, reabsorbed, or metabolized by the tubules; is constantly infused to maintain a stable plasma level; and is easy to measure. Inulin (a fructose polysaccharide) is one substance that meets the criteria for measurement of GFR. The kidney "clears" inulin from the plasma by filtering it at the glomerulus, reabsorbing nearly all of the fluid, and excreting the inulin left behind in the urine. However, the accurate determination of clearance requires constant infusion to maintain a stable plasma level. This is time consuming, inconvenient, and prone to error.

Therefore, the clearance of creatinine, a natural substance produced by muscle and released into the blood at a relatively constant rate, is commonly used as an estimate clinically. It is freely filtered at the glomerulus and is not reabsorbed by the renal tubules, but a small amount is secreted by the renal tubules, meaning creatinine clearance overestimates the GFR, but within tolerable limits. Creatinine clearance provides a good clinical measure of the GFR, because only one blood sample is required in addition to an accurately collected 24-hour volume of urine. The GFR estimated by creatinine clearance is calculated by multiplying the creatinine concentration of urine (U_{CR}) by the volume of urine per unit of time V (usually 24 hours) divided by the plasma creatinine (P_{CR}) concentration, as follows:

$$\mathrm{GFR(mL/min)} = \frac{U_{CR} \times V}{P_{CR}}$$

Cystatin C is a stable protein in serum filtered at the glomerulus and metabolized in the tubules. Serum levels of cystatin C also are a marker for estimating the GFR, particularly for mild to moderate impaired renal function. Formulas are used to estimate the GFR. Calculators for estimates of the GFR use a variety of formulas and are readily available on the internet (see an example at http://touchcalc.com/ip_epi_gfr/ip_ckd_epi). Normal GFR values are 90 to 120 mL/min.

Plasma Creatinine Concentration

A chronic decline in the GFR over weeks or months is reflected in the plasma creatinine (P_{CR}) concentration (normal value = 0.7 to 1.2 mg/dL). The P_{CR} concentration has a stable value when the GFR is stable because creatinine has a constant rate of production as a product of muscle metabolism. The amount filtered is approximately equal to the amount excreted. When the GFR declines, the P_{CR} increases proportionately. Thus, the GFR and P_{CR} are inversely related. If the GFR were to decrease by 50%, the filtration and excretion of creatinine would be reduced by 50% and creatinine would accumulate in the plasma to twice the normal value. Therefore, elevated P_{CR} values represent a decreasing GFR. In the new steady state, however, the total amount of creatinine excreted in the urine would remain the same because of the proportionate decrease in the GFR and increase in the P_{CR}.

The application of this principle is simple and useful for monitoring progressive changes in renal function. The test is most valuable for monitoring the progress of chronic rather than acute renal disease because it takes 7 to 10 days for the P_{CR} level to stabilize when the GFR declines. Serial measures can be obtained over a long time and plotted as a curve of glomerular function. Normal P_{CR} value decreases with advanced age, since older adults experience a decrease in lean muscle mass. The P_{CR} also becomes elevated during trauma or the breakdown of muscle tissue. In such instances, the value is then not useful for estimating the GFR.

Blood Urea Nitrogen

The concentration of urea nitrogen in the blood reflects glomerular filtration and urine-concentrating capacity. Because urea is filtered at the glomerulus, blood urea nitrogen (BUN) levels increase as glomerular filtration drops. Urea is reabsorbed by the blood through the permeable tubules, so the BUN value rises in states of dehydration and with acute and chronic renal failure when the passage of fluid through the tubules slows. BUN values also change as a result of altered protein intake and protein catabolism making it a poor measure of GFR. The normal range for the BUN level in adults is 10 to 20 mg/dL of blood.

Clearance and Renal Blood Flow

A clearance formula also can be devised to estimate the RPF and RBF using the PAH molecule. When PAH is administered intravenously, some of it is filtered at the glomerulus, and most of the remainder is secreted into the tubules in one circulation through the kidney. A blood sample and urine sample are obtained simultaneously to measure the amount of PAH in each sample. If all the PAH is removed from the plasma during a single pass through the kidney, the total RPF can be determined. Because the supporting and non-secreting structures of the kidney receive 10% to 15% of the effective renal blood flow (ERBF), the clearance of PAH measures only what is known as the effective renal plasma flow (ERPF), which is 85% to 90% of the true RPF

$$\text{ERBF} = \text{ERPF}$$
$$1 - \text{Hematocrit}$$
$$(1.0 - 0.45)$$

Evaluation of the biochemical components of the blood and urine provides valuable information regarding renal function.

Urinalysis

Urinalysis is a noninvasive and relatively inexpensive diagnostic procedure. The best results are obtained from a fresh, cleanly voided specimen, because decay permits changes in the composition of the urine. Urinalysis includes evaluation of the color, turbidity, protein, pH, specific gravity, sediment, and supernatant. Urine tests are listed in Table 37.3.

Urine color is normally a clear, light yellow because of urochrome and other pigments. When formed substances (crystals, blood cells, or casts) are in the urine, it appears turbid. Protein in the urine creates marked foaming when shaken, and the foam is yellow or orange when the urine contains bile pigments. Urine does not normally contain protein or bile.

Urine pH normally ranges between 5 and 6.5, but it may vary from 4.5 to 8. Urine is more alkaline after eating and then becomes less alkaline before the next meal. Because sleep is accompanied by intermittent hypoventilation, urine is more acidic on awakening. Dipstick evaluations may be falsely high when urine pH is less than 6 and falsely low when the pH is more than 7.

Specific gravity is an estimated measure of the solute concentration of the urine. The specific gravity of any solution is measured by comparing the weight of the solution with an equal volume of distilled water. Hence, specific gravity is not a true measure of the number or concentration of particles, but it correlates well with osmolality and is a useful clinical tool. Specific gravity usually is measured with a hydrometer in a cylinder of urine; the normal value is 1.010 to 1.025.

The final urine osmolality is primarily a function of ADH, which controls water reabsorption in the collecting ducts. If the kidney is unable to concentrate or dilute urine, given a stimulus, the cause is usually a malfunction of the renal tubules or inappropriate ADH secretion by the posterior pituitary gland. The state of hydration also affects the urine specific gravity, so hydration status should be evaluated before making a diagnosis. This determination is helpful for differentiating oliguria caused by intrinsic renal disease from hypovolemia as a result of dehydration.

Urine Sediment

The urine sediment is examined microscopically and may contain cells, casts, crystals, and bacteria. Epithelial cells may be seen in the microscopic field because they are shed naturally throughout the urinary tract.

Normal urine contains few or no red blood cells. If a large number of red cells are present, this is known as hematuria, and the sediment may be red or brown. An alkaline or hypotonic urine causes lysis of red cells, however, so that the cells will not be seen. Urine then will be positive for hemoglobin, and the specific gravity will be elevated. Hematuria can occur with the administration of anticoagulants and with several renal diseases.

Casts (accumulations of cellular precipitates) originate in the renal tubules, from which they take their shape. They are cylindrical with distinct borders. Casts arise primarily from the ascending limb of the distal tubule. Red cell casts indicate bleeding into the tubules or escape of red blood cells through the glomerulus; white cell casts are associated with an inflammatory process. Epithelial cell casts indicate degeneration of the tubular lumen or necrosis of the renal tubules. The type of cast identified suggests the disease process occurring in the kidney.

Numerous kinds of crystals can be observed in the urine. They may be composed of cystine, uric acid, calcium oxalate, or phosphate. They may not be initially observable, but as the urine cools, crystals will form. Crystals tend to form in a concentrated acidic or alkaline urine. Crystal formation is diagnostically significant, usually indicating inflammation, infection, or a metabolic disorder.

White blood cells (WBCs) in the urine (a condition termed pyuria) are indicative of urinary tract infection, particularly when bacteria are present. Glomerulonephritis and nephrotic syndrome also may demonstrate pyuria but usually in combination with proteinuria, red cells, and casts. The finding of WBC casts reflects a kidney infection because these casts are not formed in the bladder or prostate. If WBCs are present in the urine, a culture should be done for specific identification of bacteria and sensitivity of bacteria to antibiotics.

Other Measures

Dipsticks and reagent strips are available for detecting other substances in the urine, including glucose, bilirubin, urobilinogen, leukocyte esterase and nitrates, ketones, proteins, hemoglobin, and myoglobin.

TABLE 37.3 Renal Function Test Results

Test	Normal Value	Interpretation of Abnormal Result
Urine		
Color	Amber-yellow	Drugs and foods may change color
Turbidity	Clear	Purulent matter causes cloudiness
pH	4.6–8	Bacteria create an alkaline urine
Specific gravity	*Adults:* 1.010–1.025 *Infants:* 1.010–1.018	Represents concentrating ability or density of urine in relation to density of water (1.000) (i.e., higher when contains glucose or protein; lower with dilute urine)
Blood	Negative	Bleeding along urinary tract
Microscopic Urine		
Bacteria	None	Infection
Red blood cells	Negative	Bleeding along urinary tract
White blood cells	Negative	Urinary tract infection
Crystals	Negative	May have potential for stones
Fat	Negative	Can be associated with nephrosis
Casts	Occasional	A few are normal; may represent renal disease
Urinary Chemistry		
Bilirubin	Negative	Increases may cause dark orange color
Urobilinogen	Less than 4 mg/24 h	Increases may indicate red blood cell hemolysis
Ketones	Negative	Indicate an increase in fat metabolism
Glucose	Negative	Usually signifies hyperglycemia
Sodium	100–260 mEq/24 h	Can increase or decrease with renal disease
Potassium	25–100 mEq/24 h	Can increase or decrease with renal disease, potassium intake, aldosteronism, or diuretic use
Protein	Negative-trace	Dysfunction of glomerulus
Normal Serum Values		
Blood urea nitrogen (BUN)	7–18 mg/dL	Elevated with diseased kidneys
Creatinine	*Male:* 0.6–1.5 mg/dL *Female:* 0.6–1.1 mg/dL	Elevated with decreased glomerular filtration rate (GFR)
Cystatin C	0.8–2.1 mg/L	Early detection of decreased GFR
Potassium		Elevated in renal failure

PEDIATRIC CONSIDERATIONS

Nephrogenesis continues until 34–36 weeks of gestation and all the nephrons are present at birth. Their numbers do not increase as the kidney grows and matures. The glomerular filtration rate (GFR) in infants does not reach adult levels until 1–2 years of age, and newborns have a decreased ability to efficiently remove excess water and solutes.[8] Their shorter loops of Henle also decrease concentrating ability and produce a more dilute urine than that produced by adults. Risks for metabolic acidosis are increased during the first few months of life, while the mechanisms for excreting acid and retaining bicarbonate are maturing. These normal developmental processes result in a narrow safety margin for fluid and electrolyte balance when there is any disturbance, such as diarrhea, infection, fever, fasting for diagnostic tests, improper feeding, fluid replacement, or drug administration.[9] Newborns diurese 2–3 days after birth, which is reflected by a decrease in total body water and body weight. An increased risk of toxicity accompanies drug administration. Low birth weight infants have a delay in achieving full renal function and may not have a full GFR until 8 years of age. They also are at greater risk for low nephron numbers and chronic kidney disease as adults.[10] Tubular secretion is immature at birth and approaches adult values by 7–12 months. Maturation of tubular reabsorption continues into adolescence, with the greatest increase occurring between 1 and 3 years of age.[11]

GERIATRIC CONSIDERATIONS

Aging and Renal Function

Throughout life the kidney responds to an increased workload by compensatory hypertrophy. This hypertrophy is marked in individuals who have donated a kidney for transplant or have lost functioning nephrons from trauma or disease. The glomeruli increase in diameter, and the tubules enlarge effectively to maintain the regulatory functions of the kidney. Hypertrophy occurs more rapidly and with a larger size increase in younger individuals and in those with high protein intake.

Changes in the kidneys occur throughout life, resulting in a reduction in size and a linear decrease in RBF and GFR; however, it is less pronounced in healthy individuals. Reference values for estimated GFR are available by age group.[12] The number and size of nephrons decrease with aging, possibly related to oxidative stress, inflammation, mitochondrial dysfunction, and associated clinical conditions (e.g., hypertension and diabetes mellitus). The primary mechanism appears to be a change in the renal vasculature and perfusion patterns related to atherosclerosis that leads to a reduction in numbers of nephrons and nephrosclerosis. Tubular atrophy also occurs. The rate of nephron loss accelerates after 50 years of age. By about 75 years of age, the nephron population is reduced by 30% to 50% with loss of renal mass occurring primarily in the cortex.[13] Degenerative changes within nephrons also occur with aging. The glomerular capillaries become sclerotic, and remaining glomeruli become hypertrophic. The arcuate and interlobular arteries become tortuous, contributing to ischemia. The loss of the glomerular tuft may cause a shunt between the afferent and efferent arterioles. Although loss of juxtaglomerular nephrons still allows the vasa recta to be perfused, the combination of events contributes to a reduction in the autoregulation of blood flow and ability to excrete a concentrated urine.[14] Thus, the specific gravity of the urine in older individuals tends to be on the low side of normal.

Tubular transport changes with aging, although under normal conditions the tubules function adequately. Adaptation to stressful conditions is more difficult. Glucose, bicarbonate, and sodium are not as efficiently reabsorbed, and hyperkalemia is more common because of decreased secretion. Response to acid or base loads is delayed and prolonged. Sudden or large changes in pH or fluid load may lead to serious imbalances with increased risk of hypervolemia or hypovolemia. Acute losses or chronic fluid deficits can lead to renal insufficiency in the older adult. Administration of drugs eliminated by renal processes may require dose modifications and more astute observations for toxic side effects. Contrast agents and nonsteroidal anti-inflammatory drugs should be used with caution.[15]

The T_m for glucose reabsorption decreases with age, contributing to a greater amount of glucose in the urine. This is an important consideration when glycosuria is used for screening or monitoring the process of diabetes mellitus in older adults. These changes occur independently of disease, however, indicating a normal process of aging and relating to a decline in sodium-glucose cotransporter 2 function.[16] An age-related decline in renal activation of vitamin D decreases intestinal absorption of calcium, and older adults need more vitamin D to overcome diminishing renal function, lack of exposure to sunlight, and lower concentrations of provitamin D3 in the skin.[17]

Previous or concurrent renal disease or urinary tract obstruction may amplify age-related changes in bladder function. Bladder symptoms are common among older adults and include frequency, urgency, and nocturia. Ischemic-induced neurogenic and myogenic changes in bladder structure and function may contribute to some symptoms, as well as influences outside the urinary tract (i.e., cardiovascular disease, prostatic disease, uterine prolapse, stool impaction and hormonal changes). Changes in neurotransmission, blood flow, and uroepithelium influence the micturition reflex and bladder capacity and may lead to an overactive or underactive bladder and incomplete bladder emptying.[18,19]

SUMMARY REVIEW

Structures of the Renal System

1. The kidneys are paired structures lying bilaterally between the twelfth thoracic and third lumbar vertebrae and behind the peritoneum of the abdominal cavity.
2. The kidney is surrounded by the renal capsule and is composed of an outer cortex and an inner medulla. The cortex contains the glomerulus, proximal tubule, and parts of the distal tubule. The medulla contains the loops of Henle and collecting ducts.
3. The calyces are chambers that receive urine from the distal tubules and join to form the renal pelvis, which is continuous with the upper end of the ureter.
4. The nephron is the urine-forming unit of the kidney and is composed of the renal corpuscle (glomerulus, Bowman capsule, mesangial cells), proximal tubule, loops of Henle, distal tubule, and collecting duct.
5. The glomerulus contains loops of capillaries (afferent and efferent arterioles) supported by mesangial cells. The capillary walls serve as a filtration membrane for the formation of the primary urine.
6. The juxtaglomerular apparatus is located in the glomerulus and is composed of renin-secreting juxtaglomerular cells

(around the afferent arteriole) and sodium-sensing macula densa cells (distal tubule) and mesangial cells (between the glomerular capillaries).

7. The proximal tubule is lined with microvilli to increase the surface area and enhance reabsorption of water, solutes, and electrolytes.
8. The loops of Henle transport solutes and water, contributing to the hypertonic state of the medulla, and are important for the concentration and dilution of urine.
9. The distal tubule adjusts acid-base balance by excreting acid into the urine and forming new bicarbonate ions.
10. The ureters extend from the renal pelvis to the posterior wall of the bladder. Urine flows through the ureters and into the bladder by means of peristaltic contraction of the ureteral muscles.
11. The bladder is a bag composed of the detrusor and trigone muscles and innervated by the autonomic nervous system. When the accumulation of urine reaches 250 to 300 mL, mechanoreceptors, which respond to stretching of tissue, stimulate the micturition reflex and elimination of urine through the urethra.

Renal Blood Flow and Glomerular Filtration

1. Renal blood flows at about 1000 to 1200mL/min, or 20% to 25% of the cardiac output.
2. The GFR is the filtration of plasma per unit of time and is directly related to the perfusion pressure of RBF.
3. Blood flow through the glomerular capillaries is maintained at a constant rate in spite of a wide range of arterial pressures by autoregulation of the glomerular capillaries.
4. Renin is an enzyme secreted from the juxtaglomerular apparatus in response to decreased blood pressure and causes the generation of angiotensin II, a potent vasoconstrictor. The RAAS is thus a regulator of renal blood flow.

Kidney Function

1. The major function of the nephron is urine formation, which involves the processes of glomerular filtration, tubular reabsorption, and tubular secretion and excretion.
2. Glomerular filtration is favored by capillary hydrostatic pressure and opposed by oncotic pressure in the capillary and hydrostatic pressure in the Bowman capsule. The NFP is the balance of favoring and opposing filtration forces.
3. The GFR is approximately 120 mL/min to 140 mL/min, and 99% of the filtrate is reabsorbed.
4. The proximal tubule reabsorbs about 60% to 70% of the filtered sodium and water and 90% of other electrolytes.
5. Because most molecules are reabsorbed by active transport, the carrier mechanism can become saturated at a point known as the transport maximum. Molecules not reabsorbed are excreted with the urine.
6. The concentration or specific gravity of the final urine is a function of the level of ADH. This hormone stimulates the distal tubules and collecting ducts to reabsorb water. The countercurrent exchange system of the long loops of Henle and their accompanying capillaries establishes a concentration gradient within the renal medulla to facilitate the reabsorption of water from the collecting duct.
7. The kidney secretes or activates a number of hormones having systemic effects, including vitamin D, erythropoietin, and the natriuretic hormone urodilatin.

Tests of Renal Function

1. Creatinine, a substance produced by muscle, is measured in both plasma and urine to calculate a commonly used clinical measurement of the GFR.
2. The plasma creatinine concentration, cystatin C level, and BUN level are estimates of glomerular function. The BUN value also is an indicator of hydration status.
3. Urinalysis involves evaluation of the color, turbidity, protein, pH, specific gravity, sediment, and supernatant. The presence of bacteria, red blood cells, white blood cells, casts, or crystals in the urine sediment may indicate a renal or bladder disorder.

Pediatrics and Renal Function

1. Glomerular filtration rate reaches adult levels by 2 to 3 months of age.
2. Compared with adults, infants and children have a more dilute urine because of higher blood flow and shorter loops of Henle. Tubular maturation is complete by adolescence.
3. Children are more affected than adults by fluid imbalances resulting from diarrhea, infection, or improper feeding because of their limited ability to quickly regulate changes in pH or osmotic pressure.

Aging and Renal Function

1. As a person ages, a decrease occurs in the number and size of nephrons. Renal blood flow and glomerular filtration rate decline.
2. Tubular transport and reabsorption decrease with age. Response to acid-base changes and reabsorption of glucose are delayed. Drugs eliminated by the kidney can accumulate in the plasma, causing toxic reactions.
3. Neurogenic, myogenic, and blood flow changes in the bladder may lead to symptoms of urgency and frequency or urine retention.

REFERENCES

1. Lassén E, Daehn IS. Molecular mechanisms in early diabetic kidney disease: glomerular endothelial cell dysfunction. *Int J Mol Sci*. 2020;21(24):9456.
2. Gyimesi G, et al. Sodium-coupled glucose transport, the SLC5 family, and therapeutically relevant inhibitors: from molecular discovery to clinical application. *Pflugers Arch*. 2020;472(9):1177–1206.
3. Marsh DJ, et al. The nephron-arterial network and its interactions. *Am J Physiol Renal Physiol*. 2019;316(5):F769–F784.
4. Shaw I, et al. Pericytes in the renal vasculature: roles in health and disease. *Nat Rev Nephrol*. 2018;14(8):521–534.
5. Micanovic R, et al. Uromodulin (Tamm-Horsfall protein): guardian of urinary and systemic homeostasis. *Nephrol Dial Transplant*. 2020;35(1):33–43.
6. Wu TH, et al. Tamm-Horsfall protein is a potent immunomodulatory molecule and a disease biomarker in the urinary system. *Molecules*. 2018;23(1):200.

7. Yang WL, Fahim M, Johnson DW. Pathophysiology and significance of natriuretic peptides in patients with end-stage kidney disease. *Clin Biochem*. 2020;83:1–11.
8. Muhari-Stark E, Burckart GJ. Glomerular filtration rate estimation formulas for pediatric and neonatal use. *J Pediatr Pharmacol Ther*. 2018;23(6):424–431.
9. Zhang Y, et al. Pediatric renal ontogeny and applications in drug development. *J Clin Pharmacol*. 2019;59(Suppl 1):S9–S20.
10. Fanos V, et al. State of the art on kidney development: how nephron endowment at birth can shape our susceptibility to renal dysfunction later in life. *Am J Perinatol*. 2019;36(S 02):S33–S36.
11. Filler G, et al. How should we assess renal function in neonates and infants? *Acta Paediatr*. 2021;110(3):773–780.
12. Hallan SI, et al. Age and association of kidney measures with mortality and end-stage renal disease. *JAMA*. 2012;308(22):2349–2360.
13. Xu J, Zhou L, Liu Y. Cellular senescence in kidney fibrosis: pathologic significance and therapeutic strategies. *Front Pharmacol*. 2020;11:601325.
14. Denic A, Glassock RJ, Rule AD. Structural and functional changes with the aging kidney. *Adv Chronic Kidney Dis*. 2016;23(1):19–28.
15. Morcos R, et al. The healthy, aging, and diseased kidney: relationship with cardiovascular disease. *J Am Geriatr Soc*. 2021;69(2):539–546.
16. Cintra R, et al. Inhibition of the sodium-glucose co-transporter 2 in the elderly: clinical and mechanistic insights into safety and efficacy. *Rev Assoc Med Bras (1992)*. 2019;65(1):70–86.
17. Bhattarai HK, et al. Vitamin D, calcium, parathyroid hormone, and sex steroids in bone health and effects of aging. *J Osteoporos*. 2020;2020:9324505.
18. Birder LA. Is there a role for oxidative stress and mitochondrial dysfunction in age-associated bladder disorders? *Ci Ji Yi Xue Za Zhi*. 2020;32(3):223–226.
19. Johnson 2nd TM, Vaughan CP. Urological function and dysfunction in aging: diagnosis and treatment. *Handb Clin Neurol*. 2019;167:495–509.

38

Alterations of Renal and Urinary Tract Function

Julia L. Rogers

http://evolve.elsevier.com/Rogers/pathophysiology/

CHAPTER OUTLINE

The renal system plays a major role in homeostasis by filtering nearly 200 L of blood every 24 hours. Approximately 1 L of filtered fluid is converted into urine and excreted through micturition per day. Because the kidneys filter the blood, the renal system is directly linked to every other organ system. A variety of disorders affects renal function by inhibiting the kidney's ability to regulate plasma volume and osmolality. Disease may be limited to only the kidney and urinary tract or may include systemic diseases that cause acute kidney injury (AKI), chronic kidney disease (CKD), or difficulty eliminating urine (e.g., infection, neurologic injury, or diabetes mellitus). Infection of the kidney or urinary tract is the most common disorder affecting renal function. Stones, tumors, inflammation, or consequences of medical procedures can obstruct and/or cause injury to the upper or lower urinary tract (LUT). Renal injury, whether acute or chronic, can affect other organs and become life-threatening.

URINARY TRACT OBSTRUCTION

Urinary tract obstruction is an anatomic (structural) or functional abnormality that causes interference with the flow of urine at any site along the urinary tract (Fig. 38.1). An obstruction impedes urine flow, increases hydrostatic pressure, dilates structures proximal to the blockage, which increases risk of infection, and compromises renal function. Anatomic changes in the urinary system caused by obstruction are referred to as an **obstructive uropathy**, which may be acute or chronic, partial, or complete, and unilateral or bilateral. The severity of an obstructive uropathy is determined by the:

1. location of the obstructive lesion,
2. involvement of ureters and kidneys,
3. severity (completeness) of the blockage,
4. duration of the blockage, and
5. nature of the obstructive lesion.

Obstructions may be relieved, or partially alleviated, by correction of the obstruction, although permanent impairments such as hydronephrosis occur if a complete or partial obstruction persists over a period of weeks to months or longer.

Upper Urinary Tract Obstruction

A stricture or compression of the calyx, ureteropelvic, or ureterovesical (ureter-bladder) junction is a common cause of upper urinary tract obstructions and is commonly caused by kidney stones (calculi). Ureteral compressions or blockages can be caused from an aberrant vessel, tumor, stone, or abdominal inflammation and scarring (retroperitoneal fibrosis).[1] The most common cause in children is a congenital anomaly (see Chapter 39); in young adults, the common cause is renal calculi; and in older adults, renal calculi, ureteral strictures, and tumors are more common.

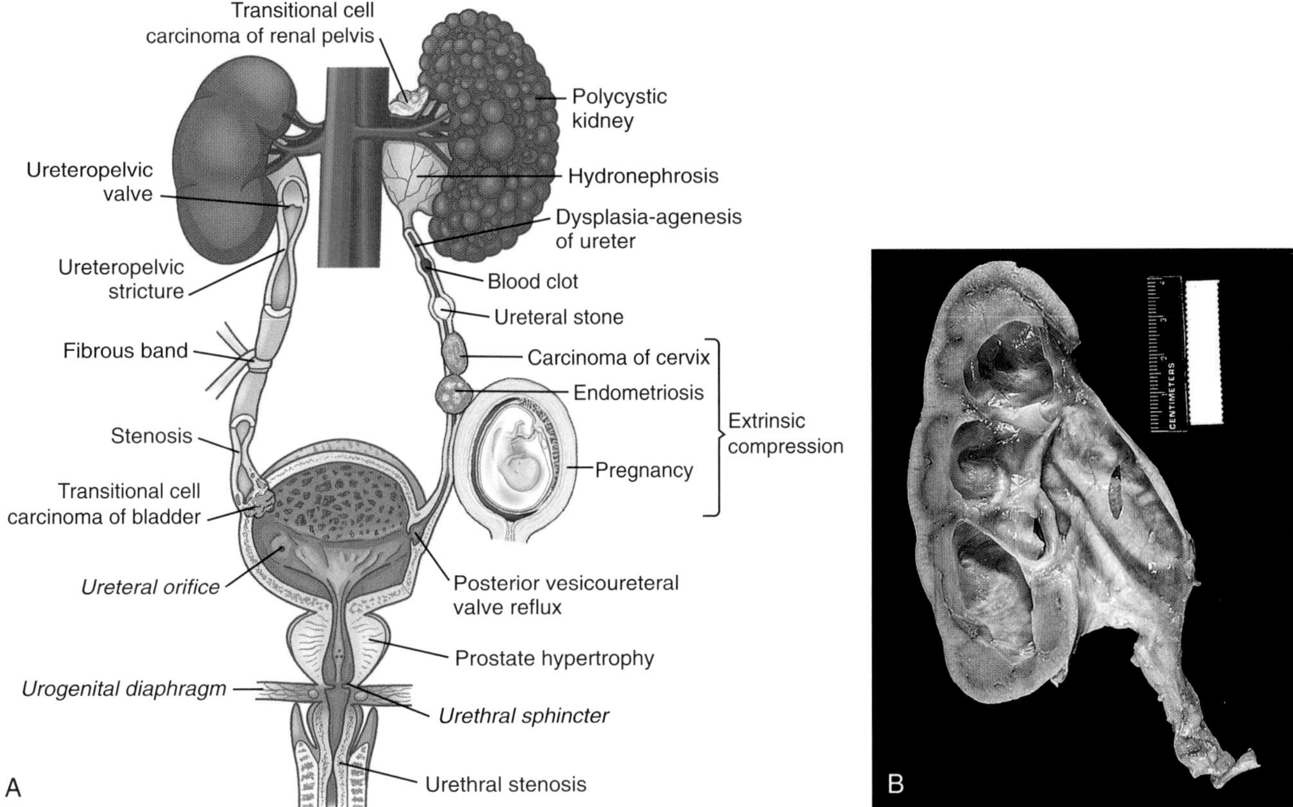

Fig. 38.1 Urinary Tract Obstruction and Hydronephrosis. **(A)** Major sites of urinary tract obstruction. **(B)** Hydronephrosis of the kidney. There is marked dilation of the renal pelvis and calyces with thinning of the overlying cortex and medulla due to compression atrophy. (B, From Kumar V, et al. *Robbins and Cotran pathologic basis of disease*, 10th edition. Philadelphia: Elsevier; 2021.)

Obstruction of the upper urinary tract causes a "backing up" of urine and dilation of the ureter, renal pelvis, calyces, and renal parenchyma proximal to the site of urinary blockage. Dilation of the ureter is referred to as **hydroureter** (accumulation of urine in the ureter). Dilation of the renal pelvis and calyces proximal to a blockage is referred to as **hydronephrosis** or **ureterohydronephrosis** (dilation of both the ureter and the pelvicaliceal system) (see Fig. 38.1B). The backup of urine into the Bowman space from an obstruction opposes the hydrostatic pressure of glomerular filtration and decreases the glomerular filtration rate (GFR).[1] Unless the obstruction is relieved, the dilation leads to tubulointerstitial fibrosis, which damages renal nephrons and can lead to CKD.

Tubulointerstitial fibrosis is the deposition of excessive amounts of extracellular matrix (collagen and other proteins) by activated inflammatory cells including macrophages and myofibroblasts with associated areas of tubular atrophy.[2] Tubulointerstitial fibrosis occurs with kidney injury including obstructive uropathies. Although deposition of extracellular matrix is a normal process of kidney repair and maintenance, activation of inflammatory cells and production of growth factors, such as transforming growth factor-beta-1 (TGF-β1), promotes the process of tubulointerstitial fibrosis and irreversible kidney damage.[3]

Apoptosis is a normal process that the body uses to replace damaged or senescent cells with new ones (see Chapter 1). An imbalance in growth factors provoked by obstruction contributes to excess cellular destruction with a transition from apoptosis to necrosis and inflammation, ultimately resulting in the loss of functioning nephrons.[4]

The magnitude of this damage, and the kidney's ability to recover normal homeostatic function, is affected by the severity and duration of the obstruction. With complete obstruction, damage to the renal tubules and compression of the renal vasculature occur in a matter of hours, and irreversible damage occurs within 3 to 4 weeks. Nevertheless, even in the face of a complete obstruction, the human kidney may recover at least partial homeostatic function provided the blockage is removed. Recovery can take up to 3 months.[5]

When there is unilateral obstruction, the body is able to partially counteract the negative consequences by a process called **compensatory hypertrophy** and **hyperfunction**. The compensatory response is guided by growth factors that cause the unobstructed kidney to increase the size and function of individual glomeruli and tubules, but not the total number of functioning nephrons. Consequently, the obstructed kidney can remain silent for a long time. Partial obstruction that is not relieved, in the absence of renal infection, leads to more subtle, but ultimately permanent impairments including loss of the kidney's ability to concentrate urine, reabsorb bicarbonate, excrete ammonia, and regulate metabolic acid-base and fluid and electrolyte balance.

The process is reversible when relief of obstruction results in recovery of function by the obstructed kidney. The ability of the body to engage in compensatory hypertrophy and hyperfunction diminishes with age. Complete bilateral obstruction causes anuria because the retrograde increase in tubular hydrostatic pressure completely opposes glomerular filtration.

Relief of upper urinary tract obstruction is usually followed by a brief period of diuresis, commonly called **postobstructive diuresis**. Postobstructive diuresis is a physiologic response and is typically mild, representing a restoration of fluid and electrolyte imbalance caused by retention of fluid related to the obstructive uropathy. Occasionally, relief of obstruction will cause rapid excretion of large volumes of water, sodium, or other electrolytes, resulting in a urine output of 200 mL/h for two consecutive hours or more than 3 L in 24 hours. Minimal normal daily urine output is approximately 720 mL/day.[6] Rapid postobstructive diuresis causes dehydration and fluid and electrolyte imbalances that must be promptly corrected. Risk factors for severe postobstructive diuresis include chronic, bilateral obstruction; impairment of one or both kidneys' ability to concentrate urine or reabsorb sodium (nephrogenic diabetes insipidus); hypertension; edema and weight gain; congestive heart failure; and uremic encephalopathy.

Nephrolithiasis

Nephrolithiasis, also commonly known as **kidney stones or renal calculi**, are masses of crystals, protein, or other substances that are a common cause of urinary tract obstruction in adults. Stones can be located anywhere along the urinary tract including in the kidneys, ureters, and urinary bladder. However, the favored sites of stone formation are in the renal calyces, renal pelvis, and bladder. Stones are unilateral in about 80% of individuals. The prevalence of kidney stones in the United States is approximately 11% in males and 7% in females with an incidence of about 1% per year.[7] The cumulative risk of recurrence at 5 years is approximately 53% overall, with a lower rate of 26% for those with a single stone episode.[8] The risk of stone formation is influenced by a number of factors, including age, sex, race, geographic location, seasonal factors, fluid intake, diet, occupation, and genetic predisposition.[9] Diseases that predispose individuals for stone formation are urinary tract infection (UTI), hypertension, atherosclerosis, metabolic syndrome, obesity, and type 2 diabetes.[10] While stones are more prevalent in males before the age of 50 years, there is increasing incidence seen in females. Geographic location influences the risk of stone formation because of indirect factors. Warmer climates with high humidity and rainfall influence a person's fluid intake and dietary patterns. Persons who regularly consume an adequate volume of water are at reduced risk when compared with persons who consume lower volumes of water.[9]

Stones are classified according to the primary minerals (salts) that make up the stones. The most common stone types include calcium oxalate or calcium phosphate (70% to 80%), struvite (magnesium–ammonium–phosphate) (5% to 10%), and uric acid (5% to 10%) (Table 38.1).[11] Cystine stones are rare (≤2%), and so are stones that are formed from the metabolic effects of some medications (e.g., atazanavir, ceftriaxone, and N-acetyl-sulfadiazine) in individuals treated for a lengthy period of time for chronic diseases.[12,13]

Stones are also classified according to location and size. *Staghorn calculi* are large and fill the minor and major calyces. *Nonstaghorn calculi* are of variable size but tend to be smaller and are located in the renal calyces, renal pelvis, or at various sites along the ureter.

Pathophysiology. Stone formation is complex and related to:

1. supersaturation of one or more salts in the urine,
2. precipitation of the salts from a liquid to a solid state (crystals),
3. growth through crystallization or agglomeration (sometimes called *aggregation*), and
4. the presence or absence of stone inhibitors (e.g., uromodulin [Tamm-Horsfall protein]).

Supersaturation is the presence of a higher concentration of a solute (salt) within a solvent (in this case, the urine) than can be dissolved. Human urine contains many ions capable of *precipitating* from solution and forming a variety of salts. The salts form crystals that are retained and grow into stones. *Crystallization* is the process by which crystals grow from a small nucleus, or nidus, to larger stones in the presence of supersaturated urine. Although supersaturation is essential for free stone formation, the urine need not remain continuously supersaturated for a stone to grow once its nucleus has precipitated from solution. Intermittent periods of supersaturation after the ingestion of a meal or during times of dehydration from limited oral intake or secondary to continued use of diuretics are sufficient for stone growth in many individuals. In addition, the renal tubules and papillae have many surfaces that may attract a crystalline nidus (known as a Randall plaque) and add biologic material (matrix), forming a stone. *Matrix* is an organic material (i.e., mucoprotein) in which the components of a kidney stone are embedded. Randall plaques start in the suburothelial layer and gradually grow until they break through into the renal pelvis. Once in continuous contact with urine, layers of calcium oxalate typically start to form on the calcium phosphate nidus (see Table 38.1).[14] The pH of the urine influences the risk of precipitation and calculus formation. An alkaline urinary pH (pH > 7.0) significantly increases the risk of calcium phosphate stone and struvite stone formation, whereas acidic urine (pH < 5.0) increases the risk of uric acid stone formation. Cystine and xanthine also precipitate more readily in acidic urine.

Substances capable of inhibiting *stone* or *crystal growth include* potassium citrate, Tamm-Horsfall protein, pyrophosphate, and magnesium.[15] These substances normally reduce the risk of calcium phosphate or calcium oxalate precipitation in the urine and prevent subsequent stone formation.

Retention of *crystal particles* occurs primarily at the papillary collecting ducts. Most crystals are flushed from the tract through the normal flow of urine. Urinary stasis (e.g., from benign prostatic hyperplasia, neurogenic bladder), anatomic abnormalities (strictures), or inflamed epithelium within the urinary tract may prevent prompt flushing of crystals from the system, thus increasing the risk of stone formation.

TABLE 38.1 Renal Calculi Prevalence and Type

Prevalence	Stone Type	
70%	**Calcium Oxalate and Phosphate**	Idiopathic hypercalciuria
50%	*Idiopathic hypercalciuria*	
20%	*Hyperuricosuria*	
15%–20%	*Unknown metabolic abnormality*	
10%	*Hypercalciuria and hypercalcemia*	
5%	*Hyperoxaluria*	
4.5%	*Enteric*	
0.5%	*Primary*	
	Frequent umbilication and Randall's plaque indicative of papillary origin.	Randall's plaque white arrow Hyperuricosuria
	Color: Brown to dark brown.	
		Hyperoxaluria
5%–10%	**Magnesium–Ammonium–Phosphate (Struvite)** Homogenous surface made of amalgamate crystals with blunt angles and edges. Color: Whitish.	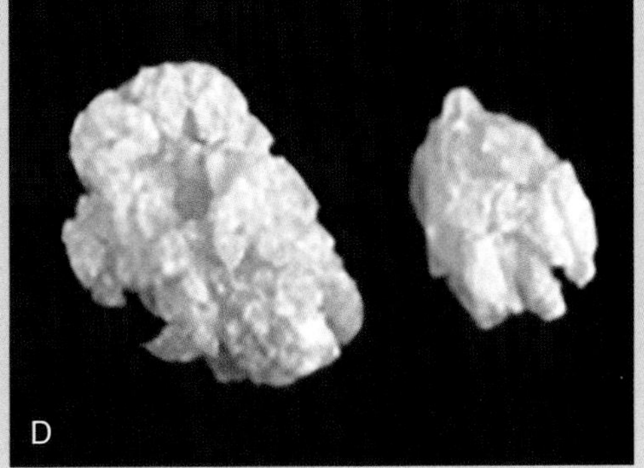

TABLE 38.1 Renal Calculi Prevalence and Type—cont'd

Prevalence	Stone Type	
5%–10%	**Uric Acid** Uric acid anhydrous: Homogeneous smooth surface. Color: Typically orange, sometimes cream, ochre or yellowish. Uric acid dihydrate ± uric acid anhydrous: Heterogeneous embossed, rough and porous surface. Color: Beige to brown–orange.	Uric acid anhydrous 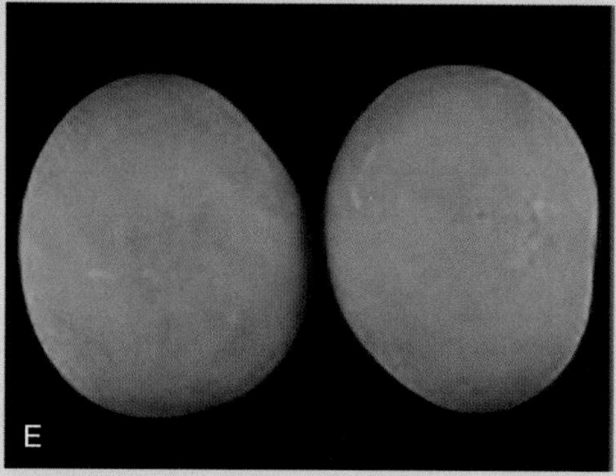 E Uric acid dihydrate ± uric acid anhydrous 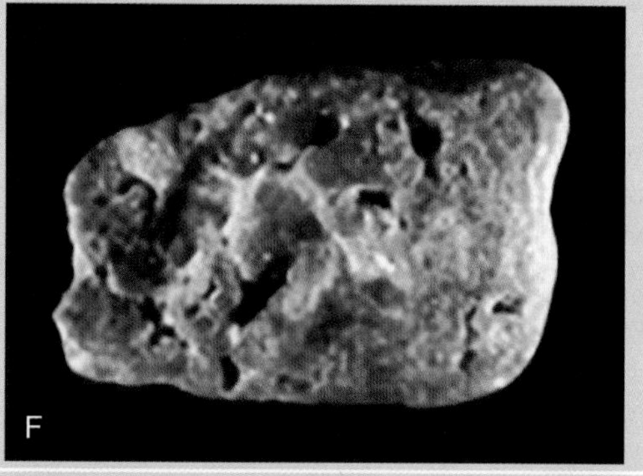 F
1%–2%	**Cystine** Smooth surface. Concentric layers at the periphery, an unorganized core. Color: Homogeneous, cream to yellowish.	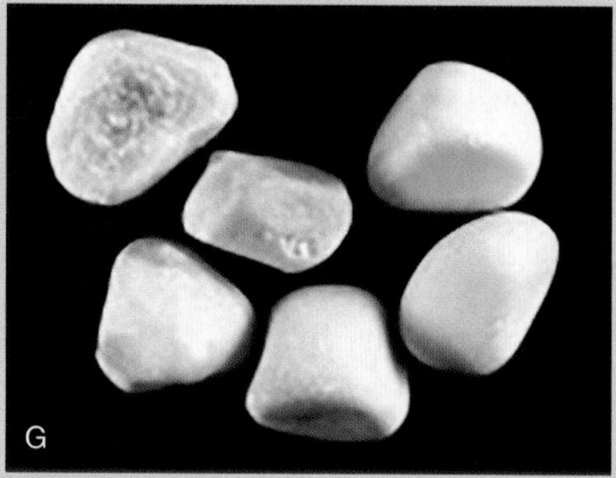 G
+5	**Unknown** Heterogeneous, irregularly rough surface. Color: Dark brown to black. Example: Drug induced (stone made of proteins and atazanavir)	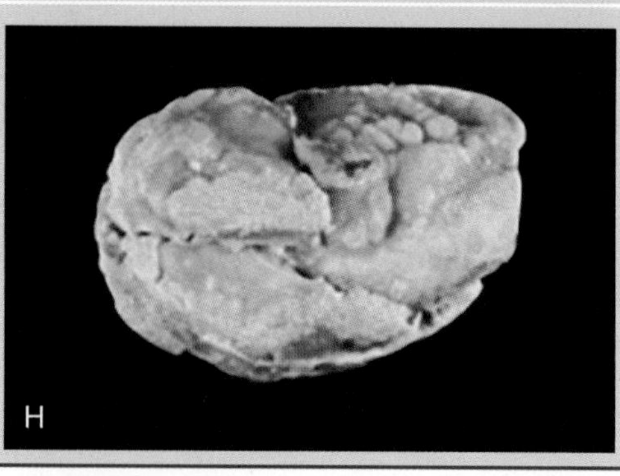 H

Pictures in right column from Daudon M, Dessombz A, Frochot V, et al. Comprehensive morpho-constitutional analysis of urinary stones improves etiological diagnosis and therapeutic strategy of nephrolithiasis. *Comptes Rendus Chimie*, 2016;19(11–12):1470–1491. https://doi.org/10.1016/j.crci.2016.05.008.

The size of a stone determines the likelihood that it will pass through the urinary tract and be excreted through micturition. Stones smaller than 5 mm have about a 50% chance of spontaneous (painful) passage, whereas stones that are larger than 1 cm have almost no chance of spontaneous passage.[16]

Both genetic and environmental factors may increase the susceptibility of calcium stones. Most affected individuals have *idiopathic calcium oxalate urolithiasis (ICOU)*, a condition the exact etiology of which has not yet been determined. Stones can form freely in supersaturated urine or detach from interstitial sites of formation (e.g., from Randall plaque). Hypercalciuria, hyperoxaluria, hyperuricosuria, hypocitraturia, mild renal tubular acidosis, crystal growth inhibitor deficiencies, and alkaline urine are associated with calcium stone formation. Hypercalciuria and hyperoxaluria are usually attributable to intestinal hyperabsorption and less commonly to a defect in renal calcium reabsorption. Hyperparathyroidism and bone demineralization associated with prolonged immobilization are also known to cause hypercalciuria.[17]

Struvite stones primarily contain magnesium, ammonium, and phosphate as well as varying levels of a matrix. Matrix forms in an alkaline urine and during infection with a urease-producing bacterial pathogen, such as a *Proteus, Klebsiella*, or *Pseudomonas*.[18] Struvite calculi may grow quite large and branch into a staghorn configuration (staghorn calculus) that approximates the pelvicaliceal collecting system. Women are at greater risk for struvite stones because they have an increased incidence of UTI.

Uric acid stones occur in persons who excrete excessive uric acid in the urine, such as those with gouty arthritis. Uric acid is primarily a product of biosynthesis of endogenous purines and is secondarily affected by consumption of purines (e.g., meat and beer) in the diet. A consistently acidic urine greatly increases this risk, including defective excretion. *Cystinuria* and *xanthinuria* are genetic disorders of amino acid metabolism, and their excess in urine can cause cystine or xanthine stone formation in the presence of acidic urine.[19]

Clinical Manifestations. Renal colic is pain related to dilation and spasms of smooth muscle related to ureteral obstruction. Moderate to severe pain often originates in the flank and radiates to the groin, and usually indicates obstruction of the renal pelvis or proximal ureter. Colic that radiates to the lateral flank or lower abdomen typically indicates obstruction in the midureter. Bothersome LUT symptoms (urinary urgency, frequency, incontinence) indicate obstruction of the lower ureter or ureterovesical junction. The pain can be incapacitating and may be accompanied by nausea and vomiting. Gross or microscopic hematuria may be present.

Evaluation and Treatment. The evaluation and diagnosis of nephrolithiasis is based on presenting symptoms and history combined with a focused physical assessment. Imaging studies determine the location of the stone, severity of obstruction, and associated obstructive uropathy. Imaging of kidney stones can include plain abdominal radiography, ultrasound, intravenous pyelography, computed tomography (CT), and magnetic resonance imaging (MRI). The history queries dietary habits, age of the first stone episode, stone analysis, and presence of complicating factors, including hyperparathyroidism or recent gastrointestinal or genitourinary surgery. Urinalysis (including pH) is obtained, and a 24-hour urine is completed to identify calcium oxalate, calcium citrate, and other significant constituents. In addition, every effort is made to retrieve and analyze stones that are passed spontaneously or retrieved through aggressive intervention. To diagnose and manage underlying metabolic disorders, additional tests are completed for those with suspected hyperparathyroidism (elevated serum calcium levels), cystine calculi, or uric acid (high purine diet) stones.

The goals of treatment are to manage acute pain, promote stone passage, reduce the size of stones already formed, and prevent new stone formation.[20] The components of treatment include:

1. managing pain (can require narcotic medication),
2. reducing the concentration of stone-forming substances by increasing urine flow rate with high fluid intake,
3. adjusting the pH of the urine (e.g., make it more alkaline with potassium citrate administration or more acid with potassium acid phosphate),
4. decreasing the amount of stone-forming substances in the urine by decreasing dietary intake or endogenous production or by altering urine pH, and
5. removing stones using percutaneous nephrolithotomy, ureteroscopy, or ultrasonic or laser lithotripsy to fragment stones for excretion in the urine.[21]

Obstructing kidney stones with a suspected proximal UTI are urologic emergencies requiring emergent decompression, stone removal, and antibiotics.[22] Prevention of recurrent stones includes increasing fluid intake to generate 2.5 L of urine per day, avoiding intake of colas and other soft drinks acidified with phosphoric acid, avoiding dietary oxalate (e.g., chocolate, beets, nuts, rhubarb, spinach, strawberries, tea, wheat bran), eating less animal protein, and limiting sodium intake. Maintaining a dietary calcium intake of 1000 to 1200 mg/day is helpful for calcium stone prevention. Potassium citrate may be used to prevent calcium stone aggregation and to raise urinary pH.[23]

Lower Urinary Tract Obstruction

Obstructions of the LUT are inherently caused by a structural or anatomic disorder or an alteration in neurologic function (neurogenic bladder). These disorders are related to alterations of urine storage in the bladder or emptying of urine through the bladder outlet. Incontinence is a common symptom associated with LUT obstructions. The types of incontinence are summarized in Table 38.2.

Anatomic Obstructions to Urine Flow

Anatomic causes of resistance to urine flow include urethral stricture, prostatic enlargement in men, pelvic prolapse (bladder and uterus) in women, and tumor compression. A urethral stricture is a narrowing of its lumen and occurs when infection, injury, or surgical manipulation produces a scar that reduces the caliber of the urethra. The severity of obstruction is influenced by its location within the urethra, its length, and the severity of the stricture. Strictures that are longer than 1 centimeter and in the proximal urethra cause more severe obstruction. They are

TABLE 38.2 **Types of Urinary Incontinence**

Type	Description
Urge incontinence (most common in older adults)	Involuntary loss of urine associated with an abrupt and strong desire to void (urgency). Often associated with involuntary contractions of the detrusor (detrusor overactivity). When associated with a neurologic disorder, this is called *detrusor hyperreflexia*. When no neurologic disorder exists, this is called *detrusor instability*. May be associated with decreased bladder wall compliance.
Stress incontinence (most common in women younger than 60 years and men who have had prostate surgery)	Involuntary loss of urine during coughing, sneezing, laughing, or other physical activity associated with increased abdominal pressure.
Mixed incontinence (most common in older women)	A combination of stress and urge incontinence.
Overflow incontinence	Involuntary loss of urine with overdistention of the bladder. Associated with neurologic lesions below S1, polyneuropathies, and urethral obstruction (i.e., an enlarged prostate) or detrusor underactivity.
Functional incontinence	Involuntary loss of urine caused by dementia or immobility.
Continuous incontinence	Continuous loss of urine related to vesicovaginal or vesico-uterine fistulas. Extreme intrinsic sphincter deficiency.
Insensible incontinence	Not clearly accompanied by either urgency or stress incontinence (i.e. increase in intra-abdominal pressure). Intrinsic sphincter deficiency. Detrusor overactivity with impaired bladder sensation.

Data from: Wyndaele M, Hashim H. Pathophysiology of urinary incontinence. *Surgery* (Oxford), 2020;38(4): 185–190.

more common in men because of a longer urethra (see Chapter 26).[24] Urethral stricture is treated with urethral dilation accomplished by using a steel instrument shaped like a catheter (urethral sound) or a series of incrementally increasing catheter-like tubes (filiforms and followers). Long, dense strictures typically require surgical repair (urethroplasty) to prevent recurrence. **Prostate enlargement** is caused by acute inflammation, benign prostatic hyperplasia, or prostate cancer (see Chapter 26). Severe **pelvic organ prolapse** (see Chapter 25) in a woman causes bladder outlet obstruction when a cystocele (the downward protrusion/herniation of the bladder into the vagina) or the uterus descends into the vagina below the level of the urethral outlet. In men, the bladder may rarely herniate into the scrotum, causing a similar type of obstruction. Each of these disorders can cause compression of the urethra with obstruction to urine flow.

Partial obstruction of the bladder outlet or urethra initially causes an increase in the force of detrusor contraction. If the obstruction persists, afferent nerves within the bladder wall are adversely affected, leading to urinary urgency and, in some cases, overactive detrusor contractions (a myogenic cause of overactive bladder). When obstruction persists, there is an increased deposition of collagen within the smooth muscle bundles of the detrusor muscle *(trabeculation)*. Ultimately, the bladder wall loses its ability to stretch and accommodate urine, a condition called **low bladder wall compliance** (loss of elasticity), and the detrusor loses its ability to contract efficiently, resulting in urine retention. This underactive bladder (UAB) syndrome can also occur as a consequence of bladder radiation treatment. Low bladder wall compliance chronically elevates intravesicular pressure, increasing the likelihood of hydroureter, hydronephrosis, impaired renal function, incontinence, and UTI.

Symptoms of obstruction include:

1. frequent daytime voiding (micturition more than every 2 hours while awake);
2. nocturia (awakening more than once each night to urinate for adults younger than 65 years of age or more than twice for older adults);
3. poor force of stream;
4. intermittency of urinary stream;
5. bothersome urinary urgency, often combined with hesitancy; and
6. feelings of incomplete bladder emptying despite micturition.

Overactive and Underactive Bladder Syndrome

Overactive bladder syndrome (OAB) is a dysfunction of urine storage with nonspecific symptoms characterized by urinary urgency, frequency, and nocturia with or without incontinence in the absence of UTI or other known pathology (e.g., neurologic disorders). OAB affects a significant number of adults (approximately 16%).[25] The specific cause is not clearly known and several mechanisms could be involved including myogenic or neurogenic alterations in sensory and motor function.[26] The symptoms are usually associated with involuntary contractions of the detrusor muscle during the bladder-filling phase, often resulting in urge incontinence and nocturia. Risk factors in women include vaginal birth with episiotomy or use of forceps, surgery for pelvic organ prolapse, and decreased estrogen associated with menopause or hysterectomy. Loss of estrogen results in thinning and loss of urethral muscle strength. Risk factors in men include enlarged prostate with urinary obstruction and surgical treatment for prostate cancer. Risk factors include the use of diuretics, antidepressants, alpha-agonists, beta-antagonists, sedatives, anticholinergics, and analgesics.

Both behavioral and pharmacologic therapy are first- and second-line treatments for OAB. Behavioral therapy includes pelvic floor (Kegel) exercises (detrusor contraction can be inhibited by pelvic floor muscle contraction providing time to get to the toilet), bladder training with timed voiding, management of fluid intake and use of caffeine and alcohol, managing constipation, and biofeedback techniques. Drug therapy to manage incontinence includes topical vaginal estrogen in women and drugs that increase urethral sphincter contraction or relax the bladder wall.

Because the parasympathetic nervous system controls detrusor muscle contraction with cholinergic (muscarinic) signals and the bladder neck consists of circular smooth muscle with α-adrenergic innervation, OAB may be managed by anticholinergic therapy (antimuscarinic) and adrenergic medications. Anticholinergics increase urethral pressure, and β_3-adrenergic agonists relax the bladder wall, increasing bladder capacity. These medications must be monitored closely for adverse side effects. When these therapies are not successful, neuromodulation therapy is considered, including intradetrusor injection of onabotulinumtoxinA (Botox) (inhibits release of acetylcholine), peripheral tibial nerve stimulation, and sacral neuromodulation. Low bladder wall compliance (loss of elasticity) may be managed by antimuscarinic drugs, intradetrusor onabotulinumtoxin A injections, and intermittent catheterization.[27] OAB syndrome should be discussed during health assessments; however, many individuals are reluctant to discuss OAB syndrome with their health care provider. Untreated OAB is an economic burden, impairs health and quality of life, and causes symptoms such as skin breakdown because of leakage, sleep disturbance, fall-related injuries, depression, prolonged hospital stays, and admission to long-term care facilities.

UAB syndrome is a voiding dysfunction characterized by the International Continence Society Working Group as bladder contraction of reduced strength and/or duration, resulting in prolonged bladder emptying or a failure to achieve complete bladder emptying, or both, within a normal time span. Symptoms include a slow urinary stream, hesitancy, and straining to void, with or without a feeling of incomplete bladder emptying and dribbling.[28] Disruption of bladder innervation can occur with spinal cord injury, stroke, multiple sclerosis, Parkinson disease, and diabetic neuropathy. Aging can be a contributing factor. The symptoms may be indistinguishable from symptoms of LUT obstruction, including weak stream, intermittency, hesitancy, and straining to void. In some cases, UAB and OAB may occur together with detrusor overactivity during storage but poor detrusor contraction in the voiding phase. Urodynamic studies are required for evaluation. Treatment depends on the cause of the disorder and may include sacral neuromodulation, drugs that increase bladder contractility, and/or drugs that induce urethral relaxation.[29]

Evaluation and Treatment. Diagnosis of LUT obstructions requires a detailed history; physical examination, including neurologic and pelvic examinations; urinalysis; and determining if pathologic causes of urgency and frequency, such as prostatic enlargement, pelvic organ prolapse, urethral strictures, and neurologic disorders or systemic disease, are present. Diaries and questionnaires are helpful to determine the pattern and severity of incontinence. However, no symptom or cluster of symptoms has been identified that accurately differentiates the various causes of these disorders. For example, symptoms such as urgency, urge incontinence, frequent urination, and nocturia may develop because of overactive bladder or either increased or decreased bladder outlet resistance. Reduced resistance is associated with the symptom of stress incontinence (incontinence with coughing or sneezing), and symptoms of increased resistance are similar to bladder outlet obstruction, including poor force of urinary stream, hesitancy, and feelings of incomplete bladder emptying. Various urodynamic tests (Box 38.1) assist with the evaluation of how efficient the bladder, sphincters, and urethra are in storing and releasing urine. An evaluation of renal function, including functional imaging studies and measurement of serum creatinine (SCr) level, is completed particularly when the obstruction is severe and associated with elevated residual urine or UTI.

BOX 38.1 Urodynamic Tests

1. *Postvoid residual urine* measures the amount of urine remaining in the bladder after urination.
2. *Uroflowmetry* provides a graphic representation of urine flow rate and voiding time (the force of the urinary stream expressed as milliliters voided per second) and evaluates the presence of obstruction.
3. *Cystometric test* uses a catheter and manometer to evaluate bladder urine volume and pressure in relation to the occurrence of involuntary bladder contraction (the leak point pressure) and the urge to void.
4. *Electromyography* uses sensors to measure detrusor and sphincter muscle contraction strength during urination.
5. *Multichannel urodynamic testing* measures pressure in both the bladder and rectum during urination.
6. *Video-urodynamic recording* takes pictures and videos of the bladder using ultrasound or x-rays during bladder filling and emptying and can demonstrate overactive bladder and detrusor sphincter dyssynergia (lack of coordination between the bladder and sphincter).

Neurogenic Bladder

Neurogenic bladder is a general term for bladder dysfunction caused by neurologic disorders (Table 38.3).[30] The types of dysfunctions are related to the sites in the nervous system that control sensory and motor bladder function (Fig. 38.2). Lesions in the upper motor neurons of the brain and spinal cord result in detrusor hyperreflexia (overactive bladder) and bladder dyssynergia (loss of coordinated neuromuscular contraction). Lesions in the sacral area of the spinal cord or peripheral nerves result in underactive, hypotonic, or atonic (flaccid) bladder function, often with loss of bladder sensation. (See Chapter 15 for upper and lower motor neuron function.)

Neurologic disorders that develop above the pontine micturition center (located near the posterior pons) result in detrusor (bladder muscle) hyperreflexia (overactivity), also known as an uninhibited or reflex bladder or neurogenic overactive bladder. This is an upper motor neuron disorder in which the bladder empties automatically (without voluntary control) when it becomes full and the urethral sphincter functions normally. Because the pontine micturition center remains intact, there is coordination between detrusor muscle contraction and relaxation of the urethral sphincter. Stroke, traumatic brain injury, dementia, and brain tumors are examples of disorders that result in detrusor hyperreflexia. Symptoms include urine leakage and incontinence.

Neurologic lesions that occur below the pontine micturition center but above the sacral micturition center (between C2 and S1) are also upper motor neuron lesions and result in **detrusor sphincter dyssynergia (detrusor hyperreflexia with vesicosphincter dyssynergia)** (loss of coordinated function between the bladder and sphincter). There is loss of pontine coordination of detrusor muscle contraction and external sphincter relaxation, so both the bladder and the sphincter are contracting at the same time (dyssynergia), causing a functional obstruction of the bladder outlet. Spinal cord injury, multiple sclerosis, Guillain-Barré syndrome, and vertebral disk problems are causes of this disorder. There is diminished bladder relaxation during storage with small urine volumes and high intravesicular (inside the bladder) pressures. The result is an OAB with symptoms of frequency, urgency, urge incontinence, and increased risk for UTI. Diagnosis includes a medical history, physical examination, urinalysis, and urodynamic testing. Detrusor sphincter dyssynergia may be managed by intermittent catheterization in combination with higher dose antimuscarinic drugs to prevent overactive detrusor contractions and associated dyssynergia, while ensuring regular, complete bladder evacuation by catheterization. Transurethral botulinum toxin A injection has shown temporary efficacy in reducing bladder outlet obstruction. Transurethral sphincterotomy can be beneficial.[31]

TABLE 38.3 Neurogenic Bladder

Cause (Symptoms)	Site of Lesion	Diseases
Detrusor hyperreflexia (urgency and urine leakage)	Lesions above C2 involve pontine micturition center (UMN disorder)	Stroke, traumatic brain injury, multiple sclerosis (MS), hydrocephalus, cerebral palsy, Alzheimer disease, brain tumors
Detrusor hyperreflexia with vesicosphincter dyssynergia (functional bladder outlet obstruction)	Lesions between C2 and S1 (UMN disorder)	Spinal cord injury C2–T12, MS, transverse myelitis, Guillain-Barré syndrome, disk problems
Acontractile detrusor, with or without urethral sphincter incompetence (stress urinary incontinence)	Lesions below S1 (cauda equina syndrome) (LMN disorder)	Myelodysplasia, peripheral polyneuropathies, MS, tabes dorsalis, spinal injury T12–S1, cauda equina syndrome, herpes simplex/zoster

LMN, Lower motor neuron; *UMN*, upper motor neuron.

Neurologic lesions involving the sacral micturition center (below S1, also termed *cauda equina syndrome*) or peripheral nerve lesions result in **detrusor areflexia** (acontractile detrusor, atonic bladder, or UAB), a lower motor neuron disorder. The atonic bladder causes retention of urine and distention with stress and overflow incontinence. There is prolonged urination time with or without a sensation of incomplete bladder emptying, usually with hesitancy, reduced sensation on filling, and a slow stream. If the *sensory innervation* of the bladder is intact, the full bladder will be sensed but the detrusor may

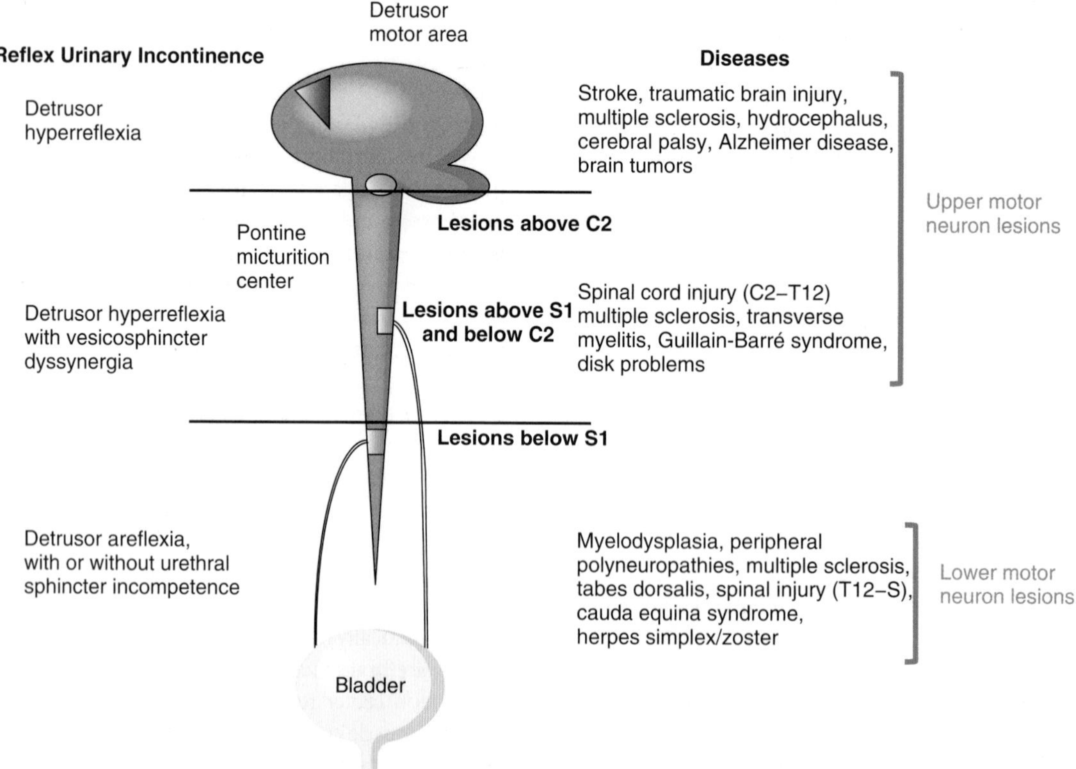

Fig. 38.2 Sites of Neurologic Injury Associated With Neurogenic Bladder. (Adapted from Doughty DB, ed. *Urinary and fecal incontinence management* concepts, 3rd edition. Philadelphia: Mosby: 2006.)

not contract. Myelodysplasia, multiple sclerosis, tabes dorsalis (deterioration of the posterior columns of the spinal cord associated with untreated syphilis), spinal cord injury, and peripheral polyneuropathies (i.e., diabetic neuropathy) are associated with this disorder.

Diagnosis includes disease history, clinical examination, urinalysis, and urodynamic studies (see Box 38.1). Bethanechol chloride (Urecholine) is a cholinergic agent (muscarinic agonist) that stimulates the bladder to empty and can be helpful in some cases. Intermittent catheterization or indwelling catheters are commonly required.

Tumors

Kidney (Renal) Tumors

Kidney (Renal) tumors were estimated at 76,080 (4%) of new cancer cases and 13,780 deaths for 2021.[32] Renal cell carcinoma (RCC) (also known as renal cell adenocarcinoma) usually occurs in men (about three times more often than in women) between 50 and 60 years of age. Risk factors include cigarette smoking, obesity, and uncontrolled hypertension. With surgical resection, 5-year survival is about 93% for stage I (encapsulated) cancer.

Pathophysiology. There are several different types of RCCs. They are classified according to subtypes and extent of metastasis. *Clear cell RCC* is the most common renal neoplasm (80% of all renal neoplasms) and represents about 2% of cancer deaths.[32,33] It occurs primarily in the proximal tubule of the renal cortex. Other types include papillary (small fingerlike growths) and chromophobe RCC (larger cells), and both occur in the distal tubules of the kidneys.[34] Confinement within the renal capsule, together with treatment, is associated with a better survival rate. The tumors usually occur unilaterally (Fig. 38.3). Renal transitional cell carcinoma (RTCC) is rare and primarily arises in the renal parenchyma and renal pelvis near the ureteral orifice. Renal adenomas (benign tumors) are uncommon but are increasing in number. The tumors are encapsulated and are usually located near the cortex of the kidney. Some tumors are unclassified because they have multiple cell types. Because the tumors can become malignant, they are usually surgically removed.

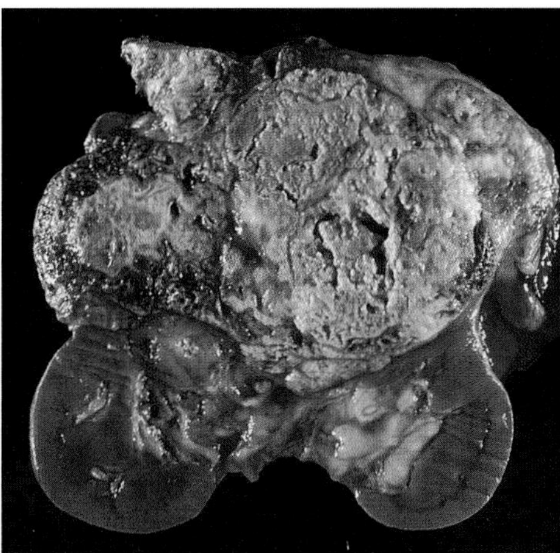

Fig. 38.3 Renal Cell Carcinoma. Renal cell carcinomas usually are spheroidal masses composed of yellow tissue mottled with hemorrhage, necrosis, and fibrosis. (From Damjanov I, Linder J, eds. *Anderson's pathology*, 10th edition. St. Louis, MA: Mosby; 1996.)

Clinical Manifestations. The classic clinical manifestations of renal tumors are hematuria, dull and aching flank pain, palpable flank mass, and weight loss, but all these symptoms occur in fewer than 10% of cases. Further, they represent an advanced stage of disease, whereas earlier stages are often silent (painless hematuria). About 25% to 30% of individuals with RCC present with metastasis.[35] The most common sites of distant metastasis are the lung, lymph nodes, liver, bone, thyroid gland, and central nervous system.

Evaluation and Treatment. Diagnosis is based on the clinical symptoms and imaging procedures. The tumor, node, metastasis (TNM) classification is used to stage RCC. Treatment for localized disease is surgical removal of the affected kidney (radical nephrectomy) or partial nephrectomy for smaller tumors, with combined use of chemotherapeutic agents. Radiofrequency ablation also may be used for early-stage tumors when surgery is not an option. Metastatic disease is treated with immunotherapy and targeted molecular therapies.[36] Survival is related to tumor grade, tumor cell type, and extent of metastasis.

Bladder Tumors

Bladder tumors represent about 4.5% of all malignant tumors with 64,280 new cases each year and 12,260 deaths.[32] The development of bladder cancer is most common in men older than 60 years. Risk factors include smoking, exposure to occupational chemicals, heavy consumption of phenacetin, uroepithelial schistosomiasis infection, or a genetic predisposition. *Transitional cell (urothelial) carcinoma* is the most common bladder malignancy, and tumors are usually superficial. More advanced tumors are muscle invasive. Less common forms are squamous cell and adenocarcinoma (cells that produce mucus).

Pathophysiology. Tumors present as flat or papillary and progress from in situ to invasive into the muscle and bladder wall (Fig. 38.4). Metastasis is usually to lymph nodes, liver, bones, or lungs. The TNM classification is used for staging bladder carcinoma. Secondary bladder cancer develops by invasion of cancer from bordering organs, such as cervical carcinoma in women or prostatic carcinoma in men.

Clinical Manifestations. Gross painless hematuria is the archetypal clinical manifestation of bladder cancer. Episodes of hematuria tend to recur, and they are often accompanied by bothersome LUT symptoms including daytime voiding frequency, nocturia, urgency, and urge urinary incontinence, particularly for carcinoma in situ. Flank pain may occur if tumor growth obstructs one or both ureterovesical junctions.

Evaluation and Treatment. Urine cytologic study (pathologic analysis of sloughed cells within the urine) is used for screening. Cystoscopy with tissue resection and biopsy is the first stage of treatment and confirms the diagnosis of bladder cancer. Use of biologic markers for bladder cancer diagnosis and treatment prognosis are available.[37] Transurethral resection or laser ablation, combined with intravesical chemotherapy or immunotherapy, is effective for superficial tumors. Radical

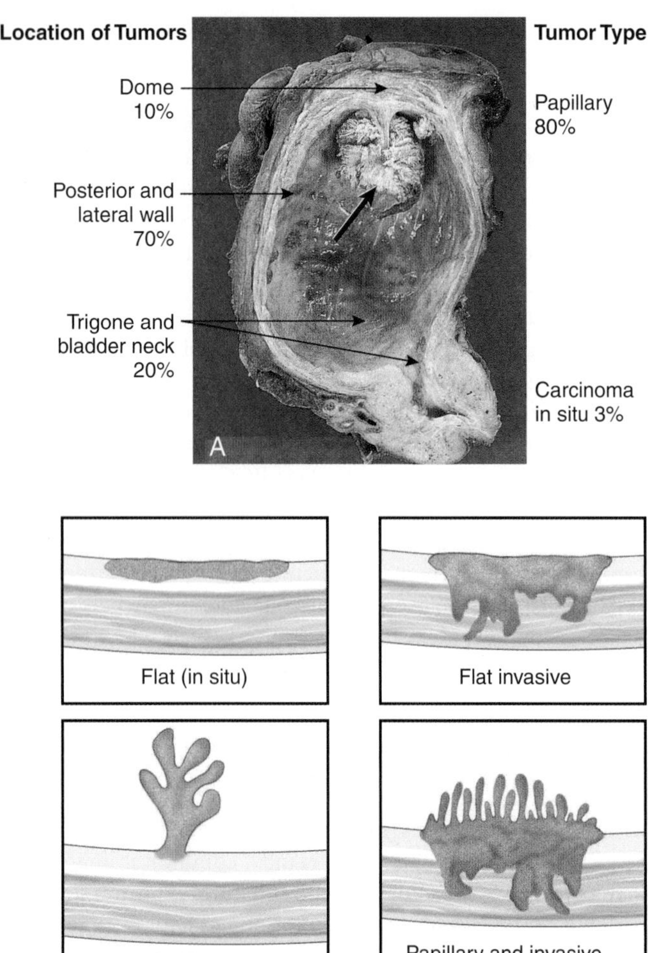

Fig. 38.4 Carcinoma of the Bladder. **(A)** Papillary transitional cell carcinoma arising in the dome of the bladder as a cauliflower-like lesion *(black arrow);* location and frequency of bladder tumor types noted. **(B)** Bladder cancer with morphologic patterns of most common tumors. (A, From Stevens A, Lowe J, Scott I, eds. *Core pathology*, 3rd edition. London: Mosby; 2009; 2009. B, Adapted from Kissane JM, ed. *Anderson's pathology*, 9th edition. St. Louis: Mosby; 1990.)

cystectomy (removal of the prostate and seminal vesicles in men and removal of the uterus, ovaries, and part of the vagina in women) with urinary diversion and adjuvant chemotherapy is required for locally invasive tumors.[38]

URINARY TRACT INFECTION

Causes of Urinary Tract Infection

A UTI is an inflammation of the urinary epithelium (mucosa) usually caused by bacteria from gut flora. UTI can occur anywhere along the urinary tract, including the urethra, prostate, bladder, ureter, or kidney. At risk are premature newborns; prepubertal children; sexually active and pregnant women; women treated with antibiotics that disrupt vaginal flora; spermicide users; estrogen-deficient postmenopausal women; individuals with indwelling catheters; and individuals with diabetes mellitus, neurogenic bladder, or urinary tract obstruction. Cystitis is more common in women because of the shorter urethra and the closeness of the urethra to the anus (increasing the possibility of bacterial contamination). Adult women have a 50% to 60% lifetime incidence of UTI.[39]

Several factors normally combine to protect against UTIs. Most bacteria are washed out of the urethra during micturition. The low pH and high osmolality of urea, the presence of Tamm-Horsfall protein or uromodulin (secreted by renal tubular cells in the distal loop of Henle), and secretions from the uroepithelium provide a bactericidal effect. The ureterovesical junction closes during bladder contraction, preventing reflux of urine to the ureters and kidneys. Both the longer urethra and the presence of prostatic secretions decrease the risk of infection in men. UTI occurs when a pathogen circumvents or overwhelms the body's natural defense mechanisms and rapidly reproduces. *Uncomplicated UTIs* are mild with a self-limiting course and occur in individuals without any functional or anatomical anomalies in the urinary tract. A *complicated UTI* develops when there is an abnormality in the urinary system or a secondary disease, syndrome, or illness that compromises an individual's defenses, such as diabetes mellitus, neurogenic bladder, urinary tract obstruction, renal transplant, or spinal cord injury.[40] UTI may occur alone or in association with pyelonephritis, prostatitis, or nephrolithiasis. Up to 30% of cases of septic shock are caused by urosepsis (a systemic response to an infection in the urogenital tract that can include symptoms of shock).[41] The mechanisms associated with UTI including bacterial and human factors are summarized in Fig. 38.5. *Recurrent UTI* is commonly defined as three or more UTIs within 12 months or two or more occurrences within 6 months. Recurrence is more common in women as compared to men. UTI may occur as a *relapse* when there is a second infection within the urinary tract caused by the same pathogen within 2 weeks of the original treatment or a *reinfection* that occurs more than 2 weeks after completion of treatment for the same or different pathogen.[40] Guidelines are available for clinical management.[42]

Types of Urinary Tract Infection

Cystitis

Cystitis is an inflammation of the bladder, which is the most common site of UTI. The appearance of the bladder through a cystoscope describes the different types of cystitis:

1. *Mild cystitis* shows a hyperemic (red) mucosa.
2. *Hemorrhagic cystitis* shows diffuse mucosal hemorrhages and occurs with more advanced inflammation.
3. *Suppurative cystitis* shows mucosal pus formation or suppurative exudates.
4. *Ulcerative cystitis* results from prolonged infection with ulcers that may lead to sloughing of the mucosa.
5. *Gangrenous cystitis* is necrosis of the bladder wall and occurs with the most severe infections.

Pathophysiology. Two factors account for the development of UTI: the virulence of the pathogen and the efficiency of host defense mechanisms. The most common infecting microorganisms are uropathic strains of *Escherichia coli*, and the second most common is *Staphylococcus saprophyticus*. Less common microorganisms include *Klebsiella, Proteus, Pseudomonas*, fungi, viruses, parasites, or tubercular bacilli. Schistosomiasis

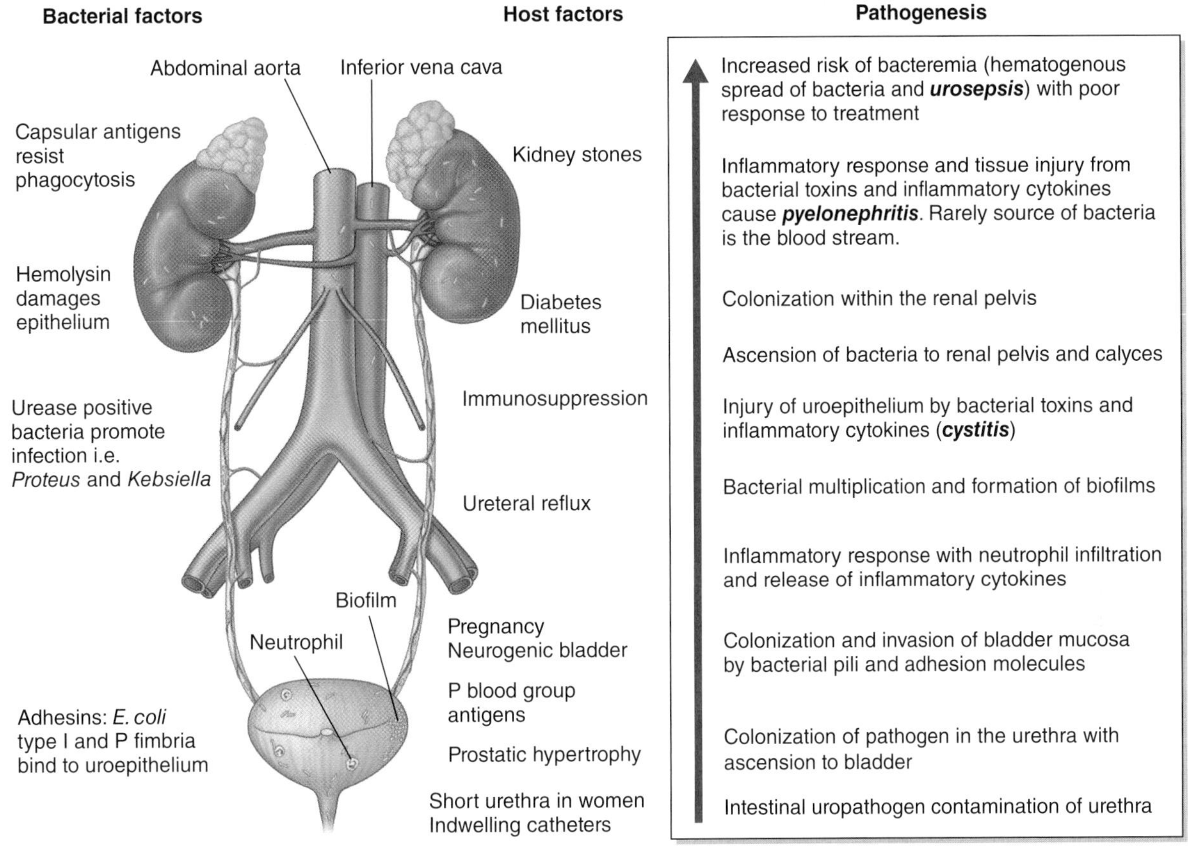

Fig. 38.5 Mechanisms of Urinary Tract Infection.

is the most common parasitic invasion of the urinary tract on a global basis, particularly Africa and areas of the Middle East, and has a strong association with bladder cancer.[43] Bacterial contamination of the normally sterile urine usually occurs by retrograde (backward) movement of gastrointestinal gram-negative bacilli into the urethra and bladder from the opening of the urethra. The microorganisms overcome normal defense mechanisms and can then move into the ureter and kidney. Uropathic strains of *E. coli* have *type-1 fimbriae* (also termed pili or fingerlike projections) that bind to receptors on the uroepithelium. Consequently, they resist flushing during normal micturition. They also can bind to latex catheters used for urinary drainage. Some women may be genetically susceptible to certain strains of *E. coli* attachment. In these cases, women have P blood group antigen (a glycolipid) that binds to *P. fimbriae* (pyelonephritis-associated fimbriae) of *E. coli* on the uroepithelium, allowing the pathogen to ascend the urinary tract. Infection initiates an inflammatory response and the symptoms of cystitis. The inflammatory edema in the bladder wall stimulates activation of stretch receptors. The activated stretch receptors initiate symptoms of bladder fullness with small volumes of urine, producing the urgency and frequency of urination associated with cystitis.

Clinical Manifestations. Clinical manifestations of cystitis are related to the inflammatory response and usually include polyuria, urinary frequency, urgency, dysuria (painful urination), and suprapubic and low back pain. Hematuria, cloudy or malodorous urine, flank pain, and mental status changes are more serious symptoms. Many individuals with bacteriuria are asymptomatic. Individuals with a complicated UTI may present with systemic symptoms such as fever, chills, mental status changes, tachycardia, hypotension, nausea, vomiting, pain, and incontinence. The elderly have the highest risk and may present with only confusion or vague abdominal discomfort.

Evaluation and Treatment. Cystitis in symptomatic individuals is diagnosed by urine culture of specific microorganisms with counts of 100,000/mL or more from freshly voided urine.[44] The standard diagnostic test for UTI is urinalysis, which is both cost-effective and noninvasive. The most accurate way to obtain a urine specimen is a midstream clean catch. Positive nitrates and leukocyte esterase on the dipstick analysis are accurate indicators of UTI. Urinalysis screening of asymptomatic bacteriuria is only recommended in women during pregnancy and for individuals prior to undergoing invasive urologic procedures.[45] Women reporting typical symptoms of uncomplicated lower UTI do not require any laboratory or diagnostic testing.[46] Risk factors, such as urinary tract obstruction, should be identified and treated.

Evidence of bacteria from urine culture and antibiotic sensitivity warrants treatment with a microorganism-specific antibiotic. Optimal therapy depends on the severity and local bacterial resistance patterns. Acute uncomplicated cystitis in nonpregnant women can be diagnosed without an office visit or urine culture. If urine culture and sensitivity are ordered, the urine specimen must be obtained before the initiation of any antibiotic therapy; 3 to 7 days of treatment is most common.[42]

Complicated UTI requires 7 to 14 days of treatment. Relapsing infection within 7 to 10 days requires prolonged antibiotic treatment. Clinical symptoms are frequently relieved, but bacteriuria may still be present. Repeat cultures are not necessary as a test for cure post-treatment. For chronic infection with a continuation of symptoms, cultures should be obtained every 3 to 4 months until 1 year after treatment for evaluation and treatment of recurrent infection. Guidelines are available for the treatment of community-acquired UTIs, uncomplicated cystitis and pyelonephritis in women, complicated cystitis, and for the prevention of catheter-associated cystitis.[47]

Painful Bladder Syndrome/Interstitial Cystitis

Interstitial cystitis/bladder pain syndrome (IC/BPS) is defined as an unpleasant sensation (pain, pressure, discomfort) perceived to be related to the urinary bladder associated with LUT symptoms of more than 6 weeks' duration in the absence of infection or other identifiable causes. It is most commonly diagnosed in women and in the fourth decade of life or after.

Pathophysiology. The cause of IC/BPS is unknown. IC/BPS can be conceptualized as a bladder pain disorder that is often associated with voiding and other systemic chronic disorders such as fibromyalgia, irritable bowel disease, chronic fatigue syndrome, Sjogren's syndrome, chronic headaches, and vulvodynia.[48] An autoimmune reaction may be responsible for the inflammatory response, which includes mast cell activation, altered uroepithelial permeability, and increased sensory nerve sensitivity. The inflammation is associated with a derangement of the glycosaminoglycan layer of the bladder mucosa that makes it more susceptible to penetration by bacteria and noxious urinary solutes.

Clinical Manifestations. Inflammation and fibrosis of the bladder wall (uroepithelium) are accompanied by pain. Bladder volume may decrease as a result of fibrosis. IC/BPS is also categorized by the presence or absence of hemorrhagic ulcers (Hunner ulcers or lesions). Absence of Hunner ulcers is a noninflammatory phenotype with little evidence of bladder etiology and presents with somatic and/or psychological symptoms that commonly result in central nervous sensitization.[49]

Evaluation and Treatment. Diagnosis of IC/PBS requires a thorough history, physical examination and urinalysis, analysis of cystoscopy findings, the presence or absence of Hunner ulcers, and the exclusion of other diagnoses. The hallmark symptom of IC/PBS is pain, including sensations of pressure and discomfort located in the suprapubic area, urethra, vulva, vagina, rectum, lower abdomen, or back lasting longer than 6 weeks. Other characteristic symptoms of IC/PBS include bladder fullness, urinary urgency, frequency (including nocturia) with small urine volume, and chronic pelvic pain. No single treatment is effective. Treatment should focus on improving quality of life through self-care practices and behavioral modifications. Oral and intravesical therapies, sacral nerve stimulation, and intradetrusor botulinum toxin A are used for symptom relief. Fulguration with laser or electrocautery and/or injection with triamcinolone should be performed if Hunner ulcers are present. Surgery is used in refractory cases.[50] Guidelines are available for the treatment of IC/BPS.[51]

Acute Pyelonephritis

Pyelonephritis is an infection of one or both upper urinary tracts (ureter, renal pelvis, and kidney interstitium). Common causes are summarized in Table 38.4. Urinary obstruction and reflux of urine from the bladder (vesicoureteral reflux) are the most common underlying risk factors, with most cases occurring in women. One or both kidneys may be involved.

Pathophysiology. Microorganisms usually associated with acute pyelonephritis include *E. coli* (most common), *Proteus*, or *Pseudomonas*. The latter two microorganisms are more commonly associated with infections after urethral instrumentation or urinary tract surgery. These microorganisms also split urea into ammonia, making an alkaline urine that increases the risk of stone formation. The infection is likely spread by ascending uropathic microorganisms along the ureters. Dissemination also may occur by way of the bloodstream. The inflammatory process primarily affects the pelvis, calyces, and medulla of the kidney. The infection causes infiltration of leukocytes with renal inflammation, renal edema, and purulent urine. In severe infections, localized abscesses may form in the medulla and extend to the cortex. The tubules are primarily affected, while the glomeruli are usually spared. Necrosis of renal papillae can develop. After the acute phase, healing occurs with fibrosis and atrophy of affected tubules. The number of bacteria decreases until the urine again becomes sterile. Acute pyelonephritis rarely causes renal failure.

TABLE 38.4 Common Causes of Pyelonephritis

Predisposing Factors	Pathologic Mechanisms
Nephrolithiasis	Obstruction and stasis of urine contributing to bacteriuria and hydronephrosis; irritation of epithelial lining with entrapment of bacteria
Vesicoureteral reflux	Chronic reflux of urine up the ureter and into kidney during micturition, contributing to bacterial infection
Pregnancy	Dilation and relaxation of ureter with hydroureter and hydronephrosis; partly caused by obstruction from enlarged uterus and partly from ureteral relaxation caused by higher progesterone levels
Neurogenic bladder	Neurologic impairment interfering with normal bladder and urethral sphincter contraction with residual urine and ascending infection
Instrumentation	Introduction of organisms into urethra and bladder by catheters and endoscopes introduced into the urinary tract for diagnostic purposes
Female sexual trauma	Movement of organisms from the urethra into the bladder with infection and retrograde spread to kidney

Clinical Manifestations. The onset of symptoms is usually acute, with fever, chills, tachycardia, nausea, vomiting, and flank or groin pain. Symptoms characteristic of UTI, including frequency, dysuria, incontinence, and costovertebral tenderness, may precede systemic signs and symptoms.[46] Older adults may have early nonspecific symptoms, such as low-grade fever, confusion, and malaise.

Evaluation and Treatment. Differentiating symptoms of cystitis from those of pyelonephritis by clinical assessment alone is difficult. The specific diagnosis is established by urine culture, urinalysis, and clinical manifestations. White blood cell casts formed in the renal tubules and flushed into the urine indicate pyelonephritis. However casts are not always present in the urine. A urine culture assay establishes a definitive diagnosis through identification of the uropathogen. A positive culture is characterized by bacteriuria of at least 10^5 CFU/mL.[44] Individuals with complicated pyelonephritis may require blood cultures and diagnostic imaging if there is no response to antibiotic treatment or if there is a suspected obstruction. Optimal therapy for acute uncomplicated pyelonephritis depends on severity and local resistance patterns.[52] Current guidelines recommend empiric therapy with a broad-spectrum antibiotic (e.g., fluoroquinolone) for patients with pyelonephritis, not requiring hospitalization. A urine specimen for culture and sensitivity must be collected prior to initiation of antibiotics.[46] A post-treatment test of cure urinalysis or urine culture in asymptomatic individuals is not performed.[42] However, follow-up urine cultures are obtained at 1 and 4 weeks after treatment if symptoms recur. Antibiotic-resistant microorganisms or reinfection may occur in cases of urinary tract obstruction or reflux. Intravenous pyelography and voiding cystourethrography are used to identify surgically correctable lesions.

Chronic Pyelonephritis

Chronic pyelonephritis is a persistent or recurrent infection of one or both of the kidneys leading to scarring. The specific cause of chronic pyelonephritis may be unknown (idiopathic) or associated with chronic UTIs, vesicoureteral reflux, or kidney stone obstructive uropathy. Other causes include drug toxicity from analgesics, such as nonsteroidal anti-inflammatory drugs (NSAIDs), ischemia, irradiation, and immune-complex diseases.

Pathophysiology. Chronic urinary tract obstruction prevents elimination of bacteria and starts a process of progressive inflammation. Alterations occur within the renal pelvis and calyces from the obstruction and inflammation (Fig. 38.6). There is destruction of the tubules and diffuse scarring, which impairs urine-concentrating ability. The lesions of chronic pyelonephritis are sometimes termed chronic interstitial nephritis because the inflammation and fibrosis are located in the interstitial spaces between the tubules.

Clinical Manifestations. The early symptoms of chronic pyelonephritis are often minimal and may include urinary frequency, dysuria, flank pain, and hypertension. Progression can lead to kidney failure, particularly in the presence of other risk factors (e.g., obstructive uropathy or diabetes mellitus). There is an inability to conserve sodium with loss of tubular function and development of hyperkalemia and metabolic acidosis. Risk for dehydration must be considered if there is loss of the ability to concentrate the urine.

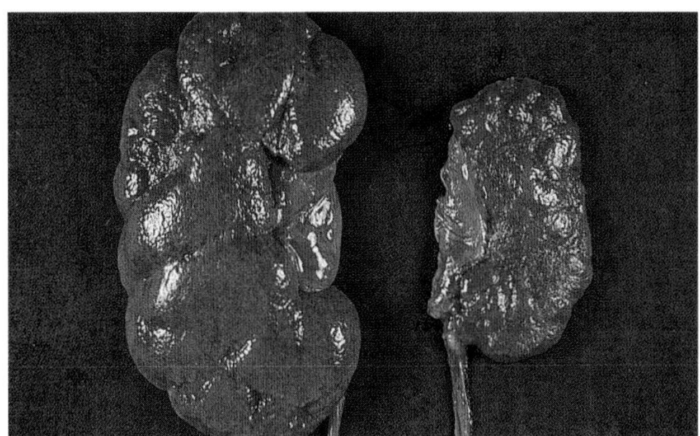

Fig. 38.6 Pyelonephritis. *(Right)* Small, shrunken, irregularly scarred kidney of an individual with chronic pyelonephritis. *(Left)* Kidney is of normal size but also shows scarring on the upper pole. From Damjanov I. *Pathology for the health professions*, 4th edition. Philadelphia: Saunders; 2012.

Evaluation and Treatment. Urinalysis, intravenous pyelography, and ultrasound are used as diagnostic tests to evaluate chronic pyelonephritis. Treatment is related to the underlying cause. Obstruction must be relieved. Antibiotics may be given, with prolonged antibiotic therapy for recurrent infection.

GLOMERULAR DISORDERS

Glomerulonephritis

Acute glomerulonephritis is an inflammation isolated to the kidney glomerulus caused by *primary glomerular injury*, including infection, immunologic responses, ischemia, free radicals, drugs, toxins, and vascular disorders. *Secondary glomerular injury* is a glomerular injury that occurs as a consequence of systemic diseases, including diabetes mellitus, hypertension, bacterial toxins, systemic lupus erythematosus, congestive heart failure, and HIV-related kidney disease.

Pathophysiology. Immune mechanisms are a major component of both primary and secondary glomerular injury. (Fig. 38.7). The injury damages the glomerular capillary filtration membrane. The most common type of immune injury is related to the presence of antigen-antibody complexes within the glomerulus (Table 38.5). Nonimmune glomerular injury is related to injury or ischemia from metabolic disorders, toxin exposure, drugs, vascular disorders, and infection. Different causes of injury may result in more than one type of glomerular lesion; thus, lesions are not necessarily disease specific (Table 38.6).

Immune injury is caused by activation of the inflammatory response (i.e., complement activation, leukocyte recruitment, and release of cytokines from leukocytes). Injury begins after the antigen-antibody complexes have deposited or formed in the glomerular capillary wall or mesangium. Complement is deposited with the antibodies and complement activation can cause cell injury or serve as a chemotactic stimulus for attraction of

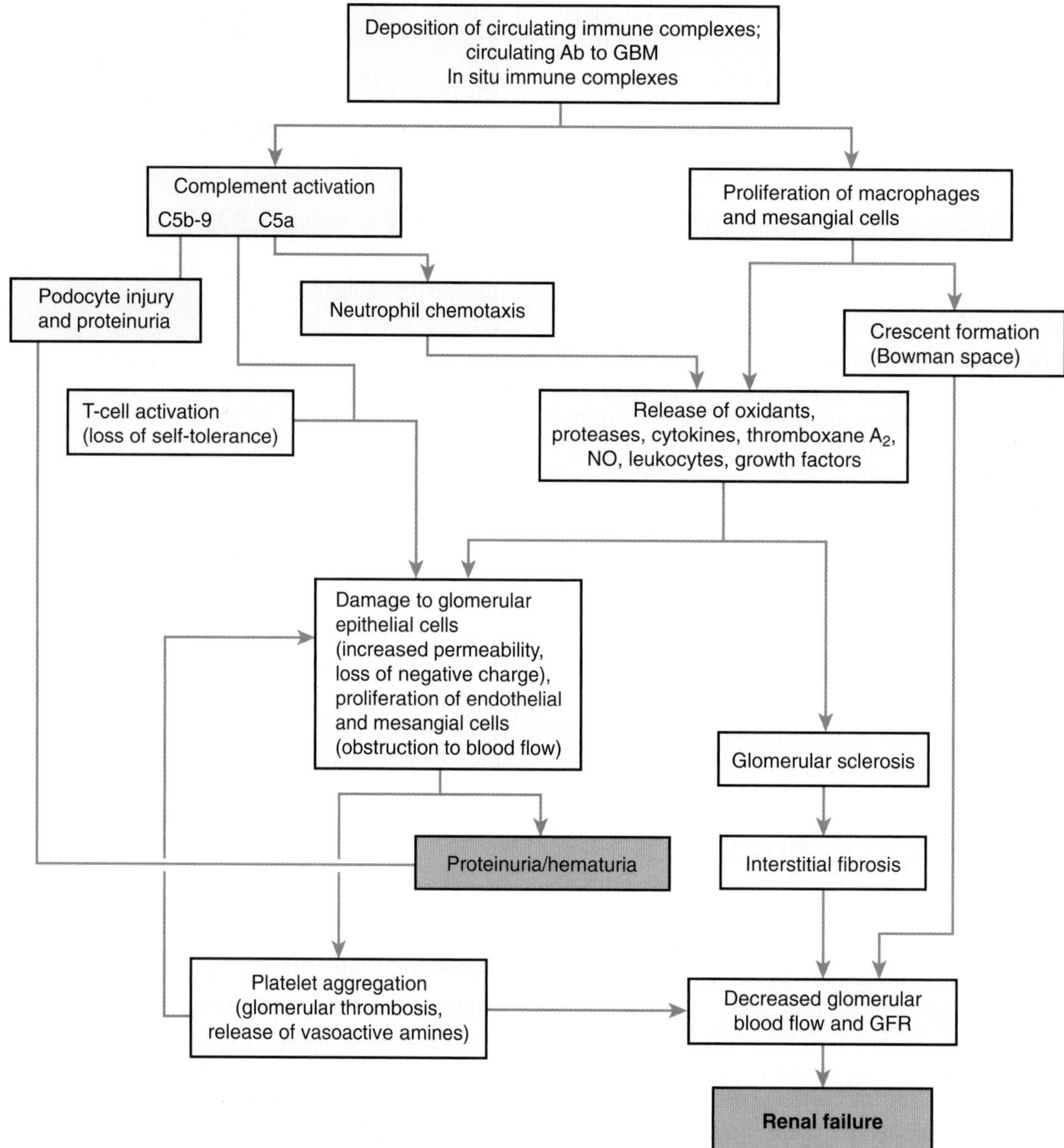

Fig. 38.7 Mechanisms of Glomerular Injury. *Ab*, Antibody; *GBM*, glomerular basement membrane; *GFR*, glomerular filtration rate; *NO*, nitric oxide.

leukocytes (neutrophils, monocytes, and T lymphocytes). These phagocytes, along with activated platelets, further the inflammatory reaction by releasing mediators that injure the glomerular filtration membrane including epithelial cells, glomerular basement membrane, and endothelial cells (podocytes and filtration slits).[53] The injury increases glomerular filtration membrane permeability and reduces glomerular membrane surface area.

There may be hypertrophy and proliferation of mesangial cells and expansion of the extracellular matrix in the Bowman space. The deposition of these substances and cell proliferation forms a crescent shape within the Bowman space that can be seen under a microscope and can assist with diagnosis if a biopsy is performed. The result of these processes is compression of glomerular capillaries, decreased glomerular blood flow, hypoxic injury, decreased driving glomerular hydrostatic pressure, alteration in the filtration membrane, and decreased GFR. Crescent formation is associated with rapidly progressive glomerulonephritis.[54]

Loss of the normal negative electrical charge across the glomerular filtration membrane and increase in filtration pore size enhance movement of proteins into the urine. Proteins are normally repelled because they also have a negative charge and thus are not filtered into the urine. Red blood cells also escape if pore size is large enough. Consequently, proteinuria and/or hematuria develop. The severity of glomerular damage and decline in glomerular function is related to the size, number, and location (i.e., focal [affecting some glomeruli] or diffuse [affecting glomeruli throughout the kidney]) of cells injured; duration of exposure; and type of antigen-antibody complexes formed.

TABLE 38.5 Immunologic Pathogenesis of Glomerulonephritis

Glomerular Injury	Mechanism
Soluble immune-complex glomerulonephritis (90%)	Formation of antibodies stimulated by the presence of endogenous or exogenous antigens results in circulating soluble antigen-antibody complexes, which are deposited in glomerular capillaries, or the in situ formation of immune complexes to planted antigens or to structural components within the glomerulus; glomerular injury occurring with complement deposition and activation and release of immunologic substances that lyse cells and increase membrane permeability; immune deposits with a microscopic appearance that fluoresce in a *granular pattern* when stained with fluorescein and viewed under ultraviolet light; severity of glomerular injury related to the number of complexes formed; a type III hypersensitivity reaction; immunoglobulin A (IgA) nephropathy and poststreptococcal glomerulonephritis are examples
Antiglomerular basement membrane glomerulonephritis (5%)	Antibodies are formed and act directly against the glomerular basement membrane (type IV collagen); immune response that causes crescent formation and a *linear pattern* of immunofluorescence; generally associated with rapidly progressive renal failure such as Goodpasture syndrome (type II hypersensitivity reaction)
Alternative complement pathway	An immune mechanism associated with circulating autoantibodies and C3 complement and membranoproliferative glomerulonephritis
Cell-mediated immunity	A delayed hypersensitivity response that damages glomerulus; actual cellular mechanism not clearly understood but may involve cytokine secretion, activation of effector cells such as macrophages or by inducing autoantibodies or immune complexes; cytotoxic CD8+ T-cell responses and failure of regulatory T cells may represent two additional types of antirenal hypersensitivity (type IV hypersensitivity); often seen in rapidly progressive glomerulonephritis

Data from Foster MH. Basement membranes and autoimmune diseases. *Matrix Biology*, 2017;57–58:149–168; Nester CM, Smith RJ. Complement inhibition in C3 glomerulopathy. *Seminars in Immunology*, 2016;28(3):241–249; Rodríguez-Iturbe B, Batsford S. Pathogenesis of poststreptococcal glomerulonephritis a century after Clemens von Pirquet. *Kidney International*, 2007;71(11):1094–1104.

TABLE 38.6 Classification of Glomerular Lesions

Lesion	Distribution When Many Glomeruli Considered
Diffuse	Relatively uniform involvement of most (>50%) or all glomeruli; most common form of glomerulonephritis
Focal	Changes in only some glomeruli (>50%), whereas others are normal
Lesion	**Distribution When Single Glomeruli Considered**
Global	A lesion involving the entire glomerulus
Segmental-local	Changes in one part of the glomerulus with other parts unaffected

Clinical Manifestations. The onset of glomerulonephritis may be sudden or insidious. A significant loss of nephron function can occur before symptoms develop. Acute glomerulonephritis may be silent, mild, moderate, or severe in symptom presentation. Severe or progressive glomerular disease causes oliguria (urine output of 30 mL/h or less), hypertension, and renal failure. Focal lesions tend to produce less severe clinical symptoms. Salt and water are reabsorbed, contributing to fluid volume expansion, edema, and hypertension.

Two distinct symptoms of more severe or rapidly progressive glomerulonephritis are (1) hematuria with red blood cell casts (the red blood cells accumulate in the kidney tubules and are washed into the urine in the form of a cast of the tubule) and (2) proteinuria exceeding 3 to 5 g/day with albumin (macroalbuminuria). Glomerular bleeding provides prolonged contact with the acidic urine and transforms hemoglobin to methemoglobin, which has a brownish color and no blood clots.

Evaluation and Treatment. The diagnosis of glomerular disease is confirmed by the progressive development of clinical manifestations and abnormal laboratory findings. Common urinalysis findings associated with glomerular disease include proteinuria, red blood cells, white blood cells, and casts. Reduced GFR during glomerulonephritis is evidenced by elevated plasma urea, cystatin C, and creatinine concentrations, or by reduced renal creatinine clearance (see Chapter 37). Microscopic evaluation from renal biopsy can provide a specific determination of renal injury and the type of pathologic lesion (i.e., the formation of glomerular crescents as previously described and location and character of glomerular lesions). Patterns of antigen-antibody complex deposition within the glomerular capillary filtration membrane have been established using light, electron, and immunofluorescent microscopy. Electron microscopy differentiates morphologic changes within the glomerular capillary wall (e.g., subendothelial and mesangial electron-dense deposits, increased mesangial matrix, mesangialization of capillary loops, and foot process fusion). Staining with fluorescein identifies complement and different antibodies (i.e., immunoglobulin G [IgG] or immunoglobulin A [IgA]) and associated configurations when viewed under ultraviolet light with light microscopy. Findings with microscopy provide information about the distribution and lesions of immune response injury and guide therapy.[55]

Reduced GFR during glomerulonephritis is evidenced by elevated plasma urea, cystatin C, and creatinine concentrations, or by reduced creatinine clearance (see Tests of Renal Function in

Chapter 37). Edema, caused by excessive sodium and water retention and or loss of plasma proteins (see Chapter 3 for the pathophysiology of edema), may require the use of diuretics or dialysis.

Management principles for treating glomerulonephritis are related to treating the primary cause, preventing or minimizing immune responses, and correcting accompanying problems. Accompanying problems include edema, hypertension, hypoalbuminemia, and hyperlipidemia. Specific treatment regimens are necessary for particular types of glomerulonephritis. Antibiotic therapy is essential for the management of underlying infections that may be contributing to ongoing antigen-antibody responses. Corticosteroids decrease antibody synthesis and suppress inflammatory responses. Cytotoxic agents (e.g., cyclophosphamide) may be used to suppress the immune response in corticosteroid-resistant cases. Anticoagulants may be useful for controlling fibrin crescent formation in rapidly progressive glomerulonephritis.

Types of Glomerulonephritis

The types of glomerulonephritis can be described according to cause, pathologic lesions determined by biopsy (Table 38.7), disease progression (acute, rapidly progressive, chronic), or clinical presentation (nephrotic syndrome, nephritic syndrome, acute or chronic renal failure). In nearly all types of glomerulonephritis, the epithelial or podocyte layer of the glomerular capillary membrane is disturbed with loss of negative charges and changes in membrane permeability. Plasma proteins (albumin) and red blood cells can escape into the urine and can cause proteinuria and/or hematuria. The mesangial matrix may be expanded, or the basement membrane thickened decreasing blood flow through the glomerular capillaries and decreasing GFR. Many types of glomerular injury occur most often in children or young adults, including acute postinfectious glomerulonephritis and minimal change nephropathy (lipoid nephrosis). Details of these diseases are presented in Chapter 39.

Complications of systemic diseases, such as diabetic nephropathy and systemic lupus erythematosus, can affect the entire nephron with significant glomerular injury. Different patterns of injury develop over the course of these diseases, and there is usually chronic progression. They are described in the next section.

TABLE 38.7 Characteristic Patterns of Glomerular Lesion

Lesion	Lesion Characteristics
Mesangial	Deposits of immunoglobulins in the mesangial matrix; mesangial cell proliferation
Membranous	Thickening of the glomerular capillary wall with immune deposits (i.e., immunoglobulin G [IgG] and complement 3 [C3])
Proliferative	Increase in the number of glomerular cells: endothelial, epithelial, mesangial
Sclerotic	Glomerular scarring from previous glomerular injury
Crescentic	Accumulation of proliferating cells within Bowman space, making the appearance of a crescent
Interstitial fibrosis	Scarring between the glomerulus and the tubules

Chronic Glomerulonephritis

Chronic glomerulonephritis encompasses several glomerular diseases with a progressive course leading to chronic kidney failure. There may be no history of kidney disease before the diagnosis. Hypercholesterolemia and proteinuria have been associated with progressive glomerular and tubular injury (Fig. 38.8). The proposed mechanism is related to those observed in glomerulosclerosis and interstitial injury, such as inflammatory processes and glomerular hyperfiltration. The primary cause may be difficult to establish because advanced pathologic changes may obscure specific disease characteristics. Diabetes nephropathy and lupus nephritis are examples of secondary causes of chronic glomerular injury. Renal insufficiency usually begins to develop after 10 to 20 years of disease, followed by nephrotic syndrome (see next section) and an accelerated progression to end-stage renal failure (ESRF). Symptom patterns vary depending on the underlying cause and the areas of the kidney that are damaged. The specific pathologic changes are identified by renal biopsy, which is best performed in the early stages of CKD to identify specific treatment options. Management of the underlying disease and use of steroids, immunosuppressive agents, dipeptidyl peptidase-4 (DPP-4) inhibitors, glucagon-like peptide-1 (GLP-1) receptor agonists, sodium-glucose co-transporter-2 (SGLT2) inhibitors, renin-angiotensin-aldosterone (RAAS) inhibitors, and angiotensin-receptor blockers (ARBs) can prolong remissions and preserve renal function (see Emerging Science Box: Renin–Angiotensin–Aldosterone System Inhibitors in Patients With COVID-19). Dialysis or kidney transplantation ultimately may be needed.

Diabetic nephropathy develops from metabolic (accumulation of advanced glycosylated end products), inflammatory (transforming growth factor-beta and protein kinase C), and macrovascular and microvascular complications related to chronic hyperglycemia (see Chapter 22). Changes in the glomerulus are characterized by podocyte injury, progressive

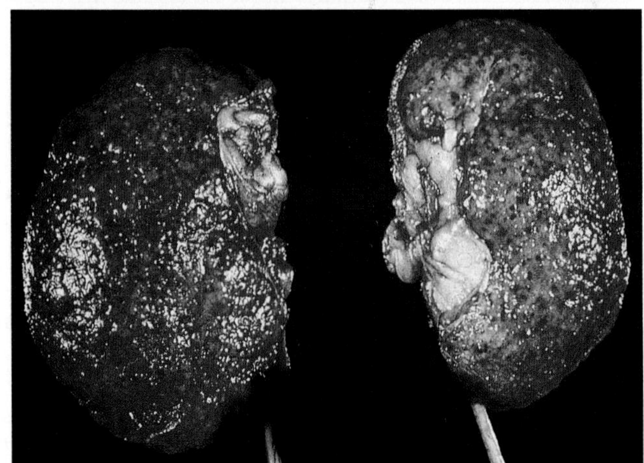

Fig. 38.8 Chronic Glomerulonephritis. The kidneys appear small, are uniformly shrunken, and have a finely granular external surface. (From Damjanov I. *Pathology for the health professions*, 4th edition. Philadelphia: Saunders, 2012.)

thickening and fibrosis of the glomerular basement membrane, expansion of the mesangial matrix (diffuse diabetic glomerulosclerosis), and nodular glomerulosclerosis (Kimmelstiel-Wilson nodules; see Fig. 38.9) with albuminuria, loss of tubular cells, and progression to chronic kidney disease. Although albuminuria is the classic phenotype of progressive diabetic renal disease, two new phenotypes have emerged (i.e., "nonalbuminuric renal impairment" and "progressive renal decline"), suggesting there can be progressive failure of renal function (i.e., declining GFR) without albuminuria. These "new" phenotypes may be the consequence of improved treatment. Work is in progress to determine if diagnostic and treatment guidelines should be modified for the management of these different phenotypes.[56] Diabetic nephropathy is the most common cause of CKD and end-stage renal disease (ESRD) for both type 1 and type 2 diabetes.[57] ESRD requires treatment with dialysis or renal transplantation.[58]

Lupus nephritis is an inflammatory complication of the chronic autoimmune syndrome systemic lupus erythematosus (see Chapter 9). The renal component of the disease may be caused by the formation of autoantibodies against double-stranded DNA and nucleosomes with glomerular deposition of the immune complexes. Immune complexes also may be formed in situ by binding to planted antigens of circulating autoantibodies. There is complement activation and a cascade of inflammatory events resulting in damage to the glomerular membrane with mesangial expansion (see Chapter 8).[59] Various glomerular lesion patterns are identifiable on biopsy, including membranous, mesangial, membranoproliferative, and diffuse proliferative glomerulonephritis; tubular fibrosis can also be present (Table 38.8). Symptom presentation is variable depending on lesion involvement and can include proteinuria, microscopic hematuria, edema, and other signs of nephrotic syndrome. Disease progression may be silent or may progress to ESRD over a period of years. Treatment includes the use of immunosuppressive agents and efforts to protect the kidney from secondary nonimmune consequences of acute injury.[60]

EMERGING SCIENCE BOX

Renin–Angiotensin–Aldosterone System Inhibitors in Patients With COVID-19

COVID-19, similar to other severe acute respiratory syndromes (SARS-CoV-1), is thought to interact with the RAAS through the angiotensin-converting enzyme 2 (ACE2). The RAAS coordinates key processes in human physiology to regulate blood pressure. The ACE2 functions as a receptor for SARS viruses and physiologically counters RAAS activation. To gain entry into the host cells, the viral surface spike (S) protein of SARS-CoV-2, the virus that causes COVID-19, binds to the ACE2 through the spike protein activation by transmembrane protease serine 2. This interaction is suggested as a potential associative factor of infectivity. However, there is currently conflicting evidence as to whether or not the use of angiotensin-receptor blockers (ARBs) and angiotensin-converting-enzyme (ACE) inhibitors may alter ACE2, which could drive disease virulence in the ongoing COVID-19 pandemic.

Data from Mancia G, et al. Renin–angiotensin– aldosterone system blockers and the risk of Covid-19. *New England Journal of Medicine*, 2020;382:2431–2440. doi:10.1056/NEJMoa2006923; Hoffmann M, et al. SARS-CoV-2 cell entry depends on ACE2 and TMPRSS2 and is blocked by a clinically proven protease inhibitor. *Cell*, 2020;181(2):271–280.e8 https://doi.org/10.1016/j.cell.2020.02.052. Vaduganathan M, et al. Renin-angiotensinaldosterone system inhibitors in patients with Covid-19. *New England Journal of Medicine*, 2020;382(17):1653–1659. doi:10.1056/NEJMsr2005760.

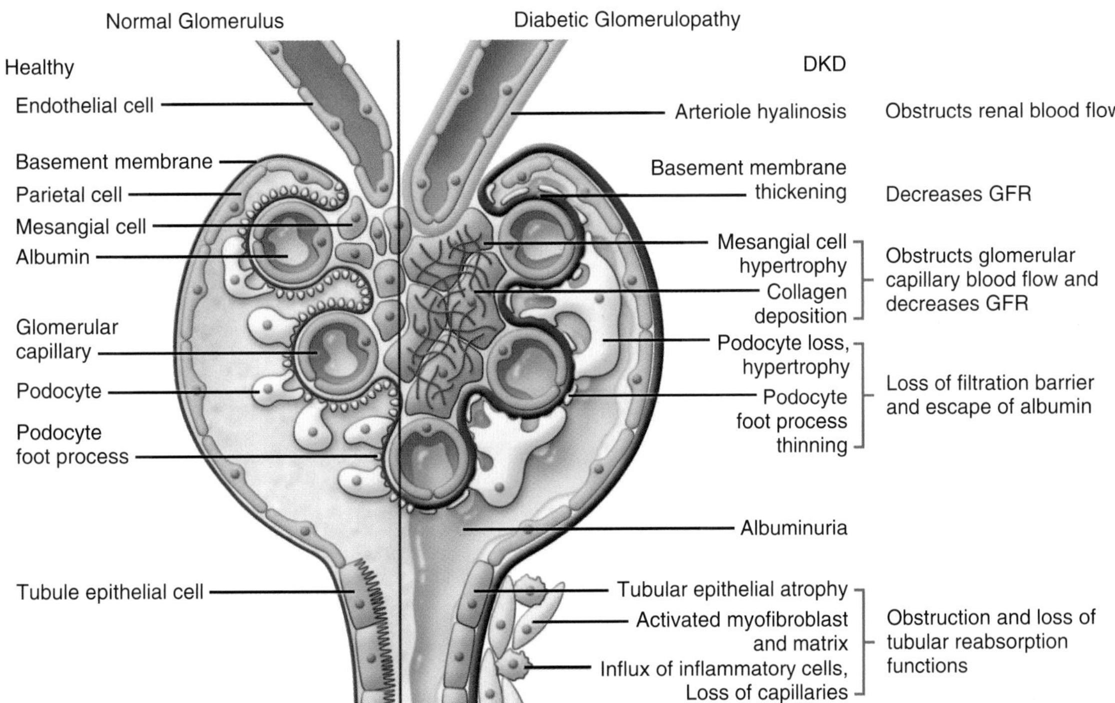

Fig. 38.9 Diabetic Glomerulopathy. (Used with permission from RReidy K, Kang HM, Hostetter T, et al. Molecular mechanisms of diabetic kidney disease. *Journal of Clinical Investigation*, 2014;124(6):2333–2340.)

TABLE 38.8 Features of the Common Types of Glomerulonephritis

Type and Cause	Histopathophysiology
Associated with Nephritic Syndrome	
Acute postinfectious glomerulonephritis (PIGN) (e.g., group A beta-hemolytic streptococci [more common in children]; staphylococcus [more common in older adults])	Subepithelial deposits of IgG and complement complexes; infiltration of neutrophils and monocytes; proliferation of mesangial and epithelial cells with occlusion of glomerular capillary blood flow and decreased glomerular filtration; usually diffuse lesions
Rapidly progressive or crescentic glomerulonephritis (a clinical syndrome): *Type I:* Formation of IgG antibodies against pulmonary capillary and glomerular basement membrane (Goodpasture syndrome); activation of complement and neutrophils; more common in young men; causes pulmonary hemorrhage and renal failure *Type II:* Mesangial immune-complex deposition (PIGN, SLE, IgA nephropathy) *Type III:* Pauci-immune, lack of antiglomerular basement membrane antibodies antibodies or immune complexes; presence of serum antineutrophil cytoplasmic (ANC) antibodies associated with systemic vasculitides (usually idiopathic); nonspecific response to glomerular injury; can occur in any severe glomerular disease	Accumulation of fibrin, macrophages, and epithelial cell proliferation into the Bowman space forms crescents and occludes glomerular capillary blood flow, decreasing glomerular filtration; antiglomerular basement membrane antibodies lead to necrotizing, proliferative glomerulonephritis, and renal failure; diffuse lesions
Mesangial proliferative glomerulonephritis Can be associated with IgA nephropathy or lupus nephritis	Deposits of immune complexes in the mesangium with mesangial cell proliferation; results in decreased glomerular blood flow and glomerular filtration; leads to hematuria/proteinuria and nephrotic syndrome
Associated with Nephrotic Syndrome	
Minimal change nephropathy (lipoid nephrosis) Glomerular basement membrane appears normal Most common cause of nephrotic syndrome in children (see Chapter 39) Usually idiopathic	Glomeruli look normal under light microscopy; electron microscopy reveals uniform diffuse effacement of epithelial (podocyte) foot processes; loss of negative charge in basement membrane and increased permeability lead to severe proteinuria and nephrotic syndrome
Focal segmental glomerulosclerosis Usually idiopathic Can be associated with HIV infection, IgA nephropathy	Focal proliferation of endothelial and mesangial cells and glomerulosclerosis from hyaline deposits in segmental parts of the glomerular membrane; there is effacement (thinning or deletion) of epithelial podocytes, with a significant increase in pore size resulting in proteinuria and nephrotic syndrome; can progress to involve entire glomerulus and development of tubulointerstitial fibrosis
Membranous nephropathy (autoimmune response to unknown renal antigen) Usually idiopathic; can be associated with systemic diseases (i.e., hepatitis B virus, hepatitis C virus, systemic lupus erythematosus, solid malignant tumors)	Diffuse thickening of glomerular basement membrane and capillary wall from deposits of antibody, complement, and release of inflammatory cytokines; increased permeability with proteinuria and leading cause of nephrotic syndrome in white adults
Membranoproliferative glomerulonephritis (MPGN) Usually idiopathic; associated with hypocomplementemia *Type I:* Activation of classical complement pathway with nephrotic syndrome (hepatitides B and C, SLE) *Type II:* Activation of alternate complement pathway with hematuria (idiopathic); no circulating immune complexes *Type III:* Activation of alternative complement pathway with nephrotic syndrome; can be familial	Mesangial cell proliferation; thickening of basement membrane; subendothelial deposits of immune-complex occlude glomerular capillary blood flow and decrease glomerular filtration; diffuse lesions
IgA Nephropathy (Berger Disease) Usually idiopathic (can be associated with cirrhosis and minimal change disease); elevated IgA plasma levels (also see Henoch-Schönlein purpura nephritis in Chapter 39)	Mesangial proliferation with deposition of IgA; release of inflammatory mediators with cellular proliferation; crescent formation, glomerulosclerosis, interstitial fibrosis, decreased GFR and hematuria; usually focal, some diffuse lesions

GBM, Glomerular basement membrane; *GFR*, glomerular filtration rate; *HIV*, human immunodeficiency virus; *IgA*, immunoglobulin A; *IgG*, immunoglobulin G; *SLE*, systemic lupus erythematosus.

Nephrotic and Nephritic Syndromes

Nephrotic and nephritic syndromes are consequences of glomerular injury and present with a pattern of clinical manifestations. **Nephrotic syndrome** is the excretion of 3.5 g or more of protein in the urine per day. It occurs when glomerular filtration of plasma proteins, particularly albumin, exceeds tubular reabsorption. *Primary causes of nephrotic syndrome* include particular types of glomerular injury including minimal change nephropathy (lipoid nephrosis) (see Chapter 39), membranous glomerulonephritis, and focal segmental glomerulosclerosis (see Table 38.8. *Secondary forms of nephrotic syndrome* occur in systemic diseases, including diabetes mellitus (see Chapter 22), amyloidosis, systemic lupus erythematosus (see Chapter 9), and IgA vasculitis (Henoch–Schönlein purpura) (see Chapter 39). Nephrotic syndrome is also associated with certain medications (e.g., NSAIDs), infections, malignancies, and vascular disorders. Familial or inherited forms of nephrotic syndrome result from genetic defects that affect the function and composition of the glomerular capillary wall (i.e., alterations in basement membrane type IV collagen [Alport syndrome] and podocyte dysfunction resulting in steroid resistance).[61] It often signifies a more serious prognosis when present as a secondary complication. Nephrotic syndrome is more common in children (see Chapter 39) than in adults and is more commonly idiopathic in adults.

Nephritic syndrome is characterized by hematuria and red blood cell casts in the urine. Hypertension, edema, and oliguria also are components of the syndrome. Proteinuria is present but is usually less severe than in nephrotic syndrome. It occurs primarily with infection-related glomerulonephritis (e.g., hepatitis B and C and acute poststreptococcal glomerulonephritis), rapidly progressive crescentic glomerulonephritis, antiphospholipid syndrome (production of antiphospholipid antibodies that cause thrombotic microangiopathy), and lupus nephritis.[59]

Pathophysiology. In nephrotic syndrome, injury to the glomerular filtration membrane leads to increased permeability and loss of an electrical negative charge. Normally, plasma proteins, which carry a negative charge, are repelled by the negative charge at the glomerular filtration membrane and thus remain in the plasma. Movement of plasma proteins, particularly albumin and some immunoglobulins, occurs across the injured membrane. The plasma proteins are then lost into the urine, resulting in decreased plasma oncotic pressure and edema (Fig. 38.10). Hypoalbuminemia results from urinary loss of albumin combined with a diminished synthesis of replacement albumin by the liver. Albumin is lost in the greatest quantity because of its high plasma concentration and low molecular weight. Decreased dietary intake of protein from anorexia, malnutrition, or accompanying liver disease may also contribute to lower levels of plasma albumin. Loss of albumin stimulates lipoprotein synthesis by the liver, causing hyperlipidemia, which can promote the progression of glomerular disease. Loss of immunoglobulins may increase susceptibility to infections. Sodium retention is common, further contributing to edema and hypertension.

Nephritic syndrome is caused by increased permeability of the glomerular filtration membrane with pore sizes large enough to allow the passage of red blood cells and protein. The pathophysiology is related to immune injury of the glomerulus, as previously described. Hypertension and uremia (accumulation of urea and other nitrogen-based metabolic products) occur in advanced stages of disease.

Clinical Manifestations. Many clinical manifestations of nephrotic and nephritic syndrome are related to loss of serum proteins and associated sodium retention (Table 38.9). The

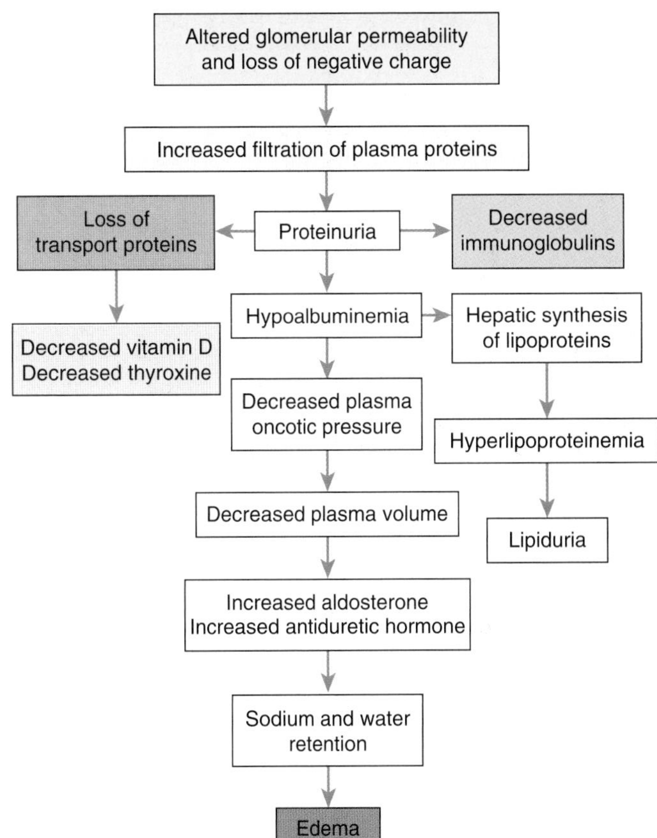

Fig. 38.10 Pathophysiology of Nephrotic Syndrome.

manifestations of both nephrotic and nephritic syndrome include edema (periorbital and pedal), hypoproteinemia, proteinuria, hyperlipidemia, lipiduria, vitamin D deficiency, and hypothyroidism. In addition, voided urine that appears foamy from protein loss is associated with nephrotic syndrome, and hematuria, hypertension, and oliguria are associated with nephritic syndrome. Vitamin D deficiency is related to loss of serum transport proteins and decreased vitamin D activation by the kidney. Hypothyroidism can result from urinary loss of thyroid-binding protein and thyroxine. Renal loss of anti-clotting factors and increased liver synthesis of clotting factors can cause hypercoagulability and may lead to thromboembolic events.[62]

Evaluation and Treatment. Nephrotic syndrome is diagnosed when the protein level in a 24-hour urine collection is greater than 3.5 g. Serum albumin level decreases (to <3 g/dL), and concentrations of serum cholesterol, phospholipids, and triglycerides increase. Fat bodies may be present and float in the urine. The presence of lipiduria (lipids within tubular cells or casts, or as free glubules) suggests a glomerular disorder.

Nephrotic syndrome is commonly treated by consuming a moderate protein restriction (i.e., 0.8 g/kg body weight/day), low-fat, salt-restricted diet, and by prescribing corticosteroids and diuretics. Glucocorticoids are used to control immune-mediated disease and may be combined with immunosuppressive drugs (e.g., rituximab). Targeted immune therapy is considered for steroid-resistant nephrotic syndrome.[63] Diuretics are used to control hypertension and eliminate fluid.

TABLE 38.9 Clinical Manifestations of Nephrotic Syndrome

Manifestations	Contributing Factors	Result
Proteinuria	Increased glomerular permeability, decreased proximal tubule reabsorption	Edema, increased susceptibility to infection from loss of immunoglobulins
Hypoalbuminemia	Increased urinary losses of protein	Edema
Edema	Hypoalbuminemia (decreased oncotic pressure, sodium and water retention, increased aldosterone and antidiuretic hormone [ADH] secretion), unresponsiveness to atrial natriuretic peptides	Soft, pitting, generalized edema
Hyperlipidemia	Decreased serum albumin; increased hepatic synthesis of very-low-density lipoproteins; increased cholesterol, phospholipids, triglycerides	Increased atherogenesis
Lipiduria	Sloughing of tubular cells containing fat (oval fat bodies); free fat from hyperlipidemia	Fat droplets that may float in urine
Decreased vitamin D	The globulin to which 1,25-dihydroxy-vitamin D_3 is attached for transport passes through the glomerulus and is lost in the urine	Decreased absorption of calcium from gut Risk for osteodystrophies
Hypothyroidism	Loss of thyroid-binding globulin and other thyroid hormone transport proteins in the urine	May be asymptomatic; may have elevated thyroid-stimulating hormone

Care must be taken to observe for hypovolemia and hypokalemia or potassium toxicity in the presence of renal insufficiency. Spironolactone may be combined with loop diuretics to suppress aldosterone activity to conserve potassium. Anticoagulants are used for prophylactic anticoagulation. Angiotensin-converting enzyme (ACE) inhibitors or ARBs lower urine protein excretion and control blood pressure.[63]

The evaluation and treatment of nephritic syndrome are similar to those described for nephrotic syndrome. Red blood cells and red blood cell casts will be found in the urine. The course of glomerulonephritis is usually more severe with nephritic syndrome. High-dose corticosteroids and cyclophosphamide represent the standard therapy for rapidly progressive crescentic glomerulonephritis. Treatment also may include supportive care with antihypertensives, diuretics, and antibiotics. The addition of plasma exchange (plasmapheresis) and dialysis may be required.

ACUTE KIDNEY INJURY

Classification of Kidney Dysfunction

Kidney injury may be acute and rapidly progressive (within hours) or may become chronic, progressing to ESRD over several months or years. The terms *renal insufficiency, renal failure, uremia*, and *azotemia* are associated with decreasing kidney function but are not specific in relation to the cause of kidney disease. Generally, **renal insufficiency** refers to a decline in renal function to about 25% of normal or a GFR of 25 to 30 mL/min. Levels of SCr and urea are mildly elevated. AKI captures the diverse nature of this syndrome, ranging from minimal or subtle changes in kidney function to complete kidney failure requiring renal replacement therapy. **Renal failure** refers to a significant loss of function. When less than 10% of kidney function remains, this is termed **ESRD**. Specific criteria for AKI are discussed in the next section. **Uremia (uremic syndrome)** is a syndrome of renal failure and includes elevated blood urea nitrogen (BUN) and creatinine levels accompanied by fatigue, anorexia, nausea, vomiting, pruritus, and neurologic changes. Uremia represents numerous consequences related to kidney failure, including retention of toxic wastes, deficiency states, electrolyte disorders, and immune activation promoting a proinflammatory state. **Azotemia** is characterized by increased BUN levels (normal is 8 to 20 mg/dL) and frequently increased SCr levels (normal is 0.7 to 1.4 mg/dL). Renal insufficiency or kidney failure causes azotemia. Both azotemia and uremia indicate an accumulation of nitrogenous waste products in the blood, a common characteristic that explains the overlap in definitions of terms.

Acute Kidney Injury

AKI is a sudden decline in kidney function with a decrease in glomerular filtration caused by a defect in the excretion of water, salts, and nitrogenous waste products, which accumulate in the blood as demonstrated by an elevation in SCr level and decrease in urine volume.[64] Classification criteria have been developed to guide the diagnosis of AKI (Table 38.10). The Kidney Disease: Improving Global Outcomes (KDIGO) developed clinical practice guidelines for AKI and is based on the Risk, Injury, Failure, Loss, End-Stage Renal Disease (RIFLE) and AKI Network (AKIN) criteria.[65] The KDIGO guideline is the commonly accepted definition and classification system for AKI clinical trials and clinical practice.[64] AKI is a complex syndrome that is classified according semi-anatomical categories (i.e., pre-renal, intrinsic, and post-renal). However, in recent years, AKI has been further differentiated into specific syndromes (i.e., hepatorenal, cardiorenal, nephrotoxic, and sepsis-associated), each having a unique pathophysiologic process and treatment course.[64]

TABLE 38.10 Criteria for Acute Kidney Injury

Category	Staging	Kidney Disease: Improving Global Outcomes (KDIGO)	Risk, Injury, Failure, Loss, End-Stage Renal Disease (RIFLE)	Acute Kidney Injury Network (AKIN)
Criteria to make diagnosis of AKI		Increased SCr by 50% in 7 days OR ≥0.3 mg/dL in 48 h	Increased SCr of >50% in <7 days	Increased SCr of 50% or more in <48 h OR ≥ 0.3 mg/dL in 48 h
Risk	Stage 1	Increased SCr of 1.5–1.9 × baseline OR ≥0.3 mg/dL within 48 h	Increased SCr of 1.5 × baseline OR GFR decrease >25% UO <0.5 mL/kg/h × 6 h	Increased SCr of 1.5–2.0 × baseline OR ≥0.3 mg/dL UO <0.5 mL/kg/h × 6 h
Injury	Stage 2	Increased SCr of 2.0–2.9 × baseline within 48 h	Increased SCr of 2 × baseline OR GFR decrease >50% UO <0.5 mL/kg/h × 12 h	Increased SCr of 2.0–3.0 × baseline UO <0.5 mL/kg/h × 12 h
Failure	Stage 3	Increased SCr of ≥3.0 × baseline within 48 h OR Increased SCr to ≥4.0 mg/dL OR Initiation of renal replacement therapy OR in individuals <18 years, with decrease in e GFR to <35 mL/min/1.73 m^2	Increased SCr of 3 × baseline OR GFR decrease >75% UO <0.3 mL/kg/h × >24 h or anuria × 12 h	Increased SCr of >3.0 × baseline OR If SCr baseline is ≥4.0 mg/dL, an increased SCr >0.5 mg/dL UO <0.3 mL/kg/h × 24 h or anuria × 12 h
Loss			Persistent AKI (complete loss of kidney function) >4 weeks requiring renal replacement therapy	
ESRD			Persistent complete loss of kidney function >3 months weeks requiring renal replacement therapy	

AKI, Acute kidney injury; *ESRD*, end-stage renal disease; *GFR*, glomerular filtration rate; *SCr*, serum creatinine; *UOP*, urine output.
Data from Kidney Disease: Improving Global Outcomes (KDIGO) Acute Kidney Injury Work Group. *Kidney Inter Suppl.* 2012;2:1–138. http://www.kdigo.org/clinical_practice_guidelines/AKI.php; Bellomo R, Kellum JA, Mehta R, et al. Acute dialysis quality initiative II: The Vicenza conference. *Current Opinion in Critical Care*, 2002;8(6):505–508; Bellomo R, Ronco C, Kellum JA, et al. Acute renal failure-definition, outcome measures, animal models, fluid therapy and information technology needs: The Second International Consensus Conference of the Acute Dialysis Quality Initiative (ADQI) Group. *Current Opinion in Critical Care*, 2004;8(4):R204–R212; Lopes JA, Jorge S. The RIFLE and AKIN classifications for acute kidney injury: A critical and comprehensive review. *Clinical Kidney Journal*, 2013;6(1):8–14. doi:10.1093/ckj/sfs160.

Pathophysiology. AKI results from ischemic injury related to extracellular volume depletion, renal hypoperfusion, exposure from chemicals, drugs, or endogenous toxins, sepsis, intra-abdominal hypertension, progressive glomerulonephritis, acute interstitial nephritis, infection, or an obstructive process. Injured, hypoxic, and ischemic tissues initiate a complex inflammatory immunopathophysiological response that results in microcirculatory and macrocirculatory disturbances in the kidney, functional impairment, and ultimately cell death.[66] The simultaneous activation of components of innate immunity, including leukocytes, coagulation factors, and complement proteins, drives kidney inflammation, glomerular and tubular damage, and breakdown of the blood-urine barrier.[66] This profound immune response is an integral part of multi-organ dysfunction associated with AKI. Alterations in kidney function may be minimal or severe.[67] AKI is an evolving clinical syndrome with multiple, often simultaneous, and overlapping causes. AKI is currently broadly classified according to the underlying pathophysiologic process as prerenal (renal hypoperfusion), intrarenal (intrinsic disorders involving renal parenchymal or interstitial tissue), or postrenal (urinary tract obstructive disorders) (Table 38.11).[68]

Prerenal AKI or inadequate kidney perfusion is the most common reason for AKI. Poor perfusion can result from hypovolemia, reduced cardiac output, renal vasomodulation/shunting, and systemic vasodilation (see Table 38.11).[69] During the early phases of hypoperfusion, protective autoregulatory mechanisms maintain GFR at a relatively constant level through afferent arteriolar dilation and efferent arteriolar vasoconstriction (mediated by angiotensin II). Tubuloglomerular feedback mechanisms also maintain GFR and distal tubular nephron flow (see Chapter 37). The GFR declines because of the decrease in glomerular filtration pressure. Failure to restore blood volume or blood pressure and oxygen delivery can cause ischemic cell injury and acute tubular necrosis (ATN) or acute interstitial necrosis, a more severe form of AKI. Reperfusion (reoxygen) injury with cell death also can occur (see Fig. 2.10 also see Chapters 32 and 48). AKI can occur with CKD if a sudden stress is imposed on already poorly functioning kidneys, hastening the progression to ESRD.

TABLE 38.11 Causes of Acute Kidney Injury

Area of Dysfunction	Possible Causes
Prerenal	**Hypovolemia** Hemorrhagic blood loss (trauma, gastrointestinal bleeding, complications of childbirth) Loss of plasma volume (burns, peritonitis) Water and electrolyte losses (severe vomiting or diarrhea, diuretics, uncontrolled diabetes mellitus) Poor oral intake **Reduced Cardiac Output** Systemic hypotension or hypoperfusion Acute myocardial infarction Heart failure Cardiac tamponade Massive pulmonary embolism **Renal Vasomodulation/Shunting (increased vascular resistance)** Iodinated contrast Medications (ACEi, aminoglycosides, ARBs, cyclosporines, NSAIDs) Hypercalcemia Increased intra-abdominal pressure (abdominal compartment syndrome) Anesthesia/Surgery **Systemic Vasodilation** Sepsis (gram negative bacteremia) Shock Systemic inflammation Cirrhosis Analphylaxis Hepatorenal syndrome
Intrarenal (Intrinsic)	**Vascular** Renal artery stenosis Renal vein thrombosis Arterial/venous cross-clamping (postischemic or nephrotoxic) **Microvascular** Vascular damage (malignant hypertension, vasculitis, atheroembolic disease) Thrombotic microangiopathies (Coagulation defects (TTP, HUS, DIC, APS), scleroderma renal crisis, preeclampsia/HELLP syndrome, drug-induced) **Glomerular** Immune-complex diseases (postinfectious glomerulonephritis, endocarditis, lupus nephritis, immunoglobulin A glomerulonephritis, Goodpasture syndrome, Wegener disease) Nephrotic-range proteinuria with associated AKI (HIV-associated nephropathy -secondary FSGS), minimal change disease with ATN/AIN) **Tubulointerstitium** ATN (surgery, ischemia (shock, surgery, hemorrhage), inflammatory (sepsis, burns), nephrotoxicity (contrast media or medications [aminoglycosides, NSAIDs, ACEi, ARBs, and antibiotics]) AIN (tumors, toxins, medications, infection, rhabdomyolysis, massive hemolysis, medications (acyclovir, sulfonamides, protease inhibitors (indinavir, azatanavir), methotrexate, ethylene glycol), myeloma-associated AKI (cast nephropathy) Bilateral acute pyelonephritis
Postrenal	**Bladder Outlet** Benign prostatic hypertrophy Bladder neck obstruction (tumor, stricture, emboli) Neurogenic bladder **Ureteral** (bilateral obstruction) Obstructive uropathy (retroperitoneal fibrosis, malignancy, nephrolithiasis) Ureteral destruction (edema, tumors, nephrolithiasis, emboli, improperly placed catheter) **Renal Pelvis** Papillary necrosis (NSAIDs) nephrolithiasis

Data from Moore PK, Hsu RK, Liu KD. Management of acute kidney injury: Core curriculum 2018. *American Journal of Kidney Disease*, 2018;72(1):136–148. doi:10.1053/j. ajkd.2017.11.021; Gameiro J, Fonseca JA, Outerelo C, et al. Acute kidney injury: From diagnosis to prevention and treatment strategies. *Journal of Clinical Medicine*, 2020;9(6):1704. doi:10.3390/jcm9061704.

ACEi, Angiotensin-converting enzyme inhibitor; *(a)HUS*, (atypical) Hemolytic uremic syndrome; *AIN*, acute interstitial nephritis; *AKI*, acute kidney injury; *APS*, antiphospholipid syndrome; *ARB*, angiotensin-receptor blocker; *ATN*, acute tubular necrosis; *DIC*, disseminated intravascular coagulation; *FSGS*, focal segmental glomerulosclerosis; *HELLP*, hemolysis, elevated liver enzymes, low platelet count) syndrome; *HIV*, human immunodeficiency virus; *NSAID*, nonsteroidal anti-inflammatory drug; *TTP*, thrombotic thrombocytopenic purpura.

Intrarenal (intrinsic) AKI can result from vascular, microvascular, glomerular, and tubulointerstitium causes (see Table 38.11). The most commonly seen cause of intrarenal AKI is ATN. Ischemic ATN most often occurs after surgery but also is associated with prerenal causes such as sepsis, obstetric complications, and severe hemorrhagic trauma or severe burns. Whereas *nephrotoxic ATN* is usually caused by exposure to radiocontrast media or nephrotoxic medications (e.g., aminoglycosides, NSAIDs, ACEi, ARBs, and antibiotics).

Hypotension associated with hypovolemia produces ischemia and the inflammatory response, generating toxic oxygen free radicals that cause cellular swelling, injury, and necrosis. Intrarenal microcirculatory vasoconstriction occurs in response to injury and inflammation and decreases blood flow. Ischemic necrosis results and tends to be patchy and may be distributed along any part of the nephron. Nephrotoxic ATN is associated with radiocontrast media and numerous antibiotics, particularly the aminoglycosides (neomycin, gentamicin, tobramycin) because these drugs accumulate in the renal cortex.[69] Other substances, such as excessive myoglobin (oxygen-transporting substance from muscles; released with crush injuries), carbon tetrachloride, heavy metals (mercury, arsenic), or methoxyflurane anesthetic, and bacterial toxins may promote kidney injury. Dehydration, advanced age, concurrent renal insufficiency, and diabetes mellitus tend to enhance nephrotoxicity. Necrosis caused by nephrotoxins is usually uniform and limited to the proximal tubules. This is due to the high surface area of the brush border (microvilli) of the proximal tubular cells and the reabsorption properties of epithelial cells, which make the proximal tubules more vulnerable to toxic injury.

Postrenal AKI is caused by an obstruction within the urinary tract that affects the kidneys bilaterally (e.g., bladder outlet obstruction, ureteral obstruction, or renal pelvis obstruction) (see Table 38.11). A pattern of several hours of anuria with flank pain followed by polyuria is a characteristic finding. The obstruction causes an increase in intraluminal hydrostatic pressure upstream from the site of obstruction with a gradual decrease in GFR.

Oliguria, or a urine output of <400 mL/24 h, occurs in AKI and can be differentiated from prerenal, intrarenal, and ATN (Table 38.12). Three mechanisms have been proposed to account for the decrease in urine volume in AKI. All three mechanisms contribute to oliguria in varying combinations and degrees throughout the course of the disease (Fig. 38.11). These mechanisms are as follows[70]:

1. *Alterations in renal blood flow.* Efferent arteriolar vasoconstriction may be produced by intrarenal release of angiotensin II or there may be a redistribution of blood flow from the cortex to the medulla. Autoregulation of blood flow may be impaired, resulting in decreased GFR. Microthrombi may obstruct blood flow. Changes in glomerular permeability and decreased GFR also may result from ischemia.
2. *Tubular obstruction.* Necrosis of the tubules causes sloughing of cells, cast formation, and obstruction to urine flow. There can be ischemic edema that results in tubular obstruction, which causes a retrograde increase in hydrostatic pressure, and opposes the hydrostatic pressure of glomerular filtration, thus reducing the GFR. Kidney failure can occur within 24 hours.
3. *Tubular backleak.* Tubular reabsorption of filtrate is accelerated as a result of increased permeability caused by

TABLE 38.12 Differentiation of Acute Oliguric Kidney Failure

	Urine Volume	Urine Specific Gravity	Urine Osmolality	Urine Sodium Concentration	Blood Urea Nitrogen (BUN)/Plasma Creatinine Ratio	FE_{Na}[a]
Normal values	800–2000 mL	1.010–1.030	500–800 mOsm	20 mEq/L	10:1–20:1	1%
Prerenal failure	<400 mL	1.016–1.020	>500 mOsm	<10 mEq/L	>20:1 BUN is elevated relative to plasma creatinine Dehydration or hypoperfusion is suspected	<1% (also seen in acute glomerulonephritis) Sodium is reabsorbed to increase plasma volume
Intrarenal failure (i.e., acute tubular necrosis)	<400 mL	1.010–1.012	<400 mOsm	>30 mEq/L	<10:1 Intrarenal damage causes reduced reabsorption of BUN	>1% (also seen in acute urinary tract obstruction and renal parenchymal disease) Sodium is lost due to tubular damage

[a] $$FE_{Na} = \frac{\text{UrineNa / plasmaNa}}{\text{Urine creatine / plasmacreatinine}} = 100$$

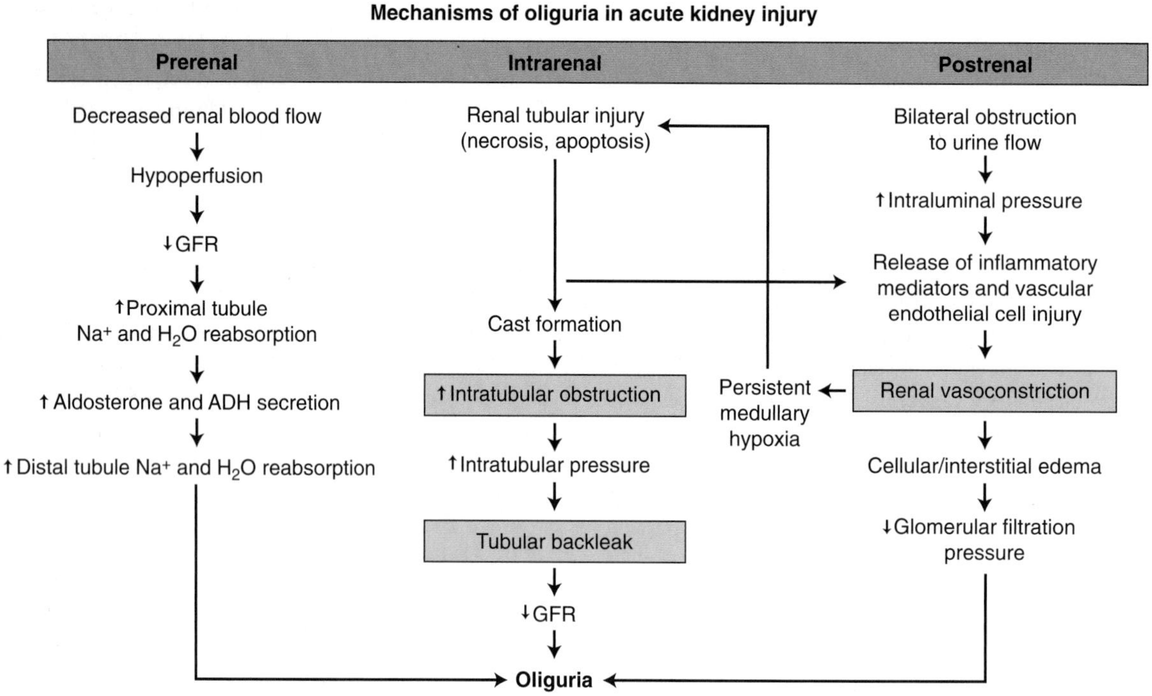

Mechanisms of oliguria in acute kidney injury

Prerenal
Decreased renal blood flow
Hypoperfusion
↓GFR
↑Proximal tubule Na^+ and H_2O reabsorption
↑Aldosterone and ADH secretion
↑Distal tubule Na^+ and H_2O reabsorption

Intrarenal
Renal tubular injury (necrosis, apoptosis)
Cast formation
↑Intratubular obstruction
↑Intratubular pressure
Tubular backleak
↓GFR

Persistent medullary hypoxia

Postrenal
Bilateral obstruction to urine flow
↑Intraluminal pressure
Release of inflammatory mediators and vascular endothelial cell injury
Renal vasoconstriction
Cellular/interstitial edema
↓Glomerular filtration pressure

Oliguria

Fig. 38.11 Acute Kidney Injury and Mechanisms of Oliguria. *ADH,* Antidiuretic hormone; *GFR,* glomerular filtration rate.

ischemia and increased tubular pressure from obstruction. The increased reabsorption of filtrate contributes to oliguria.

Oliguria begins within 1 day after a hypotensive event and lasts 1 to 3 weeks, but may regress in several hours or extend for several weeks depending on the duration of ischemia or the severity of injury or obstruction.

AKI also can present with **nonoliguric kidney failure (high output kidney failure)** and represents less severe injury, particularly with intrinsic kidney injury associated with nephrotoxins. The renal tubules have impaired reabsorption and concentration and dilution function. The urine output may be normal or high in volume, but the BUN and plasma creatinine concentrations increase. **Anuria** (urine output <50 mL/day) can occur in AKI but is uncommon in ATN. It involves both kidneys and suggests bilateral renal artery occlusion, obstructive uropathy, or acute cortical necrosis.

Clinical Manifestations. The clinical progression of AKI due to ATN, the most common cause of AKI, occurs in four overlapping phases: initiation, extension, maintenance, and recovery.[71] Each phase is described as follows:

1. The *initiation phase* occurs with the onset of renal hypoperfusion or toxicity resulting in severe cellular ATP depletion leading to acute cell injury and dysfunction (renal tubular epithelial cell injury is a key feature). Prevention of injury is possible during this phase and the next phase with therapeutic interventions, but there is a short window of opportunity.
2. The *extension phase* is initiated by continued hypoxia following the initial ischemic event and an inflammatory response. Cells continue to undergo injury and death with necrosis and apoptosis present in the outer medulla. However, in the outer cortex, where blood flow has returned to near normal levels, the proximal tubule cells undergo cellular repair during this phase.
3. The *maintenance* or *oliguric phase* is the period of established kidney injury and dysfunction after the initiating event has been resolved. Cells undergo repair, migration, apoptosis, and proliferation, which may last from weeks to months with urine output lowest during this phase. During this phase, SCr, BUN, and serum potassium levels increase; metabolic acidosis develops; there is salt and water overload; and urine output is decreased with oliguria.
4. The *recovery* or *polyuria phase* is the interval when glomerular function returns but the regenerating tubules cannot yet concentrate the filtrate. Diuresis is common during this phase, with a decline in SCr and urea concentrations and an increase in creatinine clearance. Cellular differentiation continues, epithelial polarity is reestablished, and homeostasis is established. As renal function improves, the increase in urine volume (diuresis) is progressive. The tubules are still damaged early in the recovery phase and have not recovered secretion and reabsorption functions. Polyuria can result in excessive loss of sodium, potassium, and water. Fluid and electrolyte balance must be carefully monitored, and excessive losses replaced. Serial measurements of SCr concentration provide an index of renal function during the *recovery phase.* Return to normal status may take 3 to 12 months; some individuals do not gain full recovery of a normal GFR or tubular function, and plasma creatinine concentration will remain higher than normal.

The hallmark features of AKI are increased SCr, reduced GFR, and decreased urine output. In the presence of fever, rash, joint pains, pulmonary infiltrates, abnormal urine analysis, thrombocytopenia, and hemolytic anemia, less common causes (e.g., glomerulopathy, vasculitis, and hemolytic uremic syndrome) of AKI should be considered.[67] Other manifestations of altered urine excretion include hyperkalemia, hyperphosphatemia, and metabolic acidosis. Edema and congestive heart failure can be associated with fluid retention.

A diagnostic challenge is to differentiate prerenal AKI from ATN. Urine composition may provide helpful diagnostic clues to changes in tubular function (Table 38.13). The ratios of BUN to plasma creatinine concentration and fractional excretion of sodium (the ratio of filtered sodium to excreted sodium) are helpful diagnostic indicators because the tests reflect renal tubular reabsorption ability. In prerenal AKI, tubular function is maintained, and salt, water, and urea are reabsorbed. With ATN, reabsorption and urinary concentration abilities are compromised. Other causes of renal failure also may exhibit similar clinical findings. Cystatin C, a serum protein constantly produced by nucleated cells, is freely filtered by the glomerulus, and its concentration can serve as a measure of GFR and may be useful for detecting early changes in GFR. Serial measurements of plasma creatinine concentration provide an index of renal function during the recovery phase. However, changes in SCr level occur only if more than 50% of glomerular filtration is lost. The SCr level may not reflect this decrease in glomerular filtration for 24 hours or more. Such diagnostic delays make the implementation of early therapy very difficult, contributing to disease progression and mortality.

Evaluation and Treatment. Prevention of AKI is the most important therapeutic approach and involves avoidance of hypotension, hypovolemia, and nephrotoxicity. However, once AKI has occurred, determination of the etiology of AKI is essential for appropriate management. There are recent developments in ways to assess, monitor, and evaluate AKI progression before the SCr increases. One advancement is the emergence of biomarker testing to aid in the risk assessment for moderate or severe AKI (see Emerging Science Box: Biomarkers for AKI Risk Stratification).[72] Other newer developments related to monitoring and evaluating risk progression include e-alert systems, machine-learning algorithms and artificial intelligence for AKI recognition and monitoring, as well as models based upon the renal angina index, and furosemide stress test (FST).[73]

The diagnosis of AKI is related to the cause of the disease. Therefore, a complete history must be obtained and include medications (prescribed and over the counter); recent exposure to nephrotoxic agents; recent surgery, trauma, or infection; and past medical history of cardiovascular disorders, obstructive uropathies (e.g., an enlarged prostate or kidney stones), or AKI (see Table 38.13).

Laboratory evaluation should include SCr, serum urea, electrolytes, complete blood count, liver function tests, glucose level, bone profile, urine analysis, and urine microscopic examination.[67] Other laboratory testing can provide information related to the cause such as an assessment of antineutrophil cytoplasmic antibodies (ANCA), antiglomerular basement membrane antibodies (anti-GBM), antinuclear antibodies (ANA), anti-double-stranded DNA (anti-dsDNA) antibodies, complement factors, rheumatoid factor, antistreptolysin O titer (ASOT), cryoglobulins, serum electrophoresis, immunoglobulins, serum free light chains, hepatitis, and HIV serology.[67] Diagnostic imaging should include a renal ultrasound, to exclude obstruction, and chest x-ray to determine a potential cause, such as pneumonia or vasculitis, and to evaluate volume status.[67]

Management principles directly related to physiologic alterations generally include the following[69,73]:

1. ensuring adequate hydration and volume status;
2. correcting electrolyte disturbances, particularly hyperkalemia;

TABLE 38.13 Differentiating Prerenal Acute Kidney Injury from Acute Tubular Necrosis

Prerenal	Acute Tubular Necrosis
Causes	
Hypovolemia	IV radiocontrast
Hypotension	Nephrotoxic medications
Hypoperfusion	Trauma
Clinical Manifestations	
Oliguria	Nonoliguria
Urine fractional excretion of sodium <1%	Urine fractional excretion of sodium >2%
Urine sodium concentration <20 mEq/L	Urine sodium concentration >40 mEq/L
Normal urine sediment	Urine sediment muddy-brown with granular casts, epithelial cell casts, free renal tubular epithelial cells
Response to Effective Fluid Resuscitation	
Timing of serum creatinine response to effective intravenous fluid resuscitation differentiates prerenal acute kidney injury from acute tubular necrosis.	
Responds within 48 h	Response takes at least 72 h

EMERGING SCIENCE BOX

Biomarkers for Acute Kidney Injury Risk Stratification

A novel approach to detecting acute kidney injury (AKI) early is using biomarkers. Most biomarkers are expressed prior to the rise in serum creatinine and are more sensitive and specific than urine output. Currently, biomarkers being investigated are cystatin C, chitinase-3-like protein-1 (UCHI3L1), neutrophil gelatinase-associated lipocalin (NGAL), interleukin-18 (IL-18), kidney injury molecule-1 (KIM-1), and interferon-gamma-inducible protein 10 (IP-10/CXCL-10). The biomarker with the highest sensitivity (92%) and specificity (100%) was IL-18. Second generation AKI biomarkers have obtained regulatory approval and are currently being studied in clinical trials. These markers include tissue inhibitor of metalloproteinases-2 (TIMP-2) and insulin-like growth factor-binding protein 7 (IGFBP7). Higher levels of these markers are associated with adverse outcomes.

Data from Pedroso LA, et al. Acute kidney injury biomarkers in the critically ill. *Clinica Chimica Acta,* 2020;508:170–178. doi:10.1016/j.cca.2020.05.024; Srisawat N, et al. The role of biomarkers in acute kidney injury. *Critical Care Clinics,* 2020;36(1):125–140. doi:10.1016/j.ccc.2019.08.010.

3. managing hemodynamics, including blood pressure;
4. preventing and treating infections;
5. avoiding nephrotoxic agents and drugs;
6. maintaining adequate nutrition; and
7. glucose control.

Fluid and electrolyte replacement must be carefully calculated with consideration of urine losses, insensible losses (up to 1000 mL/day), and production of endogenous water by oxidation (450 mL/day). Overhydration of individuals dilutes plasma sodium concentration and can precipitate pulmonary, cerebral, myocardial, and liver edema. A positive fluid balance is independently associated with increased mortality in individuals with AKI and contributes to worse outcomes in critically ill persons.[67] Metabolic acidosis is treated when serum bicarbonate concentration is less than 22 mEq/L.

Hyperkalemia can be managed by restricting dietary sources of potassium, using loop diuretics, and using cation exchange resins, which may be administered orally or rectally. These resins exchange potassium for another cation, such as sodium in the bowel, and the potassium is then excreted attached to the resin.[69] With severe hyperkalemia (more than 6.5 mEq/L), dialysis may be required, or potassium can be temporarily driven back into the cells by administering insulin (followed by glucose to prevent hypoglycemia), or by infusing sodium bicarbonate or administering albuterol. Insulin administered with glucose facilitates the uptake of glucose into the cell, which results in potassium shifting from the extracellular environment to the intracellular fluid. (Glucose metabolism is discussed in (see Chapters 1 and 22). Using sodium bicarbonate to cause alkalemia also shifts potassium into cells in exchange for hydrogen ions but requires consideration of hypervolemia. Careful monitoring of the electrocardiogram for peaking T waves is essential for individuals with hyperkalemia. Intravenous infusion of calcium is the most rapid method of treating cardiac effects of hyperkalemia. Calcium decreases the threshold potential and reduces the membrane excitability caused by hyperkalemia (see Chapter 3). Calcium should be used only in emergencies, however, because hypercalcemia also may cause cardiac arrest.

Azotemia is generally controlled and nutrition maintained with a low-protein, high-carbohydrate diet. Essential amino acid replacement can be given orally or parenterally. Adequate carbohydrate intake slows protein catabolism and helps prevent release of potassium from cellular breakdown. Because sepsis is a common serious and potentially fatal complication of renal failure, observation for signs of infection and early treatment with antibiotics are necessary. Drug dosage levels may require adjustment if they are metabolized or excreted by the kidneys. Recovery may take up to 1 year.

Continuous renal replacement therapy (CRRT) (mechanical removal of water, electrolytes, and toxins from the blood) is indicated for uncontrollable hyperkalemia, acidosis, or severe fluid overload. CRRT is particularly promising in critically ill individuals with multiple organ dysfunction or sepsis. According to the KDIGO guideline, CRRT is a complementary therapy in the treatment of AKI.[69] The timing and optimal dose-response relationships for CRRT are individually determined with consideration to hemodynamic status, degree of volume overload, bleeding risk, and the treating facility's availability/experience.[74]

CHRONIC KIDNEY DISEASE

CKD is the progressive and irreversible loss of renal function indicated by a decline in GFR to below 60 mL/min/1.73 m^2 for 3 months or more with implications for health. CKD is associated with systemic diseases, such as diabetes mellitus (most significant risk factor), hypertension, and systemic lupus erythematosus. CKD also is associated with intrinsic kidney diseases, such as AKI, chronic glomerulonephritis, chronic pyelonephritis, obstructive uropathies, or vascular disorders (Table 38.14).

Pathophysiology. The progression phase of the disease is characterized by a persistent state of inflammation and hypoxia and oxidative stress that contribute to the development of renal fibrosis.[75] The kidneys have a remarkable ability to adapt to the loss of nephron mass. Symptomatic changes result from increased plasma levels of creatinine, urea, and potassium. Alterations in salt and water balance usually do not become apparent until renal function declines to less than 25% of normal when adaptive renal reserves have been exhausted.[76]

TABLE 38.14 Stages of Chronic Kidney Disease

Stage	Description	Signs/Symptoms
I	Normal kidney function Normal or high GFR (>90 mL/min)	Usually none Hypertension common
II	Mild kidney damage, mild reduction in GFR (60–89 mL/min)	Subtle Hypertension Increasing creatinine and urea levels
III	Moderate kidney damage GFR 30–59 mL/min	Mild As above
IV	Severe kidney damage GFR 15–29 mL/min	Moderate As above Erythropoietin deficiency anemia Hyperphosphatemia Increased triglycerides Metabolic acidosis Hyperkalemia Salt/water retention
V	End-stage kidney disease Established kidney failure GFR <15 mL/min	Severe As above

GFR, Glomerular filtration rate.

Different theories have been proposed to account for the adaptation to the loss of renal function. The *intact nephron hypothesis* proposes that loss of nephron mass with progressive kidney damage causes the surviving nephrons to increase their capacity to maintain solute and water regulation. These nephrons are capable of a compensatory hypertrophy and expansion or hyperfunction in their rates of filtration, reabsorption, and secretion. Although the urine of an individual with CKD may contain abnormal amounts of protein and red and white blood cells or casts, the major end products of excretion are similar to those of normally functioning kidneys until the advanced stages of renal failure when there is a significant reduction of functioning nephrons.

The *particular location of kidney damage* influences loss of kidney function. For example, tubular interstitial diseases damage primarily the tubular or medullary parts of the nephron, producing problems such as renal tubular acidosis, salt wasting, and difficulty diluting or concentrating the urine. Proteinuria, hematuria, and nephrotic syndrome are more prominent when the damage is primarily vascular or glomerular. With severe or repeated injury, interstitial capillary loss, and fibroblast proliferation result in progressive glomerulosclerosis and tubulointerstitial fibrosis. These conditions contribute to CKD and ESRD. A summary of factors involved in the progression of CKD is outlined in Table 38.15 and Fig. 38.12.

The factors that contribute to the pathogenesis of CKD are complex and involve the interaction of many cells, cytokines, and structural alterations. Two factors that have consistently been recognized to advance renal disease are proteinuria and angiotensin II activity. Glomerular hyperfiltration, increased glomerular capillary permeability, and loss of negative charge may lead to proteinuria. *Proteinuria* contributes to tubulointerstitial injury by accumulating in the interstitial space of the nephron tubules. There is activation of complement proteins and other mediators and cells, such as macrophages, that promote inflammation and progressive fibrosis. *Angiotensin II* (from activation of the renin-angiotensin-aldosterone system [RAAS]) causes efferent arteriolar vasoconstriction that

TABLE 38.15 Factors Representing Progression of Chronic Kidney Failure

Factor	Characteristics
Proteinuria	Glomerular hyperfiltration of protein contributes to tubular interstitial injury by accumulating in interstitial space and promoting inflammation and progressive fibrosis.
Creatinine and urea clearance	In chronic renal failure, the GFR falls and the plasma creatinine concentration increases by a reciprocal amount; because there is no regulatory adjustment for creatinine, plasma levels continue to rise and serve as an index of changing glomerular function. As GFR declines, urea clearance increases. (Note: Urea is both filtered and reabsorbed and varies with state of hydration.)
Sodium and water balance	In chronic renal failure, sodium load delivered to nephrons exceeds normal, so excretion must increase; thus less is reabsorbed. Obligatory loss occurs, leading to sodium deficits and volume depletion. As GFR is reduced, ability to concentrate and dilute urine diminishes.
Phosphate, calcium and magnesium balance	Changes in acid-base balance affect phosphate and calcium balance. Major disorders associated with chronic renal failure are reduced renal phosphate excretion, decreased renal synthesis of 1,25-dihydroxy-vitamin D_3, and hypocalcemia. Hypocalcemia leads to secondary hyperparathyroidism, GFR falls, and progressive hyperphosphatemia, hypocalcemia, and dissolution of bone result. Hypermagnesemia tends to develop with impaired fractional excretion of magnesium in relation to declining GFR. Hypomagnesemia may develop associated with decreased intestinal absorption, alterations in parathyroid hormone and effects of medication.
Hematocrit	Because of anemia that accompanies chronic renal failure, lethargy, dizziness, and low hematocrit are common.
Potassium balance	In chronic renal failure, tubular secretion of potassium increases until oliguria develops. Use of potassium-sparing diuretics also may precipitate elevated serum potassium levels. As disease progresses, total body potassium levels can rise to life-threatening levels and dialysis is required.
Acid-base balance	In early renal insufficiency, acid excretion and bicarbonate reabsorption are increased to maintain normal pH. Metabolic acidosis begins when GFR reaches 30%–40%. Metabolic acidosis and hyperkalemia may be severe enough to require dialysis when end-stage renal failure develops.
Dyslipidemia	Chronic hyperlipidemia may induce glomerular and tubulointerstitial injury, contributing to progression of chronic renal disease.

GFR, glomerular filtration rate.

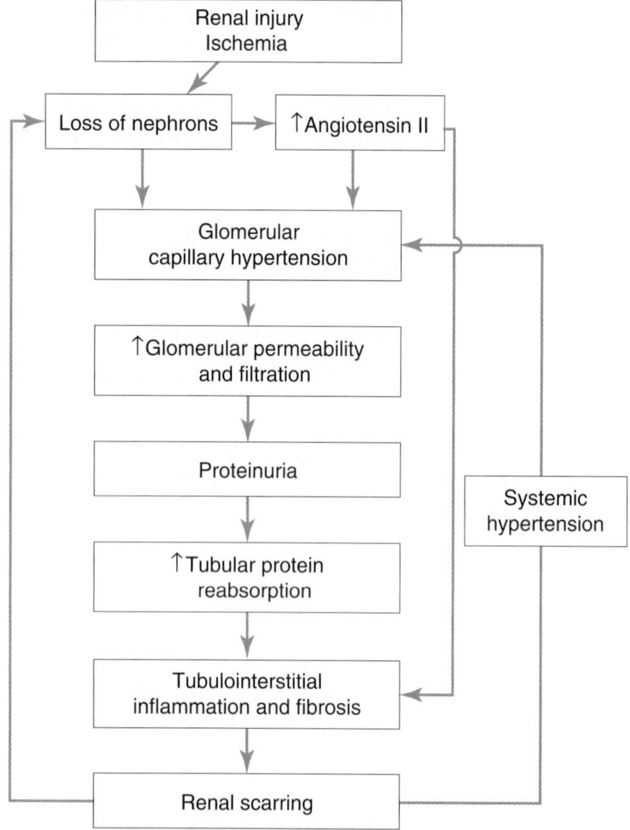

Fig. 38.12 Mechanisms Related to the Progression of Chronic Kidney Disease.

promotes glomerular hypertension, systemic hypertension, and hyperfiltration. Hyperfiltration is also associated with hyperglycemia and diabetic nephropathy. The chronically high intraglomerular pressure increases glomerular capillary permeability, contributing to proteinuria. Angiotensin II promotes the activity of inflammatory cells and growth factors that participate in tubulointerstitial fibrosis and scarring.[3]

The progression of AKI to CKD is related to incomplete or maladaptive tissue repair, setting in motion processes promoting the development of interstitial fibrosis.[77] CKD and progressive renal dysfunction are also characterized by an amplification of oxidative stress.[78] Oxidative stress accompanied by inflammation (in which the cells of the innate immune response system are mainly involved) has a significant role in the pathogenesis of CKD.[78] The effect of reactive oxidative stress (ROS) disrupts the excretory function of each section of the nephron, preventing the maintenance of intra-systemic homeostasis and leading to the accumulation of metabolic products.[78] Renal regulatory mechanisms, such as tubular glomerular feedback and the RAAS, are also affected, making it impossible for the kidney to compensate for water–electrolyte and acid-base disturbances. Without appropriate compensatory mechanisms, there is further intensification of oxidative stress resulting in the progression of CKD and a spectrum of complications such as malnutrition, calcium phosphate abnormalities, atherosclerosis, and anemia.[78] Hypertension can be used as an example. Oxidative stress in the kidney and vascular tissue causes hypertension, and hypertension promotes oxidative stress. Now add in the inflammation component. Chronic inflammation is a significant contributor to the promotion of oxidative stress.[78] Therefore, oxidative stress, along with inflammation, is a critical component of CKD-related pathologies that can adversely affect the human body (e.g., diabetes mellitus, hypertension).[78]

Clinical Manifestations. The clinical manifestations of CKD are often described using the terms *azotemia* and *uremia.* **Azotemia** is manifested by increased levels of serum urea, SCr, and other nitrogenous compounds related to decreasing kidney function. **Uremia** is the accumulation of urea and other nitrogenous compounds and toxins. Sources of toxins include the accumulation of end products of protein metabolism, alterations in fluid and electrolytes, metabolic acidosis, intestinal absorption of toxins produced by gut bacteria, and results of altered renal hormone synthesis (e.g., anemia, hyperphosphatemia, and hypocalcemia). The accumulation of toxins has systemic effects known as **uremic syndrome**.[79] The manifestations involve almost every organ system and include hypertension; anorexia; nausea; vomiting; diarrhea or constipation; malnutrition and weight loss; pruritus; edema; anemia; clotting disorders; neurologic, cardiovascular, and endocrine disease; and skin and skeletal changes. The manifestations are summarized in Table 38.16 and Fig. 38.13. Details of the systemic manifestations associated with CKD are discussed in the following sections.

Creatinine, Cystatin C, and Urea Clearance

Creatinine is constantly released from muscle and excreted primarily by glomerular filtration. In CKD, as GFR declines, the SCr level increases by a reciprocal amount to maintain a constant rate of excretion (Fig. 38.14). With continuing decline in GFR, the plasma creatinine concentration increases. Measures of SCr can serve as an index of changing glomerular function. However, SCr as an estimate of GFR is limited when there is reduced muscle mass or fluid overload. Equations including cystatin C or combined with SCr provide a better index. The clearance of *urea* follows a similar pattern, but urea is both filtered and reabsorbed. The measured urea level varies with the state of hydration; therefore, urea concentration is not a good index of GFR. However, as the GFR decreases, plasma urea concentration increase.

Fluid and Electrolyte Balance

Fluid and electrolyte and acid-base balances are significantly disturbed with CKD.[80] A summary of electrolyte and acid-base balance alterations is presented in Table 38.17.

Levels of *sodium* must be regulated within narrow limits because sodium is the major extracellular solute. In CKD, sodium and water balance is maintained very close to normal until the development of stage V ESRD (see Table 38.14). This occurs because of the increased fractional excretion of sodium, particularly in the distal nephron, in relation to decreasing GFR. Hormones including aldosterone, prostaglandins, and natriuretic peptides also modulate sodium excretion, and their levels are elevated with progressive kidney disease. Individual variation in the underlying pathology of

TABLE 38.16 Systemic Effects of Chronic Kidney Disease and Uremia

System	Manifestations	Mechanisms	Treatment
Skeletal	Spontaneous fractures and bone pain Deformities of long bones	Chronic kidney disease—mineral bone disorder: bone inflammation with fibrous degeneration related to hyperparathyroidism; bone resorption associated with vitamin D and calcium deficiency	Control of hyperphosphatemia to reduce hyperparathyroidism; administration of calcium and aluminum hydroxide antacids, which bind phosphate in the gut, together with a phosphate-restricted diet; vitamin D replacement; avoidance of magnesium antacids because of impaired magnesium excretion
Cardiopulmonary	Pulmonary edema, Kussmaul respirations	Fluid overload associated with pulmonary edema and metabolic acidosis leading to Kussmaul respirations	Angiotensin-converting enzyme (ACE) inhibitors; combination of propranolol, hydralazine, and minoxidil for those with high levels of renin; bilateral nephrectomy with dialysis or transplantation
Cardiovascular	Left ventricular hypertrophy, cardiomyopathy, and ischemic heart disease; hypertension, dysrhythmias, accelerated atherosclerosis; pericarditis with fever, chest pain, and pericardial friction rub	Extracellular volume expansion and hypersecretion of renin associated with hypertension; anemia increases cardiac workload; hyperlipidemia promotes atherosclerosis; toxins precipitate into pericardium	Volume reduction with diuretics that are not potassium sparing (to avoid hyperkalemia); lipid-lowering drugs; blood pressure–lowering strategies; dialysis
Neurologic	Encephalopathy (fatigue, loss of attention, difficulty with problem solving); peripheral neuropathy (pain and burning in the legs and feet, loss of vibration sense and deep tendon reflexes); loss of motor coordination, twitching, fasciculations, stupor, and coma with advanced uremia	Progressive accumulation of uremic toxins associated with end-stage renal disease Stroke or intracerebral hemorrhage associated with chronic dialysis	Dialysis or successful kidney transplantation
Endocrine	Restricted growth in children Higher incidence of goiter Osteomalacia	Elevated parathyroid hormone levels Decreased thyroid hormone	Endogenous recombinant human growth hormone; thyroid hormone replacement Same as skeletal above
Hematologic	Anemia, usually normochromic normocytic; platelet disorders with prolonged bleeding times	Reduced erythropoietin secretion and reduced red cell production; uremic toxins shorten red blood cell survival and alter platelet function	Dialysis; recombinant human erythropoietin (controversial) and iron supplementation; conjugated estrogens; DDAVP (1-deamino-[8-c-arginine] vasopressin); transfusion
Gastrointestinal	Anorexia, nausea, vomiting; mouth ulcers, stomatitis, urinous breath (uremic factor), hiccups, peptic ulcers, gastrointestinal bleeding, and pancreatitis associated with end-stage renal failure	Retention of metabolic acids and other metabolic waste products	Protein-restricted diet for relief of nausea and vomiting; Na^+-based alkali or alkali-inducing food
Integumentary	Abnormal pigmentation and pruritus	Retention of urochromes, contributing to sallow, yellow color; high plasma calcium levels and neuropathy associated with pruritus	Dialysis with control of serum calcium and phosphate levels
Immunologic	Increased risk of infection that can cause death; increased risk of carcinoma	Suppression of cell-mediated immunity; reduction in number and function of lymphocytes, diminished phagocytosis	Routine dialysis
Reproductive	Sexual dysfunction: menorrhagia, amenorrhea, infertility, and decreased libido in women; decreased testosterone levels, infertility, and decreased libido in men	Dysfunction of ovaries and testes; presence of neuropathies	No specific treatment

Data from Almeras C, Argilés A. The general picture of uremia. *Seminars in Dialysis*, 2009;22(4):329–333; Keane WF. The role of lipids in renal disease: Future challenges. *Kidney International Supplement*, 75:S27–S31, 2000; Thomas R, Kanso A, Sedor JR. Chronic kidney disease and its complications. *Primary Care*, 2008;35(2):329–344.

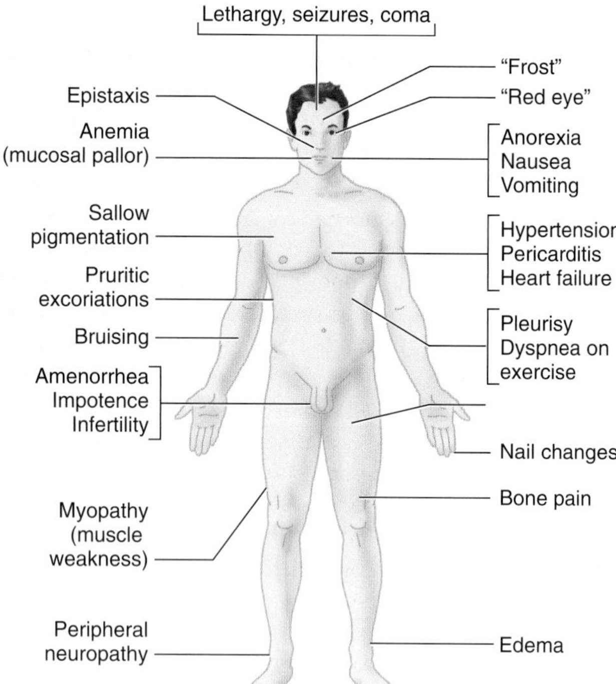

Fig. 38.13 Common Signs and Symptoms of Kidney Dysfunction. (From Goldman L, Schafer AI. *Goldman-Cecil medicine,* 25th edition. Philadelphia: Saunders; 2016; redrawn from Forbes CD, Jackson WF. *Color atlas and text of clinical medicine,* 3rd edition. London: Mosby; 2003.)

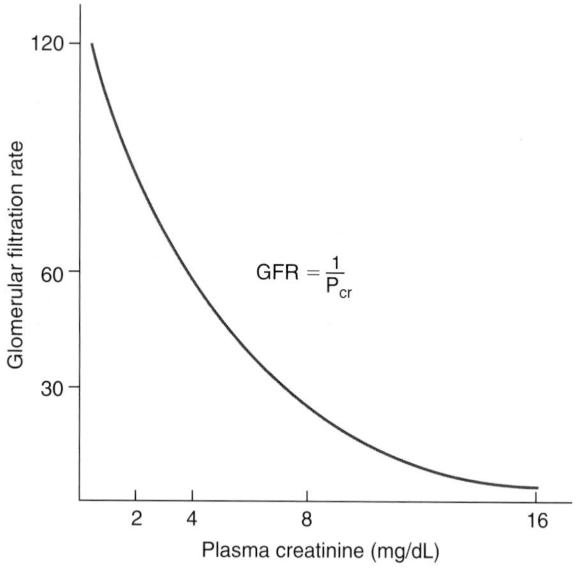

Fig. 38.14 Plasma Creatinine (P_{cr}) and Glomerular Filtration Rate (GFR).

CKD must be considered in the management of sodium intake or restriction. Sodium wasting may be present with tubulointerstitial causes of CKD, and there may also be extra renal losses of sodium from vomiting, diarrhea, or fever. Sodium retention is more likely in ESRD particularly in the presence of nephrotic syndrome or heart failure. Sodium retention contributes to hypertension, edema, heart failure, and mortality. Interdialytic water intake can cause volume overload and dilutional hyponatremia prior to dialysis. Management of salt and water balance requires individual assessment, and both hyponatremia and hypernatremia require management.[81,82]

The regulation of *water balance* and osmolality is normally achieved by urinary concentration mediated by antidiuretic hormone (ADH). As GFR is reduced, the ability to concentrate and dilute the urine diminishes. In earlier stages of renal disease, this may be caused by osmotic diuresis produced by increased fractional excretion of solutes by the remaining functioning nephrons or by a decreased tubular response to ADH. Individual nephrons can maintain water balance until severe renal failure occurs and GFR declines to 15% to 20% of normal with extensive loss of nephron and tubular function. At this stage, the urinary concentration

TABLE 38.17 Electrolyte and Acid-Base Alterations of Chronic Kidney Disease

Factor	Characteristics
Sodium and water balance	In chronic renal failure, sodium load delivered to nephrons exceeds normal, so excretion must increase; thus less is reabsorbed. Obligatory loss occurs, leading to sodium deficits and volume depletion. As GFR is reduced, ability to concentrate and dilute urine diminishes.
Phosphate, calcium and magnesium balance	Changes in acid-base balance affect phosphate and calcium balance. The major disorders associated with chronic renal failure are reduced renal phosphate excretion, decreased renal synthesis of 1,25-$(OH)_2$-vitamin D_3 (calcitriol), and hypocalcemia. Hypocalcemia leads to secondary hyperparathyroidism, GFR falls, and progressive hyperphosphatemia, hypocalcemia, and dissolution of bone result. Serum magnesium levels are elevated in late stages of renal failure related to loss of renal excretion.
Potassium balance	In chronic renal failure, tubular secretion of potassium increases until oliguria develops. Use of potassium-sparing diuretics also may precipitate elevated serum potassium levels. As disease progresses, total body potassium levels can rise to life-threatening levels and dialysis is required.
Acid-base balance	In early renal insufficiency, acid excretion and bicarbonate reabsorption are increased to maintain normal pH.
	Metabolic acidosis begins to develop when GFR decreases to 30%–40% of normal. When end-stage renal failure develops, the metabolic acidosis may be severe enough to require dialysis.

GFR, Glomerular filtration rate.

becomes fixed and approaches that of the plasma at 285 mOsm/L with a specific gravity of about 1.010.

Urinary excretion of *potassium* is related primarily to distal tubular secretion mediated by aldosterone and sodium-potassium adenosine triphosphatase (see Chapter 3). In renal failure, there is increased tubular secretion that provides effective regulation until the onset of oliguria. With hyperkalemia, larger amounts of potassium can be eliminated through the bowel.[83] Although nonoliguric patients can maintain potassium excretion with normal dietary intake, they are more prone to develop hyperkalemia with increased loading (i.e., use of salt substitutes). Use of potassium-sparing diuretics, such as spironolactone (aldactone), volume depletion, acute infection, severe acidosis, or marked hyperglycemia also may precipitate elevated levels of serum potassium. With progression of disease to ESRD, total body potassium can increase to life-threatening levels and must be controlled by dietary restriction, loop diuretics, cation exchange resins, and dialysis. Sodium polystyrene sulfonate (a nonspecific sodium-cation exchange resin in the colon), patiromer sorbitex calcium (exchanges calcium for potassium in the colon), and sodium zirconium cyclosilicate (traps potassium in the colon) are effective in managing hyperkalemia.[84] Hyperkalemia also can be a side effect of ACE inhibitors or angiotensin receptor blockers (ARB) often used to prevent diabetic nephropathy. Severe acute hyperkalemia is treated with intravenous 10% calcium gluconate or 10% calcium chloride, intravenous dextrose, and insulin, and nebulized or intravenous salbutamol (sympathetic beta$_2$ agonist, promotes Na^+-K^+-ATPase pump and intracellular movement of potassium). Renal replacement therapy may be required to manage hyperkalemia (support of renal function using hemodialysis or peritoneal dialysis).

The intake of a normal diet produces 50 to 100 mEq of hydrogen per day. These ions are secreted from the renal tubules and excreted in the urine combined with phosphate and ammonia buffers (buffering is described in Chapter 3). *Metabolic acidosis* (Chapter 3) develops when the GFR decreases to less than 20% to 25% of normal. The causes of acidosis are primarily related to decreased hydrogen ion elimination and decreased bicarbonate reabsorption. With ESRD, metabolic acidosis may be severe enough to require alkali therapy and dialysis.[85]

Calcium, Phosphate, Magnesium, and Bone

Bone and skeletal changes develop with alterations in calcium, phosphate, magnesium, and vitamin D metabolism (Table 38.18).[86] These changes begin when the GFR decreases to 25% or less. *Hypocalcemia* is accelerated by impaired renal synthesis of 1,25-dihydroxy-vitamin D_3 (calcitriol) with decreased intestinal absorption of calcium. Renal phosphate excretion also decreases, and the increased serum phosphate binds calcium, further contributing to hypocalcemia. Acidosis also contributes to a negative calcium balance. Decreased serum calcium level stimulates parathyroid hormone secretion with mobilization of calcium from bone. The combined effect of *secondary hyperparathyroidism* and *vitamin D deficiency* can result in renal osteodystrophies (i.e., *osteomalacia* and *osteitis fibrosa* with increased risk for fractures) (see Chapter 44) and vascular calcification, including coronary artery calcification. Fractional excretion of magnesium increases as compensation for the decline in GFR with the progression of CKD. With ESRD, fractional excretion of magnesium is inadequate and serum magnesium levels must be monitored considering dietary intake, intestinal absorption, alterations in parathyroid hormone, and effects of different medications. Generally, there is a tendency to develop hypermagnesemia. However, hypomagnesemia can develop in some cases and requires modification of the dialysate magnesium concentration.[87] Hypomagnesemia has been associated with osteoporosis in postmenopausal women,[88] but the effects on bone in ESRD are not clearly known.

Protein, Carbohydrate, and Fat Metabolism

Protein, carbohydrate, and fat metabolism are altered in CKD. *Proteinuria*, metabolic acidosis, inflammation, and a catabolic state contribute to a negative nitrogen balance. Levels of serum proteins diminish, including albumin, complement, and transferrin, and there is loss of muscle mass. The amount of proteinuria is also related to the extent of renal injury and predicts disease progression. Proteinuria may independently cause renal damage by promoting tubular inflammation and fibrosis from particular protein-bound fatty acids.[89] Monitoring of proteinuria using the urine albumin-to-creatinine ratio can assist in staging CKD.[90]

TABLE 38.18 Calcium, Phosphate, and Magnesium Metabolism in Chronic Kidney Disease

Kidney	Plasma	Bone
Decreased renal production of vitamin D_3	Decreased calcium absorption from gut Decreased ionized calcium Increased PTH secretion (secondary hyperparathyroidism)	Decreased calcium deposition
Decreased phosphate excretion	Elevated phosphate Formation of $CaHPO_4$	Release of calcium and phosphate Osteitis fibrosa, osteomalacia, calcium deposits in soft tissue and vascular calcification (occurs when kidney fails to respond to PTH secretion because of loss of renal mass and calcium and phosphate continues to be absorbed from bone)
Decreased magnesium excretion	Elevated magnesium in late-stage disease	Effect on bone not clearly known

$CaHPO_4$, Calcium hydrogen phosphate; *PTH*, parathyroid hormone.

Insulin resistance and glucose intolerance are common and may be related to proinflammatory cytokines and alterations in adipokines (high leptin and low adiponectin levels) that interfere with insulin action. In both nondiabetic and diabetic persons with CKD, oxidative stress can contribute to renal tubular and vascular injury as antioxidant systems become inadequate.[91]

Dyslipidemia is common among individuals with CKD. There is a high ratio of low-density lipoprotein (LDL) to high-density lipoprotein (HDL), a high level of triglycerides, and an accumulation of LDL particles with accelerated atherosclerosis and vascular calcification. Uremia causes a deficiency in lipoprotein lipase and a decreased level of hepatic triglyceride lipase. Decreased lipolytic activity results in a reduction and protection effects of the HDL level. Apolipoprotein concentration also is elevated, thereby accelerating atherogenesis.[92]

Hematologic System

Hematologic alterations include *normochromic-normocytic anemia, impaired platelet function*, and *hypercoagulability*. Inadequate production of erythropoietin decreases red blood cell production and causes anemia. Chronic inflammation, iron deficiency, and decreased half-life of erythrocytes are also contributing factors. Anemia contributes to decreased tissue oxygenation and to progression of kidney disease. Low serum levels of hemoglobin and symptoms of anemia, such as lethargy, weakness, and dizziness, are common findings. Treatment of anemia includes infusion of erythropoiesis stimulating agents (ESAs) (i.e., recombinant human erythropoietin), and intravenous iron. Hypoxia-inducible factor-prolyl hydroxylase inhibitors, oral agents that stimulate endogenous erythropoietin production and enhance iron availability, are in clinical trials and may replace ESAs.[93]

Disorders of hemostasis in CKD are primarily related to defective platelet aggregation, impaired adhesion of platelets to the vascular endothelium, and alterations in coagulation factors and in the fibrinolytic pathway. The consequence is either (1) an increased bleeding tendency (more common with later stages of CKD) manifested by bruising, epistaxis and other mucosal bleeding, gastrointestinal bleeding, and cerebrovascular hemorrhage or (2) excessive formation of thrombi (e.g., deep vein thrombosis, pulmonary embolism, and cardiovascular events), which is more common in earlier stages of CKD.[94]

Cardiovascular System

Cardiovascular disease is a major cause of morbidity and mortality in CKD. Proinflammatory cytokines, oxidative stress, metabolic derangements, dyslipidemia, uremic toxins, and anemia are significant contributors.

Hypertension is the result of excess sodium and fluid volume and arteriosclerosis. Endothelial cell dysfunction and calcium deposits lead to a loss of vessel elasticity and vascular calcification. Elevated renin concentration also stimulates the secretion of aldosterone, increasing sodium and water reabsorption.

Dyslipidemia promotes atheromatous plaque formation (see section on Protein, Carbohydrate and Fat Metabolism). The resulting vascular disease increases the risk for *ischemic heart disease, left ventricular hypertrophy, congestive heart failure, stroke*, and *peripheral vascular disease* in individuals with uremia.[95]

Pericarditis can develop from pericardial inflammation caused by the presence of uremic toxins. Accumulation of fluid in the pericardial space can compromise ventricular filling and cardiac output.[96]

Congestive heart failure can develop from fluid overload, hypertension, cardiac remodeling with hypertrophy and fibrosis (cardiorenal syndrome).[97]

Anemia increases demands for cardiac output and adds to the cardiac workload.

Pulmonary System

Pulmonary complications are associated with fluid overload causing pulmonary edema, congestive heart failure, and dyspnea. Pulmonary edema leads to respiratory acidosis causing Kussmaul respirations. Pulmonary hypertension is associated with left ventricular dysfunction or uremic-related pulmonary vascular changes.[98]

Immune System

Immune system dysregulation develops with the uremia of CKD. Chemotaxis, phagocytosis, antibody production, and cell-mediated immune responses are suppressed. Malnutrition, metabolic acidosis, and hyperglycemia may amplify immunosuppression. Release of inflammatory cytokines results in systemic inflammation. Failure of antioxidant systems also promotes inflammation. There are deficient responses to vaccination, increased risk for infection, and virus-associated cancers (e.g., human papillomavirus, hepatitis B and C viruses, Epstein–Barr virus).[99]

Neurologic System

Neurologic symptoms are common and progressive with CKD. Symptoms are related to dysfunction of lower motor and sensory neurons associated with uremic toxicity, chronic hyperkalemic depolarization, and anemia. The symptoms may include headache, pain, drowsiness, sleep disorders, impaired concentration, memory loss, and impaired judgment (known as uremic encephalopathy). In advanced stages of kidney failure, symptoms may progress to seizures and coma. Neuromuscular irritation can cause hiccups, muscle cramps, and muscle twitching. Peripheral neuropathies associated with uremic toxins also can develop with impaired sensations, particularly in the lower limbs causing decreased tendon reflexes, muscle weakness, and muscle atrophy. Symptoms improve with renal replacement therapy (i.e., hemodialysis or peritoneal dialysis) or kidney transplant.

Gastrointestinal System

Gastrointestinal complications are common in individuals with CKD. Uremic gastroenteritis can cause bleeding ulcer and significant blood loss. Nonspecific symptoms include anorexia, nausea, vomiting, constipation, or diarrhea. Uremic fetor is a form of bad breath caused by the breakdown of urea by salivary enzymes. Malnutrition is common.

Endocrine and Reproductive Systems

Endocrine and reproductive alterations develop with progression of CKD. Both males and females have a decrease in levels of circulating sex steroids. Males often experience a reduction in testosterone levels and may be impotent. Oligospermia and germinal cell dysplasia can result in infertility. Females have reduced estrogen levels, amenorrhea, anovulation, difficulty maintaining a pregnancy to term, and early menopause.[100–102]

Insulin resistance is common in uremia, and as CKD progresses, the ability of the kidney to degrade insulin is reduced and the half-life of insulin is prolonged. Individuals with diabetes mellitus and CKD need to carefully manage their insulin dosages.

CKD also causes alterations in thyroid hormone metabolism, particularly hypothyroidism, known as *nonthyroidal illness syndrome*. Uremia delays the response of thyroid-stimulating hormone receptors, and triiodothyronine (T_3) levels are often low.

Integumentary System

Skin changes are associated with other complications that develop with CKD. Anemia can cause pallor and bleeding into the skin and results in hematomas and ecchymosis. Retained urochromes manifest as a sallow skin color. Hyperparathyroidism and uremic skin residues (known as uremic frost) are associated with inflammation, irritation, and pruritus with scratching, excoriation, and increased risk for infection. Half-and-half nails (half white and half red or brown) are common.

Evaluation and Treatment. Early screening and evaluation of CKD is based on risk factors, health history, presenting signs and symptoms, and diagnostic testing. Decreased GFR (< 80) with elevated SCr and BUN concentrations are consistent with CKD. Markers of kidney damage include measurement of urine protein level, particularly albumin, and examination of urine sediment. Imaging will show small kidney size, and renal biopsy confirms the diagnosis.

Management involves promotion of adequate caloric intake with dietary restriction of protein, sodium, potassium, and phosphate. Supplementation with vitamin D or vitamin D receptor activators aids in the management of hyperphosphatemia. Maintenance of sodium and fluid balance may require fluid restriction. Management of dyslipidemias includes both pharmacological (statins and fibrates) and nonpharmacological measures (lifestyle and behavioral modifications). Erythropoietin can be used as needed to increase red blood cells. ACE inhibitors or ARBs are often used to control systemic hypertension, reduce proteinuria, provide renoprotection, and prevent progressive renal damage. CKD related to diabetic nephropathy can be significantly reduced with glycemic control. SGLT2 inhibitors are nephroprotective and provide blood pressure and hemodynamic regulation, protection from lipotoxicity, uric acid control, anti-inflammatory actions, and renal gluconeogenesis inhibition.[103] ESRD is treated with conservative care, CRRT, supportive therapy, and renal transplantation.

SUMMARY REVIEW

Urinary Tract Obstruction

1. Obstruction can occur anywhere in the urinary tract. It may be anatomic (structural) or functional. Obstruction impedes flow and dilates structures proximal to the blockage, increases risk for infection, and compromises renal function.
2. Upper urinary tract obstructions are caused by kidney stones or tumors within the kidney; or compression from a tumor, stone, or fibrosis along the ureter or at the ureter-bladder junction,
3. Complications of upper urinary tract obstruction include hydronephrosis, hydroureter, ureterohydronephrosis, and tubulointerstitial fibrosis.
4. Hypertrophy and hyperfunction of the unobstructed kidney compensate for loss of function of the kidney with obstructive disease.
5. Relief of obstruction is usually followed by postobstructive diuresis and may cause fluid and electrolyte imbalance.
6. Kidney stones are caused by supersaturation of the urine with precipitation of stone-forming substances and changes in urine pH.
7. Stones can be located in the kidneys, ureters, and urinary bladder. The most common kidney stone is formed from calcium oxalate.
8. LUT obstructions include both structural or anatomic disorders and alterations in neurologic function (neurogenic bladder), or both. They are related to urine storage and emptying.
9. Anatomic causes of resistance to urine flow include urethral stricture, prostatic enlargement in men, pelvic prolapse in women, and tumor compression.
10. Partial obstruction of the bladder can result in an increase in the force of detrusor contraction. If obstruction persists, there is deposition of collagen in the bladder wall over time, resulting in decreased bladder wall compliance and ineffective detrusor muscle contraction.
11. OAB is a dysfunction of urine storage with uncontrollable or premature contraction of the bladder that results in urgency with or without incontinence, frequency, and nocturia.
12. UAB syndrome is a voiding dysfunction resulting in prolonged bladder emptying or a failure to achieve complete bladder emptying, or both, within a normal time span.
13. A neurogenic bladder is caused by a neural lesion that interrupts innervation of the bladder.
14. Upper motor neuron lesions above the pontine micturition center result in overactive (hyperreflexive) bladder function and bladder dyssynergia (loss of coordinated neuromuscular contraction).
15. Lesions in the sacral area of the spinal cord or peripheral nerves result in underactive, hypotonic, or atonic bladder function.
16. Detrusor sphincter dyssynergia is failure of the urethrovesical junction smooth muscle to release urine during bladder contraction and causes a functional obstruction.
17. Kidney (renal) tumors include RCC (the most common), RTCC s and renal adenomas. RCC can metastasize to the

lung, lymph nodes, liver, bone, thyroid gland, and central nervous system.
18. Bladder tumors are commonly composed of transitional cells with a papillary appearance and a high rate of recurrence

Urinary Tract Infection

1. UTIs are commonly caused by the retrograde movement of bacteria into the urethra and bladder and can ascend to the kidney. UTIs are uncomplicated when the urinary system is normal or complicated when there is an abnormality. Types of UTI include cystitis, interstitial cystitis, and acute or chronic pyelonephritis.
2. Host defenses that protect against UTI include high osmolality and acidic pH of urine, mucus, uromodulin, and other antimicrobial proteins that activate the immune response, sphincters that prevent reflux, and urine flow that washes out bacteria.
3. Virulent uropathogens have pili or fimbriae, or both, that promote binding to the uroepithelium and retrograde movement in the urinary tract. Formation of biofilms enhances colonization and resists host defenses and antimicrobial therapy.
4. Cystitis is an inflammation of the bladder commonly caused by bacteria and may be mild, hemorrhagic, suppurative, ulcerative, or gangrenous.
5. Interstitial cystitis/painful bladder syndrome is a bladder pain disorder associated with LUT symptoms of more than 6 weeks' duration in the absence of infection or other identifiable causes. It is likely related to an inflammatory autoimmune reaction with a derangement of the glycosaminoglycan layer of the bladder mucosa that makes it more susceptible to penetration by bacteria and noxious urinary solutes.
6. Acute pyelonephritis is an inflammation of the upper urinary tracts (ureter, renal pelvis, and kidney interstitium). Infection due to urinary obstruction and reflux of urine from the bladder are the most common underlying risk factors. Severe infections may cause localized abscess formation.
7. Chronic pyelonephritis is an acute or chronic inflammation of the renal pelvis often related to ascending infection and obstructive uropathies leading to scarring of one or both kidneys and alteration in renal function. Untreated, chronic pyelonephritis can lead to kidney failure.

Glomerular Disorders

1. Glomerular disorders are a group of related diseases of the glomerulus that can be primary and caused by immune injury, infection, ischemia, toxins or drugs, or vascular disorders or, secondarily, caused by systemic diseases.
2. Acute glomerulonephritis commonly results from inflammatory damage to the glomerulus as a consequence of immune reactions including deposition of circulating immune complexes, antibodies reacting in situ to planted antigens, antibodies directed against the glomerular basement membrane, and complement activation.
3. Chronic glomerulonephritis is related to a variety of diseases that cause deterioration of the glomerulus and a progressive course leading to chronic kidney failure.
4. Diabetic nephropathy is the most common cause of glomerular injury progressing to CKD and is related to chronic hyperglycemia, inflammatory mediators, and microvascular and macrovascular complications.
5. Lupus nephritis is caused by the formation of autoantibodies against double-stranded DNA and nucleosomes with glomerular deposition of the immune complexes or formation of immune complexes against planted antigens in the glomerulus.
6. Nephrotic syndrome is the excretion of at least 3.5 g of protein (primarily albumin) in the urine per day primarily because of glomerular injury with increased capillary permeability and loss of membrane negative charge.
7. Nephritic syndrome is characterized by hematuria and red blood cell casts with less severe proteinuria.
8. The manifestations of both nephrotic and nephritic syndrome include edema, hypoproteinemia, proteinuria, hyperlipidemia, lipiduria, vitamin D deficiency, and hypothyroidism.

Acute Kidney Injury

1. AKI is a sudden decline in kidney function with a decrease in GFR and urine output and with an elevation in plasma creatinine and BUN levels.
2. Prerenal AKI is caused by decreased renal perfusion with ischemia, decreased GFR, and tubular necrosis.
3. Intrarenal AKI is associated with several systemic diseases but is commonly related to acute tubular necrosis.
4. Postrenal kidney injury is associated with diseases that obstruct the flow of urine from the kidneys.
5. Oliguria is urine output that is less than 400 mL/24 h and can be caused by alterations in renal blood flow, tubular obstruction, or tubular fluid backleak, or by a combination of these events.

Chronic Kidney Disease

1. CKD is the progressive loss of renal function for 3 months or more, with implications for health. Plasma creatinine levels gradually become elevated as GFR declines; sodium is lost in the urine; potassium is retained; acidosis develops; calcium, phosphate, magnesium, and vitamin D metabolism are altered; and erythropoietin production is diminished. All organ systems are affected by CKD.
2. Symptomatic changes usually do not become evident until renal function declines to less than 25%.
3. Glomerular hypertension, hyperfiltration, and chronic inflammation, oxidative stress, and fibrosis contribute to the progression of CKD. Proteinuria and angiotensin II promote the pathologic changes of chronic renal injury.
4. Uremic syndrome is a proinflammatory state with the accumulation of urea and other nitrogenous compounds as well as toxins and alterations in fluid, electrolyte, and acid-base balance that result from chronic kidney failure.
5. All organ systems are affected and contribute to disease symptoms.

REFERENCES

1. Washino S, Hosohata K, Miyagawa T. Roles played by biomarkers of kidney injury in patients with upper urinary tract obstruction. *Int J Mol Sci*. 2020;21(15):5490.
2. Meng XM. Inflammatory mediators and renal fibrosis. *Adv Exp Med Biol*. 2019;1165:381–406.
3. Rauchman M, Griggs D. Emerging strategies to disrupt the central TGF-β axis in kidney fibrosis. *Transl Res*. 2019;209: 90–104.
4. Priante G, et al. Cell death in the kidney. *Int J Mol Sci*. 2019;20(14):3598.
5. Forni LG, et al. Renal recovery after acute kidney injury. *Intensive Care Med*. 2017;43(6):855–866.
6. Singh A, et al. Post-obstructive diuresis: a cautionary tale. *Cureus*. 2019;11(12):e6328.
7. Tundo G, et al. Beyond prevalence: annual cumulative incidence of kidney stones in the United States. *J Urol*. 2021;205(6): 1704–1709.
8. Ferraro PM, et al. Risk of recurrence of idiopathic calcium kidney stones: analysis of data from the literature. *J Nephrol*. 2017;30:227–233.
9. Ferraro PM, et al. Risk of kidney stones: influence of dietary factors, dietary patterns, and vegetarian-vegan diets. *Nutrients*. 2020;12(3):779.
10. Sorokin I, et al. Epidemiology of stone disease across the world. *World J Urol*. 2017;35:1301–1320.
11. Huang Y, et al. The handling of oxalate in the body and the origin of oxalate in calcium oxalate stones. *Urol Int*. 2020;104 (3–4):167–176.
12. Chang A, Laszik ZG. The kidney. In: Kumar V, Abbas A, Aster J, eds. *Robbins & Cotran pathologic basis of disease*. ed 10. Elsevier; 2020. p 947.
13. Daudon M, et al. Comprehensive morpho-constitutional analysis of urinary stones improves etiological diagnosis and therapeutic strategy of nephrolithiasis. *C R Chim*. 2016;19(11–12):1470–1491. Available at https://doi.org/10.1016/j.crci.2016.05.008. (Accessed October 26, 2021).
14. Wiener SV, Ho SP, Stoller ML. Beginnings of nephrolithiasis: insights into the past, present and future of Randall's plaque formation research. *Curr Opin Nephrol Hypertens*. 2018;27(4): 236–242.
15. Micanovic R, et al. Uromodulin (Tamm–Horsfall protein): guardian of urinary and systemic homeostasis. *Nephrol Dial Transplant*. 2020;35(1):33–43.
16. Moran CP, Courtney AE. Managing acute and chronic renal stone disease. *Practitioner*. 2016;260(1790): 17–20, 2–3.
17. Evan AP, et al. Mechanisms of human kidney stone formation. *Urolithiasis*. 2015;43(Suppl 1):19–32.
18. Schwaderer AL, Wolfe AJ. The association between bacteria and urinary stones. *Ann Transl Med*. 2017;5(2):32.
19. Song L, Maalouf NM. Nephrolithiasis. In: Feingold KR, ed. *Endotext*. South Dartmouth, MA: MDText.com, Inc; 2000. Updated March 9, 2020. Available at https://www.ncbi.nlm.nih.gov/books/NBK279069/. (Accessed October 26, 2021).
20. Fontenelle LF, Sarti TD. Kidney stones: treatment and prevention. *Am Fam Physician*. 2019;99(8):490–496.
21. Janssen KM, et al. Effect of stone size and composition on ultrasonic propulsion ex vivo. *Urology*. 2018;111:225–229.
22. Corbo J, Wang J. Kidney and ureteral stones. *Emerg Med Clin North Am*. 2019;37(4):637–648.
23. Abou Chakra M, et al. Established and recent developments in the pharmacological management of urolithiasis: an overview of the current treatment armamentarium. *Expert Opin Pharmacother*. 2020;21(1):85–96.
24. Verla W, et al. A comprehensive review emphasizing anatomy, etiology, diagnosis, and treatment of male urethral stricture disease. *Biomed Res Int*. 2019;2019:9046430.
25. Reynolds WS, Fowke J, Dmochowski R. The burden of overactive bladder on US public health. *Curr Bladder Dysfunct Rep*. 2016; 11(1):8–13.
26. Peyronnet B, et al. A comprehensive review of overactive bladder pathophysiology: on the way to tailored treatment. *Eur Urol*. 2019;75(6):988–1000.
27. Leron E, et al. Overactive bladder syndrome: evaluation and management. *Curr Urol*. 2017;11:117–125.
28. Abrams P, et al. The standardisation of terminology in lower urinary tract function: report from the Standardisation Subcommittee of the International Continence Society. *Urology*. 2003;61(1):37–49.
29. Ko KJ, Lee CU, Lee KS. Clinical implications of underactive bladder. *Investig Clin Urol*. 2017;58(Suppl 2):S75–S81.
30. Amarenco G, et al. Diagnosis and clinical evaluation of neurogenic bladder. *Eur J Phys Rehabil Med*. 2017;53(6):975–980.
31. Stoffel JT. Detrusor sphincter dyssynergia: a review of physiology, diagnosis, and treatment strategies. *Transl Androl Urol*. 2016;5(1):127–135.
32. American Cancer Society. *Cancer Facts & Figures 2021*. Atlanta, GA: American Cancer Society; 2021. Available at https://www.cancer.org/research/cancer-facts-statistics/all-cancer-facts-figures/cancer-facts-figures-2021.html#. (Accessed October 26, 2021).
33. National Cancer Institute (NCI). *Clear cell renal cell carcinoma*. Bethesda, MD: NCI; 2020. Available at https://www.cancer.gov/pediatric-adult-rare-tumor/rare-tumors/rare-kidney-tumors/clear-cell-renal-cell-carcinoma. (Accessed October 26, 2021).
34. Muglia VF, Prando A. Renal cell carcinoma: histological classification and correlation with imaging findings. *Radiol Bras*. 2015;48(3):166–174.
35. Padala SA, et al. Epidemiology of renal cell carcinoma. *World J Oncol*. 2020;11(3):79–87.
36. Zhang T, et al. The landscape of contemporary clinical trials for untreated metastatic clear cell renal cell carcinoma. *Cancer Treat Res Commun*. 2020;24:100183.
37. Kim J, Kim WT, Kim WJ. Advances in urinary biomarker discovery in urological research. *Investig Clin Urol*. 2020;61(Suppl 1):S8–S22. Available at https://doi.org/10.4111/icu.2020.61.S1.S8. (Accessed October 26, 2021).
38. PDQ Adult Treatment Editorial Board: Bladder cancer treatment (PDQ®): health professional version. In: *PDQ cancer information summaries*, Bethesda, MD, 2021, National Cancer Institute. Updated August 27, 2021. Available at: https://www.cancer.gov/types/bladder/hp/bladder-treatment-pdq. (Accessed October 26, 2021).
39. Medina M, Castillo-Pino E: An introduction to the epidemiology and burden of urinary tract infections, *Ther Adv Urol*. 11:1756287219832172, 2019. Available at https://doi.org/10.1177/1756287219832172. (Accessed October 26, 2021).
40. Rogers J. Understanding the most commonly billed diagnoses in primary care. *Nurse Pract*. 2020;45(11):35–40.
41. Wagenlehner FM, Tandogdu Z, Bjerklund Johansen TE. An update on classification and management of urosepsis. *Curr Opin Urol*. 2017;27(2):133–137.

42. Anger J, et al. Recurrent uncomplicated urinary tract infections in women: AUA/CUA/SUFU Guideline. *J Urol*. 2019;202(2):282–289.
43. Saginala K, et al. Epidemiology of bladder cancer. *Med Sci (Basel)*. 2020;8(1):15.
44. Brubaker L, et al. American Urogynecologic Society best-practice statement: recurrent urinary tract infection in adult women. *Female Pelvic Med Reconstr Surg*. 2018;24(5):321–335.
45. Nicolle LE, et al. Clinical practice guideline for the management of asymptomatic bacteriuria: 2019 update by the Infectious Diseases Society of America. *Clin Infect Dis*. 2019;68(10):e83–e110.
46. Kang CI, et al. Clinical practice guidelines for the antibiotic treatment of community-acquired urinary tract infections. *Infect Chemother*. 2018;50(1):67–100.
47. Centers for Disease Control and Prevention (CDC). *Catheter-associated urinary tract infections (CAUTI)*. Atlanta, GA: CDC; 2009. Page last reviewed November 5, 2015. Available at https://www.cdc.gov/infectioncontrol/guidelines/cauti/index.html. (Accessed October 26, 2021).
48. Hanno PM, et al. Diagnosis and treatment of interstitial cystitis/bladder pain syndrome: AUA guideline amendment. *J Urol*. 2015;193(5):1545–1553.
49. Akiyama Y, et al. Interstitial cystitis/bladder pain syndrome: the evolving landscape, animal models and future perspectives. *Int J Urol*. 2020;27(6):491–503.
50. Osman NI, et al. A systematic review of surgical interventions for the treatment of bladder pain syndrome/interstitial cystitis. *Eur Urol Focus*. 2021;7(4):877–885.
51. Malde S, et al. Guideline of guidelines: bladder pain syndrome. *BJU Int*. 2018;122(5):729–743.
52. Gupta K, et al. International clinical practice guidelines for the treatment of acute uncomplicated cystitis and pyelonephritis in women: a 2010 update by the Infectious Diseases Society of America and the European Society for Microbiology and Infectious Diseases. *Clin Infect Dis*. 2011;52(5):e103–e120.
53. Mastrangelo A, et al. Clinical and pathophysiological insights into immunological mediated glomerular diseases in childhood. *Front Pediatr*. 2020;8:205.
54. Parmar MS, Bashir K. *Crescentric glomerulonephritis*. In: *StatPearls*. Treasure Island, FL: StatPearls Publishing; 2021. Updated August 12, 2021. Available at https://www.ncbi.nlm.nih.gov/books/NBK430727/. (Accessed October 26, 2021).
55. Sethi S, Fervenza FC. Standardized classification and reporting of glomerulonephritis. *Nephrol Dial Transplant*. 2019;34(2):193–199.
56. Pugliese G, et al. Diabetic kidney disease: new clinical and therapeutic issues. Joint position statement of the Italian Diabetes Society and the Italian Society of Nephrology on "The natural history of diabetic kidney disease and treatment of hyperglycemia in patients with type 2 diabetes and impaired renal function". *J Nephrol*. 2020;33(1):9–35.
57. Burrows NR, et al. Incidence of end-stage renal disease attributed to diabetes among persons with diagnosed diabetes — United States and Puerto Rico, 2000–2014. *MMWR Morb Mortal Wkly Rep*. 2017;66:1165–1170.
58. Selby NM, Taal MW. An updated overview of diabetic nephropathy: diagnosis, prognosis, treatment goals and latest guidelines. *Diabetes Obes Metab*. 2020;22(Suppl 1):3–15.
59. Parikh SV, et al. Update on lupus nephritis: core curriculum 2020. *Am J Kidney Dis*. 2020;76(2):265–281.
60. Kostopoulou M, Adamichou C, Bertsias G. An update on the diagnosis and management of lupus nephritis. *Curr Rheumatol Rep*. 2020;22(7):30.
61. Ha TS. Genetics of hereditary nephrotic syndrome: a clinical review. *Korean J Pediatr*. 2017;60(3):55–63.
62. Law JP, et al. Anticoagulant strategies for the patient with chronic kidney disease. *Clin Med (Lond)*. 2020;20(2):151–155.
63. Lee JM, et al. Current understandings in treating children with steroid-resistant nephrotic syndrome. *Pediatr Nephrol*. 2021;36(4):747–761.
64. Ronco C, Bellomo R, Kellum JA. Acute kidney injury. *Lancet*. 2019;394(10212):1949–1964.
65. Kidney Disease: Improving Global Outcomes (KDIGO) Acute Kidney Injury Work Group: KDIGO Clinical Practice Guideline for Acute Kidney Injury, *Kidney Int Suppl*. 2:1–138, 2012. Available at https://kdigo.org/wp-content/uploads/2016/10/KDIGO-2012-AKI-Guideline-English.pdf. (Accessed October 26, 2021).
66. Messerer DAC, et al. Immunopathophysiology of trauma-related acute kidney injury. *Nat Rev Nephrol*. 2021;17(2):91–111.
67. Gameiro J, et al. Acute kidney injury: from diagnosis to prevention and treatment strategies. *J Clin Med*. 2020;9(6):1704.
68. Bonavia A, Vece G, Karamchandani K. Prerenal acute kidney injury—still a relevant term in modern clinical practice? *Nephrol Dial Transplant*. 2021;36(9):1570–1577.
69. Moore PK, Hsu RK, Liu KD. Management of acute kidney injury: core curriculum 2018. *Am J Kidney Dis*. 2018;72(1):136–148.
70. Klein SJ, et al. Oliguria in critically ill patients: a narrative review. *J Nephrol*. 2018;31(6):855–862.
71. Basile DP, Anderson MD, Sutton TA. Pathophysiology of acute kidney injury. *Compr Physiol*. 2012;2(2):1303–1353.
72. Amaral Pedroso L, et al. Acute kidney injury biomarkers in the critically ill. *Clin Chim Acta*. 2020;508:170–178.
73. Ostermann M, et al. Controversies in acute kidney injury: conclusions from a Kidney Disease: Improving Global Outcomes (KDIGO) conference. *Kidney Int*. 2020;98(2):294–309.
74. Karkar A, Ronco C. Prescription of CRRT: a pathway to optimize therapy. *Ann Intensive Care*. 2020;10(1):32.
75. Lousa I, et al. New potential biomarkers for chronic kidney disease management—a review of the literature. *Int J Mol Sci*. 2020;22(1):43.
76. Denic A, et al. The substantial loss of nephrons in healthy human kidneys with aging. *J Am Soc Nephrol*. 2017;28(1):313–320.
77. Ullah MM, Basile DP. Role of renal hypoxia in the progression from acute kidney injury to chronic kidney disease. *Semin Nephrol*. 2019;39(6):567–580.
78. Podkowińska A, Formanowicz D. Chronic kidney disease as oxidative stress- and inflammatory-mediated cardiovascular disease. *Antioxidants (Basel)*. 2020;9(8):752.
79. Vanholder R, et al. Clinical management of the uraemic syndrome in chronic kidney disease. *Lancet Diabetes Endocrinol*. 2016;4(4):360–373. [Published correction appears in *Lancet Diabetes Endocrinol* 4(4):e4, 2016.].
80. Dhondup T, Qian Q. Electrolyte and acid-base disorders in chronic kidney disease and end-stage kidney failure. *Blood Purif*. 2017;43(1–3):179–188.
81. Combs S, Berl T. Dysnatremias in patients with kidney disease. *Am J Kidney Dis*. 2014;63(2):294–303.
82. Zhang R, et al. Hyponatremia in patients with chronic kidney disease. *Hemodial Int*. 2017;1(1):3–10.

83. Batlle D, Boobés K, Manjee KG. The colon as the potassium target: entering the colonic age of hyperkalemia treatment? *EBioMedicine*. 2015;2(11):1562–1563.
84. Desai NR, et al. Hyperkalemia treatment modalities: a descriptive observational study focused on medication and healthcare resource utilization. *PLoS One*. 2020;15(1):e0226844.
85. Bushinsky DA. Tolerance to sodium in patients with CKD-induced metabolic acidosis: does the accompanying anion matter? *Am J Kidney Dis*. 2019;73(6):858–865.
86. Felsenfeld AJ, Levine BS, Rodriguez M. Pathophysiology of calcium, phosphorus, and magnesium dysregulation in chronic kidney disease. *Semin Dial*. 2015;28(6):564–577.
87. Oliveira B, Cunningham J, Walsh SB. Magnesium balance in chronic and end-stage kidney disease. *Adv Chronic Kidney Dis*. 2018;25(3):291–295.
88. Rondanelli M, et al. An update on magnesium and bone health. *Biometals*. 2021;34:715–736.
89. Liu D, Lv LL. New understanding on the role of proteinuria in progression of chronic kidney disease. *Adv Exp Med Biol*. 2019;1165:487–500.
90. Biljak VR, et al. The role of laboratory testing in detection and classification of chronic kidney disease: national recommendations. *Biochem Med (Zagreb)*. 2017;27(1):153–176.
91. Irazabal MV, Torres VE. Reactive oxygen species and redox signaling in chronic kidney disease. *Cells*. 2020;9(6):E1342.
92. Vlad C, et al. A comprehensive review on apolipoproteins as nontraditional cardiovascular risk factors in end-stage renal disease: current evidence and perspectives. *Int Urol Nephrol*. 2019;51(7):1173–1189.
93. Haase VH. Hypoxia-inducible factor-prolyl hydroxylase inhibitors in the treatment of anemia of chronic kidney disease. *Kidney Int Suppl (2011)*. 2021;11(1):8–25.
94. Lutz J, et al. Haemostasis in chronic kidney disease. *Nephrol Dial Transplant*. 2014;29(1):29–40.
95. Dincer N, et al. The effect of chronic kidney disease on lipid metabolism. *Int Urol Nephrol*. 2019;51(2):265–277.
96. Nesheiwat Z, Lee JJ. *Uremic pericarditis*. In: *StatPearls*. Treasure Island, FL: StatPearls Publishing; 2021. Updated July 26, 2021. Available at https://www.ncbi.nlm.nih.gov/books/NBK536920/. (Accessed October 26, 2021).
97. Kaesler N, et al. Cardiac remodeling in chronic kidney disease. *Toxins (Basel)*. 2020;12(3):161.
98. Walther CP, et al. Diagnosis and management of pulmonary hypertension in patients with CKD. *Am J Kidney Dis*. 2020;75(6):935–945.
99. Espi M, et al. Chronic kidney disease-associated immune dysfunctions: impact of protein-bound uremic retention solutes on immune cells. *Toxins (Basel)*. 2020;12(5):300.
100. Rojas R, Clegg DJ, Palmer BF. Amenorrhea and estrogen disorders in kidney disease. *Semin Nephrol*. 2021;41(2):126–132.
101. Oliverio AL, Hladunewich MA. End-stage kidney disease and dialysis in pregnancy. *Adv Chronic Kidney Dis*. 2020;27(6):477–485.
102. Lundy SD, Vij SC. Male infertility in renal failure and transplantation. *Transl Androl Urol*. 2019;8(2):173–181.
103. Takata T, Isomoto H. Pleiotropic effects of sodium-glucose cotransporter-2 inhibitors: renoprotective mechanisms beyond glycemic control. *Int J Mol Sci*. 2021;22(9):4374.

39

Alterations of Renal and Urinary Tract Function in Children

Julia L. Rogers

http://evolve.elsevier.com/Rogers/pathophysiology/

CHAPTER OUTLINE

Renal and urinary disorders occur in children as well as adults. The incidence and type of renal and urinary tract disorders experienced by children vary with age and maturation. Newborn disorders may involve congenital malformations. During childhood, the kidney and genitourinary structures are continuing to develop, so renal dysfunction may be associated with mechanisms and manifestations that are different from those in adults. In addition, some renal and urinary disorders are congenital and involve structural anomalies of the kidney and urinary drainage system.

STRUCTURE AND FUNCTION OF THE URINARY SYSTEM IN CHILDREN

Development of the Urinary System

The embryonic urinary system develops as three sets of sequentially replaced organs: the pronephros, mesonephros, and metanephros. The pronephros is a nonfunctional structure that arises at the level of the cervical and upper thoracic regions during the third fetal week and connects the primitive mesonephritic duct (wolffian duct) to the cloaca. As the kidney develops, the cloaca degenerates by apoptosis and becomes part of the foundation for male sexual development. While the kidneys mature, the cloaca divides into two parts; one part becomes the rectum and the other part becomes the urogenital sinus. The urogenital sinus differentiates into the vesicourethral canal, which forms the bladder and the urethra. The development of the mesonephros and metanephros is described in Fig. 39.1. The Wilms tumor 1 *(WT1)* gene plays an important role at all stages of kidney development and maintenance of kidney function.

After glomeruli and tubules form, the tissues organize and progressively differentiate over approximately 30 days. Initial glomerular development is staggered, so there are glomeruli in various stages. A few of the first glomeruli that are formed degenerate and disappear during the later stages of fetal development. Progressive development continues into the ninth fetal month, when all metanephrogenic tissue disappears.

As the embryo develops and the vertebral column straightens, the kidneys appear to ascend to the sacral area at about 6 weeks, to the third lumbar area by the third month, and to the first lumbar area at term. The kidneys rotate 90 degrees as they ascend so that renal tissue is lateral and the collecting system is medial.

At birth, the kidneys occupy a large portion of the posterior abdominal wall, and the ureters are proportionately shorter than those of an adult. All the nephrons are present at birth, and their number does not increase as the kidney grows and matures. The kidney reaches adult size by adolescence and, because of maturation of the tubular system, increases in weight fivefold from the time of birth.

Urine formation and excretion begin by the third month of gestation, contributing to the amniotic fluid. In infancy the bladder lies close to the abdominal wall, making urinary bladder aspiration for diagnostic purposes a relatively simple procedure. The bladder descends into the pelvis with growth, changing from a cylindrical organ to the adult pyramidal shape. Although small amounts of urine are found in the bladder at birth, the newborn may not void for 12 to 24 hours.

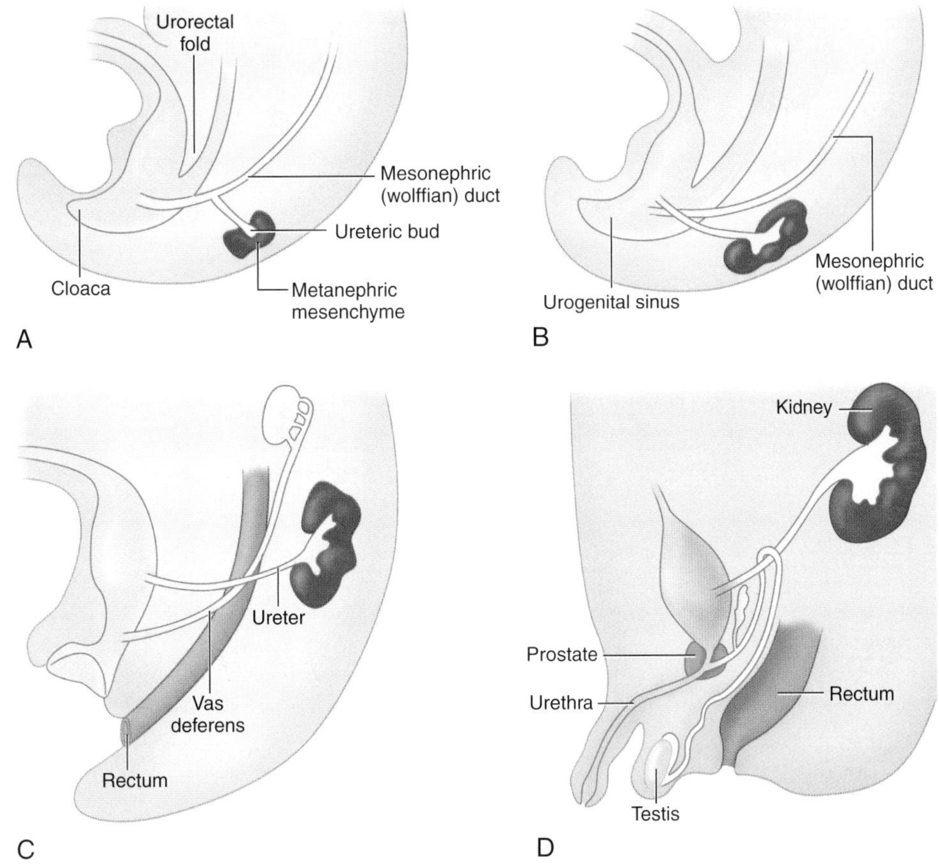

Fig. 39.1 Embryonic Development of the Kidneys. (A) Pronephros, **(B)** mesonephros, **(C)** metanephros, and **(D)** fully developed embryonic kidney (From Goldman L, Schafer AI. *Goldman's Cecil medicine*, 24th edition. Philadelphia: Saunders; 2012.)

Immediately at birth the renal blood flow and glomerular filtration rate (GFR) increase because of a decrease in vascular resistance and the need to perform excretory functions no longer performed by the placenta. Renal vascular resistance remains higher in newborns and infants, which may be attributed to increased levels of circulating renin. The resistance progressively declines during the first year of development, with an increasing fraction of the cardiac output going to the kidney. The GFR continues to increase, achieving adult levels by 2 years of age.

ALTERATIONS IN RENAL AND BLADDER FUNCTION IN CHILDREN

Congenital Abnormalities

Congenital abnormalities of the kidney and urinary tract (CAKUT) range from minor or easily correctable anomalies to those that are incompatible with life (Fig. 39.2). For example, the kidneys may fail to ascend from the pelvis to the abdomen, causing ectopic kidneys (abnormal location), which usually function normally. The lower poles of the kidneys may fuse as they ascend during fetal development, causing a single, U-shaped horseshoe kidney. Approximately one-third of individuals with horseshoe kidneys are asymptomatic, with the most common problems being infection, stone formation, hydronephrosis (from obstruction of urine flow), and rarely, renal malignancies.[1] Collectively, structural anomalies of the renal system account for approximately 40% to 50% of cases of renal failure in children in developed countries.[2] Many are linked to gene defects and may be associated with other structural malformations. (See Emerging Science Box: Promising Biomarkers to Predict Chronic Kidney Disease in Children With CAKUT.)

Some anomalies are obvious at birth, whereas others remain silent or become apparent in childhood. The following structural anomalies can be associated with urinary tract malformations:

- Low-set, malformed ears, sensorineural deafness
- Chromosomal disorders, especially trisomy 13 (Patau syndrome) and trisomy 18
- Absent abdominal muscles (prune-belly syndrome)
- Vertebral and extremity anomalies
- Imperforate anus
- Renal (nephroblastoma) and extrarenal tumors
- Ocular abnormalities (coloboma of the iris, congenital cataracts)
- Hepatic cysts or cirrhosis

Hypoplastic/Dysplastic Kidneys

During embryologic development, the ureteric duct grows into the metanephric tissue (see Fig. 39.1), triggering the formation

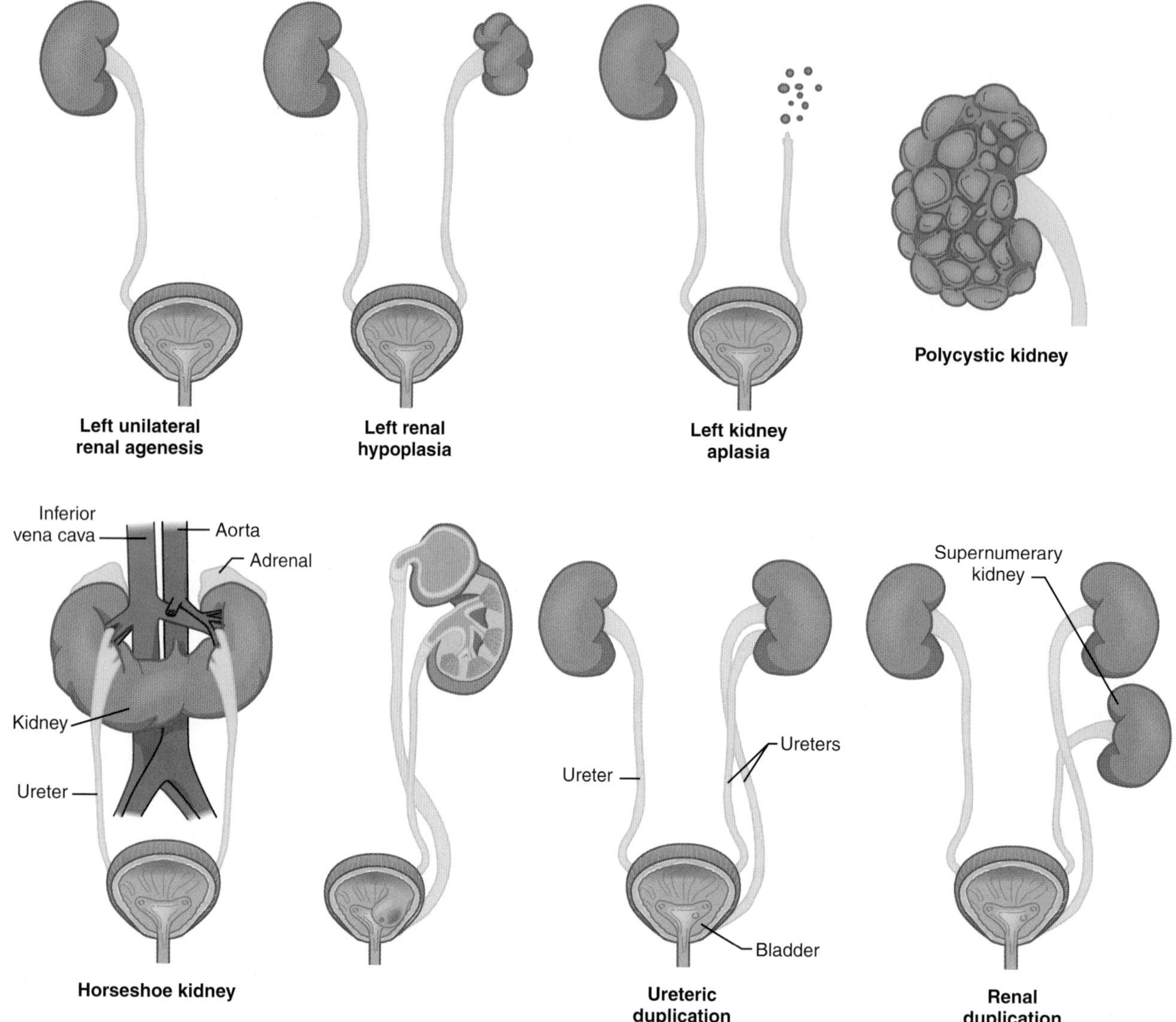

Fig. 39.2 Congenital Anomalies of the Kidney and Urinary Tract.

EMERGING SCIENCE BOX

Promising Biomarkers to Predict Chronic Kidney Disease in Children With Congenital Anomalies of Kidney and Urinary Tract

Children with congenital anomalies of kidney and urinary tract (CAKUT) have an increased risk of progressive kidney disease and developing chronic kidney disease (CKD) stage 5. There are emerging scientific studies on a promising, new peptide biomarker to predict functional deterioration on the kidneys.

Recent research studies revealed urinary trefoil family factors (TFFs) have a significant correlation with renal dysfunction in the pediatric population with CAKUT. TFF are a group of peptides, which include TFF_1, TFF_2, and TFF_3. These small peptides are mainly secreted in the mucous epithelia of the gastrointestinal system, respiratory system, urogenital system, and conjunctiva. TFFs are expressed in the entire urinary tract, with TTF_1 expression limited to the collecting ducts of medulla, and urothelium of the pelvis; TTF_2 expression within the bladder; and TTF3 has a pronounced expression in the cortex and medulla of the kidneys. Previous research has indicated that TTF_3 aids in mucosal protection, wound healing, cell proliferation, and cell migration in vivo and in vitro. TTF_3 is released when there is damage or inflammation to the kidneys, and therefore, an increase of TTF_3 levels in the urine is considered to be part of the compensatory and regenerative capacity of the kidney.

Because of the emerging research, TTFs are proving to be an instrumental peptide in determining functional deterioration on the kidneys in children with CAKUT. TTF_3 has been validated as a biomarker in a few studies with more to come. With the emergence of evidence, a urine TTF_3 should be included in the biomarker panel when assessing children with CAKUT for CKD.

Data from Anand S, et al. Urinary biomarkers as point-of-care tests for predicting progressive deterioration of kidney function in congenital anomalies of kidney and urinary tract: Trefoil family factors (TFFs) as the emerging biomarkers. *Pediatric Nephrology*, 2021;36:1465–1472. https://doi.org/10.1007/s00467-020-04841-8; McLeod DJ, et al. Longitudinal kidney injury biomarker trajectories in children with obstructive uropathy. *Pediatric Nephrology*, 2020;35:1907–1914; Stankovic A. Promising biomarkers in pediatric chronic kidney disease through the kaleidoscope of CAKUT background complexity. *Pediatric Nephrology*, 2021;36:1321–1325. https://doi.org/10.1007/s00467-020-04877-w.

of the kidneys.[3] If this growth does not occur, the kidney is absent—a condition called renal aplasia. A hypoplastic kidney is small with fewer nephrons. These conditions may be unilateral or bilateral. The occurrence may be incidental or familial. Bilateral hypoplastic kidneys are a common cause of chronic kidney disease (CKD) in children. Renal segmental hypoplasia (failure of parts of the renal cortex to develop)—the Ask-Upmark kidney—is a rare disorder and may be congenital or secondary to vesicoureteral reflux (VUR). Systemic hypertension is a common presentation.[4]

Renal dysplasia (abnormal development of renal tissue) usually results from abnormal differentiation of the renal tissues. For example, primitive glomeruli and tubules, cysts, and nonrenal tissue (such as cartilage) are found in the dysplastic kidney. Dysplasia may be secondary to antenatal obstruction of the urinary tract from ureteroceles (an outpouching of the ureter where it enters the bladder), posterior urethral valves (an obstructing membrane in the male urethra), or prune-belly syndrome (congenital absence of abdominal muscles).

Polycystic Kidney Disease

Polycystic kidney disease (PKD) is an inherited condition occurring in about 1 of 1000 live births in the United States.[5] PKD is associated with mutation of two genes: *PDK1* (autosomal dominant, chromosome 16) or *PDK2* (autosomal recessive, chromosome 4, more rare). Affected kidneys have multiple cysts that interfere with renal function. Autosomal dominant PKD (ADPKD) usually presents in late childhood or adulthood with the development of cysts. Defects in the formation of epithelial cells and their cilia result in cyst formation in all parts of the nephron. Cysts in other organs, including the liver, pancreas, and ovaries, may occur. Hypertension, aortic and intracranial aneurysms, and heart valve defects may develop. Autosomal recessive PKD (ARPKD) is often first suspected on a prenatal ultrasound. Epithelial hyperplasia and fluid secretion result in collecting duct cysts. Hepatic disease and hypertension typically accompany PKD. Renal dialysis is usually required during childhood or adolescence.

Renal Agenesis

Renal agenesis (the absence of one or both kidneys) may be unilateral or bilateral and may occur randomly or be hereditary. It may be an isolated entity or associated with anomalies in other organs.

Unilateral renal agenesis (congenital solitary functioning kidney) occurs in about 1 in 1000 live births in the United States. Males are more often affected, and it is usually the left kidney that is absent. The single remaining kidney is often completely normal so that the child can expect a normal healthy life. By the time the child is several years old, the volume of this kidney may approach twice the normal size to compensate for the absence of a second kidney. In some instances, the single kidney is abnormally formed and associated with abnormalities of its collecting system. Because the child has fewer nephrons, there is a risk of glomerular hyperfiltration injury, increasing the chance of developing proteinuria, hypertension, and CKD.[6] Extrarenal congenital abnormalities of the urogenital, skeletal, cardiac, and other systems may coexist.

Bilateral renal agenesis (also called Potter syndrome) is a rare disorder incompatible with extrauterine life. Approximately 75% of affected newborns are males. The term Potter syndrome refers to the association of a specific group of facial anomalies (wide-set eyes, parrot-beak nose, low-set ears, and receding chin). Bilateral renal agenesis results from either an abnormal development of the normal progression from pronephros to mesonephros to metanephros or an isolated bilateral failure of development of the ureteral buds from lack of growth factors. Oligohydramnios (low amount of amniotic fluid) resulting from inadequate fetal urine production leads to underdeveloped lungs. Infants with this condition rarely live more than 24 hours because of pulmonary insufficiency. Approximately 40% of affected infants are stillborn. Renal agenesis can be detected prenatally by ultrasound.

Ureteropelvic Junction Obstruction

Ureteropelvic junction (UPJ) obstruction is a partial or total blockage of the section where the renal pelvis transitions into the ureter. UPJ obstruction is the most common cause of hydronephrosis (distention of the renal pelvis and calyces with urine) in neonates. An intrinsic malformation of smooth muscle or urothelial development produces an obstruction in most cases. Extrinsic compression abnormalities are less common. Secondary ureteropelvic junction (UPJ) obstruction may be caused by kinking or secondary scarring as a complication of surgical repair. Children with UPJ obstruction have an increased risk of VUR. Diagnosis of a UPJ obstruction can be made by ultrasound. Obstruction of the distal ureter (ureterovesical junction obstruction) causes dilation of the entire ureter, renal pelvis, and calyceal system (megaureter). Megaureter can occur when a short acontractile segment of the ureter develops just above the ureterovesical junction or from ureteral reflux.[7] A ureterocele is a ballooning dilation of the ureter where it enters the bladder and impedes urine drainage. It often occurs when two ureters drain from one kidney instead of one ureter. The most commonly associated problems are hydronephrosis and infection. Open or endoscopic surgery to relieve an obstruction is performed if there is decline of renal drainage or function.[8] There is controversy about the preoperative use of continuous antibiotic prophylaxis, as in many cases, it does not prevent infection. An individualized approach is taken until the obstruction is surgically corrected.[9]

Hypospadias

Hypospadias is a congenital condition in which the cardinal feature is an ectopic urethral opening anywhere on the glans, penile shaft, base of the penis, penoscrotal junction, or in the perineum. Commonly, the urethral meatus is on the ventral side or undersurface of the penis (Fig. 39.3).[10] This is the most common anomaly of the penis, with an estimated prevalence of 64.7 cases per 10,000 male live births in the United States.[11] Partial absence of the foreskin, inguinal hernia, and cryptorchidism (undescended testes; see Chapter 26) are associated with the anomaly. The cause of this condition is multifactorial and includes genetic, endocrine, and environmental factors; advanced maternal age; low birth weight; and prematurity.[12] Chordee, or penile torsion, may

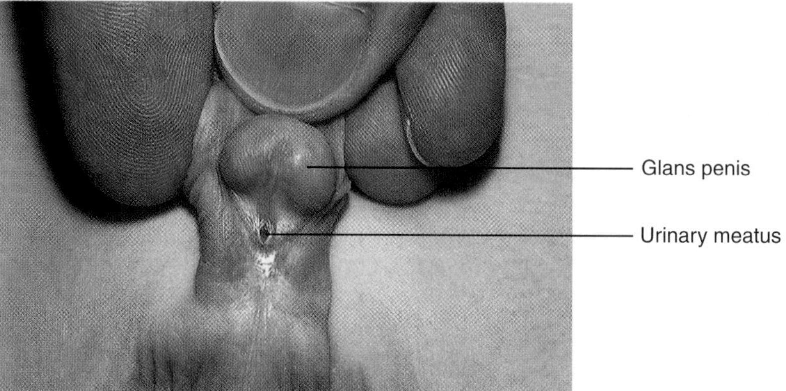

Fig. 39.3 Hypospadias. (Courtesy H. Gil Rushton MD, Children's National Medical Center, Washington, DC. From Hockenberry MJ, Wilson D. *Wong's nursing care of infants and children*, 10th edition. St. Louis: Mosby; 2015.)

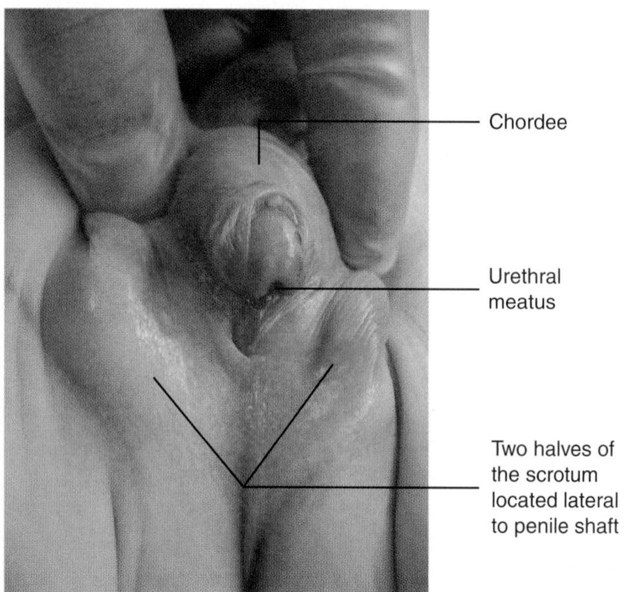

Fig. 39.4 Hypospadias With Significant Chordee. (From Kliegman RM et al., eds. *Nelson textbook of pediatrics*, 19th edition. Philadelphia: Saunders; 2011.)

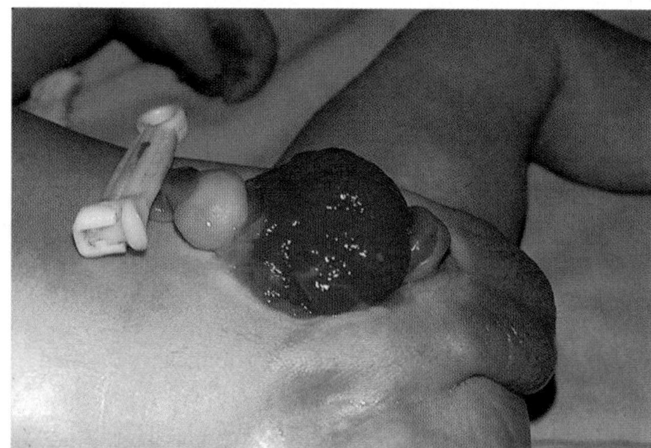

Fig. 39.5 Exstrophy of Bladder. (Courtesy H. Gil Rushton MD, Children's National Medical Center, Washington, DC. From Hockenberry MJ, Wilson D. *Wong's nursing care of infants and children*, 10th edition. St. Louis: Mosby; 2015.)

accompany cases of hypospadias. In chordee, a shortage of skin on the ventral surface causes the penis to bend or "bow ventrally" (Fig. 39.4). Penile torsion is rotation, usually in a counterclockwise direction, of the penile shaft.

The goals for corrective surgery on a child with hypospadias are (1) a straight penis when erect to facilitate intercourse as an adult, (2) a uniform urethra of adequate caliber to prevent spraying during urination, (3) a cosmetic appearance satisfactory to the individual, and (4) repair completed in as few procedures as possible. Surgery is usually performed between 6 and 12 months of age.

Epispadias and Exstrophy of the Bladder

Epispadias and exstrophy of the bladder are the same congenital defect but expressed to a different degree. The dorsal urethra is not fused in epispadias and has failed to form a tube. In males, the meatus may be small and situated behind the glans (glanular epispadias), a fissure may extend the entire length of the penis and into the bladder neck (penile epispadias), or the meatus is found near the pubic bone (penopubic epispadias). In females, a cleft along the ventral urethra usually extends to the bladder neck. The incidence of epispadias is about 1 per 117,000 births.[13] Continence is determined, in part, by the location of the defect. In children with distal epispadias, urinary incontinence rates can be up to 75%.[14] Treatment is surgical reconstruction.

Exstrophy of the bladder is a rare, extensive congenital anomaly of herniation of the bladder through the abdominal wall. The bony part of the pelvis remains open (Fig. 39.5). The posterior portion of the bladder mucosa is exposed through the abdominal opening and appears bright red. The incidence of bladder exstrophy in the United States is about 1.7 per 100,000 live births.[15]

Exstrophy of the bladder is caused by intrauterine failure of the abdominal muscles and the anterior bladder to fuse during embryonic development. The pubic rami (bony projections of the pubic bone) are not joined. This causes a waddling gait when the child first learns to walk, but most children quickly learn to compensate. The clitoris in girls is divided into two parts with the urethra between each half. The penis in boys is epispadias. Urine seeps onto the abdominal wall from the ureters, causing a constant odor of urine and excoriation of the surrounding skin. Because the exposed bladder mucosa becomes hyperemic and edematous, it bleeds easily and is painful.

The unrepaired exstrophic bladder is prone to cancerous changes as soon as 1 year after birth. Ideally, the bladder and pubic defect should be closed before the infant is 72 hours old. Surgical reconstruction is usually performed within the first year, either as a complete primary repair or as staged procedures. Staged procedures may include bladder augmentation, bladder neck reconstruction, and epispadias repair.[16] Objectives of management include preservation of renal function, attainment of urinary control, prevention of infection, and improvement of sexual function. Diagnosis is often made by prenatal ultrasound.

Bladder Outlet Obstruction

Congenital causes of bladder outlet obstruction are rare and include urethral valves and polyps. A urethral valve is a thin membrane of tissue that occludes the urethral lumen and obstructs urinary outflow, usually in the posterior urethra in males. Urethral polyps are a benign fibroepithelial growth and are very rare in children. The timing and presentation of these conditions depend on the degree of obstruction they cause. Severe obstruction may impair renal embryogenesis and lead to renal failure. Congenital urethral valves or polyps can be diagnosed with prenatal ultrasound and treated with prenatal bladder shunting or with resection during the first days of life.

GLOMERULAR DISORDERS

Glomerular disease or injury can result from genetic, immunologic, perfusion, or coagulation disorders. The most common glomerular disorders in children are glomerulonephritis, nephrotic syndrome, and hemolytic uremic syndrome (HUS). Most glomerular diseases are acquired and immunologically mediated. The disease can be acute or chronic. The likelihood of developing renal failure depends on the specific condition.

Glomerulonephritis

Acute glomerulonephritis includes several renal disorders in which inflammation of the glomeruli are secondary to an immune mechanism (Table 39.1) (other types of glomerulonephritis are described in Chapter 38 and Table 38.5). Chronic glomerulonephritis accounts for about 8% of the cases of CKD in children in the United States and is the causative factor for 15% to 29% of end-stage renal disease (ESRD) in children worldwide.[17,18]

Acute Poststreptococcal Glomerulonephritis

Acute poststreptococcal glomerulonephritis (PSGN) is caused by nephritogenic strains of *Streptococcus pyrogenes*, also called group A β-hemolytic Streptococcus (cause hemolysis on blood agar plates). PSGN is one of the most common immune complex–mediated renal diseases in children and a major cause of morbidity in group A β-hemolytic Streptococcal infections.[19] Glomerulonephritis develops with the deposition of antigen-antibody complexes or the formation of complexes in the glomerulus. The antigen-antibody complex activates complement and the release of inflammatory mediators that recruit neutrophils and macrophages and damages endothelial and epithelial cells lying on the glomerular basement membrane. Damage to the glomerular basement membrane alters membrane permeability and leads to hematuria and proteinuria.

TABLE 39.1 Primary Glomerulonephritis in Children

Classification	Findings
Cause	Poststreptococcal infection Related to other bacterial or viral infection Unknown
Immunologic mechanism	Antigen-antibody complex deposition Planted antigens with immune complex formed in situ
	Formation of antiglomerular basement membrane antibodies (rare) No immunologic cause established
Histopathology	No lesion Diffuse, focal, or segmented Membranous, proliferative, or combination of types Lobular, exudative, necrotizing, and other types Chronic with glomerular proliferation
Clinical manifestations of disease	Acute glomerulonephritis Persistent (chronic) glomerulonephritis Idiopathic nephrotic syndrome

PSGN is most common in children ages 5 to 12 years and uncommon in children before the age of 3 years.[20] Symptoms usually begin 1 to 2 weeks after an infection, such as an upper respiratory tract infection (pharyngitis, more common during cold weather), and up to 6 weeks after a skin infection (impetigo, more common during warm weather). Differential diagnosis includes systemic lupus erythematosus, endocarditis, membranoproliferative glomerulonephritis, an acute exacerbation of chronic glomerulonephritis, and other causes associated with streptococcal or staphylococcal microorganisms, or after viral diseases, such as varicella-zoster and hepatitis B and C. Confirmation of PSGN from a positive throat culture or rising antibody titer to streptococcal antigen can provide evidence of prior streptococcal infection.[20]

The onset of symptoms is abrupt, varying with disease severity. The child typically has gross or microscopic hematuria, proteinuria, edema, and renal insufficiency. Oliguria may be present. Hypertension occurs because of increased vascular volume. Acute hypertension may cause headache, vomiting, somnolence, and other central nervous system (CNS) manifestations. Cardiovascular symptoms, such as dyspnea, tachypnea, and an enlarged tender liver are related to circulatory overload and are compounded by hypertension. The most severely affected children develop acute kidney injury with oliguria. As many as half of affected children are asymptomatic.

The disease usually runs its course in 1 month, but urine abnormalities may be found for up to 1 year or longer after the onset. Most children recover completely. Treatment is supportive and symptom-specific for the acute effects of renal dysfunction and hypertension. A 10-day course of systemic antibiotic therapy with penicillin is recommended to limit the spread of the nephritogenic organisms; however, antibiotic therapy does not affect the natural history of PSGN.[20,21]

Immunoglobulin A Nephropathy

Immunoglobulin A (IgA) nephropathy is the most common form of glomerulonephritis in children worldwide and occurs more often in males. It is an autoimmune disease characterized by deposition primarily of secretory or mucosal IgA immune complexes with activation of complement proteins initiating an inflammatory response in the mesangium of the glomerulus.[22] Children with the disease have recurrent microscopic or gross hematuria concurrent with a respiratory tract infection (e.g., tonsillitis) or gastroenteritis. Most continue to have microscopic hematuria between the attacks of gross hematuria and have a mild proteinuria as well. Treatment is supportive. Some children recover completely, whereas 20% or more will eventually require dialysis and transplantation. IgA nephropathy may recur after transplantation.

Immunoglobulin A vasculitis (Henoch-Schönlein purpura nephritis) is a rare form of IgA nephropathy. It is the most common form of systemic vasculitis in children. Symptoms include palpable purpura (usually on the legs), arthralgia, abdominal pain, hematuria, and/or proteinuria. Complete recovery usually occurs, but some children progress to ESRD.[23]

Nephrotic Syndrome

Nephrotic syndrome is a group of symptoms characterized by severe proteinuria, hypoalbuminemia, hyperlipidemia, and edema. The syndrome is more common in children than in adults. When no identifiable cause is found, the condition is called primary (idiopathic) nephrotic syndrome (Fig. 39.6). If it results from a systemic disease or other causes (e.g., systemic lupus erythematosus, IgA vasculitis, malignancy [lymphoma and leukemia], and infections [hepatitis, HIV, and malaria]), it is called secondary nephrotic syndrome. Primary nephrotic syndrome is found predominantly in the preschool-age child, with a peak incidence of onset between ages 2 and 3 years. It is rare after age 6 years. Males are affected more often than females. No prevalent racial or geographic distributions are evident. The incidence is approximately 1 to 3 per 100,000 children younger than 16 years of age per year.[20]

Pathophysiology. Nephrotic syndrome is caused by increased permeability of the glomerular capillary wall, which leads to massive proteinuria and hypoalbuminemia. The most common causes of primary nephrotic syndrome in children are minimal change nephropathy (MCN) and focal segmental glomerulosclerosis (FSGS).[24] **Minimal change nephropathy (MCN, lipoid nephrosis)** is associated with an alteration in immune function and is characterized by fusion of the glomerular podocyte foot processes, which are seen by electron microscopy. The glomeruli appear normal by light microscopy. This leads to a decrease in number of functional podocytes and altered glomerular membrane integrity. The result is increased protein leakiness across the glomerular capillary wall into the urinary space. Loss of the electrical negative charge and increased permeability within the glomerular capillary wall lead to albuminuria. Hypoalbuminemia (causing decreased plasma oncotic pressure) and sodium retention contribute to edema. Hyperlipidemia leads to lipiduria (lipoprotein fat bodies in the urine) and primarily results from increased hepatic lipid synthesis and decreased plasma lipid catabolism in response to a decrease in plasma oncotic pressure.[25]

In idiopathic focal segmental glomerulosclerosis (FSGS), there is both focal (some glomeruli) and segmental (parts of glomeruli) scarring. Electron microscopy reveals segmental scarring of the glomerular tuft with loss of glomerular capillaries along with podocyte injury.[26]

Clinical Manifestations. Onset of nephrotic syndrome is often insidious, with periorbital edema as the first sign. The edema is most noticeable in the morning and subsides during the day as fluid shifts to the abdomen, genitalia, and lower extremities. Parents may notice diminished, frothy, or foamy urine output or, when edema becomes pronounced with ascites, respiratory difficulty from pleural effusion or labial or scrotal swelling (Fig. 39.7). Edema of the intestinal mucosa may cause diarrhea, anorexia, and poor absorption. Edema often masks the malnutrition caused by malabsorption and protein loss. Pallor, with shiny skin and prominent veins, also is common. Blood pressure is usually normal. Children with nephrotic syndrome are more susceptible to infections such as cellulitis, spontaneous bacterial peritonitis, and bacteremia. This occurs partially as a result of the urinary losses of immunoglobulin G causing hypoglobulinemia.[20] Irritability, fatigue, and lethargy are common. **Congenital nephrotic syndrome (Finnish type)** is caused by an autosomal recessive mutation of the *NPHS1* gene. *NPHS1* normally encodes an immunoglobulin-like protein, nephrin, at the podocyte filtration membrane. Lack of nephrin alters membrane permeability and causes heavy proteinuria, hypoproteinemia, and edema in the first 3 months of life. These babies do not respond to steroid treatment (termed steroid resistance) and require albumin infusion and diuretics to manage their fluid balance.

Evaluation and Treatment. The diagnosis of nephrotic syndrome is evident from urinalysis findings of proteinuria, hematuria, and lipiduria; hematologic evidence of hyperlipidemia and hypoalbuminemia; and assessment of edema. Diagnostic testing, including kidney biopsy, may be required to determine whether the cause is an intrinsic renal disease or a consequence of systemic disease. Basic management of nephrotic syndrome includes administering corticosteroids (prednisone) (Table 39.2); adhering to a low sodium (<1500 mg/day), well-balanced diet; performing good skin care; and, if edema becomes problematic, prescribing diuretics (furosemide, metolazone).[27] Immunosuppressive agents (i.e., cyclophosphamide) may be

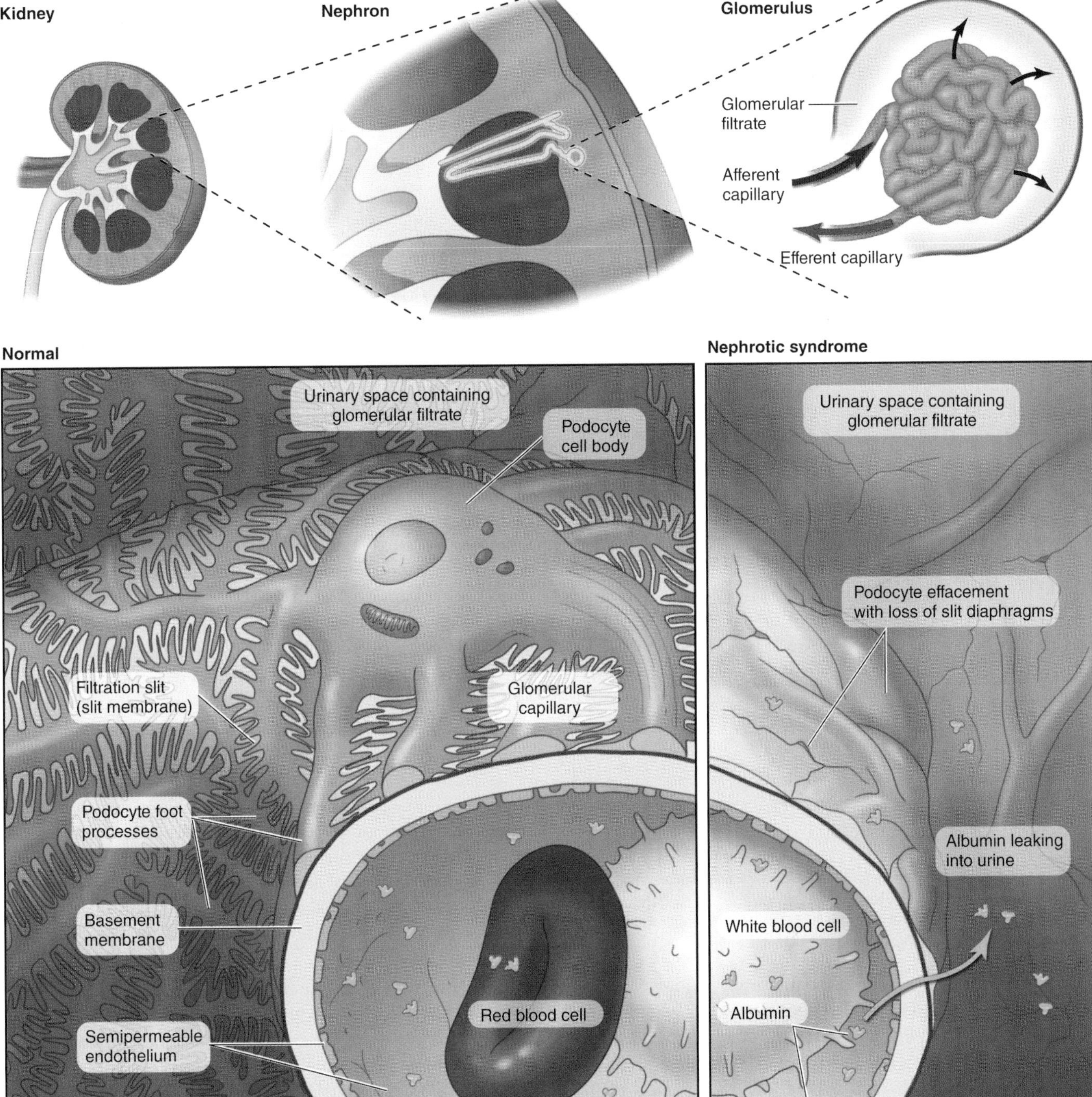

Fig. 39.6 Primary Nephrotic Syndrome. The Glomerulus and Pathogenesis of Idiopathic Nephrotic Syndrome. Within the kidney the glomerular capillary filters blood from the systemic circulation. The podocyte, glomerular basement membrane and semipermeable glomerular endothelium comprise the glomerular filtration barrier allowing the ultrafiltrate to enter the urinary space. The podocyte has extensive cellular extensions (foot processes) that interdigitate and are connected by slit membranes. In nephrotic syndrome, there is extensive effacement (thinning and shortening) of the podocytes with loss of their negative charge and loss of slit diaphragms (cell junctions between podocytes), allowing excessive serum albumin to leak into the urine causing proteinuria. The pathogenesis of idiopathic nephrotic syndrome is hypothesized to be either immune-mediated or a genetic variation in glomerular capillary structure. Numerous mutations are associated with steroid-resistant form of nephrotic syndrome that affect various parts of the podocyte itself, or other constituent proteins of the glomerular basement membrane. (Reprinted with permission from Elsevier (From Noone DG, Iijima K, Parekh R. Idiopathic nephrotic syndrome in children. *The Lancet* 2018;392(10141):61–74. https://doi.org/10.1016/s0140-6736(18)30536-1)

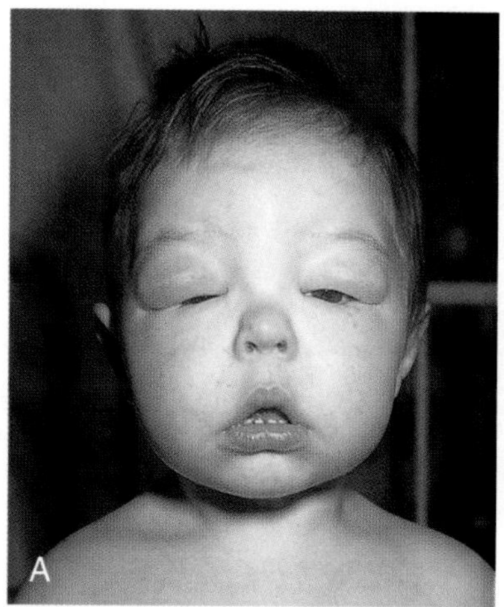

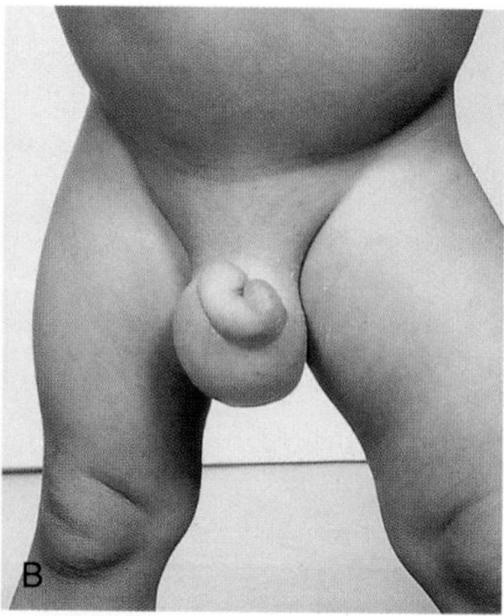

Fig. 39.7 Nephrotic Syndrome. **(A)** Facial edema. **(B)** Gross edema of scrotum and legs with abdominal distention from ascites. (From Lissauer T, Clayden G. *Illustrated textbook of paediatrics*, 4th edition. London: Mosby; 2012.)

TABLE 39.2 Corticosteroid Response in Children With Nephrotic Syndrome

Response to Corticosteroid	Outcomes
Steroid sensitive	May have just one or recurrent episodes.
Steroid dependent or frequently relapsing	May require low-dose prednisone or treatment with other immunosuppressive agents to prevent recurrence
Steroid resistant	Treatment with immunosuppressive and nonimmunosuppressive medications; risk for development of end-stage kidney disease

Data from Hodson EM, Wong SC, Willis NS, et al. Interventions for idiopathic steroid-resistant nephrotic syndrome in children. *Cochrane Database Systems Review*, 2016;10:CD003594; Larkins N, Kim S, Craig J, et al. Steroid-sensitive nephrotic syndrome: An evidence-based update of immunosuppressive treatment in children. *Archives of Disease in Childhood*, 2016;101(4):404–408.

used with children who have frequent relapses or who develop steroid toxicity or are resistant to steroid therapy (steroid-resistant nephrotic syndrome) which is more common with FSGS.[28] Long-term outcomes depend on the underlying cause of the nephrotic syndrome. Children with minimal change disease tend to do very well, whereas those with FSGS may develop ESRD.

Hemolytic Uremic Syndrome

Hemolytic uremic syndrome (HUS) is an acute disorder characterized by hemolytic anemia, thrombocytopenia (a decrease in blood platelets), and acute renal failure. HUS is a thrombotic microangiopathy and the most common cause of community acquired acute kidney injury in children. The disease occurs most often in infants and children younger than 4 years of age but has been known to occur in adolescents and adults.

Pathophysiology. HUS has been associated with bacterial and viral agents, as well as endotoxins, such as Shiga toxin-producing *Escherichia coli* (known as D^+,STEC-HUS, or diarrhea associated HUS). Potential sources of exposure include animals, unpasteurized beverages, undercooked meat, and vegetables. Genetic forms of HUS (nondiarrhea, or atypical) are rare and known as D^- disease. It is caused by other microorganisms or by an inherited abnormality in complement alternate pathway regulation (e.g., von Willebrand factor–cleaving protease).[29] A major characteristic of genetic or alternative forms of HUS is the absence of prodromal diarrhea, thus the designation D^-.

In HUS D^+ (with diarrhea), toxins are absorbed from the intestine into the blood and bind to white blood cells, which are transported to the kidney. In the kidney, white blood cells cause damage to the glomerular endothelium with activation of the coagulation cascade and aggregation of platelets. The glomerular arterioles become swollen and occluded with platelets and fibrin clots. There is decreased glomerular filtration, and the damaged glomerular membrane results in hematuria and proteinuria. Narrowed glomerular vessels damage passing erythrocytes and platelets. These damaged red blood cells and platelets are removed by the spleen, causing acute hemolytic anemia and thrombocytopenia. Fibrinolysis, the process of dissolution of a clot, acts on precipitated fibrin, causing the fibrin split products to appear in serum and urine. Varying degrees of renal vascular occlusion cause altered renal perfusion and renal insufficiency or failure.[30]

Clinical Manifestations. HUS is characterized by the triad of microangiopathic hemolytic anemia, thrombocytopenia, and renal insufficiency. A prodromal gastrointestinal illness (diarrhea with or without vomiting) or, less frequently, an upper respiratory tract infection often precedes the onset by 1 to 2 weeks. After a symptom-free 1- to 5-day period, there is sudden onset of pallor, bruising or purpura, irritability, weakness, and oliguria. Slight fever, anorexia, vomiting, diarrhea (with the stool characteristically watery and blood stained), abdominal pain, mild jaundice, and circulatory overload are accompanying symptoms. Seizures and lethargy indicate CNS involvement.

In severe cases, renal failure is apparent within the first days of onset. The renal failure causes metabolic acidosis, azotemia (accumulated nitrogenous wastes in the blood), hyperkalemia, and often hypertension.

Evaluation and Treatment. Clinical evaluation includes history of preexisting illness, presenting symptoms, and urine and blood analysis. Management is supportive with fluid and electrolyte management. Blood transfusions with packed red cells may be needed to maintain reasonable hemoglobin levels. Eculizumab, a complement inhibitor, has provided effective treatment for atypical or D^- HUS.[30] Most children recover completely. Potential long-term sequelae include renal (hypertension, proteinuria, CKD, and ESRD) and nonrenal abnormalities (diabetes mellitus, neurologic manifestations). Up to half of patients may require dialysis support during the acute phase of the disease.[20] The major causes of morbidity and mortality are due to extrarenal complications such as CNS involvement, infection, or myocardial causes.[31]

NEPHROBLASTOMA

Nephroblastoma (Wilms tumor) is a rare embryonal tumor of the kidney arising from undifferentiated mesoderm. Approximately 650 children are diagnosed each year in the United States, and most are younger than 5 years of age. The peak incidence occurs between 2 and 3 years of age and is more common in girls than boys. Nephroblastoma is less common in Asian-American children.[32]

Pathophysiology. Nephroblastoma has both sporadic and inherited origins. The sporadic form occurs in children with no known genetic predisposition. Inherited cases, which are relatively rare, are transmitted in an autosomal dominant fashion. Syndromic and nonsyndromic causes of nephroblastoma have been linked to mutation of several tumor-suppressor genes (i.e., *WT1* and *WT2* mutations; these genes are important for development of the kidney).[33]

Some children who have nephroblastoma also have other congenital anomalies. The anomalies include aniridia (lack of an iris in the eye), hemihyperplasia (an asymmetry of the body), and genitourinary malformations (i.e., horseshoe kidneys, hypospadias, ureteral duplication, polycystic kidneys).

Clinical Manifestations. Most children with nephroblastoma present with an enlarging asymptomatic abdominal mass before the age of 5 years.[34] Many tumors are discovered by the child's parent, who feels or notices abdominal swelling, usually while dressing or bathing the child. The child appears healthy and thriving. Other presenting complaints include vague abdominal pain, hematuria, anemia, and fever. Hypertension may be present, often as a result of excessive renin secretion by the tumor.[35]

Nephroblastoma may occur in any part of the kidney and varies greatly in size at the time of diagnosis. Bilateral tumors are very rare. The tumor generally appears as a solitary mass surrounded by a smooth, fibrous external capsule and may contain cystic or hemorrhagic areas. A pseudocapsule generally separates the tumor from the renal parenchyma.

Evaluation and Treatment. On physical examination, the tumor feels firm, nontender, smooth, and is confined to one side of the abdomen. If the tumor is palpable past the midline of the abdomen, it may be large or may be arising from a horseshoe or ectopic kidney.

Diagnosis is based on selected laboratory tests and surgical biopsy. Laboratory tests assist with differentiation of a nephroblastoma from a neuroblastoma (a mimicker of nephroblastoma).

Diagnostic imaging demonstrates a solid intrarenal mass and can identify the presence or absence of metastasis. The most common sites of metastasis are regional lymph nodes and the lungs, and less commonly the liver, brain, and bone. Several staging systems for nephroblastoma have been developed and serve as guides to treatment. The most widely accepted system has been developed by the Children's Oncology Group (Table 39.3). Primary treatment is usually surgical exploration and resection, including nephron sparing surgery or chemotherapy, and then surgical resection depending on stage of disease and treatment guidelines.[36] Because of the long-term side effects of radiation therapy, it is primarily used for children with higher stages of disease, recurrent disease, and metastases. In these cases, radiation therapy may be combined with chemotherapy therapy and hematopoietic stem cell transplantation. Survival is greater than 90% for localized disease and

TABLE 39.3 Staging and Survival Rates for Nephroblastoma (Wilms Tumor)

Stage	Tumor Characteristics	4 Year Survival Rates for Favorable Histology Focal Anaplastic Diffuse Anaplastic
I	Tumor limited to one kidney; renal capsule intact; cancer not spread into blood vessels or other kidney; completely resected with no biopsy	95%–100% 85%–90% 75%–80%
II	Tumor involves perirenal fat, lymphatic vessels outside kidney, or infiltrates adjacent organs; completely resected with no biopsy	95%–100% 80%–85% 80%–85%
III	Residual nonhematogenous tumor confined to abdomen and involved regional lymph nodes; biopsy before removal of kidney.	95%–100% 75%–90% 50%–70%
IV	Hematogenous metastases to organs such as lungs, liver, bone, brain, or lymph nodes away from the kidneys	85%–90% 70%–75% 30%–45%
V	Bilateral kidney tumors disease either at diagnosis or later, then staged for each kidney	95%–100% 95%–100% 65%–70%

Data from American Cancer Society Staging system of the Children's Oncology Group staging. Last revised October 17, 2018. Accessed March 7, 2022. https://www.cancer.org/cancer/wilms-tumor/detection-diagnosis-staging/staging.html

more than 70% for higher stages. Heart failure, renal failure, (see Table 39.3) and hypertension occur more frequently in long-term survivors than in the general population.[37]

BLADDER DISORDERS

Urinary Tract Infections

Urinary tract infections (UTIs) are one of the most common bacterial infections in childhood. UTIs are caused by colonization of a pathogen anywhere along the urinary tract (urethra, bladder, ureter, kidney) and occurs equally in males and females during the first year of life, with incidence in females increasing after age 1 year. During the neonatal period, children with congenital renal abnormalities and noncircumcised males are at increased risk; whereas in adolescence, sexually active females are at increased risk as a result of perineal bacteria, especially *E. coli*, ascending the urethra. An abnormal urinary tract (presence of reflux, obstruction, stasis, or stones) is a risk factor for infection.

Cystitis, or infection of the bladder, results in mucosal inflammation and congestion. This causes detrusor muscle hyperactivity resulting in dysuria, urinary urgency, frequency, and a decrease in bladder capacity.[38] It may also cause distortion of the ureterovesical junction (UVJ), leading to transient reflux of infected urine up the ureters, causing acute or chronic pyelonephritis.

Symptoms in children are nonspecific, and differentiating whether an infection is in the bladder or in the kidneys (pyelonephritis) is difficult based on symptoms alone. Infants may be asymptomatic or develop fever, lethargy, abdominal pain, vomiting, diarrhea, or asymptomatic jaundice. Children may present with fever of undetermined origin, frequency, urgency, dysuria, enuresis or incontinence in a previously dry child, flank or back pain, and sometimes hematuria. Acute pyelonephritis, an infection in the kidney, usually causes chills, high fever, and flank or abdominal pain, along with enlarged kidney(s) caused by inflammatory edema.[38] Chronic pyelonephritis may be asymptomatic.

Diagnosis of UTI is by urine culture which should be obtained prior to the initiation of antibiotic therapy. Dipstick urinalysis may be used as a screening tool and may reveal nitrites, leukocyte esterase, and blood which are used to support the diagnosis. Leukocyturia, regarded by the American Association of Pediatrics as a prerequisite to making the diagnosis, is found in most children with a UTI, but not found in all, hence the reasoning for obtaining a urine culture.[38,39] Diagnostic imaging (e.g., ultrasound, computed tomography [CT], and cystogram) and laboratory tests, in particular inflammatory markers (C-reactive protein and procalcitonin), may be necessary to rule out obstructions, infectious processes, renal scarring, or functional abnormalities.[38]

Treatment of UTI is based on presenting symptoms, the child's previous medical history, and local resistance patterns of uropathogens.[38] Children with acute cystitis are treated with a less broad-spectrum antibiotic (i.e., nitrofurantoin or trimethoprim) for a short duration (1 to 3 days).[38] Previously healthy children, with a high suspicion of acute pyelonephritis without microbe identification, are prescribed treatment with broad-spectrum antibiotics. However, once the pathogen is identified, then the antimicrobial must be tailored to cover the offending organism. With treatment, symptoms are usually relieved in 1 to 2 days, and the urine becomes sterile. A 3-to-5-day course of oral antibiotics is effective for uncomplicated UTI and 7 to 14 days for complicated UTI.[40] Longer treatment may be required if the child has a history of recurrent UTIs, congenital abnormalities of the urinary tract, or upper UTI. If there is no improvement in 2 days, the child should be reevaluated.

Vesicoureteral Reflux

Vesicoureteral reflux (VUR) is the retrograde flow of urine from the bladder into the kidney or ureters, or both. Reflux allows infected urine from the bladder to reach the kidneys. VUR is usually present in children with CAKUT, specifically congenital renal dysplasia.[38] VUR occurs more often in females and is uncommon in Black Americans. The actual incidence is unknown because VUR is often undiagnosed. An estimated 30% to 40% of children younger than 5 years who develop a UTI have VUR. Siblings of those affected have about a 27% to 51% chance of having reflux, and children with parents who had childhood reflux have almost a 70% chance of reflux.[41] Although reflux is considered abnormal at any age, the shortness of the submucosal tunnel of the ureter during infancy and childhood renders the antireflux mechanism relatively inefficient and delicate. Thus, reflux is seen commonly in association with infections during early childhood but rarely in older children and adults.

Pathophysiology. The normal distal ureter enters the bladder through the detrusor muscle and passes through a submucosal tunnel before opening into the bladder lumen via the ureteral orifice. As the bladder fills with urine, the ureter is compressed within the bladder wall, preventing reflux. *Primary reflux* results from a congenital, abnormally short submucosal tunnel and ureter that permits reflux by the rising pressure of the filling bladder (Fig. 39.8). Urine sweeps up into the ureter and then flows back into the empty bladder. The reflux perpetuates infection by preventing complete emptying of the bladder and providing a reservoir for infection. With bladder filling, the intravesical pressure can be transmitted up the ureter to the renal pelvis and calyces. The combination of reflux lower UTI is an important cause of pyelonephritis. Renal parenchymal injury, scarring, hypertension, and CKD can occur many years later, making early diagnosis and treatment important. *Secondary reflux* develops in association with acquired conditions (e.g., neurogenic bladder dysfunction, ureteral obstruction, voiding disorders, or surgery on the UVJ). Reflux may be unilateral or bilateral and is graded on a scale of I (mild) to V (severe) using the International Reflux Grading System with 95% of VUR in children ranging from grades I to III (Fig. 39.9).[38] The grades are as follows:

Grade I: reflux into a nondilated distal ureter
Grade II: reflux into the upper collecting system without dilation
Grade III: reflux into a dilated ureter or blunting of calyceal fornices
Grade IV: reflux into a grossly dilated ureter and calyces

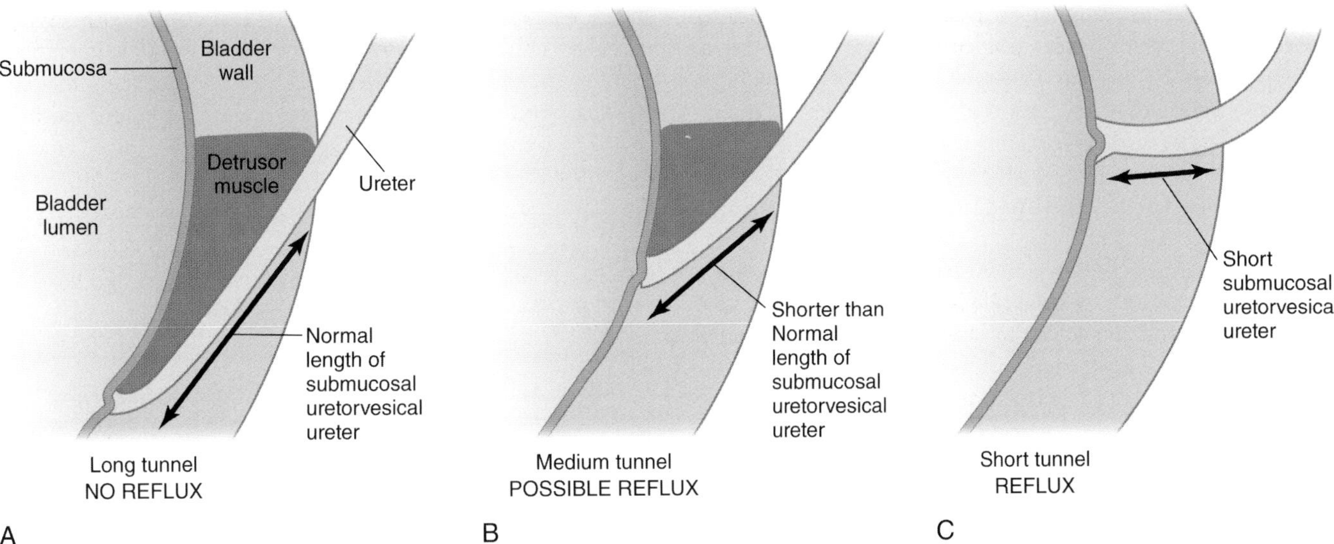

Fig. 39.8 Normal and Abnormal Configurations of the Ureterovesical Ureter. A refluxing ureterovesical ureter **(B)** and **(C)** has the same anatomic features as a nonrefluxing ureter **(A)**, except for the shorter length of the intravesical ureter, which allows reflux of urine during filling of the bladder. (Adapted from Liaw A, Cunha GR, Shen J, et al. Development of the human bladder and ureterovesical junction. *Differentiation*, 2018;103;66–73. https://doi.org/10.1016/j.diff.2018.08.004.)

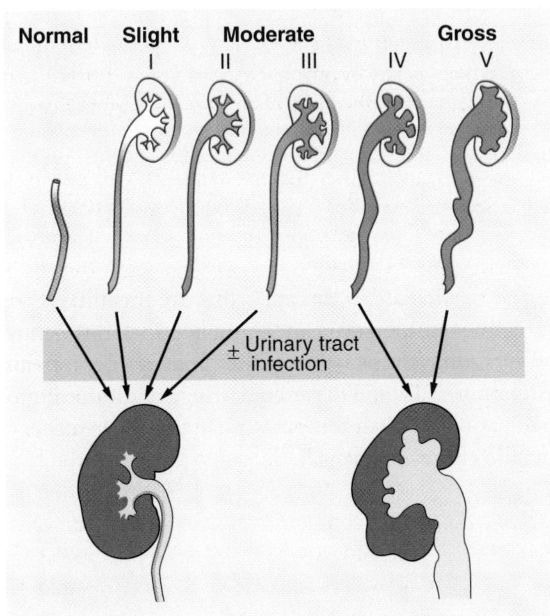

Fig. 39.9 Grades of Vesicoureteral Reflux. (Adapted from Johnson JR, Feehally J, Floege J. *Comprehensive clinical nephrology*, 5th edition. Philadelphia: Saunders; 2015.)

Grade V: massive reflux with urethral dilation and tortuosity and effacement of the calyceal details

Clinical Manifestations. Children with reflux may be asymptomatic or have recurrent UTIs, unexplained fevers, poor growth and development, irritability, and feeding problems. The family history may reveal VUR or UTIs.

Evaluation and Treatment. In addition to the history of recurrent UTI and other symptoms, a voiding cystourethrogram is the primary diagnostic procedure. While VUR spontaneously resolves in most children several years after detection, prompt treatment of UTIs in children with reflux is important to minimize the risk of pyelonephritis and renal scarring. Spontaneous remission of grades I, II, and III reflux may occur in 50% to 80% of children younger than 5 years of age. Approximately 20% of grades IV and V will resolve. Because of the spontaneous remission, treatment of children with VUR is controversial. There are three options are available: correcting the VUR with surgery, using long-term antimicrobial prophylaxis, or careful monitoring of the child. The goal is to prevent kidney infection and reduce scarring.[38,42]

URINARY INCONTINENCE

Urinary incontinence refers to the involuntary passage of urine by a child, without underlying anatomical neurological abnormalities, who is beyond the age when voluntary bladder control should have been acquired. Bladder control is accomplished by most children before the age of 5 years, although this is largely influenced by cultural beliefs and parental toilet training practices. Wetness that occurs during the day is called daytime incontinence. Nighttime wetting is called nocturnal enuresis. Functional incontinence is urinary incontinence in which no structural or neurologic abnormality can be identified.

The incidence of incontinence is difficult to determine because it is not a problem parents often discuss. The incidence of enuresis in children older than 5 years ranges from 15% to 20%. Boys are more enuretic than girls by a ratio of 2:1. Enuresis resolves at a rate of 15% per year. Daytime incontinence occurs in approximately 9% of early school-age children.[43]

Pathophysiology. A combination of factors is likely to be responsible for incontinence. A reasonable approach is to eliminate organic or physiologic causes before exploring psychological ones. Organic causes account for a minority of cases and include UTIs; neurologic disturbances; congenital defects of the meatus, urethra, or bladder neck; and allergies. Disorders that increase the normal output of urine, such as diabetes mellitus and diabetes insipidus, or disorders that impair the concentrating ability of the kidney, such as CKD or sickle cell disease, must be considered during evaluation. Other conditions that may be associated with incontinence include perinatal anoxia, CNS trauma, seizures, attention-deficit/hyperactivity disorder, developmental delay, imperforate anus, bladder trauma or surgery, obesity, and occult spinal dysraphism. Altered sleep arousal or obstructive sleep apnea may be associated with enuresis. Stressful psychologic situations, such as a new sibling, may cause incontinence or enuresis to develop. Constipation is frequently present in children with urinary incontinence.

Genetic factors contribute to some types of incontinence. At least four gene loci associated with enuresis have been identified. Urinary incontinence occurs with high frequency among parents, siblings, and other near relatives of symptomatic children. There is a high concordance rate in monozygotic twins with enuresis.[44]

Clinical Manifestations. Primary incontinence (enuresis) means the child has never been continent. Secondary incontinence (enuresis) means the child has been continent for at least 6 months before wetting recurs. A child may have daytime incontinence, enuresis, or a combination of both. Types of incontinence and clinical manifestations are defined in Table 39.4.

Evaluation and Treatment. Evaluation of incontinence includes assessment of associated conditions summarized above, use of questionnaires, drinking and voiding charts, physical examination, and urinalysis. Underlying pathology, including kidney disease, VUR, UTI, or neurogenic bladder, needs to be excluded. Radiologic and urodynamic evaluation may be required to identify anatomical abnormalities of the genitourinary tract.[38] While bladder dysfunction tends to spontaneously resolve over time, therapeutic management of incontinence begins with education. If the child and family understand the probable etiology of the child's condition, they are better able to choose and participate in therapies that are most likely to succeed. Treatment of daytime incontinence includes behavioral therapy, including timed voiding; fluid management; treatment of constipation, UTI, and other coexisting conditions if present; and medication (e.g., desmopressin). Enuresis treatment also may include enuresis alarms.[45]

TABLE 39.4 Types of Incontinence

Type	Definition
Diurnal enuresis Daytime voiding frequency	Decreased: 3 or fewer voids per day Increased: 8 or more voids per day
Dysfunctional voiding	Habitual contraction of urethral sphincter during voiding; observed by uroflow measurements; normal micturition frequency, incontinence, urinary tract infections, enuresis
Nocturnal Enuresis	Incontinence of urine while sleeping
Incontinence, continuous	Continuous leakage, not in discrete portions
Incontinence, stress	Leakage with raised intra-abdominal pressure
Urgency	Sudden, unexpected, immediate need to void
Overactive bladder	Increased detrusor contractions; urinary urgency; increased micturition frequency; and/or incontinence may or may not be present
Underactive bladder	Decreased detrusor contractions; low micturition frequency; decreased micturition frequency with use of raised intra-abdominal pressure to void
Urge incontinence	Incontinence in children with urgency

Adapted from Nieuwhof-Leppink AJ, Schroeder RPJ, van de Putte EM, et al. Daytime urinary incontinence in children and adolescents. *Lancet Child Adolescent Health*, 2019;3(7):492–501; Nevéus T, von Gontard A, Hoebeke P, et al. The standardization of terminology of lower urinary tract function in children and adolescents: Report from the Standardisation Committee of the International Children's Continence Society. *Journal of Urology*, 2006;176(1):314–324..

SUMMARY REVIEW

Structural Abnormalities

1. Congenital abnormalities of the kidney and urinary tract are related to gene alterations in about 50% of cases, range in severity from minor conditions that need no treatment to those incompatible with life, and often occur with other structural malformations.
2. A hypoplastic kidney is small, with a decreased number of nephrons. A dysplastic kidney is the result of abnormal differentiation of renal tissues.
3. Polycystic kidney disease is a cystic genetic disorder that can be autosomal dominant or autosomal recessive and results in multiple kidney cysts that interfere with renal function and cause hypertension.
4. Renal agenesis is the absence of one or both kidneys and may occur as an isolated entity or in association with other disorders.
5. Ureteropelvic junction obstruction is blockage where the renal pelvis joins the ureter or at the bladder neck or posterior urethra and is often caused by smooth muscle or urothelial malformation or by secondary scarring as a complication of corrective surgery. Complications include hydronephrosis and infection.
6. Hypospadias is a congenital anomaly in which the urethral meatus can be located anywhere on the ventral surface of the glans, the penile shaft, the midline of the scrotum, or the perineum.

7. Epispadias and exstrophy of the bladder are congenital malformations expressed to a different degree. Epispadias involves the dorsal urethra failing to form a tube. In exstrophy, the pubic bones are separated, and the posterior wall of the bladder is everted through the opening.
8. Urethral valves and polyps are congenital formations of tissue that block the urethra.

Glomerular Disorders

1. Glomerulonephritis is an inflammation of the glomeruli. The cause is unknown but is often immune mediated.
2. Acute poststreptococcal glomerulonephritis usually follows infection by nephritic strains of group A β-hemolytic streptococcus. Immune deposits or formation promote injury and increase glomerular capillary permeability leading to hematuria, proteinuria, edema, hypertension, and renal insufficiency.
3. Immunoglobulin A (IgA) nephropathy occurs with autoimmune deposition of IgA in the glomerulus, causing glomerular injury with gross hematuria. IgA vasculitis (Henoch-Schönlein purpura nephritis) is a particular form of IgA nephropathy that involves a systemic vasculitis.
4. Nephrotic syndrome is a group of symptoms characterized by severe proteinuria, hypoalbuminemia, hyperlipidemia, and edema. Metabolic, biochemical, or physiochemical disturbances in the glomerular basement membrane may lead to increased permeability to protein. Minimal change nephropathy and focal segmental glomerulosclerosis are the most common causes of nephrotic syndrome in children.
5. Hemolytic uremic syndrome is an acute thrombotic microangiopathy characterized by hemolytic anemia, thrombocytopenia, and may cause acute renal failure. Typical HUS is associated with bacterial and viral toxins, particularly Shiga toxin of *Escherichia coli* infection and diarrhea.

Nephroblastoma

1. Nephroblastoma (Wilms tumor) is an embryonal tumor of the kidney that usually presents as a solid, smooth abdominal mass between birth and 5 years of age. Survival is high after treatment by surgery, a combination of drugs, and, for advanced disease, combination chemotherapy, radiation therapy, and stem cell therapy.

Bladder Disorders

1. Urinary tract infections (UTIs) result from bacteria ascending the urethra and occur anywhere along the urinary tract. The bladder alone is infected in cystitis. The infection ascends to one or both kidneys in pyelonephritis.
2. Vesicoureteral reflux is the retrograde flow of bladder urine into the kidney or ureter, or both, increasing the risk for pyelonephritis. It can be unilateral or bilateral; primary or secondary.

Urinary Incontinence

1. Urinary incontinence is the involuntary passage of urine by a child beyond the age of 5 years when bladder control should have been acquired. It may occur during the day (daytime incontinence) or at night (nocturnal enuresis), or both. Maturational delay, UTIs, constipation, and many other physiologic and emotional factors may contribute.

REFERENCES

1. Natsis K, et al. Horseshoe kidney: a review of anatomy and pathology. *Surg Radiol Anat*. 2013;36(6):517–526.
2. Sanna-Cherchi S, et al. Genetic basis of human congenital anomalies of the kidney and urinary tract. *J Clin Invest*. 2018; 128(1):4–15.
3. Chen RY, Chang H. Renal dysplasia. *Arch Pathol Lab Med*. 2015;139(4):547–551.
4. Prasad S, Kaler AK, Sharif S. Ask-Upmark kidney: a report of 2 cases. *Int J Health Sci Res*. 2013;3(1):61–64. Available at https://www.ijhsr.org/IJHSR_Vol.3_Issue.1_Jan2013/13.pdf. (Accessed November 17, 2021).
5. Cordido A, Besada-Cerecedo L, García-González MA. The genetic and cellular basis of autosomal dominant polycystic kidney disease—a primer for clinicians. *Front Pediatr*. 2017;5:279.
6. Rosenblum S, Pal A, Reidy K. Renal development in the fetus and premature infant. *Semin Fetal Neonatal Med*. 2017;22(2):58–66.
7. Hodges SJ, et al. Megaureter. *ScientificWorldJournal*. 2012;10:603–612.
8. Timberlake MD, Corbett ST. Minimally invasive techniques for management of the ureterocele and ectopic ureter: upper tract versus lower tract approach. *Urol Clin North Am*. 2015;42(1):61–76.
9. Faiz S, et al. Role of antibiotic prophylaxis in the management of antenatal hydronephrosis, vesicoureteral reflux, and ureterocele in infants. *Cureus*. 2020;12(7):e9064.
10. Buschel H, Carroll D. Hypospadias. *Paediatr Child Health (Oxford)*. 2018;28(5):218–221. Available at https://doi.org/10.1016/j.paed.2018.03.006. (Accessed November 17, 2021).
11. Yu X, et al. Hypospadias prevalence and trends in international birth defect surveillance systems, 1980-2010. *Eur Urol*. 2019; 76(4):482–490. Available at https://doi.org/10.1016/j.eururo.2019.06.027. (Accessed November 17, 2021).
12. Dave S, et al. A retrospective population-based cohort study to evaluate the impact of an older sibling with undescended testis and hypospadias on the known maternal and fetal risk factors for undescended testis and hypospadias in Ontario, Canada, 1997-2007. *J Pediatr Urol*. 2019;15(1):41.e1–41.e9.
13. Cendron M, et al. Anatomic findings associated with epispadias in boys: implications for surgical management and urinary continence. *J Pediatr Urol*. 2018;14(1):42–46.
14. Suzuki K, et al. Epispadias and the associated embryopathies: genetic and developmental basis. *Clin Genet*. 2017;91(2):247–253.
15. Lloyd JC, et al. Contemporary epidemiological trends in complex congenital genitourinary anomalies. *J Urol*. 2013;190(4 Suppl): 1590–1595.
16. Promm M, Roesch WH. Recent trends in the management of bladder exstrophy: the Gordian knot has not yet been cut. *Front Pediatr*. 2019;7:110.
17. Vivante A, Hildebrandt F. Exploring the genetic basis of early-onset chronic kidney disease. *Nat Rev Nephrol*. 2016;12(3):133–146.
18. Ingelfinger FR, et al. World Kidney Day 2016, averting the legacy of kidney disease focus on childhood. *Clin Nephrol*. 2016;85(2): 63–69.
19. Hunt EAK, Somers MJG. Infection-related glomerulonephritis. *Pediatr Clin North Am*. 2019;66(1):59–72.
20. Kliegman RM, St. Geme J, eds. *Nelson Textbook of Pediatrics*. ed 21, Philadelphia: Elsevier; 2020.

21. Balasubramanian R, Marks SD. Post-infectious glomerulonephritis. *Paediatr Int Child Health*. 2017;37(4):240–247.
22. Chang S, Li XK. The role of immune modulation in pathogenesis of IgA nephropathy. *Front Med (Lausanne)*. 2020;7:92.
23. Dyga K, Szczepańska M. IgA vasculitis with nephritis in children. *Adv Clin Exp Med*. 2020;29(4):513–519.
24. Wang CS, Greenbaum LA. Nephrotic syndrome. *Pediatr Clin North Am*. 2019;66(1):73–85.
25. Vivarelli M, et al. Minimal change disease. *Clin J Am Soc Nephrol*. 2017;12(2):332–345.
26. Nagata M, Kobayashi N, Hara S. Focal segmental glomerulosclerosis: why does it occur segmentally? *Pflugers Arch*. 2017;469(7–8):983–988.
27. Kidney Disease Improving Global Outcomes (KDIGO) Glomerulonephritis Work Group: KDIGO clinical practice guidelines for glomerulonephritis. *Kidney Int Suppl (2011)*. 2012;2(2):139–274.
28. Lee JM, et al. Current understandings in treating children with steroid-resistant nephrotic syndrome. *Pediatr Nephrol*. 2021;36(4):747–761.
29. Raina R, et al. Atypical hemolytic-uremic syndrome: an update on pathophysiology, diagnosis, and treatment. *Ther Apher Dial*. 2019;23(1):4–21.
30. Sheerin NS, Glover E. Haemolytic uremic syndrome: diagnosis and management. *F1000Res*. 2019;8 F1000 Faculty Rev-1690.
31. Tsai HM. Atypical hemolytic uremic syndrome: beyond hemolysis and uremia. *Am J Med*. 2019;132(2):161–167.
32. PDQ Pediatric Treatment Editorial Board: *Wilms tumor and other childhood kidney tumors treatment (PDQ®): health professional version*. In: *PDQ Cancer Information Summaries*. Bethesda, MD: National Cancer Institute; 2021. Published online October 8, 2021. Available at https://www.ncbi.nlm.nih.gov/books/NBK65842/. (Accessed November 17, 2021).
33. Cotterill SJ. Wilms tumour. *Cancer Genetics Web*. Available at http://www.cancer-genetics.org/X210202.htm. (Accessed November 17, 2021).
34. American Cancer Society (ACS): *Signs and Symptoms of Wilms Tumors*. Kennesaw, GA: ACS; 2018. Last revised October 17, 2018. Available at https://www.cancer.org/cancer/wilms-tumor/detection-diagnosis-staging/signs-and-symptoms.html. (Accessed November 17, 2021).
35. Romao RL, Lorenzo AJ. Renal function in patients with Wilms tumor. *Urol Oncol*. 2016;34(1):33–41.
36. Bhutani N, Kajal P, Sharma U. Many faces of Wilms tumor: recent advances and future directions. *Ann Med Surg (Lond)*. 2021;64:102202.
37. Cozzi DA, Ceccanti S, Cozzi F. Renal function up to the 5th decade of life after nephrectomy in childhood: a literature review. *Nephrology (Carlton)*. 2018;23(5):397–404.
38. Tullus K, Shaikh N. Urinary tract infections in children. *Lancet*. 2020;395(10237):1659–1668.
39. Roberts KB. Urinary tract infection: clinical practice guideline for the diagnosis and management of the initial UTI in febrile infants and children 2 to 24 months. *Pediatrics*. 2011;128:595–610.
40. Millner R, Becknell B. Urinary tract infections. *Pediatr Clin North Am*. 2019;66(1):1–13.
41. Hunziker M, Puri P. Familial vesicoureteral reflux and reflux related morbidity in relatives of index patients with high grade vesicoureteral reflux. *J Urol*. 2012;188(4 Suppl):1463–1466.
42. Läckgren G, et al. Management of vesicoureteral reflux: what have we learned over the last 20 years? *Front Pediatr*. 2021;9:650326.
43. Abdulkadir A, et al. Prevalence of enuresis among children and adolescents: a systematic review and meta-analysis. *Sahel Medical Journal*. 2019;22:157–163. Available at http://www.doi.org/10.4103/smj.smj_41_18. (Accessed November 17, 2021).
44. von Gontard A, Heron J, Joinson C. Family history of nocturnal enuresis and urinary incontinence: results from a large epidemiological study. *J Urol*. 2011;185(6):2303–2306.
45. Gontard AV, Kuwertz-Bröking E. The diagnosis and treatment of enuresis and functional daytime urinary incontinence. *Dtsch Arztebl Int*. 2019;116(16):279–285.

40

Structure and Function of the Digestive System

Karen C. Turner

http://evolve.elsevier.com/Rogers/pathophysiology/

CHAPTER OUTLINE

The digestive system includes the gastrointestinal (GI) tract and accessory organs of digestion: the liver, gallbladder, and exocrine pancreas (Fig. 40.1). The GI system carries out at least four major functions: digestion of food, absorption of nutrients, secretion of hormones, and defense against pathogens. The digestive system breaks down ingested food, prepares it for uptake by the body's cells, absorbs fluid, and eliminates wastes. The GI tract and gut microbiome provide important immune and protective functions. Except for chewing, swallowing, and defecation of solid wastes, the movements of the digestive system (peristalsis) are all controlled by hormones and the autonomic nervous system (ANS).

Food breakdown begins in the mouth with chewing and continues in the stomach, where food is mixed with acid, mucus, and enzymes. From the stomach, the fluid and partially digested food pass into the small intestine, where bile and enzymes secreted by the intestinal cells, liver, gallbladder, and exocrine pancreas break it down into absorbable components of proteins, carbohydrates, and fats. These nutrients pass through the walls of the small intestine into underlying blood and lymphatic vessels, which carry them to the liver for storage or further processing. Ingested substances and secretions not absorbed in the small intestine pass into the large intestine, where fluid continues to be absorbed. Fluid wastes travel to the kidneys and are eliminated in the urine. Solid wastes pass into the rectum and are eliminated from the body through the anus.

THE GASTROINTESTINAL TRACT

The gastrointestinal tract (alimentary canal) is a single, hollow tube that consists of the mouth, esophagus, stomach, small intestine, large intestine, rectum, and anus (see Fig. 40.1). It carries out these digestive processes:

1. Ingestion of food
2. Propulsion of food and wastes from the mouth to the anus
3. Secretion of mucus, water, and enzymes (Box 40.1)
4. Mechanical digestion of food particles
5. Chemical digestion of food particles
6. Absorption of digested food
7. Elimination of waste products by defecation
8. Immune and microbial protection against infection

Histologically, the GI tract consists of four layers. From the inside out they are the mucosa, submucosa, muscularis, and serosa or adventitia (Fig. 40.2). These concentric layers vary in thickness, and each layer has sublayers. Neurons forming the

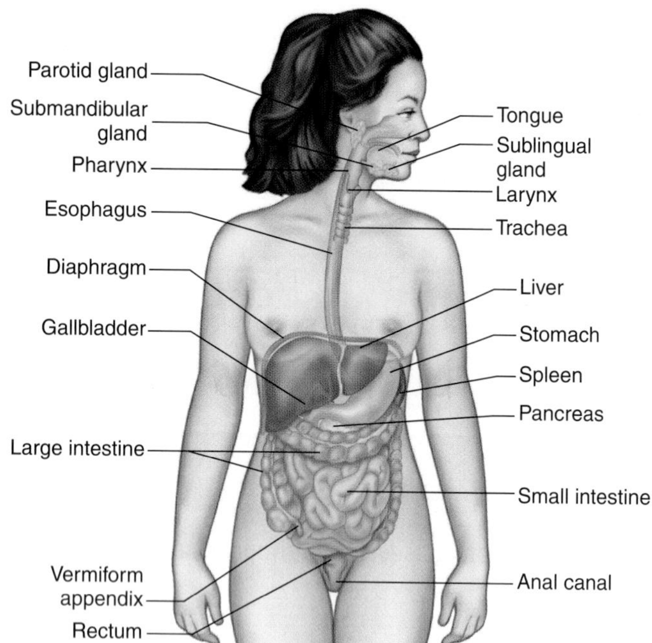

Fig. 40.1 Structures of the Digestive System. (From Patton KT, Thibodeau GA. *The Human Body in Health & Disease.* 7th ed. St Louis: Elsevier; 2018.)

BOX 40.1 Sources of Digestive Enzymes

Salivary Glands
Amylase
Lingual lipase

Stomach
Pepsin
Gastric lipase

Pancreas
Amylase
Trypsin
Chymotrypsin
Carboxypeptidase
Elastase
Lipase-colipase
Phospholipase A_2
Cholesterol esterase–nonspecific lipase

Small Intestine
Enterokinase
Disaccharidases
Maltase
Sucrase
Lactase
α,α'-1 Trehalase
Isomaltase
Peptidases
Amino-oligopeptidase
Dipeptidase

From Johnson LR. *Gastrointestinal Physiology*. 9th ed. St Louis: Mosby; 2019.

enteric nervous system are located solely within the GI tract and are controlled by local and ANS stimuli. The enteric nervous system comprises three nerve plexuses located in different layers of the GI walls (see Fig. 40.2). The submucosal (Meissner) plexus is located in the muscularis mucosae, the myenteric (Auerbach) plexus is between the inner circular and outer longitudinal muscle layers in the muscularis, and the subserosal plexus is just beneath the serosa. The neurons from the entire enteric (intramural) plexus regulate motility reflexes, blood flow, absorption, secretions, and immune response.

Mouth and Esophagus

The mouth is the site for mastication (chewing) and mixing of food with saliva. There are 32 permanent teeth in the adult mouth, and they are important for speech and mastication. As food particles become smaller and move around in the mouth, taste buds are continuously stimulated, adding to the satisfaction of eating. The tongue's surface and soft palate have thousands of taste buds that contain taste receptors. These can distinguish salty, sour, bitter, sweet, and savory (umami) tastes. Tastes and food odors, which stimulate the olfactory nerve (cranial nerve [CN] I), help to initiate salivation and the secretion of gastric juice in the stomach.

Salivation

The four pairs of salivary glands—the submandibular, sublingual, parotid, and tubarial glands (Fig. 40.3) secrete about 1 to 1.5 L of saliva per day.[1] Saliva consists mostly of water with varying amounts of mucus, sodium, bicarbonate, chloride, potassium, and salivary α-amylase (ptyalin), an enzyme that initiates carbohydrate digestion in the mouth and stomach.

The composition of saliva and other gastric juices depends on the rate of secretion (Fig. 40.4A). Aldosterone can increase the epithelial exchange of sodium for potassium, increasing sodium conservation and potassium excretion. The bicarbonate concentration of saliva sustains a pH of about 7.4, which neutralizes bacterial acids and prevents tooth decay. Saliva also contains mucin, immunoglobulin A (IgA), and other antimicrobial substances, which help prevent infection. Mucin provides lubrication. Exogenous fluoride (e.g., fluoride in drinking water) is also secreted in the saliva, providing additional protection against tooth decay.

Both the sympathetic and parasympathetic divisions of the ANS control salivation. Cholinergic parasympathetic fibers stimulate the salivary glands, and atropine (an anticholinergic agent) inhibits salivation and makes the mouth dry. β-Adrenergic stimulation from sympathetic fibers also increases salivary secretion. Hormones do not regulate salivary gland secretion, although hormones are found in saliva (e.g., cortisol, testosterone, and estradiol) and aldosterone regulates salivary sodium secretion. Changes in salivary hormones can be tested in a variety of conditions, including monitoring of fetal development during pregnancy.[2]

Swallowing

Swallowing is a complex event by which a food bolus travels from the oropharynx through the esophagus and into the stomach. Swallowing is mediated by the trigeminal nucleus, nucleus tractus solitarius, and reticular formation of the brainstem, as well as other brain regions, including the insula/claustrum and cerebellum. In addition to ensuring the sequential movement of food from the oropharynx into the esophagus, these neural pathways modulate the swallowing process to accommodate changing size and viscosity of a food bolus.[3]

Swallowing occurs in two phases: the oropharyngeal phase and the esophageal phase. During the oropharyngeal (voluntary) phase, which takes 1 or 2 seconds, the movements of the tongue and pharyngeal constrictors propel the food into the esophagus in a series of coordinated events. The following steps occur:

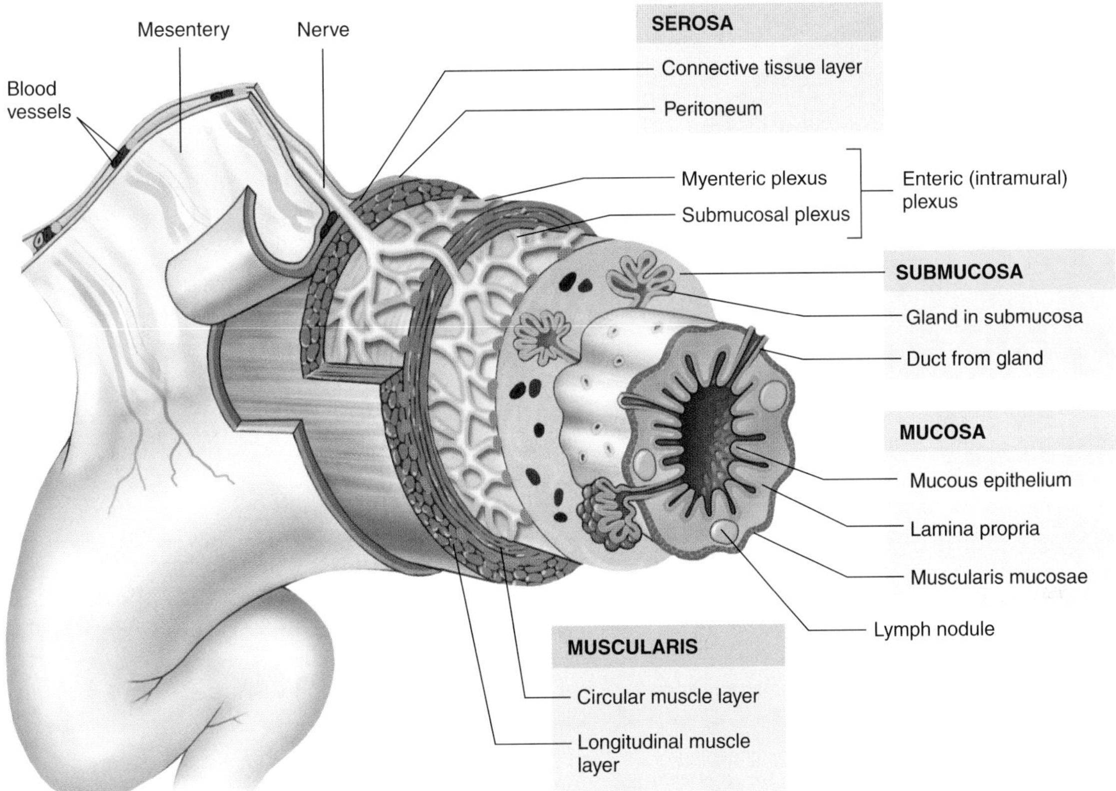

Fig. 40.2 Wall of the Gastrointestinal Tract. The wall of the gastrointestinal tract is made up of four layers with a network of nerves between the layers. This generalized diagram shows a segment of the gastrointestinal tract. Note that the serosa is continuous with a fold of serous membrane called the *mesentery*. Note also that digestive glands may empty their products into the lumen of the gastrointestinal tract by way of ducts. (From Patton KT, Thibodeau GA. *The human body in health & disease*, 7th ed. St Louis: Mosby, 2018.)

1. Food is segmented into a bolus by the tongue and forced posteriorly toward the pharynx as the tongue pushes upward against the hard palate.
2. The superior constrictor muscle of the pharynx contracts so the food cannot move into the nasopharynx.
3. Respiration is inhibited, and the epiglottis slides down to prevent the food from entering the larynx and trachea.
4. The upper esophageal sphincter (cricopharyngeal muscle) opens to allow the food bolus to pass into the esophagus, then closes again to prevent air from entering the esophagus during respiration.[4]

During the esophageal (involuntary) phase, which takes 8 to 10 seconds, the bolus is transported to the stomach by the coordinated sequential contraction and relaxation of outer longitudinal and inner circular layers of smooth muscle around the esophageal lumen. This phase proceeds as follows:

1. The bolus of food enters the esophagus.
2. Waves of muscular relaxation move along the esophagus, preparing for the movement of the bolus.
3. Peristalsis, the sequential waves of muscular contractions that travel down the esophagus, transports the food to the lower esophageal sphincter.
4. The lower esophageal sphincter relaxes, and the bolus enters the stomach, after which the sphincter muscles return to their resting tone.

The esophagus is a hollow, muscular tube approximately 25 cm long that conducts substances from the oropharynx to the stomach (see Fig. 40.1). The esophageal mucosa consists of squamous epithelium that transitions to columnar epithelium at the gastroesophageal junction. The pharynx and upper third of the esophagus contain striated muscle (voluntary) that is directly innervated by skeletal motor neurons that control swallowing. The middle third contains a mix of striated and smooth muscle, and the lower third contains smooth muscle (involuntary) that is innervated by preganglionic cholinergic fibers from the vagus nerve (CN X).

Peristalsis that immediately follows the oropharyngeal phase of swallowing is called primary peristalsis. Primary peristalsis results from the contraction of striated muscle in the upper esophagus. Increased tension in the esophageal wall stimulates stretch receptors to activate vagal afferent nerves that then elicit impulses from the swallowing center of the brain.[5] These impulses cause sequential contraction and relaxation of the smooth muscle in the mid and lower esophagus called secondary peristalsis, which propels the food bolus toward the gastroesophageal junction.

The lower esophageal sphincter (cardiac sphincter) is located near the gastroesophageal junction—the opening in the diaphragm just below where the esophagus ends at the stomach. At rest, the tonic contraction of circular muscle fibers called clasp

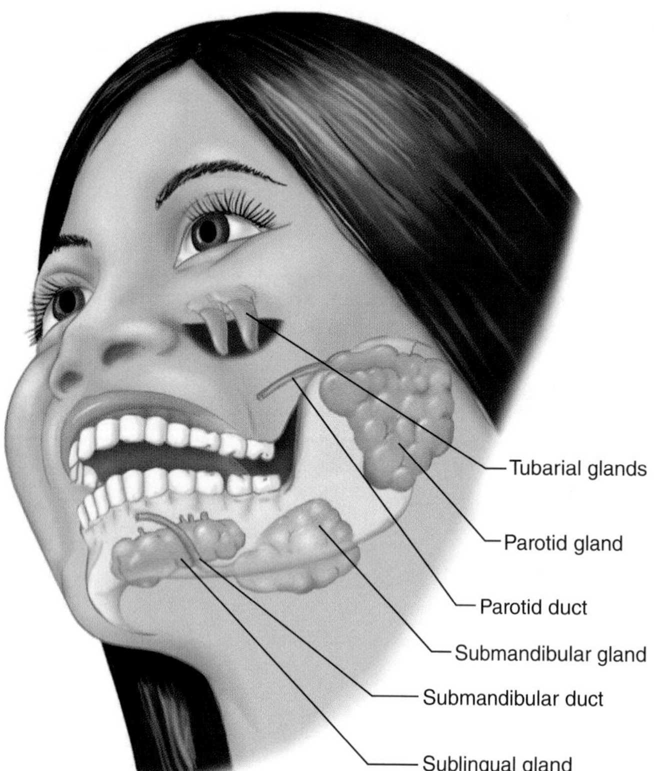

Fig. 40.3 Salivary Glands. (Adapted from Patton KT, Thibodeau GA. *The Human Body in Health & Disease.* 7th ed. St Louis: Elsevier; 2018.)

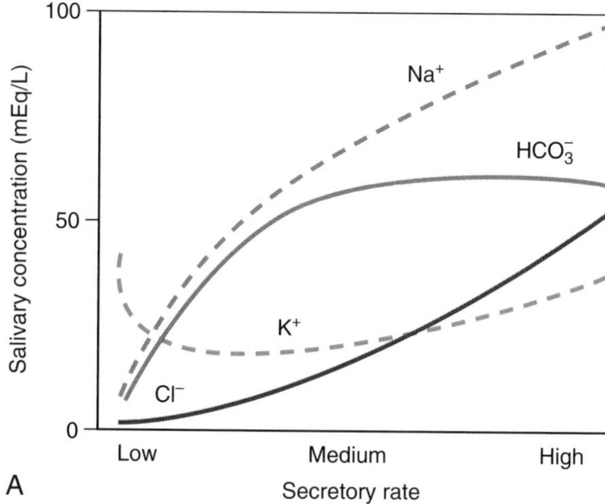

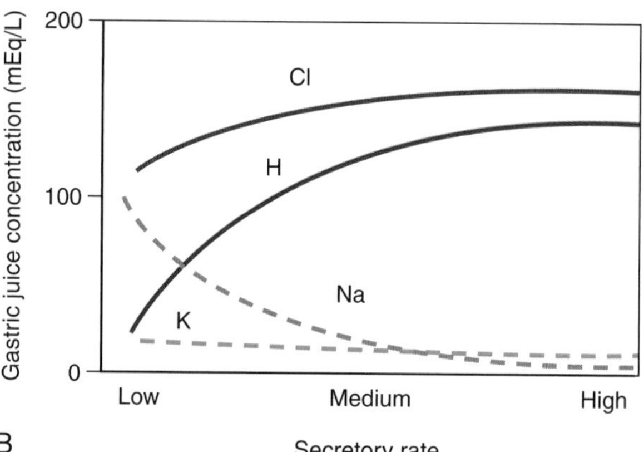

Fig. 40.4 Electrolyte Concentrations and Flow Rate. (A) Saliva. Changes in the concentrations of sodium (Na^+), potassium (K^+), chloride (Cl^-), and bicarbonate (HCO_3^-) increase the flow rate of saliva. At low rates of salivary flow (e.g., between meals), Na^+, Cl^-, and HCO_3^- are reabsorbed in the collecting ducts of the salivary glands and the saliva contains fewer of these electrolytes (i.e., is more hypotonic). At higher flow rates (e.g., when stimulated by food), reabsorption decreases and saliva is hypertonic. By this mechanism, Na^+, Cl^-, and HCO_3^- are recycled until they are released to help with digestion and absorption. (B) Gastric juice. The Na^+ concentration is lower in the gastric juice than in the plasma, whereas the hydrogen (H^+), potassium (K^+), and Cl^- concentrations are higher.

fibers in the lower esophageal sphincter prevents gastroesophageal reflex.[6] The muscle tone of the lower esophageal sphincter changes with neural and hormonal stimulation and relaxes with swallowing. Cholinergic vagal input and the digestive hormone gastrin increase sphincter tone. Nitric oxide is the main neurotransmitter involved in relaxation of the sphincter muscles.[5] Noradrenergic, noncholinergic vagal impulses relax the lower esophageal sphincter, as do the hormones progesterone, secretin, and glucagon.

The Abdominal Cavity

The abdominal cavity contains all the organs of digestion including the lower part of the esophagus, stomach, intestines, liver, gallbladder, pancreas, spleen, kidneys, adrenal glands and their blood, lymphatic supply, and innervation. The supporting structures of the abdominal cavity are the mesentery, peritoneum, and omentum. The boundaries of the abdominal cavity are the diaphragm (superior), the inferior muscular layer of the true pelvic cavity (inferior), the vertebral column (posterior), and the abdominal muscles (anterior).

The mesentery is a double fold of peritoneum composed of several contiguous segments. Classically, the segments were thought to be discontinuous and only provide structural support. Recent evidence from embryology, tissue analysis, and imaging have redefined the mesentery as an internal organ in which all abdominal digestive organs develop and maintains these organs in systemic continuity in adulthood. Organs not of "mesenteric" embryonic origin and anatomical position are described as "non-mesenteric" and includes the kidneys and adrenal glands.[7] The mesentery provides a conduit for lymphatics, blood vessels, and nerves and is continuous from the esophago-gastric to anorectal junction. It has different segments or regions generally named for the parts of the intestine to which it attaches (Fig. 40.5A and B). It is these segments that were classically thought not to be components of a single organ. The small intestinal mesentery segment is fan shaped and arises from the *mesenteric root*. The root is about 15 cm long and 20 cm wide and extends from the duodenojejunal flexure (near the left part of the second lumbar vertebrae) to the ileocolic junction (at the right sacroiliac joint). Toldt fascia provides the points of anchorage between the mesentery and the abdominal wall

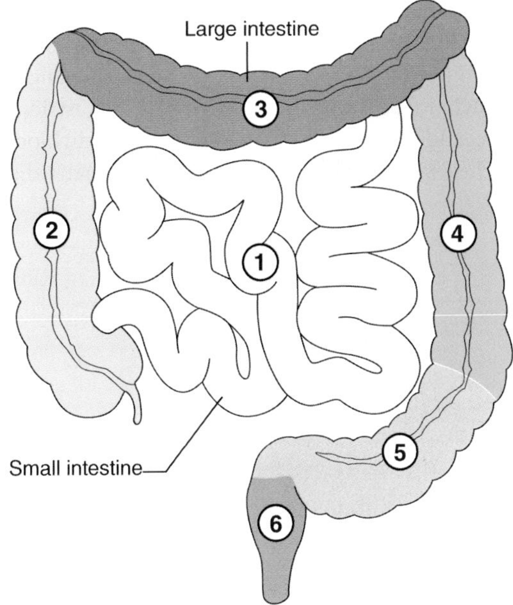

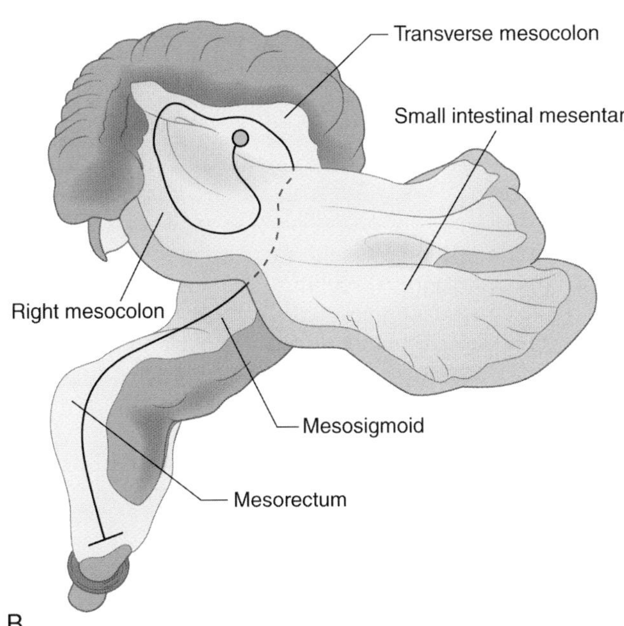

Fig. 40.5 The Mesentery Segments. **(A)** Location of the continuous mesentery: **1**. Small-intestinal mesentery—connects the loops of jejunum and ileum to the posterior abdominal wall and is a mobile structure; **2**. Right mesocolon runs flat against the right posterior abdominal wall; **3**.Transverse mesocolon—a mobile area of mesentery that lies between the colic flexures; **4**. Left mesocolon: runs flat against the left posterior abdominal wall; **5**. Mesosigmoid—has a medial portion which is flattened against the posterior abdominal wall, whereas the region of mesentery associated with the sigmoid colon itself is mobile; **6**. Mesorectum—assists in anchoring the rectum through the pelvis. **(B)** Digital representation of the intestinal mesentery. (Data from A, Cresci GAM, Izzo K. Gut microbiome. In *Adult Short Bowel Syndrome*. 2019;45–54. https://doi.org/10.1016/b978-0-12-814330-8.00004-4. B, From Coffey JC, O'Leary DP. The mesentery: structure, function, and role in disease. *Lancet Gastroenterol Hepatol*. 2016;1[3];238–247. https://doi.org/10.1016/s2468-1253(16)30026-7.)

BOX 40.2 Functions of the Mesentery

Functions of the Mesentery

Supports embryonic development of abdominal organs of digestion by providing molecular and cellular signals (mesenteric organogenesis).

Maintains abdominal digestive organs in position and in continuity with all other body systems.

Reduces friction and supports free movement, prevents twisting, and dislocation into the pelvic area.

Stores fat, regulates glycemic and lipid metabolism, and provides organs with rapid access to metabolic substrates.

Is a major source of systemic C-reactive protein when there is intestinal inflammation.

with additional support from the peritoneum and omentum. The mesenteric segments have both structural and physiologic functions (Box 40.2).[8]

The superior and inferior mesenteric arteries and veins provide the circulation to the mesentery. Innervation is provided by the superior mesenteric plexus which divides into many secondary plexuses and contains parasympathetic and sympathetic innervation to the organs associated with the mesentery. Both lymph nodes and lymph vessel are contained within the mesentery. Considering the mesentery as an organ, with both structural and functional significance, expands clinical implications of the mesentery as an organ of disease or contributing to the cause of systemic diseases. The mesentery can become a significant source of fat deposition. Excess fat is associated with metabolic syndrome and inflammation. In diseases such as Crohn disease (an autoimmune inflammatory bowel disease–see Chapter 41), the mesentery may be a source of inflammation, contributing to increased permeability and bacterial invasion making the mesentery a target for pharmacologic interventions.[9] The conceptualization is also important in selecting and interpreting different radiologic techniques and findings as well as surgical decisions about whether to remove mesenteric tissue for cancer treatment or inflammatory diseases of the intestine and other digestive organs.[8] The mesentery as an organ has been implicated in the development of systemic inflammation. Mechanisms by which the mesentery contributes to systemic inflammatory response syndrome (SIRS) and multiple organ dysfunction syndrome are under investigation.

The peritoneum is a serous membrane surrounding the organs of the abdomen and pelvic cavity. It is analogous to the pericardium around the heart and the pleura around the lungs. The *visceral peritoneum* lies on the surface of the organs, and the *parietal peritoneum* lines the wall of the body cavity. The space between these two layers is called the peritoneal cavity (peritoneal space) and normally contains a thin layer of fluid to lubricate the two layers and prevent friction during organ movement.

The omentum is an intraabdominal organ composed of a large flat layer of adipose tissue with two parts. The *greater omentum* arises from the greater curvature of the stomach and spleen, drapes over the transverse colon, and separates the abdomen into greater and lesser sacs. It has a double fold that connects the stomach to the posterior abdominal wall. The *lesser omentum* arises from the lesser curvature of the stomach and contains the only opening between the greater and lesser sacs (epiploic foramen or foramen of Winslow) providing communication between them. As an organ, the omentum has multiple functions including fat storage; protection of underlying structures; immune regulation (contains immune cells known as "milky spots"); participation in infection control; and wound healing and tissue regeneration, including activation of stem cells and neovascularization.[10]

Stomach

The stomach is a hollow, muscular organ just below the diaphragm (Fig. 40.6) that stores food during eating, secretes digestive juices, mixes food with these juices, and propels partially digested food, called chyme, into the duodenum of the small intestine. Functional areas are the fundus (upper portion), body (middle portion), and antrum (lower portion). Its major anatomic boundaries are:

- The lower esophageal sphincter, where food passes through the cardiac orifice at the gastroesophageal junction into the stomach.
- The pyloric sphincter, which relaxes as food is propelled through the pylorus (gastroduodenal junction) into the duodenum.

The stomach has three layers of smooth muscle: an outer, longitudinal layer; a middle, circular layer; and an inner, oblique layer (see Fig. 40.6).[6] These layers become progressively thicker in the body and antrum where food is mixed, churned, and pushed into the duodenum. The circular layer is most prominent, the oblique layer is the least complete, and the longitudinal layer is absent on the anterior and posterior surfaces. The interior of the stomach is lined with mucosa. When the stomach is empty, this mucosal layer sits in folds called rugae. Few substances are absorbed in the stomach. The stomach mucosa is impermeable to water but can absorb alcohol and aspirin because they are lipid soluble. The stomach's blood supply comes from a branch of the celiac artery (Fig. 40.7) and is so abundant that nearly all arterial vessels would need to be blocked before ischemic changes occur in the stomach wall. A series of small veins (short gastric, left and right gastric, and left and right gastro-omental) drain blood from the stomach toward the hepatic portal vein. Hepatic disorders

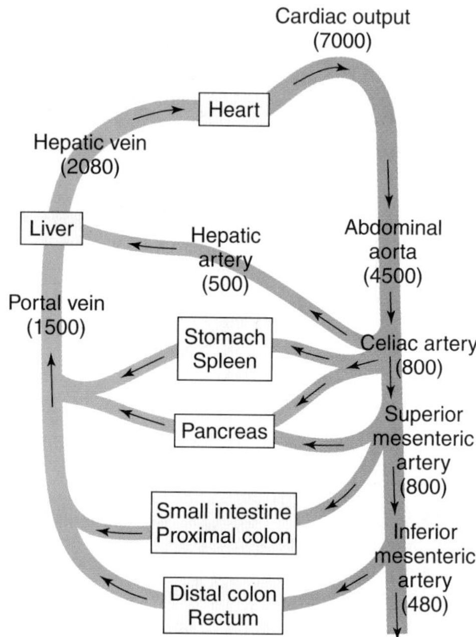

Fig. 40.7 Major Blood Vessels and Organs Supplied With Blood in the Splanchnic Circulation. Numbers in parentheses reflect approximate blood flow values (mL/min) for each major vessel in an 80-kg (176 lb) normal, resting, adult human. Arrows indicate the direction of blood flow. (Modified from Johnson LR. *Gastrointestinal Pathophysiology*. St Louis: Mosby; 2001.)

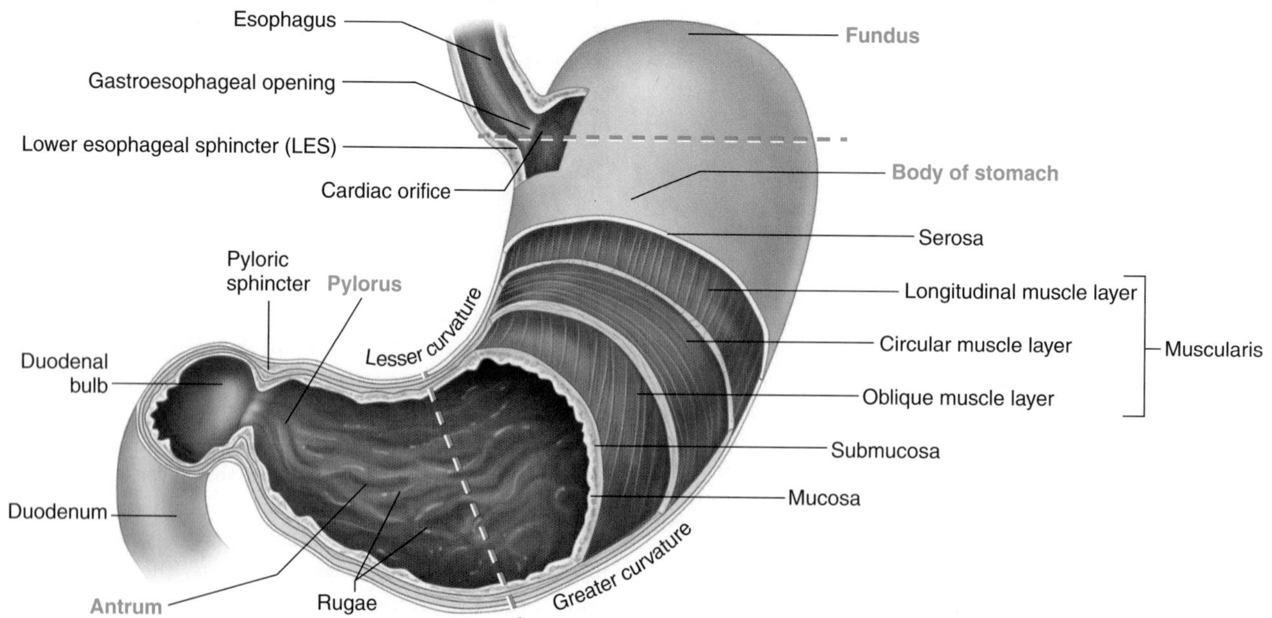

Fig. 40.6 The Stomach. A portion of the anterior wall has been excised to reveal the muscle layers of the stomach wall. Note that the mucosa lining the stomach forms folds called *rugae*. The dashed lines distinguish the fundus, body, and antrum of the stomach. (Modified from Patton KT, Thibodeau GA. *The Human Body in Health & Disease*. 7th ed. St Louis: Elsevier; 2018.)

that increase pressure in the portal vein can cause these gastric veins to dilate (varices) and bleed (see Chapter 41).

The sympathetic and parasympathetic divisions of the ANS innervate the stomach. Some of the autonomic fibers are extrinsic—that is, they originate outside the stomach. Impulses through these external autonomic fibers are controlled by nerve centers in the brain. The vagus nerve provides parasympathetic innervation and branches of the celiac plexus innervate the stomach sympathetically. The myenteric (Auerbach) plexus and submucosal (Meissner) plexus are intrinsic and part of the enteric (intramural) nervous system. They originate within the stomach and respond to local stimuli.

Gastric Motility

In its resting state, the stomach is small and contains about 50 mL of fluid. There is minimal wall tension, and the muscle layers in the fundus contract very little. Swallowing causes the fundus to relax (receptive relaxation) to receive a bolus of food from the esophagus. Relaxation is coordinated by efferent, nor-adrenergic, noncholinergic vagal fibers and is facilitated by two polypeptide hormones secreted by the GI mucosa—gastrin and cholecystokinin. (The actions of digestive hormones are summarized in Table 40.1.) These two hormones also play important roles in protecting the gastric mucosa during digestion and help to maintain the integrity of the islet cells in the pancreas.[11]

TABLE 40.1 Selected Hormones[a] and Neurotransmitters of the Digestive System

Source	Hormone/Neurotransmitter	Stimulus for Secretion	Action
Mucosa of the stomach	Gastrin	Presence of partially digested proteins in the stomach	Stimulates gastric glands to secrete hydrochloric acid, pepsinogen, and histamine; growth of gastric mucosa
	Histamine	Gastrin	Stimulates acid secretion
	Somatostatin	Acid in stomach	Inhibits acid, pepsinogen, and histamine secretion and release of gastrin
	Acetylcholine	Vagus and local nerves in stomach	Stimulates release of pepsinogen and acid secretion
	Gastrin-releasing peptide (bombesin)	Vagus and local nerves in stomach	Stimulates gastrin and release of pepsinogen and acid secretion
	Ghrelin	High during fasting	Stimulates growth hormone secretion and hypothalamus to increase appetite
Mucosa of the small intestine	Motilin	Presence of acid and fat in the duodenum	Increases gastrointestinal motility
	Secretin	Presence of chyme (acid, partially digested proteins, fats) in duodenum	Stimulates pancreas to secrete alkaline pancreatic juice and liver to secrete bile; decreases gastrointestinal motility; inhibits gastrin and gastric acid secretion
	Serotonin (5-hydroxytryptamine)	Intestinal distention; vagal stimulation; presence of acids, amino acids, or hypertonic fluids; released from enterochromaffin cells throughout intestine	Stimulates intestinal secretion, motility and sensation (i.e., pain and nausea), vasodilation; activates gut immune responses
	Cholecystokinin	Presence of chyme (acid, partially digested proteins, fats) in duodenum	Stimulates gallbladder to eject bile and pancreas to secrete alkaline fluid; decreases gastric motility; constricts pyloric sphincter; inhibits gastrin
	Enteroglucagon	Intraluminal fats and carbohydrates	Weakly inhibits gastric and pancreatic secretion and enhances insulin release, lipolysis, ketogenesis, and glycogenolysis
	Gastric inhibitory peptide (GIP)	Fat and glucose in the small intestine	Inhibits gastric secretion and emptying; stimulates insulin release
	Peptide YY	Intraluminal fat and bile acids	Inhibits postprandial gastric acid and pancreatic secretion and delays gastric and small bowel emptying
	Pancreatic polypeptide	Protein, fat, and glucose in the small intestine	Decreases pancreatic bicarbonate and enzyme secretion
	Vasoactive intestinal peptide	Intestinal mucosa and muscle	Relaxes intestinal smooth muscle

[a]The digestive hormones are not secreted into the gastrointestinal lumen, but rather into the bloodstream, where they travel to target tissues. Multiple peptide hormone genes and more than 100 hormonally active peptides are expressed in the gastrointestinal tract.

Modified from Johnson LR. *Gastrointestinal Physiology.*8th ed. St Louis: Mosby; 2014. Data from Feldman M, et al. *Sleisenger and Fordtran's Gastrointestinal and Liver Disease.* 10th ed. Philadelphia, PA: Saunders; 2015.

Food is stored in vertical or oblique layers as it arrives in the fundus, whereas fluids flow relatively quickly down to the antrum.

Gastric (stomach) motility increases with the initiation of peristaltic waves, which sweep over the body of the stomach toward the antrum. The rate of peristaltic contractions is approximately three per minute and is influenced by neural and hormonal activity. Gastrin, motilin (an intestinal hormone), and the vagus nerve increase the rate of contraction by lowering the threshold potential of muscle fibers. (The neural and biochemical mechanisms of muscle contraction are described in Chapter 43.) Motilin also impacts the brain-pancreas axis and influences insulin secretion during meals.[12] Sympathetic activity and secretin (another intestinal hormone) are inhibitory and raise the threshold potential as well as decrease gastric secretion (see Table 40.1). The rate of peristalsis is mediated by pacemaker cells that initiate a wave of depolarization (basic electrical rhythm), which moves from the upper part of the stomach to the pylorus.

Gastric mixing and subsequent emptying of gastric contents (chyme) from the stomach takes several hours. Mixing occurs as food is propelled toward the antrum. As food approaches the pylorus, the velocity of the peristaltic wave increases. This forces the contents back toward the body of the stomach. This retropulsion effectively mixes food with digestive juices, and the oscillating motion breaks down large food particles. With each peristaltic wave, a small portion of the chyme passes through the pylorus and into the duodenum. The pyloric sphincter is about 1.5 cm long and is always open about 2 mm. It opens wider during contraction of the antrum. Normally there is no regurgitation from the duodenum into the antrum.

The rate of gastric emptying (movement of chyme into the duodenum) depends on the volume, osmotic pressure, and chemical composition of the gastric contents. Larger volumes of food increase gastric pressure, peristalsis, and rate of emptying. Solids, fats, and nonisotonic solutions (i.e., hypertonic or hypotonic gastric tube feedings) delay gastric emptying. (Osmotic pressure and tonicity are described in Chapters 1 and 3.) Products of fat digestion, which are formed in the duodenum by the action of bile from the liver and enzymes from the pancreas, stimulate the secretion of cholecystokinin. This hormone inhibits food intake, reduces gastric motility, and decreases gastric emptying so that fats are not emptied into the duodenum at a rate that exceeds the rate of bile and enzyme secretion. Osmoreceptors in the wall of the duodenum are sensitive to the osmotic pressure of duodenal contents. The arrival of hypertonic or hypotonic gastric contents activates the osmoreceptors, which delays gastric emptying to facilitate formation of an isosmotic duodenal environment. The rate at which acid enters the duodenum also influences gastric emptying. Secretions from the pancreas, liver, and duodenal mucosa neutralize gastric hydrochloric acid in the duodenum. The rate of emptying is adjusted to the duodenum's ability to neutralize the incoming acidity. Peristaltic activity in the stomach is also affected by blood glucose levels. Low blood glucose levels stimulate the vagus nerve and gastric smooth muscles, increasing the rate of contraction and gastric emptying. Hyperglycemia delays gastric emptying.[13]

Gastric Secretion

Specialized cells located throughout the gastric mucosa secrete large volumes of gastric secretions, including acid, pepsinogen, mucus, enzymes, hormones, intrinsic factor, and gastroferrin. Acid converts inactive pepsinogen into the enzyme pepsin. Most of these secretions are released directly into the stomach lumen under neural and hormonal regulation. Intrinsic factor is necessary for the intestinal absorption of vitamin B_{12} (see Chapter 28), and gastroferrin facilitates the absorption of iron in the small intestine by preventing the formation of insoluble iron salts. Gastric hormones are secreted into the blood and travel to target tissues.

In the fundus and body of the stomach, the gastric glands of the mucosa are the primary secretory units (Fig. 40.8). Several of these glands empty into a common duct known as the gastric pit. The parietal cells within the glands secrete hydrochloric acid, intrinsic factor, and gastroferrin. The chief cells within the glands secrete pepsinogen, an enzyme precursor that is readily converted to pepsin in the gastric fluid, and acidic lipase. The pyloric gland mucosa, in the antrum, synthesizes and releases the hormone gastrin from G cells. Enterochromaffin-like cells secrete histamine, and D cells secrete somatostatin.

Gastric secretion is stimulated by anticipating, smelling, and tasting food which activates chemoreceptors and

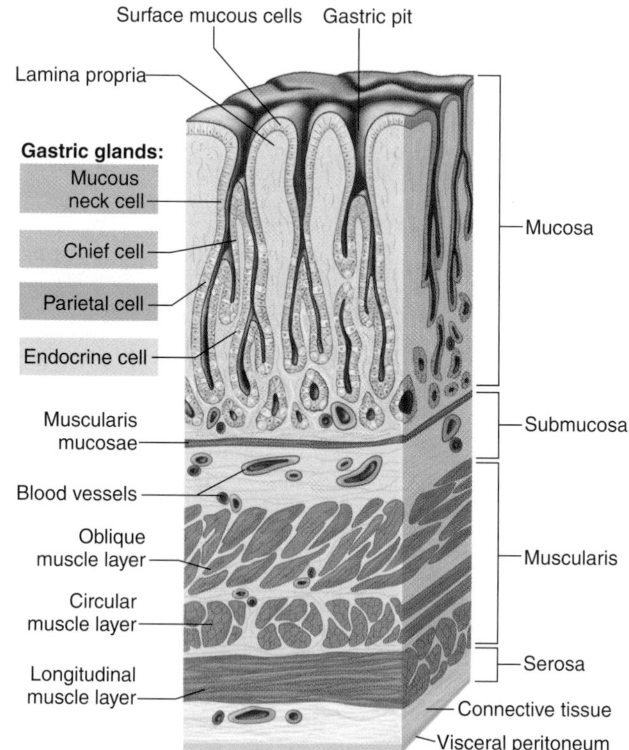

Fig. 40.8 Gastric Pits and Gastric Glands. Gastric pits are depressions in the epithelial lining of the stomach. At the bottom of each pit are one or more tubular *gastric glands*. Chief cells produce pepsinogen, which is converted to pepsin (a proteolytic enzyme); parietal cells secrete hydrochloric acid and intrinsic factor; G cells produce gastrin; endocrine cells (enterochromaffin-like cells and D cells) secrete histamine and somatostatin. (From Patton KT, et al. *Essentials of Anatomy & Physiology*. St Louis: Mosby; 2012.)

mechanoreceptors in the oral and nasal cavities. These receptors stimulate vagal fibers in the stomach.[4] It is also stimulated by gastric distention, by the actions of the hormone gastrin and paracrine pathways (e.g., histamine, ghrelin, somatostatin), and by the effects of the neurotransmitter acetylcholine (ACh) and other chemicals (e.g., ethanol, coffee, protein). Together these stimuli facilitate the process of digestion. Gastric secretion is inhibited by somatostatin, unpleasant odors and tastes, and rage, fear, or pain. Mucus covering the entire mucosa, intercellular tight junctions, bicarbonate secretion, and submucosal acid sensors form a protective barrier against acid and proteolytic enzymes, which otherwise would damage the gastric lining.

The composition of gastric juice depends on volume and flow rate (see Fig. 40.4B). The rate of secretion varies with the time of day. Generally, the rate and volume of secretion are lowest in the morning and highest in the afternoon and evening. At low secretion rates, the gastric juice contains primarily sodium chloride, with small amounts of hydrogen ion, potassium, and bicarbonate.[4] At peak rates, the gastric juice is primarily composed of hydrogen chloride. The potassium level remains relatively constant, but its concentration is greater in gastric juice than in plasma. Loss of gastric juices through vomiting, drainage, or suction may decrease body stores of sodium and potassium and result in fluid, electrolyte (e.g., hyponatremia, hypokalemia, dehydration), and acid-base imbalances (e.g., metabolic alkalosis) (see Chapter 3).

Phases of gastric secretion. There are three phases of gastric secretion: the cephalic phase, gastric phase, and intestinal phase (Fig. 40.9).

Cephalic phase. The anticipatory and sensory experiences of smelling, seeing, tasting, chewing, and swallowing food contribute to the cephalic phase of secretion. The cephalic phase is mediated by ACh produced by the vagus nerve which directly stimulates parietal cell secretion. Vagal stimulation also causes the release of gastrin-releasing peptide which stimulates G cells to produce gastrin. Hypoglycemia caused by insulin secretion by the endocrine pancreas also is a strong stimulus for gastric secretion and is mediated by the vagus nerve through sensors located in the hypothalamus.[4] Maintenance of steady serum glucose levels suppresses the gastric response to insulin.

Gastric phase. The gastric phase of secretion begins with the arrival of food in the stomach. Two major stimuli have a secretory effect: (1) distention of the stomach and (2) the presence of digested protein. The vagus and enteric nerve plexuses are stimulated by distention and contribute to gastric secretion through a local reflex. Both neural reflexes are mediated by ACh and can be blocked by atropine. As digestion proceeds, products of protein break down, stimulating the release of more gastrin from G cells.

Intestinal phase. The movement of chyme from the stomach into the duodenum initiates the intestinal phase of secretion. This phase represents a deceleration of the gastric secretory response; however, the presence of digested protein and amino acids in the duodenum continues to stimulate some gastric secretion.

Concurrently, in response to low duodenal pH and the presence of lipids, inhibitory vagal, and enteric reflexes decrease gastric motility when chyme enters the duodenum. The release of secretin and cholecystokinin stimulates pancreatic secretions and inhibits gastric secretions.

Acid. The major functions of gastric hydrochloric acid are to dissolve food fibers, act as a bactericide against swallowed

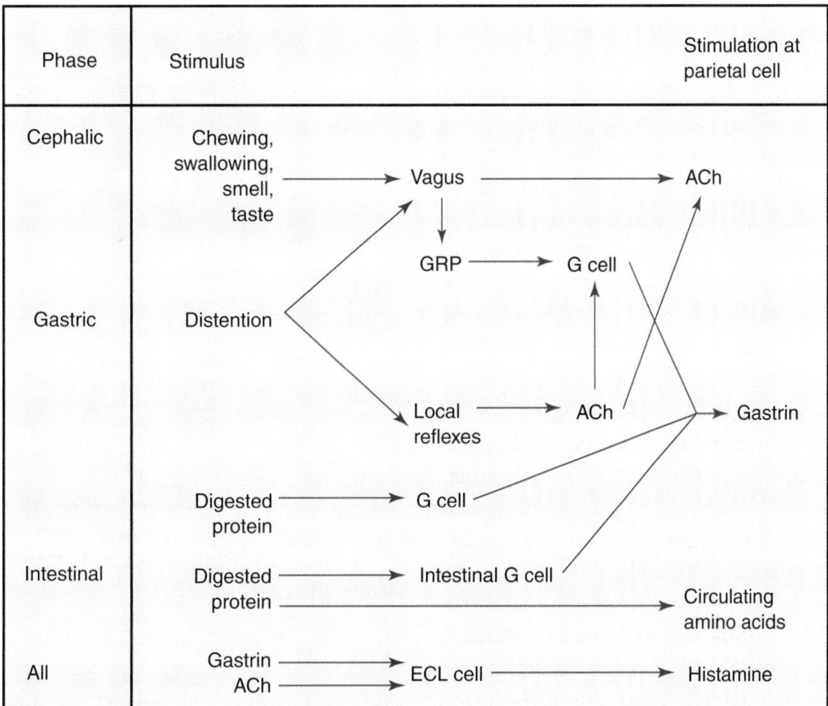

Fig. 40.9 Mechanisms for Stimulating Acid Secretion. *ACh*, Acetylcholine; *ECL*, enterochromaffin-like cell; *GRP*, gastrin-releasing peptide. (From Johnson LR. *Gastrointestinal Physiology*. 9th ed. Philadelphia, PA: Mosby; 2019.)

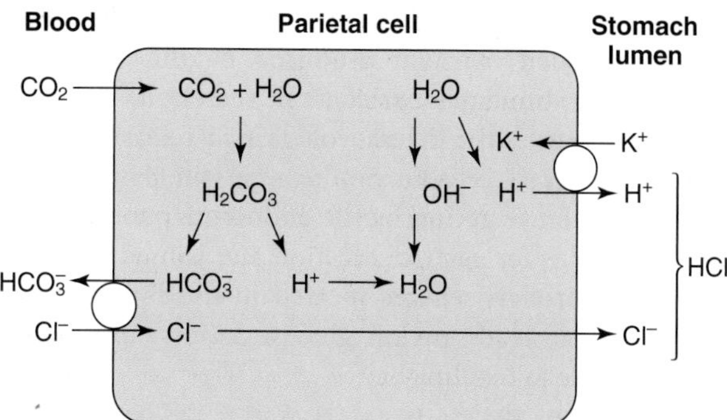

Fig. 40.10 Hydrochloric Acid Secretion by Parietal Cell.

microorganisms, and convert pepsinogen to pepsin. Gastric acid entering the duodenum facilitates the absorption of ferric iron. The production of acid by the parietal cells requires the transport of hydrogen and chloride from the parietal cells to the stomach lumen. Acid is formed in the parietal cells, primarily through the hydrolysis of water (Fig. 40.10). At a high rate of gastric secretion, bicarbonate moves into the plasma, producing an "alkaline tide" in the venous blood, which may result in a more alkaline urine.

Acid secretion is stimulated by the vagus nerve, which releases ACh and stimulates the secretion of gastrin; gastrin then stimulates the release of histamine from enterochromaffin cells (mast cells; see Chapter 7) in the gastric mucosa. Histamine stimulates acid secretion by activating histamine receptors (H_2 receptors) on acid-secreting parietal cells. Caffeine, calcium, and ghrelin also stimulate acid secretion. Acid secretion is inhibited by somatostatin, secretin, cholecystokinin, glucagon-like peptide-1, atrial natriuretic peptide, and prostaglandins.[14]

Pepsin and gastric lipase. The ACh, gastrin, and secretin stimulate the chief cells to release pepsinogen during eating. Pepsinogen is quickly converted to pepsin in the acidic gastric environment (optimum pH for pepsin activation = 2). Acid also stimulates a local cholinergic reflex and stimulates chief cells to secrete pepsin. Pepsin is a proteolytic enzyme—that is, it breaks down protein and forms polypeptides in the stomach. Once chyme has entered the duodenum, the alkaline environment of the duodenum inactivates pepsin. Gastric lipase is an acid lipase and does not require bile for activation like alkaline pancreatic and intestinal lipases and is active in an acid environment. It accounts for about 30% of fat digestion in adults and up to 50% of fat digestion in infants. It cleaves only one monoglyceride from triglyceride so is less efficient than alkaline lipase.

Mucus. The gastric mucosa is protected from the digestive actions of acid and pepsin by intercellular tight junctions, a coating of mucus called the mucosal barrier, and gastric mucosal blood flow. The quality and quantity of mucus and the tight junctions between epithelial cells make gastric mucosa relatively impermeable to acid. Prostaglandins and nitric oxide protect the mucosal barrier by stimulating the secretion of mucus and bicarbonate and by inhibiting the secretion of acid. A break in the protective barrier may occur from ischemia or by exposure to *Helicobacter pylori*, aspirin, nonsteroidal anti-inflammatory drugs (inhibit prostaglandin synthesis),

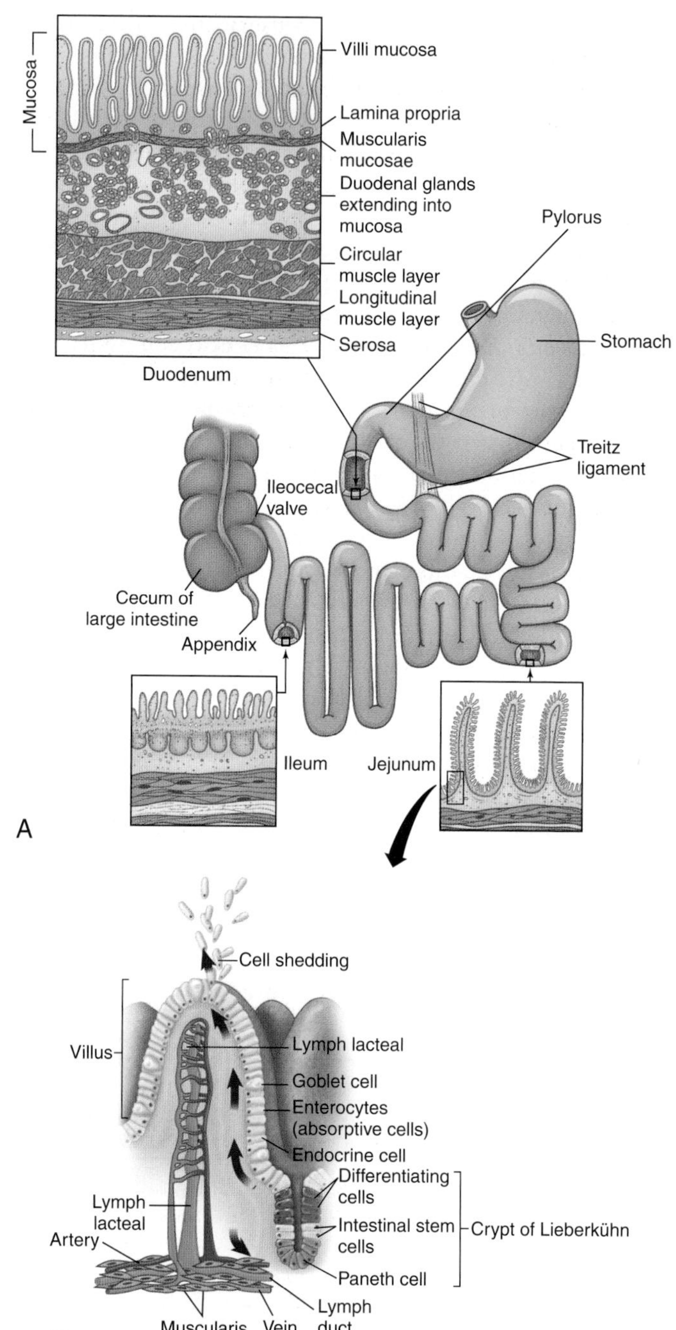

Fig. 40.11 The Small Intestine. **(A)** Segments of the small intestine. Inserts show longitudinal sections of the duodenum, jejunum, and ileum. **(B)** Anatomy of a villus. Arrows show migration and then shedding of epithelial cells.

ethanol, or regurgitated bile. Breaks cause inflammation and ulceration (see Chapter 41).

Small Intestine

The small intestine is coiled within the abdominal cavity and is about 5 to 6 m long. It is suspended in loose folds from the posterior abdominal wall by the mesentery. Functionally, it is divided into three segments: the duodenum, jejunum, and ileum (Fig. 40.11A). The duodenum begins at the pylorus and ends where it joins the jejunum at a suspensory ligament called the *Treitz ligament.* The end of the jejunum and the beginning of the ileum are not distinguished by an anatomic marker. These structures are not grossly different, but the jejunum has a slightly larger lumen than the ileum. The ileocecal valve, or sphincter, controls the flow of digested material from the ileum into the cecum of the large intestine and prevents reflux into the small intestine.

The arterial supply to the duodenum arises primarily from the gastroduodenal artery, a branch of the celiac artery. The jejunum and ileum are supplied by branches of the superior mesenteric artery (see Fig. 40.7). Blood flow increases significantly during digestion. The superior mesenteric vein drains blood from the entire small intestine and empties into the hepatic portal circulation. The regional lymph nodes and lymphatics drain into the thoracic duct, which empties into the subclavian vein.

Enteric nerves from both divisions of the ANS innervate the small intestine. Secretion, motility, pain sensation, and intestinal reflexes (e.g., relaxation of the lower esophageal sphincter) are mediated parasympathetically by the vagus nerve. Sympathetic activity inhibits motility and produces vasoconstriction. Intrinsic reflexive activity is mediated by the myenteric (Auerbach) plexus and the submucosal (Meissner) plexus of the enteric nervous system.[4]

The smooth muscles of the small intestine are arranged in two layers: a longitudinal outer layer and a thicker inner circular layer (see Figs. 40.2 and 40.11A). Circular folds of the small intestine slow the passage of food, thereby providing more time for digestion and absorption. The folds are most numerous and prominent in the jejunum and proximal ileum.

Absorption occurs through villi (sing., villus), which cover the circular folds and are the functional units of the intestine. A villus is composed of absorptive columnar cells (enterocytes) and mucus-secreting goblet cells of the mucosal epithelium (see Fig. 40.11B). Each villus secretes some of the enzymes necessary for digestion and absorbs nutrients. Near the surface, columnar cells closely adhere to each other at sites called *tight junctions.* Water and electrolytes are absorbed through these intercellular spaces. The surface of each columnar epithelial cell on the villus contains tiny projections called microvilli (sing., microvillus). Together the microvilli create a mucosal surface known as the brush border. The villi and microvilli greatly increase the surface area available for absorption. Coating the brush border is an "unstirred" layer of water that is important for the absorption of water-soluble substances including emulsified micelles of fat. The lamina propria (a connective tissue layer of the mucous membrane) lies beneath the epithelial cells of the villi and contains lymphocytes and plasma cells, which produce immunoglobulins (see The Gastrointestinal Tract and Immunity section).

Central arterioles ascend within each villus and branch into a capillary array that extends around the base of the columnar cells and cascades down to the venules that lead to the hepatic portal circulation. The opposing ascending and descending blood flow provide a countercurrent exchange system for absorbed substances and blood gases. A central lacteal, or lymphatic capillary, also is contained within each villus and is important for the absorption and transport of fat molecules (see Fig. 40.11B). The contents of the lacteals flow to regional nodes and channels that eventually drain into the thoracic duct.

Between the bases of the villi are the crypts of Lieberkühn, which extend to the submucosal layer. Undifferentiated cells arise from stem cells at the base of the crypt, and move toward the tip of the villus, maturing to become columnar epithelial secretory cells (water, electrolytes, and enzymes) and goblet cells (mucus).[15] After completing their migration to the tip of the villus, they function for a few days and then are shed into the intestinal lumen and digested. Discarded epithelial cells are an important source of endogenous protein. The entire epithelial population is replaced about every 4 to 7 days. Many factors can influence this process of cellular proliferation. Starvation, vitamin B_{12} deficiency, and cytotoxic drugs or irradiation suppress cell division and shorten the villi. Decreased absorption across the epithelial membrane can cause diarrhea and malnutrition. Nutrient intake and intestinal resection stimulate cell production.

Intestinal Digestion and Absorption

The process of intestinal digestion is initiated in the stomach by the actions of gastric hydrochloric acid and pepsin, which break down food fibers and proteins. The chyme that passes into the duodenum is a liquid with small particles of undigested food. Digestion of food components continues in the proximal portion of the small intestine by the action of pancreatic enzymes, intestinal brush-border enzymes, and bile salts. As seen in Fig. 40.12, in the proximal small intestine, carbohydrates are broken down to monosaccharides and disaccharides, proteins are degraded further to amino acids and peptides, and fats are emulsified and reduced to fatty acids and monoglycerides.

These nutrients, along with water, vitamins, and electrolytes, are absorbed across the intestinal mucosa and into the blood by active transport, diffusion, or facilitated diffusion. Products of carbohydrate and protein breakdown move into villus capillaries and then to the liver through the hepatic portal vein. Digested fats move into the lacteals and reach the liver through the portal and systemic circulation. These components are metabolized within the liver (see the Metabolism of Nutrients section). Intestinal motility exposes nutrients to a large mucosal surface area by mixing chyme and moving it through the lumen. Different segments of the GI tract absorb different nutrients. Digestion and absorption of all major nutrients and many drugs occur in the small intestine. Sites of absorption are shown in Fig. 40.13. Box 40.3 outlines the major nutrients involved in this process.

Water and electrolyte transport by the small intestine. The epithelial cell membranes of the small intestine are formed of lipids and are hydrophobic or tend to repel water. Therefore, water and electrolytes are transported in both directions (toward the capillary blood or toward the intestinal lumen) through the tight junctions and intercellular spaces rather than across cell membranes. Water diffuses passively across hydrostatic pressure and osmotic gradients established by the active transport of sodium and other substances. Approximately 85% to 90% of the water that enters the GI tract each day is absorbed in the small intestine.

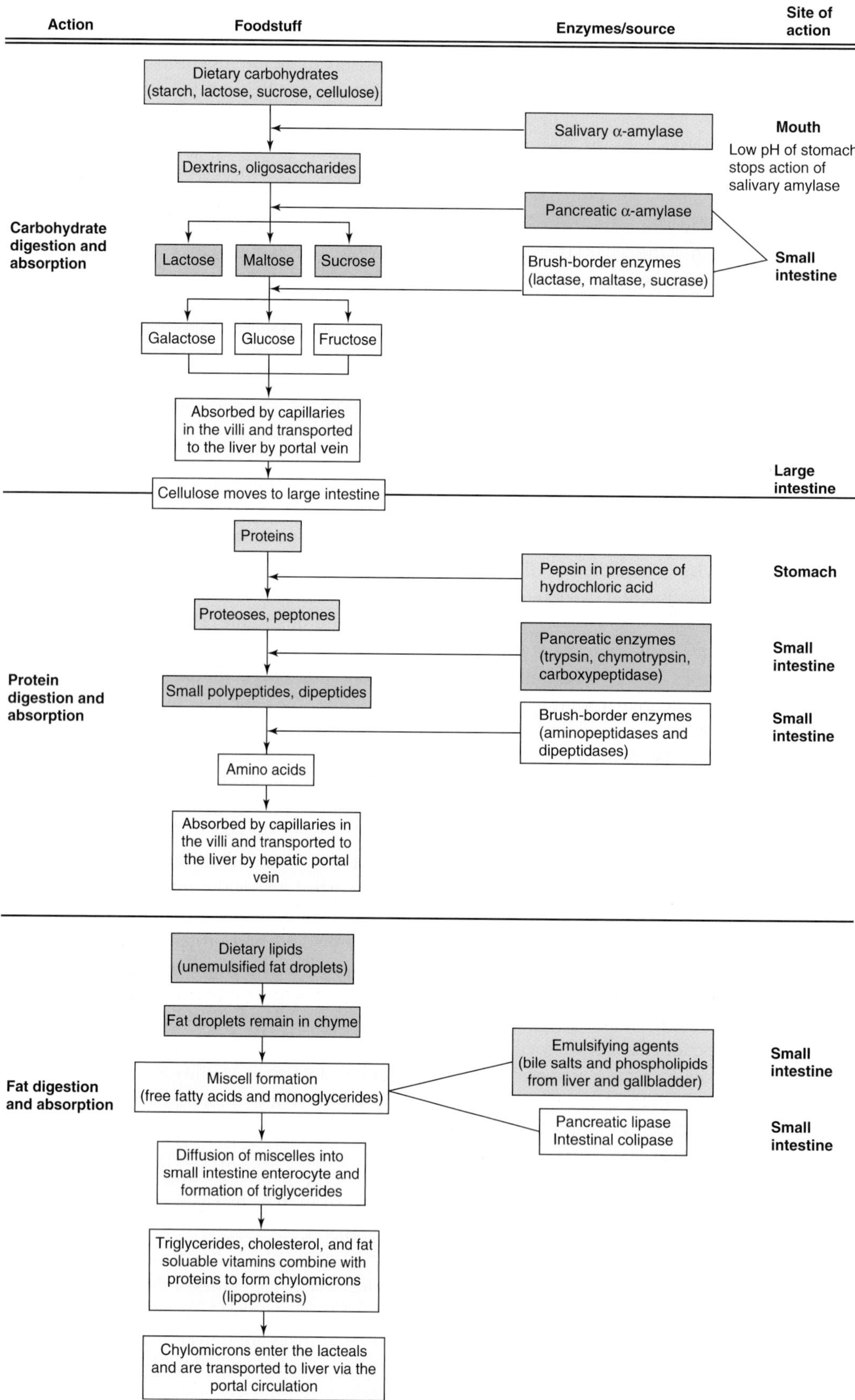

Fig. 40.12 Digestion and Absorption of Food.

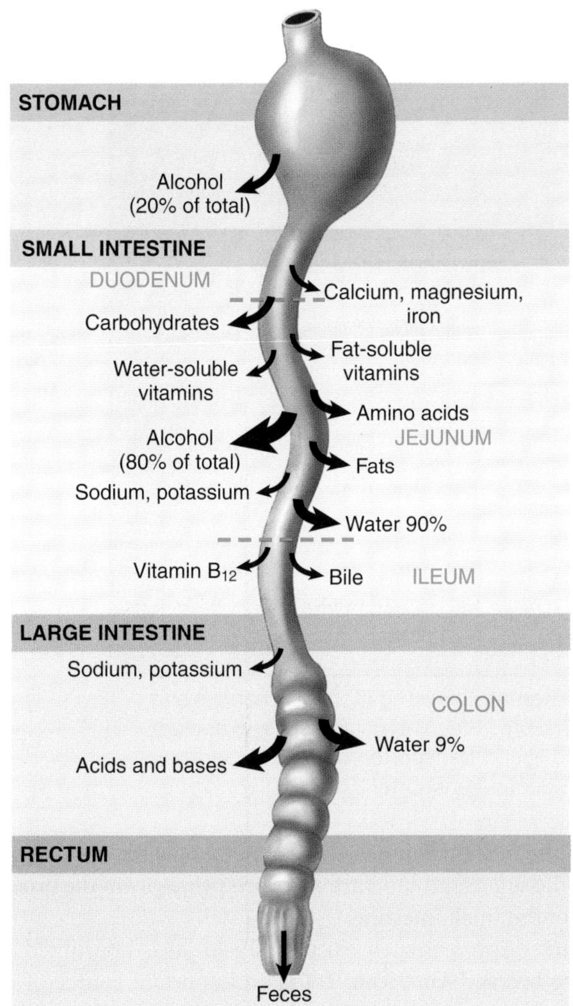

Fig. 40.13 Sites of Absorption of Major Nutrients. (Modified from Patton KT. *Anatomy & Physiology*. 10th ed. St Louis: Elsevier; 2019.)

The remaining water and electrolytes are absorbed at a constant rate in the large intestine. Sodium passes through the tight junctions and is actively transported across cell membranes. Sodium and glucose share a common active transport carrier (sodium-glucose ligand transporter1 [SGLT1]) so that sodium absorption is enhanced by glucose transport (Fig. 40.14).[16] Potassium moves passively across the tight junctions with changes in the electrochemical gradient. Chloride is actively secreted throughout the large and small intestines.

Carbohydrates. Only monosaccharides (ribose, galactose, glucose, fructose) are absorbed by the intestinal mucosa; the complex carbohydrates (polysaccharides and oligosaccharides) must be hydrolyzed to their simplest form.[4] The major disaccharides are sucrose (glucose-fructose), maltose (glucose-glucose), and lactose (glucose-galactose) (see Fig. 40.14). Salivary and pancreatic amylases break down starches to oligosaccharides by splitting α-1,4-glucosidic linkages of long-chain molecules. Approximately half of starch hydrolysis occurs in the stomach and about half in the duodenum. In the small intestine, disaccharides are hydrolyzed by brush-border enzymes (sucrase, maltase, and lactase) to their respective monosaccharides.

BOX 40.3 Major Nutrients Absorbed in the Small Intestine

Water and Electrolytes

- Approximately 85%–90% of the water that enters the GI tract is absorbed in the small intestine.
- Sodium passes through tight junctions and is actively transported across cell membranes; it is exchanged for bicarbonate to maintain electroneutrality in the ileum; sodium absorption is enhanced by cotransport with glucose.
- Potassium moves passively across tight junctions with changes in the electrochemical gradient.

Carbohydrates

- Only monosaccharides are absorbed by the intestinal mucosa; therefore complex carbohydrates must be hydrolyzed to the simplest form.
- Salivary and pancreatic amylases break down starches to oligosaccharides (lactose, maltose, sucrose) in the stomach and duodenum; brush-border enzymes hydrolyze them in the small intestine so they can pass through the unstirred water layer by diffusion.
- Fructose diffuses into the bloodstream; glucose and galactose diffuse or are actively transported.
- Cellulose remains undigested and stimulates large intestine motility.

Proteins

- From 90%–95% of protein is absorbed; major hydrolysis is accomplished in the small intestine by the pancreatic enzymes trypsin, chymotrypsin, and carboxypeptidase.
- Brush-border enzymes break down proteins into smaller peptides that can cross cell membranes. In the cytosol, they are metabolized into amino acids, specifically neutral amino acids, basic amino acids, and proline and hydroxyproline.

Fats

Digestion and absorption occur in four phases:

- Phase 1—Emulsification and lipolysis: Emulsifying agents (bile salts) cover small fat particles and prevent them from reforming into fat droplets; then lipolysis with pancreatic lipases divides them into monoglycerides and free fatty acids.
- Phase 2—Micelle formation: A spherical formation of lipid products that are water soluble.
- Phase 3—Fat absorption: Fat products move from micelles to the absorbing surface of the intestinal epithelium and enter enterocytes.
- Phase 4—Triglycerides are resynthesized and, along with cholesterol, fat-soluble vitamins, and phospholipids, combine with proteins to form chylomicrons (lipoproteins). Chylomicrons leave the enterocyte, enter the lymphatics, and travel to the portal circulation.

Minerals

- Calcium—absorbed by passive diffusion and transported actively across cell membranes bound to a carrier protein; absorption primarily in the ileum.
- Magnesium—50% absorbed by active transport or passive diffusion in the jejunum and ileum.
- Phosphate—absorbed by passive diffusion and active transport in the small intestine.
- Iron—absorbed by epithelial cells of the duodenum and jejunum; vitamin C facilitates.

Vitamins

- Absorbed mainly by sodium-dependent active transport, with vitamin B_{12} bound to intrinsic factor and absorbed in the terminal ileum.

The sugars are absorbed primarily in the duodenum and upper jejunum by facilitated diffusion mediated by glucose transporter proteins. The monosaccharides pass through the unstirred layer by diffusion. At the cell membrane, glucose

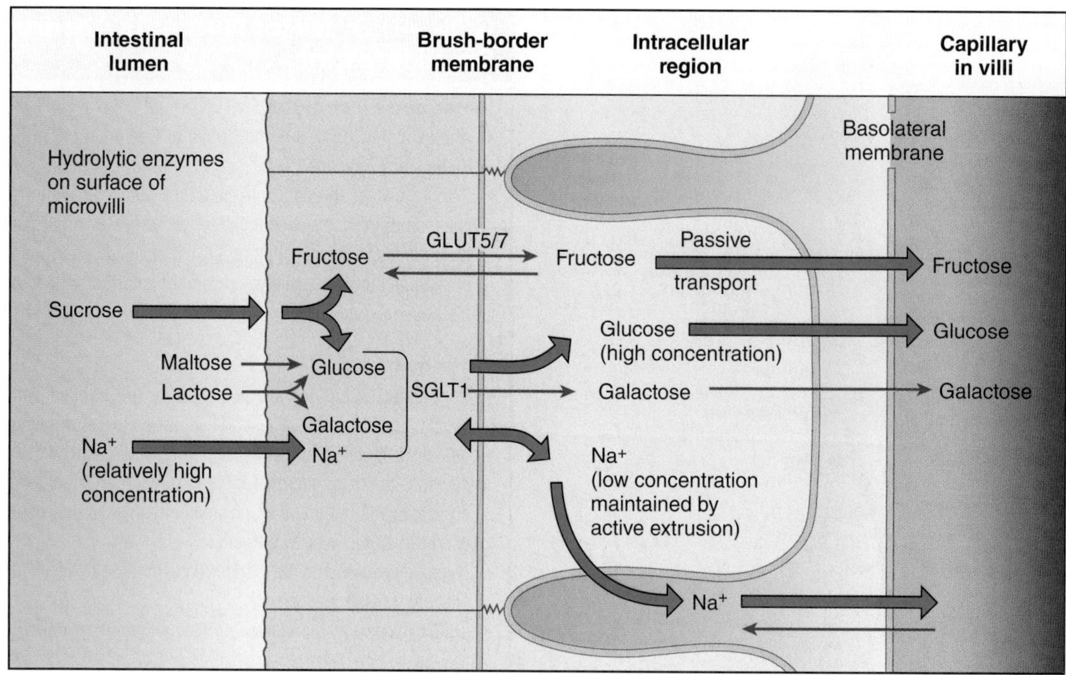

Fig. 40.14 Monosaccharides and Sodium Transport. Schematic showing monosaccharides and sodium *(Na^+)* transport through the small intestinal epithelium. Glucose, galactose, and sodium are transported into the epithelial cell by sodium-glucose ligand transporter 1 *(SGLT1)*. See text for details regarding other glucose transporters. *GLUT*, Glucose transporter.

and galactose are actively transported with a sodium carrier (SGLT1), and fructose absorption is facilitated by glucose transporter 5 (GLUT5) and GLUT7 (see Fig. 40.14).[17] Transport of all three monosaccharides from the cytosol to the bloodstream is facilitated by GLUT2. Insulin facilitates glucose transport into fat and muscle cells via glucose transporter 4 (GLUT4), but insulin is not required for the intestinal absorption of glucose.[18]

Proteins. Adults require 44 to 56g of protein per day. Approximately 20 to 30g of protein is derived endogenously from shed epithelial cells and small amounts of plasma proteins. Most ingested protein is absorbed; only 5% to 10% is eliminated in the stool.

The site of digestion of protein depends on the source of the protein. For example, casein from bovine milk precipitates in the stomach and is digested by gastric pepsin and acid, whereas the soluble proteins whey and soy pass rapidly through the stomach and are digested by pancreatic enzymes. Major protein hydrolysis is accomplished in the small intestine by the pancreatic enzymes trypsin, chymotrypsin, and carboxypeptidase (see Fig. 40.12).[4] Trypsin and chymotrypsin (endopeptidase) hydrolyze the interior bonds of the large molecules, and carboxypeptidases cleave the end amino acids (exopeptidase). Hydrolysis of proteins is also carried out by the brush-border enzymes and enzymes in the epithelial cytosol (intracellular fluid). The brush-border enzymes hydrolyze the large oligopeptides (proteins composed of three to six amino acids) into smaller peptides, which can cross cell membranes. Enzymes in the cytosol then break them down to amino acids. Amino acids are actively transported from the cytosol into the bloodstream by a sodium-dependent carrier in the basolateral membrane. There also are free amino acids that can be absorbed directly from the intestinal lumen using a membrane transport protein. Like the sugars, proteins are absorbed primarily in the proximal area of the small intestine.

Fats. Approximately 90 to 100g of fat is consumed daily by the average American. Fat is an important source of calories and is a primary structural component of cell membranes and organelles. Sources of dietary fat are reviewed in Box 40.4. Although triglycerides are the major dietary lipids, cholesterol, phospholipids, and fat-soluble vitamins also have nutritional importance. The digestion and absorption of fat occur in four phases: (1) emulsification and lipolysis, (2) micelle formation, (3) fat absorption, and (4) resynthesis of triglycerides and phospholipids.

The mechanical action of the stomach and small intestine disperses the triglyceride droplets into small particles. Emulsification is the process by which emulsifying agents (fatty acids, monoglycerides, lecithin, cholesterol, protein, bile salts) in the small intestinal lumen cover the small fat particles and prevent them from re-forming into fat droplets. Emulsified fat is then ready for lipolysis (lipid hydrolysis) by lingual and gastric lipase (acid lipases), pancreatic lipase, phospholipase, and hydrolase (alkaline lipases).[4] Lipase breaks down triglycerides to diglycerides, monoglycerides, free fatty acids, and glycerol (see Fig. 40.12). The action of alkaline lipases requires the presence of colipase, a pancreatic coenzyme that allows lipase to penetrate the triglyceride molecule. Phospholipase cleaves fatty acids from phospholipids, and cholesterol esterase breaks cholesterol esters into fatty acids and glycerol.

The products of lipid hydrolysis must be made water soluble if they are to be absorbed efficiently from the intestinal lumen. This is accomplished by the formation of water-soluble

BOX 40.4 Dietary Fat

Saturated Fatty Acid (Palmitic Acid [$C_16H_{32}O_2$])

Solid at room temperature

Each carbon atom in the chain is linked by single bonds to adjacent carbon and hydrogen atoms

Found in animal fat and tropical oils (coconut and palm oils)

Increase the blood levels of low-density lipoprotein (LDL) cholesterol ("bad" cholesterol) and also the risk of coronary artery disease

Unsaturated Fatty Acid

Soft or liquid at room temperature

Monounsaturated Fatty Acids (e.g., oleic acid [$C_{18}H_{34}O_2$])

Contain one double bond in the carbon chain

Found in plants and animals

May be beneficial in reducing blood cholesterol, glucose levels, and systolic blood pressure; do not lower high-density lipoprotein (HDL) cholesterol ("good" cholesterol) level; low HDL levels have been associated with coronary heart disease.

Polyunsaturated Fatty Acids (e.g., linoleic acid [C18H32O2])

Contain two or more double bonds in the carbon chain

Found in plants and fish oils

Omega-6 fatty acids lower total and LDL cholesterol blood levels

Omega-3 fatty acids lower blood triglyceride levels; reduce platelet aggregation and blood-clotting tendencies; are necessary for growth and development; and may prevent coronary artery disease, hypertension, cancer, and inflammatory and immune disorders

molecules known as micelles (Fig. 40.15). Micelles are formed of bile salts, the products of fat hydrolysis, fat-soluble vitamins, and cholesterol. The fats form the core of the micelle, and the polar bile salts form an outer shell, with the hydrophobic ("water-repelling") side facing the interior and the hydrophilic ("water-loving") side facing the aqueous (water-like) content of the intestinal lumen. Because the unstirred layer of the brush border is aqueous, the micelles readily diffuse through it (Fig. 40.16). The micelles maintain the fat molecules in the dissolved or solubilized form, which allows them to move more rapidly from the micelle toward the absorbing surface of the intestinal epithelium. The fat products of the micelle then readily diffuse through the epithelial cell membrane, while the bile salts remain in the lumen and proceed to the ileum, where they are absorbed into the circulation and returned to the liver via the enterohepatic circulation (see Fig. 40.22). Almost all the bile salts are recycled in this way.

When the fat products reach the inside of the epithelial cell, they are resynthesized into triglycerides and phospholipids. The triglycerides are covered with phospholipids, lipoproteins, and cholesterol to become particles called chylomicrons. The chylomicrons travel to the basolateral membrane of the columnar epithelial cells, where they are extruded into the intercellular spaces of the villus. From here they enter the lacteals and lymphatic channels and, eventually, the systemic circulation.

Minerals and vitamins. The recommended intake of calcium ranges from 1000 to 1500 mg/day. Between 500 and 600 mg is secreted or shed into the lumen with epithelial cell shedding. Not all this calcium is absorbed. Daily absorption of calcium

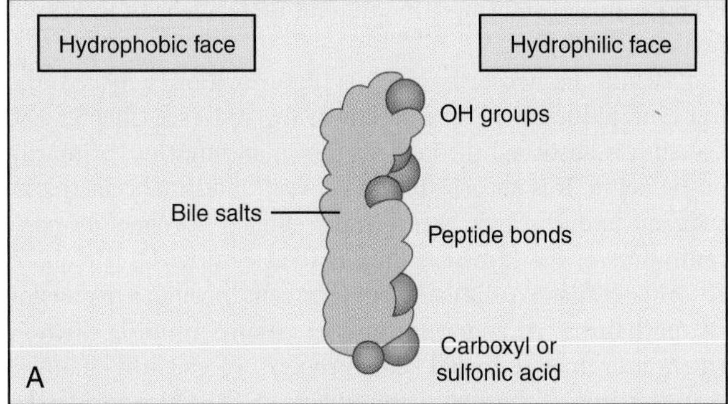

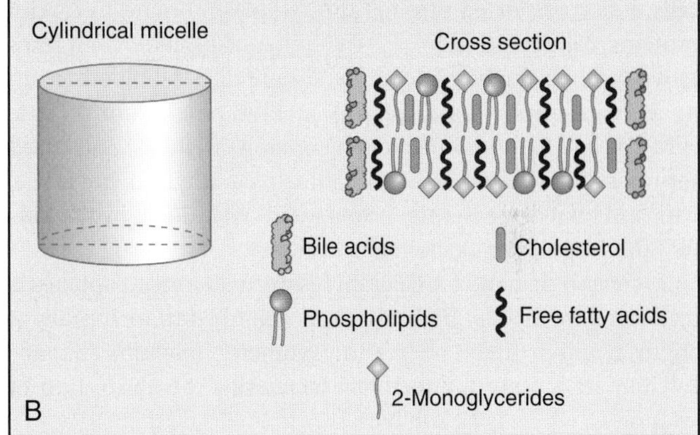

Fig. 40.15 Structure of Bile Acid and Micelle. (A) A bile salt molecule in solution. The molecule is amphipathic in that it has a hydrophilic face and a hydrophobic face. The amphipathic structure is key in the ability of the bile salts to emulsify lipids and form micelles. **(B)** A model of the structure of a bile salt–lipid mixed micelle, an emulsified fat. (From Levy MN, Koeppen BM, Stanton BA. *Principles of Physiology*. 4th ed. St Louis: Mosby; 2006.)

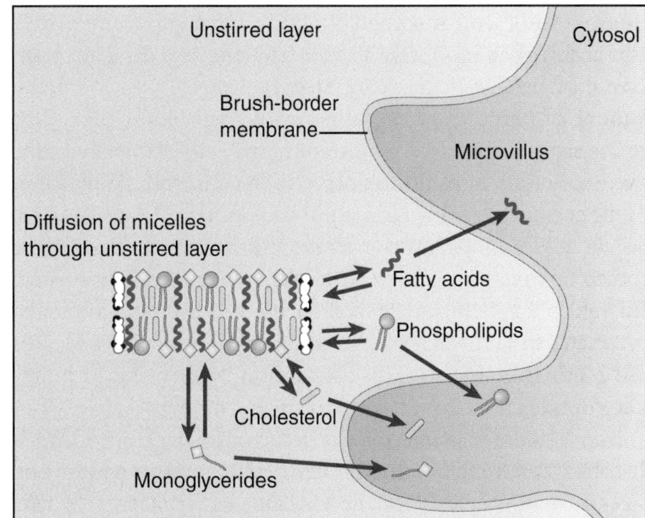

Fig. 40.16 Lipid Absorption in the Small Intestine. Micelles of bile salts and products of lipid digestion diffuse through the unstirred layer and among the microvilli. As digestive products are absorbed from free solution by epithelial cells of the villi, more digestive products dissociate from the micelles. (From Levy MN, Koeppen BM, Stanton BA. *Principles of Physiology*. 4th ed. St Louis: Mosby; 2006.)

is approximately 600 mg. This amount increases with increased intake.

Calcium homeostasis requires coordination between the intestine, kidney, bone, and parathyroid glands (see Chapter 21). Calcium is absorbed throughout the small intestine, primarily in the ileum. It is absorbed both between intestinal cells (paracellular) and through them (transcellular).[19] When its concentration in the lumen is greater than 5 mmol/L, calcium is absorbed by passive diffusion between cells through a paracellular mechanism. At concentrations less than 5 mmol/L, calcium enters intestinal epithelial cells through two calcium channels that respond to the presence of vitamin D_3. Once inside the cells, it is transported through the cytoplasm bound to carrier proteins called calbindins.[19] The calcium-protein complexes move through the basolateral membrane into the bloodstream by active transport using plasma membrane calcium-ATPase (PMCA) and the sodium/calcium exchanger (NCX1). Increased serum calcium concentration inhibits parathyroid hormone, which in turn decreases the formation of vitamin D_3 by the kidney, thus regulating calcium absorption.

Increased demand for calcium results in increased uptake, as evidenced by the fact that calcium is absorbed more rapidly in children and pregnant or lactating women.[19] Bile salts enhance calcium absorption indirectly by facilitating the absorption of vitamin D, which is fat soluble.

The recommended intake of magnesium for adults is 300 to 350 mg/day. Approximately 50% of it is absorbed by active transport or passive diffusion in the jejunum and ileum. Phosphate is also absorbed in the small intestine by passive diffusion and active transport.

The levels of iron in the body are regulated primarily by intestinal absorption and secretion. The average intake ranges from 15 to 30 mg/day. Of this amount, menstruating women absorb 1 to 1.5 mg and men absorb 0.15 to 1 mg. Generally, the amount of iron absorbed is equal to the amount required. Iron is absorbed more rapidly if a deficiency exists. A primary source of iron is heme from animal protein with a smaller amount of heme from recycling of old red blood cells. This iron is rapidly absorbed by the epithelial cells primarily in the proximal duodenum. Inorganic iron (e.g., iron in fruits, cereals, eggs, vegetables) is also readily absorbed. The presence of gastric acid and vitamin C in the duodenum reduces ferric iron to ferrous iron, which is the form more easily absorbed. Calcium phosphate and phosphoproteins (milk and antacids) in the intestinal lumen bind iron and reduce absorption. Tea also binds iron and inhibits absorption by forming iron tannate complexes.

Iron is bound to *intestinal transferrin* in the lumen and is absorbed and bound to the protein *ferritin* and to amino acid chelates in the cytosol of the enterocytes. Transport of iron across the basolateral membrane is determined by the amount of iron in the circulation. It is transported in the blood by *plasma transferrin*, a glycoprotein, and is carried to body tissues. When there is less need for iron, it remains in the enterocyte as ferritin and is carried into the lumen when the cell is sloughed from the end of the villus. Following hemorrhage, the intestinal cells require 3 days to increase their rate of iron absorption. This is because the need for iron is perceived by the precursor stem cells in the crypts of Lieberkühn, and they take 3 days to mature and migrate to the tips of the villi, where they absorb more iron. Hepcidin is a protein synthesized by the liver that inhibits apical uptake of iron by enterocytes and modulates iron trafficking (see Chapter 28).[20]

The absorption of vitamins is summarized in Table 40.2. Most of the water-soluble vitamins are absorbed passively or by sodium-dependent active transport.[4] Most vitamin B_{12} (cobalamin) is bound to intrinsic factor (making it resistant to digestion) and absorbed in the terminal ileum, although a small amount of the vitamin is absorbed in its free (unbound) form.

Intestinal Motility

The movements of the small intestine facilitate digestion and absorption. Chyme leaving the stomach and entering the duodenum stimulates intestinal movements that help blend secretions from the liver, gallbladder, pancreas, and intestinal glands. A churning motion brings the luminal contents into contact with the absorbing cells of the villi. Propulsive movements then

TABLE 40.2 Intestinal Absorption of Vitamins

Vitamin	Mechanisms of Absorption	Site of Absorption
Fat-Soluble Vitamins		
A (retinal)	Micelle formation with bile salts; lipid diffusion	Ileum
D_3 (1,25-dihydroxy-vitamin D)		
E (α-tocopherol)		
K		
Water-Soluble Vitamins		
B_1 (thiamine)	Active transport (sodium dependent)	Duodenum and jejunum
B_2 (riboflavin)	Unknown	Duodenum and jejunum
Niacin (nicotinic acid)	Passive diffusion	Jejunum
C (ascorbic acid)	Passive diffusion; active transport (sodium dependent)	Ileum
Folic acid	Active transport (sodium dependent)	Jejunum
B_{12} (cobalamin)	Active transport (intrinsic factor dependent)	Terminal ileum
B_6 (pyridoxine, pyridoxamine, pyridoxal phosphate)	Passive diffusion	Jejunum
Pantothenic acid	Passive diffusion	Duodenum and jejunum
Biotin	Unknown	Unknown

advance the chyme toward the large intestine. The two movements that promote motility are segmentation and peristalsis.

Segmentation consists of localized rhythmic contractions of the circular smooth muscles and occurs more frequently than peristalsis. The contraction waves occur at different rates in different parts of the small intestine in segments of 1 to 4 cm. Frequency is greatest (12/min) in the upper small intestine and least (8/min) in the distal part of the ileum. Segmentation divides and mixes the chyme, bringing it into contact with the absorbent mucosal surface. It also helps to propel the chyme toward the large intestine. The frequency of the segmentation is regulated intrinsically by the frequency of the basic electrical rhythm, which arises in the myenteric plexus of longitudinal smooth muscle and is controlled by the pacemaker cells of the GI tract.[4] Although the basic rate of contraction is controlled intrinsically, the force of contraction can be enhanced extrinsically by vagal stimulation.

Intestinal peristalsis is waves of contraction along short segments (about 10 cm) of longitudinal smooth muscle and propels chyme through the intestine. The intestinal villi move with contractions of the muscularis mucosae, a thin layer of muscle separating the mucosa and submucosa, with absorption promoted by the swaying of the villi in the luminal contents. The wave of contraction moves slowly (1 to 2 cm/s) to allow time for digestion and absorption.

Neural reflexes along the length of the small intestine facilitate motility, digestion, and absorption. Through reflex action, receptors in one part of the intestine transmit signals that influence the function of another part. The ileogastric reflex inhibits gastric motility when the ileum becomes distended. This prevents the continued movement of chyme into an already distended intestine. The intestinointestinal reflex inhibits intestinal motility when one part of the intestine is overdistended or its mucosa is irritated. Both of these reflexes require extrinsic innervation. The gastroileal reflex, which is activated by an increase in gastric motility and secretion, stimulates an increase in ileal motility and relaxation of the ileocecal valve. This empties the ileum and prepares it to receive more chyme. The gastroileal reflex is regulated by the hormones gastrin and cholecystokinin or through the autonomic nerves.

During prolonged fasting or between meals, particularly overnight, slow waves sweep along the entire length of the intestinal tract from the stomach to the terminal ileum. This interdigestive myoelectric complex appears to propel residual gastric and intestinal contents into the colon.

The ileocecal valve (sphincter) marks the junction between the terminal ileum and the large intestine. This valve is intrinsically regulated and is normally closed. The arrival of peristaltic waves from the last few centimeters of the ileum causes the ileocecal valve to open, allowing a small amount of chyme to pass. Distention of the upper large intestine causes the sphincter to constrict, preventing further distention or retrograde flow of intestinal contents.

Large Intestine

The large intestine is approximately 1.5 m long and consists of the cecum, appendix, colon, rectum, and anal canal (Fig. 40.17A). The cecum is a pouch that receives chyme from

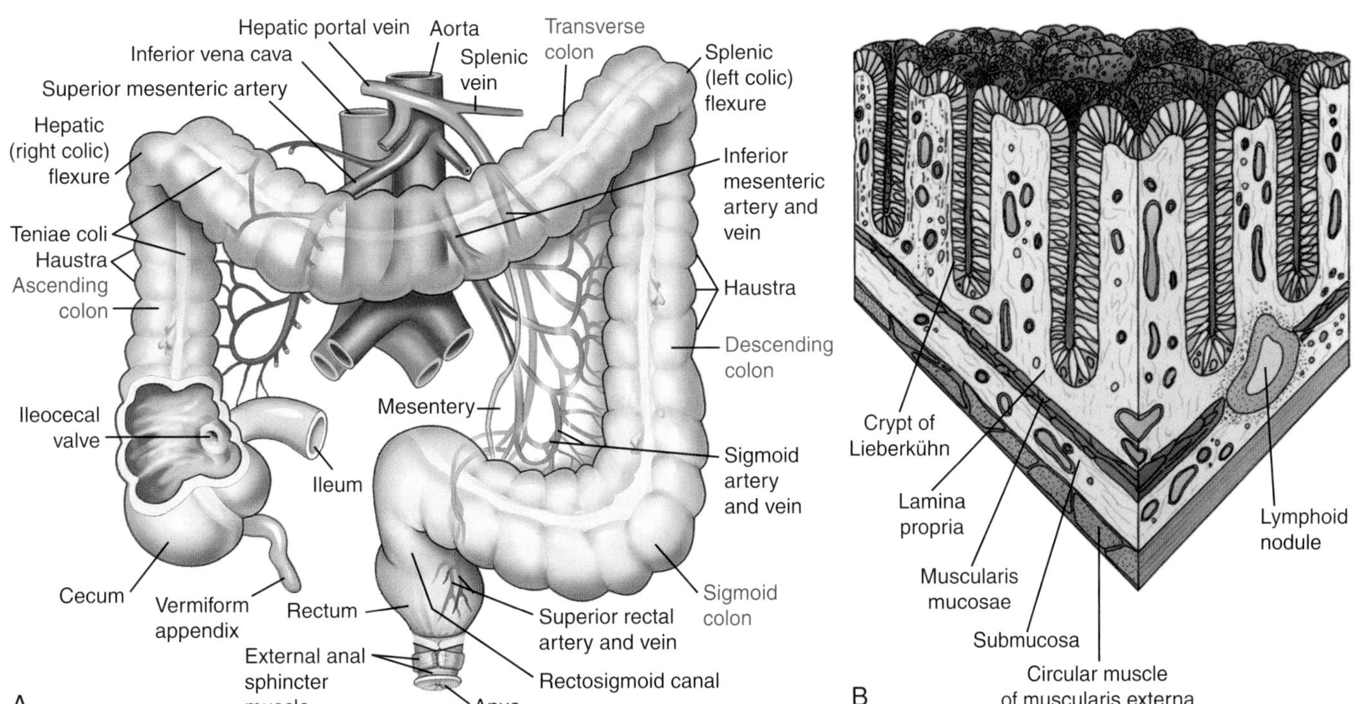

Fig. 40.17 The Large Intestine. (A) Structure of the large intestine. (B) Microscopic cross section illustrating cellular structures of the large intestine. The wall of the large intestine is lined with columnar epithelium, in contrast to the villi characteristics of the small intestine. The longitudinal layer of muscularis is reduced to become the teniae coli. (A, Modified from Patton KT, Thibodeau GA. *The Human Body in Health & Disease*. 7th ed. St Louis: Mosby; 2018; B, From Gartner LP, Hiatt JL. *Color Textbook of Histology*. 3rd ed. Philadelphia, PA: Saunders; 2007.)

EMERGING SCIENCE BOX

The Appendix in Health and Disease

The appendix has long been considered an evolutionary redundancy. However, emerging evidence suggests that it has two key functions: (1) it contains large amounts of lymphoid tissue and is important in immune function, and (2) it hosts a microbiome that continuously sheds into the intestinal lumen thus preventing intestinal dysbiosis. The appendiceal mucosa contains numerous macrophages, T, and B lymphocytes, large amounts of immunoglobulin A and immunoglobulin G generating plasma cells and is located near numerous lymphoid follicles. It plays a key role in both immune activation and tolerance. There is increasing evidence that the appendix helps to maintain tolerance to food-borne microorganisms by shifting intestinal immune cells from proinflammatory to anti-inflammatory responses. It is postulated that appendicitis occurs when proinflammatory processes (e.g., production of high levels of interferon-γ) overcome its anti-inflammatory mechanisms. With regard to its role in maintaining the intestinal microbiome, biofilms of healthy microbiota in the appendix constantly inoculate the distal ileum and proximal colon. Variations in the intestinal microbiome that result from diet, illness, and medications result in increased shedding of microorganisms from the appendix into the intestinal lumen, helping to maintain microbiome homeostasis. Recent studies suggest that individuals who have undergone appendectomy may be at some increased risk for inflammatory bowel disease and more severe complications from *Clostridium difficile* infection. In contrast, there is an emerging link between appendectomy and a decreased risk for the development of Parkinson disease. The appendix is highly innervated by the autonomic nervous system and contains a concentration of an intraneural protein called α-synuclein (α-syn). It is postulated that the complex interaction among the appendiceal microbiome, enteric nervous system, and immune system results in an autoimmune response to α-syn that spreads to the brain via the vagus nerve. Aggregates of this compound accumulate in Lewy Bodies, a hallmark of Parkinson disease.

Data from Bakx R, et al. Microbiota of children with complex appendicitis: different composition and diversity of the microbiota in children with complex compared with simple appendicitis. *Pediatr Infect Dis.* 2019;38:1054–1060; Cosentino M, et al. The vermiform appendix in Parkinson's disease: at the crossroad of peripheral immunity, the nervous system and the intestinal microbiome. *Autoimmun Rev.* 2019;18(9):102357; Girard-Madoux MJH, et al. The immunological functions of the appendix: an example of redundancy? *Semin Immunol.* 2018;36:31–44; Killinger BA, et al. The vermiform appendix impacts the risk of developing Parkinson's disease. *Sci Transl Med.* 2018;10(465):eaar5280; Killinger B, et al. The appendix in Parkinson's disease: from vestigial remnant to vital organ? *J Parkinsons Dis.* 2019;9(s2):S345–S358; Takakura W, et al. Comparing the rates of methane production in patients with and without appendectomy: results from a large-scale cohort. *Sci Rep.* 2020;10: 867; Vitetta L, et al. The vermiform appendix: an immunological organ sustaining a microbiome inoculum. *Clin Sci.* 2019;133(1):1–8.

the ileum. Attached to it is the vermiform appendix, an appendage having limited physiologic function. However, recent studies suggest it may have an important protective role in gut immunity (Emerging Science Box: The Appendix in Health and Disease). From the cecum, chyme enters the colon, which loops upward, traverses the abdominal cavity, and descends to the anal canal. The four parts of the colon are the ascending colon, transverse colon, descending colon, and sigmoid colon. Two sphincters control the flow of intestinal contents through the cecum and colon: the ileocecal valve, which admits chyme from the ileum to the cecum; and the rectosigmoid canal, which controls the movement of wastes from the sigmoid colon into the rectum. A thick (2.5 to 3 cm) portion of smooth muscle surrounds the anal canal, forming the internal anal sphincter. Overlapping it distally is the striated skeletal muscle of the external anal sphincter (anus).

In the cecum and colon, the longitudinal muscle layer consists of three longitudinal bands called teniae coli (see Fig. 40.17B). They are shorter than the colon and give it a gathered appearance. The circular muscles of the colon separate the gathered areas into outpouchings called haustra (sing., haustrum). The haustra become more or less prominent with the contractions and relaxations of the circular muscles. The mucosal surface of the colon has rugae (folds), particularly between the haustra, and crypts of Lieberkühn but no villi. Columnar epithelial cells and mucus-secreting goblet cells form the mucosa throughout the large intestine. The columnar epithelium absorbs fluid and electrolytes, and the mucus-secreting cells lubricate the mucosa.

In the large intestine, extrinsic parasympathetic innervation occurs through the vagus nerve. Vagal stimulation increases rhythmic contraction of the proximal colon from the cecum to the first part of the transverse colon. Vagal fibers reach the distal colon through the sacral parasympathetic splanchnic nerves. The internal anal sphincter is usually contracted, and its reflex response is to relax when the rectum is distended. The intrinsic myenteric plexus provides the major innervation of the internal anal sphincter but responds to sympathetic stimulation to maintain contraction and parasympathetic stimulation that facilitates relaxation when the rectum is full. Sympathetic innervation of this sphincter arises from the celiac and superior mesenteric ganglia and the sphincter nerve. The external anal sphincter is innervated by the pudendal nerve arising from sacral levels of the spinal cord. Sympathetic activity in the entire large intestine modulates intestinal reflexes, conveys somatic sensations of fullness and pain, participates in the defecation reflex, and constricts blood vessels. The blood supply of the large intestine and rectum is derived primarily from branches of the superior and inferior mesenteric arteries[21] (see Figs. 40.7 and 40.17A) and venous blood drains through the inferior mesenteric vein.

The primary type of colonic movement is segmental. The circular muscles contract and relax at different sites, shuttling the intestinal contents back and forth between the haustra, most commonly during fasting. The movements massage the intestinal contents, called the fecal mass at that point, and facilitate the absorption of water. Propulsive movement occurs with the proximal-to-distal contraction of several haustral units. Peristaltic movements also occur and promote the emptying of the colon. The gastrocolic reflex initiates propulsion in the entire colon, usually during or immediately after eating, when chyme enters from the ileum. The gastrocolic reflex causes the fecal mass to pass rapidly into the sigmoid colon and rectum, stimulating defecation. It is mediated by vagal stimulation along with gastrin and cholecystokinin.[4] Epinephrine inhibits contractile activity, as do exogenous opioids.

Approximately 500 to 700 mL of chyme flows from the ileum to the cecum per day. Most of the water is absorbed in the colon by diffusion and active transport. Aldosterone increases colon membrane permeability to sodium, thereby increasing both the diffusion of sodium into the cell and the active transport of sodium across the basolateral membrane to the interstitial fluid. (See Chapters 3 and 21 for a discussion of aldosterone secretion.) This increases the cell-to-lumen diffusion gradient for potassium. Potassium moves outward, and chloride is absorbed with sodium as the complementary anion. Chloride also enters the cell in exchange for bicarbonate. The colon does not absorb monosaccharides and amino acids, but some short-chain free fatty acids, which are produced by bacterial fermentation, are absorbed.

Absorption and epithelial transport occur in the cecum, ascending colon, transverse colon, and descending colon. By the time the fecal mass enters the sigmoid colon, the mass consists entirely of wastes, called the feces, and is composed of food residue, unabsorbed GI secretions, shed epithelial cells, and bacteria.

The movement of feces into the sigmoid colon and rectum stimulates the defecation reflex (rectosphincteric reflex). The rectal wall stretches, and the tonically constricted internal anal sphincter (smooth muscle with ANS control) relaxes, creating the urge to defecate. The defecation reflex can be overridden voluntarily by contraction of the external anal sphincter and muscles of the pelvic floor. The rectal wall gradually relaxes, reducing tension, and the urge to defecate passes. Retrograde contraction of the rectum may displace the feces out of the rectal vault until a more convenient time for evacuation. Pain or fear of pain associated with defecation (e.g., rectal fissures or hemorrhoids) can inhibit the defecation reflex. The defecation reflex is regulated by parasympathetic cholinergic fibers. Voluntary inhibition or facilitation of defecation is mediated from cortical projections onto the medulla and down to sacral segments of the cord.

Squatting and sitting facilitate defecation because these positions straighten the angle between the rectum and anal canal and increase the efficiency of straining (increasing intra-abdominal pressure). Intra-abdominal pressure is increased by initiating the Valsalva maneuver—that is, inhaling and forcing the diaphragm and chest muscles against the closed glottis to increase both intrathoracic and intra-abdominal pressure, which is transmitted to the rectum.

The Gastrointestinal Tract and Immunity

The GI tract's gut-associated lymphoid tissue (GALT) plays a major role in immune defenses by killing many pathogenetic microorganisms and preventing reaction to foreign proteins (dietary antigens) ingested in the diet. It also plays a fundamental role in modulating the systemic adaptive immune system through its interaction with resident microorganisms (microbiome) (see Chapter 8).[22] The mucosa of the intestine covers a large surface area, and mucosal secretions produce antibodies, particularly IgA, and enzymes that provide defenses against pathogenic microorganisms. Small intestinal Paneth cells, located near the base of the crypts of Lieberkühn (see Fig. 40.11B), produce defensins and other antimicrobial peptides and lysozymes important to mucosal immunity. Small intestinal Peyer patches (lymph nodules containing collections of lymphocytes, plasma cells, and macrophages) are most numerous in the ileum and produce antimicrobial peptides and IgA as a component of GALT in the small intestine (see Figs. 40.2 and 8.3). Peyer patches are important for antigen processing and immune defense (see Chapter 8).

Intestinal Microbiome

The type and number of bacterial flora vary greatly throughout the normal GI tract and among individuals. The normal flora of the GI tract are called the intestinal microbiome. There are an increasing number of bacteria from the proximal to the distal GI tract, with the highest number in the colon. Bacteria in the stomach are relatively sparse because of the secretion of hydrochloric acid that kills ingested pathogens or inhibits bacterial growth (with the exception of *H. pylori*). Bile acid secretion, intestinal motility, and antibody production suppress bacterial growth in the duodenum. In the duodenum and jejunum, there is a low concentration of aerobes, primarily streptococci, lactobacilli, staphylococci, enterobacteria, and *Bacteroides*. Anaerobes are found distal to the ileocecal valve but not proximal to the ileum. They constitute about 95% of the fecal flora in the colon and contribute one-third of the solid bulk of feces. *Bacteroides* (gram negative) and *Firmicutes* (gram positive) are the most common colon bacteria.

The microorganisms that inhabit the healthy GI tract (normal flora) generally do not have the virulence factors associated with pathogenic microorganisms. Intestinal bacteria play a role in the metabolism of bile salts, estrogens, androgens, lipids, carbohydrates, various nitrogenous substances, and drugs. They produce antimicrobial peptides, hormones, neurotransmitters, anti-inflammatory metabolites, vitamin K_2, and B vitamins; destroy toxins; prevent pathogen colonization; and alert the immune system to protect against infection. The GI microbiome also has regulatory influences on systemic innate and adaptive immune responses and inflammation, including expansion and activity of T-cell populations and systemic anti-inflammatory signaling (see Chapters 7 and 8).

Genetics, diet, environmental pollution, personal hygiene, vaccination, infection, antibiotics and other drugs, and radiation affect the normal composition of bacterial flora.[22] The intestinal tract is sterile at birth but becomes colonized within a few hours. Within 3 to 4 weeks after birth, the normal flora are established. The health of the gut microbiome in early life is a predictor of diseases such as allergy and autoimmune conditions in later life.[23] The number and diversity of bacteria decrease with aging, increasing the risk for infection and disease. Deleterious changes in the gut microbiome (dysbiosis) are associated with a large range of disorders including cardiac, pulmonary, endocrine, GI, and neurological diseases; obesity; cancer; viral and bacterial infections; sepsis; cognitive impairment; and mental health conditions. Dietary and lifestyle changes can improve the health of the intestinal microbiome. Fecal microbiota transplantation is being used to reverse GI dysbiosis for the treatment of many disorders including diabetes, cancer, and Parkinson disease.[24] With regard to GI diseases, fecal transplant has been used with considerable success for Clostridium difficile infection, as well as inflammatory bowel disease, irritable bowel disease, and liver disease.

Splanchnic Blood Flow

The splanchnic (visceral) blood flow provides blood to the esophagus, stomach, small and large intestines, liver, gallbladder, pancreas, and spleen (see Fig. 40.7). Blood flow is regulated by cardiac output and blood volume, the ANS, hormones, and local autoregulatory blood flow mechanisms. The GI circulation serves as an important reservoir of blood volume to maintain circulation to the heart and lungs when needed.

ACCESSORY ORGANS OF DIGESTION

The liver, gallbladder, and exocrine pancreas all secrete substances necessary for the digestion of chyme. These secretions are delivered to the duodenum through the sphincter of Oddi at the major duodenal papilla (of Vater) (Fig. 40.18). The liver produces bile, which contains salts necessary for fat digestion and absorption. Between meals, bile is stored in the gallbladder. The exocrine pancreas produces (1) enzymes needed for the complete digestion of carbohydrates, proteins, and fats; and (2) an alkaline fluid that neutralizes chyme, creating a duodenal pH that supports enzymatic action.

The liver also receives nutrients absorbed by the small intestine and metabolizes or synthesizes them into forms that can be absorbed by the body's cells. It then releases the nutrients into the bloodstream or stores them for later use.

Liver

The liver weighs 1200 to 1600 g and is the largest solid organ in the body. It is located under the right diaphragm and is divided into right and left lobes (Fig. 40.19). The larger, right lobe is

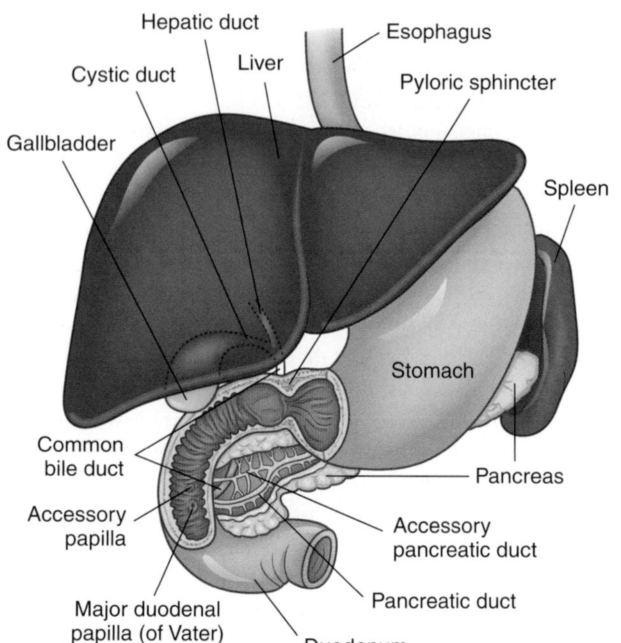

Fig. 40.18 Accessory Organs of Digestion. Location of the liver, gallbladder, and exocrine pancreas.

divided further into the caudate and quadrate lobes. The *falciform ligament* separates the right and left lobes and attaches the liver to the anterior abdominal wall. A fibrous cord that is a remnant of the umbilical vein, called the *round ligament (ligamentum teres)*, extends along the free edge of the falciform ligament, extending from the umbilicus to the inferior surface of the liver.[6] The *coronary ligament* branches from the falciform ligament and extends over the superior surface of the right and left lobes, binding the liver to the inferior surface of the diaphragm. The liver is covered by a fibroelastic capsule called the Glisson capsule, which contains blood vessels, lymphatics, and nerves. When the liver is diseased or swollen, distention of the capsule causes pain because it is innervated by sensory neurons of the lower intercostal nerves.

The metabolic functions of the liver require a large amount of blood. The liver receives blood from both arterial and venous sources. The hepatic artery is formed by the merging of superior mesenteric and splenic veins and receives blood from the inferior mesenteric, gastric, and cystic veins. The hepatic artery supplies one-third of the blood supply, while the hepatic portal vein supplies two-thirds.[6] The liver receives approximately 25% of the overall cardiac output even though it only accounts for less than 3% of the total body weight. The hepatic artery provides arterial oxygenated blood to the liver, whereas the hepatic portal vein delivers deoxygenated blood which it receives from the inferior and superior mesenteric veins, the splenic vein, and the gastric and esophageal veins (see Fig. 40.7). The blood supplied by the hepatic portal vein is rich in nutrients that have been absorbed from the intestinal tract (Fig. 40.20).

Within the liver lobes are approximately 100,000 tiny anatomic units called liver lobules which are spatially zonated between the portal and central veins (Fig. 40.21). They are formed of cords or plates of hepatocytes, which are the functional cells of the liver. These cells line up along the portocentral blood flow, so that they can metabolize nutrients, as well as produce and recycle proteins.[25] They can regenerate; therefore, damaged or resected liver tissue can regrow. Hepatocytes secrete electrolytes, lipids, lecithin, bile acids, and cholesterol into the canaliculi. Plasma proteins are also synthesized and released into the bloodstream. Hepatocyte function is adjusted temporally to meet the changing metabolic demands of daily feeding cycles.[25] Lipocytes are star-shaped cells that store lipids, including vitamin A. Small capillaries, or sinusoids, are located between the plates of hepatocytes. They receive a mixture of venous and arterial blood from branches of the hepatic artery and portal vein. Blood from the sinusoids drains to a central vein in the middle of each liver lobule. Venous blood from all the lobules then flows into the hepatic vein, which empties into the inferior vena cava. The sinusoids of the liver lobules are lined with highly permeable endothelium. This permeability enhances the transport of nutrients from the sinusoids into the hepatocytes, where they are metabolized.

The immune functions of the liver are carried out by various cells, including sinusoidal endothelial cells, Kupffer, stellate, and natural killer cells. Sinusoidal cells line the sinusoidal capillaries and, in addition to their barrier function, have immune functions including endocytosis, antigen

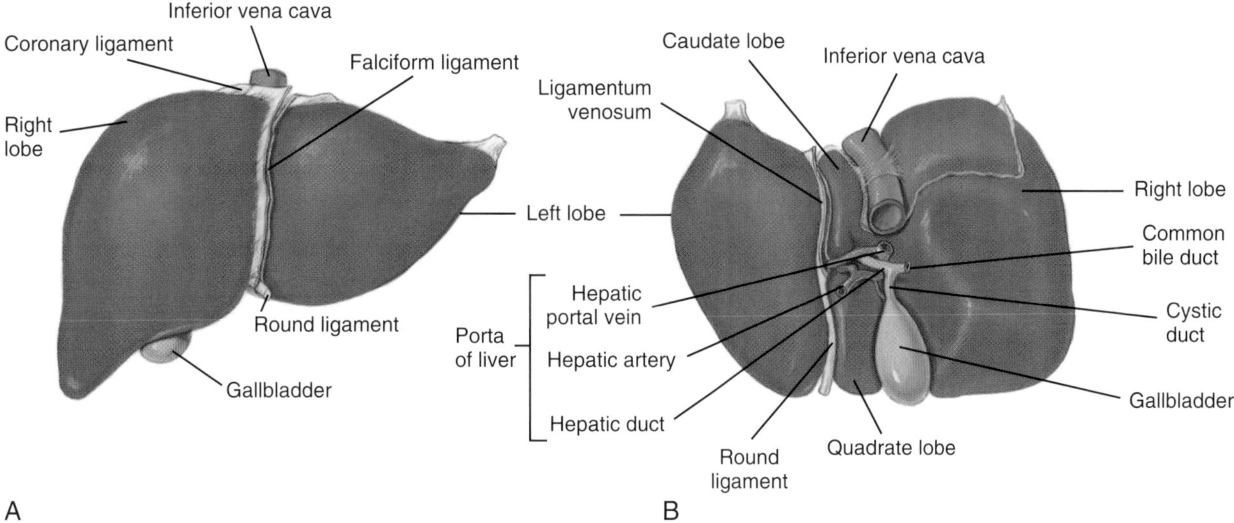

Fig. 40.19 Gross Structure of the Liver. (A) Anterior surface. (B) Visceral surface. (From Applegate E. *The Anatomy and Physiology Learning System.* 4th ed. St Louis: Saunders; 2011.)

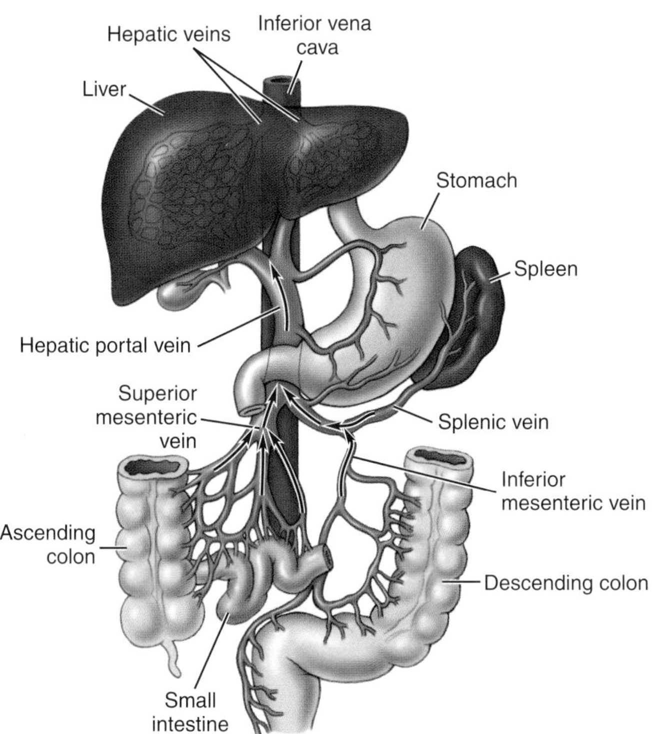

Fig. 40.20 Hepatic Portal Circulation. In this unusual circulatory route, a vein is located between two capillary beds. The hepatic portal vein collects blood from capillaries in visceral structures located in the abdomen and empties into the liver. Hepatic veins return blood to the inferior vena cava. (From Herlihy B. *The Human Body in Health and Illness.* 5th ed. St Louis: Saunders; 2015.)

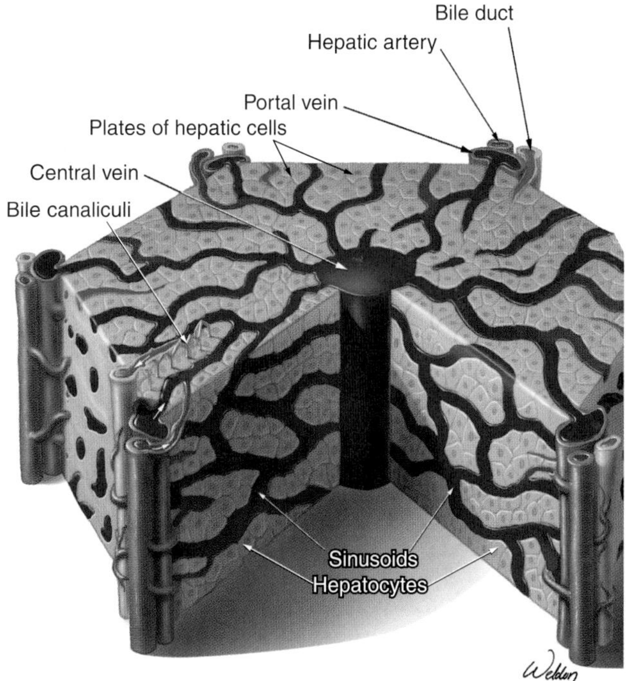

Fig. 40.21 Schematic of the Liver Lobule. A cross section of a single liver lobule shows that, in whole, it is shaped like a hexagonal cylinder. The cut away area shows the central vein in the center of the lobule, separated by cords of hepatocytes forming sinusoids from six portal areas at the periphery. The portal areas contain a portal vein, hepatic artery, and bile duct. Blood flows toward the center of the lobule, whereas bile flows toward the portal triads at the margins. Note the hepatic artery providing oxygenated blood to the hepatic sinusoids. (From Polin RA, et al. *Fetal and Neonatal Physiology.* 4th ed. St Louis: Saunders; 2011.)

presentation, and leukocyte recruitment. The sinusoids also are lined with phagocytic and bactericidal Kupffer cells (tissue macrophages), which are part of the mononuclear phagocyte system. Kupffer cells are the largest population of tissue macrophages in the body and are central to innate and adaptive immunity. They play a key role in the identification and presentation of foreign antigens to the immune system, as well as phagocytose opsonized particles and iron molecules from the blood.[26] Kupffer cells are important for healing injury to the liver and are important for bilirubin production and lipid metabolism. Stellate cells contain retinoids (vitamin A), are contractile in liver injury, regulate sinusoidal blood flow, may proliferate into myofibroblasts, participate in liver fibrosis, produce erythropoietin, can act as antigen-presenting cells, remove foreign substances from the blood, and trap bacteria. They also contribute to the mature differentiation of Kupffer cells.[27] Natural killer cells (pit cells) also are found in the sinusoidal lumen; they produce interferon-γ and are important in tumor defense (see Chapter 7). Between the endothelial lining of the sinusoid and the hepatocyte is the Disse space, which drains interstitial fluid into the hepatic lymph system.

Secretion of Bile

The liver assists intestinal digestion by secreting 700 to 1200 mL of bile per day. Bile is an alkaline, bitter-tasting, yellowish green fluid that contains bile salts (conjugated bile acids), cholesterol, bilirubin (a pigment), electrolytes, and water. It is formed by hepatocytes and secreted into the bile canaliculi. Bile canaliculi are small channels that conduct bile outward to bile ducts and eventually drain into the common bile duct (see Figs. 40.18 and 40.21). This duct empties bile into the ampulla of Vater, and then into the duodenum through an opening called the major duodenal papilla (sphincter of Oddi). Bile salts are required for the intestinal emulsification and absorption of lipids and fat-soluble vitamins, and the elimination of cholesterol. Having facilitated fat emulsification and absorption in the small intestine, most bile salts are actively absorbed in the terminal ileum and returned to the liver through the portal circulation for resecretion. The pathway for recycling of bile salts is termed the enterohepatic circulation (Fig. 40.22).

Bile has two fractional components: the acid-dependent fraction and the acid-independent fraction. Hepatocytes secrete the bile acid–dependent fraction, which consists of bile acids, cholesterol, lecithin (a phospholipid), and bilirubin (a bile pigment).[4] The bile acid–independent fraction, which is secreted by the hepatocytes and epithelial cells of the bile canaliculi, is a bicarbonate-rich aqueous fluid that gives bile its alkaline pH and facilitates buffering of chyme entering the duodenum from the stomach.

Bile salts are conjugated in the liver from primary and secondary bile acids. In addition to their role in emulsifying lipids, bile acids serve as metabolites that regulate metabolic, immune, and inflammatory pathways.[28] The primary bile acids are cholic acid and chenodeoxycholic (chenic) acid. These acids are synthesized from cholesterol by the hepatocytes. The secondary bile acids are deoxycholic and lithocholic acid.[4] These acids are formed in the small intestine by intestinal bacteria, after which they are absorbed and flow to the liver (see Fig. 40.22). The content of bile can be influenced by the intestinal microbiome such that dysbiosis can lead to formation of gallstones.[29] Both forms of bile acids are conjugated with amino acids (glycine or taurine) in the liver to form bile salts. Conjugation makes the bile acids more water soluble, thus restricting their diffusion from the duodenum and ileum. The primary and secondary bile acids together form the bile acid pool.

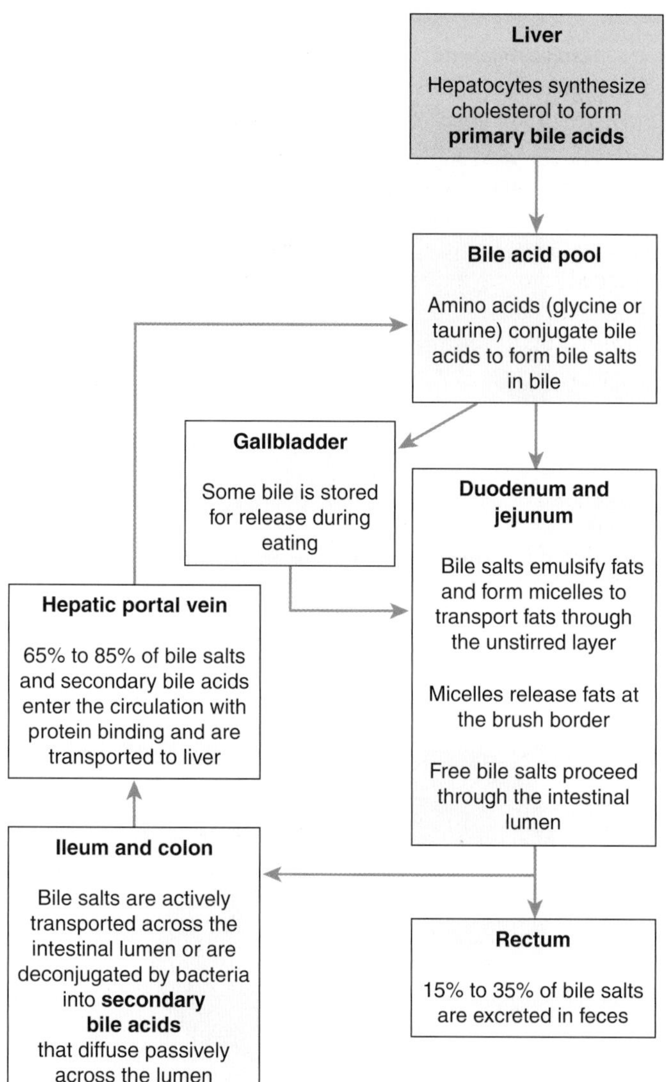

Fig. 40.22 Enterohepatic Circulation of Bile Salts.

Some bile salts are deconjugated by intestinal bacteria to secondary bile acids. These acids diffuse passively into the portal blood from both small and large intestines. An increase in the plasma concentration of bile acids accelerates the uptake and resecretion of bile acids and salts by the hepatocytes. In pregnancy, deconjugation of bile acids by intestinal bacteria is enhanced and ileal uptake of bile acids is impaired which may lead to hypercholesterolemia.[30] The cycle of hepatic secretion, intestinal absorption, and hepatic resecretion of bile acids completes the enterohepatic circulation. Disruption of the enterohepatic circulation has been linked to the development of cholestatic liver disease, inflammatory bowel disease, metabolic syndrome, and colon cancer.[28]

Most bile secretion occurs during the digestion of meals. Bile secretion is called choleresis. A choleretic agent is a substance that stimulates the liver to secrete bile. One strong stimulus is a high concentration of bile salts. Other choleretics include cholecystokinin, vagal stimulation, and secretin, which increase the rate of bile flow by promoting contraction of the gallbladder and the secretion of bicarbonate from canaliculi and other intrahepatic bile ducts.[4]

Metabolism of Bilirubin

Bilirubin is a byproduct of the destruction of aged red blood cells. It gives bile a greenish black color and produces the yellow tinge of jaundice. Aged red blood cells are absorbed and destroyed by macrophages (Kupffer cells) of the mononuclear phagocyte system, primarily in the spleen and liver. Within these cells, hemoglobin is separated into its component parts: heme and globin (Fig. 40.23). The globin component is further degraded into its constituent amino acids, which go into the amino acid pool to form new protein. The heme component is converted to biliverdin by the enzymatic cleavage of iron. The iron attaches to transferrin in the plasma and can be stored in the liver or used by the bone marrow to make new red blood cells. The biliverdin is enzymatically converted to bilirubin in the Kupffer cell and then is released into the plasma where it binds to albumin and is known as unconjugated bilirubin, or free bilirubin, which is lipid soluble. Bilirubin also has a role as an antioxidant and provides cytoprotection.

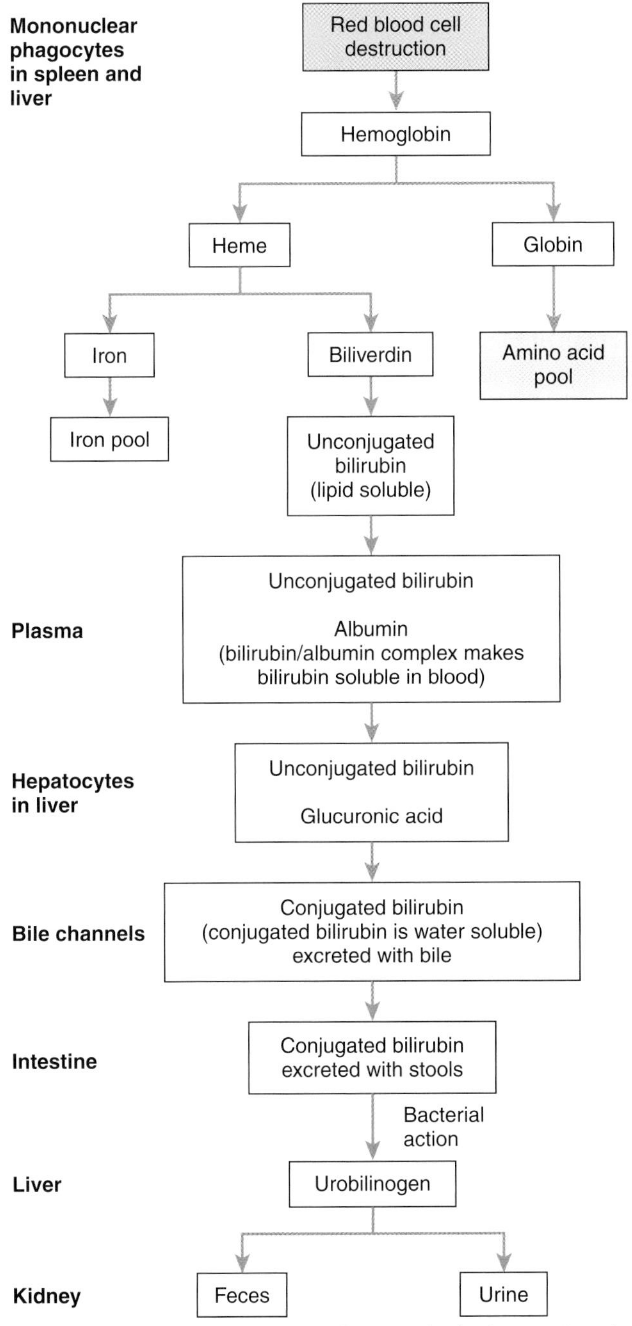

Fig. 40.23 Bilirubin Metabolism. See text for further explanation.

In the liver, unconjugated bilirubin moves from plasma in the sinusoids into the hepatocyte. Within hepatocytes, unconjugated bilirubin joins with glucuronic acid to form conjugated bilirubin. Conjugation transforms bilirubin from a lipid-soluble substance that can cross biologic membranes to a water-soluble substance that can be excreted. When conjugated bilirubin reaches the distal ileum and colon, it is deconjugated by bacteria and converted to urobilinogen. Urobilinogen is then reabsorbed in the intestines and transported to the kidney where it is excreted in the urine as urobilin, giving urine its yellow color. A small amount of urobilin is recirculated back into the liver and eliminated in feces as stercobilin (an end-product of heme metabolism), which contributes to the stool's brown pigmentation. The elimination of bilirubin is an important route for the elimination of cholesterol. Serum bilirubin levels are measured in the evaluation of numerous disorders including hepatobiliary disease, cardiovascular disease, prematurity, and cancer.

Vascular and Hematologic Functions

Because of its extensive vascular network, the liver can store a large volume of blood. The liver can release blood to maintain systemic circulatory volume in the event of hemorrhage. The liver also has hemostatic functions; it synthesizes most clotting factors (see Chapter 28). Vitamins K_1 and K_2, fat-soluble vitamins, are essential for the synthesis of the clotting factors. Because bile salts are needed for reabsorption of fats, vitamin K absorption depends on adequate bile production in the liver. Impairment of vitamin K absorption diminishes production of clotting factors and increases risk of bleeding.

Metabolism of Nutrients

Carbohydrates. The liver contributes to the stability of serum blood glucose levels by releasing glucose during hypoglycemia (low blood glucose level), absorbing glucose during hyperglycemia (high blood glucose level), and storing it as glycogen (glycogenesis) or converting it to fat. Hepatic glycogenesis is stimulated by insulin via the action of the enzyme glucokinase.[31] When all glycogen stores have been used, the liver can convert amino acids and glycerol to glucose (gluconeogenesis). Gluconeogenesis increases in diabetes and contributes to hyperglycemia. Dietary changes and hypoglycemic agents such as metformin suppress hepatic gluconeogenesis.[32]

Proteins. Protein synthesis requires the presence of all the essential amino acids (obtained only from food), as well as nonessential amino acids. Proteins perform many important functions in the body; these are summarized in Table 40.3.

Within hepatocytes, amino acids are converted to carbohydrates (keto acids) by the removal of ammonia (NH_3), a process known as deamination. The ammonia is converted to urea by the liver and passes into the blood to be excreted by the kidneys. Depending on the nutritional status of the body, the keto acids either are converted to fatty acids for fat synthesis and storage or

TABLE 40.3 Importance of Proteins in the Body

Function	Example
Contraction	Actin and myosin enable muscle contraction.
Energy	Proteins can be metabolized for energy.
Fluid balance	Albumin is a major source of plasma oncotic pressure.
Protection	Antibodies, complement, and C-reactive protein protect against infection and foreign substances.
Regulation	Enzymes control chemical reactions; hormones regulate many physiologic processes.
Structure	Collagen fibers provide structural support to many parts of the body; keratin strengthens skin, hair, and nails.
Transport	Hemoglobin transports oxygen and carbon dioxide in the blood; plasma proteins serve as transport molecules; proteins in cell membranes control movement of materials into and out of cells.
Coagulation	Hemostasis is regulated by clotting factors and proteins that balance coagulation and anticoagulation.

are oxidized by the Krebs tricarboxylic acid cycle (see Chapter 1) to provide energy for the liver cells.

The plasma proteins, including albumins and α- and β- globulins, are synthesized by the liver (gamma globulin are formed in lymph nodes and lymphoid tissue). They play an important role in preserving blood volume and pressure by maintaining plasma oncotic pressure. The liver also synthesizes several nonessential amino acids and serum enzymes that become elevated with liver injury (and other diseases):

- Aspartate aminotransferase (AST): also present in red blood cells and skeletal muscle; AST transfers an α-amino group between aspartate and glutamate.
- Alanine aminotransferase (ALT): also present in small amounts in the kidneys, heart, skeletal muscle, and pancreas; ALT transfers an amino group from alanine to α-ketoglutarate to form pyruvate and glutamate.
- Lactate dehydrogenase (LDH): catalyzes the conversion of lactate to pyruvate; LDH is widely distributed throughout the body and different isoenzymes are found in different tissues.
- Alkaline phosphatase: removes phosphate groups, particularly in an alkaline environment.
- Gamma-glutamyltransferase: transfers the gamma-glutamyl moiety of glutathione to an acceptor to form glutamate (neurotransmitter) and is a pro-oxidant.

Fats. Ingested fat absorbed by lacteals in the intestinal villi enters the liver circulation through the lymphatics, primarily as triglycerides. In the liver, the triglycerides can be hydrolyzed to glycerol and free fatty acids and used to produce metabolic energy called adenosine triphosphate (ATP), or they can be released into the bloodstream bound to proteins (lipoproteins). The lipoproteins are carried by the blood to adipose cells for storage. The liver also synthesizes phospholipids and cholesterol, which are needed for the hepatic production of bile salts, steroid hormones, components of plasma membranes, and other special molecules.

Metabolic Detoxification

The liver alters exogenous and endogenous chemicals (e.g., drugs), foreign molecules, and hormones to make them less toxic or less biologically active. This process, called metabolic detoxification or biotransformation, diminishes intestinal or renal tubular reabsorption of potentially toxic substances and facilitates their intestinal and renal excretion. In this way, alcohol, barbiturates, amphetamines, steroids, and hormones (including estrogens, aldosterone, antidiuretic hormone, and testosterone) are metabolized or detoxified, preventing excessive accumulation and adverse effects. Although metabolic detoxification is usually protective, the end products of metabolic detoxification sometimes become reactive metabolites (see Chapter 2). Reactive metabolites of alcohol metabolism, for example, are acetaldehyde and hydrogen. Acetaminophen toxicity occurs when its metabolite N-acetyl-p-benzoquinone imine (NAPQI) overwhelms the glutathione pathway. Reactive metabolites can induce oxidative stress, bind to proteins, disrupt mitochondria, interfere with bile transport, or induce autoimmune responses.[33]

Storage of Minerals and Vitamins

The liver stores certain vitamins and minerals, including iron and copper, in times of excessive intake and releases them in times of need. Iron is stored in the liver as ferritin, an iron-protein complex, and is released as needed for red blood cell production (see Chapter 28). The liver can store vitamins B_{12} and D for several months and vitamin A for several years. The liver also stores vitamins E and K.

Gallbladder

The gallbladder is a sac-like organ on the inferior surface of the liver (see Fig. 40.23). Its primary function is to store and concentrate bile between meals. The wall of the gallbladder is composed of the mucous membrane, muscularis, and serosa. During the interdigestive period, bile flows from the liver through the right or left hepatic duct into the common hepatic duct and meets resistance at the closed sphincter of Oddi (duodenal papilla), which controls flow into the duodenum and prevents backflow of duodenal contents into the pancreatobiliary system. Bile then flows through the cystic duct into the gallbladder, where it is concentrated and stored. The mucosa of the gallbladder wall readily absorbs water and electrolytes, leaving a high concentration of bile salts, bile pigments, and cholesterol. The gallbladder holds about 90 mL of bile.

Within 30 minutes after eating, the gallbladder begins to contract, forcing stored bile through the cystic duct and into the common bile duct.[4] The sphincter of Oddi relaxes, and bile flows into the duodenum through the major duodenal papilla. During the cephalic and gastric phases of digestion, gallbladder contraction is mediated by cholinergic branches of the vagus nerve. Hormonal regulation of gallbladder contraction is derived primarily from the release of cholecystokinin secreted by the duodenal and jejunal mucosa in the presence of fat. Vasoactive intestinal peptide, pancreatic polypeptide, and sympathetic nerve stimulation relax the gallbladder.

Exocrine Pancreas

The pancreas is approximately 20 cm long. Its head is tucked into the curve of the duodenum, and its tail touches the spleen. The body of the pancreas lies deep in the abdomen, behind the stomach (see Figs. 40.1 and 40.24). The pancreas is unique in that it has both endocrine and exocrine functions. The endocrine pancreas secretes hormones—insulin, glucagon, somatostatin, and pancreatic polypeptide—from cells in the pancreatic islets (see Chapter 22).

The exocrine pancreas is composed of acinar cells that secrete enzymes and networks of ducts that secrete alkaline fluids. Both have important digestive functions. The acinar cells are organized into spherical lobules, called acini, around small secretory ducts (see Fig. 40.24). Secretions drain into a system of ducts that leads to the pancreatic duct (Wirsung duct), which empties into the common bile duct at the ampulla of Vater and then through the duodenal papilla into the duodenum. In some individuals, an accessory duct (the duct of Santorini) branches off the pancreatic duct and drains directly into the duodenum at an opening called the minor duodenal papilla.

Arterial blood is supplied to the pancreas by branches of the celiac and superior mesenteric arteries (see Fig. 40.7). Venous blood leaves the head of the pancreas through tributaries to the portal vein, and the body and tail are drained through the splenic vein. All hormonal pancreatic secretions also pass through the hepatic portal vein into the liver.

Pancreatic innervation arises from parasympathetic neurons of the vagus nerve. These fibers activate postganglionic fibers, which stimulate enzymatic and hormonal secretion. Sympathetic postganglionic fibers from the celiac and superior mesenteric plexuses innervate the blood vessels, cause vasoconstriction, and inhibit pancreatic secretion.

The aqueous secretions of the exocrine pancreas are isotonic and contain potassium, sodium, bicarbonate, magnesium, calcium, and chloride. Sodium and potassium concentrations are about equal to those in the plasma. Pancreatic ductal cells secrete bicarbonate and the concentration in pancreatic juice

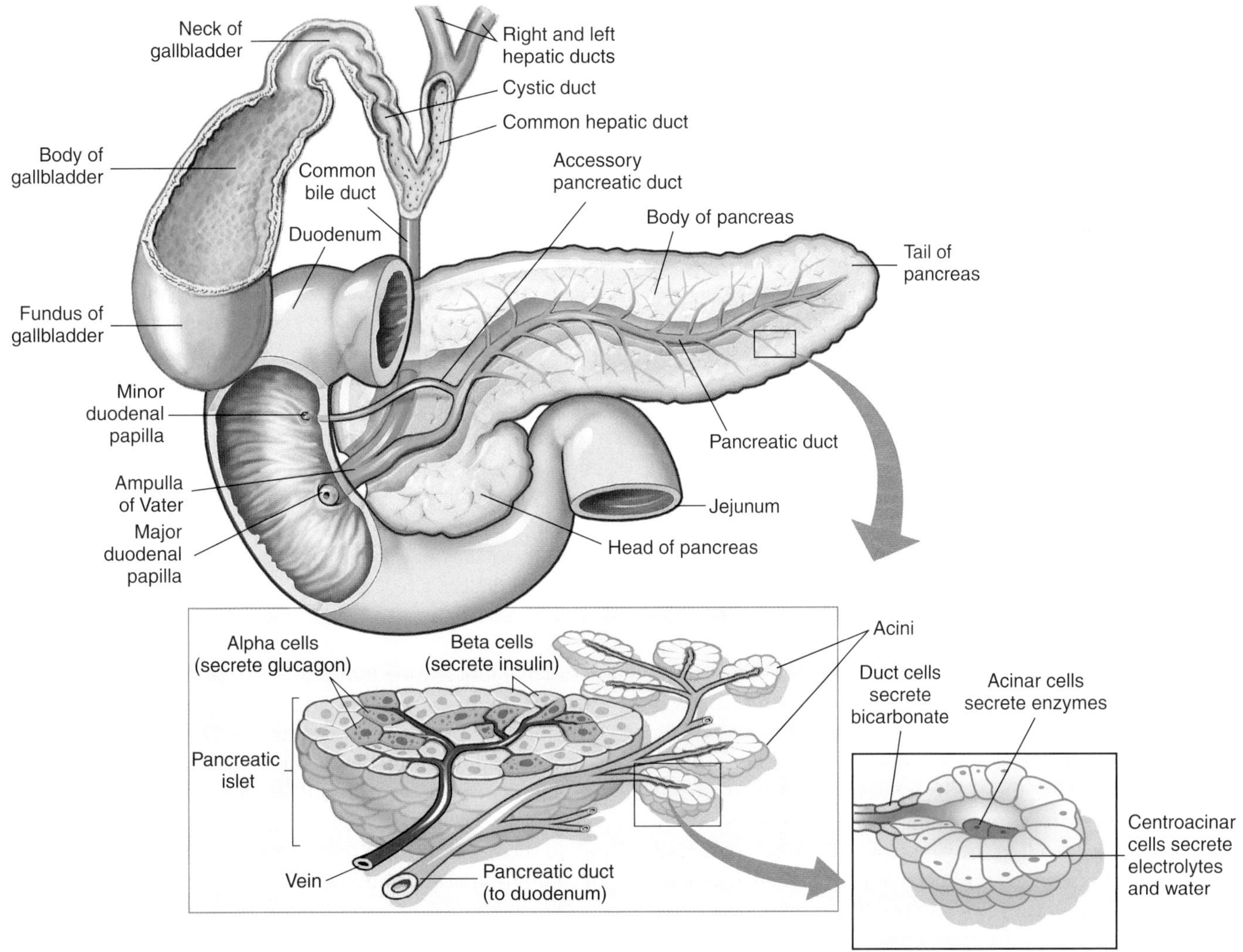

Fig. 40.24 Associated Structures of the Gallbladder, Pancreas, and Pancreatic Acinar Cells and Duct. (Modified from Thibodeau GA, Patton KT. *Anatomy & Physiology*. 6th ed. St Louis: Mosby; 2007.)

varies directly with the secretory flow rate. As bicarbonate secretion increases, chloride secretion decreases to maintain a constant anionic concentration. The highly alkaline pancreatic juice neutralizes the acidic chyme that enters the duodenum from the stomach and provides the alkaline medium needed for the actions of digestive enzymes and intestinal absorption of fat.

In the pancreas, transport of water and electrolytes through the ductal epithelium involves both active and passive mechanisms. The ductal cells actively transport hydrogen into the blood and bicarbonate into the duct lumen. Potassium and chloride are secreted by diffusion according to changes in electrochemical potential gradients. As the secretion flows down the duct, water is osmotically transported into the pancreatic juice until it becomes isosmotic. At low flow rates bicarbonate is exchanged passively for chloride, but at higher flow rates there is less time for this exchange and bicarbonate concentration increases. Because eating stimulates the flow of pancreatic juice, the juice is most alkaline when it needs to be: during digestion.

The pancreatic enzymes can hydrolyze proteins (proteases), carbohydrates (amylases), and fats (lipases) (see Fig. 40.12). The proteolytic (protein-digesting) enzymes include trypsin, chymotrypsin, carboxypeptidase, and elastase. These enzymes are secreted in their inactive forms—that is, as trypsinogen, chymotrypsinogen, procarboxypeptidase, and proelastase, respectively—to protect the pancreas from the digestive effects of its own enzymes. For further protection, the pancreas produces trypsin inhibitor, which prevents the activation of proteolytic enzymes while they are in the pancreas. Once in the duodenum, the inactive forms (proenzymes) are activated by enterokinase, an enzyme secreted by the duodenal mucosa. Trypsinogen is the first proenzyme to be activated. Its conversion to trypsin stimulates the conversion of chymotrypsinogen to chymotrypsin and procarboxypeptidase to carboxypeptidase. Each of these enzymes cleaves specific peptide bonds to reduce polypeptides to smaller peptides.

Pancreatic α-amylase is secreted in active form and digests intestinal carbohydrate by cleaving interior α-1,4-glucosidic bonds to yield glucose and maltose at an optimum pH of approximately 6.9. Pancreatic lipases hydrolyze triglycerides, cholesterol, and phospholipids to free fatty acids in the intestine.

Secretion of the aqueous and enzymatic components of pancreatic juice is controlled by hormonal and autonomic stimuli. Both parasympathetic and sympathetic innervation affect exocrine pancreatic secretion. Secretion can be stimulated by meal anticipation and ingestion, ACh, insulin, amylin, glucagon, and pancreatic polypeptide.[34] The hormone secretin stimulates the acinar and duct cells to secrete the bicarbonate-rich fluid that neutralizes chyme and prepares it for enzymatic digestion. As chyme enters the duodenum, its acidity (pH of 4.5 or less) stimulates the S cells (secretin-producing cells) of the duodenum to release secretin, which is absorbed by the intestine and delivered to the pancreas in the bloodstream. In the pancreas, secretin causes ductal and acinar cells to release alkaline fluid. Secretin also inhibits the actions of gastrin, thereby decreasing gastric hydrochloric acid secretion and motility. The overall effect is to neutralize the contents of the duodenum.

Enzymatic secretion follows, stimulated by cholecystokinin, which activates ACh from the vagus nerve and release of ACh from pancreatic stellate cells. Cholecystokinin is released in the duodenum in response to the essential amino acids and fatty acids already present in chyme. Once in the small intestine, activated pancreatic enzymes inhibit the release of more cholecystokinin and ACh. This feedback mechanism inhibits the secretion of more pancreatic enzymes. Pancreatic polypeptide is released after eating and inhibits postprandial pancreatic exocrine secretion. (See Table 40.1 for a summary of hormonal stimulation of pancreatic secretions.) Selected tests of pancreatic function are listed in Table 40.4.

TESTS OF DIGESTIVE FUNCTION

Gastrointestinal Tract

Although important diagnostic information can be obtained from an individual's medical history and presenting symptoms, numerous disease-specific tests must be performed to evaluate the structure and function of the GI tract. A description of selected studies is presented in Tables 40.4 and 40.5. Of interest in relation to infection with coronavirus 2 (SARS-nCoV-2) is the evaluation of liver function related to disease severity and fecal testing for presence of the virus (Emerging Science Box: Digestive Manifestations Related to Covid 19). Radiography and imaging techniques—including radionuclide, positron emission tomography (PET), magnetic resonance imaging (MRI), computed tomography (CT) scanning, and ultrasound—are procedures for evaluating structure and function. Plain radiographs using contrast media such as barium- or iodine-containing compounds can be used to outline the GI lumen, biliary tree and pancreatic ducts, fistulae, and arteriovenous systems. CT scanning is particularly useful for diagnosis of intestinal lesions and pancreatic or hepatic tumors or cysts. Ultrasonic scanning is a safe, simple, and relatively inexpensive technique used to detect gallstones and intraabdominal masses, particularly abscesses.

Fiberoptic endoscopy, using flexible endoscopes, allows direct visualization of the GI tract. A biopsy channel allows tissue sampling, and suction can be applied to remove GI secretions or blood. Analysis of stool, gastric secretions, tissue, and plasma provides important clues to infection, malabsorption syndromes, ulcerative lesions, and tumor growth.

Liver

A variety of diagnostic tests can be performed to evaluate liver function (Table 40.6). Imaging techniques similar to those described for the GI tract also are useful for evaluating liver structure and function. Elevated plasma levels of liver enzymes are associated with many liver diseases because of the release of cytoplasmic enzymes into the circulation when there is damage to the hepatocyte. Of particular importance are elevations of aminotransferases and LDH.

Obstruction of bile canaliculi or ducts results in regurgitation of bile back into the hepatic sinusoids and into the circulation, manifesting with elevation of conjugated bilirubin levels. Prothrombin times (a measure of clotting tendency) are

TABLE 40.4 Selected Tests of Gastrointestinal Function

Test	Normal Findings	Clinical Significance of Abnormal Findings
Stool studies	Resident microorganisms: clostridia, enterococci, *Pseudomonas*, a few yeasts	Detection of *Salmonella typhi* (typhoid fever), *Shigella* (dysentery), *Vibrio cholerae* (cholera), *Yersinia* (enterocolitis), *Escherichia coli* (gastroenteritis), *Staphylococcus aureus* (food poisoning), *Clostridium botulinum* (food poisoning), *Clostridium perfringens* (food poisoning), *Aeromonas* (gastroenteritis)
	Fat: 2–6 g/24 h	Steatorrhea (increased values) can result from intestinal malabsorption or pancreatic insufficiency
	Pus: none	Large amounts of pus are associated with chronic ulcerative colitis, abscesses, and anorectal fistula
	Occult blood: none (orthotolidine or guaiac test)	Positive tests associated with bleeding
	Ova and parasites: none	Detection of *Entamoeba histolytica* (amebiasis), *Giardia lamblia* (giardiasis), and worms
D-Xylose absorption	5-h urinary excretion: 4.5 g/L Peak blood level: >30 mg/dL	Differentiation of pancreatic steatorrhea (normal D-xylose absorption) from intestinal steatorrhea (impaired D-xylose absorption)
Gastric acid stimulation	11–20 mEq/h after stimulation	Detection of duodenal ulcers, Zollinger-Ellison syndrome (increased values), gastric atrophy, gastric carcinoma (decreased values)
Manometry (use of water-filled catheters connected to pressure transducers passed into the esophagus, stomach, colon, or rectum to evaluate contractility)	Values vary at different levels of the intestine	Inadequate swallowing, motility, sphincter function
Culture and sensitivity of duodenal contents	No pathogens	Detection of *Salmonella typhi* (typhoid fever)
Breath tests		
Glucose or D-xylose breath test	Negative for hydrogen or CO_2	May indicate intestinal bacterial overgrowth
Urea breath test	Negative for isotopically labeled CO_2	Presence of *Helicobacter pylori* infection
Lactose breath test	Negative for exhaled hydrogen	Lactose intolerance

TABLE 40.5 Selected Studies of Gastrointestinal Structure

Test	Description	Application
Plain roentgenograms	Use of high-energy electromagnetic radiation to evaluate tissue structure by radiopacity or radiolucency	Visualization of the position, size, and structure of abdominal contents
Air or barium contrast roentgenograms	Introduction of radiopaque substances into the upper or lower gastrointestinal tract	Enhanced visualization of the contours, position, and size of the gastrointestinal tract to detect umbilical hernia, ulcers, diverticula, congenital anomalies, polyps, tumors, strictures, obstructions
Endoscopy Esophagoscopy (esophagus) Gastroscopy (stomach) Duodenoscopy (duodenum) Colonoscopy (large intestine) Sigmoidoscopy (sigmoid colon)	Passage of rigid or flexible (fiberoptic) endoscope into the gastrointestinal tract for visualization or biopsy	Visualization or biopsy of inflamed hernias, polyps, ulcers, strictures, varices, tumors, sites of bleeding, mucosal or neoplastic lesions and for culture of *Helicobacter pylori* from stomach
Ultrasound	Use of piezoelectric crystal to generate sound waves that are reflected from tissue interfaces to provide an image	Imaging of abdominal organs (gallbladder, liver, pancreas, spleen), masses, stones, abscesses, structural abnormalities
Computed tomography (CT)	Use of a computer to integrate differences in absorption of a large number of x-rays to produce a cross-sectional image; may be done with contrast agents	Imaging of gallbladder, liver, pancreas, spleen, cysts, hematomas, abscesses, stones, extrahepatic bile ducts, and portal vein
Magnetic resonance imaging	Projection of differences in magnetic properties of molecules within different cells and tissues, using the field of a large magnet	Same applications as CT scan; also can detect blood flow and vessel patency

EMERGING SCIENCE BOX

Digestive Manifestations Related to COVID-19

The digestive system has emerged as a site of severe acute respiratory syndrome novel coronavirus 2 (SARS-nCoV-2) expression and may also be implicated in the severity of disease and viral transmission. To date it has been determined that SARS-nCoV-2 infects the gastrointestinal (GI) tract of about 50% of infected persons based on the high incidence of digestive symptoms, expression of angiotensin-converting enzyme 2 receptors (viral target for cellular entry in digestive system), and presence of viral RNA in the feces. Persons infected with SARS-nCoV-2 have clinical manifestations related to the alimentary canal including sore throat, dysgeusia, diarrhea, abdominal pain, nausea, vomiting, and hematochezia. Furthermore, abnormal liver function is present in up to 50% of infected persons seen on liver function testing (LFTs). Additionally, viral RNA in stools is rarely tested, but is positive in 0%–48.1% of tests.

Data from Aroniadis OC, et al. Current knowledge and research priorities in the digestive manifestations of COVID-19. *Clin Gastroenterol Hepatol.* 2020;18(8):1682–1684. Xiao F, et al. Evidence for gastrointestinal infection of SARS-CoV-2. *Gastroenterology.* 2020;158:1831–1833; Prolonged presence of SARS-CoV-2 viral RNA in faecal samples. *Lancet Gastroenterol Hepatol.* 2020; 5:434–435; Zhang C, et al. Liver injury in COVID-19: management and challenges. *Lancet Gastroenterol Hepatol.* 2020;5:428–430. Xu Z, et al. Pathological findings of COVID-19 associated with acute respiratory distress syndrome. *Lancet Respir Med.* 2020;8:420–422. Almeida JFM, et al. COVID-19 and the gastrointestinal tract: what do we already know? *Einstein (Sao Paulo).* 2020;18:eRW5909.

TABLE 40.6 Common Tests of Liver Function

Test	Normal Value	Interpretation
Serum Enzymes		
Alkaline phosphatase	35–150 units/L	Increases with biliary obstruction and cholestatic hepatitis
Gamma-glutamyl transpeptidase	Male: 12–38 units/L Female: 9–31 units/L	Increases with biliary obstruction and cholestatic hepatitis
Aspartate aminotransferase (previously serum glutamate-oxaloacetate transaminase)	Male: 8–40 units/L Female: 6–34 units/L	Increases with hepatocellular injury and injury in other tissues (e.g., skeletal and cardiac muscle)
Alanine aminotransferase (previously serum glutamate-pyruvate transaminase)	Male: 10–40 units/L Female: 9–32 units/L	Increases with hepatocellular injury and necrosis
Lactate dehydrogenase	110–220 units/L	Isoenzyme LD5 is elevated with hypoxic and primary liver injury
5′-Nucleotidase	2–11 units/L	Increases with increase in alkaline phosphatase and cholestatic disorders
Bilirubin Metabolism		
Serum bilirubin		
Unconjugated (indirect)	0.1–1 mg/dL	Increases with hemolysis (lysis of red blood cells)
Conjugated (direct)	0.1–0.4 mg/dL	Increases with hepatocellular injury or obstruction
TOTAL	<1 mg/dL	Increases with biliary obstruction
Urine bilirubin	0	Increases with biliary obstruction
Urine urobilinogen	0–4 mg/24 h	Increases with hemolysis or shunting of portal blood flow
Serum Proteins		
Albumin	3.5–5.5 g/dL	Reduced with hepatocellular injury
Globulin	2–4 g/dL	Increases with hepatitis
TOTAL	6–7 g/dL	
Albumin/globulin ratio	1.5:1 to 2.5:1	Ratio reverses with chronic hepatitis or other chronic liver disease
Transferrin	250–300 mcg/dL	Liver damage with decreased values, iron deficiency with increased values
Alpha fetoprotein	6–20 ng/mL	Elevated values in primary hepatocellular carcinoma
Blood-Clotting Functions		
Prothrombin time	10–13 s or 90%–100% of control	Increases with chronic liver disease (cirrhosis) or vitamin K deficiency
Partial thromboplastin time	22–37 s	Increases with severe liver disease or heparin therapy
Bromsulphthalein excretion	<6% retention in 45 min	Increased retention with hepatocellular injury

often prolonged with both hepatitis and chronic liver disease. In severe disease, other plasma proteins, such as albumin and globulins, may be diminished as a result of hepatocyte damage. Liver biopsies are often performed to evaluate the extent of liver involvement or degeneration with cirrhosis, hepatitis, or fatty liver disease.

Gallbladder

Evaluation of structural alterations in the gallbladder may be achieved by the use of various imaging techniques. Table 40.7 summarizes these techniques. Obstructive pathology of the bile ducts results in elevated values for both conjugated and total serum bilirubin, increased urine urobilinogen level, clay-colored stools, and development of jaundice. Fat absorption can be impaired and the prothrombin time prolonged if vitamin K is not absorbed. With inflammation of the gallbladder, the white cell count is elevated.

Exocrine Pancreas

Tests of pancreatic function are summarized in Table 40.8. Evaluation of serum lipase and urinary amylase provides particularly significant measures of pancreatic injury. Inflammation or obstruction of the pancreas results in an early increase in serum amylase levels. Serum lipase level remains elevated after serum amylase has returned to normal levels and provides greater sensitivity with delayed presentation of pancreatitis. Elevation of urine amylase level also occurs later (after 48 hours) when serum amylase may have returned to normal levels. Urinary trypsinogen 2 (available as dipstick) is used to diagnose acute pancreatitis and is comparable to serum amylase and lipase. Increased stool fat can reflect pancreatic insufficiency caused by decreased lipase secretion when biliary function is normal.

TABLE 40.7 Diagnostic Evaluation of the Gallbladder

Test	Application
Plain roentgenogram of the abdomen	Visualization of calcified gallstones
Oral cholecystogram (use of an oral contrast medium such as iopanoic acid, which is excreted with bile and concentrated in the gallbladder for visualization by radiography; may be administered as a double dose)	Visualization of gallstones; evaluation of filling and emptying of gallbladder
Intravenous cholangiography (use of intravenous contrast agents for visualization of gallbladder and bile ducts)	Diagnosis of acute gallbladder inflammation (cholecystitis) or disease of bile ducts
Cholecystography (ultrasound imaging of gallbladder and bile ducts including endoscopic ultrasound)	Preferred method for detecting gallstones; differentiation of hepatic disease from biliary obstruction; diagnosis of chronic cholecystitis
Cholescintigraphy (radioisotope imaging of gallbladder)	Diagnosis of cholecystitis in individuals allergic to iodine-containing contrast agents; diagnosis of cystic duct obstruction
Endoscopic retrograde cholangiography (instillation of contrast medium through cannulation of ampulla of Vater with a duodenoscope)	Differentiation of intrahepatic or extrahepatic obstructive jaundice Diagnosis of gallstones
Computed tomography	Diagnosis of biliary obstruction or malignancy when ultrasound is not successful
Magnetic resonance cholangiography	Diagnosis of complicated cholelithiasis or choledocholithiasis

TABLE 40.8 Selected Tests of Pancreatic Function

Test	Normal Value	Clinical Significance
Serum amylase	25–125 units/mL	Elevated levels with pancreatic inflammation
Serum lipase	20–240 units/mL	Elevated levels with pancreatic inflammation (may be elevated with other conditions; differentiates with amylase isoenzyme study)
Urine amylase	35–260 Somogyi units/h	Elevated levels with pancreatic inflammation
Secretin test	Volume: 1.8 mL/kg/h Bicarbonate concentration: >80 mEq/L Bicarbonate output: >10 mEq/L/30 s	Decreased volume with pancreatic disease as secretin stimulates pancreatic secretion
Stool fat	2–5 g/24 h	Measures fatty acids; decreased pancreatic lipase increases stool fat (malabsorption)
Fecal elastase	>200 μg/g of stool	Decreased in pancreatic insufficiency

GERIATRIC CONSIDERATIONS

Age-related change in GI function is variable among individuals and is related to health status and disease treatments, genetics, and environmental factors. Changes can begin to occur before 50 years of age. Tooth enamel and dentin wear down, making the teeth vulnerable to cavities. Teeth are lost, often as a result of periodontal (gum) disease, recession of the gums, osteoporotic bone changes, and more brittle roots that fracture easily.[35] Taste buds decline in number, and the sense of smell diminishes. Together these losses decrease the sense of taste. These oral and sensory changes make eating less pleasurable and reduce appetite in very old adults.[36] Salivation decreases, and food may not be chewed or lubricated sufficiently, making swallowing difficult. The esophagus develops decreased motility, and changes in the upper esophageal sphincter, history of stroke, and dementia may affect swallowing and contribute to gastroesophageal reflux.[35] Age diminishes gastric motility, secretion, and blood flow with increased risk for mucosal injury.[36] Acid content of gastric juice is related to gastric atrophy, which results in hypochlorhydria (insufficient hydrochloric acid), delayed gastric emptying, and compromise of the gastric mucosal barrier.[35] Decreased production of intrinsic factor leads to inadequate small intestinal absorption of vitamin B_{12} and pernicious anemia. Aging may be associated with a change in the composition of the intestinal microflora, loss of intestinal mucosal integrity, and a decline in pathogen-specific IgA with increased susceptibility to disease. GALT and overall immunity declines.[36] The ileal villi of the small intestine may become broader and shorter, perhaps because of a decrease in cell turnover. Degeneration and density of the enteric nervous system neurons can decrease intestinal absorption, motility, and blood flow, impairing nutrient absorption. Proteins, fats, minerals (including iron and calcium), and vitamins are absorbed more slowly and in lesser amounts, and absorption of carbohydrates is decreased. Intestinal transit time is delayed. Constipation is often described as a condition of old age, but it is probably caused by lifestyle factors (e.g., diet, immobility, lack of fluid intake) rather than physiologic decline, although studies demonstrate there can be alterations in both enteric and external intestinal innervation.[35]

The liver is remarkably resilient during the aging process, but abnormalities in various functions do occur. Liver aging results from alterations in the metabolic epigenome. Low-grade inflammation and cellular senescence contribute to hepatocyte, sinusoidal, stellate cell, and Kupffer cell dysfunction in the elderly.[37] The rate of liver regeneration decreases with advancing age, but the volume of the liver can be maintained. Liver blood flow and enzyme activity decrease with age and can influence the efficiency of drug and alcohol metabolism. However, liver function test results often remain within relatively normal ranges. Alterations in liver function in older individuals are usually a sign of a pathologic condition. The pancreas undergoes structural changes, such as fibrosis, fatty acid deposits, and atrophy, and there is a decline in β-cell function. Pancreatic secretion decreases, but there is usually no observable dysfunction. Aging does not cause apparent changes in the structure and function of the gallbladder and bile ducts, but the incidence of gallstones increases.

SUMMARY REVIEW

The Gastrointestinal Tract

1. The major functions of the GI tract are the mechanical and chemical breakdown of food and the absorption of digested nutrients.
2. Except for swallowing and defecation, which are controlled voluntarily, the functions of the GI tract are controlled by extrinsic and intrinsic autonomic nerves and intestinal hormones.
3. The GI tract is a hollow tube that extends from the mouth to the anus.
4. The walls of the GI tract have four layers. From the inside out they are the mucosa, submucosa, muscularis, and serosa.
5. Digestion begins in the mouth, with chewing and salivation. The digestive component of saliva is α-amylase, which initiates carbohydrate digestion.
6. The esophagus is a muscular tube that transports food from the mouth to the stomach. The tunica muscularis in the upper part of the esophagus is striated muscle, and that in the lower part is smooth muscle.
7. Food is propelled through the esophagus by peristalsis (waves of sequential relaxations and contractions of the layers of muscles).
8. Swallowing is controlled by the swallowing center in the medulla of the brain. The two phases of swallowing are the oropharyngeal phase (voluntary swallowing) and the esophageal phase (involuntary swallowing).
9. The lower esophageal sphincter opens to admit swallowed food into the stomach and then closes to prevent regurgitation of food back into the esophagus.
10. The stomach is a bag-like structure that secretes digestive juices, mixes and stores food, and propels partially digested food (chyme) through the pylorus into the duodenum.
11. The vagus nerve stimulates gastric (stomach) secretion and motility.
12. The hormones gastrin and motilin stimulate gastric emptying; the hormones secretin and cholecystokinin delay gastric emptying.
13. The stomach secretes large volumes of gastric secretions, including acid, pepsinogen, mucus, enzymes, hormones, intrinsic factor (needed for vitamin B_{12} absorption), and gastroferrin (facilitates absorption of iron).
14. The three phases of gastric secretion by the stomach are the cephalic phase (anticipation and swallowing), the gastric phase (food in the stomach), and the intestinal phase (chyme in the intestine).
15. Parietal cells produce hydrochloric acid, which dissolves food fibers, kills microorganisms, and activates the enzyme pepsin. Acid secretion is stimulated by the vagus nerve, gastrin, and histamine and is inhibited by sympathetic stimulation and intestinal hormones.
16. Chief cells in the stomach secrete pepsinogen, which is converted to pepsin in the acidic environment created by hydrochloric acid. Pepsin breaks down proteins and forms polypeptides.

17. Mucus is secreted throughout the stomach and protects the stomach wall from acid and digestive enzymes.
18. The abdominal cavity includes all the organs of digestion, and the mesentery, peritoneum and omentum.
19. The mesentery is an organ formed from a double fold of peritoneum and composed of several contiguous segments that have both structural and physiologic function.
20. The peritoneum is a double layer of membranous tissue. The visceral layer covers the abdominal organs, and the parietal layer extends along the abdominal wall. The peritoneal cavity is the space between the two layers
21. The omentum is composed of a large flat layer of adipose tissue with two parts, the greater and lesser omentum has fat storage, protective, immune, wound healing, and tissue regeneration functions
22. The small intestine is 5 m long and has three segments: the duodenum, jejunum, and ileum.
23. The duodenum lies behind the peritoneum (retroperitoneal).
24. The ileocecal valve connects the small and large intestines and prevents reflux into the small intestine.
25. Villi are small finger-like projections that extend from the small intestinal mucosa and increase its absorptive surface area.
26. Enzymes secreted by the small intestine (maltase, sucrase, lactase), pancreatic enzymes, and bile salts act in the small intestine to digest proteins, carbohydrates, and fats.
27. Digested substances are absorbed across the intestinal wall and then transported to the liver, where they are metabolized further. Carbohydrate and protein components move into villus capillaries and to the liver through the hepatic portal vein.
28. Bile salts emulsify and hydrolyze fats and incorporate them into water-soluble micelles. The fat content of the micelles diffuses through the epithelium into lacteals (lymphatic ducts) in the villi. From there, fats flow into lymphatics and into the systemic circulation, which delivers them to the liver.
29. Minerals and water-soluble vitamins are absorbed by both active and passive transport throughout the small intestine.
30. Contractions of the circular muscles (segmentation) mix the chyme, and peristaltic movements created by longitudinal muscles propel the chyme along the intestinal tract.
31. The ileogastric reflex inhibits gastric motility when the ileum is distended. The intestinointestinal reflex inhibits intestinal motility when one intestinal segment is overdistended. The gastroileal reflex increases intestinal motility when gastric motility increases.
32. The large intestine consists of the cecum, appendix, colon (ascending, transverse, descending, and sigmoid), rectum, and anal canal.
33. The teniae coli are three bands of longitudinal muscle that extend the length of the colon and give it a gathered appearance. Haustra are pouches of colon formed with alternating contraction and relaxation of the circular muscles.
34. The mucosa of the large intestine contains mucus-secreting cells and mucosal folds, but no villi.
35. The large intestine massages the fecal mass and absorbs water and electrolytes.
36. Distention of the ileum with chyme causes the gastrocolic reflex, or the mass propulsion of feces to the rectum.
37. Defecation is stimulated when the rectum is distended with feces. The tonically contracted internal anal sphincter relaxes, and if the voluntarily regulated external sphincter relaxes, defecation occurs.
38. The immune system of the GI tract consists of Paneth cells, which produce defensins and other antimicrobial peptides and lysozymes; and the lymph nodes of Peyer patches, which contain lymphocytes, plasma cells, and macrophages.
39. The largest number of intestinal bacteria (intestinal microbiome) is in the colon. The most numerous anaerobes are *Bacteroides* and *Firmicutes*. Intestinal bacteria are important for metabolism of bile salts, metabolism of selected drugs and hormones, destruction of pathogens, and prevention of pathogen colonization.
40. The intestinal tract is sterile at birth and becomes totally colonized within 3 to 4 weeks.
41. The splanchnic blood flow provides blood to the esophagus, stomach, small and large intestines, gallbladder, pancreas, and spleen.

Accessory Organs of Digestion

1. The liver, gallbladder, and exocrine pancreas secrete substances necessary for digestion. These secretions flow through an opening guarded by the sphincter of Oddi.
2. The liver sits under the diaphragm. It has digestive, metabolic, hematologic, vascular, and immunologic functions.
3. The liver is divided into the right and left lobes and is supported by the falciform, round, and coronary ligaments.
4. Plates of hepatocytes, which are the functional cells of the liver, together form anatomic units called liver lobules.
5. Hepatocytes synthesize bile and secrete it into the bile canaliculi, which are small channels between the hepatocytes. The bile canaliculi drain bile into the common bile duct and then into the duodenum through an opening called the major duodenal papilla (sphincter of Oddi).
6. Sinusoids are capillaries located between the plates of hepatocytes. Blood from the portal vein and hepatic artery flows through the sinusoids to a central vein in each lobule and then to the hepatic vein and inferior vena cava.
7. Kupffer cells, which are part of the mononuclear phagocyte system, line the sinusoids and destroy microorganisms in sinusoidal blood; they are important in bilirubin production and lipid metabolism.
8. The liver produces 700 to 1200 mL of bile per day. Bile is made up of bile salts, cholesterol, bilirubin, electrolytes, and water.
9. The primary bile acids are synthesized from cholesterol by the hepatocytes. The primary acids are then conjugated to form bile salts. The secondary bile acids are the product of bile salt deconjugation by bacteria in the intestinal lumen.
10. Most bile salts and acids are recycled. The absorption of bile salts and acids from the terminal ileum and their return to the liver are known as the enterohepatic circulation of bile.

11. Bilirubin is a pigment liberated by the lysis of aged red blood cells in the liver and spleen. Unconjugated bilirubin is fat soluble and can cross cell membranes. Unconjugated bilirubin is converted to water-soluble, conjugated bilirubin by hepatocytes and is secreted with bile.
12. The liver produces clotting factors and can store a large volume of blood.
13. The liver plays a major role in the metabolism of carbohydrates, proteins, and fats and stores minerals, vitamin B_{12}, and fat-soluble vitamins.
14. The liver metabolically transforms or detoxifies hormones, toxic substances, and drugs to less active substances. This process is known as metabolic detoxification.
15. The gallbladder is a sac-like organ located on the inferior surface of the liver. The gallbladder stores bile between meals and ejects it when chyme enters the duodenum.
16. Stimulated by cholecystokinin, the gallbladder contracts and forces bile through the cystic duct and into the common bile duct. The sphincter of Oddi relaxes, enabling bile to flow through the major duodenal papilla into the duodenum.
17. The pancreas is a gland located behind the stomach. The endocrine pancreas produces hormones (glucagon, insulin) that facilitate the formation and cellular uptake of glucose. The exocrine pancreas secretes an alkaline solution and the enzymes (trypsin, chymotrypsin, carboxypeptidase, α-amylase, lipase) that digest proteins, carbohydrates, and fats.
18. Secretin stimulates pancreatic secretion of alkaline fluid, and cholecystokinin and ACh stimulate secretion of enzymes. Pancreatic secretions originate in acini and ducts of the pancreas and empty into the duodenum through the common bile duct or an accessory duct that opens directly into the duodenum.

Tests of Digestive Function

1. Numerous diagnostic tests can evaluate structure and function (digestion, secretion, absorption) of the GI tract. Radiographs and scans are most commonly used to evaluate structure, in addition to direct observation by endoscopy. Gastric and stool analysis and blood studies provide important information about digestion, absorption, and secretion.
2. Plasma chemistry levels and imaging procedures are commonly used to diagnose alterations in liver function. Of particular importance are the enzymes LDH, AST, and ALT. Plasma bilirubin levels reflect alterations in bilirubin and bile metabolism, and prothrombin times are prolonged in hepatitis and chronic liver disease.
3. Obstructive diseases of the gallbladder are evident by elevated serum bilirubin levels, elevated urine urobilinogen levels, and increased stool fat. The serum leukocyte levels become elevated with inflammation of the gallbladder.
4. The most significant indicators of pancreatic dysfunction are serum amylase and stool fat. Both values are increased with pathology of the pancreas.

Aging and the Gastrointestinal System

1. Advancing age is often associated with the loss or deterioration of teeth, diminished senses of taste and smell, and diminished salivary secretions, all of which may make eating difficult and reduce appetite.
2. Aging reduces gastric motility and secretions, particularly of hydrochloric acid. These changes slow gastric digestion and emptying.
3. Intestinal motility and absorption of carbohydrates, proteins, fats, and minerals decrease with age.
4. Efficiency of drug and alcohol metabolism decreases with age and can be related to decreased liver perfusion and decreased liver enzymes.

REFERENCES

1. Valstar MH, et al. The tubarial salivary glands: a potential new organ at risk for radiotherapy. *Radiother Oncol.* 2021;154:292–298.
2. Alonso S, et al. Longitudinal study on steroid hormone variations during the second trimester of gestation: a useful tool to confirm adequate foetal development. *BMC Pregnancy Childbirth.* 2021;21:120.
3. Ferris L, et al. Modulation of pharyngeal swallowing by bolus volume and viscosity. *Am J Physiol Gastrointest Liver Physiol.* 2021;320(1):G43–G53.
4. Johnson LR. *Gastrointestinal physiology*. 9th ed. Philadelphia: Elsevier; 2019.
5. Nikaki K, et al. Neuronal control of esophageal peristalsis and its role in esophageal disease. *Curr Gastroenterol Rep.* 2019;21:59.
6. Standring S, ed. *Gray's Anatomy: The Anatomical Basis of Clinical Practice.* 42nd ed. Elsevier; 2020.
7. Coffey JC, et al. Mesentery—a 'new' organ. *Emerg Top Life Sci.* 2020;4(2):191–206.
8. Dalla Pria HRF, et al. The mesenteric organ: new anatomical concepts and an imaging-based review on its diseases. *Semin Ultrasound CT MR.* 2019;40(6):515–532.
9. Rivera ED, et al. The mesentery, systemic inflammation, and Crohn's disease. *Inflamm Bowel Dis.* 2019;25(2):226–234.
10. Di Nicola V. Omentum a powerful biological source in regenerative surgery. *Regen Ther.* 2019;11:182–191.
11. Zeng Q, et al. Gastrin, cholecystokinin, signaling, and biological activities in cellular processes. *Front Endocrinol.* 2020;11:112.
12. Singaram K, Gold-Smith FD, Petrov MS. Motilin: a panoply of communications between the gut, brain, and pancreas. *Expert Rev Gastroenterol Hepatol.* 2020;14(2):103–111.
13. Bharucha AE, Kudva YC, Prichard DO. Diabetic gastroparesis. *Endocr Rev.* 2019;40(5):1318–1352.
14. Engevik AC, Kaji I, Goldenring JR. The physiology of the gastric parietal cell. *Physiol Rev.* 2020;100(2):573–602.
15. Karmakar S, et al. Intestinal epithelial regeneration: active versus reserve stem cells and plasticity mechanisms. *Am J Physiol Gastrointest Liver Physiol.* 2020;318:G796–G802.
16. Dominguez Rieg JA, Rieg T. What does sodium-glucose co-transporter 1 inhibition add: prospects for dual inhibition. *Diabetes Obes Metab.* 2019;21(Suppl 2):43–52.
17. Koepsell H. Glucose transporters in the small intestine in health and disease. *Pflugers Arch.* 2020;472(9):1207–1248.
18. Wang T, et al. Current understanding of glucose transporter 4 expression and functional mechanisms. *World J Biol Chem.* 2020;11(3):76–98.
19. Areco VA, et al. Intestinal Ca2+ absorption revisited: a molecular and clinical approach. *World J Gastroenterol.* 2020;26(24):3344–3364.

20. Rauf A, et al. Hepcidin, an overview of biochemical and clinical properties. *Steroids*. 2020;160:108661.
21. Bobadilla JL. Mesenteric ischemia. *Surg Clin North Am*. 2013;93(4):925–940. ix.
22. Quiroz-Olguín G, et al. The effect of enteral stimulation on the immune response of the intestinal mucosa and its application in nutritional support. *Eur J Clin Nutr*. 2021;75:1533–1539.
23. Di Costanzo M, et al. Gut microbiome modulation for preventing and treating pediatric food allergies. *Int J Mol Sci*. 2020;21(15):5275.
24. Antushevich H. Fecal microbiota transplantation in disease therapy. *Clin Chim Acta*. 2020;503:90–98.
25. Annunziato S, Tchorz JS. Liver zonation—a journey through space and time. *Nat Metab*. 2021;3:7–8.
26. Bennett H, et al. Epigenetic regulation of Kupffer cell function in health and disease. *Front Immunol*. 2021;11:3600.
27. Bonnardel J, et al. Stellate cells, hepatocytes, and endothelial cells imprint the Kupffer cell identity on monocytes colonizing the liver macrophage niche. *Immunity*. 2019;51(4). 638–654.e9.
28. Chen ML, Takeda K, Sundrud MS. Emerging roles of bile acids in mucosal immunity and inflammation. *Mucosal Immunol*. 2019;12:851–861.
29. Wang Q, et al. Intestinal flora imbalance affects bile acid metabolism and is associated with gallstone formation. *BMC Gastroenterol*. 2020;20(1):59.
30. Ovadia C, et al. Enhanced microbial bile acid deconjugation and impaired ileal uptake in pregnancy repress intestinal regulation of bile acid synthesis. *Hepatology*. 2019;70:276–293.
31. Nozaki Y, et al. Metabolic control analysis of hepatic glycogen synthesis in vivo. *Proc Natl Acad Sci U S A*. 2020;117(14): 8166–8176.
32. Zhang X, et al. Unraveling the regulation of hepatic gluconeogenesis. *Front Endocrinol*. 2019;9:802.
33. European Association for the Study of the Liver (EASL) EASL clinical practice guidelines: drug-induced liver injury. *J Hepatol*. 2019;70(6):1222–1261.
34. Chien HJ, et al. Human pancreatic afferent and efferent nerves: mapping and 3-D illustration of exocrine, endocrine, and adipose innervation. *Am J Physiol Gastrointest Liver Physiol*. 2019;317:G694–G706.
35. Dumic I, et al. Gastrointestinal tract disorders of older age. *Can J Gastroenterol Hepatol*. 2019;2019:6757524.
36. Lerner A, McCarty MF. The aging bowel dysfunction and elderly vulnerability towards COVID-19 infection. *Life (Basel)*. 2021;11(2):97.
37. Hunt NJ, et al. Hallmarks of aging in the liver. *Comput Struct Biotechnol J*. 2019;17:1151–1161.

41

Alterations of Digestive Function

Scarlet R. Spain

http://evolve.elsevier.com/Rogers/pathophysiology/

CHAPTER OUTLINE

Disorders of the gastrointestinal (GI) tract disrupt one or more of its structures and functions. The GI tract is a continuous, hollow organ that extends from the mouth to the anus. It includes the esophagus, stomach, small intestine, large intestine, and rectum. The accessory organs of digestion include the salivary glands, liver, gallbladder, and pancreas. Structural and neural abnormalities can slow, obstruct, or accelerate the movement of intestinal contents at any level of the GI tract. Inflammatory and ulcerative conditions of the GI wall disrupt secretion, motility, and absorption. Inflammation or obstruction of the liver, pancreas, or gallbladder can alter metabolism and result in local and systemic symptoms. Many clinical manifestations of GI tract disorders are nonspecific and can be caused by a variety of impairments.

DISORDERS OF THE GASTROINTESTINAL TRACT

Clinical Manifestations of Gastrointestinal Dysfunction

Anorexia

Anorexia is the lack of desire to eat despite physiologic stimuli that would normally produce hunger (see Chapter 23). This nonspecific symptom is often associated with nausea, abdominal pain, diarrhea, psychological stress, and weight loss. Side effects of drugs and pathologic disease processes such as cancer, heart disease, renal disease, and liver disease are often accompanied by anorexia. Anorexia can lead to weight loss, protein energy malnutrition, sarcopenia, functional decline, and is often associated with cachexia.[1] The aging population exhibits a high prevalence of anorexia and is an independent predictor of morbidity and mortality in the community and in clinical care settings.[2,3]

Vomiting

Vomiting (emesis) is an involuntary, forceful emptying of stomach and intestinal contents (chyme) through the mouth. The vomiting center, called the *area postrema*, lies in the medulla oblongata. The vomiting center contains receptors that may be stimulated to cause vomiting. Stimulation of the vomiting center occurs by either irritants or indirect stimuli. Some causes of indirect stimulation involve the cerebral cortex and thalamus (e.g., anxiety and pain); the vestibular system through the eighth cranial nerve (e.g., motion sickness); and several types of intestinal, vagal, as well as differing types of sympathetic input. Examples of vomiting caused by intestinal, vagal, or sympathetic input include presence of ipecac in the duodenum after ingestion; side effects of certain drugs; distention of the stomach or duodenum; and torsion or trauma affecting the ovaries, testes, uterus, bladder, or kidney. Serotonin (5-hydroxytryptamine [5-HT]) may also stimulate the vomiting center and appears to be released from enterochromaffin cells that lie in the intestinal wall. These cells activate vagal afferents leading to the chemoreceptor trigger zone (CTZ), which leads to vomiting by triggering receptors for dopamine (D_2), opioids, acetylcholine, substance P, serotonin (5-HT type 3), and neurokinin-1.

Nausea and retching (dry heaves) are distinct events that usually precede vomiting. Nausea is a subjective experience associated with various conditions, including abnormal pain, used of opioids, and labyrinthine stimulation (i.e., motion). Specific neural pathways that cause nausea have not been identified, but hypersalivation and tachycardia are common associated symptoms. Retching is the muscular event of vomiting without the expulsion of vomitus.

Vomiting begins with deep inspiration. The glottis closes, the intrathoracic pressure decreases, and the esophagus becomes distended. Simultaneously, the abdominal muscles contract, creating a pressure gradient from abdomen to thorax. The lower esophageal sphincter (LES) and body of the stomach relax, but the duodenum and antrum of the stomach spasm. The reverse peristalsis and pressure gradient force chyme from the stomach and duodenum up into the esophagus. Because the upper esophageal sphincter is closed, chyme does not enter the mouth. When the stomach is full of gastric contents, the diaphragm is forced high into the thoracic cavity by strong contractions of the abdominal muscles. The higher intrathoracic pressure forces the upper esophageal sphincter to open, and chyme is expelled from the mouth. Then the stomach relaxes and the upper part of the esophagus contracts, forcing the remaining chyme back into the stomach. The LES then closes. The cycle is repeated if there is a volume of chyme remaining in the stomach. A diffuse sympathetic discharge causes the tachycardia, tachypnea, and diaphoresis that accompany retching and vomiting. The parasympathetic system mediates copious salivation, increased gastric motility, and relaxation of the upper and LESs.

Spontaneous vomiting not preceded by nausea or retching is called projectile vomiting. It is caused by direct stimulation of the vomiting center by neurologic lesions (e.g., increased intracranial pressure, tumors, or aneurysms) involving the brainstem (see Chapter 17), or it can be a symptom of GI obstruction (pyloric stenosis). The metabolic consequences of vomiting are fluid, electrolyte, and acid-base disturbances, including hyponatremia, hypokalemia, hypochloremia, and metabolic alkalosis (see Chapter 3). The management of nausea and vomiting includes fluid and electrolyte maintenance, use of medications, and complimentary nonpharmacologic therapies.[4]

Constipation

Constipation is difficult or infrequent defecation. It is a common problem, afflicting 24% of the United States population. Although it affects all age groups, prevalence increases with age.[5] Constipation means a decrease in the number of bowel movements per week, hard stools, straining, abdominal pain, and difficult evacuation. The definition of constipation must be individually determined because normal bowel habits range from one to three evacuations per day to one per week.

Pathophysiology. Constipation can occur as a primary or secondary condition. Chronic idiopathic or primary constipation is generally classified into three categories: functional defecation disorder, slow transit constipation (STC), and constipation-predominant irritable bowel syndrome (IBS-C). Overlap may exist between these three classifications, and the classifications are not mutually exclusive.[6] *Functional constipation* is similar between children and adults, but differences exist regarding the symptomology and pathophysiology of disease, as well as differences in required diagnostic work-up and treatment modalities.[7] Functional constipation involves a normal rate of stool passage but difficulty with stool evacuation. *STC* involves impaired colonic motor activity with symptoms of infrequent bowel movements, straining to defecate, mild abdominal distention, and palpable stool in the sigmoid colon. *IBS-C* is associated with chronic constipation and abdominal pain. The exact cause of IBS-C is poorly understood, but various factors that may contribute to the pathology of the disease include diet, genetics, colonic motility, absorption, socioeconomic status, daily behaviors, and medication use.[8] Lack of access to toilet facilities, consistent suppression of the urge to empty the bowel, pelvic floor dyssynergia, and dehydration may be other causes of primary constipation.

Secondary constipation can be caused by diet, medications, or neurogenic disorders (e.g., stroke, Parkinson disease, spinal cord lesions, multiple sclerosis, and Hirschsprung disease) in which neural pathways or neurotransmitters are diseased or degenerated, resulting in altered or delayed colon transit time. Rectal fissures, strictures, or hemorrhoids also may cause constipation. Antacids containing calcium carbonate or aluminum hydroxide, anticholinergics, iron, and bismuth tend to inhibit bowel motility causing constipation. *Opioid-induced constipation* is caused by drugs that activate μ-opioid receptors in the gut and slow transit time. Endocrine or metabolic disorders, which may also be associated with constipation, include hypothyroidism, diabetes mellitus, hypokalemia, and hypercalcemia. Pelvic hiatal hernia (herniation of the bowel through the floor of the pelvis), diverticula, irritable bowel syndrome (IBS) (constipation predominant), and pregnancy are associated with constipation. Aging may result in decreased mobility, changes in neuromuscular function, use of medications, and comorbid medical conditions causing constipation. Pain or weakness of the abdominal muscles may interfere with the generation of adequate intra-abdominal pressure needed to evacuate stool from the rectum. Depression may also impair bowel evacuation due to a sedentary lifestyle and diet changes. It is important to remember that constipation or a notable change in bowel habits can be an indication of colorectal cancer (CRC).

Clinical Manifestations. Indicators of primary or functional constipation (not including IBS-C) are guided by the Rome IV criteria. The Rome IV criteria define chronic constipation as including at least two of the following symptoms: straining with defecation at least 25% of the time; lumpy or hard stools at least 25% of the time; sensation of incomplete emptying at least 25% of the time; feeling of anorectal obstruction/blockage at least 25% of the time; manual maneuvers to facilitate stool evacuation for at least 25% of defecations; and fewer than three bowel movements per week (see Table 41.1 for Rome IV criteria).[6,8] Changes in bowel evacuation patterns, such as less frequent defecation, smaller stool volume, hard stools, difficulty passing stools (e.g., straining), a feeling of bowel fullness and discomfort, or blood in the stools, require further assessment. Straining to evacuate stool may cause engorgement of the hemorrhoidal

TABLE 41.1 Definition of Chronic Constipation According to the Rome IV Criteria

Diagnostic criteria Includes ≥2 of the following symptoms over the preceding three months:

- Straining during ≥25% of toilet visits
- Lumpy, hard feces on ≥25% of defecations
- Feeling of anorectal obstruction/blockage ≥25% of defecations
- Requirement of manual stimulation ≥25% of defecations
- Loose stools are rarely achievable without laxatives
- Symptoms do not fit the criteria for irritable bowel syndrome

veins and hemorrhoidal disease or thrombosis with rectal pain, bleeding, and itching. Passage of hard stools can cause painful anal fissures. Fecal impaction (hard, dry stool retained in the rectum) is associated with rectal bleeding, abdominal or cramping type pain, nausea and vomiting, weight loss, and episodes of diarrhea. If left untreated, fecal impaction may cause increased pressure on the intralumen of the colon that may lead to ischemia with possible perforation of the colon and even death.[9]

Evaluation and Treatment. The history, current use of medications, physical examination, and stool diaries provide precise clues regarding the nature of constipation. The individual's description of the duration of symptoms, frequency of bowel movements, stool consistency, difficult rectal evacuation, sense of incomplete evacuation, presence of blood with stools, and if evacuation was stimulated by enemas or laxatives is important. It is also important to note any abdominal pain or bloating and if any type of digital evacuation to remove stool has been performed. The clinician should also discuss comorbidities, previous GI disorders or surgeries, diet, fluid intake, and physical activity. As mentioned, sudden-onset constipation may signify a new or developing mass and requires careful evaluation for CRC. Abdominal palpation may disclose colonic distention, masses, and tenderness. Digital examination of the rectum and anorectal manometry are performed to assess sphincter tone and detect anal lesions. Colonic transit time and imaging techniques can assist in identifying the cause of constipation. Colonoscopy is used to visualize the bowel lumen directly and can help with identification of polyps, inflammatory bowel diseases (IBDs), or other suspicious lesions including tumors.

The treatment for constipation is to manage the underlying cause or disease. Lifestyle modifications can often help immensely. Management of constipation usually consists of bowel retraining, in which the individual establishes a satisfactory bowel evacuation routine without becoming preoccupied with bowel movements. The individual also may need to engage in moderate exercise and increase fluid and fiber intake. Fiber supplements and stool softeners are useful for some individuals. Many different types of laxatives are available; however, studies are lacking comparing the efficacy and safety of different categories of laxatives. Choice of laxative for an individual should be guided by a healthcare professional and should take into account individual preferences and cost.[5] Enemas can be used to establish a bowel routine, but they should not be used routinely. Biofeedback may be beneficial in some instances for forming new bowel evacuation habits. Colectomy with ileorectal anastomosis is rarely performed but may be done with individuals with severe symptoms that have not responded to other treatments.[5]

Diarrhea

Diarrhea is the presence of loose, watery stools and may be acute, persistent, or chronic. Diarrhea is defined as the passage of three or more loose or liquid stools per day, or more frequent passing of stools than what has routinely been "normal" for a specific individual.[10] Acute diarrhea is more than three loose stools developing within 24 hours and lasting less than 14 days. Persistent diarrhea is diarrhea in an individual that lasts longer than 14 to 30 days and chronic diarrhea is diarrhea that lasts longer than 4 weeks. Diarrhea can have high rates of morbidity and mortality in children younger than 5 years of age, particularly in developing countries (see Chapter 42), and in the elderly. Diarrheal disease is the second leading cause of death in children younger than age 5.[10]

Many factors determine stool volume, including water content of the colon, diet, presence of nonabsorbed food or material, and intestinal secretions. Stool volume in the normal adult averages less than 200 g/day. Stool volume in children depends on age and size. An infant may pass up to 100 g/day. The adult intestine processes approximately 9 L of luminal contents per day: 2 L are ingested, and the remaining 7 L consist of intestinal secretions. Of this volume, most of the fluid is absorbed: 90% (7 to 8 L) in the small intestine and a smaller amount 9% (1 to 2 L) in the colon. Normally, approximately 150 mL of water is excreted daily in the stool.

Pathophysiology. The intestinal mucosa is made up of a complex epithelium where absorption and secretion occur. The majority of water and electrolyte absorption occurs in the small intestine.[11] Diarrhea in which the volume of feces is increased is called *large-volume diarrhea.* It generally is caused by excessive amounts of water or secretions in the intestines. *Small-volume diarrhea*, in which the volume of feces is not increased, usually results from excessive intestinal motility and may be caused by an inflammatory disorder of the intestine, such as ulcerative colitis (UC), Crohn disease (CD), or microscopic colitis, but also can result from colon cancer or fecal impaction.

The three major mechanisms of diarrhea are osmotic, secretory, and motile.

1. Osmotic diarrhea. A nonabsorbable substance in the intestine draws excess water into the lumen of the intestine by osmosis and increases stool weight and volume, producing large-volume diarrhea. Large oral doses of poorly absorbed ions, such as magnesium, sulfate, and phosphate, can increase intraluminal osmotic pressure. Excessive ingestion of synthetic, nonabsorbable sugars (e.g., sorbitol); introduction of full-strength tube feeding formulas; and dumping syndrome associated with gastric resection draw water into the intestinal lumen. Once ingestion of the osmotic substance stops, the osmotic diarrhea will stop. Malabsorption

related to lactase deficiency, pancreatic enzyme, or bile salt deficiency, small intestine bacterial overgrowth, or celiac disease also causes osmotic diarrhea.

2. Secretory diarrhea. A form of large-volume diarrhea caused by excessive mucosal secretions of chloride or bicarbonate-rich fluid or overall inhibition of net sodium absorption. Infectious causes include viruses (e.g., rotavirus), bacterial enterotoxins (e.g., *Escherichia coli*, *Vibrio cholera*, Shiga toxin), exotoxins (e.g., overgrowth of *Clostridioides difficile* following antibiotic therapy), or small bowel bacterial overgrowth. These infections cause secretion of transmitters from enteroendocrine cells (e.g., cells found in the wall of the bowel that have numerous processes in the body), activation of afferent neurons that stimulate submucosal secretomotor neurons, and altered sodium and chloride transport that results in decreased water absorption. Certain neoplasms (e.g., gastrinoma and thyroid carcinoma) also produce hormones that stimulate intestinal secretion, causing diarrhea.
   Small-volume diarrhea is usually caused by an inflammatory bowel disorder, such as UC or CD. Inflammation of the colon causes smooth muscle contraction, cramping type pain, bowel urgency, and frequency. Small-volume diarrhea also can be caused by fecal impaction. The diarrhea caused from a fecal impaction consists of secretions of mucus of fluid produced by the colon to lubricate the impacted feces and move it toward the anal canal. These secretions flow around the impaction and cause low-volume, secretory diarrhea.
3. Motility diarrhea. Excessive motility decreases transit time and the opportunity for fluid absorption, resulting in diarrhea. This type of diarrhea is caused by resection of the small intestine (short bowel syndrome), surgical bypass of an area of the intestine, fistula formation between loops of intestine, IBS–diarrhea predominant, diabetic neuropathy, hyperthyroidism, and laxative abuse.

Clinical Manifestations. Diarrhea can be acute or chronic, depending on the cause. Systemic effects of prolonged diarrhea are dehydration, electrolyte imbalance (hyponatremia, hypokalemia), metabolic acidosis, and weight loss. Manifestations of acute bacterial or viral infection include fever, with or without vomiting or cramping pain. Most diarrhea caused by infectious organisms lasts less than 2 weeks, although some causes of bacterial gastroenteritis may last longer, such as *C. difficile, Aeromonas,* or *Yersinia enterocolitica*. Fever, cramping pain, and bloody stools accompany chronic diarrhea caused by IBD or dysentery. Steatorrhea (fat in the stools), bloating, and diarrhea are common signs of malabsorption syndromes. Diarrhea may also cause anal and perineal skin irritation.

Evaluation and Treatment. A thorough history is taken to document the onset, frequency, volume of stools, duration of diarrhea, and presence of blood in the stools. Documentation of recent travel is important to obtain in the history. Iatrogenic diarrhea is suggested if the individual has undergone abdominal radiation therapy, intestinal resection, or treatment with selected drugs (e.g., antibiotics, diuretics, antihypertensives, laxatives, anticoagulants, or chemotherapy). A thorough physical examination should be completed and can help identify underlying systemic disease. Stool studies, abdominal imaging, endoscopy, and intestinal biopsies provide more specific data, particularly for persistent diarrhea.

Treatment for diarrhea includes restoration of fluid and electrolyte balance, administration of antimotility (e.g., loperamide) and/or water-absorbent (e.g., attapulgite and polycarbophil) medications, and treatment of causal factors. Natural bran and commercial preparations of psyllium are inexpensive and effective treatments for mild diarrhea. Probiotics can be useful for preventing and treating *C. difficile*–associated diarrhea as an approach to restoring normal microflora in addition to antibiotic therapy. Fecal transplantation can be used for cases that are resistant to conventional therapies, particularly *C. difficile*–associated diarrhea. Nutritional deficiencies need to be corrected in cases of chronic diarrhea or malabsorption.[12]

Abdominal Pain

Abdominal pain is the presenting symptom of several GI diseases and can be acute or chronic. The causal mechanisms of abdominal pain are *mechanical, inflammatory,* or *ischemic*. Abdominal organs are sensitive to stretching and distention. This stretching activates nerve endings in both hollow and solid structures, causing pain. Pain accompanies rapid distention rather than gradual distention. Traction on the peritoneum caused by adhesions, distention of the common bile duct, or forceful peristalsis resulting from intestinal obstruction causes pain because of increased tension. Capsules that surround solid organs, such as the liver and gallbladder, contain pain fibers that are stimulated by stretching if these organs swell. Abdominal pain may be generalized to the abdomen or localized to a particular abdominal quadrant. The nature of the pain is often described as sharp, dull, or colicky.

Abdominal pain is usually associated with tissue injury and inflammation. Biochemical mediators of the inflammatory response, such as histamine, bradykinin, and serotonin, stimulate organic nerve endings and produce abdominal pain. The edema and vascular congestion that accompany chemical, bacterial, or viral inflammation also cause painful stretching. Hindrance of blood flow from the distention of bowel obstruction or mesenteric vessel thrombosis produces the pain of ischemia and increased concentrations of tissue metabolites stimulate pain receptors.

Abdominal pain can be parietal (somatic), visceral, or referred. Parietal pain, originating from the parietal peritoneum, is more localized and intense than visceral pain, which arises from the organs themselves. Nerve fibers from the parietal peritoneum are predominantly A-delta fibers and travel with somatic peripheral nerves to the spinal cord. Parietal pain is caused by an irritation of fibers of the peritoneal peritoneum or lining. The sensation of pain is localized to the dermatome superficial to the area of painful stimuli. Visceral pain arises from a stimulus (distention, inflammation, ischemia) causing stretching, damage, or disruption of the organ or organ tissue involved and is transmitted via sympathetic fibers. Inflammatory mediators associated with chronic low-grade inflammation can cause pain hypersensitivity, and they include neurokinins, histamine, serotonin, and proteases.[13] These mediators can activate voltage-gated sodium ion channels.[14] Pain is usually near the midline in the epigastrium, midabdomen, or lower abdomen because sensory afferents enter the spinal cord bilaterally and lack specificity. The pain is usually poorly localized, diffuse, or vague with a radiating pattern because nerve endings in abdominal organs are sparse and multisegmented. Pain arising from the stomach, for example, is experienced as a sensation of fullness, cramping, or gnawing in the midepigastric area. Referred pain is visceral pain felt at some distance from a diseased or affected organ. It is usually well localized and is felt in the skin dermatomes or deeper tissues that share a central afferent pathway with the affected organ. For example, acute cholecystitis may have pain referred to the right shoulder or scapula.

Gastrointestinal Bleeding

Upper GI bleeding is bleeding in the esophagus, stomach, or duodenum and is characterized by frank, bright red bleeding or dark, grainy digested blood ("coffee grounds") in the stool (Table 41.2). Upper GI bleeding is commonly caused by bleeding esophageal or gastric varices, peptic ulcers, arteriovenous malformations, or a Mallory-Weiss tear at the esophageal-gastric junction caused by severe retching. Upper GI bleeding may also be associated with use of nonsteroidal antiinflammatory drugs (NSAIDs), selective serotonin reuptake inhibitors, and antiplatelet and anticoagulant drugs.[15,16]

Lower GI bleeding, or bleeding from the jejunum, ileum, colon, or rectum, can be caused by polyps, diverticulitis, inflammatory disease, cancer, or hemorrhoids. **Occult bleeding** is usually caused by slow, chronic blood loss that is not obvious and results in iron deficiency anemia as iron stores in the bone marrow are slowly depleted.

Physiologic response to GI bleeding depends on the amount and rate of the loss. Acute, severe GI bleeding can be life threatening, depending on the volume and rate of blood loss, associated diseases, the age of the individual, and the effectiveness of treatment. Changes in blood pressure and heart rate are the best indicators of massive blood loss in the GI tract. During the early stages of blood volume depletion, the peripheral arteries and arterioles constrict to shunt blood to vital organs, including the brain. Signs of large-volume blood loss are postural hypotension (a drop in blood pressure that occurs with a change from the recumbent position to a sitting or upright position), lightheadedness, and loss of vision. Tachycardia develops as a compensatory response to maintain cardiac output and tissue perfusion. If blood loss continues, hypovolemic shock develops (see Chapters 32 and 48). Diminished blood flow to the kidneys causes decreased urine output and may lead to oliguria (low urine output), tubular necrosis, and renal failure. Ultimately, insufficient cerebral and coronary blood flow causes irreversible anoxia and death (Fig. 41.1).

The presentations of GI bleeding are summarized in Table 41.2. The accumulation of blood in the GI tract is irritating and increases peristalsis, causing vomiting or diarrhea, or both. Hematemesis may be present. If bleeding is from the lower GI tract, hematochezia (bloody stools) may be present. Bleeding from the upper GI tract may also be rapid enough to produce hematochezia, but generally some digestion of the blood components will have occurred, producing melena. The digestion of blood proteins originating from massive upper GI bleeding is reflected by an increase in blood urea nitrogen (BUN) levels.

The hematocrit and hemoglobin values are not the best indicators of acute GI bleeding because plasma volume and red cell volume are lost proportionately. As the plasma volume is replaced, the hematocrit and hemoglobin values begin to reflect the extent of blood loss. The interpretation of these values is modified to account for exogenous replacement of fluids and the hydration status of the tissues. Anemia associated with chronic GI bleeding is caused by iron depletion. Evaluation and treatment involve identifying and treating the source of the bleeding and replacing iron losses. Administration of blood products may be used for massive hemorrhage. Guidelines are available for the diagnosis and management of GI bleeding that may include endoscopic management with upper GI bleeds.[16–18]

TABLE 41.2 Presentations of Gastrointestinal Bleeding

Presentations	Definition
Acute Bleeding	
Hematemesis	Bloody vomitus; either fresh, bright red blood or dark grainy digested blood with "coffee grounds" appearance
Melena	Black, sticky, tarry, foul-smelling stools caused by digestion of blood in gastrointestinal tract; should be distinguished from black stools caused by dietary iron supplements, blackberries, or bismuth (e.g., Pepto-Bismol)
Hematochezia	Fresh, bright red blood passed from rectum
Occult Bleeding	Trace amounts of blood in normal-appearing stools or gastric secretions; detectable only with positive fecal occult blood test (guaiac test)

Disorders of Motility

Dysphagia

Pathophysiology. Dysphagia is difficulty swallowing or the perception of obstruction while swallowing. It can result from *mechanical obstruction* of the esophagus or from a functional disorder that impairs esophageal motility. Intrinsic obstructions originate in the wall of the esophageal lumen (e.g., esophageal dysphagia) and include tumors, strictures, and diverticular herniations (e.g., outpouchings). Extrinsic mechanical obstructions originate outside the esophageal lumen and narrow the esophagus by pressing inward on the esophageal wall. The most common cause of extrinsic mechanical obstruction is tumor.

Functional dysphagia is caused by neural or muscular disorders that interfere with voluntary swallowing or peristalsis. Disorders that affect the striated muscles of the hypopharyngeal area and upper esophagus interfere with the oropharyngeal (voluntary) phase of swallowing (oropharyngeal dysphagia). Typical causes are dermatomyositis (a muscle disease) and neurologic impairments caused by cerebrovascular accidents, Parkinson disease, multiple sclerosis, muscular dystrophy, or achalasia.

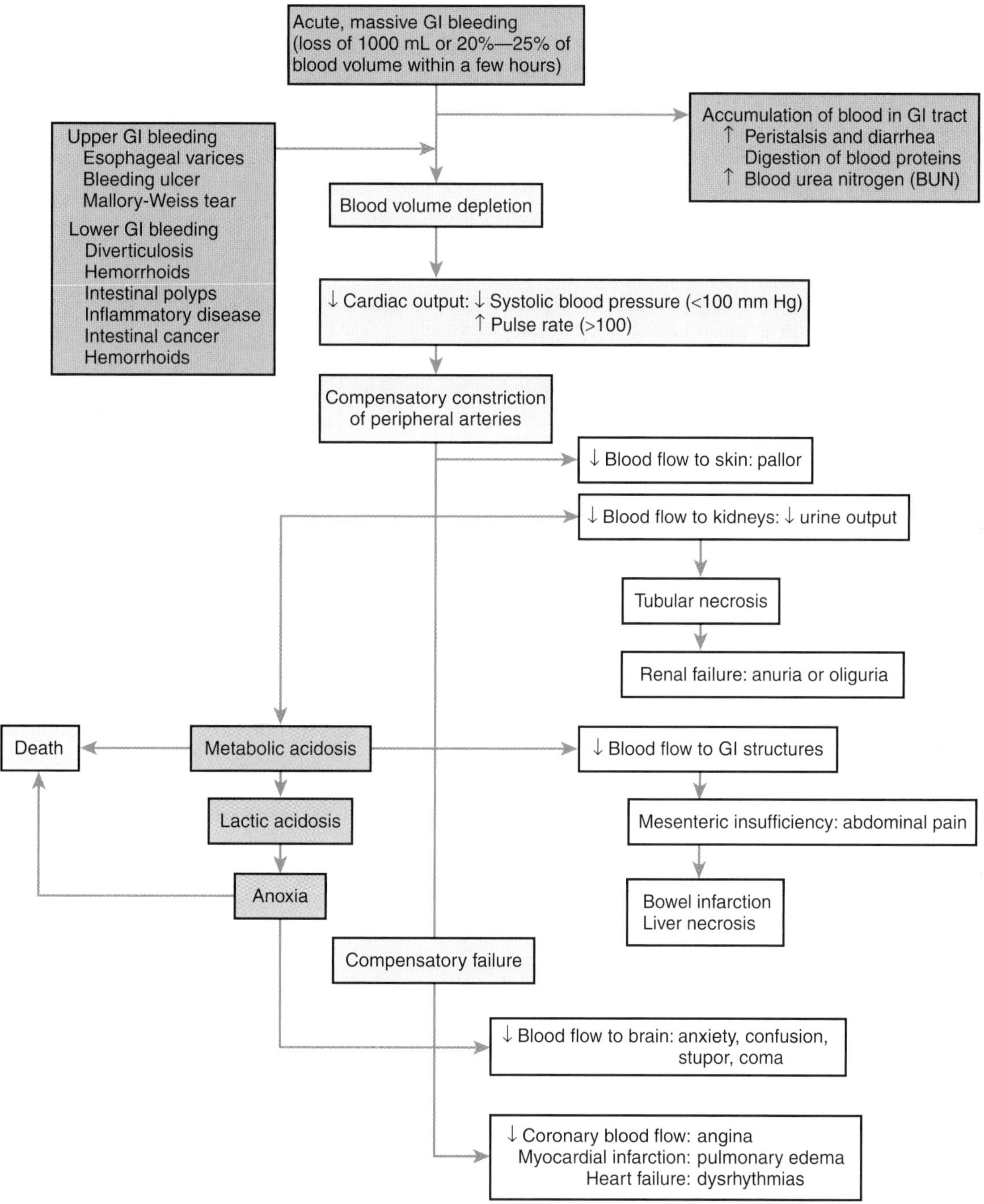

Fig. 41.1 Pathophysiology of Gastrointestinal Bleeding.

Achalasia is a rare form of dysphagia related to loss of inhibitory neurons in the myenteric plexus with smooth muscle atrophy in the middle and lower portions of the esophagus. A proposed mechanism is that myenteric neurons are attacked by a cell-mediated and antibody-mediated immune response against an unknown antigen (e.g., a virus). This leads to altered esophageal peristalsis and failure of the LES to relax, causing functional obstruction of the lower esophagus with varying severity. Food accumulates above the obstruction, distends the esophagus, and causes dysphagia. Cough and aspiration can occur. As hydrostatic pressure increases, food is slowly forced past the obstruction into the stomach. Chronic inflammation from esophageal food retention can increase risk for esophageal cancer.

Clinical Manifestations. Clinical manifestations of dysphagia vary according to the location of the obstruction. Distention and spasm of the esophageal muscles during eating or drinking may cause a mild or severe stabbing pain at the level of obstruction. Discomfort occurring 2 to 4 seconds after swallowing is associated with upper esophageal obstruction. Discomfort occurring 10 to 15 seconds after swallowing is more common in obstructions of the lower esophagus. If obstruction results from a growing tumor, dysphagia begins with difficulty swallowing solids and advances to difficulty swallowing semisolids and liquids. If motor function is impaired, both solids and liquids are difficult to swallow. Regurgitation of undigested food, an unpleasant taste sensation, vomiting, aspiration, and weight loss are common manifestations of all types of dysphagia. Aspiration of esophageal contents can lead to cough and pneumonia.

Evaluation and Treatment. Knowledge of the individual's history and clinical manifestations contributes significantly to a diagnosis of dysphagia. Imaging is used to visualize the contours of the esophagus and identify potential structural defects. Esophageal motility testing documents abnormal pressure changes associated with obstruction or loss of neural regulation. Esophageal endoscopy is performed to examine the esophageal mucosa and obtain biopsy specimens.

The individual is taught to manage symptoms by eating small meals slowly, taking fluid with meals, and sleeping with the head elevated to prevent regurgitation and aspiration. Food and medications may need to be formulated with a thickening agent so they can be swallowed. Tube feedings may be required for some individuals, particularly following stroke. Mechanical dilation of the esophageal sphincter and surgical separation of the lower esophageal muscles with a longitudinal incision (myotomy) may be an effective treatment for achalasia.[19]

Gastroesophageal Reflux Disease

Gastroesophageal reflux disease (GERD) is the reflux of acid and pepsin or bile salts from the stomach into the esophagus, causing esophagitis. The prevalence of GERD is estimated at 18% to 27% in North America.[20] Risk factors for GERD include increasing age, obesity, hiatal hernia, and drugs or chemicals that relax the LES (anticholinergics, nitrates, calcium channel blockers, nicotine). GERD may be a trigger for asthma or chronic cough. Gastroesophageal reflux that does not cause symptoms is known as *physiologic reflux*. In *nonerosive reflux disease (NERD)*, individuals have symptoms of reflux disease but no visible or minimal esophageal mucosal injury (functional heartburn).

Pathophysiology. Abnormalities in LES function, esophageal motility, and gastric motility or emptying can cause GERD. The resting tone of the LES has an average pressure of approximately 20 mm Hg that prevents gastric content from refluxing into the esophagus. Spontaneous relaxation of the LES may be triggered by gastric distention after meals and trigger acid reflux. Acid reflux may be triggered by diet and lifestyle factors such as food intake that causes delayed gastric emptying, acidic foods, and obesity. Sliding hiatal hernia facilitates reflux.[21] Vomiting, coughing, lifting, bending, and pregnancy also increase abdominal pressure, contributing to the development of reflux esophagitis.

The severity of the esophagitis depends on the composition of the gastric contents and the esophageal mucosa exposure time. If the gastric contents are highly acidic or contain bile salts and pancreatic or intestinal enzymes, reflux esophagitis can be severe. In individuals with weak esophageal peristalsis, refluxed chyme remains in the esophagus longer than usual. The refluxate causes mucosal injury and inflammation, with hyperemia, increased capillary permeability, edema, tissue fragility, and erosion (Fig. 41.2). Fibrosis and thickening may develop. Precancerous lesions (Barrett esophagus [BE]; see the Esophageal Cancer section) can be a long-term consequence. Precancerous lesions can progress to adenocarcinoma.

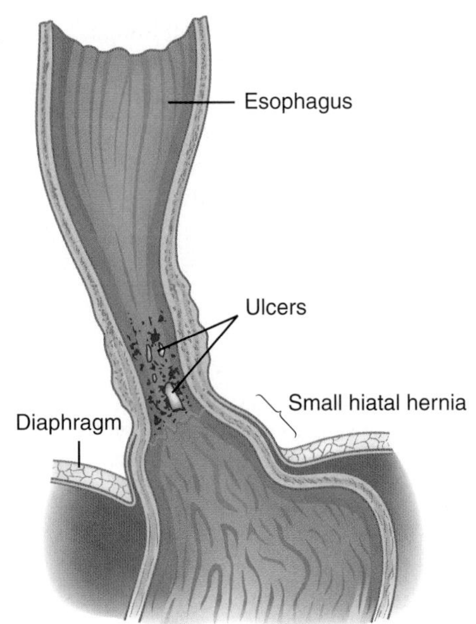

Fig. 41.2 Esophagitis With Esophageal Ulcerations.

Clinical Manifestations. The clinical manifestations of erosive reflux esophagitis are related to mucosal injury from acid regurgitation. Manifestations are heartburn (e.g., pyrosis) and acid regurgitation. Dysphagia, chest pain, chronic cough, asthma attacks (see Chapter 35), laryngitis, hoarseness, and upper abdominal pain that occurs within 1 hour of eating are less common. The symptoms worsen if the individual lies down or if intra-abdominal pressure increases (e.g., as a result of coughing, vomiting, or straining at stool). Edema, strictures, esophageal spasm, or decreased esophageal motility may result in dysphagia with weight loss. Alcohol or acid-containing foods, such as citrus fruits, can cause discomfort during swallowing.

Evaluation and Treatment. The diagnosis of GERD is based on the history and clinical manifestations. Esophageal endoscopy shows hyperemia, edema, erosion, and strictures. Dysplastic changes, such as occurs with BE (see section on esophageal carcinoma), can be identified by tissue biopsy. Impedance/pH monitoring measures the movement of stomach contents upward into the esophagus and the acidity of the refluxate. Heartburn may be experienced as chest pain, so cardiac ischemia must be ruled out.

Treatment includes once-daily proton pump inhibitors (PPIs) for 4 weeks, and continuing therapy if esophagitis or BE is present.[21] Weight reduction, smoking cessation, elevation of the head of the bed 6 inches, and avoiding tight clothing may also help to alleviate symptoms. The most common surgical treatment is laparoscopic fundoplication. Emerging surgical treatments include magnetic sphincter augmentation (a device placed around the distal esophagus and comprises titanium beads with magnets in the center that augment lower esophageal tone and thus prevent reflux), radiofrequency ablation, and transoral incisionless fundoplication.

Eosinophilic esophagitis (EoE) is an idiopathic chronic allergic/immune disease of the esophagus characterized by infiltration of eosinophils in the esophagus. EoE is most associated with atopic disease, including asthma, allergic rhinitis, eczema, and food allergies that occur in both children and adults, but the symptoms may vary by age. EoE causes many white blood cells to be found in the inner lining of the esophagus. Typically, eosinophils are not found in the esophagus, although other conditions (e.g., acid reflux disease) may contribute to the presence of eosinophils in the esophagus. Manifestations of the disease are caused by esophageal inflammation (See Chapter 42).[22] Dysphagia, decreased appetite, recurring abdominal pain, vomiting, and weight loss are common symptoms. Diagnosis is made by endoscopy with biopsy that identifies the eosinophilic infiltration and differentiates this condition from GERD. Treatment is symptomatic and includes acid inhibitors, elimination diets, and corticosteroids.[22] Other conditions associated with EoE, such as food allergies, asthma, or eczema, must also be treated appropriately (see Chapter 42).

Hiatal Hernia

Pathophysiology. Hiatal hernia is a common disorder characterized by a protrusion or bulging of an abdominal structure into the thoracic cavity. Causation is from a weakening of the diaphragm muscle.[23] (Fig. 41.3) The most common type is a sliding hiatal hernia (type 1) (see Fig. 41.3 A). In this type of hernia, the proximal portion of the stomach moves into the thoracic cavity through the esophageal hiatus. The esophageal hiatus is an opening in the diaphragm for the esophagus and vagus nerves. A congenitally short esophagus, fibrosis, excessive vagal nerve stimulation, or weakening of the diaphragmatic muscles at the gastroesophageal junction contributes to this type of hernia. Laying in the supine position causes the lower esophagus and stomach to be pulled into the thorax. As an individual stands, the organs slide back into the abdomen. Coughing, bending, tight clothing, ascites, obesity, and pregnancy accentuate the hernia in association with the resting pressure of the LES.

Paraoesophageal hiatal hernia (type 2) is a herniation of the greater curvature of the stomach through a secondary opening in the diaphragm alongside the esophagus that moves into the thorax above the diaphragm (see Fig. 41.3 B). This abnormal positioning of a portion of the stomach causes congestion of mucosal blood flow, leading to gastritis and ulcer formation. Reflux is uncommon with this type of hernia. Strangulation of the hernia is a major complication that results with occlusion of blood vessels and causes vascular engorgement with resulting edema, ischemia, and hemorrhage. Manifestations or symptoms of this type of hernia include vomiting and epigastric/retrosternal epigastric pain and is a surgical emergency.

Mixed hiatal hernia (type 3), less common, is a combination of sliding and paraoesophageal hiatal hernias (see Fig. 41.3 C). It tends to occur in conjunction with several other diseases, including reflux esophagitis, peptic ulcer, cholecystitis, cholelithiasis, chronic pancreatitis, and diverticulosis. A mixed hiatal hernia may progress to a type 4 hernia. This type of hernia involves the presence of a structure other than the stomach (e.g., omentum, colon, or small bowel) within the hernia sac.[23]

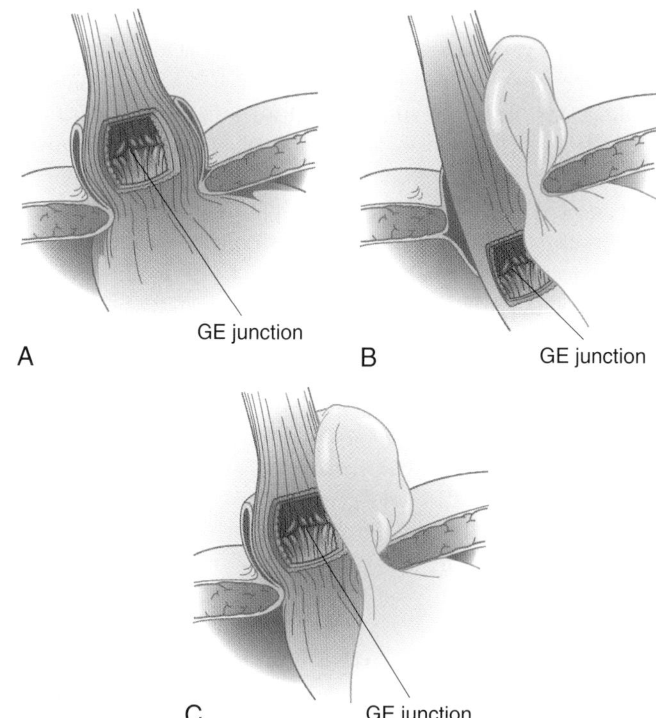

Fig. 41.3 Three Types of Hiatal Hernia. **(A)** Type I—*sliding hernia.* The visceral peritoneum remains intact and restrains the size of the hernia in sliding hiatal hernia. **(B)** Type II—*paraesophageal* or *rolling hernia.* The membrane becomes thinner or defective in a paraesophageal hernia, allowing a true peritoneal sac to protrude into the posterior mediastinum, where negative intrathoracic pressure causes it to enlarge. **(C)** Type III—*mixed hernia. GE,* Gastroesophageal. Note: Type IV—complex paraesophageal hernia is not shown. (From Townsend CM, et al. *Sabiston textbook of surgery: The biologic basis surgical practice,* 21st edition. St. Louis: Elsevier; 2022)

Clinical Manifestations. Hiatal hernias are often asymptomatic. In general, a wide variety of symptoms develop later in life; symptoms are associated with other GI disorders, including GERD, and include heartburn, regurgitation, dysphagia, and epigastric pain. Ischemia from hernia strangulation causes acute pain that may include severe chest or epigastric pain and other associated symptoms of nausea, vomiting, and GI bleeding.

Evaluation and Treatment. Many diagnostic procedures may be indicated in diagnosing a hiatal hernia. The mainstays of evaluation are upper endoscopy and barium swallows.[23] Plain chest radiographs, contrast studies, esophagogastroduodenoscopy (EGD), manometry, pH testing, and nuclear medicine studies may also be ordered. Computed tomography (CT) scan may be indicated in an urgent situation for an individual with suspected complications.[23]

Treatment for a sliding hiatal hernia is usually conservative. The individual can diminish reflux by eating small, frequent meals and avoiding the recumbent position after eating. Abdominal supports and tight clothing should be avoided, and weight control is recommended for obese individuals. Antacids may help to alleviate reflux esophagitis. Individuals who are uncomfortable at night may benefit from sleeping with the head of the bed elevated 6 inches. PPIs alleviate reflux esophagitis. Histamine 2 (H_2) receptor antagonists and antacids are typically less effective treatments. Drugs that relax the LES, such as anticholinergic type drugs, nitrates, and calcium channel blockers, are contraindicated due to delaying gastric emptying. If medical management fails to provide symptom control or a paraesophageal hiatal hernia is present, a laparoscopic fundoplication may be indicated, and permanent mesh maybe used to prevent recurrence.[24]

Gastroparesis is delayed gastric emptying in the absence of a mechanical gastric outlet obstruction. It is most associated with diabetes mellitus, surgical vagotomy, or fundoplication but may be idiopathic. The pathophysiology is not well understood but involves abnormalities of the autonomic nervous system, smooth muscle cells, enteric neurons, and GI hormones. Diabetic gastroparesis represents a form of neuropathy involving the vagus nerve. Symptoms include nausea, vomiting, abdominal pain, and postprandial fullness or bloating. Treatment options for gastroparesis are challenging due to the availability of therapies demonstrating poor evidence of efficacy or long-term safety concerns.[25] Current treatments include dietary management, prokinetic drugs, endoscopic techniques, and, in some cases, gastric electrical stimulation or surgical venting gastrostomy.[25–27]

Pyloric Obstruction

Pathophysiology. Pyloric obstruction (gastric outlet obstruction) is the consequence of diseases causing narrowing or blocking of the opening between the stomach and the duodenum. This condition can be congenital (e.g., infantile hypertrophic pyloric stenosis; see Chapter 42) or acquired. Acquired obstruction is caused by peptic ulcer disease or carcinoma near the pylorus. Duodenal ulcers are more likely than gastric ulcers to obstruct the pylorus. Ulceration causes obstruction resulting from inflammation, edema, spasm, fibrosis, or scarring. Tumors cause obstruction by growing into the pylorus.

Clinical Manifestations. Early in the course of pyloric obstruction, the individual experiences vague epigastric fullness, which becomes more distressing after eating and at the end of the day. Nausea and epigastric pain may occur as the muscles of the stomach contract in an attempt to force chyme (pulpy acidic gastric secretions) past the obstruction. These symptoms disappear when the chyme finally moves into the duodenum. As the obstruction progresses, anorexia and accompanying weight loss may occur. Severe obstruction causes gastric distention and atony (lack of muscle tone and gastric motility). Gastric distention stimulates gastric secretion, which increases the feeling of fullness. Rolling or jarring of the abdomen produces a sloshing sound called the *succussion splash.* At this stage, vomiting is a cardinal sign of obstruction. It is usually copious and occurs several hours after eating. The vomitus contains undigested food but no bile. Prolonged vomiting leads to dehydration, which is accompanied by a hypokalemic and hypochloremic metabolic alkalosis caused by loss of gastric potassium and acid. Food is not able to enter the intestine, making stools infrequent and small. Prolonged pyloric obstruction causes severe malnutrition, dehydration, and extreme debilitation.

Evaluation and Treatment. Diagnosis is based on clinical manifestations, a history of ulcer disease, and examination of residual gastric contents. Endoscopy is performed if gastric carcinoma is the suggested cause of pyloric obstruction.

Obstructions resulting from ulceration often resolve with conservative management. A nasogastric tube is used to aspirate stomach contents and relieve distention. Nasogastric suction is typically placed to decompress the stomach and to help restore normal motility. Gastric secretions that contribute to inflammation and edema can be suppressed with PPIs or H_2-receptor antagonists. Fluids and electrolytes (saline and potassium) are given intravenously to promote rehydration and correct hypokalemia and alkalosis (see Chapter 3). Severely malnourished individuals may require parenteral hyperalimentation (artificial nutrients, usually intravenous nutrition). Surgery or the placement of pyloric stents may be required to treat gastric carcinoma or persistent obstruction caused by fibrosis and scarring.[28]

Intestinal Obstruction and Paralytic Ileus

Intestinal obstruction can be caused by any condition that prevents the normal flow of chyme through the intestinal lumen (Table 41.3). Obstructions can occur in either the small or the large intestine (Table 41.4). The small intestine is more commonly obstructed because of its narrower lumen. Classifications of intestinal obstruction are summarized in Table 41.5. Intestinal obstruction is classified by cause as simple or functional. *Simple obstruction* caused by fibrous adhesions of the small intestine is the most common type of intestinal obstruction. Paralytic ileus, or *functional or pseudo-obstruction*, is a failure of normal intestinal motility often occurring after intestinal or abdominal surgery, acute pancreatitis, intestinal infection, cardiac dysfunction, or hypokalemia. Acute obstructions usually have mechanical causes, such as adhesions or hernias (Fig. 41.4). In a strangulated obstruction, blood flow is compromised, leading to intestinal ischemia and possible necrosis and perforation if left untreated. Chronic pseudo-obstruction is often idiopathic and partial obstructions are often associated with tumors or inflammatory disorders, particularly of the large intestine.[29–31]

Pathophysiology. The consequences of intestinal obstruction are related to the onset and location of the obstruction, as well as the presence and severity of associated ischemia. The major pathophysiologic alterations are presented in Fig. 41.5. The exact cause of postoperative paralytic ileus remains unknown, but it is thought to be a multifactorial and complex interaction between the autonomic and central nervous system that alters the equilibrium of the intestine, resulting in disorganized electrical activity and paralysis.[32]

Small bowel obstruction (SBO) is often caused by postoperative adhesions, tumors, CD, and hernias. SBO leads to distention caused by impaired absorption and increased secretion with the accumulation of fluid and gas inside the lumen proximal to the obstruction.[33] Distention decreases the intestine's ability to absorb water and electrolytes and increases the net secretion of these substances into the lumen. Copious vomiting or sequestration of fluids in the intestinal lumen prevents their

TABLE 41.3 Common Causes of Intestinal Obstruction

Cause	Pathophysiology
Hernia	Protrusion of intestine through weakness in abdominal muscles or through inguinal ring
Intussusception	Telescoping of one part of intestine into another; this usually causes strangulation of the blood supply; more common in infants 10–15 months of age than in adults (see Fig. 41.4D)
Torsion (volvulus)	Twisting of the intestine on its mesenteric pedicle, with occlusion of the blood supply; often associated with fibrous adhesions; occurs most often in middle-aged and elderly men
Diverticulosis	Inflamed saccular herniations (diverticula) of mucosa and submucosa through tunica muscularis of the colon; diverticula are interspersed between thick, circular, fibrous bands; most common in obese individuals older than 60 years (see Fig. 41.14)
Tumor	Tumor growth into intestinal lumen; adenocarcinoma of the colon and the rectum is the most common tumoral obstruction; most common in individuals older than 60 years
Paralytic (adynamic) ileus	Loss of peristaltic motor activity in intestine; associated with abdominal surgery, peritonitis, hypokalemia, ischemic bowel, spinal trauma, or pneumonia
Fibrous adhesions	Peritoneal irritation from surgery, trauma, or Crohn disease leads to the formation of fibrin and adhesions that attach to intestine, omentum, or peritoneum and can cause obstruction; most common in small intestine

TABLE 41.4 Large and Small Bowel Obstruction

Type of Obstruction	Cause
Small bowel obstruction	Adhesions: secondary to previous abdominal surgeries—75% Hernia: inguinal, ventral, or femoral—10% Tumors: may be associated with intussusception—10% Mesenteric ischemia—3–5% Crohn disease—<1%
Large bowel obstruction	Colon/rectal cancer—90% Volvulus—4–5% Diverticular disease—3–5% Other causes (inflammatory bowel disease, adhesions, hernia)

Data from Mizell JS, Turnage RH. Intestinal obstruction. In: Feldman M, et al, eds. *Sleisenger & Fordtran's gastrointestinal and liver disease*, 10th edition. Philadelphia: Saunders; 2016: pp 2154–2170.

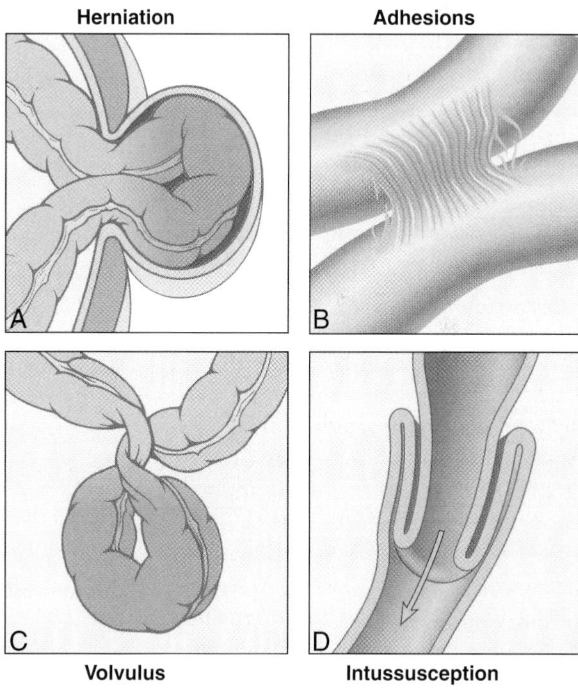

Fig. 41.4 Intestinal Obstructions. (A) Hernia. (B) Constrictions from adhesions. (C) Volvulus. (D) Intussusception. (From Kumar V, et al. *Robbins basic pathology*, 10th edition. Philadelphia: Elsevier; 2018.)

reabsorption and produces severe fluid and electrolyte disturbances. Extracellular fluid volume and plasma volume decrease, causing dehydration, increased hematocrit level, hypotension, and tachycardia. Severe dehydration leads to hypovolemic shock. Metabolic alkalosis initially develops because of excessive loss of hydrogen ions that would normally be reabsorbed from the gastric juice and vomiting. Prolonged obstruction or obstruction lower in the intestine may contribute to metabolic acidosis because bicarbonate from pancreatic secretions and bile cannot be reabsorbed. Hypokalemia from vomiting and decreased potassium absorption can be extreme, promoting acidosis and atony of the intestinal wall. Metabolic acidosis also may be accentuated by ketosis, which is the result of declining carbohydrate stores caused by starvation. In addition, lack of circulation permits the buildup of significant amounts of lactic acid, which worsens the metabolic acidosis. If pressure from the distention is severe enough, it occludes arterial circulation and causes ischemia, necrosis, perforation, and peritonitis. Fever and leukocytosis are often associated with overgrowth of bacteria, ischemia, and bowel necrosis. Bacterial proliferation and translocation across the mucosa to the systemic circulation cause peritonitis or sepsis. The release of inflammatory mediators into the circulation causes remote organ failure.

Large bowel obstruction is less common and often related to cancer. Diverticulitis, IBD, and other causes of obstruction are less common. Acute colonic pseudo-obstruction (Ogilvie

TABLE 41.5 Classifications of Intestinal Obstruction

Criteria for Classification	Definition
Onset	
Acute	Sudden onset; often caused by torsion, intussusception, or herniation
Chronic	Protracted onset; more commonly from tumor growth or progressive formation of strictures
Extent of Obstruction	
Partial	Incomplete obstruction of intestinal lumen
Complete	Complete obstruction of intestinal lumen
Location of Obstructing Lesion	
Intrinsic	Obstruction develops within intestinal lumen; examples: gut wall edema or hemorrhage, foreign bodies (gallstones), tumors, or gut wall fibrosis
Extrinsic	Obstruction originates outside intestine; examples: tumors, torsion, fibrosis, hernia, intussusception
Effects on Intestinal Wall	
Simple	Luminal obstruction without impairment of blood supply
Strangulated	Luminal obstruction with occlusion of blood supply
Closed loop	Obstruction at each end of a segment of intestine
Casual Factors	
Mechanical	Blockage of intestinal lumen by intrinsic or extrinsic lesions; usually treated surgically
Functional (paralytic ileus)	Paralysis of intestinal musculature caused by trauma, peritonitis, electrolyte imbalances, or spasmolytic agents; usually treated by decompression with suction or surgery if death of tissue

syndrome) is a pathologic massive dilation of the colon without underlying mechanical obstruction or other identified organic causes. This occurs mostly in individuals with serious comorbidities. The pathologic basis remains unclear but may be caused from a functional disturbance in the enteric nervous system.[34]

Clinical Manifestations. Signs and symptoms of *small intestine obstruction* include distention and colicky type pain, followed by nausea and vomiting. Pain usually intensifies for seconds or minutes as a peristaltic wave of muscle contraction meets the obstruction. Pain may be continuous with severe distention and then diminish in intensity. If ischemia occurs, the pain loses its colicky character and becomes more constant and severe. Sweating and tachycardia occur as a sympathetic nervous system response to hypotension. Fever, severe leukocytosis, abdominal distention, and rebound tenderness develop as ischemia progresses to necrosis, perforation, and peritonitis.

Obstruction at the pylorus causes early, profuse vomiting. Obstruction in the proximal small intestine causes mild distention and vomiting of bile-stained fluid. Lower obstruction in the small intestine causes more pronounced distention because a greater length of intestine is proximal to the obstruction. In this case, vomiting may occur later and contain fecal material. Partial obstruction can cause diarrhea or constipation, whereas complete obstruction usually causes constipation only. Complete obstruction increases the number of bowel sounds, which may be accompanied by peristaltic rushes and crampy type abdominal pain. Signs of hypovolemia and metabolic acidosis may be observed as early as 24 hours after the occurrence of complete obstruction. Distention may be severe enough to push against the diaphragm and decrease lung volume. This can lead to atelectasis and pneumonia, particularly in debilitated individuals.

Large bowel obstruction usually presents with hypogastric type pain and abdominal distention. Pain can vary from vague to excruciating, depending on the degree of ischemia and the development of peritonitis. Vomiting occurs late in the obstructive process. Small and large intestinal perforation presents with the same acute, persistent type abdominal pain, nausea, vomiting, and fever. *Acute colonic pseudo-obstruction* has the absence of mechanical obstruction and is characterized by abdominal distention, abdominal pain, nausea, and vomiting. Bowel sounds are usually present.

Evaluation and Treatment. Evaluation is based on clinical manifestations and imaging studies. Successful management requires early identification of the location and type of obstruction. Replacement of fluid and electrolytes and decompression of the lumen with gastric or intestinal suction are essential forms of therapy. Laparoscopic procedures can release adhesions. Immediate surgical intervention is required for strangulation, complete obstruction, or perforation. Colonic stents may be placed for malignant obstruction. If conservative methods are not successful, neostigmine, a parasympathomimetic, may be used for colonic pseudo-obstruction. Neostigmine increases the activation of muscarinic receptors by inhibition of the breakdown of acetylcholine. This stimulates colonic motor activity and increases intestinal transit time. Pseudo-obstruction is often managed symptomatically.[31,35]

Gastritis

Gastritis is a nonspecific inflammatory disorder of the gastric mucosa. Gastritis can present as an acute manifestation or may be chronic and often will progress to chronic gastritis if not treated in the acute phase.[36] The most common causes of gastritis

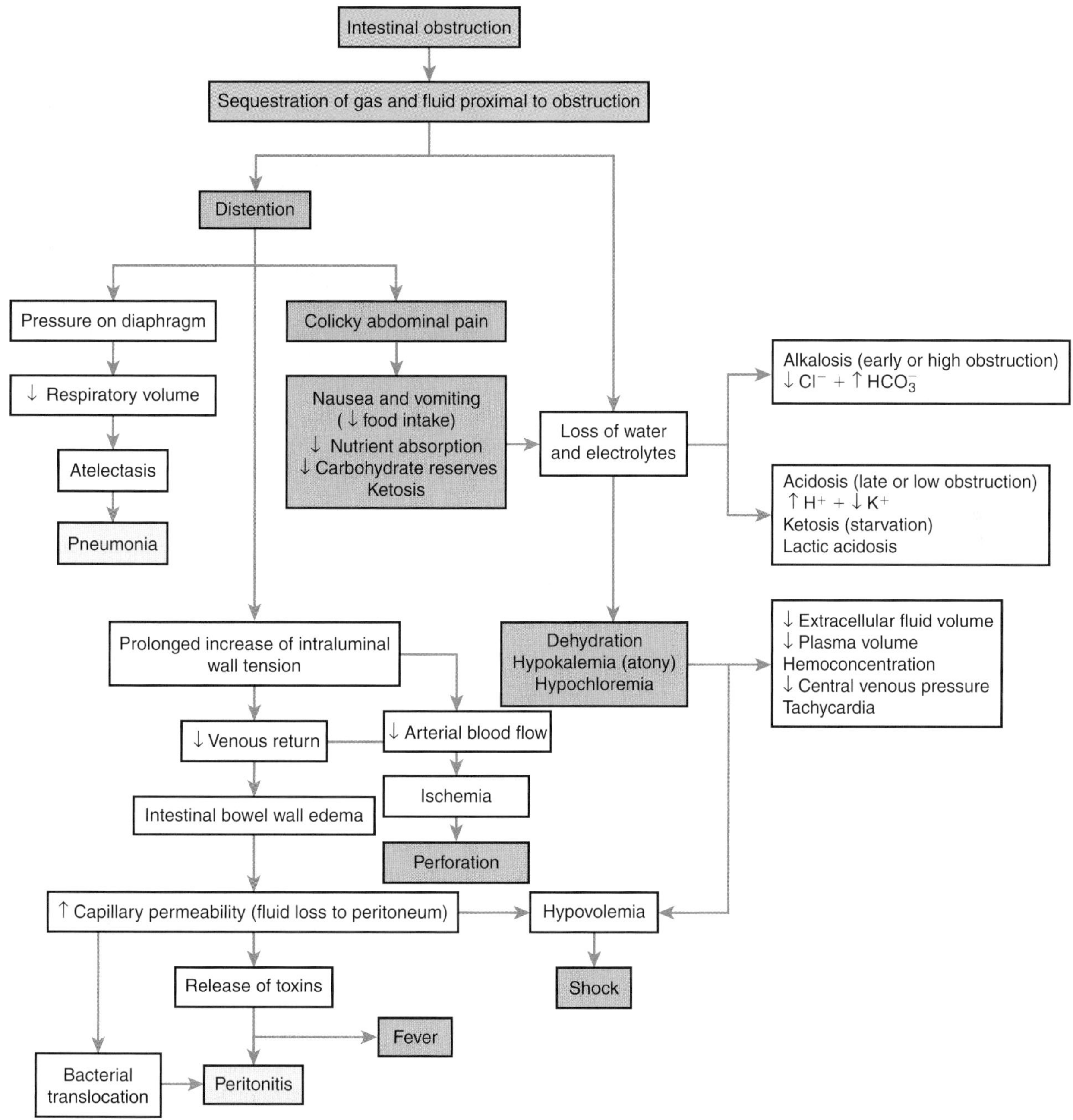

Fig. 41.5 Pathophysiology of Intestinal Obstruction.

are use of NSAIDs, *Helicobacter pylori* infection, and physiologic stress–related mucosal changes. Alcohol, digitalis, and metabolic disorders, such as uremia, also are contributing factors.

Acute gastritis is caused by injury of the protective mucosal barrier. NSAIDs (e.g., ibuprofen, naproxen, indomethacin, and aspirin) cause gastritis by inhibition of prostaglandin synthesis, which normally stimulates the secretion of mucus. Alcohol, histamine, digitalis, and metabolic disorders, such as uremia, are contributing factors. *H. pylori*–associated acute gastritis causes inflammation, increased gastric secretion in antral gastritis, decreased gastric secretion in fundal gastritis, pain, nausea, and vomiting (Box 41.1 and Fig. 41.6). The clinical manifestations of acute gastritis can include vague abdominal discomfort, epigastric tenderness, and bleeding. Healing usually occurs spontaneously within a few days. Discontinuing injurious drugs, using antacids, or decreasing acid secretion with H_2 receptor antagonist or PPIs facilitates healing.

Chronic gastritis causes chronic inflammation of the gastric mucosa which progresses to atrophic gastritis, characterized by the loss of normal mucosal glands.[36] Chronic gastritis is classified as type A immune (fundal) or type B nonimmune (antral), depending on the pathogenesis and location of the lesions. When both types of chronic gastritis occur, it is known as type AB, or pangastritis, and the antrum is more severely involved. Type C gastritis is associated with reflux of bile and pancreatic secretions into the stomach, causing chemical injury.

BOX 41.1 Pathologic Characteristics of *Helicobacter pylori*

H. pylori is a gram-negative spiral bacterium with a flagellum and is a major cause of acute and chronic gastritis, peptic ulcer disease in the duodenum and stomach, gastric adenocarcinoma, and gastric mucosa-associated lymphoid tissue (MALT) lymphoma in approximately 20% of infected individuals. *H. pylori* is transmitted through the fecal-oral route and is usually acquired in childhood. Infection is asymptomatic in approximately 70% of cases. In other cases, inflammation and immune responses promote mucosal ulcerations or prevent healing of injured tissue. Gene-environment interaction and different pathogenic strains of *H. pylori* increase risk for disease. Patterns of gastritis and development of adenocarcinoma vary by site of infection and strain of *H. pylori*. Pathogenic and virulence factors include the following:

1. An ability to colonize and adhere to gastric epithelial cells
2. The possession of flagella, which allows movement through the luminal mucous layer to a site of higher pH
3. A lipopolysaccharide membrane component evades immune protection and promotes inflammation
4. Secretion of urease that produces ammonia and carbon dioxide, resulting in a more alkaline environment and neutralization of the protective properties of hydrochloric acid
5. Release of vacuolating cytotoxin (VacA) that promotes bacterial survival and causes epithelial injury
6. The presence of cytotoxin-associated gene (CagA) strains that can escape normal immune responses and cause inflammation with release of inflammatory cytokines and reactive oxygen metabolites that damage mucosal epithelial cells and cause loss of the protective mucosal barrier; they also promote tumor development by degrading tp53 tumor suppression
7. An ability of adherent strains to suppress acid secretion to improve their survival, particularly CagA and VacA strains
8. Recruitment and activation of neutrophils, macrophages, and mast cells with release of inflammatory cytokines (tumor necrosis factor [TNF]-α, interleukin [IL]-1, IL-6, IL-8, IL-17, histamine) that promote cellular injury
9. Downregulation of antral somatostatin leading to increased gastrin, increased acid, impaired mucosal bicarbonate production, and increased mucosal exposure to acid and pepsin
10. Activation or inhibition of T- and B-cell immune responses that may contribute to mucosal injury
11. Release of cytokines and chemokines that promote gastric epithelial cell death (apoptosis) that can result in atrophy, ulcers or cell proliferation, and dysplasia or malignant growth

Data from Reshetnyak VI, Burmistrov AI, Maev IV. *Helicobacter pylori*: commensal, symbiont or pathogen? World *Journal of Gastroenterology*, 2021;27(7):545–560; Padda J, Khalid K, Cooper AC, Jean-Charles G. Association between *Helicobacter pylori* and gastric carcinoma. *Cureus*, 2021;13(5):e15165; Chmiela M, Kupcinskas J. Review: pathogenesis of *Helicobacter pylori* infection. *Helicobacter*, 2019;24(suppl 1):e12638.

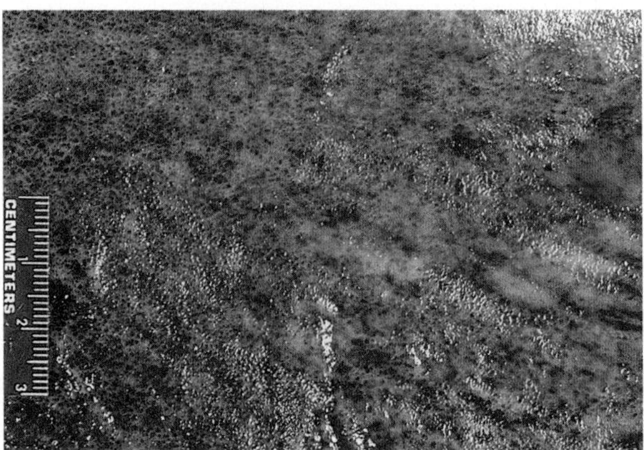

Fig. 41.6 Acute Erosive Gastritis. Acute erosive gastritis is shown in the opened stomach. The mucosa appears hyperemic, and the foci of superficial ulceration are manifested as scattered, small, red areas termed erosions. (From Kumar V, et al. *Pathologic basis of disease*, 7th edition. Philadelphia: Saunders; 2006.)

Chronic immune (fundal) gastritis (autoimmune gastritis) is the rarest form of gastritis and is a recessive, multigenetic disease. It is associated with the loss of T-cell tolerance and the development of autoantibodies to acid-secreting parietal cells. *H. pylori* infection may trigger the immune response through molecular mimicry (a mechanism of autoimmune disease with similarities between foreign and self-antigens sufficient to result in the cross-activation of autoreactive T or B cells).[37] The gastric mucosa degenerates extensively in the fundus (body) of the stomach, leading to gastric atrophy. Loss of parietal cells diminishes acid and intrinsic factor secretion. Pernicious anemia can develop from decreased vitamin B_{12} absorption (see Chapter 29). The feedback mechanism that normally inhibits gastrin secretion (i.e., loss of acid secretion) is also impaired, causing elevated plasma levels of gastrin, thus stimulating gastric secretion. Chronic fundal gastritis occurs in association with other autoimmune diseases (e.g., rheumatoid arthritis, autoimmune thyroid disease, or type 1 diabetes mellitus) and is a risk factor for gastric carcinoma, particularly in individuals who develop pernicious anemia.

Chronic nonimmune (antral) gastritis generally involves the antrum only and is more common than fundal gastritis.[38] Chronic use of alcohol, tobacco, and NSAIDs and *H. pylori* infection are contributing factors. There are high levels of hydrochloric acid secretion with an increased risk of duodenal ulcers. *H. pylori* infection also can progress to autoimmune atrophic gastritis and involve the fundus, thus becoming pangastritis.[39] There is greater risk for the development of gastric cancer in these cases.

Clinical Manifestations. Signs and symptoms of chronic gastritis often include vague symptoms, such as anorexia, fullness, nausea, vomiting, and epigastric pain. Gastric bleeding may be the only clinical manifestation of gastritis. Gastroscopic examination and biopsy may show a long-standing inflammatory process and gastric atrophy in an individual with no history of abdominal distress. Gastric secretion analysis confirms achlorhydria (the absence of hydrochloric acid) and loss of intrinsic factor. Pernicious anemia can develop because intrinsic factor is less available to facilitate vitamin B_{12} absorption. Iron deficiency may also be present. The presence of antiparietal cell antibody and elevated plasma ghrelin level are specified for atrophic gastritis. *H. pylori* infection is evidence for *H. pylori* chronic gastritis with infiltration of neutrophils and lymphocytes. Eradication of *H. pylori* is recommended for the prevention of gastric carcinoma.[40–42]

Evaluation and Treatment. Symptoms can usually be managed by eating smaller meals in conjunction with a soft, bland diet and by avoiding alcohol and NSAIDs. *H. pylori* infection is treated with antibiotics, and vitamin B_{12} is administered to correct pernicious anemia.

Peptic Ulcer Disease

A peptic ulcer is a break or ulceration in the protective mucosal lining, usually located in the stomach or proximal duodenum; however, they can be found in the esophagus (see Figs. 41.7 and 41.8). Ulcers develop when mucosal protective factors are overcome by erosive factors such as gastric acid secretion or pepsin. This causes an imbalance between the gastric mucosal protective factors and the destructive factors. Peptic ulcer disease has various causes; however, most cases are caused by *H. pylori* and NSAIDs. Additional risk factors for peptic ulcer disease include the use of the following medications: corticosteroids, bisphosphonates, potassium chloride, and fluorouracil. Smoking, alcohol consumption, and certain disease processes that can make the gastric lining a hypersecretory environment, such as Zollinger-Ellison syndrome, systemic mastocytosis, cystic fibrosis, hyperparathyroidism, and antral G-cell hyperplasia, are also risk factors.[43]

Peptic ulcers can be single or multiple, acute, or chronic, and superficial or deep. Superficial ulcerations are called *erosions* because they erode the mucosa but do not penetrate the muscularis mucosa. True ulcers extend through the muscularis mucosae and damage blood vessels, causing hemorrhage and possible perforation of the GI wall. Successful antibiotic treatment of *H. pylori* infection and the use of mucosal protecting agents during NSAID and *H. pylori* treatment have significantly reduced the incidence of peptic ulcer disease.

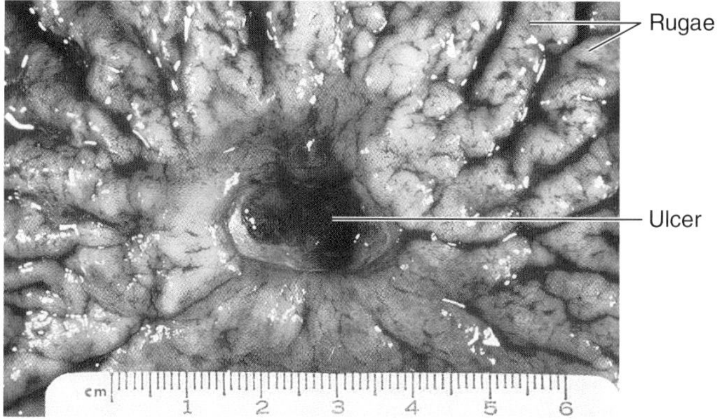

Fig. 41.7 Chronic Peptic Ulcer. Gross photograph of a chronic peptic ulcer located in the lesser curvature, straddling the antrum and corpus of the stomach. (From Damjanov I, Linder J, eds. *Anderson's pathology*, 10th edition. St. Louis: Mosby; 1996.)

Zollinger-Ellison syndrome is a rare syndrome that also is associated with peptic ulcers caused by a gastrin-secreting neuroendocrine tumor or multiple tumors of the pancreas or duodenum that release large amounts of acid. The body normally releases small amounts of gastrin after eating; gastrin then triggers the stomach to make gastric acid. Gastrin stimulates a proliferation of gastric parietal cells and chronic secretion of gastric acid. The resulting excess acid causes gastric and duodenal ulcers, gastroesophageal reflux with abdominal pain, diarrhea, bloating, burping, weight loss, and poor appetite. Diagnosis includes secretin or calcium- stimulated measures of gastrin levels, gastric pH levels less than 2, and symptomatic evidence of peptic ulcer disease. PPIs reduce gastric acid secretion, and surgical removal of tumors limits metastasis.[44]

Duodenal Ulcers

Duodenal ulcers occur with greater frequency than other types of peptic ulcers and are generally caused by *H. pylori* infection and NSAID use. Idiopathic duodenal ulcers are rare and can be associated with altered mucosal defenses, rapid gastric emptying, elevated serum gastrin levels, or acid production stimulated by smoking.[45]

Pathophysiology. Causative factors, independently or in combination, cause acid and pepsin concentrations in the duodenum to increase and penetrate the mucosal barrier, causing ulceration (Fig. 41.9). The host response to chronic stomach antral *H. pylori* infection is increased levels of gastrin resulting in increased stomach acid secretion and an increased acid load in the duodenum. The increased duodenal acid promotes gastric metaplasia in the duodenum and favors *H. pylori* colonization. Both *H. pylori* and the increased acid result in decreased duodenal bicarbonate production. In addition, *H. pylori* infection activates immune cells (T and B lymphocytes with the infiltration of neutrophils) and the release of inflammatory cytokines which damage the mucosa. *H. pylori* also produces a toxin that causes loss of protective mucosal cells, resulting in ulceration. *H. pylori* mucosal infection can promote gastric cancer, but the incidence is lower for duodenal ulcer than for gastric ulcer, and the mechanism is unknown.[46]

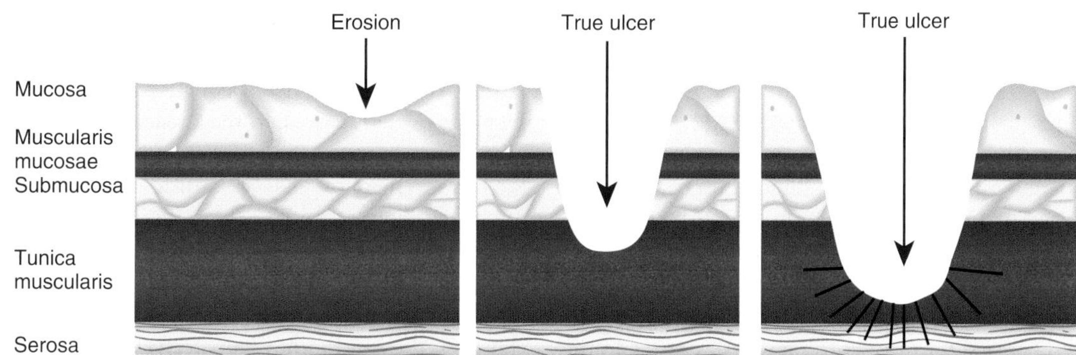

Fig. 41.8 Lesions Caused by Peptic Ulcer Disease.

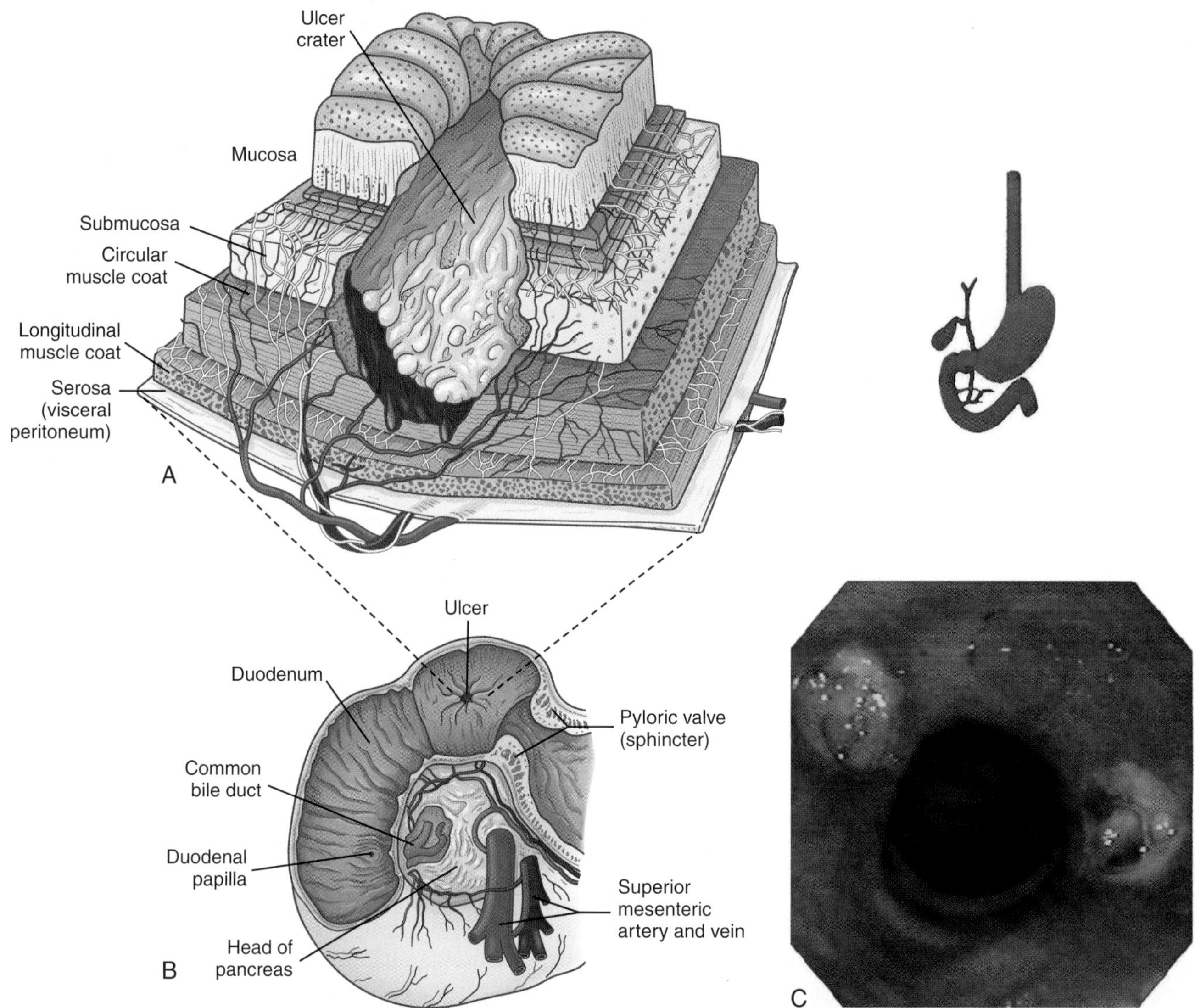

Fig. 41.9 Duodenal Ulcer. (A) A deep ulceration in the duodenal wall extending as a crater through the entire mucosa and into the muscle layers. **(B)** Sequence of ulcerations from normal mucosa to duodenal ulcer. **(C)** Bilateral (kissing) duodenal ulcers in a person using nonsteroidal antiinflammatory drugs. (C, Courtesy David Bjorkman, MD, University of Utah School of Medicine, Department of Gastroenterology, Salt Lake City, UT.)

Clinical Manifestations. The characteristic manifestation of a duodenal ulcer is chronic, intermittent pain in the epigastric area. The pain begins 2 or 3 hours after eating, when the stomach is empty. It is not unusual for pain to occur in the middle of the night and disappear by morning. Pain is relieved rapidly by ingestion of food or antacids, creating a typical pain-food-relief pattern. Some individuals with a duodenal ulcer may have no symptoms; the first manifestation may be hemorrhage or perforation, particularly with a history of NSAID or anticoagulant use. Complications of a duodenal ulcer include bleeding, perforation, and obstruction of the duodenum or outlet of the stomach. Bleeding is the most common cause of mortality, particularly among the elderly. Bleeding from duodenal ulcers causes hematemesis or melena. Perforation occurs with destruction of all layers of the duodenal wall and causes sudden, severe epigastric pain. Obstruction may be the result of edema from inflammation or scarring from chronic injury. Duodenal ulcers often heal spontaneously. However, repeat imaging is indicated if the ulcer was large, associated complications were present, or the individual has continued pain.[47]

Evaluation and Treatment. Several diagnostic approaches are used to differentiate duodenal ulcers from gastric ulcers or gastric carcinoma. Endoscopic evaluation allows visualization of lesions and biopsy. Radioimmune assays of gastrin levels are evaluated to identify ulcers associated with gastric carcinomas. *H. pylori* is detected using the urea breath test, *H. pylori*–specific serum immunoglobulin G (IgG) and IgA antibodies, and the measurement of *H. pylori* stool antigen levels. Findings from the gastric biopsy detect *H. pylori* infection and can also confirm eradication after treatment. Polymerase chain reaction testing provides additional virulence and antibiotic sensitivity profiling.[48]

The management of duodenal ulcers is aimed at relieving the causes of the ulceration. The effects associated with the hyperacidity and pepsin present in the gut should be managed with diet and pharmacotherapy. Antacids neutralize gastric contents and relieve pain. Acid secretion can be suppressed with drugs that block H_2 receptors and inhibit the secretion of acid. PPIs inhibit acid production. *H. pylori* is treated with a combination of antibiotics and PPIs, but antibiotic resistance is an increasing problem.[49] Surgical resection may be required for bleeding or perforating ulcers, obstruction, or peritonitis.

Gastric Ulcers

Gastric ulcers are ulcers of the stomach. They occur about equally in males and females, usually between the ages of 55 and 65 years. They are less common than duodenal ulcers (Table 41.6).

Pathophysiology. In general, gastric ulcers develop in the antral region, adjacent to the acid-secreting mucosa of the body. The primary defect is an abnormality that increases the mucosal barrier's permeability to hydrogen ions. Gastric secretion may be normal or less than normal, and there may be a decreased mass of parietal cells. Chronic gastritis is often associated with the development of gastric ulcers and may precipitate ulcer formation by limiting the mucosa's ability to secrete a protective layer of mucus (Fig. 41.10). Other factors include:

- Decreased mucosal synthesis of prostaglandins
- Damage to the mucosal membrane from duodenal reflux of bile and pancreatic enzymes
- Use of NSAIDs (decreases prostaglandin synthesis)
- *H. pylori* infection

A break in the mucosal barrier permits hydrogen ions to diffuse into the mucosa, where they disrupt permeability and cellular structure. A vicious cycle can be established as the damaged mucosa liberates histamine, which stimulates the increase of acid and pepsinogen production, blood flow, and capillary permeability. The disrupted mucosa becomes edematous and loses plasma proteins. Destruction of small vessels causes bleeding.

Clinical Manifestations. The clinical manifestations of gastric ulcers are similar to those of duodenal ulcers (see Table 41.6). The pattern of pain is common, but the pain of gastric ulcers also occurs immediately after eating. Gastric ulcers also tend to be chronic rather than alternating between periods of remission and exacerbation, and they cause more anorexia and vomiting than duodenal ulcers. The pain associated with eating tends to suppress food intake, resulting in weight loss. The evaluation and treatment of gastric ulcers are similar to those for duodenal ulcers. However, long-term use of PPIs is a reported risk factor for gastric cancer after *H. pylori* eradication and is related to hypergastrinemia and hyperplasia of enterochromaffin-like cells that promote the secretion of gastric acid.[50]

TABLE 41.6 Characteristics of Gastric and Duodenal Ulcers

Characteristics	Gastric Ulcer	Duodenal Ulcer
Incidence		
Age at onset	50–70 years	20–50 years
Family history	Usually negative	Positive
Sex (prevalence)	Equal in women and men	Equal in men and women
Stress factors	Increased	Average
Ulcerogenic drugs	Normal use	Increased use
Cancer risk	Increased	Not increased
Pathophysiology		
Helicobacter pylori infection	Often present (60%–80%)	Often present (95%–100%)
Abnormal mucus	May be present	May be present
Parietal cell mass	Normal or decreased	Increased
Acid production	Normal or decreased	Increased
Serum gastrin	Increased	Normal
Serum pepsinogen	Normal	Increased
Associated gastritis	More common	Usually not present
Clinical Manifestations		
Pain	Located in upper abdomen	Located in upper abdomen
	Intermittent	Intermittent
	Pain-antacid-relief pattern	Pain-antacid or food-relief pattern
	Food-pain pattern	Nocturnal pain common
Clinical course	Chronic ulcer without pattern of remission and exacerbation	Pattern of remissions and exacerbation for years

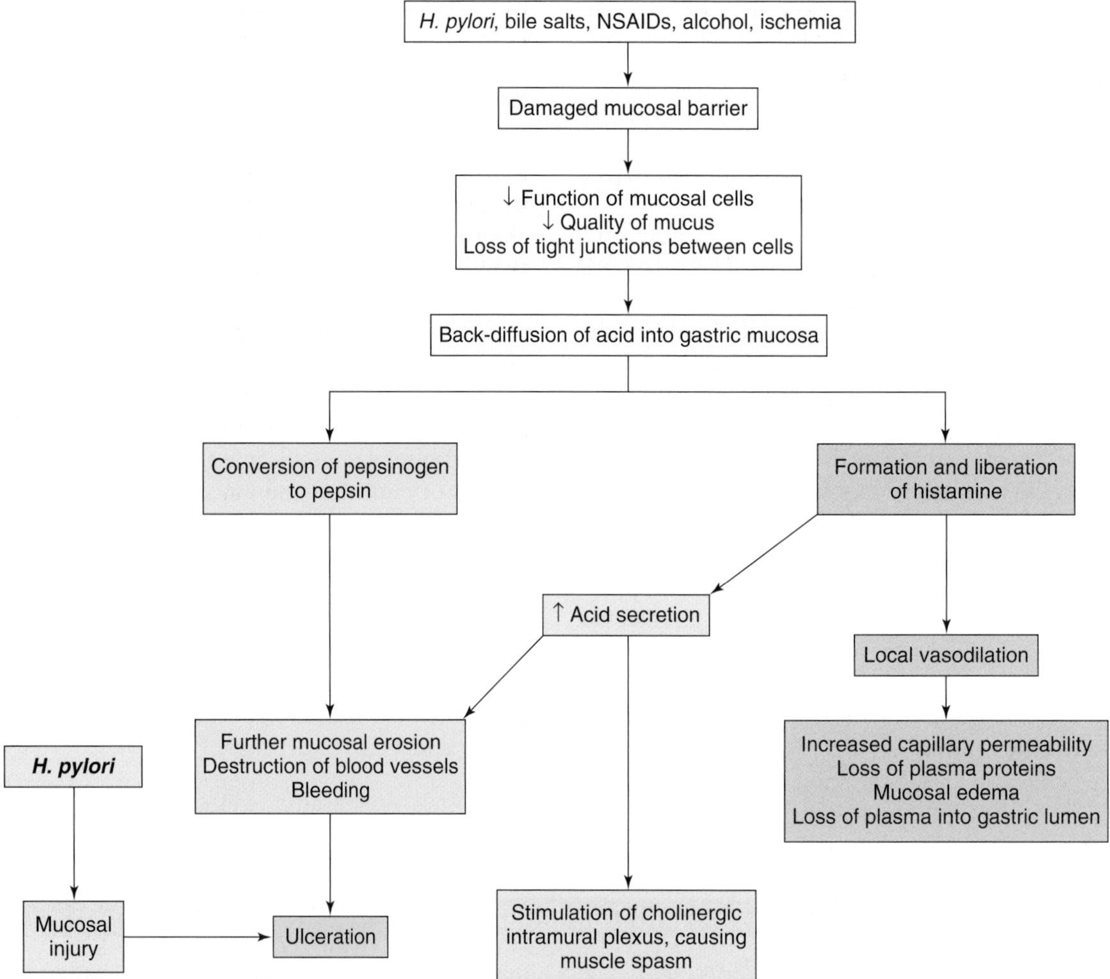

Fig. 41.10 Pathophysiology of Gastric Ulcer Formation. *NSAIDs*, Nonsteroidal antiinflammatory drugs.

Stress-Related Mucosal Disease

A stress-related mucosal disease (stress ulcer) is an acute form of peptic ulcer that tends to accompany the physiologic stress of severe illness or major trauma. Usually, multiple sites of ulceration are distributed within the stomach or duodenum. Stress ulcers may be classified as ischemic ulcers or Cushing ulcers.

Ischemic ulcers develop within hours of an event such as hemorrhage, multisystem trauma, severe burns, heart failure, or sepsis. Shock, anoxia, inflammation, and sympathetic responses cause ischemia of the stomach and duodenal mucosa, disrupting the mucosal barrier. Stress ulcers that develop as a result of burn injury are often called Curling ulcers. Cushing ulcer is a stress ulcer associated with severe brain trauma or brain surgery. Decreased mucosal blood flow and hypersecretion of acid caused by overstimulation of the vagal nuclei damage the mucosal barrier, causing erosions and ulceration.

The primary clinical manifestation of stress-related mucosal disease is bleeding, which is uncommon, but occurs more readily with the presence of coagulopathy and in the presence of more than 48 hours of mechanical ventilation. Prophylactic treatment regimens are used to prevent this disease. Stress ulcers seldom become chronic.[51]

Surgical Treatment of Ulcer

Advances in the medical treatment of peptic ulcer disease with acid suppression and eradication of *H. pylori* have reduced the number of cases requiring surgery. The most common indications for ulcer surgery are recurrent or uncontrolled bleeding and perforation of the stomach or duodenum. The primary objectives of surgical treatment are to reduce stimuli for acid secretion, decrease the number of acid-secreting cells in the stomach, and correct complications of ulcer disease.

Acute complications of gastrectomy or anastomosis are relatively uncommon except in debilitated persons. However, chronic complications are likely to develop if a large portion of the stomach has been removed. These complications and their pathophysiologic mechanisms are described in the next section.

Postgastrectomy Syndromes

Postgastrectomy syndromes are a group of signs and symptoms that occur after gastric resection for the treatment of peptic ulcer, gastric carcinoma, or bariatric surgery for extreme obesity. They are caused by anatomic and functional changes in the stomach and upper small intestine[52] and include the following conditions.

Dumping syndrome is the rapid emptying of hypertonic chyme from the surgically created residual stomach (i.e., the smaller stomach component remaining after surgical resection following gastric or bariatric surgery) into the small intestine 10 to 20 minutes after eating. It occurs with varying severity and is promoted by loss of gastric capacity, loss of emptying control when pylorus is removed, and loss of feedback control by the duodenum once removed. Rapid gastric emptying and a creation of a nonphysiologic, high osmotic gradient within the small intestine cause a sudden shift of fluid from the vascular compartment to the intestinal lumen. Plasma volume decreases and rapid distention of the intestine occurs, producing symptoms such as cramping type pain, nausea, vomiting, osmotic diarrhea, hypotension, weakness, and pallor.

Late dumping syndrome occurs 1 to 3 hours after eating a high carbohydrate meal and is related to hyperinsulinemia with hypoglycemia. The symptoms of late dumping syndrome include weakness, diaphoresis, and confusion. Most cases of dumping syndrome respond to dietary management. Individuals should eat frequent small meals high in protein and low in carbohydrates.

Alkaline (bile) reflux gastritis occurs when there is a dis ruption of the mucosal barrier in the remnant stomach. Reflux of bile and alkaline pancreatic secretions containing proteo lytic enzyme disrupts the mucosal barrier in the remnant stom ach causing inflammation. Symptoms include nausea, bilious vomiting, and sustained epigastric pain that worsen after eat ing and is not relieved by antacids. It responds somewhat to avoidance of aspirin and alcohol, but surgical correction may be required.

Afferent loop obstruction is a rare complication of Billroth gastrojejunostomy. Symptoms include intermittent severe pain and epigastric fullness after eating because of volvulus, hernia, adhesion, or stenosis of the duodenal stump on the proximal side of the gastrojejunostomy. Vomiting typically relieves symptoms. Management includes low-fat diet, but decompression or surgery revision is required for complete obstruction.

Diarrhea is related to rapid gastric emptying and osmotic attraction of water into the gut, especially after a large intake of high-carbohydrate liquids. Small, dry meals and anticholinergic drugs are effective control measures.

Weight loss is commonly caused by inadequate caloric intake because the individual cannot tolerate carbohydrates or a normal-sized meal. The stomach also is less able to mix, churn, and break down food. In the case of bariatric surgery for extreme obesity, weight loss is the intended outcome, but nutrients, including vitamins and minerals, must be monitored and supplemented to prevent deficiencies.[53]

Anemia may occur if iron malabsorption results from decreased acid secretion or lack of duodenum after a Billroth II procedure (gastrojejunostomy). Deficiencies of iron, vitamin B_{12}, or folate also may result.

Bone and mineral disorders are related to altered calcium absorption and metabolism. This causes an increased risk of fractures and deformity, and malabsorption of vitamins and nutrients, such as vitamin D.

Malabsorption Syndromes

Malabsorption syndromes interfere with nutrient absorption in the small intestine. Historically they have been classified as maldigestion or malabsorption. Maldigestion is failure of the chemical processes of digestion that take place in the intestinal lumen or at the brush border of the intestinal mucosa. Malabsorption is failure of the intestinal mucosa to absorb the digested nutrients. Often these two syndromes are interrelated or occur together, making classification difficult. In general, maldigestion is caused by deficiencies of the enzymes needed for digestion or inadequate secretion of bile salts and inadequate reabsorption of bile in the ileum. Malabsorption is the result of mucosal disruption caused by gastric or intestinal resection, vascular disorders, or intestinal disease (also see Chapter 42).

Pancreatic Exocrine Insufficiency

The pancreatic enzymes (lipase, amylase, trypsin, chymotrypsin) are required for the digestion of proteins, carbohydrates, and fats. Pancreatic insufficiency is the deficient production of these enzymes, particularly lipase, by the pancreas. Causes include chronic pancreatitis, pancreatic carcinoma, pancreatic resection, and cystic fibrosis. Significant damage to or loss of pancreatic tissue must occur before enzyme levels decrease sufficiently to cause maldigestion. Although pancreatic insufficiency causes poor digestion of all nutrients, fat maldigestion is the chief problem. Absence of pancreatic bicarbonate in the duodenum and jejunum causes an acidic pH that worsens maldigestion by precipitating bile salts and preventing activation of the pancreatic enzymes that are present. A large amount of fat in the stool (steatorrhea) is the most common sign of pancreatic insufficiency. There is also a deficit of fat-soluble vitamins (A, D, E, and K) and weight loss. Several diagnostic tests are available to diagnose pancreatic exocrine insufficiency; however, there remains confusion regarding which testing procedure demonstrates the best approach. Treatment consists of dietary management and lifestyle changes and pancreatic enzyme replacement therapy.[54]

Lactase Deficiency (Lactose Intolerance)

A deficiency of disaccharidase at the brush border of the small intestine is caused by a genetic defect in which a single enzyme, usually lactase, is lacking. Lactase deficiency inhibits the breakdown of lactose (milk sugar) into monosaccharides and therefore prevents lactose digestion and absorption across the intestinal wall. Lactase deficiency is most common in Blacks, Latinos, and Native Americans and usually does not develop until adulthood. Secondary (acquired) lactase deficiency can be caused by several diseases of the intestine, including gluten-sensitive enteropathy, enteritis, and bacterial overgrowth.

The undigested lactose remains in the intestine, where bacterial fermentation causes formation of gases. Undigested lactose also increases the osmotic gradient in the intestine, causing irritation and osmotic diarrhea. Clinical manifestations of lactose consumption with lactase deficiency are bloating, cramping type pain, diarrhea, and flatulence. The disorder is diagnosed by a lactose-tolerance test. Avoiding milk products and adhering to a lactose-free diet relieves symptoms.[55]

Bile Salt Deficiency and Malabsorption

Pathophysiology. Conjugated bile acids (BAs) (bile salts) are necessary for the digestion and absorption of fats. Bile salts are conjugated in the bile that is secreted from the liver. When bile enters the duodenum, the bile salts aggregate with fatty acids and monoglycerides to form micelles. Micelle formation makes fat molecules more soluble and allows them to pass through the unstirred layer at the brush border of the small intestinal villi (see Chapter 40). A minimum concentration of bile salts, termed the *critical micelle concentration,* is required to allow formation of micelles. Therefore conditions that decrease the production or secretion of bile result in bile salt deficiency and decreased micelle formation and fat malabsorption. These conditions include advanced liver disease, which decreases the production of bile salts; obstruction of the common bile duct, which decreases flow of bile into the duodenum (cholestasis); intestinal stasis (lack of motility), which permits overgrowth of intestinal bacteria that deconjugate bile salts; and diseases of the ileum, which prevent the reabsorption and recycling of bile salts (enterohepatic circulation).[56]

Clinical Manifestations. Clinical manifestations of bile salt deficiency are related to poor intestinal absorption of fat and fat-soluble vitamins (A, D, E, and K). Increased fat in the stools (steatorrhea) leads to diarrhea and decreased levels of plasma proteins. The losses of fat-soluble vitamins and their effects include:

- Vitamin A deficiency results in night blindness.
- Vitamin D deficiency results in decreased calcium absorption with bone demineralization (osteoporosis), bone pain, and fractures.
- Vitamin K deficiency prolongs prothrombin time, leading to spontaneous development of purpura (bruising) and petechiae.
- Vitamin E deficiency has uncertain effects but may cause testicular atrophy and neurologic defects in children.

Evaluation and Treatment. The most effective treatment for fat-soluble vitamin deficiency is TO increase consumption of medium-chain triglycerides in the diet, for example, by using coconut oil for cooking. Vitamins A, D, and K may be given parenterally. Oral bile salts are also an effective therapy.

Bile malabsorption is associated with a number is disorders, including ileal resection or inflammation, small intestinal bacterial overgrowth, and celiac disease. The accumulation of bile in the colon results in watery diarrhea known as BA diarrhea. Cholestyramine and colesevelam, which bind BA in the colon, are used for treatment. In the future, farsenoid X receptor agonists may also be effective because they regulate BA synthesis, conjugation, and transport.[57]

Inflammatory Bowel Disease

UC and CD are major types of chronic relapsing IBDs, and the cause is unknown. The prevalence of IBD is approximately 1.4 million people in the United States, with approximately 30,000 new cases annually.[58]

IBD causes an inflammation of the intestinal mucosa, which causes episodic abdominal pain, diarrhea, bloody stools, and weight loss. Inflammation and ulceration are caused by an influx of neutrophils and macrophages that produce proinflammatory cytokines, proteolytic enzymes, and free radicals (Table 41.7).[59]

Environmental factors or infections are thought to alter the barrier function of the mucosal epithelium, leading to loss of immune tolerance to normal intestinal antigens. Environmental triggers may include diet, psychological stress, viruses, and smoking.[58] There is possible loss of discrimination of potentially harmful pathogens from commensal microorganisms in the intestinal mucosa. The loss of tolerance activates immune cells. Production of proinflammatory mediators also damages the intestinal epithelium.

The risk of colon cancer has been significantly reduced with current approaches to treatment.[60] Future research is directed at an integration of these factors to refine our understanding of disease cause and trajectory, particularly interactions between genetics, the microflora, mucosa, and immune responses. The clinical manifestations of UC and CD are similar, but there are different pathologic features and extent of inflammatory involvement.

Ulcerative Colitis

Ulcerative colitis (UC) is a chronic inflammatory disease that causes ulceration of the colonic mucosa, most commonly in the rectum and sigmoid colon (Fig. 41.11). The lesions appear in susceptible individuals between 20 and 40 years of age. UC is less common in people who smoke or have had an appendectomy, and the mechanisms are not clearly known.[61]

Pathophysiology. The primary lesion of UC begins with inflammation at the base of the crypt of Lieberkühn in the large intestine. The disease begins in the rectum (proctitis) and may extend proximally to the entire colon (pancolitis). The lesions are limited to mucosal epithelium, are not transmural, and do not involve skip lesions. There is decreased secretion of mucin, which is antimicrobial and provides a protective layer against pathogens. Loss of this protection leads to increased permeability of the mucosa, increased passage of pathogens and other antigens, and stimulation of the gut immune system with an inflammatory response. There is activation of T cells and dendritic cells, triggering the production of proinflammatory cytokines and chemokines, including tumor necrosis factor (TNF)-α, interleukin (IL)-12 and IL-23, toxic oxygen free radicals, and interferon-gamma (IFN-γ), producing damage to the intestinal epithelium. In addition, there is activation

TABLE 41.7 **Features of Ulcerative Colitis and Crohn Disease**

Feature	Ulcerative Colitis	Crohn Disease
Incidence		
Age at onset	Any age; 10–40 years most common	Any age; 10–30 years most common
Family history	Less common	More common
Sex	Prevalence equal in women and men	Prevalence about equal in women and men
Cancer risk	Increased	Increased
Nicotine use	Later and less severe disease; nicotine withdrawal may cause exacerbation	Increases disease risk and greater disease severity
Pathophysiology		
Location of lesions	Large intestine, continuous lesions Left side more common	Mouth to anus, "skip" lesions common Right side more common
Inflammation	Mucosal layer involved	Entire intestinal wall involved
Granulomata	Rare	Transmural granulomata common; cobblestone appearance
Ulceration	Friable mucosa, superficial ulcers, crypt abscesses common	Deep fissuring ulcers and fistulae common
Anal and perianal fistulae	Rare	Common; abscesses
Narrowed lumen and possible obstruction	Rare	Common; obstruction
Clinical Manifestations		
Abdominal pain	Mild to severe	Moderate to severe
Diarrhea	Common; 4 times/day	May or may not be present
Bloody stools	Common	Less common
Weight loss	Less common	Common
Abdominal mass	Rare	Common
Small intestine malabsorption	None	Common
Clinical course	Remissions and exacerbations	Remissions and exacerbations
Comorbidities	Extraintestinal manifestations	Extraintestinal manifestations

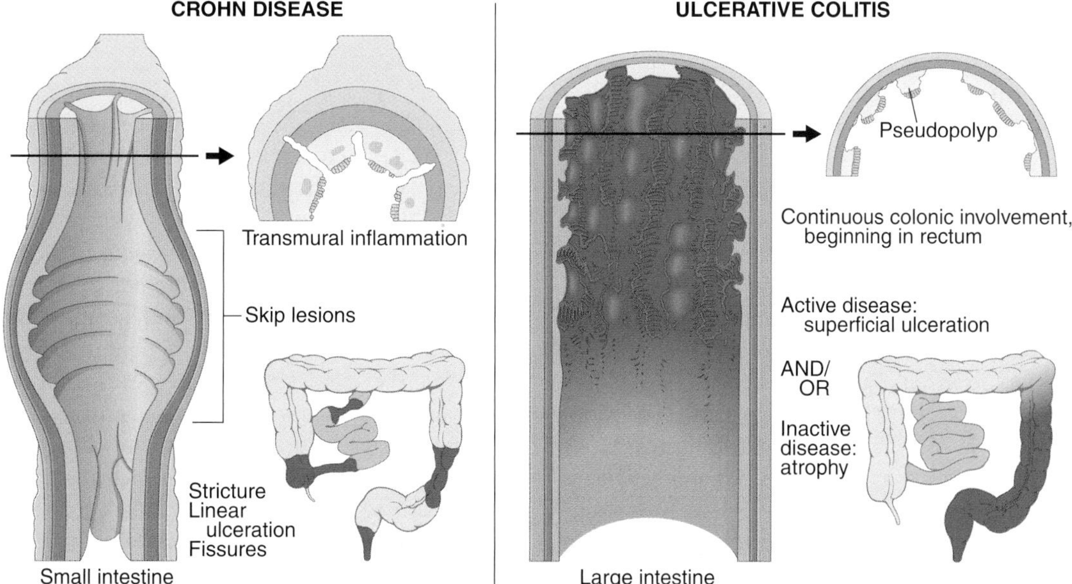

Fig. 41.11 Distribution Patterns of Crohn Disease and Ulcerative Colitis. Comparison of distribution patterns of Crohn disease and ulcerative colitis as well as different conformations of ulcers and wall thickenings. (From Kumar V, et al. *Robbins basic pathology*, 8th edition. St. Louis: Mosby; 2008.)

of vascular adhesion molecules (integrins, e.g., mucosal addressin cellular adhesion molecule-1 [MadCAM-1]) which promote the trafficking of lymphocytes into the gut, furthering potentiation of the inflammatory response. Some of these molecules have become important targets for treatment.[62]

The mucosa is inflamed and is involved in a continuous fashion. With milder inflammation, the mucosa is hyperemic and edematous and may appear dark red. In more severe inflammation, the mucosa becomes hemorrhagic, and small erosions form and coalesce into ulcers. Abscess formation, necrosis, and ragged ulceration of the mucosa ensue. Edema and thickening of the muscularis mucosae may narrow the lumen of the involved colon. Mucosal destruction and inflammation cause bleeding, cramping pain, and an urge to defecate. Frequent diarrhea, with passage of small amounts of blood and purulent mucus, is common. Loss of the absorptive mucosal surface and rapid colonic transit time cause large volumes of watery diarrhea.

Clinical Manifestations. The course of UC consists of intermittent periods of remission and exacerbation. Mild UC involves less mucosa, so the frequency of bowel movements, bleeding, and pain is minimal. Severe forms may involve the entire colon and are characterized by abdominal pain, fever, an elevated pulse rate, frequent diarrhea (10 to 20 stools/day), urgency, bloody stools, and continuous, crampy pain; dehydration, weight loss, anemia, and fever result from fluid loss, bleeding, and inflammation. Complications include anal fissures, hemorrhoids, and perirectal abscess. Severe hemorrhage is rare. Edema, strictures, or fibrosis can obstruct the colon. Perforation is an unusual but possible complication. Extraintestinal manifestations include cutaneous lesions (erythema nodosum), polyarthritis, episcleritis, uveitis, disorders of the liver, and alterations in coagulation.[63]

Evaluation and Treatment. The diagnosis of UC is based on the medical history, clinical manifestations, and laboratory, serologic, imaging, endoscopic, and histology findings. Infectious causes are ruled out by stool culture. Endoscopic evaluation shows an inflamed and hemorrhagic mucosa. Radiologic assessment may show ulceration and irregular mucosa. The laboratory data include low hemoglobin levels, hypoalbuminemia, and low serum potassium levels. The gold standard in making the diagnosis remains biopsy and histology.[63] The symptoms of UC are often similar to those of CD, making differential diagnosis challenging.

Treatment is individualized and depends on the severity of symptoms and the extent of mucosal involvement. A goal is to promote mucosal healing and avoid surgery. Mild to moderate disease is treated with 5-aminosalicylate therapy followed by steroids. Immunomodulatory agents are used for failure of first-line treatments or serious recurrent disease including TNF-α–blocking agents (e.g., tacrolimus) or antiadhesion agents (i.e., vedolizumab). New small molecule drugs are being investigated.[64] New oral agents have recently been approved (see Emerging Science Box: Oral Treatments for Ulcerative Colitis). Severe, unremitting disease can require hospital admission for administration of intravenous fluids and steroids. Extreme malnutrition may require total parenteral nutrition (TPN). Surgical resection of the colon may be performed if other forms of therapy are unsuccessful or if there are acute serious complications (sepsis, hemorrhage, perforation, or obstruction). Surgical approaches for severe UC include total proctocolectomy with end ileostomy or ileorectal anastomosis, or ileal pouch–anal anastomosis (IPAA). *Pouchitis* is a common complication of restorative proctocolectomy with IPAA performed as surgical treatment for both UC and CD. There are more frequent bowel movements, urgency to defecate, blood in the stool, incontinence, and abdominal pain. Antibiotic treatment is usually successful, and chronic symptoms may be managed with steroids or immune modulators.[65]

EMERGING SCIENCE BOX

Oral Treatments for Ulcerative Colitis

Ulcerative colitis is a chronic inflammatory condition that often requires use of medications to maintain remission and stop flare up of the disease. Historically, this disease was treated with a bottom-up approach. Emerging science demonstrates that ulcerative colitis should be treated with a top-down strategy aiming to treat the underlying severity of disease with medications that are most appropriate for the level of disease severity. Two new oral drugs have been approved and are desirable due to their oral dosing. The drugs suppress lymphocyte trafficking and several inflammatory pathways, promote mucosal healing, and have a short half-life and good safety profile. Tofacitinib is a Janus kinase inhibitor and was approved for use in the United States in 2018 for adults with moderate to severe ulcerative colitis who fail anti–tumor necrosis factor agents. Ozanimod (Zeposia) is a sphingosine 1-phosphate (S1P) receptor modulator approved in March 2020 for the treatment of moderate to severe ulcerative colitis and multiple sclerosis. These drugs still retain a side-effect profile, particularly infection, that can be significant and must be examined and prescribed by a treating provider after review of other medications and risk factors.

Data from Misselwitz B, et al. Swiss IBDnet, an official working group of the Swiss Society of Gastroenterology. Emerging treatment options in inflammatory Bowel disease: janus kinases, stem cells, and more. *Digestion.* 2020;101(suppl 1):69–82. U.S. Food and Drug Adminstration: Zeposia, 3/25/2020 and 5/27/2021. Available at https://www.accessdata.fda.gov/scripts/cder/daf/index.cfm?event=BasicSearch.process.

Crohn Disease

Crohn disease (CD) (granulomatous colitis, ileocolitis, or regional enteritis) is an inflammatory disorder that affects any part of the GI tract from the mouth to the anus. In a small percentage of cases, CD is difficult to differentiate from UC (see Table 41.7). Risk factors associated with CD include smoking, low fiber–high carbohydrate diet, medications such as NSAIDs, and an altered intestinal microbiome.[66] CD appears to have a multifactorial etiology in which both genetics and environmental factors manifest the disease. Smoking increases the risk of developing severe disease and may cause a poorer response to treatment. The inflammation is driven by a sustained immune response against luminal bacterial antigens with activation of leukocyte adhesion molecules (integrins), hyperactivity of T cells with excess production of inflammatory cytokines (e.g., IL-12, IL-23, and IL-34), and activation of cytotoxic enzymes resulting in tissue damage.[67]

Pathophysiology. Inflammation begins in the intestinal submucosa and spreads with discontinuous transmural involvement or "skip lesions" that can involve any part of the GI tract from the mouth to the perianal area. Skip lesions are distinguished by inflamed areas mixed with uninflamed areas, noncaseating granulomas, fistulas, and deep penetrating ulcers. The distal small intestine and proximal large colon are most involved. The ulcerations of CD can produce fissures that extend inflammation into lymphoid tissue. The typical lesion associated with CD is a granuloma or a mass of inflammatory tissue with a cobblestone appearance of inflamed tissue (Fig. 41.12) surrounded by ulceration. Fistula may form in the perianal area between loops of intestine and may extend into the bladder, rectum, or vagina and form intra-abdominal abscesses. Strictures may develop, promoting obstruction.[67]

Clinical Manifestations. Individuals with CD may have no specific symptoms for several years. Symptoms vary according to the location of the disease but are similar to those for UC. Diarrhea is one of the most common symptoms, and occasionally rectal bleeding is noted if the colon is involved. Weight loss and abdominal pain accompany CD. Abdominal tenderness may also be noted over the lesions. If the ileum is involved, the individual may be anemic as a result of malabsorption of vitamin B_{12}. There also may be deficiencies in folic acid and vitamin D absorption. In addition, proteins may be lost, leading to hypoalbuminemia. Extraintestinal complications are similar to those occurring in UC. Additional complications include anal fissure, perianal abscess, and fistula. Individuals with CD of long duration also are at risk for intestinal adenocarcinoma. Extraintestinal manifestations include arthropathies, skin, oral, and ocular lesions.[68]

Evaluation and Treatment. The diagnosis and treatment of CD are similar to the diagnosis and treatment of UC. Imaging of the small intestine is used in the diagnosis of CD, including either a small bowel series or a capsule endoscopy (camera pill). There are no specific biomarkers or definitive treatments for the disease. Smoking cessation is a component of therapy. Steroids are used to induce remission, and immunosuppressants (e.g., thiopurines and methotrexate) are used to sustain remission. Anti–TNF-α, antiintegrins (target the adhesion molecular inhibiting leukocyte migration), and IL inhibitors (target IL-12 and IL-23) are used for the most severe forms of the disease. Surgery may be performed to manage complications, such as fistula, abscess, or obstruction. When treatment involves surgical resection of small intestinal segments, complications related to short bowel syndrome may occur. Complications of short bowel syndrome include malabsorption, diarrhea, and nutritional deficiencies. Since malnutrition affects a significant number of individuals with CD, diet management is a significant component of the care plan.[69] Routine colonoscopy for cancer screening should be performed for long-standing colonic disease.[66]

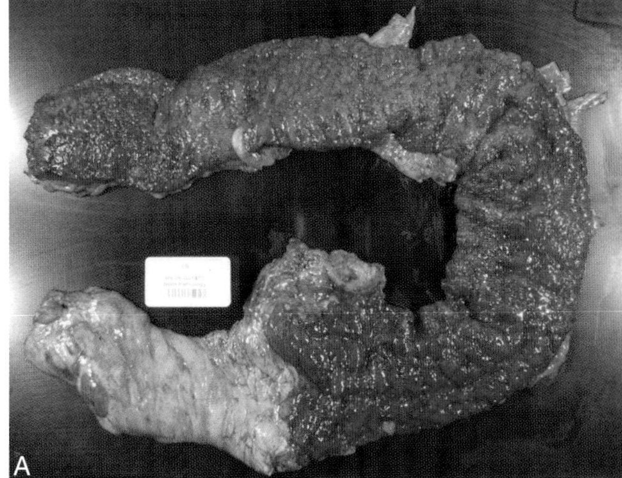

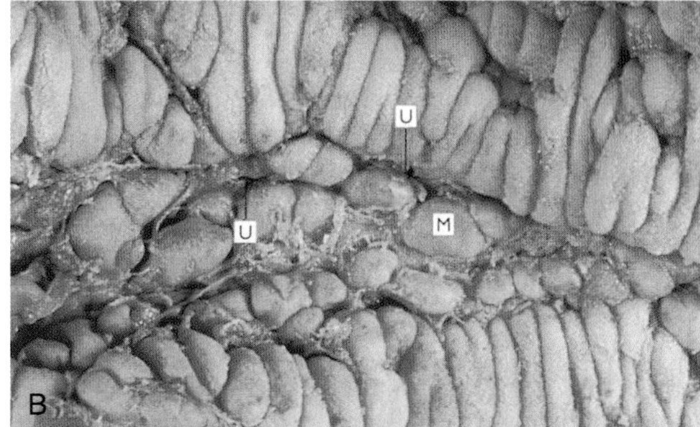

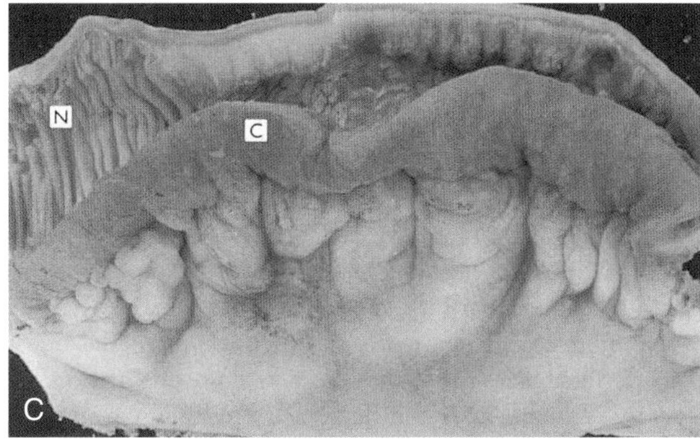

Fig. 41.12 (A) Acute ulcerative colitis. A gross specimen of subtotal ulcerative colitis showing diffuse continuous disease starting from the distal rectum and continuing up to the midportion of the ascending colon. *(B)* Crohn disease. The mucosa in Crohn disease demonstrates a cobblestone pattern as a result of fissured ulcers (U) with intervening areas of edematous mucosa *(M)*. (C) Compared with normal small bowel wall *(N)*, the Crohn segment *(C)* shows wall thickening that has caused a stenosis. (A, From Odze RD, Goldblum JR, eds. *Surgical pathology of the GI tract, liver, biliary tract, and pancreas*, 2nd edition. Philadelphia: Saunders; 2009. B and C, From Kumar V, et al. *Pathologic basis of disease*, 7th edition. Philadelphia: Saunders; 2006.)

Microscopic Colitis

Microscopic colitis is a relatively common cause of nonbloody diarrhea. Although the mucosa appears normal, there are two histologic forms: lymphocytic and collagenous. Lymphocytic colitis shows an increase in the number of intraepithelial lymphocytes in the wall of the colon. Collagenous colitis is characterized by a thickened subepithelial collagen layer, with mucosal nodularity and an alteration of the vascular mucosal pattern. Risk factors include age 50 years or older, female sex, weight loss, smoking, use of PPIs, use of NSAIDs, and use of selective serotonin reuptake inhibitors. The cause of microscopic colitis is unknown, and proposed mechanisms include autoimmunity, genetic predisposition, an immune or inflammatory response to luminal antigens, certain medications, and abnormal collagen metabolism.[70]

The symptoms of frequent daily watery diarrhea are the same for both types and may be accompanied by abdominal pain and weight loss. Diagnosis is made from biopsy. Antidiarrheal agents and budesonide (an oral antiinflammatory steroid) are the best-documented treatments. The disease is negatively associated with CRC.

Irritable Bowel Syndrome

IBS currently is considered a disorder of brain-gut interaction (previously termed a functional GI disorder) characterized by recurrent abdominal pain with altered bowel habits.[71] It is estimated that in the United States 10% to 12% of adults suffer with IBS symptoms.[72] It is more common in women, with a higher prevalence during youth and middle age. Individuals with symptoms of IBS also are more likely to have anxiety, depression, and a reduced quality of life.[73]

Pathophysiology. The pathophysiology of IBS is unknown, and there are no specific biomarkers for the disease. There is increasing evidence to explain a multisystem interaction with variables, including infection, gut microbiota, immune activation, serotonin dysregulation, psychological stress, abnormal gut function and diet, as contributing factors to the varying symptom presentations. Mechanisms of pathophysiology are summarized as follows:

- *Visceral hypersensitivity or hyperalgesia* may originate in either the peripheral or the central nervous system. The mechanism may be related to a dysregulation of the bidirectional "brain-gut axis" (alterations in gut or central nervous system processing of gut-pain information). Factors include genetic-related changes in the function of serotonin-secreting cells of gut-brain pain modulation, alterations in gut microbiota metabolite production with activation of the gut immune system, increased visceral sensitivity and permeability, and altered motility and secretion.
- *Abnormal GI permeability, motility, secretion, and sensitivity* are associated with IBS. Individuals with diarrhea-type IBS have more rapid colonic transit times and increased intestinal permeability. Those with bloating and constipation have delayed transit times and decreased intestinal permeability. The mechanism may be related to dysregulation of the brain-gut axis, alterations in the function of gut neuroendocrine cells or dorsal root ganglion neurons, or changes in the activity of mast cells (produce histamine). Sex hormones may be a contributing factor.
- *Postinflammatory (infectious or noninfectious) IBS* is associated with intestinal infection (bacterial enteritis) and low-grade inflammation. Alterations in gut microbiota, immune activation in gut tissues, and changes in intestinal permeability have been proposed.
- *Alteration in gut microbiota (dysbiosis)* influences the sensory, motor, and immune systems of the gut and interacts with higher brain centers and may contribute to symptoms of IBS. Small intestine overgrowth of normal gut bacteria may be associated with IBS symptoms in some cases. Nonabsorbable antibiotics and prebiotics and probiotics may be helpful in some individuals.
- *Psychosocial factors (epigenetic factors)*—including early life trauma or abuse or emotional stress interacting with neuroendocrine, neuroimmune, autonomic nervous system, and pain modulatory responses—contribute to the symptoms of IBS.

Clinical Manifestations. IBS symptoms may be mild or debilitating. IBS is characterized by lower abdominal pain or discomfort and bloating. IBS can be grouped as diarrhea-predominant, constipation-predominant, or mixed diarrhea/constipation. Symptoms including gas, bloating, fecal urgency, incomplete evacuation, and nausea are usually relieved with defecation and do not interfere with sleep.

Evaluation and Treatment. The diagnosis of IBS is based on signs, symptoms, personal history, and includes the exclusion of structural or biochemical causes of disease such as IBD or intestinal infection. Diagnostic procedures to rule out other causes of symptoms may include endoscopic evaluations, CT scans, abdominal ultrasound, blood tests, and lactose intolerance test. Fecal calprotectin is evaluated in those with suspected IBS and diarrhea symptoms to rule out IBD. The individual may be evaluated for food allergies, parasites, or bacterial growth. The Rome IV criteria for diagnosing IBS are presented in Box 41.2.

There is no cure for IBS, and treatment is individualized.[74] Treatment of symptoms may include laxatives, fiber, antidiarrheals, antispasmodics, prosecretory drugs, low-dose antidepressants, visceral analgesics, and serotonin agonists or antagonists and supportive care is symptom related. Alternative therapies include prebiotics and probiotics to manipulate the microflora. Hypnosis, acupuncture, yoga, cognitive behavioral therapy, and dietary interventions have been used with varying results.[75] Research continues to advance the management and understanding of the pathophysiology of this complex syndrome.

Diverticular Disease of the Colon

Diverticula are herniations or sac-like outpouchings of the mucosa and submucosa through the muscle layers, usually located in the wall of the sigmoid colon and they are more common in older adults (Fig. 41.13). They rarely occur in the small

BOX 41.2 Diagnostic Criteria[a] for Irritable Bowel Syndrome

Rome IV Criteria

Recurrent abdominal pain, on average, at least 1 day per week in the past 3 months associated with two or more of the following criteria:

- Related to defecation
- Associated with a change in frequency of stool
- Associated with a change in form (appearance) of stool

IBS subtypes include:

- IBS with predominant constipation (IBS-C)
- IBS with predominant diarrhea (IBS-D)
- IBS with mixed bowel habits (IBS-M)
- IBS unclassified (IBS-U)

[a]Criteria met for the past 3 months with symptom onset at least 6 months before diagnosis.

IBS, Irritable bowel syndrome.

Adapted from Drossman DA. Functional gastrointestinal disorders: history, pathophysiology, clinical features and Rome IV. *Gastroenterology*, 2016;150(6):1262–1297; Lacey BE et al: *Gastroenterology*, 2016;150(6): 1393–1407.

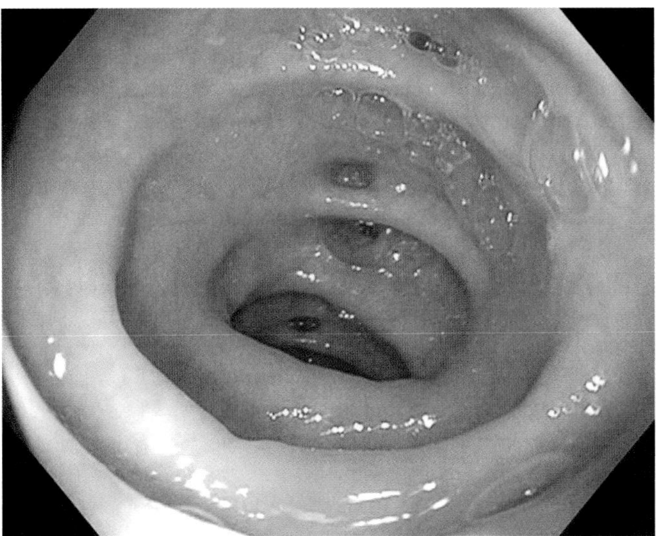

Fig. 41.13 Diverticular Disease. In diverticular disease, the outpouches of mucosa seen in the sigmoid colon appear as slit-like openings from the mucosal surface of the opened bowel. (From Townsend CM, et al. *Sabiston textbook of surgery: The biologic basis of modern surgical practice*, 21st edition. St. Louis: Elsevier; 2022.)

intestine. Diverticulosis is asymptomatic diverticular disease. Diverticulitis represents inflammation of the diverticula and occurs in approximately 10% to 15% of cases of diverticular disease of the colon.[76] The cause of diverticular disease is unknown, but it is associated with increased intracolonic pressure, abnormal neuromuscular function, and alterations in intestinal motility. Predisposing factors include older age, genetic predisposition, obesity, smoking, diet, lack of physical activity, and medication use (e.g., aspirin and NSAIDs).[77] Lack of dietary fiber may or may not contribute to diverticular disease. Altered intestinal microbiota, visceral hypersensitivity, and abnormal colonic motility also may be contributing factors.[78]

Pathophysiology. Diverticula can occur anywhere in the GI tract, particularly at weak points in the colon wall, usually where arteries penetrate the tunica muscularis. The most common sites are the left sigmoid colon (more prevalent in Western countries) and the right colon (more prevalent in Asian countries). A common associated finding of the disease is thickening of the circular muscles and shortening of the longitudinal (teniae coli) muscles surrounding the diverticula. Although not characterized as muscle hypertrophy, diverticular disease may cause increased collagen and elastin deposition and is associated with muscle thickening. This contributes to increased intraluminal pressure and herniation. According to the law of Laplace (see Chapter 34), wall pressure increases as the diameter of a cylindrical structure decreases. Therefore pressure within the narrow lumen can increase enough to rupture the diverticula, causing inflammation and diverticulitis. Bacteria and local ischemia also may be contributing factors. Complicated diverticulitis includes abscess, fistula, obstruction, bleeding, or perforation.

Clinical Manifestations. Symptoms of uncomplicated diverticular disease may be vague or absent. Cramping pain of the lower abdomen can accompany constriction of the thickened colonic muscles. Diarrhea, constipation, distention, or flatulence may occur. If the diverticula become inflamed or abscesses form, the individual develops fever, leukocytosis, and tenderness in the lower left quadrant.

Evaluation and Treatment. Diverticula are often discovered during diagnostic procedures performed for other problems. Ultrasound, sigmoidoscopy, or colonoscopy permits direct observation of the lesions. Abdominal CT is used for diagnosis of complicated cases.

An increase in dietary fiber intake often relieves symptoms by increasing bulk and lowering colonic pressure. Uncomplicated diverticulitis is usually treated with bowel rest and a clear, liquid diet, analgesia, and selective use of antibiotics. Complicated cases may require intravenous antibiotics and abscess drainage if needed. In severe cases, bowel resection surgery may be needed with or without a colostomy.[79]

Appendicitis

Appendicitis is an inflammation of the vermiform appendix, which is a projection from the apex of the cecum. Appendicitis is a medical emergency. It is the most common surgical emergency of the abdomen, usually occurring between 10 and 19 years of age (although it may develop at any age). The incidence in the United States is 10 cases per 10,000 persons.[80]

Pathophysiology. The exact mechanism of the cause of appendicitis is not well understood. Obstruction of the lumen with stool, tumors, or foreign bodies, with consequent bacterial infection, is the most common theory. The obstructed lumen does not allow drainage of the appendix, and as mucosal secretion continues, intraluminal pressure increases. The increased pressure decreases mucosal blood flow, and the appendix becomes hypoxic. The mucosa ulcerates, promoting bacterial or other microbial invasion, with further inflammation and edema. Inflammation may involve the distal or entire appendix. Gangrene develops from thrombosis of the luminal blood vessels, followed by a periappendicular abscess and perforation resulting in peritonitis in complex cases.[80,81]

Clinical Manifestations. Epigastric or periumbilical pain is the typical symptom of an inflamed appendix. The pain may be vague at first but will increase in intensity over 3 to 4 hours. It may subside and then migrate to the right lower quadrant, indicating extension of the inflammation to the surrounding tissues. Nausea, vomiting, and anorexia follow the onset of pain, and a low-grade fever is common. Diarrhea occurs in some individuals, particularly children; others have constipation. Perforation, peritonitis, and abscess formation are the most serious complications of appendicitis.

Evaluation and Treatment. In addition to clinical manifestations, there is pain with abdominal palpation and rebound tenderness, usually referred to the right lower quadrant. The white blood cell count is greater than 10,000 cells/mm^3, with increased neutrophils and C-reactive protein. Abdominal ultrasound, CT scans, and magnetic resonance imaging (MRI) (particularly for pregnant women and children) assist with diagnostic accuracy and help to rule out nonappendiceal disease. Antibiotics and appendectomy are the treatment for simple appendicitis.[82] Treatment for complicated appendicitis (perforation, abscess formation, peritonitis) also includes antibiotics and appendectomy; however, recovery may be more complicated.[80,83] There is an increased risk of colon cancer post appendectomy among individuals aged 50 to 54 years, and follow-up colonoscopy is recommended.[84]

Mesenteric Vascular Insufficiency

Mesenteric vascular insufficiency is rare, with an incidence of approximately 2 to 3 cases per 100,000 persons.[85] Three branches of the abdominal aorta supply the stomach and intestines: the celiac artery and the superior and inferior mesenteric arteries. The inferior mesenteric vein drains into the splenic vein, and the splenic vein and superior mesenteric vein join the portal vein. *Mesenteric venous thrombosis* is the least common of the causes of mesenteric vascular insufficiency. Malignancies, right-sided heart failure, and deep vein thrombosis are risk factors. Mesenteric venous thrombosis presents with abdominal pain and is treated with anticoagulants.

Acute mesenteric arterial insufficiency results in a significant reduction in mucosal blood flow to the large and small intestines.[86] Preexisting morbidities include dissecting aortic aneurysms, arterial thrombi, or emboli. Embolic obstruction is associated with atrial fibrillation, mitral valve disease, heart valve prostheses, and myocardial infarction. The superior mesenteric artery has a more direct line of flow from the aorta; therefore emboli enter it more readily than the inferior branch, causing ischemia and necrosis of the small intestine. Ischemia, infarction, and necrosis all alter membrane permeability. Initially, there is increased motility, nausea and vomiting, urgent bowel evacuation, and severe abdominal pain. Ischemia leads to decreased motility and distention. The damaged intestinal mucosa cannot produce enough mucus to protect itself from digestive enzymes. Mucosal alteration causes fluid to move from the blood vessels into the bowel wall and peritoneum. Fluid loss causes hypovolemia and further decreases intestinal blood flow. As intestinal infarction progresses, shock, fever, bloody diarrhea, and leukocytosis develop. Bacteria invade the necrotic intestinal wall, causing gangrene and peritonitis.

Chronic mesenteric ischemia (CMI) is rare. The most common etiology is atherosclerotic stenosis or occlusion of the mesenteric arteries. CMI can be associated with congestive heart failure, acute myocardial infarction, hemorrhage, thrombus formation, or any condition that decreases arterial blood flow. Chronic occlusion is often accompanied by the formation of collateral circulation. The collateral vessels may be able to nourish the resting intestine, but after eating, when the intestine requires more blood, the arterial supply may be insufficient. Ischemia develops, causing cramping abdominal pain or abdominal angina, which is a cardinal symptom reoccurring over a period of 3 months. Some individuals suffer significant weight loss because they stop eating to control the pain. Progressive vascular obstruction eventually causes continuous abdominal pain and necrosis of the intestinal tissue.

The diagnosis of acute and CMI is based on clinical manifestations, laboratory findings, and imaging studies. The diagnosis may be difficult because of the vagueness of symptoms. A bruit can often be heard over a partially occluded artery. Treatment includes aggressive rehydration and the use of antibiotics, anticoagulants, vasodilators, and inhibitors of reperfusion injury. Surgery, including percutaneous stenting or open techniques, is required to remove necrotic tissue, repair sclerosed vessels, and revascularize affected tissue. Acute occlusion is a surgical emergency, and the mortality rate is high (50% to 90%). Early diagnosis and aggressive treatment result in the best survival rates.[87,88]

DISORDERS OF THE ACCESSORY ORGANS OF DIGESTION

The accessory organs of digestion, including the liver, gallbladder, and pancreas, secrete substances necessary for digestion and in the case of the liver carry out metabolic functions needed to maintain life. Disorders of these organs include inflammatory disease, obstruction of ducts, and tumors. (Cancers of the digestive system are described at the end of this chapter.)

Common Complications of Liver Disorders

Of all the accessory organ disorders, acute or chronic liver disease leads to the most significant systemic, life-threatening complications. These complications are common to all liver disorders and include portal hypertension, ascites, hepatic encephalopathy, jaundice, and hepatorenal syndrome (HRS).

Portal Hypertension

Portal hypertension is abnormally high blood pressure in the portal venous system caused by resistance to blood flow. Pressure in this system is normally 3 mm Hg; portal hypertension is an increase to at least 10 mm Hg.

Pathophysiology. Portal hypertension is caused by disorders that obstruct or impede blood flow through any component of the portal venous system or vena cava. *Intrahepatic causes* result from vascular remodeling with shunts, thrombosis, inflammation, or fibrosis of the sinusoids, as occurs in cirrhosis of the liver, biliary cirrhosis, viral hepatitis, or schistosomiasis (a parasitic infection). *Posthepatic causes* occur from hepatic vein thrombosis or cardiac disorders that impair the pumping ability of the right side of the heart. This causes blood to collect and increases pressure in the veins of the portal system. The most common cause of portal hypertension is fibrosis and obstruction caused by cirrhosis of the liver. Long-term portal hypertension causes several pathophysiologic problems that are difficult to treat and can be fatal. These problems include varices, splenomegaly, ascites, hepatic encephalopathy, and hepatopulmonary syndrome (HPS) (see Emerging Science Box: Portal Hypertension).

Varices are distended, tortuous collateral veins. Prolonged elevation of pressure in the portal vein causes collateral veins to open between the portal vein and systemic veins. The prolonged pressure is distributed throughout the GI tract and results in transformation into varices, particularly in the lower esophagus and stomach, but also over the abdominal wall (known as the caput medusae [Medusa head]) and rectum (hemorrhoidal varices) (Fig. 41.14). The hyperdynamic circulation in the stomach and esophagus impairs mucosal defenses, promotes inflammation, and disrupts healing with increased risk of mucosal erosion, ulceration, and bleeding.[89] Rupture of varices can cause life-threatening hemorrhage.[90]

EMERGING SCIENCE BOX

Portal Hypertension

Portal hypertension is a severe complication in the progression of liver disease. Portal hypertension causes an increase in pressure gradients between the portal system and the hepatic veins and is the cause of most complications associated with liver disease. The past three decades have noted a great decline in mortality rates of individuals with portal hypertension as emerging science on the pathophysiology of this complication has helped decrease mortality. A pathogenesis-based approach to treatment has based the introduction of simvastatin for treatment to improve endothelial dysfunction and for use of its liver-protective effects. Pharmaceutical treatments also may involve use of carvedilol, a nonselective β-blocker, in place of historically used propranolol due to carvedilol having a vasodilatory effect, particularly for the prophylaxis of variceal bleeding. Emerging interventions include early transjugular intrahepatic portosystemic shunt (TIPS), esophageal stents, and balloon-occluded retrograde transvenous obliteration (BRTO).

Data from Bosch J. Portal hypertension and cirrhosis: From evolving concepts to better therapies. *Clinical Liver Disease*, 2020;15(suppl 1): S8–S12; Iwakiri Y, et al. Portal hypertension in cirrhosis: Pathophysiological mechanisms and therapy. JHEP Reports, 2021;3(4):100316.

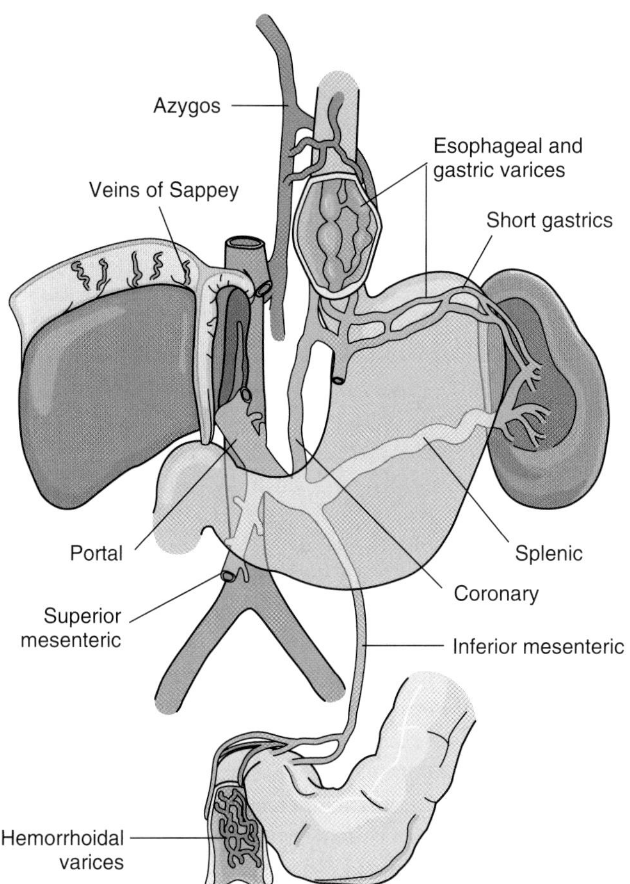

Fig. 41.14 Varices Related to Portal Hypertension. The portal vein, its major tributaries, and the most important shunts (collateral veins) between the portal and caval systems. The shunted blood returns to the systemic venous system, bypassing the liver. (From Monahan FD, et al. *Phipps' medical-surgical nursing: Concepts and clinical practice*, 8th edition. St. Louis: Mosby; 2007.)

Splenomegaly is enlargement of the spleen caused by increased pressure in the splenic vein, which branches from the portal vein. Thrombocytopenia is the most common symptom of congestive splenomegaly. The enlarged spleen can often times be palpated. HPS and portopulmonary hypertension (PPH) are respiratory complications of liver disease and portal hypertension. The pathophysiology of both is complex and involves different effects of vasoactive substances. In HPS there is pulmonary vasodilation, probably because of the increased nitric oxide synthesis, increased pulmonary venous congestion, and right-to-left shunting that induces hypoxemias. PPH is associated with vasoconstriction and arterial vascular remodeling with thickening and fibrosis of the arterial wall that increases pulmonary artery resistance. Individuals may be asymptomatic, or fatigue, dyspnea, cyanosis, and clubbing may occur with or without signs of right heart failure (jugular venous distention, ascites, and peripheral edema).

Diagnosis includes pulmonary function tests, arterial blood gas analysis, contrast echocardiography, transthoracic echocardiography, and right heart catherization. In PPH, mean pulmonary artery pressure is greater than 25 mm Hg at rest. There is no specific treatment for HPS. Treatment of PPH includes targeting the pulmonary arterial vasculature to reduce pulmonary hypertension with various medication options that include endothelin receptor antagonists, phosphodiesterase type 5 inhibitors, and prostanoids. Liver transplant may be indicated.[91]

Clinical Manifestations. Hematemesis from bleeding esophageal varices is the most common clinical manifestation of portal hypertension. Bleeding is usually from varices that have developed slowly over a period of years. Slow, chronic bleeding from varices causes anemia or melena. Acute rupture of esophageal varices causes hemorrhage and voluminous vomiting of dark-colored blood. The ruptured varices are usually painless. Rupture is caused by a combination of erosion by gastric acid and elevated venous pressure. Mortality from ruptured esophageal varices ranges from 30% to 60%. Recurrent bleeding of esophageal varices indicates a poor prognosis. Hemorrhoidal varices present as hematochezia with copious rectal bleeding.

Evaluation and Treatment. Portal hypertension is often diagnosed at the time of variceal bleeding and confirmed by upper GI endoscopy and evaluation of portal venous pressure. The individual usually has a history of jaundice, hepatitis, alcoholism, or cirrhosis. Liver elastography is an imaging test that provides a noninvasive measure of liver stiffness and can diagnose the extent of fibrosis.[92]

Emergency management of bleeding varices includes use of vasopressors and compression of the varices with an inflatable tube or balloon, sclerotherapy, variceal ligation, or portacaval shunt. Surgical construction of transjugular intrahepatic portosystemic shunts (TIPSs) and anastomosis of the portal vein to the inferior vena cava may decompress the varices. This treatment can precipitate encephalopathy. Emergency management will also include stabilization of the individual with fluid resuscitation, red blood cell replacement, and antibiotics. Liver transplantation is the most successful option for liver failure. Nonemergent or long-term management may include

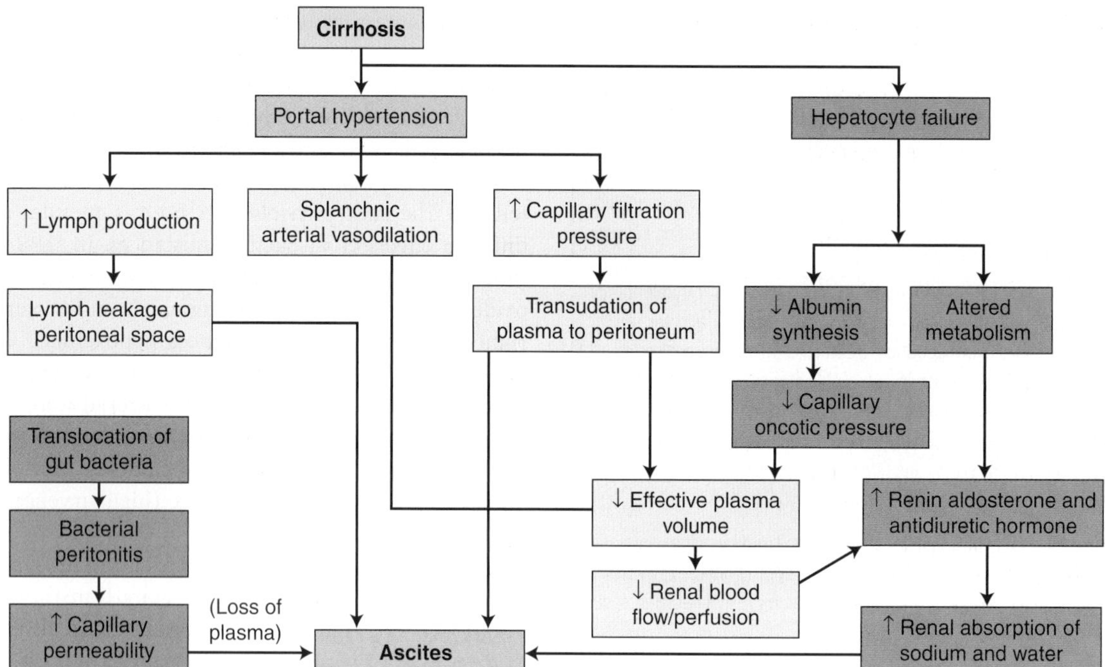

Fig. 41.15 Mechanisms of Ascites Caused by Cirrhosis.

nonselective β-blocking drugs to assist reducing the pressure in the portal venous system and to prevent variceal bleeding.[93]

Ascites

Ascites is the accumulation of fluid in the peritoneal cavity. Ascites traps body fluid in the peritoneal space, from which it cannot escape. Ascites reduces the amount of body fluid available for normal physiologic functions. Cirrhosis is the most common cause of ascites, but other causes include heart failure, constrictive pericarditis, abdominal malignancies, nephrotic syndrome, and malnutrition. Of individuals who develop ascites caused by cirrhosis, 25% die within 1 year. Continued heavy drinking of alcohol is associated with this mortality and is related to decompensated cirrhosis.

Pathophysiology. Several factors contribute to the development of ascites, including portal hypertension, splanchnic vasodilation, decreased synthesis of albumin by the liver, splanchnic arterial vasodilation, and renal sodium and water retention. Portal hypertension causes capillary hydrostatic pressure to exceed capillary osmotic pressure (see Chapter 3), pushing water into the peritoneal cavity. Portal hypertension also increases the production of hepatic lymph, which "weeps" into the peritoneal cavity. Reduced serum albumin levels reduce capillary oncotic pressure adding to the fluid shift. Splanchnic arterial vasodilation is associated with increased nitric oxide produced by the diseased liver and can decrease effective circulating blood volume, activating the renin-angiotensin-aldosterone system and antidiuretic hormone, which in turn promotes renal sodium and water retention. The sodium and water retention expands plasma volume, thereby accelerating portal hypertension and ascites formation. In addition, translocation of bacteria and release of endotoxin cause peritonitis with an inflammatory response that increases splanchnic vasodilation and mesenteric capillary permeability and fluid movement into the peritoneal cavity, promoting ascites. Fig. 41.15 summarizes the mechanisms by which cirrhosis of the liver cause ascites.

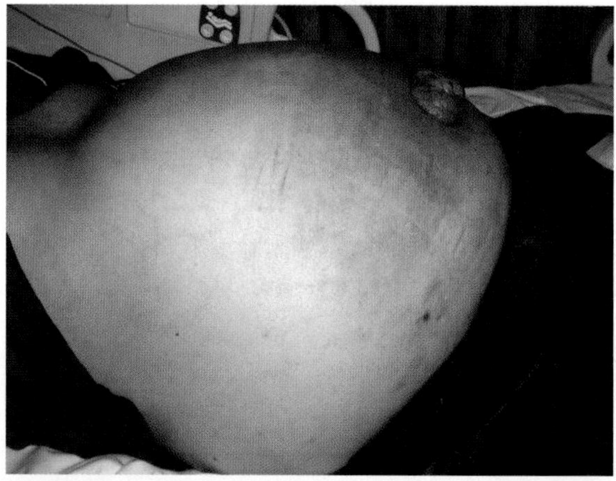

Fig. 41.16 Massive Ascites in an Individual With Cirrhosis. Distended abdomen, dilated upper abdominal veins, and inverted umbilicus are classic manifestations. (From Goldman L, Schafer AI. *Goldman's Cecil medicine*, 24th edition. Philadelphia: Saunders; 2012.)

Clinical Manifestations. The accumulation of ascitic fluid causes abdominal distention, increased abdominal girth, and weight gain (Fig. 41.16). Large volumes of fluid (10 to 20 L) displace the diaphragm and cause dyspnea by decreasing lung capacity. The respiratory rate increases, and the individual may need to assume a sitting position to relieve the dyspnea. Some peripheral edema is usually present. Dilutional hyponatremia may be noted because of excess fluid volume. Approximately 10% of individuals with ascites develop bacterial peritonitis, either spontaneously or because of paracentesis, which causes fever, chills, abdominal pain, decreased bowel sounds, and cloudy ascitic fluid.

Evaluation and Treatment. The diagnosis is usually based on clinical manifestations and identification of liver disease. Marked abdominal distention is associated with higher grades of ascites. The serum ascites albumin gradient (SAAG) from ascetic fluid analysis is the most specific diagnostic indicator for portal hypertension–related ascites. Ultrasonography, chest and abdominal x-rays, or CT scans are used to evaluate the cause and extent of the ascites and other complications of the disease. Serum electrolyte levels must be carefully monitored as the disease process puts an individual at risk for hyponatremia and hypokalemia. Spontaneous bacterial peritonitis can occur with cirrhotic ascites, the neutrophil count will be elevated in ascetic fluid, and bacterial culture guides antibiotic therapy.

The goal of treatment is to relieve discomfort. If the restoration of liver function is possible (e.g., in ascites caused by viral hepatitis), the ascites diminishes spontaneously. Dietary salt restriction and potassium-sparing diuretics can reduce ascites. Vasopressin receptor-2 antagonists are effective for dilutional hyponatremia. Albumin may be given. Paracentesis is used to aspirate ascitic fluid for bacterial culture, biochemical analysis, and microscopic examination. Maintenance of caloric and protein intake is necessary to prevent malnutrition.

Palliative paracentesis in amounts of 1 or 2 L of ascitic fluid is completed to relieve respiratory distress. However, the removal of too much fluid too quickly relieves pressure on blood vessels and carries the risk of hypotension, shock, or death. Despite repeated paracentesis, ascitic fluid reaccumulates because of the persistent portal hypertension and reduced plasma albumin levels associated with irreversible disease. Peritonitis is treated with antibiotics. Other procedures include placement of a peritoneovenous shunt and TIPS. Individuals with ascites and portal hypertension have a poor prognosis, and liver transplantation is the best treatment option.[94]

Hepatic Encephalopathy

Hepatic encephalopathy (portal system encephalopathy) is a complex neurologic syndrome characterized by impaired behavioral, cognitive, and motor function. The syndrome may develop rapidly during acute fulminant hepatitis or slowly during the course of cirrhosis and the development of portal hypertension or after portosystemic bypass or shunting.

Pathophysiology. Hepatic encephalopathy results from a combination of biochemical alterations that affect neurotransmission and brain function. Liver dysfunction and the development of collateral vessels that shunt blood around the liver to the systemic circulation permit toxins absorbed from the GI tract and normally removed by the liver, to accumulate and circulate freely to the brain. The accumulated toxins alter cerebral energy metabolism, interfere with neurotransmission, and cause edema. The most hazardous substances are end products of intestinal protein digestion, particularly ammonia, which cannot be converted to urea by the diseased liver. The digestion of blood from leaking or ruptured varices adds to the amount of ammonia present in systemic blood, as does the action of ammonia-forming bacteria in the colon. Ammonia that reaches the brain is metabolized to glutamine, with osmotic disturbances and alterations in cerebral blood flow that interfere with neurotransmitters and cause astrocyte edema or cytotoxic edema and oxidation. Disruption of the blood-brain barrier causes vasogenic edema and contributes to astrocytes swelling, brain edema, and intracranial hypertension. Excessive amounts of gamma-aminobutyric acid (GABA), an inhibitory neurotransmitter from intestinal flora, may contribute to reduced levels of consciousness. Infection, systemic inflammation, hemorrhage, and electrolyte imbalance (including zinc deficiency), constipation, and the use of sedatives and analgesics can precipitate hepatic encephalopathy in the presence of liver disease.[95]

Clinical Manifestations. Subtle changes in personality, memory loss, irritability, disinhibition, lethargy, and sleep disturbances are common initial manifestations of hepatic encephalopathy. Symptoms then can progress to confusion, disorientation to time and space, asterixis, slow speech, bradykinesia, stupor, convulsions, and coma, which are less frequent. Coma is usually a sign of liver failure and ultimately results in death. Variceal bleeding and ascites may develop concurrently. Symptoms may be episodic, recurrent, or persistent. Hepatic encephalopathy is often associated with bleeding varices and ascites.

Evaluation and Treatment. The diagnosis of hepatic encephalopathy is based on a history of liver disease, clinical manifestations, psychometric tests, and exclusion of other causes of brain dysfunction. Electroencephalography and blood chemistry tests provide supportive data. Tracking levels of serum ammonia can assist to assess treatment effectiveness and liver function, but the test is difficult to perform and may be influenced by hemolysis and severe jaundice.[96] Correction of fluid and electrolyte imbalances and withdrawal of depressant drugs metabolized by the liver are the first steps in the treatment of hepatic encephalopathy. Dietary protein is maintained to prevent malnutrition but at levels that reduce blood ammonia levels. Lactulose prevents ammonia absorption in the colon, and polyethylene glycol has also been used with success in reducing ammonia levels.[97] Neomycin eliminates ammonia-producing intestinal bacteria but can be nephrotoxic. Glutamase inhibitors reduce gut ammonia. Rifaximin (a nonabsorbable antibiotic) decreases intestinal production of ammonia and may be combined with lactulose or used alone for lactulose nonresponders. Extracorporeal liver support systems remove toxins from the blood and are an option for managing overt hepatic encephalopathy or as a bridge to liver transplantation.[96]

Jaundice

Jaundice, or icterus, is a yellow or greenish pigmentation of the skin caused by hyperbilirubinemia (plasma bilirubin concentrations greater than 2.5 to 3 mg/dL). Hyperbilirubinemia and jaundice can result from (1) extrahepatic (posthepatic) obstruction to bile flow, (2) intrahepatic obstruction, or (3) prehepatic excessive production of unconjugated bilirubin (i.e., excessive hemolysis of red blood cells) (Fig. 41.17). Jaundice in newborns is caused by impaired bilirubin uptake and conjugation (see Chapter 42).

Pathophysiology. Obstructive jaundice can result from extrahepatic or intrahepatic obstruction.[98] *Extrahepatic*

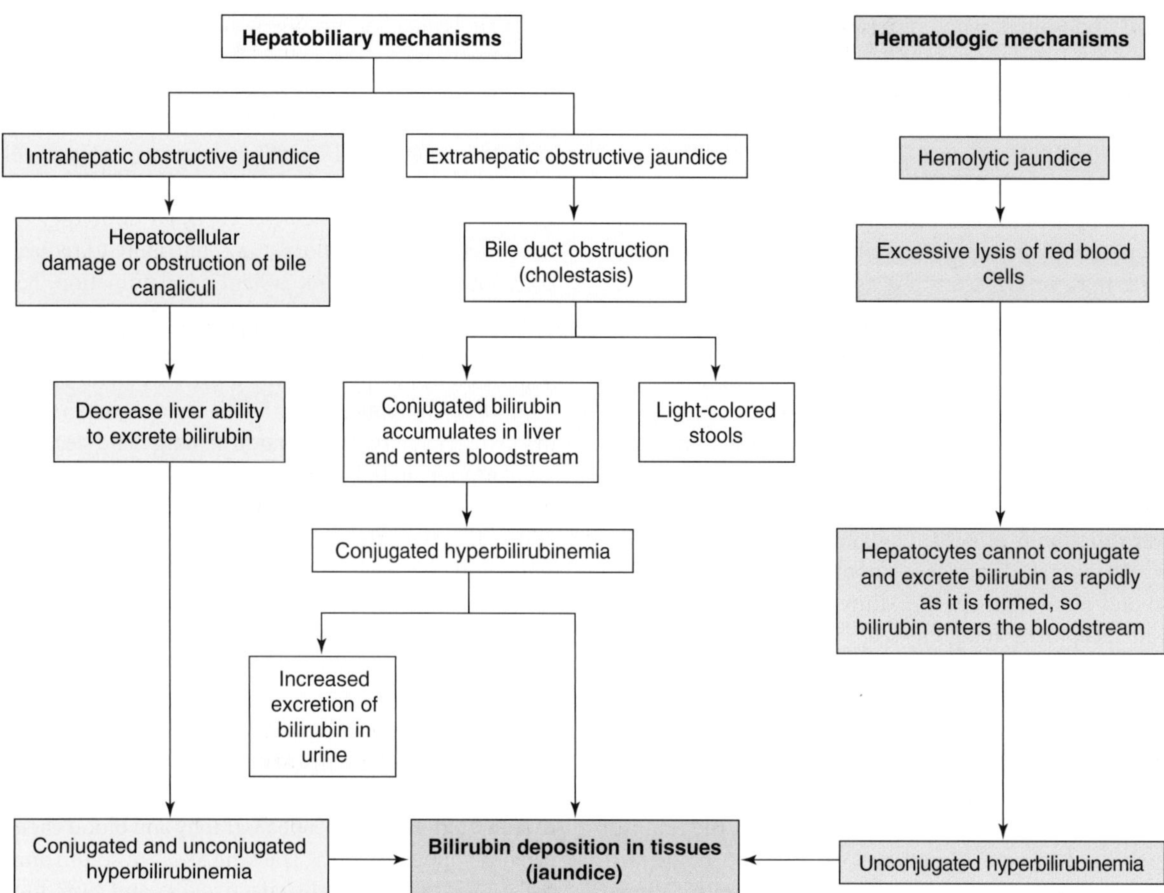

Fig. 41.17 Mechanisms of Jaundice.

obstructive jaundice develops if the common bile duct is occluded. Occlusion may be from a gallstone, tumor, or inflammation. If occluded, bilirubin conjugated by the hepatocytes cannot flow through the obstructed common bile duct into the duodenum. Therefore bilirubin accumulates in the liver and enters the bloodstream, causing hyperbilirubinemia and jaundice. *Intrahepatic (hepatocellular) obstructive jaundice* involves disturbances in hepatocyte function and obstruction of bile canaliculi. The uptake, conjugation, or excretion of bilirubin can be affected with elevated levels of both conjugated and unconjugated bilirubin. Obstruction of bile canaliculi diminishes flow of conjugated bilirubin into the common bile duct. In mild cases, some of the bile canaliculi open. Consequently, the amount of bilirubin in the intestinal tract may be only slightly decreased.

Excessive hemolysis (destruction) of red blood cells can cause hemolytic jaundice *(prehepatic* or *nonobstructive jaundice).* Increased unconjugated bilirubin is formed through metabolism of the heme component of destroyed red blood cells and exceeds the conjugation ability of the liver, causing blood levels of unconjugated bilirubin to rise. Decreased bilirubin uptake or conjugation also causes unconjugated hyperbilirubinemia, as occurs with reaction to some drugs (e.g., rifampin), and in genetic disorders, such as Gilbert syndrome. Unconjugated bilirubin is not water soluble, so it will not be excreted in the urine. The causes of jaundice are summarized in Table 41.8.

Clinical Manifestations. Conjugated bilirubin is water soluble and appears in the urine. The urine may darken several days before the onset of jaundice. The complete obstruction of bile flow from the liver to the duodenum causes light-colored stools. With partial obstruction, the stools are normal in color and bilirubin is present in the urine.

Fever, chills, and pain often accompany jaundice resulting from viral or bacterial inflammation of the liver. Yellow discoloration may first occur in the sclera of the eye and then progress to the skin as bilirubin attaches to elastic fibers. Pruritus (itching) often accompanies jaundice because bilirubin accumulates in the skin, irritating itch receptors.

Evaluation and Treatment. Laboratory evaluation of serum establishes whether elevated plasma bilirubin is conjugated or unconjugated, or both. The history and physical examination identify underlying disorders, such as cirrhosis, exposure to hepatitis virus, gallbladder or pancreatic disease, or hematologic disorders. The treatment for jaundice consists of correcting the cause.

Hepatorenal Syndrome

HRS is functional renal failure that develops as a complication of advanced liver disease. The renal failure is not caused by primary renal disease or other extrinsic factors but rather by portal hypertension, cardiac impairment, and other circulatory alterations associated with advanced liver disease, such as cirrhosis

TABLE 41.8 Three Common Types of Jaundice

Type	Mechanism	Causes
Hemolytic jaundice (predominantly unconjugated bilirubin)	Excessive destruction of erythrocytes	Membrane defect of erythrocytes Hemolytic anemias Immune reaction Severe infection Toxic substances in the circulation (e.g., snake venom) Transfusion of incompatible blood
Obstructive (cholestatic) jaundice (predominantly conjugated bilirubin)	Obstruction to passage of conjugated bilirubin from liver to intestine	Obstruction of bile duct by gallstones or tumor (extrahepatic obstructive jaundice) Obstruction of bile flow through the liver (intrahepatic obstructive jaundice) Drugs
Hepatocellular jaundice (both conjugated and unconjugated bilirubin)	Failure of liver cells (hepatocytes) to conjugate bilirubin and of bilirubin to pass from liver to intestine	Genetic defect of hepatocyte (decreased enzymes), such as occurs in premature infants (see Chapter 42) Hepatitis or biliary cirrhosis

or fulminant hepatitis with portal hypertension and decreased systemic vascular resistance. HRS is characterized by reduced renal blood flow and glomerular filtration rate.

Pathophysiology. *Type 1 HRS–acute kidney injury* occurs in less than 2 weeks and accompanies a sudden decrease in blood volume secondary to massive GI or variceal bleeding and hypotension caused by bleeding and peripheral vasodilation associated with failing liver function. Proinflammatory cytokines related to translocation of bacterial to ascetic fluid can promote systemic hypotension and reduced renal blood flow. Hypotension also can be caused by the excessive use of diuretics to treat ascites or decreased cardiac output. The decrease in blood volume and hypotension result in decreased renal perfusion, decreased glomerular filtration, and oliguria (see Chapter 38). The serum creatinine increases to a concentration of greater than 0.3 mg/dL within 48 hours or a urine output less than 0.5 mL/kg body weight for greater than 6 hours.

Type 2 HRS–nonacute kidney injury (HRS-NAKI) develops slowly and is related to ascites resistant to diuretics. Ineffective circulating blood volume causes decreased glomerular filtration and oliguria. Intrarenal vasoconstriction may result from the selective effects of vasoactive substances that accumulate in the blood because of liver failure or as a compensatory response to portal hypertension and the pooling of blood in the splanchnic circulation. Vasoconstriction also may be a compensatory response to portal hypotension and vasodilation in the splanchnic circulation. There are two categories of NAKI. HRS–acute kidney disease (HRS-AKD) is diagnosed when the estimated glomerular filtration rate is less than 60 mL/min/1.73 m^2 for less than 3 months and the percent increase in serum creatinine is less than 50% compared with a baseline value obtained within the past 3 months. The kidney usually maintains a normal structure with this condition; HRS–chronic kidney disease (HRS-CKD) is diagnosed when the estimated glomerular filtration rate is less than 60 mL/min/1.73 m^2 for more than 3 months. The kidney usually maintains a normal structure, and there is absence of other structural causes of kidney disease.[99]

Clinical Manifestations. The onset of hepatorenal manifestations may be acute or gradual. Oliguria and complications of advanced liver disease, including jaundice, ascites, peripheral edema, hypotension, and GI bleeding, are usually present. Systolic blood pressure is usually less than 100 mm Hg. Nonspecific symptoms of HRS include anorexia, weakness, and fatigue.

Evaluation and Treatment. Diagnosis of HRS is made by excluding other causes of renal failure. Despite decreased glomerular filtration, serum potassium levels do not become dangerously elevated until the terminal stages of the HRS. Serial changes in serum creatinine provide an index for estimation of GFR, and values increase to 2.5 mg/dL or higher. Guidelines are available for determining AKI or CKD.[100] The BUN level increases, and metabolic acidosis develops. Urine osmolality increases, but urine sodium concentrations are less than normal. Urine specific gravity is greater than 1.015.

The prognosis is usually poor and is related to a failing liver, requiring liver transplantation. Secondary problems, including fluid and electrolyte disorders, bleeding, infections, and encephalopathy, are treated. Vasoconstrictors and albumin are often used as first line treatment of HRS. Liver transplant reverses HRS symptoms in most individuals and may be combined with kidney transplant.[101]

Disorders of the Liver

Acute Liver Failure

Acute liver failure is a rare clinical syndrome resulting in severe impairment or necrosis of liver cells without preexisting liver disease or cirrhosis. Acetaminophen overdose is a leading cause of acute liver failure in the United States.[102] N-acetyl cysteine is an available treatment for detoxification and should be given as soon as possible, preferably within 16 hours after the acetaminophen was taken. Acute liver failure also can occur with concurrent liver disease (acute on chronic liver failure), including complication of viral hepatitis, particularly hepatitis B virus (HBV) infection; compounded by infection with the delta virus; as well as metabolic liver disorders (Wilson disease and α_1-antitrypsin deficiency; see Chapter 42). Edematous hepatocytes and patchy areas of necrosis and inflammatory cell infiltrates disrupt liver tissue. The death of hepatocytes may also be caused by viral or toxic injury or immunologic and inflammatory damage.

Acute liver failure usually develops 6 to 8 weeks after the initial symptoms of viral hepatitis or a metabolic liver disorder, or within 5 days to 8 weeks of acetaminophen overdose. Anorexia, vomiting, abdominal pain, and progressive jaundice are initial signs, followed by ascites, GI bleeding and hepatic encephalopathy as described in previous sections. Liver function tests reflect liver injury and show elevations in the levels of both direct and indirect serum bilirubin, serum transaminases, and blood ammonia. The prothrombin time is prolonged. Renal failure and pulmonary dysfunction can occur. Treatment of acute liver failure requires rapid evaluation and critical care. The hepatic necrosis is irreversible, and there can be significant mortality. Liver transplantation may be lifesaving. Artificial liver support systems can provide a bridge to transplantation or to allow the liver to recover.[103]

Autoimmune Hepatitis

Autoimmune hepatitis is a rare chronic, progressive, autoimmune inflammatory liver disease that affects genetically susceptible individuals, usually female adults, and children. The cause is unknown, but certain infections and drugs are thought to trigger the autoimmune response. Autoreactive T cells trigger secretion of proinflammatory cytotoxic cytokines. Serologically, there are two types: type 1 with positivity for antinuclear and/or anti-smooth muscle antibody, and type 2 with anti-liver kidney microsomal type 1 antibody or anti-liver cytosol type 1 antibody. There is hypergammaglobulinemia and an elevation in aspartate and alanine aminotransferase. Biopsy confirms the diagnosis and shows lymphocytic infiltration with interface (parenchymal–connective tissue interface) hepatitis. The individual may be asymptomatic or present with jaundice, fatigue, loss of appetite, amenorrhea, or acute liver failure. Most individuals respond to immunosuppressive drug therapy (e.g., corticosteroids or in combination with azathioprine) with remission within 24 months. Relapses are common with treatment withdrawal. Approximately 10% of cases require liver transplant.[104]

Cirrhosis

Cirrhosis is an irreversible inflammatory, fibrotic liver disease. The prevalence of liver disease in the United States is approximately 4.5 million, with a mortality rate of 44,358 deaths yearly.[105] Hepatitis C, alcohol-related liver disease, nonalcoholic fatty liver disease (NAFLD), and hepatitis B are the most common causes of cirrhosis[106]; however, many disorders can cause cirrhosis (Box 41.3). Cirrhosis involves the replacement of normal healthy liver tissue with scar tissue.[106] The process of cellular injury depends on the cause of cirrhosis; however, not all pathologic mechanisms are clearly understood. Structural changes result from injury (e.g., viruses or toxicity from alcohol) and fibrosis, which is a consequence of infiltration of leukocytes, and release of inflammatory mediators with activation of stellate cells which transdifferentiate into fibrogenic myofibroblasts and promote fibrotic processes. Chaotic fibrosis alters or obstructs biliary channels and blood flow, producing jaundice and portal hypertension. New vascular channels form shunts, and blood from the portal vein bypasses the liver, contributing to portal hypertension, metabolic alterations, and toxin accumulation. The process of regeneration is disrupted by hypoxia, necrosis, atrophy, and, ultimately, liver failure. The formation of fibrous bands and regenerating nodules distorts the architecture of the liver parenchyma and gives the liver a cobbly appearance (Fig. 41.18). The liver may be larger or smaller than normal and is usually firm or hard when palpated.[107]

BOX 41.3 Causes of Cirrhosis

Hepatitis viruses—B and C (common)
Excessive alcohol intake (common)
Idiopathic (common)
Nonalcoholic fatty liver disease (NAFLD), also known as nonalcoholic steatohepatitis (NASH)
Autoimmune disorders
- Autoimmune hepatitis
- Primary biliary cirrhosis
- Primary sclerosing cholangitis

Hereditary metabolic disorder
- α-Antitrypsin deficiency
- Hemochromatosis
- Wilson disease
- Glycogen or lipid storage diseases

Prolonged exposure to drugs or toxins (e.g., carbon tetrachloride, cleaning and industrial solvents, copper salts)
Hepatic venous outflow obstruction
- Budd-Chiari syndrome (blood clotting of the hepatic vein)
- Right-sided heart failure

Cirrhosis develops slowly over a period of years. Its severity and rate of progression depend on the cause. If toxins, such as alcohol metabolites, are involved, the rate of cell death and the severity of inflammation depend on the amount of toxin present. Removal of the toxin slows the progression of liver damage and enhances the process of regeneration. Complications of cirrhosis include jaundice, portal hypertension, ascites, hepatic encephalopathy, varices with GI bleeding, HRS, HPS, and portopulmonary syndrome, which have been previously described.[108] The pathophysiology of cirrhosis causes immune suppression and increases the risk for infection.[109]

Alcoholic Liver Disease

Alcoholic liver disease is related to the toxic effects of alcohol, the formation of acetaldehyde (see Chapter 2), and coexisting liver disease. In 2019, there were 24,110 deaths in the United States related to alcoholic liver disease.[110] The spectrum of alcoholic liver disease includes alcoholic fatty liver, alcoholic steatohepatitis, and alcoholic cirrhosis with progression to hepatocellular carcinoma (HCC) in some cases. The progression of liver injury is related to the amount and duration of alcohol use, and the influence of associated diseases (e.g.,

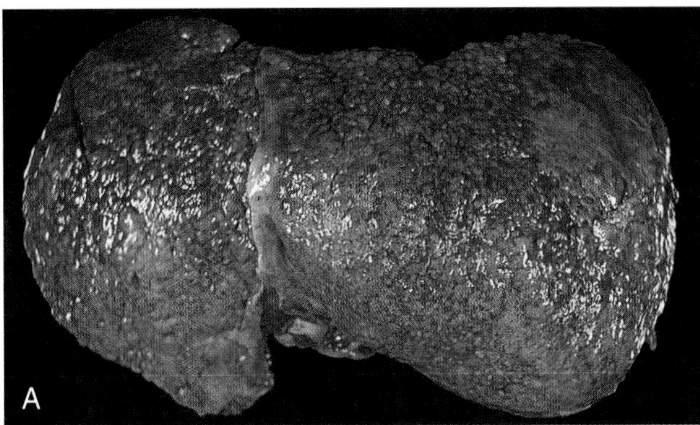

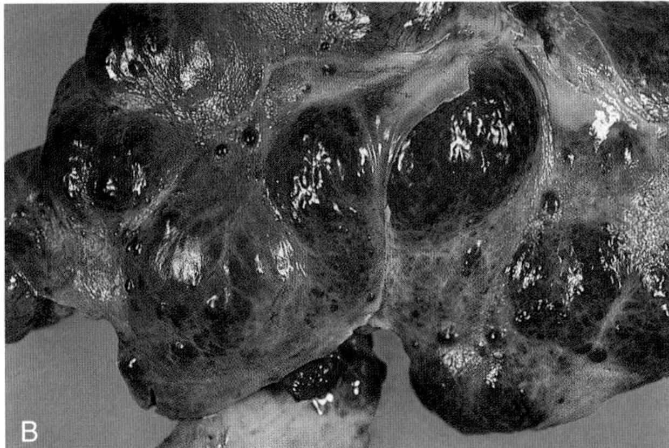

Fig. 41.18 Cirrhosis. **(A)** Micronodular cirrhosis. The nodular appearance develops from regeneration of hepatocytes projecting through fibrous bands of tissue. **(B)** Macronodular cirrhosis. (From Damjanov I, Linder J, eds. *Anderson's pathology*, 10th edition. St. Louis: Mosby; 1996.)

obesity, metabolic syndrome, and viral hepatitis). Although alcoholic cirrhosis is the most prevalent of the various types of cirrhosis, the occurrence of cirrhosis among persons with alcoholism is relatively low (approximately 25%).

Malnutrition contributes to the risk of complications and adverse outcomes associated with alcohol-related liver disease. Chronic alcohol abuse results in a catabolic state with upregulation of inflammatory mediators that suppress appetite and cause intestinal dysfunction with malabsorption of nutrients and pancreatic insufficiency. The chronic inflammatory state and altered metabolic pathways associated with alcoholic liver injury and anorexia lead to a hypermetabolic state, protein energy, caloric, and micronutrient malnutrition. The malnutrition and loss of muscle mass accelerate liver decompensation and disease progression.[111]

Pathophysiology. Alcoholic fatty liver disease (steatosis) is the mildest form of alcoholic liver disease, and there may be no symptoms. It can be caused by relatively small amounts of alcohol and is typically reversible with the cessation of drinking. The fat deposition (deposition of triglycerides) within the liver is caused primarily by increased lipogenesis, cholesterol synthesis, and decreased fatty acid oxidation by hepatocytes that occurs with increased alcohol metabolism.[112] Lipids mobilized from adipose tissue or dietary fat intake may contribute to fat accumulation.

Alcoholic steatohepatitis (alcoholic hepatitis) is a precursor of cirrhosis characterized by increased hepatic fat storage, inflammation, and degeneration and necrosis of hepatocytes with infiltration of neutrophils and lymphocytes. The inflammation and necrosis caused by alcoholic steatohepatitis stimulate the irreversible fibrosis characteristic of the cirrhotic stage of disease.

Alcoholic cirrhosis is caused by the toxic effects of alcohol metabolism in the liver, immunologic alterations, inflammatory cytokines, oxidative stress from lipid peroxidation, malnutrition, and an ongoing cycle of liver injury and regeneration. Alcohol is transformed to acetaldehyde; excessive amounts are toxic and significantly alter hepatocyte function and activate hepatic stellate cells, a primary cell involved in liver fibrosis. Enzyme and protein synthesis may be depressed or altered, and hormone and ammonia degradation is diminished. Acetaldehyde inhibits protein synthesis and export of proteins from the liver, alters metabolism of vitamins and minerals, and induces malnutrition. Kupffer cell (macrophage) activation attracts neutrophils promoting inflammation, endotoxins accumulate from translocation of gut bacteria, and cell-mediated immunity is suppressed. Cellular damage initiates an inflammatory response that, along with necrosis, results in activation of hepatic stellate cells and excessive collagen formation. Fibrosis and scarring interspersed with regenerating nodules alter the structure of the liver and obstruct biliary and vascular channels. Eventually hepatocytes lose their ability to regenerate with progression to liver failure.

Clinical Manifestations. Fatty infiltration causes no specific symptoms or abnormal liver function test results. The liver is usually enlarged and may be found during a routine examination. The individual has a history of continuous alcohol intake during the previous weeks or months.

The clinical manifestations of alcoholic steatohepatitis can be mild or severe. Nonspecific symptoms include fatigue, weight loss, and anorexia Manifestations of acute illness include nausea, anorexia, fever, abdominal pain, and jaundice. Cirrhosis is a multiple-system disease and causes hepatomegaly, splenomegaly, ascites, portal hypertension, GI hemorrhage, hepatic encephalopathy, and esophageal varices. Anemia results from blood loss, malnutrition, and hypersplenism. Pulmonary syndrome and HRS are usually late complications (Fig. 41.19). Toxic effects of alcohol also can cause testicular atrophy, reduced libido, azoospermia, and decreased testosterone levels in men. Premenopausal women with cirrhosis experience anovulation or irregular ovulation related to alterations in hormone metabolism. The presence of numerous and severe manifestations increases the risk of death. Cirrhosis increases the risk of HCC because acetaldehyde has mutagenic effects on deoxyribonucleic acid (DNA).[113]

Evaluation and Treatment. The diagnosis of alcoholic steatohepatitis or cirrhosis is based on the individual's history of alcohol use and clinical manifestations.[114] The results of liver function tests are abnormal, and serologic studies show elevated levels of serum enzymes (i.e., alanine aminotransferase, aspartate aminotransferase, and γ-glutamyltransferase) and bilirubin, decreased levels of serum albumin, and a prolonged prothrombin time that is not easily corrected with vitamin K therapy. Liver biopsy can confirm the diagnosis of cirrhosis, but biopsy is not necessary if clinical manifestations of cirrhosis are evident.

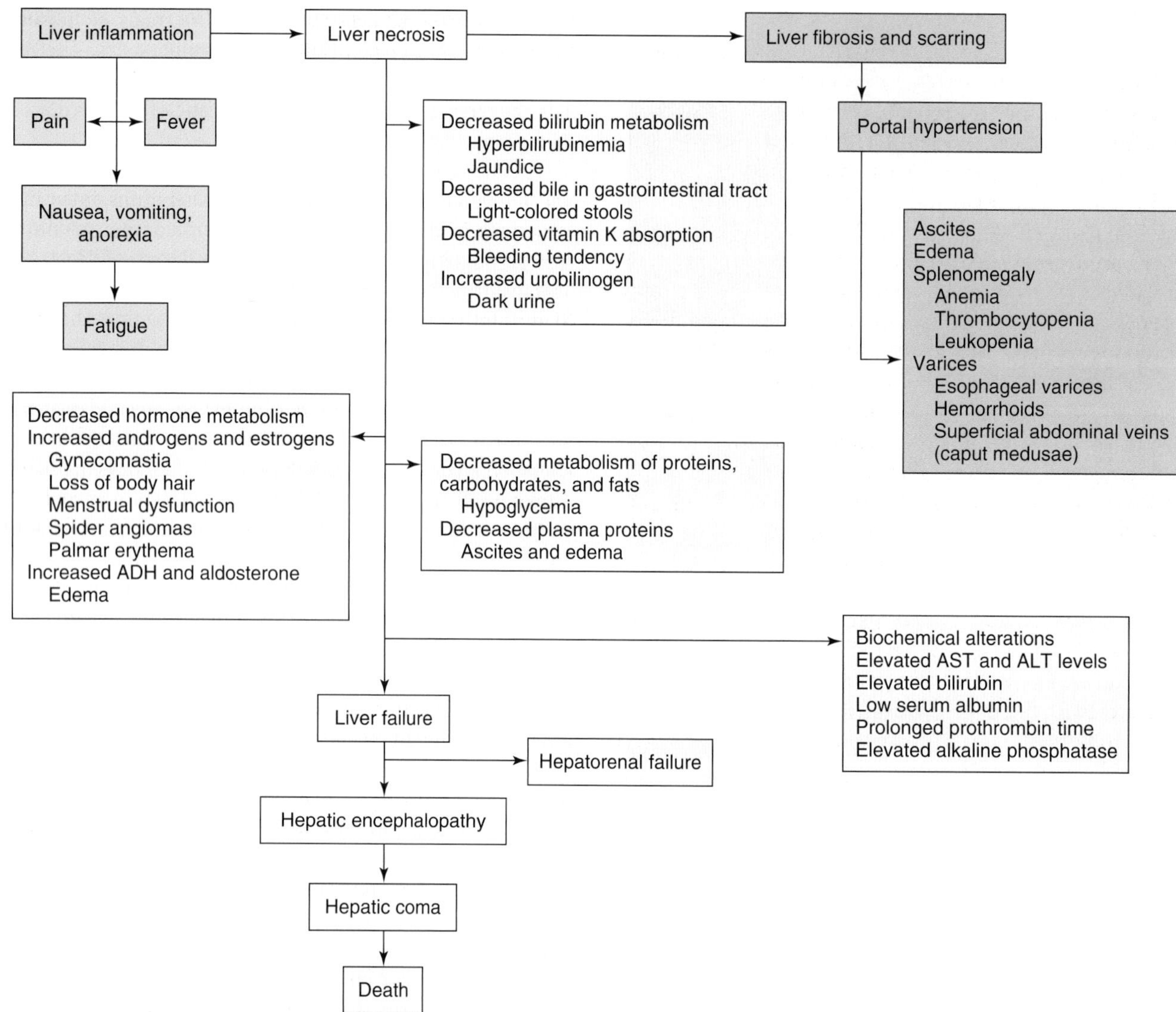

Fig. 41.19 Clinical Manifestations of Cirrhosis. *ADH*, Antidiuretic hormone; *ALT*, alanine transaminase; *AST*, aspartate transaminase.

There is no specific treatment for alcoholic steatohepatitis or cirrhosis. Rest, vitamin supplements, a nutritious diet, corticosteroids, antioxidants, drugs that slow fibrosis, and management of complications (e.g., ascites, GI bleeding, and encephalopathy) slow disease progression. Cessation of alcohol consumption slows the progression of liver damage, improves clinical symptoms, and prolongs life. Although the liver damage is irreversible, measures that halt the inflammation and destruction of liver cells prolong life, and many new drugs are being evaluated.[115] Liver transplantation is the treatment of end-stage liver disease.

Nonalcoholic Liver Disease and Nonalcoholic Steatohepatitis

Nonalcoholic fatty liver disease (NAFLD) is the infiltration of hepatocytes with fat, primarily in the form of triglycerides, that occurs in the absence of alcohol intake and inflammation. It is associated with obesity (including obese children), insulin resistance, high levels of cholesterol and triglycerides that exceed metabolic capacity, metabolic syndrome, and type 2 diabetes mellitus. NAFLD is the most common chronic liver disease in the United States. Some individuals with NAFLD will develop nonalcoholic steatohepatitis (NASH), with hepatocellular injury, inflammation, and with or without fibrosis. NASH can be difficult to distinguish from alcohol-induced liver fibrosis. There are several noninvasive biomarkers to evaluate the progression of fibrosis in NASH.[116] In some cases biopsy may be required. Alcohol consumption may also promote disease progression in NAFLD.[117] Exercise and coffee consumption are thought to be protective environmental factors.

NAFLD is usually asymptomatic and may remain undetected for years. Individuals with type 2 diabetes mellitus are at high risk for NASH, and assessment for NAFLD should be part of their care with consideration of bariatric surgery.[118] The most severe forms of NASH progress to cirrhosis and end-stage liver disease. There can be progression to HCC. The most common cause of death among individuals with NAFLD is cardiovascular disease. Treatment is individualized and includes the use of behavioral modification, dietary counseling, and regular exercise. Pharmacotherapy with insulin sensitizers, vitamin E, and lipid-lowering drugs may be considered. Pioglitazone should be considered for those with NASH, especially if fibrosis is present. Liver transplant is the only option for liver failure.[119]

Primary Biliary Cholangitis

Primary biliary cholangitis (previously called primary biliary cirrhosis) is a rare, chronic, slowly progressive, autoimmune, cholestatic liver disease that slowly destroys the bile ducts in the liver. The disease begins in the bile canaliculi and bile ducts rather than in the hepatocytes as with other liver diseases. It is caused by autoimmune T lymphocyte and highly specific antimitochondrial antibody destruction of the small intrahepatic bile ducts and primarily affects middle-aged women. Primary biliary cholangitis often accompanies other autoimmune diseases. Pathogenesis includes inflammation, destruction, fibrosis, and obstruction of the intrahepatic bile ducts. Primary biliary cholangitis can be detected by biochemical evidence of cholestatic liver disease. Test findings include the presence of antinuclear antibodies, anticentromere antibodies, and the GP210 antinuclear antibody, as well as elevated alkaline phosphatase levels for at least 6 months. Ultrasound imaging of the liver or liver biopsy assists with diagnosis. Manifestations progress insidiously from pruritus, hyperbilirubinemia, jaundice, and light or clay-colored stools to cirrhosis, portal hypertension, and encephalopathy. Life expectancy is 5 to 10 years after the onset of symptoms if the condition is not treated. Treatment with ursodeoxycholic acid (UDCA) has anticholestatic effects and slows disease progression. Obeticholic acid indirectly reduces BA synthesis and may be used in combination with or as second line therapy. It should be used with caution with severe liver disease. Other drugs used in combination with UDCA include bezafibrate (can also reduce pruritus) and budesonide.[120] Pruritus may be relieved by cholestyramine, which binds bile salts in the intestine. Liver transplantation is highly effective. Because of increased risk for cholangiocellular and gallbladder carcinoma, yearly screening is recommended.[121]

Secondary Biliary Cirrhosis

Secondary biliary cirrhosis develops when there is prolonged partial or complete obstruction of the common bile duct or its branches. The obstruction may be caused by gallstones, tumors, fibrotic strictures, or chronic pancreatitis. Biliary atresia and cystic fibrosis cause secondary biliary cirrhosis in children.

Chronic obstruction to extrahepatic bile flow increases pressure in the hepatic bile ducts and results in the accumulation of bile in the centrilobular spaces. Necrotic areas develop and are followed by proliferation and inflammation of the portal ducts that result in edema and fibrosis. Pools of bile form when the portal ducts rupture into surrounding necrotic areas. Injury is accompanied by regeneration of hepatic cells with the development of finely nodular cirrhosis.

Clinical manifestations are similar to those of primary biliary cholangitis, with jaundice and pruritus the most distressing symptoms. Right upper quadrant pain is common, and a low-grade fever may be present from bile duct inflammation (cholangitis).

Cholangiography provides the most definitive diagnosis. Laboratory tests usually show elevated conjugated bilirubin and alkaline phosphatase levels. Aminotransferase level increases if there is an accompanying cholangitis. Surgery or endoscopy relieves obstruction, prolongs survival, and diminishes or resolves symptoms. Continued obstruction leads to advanced cirrhosis and liver failure.

Viral Hepatitis

Viral hepatitis is a relatively common systemic disease that primarily affects the liver. Different strains of viruses cause different types of hepatitis. Since a widespread outbreak of hepatitis A virus (HAV) in the United States in 2016, 44,217 cases have been reported as of April 29, 2022.[122] In 2019, the estimated incidence in the United States was 3192 new cases of acute HBV and an estimated 20,700 cases after adjusting for under-ascertainment and under-reporting; 4136 new cases of hepatitis C virus (HCV) and an estimated 57,500 cases after adjusting for under-ascertainment and under-reporting.[123] Hepatitis A formerly was known as infectious hepatitis and hepatitis B as serum hepatitis. Characteristics of the different types of viruses that cause hepatitis are presented in Table 41.9. Viral hepatitis in children is presented in Chapter 42.

Pathophysiology. Hepatitis means inflammation of the liver. The five main types of viral hepatitis (A, B, C, D, and E) can cause acute, icteric illness. HBV and HCV are the most common causes. HDV occurs as a coinfection with HBV and depends on the viral coat of HB surface antigen (HBsAg) molecules on HBV for its replication in pregnant women. HEV infection can be a serious disease. The pathologic lesions of hepatitis include hepatic cell necrosis, scarring (with chronic disease), and Kupffer cell hyperplasia. In addition, infiltration by mononuclear phagocytes occurs with varying severity. Cellular injury is promoted by cell-mediated immune mechanisms, release of inflammatory mediators, and persistent inflammation.[124,125] Regeneration of hepatic cells begins within 48 hours of injury. The inflammatory process can damage hepatocytes and obstruct bile canaliculi, leading to cholestasis and obstructive jaundice. In milder cases, the liver parenchyma is not damaged. Damage tends to be most severe in cases of HBV and HCV and can progress to chronic disease.

Acute fulminating hepatitis can cause acute liver failure and severe hepatic encephalopathy, which is manifested as confusion, stupor, coma, and coagulopathy. Coinfection with HBV, HCV, HDV, and the human immunodeficiency virus (HIV) is common because they share the same route of transmission. Progression of liver disease is more rapid in these cases.

Clinical Manifestations. The clinical manifestations of the various types of hepatitis are very similar, and onset of symptoms varies with the duration of the incubation phase. The spectrum of manifestations ranges from absence of symptoms to fulminating hepatitis, with rapid onset of liver failure and coma. Acute viral hepatitis causes abnormal liver function test results. The serum aminotransferase values, aspartate transaminase (AST) and alanine transaminase (ALT), are elevated but not consistent with the extent of cellular damage. The clinical course of hepatitis usually consists of three phases, preceded by an incubation phase. The incubation phase and manifestations vary depending on the virus (see Table 41.9). The other three phases are:

TABLE 41.9 Characteristics of Viral Hepatitis

Characteristic	Hepatitis A	Hepatitis B	Hepatitis D	Hepatitis C	Hepatitis E
Size of virus	27-nm RNA virus	47-nm DNA virus	36-nm RNA virus, defective virus with HBsAg coat	30- to 60-nm RNA virus	32-nm RNA virus
Incubation phase	30 days	60–180 days	30–180 days; dependent on HBV for multiplication	35–72 days	15–60 days
Route of transmission	Fecal-oral, parenteral, sexual	Parenteral, sexual	Parenteral, fecal-oral, sexual	Parenteral	Fecal-oral
Onset	Acute with fever	Insidious	Insidious	Insidious	Acute
Carrier state	Negative	Positive	Positive	Positive	Negative
Severity	Mild	Severe; may be prolonged or chronic	Severe	Mild to severe	Severe in pregnant women
Chronic hepatitis	No	Yes	Yes	Yes	No
Age-group affected	Children and young adults	Any	Any	Any	Children and young adults
Prophylaxis	Hygiene, immune serum globulin, HAV vaccine	Hygiene, HBV vaccine	Hygiene, HBV vaccine	Hygiene, screening blood, interferon-α or combined with ribavirin; treatment also related to HCV genotype ± cirrhosis	Hygiene, safe water and meat
Treatment	None or symptomatic	Interferon-α and nucleoside/ nucleotide analogues	Interferon-α and nucleoside/ nucleotide analogues	Direct antiviral agents	Ribavirin and interferon-α for severe infection

Data from Pisano MB, Giadans CG, Flichman DM, et al. Viral hepatitis update: Progress and perspectives. *World Journal of Gastroenterology*, 2021;27(2):4018–4044.

DNA, Deoxyribonucleic acid; *HAV*, hepatitis A virus; *HBsAg*, hepatitis B surface antigen; *HBV*, hepatitis B virus; *HCV*, hepatitis C virus; *RNA*, ribonucleic acid.

1. Prodromal (preicteric) phase begins approximately 2 weeks after exposure and ends with the appearance of jaundice; marked by fatigue, anorexia, malaise, nausea, vomiting, headache, hyperalgia, cough, and low-grade fever; the infection is highly transmissible during this phase.
2. Icteric phase begins 1 to 2 weeks after the prodromal phase and lasts 2 to 6 weeks; jaundice, dark urine, and clay-colored stools are common; the liver is enlarged, smooth, and tender, and percussion or palpation of the liver causes pain; GI and respiratory symptoms subside, but fatigue and abdominal pain may persist or become more severe. This is the actual phase of illness. Individuals who develop chronic HBV, HDV, or HCV infection do not become jaundiced and may not be diagnosed.
3. Recovery phase begins with resolution of jaundice, approximately 6 to 8 weeks after exposure; symptoms diminish, but the liver remains enlarged and tender; liver function returns to normal 2 to 12 weeks after the onset of jaundice.

Chronic active hepatitis is the persistence of clinical manifestations and liver inflammation after the acute stages of HBV, HBV/HDV coinfection, and HCV infection. Liver function tests remain abnormal for longer than 6 months, and the HBsAg persists. Chronic, active HBV or HCV infection is a predisposition to cirrhosis and primary HCC. Chronic active hepatitis constitutes a carrier state, and HBV and HCV can be transmitted from mothers to infants. Prolonged HCV infection promotes systemic inflammation and is a risk factor for insulin resistance, type 2 diabetes mellitus, and cardiovascular disease.[126]

Evaluation and Treatment. The diagnosis of HAV and HCV infections is based on the presence of anti-HAV and anti-HCV antibodies. The most specific diagnostic test for HBV is serologic analysis for specific hepatitis virus antigens (i.e., HB surface antigen [HBsAg], which is the marker for HBV). There are other markers for HBV, including hepatitis B surface antibody (anti-HBs), hepatitis B envelope antigen (HBeAg), hepatitis B envelope antibody (anti-HBe), hepatitis B core antibody (anti-HBc), IgM and IgG, and HBV DNA. The assay for HDV is the measurement of total antibody to hepatitis D antigen (anti-HDV) and serum HDV ribonucleic acid (RNA). HCV RNA quantification is important for assessment of the viral load, to evaluate antiviral therapy for chronic HCV infection. HEV infection is diagnosed from the presence of serum anti-HEV IgG and HEV RNA. HEV infection is usually a self-limiting disease, except in undeveloped countries, where it causes chronic hepatitis with an increased risk in pregnant women. Liver enzyme levels and function tests also can indicate other viral liver diseases, drug toxicity, or alcoholic hepatitis.[127]

Prophylaxis and treatments for different types of viral hepatitis are summarized in Table 41.9. Physical activity may be restricted, and a low-fat, high-carbohydrate diet is beneficial if bile flow is obstructed. For chronic hepatitis, treatment is directed at suppressing viral replication before irreversible liver cell damage or hepatic carcinoma occurs. Cyclic and combination therapy may prevent drug resistance, and treatment regimens may be genotype specific. Recent advances in the development of direct-acting antiviral agents (DAAs) have broadened first line treatment options for individuals with hepatitis C, and the World Health Organization has set 2030 as the target for eliminating hepatitis B and C.[128] Coinfection of HIV and HCV is common, and interruption of HIV antiretroviral therapy is not recommended prior to HCV DAA treatment.[129]

Outbreaks of HAV have been reported in the United States, and the prevalence is tracked by state health departments. Although HAV is transferred via the fecal-oral route through food and water contamination, it is more commonly spread from person to person in the United States, and outbreaks were identified in 2016.[130] After ingestion and GI uptake, HAV replicates in the liver and is secreted into the stool and blood. To prevent the transmission of HAV, proper hand hygiene and the use of gloves for disposing of bedpans and fecal matter are imperative. HAV may be shed in the stool for up to 3 months after the onset of symptoms. Molecular procedures are available for direct surveillance of HAV in food. Direct contact with blood or body fluids of individuals should be avoided. The administration of immune globulin before exposure or early in the incubation period can prevent HAV and HBV infection. A combined vaccine is available to protect against HAV and HBV infection. To prevent outbreaks of HAV, hepatitis A vaccine is recommended for adults at risk: people who use drugs (including drugs that are not injected), people experiencing homelessness, men who have sex with men, people with liver disease, and people who are or were recently in jail or prison. These recommendations are in addition to vaccine recommendations for children.[130] Preexposure vaccination is recommended for healthcare workers, liver transplant recipients, and others who are at risk for contact with infected body fluids, particularly children. There is no vaccine for HCV or HEV in the United States.

Disorders of the Gallbladder

Obstruction and inflammation are the most common disorders of the gallbladder. Obstruction is caused by gallstones, which are aggregates of substances in the bile. The gallstones may remain in the gallbladder or may be ejected, with bile, into the cystic duct. Gallstones that become lodged in the cystic duct obstruct the flow of bile into and out of the gallbladder and cause inflammation. Gallstone formation is termed cholelithiasis. Inflammation of the gallbladder or cystic duct is known as cholecystitis.

Cholelithiasis

Cholelithiasis (gallstones) is a prevalent disorder in developed countries, where the incidence is 10% to 20% of adults in the United States. Approximately 500,000 people will develop symptoms or complication of cholelithiasis annually.[131] Risk factors include obesity, female sex, pregnancy, use of oral contraceptives, gallbladder stasis, genetics, drugs, prolonged fasting with TPN, rapid weight loss, and certain medical conditions such as CD, cirrhosis, ileal resection, or other diseases of the ileum.[131,132]

Pathophysiology. Cholelithiasis is the presence of gallstones. Gallstones form in the biliary tract as a result of impaired metabolism of cholesterol, bilirubin, and BA and hypomotility of the gallbladder.[133] All gallstones contain a supersaturated amount of cholesterol, unconjugated bilirubin, bilirubin calcium salts, fatty acids, calcium carbonates and phosphates, and mucin glycoproteins. Stones form in three locations: the gallbladder or cystic duct (cholecystolithiasis), the extrahepatic bile duct (choledocholithiasis), and rarely in the intrahepatic bile duct (hepatolithiasis). There are three types of gallstones, determined by their chemical composition: cholesterol stones (70% cholesterol and the most common type [70% to 80% prevalence]), pigmented stones (black [hard] and brown [soft] with less than 30% cholesterol), and mixed stones. Cholesterol and black stones are more commonly formed within the gallbladder, and brown stones are formed in the bile ducts. *Cholesterol gallstones* form in bile that is supersaturated with cholesterol produced by the liver. Supersaturation sets the stage for cholesterol crystal formation (cholesterol nucleation), or the formation of "microstones." More crystals aggregate on the microstones, which grow to form "macrostones." This process more commonly occurs in the gallbladder. Prolonged exposure to supersaturated bile can decrease gallbladder motility, with incomplete postprandial emptying and biliary stasis also promoting gallbladder cholesterol stone formation. The stones may lie dormant or may become lodged in the cystic or common duct, causing obstruction, and pain when the gallbladder contracts. Bile stasis in the gallbladder can cause inflammation and cholecystitis. The stones can accumulate and fill the entire gallbladder (Fig. 41.20). *Black gallstones* are rare and are associated with chronic liver disease and hemolytic disease. They are composed of calcium bilirubinate with mucin glycoproteins. *Pigmented brown gallstones* form from calcium bilirubinate and fatty acid soaps that bind with calcium They are associated with biliary stasis, bacterial infections (e.g., *E. coli*), and biliary parasites. Hepatocytes secrete bile that is supersaturated with cholesterol promoting stone formation. Several possible mechanisms are related to this process, and they are summarized in Box 41.4.

Clinical Manifestations. Cholelithiasis is often asymptomatic as it takes years for gallstones to develop, and they may be found incidentally on imaging for another condition or disease. Manifestations of disease are caused by occlusion of the ducts by sludge or gallstones. Epigastric and right hypochondrium pain and intolerance to fatty foods are the cardinal manifestations of cholelithiasis. Vague symptoms include heartburn, flatulence, epigastric discomfort, and food intolerances, particularly to fats, and they occur long before the development of complications. The pain, oftentimes referred to as biliary colic, occurs 30 minutes to several hours after eating a fatty meal. It is caused by the lodging of one or more gallstones in the cystic or common duct during contraction of the gallbladder (a physiologic response to cholecystokinin) with increases in intraluminal pressure and distention of the gallbladder wall. It can be intermittent or steady and usually occurs in the right upper quadrant, radiating to the midupper area of the back. Jaundice indicates that the stone is located in the common bile duct.

Evaluation and Treatment. The diagnosis is based on the medical history, physical examination (including circumscribed pain over the gallbladder on direct pressure), laboratory tests

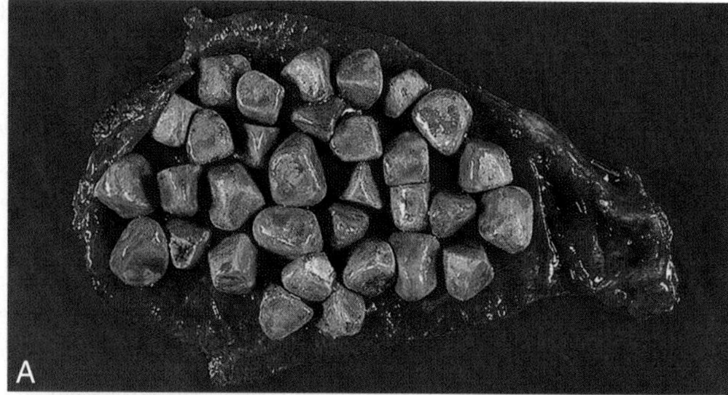

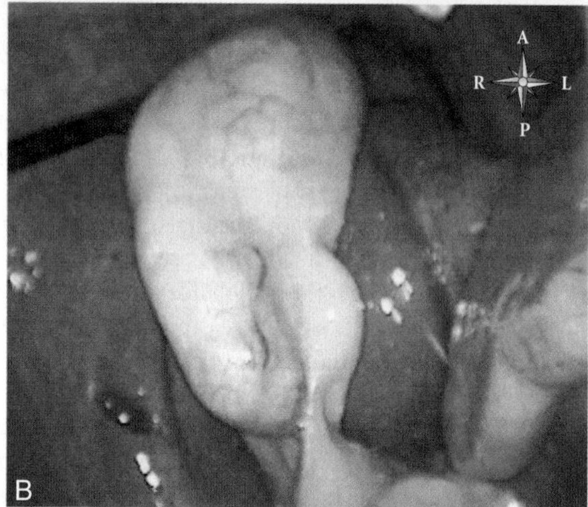

Fig. 41.20 (A) Resected gallbladder containing mixed gallstones. (B) Gallbladder before removal. (Courtesy Thompson JM, Wilson SF. *Health assessment for nursing practice*, St. Louis: Mosby, 1996.)

(leukocytosis differentiates biliary colic from acute cholecystitis), and imaging evaluation. Transcutaneous sonography identifies the gallbladder and stone(s) and outlines the intrahepatic and extrahepatic bile ducts. CT or MRI can be helpful if there are complications. Other imaging options including endosonography are used if choledocholithiasis is suspected. Acute episodic biliary colic is managed with pain control.[134] Oral BA (UDCA or chenodeoxycholic acid) may prevent or dissolve cholesterol stones, particularly when there is gallstone sludge, but the stones may recur when the drug is discontinued. Dietary factors may prevent the development of gallstones, including increasing the intake of polyunsaturated fat, monounsaturated fat, and caffeine, vitamin C, and consumption of fiber. Exercise and maintenance of normal body weight with gradual weight loss are important. Laparoscopic cholecystectomy is the preferred treatment for uncomplicated gallstones causing obstruction of the bile ducts. Large stones may be managed by extracorporeal shock wave lithotripsy prior to endoscopic removal.[135]

Cholecystitis

Cholecystitis is inflammation of the gallbladder and typically develops after a gallstone becomes lodged in the cystic duct. This disorder may have either an acute or chronic presentation. The obstruction of the cystic duct causes the gallbladder to become distended and inflamed. The pain is similar to that caused by gallstones. Pressure against the distended wall of the gallbladder decreases blood flow and may result in ischemia, necrosis, and perforation. Fever, leukocytosis, rebound tenderness, and abdominal muscle guarding are common findings. Serum bilirubin and alkaline phosphatase levels may be elevated. Cholescintigraphy (a radiotracer scan of the gallbladder) is the most sensitive imaging for cholecystitis. The acute abdominal pain of cholecystitis must be differentiated from that caused by pancreatitis, myocardial infarction, and acute pyelonephritis of the right kidney. Narcotics may be required to control pain not responding to NSAIDs, and antibiotics are prescribed to manage

BOX 41.4 Possible Mechanisms of Hepatic Supersaturated Cholesterol Formation

- An enzymatic defect (e.g., increased 3-hydroxy-3-methylglutaryl coenzyme A (HMG-CoA) reductase) increases hepatocyte synthesis of cholesterol;
- Diminished secretion of bile acids (BAs), which normally promote cholesterol solubility;
- Decreased resorption of bile salts from the ileum, which decrease the bile acid pool;
- Slower intestinal motility and increased cholesterol absorption;
- Gallbladder smooth muscle hypomotility and stasis (prolonged exposure to supersaturated bile can decrease motility with incomplete postprandial emptying, biliary stasis and time for cholesterol nucleation);
- Increased secretion of gallbladder epithelial procrystallizing agents mucin and biliary calcium;
- Genetic predisposition (*Lith* genes)—population studies suggest a 25%–30% genetic predisposition is associated with alterations in mucin secretion, hepatic cholesterol metabolism and transport, with variations among different populations (higher among Hispanic and American Indian ancestry);
- Insulin resistance increases cholesterol secretion with a higher prevalence of gallstones among obese individuals and those with metabolic syndrome and type 2 diabetes mellitus;
- Estrogen stimulates biliary cholesterol section and decreases bile acid synthesis, accounting for the increased incidence of gallstones among some women during years of reproduction and when taking estrogen supplements;
- Rapid weight loss dieting and bariatric surgery for treatment of obesity enhances hepatic secretion of cholesterol into bile caused by increased metabolism of lipid stores, reduced gallbladder emptying, and biliary stasis;
- Vitamin C deficiency as vitamin C modulates the hepatic and biliary pathways of cholesterol homeostasis by promoting the conversion of cholesterol into BAs through liver 7α-hydroxylation and prolongs cholesterol nucleation and crystallization time;
- Low fiber has a negative effect on colonic motility and increased production of secondary [lithogenic] BAs and is associated with high saturated fat and refined sugar diet;
- Some combination of the above mechanisms.

Data from Dosch AR, Imagawa DK, Jutric Z. Bile metabolism and lithogenesis: An update. *Surgical Clinics of North America*, 2019;99(2):215–229; Di Ciaula A, Wang DQ, Portincasa P. An update on the pathogenesis of cholesterol gallstone disease. *Current Opinion in Gastroenterology*, 2018;34(2):71–80; E Swarne, Srikanth MS, Shreyas A, et al. Recent advances, novel targets and treatments for cholelithiasis; A narrative review. *European Journal of Pharmacology*, 2021;908:174376; Bonfrate L, et al. Obesity and the risk and prognosis of gallstone disease and pancreatitis. *Best Practice and Research in Clinical Gastroenterology*, 2014;28(4):623–635; Di Ciaula A, Garruti G, Frühbeck G, et al. The role of diet in the pathogenesis of cholesterol gallstones. *Current Medicinal Chemistry*, 2019;26(19):3620–3638.

bacterial infection in severe cases. Acute attacks usually require laparoscopic cholecystectomy. Obstruction also may lead to reflux of bile into the pancreatic duct, causing acute pancreatitis.[136]

Disorders of the Pancreas

Pancreatitis, or inflammation of the pancreas, is a relatively rare disease and potentially serious disorder. The incidence is about equal in men and women, is more common between 50 and 60 years of age and is more likely to occur in Blacks. Risk factors include obstructive biliary tract disease (particularly cholelithiasis), alcoholism, obesity, peptic ulcers, trauma, hyperlipidemia, hypercalcemia, smoking, certain drugs, and genetic factors (hereditary pancreatitis, cystic fibrosis). The cause is unknown in 15% to 25% of cases. Pancreatitis can be acute or chronic.

Acute Pancreatitis

Acute pancreatitis is usually a mild disease and resolves spontaneously, but approximately 20% of those with the disease develop a severe, acute pancreatitis requiring hospitalization, with more than 300,000 emergency department visits per year in the United States.[137] Pancreatitis develops because of obstruction to the outflow of pancreatic digestive enzymes caused by bile and pancreatic duct obstruction. Gallstones are the leading cause of acute obstructive pancreatitis. Acute pancreatitis also results from direct cellular injury from alcohol, drugs, or viral infection.

Pathophysiology. Acute pancreatitis has an unclear pathophysiologic trigger. Both intracellular and systemic events are proposed to contribute to the disease process. Reflux of BA into the pancreatic duct from gallstone obstruction of the common bile duct and ethanol metabolites within the pancreas promote intracellular pancreatic injury, including calcium overload, alterations in heat shock proteins (HSPs), and injury to the mitochondria and endoplasmic reticulum. Intracellular calcium overload is proposed as a primary mechanism of cell injury in acute pancreatitis. Ethanol metabolites and BAs stimulate sustained pathologic calcium release from acinar endoplasmic reticulum stores, increased entry of extracellular calcium, and defects in calcium extrusion and reuptake mechanism. Intracellular calcium overload causes inappropriate intracellular trypsin activation, impaired fluid and $HCO3^-$ secretion in ductal cells, activation of the nuclear factor (NF)-κB proinflammatory pathway, and cell necrosis. Cellular injury leads to recruitment of neutrophils with release of inflammatory mediators and the formation of neutrophil extracellular traps, which further ductal obstruction and systemic inflammatory responses.[138] Trypsin activation causes autodigestion, while the activation of proinflammatory pathways leads to release of inflammatory cytokines with amplification of injury within the pancreas and systemic inflammatory responses.

Severe acute pancreatitis is also associated with sustained hypercalcemia in cases of primary hyperparathyroidism.[139] Sustained hypercalcemia increases the content of calcium in the pancreatic secretions, resulting in an accelerated transformation of trypsinogen to trypsin with cell injury, inflammation, and necrosis. HSPs are cytoprotective. They stabilize protein folding, are antioxidative and antiinflammatory, downregulate intra-acinar activation of trypsinogen and the NF-κB pathway, and are released in response to cellular stress and injury. BA and alcohol metabolites depress HSP function, contributing to the injury and inflammation of acute pancreatitis. There are increased demands for protein synthesis, and the endoplasmic reticulum is important for protein synthesis and transport, protein folding, and calcium storage. Mitochondria supply the adenosine triphosphate (ATP) for metabolism and protein synthesis. Alterations in mitochondrial function and stress to the endoplasmic reticulum contribute to the pathophysiology of acute pancreatitis. Synthesis of needed proteins and failure to recycle unneeded proteins and refold proteins (autophagy) fail and result in apoptosis (programmed cell death) and inflammation.[140–143] Paradoxically hypocalcemia is common in acute pancreatitis and is associated with severity of disease. Hypocalcemia develops from the autodigestion of mesenteric fat by pancreatic enzymes and release of free fatty acids, which form calcium salts (soaps). Transient hypoparathyroidism, and hypomagnesaemia can also contribute to hypocalcemia associated with pancreatitis.[144]

Activated trypsin activates other enzymes (chymotrypsin, lipase, and elastase) within the pancreatic acinar cells, causing autodigestion of pancreatic cells and tissues, resulting in inflammation. The autodigestion causes vascular damage, coagulation necrosis, fat necrosis (see Chapter 2), and the formation of pseudocysts (walled-off collections of pancreatic secretions). Edema within the pancreatic capsule causes compression and leads to ischemia and can contribute to necrosis (Fig. 41.21). Chronic alcohol use may also cause formation of protein plugs in pancreatic ducts and spasm of the sphincter of Oddi, resulting in obstruction. The obstruction leads to further intrapancreatic release of activated enzymes, autodigestion, inflammation, and pancreatitis.

Systemic effects of acute pancreatitis are related to the release of proinflammatory cytokines and digestive enzymes into the bloodstream. There is activation of leukocytes and complement, injury to vessel walls, and coagulation abnormalities, with the development of vasodilation, hypotension, and shock. Complications can include acute respiratory distress syndrome (ARDS), heart failure, renal failure, coagulopathies, splenic vein obstruction, intra-abdominal hypertension, and systemic inflammatory response syndrome (SIRS). Paralytic ileus from release of toxic fluid into the peritoneum and GI bleeding can occur. Translocation of intestinal bacteria to the bloodstream may cause peritonitis or sepsis. Recurrent inflammation activates pancreatic stellate cells, which transdifferentiate into fibrogenic myofibroblasts, causing pancreatic fibrosis, strictures, and duct obstruction, which can all lead to chronic pancreatitis.

Clinical Manifestations. The cardinal manifestation of acute pancreatitis is epigastric or midabdominal constant pain ranging from mild abdominal discomfort to severe, incapacitating pain. The pain may radiate to the back. Pain is caused by (1) edema, which distends the pancreatic ducts and capsule, (2) chemical irritation and inflammation of the peritoneum, (3) irritation or obstruction of the biliary tract, and (4) inflammation of nerves. Fever and leukocytosis accompany the inflammatory response. Nausea and vomiting are caused by paralytic ileus secondary to the pancreatitis or peritonitis. Jaundice can occur from

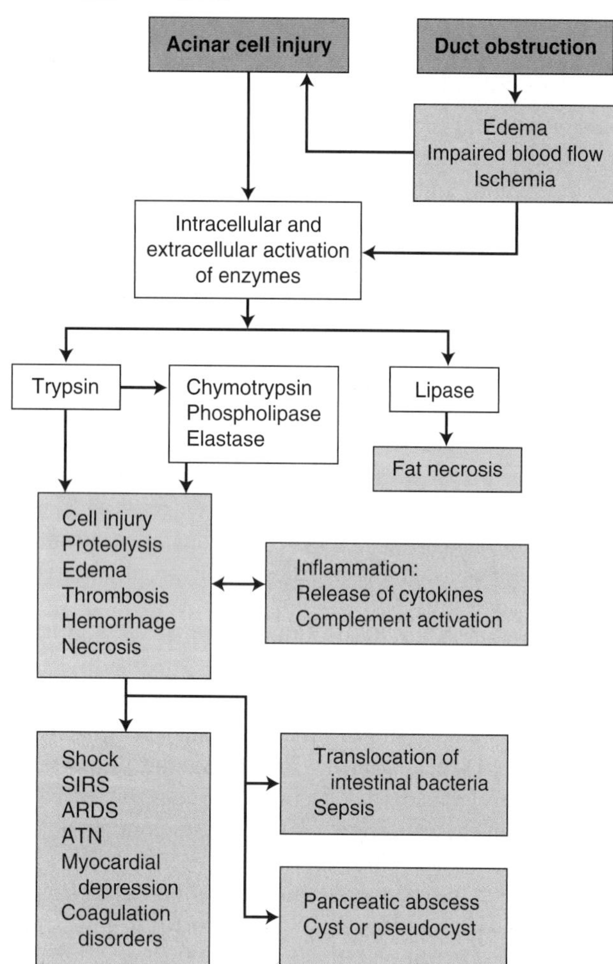

Fig. 41.21 Pathophysiology of Acute Pancreatitis. *ARDS*, Acute respiratory distress syndrome; *ATN*, acute tubular necrosis; *SIRS*, systemic inflammatory response syndrome.

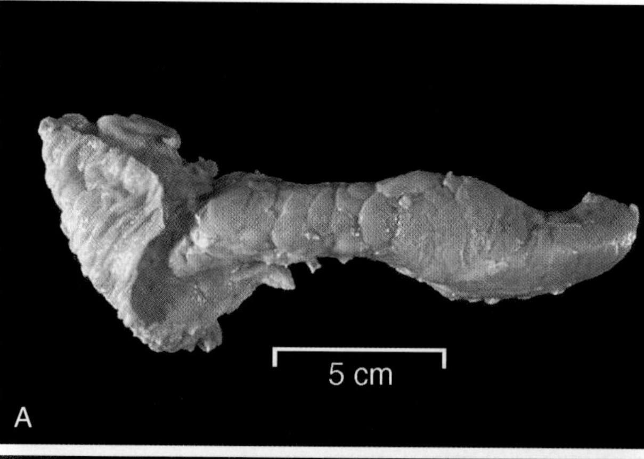

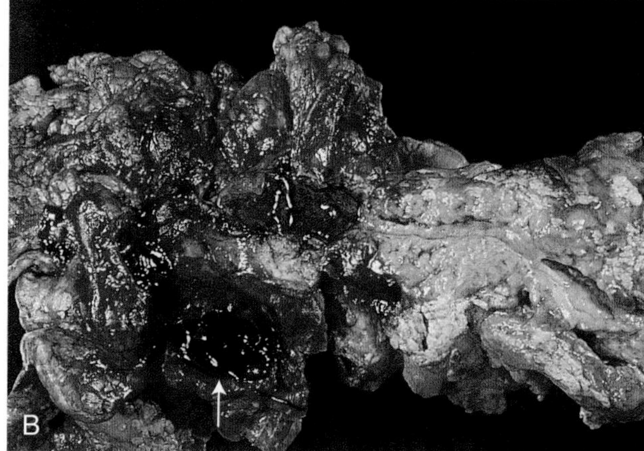

Fig. 41.22 Acute Severe Pancreatitis With Hemorrhage. **(A)** Normal pancreas. **(B)** Acute hemorrhagic pancreatitis. The pancreas has hemorrhage, fat necrosis *(white patches)*, and a pseudocyst filled with blood *(white arrow)*. (A, From Klatt EC. *Robbins and Cotran atlas of pathology*. Philadelphia: Elsevier; 2021. B, From Damjanov I, Linder J, eds. *Pathology: A color atlas*. St. Louis: Mosby; 2000.)

obstruction of the bile duct (e.g., a gallstone) or from pancreatic edema pressing on the duct. Abdominal distention accompanies bowel hypomotility and the accumulation of fluids in the peritoneal cavity. Hypovolemia, hypotension, tachycardia, myocardial insufficiency, and shock occur because plasma volume is lost as inflammatory mediators released into the circulation increase vascular permeability and dilate vessels. Tachypnea and hypoxemia develop secondary to ascites, pulmonary edema, atelectasis, or pleural effusions. Hypovolemia can decrease renal blood flow sufficiently to impair renal function and can cause renal failure. Tetany may develop as a result of hypocalcemia when calcium is deposited in areas of fat necrosis or as a decreased response to parathormone. Transient hyperglycemia also can occur if glucagon is released from damaged alpha cells in the pancreatic islets. In severe acute pancreatitis, some individuals develop flank or periumbilical ecchymosis, a sign of a poor prognosis. Multiple organ failure or SIRS accounts for most deaths of those with severe acute pancreatitis (Fig. 41.22).

Evaluation and Treatment. The diagnosis is based on clinical findings, identification of associated disorders, laboratory studies, and imaging results. The revised Atlanta classification (RAC) is used to guide diagnosis and requires two of the three following criteria be present: (1) abdominal pain suggestive of pancreatitis, (2) serum amylase and/or lipase greater than 3 times the upper limit of normal, and (3) and cross-sectional imaging (CT or MRI) findings consistent with acute pancreatitis.[145] An elevated direct bilirubin and/or alkaline phosphatase level or transabdominal ultrasound may indicate the presence of an obstructing gallstone.

The goal of treatment for acute pancreatitis is to stop the process of autodigestion and prevent systemic complications. Parenteral fluids are essential to restore blood volume, maintain perfusion, and prevent hypotension and shock. Narcotic medications may be needed to relieve pain. Epidural anesthesia was used successfully with reduced mortality in one multicenter study, but more evaluation is needed before use as routine care.[146] To decrease pancreatic secretions, oral food and fluids may be withheld initially and continuous gastric suction instituted. Nasogastric suction may not be necessary with mild pancreatitis, but it helps to relieve pain and prevent paralytic ileus in individuals who are nauseated and vomiting. Enteral feeding is usually initiated within 24 to 72 hours if ileus is not present. In severe pancreatitis, enteral nutrition with use of nasogastric or nasojejunal feeding usually is well tolerated, may decrease pancreatic enzyme secretion, prevents gut bacterial overgrowth, and maintains gut barrier function. In the presence of ileus, parenteral nutrition is started within 72 hours.[147] Drugs that decrease gastric acid production (e.g., H_2 receptor antagonists) can decrease stimulation of the pancreas by secretin. Antibiotics are used if there is documented infection.[148] Research is in progress to develop agents that target the intracellular mechanism of pancreatic injury, particularly intracellular calcium regulation.[139] The risk of mortality increases significantly with the development of infection or pulmonary, cardiac, and renal complications.

Chronic Pancreatitis

Chronic pancreatitis is a process of progressive fibrotic destruction and irreversible scarring of the pancreas. Multiple forms of the disease exist, but chronic alcohol abuse is the most common cause due to chronic changes in the structure of the pancreas related to repeated exacerbations of pancreatitis. Obstruction from gallstones, smoking, hypertriglyceridemia, and genetic factors increase the risk of chronic pancreatitis[149]; however, the disease may also be idiopathic. Toxic metabolites and chronic release of inflammatory cytokines contribute to the destruction of acinar cells and islets of Langerhans. The pancreatic parenchyma is destroyed and replaced by fibrous tissues, strictures, calcification, ductal obstruction, and pseudocysts. The cysts are walled-off areas or pockets of pancreatic juice, necrotic debris, or blood within or adjacent to the pancreas.

Continuous or intermittent abdominal pain and weight loss are common and reduce quality of life. The pain is difficult to manage, involves both peripheral and central pain sensitization (see Chapter 16), and is associated with inflammation induced by increased intraductal pressure, acinar cell injury, and parenchymal ischemia.[150] There are elevations in serum and urine pancreatic amylase and lipase, and imaging findings show pseudocysts and alterations in pancreatic structure. Manifestations of pancreatic enzyme deficiency, such as steatorrhea or a malabsorption syndrome, are present in late stages of chronic pancreatitis. To correct enzyme deficiencies and prevent malabsorption and malnutrition, oral enzyme replacements are taken before and during meals. Loss of islet cells can cause insulin-dependent diabetes and requires treatment. Osteoporosis is common in chronic pancreatitis and is related to smoking, alcohol abuse, low vitamin D, maldigestion, and malnutrition.[151] Hypocalcemia can develop from the autodigestion of mesenteric fat by pancreatic enzymes and release of free fatty acids, which form calcium salts (soaps). Transient hypoparathyroidism, and hypomagnesaemia can also contribute to hypocalcemia associated with pancreatitis.[144] Cessation of alcohol intake and smoking is essential for the management of both acute and chronic pancreatitis. Endoscopic or surgical drainage of cysts or partial resection of the pancreas may be required to relieve pain and to prevent cystic rupture. Total pancreatectomy with autologous islet cell transplant (TPAIT) may be considered for relief of intractable pain and to prevent postoperative diabetes mellitus.[152] Chronic pancreatitis is a risk factor for pancreatic cancer and requires screening.[153,154]

RISK FACTORS

Esophageal Cancer

- Age older than 50 years
- Male
- White race
- Tobacco use
- Alcoholism
- Dietary factors: deficiencies of trace elements and vitamins
- Malnutrition associated with poor economic conditions or special dietary habits (e.g., very hot drinks, fish preserved in lye; diet deficient in fruits and vegetables)
- Gastroesophageal reflux with dysplasia
- Sliding hiatal hernia
- Obesity
- Family history of barrett esophagus or esophageal adenocarcinoma

CANCER OF THE DIGESTIVE SYSTEM

Cancer of the Gastrointestinal Tract

Table 41.10 presents information on the various GI cancers by organ, percentage of deaths compared with all cancer deaths, risk factors, type of cell, and common manifestations. The biology of cancer is presented in Chapter 12.

Cancer of the Esophagus

Carcinoma of the esophagus is a rare type of cancer with an estimated incidence of 17,650 new cases and 16,080 deaths in the United States in 2019.[155]

Risk factors are summarized in the box Risk Factors: Esophageal Cancer.

Pathophysiology. Carcinoma of the esophagus includes squamous cell carcinoma and adenocarcinoma, which is more prevalent in the United States. Squamous cell carcinomas are more common in the thoracic and cervical areas of the esophagus and are associated with smoking tobacco and chronic alcohol consumption. Adenocarcinomas are associated with chronic GERD.[156] **BE** is the known precursor to adenocarcinoma. Normal squamous epithelium of the distal esophagus is replaced by specialized columnar epithelium with intestinal metaplasia, the precancerous lesion. The disease then progresses through stages from intestinal metaplasia (nondysplastic BE [NDBE]), to low-grade dysplasia (LGD), to high-grade dysplasia (HGD), to intramucosal carcinoma, and finally to invasive adenocarcinoma.[157] Both genomic and epigenomic events are associated with esophageal cancers, and mutation of the *TP53* gene and aberrant DNA methylation are early events, although the genetic landscape is diverse. The *CagA*-positive strain of *H. pylori* may be protective against esophageal carcinoma.[158] The tendency for early metastasis is related to the superficial nature of the esophageal lymphatics and the lack of symptoms until late stages of tumor progression.

Clinical Manifestations. The two frequent symptoms of esophageal carcinoma are chest pain and dysphagia. The most common type of pain is heartburn. It is initiated by eating spicy or highly seasoned foods and by assuming the recumbent position. Odynophagia (pain on swallowing) may be initiated by

TABLE 41.10 **Cancer of the Gut, Liver, and Pancreas**

Organ	Proportion of All Cancer Deaths[a]	Risks	Cell Type	Common Manifestations
Esophagus	2.6%	Malnutrition Alcohol Tobacco Chronic reflux	Squamous cell Adenocarcinoma	Chest pain Dysphagia
Stomach	1.8%	Salty food Fried red meat Nitrates-nitrosamines	Adenocarcinoma Squamous cell	Anorexia Malaise Weight loss Upper abdominal pain Vomiting Occult blood
Colon/rectum	8.7%	Polyps Long-term inflammatory bowel disease Diverticulitis Diets high in fat and refined carbohydrates; low in fiber	Adenocarcinoma (left colon grows as ring; right colon grows as mass)	Pain Mass Anemia Bloody stool Obstruction Distention
Liver	5.0%	HBV, HCV, HDV Cirrhosis Intestinal parasite Aflatoxin from moldy peanuts and corn	Hepatomas Cholangiomas	Pain Anorexia Bloating Weight loss Portal hypertension Ascites Jaundice
Pancreas	7.9%	Chronic pancreatitis Cigarette smoking Alcohol (?) Diabetic women	Adenocarcinoma (exocrine part of gland, ductal epithelium)	Weight loss Weakness Nausea Vomiting Abdominal pain Depression ± jaundice May have insulin-secreting tumors with symptoms of hypoglycemia

HBV, Hepatitis B virus; *HCV,* hepatitis C virus; *HDV,* hepatitis D virus.
[a]The percentage of all cancer deaths combined.
From the *Cancer Facts & Figures 2019.* Atlanta, GA: American Cancer Society; 2019. https://www.cancer.org/content/dam/cancer-org/research/cancer-facts-and-statistics/annual-cancer-facts-and-figures/2021/cancer-facts-and-figures-2021.pdf.

the swallowing of cold liquids. Some individuals with esophageal cancer complain of a constant retrosternal pain that radiates to the back. Dysphagia (difficulty swallowing) is usually pressure-like and may radiate posteriorly between the scapulae. Dysphagia usually progresses rapidly. Esophageal carcinoma is asymptomatic during the early stages and presents at an advanced stage. Esophageal cancer metastasizes rapidly and therefore has a poor prognosis.

Evaluation and Treatment. The stepwise progression of BE underlies the rationale for screening. Individuals who have BE risk factors are screened with an endoscopic evaluation, with biopsy if the endoscopic appearance of the distal esophagus is consistent with BE.[159] Noninvasive screening procedures have been developed, including the use of a cytosponge on a string combined with a biomarker for use in primary care settings (Cytosponge-TFF3 test).[160] Endoscopic ablative therapy is recommended for individuals with BE and LGD or HGD. Endoscopic ultrasound and CT studies of the thorax are also used for diagnosis and staging. Prevention of gastroesophageal reflux and removal of HGD are essential to the management of BE. Once-daily PPIs are recommended for chemoprevention of BE. Aspirin, and nonaspirin antiinflammatory drugs and statins may be used in selected cases to prevent HGD and adenocarcinoma.[161] It is impossible to remove all lymph nodes with the tumor, but removal of the primary lesion and the local lymph nodes can benefit the individual with esophageal cancer. If the malignancy has not spread beyond these sites, cure is likely. However, if metastasis has occurred, an incomplete resection is of little survival benefit. Treatment is combined radiation and chemotherapy.

Cancer of the Stomach

The incidence of gastric cancer is estimated at 27,510 new cases and 11,140 deaths in the United States in 2019.[155] Most cases are adenocarcinoma. Squamous cell carcinoma is very rare and accounts for only a small percentage of all gastric carcinomas. Nonenvironmental risk factors include a family history of gastric adenocarcinoma; mutations in tumor suppressor and DNA repair genes, epigenetic modulation, type A atrophic gastritis (autoimmune); pernicious anemia, which is associated with atrophy of the gastric mucosa in the same locations where gastric tumors arise. Environmental factors include *H. pylori* infection, diet, alcohol consumption, smoking, and Epstein-Barr virus (EBV)-associated gastric carcinoma in some individuals; however, the mechanism is unknown.

Pathophysiology. Gastric adenocarcinomas are associated with the many virulence factors associated with *H. pylori* infection and progresses from chronic gastritis to atrophic gastritis, intestinal metaplasia to dysplasia and intestinal-type gastric cancer. *H. pylori* generally colonizes the pyloric antrum. *H. pylori* also causes gastric B-cell mucosa-associated lymphoid tissue lymphoma (see Box 41.1). Most adenocarcinomas are sporadic and associated with consumption of heavily salted and preserved foods (e.g., nitrates in pickled or salted foods such as bacon), a low intake of fruits and vegetables, and the use of tobacco and alcohol. Dietary salt enhances the conversion of nitrates to carcinogenic nitrosamines in the stomach. Salt and nitrates converted to nitrites are caustic to the stomach, delay gastric emptying, and can cause chronic atrophic gastritis. Insufficient acid secretion by the atrophic mucosa creates a relatively alkaline environment that permits bacteria to multiply and act on nitrates. The resulting increase in nitrosamines damages the DNA of mucosal cells, further promoting metaplasia and neoplasia. Gastric adenocarcinoma usually begins in the glands of the proximal or distal stomach mucosa. Different cell types, tumor locations, and molecular subtypes contribute to the heterogeneity of gastric adenocarcinoma.[162] Duodenal reflux also may contribute to an intestinal-like metaplasia. The reflux contains caustic bile salts that destroy the mucosal barrier that normally protects the stomach. There are two types of gastric cancer, intestinal and diffuse. Intestinal is associated with the inflammation of *H. pylori* infection and other environmental factors, and diffuse is related to familial gene mutations.[163,164]

Clinical Manifestations. The early stages of gastric cancer are generally asymptomatic or produce vague symptoms such as loss of appetite, malaise, and indigestion. Later manifestations of advanced gastric cancer include unexplained weight loss, upper abdominal pain, vomiting, change in bowel habits, and anemia caused by persistent occult bleeding. The prognosis is poor because symptoms do not occur until the tumor has spread and caused distant metastases, particularly to the liver and peritoneal structures. In general, the first manifestations of carcinoma are caused by distant metastases, and the disease is already in an advanced stage (Fig. 41.23).

Evaluation and Treatment. No specific biomarkers have been identified for gastric cancer, and often it is at an advanced stage when diagnosed. Direct endoscopic visualization, lavage, and cellular examination or biopsy and imaging are used to establish the diagnosis and for staging. Screening and treatment for *H. pylori* infection constitute the best preventive approach to gastric cancer but must be done before dysplasia and metaplasia develop. Eradication of *H. pylori* has been shown to significantly reduce the risk of gastric cancer.[165] Chemotherapy and endoscopic resection are the usual treatment for early stages of disease, including lymphadenectomy, although recurrence is common. Staging is determined by histologic findings after resection. Liquid biopsy identifies molecular characteristics of the tumor and guides therapy.[164] Early diagnosis and chemotherapy, combined with radiation, improve the postsurgical outcomes. Because of the diverse cell types and molecular mechanisms involved in gastric cancer, there is resistance to the effectiveness of chemotherapy treatment (see Box 41.5). Survival at 5 years for localized disease is approximately 70% and for distant metastasis is approximately 6%.[166]

Cancer of the Small Intestine

Small intestine carcinoma is rare, with 11,790 estimated new cases and 1960 estimated deaths in 2022.[155] Adenocarcinoma is the most common tumor type usually occurring in the duodenum, followed by well-differentiated neuroendocrine tumors (most common in the ileum), sarcomas, and lymphomas. Carcinoma occurs more frequently in Familial adenomatous polyposis and CD. Symptoms are nonspecific and develop when there is obstruction (anorexia, nausea and vomiting, abdominal distention, weight loss). Tumors are usually found incidentally during abdominal surgery or with imaging for other reasons. Screening includes imaging and endoscopic surveillance. Urinary evaluation of 5-hydroxyindoloacetic acid can assist

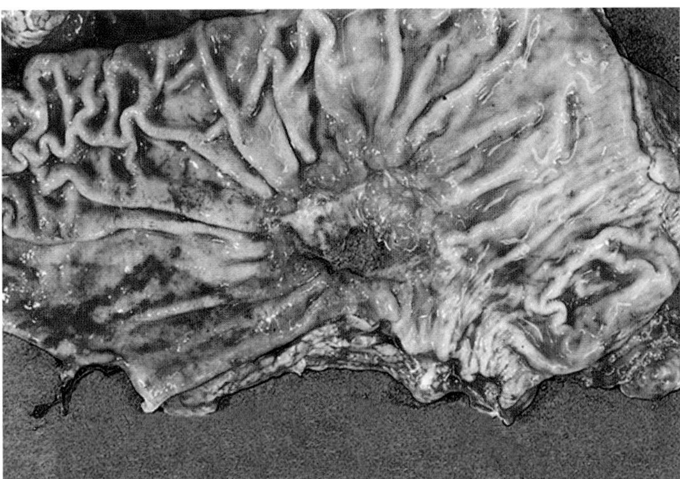

Fig. 41.23 Stomach Cancer. (From Patton KT. *Anatomy & physiology*, 10th edition. Elsevier; 2019.)

BOX 41.5 Mechanisms of Drug Resistance in Gastric Adenocarcinoma

Mechanisms proposed to reduce the effectiveness of chemotherapy for the treatment of gastric adenocarcinoma include:

- Reduced cellular drug uptake
- Enhanced drug efflux from cancer cells
- Impaired drug activation or active drug inactivation
- Spontaneous changes in molecular targets sensitive to anticancer drugs,
- Enhanced ability of cancer cells to repair drug-induced DNA damage
- Decreased function of proapoptotic factors versus upregulation of antiapoptotic genes
- Changes in the tumor cell microenvironment (blood vessels, immune cells, extracellular matrix) reducing the efficacy of antitumor agents
- Phenotypic transformations, including epithelial-mesenchymal transition (EMT) and the appearance of stemness characteristics (an ability of cells to transform into other cell types)

Data from Marin J, Perez-Silva L, Macias R, et al. Molecular bases of mechanisms accounting for drug resistance in gastric adenocarcinoma. *Cancers*, 2020;12(8):2116. https://doi.org/10.3390/cancers12082116.

RISK FACTORS

Cancer of the Colon and Rectum

- Advanced age
- Diet high in fat (especially egg consumption) and red and processed meats, low in fiber
- High consumption of alcohol
- Cigarette smoking
- Obesity
- Familial polyposis or family history of colorectal cancer
- Low levels of physical activity
- Inflammatory bowel disease
- Type 2 diabetes mellitus
- Black-American race/ethnicity

with diagnosis of well-differentiated neuroendocrine tumors. Treatment is surgical resection followed by tumor type–specific treatment.[167,168]

Cancer of the Colon and Rectum

CRC is the third most common cause of cancer and cancer death. An estimated 106,180 new cases of colon cancer and 54,040 new cases of rectal cancer, and 44,850 deaths, occurred in the United States in 2022.[155] The number of deaths has been declining over the past several years because of successful screening programs and diagnosis and treatment of *H. pylori* infection. CRC tends to occur in individuals older than 50 years, although the incidence is increasing in those younger than 50 years[169] and is rare in children. Risk factors for CRC can be reviewed in the box Risk Factors: Cancer of the Colon and Rectum. Regular use of aspirin and cyclooxygenase 2 (COX-2) selective inhibitors are associated with a decreased risk of CRC.[170]

Pathophysiology. Most CRCs are sporadic (acquired) or associated with a family history of CRC (approximately 5% to 10%). They are caused by multiple gene alterations and environmental interactions (see Chapter 6 for epigenetics and Chapter 12 for mechanisms of oncogenesis). Familial adenomatous polyposis (FAP) is a mutation of the *APC* gene (adenomatous polyposis coli, a tumor-suppressor gene) and is the most common hereditary cause of CRC. Hereditary nonpolyposis CRC (HNPCC), or Lynch syndrome, is associated with several DNA mismatch repair (MMR) genes. Both FAP and HNPCC have a rare, family-linked autosomal dominant inheritance trait that accounts for approximately 3% to 5% of CRCs.[171] Sporadic tumors are thought to involve the loss of function or mutation of tumor-suppressor genes and epigenetic modifiers. Understanding the molecular events associated with CRC is allowing more targeted detection, diagnosis, and prognosis prediction and more specific and personalized treatment approaches.[172] CRC begins with the formation of an adenoma, termed "tumor initiation." The progression to carcinoma is termed "tumor progression" and is a multistep process of genetic mutations that may take 8 to 10 years.

Colorectal polyps are closely associated with the development of cancer. A polyp, or papilloma, is a projection arising from the mucosal epithelium. The most common types of polyps are benign. However, adenomatous polyps are neoplastic (Fig. 41.24). The larger the polyp, the greater the risk of CRC. Although lesions larger than 1.5 cm occur less often, they are more likely to be malignant than those smaller than 1 cm. Thus screening colonoscopy with polypectomy is performed when polyps are found Neoplastic polyps are premalignant lesions that arise from aberrant crypt epithelial stem cells and grow and progress to CRC (Fig. 41.25). Over a period of 10 to 15 years there is progressive multistep cascade of genetic and epigenetic alterations that inactivate tumor-suppressor genes and activate oncogenes that lead to carcinoma and metastasis with a long preinvasive phase (Box 41.6 and Table 41.11).[173] There are distinct precursor lesion pathways, and they are summarized in Fig. 41.26. Because the lymphatic channels are located under the submucosae, the lesions must traverse this layer before the multistep process of metastasis can occur. Once the malignant cells of an adenoma traverse the submucosae, tumor cells enter the bloodstream and lymphatics and become invasive, spreading to other organs. However, adenomas can be detected early because the submucosa may not be penetrated for several years.

Clinical Manifestations. Symptoms of CRC depend on the location, size, and shape of the lesion and are silent in the early stages (Fig. 41.27). Tumors of the right (ascending) colon and left (descending) colon evolve into two distinct tumor types.[173] On the right side (proximal colon), the lesions extend along one wall of the cecum and ascending colon. These tumors may be silent, evolving to pain, a palpable mass in the lower right quadrant, iron deficiency anemia, fatigue, and dark red or mahogany-colored blood mixed with the stool. These tumors can become large and bulky with necrosis and ulceration, contributing to persistent blood loss and anemia. Obstruction is unusual because the growth does not readily encircle the colon. These tumors are more common in women and have a poorer prognosis with the occurrence of metastasis.

Tumors of the left, or descending, colon (distal colon) start as small, elevated, button-like masses and are more common in men. This type grows circumferentially, encircling the entire bowel wall and eventually ulcerating in the middle of the tumor as the tumor penetrates the blood supply. Obstruction is common but occurs slowly, and stools become

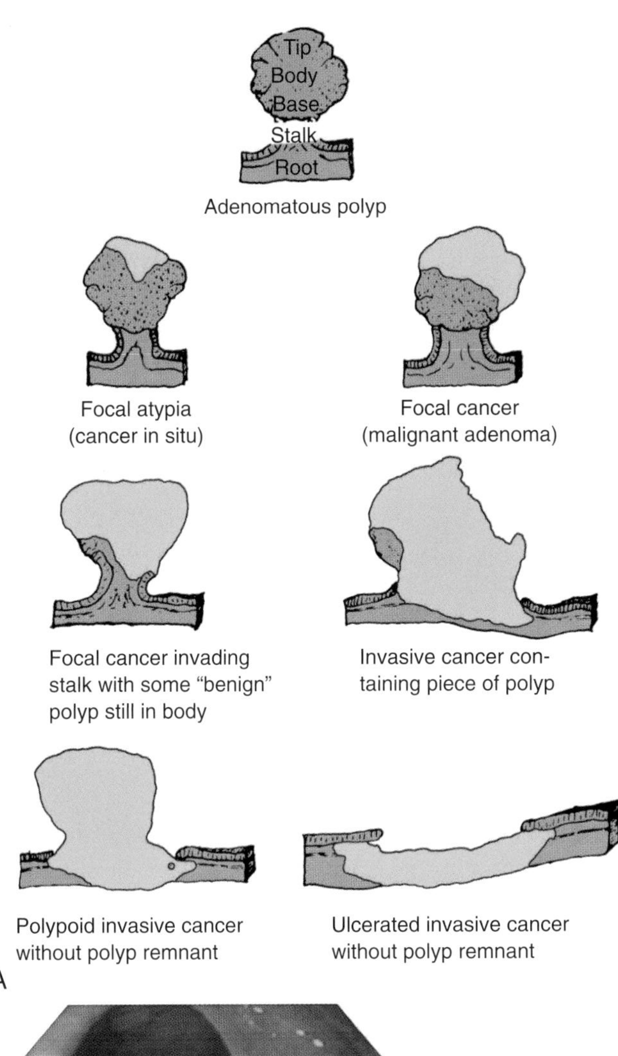

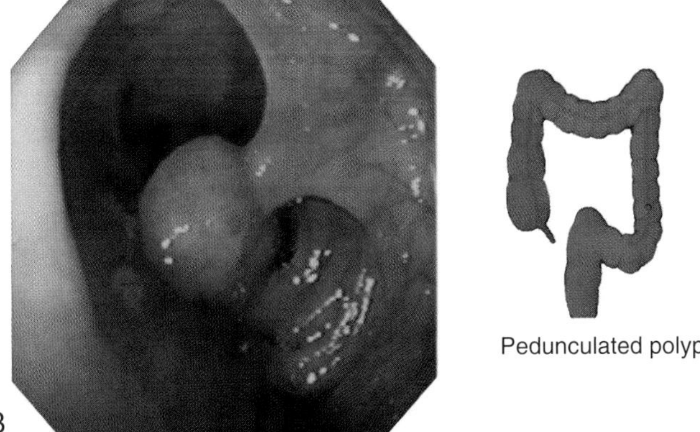

Fig. 41.24 Development of Cancer of the Colon From Adenomatous Polyps. (A) The tumor becomes invasive if it penetrates the muscularis mucosae and enters the submucosal layer. **(B)** Endoscopic image of pedunculated polyp in descending colon. (A, From del Regato JA, Spjut HJ, Cox JD. *Cancer: Diagnosis, treatment, and prognosis*, 2nd edition. St. Louis: Mosby; 1985. B, Courtesy David Bjorkman, MD, Department of Gastroenterology, University of Utah School of Medicine, Salt Lake City, UT.)

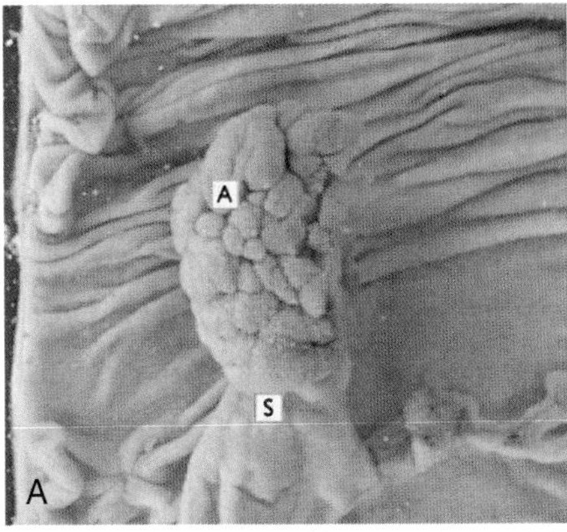

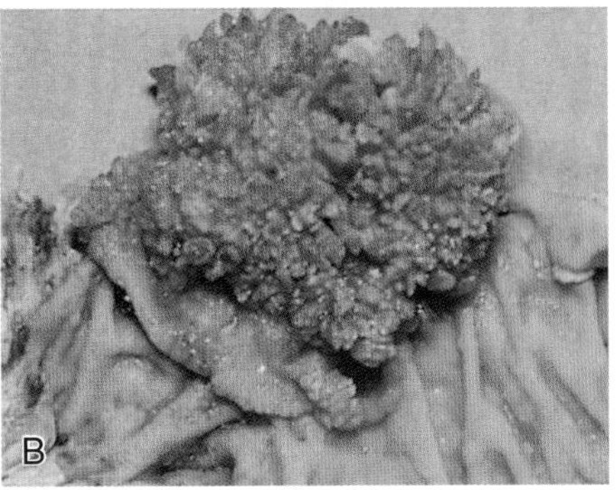

Fig. 41.25 Neoplastic Polyps. (A) Tubular adenomata *(A)* are rounded lesions 0.5 to 2 cm in size that are generally red and sit on a stalk *(S)* of normal mucosa that has been dragged up by traction of the polyp in the bowel lumen. **(B)** Villous adenomata are velvety lesions about 0.6 cm thick that occupy a broad area of mucosa generally 1 to 5 cm in diameter. (From Stevens A, et al. *Core pathology*, 3rd edition. London: Mosby; 2009.)

BOX 41.6 Common Genes Associated With Colorectal Cancer

APC (adenomatous polyposis coli): tumor suppressor; suppresses cell growth
TP53 (tumor protein 53): prevents gene mutations; a tumor suppressor gene
KRAS (V-Ki-ras2 Kirsten rat sarcoma viral oncogene homolog, proto-oncogene): promotes cell proliferation
BRAF (B-Raf proto-oncogene serine/threonine kinase): promotes cell proliferation
DCC (deleted in colon cancer): located at chromosome *18q*; tumor suppressor and apoptosis regulation
SMAD4 (Mothers against decapentaplegic homolog 4, proto-oncogene): promotes cell growth through TGF-β
TGF-β (transforming growth factor-beta): activates signaling pathways that facilitate tumor growth
EGFR (epidermal growth factor receptor): activates signaling pathways that facilitate tumor growth
COX-2 (cycloocygenase-2): promotes cell growth and inflammation.
BAX: promotes apoptosis and normal cell life cycle
DNA: (mismatch repair genes [hereditary nonpolyposis colorectal cancer/Lynch syndrome and some sporadic colorectal cancers]):
- *hMLH1* (human mutator homolog 1)
- *hMSH2* (human mutator S protein homolog 2)
- *hMSH6* (human mutator S homolog 6)
- *PMS2* (postmeiotic segregation increased 2)

LOH (loss of heterozygosity): loss of entire genome and surrounding chromosomal region narrow and pencil shaped. Manifestations include progressive abdominal distention, pain, vomiting, constipation, a need for laxatives, cramps, and bright red blood on the surface of the stool.

Systematic lymphatic distribution occurs along the aorta to the mesenteric and pancreatic lymph nodes. Liver metastasis is common and follows invasion of the mesenteric veins (left colon) or superior veins (right colon), which drain into the portal circulation.

Rectal carcinomas (approximately 20% of CRCs) are defined as tumors occurring up to 15 cm from the anal opening. Tumors of the rectum can spread through the rectal wall to nearby structures: the prostate in men and the vagina in women. Penetration occurs more readily in the lower third of the rectum because it has no serosal covering. Systemic and pulmonary metastases occur through the hemorrhoidal plexus, which drains into the vena cava.

Evaluation and Treatment. Individuals with hereditary polyposis should begin screening at an early age (10 to 12 years); colonoscopy should be used, with the removal of polyps when they are found. Specific, sensitive, and affordable molecular markers are being evaluated using liquid biopsy to assist with early diagnosis and evaluation of therapy. Carcinoembryonic antigen (CEA) is evaluated during and after cancer treatment.[174] Screening procedures for the detection of nonhereditary CRC are summarized in Box 41.7. Aspirin and celecoxib may reduce the incidence of CRC in the general population, but the risk of GI bleeding must be considered. Vitamin D, calcium, fiber, folate, dietary modification, weight control, exercise, and other nondietary lifestyle changes can reduce the risk of CRC.

The staging of CRC involves imaging and operative exploration. Physical examination of the abdomen detects liver enlargement and ascites; appropriate lymph nodes are palpated. Imaging is useful for pretreatment staging. Operative staging consists of careful exploration during surgery and biopsy of possible metastases. The National Cancer Institute's[175] tumor-node-metastasis (TNM) classification system is widely used for staging CRC (also see Chapter 12).

Treatment for all stages of cancer of the colon is surgical. Chemotherapy and radiation therapy may be given before surgery in the hope they will shrink the tumor or alter the malignant cells, or both, so that these cells will not survive after surgery. Resection and anastomosis can be performed for cancer of the ascending, transverse, descending, or sigmoid colon and upper rectum. These surgeries are performed through abdominal incisions and assisted with radiofrequency ablation. Natural defecation is preserved. Growths in the lower portion of the rectum require removal of the entire rectum with the formation of a permanent colostomy. Chemotherapy, including immunotherapy, is used to treat metastatic disease and cases with a high risk of recurrence. New therapeutic agents are improving personalized, first line therapy. Immunotherapy, vaccines, and viral vectors for the treatment of colon cancer are under continuing investigation (see Emerging Science Box: Colorectal Cancer).

TABLE 41.11 Conditions Commonly Confused With Colorectal Cancer

Condition	Significant Characteristics
Diverticulitis	Left-sided pain similar to that of appendicitis; tender lower left quadrant; associated findings: nausea, vomiting, fever, obstruction, anorexia, and leukocytosis; mucosa is intact, and perforation, peritonitis, and abscesses occur more often than in cancer; ultrasound, CT scan, MRI, and proctosigmoidoscopy are used to distinguish from cancer
Ulcerative colitis	Younger individuals with chronic attacks of bloody diarrhea, crampy abdominal pain, fever, malnutrition, and dehydration; usually involves the left colon and rectum; endoscopy, barium enema, and biopsy performed for definitive diagnosis
Crohn disease (granulomatous colitis)	Generally involves the right colon; chronic diarrhea with abdominal cramps, fever, weight loss, and often a palpable abdominal mass; difficult at times to distinguish Crohn disease from ulcerative colitis; endoscopic examination and CT scan used to distinguish from cancer
Appendicitis	Vague abdominal symptoms, often with a tender or nontender mass in the lower right quadrant; associated symptoms: mild fever and leukocytosis; CT scan used to distinguish cancer of the cecum from appendiceal abscess
Thrombosed hemorrhoids	Examination shows a tender, swollen, bluish painful mass in the anus; individual has a history of hemorrhoids

CT, Computed tomography; *MRI*, magnetic resonance imaging.

EMERGING SCIENCE BOX

Colorectal Cancer

Colorectal cancer (CRC) is heavily researched as advancements for ways to reduce risk of CRC, early detection, and effective treatment strategies are sought. In particular, advances continue to be made in targeted therapy for CRC. Targeted therapy drugs affect cancer cells specifically as opposed to general chemotherapy drugs that target healthy cells as well. Targeted therapy drugs are already being used to treat CRC, but researchers continue to examine new-targeted therapy drugs that are indicated after common gene mutations are tested. If there is a specific mutation in the *BRAF* gene; the drugs cetuximab and panitumumab may be helpful if administered with other targeted drugs. Some CRCs that have no gene mutations in *KRAS, NRAS,* and *BRAF* genes may respond well to treatment with targeted drugs trastuzumab and lapatinib or trastuzumab or pertuzumab. Vaccines for prevention of CRC are under investigation including those that target tumor cells, loading immune cells with immunostimulatory adjuvants, and genetic-based vaccines that allow antigen-presenting cells to carry antigen-specific fragments to cancer cells. Dendritic cell vaccines which prime T cells to release antiangiogenic mediators within tumor tissue are holding promise for advanced stages of CRC. Research is continuing for the advancement of these therapies and their use for the treatment of CRC.

Data from American Cancer Society. What's new in colorectal research? 2020. Obtained from www.cancer.org/cancer/colon-rectal-cancer/about/new-research.html); Chudasama R, et al. Vaccines in gastrointestinal malignancies: From prevention to treatment. *Vaccines*, 2021;9(6):647. https://doi.org/10.3390/vaccines9060647; Wooster AL, et al. Dendritic cell vaccine therapy for colorectal cancer. *Pharmacological Research*, 2021;164:105374.

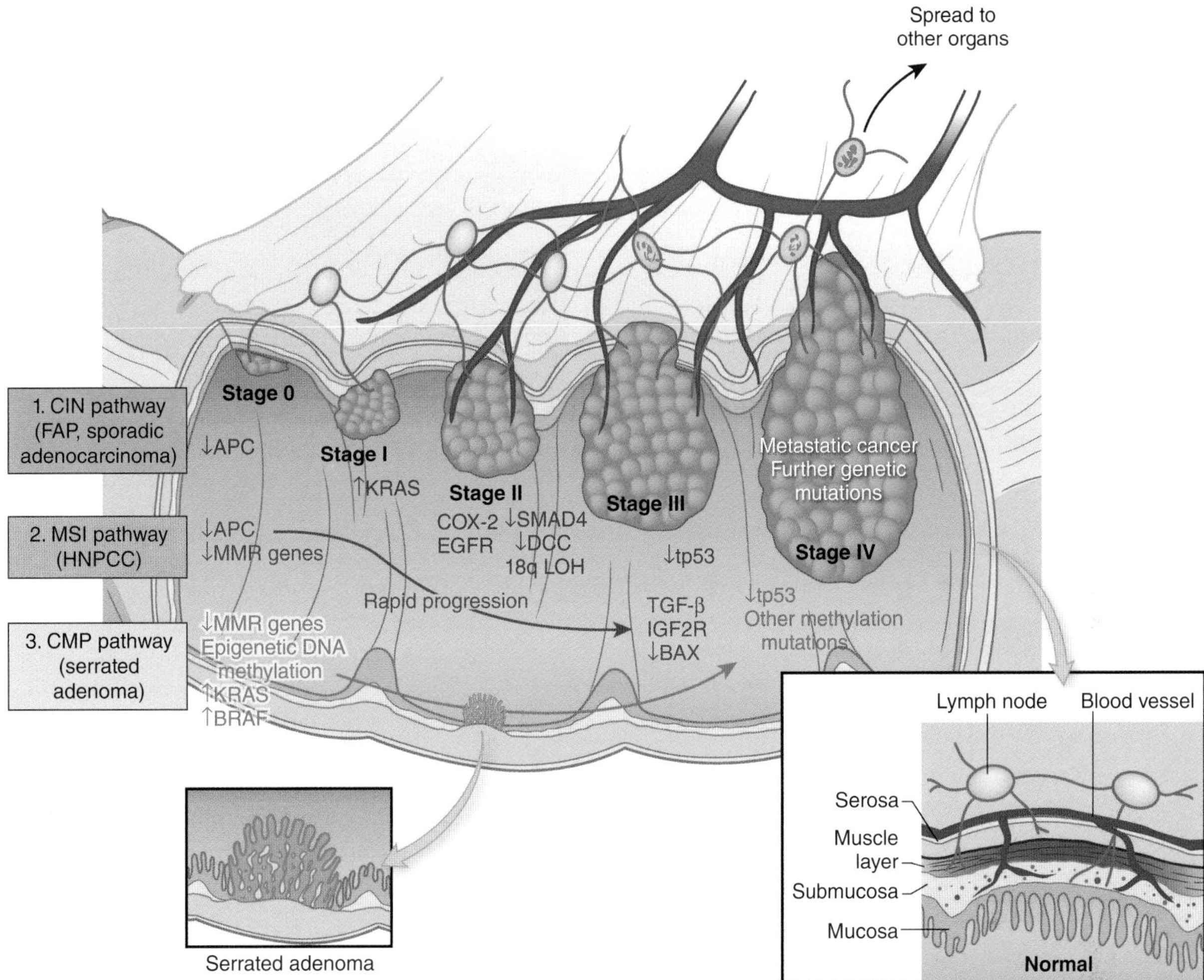

Fig. 41.26 Multistage Development of Colonic Cancer. Colorectal carcinoma develops from the sequential progression of genetic abnormalities in different pathways. These pathways overlap in many tumors. *1*, Most colonic cancers arise in the chromosomal instability (CIN) pathway with imbalances in chromosomal numbers (aneuploidy) and loss of heterozygosity. Abnormalities in oncogenes and tumor-suppressor genes activate the pathways for CRC initiation and progression. Mutations in the APC gene are the earliest known event and inactivation of APC accelerates cell cycle progression. K-ras (proto-oncogene) overexpression leads to loss of other tumor-suppressor genes SMAD4, DCC, and tp53 and transforms an adenoma into a metastatic carcinoma. tp53 loss occurs in about 35% to 45% of colorectal carcinomas and occurs less frequently in benign lesions. Growth factors cyclooxygenase 2 and epidermal growth factor receptor promote tumor growth and angiogenesis in response to inflammatory cytokines and proto-oncogenes. *2*, The microsatellite instability (MSI) pathway involves the epigenetic mutation of DNA mismatch repair (MMR) genes that encode key molecules that repair DNA, resulting in replication errors and deactivation of proteins from other downstream mutations (transforming growth factor-β, IGF2R, BAX). *3*, The epigenetic pathway, CpG island methylator phenotype (CIMP), involves early hypermethylation of DNA with gene silencing of MMR (i.e., MLH1, MSH2, MSH6). Proto-oncogenes KRAS and BRAF also are involved in this pathway. This pathway also can transform into the MSI pathway. NOTE: definitions for all abbreviations are listed in Box 41.4. (Adapted from Collins FC. *Advances in colorectal cancer research.* Bethesda, MD: National Institutes of Health; 2010. https://www.nih.gov/research-training/advances-colorectal-cancer-research.)

Resection of liver metastases or hepatic intra-arterial chemotherapy may prolong survival.

Cancer of the Accessory Organs of Digestion

Cancer of the Liver

Cancer of the liver is a leading cause of cancer death worldwide. The estimated number of new cases is 41,260 with 30,520 deaths in the United States in 2022.[155] Primary liver cancer is rare before the age of 40 years and is most common after 60 years. Cancer in the liver is usually caused by metastatic spread from a primary site elsewhere in the body. Risk factors for primary liver cancer are summarized in the box Risk Factors: Primary Liver Cancer. Risks associated with HBV and HCV infection are decreasing with antiviral therapy and HBV vaccination.

Pathophysiology. Primary carcinomas of the liver are hepatocellular or cholangiocellular. HCC is the most common (approximately 90% of liver cancers) and develops in hepatocytes. It can be nodular (consisting of multiple, discrete nodules), massive (consisting of a large tumor mass having satellite nodules),

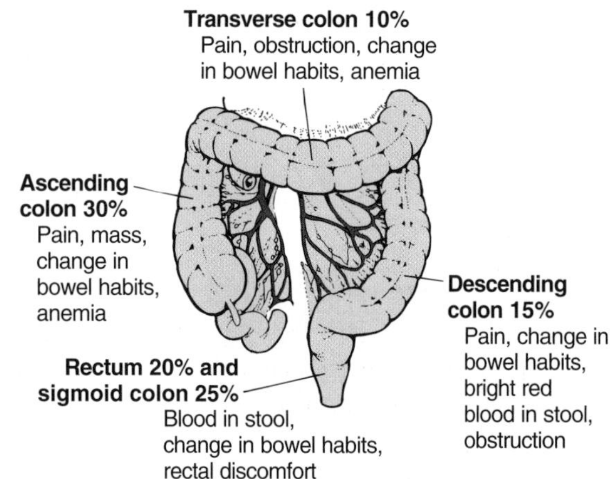

Fig. 41.27 Signs and Symptoms of Colorectal Cancer by Location of Primary Lesion. Clinical manifestations are listed under the order of frequency for each region.

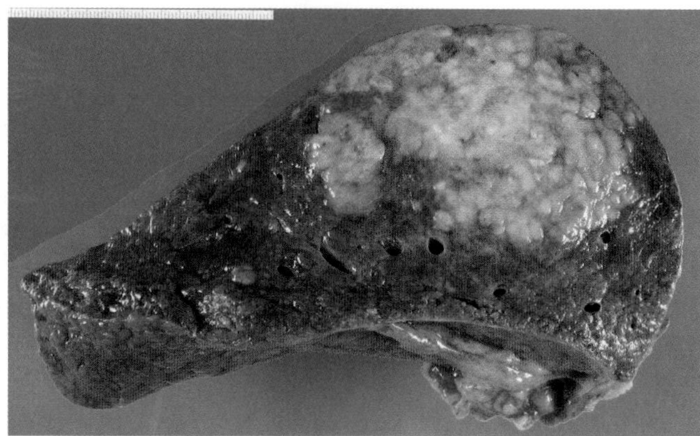

Fig. 41.28 Primary Hepatocellular Carcinoma. Macroscopically, hepatocellular carcinomas may be single or multifocal. They usually develop in a liver already affected by cirrhosis as shown in this image. Tumor appears as the light-colored mass within the top part of the liver. (From Connolly AJ, et al., eds. *Autopsy pathology: A manual and atlas*, 3rd edition. Philadelphia: Saunders; 2016.)

RISK FACTORS

Primary Liver Cancer

1. Infection and inflammation associated with HBV, HCV, and HDV, particularly in conjunction with cirrhosis, act either as a carcinogen or as a cocarcinogen in chronically infected hepatocytes;
2. Chronic alcoholic liver disease and nonalcoholic fatty liver disease that results in cirrhosis
3. Exposure to mycotoxins (e.g., aflatoxins), particularly those produced by *Aspergillus flavus*, a mold found on spoiled corn, peanuts, and grain; aflatoxins cause mutation of the *TP53* suppressor gene and activation of WNT signal transduction pathway
4. Long duration of heavy smoking (>20 years)
5. Hepatic iron overload (hemochromatosis)

BOX 41.7 Screening for Colorectal Cancer

Beginning at age 45, both asymptomatic men and women of average risk should follow one of these testing schedules:

- Yearly fecal occult blood test (gFOBT) with at least 50% sensitivity* *or*
- Yearly fecal immunochemical test (FIT) with at least 50% sensitivity,*
- Every 3 years: multitarget stool DNA test
- Flexible sigmoidoscopy every 5 years,
  Flexible sigmoidoscopy every 10 years + FIT every year
- Colonoscopy every 10 years

Data from US Preventive Services Task Force, Davidson KW, et al. Screening for colorectal cancer: US preventive services task force recommendation statement. *JAMA*, 2021;325(19):1965–1977.

or diffuse (consisting of small nodules distributed throughout most of the liver) (Fig. 41.28).[176] Chronic hepatitis B and hepatitis C and cirrhosis give rise to HCC repetitive cellular proliferation that occurs in the inflamed liver in response to alterations in immunity, growth factor and cytokine stimulation, oxidative stress–induced DNA damage, and incorporation HBV DNA in or near cancer-related genes. Numerous genetic and epigenetic alterations, including activation of oncogenes, failure of tumor-suppressor genes, and signaling pathways, combine to promote carcinogenesis.[177] NAFLD progressing to cirrhosis is a risk for HCC and may be related to metabolic syndrome, lipotoxicity, and chronic inflammation that promotes tumor angiogenesis.[178] There is extensive heterogeneity among individual risk factors and within tumor intrinsic factors, including numerous gene mutations, epigenetic modifications, and signaling molecule subclasses affecting growth and proliferation. This significant variability contributes to difficulty in prevention, early diagnosis, identification and selection of targeted treatment, and survival prognosis.[179] Because carcinoma of the liver invades the hepatic and portal veins, it often spreads to the heart and lungs. Other sites of metastases are the brain, kidney, and spleen.

Cholangiocellular carcinoma (cholangiocarcinoma) is rare (less than 1% of liver cancers) and develops in the bile ducts. It is associated with primary sclerosing cholangitis (a rare autoimmune disease often associated with UC) and is geographically associated with areas where parasitic liver fluke infestation is prevalent, such as Southeast Asia. Cholangiocellular carcinoma can occur anywhere along the bile duct and is often classified by where it is found (common bile duct, intrahepatic ducts, and in small ductules) and extend directly into the liver, usually as a solitary lesion. A combined form of HCC is known as combined (mixed) hepatocellular-cholangiocellular carcinoma. Chronic inflammation from autoimmune processes and parasitic fluke infestations are drivers of dysplasia and metaplasia. It is difficult to distinguish an invasion of cholangiocellular carcinoma from a metastatic adenocarcinoma except by neoplastic changes found in nearby ducts.[180]

Clinical Manifestations. HCC is usually asymptomatic. Manifestations are often nonspecific, can develop slowly or abruptly, and include vague abdominal symptoms, such as nausea and vomiting, fullness, pressure, a dull ache in the right upper abdominal area, and weight loss. In individuals with cirrhosis, deepening jaundice or abrupt lack of appetite is a sign of

HCC. Obstruction by the tumor can cause sudden worsening of portal hypertension and development of ascites. As the tumor enlarges, it causes pain. Cholangiocellular carcinoma is often silent in early stages and presents insidiously as pain, loss of appetite, weight loss, and gradual onset of jaundice. Some carcinomas of the liver rupture spontaneously, causing hemorrhage. Others are discovered accidentally during laboratory evaluation, imaging, or surgery for other diseases or trauma.

Evaluation and Treatment. There is no specific test for the diagnosis of liver cancer. For high-risk individuals, α-fetoprotein associated with HBV infection and abdominal ultrasound are common screening tools. Imaging is required for diagnosis supported by clinical manifestations, laboratory findings, and exploratory laparotomy. In individuals without cirrhosis, CT or ultrasonography is used to detect solid tumors, but neither can distinguish benign from malignant tumors. Biopsy is generally not performed because of risk for tumor seeding and bleeding. Several staging systems are available for HCC, including the TNM system and those that include liver function.[181]

Primary prevention may be achieved by vaccinating against HBV, preventing and treating HBV and HCV infection, screening all donated blood for the presence of HBV, and reducing contamination of food with aflatoxins.

Surgical resection for HCC and cholangiocarcinoma is possible only if the tumor is localized to a removable lobe of the liver. Surgery is hazardous and usually not undertaken if the individual has cirrhosis. Percutaneous or laparoscopic ablation and transplantation are effective for early stages of disease. Most individuals develop metastases after surgical resection, but long-term survival is possible. Chemoembolization, immunotherapy, and radiotherapy are treatment options. Targeted molecular therapy for HCC includes multikinase inhibitors (sorafenib is standard of care), anti-vascular endothelial growth factor (VEGF) antibodies (ramucirumab for second line therapy), immune checkpoint inhibitors, and combination therapies. Gene therapy and epigenic modulators are under investigation.[182] Cholangiocarcinoma is usually diagnosed at late stages and is unresectable. Systemic chemotherapy is palliative.[180] The prognosis for those with symptomatic liver cancer is poor.

Cancer of the Gallbladder

In 2022 in the United States, there were an estimated 12,130 new cases and 4400 deaths attributable to gallbladder cancer.[155] Risk factors include biliary reflux, gallstones, advancing age, female sex (2:1), obesity, anomalous pancreaticobiliary ductal junction, bacterial infection, and exposure to heavy metals. It occurs rarely before the age of 40 years and is most common between the ages of 65 and 75 years. Primary carcinoma of the gallbladder is the most common cancer of the biliary tree but is rare in the United States and associated with gallstones. Approximately 85% of people who develop gallbladder cancer have gallstones.[183] Most gallbladder cancer is caused by metastasis.

Pathophysiology. Most primary carcinomas of the gallbladder are adenocarcinomas and more rarely squamous cell carcinomas. It is the most aggressive of the biliary tract cancers, with a mean survival of approximately 2 years. The pathogenesis is not clear. Chronic inflammation due to exposure to gallstones and BA or infection may trigger genomic alterations, dysplasia, and progression to metaplasia. The molecular mechanisms involve mutation of several genes, including tumor-suppressor genes and oncogenes, DNA repair genes, and alterations in the extracellular matrix. Epigenetic modification, particularly DNA hypermethylation and hypomethylation of tumor suppressor genes and oncogenes, is common in gallbladder cancer, and its exact role in tumor initiation is under investigation.[184] Invasion of the liver and lymph nodes occurs early. Direct invasion of the stomach and the duodenum can cause pyloric obstruction, and infection often accompanies cancer of the gallbladder. Generalized peritonitis, gangrene, perforation, and liver abscesses are potential complications of infection.

Clinical Manifestations. Early stages of gallbladder carcinoma are asymptomatic, and the disease usually presents at an advanced stage. When symptoms develop, there is usually steady, upper right quadrant pain for approximately 2 months. Other manifestations include diarrhea, belching, weakness, loss of appetite, weight loss, and vomiting. Obstructive jaundice can occur if an enlarging tumor presses on the extrahepatic ducts and is a sign of an inoperable tumor.

Evaluation and Treatment. Early diagnosis of cancer of the gallbladder is rare and is often found incidentally. Therefore older adults with gallstones, particularly women, are evaluated for disease. Inflammatory disorders, such as cholangitis (bile duct inflammation) and peritonitis, often obscure an underlying malignancy. Diagnostic procedures include ultrasonography and further imaging with suspicious findings. Complete surgical resection of the gallbladder is the only effective treatment for early stages of disease, and recurrence is common. Complete removal of tumor tissue and lymph nodes with chemoradiation therapy is performed for more advanced stages. Because advanced malignancies cannot be resected, gallbladders containing stones are removed as a preventive measure. The prognosis of unresectable gallbladder cancer is extremely poor. Targeted molecular therapies, including epidermal growth factor receptor, fibroblast growth factor receptor, and VEGF receptor, and immune therapy using monoclonal antibodies are in clinical trials.[185]

Cancer of the Pancreas

Pancreatic cancer is the fourth leading cause of cancer deaths in the United States. An estimated 62,210 new cases and 49,830 deaths occurred in the United States in 2022.[155] The incidence of pancreatic cancer rises steadily with age, and it has been increasing in recent years. The cause of pancreatic cancer is not known, but there are modest risks associated with tobacco smoking, certain dietary factors (e.g., high-fat foods and processed meat), obesity, diabetes mellitus, chronic pancreatitis, family history of pancreatic cancer, Lynch syndrome gene mutation, and several oncogenic and tumor-suppressor gene mutations.[186]

Pathophysiology. Pancreatic cancer can arise from exocrine or endocrine cells. Most pancreatic tumors arise from metaplastic exocrine cells in the ducts and are called *pancreatic ductal adenocarcinomas;* they commonly arise from the head of the pancreas and are highly malignant. The *K-ras* oncogene is the most common gene mutation, and mutations also occur in tumor suppressor genes and DNA repair genes. Chronic pancreatitis and inflammatory cytokines support tumor growth. There is significant expansion of the extracellular matrix (stroma) from activation of stellate cells that contributes to therapeutic resistance. Tumors arising in small ducts invade nearby glandular tissue, penetrate the covering of the pancreas, and extend into surrounding tissues. Tumors of the head of the pancreas quickly spread to obstruct the common bile duct and portal vein (Fig. 41.29). These tumors can then infiltrate the superior mesenteric artery, the vena cava, and the aorta and form emboli. Tumors of the body and tail of the pancreas infiltrate the posterior abdominal wall. Lymphatic invasion occurs early and rapidly. Venous invasion causes metastases to the liver. Tumor implants on the peritoneal surface can obstruct veins and promote development of ascites. Tumors are staged using the TNM classification. Tumors of the endocrine pancreas are rare.

Clinical Manifestations. Early stages of pancreatic cancer are asymptomatic. When symptoms occur, there usually has been obstruction and a malignant transformation. Typically, vague upper abdominal pain that radiates to the back or shoulder develops. Nonspecific symptoms include lethargy, nausea, vomiting, bloating, and changes in bowel habits. Jaundice arises in most cases, usually caused by obstruction of the bile duct. Because obstruction impairs enzyme secretion and flow to the duodenum, pancreatic cancer causes fat and protein malabsorption, resulting in weight loss. Distant metastases are found in the cervical lymph nodes, the lungs, and the brain. Most individuals die of hepatic failure, malnutrition, or systemic diseases.

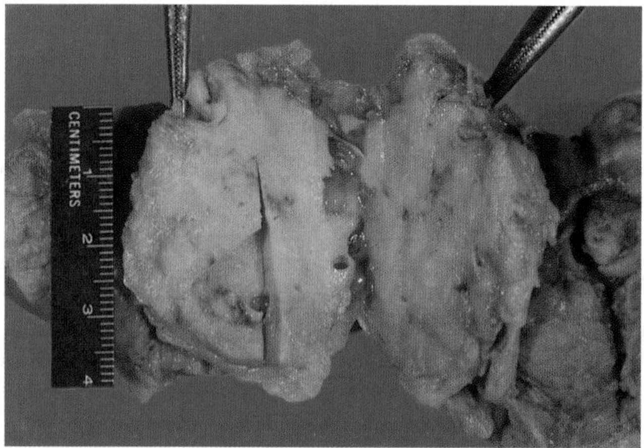

Fig. 41.29 Pancreatic Carcinoma. Adenocarcinoma of the head of pancreas. Pancreatic adenocarcinoma may arise in the head (60%), body (15%), or tail (5%) of the pancreas; in 20% of cases there is involvement of more than one segment. (From Connolly AJ, Finkbeiner WE, Ursell PC, et al. *Autopsy pathology: A manual and atlas*, 3rd edition. St. Louis: Elsevier; 2016.)

Evaluation and Treatment. The molecular pathogenic pathways associated with pancreatic cancer are very complex, and there is no specific biomarker for pancreatic cancer. Several molecular markers are under investigation, and molecular profiling can guide targeted treatment and monitor treatment response.[187] The relative rarity of the disease and vagueness of symptoms contribute to the late diagnosis. There is no specific biomarker for pancreatic cancer. The diagnosis is usually made after the tumor has spread and is nonresectable. CT and endoscopic ultrasound are used initially for diagnosis. Laparotomy is often used to establish a definitive diagnosis, evaluate the extent of disease, and determine whether palliative bypass surgery (i.e., cholecystojejunostomy and gastrojejunostomy) is needed. Pancreaticoduodenectomy (Whipple procedure) is performed to decompress duct obstruction. Many surgeons recommend a total pancreatectomy because cancer of the pancreas seldom consists of a single lesion. However, resection is difficult as the tumor often grows into adjacent large vessels. Adjuvant chemotherapy, immunotherapy, radiochemotherapy, and combination therapy may produce favorable controls in locally advanced cancer. There is no targeted therapy for the treatment of pancreatic cancer. Supportive therapy involves pain management, nutritional support, and an interdisciplinary team. Five-year survival is approximately 15% to 20% with resectable disease (a small subset) and less than 6% for metastatic disease. Screening is recommended for those with the highest risk factors, particularly those with a known family history. There is a need for new approaches for earlier diagnosis and more effective treatment.[188]

SUMMARY REVIEW

Disorders of the Gastrointestinal Tract

1. Anorexia (loss of appetite), vomiting, constipation, diarrhea, abdominal pain, and evidence of GI bleeding are clinical manifestations of many disorders and diseases of the GI tract.
2. Vomiting is the forceful emptying of the stomach effected by GI contraction and reverse peristalsis of the esophagus. It is usually preceded by nausea and retching, with the exception of projectile vomiting, which is associated with direct or indirect stimulation of the vomiting center in the brain.
3. Primary constipation is defined in three categories: functional, associated with low-residue, low-fluid diet; slow-transit, related to impaired colonic motor function; and IBS-C. Secondary constipation results from diet, neurogenic disorders and abdominal pain or muscle weakness, drugs that decrease intestinal motility, endocrine or metabolic disorders, or obstruction.
4. Diarrhea is three or more loose stools per day and can be acute, persistent, or chronic. It can be caused by excessive fluid drawn into the intestinal lumen by osmosis (osmotic

diarrhea), excessive secretion of fluids by the intestinal mucosa (secretory diarrhea), or excessive GI motility (motility diarrhea).
5. Abdominal pain is caused by stretching, inflammation, or ischemia and originates in the peritoneum (parietal pain) or in the abdominal organs (visceral pain). Visceral pain is often referred to the back.
6. GI bleeding can occur in the upper or lower GI tract. Obvious manifestations of GI bleeding are hematemesis (vomiting of blood), melena (dark, tarry stools), and hematochezia (frank bleeding from the rectum). Occult bleeding can be detected only by testing stools or vomitus for the presence of blood.
7. Dysphagia is difficulty in swallowing or perception of obstruction during swallowing. It can be caused by a mechanical obstruction or a functional neuromuscular disorder of esophageal motility.
8. Achalasia is a rare form of functional dysphagia caused by loss of esophageal innervation or relaxation of the LES that may be caused by and immune response to an unknown antigen.
9. GERD is the regurgitation of chyme from the stomach into the esophagus, causing esophagitis from repeated exposure to acids, enzymes, or bile salts in the regurgitated gastric contents. GERD is related to abnormalities in lower esophageal function, esophageal motility, and gastric motility or emptying and can cause reflux esophagitis.
10. EoE is an idiopathic chronic allergic/immune disease of the esophagus characterized by infiltration of eosinophils in the esophagus with inflammation.
11. Hiatal hernia is the protrusion of the upper part of the stomach through the hiatus (esophageal opening in the diaphragm) at the gastroesophageal junction. Hiatal hernia can be sliding, paraoesophageal, or mixed.
12. Gastroparesis is delayed gastric emptying in the absence of mechanical gastric outlet obstruction and involves abnormalities of the autonomic nervous system, smooth muscle cells, enteric neurons, and GI hormones.
13. Pyloric obstruction is the narrowing or blockage of the pylorus, which is the opening between the stomach and the duodenum. It can be caused by a congenital defect, inflammation and scarring secondary to a gastric ulcer, or tumor growth.
14. Intestinal obstruction can occur in the small or large intestine and prevents the normal movement of chyme through the intestinal tract. It is usually mechanical (i.e., caused by torsion, herniation, or tumor). Functional or pseudo-obstruction is caused by paralytic ileus and can be associated with abdominal surgery, intestinal infection, cardiac dysfunction, or hypokalemia.
15. The most severe consequences of intestinal obstruction or ileus are fluid and electrolyte losses, hypovolemia, shock, intestinal necrosis, and perforation of the intestinal wall.
16. Gastritis is an acute or a chronic inflammation of the gastric mucosa.
17. Regurgitation of bile, use of NSAIDs or alcohol, *H. pylori* infection, and some systemic diseases are associated with gastritis.
18. Chronic fundal gastritis (autoimmune gastritis) is rare and associated with autoantibodies to parietal cells and intrinsic factor, resulting in gastric atrophy and causing pernicious anemia.
19. Chronic antral gastritis is the most common and is associated with *H. pylori*, which stimulates gastrin secretion, and NSAIDs.
20. Alkaline reflux gastritis is stomach inflammation caused by the reflux of bile and pancreatic secretions from the duodenum into the stomach. These substances disrupt the mucosal barrier and cause inflammation.
21. A peptic ulcer is a circumscribed area of mucosal inflammation and ulceration caused by excessive secretion of gastric acid, disruption of the protective mucosal barrier, or both.
22. The three types of peptic ulcers are duodenal, gastric, and stress ulcers. Duodenal and gastric ulcers are associated with *H. pylori* infection and chronic use of NSAIDs.
23. Zollinger-Ellison syndrome is associated with a gastrin secreting gastrinoma, chronic secretion of gastric acid, and gastric and duodenal ulcers.
24. Duodenal ulcers, the most common peptic ulcers, are associated with increased numbers of parietal (acid-secreting) cells in the stomach, elevated gastrin levels, and rapid gastric emptying. Pain occurs when the stomach is empty, and pain is relieved with food or antacids. Duodenal ulcers tend to heal spontaneously and recur frequently.
25. Gastric ulcers develop near parietal cells, generally near the antrum, and tend to become chronic. Gastric secretions may be normal or decreased, and pain may occur after eating.
26. Stress ulcer (stress-related mucosal disease) is an acute form of peptic ulcer associated with severe illness or extensive trauma.
27. Ischemic stress ulcers develop suddenly after severe illness, systemic trauma, neural injury, or burns (Curling ulcer). Ulceration follows mucosal damage caused by ischemia (decreased blood flow to the gastric mucosa and hypersecretion of acid).
28. Cushing ulcer is a stress ulcer caused by head trauma. Ulceration follows hypersecretion of hydrochloric acid caused by overstimulation of the vagal nuclei.
29. Postgastrectomy syndromes are a group of signs and symptoms that occur after gastric resection for the treatment of peptic ulcer, gastric carcinoma, or bariatric surgery for extreme obesity. Dumping syndrome causes malabsorption by the rapid emptying of hypertonic chyme from the surgically created residual stomach into the small intestine. It causes an osmotic shift of fluid from the vascular compartment to the intestinal lumen, which decreases plasma volume and increases intestinal motility. Other syndromes include alkaline reflux gastritis, afferent loop obstruction, anemia, and bone and mineral disorders.

30. Malabsorption syndromes result in disruption of absorption of nutrients, and maldigestion is failure of the chemical process of digestion.
31. Pancreatic insufficiency causes maldigestion and malabsorption associated with insufficient amounts of the enzymes that digest protein, carbohydrates, and fats into components that can be absorbed by the intestine.
32. Lactase deficiency or production in the brush border of the small intestine inhibits the breakdown of lactose. This prevents lactose absorption and causes osmotic diarrhea.
33. Bile salt deficiency causes fat malabsorption, including fat-soluble vitamins, and steatorrhea (fatty stools). Bile salt deficiency can result from inadequate secretion of bile, excessive bacterial deconjugation of bile, or impaired reabsorption of bile salts caused by ileal disease.
34. UC is an IBD associated with immune dysregulation that causes ulceration, abscess formation, and necrosis of the colonic and rectal mucosa. Cramping pain, bleeding, frequent diarrhea, dehydration, and weight loss accompany severe forms of the disease. A course of frequent remissions and exacerbations is common.
35. CD is similar to UC, but it affects the entire GI tract, including the large and small intestines. Ulceration tends to involve all layers of the lumen. "Skip lesion" fissures and granulomas are characteristic of CD. Abdominal tenderness and pain, nonbloody diarrhea, and weight loss are the usual symptoms.
36. Microscopic colitis involves two histologic forms of the disease, lymphocytic and collagenous, with both resulting in frequent diarrhea but without ulceration.
37. IBS is a disorder of brain-gut interaction characterized by abdominal pain with altered bowel habits (diarrhea, constipation, or both).
38. Diverticula are outpouchings of colonic mucosa through the muscle layers of the colon wall. Diverticulosis is the presence of these outpouchings; diverticulitis is inflammation of the diverticula.
39. Appendicitis is caused by obstruction of the lumen leads to increased pressure, ischemia, and inflammation of the appendix. Without surgical resection, inflammation may progress to gangrene, perforation, and peritonitis.
40. Vascular insufficiency in the intestine is associated most often with acute or chronic occlusion or obstruction of the mesenteric vessels or insufficient mesenteric arterial blood flow. The resulting ischemia and necrosis produce abdominal pain, fever, bloody diarrhea, hypovolemia, and shock.

Disorders of the Accessory Organs of Digestion

1. Portal hypertension, ascites, hepatic encephalopathy, jaundice, and HRS are complications of many liver disorders.
2. Portal hypertension is an elevation of portal venous pressure to at least 10 mm Hg. It is caused by increased resistance to venous flow in the portal vein and its tributaries, including the sinusoids and hepatic vein.
3. Portal hypertension is the most serious complication of liver disease because it can cause fatal complications, such as bleeding varices, ascites, hepatic encephalopathy, and renal failure.
4. Varices are distended, tortuous, collateral veins associated with portal hypertension and can develop in the esophagus, stomach, abdominal wall, and rectum.
5. Splenomegaly is an enlargement of the spleen resulting from increased splenic vein pressure caused by portal hypertension.
6. HPS is pulmonary hypertension related to the release of vasodilators that effect pulmonary arterioles and is associated with portal hypertension and severe liver disease. PPH occurs with portal hypertension with arterial remodeling and increased arterial resistance.
7. Ascites is the accumulation and sequestration of fluid in the peritoneal cavity, often as a result of portal hypertension, decreased concentrations of plasma proteins, and sodium retention.
8. Hepatic encephalopathy (portal system encephalopathy) is impaired cerebral function caused by blood-borne toxins (particularly ammonia) not metabolized by the liver.
9. Jaundice (icterus) is a yellow or greenish pigmentation of the skin or sclera of the eyes caused by increases in plasma bilirubin concentration (hyperbilirubinemia).
10. Obstructive jaundice is caused by obstructed bile canaliculi (intrahepatic obstructive jaundice) or obstructed bile ducts outside the liver (extrahepatic obstructive jaundice). Bilirubin accumulates proximal to sites of obstruction, enters the bloodstream, and is deposited in the skin and other connective tissues.
11. Hemolytic jaundice is caused by destruction of red blood cells at a rate that exceeds the liver's ability to metabolize unconjugated bilirubin.
12. HRS is functional renal failure caused by advanced liver disease, particularly cirrhosis with portal hypertension. *Type 1 HRS-AKI* is caused by a decrease in blood flow to the kidneys that occurs in less than 2 weeks, usually as a result of massive GI hemorrhage or liver failure. *Type 2 HRS-NAKI* develops more slowly and is associated with ascites and decreased circulating blood volume. The predominant clinical manifestation is oliguria.
13. Acute liver failure can be caused by toxic overdose of acetaminophen, complications of viral hepatitis, or metabolic disorders that cause death of hepatocytes.
14. Autoimmune hepatitis may be caused by an autoimmune T cell–mediated inflammatory response with hypergammaglobulinemia, elevated transaminases, and absence of viral hepatitis. The disease may be mild or cause acute liver failure.
15. Cirrhosis is an irreversible inflammatory disease of the liver that develops slowly and causes disorganization of lobular structure, fibrosis, and nodular regeneration. Bile obstruction causes jaundice. Vascular obstruction causes portal hypertension, shunting, and varices. Cirrhosis can result from hepatitis or exposure to toxins, such as acetaldehyde (a product of alcohol metabolism). The disease causes progressive irreversible liver damage, usually over a period of years.

16. Alcoholic liver disease results from formation of acetaldehyde impairing the hepatocytes' ability to oxidize fatty acids, synthesize enzymes and proteins, degrade hormones, and clear portal blood of ammonia and toxins. The disease causes progressive fibrosis and includes steatosis, steatohepatitis, and alcoholic cirrhosis.
17. NAFLD is fat infiltration into hepatocytes, and NASH is inflammation of hepatocytes associated with obesity, hypertriglyceridemia, metabolic syndrome, and type 2 diabetes mellitus that can progress to liver failure.
18. Primary biliary cholangitis is an autoimmune disease with inflammatory destruction of intrahepatic bile ducts. Mitochondrial autoantibodies are found in this disease.
19. Secondary biliary cirrhosis develops from prolonged obstruction of bile flow (e.g., gallstones, tumors, chronic pancreatitis) with increased pressure in the hepatic bile ducts that causes pooling of bile and necrosis of tissue. Relief of obstruction alleviates symptoms of jaundice and pruritus. Continued obstruction causes cirrhosis and liver failure.
20. Viral hepatitis is an infection of the liver caused by strains of the hepatitis virus: HAV (fecal-oral transmission), HBV, HCV, HDV, and HEV (parenteral and sexual transmission). The hepatitis viruses can cause hepatic cell necrosis, Kupffer cell hyperplasia, and infiltration of liver tissue by mononuclear phagocytes. These changes obstruct bile flow and impair hepatocyte function.
21. The clinical manifestations of viral hepatitis depend on the type of virus and stage of infection. Fever, malaise, anorexia, and liver enlargement and tenderness characterize the prodromal phase (stage 1). Jaundice and hyperbilirubinemia mark the icteric phase (stage 2). During the recovery phase (stage 3), symptoms resolve. Recovery takes several weeks.
22. Chronic active hepatitis can occur with HBV and HCV with predisposition to cirrhosis and HCC.
23. Fulminant hepatitis is a complication of hepatitis B (with or without hepatitis D infection) or hepatitis C. It causes widespread hepatic necrosis and is often fatal.
24. Cholelithiasis (the formation of gallstones) is a result of bile aggregation of cholesterol crystals (cholesterol stones) or precipitates of unconjugated bilirubin (pigmented stones). Gallstones that fill the gallbladder or obstruct the cystic, or common, bile duct cause abdominal pain and jaundice.
25. Cholecystitis is an inflammation of the gallbladder. It is usually associated with obstruction of the cystic duct by gallstones.
26. Acute pancreatitis (pancreatic inflammation) is a serious but relatively rare disorder associated with biliary obstruction, toxic effects of alcohol, or unknown causes. Injury permits leakage of digestive enzymes into pancreatic tissue, where they become activated and begin the process of autodigestion, inflammation, and destruction of tissues. Release of pancreatic enzymes into the bloodstream or abdominal cavity causes damage to other organs.
27. Chronic pancreatitis is a process of progressive fibrotic destruction, irreversible scarring of the pancreas, and formation of pseudocysts resulting in functional impairment and commonly related to alcoholism or recurrent acute pancreatitis. It causes recurrent abdominal pain, digestive disorders, and malnutrition.

Cancer of the Digestive System

1. Cancer of the esophagus is rare and tends to occur in people older than 60 years. Alcohol and tobacco use, reflux esophagitis, radiation exposure, and nutritional deficiencies are associated with esophageal carcinoma. There are two types, squamous cell and adenocarcinoma, the most common. It is preceded by precancerous lesions known as BE, with progression from intestinal metaplasia to dysplasia to adenocarcinoma.
2. Dysphagia and chest pain are the primary manifestations of esophageal cancer. Early treatment of tumors that have not spread into the mediastinum or lymph nodes results in a better prognosis.
3. Gastric carcinoma is commonly an adenocarcinoma associated with *H. pylori (CagA)*, high salt intake, food preservatives (nitrates and nitrites), duodenal reflux, atrophic gastritis, and familial gene mutations.
4. Gastric cancers are commonly located in the prepyloric antrum. Clinical manifestations (weight loss, upper abdominal pain, vomiting, hematemesis, and anemia) develop only after the tumor has penetrated the wall of the stomach.
5. Cancer of the small intestine is rare and associated with FAP and CD. Tumors are usually found incidentally.
6. CRC is the third most common type of cancer and cancer death in the United States. FAP coli and HNPCC (or Lynch syndrome) are inherited forms of colon cancer. Preexisting large and numerous polyps are highly associated with sporadic (acquired) adenocarcinoma of the colon. Specific molecular pathways and gene mutations are associated with sporadic and familial CRCs.
7. Tumors of the right (ascending) colon are usually large and bulky; tumors of the left (descending, sigmoid) colon develop as small button-like masses. Manifestations of colon tumors include pain, bloody stools, and change in bowel habits.
8. Rectal carcinoma is located up to 15 cm from the opening of the anus. The tumor spreads transmurally to the vagina in women or to the prostate in men.
9. Metastatic invasion of the liver is more common than primary cancer of the liver.
10. Primary liver cancers are associated with chronic liver disease (cirrhosis and hepatitis B and C) and alterations in tumor suppressor genes and oncogenes. HCCs arise from the hepatocytes, whereas cholangiocellular carcinomas arise from the bile ducts. Primary liver cancer spreads to the heart, lungs, brain, kidney, and spleen through the circulation.
11. Cancer of the gallbladder is relatively rare and tends to occur in women older than 50 years. Adenocarcinoma is

most common. Because clinical manifestations occur late in the disease, metastases to lymph channels have usually occurred by the time of diagnosis, and the prognosis is poor.
12. Cancer of the pancreas represents approximately 2.6% of all cancers in the United States. Most tumors are adenocarcinomas that arise in the exocrine cells of ducts in the head, body, or tail of the pancreas. Symptoms may not be evident until the tumor has spread to surrounding tissues. Treatment is palliative, and mortality is nearly 100% for advanced tumors.

REFERENCES

1. Visvanathan R. Anorexia of aging. *Clin Geriatr Med.* 2015;31(3):417–427.
2. Landi F, et al. Anorexia of aging: assessment and management. *Clin Geriatr Med.* 2017;33(3):315–323.
3. Cox NJ, et al. New horizons in appetite and the anorexia of ageing. *Age Ageing.* 2020;49(4):526–534.
4. Heckroth M, et al. Nausea and vomiting in 2021: a comprehensive update. *J Clin Gastroenterol.* 2021;55(4):279–299.
5. Krogh K, Chiarioni G, Whitehead W. Management of chronic constipation in adults. *United European Gastroenterol J.* 2017;5(4):465–472.
6. Sharma A, Rao S. Constipation: pathophysiology and current therapeutic approaches. *Handb Exp Pharmacol.* 2017;239:59–74.
7. Vriesman MH, et al. Management of functional constipation in children and adults. *Nat Rev Gastroenterol Hepatol.* 2020;17(1):21–39.
8. Forootan M, Bagheri N, Darvishi M. Chronic constipation: a review of literature. *Medicine (Baltimore).* 2018;97(20):e10631.
9. Serrano Falcón B, et al. Fecal impaction: a systematic review of its medical complications. *BMC Geriatr.* 2016;16(4).
10. World Health Organization (WHO). *Diarrhoeal disease.* Geneva, Switzerland: WHO; 2017. Available at https://www.who.int/news-room/fact-sheets/detail/diarrhoeal-disease. (Accessed May 3, 2022).
11. Kelly L, Jenkins H, Whyte L. Pathophysiology of diarrhea. *Paediatr Child Health.* 2018;28(11):520–526.
12. Schiller LR, Pardi DS, Sellen JH. Chronic diarrhea: diagnosis and management. *Clin Gastroenterol Hepatol.* 2017;15(2):182–193.
13. Basso L, Bourreille A, Dietrich G. Intestinal inflammation and pain management. *Curr Opin Pharmacol.* 2015;25:50–55.
14. Coates MD, Vrana KE, Ruiz-Velasco V. The influence of voltage-gated sodium channels on human gastrointestinal nociception. *Neurogastroenterol Motil.* 2019;31(2):e13460.
15. Bindu S, Mazumder S, Bandyopadhyay U. Non- nonsteroidal antiinflammatory drugs (NSAIDS s (NSAIDs) and organ damage: a current perspective. *Biochem Pharmacol.* 2020;180:114147.
16. Cañamares-Orbís P, Lanas Arbeloa Á. New trends and advances in non-variceal gastrointestinal bleeding-series II. *J Clin Med.* 2021;10(14):3045.
17. Wilkins T, Wheeler B, Carpenter M. Upper gastrointestinal bleeding in adults: evaluation and management. *Am Fam Physician.* 2020;101(5):294–300. [Erratum in: *Am Fam Physician* 103(2):70, 2021.].
18. Laine L, et al. ACG clinical guideline: upper gastrointestinal and ulcer bleeding. *Am J Gastroenterol.* 2021;116(5):899–917.
19. Pesce M, Sweis R. Advances and caveats in modern achalasia management. *Ther Adv Chronic Dis.* 2021;12 2040622321993437.
20. Chen J, Brady P. Gastroesophageal reflux disease pathophysiology, diagnosis, and treatment. *Gastroenterol Nurs.* 2019;42(1):20–28.
21. Maret-Ouda J, Markar SR, Lagergren J. Gastroesophageal reflux disease: a review. *JAMA.* 2020;324(24):2536–2547.
22. American Academy of Allergy Asthma & Immunology (AAAAI). *Eosinophilic esophagitis (EoE).* Milwaukee, WI: AAAAI; 2020. Revised February 24, 2020. Available at https://www.aaaai.org/conditions-and-treatments/related-conditions/eosinophilic-esophagitis. (Accessed May 3, 2022).
23. Kohn G, et al. SAGES Guidelines Committee: Guidelines for the management of hiatal hernia. *Surg Endosc.* 2013;27(12):4409–4428. Available at https://www.sages.org/publications/guidelines/guidelines-for-the-management-of-hiatal-hernia/. (Accessed May 3, 2022).
24. Rochefort M, Wee JO. Management of the difficult hiatal hernia. *Thorac Surg Clin.* 2018;28(4):533–539.
25. Sullivan A, Temperley L, Ruban A. Pathophysiology, aetiology and treatment of gastroparesis. *Dig Dis Sci.* 2020;65(6):1615–1631.
26. Camilleri M, et al. Clinical guideline: management of gastroparesis. *Am J Gastroenterol.* 2013;108(1):18–37.
27. Longley KJ, Ho V. Practical management approach to gastroparesis. *Intern Med J.* 2020;50(8):909–917.
28. Castellanos A. *Gastric outlet obstruction treatment & management.* New York: Medscape Medical News, WebMD LLC; 2020. Updated April 29, 2022. Available at https://emedicine.medscape.com/article/190621-treatment#d9. (Accessed May 3, 2022).
29. Ten Broek RPG, et al. Bologna guidelines for diagnosis and management of adhesive small bowel obstruction (ASBO): 2017 update of the evidence-based guidelines from the World Society of Emergency Surgery ASBO working group. *World J Emerg Surg.* 2018;13:24.
30. Gore RM, et al. Bowel obstruction. *Radiol Clin North Am.* 2015;53(6):1225–1240.
31. Vasant DH, Lal S. Recent advances in the management of severe gastrointestinal dysmotility. *Clin Exp Gastroenterol.* 2021;14:163–172.
32. Kapoor V. *Postoperative ileus.* New York: Medscape Medical News, WebMD LLC; 2021. Updated November 1, 2021. Available at https://emedicine.medscape.com/article/2242141-overview. (Accessed May 3, 2022).
33. Paulson EK, Thompson WM. Review of small bowel obstruction; the diagnosis and when to worry. *Radiology.* 2015;275(2):332–342.
34. Haj M, Haj M, Rockey D. Ogilvie's syndrome: management and outcomes. *Medicine (Baltimore).* 2018;97(27):e11187.
35. Iiban O, et al. Neostigmine treatment protocols applied in a acute colonic pseudo-obstruction disease: a retrospective study. *Turk J Gastroenterol.* 2018;30(3):228–233.
36. Rugge M, et al. Gastritis: the clinico-pathological spectrum. *Dig Liver Dis.* 2021;53(10):1237–1246.
37. Lenti MV, et al. Autoimmune gastritis. *Nat Rev Dis Primers.* 2020;6(1):56.
38. Varbanova M, Frauenschlager K, Malfertheiner P. Chronic gastritis—an update. *Best Pract Res Clin Gastroenterol.* 2014;28(6):1031–1042.
39. Conti L, Annibale B, Lahner E. Autoimmune gastritis and gastric microbiota. *Microorganisms.* 2021;8(11):1827.

40. Liou JM, et al. Asian Pacific Alliance on Helicobacter and Microbiota (APAHAM): Screening and eradication of *Helicobacter pylori* for gastric cancer prevention: the Taipei global consensus. *Gut*. 2020;69(12):2093–2112.
41. Dore MP, Pes GM. What is new in Helicobacter pylori diagnosis. In: An overview. *J Clin Med*. 2021;10(10):2091.
42. Huang RJ, Hwang JH. Improving the early diagnosis of gastric cancer. *Gastrointest Endosc Clin N Am*. 2021;31(3):503–517.
43. Malik TF, Gnanapandithan K, Singh K. Peptic ulcer disease. In: *StatPearls*. Treasure Island, FL: StatPearls Publishing; 2021. Updated July 29, 2021. Available at https://www.ncbi.nlm.nih.gov/books/NBK534792/. (Accessed May 3, 2022).
44. Shao QQ, et al. Surgical management of Zollinger-Ellison syndrome: classical considerations and current controversies. *World J Gastroenterol*. 2019;25(32):4673–4681.
45. Lanas A, Chan FKL. Peptic ulcer disease. *Lancet*. 2017;390(10094):613–624.
46. Graham DY. History of *Helicobacter pylori*, duodenal ulcer, gastric ulcer and gastric cancer. *World J Gastroenterol*. 2014;20(18):5191–5204.
47. Crowe S. *Peptic ulcer disease (beyond the basics)*. Waltham, MA: UpToDate Inc.; 2020. Literature review current through October 2021. Last updated April 29, 2022. Available at https://www.uptodate.com/contents/peptic-ulcer-disease-beyond-the-basics. (Accessed May 3, 2022).
48. Dore MP, Pes GM. What is new in *Helicobacter pylori* diagnosis. An overview. *J Clin Med*. 2021;10(10):2091.
49. Chey WD, et al. Correction: ACG clinical guideline: treatment of Helicobacter pylori infection. *Am J Gastroenterol*. 2018;113(7):1102 [Erratum for *Am J Gastroenterol* 112(2):212–239, 2017.].
50. Cheung KS, Leung WK. Long-term use of proton-pump inhibitors and risk of gastric cancer: a review of the current evidence. *Therap Adv Gastroenterol*. 2019;12:1756284819834511.
51. Toews I, et al. Interventions for preventing upper gastrointestinal bleeding in people admitted to intensive care units. *Cochrane Database Syst Rev*. 2018;6:CD008687.
52. Davis JL, Ripley RT. Postgastrectomy syndromes and nutritional considerations following gastric surgery. *Surg Clin North Am*. 2017;97(2):277–293.
53. Toninello P, et al. Nutritional support for bariatric surgery patients: the skin beyond the fat. *Nutrients*. 2021;13(5):1565.
54. Phillips ME, et al. Consensus for the management of pancreatic exocrine insufficiency: UK practical guidelines. *BMJ Open Gastroenterol*. 2021;8(1):e000643.
55. Misselwitz B, et al. Update on lactose malabsorption and intolerance: pathogenesis, diagnosis and clinical management. *Gut*. 2019;68(11):2080–2091.
56. Johnston I, et al. New insights into bile acid malabsorption. *Curr Gastroenterol Rep*. 2011;13(5):418–425.
57. Camilleri M, Vijayvargiya P. The role of bile acids in chronic diarrhea. *Am J Gastroenterol*. 2020;115(10):1596–1603.
58. Crohn's and Colitis Foundation of America. *Fact sheet—about IBD*. New York: Author; 2019. Available at: https://www.crohnscolitisfoundation.org/sites/default/files/2019-02/Updated%20IBD%20Factbook.pdf.
59. Guan Q. A comprehensive review and update on the pathogenesis of inflammatory bowel disease. *J Immunol Res*. 2019;2019:7247238.
60. Linson EA, Hanauer SB. Epidemiology of colorectal cancer in inflammatory bowel disease—the evolving landscape. *Curr Gastroenterol Rep*. 2021;23(9):16.
61. Ungaro R, et al. Ulcerative colitis. *Lancet*. 2017;389(10080):1756–1770.
62. Du L, Ha C. Epidemiology and pathogenesis of ulcerative colitis. *Gastroenterol Clin North Am*. 2020;49(4):643–654.
63. Jansen FM, et al. Clinical management of the most common extra-intestinal manifestations in patients with inflammatory bowel disease focused on the joints, skin, and eyes. *United European Gastroenterol J*. 2020;8(9):1031–1044.
64. Ben Ghezala I, et al. Small molecule drugs in inflammatory bowel diseases. *Pharmaceuticals (Basel)*. 2021;14(7):637.
65. Rabbenou W, Chang S. Medical treatment of pouchitis: a guide for the clinician. *Therap Adv Gastroenterol*. 2021;14:17562848211023376.
66. Gajendran M, et al. A comprehensive review and update on Crohn's disease. *Dis Mon*. 2018;64(2):20–57.
67. Petagna L, et al. Pathophysiology of Crohn's disease inflammation and recurrence. *Biol Direct*. 2020;15(1):23.
68. Colia R, Corrado A, Cantatore FP. Rheumatologic and extraintestinal manifestations of inflammatory bowel disease. *Ann Med*. 2016;48(8):577–585.
69. Caio G, et al. Nutritional treatment in Crohn's disease. *Nutrients*. 2021;13(5):1628.
70. Tome J, Kamboj AK, Pardi DS. Microscopic colitis: a concise review for clinicians. *Mayo Clin Proc*. 2021;96(5):1302–1308.
71. Videlock EJ, Chang L. Latest insights on the pathogenesis of irritable bowel syndrome. *Gastroenterol Clin North Am*. 2021;50(3):505–522.
72. American College of Gastroenterology. *Irritable Bowel Syndrome*. Bethesda, MD: American College of Gastroenterology; 2021. Available at https://gi.org/topics/irritable-bowel-syndrome/#. (Accessed May 3, 2022).
73. Khlevner J, Park Y, Margolis KG. Brain-gut axis: clinical implications. *Gastroenterol Clin North Am*. 2018;47(4):727–739.
74. Lacy BE, et al. ACG Clinical Guideline: management of irritable bowel syndrome. *Am J Gastroenterol*. 2021;116(1):17–44.
75. Shapiro JM, Deutsch JK. Complementary and alternative medicine therapies for irritable bowel syndrome. *Gastroenterol Clin North Am*. 2021;50(3):671–688.
76. Wan D, Krisko T. Diverticulosis, diverticulitis, and diverticular bleeding. *Clin Geriatr Med*. 2021;37(1):141–154.
77. Copeland E, Jones A. Diverticular disease and diverticulitis: causes symptoms and treatment. *Pharm J*. May, 2019 Available at https://pharmjdev.wpengine.com/article/ld/diverticular-disease-and-diverticulitis-causes-symptoms-and-treatment. (Accessed May 3, 2022).
78. Walker MM, Harris AK. Pathogenesis of diverticulosis and diverticular disease. *Minerva Gastroenterol Dietol*. 2017;63(2):99–109.
79. Peery AF, Shaukat A, Strate LL. AGA clinical practice update on medical management of colonic diverticulitis: expert review. *Gastroenterology*. 2021;160(3). 906–911.e1.
80. Craig S. *Appendicitis*. New York: Medscape Medical News, WebMD LLC; 2018. Updated July 23, 2018. Available at https://emedicine.medscape.com/article/773895-overview#a7. (Accessed May 3, 2022).
81. Bhangu A, et al. Acute appendicitis: modern understanding of pathogenesis, diagnosis, and management. *Lancet*. 2015;386(10000):1278–1287.
82. Salminen P, et al. Five-year follow-up of antibiotic therapy for uncomplicated acute appendicitis in the APPAC randomized clinical trial. *JAMA*. 2018;320(12):1259–1265.

83. Wagner M, Tubre DJ, Asensio JA. Evolution and current trends in the management of acute appendicitis. *Surg Clin North Am.* 2018;98(5):1005–1023.
84. Mohamed I, et al. Appendicitis as a manifestation of colon cancer: should we image the colon after appendectomy in patients over the age of 40 years? *Int J Colorectal Dis.* 2019;34(3):527–531.
85. Bobadilla JL. Mesenteric ischemia. *Surg Clin North Am.* 2013;93(4):925–940. ix.
86. Ehlert BA. Acute gut ischemia. *Surg Clin North Am.* 2018;98(5): 995–1004.
87. Reintam Blaser A, Acosta S, Arabi YM. A clinical approach to acute mesenteric ischemia. *Curr Opin Crit Care.* 2021;27(2): 183–192.
88. Sardar P, White CJ. Chronic mesenteric ischemia: diagnosis and management. *Prog Cardiovasc Dis.* 2021;65:71–75.
89. Misra V, Agrawal R, Misra SP. Portal hypertensive vasculopathy—an entity worth remembering with non-neoplastic gastrointestinal lesions. *Indian J Pathol Microbiol.* 2021;64(Supplement):S32–S42.
90. Tayyem O, et al. Evaluation and management of variceal bleeding. *Dis Mon.* 2018;64(7):312–320.
91. Thomas C, et al. Portopulmonary hypertension: from bench to bedside. *Front Med (Lausanne).* 2020;7:569413.
92. Vuille-Lessard É, Rodrigues SG, Berzigotti A. Noninvasive detection of clinically significant portal hypertension in compensated advanced chronic liver disease. *Clin Liver Dis.* 2021;25(2):253–289.
93. Pfisterer N, Unger LW, Reiberger T. Clinical algorithms for the prevention of variceal bleeding and rebleeding in patients with liver cirrhosis. *World J Hepatol.* 2021;13(7):731–746.
94. Gallo A, et al. Optimal management of cirrhotic ascites: a review for internal medicine physicians. *J Transl Int Med.* 2020;8(4):220–236.
95. Häussinger D, et al. Pathomechanisms in hepatic encephalopathy. *Biol Chem.* 2021;402(9):1087–1102.
96. Rudler M, et al. Diagnosis and management of hepatic encephalopathy. *Clin Liver Dis.* 2021;25(2):393–417.
97. Hoilat GJ, et al. Polyethylene glycol versus lactulose in the treatment of hepatic encephalopathy: a systematic review and meta-analysis. *BMJ Open Gastroenterol.* 2021;8(1):e000648.
98. Fargo MV, Grogan SP, Saguil A. Evaluation of jaundice in adults. *Am Fam Physician.* 2017;95(3):164–168.
99. Subedi A, et al. A review of hepatorenal syndrome. *Cureus.* 2021;13(7):e16084.
100. Simonetto DA, Gines P, Kamath PS. Hepatorenal syndrome: pathophysiology, diagnosis, and management. *BMJ.* 2020;370:m2687.
101. Gupta K, et al. Acute kidney injury and hepatorenal syndrome in cirrhosis. *World J Gastroenterol.* 2021;27(26):3984–4003.
102. Chiew AL, et al. Interventions for paracetamol (acetaminophen) overdose. *Cochrane Database Syst Rev.* 2018;2:CD003328.
103. Tandon R, Froghi S. Artificial liver support systems. *J Gastroenterol Hepatol.* 2021;36(5):1164–1179.
104. Mieli-Vergani G, et al. Autoimmune hepatitis. *Nat Rev Dis Primers.* 2018;4:18017.
105. Centers for Disease Control and Prevention (CDC). *Chronic liver disease and cirrhosis.* Atlanta, GA: CDC; 2021. Last updated January 5, 2022. Available at https://www.cdc.gov/nchs/fastats/liver-disease.htm. (Accessed May 3, 2022).
106. American Liver Foundation. *Cirrhosis of the Liver.* West Orange, NJ: American Liver Foundation; 2021. Last updated March 30, 2022. Available at https://liverfoundation.org/for-patients/about-the-liver/diseases-of-the-liver/cirrhosis/#facts-at-a-glance. (Accessed May 3, 2022).
107. Zhou WC, Zhang QB, Qiao L. Pathogenesis of liver cirrhosis. *World J Gastroenterol.* 2014;20(23):7312–7324.
108. Ge PS, Runyon BA. Treatment of patients with cirrhosis. *N Engl J Med.* 2016;375(8):767–777.
109. Saleem S, et al. Morbidity and mortality of infections in the cirrhotic patients: a US population-based study. *Gastroenterol Hepatol Bed Bench.* 2019;12(3):233–238. 2019.
110. Centers for Disease Control and Prevention (CDC). *Chronic Liver Disease and Cirrhosis.* Atlanta, GA: CDC; 2021. Page last reviewed January 5, 2022. Available at https://www.cdc.gov/nchs/fastats/liver-disease.htm. (Accessed May 3, 2022).
111. Kamran U, et al. Nutrition in alcohol-related liver disease: physiopathology and management. *World J Gastroenterol.* 2020;26(22):2916–2930.
112. Cederbaum I. Alcohol metabolism. *Clin Liver Dis.* 2012;16: 667–685.
113. Robinson KE, Shah VH. Pathogenesis and pathways: nonalcoholic fatty liver disease & alcoholic liver disease. *Transl Gastroenterol Hepatol.* 2020;5:49.
114. Crabb DW, et al. NIAAA Alcoholic Hepatitis Consortia: Standard definitions and common data elements for clinical trials in patients with alcoholic hepatitis: recommendation from the NIAAA Alcoholic Hepatitis Consortia. *Gastroenterology.* 2016;150(4):785–790.
115. Sehrawat TS, Liu M, Shah VH. The knowns and unknowns of treatment for alcoholic hepatitis. *Lancet Gastroenterol Hepatol.* 2020;5(5):494–506.
116. Wong VWS, et al. Noninvasive biomarkers in NAFLD and NASH—current progress and future promise. *Nat Rev Gastroenterol Hepatol.* 2018;15(8):461–478.
117. Idalsoaga F, et al. Non-alcoholic fatty liver disease and alcohol-related liver disease: two intertwined entities. *Front Med (Lausanne).* 2020;7:448.
118. Lassailly G, et al. Bariatric surgery provides long-term resolution of nonalcoholic steatohepatitis and regression of fibrosis. *Gastroenterology.* 2020;159(4):1290–1301.e5.
119. Powell EE, Wong VW, Rinella M. Non-alcoholic fatty liver disease. *Lancet.* 2021;397(10290):2212–2224.
120. Mazzetti M, et al. The management of cholestatic liver diseases: current therapies and emerging new possibilities. *J Clin Med.* 2021;10(8):1763.
121. Prokopič M, Beuers U. Management of primary sclerosing cholangitis and its complications: an algorithmic approach. *Hepatol Int.* 2021;15(1):6–20.
122. Centers for Disease Control and Prevention (CDC). *Viral Hepatitis; Widespread Person-To-Person Outbreaks of Hepatitis A Across the United States.* Atlanta, GA: CDC; 2021. Page last reviewed May 2, 2022. Available at https://www.cdc.gov/hepatitis/outbreaks/2017March-HepatitisA.htm. (Accessed May 3, 2022).
123. Centers for Disease Control and Prevention (CDC). *Viral hepatitis surveillance report United States, 2019.* Atlanta, GA: CDC; 2021. Page last reviewed May 19, 2021. Available at https://www.cdc.gov/hepatitis/statistics/2019surveillance/index.htm. (Accessed May 3, 2022).
124. Wang M, Feng Z. Mechanisms of hepatocellular injury in hepatitis A. *Viruses.* 2021;13(5):861.
125. Khatun M, Ray RB. Mechanisms underlying hepatitis C virus-associated hepatic fibrosis. *Cells.* 2019;8(10):1249.

126. El-Serag HB, et al. The effects of sustained virological response to direct-acting anti-viral therapy on the risk of extrahepatic manifestations of hepatitis C infection. *Aliment Pharmacol Ther.* 2019;49(11):1442–1447.
127. Easterbrook PJ, et al. Diagnosis of viral hepatitis. *Curr Opin HIV AIDS.* 2017;12(3):302–314.
128. World Health Organization (WHO). *Combating Hepatitis B and C to Reach Elimination by 2030: Advocacy Brief.* Geneva, Switzerland: WHO; 2016. Available at https://apps.who.int/iris/handle/10665/206453. (Accessed May 3, 2022).
129. Zhang W, et al. A focused review on recent advances in the diagnosis and treatment of viral hepatitis. *Gastroenterology Res.* 2021;14(3):139–156.
130. Centers for Disease Control and Prevention (CDC). *Viral Hepatitis; Outbreaks of Hepatitis A are Occurring Across the United States.* Atlanta, GA: CDC; 2020. Page last reviewed October 19, 2020. Available at https://www.cdc.gov/hepatitis/outbreaks/HepAOutbreaks.htm. (Accessed May 3, 2022).
131. Heuman D, Mihas A, Allen J. *Gallstones (cholelithiasis).* New York: Medscape Medical News, WebMD LLC; 2019. Updated April 1, 2019. Available at https://emedicine.medscape.com/article/175667-overview#a5. (Accessed May 3, 2022).
132. Stinton LM, Shaffer EA. Epidemiology of gallbladder disease: cholelithiasis and cancer. *Gut Liver.* 2012;6(2):172–187.
133. Lammert F, et al. Gallstones. *Nat Rev Dis Primers.* 2016;2:16024.
134. Lam R, et al. Gallbladder disorders: a comprehensive review. *Dis Mon.* 2021;67(7):101130.
135. Gutt C, Schläfer S, Lammert F. The treatment of gallstone disease. *Dtsch Arztebl Int.* 2020;117(9):148–158.
136. Chung AY, Duke MC. Acute biliary disease. *Surg Clin North Am.* 2018;98(5):877–894.
137. Garg SK, et al. Incidence, admission rates, and predictors, and economic burden of adult emergency visits for acute pancreatitis. *J Clin Gastroenterol.* 2019;53(3):220–225.
138. Wan J, et al. The role of neutrophils and neutrophil extracellular traps in acute pancreatitis. *Front Cell Dev Biol.* 2021;8:565758.
139. Pallagi P, et al. Intracellular Ca2+ signalling in the pathogenesis of acute pancreatitis: recent advances and translational perspectives. *Int J Mol Sci.* 2020;21(11):4005.
140. Giri B, et al. Heat shock protein 70 in pancreatic diseases: friend or foe. *J Surg Oncol.* 2017;116(1):114–122.
141. Tran QT, et al. Role of bile acids and bile salts in acute pancreatitis: from the experimental to clinical studies. *Pancreas.* 2021;50(1):3–11.
142. Barrera K, et al. Acinar cell injury induced by inadequate unfolded protein response in acute pancreatitis. *World J Gastrointest Pathophysiol.* 2018;9(2):37–46.
143. Li J, et al. Calcium signaling of pancreatic acinar cells in the pathogenesis of pancreatitis. *World J Gastroenterol.* 2014;20(43):16146–16152.
144. Ahmed A, et al. Hypocalcemia in acute pancreatitis revisited. *Indian J Crit Care Med.* 2016;20(3):173–177.
145. Banks PA, et al. Acute Pancreatitis Classification Working Group: Classification of acute pancreatitis–2012: revision of the Atlanta classification and definitions by international consensus. *Gut.* 2013;62(1):102–111.
146. Jabaudon M, et al. Thoracic epidural analgesia and mortality in acute pancreatitis: a multicenter propensity analysis. *Crit Care Med.* 2018;46:e198–e205.
147. Mederos MA, Reber HA, Girgis MD. Acute pancreatitis: a review. *JAMA.* 2021;325(4):382–390.
148. Gardner TB. Acute pancreatitis. *Ann Intern Med.* 2021;174(2):ITC17–ITC32.
149. Pham A, Forsmark C. Chronic pancreatitis: review and update of etiology, risk factors, and management. *F1000Res.* 2018;7:F1000 Faculty Rev-607.
150. Olesen SS, et al. Towards a neurobiological understanding of pain in chronic pancreatitis: mechanisms and implications for treatment. *Pain Rep.* 2017;2(6):e625.
151. Barkin JA, Barkin JS. Chronic pancreatitis and bone disease. *J Clin Densitom.* 2020;23(2):237–243.
152. Jabłońska B, Mrowiec S. Total pancreatectomy with autologous islet cell transplantation—the current indications. *J Clin Med.* 2021;10(12):2723.
153. Beyer G, et al. Chronic pancreatitis. *Lancet.* 2020;396(10249):499–512.
154. Singh VK, Yadav D, Garg PK. Diagnosis and management of chronic pancreatitis: a review. *JAMA.* 2019;322(24):2422–2434.
155. American Cancer Society (ACS). *Cancer Facts & Figures 2022.* Atlanta, GA: ACS; 2022. https://www.cancer.org/content/dam/cancer-org/research/cancer-facts-and-statistics/annual-cancer-facts-and-figures/2022/2022-cancer-facts-and-figures.pdf. (Accessed May 3, 2022).
156. Cook MB, et al. Gastroesophageal reflux in relation to adenocarcinomas of the esophagus: a pooled analysis from the Barrett's and Esophageal Adenocarcinoma Consortium (BEACON). *PLoS One.* 2014;9(7):e103508.
157. Qumseya BJ, et al. Disease progression in Barrett's low-grade dysplasia with radiofrequency ablation compared with surveillance: systematic review and meta-analysis. *Am J Gastroenterol.* 2017;112:849–865.
158. Kuipers EJ, Spaander MC. Natural history of Barrett's esophagus. *Dig Dis Sci.* 2018;63(8):1997–2004.
159. ASGE Standards of Practice Committee Qumseya B, et al. ASGE guideline on screening and surveillance of Barrett's esophagus. *Gastrointest Endosc.* 2019;90(3). 335–359.e2.
160. Fitzgerald RC, et al. Cytosponge-trefoil factor 3 versus usual care to identify Barrett's oesophagus in a primary care setting: a multicentre, pragmatic, randomised controlled trial. *Lancet.* 2020;396(10247):333–344.
161. Shaheen NJ, et al. American College of Gastroenterology: ACG clinical guideline: diagnosis and management of Barrett's esophagus. *Am J Gastroenterol.* 2016;111(1):30–50.
162. Seeneevassen L, et al. Gastric cancer: advances in carcinogenesis research and new therapeutic strategies. *Int J Mol Sci.* 2021;22(7):3418.
163. Ajani JA, et al. Gastric adenocarcinoma. *Nat Rev Dis Primers.* 2017;3:17036.
164. Smyth EC, et al. Gastric cancer. *Lancet.* 2020;396(10251):635–648.
165. Cheung KS, Leung WK. Risk of gastric cancer development after eradication of *Helicobacter pylori. World J Gastrointest Oncol.* 2018;10(5):115–123.
166. American Cancer Society. Stomach Cancer Survival Rates 2010-2016 Data. www.cancer.org/cancer/stomach-cancer/detection-diagnosis-staging/survival-rates.html Last review March 1, 2022; Accessed May 3, 2022
167. PDQ® Adult Treatment Editorial Board. *Small Intestine Cancer Treatment (PDQ®)–Health Professional Version.* Bethesda, MD:

National Cancer Institute. Updated February 9, 2022. Available at https://www.cancer.gov/types/small-intestine/hp/small-intestine-treatment-pdq. (Accessed May 3, 2022).
168. Aparicio T, et al. Small bowel adenocarcinoma: epidemiology, risk factors, diagnosis, and treatment. *Dig Lever Dis.* 2014;46(2):97–104.
169. Burnett-Hartman AN, et al. An update on the epidemiology, molecular characterization, diagnosis, and screening strategies for early-onset colorectal cancer. *Gastroenterology.* 2021;160(4):1041–1049.
170. Friis S, et al. Low-dose aspirin or nonsteroidal anti-inflammatory drug use and colorectal cancer risk: a population-based, case-control study. *Ann Intern Med.* 2015;163(5):347–355.
171. Wells K, Wise PE. Hereditary colorectal cancer syndromes. *Surg Clin North Am.* 2017;97(3):605–625.
172. Palma S, et al. From molecular biology to clinical trials: toward personalized colorectal cancer therapy. *Clin Colorectal Cancer.* 2016;15(2):104–115.
173. Dekker E, et al. Colorectal cancer. *Lancet.* 2019;394(10207): 1467–1480.
174. Mazouji O, et al. Updates on clinical use of liquid biopsy in colorectal cancer screening, diagnosis, follow-up, and treatment guidance. *Front Cell Dev Biol.* 2021;9:660924.
175. PDQ® Adult Treatment Editorial Board. *Colon cancer treatment (PDQ®)–health professional version.* Bethesda, MD: National Cancer Institute; 2021. Updated January 21, 2022. Available at https://www.cancer.gov/types/colorectal/hp/colon-treatment-pdq. (Accessed May 3, 2022).
176. Dimitroulis D, et al. From diagnosis to treatment of hepatocellular carcinoma: an epidemic problem for both developed and developing world. *World J Gastroenterol.* 2017;23(29):5282–5294.
177. de Mattos ÂZ, et al. Current impact of viral hepatitis on liver cancer development: the challenge remains. *World J Gastroenterol.* 2021;27(24):3556–3567.
178. Orabi D, Berger NA, Brown JM. Abnormal metabolism in the progression of nonalcoholic fatty liver disease to hepatocellular carcinoma: mechanistic insights to chemoprevention. *Cancers (Basel).* 2021;13(14):3473.
179. Barcena-Varela M, Lujambio A. The endless sources of hepatocellular carcinoma heterogeneity. *Cancers (Basel).* 2021;13(11):2621.
180. Banales JM, et al. Cholangiocarcinoma 2020: the next horizon in mechanisms and management. *Nat Rev Gastroenterol Hepatol.* 2020;17(9):557–588.
181. American Cancer Society (ACS) *Liver and Cancer Stages.* Atlanta, GA: ACS; 2019. Last reviewed April 1, 2019. Available at https://www.cancer.org/cancer/liver-cancer/detection-diagnosis-staging/staging.html. (Accessed May 3, 2022).
182. Raees A, et al. Updates on the diagnosis and management of hepatocellular carcinoma. *Euroasian J Hepatogastroenterol.* 2021;11(1):32–40.
183. Rawla P, et al. Epidemiology of gallbladder cancer. *Clin Exp Hepatol.* 2019;5(2):93–102.
184. Mishra SK, Kumari N, Krishnani N. Molecular pathogenesis of gallbladder cancer: an update. *Mutat Res.* 2019;816–818: 111674.
185. Yang W, Sun Y. Promising molecular targets for the targeted therapy of biliary tract cancers: an overview. *Onco Targets Ther.* 2021;14:1341–1366.
186. Hu JX, et al. Pancreatic cancer: a review of epidemiology, trend, and risk factors. *World J Gastroenterol.* 2021;27(27):4298–4321.
187. Hamad A, et al. Neoadjuvant therapy for pancreatic ductal adenocarcinoma: opportunities for personalized cancer care. *World J Gastroenterol.* 2021;27(27):4383–4394.
188. Gupta N, Yelamanchi R. Pancreatic adenocarcinoma: a review of recent paradigms and advances in epidemiology, clinical diagnosis, and management. *World J Gastroenterol.* 2021;27(23):3158–3181.

42

Alterations of Digestive Function in Children

Corinne M. Djuric

http://evolve.elsevier.com/Rogers/pathophysiology/

CHAPTER OUTLINE

Disorders of the gastrointestinal (GI) tract and liver in children include congenital anomalies with structural and functional alterations, enzyme deficiencies, and infections. These disorders lead to impairment of normal digestive function and often affect growth and development.

DISORDERS OF THE GASTROINTESTINAL TRACT

Congenital Impairment of Motility

Congenital impairments of motility can occur throughout the GI tract. Here they are presented in order by location, starting with the mouth and esophagus, through the stomach and small intestine, and into the large intestine, rectum, and anus.

Mouth and Esophagus

Cleft lip and cleft palate. There are numerous types of congenital orofacial anomalies, the most common of which is cleft lip (CL) or cleft palate (CP), or both (CLP). In the United States, the estimated prevalence of CL with CP is about 1 in every 1600 live births. Prevalence of CL alone was 1 in every 2800 live births, and approximately 1 in every 1700 babies are born with CP. The prevalence of CP is consistent across all ethnicities. However, the prevalence of CL alone and CL with CP is highest in American Indian or Alaska Natives and lowest in African Americans in the United States. Male to female ratio of CL/P is 2:1, while male to female ratio of CP is 1:2.[1,2] CL, CP, or CL/P can be classified as nonsyndromic or syndromic. Overall, 70% of are nonsyndromic clefting disorders, which are complex genetic and environmental phenomena. Nonsyndromic occur as isolated cases without any additional physical or cognitive deficits. In contrast, 30% of clefts are syndromic. Syndromic clefting disorders are associated with single gene mutations or deletions and are associated with other congenital malformations.[3]

Pathophysiology. CL and CP are the most common craniofacial malformation of the newborn. CL, CP, and CL/P differ in their embryonic development, etiology, and genetic associations. There are a variety of cellular mechanisms, such as cell proliferation, cell migration, cell growth, cell fusion, apoptosis, epithelial-mesenchymal transition, and extracellular remodeling, that are involved in a coordinated manner during the development of lip and palate.[4] Disruption in the gene(s) involved in these processes during lip and palate development may lead to CL, CP, or CL/P.[4] Epigenetic and genetic influences include maternal use of tobacco, exposure to smoke, alcohol intake, medication use (such as anti-seizure agents, corticosteroids, anti-nausea drugs, and methotrexate), B vitamin deficiency (B_6, folic acid, B_{12}), maternal obesity, gene mutations of the amniotic band sequence, maternal exposure to viral illness or radiation, and chronic disease conditions such as diabetes.[5] CL and CP also may be syndromic, and therefore may be associated with other malformations (e.g., cardiac, skeletal, or central nervous system). Together the genetic and epigenetic factors reduce the amount of neural crest mesenchyme that migrates into the area that will develop into the face of the embryo.[4] Orofacial clefts are categorized by location, degree of lip involvement, and the presence or absence of a CP.[5]

Cleft lip is caused by the incomplete fusion of the nasomedial or intermaxillary process beginning the fourth week of embryonic development, a period of rapid development. The cleft causes structures of the face and mouth to develop without the normal restraints of encircling lip muscles. The facial cleft may affect not only the lip but also the external nose, nasal cartilages, nasal septum, and alveolar processes. The cleft is usually just beneath the center of one nostril.

The defect may occur bilaterally and may be symmetrical or asymmetrical. The more complete the CL, the greater the chance that teeth in the line of the cleft will be missing or malformed.

Cleft palate is often associated with CL but may occur without it. The fissure may affect only the uvula and soft palate or may extend forward to the nostril and involve the hard palate and the maxillary alveolar ridge. It may be unilateral or bilateral, with the cleft occupying the midline posteriorly and as far forward as the alveolar process (the ridge of bone that holds the teeth), where it deviates to the involved side. Clefts involving the palate only are usually, but not necessarily, in the midline. In some cases, the vomer (the small, thin bone separating the left and right nasal cavities) and nasal septum are partly or completely undeveloped. When these facial bones are involved, the nasal cavity may freely communicate with the oral cavity.

Clinical Manifestations. Clefts of the lip or palate, or both, are immediately recognizable disruptions of normal facial structure (Fig. 42.1). The most common type of CL is unilateral with or without a CP.[5] Feeding difficulty is the most significant clinical manifestation because of the oronasal communication and inability to generate negative pressure needed for normal sucking. There also may be swallowing and speech difficulty. Children with any cleft abnormalities have an increased risk for middle ear infections and may have recurrent otitis media.[6] Individuals with CL, CP, or CL/P may suffer appearance-related distress secondary to the facial disfiguration.[7]

Evaluation and Treatment. Prenatal diagnosis is made by ultrasound, and postnatal imaging confirms the extent of bone deformity. Soft tissue alterations are evaluated by history and physical examination. The oral palate should be carefully examined for a translucent appearance, an elevation of the palate during phonation, and possibly a bifid uvula.[5] A speech therapist should evaluate the child's speech articulation and phonology, making note of hypernasality.[5] Children with CL, CP, or CL/P require long-term complex and coordinated care.[5] The nature and extent of the cleft, the infant's condition, and the method of surgical correction proposed determine the course of treatment. Surgical correction is planned at about the third to sixth month and may be performed in stages.

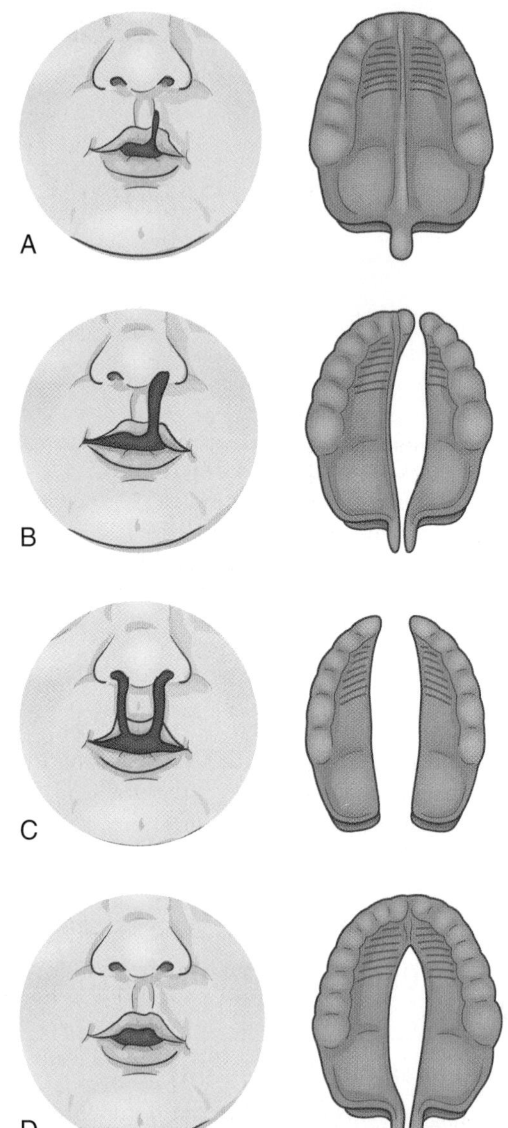

Fig. 42.1 Variations in Clefts of the Lip and Palate. **(A)** Notch in the vermilion border. **(B)** Unilateral cleft lip and palate. **(C)** Bilateral cleft lip and cleft palate. **(D)** Cleft palate.

Feeding the infant with CL usually presents no difficulty if the CL is simple and the palate intact. An infant with a complete CP requires consultation with a feeding and swallowing specialist to ensure adequate and safe nutritional intake. Bottles with nipples specialized for feeding an infant with a CP are required. Breast-feeding is encouraged and recommended; therefore, a certified lactation consultant should be offered to the mother.[5,8] An orthodontic prosthesis for the roof of the mouth may facilitate sucking for some infants. Parental education and support are required for the long-term care of children with CP. Longitudinal monitoring requires a multidisciplinary team, including an oral and maxillofacial surgeon, dentist, orthodontist, otolaryngologist, neurosurgeon, geneticist, nutritionist, speech therapist, and child development specialist.[5]

Esophageal malformations. Congenital malformations of the esophagus are rare and often occur with other congenital malformations. **Esophageal atresia (EA)**, where the esophagus ends in a blind pouch, is the most common congenital malformation involving the esophagus. **Atresia** is an absence or abnormal narrowing of a passage, in this case the esophagus, during embryonic development. EA is often accompanied by a fistula (an abnormal connection) between the esophagus and the trachea (**tracheoesophageal fistula [TEF]**). Either defect can occur alone, although isolated TEF is very rare (Fig. 42.2). Environmental risk factors include maternal exposure to methimazole (used to treat an overactive thyroid), exogenous sex hormones, infectious diseases, alcohol, or smoking; maternal diabetes; advanced maternal age; and maternal employment in agriculture or horticulture.[9] EA and TEF may be associated with congenital vertebral, anorectal, cardiovascular, renal, and limb malformations (collectively known as the VACTERL association).[10] EA and TEF also are

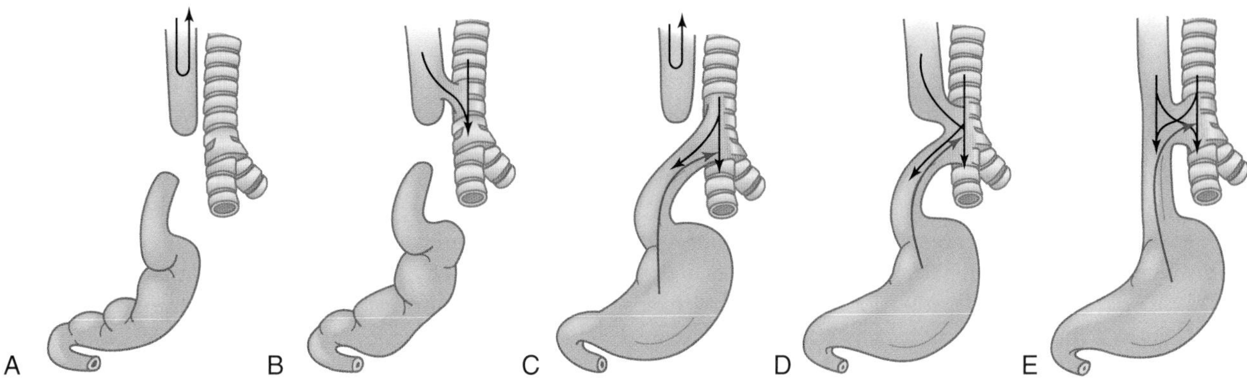

Fig. 42.2 Five Types of Esophageal Atresia and Tracheoesophageal Fistulae. **(A)** Simple esophageal atresia. The proximal esophagus and distal esophagus end in blind pouches, and there is no tracheal communication. Nothing enters the stomach; regurgitated food and fluid may enter the lungs. **(B)** Proximal and distal esophageal segments end in blind pouches, and a fistula connects the proximal esophagus to the trachea. Nothing enters the stomach; food and fluid enter the lungs from the mouth. **(C)** Proximal esophagus ends in a blind pouch, and a fistula connects the trachea to the distal esophagus. Air enters the stomach; regurgitated gastric secretions enter the lungs through the fistula. **(D)** A fistula connects both proximal and distal esophageal segments to the trachea. Air, food, and fluid enter the stomach and the lungs from the mouth; regurgitated gastric secretions enter the lungs through the fistula. **(E)** A simple tracheoesophageal fistula is present between an otherwise normal esophagus and trachea. Air, food, and fluid enter the stomach and the lungs from the mouth through the fistula; regurgitated gastric secretions enter the lungs through the fistula. Of esophageal anomalies, 85% to 90% are the type shown in (C); 6% to 8% are the type shown in (A); 3% to 5% are the type shown in (E); and fewer than 1% are the types shown in (B) and (D).

commonly present with other birth defects, such as trisomy 13, 18, or 21.

Pathophysiology. The pathogenesis of esophageal abnormalities is unknown, but viral, infectious, environmental, and genetic factors have been suggested.[11] Defective growth of endodermal cells and impaired embryonic foregut development of the trachea and esophagus lead to atresia.[12]

Clinical Manifestations. The diagnosis of EA/TEF during pregnancy increases with the findings of polyhydramnios (excessive amniotic fluid) on ultrasound. Swallowed amniotic fluid is usually absorbed into the placental circulation; therefore, if the fetus cannot swallow, amniotic fluid accumulates in the uterus. Many cases are not detected during the prenatal period. EA is diagnosed at birth on the basis of drooling, inability to swallow secretions, or choking with feeding, and respiratory distress. Confirmation is established by inability to pass a gastric tube into the stomach and radiographic evidence of the gastric tube curled up within the distal pouch. If a fistula connects the trachea with the distal esophagus, the abdomen fills with air and becomes distended, possibly interfering with breathing (see Fig. 42.2C–E). Intermittent cyanosis may result.

Pulmonary complications are compounded by reflux of air and gastric secretions into the tracheobronchial tree through the fistula, causing severe chemical irritation. Infants with EA but no fistulae have scaphoid (boat-shaped), gasless abdomens. In infants with fistulae, but without atresia (see Fig. 42.2E), the usual symptoms are recurrent aspiration, pneumonia, and atelectasis that remains unexpressed for days or even months.

Evaluation and Treatment. EA is rarely diagnosed during pregnancy and most often is detected after birth when the neonate has difficulty feeding and often has choking or vomiting. To assist the child with feeding, a tube is inserted in the baby's nose or mouth, but it cannot pass down into the stomach because of EA or TEF. An x-ray can confirm where the upper esophagus ends.[13] Infants presenting with EA are further evaluated with ultrasound, echocardiogram, and vertebral and limb radiographs.

After diagnosis, a tube should be placed into the upper pouch and continuous suction applied to reduce the risk of aspiration. The head of the bed should be elevated slightly to assist drainage of the upper pouch. The infant should not be fed orally. The surgical options for EA/TEF repair include open thoracotomy or video-assisted thoracoscopic surgery. The best radical surgical treatment for EA with TEF is primary single-staged correction comprising esophagoesophagostomy and TEF division. However, the procedure is generally performed in a staged manner for infants with unstable respiratory or cardiovascular conditions.[14]

The overall survival rate for infants with esophageal defects is greater than 90%; however, it is dependent on the extent of associated abnormalities.[15] Children will require life-long follow-up as respiratory and gastrointestinal (GI) complications occur frequently.[16,17]

Infantile hypertrophic pyloric stenosis. Infantile hypertrophic pyloric stenosis (IHPS) is an acquired narrowing and distal obstruction of the pylorus and a common cause of postprandial (after a meal) vomiting. It is the most common cause of intestinal obstruction in infancy. The etiology of IHPS is unknown, but genetic and environmental factors, bottle feeding, younger maternal age, maternal smoking, and erythromycin administration in the first two weeks of life have shown associations with the disease.[18,19]

Pathophysiology. Individual muscle fibers of the longitudinal and circular muscles thicken, so the entire pyloric sphincter becomes enlarged and inflexible.[20] The mucosal lining of the pyloric opening is folded and narrowed by the encroaching muscle. Because of the extra peristaltic effort necessary to force the gastric contents through the narrow opening, the muscle layers of the stomach may become hypertrophied as well.

Clinical Manifestations. Within 2 to 3 weeks after birth, an infant who has fed well and gained weight begins forceful, nonbilious vomiting immediately after feeding. The infant then demands to be refed. Constipation occurs because little food reaches the intestine.

In severe, untreated cases, increased gastric peristalsis and vomiting lead to dehydration and electrolyte imbalances, malnutrition, weight loss, and shock that can be life-threatening. Infants with pyloric stenosis are irritable because of hunger, and they may have esophageal discomfort caused by repeated vomiting and esophagitis. The vomitus may be blood streaked because of rupture of gastric and esophageal vessels.

Evaluation and Treatment. The diagnosis is based on the history, clinical manifestations, and findings on abdominal ultrasound. The force or "projectile" vomiting and the timing of the vomiting can help distinguish IHPS from gastroesophageal reflux (for which episodes of vomiting are not forceful and occur 10 minutes or more after a feeding). The hypertrophied pylorus is palpable as a firm, small, movable mass, approximately the size of an olive, and is felt in the right upper quadrant in 70% to 90% of infants with pyloric stenosis. A visible gastric peristaltic wave after eating is observed in some infants. The hypertrophied pyloric muscles and narrowed pyloric channel are identified with ultrasound. A fluoroscopic upper GI series may be necessary if the physical exam and ultrasound are inconclusive. Gastric decompression by nasogastric tube may be required for comfort and to clear the stomach for further evaluation and treatment.

The standard treatment for IHPS is a laparoscopic pyloromyotomy, in which the muscles of the pylorus are split and separated. Preoperative and postoperative medical management to correct fluid and electrolyte imbalance has been the key to the high success and low complication rates associated with this surgery.[21]

Obstructions of the duodenum, jejunum, and ileum. High intestinal obstruction should be considered whenever persistent vomiting occurs. With duodenal obstruction there will be upper abdominal distention, visible peristaltic waves, a decrease in the size and frequency of meconium stools, progressive weight loss, persistent vomiting, and dehydration. Congenital obstruction of the duodenum is rare and can be caused by intrinsic malformations, such as atresia (complete blockage), stenosis (partial obstruction or narrowing), or external pressure (choledochal cyst or annular pancreas). Duodenal obstruction may be partial or complete and is usually located at or near the major duodenal papilla (the opening of the common bile duct and pancreatic duct into the duodenum). The classic "double bubble" sign is seen on imaging of the abdomen and represents dilation associated with duodenal obstruction. The larger, proximal "bubble" is air in a dilated stomach. The more distal, smaller "bubble" is air in a dilated proximal duodenum. There is usually little or no air in the bowel distal to the obstruction. Double bubble also may be seen on prenatal ultrasounds.

Congenital obstructions of the jejunum and ileum can be attributable to atresia, stenosis, meconium ileus, megacolon (Hirschsprung disease), intussusception, Meckel diverticulum, intestinal duplication, or strangulated hernia. In ileal or jejunal atresia, the intestine ends blindly, proximal and distal to an interruption in its continuity, with or without a gap in the mesentery. Stenosis (narrowing of the lumen) causes dilation proximal to the obstruction and luminal collapse distal to it.

Intestinal malrotation. Intestinal malrotation is a common congenital anomaly of the small intestine. Once thought to be a disease of infancy, newer epidemiologic evidence supports presentation of intestinal rotation in children up to 17 years of age. The majority of cases (approximately 75%) will present before the age of 5.[22] Associated abnormalities are common and include duodenal, jejunal, or biliary atresia; pancreatic malformations; and heart defects.[23]

Pathophysiology. During normal embryonic development, the ileum and cecum rotate into the lower right abdominal quadrant and are fixed there by the mesentery. In malrotation, this rotation does not occur and the small intestine lacks a normal posterior attachment (Fig. 42.3). The mobile loops of intestine can twist upon themselves (volvulus), leading to symptoms of bowel obstruction. The twisting can partly or completely occlude the superior mesenteric artery, causing infarction and necrosis of the entire midgut. Additionally, abnormal periduodenal (Ladd) bands may press against and obstruct the duodenum.

Clinical Manifestations. Classic symptoms in infants are intermittent or persistent bile-stained vomiting after feedings and epigastric distention. Dehydration and electrolyte imbalance may occur rapidly. Fever usually ensues, with pain and scanty stools. Diarrhea and bloody stools are associated with progressive volvulus, vascular compression, and infarction of the intestine. Intermittent or partial volvulus may be seen in older children and adults. It may be asymptomatic or cause minor abdominal discomfort and be discovered during unrelated abdominal surgery.[24]

Evaluation and Treatment. The diagnosis of malrotation with volvulus and infarction is based on clinical manifestations. Radiographic films of the abdomen and barium studies show intestinal gas bubbles and distention proximal to the site of obstruction. Asymptomatic infants with complex birth defects of the heart, lungs, liver, spleen, or intestines should be screened for intestinal malrotation with a contrast upper GI study.[24] Ultrasound imaging has also been used with good success and avoids exposure to ionizing radiation.[25]

Treatment includes laparoscopic or open Ladd procedure to reduce the volvulus.[26] Necrotic bowel is resected and a primary anastomosis performed. An intestinal diversion

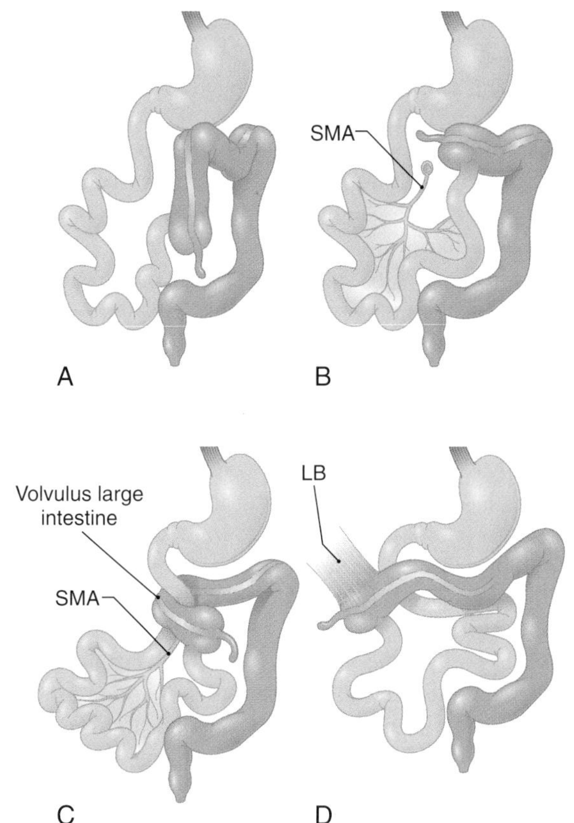

Fig. 42.3 Variations of Intestinal Malrotation. (A) Nonrotation. (B) Incomplete rotation. (C) Midgut volvulus with duodenal obstruction and obstruction of superior mesenteric artery blood flow. (D) Incomplete rotation with Ladd bands extending from the lateral and posterior abdominal wall to the subhepatic cecum. *LB*, Ladd band; *SMA*, superior mesenteric artery. (From Gilbert-Barness E, et al. *Potter's pathology of the fetus, infant and child*, 2nd edition. Philadelphia, PA: Mosby; 2007

(ostomy) may need to be created. Most children have a good outcome; however, there is risk for adhesion-related bowel obstruction in a small number of cases. Resection of large segments of the small intestine results in short bowel syndrome, a malabsorption syndrome with diarrhea, dehydration, and malnutrition.[27]

Meckel diverticulum. Diverticula are small outpouches, or sacs, that have formed and pushed outward through weak spots of the intestinal wall. Meckel diverticulum is a true diverticulum in that it contains all layers of the wall of the intestine, usually the ileum. It is a remnant of the embryonic yolk sac and is the most prevalent congenital abnormality of the small bowel. Ectopic (abnormal location) gastric mucosal cells are contained in the diverticula and may cause peptic ulcer and painless bleeding or mimic colonic diverticulitis. Often referred to as "the rule of 2 s," a Meckel diverticulum occurs in approximately 2% of the general population, is typically located within 2 feet of the ileocecal valve (on the antimesenteric border of the ileum), is 2 inches in length on average, and its clinical symptomatology often occurs before 2 years of age.

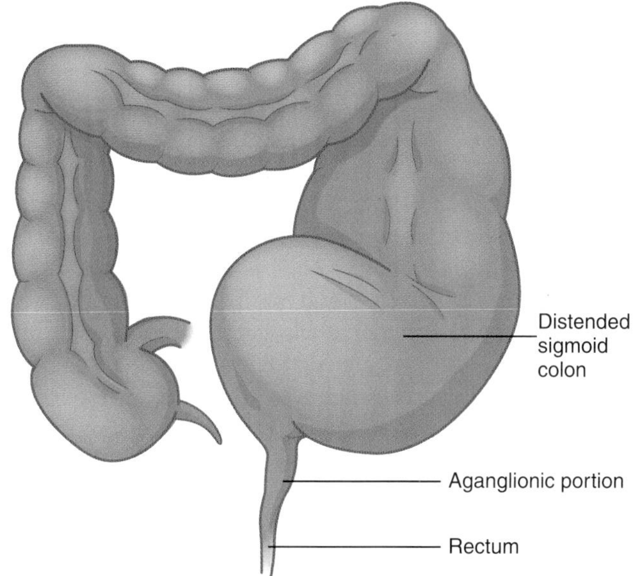

Fig. 42.4 Hirschsprung Disease.

Although most Meckel diverticula are generally asymptomatic, symptomatic Meckel diverticula can present as obstruction of the small bowel, fever, vomiting, abdominal pain, or painless rectal bleeding. Diagnosis can be made by symptom presentation and imaging studies. Radionucleotide scintigraphy shows the gastric mucosal cells in the diverticula. Treatment for symptomatic Meckel's diverticula includes laparoscopic or open surgical resection. Treating asymptomatic Meckel's diverticula remains controversial.[28]

Obstruction of Large Intestine, Rectum, and Anus

Hirschsprung disease. Hirschsprung disease, or congenital aganglionic megacolon, is a functional obstruction of the colon. It is rare but the most common cause of colon obstruction in infants. The incidence is higher in males, siblings of children with Hirschsprung disease, and children with Down syndrome or other congenital malformations.[29]

Pathophysiology. The exact cause of Hirschsprung disease is unknown, but it is associated with multiple interacting factors, including gene mutations and epigenetic mechanisms. The congenital malformation results from failure of neural crest cells to migrate into the GI tract. There is an absence of parasympathetic plexuses (Meissner and Auerbach plexuses) along variable lengths of the colon. Lacking neural stimulation, muscle layers fail to propel feces through the colon, leading to functional obstruction. This causes the proximal colon to become distended, hence the term *megacolon* is often used (Fig. 42.4). In most cases, the aganglionic segment is limited to the rectal end of the sigmoid colon. In rare cases, the entire colon lacks ganglion cells and the ileum may be involved.[30]

Clinical Manifestations. The infant typically becomes symptomatic during the first 48 hours after birth with delayed passage of meconium. Children with less severe disease may not be diagnosed until 3 years of age. Mild to severe constipation is the usual manifestation accompanied by poor feeding, poor weight gain, and progressive abdominal distention. However, diarrhea may be the first sign because only water can travel around the impacted feces.[31]

The most serious complication in the neonatal period is enterocolitis related to fecal impaction. This presents with sepsis-like symptoms of fever, abdominal distension, vomiting, and diarrhea. The intestinal inflammation is related to fecal impaction, alterations in intestinal microbiota, impaired mucosal barrier function, and innate immunity with bacterial translocation.[32,33]

Bowel dilation stretches and partly occludes the encircling blood and lymphatic vessels, causing edema, ischemia, infarction of the mucosa, and significant outflow of fluid into the bowel lumen. Copious liquid stools result. Infarction and destruction of the mucosa enable enteric microorganisms to penetrate the bowel wall and gram-negative sepsis can occur. Severe and rapid fluid and electrolyte changes may take place, causing hypovolemic or septic shock or death.

Evaluation and Treatment. Radiocontrast enema and anorectal manometry are screening tools for the diagnosis of Hirschsprung disease. The definitive diagnosis is made by rectal biopsy, showing an absence of ganglion cells in the submucosa of the colon. Surgery is the definitive treatment in all cases of Hirschsprung disease. In general, the prognosis of congenital megacolon is satisfactory for children who undergo surgical treatment. Bowel training may be prolonged; most children achieve bowel continence before puberty, but some have long-term constipation or fecal incontinence that can adversely affect their quality of life.[34]

Distal intestinal obstruction syndrome. Distal intestinal obstruction syndrome (DIOS), formerly called *meconium ileus equivalent*, is the partial or complete obstruction of the terminal ileum and proximal colon by abnormally viscous intestinal contents. The condition is unique to children with cystic fibrosis (CF).

Pathophysiology. The epithelium of the intestine secretes chloride and inhibits sodium absorption, which will force fluid into the lumen. This is a similar mechanism as is seen in the epithelium of the lungs. Defective CF transmembrane conductance regulator (CFTR) function disrupts this fluid homeostasis resulting in intestinal fluid imbalance.[35] This is coupled with insufficient pancreatic enzyme activity, causing malabsorption of fat. This leads to impaired motility that causes slow intestinal transit and altered viscosity of the bowel contents.[36] The terminal ileum or proximal colon becomes plugged with thick, sticky meconium resulting from the formation of abnormal mucus. The segment of the ileum proximal to the obstruction is distended with liquid contents, and its walls may be hypertrophied. The segment distal to the obstruction is collapsed and filled with small pellets of pale-colored stool. Meconium in the obstructed segment has the consistency of thick syrup or glue. Peristalsis fails to propel this sticky material through the ileum, so it becomes impacted.

Clinical Manifestations. Abdominal distention usually develops during the first few days after birth. The distention increases as air is swallowed. The infant does not pass meconium and begins to vomit bile-stained material within hours or days of birth. Infants with CF may have signs of pulmonary involvement, such as tachypnea, intercostal retractions, and grunting respirations. The distended abdomen shows patterns of dilated intestinal loops that feel dough-like when palpated. Some of the loops contain scattered, firm, movable masses. Despite hyperactive peristalsis, the rectal ampulla is empty.

Evaluation and Treatment. Radiologic examination confirms the presence of meconium in the ileum or ileocecum and is typically described as "bubbly" or granular in appearance. The sweat test, which measures the amount of chloride in the sweat, is performed to detect or rule out CF and is accurate in 90% of infants. In cases not complicated by volvulus or perforation, the obstruction is relieved by intestinal lavage and administration of oral laxatives. If this is not possible, the meconium is removed surgically. Survival of infants with simple meconium ileus is improving, with rates approaching 100%. Mortality of infants increases if the obstruction is complicated by peritonitis. DIOS is treated with hydration and stool softeners.[37]

Anorectal malformations. Anorectal malformations (ARMs) represent a spectrum of rare anomalies of the anus and rectum (Fig. 42.5). ARMs include anorectal stenosis, imperforate anus, anorectal atresia, and rectal atresia. Persistent cloaca (an embryonic component of the hind gut) is the most severe type of anorectal malformation and occurs exclusively in girls. The rectum, urethra, and vagina fail to develop separately; instead, they drain through a single, common channel onto the perineum.[38] Infants with anorectal malformations may have other developmental anomalies (e.g., Down syndrome, Hirschsprung disease, duodenal atresia, neurogenic bladder, and spinal malformations).

Most ARMs are identified in routine physical examination during the neonatal period. Ultrasound and magnetic resonance imaging (MRI) can assist prenatal diagnosis. Types of imperforate anus include an anal opening that is narrow or misplaced; a membrane (covering) may be present over the anal opening; the rectum may not connect to the anus; the rectum may connect to part of the urinary tract or to the reproductive system through a *fistula*; or the anal opening is not present. Treatment recommendations depend on the type of imperforate anus, the presence and type of associated abnormalities, and the child's overall health status. Infants with an imperforate anus and other anorectal malformations require surgical correction. Outcomes are affected by the type of malformation, sacral development, and presence of spinal abnormalities.[39]

Meconium Syndromes

Meconium is a substance that fills the entire intestine before birth. It is a dark greenish mass of desquamated cells, mucus, and bile that accumulates in the bowel of a fetus and is typically discharged during the first 12 to 48 hours after birth.

Meconium ileus (MI) is an intestinal obstruction in the neonatal period caused by meconium formed in utero that is abnormally thick and sticky, which leads to a partial or complete obstruction at the level of the terminal ileum. There are two forms of MI: simple and complex. In simple MI, thickened meconium accumulates and obstructs the ileum causing proximal dilatation, bowel wall thickening, and congestion. Complex MI is associated with bowel atresia, volvulus, necrosis, or

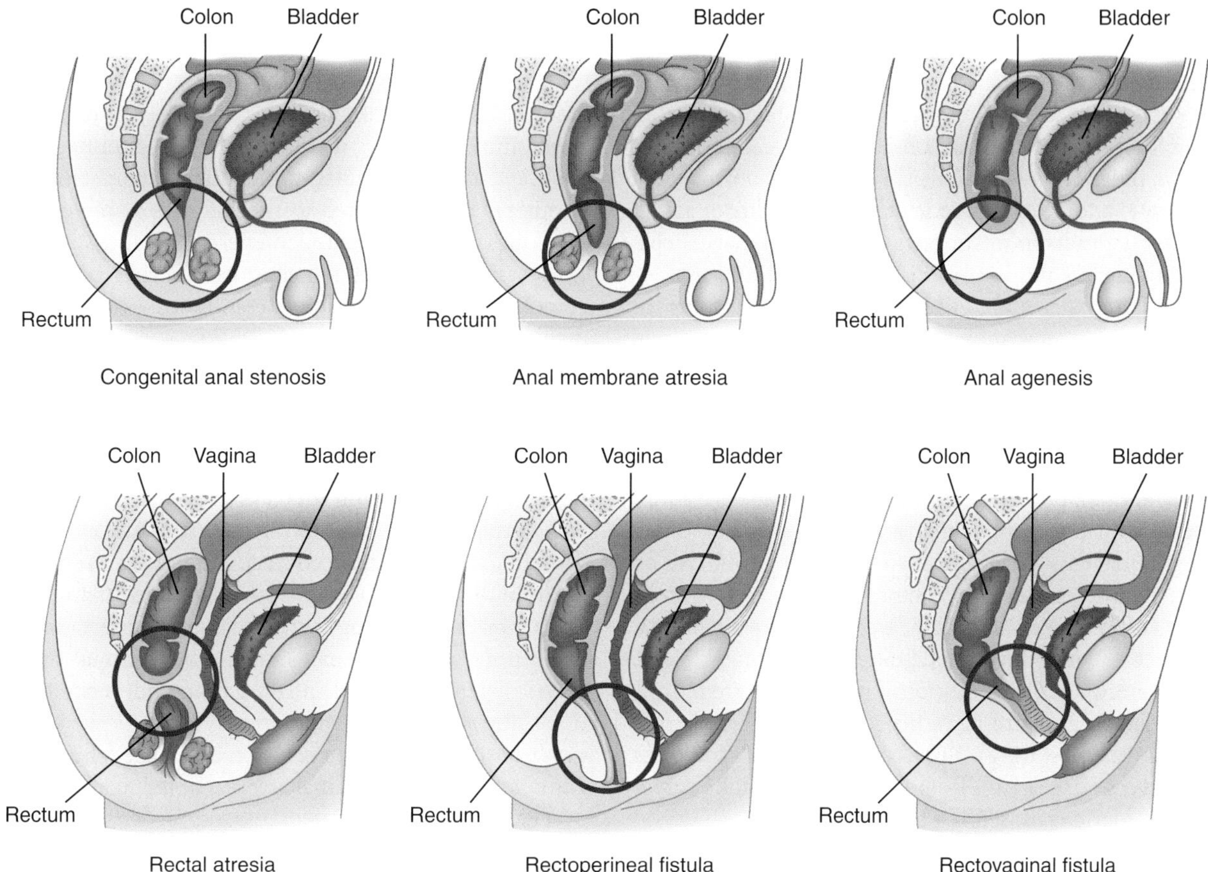

Fig. 42.5 Anorectal Stenosis and Imperforate Anus. Except for the rectovaginal fistula, all of the malformations shown occur in both males and females.

perforation and is a surgical emergency. MI occurs in up to 20% of infants with CF. It is thought to result from abnormal mucus production in the intestine or impaired pancreatic enzymes, or both.[40]

Meconium plug syndrome (MPS), also termed *functional immaturity of the colon*, is a transient disorder of the newborn colon characterized by an inability to pass meconium within 24 to 48 hours following delivery along with radiographic evidence of intestinal dilation. Plugs of meconium are found in the distal ileum and proximal colon, resulting in obstruction of passage of meconium from the rectum. There may be an association with MPS in prematurity, mothers with diabetes, and mothers who received magnesium sulfate.[41]

Meconium aspiration syndrome occurs following intestinal peristalsis, meconium release, and contamination of amniotic fluid associated with fetal hypoxia. Gasping respirations cause aspiration of the contaminated amniotic fluid deep into the fetal lung. Infants present with respiratory distress with expiratory airway obstruction, air trapping, surfactant inactivation, atelectasis, and chemical pneumonitis. Meconium aspiration also predisposes to infection and the development of persistent patent ductus arteriosus and foramen ovale.[42] The presence of meconium-stained amniotic fluid and the clinical presentation help confirm the diagnosis. Treatment includes surfactant administration, oxygen, inhaled nitric oxide, and ventilator support.[43]

Acquired Impairment of Motility

Gastroesophageal Reflux and Gastroesophageal Reflux Disease

Gastroesophageal reflux (GER) is the passage of gastric contents into the esophagus with or without regurgitation and/or vomiting.[44] GER is normal and nonpathologic in healthy infants and children. Most episodes are asymptomatic and without long-term consequence. The frequency of GER is highest in premature infants and peaks at 4 months of age in healthy infants. GER will subside in 90% of cases by 12 months of age.[45]

GER disease (GERD) is different from GER and is considered pathologic. It occurs when GER induces troublesome symptoms or complications, such as esophagitis or structuring, that affect daily functioning.[44] Children at greatest risk for complicated GERD are those with other underlying medical conditions including prematurity, neurologic impairment, EA, obesity, hiatal hernia, achalasia, chronic lung diseases, and certain genetic disorders, including CF.[44]

Pathophysiology. GERD is influenced by genetic, environmental, anatomic, hormonal, and neurogenic factors. Although transient lower esophageal sphincter relaxations (TLESRs) are the most common pathophysiologic cause of GERD, inadequate adaptation of sphincter tone to changes in abdominal pressure also may be implicated. Factors that maintain lower esophageal sphincter integrity in children include the location of the gastroesophageal junction in a high-pressure zone within the abdomen, mucosal gathering within the sphincter, and the angle at which the esophagus is inserted into the stomach. Reflux persists if any one of these pressure-maintaining factors is altered. Other mediators of GERD are esophageal peristalsis or clearance, mucosal resistance that mediates the noxiousness of the refluxate, and delayed gastric emptying. Reflux of acidic gastric contents results in inflammation of the esophageal epithelium (esophagitis) and stimulation of the vomiting reflex.

Clinical Manifestations. The clinical manifestations of GERD will differ in accordance with the age of the child. Infants with GERD will present with symptoms of irritability, sleep disturbance, excessive regurgitation, hematemesis, unexplained crying, back arching, food refusal or anorexia, and failure to thrive (FTT).[44] Children may present with decreased food intake, weight loss, and abdominal or epigastric pain. Older children and adolescents will present similarly to adults with heartburn and regurgitation.[44] Esophageal complications of GERD can be significant, such as esophagitis, hemorrhage, stricture, Barrett esophagus (see Chapter 41), and, rarely, adenocarcinoma. Extraesophageal symptoms include cough, wheezing, stridor, laryngitis, pharyngitis, dental erosions, sinusitis, recurrent otitis media, and Sandifer syndrome (a neurologic disorder characterized by unusual posturing).[44] This constellation of symptoms is often difficult to distinguish from those of cow's milk protein allergy, which may coexist with or overlap GERD.[46]

Evaluation and Treatment. The clinical manifestations are often adequate to confirm a diagnosis of GERD. Barium contrast studies may be beneficial to exclude anatomical abnormalities but are not recommended to diagnose GERD in children. There is insufficient evidence to support the use of pH metry for the diagnosis of GERD, but it can be useful to correlate troublesome symptoms and determine the efficacy of acid suppression therapy.[44]

In breast-fed babies, maternal elimination of cow's milk protein is recommended, whereas formula-fed infants may require feeding volume and frequency adjustments using extensively hydrolyzed protein or amino acid–based formulas. Using thickened feedings is recommended for treating visible regurgitation and/or vomiting in infants with GERD. Prone positioning is recommended only for infants older than 1 year of age because of the risk of sudden infant death syndrome. Lifestyle changes for children and adolescents include weight loss, smoking cessation, sleeping position changes, and avoidance of caffeine, chocolate, alcohol, and spicy foods. Medications are used to buffer or reduce gastric acid secretion, increase motility, or increase lower esophageal sphincter pressure to treat GERD. If no improvement is seen with medical management or the child has life-threatening events with reflux, an anti-reflux surgical procedure, including gastropexy and fundoplication, is performed.[44]

Eosinophilic Esophagitis. Pediatric eosinophilic esophagitis (EoE) is an emerging chronic, local, progressive antigen- immune-mediated relapsing disease caused by eosinophilic infiltration of the esophageal mucosa, belonging to a group of eosinophilic GI disorders.[47–49] EoE is an atopic inflammatory disease and often referred to as the "asthma of the esophagus" due to the similar clinical and pathophysiologic characteristics.[50] EoE is the most prevalent cause of esophagitis after GERD.[47] The incidence and prevalence of EoE have sharply increased globally within the last 20 years.[49]

Pathophysiology. The pathogenesis of EoE is complex and still not completely understood. The onset of disease involves a multitude of factors including genetics, immunity, the environment, as well as damaged mucosa and fibrosis mechanisms. Eosinophils are recruited to specific sites of the esophagus by cytokines and begin remodeling esophageal tissues. It is likely EoE is associated with T-helper cell-2 (Th2) type of immune response seen in other atopic conditions.[47] High levels of Th2 cytokines, mast cells, and interleukins 4, 5, and 13 have been found in esophageal biopsies of individuals with EoE.[47]

Clinical Manifestations. The symptoms associated with EoE are dependent on the age at presentation.[47] The typical clinical manifestations associated with EoE include dysphagia and food impaction.[47] Infants and toddlers may have feeding difficulties, such as prolonged feeding time, food refusal, or GERD-like symptoms, and in advanced stage can present as FTT.[49] School-aged children and adolescents may present with dysphagia, food impaction, and gagging with meals. It is important to identify any history of food or environmental allergens as this is a common trigger of mucosal inflammation and hence the recruitment of eosinophils.[47] Children may have atopic diathesis or a predisposition to develop one or more of the following: allergic rhinitis, hay fever, bronchial asthma, or atopic dermatitis.[49]

Evaluation and Treatment. A comprehensive evaluation of EoE can be performed by using one of the scoring systems developed. The Pediatric Eosinophilic Esophagitis Symptoms Score correlates with histologic activity, and the Pediatric Quality of Life Inventory EoE is a valid symptomatic measure in children.[49] Diagnosis is confirmed by the demonstration in biopsy specimens obtained through upper endoscopy of eosinophilic inflammation (more than 15 for high powered field) of the esophageal mucosa and other histologic features.[47] Endoscopic features change from childhood to adulthood. Chronic inflammation drives a progressive fibrosis and esophageal modeling.[49]

Therapeutic approaches to treatment include eliminating triggers, medications, dietary interventions, and esophageal dilation.[49,51] Identification, management, and elimination of food allergens and aeroallergen sensitivities is an important step in the prevention of flares.[47] Children with EoE should be advised to take small bites and chew food slowly and completely, making sure to consume fluids in between each bite. Foods lubricated with sauces may assist with food passage down the esophagus. Proton pump inhibitors can be used in the treatment for EoE, with about one-third of individuals responding to this therapy.[47] Corticosteroids are a mainstay therapeutic treatment for EoE because of the anti-inflammatory effects, which decrease esophageal fibrosis and remodeling and improve the integrity of the esophageal mucosal barrier.[49,51] Complications such as strictures, esophageal rings, and narrowing of the esophagus can occur if EoE is left untreated.[47] In some cases, EoE strictures require endoscopic dilation.[51]

Intussusception

Intussusception is the telescoping of a proximal segment of intestine into a distal segment, causing an obstruction. It is rare but the most common cause of small bowel obstruction in children in the United States. Most cases occur between 5 and 7 months of age. Intussusception is more common in males and can occur in children with polyps or tumors (lead points), CF, Meckel diverticulum, intestinal adhesions, or immediately after abdominal surgery. There is a small risk of intussusception associated with rotavirus vaccination, but the health benefits of the vaccine far exceed the risk of intussusception.[52]

Pathophysiology. In intussusception, the ileum commonly telescopes into the cecum and part of the ascending colon by collapsing through the ileocecal valve, although intussusception can occur anywhere from the duodenum to the rectum. The proximal portion of the intestine (the intussusceptum) telescopes into the distal portion (the intussuscipiens) in the direction of peristaltic flow (Fig. 42.6). The intussusceptum then drags its mesentery into the enveloping lumen, causing an intussusception. Initially, the mesentery is constricted, obstructing venous return. Compression of the mesenteric vessels between the two layers of intestinal wall and at the U-shaped angle at either end of the intussusceptum leads to venous stasis, engorgement, edema, exudation, and further vascular compression within hours. The tension of the mesentery on the intussusceptum tends to arch the bowel in a curve with its center at the mesenteric root. Edema and compression obstruct the flow of chyme through the intestine. Unless the intussusception is treated, bleeding, necrosis, and bowel perforation ensue.

Clinical Manifestations. The classic symptoms of intussusception include colicky abdominal pain, irritability, knees drawn to the chest, abdominal mass, vomiting, and bloody (currant jelly) stools. In children older than 1 year, abdominal pain is the most common symptom. In children younger than 1 year, vomiting, irritability, and bloody stools are the most common symptoms.[53]

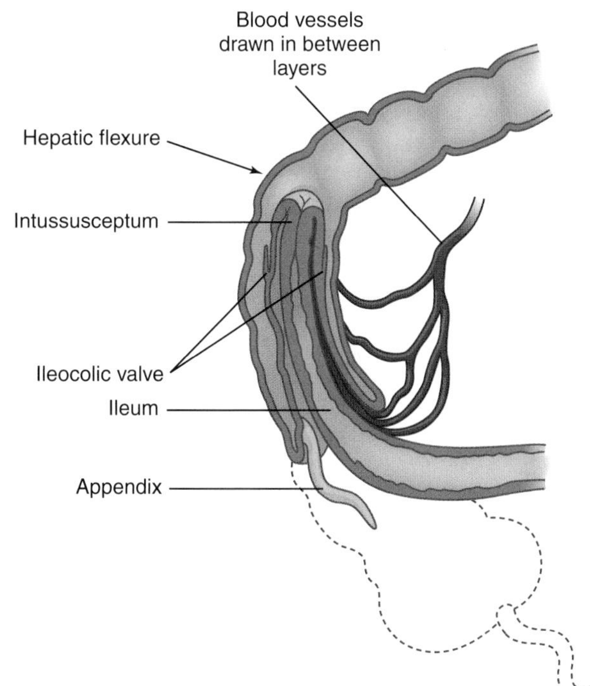

Fig. 42.6 Ileocolic Intussusception. Dotted outline indicates normal anatomy.

Intussusception has been discovered incidentally by computed tomography (CT) or MRI scan for other indications. Abdominal tenderness and distention develop as intestinal obstruction becomes more acute.

Evaluation and Treatment. The diagnosis is based on clinical manifestations, the onset of symptoms, and ultrasonographic or radiologic imaging studies. Ultrasonography is highly sensitive and specific for the diagnosis of intussusception and appears to be diagnostically superior to radiographs.[53,54]

In a stable child the obstructive area can be successfully reduced with the use of an enema (air or liquid). However, if the child is unstable or presents with peritonitis, bowel perforation, or shock, then surgical intervention is necessary.

Open laparotomy with manual reduction is commonly performed. Untreated intussusception in infants is nearly always fatal. Most infants recover if the intussusception is reduced within 24 hours. Spontaneous reduction of intussusception may occur in symptomatic or asymptomatic children.[55,56]

Appendicitis

Appendicitis is the most common cause of emergency abdominal surgery in children. The mechanisms of disease, symptoms, and treatment are similar to those for adults and can be reviewed in Chapter 41. Most cases of appendicitis will occur in the second decade of life. Children typically present differently from adults, especially children under the age of 6. This puts them at greatest risk for perforation.[57]

Impairment of Digestion, Absorption, and Nutrition

Cystic Fibrosis

CF is an autosomal recessive disease of the exocrine glands that involves multiple organ systems but mostly the GI and respiratory systems. CF causes a shortened lifespan and prognosis is determined mainly by the degree of pulmonary involvement. This section focuses on GI complications of CF. (Chapter 36 discusses the epidemiology and pulmonary involvement.)

Pathophysiology. The GI presentation of CF is caused by a dysfunction of the CF transmembrane regulator (CFTR) protein, which is located on epithelial membranes and regulates chloride and sodium ion channels. It is found throughout the airways, sweat glands, digestive tract, pancreas, hepatobiliary system, and reproductive system. The hallmark pathophysiologic triad of CF is obstruction, infection, and inflammation that are evident throughout the GI tract. The full extrapulmonary spectrum of involvement is summarized in Table 42.1.

Dysfunction of the CFTR protein results in altered sodium, chloride, and potassium resorption, all of which remain external to the surface of the epithelial membrane, with reduced clearance from tubular structures lined by affected epithelia. Maldigestion of proteins, carbohydrates, fats, and fat-soluble vitamins occurs because mucus obstruction of the pancreatic ducts blocks the flow of pancreatic enzymes, causing intestinal malabsorption and degenerative and fibrotic changes in the pancreas and GI tract. Cystic fibrosis-related diabetes (CFRD) is the most common comorbidity of CF. Pancreatic islet cells are lost, which leads to insulin and glucagon deficiency, insulin resistance, delayed gastric emptying, and altered intestinal motility.[58]

TABLE 42.1 Cystic Fibrosis—Pathophysiology, Clinical Manifestations, and Complications

Organ Involved	Secretory Dysfunction	Clinical Manifestations	Complications
Sweat Glands	Elevated concentrations of sodium and chloride in sweat	Hyponatremia; hypochloremia	Heat prostration; shock
Digestive System			
Esophagus	None	Gastroesophageal reflux	Risk for aspiration events
Intestine			
Newborn	Viscid meconium	Meconium ileus with intestinal obstruction	Meconium peritonitis
Older child and adult	Inspissated (dried out) mucofecal masses (intestinal sludging)	Partial intestinal obstruction with severe cramping pains	Gastroesophageal reflux Volvulus (obstruction), intussusception (prolapse) Distal intestinal obstruction syndrome
Pancreas (enzyme deficiency)	Inspissation and precipitation of pancreatic secretions, causing obstruction of pancreatic ducts Insulin deficiency	Absence of pancreatic enzymes, causing malabsorption of food; fatty, bulky stools Decreased vitamins A, D, E, and K absorption Growth failure Glucose intolerance	Hypoproteinemia; iron deficiency anemia; malnutrition Recurrent pancreatitis, pancreatic cysts Vitamins A, D, E, and K deficiency and rectal prolapse Decreased bone density and risk of fractures in adolescents and adults Diabetes mellitus
Liver	Inspissation and precipitation of bile in biliary system	Focal biliary cirrhosis; shrunken, "hobnail" liver	Portal hypertension with esophageal varices, hematemesis and hypersplenism Hepatic steatosis Focal biliary cirrhosis Steatorrhea from lack of bile salts
Salivary glands	Inspissation and precipitation of secretions in small ducts of submaxillary and sublingual salivary glands	Mild patchy fibrosis of salivary glands	None
Respiratory System			
Paranasal structures	Viscid mucus	Retention of mucus; clouding seen on sinus roentgenograms	Mucopyoceles (pus accumulations) with nasal deformity or orbital cavity extension
Nose	Nasal polyps	Obstruction of nasal airflow	None
Lungs	Viscid mucus in bronchioles and bronchi	Obstruction of bronchioles causing bronchiolectasis, bronchiectasis, and chronic lung infection	Hemoptysis; pneumothorax; cor pulmonale; atelectasis; chronic bacterial infection; respiratory failure
Reproductive System			
Male	Viscid genital tract secretions during embryologic development, causing failure of formation of normal vas deferens	Delayed puberty Sterility	None
Female	Distention of endocervical epithelial cells with cytoplasmic mucin	Delayed puberty Decreased fertility	Polypoid cervicitis (cervical inflammation) while taking oral contraceptives

Data from Assis DN, Freedman SD. Gastrointestinal disorders in cystic fibrosis. *Clinics in Chest Medicine*, 2016;37(1):109–118; Lavelle LP, McEvoy SH, Ni Mhurchu E, et al. Cystic fibrosis below the diaphragm: Abdominal findings in adult patients. *Radiographics*, 2015;35(3):680–695; Leeuwen L, Fitzgerald DA, Gaskin KJ. Liver disease in cystic fibrosis. *Paediatric Respiratory Reviews*, 2014;15(1):69–74; Marcdante KJ, Kliegman RM, eds. *Nelson essentials of pediatrics*, 7th edition. Philadephia: Saunders; 2014; Stalvey MS, Clines GA. Cystic fibrosis-related bone disease: Insights into a growing problem. *Current Opinion in Endocrinology, Diabetes and Obesity*, 2013;20(6):547–552.

Clinical Manifestations. Clinical manifestations are summarized in Table 42.2. Newborn screening programs have changed the standard of diagnosis for CF. Traditionally, the diagnosis of CF was based on the presence of clinical features. Early diagnosis can now be made before clinical symptoms appear, which has led to modernized and streamlined interventions.[59,60]

GI symptoms, such as meconium ileus, often precede pulmonary manifestations. Most of those with CF present early in life with pancreatic insufficiency (PI). PI is the cause of nutrient malabsorption and FTT in children with CF. Steatorrhea (fatty stools) and abdominal distention are common symptoms with potential sequelae that include DIOS, fibrotic colonopathy, intussusception, or focal biliary cirrhosis. Children who are pancreatic sufficient (PS) are at greater risk of developing pancreatitis.

Evaluation and Treatment. All states in the United States screen newborns for CF using a blood test to detect immunoreactive trypsinogen (IRT). Genetic screening and the sweat test are required for diagnosis. Evaluation of pancreatic sufficiency also is essential. The extent of pancreatic function is determined by 72-hour fecal fat measurements, which are not easily obtained. Therefore, the most common measurement of fat malabsorption is fecal elastase. A serum test for IRT also can be used to detect PI in children older than 8 years of age, and various combinations of tests, including IRT, deoxyribonucleic acid (DNA) CF, pancreatitis-associated protein (PAP), and CFTR-extended genetic analysis (EGA), are being used in some states and countries.[59,61]

The goal of treatment for PI is to reduce malabsorption of nutrients and improve growth. Most children with CF take pancreatic enzyme replacement therapy (PERT) for the rest of their lives. PERT is administered before or with every meal, snack, or enteral feeding supplementation. High doses of PERT are associated with DIOS; therefore, minimal effective doses are indicated. High-caloric, high-protein diets with frequent snacks and vitamin supplements are used to treat malnutrition. Nutritional status and growth should be carefully monitored, and growth hormone may be included with nutritional supplements.[62,63]

Celiac Disease

Celiac disease (CD), also known as *celiac sprue* or *gluten-sensitive enteropathy*, is an autoimmune disease that damages small intestinal villous epithelium when gluten (gliadin), the protein component of wheat derivatives, barley, or rye, is ingested. CD is a common multiorgan disease with a strong genetic predisposition. It is associated with certain human leukocyte antigens (HLAs): HLA-DQ2 and HLA-DQ8. Nonceliac gluten sensitivity (GS) should not be confused with CD. It presents similarly after the ingestion of products containing gluten. The individual will not have positive antibodies, nor will they exhibit the classic intestinal villous atrophy. Instead, there will be variable HLA status with similar symptoms of the disease.[64] IgE-mediated wheat allergy is a gluten-related disorder, with GI manifestation in younger children (vomiting and/or diarrhea), and dermatitis and wheezing in older children.[65]

The pathogenesis of CD is complex and involves genetic and immunologic factors. Environmental factors include early infections, gut microbiota in infants, feeding patterns, and the timing and amount of gluten. CD presents with greater frequency in children with type 1 diabetes mellitus, autoimmune thyroid or liver disease, Down syndrome, Turner syndrome, Williams

TABLE 42.2 Galactosemia, Fructosemia, and Wilson Disease

	Galactosemia	Fructosemia	Wilson Disease
Mechanism of disease	Deficiency of galactose-1-phosphate uridylyltransferase Autosomal recessive trait Cannot convert galactose to glucose Toxic accumulation of galactose in body tissues, liver, and brain	Deficiency of fructose-1-phosphate aldolase Autosomal recessive trait Cannot metabolize fructose, sucrose, or honey; occurs when breast milk is replaced with cow's milk Toxic accumulation of fructose in body tissues	Defect in copper excretion by liver Autosomal recessive: defect on chromosome 13 (ATP 7B) Impaired transport of copper into bile/blood caused by diminished transport protein (ceruloplasmin) Toxic accumulations of copper in liver, brain, kidney, corneas
Clinical manifestation	High levels of blood galactose Vomiting Hypoglycemia May have failure to thrive Symptoms of cirrhosis at 2–6 months—jaundice Intellectual disabilities if not treated Cataracts if not treated	High levels of blood fructose Vomiting Hypoglycemia May have failure to thrive Hepatomegaly Jaundice Seizures	Intention tremors Indistinct speech Dystonia Greenish yellow rings in cornea Hepatomegaly Jaundice Anorexia Renal tubular defects
Evaluation	Newborn screening Presence of reducing substances in urine when infant is receiving lactose	Detailed dietary history Liver or intestinal mucosa biopsy	Low plasma ceruloplasmin level
Treatment	Galactose-free diet	Fructose-, sucrose-, honey-free diet Vitamin C supplementation	Chelation therapy to remove copper from body Decreased dietary intake of copper Liver transplantation

syndrome, selective immunoglobulin A (IgA) deficiency, Addison disease, and in those with first-degree relatives with CD. Individuals with CD are also at greater risk for non-Hodgkin's lymphoma and, rarely, small intestinal adenocarcinoma.[66]

Pathophysiology. The major pathophysiologic characteristic of CD is an HLA-DQ2- or HLA-DQ8-induced CD4+ T-cell-mediated autoimmune injury to the small intestinal epithelial cells of genetically susceptible individuals. There are increased numbers of intraepithelial lymphocytes, atrophy and flattening of villi, crypt hyperplasia in the upper small intestine, and malabsorption of most nutrients in the presence of gluten (Figs. 42.7 and 42.8). Atrophy is caused by accelerated shedding of epithelial cells from the villi. To compensate for this loss, epithelial cell production increases, causing hypertrophy

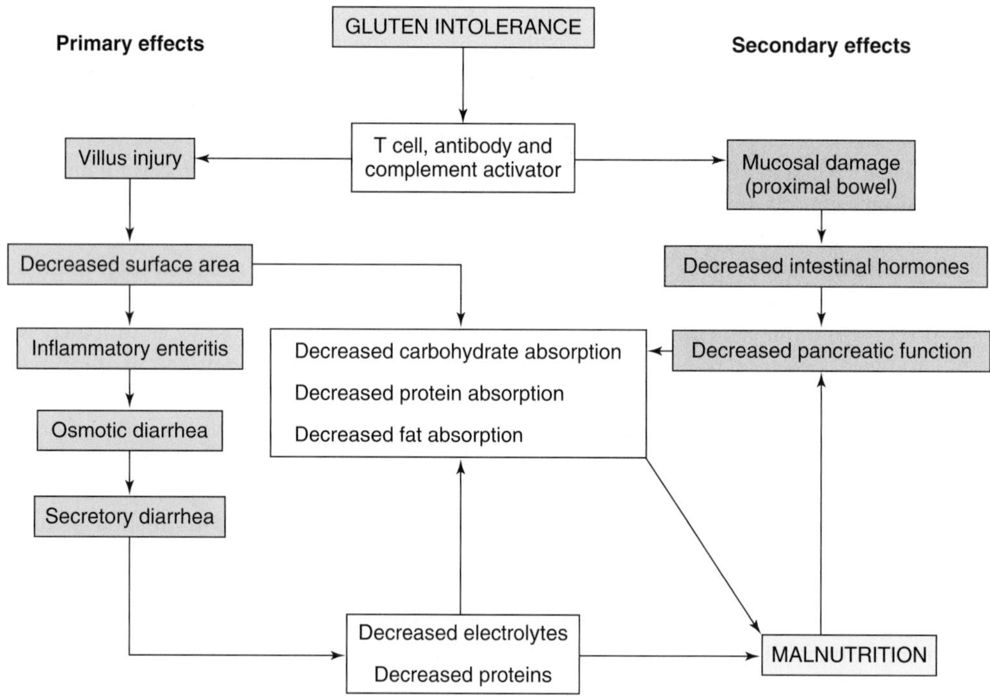

Fig. 42.7 Pathophysiology of Celiac Disease.

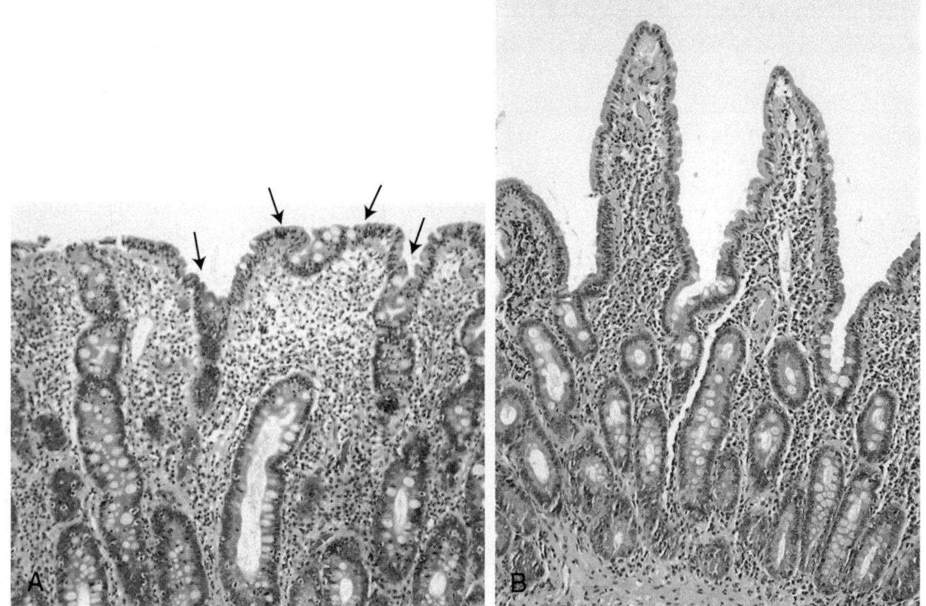

Fig. 42.8 Gluten – Sensitive Enteropathy. (A) Atrophy of villi and elongation of crypts that result in reduced surface area, loss of digestive enzymes, and malabsorption. **(B)** Recovery of normal villous structure after 6 months of gluten-free diet. (From Damjanov I, Linder J. *Pathology: A color atlas.* St. Louis, MO: Mosby; 2000.)

of the crypts and Lieberkühn. Increased cell production is not sufficient to keep pace with cell loss, and the cells are not mature enough to sustain absorptive functions. The microvilli and crush border disappear, leaving patches of bald mucosa. The loss of mucosal surface area and brush-border is pronounced in the duodenum and jejunum. The ileum may be spared. The severity of the disease correlates with the length of the small intestinal mucosa involved.[67,68]

Damage to the mucosa of the duodenum and jejunum exacerbates malabsorption. The secretion of intestinal hormones, such as secretin and cholecystokinin, may be diminished. Consequently, secretion of pancreatic enzymes and expulsion of bile from the gallbladder are reduced, contributing to malabsorption. Destruction of mucosal cells causes inflammation, and water and electrolytes are secreted, leading to watery diarrhea. Potassium loss leads to muscle weakness. Magnesium and calcium malabsorption can cause seizures or tetany. Unabsorbed fatty acids combine with calcium, and secondary hyperparathyroidism increases phosphorus excretion, resulting in bone reabsorption. Calcium is no longer able to bind oxalate in the intestine and is absorbed, which causes hyperoxaluria. Gallbladder function may be abnormal, and bile salt conjugation may decrease.

Fat malabsorption in the jejunum is the major cause of steatorrhea (fatty stools). Deficiencies of fat-soluble vitamins are common in children with CD. Vitamin K malabsorption leads to hypoprothrombinemia. There can be iron and folic acid malabsorption manifested as cheilosis, anemia, and a smooth, red tongue. Vitamin B_{12} absorption is impaired in those with extensive ileal disease. Because the absorption of folate and iron is greatest in the proximal small intestine, deficiencies of these substances are common.

Clinical Manifestations. The onset of clinical manifestations of CD are dependent on the age of the infant when gluten-containing substances are added to the diet. This can make diagnosis difficult. It is not uncommon for a person to be diagnosed later in life. Severity of symptoms can vary tremendously and depend on the age of the child. Abdominal pain, abdominal distention, anorexia, and diarrhea are early signs in most infants, which result in FTT and anemia. The stools are pale, bulky, greasy, and foul smelling, and many contain oil droplets. Some children present with constipation. Many untreated children older than 3 years of age present with non-GI symptoms related to malabsorption and malnutrition and the effect of autoantibodies on nonintestinal tissues.[69,70] Older children typically do not present with vomiting and abdominal pain; however, anorexia is prevalent. Extraintestinal manifestations of malabsorption, such as rickets, tetany, frank or occult bleeding, or anemia may be obvious. Some children will have increased nocturia. The tongue can be smooth and red, and the child may bruise and bleed easily. Hypomagnesemia and hypocalcemia cause irritability, tremor, convulsions, tetany, bone pain, osteomalacia, and dental abnormalities. If vitamin D deficiency is prolonged, rickets and clubbing of the terminal phalanges are likely. In older children, delayed puberty and infertility may be a manifestation of otherwise subtle gluten-sensitive enteropathy. There is an increased incidence of malignant disease, particularly T-cell lymphoma, in individuals who have refractory CD.[71]

Evaluation and Treatment. The diagnosis includes confirmation with serologic autoantibody measurement against tissue transglutaminase IgA (most sensitive and specific), anti-endomysium IgA, or deaminated gliadin peptides, which are more sensitive in children younger than 2 years of age. A negative genetic screening for HLA haplotypes rules out CD. If an autoantibody or genetic screen is positive, a small duodenal biopsy sample may be obtained to check for the classic mucosal changes caused by CD.[69,72] A wide variety of screening tests for malabsorption also may be useful. Even though very useful screening tools are available to diagnose CD, many children remain undiagnosed.[73–75]

Treatment consists of lifelong adherence to a gluten-free diet (GFD), which includes the elimination of wheat, rye, barley, and malt. Lactose (milk sugar) intolerance also may be present from damage to villi; therefore, lactose also may be excluded from the diet but should be resumed after treatment. Infants are routinely given fat-soluble vitamins, iron, and folic acid supplements to treat deficiencies. Most children have complete remission of symptoms with clearing of serologic markers and an excellent prognosis. Refractory CD, which is resistant to a GFD treatment, is rare and may require steroids or immunosuppressants. Steroid or immunosuppressants may be required in special cases.[76,77]

Malnutrition

Pediatric malnutrition is an imbalance between nutrient requirements (energy expenditure) and intake that results in energy, protein, and micronutrient deficits that impair growth and development. Malnutrition may involve impaired absorption, altered nutrient utilization, increased nutrient losses, or increased nutrient requirements (hypermetabolism). Severe or moderate acute or chronic illnesses can contribute to the development of malnutrition, including surgery, trauma, burns, and chronic diseases (e.g., CF, tuberculosis, chronic kidney disease, malignancies, congenital heart disease [CHD], GI diseases, and neuromuscular diseases). Malnutrition unrelated to illness develops from a lack of access to nutrients as a result of environmental factors (i.e., political/socioeconomic, inadequate food supplies, or food contaminated with parasites) or behavioral factors (e.g., anorexia nervosa). Malnutrition may be acute (less than 3 months' duration) or chronic (more than 3 months' duration).

Kwashiorkor (a deficiency of dietary protein) and **marasmus** (all forms of inadequate nutrient intake) are terms that have been used to describe types of malnutrition in children, particularly in developing countries. Collectively they are known as **protein-energy malnutrition (PEM)**. PEM describes the effects of malnutrition but not the etiology or interactions that contribute to nutrient depletion. A definition of pediatric malnutrition that includes the etiology (illness or environmental), identification of pathogenesis and chronicity, associations with inflammation, and resulting impact on functional status is more directive for defining the risk of malnutrition, planning interventions, and assessing outcomes.[78] States of long-term starvation are often the result of widespread nutritional deficiencies among children in developing countries and economically destitute populations, particularly when associated with human immunodeficiency virus (HIV) infection. Malnutrition can occur in infants or children from 1 to 4 years of age who have been weaned from breast milk to a high-starch, protein-deficient diet or switched to overdiluted commercial formulas that lack adequate protein and carbohydrates.[79–81]

Hospitalized children are at risk for malnutrition. Acute illness, trauma, surgery, or preexisting chronic diseases contribute to malnutrition and requires assessment and intervention. Acute and chronic inflammatory states also increase nutrient requirements. Treatments, including radiation therapy, chemotherapy, and longer times on mechanical ventilation, also can contribute to malnutrition with increased hospital length of stay, and increased morbidity and mortality rates.[82]

Pathophysiology. The pathogenesis of marasmus is uncertain but includes inadequate dietary proteins, carbohydrates, fats, and micronutrients over a period of months or years. There is wasting of fat and muscle. It is the most common form of PEM. Young children are most susceptible because of increased caloric requirements. Children with marasmus demonstrate greater wasting of protein and fat stores, which is presented in the clinical manifestations.

The metabolic response in Kwashiorkor is different. Kwashiorkor is the result of inadequate protein intake, but a high carbohydrate intake, and is more common where the diet is rice, corn, or beans. The liver swells with stored fat because no hepatic proteins are synthesized to form and release lipoproteins. Pancreatic atrophy and fibrosis may be present. Atrophy of intestinal villi and alterations in gut microbiota results in nutrient malabsorption and malnutrition. Malabsorption causes reduced bone density and impaired renal function. If the condition is not reversed, the prognosis is very poor and growth is severely retarded.

Children with malnutrition show stunting of gut microbiota maturation, which may delay normal development of the gut, depress intestinal immune function, and promote inflammation, leaky gut syndrome, and infection. Healthy gut bacteria also produce short-chain fatty acids, B vitamins, and vitamin K, and promotes the absorption of minerals important for maintaining the intestinal epithelium. Alterations in intestinal microbiota and immune dysregulation can cause leaky gut syndrome (compromised gut barrier) and intestinal inflammation. Atrophy of the thymus gland and tonsils with decreased T cell formation, synthesis of IgA, and impaired phagocytosis increase susceptibility for infection and poor tissue repair and regeneration.[83–85]

Clinical Manifestations. Children with marasmus have systemic muscle wasting and appear emaciated, and are weak and may have associated bradycardia, hypotension, and hypothermia. Anemia is common and can be severe. Their skin is wrinkled and loose from loss of subcutaneous fat. Metabolic processes, including liver function, are preserved, but growth is severely retarded; therefore, marasmus is characterized by low weight for height representation. Marasmus is not only characterized by muscle wasting, but children also may have diarrhea, dermatosis, low hemoglobin level, and infection. There is loss of subcutaneous fat and an absence of edema, whereas marked generalized edema is characteristic of Kwashiokor. Edema begins in the most dependent regions and proceeds toward the cranium as the process continues. The response to starvation includes low serum albumin (hypoproteinemia), increased cortisol, inability to activate antidiuretic hormone, and hypokalemia. The hair is dry, sparse, brittle, and depigmented, appearing reddish yellow. The skin can appear dry and shiny with areas of hyperpigmentation or hypopigmentation. Body weight may be normal and related to edema. Children also may have clinical manifestations of a distended abdomen, hepatomegaly, and almost normal weight for age (because of edema). Both conditions lead to delays in physical, behavioral, and cognitive development and academic performance. Finally, micronutrient deficiencies, especially with zinc, selenium, iron, and antioxidant vitamins, can lead to immune deficiency and infections. Severe vitamin A deficiency commonly results in blindness.[86–88]

Evaluation and Treatment. Evaluation of malnutrition is based on the nutritional history and clinical manifestations, including anthropometric measurements and use of appropriate growth charts. Laboratory monitoring is used to assess for macronutrient and micronutrient deficiencies, aminotransaminase alterations, the presence of inflammation, and response to refeeding. Treatment of underlying disease and provision of deficient nutrients will resolve clinical symptoms in 4 to 6 weeks. Use of antibiotics has been shown to improve recovery and decrease mortality as severe caloric restriction causes an increased susceptibility to infection. This is secondary to immunodeficiency.[85]

Developmental sequelae of malnutrition may be irreversible; therefore, early intervention is recommended. Nutritional rehabilitation and adequate hydration with appropriate environmental stimulation for infants and young children has been shown to resolve or improve cerebral shrinkage, physical growth, and psychomotor development.

Faltering Growth (Failure to Thrive)

Faltering growth (previously known as FTT) is not a diagnosis but a physical sign demonstrating that a child has a slower rate of weight gain in childhood than expected for age and sex. It is manifested as a decrease in velocity in weight gain, a low weight/height or body mass index (BMI) ratio, or a low weight/height/head circumference ratio over time. Faltering growth is a common problem and can present at any time in childhood but is usually present before 18 months of age.[89]

Pathophysiology. Faltering growth is considered a multifactorial condition that includes biologic, psychosocial, and environmental contributions that may or may not be related to illness (Box 42.1). In more than 80% of cases, an underlying medical condition is never found. Categories of faltering growth include inadequate caloric intake, inadequate caloric absorption, or excessive caloric expenditure. Infants and children are at risk if their parents or primary caregivers are unable to provide nurturance.

Clinical Manifestations. Clinical manifestations of faltering growth are delayed growth accompanied by manifestations of

BOX 42.1 Factors Associated With Faltering Growth

Poverty (food insecurity related to lack of money)
Premature birth; low birth weight
Inadequate caloric intake or caloric absorption (infant feeding problems, underlying chronic disease or malabsorption syndromes)
Incorrect preparation of formula (too diluted, too concentrated)
Mechanical feeding difficulties (oromotor dysfunction, congenital anomalies, central nervous system disorders)
Unsuitable feeding habits (food fads, excessive juice)
Behavior problems affecting eating
Disturbed parent-child relationship; parental stress, parental lack of knowledge; child neglect

Data from Krishna A, et al: Glob Health Action 8:26523, 2015; National Guideline Alliance (UK): Faltering growth–recognition and management, London, UK; 2017, National Institute for Health and Care Excellence (UK); https://www.ncbi.nlm.nih.gov/books/NBK458459/.

malnutrition or an underlying disease (e.g., diarrhea or infectious disease, or both). Infants who present with faltering growth frequently have feeding problems. Symptoms include pallid or dry, cracked skin; sparse hair; poorly developed musculature; decreased subcutaneous fat; swollen abdomen with malabsorption, diarrhea, or anorexia; and signs of vitamin deficiencies, such as rickets. Social or emotional manifestations include reduced energy level, reduced responsiveness and interaction with the environment, social isolation, spasticity and rigidity when held or touched, inability to make eye contact or smile, refusal to eat, and rejection of foods. There may be long-term adverse effects on cognitive, behavioral, and academic performance.

Evaluation and Treatment. Faltering growth is a clinical finding as opposed to a diagnosis. Therefore, serial growth measurements over time are necessary. Underlying medical conditions should be thoroughly evaluated. If illness is ruled out, a thorough review of psychosocial, emotional, and environmental components of care is necessary. Screening tools are available to assist with evaluation of nutrition status and to guide therapy, particularly in hospitalized children.

Treatment for faltering growth includes treating an underlying illness if found, increasing volume or caloric density of formula, increasing frequency of breast-feeding (if found to be insufficient), structuring meals and snacks, and adding high-calorie foods and additives. Eliminating fruit juice, soda, or excessive milk also will improve appetite and absorption of nutrients. Medications are used to stimulate appetite. Nutrient deficiencies are supplemented. If the child is unable to gain weight, an oral enteral supplement may be added to the diet or a nasogastric or gastrostomy tube can be used to supplement oral intake.

If the cause is not medical, management involves the immediate total care of the child and measures to address (1) the psychosocial and emotional problems of the caregivers and (2) parent-child interactions. Counseling, parental modeling, and long-term family support are sometimes required. Hospital admission and evaluation are recommended if the diagnosis is unclear or the child is in nutritional or emotional jeopardy. Eating patterns, food preferences, caloric intake, and family interactions can be assessed and treatment plans implemented during the hospital stay.[89]

Necrotizing Enterocolitis

Necrotizing enterocolitis (NEC) is an ischemic, inflammatory condition that causes bowel necrosis and perforation. NEC is not a specific diagnosis but a constellation of signs and symptoms with several proposed etiologies. It is the most common severe neonatal GI emergency that predominantly affects the smallest (weighing less than 1500 g) and most premature infants. The incidence and mortality of NEC have decreased over the past decade and have been attributed to improved risk assessments.[90]

Pathophysiology. The exact etiology of NEC is unclear. Factors contributing to the development of NEC include infections, abnormal bacterial colonization, intestinal ischemia, immature immune responses, exaggerated inflammatory responses, immature intestinal motility, altered microcirculatory blood flow and barrier function, perinatal stress, effects of medications, and feeding practices, including alterations in TLR4 expression (a pattern recognition receptor that triggers the NF-κB inflammatory pathway activating the innate immune system).[90]

The immature mucosal barrier delays digestion and motility is slower, allowing for the accumulation of noxious substances that damage the intestine, increase permeability, and increase the risk for infection. Translocation of intestinal bacteria and other substances contributes to injury, with inflammation, vasoconstriction of mesenteric blood flow, development of systemic inflammatory disease, multiple organ failure, and death. Immature intestinal innate immunity and an unfavorable balance between normal and pathogenic bacteria promote intestinal inflammation and release of proinflammatory cytokines. Accumulation of gas in the intestine can cause pressure that decreases blood flow, and an imbalance between vasodilator and vasoconstrictor inputs in the immature gut may lead to vasoconstriction promoting ischemia and oxidative stress, reperfusion injury, necrosis, and perforation.[91,92]

Clinical Manifestations. Manifestations of NEC usually appear suddenly and within weeks of premature birth, and sooner for term neonates. Signs and symptoms of "classic" NEC include feeding intolerance, abdominal distention and bloody stools after 8 to 10 days of age, septicemia with an elevated white blood cell count, and falling platelet levels. Unstable temperature, bradycardia, and apnea are nonspecific signs. In late preterm or term infants, NEC is more likely to be associated with other predisposing factors, such as low Apgar scores, chorioamnionitis, exchange transfusions, prolonged rupture of membranes, congenital heart defects, or neural tube defects.[93]

Evaluation and Treatment. Diagnosis is based on the clinical manifestations, laboratory results, and plain films of the abdomen. Symptoms usually progress rapidly, often within hours, from subtle signs to abdominal discoloration, intestinal perforation, and peritonitis, or even death. Abdominal radiographs show pneumoperitoneum, pneumatosis intestinalis (gas in the bowel wall), or unchanging "rigid" loops of small bowel. Systemic hypotension requires intensive medical support or bowel resection, or both. Efforts are in progress to identify predictive biologic markers for early diagnosis. Preventive strategies include encouragement of breast milk feeding, preferential feeding of human milk, judicious fluid management to prevent vascular fluid overload, and confirmation of patent ductus arteriosus (see Chapter 33). Additional treatments include administration of amino acids (i.e., arginine and glutamine supplements) to support intestinal epithelial cell growth and enteral probiotics to support normal gut bacteria. The rapid onset of symptoms makes primary prevention difficult.[94,95]

Treatments include cessation of feeding, implementation of gastric suction to decompress the intestines, maintenance of fluid and electrolyte balance, and administration of antibiotics to control sepsis. Surgical resection is the treatment of choice for perforation, and peritoneal drainage may be used as an adjunct to laparotomy. Overall mortality is high, particularly for infants who have surgery.[96]

Diarrhea

Diarrhea is an increase in the water content, volume, or frequency of stools and can be acute or chronic. Diarrhea is usually defined as three or more watery or loose stools in 24 hours. Children with acute gastroenteritis often remain mildly symptomatic for up to 4 weeks; therefore, diarrhea that persists longer than 4 weeks is considered chronic. Diarrhea is a common GI problem during infancy and early childhood and is the leading cause of death in young children, particularly among preterm infants and children in developing countries.[97] Severe, acute infectious diarrhea occurs one to three times during the first 3 years of life. Most episodes are self-limiting and resolve within 72 hours.

The pathophysiologic mechanisms of diarrhea in children are similar to those described for adults: osmotic, secretory, intestinal dysmotility, or inflammatory (see Chapter 41). Prolonged diarrhea is more dangerous in infants and children, however, because they have much smaller fluid reserves and more rapid peristalsis and metabolism than adults. Therefore, dehydration in children can develop rapidly if any disturbance:

- increases fluid secretion into the GI lumen (secretory diarrhea).
- draws fluid into the lumen by osmosis (osmotic diarrhea).
- reduces intestinal transit time with luminal fluid retention (intestinal dysmotility).
- causes inflammation that results in malabsorption and an increased luminal osmotic load from nutrients, fluid, and blood, which may increase gut motility (inflammatory diarrhea).

There are numerous causes of diarrhea in infants and children, including viral, bacterial, and systemic infections; malabsorption syndromes; autoimmune disorders; congenital malformations; and genetic disorders. Acute infection is the most common cause of childhood diarrhea worldwide.[98] Most recently, episodes of diarrhea have been associated with the COVID-19 pandemic. See Emerging Science Box: COVID-19 and the Gastrointestinal System in Children.

EMERGING SCIENCE BOX

COVID-19 and the Gastrointestinal System in Children

The severe acute respiratory syndrome coronavirus 2 (SARS-CoV-2) is primarily a respiratory pathogen that manifests as viral infectious pneumonia. That said, the pathogen can also cause gastrointestinal (GI) and hepatic symptoms. Angiotensin converting enzyme-2 (ACE-2) receptor and transmembrane serine protease 2 (TMPRSS2) are expressed in the respiratory mucosa as well as in the enterocytes of the ileum and colon. The most common GI symptoms reported in children are diarrhea, nausea, vomiting, and abdominal pain. Aspartate transferase, alanine transferase, and total bilirubin are commonly elevated in infected individuals with these symptoms. SARS-CoV-2 is believed to be transmitted through respiratory droplet and fomite contamination. However, RT-PCR positive stool samples have been found in multiple children, which raises the concern of a possible fecal-oral transmission route.

Data from Matthai J, et al. Indian Society of Pediatric Gastroenterology, Hepatology and Nutrition; Pediatric Gastroenterology Chapter of Indian Academy of Pediatrics. Coronavirus disease (COVID-19) and the gastrointestinal system in children. *Indian Pediatrics*, 2020;57(6):533–535. https://doi.org/10.1007/s13312-020-1851-5; Cha MH, et al. Gastrointestinal and hepatic manifestations of COVID-19: A comprehensive review. *World Journal of Gastroenterology*, 2020;26(19):2323–2332. https://doi.org/10.3748/wjg.v26.i19.2323; Tang A, et al. Detection of Novel Coronavirus by RT-PCR in stool specimen from asymptomatic child, China. *Emerging Infectious Diseases*, 2020;26(6):1337–1339. https://doi.org/10.3201/eid2606.200301.

Acute Infectious Diarrhea

Acute infectious diarrhea in infants and young children is usually associated with viral or bacterial gastroenteritis from contaminated food or water. Viruses include rotaviruses, noroviruses, and adenoviruses. Rotavirus is the most common cause in young children and is associated with a higher death rate in low-income countries. It is transmitted by the fecal-oral route among humans. Rotavirus vaccination is an effective preventive strategy.[98]

Pathophysiology. Numerous bacteria or parasites can contaminate food or water and cause diarrhea. Bacterial causes of diarrhea have geographic variation, and specific bacteria can be identified using molecular analysis or stool culture. *Clostridium difficile* is often associated with previous antibiotic therapy.

Clinical Manifestations. Infectious diarrhea has a rapid onset, with watery stools sometimes mixed with blood, abdominal cramping, fever, vomiting, and weight loss. Severe dehydration, acidosis, and shock can occur quickly from diarrhea and vomiting. Hemolytic uremic syndrome and renal failure can develop when diarrhea is associated with *Shigella* toxin and *Escherichia coli* infection (see Chapter 39). Other causes of acute diarrhea in the older child include antibiotic therapy, appendicitis, chemotherapy, inflammatory bowel disease (IBD), parasitic infestation, parenteral infections, and ingestion of toxic substances.

Evaluation and Treatment. Treatment of diarrhea requires evaluation of the cause through the history, stool testing for common pathogens, and laboratory analysis. Treatment of underlying illness is warranted when identified. Other treatments include hydration, electrolyte replacement, nutrition maintenance, and antibiotics if a pathogen is found. In certain children, antispasmodics may relieve abdominal cramping and selected probiotics can reduce the duration and improve morbidity and mortality. Intravenous solutions are used only when oral solutions are not tolerated. Prevention includes clean water, environmental sanitation, and good hygiene.[99]

Primary Lactose Intolerance

Lactose malabsorption, lactose intolerance, and lactase deficiency are three separate entities. Lactase deficiency refers to the lower than expected activity of lactase at the brush border of the intestine. Lactose malabsorption refers to the small bowel's inability to absorb ingested lactose due to lactase deficiency. Lactose intolerance is the clinical manifestation in which the ingestion of lactose-containing products induces symptoms. Primary lactose intolerance is an acquired deficiency and rarely manifests itself before age 5. Transient lactose malabsorption following gastroenteritis is common in children under the age of 2.[100]

The malabsorption of lactose results in osmotic diarrhea accompanied by abdominal pain, diarrhea, and flatulence. Symptoms of cow's milk allergy (CMA) are similar, which leads to misdiagnosis and inappropriate dietary modification.[101]

The diagnosis can be made through elimination of dietary lactose or by performing a hydrogen lactose breath test or an oral lactose tolerance test. Treatment consists of reducing milk consumption or supplementing the diet with oral lactase. Some children can tolerate lactose in fermented forms, such as cheese and yogurt, or by adding soy food. A diet low in fermentable oligosaccharides, disaccharides, and monosaccharides and polyols (FODMAPs) or administration of probiotics to alter intestinal flora has been found to be effective in children with lactose intolerance and irritable bowel syndrome (IBS) who have persistent symptoms. Additional sources of dietary calcium and vitamin D should be considered.[102]

DISORDERS OF THE LIVER

Disorders of Biliary Metabolism and Transport

Neonatal Jaundice

Jaundice (icterus) is a yellow pigmentation of the skin, mucus membranes, or the whites of the eyes caused by an increased level of bilirubin in the bloodstream (i.e., a total serum bilirubin [TSB] level that exceeds the 95th percentile for the infant's age in hours or greater than 20 mg/dL, except in the low birth weight population). Jaundice usually becomes clinically apparent when the serum bilirubin concentration is greater than 2 mg/dL (34 μmol/L). Physiologic jaundice (hyperbilirubinemia) of the newborn is a frequently encountered problem in otherwise healthy newborns caused by lack of maturity of bilirubin uptake and conjugation. Poor caloric intake or dehydration, or both, associated with inadequate breast-feeding also may contribute to the high levels of bilirubin. High bilirubin levels in the newborn period can be associated with hemolytic disease, metabolic and endocrine disorders, anatomic abnormalities of the liver, and infections. For older infants and children, the most common causes of unconjugated hyperbilirubinemia are hemolytic processes resulting in bilirubin overproduction.

Pathologic jaundice appears within 24 hours after birth and with TSB concentration greater than 17 mg/dL in the newborn period associated with a severe illness, or a TSB level that rises by more than 5 mg/dL during the newborn period. Risk factors for development of pathologic jaundice include preeclampsia, maternal hypertension, maternal diabetes mellitus, vaginal bleeding, fetal-maternal blood type incompatibility (ABO and Rh incompatibility, hemolytic disease in the newborn), premature birth, maternal age greater than or equal to 25 years, male gender, delayed meconium passage, glucose-6-phosphate dehydrogenase deficiency, and excessive birth trauma, such as bruising or cephalohematomas.[103]

Pathophysiology. Pathologic jaundice results from the complex interaction of factors that cause (1) increased bilirubin production (e.g., hemolysis), (2) impaired hepatic uptake or excretion of unconjugated bilirubin, or (3) delayed maturation of liver bilirubin conjugating mechanisms. The most common cause is hemolytic disease of the newborn, also called erythroblastosis fetalis (ABO blood incompatibility [see Chapters 9 and 30]). All pregnant women should be tested for ABO and Rh incompatibility. Unconjugated bilirubin (indirect bilirubin) is lipid soluble and bound to albumin in the blood, and in the free form it readily crosses the blood-brain barrier in infants. Bilirubin encephalopathy (kernicterus) is caused by the deposition of toxic, unconjugated bilirubin in brain cells and usually does not occur in healthy, full-term infants. The mechanism of injury is not clearly known. An elevated level of conjugated bilirubin is a sign of underlying disease.[104,105]

Clinical Manifestations. Physiologic jaundice develops during the second or third day after birth and usually subsides in 1 to 2 weeks in full-term infants and in 2 to 4 weeks in premature infants. After this, increasing bilirubin values and persistent jaundice indicate pathologic hyperbilirubinemia. Manifestations include yellowing of the skin, dark urine, light-colored stools, and weight loss. Premature infants with respiratory distress, acidosis, or sepsis are at greater risk for kernicterus and the development of bilirubin-induced neurologic dysfunction (BIND) (e.g., neuromotor signs, hyperexcitable neonatal reflexes, and speech and hearing impairment).[106]

Evaluation and Treatment. Jaundice is detected by clinical assessment. Both total and direct (conjugated) bilirubin levels are monitored, and the bilirubin/albumin ratio is being evaluated as a corollary to unbound serum bilirubin level for predicting neurotoxicity, particularly in premature infants. Other causes of jaundice must be eliminated to confirm physiologic jaundice. Treatment depends on the degree of hyperbilirubinemia. Physiologic jaundice is commonly treated by phototherapy and several techniques are available. Pathologic jaundice requires an exchange transfusion and treatment of the underlying disorder.[107]

Biliary Atresia

Biliary atresia (BA) is a rare congenital malformation characterized by the absence or obstruction of extrahepatic bile ducts resulting in neonatal cholestasis. The etiology of duct injury is not clear but is thought to be related to an embryonic (or congenital) abnormality or an acquired anomaly (e.g., perinatal viral or toxin-induced progressive inflammation with innate autoimmune destruction). Genetic associations have been reported in the following sequences: *GATA3, FOXA2, NODAL.* More research is needed in this area. The disease expression is a continuum in which the principal process is one of bile duct destruction. The atresia of the bile ducts is associated with inflammation, fibrosis, loss of epithelial cells, and obstruction of the bile canaliculi. Progressive obstruction leads to secondary biliary cirrhosis (see Chapter 39), portal hypertension, liver failure, and subsequent liver transplant.[108]

Jaundice is the primary clinical manifestation of BA, along with hepatomegaly and acholic (clay-colored) stools. Fat absorption is impaired because of the lack of bile salts. Abdominal distention caused by hepatomegaly and ascites may cause anorexia and faltering growth. Fat-soluble vitamin deficiencies (A, D, E, K) require supplementation. Manifestations of cirrhosis and liver failure include ascites, hypoalbuminemia, hypercoagulation, thrombocytopenia, pruritus, esophageal varices, and GI bleeding that may lead to death.

Early diagnosis of BA is essential; the best outcome is achieved when the infant is diagnosed and treated in the first 30 to 45 days of life. BA that is diagnosed late does not respond well to current surgical treatment. The diagnosis of BA is based on the clinical manifestations, abnormal liver function test results, liver biopsy results, and an intraoperative cholangiogram. Serum aminotransaminase and alkaline phosphatase levels are elevated, and conjugated (direct) serum bilirubin levels rise progressively. Surgical intervention removes the atretic biliary remnants and creates an intestinal conduit for bile drainage, also known as the hepatoportoenterostomy (HPE), or Kasai portoenterostomy (KPE) (Fig. 42.9). Even with initial restoration of bile flow, however, obliteration of intrahepatic bile ducts can continue and cirrhosis results. The vast majority of children will eventually need a liver transplant.[109]

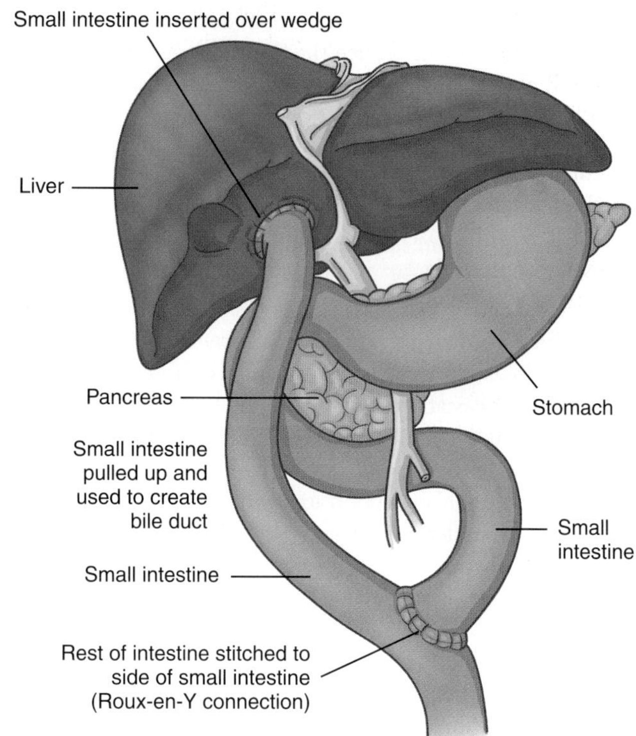

Fig. 42.9 Kasai Procedure. Surgical correction for extrahepatic biliary atresia. The jejunal segment between the liver and the bowel may be externalized, creating a double-barrel portoenterostomy.

Inflammatory Disorders

Hepatitis

Hepatitis refers to an inflammation of the liver. The condition can be self-limiting, or it can lead to cirrhosis, liver, cancer, and even death. Etiology includes toxic substances and viral, infectious, and autoimmune diseases. There are five main types of viral hepatitis. Details are presented in Chapter 41.

Hepatitis A virus. Hepatitis A virus (HAV) is transmitted through the fecal-oral route. The incubation period is 28 days and can produce either symptomatic or asymptomatic infection, which is related to the age of the infected person. Children younger than 6 years do not present with symptoms 70% of the time, whereas older children and adults typically do present with symptoms. HAV replicates in the liver and is excreted through the biliary system into the stool. Concentration of viral shedding in the stool is highest during the 2-week period before the onset of symptoms. Children can shed longer than adults, for up to 10 weeks.

Outbreaks tend to occur in day-care centers with large numbers of children who are not toilet trained, throughout a household, and sometimes through food or water contaminated with fecal matter. Vertical transmission from mother to newborn or from a transfusion, as well as from a blood transfusion infection, is rare. HAV in children is usually asymptomatic, but if symptoms do appear, they are mild and may include nausea, vomiting, and diarrhea. Jaundice is more likely to appear in older children.[110]

Almost all children recover from hepatitis A without residual liver damage, although relapse may occur. After HAV infection, the body produces antibodies and natural immunity to prevent reinfection. Vaccination programs have successfully reduced the incidence of HAV in the United States by 95%.[111]

Hepatitis B virus. Hepatitis B virus (HBV) is a world health problem. Despite immunization programs, HBV continues to be a major cause of acute and chronic liver disease and associated population morbidity and mortality. Transmission occurs through contact of infected blood and body fluids. Risk factors for HBV include infants of mothers who are chronic hepatitis B surface antigen (HBsAg) carriers, children from families who immigrated to the United States or are adopted from endemic areas, infection from HBsAg-positive household contacts, and children who abuse parenteral drugs or engage in unprotected sex. Vertical transmission (mother-to-child) and horizontal early childhood transmission continue to be the main routes of HBV transmission for children.[112]

Chronic hepatitis may develop more often in young children because their immune system is immature. Cirrhosis and hepatocellular carcinoma are rare. The most serious consequence of HBV infection is fulminant hepatitis, which occurs in 1% of cases. There is evidence that the risk of fulminant hepatitis is higher in individuals with combined infection with HBV, hepatitis D virus (HDV), hepatitis C virus (HCV), or HIV than in those with HBV infection alone. Aggressive HBV vaccination programs have reduced the incidence of HBV. To prevent perinatal transmission of HBV, immunoprophylaxis and HBV vaccination within the first 12 hours of birth are recommended, with close follow-up visits. Treatment is conservative, and antivirals are used for chronic disease. Children ages 2 to 17 years who are HBsAg seropositive for more than 6 months with elevated serum alanine transaminase (ALT) and HBV DNA levels for more than 3 months respond to treatment with antivirals. Maternal antiviral therapy during pregnancy and lactation reduces the HBV mother-to-child transmission rate.[113–115]

Hepatitis C virus. Hepatitis C Virus (HCV) in children is most commonly transmitted vertically and is enhanced by maternal coinfection with HIV. Risk factors for vertical transmission include internal fetal monitoring, mothers with high HCV viral load, prolonged rupture of membranes, and fetal anoxia. In older children, HCV transmission occurs more commonly through exposure to infected blood or contaminated materials (as in injection drug use or tattooing and body piercing) and after sexual encounters with individuals infected with HCV. Transmission from blood transfusions has become a negligible risk with universal HCV screening of blood. With vertical transmission, spontaneous resolution of HCV is high; otherwise, the disease is usually mild in children and cirrhosis is rare. Treatment is genotype specific, but because of adverse drug events, only children with persistently elevated serum aminotransferases or those with progressive liver disease are treated with antiviral drugs. Unfortunately, treatment seldom results in cure, and there is currently a need for further research and collaboration in order to guide pediatric management practice and policy.[116,117]

Hepatitis D virus. Hepatitis D Virus (HDV) is a single-strand RNA virus. Replication depends on the presence of HBV. Infection occurs simultaneously or as a superinfection; therefore, individuals with HVD infection are always mutually infected with HBV. Vertical transmission is uncommon. The prevalence in the United States is low, but HDV continues to affect parts of Europe and Asia and is a cause of progressive liver disease in children who are chronic hepatitis B surface antigen (HBsAg) carriers.[118] Treatment is based on genotype (genotype 1 is most common in the United States), but more research is currently underway for novel approaches to treatment.[119]

Chronic hepatitis. HBV and HCV are the main causes of chronic hepatitis in children. Manifestations of chronic hepatitis may include malaise, anorexia, fever, GI bleeding, hepatomegaly, edema, and transient joint pain. However, often there are no symptoms. Serum alanine aminotransferase and bilirubin levels are elevated. There may be evidence of impairment of synthetic functions of the liver: prolonged prothrombin time, thrombocytopenia, and hypoalbuminemia. The diagnosis is based on the clinical manifestations and liver biopsy results. There is no curative therapy for chronic HBV or chronic HCV. Children are treated with antiviral drugs and should continue to be monitored. Large scale clinical trials for the children with chronic hepatitis are lacking. Liver transplant may ultimately be required for these children.[120]

There is an autoimmune form of chronic hepatitis, known as *autoimmune hepatitis* (AIH) or *autoimmune primary sclerosing cholangitis* (PSC), which has an unknown etiology. The pathogenic mechanism is thought to be immunologic with loss of tolerance to hepatocyte-specific autoantigens, environmental, or genetic in nature. PSC is associated with a diagnosis of IBD. Advances are being made in identifying serologic markers to guide diagnosis and treatment. These diseases are chronic and progressive, typically presenting with elevations in the levels of bilirubin, aspartate aminotransferase-to-platelet ratio index, gamma-glutamyltransferase, and alkaline phosphatase. Children diagnosed at younger ages and those with small duct disease as compared to large duct involvement have better outcomes and less long term sequelae.[121]

Cirrhosis

Cirrhosis is fibrotic scarring of the liver, in response to inflammation and tissue damage, that results in nodular obstruction to the flow of blood and bile (see Chapter 41). Most forms of chronic liver diseases in children can progress to cirrhosis, but that is rare. The complications of cirrhosis in children are the same as those in adults: portal hypertension, the opening of collateral vessels between the portal and systemic veins, and varices. In addition, children with cirrhosis experience growth failure caused by nutritional deficits, as well as developmental delay, particularly in gross motor function because of ascites and weakness. The cause of cirrhosis may influence its severity and course (i.e., biliary atresia and hepatitis). Some types of cirrhosis can be stabilized if the cause is identified and treated early.[122]

Nonalcoholic fatty liver disease. Nonalcoholic fatty liver disease (NAFLD) is the most common cause of chronic liver disease in children. It is associated with obesity, insulin resistance, genetic predisposition, ethnicity, the gut microbiome, and environmental factors (diet and lack of exercise). NAFLD is associated with dyslipidemia, hypertension, and early cardiac dysfunction in children and can progress to cirrhosis and cardiometabolic syndrome within a few years if not treated. The rise in childhood obesity worldwide is contributing to the increasing prevalence of NAFLD. Circulating mRNAs may serve as important biomarkers for obesity and its comorbidities (See Emerging Science Box: The Role of miRNAs as Biomarkers of Obesity). The disease usually presents in prepubertal children and is predominant in males and in children of Hispanic origin. The diagnosis is made by exclusion of other causes of the disease, usually by 12 to 13 years of age. Liver biopsy is required for definitive diagnosis of nonalcoholic steatohepatitis (NASH). Compared to adults, there are differences in the extent of fat, inflammation, and fibrosis in children, and there is no standard scoring system. There also is no consensus regarding treatment. Exercise and slow, consistent weight loss with a low glycemic index diet have been shown to be more effective than a low-fat diet in lowering body weight. Pharmacologic agents are being evaluated to control insulin

EMERGING SCIENCE BOX

The Role of miRNAs as Biomarkers of Obesity

MicroRNAs or miRNAs are a class of small, non-coding RNAs that modulate gene expression at the post-transcription level. Several miRNAs have been found in research as overexpressed in obesity (miR199a, miR-122, miR-222, miR-142-3, miR-140-5p, and miR-143 to name a few). Two miRNAs have been identified as overexpressed in children with obesity and nonalcoholic fatty liver disease (NAFLD) and/or insulin resistance (miR-122 and miR-34). Also implicated in the pathogenesis of NAFLDA is miR-34a. Circulating miRNAs may prove to become a sensitive and specific biomarker for the development of obesity and obesity-associated diseases such as NAFLD.

Data from Oses M, et al. Circulating miRNAs as biomarkers of obesity and obesity-associated comorbidities in children and adolescents: A systematic review. *Nutrients,* 2019;11(12):2890. https://doi.org/10.3390/nu11122890; Torres J, et al. Role of microRNAs in alcohol-induced liver disorders and non-alcoholic fatty liver disease. World Journal of Gastroenterology, 2018;24(36):4104–4118. https://doi.org/10.3748/wjg.v24.i36.4104; Thompson MD, et al. Elevation of circulating microRNA levels in obese children compared to healthy controls. Clinical Obesity, 2017;7(4):216–221. https://doi.org/10.1111/cob.12192.

resistance, prevent the progression of liver disease, and cirrhosis. Omega-3 fatty acids, probiotics, and vitamin E may delay disease progression. Research is in progress to define the pathophysiology, noninvasive diagnostic procedures, and prevention measures.[123–125]

Portal Hypertension

Portal hypertension is an increased pressure in the portal venous system and a major cause of morbidity and mortality in children with liver disease. There are two basic causes of portal hypertension in children: (1) increased resistance to blood flow within the portal system, and (2) increased volume of portal blood flow. The second cause is rare in children and is not discussed here. Increased resistance to flow can occur anywhere in the portal circulatory system. Portal hypertension can accompany cirrhosis, intra-abdominal infections, portal vein thrombosis, congenital anomalies of the portal vein, and congenital hepatic fibrosis.

Types of Portal Hypertension

Extrahepatic portal hypertension. Extrahepatic portal hypertension causes 50% to 70% of portal hypertension in children. No specific cause can be found in approximately two-thirds of these children. Obstructions are almost always in the portal vein and are usually caused by thrombosis as a complication of abdominal trauma, pancreatitis, abdominal infections, and some systemic disorders; however, these causes are rare. Umbilical infection with or without a history of catheterization of the umbilical vein may be a cause in neonates. It also has been associated with neonatal dehydration, inflammatory bowel disease (IBD), and hypercoagulable states, such as protein C and protein S deficiencies. Life-threatening bleeding and coagulation disorders can occur. Mesoportal bypass (anastomosis of the mesenteric vein to the portal vein) restores normal physiologic portal flow to the liver and corrects portal hypertension.[126]

Intrahepatic portal hypertension. Intrahepatic portal hypertension is usually caused by fibrosis. This can lead to cirrhosis and increased resistance to portal blood flow by constricting and reducing the compliance of hepatic sinusoids. Chronic hepatitis, biliary atresia, NAFLD, and congenital hepatic fibrosis are causes of liver fibrosis in children.

The clinical manifestations of portal hypertension are (1) splenomegaly, (2) upper GI tract bleeding, (3) ascites, (4) hepatopulmonary syndrome, (5) hepatorenal syndrome, and (6) hepatic encephalopathy (see Chapter 41).

The objectives of the clinical investigation are to locate the site of the venous block and to identify the disease responsible for the portal hypertension. Thorough physical examination, laboratory evaluation, ultrasonic evaluation, endoscopic evaluation, and biopsy may be included in the diagnostic workup. Treatment in children is the same as that in adults (see Chapter 41). The outcome of portal hypertension depends almost entirely on its cause. Children with extrahepatic disease are expected to recover with little morbidity. For children with intrahepatic disease, the prognosis varies.

Metabolic Disorders

More than 5000 genetically determined metabolic pathways have been identified in liver tissue. The earliest possible identification of metabolic disorders is essential because (1) early treatment may prevent permanent damage to vital organs, such as the liver or brain; (2) precise genetic counseling may be possible with prenatal diagnosis; and (3) complications can be minimized, even if cure is not possible. Galactosemia, fructosemia, and Wilson disease are rare, treatable metabolic disorders that have hepatic clinical manifestations.[127–129] The mechanisms of disease, clinical manifestations, evaluation and treatment of these disorders are reviewed in Table 42.2.

SUMMARY REVIEW

Congenital Impairment of Motility in the Gastrointestinal Tract

1. CL and CP may occur separately or together and both defects are associated with multiple gene-environmental interactions and deficiency of B vitamins. The fissure may affect the uvula, soft palate, hard palate, nostril, and maxillary alveolar ridge, with difficulty sucking and swallowing.
2. EA, a condition in which the esophagus ends in a blind pouch, may occur with or without a TEF. As the infant swallows oral secretions or ingests milk, the pouch fills, causing either drooling, regurgitation, or aspiration into the lungs.
3. IHPS is an obstruction of the pyloric outlet caused by hypertrophy of circular muscles in the pyloric sphincter.

4. In intestinal malrotation, the small intestine lacks a normal posterior attachment during fetal development, causing volvulus (twisting of the bowel on itself) that may partly or completely occlude the GI tract and its blood vessels.
5. Meckel diverticulum is a congenital malformation of the GI tract involving all layers of the small intestinal wall. It usually occurs in the ileum.
6. Hirschsprung disease (congenital aganglionic megacolon) is caused by a malformation of the parasympathetic nervous system in a segment of the colon needed for peristalsis, resulting in colon obstruction.
7. Idiopathic intestinal pseudo-obstruction is repetitive episodes or continuous symptoms of intestinal obstruction without an obstructing lesion and may be associated with atrophy of enteric nerves and/or muscles.
8. DIOS, formerly called meconium ileus equivalent, can occur when intestinal contents become abnormally thick and obstruct the intestinal lumen. CR, pancreatic enzyme deficiency, and dehydration are common causes.
9. Malformations of the anus and rectum range from mild congenital stenosis of the anus to complex deformities.
10. MI is a newborn condition in which intestinal secretions and amniotic waste products produce a thick, sticky plug that obstructs the intestine, usually from lack of fetal digestive enzymes.

Acquired Impairment of Motility in the Gastrointestinal Tract

1. GERD is the presence of symptoms related to the return of stomach contents into the esophagus. This is caused by relaxation or incompetence of the lower esophageal sphincter that results from immaturity of the gastroesophageal sphincter. Infants are susceptible to reflux because the sphincter is not fully mature, their diet consists of liquids, and they are seldom in an upright position.
2. EoE is an emerging chronic, local, progressive antigen-immune-mediated relapsing disease caused by eosinophilic infiltration of the esophageal mucosa.
3. Intussusception is the telescoping of a proximal segment of intestine into a distal segment, causing an obstruction. It occurs most commonly in the area of the ileocecal junction.
4. Appendicitis is common in children 10 to 11 years of age, however, presentation may differ from adults in younger children.

Impairment of Digestion, Absorption, and Nutrition

1. CF is an inherited fibrocystic disease that involves mucosal chloride and sodium ion channels in many organs, including the GI tract and pancreas; CF causes pancreatic enzyme deficiency with maldigestion.
2. CD is caused by hypersensitivity to gluten protein, with autoimmune injury and loss of the villous epithelium. It results in malabsorption and growth failure.
3. Pediatric malnutrition is an imbalance between nutrient requirements and intake that results in energy, protein, and micronutrient deficits, which impair growth and development.
4. Kwashiorkor is a severe protein deficiency. Marasmus is a deficiency of all dietary nutrients, including carbohydrates.
5. Faltering growth, or FTT, is a multifactorial condition that includes biologic, psychosocial, and environmental contributions. It may or may not be related to illness, and it results in inadequate physical growth and development of a child.
6. NEC is an ischemic, inflammatory disorder in neonates, particularly premature infants, thought to result from immaturity, infection, stress, and anoxia of the bowel wall.

Diarrhea

1. Diarrhea in infants and children is three or more watery or loose stools in 24 hours. It may last up to 4 weeks in acute cases, or longer in chronic cases. It is commonly caused by viral or bacterial enterocolitis.
2. Primary lactose intolerance is the inability to digest milk sugar because of a lack of the enzyme lactase, resulting in osmotic diarrhea.

Disorders of the Liver

1. Physiologic jaundice of the newborn is caused by mild hyperbilirubinemia that subsides in 1 or 2 weeks. Pathologic jaundice is caused by severe hyperbilirubinemia and can cause brain damage (kernicterus).
2. BA is a congenital malformation of the bile ducts that obstructs bile flow and causes jaundice, cirrhosis, and liver failure.
3. Acute hepatitis is usually caused by a virus, and hepatitis A is the most common form of childhood hepatitis. Chronic hepatitis B or C usually occurs by maternal transmission.
4. Cirrhosis is fibrotic scarring of the liver and is rare in children, but it can develop from most forms of chronic liver disease.
5. Portal hypertension in children usually is caused by extrahepatic obstruction. Thrombosis of the portal vein is the most common cause of portal hypertension in children, and splenomegaly is the most common sign.
6. The most common metabolic disorders that cause liver damage in children are galactosemia, fructosemia, and Wilson disease. All three are rare and inherited as genetic traits that allow toxins to accumulate in the liver and other body tissues.

REFERENCES

1. National Center on Birth Defects and Developmental Disabilities, Centers for Disease Control and Prevention: *Facts About Cleft Lip and Palate*. Atlanta, GA: CDC; 2020. Page last reviewed: December 28, 2020. Available at https://www.cdc.gov/ncbddd/birthdefects/cleftlip.html. (Accessed December 13, 2021).
2. Mai CT, et al. National population-based estimates for major birth defects, 2010–2014. *Birth Defects Res*. 2019;111(18): 1420–1435.
3. Neela PK, et al. Association of MAPK4 and SOX1-OT gene polymorphisms with cleft lip palate in multiplex families: a genetic study. *J Dent Res Dent Clin Dent Prospects*. 2020;14(2):93–96.
4. Khan MI, Cs P, Srinath NM. Genetic factors in nonsyndromic orofacial clefts. *Glob Med Genet*. 2020;7(4):101–108.

5. Alois CI, Ruotolo RA. An overview of cleft lip and palate. *JAAPA*. 2020;33(12):17–20.
6. Lewis CW, Jacob LS, Lehmann CU. The primary care pediatrician and the care of children with cleft lip and/or cleft palate. *Pediatrics*. 2017;139(5):e20170628.
7. Paganini A, et al. A gender perspective on appearance-related concerns and its manifestations among persons born with unilateral cleft lip and palate. *Psychol Health Med*. 2021;26(6):771–778.
8. Goswami M, Jangra B, Bhushan U. Management of feeding problem in a patient with cleft lip/palate. *Int J Clin Pediatr Dent*. 2016;9(2):143–145.
9. de Jong EM, et al. Etiology of esophageal atresia and tracheoesophageal fistula: "mind the gap". *Curr Gastroenterol Rep*. 2010;12(3):215–222.
10. Forero Zapata L, Pappagallo M. Esophageal atresia and tracheoesophageal fistula. *N Engl J Med*. 2018;379(7):e11.
11. Edwards NA, et al. Developmental basis of trachea-esophageal birth defects. *Dev Biol*. 2021;477:85–97.
12. El-Gohary Y, Gittes GK, Tovar JA. Congenital anomalies of the esophagus. *Semin Pediatr Surg*. 2010;19(3):186–193.
13. Centers for Disease Control and Prevention (CDC): *Facts About Esophageal Atresia*. Atlanta, GA: CDC; 2020. Page last reviewed: October 23, 2020. https://www.cdc.gov/ncbddd/birthdefects/esophagealatresia.html. (Accessed December 13, 2021).
14. Baldwin D, Yadav D:. *Esophageal atresia*. *StatPearls*. Treasure Island, FL: StatPearls Publishing; 2021. Last updated 2021 August 1, 2021. Available at https://www.ncbi.nlm.nih.gov/books/NBK560848/. (Accessed December 13, 2021).
15. Choudhury SR, et al. Survival of patients with esophageal atresia: influence of birth weight, cardiac anomaly, and late respiratory complications. *J Pediatr Surg*. 1999;34(1):70–73.
16. Kovesi T, Rubin S. Long-term complications of congenital esophageal atresia and/or tracheoesophageal fistula. *Chest*. 2007;126(3):915.
17. Connor MJ, et al. Esophageal atresia and transitional care – step 1: a systematic review and meta-analysis of the literature to define the prevalence of chronic long-term problems. *Am J Surg*. 2015;209(4):747.
18. Galea R, Said E. Infantile hypertrophic pyloric stenosis: an epidemiological review. *Neonatal Netw*. 2018;37(4):197–204.
19. Abdellatif M, et al. Association between exposure to macrolides and the development of infantile hypertrophic pyloric stenosis: a systematic review and meta-analysis. *Eur J Pediatr*. 2019;178(3):301–314.
20. Pandya S, Heiss K. Pyloric stenosis in pediatric surgery: an evidence-based review. *Surg Clin North Am*. 2012;92(3):527–539.
21. Ismail I, et al. Laparoscopic vs. open pyloromyotomy in treatment of infantile hypertrophic pyloric stenosis. *Front Pediatr*. 2020;8:426.
22. Aboagye J, et al. Age at presentation of common pediatric surgical conditions: reexamining dogma. *J Pediatr Surg*. 2014;49(6):995–999.
23. Langer JC. Intestinal rotation abnormalities and midgut volvulus. *Surg Clin North Am*. 2017;97(1):147–159.
24. Graziano K, et al. Asymptomatic malrotation: diagnosis and surgical management: an American Pediatric Surgical Association outcomes and evidence based practice committee systematic review. *J Pediatr Surg*. 2015;50(10):1783–1790.
25. Binu V, et al. Ultrasound imaging as the first line of investigation to diagnose intestinal malrotation in children: safety and efficacy. *J Pediatr Surg*. 2021;56(12):2224–2228.
26. Ooms N, et al. Laparoscopic treatment of intestinal malrotation in children. *Eur J Pediatr Surg*. 2016;26(4):376–381.
27. El-Gohary Y, Alagtal M, Gillick J. Long-term complications following operative intervention for intestinal malrotation: a 10-year review. *Pediatr Surg Int*. 2010;26(2):203–206.
28. Hansen CC, Søreide K. Systematic review of epidemiology, presentation, and management of Meckel's diverticulum in the 21st century. *Medicine*. 2018;97(35):e12154.
29. Travassos D, van Herwaarden-Lindeboom M, van der Zee DC. Hirschsprung's disease in children with Down syndrome: a comparative study. *Eur J Pediatr Surg*. 2011;21(4):220–223.
30. McKeown SJ, et al. Hirschsprung disease: a developmental disorder of the enteric nervous system. *Wiley Interdiscip Rev Dev Biol*. 2013;2(1):113–129.
31. Arshad A, Powell C, Tighe MP. Hirschsprung's disease. *BMJ*. 2012;345:e5521.
32. Gosain A, Brinkman AS. Hirschsprung's associated enterocolitis. *Curr Opin Pediatr*. 2015;27(3):364–369.
33. Jiao CL, Chen XY, Feng JX. Novel insights into the pathogenesis of Hirschsprung's-associated enterocolitis. *Chin Med J*. 2016;129(12):1491–1497.
34. Drissi F, et al. Long-term outcome of Hirschsprung disease: impact on quality of life and social condition at adult age. *Dis Colon Rectum*. 2019;62(6):727–732.
35. Gustafsson JK, et al. Bicarbonate and functional CFTR channel are required for proper mucin secretion and link cystic fibrosis with its mucus phenotype. *J Exp Med*. 2012;209(7):1263–1272.
36. Abraham JM, Taylor CJ. Cystic fibrosis & disorders of the large intestine: DIOS, constipation, and colorectal cancer. *J Cyst Fibros*. 2017;16(Suppl 2):S40–S49.
37. Colombo C, et al. Guidelines for the diagnosis and management of distal intestinal obstruction syndrome in cystic fibrosis patients. *J Cyst Fibros*. 2011;10(Suppl 2):S24–S28.
38. VanderBrink BA, Reddy PP. Early urologic considerations in patients with persistent cloaca. *Semin Pediatr Surg*. 2016;25(2):82–89.
39. Wood RJ, Levitt MA. Anorectal malformations. *Clin Colon Rectal Surg*. 2018;31(2):61–70.
40. Dupuis A, et al. Prevalence of meconium ileus marks the severity of mutations of the Cystic Fibrosis Transmembrane Conductance Regulator (CFTR) gene. *Genet Med*. 2016;18(4):333–340.
41. Yasir M, Kumaraswamy AG, Rentea RM. *Meconium plug syndrome*. *StatPearls*. Treasure Island, FL: StatPearls Publishing; 2021. Last update August 12, 2021. Available at https://www.ncbi.nlm.nih.gov/books/NBK562320/. (Accessed December 13, 2021).
42. Glen J, Kinsella JP. Pathophysiology of meconium aspiration syndrome. In: Polin RA, ed. *Fetal and Neonatal Physiology*. ed 5 Philadelphia: Elsevier; 2017:1619–1624.
43. Vain NE, Batton DG. Meconium "aspiration" (or respiratory distress associated with meconium-stained amniotic fluid?). *Semin Fetal Neonatal Med*. 2017;22(4):214–219.
44. Rosen R, et al. Pediatric Gastroesophageal Reflux Clinical Practice Guidelines: Joint Recommendations of the North American Society for Pediatric Gastroenterology, Hepatology, and Nutrition and the European Society for Pediatric Gastroenterology, Hepatology, and Nutrition. *J Pediatr Gastroenterol Nutr*. 2018;66(3):516–554.
45. Poddar U. Gastroesophageal reflux disease (GERD) in children. *Paediatr Int Child Health*. 2019;39(1):7–12.
46. Czinn SJ, Blanchard S. Gastroesophageal reflux disease in neonates and infants: when and how to treat. *Paediatr Drugs*. 2013;15(1):19–27.

47. Iuliano S, et al. Eosinophilic esophagitis in pediatric age, state of the art and review of the literature. *Acta Biomed*. 2018;89(8-S):20–26.
48. Papadopoulou A, et al. ESPGHAN Eosinophilic Esophagitis Working Group and the Gastroenterology Committee: Management guidelines of eosinophilic esophagitis in childhood. *J Pediatr Gastroenterol Nutr*. 2014;58(1):107–118.
49. Visaggi P, et al. Eosinophilic esophagitis: clinical, endoscopic, histologic and therapeutic differences and similarities between children and adults. *Therap Adv Gastroenterol*. 2021;14 17562848209808 60.
50. Carr S, Chan ES, Watson W. Eosinophilic esophagitis. *Allergy Asthma Clin Immunol*. 2018;14(Suppl 2):58.
51. Hirano I, Furuta GT. Approaches and challenges to management of pediatric and adult patients with eosinophilic esophagitis. *Gastroenterology*. 2020;158(4):840–851.
52. Tate JE, et al. Intussusception rates before and after the introduction of rotavirus vaccine. *Pediatrics*. 2016;138(3):e20161082.
53. Mandeville K, et al. Intussusception: clinical presentations and imaging characteristics. *Pediatr Emerg Care*. 2012;28(9):842–844.
54. Li XZ, et al. Ultrasonographic diagnosis of intussusception in children: a systematic review and meta-analysis. *J Ultrasound Med*. 2021;40(6):1077–1084.
55. Gluckman S, et al. Management for intussusception in children. *Cochrane Database Syst Rev*. 2017;6(6):CD006476.
56. Kelley-Quon LI, et al. Management of intussusception in children: a systematic review. *J Pediatr Surg*. 2021;56(3):587–596.
57. Almaramhy HH. Acute appendicitis in young children less than 5 years: review article. *Ital J Pediatr*. 2017;43(1):15.
58. Moran A, et al. ISPAD Clinical Practice Consensus Guidelines 2018: management of cystic fibrosis-related diabetes in children and adolescents. *Pediatr Diabetes*. 2018;19(Suppl 27):64–74.
59. Castellani C, et al. Cystic fibrosis diagnosis in newborns, children, and adults. *Semin Respir Crit Care Med*. 2019;40(6):701–714.
60. Coverstone AM, Ferkol TW. Early diagnosis and intervention in cystic fibrosis: imagining the unimaginable. *Front Pediatr*. 2021;8:608821.
61. Sommerburg O, Hammermann J. Pancreatitis-associated protein in neonatal screening for cystic fibrosis: strengths and weaknesses. *Int J Neonatal Screen*. 2020;6(2):28.
62. Savant AP, McColley SA. Cystic fibrosis year in review 2018, part 1. *Pediatr Pulmonol 54(8)*. 2019:1117–1128.
63. Brownell JN, Bashaw H, Stallings VA. Growth and nutrition in cystic fibrosis. *Semin Respir Crit Care Med*. 2019;40(6):775–791.
64. Watkins RD, Zawahir S. Celiac disease and nonceliac gluten sensitivity. *Pediatr Clin North Am*. 2017;64(3):563–576.
65. Czaja-Bulsa G, Bulsa M. What do we know now about IgE-mediated wheat allergy in children? *Nutrients*. 2017;9(1):35.
66. Shannahan S, Leffler DA. Diagnosis and updates in celiac disease. *Gastrointest Endosc Clin N Am*. 2017;27(1):79–92.
67. Parzanese I, et al. Celiac disease: from pathophysiology to treatment. *World J Gastrointest Pathophysiol*. 2017;8(2):27–38.
68. Lebwohl B, Rubio-Tapia A. Epidemiology, presentation, and diagnosis of celiac disease. *Gastroenterology*. 2021;160(1):63–75.
69. Hujoel IA, Reilly NR, Rubio-Tapia A. Celiac disease: clinical features and diagnosis. *Gastroenterol Clin North Am*. 2019;48(1):19–37.
70. Sahin Y. Celiac disease in children: a review of the literature. *World J Clin Pediatr*. 2021;10(4):53–71.
71. Rishi AR, Rubio-Tapia A, Murray JA. Refractory celiac disease. *Expert Rev Gastroenterol Hepatol*. 2016;10(4):537–546.
72. Lindfors K, et al. Coeliac disease. *Nat Rev Dis Primers*. 2019;5(1):3.
73. Leonard MM, et al. Screening for celiac disease in a pediatric primary care setting. *Clin Pediatr (Phila)*. 2016;55(3):214–218.
74. Liu E, et al. Routine screening for celiac disease in children with Down syndrome improves case finding. *J Pediatr Gastroenterol Nutr 71(2)*. 2020(2020):252–256.
75. Roldán Martín MB, et al. Celiac disease screening in children and adolescents with type1 diabetes mellitus: what test should be performed? *Endocrinol Diabetes Nutr (Engl Ed)*. 2021;68(3):153–158.
76. Gallegos C, Merkel R. Current evidence in the diagnosis and treatment of children with celiac disease. *Gastroenterol Nurs*. 2019;42(1):41–48.
77. Rubio-Tapia A, et al. American College of Gastroenterology: ACG clinical guidelines: diagnosis and management of celiac disease. *Am J Gastroenterol*. 2013;108(5):656–677.
78. Dipasquale V, Cucinotta U, Romano C. Acute malnutrition in children: pathophysiology, clinical effects and treatment. *Nutrients*. 2020;12(8):2413.
79. Prendergast AJ, et al. Inflammatory biomarkers in HIV-infected children hospitalized for severe malnutrition in Uganda and Zimbabwe. *AIDS*. 2019;33(9):1485–1490.
80. Narayan J, John D, Ramadas N. Malnutrition in India: status and government initiatives. *J Public Health Policy*. 2019;40(1):126–141.
81. Yirga AA, et al. Factors affecting child malnutrition in Ethiopia. *Afr Health Sci*. 2019;19(2):1897–1909.
82. Beser OF, et al, TUHAMAR Study Group: Evaluation of malnutrition development risk in hospitalized children, *Nutrition* 48:40–47, 2018.
83. Fan Y, Pedersen O. Gut microbiota in human metabolic health and disease. *Nat Rev Microbiol*. 2021;19(1):55–71.
84. Pekmez CT, Dragsted LO, Brahe LK. Gut microbiota alterations and dietary modulation in childhood malnutrition - the role of short chain fatty acids. *Clin Nutr*. 2019;38(2):615–630.
85. Ibrahim MK, et al. Impact of childhood malnutrition on host defense and infection. *Clin Microbiol Rev*. 2017;30(4):919–971.
86. Pham TP, et al. Difference between kwashiorkor and marasmus: Comparative meta-analysis of pathogenic characteristics and implications for treatment. *Microb Pathog*. 2021;150:104702.
87. Aghaji AE, Duke R, Aghaji U. Inequitable coverage of vitamin A supplementation in Nigeria and implications for childhood blindness. *BMC Public Health*. 2019;19(1):282.
88. Wadhwani M, Singh R. Bilateral keratomalacia leading to blindness secondary to diet-induced vitamin A deficiency in infants. *J Pediatr Ophthalmol Strabismus*. 2020;57:e12–e14.
89. Homan GJ. Failure to thrive: a practical guide. *Am Fam Physician*. 2016;94(4):295–299.
90. Han SM, et al. Trends in incidence and outcomes of necrotizing enterocolitis over the last 12 years: a multicenter cohort analysis. *J Pediatr Surg*. 2020;55(6):998–1001.
91. Kim CS, Claud EC. Necrotizing enterocolitis pathophysiology: how microbiome data alter our understanding. *Clin Perinatol*. 2019;46(1):29–38.
92. Bazacliu C, Neu J. Pathophysiology of necrotizing enterocolitis: an update. *Curr Pediatr Rev*. 2019;15(2):68–87.
93. Ginglen JG, Butki N:. *Necrotizing enterocolitis. StatPearls*. Treasure Island, FL: StatPearls Publishing; 2021. Last update August 13, 2021. Available at https://www.ncbi.nlm.nih.gov/books/NBK513357/. (Accessed December 13, 2021).
94. Evidence-Based Medicine Group [Clinical guidelines for the diagnosis and treatment of neonatal necrotizing enterocolitis (2020)]. *Zhongguo Dang Dai Er Ke Za Zhi*. 2021;23(1):1–11. https://doi.org/10.7499/j.issn.1008-8830.2011145.

95. Neu J. Necrotizing enterocolitis: the future. *Neonatology*. 2020;117(2):240–244.
96. Meister AL, Doheny KK, Travagli RA. Necrotizing enterocolitis: it's not all in the gut. *Exp Biol Med (Maywood)*. 2020;245(2):85–95.
97. Mujuru HA, et al. Cost estimates of diarrhea hospitalizations among children <5 years old in Zimbabwe. *Vaccine*. 2020;38(43):6735–6740.
98. Posovszky C, et al. Acute infectious gastroenteritis in infancy and childhood. *Dtsch Arztebl Int*. 2020;117(37):615–624.
99. Guarino A, et al. Universal recommendations for the management of acute diarrhea in nonmalnourished children. *J Pediatr Gastroenterol Nutr*. 2018;67(5):586–593.
100. Harvey L, et al. Prevalence, cause and diagnosis of lactose intolerance in children aged 1-5 years: a systematic review of 1995-2015 literature. *Asia Pac J Clin Nutr*. 2018;27(1):29–46.
101. Heine RG, et al. Lactose intolerance and gastrointestinal cow's milk allergy in infants and children - common misconceptions revisited. *World Allergy Organ J*. 2017;10(1):41.
102. Szilagyi A, Ishayek N. Lactose intolerance, dairy avoidance, and treatment options. *Nutrients*. 2018;10(12):1994.
103. Boskabadi H, Rakhshanizadeh F, Zakerihamidi M. Evaluation of maternal risk factors in neonatal hyperbilirubinemia. *Arch Iran Med*. 2020;23(2):128–140.
104. Rathore S, Kumar VKC. R S: A critical review on neonatal hyperbilirubinemia—an Ayurvedic perspective. *J Ayurveda Integr Med*. 2020;11(2):190–196. https://doi.org/10.1016/j.jaim.2018.08.006.
105. Riordan SM, Shapiro SM. Review of bilirubin neurotoxicity I: molecular biology and neuropathology of disease. *Pediatr Res*. 2020;87(2):327–331.
106. Bratton S, Cantu RM, Stern M. *Breast milk jaundice. StatPearls*. Treasure Island, FL: StatPearls Publishing; 2021. Last update September 6, 2021. Available at https://www.ncbi.nlm.nih.gov/books/NBK537334/. (Accessed December 13, 2021).
107. Chee YY, et al. Jaundice in infants and children: causes, diagnosis, and management. *Hong Kong Med J*. 2018;24(3):285–292.
108. Kilgore A, Mack CL. Update on investigations pertaining to the pathogenesis of biliary atresia. *Pediatr Surg Int*. 2017;33(12):1233–1241.
109. Sundaram SS, et al. Biliary atresia: indications and timing of liver transplantation and optimization of pretransplant care. *Liver Transpl*. 2017;23(1):96–109.
110. Abutaleb A, Kottilil S. Hepatitis A: epidemiology, natural history, unusual clinical manifestations, and prevention. *Gastroenterol Clin North Am*. 2020;49(2):191–199.
111. Shouval D. Immunization against hepatitis A. *Cold Spring Harb Perspect Med*. 2019;9(2):a031682.
112. Indolfi G, et al. Hepatitis B virus infection in children and adolescents. *Lancet Gastroenterol Hepatol*. 2019;4(6):466–476.
113. Liu J, et al. Countdown to 2030: eliminating hepatitis B disease, China. *Bull World Health Organ*. 2019;97(3):230–238.
114. Hou J, et al. Management algorithm for interrupting mother-to-child transmission of hepatitis B virus. *Clin Gastroenterol Hepatol*. 2019;17(10). 1929–1936.e1.
115. Lin CL, Kao JH. Hepatitis B: immunization and impact on natural history and cancer incidence. *Gastroenterol Clin North Am*. 2020;49(2):201–214.
116. Karnsakul W, Schwarz KB. Hepatitis B and C. *Pediatr Clin North Am*. 2017;64(3):641–658.
117. Indolfi G, et al. Hepatitis C virus infection in children and adolescents. *Lancet Gastroenterol Hepatol*. 2019;4(6):477–487.
118. Abbas Z, et al. The severity of hepatitis D in young adults of age 18-25 years. *Cureus*. 2020;12(10):e10855.
119. Koh C, Heller T, Glenn JS. Pathogenesis of and new therapies for hepatitis D. *Gastroenterology*. 2019;156(2). 461–476.e1.
120. Defresne F, Sokal E. Chronic hepatitis B in children: therapeutic challenges and perspectives. *J Gastroenterol Hepatol*. 2017;32(2):368–371.
121. Deneau MR, et al. The natural history of primary sclerosing cholangitis in 781 children: a multicenter, international collaboration. *Hepatology*. 2017;66(2):518–527.
122. Chapin CA, Bass LM. Cirrhosis and portal hypertension in the pediatric population. *Clin Liver Dis*. 2018;22(4):735–752.
123. Fang YL, et al. Pathogenesis of non-alcoholic fatty liver disease in children and adolescence: from "two hit theory" to "multiple hit model". *World J Gastroenterol*. 2018;24(27):2974–2983.
124. Goyal NP, Schwimmer JB. The genetics of pediatric nonalcoholic fatty liver disease. *Clin Liver Dis*. 2018;22(1):59–71.
125. Selvakumar P, et al. Nonalcoholic fatty liver disease in children: hepatic and extrahepatic complications. *Pediatr Clin North Am*. 2017;64(3):659–675.
126. Khanna R, Sarin SK. Idiopathic portal hypertension and extrahepatic portal venous obstruction. *Hepatol Int*. 2018;12(Suppl 1):148–167.
127. Cerone J, Rios A. Galactosemia. *Pediatr Rev*. 2019;40(Suppl 1):24–27.
128. Koepsell H. Glucose transporters in the small intestine in health and disease. *Pflugers Arch*. 2020;472(9):1207–1248.
129. Gerosa C, et al. Liver pathology in Wilson's disease: from copper overload to cirrhosis. *J Inorg Biochem*. 2019;193:106–111.

43

Structure and Function of the Musculoskeletal System

Geri Cage Reeves and Benjamin Allan Smallheer

http://evolve.elsevier.com/Rogers/pathophysiology/

CHAPTER OUTLINE

The way an individual functions in daily life, moves about, or manipulates objects physically depends on the integrity of the musculoskeletal system. The musculoskeletal system consists of two systems: (1) the skeleton composed of bones and joints and (2) soft tissues (skeletal muscles, tendons, and ligaments). Each system contributes to mobility. The skeleton supports the body and provides leverage to the skeletal muscles so that movement of various parts of the body is possible. Contraction of the skeletal muscles and bending or rotation at the joints facilitate movements of the various body parts.

STRUCTURE AND FUNCTION OF BONES

Bones give form to the body, support tissues, and permit movement by providing points of attachment for muscles. Many bones meet in movable joints that determine the type and extent of movement possible. Bones also protect many of the body's vital organs. For example, the bones of the skull, thorax, and pelvis are hard exterior shields that protect the brain, heart, lungs, and reproductive and urinary organs, respectively.

Bone marrow is one of the sources of mesenchymal stem cells (MSCs) (Fig. 43.1). These nonhematopoietic stem cells consist of a small proportion of the stromal cell population in the bone marrow and can generate bone cells, cartilage cells, and fat cells that support the formation of blood and fibrous connective tissue. Within certain bones, the marrow cavities serve as storage sites for the hematopoietic stem cells that form both blood and immune cells. In adults, blood cells originate exclusively in the marrow cavities of the skull, vertebrae, ribs, sternum, shoulders, and pelvis. The development of blood cells is discussed in Chapter 28. Bones have a crucial role in mineral homeostasis (storing minerals [i.e., calcium, phosphate, carbonate, magnesium]), hormone homeostasis (essential for the proper performance of many delicate cellular mechanisms), and assist in maintaining normal immunologic function.

Elements of Bone Tissue

Mature bone is a rigid connective tissue consisting of cells; fibers; a homogenous, gelatinous medium termed ground substance; and large amounts of crystallized minerals, mainly calcium, that give bone its rigidity. Ground substance consists of proteoglycans and hyaluronic acid secreted by chondroblasts. The structural elements of bone are summarized in Table 43.1.

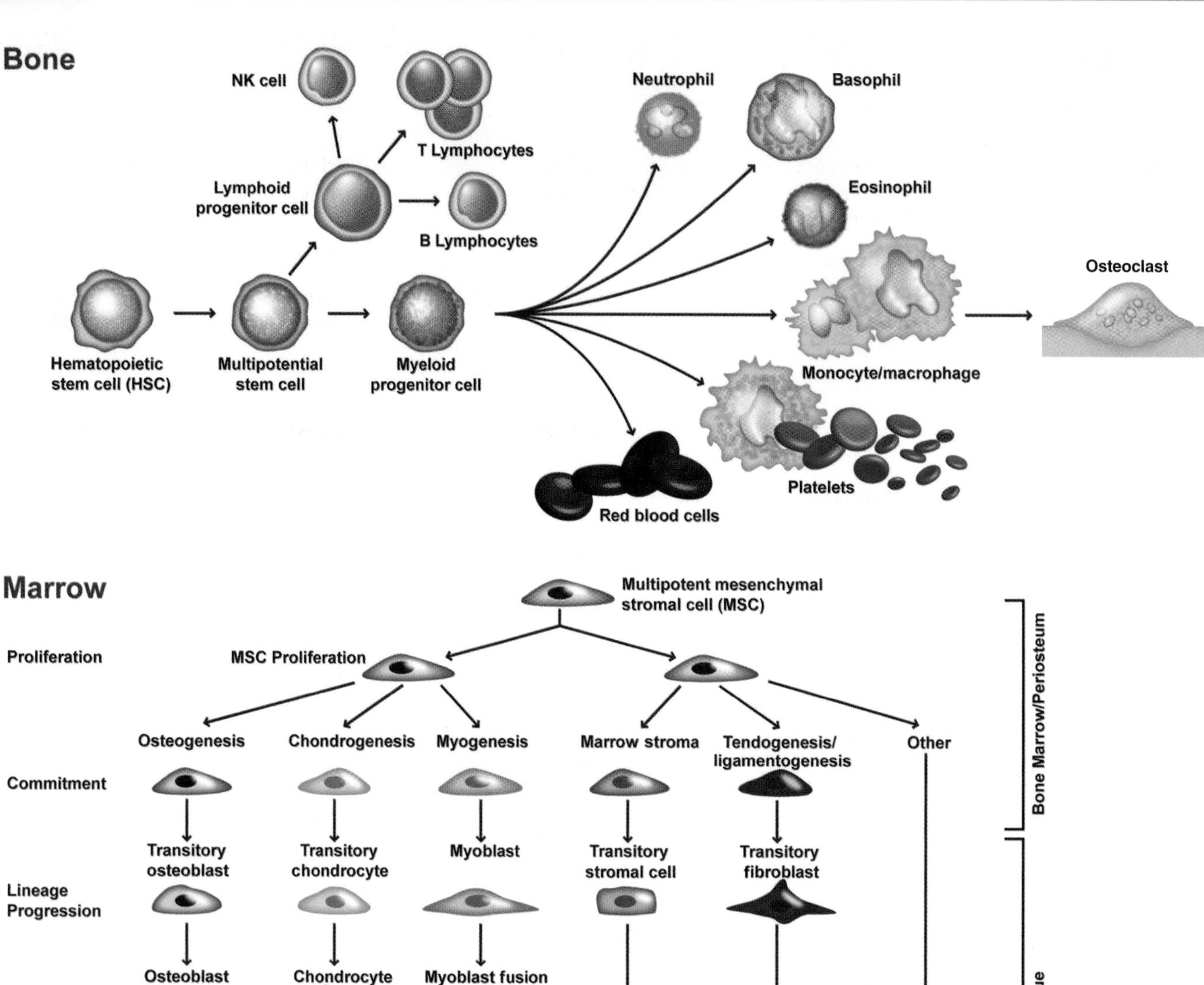

Fig. 43.1 Hematopoietic and Mesenchymal Stromal Differentiation.

Bone cells enable bone to grow, repair itself, change shape, and continuously synthesize new bone tissue and resorb (dissolve or digest) old tissue. The fibers in bone are made of collagen, which gives bone its tensile strength (the ability to hold itself together). Ground substance acts as a medium for the diffusion of nutrients, oxygen, metabolic wastes, biochemicals, and minerals between bone tissue and blood vessels.

Bone formation begins during embryonic development when MSCs begin differentiating into either chondrocytes or preosteoblasts. Endochondral ossification and intramembranous ossification are the two major mechanisms responsible for normal bone development.

Endochondral ossification occurs when mesenchymal (mesenchyme, or loose tissue found during embryonic development) stem cells begin differentiating into chondrocytes (see Fig. 43.1), which in turn develop a mineralized cartilage scaffold that allows the formation of osteoblasts. Long bones and most other bone elements are formed this way. Intramembranous ossification is responsible for the

TABLE 43.1 **Structural Elements of Bone**

Structural Elements	Function
Bone Cells	
Osteoblasts	Synthesize collagen and proteoglycans; initiate new bone formation by their synthesis of osteoid; mineralize osteoid matrix; produce receptor activator of nuclear factor-κB ligand (RANKL), which in turn stimulates osteoclast resorption of bone; also produce osteoprotegerin (OPG), which inhibits osteoclast formation by binding to RANKL
Osteoclasts	Resorb bone; major role in bone homeostasis
Osteocytes	Transform osteoblasts trapped in osteoid; signal both osteoblasts and osteoclasts; maintain bone homeostasis; synthesize new bone matrix; initiate osteoclast function; mechanosensory receptors to reduce or augment bone mass; produce sclerostin (SOST), which inhibits bone growth
Bone Matrix	
Bone morphogenic proteins (BMPs)	Subfamily of transforming growth factor-β (TGF-β) cytokine growth factors; induce and regulate bone and cartilage formation; affect all other organ systems
BMP-1	Unrelated to other BMPs (is a metalloprotease); involved in cartilage development; is actually a metalloprotease; key role in extracellular matrix (ECM) formation
BMP-2	Promotes chondrogenesis, bone formation; induces bone and cartilage formation, osteoblast differentiation, bone healing; clinically used to enhance bone formation in spine surgery
BMP-3 (osteogenin)	Inhibits bone formation
BMP-4	Osteoblast differentiation; involved in cartilage repair, endochondral bone formation; enhances chondrogenesis; regulates formation of teeth, limbs, and bone
BMP5	Involved in cartilage development
BMP-6	Found in osteoblasts; helps maintain adult joint integrity; accelerates bone repair
BMP-7	Osteogenic cell formation from mesenchymal stem cells (MSCs); enhances bone formation in spine surgery; induces formation of brown fat; has a major role in osteoblast differentiation, chondrocyte formation, fracture healing; important in renal development and repair
BMP8a	Involved in bone and cartilage development; up-regulated in fracture nonunion
BMP-9	Promotes osteoblast formation from MSCs; induces osteogenesis in mature osteoblasts
BMP10	Plays role in development of the heart
BMP12 (cartilage-derived morphogenic protein-3; CDMP-3)	Involved in tendon and ligament formation
BMP-13	Inhibits bone formation by reducing calcium mineralization; involved in cartilage development; tendon and ligament repair
BMP14	Assists in bone and tendon healing; cartilage formation
Collagen fibers	Lend support and tensile strength
Proteoglycans	Control transport of ionized materials through matrix
Glycoproteins	
Albumin	Transports essential elements to matrix; maintains osmotic pressure of bone fluid
α-Glycoproteins	Promote calcification
Laminin	Stabilizes basement membranes in bones
Osteocalcin	Vitamin K–dependent protein present in bone; inhibits calcium phosphate precipitation (attracts calcium ions to incorporate into hydroxyapatite crystals); serum osteocalcin is a sensitive marker of bone formation
Osteonectin	Binds calcium in bone; necessary for normal bone formation
Sialoprotein	Promotes calcification, osteoblast formation
Minerals	
Calcium	Crystallizes, providing bone rigidity and compressive strength

Continued

TABLE 43.1 Structural Elements of Bone—cont'd

Structural Elements	Function
Phosphate	Balance of organic and inorganic phosphate required for proper bone mineralization; regulates vitamin D, promoting mineralization
Alkaline phosphatase	Promotes mineralization
Vitamins	
Vitamin D	Assists with differentiation, mineralization of osteoblasts
Vitamin K	Increases bone calcification; reduces serum osteocalcin

Data adapted from Caetano-Lopes J, Canhão H, Fonseca JE. Osteoblasts and bone formation. *Arthritis Research and Therapy*, 2007;9 (suppl 1):S1; Hojo H, Ohba S, Yano F, et al. Coordination of chondrogenesis and osteogenesis by hypertrophic chondrocytes in endochondral bone development. *Journal of Bone and Mineral Metabolism*, 2010;28(5):489–502; Fajardo M, Liu C-J, Egol K. Levels of expression for BMP-7 and s veral BMP antagonists may play an integral role in a fracture nonunion: A pilot study. *Clinical Orthopaedics and Related Research*, 2009;467(12):3071–3078; Li Y, Shen H, Burczynski FJ, et al. Prospect of bone morphogenetic protein 13 in liver diseases. *Zhong Nan Da Xue Xue Bao Yi Xue Ban*, 2012;37(1):1–5.

development of skull and flat bones.[1] With intramembranous ossification, MSCs differentiate into a preosteoblast line that forms osteoblasts without any cartilage framework.[2]

Multiple factors influence normal bone formation, maintenance, and remodeling. Bone morphogenic proteins (BMPs) are members of the transforming growth factor-β (TGF-β) superfamily and play a major role in bone formation. This group is primarily responsible for the initiation, differentiation, and commitment of precursor cells into osteoblasts. TGF-β signals are transmitted across the plasma membrane, combine with certain proteins that act as transcription factors (Smads) and then form specific receptors known as *R-Smads*.[3] These receptors, in turn, initiate intracellular signaling, interact with other transcription factors, and regulate other factors that are important in osteoblast formation, function, and maintenance. Crosstalk between signaling pathways is critical in regulating osteoblasts.

BMPs have multiple crucial functions in the skeletal system. BMP activities are regulated at different molecular levels. The Bones Matrix section in Table 43.1 summarizes the function of several important BMPs.

Wnt genes belong to a large family of protein-signaling factors that are required for the development of body systems, including the musculoskeletal system. They play a significant role in forming bone, developing bone mass, remodeling bone, and healing fractures. Wnt signaling regulates the production and differentiation of osteoblasts and osteoclasts and affects bone mass and density, joint formation, fracture repair, bone remodeling, and some bone diseases. Other important elements responsible for bone formation and homeostasis are presented in Table 43.2.

In mature bone, the formation of new tissue begins with the production of an organic matrix by the bone cells. This bone matrix consists of ground substance, collagen, and other proteins (see Table 43.1) that take part in bone formation and maintenance.

The next step in bone formation is calcification, in which minerals are deposited and then crystallize. Minerals bind tightly to collagen fibers, producing tensile and compressional strength in bone and allowing it to withstand pressure and weightbearing.

Bone Cells

Bone contains three types of cells: osteoblasts, osteocytes, and osteoclasts (Fig. 43.2). Both osteoblasts and osteocytes originate from osteoprogenitor cells found in the MSC lineage. Osteoclasts originate from hematopoietic stem cells. Osteoblasts are the bone-forming cells. Osteocytes, the most numerous cells within bone, are osteoblasts that have become imprisoned within the mineralized bone matrix. They have multiple important duties in maintaining bone homeostasis, including synthesizing new bone matrix molecules and initiating osteoclast function. Osteoclasts primarily resorb (remove) bone during processes of growth and repair.

Osteoblasts. Originating from MSCs, osteoblasts are the primary bone-producing cells and are involved in many functions related to the skeletal system (see Table 43.1). Mature osteoblasts produce inorganic calcium phosphate, which is converted to hydroxyapatite, and an organic matrix that is composed mainly of type I collagen.[4]

Once this process is complete, osteoblasts deposit new bone in response to the bone resorbed by osteoclasts.[4] Osteoblasts are responsive to parathyroid hormone (PTH) and produce osteocalcin when stimulated by 1,25-dihydroxy-vitamin D_3. Osteoblasts are active on the outer surfaces of bones, where they form a single layer of cells. Osteoblasts initiate new bone formation by their synthesis of osteoid (nonmineralized bone matrix). Osteoblasts also mineralize the newly formed bone matrix. Stimulation of new bone formation and orderly mineralization of bone matrix occur by concentrating some of the plasma proteins (growth factors) found in the bone matrix and by facilitating the deposit and exchange of calcium and other ions at the site. Enzymes, signaling proteins, and growth factors, including BMPs and other members of the TGF-β superfamily, are critical components of bone formation, maintenance, and remodeling (see Table 43.2).

Osteocytes. Osteocytes, the most abundant cells in bone, are transformed osteoblasts trapped or surrounded in osteoid as it hardens because of minerals that enter during calcification (see Fig. 43.2B). It is the final differentiation stage for an osteoblast. The osteocyte is within a space in the hardened bone matrix called a lacuna. Osteocytes have numerous functions, including acting as mechanoreceptors and synthesizing certain matrix

TABLE 43.2 **Selected Factors Affecting Bone Formation, Maintenance, and Remodeling**

Factor	Function
Transforming growth factor-beta (TGF-β)	Superfamily of polypeptides; regulates bone formation, many other cellular processes through signaling
Platelet-derived growth factor (PDGF)	Increases number of osteoblasts
Fibroblast growth factor (FGF)	FGF-2 increases osteoblast population, but not function; inhibits alkaline phosphatase activity, osteocalcin, type I collagen, and osteopontin
Insulin-Like Growth Factor (IGF)	
IGF-1	Increases peak bone mass during adolescence; decreases osteoblast apoptosis; maintains bone matrix
IGF-2	Increases BMP-9–induced endochondral ossification
Smad proteins	Mediate signaling cascade of TGF-β, especially in embryonic bone development; play role in crosstalk between BMP/TGF-β and Wnt signaling pathways
Bone morphogenic proteins (BMPs)	Members of TGF-β superfamily of polypeptides; have many functions outside skeletal system; stimulate endochondral bone and cartilage formation and function, promote osteoblast maturation; augment bone remodeling by affecting both osteoblasts and osteoclasts
Tumor necrosis factors (TNFs)	Superfamily of cytokines; play major role in regulating bone metabolism, especially osteoclast function
Osteoprotegerin (OPG)	Inhibits bone remodeling/resorption; produced by several cells, including osteoblasts; is a decoy receptor for RANKL (binds to RANKL, inhibiting RANK/RANKL interactions, suppressing osteoclast formation and bone resorption); also may directly interfere with ability of osteoclasts' podosomes to attach to bone matrix
Receptor activator of nuclear factor-κB (RANK)	Stimulates differentiation of osteoclast precursors; activates mature osteoclasts
Receptor activator of nuclear factor-κB ligand (RANKL)	Promotes osteoclast differentiation/activation; inhibits osteoclast apoptosis
BMP antagonists	Prevent BMP signaling
Noggin	Binds BMP-2 and -4, reducing osteoblast function
Gremlin	Multiple effects in and out of skeletal system, but also binds BMP-2, -4, and -7, thus reducing BMP signaling; may play role in development of osteoporosis
Twisted gastrulation	Acts as either a BMP agonist or a BMP antagonist
Activin (a BMP-related protein)	Affects both osteoblasts and osteoclasts; may promote bone formation and fracture healing; expressed by both osteoblasts and chondrocytes; helps regulate bone mass
Annexins	Class of calcium-binding proteins; help mineralize matrix vesicles; may influence bone formation
Inhibin	Dominant over activin and BMPs; helps regulate bone mass and strength by affecting formation of osteoblasts and osteoclasts
Leptin	Plays role in bone formation and resorption
Wnt Antagonists	
Dickkopf family (Dkk)	Disrupt Wnt signaling, leading to reduced bone mass
Sclerostin	A protein secreted by osteocytes, osteoblasts, and osteoclasts; binds to BMP-6 and BMP-7; interferes with Wnt signaling pathway, inhibiting bone formation by osteoblasts
Transcription Factors	
β-Catenin pathway	Protein with multiple functions; one of most important is activation of genetic transcription factors; balance between Wnt/β-catenin signaling promotes normal bone formation/resorption
Wnts (complex signaling pathway)	Important in differentiating osteoblasts, bone formation; has overlapping effects with BMPs, helps regulate bone formation and remodeling; crosstalks with other signaling pathways
Nuclear factor of activated B cells (NF-κB)	Affects embryonic osteoclastogenesis; plays role in certain osteoclast, osteoblast, and chondroblast functions

Continued

TABLE 43.2 Selected Factors Affecting Bone Formation, Maintenance, and Remodeling—cont'd

Factor	Function
Matrix Metalloproteinases (MMPs)	
Family of endopeptidases (enzymes) that includes collagenases, gelatinases, stromelysins, matrilysins	Help maintain equilibrium of extracellular matrix (ECM); breakdown almost all components of ECM
A disintegrin and metalloproteinase (ADAM)	Proteolytic enzymes; also have cell-signaling functions, usually linked to cell membrane
A disintegrin and metalloproteinase with thrombospondin motifs (ADAMTs)	Similar to ADAMs but are secreted into circulation, are found around cells; various subgroups affect multiple tissues
Cysteine protease	Cathepsin K expressed by osteoclasts; assists in bone remodeling by cleaving proteins, such as collagen type I, collagen type II, and osteonectin
MMP Inhibitors	
Tetracyclines (especially doxycycline), bisphosphonates	Block enzymatic function of MMPs
Tissue inhibitors of metalloproteinases (TIMPs)	Balance effect of MMPs in maintaining ECM equilibrium

Data adapted from Boyce BF, Yao Z, Xing L. Functions of nuclear factor κB in bone. *Annals of the New York Academy of Sciences*, 2010;1192:367–375; Genetos DC, Wong A, Weber TJ, et al. Impaired osteoblast differentiation in annexin A2- and -A5-deficient cells. *PLoS One*, 2015;9(9):e107482; Kim Y-S, Paik IY, Rhie YJ, et al. Integrative physiology: Defined novel metabolic roles of osteocalcin. *Journal of Korean Medical Science*, 2010;25:985–991; Norrie JL, Lewandowski JP, Bouldin CM, et al. Dynamics of BMP signaling in limb bud mesenchyme and polydactyly. *Developmental Biology*, 2014;393(2):270–281; Stewart A, Guan H, Yang K, et al. BMP-3 promotes mesenchymal stem cell proliferation through the TGF-β/activin signaling pathway. *Journal of Cellular Physiology*, 2010;223(3):658–666; Wang RN, Green J, Wang Z, et al. Bone Morphogenetic Protein (BMP) signaling in development and human diseases. *Genes & Diseases*, 2014;1(1):87–105; Zhao H, Liu X, Zou H, et al. Osteoprotegerin induces podosome disassembly in osteoclasts through calcium, ERK, and p38 MAPK signaling pathways. *Cytokine*, 2014;71(2):199–206.

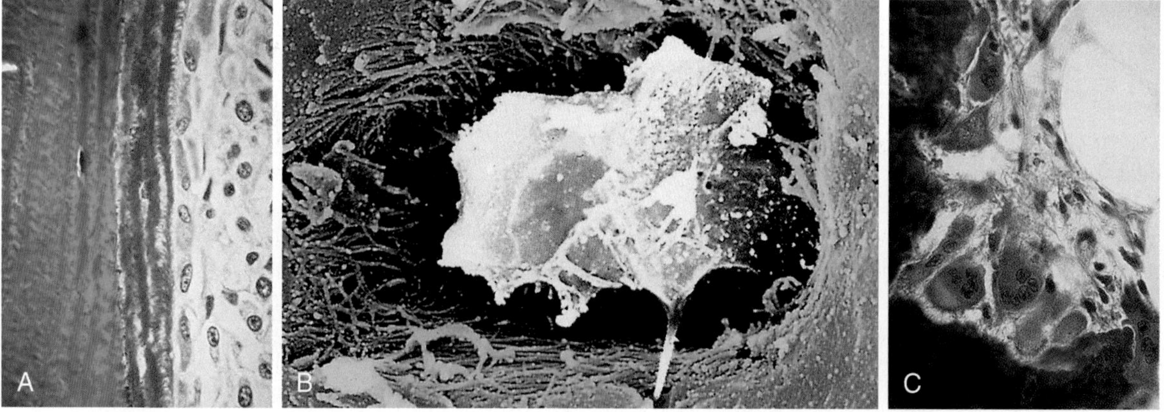

Fig. 43.2 Bone Cells. **(A)** Osteoblasts are responsible for the production of collagenous and non-collagenous proteins that compose osteoid. Active osteoblasts are aligned on the osteoid. Note the eccentrically located nuclei. **(B)** Electron photomicrograph of an osteocyte. Osteocytes reside within the lacunae of compact bone. **(C)** Osteoclasts actively resorb mineralized tissue. The scalloped surface in which the multinucleated osteoclasts rest is termed *Howship lacuna*. (A and C, From Damjanov I, Linder J, eds. *Anderson's Pathology*, 10th edition. St. Louis: Mosby; 1996; B, From Wikimedia Commons, courtesy Robert M. Hunt.)

molecules, playing a major role in controlling osteoblast differentiation and production of growth factors, and maintaining bone homeostasis.

As the major source of sclerostin, receptor activator nuclear factor κ-B ligand (RANKL), and osteoprotegerin, osteocytes are thought to be key regulators of both bone formation and bone resorption.[5] They also help concentrate nutrients in the matrix. Osteocytes obtain nutrients from capillaries in the canaliculi, which contain nutrient-rich fluids. Through exchanges among these cells, hormone catalysts, and minerals, optimal levels of calcium, phosphorus, and other minerals are maintained in blood plasma.

One of the osteocyte's primary functions is to act as a mechanoreceptor, responding to changes in weightbearing or other stressors ("loading") on bone. Lying within the lacunae are the osteocyte's primary cilia, which are likely the primary mechanoreceptors in bone. Once changes in bone, such as mechanical stress, hormonal imbalance, loading, or unloading, are detected by the osteocyte's mechanoreceptors, multiple molecular signals are produced, and the process of bone remodeling begins. Remodeling is described in the Maintenance of Bone Integrity Section.

Osteoclasts. Osteoclasts are large (typically 20 to 100 μm in diameter), multinucleated cells that develop from the hematopoietic monocyte-macrophage lineage. Osteoclasts are the major resorptive cells of bone. They migrate over bone surfaces to resorption areas that have been prepared and stripped of osteoid by enzymes, such as collagenases produced by osteoblasts in the presence of PTH, which is necessary for the resorptive process. Osteoclasts travel over the prepared bone surfaces, creating irregular, scalloped cavities known as *Howship lacunae* or *resorption bays*, as they resorb bone areas and then acidify hydroxyapatite to dissolve it.

A specific area of the cell membrane forms adjacent to the bone surface and develops multiple infoldings to permit intimate contact with the resorption bay. These infoldings, known as the ruffled border, greatly increase the surface areas of cells under their scalloped or ruffled borders. Osteoclasts resorb bone by the secretion of hydrochloric acid, acid proteases (such as cathepsin K), and matrix metalloproteinases (MMPs) that help digest collagen, along with the action of cytokines (see Table 43.2). Osteoclasts also resorb bone through the action of lysosomes (digestive vacuoles) filled with hydrolytic enzymes in their mitochondria.

Osteoclasts bind to the bone surfaces through attachments called podosomes, which are footlike structures that cluster together along a sealing membrane that forms a "belt" containing multiple proteins, enzymes, and integrin receptors. Once resorption is complete, the osteoclasts retract and loosen from the bone surface under the ruffled border through the action of calcitonin. Calcitonin binds to receptor areas of the osteoclasts' cell membranes to effectively loosen the osteoclasts from the bone surfaces. Once resorption is completed, osteoclasts disappear by the process of degeneration, either by reverting to the form of their parent cells or by undergoing cell movements away from the site, in which the osteoclast becomes an inactive or a resting osteoclast.

In addition to resorption of bone, osteoclasts assist the endocrine and renal systems in maintaining appropriate serum calcium and phosphorus levels. Osteoclasts also appear to have a role in the body's immune response.

Osteoprotegerin/Receptor Activator Nuclear Factor κ-B Ligand/Receptor Activator Nuclear Factor κ-B System

Osteoprotegerin (OPG), a glycoprotein belonging to the tumor necrosis factor (TNF) superfamily, inhibits bone remodeling and resorption, inhibiting osteoclast formation. Numerous cells, including osteoblasts and osteocytes, produce it. OPG is the key to the interaction between osteoblasts and osteoclasts. Osteoblasts and osteoclasts cooperate (a process called *coupling*) to maintain normal bone homeostasis. RANKL is an essential cytokine needed for the formation and activation of osteoclasts. Like an automobile's accelerator, RANKL increases bone loss. OPG, similar to an automobile's brakes, reduces bone loss because when it is activated, it promotes bone formation. When RANKL binds to its receptor (i.e., receptor activator nuclear factor κ-B [RANK]) on osteoclast precursor cells, it triggers their proliferation and increases bone resorption. OPG is secreted by osteoblasts and B lymphocytes and serves as a decoy by binding to RANK, preventing RANKL from binding to RANK and thus preventing bone resorption. Therefore, the overall balance between RANKL and OPG determines the amount of bone loss. The balance between RANKL and OPG is regulated by cytokines and hormones. Alterations of the RANKL/RANK/OPG system can lead to dysregulation and pathologic conditions, including primary osteoporosis, immune-mediated bone diseases, malignant bone disorders, and inherited skeletal diseases.

Bone Matrix

Bone matrix is made of the *extracellular elements* of bone tissue, specifically collagen fibers, structural proteins (e.g., proteoglycans and certain glycoproteins), carbohydrate-protein complexes, ground substance, and minerals.

Collagen fibers. Collagen fibers make up the bulk of the bone matrix. They are formed in this way:

1. Osteoblasts synthesize and secrete type I collagen and osteocalcin.
2. Collagen molecules assemble into three thin chains (alpha chains) to form fibrils.
3. Fibrils organize into the staggered pattern, with each fibril overlapping its nearest neighbor by about one-fourth its length. This creates gaps into which mineral crystals are deposited.
4. After mineral deposition, fibrils interlink and twist to form ropelike fibers.
5. The fibers join to form the framework that gives bone its tensile and supportive strength. Collagen is the most abundant macromolecule in the body, accounting for approximately one-third of all protein and providing the structural framework for nearly all tissues. Collagen is one of the extracellular components, along with proteoglycans and noncollagenous matrix proteins, of articular cartilage. To date, more than 20 types of collagen have been identified, though all their functions are not yet known. Cartilage-specific collagens include types II (the principal component), VI, IX, X, and XI. Type IX collagen is thought to be the "glue" that holds together the type II collagen scaffold of articular cartilage, helps maintain the structural integrity of cartilage, and resists tensile forces on joint cartilage. Type XI regulates the fibril diameter of type II cartilage. Degradation of type IX collagen by proteolytic enzymes has been seen in the early stages of osteoarthritis and rheumatoid arthritis. Researchers have proposed that this degradation, or "unplugging," may be the mechanism for the degenerative changes seen in osteoarthritic and rheumatoid cartilage (Table 43.3).

Proteoglycans. Proteoglycans are large complexes of numerous polysaccharides attached to a common protein core. They strengthen bone by forming compression-resistant networks between the collagen fibers. Proteoglycans also control the transport and distribution of electrically charged particles (ions), particularly calcium, through the bone matrix, thereby playing a role in bone calcium deposition and calcification. Proteoglycans are important constituents of ground substances.

TABLE 43.3 Types of Collagen in Musculoskeletal Tissues

Type of Collagen	Distribution in Musculoskeletal Tissues
I	Bone, tendon, ligament, intervertebral disk, muscle[a]
II	Cartilage, intervertebral disk
III	Skin, muscle, often with type I
IV	Basement cell membrane, muscle
V	Codistributed with type I muscle, most interstitial tissues
VI	Ubiquitous, muscle
IX	Codistributed with type II muscle
X	Cartilage growth plate
XI	Cartilage, muscle
XII	Codistributed with type I and type III muscle
XIII	Molecule has not been isolated in connective tissues to date
XIV	Codistributed with type I muscle
XV	Muscle; contains heparin sulfate proteoglycans (HSPGs)
XVII	Muscle; contains HSPGs

[a]Refers specifically to skeletal mass.

Glycoproteins. Glycoproteins are carbohydrate-protein complexes that control the collagen interactions that lead to fibril formation. They also may function in calcification. Four glycoproteins are present in bone: sialoprotein, which binds easily with calcium; osteocalcin, which binds preferentially to crystallized calcium; bone albumin, which is identical to serum albumin and possibly transports essential nutrients to and from bone cells and maintains the osmotic pressure of bone fluid; and alpha-glycoprotein (α-glycoprotein), which probably plays a significant role in calcification and also may facilitate bone resorption by activating osteoclasts (see Table 43.1).

Bone Minerals

After collagen synthesis and fiber formation, the final step in bone formation is mineralization. Mineralization has two distinct phases: (1) formation of the initial mineral deposit (initiation) and (2) proliferation or accretion of additional mineral crystals on the initial mineral deposits (growth). The majority of the minerals in the body are analogs of the naturally occurring mineral hydroxyapatite (HAP). The HAP crystals then penetrate the matrix vesicle membrane and enter the extracellular space.

As the calcium and phosphorus concentrations increase in the bone matrix, the first precipitate to form is dicalcium phosphate dihydrate (DCPD). Once DCPD precipitation begins, the remaining phases of bone crystal formation proceed until insoluble HAP is produced, with approximately 80% to 90% of the HAP incorporated into the collagen fibers. Amorphous calcium phosphate is distributed throughout the bone matrix.

Types of Bone Tissue

Bone is composed of two types of bony (osseous) tissue: compact bone (cortical bone) and spongy bone (cancellous bone) (Fig. 43.3). Cortical bone is about 85% of the skeleton; cancellous bone makes up the remaining 15%. Both types of bone tissue contain the same structural elements, with a few exceptions. In addition, both compact tissue and spongy tissue are present in every bone. The major difference between the two types of tissue is the organization of the elements.

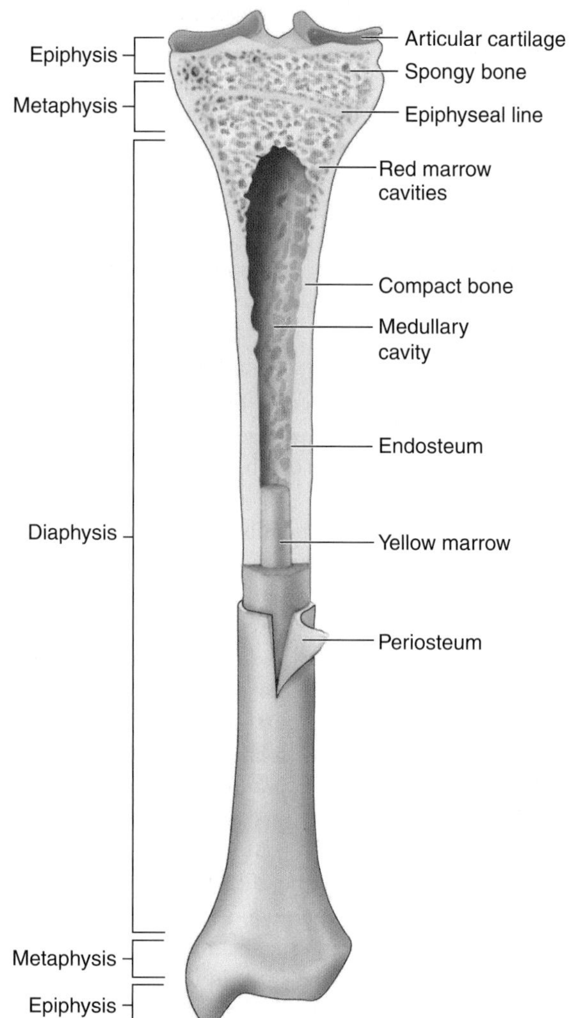

Fig. 43.3 Cross Section of Bone. Longitudinal section of long bone (tibia) showing cancellous and compact bone. (From Patton KT, Thibodeau GA. *The human body in health & disease*, 7th edition. St. Louis: Mosby; 2018.)

Compact bone is highly organized, solid, and extremely strong. The basic structural unit in compact bone is the haversian system. Each haversian system consists of:

- A central canal, called the haversian canal
- Concentric layers of bone matrix, called lamellae (sing., lamella)
- Tiny spaces (lacunae) between the lamellae
- Bone cells (osteocytes) within the lacunae
- Small channels or canals, called canaliculi (sing., canaliculus)

Spongy bone is less complex and lacks haversian systems. In spongy bone, the lamellae are not arranged in concentric layers but in plates or bars termed trabeculae (sing., trabecula) that branch and unite with one another to form an irregular meshwork. The pattern of the meshwork is determined by the direction of stress on the particular bone. The spaces between the trabeculae are filled with red bone marrow. The osteocyte-containing lacunae are distributed between the trabeculae and interconnected by canaliculi. Capillaries pass through the marrow to nourish the osteocytes.

All bones are covered with a double-layered connective tissue called the periosteum. The outer layer of the periosteum contains blood vessels and nerves, some of which penetrate to the inner structures of the bone through channels called *Volkmann canals*. The inner layer of the periosteum is anchored to the bone by collagenous fibers (Sharpey fibers) that penetrate the bone. Sharpey fibers also help hold or attach tendons and ligaments to the periosteum of bones.

Characteristics of Bone

The human skeleton consists of 206 bones that constitute the axial skeleton and the appendicular skeleton. The axial skeleton consists of 80 bones that make up the skull, vertebral column, and thorax. The appendicular skeleton consists of 126 bones that make up the upper and lower extremities, the shoulder girdle (pectoral girdle), and the pelvic girdle (os coxae) (Fig. 43.4). The skeleton contributes approximately 14% of an adult's body weight.

Bones can be classified by shape as long, flat, short (cuboidal), or irregular. Long bones are longer than they are wide and consist of a narrow tubular midportion (diaphysis) that merges into a broader neck (metaphysis) and a broad end (epiphysis) (see Fig. 43.3).

The diaphysis consists of a shaft of thick, rigid compact bone that is able to tolerate bending forces. Contained within the diaphysis is the elongated marrow (medullary) cavity. The marrow cavity of the diaphysis contains primarily fatty tissue, which is referred to as *yellow marrow*. The yellow marrow assists red bone marrow in hematopoiesis only during times of stress. The yellow marrow cavity of the diaphysis is continuous with marrow cavities in the spongy bone of the metaphysis and diaphysis. The marrow contained within the epiphysis is red because it contains primarily blood-forming tissue (see Chapter 28). A layer of connective tissue, the endosteum, lines the outer surfaces of both types of marrow cavities.

The broadness of the epiphysis allows weightbearing to be distributed over a wide area. The epiphysis is made up of spongy bone covered by a thin layer of compact bone. In a child, the epiphysis is separated from the metaphysis by a cartilaginous growth plate (epiphyseal plate). After puberty, the epiphyseal plate calcifies and the epiphysis and metaphysis merge. By adulthood, the line of demarcation between the epiphysis and metaphysis is undetectable.

In flat bones, such as the ribs and scapulae, two plates of compact bone are nearly parallel to each other. Between the compact bone plates is a layer of spongy bone. Short bones, such as the bones of the wrist or ankle, are often cuboidal. They consist of spongy bone covered by a thin layer of compact bone.

Irregular bones, such as the vertebrae, mandibles, or other facial bones, have various shapes that include thin and thick segments. The thin part of an irregular bone consists of two plates of compact bone surrounding spongy bone. The thick part consists of spongy bone surrounded by a layer of compact bone.

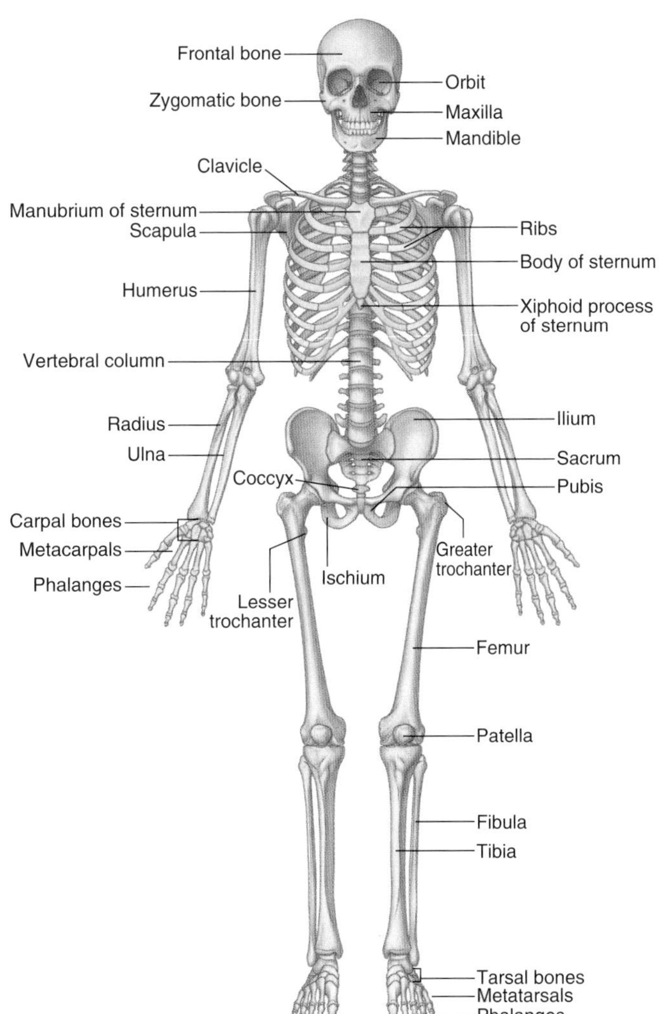

Fig. 43.4 Anterior View of the Skeleton. (From Drake R, et al. *Gray's atlas of anatomy*, 3rd edition. Philadelphia: Churchill Livingstone; 2021.)

Maintenance of Bone Integrity

Remodeling

The internal structure of bone is maintained by remodeling, a three-phase process in which existing bone is resorbed and new bone is laid down to replace it. Clusters of bone cells, termed basic multicellular units, implement remodeling. The basic multicellular units are made up of bone precursor cells that differentiate into osteoclasts and osteoblasts. Precursor cells are located on the free surfaces of bones and along the vascular channels (especially the marrow cavities).

In phase 1 (activation) of the remodeling cycle, a stimulus (e.g., hormone, drug, vitamin, physical stressor) activates the cytokine system, particularly the TNF superfamily, to form osteoclasts. Osteoclasts attach to the bone matrix by actin microfilaments and multiple other proteins that form footlike structures called *podosomes*. Once attached, the osteoclasts' integrin receptors anchor their microfilaments to the extracellular matrix, thus providing receptor pathways between the osteocyte and bone matrix. Lysosomal enzymes produced by osteoclasts "digest" bone; the osteoclasts then release the degraded bone products into the vascular system. After bone is resorbed, the osteoclast leaves behind an elongated cavity termed a *resorption cavity*. The resorption cavity in compact bone follows the longitudinal axis of the haversian system, whereas the resorption cavity in spongy bone parallels the surface of the trabeculae.

New bone formation begins as osteoblasts lining the walls of the resorption cavity express osteoid and alkaline phosphatase, forming sites for calcium and phosphorus deposition. As the osteoid mineralizes, new bone is formed. Successive layers (lamellae) in compact bone are laid down, until the resorption cavity is reduced to a narrow haversian canal around a blood vessel. In this way, old haversian systems are destroyed and new haversian systems are formed. New trabeculae are formed in spongy bone. The formation phase takes 4 to 6 months in humans.

Repair

The remodeling process can repair microscopic bone injuries, but gross injuries, such as fractures and surgical wounds (osteotomies), heal by the same stages as soft tissue injuries, except that new bone, instead of scar tissue, is the final result (see Chapter 7). The stages of bone healing are listed here and shown in Fig. 43.5:

1. *Hematoma formation:* This process occurs if vessels have been damaged, causing hemorrhage. Fibrin and platelets within the hematoma form a meshwork that is the initial framework for healing with the help of hematopoietic growth factors such as platelet-derived growth factor and TGF-β (see Table 43.2).
2. *Procallus formation:* Fibroblasts, capillary buds, and osteoblasts move into the wound to produce granulation tissue called procallus. Cartilage is formed as a precursor of bone, and types I, II, and III collagen are formed. Enzymes and growth factors, such as insulin and insulin-like growth factors, plus BMP and osteogenin, aid in this stage of healing.
3. *Callus formation:* Osteoblasts in the procallus form membranous or woven bone (callus). Enzymes increase the phosphate content and permit the phosphate to join with calcium to be deposited as a mineral to harden the callus.
4. *Replacement:* Basic multicellular units of the callus are replaced with lamellar bone or trabecular bone (see Fig. 43.5)
5. *Remodeling:* The periosteal and endosteal surfaces of the bone are remodeled to the size and shape of the bone before injury. Synthesis of other types of collagen recedes in favor of type I, which is the collagen found in bone. This final stage of healing, or remodeling, is vital because bone that has not been remodeled does not have good mechanical properties for weightbearing and mobility.

The speed with which bone heals depends on the severity of the bone disruption; the type and amount of bone tissue that need to be replaced (spongy bone heals faster). (See Emerging Science Box: Factors Affecting Bone Healing.)

STRUCTURE AND FUNCTION OF JOINTS

The site where two or more bones are attached is called a joint, or an articulation (Fig. 43.6). The primary function of joints is to provide stability and mobility to the skeleton. A joint's function depends on both its location and its structure. Generally, joints that stabilize the skeleton have a simpler structure than those that enable the skeleton to move. Most joints provide both stability and mobility to some degree.

Joints are classified based on the degree of movement they permit or on the connecting tissues that hold them together. Based on movement, a joint is classified as a synarthrosis (immovable joint), an amphiarthrosis (slightly movable joint), or a diarthrosis (freely movable joint). From connective structures, joints are classified broadly as fibrous, cartilaginous, or synovial. Each of these three structural classifications can be subdivided according to the shape and contour of the articulating surfaces (ends) of the bones and the type of motion the joint permits.

Fibrous Joints

A joint in which bone is united directly to bone by fibrous connective tissue is called a fibrous joint. These joints have no joint cavity and allow little, if any, movement.

Fibrous joints are further subdivided into three types: sutures, syndesmoses, and gomphoses. A suture has a thin layer of dense fibrous tissue that binds together interlocking flat bones in the skulls of young children. Sutures form an extremely tight union that permits no motion. By adulthood, the fibrous tissue has been replaced by bone. A syndesmosis is a joint in which the two bony surfaces are united by a ligament or membrane. The fibers of ligaments are flexible and stretch, permitting a limited amount of movement. The paired bones of the lower arm (radius and ulna) and the lower leg (tibia and fibula) and their ligaments are syndesmotic joints. A gomphosis is a special type of fibrous joint in which a conical projection fits into a complementary socket and is held in place by a ligament. The teeth held in the maxilla or mandible are gomphosis joints.

Cartilaginous Joints

There are two types of cartilaginous joints: symphyses and synchondroses. A symphysis is a cartilaginous joint in which

EMERGING SCIENCE BOX

Factors Affecting Bone Healing

Among the many factors affecting bone healing are the condition of local vasculature and surrounding soft tissues; the availability of effective treatment, including immobilization and the prevention of complications such as infection; chronic diseases (such as diabetes and cardiovascular disorders); age; gender; nutritional status; stimulants; and drugs.[1,2] Drugs administered due to an injury, such as analgesic drugs are the most controllable factor because their impact on bone healing can be taken into account with respect to choice and dosage. Primarily because of their analgesic efficacy and anti-inflammatory effect, nonsteroidal antiinflammatory drugs (NSAIDS) are at the forefront in terms of frequency of use. However, NSAIDS have been shown to have negative effects on bone healing by limiting osteogenesis and should be used for the least amount of time (up to seven days).

Data from Lisowska B, et al. Positives and negatives of nonsteroidal anti-inflammatory drugs in bone healing: The effects of these drugs on bone repair. Drug Design, Development and Therapy, 2018;12:1809–1814; Loi F, et al. Inflammation, fracture and bone repair. Bone, 2016;86:119–130.

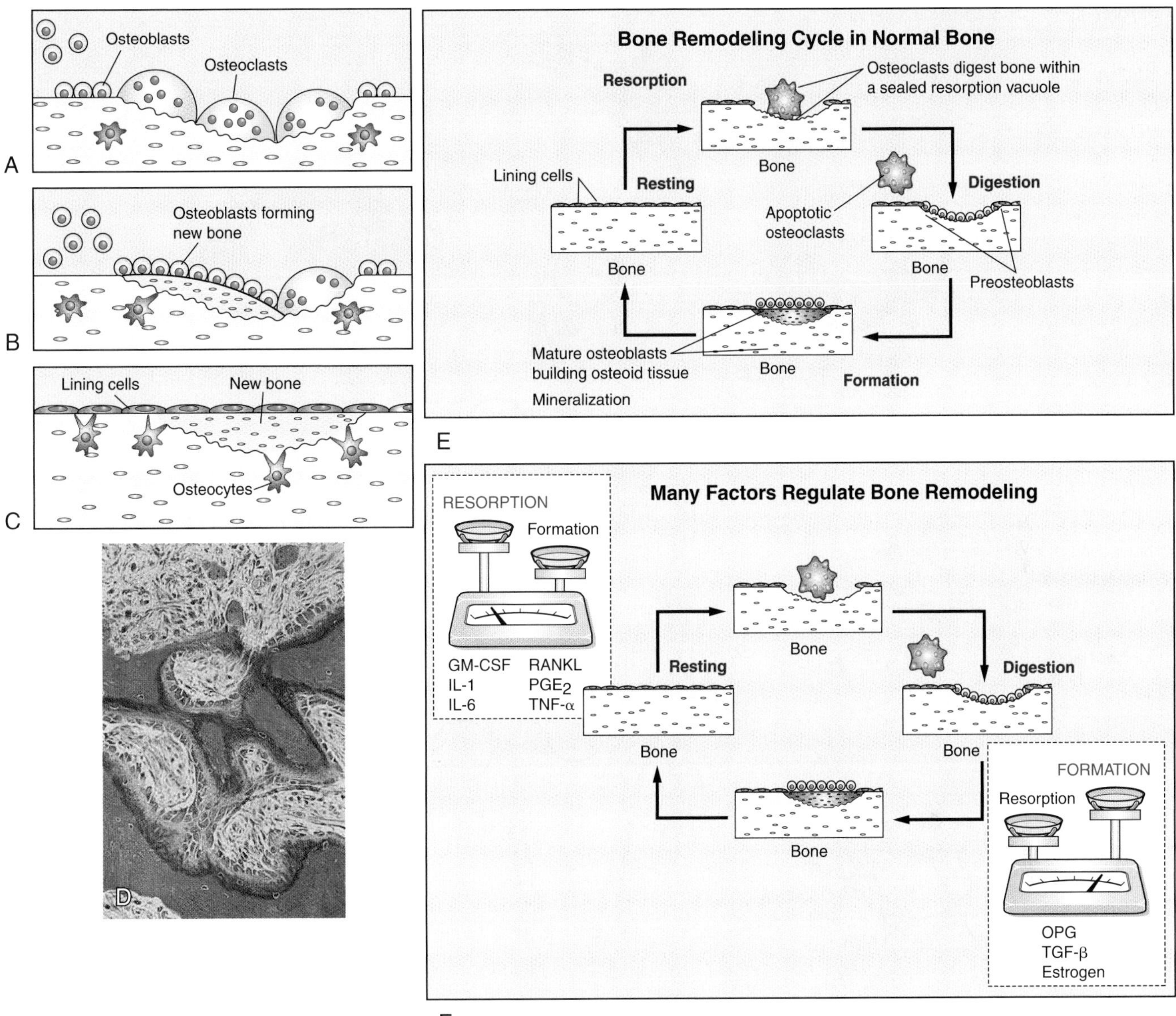

Fig. 43.5 Bone Remodeling. All bone cells participate in bone remodeling. In the remodeling sequence, bone sections are removed by bone-resorbing cells (osteoclasts) and replaced with a new section laid down by bone-forming cells (osteoblasts). Bone remodeling is necessary because it allows the skeleton to respond to mechanical loading, maintains quality control (repair and prevent microdamage), and allows the skeleton to release growth factors and minerals (calcium and phosphate) stored in the bone matrix to the circulation. The cells work in response to signals generated in the environment (see F). Only the osteoclastic cells mediate the first phase of remodeling. They are activated, scoop out bone **(A)**, and resorb it; then the work of the osteoblasts begins **(B)**. They form new bone that replaces bone removed by the resorption process **(C)**. The sequence takes 4 to 6 months. **(D)** Micrograph of active bone remodeling seen in the settings of primary or secondary hyperparathyroidism. Note the active osteoblasts surmounted on red-stained osteoid. Marrow fibrosis is present. **(E)** Bone remodeling cycle in normal bone with **(F)**. Numerous signaling factors are necessary for remodeling. Factors most important for resorption include granulocyte macrophage-colony stimulating factor *(GM-CSF)*, interleukin-1 *(IL-1)* and IL-6, receptor activator for nuclear factor-κB ligand *(RANKL)*, prostaglandin E_2 *(PGE_2)*, and tumor necrosis factor-α *(TNF-α)*. Important factors for bone formation include osteoprotegerin *(OPG)*, transforming growth factor-beta *(TGF-β)*, and estrogen. (Adapted from Nucleus Medical Art. D, From Damjanov I, Linder J, eds. *Anderson's pathology*, 10th edition. St. Louis: Mosby; 1996.)

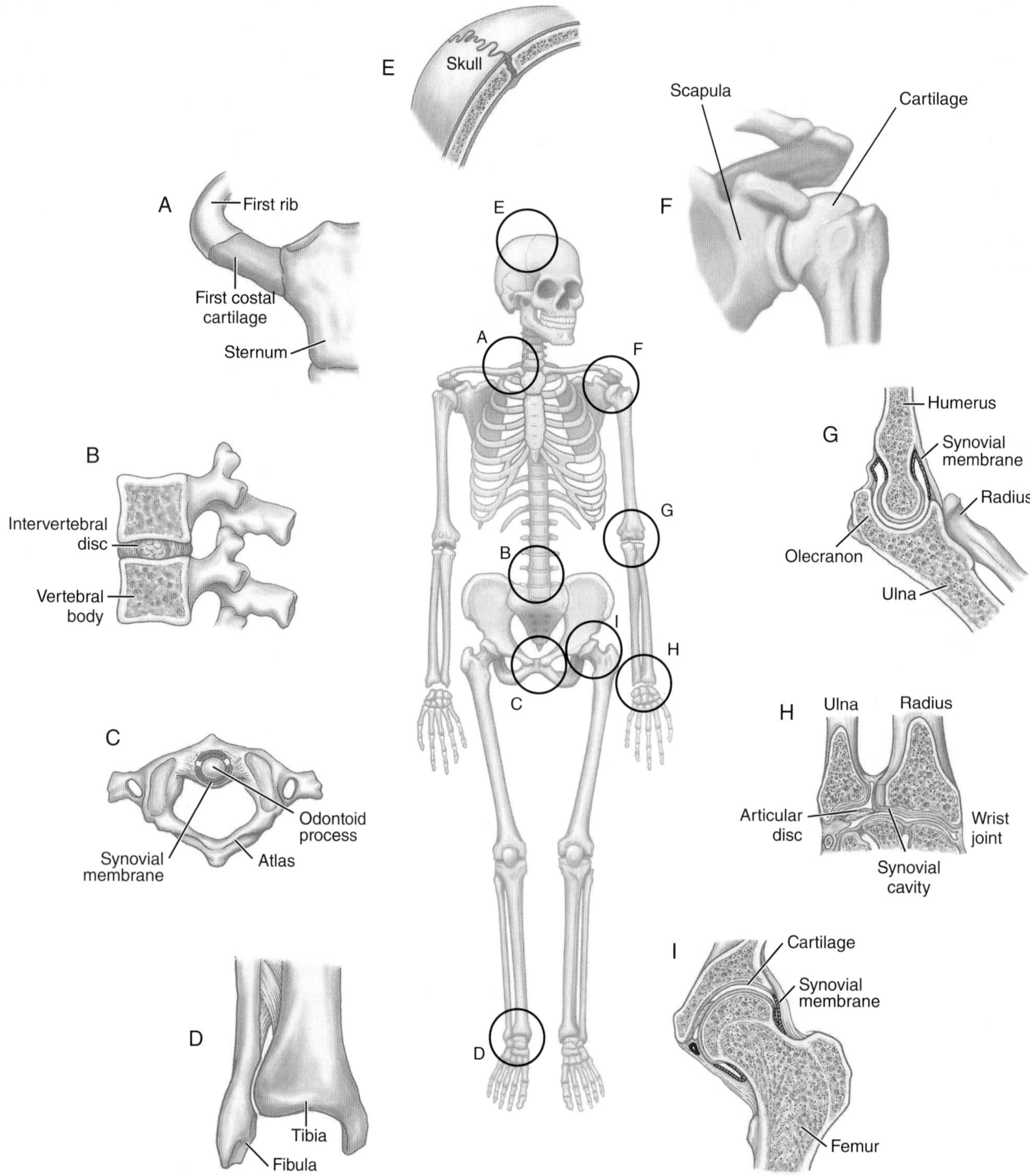

Fig. 43.6 Types of Joints. Cartilaginous (amphiarthrodial) joints, which are slightly movable, include: **(A)** a synchondrosis that attaches ribs to costal cartilage; **(B)** a symphysis that connects vertebrae; and **(C)** the symphysis that connects the two pubic bones. Fibrous (synarthrodial) joints, which are immovable, include **(D)** the syndesmosis between the tibia and fibula; **(E)** sutures that connect the skull bones; and the gomphosis (not shown), which holds teeth in their sockets. The synovial joints include **(F)** the spheroid type at the shoulder; **(G)** the hinge type at the elbow; **(H)** the gliding joints of the hand; and **(I)** the ball and socket (hip). (Adapted from Dorland. *Dorland's medical illustrated dictionary*, 32rd edition. St. Louis: Saunders; 2012.)

bones are united by a pad or disk of fibrocartilage. A thin layer of hyaline cartilage usually covers the articulating surfaces of these two bones, and the thick pad of fibrocartilage acts as a shock absorber and stabilizer. Examples of symphyses are the symphysis pubis, which joins the two pubic bones, and the intervertebral disks, which join the bodies of the vertebrae. A synchondrosis is a joint in which hyaline cartilage, rather than fibrocartilage, connects the two bones. The joints between the ribs and the sternum are synchondroses. The hyaline cartilage of these joints is called *costal cartilage*. Slight movement at the synchondroses between the ribs and the sternum allows the chest to move outward and upward during breathing.

Synovial Joints

Structure

Synovial joints (diarthroses) are the most movable and the most complex joints in the body (Fig. 43.7). A synovial joint consists of the following parts:

1. A fibrous joint capsule (articular capsule)
2. A synovial membrane that lines the inner surface of the joint capsule
3. A joint cavity (synovial cavity), a space formed by the capsule
4. Synovial fluid, which fills the joint cavity and lubricates the joint surface
5. Articular cartilage, which covers and pads the articulating bony surfaces

Joint (articular) capsule. The joint (articular) capsule is fibrous connective tissue that covers the ends of bones where they meet in a joint. Sharpey fibers firmly attach the proximal and distal capsule to the periosteum, and ligaments and tendons also may reinforce the capsule. It is composed of parallel, interlacing bundles of dense, white fibrous tissue richly supplied with nerves, blood vessels, and lymphatic vessels. Nerves in and around the joint capsule are sensitive to the rate and direction of motion, compression, tension, vibration, and pain.

Synovial membrane. The synovial membrane (synovium) is a smooth, delicate inner lining of the joint capsule found in the nonarticular portion of the synovial joint and any ligaments or tendons that traverse this cavity (Fig. 43.8). It is composed of two layers: the vascular subintima and the thin cellular intima. The vascular subintima merges with the fibrous joint capsule and is composed of loose fibrous connective tissue, elastin fibers, fat cells, fibroblasts, macrophages, and mast cells; the cellular intima consists of rows of synovial cells embedded in a fiber-free intercellular matrix and contains two types of cells—A and B. A cells (macrophages) ingest and remove (phagocytose) bacteria and particles of debris in the joint cavity; B cells (fibroblasts) are the most numerous and secrete hyaluronate, which gives synovial fluid its viscous quality. The synovial membrane is richly supplied with blood and lymphatic vessels and is capable of rapid repair and regeneration.

Joint (synovial) cavity. The joint (synovial) cavity is an enclosed, fluid-filled space between articulating surfaces of two bones, also called *joint space*. It enables two bones to move "against" one another and is surrounded by synovial membrane and filled with synovial fluid.

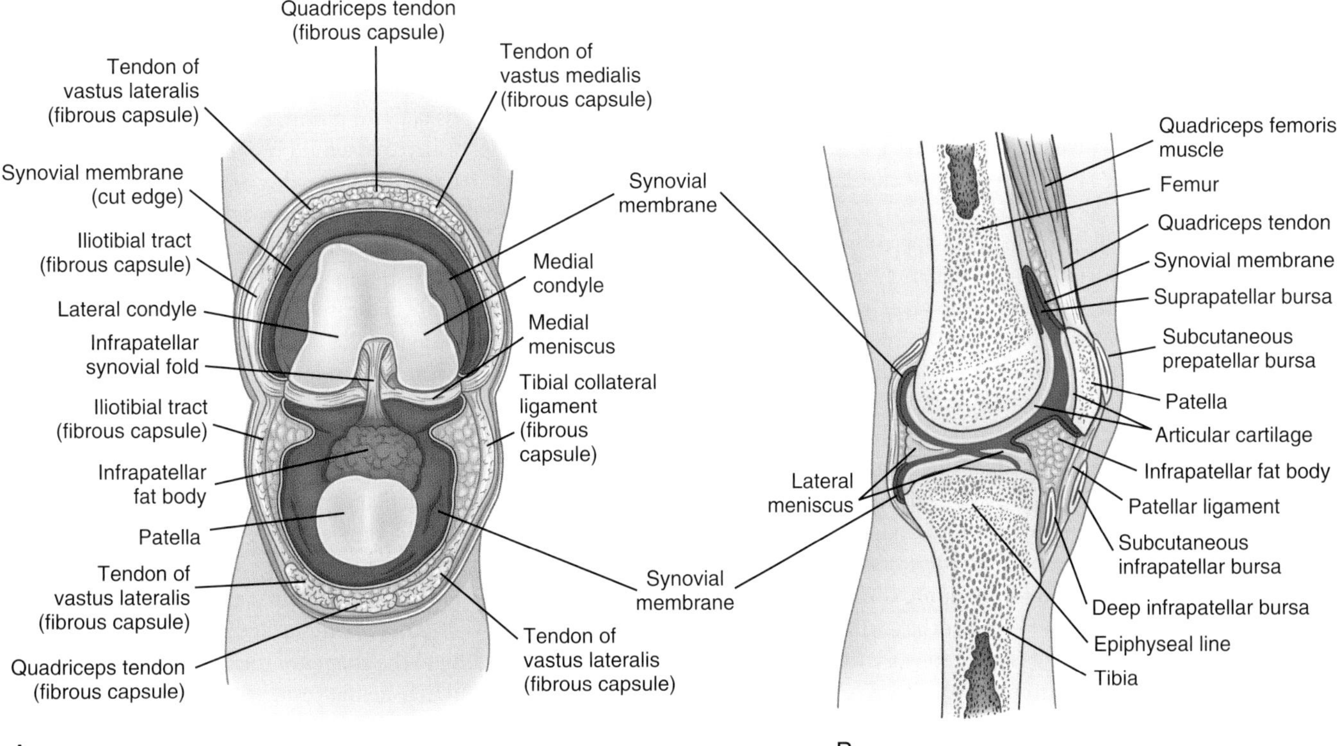

Fig. 43.7 Knee Joint (Synovial Joint). (A) Frontal view. (B) Lateral view.

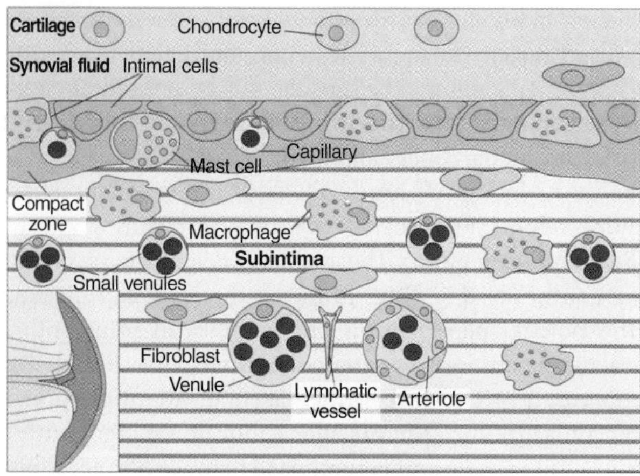

Fig. 43.8 Synovium. Note the delicate synovial lining resting on a fibroadipose subintimal lining rich in capillaries, lymphatics, and nerve endings. (Modified from Hochberg MC, et al. *Rheumatology*, 4th edition. Philadelphia: Mosby; 2008.)

Synovial fluid. Synovial fluid is superfiltrated plasma from blood vessels that lubricates the joint surfaces, nourishes the pad of the articular cartilage, and covers the ends of the bones. Hyaluronic acid in the synovial fluid gives it important biomechanical properties. It also contains free-floating synovial cells and various leukocytes that phagocytose joint debris and microorganisms. Loss of synovial fluid leads to rapid deterioration of articular cartilage.

Articular cartilage. Articular cartilage is a layer of hyaline cartilage that covers the end of each bone; it may be thick or thin, depending on the size of the joint, the fit of the two bone ends, and the amount of weight and shearing force the joint normally withstands. The function of articular cartilage is to reduce friction in the joint and to distribute the forces of weightbearing. Articular cartilage is composed of chondrocytes (cartilage cells) and an intercellular matrix consisting of type II collagen, proteoglycans, and water. The water content ranges from 60% to almost 80% of the net weight of the cartilage, and individual molecules rapidly enter or exit the articular cartilage to contribute to the resiliency of the tissue.

At the surface of articular cartilage, the collagen fibers run parallel to the joint surface and are closely compacted into a dense, protective mat. In the middle layer (the proliferative zone) of the cartilage, the fibers are arranged tangential to the surface, allowing them to deform and absorb some of the weightbearing (Fig. 43.9). In the bottom layer (the hypertrophic zone) of the cartilage, the fibers are perpendicular to the joint surface, allowing them to resist shear forces, and are embedded in a calcified layer of cartilage called the *tidemark*. The tidemark anchors the collagen fibers to the underlying (subchondral) bone. Collagen fibers are important components of the cartilage matrix because they account for approximately 60% of the dry weight and because they (1) anchor the cartilage securely to underlying bone, (2) provide a taut framework for the cartilage, (3) control the loss of fluid from the cartilage, and (4) prevent the escape of protein polysaccharides (proteoglycans) from the cartilage. The proteoglycans give articular cartilage its stiff quality and regulate the movement of synovial fluid through the cartilage. The proteoglycans are macromolecules consisting of proteins, carbohydrates (glycosaminoglycans), and hyaluronic acid. The proteoglycans give articular cartilage its stiff quality and regulate the movement of synovial fluid through the cartilage. Without proteoglycans, normal weightbearing would rapidly and completely press all the synovial fluid out of the cartilage. Proteoglycans act as a pump, permitting enough fluid to be pressed out to ensure that a fluid film is always present on the surface of the cartilage, even after hours of weightbearing. The pumping action of proteoglycans also draws synovial fluid back into the cartilage after a weightbearing load is released. Mobility and weightbearing are necessary for the pumping action of proteoglycans to occur. Nonuse of a joint quickly reduces the pumping action, changing the composition of the matrix and interfering with the nutrition of the chondrocytes. Normal articular cartilage has no blood vessels, lymph vessels, or nerves. Therefore, it is insensitive to pain and regenerates slowly and minimally after injury.[6] Regeneration occurs primarily at sites where the articular cartilage meets the synovial membrane, where blood vessels and nutrients are available. In general, it has been difficult to enhance cartilage repair, but that may be changing (see Emerging Science Box: Progress in Rebuilding Cartilage). Synovial joints are described as uniaxial, biaxial, or multiaxial according to the shapes of the bone ends and the type of movement occurring at the joint (Fig. 43.10). Usually, one of the bones is stable and serves as an axis for the motion of the other bone. The body movements made possible by various synovial joints are either circular or angular (Fig. 43.11).

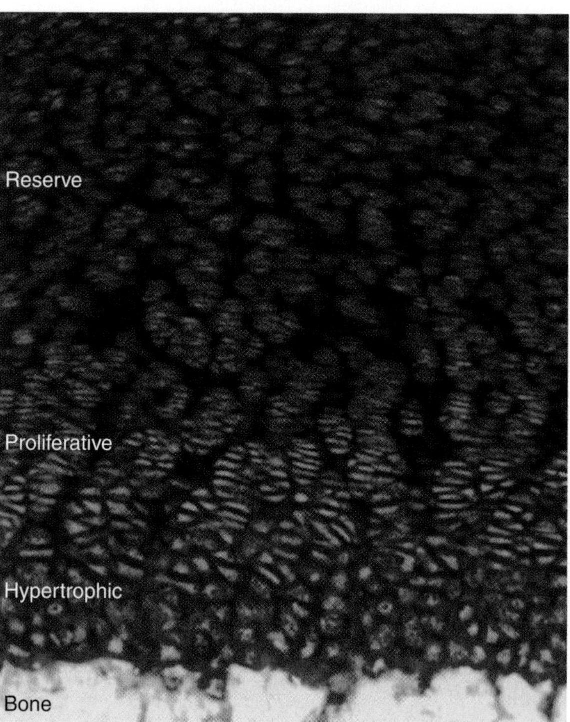

Fig. 43.9 Collagen Zones. The three collagen zones (reserve, proliferative, and hypertrophic) are distinctly shown in a growth plate. (From Hjorten R, Hansen U, Underwood RA, et al. Type XXVII collagen at the transition of cartilage to bone during skeletogenesis. *Bone*, 2007;41[4]:535.)

EMERGING SCIENCE BOX

Progress in Rebuilding Cartilage

Although much research is needed, recent evidence suggests that mesenchymal stem cell therapies may be a potential solution to rebuilding articular cartilage. Multipotent adult stem cells are largely available and accessible. It is theorized that bone marrow mesenchymal stem cells secrete proliferative and regenerative factors in the lesion site of articular cartilage (AC), thereby retarding osteoarthritis progression and promoting AC regeneration locally by trophic effects. Gene therapy (GT) also represents a novel approach to managing joint degradation. The principle of GT is the overexpression of desired gene products. GT can support AC generation by targeting different genes involved in different cellular processes, such as inhibiting inflammatory and catabolic pathways, stimulating anabolic pathways, or preventing cell senescence and apoptosis. Candidate transgene studies are currently in the exploratory phases, generally using animal models. Candidate transgenes with anti-inflammatory action include interleukin-1 (IL-1) receptor antagonist and soluble tumor necrosis factor (sTNF). GT strategies also may target the catabolic effect of matrix metalloproteinases by the delivery of tissue inhibitor of metalloproteinase.

The overexpression of growth factors has been shown to enhance matrix formation. TGF-β, in particular, was reported to aid cartilage regeneration and enhance meniscal tissue healing in vitro. GT shows promise for the future; however, to ensure safety and efficacy, thorough evaluation of the technique is necessary.

Data from Ondresik M, et al. Management of knee osteoarthritis: Current status and future trends. *Biotechnology and Bioengineering*, 2017;114(4):717–739; Zhang R, et al. Mesenchymal stem cell related therapies for cartilage lesion and osteoarthritis. *American Journal of Translational Research*, 2019;11(10):6275–6289; Kim GB, et al. Current perspectives in stem cell therapies for osteoarthritis of the knee. *Yeungnam University Journal of Medicine*, 2020;37(3):149–158.

STRUCTURE AND FUNCTION OF SKELETAL MUSCLES

Skeletal muscles arise from mesodermal progenitor cells; the most numerous are the somites. Actual formation of skeletal muscle is a complex process controlled by multiple signaling factors. A critical component of successful embryonic muscle formation (myogenesis) is protein kinase, an enzyme that adds phosphate groups to substrate proteins, thereby directing cell processes.[7] In muscle, these factors direct the formation of myoblasts. Once myoblasts are formed, they fuse with other myoblasts and form myotubes, eventually developing into muscle fibers. At birth, the muscle fibers have completed development from myoblasts. Final muscle type is determined by transcription factors that regulate both pre- and postnatal muscle development.[8]

The millions of individual fibers of skeletal muscle contract and relax to perform the work necessary to move the body (Fig. 43.12). Muscle constitutes 40% of an adult's body weight and 50% of a child's weight. Muscle is 75% water, 20% protein, and 5% organic and inorganic compounds. Thirty-two percent of all protein stores for energy and metabolism are contained in muscle. Between the ages of 30 and 60, muscle mass decreases by about 0.5 pound of muscle each year. For each 0.5 pound of muscle lost, almost 1 pound of fat typically is gained.

Whole Muscle

There are more than 350 named muscles in the body. The body's muscles vary dramatically in size and shape. They range from 2 to 60 cm in length and are shaped according to function.

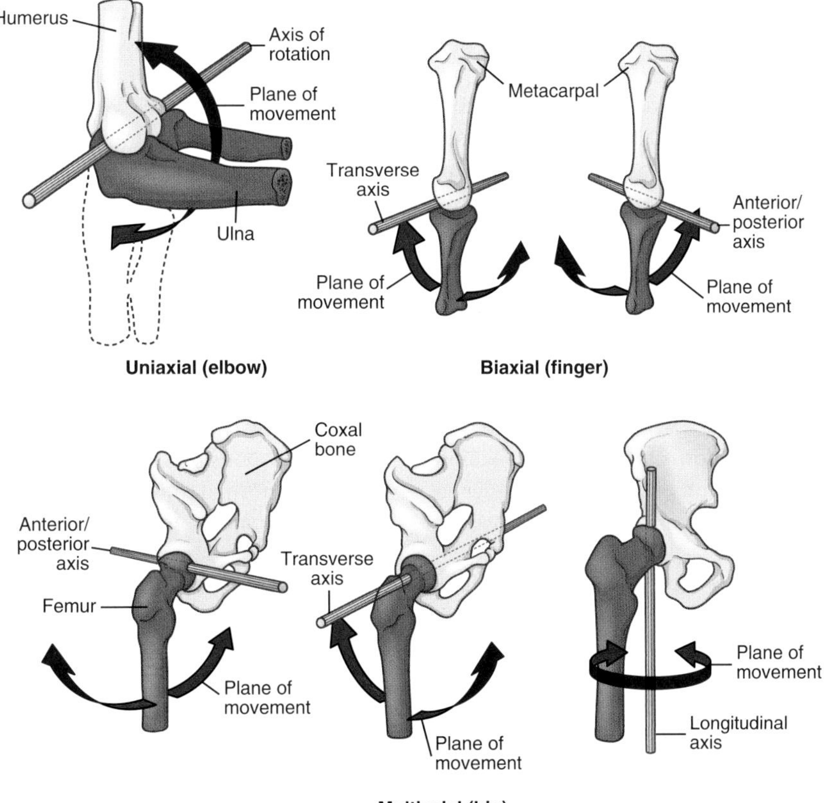

Fig. 43.10 Movements of Synovial (Diarthrodial) Joints.

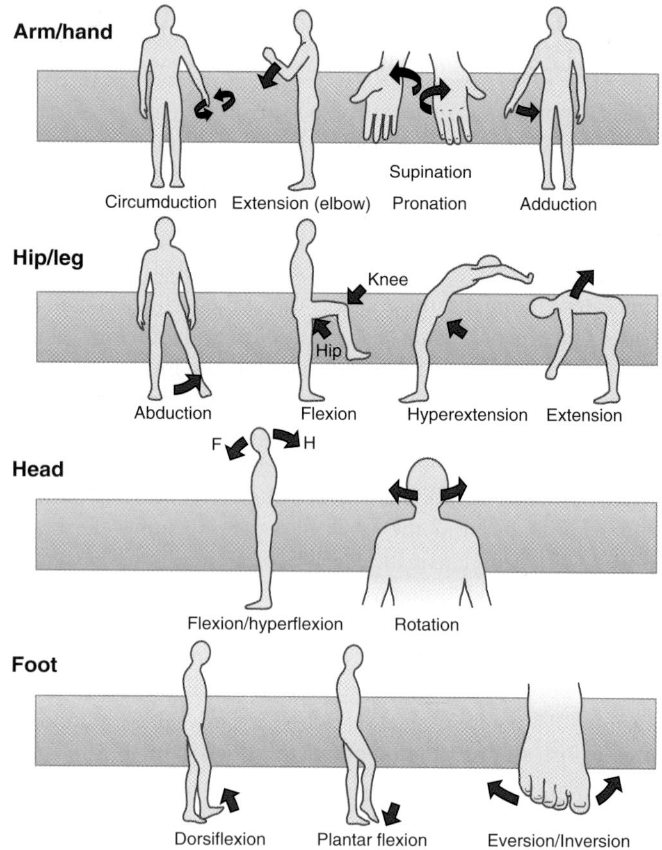

Fig. 43.11 Body Movements Made Possible by Synovial (Diarthrodial) Joints.

Fusiform muscles are elongated muscles shaped like straps that can run from one joint to another. The biceps brachii and psoas major are examples of fusiform muscles. Pennate muscles are broad, flat, and slightly fan shaped, with fibers running obliquely to the muscle's long axis. The multipennate deltoid muscle, which flexes and extends the arm, is a good example of a muscle shaped according to its function.

Each skeletal muscle is a separate organ, encased in a three-part connective tissue framework called fascia. The layers of connective tissue protect the muscle fibers, attach the muscle to bony prominences, and provide a structure for a network of nerve fibers, blood vessels, and lymphatic channels. The layers are:

1. The outermost layer, the epimysium, which is located on the surface of the muscle and tapers at each end to form the tendon (Fig. 43.13); also see the Tendons and Ligaments Section for a discussion of tendons. Tendons allow short muscles to exert power on a distant joint, whereas a thick muscle would interfere with the joint's mobility.
2. The perimysium, which further subdivides the muscle fibers into bundles of connective tissue, or fascicles.
3. The endomysium, which surrounds the muscle. It is the smallest unit of muscle visible without a microscope.

The ligaments, tendons, and fascia are made up of connective tissue that also buffers the limbs from the effects of sudden strains or changes in speed. The rapid recovery necessary for strenuous exercise is supported by the elastic property of muscle and its connective tissue.

Skeletal muscle has been designated as voluntary (controlled directly by the nervous system), striated (has a striped pattern when viewed under a light microscope), or extrafusal (to distinguish from other contractile fibers in the sensory organ of the muscle). Components that are visible on gross inspection of the whole muscle include the motor and sensory nerve fibers. These function together with the muscle, innervating portions of it and providing the electrical impulses needed for motor function.

Motor Unit

From the anterior horn cell of the spinal cord, the axons of motor nerves branch to innervate a specific group of muscle fibers. Each anterior horn cell, its axon (part of the lower motor neuron; see Chapter 15), and the muscle fibers innervated by it are called a motor unit (Fig. 43.14). The motor units are composed of lower motor neurons, which extend to skeletal muscles. Often termed the *functional unit* of the neuromuscular system, the motor unit behaves as a single entity and contracts as a whole when it receives an electrical impulse.

The whole muscle may be controlled by several motor nerve axons. These branch to innervate many motor units within the muscle. The whole muscle then may be made up of many motor units. The number of motor units per individual muscle varies greatly. In the calf, for example, 1 motor axon innervates approximately 2000 muscle fibers, out of a total of 1.2 million muscle fibers. This is a high innervation ratio of muscle fibers to axons, and it contrasts markedly with the low innervation ratio found in laryngeal muscles, where two to three muscle fibers constitute each motor unit and the innervation ratio can be of great functional significance. The greater the innervation ratio of a particular organ, the greater its endurance. Higher innervation ratios prevent fatigue, whereas lower innervation ratios allow for precision of movement.

Sensory receptors. Although muscles function as effector organs, they also contain sensory receptors and are involved in sending different signals to the central nervous system. Among these are the muscle spindles and Golgi tendon organs. Spindles are mechanoreceptors that lie parallel to muscle fibers and respond to muscle stretching. Golgi tendon organs are dendrites that terminate and branch to tendons near the neuromuscular junction. The muscle spindles, Golgi tendon organs, and free nerve endings provide a means of reporting changes in length, tension, velocity, and tone in the muscle. This system of afferent signals is responsible for the muscle stretch response and maintenance of normal muscle tone.

Muscle fibers. Each muscle fiber is a single muscle cell that is cylindrical in structure and surrounded by a membrane capable of excitation and impulse propagation. The muscle fiber contains bundles of myofibrils, the fiber's functional subunits, in a parallel arrangement along the longitudinal axis of the muscle (Fig. 43.15). At birth, the muscle fibers have completed development from precursor cells called *myoblasts.* All voluntary muscles are derived from the mesodermal layer of the embryo. Genetic transcription factors, most notably MyoD, induce skeletal muscle differentiation. Myoblasts are the main cells responsible for muscle growth and regeneration. Myoblasts are termed

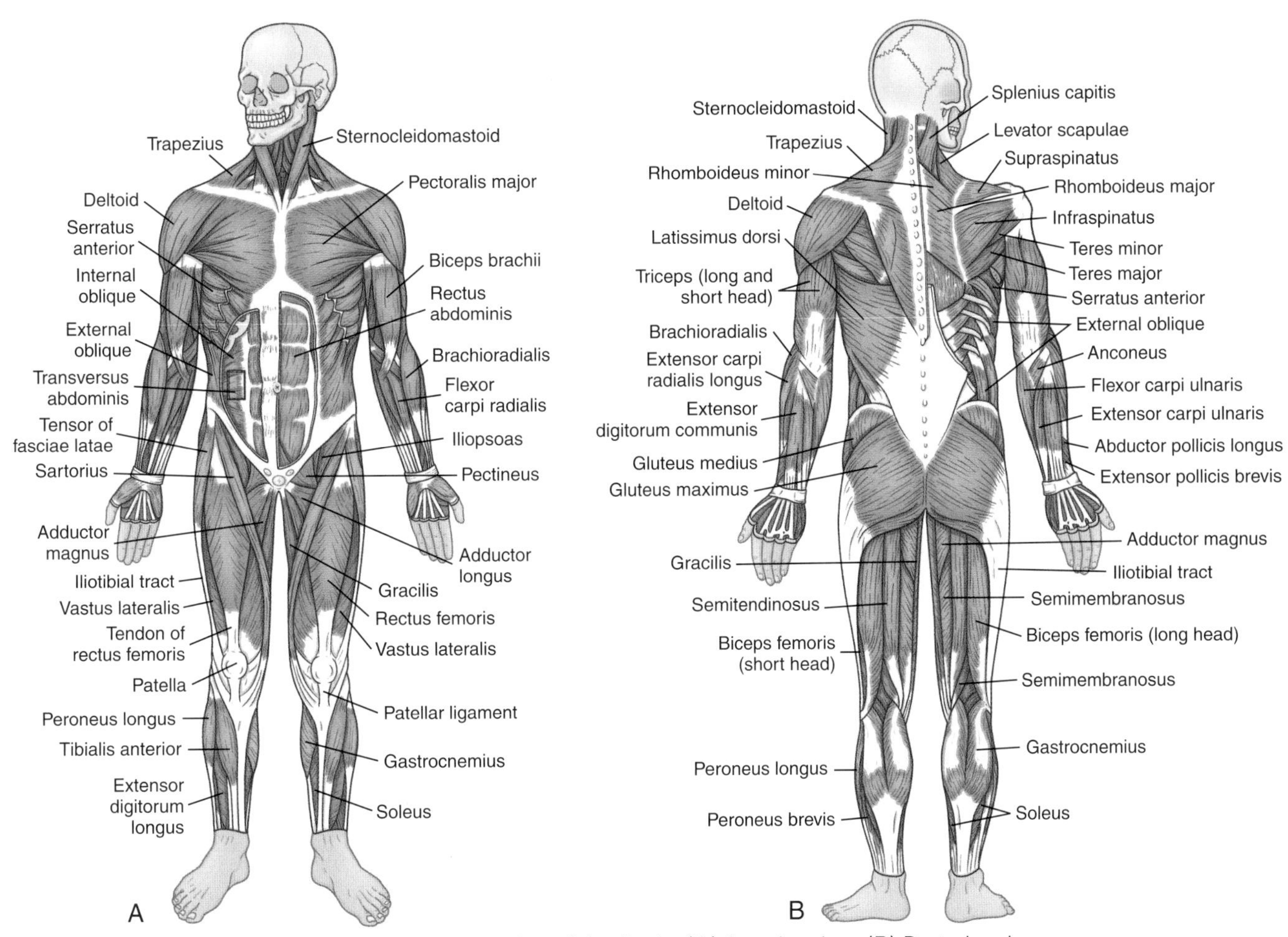

Fig. 43.12 Skeletal Muscles of the Body. (A) Anterior view. (B) Posterior view.

satellite cells when in a dormant state. Satellite cells are crucial in muscle growth, maintenance, repair, and regeneration. Once muscle is injured, satellite cells become activated and increase the number of transcriptional factors necessary to form myoblasts and assist in repair.

The type of peripheral nerve influences the muscle fiber and motor unit considerably. Whether motor nerves are fast or slow determines the type of muscle fibers in the motor unit. White muscle (type II fibers [white fast-twitch fibers]) is innervated by relatively large type II alpha motor neurons with fast conduction velocities. These fibers rely on a short-term anaerobic glycolytic system for rapid energy transfer. Red muscle (type I fibers [slow-twitch fibers]) depends on aerobic oxidative metabolism. Table 43.4 describes the specific characteristics of type I and type II fibers.

The overlap of muscle fibers that appears with staining gives a checkerboard appearance to muscle biopsy specimens. This overlap provides an equal distribution of fiber types throughout the muscle and helps to compensate for muscle fiber loss and fatigue of individual motor units during activity. Despite this, some muscles contain proportionally more of one fiber type than another. Postural muscles have more type I fibers, allowing them the high resistance to fatigue that is necessary to maintain the same position for extended periods. The ocular muscles have more type II muscle fibers, allowing them to respond rapidly to visual changes.

The number of muscle fibers varies according to location. Large muscles, such as the gastrocnemius, have more fibers (1.2 million) than smaller muscles, such as the lumbrical muscles in the hand (10,000). The diameter of muscle fibers also varies. The closely packed polygons are small (10 to 20 μm) until puberty, when they attain the normal adult diameter of 40 to 80 μm. Women usually have smaller diameter fibers than men. Small muscles, such as the ocular muscles, are 15 μm in diameter; larger, more proximal muscles are 40 μm in diameter. Fiber size can have functional significance, such as the association of larger fiber diameter with the generation of greater forces.

The major components of the muscle fiber include the muscle membrane, sarcoplasm, mitochondria, sarcotubular system, and myofibrils (see Fig. 43.15). The muscle membrane is a two-part membrane. It includes the sarcolemma, which contains the plasma membrane of the muscle cell, and the cell's basement membrane. The sarcolemma is 7.5 μm thick and is capable of propagating electrical impulses to initiate contraction. At the motor nerve end plate, where the nerve impulse is transmitted, the sarcolemma forms the highly convoluted synaptic cleft. The sarcolemma is made up of lipid molecules and protein systems. The protein systems perform special functions, such as

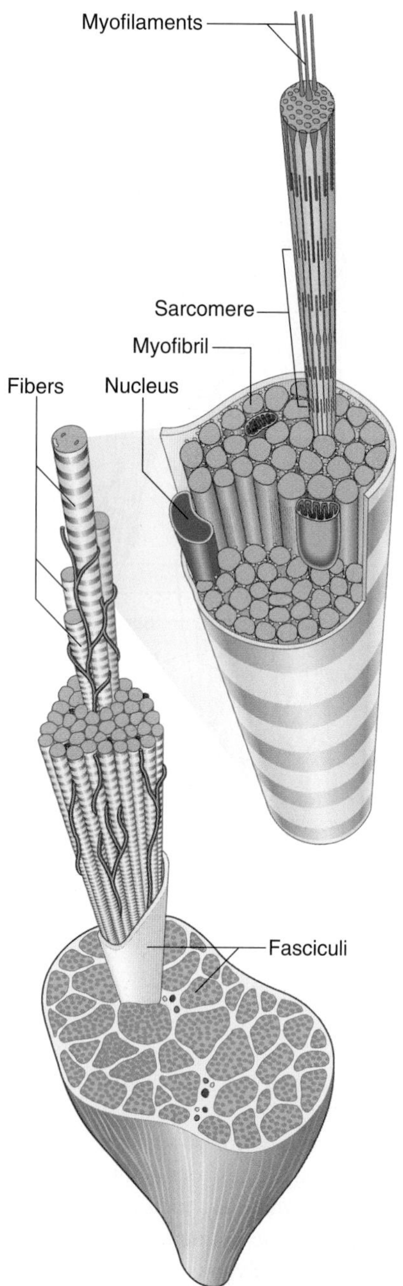

Fig. 43.13 Levels of Organization Within a Skeletal Muscle Showing Muscle Fibers and Their Coverings. (From Standring S. *Gray's anatomy*, 40th edition. Edinburgh: Churchill Livingstone; 2008)

transport of nutrients and protein synthesis. They also provide the sodium-potassium pump and include the cell's cholinergic receptor. The basement membrane is 50 μm thick and is composed primarily of proteins and polysaccharides. It also serves as the cell's microskeleton and maintains the shape of the muscle cell. The basement membrane also may function to restrict further diffusion of electrolytes once they have crossed the sarcolemma.

The sarcoplasm is the cytoplasm of the muscle cell and contains myoglobin plus the intracellular components that are common to all cells (see Chapter 1). Myoglobin is a protein found primarily in skeletal and heart muscle. Related to hemoglobin in the blood, myoglobin stores oxygen and iron in the muscle. The sarcoplasm is an aqueous substance that provides a matrix that surrounds the myofibrils. It contains numerous enzymes and proteins that are responsible for the cell's energy production, protein synthesis, and oxygen storage. The mitochondria house enzyme systems for energy production, particularly those that regulate processes such as the citric acid cycle and adenosine triphosphate (ATP) formation. Many other structures are present in the sarcoplasm. The ribosomes are composed of primarily ribonucleic acid (RNA) and participate in protein synthesis. The cell nucleus, satellite cells, glycogen granules, and lipid droplets are suspended in the sarcoplasmic matrix. Blood vessels, nerve endings, muscle spindles, and Golgi tendon organs are also directly located within this structure.

Unique to the muscle is the sarcotubular system, a network that includes the transverse tubules and the sarcoplasmic reticulum, which crosses the interior of the cell. The sarcoplasmic reticulum is constructed like the endoplasmic reticulum in other cells. The sarcoplasmic reticulum is composed of tubules that run parallel to the myofibrils. The longitudinal tubules are termed sarcotubules. In muscle cells, the sarcoplasmic reticulum contains a network of intracellular receptors known as ryanodine receptors (RyRs). In response to a nerve impulse, RyR1 (found in skeletal muscle cells) releases intracellular calcium and initiates muscle contraction at the sarcomere, a portion of the myofibril. The transverse tubules, which also contain calcium release channels and are closely associated with the sarcotubules, run across the sarcoplasm and communicate with the extracellular space. Together, the tubules of this membrane system allow for uptake and regulation of intracellular calcium, release of calcium during muscle contraction, and storage of calcium during muscle relaxation.

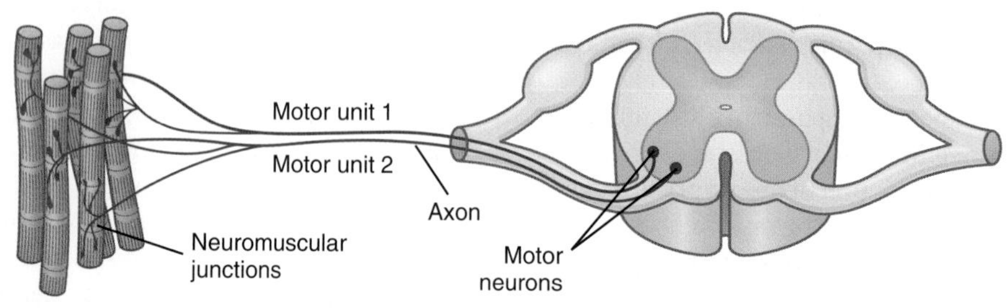

Fig. 43.14 Motor Units of a Muscle. Each motor unit consists of a motor neuron and all the muscle fibers (cells) supplied by the neuron and its axon branches.

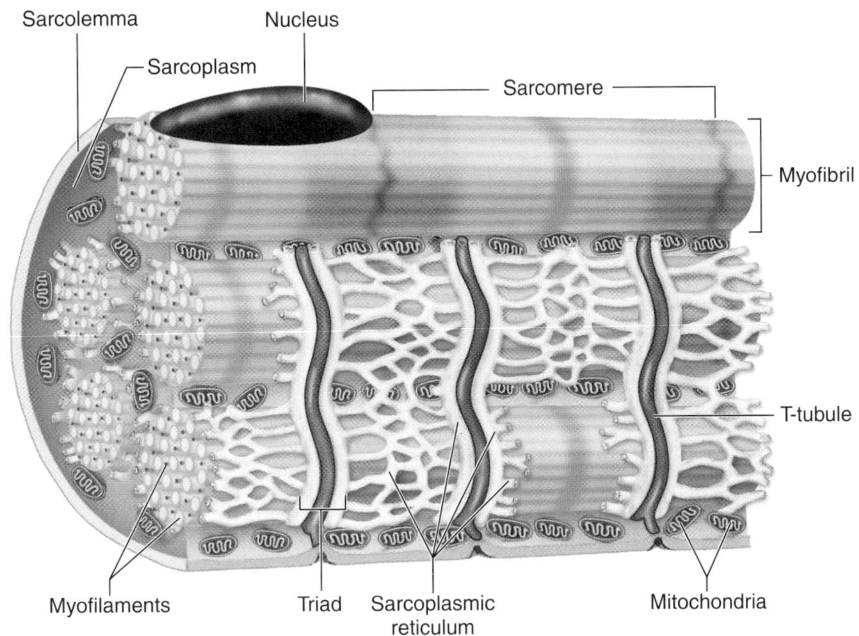

Fig. 43.15 Myofibrils of a Skeletal Muscle Fiber (Cell) and Overall Organization of Skeletal Muscle. (From Patton KT, Thibodeau GA. *Anatomy & physiology*, 9th edition. St. Louis: Mosby; 2016.)

Myofibrils. Myofibrils, the most abundant subcellular muscle component (85% to 90% of the total volume), are the functional units of muscle contraction. Each myofibril contains sarcomeres, which appear at intervals (see Fig. 43.15). Sarcomeres are composed of several proteins. The two most abundant are actin and myosin, but three other giant, muscle-specific proteins (titin, nebulin, and obscurin) play important roles in myofibril formation and function (Table 43.5).

On cross section, they are seen to be irregular polygons with a mean diameter of less than 1 µm. Each myofibril is composed of serially repeating sarcomeres, separated by Z bands, which give the muscle its striped, cross-striated appearance. Each sarcomere has a dark A band and is flanked by two light I bands (Fig. 43.16). The A band is 1.5 to 1.6 µm long and contains the thick myosin filaments. Included in the A band is a lighter zone called the *H band*, and in the center of the H band is the dark *M band*, or *M line*. The *I band*, which contains actin, is divided at the midpoint of each sarcomere by the *Z band*. Its length varies with the start of muscle contraction. The *Z disk* (made up of different layers of Z bands, depending on muscle type) marks the boundaries of the sarcomere.

Myofibrils are composed of myofilaments. Each myofilament is structured in a closely packed hexagonal arrangement, with two thin filaments for every thick filament. The thick filament, along with C protein and M line protein, is made up of myosin. Myosin has two subunits—heavy and light meromyosin, which resemble twisted golf club shafts. The thin filaments are twisted double strands consisting of actin, troponin, and tropomyosin (see Chapter 31).

Muscle proteins. Table 43.6 summarizes muscle protein distribution, location, and possible functional significance. The contractile and regulatory functions of actin, myosin, and the troponin-tropomyosin complex (associated with actin) are the most known. They also account for most of the protein found in the myofibril. The structural and regulatory processes of muscle proteins are less well understood. Alpha actin and beta actin are known to link the filaments. M protein contains the enzyme creatine kinase (CK). Creatine is released when muscle cells are damaged, making the serum creatine value an important measurement of pathologic conditions of muscles.

The most abundant proteins, actin and myosin, are also found in other cells, particularly motile cells such as platelets. The complete amino acid sequences of actin and myosin have been identified. Noteworthy is the presence of the amino acid 3-methylhistidine, found only in the thin filament, actin; 85% to 90% of 3-methylhistidine is found in skeletal muscle.

Nonprotein constituents of muscle. Nitrogen, creatine, creatinine, phosphocreatine, purines, uric acid, and amino acids all serve in the complex process of muscle metabolism. Energy is provided by glycogen and its derivatives.

Creatine metabolism and creatinine metabolism have been used to measure muscle mass. Plasma creatine is taken up by muscle and converted into the high-energy phosphate compound phosphocreatine by the enzyme CK. Creatinine is formed in muscle from creatine at a constant rate of 2% per day. Creatine excretion is increased in muscle wasting. This change reflects the reduction in total body creatine stores and the loss of muscle mass.

Inorganic compounds, anions (phosphate, chloride), and cations (calcium, magnesium, sodium, potassium) are important in the regulation of protein synthesis, muscle contraction, and enzyme systems, as well as in the stabilization of cell membranes. The total body potassium (TBK) level, measured by the K40 method, has been used to measure muscle mass, also called

TABLE 43.4 **Characteristics of Human Skeletal Muscle Type I and Type II Fibers**

Characteristics	Type I (Red) (Oxidative Fibers [OFs])	Type II (White) Type II-1A (Fast Oxidative Glycolic Fibers [FOGs])
Anatomic location	Deep axial portion of muscle	Surface portion of muscle
Fiber diameter	Small	Large
Motor neuron size	Small	Large
Contraction speed	Slow	Fast
Motor neuron type	Type I, α	Type II-A, II-B, II-X, and II-D II-A: fatigue resistant; II-B: fast fatigable; II-X and II-D: intermediate fatigability
Glycogen content (at rest)	Low	High
Oxidative capacity	High	High (for short periods)
Myosin-ATPase activity	Low	High
Metabolism	Oxidative (also most effective in removing glucose from bloodstream)	Some oxidative pathways, mostly glycolysis
Used for	Maintaining body posture, skeletal support, aerobic activity	Short, intense activity (e.g., sprinting)
Aerobic metabolic capacity	High	Low
Fatigue resistance	High	Intermediate to low
Myoglobin content	High	Low
Capillary supply	Profuse	Intermediate to low
Mitochondria	Many	Few
Intensity of contraction	Low	High
Example (most muscles are mixed)	Soleus muscle	Laryngeal
Satellite cell content	High	Low

Data from Schiaffino S, Reggiani C. Fiber types in mammalian skeletal muscles. *Physiological Reviews*, 2011;91:1447–1531; Verdijk LB, Snijders T, Drost M, et al. Satellite cells in human skeletal muscle; from birth to old age. *Age*, 2014;36(2):545–547.

lean body mass. TBK levels reflect changes in muscle mass seen during growth, malnutrition, and muscle wasting.

Components of Muscle Function

The ultimate function of muscle is to accomplish work. Although variously expressed in such measures as foot-pounds or kilogram-meters, work usually refers to the amount of energy liberated, or force exerted over a distance (Work = Force × Distance). Muscles usually contract or tense while doing work. Muscle contraction occurs on the molecular level and leads to the observable phenomenon of muscle movement.

Muscle Contraction at the Molecular Level

The four steps of muscle contraction are (1) excitation, (2) coupling, (3) contraction, and (4) relaxation. The process involves the electrical properties of all cells and the movement of ions across the plasma membrane (see Chapter 1). The muscle fiber is an excitable tissue. At rest, an electrical charge of −90 mV is continually maintained across the sarcolemma. This resting potential, generated by the separation of positive and negative charges on either side of the membrane, creates an electrochemical equilibrium caused by the selective permeability of the sarcolemma to electrolytes in the intracellular and extracellular fluids, particularly potassium and sodium.

Excitation, the first step of muscle contraction, begins with the spread of an action potential from the nerve terminal to the neuromuscular junction. The rapid depolarization of the membrane initiates an electrical impulse in the muscle fiber membrane called the muscle fiber action potential. As the action potential advances along the sarcolemmal membrane, it spreads to the transverse tubules. A receptor on the transverse tubule opens, allowing calcium to enter the cell.

The second stage, coupling, follows the depolarization of the transverse tubules. This triggers the release of calcium ions from the sarcoplasmic reticulum through RyR1 channels into the sarcoplasm. The calcium then binds to a protein on the actin filament. (Calcium affects troponin and tropomyosin, muscle proteins that bind with actin when the muscle is at rest.) In the presence of calcium, however, both these proteins are attracted to calcium ions, leaving the actin free to bind with myosin. The release of intracellular calcium ions is the critical link between a nerve impulse (electrical excitation) and muscle contraction.

Contraction begins as the calcium ions combine with troponin, a reaction that overcomes the inhibitory function of the troponin-tropomyosin system. Myosin binds to actin, forming cross-bridges. The myosin heads attach to the exposed actin-binding sites, pulling actin (the thin filament) inward. The thin filament, actin, then slides toward the thick filament, myosin.

TABLE 43.5 **Contractile Proteins of Skeletal Muscle Sarcomere**

Protein	Location	Function
Actinin	Z disk	Attaches actin to Z disks; helps coordinate sarcomere contraction; cross-links thin filaments in adjacent sarcomeres
Actin	I band (thin filaments)	Contraction; activates myosin-ATPase; interacts with myosin
α-Actin	Z disk	Main ligand of titin; links and controls filament length
β-Actin	Z disk	Regulatory and structural function; links filaments, controls filament length
Myosin	A band (thick filament)	Contraction force; two distinct types: myosin heavy chain (MyHC) and myosin light chain (MyLC); hydrolyzes ATP and develops tension
Titin[a] (largest and third most abundant muscle protein)	Half of sarcomere (from Z disk to M band)	Coordinates assembly of proteins that comprise sarcomere; regulates resting length of sarcomere; important for myofibril assembly, stabilization, and maintenance
Nebulin[a]	I band (with α-actin)	Interacts with myosin to produce contraction; binding site for actin, desmin, titin, other proteins; stabilizes and regulates length of actin filaments; plays role in assembly, structure, and maintenance of Z disks
Obscurin[a]	Surrounds sarcomere (mainly at Z disk and M band)	May mediate interaction of sarcoplasmic reticulum and myofibrils; plays role in muscle response to injury; has role in formation and stabilization of M bands and A band

[a]Also may function as molecular scaffolds for myofibril formation.
ATP, Adenosine triphosphate; *ATPase*, adenosine triphosphatase.
Data from Herzog JA, Leonard TR, Jinha A, et al. Titin (visco-) elasticity in skeletal muscle myofibrils. *Molecular and Cellular Biomechanics*, 2014;11(1):1–17; Luther PK. The vertebrate muscle Z-disc: sarcomere anchor for structure and signalling. *Journal of Muscle Research and Cell Motility*, 2009;30:171–185; Pappas CT, Krieg PA, Gregorio CC. Nebulin regulates actin filament lengths by a stabilization mechanism. *Journal of Cell Biology*, 2010;189(5):858–870; Schiaffino S, Reggiani C. Fiber types in mammalian skeletal muscles. *Physiological Reviews*, 2011;91:1447–1531.

The two ends of the myofibril shorten after contraction when the myosin heads attach to the actin molecules, forming a cross-bridge that constitutes an actin-myosin complex. ATP, located on the actin-myosin complex, is released when the cross-bridges attach. Contraction was first described by A.F. Huxley in the 1950s. It is commonly known as the cross-bridge theory because the actin and myosin proteins form cross-bridges as they contract. The useful distance of contraction of a skeletal muscle is approximately 25% to 35% of the muscle's length.

The last step, relaxation, begins as calcium ions are actively transported back into the sarcoplasmic reticulum, removing ions from interaction with troponin. The cross-bridges detach, and the sarcomere lengthens. (The cross-bridge theory of muscle contraction is discussed in Chapter 31.)

Muscle Metabolism

Skeletal muscle requires a constant supply of ATP and phosphocreatine. These substances are necessary to fuel the complex processes of muscle contraction, driving the cross-bridges of actin and myosin together and transporting calcium from the sarcoplasmic reticulum to the myofibril. Other internal processes of the muscular system that require ATP include protein synthesis, which replenishes muscle constituents and accommodates growth and repair. The rate of protein synthesis is related to hormone levels (particularly insulin), the presence of amino acid substrates, and overall nutritional status. At rest, the rate of ATP formation by oxidation of glucose or acetoacetate is sufficient to maintain internal processes, given normal nutritional status. During activity, the need for ATP increases 100-fold. The metabolic pathways for muscle activity in Table 43.7 show reactions to the immediate need for increased ATP caused by contraction. Activity lasting longer than 5 seconds expends the available stored ATP and phosphocreatine.

Stored glycogen and blood glucose are converted anaerobically to sustain brief activity without increasing the demand for oxygen. Anaerobic glycolysis is much less efficient than aerobic glycolysis, using six to eight times more glycogen to produce the same amount of ATP. With increased activity, such as intense exercise, or with ischemia, an increase in the amount of lactic acid occurs because of the breakdown of glycogen, thus causing a shift in muscle pH (see Table 43.7). This short-term mechanism buys time by allowing ATP formation despite inadequate energy stores or oxygen supply. When the anaerobic threshold is reached and more oxygen is required, physiologic changes occur, including an increase in lactic acid level and increases in oxygen consumption, heart rate, respiratory rate, and muscle blood flow.

Strenuous exercise requires oxygen, which activates the aerobic glycogen pathway for ATP formation. During maximal exercise, free fatty acid mobilization and the aerobic glycogen pathways provide ATP over an extended time. These pathways require oxygen both to maintain maximal activity and to return the muscle to the resting state. Maximal exercise increases oxygen uptake by 15 to 20 times over the resting state. When this system becomes exhausted or inadequate to respond to the need for ATP, fatigue and weakness finally force the muscle to reduce activity, with a resultant buildup of lactic acid in muscle fibers.

Sustaining maximal muscular activity accumulates an oxygen debt, which is the amount of oxygen needed to oxidize the residual lactic acid, convert it back to glycogen, and replenish ATP and phosphocreatine stores. For example, after running at maximal speed for 10 seconds, the average person has consumed 1 L of oxygen. At rest, oxygen consumption for the

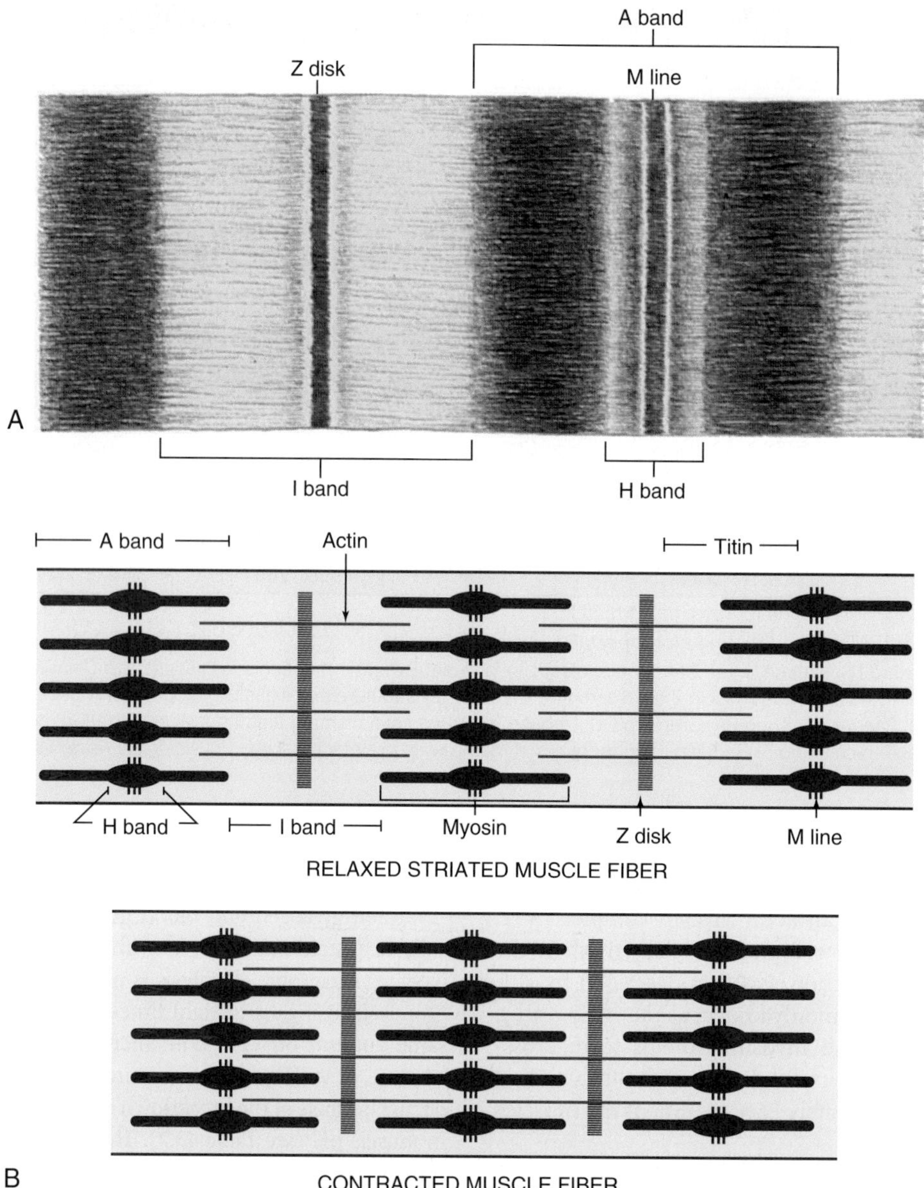

Fig. 43.16 Muscle Fibers. (A) The Z disks define the end of an individual sarcomere. The M line (which lies within the H band) is made of cross-connecting elements of the cytoskeleton. **(B)** Actin is the primary protein of the I band (thin filament). Nebulin also extends along the I band and contains binding sites for actin and myosin. Myosin (thick filament) extends through the A band. Titin extends from the Z disk to the M band, binding with myosin; strong titin anchoring within the I band is necessary for proper muscle function. During contraction, the I bands and H bands shorten, moving the Z disks closer together. (A, Modified from Thompson JM, et al. *Mosby's clinical nursing*, 5th edition. St. Louis: Mosby; 2002.)

same period is approximately 40 mL. As the person recovers, the measured oxygen debt is 4 L greater than the amount used during activity.

Oxygen consumption is measured to calculate the metabolic cost of activity in normal and diseased muscles. It is an indirect measure of energy expenditure, along with timed tests of activity, heart rate, and respiratory quotient (ratio of carbon dioxide to expired oxygen consumed). Energy expenditure is measured directly by heat production because heat is released whenever work is accomplished.

Another factor that changes energy requirements is muscle fiber type. Type II fibers rely on anaerobic glycolytic metabolism and fatigue readily. Type I fibers can resist fatigue for longer periods because of their capacity for oxidative metabolism.

Muscle Mechanics

Muscle contraction cannot be viewed in isolation. Several factors determine how force is transmitted from the cross-bridges on individual muscle fibers to accomplish whole-muscle contraction. First, when a motor unit responds to a single nerve stimulus, it develops a phasic contraction, also called a *twitch*. Because the motor unit contracts in an all-or-nothing manner, the contraction that is generated will be a maximal contraction. The central nervous system smoothly grades the force generated

TABLE 43.6 Contractile Proteins of Skeletal Muscle Fibrils

Name	Approximate Percentage of Myofibrillar Protein	Location	Function
Myosin	55	A band (thick filament)	Contraction; hydrolyzes ATP and develops tension
Actin	20	I band (thin filament)	Contraction; activates myosin ATPase and interacts with myosin
Troponin	7	Thin filament	Regulatory protein; in presence of Ca^{++}, promotes actin-myosin activation
Tropomyosin	5–7	Thin filament	Regulatory and structural function; links filaments, controls filament length
Alpha (α) actin	10	Z band	Regulatory and structural function; links filaments, controls filament length
Beta (β) actin	2	Z band	Regulatory and structural function; links filaments, controls filament length
M protein	2	M line (center of thick filaments)	Regulatory and structural function; provides enzyme creatine kinase
C protein	2	A band (thick filaments)	Possible structural role
Titin	Unknown	Z line (thick filament)	Interconnects thin filaments in Z line
Creatine kinase	Unknown	M line	Catalyzes the phosphorylation of ADP to form ATP
Desmin	Unknown	Z line	Interconnects thin filaments in Z line
Filamin[a]	Unknown	Z line	Interconnects thin filaments in Z line; stabilizes membrane
Nebulin[a]	Unknown	Z line	Determines filament length

ADP, Adenosine diphosphate; *ATP*, Adenosine triphosphate; *ATPase*, adenosine triphosphatase.
[a]Data from Ma K, Wang K: *Fed Eur Biochem Soc Lett* 532(3):273–278, 2002; Sampson LJ, Leyland ML, Dart D: *J Biol Chem* 278(43):41988–41997, 2003.

TABLE 43.7 Energy Sources for Muscular Activity

Sources	Reactions
Short-term (anaerobic) sources	ATP → ADP + P_i + Energy Phosphocreatine + ADP ⇌ Creatine + ATP Glycogen/glucose + P_i + ADP → Lactate + ATP
Long-term (aerobic) sources	Glycogen/glucose + ADP + P_i + O_2 → H_2O + CO_2 + ATP Free fatty acids + ADP + P_i + O_2 → H_2O + CO_2 + ATP Creatine kinase catalyzes reversible reaction of ATP to ADP: Creatine phosphate + ATP $\xrightleftharpoons{\text{Creatine Kinase}}$ Creatine + ATP

ADP, Adenosine diphosphate; *ATP*, adenosine triphosphate; *CO_2*, carbon dioxide; *H_2O*, water; *O_2*, oxygen; *Pi*, inorganic phosphate.
From Spence AP, Mason EE. *Human anatomy and physiology*, 4th edition. St. Paul, Minn: West Publishing; 1992.

by recruiting additional motor units and varying the discharge frequency of each active motor unit. This adding of motor units within the muscle is called repetitive discharge.

Recruitment and repetitive discharge of motor units allow the muscle to activate the number of motor units needed to generate the desired force. The total force developed is the sum of the force generated by each motor unit. If the motor units are stimulated again and the muscle unit has not been able to relax between stimulation and the next contraction, the second contraction will fuse with the first, causing physiologic tetanus (not to be confused with the disease tetanus).

Other variables, such as fiber type, innervation ratio, muscle temperature, and muscle shape, influence the efficiency of muscular contraction. The two muscle fiber types differ in their responses to electrical activity. Tetanus and duration of phasic contractions, which take microseconds to accomplish, are achieved more rapidly in type II (white fast-twitch) than in type I (red slow-twitch) muscle fibers. Low innervation ratios promote control and coordination, whereas high ratios promote strength and endurance. Muscles work best at normal body temperature, or 37°C (98.6°F). Finally, muscles with a large cross-sectional area, such as the fan-shaped pennate muscles, develop greater contractile forces than smaller diameter muscles. The initial length of a muscle and the range of shortening that occur when the muscle contracts also determine the force it can generate. The long fusiform muscles have a greater range of shortening and can contract up to 57% of their resting length. A certain amount of elongation is necessary to generate sufficient tension and muscular force. The elongation that occurs during the swing of a golf club or tennis racket is an example of how stretch improves contractile force.

Types of Muscle Contraction

During isometric (or static) contraction, the muscle maintains constant length as tension is increased (Fig. 43.17). Isometric contraction occurs, for example, when the arm or leg is pushed

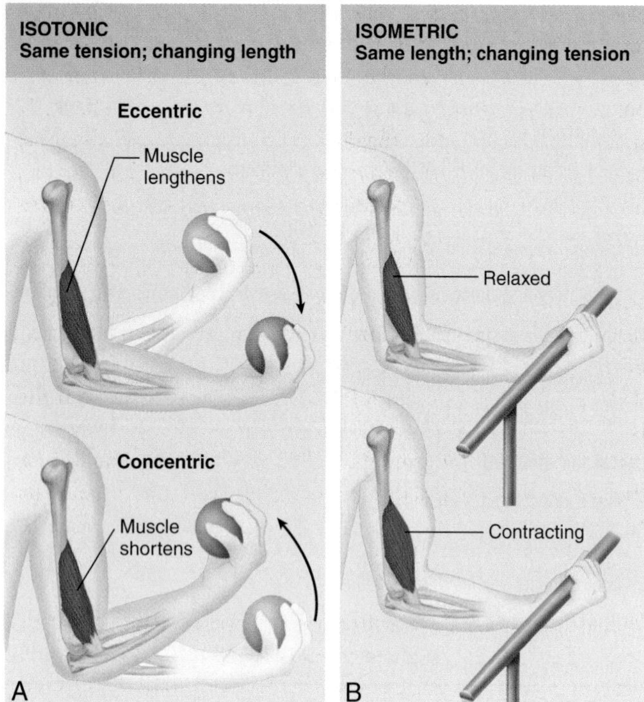

Fig. 43.17 Isotonic and Isometric Contraction. **(A)** In isotonic contraction, the muscle shortens, producing movement. **(B)** In isometric contraction, the muscle pulls forcefully against a load but does not shorten. (From Patton KT, Thibodeau GA. *Structure & function of the body*, 15th edition. St. Louis: Mosby; 2016.)

against an immovable object. The muscle contracts, but the limb does not move. Isometric contraction is also called static (holding) contraction.

During dynamic (formerly known as isotonic) contraction, the muscle maintains a constant tension as it moves. Isotonic contractions can be eccentric (lengthening) or concentric (shortening). Positive work is accomplished during concentric contraction, and energy is released to exert force or lift a weight. In contrast, during an eccentric contraction, the muscle lengthens and absorbs energy (e.g., extending the elbow while lowering a weight). Eccentric contraction requires less energy to accomplish and has been said to result in the development of pain and stiffness after unaccustomed exercise.

Movement of Muscle Groups

Muscles do not act alone but in groups, often under automatic control. When a muscle contracts and acts as a prime mover, or agonist, its reciprocal muscle, or antagonist, relaxes. To illustrate this, hold the right arm in the horizontal position in front of the body and bend the elbow; use the other hand to feel the biceps on the top and the triceps on the bottom of the arm. When the elbow is bent, the biceps are firm, and the triceps are soft. As the arm is extended, the muscles change. When the elbow is completely extended, the biceps is soft and the triceps firm. Completing this movement causes the agonist and antagonist to change automatically; only the movement is commanded, not the alternate contraction and relaxation of the specific muscle groups.

Other associated actions occur with walking; as the foot leaves the ground, the paravertebral and gluteal muscles on the opposite sides of the body contract to maintain balance. Paralysis offsets this process and decreases balance.

Tendons and Ligaments

Tendons are important musculoskeletal structures that attach muscle to bone at a site called an enthesis. Ligaments attach bone to bone, helping to form joints, as well as stabilizing them against excessive movement. Both tendons and ligaments are primarily composed of types III, IV, V, and VI collagen and fibroblasts (called *tenocytes* in tendons).

The fibroblasts in tendons are arranged in parallel rows; fibroblasts appear less organized in ligaments. Collagen fibers and fibroblasts form fascicles, with multiple fascicles then forming a whole tendon or ligament. In the proteoglycan matrix of tendons, collagen oligomeric matrix protein (COMP) assists in providing gliding and viscoelastic properties. Compared with tendons, ligament fibers typically contain a greater proportion of elastin.

Two main functions of tendons are (1) transferring forces from muscle to bone and (2) as a type of biologic spring for muscles to enable additional stability during movement. Ligaments stabilize joints by restricting movement. Although both tendons and ligaments can withstand significant distraction (stretching) force, they tend to buckle when compressive force is applied.

Both tendons and ligaments have complex structures at the attachment site of two dissimilar tissues. These complex structures and differences in mechanical and structural characteristics (either tendon and bone or ligament and bone) make healing and repair of damaged tissue complicated (see Emerging Science Box: Understanding Tendon and Ligament Repair).

EMERGING SCIENCE BOX

Understanding Tendon and Ligament Repair

Injury of tendons and ligaments is one of the greatest challenges in musculoskeletal rehabilitation. When these types of structures are damaged, attempts to engineer suitable tissue replacements have proved disappointing. The structures and intricate protein composition of tendons and ligaments are the basis for their complex biomechanical properties. One reason for a poor clinical outcome in synthetic tendon structures has been the inability to replicate any material that can bear the high mechanical stresses that occur at the interface between two dissimilar materials (i.e., either tendon and bone or ligament and bone). One promising area of investigation is finding or engineering a biodegradable material, or "scaffold," implanted with specific cells that would regenerate into a normal tendon or ligament. The scaffold must be strong enough to withstand the forces at the tissue/bone interface and then gradually break down as it is completely replaced by new cells. Currently, investigators are using synthetic polymers, silk, and collagen as scaffolds, with tendon or ligament fibroblasts and mesenchymal stem cells as the implanted cells. Once these biochemical hurdles have been overcome, the repair of damaged tendons and ligaments will be revolutionized.

Data from Jahr H, et al. Physicochemical and biomechanical stimuli in cell-based articular cartilage repair. *Current Rheumatology Reports*, 2015;17(3):22.

TESTS OF MUSCULOSKELETAL FUNCTION

Tests of Bone Function

Diagnostic procedures to evaluate bone function include gait analysis, measurement of serum calcium and phosphorus levels, and imaging studies. Most imaging techniques provide morphologic rather than functional information about bone. Plain radiographs (x-rays) remain the standard initial imaging tool for bone evaluation because bone absorbs x-ray beams better than soft tissue. Computed tomography (CT) provides multiple images that are then processed into single (two-dimensional) or multiple images taken around a single axis to form (three-dimensional) pictures. Dual-energy computed tomography (DECT) utilizes x-ray beams at two different energy levels to determine different chemical compositions of tissues, thereby expanding CT imaging to include soft tissues, bone marrow, and crystals.[9] Advances in CT technology allow for detailed visualization of bone microstructure.[10]

Magnetic resonance imaging (MRI) provides detailed anatomic information and is useful for evaluating primary or metastatic bone lesions, infection, marrow edema, bony erosions, osteonecrosis, fractures, and other pathologic changes of bone. Magnetic resonance arthrography (MRa) involves the injection of a contrast agent into the area of interest but allows better visualization of small abnormalities. Detailed functional imaging of bone can be attained with positron emission tomography (PET) scanning. A relatively new technology, MRI-PET combines MRI with functional imaging of molecular events seen with PET.

Nuclear medicine studies also provide imaging about metabolic activity in bone and soft tissue. After a small amount of radioactive tracer is injected, a special camera is used to identify bone absorption of the tracer. Bone scanning is very sensitive, but not specific about the cause of increased metabolic activity.

Dual-photon absorptiometry (DXA) is often used to measure the density of bones in the extremities and the fracture risk of vertebral bodies, femoral neck, and distal radius. Dual-photon absorptiometry allows the soft tissue components to be subtracted. New technology promises more accurate evaluation of bone.

Serum bone-specific alkaline phosphatase (BAP) is a marker of bone formation. Bone resorption is evaluated with urinary and serum measurements of cross-linked N-terminal telopeptides (NTx), a product of osteoclast bone resorption. NTx is specific for bone because the cross-links assessed are characteristic of bone collagen alone. Urine NTx is a more sensitive and specific biochemical marker of bone resorption than serum NTx.[11]

Tests of Joint Function

Procedures used to diagnose joint function include arthrography, arthroscopy, MRI, and synovial fluid analysis. Arthrography (the injection of dye into the joint) is particularly useful to diagnose tears in the fibrocartilage of the knee (meniscus) and the rotator cuff of the shoulder. Arthroscopy is the direct visualization of a joint through an arthroscope. Magnetic resonance imaging (MRI) produces images of body tissues through electromagnetic (radio) waves that alter the atoms (hydrogen ions) in the nuclei of cells being examined. When the polarized radio waves are stopped, the nuclear atoms return to their original positions, emitting energy as signals as they move back. The signals produce visible images for examination and diagnosis. MRI produces excellent contrast of soft tissues for the evaluation of musculoskeletal conditions. MRa is injection of contrast into a joint, followed by MRI evaluation.

Analysis of synovial fluid may reveal inflammatory, septic, and noninflammatory joint diseases, which cause characteristic changes in the color, clarity, viscosity, and cellular elements of the fluid. The presence of blood in the joint fluid (hemarthrosis) usually indicates joint trauma. Normal synovial fluid is sterile, so the presence of bacteria in the fluid always indicates disease. Cell fragments and fibrous tissue in the fluid are the result of inflammation or wear-and-tear on the articular surfaces.

Tests of Muscular Function

When the individual's history and physical examination disclose abnormalities, such as weakness, atrophy, muscle tenderness, cramps, and stiffness, specific tests of muscle function are in order. One of the most useful tests is the serum CK concentration. CK is found in large quantities in the muscle fibers, and when these fibers are diseased or damaged, CK leaks into the serum. Myoglobin is also detectable in the urine after acute muscle damage caused by crush injury, ischemic disorders, extreme exertion, and some inherited diseases.

Because the muscle membrane tissue is excitable and carries an electrical charge, its capacity to function can be assessed by electromyography. Using sensitive needle electrodes, the electromyogram (EMG) records the summation of action potentials of the muscle fibers in each motor unit. The EMG is often compared with the electrocardiogram (ECG), but the activity recorded on the EMG is on a much smaller scale. The amplitude of the ECG is measured in volts, the duration of impulse is recorded in seconds, and both are recorded as the heart rate (e.g., 80 V/60 seconds). EMG amplitude is recorded in millivolts and the duration is measured in milliseconds, with a frequency of about 5 to 50 action potentials per second. Motor unit potentials are measured to determine rate of firing, duration, and amplitude. Abnormalities in EMG and nerve conduction velocities help differentiate muscle diseases (myopathy) from peripheral nerve (neuropathy) and neuromuscular junction disorders. The muscle biopsy (using histologic, histochemical, and electron microscopic studies) is used to further define the presence of myopathic and neuropathic disorders, many of which can be diagnosed only by muscle biopsy. Complex myography, a relatively new technique, allows a noninvasive way to gather information on the mechanical characteristics of muscle.

A new area of evaluation is genetics. Recent advances in molecular genetics, deoxyribonucleic acid (DNA) libraries, genetic probes, and gene localization techniques have enhanced the knowledge of neuromuscular diseases, including types of muscular dystrophy, Charcot-Marie-Tooth disease, and familial amyotrophic lateral sclerosis.

GERIATRIC CONSIDERATIONS
Aging and the Musculoskeletal System

Aging of Bones

Aging is accompanied by the loss of bone tissue. Bones become less dense, less strong, and more brittle with aging. The bone remodeling cycle takes longer to complete, and the rate of mineralization also decelerates. With aging, women experience loss of bone density, accelerated by rapid bone loss during early menopause from increased osteoclastic bone resorption, fewer osteocytes, and decreased numbers of osteoblasts. By age 70 years, susceptible women have, on average, lost 50% of their peripheral cortical bone mass (see Chapter 44). Bone mass losses can lead to deformity, pain, stiffness, and high risk for fractures. Men also experience bone mass loss but at later ages and much slower rates than women. Also, initial bone mass in men is approximately 30% higher than in women; therefore, bone loss in men causes less risk of disability than that found in women. Men's peak bone mass is related to race, heredity, hormonal factors, physical activity, and calcium intake during childhood. Bone loss in both sexes is related to smoking, calcium deficiency, alcohol intake, and physical inactivity. Bone mass can be gained in healthy young women up to the third decade through participation in physical activity, intake of dietary calcium and other minerals, and use of oral contraceptives. Height is also lost with aging because of intervertebral disk degeneration and, sometimes, osteoporotic spinal fractures.

Stem cells in the bone marrow perform less efficiently with aging, predisposing older persons to acute and chronic illnesses. Such illnesses cause weakness and confusion in older persons and may increase the risk of injury or falling.

Aging of Joints

With aging, cartilage becomes more rigid, fragile, and susceptible to fraying because of increased cross-linking of collagen and elastin, decreased water content in the cartilage ground substance, and reduced concentrations of glycosaminoglycans. Decreased range of motion of the joint is related to the changes in ligaments and muscles. Bones in joints develop evidence of osteoporosis, with fewer trabeculae and thinner, less dense bones, making them prone to fractures. Intervertebral disk spaces decrease in height. The rate of loss of height accelerates at age 70 years and beyond. Tendons shrink and harden.

Aging of Muscles

The function of skeletal muscle depends on many influences that are affected by cellular factors, such as reduced mitochondrial volume associated with aging. Other influences include the nervous, vascular, and endocrine systems. In the young child, the development of muscle tissue depends greatly on continuing neurodevelopmental maturation. Muscle loss begins at about age 50; however, muscle function remains trainable even into advanced age. Maintaining musculoskeletal fitness at any age can improve overall health.

Age-related loss in skeletal muscle is referred to as **sarcopenia** and is a direct cause of the age-related decrease in muscle strength. As the body ages, muscle mass and strength decline slowly; thus, strength is maintained through the fifth decade, with a slow decline in dynamic and isometric strength evident after age 70. The amount of type II fibers also decreases. There is reduced synthesis of RNA, loss of mitochondrial function, and reduction in the size of motor units. The regenerative function of muscle tissue remains normal in aging persons. As much as 30% to 40% of skeletal muscle mass and strength may be lost from the third to ninth decades. Muscle fatigue also may contribute to loss of function with aging. Sarcopenia is thought to be secondary to progressive neuromuscular changes and diminishing levels of anabolic hormones. There is an age-related decline in the synthesis of mixed proteins, myosin heavy chains, and mitochondrial protein. Changes in these muscle proteins are related to reduced levels of insulin-like growth factor-1 (IGF-1), testosterone, and dehydroepiandrosterone (DHEA) sulfate.

Maximal oxygen intake declines with age. The basal metabolic rate is reduced, and lean body mass decreases in the aged population.

SUMMARY REVIEW

Structure and Function of Bones

1. Bones provide support and protection for the body's tissues and organs and are important sources of minerals and blood cells. Bones permit movement by providing points of attachment for muscles.
2. Mature bone is a rigid connective tissue consisting of cells (growth, repair, synthesis, and resorption of old tissue); collagen fibers (tensile strength); a homogenous gelatinous medium called *ground substance* (diffusion); and large amounts of crystallized minerals, mainly calcium (rigidity).
3. Bone formation begins with the production of an organic matrix by bone cells. Bone minerals crystallize in and around collagen fibers in the matrix, called *calcification*, giving bone its characteristic hardness and strength.
4. Bone contains three types of cells: osteoblasts, osteocytes, and osteoclasts. These allow bone tissue to be continuously synthesized, remodeled, and resorbed.
5. Osteoblasts are cells derived from osteogenic mesenchymal stem cells; they are the primary bone-producing cells and are involved in many functions related to the skeletal system. Osteoblasts initiate new bone formation by their synthesis of osteoid (nonmineralized bone matrix).
6. Osteocytes are transformed osteoblasts that are trapped or surrounded in osteoid as it hardens. They are the most numerous cells in bone. Though imbedded in the bone matrix, osteocytes have important functions in directing bone remodeling.
7. Osteoclasts are large, multinucleated cells that develop from the hematopoietic monocyte-macrophage lineage. Osteoclasts are the major resorptive cells of bone.
8. Bone matrix is made of the extracellular elements of bone tissue, specifically collagen fibers, structural proteins (e.g., proteoglycans and certain glycoproteins), carbohydrate-protein complexes, ground substance, and minerals.
9. Bones in the body are made up of compact (cortical) bone tissue and spongy (cancellous) bone tissue.
10. Compact bone is highly organized, solid, and extremely strong. The basic structural units are the haversian systems that consist of concentric layers of crystallized matrix called *lamellae*, surrounding a central canal that contains blood vessels and nerves. Dispersed throughout the concentric layers of crystallized matrix are small spaces, called *lacunae*, containing osteocytes. Smaller canals, called *canaliculi*, interconnect the osteocyte-containing spaces.

11. The crystallized matrix in spongy bone is arranged in bars or plates called *trabeculae*. Spaces containing osteocytes are dispersed between the bars or plates and interconnected by canaliculi.
12. Bone morphogenic proteins are part of the transforming growth factor-β superfamily and are involved in multiple crucial functions in the skeletal system.
13. There are 206 bones in the body, divided into the axial skeleton and the appendicular skeleton. Bones are classified by shape as long, short, flat, or irregular. Long bones have a broad end (epiphysis), broad neck (metaphysis), and narrow midportion (diaphysis) that contains the medullary cavity.
14. The internal structure of bone is maintained by remodeling, a process in which existing bone is resorbed and new bone is laid down to replace it. Clusters of bone precursor cells, called *basic multicellular units*, implement remodeling.
15. Bone injuries are repaired in stages: (1) hematoma formation occurs within hours of fracture or surgery, (2) procallus formation by osteoblasts occurs within days, (3) callus formation occurs within weeks, and (4) replacement and (5) remodeling occur within years. Remodeling restores the original shape and size to the injured bone.

Structure and Function of Joints

1. A joint, or articulation, is the site where two or more bones attach. Joints provide stability and mobility to the skeleton. Joints help move bones and muscles.
2. Joints are classified as synarthroses (immovable), amphiarthroses (slightly movable), or diarthroses (freely movable), depending on the degree of movement they allow.
3. Joints are also classified by the type of connecting tissue holding them together. Fibrous joints are connected by dense fibrous tissue, ligaments, or membranes. Cartilaginous joints are connected by fibrocartilage or hyaline cartilage. Synovial joints are connected by a fibrous joint capsule that contains a small fluid-filled space. The fluid in the space nourishes the articular cartilage that covers the ends of the bones meeting in the synovial joint.
4. Articular cartilage is a highly organized system of collagen fibers and proteoglycans. The fibers firmly anchor the cartilage to the bone, and the proteoglycans control the loss of fluid from the cartilage.

Structure and Function of Skeletal Muscles

1. *Myoblasts* are precursor cells that become muscle cells.
2. Skeletal muscle is the largest organ in the body and is made up of millions of individual fibers.
3. Whole muscles vary in size (2 to 60 cm) and shape (fusiform, pennate). They are encased in a three-part connective tissue framework, called *fascia*, that protects the muscle fibers, attaches the muscle to bone, and provides a structure for a network of nerve fibers, blood vessels, and lymphatic channels.
4. The fundamental concept of muscle function is the motor unit, defined as the muscle fibers innervated by a single motor nerve, its axon, and anterior horn cell.
5. Satellite cells are dormant myoblasts; however, when activated, they can regenerate muscle.
6. Skeletal muscle is made up of millions of individual muscle fibers, each of which is a single, cylindrical muscle cell. Muscle fibers contain bundles of myofibrils arranged in parallel along the longitudinal axis and include the muscle membrane, myofibrils, sarcotubular system, sarcoplasm, and mitochondria.
7. There are two types of muscle fibers, type I and type II, determined by motor nerve innervation.
8. Myofibrils and myofilaments contain the major muscle proteins actin and myosin, which interact to form cross-bridges during muscle contraction. The nonprotein muscle constituents provide an energy source for contraction and regulate protein synthesis and enzyme systems, as well as stabilize cell membranes.
9. Muscle contraction includes (1) excitation, (2) coupling, (3) contraction, and (4) relaxation.
10. Skeletal muscle requires a constant supply of adenosine triphosphate (ATP) and phosphocreatine to fuel muscle contraction and for growth and repair. ATP and phosphocreatine can be generated aerobically or anaerobically.
11. Motor units contract in an all-or-nothing manner, so the contraction generated will be the maximal contraction. The efficiency of muscle contraction is affected by muscle fiber type, innervation ratio, temperature, and muscle shape.
12. There are two types of muscle contraction. In isometric (static) contraction, the muscle maintains a constant length as tension is increased. In dynamic (formerly called isotonic) contraction, the muscle maintains a constant tension as it moves, either lengthening (eccentric contraction) or shortening (concentric contraction).
13. Muscles act in groups. When a muscle contracts and acts as a prime mover, or agonist, its reciprocal muscle, or antagonist, relaxes.
14. Tendons attach muscle to bone at sites called *entheses*. Ligaments attach bone to bone, helping to form joints and stabilizing them against excessive movement. Both tendons and ligaments are mostly composed of types III, IV, V, and VI collagen and fibroblasts (called tenocytes in tendons).

Tests of Musculoskeletal Function

1. Procedures used to evaluate bone function include analysis of gait, evaluation of urinary bone resorption markers, measurement of serum calcium and phosphorus levels and serum bone-specific alkaline phosphatase (BAP) level, x-ray films, angiography, bone scanning, and MRI.
2. Procedures used to evaluate joint function include arthrography, arthroscopy, MRI, and synovial fluid analysis.
3. Serum creatine kinase concentration is useful in detecting muscle damage. Electromyography is used to assess the muscle membrane's capacity to function. Genetic evaluation is useful in detecting, diagnosing, and developing specific treatment for certain inheritable muscle diseases such as muscular dystrophy.

Aging and the Musculoskeletal System

1. Bones become less dense, less strong, and more brittle with aging. The bone remodeling cycle takes longer to complete, and the rate of mineralization also decelerates.
2. With aging, cartilage becomes more rigid, fragile, and susceptible to fraying. Decreased range of motion of the joint is related to the changes in ligaments and muscles.
3. The regenerative function of muscle tissue and the trainability of muscle function remains normal in elderly persons.
4. Sarcopenia, or age-related loss of skeletal muscle, is a direct cause of decrease in muscle strength. A slow decline in dynamic and isometric strength is evident after age 70 years.
5. As much as 30% to 40% of skeletal muscle mass and strength may be lost from the third to ninth decades. Muscle fatigue also may contribute to loss of function with aging. A reduced basal metabolic rate and decreased lean body mass are also noted in the elderly population.

REFERENCES

1. Kumar V, Abbas AK, Aster JC. *Robbins & Cotran pathologic basis of disease*. ed 10, Philadelphia: Elsevier; 2020.
2. Tresguerres FGF, et al. The osteocyte: a multifunctional cell within the bone. *Ann Anat*. 2020;227:151422.
3. Wu M, Chen G, Li Yi-Ping. TGF-β and BMP signaling in osteoblast, skeletal development, and bone formation, homeostasis and disease. *Bone Res*. 2016;4:16009.
4. Hambli R. Connecting mechanics and bone remodelling process: an integrated finite element modelling. *Front Bioeng Biotechnol*. 2014;2:6.
5. Chen H, et al. The osteocyte plays multiple roles in bone remodeling and mineral homeostasis. *Med Mol Morphol*. 2015;48:61–68.
6. Camarero-Espinosa S, et al. Articular cartilage: from formation to tissue engineering. *Biomater Sci*. 2016;4:734.
7. Knight JD, Kothary R. The myogenic kinome: protein kinases critical to mammalian skeletal myogenesis. *Skelet Muscle*. 2011;1:29–46.
8. Braun T, Gautel M. Transcriptional mechanisms regulating skeletal muscle differentiation, growth and homeostasis. *Nat Rev Mol Cell Biol*. 2011;12:349–361.
9. Wong WD. Advanced musculoskeletal applications of dual-energy CT. *Radiol Clin North Am*. 2018;56(4):587–600.
10. Ito M. Recent progress in bone imaging for osteoporosis research. *J Bone Miner Metab*. 2011;29:131–140.
11. Baxter I, et al. Evaluation of urinary N-telopeptide of type I collagen measurements in the management of osteoporosis in clinical practice. *Osteoporos Int*. 2013;24(3):941–947.

44

Alterations of Musculoskeletal Function

Benjamin Allan Smallheer and Geri Cage Reeves

http://evolve.elsevier.com/Rogers/pathophysiology/

CHAPTER OUTLINE

Musculoskeletal injuries include fractures, dislocations, sprains, and strains. Metabolic disorders, infections, inflammatory or noninflammatory diseases, or tumors may cause alterations in bones, joints, and muscles. The most common disease affecting bone is osteoporosis; much attention and debate has been focused on its risk factors and pathophysiology. Soft tissue disorders—including muscle, tendon, and ligament injuries; tumors; and metabolic derangements—also affect the musculoskeletal system.

MUSCULOSKELETAL INJURIES

Trauma is referred to as the "neglected disease." It is the leading cause of death in people ages 1 to 44 years of all races and socioeconomic levels. Each year, more than 120,000 persons in the United States die from unintentional injuries.

Musculoskeletal injuries have a major impact on the affected individuals, families, and society in general because of the physical and psychological effects of limitation on mobility and daily activities, pain, and decreased quality of life. In addition, there are direct costs of diagnosis and treatments and indirect economic costs related to loss of employment and decreased productivity.

Skeletal Trauma

Fractures

A fracture is a break in the continuity of a bone. A break occurs when force is applied that exceeds the tensile or compressive strength of the bone. The incidence of fractures varies for individual bones according to age and sex with the highest incidence of fractures in young males (between the ages of 15 and 24 years) and older persons (65 years of age or older). Fractures of healthy bones, particularly the tibia, clavicle, and lower humerus, tend to occur in young persons as the result of trauma. Fractures of the hands and feet are often caused by accidents in the workplace. The incidence of fractures of the upper femur, upper humerus, vertebrae, and pelvis is highest in older adults and often is associated with osteoporosis (see the Osteoporosis section). Hip fractures, the most serious outcome of osteoporosis, have a wide variation in geographic occurrence.

Classification of fractures. There are numerous classification systems for various types of fractures, but the simplest systems describe the basic features of the broken bone. Fractures can be classified as complete or incomplete, and as open or closed (Fig. 44.1). In a complete fracture the bone is broken entirely, whereas in an incomplete fracture the bone is damaged but is still in one piece. Complete and incomplete fractures also can be called open (formerly referred to as *compound*) if the skin is open and closed (formerly referred to as *simple*) if skin remains intact. A fracture in which a bone breaks into more than two fragments is termed a comminuted fracture. Fractures are also classified according to the direction of the fracture line. A linear fracture runs parallel to the long axis of the bone. An oblique fracture occurs at a slanted angle to the shaft of the bone. (see Fig. 44.1) A spiral fracture encircles the bone, and a transverse fracture occurs straight across the bone.

Incomplete fractures tend to occur in the more flexible, growing bones of children. The three main types of incomplete fractures are greenstick, torus, and bowing fractures. A greenstick fracture perforates one cortex and splinters the spongy bone. The name is derived from the damage sustained by a young tree branch (a green stick) when it is bent sharply. The outer surface is disrupted, but the inner surface remains intact. Greenstick fractures typically occur in the metaphysis or diaphysis of the tibia, radius, and ulna. In a torus fracture, the cortex buckles but does not break. Bowing fractures usually occur when longitudinal force is applied to bone. This type of fracture is common in children and usually involves the paired radius-ulna or the fibula-tibia. A complete diaphyseal fracture occurs in one of the bones of the pair, which disperses the stress sufficiently to prevent a complete fracture of the second bone, which bows rather than breaks. A bowing fracture resists correction (reduction) because the force necessary to reduce it must be equal to the force that bowed it. Treatment of bowing fractures is also difficult because the bowed bone interferes with reduction of the fractured bone. Types of fractures are summarized in Table 44.1.

Fractures may be further classified by cause as pathologic, stress, or transchondral fractures. A pathologic (also known as insufficiency or fragility) fracture is a break at the site of a

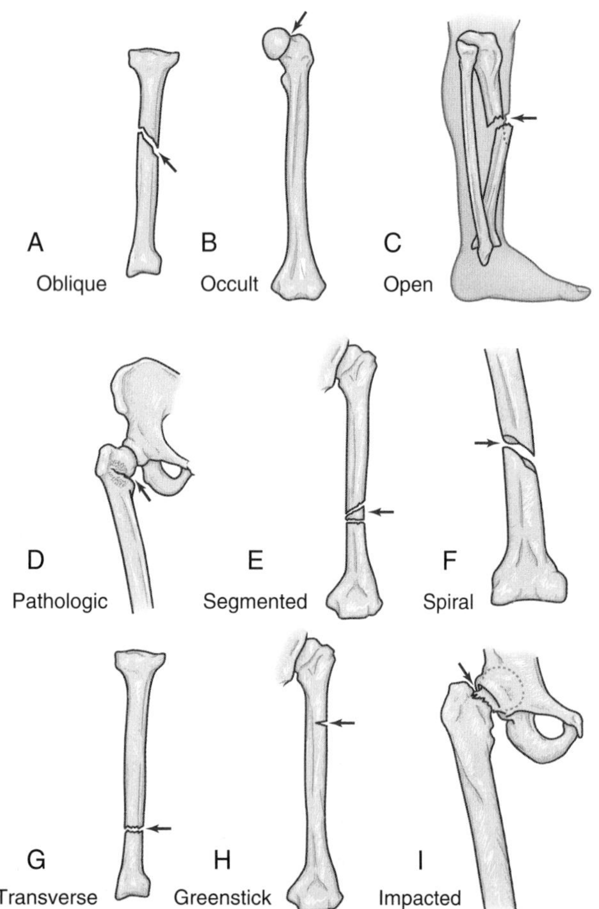

Fig. 44.1 Examples of Types of Bone Fractures. **(A)** *Oblique:* Fracture at oblique angle across both cortices. *Cause:* Direct or indirect energy, with angulation and some compression. **(B)** *Occult:* Fracture that is hidden or not readily discernible. *Cause:* Minor force or energy. **(C)** *Open:* Skin broken over fracture; possible soft tissue trauma. *Cause:* Moderate to severe energy that is continuous and exceeds tissue tolerance. **(D)** *Pathologic:* Transverse, oblique, or spiral fracture of bone weakened by tumor pressure or presence. *Cause:* Minor energy or force, which may be direct or indirect. **(E)** *Segmented:* Fracture with two or more pieces or segments. *Cause:* Direct or indirect moderate to severe force. **(F)** *Spiral:* Fracture that curves around cortices and may become displaced by twist. *Cause:* Direct or indirect twisting energy or force with distal part held or unable to move. **(G)** *Transverse:* Horizontal break through bone. *Cause:* Direct or indirect energy toward bone. **(H)** *Greenstick:* Break in only one cortex of bone. *Cause:* Minor direct or indirect energy. **(I)** *Impacted:* Fracture with one end wedged into opposite end of inside fractured fragment. *Cause:* Compressive axial energy or force directly to distal fragment. (Redrawn from Mourad L. Musculoskeletal system. In: Thompson JM, et al., eds. *Mosby's clinical nursing,* 7th edition. St. Louis: Mosby; 2002.)

TABLE 44.1 Types of Fractures

Type of Fracture	Definition
Typical Complete Fractures	
Closed	Noncommunicating wound between bone and skin
Open	Communicating wound between bone and skin
Comminuted	Multiple bone fragments
Linear	Fracture line parallel to long axis of bone
Oblique	Fracture line at an angle to long axis of bone
Spiral	Fracture line encircling bone (as a spiral staircase)
Transverse	Fracture line perpendicular to long axis of bone
Impacted	Fracture fragments pushed into each other
Pathologic	Fracture at a point where bone has been weakened by disease, for example, by tumors or osteoporosis
Avulsion	Fragment of bone connected to a ligament or tendon detaches from main bone
Compression	Fracture wedged or squeezed together on one side of bone
Displaced	Fracture with one, both, or all fragments out of normal alignment
Extracapsular	Fragment close to joint but remains outside joint capsule
Intracapsular	Fragment within joint capsule
Typical Incomplete Fractures	
Greenstick	Break in one cortex of bone with splintering of inner bone surface; commonly occurs in children and elderly persons
Torus	Buckling of cortex
Bowing	Bending of bone
Stress	Microfracture
Transchondral	Separation of cartilaginous joint surface (articular cartilage) from main shaft of bone

preexisting abnormality, resulting from force that would not fracture a normal bone. In any bone that lacks normal ability to deform and recover, these fractures can occur with normal weight bearing or activity. Rheumatoid arthritis (RA), osteoporosis, Paget disease, osteomalacia, rickets, hyperparathyroidism, and radiation therapy all cause bone to lose its normal ability to deform and recover. Pathologic fractures are generally a result of bone weakness caused by another disease, such as cancer, metabolic bone disorders, or infection. Although usually considered insufficiency fractures, breaks in the bone attributable to osteoporosis can also be referred to as pathologic fractures. Any disease process that weakens a bone (especially the cortex) predisposes the bone to pathologic fracture.

During activities that subject a bone to repeated strain, such as certain types of sports, a stress fracture can occur in normal or abnormal bone. The forces placed on the bone are cumulative, eventually causing a fracture. A fatigue fracture is caused by repetitive, sometimes abnormal stress or torque applied to a bone with a normal ability to deform and recover. Fatigue fractures usually occur in individuals who engage in a new or different activity that is both strenuous and repetitive (e.g., joggers, skaters, dancers, and military recruits). Because gains in muscle strength occur more rapidly than gains in bone strength, the newly developed muscles place exaggerated stress on the bones that are not yet ready for the additional stress. The imbalance between muscle and bone development causes micro-fractures to develop in the cortex. If the activity is controlled and increased gradually, new bone formation catches up to the increased demands and micro-fractures do not occur.

A transchondral fracture consists of fragmentation and separation of a portion of the articular cartilage. (Joint structures are defined in Chapter 43.) Single or multiple sites may be fractured, and the fragments may consist of cartilage alone or cartilage and bone. Typical sites of transchondral fracture are the distal femur, the ankle, the patella, the elbow, and the wrist. Transchondral fractures are most prevalent in adolescents.

Pathophysiology. Fracture healing is a complex process that occurs primarily in one of two ways: direct or indirect healing. Both types of healing require integration of cells, signaling pathways, and various molecules. In direct (or primary) healing, intramembranous bone formation occurs when adjacent bone cortices are in contact with one another, such as when surgical fixation devices are used. No callus formation occurs with direct bone healing. Indirect (or secondary) healing involves both intramembranous and endochondral bone formation, development of callus, and eventual remodeling of solid bone. Bone formation that begins with an underlying cartilage scaffold is termed endochondral bone formation.

A hallmark of indirect fracture healing is the formation of callus. Indirect fracture healing is most often observed when a fracture is treated with a cast. When a bone is broken, the periosteum and blood vessels in the cortex, marrow, and surrounding soft tissues are disrupted. Bleeding occurs from the damaged ends of the bone and from the neighboring soft tissue. A clot (hematoma) forms within the medullary canal, between the fractured ends of the bone, and beneath the periosteum (Fig. 44.2). Bone tissue immediately adjacent to the fracture dies. This dead tissue (along with any debris in the fracture area) stimulates vasodilation, exudation of plasma and leukocytes, and infiltration by inflammatory leukocytes, growth factors, and mast cells that simultaneously decalcify the fractured bone ends. Within 48 hours after injury, vascular tissue from surrounding soft tissue and the marrow cavity invades the fracture area, and blood flow to the entire bone increases. Bone-forming cells in the periosteum, endosteum, and marrow are activated to produce subperiosteal procallus along the outer surface of the shaft and over the broken ends of the bone (Fig. 44.3). Osteoblasts within the procallus synthesize collagen and matrix, which becomes mineralized to form callus. As the repair process continues, remodeling occurs, during which unnecessary callus is resorbed and trabeculae are formed along lines of stress as the repair tissues align with the tissue cells of the host (Fig. 44.4).

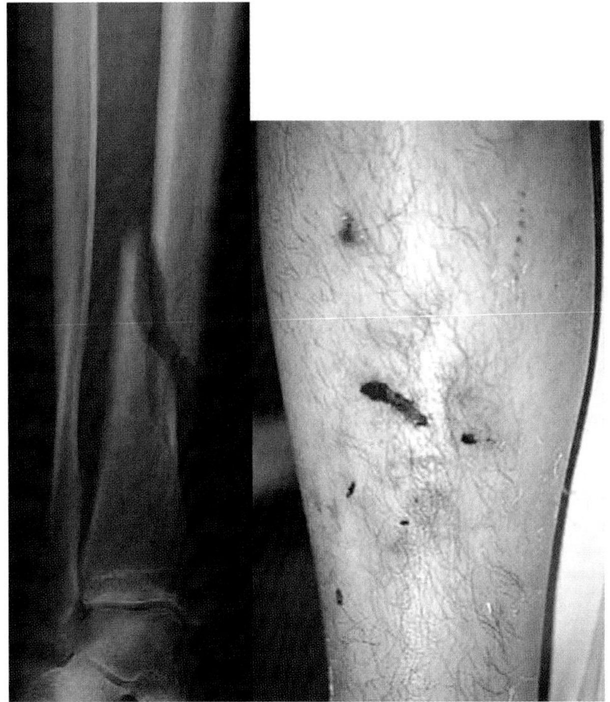

Fig. 44.2 **A fracture causes bleeding from the damaged ends of the bone and from the neighboring soft tissue.** (From Nyary T, Scammell BE. Principles of bone and joint injuries and their healing. *Surgery (Oxford)*, 2018;36(1):7–14.)

Clinical Manifestations. The signs and symptoms of a fracture include unnatural alignment (deformity), swelling, muscle spasm, tenderness, pain and impaired sensation, and decreased mobility. The position of the broken bone segments is determined by the pull of attached muscles, gravity, and the direction and magnitude of the force that caused the fracture.

Immediately after a bone is fractured, there often is numbness at the fracture site because of trauma to the nerve or nerves at the injury site. The numbness may last several minutes, during which time the injured person can continue to use the fractured bone. However, once the numbness dissipates, the subsequent pain is quite severe and may be incapacitating until relieved with medication and treatment of the fracture. Pain can be caused by muscle spasms at the fracture site, overriding of the fracture segments, or damage to adjacent soft tissues.

Pathologic fractures can cause angular deformity, painless swelling, or generalized bone pain. Stress fractures are painful because of accelerated remodeling; initially, pain occurs during activity and is usually relieved by rest. Stress fractures also cause local tenderness and soft tissue swelling. Transchondral fractures may be entirely asymptomatic or may be painful during movement. Range of motion (ROM) in the joint is limited, and movement may evoke audible clicking or crunching sounds (crepitus).

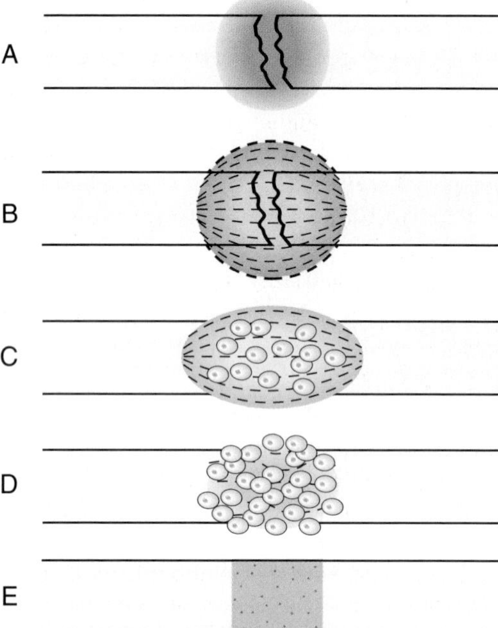

Fig. 44.3 Schematic of Bone Healing. (A) Bleeding at broken ends of the bone with subsequent hematoma formation. **(B)** Organization of hematoma into fibrous network. **(C)** Invasion of osteoblasts, lengthening of collagen strands, and deposition of calcium. **(D)** Callus formation; new bone is built while osteoclasts destroy dead bone. **(E)** Remodeling is accomplished while excess callus is reabsorbed and trabecular bone is deposited. (From Monahan FD, et al. *Phipps' medical-surgical nursing: Health and illness perspectives,* 8th edition. St. Louis: Mosby; 2007.)

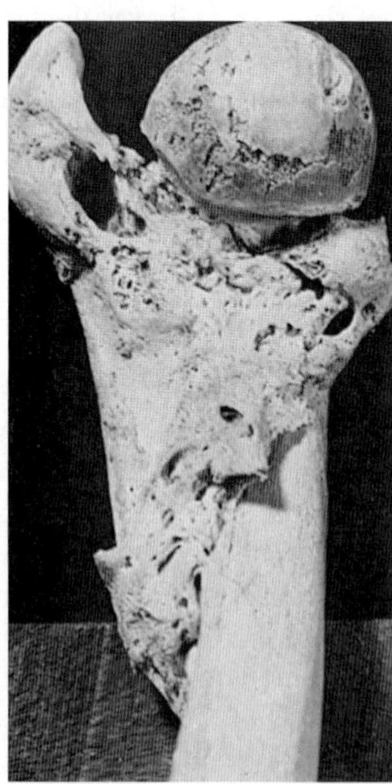

Fig. 44.4 Exuberant Callus Formation After Fracture. (From Rosai J. *Ackerman's surgical pathology*, 8th edition. St. Louis: Mosby; 1996.)

Evaluation and Treatment. Adequate immobilization with a splint or cast is often all that is required for healing of fractures that are *not* misaligned. Treatment of a displaced fracture involves realigning the bone fragments (reduction) close to their normal or anatomic position and holding the fragments in place (immobilization) so that bone union can occur. Several methods are available to reduce a fracture: closed manipulation, traction, and open reduction. Many displaced fractures can be reduced by closed manipulation and reduction. The bone is moved or manipulated into place without opening the skin. Closed reduction is used when the contour of the bone is in fair anatomic alignment and can be manually placed into normal alignment, and then maintained with immobilization. Splints and casts are used to immobilize and hold a closed reduction in place.

Traction may be used to accomplish or maintain reduction. When bone fragments are displaced (not in their anatomic position) weights may be used to apply firm, steady traction (pull) and countertraction to the long axis of the bone. Traction stretches and fatigues muscles that have pulled the bone fragments out of place, more readily allowing the distal fragment to align with the proximal fragment. Traction can be applied to the skin (skin traction) or directly to the involved bone (skeletal traction). Skin traction is used when only a few pounds of pulling force are needed to realign the fragments or when the traction will be used only for a brief time, such as before surgery, or for children with femoral fractures, for 3 to 7 days before a cast is applied. In skeletal traction, a pin or wire is drilled through the bone distal to the fracture site, and a traction bow, rope, and weights are attached to the pin or wire to apply tension and to provide the pulling force required to overcome the muscle spasm and help realign the fracture fragments (Fig. 44.5). More often, surgical repair (open reduction and internal fixation) or external fixation devices are used to realign displaced fractures.

Open reduction is a surgical procedure that exposes the fracture site; the fragments are then manipulated into alignment under direct visualization. Some form of hardware, such as a screw, plate, nail, or wire, is used to maintain the reduction (internal fixation). External fixation, a procedure in which pins or rods are surgically

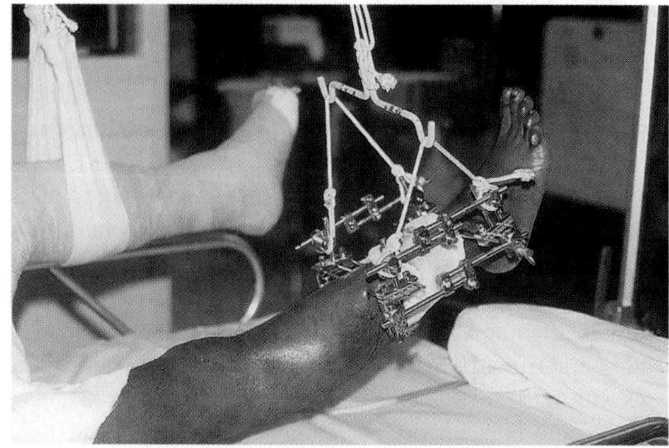

Fig. 44.5 External Fixation Device on Right Leg.

placed into uninjured bone near the fracture site and then stabilized with an external frame of bars, is another method used to treat fractures that would not be adequately stabilized with a cast (see Fig. 44.5). Bone grafts—using donor bone from the individual (autograft), a cadaver (allograft), or bone substitutes (ceramic composites, bioactive cement)—can fill voids in the bone.

Improper reduction or immobilization of a fractured bone may result in nonunion, delayed union, or malunion. Nonunion is failure of the bone ends to grow together. The gap between the broken ends of the bone fills with dense fibrous and fibrocartilaginous tissue instead of new bone. Occasionally, the fibrous tissue contains a fluid-filled space that resembles a joint and is termed a *false joint*, or *pseudoarthrosis*. Delayed union is union that does not occur until approximately 8 to 9 months after a fracture. Malunion is the healing of a bone in an incorrect anatomic position.

Dislocation and Subluxation

Dislocation and subluxation are usually caused by trauma. Dislocation is the displacement of one or more bones in a joint in which the opposing joint surfaces entirely lose contact with one another. If contact between the opposing joint surfaces is only partially lost (partial dislocation), the injury is called a subluxation.

Dislocation and subluxation are most common in persons younger than 20 years of age and are generally associated with fractures. However, they also may be the result of congenital or acquired disorders that cause (1) muscular imbalance, seen with congenital dislocation of the hip; (2) incongruities in the articulating surfaces of the bones, as occur with RA (see the Rheumatoid Arthritis section); or (3) joint instability.

The joints most often dislocated or subluxated are the joints of the shoulder, elbow, wrist, finger, hip, and knee (Fig. 44.6). The shoulder joint most often injured is the glenohumeral joint.

In the immature skeleton, a traumatic partial dislocation of the elbow joint is common ("nursemaid's elbow"). This injury is the result of the subluxation of the radial head from under the ligament holding it in place within the elbow joint. This injury is often the result of a pulling force on the hand or forearm. In adults, however, an elbow dislocation is usually associated with a fracture of the ulna or head of the radius. Traumatic dislocation of the wrist usually involves the distal ulna and carpal bones. Any one of the eight carpal bones can be dislocated after an injury. The most common cause is a fall on the hyperextended hand. Dislocation in the hand usually involves the metacarpophalangeal (MCP) and interphalangeal joints. This injury is also associated with a fall on the outstretched hand, which forces the joint into hyperextension. Dislocation of the interphalangeal joints of the fingers is a common injury in contact sports and caused by a hyperextension of the joint.

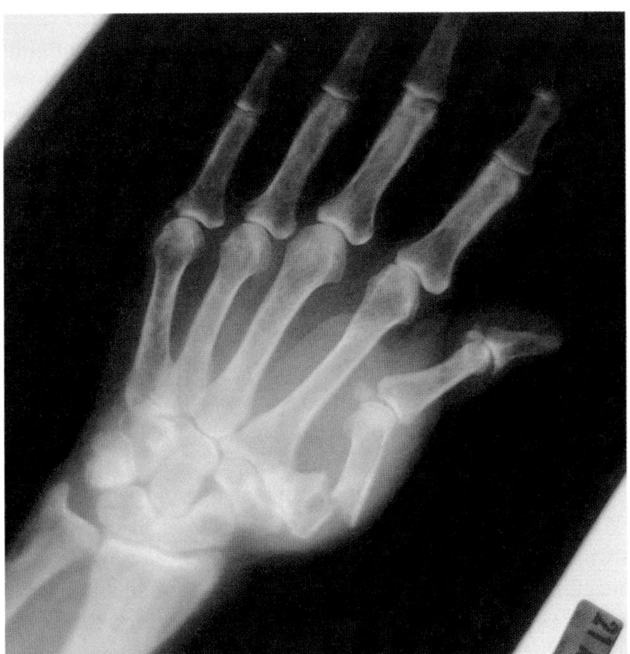

Fig. 44.6 Displaced Fracture.

Considerable trauma is needed to dislocate the hip. Anterior hip dislocation is rare in healthy individuals. It is caused by forced abduction, for example, when an individual lands on their feet from a high-altitude fall. Posterior dislocation of the hip can occur as a result of an automobile accident in which the flexed knee strikes the dashboard, causing the head of the femur to be pushed posteriorly from the hip joint.

The knee is an unstable weight-bearing joint that depends heavily on the soft tissue structures around it for support. Because of the many different types of motion (flexion, extension, rotation) the knee is capable of, it is one of the most commonly injured joints. A knee dislocation can be anterior, posterior, lateral, medial, or rotary. It is often the result of a hyperextension injury that occurs during sports activities.

Pathophysiology. Dislocations and subluxations are often accompanied by fracture because stress is placed on areas of bone not typically subjected to stress. In addition, as the bone separates from the joint, it may bruise or tear adjacent nerves, blood vessels, ligaments, supporting structures, and soft tissue. Dislocations of the shoulder may damage the shoulder capsule and the axillary nerve. Damage to axillary nerves can cause anesthesia or dysesthesia in the sensory distribution of the nerve and paralysis of the deltoid muscle. Dislocations also may disrupt circulation leading to ischemia and possible permanent disability of the affected extremity. In the hip, this can develop into avascular necrosis of the femoral head.

Clinical Manifestations. Signs and symptoms of dislocations or subluxations include pain, swelling, limitation of motion, and joint deformity. Pain may be caused by effusion of inflammatory exudate into the joint or associated tendon and ligament injury. Joint deformity is typically caused by fluid in the joint, or muscle contractions that exert pull on the dislocated or subluxated joint. Limitation of motion may also result from effusion into the joint or the displacement of bones.

Tenderness and deformity are prominent in dislocations of the fingers. Unusual muscle pull and pain often result in abnormal flexion of the fingers. A dislocated elbow is often held in a flexed position, and the joint resists active or passive movement. In most shoulder dislocations, pain is the primary symptom. Attempts to lift the arm aggravate the pain, and the ability to elevate the arm is minimal requiring the individual to support the injured arm. Pain, an abnormal gait, or an inability to bear full weight usually accompanies traumatic dislocation of the hip. The pain is constant, severe, and is felt in the thigh or inguinal region. The affected extremity may appear to be inwardly rotated, adducted, or flexed and appear shortened. In a rare anterior dislocation, the limb is not shortened, and the joint is fixed in abduction, outward rotation, and flexion.

Evaluation and Treatment. Evaluation of dislocations and subluxations is based on clinical manifestations and radiographic evaluation. Treatment consists of reduction and immobilization for 2 to 6 weeks to allow healing of damaged structures. Following the period of immobilization, exercise is necessary to restore normal ROM in the joint. Depending on the joint and severity of injury, complete healing can take months to years.

Support Structure Trauma

Sprains and Strains of Tendons and Ligaments

Tendons and ligaments support the bones and joints and can either facilitate or limit motion. Tendon and ligament injuries often accompany fractures and dislocations and can include being torn, lacerated, ruptured, or completely separated from its point of attachment to the bone. A tendon is fibrous connective tissue that attaches skeletal muscle to either bone or another structure. A ligament is a band of fibrous connective tissue that connects bones where they meet in a joint. The structural composition of tendons and ligaments are similar with their primary difference being their anatomic function and location.

Tearing or stretching of a muscle or tendon is known as a strain. Major trauma can tear or rupture a tendon at any site in the body. The most commonly injured tendons are those of the hands and feet, the knee (patellar), the upper arm (biceps and triceps), the thigh (quadriceps), the ankle, and the heel (Achilles). Traumatic rupture of tendons can be caused by excessive weight or extreme flexion. Spontaneous ruptures can occur in individuals with RA or systemic lupus erythematosus (SLE), or in individuals receiving local corticosteroid injections or taking fluoroquinolones.[1,2]

Ligament tears are known as sprains. Ligament tears and ruptures can occur at any joint but are most common in the wrist, ankle, elbow, and knee joints. A complete separation of a tendon or ligament from its bony attachment site is known as an avulsion. An avulsion is the result of abnormal stress on the ligament and is commonly seen in young athletes.

Strains and sprains are classified as first degree (mild), second degree (moderate), and third degree (severe). In first-degree injuries, the fibers are stretched but the muscle (strain) or joint (sprain) remains stable. In second-degree strains or sprains, there is more tearing of the tendon or ligament fibers, resulting in muscle weakness or some joint instability and incomplete tearing of fibers. Third-degree strains and sprains result in a full tearing of fibers, creating an inability to contract the muscle normally (strain) or cause significant joint instability (sprain).

Pathophysiology. When a tendon or ligament is torn, an inflammatory exudate develops between the torn ends. Within 3 to 4 days after the injury, collagen formation begins. As the collagen fibers interweave and connect with preexisting tendon fibers, they organize parallel to the lines of the musculotendinous unit. Eventually vascular fibrous tissue fuses the new and surrounding tissues into a single mass. Collagen fibers reconnect the tendon and bone, forming a new enthesis, or point of connection. If strong muscle contractions occur during healing, the tendon or ligament ends may separate again, which causes the tendon or ligament to heal in a lengthened shape or with an excessive amount of scar tissue, resulting in poor tendon or ligament function.[3]

Clinical Manifestations. Tendon and ligament injuries are painful and cause functional limitations. These injuries are usually accompanied by soft tissue swelling, changes in tendon or ligament contour, and dislocation or subluxation of bones. Joint swelling can typically be observed in finger and elbow sprains. Flexion deformities of a joint may be seen with extensor tendon injuries. Crepitus may also accompany tendon injuries. Pain is often the key symptom of injuries with pain radiating distal from the joint and aggravated by attempts to actively move the joint. Movement or weight bearing increases pain. Pain is generally sharp, and tenderness persists over the distribution of the tendon or ligament. Even with prompt treatment, significant injuries may result in decreased mobility, instability, and weakness of the affected joints.

Evaluation and Treatment. Evaluation is based on the mechanism of injury and the clinical manifestations. Stress radiography, x-ray, magnetic resonance imaging (MRI), arthroscopy, or arthrography may be considered. Initial treatment consists of *p*rotection, *r*est, *i*ce, *c*ompression, and *e*levation (PRICE) for the first 48 to 72 hours. Once swelling and acute pain subside, support of the affected tendon or ligament with a compression dressing or brace is often indicated to provide appropriate reinforcement while the tissues heal. Rehabilitation and early mobilization are crucial for a favorable functional outcome. In some cases of severe (third-degree) injuries, treatment may include surgical intervention to suture the tendon or ligament ends in close approximation with one another or the enthesis.

Tendinopathy, Epicondylopathy, and Bursitis

Trauma and overuse injuries can cause painful inflammation of tendons (tendonitis), or inflammation in bursal sacs (bursitis). The term *tendinopathy* includes tendinitis, tendinosis, and paratendinitis. Microvascular and increased nerve growth often occur to these areas which increases the body's transmission of pain sensations.

A bony prominence at the end of a bone where tendons or ligaments attach is termed an epicondyle. Therefore, epicondylitis is inflammation of a tendon where it attaches to a bone at its origin (epicondyle). The histopathology of common conditions, such as lateral epicondylopathy ("tennis elbow") or medial epicondylopathy ("golfer's elbow"), is a process caused by tissue degeneration rather than inflammation and is called tendinosis (Fig. 44.7).[4]

When force is sufficient to cause microscopic tears (microtears) in tissue, the result is known as tendinopathy or epicondylopathy. Microtears in the tendon, the presence of disorganized collagen fibers, and neovascularization indicate incomplete tissue repair. Initial inflammatory changes cause thickening of the tendon sheath, limited movements, and pain. Microtears cause bleeding, edema, and pain in the involved tendon or tendons.

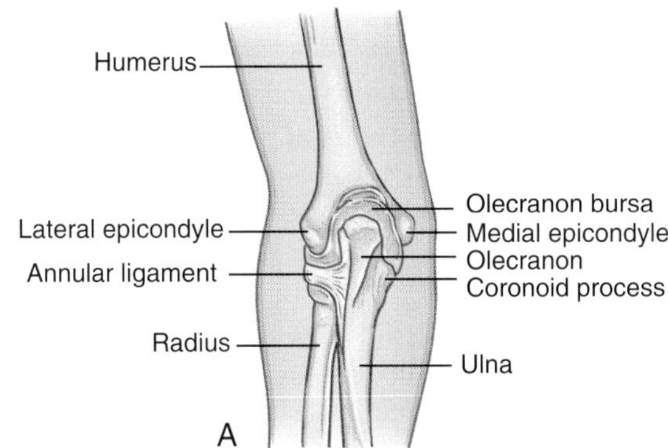

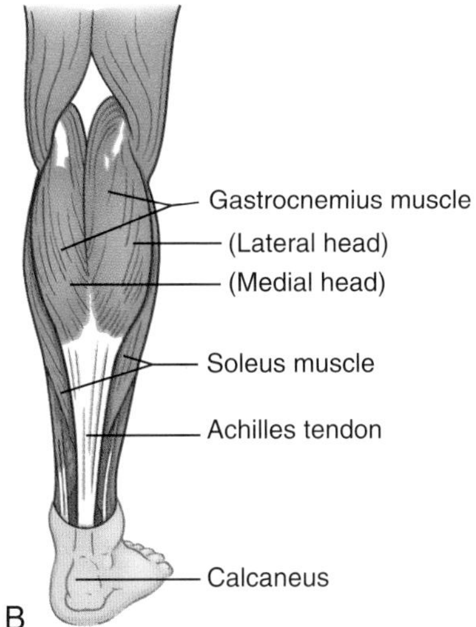

Fig. 44.7 Epicondylopathy and Tendinopathy. (A) Lateral and medial epicondyles of the distal humerus, sites of tennis elbow (lateral) and golfer's elbow (medial). **(B)** Achilles tendon, common site of tendinopathy.

Lateral epicondylopathy (tennis elbow) is caused by irritation and overstretching of the extensor carpi radialis brevis (ECRB) tendon and forearm extensor muscles, resulting in tissue degradation, loss of grip strength, and pain. Medial epicondylopathy (golfer's elbow) is the result of similar forces affecting the forearm muscles responsible for forearm flexion and pronation (see Fig. 44.7). Repetitive load-bearing activities or acute injuries that involve flexion, extension, pronation, or supination of the elbow and forearm can lead to either lateral or medial elbow symptoms.

Clinical manifestations of epicondylopathy are typically localized to one side of the joint. Localized pain and tenderness are more evident with active motion than with passive motion. With tendinopathy or tendonitis, the pain is localized over the involved tendon. Stressing the tendon with simple activities, such as lifting lightweight objects, can increase pain and weakness, limiting joint movement.

Bursae are small sacs lined with synovial membrane and filled with synovial fluid that are located between bony prominences, tendons, muscles, and ligaments (Fig. 44.8). Their primary function is to separate, lubricate, and cushion these structures. Bursae can be either "constant" (those formed

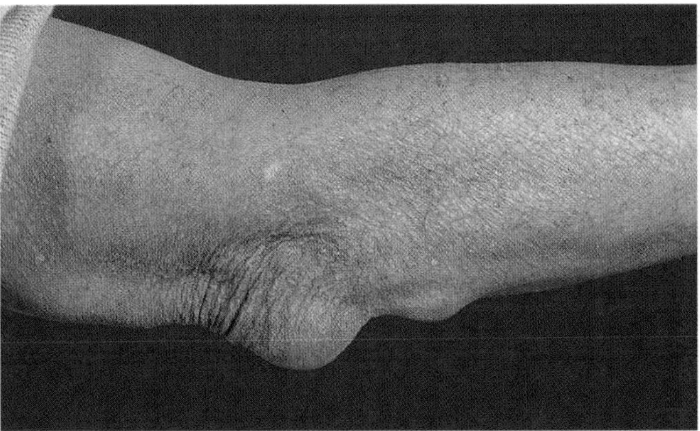

Fig. 44.8 Olecranon Bursitis. Note swelling at the point of the elbow (olecranon). A smaller, rheumatoid nodule also is present. (From Hochberg MC, et al. *Rheumatology,* 6th edition. Philadelphia: Elsevier; 2015.)

during embryologic development) or "adventitious" (bursae that develop as a result of chronic friction and degeneration of fibrous tissue between adjacent structures). When irritated or injured, these sacs become inflamed and swell. Because most bursae lie outside joints, joint movement is rarely compromised with bursitis. Acute bursitis occurs primarily during middle age years of life and is often caused by trauma. Chronic bursitis, however, can result from repeated trauma or repetitive irritation. Septic bursitis is caused by wound infection or bacterial infection of the skin overlying the bursae. Bursitis commonly occurs in the shoulder, hip, knee, and elbow but can also affect the spine, wrist, foot, and ankle.

Pathophysiology. In tendinitis, inflammatory fluid accumulates, causing swelling of the tendon and its enclosing sheath. Inflammatory changes cause thickening of the sheath, which limits movements and causes pain. Microtears cause bleeding, edema, and pain in the involved tendons or surrounding structures. At times, after repeated inflammations, calcium may be deposited in the tendon origin area, causing a calcific tendinitis.

Typical bursitis is due to inflammation that is reactive to overuse or excessive pressure. Bursitis can also be caused by infection, autoimmune diseases, crystal deposition, or acute trauma. The inflamed bursal sac becomes engorged, and the inflammation can spread to adjacent tissues (see Fig. 44.8). The inflammation may decrease with rest, ice, and aspiration of the fluid. (Inflammation is discussed in Chapter 7.)

Clinical Manifestations. Tendinopathy may be asymptomatic. Generally, however, there is localized pain that worsens with active motion, more than passive motion. With symptomatic tendinopathy, the pain is localized over the involved tendon and movement of the affected joint is limited. In bursitis, onset of pain may be gradual or sudden, but movement of the joint itself is normal. Shoulder bursitis impairs arm abduction due to pain and swelling of the bursa. Bursitis in the knee produces pain when climbing stairs, while crossing the legs is painful in bursitis of the hip. Furthermore, lying on the side of the inflamed trochanteric bursa is also very painful. Signs of infectious bursitis may include the presence of pain, warmth and erythema, severe inflammation, or an adjacent source of infection, such as

TABLE 44.2 Common Sites and Causes of Bursitis

Site	Common Causes
Shoulder (subacromial)	Repetitive overhead activities
Elbow (olecranon)	Rheumatoid arthritis (RA), gout, tuberculosis, leaning on elbow
Hip (greater trochanter)	Acute trauma, chronic stress
Ischial (weaver's bottom)	Overuse (runner, ballet dancers), lumbosacral disease, RA, osteoarthritis (OA)
Knee	
Prepatellar (housemaid knee)	Trauma, frequent kneeling, infection
Pes anserine (medial knee)	Obesity, long-distance runner, OA, type 2 diabetes
Heel (calcaneal)	Poorly fitting footwear, Achilles tendinitis

TABLE 44.3 Muscle Strain

Type	Manifestations	Treatment
First degree (example: bench press in untrained athlete)	Muscle overstretched, pain but no muscle deformity	Ice should be applied 5 or 6 times in first 24–48 hours; complete rest for up to 2 weeks, followed by gradual resumption of full weight bearing 3 times per week and range of motion daily Exercises individualized to specific injury
Second degree (example: any muscle strain with bruising and pain)	Muscle intact with some tearing of fibers, pain, swelling, mild bruising; fascia is intact	Treatment similar to that for first-degree strains, with added mild analgesia; cryokinetics (a treatment system of alternating applications of cold with progressive exercise)
Third degree (example: traumatic injury)	Caused by tearing of fascia, muscle rupture palpable, bleeding present, marked weakness, deformity	Surgery to approximate ruptured edges; immobilization and non–weight bearing status for 6 weeks, followed by an individualized rehabilitation regimen of strengthening exercises

from total joint replacement surgery. Prior corticosteroid injections or evidence of a puncture site at the joint increases the potential for infectious bursitis. Table 44.2 summarizes common sites of bursitis.

Evaluation and Treatment. Diagnosis of tendinopathy, epicondylopathy, and bursitis is primarily based on the clinical history and physical examination. Other advanced imaging, such as arthroscopy, arthrography, ultrasound, or MRI, may be used to evaluate the severity of the condition. Treatment may include temporary immobilization of the joint with a sling, splint, or cast; administration of systemic analgesics; application of ice or heat; or local injection of an anesthetic and/or a corticosteroid to reduce inflammation. Bursitis may require aspiration to drain excess fluid. Physical therapy to prevent loss of function begins after acute inflammation subsides.

Muscle Strains

Muscle strain is a general term for local muscle damage. Mild muscle strain is usually seen after traumatic or sports injuries. It is often the result of sudden, forced motion causing the muscle to become stretched beyond normal capacity. Strains often involve the tendon as well. Muscle strain may be chronic when the muscle is repeatedly stretched beyond its usual capacity. Hemorrhage into the surrounding tissue and signs of inflammation also may occur. Penetrating injuries, such as knife and gunshot wounds, can cause traumatic rupture. The incidence of muscle rupture is greater in young people. However, tendon rupture occurs with greater frequency in the older population. Regardless of the cause of trauma, muscle cells usually can regenerate. Regeneration may take up to 6 weeks, and the affected muscle should be protected during this time. Types of muscle strain, together with their manifestations and treatment, are summarized in Table 44.3.

Muscle healing occurs in three phases:

1. Destruction: the myofibers of the damaged muscle contract and necrose, beginning an inflammatory reaction; the gap between torn fibers is filled by a hematoma.
2. Repair: monocytes phagocytize the dead tissue which activate satellite cells, becoming myoblasts; myoblasts infiltrate the scar tissue; and new capillary formation begins at the site of injury.
3. Remodeling: myofibers mature, forming contractile tissue, and attach to the ends of scar tissue; regeneration may take up to 6 weeks, and the affected muscle should be protected during that time.

A late complication of localized muscle injury is abnormal bone formation in soft tissue, often called myositis ossificans or heterotopic ossification (HO). Although its exact pathophysiology remains unknown, evidence suggests the fundamental cause is the inability of mesenchymal cells to differentiate into osteoblastic stem cells, resulting in an inappropriate differentiation of fibroblasts into bone-forming cells. Though uncommon, HO may also be associated with burns, joint surgery, and trauma to the musculoskeletal system or central nervous system (CNS). HO may involve the muscle or tendons, ligaments, or bones near the muscle causing stiffness or deformity of an extremity. Radiographic evidence of HO may be seen as soft tissue calcification on plain radiographs.

Rhabdomyolysis

Once used interchangeably with the term *myoglobinuria*, rhabdomyolysis is the rapid breakdown of muscle that causes the release of intracellular contents, including the protein pigment myoglobin, into the extracellular space and bloodstream. Physical interruptions in the sarcolemma membrane, called *delta lesions*, are the route by which muscle constituents are released. (The sarcolemma membrane, the plasma membrane of the muscle cell, is described in Chapter 43.) Myoglobinuria refers to the presence of the muscle protein myoglobin in the urine.

Pathophysiology. The term rhabdomyolysis may be incorrectly used interchangeably with *crush injury* (a description of injuries resulting from the crushing of a body part), *compartment syndrome* (the consequences of increased intracompartmental pressures (ICPs) of a muscle), or *crush syndrome* (the systemic pathophysiologic events caused by rhabdomyolysis, primarily involving the kidneys and coagulation syndrome).[5] Rhabdomyolysis has many causes and can result in serious complications, including hyperkalemia (due to the release of intracellular potassium into the circulation), metabolic acidosis (from liberation of intracellular phosphorus and sulfate), acute renal failure (myoglobin precipitation in the renal tubules, obstructing flow through the nephron), and even disseminated intravascular coagulation (DIC) (likely caused by activation of the clotting cascade by sarcolemma damage and the release of intracellular components from the damaged muscles).

Clinical Manifestations. A *classic triad* of muscle pain, weakness, and dark urine is considered typical of rhabdomyolysis. Abnormally dark urine caused by myoglobinuria may be the first and only symptom; however, the presence of myoglobin in urine alone is not a reliable test to diagnose rhabdomyolysis. The renal threshold for myoglobin is low (approximately 0.5 mg/dL of urine); therefore, only 200 g of muscle need to be damaged to cause visible changes in the urine. Myoglobin is rapidly cleared, and levels may return to normal within 24 hours of injury. Along with the release of myoglobin, creatine kinase (CK) and other serum enzymes are released in massive quantities. The efflux of intracellular proteins and enzymes also includes loss of potassium, phosphate, nucleotides, creatinine, and creatine. Serum hypocalcemia is seen early during myoglobinuria and is followed by late hypercalcemia. The risk of renal failure increases proportionately to the increase in the levels of serum CK, potassium, and phosphorus.

Evaluation and Treatment. The most important and clinically useful measurement in rhabdomyolysis is the serum CK level.[6] With normal CK serum levels of 5 to 25 international units/L for women and 5 to 35 international units/L for men, a level of 1000 international units/L is used to identify rhabdomyolysis. Once CK levels exceed 15 to 20,000 international units/L, acute kidney injury is likely. Other laboratory tests may include the evaluation for hyperkalemia, which can cause life-threatening cardiac arrhythmias, and a blood urea nitrogen (BUN) to creatinine ratio, which can be decreased from a release of creatine from damaged muscle being converted to creatinine. Additional laboratory tests—such as measurement of the hemoglobin, hematocrit, and platelet levels and determination of the activated partial thromboplastin time—may be indicated in the presence of other trauma or suspected bleeding.

Maintaining adequate urinary flow and prevention of kidney failure are goals of treatment. Rapid intravenous hydration maintains adequate kidney perfusion. Other complications, such as hyperkalemia, may require temporary hemodialysis. Treatments such as using mannitol to cause an osmotic diuresis or bicarbonate to alkalinize the urine have not been shown to consistently improve outcomes.

Compartment Syndrome

Compartment syndrome is the result of increased pressure within a closed osteofascial compartment resulting in impaired circulation, decreased arterial inflow, ischemia, and edema.[7] These skeletal muscle compartments are surrounded by several layers of fibrous fascia which are not able to expand (Fig. 44.9). Common causes of compartment syndrome include conditions that increase the contents of the compartment (such as bleeding or interstitial edema after an injury), a decrease in the compartment's volume (e.g., a tight bandage or cast), or a combination of these two conditions that results in a disturbance of the muscle's microvasculature.[8] After fractures, the most common cause of compartment syndrome is soft tissue injuries. Other causes include burns, vascular injuries, crush injuries, drug overdoses, reperfusion injuries, thrombosis, bleeding disorders, infections, improperly placed casts or splints, tight circumferential bandages, penetrating trauma, intense athletic activity, and poor positioning during surgery.[7] Greater risk is found in hemophilia cases and in those with pediatric leukemia (without acute trauma).[8,9]

Pathophysiology. Any condition that disrupts the vascular supply to an extremity can cause increased pressure within the muscle compartments. This may also include prolonged pressure on a muscle compartment, such as external compression. The weight of a limb extremity can generate enough pressure to produce muscle ischemia. The increased pressure within these compartments leads to diminished capillary blood flow, edema, rising compartment pressure, and tamponade, resulting in local tissue hypoxia and necrosis (Fig. 44.10). Normal pressure within a compartment is less than 10 mmHg; acute compartment syndrome occurs when pressures reach 30 mmHg or greater. A normal intracompartmental pressure (ICP) reading, however, does not exclude acute compartment syndrome, thus ICP should be monitored serially or continuously.[10–12]

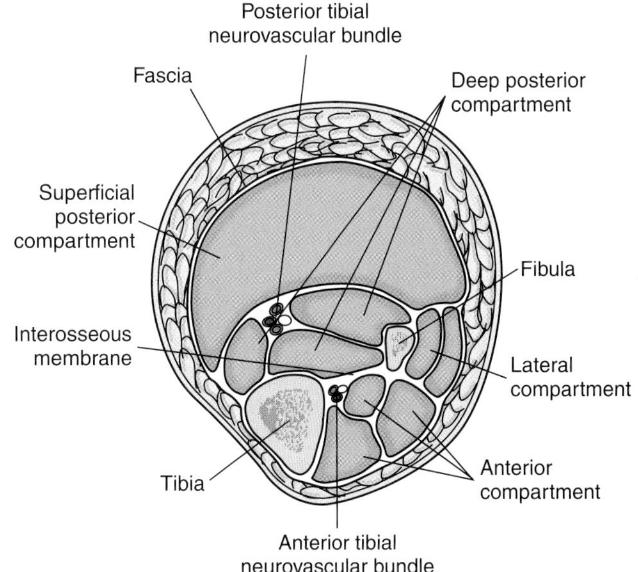

Fig. 44.9 Muscle Compartments of the Lower Leg. (From Mohahan FD, et al. *Phipps' medical-surgical nursing: Health and illness perspectives,* 8th edition. St. Louis: Mosby; 2007.)

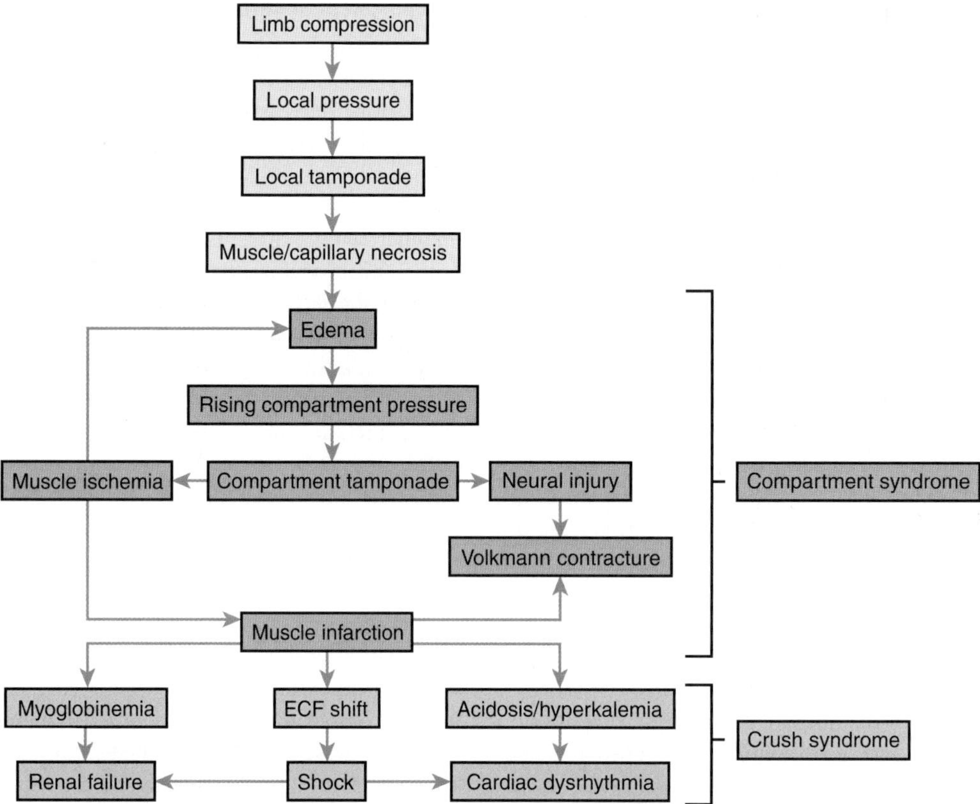

Fig. 44.10 Pathogenesis of Compartment Syndrome and Crush Syndrome Caused by Prolonged Muscle Compression. *ECF,* Extracellular fluid.

Clinical Manifestations. The compartments often affected are the anterior compartments of the leg.[7] Other common locations include the forearm, thigh, buttock, shoulder, hand, and foot.[7] It is uncommon in the abdomen.[7] Diagnosis is initiated by clinical examination with the earliest objective finding being pressure or tense feeling (swelling and rigidity) of the affected compartment. The classic symptoms of compartment syndrome are referred to as the "5 Ps": *p*ain (out of proportion to the injury); *p*allor (pale appearance); *p*aresthesia (impaired or altered sensations to the area, or both); *p*aresis (impaired function of the involved extremity); and *p*ulselessness (loss of a pulse to the area). None of these signs are truly dependable, although pain with passive extension of the fingers or toes in the affected extremity and paresthesia tend to be most suggestive of compartment syndrome.[7,13]

A condition known as Volkmann ischemic contracture can develop when compartment syndrome goes unrecognized or is not adequately treated.[14] Irreversible neurovascular damage can occur. Contracture deformities of the fingers, hand, and wrist can lead to partial or complete disability of the affected limb.

Evaluation and Treatment. Compartment syndrome is a clinical diagnosis that requires immediate treatment and surgical consultation. Delayed treatment can cause loss of limb.[15] The individual's history and physical examination findings alone can provide the necessary information to make a diagnosis of compartment syndrome. When clinical evaluation is inconclusive, the rising ICP can be directly measured by using a manometer or an electronic transducer, to confirm the diagnosis. Laboratory tests, ultrasonography, and imaging studies may help exclude other conditions but, generally, are not helpful in diagnosing compartment syndrome. Once the diagnosis is confirmed, immediate surgical intervention is warranted to relieve pressure within the compartment. Surgical intervention consists of performing an immediate fasciotomy and debridement of the affected area to decompress the compartment and allow the return of a normal blood supply. Skin grafts are often required to close the resultant opening, but vacuum-assisted wound closure devices also have been used successfully in accelerating wound closure. With delayed treatment, the limb may require amputation.[7]

Malignant Hyperthermia

Malignant hyperthermia (MH) is a potentially life-threatening hereditary musculoskeletal disorder characterized by a hypermetabolic reaction to certain volatile anesthetics or certain depolarizing muscle relaxants (e.g., succinylcholine). Nitrous oxide and xenon, although inhaled, are not halogenated or implicated in MH.[16] Other disorders associated with MH are the rare central core disease (CCD) and King-Denborough syndrome.[17]

Pathophysiology. MH is an autosomal dominant inherited disorder. The gene for the ryanodine receptor RYR1 is the location for mutations. Other genetic loci have been identified. The main concern is uncontrolled release of calcium from skeletal muscle sarcoplasmic reticulum which leads to sustained muscle contraction, depletion of adenosine triphosphate (ATP), and notably increases oxygen consumption, carbon dioxide production, and heat.[16] Depletion of ATP stores leads to membrane integrity failure and leakage of cellular potassium, CK, and myoglobin into the circulation.[18,19] The sustained elevation of calcium concentration allows excessive stimulation of aerobic and anaerobic glycolytic metabolism, causing a hypermetabolic state resulting in extremely high body temperature, respiratory and metabolic acidosis, muscle rigidity, altered cell permeability, and hyperkalemia. Rhabdomyolysis and death may result if this condition is not quickly identified and treated.

Clinical Manifestations. Common signs and symptoms are tachycardia, tachypnea, hypoxemia, hypercarbia, metabolic and respiratory acidosis, hyperkalemia, cardiac dysrhythmias, hypotension, skeletal muscle rigidity, and hyperthermia.[16]

Evaluation and Treatment. Careful and thorough preoperative assessment by the anesthesia team will help to alert care providers to the possibility of an individual being susceptible to MH. A family history of anesthetic problems and previous untoward anesthetic experiences (muscle cramping, unexplained fevers, dark urine) are criteria that require further clarification before administration of a volatile anesthetic, such as halothane, or the muscle relaxant succinylcholine. The caffeine halothane muscle contracture test is considered the most sensitive and definitive predictor of an individual developing MH. A muscle biopsy is obtained from the individual and then separately exposed to standardized amounts of halothane and caffeine. If the muscle bundles exhibit a contracture at specified limits, the individual is considered susceptible to MH. Common signs and symptoms are tachycardia, masseter muscle and skeletal muscle spasm, and elevated body temperature.

Priorities in the treatment of MH include identifying and treating the underlying disorder and preventing life-threatening renal failure. Dantrolene, a skeletal muscle relaxant, which inhibits calcium release from the sarcoplasmic reticulum and reverses the effects of MH, should be administered immediately. Once MH is suspected, all triggering agents must be discontinued, the person hyperventilated with 100% oxygen with non-triggering anesthetic agents used for patient care, and surgery ended as quickly as possible.[16] The management algorithm is presented in Box 44.1.[16,20,21] Secondary problems to be monitored and treated include electrolyte imbalance, volume depletion, acidosis, hyperuricemia, hyperkalemia, and calcium imbalance. Short-term dialysis also may be necessary. The mortality rate of MH is 3% to 5%, even when properly treated.[16]

BOX 44.1 Critical Management Algorithm for Malignant Hyperthermia

- **Stop** the triggering agent.
- **Call** for help.
- **Administer** dantrolene 2.5 mg/kg every 5 minutes until the reaction subsides up to a maximum of 10 mg/kg.
- **Increase** ventilation to lower end-tidal CO_2.
- **Cooling** measures (cool or cold isotonic crystalloid IV fluids (20 to 30 mL/kg and ice packs to exposed surfaces).
- **Treat** arrhythmias (e.g., amiodarone; avoid calcium channel blockers).
- **Laboratory** studies include arterial blood gas, electrolytes (especially potassium), creatinine kinase (CK), serum and urine myoglobin, and coagulation profile.
- **Continue** dantrolene at 1 mg/kg every 4 hours for 24–48 hours.
- **Ensure** urine output of 2 mL/kg/h (mannitol 3 g are included in each vial of dantrolene)

Hopkins PM, Girard T, Dalay S, Jenkins B, Thacker A, Patteril M, McGrady E. Malignant hyperthermia 2020: Guideline from the Association of Anaesthetists. *Anaesthesia.* 2021;76(5):655.

DISORDERS OF BONES

Metabolic Bone Diseases

Metabolic bone disease is characterized by abnormal bone strength caused by abnormalities of minerals, vitamin D, bone mass, or bone structures. Individuals of all ages may be affected by this disease. Causes of these conditions are attributed to genetics, poor diet, or hormone influence leading to altered or inadequate biochemical reactions.

Osteoporosis

Osteoporosis, or porous bone, is characterized by low bone mineral density caused by altered bone microstructure and leads to an increased risk of fractures.[22] It is a complex, multifactorial, chronic disease that often progresses silently causing impaired structural integrity of the bone, and decreased bone strength. Bone tissue can be normally mineralized in osteoporosis, but the density of bone is decreased and the structural integrity of trabecular bone is impaired. Cortical bone becomes more porous and thinner, making bone weaker and prone to fractures (Figs. 44.11 and 44.12; Box 44.2). It is the most common disease that affects bone. The World Health Organization (WHO) has defined osteoporosis as "a systematic skeletal disease characterized by low bone density and microarchitectural deterioration of bone tissue with a consequent increase in bone fragility."[23] Incidence of osteoporosis increases with age and affects over 200 million people.[22] Over 70% of those affected are over 80 years old. In the developed world, those affected are 2% to 8% of males and 9% to 38% females. Globally, osteoporosis causes approximately 9 million fractures per year.[22] Box 44.3 presents risk factors for osteoporosis. Over 50% of postmenopausal

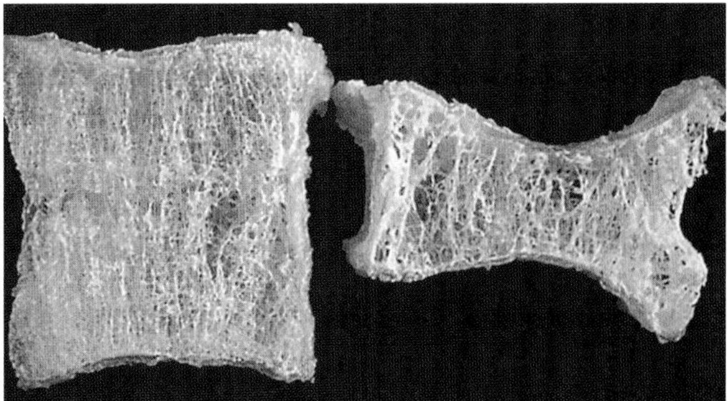

Fig. 44.11 Vertebral Body. Osteoporotic vertebral body *(right)* shortened by compression fractures compared with a normal vertebral body. Note that the osteoporotic vertebra has a characteristic loss of horizontal trabeculae and thickened vertical trabeculae. (From Kumar V, et al. *Robbins & Cotran pathologic basis of disease*, 10th edition. Philadelphia: Elsevier; 2021.)

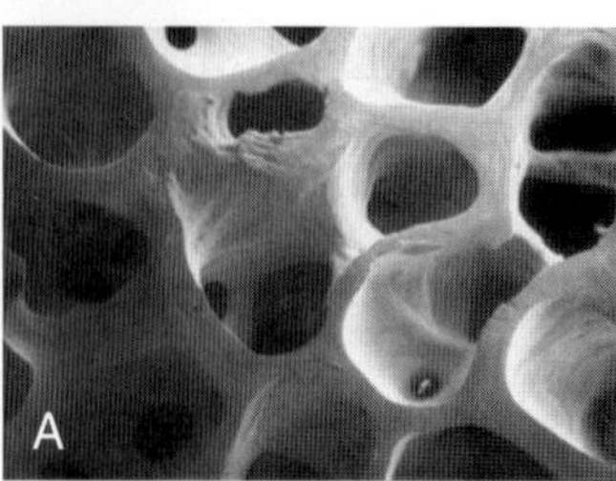

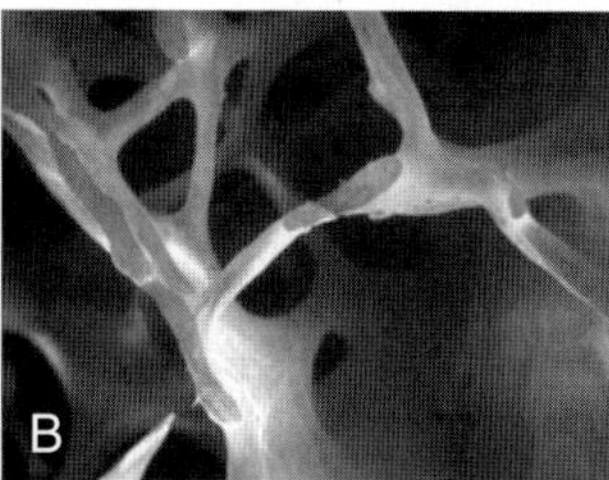

Fig. 44.12 Electron Microscopic Comparison of Normal and Osteoporotic Bone. (A) Normal trabecular structure. **(B)** Osteoporotic bone; note the loss of supporting trabeculae. (From Golob AL, Laya MB. Osteoporosis: Screening, prevention, and management. *Medical Clinics of North America,* 2015;99(3):587–606.)

BOX 44.2 Causes of Secondary Osteoporosis

- Medications such as glucocorticoids, anti-epileptics, chemotherapy, proton pump inhibitors, possibly thiazolidines
- Hyperparathyroidism
- Overtreatment of hypothyroidism
- Chronic kidney disease
- Cushing disease
- Diseases related to long-term immobilization
- Secondary amenorrhea duration longer than one year (non-estrogen hormonal therapy,
- Low body weight, excessive exercise

white women will have an osteoporotic-related fracture. Only about 33% of senior women who have a hip fracture will be able to return to independent living.[22] The risk of an osteoporotic fracture is 20% in white men, however, their 1-year mortality is twice that of women.[22] Osteoporotic fractures significantly decrease quality of life, increasing morbidity, mortality, and disability.[24] Black males and females have a decreased incidence of osteoporosis compared to white individuals but have similar fracture risks. The aging of the American population is expected to triple the number of osteoporotic fractures.[22,25,26] Due to lower exposure to sunlight and consequent lower synthesis of vitamin D, individuals who live at higher latitudes have higher fracture rates than those who live closer to the equator.[22,27]

There are two types of osteoporosis: *primary* or *idiopathic osteoporosis,* which is more common, and *secondary osteoporosis.* Primary osteoporosis is related to the aging process associated with decreasing sex hormones.[22] Secondary osteoporosis is caused by other conditions, including endocrine diseases (hormone imbalances, diabetes, hyperparathyroidism, hyperthyroidism), medications (such as heparin, corticosteroids, phenytoin, barbiturates, lithium), and other substances (including tobacco and ethanol) (see Box 44.2). Other conditions (including rheumatoid disease, human immunodeficiency virus [HIV], malignancies, malabsorption syndromes, liver or kidney disease) also increase the risk for developing osteoporosis (see Box 44.3).

Bone quality is not defined by bone mass alone (as measured by BMD) but also by the microarchitecture of the bone. Other variables include crystal size and shape, brittleness, vitality of bone cells, structure of the bone proteins, water volume, integrity of the trabecular network, vascular supply, and the ability to repair tiny cracks. Because bone density relates to the *quantity* of bone, the *quality* of bone is not accurately identified by bone density testing alone. As a result, bone density testing may not accurately identify those who will eventually be susceptible to fractures.

BOX 44.3 Risk Factors for Osteoporosis

- Increasing age
- Body weight under 128 pounds
- Smoking
- Positive family history of osteoporosis
- White or Asian race
- Early menopause
- Low levels of physical activity
- Personal history of a fracture from a ground-level fall or minor trauma after the age of 40
- Conditions affecting mobility, such as spinal cord injuries

Highest Risk for Fracture

- Advanced age
- Prior history of a fracture
- Female gender
- Use of corticosteroids
- Low body mass index
- Smoker
- Secondary osteoporosis
- Intake of alcohol

Postmenopausal osteoporosis is bone loss that occurs in middle-aged and older women. It can occur because of estrogen deficiency, as well as estrogen-independent age-related mechanisms (e.g., secondary causes such as hyperparathyroidism and decreased mechanical stimulation). Increased oxidative stress and intracellular reactive oxygen species play a significant role in the development of age-related bone loss and other age-related changes in the body. Estrogen deficiency can also increase with stress, excessive exercise, and low body weight. Postmenopausal changes result in a substantial increase in bone turnover—that is, an imbalance between the remodeling activity of osteoclasts (bone destroyers) and osteoblasts (bone formers). Increased formation and activity of osteoclasts result in increased bone resorption and is associated with a cascade of proinflammatory cytokines. Increased cytokine activation, especially tumor necrosis factor (TNF), can occur with declining estrogen levels. In addition, estrogen helps to protect against the effects of oxidative stress and osteoclast apoptosis (programmed cell death). A decrease in estrogen levels is therefore associated with *survival* of the bone-removing osteoclasts. Biologically, these processes involve the receptor activator nuclear factor κβ ligand (RANKL), transcription factors such as Forkhead proteins the Wnt and osteoprotegerin (OPG) signaling pathways, and insulin-like growth factor (IGF) (Fig. 44.13; also see Chapter 43). Other causes may include a combination of inadequate dietary calcium intake and lack of vitamin D, possibly decreased magnesium levels, lack of exercise, low body mass, and family history. IGF is known to help in fracture

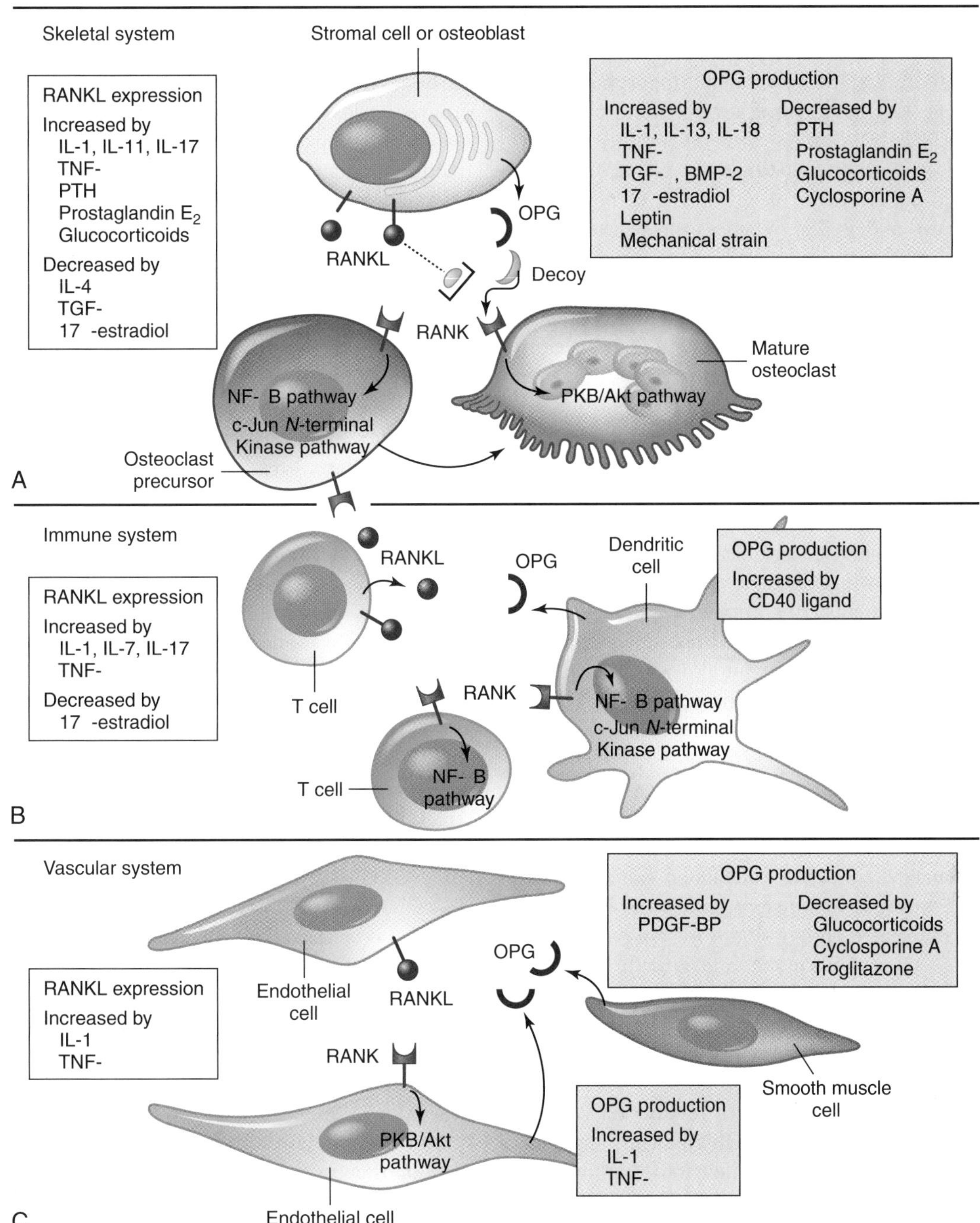

Fig. 44.13 OPG/RANKL/RANK System. Receptor activator of nuclear factor κβ ligand (*RANKL*, which is a cytokine and part of the tumor necrosis factor *[TNF]* family) and osteoprotegerin (*OPG*, which is a glycoprotein receptor antagonist) are modulated by various cytokines, hormones, drugs, and mechanical strains *(see inserts)*. **(A)** In bone, RANKL is expressed by both stromal cells and osteoblasts. RANKL stimulates the receptor RANK on osteoclast precursor cells and mature osteoclasts, and activates intracellular signaling pathways to promote osteoclast differentiation and activation and cytoskeletal reorganization and survival *(PKB/Akt pathway)* that increase resorption and bone loss. OPG, secreted by stromal cells and osteoblasts, acts as a "decoy" receptor and blocks RANKL binding to and activation of RANK. **(B)** In the immune system, RANKL is expressed and secreted by T cells. T-cell–derived RANKL also can activate RANK on osteoclasts, T cells, and dendritic cells (antigen-presenting cells), which enhances bone loss that occurs in inflammatory bone diseases such as rheumatoid arthritis. Dendritic cells may regulate these processes by secreting OPG. **(C)** In the vascular system, endothelial cells express RANKL and the RANK receptor. RANKL/RANK interactions contribute to endothelial and smooth muscle cells and can block RANKL binding. The physiologic significance of the OPG/RANKL/RANK system in endothelial and smooth muscle cells is being studied. *BMP-2*, Bone morphogenic protein 2; *IL*, interleukin; *PDGF-BP*, platelet-derived growth factor-beta polypeptide; *PTH*, parathyroid hormone; *TGFα*, tumor necrosis factor-alpha; *TGFβ*, transforming growth factor-beta. (Adapted from Hofbauer LC, Schoppet M. Clinical implications of the osteoprotegerin/RANKL/RANK system for bone and vascular diseases. *JAMA*, 2004;292(4):490–495.)

healing and collagen synthesis and improves conditions for bone mineralization. IGF levels significantly decline by age 60. Excessive phosphorus intake, chiefly through the intake of highly processed foods, hampers the calcium/phosphorus balance by interfering with parathyroid hormone and fibroblast growth factor 23 (FGF-23).

The levels of sex hormones, particularly estradiol (estrogen) and testosterone, are major determinants of bone density in both females and males. When estrogen levels drop after menopause, circulating androgens (i.e., testosterone and dihydrotestosterone) become significant effectors on bone metabolism through their influence on the stimulation of bone formation. Other factors, such as inadequate dietary calcium intake, decreases in weight-bearing exercise, and sarcopenia, also are associated with osteoporosis. (Other risk factors are identified in Box 44.3.)

Poor nutrition, insufficient intake, or malabsorption of dietary minerals (in particular calcium) are factors in the development of osteoporosis. Calcium intake and absorption from the intestine decreases with age and has also been associated with malnutrition following bariatric surgery.[28] Decreased serum levels of trace elements (zinc, copper, iron, magnesium, and manganese) have also been associated not only with lower peak bone mass in developing bone, but also with later development of osteoporosis. Vitamin deficiencies, particularly vitamins C, D, E, and K, as well as either deficiencies or excesses of protein, also contribute to bone loss.

Skeletal homeostasis depends on a very narrow range of plasma calcium and phosphate concentrations, which are maintained by the endocrine system. Therefore, endocrine dysfunction ultimately can cause metabolic bone disease. In addition to declining levels of sex steroids, the hormones most commonly associated with osteoporosis are parathyroid hormone, cortisol, thyroid hormone, and growth hormone. Excessive intake of caffeine, phosphorus, alcohol, and nicotine, along with lower body mass index has also been shown to lower bone mineral density.

Secondary osteoporosis is osteoporosis caused by other conditions, including hormonal imbalances (endocrine disease, diabetes, hyperparathyroidism, hyperthyroidism), medications (e.g., heparin, corticosteroids, phenytoin, barbiturates, and lithium), and other substances (e.g., tobacco, ethanol). Other conditions, including rheumatoid disease, HIV, malignancies, malabsorption syndrome, and liver or kidney disease, also increase the risk for developing osteoporosis (see Box 44.3 *Risk Factors:* Osteoporosis).[29] Secondary osteoporosis caused by heparin therapy is due to reduced osteoblast formation and increasing bone resorption by reducing OPG, thus increasing osteoclast formation. These effects usually resolve when therapy stops. Other medications that increase the risk of osteoporosis include glucocorticoids, proton pump inhibitors, aromatase inhibitors, lithium, methotrexate, anticonvulsants, cyclophosphamide, thiazolidinediones, and cyclosporine.

Pathophysiology. Osteoporosis develops when the remodeling cycle (coupling)—bone resorption and bone formation—is disrupted, leading to an imbalance in the coupling process. Throughout an individual's lifetime, old bone is removed (resorption) and new bone is added (formation) to the skeleton (see bone remodeling Chapter 43). In osteoporosis, old bone is being resorbed faster than new bone is being formed, causing the bones to lose density, becoming thinner and more porous. A progressive loss of bone mass may continue until the skeleton is no longer strong enough to support itself. Eventually, bones can fracture spontaneously. Studies in the field of bone biology have led to new understanding of the roles of hormones, growth and signaling factors, and cellular biology in osteoporosis.[30] Of primary importance is the osteoblast lineage, chondrocyte lineage, and osteoclast differentiation pathway, which are dependent on various processes, including proliferation, maturation, fusion, and activation. These processes, in turn, are dependent on the availability of stem cells to allow differentiation to occur and are controlled by hormones, cytokines, and paracrine stromal cell interactions. Mesenchymal stem cells (MSCs) and skeletal stem cells (SSCs) have been shown separately to give rise to osteoblasts but the relationship between these two stem cell populations needs much more study.[31]

Although hormonal influences remain important in maintaining bone health, genetic/ epigenetic factors and the role of oxidative stress are receiving increased attention as critical determinants of bone homeostasis. Thus, proper intracellular communication within bone among its molecular regulators is necessary for normal bone homeostasis. Numerous interleukins, TNF, TGF-β, prostaglandin E_2, and hormones interact to control osteoclasts (see Fig. 44.13). Normal bone homeostasis is dependent on the balance between the cytokine receptor activator of nuclear factor κβ ligand (RANKL); its receptor activator nuclear factor κβ (RANK); and its decoy receptor osteoprotegerin (OPG), a glycoprotein (see Chapter 43).[32,33]

Postmenopausal osteoporosis results from estrogen deficiency. It is characterized by increased bone resorption relative to the rate of bone formation, leading to sustained bone loss. This phenomenon can also be seen in men, as circulating estrogen, though in lower levels compared to women, is essential for modulating libido, erectile function, and spermatogenesis. Therefore, bone loss in men may be a result of male estrogen deficiency.

Increased bone resorption results from enhanced development of osteoclasts and decreased osteoclast apoptosis (see Fig. 44.13). Estrogen stimulates OPG secretion and down-regulates RANKL; drugs known as *selective estrogen response modifiers (SERMs)* also stimulate OPG production. Postmenopausal women express higher levels of RANKL on bone marrow stromal cells, T cells, and B cells than premenopausal women. Importantly, RANKL expression is increased when estrogen levels are decreased, leading to increased formation of osteoclasts while reducing osteoclast apoptosis.

Sex steroids (e.g., estrogens) exert antiapoptotic effects on osteoblasts but exert proapoptotic effects on osteoclasts. The difference in activity is determined by the length of time extracellular signal regulated kinases (ERKs) remain in the nucleus. Estrogen activates ERKs outside the nucleus; ERKs then accumulate in the nucleus and activate downstream transcription factors. Prolonged nuclear accumulation of activated ERKs converts the antiapoptotic effect of estradiol to proapoptotic. In addition to

ERKs, RANKL promotes the antiapoptotic effects on osteoclasts, thus increasing their life span. Wnt signaling induces a biochemical series of events that increases osteoblast and bone formation. Alterations in Wnt signaling account for critical pathophysiologic changes in most acquired metabolic bone diseases including postmenopausal osteoporosis, aging effects, and glucocorticoid (i.e., cortisone) excess. Agents such as parathyroid hormone and bisphosphonates, used for treatment of bone loss, exert their positive effects by altering the formation of osteoblasts or osteoclasts or by inducing osteoclast apoptosis.

Glucocorticoid-induced osteoporosis (e.g., prednisone, cortisone) is the most common type of secondary osteoporosis and is characterized by increased bone resorption and decreased bone formation. Glucocorticoids have a direct impact on bone quality by improving osteoclast survival, inhibiting osteoblast formation and function, and increasing osteocyte apoptosis. Glucocorticoids increase RANKL expression and inhibit OPG production by osteoblasts (see Fig. 44.13). The use of immunosuppressive drugs (e.g., cyclosporine A) to reduce rejection of transplanted organs also alters the OPG/RANKL/RANK system and can lead to post-transplantation osteoporosis. Overall, these alterations result in decreased thickness of the bone cortex and fewer, thinner, and more widely spaced trabeculae in the marrow. Other conditions affected by OPG/RANKL/RANK include RA, myeloma, vascular diseases, and skeletal metastases from neoplastic disorders.

Age-related bone loss begins in the third to fourth decade for women but later for men.[24,34] Trabecular bone loss begins in young adult women and men at all skeletal sites, continues throughout life, and accelerates during perimenopause in women.[34] Late onset of cortical bone loss is associated with sex steroid deficiency.[22,34] Loss of trabecular bone in men proceeds in a linear fashion with thinning of trabecular bone rather than complete loss, as is noted in women (Fig. 44.14A and B). Men have approximately 30% greater bone mass than women, which may be a factor in their later involvement with osteoporosis (Fig. 44.15). Secondary osteoporosis occurs more frequently in men than women.[22] Androgens promote OPG production, thus inhibiting the osteoclastic effect of RANKL. Since men typically have a more gradual decrease in the levels of testosterone and estradiol (and possibly progesterone), bone mass is maintained longer than in women. Reduction in physical activity in older persons also may be a major factor in the degree of bone loss. Preservation of bone mass depends on skeletal stress (mechanical) through muscle contraction and weight-bearing.

Clinical Manifestations. The specific clinical manifestations of osteoporosis depend on the bones involved. The most

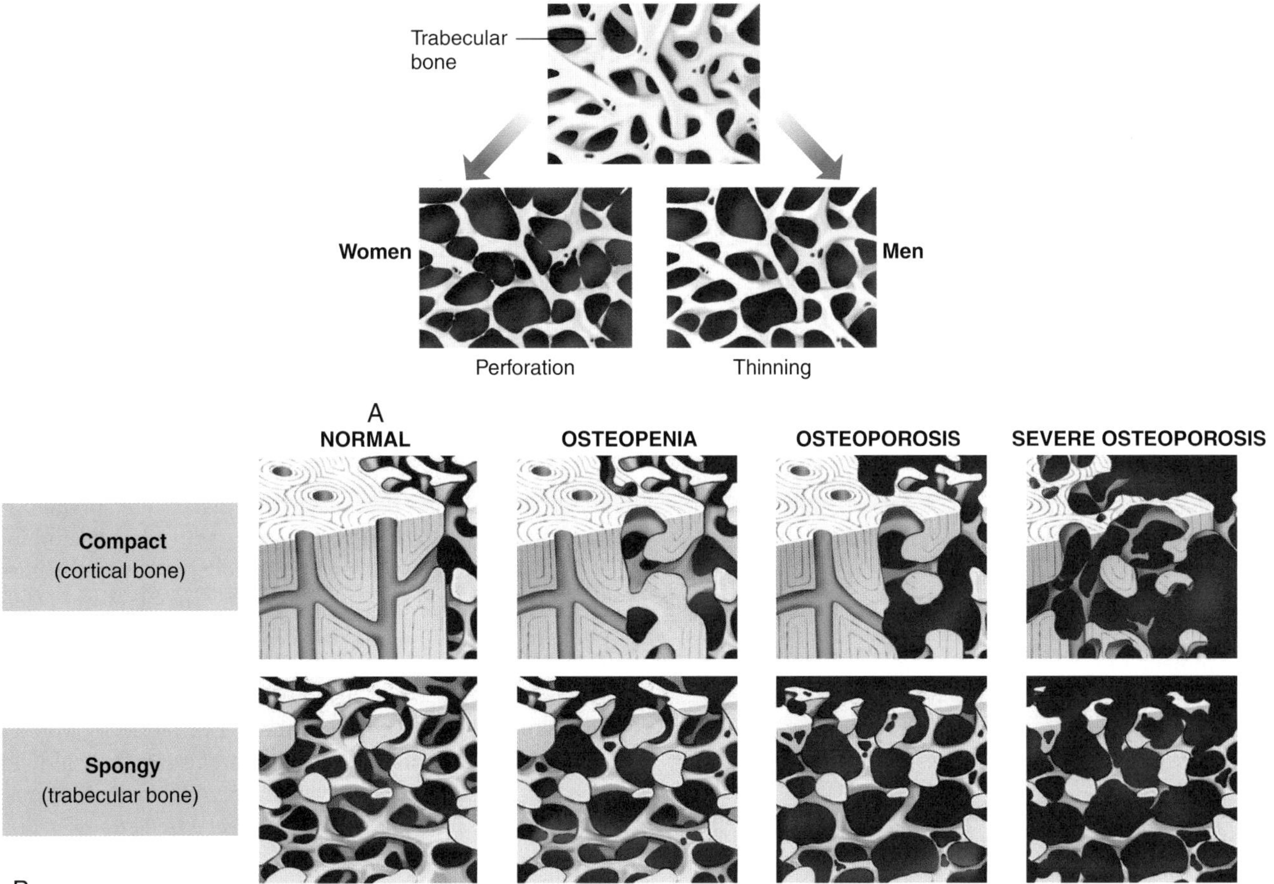

Fig. 44.14 Osteoporosis. (A) Osteoporosis in Cortical and Trabecular Bone. **(B)** Mechanism of Loss of Trabecular Bone in Women and Trabecular Thinning in Men. Bone thinning predominates in men because of reduced bone formation. Loss of connectivity and complete trabecular loss predominate in women.

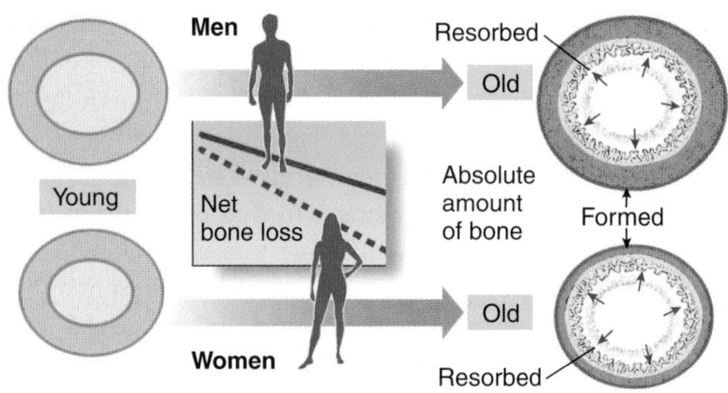

Fig. 44.15 Bone Loss in Men and Women. With aging, the absolute amount of bone resorbed on the inner bone surface and formed on the outer bone surface is greater in men than in women.

common manifestation, however, is bone deformity. Pain tends to occur only when there is a fragility fracture. Fractures are likely to occur because the trabeculae of spongy bone become thin and sparse, and compact bone becomes porous. As bone becomes more fragile, falls or bumps which would not have caused a fracture previously may now cause bone to break; this is referred to as a fragility fracture. The most common sites for osteoporosis-related fractures are the spine, femoral neck, and wrist. As the bones lose volume, they become brittle and weak and may collapse or become misshapen. Vertebral collapse causes kyphosis (hunchback) and diminishes height. Fractures of the long bones (particularly the femur and humerus), distal radius, ribs, and vertebrae are most common. The most serious fractures associated with osteoporosis are hip fractures and spinal fractures, which have a high incidence of chronic pain, disability, diminished quality of life, and premature death.[22] Fracture of the neck of the femur (intertrochanteric fracture) tends to occur in older women with osteoporosis. Fatal complications of fractures include fat or pulmonary embolism, pneumonia, hemorrhage, and shock. Approximately 20% of persons with a hip fracture die as a result of surgical complications. Osteoporosis in men, as in women, also may be related to hypogonadism, with estradiol levels being more clinically important than testosterone levels in both genders.

Evaluation and Treatment. A thorough history and physical examination helps to define risk factors from secondary causes of bone loss. Emphasis on social history includes smoking and chronic alcohol habits. A family history is obtained as is a history of previous fractures. The physical exam rarely reveals alterations until osteoporosis is advanced.[22] The USPSTF current recommendations include screening for osteoporosis with bone measurement testing to prevent osteoporotic fractures in postmenopausal women younger than 65 years at increased risk of osteoporosis, but the USPSTF does not recommend screening in men.[35]

Generally, osteoporosis is detected radiographically as increased radiolucency of bone. By the time abnormalities are detected by x-ray examination, up to 25% to 30% of bone tissue may have been lost. The best test for assessing bone mineral density is the dual x-ray absorptiometry (DXA) tests scans of the central skeleton.[36] In bones not at high risk, peripheral DXA tests and ultrasound measure density, but do not correlate well to the standard DXA scan of the hip and spine and are not as useful in diagnosis or treatment decisions.[22]

Bone density is based on the number of standard deviations that differ from the mean bone mineral density of a young-adult reference population (a T-score) (Table 44.5). When BMD measurement is not available, fracture prediction can be determined using an assessment tool developed by the WHO called Fracture Risk Assessment (FRAX) (Fig. 44.16). This tool incorporates clinical risk factors with BMD at the femoral neck to predict an individual's 10-year risk of fracture. This tool is available at http://www.shef.ac.uk/FRAX and is a downloadable computer-based questionnaire that has been developed for use in Europe, North America, Asia, and Australia.

Osteopenia is categorized as a bone density score between negative 1.0 and negative 2.5 standard deviations below normal.[22] The diagnosis of osteoporosis is made with scores below negative 2.5.[22] Severe or established osteoporosis is identified when there has been a fragility fracture associated with low bone density. The disease can be generalized as involving major portions of the axial skeleton or regional loss that involves one segment of the appendicular skeleton.

Other evaluation procedures include tests for measuring levels of serum calcium, phosphorus, and alkaline phosphatase, protein electrophoresis, as well as urinary biochemical markers to monitor bone turnover (Box 44.4). Body calcium levels also can be measured by neuron activation analysis, a procedure involving use of radioactive calcium-49, whose gamma activity can be measured with a whole-body counter. Evaluation tools are summarized in Table 44.4.

Fracture prevention and maintaining optimal bone function is a primary goal of osteoporosis treatment. Several pharmacologic treatments are available. These agents are either antiresorptive or anabolic. In women diagnosed with known osteoporosis, the recommendations to reduce the risk of fracture are to start treatment with risedronate, alendronate, zoledronic acid, or denosumab.[22] These treatments reduce fracture both at vertebral and non-vertebral sites. The FDA has approved bazedoxifene, a selective estrogen receptor modulator combined with conjugated estrogen, for the prevention, not treatment, of osteoporosis.[22] Men should be offered bisphosphonates as first-line therapy.[22] Bisphosphonates are a class of inorganic pyrophosphate derivatives that primarily work through inhibition of hydroxyapatite breakdown and reducing bone resorption by binding bone mineral. They improve osteoblast and osteocyte survival while promoting osteoclast apoptosis, thus slowing the bone remodeling process. With low tolerance of these medications, individuals can use medications such as teriparatide. Those medications shown to reduce vertebral fractures only, such as raloxifene and ibandronate, are reserved for individuals who cannot tolerate any previously mentioned medications. For both groups, secondary causes should be treated.

Adequate dietary intake of calcium, vitamin D, magnesium, and other trace minerals; adherence to a regular regimen of weight-bearing exercise; and avoidance of alcohol, tobacco, and glucocorticoids help to prevent primary osteoporosis. The role of calcium intake to prevent and treat osteoporosis is controversial. It is well accepted that oral calcium intake sufficient to maintain normal calcium balance is necessary during adolescence to ensure development of peak bone mass, and that calcium-deficient diets can aggravate bone loss associated with menopause and aging. Although recommendations have been established for young women of 1000 mg of calcium daily (particularly from dietary sources) and for postmenopausal women of 1500 mg daily (with vitamin D), it has been difficult to translate these recommendations into clear-cut clinical outcomes. A significant relationship has been observed between an individual's lifetime history of calcium intake and peak bone mineral density. Diets with higher fruit and vegetable intake correlate with higher BMD. Other nutrients that appear to have a positive impact on bone health include magnesium, vitamin K_2, and docosahexaenoic acid or DHA (from purified fish oil).

Magnesium (Mg^{++}), another mineral important for skeletal development, is an essential mineral in many biochemical and physiologic functions, including activation of enzymes, involvement in ATP synthesis and protein synthesis, regulation of membrane channels, and contraction of muscle. Mg^{++} is important to bone quality because it helps control hydroxyapatite crystal growth and thereby prevents formation of brittle bones. It seems reasonable that Mg^{++} is required for normal calcium (Ca^{++}) absorption because severe Mg^{++} deficiency results in hypocalcemia.

Regular, moderate weight-bearing exercise can slow the rate of bone loss and, in some cases, reverse demineralization because the mechanical stress of exercise stimulates bone formation. It is important to reduce the risk of falls and enhance bone quality. Therefore, an exercise program to enhance muscle strength and balance has the added benefits of reducing the risk of falls and promoting bone quality.

TABLE 44.4 Comparison of Fracture Risk Assessment Tools Not Using Bone Mineral Density

Risk Factor	FRAX	Score	OSIRIS	ORAI	OST
Age	X	X	X	X	X
Weight	X	X	X	X	X
Previous low-energy fracture	X	X	X		
Estrogen therapy		X	X	X	
Rheumatoid arthritis	X	X			
Height	X				
Parental hip fracture	X				
Smoking	X				
Alcohol	X				
Glucocorticoid therapy	X				
Secondary osteoporosis	X				
Sex	X				
Ethnicity		X			

FRAX, World Health Organization's "Fracture Risk Assessment Tool"; *ORAI*, osteoporosis risk assessment instrument; *OSIRIS*, osteoporosis index of risk; *OST*, osteoporosis self-assessment tool; *SCORE*, simple calculated osteoporosis risk estimation.

Chart from Rubin KH, Abrahamsen B, Friis-Holmberg T, et al. Comparison of different screening tools (FRAX, OST, ORAI, OSIRIS, SCORE and age alone) to identify women with increased risk of fracture. A population-based prospective study. *Bone*, 2013;56:18.

Osteomalacia

Osteomalacia is a metabolic disease characterized by inadequate and delayed mineralization of osteoid in mature compact and spongy bone. The remodeling cycle proceeds normally through osteoid formation, but mineral calcification and deposition do not occur. Bone volume remains unchanged, but the replaced bone consists of soft osteoid instead of rigid bone. The

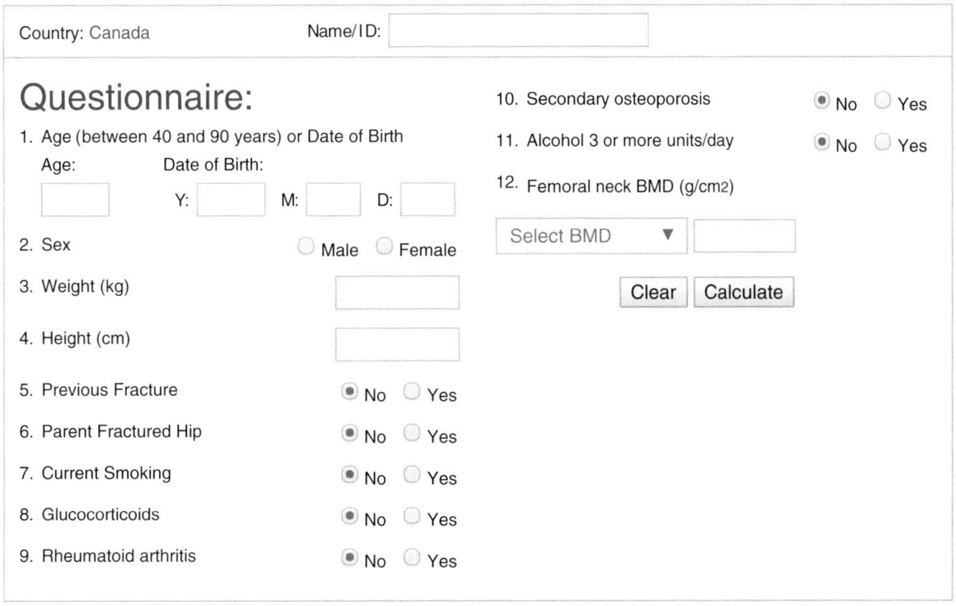

Country: Canada Name/ID:

Questionnaire:

1. Age (between 40 and 90 years) or Date of Birth
   Age: Date of Birth: Y: M: D:
2. Sex ○ Male ○ Female
3. Weight (kg)
4. Height (cm)
5. Previous Fracture ● No ○ Yes
6. Parent Fractured Hip ● No ○ Yes
7. Current Smoking ● No ○ Yes
8. Glucocorticoids ● No ○ Yes
9. Rheumatoid arthritis ● No ○ Yes
10. Secondary osteoporosis ● No ○ Yes
11. Alcohol 3 or more units/day ● No ○ Yes
12. Femoral neck BMD (g/cm2)
   Select BMD ▼

Clear Calculate

Fig. 44.16 Fracture Risk Assessment Tool: FRAX.

TABLE 44.5 T-Score Classification

T-Score	Classification
$T \geq -1.0$	Normal bone density
T between −1.0 and −2.5	Osteopenia or low bone density
$T \leq -2.5$	Osteoporosis

[a]The World Health Organization's T-score classification scale for the diagnosis of osteoporosis. *T*, T-score.
Data from National Osteoporosis Foundation. *Clinician's Guide to Prevention and Treatment of Osteoporosis*. Washington, DC: Author; 2017.

BOX 44.4 Biochemical Markers of Bone Turnover

Biochemical markers of bone turnover are useful in monitoring osteoporosis treatment. Markers of resorption include urinary N-telopeptide (NTx), C-telopeptide (CTx), and deoxypyridinoline. Markers of bone formation include bone-specific alkaline phosphatase (BSAP) and osteocalcin. However, these tests have diurnal variability within the same individual, so there must be significant changes in levels to indicate a difference in bone turnover.

result is abnormal bone matrix mineralization. Rickets is similar to osteomalacia in pathogenesis, but it occurs in the growing bones of children, whereas osteomalacia occurs in adult bone. (Rickets is described in Chapter 45.)

Both osteomalacia and rickets are rare in the United States and Western Europe but are significant health problems in Great Britain, Ethiopia, Pakistan, Iran, and India. Concomitant diseases, such as HIV, chronic kidney or liver disease, certain cancers, and impaired nutrient absorption from bariatric surgery, can result in vitamin D deficiency and secondary osteomalacia. In the United States, these conditions occur in older adults, premature infants of very low birth weight, and in individuals adhering to rigid macrobiotic vegetarian diets. Breastfed black infants who do not receive vitamin D supplementation have been shown to be at risk for developing nutritional rickets.

Many factors contribute to the development of osteomalacia, but the most important is a deficiency of vitamin D. The major risk factors in vitamin D deficiency are diets deficient in vitamin D, decreased endogenous production of vitamin D, intestinal malabsorption of vitamin D, renal tubular diseases, certain types of tumors (particularly of mesenchymal origin), and anticonvulsant therapy. Classic vitamin D deficiency is rare in the United States because of the addition of synthetic vitamin D to dairy products and bread. Still, disorders of the small bowel, kidneys, hepatobiliary system, and pancreas are causes of vitamin D deficiency in the United States. In malabsorptive disease of the small bowel, both vitamin D and calcium absorption are decreased, causing vitamin D to be lost in feces. Liver disease interferes with the metabolism of vitamin D to its more active form, and diseases of the pancreas and biliary system cause a deficiency of bile salts, which are necessary for normal intestinal absorption of vitamin D.

Pathophysiology. Crystallization of minerals in osteoid requires adequate concentrations of calcium and phosphate. When the concentrations are too low, crystallization, and hence ossification, does not proceed normally.

Vitamin D deficiency disrupts mineralization because vitamin D normally regulates and enhances the absorption of calcium ions from the intestine. A lack of vitamin D causes the plasma calcium concentrations to fall. Low plasma calcium levels stimulate increased synthesis and secretion of PTH. Although the increase in circulating PTH level raises the plasma calcium concentration, it also stimulates increased renal clearance of phosphate. When the concentration of phosphate in the bone decreases below a critical level, mineralization cannot proceed normally.

Abnormalities occur in both spongy and compact bone. Trabeculae in spongy bone become thinner and fewer, whereas haversian systems in compact bone develop large channels and become irregular. Because osteoid continues to be produced but not mineralized, abnormal quantities of osteoid accumulate, coating the trabeculae and the linings of the haversian canals. Excessive osteoid also can accumulate in areas beneath the periosteum. The excess of osteoid leads to gross deformities of the long bones, spine, pelvis, and skull.

Clinical Manifestations. Osteomalacia causes varying degrees of diffuse musculoskeletal pain and tenderness. Bone pain is typically between joints, rather than within them. Pain is noted particularly in the hips, and the individual may be hesitant to walk. Muscular weakness, particularly of the proximal muscles, is common and may contribute to a waddling gait. Facial deformities and bowed legs or "knock-knees" may be present. Bone fractures and vertebral collapse occur with minimal trauma. Low back pain may be an early complaint, but pain may also involve ribs, feet, other areas of the vertebral column, and other sites. Fragility fractures may occur. Uremia may be present in renal osteodystrophy.

Evaluation and Treatment. Laboratory data may include elevated BUN and creatinine levels, normal or low serum calcium levels, and a serum inorganic phosphate level that is usually higher than 5.5 mg. Alkaline phosphatase and PTH levels are usually elevated. Radiographic findings may show symmetric bowing deformities and fractures with callus formation, particularly in the lower extremities. These types of fractures, known as *pseudofractures*, appear as radiolucent bands perpendicular to the surface of involved bones. Bone biopsy is used in determining bone structure and remodeling.

Treatment of osteomalacia may vary, depending on its etiology, but these general principles are followed:

- Adjustment of serum calcium and phosphorus levels to normal
- Suppression of secondary hyperthyroidism
- Chelation of bone aluminum if needed
- Administration of calcium carbonate to reduce hyperphosphatemia
- Administration of vitamin D supplements (oral or infusion)
- Administration of bisphosphonate
- Implementation of renal dialysis, if indicated
- Considering renal transplant for renal osteodystrophy

Paget Disease

Paget disease of bone (PDB, or osteitis deformans), the second most common bone disease after osteoporosis, is a state of increased metabolic activity in bone characterized by abnormal and excessive bone resorption and formation (remodeling). Genetic manipulations involving the RANK–NF-κβ signaling pathways are significant in the development of Paget disease, resulting in increased osteoclast activity. Chronic accelerated remodeling eventually enlarges and softens the affected bones, causing bowing deformity, fracture, or neurologic problems.

Classic PDB arises as a consequence of disorderly bone resorption and formation. This process can occur in any bone but most often affects the axial skeleton, especially the vertebrae, skull, sacrum, sternum, pelvis, and femur. The disease process may occur in one or more bones without causing significant clinical manifestations.

Paget disease occurs with equal frequency in men more than 55 years of age and women older than 40 years of age. Its incidence almost doubles each decade after age 50 and affects men more than women in a proportion of 1.8:1. Because it is often asymptomatic, PDB is often unrecognized, making few epidemiologic data available. Autopsy data from England and Germany indicate that approximately 3% to 4% of the population older than 40 years of age has Paget disease. It is most prevalent in Australia, Great Britain, New Zealand, and the United States. Paget disease affects several members of the same family in 5% to 25% of individuals.

The cause of PDB is not yet fully known, but studies have implicated both genetic and environmental factors. About 10% to 30% of individuals with PDB have mutations of a specific gene, sequestosome-1. Researchers have identified variations in three genes associated with PDB: *SQSTM1*, *TNFRSF11A*, and *TNFRSF11B*. Implicated environmental factors include viruses, particularly the paramyxovirus family (that includes mumps, parainfluenza, and measles viruses), but no definitive microorganism has yet been identified. Interaction between genetic and environmental factors appears to increase osteoclast activity in PDB.

Pathophysiology. Paget disease begins with excessive resorption of spongy bone and deposition of disorganized bone. The trabeculae diminish, and bone marrow is replaced by extremely vascular fibrous tissue. The resorption phase of Paget disease is followed by the formation of abnormal new bone at an accelerated rate. The collagen fibers are disorganized, and glycoprotein levels in the matrix decrease. Mineralization may extend into the bone marrow. Bone formation is excessive around partially resorbed trabeculae, causing them to thicken and enlarge. Paget disease eventually progresses to an inactive phase, in which abnormal remodeling is minimal or absent. The net result of this accelerated remodeling process is increased bone fragility and an increased risk for bone tumors.

Clinical Manifestations. In the skull, abnormal remodeling is first evident in the frontal or occipital regions; then it encroaches on the outer and inner surfaces of the entire skull. The skull thickens and assumes an asymmetric shape (Fig. 44.17). Thickened segments of the skull may compress areas of the brain, producing altered mentation and dementia. Impingement of new bone on cranial nerves can cause sensory abnormalities, impaired motor function, deafness, atrophy of the optic nerve, and obstruction of the lacrimal duct. Headaches are commonly noted.

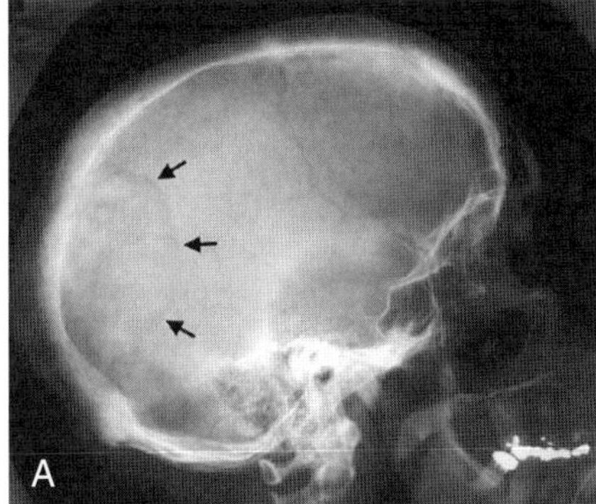

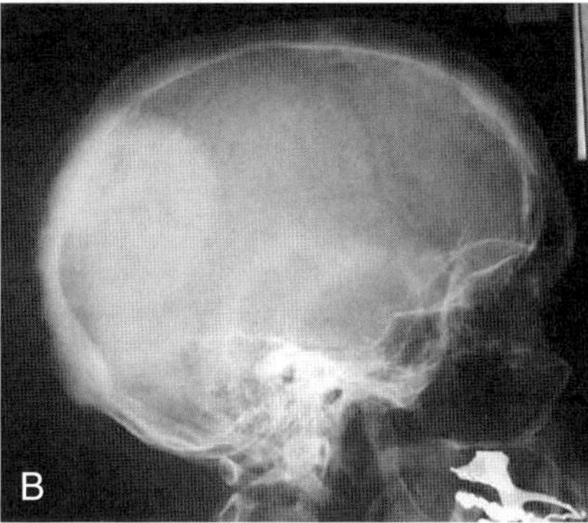

Fig. 44.17 Paget Disease of the Skull. (A) Active Paget disease of the skull with marked cortical thickening and an area of osteoporosis circumscripta (*arrows*). **(B)** The same individual several years later (after biphosphonate treatment) with the lytic lesion largely replaced by sclerotic bone. (From Walsh JP; *Med J Aust* 181[5]; 263, 2004).

Extensive alterations of the facial bones are rare except in the jaw, where sclerosis and thickening of the maxilla and mandible displace teeth and produce malocclusion. In long bones, resorption begins in the subchondral regions of the epiphysis and extends into the metaphysis and diaphysis. Warmth over the affected area, bone and joint pain, and bone deformity may be appreciated as the condition progresses. Occasionally, Paget disease affects both ends of a tubular bone. In the femur, Paget disease produces an exaggerated lateral curvature and in the tibia, anterior curvature is also exaggerated. Stress fractures are common in the lower extremities.

Clinical manifestations of Paget disease in the vertebral column depend on the level of involvement and are caused by compression of adjacent structures. In the cervical spine, cord compression can lead to spastic quadriplegia. Approximately 1% of persons with Paget disease develop osteogenic sarcoma which carries a poor prognosis.

Evaluation and Treatment. PDB is suspected when an elevated serum alkaline phosphatase level is recognized along with abnormal x-ray films that demonstrate characteristic radiographic changes. These changes include thickened cortices marked by tunneling, and accentuated trabeculae. Plain films obtained earlier in the course of illness may show bone lesions that appear lytic in nature. Radioisotope bone scan, x-rays, and CT are used to confirm the diagnosis. Serum plasma procollagen-1 N-peptide (PINP) is another serum marker that may provide a more accurate diagnosis. Evaluation of Paget disease is made on the basis of radiographic findings of irregular bone trabeculae with a thickened and disorganized pattern. Early detection and diagnosis of the extent of Paget disease is readily obtained by bone scanning which shows increased uptake of bone radionuclides. A typical V-shaped lesion in long bones and rounded areas of thinning bone in the skull are often seen on plain x-rays. Serum total alkaline phosphatase and urinary hydroxyproline levels are elevated.

Many individuals require no treatment if the disease is localized and does not cause symptoms. Treatment during active disease is focused on pain relief and prevention of deformity or fracture. Bisphosphonates (alendronate, risedronate, and pamidronate) and calcitonin (salmon and human) are the treatment of choice; a one-time infusion of zoledronic acid can provide long-term reduction of biochemical markers and even remission. Surgery is indicated if there are neurologic complications or severe bony deformities.

Infectious Bone Disease: Osteomyelitis

Osteomyelitis is a bone infection most often caused by bacteria; however, fungi, parasites, and viruses also can cause bone infection (Fig. 44.18). Multiple classification systems have been used to describe osteomyelitis; the simplest refers to the mode of infection. Exogenous osteomyelitis is an infection that enters from outside the body. Direct contamination of bones with bacteria can occur in open fractures or dislocations with an overlying skin wound. Exogenous osteomyelitis can be caused by human bites or fist blows to the mouth. Superficial animal or human bites inoculate local soft tissue with bacteria that later spread to underlying bone. Deep bites can introduce microorganisms directly onto bone. The most common infecting organism in human bites is *S. aureus*. In animal bites, the most common infecting organism is *Pasteurella multocida*, which is part of the normal oral flora of cats and dogs. In exogenous osteomyelitis, infection spreads from soft tissues into adjacent bone. Individuals that receive large doses of corticosteroids or immunosuppressive medications are particularly susceptible to chronic exogenous osteomyelitis or recurring episodes of this disease. Endogenous osteomyelitis is caused by pathogens carried in the blood from sites of infection elsewhere in the body. In hematogenous osteomyelitis, infection spreads from bone to adjacent soft tissues. Hematogenous osteomyelitis is commonly found in infants, children, and older adults. Acute hematogenous osteomyelitis is more often seen in children and is characterized by fever, pain, and voluntary immobility of the affected limb. (Osteomyelitis in children is discussed in Chapter 45.) In adults, hematogenous osteomyelitis is more common in the spine, pelvis, and small bones. Microorganisms reach the vertebrae through arteries, veins, or lymphatic vessels. The primary origin of bacteria entering the body is from cutaneous, sinus, ear, or dental infections. However, soft tissue, genitourinary, and respiratory tract infections also are sources of bacterial contamination. The spread of infection from pelvic organs (vaginal, uterine, ovarian, bladder, and gastrointestinal infections) to the vertebrae has been shown to cause iliac or sacral osteomyelitis.

Contiguous osteomyelitis occurs when infection spreads from one adjacent structure to another. The pathogens may enter the body through an exogenous route (open fractures, penetrating wounds, or surgical procedures). Intervertebral disk surgery and operative procedures involving implantation of large foreign objects, such as metallic plates can result in contiguous osteomyelitis. In addition, infections following total joint replacement surgeries can lead to osteomyelitis. The vulnerability of specific bone depends on the anatomy of its vascular supply. Other causes of osteomyelitis include metabolic and vascular diseases (diabetes, peripheral vascular disease), lifestyle risks (smoking, alcohol or IV drug abuse), and advanced age.

A new category of autoimmune, noninfectious osteomyelitis, known as chronic nonbacterial osteomyelitis (CNO), has recently been identified as a cause of chronic bone pain in children.

Staphylococcus aureus (including methicillin-resistant *Staphylococcus aureus* [MRSA]) is the primary microorganism responsible for hematogenous osteomyelitis. Other microorganisms include group B streptococcus, *Haemophilus influenzae*, *Salmonella*, and gram-negative bacteria. Group B streptococcus and *H. influenzae* tend to infect young children; *Salmonella* infection is associated with sickle cell anemia; and gram-negative infections are most common in older adults and individuals with impaired immunity. Mycobacterial, viral, and fungal infections occur in immunocompromised individuals.

Pathophysiology. Regardless of the source of the pathogen, the pathologic features of bone infection are similar to those in any other body tissue (see Chapter 7). First, the invading pathogen provokes an intense inflammatory response. Inflammation in bone is characterized by vascular engorgement, edema,

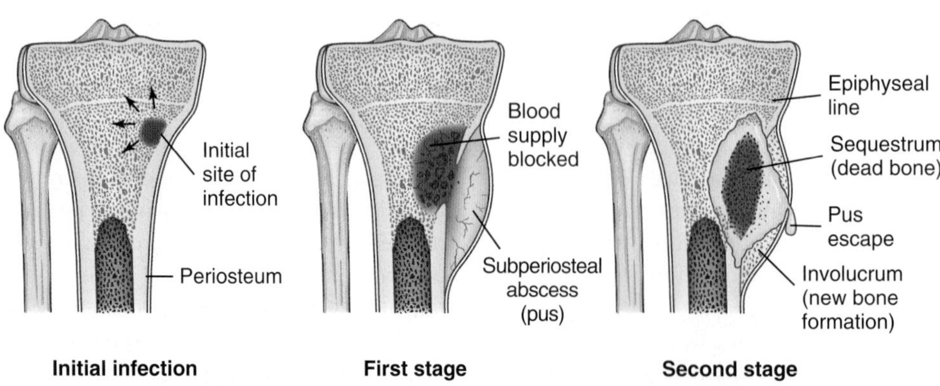

Fig. 44.18 Osteomyelitis Showing Sequestration and Involucrum.

leukocyte activity, small blood vessel thrombosis, and abscess formation. When *S. aureus* is the invading pathogen, in addition to producing toxins that destroy neutrophils, it forms colonies of microorganisms, called *biofilms*. They adhere to surfaces (such as surgical implants) and increase antibiotic resistance. Biofilms alter the normal balance between osteoblast and osteoclast activity by reducing the duration of osteoblast activity, enhancing osteoclast activity, and promoting inflammation (also see Chapter 10).

Once inflammation is initiated, the small terminal vessels thrombose and exudate seals the bone's canaliculi. Inflammatory exudate extends into the metaphysis and the marrow cavity and through small metaphyseal openings into the cortex. In children, exudate that reaches the outer surface of the cortex forms abscesses that lift the periosteum of underlying bone. Lifting of the periosteum disrupts blood vessels that enter bone through the periosteum, which deprives underlying bone of its blood supply. This leads to necrosis and death of the area of bone infected, producing sequestrum, an area of devitalized bone (Fig. 44.19). Lifting of the periosteum also stimulates an intense osteoblastic response. Osteoblasts laying down new bone can partially or completely surround the infected bone. This layer of new bone surrounding the infected bone is called an involucrum. Openings in the involucrum allow the exudate to escape into surrounding soft tissue and ultimately through the skin by way of sinus tracts. Involucrum in adults is rare because the periosteum is firmly attached to the cortex and resists displacement. Instead, infection disrupts and weakens the cortex, which predisposes the bone to pathologic fracture.

Clinical Manifestations. Clinical manifestations of osteomyelitis vary with the age of the individual, the site of involvement, the initiating event, the infecting organism, and whether the infection is acute, subacute, or chronic. Osteomyelitis is generally considered acute if diagnosed within 2 weeks after symptom onset and is associated with an abrupt onset of inflammation (see Fig. 44.19). Subacute osteomyelitis is disease that has been present from one to several months, while chronic osteomyelitis is that which has been present for many months to even years.

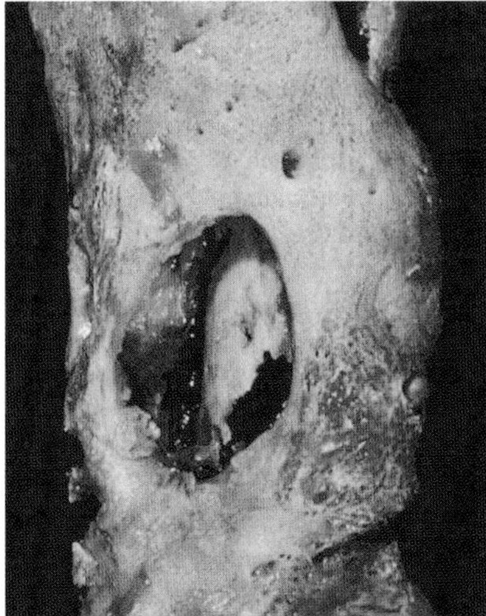

Fig. 44.19 Resected Femur in a Person With Draining Osteomyelitis. The drainage tract in the subperiosteal shell of viable new bone (involucrum) reveals the inner native necrotic cortex (sequestrum). (From Kumar V, et al. *Robbins & Cotran pathologic basis of disease,* 9th edition. Philadelphia: Saunders; 2015.)

If an acute infection is not eliminated, the disease may become subacute or chronic. In subacute osteomyelitis, signs and symptoms are usually vague. In the chronic stage, infection is silent between exacerbations. The microorganisms persist in small abscesses or fragments of necrotic bone and produce occasional exacerbations of acute osteomyelitis. The progression from acute to subacute osteomyelitis may be the result of inadequate or inappropriate therapy, or the development of drug-resistant microorganisms.

In the adult, hematogenous osteomyelitis has an insidious onset. The symptoms are usually vague and include fever, malaise, anorexia, weight loss, and pain in and around the infected areas. Edema may or may not be evident. Recent infection (urinary, respiratory, cutaneous) or instrumentation (catheterization, cystoscopy, myelography, diskography) usually precedes onset of symptoms.

Back pain is the primary symptom in vertebral osteomyelitis. Pain may be intermittent or constant, aggravated by motion, and throbbing at rest. It may radiate in a radicular distribution and is commonly accompanied by spinal tenderness and rigidity. Hip contracture can occur in the presence of soft tissue inflammation as a result of irritation of the psoas muscle.

Signs and symptoms of sacroiliac osteomyelitis are generally severe and include local pain, tenderness, and a limp. The pain may radiate to the buttock or the abdomen.

Single or multiple abscesses (Brodie abscesses) characterize subacute or chronic osteomyelitis. Brodie abscesses are painless, circumscribed lesions 1 to 4 cm in diameter, usually in the ends of long bones and surrounded by dense ossified bone matrix. The abscesses are thought to develop when the infectious microorganism has become less virulent or the individual's immune system is resisting the infection somewhat successfully.

In exogenous osteomyelitis, signs and symptoms of soft tissue infection predominate. Inflammatory exudate in the soft tissues disrupts muscles and supporting structures and forms abscesses. Low-grade fever, lymphadenopathy, local pain, and swelling usually occur within days of contamination by a puncture wound. Osteomyelitis in the hand causes exquisite tenderness over the course of tendon sheaths. The fingers are usually in a semiflexed position, and extension usually causes severe pain. Palmar swelling or symmetrical swelling of the fingers may be present.

Evaluation and Treatment. Laboratory data show an elevated white cell count and an elevated level of noncardiac C-reactive protein (CRP). Radiographic studies include radionuclide bone scanning, CT, functional imaging using a combination of radionuclide scanning (using fluorodeoxyglucose [FDG]) and single photon emission computed tomography (SPECT), positron emission tomography (PET), and MRI. MRI scanning with gadolinium contrast shows both bone and soft tissue, providing more accurate assessment of infection. MRI also shows early changes of bone marrow edema. FDG-SPECT imaging is highly sensitive for evaluating osteomyelitis of the extremities.

Treatment of osteomyelitis includes bone biopsy to identify the causative organism, use of antimicrobial agents, and surgical debridement of infected bone. Initial antibiotic therapy should be intravenous. Chronic conditions may require surgical removal of the inflammatory exudate or any involved implanted hardware followed by continuous wound irrigation with antibiotic solutions in addition to systemic treatment with antibiotics. Hyperbaric oxygen therapy of 100% oxygen, given at 2 atmospheres of pressure for 2 hours' duration per day for 30 treatments, is also beneficial for chronic refractory osteomyelitis. This therapy has been shown to stimulate healing by suppressing proinflammatory cytokines and prostaglandins.

Bone Tumors

Primary bone cancer is rare and metastatic disease commonly affects bone. Many different types of tumors involve the skeleton. Based on the tissue of origin, bone tumors are classified as osteogenic, chondrogenic, collagenic, or myelogenic. Each of the four types arises from one of the four stem cells that are ultimately derived from the primitive mesoderm (Fig. 44.20) In addition, bone tumors may be classified as being of histiocytic, notochordal, lipogenic, and neurogenic origins (Box 44.5). Chondrogenic tumors contain chondroblasts and produce an intercellular substance similar to chondroid (cartilage). Collagenic tumors contain fibrous tissue cells and produce an intercellular substance similar to the type of collagen found in fibrous connective tissue.

Tumors also are classified as benign or malignant. The criteria used to identify tumor cells as malignant are (1) an increased nuclear/cytoplasmic ratio, (2) an irregular nuclear border, (3) an excess of chromatin, (4) a prominent nucleolus, and (5) an increase in the number of cells undergoing mitosis. However, many young, rapidly growing, normal cells and cells subjected to inflammation and change in their blood supply also exhibit many of these same characteristics. (Tumor biology is described in Chapter 12.)

Epidemiology

The incidence of bone tumors varies with age. Osteosarcoma is the most common primary malignant bone tumor in children and young adults. Adolescents have the highest incidence of bone tumors, and adults between 30 and 35 years of age have the lowest incidence. After age 35, the incidence slowly increases until, at age 60, it equals the incidence in adolescents, primarily related to metastatic tumors.

Patterns of Bone Destruction

The general pathologic features of bone tumors include bone destruction, erosion or expansion of the cortex, and periosteal response to changes in underlying bone. The least amount of pathologic damage occurs with benign bone tumors that push against neighboring tissue. Because they usually have a symmetrical, controlled growth pattern, benign bone tumors tend to compress and displace neighboring normal bone tissue, which weakens the bone's structure until it is incapable of withstanding the stress of ordinary use, leading to pathologic fracture. Other tumors invade and destroy adjacent normal bone tissue by producing substances that promote resorption by increasing osteoclast activity or by interfering with a bone's blood supply. Three patterns of bone destruction by bone tumors have been identified: (1) the geographic pattern, (2) the moth-eaten pattern, and (3) the permeative pattern (Table 44.6).

Tumors that erode the cortex of the bone usually stimulate new bone formation at the interface between the surface of the bone and the periosteum. Slow erosion of the cortex usually stimulates a uniform periosteal response. Additional layers of bone are added to the exterior surface of the bone to buttress the cortex. Eventually the additional layers expand the bone's contour. Aggressive penetration of the cortex elevates the periosteum and stimulates erratic patterns of new bone formation. This may result in concentric layers of new bone, a sunburst pattern in which delicate rays of new bone radiate toward the periosteum from a single focus on the underlying surface, and rays of new bone that grow perpendicularly, creating a brush or bristle pattern.

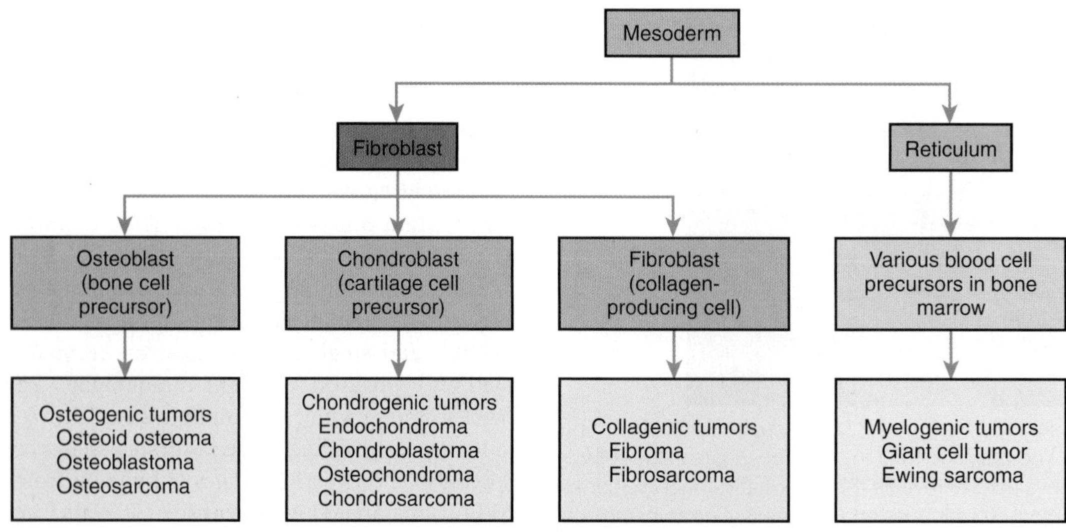

Fig. 44.20 Derivation of Bone Tumors.

BOX 44.5 World Health Organization Classification of Bone Tumors

Cartilage Tumors
Chondrosarcoma (M)
Chondroma (B)
Osteochondroma (B; but may become malignant)
Chondroblastoma (B)

Osteogenic Tumors
Osteoblastoma (B)
Osteoid osteoma (B)
Osteosarcoma (M)

Fibrogenic Tumors (Often Produce Collagen; Do Not Have a Mineralizing Matrix)
Fibrosarcoma (M)

Fibrohistiocytic Tumors (Comprised of Fibroblasts)
Benign fibrous histiocytoma (B)
Malignant fibrous histiocytoma (M)

Ewing Sarcoma
Ewing sarcoma (M)

Hematopoietic Tumors
Plasma cell myeloma (M)
Malignant lymphoma (M)

Giant Cell Tumor
Giant cell tumor (B, but can grow aggressively)
Malignancy in giant cell tumor (M; very rare tumor)

Smooth Muscle Tumors
Leiomyoma (B)
Leiomyosarcoma (M)

Miscellaneous Tumors
Adamantinoma (M; almost exclusively found in tibia)
Metastatic malignancy (M; most common skeletal malignancy)

Miscellaneous Lesions
Aneurysmal bone cyst (B)
Simple cyst (B)
Fibrous dysplasia (B; rarely can become malignant)
Osteofibrous dysplasia (B)
Langerhans cell histiocytosis (B, but can aggressively grow)
Chest wall hamartoma (B; is excessive growth of mesenchymal tissue [mostly cartilage])

Joint Lesions
Synovial chondromatosis (B; rarely becomes M)
B, Benign lesion; *M*, malignant lesion.

Data from Dorfman HD, et al. WHO classification of tumours of the bone: introduction. In: Christopher EM, et al., eds. *World Health Organization classification of tumors, International Agency for Research on Cancer (IARC) Pathology and Genetics of Tumours of Soft Tissue and Bone.* Lyon, France: IARC Press; 2002:226.

TABLE 44.6 Patterns of Bone Destruction by Bone Tumors

Type of Destruction	Pattern Seen
Geographic	Well-defined margins separated from surrounding normal bone; well-defined lytic area in affected bone
Moth-eaten	Less-defined margin not easily separated from normal bone; areas of partially destroyed bone adjacent to completely lytic areas
Permeative	Poorly demarcated margins; abnormal lytic bone merges imperceptibly with surrounding normal bone

TABLE 44.7 The Enneking Surgical Staging System for Malignant Bone Tumors

Stage	Grade	Site (T)	Metastasis (M)
IA	Low (G_1)	Intracompartmental (T_1)	None (M_0)
IB	Low (G_1)	Extracompartmental (T_2)	None (M_0)
IIA	High (G_2)	Intracompartmental (T_1)	None (M_0)
IIB	High (G_2)	Extracompartmental (T_2)	None (M_0)
IIIA	Low (G_1)	Intracompartmental or extracompartmental (T_1 or T_2)	Regional or distant (M_1)
IIIB	High (G_2)	Intracompartmental or extracompartmental (T_1 or T_2)	Regional or distant (M_1)

Diagnosis

Malignant bone tumors account for less than 0.2% of all cancers. A tumor must be identified early to allow survival of the individual and the preservation of the affected limb. However, individuals often have vague symptoms that may be attributed to minor trauma, degenerative changes, or inflammatory conditions. In addition, other conditions may obscure the diagnosis.

Thorough diagnostic studies are needed to determine the exact type and extent of bone tumor present, which also helps determine the optimal treatment regimen. Staging of any bone tumor is critical to determine future treatment and results. The American Joint Committee on Cancer (AJCC) staging system (also known as the *Enneking* or *TNM staging system*) is the most commonly used arrangement (Table 44.7). This system classifies tumors according to grade (G), tumor site (T), and metastasis (M). Benign tumors are given a numeric value of zero for their grade, whereas malignant tumors are low grade (G_1) or high grade (G_2).

Serum alkaline phosphatase levels are elevated in bone lytic tumors, and they are significantly elevated in osteosarcoma and Ewing sarcoma. Radiologic studies include plain radiologic film, technetium-99 bone scan, CT scan, and MRI, which has become the examination of choice for the local staging of bone tumors, especially the staging of peripheral osteosarcomas (see Table 44.7). MRI is also used to monitor the response of osteosarcomas to radiation or chemotherapy and to detect recurrent disease. A CT scan can evaluate involvement of osteosarcoma in flat bones when the tumor is not well-defined on a plain film, can assist in differentiating the tumor, and can locate pulmonary metastases. Radionucleotide bone scans show an increased uptake at the tumor site. Before any surgical procedure, placement of bone biopsy is critical.

Additional diagnostic studies performed for specific bone tumors include a complete blood count and erythrocyte sedimentation rate (to rule out infection, myeloma, or Ewing sarcoma) and measurement of serum levels of calcium and phosphorus to detect hypercalcemia. Serum glucose levels may be elevated in chondrosarcoma. Acid phosphatase level may be moderately elevated in bone metastases, multiple myeloma, and advanced Paget disease. Serum protein electrophoresis and immunoelectrophoresis are done to rule out multiple myeloma. Fine-needle biopsy is done, usually at the time of surgery, to determine the exact tumor type.

Types

A large number of lesions are classified as bone tumors. Bone tumors are typically classified according to their origin—osteogenic, chondrogenic, collagenic, and myelogenic tumors.

Osteogenic tumors: Osteosarcoma. Osteogenic (bone-forming) tumors are characterized by the formation of bone or osteoid tissue with a sarcomatous tissue. The tissue can have the appearance of compact or spongy bone. The most common malignant bone-forming tumor is osteosarcoma (Fig. 44.21), which is typically found in the bone marrow. Osteosarcoma occurs mostly in adolescents and young adults; 60% of osteosarcomas occur in those younger than 20 years, and it has a slightly higher incidence in males. A secondary peak incidence for osteosarcoma occurs in the 60 and older age group, primarily in individuals with a history of radiation therapy several years previously for pelvic or other malignancies.

Pathophysiology. Osteosarcoma is aggressive and has a moth-eaten pattern of bone destruction. The borders of the tumor are indistinct and merge into adjacent normal bone. Osteosarcomas contain osteoid and callus produced by anaplastic stromal cells, which are atypical, abnormal cells not seen in normal developing bone; they are neither normal nor embryonal. Many tumors are heterogeneous; for example, the osteosarcoma also may contain chondroid (cartilage) (e.g., chondroblastic sarcoma) and fibrinoid tissue (e.g., fibroblastic sarcoma) that may form the bulk of the tumor. The osteoid is deposited as thick masses or "streamers" which infiltrate the normal compact bone, destroy it, and replace it with masses of osteoid. Bone tissue produced by osteosarcomas never matures to compact bone.

Ninety percent of osteosarcomas are located in the metaphyses of long bones, especially the distal femoral metaphysis, with 50% around the knee area. The tumor typically impregnates the cortex, lifts the periosteum, and forms a soft tissue mass that is not covered by a smooth shell of new bone. Lifting of the periosteum stimulates bizarre patterns of new bone formation, called a *periosteal reaction.* Distinct osteosarcomas occur on the surface of long bones, called *parosteal, periosteal,* and *high-grade surface osteosarcomas*; dedifferentiated parosteal and central osteosarcomas also occur.

Clinical Manifestations. The most common initial symptoms are pain and swelling. The pain is initially slight and intermittent, but increases in severity and duration. Pain is usually worse at night and gradually requires medication. Often, a coincidental history of trauma is noted. Occasionally, the individual may present with a pathologic fracture.

Evaluation and Treatment. Systemic chemotherapy and surgery are the treatments of choice, with the location of the tumor and its size, grade, and pattern of metastasis dictating the type and extent of surgery. Preoperative chemotherapy has greatly increased the number of individuals qualifying for limb salvage surgery. Other agents under investigation include monoclonal antibodies, hormone antagonists, gene therapy, and other biologic agents.

Chondrogenic tumors: Chondrosarcoma. Chondrogenic (cartilage-forming) tumors produce cartilage or chondroid, a primitive cartilage or cartilage-like substance. The most common chondrogenic tumor is chondrosarcoma.

Chondrosarcoma is the second most common primary malignant bone tumor (Fig. 44.22). It is a tumor found in

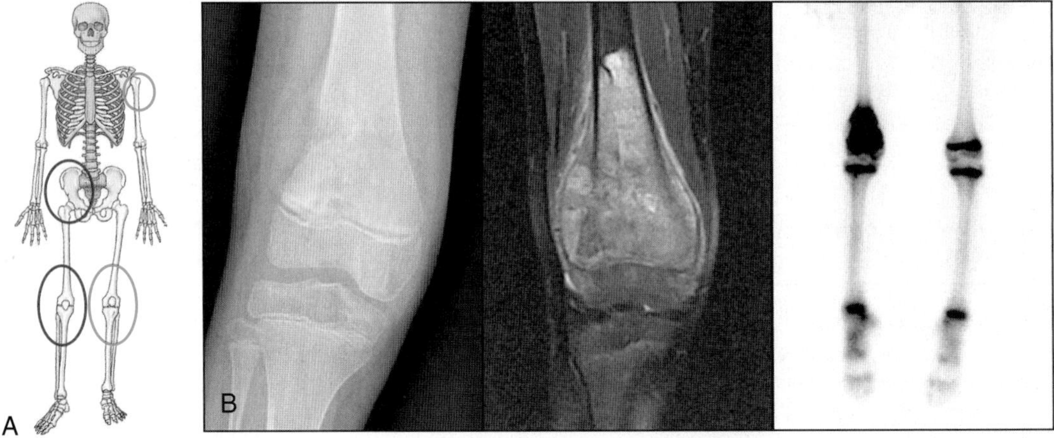

Fig. 44.21 Osteosarcoma. **(A)** Common locations of Ewing sarcoma and osteosarcoma. *blue,* Osteosarcoma; *red,* Ewing sarcoma. **(B)** Comparison of plain radiograph, MRI, and nuclear bone scan appearances of osteosarcoma of the distal femur. Note destruction of the bone cortex and soft tissue component. (A, Adapted from Bontrager KL, Lampignanno JP, eds. *Textbook of radiographic positioning and related anatomy.* St. Louis: Elsevier; 2013. B, From HaDuong JH, Martin AA, Skapek SX, et al. Sarcomas. *Pediatric Clinics of North America,* 2015;62:179–200.)

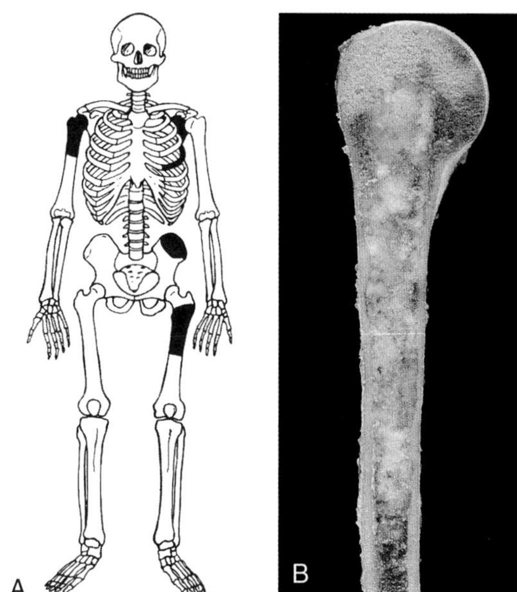

Fig. 44.22 Chondrosarcoma. **(A)** Common locations of chondrosarcoma. **(B)** Chondrosarcoma of humerus. (From Damjanov I, Linder J, eds. *Anderson's pathology,* 10th edition. St. Louis: Mosby; 1996.)

middle-aged and older adults, with peak incidence in the sixth decade of life. The tumor is found more commonly in men than in women. Chondrosarcomas that develop from a preexisting benign bone lesion (e.g., an enchondroma) are known as secondary chondrosarcomas. Individuals with certain conditions, such as multiple osteochondromas, may be at greater risk for developing secondary chondrosarcoma. Secondary chondrosarcomas are rare, occurring most often in young adults between 20 and 30 years of age, and are more common in men.

Pathophysiology. A chondrosarcoma is a large, ill-defined malignant tumor that infiltrates trabeculae in spongy bone. It produces cartilage-forming cells, without ossification, that occur normally in bone formation. It appears most often in the metaphysis or diaphysis of long bones, especially the femur or proximal humerus, and in the bones of the pelvis (see Fig. 44.22). Chondrosarcomas typically implant in surrounding tissue *(seeding).*

Clinical Manifestations. Symptoms associated with a chondrosarcoma have an insidious onset. Local swelling accompanied by a dull, intermittent pain is the usual presenting symptom. The pain gradually intensifies and becomes constant, awakening the person at night.

Evaluation and Treatment. Diagnostic studies include radiographs, which must be reviewed carefully for an accurate diagnosis. Biopsy is done at the time of surgery. Performing a bone biopsy prior to surgery can result in seeding of tumor cells and metastasis. Additionally, sufficient tumor material must be obtained to facilitate an accurate diagnosis.

Surgical excision is generally regarded as the treatment of choice because chemotherapy and radiation seem to have little effect. Many surgically treated individuals demonstrate recurrences, thus amputation becomes one treatment of choice.

Collagenic tumors: Fibrosarcoma. Collagenic (collagen-forming) tumors produce fibrous connective tissue. Fibrosarcoma is the most common collagenic tumor and can affect bone or soft tissue.

Pathophysiology. Fibrosarcomas come from fibroblasts that originate from MSCs; they represent 4% of primary malignant bone tumors. The incidence has a broad age range, but this tumor type is most common in adults between 30 and 50 years of age. The incidence is slightly greater in females. Fibrosarcoma also may be a secondary complication of radiation therapy, Paget disease, and long-standing osteomyelitis; secondary fibrosarcoma tends to be more aggressive with a poorer outcome.

Fibrosarcoma is a solitary tumor that most often affects the metaphyseal region of the femur or tibia. The tumor is composed of a firm, fibrous mass of tissue that contains collagen, malignant fibroblasts, and occasional osteoclast-like giant cells.

The tumor begins in the marrow cavity of the bone and infiltrates the trabeculae. It demonstrates a permeative growth pattern, destroys the cortex, and extends into the soft tissue. Metastasis to the lung is common.

Clinical Manifestations. Symptoms associated with the tumor have an insidious onset, which delays diagnosis. Pain and swelling are the usual presenting symptoms and usually indicate that the tumor has infiltrated the cortex. Local tenderness, a palpable mass, and limitation of motion also may be present. A pathologic fracture in the affected bone is often the reason for seeking medical help. Diagnostic studies include radiographs and MRI.

Evaluation and Treatment. Radical surgery and amputation are the treatments of choice for fibrosarcoma. Radiation therapy is generally considered ineffective treatment for this tumor.

Myelogenic tumors. Myelogenic tumors originate from various bone marrow cells. Two types of myelogenic tumors are giant cell tumor (GCT) and myeloma. Myeloma is discussed in Chapter 29.

Giant cell tumor. Giant cell tumor (GCT) is the sixth most common primary bone tumor, accounting for 4% to 5% of bone tumors. GCTs have a wide age distribution; however, they are rare in persons younger than 10 years or older than 70 years. Most GCTs are found in persons between 20 and 40 years of age. Unlike most other bone tumors, GCTs affect females more often than males.

Pathophysiology. The GCTs are generally benign, solitary, circumscribed tumors that cause extensive bone resorption because of their osteoclastic origin. There is a high rate of recurrence, but metastasis is rare. A GCT is typically located in the epiphyseal regions of the femur, tibia, radius, or humerus (Fig. 44.23). The tumor has a slow, relentless growth rate, and it is usually contained within the original contour of the affected bone. Aggressive bone resorption causes pathologic fractures. However, it may extend into the articular cartilage. When the tumor extends, it is usually covered by periosteum or periosteal bone growth; it may extend into surrounding soft tissue.

Clinical Manifestations. The most common symptoms associated with GCT are pain, local swelling, and limitation of movement.

Evaluation and Treatment. Diagnostic studies include radiographs, CT, and MRI. Cryosurgery and resection of the tumor

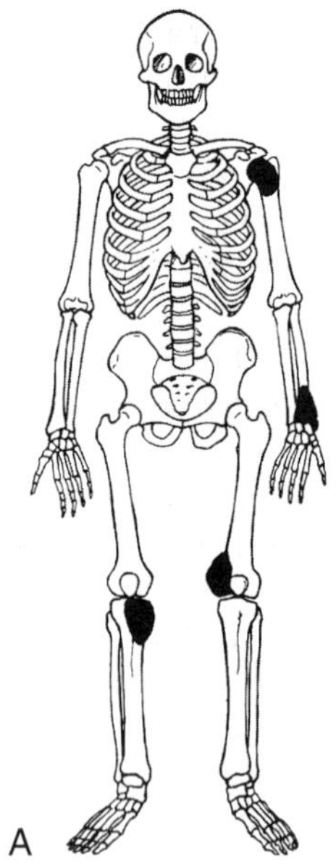

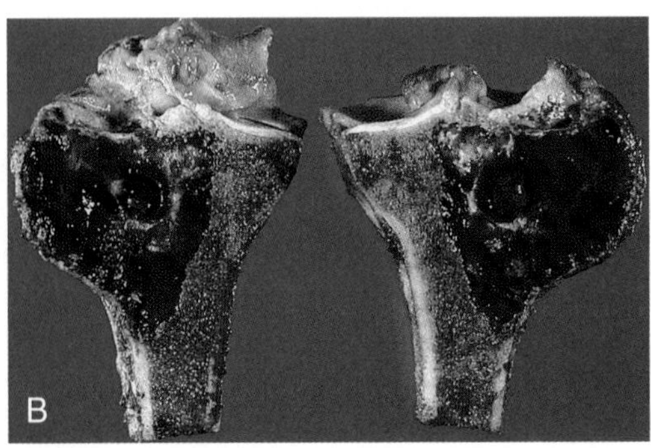

Fig. 44.23 Giant Cell Tumor of Bone. (A) Common skeletal locations. **(B)** Gross picture of cell tumor of bone (epimetaphysis). (From Damjanov I, Linder J, eds. *Anderson's pathology,* 10th edition. St. Louis: Mosby; 1996.)

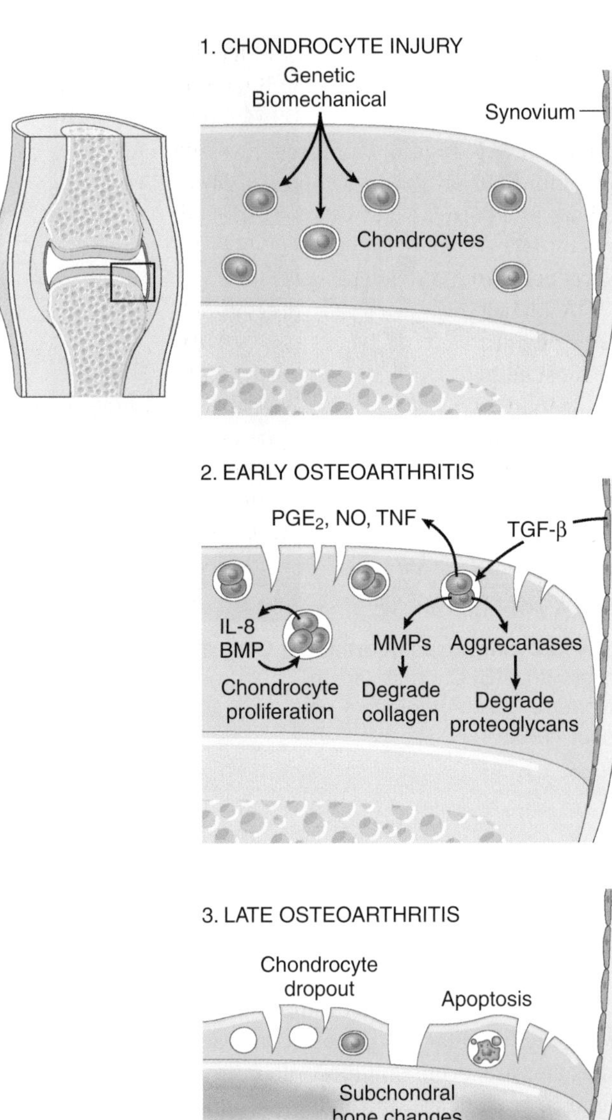

Fig. 44.24 Osteoarthritis. *(1)* Osteoarthritis (OA) is initiated by biomechanical cartilage damage, it is accelerated in genetically predisposed individuals and results in changes to the extracellular matrix, *(2)* chondrocytes may proliferate to try and repair the damaged matrix, degradation exceeds repair in early OA, *(3)* Late OA has loss of both matrix and chondrocytes with subchondral bone loss (From Kumar V, et al. *Robbins & Cotran pathologic basis of disease,* 10th edition. Philadelphia: Elsevier; 2021.)

with the use of adjuvant polymethylmethacrylate (PMMA) for bone grafts reduce recurrence and are more successful treatments than curettage and radiation. Amputation may be necessary but is not common.

DISORDERS OF JOINTS

The American College of Rheumatology (ACR) recognizes a growing body of evidence identifying and classifying joint diseases, called arthropathies. The two major categories of these disorders include noninflammatory joint disease and inflammatory joint disease. Current detection methods, through diagnostic imaging and serum and synovial fluid analysis, allow for a clearer delineation between the inflammatory and noninflammatory pathways once poorly understood.

Osteoarthritis

Osteoarthritis (OA) is the most common form of age-related joint disease involving the synovial joints. OA is characterized by pathologic changes in cartilage, bone, synovium, ligament, muscle, and periarticular fat (Fig. 44.24).[37] These changes lead to joint dysfunction, pain, stiffness, functional limitation, and loss of activities, such as walking for exercise.[37] Though the term OA implies an inflammatory disease, it is mostly considered a degenerative disease of cartilage.[38] Advancing disease shows first molecular derangement or abnormal joint tissue metabolism, followed by anatomic and/or physiologic derangements. The physiologic changes include cartilage degradation, bone remodeling, osteophyte formation (bone spurs), joint inflammation, and loss of normal joint function, and progresses to illness.[37,39]

OA is commonly found in the knees, hips, hands, and spine.[37] Globally, OA causes moderate to severe disability in 43 million people, and in the United States it is estimated that 80% of those over 65 years old have radiographic evidence of OA. 60% of this subset has symptoms.[40] Risk factors include age (33% older than 75 years have symptomatic and radiographic knee OA), female, obesity, genetics, and previous joint injury. The level of disease severity detected radiographically does not correlate well with pain and disability.[38] Those with OA have more comorbidities and are more sedentary.[37] OA is associated with comorbidities linked to lack of physical activity, medication toxicity, and the effects of inflammatory cytokines.[37,41]

OA is a heterogenous disease process and is classified into two categories: primary and secondary. *Primary OA* or *idiopathic* is the most common and is diagnosed in the absence of a predisposing trauma or disease and is associated with risk factors listed above. *Secondary OA* occurs with preexisting joint abnormality from conditions such as congenital joint disorders, inflammatory arthritis, avascular necrosis, infectious arthritis, Paget disease, osteopetrosis, osteochondritis dissecans, metabolic disorders (e.g., hemochromatosis, Wilson disease), hemoglobinopathy, Ehlers–Danlos syndrome, or Marfan syndrome.[42,43]

Pathophysiology. The primary defect in OA is degeneration and eventual loss and disordered repair of articular cartilage. The chondrocytes of the articular cartilage become damaged early in the disease process because of biomechanical stress, as well as genetic and biochemical factors (Fig. 44.25A and C). These changes lead to increased chondrocyte injury, altered chondrocyte signaling, and alterations of the extracellular matrix (ECM).[44,45] The progressive destruction of ECM is considered a hallmark.[46] The ECM is synthesized by chondrocytes, which have a key role in maintaining an equilibrium between anabolism and catabolism.[46] Although chondrocytes proliferate and continuously make proteoglycans, OA develops when degradation exceeds synthesis.[38] A phenotypic alteration to hypertrophic chondrocyte occurs, causing chondrocytes to proliferate and form clusters.[40] When collagen matrix is damaged, chondrocytes undergo apoptosis.[40] The ECM is essential for the biomechanical properties of cartilage because it provides critical elastic support to distribute pressure and shear stress with joint movement.[46] Chondrocytes secrete matrix metalloproteases

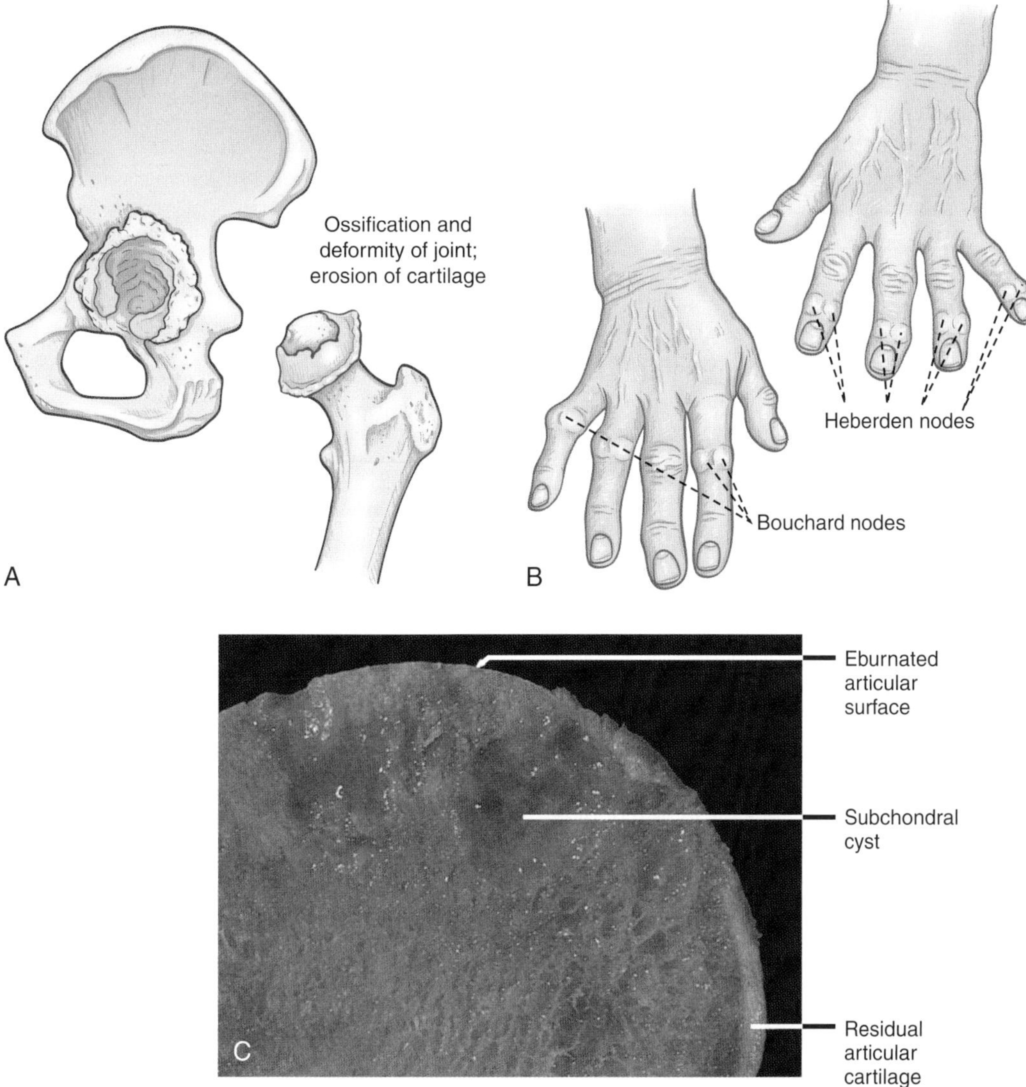

Fig. 44.25 Osteoarthritis (OA). **(A)** Cartilage, and degeneration of the hip joint from osteoarthritis. **(B)** Heberden nodes and Bouchard nodes. **(C)** Severe osteoarthritis with small islands of residual articular cartilage next to exposed subchondral bone. (C, From Kumar V, et al. *Robbins & Cotran pathologic basis of disease,* 10th edition. Philadelphia: Elsevier; 2021.)

(MMPs) that degrade type II collagen. Other involved factors include cytokines, diffusible factors from chondrocytes and synovial cells, especially TGF-β (promotes the production of MMPs), TNF, prostaglandins, and nitric oxide. Altered mineralized collagen causes subchondral bone thickening, and bone cysts infrequently occur.[40] Soft tissues are affected, such as ligaments, joint capsule, and menisci.[40] Chronic low-level inflammation can contribute to disease progression.[38] Overall, advanced disease involves chondrocyte loss and severe matrix degradation.[38]

Clinical Manifestations. Individuals with primary OA are usually asymptomatic until their 50 s.[38] If a younger person has manifestations of OA, it triggers a search for underlying causes. The triad of symptoms include joint pain (deep, achy) that worsens with use, morning stiffness, and motor restriction.[40] Other manifestations include muscle weakness, *crepitus* (grating sound or sensation by friction between bone and cartilage), and balance issues (Box 44.6).[40]

Pain is related to activity and resolves with rest, but with disease progression, pain is more constant and affects activities of daily living and eventually causes severe restrictions in function.[40] Individuals will use the following descriptors: bony swelling, joint deformity, instability, and "giving way" or "buckling," a sign of muscle weakness.[40] Joint deformities can develop with time. The types of joint deformities in the fingers are termed Bouchard nodes and Heberden nodes, which are typical features of OA (see Fig. 44.25B). Bouchard nodes are prominent osteophytes (mushroom shaped bony outgrowths) at the proximal interphalangeal (PIP) joints, whereas Heberden nodes are prominent at the distal interphalangeal joints.

Inflammation of the joint capsule leads to remodeling and a fibrous contraction of the capsule, causing the joint to become stiff and painful with movement (Fig. 44.26). Inflammation of the joint lining, known as *synovitis*, is thought to be initiated by the release of cartilage ECM into the joint, which then activates the body's complement system. Swelling also occurs in response to tissue injury. Such injuries initiate the inflammatory cascade of cytokines and chemokines, resulting in capillary permeability and interstitial fluid collection. If inflammatory exudate or blood enters the joint cavity, the total volume of synovial fluid will be increased. This condition, termed joint effusion, is attributed to (1) the presence of osteophyte fragments in the synovial cavity, (2) drainage of cysts from diseased subchondral bone, or (3) acute trauma to joint structures, resulting in hemorrhage and inflammatory exudation into the synovial cavity (see Fig. 44.25C).

ROM may become limited to some degree, depending on the extent of cartilage degeneration. Frequently, joint motion is accompanied by crepitus, creaking, or grating. Abnormal knee alignment also has been shown to increase the incidence and progression of OA. The person may begin to noticeably limp as OA of the lower extremity progresses (Fig. 44.27). Either varus or valgus disorders of the knee of more than 5 degrees have been associated with increased risk of development and progression of OA.

Evaluation and Treatment. Evaluation consists primarily of individual subjective reports, clinical assessment, and radiologic studies. The ACR classification is widely used for OA.[40] A clinical diagnosis of OA is made if the following are found: (1) pain worse with activity and better with rest, (2) age greater than 45 years,

BOX 44.6 Signs and Symptoms of Osteoarthritis

Hand
- Pain on range of motion
- Hypertrophic changes at distal and proximal interphalangeal joints (Heberden nodes and Bouchard nodes)
- Tenderness over carpometacarpal joint of thumb

Shoulder
- Pain on range of motion
- Limitation of range of motion, especially external rotation
- Crepitus on range of motion

Knee
- Pain on range of motion
- Joint effusion
- Crepitus on range of motion
- Sometimes presence of popliteal cyst (Baker cyst)
- Lateral instability
- Valgus or varus deformity

Hip
- Pain on range of motion
- Pain in buttock
- Limitation of range of motion, especially internal rotation

Foot
- Pain on ambulation, especially at first metatarsophalangeal joint
- Limited range of motion of first metatarsophalangeal joint, hallux rigidus
- Hallux valgus deformity

Spine
- Pain on range of motion
- Limitation of range of motion
- Lower extremity sensory loss, reflex loss, motor weakness caused by nerve root impingement
- Pseudoclaudication caused by spinal stenosis

Data from Sinusas K. Osteoarthritis: diagnosis and treatment. *American Family Physician*, 2012;85(1):49–56.

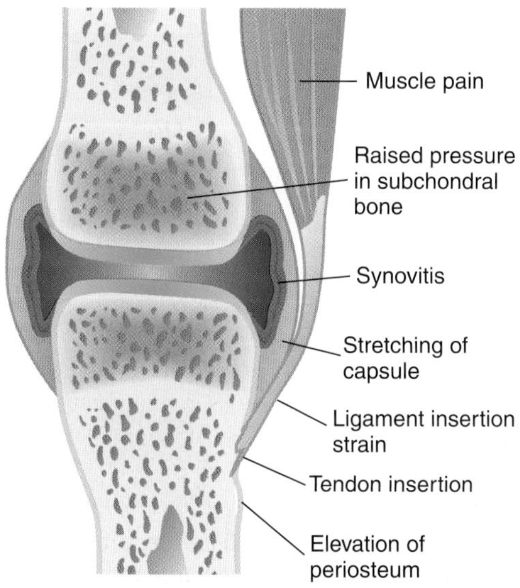

Fig. 44.26 Possible Causes of Pain in Osteoarthritis.

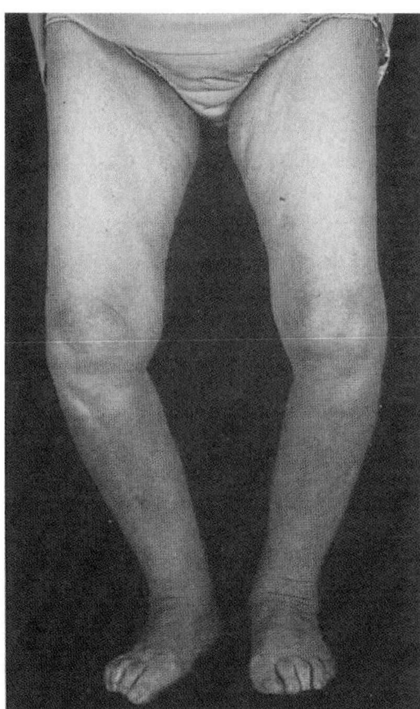

Fig. 44.27 Typical Varus Deformity of Knee Osteoarthritis. (From Doherty M. *Color atlas and text of osteoarthritis*. London: Wolfe; 1994.)

(3) morning stiffness lasting less than 30 minutes, (4) bony joint enlargement, and (5) ROM limitation.[40] There may be pain upon passive movement and tenderness at joint lines.[40] Imaging may include CT scan, arthroscopy, X-rays, and MRI, however MRI is not routinely indicated for OA workup.[40] Ultrasound can identify synovial inflammation, effusion, and osteophytes. Synovial fluid may be obtained and sent for evaluation and pathology. Normal blood evaluations include CBC, ESR, rheumatoid factor (RF), and ANA.[40] Widely used is the ACR classification.[40] A clinical diagnosis of OA is made if the following are found: (1).

Treatment is often determined by the severity of pain and immobility with the goal to minimize pain and functional loss.[40] Treatment regimens span from conservative to surgical, as well as nonpharmacologic to pharmacologic.[47–49] Lifestyle modification, particularly exercise and weight reduction, is a core management approach. Both exercise and weight loss have been shown to be two of the most important nonpharmacologic treatments in improving knee OA symptoms. Exercise can reduce pain and improve physical function in individuals with OA. Exercises to improve muscle tone, ROM, and balance; stretch the joint capsule; and reduce the fear of falling also have shown promise in reducing OA symptoms.

Although the use of biomechanical devices, such as foot wedges or alignment braces, has been shown to decrease pain, the reduction of disease progression has yet to be supported. Use of supportive devices is recommended, such as a cane, walker, brace, or other device to decrease weight bearing. Braces and foot orthoses may help correct biomechanical abnormalities, thereby reducing pain and improving mobility. Physical therapy is an important management strategy for OA. Weight loss reduces pain-associated inflammation and when combined with physical activity has a greater benefit. Dietary and nutritional recommendations include increasing intake of long-chain n-3 fatty acids, preferably by eating oily fish twice a week; aiming for a safe level of sun exposure; eating rich vitamin D dietary sources or taking vitamin D supplements ($\leq$25 μg/day); and increasing vitamin K intake by eating green, leafy vegetables. Nutraceuticals, such as chondroitin and glucosamine, have also shown success in relieving OA pain in some individuals. Pharmacologic therapies may include the use of analgesic and anti-inflammatory drug therapies to reduce swelling and pain. Acetaminophen has been shown to be less effective than nonsteroidal anti-inflammatory drugs (NSAIDs), such as ibuprofen. Because of gastrointestinal toxicity, adverse renal and cardiovascular effects, oral NSAIDs should be used very cautiously and with long-term close monitoring. Fewer systemic side effects occur with topical NSAIDs, but topical NSAIDs are less efficacious than their oral counterparts and often cause local skin irritation.[40] Intra-articular injection of corticosteroids and high-molecular-weight viscose supplements, such as hyaluronic acid, can be used as an effective treatment of acute pain. Surgical intervention may be used to improve joint movement, correct deformity or malalignment, or create a new joint with artificial implants. The key to surgery is timing because those with considerable muscle weakness may not gain postoperative functional status versus those undergoing surgery earlier.[40] Individuals with significant OA on imaging typically do poorly with partial meniscectomy.[50] For these individuals, knee arthroplasty is commonly the surgical procedure of choice.[51] More aggressive surgical procedures involve creating a new joint with artificial implants. See Emerging Science Box: Cartilage Regeneration to learn more about future treatments for damaged and/or deteriorated cartilage. Two of the most important nonpharmacologic treatments are exercise and weight loss for improving knee OA symptoms. Also considered are complementary and alternative therapies, with Tai Chi strongly recommended in the 2019 American College of Rheumatology and Arthritis guidelines.

EMERGING SCIENCE BOX

Cartilage Regeneration

Active research in the area of cartilage regeneration has revealed success in both animal and human models. This process involves first causing minor injury to the joint tissue, followed by the use of chemical signals and skeletal stem cells, to facilitate cartilage growth. Cartilage inherently has very limited ability to regenerate in adults. Therefore, the use of chemical signaling and stem cells is showing great promise for individuals with damaged and/or deteriorated cartilage. Skeletal stem cells are responsible for the production of bone, cartilage, and bone marrow. Through new and innovative emerging science, these cells are being used to regrow damaged cartilage, serving as another alternative treatment rather than joint replacement for arthritis.

Data From Vaughan, C. *Researchers find method to regrow cartilage in the joints*. Medical Xpress- Arthritis & Rheumatism; August 2020. https://medicalxpress.com/news/2020-08-method-regrow-cartilage-joints.html; Murphy MP, et al. Articular cartilage regeneration by activated skeletal stem cells. *Nature Medicine*, 2020. DOI: 10.1038/s41591-020-1013-2.

Inflammatory Joint Disease

Inflammatory joint disease, commonly called arthritis, is characterized by inflammatory damage or destruction in the synovial membrane or articular cartilage and by systemic signs of inflammation (fever, leukocytosis, malaise, anorexia, hyperfibrinogenemia).

Inflammatory joint disease can be infectious or noninfectious. In infectious inflammatory joint disease, inflammation is caused by invasion of the joint by bacteria, mycoplasmas, viruses, fungi, or protozoa. These microorganisms can invade the joint through a number of ports of entry, such as a traumatic wound, surgical incision, or contaminated needle. Additionally, these pathogens can be delivered by the bloodstream from sites of entry through the body's mucous membranes, as well as infections elsewhere in the body, such as bones, heart valves, or blood vessels. Noninfectious inflammatory joint disease, such as gout, is the more common form, and is caused by immune response to the deposition of crystals of monosodium urate (MSU) in and around the joint. RA, psoriatic arthritis, and ankylosing spondylitis (AS) are other noninfectious inflammatory diseases caused by immune and hypersensitivity reactions.

Rheumatoid Arthritis

Rheumatoid arthritis (RA) is a chronic, systemic, inflammatory autoimmune disease distinguished by joint swelling, tenderness, and destruction of synovial joints leading to disability.[52,53] (Autoimmune disease is described in Chapter 9.) RA involves synovial inflammation, joint swelling, and ankylosis and destruction of articular cartilage. RA may cause inflammation of other tissues and organs, but predominately affects the joints. The first joint tissue to be affected is the synovial membrane, which lines the joint cavity (see Chapter 43). The two primary types of synovial cells are fibroblast-like synovial cells and macrophage-like synovial cells. The joints most commonly affected are in the fingers, feet, wrists, elbows, ankles, and knees. Other joints, such as shoulders, hips, and cervical spine, also may be involved, as well as the tissues of the lungs, heart, kidneys, and skin. In addition to joint inflammation and tissue damage, RA can cause fever, malaise, rash, lymph node or spleen enlargement, and Raynaud phenomenon (transient lack of circulation to the fingertips and toes). Internationally, the incidence and prevalence of RA ranges from 0.4% to 1.3%. The incidence of RA increases with age and peaks at ages 65 to 74 years, with women having a greater lifetime risk than men (4% vs. 3%). The incidence and prevalence of RA have decreased in developing countries to approximately 1% of the adult population.[54,55]

Risk factors for developing RA include female sex, environmental factors, and genetics/epigenetics (Fig. 44.28). Cigarette smoking is a known risk factor for RA, and in those with *anti-citrullinated peptide antibodies* (ACPAs) an interaction between

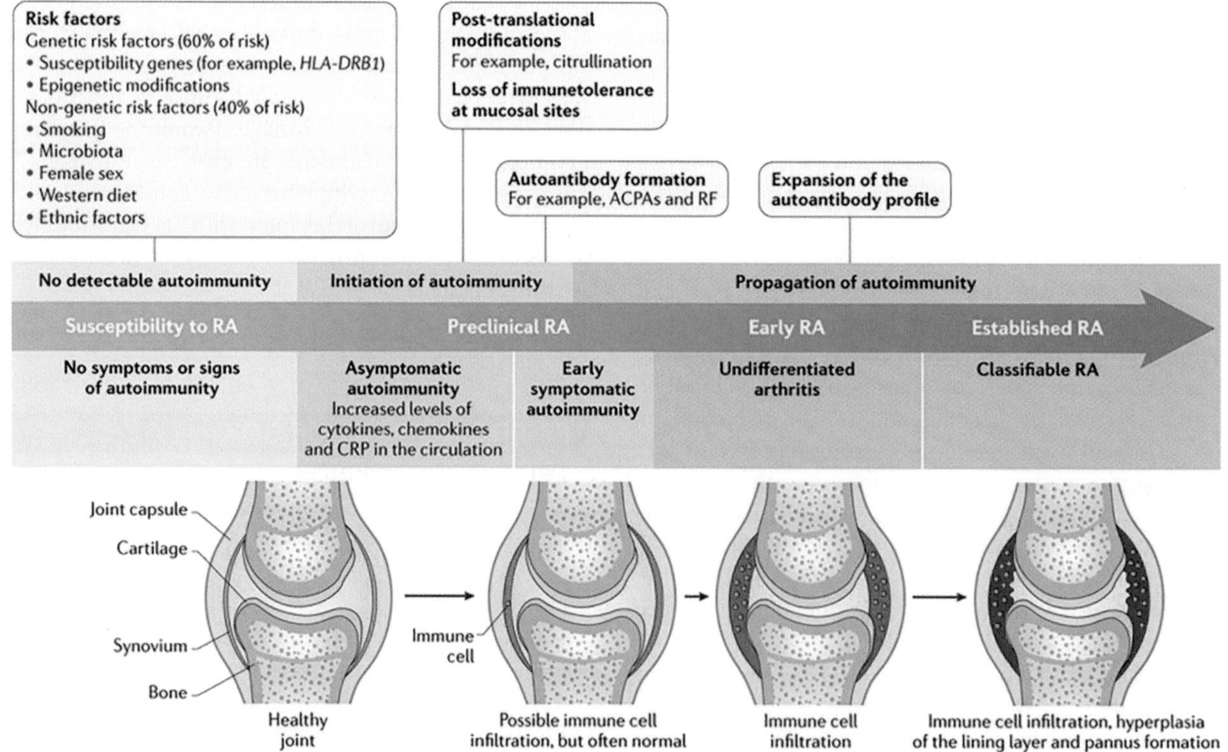

Fig. 44.28 Risk Factors, Development, and Progression of Rheumatoid Arthritis. Genetic, epigenetic, and environmental risk factors contribute to rheumatoid arthritis *(RA)*. Disease progression involves initiation and promotion of autoimmunity against modified self-proteins. These interactions can occur years before the onset of subclinical synovitis (inflammation of the synovium) and clinical symptoms. *ACPA*, Anti-citrullinated protein antibody; *CRP*, C-reactive protein; *RF*, rheumatoid factor. (From Smolen JS, Aletaha D, Barton A, et al. Rheumatoid arthritis. *Nature Reviews Disease Primers,* 2018;4:180001.)

genes and smoking has been reported.[56,57] Another risk factor is silica. A case-control study of firefighters exposed to dust at the World Trade Center collapse found an increased risk of systemic autoimmune diseases including RA.[58] Occupational exposure to textile dust was found significantly correlated with developing RA in a group of Malaysian women.[59] Periodontal disease is associated with an increased risk of developing RA.[60] The association with periodontal disease is partly mediated by the oral microbiota, such as *Porphyromonas gingivalis* and *Aggregatibacter actinomycetemcomitans*.[52] Importantly, the gut microbiota may have a role and needs further study.[61]

Pathophysiology. RA is a chronic autoimmune disease initiated by CD4$^+$ helper T cells (Fig. 44.29). The pathologic changes are mediated by antibodies against self-antigens, such as ACPAs detected in the serum of up to 70% of those with RA.[38] CD4$^+$ T cells promote inflammation. Acting together, T cells produce cytokines that stimulate other inflammatory cells and promote tissue injury. The most significant cytokines include interferon-gamma (IFN-γ) (activates macrophages and synovial cells), IL-17 (stimulates neutrophils and monocytes), TNF and IL-1 (stimulate synovial cells to secrete proteases that damage hyaline cartilage), and RANKL (activates bone resorption and erosion).

During inflammation, arginine (an α-amino acid) can be enzymatically modified into another α-amino acid, citrulline.

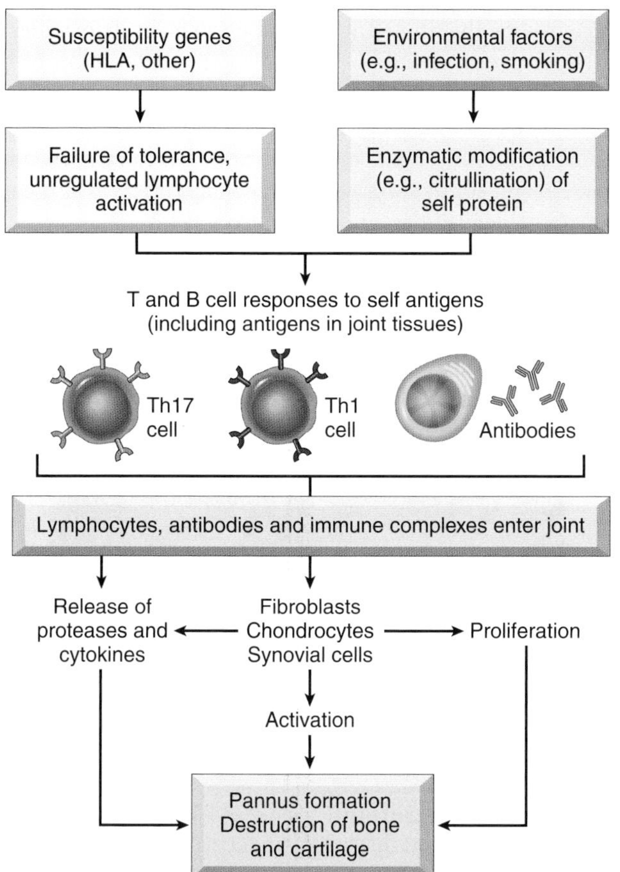

Fig. 44.29 Pathogenesis of Rheumatoid Arthritis. *HLA,* Human leukocyte antigen. (From Kumar V, et al. *Robbins & Cotran pathologic basis of disease,* 10th edition. Philadelphia: Elsevier; 2021.)

The process (citrullination) changes the structure and function of the protein. Other proteins, like fibrin and vimentin, can become citrullinated during cell death and tissue inflammation. In turn, the citrullinated proteins may act as new antigenic determinants or epitopes.

Given the strong genetic predisposition to developing RA, many genes have been studied as risk factors for RA, and some are involved in immune function. Genetic risk factors for RA have been localized to variations in the human leukocyte antigen (HLA) genes, particularly the HLA-DRB4 allele. The proteins produced from HLA genes assist the immune system with distinguishing self-proteins from proteins made by invaders such as bacteria and viruses. Investigation of epigenetic factors, such as histone deacetylases, can confer the effects of environmental triggers, such as smoking or diet (e.g., *n*-3 fatty acids, or in combination with γ-linolenic acid [GLA]), or treatment on expression levels of target genes.

Chronic inflammation results from an intricate interplay of chemokines that are powerful mediators of inflammation. Chemokines attract T cells and produce inflammatory changes With long-term or intensive exposure to the antigen, normal antibodies (immunoglobulins [Igs]) become autoantibodies—antibodies that attack host tissues (self-antigens). Because they are usually present in individuals with RA, the altered antibodies are termed rheumatoid factors (RFs). The RFs are mainly autoantibodies reactive with the Fc part of IgG antibodies. RFs bind with their target self-antigens in blood and synovial membrane, forming immune complexes (antigen-antibody complexes) (see Chapter 8).

The B lymphocytes are stimulated to produce more RFs, and the T lymphocytes eventually cause the release of enzymes that amplify and perpetuate the inflammatory response (see Fig. 44.29). Cartilage destruction is mediated by proteases, such as collagenase, which activates the synoviocytes to invade the synovium and cartilaginous matrix. In addition, RANKL is expressed by various cells in the synovium and induces osteoclast maturation and activation, thus producing increased bone resorption (also see Chapter 43).

Multiple immunoregulatory cytokines and inflammatory enzymes, such as interleukins, B cells, and collagenase, contribute to the development of an exaggerated immune response, resulting in leukocyte infiltration into the synovium. Once activated, synovial fibroblasts change to an invasive phenotype. Fibroblasts and inflammatory cells perpetuate the inflammatory process and thicken the synovial tissue, called "*pannus*" (Fig. 44.30; see Chapter 8). Eventually, this process leads to osteoclast generation resulting in bone destruction, the hallmark of RA. Inflammation may spread to the articular cartilage, fibrous joint capsule, bone, and surrounding ligaments and tendons, causing pain, joint deformity, and loss of function (Fig. 44.31).

Macrophages, components of pannus (see Figs. 44.29 and 44.30), stimulate the release of IL-1, PDGF, and fibronectin. The B lymphocytes are stimulated to produce more RFs. The newly targeted self-antigens (Igs) are in relatively constant supply and can thus perpetuate inflammation and the formation of immune complexes indefinitely. Along with the swelling and

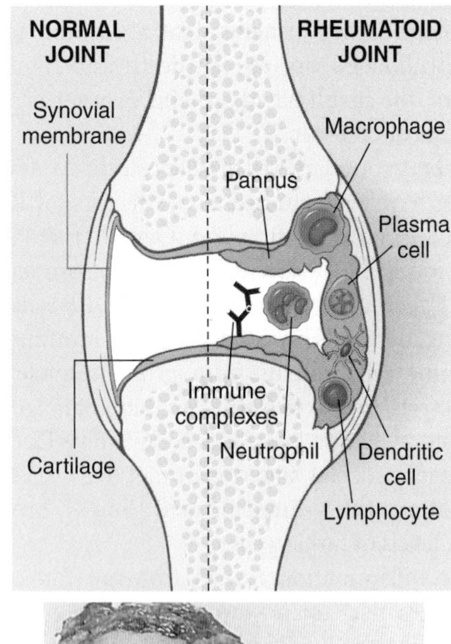

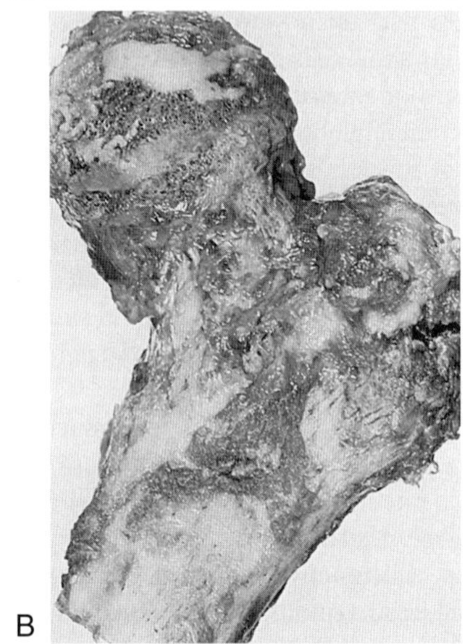

Fig. 44.30 Rheumatoid Arthritis and Pannus. Rheumatoid Arthritis. (A) Schematic view of the joint lesion. **(B)** Advanced rheumatoid arthritis involving femur. There is prominent proliferation of synovium and almost complete destruction of overlying articular cartilage. (A, Modified from Feldmann M. Development of anti-TNF therapy for rheumatoid arthritis. *Nature Reviews Immunology,* 2002;2:364. B, From Rosai J. *Ackerman's surgical pathology,* 10th edition. Philadelphia: Mosby; 2011.)

damage to the synovial membrane caused by leukocyte infiltration, the synovial membrane undergoes hyperplastic thickening as its cells proliferate and become abnormally large. As synovial inflammation progresses to involve its blood vessels, small venules become occluded by hypertrophied endothelial cells, fibrin, platelets, and inflammatory cells, which decrease vascular flow to the synovial tissue. Compromised circulation, coupled with increased metabolic needs as a result of hypertrophy and hyperplasia, causes hypoxia and metabolic acidosis. Acidosis stimulates the release of hydrolytic enzymes from synovial cells into the surrounding tissue, initiating erosion of the articular cartilage and inflammation in the supporting ligaments and tendons. Inflammation causes hemorrhage, coagulation, and fibrin deposition on the synovial membrane, in the intracellular matrix, and in the synovial fluid (see Fig. 44.30).

Clinical Manifestations. The onset of RA is usually insidious, although as many as 15% of cases have an acute onset. RA begins with general systemic manifestations of inflammation, including fever, fatigue, weakness, anorexia, weight loss, and generalized aching and stiffness. Local manifestations also appear gradually over a period of weeks or months. The joints typically become painful, tender, and stiff. Pain early in the disease is caused by pressure from swelling; later, it is caused by sclerosis of subchondral bone and new bone formation. Stiffness usually lasts for about 1 hour after arising in the morning and may be caused by synovitis. Initially, the most commonly involved joints are the MCP joints, PIP joints, and wrists, with later involvement of larger weight-bearing joints.

Widespread, symmetric joint swelling is caused by increasing amounts of inflammatory exudate (leukocytes, plasma, plasma proteins) in the synovial membrane, hyperplasia of inflamed tissues, and formation of new bone. On palpation, the swollen joint feels warm and the synovial membrane feels "boggy." The skin over the joint may have a ruddy, cyanotic hue and may look thin and shiny.

An inflamed joint may lose some of its mobility; even mild synovitis can lead to loss of ROM. Extension becomes limited and is eventually lost if flexion contractures form. Chronic synovitis weakens ligamentous structures, leading to deformities caused by the limited ROM and permanent deformities of the fingers, toes, and limbs, including ulnar deviation of the hands, boutonnière and swan neck deformities of the finger joints, plantar subluxation of the metatarsal heads of the foot, and hallux valgus (angulation of the great toe toward the other toes). Flexion contractures of the knees and hips are also common. Joint deformities cause the physical limitations experienced by persons with RA (see Fig. 44.31). Loss of joint motion is quickly followed by secondary atrophy of the surrounding muscles. With secondary muscle atrophy, the joint becomes unstable, which further aggravates joint pathology.

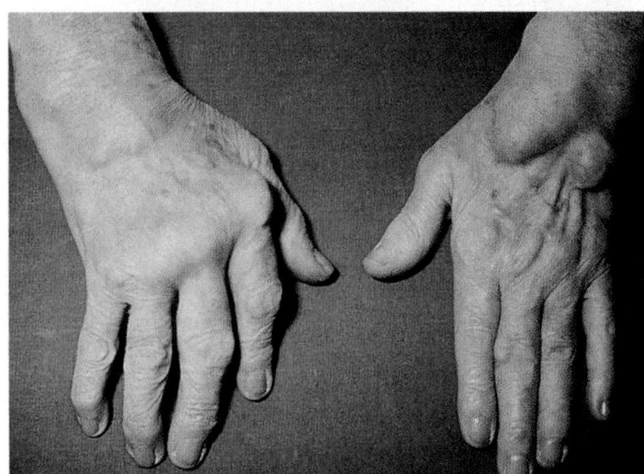

Fig. 44.31 Rheumatoid Arthritis of the Hand. Note swelling from chronic synovitis of metacarpophalangeal joints, marked ulnar drift, subcutaneous nodules, and subluxation of metacarpophalangeal joints with extension of proximal interphalangeal joints and flexion of distal joints. Note also deformed position of thumb. (From Walker BR, et al. *Davidson's principles and practice of medicine,* 22nd edition. London: Churchill Livingstone; 2014.)

Two complications of chronic RA are caused by excessive amounts of inflammatory exudate in the synovial cavity. One complication is the formation of cysts in the articular cartilage or subchondral bone. Occasionally, these cysts communicate with the skin surface (usually the sole of the foot) and begin to drain, causing a *fistula*. The second complication is rupture of a cyst or of the synovial joint itself, usually caused by strenuous physical activity that places excessive pressure on the joint. Rupture releases inflammatory exudate into adjacent tissues, thereby spreading inflammation. Both of these complications contribute to the formation of bone erosion and worsened outcomes for the individual with RA.

Extrasynovial rheumatoid nodules, the most common extra-articular manifestations, are seen in areas of pressure or trauma, and occur in up to 30% of individuals with RA. Each nodule is an aggregate of inflammatory cells surrounding a central core of fibrinoid and cellular debris. T lymphocytes are the predominant leukocytes in the nodule; B lymphocytes, plasma cells, and phagocytes are found around the periphery. Nodules are most often found in subcutaneous tissue over the extensor surfaces of elbows and fingers. Less common sites are the scalp, back, feet, hands, buttocks, and knees.

Rheumatoid nodules also may invade the skin, cardiac valves, pericardium, pleura, lung parenchyma, and spleen. These nodules are identical to those encountered in some individuals with rheumatic fever and are characterized by central tissue necrosis surrounded by proliferating connective tissue. Also noted are large numbers of lymphocytes and occasional plasma cells. Acute glaucoma may result with nodules forming on the sclera. Pulmonary involvement may result in diffuse pleuritis or multiple intraparenchymal nodules. Together, the occurrence of pulmonary nodules and pneumoconiosis (chronic inflammation of the lungs from inhalation of dust) creates Caplan syndrome. Diffuse pulmonary fibrosis may also occur as a result of immunologically mediated immune complex deposition.

Rheumatoid nodules within the heart may cause valvular deformities, particularly of the aortic valve leaflets. Pericardial effusion or other pericardial problems occur in almost 50% of individuals with RA. Lymphadenopathy of the nodes close to the affected joints may develop. Rheumatoid nodules within the spleen result in splenomegaly. Involvement of any blood vessel can result in the development of necrotizing vasculitis. Thromboses of such involved vessels may give rise to myocardial infarctions, cerebrovascular occlusions, mesenteric infarction, kidney damage, and vascular insufficiency in the hands and fingers (Raynaud phenomenon). Vascular changes are noted primarily in individuals receiving corticosteroid therapy; thus, there is some concern that the therapy may play a role in initiating these lesions. Changes in skeletal muscle are often noted in the form of nonspecific atrophy secondary to joint dysfunction.

Evaluation and Treatment. The presence of RF is a laboratory evaluation and is positive in about 45% to 75% of individuals with RA. Thus, it is not considered diagnostic of RA.[57] It is also present in connective tissue disease, chronic infections, and healthy individuals, mostly in low titers.[57] ACPA are detected in about 50% of individuals with early arthritis. These individuals are diagnosed with RA.[57] In the active phase of arthritis, acute-phase reactants, ESR and CRP may be elevated.[57] MRI and ultrasound of joints detect erosions earlier than an x-ray; MRI and ultrasound are more sensitive than clinical examination in identifying synovitis and joint effusion.[62–64] Disease-modifying, anti-rheumatic drugs (DMARDS) are initiated when the diagnosis of RA is made.[57] In 2010 the ACR and the European League Against Rheumatism (EULAR) revised their classification criteria to better identify early stages of RA.[65]

Early and aggressive treatment can decrease the systemic impact of RA, leading to a decreased development of disability and joint destruction. More recently, targeted treatment for RA has involved use of agents aimed at interrupting the pathogenesis of the disease. Known as *biologic DMARDs (bDMARDs)*, these medications affect specific processes in the development of RA and include TNF inhibitors and monoclonal antibodies. Other agents interfere with cytokine function, inhibit T-cell activation, or deplete B cells. Other treatments and therapies include NSAIDs, glucocorticoids, intra-articular steroid injections, physical and occupational therapy with therapeutic exercise, and use of assistive devices. Surgery is used to treat deformities or mechanical deficiencies of joints and can include synovectomy or joint replacement surgery.

Ankylosing Spondylitis

Ankylosing spondylitis (AS) is a chronic inflammatory disease of the axial spine. AS is characterized by stiffening and fusion (ankylosis) of the spine, sacroiliac joints, peripheral joints, digits, entheses, and dactylitis.[66] AS is part of a group of related diseases known as spondyloarthropathies. The most common features of AS are chronic back pain and progressive spinal stiffness.

The primary pathologic site is the enthesis (the point at which ligaments, tendons, and the joint capsule are inserted into bone), and the result is fibrosis, ossification, and fusion of the joint, primarily the sacroiliac joints and the vertebral column (axial skeleton). There are two subgroups of AS: (1) mainly axial disease (involving the spine and/or sacroiliac joints); and (2) peripheral disease (involving joints and/or tendons outside the spine or sacroiliac joints).

AS ranges from 9 to 30 per 10,000 persons which are lower than previous estimates.[67] Worldwide, AS has greater prevalence in men than women. It is typically diagnosed in those younger than 40 years and about 80% of individuals develop initial symptoms when they are younger than 30 years.[66] Although AS can occur in more than one person in a family, it is not a purely genetic disease and has multiple genetic and environmental factors.[68]

Pathophysiology. The exact cause of AS is unknown, but its high association with histocompatibility antigen HLA (*HLA-B27*) has been known for decades. Though many people with AS have the *HLA-B27* variation, most people with this version never develop the disorder.[68] Ongoing genetic studies are needed to clarify the role in AS. AS has an insidious onset and chronic inflammation. The hallmark is enthesitis with chronic inflammation, including CD4 and CD8 T lymphocytes and macrophages.[66] TNF-α and TGF-β, both cytokines, are important in the inflammatory process and promote progression to fibrosis and ossification at sites of enthesitis. The new enthesis, which forms on top of the old one, is called a syndesmophyte. As calcification of the spinal ligaments progresses, the vertebral bodies lose their concave anterior contour and appear square. The spine assumes the classic bamboo spine appearance of AS.

Clinical Manifestations. The most common signs and symptoms of early AS are low back pain and stiffness. Back pain typically exhibits at least four of the five following characteristics: age of onset less than 40 years, insidious onset, improvement with exercise, no improvement with rest, and pain at night with improvement upon arising.[66] Commonly seen is immobility, spinal stiffness, and postural changes, especially hyperkyphosis.[66] The thoracic spine becomes rounded, the head and neck are held forward on the shoulders, and the hips are flexed (Fig. 44.32). Complications can include chronic pain and disability, aortic regurgitation, pulmonary fibrosis, cauda equina syndrome, and mood disorders.[66]

Inflammation in the tendon insertions of the many costosternal and costovertebral muscles can cause pleuritic chest pain and restricted chest movement. The pain is usually worse on inspiration. Movement of the diaphragm is normal and full. Pressure on the anterior chest wall over the sternum, ribs, and costal cartilages may cause tenderness. Tenderness over the pelvic brim may cause discomfort at night and interfere with sleep because turning onto the iliac crests causes pain. Tenderness over the ischial tuberosities may make sitting on hard seats unbearable. Tenderness in the heels may contribute to a limp or cautious placement of the feet during walking.

Evaluation and Treatment. The diagnosis of AS is made on the basis of both clinical and radiologic findings. Clinical findings include low back pain and stiffness lasting more than 3 months that improves with exercise but is not relieved by rest, limited spine ROM in both frontal and sagittal planes, and limited chest expansion relative to normal values for age and gender. Radiologic changes of the sacroiliac joint are graded according to severity of abnormality; abnormalities include sclerosis, widening, narrowing, or ankylosis. MRI can discover sacroiliitis years before there is evidence on x-rays.

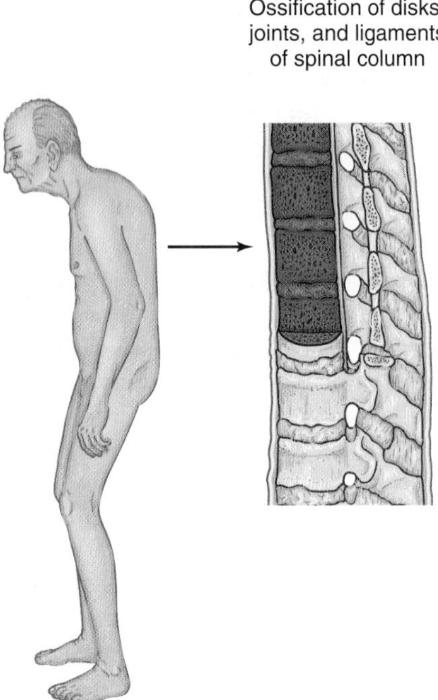

Fig. 44.32 Ankylosing Spondylitis. Characteristic posture and primary pathologic sites of inflammation and resulting damage. (Redrawn from Mourad LA. *Orthopedic disorders.* St. Louis: Mosby; 1991.)

Laboratory tests, including serum analysis for the presence of the histocompatibility antigen HLA-B27, elevated ESR, and elevated alkaline phosphatase levels are generally nonspecific but can assist the diagnosis. A normal ESR and CRP should not exclude the disease.[69–71] First-line treatment consists of NSAIDs. If NSAIDs do not provide adequate relief, they can be combined with or replaced with TNF inhibitors (TNF-Is) (certolizumab, golimumab) or B-cell depleting agents (rituximab). Local corticosteroid injections also may be used. Systemic glucocorticoids are not recommended.[66] Surgical procedures, such as osteotomy, total hip replacement, and cervical spinal fusion, and radiation therapy may be utilized to provide relief for individuals with end-stage disease or intolerable deformity. Non-pharmacologic approaches include regular exercise, postural training, and physical therapy.

Gout

Gout is a systemic disease of uric acid (UA) disturbance that results from the deposition of monosodium urate crystals (MSUs) in tissues.[72] Increased serum uric acid (SUA) above a specific threshold leads to the formation of MSU crystals in and around joints, forming insoluble precipitates of MSU. These precipitates are then deposited in connective tissues throughout the body. Many individuals, however, with hyperuricemia do not develop gout or form UA crystals. Only about 5% of people with hyperuricemia above 9 mg/dL develop gout. Thus, other factors are important to its pathophysiology, such as genetic predisposition.[72,73] The genetic basis of progression to clinical gout needs much more investigation. Other risk factors for gout or hyperuricemia include older age, male sex, obesity, a purine diet, alcohol, medications, and comorbid diseases.[74]

In the United States, gout is the most prevalent etiology of chronic inflammatory arthritis.[73,75] Every condition that causes alterations in extracellular urate concentration has the potential to trigger an acute onset of gout "flare-up." These triggers include stress (surgical procedure, recent trauma, starvation), dietary factors (e.g., fatty food, beer, wine, spirits), and drugs (e.g., aspirin, diuretics, or even allopurinol).[74]

The disease burden of gout is substantial, increasing in Western countries and those becoming westernized analogous to the obesity epidemic. Obesity and gout are aspects of the metabolic syndrome. Estimates of gout prevalence range from 2.7% to 6.7% in countries with a Western lifestyle.[76] In the United States the most recent data (2015 to 2016) of lifetime prevalence of gout is 3.9% which equates to 9.2 million people.[77]

Pseudogout mimics gout; however, it is caused by the formation and deposition of calcium pyrophosphate dihydrate (CPPD) crystals. CPPD crystals predominantly deposit in joint cartilage and intervertebral disks. The effect of either crystal is the same—the onset of a cytokine-mediated acute inflammatory response (see Chapter 9).

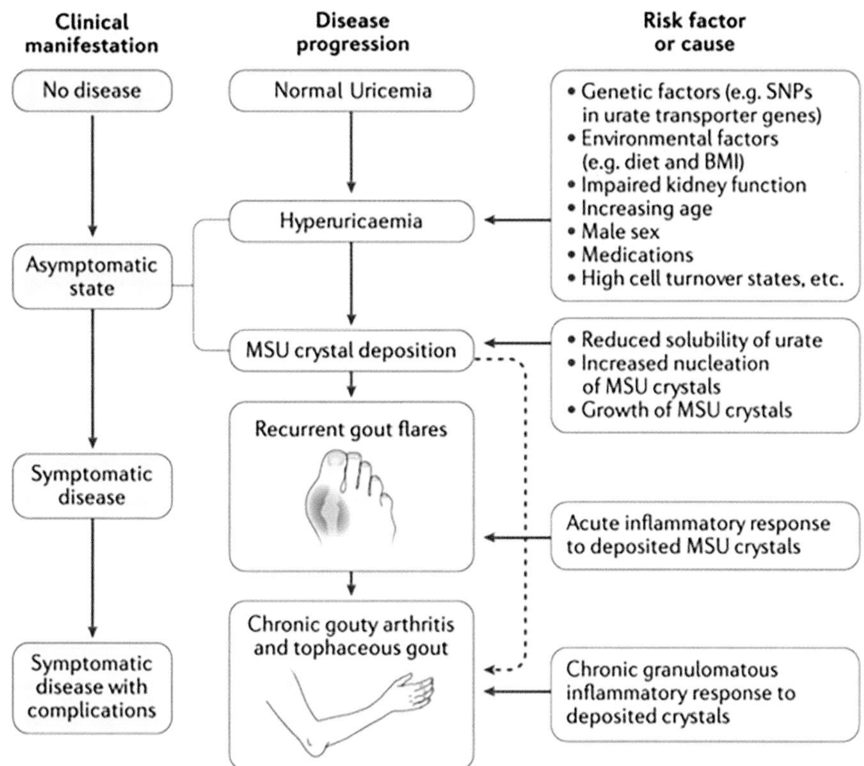

Fig. 44.33 Gout Disease Progression. Many steps occur in the transition from normal serum uric levels to clinically evident gout. Step one is hyperuricemia, caused by both lifestyle /environmental and genetic factors. Monosodium urate (MSU) crystal deposition occurs in some individuals (see text) and the clinical manifestations of gout (gout flares, chronic gouty arthritis, tophaceous gout) occur. The transition from hyperuricemia to clinically evident gout is unclear. SNP, single-nucleotide polymorphism. (From Dalbeth N, Choi HK, Joosten LAB, et al. Gout. *Nature Reviews Disease Primers*, 2019;5:69.)

Pathophysiology. Gout develops in stages (Fig. 44.33). Crystallization in synovial fluid triggers TNF-α, causing the release of chemokines and interleukins. The result of crystallization in synovial fluid is acute, painful inflammation of the joint. This inflammatory response triggers macrophages that phagocytose MSU crystals. When macrophages phagocytize MSU crystals, they form a protein scaffold known as an *inflammasome.* Inflammasomes then convert inactive interleukins of IL-1β and IL-18 into their active forms. Prolonged accumulation results in joint damage, a condition known as gouty arthritis. With time, crystal deposition in subcutaneous tissues causes the formation of small, white nodules, or tophi, that are visible through the skin.[76]

Gout flare is an acute inflammatory response to the deposited MCU crystals, and trophus is a chronic inflammatory granulomatous response to the deposited crystals.[76] The understanding of the pathophysiology of gout has progressed in the last decade. Although gout has been understood as a disorder of purine metabolism it has now become apparent that altered urate transport, both in the gut and the kidneys, is central in the pathogenesis of hyperuricemia and gout.[76] Genome-wide association studies (GWAS) have identified single-nucleotide polymorphisms (SNPs) in several loci and many are correlated with gout.[78,79] The urate transporter genes *SLC2A9* (encoding GLUT9), *SLC22A12* (encoding URAT1), *SLC17A1* (encoding NPT1), and *ABCG2* are strongly correlated with urate levels.[76] Serum urate levels are mostly regulated by the activity of these four transporters in renal transport, and of *ABCG2* in intestinal transport.[76]

MSU crystals can stimulate and perpetuate the inflammatory response. The presence of MSU crystals triggers the acute inflammatory response. Initiation of the complement system activates cytokines and interleukins, which draw neutrophils out of the circulation to begin phagocytizing the crystals. Within the joint fluid, urate crystals react particularly with neutrophils and monocytes. Tissue damage occurs, principally when the neutrophils release the contents of their phagolysosomes (Fig. 44.34). These contents also perpetuate inflammation. The joint affected by gout flare has a pronounced neutrophilic infiltration in both the synovial tissue and synovial fluid.[76] At an early phase of an acute gouty attack, synovial microtophi have been demonstrated. As the process continues, numerous microtophi may be present on the synovial membrane.

Clinical Manifestations. Individuals typically present with acute onset of joint pain. Often the involved joint is the first metatarsophalangeal joint.[74] Clinicians need to also inspect talar, subtalar, ankle, and knee as well as joints that may have OA. Tendons and bursa may also be affected. Pain is usually severe and mostly unresponsive to home remedies. Even touching the joint can cause excruciating pain. Gout flare-ups incite inflammation and can cause redness, swelling, and a warm joint. Other symptoms may be fever, general malaise, and fatigue.[75]

Tophaceous deposits are the characteristic diagnostic lesions of chronic gout. These deposits produce irregular swellings of the fingers, hands, knees, and feet. Tophi within the soft tissue commonly form lumps along the ulnar surface of the forearm, the tibial surface of the leg, the Achilles tendon, and the olecranon bursa. Each tophus consists of a deposit of urate crystals, surrounded by a granuloma made up of mononuclear phagocytes (macrophages) that have developed into epithelial and giant cells. (Granuloma formation is described and illustrated in Chapter 7.) Tophi may produce marked limitation of joint movement and can eventually cause grotesque deformities of the hands and feet (see Fig. 44.34). Although the tophi themselves are painless, they often cause progressive stiffness and persistent aching of the affected joint. Tophi in the extremities can cause nerve compression, such as carpal tunnel syndrome in the wrists, or tarsal tunnel syndrome in the ankles.

Evaluation and Treatment. MSU crystal identification is the gold standard for gout diagnosis.[74] Synovial fluid or tophus aspiration analysis is done under polarizing microscopy. Arthrocentesis may be necessary to confirm the diagnosis and rule out septic arthritis, Lyme disease, or pseudogout (calcium pyrophosphate).[80] Laboratory tests may include white blood cell count, ESR, and CRP during a flare-up, but are non-specific and do not confirm a diagnosis.[74] During a flare-up, serum urate may be normal. Hyperuricemia is helpful for the clinical diagnosis of gout in symptomatic individuals, but alone does not confirm the diagnosis.[74] In the overall population, asymptomatic hyperuricemia is common (Table 44.8). Urinary studies may also be done. Not routinely used, ultrasonography and dual-energy CT (DECT) can assist in the diagnosis.

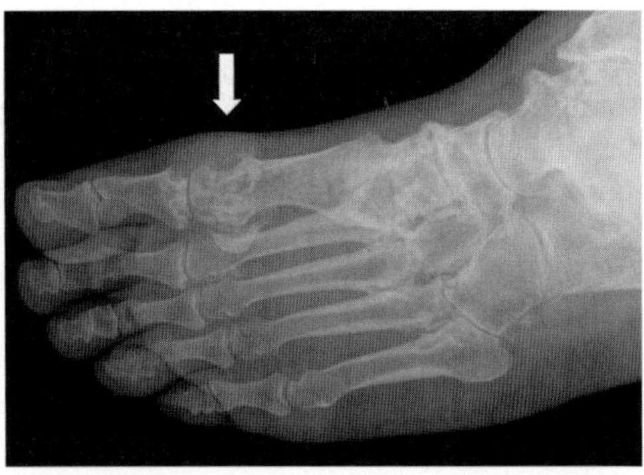

Fig. 44.34 Bone Destruction of First Metatarsal Because of Gout. (From Chhana A, Dalbeth N. Structural joint damage in gout. *Rheumatic Disease Clinics of North America*, 2014;40(2):291–309.)

TABLE 44.8 Mean Urate Concentrations by Age and Sex

Characteristic	Mean Urate Levels (mg/dL)
Prepuberty	3.5
Males (at puberty)	Steep rise to 5.2
Females (puberty to after premenopause)	Slow rise to ≈4
Females (after menopause)	4.7
Hyperuricemia	
• Males	7
• Females	6

During an acute flare-up the goal of treatment is to decrease inflammation and pain. Treatment is usually started within the first 24 hours of onset to reduce the severity and duration of the flare-up.[81] First-line treatment for gout flares are NSAIDs, colchicine, or systemic glucocorticoids. Indomethacin is not preferred because of toxicity effects.[81] Lifestyle factors are very important, and individuals should be counseled to lose weight if obese, avoid certain high-risk foods, avoid consumption of alcohol, and hydrate adequately.

DISORDERS OF SKELETAL MUSCLE

Weakness and fatigue are common symptoms of disorders of the skeletal muscles, termed myopathies. In many cases, neural, traumatic, and psychogenic causes provide an adequate explanation for the failure to generate force (weakness) or sustain force (fatigue) seen in myopathies. The pathophysiologic mechanisms in some of the metabolic and inflammatory muscle diseases have been explored, but the cause of many of the myopathies remains obscure. The complex interaction between muscles and nerves affects muscular function as well. Only inherited and acquired disorders of skeletal muscles are discussed here.

Secondary Muscular Dysfunction

Muscular symptoms arise from a variety of causes unrelated to the muscle itself. Secondary muscular phenomena (contracture, stress-related muscle tension, immobility) are common disorders that influence muscular function.

Contractures

Contractures are the lack of full passive ROM of a joint because of muscle, connective tissue, or other soft tissue limitations. The causes of these limitations can be *pathologic* or *physiologic*. A physiologic muscle contracture occurs as a result of the absence of a muscle action potential in the sarcolemma. Muscle shortening is caused by failure of the calcium pump in the presence of ATP. A physiologic contracture is seen in McArdle disease (muscle myophosphorylase deficiency) and MH. The contracture is usually temporary if the underlying pathology is reversed.

A pathologic contracture is a permanent muscle shortening caused by muscle spasm or weakness. Heel cord (Achilles tendon) contractures are examples of pathologic contractures. They are associated with plentiful ATP and occur in spite of a normal action potential. Most occurrences of pathologic contractures are seen in stroke, neuromuscular disorders such as muscular dystrophy, Charcot-Marie-Tooth disease, amyotrophic lateral sclerosis (ALS), cerebral palsy (see Chapter 45), and CNS injury. Contractures of the lower extremities are more common than those in the upper extremity. Prolonged splinting in a single position or an imbalance between agonist-antagonist muscles also can cause joint stiffness and contractures. Contractures also may develop secondary to scar tissue contraction in the flexor tissues of a joint, for example, contracture of burned tissues in the antecubital area of the forearm or the palmar surface of the hand, leading to a flexion contracture.

Stress-Induced Muscle Tension

Abnormally increased muscle tension has been associated with chronic anxiety, as well as a variety of stress-related muscular symptoms, including neck stiffness, back pain, and headache. Abnormalities in the CNS, reticular activating system, and autonomic nervous system (ANS) have been implicated. The underlying pathophysiology may be related to the fact that as a muscle contracts, the muscle spindle is activated. This gamma-feedback system produces a series of impulses that are transmitted to the brain by the sensitive 1A afferent fibers. Unconscious tension is thought to increase the activity of the reticular activating system as well. This causes increased firing of the efferent loop of the gamma fibers, producing further muscle contraction which increases muscle tension. ANS function that regulates increased blood flow to the muscle during sympathetic activity may be related to increased muscle contraction tension.

Various forms of treatment have been used to reduce the muscle tension associated with stress. Progressive relaxation training, yoga, meditation, and biofeedback are examples of stress reduction therapies.

Fibromyalgia

Fibromyalgia (FM) is a chronic musculoskeletal syndrome characterized by chronic widespread pain (CWP) primarily (but not only) from the musculoskeletal system.[82] Pain can affect the whole body from head to toe.[82] The other two most frequent symptoms are fatigue (mental and physical) and sleep disturbances, particularly non-restorative sleep.[83,84] The symptoms, however, can be complex and not explained by structural or pathologically defined causes.[82] Memory deficits can be among the severe symptoms, and depression and anxiety can affect the cognitive symptoms.[82]

FM is more common in women, and its prevalence is 2% to 3% worldwide. Debated are the etiologies, pathogenesis, diagnostic criteria, classification, and treatment. Several factors, uniquely, contribute to the development of FM: genetic predisposition, personal experiences, emotional-cognitive factors, the mind-body relationship, and a biopsychological ability to cope with stress.[82] The complex symptoms also include hypersensitivity to external stimuli, somatic symptoms, and psychiatric disorders.[82] The 2016 revisions to the 2010/2011 ACR[85] highlighted the concept of "generalized pain" which is also prominent in the ACTTION-APS Pain Taxonomy diagnostic criteria published in 2018 (Fig. 44.35).[86] The main problem to FM diagnosis is the lack of biomarkers; thus it is a clinical diagnosis.[82]

Despite much debate on the classification and pathophysiology of FM, it is recognized as a disease of the musculoskeletal system and connective tissue by the WHO.

Pathophysiology. FM has an unclear pathophysiology, and many hypothetical explanations have been proposed. One hypothesis involves nociplastic pain or pain arising from altered nociception, despite no evidence of tissue damage.[82] This type of pain conforms to FM as apart of *central sensitivity syndromes.*[82] Central sensitization is a neurophysiological process of pain amplification in the CNS. This process occurs after injuries to elicit a protective behavior and maximize the healing process. Central sensitization is also known as central hyperactivation and includes hyperalgesia, (pain perceived as hyper painful), allodynia (a normal stimulus is perceived as pain), temporal summation (perception of repetitive noxious stimulation as being increasingly painful), and hypersensitivity to external stimuli such as sounds or light.[87–90] Some studies have found diffuse pain processing in the brain is altered in FM. Individuals present with altered connectivity and a reduction in brain activity.[82,91,92] Overall, FM is becoming known as a disorder of pain regulation often classified under central sensitization.[93] Studies have suggested a link between FM and stress/stressors (such as infection including Lyme disease, psychosocial stress, sleep abnormalities, immune dysfunction, and physical or emotional trauma). The relationships continue to be researched.

Clinical Manifestations. The prominent symptom of FM is diffused, chronic pain. As discussed previously, the ACR has identified criteria for the diagnosis of FM that expand to include other non-pain symptoms not previously included. A tender point evaluation is no longer required. Instead, the use of a widespread pain index (WPI) and symptom severity inventory (SSI) is recommended. Pain often begins in one location, especially the neck and shoulders, but then becomes more generalized. Fatigue is most notable when arising from sleep and during the midafternoon. Headaches, symptoms of irritable bowel syndrome, and excess sensitivity to cold (Raynaud-like) are reported in 50% of individuals. Fatigue is profound causing a considerable effect on everyday life. Almost 25% of individuals seek psychological support for depression. Anxiety, particularly with regard to their diagnosis and future, is almost universal. Again, the only reliable finding on examination is the presence of multiple tender points.

Evaluation and Treatment. Because the manifestations of chronic, generalized pain and fatigue are present in many musculoskeletal (e.g., rheumatic) disorders, these disorders should be considered in the differential diagnosis of FM (Tables 44.9 and 44.10). The WPI and SSI are then used for diagnostic and evaluation purposes.

No single regimen of medication has proved successful for FM. Current recommendations outline a combination of both pharmacologic and nonpharmacologic therapies. Stress reduction, sleep, and exercise remain central lifestyle modifications for individuals living with FM. Medications that improve sleep may be helpful, as well as vitamin D supplementation. The use of anti-inflammatory medications has not been effective in the treatment of FM as there is no evidence of tissue inflammation. Certain CNS-active medications, most notably pregabalin, were better than placebo in controlled trials. Other medications, designed to augment the activity of neurotransmitters and the endogenous opioid system, also have been shown to provide symptom relief. A randomized trial is needed to compare current drug regimens and cannabis.[94] Two meta-analyses have shown acupuncture efficacy in improving stiffness and pain.[95,96] Some studies have shown benefits with neuromodulation techniques such as transcranial stimulation, occipital and C2 nerve stimulation, and transcutaneous electrical nerve stimulation.[93] Finally, the use of hyperbaric oxygen therapy has shown a promising impact in the management of FM and other chronic pain disorders.[97] The most

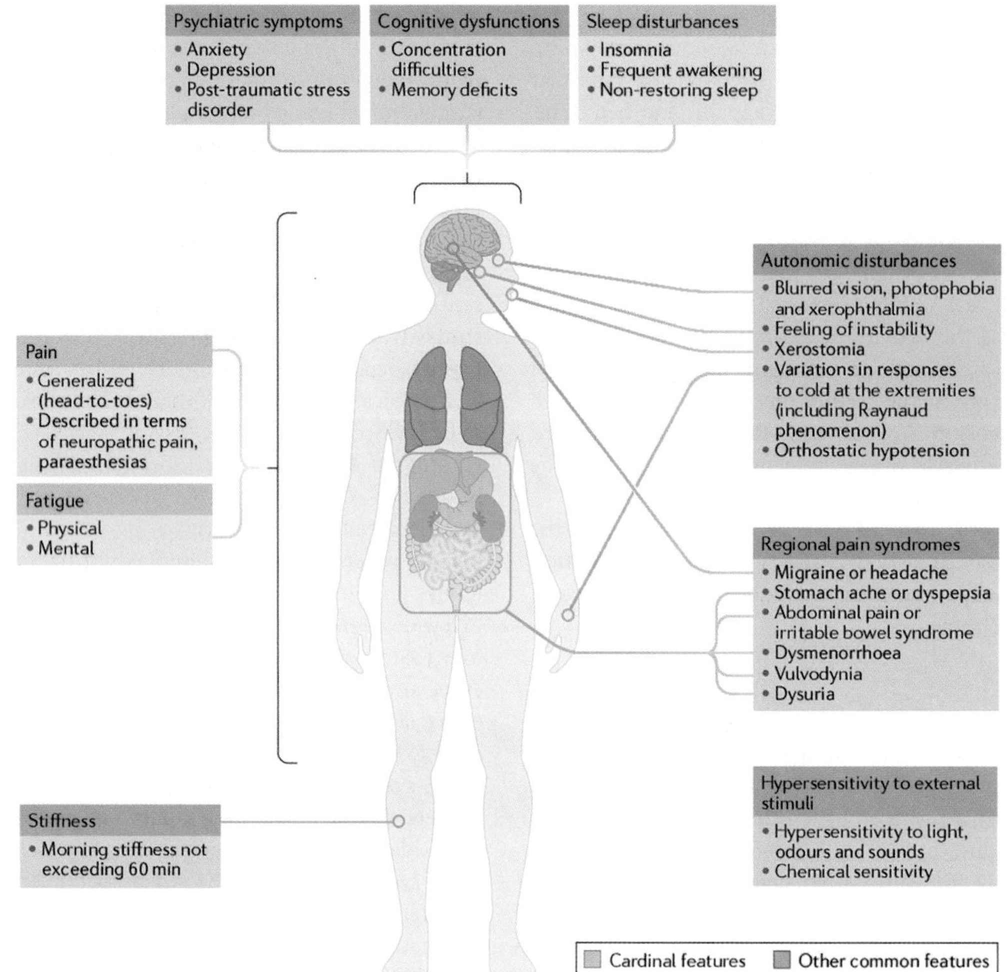

Fig. 44.35 **Main Fibromyalgia (FM) Symptoms.** The symptoms of FM are complex. They are divided into two groups: cardinal features (shown in pink) which are the main symptoms for achieving a diagnosis. Shown in grey are other common features. (From Sarzi-Puttini P, Giorgi V, Marotto D, et al. Fibromyalgia: An update on clinical characteristics, aetiopathogenesis and treatment. *Nature Reviews Rheumatology*, 2020;16:645–660.)

TABLE 44.9 Differential Diagnosis of Fibromyalgia

Differential Diagnosis	Helpful Differential Features
Rheumatoid arthritis[a]	Synovitis, serologic tests, elevated erythrocyte sedimentation rate (ESR)
Systemic lupus erythematosus	Dermatitis, serositis (renal, central erythematosus,[a] nervous system, etc.)
Polymyalgia rheumatica[a]	Elevated ESR, older adults, response to corticosteroids
Myositis	Increased muscle enzymes, weakness more than pain
Hypothyroidism[a]	Abnormal thyroid function tests
Neuropathies	Clinical and electrophysiologic evidence of neuropathy

[a]Fibromyalgia may also more commonly coexist with these conditions.
Data from Klippel JH, Dieppe PA, eds. *Rheumatology*, 2nd edition. London: Mosby-Wolfe; 1998.

TABLE 44.10 Concomitant Conditions With Fibromyalgia

Concomitant Condition	Relationship to Fibromyalgia
Depression	Present in 25%–60% of fibromyalgia cases
Irritable bowel syndrome	Present in 50%–80% of fibromyalgia cases
Migraine	Present in 50% of fibromyalgia cases
Chronic fatigue syndrome (CFS)	70% of CFS cases meet criteria for fibromyalgia
Myofascial pain	May be a localized form of fibromyalgia

Data from Klippel JH, Dieppe PA, eds. *Rheumatology*, 2nd edition. London: Mosby-Wolfe; 1998.

BOX 44.7 Educating and Providing Reassurance for Individuals With Fibromyalgia

- Stress that the illness is real, not imagined.
- Explain that fibromyalgia is presumably not caused by infection.
- Explain that fibromyalgia is not a deforming or deteriorating condition.
- Explain that fibromyalgia is neither life-threatening nor markedly debilitating, although it is an irritating presence.
- Discuss the role of sleep disturbances and the relationship of neurohormones to pain, fatigue, abnormal sleep, and mood.
- Reassure that although the cause is unknown, some information is known about the physiologic changes responsible for the symptoms.
- Use muscle "spasms" and, perhaps, "low muscle blood flow" to lay the groundwork for exercise recommendations.
- Assist the individual to use aerobic exercise to reduce stress and increase rapid eye movement (REM) sleep.

effective approach is a combination of modalities, including education, medication, exercise, and cognitive behavioral therapy. Box 44.7 lists some of these modalities.

Chronic Fatigue Syndrome

Chronic fatigue syndrome (CFS), also known as myalgic encephalomyelitis (ME), is a disabling clinical condition characterized by unexplained and persistent post-exertional fatigue and symptoms related to cognitive, immunological, endocrinological, and autonomic dysfunction.[98] Additionally, individuals may experience sore throat, headache, and tender lymph nodes. These symptoms, however, occur without a clear pathophysiologic explanation. Without a clear etiology, diagnosis of CFS is often a diagnosis of exclusion. Current research is investigating the potential impact of the immune and adrenal systems, as well as genetics and biopsychosocial involvement. As a result, CFS/ME is believed to be less of a musculoskeletal disorder and more related to hypersensitivity of the CNS, a condition known as *central sensitization*. In the WHO International Classification of Diseases version 2016, both ME and CFS were coded identically and classified as disorders of the nervous system. However, many non-expert clinicians view "fatigue syndrome" as synonymous with CFS, and classify it under mental and behavioral disorders.[98] Nonetheless, the etiology of ME/CFS is incompletely understood, complicated, and controversial.[99]

Pathophysiology. The pathophysiology of CFS remain unknown. International Consensus Criteria have recommended use of the term ME rather than CFS, because ME indicates an underlying pathophysiology. Investigators are studying alterations in the immune system. abnormal cytokine regulation, alteration of natural killer cells, B cell impairment, Igs, autoimmunity, deregulation of antiviral pathway (Oligoadenylate synthetase/RNase L pathway), neuroinflammation, changes in serotonin transmission, hypercortisolism, and genetic predisposition.[98–102] Functional MRI (fMRI) has shown lower blood perfusion to the brainstem in individuals affected by CFS supporting CNS abnormalities, immunologic dysregulation, and higher-than-normal levels of proinflammatory cytokines. Certain points within the skeletal muscle may be affected by oxidative stress reactions (see Chapter 2), accounting for the muscle pain and fatigue associated with CFS.

Clinical Manifestations. Unrestful sleep is a hallmark of CFS. Defining symptoms include debilitating fatigue made worse by physical or mental exercise (postexertional fatigue), muscle pain, noninflammatory joint pain, headaches, flulike symptoms, and memory or concentration problems. Other common symptoms include bloating, morning joint stiffness, chest or jaw pain, chills and night sweats, visual disturbances, sore throat, and tender axillary or cervical lymph nodes. Symptoms and their consequences can be severe.

Evaluation and Treatment. ME/CFS is a diagnosis made on clinical examination and after exclusion of other possible etiologies. Diagnosis of CFS is often delayed or missed because there is no biologic marker or specific laboratory test for CFS, and many CFS symptoms are shared with other illnesses. Individuals with CFS do not necessarily appear sick, and symptoms typically have a variable course. Currently, the CDC recommends considering a diagnosis of CFS if the following two criteria are met:

1. Unexplained, persistent fatigue is not due to ongoing exertion, is not substantially relieved by rest, is of new onset (not lifelong), and results in a significant reduction of previous levels of activity.
2. Four or more of the following symptoms are present for 6 months or more:

   Impaired memory or concentration
   Postexertional malaise (extreme, prolonged exhaustion and exacerbation of symptoms following physical or mental exertion)
   Unrefreshing sleep
   Muscle pain
   Multijoint pain without swelling or redness (adults)
   Headaches of a new type or severity
   Sore throat that is frequent or recurring
   Tender cervical or axillary lymph nodes

Treatment of CFS should focus on symptom management, especially management of sleep disturbances, depression, and pain. Acknowledgement and consideration of the person's individual needs is important and involves psychosocial factors as well as symptomatic and supportive care. Professional counseling, medication, diet, and activity helps CFS sufferers deal with the limitations imposed by the disease. Alternative therapies such as acupuncture, massage, and therapeutic touch can relieve anxiety.

Disuse Atrophy

Disuse atrophy describes the pathologic reduction in normal size of muscle fibers from an accelerated degradation of myofibrillar proteins. This may be associated with the normal aging process (sarcopenia), as well as following periods of prolonged immobilization and low mechanical load, such as from inactivity during bed rest, trauma (casting), space flight, or local nerve damage seen with spinal cord trauma or poliomyelitis. Disease-induced atrophy also is seen in debilitating conditions, such as cancer, acquired immunodeficiency syndrome (AIDS), renal failure, congestive heart failure, chronic obstructive pulmonary disease, and burns. Oxidative stress from lack of muscle activity reduces muscle mass through both decreased muscle protein synthesis and increased muscle protein breakdown. The effects of muscular deconditioning associated with lack of physical activity have been seen in as few as 5 days after immobility. The normal individual on bed rest loses muscle strength from baseline levels at a rate of 3% per day. Bed rest also is associated with cardiovascular, skeletal, and other organ system changes.

The most effective restorative measure for disuse atrophy is to reapply mechanical load to the muscle group, including resistance exercises, stretching, electrical stimulation, frequent forceful isometric muscle contractions and passive lengthening exercises. Artificial gravity (fusing a *human centrifuge*) has shown benefit in maintaining muscle strength. Measures to prevent atrophy include adequate nutrition, frequent forceful isometric muscle contractions, and passive lengthening exercises. If reuse is not restored within 1 year, regeneration of muscle fibers becomes impaired.

Muscle Membrane Abnormalities

Two defects of the muscle membrane (plasma membrane of the muscle fiber) have been linked to clinical syndromes: the hyperexcitable membrane seen in myotonic disorders and the intermittently unresponsive membrane seen in periodic paralyses. Although these are infrequent disorders, research into their pathologic processes has led to an improved understanding of cell membrane channelopathies (ion channels are described in Chapter 15).

Skeletal Muscle Channelopathies

Skeletal muscle channelopathies can be divided into two primary groups: (1) those presenting with myotonia (nondystrophic myotonias) and (2) those associated with episodes of weakness (periodic paralysis [PP]). In myotonic channelopathies, muscle relaxation is delayed after voluntary contractions, such as handgrip or eye closure, leading to a disabling muscle stiffness and/or weakness. PP is an autosomal dominant disorder in which depolarization of the sarcolemma is severe enough that the muscle cannot be *fired* again, resulting in paralysis or even myotonia. Myotonia can be reproduced by removing extracellular chloride, thus reducing chloride conductance across the plasma membrane. The delicate balance in which sodium diffuses into the intracellular fluid, potassium diffuses out of the intracellular fluid, and chloride is in flux, is interrupted. Because the normal diffusion processes (described in Chapter 3) stabilize the membrane, the shift in chloride ions is thought to increase membrane excitability. The chloride abnormality may explain the resting membrane hyperexcitability, but it does not explain the delayed relaxation present in myotonia and has not been detected in human myotonia. Myotonia is noted in several disorders: myotonia congenita, paramyotonia congenita, myotonic muscular dystrophy, and some forms of PP. Most are inherited disorders and are mild in symptomatology, with the exception of myotonic muscular dystrophy. Myotonia is treated by drugs that reduce muscle fiber excitability, such as sodium channel blocking agents (mexiletine, procainamide) and phenytoin.

Central core disease (CCD) is another inherited channelopathy that involves mutations in ryanodine receptors (RyR1) and affects calcium channels. In CCD, RyR1 channels are defective, and either too much or too little calcium is released from the cell's sarcoplasmic reticulum, resulting in symmetrical proximal muscle weakness. This weakness, however, is usually not progressive in nature. Classified as a neuromuscular disorder, CCD typically manifests during infancy as decreased muscle tone, delayed motor development, muscle weakness (particularly around the hip girdle), and other skeletal deformities, such as scoliosis. Thought to be the most common congenital myopathy, the pathology of CCD relates to the lack of "cores" within skeletal myofibers that do not contain mitochondria and their oxidative enzymes. Therefore, definitive diagnosis is made through muscle biopsy.

Periodic Paralysis

Periodic paralysis (PP) includes a rare group of muscle diseases caused by the inheritance of an autosomal dominant mutation of skeletal muscle calcium, sodium, or potassium channel. During an exacerbation of PP, the muscle membrane is unresponsive to neural stimuli and the resting membrane potential is reduced from −90 to −45 mV. PP can be either hyperkalemic or hypokalemic. As the name implies, PP is usually transient.

The paralysis, which leaves the individual flaccid and weak, typically affects only the skeletal muscles and not the respiratory muscles. The weakness is accompanied by a change in serum potassium levels, although in most individuals the change is negligible unless a secondary underlying condition affecting potassium distribution coexists. For this reason, cardiac dysrhythmias, although not common, have been present during attacks.

Hypokalemic PP is often triggered by thyrotoxicosis caused by alterations in potassium ion channels that are regulated by triiodothyronine (T_3). Glucose and insulin infusions and oral potassium loading are used as provocative tests; oral and intravenous potassium administration can relieve acute attacks. Treatment includes potassium-sparing diuretics and a high-salt diet. Acetazolamide, dichlorphenamide, and a low-salt diet are useful for long-term therapy.

Hyperkalemic PP is episodes of extreme muscle weakness beginning in childhood or adolescence. These episodes most often involve a temporary inability to move muscles in the arms and legs. Hyperkalemic PP is caused by an *SNC4A* genetic mutation affecting sodium channels and can be precipitated by several factors including pregnancy, alcohol, illness, exercise, and increased potassium intake. Attacks can occur without warning or can be triggered by rest after exercise, a viral illness, or certain medications, and are typically less severe than the hypokalemic form. Often a large carbohydrate-rich meal or vigorous exercise in the evening can trigger an attack upon waking the next morning. Treatment includes small carbohydrate-rich meals, light exercise, and intravenous calcium gluconate.

Metabolic Muscle Diseases

Metabolic muscle diseases are a collection of disorders caused by a genetic mutation and endocrine abnormalities that affect a muscle's metabolism. The resulting disorders in muscle metabolism lead to diseases of energy metabolism, such as glycogen storage disease, enzyme deficiencies, and abnormalities in lipid metabolism and mitochondrial function.

Endocrine Disorders

Often the systemic effects of hormonal imbalance overshadow the individual's muscular symptoms. For example, individuals with thyrotoxicosis may have signs of proximal weakness, paresis of the extraocular muscles (exophthalmic ophthalmoplegia), and, rarely, hypokalemic PP, as discussed earlier in the previous section. Hypothyroidism is often associated with a decrease in muscle mass and strength, with weak, flabby skeletal muscles and sluggish movements.

Thyroid hormone is believed to regulate muscle protein synthesis and electrolyte balance. Changes in muscle protein synthesis and electrolyte balance may therefore explain the alterations in muscle mass and contractility seen in endocrine disorders. The muscular symptoms subside with appropriate treatment of the primary hormonal disorder.

Other endocrine disorders affecting the musculoskeletal system include Dent disease (a syndrome that causes bone deformities); rickets or osteomalacia (softening of the bone because of deficiencies in vitamin D and calcium); and osteopetrosis (also known as *Albers-Schönberg disease*) caused by failure of osteoclasts to resorb bone which thereby results in increased bone mass while causing increased bone fragility, growth abnormalities, and bone marrow failure in infants as bone marrow is replaced by bony masses. Familial hypomagnesemia is an autosomal recessive disease that primarily affects the renal system causing hypomagnesemia and secondary hypocalcemia and can result in tetany and convulsions.

Diseases of Energy Metabolism

Muscles rely on carbohydrates (e.g., glycogen) and lipids (free fatty acids) for energy. When stored glycogen or lipids cannot be used because of the lack of enzymes necessary to generate ATP for muscle contraction the individual experiences cramps, fatigue, and exercise intolerance. Disorders of muscle metabolism can be self-limiting, such as McArdle disease and some lipid disorders, or they can cause widespread irreparable muscle destruction, as in acid maltase deficiency.

McArdle disease. McArdle disease, or glycogen myophosphorylase deficiency, is an autosomal recessive disease caused by an inability to metabolize glycogen. It was the first myopathy in which a single enzyme defect was identified (Fig. 44.36). Individuals with McArdle disease lack muscle phosphorylase, which is responsible for the breakdown of glycogen in muscle. As a result, a lack of glycogen breakdown can interfere with the function of muscle cells. The altered energy production manifests itself as exercise intolerance, fatigue, muscle pain, and cramps during the first few minutes of exercise. Some individuals describe a "second wind" phenomenon, in which exercise tolerance increases if they slow their pace once the initial sensation of fatigue commences. This is caused by the use of free fatty acids as a secondary source of energy. When exercise is carried to an extreme, muscle damage may occur, leading to the breakdown of muscle tissue (rhabdomyolysis), painful muscle contracture, and myoglobinuria.

Acid maltase deficiency. Acid maltase deficiency is an uncommon, autosomal recessive disorder affecting glycogen storage from an accumulation of glycogen in the lysosomes of muscle and other tissue cells. The usual pathways of glycogen degradation are preserved. However, deficiency of α-glucosidase (GAA) enzyme is responsible for the abnormality in glycogen metabolism. The infantile form, Pompe disease, is often recognized shortly after birth because of the presence of hypotonia, respiratory weakness, dysreflexia, and physiologic abnormalities such as cardiomegaly, an enlarged tongue, and hepatomegaly. The adult form tends to be less severe than the infantile form. Hypertrophy of these tissues is thought to be the result of glycogen deposition. Diagnosis of Pompe disease can be made through the evaluation of GAA activity in blood or through muscle biopsy. Previously, children with Pompe disease often died of cardiac or respiratory failure before age 2; now enzyme replacement therapy (ERT) with recombinant human acid GAA and physical therapy has shown a significant improvement in symptom presentation.

Myoadenylate deaminase deficiency. Myoadenylate deaminase deficiency (MDD), also referred to as *adenosine monophosphate deaminase deficiency*, is a fairly common, autosomal recessive, enzyme deficiency that causes changes in skeletal muscles and is associated with exercise intolerance accompanied by muscle pain and cramps, although the majority of individuals are asymptomatic. Because these individuals lack myoadenylate deaminase, they have a poor capacity for sustained energy production. Myoadenylate deaminase is the catalytic enzyme that forms phosphocreatine and ATP during exercise through a metabolic pathway that binds the purine and phosphate molecules that constitute ATP. Persons with MDD differ from those with McArdle disease in that during the ischemic exercise test, lactate production is normal when ATP and phosphocreatine

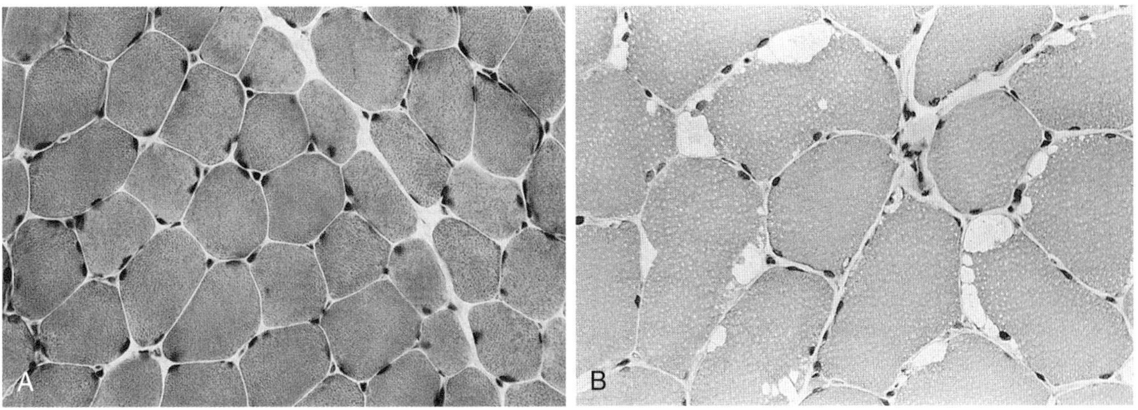

Fig. 44.36 McArdle Disease.

are synthesized. Symptoms range from minimal complaints to exercise-induced muscle pain to rhabdomyolysis. Currently, there are limited reports of successful treatments. Avoidance of rigorous exercise is generally recommended.

Lipid deficiencies. Inherited disorders of lipid metabolism are uncommon but account for severe changes in muscle metabolism. These disorders are caused by abnormalities in the transport and processing of fatty acids for energy. The lipid content of muscle cells consists of free fatty acids, which are oxidized in the mitochondria. These acids require carnitine and the enzyme carnitine palmitoyltransferase (CPT) to transport long-chain fatty acids to the mitochondria. Individuals with CPT deficiency often have mild muscular symptoms but can experience bouts of renal failure caused by rhabdomyolysis. Individuals with a deficiency of carnitine alone have progressive muscle weakness and can experience sudden exacerbations. There are two types of CPT deficiency: CPT I and CPT II deficiency. CPT I deficiency often appears during early childhood and is caused by mutations in the *CPT1A* gene. The gene mutation creates the deficiency of the enzyme CPT IA, which is found in the liver. Individuals with CPT I deficiency are at risk for liver failure, nervous system damage, seizures, coma, and sudden death. They often exhibit hepatomegaly, liver dysfunction, and elevated blood levels of carnitine. Carnitine is a natural substance acquired mostly from diet and is used by cells to process fats and produce energy. Affected individuals usually have hypoglycemia and a low level of ketones, which are produced from the breakdown of fats and used for energy. Viral infections or periods of fasting can trigger problems with CPT I deficiency, and the disorder is sometimes mistaken for Reye syndrome. Most cases of Reye syndrome are associated with the use of aspirin during viral infections. There are three main types of CPT II deficiency: a lethal neonatal form, a severe infantile hepatocardiomuscular form, and a myopathic form.[103] These three types are discussed in Table 44.11. Treatments with riboflavin, medium-chain triglycerides, oral carnitine, prednisone, and propranolol are proposed.

TABLE 44.11 Types of Carnitine Palmitoyltransferase II Deficiency

Lethal Neonatal Form	Becomes apparent soon after birth Respiratory failure, seizures, liver failure, cardiomyopathy and dysrhythmia develop Affected infants have hypoglycemia and low level of ketones (hypoketotic hypoglycemia) The brain and kidneys may be abnormal Infants usually live a few days to few a few months
Severe Infantile Hepatocardiomuscular Form	Affects the liver, heart and muscles Clinical manifestations usually appear within the first year of life Involves recurring episodes of hypoketotic hypoglycemia, seizures, hepatomegaly, cardiomegaly, and dysrhythmia Problems can be triggered by fasting or viral infections and other illnesses Affected infants may have liver failure, nervous system damage, coma, and sudden death
Myopathic Form	First episodes usually occur during childhood or adolescence Most affected individuals do not have clinical manifestations between episodes Include recurrent episodes of myalgia and weakness, and rhabdomyolysis Destruction of muscle causes the release of myoglobin by the kidneys, causing myoglobinuria Myoglobin causes urine to be red or brown Kidney failure may develop Myalgia and rhabdomyolysis may be triggered by exercise, stress, exposure to extreme temperatures, infections, or fasting

Data from U.S. Department of Health & Human Services, National Institutes of Health (USDHHS, NIH). *Genetics Home Reference: Carnitine Palmitoyltransferase I Deficiency*. Bethesda, MD: Author; 2018.

Inflammatory Muscle Diseases: Myositis

Viral, Bacterial, and Parasitic Myositis

Viral, bacterial, and parasitic infections of varying severity are known to produce inflammatory changes in skeletal muscle, a group of conditions collectively described by the term myositis. In tuberculosis and sarcoidosis, chronic inflammatory changes and granulomata are found in muscle as well as in other affected tissues. In the parasitic infection trichinellosis, *Trichinella* larvae reside in the muscles of infected animals, such as pigs, horses, and other wildlife, including cougars and black bears. After ingestion, the parasites migrate to the intestinal mucosa and from there to the lymphatic and circulatory systems.

Initial symptoms occur 1 to 2 days after consumption of infected meat and present as gastrointestinal distress (e.g., nausea, diarrhea, vomiting, abdominal pain). The more traditional trichinellosis symptoms generally occur 2 to 8 weeks after ingestion and include muscle pain and stiffness, fever, rash, itching, and headaches. Treatment includes administration of corticosteroids, such as prednisone, and anti-parasitic agents, such as albendazole. Mebendazole also may be used, though it is not available in the United States. Toxoplasmosis, a common parasitic infection, also is associated with a generalized polymyositis (PM) that responds rapidly to therapy.

In the tropics, more prevalent disorders include bacterial infections with *S. aureus* and parasites such as cysticercus, the larva of the tapeworm *Taenia solium*. Viral infections can be associated with an acute myositis. Muscle pain, tenderness, signs of inflammation, and elevation of CK are common manifestations of viral myositis. The self-limiting symptoms of muscle aches and pains during a bout of influenza may actually be a subacute form of viral myopathy.

Polymyositis, Dermatomyositis, and Inclusion Body Myositis

Idiopathic inflammatory myopathy (IIM) is a group of autoimmune disorders that typically target skeletal muscles, though cutaneous manifestations have been documented in 50% to 60% of individuals. IIMs are characterized by

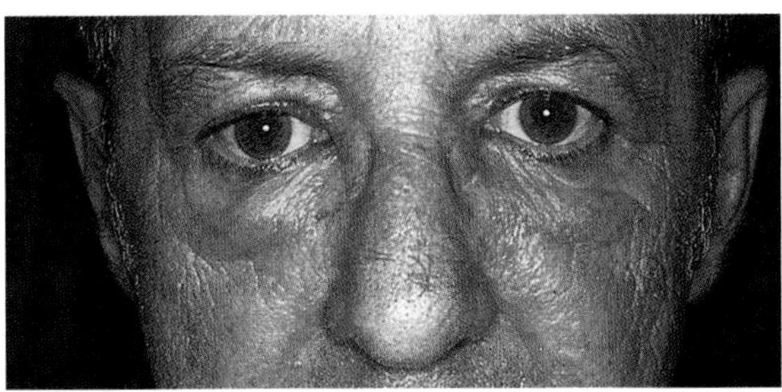

Fig. 44.37 Dermatomyositis. Heliotrope (violaceous) discoloration around the eyes and periorbital edema. (From Habif TP. *Clinical dermatology,* 3rd edition. St. Louis: Mosby; 1996.)

symmetrical proximal muscle weakness (hip and neck flexors and shoulder girdle) and myalgia that develops over weeks to months. The four principal types are PM, dermatomyositis (DM), necrotizing myopathy (NM), and inclusion-body myositis (IBM). PM and DM involve weakness of muscles such as the hips, thighs, upper arms, and neck. Although DM and PM have similar symptoms, DM is distinguished by a reddish or purplish rash on the eyelids (Fig. 44.37), elbows, knees, or knuckles. Sometimes, abnormal calcium deposits form hard bumps found under the skin (calcinosis). Inclusion body myositis involves the muscles mostly of the wrists, fingers, and the front of the thigh. Affected individuals may stumble while walking and have difficulty with grasping items. The incidence of IIM appears to be increasing, but this may simply reflect improved diagnosis. With an incidence of 5 to 22 per 100,000, it is more prevalent in nonwhite women older than age 50. The specific cause of the disorder is unknown and is thought to arise from both genetic and environmental factors. Most cases are sporadic; however, some individuals with IIM have close relatives with autoimmune disorders.

Acute clinical manifestations include many of those seen in any inflammatory process: malaise, fever, muscle swelling, pain and tenderness, lethargy, and listlessness. In adults, weakness of the shoulder and pelvic girdle muscles is a primary manifestation of PM. Both PM and DM often are associated with symmetrical proximal muscle weakness and initially can be confused with other myopathies. A thorough evaluation is required to exclude other disorders. Clinical features common to both are dysphagia, reduced esophageal motility, vasculitis, Raynaud phenomenon, cardiomyopathy, and interstitial pulmonary fibrosis. Some individuals have other coexisting collagen vascular disorders, such as RA, SLE, and progressive systemic sclerosis (formerly called *scleroderma*).

Although PM and DM have similar histories of onset, DM includes cutaneous manifestations. The two most classic signs of skin involvement are (1) a heliotrope (reddish purple) rash that generally covers the eyelids and periorbital area (see Fig. 44.37) and often includes the chest; and (2) erythematous, scaly lesions (Gottron lesions) that cover joints, such as the knees and elbows. DM is slightly more common in children and older adults, with onset before age 15 or after age 50. The adult with DM occasionally has underlying malignancies.

Additional differences between PM and DM exist. Muscle biopsy and histopathologic studies of IBM show degenerative changes of muscle, accumulation of multiple proteins within muscle fibers, and evidence of endoplasmic reticular stress with misfolding of proteins. Clinically, IBM may show weakness of the wrist and finger flexors as well as asymmetrical atrophy and quadriceps weakness. Additionally, IBM does not respond to standard pharmacologic treatment of immunosuppressants and immune-modifying agents.

The two approaches for treatment of myositis are medical treatment and lifestyle changes. Medical treatment primarily includes pharmacologic immunosuppression, although the evidence surrounding the effectiveness of this treatment is not robust. The use of pulsed intravenous glucocorticoids is followed by a 4-week oral regimen, concluding with a tapering of medication. High-dose intravenous immunoglobulin (IVIg) administration is sometimes used during active disease. Successful treatment with IVIg, azathioprine, methotrexate, mycophenolate mofetil, and cyclosporine has been reported. Lifestyle factors include exercise, rest, nutrition, and reduction of stress.

Myopathy

Myopathy is the term applied to a primary muscle disorder. Many pathologic processes affect muscles and cause loss of functional muscle cells. Myopathies affect muscle strength, tone, and bulk. Primary muscle disease is associated with marked weakness. The distribution of the weakness in myopathy is usually symmetrical and proximal, although occasionally the weakness is predominantly distal, such as in myotonic dystrophy. The weakness is associated with mild fatigue. Muscle tone is decreased, as are the tendon reflexes. Atrophy may be present. Some myopathies are associated with muscle hypertrophy as in cretinism and the familial progressive muscular dystrophies of childhood. Fasciculations are not present with myopathy because no denervation is present. No sensory changes are found. (Specific neurologic-associated myopathies are discussed in Chapter 17.)

Toxic Myopathies

Several agents, including corticosteroids, chloroquine, alcohol, phenytoin, azathioprine, organophosphates, and reverse transcriptase inhibitors have been shown to cause muscle damage known as toxic myopathy. Other contributing agents may include lipid-lowering agents and opioids, such as heroin (Box 44.8).

Alcohol, specifically, has been attributed to myopathies since the mid-nineteenth century and is associated with approximately 50% of skeletal muscle myopathies. Alcoholic toxic myopathies may have either an acute or a chronic presentation. An acute alcoholic toxic myopathy presents with muscle weakness, pain, and swelling after a large consumption of alcohol. A chronic alcoholic toxic myopathy is characterized by a progressive proximal weakness associated with long-term consumption of alcohol. The mechanisms by which alcohol affects the muscle include increasing the rate of proteolysis and amino acid oxidation and causing impaired cellular

BOX 44.8 Agents That Can Cause Toxic Myopathy

Drug Induced
Alcohol
Amiodarone (and others that inhibit CYP3A4 when combined with a statin)
Amphotericin B
AZT (zidovudine)
Azathioprine
Chloroquine
Clofibrate
Cocaine
Colchicine
Ethanol
Ipecac (withdrawn from U.S. markets)
3,4-Methylenedioxymethamphetamine (MDMA, "ecstasy")
Pentachlorophenol (PCP)
Statins
Steroids (especially with prolonged high doses; doses >25 mg/day; fluorinated steroids)

Endocrine Disorders
Adrenal disorders (Addison disease, Cushing disease)
Hyperparathyroidism
Hyperthyroidism (creatine kinase may be normal)
Hypothyroidism (creatine kinase may be mildly elevated)

Infectious disorders
Coxsackie A and B viruses
Human immunodeficiency virus (HIV)
Influenza
Lyme disease
Staphylococcus aureus muscle infection (frequent cause of pyomyositis)
Toxoplasmosis
Trichinosis

Miscellaneous
Licorice
Certain edible wild mushrooms
Lead poisoning
Organophosphates
Red yeast rice
European migratory quail (quail eat toxic hemlock, hellebore seeds)
Any medication that alters serum concentrations of sodium, potassium, calcium, phosphorus, or magnesium

Data from Kuncl RW. Agents and mechanisms of toxic myopathy. *Current Opinion in Neurology,* 2009;22(5):506–515; Valiyil R, Christopher-Stine L. Drug-related myopathies of which the clinician should be aware. *Current Rheumatology Reports,* 2010;12(3):213–220.

metabolism, gene dysregulation, and premature initiation of apoptosis.

Acute alcoholic myopathy can range from benign cramps and pain that resolves in a matter of hours to severe weakness and a markedly increased CK level associated with myoglobinuria and renal failure. Individuals are prone to repeated attacks after recovery. The first-line treatment remains abstinence from alcohol and improved nutrition. The individual with chronic alcoholic myopathy often has coexisting peripheral neuropathy that complicates the diagnosis.

Repeated intramuscular injections also have been associated with changes in muscle fibers. Local necrosis of muscle fiber and elevated CK concentration has been reported after intramuscular injections of certain cephalosporins, lidocaine, diazepam, and digoxin; these effects were not produced with injections of saline. When drugs are injected over long periods, a chronic focal myopathy develops. Proliferation of connective tissue both in the muscle fiber and in the overlying skin and subcutaneous tissue has been reported. Over time, segments of the muscles, particularly the deltoid and quadriceps, are converted into fibrotic bands. Pathophysiologic mechanisms for these changes include repeated needle trauma and infection, along with the nonphysiologic acidity and alkalinity of the injected material (see Box 44.8 for a list of some of the causes of toxic myopathy).

MUSCLE TUMORS

Rhabdomyoma

Rhabdomyoma is an extremely rare benign tumor of striated muscle that generally occurs in the tongue, neck muscles, larynx, uvula, nasal cavity, axilla, vulva, and heart. These tumors are usually treated by surgical excision and typically do not recur. When malignant, these tumors are called *rhabdomyosarcomas* (RMS).

Rhabdomyosarcoma

Rhabdomyosarcoma (RMS) is a rare malignant tumor of striated muscle, which is a subgroup of sarcoma. It is the most common soft tissue sarcoma in children and adolescents, constituting 50% of all soft tissue sarcomas and 10% of all malignant tumors occurring in children. These tumors are highly malignant and metastasize rapidly. RMSs are located in the muscle tissue of the head, neck, and genitourinary tract in 75% of cases, with the remaining 25% found in the trunk, extremities, and urinary tract.

Three types of RMS are differentiated on pathologic section: pleomorphic, embryonal, and alveolar. Each type differs from the other molecularly; they are all aggressive tumors and are typically more resistant to therapy. The pleomorphic, or spindle cell, type is considered to be one of the most highly malignant tumors of the extremities seen in adulthood but has a better outcome in children. Embryonal tumors are most commonly seen in children and appear on biopsy to resemble the shape of a tadpole or tennis racquet. Alveolar-type tumors, which appear latticelike, resemble alveolar lung tissue. They are more often found in adolescents and adults and are associated with the poorest outcomes.

The diagnosis and staging of RMS are made by the history, physical examination, serologic testing, CT, and MRI. Diagnosis is confirmed by incisional biopsy with surgical resection and by examination of the specimen by a pathologist. Staging is based on the site of origin, residual disease, lymph node involvement, and distant metastases. This information allows a diagnosis of RMS to be classified into one of the following four different groups: group I, completely resected without lymph node involvement; group II, localized disease with or without complete resection, or microscopic residual disease with or without lymph node involvement; group III, localized gross residual disease; and group IV, distant metastases. This staging is then helpful in determining prognosis and treatment.

Treatment consists of a combination of surgical excision, systemic chemotherapy, and adjunct radiation therapy. The overall survival of childhood RMS has improved over the past decades, but adult survival remains poor.

Other Tumors

Metastatic tumors in muscles are rare in spite of the extensive vascular supply of skeletal muscles. It is suggested that local pH or metabolic changes within muscles prevent metastatic involvement from other tumors. When adjacent carcinomas do cause muscle damage, it is usually related to the compression of tissue and resultant muscle atrophy.

EMERGING SCIENCE BOX

Invasive Therapies to Treat Musculoskeletal Conditions

The use of minimally invasive therapies to treat various musculoskeletal conditions continues to expand. This includes consolidation of skeletal tumors, palliation of painful skeletal lesions, and the treatment of symptomatic soft tissue lesions. The decision to treat individuals with percutaneous ablation is made through a team approach including radiologist, oncologist, and orthopedic/neurologic surgery. Through the use of PET, CT, MRI, and ultrasound, the individual is evaluated for optimal treatment planning. The structural characteristics of the tumor are evaluated and measured, the surrounding structures are mapped, and the metabolic characteristics determined. This allows for a more patient-specific treatment plan. Individuals may require either procedural sedation or general anesthesia depending on the extent of treatment and provider preference. Ablation options include cryoablation, radiofrequency ablation, and microwave ablation. Cryoablation utilizes a repeated freeze-thaw cycle while radiofrequency ablation uses high-frequency alternating current to cause ionic agitation and frictional heating in tissue. Microwave ablation uses alternating electromagnetic fields to cause oscillation of water molecules in tissue, generating cytotoxic temperatures independent of tissue conductivity. All result in targeted cellular destruction of tumor cells. As these techniques continue to be developed and specialized, persons with musculoskeletal tumors have additional treatment options available to them.

Data from Parvinian A, et al. Trends in musculoskeletal ablation: emerging indications and techniques. *Techniques in Vascular and Interventional Radiology*, 23(2):100678, 2020; Kurup AN, et al. Ablation of musculoskeletal metastases. *AJR American Journal of Roentgenology*, 209(4):713–721, 2017; Moynagh MR, et al. Thermal ablation of bone metastases. *Seminars in Interventional Radiology*, 35(4):299–308, 2018; Welch BT, et al. Percutaneous cryoablation of abdominal wall endometriosis: The Mayo Clinic approach. *Abdominal Radiology*, 45(6):1813–1817, 2020.

SUMMARY REVIEW

Musculoskeletal Injuries

1. The most common skeletal injury is a fracture. A bone can be completely or incompletely fractured. A closed fracture leaves the skin intact. An open fracture has an overlying skin wound. The direction of the fracture line can be linear, oblique, spiral, or transverse. Greenstick, torus, and bowing fractures are examples of incomplete fractures that occur in children. Stress fractures occur in normal or abnormal bone that is subjected to repeated stress. Fatigue fractures occur in normal bone subjected to abnormal stress. Normal weightbearing can cause an insufficiency fracture in abnormal bone.
2. Dislocation is complete loss of contact between the surfaces of two bones. Subluxation is partial loss of contact between two bones. As a bone separates from a joint, it may damage adjacent nerves, blood vessels, ligaments, tendons, and muscle.
3. Tendon tears are called *strains*, and ligament tears are called *sprains*. A complete separation of a tendon or ligament from its attachment is called an *avulsion*.
4. Epicondylopathy is degeneration of a tendon where it attaches to a bone. Bursitis is inflammation of the bursae (small sacs lined with synovial membrane and filled with synovial fluid). Bursitis can be inflammatory, septic, or hemorrhagic.
5. Muscle strain can range from mild injury to severe damage that can result in loss of muscle function.
6. Rhabdomyolysis can be a life-threatening complication of severe muscle trauma wherein muscle cell contents are released into the circulation. It may result in myoglobinuria, the presence of myoglobin in the urine, and is often associated with acute renal failure.
7. Compartment syndrome is the result of increased pressure within a closed osteofascial compartment resulting in impaired circulation. These skeletal muscle compartments are surrounded by several layers of fibrous fascia which are not able to expand. After fractures, the most common cause is soft tissue injuries.
8. Malignant hyperthermia (MJ) is a potentially life-threatening hereditary musculoskeletal disorder characterized by a hypermetabolic reaction to certain volatile anesthetics or certain depolarizing muscle relaxants (e.g., succinylcholine). Rarely is MH related to exercise and heat exposure.

Disorders of Bones

1. Osteoporosis is defined as low bone mineral density caused by altered bone microstructure and leads to an increased risk of fractures. It is a complex, multifactorial, chronic disease that often progresses silently causing decreased bone strength. Bone tissue can be normally mineralized in osteoporosis, but the density of bone is decreased and the structural integrity of trabecular bone is impaired.
2. In osteoporosis, old bone is being resorbed faster than new bone is being formed, causing the bones to lose density, becoming thinner and more porous. Postmenopausal osteoporosis results from estrogen deficiency. Estrogen stimulates osteoprotegerin (OPG) secretion and down-regulates

RANKL; RANKL expression is increased when estrogen levels are decreased, leading to increased formation of osteoclasts while reducing osteoclast apoptosis.

3. Glucocorticoid-induced osteoporosis (e.g., prednisone, cortisone) is the most common type of secondary osteoporosis and is characterized by increased bone resorption and decreased bone formation. Glucocorticoids increase RANKL expression and inhibit OPG production by osteoblasts, thus leading to lower bone density.
4. Osteomalacia is a metabolic bone disease characterized by inadequate bone mineralization.
5. Excessive and abnormal bone remodeling occurs in Paget disease. Sporadic Paget disease involves overexpression of RANKL.
6. Osteomyelitis is a bone infection caused most often by bacteria (e.g., *S. aureus*) that can enter bone from outside the body (exogenous osteomyelitis) or from infection sites within the body (hematogenous osteomyelitis).
7. Bone tumors originate from bone cells, cartilage cells, fibrous tissue cells, or vascular marrow cells. Each cell produces a specific type of ground substance that is used to classify the tumor as osteogenic (bone cell), chondrogenic (cartilage cell), collagenic (fibrous tissue cell), or myelogenic (vascular marrow cell). Malignant bone tumors are large, aggressively destroy surrounding bone, invade surrounding tissue, and initiate independent growth outside the site of origin. Benign bone tumors are less destructive, limit their growth to the anatomic confines of the bone, and have a well-demarcated border.

Disorders of Joints

1. Two major categories of joint diseases are noninflammatory and inflammatory joint disease. Osteoarthritis (OA) is the most common joint disease.
2. OA is an inflammatory joint disease and is characterized by pathologic changes in cartilage, bone, synovium, ligament, muscle, and periarticular fat. OA is commonly found in the knees, and less so in hips, hands, and spine. Hip and knee OA are highly prevalent and disabling.
3. The primary defect in OA is degeneration and eventual loss and disordered repair of articular cartilage. The chondrocytes of the articular cartilage become damaged early in the disease process because of biomechanical stress, as well as genetic and biochemical factors.
4. Rheumatoid arthritis (RA) is a chronic, systemic, inflammatory autoimmune disease distinguished by joint swelling, tenderness, and destruction of synovial joints leading to disability. RA is initiated by $CD4^+$ helper T cells. The pathologic changes are mediated by antibodies against self-antigens, such as anti-citrullinated peptide antibodies (ACPAs) detected in the serum of up to 70% of those with RA. $CD4^+$ T cells promote inflammation. RA is a systemic disease that affects other organs, as well as the joints.
5. AS is a chronic inflammatory joint disease of the axial spine. AS is characterized by stiffening and fusion (ankylosis) of the spine sacroiliac joints, peripheral joints, digits, and entheses, and dactylitis. The most common features of AS are chronic back pain and progressive spinal stiffness. The hallmark is enthesitis with chronic inflammation, including CD4 and CD8 T lymphocytes and macrophages.
6. Gout is a systemic disease of uric acid disturbance that results from the deposition of monosodium urate crystals (MSU) in tissues. In the United States, gout is the most prevalent etiology of chronic inflammatory arthritis. Gout develops in stages. Most people with hyperuricemia do not develop gout. For gout to develop it requires the deposition of MSU crystals. Altered urate transport, both in the gut and the kidneys, is central in the pathogenesis of hyperuricemia and gout. Identification of urate transporter genes are strongly correlated with urate levels.

Disorders of Skeletal Muscle

1. A pathologic contracture is permanent muscle shortening caused by muscle spasticity, as seen in CNS injury or severe muscle weakness.
2. Stress-induced muscle tension is presumably caused by increased activity in the reticular activating system and gamma loop in the muscle fiber. Progressive relaxation training and biofeedback have been advocated to reduce muscle tension.
3. Fibromyalgia (FM) is a chronic musculoskeletal syndrome characterized by chronic widespread pain (CWP) primarily (but not only) from the musculoskeletal system. Other most frequent symptoms include fatigue and sleep disturbances. Several factors, uniquely, contribute to the development of FM: genetic predisposition, personal experiences, emotional-cognitive factors, the mind-body relationship, and a biopsychological ability to cope with stress. One hypothesis for pathophysiology involves nociplastic pain or pain arising from altered nociception, despite no evidence of tissue damage. This type of pain conforms to FM as a part of *central sensitivity syndromes*. FM is becoming known as a disorder of pain regulation often classified under central sensitization.
4. Chronic fatigue syndrome (CFS), also known as myalgic encephalomyelitis (ME), is a disabling clinical condition characterized by unexplained and persistent post-exertional fatigue and symptoms related to cognitive, immunological, endocrinological, and autonomic dysfunction. The cause of CFS/ME is hypothesized to include immunologic alterations, chronic proinflammatory cytokines, autoantibodies, neuroinflammation, central nervous system disruptions, hypercortisolism, and genetic predisposition.
5. Atrophy of muscle fibers and overall diminished size of the muscle are seen after prolonged inactivity. Isometric contractions and passive lengthening exercises decrease atrophy to some degree in immobilized persons.
6. Hyperexcitable membranes cause the physical and electrical phenomenon of myotonia. The disorder is treated with drugs that reduce fiber excitability. Periodic paralysis is caused by an unresponsive muscle membrane and is accompanied by changes in the level of serum potassium. The biochemical defect is possibly related to changes in the muscle membrane and sarcoplasmic reticulum.
7. Metabolic muscle diseases are caused by endocrine disorders, glycogen storage disease, enzyme deficiencies, and

abnormal lipid function. The muscle depends on a complex system of carbohydrates and fats converted by enzymes to produce energy for the muscle cell. Abnormalities in these pathways can inhibit function or cause damage to the muscle fiber. These illnesses are rare, yet they account for significant functional abnormalities.
8. Viral, bacterial, and parasitic infections of muscles produce the characteristic clinical and pathologic changes associated with inflammation. These are usually treatable and self-limiting disorders.
9. Polymyositis (generalized muscle inflammation) and dermatomyositis (polymyositis accompanied with skin rash) are characterized by inflammation of connective tissue and muscle fibers, and muscle fiber necrosis. Cell-mediated and humoral immune factors have been implicated. Treatment with immunosuppressive agents is effective in many cases.
10. Primary disorders with weakness and atrophy are known as *myopathies*.
11. The most common toxic myopathy is caused by alcohol abuse. Direct toxic effects of alcohol-producing necrosis of muscle fibers and nutritional deficiency have been identified. The most effective treatment is abstinence and improved nutrition. The toxic effects of many drugs on muscle fibers cause local trauma to the muscle fibers from direct effects of the needle, secondary infection, and changes caused by nonphysiologic acidity and alkalinity in the fibers.
12. Sarcomas of muscle tissue are rare. Rhabdomyosarcoma is a rare malignant tumor of striated muscle. It has aggressive invasion and early, widespread dissemination.

REFERENCES

1. Alves C, Mendes D, Marques FB. Fluroquinolones and the risk of tendon injury: a systematic review and meta-analysis. *Eur J Clin Pharmacol.* 2019;75(10):1431–1443.
2. Persson R, Jick S. Clinical implications of the association between fluoroquinolones and tendon rupture: the magnitude of the effect with and without corticosteroids. *Br J Clin Pharmacol.* 2019;85(5):949–959.
3. Millar NL, Murrell GAC, McInnes IB. Inflammatory mechanisms in tendinopathy—towards translation. *Nat Rev Rheumatol.* 2017;13:110–122.
4. Weinreb JH, et al. Tendon structure, disease, and imaging. *Muscles Ligaments Tendons J.* 2014;4(1):66–73.
5. Genthon A, Wilcox SR. Crush syndrome: a case report and review of the literature. *J Emerg Med.* 2014;46(2):313–319.
6. Moghadam-Kia S, Oddis CV, Aggarwal R. Approach to asymptomatic creatine kinase elevation. *Cleve Clin J Med.* 2016;83(1):37–42.
7. Torlincasi AM, Lopez RA, Waseem M. *Acute compartment syndrome. StatPearls.* Treasure Island, FL: StatPearls Publishing; 2021. Last updated July 19, 2021. Available at https://www.ncbi.nlm.nih.gov/books/NBK448124/. (Accessed May 7, 2022).
8. Schmidt AH. Acute compartment syndrome. *Injury.* 2017;48(Suppl 1):S22–S25.
9. Wuarin L, et al. Clinical and radiographic predictors of acute compartment syndrome in the treatment of tibial shaft fractures: a retrospective cohort study. *BMC Musculoskelet Disord.* 2020;21(1):25.
10. Smith-Singares E, et al. Fusobacterium emphysematous pyomyositis with necrotizing fasciitis of the leg presenting as compartment syndrome: a case report. *J Med Case Rep.* 2017;11(1):332.
11. Thabet AM, et al. The impact of acute compartment syndrome on the outcome of tibia plateau fracture. *Eur J Orthop Surg Traumatol.* 2018;28(1):85–93.
12. Dunphy L, Morhij R, Tucker S. Rhabdomyolysis-induced compartment syndrome secondary to atorvastatin and strenuous exercise. *BMJ Case Rep.* 2017;2017 bcr2016218942.
13. Raza H, Mahapatra A. Acute compartment syndrome in orthopedics: causes, diagnosis, and management. *Adv Orthop.* 2015;2015:543412.
14. Maheshwar L, et al. Volkmann's ischemic contracture with atrophic non-union of ulna managed by bone shortening and transposition of radial autograft. *J Orthop Case Rep.* 2015;5(1):65–68.
15. Osborn CPM, Schmidt AH. Management of acute compartment syndrome. *J Am Acad Orthop Surg.* 2020;28(3):e108–e114.
16. Watt S, McAllister RK. *Malignant hyperthermia. StatPearls.* Treasure Island, FL: StatPearls Publishing; 2021. Last updated July 25, 2021. Available at https://www.ncbi.nlm.nih.gov/books/NBK430828/. (Accessed December 30, 2021).
17. Rosenberg H, et al. Malignant hyperthermia: a review. *Orphanet J Rare Dis.* 2015;10:93.
18. Altamirano F, et al. Is malignant hyperthermia associated with hyperglycaemia? *Br J Anaesth.* 2019;122(1):e3–e5.
19. Dirksen RT, Allen PD, Lopez JR. Understanding malignant hyperthermia: each move forward opens our eyes to the distance left to travel. *Br J Anaesth.* 2019;122(1):8–9.
20. Hopkins PM, Gupta PK, Bilmen JG. Malignant hyperthermia. *Handb Clin Neurol.* 2018;157:645–661.
21. Larach MG, et al. Malignant hyperthermia deaths related to inadequate temperature monitoring, 2007-2012: a report from the North American malignant hyperthermia registry of the Malignant Hyperthermia Association of the United States. *Anesth Analg.* 2014;119(6):1359–1366.
22. Porter JL, Varacallo M. *Osteoporosis. StatPearls.* Treasure Island, FL: StatPearls Publishing; 2021. Last updated July 18, 2021. Available at https://www.ncbi.nlm.nih.gov/books/NBK441901/. (Accessed May 7, 2022).
23. World Health Organization (WHO) Scientific Group on the Prevention and Management of Osteoporosis :. *Prevention and Management of Osteoporosis: Report of a WHO Scientific Group. WHO Technical Report Series, no. 921.* Geneva, Switzerland: WHO; 2003. Available at https://apps.who.int/iris/bitstream/handle/10665/42841/WHO_TRS_921.pdf. (Accessed May 7, 2022).
24. Varacallo MA, Fox EJ. Osteoporosis and its complications. *Med Clin North Am.* 2014;98(4):817–831. xii–xiii.
25. Kanis JA. A brief history of FRAX. *Arch Osteoporos.* 2018;13(1):118.
26. Walzak LC, Loken Thornton W. The role of illness burden in theory of mind performance among older adults. *Exp Aging Res.* 2018;44(5):427–442.
27. Pasco JA, et al. Seasonal periodicity of serum vitamin D and parathyroid hormone, bone resorption, and fractures: the Geelong Osteoporosis Study. *J Bone Miner Res.* 2004;19: 752–758.
28. Thibault R, et al. Twelve key nutritional issues in bariatric surgery. *Clin Nutr.* 2016;35(1):12–17.
29. Lewiecki EM. Osteoporosis: clinical evaluation. In: Feingold KR, ed. *Endotext.* South Dartmouth, MA: MDText.com, Inc.; 2018. Updated June 7, 2021. Available at https://www.ncbi.nlm.nih.gov/books/NBK279049/. (Accessed May 7, 2022).
30. Salhotra A, et al. Mechanisms of bone development and repair. *Nat Rev Mol Cell Biol.* 2020;21:696–711.

31. Worthley DL, et al. Gremlin 1 identifies a skeletal stem cell with bone, cartilage, and reticular stromal potential. *Cell.* 2015;160:269–284.
32. Lacey DL, et al. Osteoprotegerin ligand is a cytokine that regulates osteoclast differentiation and activation. *Cell.* 1998;93:165–176.
33. Yasuda H, et al. Osteoclast differentiation factor is a ligand for osteoprotegerin/osteoclastogenesis-inhibitory factor and is identical to TRANCE/RANKL. *Proc Natl Acad Sci U S A.* 1998;95:3597–3602.
34. Khosla S. Pathogenesis of age-related bone loss in humans. *J Gerontol A Biol Sci Med Sci.* 2013;68(10):1226–1235.
35. US Preventative Services Task Force Screening for osteoporosis to prevent fractures US Preventive Services Task Force recommendation statement. *JAMA.* 2018;319(24):2521–2531.
36. World Health Organization (WHO) Scientific Group on the Assessment of Osteoporosis at Primary Health Care Level Summary Meeting Report. Brussels, Belgium, May 5–7, 2004. Geneva, Switzerland, 2007, WHO. Available at https://www.who.int/chp/topics/Osteoporosis.pdf. (Accessed May 7, 2022).
37. Katz JN, Arant KR, Loeser RF. Diagnosis and treatment of hip and knee osteoarthritis: a review. *JAMA.* 2021;325(6):568–578.
38. Kumar V, Abbas AK, Aster JC. *Robbins & Cotran pathologic basis of disease.* ed 10 Philadelphia: Elsevier; 2020.
39. Kraus VB, et al. Call for standardized definitions of osteoarthritis and risk stratification for clinical trials and clinical use. *Osteoarthritis Cartilage.* 2015;23(8):1233–1241.
40. Sen R, Hurley JA. *Osteoarthritis. StatPearls.* Treasure Island, FL: StatPearls Publishing; 2021. Updated Aug 19, 2021. Available at https://www.ncbi.nlm.nih.gov/books/NBK482326/. (Accessed May 7, 2022).
41. Hawker G. *Osteoarthritis as a Serious Disease.* Mount Laurel, NJ: Osteoarthritis Research Society International (OARSI); 2016. Available at https://oarsi.org/sites/default/files/docs/2016/oarsi_white_paper_oa_serious_disease_121416_1.pdf. (Accessed May 7, 2022).
42. Donahue SW. Krogh's principle for musculoskeletal physiology and pathology. *J Musculoskelet Neuronal Interact.* 2018;18(3):284–291.
43. Krishnan Y, Grodzinsky AJ. Cartilage diseases. *Matrix Biol.* 2018;71–72:51–69.
44. Rahmati M, et al. Aging and osteoarthritis: central role of the extracellular matrix. *Aging Res Rev.* 2017;40:20–30.
45. Maldonado M, Nam J. The role of changes in extracellular matrix of cartilage in the presence of inflammation on the pathology of osteoarthritis. *Biomed Res Int.* 2013;2013:284873 Available at https://doi.org/10.1155/2013/284873. (Accessed May 7, 2022).
46. Shi Y, et al. A small molecule promotes cartilage extracellular matrix generation and inhibits osteoarthritis development. *Nat Commun.* 2019;10:1914.
47. Kriz J, et al. Updated strategies in the treatment of benign diseases—a patterns of care study of the German Cooperative Group on Benign Diseases. *Adv Radiat Oncol.* 2018;3(3): 240–244.
48. di Laura Frattura G, : Risk of falls in patients with knee osteoarthritis undergoing total knee arthroplasty: a systematic review and best evidence synthesis. *J Orthop.* 2018;15(3)::903–908.
49. Xing D, et al. Evidence-based guidelines for intra-articular injection in knee osteoarthritis: formulating and evaluating research questions. *Int J Rheum Dis.* 2018;21(8):1533–1542.
50. Burgess CJ, De Cicco FL. *Meniscectomy. StatPearls.* Treasure Island, FL: StatPearls Publishing; 2021. Updated July 18, 2021. Available at https://www.ncbi.nlm.nih.gov/books/NBK559105/. (Accessed May 7, 2022).
51. Abram SGF. Arthroscopic partial meniscectomy for meniscal tears of the knee: a systematic review and meta-analysis. *Br J Sports Med.* 2020;54(11):652–663.
52. Smolen JS, et al. Rheumatoid arthritis. *Nat Rev Dis Primers.* 2018;4:18001.
53. Guo Q, et al. Rheumatoid arthritis: pathological mechanisms and modern pharmacologic therapies. *Bone Res.* 2018;6:15.
54. Center for Disease Control and Prevention (CDC) *Rheumatoid Arthritis Fact Sheet (2020).* Atlanta, GA: CDC; 2020. Page last reviewed July 27, 2020. Available at https://www.cdc.gov/arthritis/basics/rheumatoid-arthritis.html. (Accessed May 7, 2022).
55. National Institutes of Health (NIH) *Rheumatoid Arthritis: Genetics Home Reference.* Bethesda, MD: NIH; 2020. Page last updated on August 18, 2020. Page last reviewed: September 1, 2013. Available at https://medlineplus.gov/genetics/condition/rheumatoid-arthritis/. (Accessed May 7, 2022).
56. Ishikawa Y, Terao C. The impact of cigarette smoking on risk of rheumatoid arthritis: a narrative review. *Cells.* 2020;9(2):475.
57. Chauhan K, et al. *Rheumatoid arthritis. StatPearls.* Treasure Island, FL: StatPearls Publishing; 2021. Updated 2021 October 7, 2021. Available at https://www.ncbi.nlm.nih.gov/books/NBK441999/. (Accessed May 7, 2022).
58. Webber MP, et al. Nested case-control study of selected systemic autoimmune diseases in World Trade Cancer rescue/recovery workers. *Arthritis Rheumatol.* 2015;67(5):1369–1376.
59. Too CL, et al. Occupational exposure to textile dust increases the risk of rheumatoid arthritis: results from a Malaysian population-based case-control study. *Ann Rheum Dis.* 2016;75(6):997–1002.
60. Hajishengalis G. Periodontitis from microbial immune subversion to systemic inflammation. *Nat Rev Immunol.* 2015;15(1):30–44.
61. Pianta A, et al. Two rheumatoid arthritis-specific autoantigens correlate microbial immunity with autoimmune responses in joints. *J Clin Invest.* 2017;127(8):2946–2956.
62. Baffour FI, et al. Sonography of active rheumatoid arthritis during pregnancy: a case report and literature review. *Radiol Case Rep.* 2018;13(6):1233–1237.
63. Mochizuki T, et al. Evaluation of factors associated with locomotive syndrome in Japanese elderly and younger patients with rheumatoid arthritis. *Mod Rheumatol.* 2019;29(5):733–736.
64. Bremander A, et al. Importance of measuring hand and foot function over the disease course in rheumatoid arthritis: an eight-year follow-up study. *Arthritis Care Res (Hoboken).* 2019;71(2):166–172.
65. Aletaha D, et al. 2010 Rheumatism classification criteria for rheumatoid arthritis: an American College of Rheumatology/European League Against Rheumatism collaborative initiative. *Arthritis Rheum.* 2010;62(9):2569–2581.
66. Wenker KJ, Quint JM. *Ankylosing spondylitis. StatPearls.* Treasure Island, FL: StatPearls Publishing; 2021. Updated August 4, 2021. Available at https://www.ncbi.nlm.nih.gov/books/NBK470173/. (Accessed May 7, 2022).
67. Wang R, Ward MW. Epidemiology of axial spondyloarthritis: an update. *Curr Opin Rheumatol.* 2018;30(2):137–143.
68. U.S. National Library of Medicine *Ankylosing Spondylitis.* Bethesda, MD: U.S. National Library of Medicine; 2022. Updated March 23, 2022 Available at https://medlineplus.gov/genetics/condition/ankylosing-spondylitis/. (Accessed May 7, 2022).
69. Aloush V, et al. Evaluating IBD-specific antiglycan antibodies in serum of patients with spondyloarthritis and rheumatoid arthritis: are they really specific? *Clin Exp Rheumatol.* 2019;37(1):32–36.
70. Rabelo CF, et al. Serum IL-6 correlates with axial mobility index (Bath Ankylosing Spondylitis Metrology Index) in Brazilian

patients with ankylosing spondylitis. *Open Access Rheumatol.* 2018;10:21–25.
71. Rahbar MH, et al. Harmonization, data management, and statistical issues related to prospective multicenter studies in ankylosing spondylitis (AS): experience from the Prospective Study of Ankylosing Spondylitis (PSOAS) cohort. *Contemp Clin Trials Commun.* 2018;11:127–135.
72. Ragab G, Elshahaly M, Bardin T. Gout: an old disease in new perspective—a review. *J Adv Res.* 2017;8(5):495–511.
73. Dalbeth N, Merriman TR, Stamp LK. Gout. *Lancet.* 2016;388(10055):2039–2052.
74. Fenando A, Rednam M, Widrich J. *Gout. StatPearls.* Treasure Island, FL: StatPearls Publishing; 2021. Updated December 7, 2021. Available at https://www.ncbi.nlm.nih.gov/books/NBK546606/. (Accessed May 7, 2022).
75. Neogi T. Gout. *Ann Intern Med.* 2016;165(1):ITC1–ITC16.
76. Dalbeth N, et al. Gout. *Nat Rev Dis Primers.* 2019;5:69.
77. Chen-Xu M, et al. Contemporary prevalence of gout and hyperuricemia in the United States and decadal trends: the National Health and Nutrition Examination Survey, 2007-2016. *Arthritis Rheumatol.* 2019;71(6):991–999.
78. Köttgen A, et al. Genome-wide association analyses identify 18 new loci associated with serum urate concentrations. *Nat Genet.* 2013;45:145–154.
79. Nakatochi M, et al. Genome-wide meta-analysis identifies multiple novel loci associated with serum uric acid levels in Japanese individuals. *Commun Biol.* 2019;2:115.
80. Sivera F, Andrés M, Quilis N. Gout: diagnosis and treatment. *Med Clin (Barc).* 2017;148(6):271–276.
81. Abhishek A, Roddy E, Doherty M. Gout—a guide for the general and acute physicians. *Clin Med (Lond).* 2017;17(1):54–59.
82. Sarzi-Puttini P, et al. Fibromyalgia: an update on clinical characteristics, aetiopathogenesis and treatment. *Nat Rev Rheumatol.* 2020;16:645–660.
83. Overman CL, et al. The prevalence of severe fatigue in rheumatic diseases: an international study. *Clin Rheumatol.* 2016;35:409–415.
84. Sandıkçı SC, Özbalkan Z. Fatigue in rheumatic diseases. *Eur J Rheumatol.* 2015;2(3):109–113.
85. Wolfe F, et al. 2016 Revisions to the 2010/2011 fibromyalgia diagnostic criteria. *Semin Arthritis Rheum.* 2016;46(3):319–329.
86. Arnold LM, et al. AAPT diagnostic criteria for fibromyalgia. *J Pain.* 2019;20(6):611–628.
87. Borchers AT, Gershwin ME. Fibromyalgia: a critical and comprehensive review. *Clin Rev Allergy Immunol.* 2015;49:100–151.
88. Ceko M, Bushnell C, Gracely RH. Neurobiology underlying fibromyalgia symptoms. *Pain Res Treat.* 2012;2012:585419.
89. Geisser ME, et al. A psychological study of auditory and pressure sensitivity in patients with fibromyalgia and healthy controls. *J Pain.* 2008;9(5):417–422.
90. Martenson ME, et al. A possible neural mechanism for photosensitivity in chronic pain. *Pain.* 2016;157(4):868–878.
91. Pujol J, et al. Mapping brain response to pain in fibromyalgia patients using temporal analysis of FMRI. *PLoS One.* 2009;4(4):e5224.
92. Jensen KB, et al. Patients with fibromyalgia display less functional connectivity in the brain's pain inhibitory network. *Mol Pain.* 2012;8:32.
93. Bhargava J, Hurley JA. *Fibromyalgia. StatPearls.* Treasure Island, FL: StatPearls Publishing; 2021. Updated October 13, 2021. Available at https://www.ncbi.nlm.nih.gov/books/NBK540974/. (Accessed May 7, 2022).
94. Farré M, et al. *Chapter e16. Cannabis use in fibromyalgia. Handbook of Cannabis and Related Pathologies: Biology, Pharmacology, Diagnosis, and Treatment.* Cambridge, MA: Academic Press; 2017:e158–e167 Available at https://doi.org/10.1016/B978-0-12-800756-3.00112-5. (Accessed May 7, 2022).
95. Deare JC, et al. Acupuncture for treating fibromyalgia. *Cochrane Database Syst Rev.* 2013;2013(5):CD007070.
96. Bai Y, et al. Efficacy of acupuncture on fibromyalgia syndrome: a meta-analysis. *J Tradit Chin Med.* 2014;34(4):381–391.
97. El-Shewy KM, et al. Hyperbaric oxygen and aerobic exercise in the long-term treatment of fibromyalgia: a narrative review. *Biomed Pharmacother.* 2019;109:629–638.
98. Rivera MC, et al. Myalgic encephalomyelitis/chronic fatigue syndrome: a comprehensive review. *Diagnostics (Basel).* 2019;9(3):91.
99. Sapra A, Bhandari P. *Chronic fatigue syndrome. StatPearls.* Treasure Island, FL: StatPearls Publishing; 2021. Updated September 18, 2021. Available at https://www.ncbi.nlm.nih.gov/books/NBK557676/. (Accessed May 7, 2022).
100. Loebel M, et al. Antibodies to β adrenergic and muscarinic cholinergic receptors in patients with chronic fatigue syndrome. *Brain Behav Immun.* 2016;52:32–39.
101. Sotzny F, et al. Myalgic encephalomyelitis/chronic fatigue syndrome—evidence for an autoimmune disease. *Autoimmun Rev.* 2018;17(6):601–609.
102. Maes M, et al. Increased IgA responses to the LPS of commensal bacteria is associated with inflammation and activation of cell-mediated immunity in chronic fatigue syndrome. *J Affect Disord.* 2012;136(3):909–917.
103. National Library of Medicine *Carnitine Palmitoyltransferase I Deficiency.* Bethesda, MD: National Library of Medicine; 2020. Updated April 1, 2014. Available at https://medlineplus.gov/genetics/condition/carnitine-palmitoyltransferase-i-deficiency/. (Accessed May 7, 2022).

45

Alterations of Musculoskeletal Function in Children

Corinne M. Djuric

http://evolve.elsevier.com/Rogers/pathophysiology/

CHAPTER OUTLINE

Musculoskeletal alterations in children can be either congenital or acquired. Both pathology and treatment can cause long-term sequelae because of the growing nature of the immature skeleton. Some disorders are acute and the child can recover completely, other disorders are chronic, and some cases are terminal. The emotional trauma of an injured or malformed child is substantial and requires that careful attention be paid to both the child and family.

MUSCULOSKELETAL DEVELOPMENT IN CHILDREN

Bone Formation

Bone formation begins at about the sixth week of gestation. It involves two phases: (1) the delivery of bone cell precursors to sites of bone formation and (2) the aggregation of these cells at primary centers of ossification, where they mature and begin to secrete osteoid (see Chapter 44). Some of the bone cell precursors are present in fetal connective tissues, whereas others migrate in blood to sites of bone formation after blood vessels have grown into the tissue.

Cellular aggregation and maturation occur in two types of fetal tissue, depending on which bones are being formed. The cranium, facial bones, clavicles, and part of the jawbone (classically called *flat bones*) arise from a fetal membrane termed the *mesenchyme*. Bones that develop on or within the mesenchyme grow by the process of intramembranous formation of bone. As the mesenchyme becomes vascularized, the immature bone cells aggregate and mature into osteoblasts that form the centers of ossification and create solid bone or osteoid.

Endochondral formation of bone is the development of new bone from cartilage (Fig. 45.1). First, mesenchymal tissue forms a cartilage anlage, which defines the shape of the bone. This is usually found by 6 weeks' gestation. Blood vessel invasion inside the anlage brings osteoprogenitor cells leading to primary centers of calcification by 8 weeks. Endochondral bone formation begins in the outer layer of the cartilage model, which consists of a layer of dense connective tissue call perichondrium. The perichondrium contains cells that develop into osteoblasts, forming a collar of bone, termed the periosteal collar, around the cartilage model. Cartilage enclosed within the periosteal collar degenerates, and capillaries from outside the perichondrium invade the degenerating cartilage cells, carrying with them osteoblast precursors from the inner layer of the perichondrium and osteoclast precursors from the blood itself.

Endochondral bone formation progresses at the primary center of ossification in the middle of the cartilage model and extends toward either end of the developing bone. At the same time, the periosteal collar thickens and becomes wider toward the epiphyses. By the end of gestation, secondary centers of ossification (the epiphyseal centers) begin to lay down bone at both ends of the cartilage model. Here, too, the cartilage within the periosteal collar degenerates, and blood vessels grow inward,

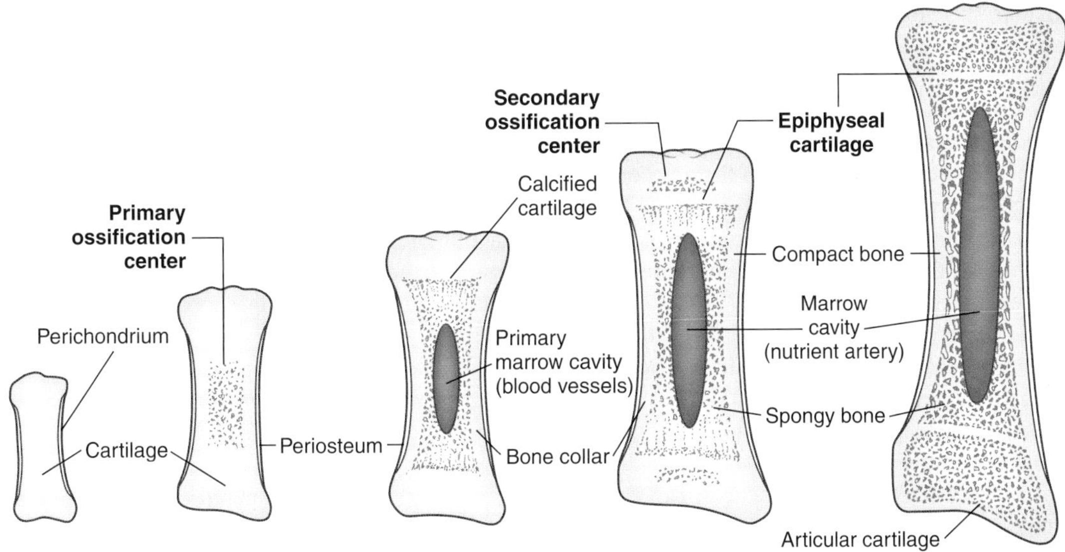

Fig. 45.1 Stages of Endochondral Bone Formation and Centers of Ossification in Long Bones.

delivering bone cell precursors. Once the osteoblasts begin to secrete osteoid, ossification spreads from the secondary centers in all directions until all the cartilage within the model is replaced by bone.

Two regions of cartilage remain at the ends of long bones: (1) articular cartilage over the free ends of the bone and (2) the physeal plate, a layer of cartilage between the metaphysis and epiphysis (see Chapter 44). The physeal plate retains the ability to form and calcify new cartilage and deposit bone until the skeleton matures approximately 1 year after sexual maturity (age 11 to 15 years in females; age 15 to 18 years in males).

Bone Growth

Until adult stature is reached, growth in the length of long bones occurs at the physeal plate through endochondral ossification. Cartilage cells at the epiphyseal side of the physeal plate multiply and enlarge. As rapidly as new cartilage cells form, cartilage cells at the metaphyseal side of the plate are destroyed and replaced by bone.

In the shaft of new bone, where growth is relatively slow, the bone produced by accretion is compact and dense. The compact bone is thickest where it has to withstand the maximal stresses, which generally occur in the middle of the shaft.

The two physes of the long bone have varying activity rates. For example, the distal physis in the femur contributes 80% of the overall length, whereas the proximal physis at the hip contributes only 20%. The more active of the two has more power to remodel deformity but also can be more sensitive to injury. The architecture of the physis also dictates its sensitivity to injury. For example, the distal femur has an undulating pattern that increases its resistance to sheer force; however, when injured, growth disturbance is highly likely. In contrast, the distal radius, which contributes 80% of overall radial length, is a flat, smooth physis that is far more resistant to traumatic injury.

Growth in the diameter of bone occurs by deposition of new bone on an existing bone surface. Bone matrix is laid down by osteoblasts on the periosteal surface and subsequently becomes calcified. At the same time, bone resorption occurs on the endosteal surface. Endosteal resorption increases the diameter of the medullary cavity, which contains marrow and spongy bone.

Many factors affect the development, physiology, and growth rate of the epiphyseal plate. Growth hormone must be secreted by the pituitary gland at a constant rate to stimulate the growth plate consistently. Other known factors affecting growth include peptide regulatory factors (e.g., fibroblast growth factor [FGF]); changes in cell-to-cell interactions through cell adhesion molecules (CAMs) and cell junctions; and complex interactions or changes in the extracellular matrix (ECM), nutrition, general health, and other hormones (e.g., thyroid hormone, adrenal and gonadal androgens, estrogens). When these factors are poorly controlled, skeletal dysplasia, such as achondroplasia, can occur.

Even after physeal closure at skeletal maturity, bone is constantly being destroyed and re-formed (see Chapter 44). This is a rapid process in young children, allowing them to heal bone injury more quickly than adults. However, by adulthood, bone turnover, or remodeling, occurs at a relatively slow rate. Peak bone mass is achieved by the middle to late 20s and slowly decreases through life; therefore ensuring appropriate intake of calcium and phosphorus, performing weight-bearing exercise, and minimizing caffeine intake are especially important for a young female if she is to avoid osteoporosis in later life. Vitamin D plays an essential role in bone homeostasis in the pediatric population. In children, low levels of vitamin D have been associated with rickets, a higher incidence of fracture, more severe fracture, and hypocalcemia that may present as seizure or tetany.[1–4]

Skeletal Development

The axial skeleton changes shape with growth (see Chapter 44). In a newborn, the entire spine is kyphosed. As the infant's ability to control the head progresses in the first 3 months of life, the cervical spine begins to arch. The normal lordotic curve of the lumbar spine begins to develop with sitting.

The appendicular skeleton grows faster during childhood than does the axial skeleton. The newborn has a relatively large head and long spine, with disproportionately shorter limbs than an adult. By 1 year of age, 50% of the total growth of the spine has occurred and is more than 70% complete by age 8.[4a] Therefore failure of the spine to grow (spinal fusion) does not limit eventual height as much as the premature fusion of the growth plates of the lower extremities. In children with congenital curvature of the spine, growth tends to worsen the deformity rather than to increase the length of the spine.

Besides getting longer, growing bones of the extremities undergo changes in rotation and alignment. In the newborn, the proximal femur is rotated forward up to 40 degrees and the tibia is rotated inward. The femur assumes its normal alignment by age 12, and tibial rotation neutralizes at 8 years of age.[6] Genu varum (bowlegs) and genu valgum (knock knees) can be normal at certain stages of growth. At birth, the newborn's legs are bowed because of stresses in utero. Genu varum peaks by 30 months, whereas genu valgum peaks by 5 to 6 years of age. If either persists past these ages, a pathologic process rather than a physiologic phase can be present. Pathologic causes of genu varum are Blount disease, rickets, skeletal dysplasia, traumatic injury, and musculoskeletal infection. Genu valgum may also persist with skeletal dysplasia, genetic predilection, benign musculoskeletal tumor, osteogenesis imperfecta (OI), or after a traumatic injury or infection.

Muscle Growth

The composition and size of muscles vary with age. In the fetus, muscle tissue contains a large amount of water and intercellular matrix. After birth, both are reduced considerably as the muscle fibers enlarge by accumulating cytoplasm. Little information is available about the numbers of fibers in a given muscle at various ages, but the total mass of muscle in the body can be estimated from the amount of creatinine excreted in the urine. The conversion of creatine to creatinine takes place only in muscle (see Chapter 44). Between birth and maturity, the number of muscle nuclei in the body increases 14 times in males and 10 times in females. Muscle fibers reach their maximal size at approximately 10 years of age in females and 14 years of age in males. Growth in length occurs at the ends of muscles, and the increase in length is accompanied by an increase in the number of nuclei in the fibers. Muscle fibers increase in diameter as the fibrils become more numerous. The fibrils themselves do not grow where the tendon and muscle meet.

A potent stimulus to the growth of a muscle is the separation of its attachments as the skeleton grows. The length of a muscle fiber is the direct consequence of its intended range of movement. The stimulus for the formation of a tendon is probably the pull of the muscle rudiment on undifferentiated connective tissue. If the normal opponents of a muscle are paralyzed, the muscle fails to grow properly and can result in contracture of a joint.

Muscle growth during adolescence is a major factor in weight gain. Gender differences in muscle size and weight are minor in childhood but become considerable with the onset of puberty. In the infant, muscle accounts for approximately 25% of total body weight, compared with 40% in the adult. The facial muscles are well developed at birth so that the infant can perform the vital functions of breathing and sucking. Other muscle groups, such as the pelvic muscles, take several years to develop fully.

MUSCULOSKELETAL ALTERATIONS IN CHILDREN

Congenital Defects

Syndactyly and Polydactyly

The most common congenital defect of the extremities is syndactyly, a condition characterized by webbed or conjoined fingers or toes (Fig. 45.2A). Simple webbing involves the soft tissue envelope alone and is best released surgically when the child is 6 months to 1 year of age. Complex syndactyly involves the fusion of the bones and nails as well as the soft tissues. It may be associated with an anomaly of bony or neurovascular units. Ideally, corrective surgery is deferred until the child is 1 to 2 years old and completed before the child enters school. Polydactyly, or supernumerary digits, is another common congenital limb anomaly. Polydactyly occurring on the hand often presents on the ulnar aspect (see Fig. 45.2B). The extra digit can vary greatly in size and shape, some appearing as fully formed digits.[7]

Anomalies on the radial aspect of the arm, such as a foreshortened or absent radius, are often associated with abnormalities of

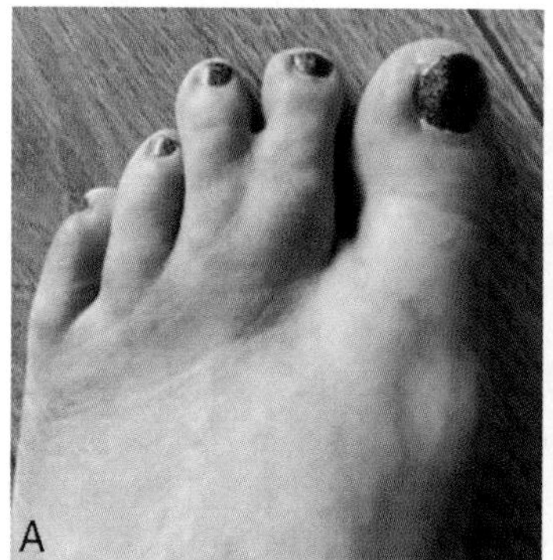

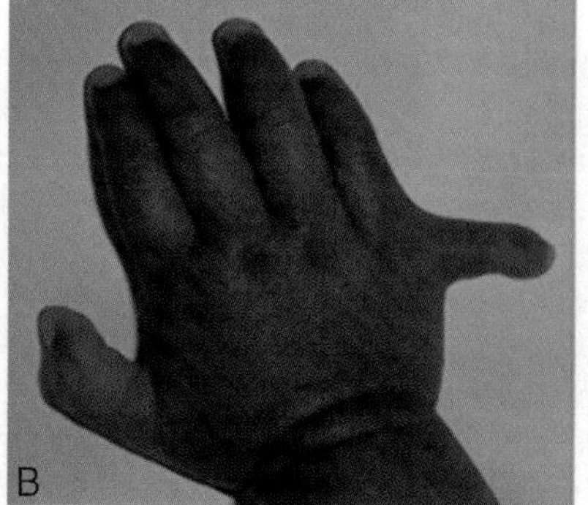

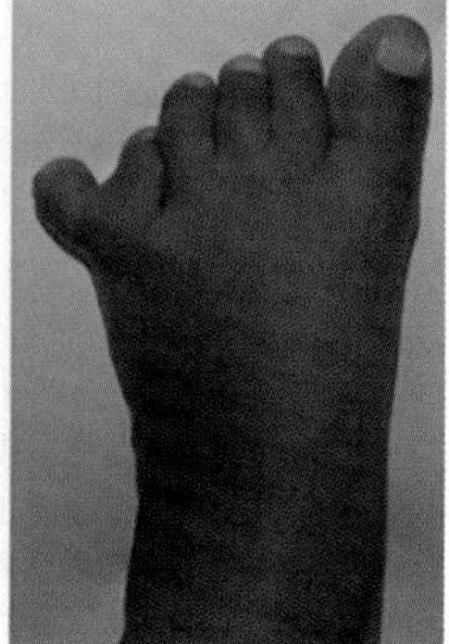

Fig. 45.2 Syndactyly and Polydactyly. **(A)** Syndactyly is the fusing together or webbing of two or more fingers or toes. **(B)** Polydactyly is the presence of extra fingers or toes.

blood, heart, or kidney. Lateral or ulnar-sided defects are less often associated with systemic anomalies and are extremely rare.

Developmental Dysplasia of the Hip

Developmental dysplasia of the hip (DDH) is an umbrella term used to describe a spectrum of disorders related to abnormal development of the hip joint that affects the proximal femur, acetabulum, or both (Fig. 45.3). Although most often present congenitally, dysplasia may develop later in the newborn or infant period and can be idiopathic or teratologic. Teratologic hips (i.e., those attributable to another disorder such as cerebral palsy (CP), Down syndrome, spina bifida, or arthrogryposis) are more difficult to treat and often need operative intervention.

Pathophysiology. By approximately 10 weeks' gestation, the femur, acetabulum, and hip joint capsule are well developed. It appears that most hip dysplasia develops within the second and third trimesters and is often the result of positioning factors, genetics, or pathology. Risk factors for DDH include family history, female gender, oligohydramnios, first pregnancy, and breech presentation (especially 34 weeks or later gestation). First pregnancies and oligohydramnios (deficient volume of amniotic fluid) are thought to limit fetal movement. Breech presentation not only limits movement but also places the hips in a position of flexion and adduction. This creates a more shallow than normal acetabulum (socket) for the head (ball) of the femur, which results in the head of the femur sliding partially or completely out of the acetabulum.

The hip of DDH can be described as dislocated (no contact between the femoral head and acetabulum), subluxated (partial contact only, maintains contact with acetabulum but not well seated within the hip joint), and acetabular dysplasia (the femoral head is located properly but the acetabulum is shallow or underdeveloped) (Fig. 45.4). Some degree of acetabular dysplasia is present in almost all cases.

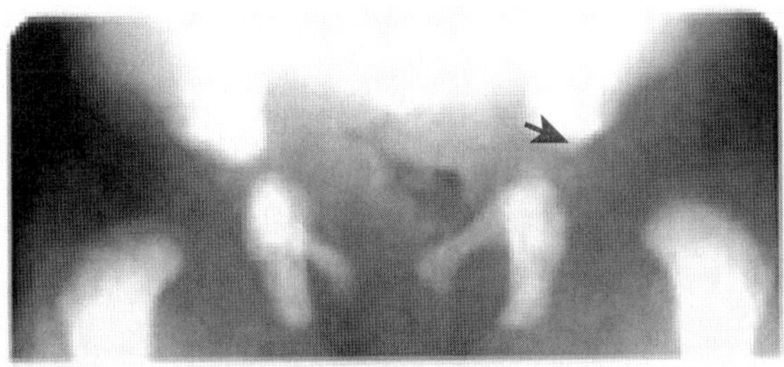

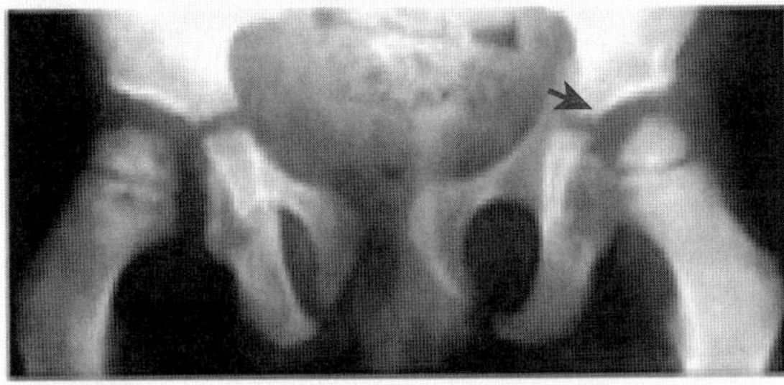

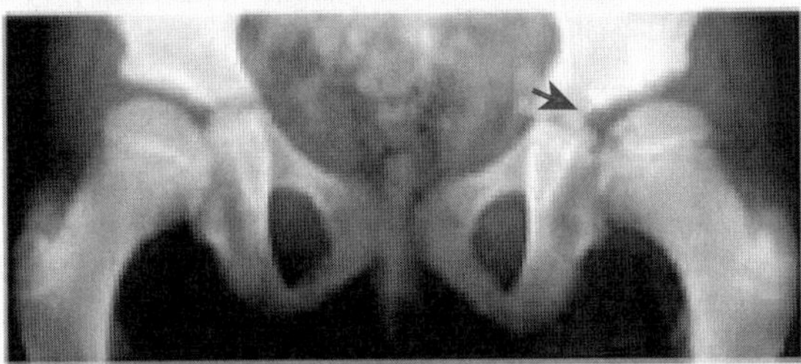

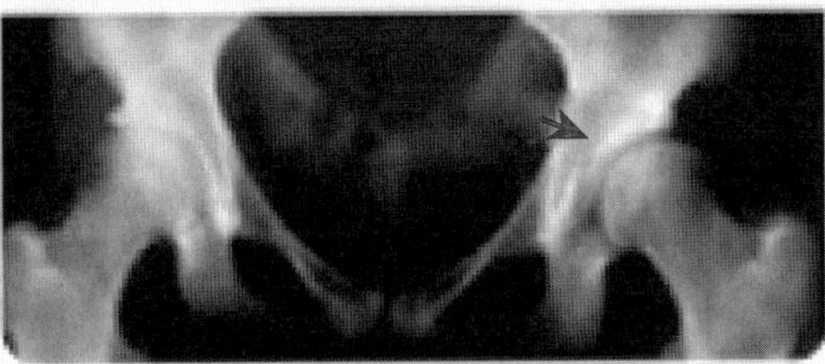

Fig. 45.3 Hip Dysplasia in Children. Developmental dysplasia of the hip (DDH) with residual acetabular dysplasia *(red arrows)*. Radiographs at birth, 3, 10, and 19 years (top to bottom) show persisting dysphasia.

Clinical Manifestations. The clinical manifestations of DDH will vary with the severity of the condition and the age of the child. Signs and symptoms that should be noted include the following:

1. Asymmetry of gluteal or thigh folds
2. Limb length discrepancy (Galeazzi sign)
3. Limitation of hip abduction
4. Positive Barlow maneuver (hip reduced, but able to be dislocated) (Fig. 45.5A)
5. Positive Ortolani sign (hip dislocated, but reducible) (see Fig. 45.5B)
6. Positive Trendelenburg gait (waddling)
7. Pain (very late)

The child also should be examined for other anomalies, such as torticollis or metatarsus adductus, which can be associated with DDH.

Evaluation and Treatment. Clinical examination is the mainstay of diagnosis and is especially important in the newborn period. The examination must be performed on a relaxed infant for accuracy. Real-time ultrasound during a hip examination is extremely valuable in the newborn period, especially in high-risk infants. The use of ultrasound allows visualization of the cartilaginous structures of the hip (the femoral head and the outer lip of the acetabulum), which are not seen on a plain roentgenogram. Radiographs are used after age 6 months when the ossific nucleus of the femoral head appears.[8]

Absolute indications for treatment include a positive Barlow sign (hip reduced but can be dislocated) (see Fig. 45.5A) or a positive Ortolani sign (hip dislocated, but reducible) (see Fig. 45.5B). Other indicators for further evaluation are limitation of abduction or apparent shortening of the femur (Galeazzi sign). Asymmetric skin folds at the groin also can be a clinical sign of hip pathology. If DDH is left untreated in the growing child, secondary changes occur. If the hip remains subluxated or dislocated, the acetabulum becomes increasingly shallow and the soft tissues shorten around the proximal femur. Subluxation leads to early osteoarthritis (OA). If the hip is dislocated, the bone acetabulum fills with soft tissue and a false acetabulum forms where the femoral head contacts the iliac crest. Adult reconstruction of a dislocated hip, even with an artificial hip, is very difficult.[5]

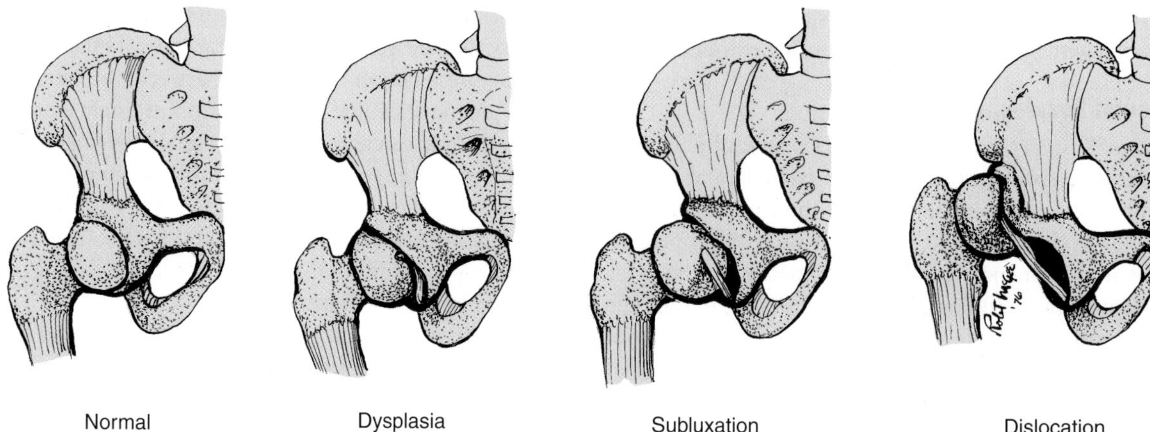

Fig. 45.4 Configuration and Relationship of Structures in Developmental Dysplasia of the Hip. (From Hockenberry MJ, Wilson DL. *Wong's nursing care of infants and children*, 10th edition. St. Louis: Mosby; 2015.)

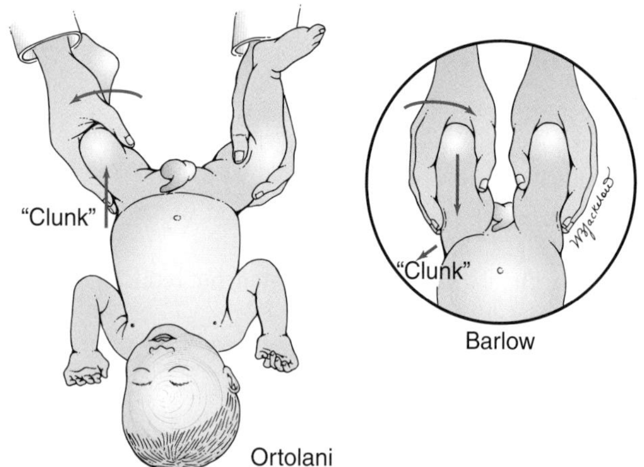

Fig. 45.5 Evaluation for Congenital Dislocation of the Hip. **(A)** Barlow maneuver *(left side)*. With one hand pressing the symphysis in front and the sacral spine in back, lateral pressure is applied to the thigh with the thumb of the other hand while pressure is applied with the palm to the knee on the side being examined. The hip that has been flexed to 90 degrees is then adducted. A positive sign is a sensation of abnormal movement, indicating dislocation of the femoral head from the acetabulum. The hands are reversed for examining the other hip. This sign and the Ortolani sign may be found only in the first weeks of life. **(B)** Ortolani maneuver *(right side)*. Sign of jerking into correct position. After Barlow maneuver (A), the hip should be abducted to about 80 degrees while the femur is lifted anteriorly with the fingers along the thigh. A positive sign is a sensation of a jerk or snap with reduction into the joint socket. (From Dains J, Baumann L, Scheibel P. *Advanced health assessment and clinical diagnosis in primary care*, 6th ed. St. Louis: Elsevier, 2019.)

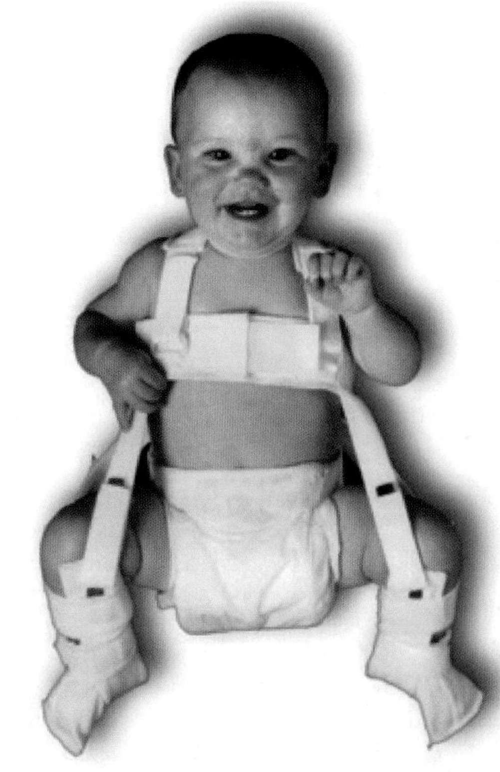

Fig. 45.6 Pavlik Harness for Bilateral Hip Dislocation. (From Wheaton Brace Co., Carol Stream, IL.)

Treatment depends on the age of the child, severity of dysplasia, and duration of dysplasia. The earlier that treatment is begun, the better the result. In children younger than 4 months old, bracing with a Pavlik harness is successful in 90% of DDH cases (Fig. 45.6). A Barlow-positive hip is easier to treat with a Pavlik harness, and success rates approach 97%.[9] An Ortolani-positive hip must be followed closely with ultrasound and examination; the success rate with Pavlik harness is 70% in this situation.[9] If a stable reduction is not attained within 2 to 3 weeks of treatment, the Pavlik harness should be abandoned and casting or surgery pursued instead. A partially reduced hip applies pressure on the rim of the acetabulum by the femoral head and can worsen dysplasia and make treatment more difficult. In older children (6 to 12 months) or those who failed bracing with a Pavlik harness, closed reduction of the hip and spica casting (casting of the trunk of the body and one or both legs) are performed using a general anesthetic. The spica cast is worn for 3 months. Children older than 12 months require surgery on the joint, the femur, or the acetabulum, or all three.

Deformities of the Foot

Congenital foot deformity is a broad category of deformities, with metatarsus adductus accounting for 75% of these anomalies. The terms used to describe foot abnormalities are summarized in Table 45.1. Metatarsus adductus is a forefoot adduction deformity associated with a normal, plantigrade hindfoot. It is believed to be secondary to intrauterine positioning. It is associated with DDH in 20% of cases; consequently, the hips of these infants must be carefully evaluated. Metatarsus adductus is usually classified by two criteria: flexibility (passively correctable vs. rigid) and degree of deformity. The degree of deformity (mild, moderate, severe) is ascertained by the heel bisection line. A mild deformity is one in which the heel bisection line passes medial to the third tow; moderate, through the third or fourth toes; and severe, lateral to the fourth toe.

Clubfoot, technically talipes equinovarus, describes a range of congenital foot deformities in which the foot turns inward and downward. It can affect one or both feet, where the heel is positioned varus (inwardly deviated) and equinus (plantar flexed) (Fig. 45.7). The clubfoot deformity can be positional (correctable passively), idiopathic, or teratologic (as a result of another syndrome, such as spina bifida).

Positional equinovarus is a deformity in which an infant's foot is in equinovarus position but does have flexibility without deep creases at the posterior ankle or midfoot. The Achilles tendon is still flexible. The foot can be passively brought to a plantigrade position and is amenable to stretching and casting. In general, conservative therapy corrects this foot without the need for surgical intervention or lengthy bracing.

Idiopathic congenital equinovarus (Fig. 45.8) is the most common pediatric deformity and occurs once in every 1000 live births. Etiology is unknown. Smoking is the major environmental factor, especially in combination with multiple gene alterations.[10] In one human fetal study, all clubfeet were associated with identifiable anterior horn cell changes in L5 and S1. Muscle biopsies of both the anterior tibialis long flexors and the peroneus brevis muscles in clubfoot reveal that at least 50% of

TABLE 45.1 Terms Used to Describe Foot Abnormalities

Term	Definition
Position[a]	
Abduction	Lateral deviation away from the midline of the body
Adduction	Lateral deviation toward the midline of the body
Eversion	Twisting of the foot outward along its long axis
Inversion	Twisting of the foot inward on its long axis
Dorsiflexion	Bending of the foot upward and backward
Plantar flexion	Bending of the foot downward and forward
Abnormality[a]	
Talipes equinovarus	Congenital abnormality of the foot (clubfoot)
Pes	Acquired deformity of the foot
Varus	Inversion and adduction of the heel and forefoot
Valgus	Eversion and abduction of the heel and forefoot
Equinus	Plantar flexion of the foot in which the heel is lower than the toes
Calcaneus	Dorsiflexion of the foot in which the heel is lower than the toes
Planus	Flattening of the medial longitudinal arch of the foot (flatfoot)
Cavus	Elevation of the medial longitudinal arch of the foot (high arch)
Equinovarus	Coexistent equinus and varus deformities
Calcaneovarus	Coexistent calcaneus and varus deformities
Equinovalgus	Coexistent equinus and valgus deformities
Calcaneovalgus	Coexistent calcaneus and valgus deformities

[a]The positions listed can all be achieved by voluntary movement of the normal foot; an abnormality exists if the foot is fixed in one or more of the positions while at rest.

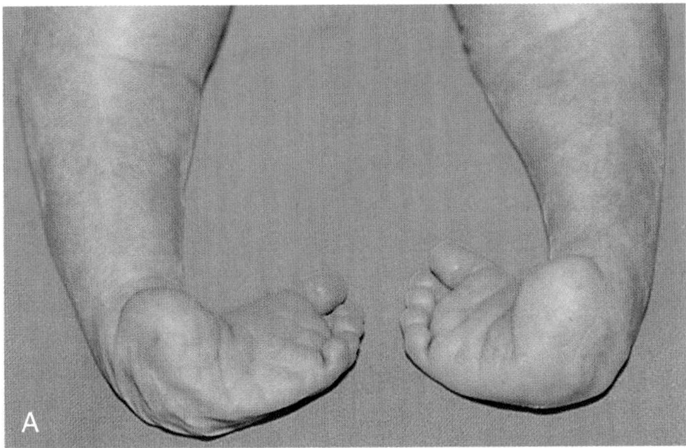

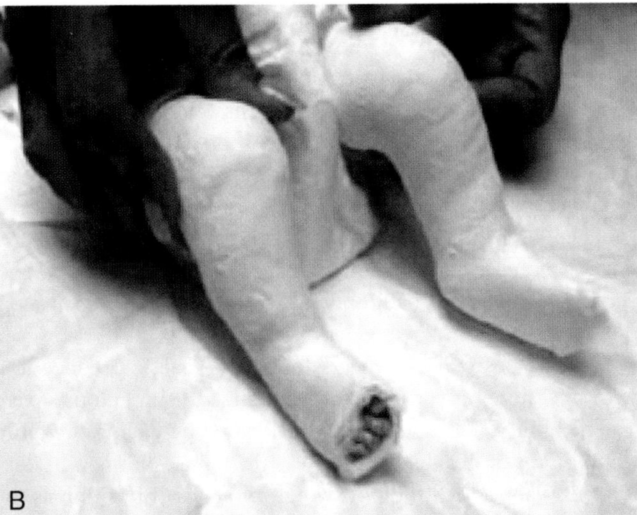

Fig. 45.7 Bilateral Clubfoot. (A) Infant with bilateral congenital talipes equinovarus. **(B)** Ponseti casting. (A, Courtesy Dr. A.E. Chudley, Section of Genetics and Metabolism, Department of Pediatrics and Child Health, Children's Hospital and University of Manitoba, Winnipeg, Manitoba, Canada. In Moore KL, et al., eds. *The developing human*, 10th edition. Philadelphia: Saunders; 2016. B, From Scher DM. The Ponseti method or clubfoot correction. *Operative Techniques in Orthopaedics*, 2005;15(4):345–349.)

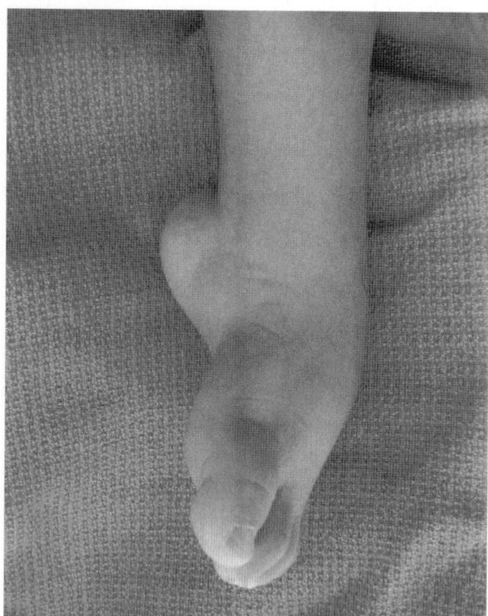

Fig. 45.8 Idiopathic Clubfoot. Idiopathic clubfoot displaying forefoot adduction (toward midline of body) and supination (upturning) and hindfoot equinus (pointed downward). Note skin creases along arch and back of heal.

cases show a decreased number of muscle fibers and/or abnormal fiber histology. The soleus often has an increase in type 1 fibers, whereas the peroneus brevis has a fiber type disproportion. The more abnormal the histopathology, the more severe the deformity, and the greater the change of recurrent deformity after treatment. The genetic component is unclear and studies are ongoing.

Teratologic equinovarus is caused by either neuromuscular, syndromic, or osteochondrodysplasia etiology. Examples of such include spina bifida and diastrophic dwarfism. The teratologic clubfoot, unlike the idiopathic type, more often fails to be corrected with Ponseti casting and may require operative intervention (see Fig. 45.7B). The surgery is often more extensive, and revision surgery is also more common (Box 45.1).

Pes planus (flatfoot) deformity is a typical parental concern. However, a flexible flatfoot is often as functional as one with a "normal" arch. The majority of babies are born with flat feet. The arch becomes more apparent with age. Significant ankle valgus, vertical talus, tarsal coalition, and skewfoot must be accurately differentiated from flexible pes planus.

Flexible pes planus appears to have a genetic predilection, with occasional association of generalized ligamentous laxity. The flexibility of the hindfoot is evaluated by having the child stand on his or her toes facing away from the examiner. In flexible pes planus, the hindfoot swings into a varus position as the planter fascia tightens in toe raise. In rigid pes planus, the hindfoot stays in valgus, and the child has more difficulty going up onto tiptoe.

There is a small subset of children with painful, flexible flat feet. For these children, careful attention to the possibility of Achilles contracture or tarsal coalition (congenital union of the hindfoot bones) must be made. In rigid flat feet, a computed tomography (CT) scan often will reveal a coalition, a bony or cartilaginous connection between the bones—if painful, this can be resected in surgery (see Box 45.1).

BOX 45.1 Ponseti Casting and Achilles Tenotomy

Ponseti casting implements toe-to-groin casts changed weekly for 6 weeks. Casting begins as early as possible after birth and culminates in a percutaneous tendo Achilles lengthening in the clinic, followed by a final cast worn for 3 weeks. In recalcitrant cases, a full surgical posteromedial release (PMR) still may be required. The need for PMR in idiopathic clubfoot has significantly decreased when this casting technique is used. Long-term results, presumably because of less scarring and more long-term flexibility, are better with Ponseti casting than with the PMR method. The hindfoot equinus portion of the deformity often requires lengthening of the Achilles tendon, which can be performed in a clinic with the use of a local anesthetic. Achilles tenotomy (complete transection of the tendon) can be safely performed with local anesthetic until 8 or 9 months after birth. After this age, a formal lengthening and repair procedure using a general anesthetic is required. Bracing is required until age 3.

Abnormal Density or Modeling of the Skeleton

Osteogenesis Imperfecta

Pathophysiology. Osteogenesis imperfecta (OI), or brittle bone disease, is an inherited bone dysplasia related to collagen, the main component of bone and blood vessels. The major errors in OI lie in the synthesis of collagen, a triple helix with two matching α chains and one β chain. Collagen is present in bone, cartilage, eye tissue, skin, and the vascular system. The severity of the OI phenotype and the related anomalies of the eye, dentition, or vascular system are all dependent on the severity of the genetic anomaly and the part of the triple helix that is affected.[11] Classification systems are based on the mode of inheritance, identifying the defective gene, protein, or mechanism (Table 45.2).[12]

Clinical Manifestations. The classic clinical manifestations of OI are osteopenia (decreased bone mass) and an increased rate of fractures. Other possible manifestations include bony deformation (bowing), triangular facies, vascular weakness (aortic aneurysm), blue sclerae, fatigue, pain, hearing loss, and poor dentition. In the most severe form of this disorder, the child is usually stillborn or dies soon after birth, although some survive into childhood. OI in its more severe forms is evident at birth because fractures and deformity have occurred in utero. The less severe forms may not become evident until the child begins to walk. Some children with this milder form then experience numerous fractures that can be mistaken for nonaccidental trauma (NAT; e.g., child abuse) until the diagnosis is made.

Evaluation and Treatment. Evaluation of OI is primarily based on the clinical manifestations. Serum alkaline phosphatase level is elevated in all forms of the disease. OI can be diagnosed prenatally by ultrasound or chorionic villi sampling. Analysis of cultured skin fibroblast collagen by electrophoresis shows a decreased quantity of collagen in 95% of individuals.

The goal of treatment of OI is to reduce the number of fractures and to prevent long bone deformities. Medications and surgical interventions are available. Biophosphonate therapy is the mainstay of pharmacologic fracture prevention, with marked improvements of bone density. Chronic bone

TABLE 45.2 Osteogenesis Imperfecta Types Caused by Defects in Genes and the Collagen-Related Proteins that They Encode

	OI Type	Defective Gene	Defective Protein	Defective Mechanism	
Autosomal dominant	I	*COL1A1*	α1(I) collagen	Collagen quantity	85%–90% of OI case types I–IV
	II	*COL1A1* or *COL1A2*	α1(I)/α2(I) collagen	Collagen structure	
	III	*COL1A1* or *COL1A2*	α1(I)/α2(I) collagen		
	IV	*COL1A1* or *COL1A2*	α1(I)/α2(I) collagen		
	V	*IFITM5*	BRIL	Matrix mineralization	10%–15% of OI cases
Autosomal recessive	VI	*SERPINF1*	PEDF	Collagen 3-hydroxylation	10%–15% of OI case types VI to unclassified
	VII	*CRTAP*	CRTAP		
	VIII	*LEPRE1*	P3H1		
	IX	*PPIB*	CyPB		
	X	*SERPINH1*	HSP47	Collagen chaperoning	
	XI	*FKBP10*	FKBP65	Telopeptide hydroxylation	
	XII	*BMP1*	BMP1/mTLD	Collagen processing	
	Unclassified	*SP7/OSX*	SP7/OSTERIX	Osteoblast development	
		WNT1	WNT1		
		TMEM38B	TRIC-B		
		CREB3L1	OASIS		

OI, Osteogenesis imperfecta.
Data from Marini JC, Reich A, Smith SM. Osteogenesis imperfecta due to mutations in non-collagenous genes: Lessons in the biology of bone formation. *Current Opinion in Pediatrics*, 2014;26(4):500–506.

pain and fatigue also are thought to be lessened with routine bisphosphonate therapy. Telescoping rods, which grow with the child, are improving in efficacy and have been shown to reduce the reoperative rate by 30%.[13] Genetic counseling for affected families should aim at primary prevention.

Rickets

Rickets is a disorder in which growing bone fails to become mineralized (ossified) prior to closure of the growth plates, resulting in "soft" bones and skeletal deformity (Fig. 45.9). Rickets results from either insufficient vitamin D, insensitivity to vitamin D, wasting of vitamin D by the kidney, or inability to absorb vitamin D and calcium in the gut. Calcipenic rickets is usually caused by insufficient dietary intake of vitamin D and/or calcium. It is the most common cause of rickets worldwide. Phosphopenic rickets is nearly always caused by wasting of vitamin D by the kidney.

Severe metabolic rickets in the immature skeleton leads to short stature and bowing of the limbs with broad, irregular growth plates. The rows of cells in the growth plate that are intended to ossify fail to do so as they reach the metaphysis, because calcification is impeded. Children with rickets are often listless and irritable. They have hypotonia and muscle weakness and may be unable to walk without support. In both forms, skeletal findings are similar, which include abnormal parietal flattening and frontal bossing of the skull, (the calvaria become soft, and the sutures may widen), costochondral junction enlargement, widening of the wrist, and lateral bowing of the femur and the tibia.

Growth is restricted, and fractures are common. Serum alkaline phosphatase is elevated in both types of rickets. Like osteogenesis

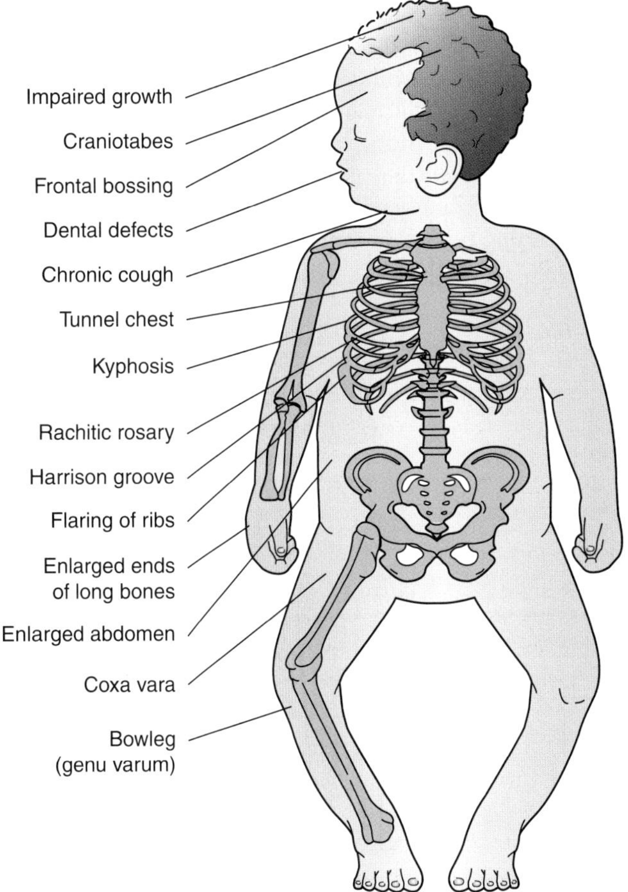

Fig. 45.9 Rickets.

imperfecta, surgical treatment of bony deformity can be required. However, medical management of calcium, phosphorous, and vitamin D levels must be optimized before surgical intervention. In addition to medical management, children may benefit from guided growth techniques to correct persistent deformity.

Scoliosis

Scoliosis is a rotational curvature of the spine most obvious in the anteroposterior plane (Fig. 45.10). It can be classified as nonstructural or structural. Nonstructural scoliosis results from a cause other than the spine itself, such as posture, leg length discrepancy, or pain. Structural scoliosis is curvature of the spine associated with vertebral rotation. Nonstructural scoliosis can become structural if the underlying cause is not found and treated. Scoliosis can also be idiopathic. Idiopathic scoliosis is classified as infantile, juvenile, or adolescent, depending on the child's age at the time of onset. In infantile scoliosis, spinal curvature develops during the first 3 years of life; in juvenile scoliosis, curvature develops between the skeletal age of 4 years and the onset of adolescence; and in adolescent scoliosis, it develops after the skeletal age of 10.

Adolescent idiopathic scoliosis is the most common form of scoliosis and affects 1% to 3% of US adolescents between 10 and 18 years of age.[14] The etiology is not completely understood; however, it is defined by a lateral curvature of the spine (Cobb angle) of at least 10 degrees (mild) in the absence of underlying congenital or neuromuscular abnormalities.[14,15] Genetic factors are thought to be a contributing factor in idiopathic scoliosis, but inheritance patterns are variable.[14]

Pathophysiology. The earliest pathologic changes occur in the soft tissue. The muscles, ligaments, and other soft tissues become shortened on the concave side of the curve. Vertebral deformity occurs as asymmetric forces are applied to the epiphyseal center of the ossification by shortened and tight soft tissues on the concave side of the curve. True curves involve not only bending but also twisting of the torso, leading to the "rib hump" seen when the child bends forward. The curves increase most rapidly during periods of rapid skeletal growth. If the curve is less than 40 degrees at skeletal maturity, the risk of progression is quite small. In curves greater than 50 degrees, the spine is biomechanically unstable, and the curve usually progresses even after the cessation of growth. Curves in the thoracic spine greater than 80 degrees result in decreased pulmonary function, whereas the most common complication of large curves in the lumbar spine is back pain. Many new treatment options are available for individuals with idiopathic scoliosis (see Emerging Science Box: Idiopathic Scoliosis).

Clinical Manifestations. The clinical manifestations of nonstructural scoliosis are mild spinal curvature with prominence of one hip or rounded shoulders. The curvature disappears with forward flexion of the spine, lying down, or traction of the head. The clinical manifestations of structural scoliosis include asymmetry of hip height, asymmetry of shoulder height, shoulder and scapular (shoulder blade) prominence, and rib prominence.

Evaluation and Treatment. Spinal curvature is usually visible or palpable, and muscles on one side of the lower back (the convex side) may be prominent or bulging. Most cases of idiopathic scoliosis are noticed during school screening programs. In girls the deformity may be noticed because clothing does not "hang" properly on the body. Diagnosis is made by roentgenographic examinations.

Treatment for nonstructural scoliosis is correction of the underlying disorder. Brace treatment is indicated for children with curves of 25 to 40 degrees who have at least 2 years of growth remaining. A rigid, low-profile thoracolumbar brace is used in most cases. Low-profile braces are worn for 18 to 23 hours per day until skeletal maturity. Bracing will only prevent progression of the curve; it will not correct the curvature.

Bracing is not effective in large curves or in skeletally mature individuals; the most effective time for bracing is in growing prepubescents with a small curve. Surgical treatment using spinal fusion with instrumentation is recommended for curves greater than 40 to 50 degrees. If surgery is indicated, it is better performed during the adolescent years while there is greater flexibility of the curves and less risk of complications.

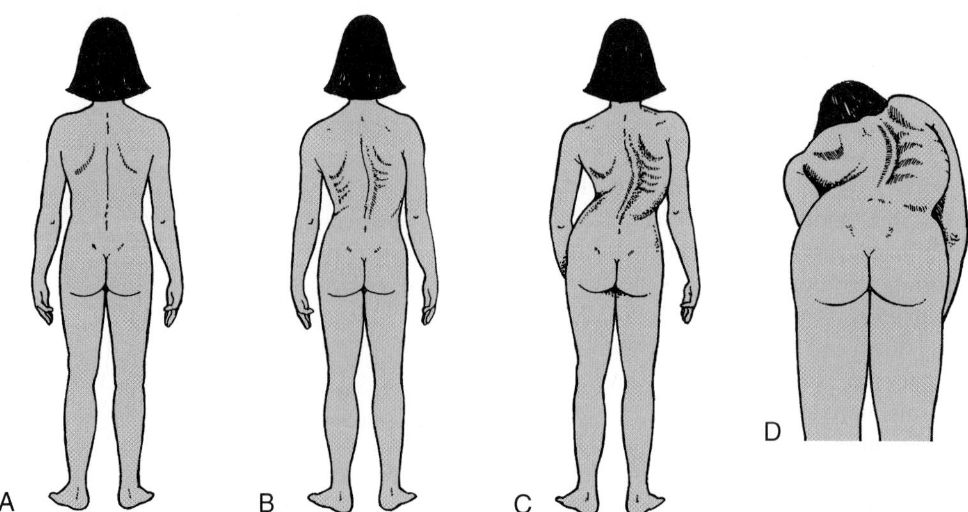

Fig. 45.10 Scoliosis in Children. Normal spinal alignment and abnormal spinal curvatures associated with scoliosis. **(A)** Normal. **(B)** Mild. **(C)** Severe. **(D)** Rotation and curvature of scoliosis.

EMERGING SCIENCE BOX

Idiopathic Scoliosis

Idiopathic scoliosis is the most common spinal disorder in the pediatric population. There are many treatment options for scoliosis, including core strengthening exercises, bracing, and surgery. The goals of treatment are to restore symmetry and optimize the individual's quality of life. Often, the severity of the scoliosis is measured objectively with the Cobb angle measurement. A Cobb angle in the range of 10–20 degrees is considered mild, 20–40 degrees is moderate, and greater than 40 degrees denotes severe scoliosis. The goals of treatment can be achieved by correcting the deformity and preventing progression of the curvature.

Exercise, such as the Schroth exercise, has proven beneficial especially for individuals with a Cobb angle of 10–30 degrees. People who practiced the exercise for more than 1 month had the best outcomes. This includes positive influence on the structural deformity and core muscle strength improvement. Interestingly, people who underwent Schroth exercise treatment perceived improved status even if the Cobb angle did not improve more than 5 degrees, which is considered the conventionally accepted threshold. This perceived improvement without significant Cobb angle improvement is leading researchers to investigate alternatives to the Cobb angle that might be more relevant.

New surgical techniques for scoliosis include robotic-assisted pedicle screw placement, vertebral body stapling, vertebral body tethering, magnetically controlled growing rods, and sublaminar polyester bands.

Data from Cheung ZB, et al. Idiopathic scoliosis in children and adolescents: emerging techniques in surgical treatment. *World Neurosurgery*, 2019;130:e737–e742. doi:10.1016/j.wneu.2019.06.207; Larson AN, et al. Minimum 20-year health-related quality of life and surgical rates after the treatment of adolescent idiopathic scoliosis. *Spine Deformity*, 2019;7(3):417–427. doi:10.1016/j.jspd.2018.09.003; Park JH, et al. Effects of the Schroth exercise on idiopathic scoli sis: a meta-analysis. *European Journal of Physical and Rehabilitation Medicine*, 2018;54(3):440–449. doi:10.23736/S1973-9087.17.04461-6; Schreiber S, et al. Patients with adolescent idiopathic scoliosis perceive positive improvements regardless of change in the Cobb angle—Results from a randomized controlled trial comparing a 6-month Schroth intervention added to standard care and standard care alone. SOSORT 2018 Award winner. *BMC Musculoskeletal Disorders*, 2019;20(1):319. doi:10.1186/s12891-019-2695-9.

Bone and Joint Infection

Osteomyelitis

Osteomyelitis is an infection of the bone. Acute osteomyelitis can affect infants and children of any age, but it occurs most often in children younger than age 5 years.[16,17] The bacterial etiology varies by age, but the most prevalent pathogen in pediatrics is *Staphylococcus aureus* (Box 45.2).[16,17,19]

Pathophysiology. Bacterial dissemination can be hematogenous (infection entering the bone through the bloodstream), contiguous (infection originating from soft tissues that spreads to the bone), or via direct inoculation (open fractures, puncture wounds, prostheses).[20] Bacteria may lodge at the end of the venous loops beneath the epiphyseal plate, and infection develops because there are no phagocytic cells present to remove the bacteria.[20]

Osteomyelitis most frequently affects the metaphyseal region of long bones (27% in the femur, 22% the tibia, 5% fibula, 12% humerus, 4% radius, and 3% the ulna) because the rich metaphyseal blood supply, with vascular loops and turbulent flow, facilitates bacterial colonization.[20]

Factors that predispose an individual to the development of osteomyelitis include sickle cell disease, prematurity, respiratory distress syndrome, trauma, sepsis, bacteremia, chronic catheterization or indwelling vascular lines, and immunodeficiency.[19,20]

Acute hematogenous osteomyelitis is the most common type of bone infection in children. The infection is initiated by bacteria that has exponential growth leading to bone resorption. A purulent exudate forms, creating a subperiosteal abscess in the metaphysis of a long bone where blood flow is sluggish and bacteria can collect.[20] With increasing pressure, the infection will rupture out of the periosteum and spread along the diaphysis of the bone. In infants younger than 1 year old, infection may go through the physis (growth plate) and into the epiphysis (Fig. 45.11). Because the periosteum is separated from an adequate blood supply, sections of the bone die; these pieces of dead bone are called sequestra. A new shell of bone can develop under the elevated periosteum and can become an involucrum. All three of these changes are apparent on radiograph. In children older than 2 years, the epiphyseal plate prevents the spread of a metaphyseal abscess into the epiphysis and the cortex of the metaphysis is thicker. These anatomic differences increase the likelihood that the metaphyseal abscess will extend into the diaphysis, and the blood supply of the bone will be disrupted. The periosteum is also more difficult to perforate in older children; this may lead to a larger subperiosteal abscess that could endanger the periosteal blood supply as well. This process results in extensive sequestrum formation and chronic osteomyelitis.[20]

BOX 45.2 Causative Microorganisms of Osteomyelitis According to Age

Newborns (0–2 months)

- *Staphylococcus aureus* (both methicillin-sensitive [MSSA] and methicillin-resistant [MRSA])
- *Escherichia coli*
- Group B *Streptococcus*
- Gram-negative enteric bacilli

Infants/Toddlers (2 months to 4 year)

- *S. aureus* (MSSA and MRSA)
- Group A β-hemolytic *Streptococcus*
- *Kingella kingae* (most common pathogen in Europe and Middle East)[18]
- *Haemophilus influenzae* (decreasingly less common secondary to immunization)

Child (5–10 years)

- *S. aureus* (MSSA and MRSA)
- Staphylococcus epidermidis
- *Salmonella*
- *Pseudomonas aeruginosa*

Adolescents (10–19 years)

- *S. aureus* (MSSA and MRSA)
- *Pseudomonas*
- *Mycobacterium tuberculosis*
- *Neisseria gonorrhoeae*

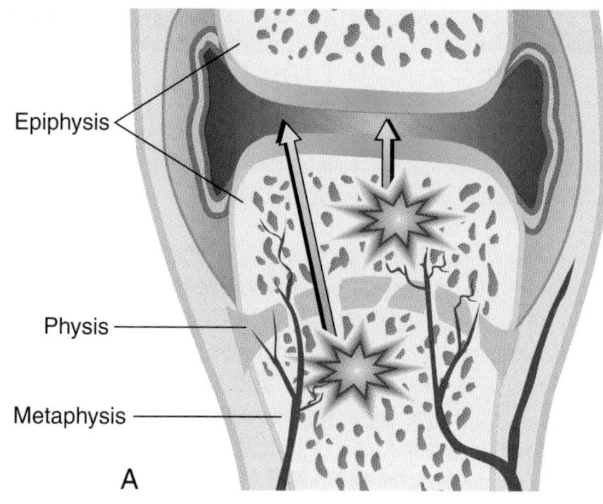

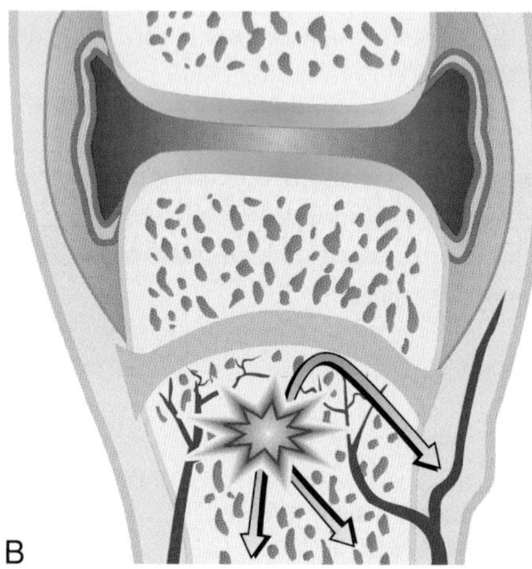

Fig. 45.11 Pathogenesis of Acute Osteomyelitis Differs with Age. **(A)** In infants younger than 1 year the epiphysis is nourished by arteries penetrating through the physis, allowing development of the condition within the epiphysis. **(B)** In children up to 15 years of age, the infection is restricted to below the physis because of interruption of the vessels.

Clinical Manifestations. Initially, osteomyelitis presents as pain, worse with ambulation, local tenderness, swelling, erythema, and warmth.[21] Children often will have fever, decreased appetite, fatigue, elevated white blood cell (WBC) count (36%), but, if both the C-reactive protein (CRP) and erythrocyte sedimentation rate (ESR) are elevated, the sensitivity for infection is 98%.[21] Blood culture is positive in 40% or less of cases, whereas bone, joint, or soft tissue cultures have a higher yield, in the range of 70%.[21]

Evaluation and Treatment. Conventional radiographs are the first step in imaging evaluation; however, radiographic bone changes are not usually apparent until 10 days after the onset of symptoms. MRI has become the recommended modality for evaluation of a child with suspected osteomyelitis.[21] Bone scans can be quite helpful with diagnosis, and in children younger than 1 year are absolutely required to define whether multiple sites are involved.

Death is rare, but serious sequelae may occur. The course of the disease and prognosis depend on the age of the child, the rapidity with which the diagnosis is established, the initiation of early treatment, and maintenance of treatment for an adequate time (typically at least 4 weeks). The most serious complications are growth arrest, osseous necrosis, and recurrence. Recurrence with presently available antibiotic regimens is approximately 1 to 2%.[22]

Septic Arthritis

Septic arthritis (SA) is a bacterial or granulomatous infection of the joint space. This is always a surgical emergency. The bacteria and the lysosomes created by WBCs fighting the bacteria can quickly destroy the articular cartilage of the joint and affect the blood supply to the epiphyseal bone nearby. Both of these complications have poor outcomes and can lead to a lifetime of disability.

SA can occur primarily or secondary to osteomyelitis that spreads from the metaphysis of the bone into the joint space (Fig. 45.12). The metaphyses of the pediatric hip, shoulder, proximal radius, and distal lateral tibia are all located within the joint capsule, and therefore osteomyelitis in these regions must be carefully monitored for secondary SA. The most common sites for SA are knees, hips, ankles, and elbows.

Children with SA present with severe joint pain, "pseudoparalysis," or marked guarding to motion of the joint; inability to bear weight; and malaise, often with anorexia. Children appear quite ill with this diagnosis. Nonpyogenic arthritis, such as juvenile idiopathic arthritis (JIA), can be difficult to distinguish clinically from SA because both can lead to malaise and elevated ESR. The Kocher criteria are often used to distinguish septic joints from joint pain of another cause. If three of the four criteria are met, there is a reported 93% probability of SA. If four of the four criteria are met, then there is a reported 99% probability of SA. However, joint aspiration is still required. The criteria include[23]:

1. WBC >12,000 cells/μL
2. Inability to bear weight on the joint
3. Fever >101.3°F (38.5°C)
4. ESR >40 mm/h

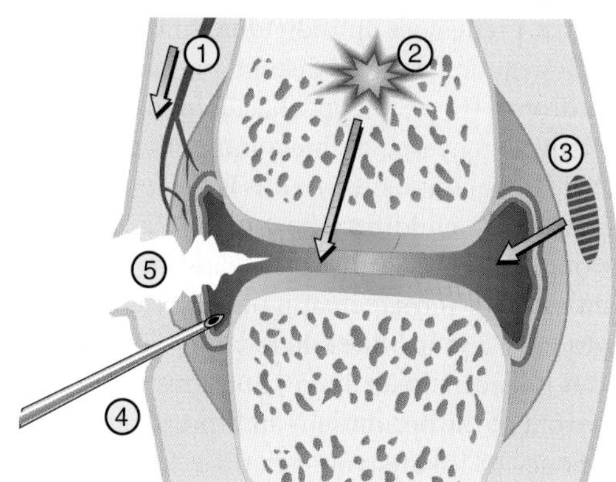

Fig. 45.12 Routes of Infection to the Joint. *(1)* Hematogenous route. *(2)* Dissemination from osteomyelitis. *(3)* Spread from an adjacent soft tissue infection. *(4)* Diagnostic or therapeutic measures. *(5)* Penetrating damage by puncture or cutting.

A 2017 retrospective chart review found that the Kocher criteria plus ultrasound were not sufficient to make a diagnosis of SA of the hip joint, and consideration should be given to add MRI to the work-up.[24] Synovial fluid aspiration and evaluation are definitive criteria for diagnosis, which should include WBC count, Gram stain, culture, and susceptibility testing.

RHEUMATOLOGIC DISORDERS

Juvenile Arthritis

Juvenile arthritides are a group of inflammatory disorders that affect children. Juvenile idiopathic arthritis (JIA) is the most common type of arthritis in children younger than the age of 16 and is the childhood form of rheumatoid arthritis (also see Chapter 44).

The International League of Associations for Rheumatology (ILAR) developed criteria for classification of juvenile arthritis[25]:

- Systemic arthritis
- Polyarthritis (rheumatoid factor [RF] positive; RF negative)
- Oligoarthritis (persistent or extended)
- Enthesitis-related arthritis
- Psoriatic arthritis
- Undifferentiated arthritis

However, JIA remains a diagnosis of exclusion (see Emerging Science Box: Serum Interleukin-18 and Systemic Juvenile Idiopathic Arthritis).

The disease must manifest before 16 years of age, the symptoms must persist for at least 6 weeks, and there can be no other explainable etiology for the symptoms.[25]

JIA has three distinct modes of onset: oligoarthritis (fewer than five joints), polyarthritis (more than five joints), and Still disease (severe systemic onset). JIA differs from adult rheumatoid arthritis in several ways:

Large joints are most commonly affected.

Chronic uveitis (inflammation of the anterior chamber of the eye) is common, especially if serum antinuclear antibodies (ANA) is positive. Slit lamp examination by a trained ophthalmologist is required every 6 months to avoid vision loss.

Serum tests may be negative for RF; RF-positive children have a worse prognosis.

Subluxation and ankylosis may occur in the cervical spine if disease progresses.

Rheumatoid arthritis that continues through adolescence can have severe effects on growth and adult morbidity.

Systemic juvenile idiopathic arthritis (sJIA) involves one or more joints and fever with at least one of the following additional symptoms: erythematous rash, hepatomegaly, splenomegaly, lymph node enlargement, or serositis. Systemic onset, or "seropositivity," of the disease is more likely consistent with lifelong arthritis. Therefore treatment is supportive, not curative. Nonsteroidal antiinflammatory drugs (NSAIDs) are a mainstay of treatment, and methotrexate is also being used with success. The goals are to minimize inflammation and deformity. Polyarthritis refers to the subgroup of JIA individuals with five or more joints affected. Inclusion in this subgroup is independent of the RF test results; however, the category can be further subdivided into RF positive and RF negative. Many children with oligoarthritis who are "seronegative" (blood tests negative for RF or ANA) will resolve their symptoms over time.

Enthesitis is common in children with JIA and refers to the inflamed and painful areas that connect a tendon or ligament to the bone. The enthesis is the area surrounding a joint where tendons or ligaments insert (Fig. 45.13).

Psoriatic arthritis is a form of JIA that is characterized by clinical diagnosis of psoriasis and arthritis plus at least two of the following criteria: dactylitis, alterations in the fingernails that typically accompany psoriasis (e.g., pitting or painless detachment from the nail bed), or a first degree relative with psoriasis. Children with symptoms that do not fall into any of the aforementioned categories or suffer from symptoms that overlap categories are diagnosed with undifferentiated arthritis. Categorization of juvenile arthritis continues to evolve and change as the categories of disease are better understood.

EMERGING SCIENCE BOX

Serum Interleukin-18 and Systemic Juvenile Idiopathic Arthritis

Interleukins (ILs) are a group of cytokines that regulate cell growth, differentiation, and motility, but are especially important in immunity and inflammation. IL-18 is a specific inflammatory cytokine. Serum IL levels may prove useful as a marker to distinguish the diagnosis of systemic juvenile idiopathic arthritis (sJIA) from other febrile diseases. A study by Xia et al. (2017) measured serum concentrations of S1000A8, S100A9, IL-6, and IL-8 from a group of individuals with various febrile conditions as well as a control group without disease. The level of IL-8 was significantly higher in the sJIA group. Another study, by Mizuta et al. (2020) suggests that levels can be used for diagnosis but also to predict the disease course and assessing remission. In people with polycyclic disease, serum IL-18 levels were elevated during flares and normalized during the inactive phase. Macrophage activation syndrome (MAS) is a severe compilation of sJIA and is characterized by a proliferation of T lymphocytes and macrophages. Yasin et al. (2020) concluded that IL-18 levels are elevated in sJIA individuals but even higher in those with active disease and a history of MAS. Furthermore, an increase in IL-18 may indicate an increase in disease action or the development of MAS.

Data from Bracaglia C, et al. Macrophage activation syndrome different mechanisms leading to a one clinical syndrome. *Pediatric Rheumatology Online Journal*, 2017;15(1):5. doi:10.1186/ s12969-016-0130-4; Mizuta M, et al. Clinical significance of interleukin-18 for the diagnosis and prediction of disease course in systemic juvenile idiopathic arthritis. *Rheumatology (Oxford)*, 2021;60(5):2421–2426. doi:10.1093/rheumatology/keaa634; Xia Y, et al. Extremely elevated IL-18 levels may help distinguish systemic-onset juvenile idiopathic arthritis from other febrile diseases. *Brazilian Journal of Medical and Biological Research*, 2017;16;50(2):e5958. doi:10.1590/1414-431X20165958; Yasin S, et al. IL-18 as a biomarker linking systemic juvenile idiopathic arthritis and macrophage activation syndrome. *Rheumatology (Oxford)*, 2020;59(2):361–366. doi:10.1093/rheumatology/kez282.

AVASCULAR DISEASE OF THE BONE

Osteochondroses

The osteochondroses are a series of avascular diseases caused by insufficient blood supply to growing bones. These childhood diseases involve areas of significant tensile or compressive stress (e.g., tibial tubercle, Achilles insertion, hip epiphysis). The pathophysiology is partial loss of blood supply, death of bone (osseous necrosis), progressive bony weakness, and then microfracture. The cause of the decreased blood supply is controversial; trauma, a change in clotting sensitivity, vascular injury, genetic predisposition, or a combination of these factors is presently considered most likely. In addition, during the years of rapid bone growth, blood supply to the growing ends of bones (epiphyses) may become insufficient, resulting in necrotic bone, usually near joints. Because bone is normally undergoing a continuous rebuilding process, the necrotic areas can self-repair over a period of weeks or months.

Use of antiinflammatory medications, modification of activities, immobilization, and rest are recommended during active stages of the disease. Reparative correction by revascularization is the rule, although years may be required for full healing, and deformity from compression during the period of osseous necrosis can persist.

Legg-Calvé-Perthes Disease

Legg-Calvé-Perthes (LCP) disease is a common osteochondrosis of the capital femoral epiphysis of the femoral head, usually occurring in children between the ages of 3 and 12 years, with a peak incidence at 6 years.[26] This self-limited disease, which runs its natural course in 2 to 5 years, is presumably created by recurrent interruption of the blood supply to the femoral head. The disorder is bilateral in 10% to 20% of children.[27] Male children are affected four to five times more often than female children, which is thought to be caused by males having a more poorly developed blood supply to the femoral head than do females of the same age.[27] The role of genetics is unclear, but LCP is more common in northern European and Japanese children and rare in Black children; family history is positive in 20% of cases. Obesity and lower socioeconomic status have been associated with LCP.[28,29]

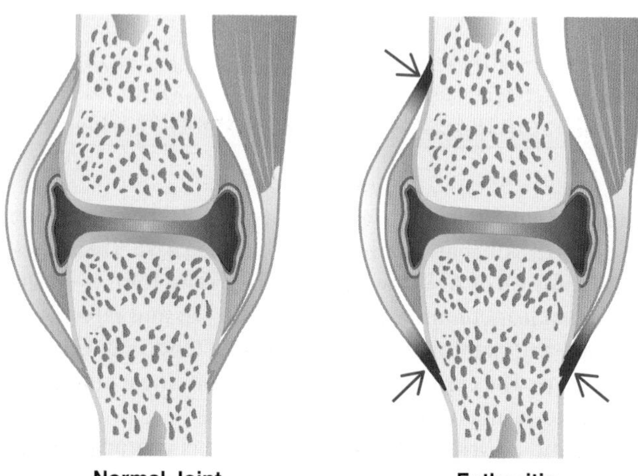

Fig. 45.13 Enthesitis.

Pathophysiology. In the initial stage of LCP, the soft tissues of the hip (synovial membrane and joint capsule) are swollen, edematous, and hyperemic, often with fluid present in the joint (Fig. 45.14). The joint space widens, and the joint capsule bulges. This first stage lasts approximately 2 weeks. Next, the anterior 50% or more of the epiphysis of the femoral head dies because of a lack of blood supply, and the metaphyseal bone at the junction of the femoral neck and capital epiphyseal plate is softened because of increased blood supply and decalcification.[30] In the fragmentation stage, the body reabsorbs the infarcted bone.[30] Granulation tissue (procallus) and blood vessels then invade the dead bone. This stage lasts several months to 1 year. Then the regenerative healing stage, which ordinarily lasts 2 to 4 years, replaces the dead bone in the femoral head by procallus, and new bone is established (see Fig. 45.14).[30] In the final stage, remodeling takes place, and the newly formed bone is organized into a live spongy bone.[30]

Clinical Manifestations. Injury or trauma precedes the onset of LCP in approximately 30% to 50% of children with the disease. For several months the child complains of a limp and pain that can be referred to the knee, inner thigh, and the groin, following the path of the obturator nerve. The pain is usually aggravated by activity but is not always relieved with rest.

The typical physical findings include spasm on rotation of the hip, limitation of internal rotation and abduction of the hip, leg length discrepancy, and hip flexion–adduction deformity. If the child is walking, an early abnormal gait termed an ***antalgic (painful) abductor lurch***, or a "Trendelenburg gait" (gluteus medius gait pattern), is apparent. If the hip pain or limp has been present for a prolonged period, muscles of the hip and thigh atrophy.

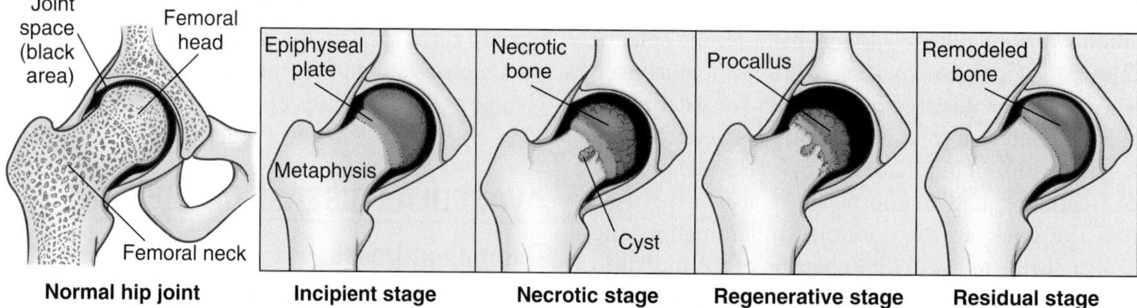

Fig. 45.14 Stages of Legg-Calvé-Perthes Disease, a Form of Osteochondrosis.

Evaluation and Treatment. Diagnosis is based on level of suspicion and confirmed by radiographic examination. However, early radiographic evidence may be normal in appearance. MRI may prove more helpful in the diagnosis because it will reveal bone marrow changes. Bone scans have the ability to reveal decreased profusion to the affected area.[31]

The goals of treatment are to preserve normal congruity of the femoral head and acetabulum and maintain spasm-free and pain-free range of motion in the hip joint. Currently, most children can be managed with antiinflammatory medications and activity modification during periods of synovitis. Serial radiographs are obtained to monitor the progress of the disease and to ensure that the femoral head remains congruent in the acetabulum. Surgery may be necessary if the femoral head becomes subluxated or incongruent with the acetabulum (Fig. 45.15). Children older than age 6 years (by bone age) have a worse prognosis attributable to poor remodeling potential. Older children require surgery more often to avoid poor congruence of the hip. Poor congruence predisposes to early OA, with nearly 50% requiring hip replacement surgery by age 40.[32]

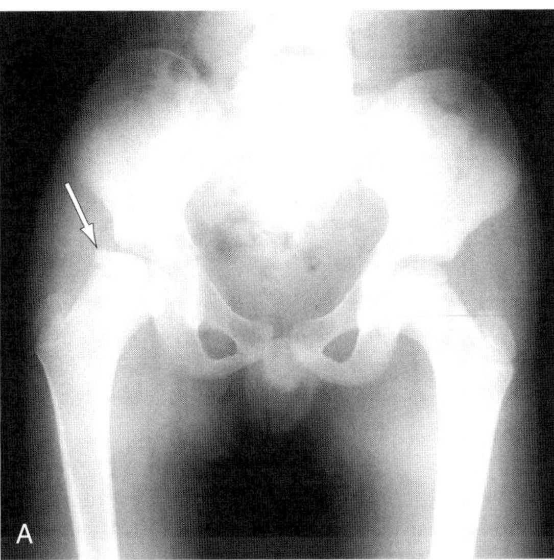

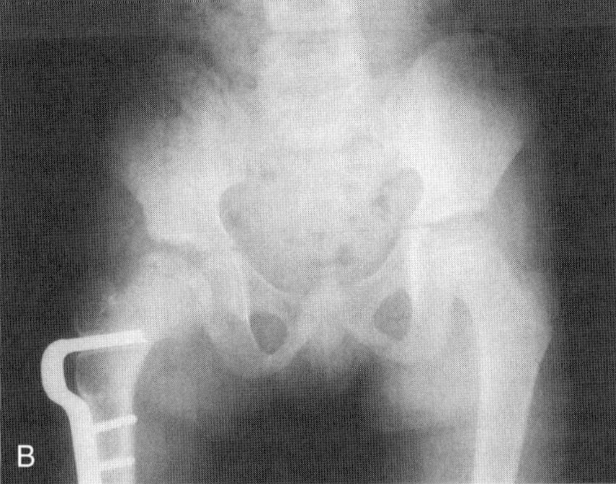

Fig. 45.15 Pelvis of a 7-Year-Old Male With Legg-Calvé-Perthes Disease. (A) The femoral head *(arrow)* is flat and extruded from the edge of the joint. This hip is at risk for early arthritis if left to revascularize and heal in this position. **(B)** Surgical replacement of the femoral head. As the Perthes heals, the ball has assumed a round shape that matches the socket well.

Osgood-Schlatter Disease

Osgood-Schlatter disease (OSD) consists of osteochondrosis of the tibia tubercle and associated patellar (kneecap) tendonitis. OSD occurs most often in children undergoing rapid growth and those who participate in sports, placing stress on the developing tubercle through patellar tendon force.[33] The disease is more prevalent in males than in females.

Pathophysiology. The severity varies from mild tendonitis to a complete separation of the anterior tibial apophysis, a part of the tibial tubercle. The mildest form of OSD causes ischemic (avascular) necrosis in the region of the bony tibial tubercle, with hypertrophic cartilage formation during the stages of repair. In more severe cases, the abnormality involves a true apophyseal separation of the tibial tubercle with avascular necrosis.[33]

Clinical Manifestations. The child complains of pain and swelling in the region around the distal patellar tendon and tibial tubercle, just below the knee, which becomes prominent and is tender to direct pressure. The pain is most severe after physical activity that involves vigorous quadriceps contraction (jumping or running) or direct local trauma to the tibial tubercle area, and is relieved with rest (Fig. 45.16A–C).[33]

Evaluation and Treatment. Radiologic evidence may indicate superficial ossicle in the patellar tendon, soft tissue swelling anterior to the tibial tuberosity, and thickening of ligamentum patellae.[33] Ultrasound, MRI, and CT are other imaging modalities used for the diagnosis of OSD. Ultrasound may show the thickened patellar tendon better than plain radiography. It can also demonstrate pretibial swelling, fragmentation of the ossification center, and excessive fluid collection in the infrapatellar bursa.[33] The goal of treatment for OSD is to decrease the stress at the tubercle. Most cases will spontaneously resolve as the skeleton matures. Treatment is typically aimed at symptom relief and includes a period of 4 to 8 weeks of restriction from strenuous physical activity, administration of antiinflammatory medications, and stretching of the quadriceps muscle. Bracing with a tubercle band can be very helpful. If the pain is not relieved, a cast or knee immobilizer is required, a situation that is particularly difficult if the condition is bilateral, which occurs in only 10% to 20% of cases. Gradual resumption of activity is permitted after 8 weeks, but return to unrestricted athletic participation requires an additional 8 weeks to allow for revascularization, healing, and ossification of the tibial tubercle. With skeletal maturity and closure of the apophysis, OSD resolves. Arthroscopic surgery is sometimes needed for unresolved lesions.[33]

The condition may recur for 12 to 18 months before complete resolution at skeletal maturity. This correlates with the closure of the apophysis.[33]

Sever Disease

Sever disease, or Calcaneal apophysitis, is the primary cause of heel pain in children between 8 and 15 years of age.[34] This injury mainly occurs during puberty with an open growth plate

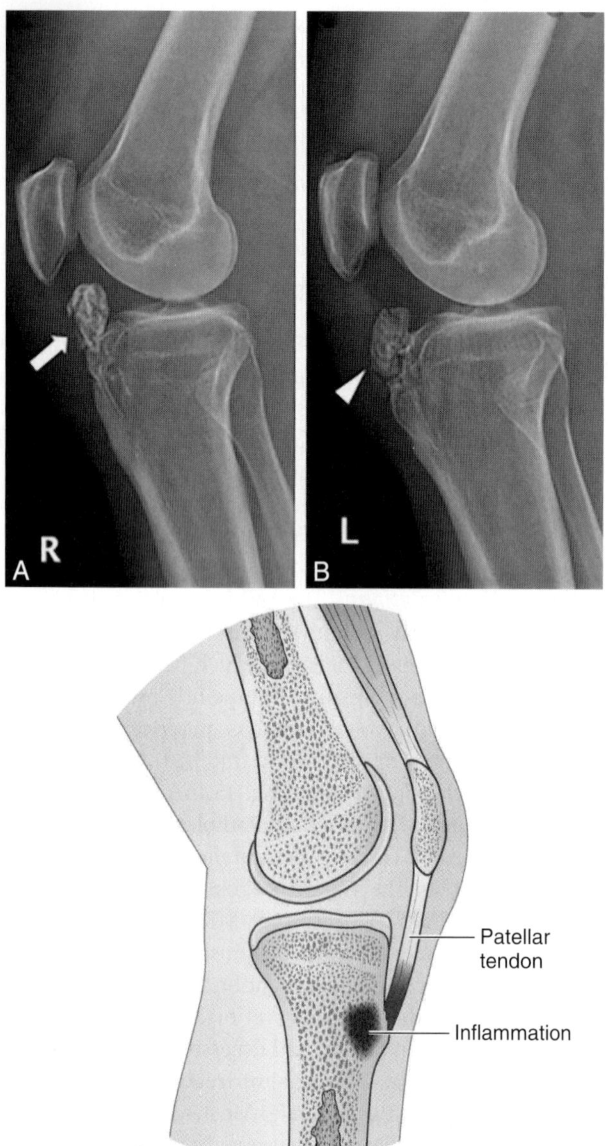

Fig. 45.16 Osgood Schlatter Lateral Plain Radiographs of Both Knees. (A) A large osseous lesion *(arrow)* is seen at the infrapatellar area of the right knee. **(B)** An osseous body *(arrowhead)* of equivalent size was partially fused to the hypertrophied tibial tuberosity of the left knee. **(C)** Clinical manifestations include pain and swelling in the region around the patellar tendon and tibial tubercle, just below the knee, which becomes prominent and is tender to direct pressure. (A and B, From Choi W, Jung K. Intra-articular large ossicle associated to Osgood-Schlatter disease. *Cureus*, 2018;10(7):e3008. doi:10.7759/ *cureus*.3008.)

in the immature calcaneus.[34] The calcaneal apophysis experiences more metabolic activity during rapid periods of growth. Similar to OSD, this condition is more common in athletic children. Repetitive motion, frequent running and jumping, and abnormal heel strike cause microinjuries that induce repetitive pain with activity, wearing unsupported footwear (e.g., sandals), or athletic footwear with cleats. Radiographic evidence is not required to make the diagnosis but may be useful to differentiate from different disease processes. MRI may be useful in severe cases.[35]

Neuromuscular Disorders

The neuromuscular disorders are a group of inherited disorders that cause progressive muscle fiber loss leading to weakness, mostly of the voluntary muscles. Common forms of neuromuscular disorders are described in Table 45.3. They cause significant disability in children, resulting in lifelong neurologic, orthopedic, and pulmonary complications. Neuromuscular disorders have different inheritance patterns and different biochemical alterations that cause each specific type, and different disorders can cause disease in different stages of life. Although the classification of neuromuscular disorders has historically been based on age of onset, rate of progression, distribution of muscular involvement, findings from muscle biopsy, and patterns of inheritance, genetic testing is increasingly being used for diagnosis and classification. Distribution of muscle weakness in common types of muscular dystrophy is depicted in Fig. 45.17.

Cerebral Palsy

Cerebral palsy (CP) is a general term that refers to nonprogressive disorders of movement and posture resulting from injury or malformation of the developing central nervous system. Although the rate of childhood CP is decreasing, it is the most common motor disability of childhood.[36,37] The resulting disability may be mild, manifesting as a stiff (spastic) gait, or severe, in which the child is in a wheelchair and needs lifelong help eating, ambulating, and communicating. Comorbid conditions, such as intellectual disability, seizures, scoliosis, and hearing or vision loss, are common, especially in children with more severe forms. The overall incidence is approximately 1 in 345 children (3 per 1000 8-year-old children) in the United States and ranges from 1 to nearly 4 per 1000 live births around the world.[37] Nearly 50% of children identified with CP have co-occurring epilepsy, and 7.5% have autism spectrum disorder.[37] Children born preterm or at a low birthweight have a higher prevalence of CP. The number of children born with CP has drastically reduced in some parts of the world by as much as 30%, likely due to a combination of comprehensive obstetric and neonatal intensive care interventions.[36]

Evaluation and Treatment. The diagnosis of CP is often made after failure to meet gross motor milestones at predicted ages. In some infants, diagnosis is made at birth or in the first months of life because the child has an underlying diagnosis, such as a major brain malformation, that is known to be associated with CP. Other children are diagnosed after a routine developmental screening reveals delays in motor and movement. By the time a child is 30 months of age, most movement delays can be found.[37] Classic patterns of motor involvement include hemiplegia, involving only one side of the body; diplegia, involving only the lower extremities; and quadriplegia, involving all four extremities. In addition to the developmental evaluation, additional tests, including brain imaging with x-ray, CT, or MRI, can be done to look for a cause of CP.[37] An electroencephalogram (EEG), genetic testing, metabolic testing or a combination of these may also be done.[37] CP is generally diagnosed during the first or second year after birth. However, with milder symptoms, it can be difficult to make a diagnosis until the child is a few years older.

TABLE 45.3 Major Neuromuscular Disorders in Children

Disease	Mode of Inheritance	Age at Clinical Onset	Usual Distribution	Rate of Progression	Intellectual Disability	Distinguishing Findings
Duchenne muscular dystrophy (DMD)	X-linked recessive	About 3 years	Hips and shoulders, quadriceps femoris, gastrocnemius (pseudohypertrophy)	Rapid	Frequent	Elevated serum enzymes (creatine phosphokinase (CPK), LDH, aspartate aminotransferase (AST), aldolase)
Spinal muscular atrophy (SMA)	Autosomal recessive	Variable depending on subtype (infant to childhood)	Proximal greater than distal, especially involving hip and shoulder girdles	Rapid	Absent	Tongue fasciculation, tremor
Facioscapulohumeral dystrophy	Autosomal dominant	In first or second decade	Shoulder girdle, neck, face, pelvic girdle (late)	Moderate	Occasional	Several distinct muscle pathologic findings
Limb girdle (LG) dystrophy	Poorly defined or recessive	Variable	Pelvic and shoulder girdles	Variable	Variable	Collection of several diseases
Myotonic dystrophy (MyD)	Autosomal dominant	Variable—birth to fifth decade	Distal extensor muscle, eyelids, face, neck, hands, pharynx	Slow, related to age at clinical onset, faster with younger individuals	Frequent	Percussion myotonia, cataracts, diabetic glucose tolerance test despite increased insulin, testicular atrophy, decreased IgG

IgG, Immunoglobulin G; *LDH*, lactate dehydrogenase.

Treatment of CP is multifaceted and focused on maximizing functional abilities. Early intervention can help the child to learn new skills and provide needed support and training to the family. Services may include counseling; home visits; occupational, physical, or speech therapy; hearing loss services; health, nutrition, social work, and assistance with service coordination; assistive technology devices and services; and transportation.[37] Children with CP should receive speech/language therapy with trials of augmentative communication devices so that underlying cognitive abilities, which may not be apparent because of motor problems, are given a chance to manifest. Physical and occupational treatments, use of orthotics, spasticity reduction (by selected dorsal rhizotomy, or with pharmacotherapies), botulinum-A (Botox) toxin injections, and surgery are commonly used approaches. In many centers, a multispecialty approach is used so that a family may, within one clinic visit, see neurology, pediatrics, orthotics, orthopedic surgery, and rehabilitation clinicians. Children with CP should be carefully followed and given all possible opportunities to flourish. Although CP is a static disorder, progressive deformity because of increased muscle tone can occur. Monitoring these children as they grow with a multispecialty approach is essential to their optimal outcome.

It is imperative within clinical practice to establish clearly defined goals for the child and family and elect interventions that address the child's specific goal based on the intervention's effect.[36]

Duchenne Muscular Dystrophy

Pathophysiology. Duchenne muscular dystrophy (DMD) is the most common of the muscular dystrophies, affecting approximately 1 in 3500 male births because of the X-linked recessive inheritance.[38] More modest mutations with residual dystrophin expression result in Becker muscular dystrophy (BMD). The onset of symptoms is typically seen later in BMD than seen in DMD; however, there are more cardiac manifestations seen in BMD.[38] Both DMD and BMD are caused by mutations in the gene that encodes dystrophin, a large membrane-stabilizing protein.[39] Dystrophin mediates anchorage of the actin cytoskeleton of skeletal muscle fibers to the basement membrane through a membrane-glycoprotein complex. Dystropin is present in normal muscle cells but absent in DMD. The lack of dystrophin causes poorly anchored fibers, which are torn apart under the repeated stress of contraction. Free calcium then enters the muscle cells, causing cell death and fiber necrosis. Disruption of the cell membrane allows the escape of creatine kinase (CK), increasing serum levels up to 10 to 100 times upper limits of normal. Marked elevations of CK levels are early identified in children suspected to have DMD and are an important diagnostic component. As muscle degenerates, there is increased endomysial connective tissue and fat; loss of striations; and concomitant hyaline, granular, and fatty degeneration of fibers. Disorganization of tendinous insertions is associated with fat accumulation in these areas (see Fig. 45.17). Although fibers regenerate in the younger child, regeneration is not able to

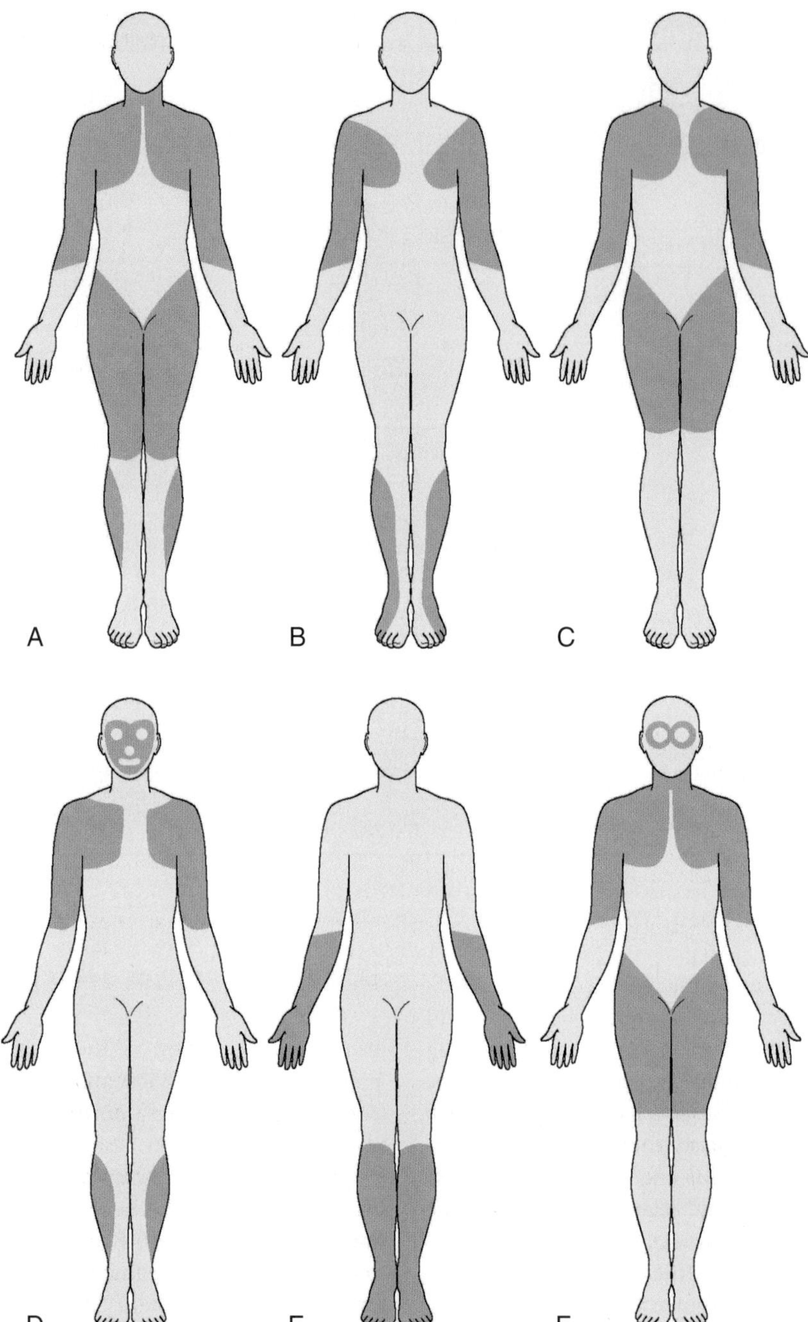

Fig. 45.17 Distribution of Muscle Weakness in Common Types of Muscular Dystrophy. **(A)** Duchenne muscular dystrophy. **(B)** Emery-Dreifuss muscular dystrophy. **(C)** Limb girdle. **(D)** Facioscapulohumeral. **(E)** Distal. **(F)** Oculopharyngeal. (From Emery-Dreifuss AE: *Lancet* 359[9307]:687–695, 2002.)

keep up with muscle cell death, resulting in progressive weakness (Fig. 45.18A).[40]

Clinical Manifestations. DMD is usually identified in children at approximately 3 to 4 years of age, when the parents first notice gait abnormalities, difficulty getting up from the ground, and frequent falls.[41] Parents also may notice enlargement of the calf muscles, which is caused by normal muscle fiber replacement with fat and connective tissue (see Fig. 45.18B and C). Muscular weakness begins in the pelvic girdle, causing a "waddling" gait. The method of rising from the floor by "climbing up the legs" (Gower sign) is characteristic and is caused by weakness of the lumbar and gluteal muscles.[39] The foot assumes an equinovarus position, and the child tends to walk on the toes because of weakness of the anterior tibial and peroneal muscles. Within 3 to 5 years, muscles of the shoulder girdle become involved.

Progressive weakness results in loss of ambulation between 12 and 15 years of age. Subsequent progression includes slowly progressive respiratory insufficiency; cardiomyopathy; and

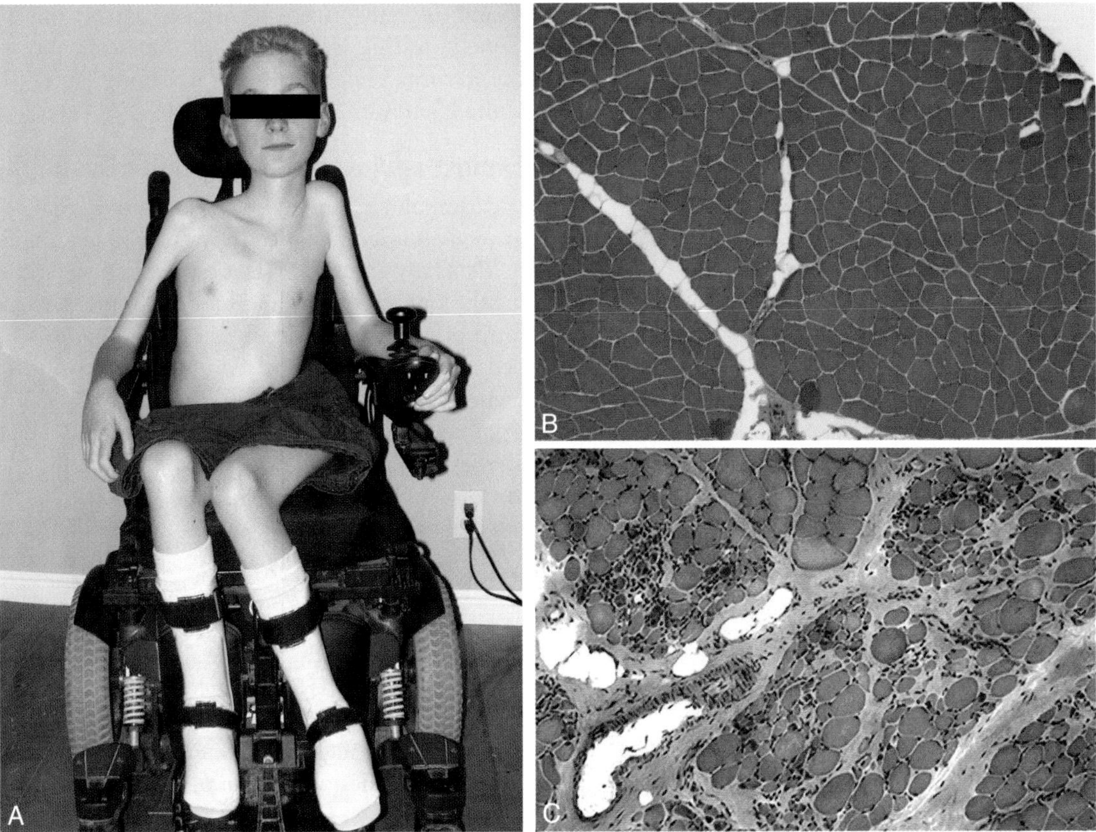

Fig. 45.18 Duchenne Muscular Dystrophy. (A) Young male with Duchenne muscular dystrophy. **(B)** Transverse section of gastrocnemius muscle from a healthy male individual. **(C)** Transverse section of gastrocnemius muscle from a male individual with Duchenne muscular dystrophy. Normal muscle fiber is replaced with fat and connective tissue. (From Jorde LB, Carey JC, Bamshad MJ. *Medical genetics*, 5th edition. Philadelphia: Mosby; 2016.)

orthopedic complications, including scoliosis. Cognitive dysfunction is a common and often overlooked aspect of DMD. Full-scale IQ is 85, which is significantly lower than the average IQ of 100, although studies suggest this decrease may be caused by specific learning disabilities rather than a true decreased intelligence. As the condition progresses, constipation and incontinence of urine and stool may develop, possibly because of smooth muscle involvement. Although the life expectancy of males with DMD continues to increase, death usually occurs from respiratory tract infection and a compromised respiratory system, with the majority living into their middle twenties. Some individuals who have chosen ventilatory support live a decade or more longer. With increased survival, cardiac complications are becoming an important contributor to mortality.

Evaluation and Treatment. Diagnosis is suggested by a high blood CK level, which can be 10 to 100 times the normal level even during infancy and before the onset of weakness. However, a high CK level does not confirm the diagnosis because many other alterations also can increase CK. Diagnosis is confirmed by genetic testing for mutations in the dystrophin gene, which is informative in 95% of cases. Muscle biopsy may be necessary in complicated cases where gene expression is not apparent on large deletion/duplication genetic testing.

Children with DMD require a multidisciplinary approach to care, including attention to heart and breathing problems, weight loss/gain, constipation, rehabilitative/developmental problems, psychosocial needs, neurologic issues, and orthopedic problems (Fig. 45.19). Maintaining function in unaffected muscle groups for as long as possible is the primary goal of treatment. Although activity fosters maintenance of muscle function, strenuous exercise may hasten the breakdown of muscle fibers. Range of motion exercises, bracing, and surgical release of contracture deformities are used to maintain normal function as long as possible. To prolong respiratory function or walking ability, or both, surgery for scoliosis is suggested when curves reach greater than 20 degrees.

Genetic counseling is recommended for all families who have children with DMD. Approximately one-third of the time, the mutation in a body with DMD is sporadic; that is, the boy is the first person in the family to develop the mutation causing DMD. Because of the X-linked inheritance, male siblings of an affected child have a 50% chance of being affected and female siblings have a 50% chance of being carriers. Prenatal diagnosis is possible, and female carriers can be identified, especially if there is a known genetic defect in another family member. Treatment with oral corticosteroids has become the standard of care and has dramatically improved outcomes.[39] Children are

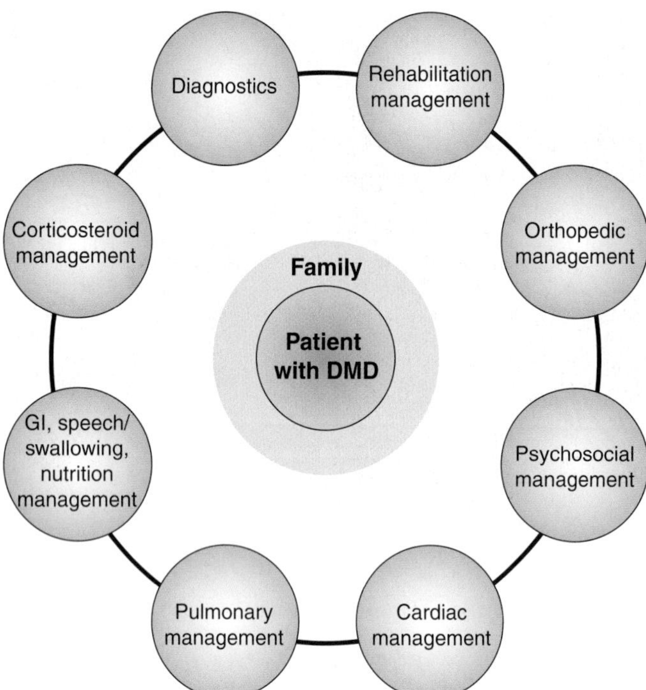

Fig. 45.19 Multisystem Approach for Evaluation and Treatment of Duchenne Muscular Dystrophy. *DMD*, Duchenne muscular dystrophy; *GI*, gastrointestinal. (Adapted from Bushby K. Diagnosis and management of Duchenne muscular dystrophy part 1: diagnosis and pharmacological and psychosocial management. 2009; Bushby K. Diagnosis and management of Duchenne muscular dystrophy part 2: implementation of multidisciplinary care. 2009. Available at www.thelancet.com/neurology. Published online November 30, 2009.)

able to walk an additional 2 to 5 years, and life expectancy has increased.[39] Complications, such as compromised pulmonary function and kyphoscoliosis ("humped" upper spine combined with scoliosis), are delayed. A gene editing tool (clustered regularly interspaced short palindromic repeats [CRISPR]) is being investigated in animals (dogs and mice) to halt disease progression as a model for humans.[42]

Families of children with DMD should receive genetic counseling for recurrence risk and prenatal screening. Various strategies to develop gene modification or gene replacement are currently in development for children with DMD.[43]

Spinal Muscular Atrophy

Spinal muscular atrophy (SMA) is a common, autosomal recessive disorder characterized by degeneration of motor neurons in the spinal cord leading to progressive muscle atrophy. Children have progressive weakness and loss of motor skills. Clues to diagnosis include tongue fasciculation (involuntary muscle twitching), a bell-shaped chest in the most severely affected infants, and tremor and quadriceps atrophy in older children. Genetically, SMA is caused by a mutation in the *SMN1* gene. Approximately 1 in 40 individuals carries the common mutation in the *SMN1* gene, making it one of the most common recessive disorders.[44]

The severity of SMA is variable, ranging from children who are never able to independently sit to children who can walk short distances. SMA is classified as types 0 through 4 and is categorized according to the onset of disease. Genetic testing is required for diagnosis and was added to the Recommended Uniform Screening Panel (RUSP) in the United States in 2018.[45]

Facioscapulohumeral Muscular Dystrophy

Facioscapulohumeral muscular dystrophy (FSHD) is a complex genetic disorder, inherited in an autosomal dominant fashion.[46]

Pathophysiology. FSHD is caused by genetic changes involving the long arm of chromosome 4. It is the third most common form of muscular dystrophy in children and is further classified into two subtypes, based on the route in which decreased methylation and a failure of epigenetic repression takes place. Approximately 95% of FSHD cases are type 1, and the other 5% are FSHD type 2.[47] Progression is usually slow and life span is normal or near normal.[46] Age at onset varies from early childhood to adulthood.

Clinical Manifestations. As the name implies, clinical manifestations begin with asymmetric weakness and atrophy of facial and scapulohumeral (shoulder girdle) muscles. The disease progresses slowly, and life span is normal or near normal. Individuals with FSHD often have weak eye closure, are not able to whistle or inflate a balloon, appear expressionless, and have scapular winging (an abnormal protrusion of the shoulder blade).[48] The most common initial physical exam finding seen in FSHD is difficulty in the abduction of the arms over the glenohumeral joint with asymmetric muscle involvement.[48] Muscle involvement gradually progresses to the distal legs and then up to the trunk.[48] FSHD generally does not involve contractures surrounding muscle groups, which differs from other dystrophies. FSHD also may be associated with mild hearing loss, retinal abnormalities, and mild cardiac problems.

Evaluation and Treatment. Diagnosis is by genetic testing, although muscle biopsies, electromyography (EMG) studies, MRI, and laboratory tests may be performed as part of the diagnostic evaluation.[49] FSHD is genetically confirmed by the presence of eight or fewer D4Z4 repeats at the 4q35 gene locus of one or more alleles. The major complications seen in FSHD are chronic pain and impaired daily functioning, which negatively impacts psychological functioning.[50] Treatment is primarily focused on supportive therapy. Administration of NSAIDs, heat treatments, physical therapy, aerobic exercise, strength training, and massage may decrease pain and inflammation.[46] Bracing may be performed for function (e.g., dorsiflexion of the feet with ankle-foot orthotics to prevent tripping or to provide support and comfort).[51]

Myotonic Muscular Dystrophy

Myotonic muscular dystrophy (MMD) is an autosomal dominant multisystem disease that occurs because of mutations in either of two genes resulting in type 1 (DM1) (dystrophia myotonica protein kinase *[DMPK]* gene on chromosome 19) and type 2 (DM2) (*ZNF9* gene on chromosome 3) MMD. DM1 may demonstrate a genetic mechanism called *anticipation*, in which children born to a mother with MMD usually have a more severe form of the disease. The childhood (infantile) subset of DM1 typically presents around age 10.

Clinical Manifestations. MMD affects the brain, skeletal and smooth muscles, eyes, heart, and endocrine system, manifesting as distal muscle weakness, learning problems, behavioral problems, intellectual disability, or a combination.[52] In addition, children can have dysphagia, constipation, cardiac dysrhythmias that, if untreated, may be life threatening, diabetes, and cataracts. Males with MMD also may manifest testicular atrophy and early male pattern baldness. A hallmark of the disease is myotonia—difficulty relaxing muscles. For example, they may have difficulty relaxing their handgrip after a handshake or opening their eyes after closing them tightly.

Children with mild disease do not develop symptoms until adolescence or older and may display mild muscle weakness (usually more pronounced in the distal muscles), cataracts, and myotonia but have normal life spans. Children with a more classic form of the disease also have onset of symptoms in the teenage years but have progressive muscle weakness, cataracts, and cardiac conduction abnormalities; they may have a shortened life span and require a wheelchair for mobility. The congenital form, the most severe, may be present at birth or become obvious over the first few years of life.[53]

Evaluation and Treatment. Diagnosis is typically made clinically and confirmed by genetic testing for the two genes known to cause MMD. In each case, an abnormal segment of deoxyribonucleic acid (DNA) causes abnormal functioning of muscle and other cells. Type 1 is more common and can present in infancy (the congenital form). Infants with MMD may have life-threatening breathing[53] and swallowing problems and developmental delay or intellectual disability, although MMD is not observed until childhood or even adolescence. Other testing, including serum CK, hepatobiliary function tests, electrodiagnostic testing, and muscle biopsy, may be added as part of the diagnostic evaluation.[54–56]

There is no curative treatment for DM; therefore the goal is to maximize individual independence with supportive management. Steroids are not useful for the treatment of DM; however, maintaining muscle function is important, including range of motion exercises, bracing, and surgical release of contractures when necessary. Children need to be followed closely by neurologists and primary care providers with treatment for the various aspects of the disease, such as dysphagia, heart dysrhythmias, and constipation, as well as other problems.[57]

MUSCULOSKELETAL TUMORS IN CHILDREN

Bone Tumors

Bone tumors are uncommon but, when cancerous, can contribute significantly to the morbidity and mortality of teenagers and young adults. Of the malignant bone tumors, osteosarcoma and Ewing sarcoma are the most common. Benign bone tumors are much more common than malignant bone tumors. However, true incidence and prevalence data are difficult to discern because most benign tumors are asymptomatic and are usually discovered accidentally during the work-up for a different issue. The most common forms of benign bone tumors are osteochondroma, nonossifying fibroma, simple bone cyst (SBC), aneurysmal bone cyst (ABC), osteoid osteoma, and fibrous dysplasia (FD) (Fig. 45.20).

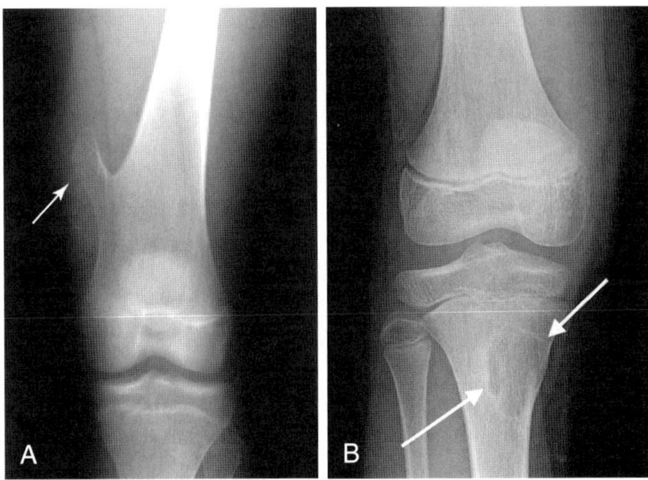

Fig. 45.20 Benign Bone Tumors. (A) Osteochondroma *(white arrow)* arising from the distal femur. **(B)** Nonossifying fibroma *(white arrows)* mostly lytic.

Benign Bone Tumors

Osteochondroma. Osteochondroma (or exostosis) is a cartilaginous bony spur on the external surface of a bone. They can occur as a solitary lesion or as an inherited syndrome of hereditary multiple exostoses (HME).[58] HME is an autosomal dominant condition with two or more exostoses occurring throughout the skeleton.

The long proposed hypothesis is that a fragment of the growth plate herniates through the periosteum, continues to grow, and results in either a sessile or pedunculated lesion, commonly in the region of the metaphysis.[59] This separation of the growth plate fragment can occur either spontaneously (primary osteochondroma), or secondarily from surgery, radiation, or fractures (secondary osteosarcoma).[59] However, recently researchers have identified genetic mutations in the gene encoding exostosin 1, suggesting that solitary osteochondromas represent true benign neoplasms.[60] HME is associated with a loss-of-function type of mutation in the tumor suppressor genes exostosin 1 and exostosin 2, which results in heparan sulfate proteoglycan (HSPG) deficiency and subsequent development of multiple osteochondromas.[60]

Osteochondromas are generally asymptomatic lesions that are incidental findings on a radiograph for noncontributory symptoms. When lesions are symptomatic, they can appear as bony protuberances because of genetic anomalies near active growth plates of the proximal humerus, distal femur, or proximal tibia. The most common presentation is a palpable mass that is painful when traumatized. Symptomatic lesions may also be secondary to fracture, malignant transformation, compression of adjacent neurovascular structures, bursal formation and/or bursitis, or palpable mass. The lesions can disturb growth plates and lead to growth disturbances. Individuals with HME are generally more severely affected, present at a younger age, and have multiple osseous deformities such as bowing of the extremities, short limbs, short stature, leg length discrepancy, coxa valgus, or genu valgus (knock knees).[58,61] Upper extremity lesions can lead to a pronounced deformity in the forearm with a very short ulnar bone. These lesions grow until skeletal maturity; growth or pain after skeletal maturity is a sign of possible malignant transformation, especially in the pelvis or scapular region. Transformation to chondrosarcoma is very rare, occurring in less than 1% of children. Osteochondromas involving the long bones (most common location) generally have a pathognomonic appearance and require no further imaging evaluation. However, radiography and MRI are useful for individuals who are symptomatic or demonstrate the need for further evaluation.[62]

Solitary osteochondroma lesions that are asymptomatic without suspicious imaging features require only follow-up. Treatment for symptomatic lesions or lesions with suspicious imaging features requires surgical resection.[63,64]

Nonossifying fibroma. Nonossifying fibromas are sharply demarcated, cortically based lesions of fibrocytes that have replaced normal bone. The lesion can occur in any bone, at any age; however, they occur ordinarily in the metaphysis of long bones, most commonly in the lower extremities on the distal femur, distal tibia, and proximal tibia.[65] These fibromas are found in approximately 30% of the population.[65] In approximately 80% of nonossifying fibroma tumors, there is cell mutation, causing activation of the RAS-MAPK (mitogen-activated protein kinase) pathway.[66]

Most fibrous cortical defects resolve spontaneously as they are obliterated by reparative ossification. In some cases, the nonossifying fibroma persists and proliferates, affecting the structural integrity of the bone.[65]

Because nonossifying fibromas are typically asymptomatic, they are incidentally noted on radiographs obtained for other symptomatology.[65] In the 1950s, when fluoride was added to drinking water, random skeletal surveys were done on hundreds of children and nonossifying fibromas were discovered in 20% to 30% of children and distributed in nearly every bone of the body. Treatment is spared until the lesion occupies more than 50% of the diameter of the width of the bone or extends 3 to 4 cm into the cortex. Quantitative CT scans help to define a large lesion clearly and are used for preoperative planning.[67]

Simple bone cyst. Simple bone cysts (SBCs) are solitary fluid-filled lesions of the central region of the metaphyseal area in children. The most common sites for a simple cyst are the proximal humerus and proximal femur.[68] With growth, these lesions may appear within the diaphysis. Affected children are typically asymptomatic until pathologic fracture or incidental discovery occurs. Lesions often heal after a fracture, but large lesions may require further intervention. Nonoperative management is the choice for mild symptoms. Surgical interventions are rarely required and are typically reserved for very large lesions that affect weight bearing.[69]

Aneurysmal bone cyst. Aneurysmal bone cysts (ABCs) are typically solitary, eccentric, blood-filled osteolytic lesions that occur in adolescence. The etiology remains controversial; many consider an ABC lesion as secondary to another process, such as giant cell tumor, or the result of a vascular malformation within the bone.[70] The lesions can be found on any bone but most often are located on the spine, femur, and tibia.[70] ABCs are locally destructive and grow aggressively. The area can be painful and edematous, causing a limp or neurologic symptom. Surgical intervention is necessary to stop their expansion and inhibit reoccurrence.[71]

Osteoid osteoma. Osteoid osteoma is a bone-forming tumor that presents as a painful lesion of the diaphysis or metadiaphysis of long bones. Involvement of the posterior elements of the spine, with resultant "splinting" scoliosis, can occur. Night pain is common, as is relief from symptoms with NSAIDs, because these tumors release prostaglandins. Advanced treatment options may be necessary for lesions causing intolerable pain, limp, or scoliosis. Radiofrequency -guided laser ablation, surgical resection, cryotherapy, and MRI-guided high-intensity focused ultrasound are options.[72]

Fibrous dysplasia. Fibrous dysplasia (FD) is a disease that causes thinning of the bone or lesion formation. Portions of the bone are replaced by fibrous tissue. FD can occur in one bone (monostotic) or in multiple bones (polyostotic). Although any bone can be affected, the long bones, ribs, and skull are the most common. A radiographic "ground-glass" appearance is present primarily in the metaphyseal or metadiaphyseal areas. Deformity can be marked and necessitate operative intervention.[73]

Malignant Bone Tumors

Malignant bone tumors are uncommon tumors in childhood, accounting for fewer than 5% of childhood malignancies and occurring mostly during adolescence. The two most common malignant bone tumors are osteosarcoma and Ewing sarcoma.

Osteosarcoma. Osteosarcoma, although very rare overall, is the most common malignant bone tumor found during childhood. Osteosarcoma originates in bone-producing mesenchymal cells and accounts for 60% of all malignant bone tumors. There is a bimodal age distribution overall, but in children, presentation usually occurs in adolescence between the ages of 13 and 16. Molecular analysis has demonstrated deletion of genetic material on the long arm of chromosome 13, leading to the identification of a tumor-suppressor gene as part of the mechanism for tumor development. The oncogene *src* also has been associated with osteosarcoma.

Pathophysiology. Osteosarcoma arises sporadically, with few cases associated with known inherited defects in cell cycle regulation, but approximately 70% of tumor specimens demonstrate a chromosomal abnormality.[74] Alterations to TP53 and RB1 tumor suppressor genes play a role in osteosarcoma.[75] Osteosarcoma occurs mainly in the metaphyses regions of long bones near sites of active physeal growth.[76] The tumor most commonly occurs at the distal femur, proximal tibia, or proximal humerus. As a tumor of mesenchymal cells, osteosarcoma makes osteoid tissue.

Osteosarcoma is a bulky tumor that extends beyond the bone into a soft tissue mass. It may encircle the bone and destroy the trabeculae of the diseased area. Osteosarcoma disseminates through the bloodstream, usually to the lung.[76] As many as 20% of children diagnosed with osteosarcoma exhibit lung metastases at diagnosis.[75] Other sites of metastatic spread include other bones and visceral organs.

Clinical Manifestations. The most common presenting complaint is pain at the site of the tumor.[77] Night pain, awakening a child from sleep, is a particularly foreboding sign. There may be swelling, warmth, and redness caused by the vascularity of the tumor.[77] Symptoms also may include cough, dyspnea, and chest pain if lung metastasis is present. If a lower extremity is involved, a child may limp or suffer a pathologic fracture.[77] Although osteosarcoma is not the result of trauma, trauma may call attention to a preexisting tumor.

Evaluation and Treatment. Diagnostic imaging (x-ray, MRI, CT, bone scan, and positron emission tomography [PET] scan) may suggest osteosarcoma, but a biopsy is confirmational.[77] Although needle biopsy is often sufficient to establish the diagnosis, tissue biopsy confirms it. The World Health Organization's (WHO's) histologic classification of bone tumors divides osteosarcoma into central, intramedullary, and surface tumors, with a number of subtypes under each group. The tumor is graded according to degree of malignancy; the higher the grade, the worse the prognosis.

Treatment is determined by the extent of the disease. Localized disease can be treated with chemotherapy with or without surgical intervention. Individuals with metastatic disease or relapse have poor prognoses. However, chemotherapy, surgery, and enrollment in clinical trial testing are options.[78]

Ewing sarcoma. Ewing sarcoma is a malignant round cell tumor of bone and soft tissue and is the second most common and most lethal malignant bone tumor that occurs during childhood.[79] The most common period of diagnosis is between 5 and 15 years of age. Ewing sarcoma is slightly more common in males than females and is linked with periods of rapid bone growth.

Pathophysiology. The pathognomonic molecular hallmark of Ewing sarcoma is a translocation between the EWS (*EWSR1* or *FUS*) gene and ETS-transcription (E26 transformation-specific or E-twenty-six) gene family (FLI*1*, *ERG*, *ETV1*, *ETV4*, or *FEV*).[80] Ewing sarcoma is most commonly located in the diaphysis of long bones or in flat bones. The most common sites include the femur, pelvis, and humerus; however, it may occur in almost any bone or soft tissue (Fig. 45.21). Arising from bone marrow, Ewing sarcoma can penetrate the cortex of the bone to form a soft tissue mass (see Fig. 45.21A and B). Metastasis occurs early and is usually apparent at diagnosis or within 1 year. The most common sites are the lung, other bones, lymph nodes, bone marrow, liver, spleen, and central nervous system, although metastasis to any organ is possible.

Clinical Manifestations. As with osteosarcoma, the most common complaint is pain, stiffness, and edema that increases in severity. A soft tissue mass is often present. Additional symptoms may include fever, malaise, and anorexia. Typically, the symptoms have been present for months preceding the presentation for treatment. However, a pathologic fracture is present upon diagnosis in 10% to 15% of cases.[81]

Evaluation and Treatment. Initial evaluation typically begins with a radiographic study. A poorly defined permeative, destructive lesion is typically seen and often times associated with a soft tissue mass. A distinctive "moth-eaten" appearance is common along with "Codman triangle" of the elevated periosteum, or multilayered "onion-skin" periosteal reaction. Diagnostic imaging of primary sites includes MRI and/or CT, with contrast is of prime importance.[82] Classification can be determined using the TNM by the American Joint Committee on Cancer (AJCC), which is based on tumor size, lymph node metastasis, distant metastasis, and tumor grade (cellular differentiation, mitotic rate, and extent of necrosis). However, the most commonly used staging system for Ewing sarcoma is classification of the tumor by grade (low grade is stage I, high grade is stage II, and distant metastasis is stage III) and compartmental status (located in the bone cortex versus extended beyond the bone cortex), which was developed by the Musculoskeletal Tumor Society (MSTS).

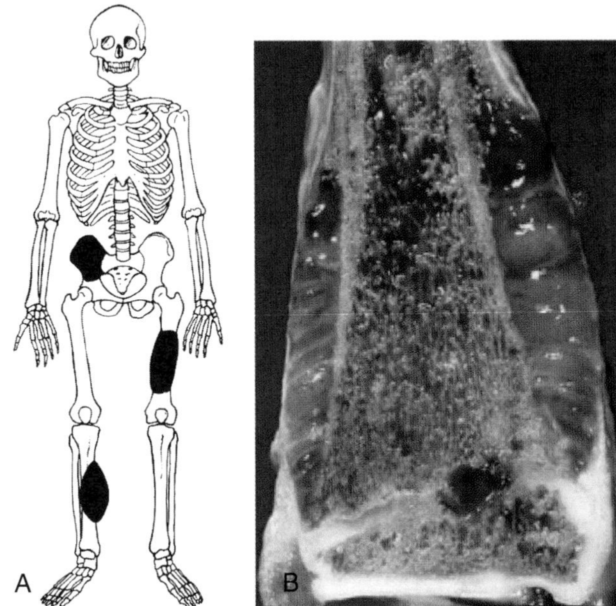

Fig. 45.21 Ewing Sarcoma (A) Most common anatomic sites. (B) Close-up view of Ewing sarcoma of the distal end of the tibia. Tumor extends into the soft tissue. (A, From Damjanov I, Linder J, eds. *Anderson's pathophysiology*, 10th edition. St. Louis: Mosby; 1996. B, Fletcher CDM. Diagnostic *histopathy of tumors*, 5th edition. Philadelphia: Elsevier.)

Biopsy is used to conclusively establish the diagnosis, which can be done with a CT-guided core-needle biopsy. The identification of t(11;22) chromosomal translocation within the tumor cells confirms the diagnosis.[83] Bone marrow aspiration with smear and bone marrow biopsy may also be considered. A serum lactate dehydrogenase (LDH) should be done because it carries prognostic significance.

The standard of treatment for Ewing sarcoma is multidrug chemotherapy and local therapy, which includes surgery and radiotherapy. Chemotherapy is continued for 12 to 18 months after resection. The major predictor of prognosis appears to be the location of the primary tumor and the presence of metastases at diagnosis.[84] Supportive care must include monitoring and treating the increased risks and adverse health outcomes associated with the current treatment for Ewing sarcoma, including severe neutropenia, recurrent fever, opportunistic infections, and mucositis.

Muscle Tumors

Most soft tissue tumors in children are benign. Only two malignant soft tissue tumors occur with any frequency:

TABLE 45.4 Classification of Tumors by Origin

Tissue	Tumor
Muscle	
Striated	Rhabdomyosarcoma
Smooth	Leiomyosarcoma
Adipose	Liposarcoma
Fibrous	Fibrosarcoma
Synovial mesothelium	Synovial sarcoma
Lymphatic structures	Lymphangiosarcoma
Blood vessels	Hemangiopericytoma
Nerve sheath	Neurogenic sarcoma

rhabdomyosarcoma (RMS) in the younger child and synovial cell sarcoma in the teenager. Both of these occur rarely. Soft tissue tumors originate from the primitive mesenchymal cells that normally give rise to muscle, tendons, blood vessels, lymphatic structures, fibrous and connective tissue, bursa, and fascia. Table 45.4 identifies the classification of soft tissue tumors according to origin. All malignant soft tissue tumors are characterized as highly aggressive tumors that invade surrounding structures and metastasize early.

Rhabdomyosarcoma (RMS) is the most common soft tissue sarcoma of childhood and accounts for approximately 50% of all soft tissue tumors.[85] RMS arises from embryonal rhabdomyoblasts that normally differentiate into mature striated muscle. RMS can develop anywhere striated muscle is located. Primary locations include the head and neck, trunk, extremities, and the genitourinary tract. Recent studies demonstrate an association between *TP53* (a tumor-suppressor gene) mutations and sporadic RMS.[86] Four major subtypes of RMS have been identified: embryonal (most common), botryoid, sclerosing and spindle cell, and alveolar.[87] Clinical manifestations of RMS are outlined in Table 45.5.

TABLE 45.5 Clinical Manifestations of Rhabdosarcoma

Location	Manifestation
Head and Neck	
Orbit	Ptosis Exophthalmos Proptosis
Paranasal sinuses	Nasal obstruction Epistaxis Swelling Chronic sinusitis
Nasopharynx	Hypernasal speech Nasal discharge Visible polypoid mass
Oropharyngeal	Dysphagia Painful mastication
Middle ear	Chronic serous otitis media Discharge from affected ear Facial nerve palsy Conduction hearing loss Visible polypoid mass
Extremities	
All locations	Deep-seated, fixed palpable mass
Retroperitoneal	
All locations	Usually asymptomatic May have vague abdominal pain Bowel or genitourinary obstruction (late) Possible palpable mass
Genitourinary	
Vaginal	Abnormal vaginal bleeding Protruding polypoid mass
Prostate	Urinary tract obstruction
Bladder	Urinary retention Straining to void Hematuria
Paratesticular	Mass in scrotum that may be painful

NONACCIDENTAL TRAUMA

In the past year, at least 1 in 7 children have experienced child abuse and/or neglect, and this is likely an underestimate.[88] In 2019, 1840 children died of abuse and neglect in the United States.[88] Maltreatment may be physical, sexual, emotional, or neglect.[88] Skeletal trauma is present in a significant number of abused children (Fig. 45.22).[89–91] Accurate and appropriate referrals to child protection agencies not only are legally mandated but also are essential for the well-being of the child.

Fractures in Nonaccidental Trauma

Children who are not yet ambulatory and present with a long bone fracture have more than a 75% chance of that fracture being caused by nonaccidental trauma (NAT).[92] An unexplained humeral fracture in children younger than 15 months of age should be considered suspicious for abuse.[93] Multiple fractures in any location without overt trauma are also strongly associated with abusive injury. Rib fractures are the most common abnormality in abused children.[93] "Corner" metaphyseal fractures are nearly always from abuse and are considered a highly specific marker for abuse in infants (Fig. 45.23).[94] Fractures highly suggestive of physical abuse include rib fractures, classic metaphyseal lesions, those unsuspected or inconsistent with the history or age of the child, multiple fractures involving more than one skeletal area, and fractures of differing ages.[93] Fractures at multiple stages of healing also suggest abuse; however, OI or other causes of systemic osteomalacia must be ruled out. The most common presentation is a transverse tibia fracture. After walking age, only 2% of long bone fractures are the result of NAT.[95]

Evaluation and Treatment. If abuse is suspected, NAT necessitates early consultation with child protective services. The

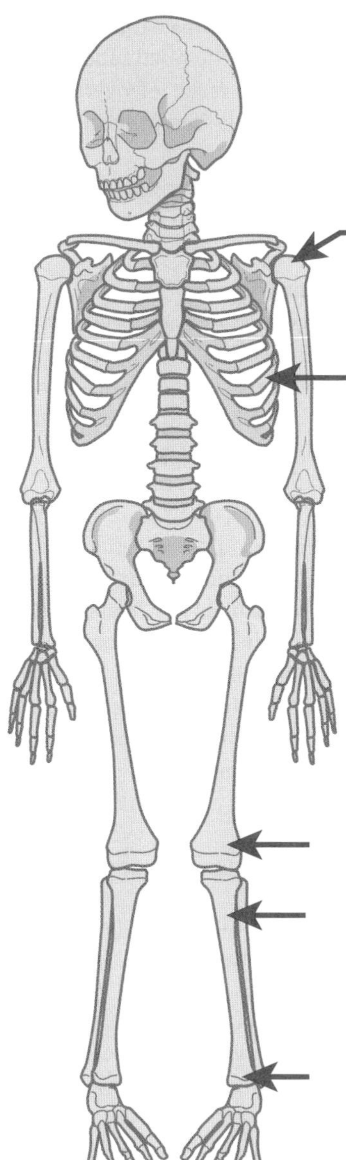

Fig. 45.22 **Rib and Metaphyseal Fractures.** Rib fractures are very common and highly specific for abuse. There is an extremely high incidence of rib and metaphyseal fractures in children who die as a result of abuse. The red arrows indicate common sites of fracture related to abuse. (Data from Radiology Assistant Radiology Assistant Educational Site, Radiological Society of the Netherlands. Available from www.radiologyassistant.nl/.)

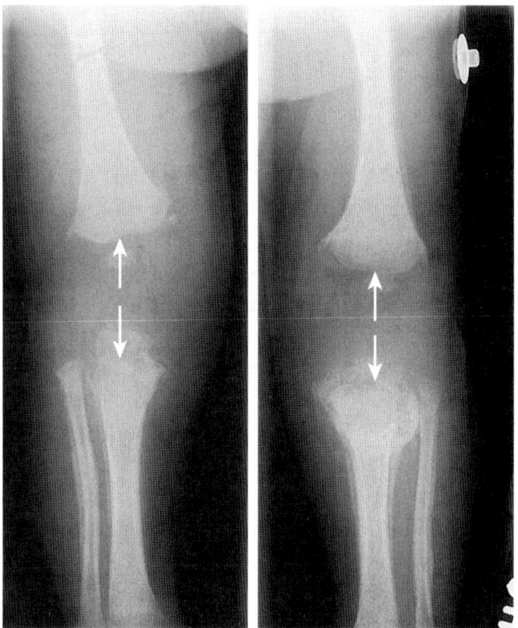

Fig. 45.23 **Corner Fracture.** Bilateral knee radiograph showing healing corner fractures of bilateral proximal tibias and distal femurs. Note the varying amount of callus formation signifying fractures at different stages of healing.

healthcare provider is legally responsible to report suspected NAT. A thorough history must be obtained for all identified injuries. The child should undergo skeletal survey (especially if younger than 2 years of age) and have a complete physical examination to evaluate for pattern bruising, burns, or multiple soft tissue injuries. The American College of Radiology (ACR) Appropriateness Criteria should be followed to rate the appropriateness of imaging and treatment procedures for specific clinical scenarios.[93] Ophthalmologic examination and brain CT should be used to evaluate for retinal or brain hemorrhage caused by shaking.

The treating healthcare provider must have a nonjudgmental attitude. The child and family involved in NAT are emotionally delicate and require not only physical but also emotional care. Social workers need to be involved early to ensure that the child receives appropriate medical care. Fortunately, fractures tend to heal quickly for those in this age group. However, neurologic injury and social disease are much more difficult to cure.

SUMMARY REVIEW

Musculoskeletal Development in Children

1. Skeletal growth and development consist of two phases: (a) delivery of bone cell precursors to sites of bone formation and (b) the aggregation of these cells at primary centers of ossification where they mature to secrete osteoid.
2. Ossification takes place in two centers in long bones: (a) the primary center, or the diaphysis (the long, central portion of the bone); and (b) the secondary center, or the epiphysis (the end portions of the bone).
3. Peak bone mass is achieved by the middle to late 20 s.
4. By 1 year of age, 50% of the total growth of the spine has occurred, and most children have achieved 50% of their adult height by 2 years of age.
5. The appendicular skeleton (extremities) grows faster during childhood than does the axial skeleton.
6. Muscle fibers reach their maximal size in females at 10 years of age and at 14 years of age in males.

Musculoskeletal Alterations in Children

1. The most common congenital defect of the upper extremities is syndactyly (webbing of the fingers or toes).
2. Polydactyly, or supernumerary digits, is another common congenital limb anomaly of the fingers or toes.
3. Developmental dysplasia of the hip (DDH) is an abnormality in the development of the femoral head, acetabulum, or both. DDH can be idiopathic or teratologic. It is a serious and disabling condition in children if not diagnosed and treated early, with best outcomes when treated before walking age.
4. Clubfoot (equinovarus) is a common deformity in which the foot is twisted out of its normal shape or position. Clubfoot can be positional, idiopathic, or teratologic. Positional is correctable passively; however, idiopathic and teratologic may require casting, bracing, or surgery.
5. Osteogenesis imperfecta (brittle bone disease) is a genetic disorder of collagen that affects primarily bones and results in fractures of many bones.
6. Rickets is a condition caused by deficiencies in vitamin D, calcium, and usually phosphorus that is characterized by the failure of bones to become mineralized (ossified) and results in skeletal deformity.
7. Scoliosis is a lateral curvature of the spinal column that can be caused by congenital malformations of the spine, neuromuscular disease, trauma, extraspinal contractures, bone infections, metabolic bone disorders, joint disease, and tumors. Nonstructural scoliosis results from a cause other than the spine itself, such as posture, leg length discrepancy, or splinting from pain. Structural scoliosis is a curvature of the spine associated with vertebral rotation.

Bone and Joint Infection

1. Osteomyelitis is a local or generalized bacterial infection of bone and bone marrow. Bacteria are usually introduced by direct extension from a nearby infection, through the bloodstream, or by trauma. Infection starts in the metaphysis, then ruptures out to spread into the diaphysis.
2. Septic arthritis is a bacterial or granulomatous infection of the joint space and is a surgical emergency. It can occur on its own, or secondary to osteomyelitis in very young children in which the metaphysis is still located within the joint capsule of certain joints.

Juvenile Idiopathic Arthritis

1. Juvenile idiopathic arthritis is an inflammatory joint disorder characterized by pain and swelling. Large joints are most commonly affected.

Avascular diseases

1. Avascular diseases of the bone are collectively referred to as *osteochondroses* and are caused by an insufficient blood supply to growing bones.
2. Legg-Calvé-Perthes disease is one of the most common osteochondroses. This disorder is characterized by epiphyseal necrosis or degeneration of the head of the femur followed by regeneration or recalcification.
3. Osgood-Schlatter disease is characterized by inflammation or partial separation of the tibial tubercle caused by chronic irritation, usually as a result of overuse of the quadriceps muscles. The condition is seen primarily in muscular, athletic adolescent males.
4. Calcaneal apophysitis or Sever disease is the primary cause of heal pain in children between 8 and 15 years of age.

Neuromuscular Disorders

1. The muscular dystrophies are a group of genetically transmitted diseases characterized by progressive atrophy of symmetrical groups of skeletal muscles without evidence of involvement or degeneration of neural tissue. There is an insidious loss of strength in all forms of the disorder with increasing disability and deformity.
2. Cerebral palsy is a general term that refers to nonprogressive disorders of movement and posture resulting from injury or malformation of the developing central nervous system. Cerebral palsy is the most common motor disability of childhood.
3. Duchenne muscular dystrophy is characterized by the absence of the membrane-stabilizing protein dystropin in muscle cells. Weakness leads to abnormal gait, frequent falls, and eventual loss of ambulation. Respiratory, cardiac, and neurologic problems are also present, requiring a multidisciplinary approach to care.
4. Spinal muscular atrophy is characterized by degeneration of motor neurons in the spinal cord leading to progressive muscle atrophy. Children have progressive muscle weakness and lack of motor skills.
5. Facioscapulohumeral muscular dystrophy involves asymmetric muscle weakness, starting in the face and then progressing to the shoulders and legs.
6. Myotonic muscular dystrophy classically presents with myotonia, or a difficulty relaxing muscles. It also can affect the brain, eyes, heart, and endocrine system.

Musculoskeletal Tumors

1. Musculoskeletal tumors may be benign (osteochondroma and nonossifying fibroma) or malignant (osteosarcoma and Ewing sarcoma).
2. Osteochondroma appears as a solitary bony protuberance near active growth plates of the proximal humerus, distal femur, or proximal tibia. Hereditary multiple exostoses is characterized by multiple bony protuberances throughout the skeleton.
3. Nonossifying fibromas are lesions in which fibrocytes have replaced normal bone. Treatment may be required if the lesions grow so large that they compromise the strength of the bone.
4. Osteosarcoma, the most common malignant childhood bone tumor, originates in bone-producing mesenchymal cells and is most often located near active growth plates, such as the distal femur, proximal tibia, or proximal humerus. It is a bulky tumor that creates osteoid tissue. Pain, especially night pain, is the most common presenting symptom. It commonly causes lung metastases. The primary treatments for osteosarcoma are surgery and chemotherapy.

5. Ewing sarcoma originates from cells within the bone marrow space and is most often located in the midshaft of long bones or in flat bones. The most common sites include the femur, pelvis, and humerus, and the most common presenting symptom is pain that increases in severity. Ewing sarcoma metastasizes to nearly every organ. The primary treatment for Ewing sarcoma is a combination of chemotherapy, radiation, and surgery.

Nonaccidental Trauma

1. Nonaccidental trauma (NAT) must be considered with any long bone injury in a preambulatory child.
2. Evidence of soft tissue injury, corner fractures, and fractures at different stages of healing is extremely helpful in making a diagnosis of NAT. The healthcare provider is legally responsible to report suspected NAT.
3. The presence of soft tissue injury, corner fractures, and multiple fractures at different stages of healing is extremely helpful for making a diagnosis of NAT. When NAT is suspected, a child must be evaluated radiographically for other fractures, head trauma, and retinal hemorrhage.
4. All social strata are at risk for NAT.
   When NAT is suspected, a child must be evaluated radiographically for other fractures, burns, multiple soft tissue injuries, and retinal hemorrhage.

REFERENCES

1. Morcuende JA, et al. Plaster cast treatment of clubfoot: the Ponseti method of manipulation and casting. *J Pediatr Orthop.* 1994;3(2):161–167.
2. Jari S, et al. Unilateral limitation of abduction of the hip: a valuable clinical sign for DDH? *J Bone Joint Surg Br.* 2002;84(1):104–107.
3. Patel RM, et al. A cross-sectional multicenter study of osteogenesis imperfecta in North America—results from the Linked Clinical Research Centers. *Clin Genet.* 2015;87(2):133–140.
4. Lee JY, So TY, Thackray J. A review on vitamin d deficiency treatment in pediatric patients. *J Pediatr Pharmacol Ther.* 2013;18(4):277–291.

4a. Simkin P. The musculoskeletal system. In Klippel JH, Dieppe PA, editors: *Rheumatology*, ed 2. London: Mosby-Wolfe; 1998.

5. Mata SG, et al. Legg-Calvé-Perthes disease and passive smoking. *J Pediatr Orthop.* 2000;20(3):326–330.
6. Principi N, et al. *Kingella kingae* infections in children. *BMC Infect Dis.* 2015;15:260.
7. Malik S. Polydactyly: phenotypes, genetics and classification. *Clin Genet.* 2014;85(3):203–213.
8. Tafazal S, Flowers MJ. Do we need to follow up an early normal ultrasound with a later plain radiograph in children with a family history of developmental dysplasia of the hip? *Eur J Orthop Surg Traumatol.* 2015;25(7):1171–1175.
9. Atalar H, et al. Indicators of successful use of the Pavlik harness in infants with developmental dysplasia of the hip. *Int Orthop.* 2007;31(2):145–150.
10. Pavone V, et al. The etiology of idiopathic congenital talipes equinovarus: a systematic review. *J Orthop Surg Res.* 2018;13:206.
11. Zaleske DJ, Doppelt SH, Mankin HJ. Endocrine abnormalities of the immature skeleton. In: Lovell WW, Winter RB, eds. *Pediatric orthopedics.* ed 2 Philadelphia: Lippincott; 1986.
12. Marini J, et al. Osteogenesis imperfect due to mutations in non-collagenous genes: lessons in the biology of bone formation. *Curr Opin Pediatr.* 2014;26(4):500–506.
13. Zeitlin L, Fassier F, Glorieux FH. Modern approach to children with osteogenesis imperfecta. *J Pediatr Orthop B.* 2003;12(2):77–87.
14. Kuznia AL, Hernandez AK, Lee LU. Adolescent idiopathic scoliosis: common questions and answers. *Am Fam Physician.* 2020;101(1):19–23.
15. Dunn J, et al. Screening for adolescent idiopathic scoliosis: evidence report and systematic review for the US Preventive Services Task Force. *JAMA.* 2018;319(2):173–187.
16. Thakolkaran N, Shetty AK. Acute hematogenous osteomyelitis in children. *Ochsner J.* 2019;19(2):116–122.
17. Iiadis AD, Ramachandran M. Paediatric bone and joint infections. *EFORT Open Rev.* 2017;2(1):7–12.
18. Peltola H, Pääkkönen M. Acute osteomyelitis in children. *N Engl J Med.* 2014;370(4):352–360.
19. Dartnell J, Ramachandran M, Katchburian M. Haematogenous acute and subacute paediatric osteomyelitis: a systematic review of the literature. *J Bone Joint Surg Br.* 2012;94(5):584–595.
20. Popescu B, et al. Acute hematogenous osteomyelitis in pediatric patients: epidemiology and risk factors of a poor outcome. *J Int Med Res.* 2020;48(4): 300060520910889.
21. Jaramillo D, et al. Hematogenous osteomyelitis in infants and children: imaging of a changing disease. *Radiology.* 2017;283(3):629–643.
22. Funk SS, Copley LA. Acute hematogenous osteomyelitis in children: pathogenesis, diagnosis, and treatment. *Orthop Clin North Am.* 2017;48(2):199–208.
23. Kocher MS, et al. Validation of a clinical prediction rule for the differentiation between septic arthritis and transient synovitis of the hip in children. *J Bone Joint Surg Am.* 2004;86:1629–1635.
24. Nguyen A, et al. Kocher criteria revisited in the era of MRI: how often does the Kocher criteria identify underlying osteomyelitis? *J Pediatr Orthop.* 2017;37(2):e114–e119.
25. Petty RE, et al. International League of Associations for Rheumatology classification of juvenile idiopathic arthritis: second revision, Edmonton, 2001. *J Rheumatol.* 2004;31: 390–392.
26. Leroux J, Abu Amara S, Lechevallier J. Legg-Calvé-Perthes disease. *Orthop Traumatol Surg Res.* 2018;104(1S):S107–S112.
27. Loder RT, Skopelja EN. The epidemiology and demographics of Legg-Calvé-Perthes' disease. *ISRN Orthop.* 2011;2011:504393.
28. Wiig O, et al. The outcome and prognostic factors in children with bilateral Perthes' disease: a prospective study of 40 children with follow-up over five years. *Bone Joint J.* 2016;98-B(4):569.
29. Neal DC, et al. Prevalence of obesity in patients with Legg-Calvé-Perthes disease. *J Am Acad Orthop Surg.* 2016;24(9):660.
30. Dustmann HO. [Etiology and pathogenesis of epiphyseal necrosis in childhood as exemplified with the hip]. *Z Orthop Ihre Grenzgeb.* 1996;134(5):407–412. German.
31. Dillman JR, Hernandex RJ. MRI of Legg-Calve-Perthes disease. *AJR Am J Roentgenol.* 2009;193(5):1394.
32. Ibrahim T, Little DG. The pathogenesis and treatment of Legg-Calvé-Perthes disease. *JBJS Rev.* 2016;4(7):e4.
33. Circi E, Atalay Y, Beyzadeoglu T. Treatment of Osgood–Schlatter disease: review of the literature. *Musculoskelet Surg.* 2017;101:195–200.
34. Ramponi DR, Baker C. Sever's disease (calcaneal apophysitis). *Adv Emerg Nurs J.* 2019;41(1):10–14.
35. Ogden JA, et al. Sever's injury: a stress fracture of the immature calcaneal metaphysis. *J Pediatr Orthop.* 2004;24(5):488.

36. Novak I, et al. State of the evidence traffic lights 2019: systematic review of interventions for preventing and treating children with cerebral palsy. *Curr Neurol Neurosci Rep*. 2020;20(2):3.
37. Centers for Disease Control and Prevention (CDC) *National Center on Birth Defects and Developmental Disabilities (NCBDDD)*. Atlanta, GA: CDC; 2021. Page last reviewed October 15, 2021. Available at https://www.cdc.gov/ncbddd/index.html. (Accessed December 31, 2021).
38. Mah JK, et al. A systematic review and meta-analysis on the epidemiology of Duchenne and Becker muscular dystrophy. *Neuromuscul Disord*. 2014;24(6):482–491.
39. Birnkrant DJ, et al. Diagnosis and management of Duchenne muscular dystrophy, part 1: diagnosis, and neuromuscular, rehabilitation, endocrine, and gastrointestinal and nutritional management. *Lancet Neurol*. 2018;17(3):251–267.
40. Stevens A, Lowe J. *Pathology*. London: Mosby-Wolfe; 1995.
41. Ciafaloni E, et al. Delayed diagnosis in Duchenne muscular dystrophy: data from the Muscular Dystrophy Surveillance, Tracking, and Research Network (MD STARnet). *J Pediatr*. 2009;155(3):380–385.
42. Bengtsson NE, et al. Muscle-specific CRISPR/Cas9 dystrophin gene editing ameliorates pathophysiology in a mouse model for Duchenne muscular dystrophy. *Nat Commun*. 2017;8:14454.
43. Wein N, Alfano L, Flanigan KM. Genetics and emerging treatments for Duchenne and Becker muscular dystrophy. *Pediatr Clin North Am*. 2015;62(3):723–742.
44. Sugarman EA, et al. Pan-ethnic carrier screening and prenatal diagnosis for spinal muscular atrophy: clinical laboratory analysis of >72,400 specimens. *Eur J Hum Genet*. 2012;20(1):27.
45. Chien YH, et al. Presymptomatic diagnosis of spinal muscular atrophy through newborn screening. *J Pediatr*. 2017;190:124.
46. Hamel J, Tawil R. Facioscapulohumeral muscular dystrophy: update on pathogenesis and future treatments. *Neurotherapeutics*. 2018;15(4):863–871.
47. van der Maarel SM, Frants RR. The D4Z4 repeat-mediated pathogenesis of facioscapulohumeral muscular dystrophy. *Am J Hum Genet*. 2005;76(3):375–386.
48. Statland JM, Tawil R. Facioscapulohumeral muscular dystrophy. *Continuum (Minneap Minn)*. 2016;22(6, Muscle and Neuromuscular Junction Disorders):1916–1931.
49. Ricci G, Zatz M, Tupler R. Facioscapulohumeral muscular dystrophy: more complex than it appears. *Curr Mol Med*. 2014;14(8):1052–1068.
50. Morís G, et al. Chronic pain has a strong impact on quality of life in facioscapulohumeral muscular dystrophy. *Muscle Nerve*. 2018;57(3):380–387.
51. Lu J, et al. Management strategies in facioscapulohumeral muscular dystrophy. *Intractable Rare Dis Res*. 2019;8(1):9–13.
52. Callus E, et al. Neuropsychological and psychological functioning aspects in myotonic dystrophy type 1 patients in Italy. *Front Neurol*. 2018;9:751.
53. Echenne B, Bassez G. Congenital and infantile myotonic dystrophy. *Handb Clin Neurol*. 2013;113:1387–1393.
54. Achiron A, et al. Abnormal liver test results in myotonic dystrophy. *J Clin Gastroenterol*. 1998;26(4):292–295.
55. Khoshbakht R, et al. Correlation between distribution of muscle weakness, electrophysiological findings and CTG expansion in myotonic dystrophy. *J Clin Neurosci*. 2014;21(7): 1123–1126.
56. Pongratz D, et al. [Diagnostic value of muscle biopsy findings in myotonic dystrophy (Curschmann-Steinert) (author's transl)]. *Klin Wochenschr*. 1979;57(5):215–224. German.
57. Johnson NE. Myotonic muscular dystrophies. *Continuum (Minneap, Minn)*. 2019;25(6):1682–1695.
58. Murphey MD, et al. Imaging of osteochondroma: variants and complications with radiologic-pathologic correlation. *Radiographics*. 2000;20(5):1407–1434.
59. Garcia RA, Inwards CY, Unni KK. Benign bone tumors—recent developments. *Semin Diagn Pathol*. 2011;28(1):73–85.
60. Pacifici M. The pathogenic roles of heparan sulfate deficiency in hereditary multiple exostoses. *Matrix Biol*. 2018;71–72:28–39.
61. Mavrogenis AF, Papagelopoulos PJ, Soucacos PN. Skeletal osteochondromas revisited. *Orthopedics*. 2008;31(10). orthosupersite.com/view.asp?rID=32071.
62. Bernard SA, et al. Improved differentiation of benign osteochondromas from secondary chondrosarcomas with standardized measurement of cartilage cap at CT and MR imaging. *Radiology*. 2012;255(3):857.
63. Heyworth PB, Rashid M. Regression of a solitary osteochondroma of the distal humerus in a toddler following trauma. *Radiol Case Rep*. 2019;14(2):187–189.
64. Aiba H, et al. Spontaneous shrinkage of solitary osteochondromas. *Skeletal Radiol*. 2018;47(1):61–68.
65. Graham P. Nonossifying fibroma of the distal femur. *Orthop Nurs*. 2020;39(6):418–419.
66. Bovée JV, Hogendoorn PC. Non-ossifying fibroma: a RAS-MAPK driven benign bone neoplasm. *J Pathol*. 2019;248(2):127–130.
67. Goldin AN, Muzykewicz DA, Mubarak SJ. Nonossifying fibromas: a computed tomography-based criteria to predict fracture risk. *J Pediatr Orthop*. 2020;40(2):e149.
68. Mascard E, Gomez-Brouchet A, Lambot K. Bone cysts: unicameral and aneurysmal bone cyst. *Orthop Traumatol Surg Res*. 2015;101(1 Suppl):S119–S127.
69. Wright JG, et al. A randomized clinical trial comparing intralesional bone marrow and steroid injections for simple bone cysts. *J Bone Joint Surg Am*. 2008;90:722–730.
70. Abrar WA, et al. Aneurysmal bone cysts of spine: an enigmatic entity. *Neurol India*. 2020;68(4):843–849.
71. Dorman JP, et al. Surgical treatment and recurrence rate of aneurismal bone cysts in children. *Clin Orthop*. 2004;421:205–211.
72. Paulin E, et al. An update for the treatment of osteoid osteoma. *Rev Med Suisse*. 2019;15(659):1462–1465. French.
73. Siegal GP, Bianco P, Dal Cin P. Fibrous dysplasia. In: Fletcher CD, ed. *WHO classification of tumours of soft tissue and bone*. ed 4 Lyons: International Agency for Research on Cancer; 2013. p. 352.
74. Hayden JB, Hoang BH. Osteosarcoma: basic science and clinical implications. *Orthop Clin North Am*. 2006;37:1–7.
75. Rathore R, Van Tine BA. Pathogenesis and current treatment of osteosarcoma: perspectives for future therapies. *J Clin Med*. 2021;10(6):1182.
76. Yang C, et al. Bone microenvironment and osteosarcoma metastasis. *Int J Mol Sci*. 2020;21(19):6985.
77. American Cancer Society (ACS) *Signs and symptoms of osteosarcoma*. Atlanta, GA: ACS; 2020. Last revised October 8, 2020. Available at https://www.cancer.org/cancer/osteosarcoma/detection-diagnosis-staging/signs-and-symptoms.html. (Accessed December 31, 2021).
78. Kager L, Tamamyan G, Bielack S. Novel insights and therapeutic interventions for pediatric osteosarcoma. *Future Oncol*. 2017;13(4):357–368.
79. Ludwig JA. Ewing sarcoma: historical perspectives, current state-of-the-art, and opportunities for targeted therapy in the future. *Curr Opin Oncol*. 2008;20(4):412–418.

80. Renzi S, et al. Ewing-like sarcoma: an emerging family of round cell sarcomas. *J Cell Physiol.* 2019;234(6):7999–8007.
81. Balamuth NJ, Womer RB. Ewing's sarcoma. *Lancet Oncol.* 2010;11(2):184–192.
82. Biermann JS, et al. NCCN guidelines insights: bone cancer, version 2.2017. *J Natl Compr Canc Netw.* 2017;15(2):155–167.
83. Burchill SA. Ewing's sarcoma: diagnostic, prognostic, and therapeutic implications of molecular abnormalities. *J Clin Pathol.* 2003;56(2):96–102.
84. Carvajal RL, Meyers P. Ewing's sarcoma and primitive neuroectodermal family of tumors. *Hematol Oncol Clin North Am.* 2005;19(3). 501–525, vi–vii.
85. Skapek SX, et al. Rhabdomyosarcoma. *Nat Rev Dis Primers.* 2019;5(1):1.
86. Lugo-Vicente H. Molecular biology and genetics affecting pediatric solid tumors. *Bol Asoc Med P R.* 2000;92(4–8):72–82.
87. Hicks J, Flaitz C. Rhabdomyosarcoma of the head and neck in children. *Oral Oncol.* 2002;38(5):450.
88. Centers for Disease Control and Prevention (CDC) National Center for Injury Prevention and Control, Division of Violence Prevention. *Violence prevention.* Atlanta, GA: CDC; 2021. Page last reviewed September 28, 2021. Available at https://www.cdc.gov/violenceprevention/. (Accessed December 31, 2021).
89. Lane WG, et al. Racial differences in the evaluation of pediatric fractures for physical abuse. *JAMA.* 2002;288(13): 1603–1609.
90. Swoboda SL, et al. Skeletal trauma in child abuse. *Pediatr Ann.* 2013;42(11):e245–e252.
91. Wood JN, et al. Evaluation for occult fractures in injured children. *Pediatrics.* 2015;136(2):232–240.
92. Rex C, Kay PR. Features of femoral fractures in nonaccidental injury. *J Pediatr Orthop.* 2000;20(3):411–413.
93. Expert Panel on Pediatric Imaging ACR Appropriateness Criteria® suspected physical abuse-child. *J Am Coll Radiol.* 2017;14(5S):S338–S349.
94. Adamsbaum C, et al. Classic metaphyseal lesions among victims of abuse. *J Pediatr.* 2019;209 154–159.e2.
95. Thomas SA, et al. Long-bone fractures in young children: distinguishing accident injuries from child abuse. *Pediatrics.* 1991;88(3):471–476.

46

Structure, Function, and Disorders of the Integument

Corinne M. Djuric and Karen C. Turner

http://evolve.elsevier.com/Rogers/pathophysiology/

CHAPTER OUTLINE

The skin is the largest organ of the body, accounting for about 20% of the body's weight. Combined with the accessory structures of hair, nails, and glands, it forms the integumentary system. The skin's primary function is environmental protection by serving as a barrier against microorganisms, ultraviolet (UV) radiation, loss of body fluids, and the stress of mechanical forces. The skin regulates body temperature within a very narrow range and is involved in immune surveillance and the activation of vitamin D. Touch and pressure receptors provide important protective functions and pleasurable sensations. The microbiome of the skin protects against pathologic bacteria.

STRUCTURE AND FUNCTION OF THE SKIN

Layers of the Skin

The skin is formed of three major layers: (1) a superficial, or outer, layer of epidermis; (2) a deeper layer of dermis (the true skin); and (3) the subcutaneous layer (hypodermis), the lowest lying layer of connective tissue that contains macrophages, fibroblasts, fat cells, nerves, fine muscles, blood vessels, lymphatics, and hair follicle roots (Fig. 46.1). Each skin layer contains cells that represent progressive stages of skin cell differentiation and function. These are summarized in Table 46.1.

Epidermis

The **epidermis** is a defensive barrier that continually renews itself. The thickness of the epidermis varies from 0.05 mm on the eyelids to 1.5 mm on the palms of the hands and soles of the feet, and averages about 0.12 mm. The epidermis is made up of several distinct layers (see Fig. 46.1B) that ensure continual renewal of the skin. The epidermis is formed primarily of keratinocytes embedded in a lipid matrix. These cells are named for the substances they produce. **Keratinocytes** produce **keratin**, a protein that provides protection from mechanical stress and is the main constituent of skin, hair, and nail cells. Keratinocytes are formed in the **basal layer** (**stratum basale**) move upward and differentiate, forming the **spinous layer** (**stratum spinosum**). In the **granular layer** (**stratum granulosum**) surface keratin formation begins. This layer is specifically important because it discharges Odland bodies (lamellar granules) that contribute to stratum corneum cell cohesion and form a barrier to water loss. In the **stratum corneum**, cells become flattened, stacked, and cornified as they ascend to the skin surface, where the cells are continuously shed. The **stratum lucidum** lies between the stratum corneum and the stratum granulosum but is only seen in the thicker skin on the palms of the hands and the soles of the feet. Cornification, or keratinization, prevents dehydration of deeper skin layers and loss of body water. The average turnover of the epidermis is about 30 days.

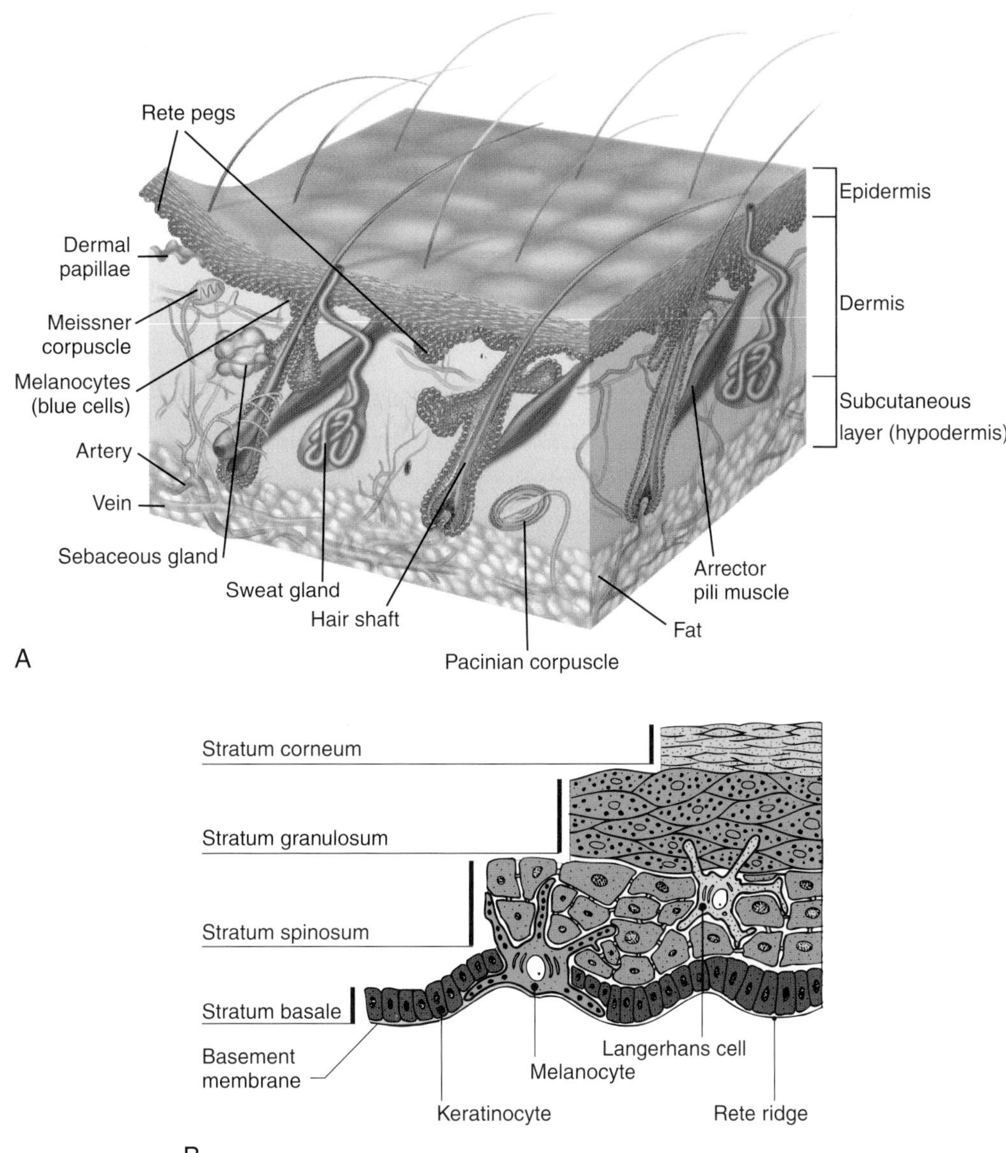

Fig. 46.1 Structure of the Skin. (A) Cross section showing major skin structures. **(B)** Layers of the epidermis. A, From Kumar V, et al. *Robbins & Cotran pathologic basis of disease*, 10th edition. Philadelphia: Saunders; 2021. B, From Gawkrodger D, Ardern-Jones M. *Dermatology*, 5th edition. Philadelphia: Churchill Livingstone; 2012.

The epidermis has three additional types of cells that facilitate its function: melanocytes, Langerhans cells, and Merkel cells. The melanocytes are usually located near the base of the epidermis (see Fig. 46.1B). They synthesize and secrete the pigment melanin with exposure to UV light in response to melanocyte-stimulating hormone (MSH). Melanin in the epidermis provides a shield against UV radiation and determines skin color. Vitiligo is thought to be an autoimmune-related loss of melanocytes resulting in the depigmentation of patches of skin (see "patch" in Table 46.3). Langerhans cells migrate to the epidermis from the bone marrow. Langerhans cells (a type of dendritic cell) and dermal dendritic cells initiate an immune response by presenting processed antigen to T cells, thus providing a defense against environmental antigens. Merkel cells are touch receptors and function as slowly adapting mechanoreceptors when stimulated by deformation of the epidermis. They are most numerous around hair follicles.

Dermis

The dermis is 1 to 4 mm thick and is composed of three types of connective tissue: (1) collagen, (2) elastin, and (3) reticulin. The haphazard arrangement of connective tissue allows the skin to be mobile and to stretch and contract with body movement. Hair follicles, sebaceous glands, sweat glands, blood vessels, lymphatic vessels, and nerves are contained in the dermis. The conelike projections of the papillary dermis interface with the epidermis. The papillae provide texture to the surface of the skin by forming *rete pegs*.

The cells of the dermis include fibroblasts, mast cells, and macrophages. Fibroblasts secrete the connective tissue matrix

TABLE 46.1 Layers of the Skin

Structure	Cell Types	Characteristics
Epidermis	Keratinocytes	Most important layer of skin; normally very thin (0.12 mm) but can thicken and form corns or calluses with constant pressure or friction; includes rete pegs that extend into papillary layer of dermis
	Langerhans (dendritic) cells	Antigen presenting cells and immune functions
Stratum corneum	Keratinocytes	Tough superficial layer covering the body
Stratum lucidum	Keratinocytes	Clear layers of cells containing eleidin, which becomes keratin as cells move up to corneum layer
Stratum granulosum	Keratinocytes	Keratohyalin gives granular appearance to this layer
	Melanocytes	
Stratum spinosum	New keratinocytes	Polygonal shaped with spinous processes projecting between adjacent keratinocytes
Stratum basale (germinativum)	Keratinocytes	Basal layer where keratinocytes divide and move upward to replace cells shed from surface
	Melanocytes	Melanocytes synthesize pigment melanin
	Merkel cells	Mechanoreceptors for light touch
Dermis	Macrophages	Irregular connective tissue layer with rich blood, lymphatic, and nerve supply; contains sensory receptors and sweat glands (apocrine, eccrine, sebaceous), macrophages (phagocytic and important for wound healing), and mast cells (release histamine and have immune functions) (see Chapter 7)
Papillary layer (thin)	Mast cells	
Reticular layer (thick)	Histiocytes	Wandering macrophages that collect pigments and inflammatory debris
Subcutaneous Layer (Hypodermis)		Subcutaneous tissue or superficial fascia of varying thickness that connects overlying dermis to underlying muscle; contains macrophages, fibroblasts, fat cells, nerves, blood vessels, lymphatics, and hair follicle roots

and collagen. Mast cells release histamine and play a role in hypersensitivity reactions in the skin. Macrophages are phagocytic and participate in immune responses.

Subcutaneous Layer

The third layer of the skin is subcutaneous tissue (hypodermis) and consists of adipose tissue. The lobules are separated by fibrous walls (septa) of collagen and large blood vessels. Dermal collagen is continuous with the collagen found in the subcutaneous tissue.

Dermal Appendages

The dermal appendages include the nails, hair, sebaceous glands, and the eccrine and apocrine sweat glands. The fingernails and toenails are protective keratinized plates. They are composed of (1) the proximal nail fold, (2) the eponychium (cuticle), (3) the matrix from which the nail grows and its nail root, (4) the hyponychium (nail bed), (5) the nail plate, and (6) the paronychium (lateral nail fold) (Fig. 46.2). Nail growth continues throughout life at 1 mm or less per day.

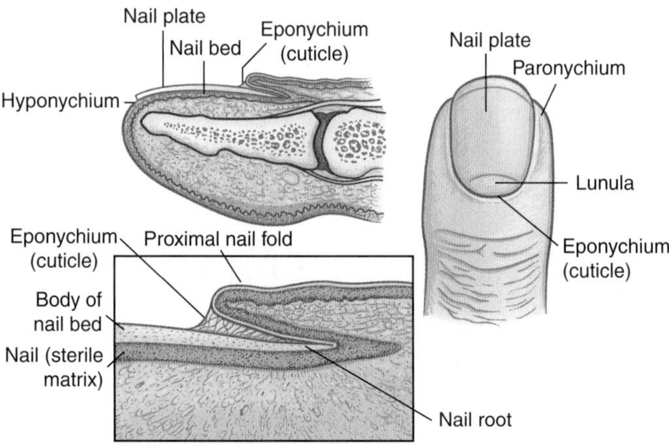

Fig. 46.2 Structures of the Nail. (Redrawn from Thompson JM, et al. *Mosby's clinical nursing*, 5th edition. St. Louis: Mosby; 2002.)

Hair color, density, grain, and pattern of distribution vary among people and depend on age, sex, and race. Hair follicles arise from the matrix (or bulb) located deep in the dermis. They extend from the dermis at an angle and have an erector pili muscle attached near the mid-dermis that straightens the follicle when contracted, causing the hair to stand up. Hair growth begins in the bulb, with cellular differentiation occurring as the hair progresses up the follicle. Hair is fully hardened, or cornified, by the time it emerges at the skin surface. Hair color is determined by melanin-secreting follicular melanocytes. Hair growth is cyclic, with periods of growth and rest that vary over different body surfaces. Changes in hair color and distribution also occur. Graying is caused by loss of melanocytes from hair bulbs. A byproduct of hair growth is the production of hydrogen peroxide, which is normally degraded by catalase. With aging, there is a decrease in catalase and accumulation of hydrogen peroxide and oxidative stress with damage to and loss of melanocytes.[1]

Hair follicles and sebaceous glands are integrated units (see Fig 46.1A). The sebaceous glands open onto the surface of the skin through a canal. They are found in greatest numbers on the face, chest, and back, with modified glands on the eyelids, lips, nipples, glans penis, and prepuce. Sebaceous glands secrete sebum, composed primarily of lipids, which oils the skin and hair and prevents drying. Androgens stimulate the growth of sebaceous glands, and their enlargement is an early sign of puberty.

The eccrine sweat glands are distributed over the body, with the greatest numbers in the palms of the hands, soles of the feet, and forehead. They are important in thermoregulation and cooling of the body through evaporation. The apocrine sweat glands are fewer in number but produce significantly more sweat than the eccrine glands. They are located near the bulb of hair follicles in the axillae, scalp, face, abdomen, and genital area. Their ducts open into the hair follicle. The interaction of sweat with commensal (normal) flora bacteria contributes to the odor of perspiration.

Blood Supply and Innervation

The blood supply to the skin is limited to the papillary capillaries, or plexus, of the dermis. These capillary loops are supplied by a deeper cutaneous arterial plexus. Branches from the deep plexus also supply hair follicles and sweat glands. A subpapillary network of veins drains the capillary loops. Arteriovenous anastomoses in the dermis facilitate the regulation of body temperature. Heat loss is regulated by (1) variations in skin blood flow through the opening and closing of arteriovenous anastomoses and (2) the evaporative heat loss of sweat. The sympathetic nervous system regulates both vasoconstriction and vasodilation of hair-bearing skin through α-adrenergic receptors in the skin. Non–hair-bearing skin (glabrous skin) of the palms, soles, and lips has the most arterio-venous anastomoses and is innervated solely by sympathetic vasoconstrictors with passive vasodilation.[2] The lymphatic vessels of the skin arise in the papillary dermis and drain into larger subcutaneous trunks, removing cells, proteins, and immunologic mediators.

Tests of Skin Function

Initial diagnostic evaluations of skin disorders are completed by gathering historical information, performing a physical examination, and observing the distribution and characteristics of the presenting lesions. Additional diagnostic studies are summarized in Table 46.2.

Clinical Manifestations of Skin Dysfunction

Lesions

Lesions of the skin are readily observable and easily assessed for distribution and structure. Identification of the morphologic structure of the skin, including differentiation between primary and secondary lesions, and assessment of the appearance of the skin in combination with obtaining a health history, are essential to identify underlying pathophysiology. Tables 46.3 and 46.4 describe and illustrate primary and secondary lesions of the skin. Special skin lesions are described in Table 46.5. Clinical manifestations of vascular skin lesions are described in Table 46.6.

Pressure injury. Pressure injury is defined by the National Pressure Injury Advisory Panel (NPIAP) as localized damage to the skin and underlying soft tissue usually over a bony prominence or a medical device. The injured skin and soft tissue can remain intact or present as an ulceration. The injury is a direct result of pressure, shear, or a combination of both.[3,4] Pressure that consistently interrupts normal blood flow to and from the skin or underlying tissues is the most common cause. Pressure injuries have substantial financial implications to healthcare organizations and are a major part of quality-of-care indicators. The risks for pressure injury are summarized in Box 46.1.

TABLE 46.2 Summary of Skin Diagnostic Procedures

Test	Purpose
Dermoscopy	Magnified illumination of the skin using a liquid medium and transparent plate to examine skin lesions
Reflectance confocal microscopy	High resolution assessment of cellular details and microstructures of the skin for evaluation of skin cancer
Skin biopsy	Histologic examination of tissue to determine differential diagnosis of cellular structure (i.e., benign growths vs. carcinoma, chronic infections, blistering diseases, and vasculitis)
Microscopic immunofluorescence	Identification of antibodies, immunoglobulins, and complement components for diseases such as pemphigus, vasculitis, and discoid lupus erythematosus using fluorescent light on slide-mounted biopsy specimens
Gram stain	Differentiation of gram-positive from gram-negative bacteria according to stain absorption
Culture	Identification of chronic bacterial and fungal infections by incubating skin specimens in culture media
Wood lamp examination	Examination of skin or hair to identify fungus that fluoresces bright yellow-green under ultraviolet light
Patch and scratch tests	Application of suspected allergens to skin by patch or scratch for evaluation of immune system responses to known allergens and evaluation of cell-mediated immune function (*Candida albicans*, skin fungus, chemicals, aeroallergens, and foods)
Skin scrapings	Application of potassium hydroxide and low heat to skin scrapings on a glass slide to identify dermatophytes and *C. albicans*
Side lighting	Indirect lighting of the skin using light to the side of the lesions to evaluate patterns of depression and elevation of skin lesions
Diascopy	Use of glass or clear plastic pressed on the skin to differentiate erythema caused by dilated capillaries (blanching) from extravasation of blood (no blanching)
Tzanck smear	A microscopic examination of cellular material from skin lesions to help diagnose vesicular diseases, including herpes simplex virus and varicella-zoster virus

TABLE 46.3 Primary Skin Lesions

Macule

A flat, circumscribed area that is a change in the color of the skin; less than 1 cm in diameter

Examples: Freckles, flat moles (nevi), petechiae, measles, scarlet fever

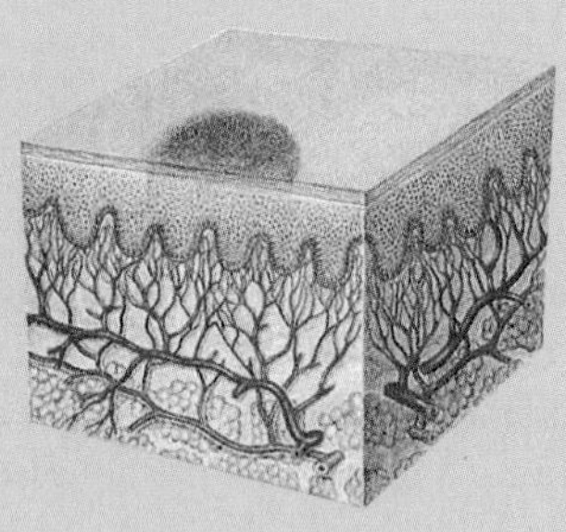

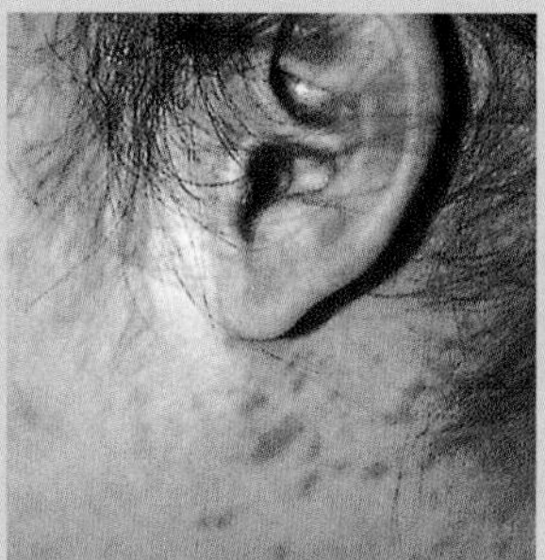

Macules[a]

Plaque

Elevated, firm, and rough lesion with flat top surface greater than 1 cm in diameter

Examples: Psoriasis, seborrheic and actinic keratoses

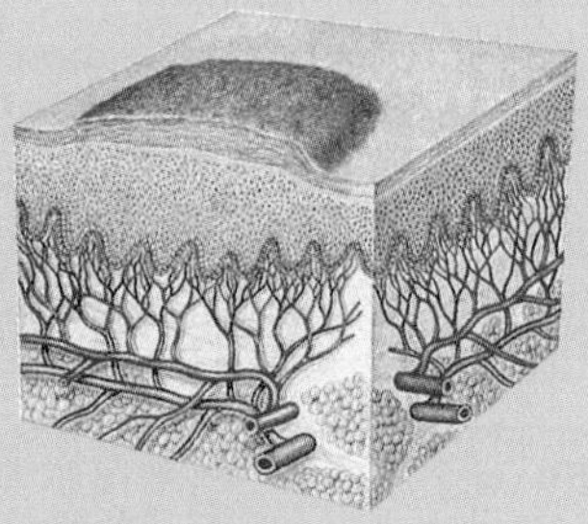

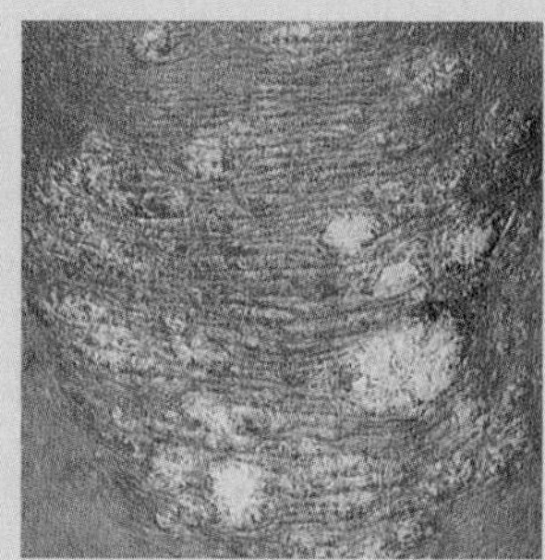

Plaque[d]

Papule

An elevated, firm, circumscribed area less than 1 cm in diameter

Examples: Wart (verruca), elevated moles, lichen planus, fibroma, insect bite

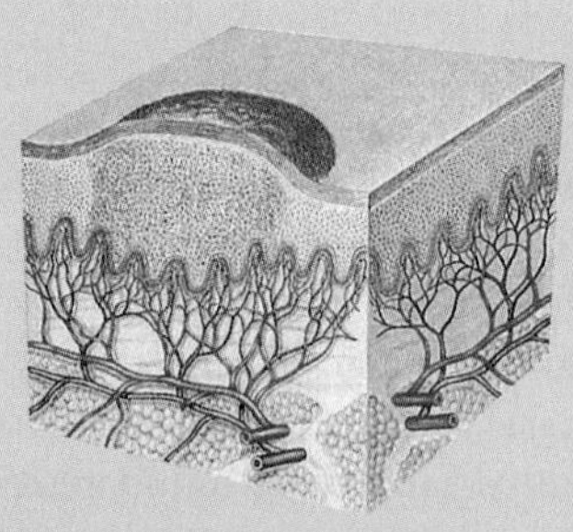

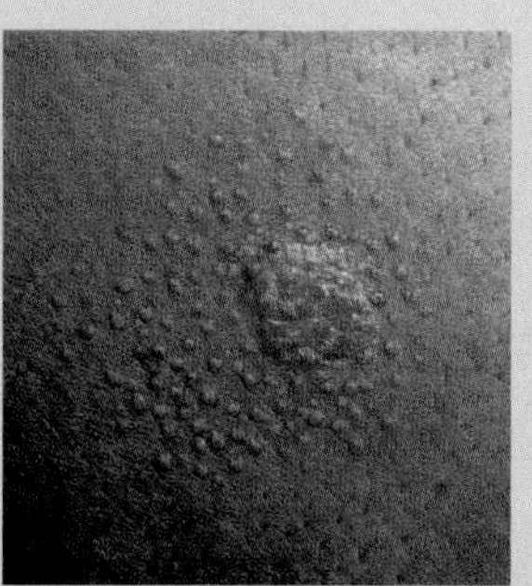

Lichen Planus[b]

Wheal

Elevated, irregularly shaped area of cutaneous edema; solid, transient; variable diameter

Examples: Insect bites, urticaria, allergic reaction

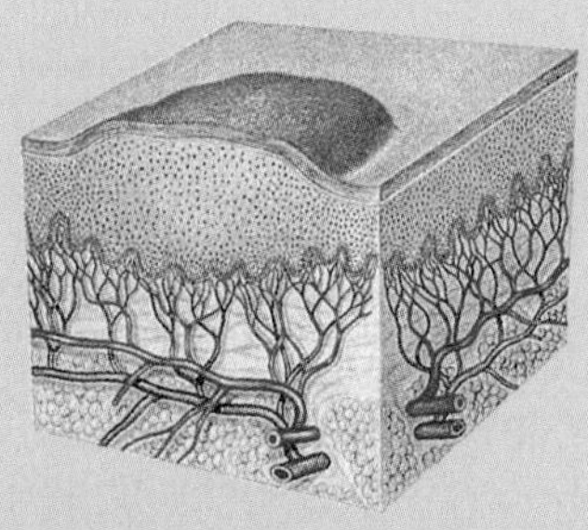

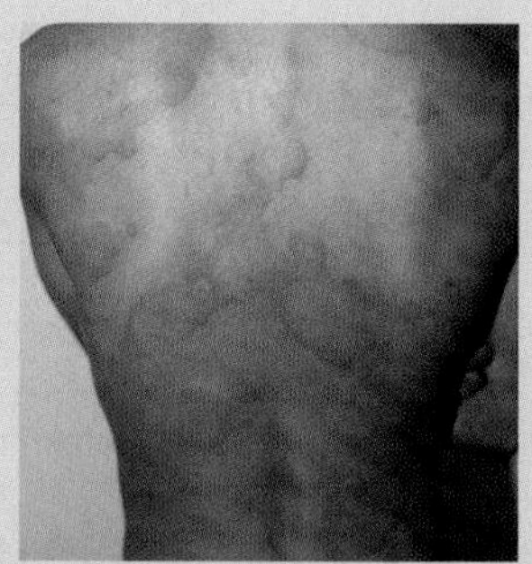

Wheal[e]

Patch

A flat, nonpalpable, irregular-shaped macule more than 1 cm in diameter

Examples: Vitiligo, port-wine stains, mongolian spots, café au lait spots

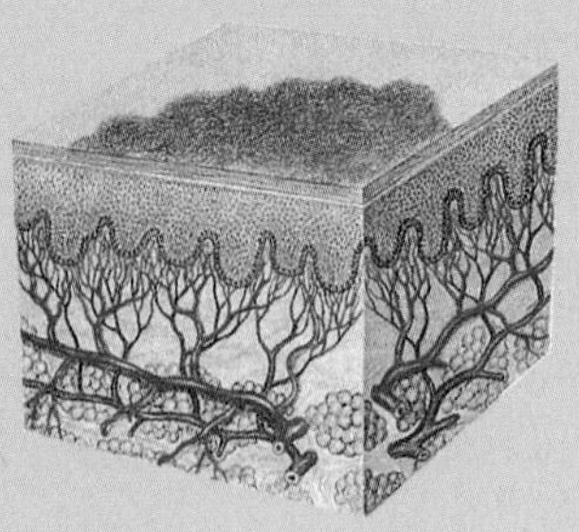

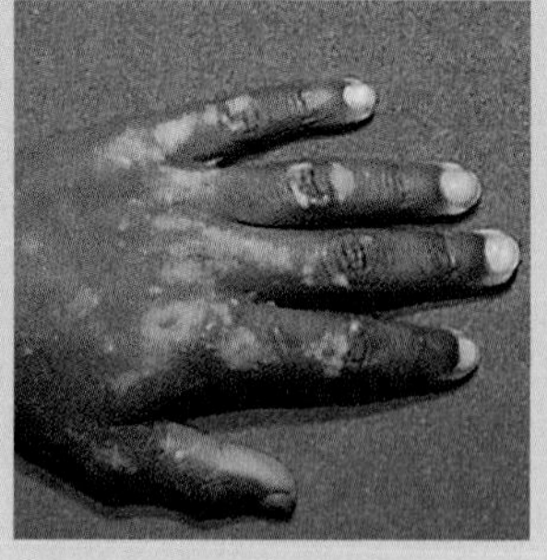

Vitiligo[c]

Nodule

Elevated, firm, circumscribed lesion; deeper in dermis than a papule; 1-2 cm in diameter

Examples: Erythema nodosum, lipomas

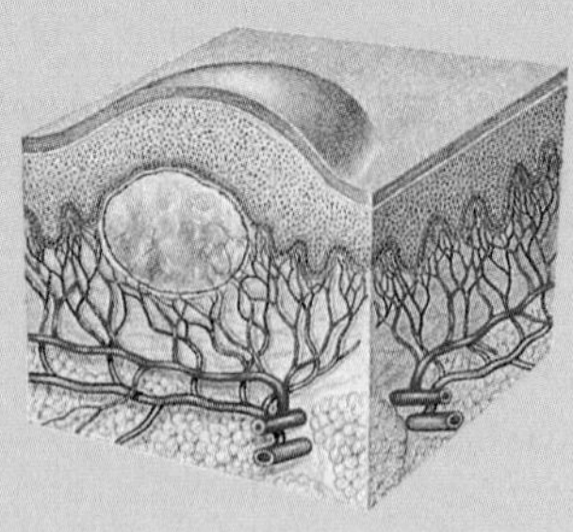

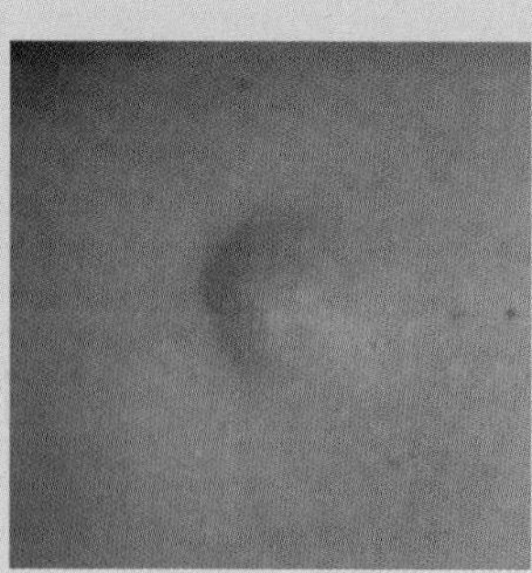

Lipoma[f]

TABLE 46.3 Primary Skin Lesions—cont'd

Tumor

Elevated, solid lesion; may be clearly demarcated; deeper in dermis; more than 2 cm in diameter

Examples: Neoplasms, benign tumor, lipoma, neurofibroma, hemangioma

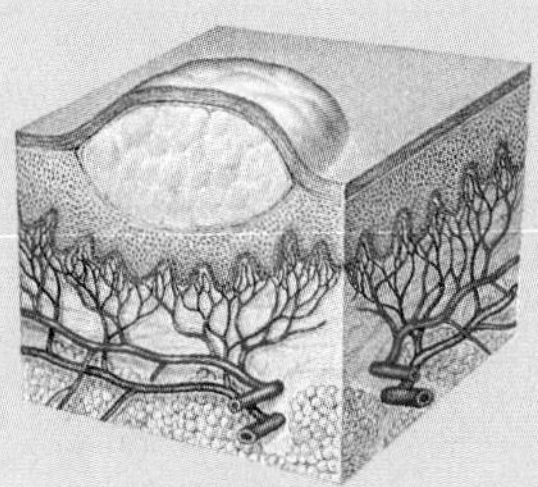
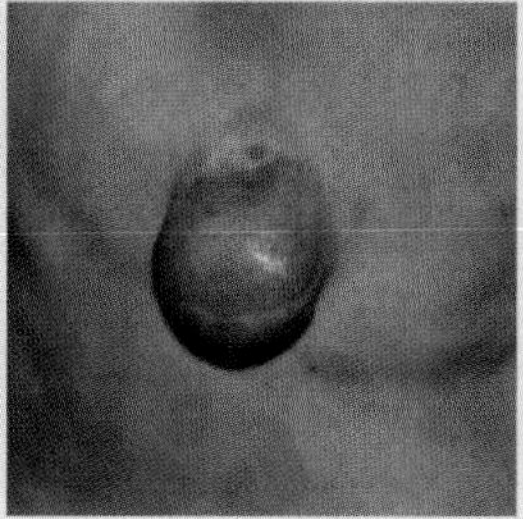

Neurofibroma[f]

Pustule

Elevated, superficial lesion; similar to a vesicle but filled with purulent fluid

Examples: Impetigo, acne

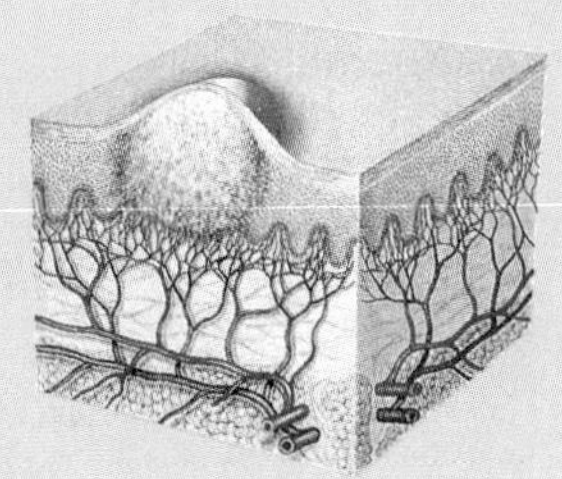
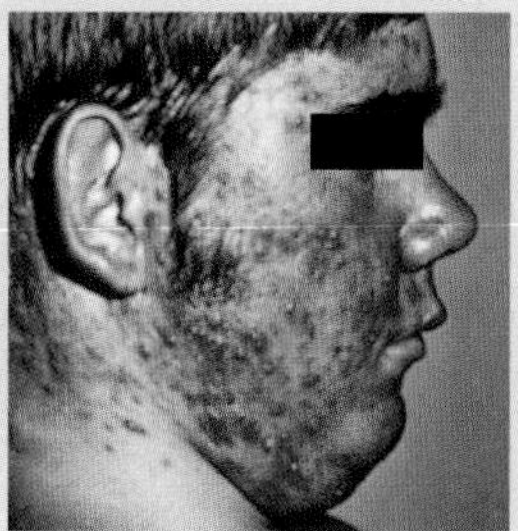

Acne[c]

Vesicle

Elevated, circumscribed, superficial; does not extend into dermis; filled with serous fluid; less than 1 cm in diameter

Examples: Varicella (chickenpox), herpes zoster (shingles), herpes simplex

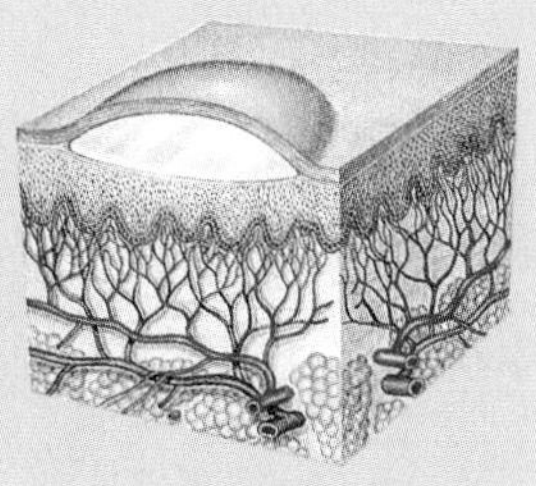
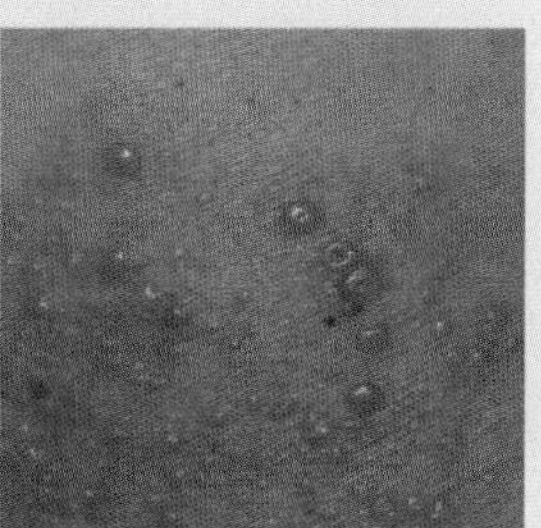

Vesicles[g]

Cyst

Elevated, circumscribed, encapsulated lesion; in dermis or subcutaneous layer; filled with liquid or semisolid material

Examples: Sebaceous cyst, cystic acne

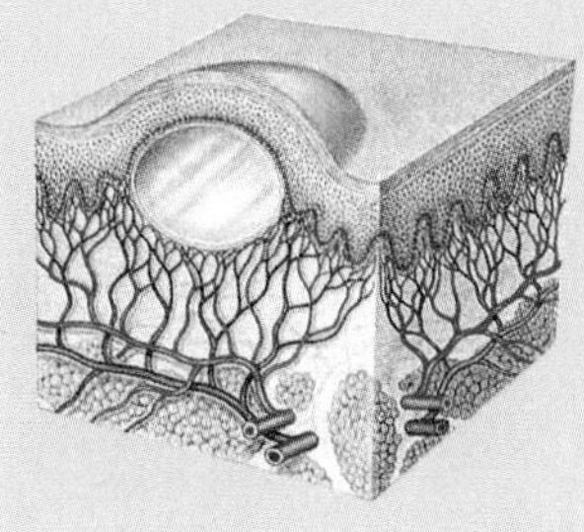
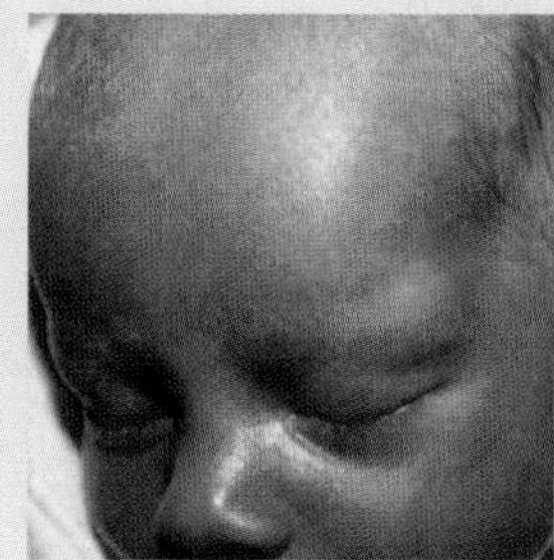

Sebaceous Cyst[c]

Vesicle more than 1 cm in diameter

Examples: Blister, pemphigus vulgaris

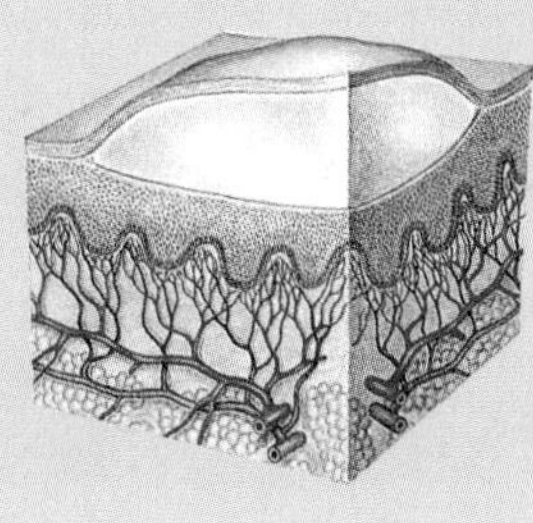
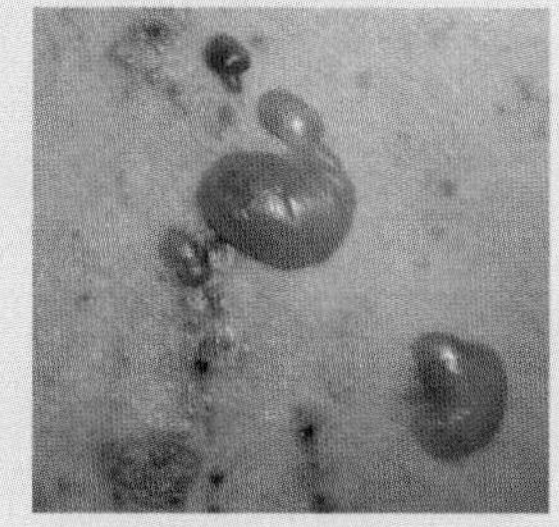

Bulla[h]

Telangiectasia

Fine (0.5-1 mm), irregular red lines produced by capillary dilation; can be associated with acne rosacea (face), venous hypertension (spider veins in legs), systemic sclerosis, or developmental abnormalities (port wine birthmarks)

Example: Telangiectasia in rosacea

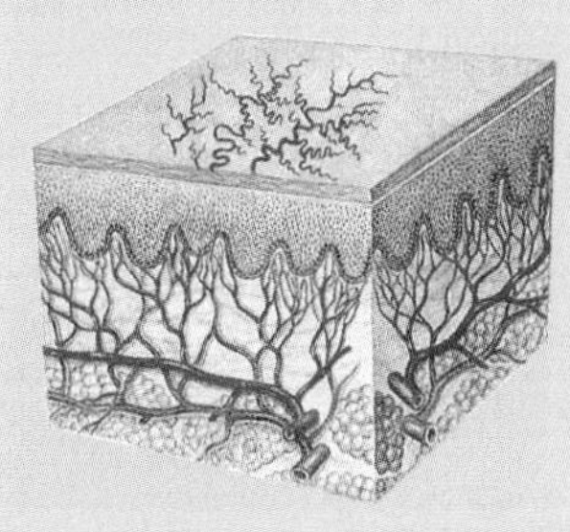
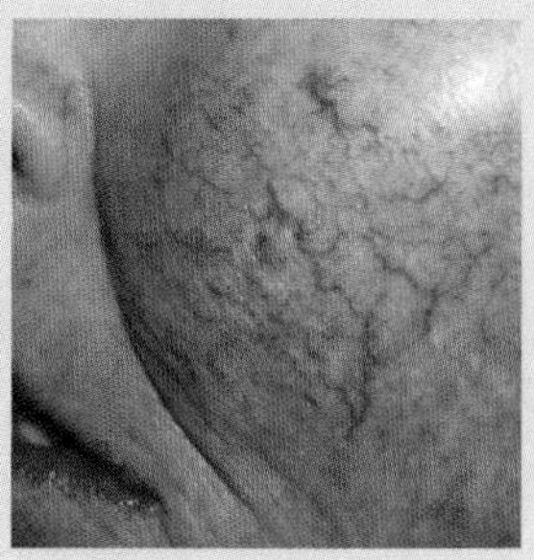

Telangiectasia[e]

[a]Farrar WE, et al. *Infectious diseases*, 2nd edition. London: Gower; 1992.
[b]James WD, et al. *Andrews' diseases of the skin*, 11th edition. Philadelphia: Saunders; 2011.
[c]Weston WL, Lane AT. *Color textbook of pediatric dermatology*, 3rd edition. Philadelphia: Mosby; 2002.
[d]Habif TP. *Clinical dermatology: A color guide to diagnosis and therapy*, 5th edition. Philadelphia: Mosby; 2010.
[e]Bolognia JL, et al. *Dermatology*, 3rd edition. Philadelphia: Saunders; 2012.
[f]Weston WL, et al. *Color textbook of pediatric dermatology*, 4th edition. Philadelphia: Mosby; 2007.
[g]Black MM, et al. *Obstetric and gynecologic dermatology*, 3rd edition. Philadelphia: Mosby; 2008.
[h]Marks JG, Miller JJ. *Lookingbill & Marks' principles of dermatology*, 4th edition. London: Saunders; 2006.

TABLE 46.4 Secondary Skin Lesions

Scale

Heaped-up, keratinized cells; flaky skin; irregular shape; thick or thin; dry or oily; variation in size

Examples: Flaking of skin with seborrheic dermatitis after scarlet fever, or flaking of skin after a drug reaction; dry skin

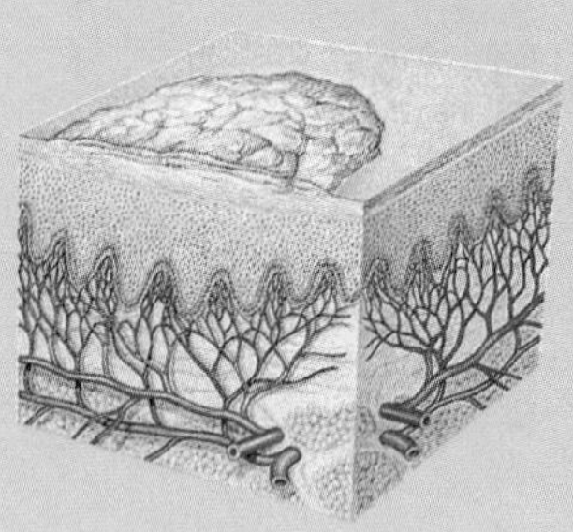

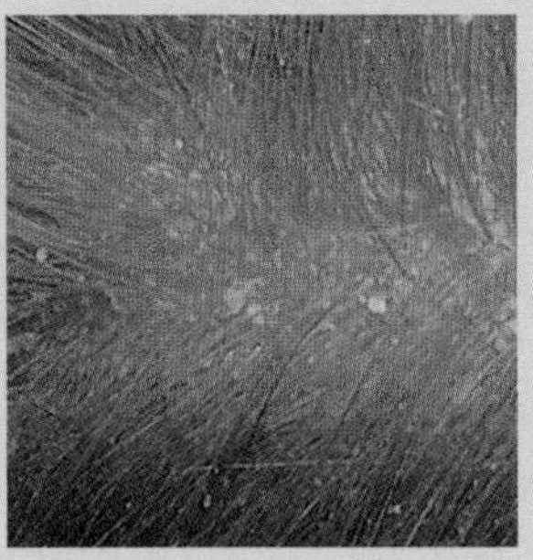

Fine Scaling[a]

Scar

Thin to thick fibrous tissue that replaces normal skin after injury or laceration to the dermis

Examples: Healed wound or surgical incision

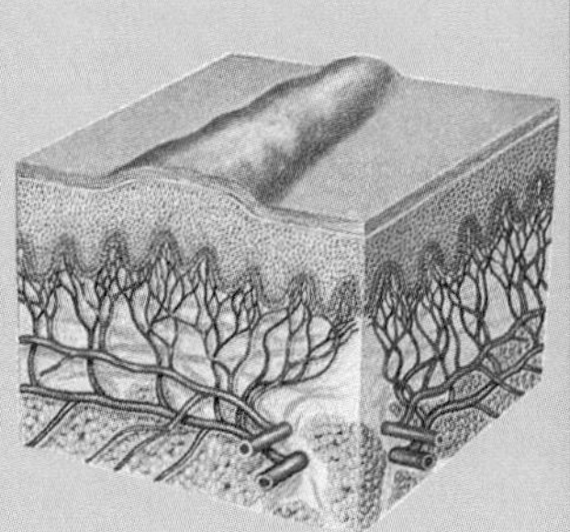

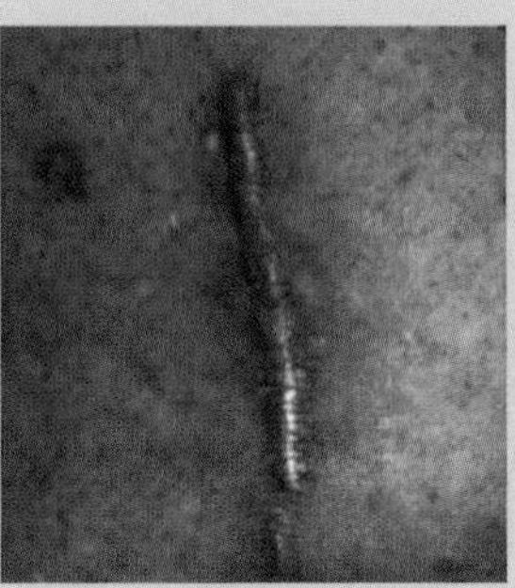

Hypertrophic Scar[d]

Lichenification

Rough, thickened epidermis secondary to persistent rubbing, itching, or skin irritation; often involves flexor surface of extremity

Example: Chronic dermatitis

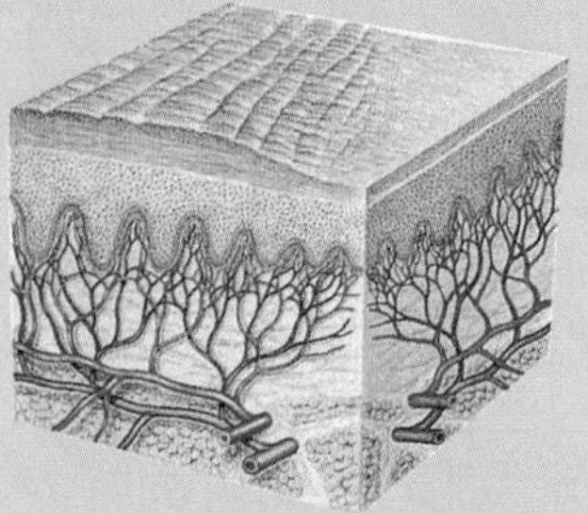

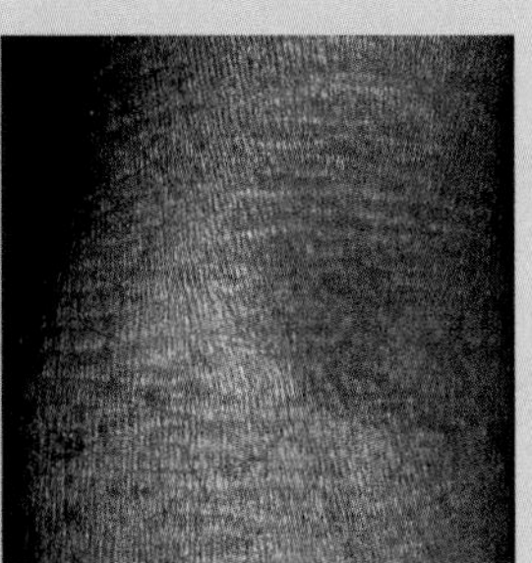

Atopic Dermatitis of Arm[b]

Excoriation

Loss of epidermis; linear, hollowed-out, crusted area

Examples: Abrasion or scratch, scabies

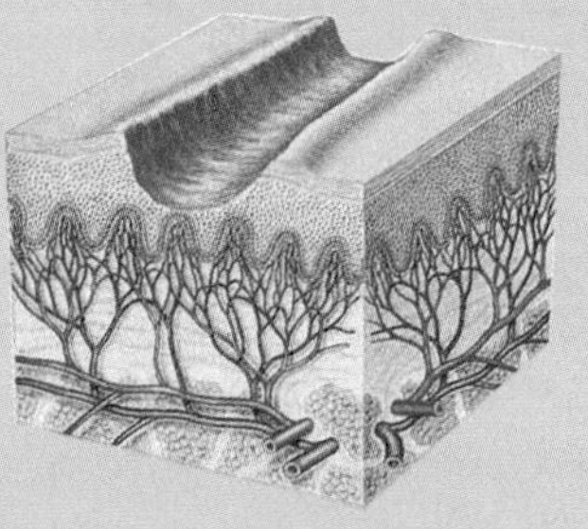

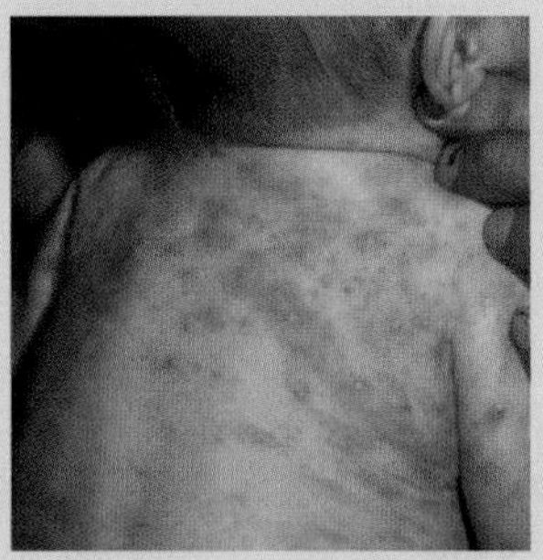

Scabies[c]

Keloid

Irregularly shaped, elevated, progressively enlarging scar; grows beyond boundaries of wound; caused by excessive collagen formation during healing

Examples: Keloid formation after surgery

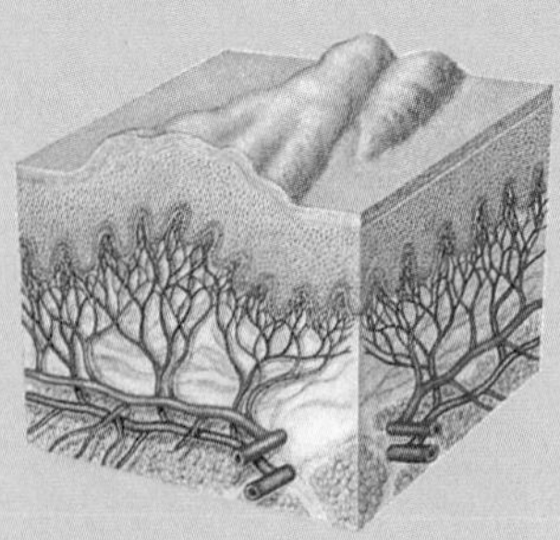

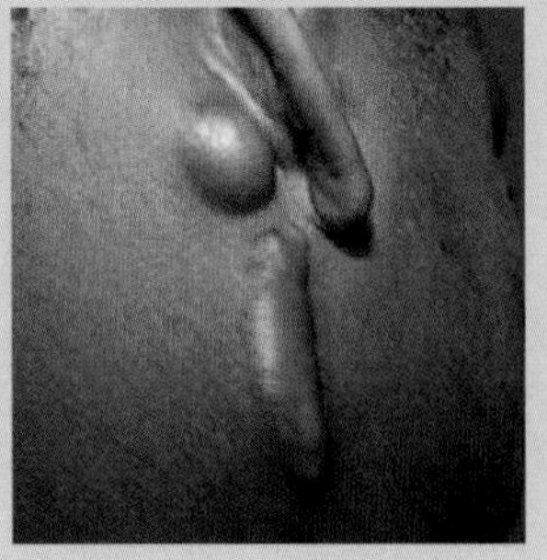

Keloid[c]

Fissure

Linear crack or break from the epidermis to the dermis; may be moist or dry

Examples: Athlete's foot, cracks at the corner of mouth, anal fissure, dermatitis

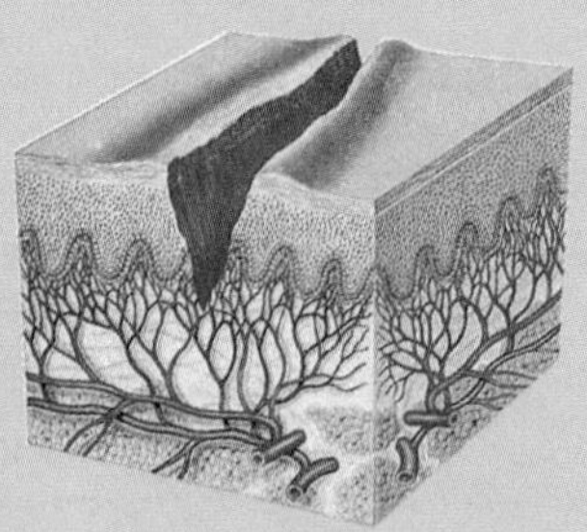

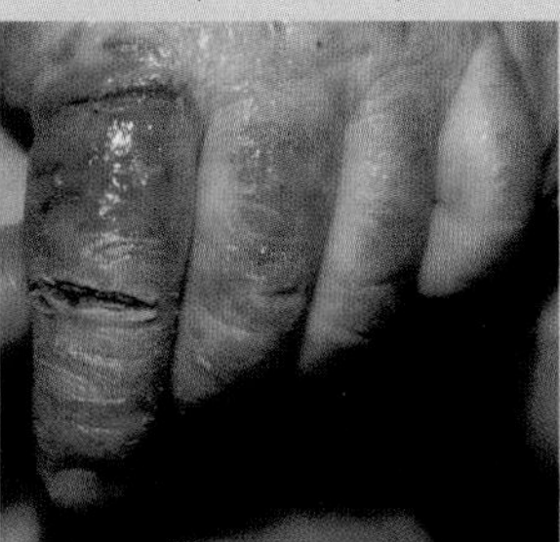

Fissures From Infected Dermatitis[c]

TABLE 46.4 **Secondary Skin Lesions—cont'd**

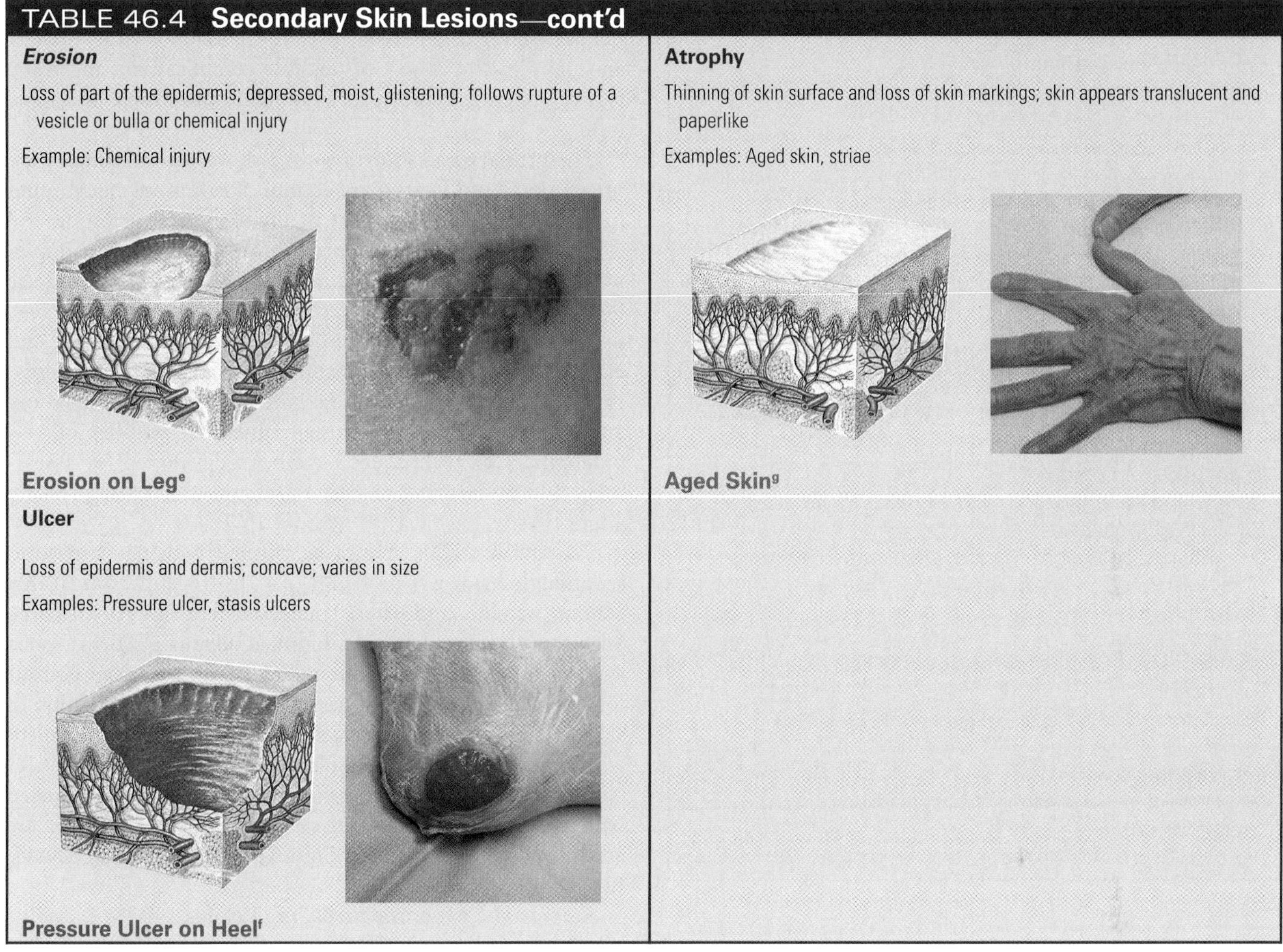

Erosion Loss of part of the epidermis; depressed, moist, glistening; follows rupture of a vesicle or bulla or chemical injury Example: Chemical injury **Erosion on Leg**[e]	**Atrophy** Thinning of skin surface and loss of skin markings; skin appears translucent and paperlike Examples: Aged skin, striae **Aged Skin**[g]
Ulcer Loss of epidermis and dermis; concave; varies in size Examples: Pressure ulcer, stasis ulcers **Pressure Ulcer on Heel**[f]	

[a]Baran R, et al. *Color atlas of the hair, scalp, and nails.* St. Louis: Mosby; 1991.
[b]Ud-Din S, Bayat A. New insights on keloids, hypertrophic scars, and striae. *Dermatologic Clinics*, 2014;32(2):193–209.
[c]Weston WL, et al. *Color textbook of pediatric dermatology*, 4th edition. St. Louis: Mosby; 2007.
[d]Nouri K, Leal-Khouri S. *Techniques in dermatologic surgery*. Philadelphia: Mosby; 2003.
[e]Bolognia JL, et al. *Dermatology*, 3rd edition. Philadelphia: Saunders; 2012.
[f]Robinson JK, et al. *Surgery of the skin*, 3rd edition. Philadelphia: Saunders; 2015.
[g]Seidel HM, et al. *Seidel's guide to physical examination*, 8th edition. St. Louis: Mosby; 2015.

TABLE 46.5 **Special Skin Lesions**

Type	Clinical Manifestations
Comedone	A plug of sebaceous and keratin material lodged in the opening of a hair follicle; an open comedone has a dilated orifice (blackhead), and a closed comedone has a narrow opening (whitehead)
Burrow	A narrow, raised, irregular channel caused by a parasite

TABLE 46.6 **Vascular Skin Lesions**

Type	Clinical Manifestation
Hemangioma	Bright red, superficial collection of blood vessels
Petechiae	Circumscribed area of blood less than 0.5 cm in diameter
Purpura	Circumscribed area of blood greater than 0.5 cm in diameter
Telangiectasia	Dilated, superficial blood vessels

Pressure injuries usually develop over bony prominences, such as the sacrum, heels, ischia, and greater trochanters. Continuous pressure on tissue between the bony prominence and a resistant outside surface distorts capillaries and occludes the blood flow and oxygen supply. Pressure injury also can occur in soft tissues from medical devices—for example, from nasal cannulas or endotracheal tubes. If the pressure is relieved within a few hours, a brief period of reactive hyperemia (redness related to vasodilation) occurs and there may be no lasting tissue damage. If the pressure continues unrelieved, the endothelial cells lining the capillaries become disrupted with platelet aggregation, forming microthrombi that block blood flow and cause anoxic

BOX 46.1 Pressure Injury Risk Factors

Prolonged Pressure/Immobilization

Lying in bed or sitting in chair or wheelchair without changing position or relieving pressure over an extended period

- Lying for hours on hard x-ray and operating tables
- Neurologic disorders (coma, spinal cord injuries, peripheral neuropathy, cognitive impairment, or cerebrovascular disease)
- Fractures or contractures
- Debilitation: elderly persons in hospitals and nursing homes
- Pain
- Sedation

Shearing forces

- Turning by dragging on coarse bed sheets

Disease/Tissue Factors

Thin or fragile skin
Impaired perfusion; ischemia
Fecal or urinary incontinence; prolonged exposure to moisture
Malnutrition, dehydration
Chronic diseases accompanied by anemia, edema, renal failure, malnutrition, peripheral vascular disease, or sepsis
Previous history of pressure ulcers

Additional Risk Factors for the Critically Ill

Norepinephrine infusion
Acute Physiology and Chronic Health Evaluation (APACHE II) score
Anemia
Age greater than 40 years
Multiple organ system disease or comorbid complications
Length of hospital stay
Use of ventilators or extracorporeal membranous oxygenation support

Data from Cowan L, Broderick V, Alderden JG. Pressure injury prevention considerations for older adults. *Critical Care Nursing Clinics of North America*, 2020;32(4):601–609; Alderden JG, Shibily F, Cowan L. Best practice in pressure injury prevention among critical care patients. *Critical Care Nursing Clinics of North America*, 2020;32(4):489–500.

necrosis of surrounding tissues. Shearing and friction are mechanical forces moving parallel to the skin (dragging) and can extend to the bony skeleton, causing detachment and injury of tissues. Individuals with darkly pigmented skin are at greater risk for developing pressure injuries because early signs of skin damage may not be clearly visible.[5] Pressure injuries are staged or graded, and there are several scales available. One classification scheme is available from the National Pressure Advisory Panel at https://npuap.org/page/PressureInjuryStages. The stages are illustrated in Fig. 46.3 and summarized in Box 46.2.

Superficial damage results in a layer of dead tissue that forms as an abrasion, blister, erosion, or non-blanchable red/darkened skin or as a reddish blue discoloration when there is deeper tissue damage. Superficial lesions are more common on the sacrum as a result of shearing or friction forces (forces parallel to the skin). Deep lesions develop closer to the bone because of tissue distortion and vascular occlusion from pressure perpendicular to the tissue (over the heels, trochanter, and ischia). Bacteria colonize the dead tissue, and infection is usually localized and self-limiting. Proteolytic enzymes from bacteria and macrophages dissolve necrotic tissues and cause a foul-smelling discharge that resembles, but is not, pus. The necrotic tissue initiates an inflammatory response with potential pain, fever, and leukocytosis. If the lesion is large, toxicity and pain lead to a host of possible complications, including loss of appetite, debility, local/systemic infections, and renal injury.

The primary goals for those at risk for pressure injury are prevention and early detection. Preventive techniques include frequent assessment of the skin, repositioning and turning of the individual, promotion of movement, implementation of pressure reduction (type of positioning and use of specialty beds), pressure removal (positioning interval), use of pressure distribution devices (positioning aids), and elimination of excessive moisture and drainage (use of moisture wicking products). Adequate nutrition, oxygenation, and fluid balance must be maintained.[6] A number of new bioengineering techniques have been developed for assessment and monitoring of tissue pressure and tissue pressure alterations.[7]

Superficial lesions should be covered with flat, moisture-retaining but not wet dressings (e.g., hydrogel dressings) that cannot wrinkle and cause increased pressure or friction. Successful healing requires continued adequate relief of pressure, debridement of necrotic tissue, opening of deep pockets for drainage, and repair of damaged tissue by construction of skin flaps for large, deep ulcers. Infection requires treatment with antibiotics, and pain should be controlled.[8] Many advances have been made in the treatment of deep wounds associated with pressure injury.[9] Skin tissue engineering techniques are advancing the treatment of skin deficits (see Emerging Science Box: Skin Engineering).

Keloids and hypertrophic scars. Keloids and hypertrophic scars both result from abnormal wound healing related to excessive inflammation and tissue remodeling. A genetic susceptibility is likely. **Keloids** are rounded, firm elevated scars with irregular claw-like margins that extend beyond the original site of injury (see Table 46.4C and Fig. 46.4). They are most common in darkly pigmented skin types and generally appear weeks to months after a stable scar has formed. Keloids have excessive and disorganized deposition of fibroblast-derived extracellular matrix proteins, particularly types I and III collagen with persistent inflammation and fibrosis. Macrophages have a role in release of proinflammatory cytokines and growth factors that promote keloid formation.[10] The fibroblasts have high metabolic and mitotic rates. Keloids first appear as pink or red, firm, well-defined rubbery plaques that persist for several months after trauma. Later, uncontrolled overgrowth causes extension beyond the site of the original wound, and the tumor becomes smoother, irregularly shaped, hyperpigmented, and harder. Keloids can cause pain and pruritus. Numerous options are available for prevention and treatment.[11]

Hypertrophic scars are elevated erythematous fibrous lesions that do not extend beyond the border of injury and primarily contain type III collagen (see Table 46.4D and Fig. 46.4). Hypertrophic scars appear within 3 to 4 months after injury and usually regress within 1 year. Excessive or poorly aligned tension on a wound, introduction of foreign material into the skin, infection, and certain types of trauma (e.g., burns) are all provocative factors. Those

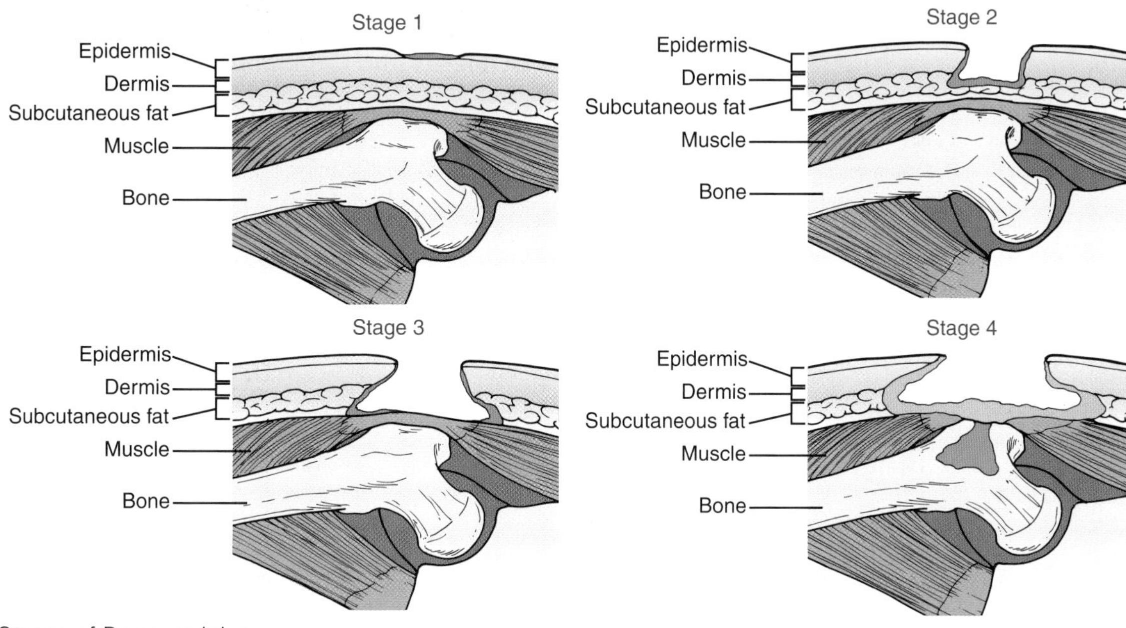

Fig. 46.3 Stages of Pressure Injury.

parts of the body at risk include shoulders, back, chin, ears, and lower legs. Like keloids, hypertrophic scars are caused by abnormal wound healing with inflammation, increased macrophage activity, excessive fibroblast activity and collagen formation, and loss of control of normal tissue repair and regeneration.[12]

Pruritus

Pruritus, or itching, is a symptom associated with local events in the skin such as dry skin (xerosis), eczema, psoriasis, or insect infestations, or it can be a manifestation of systemic disease (e.g., chronic renal failure, cholestatic liver disease, thyroid disorders, iron deficiency, neuropathies, or malignancy) or the use of medications such as opiate drugs. It may be acute (mosquito bite) or chronic (neuropathic itch), localized or generalized, and migratory (moves from one location to another). Multiple stimuli can produce itching, and there is interaction between itch and pain sensations. There are many itch mediators, including histamine, serotonin, prostaglandins, bradykinins, neuropeptides, acetylcholine opioids; and itch modulators, including interleukin-2 and -31 (IL-2 and IL-31), substance P, proteinases, and nerve growth factor.[13] Small unmyelinated type C nerve fibers and thinly myelinated Aδ fibers in the epidermis transmit itch sensations, and specific spinal pathways carry itch sensations to the brain.

Central nervous system mechanisms also can modulate itching, which is less perceptible when the mind is distracted by other stimuli. How the central nervous system influences the itch sensation is unclear, but it may be related to dampened central inhibition of itch pathway neurons. *Neuropathic itch* (itch without pruritogenic stimuli) is related to pathology along an afferent pathway. *Psychogenic itch* is associated with psychologic disorders (e.g., depression and obsessive compulsive disorder). Chronic itching is an unpleasant sensation that may or may not be relieved by scratching—often done so intensely that trauma to the skin occurs, resulting in infection, skin thickening (lichenification), and scarring. Both central and peripheral sensitization occurs.[14] Management of pruritus is challenging and depends on the cause; the primary condition must be treated. Both topical and systemic therapies are used.

BOX 46.2 Pressure Injury Stages

Stage 1: Non-blanchable erythema of intact skin usually over a bony prominence; darkly pigmented skin may appear differently; color changes do not include purple or maroon discoloration.

Stage 2: Partial-thickness skin loss with exposed dermis (erosion or intact or ruptured blistering) involving epidermis or dermis presenting as a shallow open ulcer with a red-pink, viable wound bed, without slough. Deeper tissues are not visible.

Stage 3: Full-thickness skin loss involving damage or necrosis of subcutaneous tissue that may extend to, but not through, underlying fascia. Adipose tissue visible in the ulcer, granulation tissue and rolled wound edges (epibole) are often present.

Stage 4: Full-thickness skin and tissue loss with exposure of muscle, bone, or supporting structures (tendons or joint capsules); can include undermining and tunneling.

Unstageable Pressure Injury: Obscured full-thickness skin and tissue loss; the extent of the damage cannot be determined due to being obscured by devitalized tissue

Deep Tissue Pressure Injury (DTPI): persistent, non-blanchable deep red, maroon, or purple discoloration; skin is intact; pain and/or temperature changes can precede the color changes; may be difficult to discern in darkly pigmented skin

Medical Device Related Pressure Injury: a direct result from the use of a medical device such as an indwelling urinary catheter; the injury mimics the pattern or shape of the device; the injury should be stages via the aforementioned staging system, but with correctly identified etiology

Mucosal Membrane Pressure Injury: injury to mucous membranes from a medical device in the anatomical location of the injury; these injuries cannot be staged

Data from: Pressure ulcers get new terminology and staging definitions. *Nursing*, 2017;47(3):68–69. Stages available at: https://cdn.ymaws.com/npiap.com/resource/resmgr/online_store/npiap_pressure_injury_stages.pdf.

EMERGING SCIENCE BOX

Skin Engineering

Replacing skin deficits can be traced back in literature as far back as the 16th century. Partial or split-thickness as well as full-thickness skin graft techniques continue to be commonplace in healthcare today. Synthetic products (skin substitutes) include biologic, synthetic, or biosynthetic options and work as skin equivalents specifically in the management of acute and chronic wound care. Although extremely useful and successful, synthetic products have yet to produce skin appendage substitutes such the microvascular networks, sweat glands, and hair follicles, which are critical for regulating body temperature and mediating the sensation of touch and pain.

Over the past decade, stem cell research has afforded scientists the ability to grow human skin, complete with hair follicles and sebaceous glands in a mouse model. The skin grows in tiny and odd shaped clusters called organoids from human pluripotent stem cells. Organoids are in vitro biological complexes with 3D structures that contain one or more cell types and partially recapitulate the structure and function of their in vitro counterparts. In approximately 4–5 months of incubation, an organoid of stratified epidermis, dermis, pigmented hair follicles complete with sebaceous glands, sensory neurons, and Schwann cells emerge. The resulting organoid has been equated to the facial skin of human fetuses in the second trimester of development. Progress has also been made in the use of 3-D bioprinting for the development of pre-vascularized skin substitutes that permit rapid perfusion and enhance the deposition of collagen and increased dermal thickness. The use of nanoparticles has allowed the integration of angiogenic and growth factors and antibiotics to support the microenvironment. This research may prove to be the future of disease modeling and use of skin substitutes for treatment of burns, ulcers and reconstructive surgery.

Data from He J, et al. Organoid technology for tissue engineering. *Journal of Molecular Cell Biology*, 2020;12(8):569–579; Lee J, et al. Hair-bearing human skin generated entirely from pluripotent stem cells. *Nature*, 2020;582(7812):399–404; Phua QH, et al. Translational stem cell therapy: Vascularized skin grafts in skin repair and regeneration. *Journal of Translational Medicine*, 2021;19(1):83; Sharma P, et al. Stem cells and growth factors-based delivery approaches for chronic wound repair and regeneration: A promise to heal from within. *Life Sciences*, 2021;268:118932.

EMERGING SCIENCE BOX

COVID-19 and Cutaneous Manifestations

The novel coronavirus of 2019 (COVID-19) causes severe acute respiratory system disease in humans. Cutaneous manifestations in individuals with COVID-19 have been identified with variance across age groups, different populations, and morphology of presentation. The incidence and timing of presentation is difficult to discern. The American Academy of Dermatology and the International League of Dermatology Societies collaborated to form The American Academy of Dermatology's COVID-19 Registry. This registry was created for healthcare providers to report cases so that data can be complied, examined, and used to further understand COVID-19 related dermatoses.

In individuals with confirmed COVID-19 positive tests, the most common dermatoses in the literature include macular or maculopapular lesions (morbilliform), pernio (chillblain)-like rash, urticarial, vesicular lesions, and retiform purpura (vascular lesions). Pernio is a disorder separate from COVID-19 that presents with red to violet or blue macules, papules or nodules that typically present on the digits (known as Covid toes or fingers) and is more common in younger individuals and milder disease. It is related to vasospasm and a probable type 1 interferon reaction to viral infection. Macular or maculopapular (morbilliform) lesions, the most common type, are red with flat or raised borders. These occur early and are more commonly found on the trunk and with more severe disease. Urticaria is common and may be related to activation of mast cells with viral infection. Vesicular lesions may be associated with herpes virus co-infection. Retiform purpura is a vaso-occlusive response associated with severe disease and the elderly. An erythema-multiforme-like pattern and Stevens-Johnson syndrome were most frequently linked to hydroxychloroquine treatment. There have been reports of infants born to COVID-19 positive mothers with diffuse maculopapular rash.

Data from Conforti C, et al. Cutaneous manifestations in confirmed COVID-19 patients: A systematic review. *Biology (Basel)*, 2020;9(12):449; Freeman EE, et al. The spectrum of COVID-19-associated dermatologic manifestations: an international registry of 716 patients from 31 countries. *Journal of the American Academy of Dermatology*, S0190-9622(20)32126-5, 2020. Advance online publication. https://doi-org.pnw.idm.oclc.org/10.1016/j.jaad.2020.06.1016; Tan SW, et al. Skin manifestations of COVID-19: A worldwide review. *JAAD International*, 2021;2:119–133; Sharma S, et al. Cutaneous manifestations and dermatological sequelae of Covid-19 infection compared to those from other viruses. *Australasian Journal of Dermatology*, 2021;62(2):141–150. doi:10.1111/ajd.13561. Epub ahead of print. PMID: 33595840.

DISORDERS OF THE SKIN

Disruptions of the skin integrity may be precipitated by trauma, abnormal cellular function, infection, immune responses, inflammation, and systemic diseases. Many skin disorders are benign and self-limiting, whereas others are severe and life-threatening. Many rashes and skin lesions have been described in association with COVID-19 viral infections (see Emerging Science Box: COVID-19 and Cutaneous Manifestations).

Inflammatory Disorders

The most common inflammatory disorders of the skin are eczema and dermatitis. **Eczema** and **dermatitis** are general terms that describe a particular type of inflammatory response in the skin and are often used interchangeably. Eczematous disorders are generally characterized by pruritus, lesions with indistinct borders, and epidermal changes. These lesions can appear as erythemic papules or scales; they can present in an acute, subacute, or chronic phase. Edema, serous discharge, and crusting occur with continued irritation and scratching.

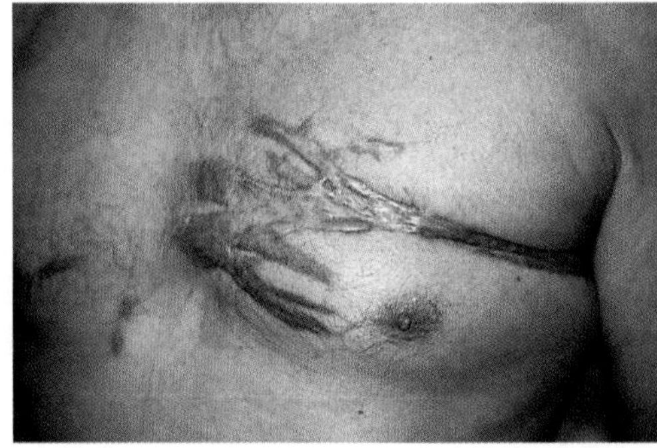

Fig. 46.4 Keloid. (Courtesy Department of Dermatology, University of Utah School of Medicine, Salt Lake City, UT.)

In chronic eczema, the skin becomes lichenified, leathery, and hyperpigmented from recurrent irritation and scratching. Eczematous inflammations need to be differentiated from other epidermal rashes and dermatoses, particularly psoriasis.

Allergic Contact Dermatitis

Allergic contact dermatitis (ACD) is a common form of T-cell–mediated or delayed hypersensitivity (see Chapter 9 for different types of allergic responses). The response is a consequence of alterations in skin barrier function with reaction to the exogenous agent; release of cytokines, chemokines, and cytotoxins from keratinocytes; Langerhans cells; and natural killer cells and neuronal responses, such as pruritis. Genetic susceptibility involves several genes, including loss of function mutations in the gene encoding the epidermal protein filaggrin, which binds keratin filaments and provides a skin barrier.[15]

Various allergens (e.g., microorganisms, chemicals, foreign proteins, latex, drugs, metals) can form a sensitizing antigen. Contact with the oil of the poison ivy plant, urushiol, is a common example (Fig. 46.5).When the allergen contacts the skin, it is bound to a carrier protein, forming the sensitizing antigen. The Langerhans cells process the antigen and present it to T cells. T cells then become sensitized to the antigen, inducing the release of inflammatory cytokines and chemokines, leading to leukocyte infiltration and antigen-specific inflammation resulting in the symptoms of dermatitis.[16] Latex allergy can be either a type IV delayed hypersensitivity reaction to chemicals used in latex rubber processing or a type I immediate hypersensitivity reaction with immunoglobulin E (IgE) antibodies formed in response to latex rubber protein.[17]

The manifestations of allergic contact dermatitis include erythema and edema with pruritic (itching) vesicular lesions, typically seen in the areas of allergen contact. The pattern of distribution provides clues to the source of the antigen (e.g., hands exposed to chemical solutions or boundaries from rings, necklaces, or bracelets). The antigen must be removed for the inflammatory response to resolve and tissue repair to begin. Treatment may require topical or systemic steroids.

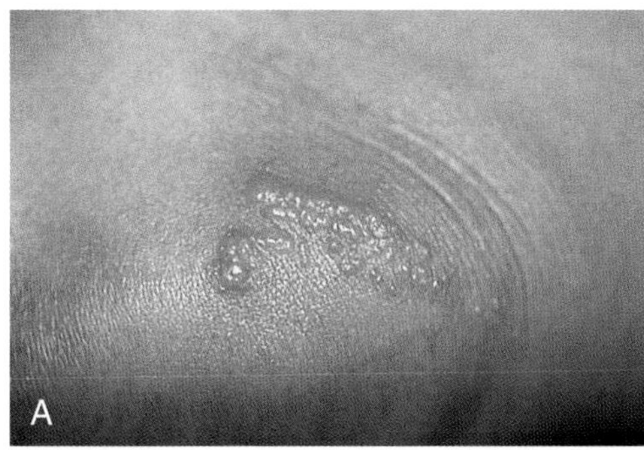

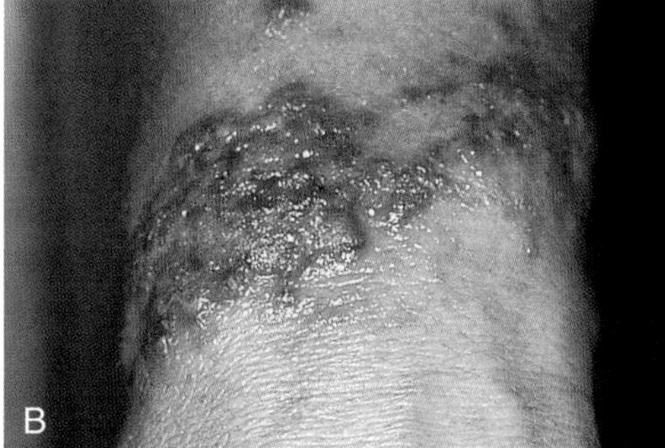

Fig. 46.5 Poison Ivy. (A) Poison ivy on knee. **(B)** Poison ivy dermatitis. (Courtesy Department of Dermatology, University of Utah School of Medicine, Salt Lake City, UT.)

Irritant Contact Dermatitis

Irritant contact dermatitis (ICD) is a localized, nonspecific inflammatory dermatitis caused by the direct cytotoxic action of the offending physical or chemical agent. Unlike ACD, ICD is not mediated by the immune system. The severity of the inflammation is related to the concentration of the irritant, length of exposure, disruption of the skin barrier and age. Irritation can occur from almost anything, especially if the epidermal barrier is compromised in any way. Common irritants include water (from frequent hand washing), detergents, solvents, acids, alkalis, fiberglass, dust, metal salts, insecticides, herbicides, dyes, fragrances, and preservatives. Irritant contact dermatitis is the most common type of occupational dermatitis, particularly in hairdressers, bakers, cooks, mechanics, industry workers, healthcare workers, and housekeepers. The hands are the primary site of involvement. The skin lesions are similar in appearance to ACD but range from mild pruritic xerosis and erythema to more severe formation of eczematous skin changes, vesicle and bullae formation, or even tissue necrosis. Patch testing can help to differentiate irritant from allergic contact dermatitis. Removing the source of irritation and using topical agents provide effective treatment.[18]

Atopic Dermatitis

Atopic dermatitis (atopic eczema) is common in individuals with a history or family history of atopy eczema, asthma, and/or allergic rhinitis) and is associated with IgE antibodies. It is more common in infancy and childhood, but some individuals are affected throughout life. Specific details of this disorder are presented in Chapter 47.

Stasis Dermatitis

Stasis dermatitis (or stasis eczema) usually occurs on the lower extremities as a result of venous hypertension, incompetent venous valves, calf muscle pump failure, or any combination of these. It is associated with edema, varicosities, phlebitis, and vascular trauma (Fig. 46.6). The lesions must be different from

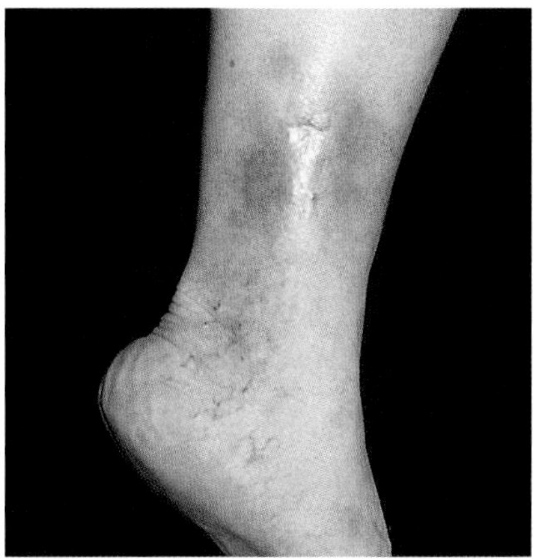

Fig. 46.6 Stasis Ulcer. (Courtesy Department of Dermatology, University of Utah School of Medicine, Salt Lake City, UT.)

those caused by arterial occlusive disease, diabetic neuropathy, malignancy, pyoderma gangrenosum, and other inflammatory ulcers. Pooling of venous blood traps neutrophils that may release oxidants and proteolytic enzymes. Increased venous pressure widens interendothelial pores and, coupled with the deposition of red blood cells, fibrin, and other macromolecules, makes them unavailable for repair while promoting inflammation.[19]

Erythema and pruritus develop initially, followed by scaling, telangiectasia, and hyperpigmentation, specifically called hemosiderin staining. As the disease progresses, vascular permeability increases, causing the chronic release of fibrin, cytokines, leukocytes, and inflammatory mediators which can lead to tropic skin changes, lipodermatosclerosis, and ulcerations, particularly above the medial or lateral malleolus. Ulcerations are typically difficult to treat, and re-ulceration frequently occurs. Preventive treatment includes elevating the legs as often as possible, not wearing tight clothes around the legs, and not standing for long periods. Defined infections are treated with antibiotics. Chronic lesions with ulceration are treated with moist dressings, external compression/dressings, and vein ablation surgery. New treatments include biologics, such as bilayer living skin construct, fibroblast derivatives, and extracellular matrices. Non-biologic products such as poly-*N*-acetyl glucosamine have been beneficial in clinical trials.[20]

Seborrheic Dermatitis

Seborrheic dermatitis is a common, chronic, relapsing, inflammation of the skin occurring in areas rich in sebaceous gland activity such as the scalp, eyebrows, eyelids, ear canals, nasolabial folds, axillae, chest, or back (Fig. 46.7). The cause is unknown, but proposed etiologies include genetic predisposition, *Malassezia* fungal infection, immunosuppression, and epidermal hyperproliferation. The lesions develop from infancy to old age with periods of remission and exacerbation. The most commonly recognized and most mild form of seborrheic dermatitis is scalp dandruff. In more severe disease, lesions appear as pruritic erythematous plaques with greasy white or yellow scales.

Topical therapy includes antifungal shampoos, calcineurin inhibitors (immunomodulating agents that reduce inflammation), and low-dose steroids for acute flares. Nonpharmacologic topical preparations may be used to control facial symptoms. Corticosteroids should not be used for maintenance therapy.[21]

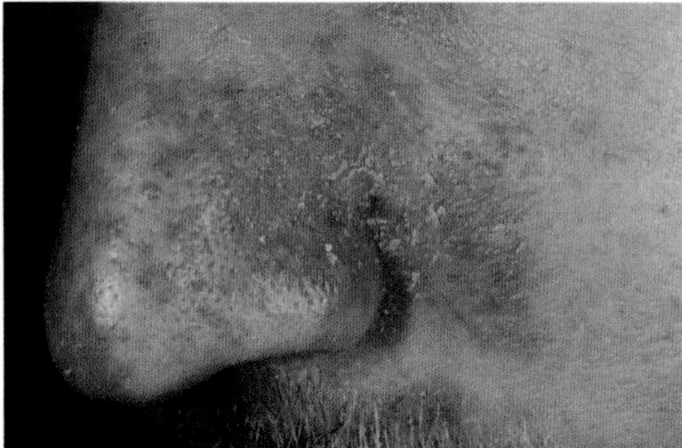

Fig. 46.7 Seborrheic Dermatitis. (Courtesy Department of Dermatology, University of Utah School of Medicine, Salt Lake City, UT.)

Papulosquamous Disorders

Psoriasis, pityriasis rosea, lichen planus, acne vulgaris, hidradenitis suppurativa, acne rosacea, and lupus erythematosus are characterized by papules, scales, plaques, and erythema. Collectively they are described as **papulosquamous disorders**.

Psoriasis

Psoriasis is a chronic, relapsing, proliferative, immune mediated inflammatory disorder that involves the skin, scalp, and nails, often accompanied by systemic comorbidities. The prevalence of psoriasis is between 0.5% and 11% in adults and is more prevalent in high-income countries and regions with older populations.[22] Genetic risk factors are predominant, and several alleles have been identified. Environmental factors, such as skin trauma or infection and smoking, can promote exacerbations. The onset is generally established by 40 years of age, but it can occur in children. The onset of psoriasis later in life is less familial and more secondary to comorbidities, such as obesity, smoking, hypertension, and diabetes.

The inflammatory cascade of psoriasis involves complex interactions between macrophages, fibroblasts, dendritic cells, natural killer cells, T-helper cells, and regulatory T cells. These immune cells lead to the secretion of numerous inflammatory mediators, such as tumor necrosis factor-α (TNF-α), and other cytokines, including IL-12, IL-17, and IL-23, that promote keratinocyte proliferation, angiogenesis, and infiltration of other immune cells into the lesions of psoriasis. IL-23–mediated activation of the T-helper cell 17 pathway is thought to be a predominant mechanism of disease. These inflammatory markers are the target for several therapeutic drugs known as biologic agents.[23]

Both the dermis and the epidermis are thickened because of cellular hyperproliferation, altered keratinocyte differentiation, and expanded dermal vasculature. Epidermal shedding time escalates to 3 to 4 days from the norm of 14 to 20 days. Cell maturation and keratinization are bypassed, and the epidermis thickens and plaques form. The loosely cohesive keratin gives the lesion a silvery appearance. Capillary dilation and increased vascularization occur from release of angiogenic factors, such as vascular endothelial growth factor (VEGF), and accommodate the increased cell metabolism and causes erythema. The disease can be mild, moderate, or severe, depending on the size, distribution, and inflammation of the lesions. Psoriasis is marked by remissions and exacerbations.

The clinical features depend on the types of psoriasis. The variants include plaque (psoriasis vulgaris), inverse, guttate, pustular, and erythrodermic. **Plaque psoriasis** is the most common. The typical plaque psoriatic lesion is a well-demarcated, thick, silvery, scaly, erythematous plaque surrounded by normal skin that can appear anywhere on the body (Fig. 46.8). Small, erythematous papules enlarge and coalesce into larger inflammatory lesions on the face, scalp, elbows, knees, and sites of

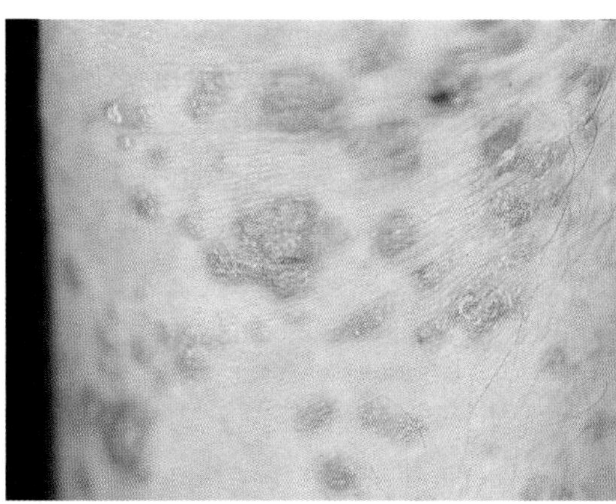

Fig. 46.8 Plaque Psoriasis. Typical oval plaque with well-defined borders and silvery scale. (Courtesy Department of Dermatology, University of Utah School of Medicine, Salt Lake City, UT.)

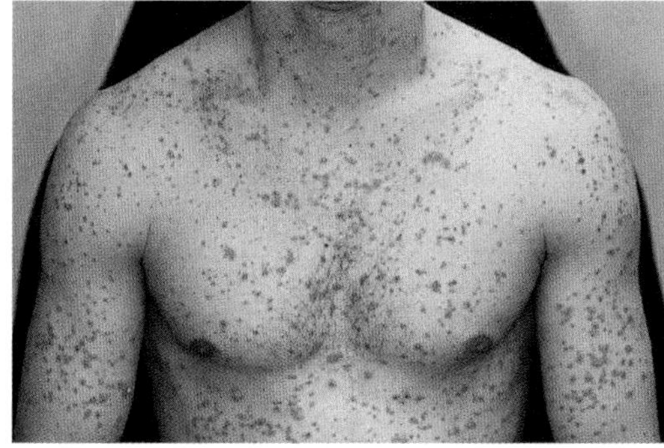

Fig. 46.9 Guttate Psoriasis After Streptococcal Infection. Numerous uniformly small lesions may abruptly occur after streptococcal pharyngitis. (Courtesy Department of Dermatology, University of Utah School of Medicine, Salt Lake City, UT.)

trauma (Koebner phenomenon). Pruritus is common with moderate to severe psoriasis or during exacerbation.

Other types of psoriasis are less common. Inverse psoriasis is rare and involves lesions that develop in skin folds (e.g., the axilla or groin). Often misdiagnosed as fungal infections, they are large, smooth, dry, and deep red. In guttate psoriasis, small papules appear suddenly on the trunk and extremities a few weeks after a streptococcal respiratory tract infection (Fig. 46.9). Guttate psoriasis may resolve spontaneously in weeks or months. Pustular psoriasis appears as blisters of noninfectious pus (collections of neutrophils) that develop over areas of plaque psoriasis. Erythrodermic (exfoliative) psoriasis is characterized by widespread red, scaling lesions that cover a large body surface area (BSA) and is often accompanied by pruritus or pain associated with constitutional symptoms (fever, chills, fatigue) and skin infections.

Psoriatic arthritis (PA) is associated with the proinflammatory cytokines that cause psoriatic skin lesions. Approximately 70% of individuals presenting with PA have a history of psoriasis. There are several phenotypes, including asymmetric arthritis of the major joints, enthesitis (inflammation of ligaments and tendons), dactylitis (involvement of finger and toes), and nail disease. Psoriatic nail disease can occur in all psoriasis subtypes with pitting, onycholysis, subungual hyperkeratosis, and nail plate dystrophy.

Psoriasis also is a risk factor for a number of comorbidities, including uveitis; inflammatory bowel disease; metabolic syndrome, including hypertension, insulin resistance, dyslipidemia, and abdominal obesity; depression and anxiety; chronic obstructive pulmonary disease; and increased risk for atherosclerosis, cardiovascular disease, and stroke that is independent of traditional risk factors for these diseases.[24] The underlying mechanisms are thought to be related to increased levels of systemic proinflammatory mediators and chemokines, which are central to the chronic inflammation, oxidative stress, and angiogenesis of psoriasis.

Treatment is individualized and related to maintaining skin moisture, reducing epidermal cell turnover and pruritus, promoting immunomodulation, preventing and managing comorbidities, and assuring support systems to maintain quality of life. Mild psoriasis is treated with topical corticosteroids, vitamin D analogues, emollients, keratolytic agents (e.g., salicylic acid), and ultraviolet light therapy. Systemic therapy is indicated for moderate to severe disease or with the presence of psoriatic arthritis and includes methotrexate, acitretin, cyclosporine (short term) and biologics that target TNF-α, IL-17, and IL-23.[25,26]

Pityriasis Rosea

Pityriasis rosea is an acute and self-limiting inflammatory disorder that occurs more often in young adults. The cause is thought to be a herpes-like virus (e.g., human herpesvirus 6 [HHV6-roseola] and HHV7).[27] Pityriasis rosea begins as a single lesion (herald patch) (Fig. 46.10) that is circular, demarcated, and salmon-pink, approximately 3 to 10 cm in diameter, and usually located on the trunk. Early lesions are maculopapular, followed by lesions that develop within 14 to 21 days and extend over the trunk and upper part of the extremities, although rarely on the face. The small, erythematous, rose-colored papules expand into characteristic oval lesions that are bilateral, symmetrically distributed, and have raised, scaly borders. The pattern of distribution

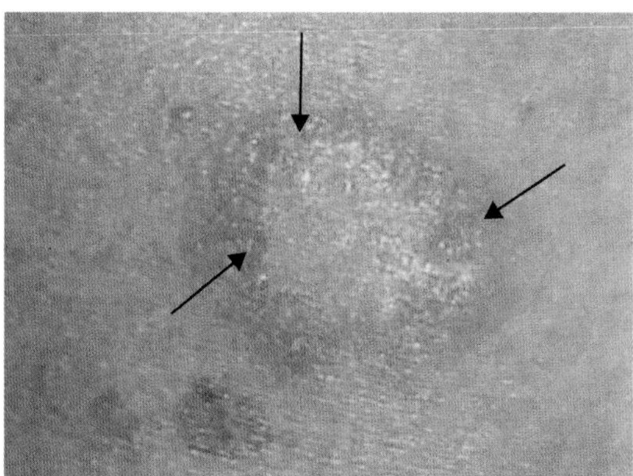

Fig. 46.10 Pityriasis Rosea Herald Patch. A collarette pattern has formed around the margins *(arrows)*. (Courtesy Department of Dermatology, University of Utah School of Medicine, Salt Lake City, UT.)

on the back follows the skin lines around the trunk and resembles a drooping pine tree. The scales are slough from the margin of the lesions, forming a collarette pattern. Pruritis is the most common symptom. Occasionally headache, fatigue, or sore throat precedes the development of the lesions. One study has found an increased risk for miscarriage or premature delivery associated with pityriasis rosea infection.[28]

The diagnosis of pityriasis rosea follows the clinical appearance of the lesion. Secondary syphilis, psoriasis, drug eruption, nummular eczema, and seborrheic dermatitis are among the differential diagnosis considerations. The disorder is usually self-limiting and resolves in a few months with symptomatic treatment for pruritus or cosmetic concerns. Ultraviolet light (with some risk for hyperpigmentation) or systemic corticosteroids have been used to control pruritus. Acyclovir and erythromycin also may be used for treatment.[27]

Lichen Planus

Lichen planus (LP) is a benign autoimmune inflammatory disorder of the skin, nail, and mucous membranes with multiple clinical variations. The age of onset is usually between 30 and 70 years. The cause is unknown, but T cells, adhesion molecules, inflammatory cytokines, perforin, and antigen-presenting cells are involved. LP also is linked to numerous drugs and to the hepatitis C virus. The disorder begins with non-scaling, purple-colored, flat-topped, polygonal pruritic papules 2 to 4 mm in size, usually located symmetrically on the wrists, ankles, lower legs, and genitalia (Fig. 46.11). New lesions are pale pink and evolve into a dark violet color. Persistent lesions may be thickened and red, forming hypertrophic lichen planus.[0] Nail lichen planus manifests as thinning and splitting of nails. Part, or all, of the nail may be shed.

Oral lesions (oral lichen planus) appear as lacy white rings that must be differentiated from leukoplakia or oral candidiasis. Lesions may be precancerous in about 2% of cases.[29] Fine lines, known as *Wickham striae*, can be seen throughout the oral lesions on magnification. Oral lesions do not commonly ulcerate, but if present, they are painful and require treatment.

Pruritus is the most distressing symptom. The lesions are self-limiting and may last for months or years, with an average duration of 6 to 18 months. Post-inflammatory hyperpigmentation is a common consequence of the lesion. Approximately 20% of individuals have a recurrence. The diagnosis is made by the clinical appearance and the histopathology of the lesion. Treatment is individualized and includes topical, intralesional, or systemic corticosteroids, topical retinoids, immunomodulators (or both), and topical light therapy.[30]

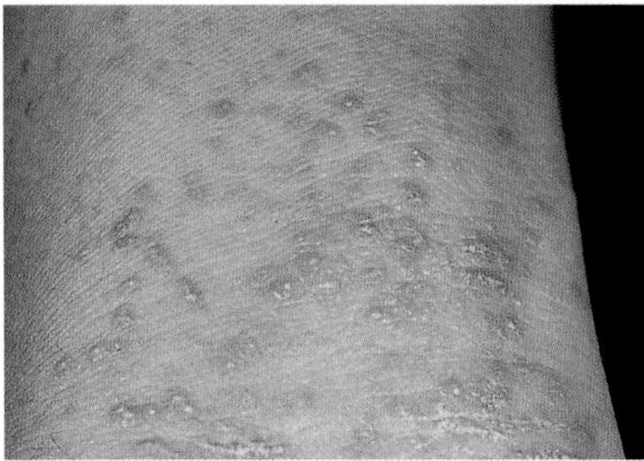

Fig. 46.11 Hypertrophic Lichen Planus on Arms. (Courtesy Department of Dermatology, University of Utah School of Medicine, Salt Lake City, UT.)

Acne Vulgaris

Acne vulgaris is an inflammatory disorder of the pilosebaceous follicle (the sebaceous gland contiguous with a hair follicle) that usually occurs during adolescence. Details of this disorder are presented in Chapter 47.

Hydradenitis Suppurativa (Inverse Acne)

Hydradenitis suppurativa (inverse acne) is a chronic, inflammatory, recurring scarring disease of the pilosebaceous follicular ducts involving areas of skin where there are folds and hair follicles (Fig. 46.12). The incidence is unknown but is estimated at 1% to 4% of the population and is more common in females. The pathogenesis of the disease is complex and includes a combination of genetic, hormonal, immune, and environmental factors. Aggravating factors include smoking (the most significant factor, as nicotine activates keratinocytes, fibroblasts, and immunocytes), tight clothing, heat, perspiration, shaving of prone areas, obesity, and stress.[31] An aberrant response to commensal follicular bacteria results in inflammatory cytokine production with follicular hyperkeratosis and occlusion of the pilosebaceous unit causing peri folliculitis, abscess formation, sinus tracts, and scarring. The sweat glands are not primarily involved.

The lesions present as deep, firm painful subcutaneous nodules that tract and rupture horizontally under the skin. They are different from furuncles because furuncles extend vertically and discharge onto the skin. Sites of involvement include apocrine gland–rich areas (e.g., the axillae, groin, perianal region, and perineum). Other areas include the neck, adjacent scalp, back, buttocks, scrotum or labia, and inframammary or mammary region in women. Lesions may be minimal or severe, with

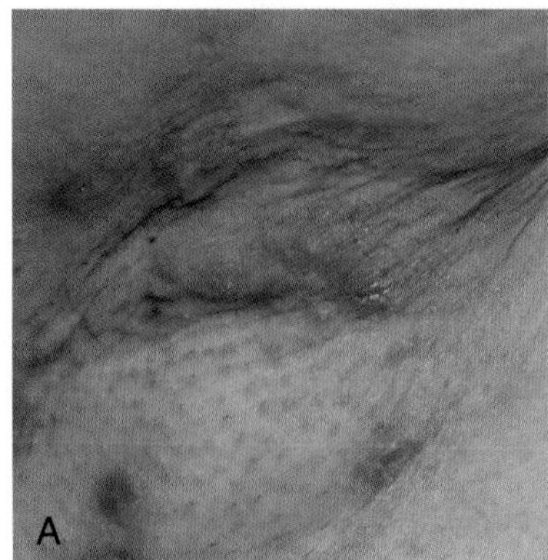

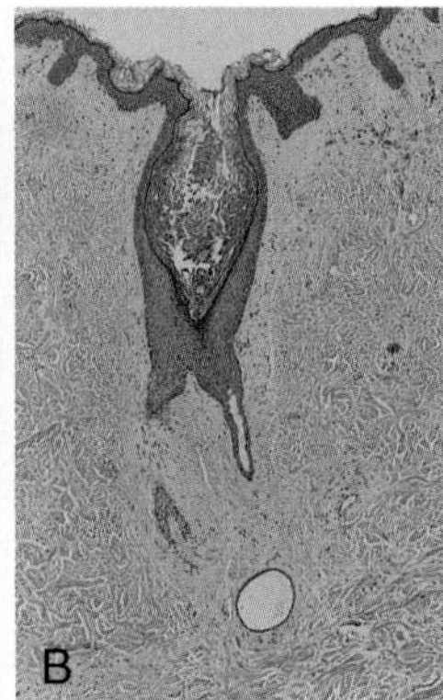

Fig. 46.12 Hydradenitis Suppurative. (A) Characteristic painful pustules and draining sinus tract. **(B)** Histology shows follicular plugging and connection to a dilated apocrine duct. (A, Courtesy Kalman Watsky, MD; from Bolognia JL Jorizzo JL, Schaffer JV, eds. *Dermatology*, 3rd edition. Philadelphia: Saunders; 2012. B, From Bolognia JL, Jorizzo JL, Rapinin RP, eds. *Dermatology*, 2nd edition. Philadelphia: Saunders; 2008.)

multiple draining fistulas. Complete, spontaneous resolution is rare. The disease can recur for years with negative effects on quality of life. Treatment includes smoking cessation, anti-inflammatories, antibiotics, immunotherapy, combination therapy, and incision and drainage of nodules.[32]

Acne Rosacea

Acne rosacea is a chronic inflammation of the skin that develops in middle-aged adults and occurs more commonly in women and those with fair skin. There are four subtypes of lesions, and they may occur singly or in combination: erythematotelangiectatic, papulopustular, phymatous (nodular), and ocular (eyelids and ocular surface). The exact cause is unknown, but genetic factors, immune dysregulation, and neurovascular dysregulation are involved. There is a familial tendency, and several genes have been identified. Factors that trigger immune responses, such as neurovascular dysregulation and infection, include chronic sun exposure and damage, heat, drinking alcohol or hot beverages, hormonal fluctuations, and stress. *Demodex folliculorum* (mites) and microorganisms residing on their surface are associated with the pathogenesis of rosacea.[33] The most common lesions are erythema, papules, pustules, and telangiectasia. They occur in the middle third of the face, including the forehead, nose, cheeks, and chin (Fig. 46.13). Neurovascular dysregulation is associated with chronic, inappropriate vasodilation, resulting in flushing, a burning sensation, and sun sensitivity. Sebaceous hypertrophy, fibrosis, and telangiectasia may be severe enough to produce an irreversible bulbous appearance of the nose, known as rhinophyma. Disorders of the eye often accompany rosacea or can occur independently of other manifestations, particularly conjunctivitis and keratitis, which can result in visual impairment.[34]

Treatment includes photoprotection (sunscreen, wide-brimmed hat), along with avoidance of other triggers. Both topical and systemic therapies may be effective. Laser therapy can be effective for removing telangiectasias. Surgical excision of excessive tissue may be required for rhinophyma.[35]

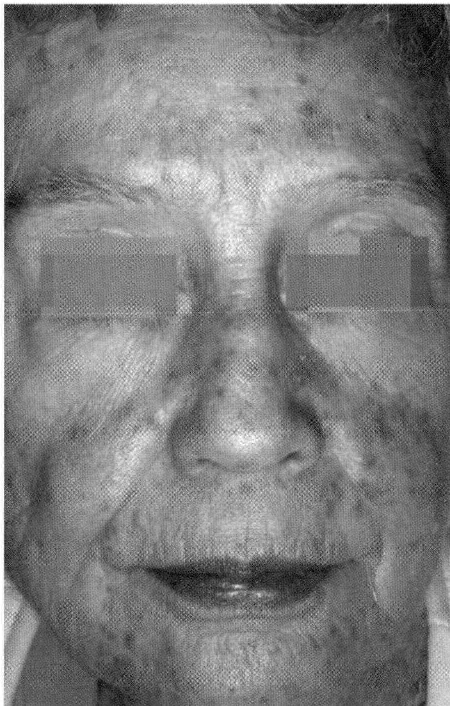

Fig. 46.13 Granulomatous Rosacea. Pustules and erythema occur on the forehead, cheeks, and nose. (From Dinulos GH. *Habif's clinical dermatology*, 7th edition. Philadelphia: Saunders.)

Lupus Erythematosus

Lupus erythematosus is a systemic inflammatory, autoimmune disease with cutaneous manifestations (see Chapter 9). Cutaneous lupus erythematosus (CLE) is limited to the skin but can progress to systemic lupus erythematosus (SLE).

Cutaneous lupus erythematosus. Cutaneous lupus erythematosus (CLE) usually occurs in genetically susceptible adults, particularly women in their late thirties or early forties, but people of any age can be affected. Three subtypes of CLE have been described with specific manifestations of the disease: acute, subacute, and chronic. The lesions may be single or multiple and vary in size (Fig. 46.14). Often the lesions are located on light-exposed areas of the skin, and photosensitivity is common. The face is the most common site of lesion involvement, with a butterfly pattern of distribution found over the nose and cheeks. The characteristic clinical manifestations of the different categories of CLE are summarized in Table 46.7.

The cause is unknown but is related to genetic and environmental factors and an altered immune response to an unknown antigen or to UV B wavelengths. There is development of self-reactive T and B cells, a decreased number of regulatory T cells, infiltration of neutrophils, and increased levels of proinflammatory cytokines. Autoantibodies and immune complexes infiltrate the dermal-epidermal junction and cause tissue damage and inflammation.[36] Exacerbation of manifestations can

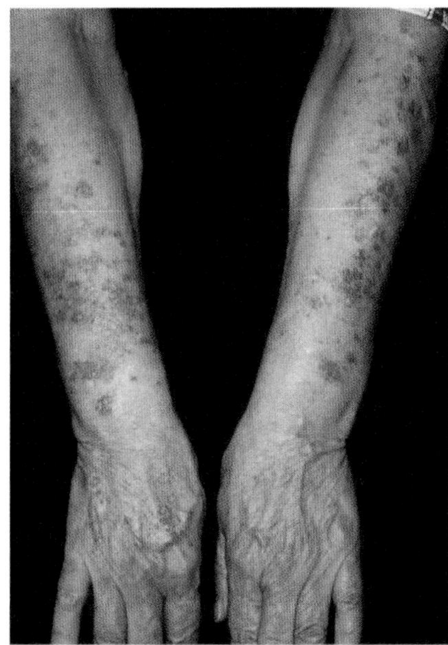

Fig. 46.14 Subacute Cutaneous Lupus (Discoid Lupus Erythematosus). (Courtesy Department of Dermatology, University of Utah School of Medicine, Salt Lake City, UT.)

TABLE 46.7 Categories and Manifestations of Cutaneous Lupus Erythematous

Category of Dle	Clinical Manifestations
Acute	
Localized	Butterfly pattern of erythema over bridge of nose and malar areas of face (malar rash); may have fine surface scales and underlying edema; scalp areas may develop alopecia; lasts for hours to days
Generalized	Diffuse or papular erythema of face, upper trunk, or extremities; develops quickly and lasts hours to days
Subacute	Erythematous macules and papules that evolve into *papulosquamous* or *annular* plaques developing on sun-exposed areas of the upper body (V area of neck, upper chest, back, shoulders, extensor surface of arms and hands); can be associated with reaction to drugs; may be accompanied by mild systemic disease
Chronic	Classic discoid lupus erythematosus is the most common form; lesions are red to purple macules or papules with a superficial brownish scale involving head, scalp and neck; scale can penetrate hair follicle leaving a carpet-tack appearance when removed; may have residual scarring, dermal atrophy hypopigmentation, alopecia, and telangiectasia; Raynaud phenomenon occurs in some individuals

Data from Data from Hejazi EZ, Werth VP. Cutaneous lupus erythematosus: An update on pathogenesis, diagnosis and treatment. *American Journal of Clinical Dermatology*, 2016;17(2):135–146; Lenormand C, Lipsker D. Lupus erythematosus: Significance of dermatologic findings. *Annales de Dermatologie et de Venereologie*, 2021;148(1):6–15.

occur with UV exposure, certain drugs (e.g., hydrochlorothiazide and proton pump inhibitors) and smoking. Skin biopsy with immunofluorescent observation reveals lumpy deposits of immunoglobulins, including IgM, IgG, and C3. The revised Cutaneous Lupus Erythematous Disease Area and Severity Index (CLASI) can be used to assess disease severity.[37] Individuals with CLE must use sunscreen and sun protection because direct sun exposure initiates or exacerbates lesions (see Fig. 46.14).

The early lesion is asymmetric, a 1 to 2 cm raised red plaque with a brownish scale. The scale penetrates the hair follicle and leaves a visible follicle opening (carpet-tack appearance) when removed. The lesions persist for months and then resolve spontaneously or atrophy, causing a depressed scar. Healed lesions may have residual telangiectasia and hypopigmented scarring. Treatment options include sun protection and use of topical steroids, calcineurin inhibitors, antimalarial drugs (e.g., hydroxychloroquine sulfate), and targeted immunotherapy. These medications must be used with caution to prevent serious side effects.[38]

Vesiculobullous Diseases

Vesiculobullous skin diseases share a common characteristic of vesicle, or blister, formation. Two such diseases are pemphigus and erythema multiforme.

Pemphigus

Pemphigus (meaning to blister or bubble) is a group of rare, life-threatening autoimmune diseases of the intradermal skin and oral mucous membranes with formation of autoantibodies against desmoglein, an adhesion molecule (Fig. 46.15). **Bullous pemphoid** is the formation of autoantibodies against hemidesmosome adhesion molecules that attach keratinocytes to the basement membrane causing subepidermal blistering. The cause of antibody formation is unknown. Pemphigus can occur in all age groups but is more prevalent in persons between 40 and 50 years of age. There is a genetic predisposition, as well as environmental (viral infections, drug-induced, dietary intake, or physical effects, such as radiation or surgery) and endogenous (emotional or hormonal stressors) influences. There are four main groups of pemphigus:

- **Pemphigus vulgaris** is the most common form and is caused by circulating immunoglobulin G (IgG) autoantibodies and C3 complement bind to the desmoglein-3 adhesion molecules, resulting in the destruction of cell-to-cell adhesion (acantholysis) at the desmosomal cell junction in the suprabasal layer of the epidermis with fluid accumulation and the resulting symptom of blister formation. With rupture, the lesion can evolve into painful erosions in the skin or mucosal surface and leads to increased risk of water loss, electrolyte imbalance, and infections.[39] Oral lesions precede the onset of skin blistering, which is more prominent on the face, scalp, and axilla.
- **Pemphigus foliaceus** is a milder form of the disease and involves demsmoglen-1 with acantholysis at the subcorneal level with blistering, erosions, scaling, crusting, and erythema, usually of the face and chest. Oral mucous membranes are not involved.
- **Paraneoplastic pemphigus** is the most severe form of pemphigus and is associated with lymphoproliferative neoplasms. Internal organs, including lungs, thyroid, kidney, smooth muscle, and the gastrointestinal tract, are also involved, leading to the term paraneoplastic autoimmune multiorgan syndrome. In contrast to pemphigus vulgaris, the lesions develop

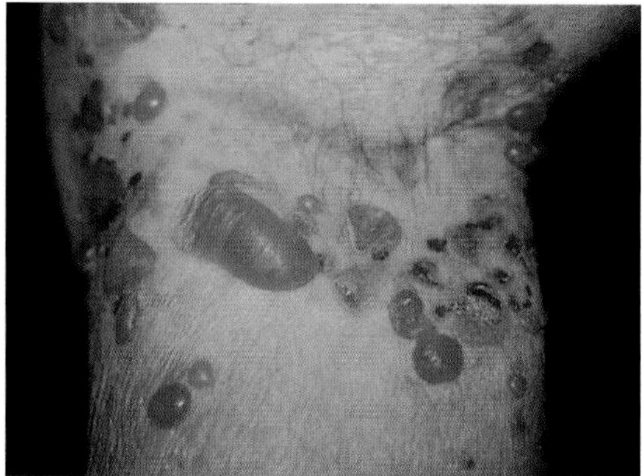

Fig. 46.15 Pemphigus. Generalized eruption with blisters arising from an edematous erythematous annular base. (Courtesy Department of Dermatology, University of Utah School of Medicine, Salt Lake City, UT.)

from inflammatory papules or macules rather than normal skin.

- IgA pemphigus is the most benign form of pemphigus characterized by tissue-bound and circulation of IgA antibodies targeting desmosomal or nondesmosomal cell surface components in the basement membrane of the epidermis. Acantholysis is not as severe as that in pemphigus vulgaris, but there is still vesicle or pustule formation with erythematous plaques with crusts.

The diagnosis of pemphigus is made from the clinical, histologic findings of autoantibodies at the site of blister formation and positive direct immunofluorescence microscopy. The clinical course of the disease may range from rapidly fatal to relatively benign. The primary treatment for pemphigus is systemic corticosteroids in combination with adjuvant immunosuppressants.[40]

Erythema Multiforme

Erythema multiforme (EM) is an uncommon syndrome characterized by inflammation of the skin and/or mucous membranes. EM is often associated with a T-cell-mediated type IV hypersensitivity reaction to a microorganism, particularly viral infections (e.g., herpes simplex virus, Epstein-Barr virus, histoplasmosis, and *Mycoplasma pneumoniae*) or related to drug reactions. Erythema multiforme major has moderate to severe mucosal involvement and some systemic symptoms, such as fever, weakness, and arthralgia. Erythema multiforme minor is characterized by inflammation of the skin without (or with very minor) mucosal disease and without associated systemic symptoms. Both EM minor and major have characteristic "bull's-eye" or "target" lesions develop on the skin surface with a central dusky region surrounded by concentric rings or alternating edema, and inflammation commonly over the extensor surfaces of the limbs. The lesions usually occur suddenly in groups over a period of 2 to 3 weeks. Urticarial plaques, 1 to 2 cm in diameter, can develop without the target lesion (Fig. 46.16). EM major includes mucous membrane lesions and erythematous plaques which can be quite painful. Single or multiple vesicles or bullae may arise on a part of the plaque, accompanied by pruritus and burning. EM is usually self-limiting, and the lesions heal within a few weeks.[41]

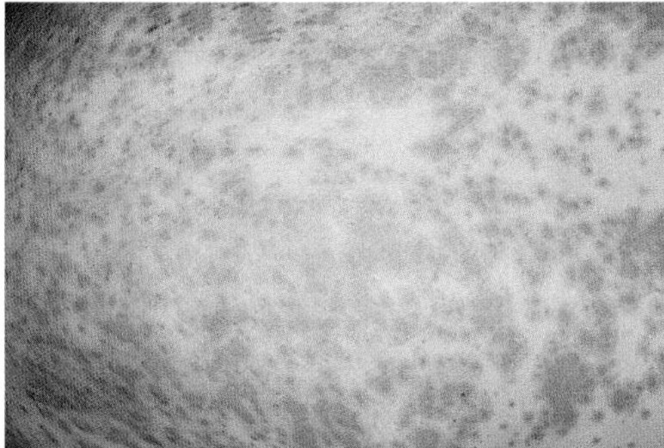

Fig. 46.16 Erythema Multiforme Caused by Doxepin. (Courtesy Department of Dermatology, School of Medicine, University of Utah.)

Stevens-Johnson Syndrome and Toxic Epidermal Necrolysis

Stevens-Johnson syndrome (SJS) and toxic epidermal necrolysis (TEN) are the same disease with a continuum of symptoms based on clinical presentation and severity. Both conditions are rare, distinct from EM, and are type IV hypersensitivity reactions to drugs. They are associated with severe mucocutaneous drug reactions with extensive keratinocyte cell death, extensive bullous epidermal detachment, mucositis, and organ involvement. SJS is less severe and involves <10% of the BSA. TEN involves >30% of the BSA. SJS/TEN overlap describes individuals with between 10% and 30% of BSA. The mechanism of cell injury is not completely understood, but involves cytotoxic T lymphocytes (CTLs), human leukocyte antigen (HLA), and the major histocompatibility complex (MHC).[42]

Prodromal symptoms of SJS/TEN include fever, headache, malaise, sore throat, and cough, which develop in approximately one third of cases. Vesicles and bullae form and the skin begins to slough as the disease progresses. Secondary erosions and crusts then develop. Mucosal involvement may be extensive and involve the mouth, air passages, esophagus, urethra, and conjunctiva. Blindness can result from corneal ulcerations. Difficulty eating, breathing, and urinating may develop, with severe manifestations. Severe cases of the disease can be fatal as the complications of extensive skin detachment can include acute kidney injury, bacteremia, multiorgan system failure, sepsis, and death.

Establishing a medication history is vital to the diagnosis of SJS/TENS. Skin biopsy findings are supportive, but not independently diagnostic. Any ongoing drug therapy should be withdrawn and reevaluated, and underlying infections should be treated. Treatment is individualized according to severity and, in severe cases, requires the care of a burn unit. Mortality can be as high as 25%. Ophthalmic, kidney, and lung involvement require special care. In mild cases, resolution occurs in 8 to 10 days, usually without scarring. Mucosal lesions may take 6 weeks to heal.[43]

Infections

Cutaneous infections are common forms of skin disease. They generally remain localized, although serious complications can develop with systemic involvement that can be life-threatening. The types of skin infection include bacterial, viral, and fungal. The microbiome (normal flora) of the skin consists of aerobes, yeast, and anaerobes and often provides protection against pathogens that cause skin infections, including *Staphylococcus* and *Streptococcus*.[44]

Bacterial Infections

Most acute bacterial skin and skin-structure infections are caused by local invasion of pathogens. Coagulase-positive *Staphylococcus aureus* and, less often, beta-hemolytic streptococci are the common causative microorganisms. Community-acquired methicillin-resistant *Staphylococcus aureus* (CA-MRSA) is also a cause of serious skin infection, particularly skin abscesses (Box 46.3).

BOX 46.3 Community-Acquired Methicillin-Resistant *Staphylococcus aureus*

Community-acquired methicillin-resistant *Staphylococcus aureus* (CA-MRSA) is a serious skin and soft tissue infection that includes abscesses, cellulitis, and necrotizing fasciitis and can serve as a source for bloodstream infections. Infections are documented among healthy individuals who have no known risk factors, that is, no recent hospitalization, surgical procedures, or prolonged antibiotic treatment. Outbreaks have been documented among athletic teams, among prisoners, in daycare centers, and homeless shelters. CA-MRSA strains are epidemiologically and clonally different from hospital or nursing home acquired MRSA, although CA-MRSA onset in hospitals is emerging. The most common tests involve genotyping for the staphylococcal chromosomal cassette mec (SCCmec) type IV that encodes resistance to methicillin and Panton-Valentine leukocidin and other genes that encode virulence toxins. The USA300-0114 strain has been epidemic in the United States and is difficult to treat with the development of biofilm formation. It is spreading internationally and has caused life-threatening pneumonia, osteomyelitis, and septic arthritis. Virulence factors include toxins (hemolysins and leukocidins), immune-evasive surface factors (e.g., capsule and protein A) and enzymes that promote tissue invasion (e.g., hyaluronidase). CA-MRSAs are more sensitive to antibiotic treatment and there is a wider choice of antibiotic treatment options for CA-MRSA compared with hospital-acquired MRSA. CA-MRSA is usually susceptible to a variety of oral non–beta-lactam antibiotics, including trimethoprim-sulfamethoxazole, clindamycin, tetracyclines, and linezolid. Parenteral therapy with vancomycin or daptomycin can also be considered. Ceftaroline has been effective for both skin and systemic infections. Dalbavancin, oritavancin, and tedizolid are options for drug resistant strains. Mupirocin may be used to clear MRSA from nasal secretions if cultures show contamination in the nose. New drugs are under investigation. Preventive measures include practicing good hand hygiene, applying antiseptics, covering cuts and abrasions, using antibacterial soaps for showers after contact sports, avoiding sharing towels and razors, and frequently washing towels. Development of a vaccine is a priority for prevention.

Data from Chalmers SJ, Wylam ME. Methicillin-resistant *Staphylococcus aureus* infection and treatment options. *Methods in Molecular Biology*, 2020;2069:229–251.

Folliculitis. Folliculitis is an inflammation of the hair follicle and is typically infectious, caused by bacteria, viruses, parasites, or fungi; *S. aureus* is a common culprit. Noninfectious causes include trauma or plugging of the follicle. The infection develops from proliferation of the microorganism around the opening and inside the follicle. Inflammation is caused by the release of chemotactic factors and enzymes from the bacteria. The lesions appear as papules or pustules with a surrounding area of erythema. Lesions are most prominent on the scalp and extremities but can occur on any hair-bearing area. Prolonged skin moisture, occlusive clothing, topical agents, skin trauma (e.g., shaving facial hair), and poor hygiene are associated contributing factors to the development of folliculitis. Cleaning with soap and water and topical antibiotics are effective treatments.

Furuncle, or "boil" is an inflammatory nodule involving a hair follicle. It may develop from a preceding folliculitis that spreads through the follicular wall into the surrounding dermis. The invading microorganism is usually *S. aureus*, including CA-MSRA. Any skin area with hair can be affected. The initial lesion is a well-circumscribed firm, red, painful nodule 1 to 5 cm in diameter (Fig. 46.17). Within a few days, the erythematous nodules change to a large, fluctuant, and tender cystic

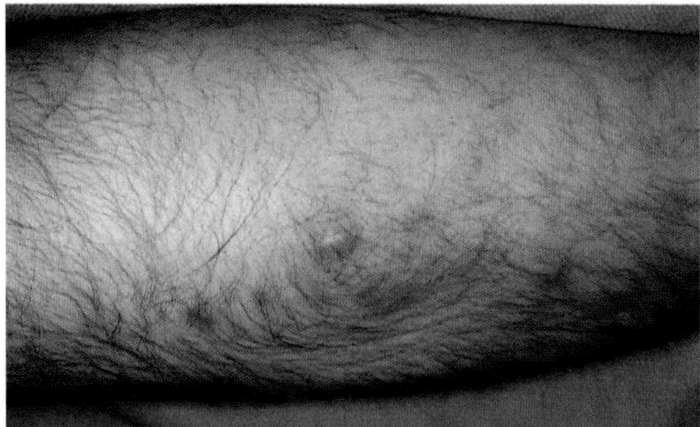

Fig. 46.17 Furuncle of the Forearm. (Courtesy Department of Dermatology, University of Utah School of Medicine, Salt Lake City, UT.)

nodule that may be accompanied by cellulitis. No systemic symptoms are present, and the lesion may drain large amounts of pus and necrotic tissue.

A carbuncle is a coalescence of several furuncles and usually occur on the back of the neck, the upper back, and the lateral thighs. The lesion begins in the subcutaneous tissue and lower dermis as a firm mass that evolves into an erythematous, painful, swollen abscess that drains through many openings. Chills, fever, and malaise can occur during the early stages of lesion development.

Furuncles and carbuncles are treated with warm compresses to provide comfort and promote localization and spontaneous drainage. Abscess formation, recurrent infections, extensive lesions, or lesions associated with cellulitis or systemic symptoms require incision and drainage and are treated with topical or systemic antibiotics.[45]

Cellulitis. Cellulitis is an infection of the dermis and subcutaneous tissue usually caused by group A *Streptococcus*, *Streptococcus* pyogenes, or *Staphylococcus aureus* (including methicillin-resistant strains). Cellulitis can occur as an extension of a skin wound, as an ulcer, or from a furuncle or carbuncle. Risk factors include diabetes mellitus, edema, peripheral vascular disease, tinea pedis, insect bites, and immune suppression from disease or medications. The infected area is erythematous, warm, edematous, painful, and without a distinct border. It can extend to the lymphatic system and the blood causing systemic infection.

Cellulitis must be differentiated from necrotizing fasciitis. Necrotizing fasciitis is a rare, rapidly spreading infection. It is commonly caused by *Streptococcus pyogenes*, which resists phagocytosis and releases toxins. Infection starts in the fascia, muscles, and subcutaneous fat, with subsequent necrosis of the overlying skin and can progress to sepsis and death without early diagnosis and treatment. Treatment requires antibiotics and often surgical debridement to prevent toxic shock syndrome.[46]

Erysipelas. Erysipelas is an acute, nonpurulent, superficial infection of the upper dermis and superficial lymphatics most often caused by beta-hemolytic streptococci. The face, ears, and lower leg are common sites of involvement. Similar to cellulitis, erysipelas is nearly always unilateral. Systemic manifestations such as chills, fever, and malaise often precede the onset of lesions by hours to days. The initial lesions appear as firm, red spots that enlarge and coalesce to form a clearly circumscribed, advancing, bright red, hot lesion with a raised border. There is a clear demarcation between involved and uninvolved skin, which differs from the presentation of cellulitis. Vesicles may appear over the lesion and at the border. Pruritus, burning, and tenderness are present. Cold compresses provide symptomatic relief, and systemic antibiotics are required to arrest the infection.[44]

Impetigo. Impetigo is a superficial infection of the skin that is caused by coagulase-positive *Staphylococcus* or beta-hemolytic streptococci. The disease occurs in adults but is more common in children (see Chapter 47).

Lyme disease. Lyme disease is a multisystem inflammatory disease caused by the spirochete *Borreliella burgdorferi*. It is transmitted by the bite of the *Ixodes* tick, and it is the most frequently reported vector-borne illness. The highest incidence of Lyme disease is among children. The microorganism is difficult to culture; escapes immune defenses through antigenic variation; blocks complement-mediated killing; impedes release of antimicrobial peptides, leukocyte chemotaxis, and antimicrobial killing; and hides in tissue. It spreads to other tissues by entering capillary beds.

Symptoms of the disease occur in three stages, although about half of infected individuals are symptom free. Early localized infection occurs soon after the bite (within 3 to 32 days), presenting with the erythema migrans (bull's-eye rash). This commonly appears at the site of tick attachment. Erythema migrans is a T-cell–mediated response. Within days to weeks after the onset of the illness, there is *disseminated infection*, with secondary erythema migrans, usually with myalgias, arthralgias, and more rarely, meningitis, neuritis, or carditis. Late Lyme disease syndrome, or *chronic Lyme disease*, may develop months to years after the initial infection and antibiotic therapy. Symptoms include arthritis, typically involving one or a few large joints; encephalopathy, polyneuropathy, and heart failure are less prominent but can also occur. *Post-treatment Lyme disease syndrome* is the persistence of pain, fatigue, insomnia, depression, and/or difficulty thinking that lasts for 6 months or more with the absence of an identifiable infection.

The diagnosis of Lyme disease is based on the clinical presentation and history of the tick bite, if known. Serologic tests are used to confirm the diagnosis, although there is a delayed antibody response and the test may be negative during the first 3 weeks after infection. Antibiotics (e.g., doxycycline [not used in children younger than 8 years or in pregnant or breast-feeding women], amoxicillin, or cefuroxime) are used for treatment.[47] Reinfection can occur. There is currently no vaccine for Lyme disease.[48]

Viral Infections

Herpes simplex virus. Skin infections with herpes simplex virus (HSV) are commonly caused by two types of HSV: HSV-1 and HSV-2. Either type can occur in different parts of the body, including oral and genital locations. Encephalitis is a rare manifestation. Their differences are distinguished by laboratory tests. HSV-1, transmitted by contact with infected oral secretions, is generally associated with oral infections (cold sore or fever blister) or infection of the cornea (herpes keratitis) or mouth (gingivostomatitis), but it can also cause genital herpes. With initial (primary) infection, the virus infects epithelial cells, embeds in sensory nerve endings, and moves by retrograde axonal transport to the dorsal root ganglion, where the virus develops lifelong latency by inhibiting apoptosis of target cells. The incubation period ranges from 2 to 14 days. During the secondary phase, the lesions occur at the same site from reactivation of the virus. The virus travels down the peripheral nerve to the site of the original infection, where it is shed. Exposure to ultraviolet light, skin irritation, fever, fatigue, or stress may cause reactivation.

The lesions for HSV-1 appear as clusters of inflamed and painful vesicles on an erythematous base (e.g., within the mouth, over the tongue, on the lips, around the nose) (Fig. 46.18). Increased sensitivity, paresthesias, pruritus, and mild burning may occur before the onset of the lesions. The vesicles rupture, forming a crust. Lesions may last 2 to 6 weeks but usually resolve within 2 weeks. HSV-1 disease can be severe, especially in the immunocompromised host. Encephalitis, meningitis, respiratory tract infections, and esophagitis are rare.[49]

Genital infections are more commonly caused by HSV-2. The virus is spread by skin-to-skin mucous membrane contact during viral shedding. Risk of infection is high in immunosuppressed persons or in persons who have sexual contact with infected individuals and among individuals who are asymptomatic. Vertical transmission from mother to neonate is associated with significant neonatal neurologic morbidity and mortality.[50] The initial infection is asymptomatic. With recurrent exposure, the lesions begin as small vesicles that progress to ulceration within 3 to 4 days with pain, itching, and weeping. Treatment is

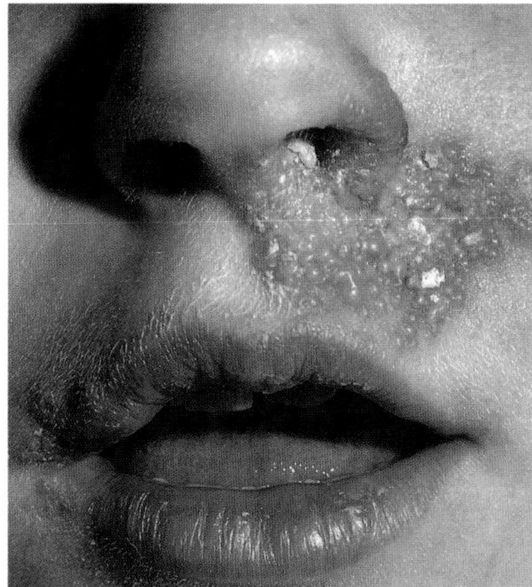

Fig. 46.18 Herpes Simplex. Typical presentation with tense vesicles appearing on the lips and extending onto the skin. (From *Habif TP. Clinical dermatology: A color guide to diagnosis and therapy*, 4th edition. St. Louis: Mosby; 2004.)

symptomatic and includes topical or oral antiviral agents, topical lidocaine, and nerve blocks. Long-term suppression of HSV-1 and HSV-2 may be attempted with daily antiviral dosing. Progress is being made with prophylactic vaccines to prevent HSV infection.[51]

Varicella-zoster virus. Varicella (chickenpox) and herpes zoster (shingles) (see Chapter 47), also known as human herpesvirus 3, are caused by the same herpesvirus and spread via airborne droplets or via direct contact with the actively viral shedding lesions. Varicella-zoster virus (VZV) is highly infectious and enters the body via the respiratory tract, followed by rapid spread from the pharyngeal lymphoid tissue to circulating T lymphocytes, then enters the skin 10 to 21 days later. The virus remains latent in trigeminal and dorsal (sensory) root ganglia, followed years later by reactivation of the virus to cause herpes zoster (HZ). HZ has initial symptoms of pain and paresthesia localized to the affected dermatome (the cutaneous area innervated by a single spinal nerve; see Chapter 15), followed by vesicular eruptions, then crusting (Fig. 46.19). The thoracic or lumbar dermatome are the most common sites affected, but HZ can appear on any dermatome. If the ophthalmic branch of the trigeminal nerve is affected, it should be considered a medical emergency as it is sight-threatening. The rash does not typically cross the body's midline, although two or even three dermatomes adjacent may be affected. Local symptoms are alleviated with compresses, calamine lotion, baking soda, topical lidocaine, or nerve blocks.[52] Approximately 15% to 20% of individuals experience postherpetic neuralgia (PHN), particularly those older than age 60. There is no cure for herpes zoster. The varicella vaccine is safe and effective in children and adults to prevent chicken pox. The herpes zoster vaccine is given to adults 60 years and older to prevent shingles.[52]

Warts. Warts (verrucae) are benign lesions of the skin caused by the many different types of human papillomavirus (HPV) that infect the stratified epithelium of skin and mucous membranes. The lesions can occur anywhere. Lesions can be flat, round, or fusiform and are typically elevated with a rough, grayish surface. Warts are transmitted by direct contact. Specific viruses are associated with specific kinds and locations of lesions. HPV 1 commonly affects the pressure points on the plantar surface of the feet producing plantar warts. Common warts (verruca vulgaris) occur most often in children and are usually on the fingers (Fig. 46.20). Spontaneous remission occurs more readily in children (within about 2 years) than adults (several years or longer). Both topical and systemic retinoids have been used for treatment.[53]

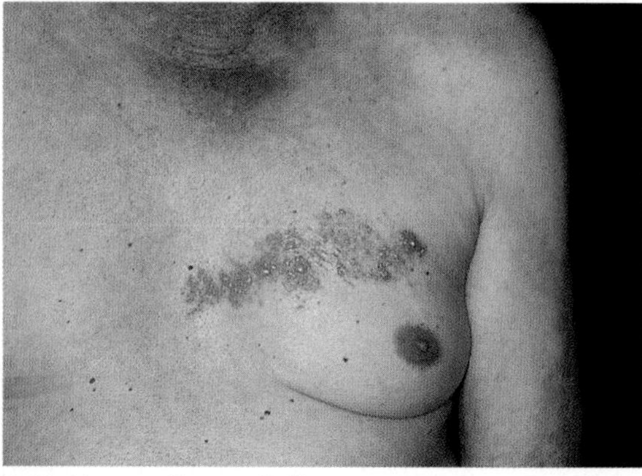

Fig.46.19 Herpes Zoster. Diffuse involvement of a dermatome. (Courtesy Department of Dermatology, University of Utah School of Medicine, Salt Lake City, UT.)

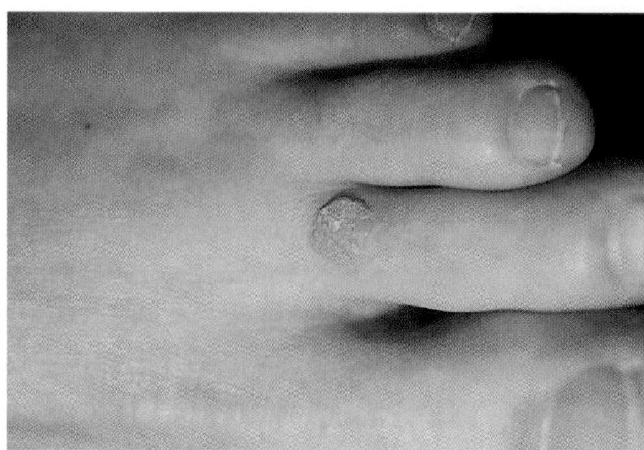

Fig. 46.20 Verruca Vulgaris (Near Toes). (Courtesy Department of Dermatology, University of Utah School of Medicine, Salt Lake City, UT.)

Condylomata acuminata (venereal warts) are caused by HPV types 6 and 11. These warts are sexually transmitted and highly contagious. The cauliflower-like lesions occur in moist areas, along the glans of the penis, vulva, and anus (see Chapter 27). Oncogenic types of HPV (e.g., 16 and 18) are a primary cause of cervical and other types of cancer and are preventable by prophylactic vaccination.[54]

Fungal infections. The fungi causing superficial skin infections are called dermatophytes, and they thrive on keratin (stratum corneum, hair, nails). Fungal disorders are known as *mycoses;* when caused by dermatophytes, the mycoses are termed *tinea* (dermatophytosis or ringworm).

Tinea infections. Tinea infections are transmitted via direct contact with the causative organism, either through person to person contact or via non-living object (fomite), such as walking barefoot on a locker room floor. They are classified according to their location on the body. Fig. 46.21 shows the location and extension of tinea pedis. The most common sites are summarized in Table 46.8. Tinea is diagnosed by culture, microscopic examination of skin scrapings prepared with potassium hydroxide (KOH) wet mount, or observation of the skin with an ultraviolet light (Wood lamp) and dermoscopy. The spores fluoresce blue-green when exposed to ultraviolet light. Cultures establish the diagnosis for a particular type of fungus. Fungi have characteristic spores and filaments, known as *hyphae*, that are more prominent when prepared in potassium hydroxide.[55] Treatment is related to the type of fungi and includes both topical and systemic antifungal medication.

Candidiasis. Candidiasis is caused by the yeastlike fungus *Candida albicans* and normally can be found on mucous membranes, on the skin, in the gastrointestinal tract, and in the vagina. *C. albicans* can change from a commensal (normal) microorganism to a pathogen, particularly in the critically ill and those who are immunosuppressed.

Factors that predispose to *C. albicans* infection include (1) local environment of moisture, warmth, maceration, or occlusion; (2) systemic administration of antibiotics; (3) pregnancy; (4) diabetes mellitus; (5) Cushing disease; (6) debilitated states; (7) infants younger than 6 months of age (as a result of decreased immune reactivity); (8) immunosuppression; and (9) certain neoplastic diseases of the blood and monocyte/macrophage system.

The commensal bacteria on the skin, mainly cocci, inhibit proliferation of *C. albincans*. Cell-mediated immunity plays a major role in the defense against infections. *C. albincans* can activate the complement system by the alternative pathway resulting in abscess. Candidiasis affects only the outer layers of mucous membranes and skin, and occurs in the mouth, vagina, uncircumcised penis, nail folds, interdigital areas, and large skin folds (inframammary area, intertriginous area, perianal region, and abdominal creases). Table 46.9 lists the points of differentiation of various sites of candidiasis habitation. *C. albincans* is highly adaptable in the human host environment, thus promoting its infection and colonization.[56] Invasive candidiasis can affect the blood, heart, brain, eyes, bones, and other parts of the body and is a serious infection associated with high morbidity and mortality.[57]

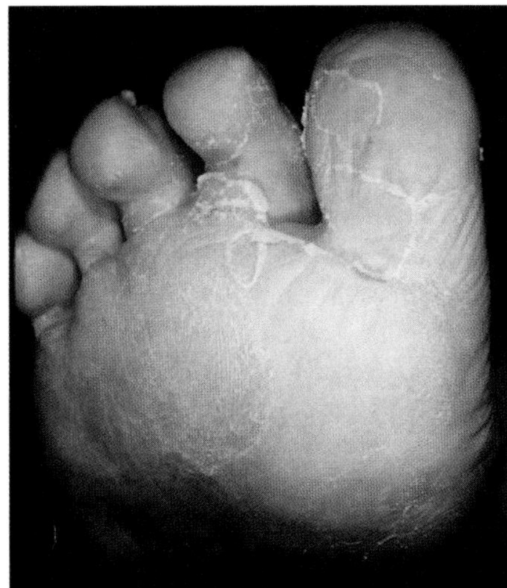

Fig. 46.21 Tinea Pedis. Inflammation has extended from the web area onto the dorsum of the foot. (Courtesy Department of Dermatology, University of Utah School of Medicine, Salt Lake City, UT.)

TABLE 46.8 Common Sites of Tinea Infections

Site	Clinical Manifestations
Tinea capitis (scalp)	Scaly, pruritic scalp with bald areas; hair breaks easily
Tinea corporis (skin areas, excluding scalp, face, hands, feet, groin; also known as "ringworm")	Circular, clearly circumscribed, mildly erythematous scaly patches with slightly elevated ringlike border; some forms are dry and macular, and other forms are moist and vesicular with satellite pustules
Tinea cruris (groin, also known as "jock itch")	Small, erythematous, and scaling vesicular patches with well-defined borders that spread over inner and upper surfaces of thighs; occurs with heat and high humidity
Tinea pedis (foot; also known as "athlete's foot")	Occurs between toes and may spread to soles of feet, nails, and skin or toes; slight scaling; macerated, painful skin, occasionally with fissures and vesiculation
Tinea manuum (palmar surface of the hand)	Dry, scaly, erythematous, annular lesions, or moist, vesicular lesions that begin with clusters of intensely pruritic, clear vesicles; often associated with fungal infection of feet
Tinea unguium or onychomycosis (nails)	Superficial or deep inflammation of nail that develops yellow-brown accumulations of brittle keratin over all or portions of nail

TABLE 46.9 Sites of Candidiasis

Site	Risk Factors	Clinical Manifestations
Vagina (vulvovaginitis, most common)	Heat, moisture, occlusive clothing Systemic glucocorticoid therapy Systemic antibiotic therapy Increased estrogen levels (contraception, pregnancy) Diabetes mellitus Immunocompromise (disease or therapy) Sexual intercourse with infected male	Vaginal *itching*, white, watery, or creamy *discharge* Red, swollen vaginal and labial membranes with erosions Lesions may spread to anus and groin
Penis (balanitis)	Uncircumcised Sexual intercourse with infected partner	Pinpoint, red, tender papules and pustules on glans and shaft of penis
Mouth (oropharyngeal)	Diabetes mellitus Immunocompromise (disease or therapy) Inhaled steroid therapy Bottle fed infants Older adults who wear dentures	Red, swollen, painful tongue and oral mucous membranes Localized erosions and plaques appear with chronic infection
Skinfolds (intertrigo)	Heat and moisture Diabetes mellitus Immunocompromise (disease or therapy) Obesity Bedridden	Pruritic and erythematous plaques with satellite papules and pustules Abdominal, inguinal, and breast skin fold.

Vascular Disorders

Vascular abnormalities are commonly associated with skin diseases; they may be congenital or may involve vascular responses to local or systemic vasoactive substances. Blood vessels may increase in number, dilate, constrict, or become obliterated by disease processes.

Cutaneous Vasculitis

Vasculitis (angiitis) is an inflammation of the blood vessel wall that can result in bleeding aneurysm formation, or occlusion with ischemia or infection of surrounding tissue. The extensive vascular bed in the skin results in vasculitic syndromes that may be localized and self-limiting or generalized with multiorgan involvement. The initiating site may be the blood, the vessel wall, or the adjacent tissue. Small vessels are usually affected.

Cutaneous small vessel vasculitis (CSVV) develops from the deposit of immune complexes in small blood vessels as a toxic response to drugs (penicillin, cephalosporins, phenytoin, allopurinol, sulfonamides), allergens, streptococcal or viral infection (such as hepatitis B or C), or as a component of systemic vasculitic syndromes. The deposits activate complement, which is chemotactic for polymorphonuclear leukocytes (neutrophils), and proinflammatory cytokines. This results in palpable purpura and/or petechiae lesions. The lower extremities and feet are the chief sites affected. The lesion may initially present with burning, pruritis, and pain. The pattern of skin involvement may progress from purpura to hemorrhagic bullae with necrosis and ulcerations from occlusion of the vessel (Fig. 46.22). Lesions appear in clusters and persist for 1 to 4 weeks. The disease may be self-limiting and occur as a single episode. Biopsy and direct immunofluorescence confirm the diagnosis. Treatment includes avoiding triggering drugs and anti-inflammatory agents.[58]

Urticaria

Urticaria (hives) is a circumscribed area of raised erythema and edema of the dermis. Urticarial lesions are most commonly associated with type I hypersensitivity reactions to drugs (penicillin, aspirin), certain foods (strawberries, shellfish, food dyes), environmental exposure (pollen, animal dander, insect bites), systemic diseases (intestinal parasites, lupus erythematosus), or physical agents (heat or cold) (see Chapter 9). The lesions are mediated by IgE-stimulated histamine release from sensitized mast cells, basophils, or both, which causes the endothelial cells of skin blood vessels to contract increasing permeability. The leakage of fluid from the vessel appears as wheals, welts, or hives, and there may be few or many that are distributed over the entire body (Fig. 46.23). IgG antibody directed against the IgE receptor and other inflammatory and vasodilatory substances, such as serotonin, leukotrienes, prostaglandins, and kinins also may be mediators of urticaria. Most lesions resolve spontaneously within 24 hours, but new lesions may appear. Antihistamines are commonly used for treatment and all possible causes of the reaction should be removed.

Chronic urticaria (recurrent wheals for more than 6 weeks) is either idiopathic or autoimmune in origin, rarely because of allergy, and involves inappropriate activation of mast cells. Angioedema (welts or swelling deeper within the skin or mucous membranes of the face and oropharynx) is associated with both groups and more commonly affects the eyes and mouth, which can result in life-threatening respiratory compromise. Treatment includes antihistamines, steroids, and immunosuppressive agents with varying results.[59]

Scleroderma

Scleroderma is a connective tissue disease associated with immune dysregulation, vascular alterations, and progressive fibrosis. There are two categories of scleroderma. Localized scleroderma or morphea is usually more benign and self-limiting and is confined to the skin and /or underlying tissues. Systemic sclerosis is characterized by cutaneous sclerosis with organ involvement. Both disease types can vary in severity and rate of progression.[60]

Localized scleroderma (morphea) means sclerosis of the skin and underlying tissue. The disease is rare, more common in females, and the cause is unknown. Genetic predisposition, autoimmunity, and an immune reaction to a toxic substance are possible igniting mechanisms of the disease. T helper cells (Th1 and Th17) and their cytokines are associated with fibroblast proliferation and fibrosis. Several autoantibodies also have been

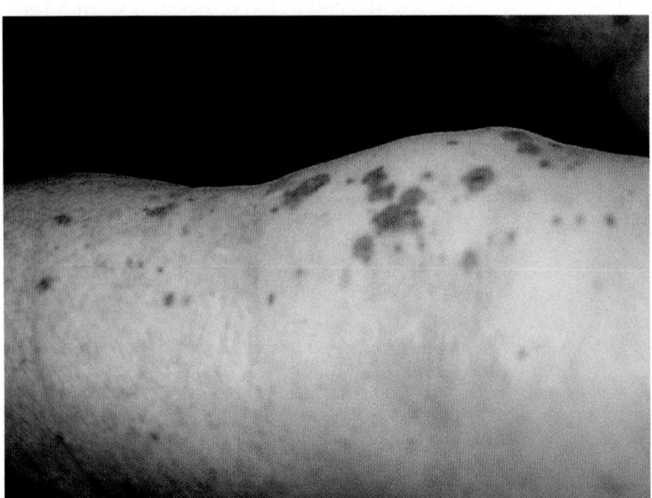

Fig. 46.22 Vasculitis of the Leg. (Courtesy Department of Dermatology, School of Medicine, University of Utah.)

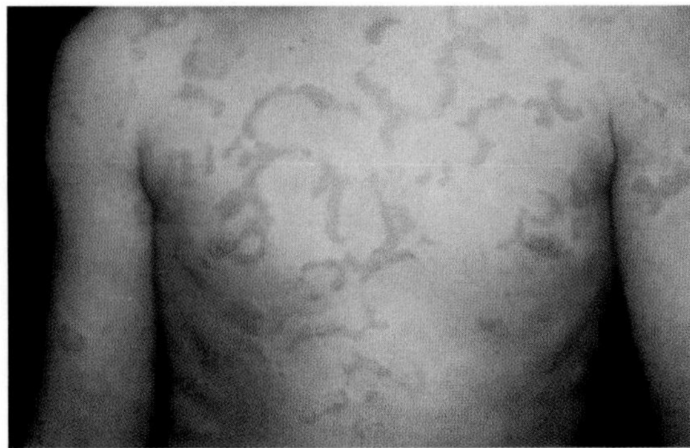

Fig. 46.23 Urticaria. (Courtesy Department of Dermatology, School of Medicine, University of Utah.)

identified, including antinuclear antibody (ANA), antihistone antibody (AHA), anti-endothelial cell antibodies and single-stranded DNA antibodies (ss-DNA ab). There are subtypes of localized scleroderma, but all involve thickening of the skin.[61] Localized scleroderma is differentiated from the systemic form of the disease by the absence of the following: sclerodactyly, Raynaud phenomenon, abnormalities of the nail bed capillaries, or internal organ involvement.

Systemic scleroderma (SSc) involves the connective tissues of the skin and internal organs, including the lungs, kidneys, gastrointestinal tract, and blood vessels.[60] Fibrosis occurs in the papillary and reticular dermis and in the subcutaneous tissue and deep fascia. There are massive deposits of type I collagen with progressive fibrosis accompanied by inflammatory reactions. Vascular changes in the capillary network with a decrease in the number of capillary loops, dilation of the remaining capillaries, formation of perivascular infiltrates, and development of occlusion and ischemia are an early manifestation.

The cutaneous lesions are most often on the face, hands, neck, and upper chest, although the entire skin can be involved. The skin is hard, hypopigmented, taut, shiny, and tightly connected to the underlying tissue. The tightness of the facial skin projects an immobile, masklike appearance, and the mouth may not open completely. The nose may assume a beaklike appearance. The hands are shiny and sometimes red and edematous (Fig. 46.24). The fingers become tapered and flexed, often with contractures, depressed scars, and loss of fingertips from atrophy. Progressive fibrosis of internal organs occurs, and death is caused by subsequent respiratory failure, cardiac dysrhythmias and heart failure, renal failure, or esophageal or intestinal obstruction or perforation. The clinical features of systemic scleroderma are summarized in Box 46.4.

Suitable clothing and a warm environment are essential for protecting the hands. Trauma and smoking should be avoided. Treatment is individualized and based on the severity and progression of the disease and includes anti-inflammatory, immunosuppressive, antifibrotic, and stem cell therapy.[62]

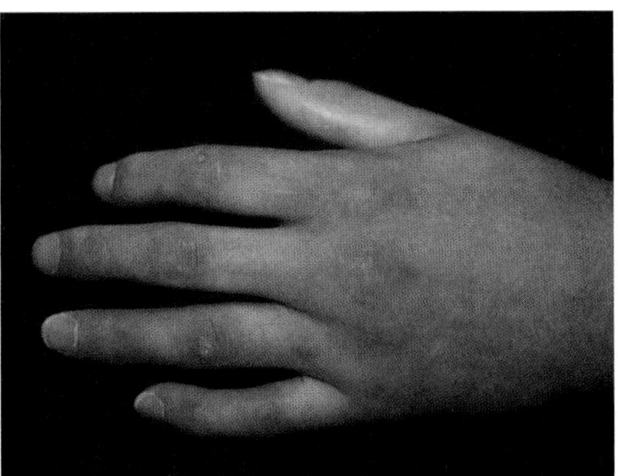

Fig. 46.24 Scleroderma. Note inflammation and shiny skin. (Courtesy Department of Dermatology, School of Medicine, University of Utah.)

BOX 46.4 Clinical Features of Systemic Scleroderma

- Raynaud phenomenon—episodes of arteriolar vasoconstriction or spasm in response to cold or stress, often a sentinel sign of disease.
- Non pitting edema of both hands
- Skin thickening of the fingers of both hands
- Sclerodactyly—tightening of skin over the fingers and toes leading to tapering of the digits with scarring and tissue atrophy
- Abnormal nail fold capillaries
- Facial skin thickening
- Telangiectasias—dilation of capillaries causing small weblike (0.5 cm) red marks on skin surface
- Pulmonary arterial hypertension and/or interstitial lung disease
- Esophageal changes—swallowing difficulty related to acid reflux and increased esophageal fibrosis
- Pericardial or myocardial disease
- Arthralgias and myalgias
- Kidney disease

Data from D'Silva KM, Bolster B. Systemic sclerosis: a comprehensive approach to diagnosis and management. *Physician Assistant Clinics*, 2021;6(1):159–175.

Benign Tumors

Most benign tumors of the skin are associated with aging. Benign tumors include seborrheic keratosis, keratoacanthoma, actinic keratosis, and moles.

Seborrheic Keratosis

Seborrheic keratosis is a benign proliferation of cutaneous basal cells that produces flat or slightly elevated lesions that may be smooth or warty in appearance. The pathogenesis is unknown. These benign tumors are usually seen in people over the age of 50 but can also appear in young adults. The lesions can occur singularly or in multiples on the chest, back, and face. The color varies from tan to waxy yellow, flesh colored, or dark brown to black. Lesion size varies from a few millimeters to several centimeters, and they are often oval and greasy-appearing, with a hyperkeratotic scaly "stuck on" appearance (Fig. 46.25). Cryotherapy with liquid nitrogen, shave excisions, and laser therapy are effective treatments. 40% hydrogen peroxide may be an alternative for facial lesions.[63]

Keratoacanthoma

A keratoacanthoma is a benign, self-limiting tumor of squamous cell differentiation arising rapidly from hair follicles. It usually occurs on sun-damaged skin of elderly and fair skinned individuals who smoke. The incidence is highest among males by nearly three times. The most commonly affected sites are the face, back of the hands, forearms, neck, and legs (Fig. 46.26). The lesion develops in stages (proliferative, mature, and involution) over a period of 1 to 2 months with a histologic pattern resembling that of squamous cell carcinoma (SCC). However, there is debate as to the relationship between KA and SCC about whether they are two distinct pathologies, or if KA is a clinical precursor to SCC and metastasis.[64]

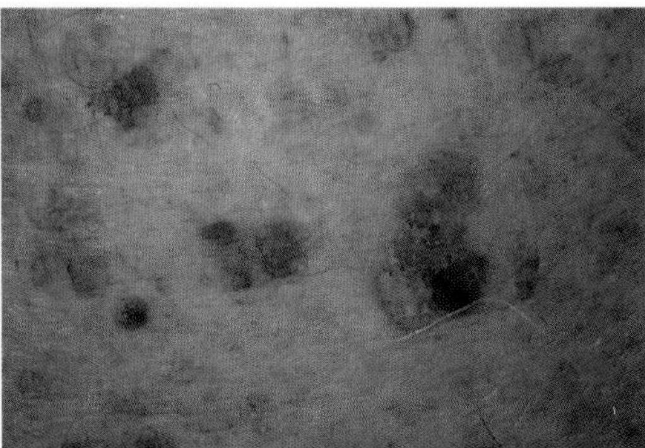

Fig. 46.25 Seborrheic Keratosis. Typical lesion is broad and flat with a comparatively smooth surface. (Courtesy Department of Dermatology, School of Medicine, University of Utah.)

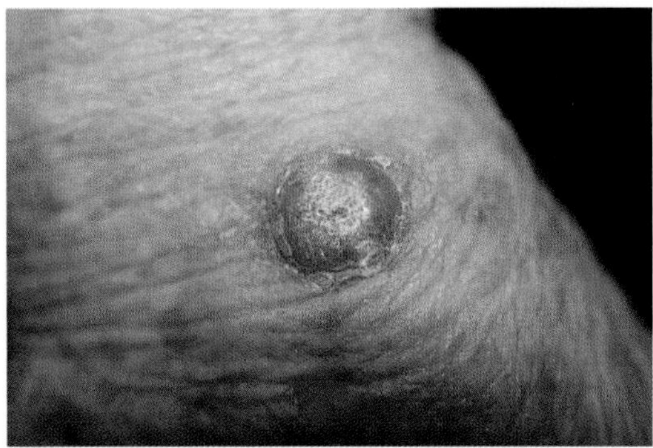

Fig. 46.26 Keratoacanthoma. Classic presentation of a fully developed tumor. Round, smooth, dome-shaped mass with a central keratin-filled crater. (Courtesy Department of Dermatology, School of Medicine, University of Utah.)

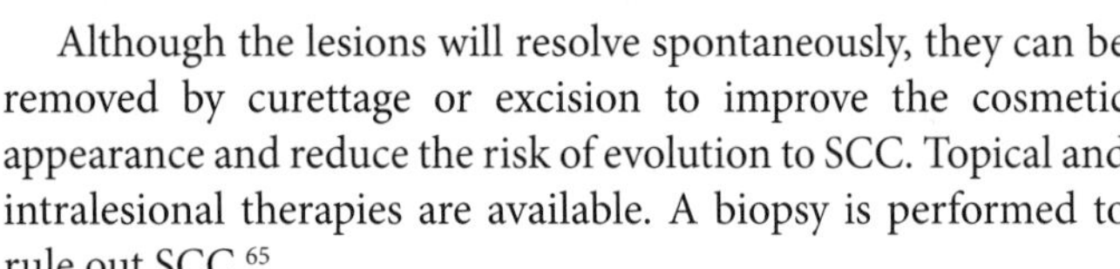

Although the lesions will resolve spontaneously, they can be removed by curettage or excision to improve the cosmetic appearance and reduce the risk of evolution to SCC. Topical and intralesional therapies are available. A biopsy is performed to rule out SCC.[65]

Actinic Keratosis

Actinic keratosis (AK), or solar keratosis, is a lesion composed of aberrant proliferations of epidermal keratinocytes caused by prolonged exposure to ultraviolet radiation. The prevalence is highest in individuals with unprotected, light-colored skin, immunosuppression, older age, and genetic predisposition. It is rare in those with dark-colored skin. The lesions may be single or multiple and appear as pink, red, or brownish patches, papules, or plaques (Fig. 46.27). Surrounding areas may have telangiectasias. AKs may evolve to SCC.[66] Dermoscopy and biopsy aid in the evaluation and differentiation between AK and SCC. The lesions should continue to be evaluated for progression to or development of SCC. Treatment options include cryoablation, photodynamic therapy, laser surgery, and topical therapies. Continuous sun protection is important.[67]

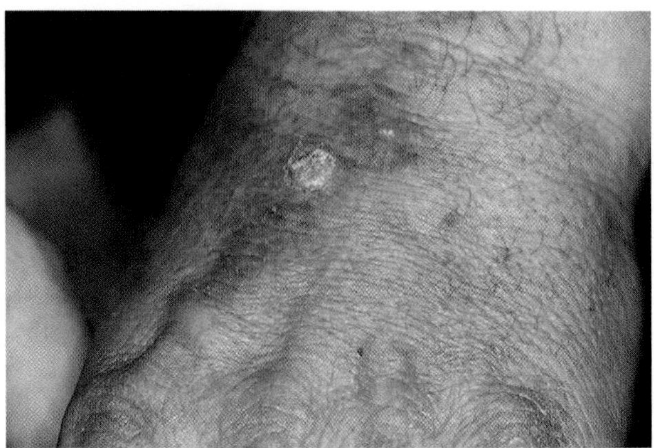

Fig. 46.27 Actinic Keratosis. (Courtesy Department of Dermatology, School of Medicine, University of Utah.)

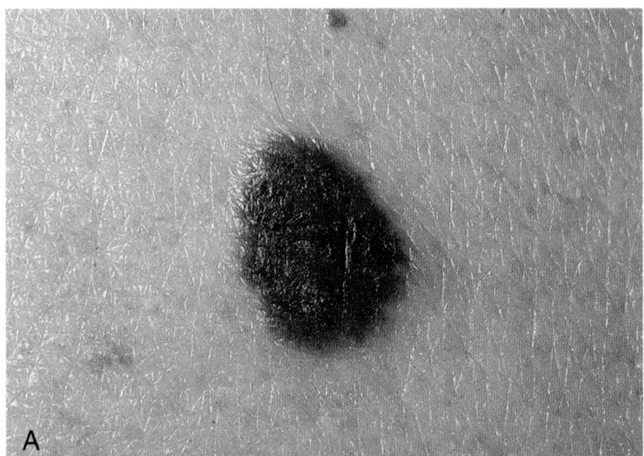

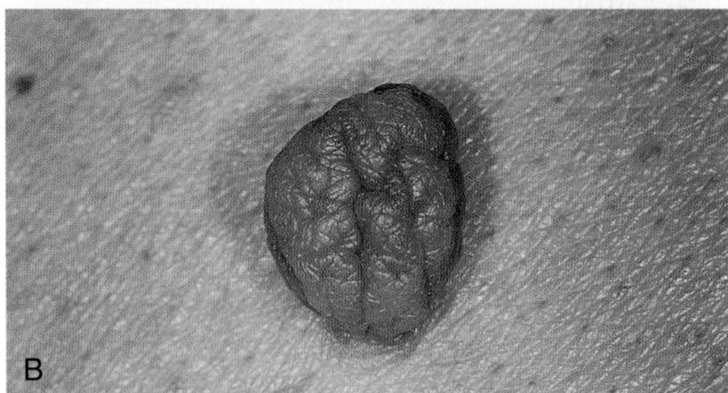

Fig. 46.28 Nevi. (A) Junction nevus: slightly raised, dark, and uniform. **(B)** Dermal nevus: pedunculated with a soft, flabby, wrinkled surface. (From Habif TP. *Clinical dermatology: A color guide to diagnosis and therapy*, 5th edition. Philadelphia: Mosby; 2010.)

Nevi (Moles)

Nevi (moles) are benign pigmented or nonpigmented lesions (Fig. 46.28). Melanocytic nevi, formed from melanocytes, may be congenital or acquired and small (less than 1 cm) or large (greater than 20 cm). During the early stages of nevi development, the cells accumulate at the junction of the dermis and epidermis (junctional nevi) and are macular lesions. Over time, the cells move deeper into the dermis and the nevi become nodular and symmetric without irregular borders (compound nevi). Nevi may appear on any part of the skin, may vary in size, may occur singly or in groups, and may undergo transition to malignant melanoma. Nevi irritated by clothing or trauma or large lesions may be excised. Multiple and changing moles require regular evaluation.[68]

Skin Cancer

Cutaneous basal cell carcinoma (BCC) and SCC are collectively known as nonmelanoma skin cancers, which are the most prevalent forms of cancer. Malignant melanoma is the most serious type of skin cancer and the most common cause of death from skin cancer.[69] Important trends related to skin cancer are described in Box 46.5.

Chronic exposure to UV radiation causes most skin cancers. Lesions are most common on the face, neck, hands, and other areas subject to intense, repetitive sunlight exposure. Protection from the sun and avoidance of tanning beds, particularly during childhood, significantly reduce the risk of skin cancer in later years. Genetic mutations in oncogenes and tumor-suppressor genes (see Chapter 12) are associated with skin cancers. This leads to loss of keratinocyte repair functions and apoptosis resistance of DNA-damaged cells.[70] Dark-skinned persons and those who avoid sunlight are significantly less likely to develop these malignant tumors. In dark-skinned persons, basal cells contain more of the pigment melanin, a protective factor against sun exposure.

Basal Cell Carcinoma

Basal cell carcinoma (BCC) of the skin is the most common cancer in the world. BCC is thought to be caused by UV radiation exposure and is also associated with arsenic in food or water, radiation therapy, and long-term immunosuppressive therapy. BCC is a surface epithelial tumor originating from undifferentiated basal or stem cells. It arises from mutation in the TP53 tumor-suppressor gene, leading to loss of keratinocyte repair functions and apoptosis resistance of DNA-damaged cells. BCC is primarily associated with the Sonic Hedgehog signaling axis with disinhibition of the PTCH1 gene and overexpression of the signaling pathway.[71]

BCCs have numerous subtypes, including superficial, nodular, morpheaform (sclerosing), and combinations of these. Thus, they can have very different clinical presentations (Fig. 46.29). The lesion often begins as a nodule (greater than 5 mm) that is pearly or ivory in appearance and slightly elevated above the skin surface with small blood vessels on the surface (telangiectasias). The tumors grow upward and laterally or downward to the dermal-epidermal junction. They usually have depressed centers and rolled borders. As the lesion grow, it often ulcerates, develops crusting, and becomes firm to the touch. If left untreated, basal cell lesions invade surrounding tissues and, over months or years, can destroy a nose, eyelid, or ear. Metastasis is rare because these tumors do not invade blood or lymph vessels.

Treatment includes complete surgical excision (micrographic surgery with histologic analysis), radiotherapy, curettage, cryotherapy, photodynamic therapy, and topical applications of imiquimod or 5-fluorouracil. If left untreated, basal cell lesions invade surrounding tissues and, over months or years, destroy tissue (i.e., nose, eyelid, or ear). These are known as locally advanced basal cell carcinomas (laBCC). Metastatic spread is rare because these tumors do not invade blood or lymph vessels. In laBCC or inoperable tumors, the Smoothened receptor in the Sonic Hedgehog pathway can be inhibited using targeted drugs.[72]

BOX 46.5 Important Trends for Skin Cancer

Nonmelanoma skin cancer was reported at more than 5.4 million cases among 3.3 million people in the United States in 2012, the most recent year new statistics available.

Greater in women younger than age 40 years; greater in men after age 40 years; 40 times more prevalent in whites than in blacks; increases steadily with age; increasing among young individuals with chronic exposure to artificial UV radiation

Majority of cases are highly curable basal or squamous cell cancers, and the most serious is malignant melanoma with an estimated 106,110 new cases and 101,280 cases of in situ melanoma in 2021; it represents 1% of all skin cancer cases but causes about 79% of all skin cancer deaths.

Mortality

Total estimated deaths in 2016 were 10,130 from melanoma and approximately 3520 from other nonepithelial types of skin cancer.

Risk Factors

Excessive exposure to ultraviolet radiation from the sun

Exposure to artificial UV radiation, particularly in ages less than 25 years

Fair complexion, blue eyes, blonde hair

Occupational exposure to coal tar, pitch, creosote, arsenic compounds, and radium

Exposure to human papillomavirus and human immunodeficiency virus

Immunosuppression

Family history of skin cancer

Skin cancer is negligible in blacks because of heavy skin pigmentation

Warning Signals

Any change on the skin, especially a change in the size or color of a mole or other darkly pigmented growth or spot

Prevention and Early Detection

Avoidance of artificial UV radiation and sun when ultraviolet light is strongest (e.g., 10 a.m. to 3 p.m.); use of protective clothing and sunscreen preparations, especially those containing ingredients such as *para*-aminobenzoic acid (PABA); prevention for all types of skin cancer should begin in childhood

Routine visual screening for skin cancer may be a benefit for those at highest risk.

Survival

For basal cell and squamous cell cancers, cure is highly likely with early detection and treatment; malignant melanoma metastasizes quickly, accounting for a lower 5-year survival rate

Data from American Cancer Society. *Cancer Facts and Figures 2021.* Atlanta: The Society; 2021; Carr S, Smith C, Wernberg J. Epidemiology and risk factors of melanoma. *Surgical Clinics of North America,* 2020;100(1):1–12.

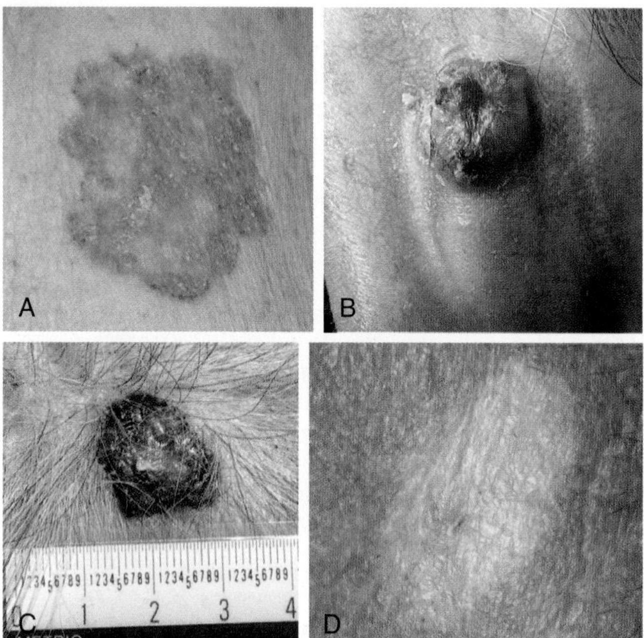

Fig. 46.29 Types of Basal Cell Carcinoma. **(A)** Superficial. **(B)** Nodular. **(C)** Pigmented. **(D)** Morpheaform-recurrent tumor. (A and D from Bolognia JL, et al. *Dermatology*, 3rd edition. Philadelphia: Saunders; 2012. B and C from James WD, et al. *Andrews' diseases of the skin: Clinical dermatology*, 11th edition. Philadelphia: Saunders; 2009.)

Squamous Cell Carcinoma

Squamous cell carcinoma (SCC) of the skin is a malignant tumor of the epidermis and is the second most common human cancer. Two types are characterized: in situ and invasive. Chronic UV radiation exposure causes SCC via mutation of the TP53 gene and other oncogenic signaling; however, it is unclear as to how UV light produces the alterations in DNA, DNA repair, and resistance to apoptosis.[71] Other risk factors include genetic predilection, chronic arsenic exposure, exposure to x-rays and gamma rays, immunosuppression, and light-colored skin. Areas typically affected include sun-exposed skin of the head, neck, and hands.

Keratoacanthoma is a benign dome shaped epidermal tumor that originates from the pilosebaceous unit of the skin. It may spontaneously resolve or transform into SCC.[73]

In situ SCC is usually confined to the epidermis (intraepidermal) but may extend into the dermis. Bowen disease is a dysplasia of the epidermis or carcinoma in situ found on unexposed areas of the body, such as the glans penis (erythroplasia of Queyrat). The lesions are flat and red with scaly patches. These lesions may enlarge to more than 1 cm in diameter, rarely invading surrounding tissue, very rarely metastasize, and are associated with HPV. Other cellular components of the skin (e.g., sweat glands, hair follicles) can give rise to SCC, but these cancers are relatively uncommon. Invasive SCC can arise from premalignant lesions of the skin. Premalignant lesions include AK, leukoplakia (whitish discolored areas), scars, radiation-induced keratosis, tar and oil keratosis, and chronic ulcers. It rarely arises from normal-appearing skin (de novo). Invasive SCC grows more rapidly than BCC; it penetrates the basement membrane between epidermis and dermis and can spread to regional lymph nodes with metastasis. The tumors are firm and increase in elevation and diameter. The surface may be granular and bleed easily (Fig. 46.30).

SCC is the most common cause of *lip cancer* and is more prevalent in older white men. The lower lip is the most common site. Long-term environmental exposure results in dryness, chapping, hyperkeratosis, and predisposition to malignancy. Immunosuppression, pipe smoking, and chronic alcoholism increase the risk for lip cancer. The most common lesion is termed *exophytic* and usually develops in the outer part of the lip along the vermilion border. The lip becomes thickened and evolves to an ulcerated center with a raised border (Fig. 46.31). These lesions have an irregular surface, follow cracks in the lip, and tend to extend toward the inner surface and progress slowly. Early diagnosis and surgical resection are usually curative.[74]

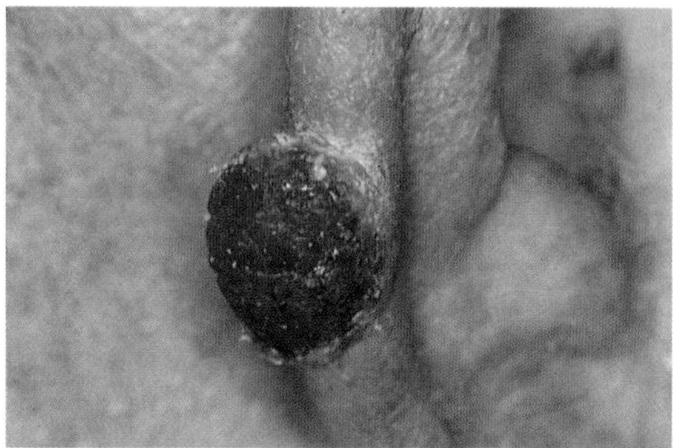

Fig. 46.30 Squamous Cell Carcinoma. The sun-exposed ear is a common site for squamous cell carcinoma. (Courtesy Department of Dermatology, School of Medicine, University of Utah.)

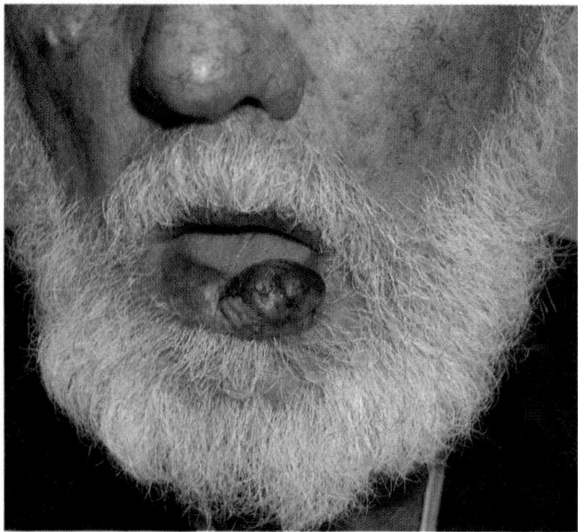

Fig. 46.31 Lip Cancer. Biopsy confirmed squamous cell carcinoma. Lip vermilion shows diffuse actinic keratosis. (From Bagheri SC, Khan HA, Cuzalina A. *Current therapy in oral and maxillofacial surgery*. Philadelphia: Saunders; 2012.)

For small, low-risk, superficial SCC, treatment includes cryotherapy, 5-FU, and photodynamic therapy. For advanced SCC, complete microsurgical excision with histologic analysis and radiotherapy with consideration of immunotherapy and adjuvant chemotherapy is recommended.[75]

Cutaneous Melanoma

Cutaneous melanoma is a malignant tumor of the skin originating from the transformation of melanocytes. Melanocytes are cells that arise from neural crest tissue and synthesize the pigment melanin. They are located in the basal layer of the skin and arise in mucosal tissue and the uveal tract. Melanoma is the most serious skin cancer, and its incidence increases with age. Risk factors include a personal or family history, or both; UV radiation exposure (including sun bed use before age 30 years); immunosuppression; fair hair; light skin with repeated sunburns; freckles; younger females and older males; geographic location; past pesticide exposure; and three or more clinically atypical (dysplastic) nevi.[76] Multiple melanocytic nevi are associated with nonchronic sun-damage melanomas and BRAF mutations and occur more commonly on the trunk and extremities. Discovering melanoma at an early stage increases 5-year survival.

Cutaneous melanomas arise as a result of malignant degeneration of melanocytes located either along the basal layer of the epidermis or in a benign melanocytic nevus. There are four major subtypes of melanoma associated with cumulative solar damage and based on their histologic growth patterns: superficial spreading melanoma (SSM), primary nodular melanoma (PNM), lentigo malignant melanoma (LMM), and acral lentiginous melanoma (ALM) (Fig. 46.32). SSM is the most common subtype of melanoma and is most likely to be associated with a preexisting nevus. Their growth is radial (or lateral) and evolves over time to vertical (invasive) growth. Typically, these lesions are asymmetrical with a variable pigment of color (red, tan, black, brown, grey, and white). PNM are vertically growing lesions that are aggressive. Rare and difficult to diagnose subtypes include desmoplastic melanoma, which resembles a scar, and amelanotic (nonpigmented) melanoma tumor with pigment loss as the tumor progresses.[77]

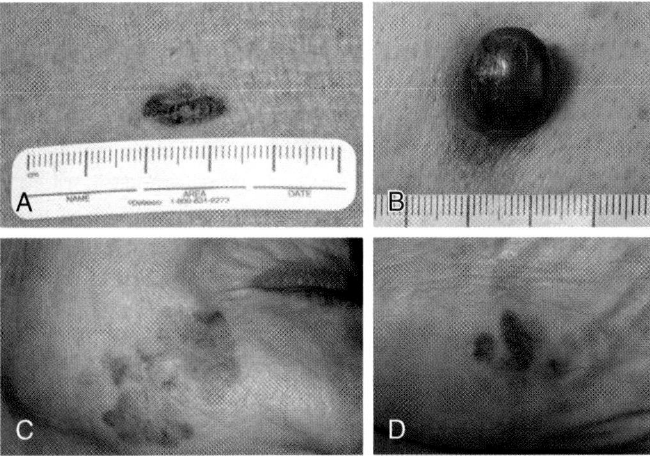

Fig. 46.32 Types of Melanoma. **(A)** Superficial spreading melanoma. **(B)** Nodular melanoma. **(C)** Lentigo malignant melanoma. **(D)** Acral lentiginous melanoma on plantar surface of foot. (From Bolognia JL, et al. *Dermatology essentials.* Philadelphia: Saunders; 2014.)

LMM is frequently found in the elderly and often confused with age spots (lentigines). Most commonly arising from sun-damaged areas of the skin, LMM present as a macule that gradually evolves into a palpable lesion. These lesions transform slowly and can be present for 10 to 50 years before the vertical growth phase begins. ALM are rare and occur on non–hair-bearing surfaces such as the palms of the hands and the soles of the feet, as well as in mucous membranes. ALM are more commonly seen in African American and Asian persons.[77] The clinical characteristics of subtypes of melanomas are summarized in Table 46.10.

The pathogenesis of malignant melanoma is complex. There is an accumulation of genetic mutations that activate oncogenes, inactivate tumor suppressor genes, and impair DNA repair genes. Most familial melanomas are associated with cyclin-dependent kinase 4 gene (CDK4) and cyclin-dependent kinase inhibitor 2A gene (p16/CDKN2A) located on chromosome 9p21, both of which function to suppress cellular growth. The CDKN2A gene encodes two potent tumor-suppressor proteins that are cell-cycle inhibitors. Both CDNKN2A and CDK4 are highly penetrant susceptibility genes and result in melanomas. A number of proto-oncogenes have been identified, including BRAF point mutations (the most common), NRAS, and genes involved in the regulation of mitogen-activated protein kinase (MAPK) and other signaling pathways. Melanomas have a high mutation rate stimulated by ultraviolet radiation (UVR), making gene sequencing difficult.[78]

The relationship between nevi and melanoma makes it important for the clinician to understand the various forms of nevi (see Fig. 46.32). Most nevi never become suspicious, but suspicious pigmented nevi need to be evaluated and removed. Indications for biopsy include any color change, size change, irregular notched margin, itching, bleeding or oozing, nodularity, scab formation, ulceration or an unusual pattern of presentation, or a de novo nevi. The ABCDE rule is used as a guide: **A**symmetry, **B**order irregularity, **C**olor variation, **D**iameter larger than 6 mm, and **E**levation or **E**volving, which includes raised appearance or rapid enlargement.[79] Staging of melanoma is determined by vertical lesion thickness (depth of **t**umor), lymph **n**ode involvement, presence of ulceration, and presence of **m**etastasis (TNM staging). Criteria established by the American Joint Committee on Cancer is used to guide treatment and is summarized in Box 46.6.

Prognostic factors include the thickness of the lesion, mitotic index, immunohistochemical assessment, ulceration, and metastasis (e.g., number of lymph nodes or viscera involved). Efforts are in progress to refine the morphologic classifications by adding subgroups that include molecular markers for proto-oncogene mutations and specific signaling pathways.[80]

Early detection of cutaneous melanomas can have a major effect on achieving a surgical cure and decreasing morality from metastatic disease. Local excision biopsy is completed for suspicious lesions. Melanoma with no evidence of metastatic disease involves wide surgical excision of the primary lesion site. A lymph node biopsy of the peripherally draining lymph node (sentinel node) is warranted for lesions greater than 1 mm deep

TABLE 46.10 Clinical Characteristics and Subtypes of Cutaneous Melanoma

Characteristic	Description
Lentigo Malignant Melanoma	
Frequency	5%–15% of cutaneous melanomas
Age at diagnosis	50–80 years old, mean age 65 years
Primary location	Head, neck, dorsum of hands (sun-exposed areas)
Pigmentation according to thickness	
<1.5 mm (levels I and II)	Tan and brown
>1.5 mm (level III)	Tan, brown, and blue-black
>1.5 mm (levels IV and V)	Nodule formation
Superficial Spreading Melanomas	
Frequency	50%–75% of cutaneous melanomas
Age at diagnosis	20–60 years old
Primary location	Legs of females; upper back of both genders
Pigmentation according to thickness	
<1.5 mm (levels I and II)	Tan and brown
>1.5 mm (level III)	Tan, brown, and blue-black
>1.5 mm (levels IV and V)	Nodule formation
Acral-Lentiginous Melanoma	
Frequency	5% –8% in whites; 30%–75% in blacks, Hispanics, Asians
Age at diagnosis	20–60 years old, male more common
Primary location	Palms, soles of feet, mucous membranes
Pigmentation at any thickness	Blue-black irregular macules, papules, or nodules
Primary Nodular Melanoma (usually invasive at diagnosis)	
Frequency	15%–35% of cutaneous melanomas
Age at diagnosis	20–60 years old, mean age 53 years
Primary location	Trunk, head, or neck
Pigmentation according to thickness	
>1.5 mm (level III)	Small nodule (any hue)
>1.5 mm (levels IV and V)	Large nodule (any hue)

Data from Johnston RB. *Weedon's skin pathology essentials*, 2nd edition. Elsevier; 2017; Longo C, Pellacani G. Melanomas. *Dermatologic Clinics*, 2016;34(4):411–419.

and, if positive, regional lymphadenectomy is performed. Lesions on the extremities have the best surgical prognosis. Radiation therapy, chemotherapy, and immunotherapy are used to treat metastatic disease and have demonstrated long-term improvement in disease outcome. Promising new immunotherapies are used for advanced disease, including checkpoint inhibitors, programmed cell death protein 1 (PD-1) receptor antibody, anti-CTLA4 antibody, and targeted therapy, including *BRAF* and/or mitogen-activated protein kinase kinase (MEK) inhibition, *C-kit* gene inhibitors of tyrosine kinases, and platelet derived growth factor. Vaccines, cell therapy, and biomarkers to assess treatment effectiveness are under continuing investigation. Prevention of melanoma includes avoidance of UVR exposure through use of protective clothing and sunscreens, as well as avoidance of artificial UVR exposure.[81]

BOX 46.6 Tumor, Node, Metastasis Staging Criteria for Melanoma

Stage 0: carcinoma in situ (TisN0M0)
Stage I A/B: includes lesions up to 2 mm with no nodal or distant metastases (T1aN0M0, T1bN0M0, T2aN0M0).
Stage II A/B/C: includes larger lesions, greater than 2 mm without positive nodes or distant metastases (T2bN0M0, T3aN0M0, T3bN0M0, T4aN0M0, T4bN0M0).
Stage III: includes lesions of any size with positive lymph nodes (TxN1M0, TxN2M0, TxN3M0).
Stage IV: includes lesions of any size with distant metastases (TxNxM1).

Data from Keung EZ, Gershenwald JE. The eighth edition American Joint Committee on Cancer (AJCC) melanoma staging system: Implications for melanoma treatment and care. *Expert Review of Anticancer Therapy*, 2018;18(8):775–784.

Merkel Cell Carcinoma

Merkel cell (a skin mechanoreceptor) carcinoma is a very rare aggressive cutaneous carcinoma usually localized to the head and neck. Risk factors include ultraviolet radiation, Merkel cell polyomavirus infection, immunosuppression, male, and age older than 50 years. The lesions appear as nodules or skin-colored or purple dome-shaped papules or plaques, usually on sun-exposed areas of the skin. Treatment includes wide excision and adjuvant radiotherapy. Targeted therapies, including checkpoint inhibitors, are improving outcomes. Mortality is high for metastatic lesions.[82]

Kaposi Sarcoma

Kaposi sarcoma (KS) is a vascular malignancy associated with immunodeficiency states. Human herpesvirus type 8 (HHV8 also known as Kaposi sarcoma herpes virus [KSHV]) is the etiological agent and is found in all lesions of KS. HHV8 is also associated with primary effusion lymphoma and multicentric Castleman's disease. Four forms of KS have been described: classic (more benign and more common in men), epidemic (rapidly progressive and associated with AIDS), endemic (associated with HPV and occurring in equatorial Africa), and iatrogenic (associated with immunosuppressant treatment, including organ transplant). Genetic and environmental cofactors determine disease progression. The virus can remain latent and avoid immune surveillance or have lytic reactivation and spread to new hosts.[83]

Saliva is thought to be the primary route of transmission, however KSHV has also been detected in breast milk, semen, and blood. The endothelial cell is the progenitor of KS with inflammation, angiogenesis, and cellular proliferation. Infection with KSHV is lifelong because the virus can establish latency in endothelial cells and B cells. The viral genome is replicated with the host genome during normal cell division.[84] The lesions

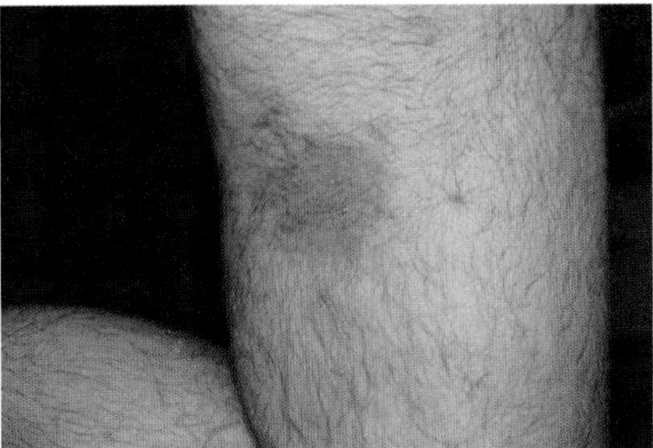

Fig. 46.33 Kaposi Sarcoma. The purple lesion commonly seen on the skin. (Courtesy Department of Dermatology, University of Utah School of Medicine, Salt Lake City, UT.)

emerge as red, purple, or brown macules and develop into plaques and nodules. They tend to be multifocal rather than spreading by metastasis. The lesions initially appear over the lower extremities in the classic form (Fig. 46.33). The rapidly progressive form associated with AIDS tends to spread symmetrically over the upper body, particularly the face and oral mucosa. The lesions are often pruritic and painful. Most individuals with epidemic KS have involvement of lymph nodes, particularly in the gastrointestinal tract and lungs. Organ involvement is much less common in the classic form than in the epidemic form. The rapidly progressive form has a poor prognosis and shorter survival rates than the classic form. (See Chapter 10 for a further discussion of AIDS.)

Diagnosis is by medical history, physical examination, and skin biopsy, with a high index of suspicion for those with immunodeficiency. Local lesions can be removed or treated topically. Multiple disseminated lesions may be treated with a combination of α-interferon, radiotherapy, and cytotoxic drugs. Antiangiogenic agents are being tested. Individuals receiving highly active antiretroviral therapy (HAART) have a markedly reduced incidence of KS.[85]

Primary Cutaneous Lymphomas

Primary cutaneous lymphomas are cutaneous T-cell and B-cell neoplasms present in the skin without evidence of extracutaneous disease at the time of diagnosis (see Chapter 29) for classification and general pathophysiology of lymphomas). Cutaneous lymphomas develop from clonal expansion of B cells, T-helper cells, and rarely, T-suppressor cells. Cutaneous lymphomas are more common in men and generally present after age 50; 75% of cases are T-cell lymphomas and 25% are B-cell lymphomas.[86] Mycosis fungoides is the most prominent subtype of cutaneous T cell lymphoma (CTCL). Mycosis fungoides can present as focal or widespread erythematous patches or plaques, follicular papules, comedone-like lesions, and tumors (Fig. 46.34) Lesions are pruritic and cause considerable distress and debilitation. There may be patches of alopecia. The lesions progress over a period of months or years. Involvement of other organs can occur in advanced stages of the disease. Sézary syndrome (a leukemic variant) and primary cutaneous

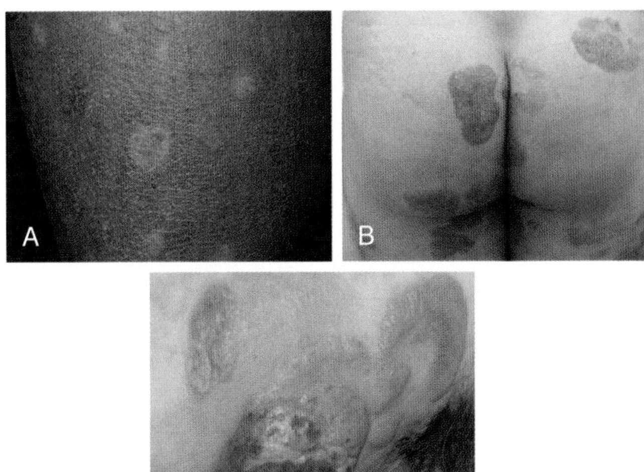

Fig. 46.34 Mycosis Fungoides. **(A)** Hypopigmented patches of mycosis fungoides. **(B)** Plaques of mycosis fungoides. **(C)** Tumors of mycosis fungoides combined with patches. (Courtesy of Ellen Korn, M.D. In James WD, Berger TG, Elston DM. *Andrews' diseases of the skin: Clinical dermatology*, 11th edition. Philadelphia: Saunders; 2011.)

CD30-positive lymphoproliferative disorders are most aggressive. Cutaneous B-cell Lymphomas (CBCL) are less common than CTCL and include primary cutaneous marginal zone lymphoma, primary cutaneous follicle center lymphoma, primary cutaneous diffuse large B-cell lymphoma (leg type), and Epstein-Barr virus (EBV)—positive mucocutaneous ulcer.[87]

The differential diagnosis of the different types of cutaneous lymphomas is based on clinical manifestations, histologic, immunologic, and cytogenetic features, and response to appropriate treatment. Treatment is based on the clinical presentation and staging of the disease and includes topical therapy, immunotherapy, chemotherapy, radiation therapy, and phototherapy.[88]

Cold Injury

Exposure to extreme cold includes a spectrum of injuries[89]:

- *Frostnip*—mild and completely reversible cold injury characterized by skin pallor and numbness, no permanent tissue damage (Fig. 46.35)
- *Chilblains*—more serious than frostnip; violaceous skin color with plaques or nodules, pain, and pruritus, but no ice crystal formation; repetitive exposure to damp cold (above freezing point); chronic vasculitis can develop; permanent damage is uncommon
- *Frostbite*—tissues freeze and form ice crystals at temperatures below −2°C (28°F); progresses from distal to proximal and potentially reversible
- *Flash freeze*—rapid cooling with intracellular ice crystals associated with contact with cold metals or volatile liquids

The most common areas affected are fingers, toes, ears, nose, and cheeks. Skin damage can range from mild to severe. Initially, the body responds with alternating cycles of vasoconstriction and vasodilation—the hunting reflex. The mechanism of injury

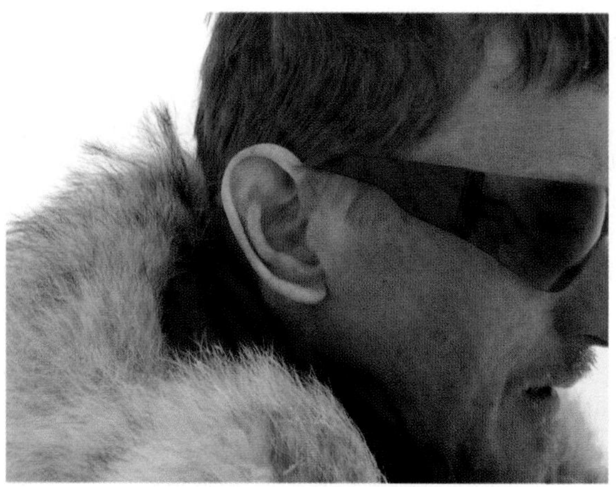

Fig. 46.35 Frostnip on an ear. (Courtesy Ian Davis. From Auerbach, PS. *Wilderness medicine*, 6th edition. Philadelphia: Elsevier; 2012.)

is complex but is related to direct cold injury to cells, indirect injury, cell death from extracellular and intracellular ice crystal formation, impaired circulation with anoxia because of thrombosis in the exposed area, and re-perfusion injury. Mild frostbite causes pallor and pain, followed by redness and discomfort during rewarming, with no tissue damage. Frostbite occurs when tissues freeze slowly with ice crystal formation. Frozen skin becomes white or yellowish and has a waxy texture. There is numbness and no sensation of pain. Frostbite injury is related to direct cold injury to cells, indirect injury from ice crystal formation, and endothelial cell damage. During rewarming, there is indirect injury related to progressive microvascular thrombosis followed by reperfusion injury with the release of inflammatory mediators (including thromboxanes, prostaglandins, bradykinins, and histamines) with impaired circulation and anoxia to the exposed area. Cyanosis and mottling develop, followed by redness, edema, and burning pain on rewarming in more severe cases. Edema can cause capillary compression and vascular stasis. Within 24 to 48 hours, vesicles and bullae appear that resolve into crusts that eventually slough, leaving thin, newly formed skin. Frostbite may be classified by depth of injury: first degree, second degree, third degree, and forth degree.[90]

- *First degree:* superficial, characterized by a numb central white area surrounded by erythema and edema; includes partial skin freezing without bullae
- *Second degree:* full-thickness skin freezing with bullae and surrounding erythema and edema; develops within 24 hours of exposure; there is no tissue loss
- *Third degree:* full-thickness and subcutaneous freezing with tissue necrosis; hemorrhagic vesicle formation; black eschar develops in one to several weeks
- *Fourth-degree:* extends past the subcutaneous level of the skin to muscle and bone; complete tissue necrosis with clear line of demarcated tissue loss

A prediction tool has been developed for frostbite of the hands and feet. It is based on the appearance of the lesions after the affected area has been treated in warm water.[91]

Grade 1: no cyanosis; no amputation or sequelae likely
Grade 2: distal cyanosis; soft tissue amputation as well as nail sequelae likely
Grade 3: distal and intermediate cyanosis; bone amputation of the digit and functional sequelae likely
Grade 4: cyanosis over the proximal areas of the hands or feet (carpal or tarsal bones); bone amputation of the limb and functional sequalae likely

Frostbite can develop in minutes. Risk factors for frostbite includes any activity that would increase heat loss or decrease the body's ability to produce heat. Examples of heat loss through convection include exposure to wind. Conductive heat loss can develop via contact with metal or water. Concomitant medical conditions that increase risk include peripheral arterial disease, diabetes, mental illness, alcohol abuse, dehydration, and malnutrition. Environmental conditions that increase risk include wind and higher altitudes.[91]

Imaging is important for determining the precise severity, depth, and level of tissue injury, the proper demarcation of dead tissue and for monitoring response to treatment. Immediate treatment of frostbite is removal of wet clothing and covering affected areas with other body surfaces and warm clothing. The area should not be rubbed or massaged. Rewarming for severe frostbite should occur with immersion in a warm water bath (40°C to 42°C [104°F to 107.6°F]) until frozen tissue is thawed. Pain is severe and should be treated with potent analgesics. Antibiotics may be given. Vasodilators, thrombolytics, hyperbaric oxygen, and sympathectomy may improve healing responses. Debridement or amputation of necrotic tissue occurs when there is a clear line of demarcation.

DISORDERS OF THE HAIR

Alopecia

Alopecia means partial or complete loss of hair from an area of the body where it normally grows. Hair loss occurs when there is disruption in the growth phase of the hair follicle. Hair loss can be associated with systemic disorders such as hypothyroidism and iron deficiency, chemotherapy for cancer, malnutrition, compulsive hair pulling (trichotillomania), traction on hair from braiding and ponytails, use of hair treatment chemicals, hormonal alterations, peripheral arterial disease, medications, and immune reactions.

Androgenic Alopecia

Androgenic alopecia, or localized hair loss, occurs in about 80% of men by 80 years of age. It is not a disease but rather a variation in the androgen receptor (AR) gene and a predisposed response to androgens that clusters in families. Within the distribution of hair over the scalp, androgen-sensitive hair follicles are on top and androgen-insensitive follicles are on the sides and back. In genetically predisposed men, the androgen-sensitive follicles are transformed into vellus follicles. The normal hair is shed and replaced by vellus hair which is fine, light, and short. Male-pattern baldness begins with frontotemporal recession and progresses to loss of hair over the top of the scalp.[92] Minoxidil may be used to stimulate hair growth. It relaxes smooth muscle around hair follicles and hair follicle perfusion increases, extending the anagen phase of hair growth and delaying conversion from terminal to vellus hair. Finasteride (a 5α-reductase inhibitor) may reduce the effect of androgens on hair follicles. Options are available for non-medical treatment including low level laser therapy and microneedling.[93]

Female-Pattern Alopecia

Female pattern alopecia, formerly known as androgenetic alopecia, is the slow progressive thinning and loss of terminal hair over the central part of the scalp. Prevalence increases with advancing age. Contrary to male-pattern baldness, there is usually no loss of hair along the frontal hairline but the hairs are shorter and thinner (follicular miniaturization). The mechanism of hair loss is unknown but related to genetic and hormonal changes. The role of androgens is not clearly known. Treatment includes topical minoxidil and light therapy.[94]

Alopecia Areata

Alopecia areata is an autoimmune T-cell–mediated or natural killer cell mediated chronic inflammatory disease with loss of immune privilege in hair follicles. Exposure to self-antigens promotes infiltration of inflammatory cells, release of interferon gamma and other cytokines, and inflammation and apoptosis that disrupts the normal hair cycle, resulting in inhibition of hair growth.[95,96] There is a rapid onset of hair loss in multiple areas of the scalp, usually in round patches. The eyebrows, eyelashes, beard, and other areas of body hair can be involved. The cause is not completely understood, but stressful events, genetic susceptibility, and metabolic disorders (e.g., Addison disease, thyroid disease, and lupus erythematosus) are associated with alopecia areata.

The affected areas have round or oval hair loss that may coalesce. The skin is smooth or may have short shafts of poorly developed hair that breaks at the surface ("exclamation point" hairs) with white shafts. Regrowth occurs within 1 year, but hair loss may recur at the same site. Permanent regrowth of hair usually occurs but is unpredictable. Some individuals will progress to total loss of scalp hair (alopecia totalis) or loss of all body hair (alopecia universalis). The diagnosis is made by observation of the pattern of hair loss. Biopsy may show a lymphocytic infiltrate around the follicle. There are several treatments for alopecia areata, including corticosteroids and topical immunotherapy, but long-term effectiveness is difficult to achieve.[97]

Hirsutism

Hirsutism occurs in women and is the abnormal growth and distribution of terminal hair on the face, body, and pubic area in a male pattern. There is also frontotemporal hair recession. These areas of hair growth are androgen sensitive. Variations of hair growth in women are great, and a male pattern may be normal. The development of hirsutism is usually a result of an underlying endocrine disorder such as polycystic ovarian syndrome (PCOS), adrenal hyperplasia, or adrenal tumors. These disorders require specific treatment. If no hormonal pathologic conditions exist, treatment may include cosmetic removal of hair, suppression of excessive androgen production, or blockage of peripheral androgen receptors.[98]

DISORDERS OF THE NAIL

Paronychia

Paronychia is an acute or chronic inflammation of the lateral and/or proximal nail fold. One or more fingers or toes may be involved. Individuals whose hands are frequently exposed to moisture are at greatest risk, along with habits such as nail biting, nail picking, thumb sucking, and excessive manicuring. Acute paronychia is manifested by the rapid onset of painful inflammation of the cuticle, usually after minor trauma. An abscess may develop requiring incision and drainage for relief of pain. The skin around the nail becomes more edematous and painful with progressive infection. Pus may be expressed from the proximal nail fold, and an abscess may develop. The nail plate is usually not affected, although it can become discolored with ridges. Typically, organisms present in the skin's normal flora such as *S. aureus* and *S. pyogenes* will be the culprit. Occasionally *Proteus vulgaris* and *Candida* will be present.

Chronic paronychia develops slowly and has been present for more than six weeks. There is tenderness and swelling around the proximal or lateral nail folds that tends to affect more than one nail. It is typically caused by repeated exposure to irritants or allergens that entices infiltrating organisms, such as those encountered by health care workers, food handlers, and farmers. Prevalence of chronic paronychia is also associated with other inflammatory skin disorders.[99]

Treatment includes prevention by keeping the hands dry. Oral antifungals are not effective because they do not penetrate the affected tissues. Therapy includes warm soaks, oral antibiotics and topical application of anti-inflammatory agents and antifungals, steroids, or calcineurin inhibitors.

Onychomycosis

Onychomycosis is a chronic infection of the toenails or fingernails caused by fungi, dermatophyte, yeasts, or nondermatophyte molds or mixed infections. Dermatophyte infection is the most common, typically caused by Trichophyton mentagrophytes and Trichophyton rubrum. Candida species are the most common yeasts. Transmission requires direct contact with the offending agent. Many times, infection from the toenails will transfer to the fingernails through nail picking or biting. Presentation varies, but discoloration, hyperkeratosis, splitting, and nail plate destruction are common. The most common pattern is a nail plate that turns yellow or white and becomes elevated with the accumulation of hyperkeratotic debris within the plate. Fungal infections of the nail are differentiated from psoriasis, lichen planus, and trauma by culture, microscopy and polymerase chain reaction. There is absence of pitting on the nail surface, which is characteristic of psoriasis. Treatment is difficult because topical or systemic antifungal agents do not penetrate the nail plate readily. Systemic antifungal drugs are effective and topical drugs are available; when used in combination the potential for success improves. Rarely, surgical excision of the nail may be required. Education is essential to preventing recurrence.[100]

GERIATRIC CONSIDERATIONS

Aging and Changes in Skin Integrity

- Skin becomes thinner, dryer, and more wrinkled with loss of pigmentation. These changes are accelerated by exposure to ultraviolet light exposure, air pollution, tobacco smoke, poor nutrition, and gravity.
- DNA repair of damaged skin decreases.
- Keratinocyte atrophy and cells contain less moisture and change shape.
- A loss of epidermal rete pegs occurs, which weakens the connection to the dermis and gives skin a smooth, shiny, and wrinkled appearance with an increased likelihood of tearing from shearing forces.
- The dermis thins, producing translucent, paper-thin quality that is more susceptible to tearing.
- Dermal fibroblasts age and release proinflammatory mediators and disrupt collagen synthesis with loss of extracellular matrix. The dermis becomes more permeable and less able to clear noxious substances, so they accumulate, cause irritation, and delay wound healing. There is a loss of elastin, contributing to wrinkling.
- There is a loss of flexibility of collagen fibers, so skin cannot stretch and regain shape as readily.
- The barrier function of the stratum corneum is diminished, increasing the risk for injury and infection.
- A significantly decreased number of Langerhans cells reduces the skin's immune response.
- The dermoepidermal border flattens, shortening and reducing the number of capillary loops.

Other Skin Changes With Aging

- Wound healing declines as a result of decreased estrogen in both men and women, decreased blood flow, and a slower rate of basal cell and fibroblast turnover.
- There are fewer melanocytes; pigmentation becomes irregular, giving decreased protection from ultraviolet radiation and leading to graying of hair.
- Atrophy of eccrine, apocrine, and sebaceous glands causes dry skin.
- Pressure and touch receptors and free nerve endings decrease in number, causing reduced sensory perception.
- With compromised temperature regulation, loss of cutaneous vasomotion, and decreased eccrine sweat production, there is an increased risk of heat stroke and hypothermia.
- Loss of hair stem cells results in thinner finer hair.
- The nail plate thins, and nails are more brittle.

Data from Chambers ES, Vukmanovic-Stejic M. Skin barrier immunity and ageing. *Immunology*, 2020;160(2):116–125; Heinz A. Elastic fibers during aging and disease. *Ageing Research Reviews*, 2021;66:101255; Krutmann J, Schikowski T, Morita A, Berneburg M. Environmentally-induced (extrinsic) skin aging: Exposomal factors and underlying mechanisms. *Journal of Investigative Dermatology*, 2021;141(4 S):1096–1103. doi: 10.1016/j.jid.2020.12.011.; Millyard A, Layden JD, Pyne DB, Edwards AM, Bloxham SR. Impairments to thermoregulation in the elderly during heat exposure events. *Gerontology and Geriatric Medicine*, 2020;6:2333721420932432; Pilkington SM, et al. Inflammaging and the skin. *Journal of Investigative Dermatology*, 2020;21:S0022–202X(20)32294-6; Wlaschek M, Maity P, Makrantonaki E, Scharffetter-Kochanek K. Connective tissue and fibroblast senescence in skin aging. *Journal of Investigative Dermatology*, 2021;Feb 6:S0022-202X(20)32351-4.

SUMMARY REVIEW

Structure and Function of the Skin

1. Skin is the largest organ of the body and equals 20% of body weight. Its major functions are to provide a protective barrier and to regulate body temperature.
2. The skin has three layers—the epidermis (outermost layer), dermis, and hypodermis (subcutaneous layer).
3. The epidermis is a continually renewing defensive layer that contains distinct layers with melanocytes, keratinocytes, Langerhans cells, and Merkel cells.
4. The dermis is composed of connective tissue elements, hair follicles, sweat glands, sebaceous glands, blood vessels, nerves, and lymphatic vessels.
5. The subcutaneous layer (hypodermis) contains connective tissue, fat cells, fibroblasts, and macrophages.
6. The dermal appendages include the nails, hair, sebaceous glands, and eccrine and apocrine sweat glands.
7. The papillary capillaries provide the major blood supply to the skin, arising from deeper arterial plexuses.
8. Heat loss and heat conservation are regulated by arteriovenous anastomoses that lead to the papillary capillaries in the dermis and evaporative loss of sweat.
9. Clinical manifestations of skin dysfunction include lesions, keloids and hypertrophic scars, and pruritus.
10. Pressure injury is localized damage to the skin that results from unrelieved pressure and shearing forces that occlude capillary blood flow, with resulting ischemia and necrosis. Areas at greatest risk are pressure points over bony prominences, such as the greater trochanters, sacrum, ischia, and heels.
11. Keloids are sharply elevated scars that extend beyond the border of traumatized skin. Hypertrophic scars are elevated fibrous lesions that do not extend beyond the border of injury. Both are caused by excess fibroblast activity and abnormal wound healing.
12. Pruritus, or itching, is associated with many skin disorders. It can be acute or chronic, localized or generalized, and migratory.

Disorders of the Skin

1. The most common inflammatory disorders of the skin are eczema and dermatitis. Eczema is characterized by pruritus, lesions with indistinct borders, and epidermal changes. There are multiple types of dermatitis.
2. Allergic contact dermatitis is a form of delayed hypersensitivity that develops with sensitization to allergens, such as metal, chemicals, or plant oils.
3. Irritant contact dermatitis develops from prolonged exposure to chemicals, such as acids or soaps, with disruption of the skin barrier.

4. Atopic or allergic dermatitis is associated with a family history of asthma or allergic rhinitis and is associated with elevated IgE levels. It is more common in infancy and childhood.
5. Stasis dermatitis, or stasis eczema, occurs on the lower extremities as a result of venous hypertension, chronic venous stasis, venous value reflux, calf muscle pump dysfunction, and edema. The disease can progress into ulcerations that are difficult to treat and lipodermatosclerosis.
6. Seborrheic dermatitis ranges from the fine white scale of dandruff to greasy, scaly, white or yellowish, inflammatory plaques. This typically occurs in areas rich in seborrheic glands such as the scalp, eyebrows, eyelids, ear canals, chest, axillae, and back. The cause is unknown but a genetic predisposition, *Malassezia* fungal infection, immunosuppression, and epidermal hyperproliferation have been implicated.
7. Papulosquamous disorders are characterized by papules, scales, plaques, and erythema and include psoriasis, pityriasis rosea, lichen planus, acne vulgaris, hidradenitis suppurative, acne rosacea, and lupus erythematosus.
8. Psoriasis is a chronic inflammatory skin disease associated with a complex inflammatory cascade involving multiple immune cells resulting in cellular proliferation of both the epidermis and the dermis; it is characterized by scaly, erythematous, pruritic plaques.
9. Pityriasis rosea is a self-limiting inflammatory disease characterized by oval lesions with scales around the edges; it is located along skin lines of the trunk and may be caused by a herpes-like virus.
10. Lichen planus is an autoimmune, papular, violet-colored inflammatory lesion of unknown origin manifested by severe pruritus.
11. Acne vulgaris is an inflammation of the pilosebaceous follicle.
12. Hidradenitis suppurativa (inverse acne) is an inflammatory disease involving the deep sections of apocrine glands. The lesions present in apocrine-gland rich areas as deep, firm painful subcutaneous nodules, often with sinus tracts, and rupture horizontally under the skin.
13. Acne rosacea develops on the middle third of the face with hypertrophy and inflammation of the sebaceous glands and is associated with altered innate immune responses.
14. Cutaneous lupus erythematosus manifests with inflammatory lesions, usually occurring in sun-exposed areas with a butterfly distribution over the nose and cheeks. The cause is unknown but is related to genetic and environmental factors and an altered immune response.
15. Pemphigus is a group of rare, blistering, life-threatening autoimmune diseases of the skin and oral mucous membranes. There are four main subtypes: pemphigus vulgaris (most common), pemphigus foliaceus, paraneoplastic pemphigus, and IgA pemphigus.
16. Erythema multiforme is an uncommon syndrome characterized by inflammation of the skin and/or mucous membranes. EM is an immune-mediated condition caused by an immunologic reaction to a drug or microorganisms. Lesions appear target-like, with alternating rings of edema and inflammation.
17. Stevens-Johnson syndrome (severe mucocutaneous bullous form involving up to 10% of the body surface area) and toxic epidermal necrolysis (severe mucocutaneous bullous form involving 30% or more of the body surface area) are the same disease with a continuum of symptoms. Both are type IV hypersensitivity reactions to drugs and are medical emergencies.
18. Cutaneous infections generally remain localized and can be bacterial, viral, and fungal in origin.
19. Folliculitis is a bacterial infection involving the hair follicles.
20. A furuncle is an infection of the hair follicle that extends to the surrounding tissue.
21. A carbuncle is a coalescence of furuncles.
22. Cellulitis is a diffuse infection of the dermis and subcutaneous tissue usually caused by *S. pyogenes* or CA-MRSA.
23. Erysipelas is a superficial infection of the dermis typically caused by beta-hemolytic streptococci.
24. Impetigo is a superficial infection of the skin caused by coagulase positive *S. aureus* or alpha-hemolytic streptococci. It occurs more commonly in children.
25. Lyme disease is an immune response caused by the spirochete *Borrelia burgdorferi*. It is transmitted by tick bites and often presents with migrating erythematous bull's eye lesions that can progress to chronic myalgias, arthralgias, and neurologic manifestations.
26. HSV-1 causes cold sores but can infect the cornea, mouth, and labia. HSV-2 commonly causes genital lesions and is usually spread by sexual contact.
27. Herpes zoster (shingles) and varicella (chickenpox) are both caused by the same varicella-zoster virus, with herpes zoster manifesting years after the initial infection from latent harboring of the virus.
28. Warts are benign, rough, elevated lesions caused by human papillomavirus. Condylomata acuminata, or venereal warts, are spread by sexual contact.
29. Tinea infections (fungal infections) can occur anywhere on the body and are classified by location (i.e., tinea pedis, tinea corporis, tinea capitis).
30. Candidiasis is a yeastlike fungal infection caused by *C. albicans* occurring on the skin, mucous membranes, in the gastrointestinal tract, and the vagina.
31. Cutaneous vasculitis is an inflammation of skin blood vessels related to immune complex deposition, with purpura, ischemia, and necrosis resulting from vessel necrosis.
32. Urticarial lesions are commonly associated with type I hypersensitivity responses and appear as wheals, welts, or hives.
33. Localized scleroderma is an autoimmune-mediated fibrosis that primarily affects the skin.
34. Systemic scleroderma is an autoimmune-mediated sclerosis of the skin that may also affect systemic organs and cause renal failure, bowel obstruction, or cardiac dysrhythmias.
35. Seborrheic keratosis is a benign proliferation of basal cells that produces elevated, smooth, or warty lesions of varying size. It is most common among the elderly population.

36. Keratoacanthoma arises from hair follicles on sun-exposed areas. Three stages of development over a period of 1 to 2 months characterize the lesion. Lesions resolve spontaneously or can be removed.
37. Actinic keratosis is a rough, poorly defined papule that develops in sun-exposed individuals with fair skin. The lesion may become malignant in the form of a squamous cell carcinoma.
38. Nevi (moles) arise from melanocytes and may be pigmented or nonpigmented. They occur singly or in groups and may undergo transition to malignant melanoma.
39. Skin cancer is usually caused by chronic exposure to ultraviolet radiation and is the most common cancer in the world.
40. Basal cell carcinoma is the most common skin cancer and occurs most often on ultraviolet-exposed areas with different subtypes and morphologic presentations.
41. Squamous cell carcinoma is a tumor of the epidermis with uncontrolled growth of keratinocytes associated with sun exposure and can be localized (in situ) or invasive.
42. Cutaneous melanoma is a malignant tumor that arises from melanocytes. If it is not excised early, metastasis occurs through the lymph nodes.
43. Kaposi sarcoma is an endothelial cell vascular malignancy associated with immunodeficiency states and herpesvirus 8.
44. Primary cutaneous lymphomas are clonal expansions of T-cell and B-cell lymphocytes. Mycosis fungoides is the most common T-cell lymphoma.
45. Cold injury usually occurs on the face and digits, with direct injury to cells and impaired circulation.

Disorders of the Hair

1. Androgenic alopecia is an inherited form of baldness with hair loss in the central scalp and recession of the frontotemporal hairline that occurs in men.
2. Female-pattern alopecia is a thinning of the central hair of the scalp in women and is associated with endocrine disorders.
3. Alopecia areata is patchy loss of hair associated with an autoimmune process and triggered by stress or metabolic diseases; it is usually reversible.
4. Hirsutism is a male pattern of terminal hair growth in women that may be normal or the result of excessive secretion of androgenic hormones.

Disorders of the Nail

1. Paronychia is an inflammation of the lateral or proximal nail fold that can be acute or chronic. It is usually caused by staphylococci, streptococci, or fungi.
2. Onychomycosis is a fungal, yeast, or dermophyte infection of the nail plate.

Aging and Changes in Skin Integrity

1. Skin becomes thinner, drier, and more wrinkled.
2. Wound healing decreases.
3. Fewer melanocytes mean pigmentation becomes irregular, providing less protection from ultraviolet light.

REFERENCES

1. Park AM, Khan S, Rawnsley J. Hair biology: growth and pigmentation. *Facial Plast Surg Clin North Am*. 2018;26(4):415–424.
2. Francisco MA, Minson CT. Cutaneous active vasodilation as a heat loss thermoeffector. *Handb Clin Neurol*. 2018;156:193–209.
3. National Pressure Injury Advisory Panel (NPIAP) *NPIAP pressure injury stages*. Westford, MA: NPIAP; 2016. Available at https://cdn.ymaws.com/npiap.com/resource/resmgr/online_store/npiap_pressure_injury_stages.pdf. (Accessed January 9, 2021).
4. Edsberg LE, et al. Revised national pressure ulcer advisory panel pressure injury staging system: revised pressure injury staging system. *J Wound Ostomy Continence Nurs*. 2016;43(6):585–597.
5. Oozageer Gunowa N, et al. Pressure injuries in people with darker skin tones: a literature review. *J Clin Nurs*. 2018;27(17–18):3266–3275.
6. Munoz N, et al. The role of nutrition for pressure injury prevention and healing: the 2019 International Clinical Practice Guideline Recommendations. *Adv Skin Wound Care*. 2020;33(3):123–136.
7. Bader DL, Worsley PR. Technologies to monitor the health of loaded skin tissues. *Biomed Eng Online*. 2018;17(1):40.
8. Roufogalis AL, Hutchinson ML. Best practices in pressure injury treatment. *Crit Care Nurs Clin North Am*. 2020;32(4):501–520.
9. Oliveira A, et al: Therapeutic advances in wound healing, *J Dermatolog Treat*. Published online February 26, 2020. Available at https://doi.org/10.1080/09546634.2020.1730296. (Accessed January 9, 2021).
10. Wang ZC, et al. The roles of inflammation in keloid and hypertrophic scars. *Front Immunol*. 2020;11:603187.
11. Betarbet U, Blalock TW. Keloids: a review of etiology, prevention, and treatment. *J Clin Aesthet Dermatol*. 2020;13(2):33–43.
12. El Ayadi A, Jay JW, Prasai A. Current approaches targeting the wound healing phases to attenuate fibrosis and scarring. *Int J Mol Sci*. 2020;21(3):1105.
13. Kahremany S, et al. Advances in understanding the initial steps of pruritoceptive itch: how the itch hits the switch. *Int J Mol Sci*. 2020;21(14):4883.
14. Cevikbas F, Lerner EA. Physiology and pathophysiology of itch. *Physiol Rev*. 2020;100(3):945–982.
15. Brites GS, et al. Allergic contact dermatitis: from pathophysiology to development of new preventive strategies. *Pharmacol Res*. 2020;162:105282.
16. Brar KK. A review of contact dermatitis. *Ann Allergy Asthma Immunol*. 2021;126(1):32–39.
17. Nucera E, et al. Latex allergy: current status and future perspectives. *J Asthma Allergy*. 2020;13:385–398.
18. Hollins LC, Flamm A. Occupational contact dermatitis: evaluation and management considerations. *Dermatol Clin*. 2020;38(3):329–338.
19. Bonkemeyer Millan S, Gan R, Townsend PE. Venous ulcers: diagnosis and treatment. *Am Fam Physician*. 2019;100(5):298–305.
20. Raffetto JD, et al. Why venous leg ulcers have difficulty healing: overview on pathophysiology, clinical consequences, and treatment. *J Clin Med*. 2020;10(1):29.
21. Piquero-Casals J, et al. Topical non-pharmacological treatment for facial seborrheic dermatitis. *Dermatol Ther (Heidelb)*. 2019;9(3):469–477.
22. Parisi R, et al. National, regional, and worldwide epidemiology of psoriasis: systematic analysis and modelling study. *BMJ*. 2020;369:m1590.

23. Honma M, Hayashi K. Psoriasis: recent progress in molecular-targeted therapies. *J Dermatol.* 2021;48(6):761–777.
24. Kovitwanichkanont T, Chong AH, Foley P. Beyond skin deep: addressing comorbidities in psoriasis. *Med J Aust.* 2020;212(11):528–534.
25. Brownstone ND, et al. Biologic treatments of psoriasis: an update for the clinician. *Biologics.* 2021;15:39–51.
26. Ibrahim S, et al. Practical compendium for psoriasis management. *Dermatol Ther.* 2020;33(2):e13243.
27. Mahajan K, et al. Pityriasis rosea: an update on etiopathogenesis and management of difficult aspects. *Indian J Dermatol.* 2016;61(4):375–384.
28. Drago F, et al. Evidence of human herpesvirus-6 and -7 reactivation in miscarrying women with pityriasis rosea. *J Am Acad Dermatol.* 2014;71:198–199.
29. González-Moles MÁ, Ramos-García P, Warnakulasuriya S. An appraisal of highest quality studies reporting malignant transformation of oral lichen planus based on a systematic review. *Oral Dis.* 2021;27(8):1908–1918.
30. Rotaru D, et al. Treatment trends in oral lichen planus and oral lichenoid lesions. *Exp Ther Med.* 2020;20(6):198.
31. Narla S, Lyons AB, Hamzavi IH. The most recent advances in understanding and managing hidradenitis suppurativa. *F1000Res.* 2020;9(F1000 Faculty Rev-1049).
32. Giuffrida R, et al. Novel therapeutic approaches and targets for the treatment of hidradenitis suppurativa. *Curr Pharm Biotechnol.* 2021;22(1):59–72.
33. Kim HS. Microbiota in rosacea. *Am J Clin Dermatol.* 2020;21(Suppl 1):25–35.
34. Tavassoli S, Wong N, Chan E. Ocular manifestations of rosacea: a clinical review. *Clin Exp Ophthalmol.* 2021;49(2):104–117.
35. Thiboutot D, et al. Standard management options for rosacea: the 2019 update by the National Rosacea Society Expert Committee. *J Am Acad Dermatol.* 2020;82(6):1501–1510.
36. Garelli CJ, et al. Current insights in cutaneous lupus erythematosus immunopathogenesis. *Front Immunol.* 2020;11:1353.
37. Albrecht J, et al. The CLASI (Cutaneous Lupus Erythematosus Disease Area and Severity Index): an outcome instrument for cutaneous lupus erythematosus. *J Invest Dermatol.* 2005;125(5):889–894.
38. Little AJ, Vesely MD. Cutaneous lupus erythematosus: current and future pathogenesis-directed therapies. *Yale J Biol Med.* 2020;93(1):81–95.
39. Yang M, et al. The pathogenesis of bullous skin diseases. *J Transl Autoimmun.* 2019;2:100014 Erratum in: *J Transl Autoimmun* 3:100041, 2020.
40. Di Lernia V, et al. Pemphigus vulgaris and bullous pemphigoid: update on diagnosis and treatment. *Dermatol Pract Concept.* 2020;10(3):e2020050.
41. Trayes KP, Love G, Studdiford JS. Erythema multiforme: recognition and management. *Am Fam Physician.* 2019;100(2):82–88.
42. Hasegawa A, Abe R. Recent advances in managing and understanding Stevens-Johnson syndrome and toxic epidermal necrolysis. *F1000Res.* 2020;9(F1000 Faculty Rev-612).
43. Noe MH, Micheletti RG. Diagnosis and management of Stevens-Johnson syndrome/toxic epidermal necrolysis. *Clin Dermatol.* 2020;38(6):607–612.
44. Clebak KT, Malone MA. Skin infections. *Prim Care.* 2018;45(3):433–454.
45. Lin HS, et al. Interventions for bacterial folliculitis and boils (furuncles and carbuncles). *Cochrane Database Syst Rev.* 2021;2(2):CD013099.
46. Bystritsky RJ. Cellulitis. *Infect Dis Clin North Am.* 2021;35(1):49–60.
47. Centers for Disease Control and Prevention (CDC), National Center for Emerging and Zoonotic Infectious Diseases (NCEZID), Division of Vector-Borne Diseases (DVBD) *Lyme disease, treatment.* Atlanta, GA: CDC; 2021. Page last reviewed November 29, 2021. Available at https://www.cdc.gov/lyme/treatment/index.html. (Accessed January 9, 2022).
48. Kullberg BJ, et al. Lyme borreliosis: diagnosis and management. *BMJ.* 2020;369:m1041.
49. Petti S, Lodi G. The controversial natural history of oral herpes simplex virus type 1 infection. *Oral Dis.* 2019;25(8): 1850–1865.
50. Samies NL, James SH. Prevention and treatment of neonatal herpes simplex virus infection. *Antiviral Res.* 2020;176:104721.
51. Kim HC, Lee HK. Vaccines against genital herpes: where are we? *Vaccines (Basel).* 2020;8(3):420.
52. Andrei G, Snoeck R. Advances and perspectives in the management of varicella-zoster virus infections. *Molecules.* 2021;26(4):1132.
53. Oren-Shabtai M, et al. Topical and systemic retinoids for the treatment of cutaneous viral warts: a systematic review and meta-analysis. *Dermatol Ther.* 2021;34(1):e14637.
54. Kombe Kombe AJ, et al. Epidemiology and burden of human papillomavirus and related diseases, molecular pathogenesis, and vaccine evaluation. *Front Public Health.* 2021;8:552028.
55. Leung AK, et al. Tinea corporis: an updated review. *Drugs Context.* 2020;9 2020-5-6.
56. Singh DK, Tóth R, Gácser A. Mechanisms of pathogenic *Candida* species to evade the host complement attack. *Front Cell Infect Microbiol.* 2020;10:94.
57. Gonzalez-Lara MF, Ostrosky-Zeichner L. Invasive candidiasis. *Semin Respir Crit Care Med.* 2020;41(1):3–12.
58. Morita TCAB, et al. Update on vasculitis: overview and relevant dermatological aspects for the clinical and histopathological diagnosis - part II. *An Bras Dermatol.* 2020;95(4):493–507.
59. Martina E, et al. Novel therapeutic approaches and targets for treatment of chronic urticaria: new insights and promising targets for a challenging disease. *Curr Pharm Biotechnol.* 2021;22(1):32–45.
60. Orlandi M, et al. One year in review 2020: systemic sclerosis. *Clin Exp Rheumatol.* 2020;38(Suppl 125):S3–S17.
61. Wolska-Gawron K, Bartosińska J, Krasowska D. MicroRNA in localized scleroderma: a review of literature. *Arch Dermatol Res.* 2020;312(5):317–324.
62. McMahan ZH, Volkmann ER. An update on the pharmacotherapeutic options and treatment strategies for systemic sclerosis. *Expert Opin Pharmacother.* 2020;21(16):2041–2056.
63. Murphy EC, Friedman AJ. Hydrogen peroxide topical solution, 40% (w/w) for the treatment of seborrheic keratoses: a review. *Skin Therapy Lett.* 2020;25(1):1–4.
64. Kossard S. Keratoacanthoma, committed stem cells and neoplastic aberrant infundibulogenesis integral to formulating a conceptual model for an infundibulocystic pathway to squamous cell carcinoma. *J Cutan Pathol.* 2021;48(1):184–191.
65. Kiss N, et al. Intralesional therapy for the treatment of keratoacanthoma. *Dermatol Ther.* 2019;32(3):e12872.
66. Puig S, et al. Review of clinical evidence over 10 years on prevention and treatment of a film-forming medical device containing photolyase in the management of field cancerization in actinic keratosis. *Dermatol Ther (Heidelb).* 2019;9(2):259–270.

67. Dianzani C, et al. Current therapies for actinic keratosis. *Int J Dermatol.* 2020;59(6):677–684.
68. Fried L, et al. Technological advances for the detection of melanoma: advances in diagnostic techniques. *J Am Acad Dermatol.* 2020;83(4):983–992.
69. American Cancer Society (ACS) *Key statistics for melanoma skin cancer.* Atlanta, GA: ACS; 2021. Available at https://www.cancer.org/cancer/melanoma-skin-cancer/about/key-statistics.html. (Accessed January 9, 2022).
70. Khandelwal AR, et al. Cutaneous cancer biology. *Otolaryngol Clin North Am.* 2021;54(2):259–269.
71. Fania L, et al. Basal cell carcinoma: from pathophysiology to novel therapeutic approaches. *Biomedicines.* 2020;8(11):449.
72. Leavitt E, Lask G, Martin S. Sonic hedgehog pathway inhibition in the treatment of advanced basal cell carcinoma. *Curr Treat Options Oncol.* 2019;20(11):84.
73. Nagarajan P. Differentiating keratoacanthoma from squamous cell carcinoma—in quest of the holy grail. *J Cutan Pathol.* 2020;47(4):418–420.
74. Toprani SM, Kelkar Mane V. A short review on DNA damage and repair effects in lip cancer. *Hematol Oncol Stem Cell Ther.* 2021;14(4):267–274.
75. McMullen CP, Ow TJ. The role of systemic therapy in advanced cutaneous squamous cell carcinoma. *Otolaryngol Clin North Am.* 2021;54(2):343–355.
76. Carr S, Smith C, Wernberg J. Epidemiology and risk factors of melanoma. *Surg Clin North Am.* 2020;100(1):1–12.
77. Chacón M, et al. Uncommon subtypes of malignant melanomas: a review based on clinical and molecular perspectives. *Cancers (Basel).* 2020;12(9):2362.
78. Pilla L, et al. Molecular and immune biomarkers for cutaneous melanoma: current status and future prospects. *Cancers (Basel).* 2020;12(11):3456.
79. Marghoob NG, Liopyris K, Jaimes N. Dermoscopy: a review of the structures that facilitate melanoma detection. *J Am Osteopath Assoc.* 2019;119(6):380–390.
80. Yang K, et al. Current molecular markers of melanoma and treatment targets. *Int J Mol Sci.* 2020;21(10):3535.
81. PDQ® Adult Treatment Editorial Board *Melanoma treatment (PDQ®)—health professional version.* Bethesda, MD: National Cancer Institute; 2021. Updated July 23, 2021. Available at https://www.cancer.gov/types/skin/hp/melanoma-treatment-pdq. (Accessed January 9, 2022).
82. Walsh NM, Cerroni L. Merkel cell carcinoma: a review. *J Cutan Pathol.* 2021;48(3):411–421.
83. Aneja KK, Yuan Y. Reactivation and lytic replication of Kaposi's sarcoma-associated herpesvirus: an update. *Front Microbiol.* 2017;8:613.
84. Cesarman E, et al. Kaposi sarcoma. *Nat Rev Dis Primers.* 2019;5(1):9.
85. Ceccarelli M, et al. The treatment of Kaposi's sarcoma: present and future options, a review of the literature. *Eur Rev Med Pharmacol Sci.* 2019;23(17):7488–7497.
86. American Cancer Society (ACS) *Types of lymphoma of the skin.* Atlanta, GA: ACS; 2018. Last revised March 29, 2018. Available at https://www.cancer.org/cancer/skin-lymphoma/about/types-of-skin-lymphoma.html. (Accessed January 9, 2022).
87. Vitiello P, et al. Primary cutaneous B-cell lymphomas: an update. *Front Oncol.* 2020;10:651.
88. Kamijo H, Miyagaki T. Mycosis fungoides and Sézary syndrome: updates and review of current therapy. *Curr Treat Options Oncol.* 2021;22(2):10.
89. Mohr WJ, Jenabzadeh K, Ahrenholz DH. Cold injury. *Hand Clin.* 2009;25(4):481–496.
90. Gao Y, et al. Research progress in the pathogenic mechanisms and imaging of severe frostbite. *Eur J Radiol.* 2021;137:109605.
91. Joshi K, et al. Frostbite: current status and advancements in therapeutics. *J Therm Biol.* 2020;93:102716.
92. Tai T, Kochhar A. Physiology and medical treatments for alopecia. *Facial Plast Surg Clin North Am.* 2020;28(2):149–159.
93. Katzer T, et al. Physiopathology and current treatments of androgenetic alopecia: going beyond androgens and anti-androgens. *Dermatol Ther.* 2019;32(5):e13059.
94. Bertoli MJ, et al. Female pattern hair loss: a comprehensive review. *Dermatol Ther.* 2020;33(6):e14055.
95. Ito T, et al. Understanding the significance of cytokines and chemokines in the pathogenesis of alopecia areata. *Exp Dermatol.* 2020;29(8):726–732.
96. Bertolini M, et al. Hair follicle immune privilege and its collapse in alopecia areata. *Exp Dermatol.* 2020;29(8):703–725.
97. Sterkens A, Lambert J, Bervoets A. Alopecia areata: a review on diagnosis, immunological etiopathogenesis and treatment options. *Clin Exp Med.* 2021;21(2):215–230.
98. Matheson E, Bain J. Hirsutism in women. *Am Fam Physician.* 2019;100(3):168–175.
99. Barger J, et al. Fingertip infections. *Hand Clin.* 2020;36(3):313–332.
100. Gupta AK, et al. Onychomycosis: a review. *J Eur Acad Dermatol Venereol.* 2020;34(9):1972–1990.

47

Alterations of the Integument in Children

Noreen Heer Nicol and Judith O'Haver

http://evolve.elsevier.com/Rogers/pathophysiology/

CHAPTER OUTLINE

Children frequently develop alterations of the skin, which range in severity. Cutaneous manifestations may provide information for other systemic concerns and provide clinical clues to assist with diagnostic dilemmas. Some skin diseases resolve spontaneously and require no treatment. Diagnosis is commonly made from the history, appearance, and distribution of the lesion or lesions. Common skin diseases of childhood are presented here.

ACNE VULGARIS

Acne vulgaris is the most common skin disease and occurs primarily between the ages of 12 and 25 years. Acne tends to occur in families, and genetic susceptibility may determine the severity of the disease.

Acne develops at distinctive pilosebaceous units, known as *sebaceous follicles*. Located primarily on the face and upper parts of the chest and back, these follicles have many large sebaceous glands, a small vellus hair (very short, nonpigmented, and very thin hair), and a dilated follicular canal that is visible as a pore on the skin surface. Acne lesions may be noninflammatory or inflammatory (cystic) (Fig. 47.1). In noninflammatory acne, the comedones are open (blackheads) and closed (whiteheads), with the accumulated material causing distention of the follicle and thinning of follicular canal walls. Inflammatory (including cystic) acne develops in closed comedones when the follicular wall ruptures, expelling sebum into the surrounding dermis and initiating inflammation (see Fig. 47.1). Pustules form when the inflammation is close to the surface; papules and cystic nodules can develop when the inflammation is deeper, causing mild to severe scarring. Both types of lesions may exist in the same individual.

The causal mechanism is not completely understood. The pathophysiology includes (1) hyperkeratinization of the follicular epithelium; (2) altered sebum production, including hyperseborrhea and dysseborrhea; (3) follicular proliferation of anaerobic *Cutibacterium acnes* (*C. acnes*, previously known as *Propionibacterium acnes*); and (4) inflammation and rupture of a follicle due to accumulated debris and bacteria. *C. acnes* strains shift from being symbiotic to a pathogenic strain of bacteria and shift from being noninflammatory to inflammatory. The main hormones responsible for the development of acne vulgaris include androgens, insulin, and insulin-like growth factor-1; additional hormones have also been identified.[1] Androgens (dehydroepiandrosterone sulfate and testosterone) that are synthesized in increasing amounts during puberty increase the size and productivity of the sebaceous glands, promoting comedome formation. Rupture of comedomes causes release of inflammatory mediators and proliferation of inflammatory *C. acnes* strains in susceptible individuals. Scarring results from chronic inflammation and lesions below the reticular dermis.[2]

The treatment of acne should be individualized, according to severity. Combinations of topical products that contain retinoids, benzoyl peroxide, and antimicrobial agents, remain preferred. Retinoids are anticomedogenic and comedolytic, have anti-inflammatory effects, and target multiple pathogenic microorganisms associated with acne. Benzoyl peroxide is antimicrobial, with some keratolytic effects. Recognition that acne is an inflammatory condition, not an infectious one, has led to a call for reduction in oral antibiotic use to avoid antibiotic resistance and to promote future effectiveness of the drugs. Use of oral antibiotics with a narrower spectrum of activity is

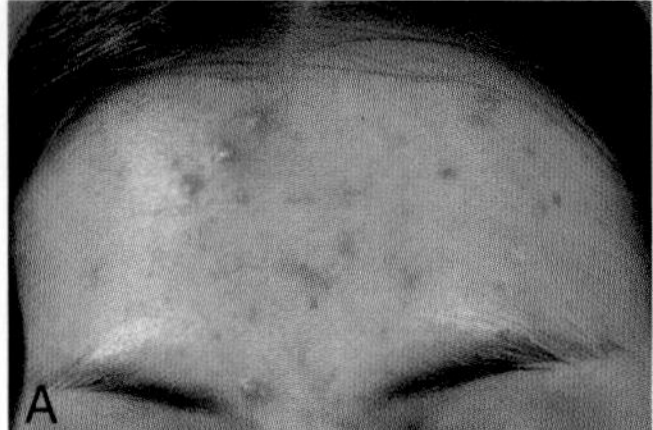
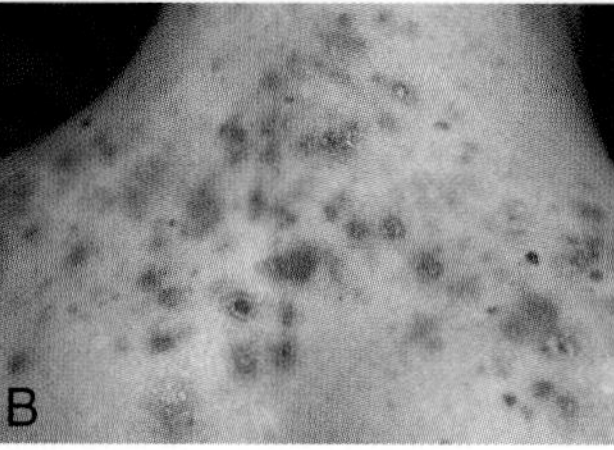

Fig. 47.1 Acne. (A) Inflammatory papules and pustules. (B) Severe nodular cystic acne. (From Nelson WE, Behrman RE, Kliegman RM, et al., eds. *Nelson textbook of pediatrics*, 21st edition. Philadelphia: Elsevier; 2020.)

another strategy.[3] Use of systemic therapies, including oral contraceptives, corticosteroids, and isotretinoin (requires pregnancy prevention and monthly monitoring), may be limited by side effects. Acne surgery, including comedone extraction, intralesional steroids, and cryosurgery, is useful in selected individuals. Special consideration must be given to treatment for those with darker skin because they have greater risk for hyperpigmentation and keloidal scarring. Severe scarring may be treated with dermabrasion, lasers, and resurfacing techniques. Laser and light modalities, although not sufficiently studied for first-line use, show promise for the future. The relationship between nutrition and acne, allowing the identification of a certain number of potential triggers, such as dairy products, hyperglycemic load, and the excessive intake of whey proteins is still unclear.[3] Psychologic support is important because acne negatively affects quality of life, self-esteem, and mood in adolescents and is associated with an increased risk of anxiety, depression, and suicidal ideation. Guidelines are available for the treatment of acne.[4]

Acne conglobata is a rare yet highly inflammatory form of acne, with communicating cysts and abscesses beneath the skin that can cause scarring and disfigurement. The bacterium involved in acne vulgaris–Propionibacterium acnes–may also play a role in acne conglobate by changing the bacteria's reactivity as an antigen. Hypersensitivity to the bacterium antigens results in an immunological response that leads to a chronic inflammatory state. Androgens and anabolic steroids, as well as exposure to thyroid medications and halogenated aromatic hydrocarbons, may result in the formation of acne conglobate. Attempts to hide the disease with clothing may lead to excessive warmth and humidity in the area of the acne, and these conditions can worsen the disease.[5] This type of acne requires the use of systemic and combination therapies to prevent drug resistance, and severe scarring may require treatment.

DERMATITIS

Atopic Dermatitis

Atopic dermatitis (AD), also known as atopic eczema, is the most common cause of eczema in children. Onset is usually from 2 to 6 months of age, and most cases develop within the first 5 years of life; however, AD can affect individuals of any age.

The cause of this chronic relapsing form of pruritic eczema involves an interplay of genetic predisposition. Atopic comorbidities of asthma, allergic rhinitis, and food allergies are well recognized in persons with AD. The skin barrier function is altered and associated with filaggrin gene mutations and filaggrin deficiency (proteins that bind keratin in the epidermis); reduced ceramide (a stratum corneum lipid) levels; decreased antimicrobial peptides; altered innate immunity; and altered immune responses to allergens, irritants, and microbes. There is an altered skin microbiome with formation of biofilm by *Staphylococcus aureus*, that may act as super-antigens, causing exacerbations of eczema. Although AD is predominantly associated with type 2 immune responses, activation of T-cell cytokine pathways have been reported,[6] resulting in new therapeutic targets using novel biologic therapy.[7]

AD has a constellation of clinical features, including severe pruritus and a characteristic eczematoid appearance with redness, edema, and scaling. The skin becomes increasingly dry, itchy, sensitive, and easily irritated because the barrier function of the skin is impaired. Itching is the hallmark of AD; rubbing and scratching to relieve the itch are responsible for many of the clinical skin changes of AD. In young children, a rash appears primarily on the face, scalp, trunk, and extensor surfaces of the arms and legs (Fig. 47.2A). In older children and adults, the rash tends to be found on the neck, antecubital and popliteal fossae, and hands and feet. Individuals with AD also tend to develop viral, bacterial, and fungal skin infections in the eczematous areas. Another common manifestation is secondary creases in the skin below the lower eyelids, known as Dennie-Morgan fold (see Fig. 47.2B); it may be related to skin edema and chronic spasm of Mullër eyelid muscles, resulting from hypoxia linked to poor blood circulation. This sign may be accompanied with dark eye circles, caused by accumulation of blood and other fluids in the infraorbital groove and an associated allergic rhinitis.[8] There are no specific laboratory features of AD that can be used for diagnostic and treatment purposes. Most affected individuals show increased serum levels of immunoglobulin E (IgE), eosinophils (eosinophilia), and positive skin test results to a variety of common food and inhalant allergens.

Management of individuals with AD includes accurate diagnosis, comprehensive evaluation of triggers, response to treatment, management of confounding factors (sleep disruption), and education provided to individuals and caregivers. Successful AD management strategies are published in national and international treatment guidelines. Treatment is implemented in a stepwise approach, tailored to the individuals.[7,9] Avoidance of triggers and promotion of skin hydration, including soaking baths and consistent use of an emollient moisturizer, are the cornerstone to good therapy.[10] Topical anti-inflammatory agents, such as corticosteroids, calcineurin inhibitors, and phosphodiesterase type 4 inhibitors, are first-line treatment options during active flare-ups of eczema at all levels of severity. Sedating antihistamines, as well as topical and oral antibiotics and bleach baths, may be added as indicated. Therapy is increased for moderate to severe AD, which may include systemic immunomodulator therapy, biologic agents, and wet wrap therapy.[7,9–11]

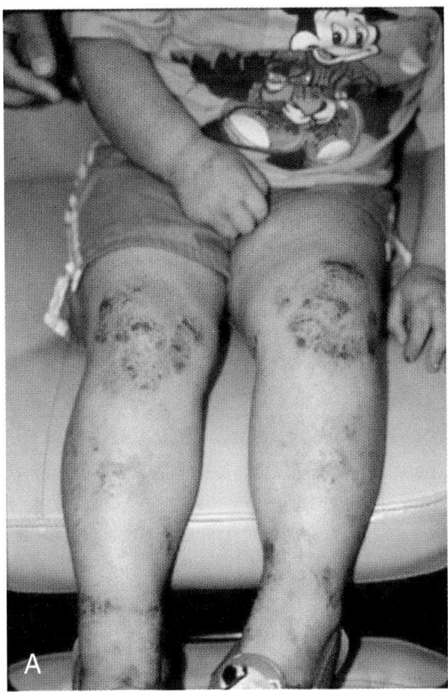

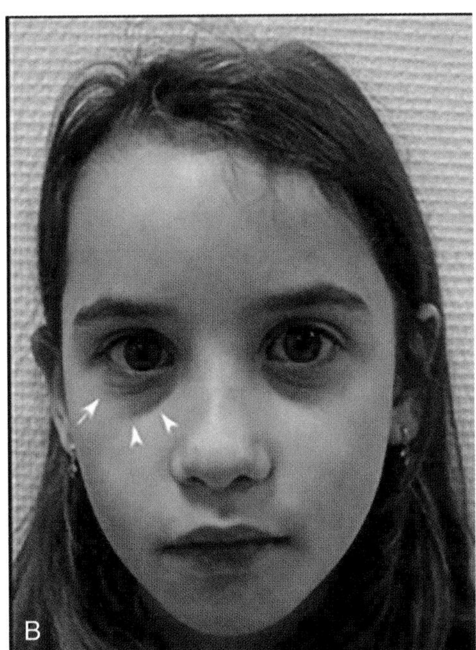

Fig. 47.2 Atopic Dermatitis. (A) Characteristic lesions with crusting from irritation and scratching over knees and around ankles. **(B)** Dennie-Morgan fold (*white arrows*) with dark eye circles. (A, Courtesy Department of Dermatology, School of Medicine, University of Utah, Salt Lake City, UT. B, From Blanc S, Bourrier T, Albertini M, et al. Dennie–Morgan fold plus dark circles: Suspect atopy at first sight. *Journal of Pediatrics*. 2015;166[6]:1541.)

Contact Dermatitis

Contact dermatitis is an umbrella term that describes an eczematous eruption, resulting from either delayed hypersensitive reaction to an allergen (allergic contact dermatitis) or direct irritation to the skin from an irritating substance (irritant contact dermatitis).[12] This results in nonspecific intracellular edema and inflammation. Key management requires the identification and elimination of future exposure to the specific allergen or irritant.

Allergic Contact Dermatitis

Allergic contact dermatitis is caused by delayed hypersensitivity reaction to contact with the allergen, which is a T-cell mediated, type IV delayed immune response. Common allergens in children are nickel exposure from metals in jewelry and snaps, as well as topical products and plants.

Clinical manifestations of allergic contact dermatitis are often localized, pruritic, and rash with discrete border and shape. Skin lesions are usually in the distribution of the contacting allergen and may appear as erythematous papular lesions, blisters, vesicles, or just erythematous linear rash. Lesions appear a day or two after exposure to allergen and may last for weeks, without further exposure. Patch testing is the gold standard for diagnosis. Treatment includes topical therapies[12] and avoidance of allergens.

Irritant Contact Dermatitis

Irritant contact dermatitis may occur at any age and be due to anything that is irritating to the individual. Irritants include topical use of almost anything used on the skin, including cleansers, moisturizers, antiseptics, shampoos, and others. It is common in young infants due to skin sensitivity and exposure to primary irritants. Irritant contact dermatitis due to irritation in the diaper area is frequently referred to as diaper dermatitis.[13] It is one common form of irritant contact dermatitis and initiated by a combination of factors including prolonged exposure to and irritation by urine wetness and feces, as well as maceration by wet diapers, airtight plastic diaper covers, or use of diaper wipes. Disposable diaper designs have decreased the incidence of diaper dermatitis in infants. Diapers with a mesh-like, aperture top sheet may represent a better way to mitigate known causes of diaper dermatitis through their superior ability to absorb fecal matter.[14] Often, diaper dermatitis is secondarily infected with *Candida albicans*. The resulting inflammation affects the lower aspect of the abdomen, genitalia, buttocks, and upper portion of the thigh.

The lesions vary from mild erythema to erythematous papular lesions and can affect overall infant health.[12] Candidal (monilial) diaper dermatitis is usually very erythematous, with sharp margination and pustulovesicular satellite lesions (Fig. 47.3).

Treatment involves frequent diaper changes to keep the affected area clean and dry or regular exposure of the perineal area to air and to use of superabsorbent diapers.[14] Topical protection of the skin can be obtained by using a product containing petrolatum or zinc oxide, or both. Cleaning should be limited to gentle washing with water, using a soft washcloth or cotton balls, without using diaper wipes, and using fragrance-free products. Additionally, for allergic dermatitis, low-potency topical corticosteroids to the groin or diaper area are indicated. Topical antifungal medication is used to treat *C. albicans* when present.

INFECTIONS OF THE SKIN

Infectious diseases caused by bacteria, viruses, and fungi constitute the major forms of skin disease. Breaks in the skin integrity, particularly those that inoculate pathogens into the dermis and epidermis, may cause or exacerbate infections. Most infections tend to occur superficially; however, systemic signs and symptoms develop occasionally and can be life-threatening in immunosuppressed children.

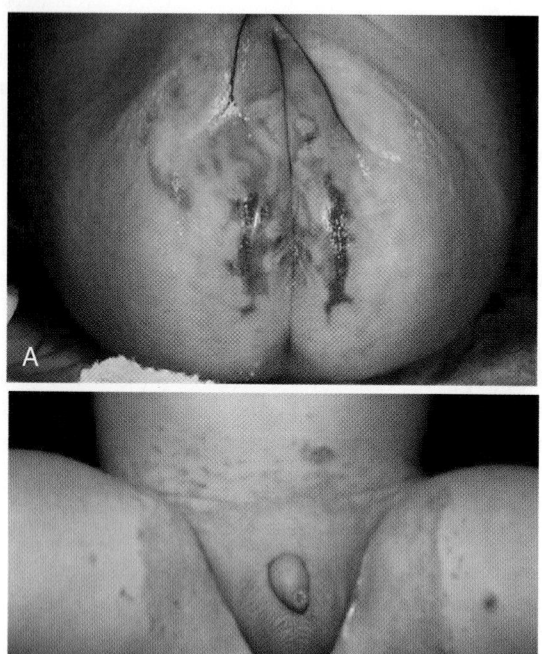

Fig. 47.3 Irritant Contact Dermatitis (ICD) in Diaper Area. **(A)** ICD in diaper area with erosions. **(B)** ICD in diaper area with *Candida albicans* secondary infection. (Courtesy Department of Dermatology, School of Medicine, University of Utah, Salt Lake City, UT.)

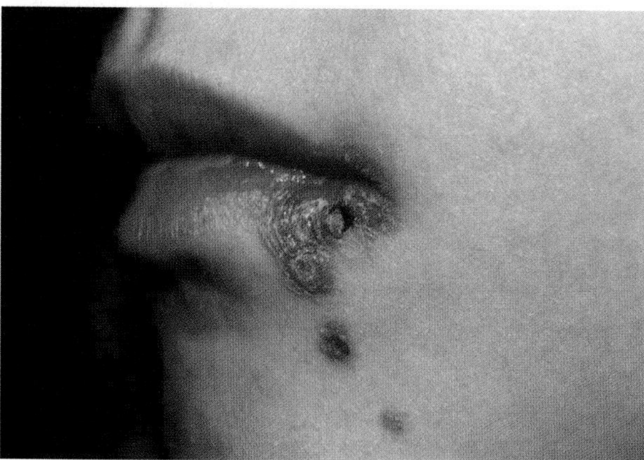

Fig. 47.4 Impetigo. Multiple crusted and oozing lesions of impetigo. (From Kliegman RM, Nelson WE, eds. *Nelson textbook of pediatrics*, 19th edition. Philadelphia: Saunders; 2011.)

Bacterial Infections

Impetigo

Impetigo is the most common bacterial skin infection in children 2 to 5 years of age and is highly contagious. *S. aureus* and, less commonly, *Streptococcus pyogenes* cause impetigo.[15] The mode of transmission is by both direct and indirect contact. The disease is more common in mid- to late summer, with a higher incidence in hot, humid climates. Impetigo is particularly infectious among people living in crowded conditions with poor sanitary facilities or in settings such as day-care facilities. It affects children in good health, but conditions such as anemia and malnutrition are predisposing factors.

Bacterial invasion occurs through minor breaks in the cutaneous surface or as a secondary infection of a preexisting dermatosis or infestation. The staphylococci produce bacterial toxins *(exfoliative toxins [ETs])* that cause a disruption in the skin barrier with blister formation. There are two types of impetigo: nonbullous or vesicular and, more rarely, bullous (caused only by *S. aureus*), in which blisters enlarge or coalesce to form bullae. Both forms of impetigo begin as vesicles that rupture to form a honey-colored crust (Fig. 47.4). The lesions are often located on the face, around the nose and mouth, but the hands and other exposed areas are also involved.

Impetigo is clinically characterized by crusted erosions or ulcers that may arise as a primary infection or as a secondary infection of other pre-existing dermatosis or infestation. Resistance patterns in a wide range of pathogens against oral or topical antibiotics and antiseptics, used for the treatment of dermatological conditions such as impetigo, have been reported. When making treatment decisions for impetigo, methicillin-resistant *Staphylococcus aureus* (MRSA) and other antimicrobial resistance has to be considered. Many treatment options exist, including bleach baths and topical antibiotics, such as mupirocin, fusidic acid, retapamulin, and ozenoxacin.[15] For extensive or complicated impetigo, systemic antibiotics may be warranted, but β-lactam antibiotics should be avoided if MRSA is suspected. Prompt treatment avoids complications, such as glomerulonephritis, necrotizing fasciitis, and septic shock syndrome. Lesions usually resolve in 2 to 3 weeks, without scarring. Using good handwashing techniques and isolating the infected child's washcloth, towels, drinking glass, and linen are important for prevention.

Staphylococcal Scalded-Skin Syndrome

Staphylococcal scalded-skin syndrome (SSSS), also known as Ritter disease, is considered a pediatric emergency. It is the most serious staphylococcal infection that affects the skin and often may occur in infants and younger children under age 5.[16,17] SSSS is caused by virulent group II strains of staphylococci that produce an exfoliative toxin. The toxin attacks desmoglein and keratinocyte adhesion molecules and causes a separation of the skin just below the granular layer of the epidermis with blister formation. The toxin is usually produced at body sites other than the skin and arrives at the epidermis through the circulatory system. Staphylococci typically are not found in the skin lesions themselves. Adults have circulating antistaphylococcal antibodies and are better able to metabolize and excrete the toxin. Neonates are at the highest risk because of their lack of immunity, with no prior exposure to the toxin.

The clinical symptoms begin with fever, malaise, rhinorrhea, and irritability, followed by generalized erythema with exquisite tenderness of the skin. The severity may vary from a few lesions to systemic exfoliation. There may be an associated impetigo, but the infection often begins in the throat or chest. The erythema spreads from the face and trunk to cover the entire body, except for the palms, soles, and mucous membranes. The diagnosis is mainly clinical, based on the findings of tender erythroderma, bullae, and desquamation with a scalded appearance, especially in friction zones, periorificial scabs/crusting, positive Nikolsky sign, and absence of mucosal involvement. Within 48 hours, blisters and bullae may form, giving the child the appearance of being scalded. The pain is severe (Fig. 47.5). Fluid loss from ruptured blisters and water evaporation from denuded areas may cause dehydration. Perioral and nasolabial crusting, as well as fissures develop. In severe cases, the skin of the entire body may slough. When secondary infection can be prevented, healing of the involved skin occurs in 10 to 14 days, usually without scarring.[17]

Although generally a clinical diagnosis, culture and histologic or exfoliative cytologic studies should be initiated prior to treatment. Prompt empiric treatment with intravenous antistaphylococcal antibiotic, such as nafcillin, oxacillin, or flucloxacillin, is essential until cultures are available to guide therapy. Ophthalmology is consulted for eye involvement to prevent scarring. When SSSS infection is confirmed, treatment with intravenous antibiotics begins, as well as fluid and electrolyte management. The skin should be treated in the same manner as a severe burn, with meticulous aseptic technique. Special care is required when the lips and eyelids are involved. Infection control practices are important for prevention.[17]

Fungal Infections

Dermatophyte infections

Dermatophyte infections of keratin-containing skin and skin structures result in tinea capitis (scalp), tinea corporis (body), tinea pedis (foot), and tinea unguium (nails). These fungal infections are some of the most common worldwide. The three dermatophyte genera include *Trichophyton*, *Microsporum*, and *Epidermophyton*. Most of the dermatophyte species are parasitic and can cause disease in either humans or animals, often being adapted to a single or narrow range of host species.[18]

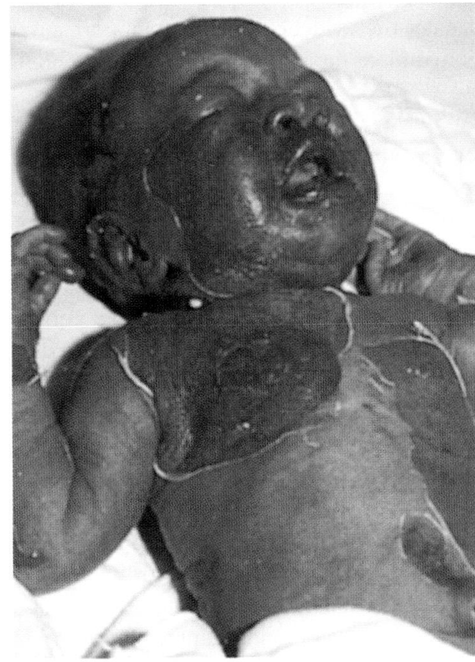

Fig. 47.5 Staphylococcal Scalded-Skin Syndrome (SSSS). The skin lesions, showing desquamation and wrinkling of the skin margins, appeared 1 day after drainage of a staphylococcal abscess. (From Kliegman RM, et al. *Nelson textbook of pediatrics*, 19th edition. St. Louis: Saunders; 2011.)

Tinea Capitis

Tinea capitis, a fungal infection of the scalp (scalp ringworm), is the most common fungal infection of childhood. It rarely affects infants and is seen in children between 2 and 10 years of age. The primary microorganism responsible for this disease in North America is *Trichophyton tonsurans*, and less commonly *Microsporum* is involved.[18,19] There is direct human transmission of *T. tonsurans* in crowded areas, the most prevalent environment of the fungus, and from contact with animals like infected cats and dogs.[20] The lesions are often circular and manifested by the presence of scales and broken hairs 1 to 3 mm above the scalp, leaving a partial area of alopecia from 1 to 5 cm in diameter (Fig. 47.6). A slight erythema and scaling, with raised borders, can be observed.

Diagnosis is best confirmed by dermoscopy, potassium hydroxide (KOH) examination of the scale from a scraping, and fungal culture. The most efficient method of sample collection[20] is the hairbrush collection method or by carefully removing broken hair stubs with forceps. Tinea capitis always requires systemic treatment because topical antifungal agents do not penetrate the hair follicle. Several oral antifungal agents are available for treatment.[18,19]

Tinea Corporis

Tinea corporis (ringworm) is a common superficial dermatophyte infection in children. The organisms most commonly responsible for this disease are *Microsporum canis* and *Trichophyton mentagrophytes*. As in tinea capitis, contact with infected kittens and puppies is a common source of the disorder. Tinea corporis preferentially affects the nonhairy parts of the face, trunk, and limbs. Lesions are often erythematous (round or oval scaling patches that spread peripherally with clearing in the center), creating the ring appearance, which is why this disease is commonly referred to as *ringworm*. The lesions are distributed

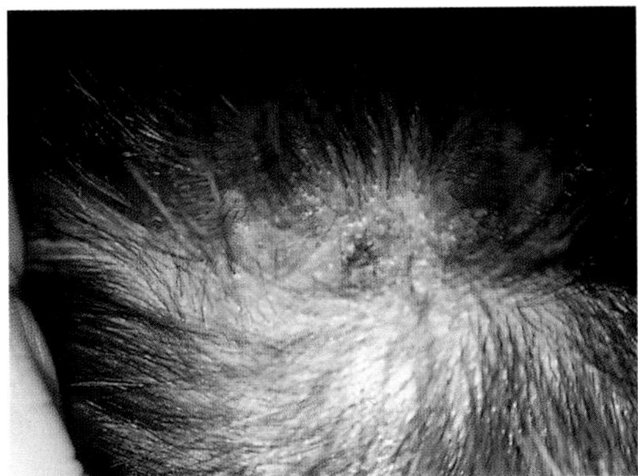

Fig. 47.6 Tinea Capitis. (Courtesy Department of Dermatology, School of Medicine, University of Utah, Salt Lake City, UT.)

asymmetrically, and multiple lesions, when present, overlap. Transmission occurs by direct contact with an infected lesion and through indirect contact with personal items used by the infected person. At times, a Majocchi granuloma develops as organisms (typically *T. rubrum*) penetrate along hair follicles to the level of the dermis, producing follicular-based pustules or nodules.[18] KOH examination of the scale from the border of the lesions or fungal culture confirms the diagnosis. Current diagnosis is critical as guessing and the inappropriate treatment of fungal disease with topical corticosteroids worsens this condition. Cutaneous lesions generally respond well to topical therapy; however, for hair or nail involvement, oral treatment is usually warranted.

Candida

Candida comprises the genus that causes the most frequent fungal infections in humans. A wide range of yeasts that reproduce via budding, often by forming long chains called pseudohyphae, are contained in this genus. There are at least 15 distinct species of Candida, the most common of which is *Candida albicans*, which comprises about 50% of Candida infections and is found normally colonized on the skin, mouth, intestinal tract, and vagina.[18]

Oral candidiasis, also known as oral thrush, is the term used to describe the presence of *C. albicans* in the mucous membranes of the mouths. It is commonly encountered in the newborn period where infants can acquire this infection in utero or postnatally, via passage through the vaginal canal.[18] It occurs in immunocompromised individuals of all ages. *C. albicans* penetrates the epidermal barrier more easily than other microorganisms because of its keratolytic proteases, other enzymes, and evasion of neutrophil killing. Oral thrush is characterized by the formation of white plaques or spots in the mouth that lead to shallow ulcers, caused by keratolytic proteases from the microorganism. The tongue may have a dense, white covering. The underlying mucous membrane is red and tender and may bleed when the plaques are removed. The prevalence of oral candidiasis is much higher in bottle-fed versus breast-fed infants.[18] The disease is often accompanied by fever and gastrointestinal irritation. The infection commonly spreads to the groin, buttocks, and other parts of the body. Treatment may be difficult and includes oral antifungal washes, such as nystatin oral suspension. Simultaneous treatment of a *Candida* nipple infection or vaginitis in the mother is helpful in reducing the *C. albicans* surface colonization of the infant. Feeding bottles and nipples should be sterilized to prevent reinfection.

Viral Infections

Molluscum Contagiosum

Molluscum contagiosum is a benign self-limiting skin disease, caused by infection with a pox virus. The virus is spread from person-to-person direct contact, auto inoculation, or through contaminated fomites.[21,22] It occurs worldwide, primarily in children and more often in warm climates.[23] Molluscum contagiosum virus (MCV) is the sole member of the *Molluscipoxvirus* genus and the causative agent of molluscum contagiosum. The lesions of molluscum are discrete, slightly umbilicated, dome-shaped papules 1 to 5 mm in diameter that appear anywhere on the skin or conjunctiva (Fig. 47.7). There is generally no inflammation surrounding molluscum lesions, unless they are traumatized, or secondary infection occurs. Scarring may occur with healing. Generally mollusca are diagnosed clinically and do not require biopsy or other diagnostic procedures. Most lesions are self-limiting and clear in 6 to 9 months; however, some may persist for 3 to 4 years.[23]

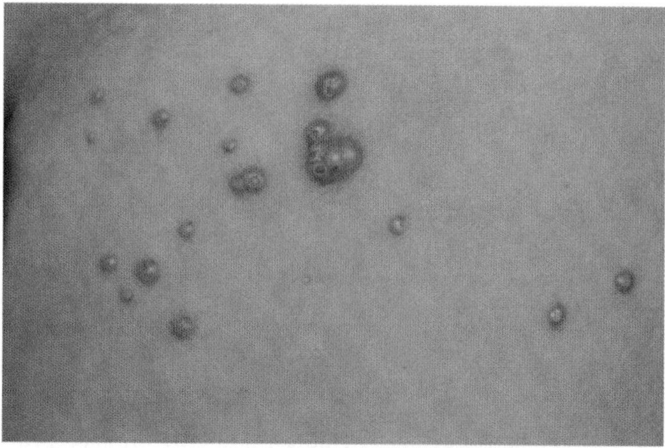

Fig. 47.7 **Molluscum Contagiosum.** Waxy pink globules with umbilicated centers. (From Habif TP. *Clinical dermatology: A color guide to diagnosis and therapy*, 4th edition. St. Louis: Mosby; 2004.)

Treatment is not necessary and usually initiated to alleviate discomfort and itch, to prevent secondary infection, to prevent trauma to lesions and bleeding, to limit the spread of the lesions, and for the social stigma or cosmetic reasons related to the infection. Although many options for treatment have been tried,[22] to date, the evidence does not support any treatment (destruction, oral, or topical) as superior to placebo.[23]

Verruca Vulgaris

Warts (verruca vulgaris) are benign lesions caused by human papillomavirus (HPV), with 189 subtypes identified. Clinical manifestations/locations have been correlated to specific subtypes. Although they may occur in any part of the body, they favor areas of epithelial disruption and mucosa. They may be spread by direct and indirect contact. Malignant transformation may occur in in immunocompromised individuals, genital warts, high-risk subtypes, or those subtypes implicated in epidermodysplasia verruciformis. This is a clinical diagnosis and does not require biopsy, unless concern for malignancy exists. Generally, warts resolve spontaneously over several years. Treatment is dependent on individual preference, type of wart, location, size, and number. Elective treatments may require multiple sessions. Treatment may be poorly tolerated or result in scarring. Generally, first-line treatment is application of salicylic acid, which is available without prescription.[24,25] Intralesion immunotherapy is an emerging alternative therapy.[26]

Rubella (German or 3-Day Measles)

Rubella is a common communicable disease of children and young adults, caused by an enveloped, positive-stranded RNA

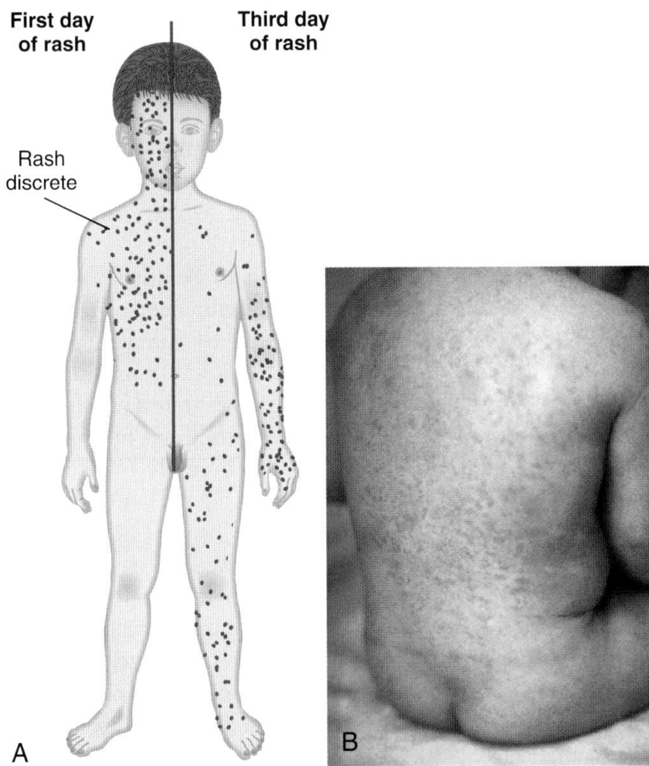

Fig. 47.8 Rubella (3-Day Measles). (A) Typical distribution of full-blown maculopapular rash with tendency to coalesce. (B) Rash of rubella. (From Centers for Disease Control and Prevention: Image Bank, Figure #712. https://www.cdc.gov/rubella/about/photos.html. Accessed April 12, 2022.)

virus and classified as a Rubivirus in the Togaviridae family. Rubella is transmitted primarily through direct or droplet contact from nasopharyngeal secretions. Humans are the only natural hosts. In temperate climates, infections usually occur during late winter and early spring.[27] This disease is mild in most children. The incubation period ranges from 12 to 23 days. Prodromal symptoms include enlarged cervical and postauricular lymph nodes, low-grade fever, headache, sore throat, rhinorrhea, and cough. A faint-pink to red confluent maculopapular rash develops on the face, with spread to the trunk and extremities 1 to 4 days after the onset of initial symptoms (Fig. 47.8). The rash is thought to be the result of virus dissemination to the skin. The rash subsides after 2 to 3 days, usually without complication. People infected with rubella are most contagious when the rash is erupting, but they can be contagious from 7 days before and 7 days after the rash appears (Table 47.1).[27] There is no specific antiviral treatment for rubella, and most therapy is supportive. Antibiotic therapy is initiated if secondary bacterial infections develop. Recovery is usually spontaneous, although lymph nodes may remain enlarged for weeks.

Vaccination for rubella is usually given in combination with mumps and measles (rubeola) (MMR). The Centers for Disease Control and Prevention vaccine recommendations are available at https://www.cdc.gov/vaccines/schedules/hcp/child-adolescent.html. The measles, mumps, and rubella (MMR) vaccine has an outstanding safety record and is highly efficacious.[28] High coverage with MMR has led to the elimination of endemic measles, rubella, and congenital rubella syndrome in the United States. The biggest challenges to global measles and rubella control and elimination are insufficient vaccination

TABLE 47.1 Differential Presentation of Viral Diseases Producing Rashes

Viral Disease	Incubation	Prodromal Symptoms	Duration/Characteristics	Clinical Symptoms
Rubella (German measles; rubivirus)	14–21 days	1–2 days Mild fever Malaise Respiratory symptoms	1–3 days Pink-red maculopapular rash Face and trunk	Enlarged and tender occipital and periauricular lymph nodes
Rubeola (measles; paramyxovirus)	7–12 days	2–5 days Fever Cough Respiratory symptoms	3–5 days Purple-red to brown maculopapular papules Face, trunk, extremities	Koplik spots[a] 1–3 days before rash Rash develops when fever subsides
Roseola (exanthema subitum; human herpesvirus 6 and 7)	5–15 days	2–5 days High fever	1–3 days Pink-red macular papules Neck and trunk	
Varicella (chickenpox; varicella- zoster virus)	11–20 days	1–2 days Low-grade fever Cough May be asymptomatic	Red papules, vesicles, pustules in clusters	Eruption of new lesions for 4–5 days Occasional ulcerative lesion in mouth
Hand, foot, and mouth disease (coxsackie A virus and enterovirus A71)	4–6 days	Fever, sore throat, anorexia	3–7 days Gray thick-walled vesicles 3–6 mm in diameter with a red or noninflamed base, commonly on palms, soles and sides of feet, and mouth mucosa	None or fever, diarrhea, sore throat

[a]Koplic spots: clusters of white lesions on the lower buccal mucosa.

coverage globally and increasing hesitancy.[28] The MMR vaccine has rarely been associated with adverse neurologic events. A common misconception is that inoculation with MMR can cause autism; however, studies conclude that MMR immunization does not cause autism.[28] Lack of vaccination, however, leads to loss of herd immunity and significant morbidity and mortality with pneumonia, croup, and encephalitis being causes of death worldwide. Women of childbearing age are immunized if their rubella hemagglutination-inhibition titer is low. Pregnancy should be avoided for 3 months after vaccination because the attenuated virus in the vaccine may remain viable for this period. Pregnancy in women who have rubella early in the first trimester has been associated with congenital defects.

Rubeola

Rubeola is a highly contagious, acute viral disease of childhood. Transmitted by direct contact with droplets from infected persons, rubeola is caused by an RNA-containing paramyxovirus with an incubation period of 7 to 12 days, during which there are no symptoms.[29] The virus enters the respiratory tract, attaches to alveolar macrophages, amplifies in local lymphatic tissue, and progresses to systemic disease. Prodromal symptoms include high fever (up to 40.5°C [104.9°F]), malaise, enlarged lymph nodes, rhinorrhea, conjunctivitis, and barking cough. Characteristic pinpoint white spots, surrounded by an erythematous ring, develop over the buccal mucosa and are known as *Koplik spots.* These spots appear 2 to 3 days after viral symptoms begin and precede the body rash by 1 to 2 days. Within 3 to 4 days, an erythematous maculopapular rash develops over the head and spreads distally over the trunk, extremities, hands, and feet. Early lesions blanch with pressure, followed by a brownish hue that does not blanch as the rash fades. The rash then subsides within 3 to 5 days.[29]

Complications associated with measles may be caused by the primary infection or by a secondary bacterial infection. Measles encephalitis occurs rarely, and most children recover completely; only a small minority of children develop permanent brain damage or die. Bacterial complications include otitis media and pneumonia, usually caused by group A hemolytic *Streptococcus, Haemophilus influenzae*, or *S. aureus* infection.

Measles is prevented by vaccination, as discussed in rubella section above. There is no specific viral treatment for measles, and supportive and care therapy is the same as that recommended for rubella.

Roseola Infantum (Exanthema Subitum, Sixth Disease)

Roseola Infantum is a common viral illness of childhood, also known as exanthema subitum and sixth disease. It is caused by a primary infection with human herpesvirus 6 (HHV-6) and caused less frequently by human herpesvirus 7 (HHV-7). The disease presents in children ages 6 to 12 months, with 90% of cases occurring in children younger than 2 years. Caused by the B variant of HHV-6, individuals with the virus classically present with an acute onset of a high-grade fever up to 40°C (104°F) for 3 to 5 days.[30] As the fever diminishes, a nonpruritic, pink papular rash appears, primarily over the trunk and neck and lasts about 24 hours. Children usually feel well, eat normally, and have few other symptoms, after fever subsides. It is a self-limited illness that is treated symptomatically.

Chickenpox

Chickenpox (varicella) is a highly contagious viral illness caused by the varicella-zoster virus and is spread by close person-to-person contact and by airborne droplets. Introduction of an infected person into a household results in a 90% possibility of susceptible persons developing the disease within the incubation period, usually 14 days. Vesicular lesions occur in the epidermis as infection occurs within keratinocytes. An inflammatory infiltrate is often present. Vesicles eventually rupture, followed by crust formation or the development of transient ulcers on mucous membranes. Children are contagious for at least 1 day before development of the lesions. Transmission of the virus may occur until approximately 5 to 6 days after the onset of the first skin lesions in healthy children. In immunocompromised children, the virus is recoverable for a longer period, but infected children must be considered contagious for at least 7 to 10 days.

Normally, children who develop chickenpox have no prodromal symptoms. The first sign of illness may be pruritus or the appearance of vesicles, usually on the trunk, scalp, or face. The rash later spreads to the extremities. Characteristically, lesions can be seen in various stages of maturation with macules, papules, and vesicles present in a particular area at the same time (Fig. 47.9). The vesicular lesions are superficial and rupture easily. New lesions will erupt for 4 to 5 days, until there are approximately 100 to 300 in different stages of development. The vesicles become crusted, and over time only the crust remains, although there may be an occasional vesicle on the palm later in the disease. Although uncommon, ulcerative lesions are sometimes seen in the mouth and, less commonly, on the conjunctiva and pharynx. Fever usually lasts 2 to 3 days, with body temperature ranging from 38.5°C to 40°C (101.3° to 104°F).

Complications are rare in children but more common in adults. They can include transient hematuria (from rupture of vesicles in the bladder), epistaxis, laryngeal edema, and varicella pneumonia. One case of chickenpox produces almost complete immunity against a second attack. Rarely, the fetus may be malformed (congenital varicella syndrome) if chickenpox develops in the first half of pregnancy. Infants whose mothers have chickenpox at any stage of pregnancy have a higher risk of developing herpes zoster during the first few years of life.[31] Varicella-zoster immunoglobulin should be administered to neonates whenever the onset of maternal disease is between 5 days before delivery and 2 days after delivery.

Uncomplicated chickenpox requires no specific therapy. Baths, wet dressings, and oral antihistamines occasionally help relieve pruritus and prevent secondary infection from developing as a result of scratching. Oral antibiotics should be given if secondary bacterial infection is present. Zoster immune globulin may be administered to immunodeficient individuals if given within 72 hours after exposure to chickenpox. Oral acyclovir may be valuable in immunosuppressed or other select groups of children. The varicella vaccine and subsequent booster protects against varicella.[32] Herpes zoster is a vesicular eruption from a recurrence of the latent varicella virus, along the distribution of a dorsal root ganglion (see Chapter 46).

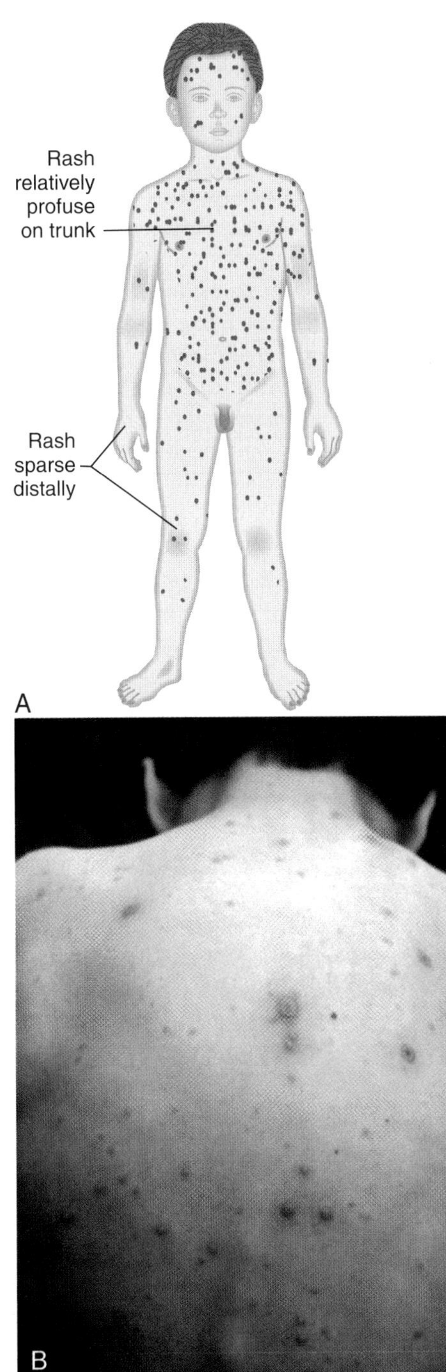

Fig. 47.9 Chickenpox. (A) Pattern of generalized, polymorphous eruption. (B) Chickenpox lesions. (From Centers for Disease Control and Prevention: Image Bank, Figure #6121. https://phil.cdc.gov/details.aspx?pid=6121. Accessed April 12, 2022.)

Hand, Foot, and Mouth Disease

Hand, foot, and mouth disease (HFMD) is a contagious viral disease primarily of children under 5 years of age. It is commonly caused by coxsackie virus and enterovirus A71. The infection manifests as fever; vesicular ulcerous lesions in the mouth; and vesicular rashes on the hands, feet, and buttocks. Atypical presentations may mimic other infections and be misleading but generally have not been associated with worse outcomes. A small number of children may experience severe complications, such as meningitis, encephalitis, acute flaccid paralysis, and neurorespiratory syndrome. The disease is self-limiting with supportive care. Research is in progress to develop a preventive vaccine.[33,34]

Erythema Infectiosum (Fifth Disease)

Erythema infectiosum (fifth disease) is caused by infection with B19 parvovirus. The infection is characterized by a mild fever, headache, sore throat, pruritus, and arthralgia, followed by a blotchy, macular, lacy rash on the cheeks (slapped-cheek), which spreads to the trunk and limbs and may last for up to 6 weeks. Symptoms are usually self-limiting. Diagnosis is related to symptoms and can include immunologic assays or a polymerase chain reaction test to identify the virus. Treatment is symptomatic and includes nonsteroidal anti-inflammatory drugs for arthralgias and antihistamines for pruritus. Infection in women less than 20 weeks pregnant can lead to miscarriage and requires special care. The virus causes severe fetal anemia, and pregnancy loss is due to suppression of erythroid progenitor cells.[35] A new viral rash was seen with the emergence of the coronavirus. It has been called COVID toes and may be the only sign of the coronavirus infection. The rash presents as erythematous or purplish in color and usually develops on the toes (see the box Emerging Science Box: Coronavirus Rash).

EMERGING SCIENCE BOX

Coronavirus Rash

The COVID-19 pandemic has differing presenting symptoms in children as compared to adults.

The pediatric population has increased cutaneous manifestations as the initial, and sometimes only, symptom of the virus. Cutaneous manifestations that have been observed in adults and children include urticaria, maculopapular rash, or vesicular rash; however, chilblains, erythema multiforme, urticaria, and Kawasaki disease-like inflammatory multisystemic syndrome are more frequently observed in children and teenagers. The lesions most common were the chilblains, often times referred to "COVID toes." Microscopic features of COVID-19 chilblains include three main components: a background area, globules, and reticular network. The background area is variously described as red, purple, brown, or grey with globules that are usually red to purple in color, and finally, a grey–brown reticular network located peripherally within the background area. While there is not a specific pathogenesis currently related to the skin manifestations observed in the pediatric population, there are similarities to rashes caused by other viral infections. A temporospatial association exists between COVID-19 and a severe multisystemic condition named pediatric inflammatory multisystem syndrome. Inflammatory markers (e.g., CRP, erythrocyte sedimentation rate, neutrophil count, and ferritin) were elevated in pediatric cases, along with pancytopenia.

Data from Andina D, et al. ESPD Group for the Skin Manifestations of COVID-19. Skin manifestations of COVID-19 in children: Part 1. *Clin Exp Dermatol.* 2021 Apr;46(3):444–450. https://doi. org/10.1111/ced.14481. Epub 2020 Nov 12. PMID: 33180982; Andina D, et al. ESPD Group for the Skin Manifestations of COVID-19. Skin manifestations of COVID-19 in children: Part 2. *Clin Exp Dermatol.* 2021 Apr;46(3):451–461. https://doi. org/10.1111/ced.14482. Epub 2020 Nov 9. PMID: 33166429; Singh H, et al. Cutaneous Manifestations of COVID-19: A Systematic Review. *Adv Wound Care (New Rochelle).* 2021 Feb;10(2):51–80. https://doi. org/10.1089/wound.2020.1309. Epub 2020 Oct 19. PMID: 33035150; PMCID: PMC8020517.

INSECT BITES AND PARASITES

Insect bites and infestations are common causes of skin disorders in children and adults. Skin damage occurs by various mechanisms, including trauma of bites and stings, allergic reactions, transmission of disease, injection of substances that cause local or systemic reactions, and inflammatory reactions resulting from embedded and retained insect mouth parts and scratching of the skin. Anaphylactic reactions are treated with epinephrine (adrenaline), and children with a history of anaphylactic reaction should be provided with epinephrine autoinjectors (i.e., an EpiPen). Skin testing and subcutaneous immunotherapy can be considered for subsequent stings and bites. Papular urticaria is a chronic inflammatory skin eruption, caused by exposure to arthropod bites usually associated with flea bites or mosquitos and is usually seen in younger children primarily in tropical environments. Generally the lesions are papular, but wheals vesicles, blisters, and scabs have been reported.[36]

Scabies

Scabies is a parasitic infestation of the skin caused by the mite, *Sarcoptes scabiei* (Fig. 47.10A). The pregnant mite burrows into the epidermis of its human host and lays eggs, which hatch in 48 to 72 hours and create new burrows. They reach adulthood in 1 to 14 days. They then mate, and the cycle is repeated. It is transmitted by close personal contact. Scabies is often epidemic in areas of overcrowded housing, with poor sanitation, and in children. Immunocompromised individuals are at greater risk. Scabies can facilitate *S. pyogenes* and *S. aureus* skin coinfections, with systemic complications. The scabies mite has adapted mechanisms to overcome host defenses.

Symptoms appear 3 to 5 weeks after infestation. The primary lesions are burrows, papules, and vesicular lesions, with intense pruritus that worsens at night. Pruritus is thought to be related to immune and inflammatory responses. In older children and adults, the lesions occur in the webs of fingers; in the axillae; in the creases of the arms and wrists; along the belt line; and around the nipples, genitalia, and lower buttocks. Infants and young children have a different pattern of distribution, with involvement of the palms, soles, head, neck, and face (see Fig. 47.10B). Secondary infections and crusting develop as a result of scratching and eczematous changes.

Diagnosis of scabies is made by observation of the tunnels and burrows and by microscopic examination of scrapings of the skin to identify the mite, its eggs, or its feces. Treatment involves the application of a scabicide, which is curative. All clothing and linens should be washed and dried in hot cycles, dry-cleaned, or kept in a sealed bag for 48 to 72 hours.[37,38]

Fleas and Bedbugs

Fleas and bedbugs are blood-sucking arthropod parasites, which bite human hosts and cause a variety of skin lesions. Bites from these insects produce pruritic, erythematous-edematous papules in a linear array or in a classic pattern of three bites, often coined the breakfast, lunch, and dinner sign (Fig. 47.11). Bed-bug bites appear as a small dot and are often unnoticed. Previous sensitization to their saliva can cause the intense erythematous papular and pruritic reactions (Fig. 47.12). Secondary infections may occur because of the scratching associated with the bites. Prevention is

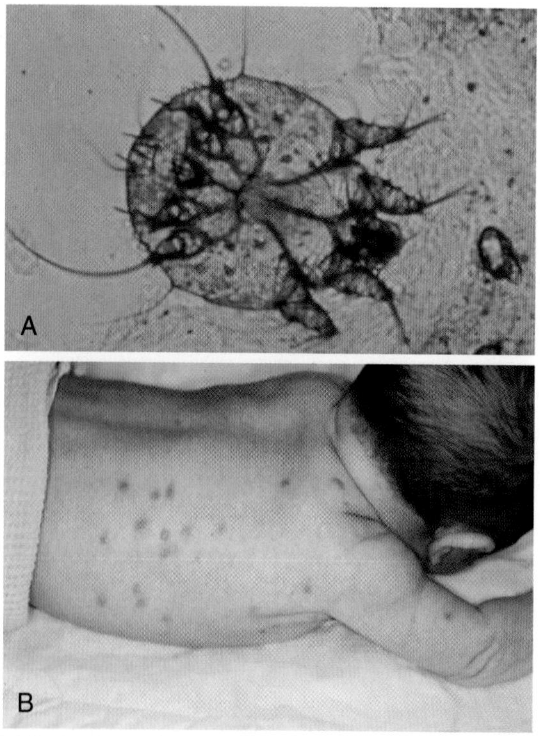

Fig. 47.10 Scabies. **(A)** Scabies mite, as seen clinically when removed from its burrow. **(B)** Characteristic scabies bites. (Courtesy Department of Dermatology, School of Medicine, University of Utah, Salt Lake City, UT.)

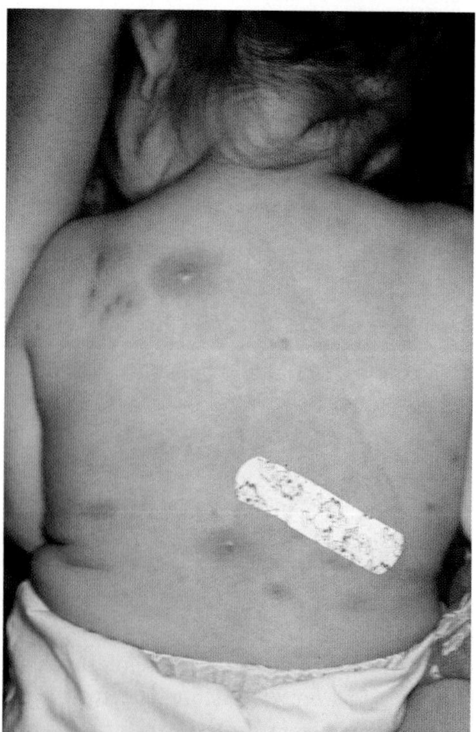

Fig. 47.11 Fleabites. Fleabite producing an urticarial wheal with central puncture.

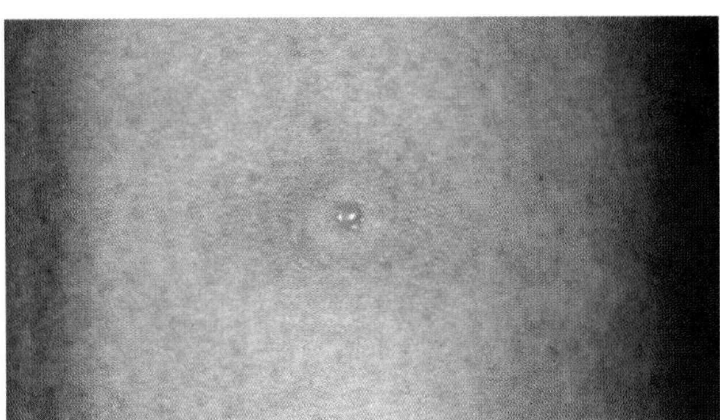

Fig. 47.12 Bullous Bed Bug Bites. (Courtesy Department of Dermatology, School of Medicine, University of Utah, Salt Lake City, UT.)

focused on environmental control of the offending insects, both indoor and outdoor. Reactions to bites are treated with symptomatic measures to control itching and prevent infection.[39]

Pediculosis (Lice Infestation)

The three known types of human lice are (1) the head louse *(Pediculus human capitis)*, (2) the body louse *(Pediculus humanas corporis)*, and (3) the crab or pubic louse *(Phthirus pubis)*. They are parasites and survive by sucking blood from the host. Their mouth is shaped for piercing and sucking and are attached to the skin of the host while the louse is feeding. When piercing the skin, the louse secretes toxic saliva, and the mechanical trauma and toxin produce a pruritic dermatitis.[40]

Pediculosis human capitus are ectoparasites. They reproduce by attaching to the hair shaft close to the scalp and laying eggs (nits). The nits hatch in 7 to 10 days.[41,42] This is commonly spread by head-to-head contact. As a result, children are more often infected. Initially, the person may be asymptomatic; however, over time may be more pruritic. Diagnosis is usually made by presence of live lice or adherent nits on the scalp. Treatment should be reserved for confirmed cases of active lice. Lindane is no longer recommended for treatment in the United States due to safety and efficacy concerns, with recommendations for safer alternatives that are both available with and without prescription. Manual removal of nits is advisable but not mandated for treatment.[41,42] OTC products are first-line recommendations, and prescription treatments are also available.[43] All close contacts should be treated at the same time to prevent spread of the infestation.[44] The Center for Disease Control has a helpful fact sheet for families, which addresses housekeeping recommendations to prevent the spread of lice to close contacts.[45]

Body lice and pubic lice are ectoparasites, require blood meals about five times per day, and have been implicated in transmission of disease. They differ from head lice as they do not reside on the host's body but infest clothes, primarily seams, and migrate to the host for meals. Because of their migration and infestation in clothing, infections are more problematic in impoverished and densely populated areas. Transmission may occur directly or via fomites. Lesions are pruritic and present as erythematous macules, papules, or papular urticaria with a central punctum. Iron deficiency anemia has been reported with this infestation due to their feeding cycle. Environmental control of the contaminated articles is mandated. Secondary infections are treated with antibiotics. Resistance has been reported with current available therapies, necessitating further research to control this infestation in populations.[46]

VASCULAR ANOMALIES

Vascular anomalies are a group of common and rare disorders of blood-vessel growth. These lesions may be further classified by their presentation and associated deformities. The International Society for the Study of Vascular Anomalies (ISSVA) revised their classification of vascular disorders in 2018. Lesions classified as benign vascular tumors included infantile hemangioma, congenital hemangioma, tufted angioma, spindle-cell and epithelioid hemangioma, and pyogenic granuloma. Additional classifications include locally aggressive or borderline vascular tumors and malignant vascular tumors. The committee also classified capillary malformations, lymphatic malformations, venous malformations, and combined malformations. The classifications have been expanded to include the known causal genes for these malformations, which has further defined these disorders.[47]

Infantile Hemangiomas

Infantile hemangiomas have glucose transporter protein-1 (GLUT1)-positive endothelial cells. It is proposed that in utero episodes of hypoxia may lead to upregulation of GLUT-1 and angiogenic cytokines, contributing to hemangioma formation. They consist of proliferating endothelial-like cells with disorganized angiogenesis, overexpression of growth factors, and a variable rate of growth. Many of these lesions resolve over time and require no treatment, however, lesions that are disfiguring or life threatening may require systemic therapy.[48] Lesions are usually classified as superficial (little or no subcutaneous involvement) (Fig. 47.13), deep (located in deeper tissues and may appear blue on surface skin) (Fig. 47.14), or combined (both components evident). Additionally, they are categorized as localized (well defined focal lesions), segmental (usually plaque like, >5 cm in diameter and in a anatomic region), indeterminate,

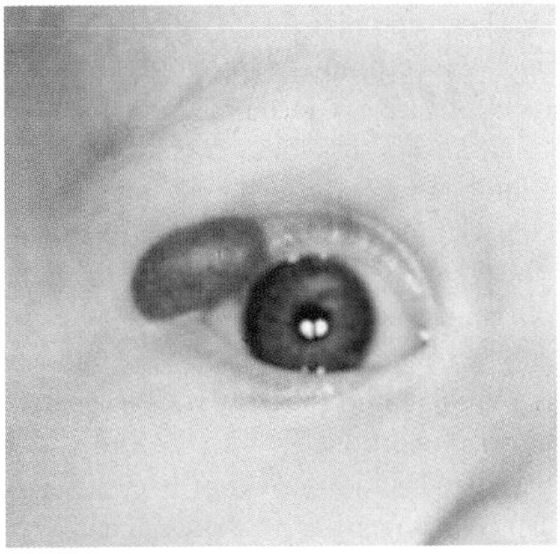

Fig. 47.13 Superficial (Capillary) Hemangioma. (Courtesy Department of Dermatology, School of Medicine, University of Utah, Salt Lake City, UT.)

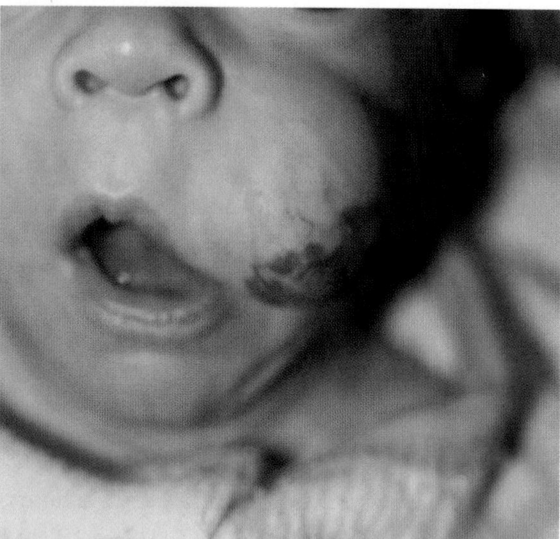

Fig. 47.14 Deep Hemangioma. (Courtesy Department of Dermatology, School of Medicine, University of Utah, Salt Lake City, UT.)

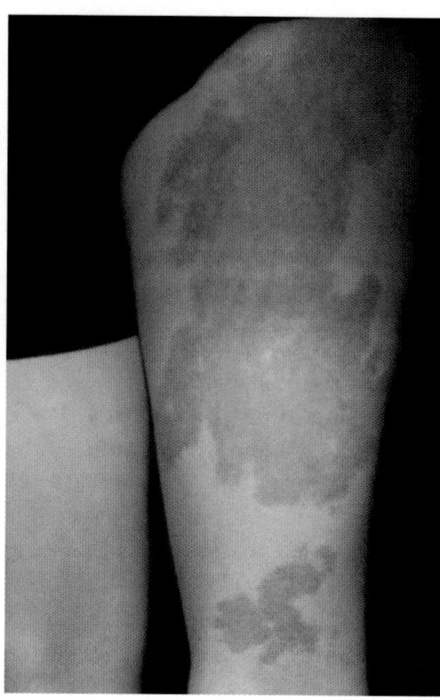

Fig. 47.15 Port-Wine Hemangioma. Port-Wine hemangioma in a child caused by malformation of dermal capillaries. (Courtesy Department of Dermatology, School of Medicine, University of Utah, Salt Lake City, UT.)

or multifocal (multiple lesions). Life-threatening lesions usually occur in the beard distribution, with concern for airway obstruction or greater than five discrete lesions and with concern for liver involvement, cardiac failure, and hypothyroidism. Functional impairment if the lesion is periocular may result in vision alterations, or if it occurs on lip or oral cavity may result in feeding impairment. Additionally, these lesions may be disfiguring if large or located on the face, scalp, or breast. Infantile hemangiomas, if segmental on the face or scalp, may be associated with systemic anomalies known as PHACE syndrome ([P]osterior fossa and other structural brain malformations; large [H]emangiomas of the face, neck, and/or scalp; anatomical anomalies of the cerebral or cervical [A]rteries; [C]ardiac anomalies/[C]oarctation of the aorta; and [E]ye abnormalities) or in the pelvic area associated with LUMBAR syndrome ([L]ower body hemangioma, [U]rogenital abnormalities / ulceration, [M]yelopathy, [B]ony deformities, [A]norectal malformations / arterial anomalies, and [R]ectal anomalies), requiring further imaging and multidisciplinary care.[49] Infantile hemangiomas grow rapidly in the first 3 months of life, and most of the growth has been completed by 5 months of age.[48,49] Clinical practice guidelines recommend propranolol as the systemic drug of choice for larger and more problematic lesions with topical treatment, using timolol for smaller, superficial lesions. Propranolol inhibits tumor growth and angiogenesis and promotes vasoconstriction. Surgery and laser treatment are usually considered for residual skin changes post-involution and are not usually first-line therapy.[49,50]

Cutaneous vascular malformations are rare anomalies of blood vessels present at birth but may not be apparent for several years. They grow proportionately with the child.[51] Vascular malformations may demonstrate rapid growth, particularly during the hormonal changes of puberty or pregnancy and in association with trauma. These lesions are classified as low flow or high flow. *Low-flow malformations* involve capillaries, veins, and lymphatics. *High-flow malformations* involve arteries. In addition to locations within the skin, they may involve the gastrointestinal tract (blue rubber bleb nevus syndrome), bone, the eye, and vascular malformation of the brain (Maffucci syndrome, Sturge-Weber syndrome). *Overgrowth syndromes* can occur with either high- or low-flow malformations, with overgrowth of the underlying structures (i.e., legs, arms, facial bones). The most common capillary malformations are port-wine stain (nevus flammeus) and salmon patches (nevus simplex).

Port-wine (nevus flammeus) stains are congenital vascular malformations of the dermal capillaries that involve both genetic and molecular alterations in capillary endothelial cells.[52] The lesions are flat and their color ranges from pink to dark reddish purple, and they do not fade with age. Involvement of the face and other body surfaces is common, and the lesions may be large and may become darker and thicker over time (Fig. 47.15). During adolescence and later adult years, the port-wine stain may become papular and cavernous. The pulsed-dye laser is the treatment of choice to successfully lighten the color and flatten the more nodular and cavernous lesions. **Sturge-Weber syndrome** is a port-wine stain distributed along the ophthalmic branch of the trigeminal nerve and is associated with the leptomeninges of the brain and choroid, glaucoma, seizures, stroke, and intellectual disability. These capillary malformations are associated with a mutation in the *GNAQ* gene (guanine nucleotide-binding protein G, q polypeptide).[53]

Salmon patches (nevus simplex) are macular pink or lilac lesions present at birth and located on the occipital scalp, forehead, upper eyelids, or nasolabial fold. They are a more superficial variant of nevus flammeus and one of the most common congenital malformations in the skin. The pink color results from distended dermal capillaries and 95% of patches fade by 1 and 3 years of age. Those located at the occipital scalp may persist for a lifetime but generally do not present a cosmetic problem.

OTHER SKIN DISORDERS

Psoriasis

Psoriasis is a chronic, relapsing autoimmune-mediated inflammatory disease affecting the skin and nails. Onset of disease can occur in children, but the differences in pathogenesis between children and adults is not clearly determined. T-cell-mediated interleukin 17 cytokines are involved in keratinocyte proliferation and inflammatory responses. In adults, the disease is also associated with joint disease and multiple comorbidities (see Chapter 46).[54,55] Morphology and distribution may vary with the age at presentation. Infants and toddlers may present with refractory diaper dermatitis.[56]

Older children may present with plaque or guttate lesions, with less common phenotypes to include pustular, erythrodermic, inverse and drug-induced psoriasis. Identified triggers include trauma to the skin, infection (primarily streptococcus), emotional stress, and medications. Overweight and obesity have emerged as risk factors in the development of psoriasis.[57] Diagnosis is usually made clinically. Unique to psoriatic lesions is the presence of the Auspiz sign, which is the presence of punctuate bleeding when the scale is scraped off the lesions. Additionally, the lesions are often present in areas of trauma (Koebner phenomena). Guidelines are available for the care of psoriasis in children, and studies are in progress for targeted treatment unique to children.[58,59] Psoriasis has a detrimental impact on quality of life, and control of exacerbation triggers and psychosocial support is recommended as part of an ongoing treatment plan.[53]

Newborn Rashes

Miliaria

Miliaria presents as a self-limited eruption, occurring in infants due to the occlusion of the sweat ducts, causing an outflow obstruction and entrapment of the sweat within the skin. The types are distinguished depending on the anatomic level of the obstruction, with the more superficial obstruction presenting as noninflammatory pinpoint vesicles usually found in intertriginous folds known as miliaria crystallina and the deeper obstruction presenting as erythematous papules or papulovesicles on the trunk, arms, or intertriginous folds. Removal of the occlusion resolves in resolution of symptoms. Generally, this can be due to tight-fitting garments or swaddling, overbundling, fever, or warm climates. Loose-fitting clothes, cool baths, and cool environments will improve this condition (Fig. 47.16).[60]

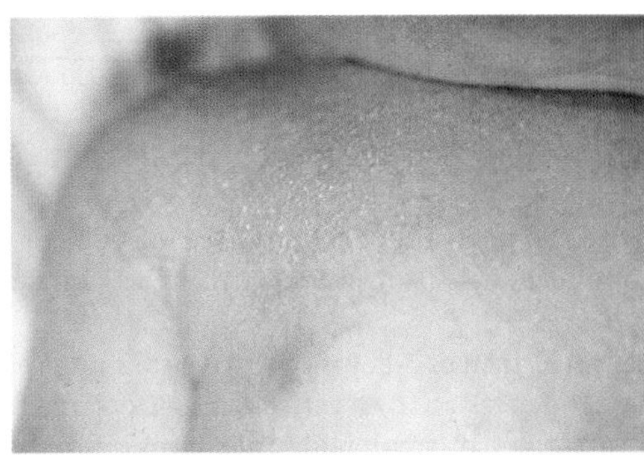

Fig. 47.16 Miliaria Rubra. Note discrete erythematous papules or papulovesicles. (Courtesy Department of Dermatology, School of Medicine, University of Utah, Salt Lake City, UT.)

Erythema Toxicum Neonatorum

Erythema toxicum neonatorum (toxic erythema of the newborn) is a benign, erythematous accumulation of macules, papules, or pustules that appears at birth or 3 to 4 days after birth. The lesions first appear as a blotchy, macular erythematous rash. The macules vary from 1 mm to 1 cm in diameter. When papules or pustules develop, they are light yellow or white and 1 to 3 mm in diameter. There may be a few or several hundred lesions, and any body surface can be affected, with the exception of the palms and soles, where there are no pilosebaceous follicles. The cause of the lesion is unknown but may be related to an innate immune response to the first commensal microflora, with release of inflammatory mediators. It is self-limiting and resolves spontaneously within a few weeks after birth. No treatment is required.[61]

SUMMARY REVIEW

Acne Vulgaris

1. Acne vulgaris is a common disorder related to obstruction of pilosebaceous follicles and proliferation of *Cutibacterium acnes*, with follicular occlusion and inflammation primarily of the face, neck, and upper trunk. It is characterized by both noninflammatory and inflammatory lesions. Treatment is dependent on severity.

Dermatitis

1. AD is an alteration in the skin barrier. It occurs as red, scaly lesions on the face, cheeks, and flexor surfaces of the extremities in infants and young children. AD is associated with inflammatory cytokines. Successful AD management strategies are implemented in a stepwise approach tailored to the individuals and are severity-based. Contact dermatitis is an eczematous eruption resulting from either delayed hypersensitive reaction to an allergen (allergic contact dermatitis) or direct irritation to the skin from an irritating substance (irritant contact dermatitis). Diaper dermatitis is a type of irritant contact dermatitis that develops from prolonged exposure to urine and feces and may become secondarily infected with *Candida albicans*.

Infections of the Skin

1. Impetigo is a contagious bacterial disease occurring in two forms: bullous and vesicular. The toxins from the bacteria produce a weeping lesion with a honey-colored crust.
2. SSSS (Ritter disease) is a staphylococcal skin infection that produces an exfoliative toxin with painful blisters and bullae formation over large areas of the skin, requiring emergency care and systemic antibiotic treatment.

3. Tinea capitis (scalp ringworm) and tinea corporis (ringworm) are fungal infections of the scalp and body caused by dermatophytes.
4. Thrush is a fungal infection of the mouth caused by *Candida albicans*.
5. Molluscum contagiosum is a poxvirus infection of the skin that produces pale papular lesions filled with viral and cellular debris.
6. Rubella (German or 3-day measles) is a communicable viral disease characterized by fever, sore throat, enlarged cervical and postauricular lymph nodes, and a generalized maculopapular rash that lasts 1 to 4 days.
7. Rubeola (red measles) is a viral contagious disease with symptoms of high fever, enlarged lymph nodes, conjunctivitis, and a red rash that begins on the head, spreads to the trunk and extremities, and lasts 3 to 5 days. Both bacterial and viral complications may accompany rubeola.
8. Roseola (exanthema subitum) is a benign disease of infants with a sudden onset of fever that lasts 3 to 5 days, followed by a rash that lasts 24 hours.
9. Chickenpox (varicella) is a highly contagious disease caused by the varicella-zoster virus. Vesicular lesions occur on the skin and mucous membranes. Individuals are contagious from 1 day before the development of the rash until about 5 to 6 days after the rash develops.
10. Hand, foot, and mouth disease (HFMD) is a contagious viral disease commonly caused by coxsackievirus and enterovirus that manifests with fever, vesicular ulcerous lesions in the mouth, and vesicular rashes on the hands, feet, and buttocks.
11. Erythema infectiosum (fifth disease) is an infection caused by B19 parvovirus that usually causes mild symptoms of fever, headache, pruritus, and arthralgias followed by a rash on the cheeks spreading to the trunk and limbs.

Insect Bites and Parasites

1. Scabies is a pruritic lesion caused by the itch mite, which burrows into the skin and forms papules and vesicles. The mite is very contagious and is transmitted by direct contact.
2. Flea and bedbugs are blood-sucking parasites and their bites can produce pruritic, erythematous-edematous papules.
3. Pediculosis (lice infestation) is caused by blood-sucking parasites that secrete toxic saliva and damage the skin to produce pruritic dermatitis. Lice are spread by direct contact and are recognized by the ova or nits that attach to the shafts of body hairs.

Infantile Hemangiomas

1. Infantile hemangiomas are benign tumors that form from the rapid growth of vascular endothelial cells and result in formation of extra blood vessels that can be superficial or deep or a combination of both. Location and distribution affect treatment considerations and concern for PHACES or LUMBAR syndromes.

Other Skin Disorders and Newborn rashes

1. Psoriasis is a chronic relapsing autoimmune mediated inflammatory disease affecting the skin and nails which has also been associated with joint disease and multiple comorbidities.
2. Miliaria is characterized by a vesicular eruption that results from obstruction of the sweat duct opening in infants. In miliaria crystallina, ductal rupture occurs within the stratum corneum and appears as 1- to 2-mm clear vesicles without erythema. In miliaria rubra (prickly heat), the ductal rupture occurs in the lower epidermis, attracts inflammatory cells, and appears as 2- to 4-mm discrete erythematous papules or papulovesicles
3. Erythema toxicum neonatorum is a benign accumulation of macules, papules, and pustules that spontaneously resolves within a few weeks after birth.

REFERENCES

1. Cong TX, et al. From pathogenesis of acne vulgaris to anti-acne agents. *Arch Dermatol Res*. 2019;311(5):337–349.
2. Kurokawa I, Nakase K. Recent advances in understanding and managing acne. *F1000Res*. 2020;9 F1000 Faculty Rev-792.
3. Habeshian KA, Cohen BA. Current issues in the treatment of acne vulgaris. *Pediatrics*. 2020;145(Suppl 2):S225–S230.
4. Conforti C, et al. An overview of treatment options for mild-to-moderate acne based on American Academy of Dermatology, European Academy of Dermatology and Venereology, and Italian Society of Dermatology and Venereology guidelines. *Dermatol Ther*. 2020;33(4):e13548.
5. Hafsi W, Badri T. *Acne conglobata. StatPearls*. Treasure Island FL: StatPearls Publishing; 2020. Last Updated December 21, 2021. Available at https://www.ncbi.nlm.nih.gov/books/NBK459219/. (Accessed February 12, 2022).
6. Nakahara T, et al. Basics and recent advances in the pathophysiology of atopic dermatitis. *J Dermatol*. 2021;48(2):130–139.
7. Brar KK, Nicol NH, Boguniewicz M. Strategies for successful management of severe atopic dermatitis. *J Allergy Clin Immunol Pract*. 2019;7(1):1–16.
8. Blanc S, et al. Dennie-Morgan fold plus dark circles: suspect atopy at first sight. *J Pediatr*. 2015;166(6):1541.
9. Nicol NH. Step-wise treatment of atopic dermatitis: basics and beyond. *Pediatr Nurs*. 2020;46(2):92–98.
10. Hebert AA, et al. Efficacy of nonprescription moisturizers for atopic dermatitis: an updated review of clinical evidence. *Am J Clin Dermatol*. 2020;21(5):641–655.
11. Nicol NH, Boguniewicz M. Wet wrap therapy in moderate to severe atopic dermatitis. *Immunol Allergy Clin North Am*. 2017;37(1):123–139.
12. Brar KK. A review of contact dermatitis. *Ann Allergy Asthma Immunol*. 2021;126(1):32–39.
13. Neale H, et al. Pediatric allergic contact dermatitis. Part I: clinical features and common contact allergens in children. *J Am Acad Dermatol*. 2021;84(2):235–244.
14. Gustin J, et al. The impact of diaper design on mitigating known causes of diaper dermatitis. *Pediatr Dermatol*. 2018;35(6):792–795.
15. Galli L, et al. Common community-acquired bacterial skin and soft-tissue infections in children: an intersociety consensus

on impetigo, abscess, and cellulitis treatment. *Clin Ther*. 2019;41(3):532–551.
16. Ross A, Shoff HW. *Staphylococcal scalded skin syndrome. StatPearls*. Treasure Island, FL: StatPearls Publishing; 2021. Last update August 1, 2021. Available at http://www.ncbi.nlm.nih.gov/books/NBK448135/. (Accessed February 12, 2022).
17. Leung AKC, Barankin B, Leong KF. Staphylococcal-scalded skin syndrome: evaluation, diagnosis, and management. *World J Pediatr*. 2018;14(2):116–120.
18. Alter SJ, et al. Common child and adolescent cutaneous infestations and fungal infections. *Curr Probl Pediatr Adolesc Health Care*. 2018;48(1):3–25.
19. Gupta AK, et al. Tinea capitis in children: a systematic review of management. *J Eur Acad Dermatol Venereol*. 2018;32:2264–2274.
20. Grigoryan KV, et al. Pediatric tinea capitis caused by *Trichophyton violaceum* and *Trichophyton soudanense* in Rochester, Minnesota, United States. *Int J Dermatol*. 2019;58(8):912–915.
21. Centers for Disease Control and Prevention (CDC) *Molluscum contagiousum*. Atlanta, GA: CDC; 2015. Available at https://www.cdc.gov/poxvirus/molluscum-contagiosum/index.html. (Accessed February 12, 2022).
22. Silverberg NB. Pediatric molluscum: an update. *Cutis*. 2019;104(5):301–305. E1–E2.
23. van der Wouden JC, et al. Interventions for cutaneous molluscum contagiousum. *Cochrane Database Syst Rev*. 2017;5(5):CD004767.
24. Aboud AM, Nigam PK. *Wart. StatPearls*. Treasure Island, FL: StatPearls Publishing; 2021. Last update August 11, 2021. Available from: https://www.ncbi.nlm.nih.gov/books/NBK431047/. (Accessed February 12, 2022).
25. Gerlero P, Hernandez-Martin A. Treatment of warts in children: an update. *Actas Dermosifiliogr*. 2016;107(7):551–558.
26. Fields JR, Saikaly SK, Schoch JJ. Intralesional immunotherapy for pediatric warts: a review. *Pediatr Dermatol*. 2020;37(2):265–271.
27. Centers for Disease Control and Prevention (CDC) *Rubella*. Atlanta, GA: CDC; 2020. Page last reviewed December 31, 2020. Available at https://www.cdc.gov/rubella/index.html. (Accessed February 12, 2022).
28. Bankamp B, et al. Successes and challenges for preventing measles, mumps and rubella by vaccination. *Curr Opin Virol*. 2019;34:110–116.
29. Centers for Disease Control and Prevention (CDC) *Rubeola*. Atlanta, GA: CDC; 2020. Page last reviewed November 5, 2020. Available at https://www.cdc.gov/measles/. (Accessed February 12, 2022).
30. Aimola G, et al. Current understanding of human herpesvirus 6 (HHV-6) chromosomal integration. *Antiviral Res*. 2020;176:104720.
31. Smith CK, Arvin AM. Varicella in the fetus and newborn. *Semin Fetal Neonatal Med*. 2009;14(4):209–217.
32. Andrei G, Snoeck R. Advances and perspectives in the management of varicella-zoster virus infections. *Molecules*. 2021;26(4):1132.
33. Esposito S, Principi N. Hand, foot and mouth disease: current knowledge on clinical manifestations, epidemiology, aetiology and prevention. *Eur J Clin Microbiol Infect Dis*. 2018;37(3):391–398.
34. Li ML, et al. Enterovirus A71 vaccines. *Vaccines (Basel)*. 2021;9(3):199.
35. Attwood LO, Holmes NE, Hui L. Identification and management of congenital parvovirus B19 infection. *Prenat Diagn*. 2020;40(13):1722–1731.
36. Bilò MB, et al. Hymenoptera venom allergy: management of children and adults in clinical practice. *J Investig Allergol Clin Immunol*. 2019;29(3):180–205.
37. Arlian LG, Morgan MS. A review of *Sarcoptes scabiei:* past, present and future. *Parasit Vectors*. 2017;10(1):297.
38. Chandler DJ, Fuller LC. A review of scabies: an infestation more than skin deep. *Dermatology*. 2019;235:79–90.
39. Peres G, et al. Breakfast, lunch and dinner sign: a hallmark of flea and bedbug bites. *An Bras Dermatol*. 2018;93(5):759–760.
40. Amanzougaghene N, et al. Where are we with human lice? A review of the current state of knowledge. *Front Cell Infect Microbiol*. 2020;9:474.
41. Devore CD, Schutze GE. Council on School Health and Committee on Infectious Diseases: Head lice. *Pediatrics*. 2015;135:e1355–e1365.
42. Koch E, et al. Management of head louse infestations in the United States—a literature review. *Pediatr Dermatol*. 2016;33(5):466–472.
43. Mumcuoglu KY, et al. International recommendations for an effective control of head louse infestations. *Int J Dermatol*. 2021;60(3):272–280.
44. Feldmeier H. Treatment of pediculosis capitus: a critical appraisal of the current literature. *Am J Clin Dermatol*. 2014;15:401–412.
45. Centers for Disease Control and Prevention (CDC) *Parasites: head lice*. Atlanta, GA: CDC; 2013. Page last reviewed September 24, 2013. Available at. http://www.cdc.gov/parasites/lice/head. Accessed February 12, 2022.
46. Nyers ES, Elston DM. What's eating you? Human body lice (*Pediculus humanus corporis*). *Cutis*. 2020;105(3):118–120.
47. International Society for the Study of Vascular Anomalies (ISSVA) *Classification of vascular anomalies*. Milwaukee, WI: ISSVA; 2018. Available at https://www.issva.org/UserFiles/file/ISSVA-Classification-2018.pdf. (Accessed February 12, 2022).
48. Pam N, Kridin K, Khamaysi Z. Propranolol for infantile hemangioma: evaluating efficacy and predictors of response and rebound growth. *Dermatol Ther*. 2021;34(3):e14936.
49. Krowchuk DP, et al. Clinical practice guideline for the management of infantile hemangiomas. *Pediatrics*. 2019;143(1):e20183475.
50. Léauté-Labrèze C, Harper JI, Hoeger PH. Infantile haemangioma. *Lancet*. 2017;390(10089):85–94.
51. Zhang B, Ma L. Updated classification and therapy of vascular malformations in pediatric patients. *Pediatr Investig*. 2018;2(2):119–123.
52. Nguyen V, et al. The pathogenesis of port wine stain and Sturge Weber syndrome: complex interactions between genetic alterations and aberrant MAPK and PI3K activation. *Int J Mol Sci*. 2019;20(9):2243.
53. Sabeti S, et al. Consensus statement for the management and treatment of port-wine birthmarks in Sturge-Weber syndrome. *JAMA Dermatol*. 2021;157(1):98–104.
54. Burden Burden-The E, et al. A systematic review of diagnostic criteria for psoriasis in adults and children: evidence from studies with a primary aim to develop of validate diagnostic criteria. *Br J Dermatol*. 2018;178:1035–1043.
55. Lavaud J, Mahé E. Proactive treatment in childhood psoriasis. *Ann Dermatol Venereol*. 2020;147(1):29–35.
56. Phan K, Lee G, Fischer G. Pediatric psoriasis and association with cardiovascular and metabolic comorbidities: systematic review and meta-analysis. *Pediatr Dermatol*. 2020;37(4):661–669.

57. Menter A, et al. Joint American Academy of Dermatology–National Psoriasis Foundation guidelines of care for the management and treatment of psoriasis in pediatric patients. *J Am Acad Dermatol.* 2020;82(1):161–201. Erratum in: *J Am Acad Dermatol* 82(3):574, 2020.
58. Cordoro KM, et al. Skin-infiltrating, interleukin-22-producing T cells differentiate pediatric psoriasis from adult psoriasis. *J Am Acad Dermatol.* 2017;77(3):417–424.
59. Tollefson MM. Diagnosis and management of psoriasis in children. *Pediatr Clin North Am.* 2014;61(2):261–277.
60. Chadha A, Jahnke M. Common neonatal rashes. *Pediatr Ann.* 2019;48(1):e16–e22.
61. Schoch JJ, et al. The infantile cutaneous microbiome: a review. *Pediatr Dermatol.* 2019;36(5):574–580.

48

Shock, Multiple Organ Dysfunction Syndrome, and Burns in Adults

Mary C. Selzer, Dennis J. Cheek, and Julia L. Rogers

http://evolve.elsevier.com/Rogers/pathophysiology/

CHAPTER OUTLINE

Shock is a life-threatening condition that occurs when the circulatory system fails to perfuse tissues, cells, and organs adequately, resulting in widespread impairment of cellular metabolism and tissue function. Tissue perfusion is defined as the adequacy of blood flow through the small vessels to maintain tissue function.[1] Inadequate tissue perfusion occurs when there is decreased delivery of blood, oxygen, and nutrients to cells and tissues and increased oxygen consumption, such as from a decrease in cardiac output, a reduction in blood volume or hemoglobin level, or a significant reduction in blood pressure. Multiple etiologies exist for shock, but shock from any cause will progress to organ failure and death unless physiologic mechanisms reverse the process or clinical intervention succeeds in stopping the progression. Untreated, shock overwhelms the body's compensatory mechanisms and results in organ dysfunction that may progress to multisystem organ failure.

Multiple organ dysfunction syndrome (MODS) is progressive and involves the failure of two or more organ systems after a severe illness or injury. The disease process is initiated and perpetuated by uncontrolled systemic inflammatory and stress responses and is characterized by a hypermetabolic and hyperdynamic state that persists as organ dysfunction develops. For many years the syndrome was referred to as *multiple organ failure* or *multiple systems organ failure*. Gradually it was recognized that the term *organ dysfunction* more accurately describes the syndrome as a process of physiologic deterioration.

Major burns result in extensive immediate tissue injury and thus are a form of trauma with wide-reaching effects on all organ systems. The cause of injury may be thermal contact, flame, chemical agents, or electrical agents; each cause requires a different approach in diagnosis and treatment. Closely associated with thermal burns is smoke inhalation injury, which accounts for about 25% of all burn unit admissions. As a multiorgan problem, thermal injuries can have an overwhelming effect on survival of the burned individual. Regardless of the cause of burns, the result is a final common pathway of physiologic response dependent on the extent of burn surface involvement and the depth of tissue destruction.

SHOCK

Shock can be classified by type, principal pathophysiologic process, or clinical manifestations. Classification by type is perhaps the most useful because it suggests the cause and pathophysiologic process of the underlying disorder, which must be treated to prevent the irreversible cellular alterations and impairment of cellular metabolism. Shock is classified as 1) distributive [septic (caused by infection), anaphylactic (caused by hypersensitivity), and neurogenic or vasogenic (caused by alterations in vascular smooth muscle tone)]; 2) cardiogenic (caused by heart failure); 3) hypovolemic [hemorrhagic (caused by insufficient intravascular fluid volume)]; or 4) obstructive. These four types of shock are not exclusive, and many individuals have multifactorial shock.

Cellular Alterations and Impairment of Cellular Metabolism

The body consists of many organs, tissues, and cells that may function or malfunction at different stages of metabolic impairment. The common pathway in all types of shock is impairment of

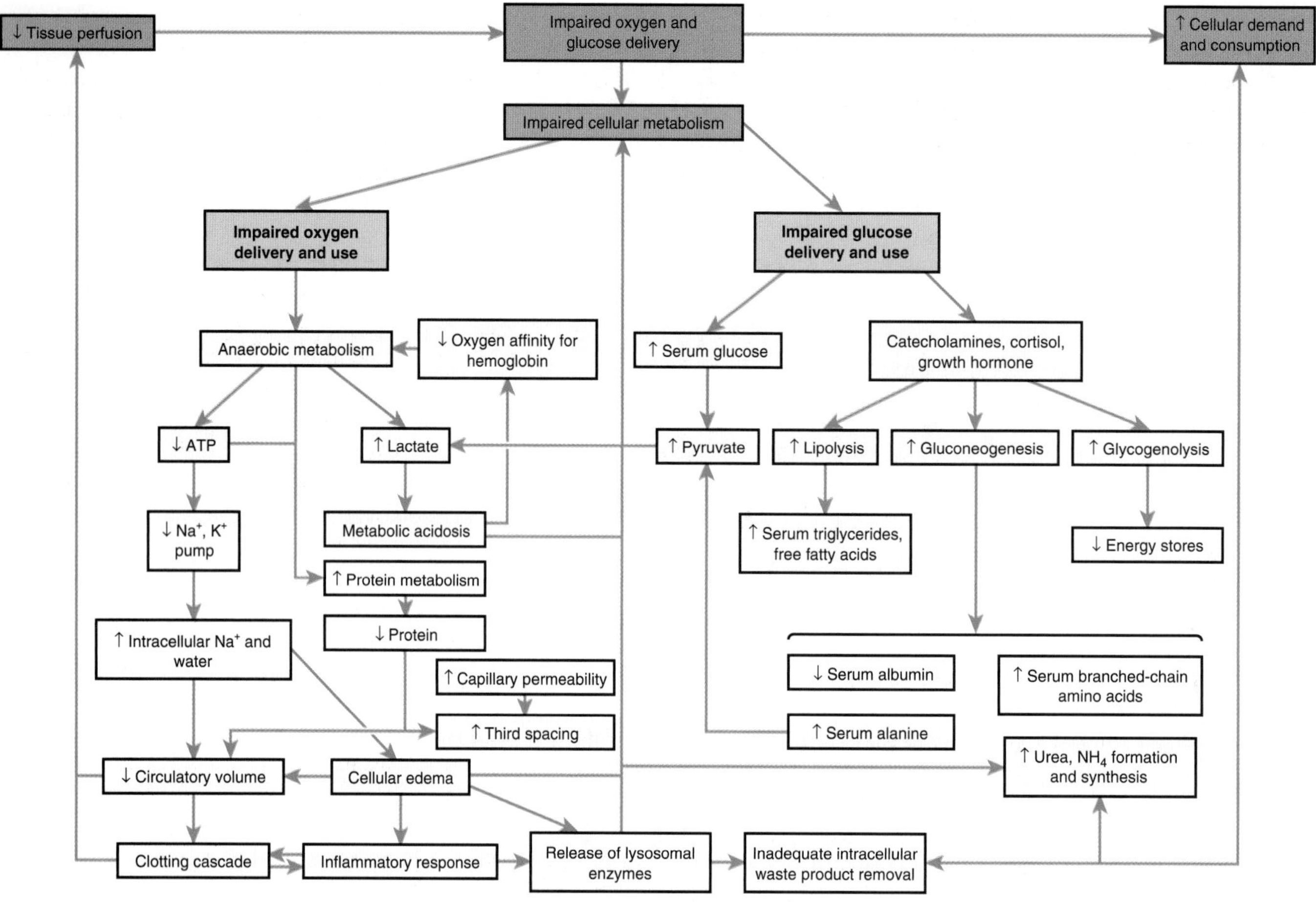

Fig. 48.1 Impairment of Cellular Metabolism by Shock. *ATP,* Adenosine triphosphate.

cellular metabolism, attributable to decreased delivery of oxygen and nutrients, frequently coupled with an increased demand and consumption of oxygen and nutrients and a decreased removal of cellular waste products.[2] In septic shock, for example, a deficiency in cellular metabolism and the buildup of lactic acid may precede the decreased tissue perfusion. Fig. 48.1 illustrates the pathophysiology of shock at the cellular level.

Impairment of Oxygen Delivery, Increased Oxygen Consumption, and Volume Changes

Normal tissue perfusion allows for the delivery of more oxygen to the capillary beds and cells than is consumed at the cellular level. In all types of shock, the cells do not receive adequate amounts of oxygen because of decreased delivery or increased cellular consumption, or both, and therefore are unable to use oxygen normally (see Fig. 48.1). In cardiogenic shock, cardiac output, either stroke volume or heart rate, is too low to deliver adequate oxygen to the cell. In hypovolemic shock, oxygen delivery is impaired by inadequate numbers of red blood cells or hemoglobin (which carries oxygen) and insufficient blood volume. In neurogenic, anaphylactic, and septic shock, systemic vascular resistance (SVR) becomes very low because of vasodilation, resulting in inadequate perfusion pressure in the capillaries. Thus the pressure needed to drive oxygen and nutrients across cell membranes is inadequate. In septic shock, hypoxia is worsened both by increased inflammatory responses (such as fever), which raise the cell's oxygen demands and consumption rate, and by direct toxic and inflammatory chemical disruption of cellular metabolism, which impairs the cell's ability to use oxygen. In particular, each molecule of hemoglobin is normally capable of carrying four molecules of oxygen, but it delivers only one molecule of oxygen at the capillary bed for delivery to the cells; however, as tissue perfusion decreases and oxygen needs increase, two molecules of oxygen will be extracted to meet needs. When this compensatory mechanism is exhausted, cellular demand becomes abnormally greater than delivery. Without oxygen, the result of poor delivery and increased consumption, the cells shift from aerobic to anaerobic metabolism, resulting in lactic acid production at the cellular level.

Both positive compensatory mechanisms, such as lysosomal enzyme and cytokine release, and negative compensatory mechanisms, such as anaerobic metabolism and decreased intravascular volume in any shock state, further impair oxygen delivery and use. Concurrently in the inflammatory state of sepsis, diffusion across capillary membranes is slowed because blood flow in the capillary beds becomes sluggish as a result of decreased fluid volume and increased blood viscosity. Sluggish capillary flow decreases tissue perfusion, which may result in microvascular clot formation, and activation of the clotting cascade may begin (see Chapter 28). Microemboli formation and platelet aggregation account for common complications of shock caused by blocked tissue perfusion to end organs, such as the kidneys (causing acute tubular necrosis) or the lungs (causing acute respiratory distress syndrome [ARDS]). Disseminated intravascular coagulation (DIC) may be activated by the inflammatory response along with clotting cascade abnormalities.[3]

Anaerobic metabolism results in disruption of electrolyte and lysosomal enzymatic processes, thus changing the normal ionic and osmotic levels in cells governed by the physical law of diffusion. Diffusion of nutrients and wastes into and out of the cell takes longer, and cellular metabolism is further distorted. Anaerobic metabolism is a less efficient method of extracting energy from carbon bonds, and the cell begins to use adenosine triphosphate (ATP) faster than it can be replaced. Without ATP the cell loses its ability to maintain an electrochemical gradient across its selectively permeable membrane. Specifically, the cell cannot operate the sodium-potassium pump. Sodium and chloride accumulate inside the cell and potassium exits the cell. Cells of the nervous system and myocardium are profoundly and immediately affected. The resting potentials of these cells are reduced, and the action potentials decrease in amplitude (see Chapter 1). Myocardial depressant factor is released, which decreases the contractility of the heart. A variety of clinical manifestations of impaired central nervous system and myocardial function results. As sodium moves into the cell, water follows. Throughout the body, the water drawn from the interstitium into the cells is "replaced" by water that is in turn drawn out of the vascular space, often called "third spacing" of fluid. This results in further decreases in circulatory volume. Within the cells, water causes cellular edema that disrupts cellular membranes, releasing lysosomal enzymes that injure the cells internally and then leak into the interstitium.

In addition to decreasing ATP stores, anaerobic metabolism affects the pH of the cell, and metabolic acidosis develops, which is indirectly measured by increasing lactate levels in the blood. A compensatory mechanism is initiated that enables cardiac and skeletal muscles to use pyruvate, of which lactic acid is the byproduct, as a fuel source, but only for a limited time. The decreasing pH of the cell that is functioning under anaerobic conditions has serious consequences. Enzymes necessary for cellular function dissociate under acidic conditions. Enzyme dissociation stops cell function, repair, and division. As lactic acid is released systemically, blood pH drops, reducing the oxygen-carrying capacity of the blood, and the heart's ability to pump. Therefore less oxygen is delivered to the cells and further hypoxia results in metabolic acidosis, which triggers more lysosomal enzyme release caused by disruption of lysosomal membrane integrity. Lysosomal enzymes released during shock injure the cell that released them and injure adjacent cells. By damaging the mechanisms of surrounding cells, lysosomal enzymes extend areas of impaired metabolism and cellular injury.

Intravascular fluid loss into the intracellular and interstitial spaces, described as "third spacing" earlier, is amplified when serum albumin and other plasma proteins are consumed for fuel, which results in decreased intravascular osmotic pressure, shift of fluid to the interstitial or extracellular spaces, and decreased circulatory volume, which can cause a relative hypovolemic state. Decreased intravascular volume causes decreased cardiac output in septic, neurogenic, and anaphylactic shock states, but it is the decreased mechanical ability to eject volume from the heart pump that reduces cardiac output in cardiogenic shock. In individuals with anaphylactic, neurogenic, or septic shock and an already dilated vasculature, hypotension worsens as a result of decreased circulatory volume.

Impairment of Glucose Delivery and Use

Impaired glucose use can be caused by either impaired glucose delivery or impaired glucose uptake by the cells (see Fig. 48.1). The reasons for inadequate glucose delivery are the same as those enumerated for inadequate oxygen delivery. In addition, in septic and anaphylactic shock, glucose metabolism and consumption may be increased or disrupted because of fever or bacteria, and glucose uptake can be prevented by the presence of vasoactive toxins, endotoxins, histamine, and kinins.

Some of the compensatory mechanisms activated by shock contribute to decreased glucose uptake and use by the cells. High serum levels of cortisol, growth hormone, and catecholamines account for hyperglycemia and insulin resistance, tachycardia, increased SVR, and increased cardiac contractility. Cells shift to glycogenolysis, gluconeogenesis, and lipolysis to generate fuel for survival (see Chapter 1). Except in the liver, kidneys, and muscles, the body's cells have extremely limited stores of glycogen. In fact, total body stores can fuel the metabolism for only about 10 hours. The depletion of fat and glycogen stores is not itself a cause of organ failure, but the energy costs of glycogenolysis and lipolysis are considerable and contribute to the cellular failure.

Impairment of Protein Metabolism and Depletion of Protein Stores

The depletion of protein is, however, a cause of organ failure. When gluconeogenesis causes proteins to be used for fuel, these proteins are no longer available to maintain cellular structure, function, repair, and replication. The breakdown of protein occurs in starvation states, hyperdynamic metabolic states, and septic shock. Under anaerobic metabolism, protein breakdown liberates alanine, which is converted to pyruvate. Pyruvic acid is changed into lactic acid, leading to an increased affinity for oxygen to bind to hemoglobin with resultant hypoxia and metabolic acidosis.

As proteins are metabolized anaerobically, ammonia and urea are produced. Ammonia is toxic to living cells. Uremia develops, and uric acid further disrupts cellular metabolism. Proteins are broken down preferentially. Serum albumin and other plasma proteins are consumed for fuel first. Serum protein consumption decreases capillary osmotic pressure and contributes to the development of interstitial edema, creating another negative compensatory outcome that decreases circulatory volume. In septic shock, plasma protein breakdown includes breakdown of immunoglobulins, thereby impairing immune system function when it is most needed.

Muscle wasting caused by protein breakdown weakens skeletal and cardiac muscle. Skeletal muscle wasting impairs the muscles that facilitate breathing. Muscle wasting therefore alters the actions of both heart and lungs. The delivery of oxygen and glucose to the cells is directly reduced, as is the removal of metabolic waste products, such as the formation of carbon dioxide and lactic acid, causing metabolic acidosis with resultant inability of muscles, organs, and tissues to function mechanically and electrically.

The metabolic wastes that accumulate in the cell and interstitial spaces are toxic to the cells and further disrupt cellular function and membrane integrity.

Types of Shock, Clinical Manifestations, and Treatment

Each type of shock (distributive, cardiogenic, hypovolemic, and obstructive) involves numerous clinical manifestations, signs, and symptoms that also may characterize other conditions, making diagnosis difficult. If there are overlapping shock states that occur simultaneously, it can be difficult to determine the etiology of shock based only on clinical manifestations, therefore an individual's history, risks, and situation are correlated with the specificity of the shock state suspected or anticipated.

The initial management for shock is to discover, diagnose, and correct or remove the underlying cause. Although this seems a simple tenet, it is one that is not always executed. Thus, treatment for cardiogenic shock begins with diagnosis and treatment of heart failure or at least enhancement of cardiac output. In hypovolemic shock, hemorrhage and other causes of fluid loss must be stopped and replaced. In neurogenic shock, as a result of spinal cord trauma, stabilization of the spine and surrounding tissue is an initial approach, followed by treatment to counteract the vasodilatory effect and decreased blood pressure related to the parasympathetic control below the level of spinal cord injury. For anaphylactic shock, antigens must be identified, removed, or neutralized. Management for septic shock begins with identification and eradication of the infective agent, with blood cultures followed by administration of antimicrobials and fluids.

Simultaneous to correcting the underlying cause or condition, treatment is directed at targeting improvement of microcirculatory tissue perfusion.[3] Optimizing oxygenation is an absolute necessity in all shock states. The goal has a dual purpose to both optimize oxygen delivery and reduce oxygen consumption. Intravenous fluid or blood products are administered to expand intravascular volume and thereby improve tissue perfusion by increasing blood pressure, hemoglobin level, and cardiac output, except in cases of cardiogenic shock, which requires diuresis to reduce preload, so that the pump is not overloaded, or augmentation therapies to increase cardiac output. Effective glucose level control in various shock states has been shown to improve outcomes. Hyperglycemia, caused by insulin resistance in the liver and muscle, is a common finding in the critically ill. This is most likely an adaptive response providing glucose for the brain, cell nourishment and production, and wound healing; it also causes the increase in circulating corticosteroids produced in the stress response. The extent of appropriate glucose level control has been evaluated in recent years, leading to more aggressive treatment with continuous, titrating insulin infusions to maintain blood glucose levels closer to normal, thus promoting normal cellular function and healing.[4]

Once cellular and organ dysfunction and physiologic derangement are established, risk of morbidity and mortality increases in all shock states. Prevention and early treatment offer the best prognosis.

Distributive Shock

Distributive shock (vasodilatory shock) is characterized by severe peripheral vasodilation and has several etiologies, including sepsis, systemic inflammatory response syndrome (SIRS), neurogenic or vasogenic, anaphylaxis, drug and toxin induced, and endocrine.

Septic shock. Septic shock is the endpoint of a physiologic state of hypoperfusion with profound underlying circulatory, cellular, and metabolic abnormalities.[5] Septic shock is a subset of sepsis, a life-threatening organ dysfunction caused by a dysregulated host response to infection.[5] Sepsis often begins with an infection entering the bloodstream, causing bacteremia, leading to progressive dysfunction. Septic shock is associated with an intense proinflammatory and immunosuppressive response with multiorgan dysfunction.[6] Sepsis, the most common cause of distributive shock, is associated with high morbidity and mortality and accounts for one of the largest causes of death and healthcare expenditures worldwide.[7]

Pathophysiology. Septic shock is commonly caused by gram-positive bacteria (e.g., Pneumococcus, Enterococcus), gram-negative bacteria (e.g., Pseudomonas, Klebsiella, Enterobacter), viruses (e.g., Coronavirus), and fungi (e.g., Candida). Antibiotic resistant organisms (e.g., methicillin-resistant staphylococcus) are linked to healthcare-associated infections and are a major factor determining clinical unresponsiveness to treatment and rapid evolution to sepsis and septic shock.[8] The largest contributors to sepsis cases and sepsis-related mortality across all ages are diarrheal diseases and lower respiratory infections.[9] The most commonly identified sources of infections in the intensive care setting associated with sepsis are respiratory tract, abdomen, urinary, wound/skin, catheter, and bloodstream.[10]

Advances in antibiotic therapy and broad-spectrum use of antibiotics in the treatment of sepsis have led to a significant increase in antibiotic-resistant infections, many of which may be hospital-acquired, but are frequently not reported to institutions such as the Centers for Disease Control and Prevention (CDC). Even when properly treated with available therapies, morbidity and mortality are extremely high. Prognosis is significantly affected by the source and virulence of the infectious microorganism, which has prompted the expansion of efforts by the CDC and its partners to describe the epidemiology of sepsis, prevent infections that lead to sepsis, and educate clinicians and individuals about reducing the risk for sepsis.[11] Sepsis outcomes depend on the person's health before infection and the degree of organ dysfunction after infection.[12]

The nidus of infection in sepsis may be readily discernible or extremely difficult to locate (Fig. 48.2). Bacteria, viruses, and fungi enter the bloodstream to produce bacteremia in one of two ways: (1) directly from the site of infection or (2) indirectly from toxic substances released by the bacteria directly into the bloodstream. These toxic substances, which act as triggering molecules, include endotoxins released by gram-negative microorganisms, lipoteichoic acids and peptidoglycan released by gram-positive microorganisms, and superantigens.[6] The triggering molecules activate the immune

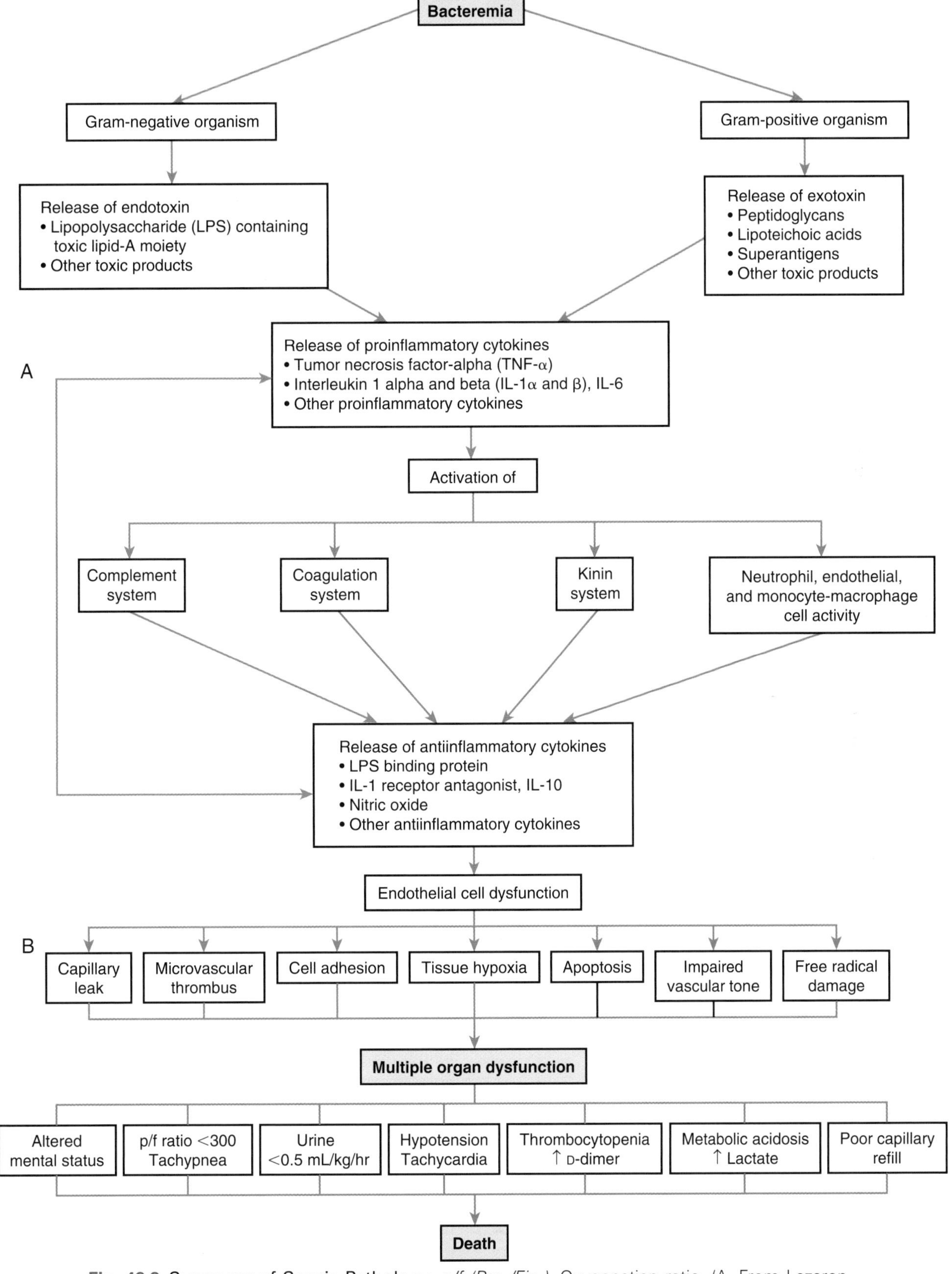

Fig. 48.2 **Summary of Sepsis Pathology.** *p/f (Pao_2/Fio_2)*, Oxygenation ratio. (A, From Lazaron V, Barke RA. Gram-negative bacterial sepsis and the sepsis syndrome. *Urologic Clinics of North America*, 1999;26[4]:687. B, Copyright 2003, Eli Lilly and Company. All rights reserved. Reprinted with permission from Eli Lilly and Company.)

EMERGING SCIENCE BOX

Pro-Inflammatory and Anti-Inflammatory Responses in Sepsis

Despite improvements in the understanding of the pathophysiology of sepsis and the implementation of improved supportive therapeutic strategies, no specific treatment for sepsis has been approved. Multiple research trials have explored therapeutics aimed at modulating the well-described hyperinflammatory phase of sepsis in which there is an overwhelming release of inflammatory cytokines resulting in fever, shock, and cardiopulmonary failure. These trials have included powerful anti-inflammatory medication such as corticosteroids and other anti-immune drugs, but to date, none have significantly impacted morbidity or mortality. In fact, evidence has emerged that mortality in sepsis more often is due to an immunosuppressed state with secondary infections that are associated with organ injury and failure. This immunosuppressed state (immune paralysis) includes decreased neutrophil and macrophage activity, loss of antigen recognition, apoptosis of lymphocytes, expansion of myeloid-derived suppressor cells (MDSCs), and adaptive immune cell dysfunction that may persist for weeks or months after the initial septic event. Any conditions that are associated with cellular metabolic dysfunction of immune cells such as hyperlipidemia, diabetes, and obesity make immune paralysis worse and are linked to higher sepsis-related morbidity and mortality. These immune changes have been termed the compensatory anti-inflammatory response syndrome (CARS) and were once thought to follow after the hyperinflammatory phase of sepsis. However, newer research suggests that immunosuppression occurs simultaneously with the hyperinflammatory response, thus leading to the term mixed antagonist response syndrome. Activation of pro-inflammatory and anti-inflammatory pathways at the same time may lead to chronic inflammatory and infectious organ injury, along with a prolonged catabolic syndrome in septic individuals. Some researchers are now exploring if measurable decreases in immune function can be used to predict sepsis outcomes, while others suggest that immune stimulant therapies, rather than anti-inflammatory medications, should be tested for the treatment sepsis.

Data from Cao C, et al. Pathological alteration and therapeutic implications of sepsis-induced immune cell apoptosis. *Cell Death and Disease*, 2019;10:782; Koutroulis I, et al. Sepsis immunometabolism: From defining sepsis to understanding how energy production affects immune response. *Critical Care Explorations*, 2019;1:e0061; Misra AK, et al. Biomarkers of immunosuppression. *Critical Care Clinics*, 2020;36(1):167–176; Pons S, et al. Immune consequences of endothelial cells' activation and dysfunction during sepsis. *Critical Care Clinics*, 2020;36(2):401–413; Remy KE, et al. Immunotherapies for COVID-19: Lessons learned from sepsis. *Lancet Respiratory Medicine*, 2020;8 946–949; Steinhagen F, et al. Immunotherapy in sepsis—brake or accelerate? *Pharmacology & Therapeutics.*, 2020;208:107476; Wakeley ME, et al. Check point inhibitors and their role in immunosuppression in sepsis. *Critical Care Clinics*, 2020;36(1):69–88.

system and cause the host to initiate both a proinflammatory and anti-inflammatory response (see the box Emerging Science Box: Pro-Inflammatory and Anti-Inflammatory Responses in Sepsis) (see Chapter 7). Inflammatory mediators are released and include polymorphonuclear leukocytes, macrophages, monocytes, and platelets. Box 48.1 lists the proinflammatory and anti-inflammatory mediators released.[3,15,16] Presumably the end result is a mixed antagonistic response syndrome as proinflammatory and anti-inflammatory mediators respond, intensify, and lead the host into MODS.

Clinical manifestations. Clinical manifestations common in septic shock are fever, tachycardia, tachypnea, and elevations

BOX 48.1 Pro-Inflammatory and Anti-Inflammatory Mediators Released During Immune Response to Sepsis

The pro-inflammatory mediators released include cytokines (interleukins [IL-1, IL-2, IL-6, IL-8, and IL-15], tumor necrosis factor-alpha [TNF-α], and granulocyte cell–stimulating factor)[13,14]; complement and complement cascade activation factors; kinins; arachidonic acid metabolites (prostaglandins, prostacyclin, leukotrienes, and thromboxane); soluble adhesion molecules; platelet-activating factor; endorphins; vasoactive neuropeptides; histamine; serotonin; monocyte chemoattractant proteins 1 and 2; proteolytic enzymes (e.g., elastase and lysosomal enzymes); protein kinase; tyrosine kinase; CD14; toxic oxygen metabolites (e.g., superoxide, hydroxyl radical, hydrogen peroxide, peroxynitrite); neopterin; and clotting cascade activation factors. Proinflammatory cytokines can cause fever, hypotension, leukocytosis, induction of other proinflammatory cytokines, and the simultaneous activation of coagulation and fibrinolysis. Anti-inflammatory mediators released include lipopolysaccharide-binding protein; IL-1 receptor antagonist; soluble CD14; type 2 IL-1 receptor; leukotriene B_4 receptor antagonist; IL-4, IL-10, and IL-13; soluble tumor necrosis factor receptor; transforming growth factor-β (TGF-β); epinephrine; and nitric oxide.[3,15,16]

in immune responses, such as leukocytosis. Elevated circulating blood glucose level, cyanosis, mottling, decreased urine output, and hypotension with altered mental status may be present in any shock state. Subjective complaints often are nonspecific and general, such as chief complaints of weakness, malaise, or shortness of breath. Clinical criteria for septic shock includes (1) hypotension, (2) requiring vasopressors to maintain a mean arterial pressure >65 mmHg, and (3) a serum lactate of >2 mmol/L despite adequate volume resuscitation.[5] Other manifestations of septic shock are persistent low arterial pressure, low tissue perfusion, low SVR from vasodilation, and an alteration in oxygen extraction by all cells (see Comments column in Table 48.1). Two main mechanisms contribute to lactic acid accumulation in sepsis: tissue hypoxia and epinephrine-induced stimulation of aerobic glycolysis.[17] Low-flow states of prolonged shock causing tissue hypoxia with lactic acidosis increase nitric oxide synthesis, activate ATP-sensitive and calcium-regulated potassium channels (K_{ATP} and K_{Ca}, respectively) in vascular smooth muscle (see Chapter 32), and lead to depletion of ADH (vasopressin) (Fig. 48.3). Tachypnea is a compensatory mechanism to increase oxygen. Tachycardia, in the initial stages of sepsis, supports cardiac output to remain normal or become elevated, although myocardial contractility is reduced. Sustained tachycardia is deleterious to improving cardiac output, especially when underlying comorbid states of heart disease exist. Temperature instability, ranging from hyperthermia to hypothermia, may indicate deterioration of the immune response, or may partially be caused by latent vasoconstriction or a vasopressor drug effect. Effects on other organ systems may result in deranged renal function, gastrointestinal mucosa changes, and ischemia that lead to translocation of bacteria from the gut, jaundice related to liver dysfunction, and clotting abnormalities that cause microemboli formation. Although deterioration of mental status and tachypnea are attributable to the low tissue perfusion described, complications such as stroke and ARDS often contribute to the distribution of these microemboli lodging in the microcirculation of the end organs, such as the brain, splanchnic organs, and pulmonary vascular system.

TABLE 48.1 Definitions of Septic Shock Components

Term	Basic Definition	Comments
Infection	A pathologic process that results from an invasion of a normal part of the body by pathogenic or potentially pathogenic microorganisms	Suspicion of infection necessitates immediate identification of possible pathogens, bacteria, fungi, or viruses with blood culture(s). Without benefit of microbiologic confirmation, clinical judgment should be used to identify signs, symptoms, and risk stratification of potential infection to promote early identification. SIRS criteria may still be used to screen for infection (see *What's New?* Sepsis and Septic Shock).
Bacteremia	Presence of viable bacteria in the blood	Insufficient to make a diagnosis of sepsis, especially in the absence of organ dysfunction.
Organ dysfunction	Abnormality or impairment of normal organ function, with or without direct insult or damage to the organ	Indirect insult of organ perfusion is caused by the septic cascade and hypoperfusion. Organ dysfunction can be represented by an increase in the Sequential Organ Failure Assessment (SOFA) score by 2 points or more when evaluating 6 organ systems. Evidence of 2 of 3 quickSOFA (qSOFA) criteria: respiratory rate of 22/min or greater; altered mentation, Glasgow Coma Scale <15 (new/worsening from baseline); or systolic blood pressure of 100 mmHg or less is considered positive for organ dysfunction. The quickSOFA (qSOFA) is not as predictive as the full SOFA score in the intensive care setting; however, it is superior to SOFA when applied to individuals outside the intensive care unit.
Sepsis	Life-threatening organ dysfunction caused by a dysregulated host response to infection	Common organ systems showing dysfunction are the respiratory, hematologic, cardiac, renal, hepatic, and central nervous systems. Additional clinical signs, symptoms, biomarkers, and variables that may be used to identify inflammation, inadequate tissue perfusion, and organ dysfunction: 1. General variables a. Fever >38°C (100.4°F) or hypothermia <36°C (96.8°F) b. Tachycardia, heart rate >90 beats/min c. Tachypnea d. Progressive deterioration of mental status e. Altered mental status f. Significant edema or positive fluid balance (>20 mL/kg over 24 h) g. Hyperglycemia (blood glucose >140 mg/dL) in the absence of diabetes 2. Inflammatory variables a. Leukocytosis or leukopenia (WBC > 12,000/mm^3, < 4000/mm^3, or > 10% bands) b. CRP > 2 SD above the normal value c. PCT > 2 SD above the normal value 3. Hemodynamic variables a. Arterial hypotension (SBP <90 mmHg; MAP <70 mmHg, or an SBP decrease >40 mmHg) b. $S\bar{v}O_2$ > 70% c. Cardiac index >3.5 L/min 4. Organ dysfunction variables a. Arterial hypoxemia (Pao_2/Fio_2 < 300 mmHg) b. Acute oliguria (urine output <0.5 mL/kg/h or 45 mL for at least 2 h) c. Creatinine increase >0.5 mg/dL d. Coagulation abnormalities (INR > 1.5 or PTT > 60 s) e. Ileus f. Thrombocytopenia (platelet count <100,000/m^3) g. Hyperbilirubinemia (plasma total bilirubin >4 mg/dL or 70 mmol/L) 5. Tissue perfusion variables a. Hyperlactatemia (>1 mmol/L) b. Decreased capillary refill or mottling
Septic shock	A subset of sepsis in which particularly profound circulatory, cellular, and metabolic abnormalities are associated with a greater risk of mortality than with sepsis alone	Clinically identified by a vasopressor requirement to maintain a mean arterial pressure of 65 mmHg or greater and serum lactate level greater than 2 mmol/L (>18 mg/dL) in the absence of hypovolemia.

CRP, Plasma C-reactive protein; *INR*, international normalized ratio; *MAP*, mean arterial pressure; *Pao_2/Fio_2*, partial pressure of oxygen in arterial blood/fraction of inspired oxygen; *PCT*, plasma procalcitonin; *PTT*, partial thromboplastin time; *SBP*, systolic blood pressure; *SD*, standard deviation; *SIRS*, systemic inflammatory response syndrome; $S\bar{v}O_2$, saturation of hemoglobin with oxygen; *Temp*, core temperature; *WBC*, white blood cell(s).
Data from 2 Dellinger RP, Levy MM, Rhodes A, et al. Surviving sepsis campaign: international guidelines for management of severe sepsis and septic shock: 2012. *Critical Care Medicine*, 2013;41(2):580–637; Levy MM, Fink MP, Marshall JC, et al. 2001 SCCM/ESICM/ACCP/ATS/SIS International Sepsis Definitions Conference. *Critical Care Medicine,* 2003;312:1250; Opal SM. Severe sepsis and septic shock: Defining the clinical problem. *Scandinavian Journal of Infectious Diseases*, 2003;35(9):529; Seymour C. *JAMA*, 2016;315(8):762–774; Shankar-Hari M, Phillips GS, Levy ML, et al. Developing a new definition and assessing new clinical criteria for septic shock: For the third international consensus definitions for sepsis and septic shock (Sepsis-3). *JAMA*, 2016;315(8):775–787; Singer M, Deutschman CS, Seymour CW, et al. The third international consensus definitions for sepsis and septic shock (Sepsis-3). *JAMA*, 2016;315(8):801–810.

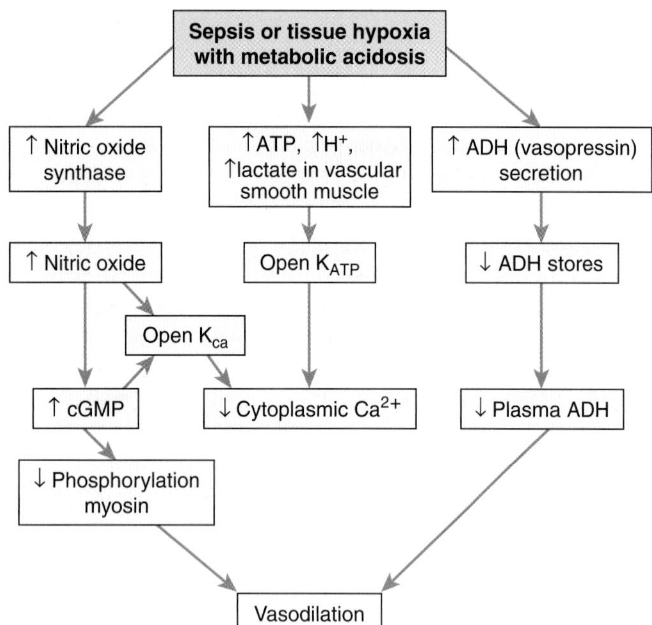

Fig. 48.3 Mechanisms of Vasodilation in Shock. Vasodilatory shock is caused by the inappropriate activation of vasodilatory mechanisms and the failure of constrictor mechanisms. Unregulated nitric oxide, by regulating guanylate cyclase and generating cyclic guanosine monophosphate *(cGMP)*, causes dephosphorylation of myosin and, thus, vasodilation. Nitric oxide synthesis and metabolic acidosis activate the potassium channels (K_{ATP} and K_{ca}) in the plasma membrane of vascular smooth muscle. The resulting hyperpolarization (see Chapter 3) of the membrane presents the calcium that mediates norepinephrine-induced and angiotensin II–induced vasoconstriction from entering the cell. Therefore hypotension and vasodilation stubbornly persist despite high plasma levels of these hormones. In contrast, and unexpectedly, the plasma level of antidiuretic hormone *(ADH)* (vasopressin) is low despite the presence of hypotension. The early, massive release of ADH may result in future depletion.

Evaluation and treatment. The 2021 international guidelines for management of sepsis and septic shock recommend hospitals and health care systems use a performance improvement program that includes screening for sepsis in acutely ill and high-risk individuals.[19] The quickSOFA (qSOFA) is no longer recommended as a single screening tool, but can be utilized to identify the presence of three variables to predict death and prolonged ICU stay in patients with known or suspected sepsis, which include altered mentation with a Glasgow Coma Score of < 15, respiratory rate ≥22 breaths/min, and systolic blood pressure ≤100 mm Hg.[5] Other screening tools include systemic inflammatory response syndrome (SIRS), Sequential Organ Failure Assessment (SOFA) criteria, National Early Warning Score (NEWS), or Modified Early Warning Score (MEWS). Standard operating procedures for sepsis are now considered "usual care" which includes components of the sepsis bundle, early identification, lactate, cultures, antibiotics, and fluids.[19]

Laboratory testing includes serum lactate (a biomarker of tissue hypoxia and dysfunction), blood cultures to determine bacteremia, urinalysis with culture if UTI suspected, complete blood count, comprehensive metabolic panel, procalcitonin (elevated level indicates a nonspecific proinflammatory response seen in bacterial infection), and C-reactive protein (CRP).[18] CRP is an acute phase reactant protein produced by the liver, mainly in response to interleukin-6 produced by inflammation of any type. CRP is most sensitive to acute phase reactants; consequently, its level rises rapidly during inflammation. Similar to procalcitonin, CRP is nonspecific to types of inflammation, but may be used to trend severity of infection and response to treatment, especially in occult and resistant infections, such as osteomyelitis. Diagnostic imaging studies include chest x-ray to rule out pneumonia, abdominal computed tomography (CT) to rule out intraabdominal process, and echocardiogram to rule out infectious endocarditis.

Treatment management needs to begin immediately. Fluid resuscitation should be initiated within the first 3 hours using IV crystalloids at a minimal rate of 30 ml/kg.[19] Fluid volume increases cardiac output (CO) and MAP; however, excess volume can cause pulmonary edema, acute kidney injury, and increase mortality, but this should not preclude adequate volume resuscitation. Therefore, it is important to monitor fluid volume status.[18] Fluid administration beyond the initial resuscitation is given as repeated small boluses and should be guided by careful assessment of intravascular volume status and organ perfusion through the use of dynamic measures including CO measurement combined with passive leg raising, fluid challenges against stroke volume (SV), systolic pressure or pulse pressure, and increases of SV in response to changes in intrathoracic pressure.[19] Albumin is suggested if large volumes of crystalloid have been infused.

The Surviving Sepsis Guidelines recommend the initiation of broad-spectrum antibiotics within 1 hour of presentation, after obtaining a full screen for infectious agents through blood, urine, and sputum cultures.[19] The initiation of empiric antibiotics should be directed toward gram-positive and gram-negative bacteria with consideration given to an individual's comorbidities, presentation, and risk of methicillin resistant Staphylococcus aureus (MRSA). Individuals with an increased risk for multidrug resistant (MDR) organisms, two antimicrobials with gram-negative coverage are recommended.[19] Antimicrobial therapy should be narrowed once cultures identify causative pathogen(s) and susceptibilities or discontinued if a non-infectious syndrome is demonstrated.[19,20] Monitoring serial procalcitonin levels, a precursor hormone to calcitonin, may be used to guide cessation of antibiotic therapy along with clinical evaluation.[19,20] Procalcitonin levels are not recommended as an indicator to start antibiotics; however, if levels are monitored sequentially at the start of empirical antibiotics and then drop, discontinuation or de-escalation may be clinically indicated.[19,20] The precise role of procalcitonin remains to be defined. Seeking to decrease use of antibiotics in the critically ill, and thereby prevent resistance to antibiotics, is an important strategy in treating infection. Adequate source control also is important and includes removal of any potentially infected intravascular access device after establishing another access site and following initial resuscitation.

Pharmacologic hemodynamic support and adjunctive therapy to maintain tissue perfusion include vasoactive agents.

Norepinephrine is the initial vasopressor of choice.[18,19] Dopamine or epinephrine can be used as alternatives if norepinephrine is not available; however, these are less preferred because of potential tachycardia, dysrhythmias, or reduction in splanchnic blood flow. Dobutamine, an inotropic agent, should be used if myocardial dysfunction is present or hypoperfusion remains after adequate intravascular volume and arterial blood pressure are achieved. When an inadequate MAP is obtained using norepinephrine, then vasopressin is added as a second agent in lieu of increasing the norepinephrine. If the MAP levels remain inadequate despite these two agents, then epinephrine is added as a third vasopressor.[19]

Sepsis induced hypoxic respiratory failure may require ventilation support. The use of high flow nasal oxygen over noninvasive ventilation is recommended.[19] Intravenous corticosteroids are suggested in septic shock to help replace intrinsic loss of cortisol, but only when hemodynamic stability is not obtained with adequate fluid resuscitation and vasopressor therapy.[19] Other supportive therapies in the treatment of septic shock include blood product administration to maintain hemoglobin levels above 7 g/dL, maintenance of targeted tidal volume (6 mL/kg) when mechanically ventilated with plateau pressure less than 30 cm H_2O, utilization of sedation and analgesic protocols when needed, and avoidance of neuromuscular blockers if possible. The initiation of insulin therapy should begin with a glucose level of > 180 mg/dL with a glucose target range of 140-180 mg/dL.[19] If renal dialysis is required, intermittent hemodialysis and continuous venovenous hemofiltration are considered equivalent. Bicarbonate therapy is contraindicated for the purpose of treating hypoperfusion lactic acidemia unless the pH is <7.2 and acute kidney injury is present. Use of low-molecular-weight heparin over low-dose unfractionated heparin is recommended for deep vein thrombosis prophylaxis, or mechanical compression if other agents are contraindicated. Stress ulcer prophylaxis with H2-receptor antagonists or proton pump inhibitors should be initiated if there is a risk of gastrointestinal bleeding.[19,23] Digestive tract decontamination and selective oropharyngeal decontamination are recommended in the prevention of ventilator-acquired pneumonia.[24,25] It is important to provide open communication with the patient and family regarding the disease process, discussing advance directives, peer support programs, post-critical illness follow-up programs, and post-hospital rehabilitation programs.[19,21]

Anaphylactic shock. Anaphylactic shock is the outcome of a widespread hypersensitivity to an allergen that triggers a reaction known as *anaphylaxis*. An allergen (usually a protein) is an antigen to which an individual mounts an immune response; this

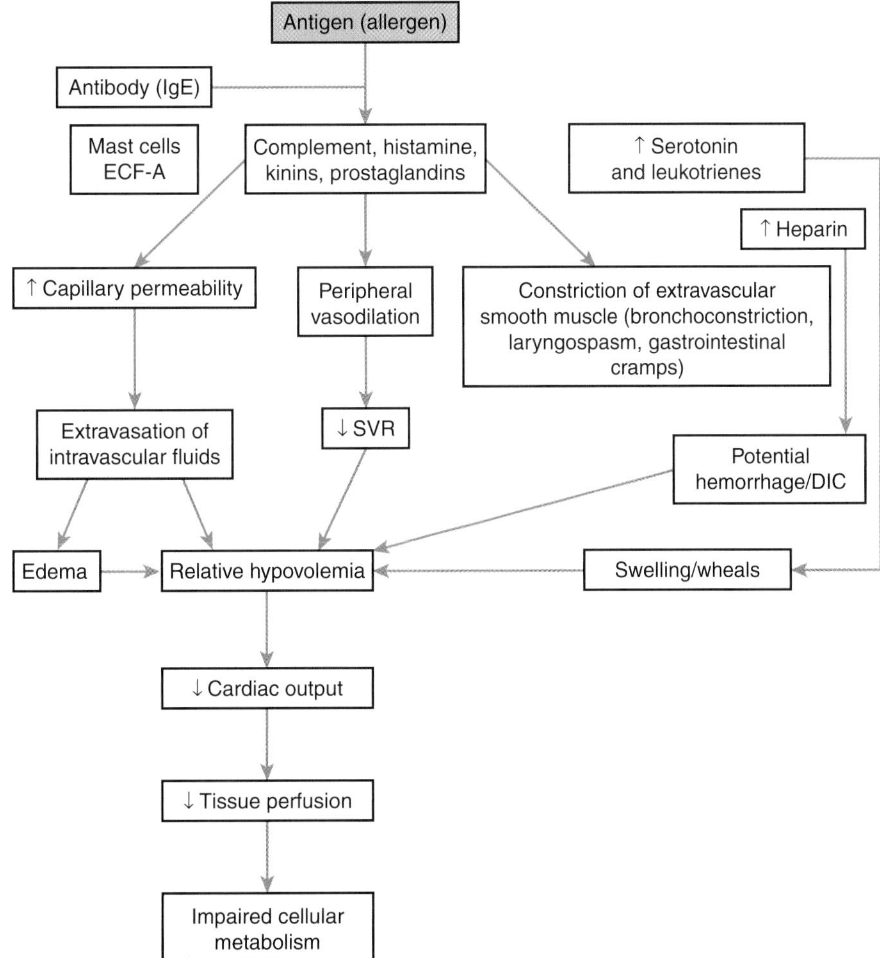

Fig. 48.4 Anaphylactic Shock. *DIC*, Disseminated intravascular coagulation; *ECF-A*, eosinophil chemotactic factor of anaphylaxis; *IgE*, immunoglobulin E; *SVR*, systemic vascular resistance.

response is an example of hypersensitivity. (see Chapters 8 and 9, for discussions of immunity, inflammation, and hypersensitivity.) Immunologic causes are related to the inflammatory and vasodilatory effects triggered by a pathologic allergic reaction to an antigen. An interaction occurs between an allergen and the allergen-specific immunoglobulin E (IgE)/high-affinity receptor (FcεRI) complex expressed on effector cells, predominantly mast cells and basophils.[27] *Anaphylactoid* type reactions, which are non-immunologic and are not IgE mediated in origin, can be related to drugs (e.g., opioids), ethanol, cold, heat, sunlight, and exercise.[27] Physiologic alterations related to the inflammatory and immune response, similar to neurogenic shock, are massive; vasodilation, peripheral pooling, and relative hypovolemia lead to decreased tissue perfusion and impaired cellular metabolism (Fig. 48.4). Anaphylactic shock is often severe and has immediate symptoms, including an itchy rash, throat swelling, and low blood pressure, related to the massive vasodilation and systemic inflammation that may progress to death in minutes if emergency treatment is not rendered.

Some allergens known to cause hypersensitivity reactions include foods (e.g., hen's eggs, cow's milk, wheat, shellfish, and peanuts), venom (e.g., bee stings, red ant bites, and snakebites), seminal fluid, latex, pollens, medications (nonsteroidal anti-inflammatory drugs [NSAIDs], dextrans), and contrast dye. Once in the body, the allergen or antigen causes immune inflammatory responses that range from mild to life-threatening or fatal.[27] Vascular effects of this response include vasodilation and increased vascular permeability, resulting in peripheral pooling and tissue edema. Extravascular effects include constriction of extravascular smooth muscle, such as the smooth muscle found in the walls of airways (e.g., the larynx and bronchioles; see Chapter 34), which may cause the extreme bronchoconstriction commonly associated with asthma and other severe allergic reactions.

Symptoms often affect multiple organ systems, including gastrointestinal (e.g., nausea, abdominal pain, vomiting, diarrhea), cutaneous (e.g., erythema, pruritus, urticaria, or angioedema), respiratory (e.g., shortness of breath, cough, rhinorrhea, tightening of throat, difficulty swallowing, wheezing), cardiovascular (e.g., diaphoresis, pallor, hypotension), or hematologic (e.g., fever, hemolysis). Other ominous clinical manifestations of anaphylactic shock may be anxiety, confusion, or impaired mentation. A precipitous decrease in blood pressure may account for altered mental status and may result in oliguria. Treatment begins with removal of the antigen (if possible) and assessment of airway, breathing, circulation, mental status, and skin. Epinephrine is administered to decrease mast cell and basophil degranulation, cause vasoconstriction, and reverse airway constriction.[27] Provide high flow oxygen to individuals with respiratory distress and those requiring further doses of epinephrine. Volume expanders or crystalloids (e.g., Lactated Ringer solution) are given intravenously to reverse the relative hypovolemia and cardiovascular instability. Antihistamines and corticosteroids are given to stop the inflammatory reaction.

The World Allergy Organization (WAO) updated guidelines in 2020 for assessment and management of anaphylaxis.[27] The guidelines include recommendations for validation of the clinical criteria for diagnosis, severity grading, diagnostic evaluation, use of epinephrine, and education. The emphasis on management of severe cases is shifting toward identification of triggers, determination of genetic predispositions, prevention of recurrence, development of tests to distinguish clinical risk from asymptomatic sensitization, and immune modulation to prevent anaphylaxis.

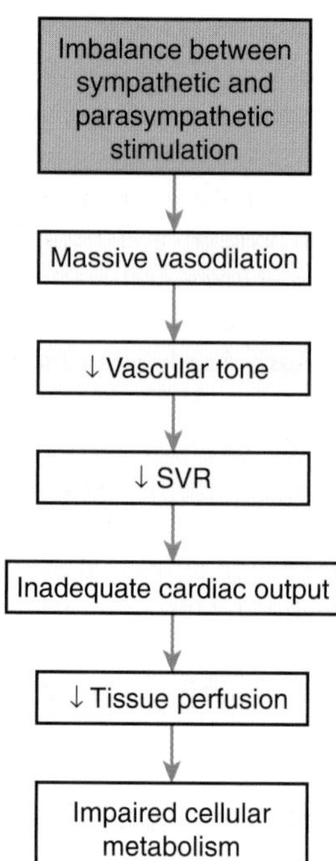

Fig. 48.5 Neurogenic Shock. *SVR,* Systemic vascular resistance.

Neurogenic shock. Neurogenic shock, also called vasogenic shock, refers to a widespread and massive vasodilation that results from an imbalance between parasympathetic and sympathetic stimulation of vascular smooth muscle (see Chapter 32). Occasionally, parasympathetic overstimulation or sympathetic understimulation persists, causing vasodilation and low blood pressure for an extended period. Extreme, persistent vasodilation leads to neurogenic shock (Fig. 48.5). Neurogenic shock creates a "relative hypovolemia." Blood volume has not changed, but the amount of space containing the blood has increased, causing the SVR to decrease drastically as a result of vasodilation.[28] Thus, pressure in the vessels is inadequate to drive oxygen and nutrients across capillary membranes and delivery to the cells is impaired, leading to impaired cellular metabolism.

Neurogenic shock can be caused by any factor that stimulates parasympathetic activity or inhibits sympathetic activity of vascular smooth muscle. Parasympathetic stimulation automatically inhibits sympathetic activity and vice versa (see Chapter 32). Normally, sympathetic stimulation maintains muscle tone. If sympathetic stimulation is interrupted or inhibited, vasodilation occurs. Therefore, trauma to the spinal cord or medulla, conditions that interrupt the supply of oxygen to the medulla, or conditions that deprive the medulla of glucose (e.g., insulin reactions) can cause neurogenic shock by interrupting sympathetic activity.[29] Depressive drugs, anesthetic agents, and severe emotional stress and pain are other causes of neurogenic shock.

The clinical hallmark of neurogenic shock is a very low SVR, along with other indicators of excessive parasympathetic activity. Bradycardia is the most obvious manifestation, especially in the early stages. Bradycardia may cease when compensatory mechanisms, particularly an increase in sympathetic system activity, have been initiated. The ejection fraction remains high, indicating a healthy myocardium, whereas central venous pressure decreases as the veins dilate. Neurogenic shock causes fainting if blood pressure decreases to the point at which cerebral metabolism is not sufficient to support consciousness. Most episodes of fainting are *not* shock; however, rarely do such episodes progress to shock. By allowing the blood pressure to equalize from head to toe as the individual becomes prone, fainting can actually prevent shock.

Cardiogenic Shock

Cardiogenic shock results from the inability of the heart to pump adequate blood to tissues and end organs.[30] Cardiogenic shock is a state of inadequate systemic tissue perfusion caused by a depression in contractility, despite adequate left ventricular filling pressure and intravascular volume. It is caused by extensive myocardial damage and appears to be aggravated by a systemic inflammatory response. The result is hypotension with metabolic acidosis and often has a fatal outcome; however, medical treatment, revascularization after acute myocardial infarction (MI), and hypothermia in the treatment of post–cardiac arrest states have been shown to improve outcomes.[31] Overall, hospital mortality because of cardiogenic shock has decreased from approximately 90% in the 1970s to a recent estimate of 40% to 50%.[31] Pathologic conditions that reduce contractility, cause pump failure, impair diastolic filling, or cause obstruction can lead to cardiogenic shock. Decreased contractility and pump failure can result from (1) acute myocardial infarction (AMI), cardiomyopathy, sepsis, myocarditis, pericarditis, aneurysm, dysrhythmias, contusion, metabolic abnormalities, and papillary muscle rupture; (2) impaired diastolic filling related to dysrhythmias; and (3) obstruction attributable to pulmonary embolism, cardiac tamponade, valvular disorders, tumors, and wall rupture or defects.[32] Dysrhythmias or conditions related to post–cardiopulmonary resuscitation reduce cardiac function and output, and may be associated with any of the previous pathologies mentioned.

As cardiac output decreases, compensatory adaptive responses are activated, such as the renin-angiotensin, neurohormonal, and sympathetic nervous systems, that lead to fluid retention, systemic vasoconstriction, and tachycardia.[33] Systemic inflammation appears to play an important role in the pathogenesis and outcome of cardiogenic shock. Activation of the inflammatory response causes pathological vasodilation, releasing nitric oxide synthase and peroxynitrite, which have cardiotoxic inotropic effects. Activation of inflammatory cytokines (interleukins and tissue necrosis factor α [TNF⊠α]) and the complement system are additional systemic inflammatory mediators that result in vasodilation and contribute to increased mortality.[32,33] Increases in contractility, heart rate, and blood pressure are maintained in mild shock states through vasoconstriction in response to catecholamine release from the adrenals. Vasoconstriction increases vascular resistance to normalize blood pressure and improves cardiac performance by returning more blood volume and increasing perfusion to the heart; however, this increases myocardial demand and consumption of oxygen and nutrients by the heart. Increasing myocardial requirements burden the already failing heart, which can no longer pump an adequate volume of blood with sufficient force to perfuse the tissues. Thus increased coronary, tissue, and cellular ischemia further deteriorates myocardial function and shock.

Morbidity and mortality caused by cardiogenic shock is reduced by use of percutaneous intravascular interventions to open coronary arteries; temporary mechanical circulatory support (e.g., intraaortic balloon pump [IABP]; transvalvular pump giving only left-sided support [Impella]; or extracorporeal membrane oxygenation [ECMO]), cardiosupportive drug regimens, and mild hypothermia, which has been shown to increase contractility while decreasing oxygen demand and metabolism, also have shown improved outcomes.[33,34] Following MI, reperfusion and revascularization can be achieved with treatment modalities that include fibrinolytic therapies (medications that disintegrate the coronary thrombus) and percutaneous interventions (balloon angioplasty, stent placement, and thrombectomies). Surgery (coronary artery bypass, ventriculoplasty, ventricular assistive device [VAD], or heart transplant) is also utilized to open the coronary vessels during an acute myocardial infarction or to replace irreparable heart muscle. Cardiovascular supportive drugs and fluid regimens are initiated to maintain adequate blood pressure and essential fluid and electrolyte balance, as well as to optimize coronary perfusion to the myocardium. Mechanical assist devices, specifically intraaortic balloon pumps and percutaneous or VADs, are used to support cardiac output temporarily until the individual improves or until transplantation is possible.[35]

Implantable VADs, pacemakers, or internal defibrillator devices are sometimes used as permanent treatment for those who survive cardiogenic shock. Continuous hemodynamic monitoring should be employed to evaluate vascular volume and pressures, optimize fluid levels, and monitor drug administration with the goal of improving cardiac output and tissue perfusion.[33]

The clinical manifestations of cardiogenic shock are caused by inadequate perfusion to the heart and end organs (Fig. 48.6). Subjective complaints of chest pain, dyspnea, and faintness, along with feelings of impending doom, are often present. Classic observable signs and symptoms of tachycardia, tachypnea, hypotension, jugular venous distention, dysrhythmia, and low measured cardiac output are hallmarks. Cyanosis; skin mottling; rapid, faint, or irregular pulses; low urine output; and occasional peripheral edema are additional signs and symptoms of end-organ hypoperfusion. Myocardial dysfunction from fluid overload may result in extra heart sounds, pulmonary edema, hypoxemia, and elevated end-organ laboratory values. The amount of brain natriuretic peptide, produced when the heart stretches in relation to increased volume with decreased cardiac output, is increased to help the diuresis of fluid volume excess.[36] Pulmonary edema increases as volume accumulates and expands from the heart into the lungs as evidenced by

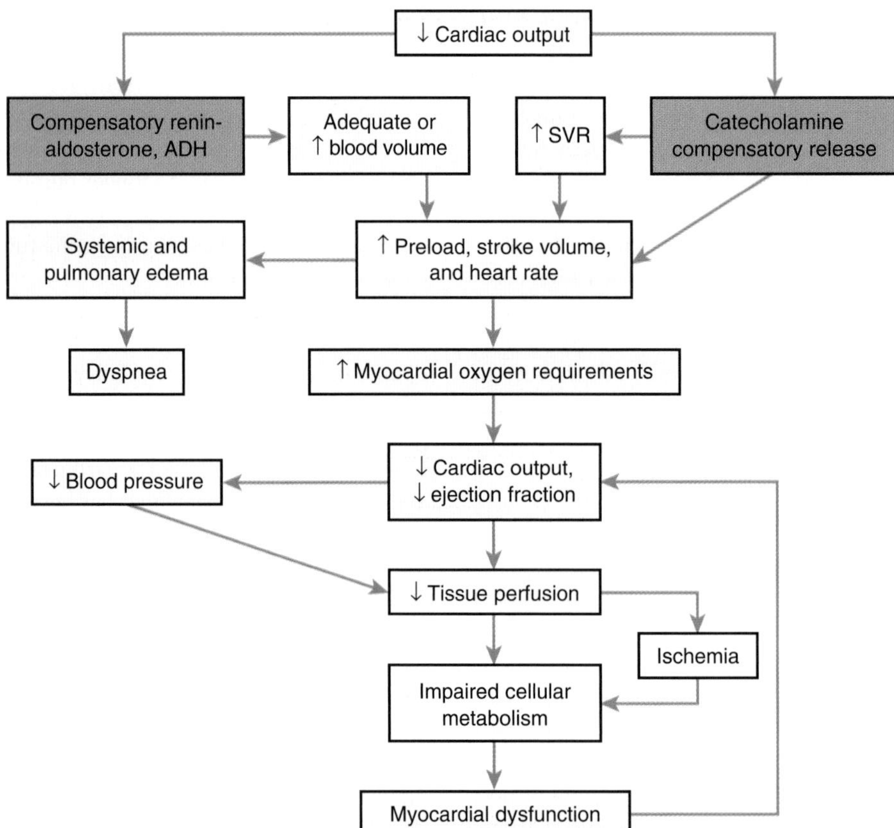

Fig. 48.6 Cardiogenic Shock. Shock becomes life-threatening when compensatory mechanisms *(orange boxes)* cause increased myocardial oxygen requirements. *ADH,* Antidiuretic hormone; *SVR,* systemic vascular resistance.

audible crackles and wheezes, as well as abnormal vascular congestion on chest radiography. Metabolic abnormalities involving electrolyte imbalances, metabolic acidosis, and elevated levels of inflammatory markers may result from or concur with the cardiac cascade of shock.

Hypovolemic Shock

Hypovolemic shock is caused by reduced intravascular volume (preload) from loss of whole blood (hemorrhage), plasma (burns), or interstitial fluid (diaphoresis, diabetes mellitus, diabetes insipidus, emesis, or diuresis) in large amounts, which reduces cardiac output. Hypovolemic shock is categorized as hemorrhagic, the loss of whole blood or plasma, and nonhemorrhagic, caused by the loss of interstitial fluid other than blood. Nonhemorrhagic losses can cause an indirect "relative" hypovolemia by promoting diffusion of plasma from the intravascular to the extravascular space. Hypovolemic shock begins to develop when intravascular volume has decreased by about 15%. Hemorrhagic shock can be related to blunt or penetrating trauma (fractures) and upper or lower gastrointestinal (GI) bleeding. Nonhemorrhagic shock can be caused from GI losses (diarrhea or vomiting), skin losses (burns, Stevens-Johnson syndrome), renal losses (diuresis, hypoaldosteronism), or third spacing (crush injury, cirrhosis).

Hypovolemia is offset initially by compensatory mechanisms (Fig. 48.7). Heart rate and vasoconstriction increase as a result of catecholamine release by the adrenals. This boosts cardiac output and tissue perfusion pressures. Compelled by a decrease in capillary hydrostatic pressures, interstitial fluid moves into the vascular compartment. The liver and spleen add to blood volume by disgorging stored red blood cells and plasma. In the kidneys, renin (through several intermediaries) stimulates aldosterone release and the retention of sodium (and hence water), whereas antidiuretic hormone (ADH, or vasopressin) from the posterior pituitary gland increases water retention. Data on the compensation of ADH, however, show that as shock worsens, ADH in plasma decreases. Eventually, hypovolemic shock results in extreme vasoconstriction and increased SVR and afterload in order to improve blood pressure and perfusion to core organs.

These compensatory mechanisms are, however, finite. If the initial fluid or blood loss is great or if loss continues, compensation fails, resulting in decreased tissue perfusion. Nutrient delivery to the cells is impaired, and cellular metabolism fails. Mortality from traumatic hemorrhagic shock ranges from 10% to 31%. Prompt control of hemorrhage, if present, is the treatment of choice. Fluid replacement is essential, but the type of fluid to be used and the rate of replacement are controversial.[37,38]

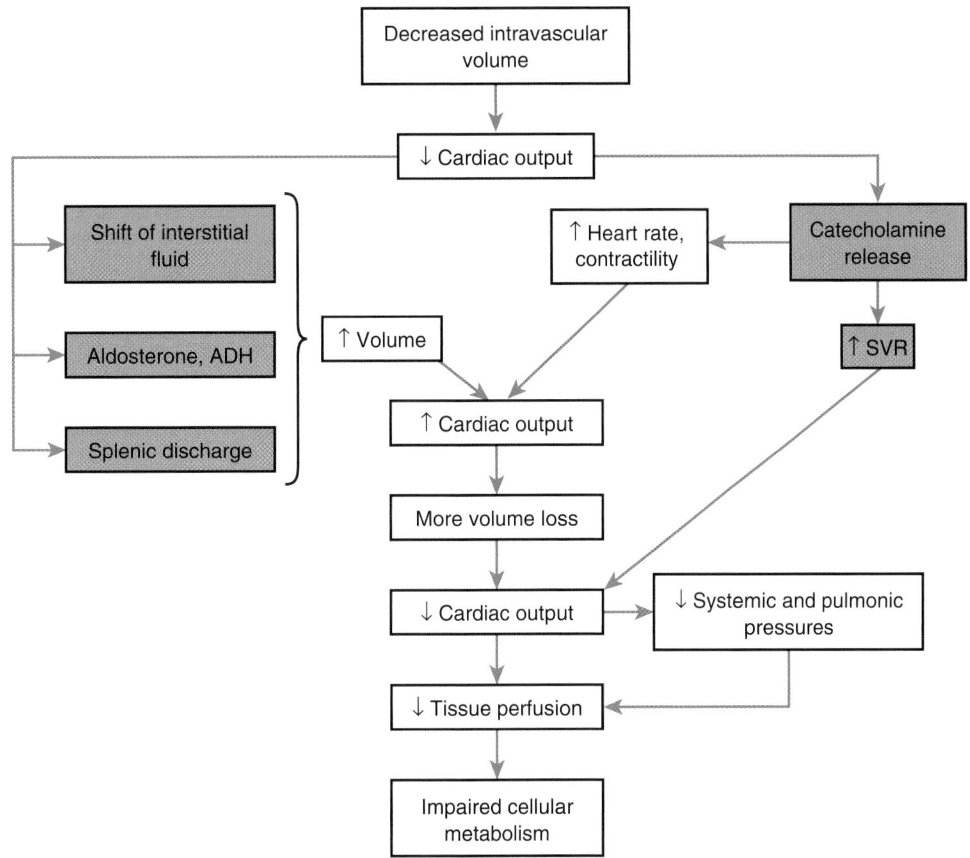

Fig. 48.7 Hypovolemic Shock. This type of shock becomes life-threatening when compensatory mechanisms *(orange boxes)* are overwhelmed by continued loss of intravascular volume. *ADH*, Antidiuretic hormone; *SVR*, systemic vascular resistance.

The clinical manifestations of hypovolemic shock include high SVR, pallor and cool extremities, increased thirst, oliguria, low systemic and pulmonary preloads, and rapid heart rate.

Obstructive Shock

Obstructive shock is a form of shock that is commonly combined with cardiogenic shock (see section on cardiogenic shock). Obstructive shock is associated with a mechanical obstruction to and/or from the heart generally within the great vessels, which causes an inadequate cardiac output. Common causes include pulmonary embolism, cardiac tamponade, and tension pneumothorax.[39,40] The clinical manifestations are specific to the related cause, but also may be accompanied by disturbances of consciousness, centralization, oliguria, hypotension, and tachycardia.[39] See chapter 35 for further information on these causes. Obstructive shock is a potentially life-threatening condition due to hemodynamic instability. This requires an expeditious and purposeful diagnosis and a rapid and directed treatment plan.[39]

MULTIPLE ORGAN DYSFUNCTION SYNDROME

Multiple organ dysfunction syndrome (MODS) is the progressive dysfunction of two or more organ systems resulting from an uncontrolled inflammatory response to a severe illness or injury. The organ dysfunction can progress to organ failure and death. In 2016, an international consensus conference developed an updated set of definitions for sepsis and related disorders (see Table 48.1). MODS is the end stage of a variety of injuries that terminate in a severe, systemic inflammatory and cell stress response, including apoptosis.[41]

MODS was first recognized as a distinct clinical syndrome in the early 1970s when advances in resuscitation and support technologies allowed many individuals to survive life-threatening illness or trauma only to die of complications of their disease. Today MODS remains a leading cause of mortality in surgical intensive care units (ICUs). Mortality for individuals with MODS increases progressively from 54% with two failing organ systems to 100% with five failing organ systems. Moreover, mortality has not improved much over the past 15 to 20 years in the medical community, but restrictive transfusion protocols in the surgical populations have demonstrated modest reduction in mortality.[42–45]

Although sepsis and septic shock are the most common causes, MODS can be initiated by any severe injury or disease process that activates a massive systemic inflammatory response by the host. Documented clinical infection is not necessary for its development. Other common triggers are severe trauma, major surgery, burns, circulatory shock, acute pancreatitis, acute renal failure, ARDS, blood transfusion, heat stroke, liver

BOX 48.2 Other Common Triggers of Multiple Organ Dysfunction Syndrome

Severe trauma	Heat stroke
Major surgery	Liver failure
Burns	Mesenteric ischemia
Circulatory shock	Propofol infusion syndrome
Acute pancreatitis	Persistent inflammatory foci
Acute renal failure	Necrotic tissue
Acute respiratory distress syndrome	Disseminated intravascular coagulation (DIC)
Blood transfusion	

failure, mesenteric ischemia, propofol infusion syndrome, persistent inflammatory foci, DIC, and tissue necrosis (Box 48.2). MODS is the major cause of death following septic shock, trauma, burn injuries, and ARDS. People at greatest risk for developing MODS are older adults and persons with significant tissue injury or preexisting disease.[5] The SOFA system (see Table 48.1), a clinically useful sepsis staging system, stratifies individuals with disease by baseline risk of adverse outcomes and potential to respond to therapy.[5]

Pathophysiology. In primary MODS, the organ injury is directly associated with a specific insult, most often ischemia or impaired perfusion from an episode of shock or trauma, thermal injury, soft tissue necrosis, or invasive infection.[46] This decreased perfusion is local (in the injured organs themselves) and generalized. The generalized hypoperfusion in primary MODS usually cannot be detected clinically. As a result of the insult, a stress response is initiated and stress hormones, catecholamines in particular, are released. The inflammatory and stress responses are not as evident because they are in secondary MODS. In primary MODS during the inflammatory response, presumably neutrophils and macrophages are "primed" by cytokines.[46] Any second insult, such as additional tissue injury, infection, or organ ischemia, may then activate the primed cells to produce an exaggerated response of secondary MODS (Fig. 48.8).[46,47]

The progressive organ dysfunction of secondary MODS is the result of an excessive inflammatory reaction, after a latent period following the initial injury, in organs distant from the site of the original injury. It is postulated that the resulting organ trauma is caused by the host response to a second insult rather than being a direct result of the primary injury. The second insult is often mild but produces an immense disproportionate response because of the previous priming of leukocytes. The interaction of injured organs then leads to a self-perpetuating inflammation.

Secondary MODS is initiated by the delayed postinjury insult as primed macrophages release a barrage of mediators, particularly the cytokines TNF and IL-1. These mediators damage the endothelium throughout the body. If a gram-negative bacterial infection is present, endotoxin released from the bacteria also causes severe damage to endothelial cells. Normal endothelial cells have little interaction with leukocytes, but when stimulated by TNF, IL-1, IL-6, or endotoxin, they change to a proinflammatory state and express adhesion molecules that mediate adhesion of neutrophils. The adhered neutrophils then migrate through the endothelium, aggregate in the area of damaged tissue, and amplify the inflammation. The activated endothelial cells increase production and release of nitric oxide (endothelium), a potent vasodilator, which is considered an important factor in blood flow changes and loss of vascular tone noted in systemic inflammation.[48] The injured endothelium also becomes much more permeable, allowing fluid and protein to leak into the interstitial spaces. An important function of normal endothelium is anticoagulation. When damaged, the endothelium loses much of its ability to prevent blood clotting, allowing microvascular thrombi to develop.

The postinjury insult also activates the neuroendocrine system, resulting in a second, more extensive stress response. The normal function of the stress response is to maintain basal and stress-related homeostasis[49]; however, homeostasis cannot be maintained in MODS. In fact, the endocrine response becomes excessive and injurious. There is an early increase in the levels of circulating catecholamines that contributes to many of the clinical manifestations of MODS, such as tachycardia, hypermetabolism, and increased oxygen consumption. Cortisol, glucagon, insulin, human growth hormone, ADH (which may become depleted), and endorphin levels also are increased. Many of these hormones contribute to the extreme catabolic state of MODS, and endorphins, which are vasodilators, decrease SVR. The sympathetic nervous system, to compensate for complications resulting from the injury (e.g., fluid loss, hypotension), also is stimulated. The stimulation persists throughout the period of critical illness.[49] The stress response can be amplified by a number of factors, including pain, anxiety, psychosis, and hyperthermia. (The stress response is discussed in detail in Chapter 11.)

Because of endothelial cell dysfunction and the release of mediators, four major plasma cascades are activated: complement, kallikrein-kinin, coagulation, and fibrinolytic.[50,51] Complement components, particularly the anaphylatoxins C3a and C5a, cause vasodilation by stimulating release of histamine from mast cells. They also have strong chemotactic properties. C5a, especially, causes adhesion and the activation and degranulation of neutrophils. Complement is thought to be a powerful trigger for the exaggerated inflammatory response. Activation of the kinin system results in the production of bradykinin, a very potent vasodilator known to decrease SVR. Coagulation mechanisms also are activated and, because tissue injury and endothelial dysfunction are extensive, microvascular thrombosis occurs throughout the body, resulting in impaired microvascular circulation and organ ischemia. Concurrently, fibrinolytic mechanisms are activated. The tendency toward clotting, however, is greater, resulting in a net procoagulant state that can lead to the development of DIC. The overall effect of the activation of the plasma cascades is a hyperinflammatory and hypercoagulant state that contributes to vasodilation, vasopermeability, cardiovascular instability, endothelial dysfunction, and clotting abnormalities.[46,51,52]

Once cytokines and other mediators have been released and the plasma enzyme cascades have been activated, a massive systemic inflammatory response develops. It involves several types of inflammatory cells, particularly neutrophils, macrophages,

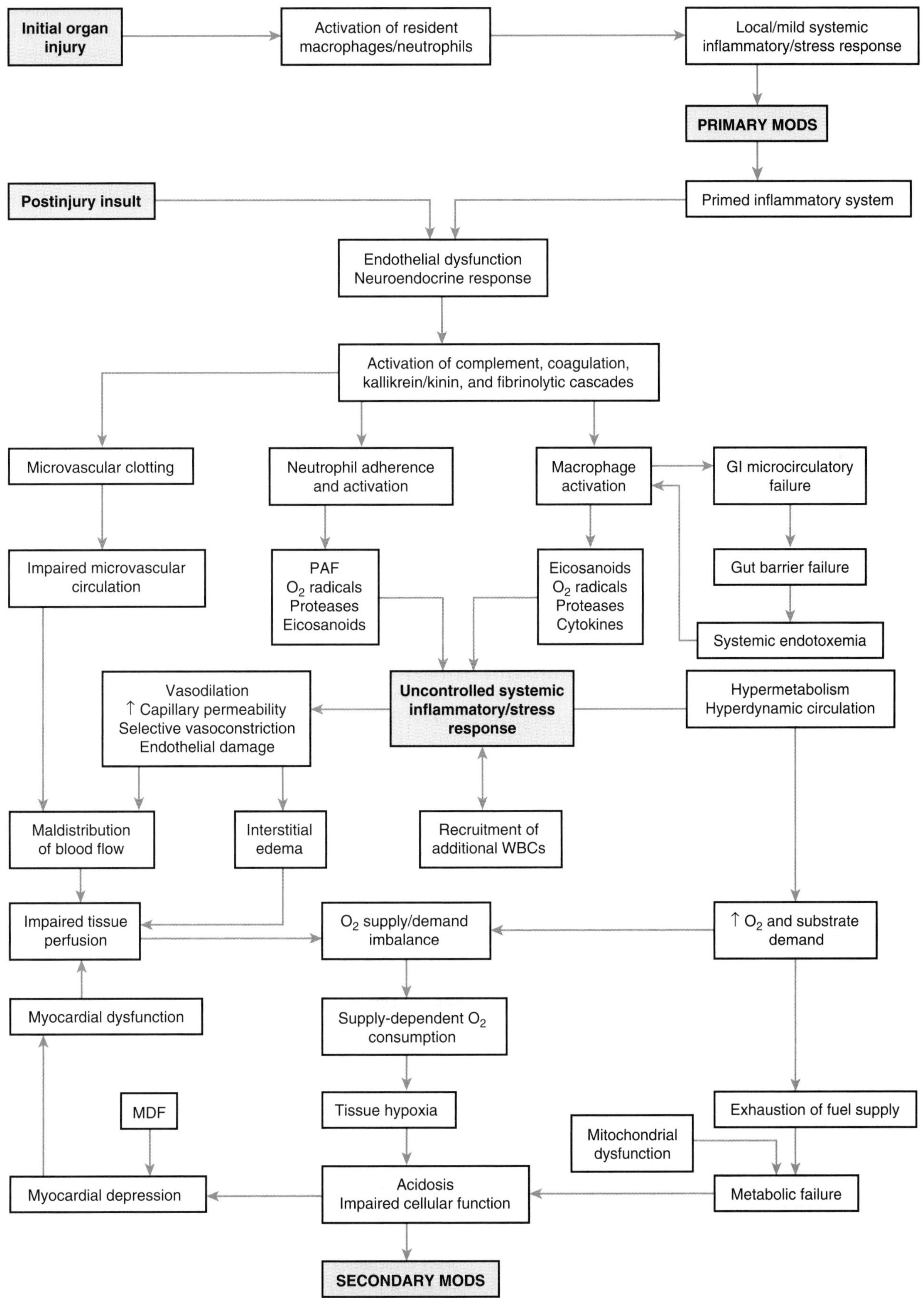

Fig. 48.8 Pathogenesis of Multiple Organ Dysfunction Syndrome. *GI*, Gastrointestinal; *MDF*, myocardial depressant factor; *MODS*, multiple organ dysfunction syndrome; *PAF*, platelet-activating factor; *WBCs*, white blood cells.

and mast cells. These cells, having been primed by their response to the initial organ injury, now pour large amounts of chemical mediators into tissues and into the systemic circulation.

Neutrophils have tremendous inflammatory potential. The accumulation of activated neutrophils in organs is thought to play a key role in the pathogenesis of MODS.[53] When neutrophils adhere to the endothelium, they undergo a "respiratory burst" (oxidative burst) and release oxygen free radicals. The respiratory burst occurs as the activated neutrophil experiences a sudden increase in oxidative metabolism, producing large quantities of highly toxic oxygen free radicals. These reactive oxygen species (ROS) cause oxidative stress. The primary ROS produced are superoxide, hydrogen peroxide (H_2O_2), hydroxyl radical (OH^-), and singlet oxygen (O). Oxygen free radicals are extremely damaging to vascular endothelium and tissue cells, attacking deoxyribonucleic acid (DNA), cross-linking membrane structures, and inducing membrane peroxidation reactions that disorganize cell membranes and lead to tissue necrosis (also see Chapter 2).[3]

Other important mediators released by neutrophils are proteases, particularly collagenase and elastase. Proteases directly damage endothelium and neighboring cells, resulting in increased capillary permeability and organ damage. When activated, neutrophils also release platelet-activating factor (PAF), a mediator that damages endothelium, stimulates clot formation, and activates increasing numbers of phagocytes. Finally, neutrophils release arachidonic acid metabolites (eicosanoids) as a result of lipid peroxidation of their cell membranes. Of the arachidonic acid metabolites (prostaglandins, thromboxanes, leukotrienes), two are particularly important in the pathogenesis of organ hypoperfusion: prostacyclin (PGI_2) and thromboxane A_2 (TXA_2). TXA_2 is a powerful vasoconstrictor, and PGI_2 is a potent vasodilator. When released in varying amounts in different organ beds, they are largely responsible for the maldistribution of blood flow characteristic of MODS. In total, neutrophils produce at least 50 to 60 toxins.[54,55] Collectively, products released by neutrophils cause endothelial dysfunction, systemic vasodilation, selective vasoconstriction (vasoconstriction of certain organ beds or parts of organ beds), increased vascular permeability, and microvascular coagulation.

Macrophages, present in most tissues, are activated by endotoxin, complement, and monocyte chemotactic substances.[56] Macrophages share a key role in the development of the unregulated inflammation of secondary MODS with the neutrophils. Like neutrophils, they produce oxygen free radicals, proteases, cytokines, nitric oxide, and arachidonic acid metabolites. It has been reported that excessive or prolonged stimulation of macrophages leads to the overproduction of cytokines and nitric oxide that initiate the cycle of harmful effects in MODS.[3,56] TNF and IL-1, which share many of the same functions and act synergistically, are the major cytokines that mediate inflammation.[56,57] TNF has potent metabolic effects, including fever, anorexia, hyperglycemia, hypermetabolism, and weight loss. It activates neutrophils, damages endothelial cells, and potentiates hypotension and shock. IL-1 also has metabolic effects, inducing fever, hypermetabolism, and muscle wasting. Normally, TNF activates cytokines, the coagulation system, fibrinolysis, and neutrophils. With the exception of neutrophil activation, IL-1 causes similar activation in individuals with cancer.[54] In the pathogenesis of MODS, the cytokines are linked to all cellular, hemodynamic, and metabolic alterations.

The gastrointestinal mucosa is particularly vulnerable to inflammatory mediators released by macrophages and neutrophils. Under normal circumstances the gut mucosa serves as a barrier to prevent bacteria in the gastrointestinal tract from entering the systemic circulation. Damage to the mucosa results in microcirculatory failure of the gut and consequent loss of the gut barrier function. The loss of intestinal barrier function leads to the systemic spread of bacteria or endotoxin, or both, from the gut (systemic endotoxemia). This phenomenon is called *translocation of bacteria*. The idea that the gut acts as a reservoir of bacteria and endotoxin that can initiate or perpetuate the development of MODS is known as the gut hypothesis. The gut hypothesis provides a possible explanation for the fact that an infectious focus is not always found in individuals with MODS. Although this hypothesis has been substantiated by animal studies and has much support, the evidence from human studies is inconclusive.[58] The numerous inflammatory processes operating in MODS cause maldistribution of blood flow and hypermetabolism. Maldistribution of blood flow refers to the uneven distribution of flow to various organs and between the large vessels and capillary beds of the body. It is caused by generalized vasodilation, increased capillary permeability, selective vasoconstriction, endothelial dysfunction, and impaired microvascular circulation. It is a major factor in the pathophysiology of MODS.[51] The alterations in blood flow—which can occur at the cellular, organ, or regional level—lead to impaired tissue perfusion and a decreased supply of oxygen to the cells. The organs most severely affected by hypoperfusion are the lungs, splanchnic bed, liver, and kidneys. Despite supernormal systemic blood flow, oxygen delivery to the tissues decreases. Several factors contribute to the problem. First, blood is shunted past selected regional capillary beds. Shunting, caused by loss of autoregulation in some organs, may be an early indicator of progression of sepsis into MODS.[59] This occurs because inflammatory mediators, particularly TXA_2, override the normal vascular control mechanisms to cause selective vasoconstriction and because injured endothelial cells are unable to respond to normal vasodilator mediators. Second, interstitial edema, resulting from microvascular permeability, contributes to decreased oxygen delivery to cells by increasing the distance oxygen must travel to reach the cells. Third, capillary obstruction occurs because of the formation of microvascular thrombi and the aggregation of leukocytes.[3,56]

Hypermetabolism, with accompanying alterations in carbohydrate, fat, and lipid metabolism, is initially a compensatory measure to meet the body's increased demands for energy. Eventually, however, hypermetabolism becomes detrimental, placing enormous demands on the heart. Hypermetabolism is the result of (1) the neuroendocrine response to stress with the release of catecholamines and cortisol, and (2) the action of TNF and IL-1. With increased metabolism the calorie requirements are markedly increased,[60] and the cardiac output increases to 1.5 to 2 times normal.[61,62] The alterations in metabolism affect all aspects of substrate use. Most important is the catabolism of protein, primarily of skeletal muscle and visceral organs. The extreme catabolism of protein can rapidly deplete lean body mass. Hyperglycemia occurs as gluconeogenesis by the liver increases and glucose use by the cells decreases. Fatty acids are mobilized from adipose tissue. The net result of the hypermetabolism is depletion of oxygen and fuel supplies.

Myocardial depression also accompanies MODS. The cause remains unclear, but possible explanations are the effects of myocardial depressant factor (MDF), TNF, and IL-1 on cardiac contractility; alterations in α-adrenergic receptors in the heart; and hypoxia of the myocardium.[63]

The decreased oxygen delivery to the cells (resulting from the maldistribution of blood flow) and the increased oxygen needs of the cells (resulting from hypermetabolism) combine to create an imbalance in oxygen supply and demand. This imbalance is critical in the pathogenesis of MODS because it results in a pathologic condition known as supply-dependent oxygen consumption. Ordinarily the amount of oxygen consumed by the cells depends only on the needs of the cells because there is an adequate reserve of oxygen that can be delivered if required. In MODS, however, the reserve has been exhausted and the amount of oxygen consumed becomes dependent on the amount the circulation is able to deliver. Because the amount is inadequate in MODS, the tissues become hypoxic. Compounding the hypoxic damage to cells is a phenomenon called *reperfusion injury* (see Chapter 2). Much of the organ damage in MODS occurs with the reestablishment of blood flow after a period of ischemia. During the ischemic episode, energy stores and ATP are depleted, and the enzyme *xanthine dehydrogenase* is converted to *xanthine oxidase*. With reperfusion of the ischemic tissue, oxygen free radicals are formed from oxygen by the action of xanthine oxidase, and they attack the already damaged tissues. Consequently, although reperfusion is necessary to restore oxygen supply to ischemic organs, it can increase the extent of injury. Therefore because of supply-dependent oxygen consumption and reperfusion injury, already compromised tissues become increasingly hypoxic. The result is cellular acidosis, impaired cellular function, and ultimately multiple organ failure.

Clinical manifestations. In MODS, the organs that show clinical manifestations of failure are not always the organs involved as part of the initial injury, and there is usually a lag time between the initial insult and the development of systemic organ failure. The development of primary MODS is difficult to monitor, but there is a well-established general pattern in the clinical development of secondary MODS.[46] Following the inciting event and aggressive resuscitation of an individual for approximately 24 hours, the individual develops low-grade fever, tachycardia, tachypnea, dyspnea, altered mental status, and a general hyperdynamic and hypermetabolic state (Box 48.3). Following this, the lungs begin to fail, and ARDS may appear within 24 to 72 hours (see discussion of ARDS in Chapter 35). Between days 7 and 10, the hypermetabolic and hyperdynamic state intensifies; bacteremia with enteric organisms is common; and signs of hepatic, intestinal, and renal failure develop. During days 14 to 21, renal failure and liver failure become more severe. Hematologic failure and myocardial failure are usually later manifestations. Encephalopathy, characterized by mental status changes ranging from confusion to deep coma, may occur at any time. This sequence can evolve rapidly, with death occurring between 14 and 21 days later, or it can evolve over weeks. Individuals can recover from either the slowly or the rapidly evolving course.

The clinical manifestations of failure of individual organs in MODS are caused by inflammatory mediator damage, tissue hypoxia, and hypermetabolism. Respiratory failure progresses early to ARDS and is characterized by tachypnea, pulmonary edema with crackles and diminished breath sounds, use of accessory muscles, and hypoxemia. Liver failure, although early in its development, is not clinically detectable until the later stages of MODS, when jaundice, abdominal distention, liver tenderness, muscle wasting, and hepatic encephalopathy appear. All aspects of metabolism, substance detoxification, and immune response are impaired. Albumin and clotting factor synthesis decreases, protein wastes accumulate, and liver tissue macrophages (Kupffer cells) no longer function effectively.

The gastrointestinal system is very sensitive to ischemic and inflammatory injury. Clinical manifestations of bowel involvement are hemorrhage, ileus, stress ulcers, malabsorption, diarrhea or constipation, vomiting, anorexia, abdominal pain, and pancreatitis. Intolerance to enteral feeding may develop. Adding to damage caused by injury to the bowel is bacterial translocation into the bloodstream resulting from the loss of the gut barrier function. The overwhelmed liver is unable to clear the bacteria from the systemic circulation. Thus regardless of whether infection or some other injury was the precipitating cause of MODS, once intestinal bacteria enter the systemic circulation, it is likely that sepsis will be a problem. Renal failure develops at about the same time and is marked by progressive oliguria, azotemia, and edema. If renal shutdown is severe, anuria, hyperkalemia, and metabolic acidosis occur.

The first manifestations of cardiac failure are similar to those of septic shock: tachycardia, bounding pulse, increased cardiac output, fall in SVR, hypotension, warm skin, and supraventricular dysrhythmias. In the terminal stages, profound hypotension and ventricular dysrhythmias may develop. Changes in central nervous system function may be noted. Ischemia and inflammation are responsible for the changes, which include apprehension, confusion, disorientation, restlessness, agitation, headache, decreased cognitive ability and memory, and decreased level of consciousness. When ischemia is severe, seizures and coma can occur.

Evaluation and treatment. Because there is no specific therapy for MODS, early detection or prevention is extremely important so that supportive measures are initiated instantly.[64] Frequent assessment of the clinical status of individuals at known risk is essential. Unfortunately, there is no way to determine with certainty when an organ is failing. Indicators of organ dysfunction are presented in Table 48.1.

BOX 48.3 Clinical Manifestations of Organ Dysfunction

Pulmonary
- Acute respiratory distress syndrome (ARDS) pattern of respiratory failure (dyspnea, patchy infiltrates, refractory hypoxemia, respiratory acidosis, abnormal O_2 indices)
- Pulmonary hypertension

Gastrointestinal
- Abdominal distention and ascites
- Intolerance to enteral feedings
- Paralytic ileus
- Upper and lower gastrointestinal bleeding (guaiac-positive stools)
- Diarrhea
- Ischemic colitis
- Mucosal ulceration
- Decreased bowel sounds
- Bacterial overgrowth in stool

Liver
- Increased serum bilirubin level (hyperbilirubinemia)
- Increased liver enzyme levels (serum aspartate transaminase [SAST], serum alanine aminotransferase [SALT], lactic dehydrogenase [LDH], alkaline phosphatase)
- Increased serum ammonia level
- Decreased serum transferrin level
- Jaundice
- Hepatomegaly

Gallbladder
- Right upper quadrant tenderness or pain
- Abdominal distention
- Unexplained fever
- Decreased bowel sounds

Metabolic/Nutritional
- Decreased lean body mass
- Muscle wasting
- Severe weight loss
- Negative nitrogen balance
- Hyperglycemia
- Hypertriglyceridemia
- Increased serum lactate levels
- Decreased serum albumin, serum transferrin, prealbumin, retinol-binding protein

Renal
- Increased serum creatinine level and blood urea nitrogen
- Oliguria, anuria, or polyuria consistent with prerenal azotemia or acute tubular necrosis
- Urinary indices consistent with prerenal azotemia or acute tubular necrosis

Cardiovascular

Hyperdynamic
- Decreased pulmonary capillary wedge pressure
- Decreased systemic vascular resistance
- Decreased right atrial pressure
- Decreased left ventricular stroke work index
- Increased oxygen consumption
- Increased cardiac output, cardiac index, heart rate

Hypodynamic
- Increased systemic vascular resistance
- Increased right atrial pressure
- Increased left ventricular stroke work index
- Decreased oxygen delivery and consumption
- Decreased cardiac output and cardiac index

Central Nervous System
- Lethargy
- Altered level of consciousness
- Fever
- Hepatic encephalopathy

Coagulation and Hematologic
- Thrombocytopenia
- Disseminated intravascular coagulation

Immune
- Infection
- Decreased lymphocyte count
- Anergy

Data from Thelan LA, et al. *Critical care nursing: Diagnosis and management*, 6th edition. St. Louis: Mosby; 2010.

Several systems for scoring severity of illness also have been developed. Commonly used systems are the Acute Physiology and Chronic Health Evaluation II and III (APACHE II and APACHE III), the logistic organ dysfunction score (LODS), the SOFA, the MODS score, and the predisposition, infection (or insult), response, and organ dysfunction (PIRO) staging system.[65]

Once organ failure develops, monitoring of laboratory values and hemodynamic parameters is necessary to assess the degree of clinical impairment.

The therapeutic management of MODS consists of prevention and support. Prevention of the syndrome is essential! First, if possible, the initial source of inflammation must be eliminated or controlled. Next, a second insult must be avoided. It is paramount to remove any potential site of infection by debriding necrotic tissue, draining abscesses, reducing the number of invasive procedures performed, and removing hematomas. Nosocomial infections from contaminated lines and catheters are of concern and must be prevented. Nosocomial infection rates of 15% to 25% have been reported in critically ill individuals.[66] Early reduction of long-bone fractures and surgical repair of injured tissues also are important preventive measures.

The goals of therapy are to control infection, provide adequate tissue oxygenation, restore intravascular volume, and support the function of individual organs.[24,67–69]

After the initial injury has been aggressively treated and sources of infection have been removed, antibiotics usually are administered. The choice of agents is based on the individual's disease process, but the regimen is usually a combination of antibiotics that covers both gram-negative and gram-positive organisms.

Because oxygen is not stored in the tissues, it must be continuously delivered. Maintaining an arterial oxygen saturation of

88% to 92% is recommended; current literature supports using a restrictive transfusion strategy (transfuse only if hemoglobin is <7 g/day or <8.0 if the individual has ischemic or current acute coronary syndrome).[42,70,71]

Mixed venous oxygen saturation greater than or equal to 70% is recommended. For oxygen delivery blood transfusions may be necessary to ensure an adequate hemoglobin level. To deliver oxygen to the organs in the face of profound systemic vasodilation, fluid volume must be restored. Therefore, aggressive fluid therapy is initiated early. Usually large volumes of isotonic crystalloid solutions are administered, although colloids (often albumin) also may be added to maintain adequate preload and circulation volume.[42,70,71]

Finally, support for individual organ systems must be provided. Respiratory failure is treated with mechanical ventilation with low tidal volumes, high oxygen concentrations, and positive end-expiratory pressures (PEEPs).[72]

To provide adequate nutrition and metabolic support, the failing gastrointestinal system is supported with enteral feedings. It is now well recognized that enteral feedings help preserve gut microbial barrier function, and thus are preferred to parenteral feedings.[73] However, if the individual is unable to tolerate the amount of enteral feeding required to meet the enormous metabolic demands, hyperalimentation may be added. Ideally the feeding formula is carefully calculated to meet the individual's nutritional requirements. Glucose level control (140 to 180 mg/dL) is recommended.[73] Once renal failure is established, dialysis or continuous hemofiltration may be required to maintain fluid and electrolyte balance. To support the failing cardiovascular system, inotropic drugs, such as low-dose dopamine and dobutamine, or vasopressors, such as norepinephrine, may be required to maximize cardiac contractility and maintain cardiac output. Although steroids have antiinflammatory effects, their use is controversial because studies showing benefit and injury are both published; however they have been shown to be effective in adults with septic shock. Obtaining an adrenocorticotropic hormone (ACTH) level is not recommended. Deep vein thrombosis prophylaxis also is important.[23]

Scientific knowledge gained about MODS and inflammatory mediators has led to many investigational therapies. Novel molecular approaches targeting a variety of interdependent mediators of MODS are being investigated.

THERMAL INJURY AND BURNS

Major thermal injury is a source of massive tissue injury and destruction that has wide-reaching effects on virtually all organ systems. Burn is a generic term used to describe cutaneous injury caused by thermal contact (friction, cold, heat), radiation, chemicals, or electrical causes.[74] In addition to cutaneous injury, burns are often associated with smoke inhalation injury or other traumatic injuries that aggravate the local and systemic problems of burns. Pulmonary injury, both primary and secondary, is common in this population and often requires ventilator support. The clinical significance of a thermal injury is dependent on the depth of the burn, the percentage of body surface area involved, the injuries caused internally from inhalation, and the timeliness of treatment. This model of multisystem injury provides an opportunity to examine the interaction of shock, inflammation, and immunocompromise in a clinical setting.

Epidemiology and Etiology

Burns are the fourth most common trauma worldwide.[75] Over 450,000 individuals seek care every year in the United States for burn injuries with approximately 10% requiring hospitalization.[75] Individuals between 20 and 59 years of age have the highest prevalence of burns accounting for 55% with young children accounting for 24%.[75] Deaths consequent to burn injuries decreased more than 50%, from 9000 in 1971[76] to 3275 annually.[75] This clinical progress is the result of several factors, such as ongoing research in burn physiology and burn care,[77] a nationally increased focus on fire safety and burn prevention, the establishment of regional burn centers, the use of smoke detectors, regulation of consumer product safety, and occupational safety mandates. A decrease in hospitalization is a result of a shift to outpatient care and improved prehospital and emergency treatment, as well as an improvement in burn assessment and delivery of care.[78] This may reduce medical transport and treatment costs. Worldwide expansion of telemedicine has occurred at an increasing rate over the past decade. These advances in care are changing measures of healthcare value from burn survival to functional outcomes in burn survivors. In fact, worldwide, digital health communications are becoming common in burn centers due to improved convenience, accuracy, efficiency, productivity, and clinical decision-making.[79]

The causes of burn injury may be thermal or nonthermal, such as chemical, electrical, or radioactive. Thermal burns may result from thermal contact, flame, or scald. Adherent materials (e.g., asphalt, tar, or plastic) may likewise produce a serious contact burn. Chemical injuries are a result of contact with substances that are directly toxic to the skin or the lining of the respiratory or alimentary tract. Such chemicals are often acidic, alkali, or organic agents, termed vesicants, which cause blistering of the epithelial surfaces. Electrical burns may be the result of the conduction of electrical current through the body with heating of tissue or flash over the body surface associated with an electrical discharge. Quality of life can be mildly to severely affected by a burn but can improve with proper and expeditious intervention.

Burn Wound Depth

The classification of burn wound depth is usually based on the physical appearance and the symptoms associated with the affected skin (see Chapter 46 on the structure and function of the integumentary system). The definitive diagnosis is determined by the histologic depth of tissue necrosis. Such historic evaluation, unfortunately, necessitates a skin biopsy. Because of the invasive nature of biopsy, clinical depth assessment is used and the ultimate fate of the wound determines final diagnosis. Advances in Laser Doppler Imaging (LDI) have been validated for determining burn wound depth.[79] LDI is a non-invasive mechanical extension of the clinical physical exam to assess burn injuries and guide the health care provider in the decision to perform surgical excision or grafting.[79]

TABLE 48.2 **Depth of Burn Injury**

	FIRST DEGREE	SECOND DEGREE		THIRD DEGREE
Characteristic		**Superficial Partial Thickness**	**Deep Partial Thickness**	**Full Thickness**
Morphology	Destruction of epidermis only	Destruction of epidermis and some dermis	Destruction of epidermis and dermis, leaving only skin appendages	Destruction of epidermis, dermis, and underlying subcutaneous tissue
Skin function	Intact	Absent	Absent	Absent
Tactile and pain sensors	Intact	Intact	Intact but diminished	Absent
Blisters	Present only after first 24 h	Present within minutes, thin walled and fluid filled	May appear as fluid-filled blisters; often is layer of flat, dehydrated "tissue paper" that lifts off in sheets	Blisters rare; usually is a layer of flat, dehydrated "tissue paper" that lifts off easily
Appearance of wound after initial debridement	Skin peels at 24–48 h, normal or slightly red underneath	Red to pale ivory, moist surface	Mottled with areas of waxy white, dry surface	White, cherry red, or black; may contain visible thrombosed veins; dry, hard leathery surface
Healing time	3–5 days	21–28 days	30 days to many months	Will not heal; may close from edges as secondary healing if wound is small
Scarring	None	May be present; low incidence influenced by genetic predisposition	Highest incidence because of slow healing rate promoting scar tissue development; also influenced by genetic predisposition	Skin graft; scarring minimized by early excision and grafting; influenced by genetic predisposition

First-degree burns are superficial and involve only the epidermis without penetration or injury to the underlying dermal or subcutaneous tissue (Table 48.2).[75] The skin maintains water vapor and bacterial barrier functions. Many sunburns are first-degree injuries caused by exposure of the skin to ultraviolet radiation from the sun. Initially there is local pain and erythema, and since the barrier remains intact, the area is dry (no blisters).[75] An extensive first-degree burn may cause systemic responses such as chills, headache, localized edema, and nausea or vomiting. Minimal treatment (analgesic and moisturizer) or no treatment of extensive first-degree burns is required unless the person is elderly or an infant, in which case severe nausea and vomiting may lead to inadequate fluid intake and dehydration. Therapy consists of intravenous hydration until the nausea and vomiting subside 24 to 72 hours after burn injury. Comfort measures for previously healthy children or adults with extensive first-degree burns consist of aspirin for adults or acetaminophen for children every 4 hours in age-appropriate doses and frequent application of a water-soluble lotion.[75] First-degree burns heal in 3 to 5 days without scarring.

Second-degree burns describe two categories of burn depth with markedly different characteristics. Both of these are partial-thickness injuries, but they evoke vastly different responses. The hallmark of superficial partial-thickness injury is the appearance of thin-walled, fluid-filled blisters that develop within just a few minutes after injury. Blisters form due to the breech of the epidermal barrier. As blisters break or are removed, nerve endings are exposed to air (Fig. 48.9), causing severe pain, another dominant characteristic of superficial injury. Tactile and pain sensors remain intact throughout healing, with each wound care procedure causing substantial pain. Wounds heal in 3 to 4 weeks if the individual is adequately nourished and no complications develop (Fig. 48.10). Scar formation is unusual with this injury; however any wound that requires more than the usual healing time has a higher chance of forming a hypertrophic scar.[75] The amount of scarring that develops is a genetically determined trait and is not predictable during the early course of treatment.

Deep partial-thickness burns involve the entire dermis, sparing skin appendages such as hair follicles and sweat glands (see Table 48.2). The burn often looks waxy white and is surrounded by margins of superficial partial-thickness injury. The injury is often clinically indistinguishable from a full-thickness injury (Fig. 48.11), but by 7 to 10 days after burn injury, skin buds and hair will appear from hair follicles, indicating that skin appendages remain. These wounds take weeks to heal, and current therapy consists of surgical removal of the burn wound (excision) followed by application of the person's own unburned skin from another body area (autograft). Wounds that heal slowly produce more scar tissue and continue to be a potential source of infection until closed. In the presence of relative surgical contraindications, such as cardiopulmonary failure, deep partial-thickness wounds are not surgically treated but are allowed to heal naturally. The fate of partial-thickness burns can be affected by treatment, such as topical antibiotics, or by the condition of biologic membranes.[80] The ultimate healing of deep partial-thickness burns commonly results in hypertrophic scarring with poor functional and cosmetic results.

Third-degree burns, or full-thickness injuries, involve destruction of the entire epidermis, dermis, and often the

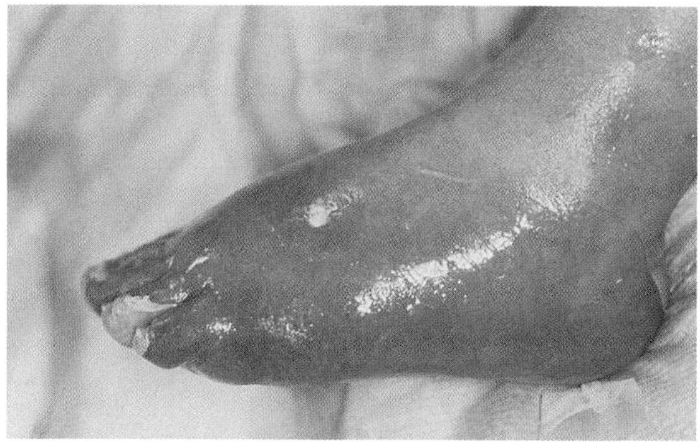

Fig. 48.9 Superficial Partial-Thickness Injury. Scald injury following debridement of overlying blister and nonadherent epithelium. (Courtesy University of Utah Burn Center.)

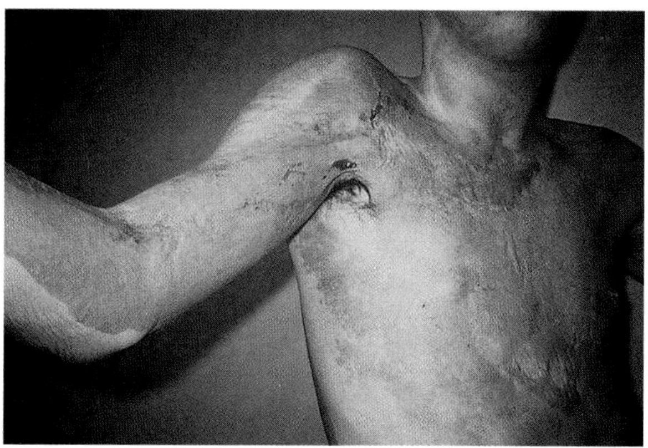

Fig. 48.10 Axillary Burn Scar Contracture. Note the blanching of the anterior axillary fold and small ulceration, both indicating the diminished range of motion. (Courtesy University of Utah Burn Center.)

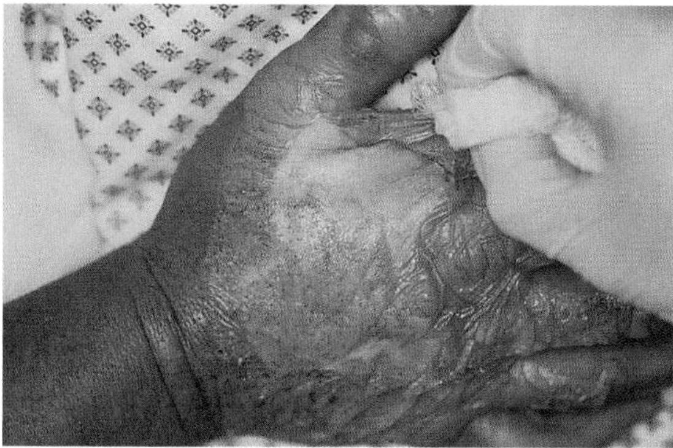

Fig. 48.11 Deep Partial-Thickness Wound. Note pale appearance and minimal exudate. (Courtesy University of Utah Burn Center.)

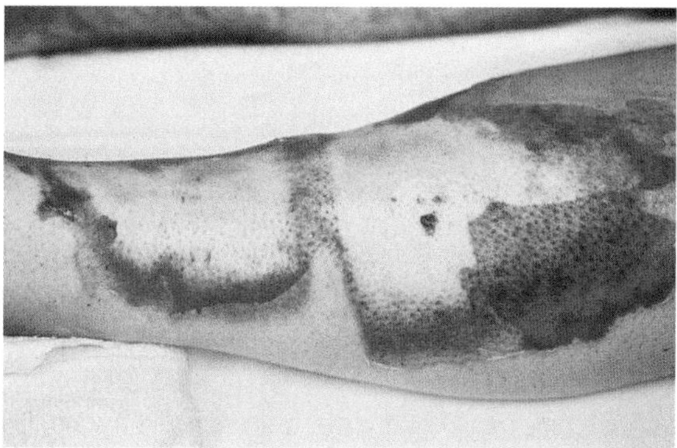

Fig. 48.12 Full-Thickness Thermal Injury. The wound is dry and insensate. (Courtesy University of Utah Burn Center.)

underlying subcutaneous tissue (fat) (see Table 48.2). On occasion, all underlying subcutaneous tissue is destroyed and muscle or bone may be involved. Full-thickness wounds often appear relatively innocuous when their color is white and the delineation between normal and burned skin is not accompanied by a marked color change. Elasticity of the dermis is absent, leaving the wound dry and leathery in appearance and texture (Fig. 48.12). As marked edema develops, distal circulation may be compromised in areas of circumferential burns. Escharotomies (cutting through burned skin) are performed to release underlying pressure. Full-thickness burns are painless because all nerve endings have been destroyed by the injury.[75]

Fourth-degree burns extend beyond the epidermis, dermis, subcutaneous tissue into the muscle, bone, or tendon and generally require extensive surgical repair with flaps or even amputation.[75] Burns to this extent are painless because all of the vasculature and nerves of the dermis are destroyed.

The extent of the total body surface area (TBSA) burn is estimated using either the "rule of nines" (Fig. 48.13) or the Lund and Browder chart (Fig. 48.14). Areas of partial-thickness and full-thickness injury are marked on the diagram (see Fig. 48.14). First-degree burns are not included in the TBSA estimate. The surface area of the palm, including palmar finger surface, averages 1% of the body surface area over a wide range of ages; thus, it can be used to estimate burn areas of irregular size and shape.[81]

Severity of burn injury is a combination of many factors, including age, medical history, extent and depth of injury, and body area involved. The American Burn Association has defined criteria to assist healthcare professionals in identifying individuals who require care at a specialized burn center (Box 48.4). The multidisciplinary burn center is recommended for those persons who are at high risk for morbidity, mortality, or permanent functional loss.

Pathophysiology and clinical manifestations. Burn injury results in dramatic changes in many physiologic functions of the body within the first few hours after the event. The effect of burn depends on two factors: first, the extent of body surface involved; and second, the depth of cutaneous injury (see the box Emerging Science Box: Pathophysiology of the Burn Wound). Body surface burn extent is described by the percentage of TBSA injured. Burns exceeding 20% of TBSA in most adults are considered to be major burn injuries and are associated with massive evaporative water losses and flux of large amounts of fluid and electrolytes in the tissues, manifested as generalized edema and circulatory hypovolemia. Depth of cutaneous injury has been categorized in many ways but always depends on the severity of injury of epidermal and dermal elements of the skin and whether the alteration is a permanent or reversible injury.

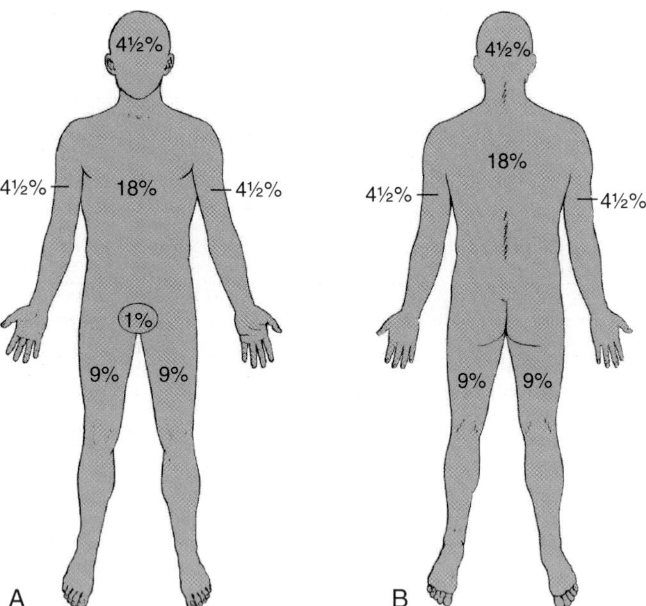

Fig. 48.13 Rule of Nines. A commonly used assessment tool with estimates of the percentages (in multiples of 9) of the total body surface area burned. **(A)** Adults (anterior view). **(B)** Adults (posterior view).

With a major burn injury, a systemic pathophysiology ensues that requires therapeutic intervention to sustain life. The immediate (acute) physiologic consequences of a major burn injury center around the profound, life-threatening hypovolemic shock that occurs in conjunction with cellular and immunologic disruption within a few hours of injury (Fig. 48.15). Burn shock is a phenomenon consisting of both a hypovolemic cardiovascular component and a cellular component. Hypovolemia associated with burn shock results from massive fluid losses from the circulating blood volume. The losses are caused by an increase in capillary permeability that persists for approximately 24 hours after burn injury. Fluid resuscitation is the administration of intravenous fluids given in an effort to restore the circulating blood volume during the period of increasing capillary permeability. Isotonic crystalloids have traditionally been used for resuscitation; however, many burn centers are now using oncotic fluids. The use of albumin or plasma is used to reduce excessive volume, which increases the risk of respiratory insufficiency, cardiac failure, and compartment syndromes.[75,82] In addition to hypovolemia, most other organ systems are affected. Cardiac contractility is diminished during the initial 24-hour resuscitation period with shunting of blood away from the liver, kidney, and gut. This is often termed the *ebb phase* of the response to trauma and can be seen with other severe injuries.[83] Normal blood volume does not result in restoration of normal cardiac output because of a phenomenon known as *myocardial depression.* The decrease in perfusion of viscera results in a decrease in their function. This may be an explanation for decreased gut barrier function seen in thermal injury.[74] Other mechanisms include hypoxia and inflammation with histologic damage of intestinal mucosa.[84]

There also is evidence that cellular metabolism is disrupted when the burn wound is created, resulting in altered cell membrane permeability and loss of normal electrolyte homeostasis. This cellular defect may be the pathophysiologic process responsible for the genesis of burn shock. There are numerous circulating factors in burn serum that may play a role in these cellular processes. Although the cardiovascular and systemic responses are intricately interwoven into the cellular response, these responses are presented here as discrete entities for purposes of description.

Cardiovascular and Systemic Response to Burn Injury

The clinical manifestations of burn shock are the result of more than simple loss of extracellular fluid at the burn wound site. Hypovolemia and numerous local mediators in the burn wound, as well as systemic signals, result in alteration of cellular function throughout the body.[83] The restoration of normal intravascular volume with either saline solutions or colloid materials (e.g., albumin, blood, or dextrans) does not reverse changes such as increases in pulmonary vascular resistance or myocardial contractility.[85–87] This is reflected in cardiac output with precipitous decreases that often result in inadequate perfusion of most tissues at the capillary level, which is the hallmark of burn shock. Fluid infusion, likewise, does not return cardiac output to preburn levels.[88,89] These findings led to the postulation of a specific MDF.[85,90,91] Other causes also have been suggested, such as reactive oxygen free radicals that attack cell membranes and other subcellular organelles as a result of first ischemia and then reperfusion of tissues during burn shock and resuscitation.[92] A third factor may be the level of nitric oxide (NO) after burn injury, which could have a direct myocardial depressant effect.[83] Burn trauma increases NO levels primarily through upregulation of inducible nitric oxide synthase (iNOS). Increased levels of NO lead to oxidative stress causing DNA breakage and activation of a protein complex that controls transcription of DNA, cytokine production, cell survival, and regulation of inflammatory responses (nuclear factor κ B [NFκB]). Inflammatory cytokines (e.g., tissue necrosis factor alpha [TNFα]) also promote iNOS activity, which leads to a persistent elevation of NO levels, contributing to cytotoxicity and cardiac dysfunction.[83] The elevation of NO causes the formation of compounds that alter mitochondrial respiration and compete with calcium for binding sites on contractile proteins (myosin and actin), which can severely depress cardiac function.[83] Regardless of the contribution of these mechanisms, fluid resuscitation eventually results in improved outcome of the massively burned person. This resuscitation involves infusion of intravenous fluid at a rate faster than the loss of circulatory vascular volume for a period of about 24 hours from the time of burn injury and may require up to 30 L in a major burn. Resuscitation from burn shock can be accomplished using any of a number of infusion protocols. The most frequently used protocol is the Parkland formula.[93,94] Lactated Ringer solution is used because it closely approximates extracellular fluid, the repository of fluid leaving the circulatory system during this phase of extensive edema formation (Table 48.3). The use of electrolyte-free fluids, such as D_5W, results in life-threatening hypovolemia and hyponatremia.

Area	Birth 1 yr.	1-4 yr.	5-9 yr.	10-14 yr.	15 yr.	Adult	2°	3°	Total	Donor Areas
Head	19	17	13	11	9	7				
Neck	2	2	2	2	2	2				
Ant. Trunk	13	13	13	13	13	13				
Post. Trunk	13	13	13	13	13	13				
R. Buttock	$2\frac{1}{2}$	$2\frac{1}{2}$	$2\frac{1}{2}$	$2\frac{1}{2}$	$2\frac{1}{2}$	$2\frac{1}{2}$				
L. Buttock	$2\frac{1}{2}$	$2\frac{1}{2}$	$2\frac{1}{2}$	$2\frac{1}{2}$	$2\frac{1}{2}$	$2\frac{1}{2}$				
Genitalia	1	1	1	1	1	1				
R. U. Arm	4	4	4	4	4	4				
L. U. Arm	4	4	4	4	4	4				
R. L. Arm	3	3	3	3	3	3				
L. L. Arm	3	3	3	3	3	3				
R. Hand	$2\frac{1}{2}$	$2\frac{1}{2}$	$2\frac{1}{2}$	$2\frac{1}{2}$	$2\frac{1}{2}$	$2\frac{1}{2}$				
L. Hand	$2\frac{1}{2}$	$2\frac{1}{2}$	$2\frac{1}{2}$	$2\frac{1}{2}$	$2\frac{1}{2}$	$2\frac{1}{2}$				
R. Thigh	$5\frac{1}{2}$	$6\frac{1}{2}$	8	$8\frac{1}{2}$	9	$9\frac{1}{2}$				
L. Thigh	$5\frac{1}{2}$	$6\frac{1}{2}$	8	$8\frac{1}{2}$	9	$9\frac{1}{2}$				
R. Leg	5	5	$5\frac{1}{2}$	6	$6\frac{1}{2}$	7				
L. Leg	5	5	$5\frac{1}{2}$	6	$6\frac{1}{2}$	7				
R. Foot	$3\frac{1}{2}$	$3\frac{1}{2}$	$3\frac{1}{2}$	$3\frac{1}{2}$	$3\frac{1}{2}$	$3\frac{1}{2}$				
L. Foot	$3\frac{1}{2}$	$3\frac{1}{2}$	$3\frac{1}{2}$	$3\frac{1}{2}$	$3\frac{1}{2}$	$3\frac{1}{2}$				
						TOTAL				

Cause of Burn ______________________

Date of Burn ______________

Time of Burn ______________

Age ______________

Sex ______________

Weight ______________

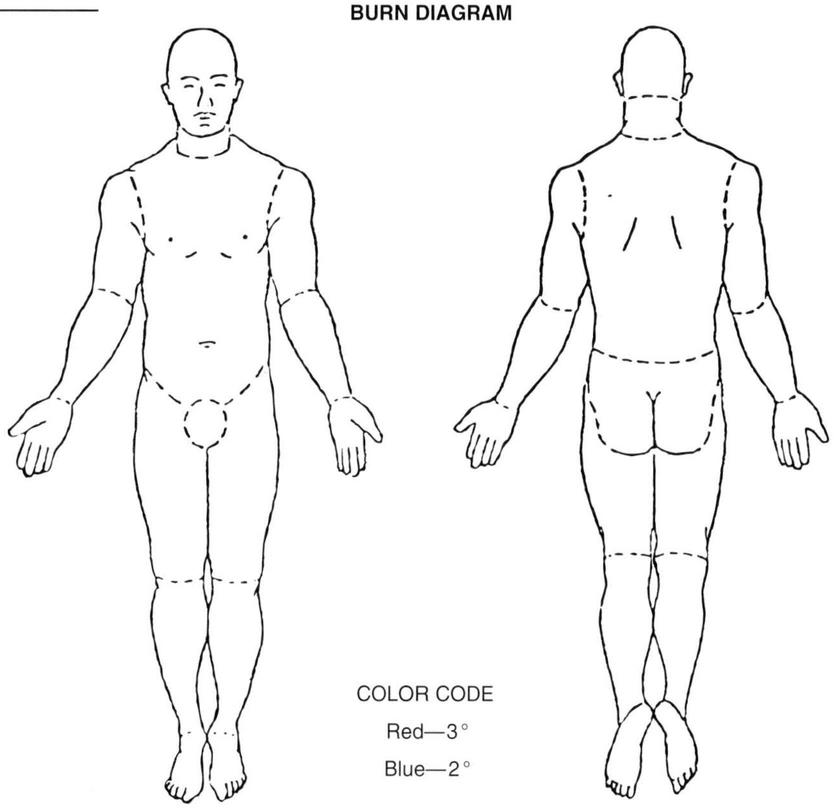

BURN DIAGRAM

COLOR CODE

Red—3°

Blue—2°

Fig. 48.14 Lund and Browder Chart. Regional differences in body surface area are calculated based on age. (Courtesy University of Utah Burn Center.)

BOX 48.4 Burn Center Referral Criteria

A burn center may treat adults or children, or both. Burn injuries that should be referred to a center include the following:

1. Partial-thickness burns greater than 10% total body surface area (TBSA).
2. Burns that involve the face, hands, feet, genitalia, perineum, or major joints.
3. Third-degree burns in any age group.
4. Electrical burns, including lightning injury.
5. Chemical burns.
6. Inhalation injury.
7. Burn injury in individuals with preexisting medical disorders that could complicate management, prolong recovery, or affect mortality.
8. Burns and concomitant trauma (such as fractures) in which the burn injury poses the greatest risk of morbidity or mortality. If the trauma poses the greater immediate risk, the individual's condition may be stabilized initially in a trauma center before being transferred to a burn center. Physician judgment will be necessary in such situations and should be in concert with the regional medical control plan and triage protocols.
9. Burns in children; children with burns should be transferred to a burn center verified to treat children. In the absence of a regional pediatric burn center, an adult burn center may serve as a second option for the management of pediatric burns.
10. Burn injury in individuals who will require special social, emotional, or rehabilitative intervention.

From *Resources for Optimal Care of the Injured Patient.* Chicago, IL: Committee on Trauma, American College of Surgeons; 2014.

The massive edema associated with burn shock is inevitable with fluid resuscitation, and failure to administer resuscitation fluid results in irreversible hypovolemic shock and death. The edema occurs in unburned as well as burned areas (Fig. 48.16). This often leads to mechanical airway obstruction, necessitation of tracheal intubation, and increased severity of the interstitial pulmonary edema associated with inhalation injury.

The most reliable criterion for adequate resuscitation of burn shock is urine output. The individual is in hypovolemic shock and will, as a compensatory mechanism, decrease or stop urine output in an effort to preserve circulation volume. The adult receiving sufficient intravenous fluids will excrete urine amounting to 30 to 50 mL/h; children will produce 0.5 to 1 mL/kg/h (see Chapter 49). If the individual does not have adequate urine output, it often indicates inadequate fluid resuscitation. Fluid resuscitation remains a challenge. The massive amount of intravenous fluid required by burned individuals during the shock phase is often intimidating to the person unfamiliar with burns. It is reported in the literature that excessive fluid resuscitation in burn injury individuals can result in "fluid creep."[95] Fluid creep occurs when the fluid volume delivered exceeds the formula predictions (e.g., Parkland formula). Common concerns are that massive fluid administration will result in pulmonary edema, respiratory distress, cardiac dysfunction, conversion of superficial to deep burns, need for fasciotomies in unburned limbs, and abdominal compartment syndrome.[96] The primary goal of resuscitation in burn victims is to maintain adequate end-organ perfusion. Severe burns result in hypovolemic shock and dramatic loss of body fluid during the resuscitation period through third spacing, exudation, and evaporation.

EMERGING SCIENCE BOX

Pathophysiology of the Burn Wound

Individuals with a severe burn wound require management of both the wound itself and the deleterious systemic consequences that accompany it. Recent research is providing new insights into the pathophysiologic impact of burn injury to the skin and other tissues. For example, immediately after a burn injury, the wound can be divided into three zones: coagulation, ischemia (stasis), and hyperemia. Each of these zones is characterized by cellular autophagy and apoptosis, inflammation, and thrombus formation. Numerous inflammatory cytokines and cells contribute to tissue injury, while at the same time, they trigger the release growth factors and initiate the wound healing process. The types, amounts, and locations of these inflammatory chemicals and growth factors impact the effectiveness of tissue recovery and the amount of scar that is generated. Systemic complications such as metabolic and immune dysregulation along with infection also impact the rate and effectiveness of wound healing. Efforts toward balancing the positive and negative roles of inflammation in burn wound recovery include administration of opioids, modified gels, and new types of topical anti-inflammatories. One factor of particular interest to researchers is the impact of oxidative stress on burn wound tissues and distant organ injury. Trials of antioxidant therapies and dietary changes have produced some positive results, although more research is needed. The role of genes in the host response to burn injury is also being explored. For example, there is evidence that expression of the melanocortin 1 receptor gene and the pyrin domain containing receptor 3 gene are important factors in wound healing. The role of stem cells in wound healing is also being explored. An understanding of these complex pathways may lead to improved burn wound treatment and recovery.

Data from Abbas OL, et al. Comparative analysis of mesenchymal stem cells from bone marrow, adipose tissue, and dental pulp as sources of cell therapy for zone of stasis burns. *Journal of Investigative Surgery*, 2019;32(6):477–490; Fang, X., et al. Identification of key genes associated with changes in the host response to severe burn shock: A bioinformatics analysis with data from the gene expression omnibus (GEO) database. *Journal of Inflammation Research*, 2020;13:1029–1041; Jeschke MG, et al. Burn injury. *Nature Reviews Disease Primers*, 2020;6(1):11; Roshangar L, et al. Skin burns: Review of molecular mechanisms and therapeutic approaches. *Wounds*, 2019;31(12):308–315; Vinaik R, et al. NLRP3 inflammasome activity is required for wound healing after burns. *Translational Research*, 2020;217:47–60; Wang P, et al. In situ formed anti-inflammatory hydrogel loading plasmid DNA encoding VEGF for burn wound healing. *Acta Biomaterialia*, 2019;100:191–201.

The endpoint of burn shock is defined as the state in which the individual is able to maintain adequate urine output for 2 hours with the intravenous fluid administration rate equal to the individual's calculated maintenance rate. As burn shock ends, fluid administered remains in the circulating volume and is reflected as an increase in urine output. The mechanism whereby capillary integrity is restored is unknown but usually occurs about 24 hours after burn injury (Fig. 48.17). After the individual has reached the endpoint of burn shock, the term used to describe the vascular status of the individual is capillary seal. In individuals with large burns, colloid-containing fluids may be given to help maintain oncotic pressure during the resuscitation phase and afterward to enhance the mobilization

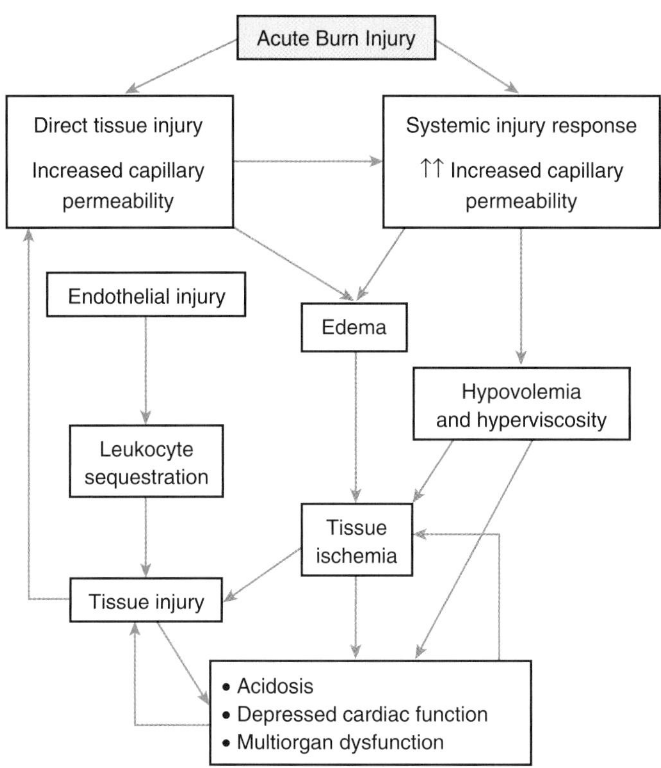

Fig. 48.15 Immediate Cellular and Immunologic Alterations of Burn Shock.

TABLE 48.3 Electrolyte Content of Ringer Lactate Solution and Extracellular Fluid

Electrolyte	Extracellular Fluid[a] (mEq/L)	Lactated Ringer Solution[b] (mEq/L)
Sodium	135–145	130
Potassium	3.2–4.5	4
Chloride	95–105	109
Lactate (bicarbonate)	24–28	28

[a]Normal values may vary slightly between laboratories.
[b]Plus 80–100 mL of free water per liter.

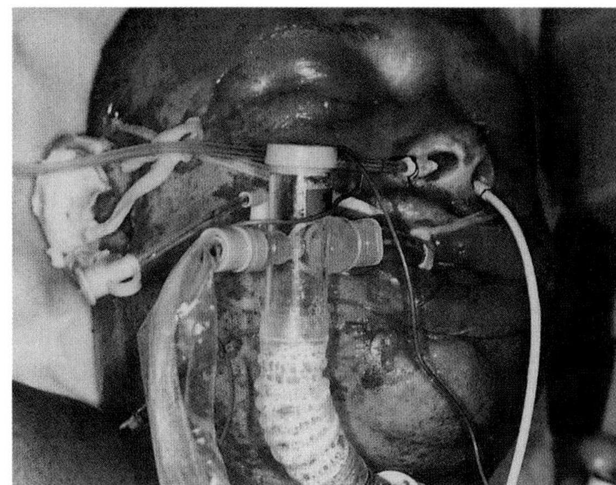

Fig. 48.16 Edema Related to Burn Injury. Superficial facial burns can result in marked swelling, requiring prompt endotracheal intubation to maintain the airway. (Courtesy University of Utah Burn Center.)

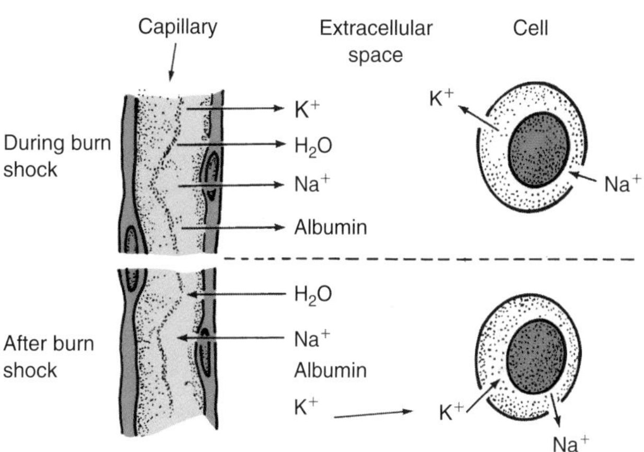

Fig. 48.17 Direction of Fluid and Electrolyte Shifts Associated With Burn Shock. (Courtesy University of Utah Burn Center.)

of interstitial fluid and diuresis.[97] Efforts to decrease burn edema and fluid resuscitation volumes can involve the use of hypertonic fluid resuscitation as well.[98]

Cellular Response to Burn Injury

In addition to capillary endothelial permeability changes resulting in vascular fluid losses, transmembrane potential changes occur in cells not directly damaged by heat. The normal potential of −90 mV decreases to nearly −70 mV, with an increase in the levels of intracellular sodium and water. Such membrane potential changes may be caused by a circulating shock factor.[99] Apoptosis is central to the cellular responses to burn injury.[74] Other changes can be categorized as (1) a metabolic response to the burn injury or (2) an immunologic response to the burn injury.

Metabolic response. The metabolic changes after a burn injury were described in 1967 by Welt and associates as "sick cell syndrome."[100] This was considered to be a cell membrane transport defect related to an alteration in the steady-state composition characterized by high intracellular concentrations of sodium. Trunkey and colleagues[101] found a marked decrease in primate muscle extracellular water and an increase in intracellular sodium and water during hypovolemic shock. In addition, other researchers demonstrated an associated decrease in resting membrane potential, a decrease in amplitude of the action potential, and a prolongation of the repolarization and depolarization times in association with a decreased intracellular potassium concentration.[102,103] The cellular dysfunction of burn injury extends beyond the transmembrane potential disruption and the sodium-potassium pump impairment to include a loss of intracellular magnesium and phosphate[104] and elevated serum lactic acid dehydrogenase (LDH) levels.[105] Thus impairment of basic cellular function may be the underlying cause of the diminished membrane potentials. The data suggest a decrease in the efficiency of the pump. The failure of rapid intravascular volume repletion to restore membrane potential completely suggests other pathways for cellular metabolic derangement.[106]

Metabolic reactions to the stress of a major burn injury involve the response of the sympathetic nervous system and other homeostatic regulators. Catecholamines are found in elevated amounts in both the serum and urine of burned individuals. Cortisol, glucagon, and insulin levels are elevated, with a corresponding increase in gluconeogenesis, lipolysis, and proteolysis. Changes in lipid metabolism are reflected as an elevation in the level of plasma free fatty acids (FFAs) and a decrease in the levels of plasma cholesterol and phospholipids.[107] Herndon and colleagues[108] found that the use of propranolol, a nonselective β_1- and β_2-blocker, could attenuate symptoms of the hypermetabolic response, including a decrease in heart rate and lipolysis. Glucose and lactate kinetics are altered after burn injury. Although tissue hypoxia produces lactic acidosis, its persistence in the presence of adequate tissue perfusion suggests an increased rate of glycogenolysis.[109] A small study conducted by Akcay and colleagues[110] showed that growth hormone levels are diminished in major burn injuries and appear to improve survival but more clearly affect wound healing.[111]

The initial 72 to 96 hours following a burn is termed the *ebb phase*, which is a state of hypometabolism. This phase is caused by intracellular processes and characterized by a decreased metabolic rate, depleted intravascular volume, poor tissue perfusion, and low cardiac output. Following the *ebb phase*, a hypermetabolic state, the *flow phase*, is initiated and persists until wound closure (up to 36 months after initial injury).[74] A hypermetabolic response causes an increase in blood pressure, peripheral insulin resistance, as well as breakdown of glycogen, proteins, and lipids caused by stress hormones such as catecholamines, glucocorticoids (produced by the adrenal glands), and glucagon (produced by the pancreas).[74]

The metabolic rate increases with burn size in a curvilinear relationship, with oxygen consumption rarely exceeding two times basal levels. Evaporative water loss and surface cooling are not the primary stimulus for the hypermetabolic state; rather, the hypermetabolism is related to an increase and resetting of the thermal regulatory set point. The results of these effects are increased resting energy expenditure, elevated core temperature (38.5°C [101.3°F] is typical), total body protein loss, muscle wasting, and increased stimulated synthesis of acute-phase proteins, resulting in organ catabolism associated with organ dysfunction and death.[74,75] A reflex arc mobilizes neural or hormonal afferent stimuli to the hypothalamus, producing a catecholamine response clinically manifested as hypermetabolism, hyperthermia, and hyperglycemia. Evidence also exists that the burn wound itself directly mediates the response to injury at both the local and systemic levels. Cytokines, oxygen free radicals, chemotactic substances, and eicosanoids contribute to the systemic inflammatory response and hypermetabolic state. The inflammatory response to the wound level is magnified into a generalized systemic inflammatory response that is often deleterious. Vasodilation, increased capillary permeability, and edema occur to facilitate healing of the local area. The distribution of the peripheral circulation after burn injury transports heat and glucose preferentially to the wound. The energy cost of these reparative and transport processes is reflected in the increased metabolism and hyperdynamic circulation (Fig. 48.18).[74]

The extensive evaporative water loss that occurs in burn tissue is a heat-consuming process, and the energy of evaporation is provided by increased visceral heat production. The signal for the response is unknown because individuals whose wounds have been denervated continue to have a **posttraumatic hypermetabolic response**. Hypothalamic function alterations result in the elevation of human growth hormone (hGH) serum levels in the presence of hyperglycemia, a finding opposite that in normal states.[112] Further, the hypermetabolic rate is not decreased during rest, sleep, or warmth.

Evidence of hepatic response to burn injury is characterized by alterations in the clotting factors.[113] A hypercoagulable state develops as manifested by an elevated plasma fibrinogen concentration in the presence of shortened prothrombin time (PT) and activated partial thromboplastin time (PTT).[114]

In summary, extensive burn injury initiates the most marked alterations in body metabolism associated with any illness (Fig. 48.19). Much of the work explaining this response has been conducted by Wilmore,[115,116] who reported that the persistent tachycardia, hyperpnea, hyperpyrexia, and marked body wasting seen in burn injury reflect heightened metabolic activity and accelerated body catabolism. The development of decreased bone density can last long after discharge from the hospital.[117] These systemic alterations occur as a result of the cutaneous inflammatory process and are thought to facilitate wound repair. The neural component of this alteration is in response to a sympathetic reaction that releases catecholamines in large amounts.

Immunologic response. The immunologic response to burn injury is immediate, prolonged, and severe. The result in individuals surviving burn shock is immunosuppression with increased susceptibility to potentially fatal systemic burn wound sepsis. Several cytokines have been identified in the immediate postburn period. Interkeukin-1 (IL-1) is detected in the serum of burned individuals. The level of IL-1 correlates inversely with burn survival; low levels may be associated with a higher mortality.[118] Fatal burn injury has often shown decreased levels of IL-2, which may result in decreased T helper 1 (Th1) lymphocytes. Th1 cells produce IL-2, interferon-gamma, and TNF, which help to initiate cellular immunity and immunoglobulin G (IgG) production. IL-4 is elevated after burn injuries and causes a shift in the T-helper cell production from Th1 to Th2 lymphocytes. Th2 cells secrete IL-4, which promotes further conversion of nonspecific Th cells to Th2 cells. Th2 cells also produce other cytokines and antibodies.[119] IL-6 levels increase quickly after burn injury and remain elevated for several weeks. The level of IL-6 correlates with the extent of burn injury.[120] IL-6, together with platelet activation factor, activates polymorphonuclear neutrophils, causing infiltration of neutrophils into burned tissue and adhesion to vascular endothelial surfaces.[121,122] IL-8 levels are elevated after burn injury with significantly greater elevations

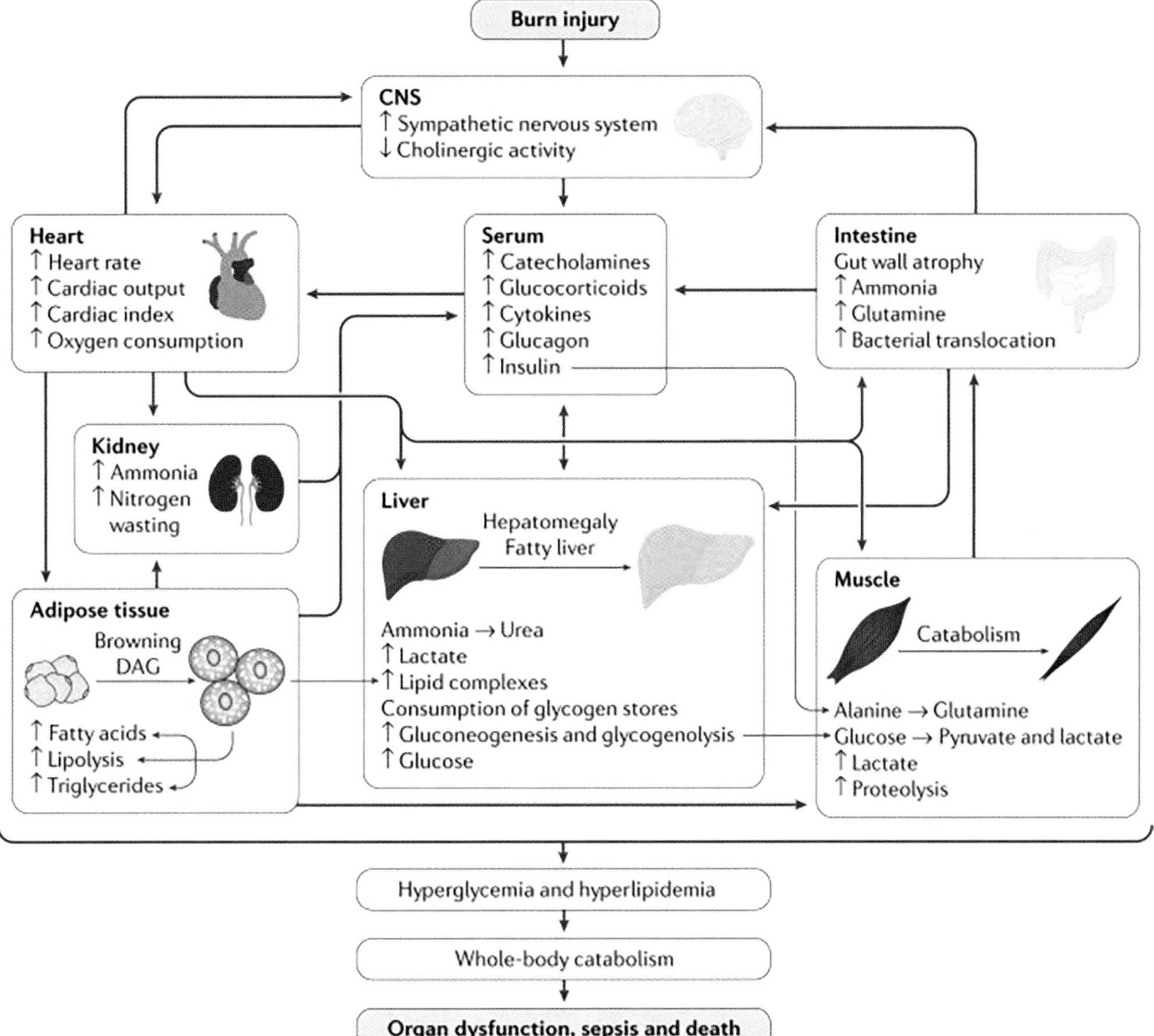

Fig. 48.18 Hypermetabolic State in Burn Injury. Severe burn injury induces a unique and remarkably complex response that involves the release of stress hormones and pro-inflammatory mediators. The immediate response leads to a hypometabolic response that lasts for ~72 to 96 hours (ebb phase), but then rapidly turns into the flow phase that can persist for years after the initial injury. Stress mediators, such as catecholamines, glucocorticoids, and cytokines, are released into the system and cause a plethora of systemic responses. The heart goes into a hyperdynamic overdrive, increasing circulation and blood flow to increase oxygen and nutrient delivery. However, increased stress signaling causes changes in organ function and metabolic demand. Protein is degraded to deliver energy for hepatic function, the gut develops mucosal atrophy to absorb more nutrients but also enable bacterial translocation. The kidneys are hyperperfused but oxygen delivery is decreased, leading to acute kidney injury and stress signals from the kidney. The interplay between these organs accumulates, leading to metabolic and inflammatory overdrive that subsequently causes white adipose tissue to change to brown adipose tissue. Brown adipose tissue releases energy and induces substantial lipolysis with the accompanying expression of lipotoxic intermediates, such as triglycerides, free fatty acids, and diacylglycerols *(DAG)*, all of which are transferred to the liver. The liver is unable to metabolize all of the accumulating substances and develops hepatomegaly. In turn, hyperlipidemia and hyperglycemia with insulin resistance is present, which worsens the hypermetabolic and inflammatory state. If hypermetabolism cannot be diminished or decreased, holistic catabolism ensues and, subsequently, multiple organ failure and death. *CNS*, Central nervous system. (From Jeschke MG, van Baar ME, Choudhry MA, et al. Burn injury. *Nature Reviews Disease Primers*, 2020;6[1]:11. doi:10.1038/s41572-020-0145-5)

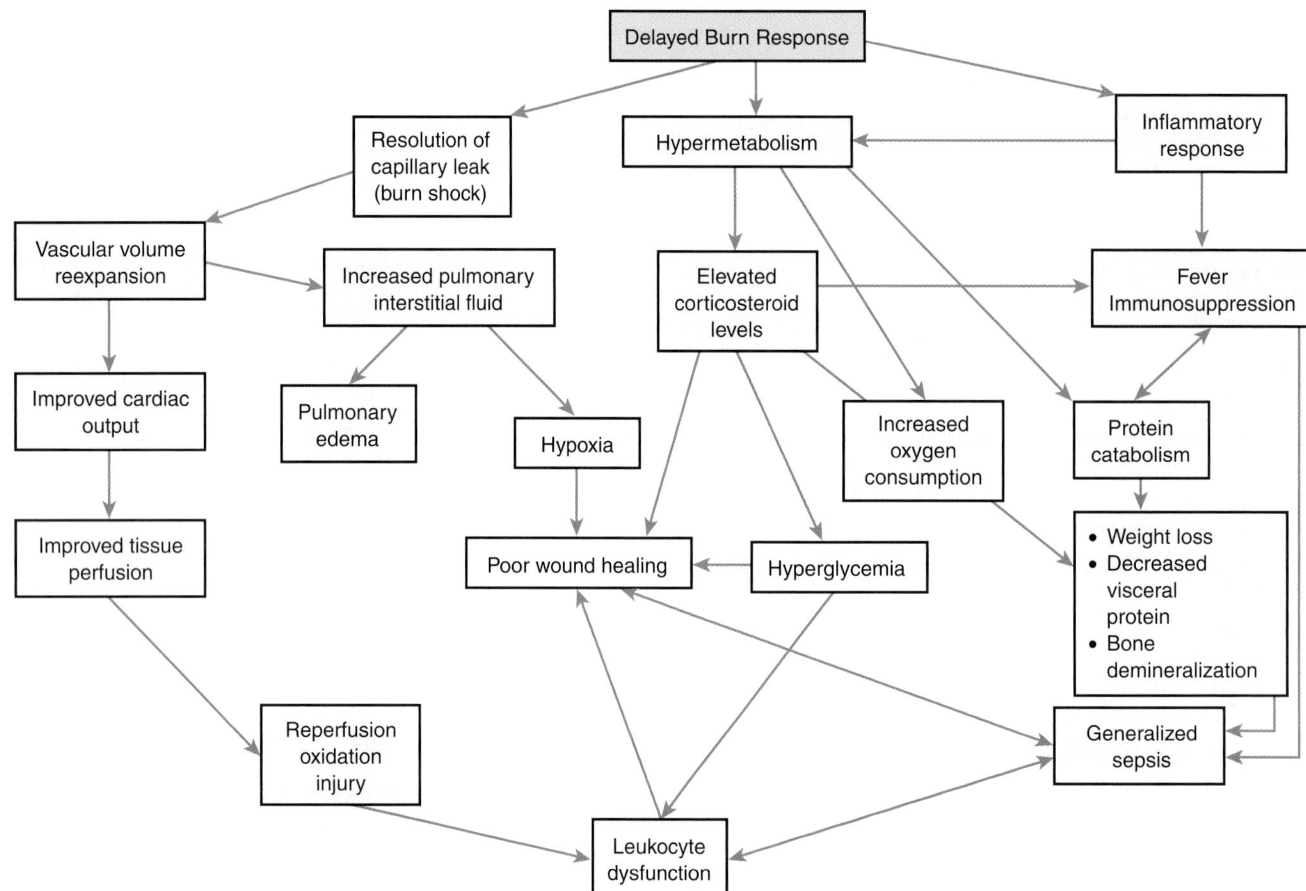

Fig. 48.19 Physiologic Alterations in Inflammatory Burn Injury Response.

in individuals with a TBSA burn of 40% or higher. IL-8 activity may play a role in the strong and persistent activation of neutrophils noted in people with large burns.[123] Burn blister fluid contains large amounts of IL-6 and IL-8 in addition to substances such as epidermal growth factor, platelet-derived growth factor, and transforming growth factor.[124]

Macrophages, platelets, neutrophils, and vascular endothelial cells release prostaglandins and leukotrienes, which are the byproducts of arachidonic acid metabolism. These chemical mediators cause peripheral vasodilation, pulmonary vasoconstriction, increased capillary permeability, and local tissue ischemia in the burn wound.

A host of chemicals found in burn plasma in altered concentrations also may play a role in burn shock. These include vasoactive amines (histamine, serotonin), products of complement activation (C3a, C5a), prostaglandins, kinins, endotoxin, and metabolic hormones (catecholamines, glucocorticoids). A decrease in complement components C3a and C5a in the circulation after burn injury suggests a nonspecific activation of the complement system.[125] Activation of the complement system in injured tissue results in an inflammatory response caused by release of histamine and serotonin by C3a and C5a, because histamine and serotonin alter capillary permeability and participate in the mechanism of burn shock along with kinin polypeptides and other chemical mediators. Prostaglandins function in the inflammatory process by regulating the metabolism of cells of inflammation (see Chapter 7).

Burn shock can induce changes in the integrity of the intestinal wall, facilitating bacterial translocation and endotoxemia.[126] Bacterial translocation from the gut may be a mechanism of infection leading to septic shock after burn injury and other major trauma.[127] Circulating endotoxin is correlated with the development of MODS and death after major burn injury.[128]

White blood cells are also altered at this time, when their need to inhibit sepsis is vital. Natural resistance to infection in burn wounds is a function of the nonspecific immune system; that is, resistance to microorganisms that infect wounds rests almost solely on the ability of phagocytic cells (i.e., granulocytes, macrophages) to leave the bloodstream, migrate to the site of infection, and ingest and kill microorganisms.[129] Normally opsonins render bacteria susceptible to phagocytosis, but the burn injury triggers a consumptive opsoninopathy. Burn serum contains an inhibitor of C3 conversion that leads to decreased opsonization and polymorphonuclear (PMN) dysfunction.[130,131]

Individuals with altered immunocompetence before burn injury are at additional risk for complications. Opportunistic infections, such as fungal sepsis, can increase a hospital stay and ICU costs.[132] Included in this group are individuals at the extremes of age and those with cardiac disease, malnutrition, immunodeficiency disease, and a history of alcohol or drug abuse.[133,134] Additional risk factors include diabetes mellitus and pulmonary or renal dysfunction.

Evaporative Water Loss

One of the major purposes of intact skin is to serve as a barrier to evaporative water loss (EWL) from the body. With major burn injury, this ability of the skin to regulate evaporative water loss is totally disrupted. In a classic 1962 study, Moncrief and Mason[135] attempted to determine the magnitude of such a loss and determined that daily evaporative water loss was in the range of 20 times normal in the early phase of injury, with gradual decreases as wound closure is achieved. Further studies indicated that insensible water loss through burned skin is not from evaporation of water from sweat glands but rather from water vapor formed within the body and lost through the skin.[136,137]

Calculation of the amount of fluid lost by evaporative water loss includes losses from all sources. Normally the skin is the major source of insensible loss (75%) and the lungs are minor sources (25%), with a total loss of only approximately 600 to 800 mL/day. This changes dramatically with burns, because not only does skin loss increase but also lung loss increases by hypermetabolism and hyperventilation, especially in an intubated individual. Total evaporative losses exceed many liters per day in an adult with large burn wounds. Replacement of the loss is mandatory to prevent volume deficit.

Evaluation and treatment. Burn recovery can be long and difficult, with complications often the rule rather than the exception. The goal of burn management is wound closure in a manner that promotes survival. Scar formation with contractures is often a consequence of healing in deep partial-thickness and full-thickness burns (Fig. 48.20; see also Fig. 48.10). Assessment of tissue viability can be difficult in complex extremity injury; pyrophosphate nuclear scanning can assist in evaluation.[138] Early intervention may have effects on tissue survival as is evident in the zone of stasis and application of cerium nitrate.[139] The advancement in survival and outcome can be as simple as using antibiotic catheters to reduce catheter-associated bloodstream infections[140] or improving glycemic management during ICU treatment.[141] Advances in care systems have shown the value of advanced practice nurses in a collaborative role in the burn ICU and emergency departments.[142] The three essential elements of survival of major burn injury are (1) meticulous wound management, (2) adequate fluids and nutrition, and (3) early surgical excision and grafting. Current therapy for deep partial- and full-thickness burn injury includes surgical removal of the burn tissue (excision) followed by grafting of the person's unburned skin (autograft) onto the excised wound. Techniques of early wound care, such as the use of amniotic membrane,[143] may well affect the nature of burn scarring. Satisfactory wound closure with cultured epithelial autograft (Fig. 48.21) has been inconsistent and costly.[144,145] Early enthusiasm for synthetic dermal replacement has been tempered by a high rate of dermal graft loss and slow epidermal engraftment.[146,147] Such advancements in skin replacement technology include sheets of acellular dermal matrix that can be used with thin, meshed autografts or cultured epithelial autografts.[148,149]

This concept also is being used on the donor site, and glycosaminoglycan hydrogels may supplement donor site wound dressings, and even topical gene therapy or stem cell applications.[150–152] Scar reduction or prevention is a challenging problem that is being addressed with pulsed-dye laser treatment.[153] Current research also is directed toward therapies to modulate hypermetabolic and inflammatory responses. Nutritional therapy is focused on early enteral feeding to reduce the potential of gut-mediated sepsis. Ongoing clinical trials using anabolic agents (e.g., recombinant human growth hormone) and pharmacologic agents that modulate inflammatory and endocrine mediators (e.g., ibuprofen, propranolol) show promise in the treatment of severe burn injuries.[154] Recent clinical data on vitamin C suggests that vitamin C might have a beneficial effect in individuals with burn injury.[155] However, there is conflicting data on renal safety.[156,157] Altered body image is a significant hurdle to those with facial burns. A framework for aiding individuals can often be useful for those reintegrating into the community.[158] Burn pain is almost always acute, and treatment strategies usually differ from strategies for chronic pain. The understanding and management of burn pain is key to recovery.[159,160] In addition to opioid-based agents, newer treatment approaches may include antianxiety agents, hypnosis, and relaxation techniques,[161] as well as virtual reality systems.[162,163]

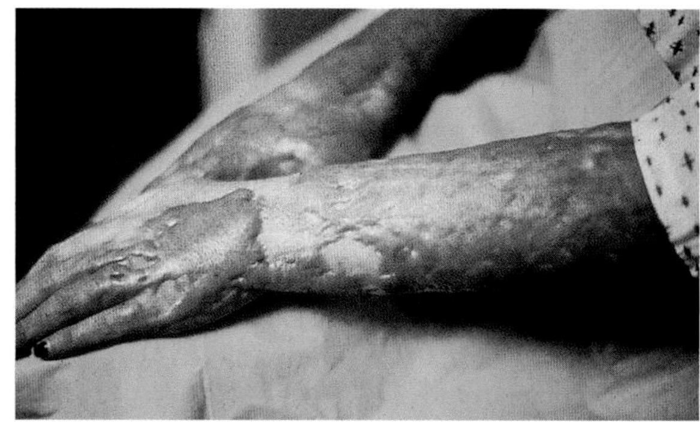

Fig. 48.20 Hypertrophic Scarring. Deep partial-thickness thermal injury can result in extensive hypertrophic scarring. (Courtesy University of Utah Burn Center.)

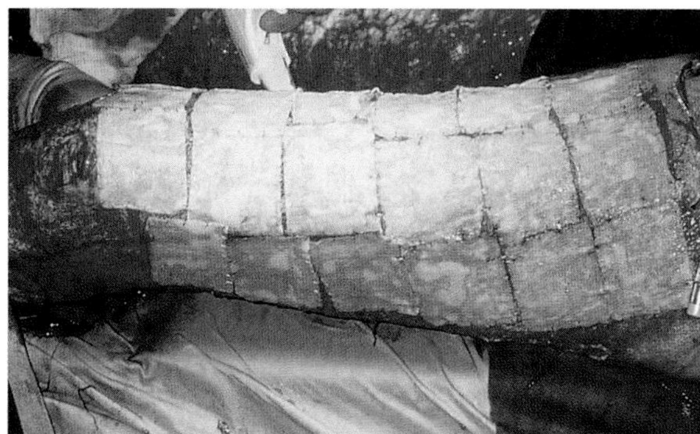

Fig. 48.21 Application of Cultured Epithelial Autografts. The thin sheets of keratinocytes are attached to gauze backing to allow application onto the clean, excised thigh. (Courtesy University of Utah Burn Center.)

SUMMARY REVIEW

Shock

1. Shock occurs when the cardiovascular system fails to perfuse tissue, cells, and organs adequately, causing a widespread impairment of cellular metabolism and tissue function. It is a downward physiologic spiral that, if not reversed, can lead to MODS.
2. The classifications of shock: (1) distributive, anaphylactic, neurogenic, or vasogenic; (2) cardiogenic; (3) hypovolemic; and (4) obstructive.
3. The final common pathway in all types of shock is impaired cellular metabolism with cells switching from aerobic to anaerobic metabolism. Energy stores drop, and cellular mechanisms relative to membrane permeability, action potentials, and lysozyme release fail.
4. Anaerobic metabolism results in activation of the inflammatory response, decrease in circulatory volume, and decrease in pH.
5. Impaired cellular metabolism results in cellular inability to use glucose because of impaired glucose delivery or impaired glucose intake, resulting in a shift of glycogenolysis, gluconeogenesis, and lipolysis for fuel generation.
6. Glycogenolysis is affected for up to 10 hours. Gluconeogenesis results in the use of proteins necessary for structure, function, repair, and replication that leads to more impaired cellular metabolism. Lipolysis is ineffective because of a lack of transport serum proteins.
7. Gluconeogenesis contributes to lactic acid, uric acid, and ammonia buildup; interstitial edema; and impairment of the immune system, as well as general muscle weakness leading to decreased respiratory function and cardiac output.
8. Distributive shock (vasodilatory shock) is characterized by severe peripheral vasodilation and has several etiologies, including sepsis, systemic inflammatory response syndrome, neurogenic or vasogenic, anaphylaxis, drug and toxin induced, and endocrine.
9. Septic shock begins with impaired cellular metabolism caused by uncontrolled septicemia. The infecting agent triggers the inflammatory and immune responses. It is part of a continuum known as *SIRS*. Mortality for septic shock is very high.
10. Anaphylactic shock is the outcome of a widespread hypersensitivity to an allergen that triggers anaphylaxis. The inflammatory response is triggered, and massive vasodilation with fluid shift into the interstitium follows. The relative hypovolemia leads to impaired cellular metabolism.
11. Neurogenic (vasogenic) shock results from massive vasodilation that occurs from an imbalance between parasympathetic and sympathetic stimulation of vascular smooth muscle. It causes a relative hypovolemia (even though cardiac output may be high), and results in impaired cellular metabolism.
12. Cardiogenic shock results from persistent hypotension and tissue hypoperfusion caused by cardiac dysfunction in the presence of adequate intravascular volume and left ventricular filling pressure.
13. Hypovolemic shock is caused by loss of whole blood, plasma, or interstitial fluid in large amounts. The use of compensatory mechanisms may be vigorous, but tissue perfusion ultimately decreases and results in impaired cellular metabolism.

Multiple Organ Dysfunction Syndrome

1. MODS is the progressive dysfunction of two or more organ systems resulting from a systemic inflammatory response after a severe illness or injury. The inflammatory response can be triggered by sepsis, necrotic tissue, trauma, burns, ARDS, acute pancreatitis, major surgery, circulatory shock, DIC, acute renal failure, blood transfusion, heat stroke, liver failure, mesenteric ischemia, propofol infusion syndrome, persistent inflammatory foci, and other severe injuries.
2. Primary MODS is the immediate local or mild systemic response to the triggering event or illness. It primes the inflammatory system.
3. Secondary MODS is the uncontrollable, excessive systemic inflammatory response that develops after a latent period and results in organ dysfunction.
4. People at greatest risk for developing MODS are older adults, those with significant tissue injury or preexisting disease, and those in whom resuscitation from the initiating illness or injury has been delayed or inadequate.
5. MODS is a leading cause of mortality in surgical ICUs. Mortality for individuals with MODS increases progressively from 54% with two failing organ systems to 100% with five failing organ systems.
6. Multiple organ dysfunction involves the stress response; release of complement, coagulation, and kinin proteins; changes in the vascular endothelium; and numerous inflammatory processes mediated by substances released by activated neutrophils and macrophages. The accumulation of activated neutrophils in organs is thought to play a key role in the pathogenesis of MODS, as well as macrophages.
7. The consequences of the release of inflammatory mediators in MODS are vasodilation, increased vasopermeability, and selective vasoconstriction resulting in maldistribution of blood flow; hypermetabolism; myocardial depression; and hypoxic injury to cells. Cellular hypoxia and acidosis impair cellular metabolism, leading to organ dysfunction.
8. Clinical manifestations of the development of MODS are general during the first 24 hours: low-grade fever, tachycardia, tachypnea, dyspnea, and altered mental status. Over the next several days, beginning with the lungs, individual organ systems show signs of failure.
9. Because there is no specific therapy for MODS, early detection is extremely important so that supportive measures can be initiated as soon as possible.
10. At present the therapeutic management of MODS consists of prevention or removal of triggering mechanisms and support of individual organs. Recent scientific knowledge about inflammatory mediators has led to many promising future therapies for MODS.

Thermal Injury and Burns

1. Burns are classified according to depth and extent of injury.
2. First-degree burns involve the superficial skin without loss of protective function.
3. Second-degree burns are superficial (blister formation) or superficial involving partial skin thickness with a waxy white appearance and no involvement of dermal appendages.
4. Third-degree burns involve full skin thickness and often underlying tissues. They are painless and can be life-threatening as a result of hypovolemic shock and metabolic and immunologic responses.
5. The TBSA burned is estimated using either the rule of nines or the Lund and Browder chart.
6. Hypovolemia associated with burn shock is caused by increased capillary permeability with massive fluid losses from blood volume.
7. Altered cell membrane permeability and loss of electrolyte homeostasis contribute to burn shock.
8. Cardiac contractility is decreased during the first 24 hours with shunting of blood away from the liver, kidney, and gut.
9. Fluid resuscitation, such as with lactated Ringer solution, involves infusion of fluid at a rate faster than the loss of circulating volume.
10. The most reliable criterion for adequate resuscitation of burn shock is urine output.
11. *Capillary seal* is the term used to indicate the end of burn shock.
12. Transmembrane potentials are altered in cells not directly damaged by heat, with impairment of the sodium-potassium pump and loss of magnesium and phosphate.
13. The stress of a major burn activates the sympathetic nervous system with release of catecholamines, cortisol, glucagon, and insulin.
14. Burn injury produces a hypermetabolic state that persists until wound closure and is related to a higher thermal regulatory set point.
15. The local inflammatory response at the burn site releases cytokines, oxygen free radicals, chemotactic factors, and eicosanoids, which lead to a systemic inflammatory response and contribute to hypermetabolism.
16. A posttraumatic hypermetabolic response is associated with increased visceral heat production.
17. Alterations in clotting factors produce a hypercoagulable state following major burns.
18. The immune response following a burn is immediate, prolonged, and severe.
19. Numerous alterations in inflammatory cytokines are evident in the immediate burn period, affecting cellular immunity, antibody production, and attraction of neutrophils and contributing to the vasodilation and increased capillary permeability associated with burn shock.
20. White blood cells are altered, and there is decreased opsonization and phagocytosis, contributing to the development of sepsis.
21. Changes in intestinal wall integrity lead to translocation of bacteria, endotoxemia, and septic shock.
22. Loss of intact skin with a major burn results in significant evaporative water loss contributing to hypovolemia.
23. Treatment of major burns involves meticulous wound management, adequate fluids and nutrition, early surgical excision and grafting, modulation of the hypermetabolic state, and pain management.

REFERENCES

1. *Mosby's dictionary of medicine: nursing and health professions*, ed 10, St. Louis, 2021, Elsevier.
2. Bonanno FG. Shock—a reappraisal: the holistic approach. *J Emerg Trauma Shock*. 2012;5(2):167–177.
3. Edul VS, Dubin A, Ince C. The microcirculation as a therapeutic target in the treatment of sepsis and shock. *Semin Respir Crit Care Med*. 2011;32(5):558–568.
4. Schmeltz LR. Management of inpatient hyperglycemia. *Lab Med*. 2011;42(7):427–434.
5. Singer M, et al. The third international consensus definitions for sepsis and septic shock (Sepsis-3). *JAMA*. 2016;315:801–810.
6. Cecconi M, et al. Sepsis and septic shock. *Lancet*. 2018;392(10141):75–87.
7. Fleischmann C, et al. Assessment of global incidence and mortality of hospital-treated sepsis. Current estimates and limitations. *Am J Respir Crit Care Med*. 2016;193:259–272.
8. World Health Organization (WHO). Sepsis, Geneva, Switzerland, 2020, WHO. Published August 26, 2020. Available at https://www.who.int/news-room/fact-sheets/detail/sepsis. (Accessed February 13, 2022).
9. Rudd KE, et al. Global, regional, and national sepsis incidence and mortality, 1990–2017: analysis for the Global Burden of Disease Study. *Lancet*. 2020;395(10219):200–211.
10. Sakr Y, et al. Sepsis in intensive care unit patients: worldwide data from the Intensive Care Over Nations Audit. *Open Forum Infect Dis*. 2018;5(12):ofy313.
11. Novosad SA, et al. Epidemiology of sepsis: prevalence of health care factors and opportunities for prevention. *MMWR Morb Mortal Wkly Rep*. 2016;65(33):864–869.
12. Shankar-Hari M, et al. Evidence for a causal link between sepsis and long-term mortality: a systematic review of epidemiologic studies. *Crit Care*. 2016;20:101.
13. Boyd JH, Russell JA, Fjell CD. The meta-genome of sepsis: host genetics, pathogens and the acute immune response. *J Innate Immun*. 2014;6:272–283.
14. Hotchkiss RS, Karl IE. The pathophysiology and treatment of sepsis. *N Engl J Med*. 2003;348:138–150.
15. Kleinpell RM, Graves BT, Ackerman MH. Incidence, pathogenesis, and management of sepsis: an overview. *AACN Adv Crit Care*. 2006;17(4):385–393.
16. Papathanassoglou ED, et al. Association of proinflammatory molecules with apoptotic markers and survival in critically ill multiple organ dysfunction patients. *Biol Res Nurs*. 2003;5(2):129–141.
17. Kraut JA, Madias NE. Lactic acidosis: current treatments and future directions. *Am J Kidney Dis*. 2016;68(3):473–482.
18. Font MD, Thyagarajan B, Khanna AK. Sepsis and septic shock—basics of diagnosis, pathophysiology and clinical decision making. *Med Clin North Am*. 2020;104(4):573–585.
19. Evans, L., Rhodes, A., Alhazzani, W., et al. Critical Care Medicine. 2021;49(11): e1063-e1143. https://journals.lww.com/ccmjournal/ toc/2021/11000. doi: 10.1097/CCM.0000000000005337.
20. Pepper DJ, et al. Procalcitonin-guided antibiotic discontinuation and mortality in critically ill adults: a systematic review and meta-analysis. *Chest*. 2019;155(6):1109–1118.

21. Dellinger R, et al. Surviving Sepsis Campaign: international guidelines for management of severe sepsis and septic shock: 2012. *Crit Care Med.* 2013;41(2):580–637.
22. Rhodes A, et al. Surviving Sepsis Campaign: international guidelines for management of sepsis and septic shock: 2016. *Intensive Care Med.* 2017;43(3):304–377.
23. Nguyen HB, et al. Early goal-directed therapy in severe sepsis and septic shock: insights and comparisons to ProCESS, ProMISe, and ARISE. *Crit Care.* 2016;20(1):160.
24. Friswell AC. Surviving Sepsis Campaign previews updated guidelines for 2012. *Pulmon Rev.* 2012;17(5):1–5.
25. Gauer R, Forbes D, Boyer N. Sepsis: diagnosis and management. *Am Fam Physician.* 2020;101(7):409–418.
26. Cardona V, et al. World Allergy Organization anaphylaxis guidance 2020. *World Allergy Organ J.* 2020;13(10):100472.
27. Ruiz IA, et al. Incidence and natural progression of neurogenic shock after traumatic spinal injury. *J Neurotrauma.* 2018;35(3):461–466.
28. Yue JK, et al. Vasopressor support in managing acute spinal cord injury: current knowledge. *J Neurosurg Sci.* 2019;63(3):308–317.
29. van Diepen S, et al. Contemporary management of cardiogenic shock—a scientific statement. *Circulation.* 2017;136:e232–e268.
30. Thiele H, et al. Management of cardiogenic shock complicating myocardial infarction: an update 2019. *Eur Heart J.* 2019;40(32): 2671–2683.
31. Vahdatpur C, Collins D, Goldberg S. Cardiogenic shock. *J Am Heart Assoc.* 2019;8(8):e011991.
32. Chioncel O, et al. Epidemiology, pathophysiology and contemporary management of cardiogenic shock - a position statement from the Heart Failure Association of the European Society of Cardiology. *Eur J Heart Fail.* 2020;22(8):1315–1341.
33. Uriel N, et al. Mechanical unloading in heart failure. *J Am Coll Cardiol.* 2018;72:569–580.
34. Jones TL, Nakaumura K, McCabe JM. Cardiogenic shock: evolving definitions and future directions in management. *Open Heart.* 2019;6(1):e000960.
35. Omland T. Advances in congestive heart failure management in the intensive care unit: B-type natriuretic peptides in evaluation of acute heart failure. *Crit Care Med.* 2008;36(1):S17–S27.
36. Kislitsina ON, et al. Shock-classification and pathophysiological principles of therapeutics. *Curr Cardiol Rev.* 2019;15(2):102–113.
37. Jentzer JC, Hollenberg SM. Vasopressor and inotrope therapy in cardiac critical care. *J Intensive Care Med.* 2021;36(8):843–856.
38. Pich H, Heller A. [Obstructive shock]. *Anaesthesist.* 2015;64(5): 403–419. [Article in German].
39. Smith LS, Hernan LJ. *Pediatric critical care.* ed 4 St. Louis: Mosby; 2011.
40. Chen P, Billiar T. Gut microbiota and multiple organ dysfunction syndrome (MODS). *Adv Exp Med Biol.* 2020;1238:195–202.
41. van Wessem KJP, Hietbrink F, Leenen LPH. Attenuation of MODS-related and ARDS-eelated mortality makes infectious complications a remaining challenge in the severely injured. *Trauma Surg Acute Care Open.* 2020;5(1):e000398.
42. Cable CA, et al. RBC transfusion strategies in the ICU: a concise review. *Crit Care Med.* 2019;47(11):1637–1644.
43. Owattanapanich N, et al. Risks and benefits of hypotensive resuscitation in patients with traumatic hemorrhagic shock: a meta-analysis. *Scand J Trauma Resusc Emerg Med.* 2018;26(1):107–127.
44. Patel SV, et al. Risks associated with red blood cell transfusion in the trauma population, a meta-analysis. *Injury.* 2014;45(10): 1522–1533.
45. Osterbur K, et al. Multiple organ dysfunction in humans and animals. *J Vet Intern.* 201428(4):1141–1151.
46. Abraham E, Singer M. Mechanism of sepsis-induced organ dysfunction. *Crit Care Med.* 2007;35(10):2408–2416.
47. Shapiro NI, et al. The association of endothelial cell signaling, severity of illness, and organ dysfunction in sepsis. *Crit Care.* 2010;14(5):R182–R192.
48. Van den Berghe G. The 2016 ESPEN Sir David Cuthbertson lecture: interfering with neuroendocrine and metabolic responses to critical illness: from acute to long-term consequences. *Clin Nutr.* 2017;36(2):348–354.
49. Aird WC. The role of the endothelium in severe sepsis & MODS. *Blood.* 2003;101:3756–3777.
50. Fry DE. Sepsis, systemic inflammatory response, and multiple organ dysfunction: the mystery continues. *Am Surg.* 2012;78(1):1–8.
51. van Meurs M, et al. Early organ-specific endothelial activation during hemorrhagic shock and resuscitation. *Shock.* 2008;29(2):291–299.
52. Souto FO, et al. Essential role of CCR2 in neutrophil tissue infiltration and multiple organ dysfunction in sepsis. *Am J Respir Crit Care Med.* 2011;183(2):234–242.
53. Kimura F, et al. Immunosuppression following surgical and traumatic injury. *Surg Today.* 2010;40(9):793–808.
54. Baue AE. Mediators or markers of injury, inflammation, and infection (harbingers of doom or predictors of disaster) and biologic puzzles or ambiguities. *Arch Surg.* 2007;142(1):89–93.
55. Cohen HE, Mosser DM. Extrinsic and intrinsic control of macrophage inflammatory responses. *J Leukoc Biol.* 2013;94(5): 913–919.
56. Opal SM, van der Poll T. Endothelial barrier dysfunction in septic shock. *J Intern Med.* 2015;277(3):277–293.
57. Otani S, Coopersmith CM. Gut integrity in critical care. *J Intensive Care.* 2019;20(7):17–24.
58. Gando S. Microvascular thrombosis and multiple organ dysfunction syndrome. *Crit Care Med.* 2010;38(2):S35–S42.
59. Awad SS. State-of-the-art therapy for severe sepsis and multisystem organ dysfunction. *Am J Surg.* 2003;186(Suppl):23S–30S.
60. Schmidt H, et al. Autonomic dysfunction predicts both 1- and 2-month mortality in middle-aged patients with multiple organ dysfunction syndrome. *Crit Care Med.* 2008;36(3):967–970.
61. Schmidt H, et al. Relation of impaired interorgan communication and parasympathetic activity in chronic heart failure and multiple-organ dysfunction syndrome. *J Crit Care.* 2014;29(3):367–373.
62. Fernandes Jr CJ, de Assuncao MSC. Myocardial dysfunction in sepsis: a large, unsolved puzzle. *Crit Care Res Pract.* 2012;2012:896430.
63. Sauaia A, et al. Validation of postinjury multiple organ failure scores. *Shock.* 2009;31(5):438–447.
64. de Grooth HJ, et al. SOFA and mortality endpoints in randomized controlled trials: a systematic review and meta-regression analysis. *Crit Care.* 2017;21(1):38–49.
65. Leistner R, et al. Costs and prolonged length of stay of central venous catheter-associated bloodstream infections (CVC BSI): a matched prospective cohort study. *Infection.* 2014;42(1):31–36.
66. Rivers E, et al. Early goal-directed therapy in the treatment of severe sepsis and septic shock. *N Engl J Med.* 2001;345:1368–1377.
67. Levy MM. Early goal-directed therapy: what do we do now? *Crit Care.* 2014;18(6):705.
68. Jaehne AK, Salem D, Garces JD. Early goal-directed therapy in the treatment of sepsis: the times have changed but not the therapy and benefit to patients. *Intensive Care Med.* 2015;41(9):1728–1729.
69. Simon GI, et al. Outcomes of restrictive versus liberal transfusion strategies in older adults from nine randomised

controlled trials: a systematic review and meta-analysis. *Lancet Haematol.* 2017;4(10):e465–e474.
70. Holst LB, et al. Restrictive versus liberal transfusion strategy for red blood cell transfusion: systematic review of randomised trials with meta-analysis and trial sequential analysis. *BMJ.* 2015;350:h1364–h1399.
71. Thompson BT, Bernard GR. ARDS network (NHLBI) studies-successes and challenges in the ARDS clinical research. *Crit Care Clin.* 2011;27(3):459–468.
72. Taylor BE, et al. Guidelines for the provision and assessment of nutrition support therapy in the adult critically ill patient: Society of Critical Care Medicine (SCCM) and American Society for Parenteral and Enteral Nutrition (A.S.P.E.N). *Crit Care Med.* 2016;44(2):390–438.
73. Jeschke MG, et al. Burn injury. *Nat Rev Dis Primers.* 2020;6:11.
74. Greenhalgh DG. Management of burns. *N Engl J Med.* 2019;380(24):2349–2359.
75. Brigham PA, McLoughlin E. Burn incidence and medical care use in the United States: estimates, trends, and data sources. *J Burn Care Rehabil.* 1996;17(2):95–107.
76. Sen S, Greenhalgh D, Palmieri T. Review of burn research for the year 2010. *J Burn Care Res.* 2012;33(5):577–586.
77. Saffle JR, Edelman L, Morris SE. Regional air transport of burn patients: a case for telemedicine? *J Trauma.* 2004;57(1):57–64.
78. Asif M, et al. The added benefit of combining laser Doppler imaging with clinical evaluation in determining the need for excision of indeterminate-depth burn wounds. *Cureus.* 2020;12(6):e8774.
79. Hosseini SN, et al. Xenoderm versus 1% silver sulfadiazine in partial-thickness burns. *Asian J Surg.* 2009;32(4):234–239.
80. Sheridan RL, et al. Planimetry study of the percent of body surface represented by the hand and palm: sizing irregular burns is more accurately done with the palm. *J Burn Care Rehabil.* 1995;16(6):605–606.
81. Navickis RJ, Greenhalgh DG, Wilkes MM. Albumin in burn shock resuscitation: a meta-analysis of controlled clinical trials. *J Burn Care Res.* 2016;37(3):e268–e278.
82. Guillory AN, et al. Cardiovascular dysfunction following burn injury: what we have learned from rat and mouse models. *Int J Mol Sci.* 2016;17(1):53.
83. Chen C, et al. Myosin light chain kinase mediates intestinal barrier disruption following burn injury. *PLoS One.* 2012;7(4):e34946.
84. Baxter CR, Cook WA, Shires GT. Serum myocardial depressant factor of burn shock. *Surg Forum.* 1966;17:1–2.
85. Demling RH, Will JA, Belzer FO. Effect of major thermal injury on the pulmonary microcirculation. *Surgery.* 1978;83(6): 746–751.
86. Horton JW, et al. Calcium antagonists improve cardiac mechanical performance after thermal trauma. *J Surg Res.* 1999;87(1):39–50.
87. Aikawa N, Martyn JA, Burke JF. Pulmonary artery catheterization and thermodilution cardiac output determination in the management of critically burned patients. *Am J Surg.* 1978;135(6):811–817.
88. Dobson EL, Warner GF. Factors concerned in the early stages of thermal shock. *Circ Res.* 1957;5(1):69–74.
89. Lefer AM, Martin J. Origin of myocardial depressant factor in shock. *Am J Physiol.* 1970;218(5):1423–1442.
90. Rosenthal SR, Hawley PL, Hakim AA. Purified burn toxic factor and its competition. *Surgery.* 1972;71(4):527–536.
91. Horton JW, Burton KP, White DJ. The role of toxic oxygen metabolites in a young model of thermal injury. *J Trauma.* 1995;39(3):563–569.
92. Vivó C, Galeiras R, del Caz MD. Initial evaluation and management of the critical burn patient. *Med Intensiva.* 2016;40(1):49–59.
93. Jennes S, et al. Management of burn wounds of the head and neck region. *B-ENT.* 2016;12(Suppl 26/1):107–126. Available at http://www.b-ent.be/en/management-of-burn-wounds-of-the-head-and-neck-region-16242. (Accessed February 13, 2022).
94. Shah A, et al. Fluid volumes infused during burn resuscitation 1980–2015: a quantitative review. *Burns.* 2020;46(1):52–57.
95. Gurney JM, Kozar RA, Cancio LC. Plasma for burn shock resuscitation: is it time to go back to the future? *Transfusion.* 2019;59(S2):1578–1586.
96. Gus E, Cleland H. Burn fluid resuscitation formulae: concept and misconception. *Injury.* 2021;52(4):780–781.
97. Belba MK, Petrela EY, Belba GP. Comparison of hypertonic vs isotonic fluids during resuscitation of severely burned patients. *Am J Emerg Med.* 2009;27(9):1091–1096.
98. Evans JA, Darlington DN, Gann DS. A circulating factor(s) mediates cell depolarization in hemorrhagic shock. *Ann Surg.* 1991;213(6):549–556.
99. Welt LG. Membrane transport defect: the sick cell. *Trans Assoc Am Physicians.* 1967;80:217–226.
100. Trunkey DD, et al. The effect of hemorrhagic shock on intracellular muscle action potentials in the primate. *Surgery.* 1973;74(2):241–250.
101. Cunningham Jr JN, Shires GT, Wagner Y. Changes in intracellular sodium and potassium content of red blood cells in trauma and shock. *Am J Surg.* 1971;122(5):650–654.
102. Rosenthal SR, Tabor H. Electrolyte changes and chemotherapy in experimental burn and traumatic shock and hemorrhage. *Arch Surg.* 1945;51:244.
103. Turinsky J, Gonnerman WA, Loose LD. Impaired mineral metabolism in postburn muscle. *J Trauma.* 1981;21(6):417–423.
104. Deets DK, Glaviano VV. Plasma and cardiac lactic dehydrogenase activity in burn shock. *Proc Soc Exp Biol Med.* 1973;142(2):412–416.
105. Button B. Evidence of circulating membrane depolarization factor(s) in hemorrhagic shock. *Shock.* 1994;1(Suppl):15.
106. Okamoto R, Glaviano VV, Pindok M. Myocardial lipases and catecholamines in burn shock. *Proc Soc Exp Biol Med.* 1971;137(1):347–353.
107. Herndon DN, et al. Long-term propranolol use in severely burned pediatric patients: a randomized controlled study. *Ann Surg.* 2012;256(3):402–411.
108. Wilmore DW, Aulick HL, Goodwin CW. Glucose metabolism following severe injury. *Acta Chir Scand Suppl.* 1980;498:43–47.
109. Akcay MN, et al. The effect of growth hormone on 24-h urinary creatinine levels in burned patients. *Burns.* 2001;27(1):42–45.
110. Ikezu T, et al. A unique mechanism of desensitization to lipolysis mediated by beta(3)-adrenoceptor in rats with thermal injury. *Am J Physiol.* 1999;277(2 Pt 1):E316–E324.
111. Wilmore DW, et al. Alterations in hypothalamic function following thermal injury. *J Trauma.* 1975;15(8):697–703.
112. Holder IA, Neely AN. Hageman factor dependent activation and its relationship to lethal *Pseudomonas aeruginosa* burn wound infections. *Agents Actions Suppl.* 1992;38(Pt 3):329–342.
113. McManus WF, Eurenius K, Pruitt BA. Jr: Disseminated intravascular coagulation in burned patients. *J Trauma.* 1973;13(5):416–422.
114. Wilmore DW, ed. *The metabolic management of the critically ill.* ed 2 New York: Plenum; 1990.
115. Wilmore DW, Aulick LH. Metabolic changes in burned patients. *Surg Clin North Am.* 1978;58(6):1173–1187.
116. Edelman LS, et al. Sustained bone mineral density changes after burn injury. *J Surg Res.* 2003;114(2):172–178.

117. Wright K, et al. Burn-activated neutrophils and tumor necrosis factor-alpha alter endothelial cell actin cytoskeleton and enhance monolayer permeability. *Surgery*. 2000;128(2):259–265.
118. Goebel A, et al. Injury induces deficient interleukin-12 production, but interleukin-12 therapy after injury restores resistance to infection. *Ann Surg*. 2000;231(2):253–261.
119. Nishiura T, et al. Gene expression and cytokine and enzyme activation in the liver after a burn injury. *J Burn Care Rehabil*. 2000;21(2):135–141.
120. Biffl WL, et al. Interleukin-6 delays neutrophil apoptosis via a mechanism involving platelet-activating factor. *J Trauma*. 1996;40(4):575–578.
121. Choi M, et al. Preventing the infiltration of leukocytes by monoclonal antibody blocks the development of progressive ischemia in rat burns. *Plast Reconstr Surg*. 1995;96(5):1177–1185.
122. Iocono JA, et al. Interleukin-8 levels and activity in delayed-healing human thermal wounds. *Wound Repair Regen*. 2000;8(3):216–225.
123. Ortega MR, Ganz T, Milner SM. Human beta defensin is absent in burn blister fluid. *Burns*. 2000;26(8):724–726.
124. Heideman M, Kaijser B, Gelin LE. Complement activation and hematologic, hemodynamic, and respiratory reactions early after soft-tissue injury. *J Trauma*. 1978;18(10):696–700.
125. Grzybowski J, et al. Antidietary antigen antibodies in the sera of patients with burns as a potential marker of gut mucosa integrity failure. *J Burn Care Rehabil*. 1992;13(2 Pt 1):194–197.
126. Deitch EA, Berg R. Bacterial translocation from the gut: a mechanism of infection. *J Burn Care Rehabil*. 1987;8(6):475–482.
127. Yao YM, et al. The association of circulating endotoxaemia with the development of multiple organ failure in burned patients. *Burns*. 1995;21(4):255–258.
128. Benhaim P, Hunt TK. Natural resistance to infection: leukocyte functions. *J Burn Care Rehabil*. 1992;13(2 Pt 2):287–292.
129. Alexander JW, et al. Consumptive opsoninopathy: possible pathogenesis in lethal and opportunistic infections. *Ann Surg*. 1976;184(6):672–678.
130. Bjornson AB, Altemeier WA, Bjornson HS. Changes in humoral components of host defense following burn trauma. *Ann Surg*. 1977;186(1):88–96.
131. Cochran A, et al. Systemic *Candida* infection in burn patients: a case-control study of management patterns and outcomes. *Surg Infect (Larchmt)*. 2002;3(4):367–374.
132. Goff DR, et al. Cardiac disease and the patient with burns. *J Burn Care Rehabil*. 1990;11(4):305–307.
133. McGill V, et al. The impact of substance use on mortality and morbidity from thermal injury. *J Trauma*. 1995;38(6):931–934.
134. Moncrief JA, Mason AD. Jr: Water vapor loss in the burned patient. *Surg Forum*. 1962;13:38–41.
135. Moncrief JA. Burns. In: Schwartz SI, ed. *Principles of surgery*. ed 2 New York: McGraw-Hill; 1974.
136. Roe CF, Kinney JM. Water and heat exchange on third-degree burns. *Surgery*. 1964;56:212–220.
137. Affleck DG, et al. Assessment of tissue viability in complex extremity injuries: utility of the pyrophosphate nuclear scan. *J Trauma*. 2001;50(2):263–269.
138. Eski M, et al. Cerium nitrate treatment prevents progressive tissue necrosis in the zone of stasis following burns. *Burn*. 2012;38(2):283–289.
139. Weber JM, et al. Incidence of catheter-associated bloodstream infection after introduction of minocycline and rifampin antimicrobial-coated catheters in a pediatric burn population. *J Burn Care Res*. 2012;33(4):539–543.
140. Lee J, et al. Computerized insulin infusion programs are safe and effective in the burn intensive care unit. *J Burn Care Res*. 2012;33(3):e114–e119.
141. Zaletel CL. Factors affecting fluid resuscitation in the burn patient: the collaborative role of the APN. *Adv Emerg Nurs J*. 2009;31(4):309–320.
142. Fraser JF, et al. A randomized controlled trial of amniotic membrane in the treatment of a standardized burn injury in the merino lamb. *Burns*. 2009;35(7):998–1003.
143. Ronfard V, et al. Long-term regeneration of human epidermis on third degree burns transplanted with autologous cultured epithelium grown on a fibrin matrix. *Transplantation*. 2000;70(11):1588–1598.
144. Williamson JS, et al. Cultured epithelial autograft: five years of clinical experience with twenty-eight patients. *J Trauma*. 1995;39(2):309–319.
145. Fitton AR, Drew P, Dickson WA. The use of a bilaminate artificial skin substitute (Integra) in acute resurfacing of burns: an early experience. *Br J Plast Surg*. 2001;54(3):208–212.
146. Peck MD, et al. A trial of the effectiveness of artificial dermis in the treatment of patients with burns greater than 45% total body surface area. *J Trauma*. 2002;52(5):971–978.
147. Carsin H, et al. Cultured epithelial autografts in extensive burn coverage of severely traumatized patients: a five year single-center experience with 30 patients. *Burns*. 2000;26(4):379–387.
148. Wainwright D, et al. Clinical evaluation of an acellular allograft dermal matrix in full-thickness burns. *J Burn Care Rehabil*. 1996;17(2):124–136.
149. Branski LK, et al. A review of gene and stem cell therapy in cutaneous wound healing. *Burns*. 2009;35(2):171–180.
150. Curinga G, et al. Comments on "Platelet-rich plasma in burns". *Burns*. 2010;36(6):944–945.
151. Pallua N, Wolter T, Markowicz M. Platelet-rich plasma in burns. *Burns*. 2010;36(1):4–8.
152. Liew SH, Murison M, Dickson WA. Prophylactic treatment of deep dermal burn scar to prevent hypertrophic scarring using the pulsed dye laser: a preliminary study. *Ann Plast Surg*. 2002;49(5):472–475.
153. Baxter CR. Fluid volume and electrolyte changes of the early postburn period. *Clin Plast Surg*. 1974;1(4):693–703.
154. Fowler AA, et al. Effect of vitamin C infusion on organ failure and biomarkers of inflammation and vascular injury in patients with sepsis and severe acute respiratory failure: the CITRIS-ALI randomized clinical trial. *JAMA*. 2019;322:1261–1270.
155. Buehner M, et al. Oxalate nephropathy after continuous infusion of high-dose vitamin C as an adjunct to burn resuscitation. *J Burn Care Res*. 2016;37:e374–e379.
156. Kahn SA, Beers RJ, Lentz CW. Resuscitation after severe burn injury using high-dose ascorbic acid: a retrospective review. *J Burn Care Res*. 2011;32:110–117.
157. Sainsbury DC. Body image and facial burns. *Adv Skin Wound Care*. 2009;22(1):39–44.
158. Connor-Ballard PA. Understanding and managing burn pain: part 1. *Am J Nurs*. 2009;109(4):48–56.
159. Connor-Ballard PA. Understanding and managing burn pain: part 2. *Am J Nurs*. 2009;109(5):54–62.
160. Jellish WS, et al. Effect of topical local anesthetic application to skin harvest sites for pain management in burn patients undergoing skin-grafting procedures. *Ann Surg*. 1999;229(1):115–120.
161. Mackey SP, et al. Return to work after burns: a qualitative research study. *Burns*. 2009;35(3):338–342.
162. Konstantatos AH, et al. Predicting the effectiveness of virtual reality relaxation on pain and anxiety when added to PCA morphine in patients having burn dressings changes. *Burns*. 2009;35(4):491–499.

49

Shock, Multiple Organ Dysfunction Syndrome, and Burns in Children

Mary A. Mondozzi, Dennis J. Cheek, and Mary Fran Hazinski

http://evolve.elsevier.com/Rogers/pathophysiology/

CHAPTER OUTLINE

This chapter reviews shock, multiple organ dysfunction syndrome (MODS), and burns in children. It focuses on the assessment and care of children but also notes many of the differences between these conditions in children and adults.

SHOCK AND MULTIPLE ORGAN DYSFUNCTION SYNDROME

Shock is a condition of acute and progressive circulatory dysfunction that results in inadequate delivery of oxygen and nutrients to the tissues. Shock in children is most often categorized as hypovolemic, distributive, cardiogenic, or obstructive. Contributing factors may include severe dehydration, hemorrhage, progressive heart failure, or sepsis; in fact, all infants under 3 months of age presenting in shock should be considered septic until proven otherwise.[1] Shock may also complicate the care of the child with congenital heart disease (CHD), pulmonary hypertension (cor pulmonale), drug toxicity, electrolyte or acid-base imbalance, dysrhythmias, obstruction to blood flow (e.g., pulmonary embolus, cardiac tamponade), or multiple organ failure.

In children, shock is present when there are signs of poor systemic perfusion, regardless of the blood pressure (shock may be present with normal, high, or low blood pressure.) When the systolic blood pressure is adequate for age, but there are signs of inadequate tissue perfusion (e.g., tachycardia, diminished peripheral pulses, abnormal capillary refill), the child is in compensated shock. In this child, although the systolic blood pressure may be normal, the diastolic or mean arterial pressure is typically low.[2] When the compensatory mechanism fails, systolic hypotension, which is associated with inadequate tissue perfusion, ensues. In addition to hypotension and inadequate tissue perfusion, the child in hypotensive (formerly called *decompensated*) shock will present with clinical signs of decreased mental status, decreased urine output, diminished peripheral pulses, metabolic acidosis, and increased respirations.[1] Hypotension in pediatrics is defined by the AHA Pediatric Advanced Life Support guidelines and training materials as less than the fifth percentile for age.[3]

Shock causes tissue ischemia (inadequate blood flow) and hypoxia (inadequate oxygen delivery) that leads to acidosis and cell dysfunction. Oxygen delivery may be inadequate because arterial oxygen content or cardiac output is low or because there are increased tissue oxygen requirements or impaired cellular use of oxygen. Ischemia and tissue hypoxia are primary insults to cells. Restoration of adequate blood flow and oxygen delivery may trigger the development of *reperfusion injury*, a secondary problem characterized by an exaggerated inflammatory response that may produce cellular death and organ failure.

Multiple organ dysfunction syndrome (MODS) is the concurrent failure of at least two organs resulting from a single cause,[4] most often from a systemic inflammatory response syndrome (SIRS), associated with acute insults such as sepsis or trauma. MODS also can complicate chronic diseases, such as cancer and CHD as well as more acute insults including drowning, acute respiratory distress syndrome (ARDS), liver failure, pancreatitis, or cardiac arrest. Finally, MODS can result from treatments such as chemotherapy, surgical correction of CHD, or organ transplantation.[1,5–7] Children with chronic diseases have both an increased risk of and increased mortality from MODS.

MODS may be either primary or secondary. Primary MODS is directly attributable to an insult and typically occurs soon

(3 to 7 days) after the insult. Secondary MODS typically occurs later and may be associated with more sequential development of organ dysfunction. New or progressive MODS (NPMODS) is a recently defined problem that can develop with severe sepsis. It is defined as a dysfunction of one or fewer organs on day 1 of sepsis recognition with subsequent development of two or more concurrent organ failures at any time during treatment.[4,7,8]

Types of Shock

Shock is categorized by type as follows[1,3]:

1. *Hypovolemic shock:* caused by inadequate intravascular volume relative to the vascular space (e.g., gastrointestinal [GI] losses, renal losses, hemorrhage, third spacing, and/or burns)
2. *Cardiogenic shock:* results from impairment of myocardial function (e.g., CHD, arrhythmia, cardiomyopathy, myocarditis, or anemia)
3. *Distributive shock* (including septic, anaphylactic, and neurogenic): results from inappropriate distribution of blood flow, increased capillary permeability, and myocardial dysfunction (e.g., septic or anaphylactic shock) or central nervous system injury (e.g., neurogenic or spinal shock)
4. *Obstructive shock:* caused by a mechanical obstruction to blood flow into and through the heart and great vessels (e.g., cardiac tamponade, pulmonary embolus, tension pneumothorax, or obstructive congenital heart lesions such as critical aortic stenosis), resulting in low cardiac output

An etiologic classification of shock is helpful because it suggests the initial therapy required. However, the etiologic classification is an oversimplification because any child with late or progressive shock is likely to demonstrate widespread cardiovascular dysfunction that may include inappropriate intravascular volume relative to the vascular space, poor myocardial function, and maldistribution of blood flow.[1] Severe shock of any kind may be followed by complications such as reperfusion injury, MODS, or NPMODS.[4] Children with septic shock demonstrate elements of hypovolemic and cardiogenic shock in addition to the complications of infection and maldistribution of blood flow. Thus, healthcare providers must assess and support all aspects of cardiovascular function and oxygen delivery during the treatment of any form of shock.[1]

Assessment of Shock

Signs of shock in children may initially be subtle; thus, detection of shock and evaluation of response to therapy typically requires careful, repeated assessments over time. Inadequate cardiac output causes signs of inadequate blood flow to some tissue beds and evidence of organ system dysfunction (Box 49.1). Critical parameters to evaluate include assessment of consciousness, breathing, and color. This initial assessment is described in the Pediatric Advanced Life Support course.[9]

Through this assessment, the provider determines if the child appears stable, in no acute distress, or in need of immediate intervention. More detailed assessment will reveal evidence of inadequate organ function resulting from inadequate organ perfusion.

BOX 49.1 Clinical Manifestations of Shock in Newborns, Infants, and Children

Signs of Shock in Infants and Children

- Change in responsiveness (initial irritability followed by lethargy)
- Tachypnea
- Mottled color, pallor (distributive shock may be associated with flushed skin)
- Tachycardia
- Cool skin, prolonged capillary refill (distributive shock may cause "flash" [instantaneous] refill)
- Diminished intensity of peripheral pulses (may also vary in intensity)
- Metabolic (lactic) acidosis (serum lactate >4 mmol/L is typically well above normal for arterial or venous blood)
- Decreased central venous oxygen saturation (more than 25%–30% below arterial oxygen saturation)
- LATE: Hypotension, bradycardia

Nonspecific Signs of Distress in Newborns

- Jitteriness or lethargy with decreased tone
- Change in oxygen requirements
- Apnea
- Bradycardia or decreased heart rate variability
- Temperature instability, hypothermia
- Glucose instability, hypoglycemia
- Feeding intolerance (e.g., increased residual volume)

The child's level of *consciousness* and *responsiveness* often provide valuable information about the severity of illness. The healthy infant should orient to faces, make eye contact, and track bright objects across a visual field. The healthy toddler is reluctant to be separated from parents or examined by strangers, and the healthy child is alert and responds to questions. By comparison, the critically ill infant or child is often extremely irritable; lethargy indicates severe deterioration in the child's level of consciousness. A decreased response to painful stimulus is abnormal and usually indicates severe cardiorespiratory or neurologic compromise.[9,10]

The infant or child normally breathes without evidence of distress or increased effort, such as retractions or nasal flaring. An extremely rapid respiratory rate (tachypnea), increased depth of respirations (hyperpnea), or evidence of increased respiratory effort (e.g., retractions, grunting) may indicate the presence of heart failure or shock. The development of apnea or inadequate respiratory rate or effort generally indicates deterioration and the need for immediate support of airway, oxygenation, and ventilation.

If perfusion is adequate and the ambient temperature is warm, the child's *color* will be consistent over the surface of the skin, and lips, nailbeds, and mucous membranes will be pink. Children who are in a cold environment, those who have undergone hypothermic surgery or a procedure in a cold room, and children in shock often demonstrate mottling (a marbled or "blotchy" appearance to the skin).[1,9]

Pallor also may be observed when perfusion is poor (Fig. 49.1). Children with sepsis occasionally demonstrate flushed, bright red (plethoric) skin.[1,9,11]

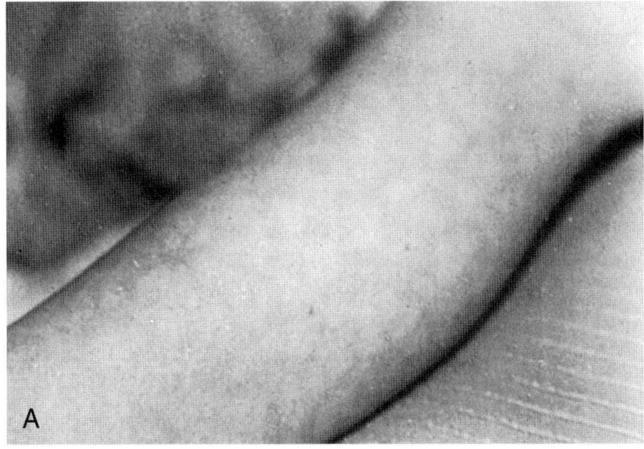

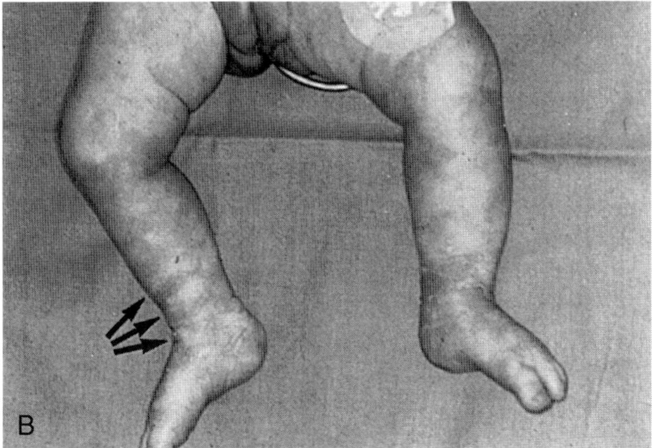

Fig. 49.1 Mottling of Skin Caused by Poor Systemic Perfusion. **(A)** Mottling of skin color often indicates inadequate tissue oxygenation; this may result from hypoxemia or poor systemic perfusion. This child developed myocardial dysfunction and signs of cardiogenic shock. **(B)** Mottled skin color is often associated with other signs of compromise of skin perfusion, including delayed capillary refill. The skin over this infant's right ankle was blanched using three fingers *(arrows)*, and the skin failed to perfuse for more than 5 seconds. This infant suffered from septic shock. (From Hazinski MF. Cardiovascular disorders. In: Hazinski MF, ed. *Nursing care of the critically ill child,* 2nd edition. St. Louis: Mosby; 1992.)

If perfusion is adequate and the ambient temperature is warm, the child's capillary refill is normally brisk (<2 seconds). Prolonged capillary refill (>2 seconds) may indicate a compromise in systemic perfusion (see Fig. 49.1B) and the development of shock.[1,9]

Septic shock may be associated with vasodilation that produces instantaneous (flash) capillary refill or may be associated with vasoconstriction and delayed capillary refill.[2]

The child's *vital signs* must be evaluated in light of the child's age and clinical condition. Normal vital signs are not always appropriate for the seriously ill or injured child (Box 49.2 and Table 49.1).[10]

The child's heart rate should be appropriate for age and clinical condition. The child in shock is often tachycardic. The tachycardia may be primary (i.e., associated with a tachydysrhythmia) or secondary to stress (i.e., sinus tachycardia). If the heart rate is extremely rapid, especially in the child with decreased myocardial function, tachycardia may be the cause rather than the symptom of shock. In general, if the ventricular rate exceeds 200 to 220 beats/min in the infant or 160 to 180 beats/min in the child, ventricular diastolic filling time and coronary artery perfusion time are significantly reduced, and stroke volume falls. Cardiac output can then fall, leading to signs of heart failure or shock. Once supraventricular or ventricular tachycardia produces signs of shock, urgent treatment is required.[12]

BOX 49.2 Estimating Blood Pressure in Children 1–10 Years of Age

Typical systolic BP for 1–10 years of age: The typical systolic blood pressure for a child 1 to 10 years of age of normal height may be estimated by adding 90 mmHg to twice the child's age in years (90 mmHg + [2 × age in years]).

Hypotensive systolic BP for 1–10 years of age: A systolic pressure less than 70 mmHg plus twice the child's age in years (<70 mmHg + [2 × age in years]) is considered hypotensive for children 1 to 10 years of age because this blood pressure corresponds to the 5th percentile systolic blood pressure for age (i.e., only 5% of normal, healthy children of average height demonstrate a systolic blood pressure lower than that number).

Hypotensive mean arterial pressure for 1–10 years of age: A mean arterial pressure less than 40 mmHg + (1.5 × age in years) is consistent with hypotension because this mean arterial pressure corresponds to the 5th percentile mean arterial pressure in children of average height.

Data from Kadec KD, McBride ME, et al. *2020 AHA pediatric advanced life support provider manual.* Dallas, TX: American Heart Association; 2020.

Bradycardia, an abnormally low heart rate, can cause a fall in cardiac output, or it can be a symptom of deterioration. In children, a fall in heart rate typically produces a commensurate fall in cardiac output.[13] The most common cause of bradycardia in young children is hypoxia.[14]

If the infant or child develops bradycardia with poor perfusion, the provider must immediately assess and support the child's airway, oxygenation, and ventilation, and be prepared to initiate chest compressions if the heart rate and systemic perfusion do not improve.[12]

Bradycardia often indicates impending cardiovascular collapse and is the most common terminal cardiac rhythm observed in children.[14] In neonates, especially preterm neonates, a *lack of heart rate variability* is a nonspecific sign of compromise, such as sepsis.[15]

The child's stroke volume may be altered by conditions affecting ventricular preload, compliance, contractility, and afterload (Table 49.2). Providers must evaluate and optimize each of these variables in the treatment of shock (see Chapter 48).

The child's *blood pressure* must be appropriate for age and clinical condition. Shock may be present despite a systolic blood pressure within the normal range for age. When hypovolemic or cardiogenic shock is present, compensatory vasoconstriction may initially maintain the systolic blood pressure, although the mean and diastolic arterial pressures may fall. The development of systolic hypotension in the child with hypovolemic or cardiogenic shock indicates severe shock, and rapid deterioration may follow. In septic shock, by comparison, a fall in systolic or diastolic blood pressure may develop relatively early in the clinical course. In all children, the development of systolic, diastolic, or

TABLE 49.1 Typical Pediatric Vital Signs

	Heart Rates		
Age	Awake Heart Rate (per min)	Sleeping Heart Rate (per min)	Respiratory Rate[a] (Breaths/min)
Newborn	100–205	90–160	30–60
Infant (6 mo)	100–180	90–160	30–53
Toddler	98–140	80–120	27–37
Preschooler	80–120	65–100	20–28
School-age child	75–118	58–90	18–25
Adolescent	60–100	50–90	12–20

Typical Blood Pressures

Age	Systolic Blood Pressure (mmHg)[b] For 1–10 Years of Age Estimated by 70 mmHg + 2 × age (Years)	Diastolic Blood Pressure (mmHg)[b]	Mean Arterial Pressure (mmHg)[c] Estimated by 40 mmHg + 2 × Patient Age (Years)	Systolic Hypotension (mmHg)[d]
Birth (12 h, <1000 g)	39–59	16–36	28–42[e]	<40–50
Birth (12 h, 3-kg weight)	60–76	31–45	48–57	<50
Newborn (96 h)	67–84	35–53	45–60	<60
Infant (1–12 mo)	72–104	37–56	50–62	<70
Toddler (1–2 years)	86–106	42–63	49–62	<70+(2×age in years)
Preschool (3–5 years)	89–112	46–72	58–69	<70+(2×age in years)
School-age child (6–9 years)	97–115	57–76	66–72	<70+(2×age in years)
Preadolescent (10–12 years)	102–120	61–80	71–79	<90
Adolescent (13–15 years)	110–131	64–83	73–84	<90

From Hazinski MF. Children are different. In: Hazinski MF, ed. *Nursing care of the critically ill child,* 3rd edition. St. Louis: Mosby; 2013.

NOTE: Always consider person's normal range and clinical condition. Heart and respiratory rates normally increase with fever or stress.

[a]Respiratory rates from Fleming S, Thompson M, Stevens R, et al. Normal ranges of heart rate and respiratory rate in children from birth to 18 years of age: A systematic review of observational studies. *Lancet,* 2011;377(9770):1011–1018.

[b]Systolic and diastolic blood pressure ranges assume 50th percentile for height for children 1 year and older, and are consistent with the Pediatric Advanced Life Support course (Chameides L, Ralston M, American Academy of Pediatrics, et al. *Pediatric advanced life support provider manual.* Dallas, TX: American Heart Association; 2011).

[c]Mean arterial pressures (Diastolic pressure+[Difference between systolic and diastolic pressures ÷ 3]) for 1 year and older, assuming 50th percentile for height.

[d]Threshold for hypotension in children 1 to 10 years old from Pediatric Advanced Life Support course (Chameides L, Ralston M, American Academy of Pediatrics, et al. *Pediatric advanced life support provider manual.* Dallas, TX: American Heart Association; 2011).

[e]Approximately equal to postconception age in weeks (may add 5 mmHg).

mean arterial pressure indicates hypotensive shock, and urgent treatment is needed.[1,2]

The central venous pressure (CVP) is normally 0 to 5 mmHg. The pulmonary artery wedge pressure (PAWP, also called *pulmonary artery occlusion pressure* [*PAOP*]) is normally 5 to 8 mmHg or less, although pulmonary artery catheters are now rarely used in children. Inadequate CVP or PAWP may indicate hypovolemia, whereas high pressures typically result from heart failure or cardiogenic shock. Note that in the absence of tricuspid valve disease, tension pneumothorax, or influence from positive pressure ventilation, the CVP reflects the right ventricular end-diastolic pressure (RVEDP). The RVEDP may differ substantially from the left ventricular end-diastolic pressure.

A central venous catheter enables the evaluation of CVP and provides a route for rapid volume administration. In addition, a CVP catheter in the superior vena cava (SVC) enables the evaluation of the central venous oxygen saturation ($ScvO_2$). The $ScvO_2$ is used as a surrogate for the mixed venous oxygen saturation (which would require a sampling of blood from the pulmonary artery). If cardiac output is adequate and oxygen consumption is normal, the $ScvO_2$ will be no more than 25% to 30% below the arterial oxygen saturation. This typical arteriovenous oxygen saturation difference is still present in the child with cyanotic heart disease, provided the cardiac output and oxygen consumption are normal. A widening difference between the arterial and central venous oxygen saturation often indicates a decrease in cardiac output.

A fall in $ScvO_2$ can indicate a fall in oxygen delivery (caused by decreased arterial oxygen content or decreased cardiac output, or both), an uncompensated rise in oxygen consumption,

TABLE 49.2 Factors Affecting Cardiovascular Performance in Children

Factor	Comments
Heart rate	Major factor affecting cardiac output in children. Normally more rapid in children than in adults. Because the *stroke volume* is smaller in children than in adults, the *cardiac output* of the child is more closely related to heart rate than to stroke volume. *Tachycardia* is expected in the seriously ill or injured child, so a relatively normal heart rate may indicate deterioration. The most common cause of *bradycardia* in young children is hypoxia; bradycardia is an ominous sign if present in association with poor perfusion. Urgent treatment is required once bradycardia or supraventricular or ventricular tachycardia produces signs of shock.
Stroke volume	Averages 1.5 mL/kg; affected by conditions altering ventricular preload, compliance, contractility, and afterload.
Ventricular end-diastolic pressure (VEDP)	Optimal VEDP for children in shock is unknown. Bolus resuscitation is linked to improved survival in children with *septic* shock, provided caregivers titrate the fluid and cease bolus fluid administration if signs of hypervolemia or new or progressive signs of heart failure (rales, hepatomegaly) develop.
Ventricular compliance or distensibility	Can be affected by congenital heart defects such as atrial septal defects (ASDs) and complex congenital heart defects or surgical interventions for these defects. If compliance is low, such as in newborns and infants, relatively small quantities of volume administration may increase VEDP. Hypoplastic ventricles are often noncompliant. Hypertrophied ventricles, present in children with severe pulmonary stenosis or aortic stenosis, may become fibrotic and noncompliant. Increased compliance may be present in early septic shock.
Contractility	Contractility probably similar in normal newborns, infants, children, and adults. Newborn myocardium does have fewer contractile proteins and higher water content than adult myocardium, but the clinical significance of this is probably minimal.
Afterload	Newborn myocardium *can* adapt to mild, nonacute increases in afterload. Afterload may be increased in children with systemic vasoconstriction or pulmonary hypertension (constrictors include alveolar hypoxia, acidosis, hypothermia, and alveolar distention). Some uncorrected congenital heart defects may increase afterload. Coarctation of the aorta and aortic stenosis increase left ventricular afterload. Pulmonary stenosis increases right ventricular afterload. Afterload may be decreased in septic shock.
Oxygen delivery and consumption	Highest per kilogram body weight during the neonatal period and infancy. The young child requires a higher cardiac output and oxygen delivery per kilogram than the adult. Increased oxygen consumption occurs in critically ill newborns exposed to cold because they cannot shiver to generate heat. Other causes of increased oxygen consumption in children and infants include fever, sepsis, trauma, pain, and seizures.

or both. If a CVP catheter is in place in the SVC, resuscitation of a child in septic shock may target a central venous oxygen saturation (SvO_2) of 70% or greater.[16]

Shock compromises renal perfusion, so despite adequate fluid intake, urine volume decreases, typically falling to less than 2 mL/kg/h in infants, less than 1 mL/kg/h in children, and less than 0.5 mL/kg/h in adolescents. Liver enzymes may be elevated if hepatic perfusion is reduced. The development of metabolic acidosis and a rise in serum lactate to greater than 4 mg/dL indicate that blood flow to some tissues is inadequate to support aerobic metabolism.

Infants have high glucose needs and low glycogen stores that may be rapidly depleted during stress. For this reason, *hypoglycemia* (glucose ≤60 mg/dL) may be observed in seriously ill or injured infants and may be associated with cardiovascular or neurologic deterioration.[17,18]

Severe physiologic stress, such as cardiac surgery, shock, sepsis, MODS, or NPMODS can produce *critical illness hyperglycemia* (CIH), a transient glucose concentration >150 mg/dL. CIH has been documented in adults and children. It is produced by a relative insulin-resistant state associated with high levels of endogenous catecholamines and hydrocortisone secretion, with resultant gluconeogenesis and glycogenolysis. Glucose uptake by the liver is increased, while glucose uptake by peripheral tissues is decreased. Inflammatory mediators can contribute to the relative insulin resistance.[1,18,19] In children, the serum glucose is often elevated in the first 12 to 18 hours after initial insult (such as injury, shock, sepsis or MODS development, or cardiac surgery) that then falls to normal ranges. Although CIH has been associated with poor survival in critically ill children,[20,21] it is not clear if the hyperglycemia is the cause or the marker of poor outcomes.[19] An international pediatric study found that aggressive treatment of the hyperglycemia (i.e., tight glycemic control to 80 to 110 mg/dL) did not improve outcomes and did result in episodes of hypoglycemia.[22]

Hypovolemic Shock

Hypovolemic shock, the most common type of shock in children, is caused by a reduction in the intravascular volume relative to the vascular space. Intravascular volume loss (e.g., dehydration or hemorrhage) and trauma are the most common causes of hypovolemic shock in children.

Pathophysiology. Hypovolemia can develop rapidly in children. When hypovolemia is mild or moderate, such as with 5% to 10% dehydration or mild hemorrhage, compensatory adrenergic vasoconstriction redistributes blood from the skin, the mesenteric (gut), and renal circulations to maintain blood flow to the heart and brain. The blood pressure is typically adequate with mild hypovolemic shock. Hypotension is a sign of severe, decompensated hypovolemic shock and may not develop unless intravascular volume loss is rapid or severe.[1,2]

Relative hypovolemia may result from vasodilation and a redistribution of blood volume or from increased capillary permeability, which can be associated with sepsis, burns, anaphylaxis, or neurogenic shock, as well as with β_2-adrenergic drug toxicity. The translocation of extravascular fluid to a location that is neither intravascular nor intracellular, as in edema, is termed "third spacing" of fluids.[18]

There are compensatory responses to regain homeostasis. Significant dehydration, hypovolemia, and low cardiac output stimulate adrenergic and renal compensatory mechanisms characterized by the "fight-or-flight" response. These include tachycardia and redistribution of blood from the skin, gut, and kidney to the brain and heart. Reduced renal perfusion stimulates the renin-angiotensin-aldosterone system, resulting in renal sodium and water retention. Decreased atrial stretch stimulates the secretion of antidiuretic hormone (ADH, also known as *arginine vasopressin* [*AVP*]) and produces free water retention by the kidneys.[1] These mechanisms are similar in adults and children and may help restore or maintain intravascular volume over time. Neonatal and young infant kidneys, however, are incapable of excreting concentrated urine, so these compensatory mechanisms are relatively ineffective during the first weeks of life.[18]

Compensatory mechanisms cannot be maintained indefinitely. Systemic vasoconstriction increases left ventricular afterload and myocardial oxygen consumption and may produce tissue ischemia. Prolonged tachycardia may impair subendocardial blood flow and increase myocardial oxygen consumption; both may ultimately contribute to myocardial ischemia.[1] Extreme tachypnea increases oxygen demand and reduces effective ventilation. A severe compromise in blood flow and systemic perfusion contributes to cerebral, renal, or hepatic ischemia and possible organ failure.

Clinical Manifestations. The child with hypovolemic shock demonstrates signs of inadequate blood flow to some tissue beds and some evidence of organ system dysfunction (see Box 49.1). The infant or child may be irritable or lethargic. Respirations will be rapid and may be labored if the shock is severe or associated with myocardial failure. The skin will be mottled, although pallor also may be observed. A prolonged capillary refill time (>2 seconds) is consistent with the development of shock.[1,2,10] The child in hypovolemic shock is often tachycardic. Bradycardia in the child with shock indicates impending cardiovascular collapse and is the most common terminal cardiac rhythm observed in children.[1,12]

When hypovolemic shock is present, compensatory vasoconstriction may initially maintain the systolic blood pressure, although the mean arterial pressure may fall. The development of systolic hypotension often indicates severe shock, and rapid deterioration may follow. The CVP is typically less than 5 to 8 mmHg unless heart failure or pulmonary hypertension is present.

Hypovolemic shock compromises renal perfusion, so urine volume decreases despite adequate fluid intake. Liver enzymes may be elevated if hepatic perfusion is reduced. The development of metabolic acidosis and a rise in serum lactate indicate that blood flow to some tissues is inadequate to support aerobic metabolism.

Hypoglycemia (glucose ≤60 mg/dL) may be observed in seriously ill or injured infants, especially if intake has been compromised, and may be associated with cardiovascular or neurologic deterioration. As noted, *critical illness hyperglycemia, CIH* (glucose>150 mg/dL) may transiently develop in critically ill or injured children.

Clinically significant dehydration is associated with weight loss (Table 49.3). Fluid intake and output records (or reports from parents or primary caretakers) reveal a history of inadequate fluid intake or excessive fluid losses. The child with significant dehydration demonstrates dry mucous membranes, a sunken fontanel (in infants), and poor skin turgor (Table 49.4).[18]

Moderate isotonic dehydration produces signs of peripheral circulatory compromise, and severe isotonic dehydration will produce hypotension. The blood urea nitrogen (BUN) and urine specific gravity are usually elevated. The serum sodium concentration and osmolality are affected by the type and severity of dehydration present; in turn, they can affect the clinical presentation. Hypotension typically develops with greater than 10% isotonic or hypotonic dehydration in the infant or child, or greater than 6% to 7% dehydration in the adolescent.[18]

Hemorrhage is another potential cause of hypovolemic shock. To appreciate the significance of any blood lost or drawn for laboratory analysis, the total blood loss should be considered as a percentage of the child's circulating blood volume (Table 49.5).[10]

Tachycardia, peripheral vasoconstriction, and altered level of consciousness may be the only early signs of internal hemorrhage in the child with trauma (Table 49.6). Acute blood loss (hemorrhage) may not cause hypotension until an estimated 25% to 30% of intravascular volume is lost (i.e., an acute intravascular or blood loss of 16 to 24 mL/kg).[23–25] Once hypotension develops in the child with hemorrhage, cardiovascular collapse is imminent; immediate, rapid intravascular volume expansion is required, and surgical intervention may be needed.

Redistribution of blood volume associated with systemic vasodilation, high capillary pressure or transudative fluid losses, or capillary leak may produce a relative hypovolemia and signs of poor systemic perfusion in the absence of evidence of absolute volume loss. For example, children with end-stage hepatic failure may demonstrate a relative hypovolemia associated with ascites and hepatorenal syndrome. Maldistribution of blood flow with distributive shock (e.g., septic shock, neurogenic shock, or severe burns) also will produce signs of relative hypovolemia because intravascular volume is inadequate relative to the vascular space.

Evaluation and Treatment. Early detection is critical to optimize treatment for shock. Specific treatment of hypovolemic shock is volume resuscitation. Volume resuscitation is designed to restore intravascular volume relative to the vascular space and to optimize ventricular preload. The specific fluid selected and route of administration are determined by the child's clinical condition. In general, isotonic crystalloids (isotonic salt-containing solutions, such as normal saline or lactated Ringer solution) or colloids (protein-containing fluids, such as albumin or blood) are administered in boluses of 20 mL/kg given over 5 to 20 minutes. Modifications in bolus volume and rate of

TABLE 49.3 Dehydration and Hypovolemia

Type of Dehydration	Clinical Indicators
Isotonic dehydration	Fluid output exceeds intake. Loss of free water is proportional to loss of sodium, so serum sodium concentration remains normal. Fluid loss is from intravascular and extravascular compartments. Compromises peripheral perfusion when the young child has lost approximately 10% (100 mL/kg) of body weight. Compromises systemic perfusion in the adolescent with acute fluid loss equivalent to 5%–6% of body weight. Can produce hypotension (decompensated shock) when the young child has lost about 15% (150 mL/kg) of body weight. Can produce hypotension in the adolescent with a fluid loss equivalent to about 7%–9% of body weight because body water constitutes a smaller percentage of body weight in older children and adults than in young children.
Hypotonic/hyponatremic dehydration	Associated with a proportionately greater loss of sodium than free water; thus the serum sodium falls. Resultant acute fall in serum osmolality produces an acute extravascular fluid shift and further loss of extravascular volume. Fluid loss in hypotonic dehydration is primarily from the intravascular compartment; thus a compromise in systemic perfusion will be observed after even small quantities of fluid loss. Poor peripheral perfusion can develop in a child with a fluid loss equivalent to about 5% (50 mL/kg) of body weight. Adolescents with hyponatremic dehydration may demonstrate a compromise in peripheral perfusion with a fluid loss equivalent to approximately 3% of body weight. Hypotension often is observed when fluid loss is equal to approximately 10% (100 mL/kg) of body weight. Hypotension in an adolescent is observed when the fluid loss equals approximately 5%–6% of body weight.
Hypertonic/hypernatremic dehydration	Free water deficit is proportionately greater than the deficit of sodium, so serum sodium concentration rises, increasing serum osmolality and producing an intravascular shift of free water. For this reason the child with hypernatremic dehydration is likely to maintain intravascular volume and systemic perfusion until relatively large quantities of fluid are lost. Compromise in systemic perfusion is not likely to be observed in the *child* with hypernatremic dehydration until *severe* dehydration is present with a fluid loss equivalent to about 10% of body weight (or 5%–6% of body weight in the adolescent). Hypotension may not be observed until the fluid loss approximates 15% or more of body weight (7%–9% or more of body weight in the adolescent). Hypotension in the child with hypertonic/hypernatremic dehydration indicates a substantial fluid deficit. However, the deficit must be replaced carefully to correct shock and avoid rapid lowering of serum sodium concentrations.

Data in part from Roberts KB. Fluid and electrolytes: parenteral fluid therapy. *Pediatrics in Review*, 2001;22(11):380–387; Roberts KE. Fluid, electrolyte and endocrine problems. In: Hazinski MF, ed. *Nursing care of the critically ill child*, 3rd edition. St. Louis: Mosby; 2013.

TABLE 49.4 Severity of (Isotonic) Dehydration Based on Clinical Examination[a]

Clinical Parameters	Mild	Moderate	Severe
Approximate body weight loss			
• Infant	5% (50 mL/kg)	10% (100 mL/kg)	15% (150 mL/kg)
• Adolescent	3% (30 mL/kg)	5%–6% (50–60 mL/kg)	7%–9% (70–90 mL/kg)
General appearance	Alert, restless, thirsty	Lethargic, postural dizziness	Limp, coma, cold and cyanotic extremities
Radial pulse	Full	Thready, weak, rapid	Feeble, not palpable
Respiration	Normal	Deep	Deep, rapid
Skin elasticity	Pinch retracts immediately	Pinch retracts slowly	Pinch retracts very slowly (>2 sec)
Eyes	Normal	Sunken	Very sunken
Tears	Present	Diminished	Absent
Mucous membranes	Moist	Dry	Very dry (parched)
Urine output	Normal	↓	↓ or absent
Capillary refill time	<2 sec	>2 sec	Prolonged
Heart rate	Varies with age	Varies with age	Varies with age
Blood pressure	Normal	Normal	Reduced

Modified from Perkin RM, et al. Shock, cardiac arrest and resuscitation. In: Hazinski MF, ed. *Nursing care of the critically ill child*, 3rd edition. St. Louis: Mosby; 2013.

[a]The interpretation of the assessments must be appropriately modified for age and type of dehydration (hypotonic or hypertonic).

administration are made if hypovolemic shock is present in a child with myocardial dysfunction: smaller fluid boluses (5 to 10 mL/kg) are administered over about 10 to 20 minutes. If septic shock with hypotension is present and critical care is available, up to 2 to 3 boluses of 10 to 20 mL/kg are administered over 5 to 20 minutes.[3,16] Hypotonic fluids should not be administered.[1,17] Administration of packed red blood cells (PRBCs) (10 mL/kg) is generally reserved for the child with hemorrhagic shock (see Table 49.6). After each bolus, it is important to reassess systemic perfusion and administer additional fluids if indicated. Providers should halt bolus fluid administration immediately if the child develops signs of hypervolemia or new or worsening heart failure (e.g., new or worsening hepatomegaly, respiratory distress, or rales).

During treatment of shock caused by dehydration, providers must avoid acute or severe alterations in the serum sodium concentration.[1,18,26] Acute changes in serum sodium alter the serum osmolality and result in fluid shifts into and out of the vascular spaces. Such fluid shifts can be associated with neurologic complications including seizures, cerebral edema, and intracranial hemorrhage.[18]

TABLE 49.5 Estimation of Pediatric Circulating Blood Volume

Age of Child	Blood Volume (mL/kg Body Weight)
Newborn	80–85
Infant	75–80
Child	70–75
Adolescent	65–70

From Hazinski MF. Children are different. In: Hazinski MF, ed. *Nursing care of the critically ill child*, 3rd edition. St. Louis: Mosby; 2013.

Administration of blood or blood component therapy may be needed to treat hemorrhage. A "normal" hematocrit does not rule out the possibility of hemorrhage in the injured person; the hematocrit typically falls in a person who has sustained whole blood loss after the blood loss is replaced with crystalloids or colloids. When blood loss is significant, 10 mL/kg boluses of PRBCs are administered as needed to replace blood loss and maintain hemoglobin and hematocrit.[17]

The optimal hemoglobin threshold for transfusion in critically ill children is unknown. The Pediatric Critical Care Transfusion and Anemia Expertise Initiative (TAXI) recommends critically ill children with a hemoglobin concentration of less than 5 g/dL receive PRBC transfusion; children with a hemoglobin concentration of >5 g/dL but <7 g/dL, the decision is based on clinical judgment; and children with a hemoglobin concentration of greater than 7 g/dL no PRBC transfusion be given.[27] However, higher hemoglobin and hematocrit thresholds may be necessary for unstable children with cardiac or respiratory disease, cyanotic CHD, and those with hemodynamic instability.[27]

Cardiogenic Shock

Cardiogenic shock is present when impaired myocardial function compromises cardiac output. In children, cardiac failure is most commonly due to CHD, cardiomyopathies, myocarditis, or arrhythmias.[2]

This form of shock is observed:

1. Following cardiovascular surgery or with inflammatory disease of the heart (e.g., cardiomyopathy and myocarditis)
2. With drug toxicity or severe electrolyte or acid-base imbalances
3. As a complication of any form of shock, and early in septic shock

Pathophysiology. In the early stages of cardiogenic shock, adrenergic compensatory mechanisms produce tachycardia,

TABLE 49.6 Classification of Pediatric Hemorrhagic Shock in Trauma Patients Based on Clinical Evaluation

System	Mild Hemorrhage, Compensated Shock, Simple Hypovolemia (<30%)	Moderate Hemorrhage, Decompensated Shock, Marked Hypovolemia (30%–45%)	Severe Hemorrhage, Cardiopulmonary Failure, Profound Hypovolemia (>45%)
Cardiovascular	Tachycardia Weak peripheral pulses, strong central pulses Low to normal blood pressure (systolic BP >70 mmHg+[2×age in years]) Mild acidosis	Moderate tachycardia Thready peripheral pulses, weak central pulses Frank hypotension (systolic BP <70 mmHg+[2×age in years]) Moderate acidosis	Severe tachycardia Absent peripheral pulses, thready central pulses Profound hypotension (systolic BP <50 mmHg) Severe acidosis
Respiratory	Mild tachypnea	Moderate tachypnea	Severe tachypnea
Central nervous system	Irritable, confused	Agitated or lethargic	Obtunded, comatose
Skin	Cool extremities, mottling Poor capillary refill (>2 s)	Cool extremities, pallor Delayed capillary refill (>2 s)	Cool extremities, cyanosis Prolonged (>5 s) capillary refill
Kidneys	Mild oliguria, increased specific gravity	Marked oliguria, increased blood urea nitrogen (BUN)	Anuria

From Soud T, Pieper P, Hazinski MF. Pediatric trauma. In: Hazinski MF, ed. *Nursing care of the critically ill child*, 2nd edition. St. Louis: Mosby; 1992.

peripheral vasoconstriction, and constriction of the splanchnic arteries to divert blood flow from the skin, gut, and kidneys to maintain flow to the heart and brain.[1–3] These compensatory mechanisms may initially be sufficient to maintain the systolic blood pressure and effective coronary and cerebral blood flow. However, tachycardia and systemic arterial constriction increase myocardial oxygen consumption. In addition, reduction in gut and kidney blood flow may produce hepatic, mesenteric, or renal ischemia or failure. Decreased renal perfusion stimulates the renin-angiotensin-aldosterone system, as described for hypovolemic shock.[1]

A fall in the mean arterial pressure or pulse pressure reduces stimulation of the baroreceptors in the carotid sinuses and aortic arch. This reduced baroreceptor activity removes inhibition from the vasomotor center in the medulla, resulting in increased adrenergic stimulation.[1] If myocardial dysfunction progresses, cardiac output and blood pressure ultimately fall. Myocardial ischemia then exacerbates myocardial dysfunction, and multisystem organ failure may result from persistent or severe organ ischemia.

Clinical Manifestations. The child with cardiogenic shock demonstrates signs of inadequate systemic perfusion despite evidence of adequate intravascular volume or even relative hypervolemia. This form of shock is generally associated with low cardiac output. The child's extremities are cool to touch (the extremities will cool from peripherally to proximally), with delayed capillary refill despite a warm, ambient temperature.[1] The skin may be mottled (see Fig. 49.1). If myocardial function is severely compromised, peripheral pulses may be diminished in intensity (dampened) or they may vary in intensity (pulsus alternans).

Evidence of systemic venous congestion, including high CVP, hepatomegaly, and periorbital edema, is typically present in cardiogenic shock, particularly if right ventricular failure is involved. The presence of venous congestion is considered "wet," the absence is described as "dry"; hypoperfusion is considered "cold," whereas normal perfusion is "warm."[28]

Evidence of pulmonary edema may be identified on a chest radiograph or clinical assessment (including signs of respiratory distress, reduced lung compliance during hand ventilation, or frothy pink sputum suctioned from the endotracheal tube) if left ventricular failure is present. The cardiac silhouette on the chest radiograph is usually enlarged, unless concurrent hypovolemia is present.

A low cardiac output may be documented by invasive or noninvasive devices. The $ScvO_2$ will be more than 25% to 30% below the arterial oxygen saturation. Signs of low cardiac output and cardiogenic shock can be similar to signs of cardiac tamponade. Although some classic signs, including muffled heart tones, or pulsus paradoxus, may be observed with tamponade, these signs may be difficult to appreciate if cardiac output and blood pressure are severely compromised. Therefore, if cardiogenic shock is suspected in a child after cardiovascular surgery or in any child at risk for the development of pericardial effusion, tamponade should be ruled out through an echocardiogram.

In infants following surgery for CHD, a low cardiac output syndrome score (LCOSS) can be calculated by assigning one point each for tachycardia (>20% higher than post induction heart rate in operating room), oliguria (<1 mL/kg/h), toe temperature less than 30°C (86°F), need for volume administration of >30 mL/kg/day, decreased near infrared spectrometry (NIRS) measurements (cerebral NIRS <50% and renal NIRS <75% of arterial saturation), arterial lactate >2 mmol/L, and need for vasoactive/inotropes beyond milrinone at 0.5 μg/kg/min. The score is assessed at ICU admission, 8, 12, and 24 hours postoperatively. Morbidity and resource utilization can be significantly higher among infants with peak LCOSS ≥4 and those with a cumulative LCOSS ≥7.[29]

Evaluation and Treatment. Treatment targeting cardiogenic shock requires titration of fluid boluses as needed to optimize cardiac preload. These boluses of 5 to 10 mL/kg of isotonic crystalloid are delivered over about 10 to 20 minutes and should be stopped immediately if the child develops signs of hypervolemia or new or worsening heart failure (e.g., new or worsening hepatomegaly, respiratory distress, or rales). Vasoactive drugs are needed to improve myocardial function and inodilators; vasodilators or vasoconstrictors may be needed to support systemic perfusion. Table 49.7 summarizes drug therapy for children in shock.[1]

Distributive/Septic Shock

With distributive (septic, anaphylactic, and neurogenic) shock, vasodilation and increased capillary permeability are typically present, and blood flow is unregulated throughout the skin and organ systems, so a normal cardiac output is likely to be inadequate to maintain sufficient perfusion of all tissue beds. Neurogenic shock is a form of hypovolemic and vasogenic (maldistributive) shock. It is caused by a loss of vasomotor tone after severe head or spinal cord injury. Massive vasodilation and loss of sympathomimetic tone result in a relative hypovolemia and hypotension. The loss of sympathetic tone prevents compensatory tachycardia.

Sepsis and its complications result from activation of biochemical and physiologic cascades that lead to the formation or activation of cytokines and other mediators that produce vasodilation, increased capillary permeability, maldistribution of blood flow, and cardiovascular and cellular dysfunction.[1] Sepsis and its complications may result in MODS or NPMODS and are leading causes of death in noncoronary intensive care units. In 2005, in the United States, there were more than 75,000 pediatric hospitalizations involving severe sepsis, with an overall mortality of 8.9% to 24%.[30]

In Hartman and colleagues,[30,31] hospital data from seven states provide the most detailed information regarding causes of pediatric sepsis in the United States. In 2013, this group reported data through 2005 and in a subsequent 2019, reported on data from 2005 through 2011.[31] In this data set, an infecting microorganism was identified in less than 40% of infants and children with severe sepsis.[30] The most common sites of identified infection were respiratory tract (roughly 50%) and bacteremia (about 20%).[30] In a more recent series from the Children's Hospital Association of nearly 50,000 children with pediatric severe sepsis from 2004 to 2012,[32] approximately two-thirds of children with severe sepsis

TABLE 49.7 Pediatric Vasoactive Drugs for the Treatment of Shock[a]

Dose	Effects	Cautions
Sympathomimetics		
Dobutamine: 2–20 μg/min	Selective β-adrenergic effects, increases cardiac contractility and also increases heart rate (this latter effect is variable); β_2 effects produce peripheral vasodilation; no dopaminergic or α-adrenergic effects	Extreme tachyarrhythmias have been reported, particularly in infants; hypotension may develop; may produce pulmonary vasoconstriction
Dopamine: 1–5 μg/kg per min	Dopaminergic effects predominate, including increase in glomerular filtration rate and urine volume	Can produce extreme tachyarrhythmias; can result in increase in pulmonary artery pressure; inhibits thyroid-stimulating hormone and aldosterone secretion
Dopamine: 2–10 μg/kg per min	Dopaminergic effects persist and β_1 effects are seen, especially an increase in heart rate	As Dopamine 1–5
Dopamine: 8–20 μg/kg per min	α-Adrenergic effects dominate	As Dopamine 1–5
Epinephrine: 0.05–0.15 μg/kg per min	Endogenous catecholamine, which produces α, β_1, and β_2 adrenergic effects; at low doses, β_1 effects dominate	Will increase myocardial work and oxygen consumption at any dose; splanchnic constriction will occur at even low doses
Epinephrine: 0.2–0.3 μg/kg per min	α-Adrenergic (vasoconstrictive) effects dominate	As Epinephrine 0.05–0.15
Isoproterenol: 0.05–0.1 μg/kg per min	β-Adrenergic effects; β_1 effects may result in rapid increase in heart rate; β_2 effects may produce peripheral vasodilation and also may effectively treat bronchoconstriction	Monitor for tachyarrhythmias, hypotension; will increase myocardial oxygen consumption
Norepinephrine: 0.05–1 μg/kg per min	Endogenous catecholamine with α- and β-adrenergic effects; produces potent peripheral and renal vasoconstriction; can increase blood pressure	May cause tachyarrhythmias, increased myocardial work, and increased oxygen consumption; may result in hepatic and mesenteric ischemia
Vasopressin		
Vasopressin: 0.2–2 milliunits/kg per min (0.0002–0.002 unit/kg per min)	Antidiuretic hormone analog that acts on vasopressin receptors; produces peripheral and splanchnic vasoconstriction; also used to treat GI hemorrhage for this reason	May cause hypertension, bradycardia
Phosphodiesterase Inhibitor/Inodilator		
Milrinone: loading dose, 0.05 mg/kg (50 μg/kg) over 10–60 min; infusion, 0.25–0.75 μg/kg per min	Nonadrenergic inotropic agent that produces phosphodiesterase inhibition and increase in intracellular cyclic adenosine monophosphate (cAMP); intracellular calcium uptake also is delayed; these effects result in improved cardiac contractility and vasodilation	Monitor for arrhythmias (especially accelerated junctional rhythm, junctional tachycardia, and ventricular ectopy); may produce hypotension (especially if person is hypovolemic), liver and GI dysfunction, thrombocytopenia, and abdominal pain; experience in children is limited and recent Reduce dose when renal dysfunction present
Vasodilators		
Nitroglycerin: 0.25–0.5 μg/kg per min; increase as tolerated to maximum 10 μg/kg/min (adolescents, 5 μg/min; Note not per kg per min)	Arterial and venodilator	Is absorbed by polyvinyl chloride tubing; use special infusion set
Nitroprusside: 0.3–0.5 μg/kg per min; titrate up to 8 μg/kg per min (max. infusion dose: 8–10 μg/kg per min)	Arterial and venodilator	Light sensitive; use special infusion set or cover tubing when infusion slow; may produce thiocyanate and cyanide toxicity, particularly for higher doses or prolonged infusion

Modified from Perkin RM, et al. Shock, cardiac arrest and resuscitation. In: Hazinski MF, ed. *Nursing care of the critically ill child,* 3rd edition. St. Louis: Mosby; 2013: p 120 and Kadec KD, McBride ME, et al. 2020 *AHA pediatric advanced life support provider manual.* Dallas, TX: American Heart Association; 2020.

GI, Gastrointestinal.

[a]Infusion rate=mL/h=Weight (kg)×Dose (μg/kg/min)×60 min/h concentration (μg/mL).

had chronic disease. Among these children, bloodstream infections were most common (67.8%), with a high incidence of respiratory (57.2%) sites of infection. Genitourinary infections were identified in one-fifth, with device infection, cardiovascular infection, and abdominal infections as additional sources.

An international series characterizing children with septic shock has been published by the Pediatric Acute Lung Injury and the Sepsis Investigators Network.[33] In this series, an infectious microorganism was identified in 65% of children, with respiratory (40%) and bloodstream (19%) infections the most frequent sources.

The microorganisms that cause sepsis vary according to age, immune function, and location. In the two large pediatric series from the United States, the most commonly reported infecting microorganisms were staphylococcus, streptococcus, and fungal infections, with fewer gram-negative and viral infections.[30,32] Fungal infections were much more common among children with cancer. When viral infections were documented, concomitant bacterial infections were nearly always present.[30] In the international series of children with severe sepsis, gram-negative (28%) and gram-positive (27%) microorganisms are identified approximately equally, followed by viruses (21%) and fungi (21%).[33]

Prevention of hospital-acquired infections can substantially reduce the risk of infection, sepsis, and its complications.[34] Clinicians must be aware of the common pathogens in various populations.

Factors associated with risk for the development of sepsis include extremes of age (risk highest among infants, young children, and older adults)[1,30,32]; chronic diseases; invasive catheters, surgical incisions, or wounds or burns; immunocompromise; and long-term antibiotic therapy.[32,35] As noted earlier in data from children's hospitals, two-thirds of children with severe sepsis had a chronic disease.[32]

It is now clear that genetic characteristics of the child, as well as of the invading microorganisms, alter the outcome of infections, sepsis, and septic shock.[36,37] Certainly, infectious diseases, such as meningococcal disease, can vary widely in invasiveness and severity of clinical consequences.[38]

Both pro-inflammatory and anti-inflammatory cytokines serve essential protective functions in fighting infection and modulating the immune response. Sepsis is caused by the effects of the invading microorganism and its toxins, and most effects that contribute to septic shock result from a disruption in the balance between *pro-inflammatory* mediators (including tumor necrosis factor-alpha [TNF-α], interleukin [IL]-1, IL-6, and IL-8; platelet-activating factor; arachidonic acid metabolites; nitric oxide; and many kinins) and *anti-inflammatory* mediators (IL-4, IL-10, IL-11, and IL-13; transforming growth factor-beta; colony-stimulating factors; soluble tumor necrosis factor receptor; IL-1 receptor antagonist; and activated protein C).[1] Extremely high levels of pro-inflammatory mediators, such as TNF, nitric oxide, and platelet-activating factor, can become destructive, even when they eradicate the triggering microorganism.[1,36]

High pro-inflammatory cytokine levels have been implicated in the development of sepsis-induced disseminated intravascular coagulation, pulmonary injury, and microcirculatory disruptions, similar to those observed with burns, severe trauma, shock reperfusion syndromes, post cardiac arrest, and MODS.[36] Tumor necrosis factor levels have been directly related to mortality in newborns and children with meningitis and sepsis,[1] and interleukin-8 levels have been shown to be reliable predictors of pediatric sepsis mortality.[37]

An increase in plasma nitric oxide concentration contributes to vasodilation, hypotension, and decreased myocardial function that develop during adult sepsis. However, infants with sepsis often demonstrate pulmonary vasoconstriction from shock-induced acidosis and hypoxia and may benefit from administration of inhaled nitric oxide or other vasodilators.[39]

During sepsis, the endothelium becomes a secretory organ, changing from the normal profibrinolytic and anticoagulant state to an antifibrinolytic and procoagulant one.[39] This change can lead to the development of microthrombi in some areas of the microcirculation, further contributing to the maldistribution of blood flow. Mediators that regulate coagulation pathways have been implicated in the sepsis process.[39] Activated protein C normally curtails the inflammatory process once the invading microorganism is destroyed, and a deficiency in activated protein C is a marker for severe sepsis in all ages.[40] Although administration of activated protein C improved survival in one study of adults with severe sepsis,[41] subsequent adult studies failed to replicate this result.[42] A study in children was halted because the activated protein C produced excessive bleeding complications.[39,42]

C-reactive protein (CRP) binds to both bacteria and macrophages and activates the complement system. The complement system is a series of proteins that helps macrophages eliminate (opsonize) invading microorganisms; these proteins also participate in the clotting cascade. CRP concentration normally rises with infection and falls when the infection is adequately treated with antibiotics, so it is a useful component to monitor response to infection. Ferritin is released when macrophages are activated in response to sepsis, injury, and inflammation. In a small sample of children with severe sepsis, mortality was highest (46.5%) among those with both a CRP ≥4.08 mg/dL and a ferritin ≥1980 ng/mL and lowest (0%) among those with a CRP and ferritin below said thresholds.[43]

There is clear interaction among catecholamines, adrenoreceptors, and glucocorticoids contributing to CIH. Endogenous glucocorticoids decrease activation of pro-inflammatory mediators, and the pro-inflammatory mediators contribute to a relative insulin resistance. The glucocorticoids modulate vasomotor tone by enhancing cardiovascular and vasomotor response to catecholamines.[44]

Critically ill children may have absolute or relative adrenal insufficiency, caused by adrenal hemorrhage, decreased renal perfusion, inhibition of corticosteroid production by TNF, or actual adrenal disease, with inadequate adrenal stress response or decreased response to circulating glucocorticoids.[45,46] When sepsis is present and the child fails to respond to initial fluid therapy and vasoactive support, providers should rule out adrenal insufficiency and consider hydrocortisone administration.[47]

Septic shock

Clinical Manifestations. Sepsis and its complications produce a cascade of physiologic and biochemical changes. The clinical progression of sepsis in children was initially defined in 2005 by an international consensus panel (Box 49.3).[48] These definitions have been further refined by the Pediatric Collaborative Group of the Society of Critical Care Medicine, with decreased focus on identification of the SIRS or sepsis, and increased focus on immediate recognition and treatment of septic shock.[47] These definitions and criteria have not been validated in newborns and are found in only about half of newborns with culture-positive sepsis.[15]

Systemic inflammatory response syndrome (SIRS) represents a nonspecific response to a variety of insults, including trauma, burns, pancreatitis, or infection. SIRS is present when the child demonstrates two or more of the following as an acute change from baseline: change in temperature, specifically fever (greater than 38.5°C [101.3°F]) or hypothermia (less than 36°C [96.8°F]); change in heart rate (tachypnea or, in infants, bradycardia); change in respiratory rate (or need for mechanical ventilation); or change in white blood cell (WBC) count (including leukocytes, leukopenia, or an increase in the percentage of immature or band forms of WBCs).[48] These clinical signs must be interpreted in light of the child's baseline organ and system function.

Sepsis is a systemic response to infection. It is present when manifestations of SIRS are observed in conjunction with suspected infection. Positive cultures are not necessary for the diagnosis, but suspicion of infection is required.[48]

Septic newborns are more likely to demonstrate a decrease in heart rate variability rather than overt tachycardia or bradycardia. Fever is uncommon in newborns, and hypothermia may relate more to inadequate temperature support rather than hypothermia. Finally, no complete blood count (CBC) variable has been shown to reliably identify septic newborns.[15]

Severe sepsis is present when the child with sepsis (SIRS+suspected infection) develops cardiovascular or pulmonary dysfunction, or if the child has sepsis and evidence of two or more other organ dysfunctions.[48] The dysfunctional organ should be separate from the site of suspected infection and not explained by effects of drug therapy or other acute effects.[48] This important distinction helps separate signs of severe sepsis from signs of simple pneumonia with respiratory failure.

Septic shock is present when the septic child develops cardiovascular dysfunction characterized by hypotension or three or more signs of altered perfusion.[47]

Experts have proposed simplified consensus criteria for the recognition of pediatric septic shock. Kissoon, Orr, and Carcillo[49] suggested a simplified triad of fever, tachycardia, and vasodilation as diagnostic for pediatric sepsis, with septic shock likely when an altered level of consciousness is added to this triad. Carcillo and colleagues[39,49] distilled the international consensus definitions of septic shock to include suspected infection with hypo- or

BOX 49.3 Potential Clinical Findings in Infants and Children With Septic Shock

Potential Alterations in Temperature

Core body temperature of >38.5°C (101.3°F) or <36°C (96.8°F)

Hypotension

Systolic blood pressure less than

- 60 mmHg in infant newborn to 1 months
- 70 mmHg in infant 1 month to 1 year
- 70+2 (age in years) for children 1–10 years of age

Potential Alterations in Heart Rate

Tachycardia in the absence of external stimulus, chronic drugs, or painful stimuli, defined as follows:

- Newborn to 1 year: >180 beats/min
- 2–5 years: >140 beats/min
- 6–12 years: >130 beats/min
- 13 to <18 years: >110 beats/min

Otherwise unexplained persistent elevation in heart rate over a 0.5- to 4-h time period

For children younger than 1 year: bradycardia, in the absence of external vagal stimulus, β-blocker drugs, or congenital heart disease, defined by one of the following rates:

- Newborn to 1 month: <100 beats/min
- 1 month to 1 year: <90 beats/min

Otherwise unexplained persistent depression in neonatal heart rate over a 30-minute time period. Lack of neonatal heart rate variability has also been associated with other signs of clinical deterioration.

Potential Alterations in Respiratory Rate

Mean respiratory rate >95th percentile normal for age, as follows:

- Newborn to 1 week: >50 beats/min
- 1 week to 1 month: >40 beats/min
- 1 month to 1 year: >34 beats/min
- 2–5 years: >22 beats/min
- 6–12 years: >18 beats/min
- 13 to <18 years: >14 beats/min
- Mechanical ventilation for an acute process not related to underlying neuromuscular disease or the receipt of general anesthesia

Potential Alterations in Capillary Refill: either prolonged (>2 s) or "flash" (instantaneous)

Potential Alterations in Mental Status: Agitated or with decreased responsiveness

Potential Alterations in Pulse: Decreased/weak or bounding

Potential Alterations in Skin

- Mottled
- Ruddy/red
- Petechiae or purpura

Modified from Perkin RM, et al. Shock, cardiac arrest and resuscitation. In: Hazinski MF, ed. *Nursing care of the critically ill child,* 3rd edition. St. Louis: Mosby; 2013; Goldstein B, Giroir B, Randolph A, et al. International pediatric sepsis consensus conference: Definitions for sepsis and organ dysfunction in pediatrics. *Pediatric Critical Care Medicine*, 2005;6(1):2–8; and Davis AL, Carcillo JA, Aneja RK, et al. American College of Critical Care Medicine clinical practice parameters for hemodynamic support of pediatric and neonatal septic shock. *Critical Care Medicine,* 2017;45(6):1061–1093. doi:10.1097/CCM.0000000000002425; Weiss SL, Peters MJ, Alhazzani W, et al. Executive summary: Surviving sepsis campaign international guidelines for the management of septic shock and sepsis-associated organ dysfunction in children. *Intensive Care Medicine,* 2020;46(suppl 1):1–9. doi:10.1007/s00134-019-05877-7.

hyperthermia and clinical signs of inadequate perfusion. These signs of inadequate perfusion include any of the following: decreased level of conscious or change in mental status; prolonged (>2 seconds) capillary refill; abnormal pulses (either diminished or bounding with wide pulse pressure); mottled, cool extremities; or decreased urine output. Hypotension is not required for the diagnosis but, if present, is confirmatory.[39,49]

In 2017, the American College of Critical Care Medicine (ACCM) recommended that every hospital caring for children establish tools for identifying infants and children with the likelihood of septic shock and trigger bundled protocols for immediate resuscitation and stabilization.[47] The ACCM Pediatric Collaborative proposed a simplified sample list of eight potential triggers (Box 49.4) in the child presenting with "concern for infection or temperature abnormality." These eight criteria include: abnormal temperature, hypotension, tachycardia, tachypnea, abnormal capillary refill, abnormal mental status, abnormal pulse, and abnormal skin. Presence of three or more of these eight criteria, or two or more of these eight in a high-risk individual (i.e., one with malignancy, bone marrow or solid organ transplant, immunodeficiency, immunocompromise, immunosuppression, cerebral palsy, developmental delay, or indwelling catheter) is consistent with sepsis/septic shock and should trigger immediate (within 15 minutes) clinical assessment and activation of the resuscitation bundle of interventions. Hypotension itself is an immediate trigger for such escalation of care.[47]

BOX 49.4 Society of Critical Care Medicine Pediatric Collaborative Sample Findings to Trigger Septic Shock Resuscitation and Stabilization Bundles of Care

While assessing vital signs, obtaining history and performing physical examination (including evaluation of mental status, skin perfusion, pulses and capillary refill), identify any of the following potential triggers

- Temperature abnormality
- Hypotension (child immediately requires activation of septic shock resuscitation and stabilization bundle)
- Tachycardia
- Tachypnea
- Capillary refill abnormality
- Mental status abormality
- Pulse abnormality
- Skin abnormality

The child meets criteria for activation of septic shock resuscitation and stabilization bundle if hypotension is present, OR 3 or more of the above triggers are present, OR 2 or more of the above triggers are present in a high-risk individual (i.e., one with malignancy, bone marrow or solid organ transplant, immunodeficiency, immunocompromise, immunosuppression, cerebral palsy, developmental delay, or indwelling catheter).

From Davis AL, Carcillo JA, Aneja RK, et al. American College of Critical Care Medicine clinical practice parameters for hemodynamic support of pediatric and neonatal septic shock. *Critical Care Medicine,* 2017;45(6):1061–1093. doi:10.1097/CCM.0000000000002425; Weiss SL, Peters MJ, Alhazzani W, et al. Executive summary: Surviving sepsis campaign international guidelines for the management of septic shock and sepsis-associated organ dysfunction in children. *Intensive Care Medicine,* 2020;46(suppl 1):1–9. doi:10.1007/s00134-019-05877-7.

Infants and children with septic shock may have a high, normal, or low cardiac output. Preterm newborns may maintain cardiac output but demonstrate severe vasodilation.[50] Unlike adults, who typically present with vasodilation, hypotension, and normal or high cardiac output, approximately half of children with septic shock present with severe peripheral vasoconstriction, high systemic vascular resistance, and low cardiac output.[39,49] Among children with CHD, sepsis is most likely to produce a decrease in cardiac output and perfusion and, postoperatively, is more likely to lead to the development of MODS.[35]

The terms *warm* and *cold septic shock* are imprecise terms and should be used only in conjunction with other descriptions of systemic perfusion and cardiovascular function.[51] Warm shock is typically associated with peripheral vasodilation, warm skin with flash/immediate capillary refill, bounding pulses, and wide pulse pressure. Cold shock is typically associated with peripheral vasoconstriction, cold skin with prolon-ged capillary refill, and decreased peripheral pulses; these characteristics are present in almost half of children who present with septic shock.[51] Cardiac output may be low, normal, or high regardless of skin temperature, perfusion, and pulses; these characteristics alone will not identify the cardiovascular support required.

Evaluation and Treatment

Resuscitation and stabilization bundle of care. The child with septic shock has hypovolemia, poor perfusion, and maldistribution of blood flow that requires immediate (within 15 minutes of identification of signs of septic shock) clinician assessment and activation of the *resuscitation bundle of care.* Within the next 5 minutes, providers should establish intravenous or intraosseous access; and within 15 to 30 minutes, clinicians should initiate appropriate bolus fluid resuscitation. Clinicians should also obtain a blood sample for culture and sensitivity *if* it does not delay antibiotic administration and correct hypocalcemia and hypoglycemia.

Within 60 minutes of the septic shock diagnosis, clinicians should administer broad-spectrum empiric antibiotics and, for fluid-refractory septic shock, initiate and titrate vasoactive drugs.[26,47] Therapeutic goals include restoring systemic perfusion and blood pressure; normalizing heart rate, improving capillary refill, pulses, and urine output; maintaining adequate oxygen delivery; and controlling/eliminating the infection.[3,16,26,47,49,52,53]

For fluid resuscitation, the 2020 Surviving Sepsis International Guidelines now provide caveats regarding recommendations for fluid resuscitation for septic shock based on the presence or absence of hypotension and the availability of critical care resources within the system caring for the infant or child.[16]

For the child in septic shock WITH availability of critical care resources: Within the first hour, administer up to 2 to 3 fluid boluses of 10 to 20 mL/kg of isotonic crystalloid, titrated to clinical response (e.g., improve blood pressure and systemic perfusion, normalize heart rate, and improve urine output). Assessment is needed after each bolus to determine the tolerance of the bolus and the need for further boluses. Cease fluid bolus administration if new or worsening signs of fluid overload/heart failure (new or worsening rales, crackles, or hepatomegaly) develop.[3,16]

For the child with septic shock and hypotension WITHOUT availability of critical care resources: In the first hour, begin fluid bolus administration. Provide up to two fluid boluses of 10- to 20 mL/kg of isotonic crystalloid, titrated to patient response, as noted previously. Up to 40 mL/kg can be administered within the first hour. Halt fluid administration if signs of fluid overload/new or worsening heart failure develop.[3,16]

For the infant or child with septic shock but no hypotension WITHOUT availability of critical care resources: The 2020 Surviving Sepsis International Guidelines recommend against bolus fluid administration for these individuals. Instead, they recommend that providers begin maintenance fluid administration.[3,16] As noted, initiation of vasoactive drug administration is necessary within 60 minutes of the diagnosis of septic shock if shock persists despite bolus fluid administration. The evidence for the selection of an initial vasoactive agent is extremely limited. In a small, randomized prospective trial in children with septic shock, the use of epinephrine was associated with higher survival (14% vs. 7%) than the use of dopamine.[54] However, experts agree that the doses of epinephrine used in this study were likely to produce a greater physiologic effect than the doses of dopamine used in the study, so many questions remain.[55] The 2017 ACCM review and the 2020 Surviving Sepsis International review identified no evidence regarding the use of norepinephrine in pediatric septic shock.[47]

Considering the evidence limitations, pediatric experts authoring both the ACCM and the Surviving Sepsis International Guidelines reported their clinical preference (e.g., expert opinion) for use of epinephrine in persons with septic shock, myocardial dysfunction and low cardiac output, and their clinical preference for use of norepinephrine for children with septic shock and vasodilation.[16,47] If central venous access is not available, epinephrine and dopamine can be administered via peripheral intravenous catheter with great caution to monitor for tissue extravasation.[47]

In a small, but seminal, 1991 study of children with septic shock, Carcillo, Davis, and Zaritsky[52] showed that rapid fluid resuscitation within the first hour of therapy was associated with significantly higher survival than less aggressive fluid resuscitation. As a result, until recently, clinicians administered multiple (2 to 3 or more) fluid boluses in the first hours of resuscitation to children in septic shock. However, experts now agree that during resuscitation of the child in septic shock, clinicians must focus both on the importance of treating hypovolemia and on the importance of preventing the development of hypervolemia or new or worsening heart failure.[3,16] This is the reason for the modified recommendations to administer *up to* 2 to 3 fluid boluses of 10 to 20 mL/kg (rather than 2 to 3 or more boluses of 20 mL/kg) and re-emphasis on the need for careful evaluation of the child's response to each fluid bolus, halting bolus fluid administration if signs of hypervolemia or new or worsening heart failure develop (e.g., new or worsening signs of respiratory distress, rales, or hepatomegaly).[16]

A positive response includes evidence of improved cardiac output and systemic perfusion. These recommendations are consistent with those of the AHA Pediatric Advanced Cardiac Life Support guidelines.[3]

As noted, clinicians must administer broad-spectrum empiric antibiotics within 60 minutes of identification of septic shock. Note that this 60-minute interval begins as soon as the child is diagnosed; this diagnosis and start of the 60-minute interval may occur in the prehospital setting. Emergency surgical consultation is indicated if infection source control is likely to require surgical intervention.

Within 60 minutes, if the child is at risk for absolute adrenal insufficiency, or the shock is refractory to fluid and vasoactive drug administration, clinicians should consider the administration of hydrocortisone.[47]

The *stabilization bundle of care* requires multimodal monitoring of cardiac and pulmonary function, as well as monitoring and support of other organ system functions to guide fluid, hormone (e.g., hydrocortisone), vasoactive, and renal therapies. Cardiovascular targets include a normal perfusion pressure (i.e., difference between mean arterial pressure and CVP [MAP-CVP] of 55 mmHg+1.5×age in years), an $ScvO_2$ greater than 70%, and/or a cardiac index of 3.3 to 6.0 L/min/m^2.[47]

Frequent monitoring of serum lactate is helpful, as a fall in serum lactate should accompany improvement in systemic perfusion. Early use of renal replacement therapies aids in hemodynamic support and maintenance of appropriate intravascular volume.[1,47]

An algorithm for the treatment of septic shock, based on the recommendations of the ACCM and the Pediatric Advanced Life Support course, is presented in Fig. 49.2.

Performance bundle of care. Every system caring for infants and children in septic shock must establish a process of continuous quality of improvement. This requires an organized system to monitor not only the treatment provided but also the interval required to identify the individual in septic shock and initiate appropriate resuscitation and stabilization. Such continuous quality improvement programs are designed to identify barriers to timely treatment and ensure that treatment adheres to best practice guidelines (e.g., ACCM and AHA PALS Guidelines). Implementation of the ACCM consensus recommendations for hemodynamic support of children with septic shock has been associated with decreased mortality (from 35% to 40% mortality to 2% to 8% mortality).[47,49] In fact, for every hour of delay in the restoration of normal blood pressure for age and restoration of capillary refill less than 3 seconds, mortality from pediatric septic shock can double.[39,47,49] Ames et al. published an excellent editorial summarizing important steps for improving outcomes of septic shock.[56]

Neurogenic Shock

Clinical Manifestations. Signs of neurogenic shock in the child with a recent, severe spinal cord injury include warm skin and hypotension with a low diastolic blood pressure. Signs of poor systemic perfusion also are observed (see Assessment of Shock), although the loss of sympathetic nervous system tone prevents the typical tachycardic response.

Evaluation and Treatment. Treatment of neurogenic shock includes positioning to enhance venous return, bolus fluid therapy as needed to support cardiac output, and administration of vasopressors to treat fluid-refractory hypotension. Supplementary warming or cooling is likely to be needed to support normothermia.[26]

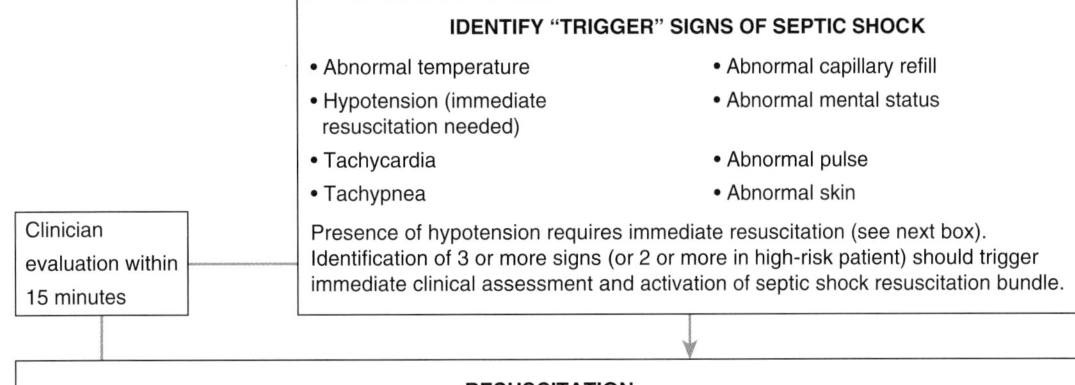

RESUSCITATION

Give oxygen and support airway, breathing and oxygenation; provide early intubation and mechanical ventilation

Begin resuscitation and treat infection

- *Within 15 minutes*: Establish IV/IO access; draw blood samples including for blood culture and sensitivity *if it will not delay* fluid and antibiotic administration
- *Within 30 minutes*: Give 10–20 mL/kg bolus of isotonic crystalloid; reassess, give up to 2–3 boluses if signs of shock persist. STOP bolus fluid administration if signs of hypervolemia or new or worsening heart failure develop (hepatomegaly, crackles, rales)
- *Within 60 minutes*: Give antibiotics. If shock is refractory to fluid administration, begin vasoactive infusion. Epinephrine or dopamine may be given via peripheral IV if no central venous catheter in place; watch carefully for extravasation.

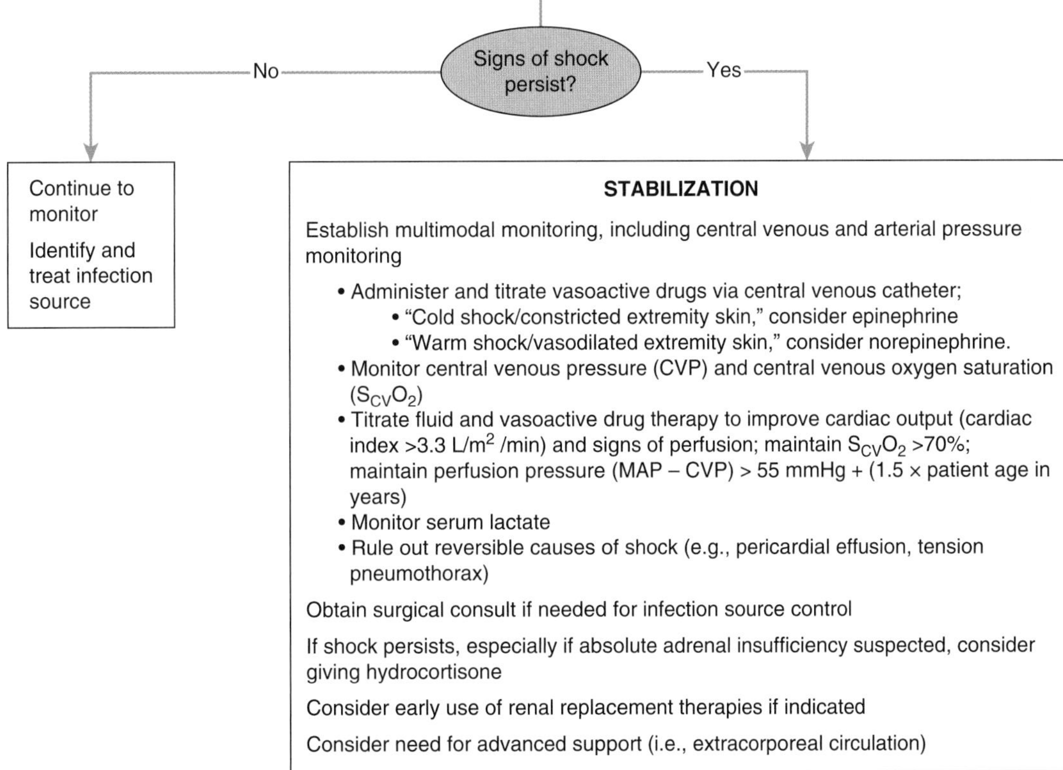

Fig. 49.2 Hemodynamic Support in Pediatric Septic Shock When Critical Care Is Available. *BSA*, Body surface area; *IO*, intake/output; *IV*, intravenous. (Modified from Perkin RM, et al. Shock, cardiac arrest and resuscitation. In: Hazinski MF, ed. *Nursing care of the critically ill child*, 3rd edition. St. Louis: Mosby; 2013:126. Updated to include information from: Davis AL, Carcillo JA, Deymann AJ, et al. The American College of Critical Care Medicine clinical practice parameters for hemodynamic support of pediatric and neonatal septic shock: Executive summary. *Pediatric Critical Care Medicine*, 2017;18:884–890.)

Obstructive Shock

Pathophysiology. Obstructive shock is inadequate cardiac output caused by an impediment to blood flow to or from the heart into the pulmonary or systemic circulation. Causes of obstructive shock in children include congenital heart defects (such as critical aortic stenosis and those with ductal-dependent pulmonary or systemic blood flow), tension pneumothorax, and pulmonary embolus. Obstruction to blood flow results in low cardiac output and circulatory collapse, typically with signs of peripheral vasoconstriction as adrenergic stimulation diverts blood flow from the skin, gut, and kidney to the heart and brain. Signs of systemic or pulmonary venous obstruction are observed.

Clinical Manifestations. Additional clinical manifestations of obstructive shock are based on the cause of the obstruction. For example, the newborn with ductal-dependent pulmonary blood flow develops profound hypoxemia when the ductus arteriosus begins to constrict. If a newborn has ductal-dependent systemic blood flow, systemic pulses become faint or absent, extremities become cold and pale, and signs of pulmonary venous congestion can develop when the ductus arteriosus begins to close. Tension pneumothorax produces signs of systemic venous obstruction and congestion, decreased breath sounds and decreased chest expansion on the side of the pneumothorax, and shift of the mediastinum to the contralateral chest. Significant hypoxemia is present. When cardiac tamponade is the cause of the obstruction, signs of systemic or pulmonary edema, or both, develop with low cardiac output. Additional signs can include muffled heart sounds and pulsus paradoxus, although low cardiac output may severely decrease the quality of all pulses. When pulmonary embolus is the cause of the obstruction, hypoxemia, severe respiratory distress/shortness of breath, hypoxemia, and signs of right ventricular failure are observed.[1,23]

Evaluation and Treatment. Treatment of obstructive shock requires restoration of systemic oxygenation and perfusion with elimination of the obstruction to flow. To support systemic oxygenation and perfusion, providers must establish and maintain an adequate airway and support oxygenation and ventilation. Diagnostic studies are limited to those essential to the establishment of the diagnosis. Elimination of the cause of obstruction may require administration of prostaglandin E_1 (to reopen a constricted ductus arteriosus in newborns with ductal-dependent CHD), interventional cardiac catheterization for treatment of other defects causing obstruction, needle decompression of a tension pneumothorax or cardiac tamponade, or fibrinolytic therapy and fibrinolytics (and possible embolectomy) for treatment of massive pulmonary embolus.[1,26]

If cardiac tamponade is present, bolus fluid administration may transiently improve cardiac output while preparations are made for pericardiocentesis. However, this should not delay definitive therapy.

Reperfusion and Inflammatory Injury

Reperfusion (reoxygenation) injury is cell damage caused by the restoration of blood flow and oxygen delivery to cells that have been exposed to injurious, but nonlethal, hypoxic conditions.[57]

Pathophysiology. Ischemia causes changes in transmembrane permeability to sodium and calcium and damage to intracellular organelles.[58] This damage triggers a pro-inflammatory and procoagulant response that can be very similar to that caused by septic shock (described previously).

Restoration of oxygen delivery to extremely ischemic tissues produces highly reactive oxygen intermediates (e.g., free oxygen radicals and superoxide) that damage cell membranes, denature proteins, and disrupt chromosomes (see Chapter 2).[58] The amount of free oxygen radicals produced is directly related to the severity and duration of the ischemic period. The reperfusion process is most likely to affect endothelial cells of the microvasculature, compromising organ perfusion after shock resuscitation.[57,58]

An ischemic insult activates WBCs, priming monocytes and macrophages and contributing to the release of inflammatory mediators or cytokines, including TNF, IL-1, IL-6, IL-8, and platelet-activating factors. These cytokines in turn contribute to vasodilation, increased capillary permeability, and altered platelet function. The ultimate result is a maldistribution of blood flow and a compromise in organ perfusion and function.[57,58] The role of these mediators is summarized in Chapter 8; Chapter 48 includes a more comprehensive discussion of MODS.

Clinical Manifestations. Signs of organ dysfunction include, but are not limited to, lactic acidosis, oliguria, and an acute alteration in level of consciousness (e.g., decrease in Glasgow Coma Scale score of 1 point or more from baseline); hypoxemia, hypotension, poor capillary refill, or shock plus signs of coagulopathy; respiratory, renal, or hepatic dysfunction; or neurologic dysfunction. CIH also may be present. Gut injury and inflammation may enable translocation of gram-negative bacteria or endotoxin into the bloodstream and may contribute to GI bleeding.[59]

Several predictive and descriptive scoring systems are available to characterize the severity of illness in critically ill children with organ dysfunction. Outcome scores include the Pediatric Logistic Organ Dysfunction (PELOD) scoring system[60] and the Pediatric Multiple Organ Dysfunction Score (P-MODS).[60–62] These scoring systems may be useful in conjunction with other factors such as prognostic indicators when they are applied for several days. Important differences exist between neonates and children in terms of mortality associated with specific organ failures and with specific PELOD scores.[61]

Evaluation and Treatment. [63]The best available model of pediatric reperfusion injury is the child who survives cardiac arrest. "Bundled" post-cardiac arrest care, including meticulous targeted temperature management (strict continuous monitor-ing and maintaining of central body temperature as either hypothermic [32° to 34°C/89.6° to 93.2°F] or "normothermic," [36°C/96.8°F] with control of temperature to prevent or promptly treat fever), as well as protocol-based support of cardiorespiratory function and function of other organ systems, has been shown to substantially increase neurologically intact survival to hospital discharge in adults who survive cardiac arrest.[64] Such a "bundled" approach is now pursued with children. This care typically requires the transfer of the child to a medical center with appropriate pediatric critical care expertise.[1,63]

Fever typically develops following resuscitation from cardiac arrest and is associated with unfavorable neurologic outcome.[65] Therapeutic hypothermia suppresses pro-inflammatory mediators and may enhance anti-inflammatory mediators.[66,67] Mild to moderate induced hypothermia (to 32° to 34°C [89.6° to 93.2°F]) was associated with increased survival in neurologic outcome in neonates with hypoxic-ischemic encephalopathy[68] and in comatose, hemodynamically stable adults following resuscitation from cardiac arrest.[69] However, the control groups in these neonatal and adult hypothermia studies were febrile, so that may have lowered survival in the control group. Three recent large, multicentered randomized clinical trials comparing strict maintenance of normothermia (36°C [96.8°F]) to moderate therapeutic hypothermia (33°C [91.4°F]) demonstrated neither benefit nor harm to the use of cooling in adults[70] or children with out-of-hospital cardiac arrest[71] or in-hospital cardiac arrest.[72] For this reason, the AHA PALS guidelines recommend strict control of temperature either in the hypothermic (to 32° to 34°C [89.6° to 93.2°F]) or normothermic (36°C [96.8°F]) range for the child who remains comatose following resuscitation from cardiac arrest.[3]

Support of airway, oxygenation, and ventilation includes oxygen administration and intubation and support of ventilation to maintain arterial oxygen saturation at 94% to 99% and avoid hypoxemia. Of course, if cyanotic heart disease is present (e.g., single ventricle), the arterial oxygen saturation is typically maintained at 65% to 75%. Support of ventilation is titrated to maintain a $PaCO_2$ within the child's normal range.

Continuous monitoring of blood pressure is indicated. Hypotension during post-cardiac arrest care can contribute to a worse neurologic outcome, so it must be promptly detected and aggressively treated. Titration of inotropic and vasoactive drugs is typically required (see Table 49.7), and bolus fluid administration may be needed. Additional treatment of shock has been summarized earlier in this chapter. If the child remains hemodynamically unstable with conventional management of shock, mechanical support of circulation should be considered in the appropriate setting.

Prevention of secondary neurologic insult requires targeted temperature management with strict maintenance of normothermia and prevention or aggressive treatment of fever. In addition to the support of airway, ventilation, and circulation, careful maintenance of fluid and electrolyte balance is imperative. If renal failure develops, early use of renal replacement therapies is indicated. If seizures develop, they must be managed aggressively.[73]

A thorough presentation of pediatric reperfusion injury and post-resuscitation care is beyond the scope of this chapter. The reader is referred to a comprehensive 2019 AHA Scientific Statement, Pediatric Post-Cardiac Arrest Care (see the box Emerging Science Box: Therapies for Shock and Sepsi).[63]

EMERGING SCIENCE BOX

Therapies for Shock and Sepsis

Prevention of shock is important. Prevention of trauma (injury prevention) and treatment of dehydration can eliminate the two leading causes of hypovolemic shock in children. The incidence of septic shock from hospital-acquired infections, such as ventilator-associated pneumonia or catheter-related bloodstream infections, is decreasing with the use of quality improvement approaches.[29]

Advances in shock therapy show promise for continued improvement in treatment. There is a better understanding of resuscitation goals with an appreciation of the need to target adequate, rather than "normal", cardiac output and oxygen delivery during resuscitation. Second, technological improvements are increasing our ability to assess cardiac output.

Trauma resuscitation also has become more targeted in adults and children. In the prehospital setting, prehospital fluid resuscitation is reserved for children with signs of shock. If penetrating trauma is associated with hypovolemic shock, the child requires urgent transport and surgical intervention, rather than attempts to aggressively treat the shock at the site of injury.

Because massive transfusions can produce immunologic and coagulation complications, the surgical approach to trauma has changed to include staged surgical repair of significant injuries (e.g., liver and bowel injuries). The initial surgery is performed to stabilize the child, and, if needed, subsequent procedures repair the injury. This multistage approach, based on battlefield experiences, reduces the volume of blood products administered and has been linked with reduced morbidity and mortality.[24]

Major advances have been made in understanding the pathophysiology of septic shock and MODS in children. These advances are beginning to be applied to modify clinical evaluation and treatment.[75] Patterns of alterations in biomarkers of sepsis—so-called biomarker signatures—may enable the identification of children at high risk for sepsis, in order to provide more careful monitoring and early intervention. In addition, if alterations in concentrations of biomarkers can be identified at the time they occur, modulation of biomarker activity may be possible using strategies such as receptor antagonists.

It soon may be possible to tailor sepsis and other critical therapies through the use of genetic profiling of the microorganism[33] and of the child.[32,75] Prospective identification of genetic markers for risk of sepsis and responsiveness to therapy may enable individual tailoring of surveillance and interventions to maximize survival and minimize risks from those therapies that are unlikely to be effective.

Finally, several devices are available that enable noninvasive or minimally invasive calculation of cardiac output and index, stroke volume, and circulating blood volume in children.[2] As providers gain experience with the use of such devices and more published data are available about their reliability in children, there will be more tools to confirm clinical assessment and monitor response to therapy.

Systems of continuous quality improvement are essential to identify barriers to, or delays in, appropriate treatment and enable improvement in survival from shock, particularly septic shock.

BURNS

Management of pediatric burn injuries requires an understanding of the differences that exist in this population related to the etiology of injury, growth and development, physiology, and clinical course. In 1988, the American Burn Association established criteria to guide the transfer of an individual to a specialized burn center (see Chapter 48). These criteria remain a standard in burn care and are based on complex management issues related to the treatment of acute burns within the first 24-hour post-burn injury.

Burn injuries in children often are preventable and are frequently the result of curiosity, inability to escape the burning agent, inadequate supervision, or nonaccidental burn trauma. Scald injuries (e.g., hot water and grease) are most common among young children, whereas flame burns are more prevalent among older children.[74] A child exposed to hot tap water at 60°C (140°F) for 3 seconds will sustain a third-degree burn.[75]

A child's skin is thinner and thus more susceptible to injury than an adult's. The extent of injury is determined by the temperature of the burning agent and the duration of exposure. Because very young children may be unable to escape the heat source, the depth of the injury is likely to be greater. The kitchen tends to be a common site for burn injury and often involves pulling over dishes or appliances containing hot liquids. Tap water burns from the bathroom, compared to other scald burns, are likely to be more severe and cover a greater surface area of the body. These are common burn injury sources for children 5 years of age and younger.

Children 3 to 9 years of age are most often injured by flame during fire play. Lighters and matches ignite clothing and cause house fires. Young children may run when clothing ignites and this increases the severity of injury. Inhalation injury significantly increases mortality for pediatric patients with a severe burn injury.[76] Escape from a burning residence or motor vehicle is often delayed because young children cannot cognitively comprehend the circumstances or physically remove themselves from the danger. Flame burns involving flammable liquids, especially gasoline, are more common in older children.

Although flame and scald burns account for the majority of thermal injuries in children, electrical burns result from direct contact with high- or low-voltage current. Most commonly, these injuries occur as a result of risk-taking behavior on the part of young males. Trauma from contact with electrical energy results from the passage of current through vital organs, muscle compartments, and nerve or vascular pathways. Very young children are at risk for injury from chewing on electrical cords or inserting objects into electrical outlets (Fig. 49.3). Lightning strikes also account for some electrical injuries. Chemical burns occur most often in an industrial setting for the adult. At home, children may be burned by swallowing corrosive agents such as cleaning products. The type of causative agent has important implications for the evaluation, treatment, and prognosis of the child.

Although child abuse can occur at any age, young children are particularly vulnerable to serious injury. Approximately 3% to 24% of children who have sustained a burn injury are referred to child protective services for suspicion of abuse.[77] Burns that may suggest nonaccidental trauma include (1) patterned burns, (2) forced immersion burn patterns with sharp stocking or glove demarcation and sparing of flexed protected areas, (3) splash/spill burn patterns not consistent with history or developmental level, and (4) contact burns with well-defined margins of the object.[78] Abuse is suggested with (1) historical inconsistencies and physical examination; (2) incompatible burn and developmental level; (3) bilateral or mirror image burns; (4) localized burns to genitals, buttocks, and perineum (especially at toilet-training stage); (5) evidence of excessive delay in seeking treatment; and (6) presence of other forms of injury.[78] Forced immersion in hot water typically presents with deep symmetric injuries lacking any evidence of splash wounds (Fig. 49.4). By contrast, a pull-down splash burn usually has a triangular pattern with immediate skin contact reflected as the area of greatest burn injury. The burn injury then forms an arrow pointing downward. Contact burns also may be intentionally inflicted by contact with cigarettes or other hot objects, such as curling irons. Young children often sustain burns to the palms of their hands while inadvertently grasping a hot object. If a burn occurs to the back of the hand, this lends cause for suspicion. The provider must rule out diseases or conditions that mimic burn injury, such as diaper dermatitis, scalded skin syndrome, or impetigo, when assessing for abuse.

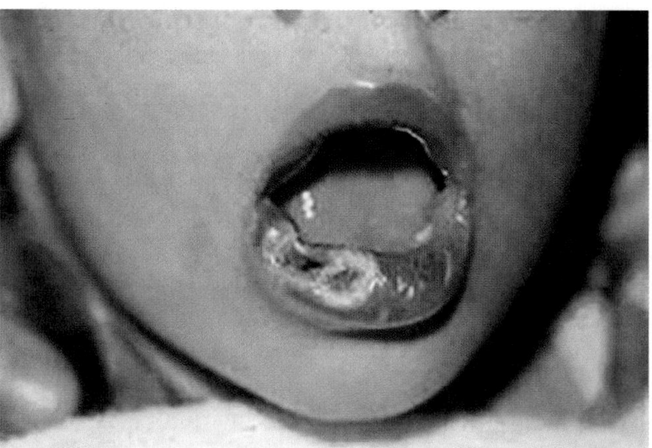

Fig. 49.3 Commissure Burn Resulting from Biting an Electrical Wire. (Courtesy Mary Fran Hazinski.)

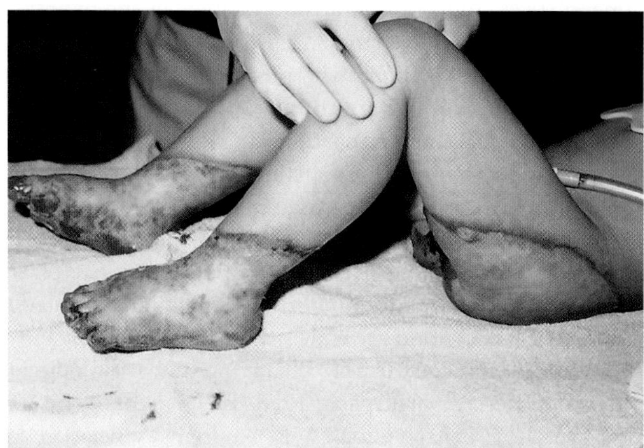

Fig. 49.4 Burn Pattern Typically Seen After Forced Immersion in Hot Water.

Severity of Injury

The severity of burn injury is assessed based on the percentage of the total body surface area (TBSA) involved. Use of the standard Rule of Nines results in inaccurate calculation of the percentage of TBSA involved in children. Although the infant's trunk and arms are of roughly the same proportion as the adult's, the head and neck make up 18% of TBSA and each lower extremity is 14% of TBSA. A modified Rule of Nines deducts 1% from the head and adds 0.5% to each leg for each year of life after 2 years (Fig. 49.5).[79] Various charts are available that assign body proportions to children of different ages. These are generally used in pediatric burn facilities and accurately compute the extent of burn injury.

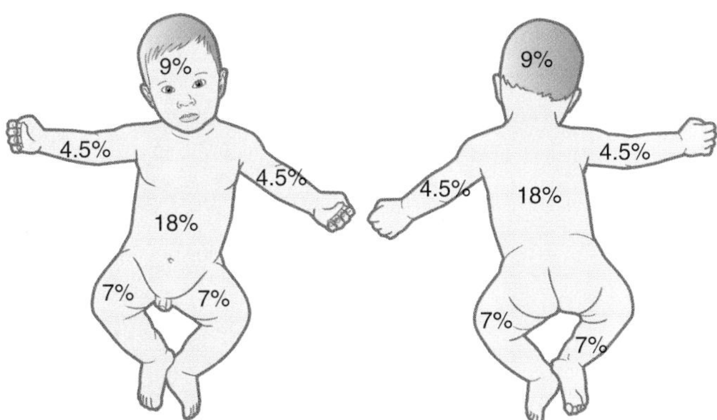

Fig. 49.5 Rule of Nines for Pediatric Burns. (Adapted from American Burn Association. *Pediatric burn injuries. Advanced burn life support provider manual 2018 update.* Chicago, IL: American Burn Association; 2018.)

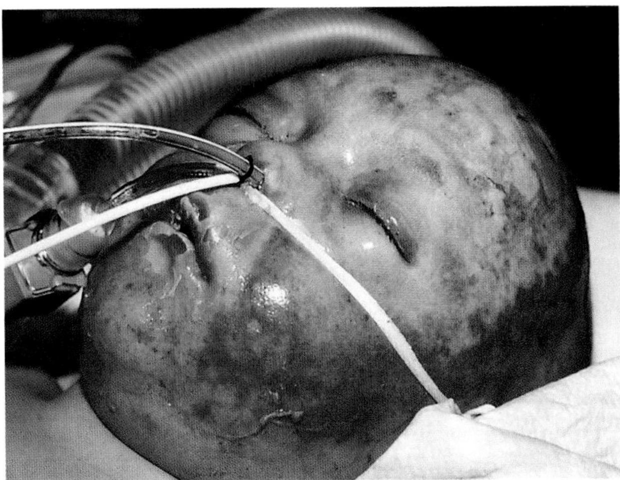

Fig. 49.6 Areas of Indeterminate Depth of Injury in a Young Child.

Because burn trauma represents a three-dimensional wound, the severity of injury is assessed also in relation to the depth of injury. The etiology of the burn and the duration of contact with the burning agent are important considerations in determining the depth of injury. In general, the more intense the heat source and longer the contact, the deeper the resulting injury; however, infant skin is extremely fragile and more likely to sustain a deeper burn. This makes the estimation of the depth of burn difficult in very young children, especially following scald injuries (Fig. 49.6). Intentionally inflicted burns tend to be more severe because contact with the burning agent is prolonged. Electrical injuries also may mask the extent of damage on initial assessment. Visible tissue damage may appear minimal despite severe injury to underlying structures.

Another important factor in assessing the severity of injury is the victim's age. Children younger than 2 years have a significantly higher risk for associated morbidity and mortality after sustaining a burn injury. They have not achieved maturity of the immune system and are at increased risk for infection and sepsis. In addition, very young children are intolerant of rapid fluid shifts and demonstrate immature renal function, negatively affecting their ability to retain sodium and water (see Shock).

The areas of the body injured are another consideration when assessing the severity of the burn. Burns of the hands, feet, perineum, and across joints carry the potential for scar formation and contracture that may interfere with function as well as growth and development. Specialized care is required to preserve maximal function. In addition, burns to the face and neck may result in airway compromise as well as deformity caused by damage to delicate cartilage of the nose and ears.

Other associated trauma or injuries due to the circumstances of the burn should always be investigated. Initially, burns do not bleed. Bloody drainage to an area of the body, even with a burn, suggests another source of trauma. Fractures may result from jumping from a window to escape a house fire. Electrical injuries and motor vehicle accidents often result in associated trauma. Any suspicion of nonaccidental burns should alert the burn team to assess for other injuries.

Pathophysiology, Clinical Manifestations, and Treatment

Major burn trauma involves all body systems, and the consequences of injury include shock, infection, hypermetabolism, organ failure, and functional limitations. These effects can be magnified in the pediatric population as a result of physiologic immaturity and age-related variation in treatment modalities. Along with recognition of changes in the pathophysiology with a burn injury, clinical manifestations are apparent in all organ systems. Although the cutaneous trauma is the initiator of the chain of responses, it is important to consider all of the likely consequences of the injury. An awareness of the changing patterns of convalescence and the development of complications assists in the identification and early treatment of potential sequelae.

Integument

The local response manifested in the area of trauma includes a reduction of tissue perfusion, cellular destruction, and an inflammatory response. Progressive injury caused by dermal ischemia may result from ineffective initial management, especially inadequate or delayed fluid resuscitation. An increase in the permeability and hydrostatic pressure of the capillaries results in the shift of fluid, proteins, and electrolytes into the interstitial spaces. A diminishing intravascular oncotic pressure further enhances these shifts and results in edema formation. Marked edema can result, not only in the area of injury but also in unburned areas. Complications arising from edema are caused by both local and systemic capillary leak.[80] Loss of substantial areas of skin has immediate and profound physiologic effects. Although these losses are maximal in the immediate post burn period, they persist until wound closure.

Circulatory alterations also occur in the area of injury. Reduced blood flow and capillary stasis result from hemoconcentration, the release of thromboplastin and clot-activating factors from heat-damaged cells, reduced cardiac output, and edema formation. Circulation in the area of partial-thickness wounds ceases for 24 to 48 hours after injury, after which it is usually restored. Vascular supply in the area of full-thickness injuries is completely occluded and is not restored until granulation tissue forms or the wound is surgically repaired. The dry, leathery eschar provides an ideal environment for bacterial growth. Infection, trauma, or applying ice to the burn area may convert a partial-thickness injury to a full-thickness one, especially in young children, who have thinner, more delicate skin.

Vitamin D, an essential factor for the proper formation of bone during growth and development, is an important nutrient in children to facilitate intestinal absorption of calcium. Even though vitamin D plays no direct role in burn wound healing, a deficiency of this vitamin has been associated with adverse effects on the skeletal system, as well as on the immune system, which can lead to an increased risk of infection. Vitamin D production may be compromised in burned children, demonstrated by a high incidence of low serum vitamin D levels. Burn-wound scarring and lack of sunlight may limit cutaneous vitamin D biosynthesis.[81]

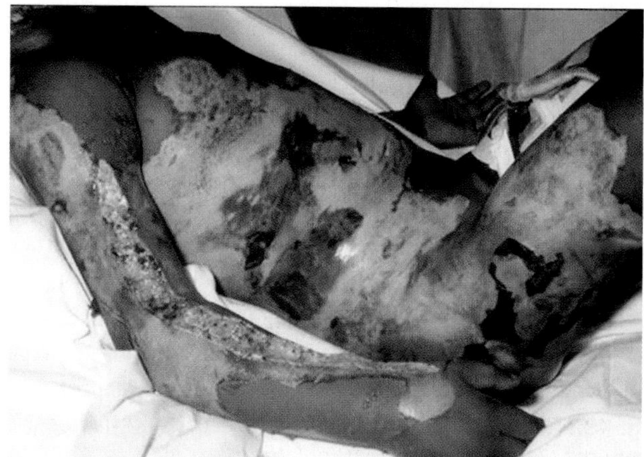

Fig. 49.7 Escharotomy in a Severely Burned Arm. (Courtesy Mary Fran Hazinski.)

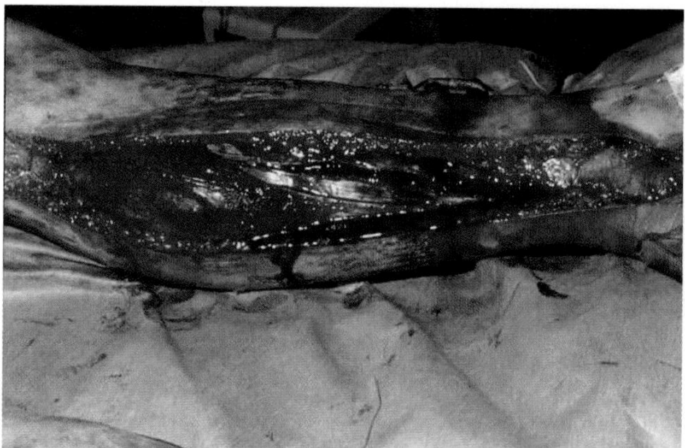

Fig. 49.8 Fasciotomy in a Severely Burned Arm. (Courtesy Mary Fran Hazinski.)

Cardiovascular System

The marked reduction in cardiac output immediately following injury is accompanied by an initial increase in systemic vascular resistance. As fluid is lost into the interstitial spaces, a further reduction in cardiac output occurs, accompanied by vasodilation. Because the infant maintains cardiac output by increasing heart rate preferentially to stroke volume, extremely elevated heart rates result in a decreased filling time and a further reduction in cardiac output.[82] An adequate resuscitation returns cardiac output to normal levels in approximately 24 to 36 hours. Without fluid replacement, cardiac output continues to decrease and results in organ failure and death.

The inefficient and labile peripheral circulation of the infant further complicates management of the burn shock phase of treatment. Related to circumferential full-thickness burns, the rapid fluid shift to the interstitial space and drying of the eschar results in compromised circulation and a resultant tourniquet effect in the extremities. This fluid shift in the torso results in compromised circulation as well as reduced muscle movement impeding respiratory effort. An escharotomy is a procedure that relieves pressure, restores circulation, and improves muscular and respiratory effort (Fig. 49.7). As muscular edema intensifies (frequently seen in electrical injuries) blood vessels and nerves become entrapped because the fascia cannot expand to accommodate the massive edema. Release of pressure is required by a fasciotomy to restore blood flow and preserve nerve function (Fig. 49.8).

A higher risk of chest constriction and impairment of respiratory excursion may result because of the increased pliability of the rib cage, especially in very young children. Excessive fluid volume and burns to the chest or abdomen decrease compliance and can contribute to a serious complication (increased intra-abdominal pressure) that may have an underestimated incidence in burned individuals. Although children with increased intra-abdominal pressure readings tended to be younger, larger TBSA injuries and full-thickness components were significantly associated with elevated pressures and can result in tissue ischemia.[83] Increased intra-abdominal pressure has the potential to impair hemodynamics, renal function, hepatic malperfusion, and pulmonary dysfunction. Despite maintaining cardiac output with fluid replacement, renal function remains impaired in the presence of increased intra-abdominal pressure. Intra-abdominal pressure, as a stressor, can stimulate the neuroendocrine system and elicit stress reactions directed at neutralizing the initial insult of the burn. Increases in the production and release of catecholamines, glucocorticoids, inflammatory mediators such as tumor necrosis factor (TNF-α), and insulin resistance support the clinical finding of profoundly altered cardiovascular, pulmonary, and renal function.[84,85]

Pulmonary System

The clinical manifestations of burn injury related to the pulmonary system include a variety of complications ranging from inhalation injury, pulmonary edema, and respiratory failure to aspiration of gastric contents and pneumonia. Inhalation injury has a negative, prolonged effect on pulmonary function that is associated with, and remains, a major determinant of increased morbidity and mortality.[86]

Anatomic differences in the pediatric airway affect the response to pulmonary complications, as well as therapeutic interventions. The infant airway is positioned anteriorly, making visualization of the cords more difficult. The difficult visualization is further compounded by the relatively large tongue and slanting vocal cords. A small degree of edema results in greatly increased work of breathing in the child (Fig. 49.9). These considerations are particularly important during the resuscitation phase when progressive edema threatens to obstruct the airway. Significant edema results in impairment of respiratory function unless an artificial airway is inserted (Fig. 49.10). Malposition of an endotracheal tube may result in inadvertent extubation, intubation of the bronchi, and atelectasis. Because of the relatively short length of the infant trachea, alterations of the position of the head and neck can affect tube position despite maintenance of the tube position at the teeth.[87–89]

Infants and children compensate for pulmonary compromise by increasing the respiratory rate. However, because the child possesses fewer type I muscle fibers, fatigue related to the

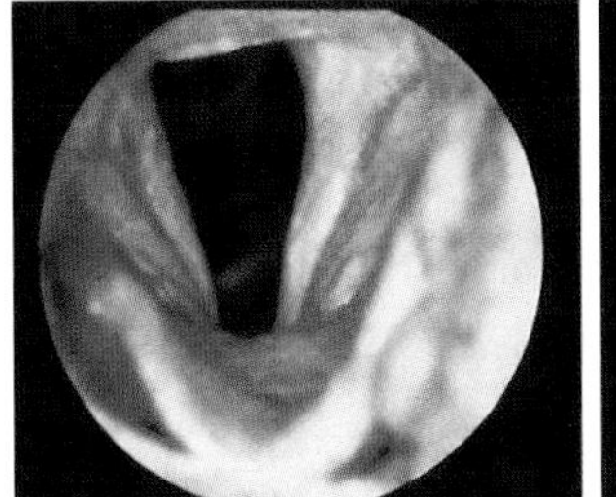
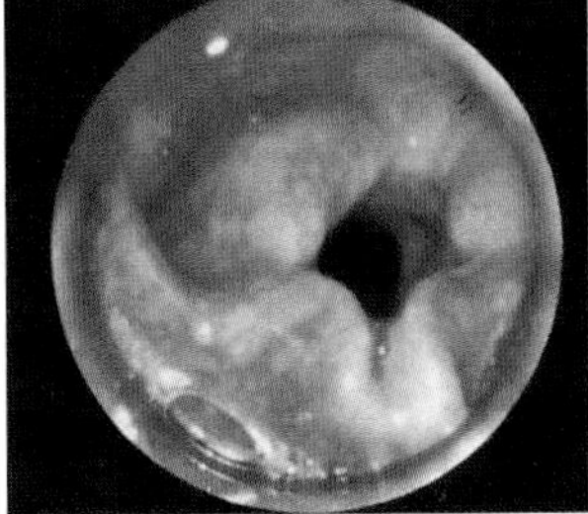

Fig. 49.9 Airways. Adult airway *(left)*; smaller pediatric airway *(right)*.

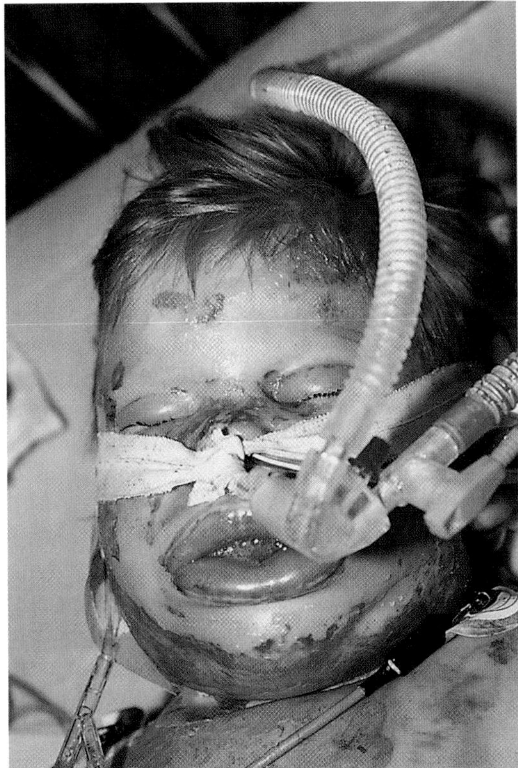

Fig. 49.10 Severe Facial Edema During Burn Shock.

increased work of breathing results in more rapid desaturation than in adults. The soft cartilage of the pediatric airway is prone to collapse in the presence of partial obstruction. Children with burns are at increased risk for these events made more complex by underlying respiratory disease or injury.

Smoke inhalation causes pulmonary parenchymal damage, resulting in decreased pulmonary compliance and increased airway resistance. Several ventilator models are found to be used to compensate for this pulmonary damage. However, for conventional models, conflicting evidence exists. In one research study, high tidal volumes decreased ventilator days and atelectasis, but increased pneumothorax, as compared to low tidal volumes. Mortality was not affected. Non-conventional ventilators include high-frequency percussive ventilation (HFPV) and high-frequency oscillatory ventilation (HFOV). HFPV requires high frequency small tidal volumes, low-frequency breathing rates and a low-pressure circuit, which may improve gas exchange and airway pressure. Outcomes, when compared to conventional ventilation, offered less incidence of pneumonia, lower peak inspiratory pressure, and decreased work of breathing. HFOV provides high respiratory rates with low tidal volumes, which generates a high flow of O_2 without a substantial increase in airway pressure. HFOV demonstrates improved oxygenation. Clinicians are vigilant for post-extubation stridor and pulmonary damage due to ventilation during the course of treatment.[76]

Additional non-ventilatory measures include pronation and extracorporeal membrane oxidation (ECMO) of the individual. Pronation reduces the work of breathing because the masses of the heart and bronchial tree are inverted, allowing for better expansion of the lungs.[88] ECMO is a treatment being used more often for persons with burns demonstrating acute hypoxemic respiratory failure and hemodynamic instability when other medical management options have been exhausted. With ECMO, the person's blood from the body is redirected to the device, oxygenated, and CO_2 removed before it is returned to the body. Even though studies on the safety of ECMO in the pediatric population are limited, value has been found in this treatment modality, and it should be considered as an added level of support. After inhalation injury, ECMO may provide time for organ function recovery, therefore increasing the tendency for survival.[89]

The consequences of metabolic and physiologic changes occurring during the acute phase of injury remain apparent during convalescence. Severe burns result in a decrease in pulmonary function from restrictive and obstructive pulmonary disease evidenced by a reduction in pulmonary volumes and maximum voluntary ventilation lasting up to 8 years. At times, chest wall scarring in children caused by burns severely limits thoracic cage excursion.

Burn Shock

The pathophysiologic responses of burn injury result in hypovolemia and extracellular sodium depletion in the burn-injured individual. Manifestations for adults are discussed in Chapter 48. Hypotension is a late sign of shock in the child. A complete circulatory assessment, including heart rate and peripheral parameters, is a more reliable measure. Urine output reflects end-organ perfusion and is therefore the most accurate monitor of adequate fluid resuscitation. A urine output in pediatric patients weighing 30 kg or less is 1 mL/kg per hour, and in children weighing greater than 30 kg is 0.5 mL/kg per hour (the same as in adults), are the suggested endpoints associated with many resuscitation formulas. Fluid is titrated to maintain the output within the parameters.[79]

The fluid of choice for burn shock resuscitation should approximate the fluid lost from the circulating volume, for example, lactated Ringer solution. Children require more fluid resuscitation for smaller burns than do adults as a result of their limited physiologic reserves. The child's relatively greater ratio of body surface area to weight results in increased evaporative water losses and proportionately more fluid during resuscitation. The need for large volumes of fluid during resuscitation causes a decrease in the concentration of plasma proteins and worsening edema formation; therefore, colloid replacement during burn shock resuscitation remains controversial.[90] A component for maintenance fluid *must* be included in the calculation of fluid needs during resuscitation. Maintenance fluids represent the body requirements in the absence of burn injury.

Successful resuscitation depends on the establishment of intravenous access. Although this is usually accomplished by peripheral or central venous cannulation, circulatory collapse may preclude timely administration of fluid replacement. Cannulation of veins in the pediatric population is further complicated by small vessels and increased subcutaneous fat. Children are good candidates for intraosseous cannulation when traditional venous access techniques fail. Blood, drugs, and fluids are readily absorbed by red marrow that drains into medullary venous channels and thus to the systemic circulation. This technique is most effective in children younger than 5 years because red marrow is steadily replaced by yellow marrow in the limbs, making infusion more difficult, hence decreasing the infusion rate.[91] Complications are minimal with proper care and removal as soon as other access is available.

Fluid Resuscitation

Fluid resuscitation is generally required for children with burn injuries of 15% TBSA or greater. Fluid is administered to compensate for fluid and electrolytes extravasating into the interstitial spaces. This replacement restores circulating volume, improves perfusion, and alleviates organ dysfunction associated with impaired circulation.

Various protocols have been proposed as guidelines for fluid administration. It is important to remember that any regimen serves merely as a guideline and will require adjustment based on the individual response of each child. Because the linear relationship between weight and surface area does not exist in children (surface area varies to weight as a two-thirds function), use of adult formulas results in under- or over-resuscitation.[90] A commonly used protocol is a modification of the Parkland formula. Children also tend to require relatively more fluids than adults because children have higher evaporative losses because of their body surface area-to-weight ratio. Evaporative fluid loss can be a significant contributor to hypovolemia in the burned child. This evaporative fluid loss continues until the burn wounds are closed. Although there are specific differences in fluid resuscitation principles between adults and children, some aspects are similar. As in adults, inhalation injury increases the magnitude of TBSA injury; therefore, children with burns and inhalation injury require more fluids.[92]

Research suggests that in practice, in the acute phase of the burn injury, children receive far more fluid than calculated by the modified Parkland formula guidelines that can result in a condition called *fluid creep*. Onset may occur from an excess of resuscitation fluids, vasodilation from an increased use of opiates, and a decrease in venous return from an increase in thoracic pressure from ventilator support resulting in increased abdominal pressure. Adequate fluid resuscitation to support organ perfusion and avoidance of over-resuscitation controls fluid creep.[92] With increased intraabdominal pressure, decompressive laparotomy is a procedure that may be used.

Renal System

Loss of circulating volume into the interstitial spaces results in reduced renal blood flow and decreased glomerular filtration. An important measure of the adequacy of volume replacement is urine excretion. Sufficient volume replacement maintains urine output during resuscitation. Approximately 36 hours after injury, edema fluid begins to mobilize and output increases.

Children younger than 2 years of age lack the ability to concentrate urine because of the immaturity of the renal system and are, therefore, at increased risk for dehydration. In addition, the child has a relatively larger body surface area in relation to weight than the adult. Combined with limited physiologic reserves, increased fluid requirements are necessary for children during burn shock resuscitation and to compensate for evaporative water losses.[93]

Myoglobin, evidence of a pink to red pigment in the urine, is the result of the breakdown of muscle tissue and hemolysis of red blood cells. This is especially common after extensive electrical injuries and destroyed muscle from deep thermal injury. The release of myoglobin may occlude the kidney tubules and result in renal failure.

Gastrointestinal System

The GI system plays an important role in the pathophysiology of burns. Alterations in blood flow result in decreased perfusion to the GI tract. Ischemia may cause erosion and necrosis of GI tissue. The GI response to a burn injury often includes mucosal atrophy, changes in digestive absorption, and increased intestinal permeability. Depending on the proportion of burn size, atrophy of the GI tract mucosa can occur immediately after injury. The atrophy results in gut barrier dysfunction, leading to increased bacterial translocation and ultimately sepsis.[94]

Paralytic ileus occurs often after major burn injuries. Although digestion ceases in the stomach and the large bowel, the small intestine maintains motility and absorptive capacity. Intestinal motility returns as fluid losses are replaced unless irreversible necrosis of the bowel has occurred as a result of insufficient perfusion.

Immune Function

Burn trauma, induced immunosuppression, results in increased susceptibility to infection and sepsis. Although the exact mechanisms responsible for this immunosuppression remain obscure, it is clear that complex interactions of the hypermetabolic response, nutritional support, bacterial translocation, and defects in both innate and acquired immune function are involved (Fig. 49.11). In addition, young children are at increased risk for microbial invasion caused by an immature immune system and limited antibody production.

Deitch reported that wound- or gut-derived endotoxemia may be one of the mediators of the hypermetabolic response observed after thermal injury, and this finding remains undisputed.[95] When bacteria translocate from the gut or from the burn wound, endotoxins may affect immunologic response as inflammatory mediators are released. A further complication in the activation of inflammatory mediators is the formation of toxic metabolites or reactive oxygen species (ROS). These ROS, such as hydrogen peroxide, nitrous oxide, and superoxide anion, are produced in enormous amounts following a burn injury and are harmful.[85]

Factors such as age and the severity of the burn injury may also affect circulating immunoglobulins. Therapeutic interventions such as multiple transfusions, surgical procedures, and antibiotic and anesthetic administration also introduce elements that confound the evaluation of immunosuppressive effects. The immune system is activated systemically after a large burn injury with extensive tissue necrosis and may become ineffective or even self-destructive. Infections in burns may result in the loss of some components of innate immune function.[96] An additional aspect of the immunopathologic consequence of a burn is the role of immunomodulatory cytokines that are suggested to regulate innate regulatory lymphocytes. The systemic inflammatory response increases pro-inflammatory cytokine production by the peripheral blood mononuclear cells. In children with moderate to severe burn injury, cytokines have been found to increase inflammation by enhancing catabolism and hypermetabolism. In this immunomodulatory process, the pro-inflammatory function of cytokines enhances protection from sepsis recalling that the anti-inflammatory function supports tissue repair.[96]

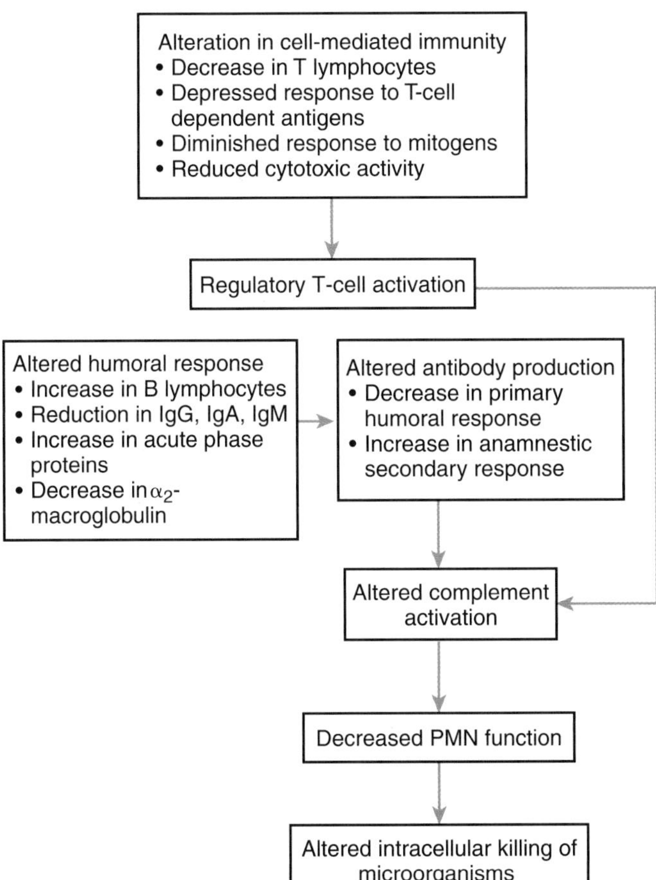

Fig. 49.11 Altered Immune Function After Thermal Injury. Cell-mediated immunity, antibody production, humoral response. *PMN*, Polymorphonuclear leukocyte.

Infection

Whereas shock and pulmonary compromise present the most immediate threat after burn trauma, local and systemic infections become the primary complication during healing. The burn wound initially is relatively free of pathogens; however, dead, avascular tissue and wound exudate provide a fertile environment for bacterial growth. Colonization of the wound is apparent by the fifth post burn day. Gram-positive microorganisms are usually recovered from cultures first, followed by opportunistic gram-negative bacteria.[97] The impaired vascular supply to burned tissue enhances the proliferation of pathogenic microorganisms. Bacterial invasion results in thrombosis and a further impairment of circulation enough to convert a partial-thickness injury to a full-thickness wound.

Improvements in treatment have resulted in a reduction in wound infection. Aggressive excision and grafting of the wounds, the development of microorganism-specific topical antimicrobials, and improved nutritional support have contributed to this trend. However, the incidence of septicemia remains relatively constant. The burn wound serves as the site of primary invasion for most instances of local or generalized infection. Because the burned child is immunosuppressed for many weeks after injury, maintaining the burn wound at low contamination levels by strict infection control measures, meticulous wound care, and routine quantitative culture samples assists in controlling infection caused by wound flora.[98]

Metabolism. Complex metabolic alterations are observed after burn injury. The extent of metabolic derangement is proportional to the magnitude of TBSA burn sustained. Wilmore demonstrated the linear increase in metabolic rate up to 2½ times normal resting energy expenditure (REE).[99] As the burn injury approaches 50% TBSA, a plateau is reached, limiting further physiologic response to the trauma or other challenges such as infection.

A biphasic pattern of physiologic response is evident in thermally injured children. The initial ebb phase occurs during the immediate post burn period and continues for 3 to 5 days. This phase is characterized by reduced oxygen consumption, impaired circulation, and cellular shock. After the resolution of the shock and the restoration of circulating volume, the metabolic response shifts to a catabolic (flow) phase (Table 49.8). A

TABLE 49.8 **Metabolic Alterations Following Injury**

Response	Dominant Factors	Clinical Findings
Ebb Response	Loss of plasma volume	Hyperglycemia
	Shock	Decreased oxygen consumption
	Low plasma insulin levels	Depressed resting energy expenditure
		Decreased blood pressure
		Cardiac output below normal
		Decreased body temperature
Flow Response		
Acute phase	Elevated catecholamines	Catabolic
	Elevated glucagons	Hyperglycemia
	Elevated glucocorticoids	Increased respiratory rate
	Normal or elevated insulin levels	Increased oxygen consumption
		Increased body temperature
	High glucagon/ insulin ratio	Redistribution of polyvalent cations such as zinc and iron
		Mobilization of metabolic reserves
		Increased urinary excretion of nitrogen, sulfur, magnesium, phosphorus, potassium
		Accelerated gluconeogenesis
Adaptive phase	Stress hormone response subsiding	Anabolic
		Normoglycemia
		Energy turnover diminished
		Convalescence

From Gottschlich M, Alexander JW, Bower RH. In: Rombeau JL, Caldwell MD, eds. *Enteral and tube feeding.* Philadelphia: Saunders; 1990.

state of hypermetabolism ensues, characterized by increased oxygen consumption and elevation of catecholamines, glucocorticoids, and glucagon.

Increased blood flow to the wound supplies additional glucose necessary for tissue repair. Insulin levels are usually normal or even elevated but are inappropriately low in relation to glucagon. Catecholamines and glucocorticoids act as antagonists to insulin. This effect combined with a tissue resistance to insulin stimulates glycogenolysis and gluconeogenesis, thus increasing glucose flow from the liver.[100] In the child, glycogen stores for meeting the increased energy demands of the burn are limited. The initiation of protein and lipid catabolism for glycogenesis is accelerated. This prolonged metabolic dysfunction may lead to loss of lean body mass and increased morbidity.[101] Metabolic rates slowly return to normal with wound closure. However, a reactivation of the hypermetabolic response may occur with sepsis or organ failure.

Hypermetabolism

The hypermetabolic response after burn injury profoundly alters the production and use of nutrients. Because of these phenomena, caloric requirements increase dramatically. Advances in burn care have allowed the performance of indirect calorimetry and assessment of metabolic rate at the bedside. Nutritional support must have an increased metabolic rate factored in (increased by 10% to 20%) because of fluctuations in energy use associated with activity. Current recommendations suggest 1.5 to 2 g protein/kg/day for adults and up to 2.5 to 4 g protein/kg/day for children.[101]

In addition to age, body composition has been found to significantly affect the post burn course. Studies suggest that obese children with burns have a longer hospital stay, a greater need for ventilatory support, more severe muscle wasting, and greater insulin resistance.[101] However, the heightened nutrient requirements of the burned child preclude a reduction in nutritional support during the acute phase of recovery. Aggressive nutritional therapy is critical to the recovery of these children, and programs designed to achieve ideal body weight should not be instituted until wound healing is achieved.

The metabolism of many micronutrients is greatly affected by burn injury. Micronutrient supplementation is necessary because vitamin and mineral requirements increase with the severity of the burn related to heightened protein synthesis, enhanced caloric expenditure, and increased micronutrient losses. Hypermetabolism results in a rapid turnover in vitamins and trace minerals important in the wound healing and immune response. A deficiency of specific nutrients interferes with carbohydrate and nucleic acid metabolism, collagen formation, and immune function.

The thermoregulatory response after burn injury results in an elevation in core body temperature. The ideal resting temperature for burned patients is about 38°C (100.4°F). Due to the loss of the skin barrier, burn injury impairs thermoregulation by reducing the body's ability to retain heat and water. A temperature lower than 38°C (100.4°F) may indicate overwhelming sepsis or a weakened temperature control function. Disproportionate heat loss by convection and evaporation require enhanced methods to preserve body heat.[102]

The pediatric surface area to mass ratios can be nearly three times that of adults, leading to greater evaporative fluid loss in pediatric patients. Neonates, infants, and children also have higher blood volumes relative to their mass, averaging ~80 mL/kg body weight compared to the adult average of 70 mL/kg. Therefore, fluid resuscitation in the pediatric patient requires larger volumes per unit of body weight. Dextrose is often coadministered to those under 20 kg (44 lb) to avoid hypoglycemia. Enhanced evaporative loss and need for isotonic fluids then increases the risk of hypothermia in this population. Burn-associated fluid and protein loss, a decrease in blood volume, and SIRS can result in renal and hepatic system dysfunction and are significant concerns in both the pediatric and adult burn patient.[102] Therapeutic interventions, such as operative procedures, dressing changes, and transport, present situations requiring increased diligence to prevent inadvertent cooling. Infants are at increased risk for a precipitous drop in core body temperature caused by an inability to regulate heat loss by shivering. Infants and children are especially vulnerable because of the large surface area relative to metabolically active tissue.[93]

Nutritional Support

Compared to sepsis and trauma, burn hypermetabolism (BHM) has an increased degree and extended duration that can persist long after the burn injury. In the immediate post burn state with the "ebb phase," metabolism decreases and tissue perfusion is reduced. A short time afterward, the "flow phase" begins with a state of BHM and hyperdynamic circulation, manifested in an increase in oxygen consumption with an REE of 10% above normal. Unless BHM is reversed with appropriate nutritional intervention, muscle mass is lost, immune response is compromised, and wound healing is delayed.[101] Adenosine triphosphate (ATP) turnover and mitochondrial oxygen consumption account for a substantial part of BHM. Evidence that supports this theory considers the presence of abnormal levels of the uncoupling protein 1, a mitochondrial transmembrane protein and principal mediator of thermogenesis, in the adipose tissue of burn patients.[103] The catecholamines, namely epinephrine, cortisol, and glucagon, mediate BHM. It follows that protein synthesis and lipogenesis are then limited. Protein breakdown becomes a substantial energy source.[101]

Early and ample enteral feeding (EF) is particularly essential to prevent the complications of BHM such as weight loss, particularly muscle mass loss and immune dysfunction. EF supports GI mucosa function, reducing the risk of Curling's ulcer. Considered together, these factors support a reduced length of stay. The metabolic state in severe burns is extremely complex and requires additional investigation.[101]

Wound Management

The goals of wound management include prevention of infection, removal of devitalized tissue, and closure of the wound (see Emerging Science Box: Advances in Burn Wound Care). Burns that are clearly deep dermal or full-thickness injuries are surgically excised as soon as the child is hemodynamically stable after resuscitation. Early excision reduces the incidence of wound infection and systemic sepsis.[104] Coverage of the excised wound is necessary to achieve wound closure. The choice of a coverage technique depends on the availability of donor skin.

Split-thickness sheet grafts are selected for areas of maximal functional and cosmetic results (Fig. 49.12). Children with very large burn injuries often do not have enough unburned skin available to facilitate the use of the sheet graft. In these cases, the surgeon uses a meshing technique to expand the available skin and increase the size of the graft. The pattern created heals by the migration of epithelium from the meshed edges. Scar formation is increased, and the mesh pattern remains clearly visible (Fig. 49.13). The color, texture, vascularity, thickness, and hair-bearing nature of the skin vary from one area to another. Site selection and depth of donor sites require careful consideration. Skin grafts for the face should be taken, if possible, from above the nipple line or from the scalp for best color match.[105]

Scar Maturation

In normal epidermal healing, minimal disruption in skin color, texture, and thickness occurs. However, burn wounds that extend into the dermis are repaired through scar formation and may result in an overgrowth of dermal constituents (Fig. 49.14A). Accelerated collagen synthesis most likely begins with high levels of activity in granulation tissue. The hypertrophic scar consists of hypercellular and disorganized connective tissue that is erythematous, raised, and pruritic. Normal dermis contains thick fibers and fiber bundles running parallel to the surface. In the hypertrophic scar, the collagen is degraded, resulting in disorganized bundles that are cross-linked tightly and lack pliability.[106] As the hypertrophic scar matures, collagen begins to orient in a more parallel fashion, and vascularity decreases (see Fig. 49.14B). Collagen synthesis is very active soon after wound closure, and alteration of

EMERGING SCIENCE BOX

Advances in Burn Wound Care

Although advances in burn care have led to a decrease in morbidity and mortality for the burn patient, those with deep partial and full thickness injuries may still require excision and surgical intervention. With large burns, donor site availability may be limited. In an effort to address this limitation, novel developments and techniques for approaching epidermal replacement shows promise. Recent studies of skin grafting with the use of an autologous skin cell suspension (ASCS) using a harvesting and processing device (ReCell, Avita Medical, Valencia, CA) have resulted in positive outcomes for these persons in the arena of skin repair. With the use of the ReCell device, the ASCS promotes rapid epidermal regeneration and re-epithelialization while requiring significantly less donor site skin. During surgery, the ReCell device is used to prepare a solution of the person's harvested skin. The regenerative epidermal suspension is then immediately applied without having to culture the skin cells. It is sprayed directly on the acute partial thickness wound or used in combination with a meshed autograft for full thickness burn wounds. It is FDA approved for individuals over 18 years of age. Pediatric patients bring a set of challenges to skin grafting and morbidity of donor sites. ReCell is approved under "compassionate use" for the pediatric patient who has sustained burn injuries and does not have available donor sites for autologous split thickness skin grafting.

Data from Holmes Iv JH, et al. A comparative study of the ReCell® device and autologous split-thickness meshed skin graft in the treatment of acute burn injuries. *Journal of Burn Care & Research,* 2018;39(5):694–701; Nannassay AD, et al.: The use of an autologous cell harvesting and processing device to decrease surgical procedures and expedite healing in two pediatric patients. *Wounds,* 2019;31(12): 316–321.

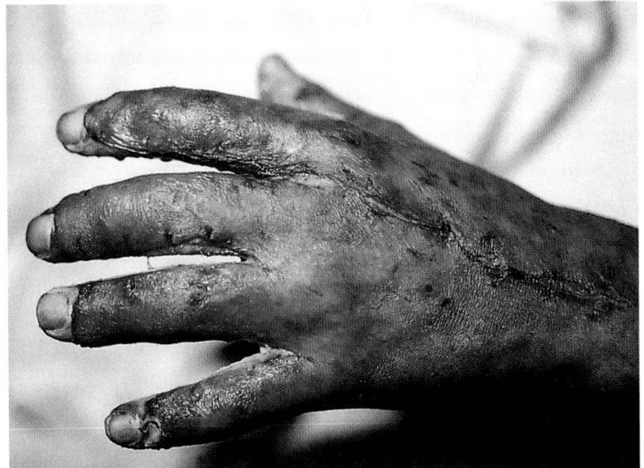

Fig. 49.12 Split-Thickness Sheet Graft.

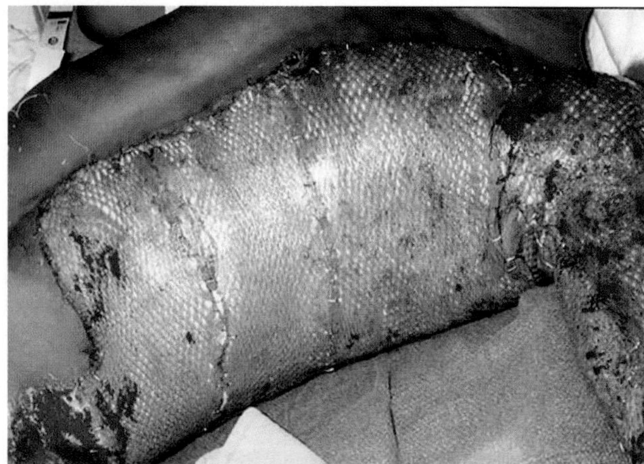

Fig. 49.13 Meshed Autograft. (Courtesy Mary Fran Hazinski.)

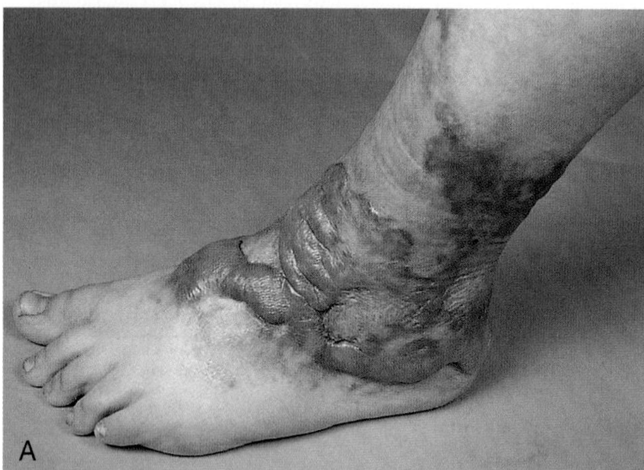

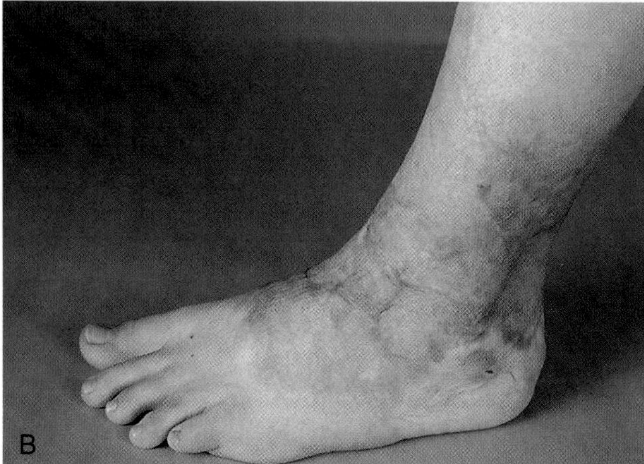

Fig. 49.14 Scar Maturation. (A) Immature hypertrophic scar. **(B)** Flat, mature scar after pressure therapy.

the scar can be accomplished before strong cross-linking of the collagen is established.

Although the duration of wound healing varies among individuals, the length of time required to achieve wound closure is the most reliable predictor of hypertrophic scarring. Deeper burns demonstrate increased scarring caused by the formation of granulation tissue and prolonged healing time. Scarring that extends beyond the edges of the initial wound is termed keloids. While keloids can develop in any burn wound, it more commonly develops in darker-pigmented skin.[106] Although age has not been found to be a predictor of hypertrophic scar formation, younger individuals are more susceptible to trauma and have greater skin tension and an accelerated rate of collagen synthesis. Increased tension with resultant trauma stimulates inflammation, which in turn results in the formation of additional collagen.

Scar tissue is metabolically active and highly vascular. Collagen is deposited in random patterns, and contraction of the scar can result in disabling deformities. The scar is active as long as it is raised, red, and firm. Scar maturation requires 1 to 2 years and depends on individual differences and compliance with the rehabilitation program. The mature scar is characterized by increased suppleness, flattening, and pigmented color.

Scar tissue does not grow and expand like normal tissue. Although massage therapy offers some benefit in stretching, functional limitation may develop as the child grows. This is particularly evident over joints. Reconstructive surgery is often necessary to restore anatomic integrity and to promote independent function.

Itching may occur at any time during burn wound healing and may last for many years after the burn has healed. As a complication, it can lead to graft loss and skin breakdown since the area may be scratched away in an effort to obtain relief. Moisturizing lotions, silicone gel sheets, and massage may lend relief. When examining medication, the combination of H_1 and H_2 antagonists may be used to control itching.[107]

Comfort Management

Pain is multidimensional and includes physical, emotional, cognitive, and cultural factors. Emotional factors are more important in the child's perception of pain than in adults. When considering pain and anxiety management, background pain and fear of pain are important considerations. Fear or anxiety may exponentially increase the sensation of pain in children. Also important is the challenge for a pediatric burn patient because children have distinct anatomic, physiological, and psychological characteristics. Post-traumatic stress disorder is demonstrated in 30% of severely burned children six months after injury. In combination with the previously mentioned characteristics, burn injury can affect medication response and elimination in children.[108] Both pharmacologic and nonpharmacologic interventions are important in treating persons with burns. The measurement of pain is particularly challenging in young infants, who lack the language skills to express pain. A variety of tools, from physiologic monitors to behavioral analyses, functional ability assessments, and analog scales have been developed to measure pediatric pain. The quality of pain control in burn centers has improved along with the ability to assess pain in the pediatric population.

Recovery From Burn Injury

Rehabilitation becomes the major focus of care once wound coverage has been achieved and continues until all reconstructive procedures have been completed. This phase may extend over many years in the pediatric population. Children require specialized management to ensure optimal functional and cosmetic results. Scar and contracture management is necessary for prolonged periods because of changes in body composition as the child grows and matures. Very young children present unique challenges because the small body size can be difficult to fit with pressure garments and splints, growth is rapid, and cooperation with the rehabilitation program is limited.

Infant skin is thinner, and the epidermis is more loosely connected to the dermis. This increases the risk of blistering, chafing, and rash formation. The infant also produces less sebum and sweat, further exacerbating the propensity to skin irritation. Because scar tissue contains no sweat glands, these characteristics of the skin in growing children compound the difficulty in maintaining pressure on maturing scars while cooling the body.

Positioning and splinting to prevent contracture formation, as well as rehabilitative aspects of therapy, are instituted on admission and continue throughout the hospitalization. Physical therapy and occupational therapy provide exercise to maintain range of motion and function. Psychosocial support is very important for the child and the family. The information provided should be consistent and honest to allow clarification of concerns. In addition to the functional aspects of rehabilitation, attention must be directed to psychosocial needs and community reintegration.

A method to facilitate the transition from the hospital to the community is a school reentry program offered by many burn centers. These programs provide education for teachers and peers about the injury, appearance, and abilities of the returning child.

SUMMARY REVIEW

Shock and Multiple Organ Dysfunction Syndrome

1. Shock in children is present when there are signs of poor systemic perfusion, regardless of blood pressure.
2. Hypovolemic shock is the most common type of shock in children and most frequently results from dehydration and trauma. Hypovolemic shock also may result from expansion of the vascular space, producing inadequate intravascular volume relative to the vascular space.
3. Hypotension is a sign of severe (preterminal), decompensated shock, referred to as *hypotensive shock.*
4. Clinical manifestations of hypovolemic shock include inadequate systemic perfusion associated with intravascular fluid loss. Adrenergic compensatory mechanisms can produce tachycardia, redistribution of blood flow, peripheral vasoconstriction, cool extremities, delayed capillary refill, and oliguria.
5. Neurogenic shock is caused by a loss of vasomotor tone after severe injury to the spinal cord.
6. Clinical manifestations of neurogenic shock include warm skin, hypotension with a low diastolic blood pressure, and poor systemic perfusion. Tachycardia is not present.
7. Cardiogenic shock, with decreased cardiac output, is observed most commonly after cardiovascular surgery or with inflammatory diseases of the heart, such as cardiomyopathy and myocarditis. It is also found in children with obstructive CHD and those with drug toxicity or severe electrolyte or acid-base imbalances.
8. Clinical manifestations of cardiogenic shock include inadequate systemic perfusion despite adequate intravascular volume. Cardiac output is typically low. Adrenergic compensatory mechanisms, including peripheral vasoconstriction and decreased urine volume, are similar to those found in hypovolemic shock.
9. Once septic shock is present, immediate treatment is urgently needed. Therapy in the first hour includes rapid identification, resuscitation, and stabilization including fluid resuscitation (up to 2 to 3 boluses of 10 to 20 mL/kg administered in the first hour of therapy, if critical care resources are present). If the child does not respond to volume administration alone, vasoactive support must be initiated within the first hour of treatment. Antibiotics also must be administered within the first hour. Goals of therapy are to rapidly normalize the heart rate and blood pressure for age and to normalize capillary refill to less than 3 seconds. Fluid and vasoactive therapy should support high cardiac output and oxygen delivery, maintaining the $S_{CV}O_2$ at approximately 70%.
10. Sepsis is a systemic response to infection. It is present when manifestations of SIRS are observed. SIRS is present when the child demonstrates two or more of the following as an acute change from baseline values: altered temperature, altered heart rate, altered respiratory rate, and alteration in the WBC count. The newborn often develops hypothermia rather than fever as a sign of infection and may develop bradycardia instead of tachycardia.
11. Severe sepsis is present when there is evidence of SIRS and signs of organ dysfunction, hypoperfusion, or hypotension.
12. The development of septic shock is heralded when the child with severe sepsis develops signs of cardiovascular dysfunction. The child may become hypotensive despite adequate fluid resuscitation or require vasopressors to maintain blood pressure.
13. Reperfusion and inflammatory injury stimulate free oxygen radicals that can damage cell membranes, denature proteins, and disrupt chromosomes. This process likely affects endothelial cells and the microvasculature, causing MODS.
14. Lactic acidosis (i.e., rise in serum lactate) may be the most sensitive indicator of inadequate systemic perfusion in children; effective shock therapy should eliminate lactic acidosis.
15. The general goals of treatment for shock are maximization of oxygen delivery and minimization of oxygen demand. This requires the support of airway, oxygenation, and ventilation.

Support of cardiovascular function requires support of appropriate heart rate and rhythm, adequate intravascular volume, good myocardial function, and appropriate vascular resistance and distribution of blood flow. The child should be kept warm, but fever must be treated promptly.

16. The signs of shock should lessen or disappear if management of shock is effective. The warmth of the child's extremities, briskness of capillary refill, quality of peripheral pulses, level of consciousness and responsiveness, urine volume, oxygenation, ventilation, and acid-base status should improve throughout shock therapy.

Burns

1. Burns in children are often the result of curiosity, inability to escape the burning agent, inadequate supervision, or nonaccidental trauma.
2. Scald injuries are commonly seen in young children and result from exposure to hot water, grease, or other hot liquids, whereas flame burns are more prevalent among older children.
3. A child's skin is thinner and thus more susceptible to injury than adult skin. The kitchen and bathroom are common sites of burn injury.
4. Approximately 3% to 24% of children who have sustained a burn injury are referred to child protective services for suspicion of abuse.
5. Flame burns involving flammable liquids, most notably gasoline, are more common in older children. Risk-taking behaviors in young males can lead to electrical burns. Children may be exposed to chemical injury by swallowing caustic agents at home.
6. Use of the standard Rule of Nines results in inaccurate calculation of the percentage of TBSA in children. A modified Rule of Nines deducts 1% from the head and adds 0.5% to each leg for each year of life after 2 years of age.
7. Major burn trauma involves all body systems, and the consequences of injury include shock, infection, hypermetabolism, organ failure, and functional limitations. These effects can be magnified in the pediatric population as a result of physiologic immaturity and age-related variation in treatment modalities.
8. Applying ice, infection, or trauma to the burn area may convert a partial-thickness injury to a full-thickness one, especially in young children, who have thinner, more delicate skin.
9. Marked reduction in cardiac output occurs immediately after injury and is accompanied by an initial increase in systemic vascular resistance. The inefficient and labile peripheral circulation of the infant complicates management of the burn shock phase of treatment. A higher risk of chest constriction and impairment of respiratory excursion may result because of the increased pliability of the rib cage, especially in very young children. Younger children are also more susceptible to developing increased intra-abdominal pressure.
10. Inhalation injury significantly increases mortality for pediatric patients with a severe burn injury.
11. Children require more fluid resuscitation for smaller burns than does the adult population as a result of limited physiologic reserves. The child incurs increased evaporative water loss, leading to proportionately more fluid during resuscitation. Large volumes of fluid during resuscitation worsen edema formation; therefore, colloid replacement during burn shock resuscitation remains controversial.
12. Children younger than 2 years lack the ability to concentrate urine because of the immaturity of the renal system and are therefore at increased risk for dehydration. Because children have a relatively larger body surface area in relation to weight than adults, they require proportionately increased fluid during burn shock resuscitation to compensate for evaporative water losses.
13. A biphasic pattern of physiologic responses is evident in the burn-injured child. The initial ebb phase occurs during the immediate post burn period and continues for 3 to 5 days. This phase is characterized by reduced oxygen consumption, impaired circulation, and cellular shock. After this phase and the restoration of volume, the metabolic response shifts to a catabolic, or flow, phase. This phase is characterized by hypermetabolism with an increased oxygen consumption and elevation of catecholamines, glucocorticoids, and glucagon.
14. Limited glycogen stores in burn injured children affect the ability to meet increased energy demands. This prolonged metabolic dysfunction may lead to loss of lean body mass and increased morbidity.
15. Although age was not found to be a predictor of hypertrophic scarring, children have greater skin tension and an accelerated rate of collagen synthesis that produces scarring easier. While the duration of burn healing varies among individuals, time to healing has been found as a predictor of hypertrophic scarring.
16. Children require specialized management to ensure optimal functional and cosmetic results. Long-term scar and contracture management is necessary because of changes in body composition as the child grows and matures.

REFERENCES

1. Perkin RM, et al. Shock, cardiac arrest and resuscitation. In: Hazinski MF, ed. *Nursing care of the critically ill child.* ed 3 St. Louis, MO: Mosby; 2013.
2. Kadec KD, et al. *Part 9: systematic recognizing shock. 2020 AHA pediatric advanced life support provider manual (student workbook).* Dallas, TX: American Heart Association; 2020.
3. Kadec KD, et al. *2020 AHA pediatric advanced life support provider manual (student workbook).* Dallas, TX: American Heart Association; 2020.
4. Lin JC, et al. New or progressive multiple organ dysfunction syndrome in pediatric severe sepsis: a sepsis phenotype with higher morbidity and mortality. *Pediatr Crit Care Med.* 2017;18(1):8–16.
5. Upperman JS, et al. Specific etiologies associated with the multiple organ dysfunction syndrome in children, part 1. *Pediatr Crit Care Med.* 2017;18:S50–S57.

6. Upperman JS, et al. Specific etiologies associated with the multiple organ dysfunction syndrome in children, part 2. *Pediatr Crit Care Med.* 2017;18:S58–S66.
7. Watson RS, et al. Epidemiology and outcomes of pediatric multiple organ dysfunction syndrome. *Pediatric Crit Care Med.* 2017;18:S4–S16.
8. Typpo KV, Lacroix JR. Monitoring severity of multiple organ dysfunction syndrome: new and progressive multiple organ dysfunction syndrome, scoring systems. *Pediatr Crit Care Med.* 2017;18:S17–S23.
9. Kadec KD, et al. *Part 4: systematic approach to the seriously ill or injured child. 2020 AHA pediatric advanced life support provider manual (student workbook).* Dallas, TX: American Heart Association; 2020.
10. Hazinski MF. Children are different. In: Hazinski MF, ed. *Nursing care of the critically ill child.* ed 3 St. Louis, MO: Mosby; 2013.
11. Samson RA, et al. *Pediatric advanced life support provider manual.* Dallas, TX: American Heart Association; 2016.
12. Kadec KD, et al. *Part 12: managing arrhythmias. 2020 AHA pediatric advanced life support provider manual (student workbook).* Dallas, TX: American Heart Association; 2020.
13. Rudolph AM. *Congenital diseases of the heart.* Chicago, IL: Year Book Medical; 1974.
14. Kadec KD, et al. *Part 11: recognizing arrhythmias. 2020 AHA pediatric advanced life support provider manual (student workbook).* Dallas, TX: American Heart Association; 2020.
15. Wynn JL, et al. Time for a neonatal-specific consensus definition for sepsis. *Pediatr Crit Care Med.* 2014;15:523–528.
16. Weiss SL, et al. Executive summary: surviving sepsis campaign international guidelines for the management of septic shock and sepsis-associated organ dysfunction in children. *Intensive Care Med.* 2020;46(Suppl 1):1–9.
17. Kadec KD, et al. *Part 10: managing shock. 2020 AHA pediatric advanced life support provider manual (student workbook).* Dallas, TX: American Heart Association; 2020.
18. Roberts KE. Fluid, electrolyte and endocrine problems. In: Hazinski MF, ed. *Nursing care of the critically ill child.* ed 3 St. Louis, MO: Mosby; 2013.
19. Doctor A, et al. Pediatric multiple organ dysfunction syndrome: promising therapies. *Pediatr Crit Care Med.* 2017;18:S67–S82.
20. Nayak PP, et al. Early change in blood glucose concentration is an indicator of mortality in critically ill children. *Intensive Care Med.* 2012;39(1):123–128.
21. Bhutia TD, Lodha R, Kabra SK. Abnormalities in glucose homeostasis in critically ill children. *Pediatr Crit Care Med.* 2013;14(1):e16–e25.
22. Agus MS, et al. HALF-PINT Study Investigators and the PALISI Network: Tight glycemic control in critically ill children. *N Engl J Med.* 2017;376(8):729–741.
23. Samson RA, et al. Recognition of shock. In: Samson RA, ed. *Pediatric advanced life support provider manual.* Dallas, TX: American Heart Association; 2016.
24. American College of Surgeons *Advanced trauma life support student manual.* ed 9 Chicago, IL: American College of Surgeons; 2012.
25. Armstrong A, Unni P, Pietsch JB. Pediatric trauma. In: Hazinski MF, ed. *Nursing care of the critically ill child.* ed 3 St. Louis, MO: Mosby; 2013.
26. Samson RA, et al. Management of shock. In: Samson RA, ed. *Pediatric advanced life support provider manual.* Dallas, TX: American Heart Association; 2016.
27. Valentine SL, et al. Consensus recommendations for RBC transfusion practice in critically ill children from the Pediatric Critical Care Transfusion and Anemia Expertise Initiative. *Pediatr Crit Care Med.* 2018;19(9):884–898.
28. Mendelson J. Emergency department management of pediatric shock. *Emerg Med Clin North Am.* 2018;36(2):427–440.
29. Ulate KP, et al. An elevated low cardiac output syndrome score is associated with morbidity in infants after congenital heart surgery. *Pediatr Crit Care Med.* 2017;18:26–33.
30. Hartman ME, et al. Trends in the epidemiology of pediatric severe sepsis. *Pediatr Crit Care Med.* 2013;14:686–693.
31. Hartman ME, et al. Comparative epidemiology of pediatric severe sepsis. *Intensive Care Med.* 2019;34(6):472–479.
32. Ruth A, et al. Pediatric severe sepsis: current trends and outcomes from the pediatric health information systems database. *Pediatr Crit Care Med.* 2014;15:828–838.
33. Weiss SL, et al. Global epidemiology of pediatric severe sepsis: the sepsis prevalence outcomes, and therapies study. *Am J Resp Crit Care Med.* 2015;191(10):1147–1157.
34. Trimarchi T. Fundamentals of patient safety and quality improvement. In: Hazinski MF, ed. *Nursing care of the critically ill child.* ed 3 St. Louis, MO: Mosby; 2013.
35. Wheeler DS, et al. Sepsis in the pediatric cardiac intensive care unit. *World J Pediatr Congenit Heart Surg.* 2011;2:393–399.
36. Nadel S. Severe pediatric sepsis. *Expert Rev Anti Infect Ther.* 2012;10(2):111–114.
37. Wong HR. Genetics and genomics in pediatric septic shock. *Crit Care Med.* 2012;40:1618–1626.
38. Brandtzaeg P, van Deuren M. Classification and pathogenesis of meningococcal infections. *Methods Mol Biol.* 2012;799:21–35.
39. Aneja RK, Carcillo JA. Differences between adult and pediatric septic shock. *Minerva Anesthesiol.* 2011;77:986–992.
40. Haley M, et al. Activated protein C in sepsis: emerging insights regarding its mechanism of action and clinical effectiveness. *Curr Opin Infect Dis.* 2004;17(3):205–211.
41. Bernard GR, et al. Efficacy and safety of recombinant human activated protein C for severe sepsis. *N Engl J Med.* 2001;344(10):699–709.
42. Martí-Carvajal AJ, et al. Human recombinant protein C for severe sepsis and septic shock in adult and paediatric patients. *Cochrane Database Syst Rev.* 2012(12):CD004388.
43. Carcillo JA, et al. A systemic inflammation mortality risk assessment contingency table for severe sepsis. *Pediatr Crit Care Med.* 2017;18:143–150.
44. Batzofin BM, Sprung CL, Weiss YG. The use of steroids in the treatment of severe sepsis and septic shock. *Best Pract Res Clin Endocrinol Metab.* 2011;25(5):735–743.
45. Hebbar KB, Petrillo T, Fortenberry JD. Adrenal insufficiency and response to corticosteroids in hypotensive critically ill children with cancer. *J Crit Care.* 2012;27(5):480–487.
46. Karaguzel G, et al. The effects of three specific conditions related to the critical care on adrenal function in children. *Intensive Care Med.* 2012;38(10):1689–1696.
47. Davis AL, et al. American College of Critical Care Medicine clinical practice parameters for hemodynamic support of pediatric and neonatal septic shock. *Crit Care Med.* 2017;45(6):1061–1093.
48. Goldstein B, Giroir B, Randolph A. International Pediatric Sepsis Consensus Conference: definitions for sepsis and organ dysfunction in pediatrics. *Pediatr Crit Care Med.* 2005;6:2–8.
49. Kissoon N, Orr RA, Carcillo JA. Updated American College of Critical Care Medicine—pediatric advanced life support

guidelines for management of pediatric and neonatal septic shock: relevance to the emergency care clinician. *Pediatr Emerg Care*. 2010;26(11):867–869.
50. Saini SS, Kumar P, Kumar RM. Hemodynamic changes in preterm neonates with septic shock: a prospective observational study. *Pediatr Crit Care Med*. 2014;15:443–450.
51. Ranjit S, Aram G, Kissoon N, et al. Multimodal monitoring for hemodynamic categorization and management of pediatric septic shock: a pilot observational study. *Pediatr Crit Care Med*. 2014;15:e17–e26.
52. Carcillo JA, Davis AL, Zaritsky A. Role of early fluid resuscitation in pediatric septic shock. *JAMA*. 1991;266(9):1242–1245.
53. de Oliveira CE, et al. ACCM/PALS haemodynamic support guidelines for paediatric septic shock: an outcomes comparison with and without monitoring central venous oxygen saturation. *Intensive Care Med*. 2008;34:1065–1075.
54. Ventura AM, et al. Double-blind prospective randomized controlled trial of dopamine versus epinephrine as first-line vasoactive drugs in pediatric septic shock. *Crit Care Med*. 2015;43:2292–2302.
55. Maconochie IK, et al. Pediatric Life Support: 2020 International Consensus on Cardiopulmonary Resuscitation and Emergency Cardiovascular Science Care with Treatment Recommendations. *Resuscitation*. 2020;156:A120–A155.
56. Ames SG, et al. The path to great pediatric septic shock outcomes. *Crit Care*. 2018;22:224–228.
57. Banz Y, Rieben R. Role of complement and perspectives for intervention in ischemia-reperfusion damage. *Ann Med*. 2012;44:205–217.
58. Francischetti I, et al. Leukocytes and the inflammatory response in ischemia-reperfusion injury. *Rev Bras Cir Cardiovasc*. 2010;25(4):575–584.
59. Proulx F, et al. The pediatric multiple organ dysfunction syndrome. *Pediatr Crit Care Med*. 2009;10:12–22.
60. Lacroix J, Cotting J, for the Pediatric Acute Lung Injury and Sepsis Investigators (PALISI) Network Severity of illness and organ dysfunction scoring in children. *Pediatr Crit Care Med*. 2005;6(Suppl 3):S126–S134.
61. Bestati N, et al. Differences in organ dysfunctions between neonates and older children: a prospective, observational, multicenter study. *Crit Care*. 2010;14:R202.
62. Leteurtre S, et al. Daily estimation of the severity of multiple organ dysfunction syndrome in critically children. *CMAJ*. 2010;182(11):1181–1187.
63. Topjian AA, et al. Pediatric post-cardiac arrest care: a scientific statement from the American Heart Association. *Circulation*. 2019;140(6):e194–e233.
64. Tømte O, et al. Strong and weak aspects of an established post-resuscitation treatment protocol—a five-year observational study. *Resuscitation*. 2011;82:1186–1193.
65. Bembea MM, et al. Temperature patterns in the early postresuscitation period after pediatric in-hospital arrest. *Pediatr Crit Care Med*. 2010;11(6):723–730.
66. Pietrini D, et al. Neuroprotection and hypothermia in infants and children. *Curr Drug Targets*. 2012;13(7):925–935.
67. Polderman KH. Mechanisms of action, physiological effects, and complications of hypothermia. *Crit Care Med*. 2009;37(Suppl):S186–S202.
68. Shankaran S, et al. Whole body hypothermia for neonates with hypoxic-ischemic encephalopathy. *N Engl J Med*. 2005;353: 1574–1584.
69. Hypothermia After Cardiac Arrest Study Group Mild therapeutic hypothermia to improve the neurologic outcome after cardiac arrest. *N Engl J Med*. 2002;346(8):549–556.
70. Nielsen N, et al. Targeted temperature management at 33íC versus 36íC after cardiac arrest. *N Engl J Med*. 2013;369:2197–2206.
71. Moler FW, et al. Therapeutic hypothermia after out-of-hospital cardiac arrest in children. *N Engl J Med*. 1898;372(20):908–2015.
72. Moler FW, et al. Therapeutic hypothermia after in-hospital cardiac arrest in children. *N Engl J Med*. 2017;376(4):318–329.
73. Samson RA, et al. Post-cardiac arrest care. In: Samson RA, ed. *Pediatric advanced life support provider manual*. Dallas, TX: American Heart Association; 2016.
74. Safe Kids Worldwide (SKW) *A parent's guide to child safety*. Washington, DC: SKW; 2020. Available at https://www.safekids.org/sites/default/files/a_parents_guide_to_child_safety.pdf. (Accessed May 4, 2022).
75. American Burn Association *Scald statistics and data resources*. Chicago, IL: American Burn Association; 2018. Available at http://www.ameriburn.org/wp-content/uploads/2018/12/nbaw2019_statsdataresources_120618-1.pdf. (Accessed May 4, 2022).
76. Sen S. Pediatric inhalation injury. *Burns Trauma*. 2017;5:31.
77. Pawlik MC, et al. Children with burns referred for child abuse evaluation: burn characteristics and co-existent injuries. *Child Abuse Negl*. 2016;55:52–61.
78. Collier ZJ, Roughton MC, Gottlieb LJ. Negligent and inflicted burns in children. *Clin Plast Surg*. 2017;44(3):467–477.
79. American Burn Association *Pediatric burn injuries. Advanced burn life support provider manual 2018 update*. Chicago, IL: American Burn Association; 2018.
80. Rae L, Fidler P, Gibran N. The physiologic basis of burn shock and the need for aggressive fluid resuscitation. *Crit Care Clin*. 2016;32(4):491–505.
81. Al-Tarrah K, et al. Vitamin D status and its influence on outcomes following major burn injury and critical illness. *Burns Trauma*. 2018;6:11.
82. Helvig E. Pediatric burn injuries. *AACN Clin Issues Crit Care Nurs*. 1993;4(2):433–442.
83. Strang SG, et al. A systematic review on intra-abdominal pressure in severely burned patients. *Burns*. 2014;40: 9–16.
84. Culnan D, et al. Significance of the hormonal, adrenal, and sympathetic responses to burn injury. In: Herndon DN, ed. *Total burn care, Edinburg.* : Elsevier; 2018.
85. Nielson CB, et al. Burns: pathophysiology of systemic complications and current management. *J Burn Care Res*. 2017;38(1):e469–e481.
86. Bittner EA, et al. Acute and perioperative care of the burn-injured patient. *Anesthesiology*. 2015;122(2):448–464.
87. Trout S, et al. Influence of head and neck position on endotracheal tube tip position on chest x-ray examination: a potential problem in the infant undergoing intubation. *J Burn Care Rehabil*. 1994;15(5):405–407.
88. Walker PF, et al. Diagnosis and management of inhalation injury: an updated review. *Crit Care*. 2015;19:351.
89. Thompson KB, et al. Extracorporeal membrane oxygenation support for pediatric burn patients: is it worth the risk? *Pediatr Crit Care Med*. 2020;21(5):469–476.
90. Romanowski KS, Palmieri TL. Pediatric burn resuscitation: past, present, and future. *Burns Trauma*. 2017;5:26.
91. Tintinalli JE, et al. *Emergency medicine: a comprehensive study guide*. New York: McGraw-Hill; 2004.

92. Greenhalgh DG. Management of burns. *N Engl J Med.* 2019;380:24.
93. Lopez ON, et al. Special considerations of age: the pediatric burned patient. In: Herndon DN, ed. *Total burn care.* Edinburg: Elsevier; 2018.
94. Earley ZM, et al. Burn injury alters the intestinal microbiome and increases gut permeability and bacterial translocation. *PLoS One.* 2015;10(7):e0129996.
95. Deitch EA. Nutritional support of the burn patient. *Crit Care Med.* 1995;11(3):735.
96. Devine RA, et al. The systemic immune response to pediatric thermal injury. *Int J Burns Trauma.* 2018;8(1):6–16.
97. Lachiewicz AM, et al. Bacterial infections after burn injuries: impact of multidrug resistance. *Clin Infect Dis.* 2017;65(12):2130–2136.
98. Norbury W, et al. Infection in burns. *Surg Infect (Larchmt).* 2016;17(2):250–255.
99. Wilmore DW. Nutrition and metabolism following thermal injury. *Clin Plast Surg.* 1974;1(4):603–619.
100. Auger C, Samadi O, Jeschke MG. The biochemical alterations underlying post-burn hypermetabolism. *Biochim Biophys Acta Mol Basis Dis.* 2017;1863(10 Pt B):2633–2644.
101. Clark A, et al. Nutrition and metabolism in burn patients. *Burns Trauma.* 2017;5:11.
102. Mathias E, Srinivas Murthy M. Pediatric thermal burns and treatment: a review of progress and future prospects. *Medicines (Basel).* 2017;4(4):91.
103. Porter C, et al. The metabolic stress response to burn trauma: current understanding and therapies. *Lancet.* 2016;388(10052):1417–1426.
104. Rowan MP, et al. Burn wound healing and treatment: review and advancements. *Crit Care.* 2015;19:243.
105. Aly MEI, et al. Operative wound management. In: Herndon DH, ed. *Total burn care.* Edinburg: Elsevier; 2018.
106. Finnerty CC, et al. Hypertrophic scarring: the greatest unmet challenge after burn injury. *Lancet.* 2016;388(10052):1427–1436.
107. Baker RU, et al. Burn wound itch control using H1 and H2 antagonists. *J Burn Care Rehabil.* 2001;22(4):263.
108. Fagin A, Palmieri TL. Considerations for pediatric burn sedation and analgesia. *Burns Trauma.* 2017;5:28.

GLOSSARY

A

Absolute polycythemia Excessive red blood cell production; a physiologic response resulting from increased erythropoietin secretion in response to chronic hypoxia or as a symptom of polycythemia vera.

Absorption atelectasis See Atelectasis.

Acid maltase deficiency (glycogen storage disease type II or Pompe disease) An autosomal recessive metabolic disorder that damages muscle and nerve cells throughout the body by an accumulation of glycogen in the lysosome attributable to deficiency of the lysosomal acid α-glucosidase enzyme. The buildup of glycogen causes progressive muscle weakness (myopathy) throughout the body and affects various body tissues, particularly in the heart, skeletal muscles, liver, and nervous system.

Acne A common skin disease characterized by pimples on the face, chest, and back. It occurs when the pores of the skin become clogged with oil, dead skin cells, and bacteria.

Acne conglobate Severe cystic acne characterized by cystic lesions, abscesses, communicating sinuses, and thickened, nodular scars; usually does not affect the face.

Acne rosacea A chronic form of dermatitis of the face in which the middle portion of the face appears red with small red lines caused by dilation of capillaries.

Acne vulgaris An inflammatory eruption of the sebaceous follicles usually occurring on the face, upper back, and chest that consists of blackheads, cysts, papules, and pustules.

Noninflammatory acne Open comedones caused by the enlargement and dilation of a plug resulting from the accumulation of oil and dead skin cells inside the hair follicle and by closed comedones that form if the hair follicle pore remains closed; they appear as a tiny, sometimes pink bump in the skin.

Acquired immunodeficiency syndrome (AIDS) See Immune deficiency.

Acquired sideroblastic anemia See Anemia.

ACTH deficiency A condition characterized by decreased or absent production of adrenocorticotropic hormone (ACTH) by the pituitary gland, resulting in a reduction in the secretion of adrenal hormones and subsequent weight loss, lack of appetite, weakness, nausea, vomiting, and low blood pressure.

Actinic keratosis A condition in which a premalignant small, reddish, rough spot appears on skin chronically exposed to the sun.

Acute chest syndrome A syndrome occurring in association with sickle cell disease defined by a new infiltrate on chest radiograph; associated with one or more new symptoms: fever, cough, sputum production, dyspnea, or hypoxia. It occurs most commonly in the 2- to 4-year-old age group and declines in incidence with age.

Acute colonic pseudo-obstruction (Ogilvie syndrome) A massive dilation of the large bowel that occurs in critically ill persons and immobilized older adults. It is characterized by significant dilation of the cecum and absence of mechanical obstruction and is related to excessive sympathetic motor input or decreased parasympathetic motor input.

Acute confusional state (ACS) A form of delirium caused by interference with the metabolic or other biochemical processes essential for normal brain functioning. Symptoms may include disturbances in cognition and levels of awareness, short-term memory deficit, retrograde and anterograde amnesia, and disturbances in orientation, accompanied by restlessness, apprehension, irritability, and apathy. The condition may be associated with an acute physiologic state, delirium, toxic psychosis, or acute brain syndrome.

Acute coronary syndrome A classification encompassing clinical presentations ranging from unstable angina through infarction.

Acute cystitis An inflammation of the bladder, which is the most common site of urinary tract infection.

Acute epiglottitis An infection that causes inflammation of the epiglottis and surrounding tissues and may lead to upper airway blockage.

Acute gastritis An inflammatory disorder of the gastric mucosa, usually caused by injury of the protective mucosal barrier by drugs, chemicals, or *Helicobacter pylori* infection.

Acute glomerulonephritis See Glomerulonephritis.

Acute gouty arthritis An abrupt pain of a joint, most often the great toe, which is swollen, hot, and shiny secondary to an attack of gout.

Acute idiopathic thrombotic thrombocytopenic purpura (TTP) See Thrombocytopenia.

Acute leukemia See Leukemia.

Acute liver failure (fulminant liver failure) A rare clinical syndrome resulting from severe impairment or necrosis of liver cells without preexisting liver disease or cirrhosis. Acetaminophen overdose is the leading cause.

Acute lung injury (ALI)/acute respiratory distress syndrome (ARDS) A spectrum of acute lung inflammation and diffuse alveolocapillary injury.

Acute lymphoblastic leukemia (ALL) See Leukemia.

Acute mesenteric ischemia Caused by acute occlusion of the mesenteric artery that results in a significant reduction in mucosal blood flow to the large and small intestines. Aortic aneurysms, arterial thrombi, or emboli can be causes.

Acute mountain sickness (AMS) The presence of a combination of nonspecific symptoms that appear within a few hours after ascent to altitude, and may include headache, loss of appetite, nausea, vomiting, weakness, lassitude, dizziness, and difficulty sleeping.

Acute myelogenous leukemia (AML) See Leukemia.

Acute orthostatic hypotension An abnormal decrease in blood pressure when a person stands. This may lead to fainting.

Acute otitis media (AOM) An infection of the middle ear space, behind the eardrum (tympanic membrane); characterized by pain, dizziness, and partial loss of hearing.

Acute pancreatitis Inflammation of the pancreas resulting from obstruction to the outflow of pancreatic digestive enzymes caused by bile duct or pancreatic duct obstruction (e.g., gallstones). Usually a mild disease and resolves spontaneously.

Acute poststreptococcal glomerulonephritis (PSGN) See Glomerulonephritis.

Acute pyelonephritis Acute inflammation of the renal parenchyma and pelvis characterized by small cortical abscesses and yellowish streaks in the medulla resulting from the accumulation of pus in the collecting tubules and interstitial tissue.

Acute renal failure (acute renal injury) A sudden decline in kidney function with a decrease in glomerular filtration and accumulation of nitrogenous waste products in the blood as demonstrated by an elevation in plasma creatinine and blood urea nitrogen levels.

Acute respiratory distress syndrome (ARDS) Capillaries or alveoli of the lungs are damaged as a result of infection, injury, blood loss, or inhalation injury-causing fluid to leak from the capillaries into the alveoli, resulting in pulmonary edema and collapse of some alveoli.

Acute tubular necrosis (ATN) The kidney undergoes ischemic or nephrotoxic injury because of severe hypotension, aminoglycosides, or radiocontrast agents and produces granular and epithelial cell casts in urine.

Acute urethral syndrome The bladder is irritated and the typical symptoms of a urinary tract infection are present in the absence of an infection.

Adenocarcinoma Tumor arising from epithelial cells with a glandular or glandlike pattern.

Adenocystic tumor (cylindroma) Rare bronchial gland tumors that arise predominantly in the trachea or large airways and cause obstruction.

Adenomyosis The presence of islands of endometrial glands surrounded by benign endometrial stroma within the uterine myometrium.

Adenosine deaminase (ADA) deficiency See Immune deficiency.

Adrenarche Growth of axillary and pubic hair and other physiologic changes induced by hyperactivity of the suprarenal cortex and adrenocortical secretion of androgenic hormones in early puberty.

Agammaglobulinemia See Immune deficiency.

Ageusia Loss of the sense of taste.

Agoraphobia A mental disorder characterized by an irrational fear of leaving the familiar setting of home, or venturing into the open; it is so pervasive that a large number of external life situations are entered into reluctantly or are avoided; often associated with panic attacks.

Agranulocytosis See Immune deficiency.

Akinesia Slowness or loss of normal motor function resulting in impaired muscle movement.

Akinetic mutism (AM) A syndrome characterized by the inability to speak, loss of voluntary movement, and apparent loss of emotional feeling. It is related to lesions of the upper brainstem.

Albright syndrome (Albright–McCune–Sternberg syndrome) A syndrome characterized by polyostotic fibrous dysplasia, patchy dermal pigmentation, and endocrine dysfunction.

Alcoholic cirrhosis See Cirrhosis.

Alcoholic fatty liver (steatosis) The mildest form of alcoholic liver disease; can be caused by chronic ingestion of relatively small amounts of alcohol, may be asymptomatic, and is reversible with cessation of drinking.

Alcoholic hepatitis (steatohepatitis) A precursor of cirrhosis characterized by inflammation; degeneration and necrosis of hepatocytes; infiltration of neutrophils, macrophages, and lymphocytes; immunologic alterations; and lipid peroxidation.

Algor mortis Postmortem reduction of body temperature.

Alkaline reflux gastritis Inflammation of the stomach caused by reflux of bile and alkaline pancreatic secretions that contain proteolytic enzymes and disrupt the mucosal barrier in the remnant stomach.

Allergic contact dermatitis Contact dermatitis attributable to allergic sensitization.

Allodynia A condition in which pain arises from a stimulus that would not normally be experienced as painful.

Allostasis Long-term or chronic exaggerated responses to stress.

Alogia Inability to speak because of mental deficiency, mental confusion, or aphasia.

Alopecia Loss of hair.

Alopecia areata An autoimmune T-cell-mediated chronic inflammatory disease directed at hair follicles that results in baldness, usually in round patches.

Alpha-thalassemia major See Anemia.

Alpha-thalassemia minor See Anemia.

Alzheimer disease (dementia of Alzheimer type [DAT], senile disease complex) A degenerative disease characterized by amyloid plaques and fibrillary tangles in the cortex and atrophy and widened sulci in the frontal and temporal lobes.

Amblyopia Poor vision caused by abnormal development of visual areas of the brain in response to abnormal visual stimulation during early development.

Amenorrhea Lack of menstruation; most common causes (aside from pregnancy) are chromosomal abnormalities, hypothalamic dysfunction, polycystic ovarian syndrome, hyperprolactinemia, hypothyroidism, malnutrition, and ovarian failure.

Amyotrophic lateral sclerosis (ALS) (sporadic motor system disease, sporadic motor neuron disease, motor neuron disease, Lou Gehrig disease) A disease that breaks down tissues in the nervous system (a neurodegenerative disease); it is of unknown cause and affects the nerves responsible for movement.

Anaphylactic shock A state of shock caused by a severe allergic reaction that lowers blood pressure and results in urticaria, breathing difficulties, and possibly death.

Anaphylactoid purpura (allergic purpura, Henoch–Schönlein purpura) Nonthrombocytopenic purpura attributable to immune hypersensitivity to foods, drugs, and insect bites.

Anemia Hemoglobin concentration is less than normal because of a deficiency in red blood cells, a low level of hemoglobin in cells, or both; it manifests as pallor of the skin and mucous membranes, weakness, dizziness, easy fatigability, and drowsiness caused by oxygen deficiency.

Hereditary spherocytosis (congenital hemolytic anemia, congenital acholuric jaundice) A defect in the cell membrane of red blood cells that causes thickened, fragile red blood cells that are susceptible to spontaneous hemolysis and results in chronic anemia, jaundice, fever, and abdominal pain.

Congenital hemolytic anemias .

Alpha-thalassemia major Thalassemia in which all four α chains of hemoglobin are defective, resulting in a fatal condition because oxygen cannot be released to the tissues.

Alpha-thalassemia minor Thalassemia in which two α chains of hemoglobin are defective.

Beta-thalassemia major (Cooley anemia) Thalassemia in which α-chain synthesis and β-chain synthesis are uncoupled; β-chain production is depressed moderately in the heterozygous form, beta-thalassemia minor, and severely in the homozygous form, beta-thalassemia major, resulting in erythrocytes that have a reduced amount of hemoglobin and accumulations of free α chains.

Beta-thalassemia minor See above.

Glucose-6-phosphate dehydrogenase (G6PD) deficiency An inherited condition that is asymptomatic in the absence of exposure to particular substances such as certain medicines, mothballs, or severe infections; with exposure the red blood cells undergo destruction, producing excessive bilirubin that overloads the liver and causes jaundice.

Hemoglobin H disease A form of alpha-thalassemia in which a hemoglobin H gene is expressed but cannot bind oxygen.

Sickle cell anemia (sickle cell disease [SCD]) An inherited autosomal recessive disorder of the blood caused by abnormal hemoglobin that distorts red blood cells and makes them fragile and prone to rupture and can cause anemia, joint pain, fever, leg ulcers, and jaundice.

Sickle cell trait An inherited condition in which an individual carries only one gene for sickle cell disease and is without symptoms.

Sickle cell–Hb C disease A heterozygous form in which the child simultaneously inherits a hemoglobin C gene from another parent.

Sickle cell–thalassemia disease A heterozygous form in which the child simultaneously inherits a thalassemia gene from another parent.

Thalassemia A potentially fatal genetic disorder in which hemoglobin molecules are abnormal, resulting in severe anemia; enlarged heart, liver, and spleen; and skeletal deformation.

Macrocytic anemia (megaloblastic anemia) A condition characterized by erythrocytes that are larger than normal; associated with deficiency of vitamin B_{12} or folic acid caused by inadequate intake or insufficient absorption secondary to alcoholism or drugs that inhibit DNA replication.

Pernicious anemia An autoimmune disorder that causes a deficiency in intrinsic factor, resulting in the inability to absorb vitamin B_{12} and a subsequent increase in the production of abnormal erythrocytes.

Microcytic-hypochromic anemia A condition in which red blood cells are smaller than normal as a result of iron deficiency.

Acquired sideroblastic anemia A heterogeneous group of disorders characterized by anemia of varying severity caused by a defect in mitochondrial heme synthesis; occurs as a primary disorder with no known cause (idiopathic) or is associated with other myeloproliferative or myelodysplastic disorders.

Hereditary sideroblastic anemia Heterogeneous group of rare disorders characterized by anemia of varying severity caused by a defect in mitochondrial heme synthesis; occurs almost exclusively in males, suggesting a predominant recessive X-linked transmission.

Hypoplastic anemia A condition in which anemia results from greatly depressed, inadequately functioning bone marrow and smaller-than-normal erythrocytes.

Iron deficiency anemia (IDA) An insufficient dietary intake or absorption of iron, resulting in decreased incorporation of hemoglobin into red blood cells and subsequent feelings of fatigue, weakness, and shortness of breath as well as pale earlobes, palms, and conjunctivae.

Reversible sideroblastic anemia Associated with alcoholism; results from nutritional deficiencies of folate.

Sideroblastic anemia (SA) Refractory anemia of varying severity that is caused by altered mitochondrial metabolism and is marked by sideroblasts in the bone marrow.

Normocytic-normochromic anemia (NNA) Erythrocytes are of normal size and hemoglobin content but of insufficient number; usually caused by hereditary spherocytosis, drug-induced anemia, and anemia secondary to malignancies.

Anemia of chronic disease (ACD) A mild to moderate anemia resulting from decreased erythropoiesis in individuals with conditions of chronic systemic disease or inflammation.

Aplastic anemia Decreased bone marrow production of adequate amounts of new red blood cells; results from an autoimmune disorder or exposure to radiation or substances such as benzene or certain drugs.

Aplastic crisis Temporary loss of bone marrow causes erythropoiesis, resulting in an acute fall in hemoglobin levels and subsequent anemia.

Atrial septal defect (ASD) An abnormal communication between the atria; isolated ASD occurs in about 5% to 10% of all congenital cardiac defects.

Autoimmune hemolytic anemia (AIHA) A form of hemolytic anemia involving autoantibodies against red blood cell antigens.

Cold agglutinin autoimmune hemolytic anemia Acquired disorder caused by autoantibodies against antigens normally on the surface of erythrocytes; mediated by immunoglobulin M (IgM) antibodies that optimally bind to and agglutinate erythrocytes in colder portions of the body (e.g., fingers, toes), and occurs less often than warm antibody hemolysis, affecting mostly middle-aged and older adults.

Cold hemolysin autoimmune hemolytic anemia (paroxysmal cold hemoglobinuria) A disorder in which exposure to cold initiates acute and severe intravascular hemolysis that, unlike cold agglutinin anemia, results in hemoglobinuria. The chronic form of this anemia is extremely rare, but an acute form of paroxysmal cold hemoglobinuria is frequently observed in autoimmune hemolytic anemia of childhood.

Drug-induced hemolytic anemia A form of immune hemolytic anemia usually resulting from an allergic reaction against foreign antigens (e.g., antibiotics) that have attached to the surface of red blood cells.

Fanconi anemia A genetic disease affecting bone marrow that is characterized by pancytopenia, hypoplasia of the bone marrow, congenital anomalies, and pigment changes of the skin and that predisposes the individual to myelodysplasia and to acute myeloid leukemia or cancers of the mouth, esophagus, intestinal and urinary tracts, and reproductive organs.

Hemolytic anemia A condition in which red blood cells are destroyed in response to certain toxic or infectious agents or in certain inherited blood disorders and the rate of breakdown exceeds the body's ability to compensate.

Hemolytic disease of the newborn (HDN) (erythroblastosis fetalis) A condition that affects a fetus or newborn in which red blood cells break down because of antibodies made by the mother that are directed against the infant's red cells, potentially resulting in anemia, heart failure, jaundice, and brain damage.

Posthemorrhagic anemia A type of normocytic-normochromic anemia that is caused by sudden blood loss in an individual with normal iron stores and triggers a compensatory response in which water and electrolytes from tissues and interstitial spaces are used to expand plasma volume and accelerate the formation and development of blood cells.

Warm autoimmune hemolytic anemia The most common form of autoimmune hemolytic anemia; caused by IgG that binds to erythrocytes at normal body temperature; often secondary to other diseases, especially lymphomas, chronic lymphocytic leukemia, other neoplastic disorders, or systemic lupus erythematosus.

Anencephaly Anomaly in which the soft, bony component of the skull and much of the brain are missing.

Angelman syndrome (happy puppet syndrome) An inherited syndrome of jerky puppet like movements, frequent laughter, mental and motor retardation, peculiar open-mouthed facies, and seizures.

Angina pectoris Chest pain caused by reduced cardiac blood flow and myocardial ischemia.

Anhedonia Absence of pleasure from the performance of acts that would ordinarily be pleasurable.

Ankylosing spondylitis (AS, spondyloarthritis) Chronic inflammation of the spine and sacroiliac joints with gradual fusion of the vertebrae that immobilizes the spine.

Anorexia nervosa (AN) A disorder with both psychologic and physiologic components that begins with dieting to lose weight and manifests into an inappropriate self-control behavior; continued restrictive eating may lead to starvation and eventually death.

Anorgasmia (orgasmic dysfunction) The inability of the woman to reach or achieve orgasm.

Anuria Urine output less than 50 mL/day.

Anxiety disorder A group of disorders involving various manifestations of anxiety that are grouped together and include panic disorder, specific phobia, social phobia, obsessive-compulsive disorder (OCD), posttraumatic stress disorder (PTSD), acute stress disorder, generalized anxiety disorder (GAD), and anxiety disorders secondary to medical conditions or substance-induced or not otherwise specified.

Aplastic anemia See Anemia.

Aplastic crisis See Anemia.

Appendicitis Inflammation of the appendix as a result of blockage of the opening from the appendix into the cecum; the appendix wall becomes infected and ruptures, allowing the infection to spread throughout the abdomen and cause pain, anorexia, fever, nausea, vomiting, and diarrhea.

Apraxia A disorder of voluntary movement consisting of impairment of the performance of skilled or purposeful movements; results from acquired cerebral disease.

Arcus senilis A gray to white ring at the periphery of the cornea; caused by deposits of cholesterol in the cornea or hyaline degeneration and occurs primarily in older persons.

Areflexia Absence of reflexes.

Arterial ischemic stroke (pediatric arterial ischemic stroke) A rare disorder in children resulting from embolism, arteriopathy, or, rarely, sinovenous thrombosis and leading to a decreased flow of blood and oxygen to areas of the brain.

Asbestosis Pulmonary inflammation and fibrosis resulting from inhalation of hydrous silicates of various metals in fibrous form.

Aseptic meningitis A form of inflammation of the meninges and subarachnoid space surrounding the brain and spinal cord without evidence of bacterial infection; may be associated with viral infection, systemic disease, or drugs.

Aspiration pneumonitis A condition caused by the abnormal entry of fluids, particulate matter, or secretions into the lower airways that can lead to chemical pneumonitis from entry of toxic material such as gastric acid, from bacterial infection, or by mechanical obstruction of the lower airways.

Asthma A chronic inflammatory disorder of the airways involving bronchial hyper responsiveness and airway obstruction marked by periodic attacks of wheezing, shortness of breath, a tight feeling in the chest, and a cough that produces mucus because of an allergic reaction triggered by certain drugs, irritants, viral infection, exercise, or emotional stress.

Asymptomatic bacteriuria The presence of bacteria in the urine without evidence of infection.

Ataxia-telangiectasia (AT) See Immune deficiency.

Ataxic cerebral palsy A form of cerebral palsy associated with damage to the cerebellum and resulting in gait disturbances and instability; at birth the infant may have hypotonia, but develops stiffness of the trunk muscles later in infancy.

Atelectasis Part of or an entire lung collapses and the alveoli deflate as a result of surgery, smoking, or blockage of a bronchiole.

Absorption atelectasis Collapse of lung tissue resulting from gradual absorption of air from obstructed or hypoventilated alveoli or from inhalation of concentrated oxygen or anesthetic agents.

Compression atelectasis Air pressure in the pleural space pushes against the already recoiled lung, causing compression atelectasis, and against the mediastinum, compressing and displacing the heart and great vessels.

Surfactant impairment Decreased production or inactivation of surfactant, which is necessary to reduce surface tension in the alveoli and causes lung collapse during expiration; can occur because of premature birth, acute respiratory distress syndrome, anesthesia, or mechanical ventilation.

Atherosclerosis A type of arteriosclerosis in which the inflammatory changes of thickening and hardening of the walls of large- and medium-sized arteries are caused by an atheroma or plaque of lipids, cells, and connective tissue in the tunica intima.

Atopic dermatitis (AD) (allergic dermatitis) A chronic hereditary skin disease characterized by intense itching and inflamed skin that causes redness, swelling, cracking, crusting, and scaling.

Atrial septal defect (ASD) A congenital heart disease involving the interatrial septum of the heart that separates the right and left atria, resulting in misdirected blood flow between the two sides of the heart.

Atrioventricular canal (AVC) defect A large hole is present in the center of the heart where the wall between the atria joins the wall between the ventricles, and the tricuspid and mitral valves are formed into a single large valve that crosses the defect.

Atypical ductal hyperplasia (ADH) Abnormal proliferating cells in breast ducts.

Atypical hyperplasia Increased number of cells with some variation in cellular structure but without sufficient qualitative or quantitative features of carcinoma.

Atypical lobular hyperplasia (ALH) Abnormal proliferating cells in breast lobules.

Autoimmune hemolytic anemia (AIHA) See Anemia.

Autoimmune neonatal thrombocytopenia See Thrombocytopenia.

Autoimmune vascular purpura (allergic purpura) Purpura caused by antibody-mediated injury of blood vessel walls, typically arterioles and capillaries. The reaction is directed to foreign proteins or chemicals in the blood (microorganisms, drugs, or other chemicals) that deposit on the vessel walls.

Autonomic hyperreflexia (dysreflexia) A syndrome resulting from afferent stimuli that cause intense sympathetic discharge originating with spinal cord injury above the major splanchnic outflow; characterized by hypertension, bradycardia, sweating of the forehead, severe headache, and piloerection on distention of the bladder and rectum.

Autosomal agammaglobulinemia See Immune deficiency.

Autosomal dominant polycystic kidney disease (ADPKD) A progressive disease characterized by the formation of multiple cysts of varying size scattered diffusely throughout both kidneys, resulting in compression and destruction of renal parenchyma, usually with hypertension, gross hematuria, and uremia leading to progressive renal failure.

Autosomal hyper-IgM syndrome See Immune deficiency.

Azotemia Kidney dysfunction characterized by increased serum urea levels and frequently associated with increased creatinine levels.

B

Bacterial pneumonia An acute or chronic disease marked by inflammation of the lungs caused by bacterial infection.

Bacterial tracheitis A condition in which the larynx, trachea, and bronchi are inflamed and present with signs similar to those of epiglottitis and croup; may result in airway obstruction secondary to subglottic edema or sloughing of the epithelial lining or the mucopurulent membrane within the trachea.

Bacterial vaginosis (BV) A condition caused by an overgrowth of normal vaginal bacteria, causing vaginal discharge with a foul odor.

Balanitis Inflammation of the glans penis caused by irritation by environmental substances, physical trauma, or infection.

Bare lymphocyte syndrome See Immune deficiency.

Barrett esophagus Chronic peptic ulceration of the esophagus; formation of precancerous lesions with possible progression to adenocarcinoma.

Bartholinitis (Bartholin cyst) Inflammation of one or both ducts that lead from the introitus (vaginal opening) to the Bartholin/greater vestibular glands.

Basal cell carcinoma A surface epithelial tumor of the skin originating from undifferentiated basal or germinative cells.

B-cell neoplasm See Lymphoma.

Becker muscular dystrophy A general term for a number of late-onset X-linked recessive hereditary, progressive degenerative disorders affecting skeletal muscles, and often other organ systems.

Beckwith–Wiedemann syndrome An inherited disorder characterized by exomphalos, macroglossia, and gigantism; often associated with visceromegaly, adrenocortical cytomegaly, and dysplasia of the renal medulla.

Benign breast disease (BBD) A spectrum of noncancerous changes in ducts and lobules of the breast, including irregular lumps, cysts, sensitive nipples, and itching.

Benign prostatic hyperplasia (BPH) Enlargement of the prostate gland, which may press against the urethra and bladder, interfering with urine flow.

Beta-thalassemia major (Cooley anemia) See Anemia.

Beta-thalassemia minor See Anemia.

Biliary atresia A condition in newborn children in which the biliary tract is blocked or absent, causing bile accumulation and progressive liver failure.

Biliary cirrhosis See Cirrhosis.

Bipolar disorder Psychiatric disorder characterized by alternating mania or hypomania and depression, often with periods of normal mood in between, and changes in energy and behavior according to mood.

Blast injury Tissue damage from compressive waves of air against the body followed by waves of decreased pressure.

Blepharitis Inflammation of the eyelids.

B-lymphocyte deficiency See Immune deficiency.

Bradycardia An abnormally low heart rate, which can cause a fall in cardiac output or can be a symptom of deterioration.

Bradykinesia Decreased spontaneity and movement; a feature of extrapyramidal disorders, such as Parkinson disease.

Brainstem gliomas A group of tumors located in the brainstem that are usually classified as high grade and result in the sudden onset of symptoms including headaches, vomiting, and visual disturbances.

Bronchial carcinoid tumor An obstructing tumor of the trachea or large bronchi that may cause paraneoplastic symptoms.

Bronchiectasis Dilation of the bronchi in response to obstruction, necrotizing pneumonias, cystic fibrosis, or Kartagener syndrome (a hereditary syndrome consisting of dextrocardia, bronchiectasis, and sinusitis).

Bronchiolitis Inflammation of the bronchioles usually caused by viral infection.

Bronchiolitis obliterans Partial or complete obliteration of bronchioles and some bronchi by granulation and fibrotic tissue masses.

Bronchiolitis obliterans with organizing pneumonia (BOOP) Obstruction of the bronchioles and alveolar ducts by fibrous granulation tissue that is further complicated by the development of pneumonia.

Bronchopulmonary dysplasia (BPD) A condition most often found in premature infants in which chronic pulmonary insufficiency occurs because of long-term artificial pulmonary ventilation.

Bruton agammaglobulinemia See Immune deficiency.

Bulbar palsy A form of palsy resulting from impaired function of the cranial nerves from degeneration of the motor neurons of primarily the brainstem; manifested as weakness and wasting of the various bulbar muscles, resulting in difficulty articulating words (dysarthria) and difficulty swallowing (dysphagia); fluid regurgitation is a major symptom and can cause aspiration.

Bullous pemphigoid (BP) A more benign autoimmune disease than pemphigus vulgaris, with blistering of the subepidermal skin layer.

Burkitt lymphoma See Lymphoma.

Burn shock A phenomenon consisting of both a hypovolemic cardiovascular component and a cellular component; results from massive fluid losses from the circulating blood volume.

Bursitis A trauma or overuse injury that can cause painful inflammation in the bursal sacs.

C

C1 deficiency See Immune deficiency.

C2 deficiency See Immune deficiency.

C3 deficiency See Immune deficiency.

C3 receptor deficiency See Immune deficiency.

C4 deficiency See Immune deficiency.

C9 deficiency See Immune deficiency.

Cachexia Illness and malnutrition seen in individuals with cancer that results in wasting and eventual death.

Calculi or urinary stone (urolithiasis) Masses of crystals, protein, or other substances that are a common cause of urinary tract obstruction in adults.

Candidiasis A fungal infection caused by an overgrowth of normal *Candida albicans* found in the skin and mucous membranes of the mouth, respiratory tract, or vagina.

Caplan syndrome Formation in coal workers of intrapulmonary nodules in pneumoconiosis that are histologically similar to subcutaneous rheumatoid nodules associated with rheumatoid arthritis.

Carbuncles A condition in which a bacterial infection of the hair follicle or sebaceous gland ducts becomes painful and discharges pus through various openings.

Carcinoma in situ (CIS) Preinvasive epithelial malignant tumors of glandular or squamous cell origin.

Carcinoma Epithelial cell tumor.

Cardiogenic shock A condition resulting from decreased cardiac output caused by heart disease in which the heart is unable to pump blood through the body, usually because of myocardial infarction.

Cardiomyopathy(ies) A diverse group of diseases primarily affecting the myocardium and resulting from tissue remodeling caused by myocardial and neurohumoral responses to ischemic and hypertensive alterations.

Cavernous (congenital) hemangioma A birthmark that is similar to the strawberry hemangioma but is more deeply rooted and may appear as a red-blue spongy mass of tissue filled with blood.

Cellulitis An infection of the dermis and subcutaneous tissue usually caused by *Staphylococcus*, CA-MRSA, or group B streptococci.

Central core disease (CCD) An autosomal dominant congenital myopathy characterized by hypotonia, delay of motor development in infancy, and nonprogressive or slowly progressive muscle weakness; on biopsy the central core of muscle fibers stains abnormally, myofibrils are abnormally compact, and there is virtual absence of mitochondria and sarcoplasmic reticulum; histochemically, the cores are devoid of oxidative enzyme, phosphorylase, and ATPase activity.

Central precocious puberty A condition in which puberty begins prematurely with normal changes in the hypothalamus-pituitary-gonad (HPG) axis and with premature development of secondary sexual characteristics and premature closure of the epiphysis of long bones, resulting in lifelong short stature.

Centriacinar emphysema See Emphysema.

Cerebellar astrocytoma Brain tumor of the right or left cerebellar hemisphere that causes motor symptoms on the same side as the tumor.

Cerebral palsy (CP) A developmental brain injury that occurs before or shortly after birth and causes muscular impairment affecting motor function and also may alter speech and learning abilities.

Cerebrovascular accidents (CVAs) The leading cause of disability, the third leading cause of death in women, and the fifth leading cause of death in men in the United States; classified pathophysiologically as ischemic, hemorrhagic, or cryptogenic.

Cervical dysplasia (cervical intraepithelial neoplasia [CIN]) A condition characterized by the appearance of abnormal cervical cells that are considered precancerous.

Cervicitis Inflammation of the mucous membrane of the uterine cervix caused by infection, typically by chlamydia, genital herpes, or gonorrhea.

Chediak-Higashi syndrome See Immune deficiency.

Cheyne-Stokes respiration An abnormal pattern of breathing in which tidal volume gradually increases followed by a gradual decrease and a period of apnea before returning to a normal respiratory pattern.

Chickenpox An infectious viral disease that is spread by direct contact or through the air by coughing or sneezing; it causes a blister-like rash that first affects the face and trunk and then can spread over the rest of the body; symptoms include severe itching, fatigue, and fever.

Childhood absence epilepsy (petit mal seizures, nonconvulsive epilepsy) A type of generalized epilepsy; age of onset is 4 to 10 years.

Chlamydia A sexually transmitted bacterial infection that can cause infertility and blindness.

Choking asphyxiation Obstruction of the internal airways.

Cholangiocellular carcinoma (cholangiocarcinoma) Primary carcinomas of the liver that develop in the bile ducts.

Cholecystitis Inflammation of the gallbladder commonly caused by impaction of a gallstone that causes right upper quadrant pain and possibly a rupture and abscess in the gallbladder.

Cholelithiasis The presence or formation of gallstones in the gallbladder or bile ducts.

Chondrosarcoma A cancer of the cartilage that usually occurs in the pelvic bones, shoulder bones, and the upper part of the arms and legs.

Chronic active hepatitis The persistence of clinical manifestations and liver inflammation after the acute stages with consistently abnormal liver function tests and persistent hepatitis B surface antigen (HBsAg) creating a predisposition to cirrhosis and primary hepatocellular carcinoma.

Chronic bronchitis Particularly as a cause of chronic cough in smokers.

Chronic gastritis Tends to occur in older adults with chronic inflammation, mucosal atrophy, and epithelial metaplasia; may be immune (fundal) or nonimmune (antral), depending on the pathogenesis and location of the lesions.

Chronic glomerulonephritis See Glomerulonephritis.

Chronic granulomatous disease (CGD) See Immune deficiency.

Chronic kidney disease (CKD) Progressive loss of renal function associated with systemic diseases such as hypertension, diabetes mellitus, systemic lupus erythematosus, or intrinsic kidney disease, including kidney stones, acute kidney injury, chronic glomerulonephritis, chronic pyelonephritis, obstructive uropathies, or vascular disorders.

Chronic leukemia See Leukemia.

Chronic lymphocytic leukemia (CLL) See Leukemia.

Chronic mesenteric ischemia Development of regions of compromised blood flow in the mesenterium secondary to atherosclerosis (most common), congestive heart failure, dysrhythmias, hemorrhage, thrombus formation, aortic aneurysm, or any condition that decreases arterial blood flow. Chronic occlusion is often accompanied by formation of collateral circulation that may be able to nourish the resting intestine.

Chronic mucocutaneous candidiasis See Immune deficiency.

Chronic myelogenous leukemia (CML) See Leukemia.

Chronic obstructive pulmonary disease (COPD) Any of a group of irreversible respiratory diseases (chronic bronchitis, emphysema, α_1-antitrypsin deficiency) that are characterized by airflow obstruction or limitation.

Chronic pancreatitis Inflammation of the pancreas resulting from repeated exacerbations of acute pancreatitis that lead to chronic changes; associated with obstruction from gallstones, autoimmune disease, gene mutations, smoking, occupational chemical exposure, and obesity.

Chronic pyelonephritis Persistent or recurrent infection of the kidney leading to scarring.

Chronic relapsing thrombotic thrombocytopenic purpura (TTP) See Thrombocytopenia.

Chronic venous insufficiency (CVI) Persistent ambulatory lower extremity venous hypertension.

Cirrhosis Degeneration of liver tissue resulting in fibrosis with nodule and scar formation that compromises liver function.

Alcoholic cirrhosis Destructive inflammation of the liver caused by the toxic effects of alcohol metabolism, immunologic processes, lipid peroxidation, and malnutrition.

Biliary cirrhosis A form of alcoholic cirrhosis in which damage and inflammation leading to cirrhosis begin in bile canaliculi and bile ducts, rather than in the hepatocytes.

Primary biliary cirrhosis A T-lymphocyte- and antibody-mediated destruction of the small intrahepatic bile ducts.

Cloacal exstrophy Family of congenital anomalies with two exstrophied bladder units separated by an exstrophied segment of intestine, which is usually cecum, receiving the ileum superiorly and continuing distally to a blind-ending microcolon.

Clubfoot Describes a range of foot deformities in which the foot turns inward and downward.

Cluster headache One of a group of rare disorders referred to as *trigeminal autonomic cephalalgia*; they occur in clusters (up to eight attacks per day) on one side of the head primarily, with pain that is severe, stabbing, and throbbing.

Coal worker pneumoconiosis (coal miner lung, black lung) Mild to severe pneumoconiosis (pulmonary fibrosis) caused by coal dust (coal, silica, quartz) deposits in the lung; symptoms initially present as a productive cough and wheezing but may advance to chronic bronchitis and emphysema.

Coarctation of the aorta (COA) A condition in which the aorta narrows in the area where the ductus arteriosus inserts; narrowing usually occurs preductal in children and postductal in adults.

Cold agglutinin autoimmune hemolytic anemia See Anemia.

Cold hemolysin autoimmune hemolytic anemia (paroxysmal cold hemoglobinuria) See Anemia.

Combined T- and B-lymphocyte deficiency See Immune deficiency.

Common variable immune deficiency See Immune deficiency.

Communicating (extraventricular) hydrocephalus A disorder in which the cerebrospinal fluid pathways are intact but cerebrospinal fluid absorption is impaired.

Community-acquired pneumonia (CAP) A major cause of morbidity and mortality in children, particularly in developing countries.

Complement deficiency See Immune deficiency.

Complete precocious puberty Refers to the early onset and progression of all pubertal features (i.e., thelarche, pubarche, and menarche).

Complex febrile seizure Seizures with characteristic features similar to those of simple febrile seizure with a longer duration and focal characteristics; occur more than once in a 24-hour period.

Complex regional pain syndrome (CRPS) Diffuse persistent pain usually in an extremity often associated with vasomotor disturbances, trophic changes, and limitation or immobility of joints; frequently follows a local injury.

Compression atelectasis See Atelectasis.

Compressive syndrome (sensorimotor syndrome; crush syndrome) A shocklike state that follows release of a limb (or limbs) or the trunk and pelvis after a prolonged period of compression, such as by a heavy weight; characterized by suppression of renal function, probably the result of damage to the renal tubules by myoglobin from the damaged muscles.

Congenital (infantile) nephrotic syndrome (Finnish type) A very rare form of nephrotic syndrome caused by a defect in a kidney protein resulting in excessive amounts of protein excreted in the urine.

Congenital adrenal hyperplasia A group of autosomal recessively inherited disorders associated with a deficiency of one of the enzymes involved in cortisol biosynthesis, resulting in elevation of ACTH levels and overproduction and accumulation of cortisol precursors proximal to the block; androgens are produced in excess, causing virilization. The most common disorder is the 21-hydroxylase deficiency, caused by mutation in the cytochrome P450 21-hydroxylase gene *(CYP21)* on chromosome 6p.

Congenital aganglionic megacolon (Hirschsprung disease) A congenital defect in which the nerves that innervate the anus through the wall of the bowel are absent, resulting in enlargement of the bowel superior to the point where the nerves are missing and a subsequent decrease in peristalsis that results in chronic constipation.

Congenital hydrocephalus Excessive accumulation of cerebrospinal fluid present at birth and characterized by increased intracranial pressure (ICP). This increase may be caused by a blockage within the ventricular system in which the cerebrospinal fluid (CSF) flows, an imbalance in the production of CSF, or a reduced reabsorption of CSF that results in ventricular enlargement and increased ICP.

Congenital hydrocephalus Lack of secretion of thyroid hormone.

Congestive splenomegaly Enlargement of the spleen accompanied by ascites, portal hypertension, and esophageal varices; most commonly seen in those with hepatic cirrhosis.

Consumptive thrombohemorrhagic disorders Heterogeneous group of conditions that demonstrate the entire range of hemorrhagic and thrombotic pathologic conditions.

Contact dermatitis An allergic response to an environmental antigen binding to specific carrier proteins contained in an individual's skin.

Contrecoup injury Brain injury resulting from the brain hitting the inside of the skull on the side opposite the site of blunt force trauma.

Cor pulmonale Right-sided heart failure caused by prolonged pulmonary hypertension.

Coronary artery disease (CAD) Narrowing of the lumen of one or more of the coronary arteries, usually attributable to atherosclerosis, leading to myocardial ischemia; can cause congestive heart failure, angina pectoris, or myocardial infarction.

Craniopharyngioma A brain tumor that develops in the pituitary gland and most often affects children, causing headache, seizure, diabetes insipidus, early onset of puberty, and delayed growth.

Craniosynostosis (craniostenosis) (see Syndromic craniosynostosis) Premature ossification of the skull and closure of the sutures, resulting in abnormal skull expansion and asymmetrical skull growth.

Cri du chat syndrome A hereditary congenital syndrome characterized by hypertelorism, microcephaly, severe mental deficiency, and a plaintive catlike cry; caused by deletion of the short arm of chromosome 5.

Crohn disease (CD) An autoimmune condition in which the intestines and possibly other regions of the digestive system are chronically inflamed and ulcerated, causing chronic diarrhea, disrupted digestion, and subsequent difficulty eating and digesting food.

Croup A viral infection that involves the larynx, trachea, and the airways leading to the lungs and that can result in serious breathing difficulties, hoarseness, sore throat, and a hacking cough.

Cryptorchidism The scrotum of one or both testes is absent because of failure of the testis to descend from the abdominal position during fetal development.

Curling ulcer Ischemic ulcers of the stomach and duodenal mucosa that develop within hours after an event, such as hemorrhage, multisystem trauma, severe burns, heart failure, or sepsis.

Cushing disease Adrenal hyperplasia caused by an ACTH-secreting basophil adenoma of the pituitary.

Cushing syndrome Increased synthesis and secretion of cortisol from a tumor of the adrenal cortex; caused by administration of glucocorticoid drugs or by the presence of an ACTH-secreting tumor of the anterior lobe of the pituitary gland (Cushing disease), resulting in weight gain, glucose intolerance, and muscle wasting.

Cushing ulcer A stress ulcer associated with severe head trauma or brain surgery.

Cyclic neutropenia See Immune deficiency.

Cylindrical bronchiectasis A reversible bronchial dilation with symmetrically dilated airways, as can be seen after pneumonia.

Cystic fibrosis (CF) A genetic disorder of the exocrine glands caused by a mutation in the CF transmembrane regulator gene, resulting in impairment in chloride transfer across cell membranes and subsequent chloride and water accumulation in organs and in thickened secretions that block ducts and form cysts.

Cystitis A condition characterized by acute or chronic inflammation of the urinary bladder, usually caused by bacterial infection of the urethra; symptoms include frequent burning on urination, blood in the urine, pain in the pubic area, chills and fever, back pain, and nausea. See Painful bladder syndrome/interstitial cystitis (PBS/IC) for further information.

D

Dandy–Walker malformation Congenital defect of midline cerebellar structures and the fourth ventricle in which hydrocephalus is caused by atresia of the foramina of Luschka or Magendie, which normally allow the fourth ventricle to empty into the areas surrounding the brain, leading the ventricular flow of CSF into a "blind pouch."

Dawn phenomenon Abrupt increases in fasting levels of plasma glucose between 5 and 9 AM, in the absence of antecedent hypoglycemia; occurs in diabetic persons receiving insulin therapy.

Decompression sickness (DCS) (caisson disease) Gas embolism created when a person under water returns to the surface too quickly, resulting in cellular hypoxia, joint and muscle pain, and tissue necrosis.

Deep venous thrombosis (DVT) A blood clot or thrombus in a deep vein, usually of the leg.

Degenerative disk disease (DDD) Intervertebral disk tissue is replaced by fibrocartilage during aging; functional capacity is rarely altered.

Demyelinating polyneuropathy A type of polyneuropathy in which the peripheral nerve myelin is primarily affected; can be familial (Charcot-Marie-Tooth disease, type 1) or acquired (Guillain-Barré syndrome); motor nerve conduction is slowed or blocked.

Dermatitis herpetiformis Pruritic chronic dermatitis with successive groups of symmetrical, erythematous, papular, vesicular, eczematous, or bullous lesions; usually associated with asymptomatic gluten-sensitive enteropathy.

Detrusor areflexia A lower motor neuron disorder that results in underactive, hypotonic, or atonic bladder function with retention of urine and distention.

Detrusor hyperreflexia (uninhibited or reflex bladder) Upper motor neuron disorders in which the bladder empties automatically when it becomes full and the external sphincter functions normally.

Developmental dysplasia of the hip (DDH) A condition in which the hip joint of babies or young children is malformed, with the ball being completely out of the socket or the socket being too shallow to support the ball.

Diabetes Diseases having in common the triad of symptoms of polyuria, weight loss, and significant glucosuria.

Diabetes insipidus A disease caused by a deficiency in or resistance to antidiuretic hormone that is characterized by excretion of large amounts of dilute urine because of a decrease in water reabsorption in the kidney.

Gestational diabetes mellitus (GDM) Carbohydrate intolerance of variable severity with onset during pregnancy.

Maturity-onset diabetes of youth (MODY) A non–insulin-requiring diabetes in lean individuals typically younger than 25 with evidence of autosomal dominant inheritance.

Type 1 diabetes mellitus A disorder of carbohydrate metabolism characterized by a decrease in insulin production, resulting in hyperglycemia, ketoacidosis, and eventually renal failure and coronary artery disease.

Type 2 diabetes mellitus A condition of glucose intolerance that normally appears first in adulthood and is exacerbated by obesity and an inactive lifestyle.

Diabetic nephropathy A progressive kidney disease caused by diabetes-induced angiopathy of capillaries in the glomeruli that causes nodular glomerulosclerosis.

Diabetic neuropathy Combined sensory and motor disorder often seen in older diabetic persons as a result of microvascular injury involving small blood vessels that supply nerves.

Diabetic retinopathy Damage to the retina caused by an over accumulation of glucose or fructose that damages the blood vessels in the retina; in advanced stages, lack of oxygen in the retina causes fragile blood vessels to grow along the retina and in the vitreous fluid of the eye that may bleed and cause blurred vision.

Diaper dermatitis A type of dermatitis characterized by inflammation of the skin in the diaper area in infants caused by exposure of the skin to feces and urine.

Diastolic heart failure A condition in which heart contractions are normal but the ventricle does not relax completely; therefore less blood enters the heart.

Diffuse brain injury (diffuse axonal injury) Injury to neuronal axons in many areas of the brain caused by stretching and shearing forces received during brain injury.

DiGeorge syndrome See Immune deficiency.

Dilated cardiomyopathy (congestive cardiomyopathy) A condition in which all four chambers of the heart are enlarged and weakened, resulting in progressive congestive heart failure and the need for heart transplantation.

Discoid (cutaneous) lupus erythematosus (DLE) See Lupus erythematosus.

Dislocation The temporary displacement of a bone from its normal position in a joint.

Disorders of desire (hypoactive sexual desire, decreased libido) The most common sexual dysfunction in women; prevalence increases with age and may be a biologic manifestation of depression, alcohol or other substance abuse, prolactin-secreting pituitary tumors, or testosterone deficiency.

Disseminated intravascular coagulation (DIC) An acquired clinical syndrome characterized by widespread activation of coagulation resulting in the formation of fibrin clots in medium and small vessels (microvasculature) throughout the body.

Distal intestinal obstruction syndrome (DIOS) A syndrome seen in cystic fibrosis secondary to impaction with feces and inspissated mucus.

Diverticulitis Inflammation of the herniations or saclike outpouchings of mucosa through the muscle layers of the colon wall.

Diverticulosis The presence of multiple bulging sacs pushing outward from the wall of the large intestine that may become infected and rupture, causing abdominal pain, tenderness, and fever.

Down syndrome Trisomy or translocation of chromosome 21, resulting in intellectual disability; distinctive facial appearance with a low nasal bridge, epicanthal folds, protruding tongue, and flat, low-set ears; poor muscle tone (hypotonia); and short stature. Congenital heart defects, reduced ability to resist respiratory tract infections, and increased risk for leukemia are common.

Drug-induced hemolytic anemia See Anemia.

Duchenne muscular dystrophy (DMD) An X-linked genetic disorder in which fat and fibrous tissue infiltrate and weaken muscle tissues such as in the legs and pelvis, lungs, and heart; usually results in death before adulthood.

Dumping syndrome Rapid emptying of hypertonic chyme from a surgically created residual stomach causing nausea, vomiting, bleeding, and diarrhea about 20 minutes after a meal.

Duodenal ulcer Most common type of peptic ulcer; usually associated with altered mucosal defenses, rapid gastric emptying, elevated serum gastrin levels, or acid production stimulated by smoking.

Dysfunctional uterine bleeding (DUB) Heavy or irregular bleeding in the absence of organic disease, such as submucous fibroids, endometrial polyps, blood dyscrasias, pregnancy, infection, or systemic disease.

Dyskinetic cerebral palsy Extreme difficulty in fine motor coordination and purposeful movements resulting from injury to the basal ganglia or thalamus.

Dysphoric mood Mood of general dissatisfaction, restlessness, depression, and anxiety; a feeling of unpleasantness or discomfort.

Dysplasia (atypical hyperplasia) Abnormal changes in the size, shape, and organization of mature cells; considered a form of atypical hyperplasia.

Dyspraxia The partial inability to perform purposeful or skilled motor acts in the absence of paralysis, sensory loss, abnormal posture and tone, abnormal involuntary movement, incoordination, or inattentiveness.

Dysrhythmias (arrhythmias) Disturbances of cardiac rhythm and the most common complication of acute MI.

Dyssynergia Development of lesions in the upper motor neurons of the brain and spinal cord; results in loss of coordinated neuromuscular contraction and overactive or hyper reflexive bladder function.

E

Eczema Most common inflammatory disorder of the skin; generally characterized by pruritus, lesions with indistinct borders, and epidermal changes.

Eisenmenger syndrome A progressively developing condition in which a congenital heart defect such as ventricular septal defect is left untreated and causes a reversed right-to-left shunt secondary to increased pressures on the right side of the heart because of pulmonary hypertension.

Embryonic tumor A tumor originating in the gestational period that contains predominantly immature blast cells that cannot differentiate into mature functional cells.

Emphysema Pulmonary inflammation resulting in increased work of breathing or physiologic dead space and abnormal permanent enlargement of gas-exchange airways (acini) accompanied by destruction of alveolar walls without obvious fibrosis.

Centriacinar emphysema Diminished pulmonary function resulting from septal destruction in the respiratory bronchioles and alveolar ducts, usually in the upper lobes of the lung.

Panacinar emphysema Destruction of the entire acinus, with damage more randomly distributed and involving the lower lobes of the lung. It tends to occur in older adults and in those with α_1-antitrypsin deficiency.

Empyema (infected pleural effusion) A condition in which purulent fluid is persistently discharged into the pleural space as a result of complications of bacterial infections.

Encephalitis Inflammation of the brain usually caused by a virus.

Endometriosis A condition that is common in women of reproductive age in which the tissue lining the uterus is found outside of the uterus, resulting in pain and infertility.

End-stage kidney disease (ESKD) A condition in which there is significant loss of renal function; usually less than 10% of renal function remains.

Eosinophilic esophagitis Rare, idiopathic inflammatory disease of the esophagus characterized by infiltration of eosinophils; associated with atopic disease, including asthma and food allergies.

Ependymoma Intracranial tumor that is most commonly found in children and typically arises from the inner lining of the fourth ventricle and the spinal canal.

Epididymitis A painful condition in which the epididymis becomes inflamed, usually because of a secondary bacterial infection that is triggered by a variety of underlying conditions such as urinary tract or sexually transmitted infections.

Epilepsy A group of chronic neurologic disorders with paroxysmal brain dysfunction from excessive neuronal discharge; symptoms vary widely from complex behavioral abnormalities to focal convulsions, to momentary spells of impaired consciousness.

Epispadias A birth defect in which the urethra opens on the upper penile surface.

Erysipelas A highly contagious bacterial infection that produces shiny, red, swollen areas and fever and can lead to blood poisoning and pneumonia.

Erythema multiforme A skin disease that is caused by allergies, seasonal changes, or drug sensitivities, resulting in the formation of red macules, papules, or subdermal vesicles on the skin and mucous membranes.

Erythema toxicum neonatorum A temporary eruption of redness of the skin, small papules, and occasionally pustules in newborns that is associated with contact dermatitis or hypersensitivity to milk or other allergens.

Erythrodermic (exfoliative) psoriasis See Psoriasis.

Erythromyalgia Chronic disorder characterized by warmth, pain, and redness, occurring primarily in the feet and lower legs.

Essential (primary) thrombocythemia (ET) Excessive production of platelets (platelet count greater than 400,000/mm^3 of blood); may be primary or secondary (reactive) and is usually asymptomatic until the count exceeds 1 million/mm^3 of blood when intravascular clot formation (thrombosis), hemorrhage, or other abnormalities can occur.

Ewing sarcoma A malignant neoplasm of bone, primarily those of the extremities, including the shoulder girdle, with a predilection for the metaphysis; histologically presents as conspicuous foci of necrosis in association with irregular masses of small, regular, rounded, or ovoid cells.

Exstrophy of the bladder A congenital defect in which the lower abdominal wall is malformed and ruptures.

Extrapyramidal/nonspecific cerebral palsy Any of a group of clinical disorders considered to be due to malfunction in the extrapyramidal system and marked by abnormal involuntary movements; included are parkinsonism, athetosis, and chorea.

F

Facioscapulohumeral muscular dystrophy (FSHD) An autosomal dominant genetic disorder that begins in childhood and causes muscle wasting and weakness, primarily in the face, shoulder, and arms.

Factor H deficiency See Immune deficiency.

Factor I deficiency See Immune deficiency.

Failure to thrive (FTT) Also called *growth faltering*, it is a physical sign demonstrating that a child is receiving inadequate nutrition for optimal growth and development. FTT is manifested as a deceleration in weight gain, a low weight/height ratio, a low weight/height/head circumference ratio, or a low body mass index (BMI).

Fanconi anemia See Anemia.

Fetal alcohol syndrome (FAS) A syndrome of altered prenatal growth and morphogenesis that occurs in infants born to women who were chronically alcoholic during pregnancy; it includes maxillary hypoplasia, prominence of the forehead and mandible, short palpebral fissures, microphthalmia, epicanthal folds, severe growth retardation, intellectual disability, and microcephaly.

Fibromyalgia A condition in which muscles, tendons, and joints are painful, stiff, and tender; often accompanied by restless sleep, fatigue, anxiety, depression, and disturbances in bowel function.

Fibrosarcoma A malignant tumor of fibrous connective tissue that usually is derived from immature proliferating fibroblasts.

Fibrous dysplasia (FD) A genetic disorder in which tumor-like growths or lesions form in one or more bones and replace the medullary bone with fibrous tissue, resulting in expansion and weakening of the bone.

Florid hyperplasia Rapid and unexpected cell growth in the lining of the breast ducts.

Focal segmental glomerulosclerosis (FSGS) A condition in which glomerular capillaries with thickened basement membranes and increased mesangial matrix collapse in segments. Usually presents as nephrotic syndrome.

Frontotemporal dementia (FTD) (Pick disease) Progressive circumscribed cerebral atrophy; a rare type of cerebrodegenerative disorder manifested primarily as dementia, in which there is striking atrophy of portions of the frontal and temporal lobes.

FSH deficiency A condition characterized by decreased or absent production of follicle-stimulating hormone (FSH), resulting in a decline in spermatogenesis/oogenesis and associated infertility.

Furuncles A staphylococcal infection produces painful pus-filled inflamed hair follicles and involves surrounding skin and subcutaneous tissue.

Fusiform aneurysm (giant aneurysm) A large aneurysm that stretches to affect the entire circumference of the arterial wall.

G

Galactorrhea (inappropriate lactation) A condition in which milk-like fluid is secreted from the breast because of hormonal alterations that are not associated with childbirth or nursing.

Ganglioneuroblastoma An embryonal aggressive tumor of intermediate cellular differentiation that originates outside the central nervous system (CNS) in the developing sympathetic nervous system.

Ganglioneuroma A benign neoplasm composed of mature ganglionic neurons scattered within a stroma of neurofibrils and collagenous fibers.

Gangliosidosis Any disease characterized by abnormal accumulation of specific gangliosides within the nervous system (e.g., Tay-Sachs disease).

Gastroesophageal reflux disease (GERD) The reflux of acid and pepsin from the stomach to the esophagus that causes esophagitis.

General adaptation syndrome (GAS) The sum of all nonspecific reactions of the body to prolonged systemic stress, comprising alarm, resistance, and exhaustion.

Generalized anxiety disorder (GAD) An anxiety disorder characterized by an excessively anxious mood lasting at least 1 month that interferes with daily functioning and may be accompanied by jitteriness, sweating, feelings of catastrophe concerning one's family or self, and irritability.

Generalized neuropathy A functional disturbance or pathologic change in the cell body of one type of peripheral neuron.

Genital herpes A sexually transmitted viral infection that is caused primarily by herpes simplex virus type 2 and is characterized by painful lesions in the genital and anal regions.

Gestational diabetes mellitus (GDM) See Diabetes.

GH deficiency A condition characterized by decreased or absent production of growth hormone (GH), resulting in a decline in insulin-like growth factor 1 and dwarfism if the deficiency is prepubertal.

Glaucoma A disease of the eye characterized by increased intraocular pressure, excavation, and atrophy of the optic nerve; produces defects in the field of vision and eventual blindness.

Glomerulonephritis Inflammation of the renal glomeruli that may not produce symptoms or may present with hematuria and proteinuria.

- **Acute glomerulonephritis** An inflammatory disease of both kidneys predominantly affecting children from ages 2 to 12.
- **Acute poststreptococcal glomerulonephritis (PSGN)** A kidney disease secondary to infection with Streptococci in which bacterial antigens complex with antibodies in the blood, deposit in the kidneys, and initiate an immune complex–mediated hypersensitivity reaction.
- **Chronic glomerulonephritis** A slowly progressive glomerulonephritis most often associated with other systemic disease, including diabetes, malaria, hepatitis, or systemic lupus erythematosus, that generally leads to irreversible renal failure.
- **Membranoproliferative glomerulonephritis (MPGN)** A chronic, slowly progressive glomerulonephritis in which the glomeruli are enlarged as a result of proliferation of mesangial cells and irregular thickening of the capillary walls, which narrows the capillary lumina.
- **Membranous glomerulonephritis** A slowly progressive disease of unknown origin or that occurs secondary to autoimmune conditions, infections, specific drugs, or malignant tumors that is caused by immune complexes formed from the binding of antibodies to antigens of the glomerular basement membrane (GBM) or antigens transported from the systemic circulation and implanted in the GBM.
- **Membranous nephropathy (membranous glomerulonephritis)** Membranous nephropathy is caused by subepithelial deposition of antibodies (IgG4 subclass) to antigens (M-type phospholipase A2 receptor [PLA2R] protein) located on glomerular podocytes and activation of complement-mediated inflammation with injury and release of inflammatory mediators by mesangial and epithelial cells, resulting in increased membrane permeability, thickening of the glomerular membrane, and ultimately glomerular sclerosis.
- **Mesangial proliferative glomerulonephritis** Deposition of immune complexes in the mesangium with mesangial cell proliferation and expansion reducing blood flow and altering filtration membrane permeability with development of hematuria, proteinuria, hypertension, and uremia (nephritic syndrome); associated with IgA nephropathy, lupus nephritis, or early diabetic nephropathy.
- **Rapidly progressive (crescentic) glomerulonephritis (RPGN) (subacute or extracapillary glomerulonephritis)** Develops over days to weeks, primarily affects adults in their fifties and sixties, and may be idiopathic or associated with a proliferative glomerular disease (diffuse proliferation of extracapillary cells), such as lupus or poststreptococcal glomerulonephritis.

Glucose-6-phosphate dehydrogenase (G6PD) deficiency See Anemia.

Gluten-sensitive enteropathy (celiac sprue) A condition characterized by mucosal inflammation and villous atrophy in the gastrointestinal tract formed in response to a genetic predisposition for an immune response to gluten and similar proteins.

Gonorrhea A sexually transmitted disease caused by the bacteria gonococci that invade the mucous membranes of the genitals and urinary tract and in women the cervix, fallopian tubes, and ovaries, causing chronic pelvic pain or infertility.

Gout A disorder of uric acid metabolism that causes painful inflammation of the joints, commonly the big toe, and arthritic attacks resulting from elevated levels of uric acid in the blood and the deposition of negatively birefringent urate crystals around the joints.

Gouty arthritis Inflammation of the joints in gout.

Graft rejection Immunologic rejection of transplanted tissue or organs based on antigen differences between the donor and recipient.

- **Acute graft rejection** Cell-mediated immune rejection that occurs within days to months after transplantation; immune response is usually against unmatched human leukocyte antigen (HLA) antigens and develops after transplantation.
- **Chronic graft rejection** Slow, progressive organ failure after a period of months or years of normal function by a developing weak cell-mediated immune response against minor histocompatibility antigens on the endothelial cells lining the blood vessels of the grafted tissue.
- **Hyperacute graft rejection** Immediate rejection of a graft because of preexisting antibodies against antigens expressed on the grafted tissue or organ.

Graft-versus-host disease (GVHD) Condition in which mature T cells in a transplanted graft (e.g., transfused blood) are capable of a destructive cell-mediated reaction against unmatched histocompatibility antigens on the tissues in the graft recipient.

Granuloma inguinale A bacterial-induced disease, also called *donovanosis*, that is thought to be transmitted primarily by anal rather than vaginal intercourse and causes painless genital ulcers like syphilis but progresses to destroy the internal and external genital tissue.

Graves disease Autoimmune hyperthyroidism caused by antibodies that continuously activate thyroid-stimulating-hormone receptors, resulting in uncontrolled production of thyroxine and characterized by an enlarged thyroid gland, protrusion of eyeballs, a rapid heartbeat, and nervous excitability.

Guillain-Barré syndrome (GBS) (Landry-Guillain-Barré syndrome, idiopathic polyneuritis, acute inflammatory polyradiculopathy, acute autoimmune neuropathy) An acute, immune-mediated disorder of peripheral nerves, spinal roots, and cranial nerves that commonly presents as a rapidly progressive, areflexic, relatively symmetrical ascending weakness of the limb, truncal, respiratory, pharyngeal, and facial musculature, with variable sensory and autonomic dysfunction; typically reaches its peak activity within 2 to 3 weeks, followed by a plateau period of similar duration, and gradual but complete recovery in most cases; often preceded by a respiratory tract or gastrointestinal tract infection and is associated with albuminocytologic dissociation of the cerebrospinal fluid.

Guttate psoriasis See Psoriasis.

Gynecomastia Abnormal breast tissue development on adolescent boys or men as a result of an imbalance in hormones.

H

Heat exhaustion Occurs when sufficient salt and water loss results in hemoconcentration with hypotension occurring secondary to fluid loss (hypovolemia), and the individual feels weak, is nauseated, and can suddenly collapse.

Heat stroke A life-threatening condition associated with high environmental temperatures and humidity causing core body temperature to rise as a result of thermoregulatory failure.

Hematemesis Accumulation of blood in the gastrointestinal tract causing irritation, increased peristalsis, and vomiting.

Hematochezia Rapid bleeding from the upper GI tract producing bright red stools.

Hemochromatosis Disorder of iron metabolism characterized by excessive absorption of ingested iron, saturation of iron-binding protein, and deposition of hemosiderin in tissue, particularly in the liver, pancreas, and skin; cirrhosis of the liver, diabetes (bronze diabetes), bronze pigmentation of the skin, and eventually heart failure may occur; also can result from administration of large amounts of iron orally, by injection, or in forms of blood transfusion therapy.

Hemoglobin H disease See Anemia.

Hemolytic anemia See Anemia.

Hemolytic disease of the newborn (HDN) (erythroblastosis fetalis) See Anemia.

Hemolytic jaundice (prehepatic jaundice, nonobstructive jaundice) Jaundice resulting from excessive hemolysis of red blood cells.

Hemolytic-uremic syndrome (HUS) A condition in which platelets aggregate within the kidney's small blood vessels, resulting in reduced blood flow to the kidney and subsequent kidney failure and destruction of the red blood cells; occurs usually after exposure to Shiga-like toxin from a strain of *E. coli*.

Hemophilia A (classic hemophilia) A genetic disorder in which a mutation in factor VIII causes prolonged clotting time, decreased formation of thromboplastin, and diminished conversion of prothrombin.

Hemophilia B (Christmas disease) A genetic disorder similar to hemophilia A in terms of symptoms but with a mutation in the factor IX gene.

Hemophilia C (factor XI deficiency) A genetic disorder characterized by a deficiency in factor XI, resulting in a mild form of hemophilia.

Hemorrhagic stroke (spontaneous intracranial hemorrhage) Stroke usually caused by hypertension that results in bleeding in the brain and typically increases intracranial pressure and may lead to death.

Henoch–Schönlein purpura nephritis Inflammation of the blood vessels causing bleeding into the skin, mucous membranes, internal organs, and other tissues; pain and inflammation in the joints; abdominal pain; gastrointestinal bleeding; inflammation of the kidneys; subcutaneous edema; encephalopathy; and inflammation of the testis.

Heparin-induced thrombocytopenia (HIT) See Thrombocytopenia.

Hepatic encephalopathy A condition that is usually caused by liver cirrhosis and portal hypertension in which toxins produced by the gut pass into the systemic circulation and damage brain cells, resulting in impaired cognition, tremor, and a decreased level of consciousness.

Hepatitis B virus One of six types of hepatitis virus that cause liver infection; it is most commonly sexually transmitted.

Hepatocellular carcinoma (hepatocarcinoma; HCC) Primary carcinoma of the liver developing in hepatocytes.

Hepatopulmonary syndrome Intrapulmonary vasodilation, intrapulmonary shunting, and hypoxia and portopulmonary hypertension (pulmonary vasoconstriction and vascular remodeling) are common respiratory complications of advanced liver disease and portal hypertension.

Hepatorenal syndrome (HRS) Acute renal failure occurs because of a decrease in renal blood flow secondary to liver disease.

Hereditary angioedema An inherited, autosomal dominant disease characterized by the episodic appearance of nonpitting edema, most often affecting the limbs, but capable of involving other parts of the body, including mucosal surfaces such as those of the intestine (causing abdominal pain) or respiratory tract (causing asphyxia); associated with deficiency of inhibitor of the first component of complement pathway (C1 esterase inhibitor).

Hereditary hemochromatosis (HH) Autosomal recessive chronic liver disease caused by excessive intestinal absorption of elemental iron; characterized by elevated serum iron saturation, transferrin, and ferritin levels; improves with phlebotomy; increased risk of developing cirrhosis, liver cancer, and liver failure.

Hereditary sideroblastic anemia See Anemia.

Hereditary spherocytosis See Anemia.

Hiatal hernia An anatomic abnormality in which the esophageal hiatus is larger than normal, causing part of the stomach to protrude through the diaphragm and up into the esophagus or chest.

High altitude cerebral edema (HACE) An increase in severity of symptoms or signs of neurologic dysfunction, such as ataxia or altered consciousness, related to high altitude.

High altitude pulmonary edema (HAPE) A noncardiogenic pulmonary edema associated with pulmonary hypertension and elevated capillary pressure related to high altitude illness.

Hirsutism Abnormal growth and distribution of androgen-sensitive hair growth on the face, body, and pubic area in a male pattern that occurs in women.

Hodgkin lymphoma (HL) See Lymphoma.

Hormonal hyperplasia Growth of cellular layers chiefly in estrogen-dependent organs, such as the uterus and breast. After ovulation, for example, estrogen stimulates the endometrium to grow and thicken for reception of the fertilized ovum.

Huntington disease (HD) An autosomal dominant disease causing a progressive increase in involuntary, jerky, dyskinetic movements; mental deterioration; and premature death.

Hyaline membrane disease (HMD) A type of respiratory distress syndrome of the newborn in which there is formation of a hyaline-like membrane lining the terminal respiratory passages; extensive atelectasis is attributed to lack of surfactant.

Hydrocele A collection of fluid within the tunica vaginalis that is the most common cause of scrotal swelling.

Hydrocephalus ex vacuo Hydrocephalus attributable to loss or atrophy of brain tissue; less commonly associated with raised intracranial pressure and dilation of the cerebral ventricles.

Hydrops fetalis Edema formation in the fetal subcutaneous tissue because of an enzyme deficiency or any one of several other disorders.

Hyperosmolar hyperglycemic nonketotic syndrome (HHNKS) A complication seen in diabetes mellitus in which very marked hyperglycemia occurs, causing osmotic shifts in water in brain cells, and resulting in coma. It can be fatal or lead to permanent neurologic damage.

Hypersensitive pneumonitis (extrinsic allergic alveolitis) An allergic, inflammatory disease of the lungs caused by inhalation of organic particles or fumes.

Hypertrophic cardiomyopathy A genetic disorder caused by various mutations that thicken the heart muscle, possibly leading to obstruction of blood flow and heart dysfunction; this is a common cause of sudden death in young athletes.

Hypogammaglobulinemia See Immune deficiency.

Hypoplastic anemia See Anemia.

Hypoplastic left heart syndrome (HLHS) A condition in which the left side of the heart, including the aorta, aortic valve, left ventricle, and mitral valve, is underdeveloped and blood returning from the lungs flows through an opening in the atrial septum and the right ventricle pumps the blood into the pulmonary artery and then into the aorta.

Hypospadias A birth defect in which the urethral opening is abnormally placed, opening anywhere from the tip of the glans penis to the shaft, or to the junction of the penis and scrotum or perineum in males; usually opens in the vagina in females.

Hypotonia Decreased muscle tone; a condition in which passive movement of a muscle occurs with little or no resistance. A symptom of cerebellar and pure pyramidal tract damage, it is thought to be caused by decreased muscle spindle activity secondary to decreased excitability of neurons.

Hypovolemic shock Caused by loss of whole blood (hemorrhage), plasma (burns), or interstitial fluid (diaphoresis, diabetes mellitus, diabetes insipidus, emesis, or diuresis) in large amounts.

Hypoxemia Reduced oxygen levels in the blood, which contributes to cardiovascular dysfunction by causing dilation of arterioles, capillaries, and venules and leads to decreased vascular resistance and increased flow.

I

Iatrogenic pneumothorax See Pneumothorax.

Icterus neonatorum (neonatal jaundice) Jaundice in newborn infants caused by functional immaturity of the liver; usually subsides within the first few days of life.

Idiopathic pulmonary fibrosis (IPF) An excessive amount of fibrous or connective tissue in the lung.

Idiopathic thrombocytopenic purpura (autoimmune or primary thrombocytopenic purpura) See Thrombocytopenia.

IgA nephropathy (Berger disease) The most common form of idiopathic acute glomerulonephritis in developed countries, especially Asia; cause is unknown.

IgA pemphigus The most benign form of pemphigus characterized by tissue-bound and circulating IgA antibodies targeting desmosomal or nondesmosomal cell surface components in the basement membrane of the epidermis.

IgG subclass deficiency See Immune deficiency.

IL-7 receptor deficiency See Immune deficiency.

Immune deficiency A group of disorders in which one or more components of the immune or inflammatory response is impaired, resulting in increased susceptibility to infections. Primary (congenital) immune deficiencies result from genetic defects, and secondary immune deficiencies result from nongenetic factors, such as infections and other physiologic or pathophysiologic conditions. Primary immune deficiencies include:

B-lymphocyte deficiency A group of disorders in which B-cell development is defective, resulting in lower levels of circulating immunoglobulins and increased susceptibility to infections in which antibodies are the primary protective mechanism. These include:

Agammaglobulinemia A condition in which no antibodies are produced.

Autosomal agammaglobulinemia An autosomal recessive form of agammaglobulinemia resulting from mutations in the B-cell receptor.

Autosomal hyper-IgM syndrome Inability to class-switch resulting from mutations in CD40 on B cells.

Bruton agammaglobulinemia A defect in B-cell development results in lower levels of circulating immunoglobulins and increased susceptibility to infections in which antibodies are the primary protective mechanism.

Common variable immune deficiency The most commonly diagnosed immune deficiency; hypogammaglobulinemia of IgG and other antibody classes; normal numbers of B cells, with or without associated T-cell defects.

Hypogammaglobulinemia A condition in which immunoglobulin levels are much lower than normal.

IgG subclass deficiency Deficiencies in certain subclasses of antibody.

Selective IgA deficiency Failure to produce IgA, with or without diminished production of other classes of antibody.

X-linked hyper-IgM syndrome Inability to class-switch resulting from a defect in activation-induced cytidine deaminase (AICD).

Combined T- and B-lymphocyte deficiency A group of immune deficiencies in which both T and B lymphocytes are defective. The most severe of these deficiencies is called *severe combined immune deficiency (SCID)*. These include:

Adenosine deaminase (ADA) deficiency A form of SCID caused by an autosomal recessive mutation in the enzyme ADA, leading to death of rapidly dividing cells, particularly lymphocytes.

Ataxia-telangiectasia (AT) An autosomal recessive disorder resulting from a large variety of sporadic mutations in the *ATM* gene; often associated with ataxia (unsteady gait), telangiectasia (dilation of capillaries), and variable effects on both B and T cells.

Bare lymphocyte syndrome Forms of SCID characterized by an inability of lymphocytes and macrophages to present antigen because of defects in class I (major histocompatibility complex (MHC) class I deficiency) or class II (MHC class II deficiency) MHC antigen expression.

IL-7 receptor deficiency A form of SCID resulting from mutations in the IL-7 receptor, which is necessary for maturation of T cells.

JAK3 deficiency A form of SCID resulting from mutations in JAK3, which encodes an enzyme (a tyrosine kinase) associated with the receptor for IL-2.

Purine nucleoside phosphorylase (PNP) deficiency A form of SCID resulting from a mutation in the enzyme PNP.

RAG-1 and RAG-2 deficiencies Autosomal recessive mutations in recombination-activating gene (RAG-1 or RAG-2) enzymes that are necessary for genetic rearrangement of antibody and T-cell receptor variable regions.

Reticular dysgenesis The most severe form of SCID in which a common stem cell for all white blood cells is absent; therefore T cells, B cells, and phagocytic cells never develop.

Wiskott-Aldrich syndrome (WAS) An X-linked recessive trait resulting in chronic eczema with chronic suppurative otitis media, anemia, thrombocytopenic purpura, poor antibody response to polysaccharide antigens, and dysfunctions of cell-mediated immunity.

X-linked SCID A form of SCID with arrested maturation of T and natural killer (NK) cells and the production of immature B cells as a result of a defect in the IL-2 receptor gamma chain (IL-2Rγ), which is shared with many other cytokine receptors.

Complement deficiency A group of conditions in which specific proteins of the complement system are absent or suboptimal, resulting in diminished complement activity. These include:

C1 deficiency A deficiency of the first component of the classical pathway.

C2 deficiency A deficiency with an increased risk for recurrent respiratory tract infections with encapsulated bacteria and a systemic lupus erythematosus–like syndrome that may be complicated by kidney disease (glomerulonephritis).

C3 deficiency The most severe complement defect; an associated deficit of C3b, which is a major opsonin, results in a risk for recurrent life-threatening infections with encapsulated bacteria.

C3 receptor deficiency Deficiencies in the complement receptor for C3 result in recurrent bacterial infections, particularly of the skin.

C4 deficiency Results in an increased risk for recurrent respiratory tract infections with encapsulated bacteria and a systemic lupus erythematosus–like syndrome that may be complicated by kidney disease (glomerulonephritis).

C9 deficiency The most common terminal pathway defect and generally asymptomatic.

Factor H deficiency A deficiency of complement factor H resulting in increased destruction of C3 and a secondary C3 deficiency.

Factor I deficiency A deficiency of complement factor I resulting in increased destruction of C3 and a secondary C3 deficiency.

Mannose-binding lectin (MBL) deficiency A defect of the lectin pathway of complement activation resulting in an increased risk of infection with microorganisms that have polysaccharide capsules rich in mannose.

Properdin deficiency An X-linked defect in the alternative pathway of complement activation resulting in recurrent meningococcal infections.

Phagocytic deficiency A group of conditions in which phagocytes are diminished, resulting in increased bacterial infections. These include:

Chediak-Higashi syndrome A lethal, progressive, autosomal recessive, systemic disorder associated with oculocutaneous albinism, massive leukocyte inclusions (giant lysosomes), histiocytic infiltration of multiple body organs, development of pancytopenia, hepatosplenomegaly, and recurrent or persistent bacterial infections.

Chronic granulomatous disease (CGD) Both X-linked and autosomal forms of mutations of the nicotinamide adenine dinucleotide phosphate + hydrogen (NADPH) oxidase complex, resulting in diminished production of hydrogen peroxide and other oxygen products necessary for the bactericidal activity of myeloperoxidase.

Cyclic neutropenia An autosomal dominant mutation in the *ELA2* gene resulting in periods of neutropenia lasting a few days to weeks.

Severe congenital neutropenia Inadequate numbers of neutrophils resulting in a variety of recurrent and severe bacterial infections beginning early in life.

Secondary immune deficiencies .

Acquired immunodeficiency syndrome (AIDS) An epidemic, transmissible retroviral disease caused by infection with the human immunodeficiency virus (HIV), resulting in destruction of T-helper cells, suppression of both antibody and cellular immune responses, and development of life-threatening infections with opportunistic organisms.

Agranulocytosis Complete absence of granulocytes in the blood is usually secondary to arrested hematopoiesis in the bone marrow or massive cell destruction in the circulation.

Qualitative leukocyte disorder A group of conditions with various disruptions of leukocyte function.

Quantitative leukocyte disorder A group of conditions, frequently associated with infections and leukemias, with decreased production of leukocytes in the bone marrow or accelerated destruction of leukocytes in the circulation.

Transient hypogammaglobulinemia of infancy A period at 6 to 8 months when the newborn may not have produced adequate amounts of antibody to replace maternal antibody; in some infants this may lead to a period of increased susceptibility to infections.

T-lymphocyte deficiency A group of disorders in which T-cell development is defective, resulting in lower levels of cellular immunity. Diminished T-helper cell function may also decrease the production of antibody. These include:

Chronic mucocutaneous candidiasis A primary defect of T-lymphocyte response to a specific infectious agent, the yeast *C. albicans*.

DiGeorge syndrome A genetic disorder caused by deletion of a piece of chromosome 22 that results in cardiac defects, abnormal facies, thymic aplasia, cleft palate, and hypocalcemia.

Immune thrombocytopenic purpura See Thrombocytopenia.

Imperforate anus A congenital defect in which the anal opening is absent because of the presence of a membranous septum or complete absence of the anal canal.

Impetigo A contagious bacterial infection that produces superficial red blisters that rupture and produce thick yellow crusts that commonly occur on the face but can spread to other regions of the body easily.

Infectious mononucleosis (IM) A disease caused by the Epstein-Barr virus or the cytomegalovirus that is transmitted by exchanging saliva or blood or by coughing and sneezing and acts by infecting the B cells and atypical T cells, resulting in fever, sore throat, and fatigue.

Infective endocarditis (IE) A general term used to describe infection and inflammation of the endocardium, especially the cardiac valves.

Infertility The inability to conceive after 1 year of unprotected intercourse with the same, opposite-sex partner.

Intracerebral hematoma (intraparenchymal hemorrhage) Blood accumulation that partially clots inside the brain, usually in the frontal and temporal lobes.

Intraductal papilloma Array of papillary cells that grow from the wall of a cyst into the lumen of the duct; growth occurs within a dilated duct often near or beside the nipple, causing benign nipple discharge.

Intrarenal (intrinsic) acute kidney injury (AKI) A sudden decline in kidney function with a decrease in glomerular filtration and an accumulation of nitrogenous waste products in the blood (elevation in plasma creatinine and blood urea nitrogen levels); may result from ischemic acute tubular necrosis (ATN), nephrotoxic ATN (i.e., exposure to radiocontrast media or antibiotics), acute glomerulonephritis, vascular disease (malignant hypertension, disseminated intravascular coagulation, and renal vasculitis), allograft rejection, or interstitial disease (drug allergy, infection, tumor growth).

Invasive breast carcinoma A malignant invasive epithelial lesion derived from the terminal duct lobular area.

Invasive carcinoma of the cervix Invasion of cervical carcinoma into adjacent tissues, such as ureters and structures of the lateral pelvic wall, the vaginal stroma and epithelium, and the lower uterine segment and myometrium.

Inverse psoriasis See Psoriasis.

Iron deficiency anemia (IDA) See Anemia.

Irritable bowel syndrome (IBS) A chronic noninflammatory disease with a psychophysiologic basis; characterized by abdominal pain, diarrhea or constipation, or both; no detectable pathologic change.

Irritative syndrome (radicular syndrome) A combination of changes usually seen with compromise of a spinal root within the intraspinal canal; these include neck or back pain and, in the affected root distribution, dermatomal pain, paresthesias, or both; decreased deep tendon reflexes; and occasionally myotomal weakness.

Isolated systolic hypertension Loss of elasticity of the arteries resulting in an increase in cardiac output or stroke volume, a systolic blood pressure consistently greater than 160 mmHg, and a diastolic pressure less than 90 mmHg.

J

JAK3 deficiency See Immune deficiency.

Jaundice (icterus) Yellowish brown staining of the skin and the conjunctivae caused by high bilirubin levels in blood secondary to excessive erythrocyte breakdown, obstruction in or around the liver, or liver disease.

Juvenile idiopathic arthritis (JIA) Chronic pauciarticular arthritis and destruction of joints beginning in childhood and often going into remission at puberty.

Juvenile myoclonic epilepsy A type of epilepsy that occurs in adolescents and young adults, usually on awakening, and is characterized by jerks of the neck, shoulders, and arms and by clonic-tonic seizures.

K

Kaposi sarcoma (KS) A rare cancer of connective tissue caused by herpesvirus 8 (HHV8) in which many bluish red nodules appear on the skin, especially skin of the lower extremities; occurs in a particularly virulent form in individuals with AIDS.

Kawasaki disease A vascular disease characterized by an inflamed heart and vessels; a coronary artery aneurysm, thickening, and stenosis; a fever that lasts at least 5 days; and at least four of the following: inflammation with reddening of the whites of the eyes; red, swollen hands or feet or peeling skin; rash; swollen lymph glands in the neck; inflamed lips or throat; or red "strawberry" tongue.

Klinefelter syndrome Smallness of testes with fibrosis and hyalinization of seminiferous tubules, variable degrees of masculinization, azoospermia, infertility, and increased levels of urinary gonadotropins; associated typically with an XXY chromosome complement although variants include XXYY, XXXY, and XXXXY.

Kwashiorkor A condition in which children do not receive enough protein in their diet, resulting in a swollen and severely bloated abdomen secondary to decreased albumin levels in the blood, skin changes resulting in a reddish discoloration of the hair and skin in dark-skinned children, severe diarrhea, fatty liver, muscle atrophy, and restricted development.

L

Lactase deficiency A condition in which insufficient lactase is present in the small intestine to digest lactose, resulting in lactose intolerance characterized by diarrhea, bloating, and gas in response to exposure to lactose.

Lactose intolerance A condition caused by lactase deficiency in which lactose is not metabolized, making it impossible for the small intestine to absorb it and causing excessive gas production and diarrhea when exposed to lactose-containing foods.

Lambert-Eaton myasthenic syndrome A generalized disorder of neuromuscular transmission caused by a defect in the release of acetylcholine from the presynaptic nerve terminals; often associated with small cell carcinoma of the lung, particularly in elderly men with a long history of cigarette smoking; weakness tends to affect solely axial muscles, girdle muscles, and less often the limb muscles; autonomic disturbances, dry mouth, and impotence are common; the deep tendon reflexes are unelicitable; caused by loss of voltage-sensitive calcium channels located on the presynaptic motor nerve terminal.

Laryngomalacia A congenital anomaly caused by a developmental delay in the laryngeal cartilage and supporting structures of the larynx that causes the cartilage to be floppy and fold in on itself during inspiration, producing high-pitched, coarse, and low-pitched sounds.

Left heart failure (congestive heart failure) Inability of the left ventricle to maintain its circulatory load, with a corresponding rise in pressure in the pulmonary circulation usually with pulmonary congestion and ultimately pulmonary edema.

Legg-Calvé-Perthes disease Blood supply to the head of the femur near the hip joint is interrupted, resulting in osteonecrosis of the corresponding epiphysis.

Lennox-Gastaut syndrome A generalized myoclonic epilepsy that occurs in children between 1 and 5 years of age as a result of various cerebral afflictions such as perinatal hypoxia, hemorrhage, encephalitis, and metabolic disorders of the brain; it is characterized by mental retardation, personality disorders, and generalized tonic seizures.

Leukemia A clonal malignant disorder of leukocytes in the bone marrow and usually, but not always of the blood; uncontrolled proliferation of malignant leukocytes, causing an overcrowding of bone marrow and decreased production and function of normal hematopoietic cells.

- **Acute leukemia** Characterized by undifferentiated or immature cells, usually a blast cell, and the onset of disease is abrupt and rapid.
- **Acute lymphoblastic/lymphocytic leukemia (ALL)** Excessive production and proliferation of malignant and immature white blood cells (lymphoblasts) in the bone marrow that progresses rapidly if left untreated.
- **Acute myelogenous leukemia (AML)** Excessive number of immature myeloid cells (myeloblasts) in the blood and bone marrow, overcrowding the marrow and decreasing the function of other cells.

Chronic leukemia Slow-growing cancer with many immature lymphocytes in the blood and bone marrow; the predominant cell is more differentiated but does not function normally.

- **Chronic lymphocytic leukemia (CLL)** Malignant transformation and progressive accumulation in the marrow of monoclonal B lymphocytes; rarely are CLL malignancies of T-cell origin.
- **Chronic myelogenous leukemia (CML)** Production of heterogeneous myeloid cells in the bone marrow, the majority of which express the Philadelphia chromosome; CML is considered a myeloproliferative disorder.

Leukocytosis A leukocyte count that is higher than normal.

LH deficiency A condition characterized by decreased or absent production of luteinizing hormone (LH), resulting in a decline in sex steroid production in testes/ovaries and associated infertility.

Lichen planus A recurrent rash of small, flat-topped bumps and rough scaly patches appearing on the skin, in the lining of the mouth, and in the vagina in response to inflammation or an allergy to a specific medication.

Localized scleroderma (morphea) Rare and idiopathic sclerosis of the skin, usually with childhood onset.

Locked-in syndrome Quadriplegia and mutism with intact consciousness and preservation of some eye movements; usually results from a vascular lesion of the anterior pons.

Lupus erythematosus Any of a group of autoimmune connective tissue disorders that commonly produce red scaly lesions and are accompanied by fever, malaise, myalgia, fatigue, and weight loss.

Discoid (cutaneous) lupus erythematosus (DLE) Lupus erythematosus limited to the skin; can progress to systemic lupus erythematosus.

Systematic lupus erythematosus A chronic, multisystem, inflammatory disease; is one of the most common, complex, and serious of the autoimmune disorders.

Lyme disease (borreliosis) Tick-borne spirochete bacterial infection that is characterized by a rash in the area of the bite, headache, neck stiffness, chills, fever, myalgia, arthralgia, malaise, fatigue, and possible development of arthritis in large joints.

Lymphadenopathy An alteration of lymphoid function characterized by enlarged lymph nodes.

Lymphoblastic lymphoma (LL) See Lymphoma.

Lymphogranuloma venereum (LGV) A sexually transmitted bacterial infection that enters the body through breaks in the skin or across the epithelial cell layer of mucous membranes and primarily targets the lymphatics and lymph nodes.

Lymphoma Diverse group of neoplasms arising from cell proliferation in lymphoid tissue.

- **B-cell neoplasm** A group of lymphomas including myelomas that originate from B cells at various stages of differentiation; previously part of non-Hodgkin lymphoma.
- **Burkitt lymphoma** An aggressive malignancy of the B lymphocytes characterized by a large osteolytic lesion in the facial bones and associated with Epstein-Barr virus infection.
- **Hodgkin lymphoma (HL)** A neoplasm of lymphoid tissue that progresses from one group of lymph nodes to another; the lymph nodes, spleen, and liver become enlarged with the presence of Reed–Sternberg cells and is often accompanied by anemia, fever, and eventually death if not treated at an early stage; also referred to as *Hodgkin disease*.
- **Lymphoblastic lymphoma (LL)** A progressive neoplasm arising in the thymus; most are of T-cell origin; a variant of acute lymphoblastic leukemia; common cause of non-Hodgkin lymphoma (NHL) in children.
- **Lymphoplasmacytic lymphoma** Also called *Waldenström macroglobulinemia*.
- **Mucosa-associated lymphoid tissue (MALT) lymphoma** A low-grade B-cell lymphoma linked to infection with *H. pylori*.
- **Mycosis fungoides** Most common cutaneous T-cell lymphoma; present as focal or widespread erythematous patches or plaques, follicular papules, comedone-like lesions, and tumors.
- **NK-cell neoplasm** A group of lymphomas that originate from natural killer (NK) cells at various stages of differentiation; previously part of non-Hodgkin lymphoma.
- **Non-Hodgkin lymphoma (NHL)** A group of malignancies of lymphoid tissue reclassified as B-cell, T-cell, and NK-cell lymphomas with varied biologic and clinical features.
- **T-cell neoplasm** A variety of lymphomas that originate from T cells at various stages of differentiation; previously part of non-Hodgkin lymphoma.
- **Waldenström macroglobulinemia** A rare type of slow-growing plasma cell tumor that secretes a monoclonal IgM molecule; also called *lymphoplasmocytic lymphoma*.

Lymphoplasmacytic lymphoma See Lymphoma.

Lysosomal storage diseases A group of more than 30 disorders that result from impaired lysosomal function, leading to mucopolysaccharidoses, lipid storage disorders, mucolipidoses, leukodystrophies, and glycoprotein storage disorders.

M

Macrocytic anemia (megaloblastic anemia) See Anemia.

Major (unipolar) depression Severely depressed mood and loss of pleasure that may begin suddenly or slowly; it persists for at least 2 weeks and may recur throughout life.

Malignant hyperthermia An inherited life-threatening disorder that causes muscle rigidity, a hypermetabolic state, tachycardia, and increased body temperature in response to administration of general anesthesia.

Malnutrition Lack of nourishment from inadequate amounts of calories, protein, vitamins, or minerals; caused by improper diet, alterations in digestion or absorption, chronic disease, or a combination of these factors.

Mannose-binding lectin (MBL) deficiency See Immune deficiency.

Marasmus A childhood disorder characterized by protein and energy malnutrition, resulting in dry skin, loss of adipose tissue from normal areas of fat deposits such as buttocks and thighs, and behavior that is fretful and irritable.

Maturity-onset diabetes of youth (MODY) See Diabetes mellitus.

McArdle disease A metabolic disorder involving an enzyme defect that causes deficiency of muscle phosphorylase, which helps break down glycogen, and consequently this disorder causes an energy deficit in the muscles, resulting in muscle pain and cramping.

Meconium ileus Obstruction with thickened meconium in the intestine of a newborn child as a result of a lack of trypsin and associated with cystic fibrosis of the pancreas.

Medulloblastoma A malignant cerebellar tumor near the fourth ventricle that is most often found in children and consists of neoplastic cells that resemble the undifferentiated cells of the neural tube.

Melanoma A malignant tumor of the skin originating from the transformation of melanocytes.

Membranoproliferative glomerulonephritis (MPGN) See Glomerulonephritis.

Membranous glomerulonephritis See Glomerulonephritis.

Membranous nephropathy (membranous glomerulonephritis) See Glomerulonephritis.

Ménière disease (endolymphatic hydrops) Dilation of the membranous labyrinth of the inner ear that is thought to be due to impaired absorption of endolymph in the endolymphatic sac; the pathologic finding in Ménière disease.

Ménière syndrome An affliction characterized clinically by vertigo, nausea, vomiting, tinnitus, and fluctuating and progressive sensory hearing loss associated with endolymphatic hydrops.

Meningioma A slow-growing mass of the meninges that is usually benign but increases intracranial pressure.

Meningocele Neural tube defect in the skull or spinal column that forms a cyst filled with cerebrospinal fluid through which the meninges of the brain protrude.

Mesangial proliferative glomerulonephritis See Glomerulonephritis.

Mesenteric venous thrombosis A condition in which a blood clot obstructs one of the mesenteric veins and compromises the intestinal blood supply; can result in intestinal gangrene and tissue death.

Mesothelioma A type of cancer that is usually associated with previous exposure to asbestos, which affects the pleura, the lining of the abdominal cavity, the pericardium, and most internal organ coverings.

Metabolic acidosis A condition in which the concentration of non–carbonic acids increases or bicarbonate (base) is lost from the extracellular fluid or cannot be regenerated by the kidney.

Metabolic syndrome A condition of unknown cause that presents with symptoms of insulin resistance, obesity, hypertension, dyslipidemia, and systemic inflammation.

Metatarsus adductus A foot deformity in which the front half of the foot bends inward, possibly because of the infant's position in the uterus.

Methicillin-resistant *Staphylococcus aureus* (MRSA) An infection that carries the extrachromosomal gene *mecA* for resistance to methicillin and has less sensitivity to inhibition by antibiotics.

MHC class I deficiency See Immune deficiency.

MHC class II deficiency See Immune deficiency.

Microcephaly A defect in which failure of normal brain growth causes delayed skull growth and production of a small head.

Microcytic-hypochromic anemia See Anemia.

Microscopic colitis A relatively common cause of diarrhea; occurs primarily in females and older adults.

Migraine headache A headache that usually begins in the temporal region unilaterally after vascular changes of cranial arteries and may cause irritability, nausea, vomiting, constipation or diarrhea, and photophobia.

Mild concussion (mild traumatic brain injury) Temporary axonal disturbances without the loss of consciousness in response to a violent blow, jarring, shaking, or other closed-head injury.

Miliaria A skin disease caused by partially obstructed sweat glands that results in small and itchy rashes usually located in skinfolds and on areas of the body that may rub against clothing, such as the back, chest, and stomach.

Minimal change nephropathy (MCN) The foot processes of the renal capillary basement membrane are fused and deformed because of a T-cell disorder that reduces the anion component of the basement membrane and allows proteins to leak into the renal tubule.

Minimally conscious state (MCS) A condition in which a severely brain-damaged person is capable of deliberate behavior distinguishable from unconscious reflexive actions.

Mitral valve prolapse syndrome The mitral valve cannot close properly because of one or both flaps being too large, possibly resulting in mitral valve regurgitation.

Mixed precocious puberty Development of some secondary sex characteristics of the opposite sex (virilization of a girl or feminization of a boy); usually evident at birth and rare in older children.

Molluscum contagiosum A viral infection of the skin occurring in young children that affects the body, arms, and legs; it is spread through direct contact, saliva, or shared articles of clothing and is considered a sexually transmitted disease in adults, affecting the genitals, lower abdomen, buttocks, and inner thighs.

Monoclonal gammopathy of undetermined significance (MGUS) Production of monoclonal antibodies by noncancerous plasma cells that accumulate in the blood.

Motility diarrhea Diarrhea caused by excessive motility decreases transit time, mucosal surface contact, and fluid absorption secondary to resection of the small intestine (short bowel syndrome), surgical bypass of an area of the intestine, fistula formation between loops of intestine, irritable bowel syndrome–diarrhea predominant, diabetic neuropathy, hyperthyroidism, and laxative abuse.

Moyamoya disease An abnormality of the blood vessels that supply the frontal region of the brain in which vessels constrict or become completely occluded, resulting in diminished blood flow. The body attempts to compensate by growing new vessels at the base of the brain, which appear as a puff of smoke on angiography.

Mucoepidermoid carcinoma A tumor of the main or lobar bronchi lumen that may extend into the peribronchial tissue.

Mucolipidosis (ML) Accumulation of both carbohydrates and lipids.

Mucopolysaccharidosis Carbohydrate excess disorders.

Mucopurulent cervicitis (MPC) Inflammation of the cervix with purulent endocervical exudate that may be asymptomatic or cause abnormal vaginal discharge and vaginal bleeding.

Mucosa-associated lymphoid tissue (MALT) lymphoma See Lymphoma.

Multiple myeloma (MM) Most common and most aggressive plasma cell tumor; a clonal plasma cell cancer characterized by the slow proliferation of malignant cells as tumor cells form masses in the bone marrow that usually result in destruction of the bone; most secrete large amounts of monoclonal proteins that resemble intact immunoglobulins.

Multiple organ dysfunction syndrome (MODS) Progressive disease often involving the ultimate failure of two or more organ systems after a severe illness or injury; disease process is initiated and perpetuated by uncontrolled systemic inflammatory and stress responses and is characterized by a hypermetabolic and hyper dynamic state that persists as organ dysfunction develops.

Multiple papilloma (diffuse papillomatosis) A minimum of five papillomas within a localized segment of breast tissue.

Multiple sclerosis (MS) Chronic demyelinating disease of the central nervous system that causes inflammation and scarring of myelin sheaths.

Muscular dystrophy A general term for a number of hereditary, progressive degenerative disorders affecting skeletal muscles, and often other organ systems.

Myasthenia gravis Neuromuscular disorder caused by an autoimmune response in which antibodies to acetylcholine receptors impair neuromuscular transmission.

Mycosis fungoides See Lymphoma.

Myelodysplastic syndrome (MDS) A group of hematologic conditions characterized by ineffective production of blood cells, resulting in anemia that requires chronic blood transfusion.

Myoadenylate deaminase deficiency (MDD) A genetic disorder in which an enzyme deficiency prevents the conversion of adenosine monophosphate (AMP) to inosine monophosphate, resulting in increased AMP loss and the inability to synthesize adenosine triphosphate for energy.

Myocardial infarction A heart condition of sudden onset in which muscle tissue dies because of a lack of blood flow, resulting in varying degrees of chest pain or discomfort, weakness, sweating, nausea and vomiting, and possibly loss of consciousness.

Myositis ossificans A condition in which bone is deposited in muscle tissue, causing pain and swelling.

Myositis Inflammation of a muscle, usually a voluntary muscle, resulting in pain, tenderness, and sometimes spasm in the affected area.

Myxedema Cutaneous edema caused by deposition of connective tissue (e.g., glycosaminoglycans and hyaluronic acid) and associated with hypothyroidism and Graves disease; characterized by dry skin, pretibial myxedema, swelling around the lips and nose, mental deterioration, and a decrease in basal metabolic rate.

N

Necrotizing enterocolitis (NEC) A condition of extensive ulceration and necrosis of the ileum and colon in premature infants during the neonatal period.

Necrotizing fasciitis A rare, rapidly spreading inflammation starting in the fascia, muscles, and subcutaneous fat with subsequent necrosis of the overlying skin; it is initiated by bacterial infection and treated with antibiotics; often requires surgical débridement.

Neonatal alloimmune thrombocytopenic purpura (NATP) See Thrombocytopenia.

Neonatal purpura fulminans A fatal syndrome found in neonates who are homozygous or double heterozygous for types I and II protein deficiency.

Nephritic syndrome A disorder of the glomerular filtration membrane in which plasma proteins and red blood cells pass into the urine, resulting in mild proteinuria, hematuria, and mild hypertension.

Nephroblastoma (Wilms tumor) A malignant renal tumor of young children that compresses the normal kidney parenchyma, causing an abdominal mass, blood in the urine, and fever and may be associated with anorexia, vomiting, and malaise; often inherited as an autosomal dominant trait.

Nephrotic syndrome A disorder of the glomerular filtration membrane that permits proteins to pass into the urine, resulting in proteinuria, hypoalbuminemia, hyperlipidemia, and systemic edema.

Neural tube defect (NTD) Lack of closure of the neural groove caused by an arrest of the normal development of the brain and spinal cord during the first month of embryonic development.

Neuroblastoma A malignant tumor containing neuroblast cells that originate in the autonomic nervous system or the adrenal medulla; is most common in infants and young children.

Neurogenic shock (vasogenic shock) A type of shock caused by the sudden loss of the sympathetic nervous system signals to the smooth muscle in vessel walls, causing the vessels to relax and a decrease in peripheral vascular resistance and blood pressure.

Neuroleptic malignant syndrome Hyperthermia with autonomic and extrapyramidal side effects caused by the administration of neuroleptic drugs.

NK-cell neoplasm See Lymphoma.

Nonalcoholic fatty liver disease (NAFLD) Accumulation of fat in hepatocytes, primarily in the form of triglycerides, occurring either in the absence of alcohol or with little alcohol intake; causes progressive inflammation and scarring that is usually asymptomatic for years.

Nonalcoholic steatohepatitis (NASH) A more serious form of nonalcoholic fatty liver disease resulting from hepatocellular injury, inflammation, and fibrosis; this condition is difficult to distinguish from alcohol-induced liver fibrosis; may progress to cirrhosis, end-stage liver disease, and an increased risk for hepatocellular carcinoma.

Nonbacterial infectious cystitis See Painful bladder syndrome/interstitial cystitis (PBS/IC).

Nonbacterial prostatitis Prostatitis causes chronic pain that disappears and returns without warning but shows no signs of bacterial infection in the prostatic fluid even though the semen and other fluids from the prostate contain immune cells that the body produces in response to infection.

Non-Hodgkin lymphoma (NHL) See Lymphoma.

Noninfectious cystitis See Painful bladder syndrome/interstitial cystitis (PBS/IC).

Noninflammatory acne See Acne.

Noninflammatory joint disease A disease in which alterations in the structure or mechanics of the joint result in pain during motion.

Nonoliguric renal failure Excretion of more than 500 mL/day of urine concurrent with renal failure; although adequate volume of urine is excreted, renal tubules have impaired reabsorption and concentration and dilution function so that filtration is defective, resulting in accumulation of uremic toxins in the blood.

Nonossifying fibroma (fibrous cortical deficit) A benign fibrous tissue tumor forms in the metaphysis of any of the long bones but usually occurs in the thigh and shin bones in children and adolescents.

Nonpuerperal hyperprolactinemia The presence of excessive amounts of prolactin (the pituitary hormone that stimulates milk production) in the blood not related to pregnancy or childbirth; most common cause of galactorrhea.

Nonsyndromic craniosynostosis (see Craniosynostosis) The premature closure of one or more of the cranial sutures during the first 18 to 20 months of an infant's life, but an isolated defect unrelated to syndrome.

Normocytic-normochromic anemia (NNA) See Anemia.

O

Obesity hypoventilation syndrome (pickwickian syndrome) A condition of severely overweight individuals related to the inability to breathe rapidly or deeply enough to maintain adequate blood oxygen levels; characterized by obstructive sleep apnea, somnolence, hypoventilation, erythrocytosis, and heart failure.

Obsessive-compulsive disorder (OCD) An anxiety disorder characterized by obsessive thoughts and repetitive compulsive actions, such as cleaning, checking, or counting.

Obstructive jaundice Jaundice related to extrahepatic or intrahepatic obstruction.

Obstructive pulmonary disease Airway obstruction that is worse with expiration so that more force or more time is required to expire a given volume of air and emptying of the lungs is slowed; characterized by shortness of breath (dyspnea) and wheezing.

Obstructive sleep apnea syndrome (OSAS) A disorder of sleep characterized by airway obstruction and episodes of apnea accompanied by snoring.

Obstructive uropathy The blockage of urine flow, often by ureteral or kidney stones, resulting in the reflux of urine and subsequent injury to kidneys.

Onychomycosis A fungal infection of the fingernails or toenails that causes thickening, roughness, and splitting of the nails.

Oophoritis Inflammation of the ovaries.

Open pneumothorax (communicating pneumothorax) See Pneumothorax.

Optic glioma Tumor originating from glial cells in the brain that affects the optic nerve; commonly seen in children with neurofibromatosis.

Organic brain syndrome A constellation of physical brain disorders with psychologic or behavioral signs and symptoms and grouped according to symptoms rather than etiology.

Orthopnea Shortness of breath (dyspnea) that occurs when an individual lies flat and is common in individuals with heart failure.

Orthostatic (postural) hypotension A sudden drop in blood pressure when a person assumes a standing position, resulting in dizziness, lightheadedness, blurred vision, and temporary loss of consciousness.

Osmotic diarrhea Nonabsorbable substance in the intestine draws water into the lumen by osmosis, resulting in large-volume diarrhea;

caused by drinking solutions with excessive sugars, salt, or vitamin C; maldigestion syndromes.

Osteoarthritis (OA) Inflammatory degenerative joint disease in which synthesis and degradation of the articular cartilage in the movable joints are altered, resulting in wearing and destruction of cartilage.

Osteochondrosis (Osgood-Schlatter disease) A condition in children that results from the tendons pulling on the epiphysis of long bones, causing pain just below the knee, irritation and swelling, and possibly abnormal bone growth.

Osteogenesis imperfecta (brittle bone disease) A genetic disease in which collagen production is deficient, making the bones abnormally fragile and causing recurring fractures with only minimal trauma, deformity of long bones, a bluish coloration of the sclerae, and often the development of otosclerosis.

Osteoid osteoma A benign tumor in one of the bones of the lower extremities that is painful and is characterized by vascularized connective tissue and osteoid material that is surrounded by a large zone of thickened bone.

Osteomalacia A disease in which vitamin D or calcium deficiency or excessive renal phosphate loss causes a softening of the bones with accompanying pain and weakness.

Osteomyelitis A bacterial infection of the bone and bone marrow that occurs through open fractures, penetrating wounds, surgical operations, or by infiltration of the bloodstream; causes pain, high fever, and formation of an abscess at the site of infection.

Osteoporosis A disease in which the bones become porous and weakened, making bones easily fracture and slow to heal.

Overactive bladder syndrome (OAB) A chronic syndrome of overactivity of the detrusor muscle; characterized by urgency with involuntary detrusor contractions during the bladder filling phase.

Oxygen toxicity An iatrogenic inflammatory condition caused by prolonged exposure to high concentrations of supplemental oxygen resulting from damage to alveolocapillary membranes, disruption of surfactant production, and interstitial and alveolar edema; caused by oxygen free radicals.

P

Paget disease of bone (PDB or osteitis deformans) A bone disorder in which excessive bone remodeling causes enlarged, deformed bones that can weaken the bone integrity and result in bone pain, arthritis, deformities, or fractures.

Painful bladder syndrome/interstitial cystitis (PBS/IC) (see Cystitis) A condition occurring in women ages 20 to 40 years who have symptoms of cystitis, such as frequency, urgency, dysuria, and nocturia, for more than 6 weeks' duration; usually related to bacterial infection.

Nonbacterial infectious cystitis Cystitis with negative urine cultures and no other known etiology; most common in immunocompromised individuals and related to viral, mycobacterial, chlamydial, or fungal infection.

Noninfectious cystitis Cystitis without evidence of infection; usually autoimmune or related to exposure to radiation or chemotherapy treatment for pelvic or urogenital cancers.

Panacinar emphysema See Emphysema.

Pancreatic insufficiency A condition in which the pancreas does not secrete enough hormones and digestive enzymes for normal digestion to occur, resulting in malabsorption, malnutrition, vitamin deficiencies, and weight loss.

Pancreatitis Inflammation of the pancreas, usually resulting in abdominal pain.

Panhypopituitarism A condition in which the secretion of all anterior pituitary hormones is inadequate or absent; caused by a variety of disorders that result in destruction or loss of function of all or most of the anterior pituitary gland.

Panic disorder A psychologic disorder that is characterized by recurrent attacks of anxiety or terror and usually results in the development of one or more phobias.

Papulosquamous disorder Collective reference to inflammatory disorders characterized by papules, scales, plaques, and erythema, including psoriasis, pityriasis rosea, and lichen planus.

Paraesophageal hiatal hernia Herniation of the greater curvature of the stomach through a secondary opening in the diaphragm.

Paralytic ileus Also known as *functional obstruction*, it is a failure of motility after intestinal or abdominal surgery, acute pancreatitis, or hypokalemia.

Paraneoplastic pemphigus See Pemphigus.

Paraphimosis A condition in which the foreskin becomes trapped behind the glans penis and cannot return to its normal flaccid position covering the glans penis.

Parkinson disease Degeneration of the basal ganglia dopaminergic nigrostriatal pathway that causes hypokinesia, tremor, and muscular rigidity.

Parkinsonism (Parkinson syndrome, parkinsonian syndrome) A neurologic condition characterized by tremors, rigidity, hypokinesia, and postural instability as a result of degeneration of the corpus striatum or substantia nigra caused by Parkinson disease and other conditions related to toxins or metabolic conditions.

Paronychia An acute or chronic infection of the cuticle. One or more fingers or toes may be involved.

Paroxysmal nocturnal dyspnea (PND) Attacks of breathing discomfort, shortness of breath, and coughing that occur at night with varying intensity so that individuals must sit up or stand to relieve dyspnea; may occur in individuals with heart failure or lung disease.

Partial obstruction of the bladder outlet or urethra Partial obstruction related to deposition of collagen within the smooth muscle bundles of the detrusor muscle; causes an increase in the force of detrusor contraction.

Partial precocious puberty The partial development of appropriate secondary sex characteristics alone or in combination.

Pediculosis pubis A contagious condition, also known as *crabs* or *crab lice*, that is an infestation of the pubic hair in which the louse feeds on human blood and multiplies rapidly.

Pelvic inflammatory disease (PID) Inflammation of the female genital tract caused by microorganisms, typically those that are sexually transmitted such as chlamydia and gonococci; characterized by severe abdominal pain, high fever, vaginal discharge, and possibly infertility.

Pelvic organ prolapse (POP) Bladder outlet obstruction in women caused most commonly by a cystocele (the downward protrusion of the bladder into the vagina) that descends below the level of the urethral outlet.

Pemphigus A category of autoimmune skin diseases marked by groups of itching blisters and raw sores on the skin and mucous membranes.

Paraneoplastic pemphigus The most severe form of pemphigus; is associated with lymphoproliferative neoplasms and affects internal organs, including lungs, thyroid, kidney, smooth muscle, and gastrointestinal tract.

Pemphigus foliaceus A milder form of pemphigus involving loss of cell-to-cell adhesion (acantholysis) at the subcorneal level with blistering, erosions, scaling, crusting, and erythema usually of the face and chest.

Pemphigus vulgaris The most common form of pemphigus with acantholysis at the suprabasal level and initiated by IgG autoantibodies against the desmoglein adhesion molecules, resulting in acantholysis in the epidermis with fluid accumulation and blister formation; oral lesions precede the onset of skin blistering.

Pericarditis The pericardium is infected by a virus, bacteria, parasite, or fungus and becomes inflamed, resulting in pain and fluid and blood components entering into the pericardial space.

Perihepatitis (Fitz-Hugh–Curtis syndrome) A complication of pelvic inflammatory disease secondary to gonococci bacteria traveling up the peritoneum to the upper abdomen and causing inflammation.

Periodic paralysis One of a group of diseases in which muscular weakness or flaccid paralysis occurs without loss of consciousness, speech, or sensation.

Peripheral artery disease (PAD) Any of a group of diseases caused by the obstruction of large peripheral arteries secondary to atherosclerosis, inflammatory processes, embolism, or thrombus formation that causes ischemia.

Pernicious anemia See Anemia.

Pes planus (flatfoot) A condition in which the arch of the foot never develops or it collapses and contacts the ground.

Peyronie disease (bent nail syndrome) A condition in which fibrous plaques grow in the soft tissue of the penis because of injury of the internal cavity of the penis that is accompanied by bleeding and scar tissue formation at the tunica albuginea of the corpora cavernosa.

Phagocytic deficiency See Immune deficiency.

Phenylketonuria (PKU) A genetic disorder in which the body lacks the enzyme necessary to metabolize the amino acid phenylalanine to tyrosine, resulting in accumulation of phenylalanine and subsequent brain damage and progressive mental retardation.

Pheochromocytoma A tumor of the adrenal medulla that causes the chromaffin cells to secrete increased amounts of epinephrine or norepinephrine.

Phimosis The foreskin of the penis of an uncircumcised male cannot be fully retracted.

Pick disease Progressive atrophy of the cerebral convolutions in a limited area (lobe) of the brain, with clinical manifestations and course similar to those of Alzheimer disease.

Pityriasis rosea A skin disorder, thought to be caused by a virus, in which patches of ovular pink rash appear primarily on the trunk and extremities.

Plaque psoriasis See Psoriasis.

Pneumoconiosis A chronic disease of the lungs typically seen in miners, sandblasters, and metal grinders that is caused by repeated inhalation of dust particles, including iron oxides, silicates, and carbonates, that collect in the lungs and become sites for the formation of fibrous nodules that eventually replace lung tissue.

Pneumonia An infection of one or both lungs caused by a bacterium, virus, fungus, or other organism that enters the body through respiratory passages and causes high fever, chills, chest pain, difficulty breathing, cough with sputum, and possibly bluish skin from insufficiently oxygenated blood.

Pneumothorax The collapse of a lung and subsequent escape of air into the pleural cavity between the lung and the chest wall that is caused by trauma, environmental factors, or spontaneous occurrence and results in a sudden pain in the chest.

Iatrogenic pneumothorax The presence of air or gas in the pleural space caused by a rupture in the visceral pleura (which surrounds the lungs) or the parietal pleura and chest wall; is most commonly caused by transthoracic needle aspiration.

Open pneumothorax (communicating pneumothorax) Spontaneous and traumatic pneumothorax in which air pressure in the pleural space equals barometric pressure because air that is drawn into the pleural space during inspiration (through the damaged chest wall and parietal pleura or through the lungs and damaged visceral pleura) is forced out during expiration.

Primary (spontaneous) pneumothorax Occurs unexpectedly in healthy individuals (usually men) between ages 20 and 40 years; is most often caused by the spontaneous rupture of blebs on the visceral pleura.

Secondary (traumatic) pneumothorax Spontaneous or secondary pneumothorax beginning with sudden pleural pain, tachypnea, and possibly mild dyspnea.

Tension pneumothorax The site of pleural rupture acts as a one-way valve, permitting air to enter on inspiration, but preventing its escape by closing during expiration and leading to air pressure in the pneumothorax exceeding barometric pressure.

Polycystic ovary syndrome (PCOS) A hormonal condition in which multiple ovarian cysts form because of elevated levels of androgens, resulting in hirsutism, obesity, menstrual abnormalities, infertility, and enlarged ovaries.

Polycythemia vera A chronic, progressive disease that is characterized by overgrowth of the bone marrow, excessive red blood cell production, and an enlarged spleen and causes headache, inability to concentrate, and pain in the fingers and toes.

Pompe disease See Acid maltase deficiency.

Port-wine (nevus flammeus) stain A birthmark caused by superficial and deep dilated capillaries in the skin that produce a reddish to purplish discoloration of the skin, usually on the face, but can occur anywhere on the body.

Postconcussive syndrome Physical and personality changes that may occur after concussion of the brain, including amnesia, headache, dizziness, tinnitus, irritability, fatigability, sweating, heart palpitations, insomnia, and difficulty concentrating.

Posthemorrhagic anemia See Anemia.

Postobstructive pulmonary edema (POPE) (negative pressure pulmonary edema) A rare life-threatening complication that can occur after relief of upper airway obstruction (e.g., postextubation laryngospasm after anesthesia induction, epiglottitis, laryngeal tumor, or obstructive tonsils).

Postrenal acute kidney injury Rare complication of urinary tract obstruction that affects the kidneys bilaterally (e.g., bilateral ureteral obstruction, bladder outlet obstruction–prostatic hypertrophy, tumors or neurogenic bladder, and urethral obstruction); obstruction causes an increase in intraluminal pressure upstream from the site of obstruction.

Postthrombotic syndrome (PTS) A syndrome that follows a vascular thrombosis, such as persistent edema.

Posttraumatic stress disorder (PTSD) A psychologic disorder that may develop in individuals who have experienced or witnessed traumatic events; is characterized by recurrent flashbacks of the traumatic event, nightmares, irritability, anxiety, fatigue, forgetfulness, and social withdrawal.

Potter syndrome A syndrome of renal agenesis with hypoplastic lungs and associated neonatal respiratory distress, hemodynamic instability, acidosis, cyanosis, edema, and characteristic (Potter) facies; death usually occurs from respiratory insufficiency, which develops before uremia.

Poverty of content A disorder, also called *poverty of speech content*, that is characterized by disorganized speech that conveys little information and may be vague or contain repetitive or obscure phrases.

Prader-Willi syndrome A rare genetic disorder caused by gene deletions on paternal chromosome 15 that result in short stature, hypotonia, small hands and feet, obesity, mild to moderate mental retardation, and hypogonadism.

Precocious puberty A condition in which a boy or girl undergoes the changes associated with puberty at an unexpectedly early age; often caused by a pathologic process that increases the secretion of estrogens or androgens.

Premenstrual dysphoric disorder (PMDD) Recurrence in the luteal phase of the menstrual cycle of distressing physical, psychologic, or behavioral changes that impair interpersonal relationships or interfere with usual activities.

Premenstrual syndrome (PMS) A group of symptoms that occur in many women from 2 to 14 days before menstruation begins, including abdominal bloating, breast tenderness, headache, fatigue, irritability, depression, and emotional distress.

Prerenal acute kidney injury Rapid development of renal hypoperfusion with the elevation of serum creatinine and urea levels.

Presbyopia A form of farsightedness usually accompanying advanced age in which the lens loses elasticity and becomes unable to accommodate and focus light for near vision.

Priapism A painful condition in which the erect penis maintains an erection in the absence of physical and psychologic stimulation.

Primary (congenital) immune deficiency See Immune deficiency.

Primary (spontaneous) pneumothorax See Pneumothorax.

Primary accidental hypothermia Unintentional drop in core body temperature below 35°C (95°F) of a previously healthy person attributable to the changes that occur with cold temperatures.

Primary adrenal insufficiency (Addison disease) Adrenal hypofunction resulting in bronzelike pigmentation of the skin, severe prostration, progressive anemia, low blood pressure, diarrhea, and digestive disturbance.

Primary amenorrhea Continued absence of menarche and menstrual function by 14 years of age without the development of secondary sex characteristics or by age 16 years if these changes have occurred.

Primary biliary cirrhosis See Cirrhosis.

Primary dysmenorrhea Painful menstruation because of a functional disturbance rather than because of inflammation, growths, or anatomic factors.

Primary gout Acute episodes of urate crystal–induced synovitis resulting from abnormality of purine metabolism; lower-than-normal urinary excretion of urate leads to hyperuricemia and acute episodes of joint inflammation.

Primary hyperaldosteronism (Conn disease, primary aldosteronism) An adrenocortical disorder caused by excessive secretion of aldosterone and characterized by headaches, nocturia, polyuria, fatigue, hypertension, potassium depletion, hypokalemic alkalosis, hypervolemia, and decreased plasma renin activity; may be associated with small benign adrenocortical adenomas.

Primary hyperparathyroidism Usually the result of a benign parathyroid tumor that secretes parathyroid hormone and increases circulating calcium levels; this condition is accompanied by hypercalcemia, nausea, vomiting, lethargy, depression, muscular weakness, and an altered mental state.

Primary hypertension (essential hypertension, idiopathic hypertension) Elevated blood pressure of unknown etiology accompanied by increased total peripheral vascular resistance as a result of vasoconstriction, increased cardiac output, or both.

Primary multiple organ dysfunction syndrome (MODS) Multiple organ injury directly associated with a specific insult, most often ischemia or impaired perfusion from an episode of shock or trauma, thermal injury, soft tissue necrosis, or invasive infection with decreased local perfusion in the injured organs.

Primary syphilis A stage of syphilis infection that occurs after an incubation period of 10 to 90 days and is characterized by a primary sore or chancre that develops at the point of initial exposure and lasts 4 to 6 weeks.

Prinzmetal angina A form of angina pectoris characterized by pain that is not precipitated by cardiac work; it is of longer duration and usually more severe and is associated with unusual electrocardiographic results including elevated ST segments.

Progressive bulbar palsy (see Bulbar palsy) A slowly progressive neurodegenerative disorder of the motor neurons of the cerebral cortex, spinal cord, and brainstem, resulting in progressive symptoms of bulbar palsy that may advance to loss of ability to manipulate food in the mouth, inability to swallow, choking, and emotional changes; may lead to aspiration of food and fluid and death from pneumonia.

Progressive spinal muscular atrophy A progressive degenerative disorder of the motor neurons of the spinal cord causing muscular weakness and wasting, typically beginning in the distal portions of the limbs and spreading proximally.

Prolactinoma The most common type of anterior pituitary tumor; produces visual disturbances and prolactin excess that results in infertility and changes in menstruation in females and in impotence, loss of libido, and infertility in males.

Properdin deficiency See Immune deficiency.

Prostatitis Inflammation of the prostate gland caused by urinary tract infection.

Protein C deficiency A disorder characterized by a lack of anticoagulant activity and an increased tendency to form blood clots because of decreased degradation of factor Va and factor VIIIa secondary to thrombosis, deep vein thrombosis, pulmonary embolism, thrombophlebitis, neonatal purpura fulminans, and disseminated intravascular coagulation.

Protein S deficiency A disorder characterized by a lack of anticoagulant activity and an increased tendency to form blood clots because of decreased degradation of factor Va and factor VIIIa.

Pseudothrombocytopenia See Thrombocytopenia.

Psoriasis A noncontagious autoimmune skin disorder in which the skin becomes scaly and inflamed when cells in the outer layer of skin reproduce faster than normal and accumulate as plaques on the skin surface.

- **Erythrodermic (exfoliative) psoriasis** Widespread red, scaling lesions that cover a large body surface area; often accompanied by itching or pain associated with constitutional symptoms (fever, chills, fatigue) and skin infections.
- **Guttate psoriasis** Sudden appearance of small papules on the trunk and extremities, occasionally after a streptococcal respiratory tract infection in children.
- **Inverse psoriasis** Rare development of large, smooth, dry, and deep red lesions in skinfolds (i.e., axilla or groin).
- **Plaque psoriasis** Most common form of psoriasis; begins with well-demarcated, thick, silvery, scaly erythematosus inflammatory lesions with epidermal hyper proliferation and the presence of activated T lymphocytes that may become mild, moderate, or severe, depending on the size, distribution, and inflammation of the lesions.
- **Pustular psoriasis** Blisters of noninfectious pus that develop over areas of plaque psoriasis.

Pulmonary artery hypertension (PAH) Increased blood pressure in the pulmonary artery attributable to vasoconstriction that may eventually lead to fibrosis, increased workload, hypertrophy of the right ventricle, and right heart failure; etiology may be idiopathic, familial, or associated with other diseases.

Pulmonary embolism (PE) Dislodgement of a blood clot from its site of origin and embolization to the arterial blood supply of one of the lungs, resulting in shortness of breath and difficulty breathing, rapid breathing that is painful, cough, and (in severe cases) hypotension, shock, loss of consciousness, and death.

Pulmonary stenosis A condition in which the opening into the pulmonary artery from the right ventricle narrows.

Pure red cell aplasia (PRCA) An acquired or congenital condition in which the bone marrow lacks red blood cell precursors even though megakaryocytes and white blood cell precursors are usually present at normal levels.

Purine nucleoside phosphorylase (PNP) deficiency See Immune deficiency.

Pustular psoriasis See Psoriasis.

Pyloric stenosis A congenital abnormality in which the pylorus is narrow, resulting in poor feeding, weight loss, and progressively worsening vomiting.

Pyramidal/spastic cerebral palsy Palsy resulting from damage or defects in the brain's corticospinal pathways (upper motor neuron) in either one or both hemispheres.

Q

Qualitative leukocyte disorder See Immune deficiency.

Quantitative leukocyte disorder See Immune deficiency.

R

RAG-1/RAG-2 deficiencies See Immune deficiency.

Rapidly progressive (crescentic) glomerulonephritis (RPGN) See Glomerulonephritis.

Raynaud disease A condition in which the blood vessels spasm because of inadequate blood supply, resulting in discoloration of the fingers and/or toes after exposure to changes in temperature or emotional events.

Raynaud phenomenon A condition caused by the temperature-dependent deposition of immune complexes in the capillary beds of the peripheral circulation, which blocks the circulation and causes localized pallor and numbness, followed by cyanosis and eventually gangrene if the circulation is not restored.

Rectocele A condition caused by childbirth or hysterectomy in which the region between the rectum and vagina bulges toward the vagina, resulting in a sense of pressure or protrusion within the vagina, the feeling of incomplete emptying of the rectum, difficulty passing stool, discomfort or pain during evacuation or intercourse, constipation, vaginal bleeding, fecal incontinence, prolapse of the bulge through the opening of the vagina, or rectal prolapse through the anus.

Refeeding syndrome Metabolic disturbances that occur upon initiating parenteral or enteral nutritional therapy to individuals who are severely malnourished; starvation results in movement of phosphate, magnesium, and potassium ions out of the cells and into the plasma and refeeding increases insulin levels and stimulates movement of glucose and these ions back into the cells, resulting in dangerously low levels in the plasma (hypophosphatemia, hypomagnesemia, hypokalemia, hyponatremia, hypocalcemia, and vitamin deficiency) and other potentially fatal metabolic complications.

Relative polycythemia A relative increase in the number of red blood cells caused by loss of the fluid portion of the blood.

Renal agenesis Only one functional kidney is present at birth.

Renal calculi (nephrolithiasis) Also called *urinary stones (urolithiasis)*; masses of crystals, protein, or other substances that can be located in the kidneys, ureters, and urinary bladder and are a common cause of urinary tract obstruction in adults.

Renal cell carcinoma (RCC) The most common renal neoplasm (approximately 80% of all renal neoplasms).

Renal dysplasia Abnormal tissue development in one or both kidneys.

Respiratory acidosis occurs when there is alveolar hypoventilation. Carbon dioxide is retained, increasing [H^+] (as H_2CO_3), thus decreasing the ratio of HCO_3^- to Pco_2 and producing acidosis.

Respiratory alkalosis Occurs when there is alveolar hyperventilation and decreased concentration of plasma carbon dioxide (termed *hypocapnia*), thus increasing the ratio of HCO_3^- to Pco_2 (H_2CO_3).

Respiratory distress syndrome (RDS) of the newborn A condition, also known as *hyaline membrane disease (HMD)*, that is a type of respiratory distress in newborns, most often in prematurely born infants, those born by cesarean section, or those having a diabetic mother; the immature lungs do not produce enough surfactant to retain air so the air spaces empty completely and collapse after exhalation.

Reticular dysgenesis See Immune deficiency.

Retinoblastoma An autosomal dominant or sporadic disorder in which a malignant tumor forms in the retina of one or both eyes; typically found in infants.

Reversible sideroblastic anemia See Anemia.

Rhabdomyolysis A potentially fatal condition in which skeletal muscle breaks down as a result of injury such as physical damage to the muscle, high fever, metabolic disorders, excessive exertion, convulsions, or anoxia of the muscle for several hours; large amounts of myoglobin are usually excreted.

Rheumatic fever An inflammatory disease that is associated with recent streptococcal infection and causes inflammation of the joints, fever, jerky movements, nodules under the skin, and skin rash and often is followed by serious heart damage or disease secondary to antibodies that react both with streptococcal antigens and with those of the heart valve.

Rheumatic heart disease (RHD) Sequela to rheumatic fever in which heart valves are repeatedly inflamed, developing fibrosis and thickening that can result in valve deformities, stenosis, or regurgitation.

Rheumatoid arthritis An autoimmune disease that causes chronic inflammation of the joints and the tissue around the joints and other organs.

Rickets A bone disease that is caused by a deficiency of vitamin D or calcium and manifests in children as softening of bones, abnormal growth of bones, and enlargement of cartilage at the ends of long bones.

Ringed sideroblast An erythroblast in which one-third or more of the nucleus is encircled by 10 or more siderotic granules that may be caused by antituberculous drugs and alcohol abuse.

Roseola A viral disease in infants and young children that causes fever and a spotty rash that appears shortly after the fever has subsided.

Rotavirus A viral infection seen in young children that causes diarrhea by attacking the lining of the small intestine, resulting in the inability to absorb fluid and electrolytes.

Rubella An infectious viral disease of children and young adults that is spread by a droplet spray from the respiratory tract of an infected individual; the disease causes a rash that lasts about 3 days with tender and swollen lymph nodes behind the ears.

Rubeola An infectious viral disease of young children, also known as *measles*, that is spread by a droplet spray from the nose, mouth, and throat of individuals in the infective stage and causes a rash, white spots in the mouth, a rash on the face that spreads to the rest of the body, and fever.

Russell-Silver syndrome (Russell-Silver dwarfism) A growth disorder manifesting as retardation, proportionate short stature, leg length discrepancy, and a small, triangular-shaped face.

S

Saccular aneurysm (berry aneurysm) A localized, progressively growing sac that affects only a portion of the circumference of the arterial wall and may be the result of congenital anomalies or degeneration.

Saccular bronchiectasis (see Bronchiectasis) Bronchiectasis resulting in dilated bronchi that become balloon-like.

Salmon patches (nevus simplex) Patches, also known as *stork bites*, of small, pink, flat spots that are small, dilated blood vessels visible through the skin and are usually found on the forehead, eyelids, and upper lip; between the eyebrows; and on the back of the neck.

Salpingitis Inflammation of one of the two fallopian tubes caused by infection spreading from the vagina or uterus.

Sarcoma Tumor of the connective tissue cells.

Sarcopenia Age-related loss in skeletal muscle, which is a direct cause of the age-related decrease in muscle strength.

Scabies Skin infestation with the itch mite, *Sarcoptes scabiei*, acquired through close contact with an infected person or contaminated clothing that produces intense itching.

Schizophrenia A psychotic disorder characterized by delusions, hallucinations, loosening of associations, disturbances in mood and sense of self and relationship to the external world, and bizarre, purposeless behavior.

Sclerosing adenosis A condition in which the number of acini per terminal duct is more than twice the number of normal terminal ducts and is associated with a significantly increased risk of subsequent breast carcinoma.

Scoliosis A condition in which the spine is curved sideways to varying degrees; occurs because of either physiologic curvature or functional curvature in which contraction of the paraspinal muscles of the back creates a vertebral curve.

Seborrheic dermatitis Scaly, flaky, itchy, and red skin on the scalp, face, and trunk because of a yeast infection.

Seborrheic keratosis A benign proliferation of cutaneous basal cells that produces smooth or warty elevated lesions; seen primarily in older people and presents as multiple lesions on the chest, back, and face.

Secondary (acquired) immune deficiency See Immune deficiency.

Secondary (traumatic) pneumothorax See Pneumothorax.

Secondary amenorrhea Menstruation begins at puberty but then is subsequently suppressed for three or more cycles or for 6 months in women who previously menstruated.

Secondary dysmenorrhea Altered menstruation because of inflammation, infection, tumor, or anatomic factors.

Secondary generalization The process by which a simple partial seizure involving one hemisphere becomes a generalized seizure involving the second hemisphere.

Secondary hyperparathyroidism A condition of elevated levels of parathyroid hormone resulting from disease such as renal failure in which parathyroid hormone concentration is elevated in response to vitamin D deficiency.

Secondary hypertension A condition of elevated blood pressure that is associated with other conditions, primarily with renal disease by a renin-dependent mechanism or a fluid volume-dependent mechanism.

Secondary hypothermia Depressed body temperature as a consequence of a serious systemic disorder, for example, endocrine disorders.

Secondary MODS The result of an excessive inflammatory reaction, after a latent period following the initial injury, in organs distant from the site of the original injury. It is postulated that the resulting organ trauma is caused by the host response to a second insult rather than being a direct result of the primary injury.

Secondary septic arthritis A bacterial infection in the joints, causing them to become inflamed and the bacteria to proliferate.

Secondary syphilis The most contagious stage of syphilis infection; characterized by a skin rash that appears on the trunk and extremities 1 to 6 months after the primary infection and possibly mucous patches on the genitals or inside the mouth.

Selective IgA deficiency See Immune deficiency.

Sepsis Severe physiologic stress typically caused by an infection; its complications result from activation of biochemical and physiologic cascades that lead to the formation or activation of cytokines and other mediators that produce vasodilation, increased capillary permeability, maldistribution of blood flow, and cardiovascular and cellular dysfunction.

Septic shock A condition caused by systemic infection that results in decreased tissue perfusion and oxygenation and can lead to multiple organ dysfunction syndrome and death.

Serum sickness A form of hypersensitivity caused by injection of soluble antigen such as antiserum, which activates a type III hypersensitivity response (formation of soluble circulating antigen-antibody [IgG or IgM] complexes) that activates the complement system.

Severe combined immune deficiency (SCID) See Immune deficiency.

Severe congenital neutropenia See Immune deficiency.

Shock A condition in which the circulatory system is unable to provide adequate circulation to the body tissues because of inadequate pumping by the heart, a reduction in blood volume, or a reduction in blood pressure; it results in slowing of vital functions and possibly death.

Short bowel syndrome A group of malabsorption conditions resulting from massive resection of the small bowel, the degree and kind of malabsorption depending on the site and extent of the resection; it is characterized by diarrhea, steatorrhea, and malnutrition.

Sickle cell anemia See Anemia.

Sickle cell disease (SCD) See Anemia.

Sickle cell trait See Anemia.

Sickle cell–Hb C disease See Anemia.

Sickle cell–thalassemia disease See Anemia.

Sideroblastic anemia (SA) See Anemia.

Silicosis Inflammation of the lung resulting from the inhalation of free silica (silicon dioxide) and silica-containing compounds, which occurs in mining and related industries.

Simple febrile seizure Benign and most common form of childhood seizure.

Simple fibroadenoma Benign solid tumors composed of both fibrous and glandular tissue.

Sliding hiatal hernia The most common type of hernia, occurring when the proximal portion of the stomach moves into the thoracic cavity through the esophageal hiatus, an opening in the diaphragm for the esophagus and vagus nerves.

Small cell lung carcinoma (SCLS) The most common type of neuroendocrine lung tumor; mostly arise from the central part of the lung.

Smallpox (variola) An infectious viral disease that is caused by a poxvirus and result in high fever, aches, and widespread eruption of large sores that leave scars.

Smoldering myeloma A condition in which abnormal plasma cells produce a monoclonal protein, but no symptoms or complications of myeloma are present and may not be present for several years.

Solitary plasmacytoma A solitary tumor of malignant plasma cells that may result in a single lytic bone lesion or may be in the tissues (extramedullary plasmacytoma).

Spina bifida occulta The mildest form of congenital disorder of incomplete closure of the embryonic neural tube; the outer part of some vertebrae may not be completely closed, but the defect is not apparent to the unaided eye and usually causes no serious neurologic dysfunctions.

Spinal stenosis Narrowing of the spinal canal as a result of congenital anomaly or spinal degeneration, resulting in pain, paresthesias, and neurogenic claudication.

Spondylolisthesis Forward displacement of one of the lower lumbar vertebrae over the vertebra below it or over the sacrum.

Sprain A ligament tear, which occurs most commonly in the wrist, ankle, elbow, and knee joints.

Squamous cell carcinoma (SCC) A tumor of the epidermis and the second most common human cancer.

Stable angina A condition in which ischemic attacks occur at predictable frequencies and duration after activities that increase myocardial oxygen demands such as exercise and stress.

Staphylococcal scalded-skin syndrome (SSSS) A disease in infants that is caused by a staphylococcal infection with release of an exfoliative toxin that results in peeling of large areas of skin.

Stevens–Johnson syndrome An inflammatory eruption of circular lesions that can cover the majority of the skin and mucous membranes and usually occurs after a respiratory tract infection or as an allergic reaction to drugs or other substances.

Strabismus The deviation of one eye from the other when a person is looking at an object; it results in failure of the two eyes to simultaneously focus on the same image and therefore loss of binocular vision.

Strawberry hemangioma A red birthmark caused by densely packed blood vessels that usually appears on the face, scalp, back, and chest and disappears during childhood.

Stress ulcer Acute peptic ulcer that occurs in association with various other pathologic conditions, including burns, cor pulmonale, intracranial lesions, and surgical operations.

Structural scoliosis A side-to-side curvature of the spine.

Subacute thyroiditis (subacute granulomatous thyroiditis, de Quervain thyroiditis) A painful inflammation of the thyroid that develops suddenly in a person who has had a viral infection, such as mumps or an upper respiratory tract illness. Pain radiates throughout the neck and individuals feel ill and feverish.

Subglottic stenosis Narrowing of the airway below the larynx caused by a congenital anomaly or acquired narrowing secondary to injury, possibly resulting in respiratory distress, cyanotic episodes, or recurrent lung infections.

Subluxation An injury in which the contact between two joint surfaces is only partially lost.

Sudden infant death syndrome (SIDS) A syndrome, also known as *crib death*, that is characterized by the sudden, unexpected, and unexplained death of an apparently healthy infant less than 1 year of age.

Superior vena cava syndrome (SVCS) Restriction of the blood flow through the superior vena cava secondary to compression by malignancies or lymphadenopathy.

Sydenham chorea (St. Vitus dance) A postinfectious chorea appearing several months after a streptococcal infection with subsequent rheumatic fever. The chorea typically involves the distal limbs and is associated with hypotonia and emotional lability.

Symphysis Fibrocartilaginous joint; a type of joint in which the apposed bony surfaces are firmly united by a plate of fibrocartilage.

Synchondrosis A cartilaginous joint creating a union between two immovable bones, such as the synchondroses of the cranium, the pubic symphysis, the sternum, and the manubrium.

Syndesmosis A fibrous union in which two bones are connected by interosseous ligaments, such as the anterior and the posterior ligaments in the radioulnar and tibiofibular articulations; is usually converted into bone before adult life.

Syndrome of inappropriate antidiuretic hormone (ADH) secretion (SIADH) A condition in which the release of ADH from the posterior pituitary is elevated relative to serum sodium levels, resulting in increased water reabsorption by the kidneys and fluid overload.

Syndromic craniosynostosis (see Craniosynostosis) Synostosis that occurs as part of a genetic syndrome; usually associated with various dysmorphisms involving the face, skeleton, and nervous system and usually accompanied by developmental delay.

Syphilis A chronic infectious disease that is transmitted by direct contact, usually in sexual intercourse, or passed from mother to child in utero, and progresses through three stages characterized by chancres, ulcerous skin eruptions, and systemic infection that leads to damage to the cardiovascular and nervous systems.

Systemic inflammatory response syndrome (SIRS) A generalized inflammatory response that may lead to depressed cardiac function and decreased organ perfusion.

Systemic lupus erythematosus (see Lupus erythematosus) A chronic, multisystem, inflammatory disease and one of the most common, complex, and serious of the autoimmune disorders.

Systolic heart failure A condition in which the heart muscle contracts so weakly that insufficient oxygenated blood is pumped throughout the body.

T

Tay-Sachs disease (GM2 gangliosidosis) A fatal autosomal recessive lysosomal storage disorder in which the lysosomal enzyme hexosaminidase A (HexA) is deficient, leading to accumulation of gangliosides in the brain and nerve tissue, mental retardation, convulsions, blindness, and premature death.

T-cell neoplasm See Lymphoma.

Tension pneumothorax See Pneumothorax.

Tertiary syphilis The most severe stage of syphilis, which can begin as early as 1 year after the initial infection but can take up to 10 years to manifest and is characterized by gummas—soft, tumor-like growths found in the skin and mucous membranes and often in the skeleton—joint deformity, neurosyphilis, and cardiovascular syphilis.

Tethered cord syndrome A group of neurologic disorders related to malformation of the spinal cord in which the cord becomes abnormally attached or tethered as a result of scar tissue that develops as the cord transcends the vertebral canal with growth; tethering may decrease blood flow.

Tetralogy of Fallot A congenital condition that is characterized by four malformations including ventricular septal defect, misplacement of the origin of the aorta, narrowing of the pulmonary artery, and enlargement of the right ventricle.

Thalassemia See Anemia.

Thromboangiitis obliterans (Buerger disease) Inflammation of the medium-sized arteries and veins because of thrombotic occlusion, resulting in ischemia and gangrene.

Thrombocythemia A chronic disorder of sustained megakaryocyte proliferation that increases the number of circulating platelets and results in megakaryocytic hyperplasia, splenomegaly, and complications by hemorrhagic and thrombotic episodes.

Thrombocytopenia A reduced number of circulating platelets.

Acute idiopathic thrombotic thrombocytopenic purpura A form of thrombocytopenic purpura (TTP) characterized by thrombotic microangiopathy in which platelets aggregate and cause occlusion of arterioles and capillaries within the microcirculation, leading to increased platelet consumption and organ ischemia.

Autoimmune neonatal thrombocytopenia Destruction of platelets in a fetus/neonate by antiplatelet antibodies produced in the mother against her own platelet antigens (autoimmune) that are shared with the child, and the antibodies are transported across the placenta and destroy the child's platelets.

Chronic relapsing thrombotic thrombocytopenic purpura A rare familial form of TTP characterized by recurring episodes of thrombocytopenia; usually seen in children.

Heparin-induced thrombocytopenia (HIT) A form of drug-induced thrombocytopenia caused by IgG antibodies against the heparin–platelet factor 4 complex leading to platelet activation and thrombocytopenia.

Idiopathic thrombocytopenic purpura (autoimmune or primary thrombocytopenic purpura) The most common cause of thrombocytopenia, secondary to increased immune-mediated platelet destruction; can be acute or chronic.

Immune thrombocytopenic purpura A condition in which the number of platelets in the blood is reduced by the production of antibodies against platelets, resulting in ecchymoses and hemorrhage from mucous membranes, anemia, and extreme weakness.

Neonatal alloimmune thrombocytopenic purpura (NATP) A condition in which fetal platelets have an antigen from the father that is absent in the mother, and the mother forms antibodies that cross the placenta and destroy the fetal platelets.

Pseudothrombocytopenia An artificially low platelet count in anticoagulated blood caused by cooling of the blood and autoagglutination of platelets.

Thrombotic thrombocytopenic purpura (TTP) Altered blood coagulation caused by an enzymatic deficiency that is characterized by a reduced number of platelets in the blood, the formation of blood clots in tissue arterioles and capillaries, and neurologic damage.

Thrombophilia Genetic or acquired abnormality of the coagulation system with an increased risk for thrombosis.

Thrombotic thrombocytopenic purpura (TTP) See Thrombocytopenia.

Thrush A yeast infection of the mouth and throat that presents as creamy white curdlike patches on the tongue, inside the mouth, and on the back of the throat and that is commonly associated with yeast infection of the esophagus.

Thyrotoxicosis Excessive concentrations of thyroid hormones in the body that are marked by increased metabolic rate, heat intolerance, goiter, reproductive disorders, excessive sweating, and other alterations in systemic function.

Tinea capitis Fungal infections of the skin classified according to their location on the body.

Tinea corporis (ringworm) A fungal infection of the scalp; much more common in children than in adults.

Tinea infection One of a group of fungal skin infections that include athlete's foot, folliculitis, jock itch, ringworm, and pityriasis versicolor.

Tinea pedis Chronic, superficial fungal infection of the skin of the foot common in adults.

Tinea unguium A fungal infection of the nails.

Tinnitus A condition in which the person hears ringing, buzzing, or other sounds without an external cause.

T-lymphocyte deficiency See Immune deficiency.

Tophaceous gout A form of purine metabolism disorder characterized by the formation of chalky deposits of sodium biurate under the skin and in the joints.

Toxic epidermal necrolysis (TEN) A rare adverse reaction to certain drugs in which a large portion of the skin becomes intensely red, may develop blisters, and exfoliates.

Toxoplasmosis A protozoan infection that is the most common opportunistic infection and occurs in one-third of persons with HIV.

Tracheomalacia (tracheobronchomalacia) A congenital or acquired condition characterized by weakness of the tracheal support cartilage, resulting in tracheal collapse when increased airflow is needed.

Trachoma (granular conjunctivitis or Egyptian ophthalmia) A contagious, chronic inflammation of the mucous membranes of the eyes, caused by *Chlamydia trachomatis.*

Transcortical dysphasia (transcortical sensory dysphasia, mixed transcortical dysphasia, isolated speech center) A type of aphasia with poor comprehension, but fluent grammatically correct speech. Those with transcortical dysphasia can communicate well and are capable of good repetition.

Transient hypogammaglobulinemia of infancy See Immune deficiency.

Transient ischemic attack (TIA) A brief episode in which the brain receives insufficient blood supply; symptoms depend on the site of the blockage.

Transposition of the great arteries (TGAs) The aorta arises from the right ventricle and the pulmonary artery arises from the left ventricle.

Traumatic (dissecting) aneurysm Aneurysm caused by weakening of arterial walls, by a penetrating missile, or after neurosurgery or neuroimaging following an injury.

Trichomoniasis A sexually transmitted bacterial infection of the urethra in males and the vagina in females that can cause urethral and bladder infection in males and urinary tract infection and painful, malodorous vaginitis in women.

Tricuspid atresia Congenital absence of the tricuspid orifice, circulation being made possible by the presence of an atrial septal defect.

True aneurysm Localized dilation of an artery with an expanded lumen lined by stretched remnants of the arterial wall.

Truncus arteriosus A congenital defect in which a large great vessel arises from a ventricular septal defect and does not divide into the aorta and pulmonary artery, resulting in one vessel carrying blood both to the body and to the lungs.

TSH deficiency A condition characterized by decreased or absent production of thyroid-stimulating hormone (TSH), resulting in a decline in thyroid hormone level and subsequent symptoms such as fatigue, cold intolerance, weakness, depression, muscle aches, weight gain, and constipation.

Tuberculosis (TB) An infectious disease of humans caused by *Mycobacterium tuberculosis* that results in the formation of tubercles on the lungs and other tissues of the body.

Tuberous sclerosis complex (TSC) An inherited disease caused by mutation of the *hamartin* and *tuberin* genes and resulting in malformation of the brain, retina, and viscera and development of epileptic seizures, mental retardation, and skin nodules on the face.

Turner syndrome Gonadal dysgenesis with short stature, undifferentiated (streak) gonads, and variable abnormalities such as webbing of the neck, low posterior hair line, increased carrying angle of elbow, cubitus valgus, and cardiac defects. The genotype is XO (45, X) or X/XX or X/XXX mosaic. The phenotype is female.

Type 1 diabetes mellitus See Diabetes.

Type 2 diabetes mellitus See Diabetes.

U

Ulcerative colitis Chronically inflamed and ulcerated mucosal and submucosal lining of the large intestine, resulting in abdominal pain, diarrhea, and rectal bleeding.

Unclassified epileptic seizure Seizure disorders that do not fit neatly into a classified grouping. These seizures characteristically have a wide variety of abnormal clinical activity. Examples of this activity include rhythmic eye movements, chewing, and swimming movements. These activities are commonly seen in neonatal seizures.

Undifferentiated large cell anaplastic cancer A cancer of epithelial origin that has lost all evidence of differentiation and may have arisen from a stem cell.

Unilateral neglect syndrome Hemiapraxia with failure to pay attention to body grooming and stimuli on one side but not the other; usually caused by a lesion in the central nervous system.

Unstable angina A condition in which unprovoked ischemic attacks occur at unpredictable frequencies and may increase in severity.

Upper airway obstruction (UAO) Infections, foreign body aspiration, angioedema, obstructive sleep apnea, and trauma in children.

Uremia Syndrome of renal failure resulting in elevated blood urea and creatinine levels.

Uremic syndrome A complex of symptoms resulting from the accumulation of urea and other nitrogenous compounds and toxins in the blood, leading to alterations in levels of fluid and electrolytes, metabolic acidosis, anemia, hyperphosphatemia, and hypocalcemia; symptoms include hypertension, anorexia, nausea, vomiting, diarrhea or constipation, malnutrition and weight loss, pruritus, edema, anemia, and neurologic, cardiovascular disease, and skeletal changes.

Ureterohydronephrosis Dilation of both the ureter and the pelvicaliceal system.

Ureteropelvic junction (UPJ) obstruction An impediment to the drainage of urine from the kidney, usually attributable to partial or intermittent blockage of the renal collecting system at the junction of the renal pelvis and ureter.

Urethral atresia Congenital absence or closure of a normal body opening or tubular structure; congenital imperforation of the urethra.

Urothelial (transitional cell) carcinoma The most common bladder malignancy, appearing on the inner lining of the bladder.

Urticaria Hives; a dermal (skin) manifestation of type I allergic reactions.

Usual ductal hyperplasia (UDH) Description of normal hyperplasia of cells that line the ducts in the normal breast; additional layers of benign cells are present, but with normal cellular structure and arrangement.

Uterine prolapse Descent or herniation of the uterus into or beyond the vagina because of weakness of the pelvic musculature, ligaments, and fascia or obstetric trauma and lacerations sustained during labor and delivery.

V

Vacuolar myelopathy HIV-induced loss of myelin and spongy degeneration of the spinal cord that may cause spastic paraparesis, sensory ataxia in lower limbs, and unsteady gait.

Vaginismus A form of sexual dysfunction that is caused by a psychologic disorder or vaginal inflammation in which the muscles at the entrance to vagina contract and prevent sexual intercourse.

Vaginitis Infection of the vagina usually caused by a fungus that may cause itching or burning and a discharge.

Vaginosis Vaginal irritation without white blood cells or other indication of infection.

Varicocele A painful condition in which the veins in the scrotum that develop in the spermatic cord enlarge, and if the valves that regulate blood flow from these veins become dysfunctional, blood does not leave the testis, thereby causing swelling in the veins above and behind the testis.

Varicose bronchiectasis A condition in which the bronchi become large and balloon-like.

Venous angioma Abnormal veins, usually near the ventricular wall, that form as a congenital anomaly.

Venous stasis ulcer A condition affecting the lower leg in which leaky valves, obstructions, or regurgitation in veins impairs blood flow back to the heart, resulting in pooling of blood in the lower leg and subsequent tissue damage.

Ventricular septal defect (VSD) A congenital malformation in which the wall between the left and right ventricles has a hole that allows blood to travel between the left and right ventricles, potentially leading to congestive heart failure.

Vesicoureteral reflux (VUR) Reflux of urine from the bladder into the ureter.

Vestibular nystagmus Involuntary rapid movement of the eyeball that is due to disturbance of the vestibular system; eye movements are rhythmic, with slow and fast components.

Vitiligo An autoimmune-related loss of melanocytes resulting in the depigmentation of patches of skin.

von Willebrand disease An inherited disease in which the von Willebrand factor proteins that are made in the blood vessel walls and function to control platelet activity are abnormal or absent, resulting in a tendency to hemorrhage.

Vulvodynia Also referred to as *vulvitis, vestibulitis*, or *vulvovestibulitis*; chronic pain and inflammation of the vulva or vestibule, or both.

W

Waldenström macroglobulinemia See Lymphoma.

Wallerian degeneration The degeneration of a nerve fiber that has been separated from its nutritive center by injury or disease; characterized by segmentation of the myelin and resulting in atrophy and destruction of the axon.

Warm autoimmune hemolytic anemia See Anemia.

Wilms tumor See Nephroblastoma.

Wilson disease A genetic disease in which the ability to metabolize copper is impaired, resulting in an accumulation of copper deposits in organs such as the brain, liver, and kidneys and subsequent organ dysfunction and failure.

Wiskott–Aldrich syndrome (WAS) See Immune deficiency.

X

Xanthelasma A planar xanthoma involving the eyelid(s).

X-linked hyper-IgM syndrome See Immune deficiency.

X-linked SCID See Immune deficiency.

Z

Zika virus A single-stranded RNA virus from the Flaviviridae family, genus *Flavivirus*, that is predominantly transmitted through bites from infected mosquitos; infection during pregnancy has been associated with severe fetal infection and associated CNS abnormalities.

Zollinger–Ellison syndrome The association of atypical, intractable, sometimes fulminating peptic ulcers with extreme gastric hyperacidity and benign or malignant gastrinomas in the pancreas.

INDEX

Page numbers followed by *f*, indicate figures, *t*, tables, or *b*, boxes respectively. Syndromes and disorders appear in boldface.

B

E

I

L

M

N

Q

R

S

U

W

X

Y

Z

COMMON LABORATORY VALUES

CONSTITUENT	NORMAL MEAN VALUE AND SOME RANGES	NORMAL RANGE IN SI UNITS
Electrolytes	Total, 1% of plasma weight	
Na^+	136–145 mEq/L	136–145 mmol/L
K^+	3.5–5 mEq/L	3.5–5 mmol/L
Ca^{++} (serum)	9–10.5 mg/dL	2.25–2.62 mmol/L
Mg^{++}	1.3–2.1 mg/dL	0.65–1.05 mmol/L
Cl^-	98–106 mEq/L	98–106 mmol/L
HCO_3^- (venous)	23–29 mEq/L	23–29 mmol/L
Phosphate (mostly HPO_4^-)	3–4.5 mg/L	1–1.5 mmol/L
Proteins		
Total Proteins	6.4–8.3 g/dL	64–83 g/L
Albumin	3.5–5 g/dL	35–50 g/L
Gamma globulin	0.7–1.7 g/dL	7–17 g/L
Globulins	2.3–3.4 g/dL	23–34 g/L
Fibrinogen	200–400 mg/dL	2–4 g/L
Troponin I	< 0.03 ng/mL	< 0.03 ng/mL
C-Reactive Protein (CRP)	<1.0 mg/dL	<10.0 mg/L
Procalcitonin[a] (PCT)		
Blood Gases		
pH (arterial)	7.35–7.45	7.35–7.45
PCO_2 content (arterial)	35–45 mmHg	35–45 mmHg
PO_2 content (arterial)	80–100 mmHg	80–100 mmHg
HCO_3^- (arterial)	21–28 mEq/L	21–28 mmol/L
Lipids		
Total Cholesterol	<200 mg/dL	<5.20 mmol/L
LDL	<130 mg/dL	
HDL	>45 mg/dL	>0.75 mmol/L (males)
	>55 mg/dL	>0.91 mmol/L (females)
Triglycerides (after 12 hr fast)	<180 mg/dL	0.45–1.81 mmol/L (males)
		0.40–1.52 mmol/L (females)
Waste Products		
Urea (BUN)	10–20 mg/dL	3.6–7.1 nmol/L
Uric acid (serum)	2.7–8.5 mg/dL	0.16–0.51 µmol/L
Creatinine	0.6–1.2 mg/dL	53–106 µmol/L
Creatinine clearance	107–139 mL/min	1.78–2.32 mL/s (males)
	87–107 mL/min	1.45–1.78 mL/s (females)
Bilirubin (total)	0.3–1.0 mg/dL	5.1–17 µmol/L
Bilirubin, direct (conjugated)	0.1–0.3 mg/dL	1.7–5.1 µmol/L
Bilirubin, indirect (unconjugated)	0.2–0.8 mg/dL	5.1–17 µmol/L
Hematology Values		
Leukocyte (white blood cell count)	5000–10,000/mm^3	5–10 × 10^9/L
Lymphocyte	20%–40% of leukocyte differential	1000–4000 × 10^6/L
Monocyte and macrophage	2%–8% of leukocyte differential	100–700 × 10^6/L
Eosinophil	1%–4% of leukocyte differential	50–500 × 10^6/L
Neutrophil (segmented)	55%–70% of leukocyte differential	2500–8000 × 10^6/L
Basophil	0.5–1% of leukocyte differential	25–100 × 10^6/L
Platelet	150,000–400,000/mm^3	150–400 × 10^9/L
Erythrocyte (red blood cell count)	4.2–6.1 million/mm^3	4.2–6.1 × 10^{12}/L
Hematocrit	36%–52%	0.40–0.54 g/L
Hemoglobin	12–18 g/dL	7.4–11.2 mmol/L
Mean corpuscular volume	80–96 mcm^3	80–96 fL

Continued